# CANCER NURSING
## Principles and Practice

## FOURTH EDITION

### EDITED BY

**Susan L. Groenwald, RN, MS**

Assistant Professor of Nursing, Complemental
Department of Medical Nursing
Rush University College of Nursing

Rush Presbyterian St. Luke's Medical Center
Chicago, Illinois

**Michelle Goodman, RN, MS, OCN®**

Assistant Professor of Nursing
Rush University College of Nursing
Oncology Clinical Nurse Specialist
Section of Medical Oncology
Rush Cancer Institute

Rush Presbyterian St. Luke's Medical Center
Chicago, Illinois

**Margaret Hansen Frogge, RN, MS**

Assistant Professor, Associate Faculty
Rush University College of Nursing

Rush Presbyterian St. Luke's Medical Center
Chicago, Illinois

Vice President, Strategic Development
and System Integration

Riverside Medical Center
Kankakee, Illinois

**Connie Henke Yarbro, RN, MS, FAAN**

Editor, *Seminars in Oncology Nursing*

Clinical Associate Professor
Division of Hematology/Oncology
Adjunct Clinical Assistant Professor
Sinclair School of Nursing

University of Missouri, Columbia
Columbia, Missouri

**JONES AND BARTLETT PUBLISHERS**
*Sudbury, Massachusetts*
Boston    London    Singapore

*Editorial, Sales, and Customer Service Offices*

Jones and Bartlett Publishers
40 Tall Pine Drive
Sudbury, MA 01776
508-443-5000
info@jbpub.com
http://www.jbpub.com

Jones and Bartlett Publishers International
Barb House, Barb Mews
London W6 7PA
UK

**Library of Congress Cataloging-in-Publication Data**

Cancer nursing: principles and practice / edited by Susan L.
    Groenwald . . . [et al.].—4th ed.
        p.   cm.
    Includes bibliographical references and index.
    ISBN 0-7637-0219-6
    1. Cancer—Nursing.   I. Groenwald, Susan L.
    [DNLM: 1. Neoplasms—nursing.   WY 156 C2197 1997]
RC266.C356   1997
610.73′698—DC21
DNLM/DLC
for Library of Congress                                                96-48548
                                                                         CIP

The selection and dosage of drugs presented in this book are in accord with standards accepted at the time of publication. The authors, editors, and publisher have made every effort to provide accurate information. However, research, clinical practice, and government regulations often change the accepted standard in this field. Before administering any drug, the reader is advised to check the manufacturer's product information sheet for the most up-to-date recommendations on dosage, precautions, and contraindications. This is especially important in the case of drugs that are new or seldom used.

*Senior Production Administrator:* Mary Sanger
*Editorial Production Service:* Editorial Services of New England (ESNE)
*Typesetting:* Modern Graphics, Inc.
*Cover Design:* Hannus Design Associates
*Printing and Binding:* World Color Book Services

Printed in the United States of America
01 00 99 98 97   10 9 8 7 6 5 4 3 2 1

*"Any one cell, embodying as it does the record of a billion years of evolution, represents more an historical than a physical event. You cannot expect to explain such a wise old bird in a few simple words."*

MAX DELBRUCHT
California Institute of Technology

## DEDICATION

To our colleagues in cancer nursing . . .
Who strive to meet the challenges imposed by the manifestations of wayward cells, and . . .
Who care for the complex human beings who live with those manifestations

SLG, MHF, MG, CHY

# Contributors

**Barbara A. Barhamand, RN, MSN, AOCN**
Oncology Clinical Nurse Specialist/Practice Manager
Hematology-Oncology Consultants Ltd.
Naperville, IL

**Andrea M. Barsevick, RN, DNSc**
Director of Nursing Research
Fox Chase Cancer Center
Philadelphia, PA

**Karen Belford, RN, MS, OCN®, CCRN**
Clinical Instructor, Department of Nursing Education
Memorial Sloan-Kettering Cancer Center
New York, NY

**Connie Yuska Bildstein, RN, MS, CORLN**
Vice President of Operations
Northwestern Memorial Home Health
Care/Services, Inc.
Chicago, IL

**Carol Blendowski, RN, BS, OCN®**
Oncology Clinical Nurse
Rush Cancer Institute
Rush Presbyterian St. Luke's Medical Center
Chicago, IL

**Karen Smith Blesch, RN, PhD**
Documentation Specialist
Hoffman-LaRoche
Nutley, NJ

**Debra L. Brock, RNC, MSN, CS, AOCN, ANP**
Nurse Practitioner
Nashville Family Medicine
Nashville, IN

**Patricia Corcoran Buchsel, RN, MSN**
Senior Research Associate
University of Washington
Transplantation Consultant
Issaquah, WA

**Dawn Camp-Sorrell, RN, MSN, AOCN, FNP**
Oncology Nurse Practitioner
University of Alabama at Birmingham Hospital
Birmingham, AL

**Brenda Cartmel, PhD**
CPS/CARET: Yale University
Occupational Health Center
Groton, CT

**David Cella, PhD**
Associate Professor of Psychology and Social Sciences
Director, Psychosocial Oncology
Rush Presbyterian St. Luke's Medical Center
Chicago, IL

**Dianne D. Chapman, RN, MS, OCN®**
Coordinator, Comprehensive Breast Center
Genetic Counselor
Rush Inherited Susceptibility for Cancer (RISC)
Program
Rush Cancer Institute
Rush Presbyterian St. Luke's Medical Center
Chicago, IL

**Rebecca F. Cohen, RN, EdD, MPA, CPHQ**
Associate Professor
Rockford College, Department of Nursing
Rockford, IL

**JoAnn Coleman, RN, MS, CRNP, OCN®**
Case Manager for Pancreas and Biliary Surgery
Department of Surgical Nursing
Johns Hopkins Hospital
Baltimore, MD

**Mary Cunningham, RN, MS**
Clinical Nurse Specialist
Department of Neuro-Oncology
Pain and Symptom Management Section
M.D. Anderson Cancer Center
Houston, TX

**Diane Scott Dorsett, RN, PhD, FAAN**
Director, Comprehensive Cancer Support Services
San Francisco, CA

**Jan M. Ellerhorst-Ryan, RN, MSN, CS**
Oncology/HIV Clinical Nurse Specialist
Vitas Health Care Corporation
Cincinnati, OH

**Jayne I. Fernsler, RN, DSN, AOCN**
Associate Professor
College of Nursing
University of Delaware
Newark, DE

**Ann T. Foltz, RN, DNS**
Breast and Cervical Cancer Program Director
Louisiana Office of Public Health
New Orleans, LA

**Susan M. Fox, RN, MS, OCN®**
Oncology Research Nurse
Indiana University Cancer Pavilion
Indianapolis, IN

**Marilyn Frank-Stromborg, EdD, JD, NP, FAAN**
Professor and Acting Chair
School of Nursing
Northern Illinois University
Dekalb, IL

**Margaret Hansen Frogge, RN, MS**
Assistant Professor, Associate Faculty
Rush University College of Nursing
Rush Presbyterian St. Luke's Medical Center
Chicago, IL
Vice President, Strategic Development and
System Integration
Riverside Medical Center
Kankakee, IL

**Annette Galassi, RN, MA, CANP, AOCN**
Adult Nurse Practitioner
Instructor in Medicine
Lombardi Cancer Center
Georgetown University Medical Center
Washington, DC

**Barbara Holmes Gobel, RN, MS**
Oncology Clinical Nurse Specialist
Gottlieb Memorial Hospital
Melrose Park, IL
Instructor, Complemental
Rush University College of Nursing
Chicago, IL

**Michelle Goodman, RN, MS, OCN®**
Assistant Professor of Nursing
Rush University College of Nursing
Oncology Clinical Nurse Specialist
Section of Medical Oncology
Rush Cancer Institute
Rush Presbyterian St. Luke's Medical Center
Chicago, IL

**Susan L. Groenwald, RN, MS**
Assistant Professor of Nursing, Complemental
Rush University College of Nursing
Rush Presbyterian St. Luke's Medical Center
Chicago, IL

**Carol Guarnieri, RN, MSN, AOCN**
Oncology Clinical Nurse Specialist
Samitivej Srinakarin Hospital
Bangkok, Thailand

**Irene Stewart Haapoja, RN, MS, OCN®**
Oncology Clinical Nurse Specialist
Rush Cancer Institute
Rush Presbyterian St. Luke's Medical Center
Chicago, IL

**Mel Haberman, RN, PhD, FAAN**
Director of Research
Oncology Nursing Society
Pittsburg, PA
Assistant Staff Scientist
Fred Hutchinson Cancer Research Center
Seattle, WA

**Lynne Hagan, RN, BSN, CETN**
Enterostomal Therapy
USC Kenneth Norris, Jr. Cancer Hospital
Los Angeles, CA

**Gloria A. Hagopian, RN, EdD**
Associate Professor of Nursing
Department of Adult Health Nursing
University of North Carolina, Charlotte
Charlotte, NC

**Pamela J. Haylock, RN, MA, ET**
Cancer Care Consultant
Kerrville, TX

**Jeanne Held-Warmkessel, RN, MSN, CS, AOCN**
Instructor, Roxborough Memorial Hospital
School of Nursing
Philadelphia, PA

**Laura J. Hilderley, RN, MS**
Clinical Nurse Specialist, Radiation Oncology
Radiation Oncology Services of Rhode Island
Warwick, RI

**Linda Hoebler, RN, MSN**
Oncology Clinical Nurse Specialist
Allegheny General Hospital
Pittsburgh, PA

**Rebecca J. Ingle, RN, MSN, FNP, AOCN**
Oncology Clinical Specialist
The Dan Rudy Cancer Center
Saint Thomas Hospital
Adjunct Instructor of Nursing
Vanderbilt University School of Nursing
Nashville, TN

**Joanne K. Itano, RN, PhD, OCN®**
The University of Hawaii at Manoa
School of Nursing
Honolulu, HI

**Barbara Hansen Kalinowski, RN, MSN, OCN®**
Clinical Research Nurse
Joint Center for Radiation Therapy
Boston, MA

**Marsha A. Ketcham, RN, OCN®**
Senior Research Nurse
Arizona Cancer Center
Tucson, AZ

**Paula Klemm, RN, DNSc, OCN®**
Assistant Chair
University of Delaware, College of Nursing
Newark, DE
Clinical Nurse
Department of GYN/OB
Johns Hopkins Hospital
Baltimore, MD

**Linda U. Krebs, RN, PhD, AOCN**
Nursing Oncology Program Leader and
Senior Instructor
University of Colorado Cancer Center
University of Colorado School of Nursing
Denver, CO

**Luana Lamkin, RN, MPH, OCN®**
Senior Vice President
Rose Medical Center
Denver, CO

**Jennifer Lang-Kummer, RN, MN, CS, FNP**
Oncology Case Management Services
Pitt County Memorial Hospital
Adjunct Assistant Professor of Nursing
East Carolina University
Greenville, NC

**Paul J. LeMarbre, MD**
Medical Oncology/Hematology
Waukesha Memorial Hospital
Waukesha, WI

**Julena Lind, RN, MN, MA, PhD(c)**
Assistant Professor of Clinical Nursing
University of Southern California
Los Angeles, CA

**Lois J. Loescher, RN, MS**
Senior Research Specialist,
Cancer Prevention and Control
Arizona Cancer Center
Tucson, AZ

**Jeanne Martinez, RN, MPH**
Clinical Nurse Manager
Northwestern Hospice Program
Chicago, IL

**Mary B. Maxwell, RN, C, PhD**
Clinical Specialist/Nurse Practitioner in Oncology
Veterans' Affairs Medical Center
Adjunct Assistant Professor of Nursing
Oregon Health Sciences University
Portland, OR

**Katherine McDermott, RN, MPA, OCN®**
Clinical Nurse Specialist
Division of Nursing
Memorial Sloan-Kettering Cancer Center
New York, NY

**Mary Ellen McFadden, RN, MLA, OCN®**
Clinical Support Specialist
Amgen
Baltimore, MD

**Deborah B. McGuire, RN, PhD, FAAN**
Edith Folsom Honeycutt Chair in Oncology Nursing
Associate Professor
Nell Hodgson Woodruff School of Nursing
Emory University
Atlanta, GA

**Joan C. McNally, RN, MSN, OCN,® CRNH**
Director, Health Care Services
Karmanos Cancer Institute Home Care
and Hospice Programs
Detroit, MI

**Mary Ann Miller, RN, PhD**
Associate Professor, College of Nursing
University of Delaware
Newark, DE

**Ida Marie (Ki) Moore, RN, DNSc**
Assistant Professor
College of Nursing
University of Arizona
Tucson, AZ

**Theresa A. Moran, RN, MS**
AIDS/Oncology Clinical Nurse Specialist
University of California, San Francisco/
San Francisco General Hospital
Assistant Clinical Professor
Department of Physiological Nursing
University of California
San Francisco, CA

**Judie Much, MSN, CRNP, AOCN**
Oncology Clinical Nurse Specialist
Psychosocial Support Nurse
Fox Chase Cancer Center
Philadelphia, PA

**Lillian M. Nail, RN, PhD, FAAN**
Associate Professor
Associate Dean for Research
University of Utah College of Nursing
Salt Lake City, UT

**Cathleen A. O'Conner-Vaccari, RN, MSN, OCN®**
Manager/Clinical Nurse Specialist
Memorial Sloan-Kettering Cancer Center
New York, NY

**Sharon Saldin O'Mary, RN, MN, OCN®**
Director of Hospice Services
Nations Health Care Hospice
San Diego, CA

**Diane M. Otte, RN, MS, ET, OCN®**
Alegent Health
Administrative Director, Cancer Center
Immanuel Medical Center
Omaha, NE

**Lawrence F. Padberg, PhD**
Vice President for Planning and
Enrollment Management
Marymount University
Arlington, VA

**Rose Mary Padberg, RN, MA, OCN®**
Nurse Consultant
Division of Cancer Prevention and Control
National Cancer Institute
National Institutes of Health
Bethesda, MD

**Patricia A. Piasecki, RN, MS**
Clinical Coordinator, Orthopedic Oncology
Rush Presbyterian St. Luke's Medical Center
Chicago, IL

**Sandra Purl, RN, MS, AOCN**
Oncology Clinical Nurse Specialist
Lutheran General Hospital
Park Ridge, IL

**Mary Reid, RN, MSPH**
Research Specialist
Department of Family and Community Medicine
University of Arizona
Tucson, AZ

**Mary Beth Riley, RN, MS**
Oncology Clinical Specialist
Rush Cancer Institute
Rush Presbyterian St. Luke's Medical Center
Chicago, IL

**Kimberly Rohan, RN, MS, OCN®**
Patient Services Coordinator
Edward Hospital
Naperville, IL

**Kathleen S. Ruccione, RN, MPH**
Division of Hematology/Oncology
Children's Hospital of Los Angeles
Los Angeles, CA

**Valinda Rutledge, RN, MSN, MBA**
Administrator
Brandon Regional Medical Center
Brandon, FL

**Vivian R. Sheidler, RN, MS**
Clinical Nurse Specialist—Neuro-Oncology
Johns Hopkins Oncology Center
Baltimore, MD

**Carol A. Sheridan, RN, MSN, AOCN**
Clinical Support Specialist
Amgen
New York, NY

**Joy Stair, RN, MS**
Director, Oncology Services
McAuley Cancer Care Center
St. Joseph Mercy Hospital
Ann Arbor, MI

**Carole Sweeney, RN, MSN, OCN®**
Fox Chase Cancer Center
Philadelphia, PA

**Karen N. Taoka, RN, MN, AOCN**
Clinical Nurse Specialist
The Queens Medical Center
Honolulu, HI

**Elizabeth Johnston Taylor, RN, PhD**
Assistant Professor
University of Southern California
Department of Nursing
Los Angeles, CA

**David C. Thomasma, PhD**
The Fr. Michael I. English S.J. Professor
of Medical Ethics
Director, Medical Humanities Program
Loyola University of Chicago Medical Center
Maywood, IL

**Peter V. Tortorice, Pharm D, BCPS**
Oncology Clinical Pharmacist
Illinois Masonic Cancer Center
Chicago, IL

**Steven Wagner, RN, BSN**
Nurse Clinician
Northwestern Hospice Program
Chicago, IL

**Janet Ruth Walczak, RN, MSN**
Clinical Nurse Specialist
The Johns Hopkins Oncology Center
Clinical Associate
The Johns Hopkins University, School of Nursing
Baltimore, MD

**Vera S. Wheeler, RN, MN, OCN®**
Consultant, Cancer Nursing and Biotherapy
Vancouver, WA

**Rita Wickham, RN, PhD(c), AOCN**
Assistant Professor, College of Nursing
Rush University
Rush Presbyterian St. Luke's Medical Center
Chicago, IL

**Debra Wujcik, RN, MSN, AOCN**
Clinical Director
Affiliate Network Office
Vanderbilt Cancer Center Clinical Trials Office
Adjunct Instructor
Vanderbilt University School of Nursing
Nashville, TN

**Connie Henke Yarbro, RN, MS, FAAN**
Editor, *Seminars in Oncology Nursing*
Clinical Associate Professor
Division of Hematology/Oncology
Adjunct Clinical Assistant Professor
Sinclair School of Nursing
University of Missouri–Columbia
Columbia, MO

**John W. Yarbro, MD, PhD**
Professor Emeritus, School of Medicine
University of Missouri–Columbia
Columbia, MO
Editor, *Seminars in Oncology*

# The Editors

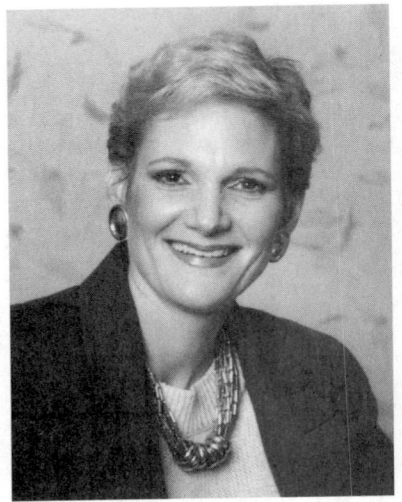

Susan L. Groenwald

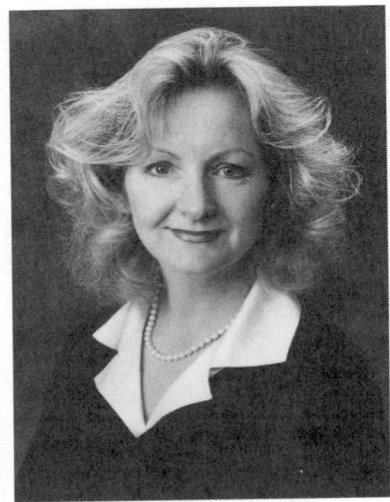

Michelle Goodman

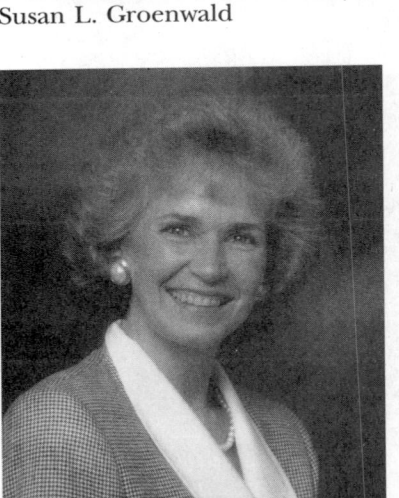

Margaret Hansen Frogge

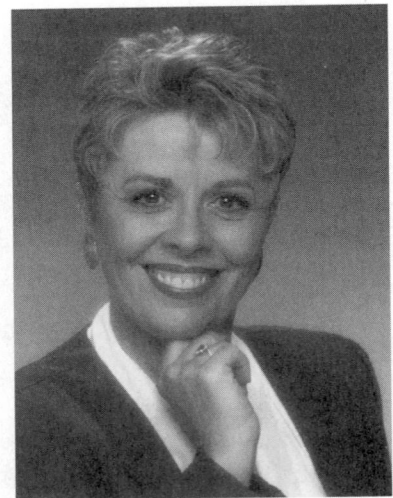

Connie Henke Yarbro

# Preface

The publication of this text marks the tenth anniversary of the first edition of *Cancer Nursing: Principles and Practice.* The preface to that first edition quoted Vincent DeVita at his swearing-in as Director of the National Cancer Institute (*The Cancer Letter,* 1980:4): "What we now know of the cancerous process and what we do to prevent, diagnose, and treat it will be outmoded and radically different by the end of the 80s." What foresight! Since the 1980s when work first began on the first edition of this text, the "war on cancer" has been waged by scientists around the world, resulting in a veritable avalanche of scientific findings about how cancer develops and progresses. The amount of information garnered over the past two decades is without parallel in the history of biomedical research. This knowledge gives new hope for saving lives through new methods of preventing and detecting cancer, provides the blueprint for new medical and nursing therapies that will extend and save lives, and offers information with which to improve the quality of life for those diagnosed with cancer.

With this increase in knowledge come new challenges to oncology nurses. Many cancer patients either receive treatment as outpatients or are discharged after a short hospital stay; as a result, they must care for themselves or their families must participate in complex care in the home. A greater number of people are living with cancer as a chronic disease, with increased physical, psychological, social, and economic needs. Within the next two decades, knowledge gleaned from the Human Genome Project will lead to predictions of likely cancers in specific populations, forcing difficult social and ethical issues. The explosion of knowledge within a sociopolitical environment in which change is exponential, faster is better, lower costs are mandated, and the population is aging provides even more challenges.

In the midst of these formidable challenges, nurses are poised to provide leadership in cancer care in the twenty-first century. Nurses are responsible for maintaining focus on the human being, whose life is the central focus of all biomedical research and knowledge. Nurses are advocates for access to care by the poor and underserved, play an important role in the ethical conduct of research, are dedicated to the provision of quality care, and provide the bridge of communication among disciplines and across care settings.

The magnitude, scope, and velocity of change in the health care arena demand that nurses have a broad, in-depth theory base for their practice as they are challenged with greater responsibility despite increasingly limited resources and support. This text was written to fill nurses' need for comprehensive information that is readily available. We believe that we are providing nurses with the most comprehensive cancer nursing text available, with the necessary science and theory base—as well as information for clinical practice, education, administration, and research—to face the challenges of the future. This has been and continues to be our commitment into the twenty-first century.

This fourth edition reflects the massive changes in knowledge about the biology of cancer and recognizes the changes in both systems and settings for the delivery of care. We have thoroughly updated all chapters, especially to reflect the changes in the environment in which care is provided.

An endeavor such as this is a daunting task. We are profoundly grateful to our outstanding contributors, who shared their knowledge and expertise in these pages amidst their own increasing responsibilities and scanty time; to our families, who had to live without us much of the time the book was in production; to the people at Jones and Bartlett for their continuing commitment to oncology nursing; to Rojean Wagner, Amy Lewis, Sarah Kimnach, and Penny Stratton at Editorial Services of New England for their patience and their commitment to excellence in preparing the final product; and to our readers, who tell us that this book is the "Bible" for their practices. We are awed by the compliment.

At the end of the day, it is the patients—the recipients of the knowledge we acquire and apply to their care—who will be the judge of whether progress has been made in the "war on cancer." This book is one small contribution to that important effort.

SUSAN L. GROENWALD
MARGARET H. FROGGE
MICHELLE GOODMAN
CONNIE HENKE YARBRO

# Contents

# PART I

# The Cancer Problem

**Chapter 1**

Milestones in Our Understanding of Cancer

**Chapter 2**

Biology of Cancer

**Chapter 3**

Carcinogenesis

**Chapter 4**

Cancer Control and Epidemiology

# Chapter 1

# Milestones in Our Understanding of Cancer

John W. Yarbro, MD, PhD

## INTRODUCTION

Cancer represents such a fundamental biological problem that its understanding requires an understanding of biology itself. Multicellular life forms depend for their very existence on the meticulous balance and regulation of reproduction, growth, development, tissue repair, response to injury, and regeneration. Cancer results from an imbalance, a perversion really, of these very mechanisms essential to life itself. It is no surprise, then, that a listing of the historical milestones related to cancer reads very much like a listing of the significant events in the history of medicine.

Cancer has been a challenge to physicians since the time of the Egyptians, Greeks, and Romans. Speculations as to its cause recorded in past centuries showed remarkable insights, as, for example, the relationship of nulliparity in nuns to breast cancer and of tobacco to nasal tumors only a few years after it was imported to London from the colonies. The notion of a cancer research plan was not invented by the National Cancer Institute; such a plan was formulated two centuries ago in Europe.

In spite of remarkable progress and the evolution of much useful knowledge, however, it has not been until the last two decades that a genuine understanding of the mechanisms of cancer has been possible because such an understanding demanded the technology to unravel and study in detail the genetic systems that lie at the heart of neoplastic growth. The story of our evolving knowledge is a fascinating one, even limited to its bare outline as is done here.

## "THERE IS NO TREATMENT"

The earliest description of cancer appears in the Edwin Smith Papyrus from Egypt in the seventeenth century B.C. After providing the oldest written description of a patient with cancer, the physician advises, "Thou should say concerning him . . . 'There is no treatment.' "[1,p.21]

A thousand years later, Hippocrates, the Father of Medicine, formulated his rules for medical practice in a series of Aphorisms. His cardinal aphorism, "Primum non nocere" (First, do no harm), is as valid today as it was in the fifth century B.C. It is widely believed that the Greek word for crab, *karkinos*, was first applied to cancer by Hippocrates. Aphorism number 38 states, "It is better not to apply any treatment in cases of occult cancer; for if treated, the patients die quickly; but if not treated they hold out for a long time."[1,p.23] More times than we like to admit, this aphorism is forgotten today.

Celsus, the great first-century Roman physician, compiled an encyclopedia of medicine, *De medicina*, containing many accurate clinical descriptions of cancer. Careful distinctions were made between benign and ma-

lignant disease along with treatment recommendations. His treatment was like that of Hippocrates. He noted:

> After excision, even when a scar has formed, none the less the disease has returned, and caused death; while at the same time the majority of patients, though no violent measures are applied in the attempt to remove the tumor but only mild applications in order to soothe it, attain a ripe old age in spite of it.[1,p.26]

Galen, the second-century Roman physician, was the central medical authority for over a thousand years because the church preserved hundreds of his writings and endorsed his views. His effect on the practice of medicine was immense long after the medieval period. He viewed cancer much as Hippocrates did, and his views set the pattern for cancer management for centuries.

The Middle Ages saw little progress in Europe, although medicine flourished in Byzantium and Arabia, where civilization persisted after the fall of Rome. The approach to cancer treatment remained Hippocratic (or Galenic) for the most part. There are, however, descriptions of attempts at radical surgery, such as the following byzantine procedure cited by Shimkin:

> I personally am in the habit of operating for cancer arising in the breast thusly: I make the patient lie down; then I incise the healthy part of the breast beyond the cancerous area and I cauterize the incised parts until the blood ceases by the formation of a coating. Then I again incise and excise the breast from its depth and I again cauterize the incised areas. And I repeat this procedure often, first cutting then cauterizing until bleeding stops.[1,p.33]

There was, of course, no mention of anesthesia.

## "THERE IS NO IMPROPRIETY IN REMOVING IT"

The advent of the Renaissance signaled the beginning of medical progress in Europe. With Galileo and Newton in the seventeenth century, there began what can legitimately be called the scientific method. William Harvey's *De Motu Cordis* in 1628, describing the circulation of the blood, provides the beginning of scientific cardiology. In 1761 Giovanni Morgagni of Padua was the first to correlate the clinical course of cancer to the gross pathological findings at autopsy, laying the foundation for scientific oncology.

Finally, in the eighteenth century, the great Scot surgeon, John Hunter, provided descriptions of the surgery of cancer that would bring nods of approval from modern surgeons:

> Great attention should be paid to the tumor, whether it is moveable or not, for as the disease is further extended so the parts are more united to the tumor. If the tumor is not only moveable but the part naturally so, then there is no impropriety in removing it. . . . [I]f any consequent can-

cers easy of extirpation are found, they may be safely removed also. But it requires very great caution to know if any
of these consequent tumors are within proper reach for we
are apt to be deceived in regard to the lymphatic glands,
which often appear moveable when, on extirpation, a chain
of them is found to run far beyond out of our reach which
renders the operation unsuccessful.[1,p.85]

A century was to pass before the development of anesthesia allowed the great surgeons of the nineteenth century
to develop radical cancer operations such as the classic
radical mastectomy, the principles of which can be recognized in the lectures of John Hunter.

## "CAUTIONS AGAINST THE IMMODERATE USE OF SNUFF"

The Egyptians blamed cancers on various gods. Hippocrates explained all diseases as resulting from an imbalance
of the four humors, in the case of cancer an excess of
black bile. For over a thousand years Galen and others
echoed Hippocrates. Then, as Europe entered the Age
of Reason, Bernardino Ramazzini, an Italian physician,
noted the high incidence of breast cancer in nuns and
hypothesized this was in some way related to their celibate
lifestyle.[1,p.92] The age of cancer epidemiology had begun.

John Hill of London was the first to recognize the
dangers of tobacco.[1,p.93;2] In 1761, only a few decades
after tobacco became popular in London, he published
a description of his observations entitled *Cautions Against
the Immoderate Use of Snuff*, which was subtitled "Founded
on the known Qualities of the Tobacco Plant and the
Effects it must produce when this Way taken into the
Body and Enforced by Instances of Persons who have
perished miserably of Diseases, occasioned, or rendered
incurable by its Use."[2,p.19]

The oft-cited description of scrotal cancer in chimney
sweeps by Percival Pott of St Bartholomew's Hospital in
London[3] was, according to Shimkin,[1,p.95] the third in a
series of reports that launched the field of cancer epidemiology. It has remained, however, the most frequently
cited example and has influenced our view of cancer
epidemiology and etiology. As we shall see, however, it is
the "immoderate use of snuff" that is our major cancer
problem today.

## "WE MIGHT SUPPRESS IT COMPLETELY IN AN EARLY STAGE"

At the beginning of the nineteenth century a committee
of English physicians and surgeons formed to investigate
the nature of cancer formulated thirteen questions, the
research significance of which would be instantly recog-

nized by any cancer scientist today.[4] Many of these questions were quite profound:

Are there premalignant lesions? If so, "though we are unable
to cure cancer in an advanced stage, we might extinguish
the disposition to it or suppress it completely in an early
stage."

"Are there any proofs of cancer being an hereditary disease?"

Is cancer infectious? Do some diseases degenerate into cancer?

"May cancer be regarded at any period or under any circumstances as merely a local disease?"

"Are brute creatures subject to any disease resembling cancer in the human body?" If so, investigation of cancer in
animals "may lead to much philosophical amusement and
useful information; particularly it may teach us how far the
prevalence or frequency of cancer may depend upon the
manners and habits of life."

This systematic approach to cancer biology laid the
foundation for scientific progress in the nineteenth century. For those of us who watched the National Cancer
Plan evolve after the passage of the National Cancer Act,
such a systematic set of questions strikes a familiar cord,
especially in view of the fact that some of the questions
asked in 1800 were the same ones asked again after nearly
two centuries.

The nineteenth century saw the birth of scientific
oncology as science shifted from anatomy to pathology.
Early in the century a microscope of sufficient quality
for research on tissues became available. The German
physiologist Johannes Müller applied this instrument to
cancer research and began to correlate cellular pathology
with clinical symptoms. He established a *cellular* basis for
tumor description. Subsequently, this work was carried
on by the man usually described as the founder of cellular
pathology, Rudolf Virchow of Berlin, who provided the
scientific basis for the modern pathological study of cancer. As Morgagni had correlated the gross autopsy findings with the clinical history of illness, so now the
microscopic findings were similarly correlated.

Rudolph Virchow established the microscopic basis
for the characterization of cancer. But even Virchow failed
to recognize the cellular nature of metastasis. He felt that
circulating cancer cells in the blood would be trapped
by the lungs, and he concluded:

The manner in which the metastatic diffusion takes place
seems, on the contrary, to render it probable that the trans-
ference takes place by means of certain fluids, and that these
possess the power of producing an infection which disposes
different parts to a reproduction of a mass of the same
nature as that which originally existed. . . . There are, however, many facts, which speak but little in favor of the infection's taking place by means of really detached cells, for
example, the circumstance that certain processes advance
in a direction contrary to that of the current of lymph, so
that after cancer of the breast, disease of the liver takes place

whilst the lung remains unaffected. Here it seems pretty probable that juices are taken up, which occasion a further propagation.[5,pp.219,460]

Wilhelm Waldeyer of Berlin did not agree that cancer metastases resulted from some kind of noncellular infectious substance; he felt *embolic* transfer through the blood or lymph channels was the mechanism.[6] The pathological basis of malignancy began to be understood, and pathology began to replace anatomy as the key basic science.

## "THIS IS NO HUMBUG!"

Soporific and narcotic agents had been used for centuries to control the pain of surgery. The effect of nitrous oxide (laughing gas) had been noted and led to its social use at parties in the nineteenth century. The suggestion that it might reduce surgical pain was not followed up. Hypnotism had been used to control pain, but this had not been accepted by the medical profession. Dr. Crawford Long of Georgia used sulfuric ether in 1842 but did not report his work. A dentist, Horace Wells, attempted to demonstrate laughing gas as an anesthetic before a medical school class at Harvard, but the patient cried out and the dentist was booed and hissed.[7]

Finally, in 1846 anesthesia was shown to work. John C. Warren, a Boston surgeon, had trained under Astley Cooper in London, and Cooper had been a student of the great Scot surgeon John Hunter, who had studied with Percival Pott. In 1846 Warren performed the first reported operation on a patient anesthetized with ether by a dentist, William Thomas Morton. The absence of pain in his patient led Warren to observe "Gentlemen, this is no humbug!"[7]

Oliver Wendell Holmes coined the term *anesthesia*. Prior to this time, the notion of anesthesia had bordered on quackery, and it was not immediately accepted. The Calvinist church fathers in England decried its use for childbirth, citing the biblical admonition that women must bring forth children in pain. But Queen Victoria elected to use chloroform anesthesia during the birth of one of her many children, and this brought about general public acceptance.[7] Anesthesia allowed the rapid progress in surgery that caused the next hundred years to be called "the century of the surgeon."[8]

## "THERE IS NO SUCH THING AS AN INEVITABLE INFECTION"[9,p.51]

Eight years after John Warren concluded that anesthesia was "no humbug," Florence Nightingale led a party of 38 nurses on a mission of mercy to the Crimean War.

When she returned to England in 1856, the care of the sick and the operation of hospitals were never to be the same again. She described nursing as the "finest of the fine arts";[9,p.68] she noted its uniqueness by observing that "nursing and medicine should never be mixed up. It spoils both";[9,p.68] she demanded influence for nurses: "[D]octors are very liable to imagine they must have the control of the whole staff";[9,p.54] she echoed Hippocrates' cardinal aphorism, relating it to hospitals: "[A] first requirement is that a hospital should do the sick no harm";[9,p.49] and she advocated preventive medicine policies far ahead of her time when she said she wanted to "inoculate the country with the view of preventing instead of cure."[9,p.39]

Nursing is, of course, older than Florence Nightingale. There were many unnamed and unrecognized women (can we doubt that they were women?) who, from the beginning, gave to the sick that solicitude, understanding, and attention to the *human* response to illness that is the essence of nursing. But Florence Nightingale gave the hospital the *professional* nurse and began that tradition of scholarship and dedication that continues today in oncology nursing. She identified the uniqueness in the practice of nursing that was not the same as the practice of medicine, and she based the professionalism of nursing on that uniqueness.

## "AMPUTATION OF THE SHOULDER JOINT MIGHT ERADICATE THE DISEASE"

There were great surgeons before the discovery of anesthesia. Such names as John Hunter, Astley Cooper, and John Warren come to mind. But when anesthesia became available at midcentury, there emerged the giants whose work so rapidly advanced the art that the next hundred years became known as "the century of the surgeon."[8] Three surgeons stand out because of their contributions to the art of cancer surgery: Bilroth in Germany, Handley in London, and Halsted at Johns Hopkins. Their work led to the "cancer operation" designed to remove all of the tumor en bloc as well as the lymph nodes that normally drained the region where the tumor was located.

William Stewart Halsted, professor of surgery at Johns Hopkins University, developed the radical mastectomy during the last decade of the nineteenth century. His work was based in part on that of W. Sampson Handley, the London surgeon who believed that cancer spread centrifugally through the lymphatics in continuity with the original growth.[10] Halsted's concept of the natural history and biology of cancer and its treatment are best described in his own words:

We believe with Handley that cancer of the breast in spreading centrifugally preserves in the main continuity with the original growth. . . . Although it undoubtedly occurs, I am not sure that I have observed from breast cancer, metastasis which seemed definitely to have been conveyed by way of the blood vessels. . . . [T]here comes to the surgeon an encouragement to greater endeavor. . . . [W]e must remove not only a very large amount of skin and a much larger area of subcutaneous fat and fascia, but also strip the sheaths from the upper part of the rectus, the serratus magnus, the subscapularis, and at times from parts of the latissimus dorsi and teres major. Both pectoral muscles are, of course, removed. . . . It must be our endeavor to trace more definitely the routes traveled in metastasis to bone, particularly the humerus, for it is even possible in cases of involvement of this bone that amputation of the shoulder joint plus a proper removal of the soft parts might eradicate the disease. So too it is conceivable that ultimately, when our knowledge of the lymphatics traversed in cases of femur involvement becomes sufficiently exact, amputation at the hip joint may seem indicated.[11,p.4]

The Halsted and Handley doctrine stated simply that cancer is contained within anatomical compartments and can be cured by radical resection en bloc of these compartments. This became the basis of the "cancer operation" for almost a century until it was called into question by the work of two twentieth-century surgeons.

## "THE SEED AND THE SOIL"

At the same time Halsted and Handley were developing their radical operations based on their interpretation of the spread of breast cancer, another surgeon was asking, "What is it that decides which organs shall suffer in a case of disseminated cancer?" Stephen Paget wrote, "I have collected 735 fatal cases of cancer of the breast in each of which a necropsy was made and recorded," and he concluded that cancer cells spread by way of the bloodstream and further that the disproportion of metastases to certain organs "cannot be due to chance."[12,p.572] In a brilliant leap of logic he drew an analogy between cancer metastasis and seeds, which "are carried in all directions, but they can only live and grow if they fall on congenial soil."

Paget had concluded that cells from a primary tumor are able to grow in only certain other organs—not in any organ in which they happen to come to rest. This accurate but highly sophisticated hypothesis was confirmed by the techniques of modern molecular biology almost a hundred years later.[13] Paget, on the basis of careful pathological examination at hundreds of autopsies, drew the correct conclusion, whereas others viewing the same autopsy material, including Virchow and Halsted, drew the wrong conclusion. The implications for the treatment of cancer are substantially different—indeed, in some ways quite the opposite—because this is the element in the new biological understanding of cancer that is integral to the breast conservation surgery introduced in recent years.

## "ALL VESTIGES OF HER PREVIOUS CANCEROUS DISEASE HAD DISAPPEARED"

The end of the nineteenth century saw publication of a second seminal but neglected paper. Thomas Beatson graduated from the University of Edinburgh in 1874 and developed an interest in lactation and ovarian function because he lived near a large sheep farm in rural Scotland. In 1878 he investigated the effect on the breasts of removing the ovaries of rabbits and found that lactation continued so long as the young were suckling but that the breasts atrophied and became fatty after suckling ceased. Here is the way he described his thoughts in a lecture to the Edinburgh Medico-Chirurgical Society in 1896:

> This fact seemed to me of great interest, for it pointed to one organ holding control over the secretion of another and separate organ. . . . I was struck by the local proliferation of epithelium seen in lactation. Here was the very thing characteristic of carcinoma of the breast, and indeed, of the cancerous process everywhere, but differing from it in that it was held in control by another organ.[14,p.105]

Because the breast was "held in control" by the ovaries, he decided to test oophorectomy in advanced breast cancer. The first patient he treated presented with a massive local recurrence. Regression of the recurrent tumor began five weeks after the operation, and by eight months "all vestiges of her previous cancerous disease had disappeared."[14,p.106] His second case had a far-advanced inoperable primary breast cancer, and oophorectomy led to a good partial remission. His third case, also an advanced inoperable primary tumor, showed continued progression after oophorectomy.

These cases led him to speculate that "the ovaries may be the exciting cause of carcinoma"[14,p.106] in women with breast cancer, an observation of particular note in view of our present large trials of tamoxifen as a preventive in breast cancer. Here, for the first time, was an experimental observation that illustrated the potential for *systemic* treatment of cancer.

A half century after Beatson, Charles Huggins, a urologist at the University of Chicago, reported dramatic regression of metastatic prostate cancer following castration.[15,16] In 1966 Huggins received the Nobel Prize.

## "A NEW KIND OF RAY" ("UBER EINE NEUE ART VON STRAHLEN")

In 1896, exactly halfway through the century of the surgeon, a remarkable lecture was presented by Wilhelm Conrad Roentgen, a German physics professor from Würzburg. This lecture was to provide the clinician with a second modality of cancer therapy. Actually, the lecture was published before it was delivered because the editor of the journal recognized its major importance and rushed it into print. The paper was entitled "Uber eine neue Art von Strahlen" ("Concerning a new kind of ray"), which Roentgen called the *x-ray*, "*x*" being the algebraic symbol for the unknown.[17]

There was immediate worldwide excitement. Roentgen's experiments were confirmed and their significance immediately recognized. Within months, systems were being devised to use x-rays for diagnosis. This was not surprising, but what was remarkable was that within three years radiation was used in the treatment of cancer. In 1901 Roentgen received the first Nobel Prize awarded in physics.

Radiation therapy began as brachytherapy with radium and as external beam therapy with relatively low-voltage diagnostic machines. It was in France that the major breakthrough took place when it was discovered that delivering radiation over a protracted period of time by use of daily fractions would greatly improve therapeutic response.[18]

## "FROM A BIT INOCULATED INTO BREAST MUSCLE OF A SUSCEPTIBLE FOWL"

The nineteenth century had begun with 13 questions. The twentieth century opened with three important answers: in the short span of 13 years, radiation, viral, and chemical carcinogenesis were clearly demonstrated. These three discoveries changed the entire focus of cancer research.

Radiation was recognized as a carcinogen only seven years after Roentgen's discovery of x-rays,[19] and a few years later a relationship to leukemia was recognized.[20] Early workers must have received massive doses of radiation to make the clinical association between radiation and cancer so obvious that it was noticed in such a short time. By comparison, the excess cancer deaths in the Hiroshima and Nagasaki populations were only about 8%, and leukemia was seen at an incidence of only about 1.5 cases per million people per year per rad of dose.[21]

In 1911 Peyton Rous, at the Rockefeller Institute, described a sarcoma in chickens caused by what later became known as the Rous sarcoma virus.[22] He ground up a tumor of chickens and passed it through a paper filter to remove the cells. He then injected this cell-free filtrate into chickens. "From a bit inoculated into the breast muscle of a susceptible fowl there develops rapidly a large firm growth; metastasis takes place to the viscera; and within four weeks the host dies."[22,p.1445] Since neither bacteria nor cells could pass through the filter, the idea that cancer might be caused by a virus was given firm experimental support. A half century later, the Rous virus was the source of the first well-characterized oncogene.

In 1915 cancer was induced in laboratory animals for the first time by coal tar applied to rabbit skin, at Tokyo University by Yamagiwa and Ichikawa.[23] The field of chemical carcinogenesis was launched with a firm scientific foundation and a research technique. This was a century and a half after the most destructive chemical carcinogen known to man, tobacco, was first identified by the astute clinician John Hill. The aniline dyes had been found to be related epidemiologically to bladder cancer in humans.[24] The first potent synthetic laboratory carcinogen, dibenzanthracene, was discovered in 1930.[25] It was to be many years until we "rediscovered" tobacco as a carcinogen.[26–28]

## "WE GOT IT ALL"

For the second half of the century of the surgeon, cancer surgery was synonymous with the Halsted radical resection of a cancer and its draining lymph node groups, in the hope of removing the tumor before it spread. The most welcome words a patient could hear after an operation were "We got it all." Radiation therapy was viewed as a means of eradicating local and regional disease that was not resectable by the surgeon. Systemic therapy was virtually nonexistent. The "seed and soil" concept of Paget was forgotten.

Based on several good experiments, cancer was thought to be caused by chemicals or radiation. But the idea was widely held that a single change in the cell somehow transformed it to a malignant growth, and this clouded the thinking. Lymph nodes were thought to trap cancer cells, and the notion of regional spread and anatomic containment formed the basis for therapeutic strategy. The clinical behavior of cancer was well understood, but not in modern terms. Progress was held back by the failure to understand multistage carcinogenesis and to grasp the relationship of clonal selection during progression to the metastasis of cancer. A key discovery was made by Peyton Rous.

## "THESE TEND TOWARD MALIGNANCY FROM THE BEGINNING AND ATTAIN IT BY A CONTINUOUS SERIES OF ALTERATIONS"

In 1935 Peyton Rous, still at the Rockefeller Institute, was studying the manner in which a benign neoplasm, virus-induced rabbit papilloma, transformed into a malignant lesion. He reported:

> The early stages of the cancerous change cannot be comprehensively described without inclusion of the entire course of events in vigorous papillomas. These tend toward malignancy from the beginning and attain it by a continuous series of alterations. . . . Often the alterations which lead to carcinosis do not stop when malignancy has been

achieved, but go further until a state of great anaplasia has been attained. The postcancerous changes appear to be no separate course of events, but only a continuation of what was long since begun. These facts might be taken to indicate that the virus is the immediate cause for the carcinosis; yet they are compatible with the assumption that it merely provides an essential, preliminary cell disturbance.[29,p.537]

In a subsequent paper Rous reported his research with another model of carcinogenesis, the induction of skin cancers by the application of coal tar. It was in this paper that he most clearly defined the difference between what he termed *initiation* and *promotion:*

> Tarring provides them with the conditions needed for growth, but after it is discontinued the tumors all more or less gradually disappear unless some other aid is forthcoming. . . . Chloroform has a marked effect to cause latent neoplastic cells to form tumors, as we discovered by accident. Occasionally the external auditory canal of ears long previously painted with methylcholanthrene and still carrying growths became infested with mites. To kill them chloroform was dropped into the canal and in several instances, through a technician's error, it was used for nearly 2 months and allowed to spread to the surface of the ear. There the skin became swollen and pink and many additional tumors arose and grew rapidly. . . . It seems certain that many agents and influences which have no actual carcinogenicity will be found to stimulate the multiplication of latent neoplastic cells. . . . [T]his is distinct from carcinogenic power.[30,p.111]

These classic experiments, confirmed by Berenblum and Shubik[31] using croton oil as the promoter, formed the prototype for the way carcinogenesis was conceptualized. This led to the concept of *initiation* by one agent followed by *promotion* by another and finally *progression* of the tumor to a more malignant form. The initiator was viewed as able to cause cancer but only after a prolonged time. The promoter alone was viewed as not always capable of causing cancer but able to potentiate the effects of the initiator. The term *progression* was said by Rous to designate "the process by which tumors go from bad to worse."[32]

Foulds codified and expanded the concept of multistage carcinogenesis.[33] Progression to the metastatic phenotype has subsequently been well elucidated in modern biological terms by Fidler.[34] Evidence was obtained 20 years after Rous's work indicating that the first stage, *initiation*, is characterized by damage to DNA while the second stage, *promotion*, does not usually involve damage to DNA but, rather, stimulation of cellular proliferation. Promotion is reversible and exhibits a distinct dose response and measurable threshold that may be important in regard to environmental carcinogenesis. The third stage, *progression*, leads to morphological change and increased grades of malignant behavior, such as invasion, metastasis, and drug resistance. The highly malignant character that the cancer has attained at the time of diagnosis is the result of progression. In 1966, 55 years after his 1911 paper, Peyton Rous was awarded the Nobel Prize.

## "THE CLINICAL RESULTS WERE SOMETIMES DRAMATIC"

The century of the surgeon had begun in 1846. Fifty years later Roentgen presented his famous lecture on the x-ray. Exactly 100 years after the beginning of the century of the surgeon, the first anticancer activity of a chemical was reported. Paul Ehrlich, the German scientist who developed arsphenamine for the treatment of syphilis, is called the "father of chemotherapy," but today the term *chemotherapy* is usually applied to cytotoxic agents used in the treatment of cancer. Nitrogen mustard was the first such agent.

Nitrogen mustard was developed by the chemical warfare research division of the U.S. Army in the course of a search for agents more effective than the mustard gas used in World War I. It proved to have remarkable activity against the lymphomas. "Indeed, the results were sometimes dramatic."[35] This agent served as the model for a long series of alkylating agents that killed rapidly proliferating cancer cells by damaging their DNA.

Two years later Sidney Farber of Boston reported the efficacy of aminopterin (the predecessor of methotrexate).[36] Subsequently, Hitchings and Elion developed the antimetabolite 6-mercaptopurine,[37] and Charles Heidelberger developed 5-fluorouracil.[38] The era of chemotherapy had begun. The first cure of metastatic cancer was obtained in 1956 by the use of methotrexate in choriocarcinoma.[39] In 1988 Hitchings and Elion received the Nobel Prize.

## "CARCINOGENS ARE MUTAGENS"

It was not until 1944 that DNA was demonstrated to be the chemical mediator of heredity.[40] The Nobel Prize–winning discovery of the helical structure of DNA by Watson and Crick followed.[41] Classic work by the Millers had led to the understanding that covalent binding within the cell was essential for carcinogenic activity, and the active metabolites of carcinogens were later identified as electrophilic reactants that bind to DNA.[42] Carcinogens were found to be converted by a series of metabolic steps into free radicals, that is, compounds with a single unpaired electron that are highly reactive with molecules rich in electrons, such as DNA. Compounds called *antioxidants* inhibit carcinogenesis because they react with free radicals before the free radicals damage DNA.

A key discovery was made by Ames, who developed a classic assay system to measure carcinogens.[43] The assay, which employs bacteria, is based on the fact that most carcinogens are mutagens, that is, they damage DNA. The Ames system requires the addition of liver enzymes in order to convert the chemicals to be tested into their active form. The metabolism of a carcinogen leads to the final active chemical, called the *proximate carcinogen,* that reacts with the DNA.

The Ames assay, of course, only identifies mutagens. And whereas "carcinogens are mutagens,"[43,p.2281] not *all* carcinogens are mutagens and not all mutagens are carcinogens. To prove carcinogenicity, substantially more than merely a positive Ames assay is required. In smokers, for instance, it is possible to directly identify the carcinogen bound to DNA, the so-called hydrocarbon adducts.[44] The proximate carcinogen exerts its effect by binding to DNA and mutating it directly or by causing errors to be made when the host cell tries to repair the damaged DNA. However, many of the lesions produced by carcinogens are repaired. The best evidence for this is the extraordinary incidence of skin cancer in patients with xeroderma pigmentosum, a disease in which patients are unable to repair DNA damage from ultraviolet light.[45]

Cancer biology was beginning to take form, but, as we shall see, the problems were exceedingly complex. An important next step was to correct the idea of anatomical containment, and this was done in the clinic rather than in the laboratory.

## "I'M NOT SAYING IT. THE DATA ARE SAYING IT"

Our recognition of the futility of radical surgery in the management of cancer began with randomized trials in breast cancer and malignant melanoma. Two surgeons, Fisher[46,47] and Veronesi,[48–50] led the way to the overthrow of the classic "cancer operation" by their demonstration that survival in breast cancer and melanoma is independent of the extent of surgical resection. The Halsted radical mastectomy was relegated to the ash heap of history, and the whole question of the "cancer operation" was thrown open to experimental trial. This not only forced a recognition that our treatment methods must change but, of greater importance, led to the reevaluation of our notion of the anatomic containment of cancer and to an understanding that it is our *biology,* not our anatomy, that restricts cancer spread.

This revolution was not easily accepted. I will always recall Dr. Bernard Fisher's calm response from the podium at a surgical society meeting when an irate questioner challenged his data by almost shouting, "You're saying we don't have to remove the lymph nodes to cure the cancer?" Dr. Fisher's answer: "I'm not saying it. The data are saying it."

What was not understood by those for whom anatomy was central to cancer spread was that the cancer cells had spread throughout the body from the time the first capillaries had been attracted into the growing tumor by angiogenesis factor secreted by the tumor cells. The initial capillary membranes growing into minute tumors are incomplete. Tumor cells spread into the bloodstream from the very beginning but are unable to establish metastatic deposits because the cells have not yet evolved the capacity to proliferate outside the site of the primary tumor. The most dramatic modern clinical example of this principle occurs when ovarian carcinomatosis is treated by shunting the ascitic fluid and cells into the jugular vein: there are no systemic metastases even though ovarian cancer cells flow throughout the body in huge numbers.[51]

Rous had observed experimental tumor cells "going from bad to worse," and it was this change that made metastasis possible, not the breakdown of some anatomic barrier. Time is indeed a factor, as simple clinical experience has long indicated; however, the time is required not to overcome some anatomic containment but to allow evolution of the cells of the primary tumor into subclones capable of metastatic growth. This is an important distinction because it has implications for alternate therapeutic strategies. Establishing the genetic basis of this biological behavior, however, required the elucidation of the genes that cause cancer, the oncogenes.

## "CARCINOGENS, IRRADIATION, AND THE NORMAL AGING PROCESS ALL FAVOR THE PARTIAL OR COMPLETE ACTIVATION OF THESE GENES"

Researchers in chemical carcinogenesis were identifying mutagens, but the target genes of the mutagens were unknown. Virologists were identifying cancer-causing viruses, but their mechanism of carcinogenesis was obscure. These two separate lines of research were to intersect dramatically.

Increasing numbers of oncogenic viruses were discovered in animal systems. They were originally called *type C viruses* and later *retroviruses;* the latter term applied because they were RNA viruses that were converted to DNA by the enzyme reverse transcriptase. Retroviral DNA is then incorporated into the chromosomes of the infected cell; thus, retroviruses add their genes to the cell and in this way influence the cell's behavior.

Huebner and Todaro focused attention on the word *oncogene* in 1969 when they proposed that RNA viruses somehow placed viral genes in the human genome that were then genetically transmitted:

> It is postulated that the viral information (the virogene), including that portion responsible for transforming a normal cell into a tumor cell (the oncogene), is most commonly transmitted from animal to progeny animal and from cell to progeny cell in a covert form. Carcinogens, irradiation, and the normal aging process all favor the partial or complete activation of these genes.[52]

This was an attempt to identify the targets of carcinogens as retroviral genes inserted into the genome. Their theory was incorrect except in the isolated cell systems, but their notion of the oncogene as the target of mutagens persisted.

The basic experiments in retroviral carcinogenesis used animal systems and cell culture systems to demonstrate that the intact virus and isolated genes were able to induce malignant transformation. This allowed the identification of the specific genes of oncogenic viruses that were capable of causing cancer. These genes were called *oncogenes*. A host of retroviruses that caused animal cancers and transformed cells in culture were identified, and each was found to contain an essential cancer-causing gene that was named after the virus.

Genes are usually designated by a three-letter code in lowercase italics, sometimes preceded by a *v*- for a viral gene or a *c*- for a cellular gene. The abbreviation for the gene often relates to the system in which it was first discovered; for example, *ras* was discovered in a rat sarcoma, *sis* was discovered in a simian sarcoma. Some genes such as *erbB* or *Ha-ras* have names that do not fit this system exactly. Some authors designate human genes using uppercase italic letters so that human homologue of the animal gene *myc* is sometimes written as *MYC*. Genes are also designated by letters describing the disease in which they were discovered: *RB* for retinoblastoma gene, *WT* for Wilms' tumor gene, *DCC* for deleted in colon cancer, and so on. Some writers use the term *proto-oncogene* for normal genes before they are modified (mutated) to become oncogenes. Other writers use the term *oncogene* as a general term for both the normal and the mutated gene.

Two discoveries led to a better understanding of how oncogenes relate to growth factors. It was found that the gene *v-sis* of the simian sarcoma virus coded for a protein that was very similar to platelet-derived growth factor (PDGF),[53,54] which is released by blood platelets in a clot to stimulate scar formation. Second, the gene *v-erbB* of the chicken erythroblastosis virus was found to be very similar to the gene coding for the epidermal growth factor receptor.[55] This provided strong support for the hypothesis that the oncogenes found in retroviruses were the same as the growth factor and growth factor receptor genes found in normal cells.

It is now known that experimental retroviruses obtain their oncogenes by capture of normal genes from the host cell. The retroviral carcinogenesis experiments did not lead, as was first hoped, to identification of a large number of retroviruses that caused human cancer. Among the human retroviruses, HTLV-1 has been clearly implicated in adult T-cell leukemia/lymphoma (ATLL), which is a malignancy of mature T4 lymphocytes endemic in Japan, the Caribbean, parts of Africa, and the southeastern United States.[56] Transmission of the virus is by sexual contact or through contaminated blood. The story on the retrovirus HIV in AIDS-related tumors is interesting but not yet complete.[58]

Retroviral oncogene research did, however, allow the identification of many human oncogenes that code for normal growth-promoting substances and improved our understanding of the way in which oncogenes promote normal and neoplastic growth. Oncogenes have been identified for many cell signals in addition to growth factors and growth factor receptors. These include signal amplification and transmission within the cell and signal reception within the nucleus.[58]

We now know that it is the human growth control genes, first identified as oncogenes in retroviruses, that are the long-sought-after targets of the mutating chemicals and radiation that contribute certain critical lesions leading to human cancer. But mutated oncogenes alone are not sufficient to cause human malignancies. Fusing a cancer cell with a normal cell will lead to suppression of malignant growth,[59] indicating that there are genes that suppress growth. These suppressor genes were first demonstrated as the targets of the oncogene products of the DNA viruses.

## "THE FIRST DEMONSTRATION OF A PHYSICAL LINK BETWEEN AN ONCOGENE AND AN ANTIONCOGENE"[60]

The DNA viruses are involved in several tumors. Unlike the retroviruses, the oncogenes of DNA viruses are not recently captured cellular genes, and thus they do not have such a close structural relationship to human genes. Their products do, however, react with the products of human genes. The first demonstration of this was the interaction of a protein of adenovirus with the *RB* gene product.[60]

The mechanisms of carcinogenesis by the DNA viruses are more complex than is the case for the retroviruses. Three examples illustrate this complexity. The polyomavirus produces an oncogenic protein that binds to a cellular oncogene protein product (c-src). This binding alters the c-src protein so that it resembles that of the protein produced by the retroviral *v-src* of the Rous sarcoma virus. It would seem that the polyoma virus achieves the same end point as the Rous sarcoma virus, but by a somewhat different mechanism.

A second example is illustrated by the Epstein-Barr virus (EBV), a herpes virus. A characteristic chromosomal translocation is seen in patients with Burkitt's lymphoma that activates the *c-myc* gene located on chromosome 8. This is the same proto-oncogene activated by the chicken myeloid leukemia retrovirus, but the mechanism of activation by the DNA virus is different from that of the retrovirus.

The third example involves three viruses (simian virus 40, papilloma, and adenovirus), all of which transform cells by producing oncogenic proteins that bind to normal cellular proteins and block their function. The function of the affected cellular proteins is to "turn off" cellular proliferation, and they are of very special interest because they are the products of antioncogenes (cancer-suppressor genes). It is these cancer-suppressor genes that have recently produced the greatest research excitement.

Work with the oncogenes of the DNA viruses led to

discovery of several viruses causing human cancer and to a better understanding of normal cellular control mechanisms because the products of DNA oncogenes interacted with and blocked the action of normal growth-regulating cellular proteins.

## "GENES I HAVE CALLED ANTIONCOGENES"[61]

Oncogenes code for proteins that induce malignant growth by "turning on" cell division. There are proteins with an opposite function, to "turn off" cell growth. These suppressor proteins were discovered because the oncogenic DNA viruses had oncogenes whose products bound to and inactivated them. Since the genes coding for these proteins had an opposite function to that of oncogenes, they were called *antioncogenes;* because they suppressed malignant growth, they were also called *cancer-suppressor genes.* The absence of the protein product of one of these genes leads to a cell in which the effect of a growth-promoting factor goes unopposed. It is thought that most human cancers result from a combination of genetic changes that must include both the absence of the protein products of cancer-suppressor genes and the presence of abnormal products of oncogenes.

It is likely that for each "up-regulating" function coded by an oncogene there is a balancing "down-regulating" function coded by a cancer-suppressor gene. For example, to balance the protein kinases that activate molecules by phosphorylation, there exists a set of protein phosphorylases that inactivate the same molecule by dephosphorylation.[62-64] This down-regulating antioncogene system is at least as complicated as the up-regulating oncogene system, but it is only beginning to be understood.

The scientific basis for our understanding of this mechanism was laid in 1971 when Alfred Knudson argued, on the basis of a statistical model, that one of the two mutations required for the development of familial retinoblastoma was inherited and the second occurred in the retinal cells of the affected eye. In the nonheritable form both mutations occurred in the same cell after birth, with neither mutation being inherited.[65] The gene has been identified on chromosome 13 and named the *retinoblastoma gene (RB).* The inheritance is dominant, but both copies of the gene must be absent or damaged for a cell to be transformed, so we know that the function of the gene is to *prevent* malignant growth. Proof of this is that when the retinoblastoma gene is introduced into cultured retinoblastoma cells, the malignant growth pattern is suppressed.[66]

Transcription factors are proteins that bind specifically to DNA and initiate expression of a set of genes controlled by the binding site. The *myc* oncogene produces a transcription factor that stimulates cell division. The *RB* antioncogene product binds to the *myc* oncogene product and blocks its action, which is presumed to be a normal physiological control function since mutant RB protein does *not* bind myc protein.[67] The conclusion is that the protein product of the *RB* antioncogene down-regulates cell division by binding to a growth-stimulating normal cellular protein.[68-70] In tumor cells, presumably, the failure of the mutant RB protein to bind the *myc* or another transcription factor contributes to transformation.

RB protein is regulated by the master cell cycle control enzyme cdc2 kinase.[71] As a suppressor of cell division, the *RB* gene product competes with stimulating factors, such as cyclin A, for the same transcription factors.[72] When the *RB* gene is mutated, its normal suppression of cell division is absent, thus allowing neoplastic growth.[73] *RB* is commonly mutated in several human cancers, although it was first discovered in retinoblastoma.

## "THERE ARE TOO MANY MUTATIONS IN HUMAN CANCERS"

As human cancers were being studied for mutations of the oncogenes and cancer-suppressor genes, it became clear that the number of such mutations was exceedingly large in all human tumors—too large, in fact, to be explained by the simple action of carcinogens on human cells:

> The dilemma is that there are too many mutations in human tumors. . . . The spontaneous mutation rate in somatic cells is not sufficient to account for these multiple mutations. If the multiple mutations in tumors are causally associated with and not just an accompaniment of cancer, then I argue that an early step in tumor progression is one that induces a mutator phenotype.[74,p.3075]

How is this mutator phenotype produced? One of the most important of the cancer-suppressor genes, and the one that appears to be the most commonly altered in human cancer, is the gene located at chromosome 17p13 that codes for a protein designated p53.[75] The *p53* gene is the most frequently mutated gene in human cancer, being altered in as many as half of the common neoplasms.[76-78] This gene codes for a transcription factor that, in the form of a dimer or tetramer, binds specifically[79] to DNA and mediates RNA synthesis. Originally identified in cells transformed by simian virus 40 and thought to be an oncogene product because mutant forms exerted a dominant transforming effect on cells, *p53* finally has been recognized as a cancer-suppressor gene product. Addition of the *p53* gene to cultures of prostate cancer suppresses malignant growth.[80]

## "THE GUARDIAN OF THE GENOME"

The *p53* cancer-suppressor gene is the most important one so far discovered. Not only is it the most frequently mutated, but when it is not mutated, as is the case in some sarcomas, there is another abnormal gene activated that blocks the p53 protein.[81]

What is the normal function of *p53*? Several observations provide clues. When cellular DNA is damaged by radiation or radiomimetic drugs, p53 protein accumulates and the cells are arrested in G1 so that they do not enter mitosis until the DNA is repaired.[82,83] When normal *p53* genes are inserted into cancer cells, they may induce programmed cell death (apoptosis).[84,85] There is a cancer family syndrome, the Li-Fraumeni syndrome, in which *p53* is inherited in mutant form, and a cancer-prone strain of mice has been developed with a mutated *p53* gene. Such patients and such mice develop normally, suggesting that *p53* has no role in normal cell development; but these patients and mice are at high risk of developing many different forms of cancer, and fibroblasts from patients with the Li-Fraumeni syndrome are genetically unstable.[86,87] These observations suggest that the protein product of *p53* is the "guardian of the genome."[88,p.15] Its normal function may be to detect the presence of damaged DNA and arrest the cell cycle in G1 until the damage is repaired or, if not repaired, to induce cell suicide (apoptosis).

This hypothesis is consistent with the known observations regarding *p53*. DNA viruses must knock out *p53* in order to move the cell into S phase, which they need for their own replication; thus, DNA viruses produce proteins that inactivate the p53 protein. It explains why inherited mutant *p53* allows normal development but predisposes to an increased risk of malignancy. It explains the very high rate of mutation of cancer cells, which seems to be essential to the evolution of enough abnormal clones to promote transformation. Finally, it explains the susceptibility of cancer cells to radiation and chemotherapy since cancer cells often have mutant *p53* and they are unable to arrest in G1 to repair DNA damage done by treatment.

## "AN IMPORTANT SAFEGUARD AGAINST TUMOR DEVELOPMENT"[89,p.88]

*Apoptosis* is cell suicide, better known as programmed cell death. It results from a specific set of genetically determined events leading to the death of the cell and its degeneration and resorption by surrounding cells. The concept of apoptosis is not new. The term was coined a quarter century ago to describe a kind of cell death that is different from necrosis. There is no release of cell contents to excite inflammation. Adjacent cells, not professional phagocytes, ingest the cell debris.[90] The name of the phenomenon was derived from the Greek *apo*, meaning "apart," and *ptosis*, meaning "fallen."

Our understanding that multicellular life forms can live only if there is a proper balance between the different cell types of their bodies should, perhaps, have led us to the concept of apoptosis sooner. After all, the notion that some cells must die so that the whole organism can survive is hardly new. White blood cells sacrifice themselves in fighting infection; lymphocytes throw themselves against a foreign invader; skin cells protect for a few days and are discarded. It is only recently, however, that the importance of apoptosis in cancer development has been appreciated.

The sequential reactions of apoptosis are set in motion by a signal sent to the cell, or sometimes by the loss of a signal that is normally present. The cell no longer needed by the body, or perhaps dangerous to the body, then quietly dies. Drugs may induce apoptosis, as first observed when glucocorticoids were found to activate an endogenous endonuclease in thymocytes.[91]

When DNA is damaged beyond repair, the cell with the damage represents a danger to the host because it will have many, possibly hazardous, mutations. A system exists that checks the DNA to be sure it is undamaged before a cell is allowed to reproduce. This system involves the gene *p53*, the guardian of the genome described previously. When *p53* is mutated it cannot signal the cell to enter apoptosis, and the result is a proliferation of mutant cells, leading to malignant growth.

Another gene related to apoptosis is *bcl-2*, first described in nodular lymphoma. This is one of a family of genes that control apoptosis. A protein called Bax directly initiates apoptosis in lymphocytes, and the protein product of *bcl-2* exerts its antiapoptotic action by forming heterodimers with Bax.[92] Activation of the *bcl-2* gene in lymphoma confers resistance to apoptosis, giving the lymphoma cells a kind of immortality. Further, since cytotoxic cell killing by chemotherapy is dependent on apoptosis of cells whose DNA is damaged by the drugs, lymphocytes with activated *bcl-2* genes are resistant to the chemotherapeutic agents commonly used in lymphoma.[93]

The progression of tumors to increasing degrees of malignant potential is related to the failure of apoptosis. As tumors grow, regions of hypoxia develop. Hypoxia normally induces apoptosis, but in the presence of a defective *p53* gene or if *bcl-2* is activated, apoptosis is blocked. Thus, hypoxia acts to select cells with defective apoptosis and is a factor in tumor progression.[89]

It now appears that the primary mechanism by which most chemotherapeutic agents induce cell kill is by causing cell damage, especially genetic damage, that results in the induction of apoptosis.[94] Resistance to apoptosis, therefore, represents the most potent form of tumor cell resistance to chemotherapy. In this light, then, the inactivation of *p53* as a late step in tumor progression takes on great significance, although pathways to apoptosis independent of *p53* have been described.[95]

## CONCLUSION

The story is far from complete, but the pieces are beginning to fit together in a pattern that allows an appreciation of how cancer violates the fundamental biological processes of multicellular life forms. In one sense cancer can be viewed as a further step in evolution. Cells scheduled to die in the interest of the host evolve the capacity to escape host regulation and grow independently. They ultimately die, of course, when they kill the host, but as they begin their mutant lives we can see the biological control mechanisms that are being circumvented as the cells attempt to avoid programmed cell death. Indeed, our understanding of many fundamental biological mechanisms has resulted from our study of cancer. The cell cycle itself, fundamental to all living cells, is likely the target of mutations in essentially every malignant growth.[96]

We can expect many new and exciting discoveries in the very near future in regard to the biology of cancer, and we can expect that this new biology will have important implications in the management of our patients with cancer.[97,98] New targets for therapy are being identified, such as the enzyme telomerase, which is probably essential to the immortality of neoplastic cells.[99] There are likely to be a number of significant milestones added to our story before the decade is over.

## REFERENCES

1. Shimkin MB: *Contrary to Nature*. DHEW publication No. (NIH) 76-720. Washington, DC, 1977

2. Redmond DE Jr: Hill cautions against snuff in 1761. *N Engl J Med* 282:18–23, 1970

3. Pott P: *Chirurgical Observations Relative to the Cataract, ye Polypus of the Nose, the Cancer of the Scrotum, the Different Kinds of Ruptures, and the Mortification of the Toes and Feet*. London, Hawkes, Clarke, and Collins, 1775.

4. Shimkin MB: Thirteen questions: Some historical outlines for cancer research. *J Natl Cancer Inst* 19:295–328, 1957

5. Virchow R: *Cellular Pathology*. Translated from the second edition by Frank Chance. London, John Churchill, 1860, pp 219, 460

6. Triolo VA: Nineteenth century foundations of cancer research: Advances in tumor pathology, nomenclature, and theories of oncogenesis. *Cancer Res* 25:75–106, 1965

7. Lyons AS, Petrucelli RJ: *Medicine, An Illustrated History*. New York, Abrams, 1978, pp 527–532

8. Thorwald J: *The Century of the Surgeon*. New York, Pantheon, 1956

9. Baly M: *As Miss Nightingale Said*. London, Scutari Press, 1991

10. Handley WS: The pathology of melanotic growths in relation to their operative treatment. *Lancet* 1:927–933, 1907

11. Halsted WS: The results of radical operations for the cure of carcinoma of the breast. *Ann Surg* 46:1–19, 1907

12. Paget S: The distribution of the secondary growths in cancer of the breast. *Lancet* 1:571–573, 1889

13. Fiddler IJ, Hart IR: Biological diversity in metastatic neoplasms: Origins and implications. *Science* 217:998–1003, 1982

14. Beatson GT: On the treatment of inoperable cases of carcinoma of the mamma: Suggestions for a new method of treatment with illustrative cases. *Lancet* 2:104–107, 1896

15. Huggins CB, Hodges CV: Studies on prostatic cancer: I. The effect of castration, of estrogen, and of androgen injection on serum phosphatase in metastatic carcinoma of the prostate. *Cancer Res* 1:293–297, 1941

16. Huggins CB: Endocrine-induced regression of cancers. *Science* 156:1050–1054, 1967

17. Roentgen WC: Uber eine neue Art von Strahlen. *Sitzungsber. phys.-med, Gesellsch. Wurzb* 132–141j, 1895

18. Coutard H: Roentgen therapy of epitheliomas of the tonsillar region, hypopharynx, and larynx from 1920 to 1926. *Am J Roentgenol* 28:313–331, 1932

19. Frieben A: Demonstration lines cancroids des rechten Handruckens, das sich nach langdauernder Einwirkung von Roentgenstrahlen entwichelt hatte. *Fortschr Geb Rontgenstr* 6:106, 1902

20. Von Jagic N, Scwarz G, von Siebenrock L: Blutbefunde bei Roentgenologon. *Berl Klin Wochenschr* 48:1220–1222, 1911

21. Preston DL, Kato H, Kopecky KJ, et al: Studies on the mortality of A-bomb survivors: 8. Cancer mortality, 1950–1982. *Radiat Res* 111:151–178, 1987

22. Rous P: Transmission of a malignant new growth by means of a cell free filtrate. *JAMA* 56:198, 1911 (reprinted *JAMA* 250:1445–1446, 1983)

23. Yamagiwa K, Ichikawa K: Experimentelle Studie uber die Pathogenese der Epitheliageschwulste. *Mitteilungen Med Facultat Kaiserl Univ Tokyo* 15:295, 1915

24. Rehn L: Blasengeschwulste bei Fuchsin-Arbeitern. *Arch Klin Chir* 50:588, 1895

25. Kennaway EL, Hieger I: Carcinogenic substances and their fluorescence spectra. *Br J Med* 1:1044, 1930

26. Wynder EL, Graham EA: Tobacco smoking as a possible etiologic factor in bronchiogenic carcinoma: A study of 684 proved cases. *JAMA* 143:329–336, 1950

27. Doll R, Hill AB: Smoking and carcinoma of the lung: Preliminary report. *Br Med J* 2:739–748, 1950

28. Levin ML, Goldstein H, Gerhardt PR: Cancer and tobacco smoking: A preliminary report. *JAMA* 143:336–338, 1950

29. Rous P, Beard JW: The progression to carcinoma of virus induced rabbit papillomas (Shope). *J Exp Med* 62:523–548, 1935

30. Friedewald WF, Rous P: The initiating and promoting elements in tumor production: An analysis of the effects of tar, benzpyrene, and methylcholanthrene on rabbit skin. *J Exp Med* 80:101–125, 1944

31. Berenblum I, Shubik P: The role of croton oil applications associated with a single painting of a carcinogen in tumor induction of the mouse's skin. *Br J Cancer* 1:379–382, 1947

32. Rous P, Kidd JG: Conditional neoplasms and subthreshold neoplastic states. *J Exp Med* 73:365–389, 1941

33. Foulds L: The experimental study of tumor progression: A review. *Cancer Res* 14:327–339, 1954

34. Fidler IJ: Critical factors in the biology of human metastasis. *Am Surg* 61:1065–1066, 1995

35. Goodman LS, Wintrobe MW, Dameshek W, et al: Nitrogen mustard therapy. *JAMA* 132:126–132, 1946 (reprinted *JAMA* 251:2255–2261, 1984)

36. Farber S, Diamond LK, Mercer RD, et al: Temporary remissions in acute leukemia in children produced by folic acid antagonist 4-aminopteroylglutamic acid (aminopterin). *N Engl J Med* 238:787–793, 1948

37. Elion GB: The purine path to chemotherapy. *Science* 244:41–47, 1989

38. Heidelberger C: Fluorinated pyrimidines, a new class of tumor inhibitory compounds. *Nature* 179:663–666, 1957

39. Li MC, Hertz R, Spencer DB: Effect of methotrexate therapy upon choriocarcinoma and chorioadenoma. *Proc Soc Exp Biol Med* 93:361–366, 1956

40. Avery OT, McCarty M, MacLeod CM: Studies on the chemical nature of the substance inducing transformation of pneumococcal types: Induction of transformation by desoxyribonucleic acid fraction from pneumococcus type III. *J Exp Med* 79:137–158, 1944

41. Watson JD, Crick FHC: Molecular structure of nucleic acids: A structure for deoxyribose nucleic acid. *Nature* 171: 737–738, 1953

42. Miller EC: Some current perspectives on chemical carcinogenesis in humans and experimental animals: Presidential Address. *Cancer Res* 38:1479–1496, 1978

43. Ames BN, Durston WE, Yamasaki E, et al: Carcinogens are mutagens: A simple test system combining liver homogenates for activation and bacteria for detection. *Proc Natl Acad Sci U S A* 70:2281, 1973

44. Perera FP, Weinstein IB: Molecular epidemiology and carcinogen-DNA adduct detection: New approaches to studies of human cancer causation. *J Chronic Dis* 35: 581–600, 1982

45. Hall EJ: Principles of carcinogenesis: Physical, in DeVita VT Jr, Hellman S, Rosenberg SA (eds): *Cancer: Principles and Practice of Oncology, 4th ed.* Philadelphia, Lippincott, 1993, pp 213–227

46. Fisher B, Redmond C, Fisher ER, et al: Ten year results of a randomized clinical trial comparing radical mastectomy and total mastectomy with or without radiation. *N Engl J Med* 312:674–681, 1985

47. Fisher B, Bauer M, Margolese R, et al: Five year results of a randomized clinical trial comparing total mastectomy and segmental mastectomy with or without radiation in the treatment of breast cancer. *N Engl J Med* 312:665–673, 1985

48. Veronesi U, Valagussa P: Inefficacy of internal mammary node dissection in breast cancer surgery. *Cancer* 47:170–175, 1981

49. Veronesi U, Adamus J, Bandiera DC, et al: Inefficacy of immediate node dissection in stage 1 melanoma of the limbs. *N Engl J Med* 297:627–630, 1977

50. Veronesi U, Cascinelli N, Adamus J, et al: Thin stage I primary cutaneous malignant melanoma: Comparison of excision with margins of 1 or 3 cm. *N Engl J Med* 318: 1159–1162, 1988

51. Tarin D, Vass AC, Kettlewell MG, et al: Absence of metastatic sequelae during long term treatment of malignant ascites by peritoneo-venous shunting. *Invasion Metastasis* 4:1–12, 1984

52. Huebner RJ, Todaro GJ: Oncogenes of RNA tumor viruses as determinants of cancer. *Proc Natl Acad Sci U S A* 64: 1087–1094, 1969

53. Waterfield MD, Scrace GT, Whittle N, et al: Platelet derived growth factor is structurally related to the putative transforming protein p28-sis of simian sarcoma virus. *Nature* 304: 35–39, 1983

54. Doolittle RF, Hunkapiller MW, Hood LE, et al: Simian sarcoma virus onc gene *v-sis* is derived from the gene (or genes) encoding a platelet derived growth factor. *Science* 221:275–276, 1983

55. Xu YH, Ishii AJ, Clark M, et al: Human epidermal growth factor receptor cDNA is homologous to a variety of RNAs overproduced in A431 carcinoma cells. *Nature* 309:806–810, 1984

56. Poiesz BJ, Ruscetti FW, Gazdar AF, et al: Detection and isolation of type C retrovirus particles from fresh and cultured lymphocytes of a patient with cutaneous T-cell lymphoma. *Proc Natl Acad Sci U S A* 77:7415–7419, 1980

57. Blattner WA: Human retroviruses and malignancy, in Brugge J, Curran T, Harlow E, McCormick F (eds): *Origins of Human Cancer.* Cold Spring Harbor, NY, Cold Spring Harbor Laboratory Press, 1991, pp 199–209

58. Weinberg RA: Growth factors and oncogenes, in RA Weinberg (ed): *Oncogenes and the Molecular Origins of Cancer.* Cold Spring Harbor, NY, Cold Spring Harbor Laboratory Press, 1989, pp 1–16

59. Pereira-Smith OM, Smith JR: Evidence for the recessive nature of cellular immortality. *Science* 221:964–966, 1983

60. Whyte P, Buchkovich KJ, Horowitz JM, et al: Association between an oncogene and an anti-oncogene: The adenovirus E1A proteins bind to the retinoblastoma gene product. *Nature* 334:124–129, 1988

61. Knudson AG: Hereditary cancer: Oncogenes and anti-oncogenes. *Cancer Res* 45:1437–1443, 1985

62. Hunter T: Protein-tyrosine phosphatases: The other side of the coin. *Cell* 58:1013–1016, 1989

63. Marx J: Biologists turn on to "off-enzymes." *Science* 251: 744–746, 1991

64. Shen SH, Bastien L, Posner BI, et al: A protein tyrosine phosphatase with sequence similarity to the SH2 domain of the protein tyrosine kinases. *Nature* 352:736–739, 1991

65. Knudson A: Mutation and cancer: Statistical study of retinoblastoma. *Proc Natl Acad Sci U S A* 68:820, 1971

66. Huang HJS, Yee JK, Shew JY, et al: Suppression of the neoplastic phenotype by replacement of the *RB* gene in human cancer cells. *Science* 242:1563–1566, 1988

67. Rustgi AK, Dyson N, Bernards R: Amino-terminal domains of c-myc and N-myc proteins mediate binding to the *retinoblastoma* gene product. *Nature* 352:541–544, 1991

68. Mihara K, Cao XR, Yen A, et al: Cell cycle dependent regulation of phosphorylation of the human *retinoblastoma* gene product. *Science* 246:1300–1303, 1989

69. Huang S, Lee WH, Lee EY: A cellular protein that competes with SV40 T antigen for binding to the *retinoblastoma* gene product. *Nature* 350:160–162, 1991

70. Bandara LR, La Thangue NB: Adenovirus E1a prevents the *retinoblastoma* gene product from complexing with a cellular transcription factor. *Nature* 351:494–497, 1991

71. Wagner S, Green MR: A transcriptional tryst. *Nature* 352: 189–190, 1991

72. Bandara LR, Adamczewski JP, Hunt T, et al: Cyclin A and the *retinoblastoma* gene product complex with a common transcription factor. *Nature* 352:249–251, 1991

73. Marx J: The cell cycle: Spinning further afield. *Science* 252: 1490–1492, 1991

74. Loeb LA: Mutator phenotype may be required for multistage carcinogenesis. *Cancer Res* 51:3075–3079, 1991

75. Levine AJ, Momand J, Finlay CA: The *p53* tumour suppressor gene. *Nature* 351:453–456, 1991

76. Vogelstein B: Cancer: A deadly inheritance. *Nature* 348: 681–682, 1990

77. Hollstein M, Sidransky D, Vogelstein B, et al: *p53* Mutations in human cancers. *Science* 253:49–53, 1991

78. Chiba I, Takahashi T, Nau MM, et al: Mutations in the *p53* gene are frequent in primary, resected non-small cell lung cancer: Lung Cancer Study Group. *Oncogene* 5:1603–1610, 1990

79. Kern SE, Kinzler KW, Bruskin AM, et al: Identification of

p53 as a sequence specific DNA binding protein. *Science* 252:1708–1711, 1991

80. Isaacs WB, Carter BS, Ewing CM: Wild type *p53* suppresses growth of human prostate cancer cells containing mutant *p53* alleles. *Cancer Res* 51:4716–4720, 1991

81. Oliner JD, Kinzler KW, Meltzer PS, et al: Amplification of a gene encoding a p53-associated protein in human sarcomas. *Nature* 358:80–83, 1992

82. Maltzman W, Czyzyk L: UV irradiation stimulates levels of *p53* cellular tumor antigen in nontransformed mouse cells. *Mol Cell Biol* 4:1689–1694, 1984

83. Kastan MB, Onyekwere O, Sidransky D, et al: Participation of p53 protein in the cellular response to DNA damage. *Cancer Res* 51:6304–6311, 1991

84. Shaw P, Bovey R, Tardy S, et al: Induction of apoptosis by wild-type *p53* in a human colon tumor-derived cell line. *Proc Natl Acad Sci U S A* 89:4495–4499, 1992

85. Yonish-Rouach E, Resnitzky D, Lotem J, et al: Wild-type *p53* induces apoptosis of myeloid leukaemic cells that is inhibited by interleukin-6. *Nature* 352:345–347, 1991

86. Donehower LA, Harvey M, Slagle BL, et al: Mice deficient for *p53* are developmentally normal but susceptible to spontaneous tumours. *Nature* 356:215–221, 1992

87. Bischoff FZ, Yim SO, Pathak S, et al: Spontaneous abnormalities in normal fibroblasts from patients with Li-Fraumeni cancer syndrome: Aneuploidy and immortalization. *Cancer Res* 50:7979–7984, 1990

88. Lane DP: *p53*, Guardian of the genome. *Science* 358:15–16, 1992

89. Graeber TG, Osmanian C, Jacks T, et al: Hypoxia-mediated selection of cells with diminished apoptotic potential in solid tumors. *Nature* 379:88–91, 1996

90. Kerr JFR, Wyllie AH, Currie AR: A basic biological phenomenon with wide-ranging implications in tissue kinetics. *Br J Cancer* 26:239–244, 1972

91. Wyllie AH: Glucocorticoid induced thymocyte apoptosis is associated with endogenous endonuclease activation. *Nature* 284:555–559, 1980

92. Yin XM, Oltvai ZN, Korsmeyer SJ: BH1 and BH2 domains of Bcl-2 are required for inhibition of apoptosis and heterodimerization with Bax. *Nature* 369:321–323, 1994

93. Miyashita T, Reed JC: Bcl-2 oncoprotein blocks chemotherapy induced apoptosis in a human leukemia cell line. *Blood* 81:151–157, 1993

94. Thompson CB: Apoptosis in the pathogenesis and treatment of disease. *Science* 267:1456–1462, 1995

95. Clarke AR, Pirdie CA, Harrison DJ, et al: Thymocyte apoptosis induced by *p53*-dependent and independent pathways. *Nature* 362:849–852, 1993

96. Clurman BE, Roberts JM: Cell cycle and cancer. *J Natl Cancer Inst* 87:1499–1501, 1995

97. Yarbro JW: Breast cancer: The new biology in conflict with the old dogma. *Semin Oncol Nurs* 1:157–162, 1985

98. Yarbro JW: The new biology of cancer: Future clinical applications. *Semin Oncol* 16:254–259, 1989

99. Rhyu M: Telomeres, telomerase, and immortality. *J Natl Cancer Inst* 87:884–894, 1995

# Chapter 2

# Biology of Cancer

Paul J. LeMarbre, MD

Susan L. Groenwald, RN, MS

## INTRODUCTION

This world we see is one of wonder, but it is also more bewildering. There are areas of thriving populations with endless streams of moving vehicles; there are desolate expanses where little changes. Heroic sentinels guard the frontiers and sacrifice their lives to protect the masses. Death is encountered daily, but new life springs forth in its place.

It is a world where communication is highly valued, though positive and negative messages bombard the inhabitants incessantly. It is a realm of magnificent balance, except for those rare times that obstinate and self-seeking members arise from a tragic imbalance—this is the world of the human cell.

The fundamental goals of cancer research are to discern the causes of cancer cell development, the nature of biochemical mechanisms that result in the growth and spread of cancer, and, finally, the means to correct abnormal mechanisms and eradicate the cancer cell population. Our knowledge about the scope of cancer development is mounting ever faster; this chapter will review the general features of cancer cells and those factors that favor their growth and eventual spread.

## RESEARCH MODELS

### Limitations of Study of Human Tissues

A major technical difficulty in studying cancer cells is that researchers cannot be sure of the actual normal cell counterpart for a cancer cell in a given tissue. Human tissues are composed of multiple subpopulations of heterogeneous cells (various parenchymal cells with different appearances and stages of differentiation, vascular and lymphatic cells, connective tissue cells, and immune system cells); to identify the immediate normal precursor of a cancer cell, or to identify a true cancer cell or even a small population of cancer cells in a tissue, is exceedingly difficult. With the development of sophisticated laboratory techniques such as the polymerase chain reaction and monoclonal antibodies, the ability to isolate individual cells in a large population will soon be at hand.

### Transformed Cell Models

Even with the limitations mentioned, researchers have long relied on cell culture models to examine the various aspects of cell growth and development. Stable continuous cell lines from animals, and at times human cell lines, are utilized as "normal" prototypes. Cell lines can be developed from a single cell to provide a certain level of uniformity. The culture environment can be defined and modified. Cell lines may or may not become continuous; they do so when they develop the ability to propagate indefinitely in tissue culture (Figure 2-1).[1] Many normal cell lines will cease growing and die after a span of time, and this phenomenon is believed to be related to a "programmed" or defined number of cell divisions that a normal cell will make before it stops proliferating (*senescence*). Occasionally a cell line will continue to grow indefinitely; this pattern of prolonged growth is more likely to occur if the cells are exposed to carcinogenic agents (chemical, viral, or radiation), and the cells are thus considered to be *transformed*. The value of transformed cells in culture is that they often resemble neoplastic cells and can be studied experimentally; more practically, they represent a self-renewing population that saves researchers time and effort.

Normal cells typically will grow in a continuous single layer on a plastic surface, stopping at the boundaries of the chamber; at that point the population stabilizes and cell loss approximates cell growth. Transformed cells will grow in multiple layers or clusters, reaching higher densities in culture. If transformed cells are added to a normal monolayer, they typically form crisscrossing colonies or clusters on top of the monolayer. Transformed cells often will require fewer nutrients in the surrounding media; they have less contact inhibition, altered antigenicity, and the ability to flourish in semisolid media, suspended without a surface for growth (normal cells would not survive in culture in this way).[2] The most demanding criterion for transformation is the ability to form tumors when injected into nude (athymic, and thus with much weakened immune systems) mice. Not all transformed cells will exhibit every criterion.

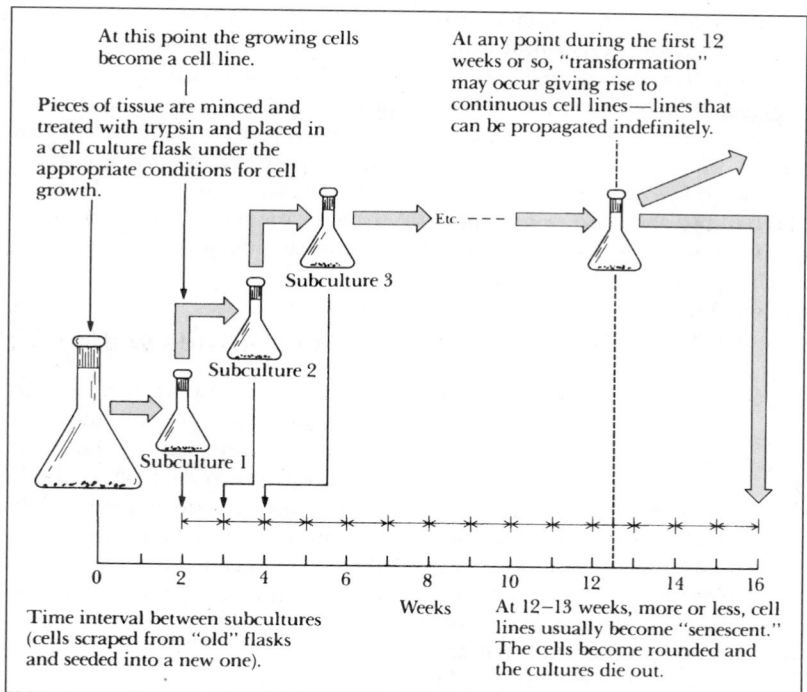

At this point the growing cells become a cell line.

Pieces of tissue are minced and treated with trypsin and placed in a cell culture flask under the appropriate conditions for cell growth.

At any point during the first 12 weeks or so, "transformation" may occur giving rise to continuous cell lines—lines that can be propagated indefinitely.

Subculture 3

Etc. ---

Subculture 2

Subculture 1

Time interval between subcultures (cells scraped from "old" flasks and seeded into a new one).

Weeks

At 12–13 weeks, more or less, cell lines usually become "senescent." The cells become rounded and the cultures die out.

**FIGURE 2-1**   How cell lines and continuous cell lines are derived. Continuous cell lines arise from normal cells by some kind of spontaneous change or "transformation." Except for their immortality, continuous cell lines behave like normal cells in culture. Transformed cells derive from continuous cell lines that have been exposed to radiation, chemical carcinogens, or oncogenic viruses and subsequently behave like cancer cells. (Reprinted with permission from Kupchella CE: *Dimensions of Cancer.* Belmont, CA, Wadsworth, 1987. Copyright © 1987 by Wadsworth, Inc.)

Unless researchers have access to actual human tumor cells that successfully endure in culture, transformed cells provide the best opportunity for investigation of cellular processes and behavior since they approximate the nature of malignant cells. Nevertheless, there are significant differences between the plastic microwells containing special media in the laboratory and the living tissue milieu of the human body; extrapolation from cell culture to cells in vivo may be inaccurate or incomplete, yet transformed cells in vitro are still a useful tool. For purposes of further discussion we will assume that transformed cells and cancer cells are essentially identical.

## DIFFERENCES IN THE FEATURES OF NORMAL AND CANCER CELLS

The primary difference between cancer cells and normal cells relates to abnormal growth regulation—cancer cells will grow even at the expense of outstripping their blood supply and destroying the host. Rapidity of growth is not a discriminating factor as many normal cellular processes (such as benign inflammatory lesions) have faster dou-

bling times than most cancer cells. Typically, cancerous tissues lack the structural and organizational integrity of normal counterparts.

Tumor doubling times are variable, but an average of two months is generally accepted. Normally a cellular mass grows to a certain volume and then stabilizes, with cell loss or death balancing new cell growth. In cancer, masses continue to expand beyond normal boundaries, with continued cell division overbalancing any cell loss. Cancer cells have a number of unusual characteristics that favor vigorous growth. These will be reviewed next.

### Immortality of Cancer Cells

The property of senescence limits normal cells to about 50 population doublings in culture; a small percentage of animal cells (less so human cells) continues indefinitely beyond this barrier and are determined to be "immortal." A potential counting mechanism to limit the number of doublings involves *telomeres*, which are DNA segments at the ends of chromosomes. Telomeres protect the chromosomal ends from damage, and the telomere length shortens a little bit with each chromosomal replication (during the phase of DNA synthesis). Once the telomere shrinks below a certain level or threshold, a signal is sent to the cell to enter senescence. If the cell continues to divide it will die. Many cancers contain an enzyme, *telomerase*, which replaces the segments trimmed away during cell division, enabling the cell to replicate indefinitely.[3]

In cells that transform while in cell culture external factors such as the media bathing them do not change. Thus, the likelihood is that a genetic mutational change has occurred, enabling the particular cells to have a growth advantage. A parallel situation, with multiple genetic changes, provides immortality for cancer in the human body.

## Loss of Contact Inhibition

As normal cells expand to form a monolayer in culture, a uniform "carpet" can be seen on the culture surface by microscopy. If a cut is made in the layer of cells, the damaged cells will disintegrate and other cells will develop, eventually restoring the monolayer to its original state. It has been assumed that this proliferation pattern demonstrates a cessation of growth when cells actually touch each other—this has been called *contact inhibition of growth*.[4] One salient reason to explain why normal cells do not form multilayers is the requirement for optimal utilization of nutrients; access to nutrients may well be compromised when normal cells crowd each other. The term *density-dependent growth*[5] has replaced the term *contact inhibition*.

Cancer cells have a different pattern of growth in culture as they pile on each other and form irregular masses of cells extending upward in the culture media. There typically appears to be no contact inhibition between cells, for a number of reasons: transformed cells are held less firmly to each other and also seem to move about with greater frequency; they also often have fewer requirements for growth substances in the surrounding media and therefore have a different density dependence than normal cells.

## Diminished Growth Factor Requirements of Cancer Cells

It has been known for a long time that cells in culture generally require some type of serum in their growth media for optimal results; undoubtedly the serum component provides necessary growth factors for the cells. Growth factors provided by serum have profound influences on normal cell development. Typically the growth factor binds with a receptor on the cell surface, which in turn activates the intracytoplasmic portion of the receptor, which is often an enzyme. As an example, this activated enzyme could have the capacity to add phosphate groups to other proteins (a protein kinase) and could start a cascade of biochemical reactions in order to send a message to the nucleus (a process called *signal transduc-*

*tion*), where an effect on gene function will take place. The cell consequently might secrete a factor that can stimulate itself (the *autocrine hypothesis*) or other cells around it. On occasion, an abnormal growth factor receptor on the surface of a transformed cell can activate the signal pathway spontaneously without exposure to a growth factor. Alternatively, transformed cell lines may grow in media without serum, suggesting that they can synthesize and secrete their own growth factors.

## Ability to Divide without Anchorage

The vast majority of normal cells require a surface on which to grow and generally cannot survive in a suspension or in a semisolid system such as agar. The situation is reminiscent of the physical supports in normal body tissue that provide a growth surface. This property of normal cells is called *anchorage-dependent growth*. Transformed cells can exist in a suspension or gel; this unique property is most closely associated with the ability to form tumors.[6]

## Loss of Restriction Point in the Cell Cycle

Cellular proliferation occurs as the result of two coordinated events: the duplication of DNA within the cell, and mitosis (the division of the cell into two daughter cells with identical complements of DNA). These two events make up what is known as the *cell cycle* (Figure 2-2). Control of the cell cycle resides in the cell nucleus, where various growth-related messages are funneled; a "decision" is then made by the cell whether to proceed through the cell cycle to form two daughter cells.

The cycle is made up of four stages. In the $G_1$ (or gap 1) phase, the cell enlarges and synthesizes proteins in preparation for copying its DNA. The exact duplication of DNA takes place in the S phase, and this is followed by $G_2$ (gap 2), where further protein synthesis heralds the onset of mitosis. In the M phase (or mitosis), equal divisions of chromosomes and cellular constituents are apportioned to the new daughter cells; they enter $G_1$ again, where they can begin the growth sequence anew, or they may divert themselves into a resting or quiescent state called $G_0$. Most of the cells in the adult body are in $G_0$, unless summoned to take the place of cells that are lost for whatever reason. Cells that are usually metabolically active, such as granulocytes and the epithelium of the gastrointestinal tract, are often in cycle.

A critical step in the cell cycle occurs late in $G_1$, when the cell has to decide if it will go through with the entire sequence or delay and rest—a sort of "point of no return." This threshold is called the *restriction point*. Sitting at the restriction point as the master brakeman to prevent the cycle from proceeding further is a protein called pRb (the product of the "retinoblastoma gene"). In order to release the "brake," a complex made up of a cyclin (a member of a protein family involved in regulation of

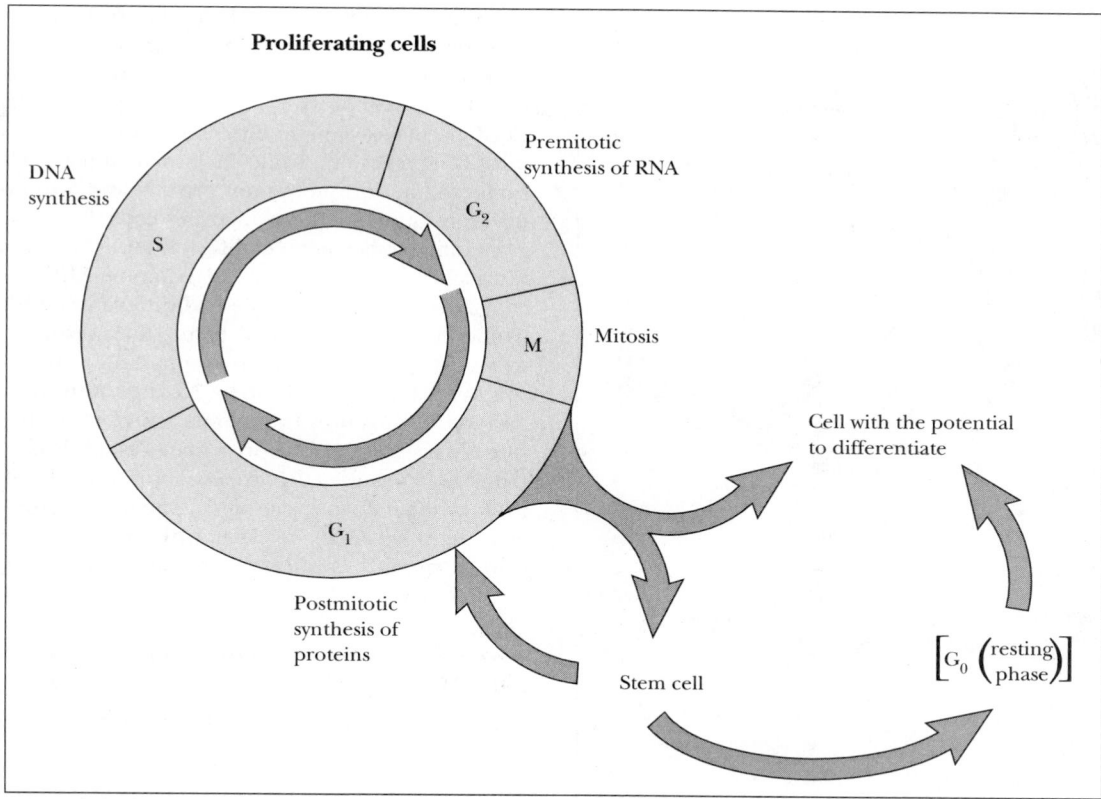

**FIGURE 2-2** The cell cycle.

the cell cycle) and a cyclin-dependent kinase transfers phosphate groups to pRb and temporarily inhibits the pRb effect.[7]

Normal cells will often leave $G_1$ and enter $G_0$ at the restriction point if there is a shortage of nutrients or growth factors. Many cancer cells lack this degree of control, particularly if they have too little of the pRb protein. This could also be a potential weakness for tumor cells exposed to chemotherapy because they do not have the option of slipping into $G_0$ to shield themselves from cytotoxins.[8]

## DIFFERENCES IN THE APPEARANCE OF NORMAL AND CANCER CELLS

Normal cells generally have a well-organized cytoskeleton composed of bundles of microfilaments and microtubules. The bundles consist of polymerized subunits of proteins that provide the structure and shape of the cell (Figure 2-3a). Transformed cells contain the subunits of proteins though they are not polymerized, causing transformed cells to have variable sizes and shapes (*pleomorphism*) (Figure 2-3b). There are a number of other important differences in the appearance of cancer cells and normal cells: the nuclei of cancer cells stain darker

(*hyperchromatism*) (Figure 2-3c); they are disproportionately larger (Figure 2-3d); and cancer cells frequently exhibit a variety of abnormal mitotic figures (Figure 2-3e). Occasionally the microscopic picture of a group of malignant tumor cells is indistinguishable from a population of benign cells; in this case the biological behavior of the cell population determines how the process is diagnosed.

## DIFFERENCES IN DIFFERENTIATION OF NORMAL AND CANCER CELLS

Following egg fertilization every somatic cell division will provide the daughter cells with an exact copy of the human genome, contained in 46 chromosomes. As a human matures, different cells must pursue various paths to provide for organ development and a reserve pool of uncommitted cells, which may develop into specific tissues at a later time. Embryonic cells necessarily are vigorous and possess certain characteristics that empower them with growth advantages compared with adult cells. They can migrate extensively, secrete factors to develop a new blood supply, and liberate enzymes to break down tissue barriers. Adult cells that activate embryonic programs of gene expression or inactivate portions of

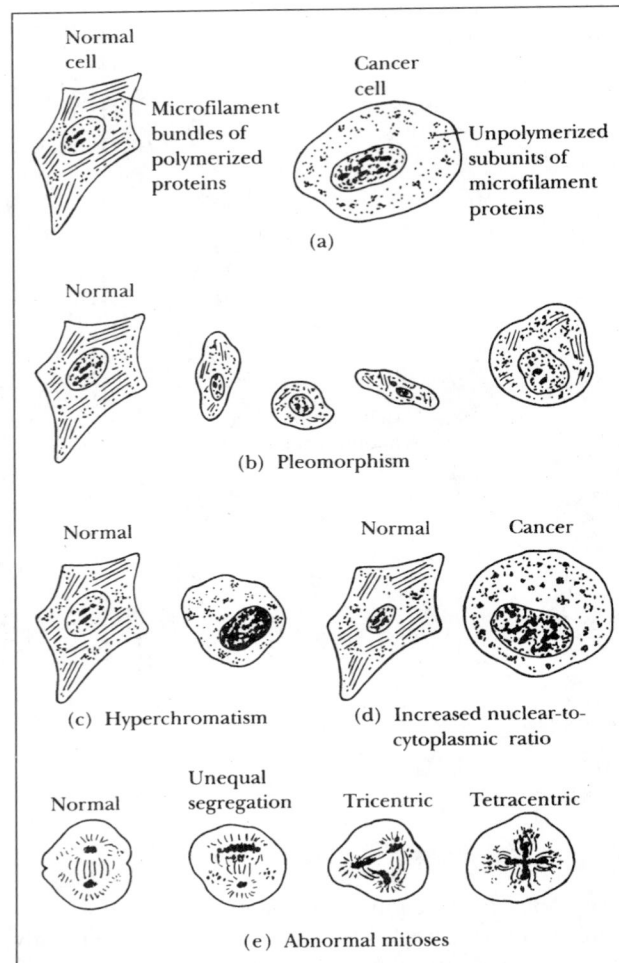

Normal cell
Cancer cell

Microfilament bundles of polymerized proteins

Unpolymerized subunits of microfilament proteins

(a)

Normal

(b) Pleomorphism

Normal

Normal    Cancer

(c) Hyperchromatism

(d) Increased nuclear-to-cytoplasmic ratio

Normal     Unequal segregation    Tricentric    Tetracentric

(e) Abnormal mitoses

**FIGURE 2-3**   Differences in appearance of normal cells and cancer cells.

the adult program may behave like malignant tumor cells.[9]

Different organs have disparate potentials for cell renewal and specific functions: nerve cells are very slow to recover from injury, whereas the liver can virtually replace itself if a major portion is resected. Each cell has the same DNA content, but only a portion of the total gene pool in a cell is expressed. As a cell assumes a distinct "personality" distinguishing it in structure and function from other cells, it is considered to be "differentiated." In a differentiated cell, particular genes are activated, leading to specific messenger RNA molecules that are translated into specific proteins; these proteins will then determine the fate of that cell. As a cell becomes more differentiated, its repertoire may be more restricted and attuned to its organ of residence; it also may lose the ability to replicate.

The process of differentiation for embryonic cells involves influences from the extracellular environment, including soluble factors. Growth factors may arise from neighboring cells or from the extracellular matrix. Fibroblast growth factors can induce mesodermal differentiation in early embryos through an interaction with membrane receptors.[10] Transforming growth factor-beta (TGF-β) may stimulate differentiation in some cells and inhibit it in others, while in human tumor cell populations it may inhibit tumor growth and promote more differentiation in the remaining cells.[11] An example of a membrane-permeable differentiating agent that acts intracellularly is retinoic acid (vitamin A).[12]

Cancer cells tend to be less differentiated than cells from surrounding normal tissue. Some cancer cells are so poorly differentiated (or anaplastic) that the tissue origin cannot be ascertained. Normal cells may undergo a gradual transition to malignancy, passing through the stages of *metaplasia* (the presence of a mildly less differentiated-appearing cell), *dysplasia* (deranged cell growth with variable shape, size and appearance), *carcinoma in situ* (literally cancer in place, with no evidence of extension or spread), and finally invasive cancer.[13]

## DIFFERENCES IN THE CELL SURFACES OF NORMAL AND CANCER CELLS

The cell membrane is the complex covering of animal cells that determines what molecules can enter and leave the cell. It is the element of both cell contact and cell adhesion. The most elementary cell membrane consists of two layers of lipid molecules (called a *lipid bilayer*). Various proteins and *glycoproteins* (proteins with sugars attached) are embedded in the lipid bilayer. Some of the proteins reside exclusively on the membrane surface (*peripheral proteins*); others are found partly or completely embedded in the membrane (*integral proteins*). The cell membrane is a loose structure, with many fluidlike properties, as proteins and glycoproteins move both laterally and between the layers, albeit slowly. The fluid nature of the membrane and the existence of mobile proteins within the membrane and on the surface was described by Singer and Nicolson[14] as the *fluid mosaic model*.

The cell surface and membrane are particularly important in cancer biology because they are involved in anchorage dependence, cell adhesion, and invasiveness, not to mention literally hundreds of biochemical interactions. Research has shown that a variety of changes occur in the surface of a cancer cell. Some new molecules appear, some molecules that normally appear are lost, and other molecules are changed.[15,16] Figure 2-4 summarizes these changes.

### Glycoprotein Alterations

Cell transformation is almost always associated with profound changes in cell-surface glycoproteins. Most of the changes are related to a lower protein content. The glyco-

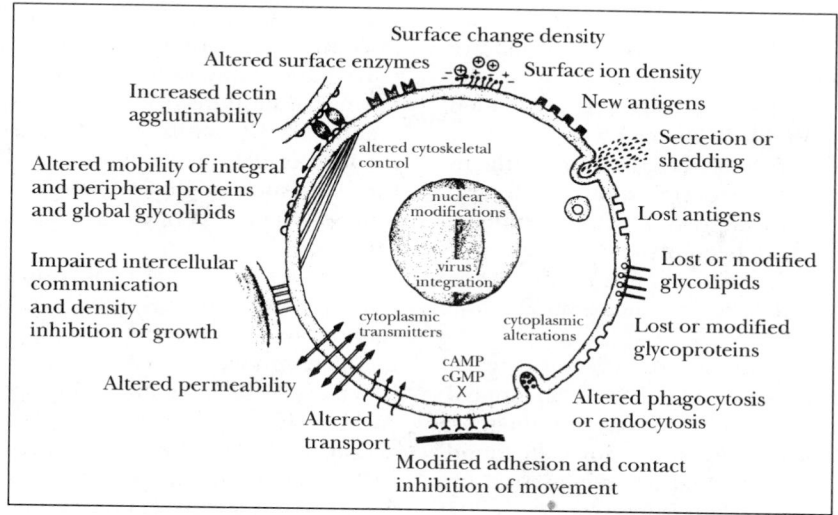

**FIGURE 2-4**   Summary of the cell surfaces and cell surface–related alterations generally seen in cancer cells. (Adapted from Nicolson GL: Transmembrane control of the receptors on normal and tumor cells: II. Surface changes associated with transformation and malignancy. *Biochim Biophys Acta* 458:16, 1976.)

proteins that remain are altered, mostly by becoming simpler. Evidence shows that the mechanism by which polysaccharides are made and attached to proteins is deranged in transformed cells.[17]

## Fibronectin

Fibronectin is a large glycoprotein found on normal cell surfaces. Together with various proteoglycans, collagen, and elastin, fibronectin forms the matrix in which cells are embedded and that anchors cells in place within tissues. It also serves as an organizing grid for the integral proteins of the cell surface.[18] For many cell types to grow in culture, fibronectin must be present in the serum component.

Cancer cells and transformed cells have low levels of fibronectin, causing them to attach poorly to the surface of the culture vessel; they do continue to grow, however. Hynes[18] suggests that the reason cancer cells have low levels of fibronectin is that they either stop making it or make a defective form of it. Addition of fibronectin to cultures of some tumor cells causes normalization of cell adhesion, flattens cells, and restores contact inhibition of cell movement. Growth control is not restored, though.[5] The lack of fibronectin in cancer cells is an important factor in the process of metastasis.

## Proteases

Transformed cells secrete a variety of protein-degrading enzymes. Research indicates that proteases are involved in metastasis by providing avenues through extracellular matrices and not by contributing to the transformation process itself.[19,20] Proteolytic enzymes may degrade both the attachment proteins and the components of the extracellular matrix.[21] In addition to producing their own proteolytic enzymes, tumor cells may also induce adjacent host cells to secrete enzymes.

Since the quantity and interactions of extracellular matrices differ, it is most likely that a variety of proteolytic enzymes are involved in the degradation of the matrices. Proteolytic enzymes that have been implicated in matrix destruction include collagenases, plasminogen activators, stromelysin, cathepsin D, and procoagulants.[22–26]

## Glycolipid Alterations

Cell-surface changes in glycolipids are another attribute of transformation. In general the content and complexity is reduced in transformed cell membranes. In particular it is evident that glycosphingolipid interacts with receptor proteins on the surface of normal cells to inhibit their responsiveness to growth factors.[27] Transformed cells have less and/or altered glycosphingolipids on their cell surfaces, thus increasing their responsiveness to growth factors. Glycosphingolipids also have been shown to serve as components of surface markers involved in cell-cell recognition.

## Cell-Surface Antigens

Many of the proteins and glycoproteins on the surface of the cell can be detected by immunologic assay and are referred to as *surface antigens*. When cells are transformed, new molecules form on the surface. If the cell is transformed by a virus, the antigens that result are determined by the virus in that the same antigen is found in different cell types transformed by the same virus. When cells are transformed by radiation or chemical carcinogens, the tumor antigens formed in these cells do not depend upon the agent involved but vary with the cell type.

In animals and transformed cells, tumor antigens have been identified that are not found on any normal cells; these are *tumor-specific antigens*. In human tumors, antigens do not show this degree of specificity. The great majority of human tumor antigens are *tumor-associated antigens* that have relative rather than absolute specificity.

Tumor-associated antigens are of two basic types: *tumor-associated transplantation antigens* (TATAs) appear on the surface of cells transformed by carcinogens; *oncofetal antigens (embryonic antigens)* are normally found exclusively on embryonic cells that are reexpressed on certain tumors. Examples of oncofetal antigens are alpha-fetoprotein (AFP), found in hepatomas and some testicular, pancreatic, and gastrointestinal tract tumors; and carcinoembryonic antigen (CEA), found in cancers of the gastrointestinal tract, pancreas, liver, lung, and breast.

Tumor-associated antigens are used clinically as markers for detection of tumors, assessment of patient prognosis, and evaluation of treatment measures.[28]

## Altered Permeability and Membrane Transport

Transformed cells transport materials across the cell membrane at higher rates than do normal cells. Materials that show enhanced uptake include glucose, other sugars, and amino acids. The mechanism of increased glucose transport has been shown to be production of a glucose transporter protein in transformed cells.[29]

## BIOCHEMICAL DIFFERENCES BETWEEN NORMAL AND CANCER CELLS

A number of biochemical substances that are altered, missing, abnormally secreted, or secreted in increased amounts by tumor cells affect cell growth and how cells interact with each other. The following are some of the more important biochemical differences between normal and cancer cells.

## Cyclic AMP and Cyclic GMP

*Cyclic adenosine monophosphate* (cAMP) participates in the regulation of a large number of intracellular biochemical reactions. Research has shown that cAMP levels are generally high in resting normal cells and low in dividing cells, including cancer cells.[30] In addition, cAMP reduces the rate of division of certain normal and transformed cells in culture. Some traits of transformation such as roundedness and diminished adhesiveness can be restored to normal when transformed cells are prevented from degrading cAMP, causing the cAMP levels in the cell to rise toward normal.[31] Since cAMP regulates the transport of nutrients such as glucose, amino acids, and phosphate into cells, it may act by controlling the availability of these substances.

Researchers have attempted to cause cell differentiation in culture systems using a triggering agent such as retinoic acid or interferon coupled with a substance that increases intracellular cAMP. The accumulation of cAMP is achieved either by increasing synthesis with an agent such as cholera toxin or by decreasing the degradative action of phosphodiesterase on cAMP with an inhibitor such as isobutyl methylxanthine.[32,33] Unfortunately, cAMP is only a weak inducer of differentiation without the triggering agents; no significant clinical results have been seen yet with this strategy.[34]

A related substance, *cyclic guanosine monophosphate* (cGMP), also restricts growth. cGMP varies opposite cAMP; that is, cell division is associated with low cAMP and high cGMP levels.[35]

## Nutrients

Cancer cells in culture have been shown to take up nutrients such as amino acids and sugars at greatly increased rates over those of untransformed cells of the same type. This increased transport may be associated with alteration of transport sites on or within the surface membrane of cancer cells.

## Growth Factors

Growth factors are polypeptides that influence cell function positively and negatively by initially binding to specific receptors in the cell membrane, and consequently setting off an activation of intracellular signal transduction. The effects of this signal to the nucleus are far-reaching and involve major regulatory pathways in normal and transformed cells. The latter cells have capabilities to make their own growth factors (autocrine stimulation),[36] to utilize abnormal receptors that can cause activation without the presence of a growth factor, and to bypass inhibitory pathways.[37,38] Normal and transformed cells can also benefit from adjacent cells that liberate growth factors (*paracrine stimulation*).[39] Platelets, when activated, are a rich source of growth factors, including platelet-derived growth factor (PDGF), transforming growth factor-alpha (TGF-α), and transforming growth factor-beta (TGF-β).[40] Transformed cells often will proliferate with growth factor levels that are too low for normal cell proliferation, as the normal cells will enter a resting state.[41]

Considerable attention has recently been directed toward growth factor receptors. High levels of epidermal growth factor (EGF) receptors on cells from cancers of the breast and bladder indicate a worse prognosis,[42] and increased expression of HER2/NEU receptors in breast carcinoma also increases the risk of recurrence.[43] Efforts to block these receptors in clinical trials are under way.

The following are a number of growth factors that are of interest in cancer biology.

### Epidermal growth factor (EGF)

EGF has multiple effects on cell proliferation and other cell functions. It has a role in normal breast development[44] but can inhibit hair follicle cells.[45] EGF binds to a specific receptor, which has protein tyrosine kinase activity.[46] High levels of EGF receptors are noted on many epithelial carcinomas, and mutant EGF receptors have been found on high-grade glioblastomas.[47] A number of monoclonal antibodies have been made that interact with the receptor and are currently being studied.

### Transforming growth factor-alpha (TGF-α)

TGF-α is quite similar to EGF and binds avidly to the same receptor. TGF-α normally is expressed by many types of epithelial cells and is angiogenic, stimulating endothelial cell proliferation.[48]

### Transforming growth factor B (TGF-β)

Originally identified as transforming substance[49] this molecule regulates many cellular processes involved in normal development and healing. It is produced by most cells. TGF-β inhibits the growth of many normal and transformed cells, and the development of a tumor may represent an escape from TGF-β influence.[50] Differentiation of certain cell types may occur due to TGF-β,[51] and it can also activate macrophages as well as increasing adhesion of cells to matrix proteins.[52] Hypotheses regarding its mechanism of action include inhibition of the oncogene c-myc[53] and reducing phosphorylation of pRb, thus providing more control of the $G_1$ phase in the cell cycle.[54]

### Platelet-derived growth factor (PDGF)

Platelet activation leads to the secretion of PDGF, and receptors normally are located on fibroblasts and smooth muscle cells.[40] PDGF is produced by some tumor cells that lack a receptor for it.[55] Combined with another growth factor such as EGF or insulin-like growth factor 1, PDGF can stimulate cell division in cultures; it cannot accomplish this effect alone.[56] PDGF appears to play a role in the development and support of brain tumors such as astrocytomas.[57]

### Basic fibroblast growth factor (bFGF)

Basic fibroblast growth factor is believed to be a vital substance in embryogenesis, and cellular targets include members of the mesoderm and ectoderm. Understandably, bFGF has strong angiogenic properties[58] and can bind heparin (thus giving rise to the title *heparin-binding growth factor*). This molecule acts also through a cell-surface receptor with tyrosine kinase activity.

### Insulin-like growth factors (IGF-I and IGF-II)

The insulin-like growth factors resemble proinsulin[59] and have growth stimulatory effects on a wide variety of human cell lines, both normal and malignant. IGF-I is also known as *somatomedin C* and mediates the effect of human growth hormone. Their receptors are similar to the insulin receptor and thus are difficult to assess on transformed cells due to the widespread nature of insulin receptors. In cell culture virtually all cancer cells are stimulated by IGF-I.[60] A monoclonal antibody to the IGF-I receptor is available, but concern exists regarding potential effects on normal cells. IGF-I is reputed to be involved in autocrine and paracrine pathways.[61]

### C-ERBB 2 (or HER2/NEU) receptor

Although technically not a growth factor, this receptor is very similar to the EGF receptor and is amplified in many adenocarcinomas, including breast carcinoma.[62] The presence of this receptor may well be a poor prognostic indicator in breast cancer and potentially indicates a more resistant phenotype with regard to chemotherapy.[63] Monoclonal antibody trials against this receptor are ongoing.

## GENETIC DIFFERENCES BETWEEN NORMAL AND CANCER CELLS

Considerable evidence supports the concept that neoplasms arise from a single altered cell that acquires an inheritable and selective growth advantage over other cells.[64] The initial change in a transformed cell is an alteration in a regulatory gene by a carcinogen. With each ensuing cell division, a cohort of cells inherits the defect, and if not already transformed, these cells have the capacity for greater genetic instability and further alterations. Thus, sequential genetic changes may occur in a portion of the total population, and eventually an invasive phenotype will emerge.

The regulatory genes that govern normal cell growth likely represent only a small percentage of our genetic material; when one of these regulatory genes becomes altered and has the capacity to contribute to the development of a malignant clone it is called an *oncogene*. The normal precursor gene (before it is altered) is called a *proto-oncogene*. This latter terminology is semantically unfortunate because a proto-oncogene is actually a normal gene involved in the natural growth process of a cell; these genes appear to be vital for normal tissue development. When they go awry, however, profound changes in cell behavior may evolve.

A powerful example of the sequential nature of genetic alteration occurs naturally in the syndrome of familial adenomatous polyposis (FAP). Individuals with this autosomal dominant condition develop numerous polyps throughout the colon at an early age. Many will develop colon cancers. As Vogelstein and colleagues have elucidated,[65] a series of genetic events needs to take place before an invasive cancer develops, an example of the "multiple hit hypothesis." Individuals with FAP were found to have an inherited deletion in the long arm of chromosome 5q of a gene now known as the *FAP* gene (or adenomatous polyposis coli [*APC*] gene).[66] The loss of this gene, which is believed to be a growth-suppressor gene, allows for the growth of numerous polyps. Next, mutations of the *K-ras* gene were noted in 90% of adenomatous polyps larger than 1 cm in diameter but in less than 10% of adenomas smaller than 1 cm. Further genetic mutations followed over time, including a loss of the protective effects of the "deleted in colon cancer," or *DCC,* gene and the *p53* gene. The *DCC* gene is located on chromosome 18, and the gene product shows structural similarity to cell adhesion molecules; expression of the gene product is reduced or absent in 70%–75% of colorectal carcinomas.[67] The *p53* gene exerts a major controlling influence over cell growth in general, and loss of the *p53* effect in colorectal cancer leads to a more aggressive malignancy.

Numerous other genetic changes have been found in colorectal cancers, in addition to the pivotal genes just described. It is evident that a number of different pathways may lead to the development of a malignant cell, but two themes hold true in the development sequence. First, multiple mutations are generally necessary for a cell to achieve a malignant character; second, cells progressively become more unstable with each genetic change, and the rate of further genetic alterations may actually increase.

The question arises: Why don't we all get cancer at a young age if these mutations are possible, given the trillions of cell divisions we encounter? Fortunately, we have mechanisms to deal with abnormal cells early in their development. Each human cell has the capacity to program itself for cell death in the event of serious damage or loss of regulation; this action is called *apoptosis.* Interestingly, the *p53* suppressor gene is intimately involved in the mechanism of apoptosis, and loss of this gene effect is a critical development. A second protective mechanism involves DNA repair genes that encode proteins able to rapidly fix damaged DNA.[68] These so-called *mismatch repair genes* recognize areas in DNA where nucleotide base pairs are mistakenly aligned. Normally in complementary strands of DNA adenine (A) is paired with thymidine (T), and guanine (G) is paired with cytosine (C). A mismatch rarely will occur during copying such that an adenine is paired with a cytosine, for example. The mismatch repair proteins can correct the mistake and align the nucleotides appropriately once again.

Mutations may involve the p53 protein (a relatively common development in human cancers). Recently specific mutations in chromosomes 2, 3, and 7 have been found, which have a negative impact on the mismatch repair gene system. The syndrome of hereditary nonpolyposis colorectal carcinoma (*Lynch syndrome*) is a clinical example of defective mismatch repair genes. Multiple carcinomas, including endometrial, stomach, ovarian, small bowel, and ureteral cancers, develop at an early age in this syndrome.[68]

In the last two years, two new growth-suppressor genes, *BRCA1* and *BRCA2,* have been located on chromosomes 17 and 13, respectively; mutations in these two genes are associated with lifetime risks of breast cancer up to 80%.[69,70] These gene mutations are inherited randomly (there is a 50% chance of passing it on to a child) and can be diagnosed with blood testing. Particularly at risk are individuals in families with a prominent history of early bilateral breast cancer and ovarian cancer.

## THE CLINICAL PROBLEM OF METASTASIS

Although many primary tumors are treated successfully with surgery, radiation therapy, or chemotherapy (or combinations of these modalities), all too frequently the local tumor appears to be resolved, but months or years later a recurrence is found far from the original site. Most cancer deaths are related to the uncontrolled progression of metastasis. As distressing as a new diagnosis of cancer is for an individual, the knowledge of a metastatic recurrence is even more ominous. Typically, microscopic colonies of cancer cells are already present in other areas when the first symptoms of cancer alert an individual to a functional change at a specific site.

Knowledge about the metastatic process has lagged behind other aspects of cancer biology until the last decade. Presently, there is great momentum to examine various steps in the metastatic continuum and to design treatment strategies to complement conventional therapies. With the collaboration of cell and molecular biologists, geneticists, and clinicians, we are likely to see positive results in our efforts to interrupt metastatic mechanisms.

## FACTORS CONTRIBUTING TO METASTATIC POTENTIAL

Historically, it has been assumed that only a very small fraction of cancer cells are able to initiate and accomplish a successful metastatic deposit,[71] although recently this has come into question (see later section on Extravasation). The metastatic process is selective, favoring the survival of certain tumor cell subpopulations already existing in a heterogeneous group of cells constituting a primary tumor.[72]

The property of abnormal proliferation in transformed cells does not guarantee invasion and metastasis. Tumorigenicity and metastasis have both overlapping and separate features. For invasion and metastasis to occur, imbalances in motility and proteolysis leading to tissue barrier breakdown are required, in addition to loss of growth control.[73] Tumor cells must also avoid the dynamic assaults of the immune system to succeed in establishing distant colonies. Finally, *angiogenesis* (new blood vessel formation) is necessary for expansion of the primary tumor as well as establishment of viable metastases. The following is a glance at tumor cell and host factors that contribute to the metastatic potential of a tumor.

## Tumor Cell Factors

### Oncogenes

Progression of tumors from benign to malignant is associated with structural alterations in genes and with changes in gene expression. There exists a question as to whether the genes controlling abnormal cell proliferation are the same as the genes involved in conferring an ability to metastasize. Current evidence supports the concept that separate mechanisms underlie these two characteristics of transformed cells. In a situation where mutated *ras* oncogene sequences are introduced (or *transfected*) into mouse fibroblasts, numerous metastases were noted.[74] The resultant metastatic cells were not any more sensitive to immune lysis by natural killer (NK) cells or macrophages in culture compared with control cells, suggesting that the transformed cells were more aggressive but not more proliferative. Similar results with *ras* family oncogenes have been seen in transfection studies with human epithelial cells.[75] In contrast, with other cell types, *ras* oncogene transfection induces transformation but no metastatic capability.[76,77] Other oncogenes have induced experimental metastatic potential, including mutations in the vitally important *p53* gene.[78] Thus it appears that invasion and metastasis have at least somewhat different genetic controls than those for proliferation alone.

There are also candidates for metastasis-suppressor genes. Among them is the *NM23* gene, which was initially identified as having generally low expression in many metastatic cell lines, with normal expression in nonmetastatic counterparts.[79] This observation supported previous experiments where cell fusions were performed, and fusion of normal cells with metastatic cells gave rise to nonmetastatic tumorigenic cells.[80]

### Heterogeneity

That tumors consist of heterogeneous populations of malignant cells was first demonstrated by Fidler and Kripke[81] in the B16 melanoma system. Various clones of cells isolated from the same tumor have been shown to differ in a wide variety of cell characteristics, including chromosome number, hormone receptors, cell-surface enzymes, morphology, growth properties, response to therapy, and metastatic potential.[82] Tumor cells are heterogeneous within the same tumor, among cancers of different histological origins, and among tumors of the same histological origin but in different individuals.

Tumor cell heterogeneity has important implications. For example, even if a 99.99% cell kill is achieved in the treatment of a 1-cm tumor (which consists of 1 billion, or $10^9$ cells), a significant number ($10^5$) of nonresponsive cells will remain. This resistant population may then continue to prosper, and unfortunately the cells may be even more unstable genetically than the original heterogeneous population (resulting in more rapid development of further genetic mutants). This disturbing tendency of resistant cells explains why conventional cancer treatments often fail in the face of metastatic disease, even when it initially appears that a tumor is responding. The concept of tumor cell heterogeneity also explains why one person's tumor may grow to a massive size without ever metastasizing.

### Production of angiogenic factors

Once a tumor has been initiated, any subsequent increase in cell population must be preceded by an increase in new capillaries that converge on the tumor.[82] The stimulus for and development of these new capillaries are initiated and supported by a group of peptide proteins called *angiogenic factors*. These polypeptides include FGF, angiogenin, TGF, and tumor necrosis factor.[83] Angiogenic factors appear to stimulate locomotion and mitosis of vascular endothelium, and to release endothelial growth factors, thus stimulating capillary proliferation.

### Motility

Motility is a central theme in the metastatic process. Tumor cells must leave the primary site, break through tissue barriers to gain entrance into lymphatic channels or blood vessels, and then find a distant site to once again traverse a blood vessel wall and locate a niche in a new tissue. Chemotactic mechanisms will draw a cell out of the primary mass, but these attracting substances give direction and do not confer motility. Motility factors produced by tumor cells and neighboring tissue cells stimulate tumor cells to move toward new destinations.[84] Motility factors are produced in human tumor cells as demonstrated in bladder cancer patients; in assays of urine specimens collected over 24 hours, the higher the pathological grade of an individual's bladder tumor, the higher the level of motility factors found in the urine.[85]

### Specific cell-surface receptors

Cells express specific surface receptors that recognize a vast array of proteins in their extracellular environment, including matrix proteins. One family of cell-surface receptors, the integrins, serves as the recognition sites for fibronectin and other components of the extracellular matrix.[86] Laminin receptors, which bind to laminin in the tissue basement membrane, are augmented in actively invading tumor cells and may play a crucial role in breaching this tissue barrier.[87]

## Host Factors

### Deficient immune response

Throughout one's lifetime the immune system continues to seek out threats to health, including microorganisms and damaged or abnormal cells. An invasive tumor will meet immune cells in the primary site environment and in virtually any other location where a metastatic cell attempts to land. For many years there has been a popular theory of immune surveillance: malignant cells develop randomly and often, but immune cells destroy them before they can gain enough numbers or protection to survive. Cells reputed to be involved in this surveillance are cytotoxic T cells, NK cells, and activated macrophages.[88] Cytotoxic T cells are capable of interacting with tumor-associated antigens on tumor cells and require prior sensitization to these antigens. Natural killers are large, granular lymphocytes that can naturally lyse a broad range of tumor cell targets even if there has been no prior exposure to the tumor cells. Macrophages are the tissue-based counterpart to the blood monocyte; they have a natural antitumor activity that is enhanced when they are "activated" by various substances. Interleukin-2 can heighten the antitumor actions of cytotoxic T cells and NK cells,[89] while gamma-interferon is a classic activator of macrophages.

How tumors escape immune destruction is still somewhat mysterious, but a number of potential mechanisms are known. Tumor cells may develop variants (in their tendency toward heterogeneity) that have no recognizable antigenic structures. Alternatively, tumor cells may undergo *antigenic modulation*, where antigens are shed into the circulation or hidden in an unstable tumor cell membrane. Antigens shed into the circulation can block T-cell function.[90] Tumor cells can secrete immunosuppressive substances such as TGF-β, while host inflammatory cells also may liberate immunosuppressants,[91] including granulocyte-macrophage colony-stimulating factor (GM-CSF).[92] Chemotherapy and radiation treatments also may depress the immune system in general. Sanctuaries such as the brain and the central nervous system allow tumor cells to hide from the immune system and cytotoxic agents. Dense, fibrous tissue stroma around a tumor deposit may shield the cells from immune cells as the circulation to this area may be underdeveloped.

Once a primary tumor gains a foothold in a tissue, it may be impossible for the immune system to keep up with the rapid proliferation of cancer cells. In culture systems it usually takes from 4 to a 100 normal immune cells to kill a single cancer cell, thus indicating that "the numbers game" needs to be heavily weighted on the side of the immune system in order to see tumor rejection.

In advanced stages of cancer, a general immunosuppression is not uncommon. Reactivity to common antigens (such as mumps, *Candida,* and *Trichophyton*) by skin testing may be lost, a defect that is related to deficient recall T-cell function. The most common patterns of immunologic deficiency that have been associated with tumor stage and grade include the following.[93,94]

1. decreased lymphocyte counts in association with relative monocytosis
2. decreased inflammatory cell chemotaxis
3. decreased antigen processing and presentation
4. decreased proliferative responses to antigen and nonspecific stimulants
5. decreased NK function
6. decreased helper and cytotoxic T-cell function
7. increased suppressor T-cell function
8. variable macrophage-mediated cytotoxicity
9. increased macrophage suppressor function
10. variable effects on cytokine synthesis

Finally, the lack of nutrition experienced by many individuals with advanced cancer contributes to the immune suppression.

### Intact hemostatic mechanism

Normal platelet function is required for optimal tumor cell metastasis. Gasic et al[95] demonstrated that a reduction in platelet number correlates with a decrease in experimental tumor metastases. It has been further documented that platelets play a central role in the metastatic process, though the exact role is still unclear.[96,97] Platelets may aid tumor cells in attaching to vessel walls, and tumor cells may directly activate platelets.[98] Antiplatelet agents can greatly inhibit experimental metastases in mice.[99,100]

## THE METASTATIC SEQUENCE

From the initial cell division of a malignant clone will arise a pair of cells that will reside in a specific site. This primary location may be in the bloodstream for leukemic cells, in the bone marrow for a myeloma, or in the parenchyma of an organ for a solid tumor. In the majority of human malignancies the growth of a tumor restricted to its primary site is not fatal; the process of tumor spread to distant body locations is a more dangerous threat to the general functions of the body and to the life process itself. Unfortunately, 60% of patients have microscopic or macroscopic metastases at the time of diagnosis.[101] Identification of those individuals harboring metastases remains a formidable clinical challenge since the presence of residual disease after treatment of the primary site will generally require the need for systemic treatment.

The intricate and complicated process of metastasis may begin very early in the development of the primary tumor. Breast carcinomas smaller than 0.125 cm$^3$ may liberate cells to travel in lymphatic and vascular channels.[102] Cells of high metastatic potential exist early in the heterogeneous population of a tumor, and may be selectively favored as they successfully escape and form distant outposts while their local counterparts compete for nutrients in a more crowded microenvironment.[103]

Although the metastatic sequence is a continuum of integrated events, an understanding of the most important facets is facilitated by dividing the process into specific steps[104] (see Figure 2-5):

1. tumor growth and neovascularization
2. tumor cell invasion of the basement membrane and other extracellular matrices
3. detachment and embolism of tumor cell aggregates
4. arrest in distant organ capillary beds
5. extravasation
6. proliferation within the organ parenchyma

## Tumor Growth and Neovascularization

A basic and necessary biological property of human tissue is the requirement for adequate blood circulation to pro-

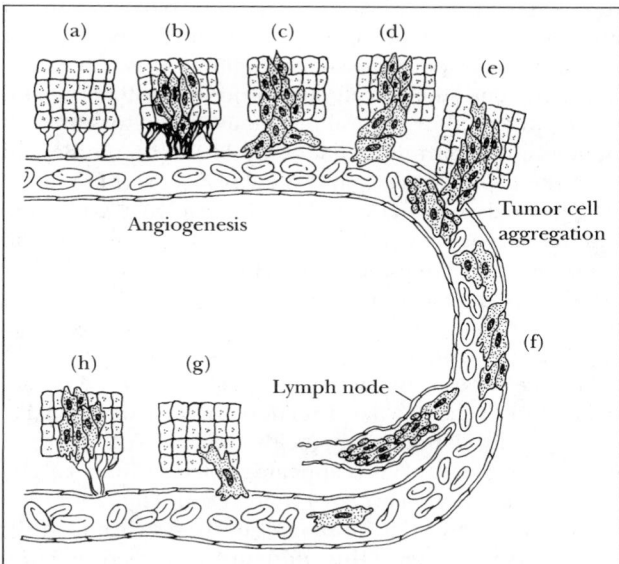

**FIGURE 2-5** The metastatic sequence. (a) Normal tissue; (b) angiogenesis and growth of tumor; (c) attachment of tumor cells to epithelial basement membrane; (d) invasion of the basement membrane by tumor cells; (e) tumor cell dissemination into lymphatic and circulatory systems; (f) arrest of tumor cells on capillary wall or in lymph node; (g) extravasation of tumor cells from capillary into target tissue; (h) angiogenesis and growth of the secondary tumor into a clinically detectable mass.

vide oxygen, nutrients, and growth factors. The formation of new blood vessels (or *angiogenesis*) is an integral part of embryology; similarly, an organizing population of tumor cells requires the development of new blood vessels. While not sufficient alone to guarantee a viable metastatic result, angiogenesis is a natural beginning. Malignant cells (and normal cells of the surrounding tissue, such as fibroblasts and macrophages) are able to elaborate substances that encourage nearby native blood vessels to form new branches extending toward the enlarging tumor mass.[58] Endothelial cells in the native vessels are stimulated to break through the endothelial basement membrane and to form new channels across parenchymal stroma, finally reaching the tumor and forming a network within it.[105] The amount of neovascularization in tumors is now thought to have considerable prognostic potential, particularly in breast carcinoma. Microvessels can be stained with an antibody to Factor VIII (a protein found only on endothelial cells) and then counted per high-power microscopic field. If microvessel counts ranged from 0 to 33 per field, 14% of breast cancer patients developed metastases, while those individuals with a score of more than 100 all developed metastases.[106]

The process of tumor angiogenesis relies on the presence of various biological substances, both stimulatory and inhibitory; in fact, the relative balance of these various factors apparently determines whether angiogenesis will develop. Examples of stimulatory compounds for angiogenesis include EGF, TGF-α,[107] beta fibroblast growth factor,[108] angiogenin,[109] and interleukin-8.[110] Many of these angiogenic factors are produced by local tissue macrophages and some by the tumor cells themselves. Two unique substances involved in angiogenesis are platelet-derived endothelial cell growth factor (PD-ECGF) and vascular endothelial growth factor (VEGF). PD-ECGF, which also has enzymatic activity as a thymidine phosphorylase, has been found in increased amounts in colon carcinoma tissue; this substance correlates with the stage of colon carcinoma and is an independent variable in determining prognosis.[111] VEGF, which promotes growth and chemotaxis of endothelial cells in vitro, is overexpressed in many tumors. Most important, VEGF may be the final pathway through which other angiogenic agents exert their influence.[112]

Inhibitory angiogenic compounds are as important as the stimulatory agents and include TGF-β$_1$, alpha interferon, and angiostatin. TGF-β$_1$ inhibits the proteolysis necessary for the formation of viable and effective endothelial sprouts emanating from parent vessels.[113] Alfa-interferon was the first antiangiogenic substance to be used in a clinical trial in 1989 as it was employed in the treatment of a life-threatening angioma.[114] Angiostatin, a fragment of the plasminogen molecule, will generally halt the multiplication of endothelial cells.[114]

Once the balance between stimulators and inhibitors is tipped in favor of endothelial cell growth, the new and immature tumor vessels are apt to be somewhat disorganized, with prominent gaps in their walls. These gaps allow tumor cells in the vicinity to gain entrance and potentially travel away from the primary site.[73]

## Invasion of Surrounding Tissue

As an early tumor develops, it is initially surrounded by the tissue of its native organ. The substance of the tissue is composed of interstitial stroma and basement membrane.[21,115] The stroma provides general support, and the basement membrane represents an acellular association of structural proteins and proteoglycans that anchors normal cells and provides tissue organization.[116] Important components of the basement membrane include type IV collagen, laminin, and fibronectin.[117]

Normal tissue cells (other than white and red blood cells) adhere to each other and to the extracellular matrix, and have no tendency to invade a basement membrane. Even benign tumors generally respect the tissue barriers around them. Of more interest is the apparent presence of cell-surface molecules on normal cells that provide an identity as to where each cell belongs in a tissue; this has been likened to an "area code" that surrounding cells recognize. These molecules determine general adhesion to other cells and the anchoring relationship to particular basement membranes.[116] One particular intercellular adhesion molecule is E-cadherin, which is often lost on cancer cells and, if lacking, appears to be related to a cancer cell's ability to escape its local position and invade tissue.[116]

Cell-surface molecules, involved in anchorage to basement membrane are called *integrins;* unless cultured cells can attach to a surface via these molecules, they will not be able to reproduce and eventually will undergo apoptosis.[118] In order for normal cells to survive and flourish they must have the right matrix code and the correct integrin. Cancer cells overcome this frailty by developing mechanisms to survive away from their normal position along a basement membrane.

As an invasive tumor develops, the integrity of the basement membrane is compromised. Whether the cancer cells are able to break through this barrier is dependent on another dynamic tension that is played out between a cast of proteolytic enzymes and their respective inhibitors. Cancer cells will often have enhanced receptors for laminin, which allows them to begin an interaction that will eventually disintegrate the barrier.[119] An association with tumor aggressiveness has been noted for various degradative enzymes including matrix metalloproteinases (MMPs)[120] and heparinases.[121] Of the metalloproteinases, type IV collagenase is a key enzyme, and it has been overexpressed in invasive cell lines but not in noninvasive lines.[122] As the process of basement membrane deterioration progresses, an immune response may develop as tumor cells release chemoattractants for monocytes and lymphocytes. The interaction of these cells will eventually lead to the elaboration of growth factors, interferons, interleukins, and TNF-α, all of which have various actions to either impede or facilitate the process of invasion. The resulting inflammatory milieu will often result in a dense, fibrous reaction around the tumor called *desmoplasia,* a development that causes tumors to become firmer and more easily appreciated on physical examination.

The human body has many inhibitory mechanisms to control biochemical pathways, and the process of tissue breakdown by proteolysis is no exception. Tissue inhibitors of metalloproteinases (TIMPs) and plasminogen activator inhibitors (PAIs) represent the two most important families of inhibitors.[123] The TIMP members are regulated by TGF-β and other cytokines, and they are made in endothelial cells and some tumor cells.[124] Of the TIMPs, the specific type TIMP-2 is able to bind to both latent and activated forms of type IV collagenase; this inhibitor can essentially abolish the hydrolytic activity of all members of the metalloproteinase family.[125] In addition, TIMP-2 has the capability to inhibit growth factor–stimulated proliferation of transformed cells in culture.[126] The net effect on tumor invasiveness is determined by the relative strengths of degradative enzymes and their inhibitors, such that a small tumor may remain noninvasive until the balance is tipped toward proteolysis. In a series of breast cancer patients a significant association was noted between the TIMP/MMP ratio and the aggressiveness of the tumor cells.[127]

Despite separating angiogenesis and tumor cell invasion as biological concepts, there are many parallels in these two processes. Endothelial cells, in order to form new vessel sprouts, must degrade the vascular basement membrane and intrude into the perivascular space, just as tumor cells invade and pass through local tissue barriers. Migrating endothelial cells also produce proteinases and can be deterred by natural proteinase inhibitors.[128] Both tumor cells and endothelial cells need to be motile and have the capacity to expand their respective numbers.

The final phase of tumor invasion involves the locomotion of cells as they push through tissue on their way to achieving an avenue for distant spread. The stimulus for movement appears to reside in various chemoattractants in tissue, including complement-derived materials, collagen peptides, and other connective tissue components.[129] Tumor cells can actually form pseudopodia to penetrate tissue and "sense" what direction the cell should take, while physically pulling the cell forward.[130] Yet the presence of chemoattractants appears to be insufficient alone to cause a cell to leave its home roost. This abnormal motility is based on a substance secreted by tumor cells that favors movement; this substance is termed *autocrine motility factor* (AMF). AMF can induce a generally heightened migrational behavior and also cause the rapid development of pseudopodia with enriched content of laminin and fibronectin matrix receptors.[130] A newly discovered gene on chromosome 8 appears to encode a glycoprotein capable of inducing a strong motility response;[131] although the glycoprotein in question has been called "autotaxin," it appears to be AMF.

Providing further evidence for crossover mechanisms between angiogenesis and motility, dividing endothelial cells can release proteins such as interleukin-6 into the microenvironment to stimulate proliferation and motility of tumor cells,[114] while local growth factors such as GM-CSF and IGFs can direct tumor cell migration.[132,133] The ability to utilize host factors that might have deleterious effects on tumor cells (such as GM-CSF) reflects the versatility and flexibility of successful clones of metastatic tumor in overcoming their microenvironment.

The development of new blood vessels, the breakdown of local basement membrane by tumor cells, and the eventual entrance of tumor cells into the local vasculature by degrading the vascular basement membrane all have similar mechanisms. The fluctuations of growth factors, cytokines, and proteolytic enzymes will determine whether a tumor cell can break away and successfully traverse the distance to enter the lumen of a blood vessel or lymphatic duct.

## Detachment and Embolism of Tumor Cell Aggregates

Tumor cells may continually press on through local tissue while maintaining continuity with the primary tumor (direct extension) or may achieve a foothold in a vessel of lymphatic or circulatory origin. Once in a vessel the cells may localize at the entry site or disseminate to other destinations. Direct extension may cause various situations and symptoms dependent on the organs involved. Lung carcinomas may obliterate bronchial passages, thus denying a segment ventilation or trapping secretions behind the tumor and causing a postobstructive pneumonia. Breast carcinomas may involve the skin, causing ulceration, or the chest wall, causing pain due to nerve compression. Malignancies of colon or ovarian origin may release cells from the outer edge of the tumor into the peritoneal cavity, where they may float randomly and implant on the surface of various organs. Patients are then at risk for ascites or chronic bowel obstruction. Similar fluid accumulation can occur in other serous cavities such as the pleural and pericardial spaces, often due to direct extension.

A common pathway of tumor dissemination involves the lymphatic system, where tumor cells can enter easily through natural openings in lymphatic ducts. Moving through the ducts, the invading cells may stagnate in the first lymph node they reach or may pass through to other nodes or into small blood vessels (lymph nodes are well vascularized). Certain tumors have strong tendencies to spread locally via lymphatics long before they ever metastasize (squamous cell carcinomas of head and neck, Hodgkin's disease), while others typically involve the bloodstream early (melanoma, small-cell carcinoma of lung).

Eventually the natural history of a malignant clone will likely involve a hematogenous phase where cells can travel to virtually any organ. In the bloodstream foreign cells are at risk due to mechanical forces and attack by the immune system. A relative protective effect occurs if tumor cells form aggregates either with each other or with platelets, as it is less likely that immune cells will be able to penetrate the conglomerate and injure individual tumor cells.

## Arrest in Distant Organ Capillary Beds

Unless circulating tumor cells are able to stop safely in capillary beds, they may circulate indefinitely until they die. In order to maximize the ability to arrest in a blood vessel, malignant cells may secrete substances that cause platelets to aggregate around them, resulting in a larger, stickier mass. In turn, platelets elaborate growth factors that favor continued survival of the adjoining tumor cells.[116]

Whether or where circulating neoplastic cells land depends on certain factors that are not entirely clear. Some tumors spread to the first organ anatomically linked to the tumor bed, but 40%–50% of malignancies do not follow this pattern.[101] Paget postulated a "seed" (the tumor cell) and "soil" (appropriate metastatic site) hypothesis where a selective process occurs.[134] More recently, there has been evidence that molecular determinants on the surface of tumor cells (the area code hypothesis) influence what organs or sites certain tumors will favor, as corresponding codes may exist on the microvasculature of distant organs.[116] Thus it is not so mysterious why prostate carcinoma cells so often go to bone and ocular melanomas arrive in the liver, while typically sparing other organs.

In addition to selective target tissue adhesion, specific chemotactic factors or growth factors may lure circulating malignant cells to a particular site.[135] Neoplastic cells with higher affinity for laminin tend to metastasize to lung tissue, whereas other tumor cells with a higher affinity for fibronectin favor settlement in the liver.[135] Specific chemotactic substances have been isolated from various organ sources, including lung, brain, bone, and liver; for instance, melanoma cells that had metastasized to the brain were found to respond in culture preferentially to brain-derived chemotactic factors.[136]

## Extravasation

Historically, it has been estimated from experimental systems that approximately 1 in 10,000 circulating tumor cells will successfully arrest and penetrate the vessel wall to establish a niche in another organ.[137] Negotiating a passage through the vessel wall is called *extravasation*. Recently Holzman[138] has shown with the use of a video-microscope that metastatic cells in large numbers (up to 80%) can extravasate into liver parenchyma within one to three days; this observation raises the issue that local parenchymal factors may primarily determine the fate of an extravasated cell. The proteolytic process of degrading the endothelial basement membrane is essentially the same as the neoplastic cell used to gain entrance into the vascular system in the first place.

## Proliferation within the Organ Parenchyma

As a metastatic focus develops in a new tissue site it is assumed that some positive influences enabled this new colony to arrive in this particular spot. The process that originally secured tumor growth in the primary site must take place all over again, yet it is likely that the new microenvironment is somewhat different. The nature of this new microenvironment may have been underestimated. As an example, melanoma cells with high levels of TIMP (which would be expected to metastasize poorly) metastasized very well with excellent extravasation, but they formed fewer and smaller metastases, suggesting that metalloproteinases are important in determining cell growth after extravasation.[138]

The immune profiles of primary and metastatic sites may also be quite different, as recently the levels of interleukin-4 and tumor necrosis factor-alpha were found to be higher in the primary site of human colon carcinomas compared with metastatic sites.[139] Once a malignancy has demonstrated the capacity to successfully complete the process of metastasis, overcoming all the natural obstacles in place, there would appear to be no significant reason that further metastases could not develop naturally; hence the profoundly worrisome situation we face when a tumor presents with metastasis.

## GENETIC CONTROL OF THE METASTATIC CONTINUUM

The search for oncogenes related to tumorigenicity (the growth enhancement underlying tumor development) has proceeded faster than the identification of genes related to the development of metastatic potential. Many genes have been implicated recently in the formation of a metastatic phenotype, including the *ras* family.[140] Yet current evidence suggests that invasion and metastasis require activation of a set of effector genes over and above those required for unrestrained growth alone.[112] A metastasis suppressor gene, *NM23*, may be a most important factor in determining metastatic potential. Melanoma cell lines that were highly metastatic were found to have much reduced *NM23* RNA levels compared with melanoma cells of low metastatic potential.[79] In a clinical setting breast carcinoma patients with positive lymph node involvement also had low *NM23* RNA levels in their tumors. In addition, patients with negative nodes but low *NM23* RNA levels had a worse prognosis.[141] To date, however, the exact nature of the gene's actions requires further elucidation.[142]

## ANTIMETASTASIS THERAPY

The most useful reason to divide the metastatic process into discrete steps is to focus on specific areas where the continuum might be disrupted. Indeed, the notion that treatment of cancer in general might be more successful with agents to interrupt metastasis is becoming more attractive. Failure of one step in the metastatic process may be enough to provide a survival advantage or to maximize the current effects of conventional systemic treatment. The fact that many cancers are metastatic at the time of diagnosis still persists, however; screening strategies and detection of tiny amounts of disease thus become more urgent. Identification of successful adjuvant programs continues to occur, and the combination of systemic therapy and antimetastasis therapy is a logical development. Potentially fruitful avenues of investigation include the following concepts.

### Prevention of Tumor Invasion

Since neoplastic cells will invade all primary site tissue barriers, including the local endothelial basement membranes as well as the basement membranes of the target organ, an inhibitor of proteinase activity would be a likely candidate to interrupt the metastatic cascade. Inhibitors both general and specific are known, yet it seems unlikely that a total blockade of the various degradative enzyme systems will be accomplished by one agent. If such a blockade were possible, it may well have a major impact on white blood cell function. Nevertheless, proteinase inhibitors will likely be studied clinically in the near future.

### Antiadhesive Therapy

Since malignant cells often initiate an interaction with the surrounding stroma, utilizing laminin and fibronectin receptors to promote invasion, an inhibitor of this reaction could block metastasis very early in the process. Certain synthetic peptides with a sequence of Arg-Gly-Asp (or the so-called RGD sequence) are capable of blocking tumor cell adhesion reactions and decreasing metastases in experimental animals.[143]

### Monoclonal Antibodies

Monoclonal antibodies are pure preparations of a specific antibody (usually of mouse origin) directed against a particular cell or cell structure. These antibodies can be used to block certain functions, to alert the immune system to the presence of a specific cell, to provide potential early diagnosis of micrometastases, or to deliver toxic substances to a cancer cell. Trials with monoclonal antibodies against cell-surface receptors, including adhesion molecules, are already under way.[144]

## Modulation of Tumor Vascularization

One of the most promising areas for future trials involves the area of angiogenesis inhibition. It is very likely that a successful blockade of tumor blood vessel formation would significantly affect the frequency of metastases and the success of conventional treatment. There are currently a number of promising agents. Razoxane (ICRF-159) appears to be able to restore the structure and integrity of capillary vessels within tumors, leading to a reduced rate of tumor cell entry. Administration of Razoxane to mice bearing Lewis lung carcinomas resulted in a decrease in the incidence of metastases.[145] In 1992 the first antiangiogenic drug, TNP-470, entered clinical trials, and others have since been tested.[114] TNP-470 selectively inhibits proliferation and migration of endothelial cells, while alfa-interferon, interleukin-2, marimastat, pentosan polysulfate, and platelet factor-4 are currently in use.[114] An interesting development is the current use of thalidomide as an antiangiogenic agent. Developed in the 1950s as a sedative (women who ingested thalidomide often had babies with poorly developed limbs), thalidomide inhibits angiogenesis induced by basic fibroblast growth factor,[146] though the exact mechanism is unknown.

Another promising agent in the antiangiogenic arsenal is CAI, a substance with additional antiproliferative properties.[147] CAI suppresses endothelial cell growth, tumor cell migration to autotoxins and type IV collagen, tumor cell adhesion, and growth of human tumors in nude mice. The mechanism of action appears to be an inhibition of receptor-mediated calcium influx into cells, thereby downgrading second messenger pathways.[147] Disease stabilization has been noted in approximately half the patients currently in trials.[127] Finally, a popular antihypertensive medication, captopril, appears capable of inhibiting chemotaxis and migration of endothelial cells in the rat cornea. This effect was mediated by endothelial metalloproteinases and was associated with decreased growth in experimental fibrosarcomas.[148] Since captopril already is well tolerated in patients, clinical trials utilizing this agent in cancer patients may soon take place.

Theoretically, abrogation of neovascularization may be the most attractive new area for investigation since the only natural processes likely to be affected would be wound healing and menstruation. Ultimately, the best results will likely be achieved if antiangiogenic agents are coupled with conventional treatments.

## Anticoagulation Therapy

An intact hemostatic system, especially the platelet component, is associated with the process of metastasis. As noted previously, tumor cell aggregates often contain platelets, and this association likely favors the arrest of tumor masses in small blood vessels. There has been a long history of efforts to modify the hemostatic mechanism in order to change the course of cancer, using both anticoagulants and antiplatelet agents. The rationale is summarized by Olden and colleagues:[149]

- Agents that inhibit platelet aggregation decrease cancer metastasis in some experimental tumors.

- Intravenous injection of intact tumor cells induces a decrease in platelet count.

- Emboli containing fibrin, platelets, and tumor cells can be detected in the circulation shortly after release of tumor cells into the circulation.

Heparin has myriad biological properties, including binding to adhesion molecules such as laminin, fibronectin, and type IV collagen.[150] Based on these observations, efforts to inhibit experimental tumors with heparin have been successful.[151] Antiplatelet agents such as prostacyclin[98] can prevent platelet activation and secretion as well as inhibiting experimentally induced metastases in mice. Clinical trials utilizing heparin and conventional cancer treatment have suggested an additive effect, especially in small-cell carcinoma of the lung.[152]

## Genetic Manipulation

Should certain genes such as *NM23* be found to have a significant impact on the metastatic character of cancer cells, it will be possible in the near future to place normal copies of missing or replace abnormal *NM23* genes in tumor cells. This approach is logical for tumor-suppressor genes that may be low in content or absent in tumor cells; alternatively, if the specific gene product is isolated, this substance might be administered to achieve the same effect. Weakened viruses can carry specific human tumor-suppressor genes (such as *p53*) and insert them into tumor cells that lack the gene; this approach is one example of "gene therapy," and despite technical obstacles that are yet to be solved, the concept is sound. Perhaps more than any other type of treatment, the modification of an abnormal genetic state back to normal function is the most natural and exciting approach to the conquest of cancer.

## CONCLUSION

The potential for success in interrupting the metastatic continuum seems brighter today than even several years ago. Despite a lack of knowledge regarding biochemical mechanisms related to metastasis, the mysteries of this process are unraveling. It is inevitable that treatment options will include new agents to abrogate various steps in the metastatic cascade. As part of a combined treatment plan with conventional therapies, the future applications are both ample and exciting.

With issues of tumor cell heterogeneity and our continuing difficulties in achieving early diagnosis of common neoplasms, the struggle against cancer will continue. We still need to know how to predict the metastatic potential of a tumor at the time of diagnosis, the degree of silent metastasis, and how to tell when a tumor is completely eradicated. With the continued collaboration of basic scientists and clinical caregivers, each of whom has a passion for truth and excellence, the answers will be found.

# REFERENCES

1. Kupchella CE: *Dimensions of Cancer.* Belmont, CA, Wadsworth, 1987, p 152
2. Ruddon R: *Cancer Biology.* New York, Oxford University Press, 1981
3. Greider C, Blackburn E: Telomeres, telomerase and cancer. *Sci Am* 274:92–97, 1996
4. Abercrombie M: The contact behavior of invading cells, in *Cellular Membranes and Tumor-Cell Behavior.* Baltimore, Williams and Wilkins, 1975, pp 21–37
5. Pitot H: *Fundamentals of Oncology* (ed 3). New York, Dekker, 1986
6. Oppenheimer S: *Cancer: A Biological and Clinical Introduction* (ed 2). Boston, Jones and Bartlett, 1985
7. Weinberg R: How cancer arises. *Sci Am* 275:62–70, 1996
8. Tannock I: Biologic properties of anticancer drugs, in Tannock I, Hill R (eds): *The Basic Science of Oncology.* New York, Pergamon Press, 1987, pp 278–291
9. Mintz B, Fleischman R: Teratocarcinomas and other neoplasms as developmental defects in gene expression. *Adv Cancer Res* 34:211–278, 1981
10. Rifkin D, Moscatelli D: Recent developments in the cell biology of basic fibroblasts growth factor. *J Cell Biol* 109:1–6, 1989
11. Twardzik D, Ranchalis J, McPherson J: Inhibition and promotion of differentiation-like phenotype of a human lung carcinoma in athymic nude mice by natural and recombinant forms of transforming growth factor–beta. *J Natl Cancer Inst* 81:1182–1185, 1989
12. Sporn M, Roberts A, Goodman D: *The Retinoids,* vol 2. New York, Academic Press, 1984, pp 56–57
13. Correa P: Morphology and natural history of precursor lesions, in Schottenfeld D, Fraumeni J (eds): *Cancer Epidemiology and Prevention.* Philadelphia, Saunders, 1982, pp 90–118
14. Singer S, Nicolson G: The fluid mosaic structure of cell membranes. *Science* 175:720–731, 1972
15. Nicolson GL: Transmembrane control of the receptors in normal and tumor cells: II. Surface changes associated with transformation and malignancy. *Biochim Biophys Acta* 458:1–72, 1976
16. Nicolson G, Poste G: The cancer cell: Dynamic aspects and modifications in cell-surface organization. Parts 1 and 2. *N Engl J Med* 295:197–203, 253–258, 1976
17. Smets L, Van Beek W: Carbohydrates of the tumor cell surface. *Biochim Biophys Acta* 738:237–249, 1984
18. Hynes R: Fibronectins. *Sci Am* 254:42–51, 1986
19. Quigley J: Proteolytic enzymes of normal and malignant cells, in Hynes R (ed): *Surfaces of Normal and Malignant Cells.* Chichester, England, Wiley, 1979, pp 247–285
20. Sloane B, Robinson D, Honn K: Role for cathepsin B and cystatins in tumor growth and progression. *Biol Chem Hoppe Seyler* 371:193–198, 1990 (suppl)
21. Liotta L: Tumor invasion and metastases—role of the extracellular matrix: Rhoads Memorial Award Lecture. *Cancer Res* 46:1–7, 1986
22. Goldfarb R: Proteolytic enzymes in tumor invasion and degradation of host extracellular matrices, in Honn K, Powers W, Sloane B (eds): *Mechanisms of Cancer Metastasis: Potential Therapeutic Implications.* Boston, Martinus Nijhoff, 1986, pp 341–375
23. Testa J, Quigley J: The role of urokinase-type plasminogen activator in aggressive tumor cell behavior. *Cancer Metastasis Rev* 9:353–367, 1990
24. Sloane B, Rozhin J, Ryan R, et al. Cathepsin D–like cysteine proteinases and metastasis, in Honn K, Powers W, Sloane B (eds): *Mechanisms of Cancer Metastasis: Potential Therapeutic Implications.* Boston, Martinus Nijhoff, 1986, pp 377–398
25. Rochefort H, Capony F, Garcia M, Cathepsin D: A protease involved in breast cancer metastasis. *Cancer Metastasis Rev* 9:321–331, 1990
26. Gordon S: Cancer cell procoagulants and their possible role in metastasis, in Honn K, Powers W, Sloane B (eds): *Mechanisms of Cancer Metastasis: Potential Therapeutic Implications.* Boston, Martinus Nijhoff, 1986, pp 159–172
27. Hakomori S: Glycosphingolipids. *Sci Am* 254:44–53, 1986
28. Herlyn M, Menrad A, Koprowski H: Structure, function and clinical significance of human tumor antigens. *J Natl Cancer Inst* 82:1883–1890, 1990
29. Birnbaum M, Haspel H, Rosen O: Transformation of rat fibroblasts by FSV rapidly increases glucose transporter gene transcription. *Science* 235:1495–1497, 1987
30. Pastan I, Johnson G, Anderson W: Role of cyclic nucleotides in growth control. *Annu Rev Biochem* 44:491–522, 1975
31. Levitzki A: From epinephrine to cyclic AMP. *Science* 241:800–806, 1988
32. Fontana J, Munoz M, Durham J: Potentiation between intracellular cyclic-AMP–elevating agents and inducers of leukemic cell differentiation. *Leuk Res* 9:1127–1132, 1985
33. Lando M, Abemayor E, Verity M, et al: Modulation of intracellular adenosine monophosphate levels and the differentiation response of human neuroblastoma cells. *Cancer Res* 50:722–727, 1990
34. Young C, Warrel R: Differentiating agents, in DeVita V, Hellman S, Rosenberg S (eds): *Cancer: Principles and Practice of Oncology* (ed 4). Philadelphia, Lippincott, 1993, pp 2636–2646
35. Watson J, Hopkins N, Roberts J: *Molecular Biology of the Gene.* Vol 2, *Specialized Aspects* (ed 4). Menlo Park, CA, Benjamin/Cummings, 1987, pp 747–1163
36. Todaro G, DeLarco E: Growth factors produced by sarcoma virus–transformed cells. *Cancer Res* 38:4147–4153, 1978
37. Sporn M, Roberts A: Autocrine growth factors and cancer. *Nature* 313:745–747, 1985
38. Kimchi A, Wang X-F, Weinberg R, et al: Absence of TGF-β receptors and growth inhibitory responses in retinoblastoma cells. *Science* 240:196–198, 1988
39. Goustin A, Leof E, Shipley G, et al: Growth factors and cancer. *Cancer Res* 46:1015–1029, 1986

40. Devel T: Polypeptide growth factors: Roles in normal and abnormal cell growth. *Annu Rev Cell Biol* 3:443–492, 1987

41. Waterfield M: The role of growth factors in cancer, in Frank L, Teich N (eds): *Introduction to the Cellular and Molecular Biology of Cancer.* Oxford, Oxford University Press, 1986, pp 27–39

42. Harris A, Nicholson S, Sainsbury J, et al: Epidermal growth factor receptor: A marker of early relapse in breast cancer and tumor stage progression in bladder cancer—interactions with NEU, in Furth M, Greaves M (eds): *The Molecular Diagnostics of Human Cancer,* vol 7. Cold Spring Harbor, NY, Cold Spring Harbor Laboratory Press, 1989, pp 353–357

43. Wright C, Angus B, Nicholson S, et al: Expression of c-*ERBB-2* oncoprotein: A prognostic indicator in human breast cancer. *Cancer Res* 49:2087–2090, 1989

44. Vonderhaar B: Local effects of EGF, α-GF, and EGF-like growth factors on lobuloalveolar development of the mouse mammary gland in vivo. *J Cell Physiol* 132:581–584, 1987

45. Thorburn G, Waters M, Dolling M, et al. Fetal maturation and epidermal growth factor. *Proc Aust Phys Pharmacol Soc* 12:11–15, 1981

46. Carpenter G, Wahl M: The epidermal growth factor family, in Sporn M, Roberts A (eds): *Peptide Growth Factors and Their Receptors,* vol 1. Berlin, Springer-Verlag 1990, pp 69–171

47. Humphrey P, Wong A, Vogelstein B, et al: Anti-synthetic peptide antibody reacting at the fusion junction of deletion-mutant epidermal growth factor receptors in human glioblastoma. *Proc Natl Acad Sci U S A* 87:4207–4211, 1990

48. Schreiber A, Winkler M, Derynck R: TGF-α: A more potent angiogenic mediator than EGF. *Science* 232:1250–1254, 1986

49. DeLarco J, Todaro G: Growth factors from murine sarcoma virus–transformed cells. *Proc Natl Acad Sci U S A* 75:4001–4005, 1978

50. Kimchi A, Wang X-F, Weinberg R, et al: Absence of TGF-β receptors and growth inhibitory responses in retinoblastoma cells. *Science* 240:196–198, 1988

51. Sporn M, Roberts A: Transforming growth factor-β: Multiple actions and potential clinical applications. *JAMA* 262:938–941, 1989

52. Massague J: The transforming growth factor-β family. *Annu Rev Cell Biol* 6:597–641, 1990

53. Pietenpol J, Stein R, Moran E, et al: TGF-β inhibition of c-*myc* transcription and growth in keratinocytes is abrogated by viral transforming proteins with pRb binding domains. *Cell* 61:777–785, 1990

54. Laiho M, DeCaprio J, Ludlow J, et al: Growth inhibition by TGF-β linked to suppression of retinoblastoma protein phosphorylation. *Cell* 62:175–185, 1990

55. Rozengurt E, Sinnet-Smith J, Taylor-Papadimitriou J: Production of PDGF-like growth factor by breast cancer cell lines. *Int J Cancer* 36:247–252, 1985

56. Pledger W, Stiles C, Antoniades H, et al: An ordered sequence of events is required before BALB/c 3T3 cells become committed to DNA synthesis. *Proc Natl Acad Sci U S A* 75:2839–2843, 1978

57. Maxwell M, Nabers, Wolfe H, et al: Coexpression of platelet-derived growth factor (PDGF) and PDGF-receptor genes by primary human astrocytomas may contribute to their development and maintenance. *J Clin Invest* 86:131–135, 1990

58. Folkman J, Klagsbrun M: Angiogenic factors. *Science* 235:442–447, 1987

59. Blundell T, Humbel R: Hormone families: Pancreatic hormones and homologous growth factors. *Nature* 287:781–787, 1980

60. Mendelsohn J, Lippman M: Principles of molecular biology of cancer: Growth factors, in DeVita V, Hellman S, Rosenberg S (eds): *Cancer: Principles and Practice of Oncology* (ed 4). Philadelphia, Lippincott, 1993, pp 114–133

61. Clemmons D: Structural and functional analysis of insulin-like growth factors. *Br Med Bull* 45:465–480, 1989

62. Paik S, Fisher E, Fisher B, et al: Pathologic findings from National Surgical Adjuvant Breast Project (Protocol B-06), prognosis significance of ERBB-2 protein overexpression in primary breast cancer. *J Clin Oncol* 8:103–112, 1990

63. Hancock M, Langton B, Chan T, et al: A monoclonal antibody against C-ERB 132 protein enhances the cytotoxicity of *cis*-diamminedichloroplatinum against human breast and ovarian tumor cell lines. *Cancer Res* 51:4575–4580, 1991

64. Nowell P: The clonal evolution of tumor cell populations. *Science* 194:23–28, 1976

65. Vogelstein B, Fearon E, Hamilton S, et al: Genetic alterations during colorectal tumor development. *N Engl J Med* 319:525–532, 1988

66. Kinzler K, Nilbert M, Su L, et al: Identification of FAP locus genes from chromosome 5q21. *Science* 253:661–665, 1991

67. Goyette M, Cho K, Fashing C, et al: Progression of colorectal cancer is associated with multiple tumor suppressor gene defects but inhibition of tumorigenicity is accomplished by correction of any single defect via chromosome transfer. *Mol Cell Biol* 12:1387–1395, 1992

68. Lynch H, Smyrk T: Hereditary nonpolyposis colorectal cancer (Lynch syndrome): An updated review. *Cancer* 78:1149–1167, 1996

69. Miki Y, Swenson J, Shattuck-Eidens D, et al: A strong candidate for the breast and ovarian cancer susceptibility gene *BRCA1. Science* 266:66–71, 1994

70. Wooster R, Neuhausen S, Mangion J: Localization of breast cancer susceptibility gene *BRCA2* to chromosome 13q 12–13. *Science* 265:2088–2090, 1994

71. Weiss L: Metastatic inefficiency: Causes and consequences. *Cancer Rev* 3:1–24, 1986

72. Fidler I, Hart I: Biologic diversity in metastatic neoplasms: Origins and implications. *Science* 217:998–1003, 1982

73. Liotta L, Steeg P, Stetler-Stevenson W: Cancer metastasis and angiogenesis: An imbalance of positive and negative regulation. *Cell* 64:327–336, 1991

74. Thorgeirsson U, Turpeenniemi-Hujanen T, Williams J, et al: NIH 3T3 cells transfected with human tumor DNA containing activated *ras* oncogenes express the metastatic phenotype in nude mice. *Mol Cell Biol* 5:259–262, 1985

75. Ura H, Bonfil R, Reich R, et al: Expression of type IV collagenase and procollagen genes and its correlation with the tumorigenic, invasive and metastatic abilities of oncogene-transformed human bronchial epithelial cells. *Cancer Res* 49:4615–4621, 1989

76. Muschel R, Williams J, Lowy D, et al: Harvey *ras* induction of metastatic potential depends upon oncogene activation and the type of recipient cell. *Am J Pathol* 121:1–8, 1985

77. Tuck A, Wilson S, Chambers A: *Ras* transfection and expression does not induce progression from tumorigenicity to metastatic ability in mouse LTA cells. *Clin Exp Metastasis* 8:417–431, 1990

78. Pohl J, Goldfinger N, Rader-Pohl A, et al: *P53* increases experimental metastatic capacity of murine carcinoma cells. *Mol Cell Biol* 8:2078–2081, 1988

79. Steeg P, Bevilacqua G, Kopper L, et al: Evidence for a novel gene associated with low tumor metastatic potential. *J Natl Cancer Inst* 80:200–204, 1988

80. Sidebottom E, Clark S: Cell fusion segregates progressive growth from metastasis. *Br J Cancer* 47:399–405, 1983

81. Fidler IJ, Kripke ML: Metastasis results from pre-existing variant cells within a malignant tumor. *Science* 197:893–895, 1977

82. Folkman J, Watson K, Ingber D, et al: Induction of angiogenesis during the transition from hyperplasia to neoplasia. *Nature* 339:58–61, 1989

83. Schroder M, Risau W, Hallmann R, et al: Tumor necrosis factor type, a potent inhibitor of endothelial cell growth in vitro, is angiogenic in vivo. *Proc Natl Acad Sci U S A* 84:5277–5281, 1986

84. Liotta L, Mandler R, Murano G, et al: Tumor cell autocrine motility factor. *Proc Natl Acad Sci U S A* 83:3302–3306, 1986

85. Guirguis R, Schiffman E, Liu B, et al: Detection of autocrine motility factor(s) in urine as markers of bladder cancer. *J Natl Cancer Inst* 80:1203–1211, 1988

86. Ruoslahti E, Giancotti F: Integrins and tumor cell dissemination. *Cancer Cells* 1:119–126, 1989

87. Rao C, Margulies L, Trakla S, et al: Isolation of a subunit of laminin and its role in molecular structure and tumor cell attachment. *J Biol Chem* 257:9740–9744, 1982

88. Karre K, Ljunggren H, Piontek G, et al: Selective rejection of H-2-deficient lymphoma variants suggests alternative immune defence strategy. *Nature* 319:675–678, 1986

89. Rosenberg S, Lotze M, Muul L, et al: A progress report on the treatment of 157 patients with advanced cancer using lymphokine-activated killer cells and interleukin-2 or high-dose interleukin-2 alone. *N Engl J Med* 316:889–897, 1987

90. Takahashi K, Ono K, Hirabayashi Y, et al: Escape mechanisms of melanoma from immune system by soluble melanoma antigen. *J Immunol* 140:3244–3248, 1988

91. Bast R Jr: Effects of cancers and their treatment on host immunity, in Holland J, Frei E (eds): *Cancer Medicine*. Philadelphia, Lea and Febiger, 1982, pp 1134–1173

92. Lopez D, Fu Y-X, Watson G: Modulation of immune responses by tumor-derived factors. *Proc Am Assoc Cancer Res* 31:236, 1990 (abstr)

93. Haskill S (ed): *Tumor Immunity in Prognosis. The Role of Mononuclear Cell Infiltration*. New York, Dekker, 1982

94. Krieder J, Bartlett G, Butkiewicz B: Relationship of tumor leucocytic infiltration to host defense mechanisms and prognosis. *Cancer Metastasis Rev* 3:53–74, 1987

95. Gasic G, Gasic T, Stewart C: Antimetastatic effects associated with platelet reduction. *Proc Natl Acad Sci U S A* 61:46–52, 1968

96. Gasic G: Role of plasma, platelets and endothelial cells in tumor metastasis. *Cancer Metastasis Rev* 3:99–114, 1984

97. Gasic G, Tuszynski G, Gorelik E: Interaction of the hemostatic and immune systems in the metastatic spread of tumor cells. *Int Rev Exp Pathol* 29:173–208, 1984

98. Honn K, Cicone B, Skoff A: Prostaglandin: A potent antimetastatic agent. *Science* 212:1270–1272, 1981

99. Agarwal K, Parks R: Forskolin: A potential antimetastatic agent. *Int J Cancer* 32:801–804, 1983

100. Gorelik E, Wiltrout R, Okumura K, et al: Role of NK cells in the control of metastatic spread and growth of tumor cells in mice. *Int J Cancer* 30:107–112, 1982

101. Liotta L, Kohn E: Cancer invasion and metastases. *JAMA* 263:1123–1126, 1990

102. Koscielny S, Tubiana M, Valleron A-J: A simulation model of the natural history of breast cancer. *Br J Cancer* 52:515–524, 1985

103. Fidler I, Hart I: Biologic diversity in metastatic neoplasms: origins and implications. *Science* 217:998–1001, 1982

104. Fidler I: Critical factors in the biology of human metastasis: Twenty-eighth G. H. A. Clowes Memorial Award Lecture. *Cancer Res* 50:6130–6138, 1990

105. Ausprunk D, Folkman J: Migration and proliferation of endothelial cells in preformed and newly formed blood vessels during angiogenesis. *Microvasc Res* 14:53–65, 1977

106. Weidner N, Semple J, Welch W, et al: Tumor angiogenesis and metastasis—correlation in invasive breast carcinoma. *N Engl J Med* 324:1–8, 1991

107. Schreiber A, Winkler M, Derynck R: Transforming growth factor-α: A more potent angiogenic mediator than epidermal growth factor. *Science* 232:1250–1253, 1986

108. Cozzolino F, Torcia M, Lucibello M, et al: Interferon-α and interleukin-2 synergistically enhance β fibroblast growth factor synthesis and induce release, promoting endothelial cell growth. *J Clin Invest* 91:2504–2512, 1993

109. Soncin F: Angiogenin supports endothelial and fibroblast cell adhesion. *Proc Natl Acad Sci U S A* 89:2232–2236, 1992

110. Koch A, Polverini P, Kunkel S, et al: Interleukin-8 as a macrophage-derived mediator of angiogenesis. *Science* 258:1798–1801, 1992

111. Takebayashi Y, Akiyama S, Akiba S, et al: Clinicopathologic and prognostic significance of an angiogenic factor, thymidine phosphorylase, in human colorectal carcinoma. *J Natl Cancer Inst* 88:1110–1117, 1996

112. Folkman J: What is the role of thymidine phosphorylase in tumor angiogenesis? *J Natl Cancer Inst* 88:1091–1092, 1996 (editorial)

113. Liotta L, Stetler-Stevenson W: Principles of molecular biology of cancer: Cancer metastasis, in DeVita V, Hellman S, Rosenberg S (eds): *Cancer: Principles and Practice of Oncology* (ed 4). Philadelphia, Lippincott, 1993, pp 134–149

114. Folkman J: Fighting cancer by attacking its blood supply. *Sci Am* 275:150–154, 1996

115. Liotta LA: Tumor invasion: Role of the extracellular matrix. *Cancer Res* 46:1–7, 1986

116. Ruoslahti E: How cancer spreads. *Sci Am* 275:72–77, 1996

117. Martinez-Hernandez A, Amenta P: The basement membrane in pathology. *Lab Invest* 48:656–677, 1983

118. Ruoslahti E, Reed J: Anchorage dependence, integrins, and apoptosis. *Cell* 77:477–478, 1994

119. Castronovo V, Colin C, Claysmith A, et al: Immunodetection of the metastasis-associated laminin receptor in human breast cancer cells obtained by fine needle aspiration biopsy. *Am J Pathol* 137:1373–1381, 1990

120. Liotta L, Tryggvason K, Garbisa S, et al: Metastatic potential correlates with enzymatic degradation of basement membrane collagen. *Nature* 284:67–68, 1980

121. Nakajima M, Morikawa K, Fabra A, et al: Influence of organ environment on extracellular matrix degradative activity and metastases of human colon carcinoma cells. *J Natl Cancer Inst* 82:1890–1898, 1990

122. Schwartz G, Wang H, Lampen N, et al: Defining the invasive phenotype of proximal gastric cancer cells. *Cancer* 73:22–27, 1994

123. Gottesman M: The role of proteases in cancer. *Semin Cancer Biol* 1:97–160, 1990

124. Boone T, Johnson M, DeClerck Y, et al: cDNA cloning and expression of a metalloproteinase inhibitor related to

tissue inhibitor of metalloproteinases. *Proc Natl Acad Sci U S A* 87:2800–2804, 1990

125. Goldberg G, Marmer B, Grant G, et al: Human 72-kDA type IV collagenase forms a complex with a tissue inhibitor of metalloproteinase inhibitor. *Proc Natl Acad Sci U S A* 86: 8207–8211, 1989

126. Corcoran M, Stetler-Stevenson W: Tissue inhibitor of metalloproteinase-2 stimulates fibroblast proliferation via a cAMP-dependent mechanism. *J Biol Chem* 270:13453–13459, 1995

127. Allesandro R, Kohn E: Molecular genetics of cancer-tumor invasion and angiogenesis. *Cancer* 76:1874–1877, 1995

128. Moses M, Sudhalter J, Langer R: Identification of an inhibitor of neovascularization from cartilage. *Science* 248: 1408–1410, 1990

129. Lam W, Delikatny J, Orr F, et al: The chemotactic response of tumor cells: A model for cancer metastasis. *Am J Pathol* 104:69–76, 1981

130. Guirguis R, Margulies I, Taraboletti G, et al: Cytokine-induced pseudopodial protrusion coupled to tumor cell migration. *Nature* 329:261–265, 1987

131. McCann J: Clues about metastasis may lead to better cancer drugs. *J Natl Cancer Inst* 87:636–638, 1995

132. Kohn E, Francis E, Liotta L: Heterogeneity of the motility responses in malignant tumor cells: A biological basis for the diversity and homing of metastatic cells. *Int J Cancer* 46:287–292, 1990

133. Kohn E, Hollister G, Savarese D: Recombinant granulocyte-macrophage colony-stimulating factor induces locomotion in human melanoma cells. *Proc Am Assoc Cancer Res* 31:61, 1990 (abstr)

134. Paget S: The distribution of secondary growth in cancer of the breast. *Lancet* 1:571–573, 1889

135. Nicholson G: Molecular mechanisms of cancer metastasis: Tumor and host properties and the role of oncogenes and suppressor genes. *Curr Opin Oncol* 3:75–92, 1991

136. Hujanen E, Terranova V: Migration of tumor cells to organ-derived chemoattractants. *Cancer Res* 45:3517–3521, 1985

137. Weiss L: Metastatic inefficiency: Causes and consequences. *Cancer Rev* 3:1–24, 1986

138. Holzman D: New view of metastasis is spreading. *J Natl Cancer Inst* 88:1336–1338, 1996

139. Barth R, Camp B, Martuscello T, et al: The cytokine environment of human colon carcinoma. *Cancer* 78:1168–1178, 1996

140. Bonfil D, Reddel R, Ura H, et al: Invasive and metastatic potential of a V-HA-RAS transformed human bronchial epithelial cell line. *J Natl Cancer Inst* 81:587–594, 1989

141. Hennessy C, Henry J, May F, et al: Expression of the anti-metastatic gene *nm23* in human breast cancer: Association with good prognosis. *J Natl Cancer Inst* 83:281–285, 1991

142. Myeroff L, Markowitz S: *NM23:* Into the basement (membrane). *J Natl Cancer Inst* 86:1815–1817, 1994 (editorial)

143. Humphries M, Olden K, Yamada K: A synthetic peptide from fibronectin inhibits experimental metastasis of murine melanoma cells. *Science* 233:467–470, 1986

144. Baselga J, Tripathy D, Mendelsohn J, et al: Phase II study of weekly intravenous recombinant humanized anti-p185 HER-2 monoclonal antibody in patients with HER-2/neu overexpressing metastatic breast cancer. *J Clin Oncol* 14: 737–744, 1996

145. James S, Salsbury A: Effect of ICRF 159 on tumor blood vessels and its relationship to the antimetastatic effect in the Lewis lung carcinoma. *Cancer Res* 34:839–842, 1974

146. Ziegler J: Angiogenesis research enjoys growth spurt in the 1990's. *J Natl Cancer Inst* 88:786–788, 1996

147. Kohn E, Liotta L: L651582: A novel antiproliferative and antimetastatic agent. *J Natl Cancer Inst* 82:54–60, 1990

148. Volpert O, Ward W, Lingen M, et al: Captopril inhibits angiogenesis and slows the growth of experimental tumors in rats. *J Clin Invest* 98:671–679, 1996

149. Olden K, White S, Mohla S, et al: Experimental approaches for the prevention of hematogenous metastasis. *Oncology* 3:83–91, 1989

150. Charonis A, Skubitz A, Koliakos G, et al: A novel synthetic peptide from the B1 chain of laminin with heparin-binding and cell adhesion–promoting activities. *J Cell Biol* 107: 1253–1260, 1988

151. Villaneuva G, Nakajima M, Nicolson G: Heparin derivatives as inhibitors of heparinase from metastatic melanoma cells. *Ann N Y Acad Sci* 556:496–498, 1989

152. Zacharski L, Henderson W, Rickles F, et al: Effect of warfarin anticoagulation on survival in carcinoma of the lung, colon, head and neck and prostate. *Cancer* 53:2046–2052, 1984

# Chapter 3

# Carcinogenesis

**John W. Yarbro, MD, PhD**

## INTRODUCTION

Cancer represents the most fundamental biological challenge to a multicellular organism because it is the process by which some of the cells of the organism attempt to destroy the organism itself. Normally, all of the body's cells are held under rigid growth control except for tissue repair and normal growth. Control of cell division is carefully maintained by two opposing sets of genes, one set promoting growth and the other set inhibiting growth. These genes were discovered initially not as "growth" genes but as "cancer" genes, and their names reflect this: *oncogenes* are growth-promoting genes, and *cancer-suppressor genes* are growth-inhibitory genes. Carcinogenesis is the process by which these genes are damaged to the extent that clones of cells lose the normal control mechanisms of growth and proliferate out of control.

Cancer develops and evolves by the process of *clonal selection*. Stated simply, an initial mutation in the genome of a cell may confer a survival advantage on that cell. If one of the progeny of that cell is hit by a second mutation that also confers a survival advantage, this new clone grows even more vigorously. A sequence of such events leads first to the selection of a clone with the characteristics of a neoplasm and later allows that neoplastic clone to progress to ever greater stages of virulence characterized by invasion, metastatic spread, drug resistance, and other characteristics that ultimately lead to the death of the host. This is Darwinian evolution, natural selection, on a clonal basis within a single organism. It is a perversion of the normal growth and repair mechanisms. Step by step, cancer overcomes a complex set of protective growth controls. The large number of mutations required to develop cancer indicates that genetic instability (an increased mutation rate) is an early change in the evolving cancer cell.

Damage to the genome may result from exposure to chemicals such as those in tobacco, radiation such as radon from natural sources or medical radiation, asbestos, or various types of viruses. In all cases the final common path of action of such agents is through oncogenes and cancer-suppressor genes. Specifically, oncogenes must be mutated or relocated so as to be activated, and cancer-suppressor genes must be mutated or lost so as to be inactivated. Many times, although exactly how frequently is uncertain, an individual may inherit a defective cancer-suppressor gene from a parent. Oncogenes usually act as dominant genes, that is, only one gene of each pair needs to be mutated to have an effect; cancer-suppressor genes usually act as recessive genes, that is, both genes of a pair must be mutated or lost to abolish their cancer-suppressor effect.

Cancer may be thought of as a defect in the control of the cell cycle that allows continuous operation of the cell cycle engine.[1] Normally this engine is regulated by a series of enzymes, the cyclin-dependent kinases (Cdks), that associate with specific substrates, the cyclins, to form complexes that regulate the movement of the cell through a series of regulatory "checkpoints" in the cell cycle. Some cancer-suppressor genes code for proteins essential to the operation of these checkpoints. For example, the gene *ATM*, which is mutated in ataxia telangiectasia, codes for a protein that regulates two checkpoints; when this protein is absent, the patient is at increased risk for developing cancer.[2]

Cancer may also be thought of as being related to a defect in programmed cell death (apoptosis), which is a mechanism by which defective cells are disposed of. Apoptosis is an ancient mechanism that is operative even in unicellular organisms.[3] Mutant cells with defective DNA are induced to undergo a process of cell death. This process is defective in cancer cells. A cancer family syndrome, the Li-Fraumeni syndrome, has a defect in a gene, *p53*, which induces apoptosis in cells with severely mutated DNA.

The cancer cell is immortal because it reproduces in an uncontrolled manner, because it does not undergo normal programmed cell death, and because it seems to lack the normal "biological clocks" located at the ends of chromosomes that limit the number of times a chromosome may replicate. The ends of chromosomes have structures called *telomeres*, which are not completely copied when the chromosome is duplicated during cell division. The result is that with age the telomeres grow progressively shorter until the chromosome can no longer replicate. Only germ cells in the testis and ovary have an enzyme, telomerase, that prevents aging by duplicating the telomeres. Cancer cells also develop this enzyme, which contributes to their immortality.[4]

Discovery of new cancer-related genes has greatly accelerated in the past few years, and previously obscure molecular events in carcinogenesis are being elucidated in great detail. The genes associated with inherited cancer are being identified and are often the same genes that are damaged in the process of carcinogenesis. These discoveries offer the potential for identification of high-risk populations and improved cancer prevention.

## STAGES OF CARCINOGENESIS

It has been customary in the past to divide carcinogenesis into three stages—initiation, promotion, and progression—based on the pioneering work of Peyton Rous described in chapter 1. Rous coined these three terms based on a series of experiments in skin carcinogenesis: *initiation*, which indicates some primary change in the target produced by a carcinogen; *promotion*, which means some secondary effect of an agent (the promoter), which alone might not be able to induce a malignancy; and *progression*, which designates "the process by which tumors go from bad to worse."[5–7] Foulds codified and expanded this concept of multistage carcinogenesis.[8] Progression to the metastatic phenotype has subsequently been well elucidated by Fidler.[9]

In humans carcinogenesis is much more complex than in well-studied animal laboratory models. The distinction between the three stages is blurred, and there are many more steps. More than one type of initiating event is probably common. In some cases it is likely that initiators act as their own promoters, that is, they are complete carcinogens. In other cases an initiator may be a complete carcinogen for one organ and an incomplete carcinogen for another organ. The line between promotion and progression is indistinct. Even when we understand a great deal about the carcinogen, it does not seem to fit the laboratory model exactly. For example, in lung cancer, cigarette tars seem to act as both initiators and promoters, but unlike the laboratory model, where initiation is irreversible, in humans the smoker who quits returns to the normal low incidence pattern in 10 to 15 years. These complexities are discussed in detail in an excellent review.[10]

Carcinogenesis is ordinarily classified as chemical, viral, physical, or familial, even though it is likely that human carcinogenesis involves a combination of factors. Carcinogenesis can also be classified as occupational, dietary, environmental, lifestyle, and so forth.

## CHEMICAL CARCINOGENESIS

In 1915 cancer was induced chemically in laboratory animals for the first time when coal tar was applied to rabbit skin at Tokyo University by Yamagiwa and Ichikawa.[11] Perhaps because the English physician Percival Pott had noted in 1775 that soot caused scrotal cancer in chimney sweeps, the chemical carcinogenesis theory became the leading theory of cancer causation. Preceding Pott's often-cited observation the single most destructive chemical carcinogen yet to be found, tobacco, was identified by John Hill,[12] an astute clinician, only a few decades after it was introduced into common usage in London. From that date, 1761, until 1950, when we "rediscovered" tobacco as a carcinogen,[13–15] the only chemicals discovered to be significant carcinogens in humans were the aniline dyes, which caused bladder cancer.[16] The first potent synthetic carcinogen, dibenzanthracene, was discovered in 1930.[17] Subsequently, many other chemicals were developed that caused cancer in various animal systems but not many in humans.

The large number of active chemicals discovered raised questions about how they caused cancer since they seemed to have no common chemical structure. Classic work by the Millers led in 1951 to the understanding that covalent binding within the cell was essential for carcinogenic activity; the active metabolite of the carcinogen was later identified to be an electrophilic reactant that bound to DNA.[18] Carcinogens are converted by a series of metabolic steps into free radicals, that is, compounds with a single unpaired electron. Free radicals are electrophilic, that is, highly reactive with macromolecules that are rich in electrons, such as DNA. Compounds called *antioxidants* inhibit carcinogenesis because they react with free radicals before the free radicals damage DNA.

Because different organisms have different metabolic systems, potential carcinogens are metabolized in one way in some organisms and in other ways in other organisms, with the result that some chemicals are carcinogenic for one species but not for another. There may be as yet unidentified metabolic differences that render some people more sensitive than others to certain carcinogens. Ames developed a classic assay system to measure carcinogens. The assay employs bacteria and is based on the fact that most carcinogens are mutagens, that is, they damage DNA.[19] The Ames system requires the addition of liver microsomes in order to metabolize the chemicals to be tested into active carcinogens. The metabolism of a carcinogen leads to the final active chemical, called the *proximate carcinogen,* that reacts with the DNA.

In smokers it is possible to directly identify the carcinogen bound to DNA, the so-called hydrocarbon adducts.[20] The proximate carcinogen exerts its effect by binding to DNA and mutating it directly or by causing errors to be made when the host cell tries to repair the damaged DNA. However, most of the lesions produced by carcinogens are repaired.

The specific targets of carcinogens are the oncogenes and cancer-suppressor genes, the "on" and "off" switches for cell growth. These have been identified in some cancers. In systems in which known chemical carcinogens and radiation induce malignant transformation, it is possible to identify mutated cellular oncogenes.[21,22] Further, specific and consistent point mutations have been demonstrated in some human malignancies.[23] Movement of an oncogene to a different site on the same or another chromosome, which may cause activation, has also been demonstrated.[24] In a few cases the specific structural change in the protein that leads to malfunction has been elucidated.[25]

In spite of the vast array of chemicals discovered to cause cancer in animals, there still remain few chemicals (other than tobacco) for which there is strong evidence of causation of the common cancers in man. Occasional industrial chemicals have been documented, such as benzene, 2-naphthylamine, vinyl chloride, and some metals, but after extensive study the best estimate is that only 4% of all cancer deaths in the United States are due to occupational causes.[26] Cancer chemotherapeutic agents are carcinogenic, and cured cancer patients are at risk for leukemia and some other tumors.

## FAMILIAL CARCINOGENESIS

A variety of sources estimate that up to 15% of all human cancers may have a hereditary component. Breast cancer, for example, is estimated to have a familial component in about 13% of cases.[27] The list of familial syndromes has begun to expand rapidly in recent years as the new techniques of molecular biology have been applied to the isolation of genes that, when inherited, increase the risk of cancer. In some cases the syndromes have been known on a clinical basis for many years; in other cases identification of genes from cancer patients has led to the description of new family syndromes.

Genes have now been isolated for several of the classic family cancer syndromes: *RB1* in retinoblastoma; *WT1* in Wilms' tumor; *NF1* and *NF2* in neurofibromatosis types 1 and 2; *APC* in familial polyposis associated with colon cancer; *RET* in syndromes of multiple endocrine neoplasias associated with tumors of the pituitary, parathyroid, and thyroid, and with pheochromocytoma and islet cell tumors; *VHL* in the von Hippel–Lindau syndrome associated with hemangioblastoma, pheochromocytoma, and renal cell cancer; *FACC* in Fanconi's anemia associated with leukemia and several other malignancies; *ATM* in ataxia telangiectasia associated with leukemia, lymphoma, and breast and ovarian cancer; *BLM* in Bloom syndrome associated with leukemia and several other tumors; *p53* in the Li-Fraumeni syndrome associated with multiple cancers; *RAD2* in xeroderma pigmentosum associated with skin cancer and leukemia; *MSH2, MLH1, PMS1,* and *PMS2* in hereditary nonpolyposis colorectal cancer (HNPCC), also known as Lynch syndromes types I and II; and *CDKN2* in the dysplastic nevus syndrome associated with melanoma.

The long-recognized familial pattern in breast cancer has led to the isolation of *BRCA1*, associated with breast and ovarian cancer, and *BRCA2*,[28] associated with breast cancer. This will allow the identification of families at risk. Both genes are extremely large and have an extensive variety of mutations that will make screening difficult. There is no clue to their function.

Familial carcinogenesis is based in large part on a group of genes that, when mutated, cause cancer by their *absence*, that is, they seem to *prevent* cancer when they are functioning normally. These protective genes are the *cancer-suppressor genes*. The scientific basis for our understanding of familial cancer began in 1971 when Alfred Knudson argued, on the basis of a statistical model, that one of the two mutations required for the development of familial retinoblastoma was inherited and the second occurred in the retinal cells of the affected eye. In the nonheritable form both mutations occurred in the same cell after birth with neither mutation being inherited.[29] This model was derived from the observation that acquired retinoblastoma occurred as a single tumor, whereas children with hereditary retinoblastoma had multiple primary tumors, indicating an inherited genetic predisposition in all the cells of the retinal tissue. The gene has been identified and named the *retinoblastoma gene (RB1)*. The inheritance is dominant, but both copies of the gene must be absent or damaged for a cell to be transformed. When the retinoblastoma gene is introduced into cultures of retinoblastoma cells, the malignant growth pattern is suppressed.[30] This confirmed in humans the classic laboratory observation that fusing a cancer cell with a normal cell will lead to suppression of malignant growth.[31] Analysis of chromosome 13 in hereditary cases of retinoblastoma revealed that the chromosome lost during tumorigenesis was the one from the nonaffected parent, whereas the one retained was from the affected parent,[32] proving dominant inheritance.

Subsequently, the mechanism discovered in retinoblastoma was found in other cancers such as Wilms' tumor. Of further interest, loss of the retinoblastoma gene was described in bladder cancer and breast cancer, which implied that genes associated with familial cancer might be a target for mutagens involved in nonhereditary cancers. For example, strong evidence has been presented for a role of the same cancer-suppressor gene associated with familial polyposis as the target for mutagenesis in a large proportion of colon cancer cases. Weinberg[33] has reviewed the implications of the negative regulation exerted on cells by genes such as the retinoblastoma gene and has emphasized the importance of the loss of the normal copy of a gene by the process of mitotic recombination. This is referred to as *loss of heterogeneity* or *reduction to homozygosity* because the cell becomes homozygous for the abnormal gene, thus losing its ability to prevent malignant growth. This process is important in carcinogenesis.

Up to 5% of colorectal cancers are due to the HNPCC syndrome, characterized by an early-age onset of predominantly proximally located tumors.[34] This hereditary syndrome results from a defect in the DNA mismatch repair (MMR) system, a system that copy edits newly synthesized DNA and repairs any errors made at the time of synthesis. An inherited mutation of any one of four genes can lead to malfunction of the MMR system and the genomic instability that allows the mutations that transform the colonic mucosa. Some families with the syndrome have an excess only of colorectal cancers (Lynch syndrome I); others also have an excess of endometrial adenocarcinoma and, to a lesser extent, cancers of the stomach, ovary, and other sites (Lynch syndrome II).[35]

## PHYSICAL CARCINOGENESIS

Physical carcinogens are agents that damage the same oncogenes and cancer-suppressor genes that are attacked by chemicals, but they exert their action by physical rather than chemical means. In some cases the nature of the reaction is known, as, for example, ionizing radiation, which releases sufficient energy to alter DNA. In other cases the mechanism is obscure, as, for example, asbestos, which may act as a promoter by an as yet unknown method.

Radiation was recognized as a carcinogen only four years after Roentgen's discovery of x-rays.[36] Only a few years later a relationship to leukemia was recognized.[37] Early workers in radiation must have received very large doses to make the association between radiation and cancer so obvious that it would be noticed in such a short time. The excess cancer deaths in the Hiroshima and Nagasaki populations were only about 8%, and leukemia was seen at an incidence of only about 1.5 cases per million people per year per rad of dose.[38]

There are two forms of radiation that induce cancer: ultraviolet radiation and ionizing radiation.

## Ultraviolet Radiation

Ultraviolet radiation (UVR) from the sun induces a change in DNA, pyrimidine dimer formation, that, if not properly repaired, leads to malignant transformation. The basal cell and squamous cell carcinomas of the exposed areas of the skin are the result, and these tumors are quite common, with nearly half a million cases each year. Melanoma is also linked to ultraviolet exposure, though not as tightly as basal and squamous cancers. The most active carcinogenic wavelength of UVR is 280–320 nm, which is referred to as ultraviolet B (UVB).

The most dramatic example of UVB carcinogenesis is seen in patients with xeroderma pigmentosum, an autosomal recessive disease in which DNA repair of UVR damage is defective.[39] These patients are hypersensitive to sunlight and have a high incidence of skin cancer, including melanoma.

Appropriate preventive techniques include avoidance of direct sunlight and the use of sunblocks that block out UVB radiation. That such measures will be effective is indicated by the protective effect of living in climates with low levels of sunlight, of skin pigmentation that blocks out UVB, and of occupations that minimize sun exposure.

## Ionizing Radiation

Life evolved in an environment high in radiation; indeed, radiation-induced mutation no doubt accelerated evolution. There are effective mechanisms to repair the damage that results when high-energy radiation interacts with DNA. Ordinarily these mechanisms are very efficient. They are not, however, perfect, and ionizing radiation leads to permanent mutations in DNA. When these mutations involve oncogenes or cancer-suppressor genes, transformation of a cell to malignant growth may occur. As with chemical carcinogenesis, there are multiple steps. Furthermore, radiation and chemicals interact synergistically, and familial susceptibilities may play a role. In a hereditary melanoma syndrome, known as the *familial dysplastic nevus syndrome* (FDNS), individuals have multiple nevi with a strong tendency to evolve into melanoma. Cultured cells from these individuals have an increased sensitivity to radiation-induced genetic damage.[40]

In the United States the average annual exposure of an individual to radiation from all sources is 360 mrem, 82% of which is from natural sources. Clearly the largest portion of our radiation dose is unavoidable.[41] Women who as children received radiotherapy for Hodgkin's disease have a 75-fold increased risk for breast cancer.[42] The use of alkylating agents potentiates the carcinogenic effect of radiation, especially in the development of leukemia.

Recent interest has focused on the radon isotope, for which the home seems to be the major site of exposure. There are substantial geographic variations influencing radon dose. Basements may allow more radon to enter a house, and good insulation may prevent dispersal of radon into the atmosphere. It is estimated that approximately 3% of all cancer deaths are due to natural radiation (excluding radon). At the present too little is known about radon effects to draw firm conclusions or to make useful recommendations for prevention, but it is estimated that radiation from natural radon contributes about 10% of lung cancer deaths, bringing the total of cancer deaths due to natural radiation to approximately 5%.[43] Many uncertainties exist in such estimates.

From the standpoint of prevention, there seems little more to be done than is already being done: minimizing exposure to man-made radiation hazards. It is notable, however, that stopping smoking provides the greatest potential for prevention of radiation-induced cancer of the lung, since radon exposure acts synergistically with tobacco smoke. Smokers exposed to radon as miners had ten times the incidence of lung cancer as did nonsmokers because radiation acts synergistically with tobacco smoke.[44] The risk of medical radiation exposure has probably been exaggerated except in the case of therapeutic radiation. The large unavoidable radiation doses from our natural environment dwarf the small medical exposure. Still, radiation is carcinogenic, and every attempt should be made to minimize our exposure consistent with effective diagnosis and therapy. Of particular public concern is exposure from mammography. This has undoubtedly been exaggerated, and the new techniques provide very low exposures to the breast. Present recommendations of the American Cancer Society for mammography seem reasonable and likely to save many more lives than are placed at risk by such a low level of radiation.

## Asbestos

Asbestos, the major carcinogenic fiber, is believed to be related to about 2000 cases of mesothelioma annually[44] in the United States. Actually, asbestos causes more bronchogenic cancers than mesotheliomas, perhaps 6000, because of its synergism with tobacco smoke. Lung cancer is rare in asbestos workers who do not smoke. There is a long latent period between exposure and the onset of mesothelioma. Furthermore, the exposure may sometimes be so brief that the patient cannot remember when it occurred unless questioned closely. The mechanism of action of the asbestos fiber is unknown.

Data do not support an association between gastrointestinal cancer and asbestos, an observation of some importance since asbestos-lined cement pipes carry much of the nation's water supply.[15] Physical properties such as crystal type and particle size play a major role in the physical carcinogenic properties of asbestos. Epidemiological studies indicate that only certain forms of asbestos increase the risk of mesothelioma.[45] Estimating the risk of exposure to asbestos is much more complicated than estimating risk from a soluble mutagenic carcinogen, and the linear dose-response model probably cannot be applied.

## VIRAL CARCINOGENESIS

In 1911 Peyton Rous, at the Rockefeller Institute, described a sarcoma in chickens caused by what later became known as the Rous sarcoma virus (RSV).[46] This virus was the source of the first well-characterized oncogene. Huebner and Todaro had coined the word *oncogene* in 1969.[47] The original concept of viral transmission proposed by early workers has been found to be extremely rare, but the work on possible cancer viruses led to the discovery of *human* genes associated with cancer.

The epidemiological evidence for the viral etiology of cancer is strongest for a relationship between hepatitis B virus (HBV) and hepatocellular carcinoma and between human T-cell leukemia virus type 1 (HTLV-1) and T-cell lymphoma.[48] Both have a geographic distribution of cancer prevalence and viral infection as well as case-by-case associations. The association between Burkitt's lymphoma and Epstein-Barr virus (EBV) in Africa is likewise strong except that there seems to be a need for an associated immunodeficiency. Similarly, the association between EBV and high-grade lymphoma in Western countries seems to require that an immunodeficiency state be present, either congenital or induced by human immunodeficiency virus (HIV) or a drug such as cyclosporin. There is evidence of a role for viruses in other cancers: EBV and nasopharyngeal carcinoma in Chinese, and herpes simplex virus type 2 (HSV-2) and human papillomavirus (HPV) in cervical carcinoma.

Among the human retroviruses, HTLV-1 has been clearly implicated in adult T-cell leukemia (ATL), a malignancy of mature T4 lymphocytes that is endemic in Japan, the Caribbean, parts of Africa, and the southeastern United States.[49] A small proportion of individuals with Sézary syndrome and mycosis fungoides also have evidence of HTLV-1. In ATL-endemic regions, only a small proportion of infected individuals, less than 1%, develop ATL. Transmission of the virus is by sexual contact, by mother's milk, and through contaminated blood, and the latency period between infection and ATL varies from a few years up to 40 years. The mechanism of carcinogenesis may be insertion of the virus into the host genome in such a way as to activate host proto-oncogenes; or, as is the case with HPV, there may be HTLV-coded proteins that interfere with the cell cycle.[50]

Hairy-cell leukemia (HCL) is a disease of B lympho-cytes for the most part, but a small portion of cases manifest T lymphocytes. HTLV-2 has been isolated from the T-cell variety of HCL.

HBV is endemic in Asia and Africa, where large numbers of people are chronic carriers, as high as 10% of the population. Epidemiological studies have established HBV to be etiologic in hepatocellular carcinoma (HCC).[51] There is growing evidence that the hepatitis C virus may also induce hepatoma.[52] In China alone between .5 million and 1 million cases of HCC occur annually; this may be the most common cancer in the world today. HBV transforms the hepatocyte not because it has an oncogene but because it integrates copies of itself at random sites into the host DNA and by chance may cause inappropriate activation of a proto-oncogene to initiate a clone of malignant cells. There is a mean duration of 35 years from the time of HBV infection to the onset of the HCC.[53] Other factors may increase risk, though these are not proven. HCC may be induced by a mechanism that does not involve HBV, such as the natural carcinogen aflatoxin, which may be important in the United States, where both chronic HBV infection and HCC are not very common.

EBV, a double-stranded DNA virus of the herpes family, causes infectious mononucleosis in the United States and Burkitt's lymphoma in Africa. It infects B lymphocytes and stimulates their proliferation. If host immunity is intact, a T-lymphocyte response is generated against an EBV protein expressed on the B-cell membrane and the proliferating B-cells are brought under control. For some reason in Africa, perhaps because of the effect of chronic malaria on the immune system, a B-cell clone may emerge uncontrolled, and this leads to Burkitt's lymphoma, a monoclonal malignancy. Chromosome 8, which contains the *c-myc* oncogene, exchanges genetic material with chromosome 14, or sometimes chromosome 2 or 22, where genes necessary for antibody synthesis are located. The presumption is that the *c-myc* oncogene is activated when the immune genes are stimulated.

Burkitt's lymphoma is rare in Western countries; when it is seen, EBV is only occasionally present. An inherited immune deficiency has been described that is X-linked in which EBV induces a polyclonal lymphoma.[54] Individuals who have AIDS or those immunosuppressed for organ transplantation are also at risk for polyclonal lymphomas associated with EBV.[51,53]

The Chinese, no matter where they live, are at increased risk for nasopharyngeal carcinoma. Their tumors are associated with the EBV genome within the tumor cell. There are other causes of this tumor in other races, but the Chinese seem to have a unique association with EBV. The EBV genome is actively transcribed in these tumors in the same way as in latently infected lymphocytes,[55] providing strong evidence for an etiologic role.

Hodgkin's disease has been suspected of being related to EBV, but the data are conflicting. In some cases the disease may be preceded by an altered antibody pattern against EBV.[56]

The HPVs are double-stranded circular DNA viruses that infect squamous epithelium. There are many strains, some of which cause the common human wart. HPVs are difficult to study because they cannot be grown in the laboratory. Two independent transforming oncogenes have been identified, and the protein product of one of these genes has recently been shown to bind specifically to the protein product of the retinoblastoma gene.[57] This provides strong support for the hypothesis that transformation results when the infecting HPV codes for a protein that blocks the product of a cancer-suppressor gene.

HPV is etiologic in genital warts. Cervical cancer is associated with promiscuity. DNA from strains HPV-16 or HPV-18 is found in 70% of all cervical carcinomas, and the morphological changes of cervical dysplasia are linked to HPV infection.[58] Thus, there are strong data supporting an etiologic role for some strains of HPV in cervical cancer. To a lesser extent there are associations with all genital cancer, including cancer of the penis and prostate.

## BACTERIAL CARCINOGENESIS

One of the most exciting developments in the mechanism of carcinogenesis is the discovery of a relationship between the bacteria *Helicobacter pylori* and the B-cell lymphoma unique to the gastric mucosa, the mucosa-associated lymphoid tissue (MALT) lymphoma. *H pylori* grows in the stomach and is responsible for gastric and duodenal ulcers. For many years it was suspected that there was some kind of relationship between chronic ulcer disease and the development of malignancy. A relationship between *H pylori* and MALT lymphoma has now been noted,[59] and resolution of the lymphoma was observed[60] after treatment with antibiotics to eradicate the bacteria. This striking observation has been confirmed.[61] It is noteworthy that when the tumor is monoclonal it will regress but will later relapse when only antibiotic therapy is used.[62]

The exact pathogenesis of this unique mechanism of carcinogenesis is not yet clear, but it seems reasonable to suggest that there is an initial polyclonal lymphoid proliferation driven by antigens from *H pylori*. Subsequently, mutations lead to a monoclonal population of lymphocytes that may or may not still be antigen-driven in their proliferation. At some point a monoclonal population emerges that is antigen-independent and able to proliferate autonomously. Thus, the early proliferation is reversible by eradication of the bacteria with antibiotics, whereas the later tumor is not and requires conventional anticancer therapy.

This exciting observation provides a model for carcinogenesis by a mechanism that is initially reversible and later autonomous. It illustrates the potential for modification of the process of carcinogenesis when the precise molecular events are understood.

## COLON CANCER AS A MODEL OF HUMAN CARCINOGENESIS

The work of many investigators, especially Vogelstein at Johns Hopkins, has provided the best insight so far into the pathogenesis of a common tumor, colon cancer.[63] These investigations reveal the complexity of the process of carcinogenesis in humans.

Adenomatosis polyposis coli, a familial syndrome, has long been known to be associated with such a high incidence of colorectal cancer that the treatment of choice is total colectomy. Recently the gene *APC* has been shown to be mutated in all cases of this syndrome, providing a clue to the pathogenesis since the product of this gene seems to be involved in negatively regulating certain intracellular pathways associated with growth signals.[64]

In HNPCC (also known as Lynch syndromes types I and II), a second form of familial colorectal cancer, four genes have now been identified that provide a better understanding of the mechanism of carcinogenesis. Loeb had observed that the high incidence of mutations in cancer suggested that an increased mutation rate was directly involved in the multistage process of carcinogenesis.[65] The genes associated with HNPCC are directly related to the development of a high mutation rate because they function to "proofread" newly synthesized DNA and correct any mistakes that are made during synthesis. When mutated, these genes lead to a high mutation rate that promotes the sequence of events necessary for carcinogenesis to take place.[66] Why this inherited defect in DNA repair leads preferentially to colorectal tumors is not yet clear.

In nonfamilial colorectal cancer the sequence of events required for carcinogenesis and progression has been worked out more completely than for any other neoplasm. The complete sequence involves more than a half dozen steps. A gene at 5q21, called *mutated in colorectal cancer* (*MCC*), is mutated in a substantial number of colorectal cancers.[67] A second gene in the same location, *APC*, is mutated in a substantial number of spontaneous colorectal cancers, as it is in all individuals with familial polyposis.[68] One of these genes is altered as the first step in colorectal carcinogenesis leading to increased cell proliferation and polyp formation. The next step is presumed to involve demethylation of DNA, a nongenetic change that alters DNA function. The third step is mutation of the *K-ras* proto-oncogene on 12p. Next there is a loss of a gene called *deleted in colorectal cancer* (*DCC*), located on 18q.[69] Finally, there is a mutation of the cancer-suppressor gene *p53*, located at 17p, leading to genetic instability and progression to frank malignancy with invasion and metastasis.[70] Addition of normal chromosomes 5 and 18 to colon cancer cell cultures reverses malignant growth.[71]

In colorectal cancer, then, two familial syndromes have been matched with their genes, and many of the genes mutated in the sporadic (nonhereditary) tumors have been identified. One of the genes associated with familial cancer, *APC*, is also sometimes mutated in sporadic cancer. Some of the functions of the involved genes have been elucidated and provide clues as to why there is loss of control of cell division. Specific chemical and physical agents that are etiologic have not been identified in colorectal cancer as is the case with bronchogenic cancer, but there are a few epidemiological associations that may be important in identifying the mutagens leading to colorectal cancer.

# CONTROVERSIES IN CARCINOGENESIS

## Estrogens and Carcinogenesis

One of the most controversial topics in carcinogenesis is the role of estrogens. Animal models and human studies have clearly shown that without estrogen, breast cancer will not develop. That estrogen is in some way related to breast cancer is not the issue. The central practical issues are two: First, does postmenopausal estrogen replacement therapy increase breast cancer risk? Second, does oral contraceptive use increase breast cancer risk?

A host of case-control studies have provided copious data to support either a yes or no answer to the first question. The only controlled randomized trial, however, showed that after ten years the placebo group had more breast cancer than the group treated with hormone replacement.[72] In view of the known benefits of postmenopausal estrogen in the prevention of osteoporosis and reduction of cardiovascular risk by up to half,[73] any decision as to a contraindication of estrogen based on a hypothetical or poorly documented breast cancer risk must be carefully evaluated. It is likely that replacement therapy has a weak effect, if any, and does not substantially alter breast cancer incidence, although an association with endometrial cancer seems well established.[74] Tamoxifen, which has an antiestrogenic action on the breast, has an estrogenic effect on the endometrium, explaining the slight increase in endometrial carcinoma with the use of this agent.

The role of contraceptives in breast cancer risk likewise is controversial and not clearly established, with most studies showing no relationship.[73,74] It is possible that long-term use before the first pregnancy may increase risk,[75] and this is obviously an important question to answer because this is a frequent pattern of use. At present the issue is unresolved, although the preponderant opinion is that contraceptives are safe.

## Involuntary (Passive) Smoking

Blum has reviewed the evidence for passive or involuntary smoking as etiologic in lung cancer.[76] There are insufficient data to allow a firm conclusion, but spousal exposure provides some information. Lung cancer mortality may be about one-third higher in spouses of smokers than in spouses of nonsmokers. This has served as the basis for estimates that exposure of nonsmokers in proximity to smokers may account for up to 20% of nonsmoker lung cancer deaths each year, or about 2400 deaths. The sex of the spouse may be a factor as well, since according to a report by the surgeon general[77] the sexes may differ in their sensitivity to tobacco smoke.

## Environmental Carcinogenesis

Perhaps the most popular subject for the lay press is environmental carcinogenesis. The term *environmental* is subject to a great deal of confusion. Its original use was intended to include all cancers that were not hereditary, that is, all cancers due to viruses, lifestyle, tobacco, diet, and a host of other causes. When the statement was made that "85% of cancer is environmental," this was misinterpreted in the lay press to mean contaminated air, water, and food. Often it has been further limited in the media to exclude natural carcinogens in our environment so that the focus has been on man-made chemicals. This has led to the mistaken notion that we can virtually eliminate cancer if we eliminate man-made cancer-causing chemicals from the air we breathe, the water we drink, and the food we eat.

Such a notion is incorrect. Ames has described what he believes are the mistaken assumptions made by those who argue that environmental pollutants represent our highest priority in cancer prevention.[78] He points out the dangers of this approach. When we focus our attention on trivial or even nonexistent dangers, our attention is diverted from significant and real dangers. There are over half a million deaths each year from tobacco, a number that dwarfs the insignificant number of deaths that result from the pollutants that receive so much emphasis in the media.

A preferred interpretation of the term *environmental* would focus on our *personal* environment or, in usual terminology, our lifestyle. It is the tobacco we abuse, the food we eat, and other lifestyle choices that have increased our risk of cancer more than everything else combined. The enemy is not the chemical plant down the street but ourselves. Tobacco is directly related to over 30% of cancer deaths. If tobacco-caused cancers are excluded, the death rate from cancer is actually decreasing.

## Diet and Carcinogenesis

Doll and Peto have suggested that perhaps one-third of all cancers could be explained by dietary factors.[79] This would suggest that up to 50% of breast cancer and 90% of colon cancer in the United States could be prevented by a change in diet. Their estimated range was, however, very wide (10%–70%). Although it may be true that there is a strong dietary relationship, radical changes would be required early in life to effect substantial reductions in incidence.

In Japan cancer of the stomach is common and cancers of the colon and the breast uncommon. When Japanese move to the United States, they rapidly develop our pattern of common colon cancer and uncommon stomach cancer. Several generations later they develop our pattern of common breast cancer. This has become a classic epidemiological observation, and most investigators assume the explanation is the change in diet. Willett[80] has critically reviewed the data on dietary risk factors for colon and breast cancer. He notes the striking correlation between the amount of fat a nation consumes and the incidence of colon cancer and breast cancer, as well as a similar correlation between meat consumption and colon cancer.

The notion that fat intake may be related to breast cancer has persisted, but there has been an inability to provide individual, as compared with national, statistics relating breast cancer to fat intake. This has led to a wide acceptance that the relationship is not to fat but to total calories, and especially to total calories consumed early in life. Willett[80] has interpreted the correlation of height to breast cancer as supporting this hypothesis; in nations where malnutrition is present in some groups, breast cancer incidence is lower in short women; such a relationship is not seen in the United States and Scandinavia. However, the analysis of data from seven prospective studies in four countries showed no evidence of a positive association between total dietary fat and the risk of breast cancer.[81] Further, the delay of several generations in Japanese immigrants in the development of increased breast cancer suggests that the issue is more complex than diet alone.

The role of fat in colon cancer is supported by both the rapid change in incidence with dietary change and the potential relationship of fat consumption to bile acids, which are known to be mutagenic. In Japan since 1945 the improved diet has been associated with an increase in colon cancer but not yet an increase in breast cancer.[80] The well-documented relationship of meat consumption to colon cancer likely reflects animal fat consumption. The role of fiber in colon cancer has repeatedly been postulated to relate to altered transit time, altered bacterial flora in the colon, and altered exposure of the colonic mucosa to potentially carcinogenic bacterially modified bile acids. Epidemiological studies have suggested an inverse relationship between dietary fiber and colon cancer, and animal studies suggest the type of fiber may be important.[82] Human studies have shown that wheat bran and cellulose, but not oat bran, are associated with lower stool mutagens by the Ames assay and reduced secondary bile acids.[83]

Stomach cancer has been suggested to be related to the intake of food that is cured, smoked, pickled, salted, or otherwise preserved, but not refrigerated. Some special methods of food preparation have also been incriminated. Long-term use of refrigeration seems particularly important in reducing the incidence of stomach cancer.[84]

The nature of the effect of fruits and vegetables is unclear. There has been speculation that the antioxidant effect of vitamin C might play a role, but this has not been well established. Many food preservatives have an antioxidant effect and may actually antagonize possible carcinogens such as nitrites. Alcohol has been well documented as a risk factor in head and neck cancer and more recently has been incriminated in breast cancer,[85] although this observation is controversial.

The actions to be taken on the basis of these observations are far from clear. The potential for substantial reduction in cancer incidence by dietary modification alone seems remote, given the extreme changes that may be required and the difficulty of changing the eating habits of most people. Even reduction in alcohol consumption may not be effective unless it takes place early in life. Nonetheless, a prudent diet that is rich in fruits, fiber, and cruciferous vegetables and low in animal fat is desirable for many health reasons and may perhaps reduce the risk of cancer.

## CONCLUSION

Modern techniques of molecular biology have allowed replacement of the classic initiation-promotion-progression sequence of carcinogenesis with a detailed list of the genes that must be mutated to transform a normal tissue into a malignant neoplasm. There is a rapidly growing list of the genes involved in this complex process, and their discovery has major implications for all aspects of cancer care, including identification of high-risk groups, genetic counseling, diagnosis and follow-up using tumor-specific markers, treatment targeted to unique genetically determined tumor characteristics, and primary prevention based on a better understanding of the steps in the process of carcinogenesis.

## REFERENCES

1. Clurman BE, Roberts JM: Cell cycle and cancer. *J Natl Cancer Inst* 87:1499–1501, 1995
2. Carr AM: Checkpoints take the next step. *Science* 271: 314–315, 1996
3. Ameisen JC: The origin of programmed cell death. *Science* 272:1278–1279, 1996
4. Rhyu MS: Telomeres, telomerase, and immortality. *J Natl Cancer Inst* 87:884–894, 1995
5. Rous P, Beard JW: The progression to carcinoma of virus induced rabbit papillomas (Shope). *J Exp Med* 62:523–548, 1935
6. Rous P, Kidd JG: Conditional neoplasms and subthreshold neoplastic states. *J Exp Med* 73:365–389, 1941
7. Friedewald WF, Rous P: The initiating and promoting elements in tumor production: An analysis of the effects of tar,

benzpyrene, and methylcholanthrene in rabbit skin. *J Exp Med* 80:101–126, 1944

8. Foulds L: The experimental study of tumor progression: A review. *Cancer Res* 14:327–339, 1954

9. Fidler IJ: Critical factors in the biology of human cancer metastasis. *Am Surg* 61:1065–1066, 1995

10. Shields PG, Harris CC: Principles of carcinogenesis: Chemical, in DeVita VT Jr, Hellman S, Rosenberg SA (eds): *Cancer: Principles and Practice of Oncology* (ed 4). Philadelphia, Lippincott, 1993, pp 200–212

11. Yamagiwa K, Ichikawa K: Experimentelle Studie uber die Pathogenese der Epitheliageschwulste. Tokyo, *Mitteilungen Med Facultat Kaiserl Univ Tokyo* 15:295, 1915

12. Redmond DE Jr: Hill cautions against snuff in 1761. *N Engl J Med* 282:18–23, 1970

13. Wynder EL, Graham EA: Tobacco smoking as a possible etiologic factor in bronchiogenic carcinoma: A study of 684 proved cases. *JAMA* 143:329–336, 1950

14. Doll R, Hill AB: Smoking and carcinoma of the lung: Preliminary report. *Br Med J* 2:739–748, 1950

15. Levin ML, Goldstein H, Gerhardt PR: Cancer and tobacco smoking: A preliminary report. *JAMA* 143:336–338, 1950

16. Rehn L: Blasengeschwulste bei Fuchsin-Arbeitern. *Arch Klin Chir* 50:588, 1895

17. Kennaway EL, Hieger I: Carcinogenic substances and their fluorescence spectra. *Br J Med* 1:1044, 1930

18. Miller EC: Some current perspectives on chemical carcinogenesis in humans and experimental animals: Presidential address. *Cancer Res* 38:1479–1496, 1978

19. Ames BN, Durston WE, Yamasaki E, et al: Carcinogens are mutagens: A simple test system combining liver homogenates for activation and bacteria for detection. *Proc Natl Acad Sci U S A* 70:2281, 1973

20. Perera FP, Weinstein IB: Molecular epidemiology and carcinogen-DNA adduct detection: New approaches to studies of human cancer causation. *J Chronic Dis* 35:581–600, 1982

21. Sukumar S, Pulciani S, Doniger J, et al: A transforming *ras* gene in tumorigenic guinea pig cell lines initiated by diverse chemical carcinogens. *Science* 223:1197–1199, 1984

22. Guerrero I, Villasante A, Corces V, et al: Activation of a *c-K-ras* oncogene by somatic mutation in mouse lymphomas induced by gamma radiation. *Science* 225:1159–1162, 1984

23. Bos JL, Toksoz D, Marshall CJ, et al: Amino acid substitutions at codon 13 of the *N-ras* oncogene in human acute myeloid leukaemia. *Nature* 315:726–730, 1985

24. Dalla-Favera R, Martinotti S, Gallo RC, et al: Translocation and rearrangements of the *c-myc* oncogene locus in human undifferentiated B-cell lymphoma. *Science* 219:963–967, 1983

25. Tong L, de Vos AM, Milburn MV, et al: Structural differences between a *ras* oncogene protein and the normal protein. *Nature* 337:90–93, 1989

26. Doll R, Peto R: *The Causes of Cancer.* New York, Oxford University Press, 1981

27. Lynch HT, Albano WA, Heieck JJ: Genetic biomarkers and the control of breast cancer. *Cancer Genet Cytogenet* 13:43–92, 1984

28. Wooster R, Bignell G, Lancaster J, et al: Identification of the breast cancer susceptibility gene *BRCA2*. *Nature* 378:789–792, 1995

29. Knudson A: Mutation and cancer: Statistical study of retinoblastoma. *Proc Natl Acad Sci U S A* 68:820, 1971

30. Huang HJS, Yee JK, Shew JY, et al: Suppression of the neoplastic phenotype by replacement of the *RB* gene in human cancer cells. *Science* 242:1563–1566, 1988

31. Pereira-Smith OM, Smith JR: Evidence for the recessive nature of cellular immortality. *Science* 221:964–966, 1983

32. Cavenee WK, Hansen MF, Nordenskold M, et al: Genetic origin of mutations predisposing to retinoblastoma. *Science* 228:501–503, 1985

33. Weinberg RA: The *RB* gene and the negative regulation of cell growth. *Blood* 74:529–532, 1989

34. Marra G, Boland CR: Hereditary nonpolyposis colorectal cancer: The syndrome, the genes, and historical perspectives. *J Natl Cancer Inst* 82:1114–1125, 1995

35. Boland CR, Troncale FJ: Familial colonic cancer without antecedent polyposis. *Ann Intern Med* 100:700–701, 1984

36. Frieben A: Demonstration lines cancroids des rechten Handruckens, das sich nach langdauernder Einwirkung von Roentgenstrahlen entwichelt hatte. *Fortschr Geb Rontgenstr* 6:106, 1902

37. von Jagic N, Scwarz G, von Siebenrock L: Blutbefunde bei Roentgenologon. *Berl Klin Wochenschr* 48:1220–1222, 1911

38. Preston DL, Kato H, Kopecky KJ, et al: Studies on the mortality of A-bomb survivors: 8. Cancer mortality, 1950–1982. *Radiat Res* 111:151–178, 1987

39. Cleaver JE: Defective repair replication of DNA in xeroderma pigmentosum. *Nature* 218:652–656, 1968

40. Standford KK, Parshad R, Green MH, et al: Hypersensitivity to $G_2$ chromatid radiation damage in familial dysplastic nevus syndrome. *Lancet* 2:1111–1116, 1987

41. National Council on Radiation Protection Measurements (NRCP): *Ionizing Radiation Exposure of the Population of the United States.* NCRP Report No. 93. Bethesda, MD, NCRP, 1987

42. Bhatia S, Robison LL, Oberlin O, et al: Breast cancer and other second neoplasms after childhood Hodgkin's disease. *N Engl J Med* 334:745–751, 1996

43. Darby S: Contribution of natural ionizing radiation to cancer mortality in the United States, in Brugge J, Curran T, Harlow E, McCormick F (eds): *Origins of Human Cancer.* Cold Spring Harbor, NY, Cold Spring Harbor Laboratory Press, 1991, pp 183–190

44. Nicholson WJ, Perbep G, Selikoff IJ: Occupational exposure to asbestos: Population at risk and projected mortality. *Am J Ind Med* 3:258–311, 1987

45. Mossman BT, Gee JBL: Asbestos related diseases. *N Engl J Med* 320:1721–1730, 1989

46. Rous P: Transmission of a malignant new growth by means of a cell free filtrate. *JAMA* 56:198, 1911

47. Huebner RJ, Todaro GJ: Oncogenes of RNA tumor viruses as determinants of cancer. *Proc Natl Acad Sci U S A* 64:1087–1094, 1969

48. Henderson BE: Establishment of an association between a virus and a human cancer. *J Natl Cancer Inst* 81:320–321, 1989

49. Poiesz BJ, Ruscetti FW, Gazdar AF, et al: Detection and isolation of type C retrovirus particles from fresh and cultured lymphocytes of a patient with cutaneous T-cell lymphoma. *Proc Natl Acad Sci U S A* 77:7415–7419, 1980

50. Franchini G: Molecular mechanisms of human T-cell leukemia/lymphoma virus type I infection. *Blood* 86:3619–3639, 1995

51. Beasly RP, Linn CC, Hwang L, et al: Hepatocellular carcinoma and hepatitis B virus: A prospective study of 22,707 men in Taiwan. *Lancet* 2:1129–1133, 1981

52. Tanaka K, Ikematsu H, Kashiwagi S: Hepatitis C virus infection and risk of hepatocellular carcinoma among Japanese: Possible role of Type 1b(II) infection. *J Natl Cancer Inst* 88: 742–746, 1996

53. Howley PM: Principles of carcinogenesis: Viral, in DeVita VT Jr, Hellman S, Rosenberg SA (eds): *Cancer: Principles and Practice of Oncology* (ed 4). Philadelphia, Lippincott, 1993, pp 182–199

54. Purtilo DT, Sakamoto K, Barnabai V, et al: Epstein-Barr virus induced diseases in boys with the X-linked lymphoproliferative syndrome (XLP): Updates on studies of the registry. *Am J Med* 73:49–56, 1982

55. Pagano JS: Epstein-Barr virus transcription in nasopharyngeal carcinoma. *J Virol* 48:580–590, 1983

56. Mueller N, Evans A, Harris NL, et al: Hodgkin's disease and Epstein-Barr virus: Altered antibody pattern before diagnosis. *N Engl J Med* 320:689–695, 1989

57. Dyson N, Howley PM, Munger K, et al: The human papilloma virus-16 E7 oncoprotein is able to bind to the retinoblastoma gene product. *Science* 243:934–936, 1989

58. zur Hausen H: Molecular pathogenesis of cancer of the cervix and its causation by specific HPV types. *Curr Top Microbiol Immunol* 186:131–156, 1994

59. Stolte M: *Helicobacter pylori* gastritis and gastric MALT lymphoma. *Lancet* 339:745–746, 1992

60. Wotherspoon AC, Doglioni C, Diss TC, et al: Regression of primary low-grade B-cell gastric lymphoma of mucosa associated lymphoid tissue type after eradication of *Helicobacter pylori*. *Lancet* 342:575–577, 1993

61. Weber DM, Dimopoulos MA, Anandu DP, et al: Regression of gastric lymphoma of mucosa-associated lymphoid tissue with antibiotic therapy for *Helicobacter pylori*. *Gastroenterology* 107:1835–1838, 1994

62. Carlson SJ, Yokoo H, Vanagunas A: Progression of gastritis to monoclonal B-cell lymphoma with resolution and recurrence following eradication of *Helicobacter pylori*. *JAMA* 275: 937–939, 1996

63. Vogelstein B: Cancer: A deadly inheritance. *Nature* 348: 681–682, 1990

64. Peifer M: Regulating cell proliferation: As easy as *APC*. *Science* 272:974–975, 1996

65. Loeb LA: Mutator phenotype may be required for multistage carcinogenesis. *Cancer Res* 51:3075–3079, 1991

66. Rhyu MS: Molecular mechanisms underlying hereditary nonpolyposis colorectal carcinoma. *J Natl Cancer Inst* 88: 240–251, 1996

67. Kinzler KW, Nilbert MC, Vogelstein B, et al: Identification of a gene located at chromosome 5q21 that is mutated in colorectal cancers. *Science* 251:1366–1370, 1991

68. Nishisho I, Nakamura Y, Miyoshi Y, et al: Mutations of chromosome 5q21 in FAP and colorectal cancer patients. *Science* 253:665–669, 1991

69. Fearon ER, Cho KR, Nigro JM, et al: Identification of a chromosome 18q gene that is altered in colorectal cancers. *Science* 247:49–56, 1990

70. Kern SE, Vogelstein B: Genetic alterations in colorectal tumors, in Brugge J, Curran T, Harlow E, McCormick F (eds): *Origins of Human Cancer*. Cold Spring Harbor, NY, Cold Spring Harbor Laboratory Press, 1991, pp 557–585

71. Tanaka K, Oshimura M, Kikuchi R, et al: Suppression of tumorigenicity in human colon carcinoma cells by introduction of normal chromosome 5 or 18. *Nature* 349:340–342, 1991

72. Nachtigall LE, Nachtigall RD, Beckman EM: Estrogen replacement therapy II: A prospective trial on the relationship of breast cancer and cardiovascular and metabolic problems. *Obstet Gynecol* 54:74–79, 1979

73. Barrett-Connor E: Postmenopausal estrogen replacement and breast cancer. *N Engl J Med* 321:319–320, 1989

74. Thomas DB: Do hormones cause breast cancer? *Cancer* 53: 595–604, 1984

75. Pike MC, Henderson BE, Casagrande JT, et al: Oral contraceptive use and early abortion as risk factors for breast cancer in young women. *Br J Cancer* 43:72–76, 1981

76. Blum A: Curtailing the tobacco pandemic, in DeVita VT Jr, Hellman S, Rosenberg SA (eds): *Cancer: Principles and Practice of Oncology* (ed 4). Philadelphia, Lippincott, 1993, pp 480–491

77. U.S. Department of Health and Human Services, Office of Smoking and Health: *The Health Consequences of Smoking: Cancer.* Report of the Surgeon General. DHHS publication No. (PHS) 82-50179. Washington, DC, 1982, p 38

78. Ames BN: What are the major carcinogens in the etiology of human cancer? Environmental pollution, natural carcinogens, and the causes of human cancer: Six errors, in DeVita VT, Hellman S, Rosenberg SA (eds): *Important Advances in Oncology* (ed 3). Philadelphia, Lippincott, 1989, pp 210–235

79. Doll R, Peto R: The causes of cancer: Quantitative estimates of available risks of cancer in the United States today. *J Natl Cancer Inst* 66:1191–1308, 1981

80. Willett W: The search for the causes of breast and colon cancer. *Nature* 338:389–394, 1989

81. Hunter DJ, Spiegelman D, Adami HO, et al: Cohort studies of fat intake and the risk of breast cancer: A pooled analysis. *N Engl J Med* 334:356–361, 1996

82. Wynder EL, Reddy BS: Dietary fat and fiber and colon cancer. *Semin Oncol* 10:264–272, 1983

83. Reddy B, Engle A, Katsifis S, et al: Biochemical epidemiology of colon cancer: Effect of types of dietary fiber on fecal mutagens, acid, and neutral sterols in healthy subjects. *Cancer Res* 49:4629–4635, 1989

84. Caggon D, Barker DJP, Cole RB, et al: Stomach cancer and food storage. *J Natl Cancer Inst* 81:1178–1182, 1989

85. Willett WC, Stampfer MJ, Colditz GA, et al: Moderate alcohol consumption and the risk of breast cancer. *N Engl J Med* 314:1174–1180, 1987

# Chapter 4

# Cancer Control and Epidemiology

**Brenda Cartmel, PhD**

**Mary Reid, RN, MSPH**

# INTRODUCTION

Epidemiology is "the study of the distribution and determinants of disease frequency."[1] Cancer epidemiology examines the frequency of cancer in populations, the role of certain risk factors that contribute to cancer rates, and the interrelationships or associations that exist between the host, the environment, and the other conditions that may contribute to the development or inhibition of cancer. The first section of this chapter will review basic epidemiological concepts. These will help the reader to better understand current clinical research; to identify groups at higher risk for cancer development; to review current medical literature; and to develop relevant research hypotheses related to the field of cancer epidemiology. This information should serve as a basis for understanding the major issues involved in cancer research design, assessment, and estimation of cancer risks. A brief glossary of fundamental terms used in the field of epidemiology is given in Table 4-1. These definitions will be helpful in understanding discussions found later in this chapter on research study considerations and cancer risk factors. Table 4-2 provides the rates and ratios commonly used in epidemiology, and Table 4-3 shows the 2 × 2 table used in calculating relative risks and odds ratios.

Subsequent sections of this chapter will discuss causes of cancer and host characteristics that influence cancer susceptibility, cancer control and related issues, and, finally, the application of epidemiologic principles and cancer prevention and control issues in nursing practice.

# BASIC CONSIDERATIONS IN EPIDEMIOLOGICAL RESEARCH

Five primary components are considered in evaluating the design of an epidemiological research project:

- study design

- definition of the population of patients or subjects to be used in the study

- eligibility criteria used to select study participants

- definitions of the disease and exposures related to the research hypothesis

- statistical plan measuring the association between the exposure and the disease

- identification of potential sources of bias and confounding

While it is important that these issues be resolved before a protocol is initiated, it is equally important that the entire research team understand these issues and that there be constant evaluation during the course of data collection.

## Study Designs

Several standard study designs are used in epidemiological research. Although the general features of all of these designs will be covered, the primary emphasis of this section is on those designs most commonly used in clinical cancer research: the case-control and clinical trial study designs. The major study designs are experimental, ecological, cross-sectional, case-control, cohort, and clinical trials studies.

In selecting the appropriate study design, certain factors must be considered. These include the frequency of the disease or condition in the general population and the defined population to be studied, the length of time the disease takes to develop, and the anticipated size of the study sample. The size of the study sample is often affected by the monies available to complete the project, the time allowed for subject recruitment, the diagnostic characteristics of the disease, and the qualities of the exposure that is being tested.

### Experimental studies

An experimental study design tests a research hypothesis. It attempts to control the variability of all factors except for the exposure of interest. These studies, which typically use animal models in laboratory settings, are conducted when a research hypothesis is being developed. They generally determine the biological plausibility of the hypothesis. Once substantial, consistent evidence has accumulated from experimental studies, other study designs may be employed to further investigate the hypothesis in free-living human populations.

### Ecological studies

The next step in investigating a hypothesis may be conducting ecological or correlational studies. In this design, trends are examined in disease distribution among humans across ecological or geographic areas. Each geographic area may represent differences in exposures. For example, cancer rates are often evaluated across different countries, or regions of a country, to investigate the effects of nutrient or natural environmental exposures, such as soil selenium or radon, on disease rates.

### Cross-sectional studies

The cross-sectional study is another design that allows an investigator to assess the rates of disease and exposure in a population. In this study design a onetime view of a population is taken, and the rates of existing (prevalent) cases of the disease, the degree of exposure, and other

**TABLE 4-1** Glossary of Epidemiological Terms

| | |
|---|---|
| Association | *Statistical association* refers to the strength of the relationship between two variables. In epidemiological terms, association imitates the degree to which the rate of disease in persons with a specific exposure is either higher or lower than the rate of disease in persons without the exposure. The strength of this dependence is greater than what would be expected by chance. |
| | *Causal association* is a biological association between the occurrence of an exposure and presence of a disease. The available evidence indicates that the presence of the exposure increases the probability of the presence of the disease. Changes in the frequency or quality of an exposure or characteristic would result in a corresponding change in the frequency of the disease or outcome of interest. |
| Bias | *Selection bias* results from a systematic difference in the manner by which the case and the comparison groups are selected for participation in the study. This bias may produce spurious associations due to the differential inclusion or exclusion of subjects from the disease or exposure groups. |
| | *Misclassification bias* is a systematic error that occurs when the measurement of either the exposure (risk factor) or the disease condition is systematically different for the groups being compared (e.g., the disease outcome between the exposed and unexposed groups was evaluated by separate physicians using different criteria). |
| Confounding | The systematic overestimation or underestimation of the effect of an exposure because the influence of a disease risk factor has not been taken into account. A *confounding variable* is a risk factor for the disease being studied that is associated with the exposure being studied and is not an intermediate step between the exposure and the disease.[2] |
| Epidemiology | A field in medical science concerned with the study of the frequency and distribution of disease in the population, and which also explores the relationship between exposures and development of diseases. |
| Incidence | The number of *new* events or cases of disease that occur in a defined population at risk within a specified period of time. Incidence rates can be used to evaluate the changing patterns of disease frequency within a population and to assess the effectiveness of screening programs and treatment modalities on disease development. |
| Population | The number of persons in a defined group who are capable of developing the disease. Can also refer to the general population; a population specifically defined by geographic, physical, or social characteristics, or risk; the sampling population; and the study population. |
| Power | The probability that a study will have the statistical strength to detect relationships that exist between exposures and disease. The power of a study can be maximized by controlling factors such as sample sizes, measurement error, and bias. |
| Prevalence | The number of *new and existing* cases of a given disease or condition in a defined population within a specified period of time. *Point prevalence* refers to prevalence at one point in time. *Period prevalence* refers to prevalence between two points in time. Prevalence rates can be used to compare disease frequencies across populations and to assess the magnitude of effect of certain diseases on the health status of a population. |
| Rates and ratios | These calculations are used to compare the frequencies of diseases in a population. Commonly used rates and ratios are given in Table 4-2, which lists the rate names, the numerator and denominator values, and the population factor used to express the rate in a standard format. |
| Risk measures | *Attributable risk* is the arithmetic or absolute difference between the exposed group and the nonexposed group in the incidence rates or the death rates. It estimates the number of disease cases that can be attributed to or explained by the exposure (e.g., the majority of lung cancer cases can be attributed to exposure to cigarette smoking). |
| | The relative risk and the odds ratio are calculated using a standard $2 \times 2$ table that separates the exposed and nonexposed groups by disease status (see Table 4-3). |
| | *Relative risk (RR)* is a ratio comparing the rates of a disease among the exposed group and the nonexposed group that serves as a measure of the association between the disease and the exposure. The RR is generally used in cohort studies. The formula for calculating it is: $$\frac{a/(a + b)}{c/(c + d)}$$ |
| | *Odds ratio (OR)* approximates the relative risk by comparing the rates of disease among the exposed and nonexposed groups. The OR is generally used in case-control studies with smaller sample sizes. The formula for calculating it is: $$\frac{ad}{cb}$$ |
| | Both the RR and the OR are expressed as ratios (e.g., an OR of 1.0 means the rate of disease among the exposed group equals that of the nonexposed group). |

**TABLE 4-1**   Glossary of Epidemiological Terms (continued)

| | |
|---|---|
| Sensitivity | Measures the probability that a screening test will correctly classify an individual as *positive* for a disease when he or she actually does have the disease. |
| Specificity | Measures the probability that a screening test will correctly classify an individual as *negative* for a disease when he or she actually does not have the disease. |
| Validity | *Internal validity* is the extent to which the subjects in an epidemiological study are truly comparable with respect to general characteristics (e.g., if most of the cases are from an urban setting and the controls are mainly from a rural setting, the two groups are not comparable; evaluation of the exposure-disease relationship may be affected by these differences). Internal validity is essential for the interpretability and reliability of a study.<br><br>*External validity*, or generalizability, is the extent to which the study population can be compared with a larger population (e.g., the general population). External validity must be assessed before study results can be applied to a broader population (e.g., a study that uses as its population a specific profession, such as nurses, may yield results that are not relevant to all women in that general population; while the study may have strong internal validity, the participating nurses may not be representative of the women in the general population or in the nursing profession). |

**TABLE 4-2**   Rates and Ratios Commonly Used in Epidemiology

| Rate Name | Rate Description | Population Factor |
|---|---|---|
| Crude birth rate | $\dfrac{\text{Number of live births}}{\text{Average or midyear population}}$ | per 1000 |
| Fertility rate | $\dfrac{\text{Number of live births}}{\text{15–41-year-old women at midyear}}$ | per 1000 |
| Crude mortality rate | $\dfrac{\text{Total number of deaths}}{\text{Total population at midyear}}$ | per 1000 |
| Age-specific mortality rate | $\dfrac{\text{Deaths in specific age-group}}{\text{Midyear population in age-group}}$ | per 100,000 |
| Cause-specific mortality rate | $\dfrac{\text{Deaths from a specific cause}}{\text{Total midyear population}}$ | per 100,000 |
| Infant mortality rate | $\dfrac{\text{Deaths of children less than 1 year of age}}{\text{Number of live births}}$ | per 1000 |
| Neonatal mortality rate | $\dfrac{\text{Deaths in infants younger than 28 days}}{\text{Number of live births}}$ | per 1000 |
| Case fatality rate | $\dfrac{\text{Number of deaths from a disease in a given period of follow-up}}{\text{Number of diagnosed cases of disease at start of follow-up period}}$ | per 1000 |
| Proportional mortality rate | $\dfrac{\text{Number of deaths from a given cause}}{\text{Number of deaths from all causes}}$ | per 1000 |
| Morbidity rate | $\dfrac{\text{Number of cases of the disease that develop in a given period}}{\text{Total population at midperiod}}$ | per 100,000 |

demographic characteristics of interest are measured. While cross-sectional studies cannot establish a causal relationship between the exposure and the disease, they do provide descriptive statistics for the population, that is, the prevalence rates for the disease in that population, and are often used as the preliminary step in planning cohort studies.

### Case-control studies

The case-control study design should be considered if at least one of the following criteria is met:

- The disease is rare in the general or source population (such as most forms of cancer).

- The investigation is preliminary.

- Time and funding limitations prohibit the use of other, larger, more expensive study designs.

The information gained from case-control studies does not establish a causal relationship between the disease and the exposure, but it does explore the concurrent association between the two. If the strength of this associa-

**TABLE 4-3** 2 × 2 Table Used in Calculating Relative Risks (RR) and Odds Ratios (OR)

|  | Diseased | Not Diseased |
|---|---|---|
| Exposed | a | b |
| Nonexposed | c | d |

tion is significant and is supported by other studies, this information can be used to justify the use of larger cohort studies or clinical trials that can establish causative relationships.

Subjects in case-control studies are recruited on the basis of disease status. Cases of the disease in question, either preexisting or newly developed, are compared with noncases, or control subjects, on the basis of the exposure being investigated. *Control subjects* are defined as people who do not have the disease at present but who, if the disease did develop, would have the same opportunity to be diagnosed as the case subjects. The selection of an appropriate control group is the major challenge of case-control studies and is often the source of selection bias introduced into the study.[3]

An example of the use of the case-control study design is a study examining the association between malignant melanoma and the use of sun beds and sunlamps.[4] The case group consisted of 583 individuals diagnosed with melanoma; the control group was composed of 608 subjects who did not have melanoma. The control subjects were randomly selected from property tax rolls. Each group was evaluated for exposure, which in this case was the use of sun beds or sunlamps. The calculated odds ratio, comparing the rate of exposure among the diseased group with that among the nondiseased, found that the exposed subjects, that is, those who reported using sun beds or sunlamps, had a 1.45–1.88-fold increase in the risk of developing melanoma. This difference was seen in both the male and the female subjects.

Demographic differences between cases and controls should be minimized. To make the two groups comparable, some investigators have used a technique called *matching*, in which certain demographic characteristics of the cases are matched to those of the controls. For example, if a case subject is female, 45 years old, white, and from a low-income household, a control subject would be selected with basically the same characteristics. The advantage of matching, and analyzing the data in pairs of subjects, is that fewer subjects are required in each group to see a relationship between the exposure and the disease, if such a relationship exists. This is useful in situations where there are small numbers of cases of the disease available for study and efficiency is a major issue. Matching is also a means for controlling potential confounding introduced by the selection of the control group. The major disadvantage of matching is that any variable used in matching cannot be studied in relation to the disease. If little is actually known about the relationship between disease and exposure, the investigator may not want to limit the opportunities to study all possible variables. The melanoma study[4] used matching to control the potential confounding variables of age, sex, and residence municipality. The resulting groups contained similar proportions of each variable. A commonly used alternative to matching is the recruitment of more than one control subject per case subject. For example, two to four control subjects may be recruited for each case subject. This technique affords an increase in statistical power without limiting the variables that can be investigated. In this scenario the baseline characteristics of both groups would be assessed for comparability. Ideally, the age ranges, racial differences, socioeconomic status (SES), and other known potential confounding variables should not be significantly different between the groups. The association seen between an exposure and the disease can be clouded by extraneous variables that are poorly distributed between the case and control groups.

Another classic example of the case-control design is a study of endometrial cancer and the use of postmenopausal estrogens.[5] In this study, women with endometrial cancer constituted the case group, while women from the same hospital who had other gynecologic ailments were recruited into the control group. Matching was not implemented. The increase in risk of cancer related to exposure to the postmenopausal estrogens was dramatic (OR = 11.28). Critics of the study stated that the two subject groups did not have comparable SESs and that selection bias explained the elevated risk. The study was redesigned and a new control group recruited. The resulting odds ratios, after an attempt to control the selection bias, still showed that estrogens significantly increased a woman's risk of developing endometrial cancer (OR = 2.30–2.69).

### Cohort studies

Once an association between a disease and an exposure has been established, a cohort study may be initiated to test the research hypothesis. The cohort, or group of subjects, that is included in this type of study design represents individuals who do not have the disease of interest. An initial cross-sectional study or assessment of a population can identify and eliminate all active cases of the disease. Once the cohort is selected, the exposures of interest are assessed and the subjects monitored for a designated period of time to record development of the disease.

Cohort studies can be retrospective, prospective, or ambidirectional. *Retrospective* studies use a previously defined cohort, and, through the review of records, identify individuals who developed the disease and assess the level of exposure. While retrospective studies are often less time-consuming and less expensive than the other cohort designs, the quality of the information collected on the disease and exposure is constrained by the quality of the records available. Many occupational cohort studies are conducted retrospectively.

In *prospective* studies a current population of disease-free individuals is selected and the exposure(s) measured. This study population is then followed into the future and evaluated for development of the disease. The rate of new cases is compared between levels of exposure to establish the disease-exposure relationship. While prospective studies often require several years of subject follow-up and are generally expensive to complete, they offer the opportunity to establish definitively a causative relationship between the exposure and the disease. In addition, the effect of multiple risk factors on disease development may be investigated.

The Framingham Heart Study[6] is one of the best-known examples of this type of cohort design. The residents of Framingham, Massachusetts, were selected for this prospective study, which examined the risk factors for cardiovascular disease. All eligible subjects were examined extensively for presence of heart disease, and potential risk factors were evaluated, such as family history, nutrition, exercise, smoking status, and alcohol consumption. Monitoring of these subjects for the development of heart disease and/or a cardiovascular-related event has continued to date and now includes a cohort of offspring of the original participants. Significant information on the multiple risk factors and treatment modalities of heart disease has been produced by this study.

The last type of cohort study is the *ambidirectional* cohort study, which starts with a previously established cohort and continues subject follow-up into the future. This design carries the same advantages and disadvantages as the retrospective and prospective designs combined.

The study of the Vietnam veteran's postservice mortality is an example of the ambidirectional cohort design.[7] A cohort of Vietnam veterans was identified retrospectively from service records. The subjects were then followed prospectively through 1983 to determine the vital status and causes of deaths of the cohort. These rates were compared with mortality rates of veterans from World War II and the Korean War. While the death rates for Vietnam veterans were slightly elevated in the first five years following the end of active service, the overall death rates were not significantly different.

## Clinical trials and intervention studies

The final study design to be discussed here is the clinical trial or intervention study. This design tests the effect of an intervention on the rates of disease development. Two groups of subjects are created within the study population; a treatment group (receiving the treatment) and a control group (receiving the placebo or the current therapy). For example, to test the effect of a drug or nutritional supplement on the rates of cancer development, subjects are randomly assigned to one of the two groups and monitored over the time period of the study for the development or recurrence of the cancer. The design is called *double-blind* when the assignment of the treatment group is kept from the subject and the immediate clinical personnel. This controls the potential biasing effects on subject participation, disease diagnosis, and monitoring that can occur when participants and/or clinical staff know the group assignments. A major benefit of a double-blind, placebo-controlled clinical trial is that the random assignment of treatment groups helps to distribute potential confounding variables evenly between the two groups, thus minimizing their effects on the measurement of the association between the exposure and the disease. If this control of confounding is successful and the primary difference between the two treatment groups is the intervention, then a clinical trial can definitively evaluate the efficacy of the intervention.

An example of a clinical trial is the Physicians' Health Study,[8] which randomized 22,071 licensed physicians into an expanded design to test the effectiveness of aspirin on decreasing the rates of heart attacks and the effect of beta-carotene on inhibiting the development of cancer. After five years the aspirin arm of the trial was stopped because a significantly lower risk of heart attack was observed among the subjects receiving aspirin. The beta-carotene arm of the trial was discontinued in December 1995; no effect of beta-carotene was observed on cancer incidence.[9]

A major limitation of the clinical trial design is that several years of subject follow-up may be required before significant changes in the rate of disease development are observed among treatment groups. The length of follow-up will depend on several factors, one of which is the strength of the effect the treatment has on the risk of the disease. Long-term studies raise patient management issues, such as maintaining active participation of subjects, monitoring subject deaths, and tracking subjects who move from the study area. These factors, if unevenly distributed among the treatment groups, may confound the results of the project.

## Defining the Population

In addition to defining the type of study design appropriate for testing a research hypothesis, it is also important to define the source population for study subjects and the actual study population. This clarifies to whom the research results can be generalized (external validity), whether the study population represents the general population and the source population, and the overall characteristics of eligible subjects. The *source population* for the study is the larger group or population from which the study subjects are recruited. This could include, for instance, residents in a certain city or neighborhood, university students, or all subjects attending a particular hospital. The source population is usually a subgroup of the general population.

The study population is the group of subjects actually recruited into the project from the source population. Recruitment into the study population, based on the defined eligibility criteria, is planned to access all potential subjects within the source population. In reviewing sources of bias that may have been introduced into the study, it is important to review the type of subjects who were part of the source population but were not eligible or not approached for recruitment. For example, if subjects were recruited from phone interviews, one could conclude that only subjects with telephones were eligible. Since the presence of a telephone in the household could be related to SES, the study population could be biased toward recruiting subjects with a higher SES. Because of this selection bias, and the recruitment of a homogeneous group of subjects with respect to SES, the relationship of SES to the disease may be impossible to evaluate and may affect the results of the study.

### Eligibility criteria

The selection of the study population is based on established eligibility criteria. These are designed to create a population of subjects with a sufficient prevalence of the disease to test the hypothesis efficiently, and for whom the intervention is considered safe. Examples of commonly used eligibility criteria in cancer research are age, race, gender, disease stage, life expectancy, absence of other cancers or chronic diseases, exposure to certain drugs or treatments, and current health status.

### Defining the disease and the exposure

The disease should be defined as specifically as possible, including pathological criteria, specific blood chemistries, histological characteristics, specific test results, and physical symptoms according to current medical practice. Clear disease definition helps to control potential misclassification bias. Even with a definition, disease status may need to be confirmed by an external reviewer, further controlling bias.

Equally important as defining the disease is clarifying the definition of the exposure used in the study. An *exposure* is considered as a contact that a subject has had with the variable of interest that may influence the development of or improvement in disease status. Exposures can include a broad range of variables, from environmental conditions, medications, nutrients, genetic influences, and health care accessibility to types of exercise. The characteristics of the exposure that are most important to clarify are the *dose* of the exposure, the *duration* or length of time of the exposure, and *characteristics* that are specific to the exposure, such as latency effects and effects that are synergistic with other exposures.

*Dose* refers to a standardized, measured amount of exposure issued (e.g., standard milligrams, as in the case of drugs), gray (Gy) for radiation, number of packs of cigarettes per year, drinks of alcohol per day, and so on. It is important to assess whether the dose is constant throughout the exposure or whether certain variables or conditions have affected the dose over time.

## Statistical Plan

In addition to calculating the rates and ratios of a disease as it develops in a population, epidemiological research affords the investigator the ability to examine the relationships of the disease to defined exposures. A major goal of epidemiological research is to make inferences to the larger population based on information obtained from the study population.[3] The validity of these inferences relies on the assumption that the study population is a representative sample of the larger group.

While risk estimates are useful, other statistical tests afford the opportunity to examine more closely the disease-exposure association. A t-test will evaluate whether the means or averages between two groups are significantly different. The chi-square test will evaluate the differences between the proportions observed and expected between groups.

## Potential Sources of Bias and Confounding

The potential sources of bias and confounding in a study are examined to determine if the differences seen between the two groups can be explained by influences other than the research hypothesis. If both of these issues have been well controlled in the study design, and the role of chance is sufficiently small, then the possibility that the hypothesis is correct increases.

## Data Sources

There are several data sources and systems in the United States relating to cancer and risk factors for cancer that can be accessed by investigators (Table 4-4). These sources are frequently useful to gain preliminary data to formulate or support a hypothesis, as well as to provide a means of examining national, regional, or temporal differences in cancer or risk factors for cancer.

**TABLE 4-4**   Data Sources for Epidemiological Research

| Source | Description |
| --- | --- |
| National Health Interview Survey (NHIS) | Annual survey started in 1957. Household interviews are conducted in approximately 50,000 households representative of the civilian noninstitutionalized population. Provides data on the incidence of illness and accidental injuries, prevalence of chronic diseases and impairments, disability, physician visits, hospitalizations, and other health topics, and on the relationship between demographic and socioeconomic characteristics and health characteristics. The questionnaires change with time to focus on current health topics. |
| National Health and Nutrition Examination Survey (NHANES) | NHANES III was begun in 1988. Ultimately, 45,000 people representative of the U.S. population will be selected to participate. Participants undergo physical examinations and clinical and laboratory testing. For example, data are collected on blood pressure, serum cholesterol, and body measurements. Dietary assessment is also conducted as part of the survey. |
| Behavioral Risk Factor Surveillance System | Started in 1984, this system is coordinated by the Centers for Disease Control and Prevention (CDC), but the telephone interviews used as the survey methodology are conducted by the participating states—currently, 45 states and the District of Columbia. The survey's purpose is to collect information regarding the prevalence of self-reported health behaviors that relate to the ten leading causes of death, including cigarette smoking, hypertension, obesity, seat belt use, physical inactivity, and alcohol use. Several of these behaviors are risk factors for cancer. This system provides a means of assessing change in these behaviors over time or in response to an intervention. |
| National Vital Statistics System | This system provides data on births, deaths, marriages, and divorces. Annual data are produced for the United States, the individual states, counties, and other local areas. Cause of death is included in this system, (e.g., breast cancer mortality rates can be compared for differing counties within a state, or over time within a specific location). |
| Surveillance, Epidemiology, and End Results (SEER) Program | This is the principal source of cancer incidence and survival data for the United States. The participating areas are Seattle (Puget Sound), Utah, San Francisco, New Mexico, Hawaii, Iowa, Detroit, Connecticut, and Atlanta (including ten rural counties), which include approximately 9.6% of the U.S. population. For each newly diagnosed cancer case, data collected include selected patient demographics, primary site, morphology, diagnostic confirmation, extent of disease, and first course of cancer-directed therapy. Active follow-up of all living patients is conducted to help ascertain survival time. |
| National Death Index | This system aids investigators in ascertaining mortality. A computerized database contains identifying information on all deaths reported by the state vital statistics offices. An investigator can determine if a study subject has died and, if relevant, where and how to obtain a copy of the death certificate. |
| Decennial census | The goal of the 10-yearly census conducted in the United States is to count each person according to "usual place of residence." A limited amount of information is requested from each person; a sample of persons is then asked to complete a more detailed questionnaire. Detailed population numbers by age, sex, and ethnicity are important to the epidemiologist, since they are used in the denominator of calculations of population rates. The demographic data from the census can be used to give a population profile of areas of research interest. |

## ENVIRONMENTAL FACTORS ASSOCIATED WITH CANCER CAUSATION

### How Do We Decide What Causes Cancer?

It is important to recognize that inference regarding causality cannot be made from a single study. Information from many sources must be drawn on to infer causality. The criteria to be considered are the following:

- the magnitude of association between the exposure and the disease

- consistency of findings from all studies

- biological credibility

- temporal association between the risk factor and the disease

### Tobacco

Tobacco use is still the most important known cause of cancer in the United States. Tobacco causes about 30% of cancer deaths, and cigarette smoking causes 90% of lung cancers.[10]

Active tobacco use has been linked to many cancer types: lung, oropharyngeal, bladder, pancreatic, cervical, and kidney,[11,12] and a clear linear relationship exists between the number of cigarettes smoked and the risk of lung and oropharyngeal cancers.

There is a gradual decrease in the ex-smoker's risk of dying from lung cancer; eventually the risk is almost equivalent to that of a nonsmoker.[13] The rate of decline of the risk after cessation of smoking is determined by the cumulative smoking exposure prior to cessation, the age when smoking began, and the degree of inhalation.[14]

Study results regarding passive smoking as a risk factor for lung cancer are inconsistent, with some studies showing a positive relationship between lung cancer and exposure to sidestream smoke[15,16] and others showing no relationship.[17] Blot and Fraumeni[18,19] combined data from existing studies and estimated an overall increase in risk for lung cancer of 30% for nonsmoking women married to smokers and an increased risk of 70% associated with heavy passive smoking. A review of recently published epidemiological studies supports the causal association between environmental tobacco smoke and lung cancer.[20]

The use of smokeless tobacco (chewing tobacco and snuff) is increasing among U.S. male youth, especially among whites.[21] This practice has been linked to both oral cancer and cancer of the tongue.[22]

The overall smoking prevalence is decreasing in the United States,[23] and this is reflected in declining lung cancer rates among young men and women.[24] However, the decrease in smoking prevalence is not uniform among all groups within society. For the period 1974–1987, smoking prevalence in women aged 20 and over declined more slowly (31.5% to 26.8%) than for men (43.4% to 31.7%), with the smoking prevalence for women aged 20–24 not changing significantly. Smoking prevalance declined from 1974 to 1985 in white adolescents, but no significant declines occurred during the period 1985–1991. In contrast, smoking prevalance declined through the entire 1974–1991 period in black adolescents. The reasons for these differences are unclear.[25]

It is believed that the lung cancer mortality rate for white men in the United States has now peaked, but the projected peak for mortality rates in women will not occur until the year 2010.[26,27] Similarly, lung cancer mortality for African-Americans is not expected to fall until after the year 2000.[27] However, even with the predicted declines in mortality rates, the absolute number of lung cancer deaths will continue to rise[28] because of the increasing size of the population.

Prevention of smoking has an impact not only on cancer rates but also on the prevalence of other common diseases, such as heart and respiratory disease. It was estimated that, in 1988, there were twice as many deaths from heart disease and respiratory disease caused by smoking as there were deaths from cancers caused by smoking.[29] Therefore, prevention and cessation of smoking in the United States is a major public health goal.

### Diet

Interest and research in the role of diet in cancer has flourished in recent years, with many micronutrients and some macronutrients being investigated for adverse or protective effects against cancer, in both human and animal studies. The impetus for many of these studies came from the results of ecological studies; for example, a high correlation was found between national per capita daily meat consumption and country-specific colon cancer incidence rates.[30]

Case-control and cohort studies of diet and cancer present several methodological problems:

1. Accurate assessment of dietary intake is very difficult, especially in large epidemiological studies. In epidemiology, the two most frequently used methods of dietary assessment are single or multiple 24-hour recall of dietary intake and the food frequency questionnaire. In the latter method, subjects are asked how many times they ate numerous foods with reference to a given time period, such as the last year. The validity of these instruments varies with the nutrient of interest. Dietary assessment, including the previously described methods, has been thoroughly described by Willett.[31]
2. Individual nutrients are often highly correlated because they are strongly related to calorie intake. This makes the assessment of the role of a single nutrient problematic. Statistical methods have been developed to adjust for calorie intake in an attempt to address this problem.[32]
3. Frequently, the range of nutrient intake within the study population is narrow, making it less likely that a nutrient effect will be observed. For example, this problem has been suggested as a possible reason for the lack of association between fat and breast cancer in the large Nurses' Health Study.[33]
4. Recall bias may be present if dietary assessment is being conducted after the presentation of the disease, as in a case-control study. This means that individuals' recall of their past diet might be affected by their knowledge that they have the disease.

To avoid the problems associated with self-reported dietary intake methods, direct assessment of some micronutrients has been developed, involving measuring the serum micronutrient levels.[34] However, this type of measurement has disadvantages; for example, in a case-control study the disease may affect blood micronutrient levels. Serum markers of intake of most macronutrients are not currently available, thus limiting this methodology.

Diet may be of great importance in cancer prevention, for it has been proposed as a contributing factor in 20%–70% of cancer deaths[10,35] and is a modifiable risk factor.

Some current issues regarding diet and cancer are discussed next.

***Colon cancer and fat intake***   Ecological studies comparing many countries have shown a strong association between per capita meat consumption[30] or dietary fat[36] and incidence of colorectal cancer. However, a causal association cannot be assumed from such studies. Results from case-control and cohort studies generally have supported high fat intake as a risk factor for colon cancer.[37–40] Difficulties can arise in the interpretation of such results because it is often difficult to separate the effects of fat, protein, and total calories,[39,40] dietary factors that are generally highly correlated.

*Colon cancer and fiber intake*   A majority of studies of differing epidemiological designs supports the hypothesis that high fiber intake is protective for colon cancer,[41] although not all studies are supportive. Vegetables as well as cereals are sources of fiber; in studies where the source of fiber has been examined, fiber from vegetables appears protective against colon cancer, whereas the data for cereal fiber are less supportive of a protective effect. These differences may be due to the difference in composition of fiber in cereals and vegetables or to the lack of a large range in cereal fiber intake, or these results may indicate that it is some other chemical or nutrient in vegetables that is protective against colon cancer.[41]

*Colon cancer and calcium intake*   A protective role of high calcium intake against colon cancer has been reported in several studies[42-44] but not in all.[38,45] Data from supportive studies suggest that to reduce the risk of colon cancer, calcium intake for females should be 1500 mg and for males 1800 mg.[46] These recommended intakes are similar to those suggested to prevent other disease states, such as osteoporosis and hypertension.

*Breast cancer and fat intake*   Ecological studies that use data from many countries show a strong positive relationship between per capita fat intake and breast cancer mortality rates.[30] However, case-control and cohort studies give conflicting results. In a combined analysis of 12 case-control studies of dietary factors and breast cancer, Howe[47] reported an association between high fat intake and breast cancer in postmenopausal women.

Two of the largest cohort studies, the Nurses' Health Study[33,48] and the Iowa Women's Study,[49] show no relationship between dietary fat intake and breast cancer risk; however, some researchers suggest this may be because the range of fat intake in such studies was too small. Current dietary recommendations are for women to reduce fat intake to less than 30% of calories. In Willett's study[48] the range of fat intake was 32%–44% of calories.

*Cancer, micronutrients, and intake of fruits and vegetables*   One of the most consistent dietary findings in analytic epidemiological studies with regard to cancer is a protective effect of fruits and vegetables.[50] What particular nutrient, nonnutrient, or combination in fruits and vegetables is protective against cancer is still under investigation. Nonnutrient compounds that may have a protective effect, such as indoles and dithiolethiones, have been summarized by Wattenberg.[51] The role of several micronutrients in cancer prevention, including the carotenoid beta-carotene, vitamin A, vitamin E, and selenium, has been extensively investigated. Relatively high levels of these four micronutrients have been found to be associated with lower cancer risk in many studies, although, again, not all study results are in agreement. The role of micronutrients in cancer prevention has been reviewed by Moon and Micozzi.[52]

Micronutrient or pharmacological compounds are used in the majority of cancer prevention clinical trials.

Clinical trials involving diet and cancer are designed to investigate the effect of an isolated nutrient or a combination of nutrients on cancer incidence. Three large cancer chemoprevention trials that investigated the efficacy of beta-carotene in cancer prevention have recently been completed:

1. The Alpha-Tocopherol and Beta-Carotene Cancer Prevention Study (ATBC), in which the effect on lung cancer incidence of two micronutrients, alpha-tocopherol (vitamin E) and beta-carotene, both alone and in combination, was investigated in a high-risk population of 29,000 Finnish male smokers.[53]
2. The Carotene and Retinol Efficacy Trial (CARET), in which the effect of two micronutrients, retinol (vitamin A) and beta-carotene in combination, on lung cancer incidence was investigated in a high-risk population of 18,000 male and female smokers and male asbestos-workers.[54]
3. The Physicians' Health Study (PHS), in which the effect of beta-carotene on incidence of all cancer was investigated in 22,000 male physicians.[9]

Surprisingly, two of the three studies (ATBC and CARET) suggested an 18%–28% increase in lung cancer risk in the group receiving beta-carotene. In comparison, the PHS showed no difference in cancer incidence between the two intervention groups for cancer at any site. These results are contrary to expectation based on animal laboratory studies, thus emphasizing the importance of randomized intervention trials in which the effect of a single nutrient can be assessed.

The goal of other cancer prevention trials involving diet is to change the intake of a macronutrient in the intervention arm while having minimal effect in the non-intervention arm. Two examples of such ongoing trials are the Women's Health Initiative[55] and the Wheat Bran Fiber Study.[56] The Women's Health Initiative has a complex trial design that involves an intervention in which women lower their fat intake to less than 20% of total calories. Other interventions include hormone replacement therapy and calcium supplementation. Among the outcomes to be assessed are breast cancer and colon cancer. In the Wheat Bran Fiber Study, participants who have had a history of adenomatous polyps, a precancerous lesion of the colon, are randomized to either receive a high-bran (13.5 g) supplement or a placebo supplement that has a low fiber content. The outcome of the trial is the occurrence of a new adenomatous polyp. Greenwald et al[57] provide a review of selected human chemoprevention trials funded by the National Cancer Institute. The reader may also refer to chapter 6, for more information on this topic.

Dietary intake has an impact not only on cancer but on many other chronic diseases as well, such as heart disease and diabetes, where its role is more fully understood. Even without proof of the role of a specific nutrient in cancer causation, there may be sufficient knowledge from a public health perspective to recommend that Americans change some aspect of their diet. For example, the role of fat in breast cancer is still controversial, but there exists sufficient knowledge concerning the role of fat in obesity, heart disease, and colon cancer that recommendations to reduce fat intake have been made to the American public.

Several groups, such as the National Research Council, have published recommendations for an optimal diet. Their recommendations include eating at least five servings of fruit and vegetables a day, reducing fat intake to 30% or less of calories, maintaining protein intake at moderate levels, and balancing food intake and physical activity to maintain appropriate body weight.[58] The role of health professionals is to encourage their patients to follow such guidelines and to help them avoid being influenced by the results of isolated studies of diet and its relationship to cancer.

### Alcohol

Alcohol has been causally linked to cancers of the oral cavity, pharynx, larynx, esophagus, and liver, and may be linked to cancers of the breast and rectum.[59,60] It is estimated that 3% of cancer deaths are attributable to alcohol.[10] For most cancer sites, alcohol appears to act synergistically with smoking.

Cancers at most sites do not appear to be associated with any particular type of alcohol. Rectal cancer is the exception, for it appears to be associated specifically with beer consumption.[61] Nitrosamines, which are found in beer, have been suggested as a possible cause of the association between rectal cancer and beer consumption.[62]

Studies regarding the relationship between alcohol and breast cancer suggest a positive but weak association. However, both the level of alcohol consumption required to significantly increase breast cancer risk [59] and the age at which exposure to alcohol is important[63] are unclear. If a causal association is shown, alcohol would present one of the only known avoidable causes of breast cancer. However, if increased risk of breast cancer is shown to be associated with moderate to low levels of alcohol intake, as some studies have shown, women will have to weigh the personal benefits of abstaining from alcohol to reduce breast cancer risk against the risk of increasing their risk of heart disease,[64] as moderate alcohol intake has been shown to be associated with a reduced risk of heart disease in women.[65]

### Physical activity

As with dietary assessment, accurate measurement of physical activity in epidemiological studies has proved to be difficult, and many questionnaires have been developed in an attempt to improve assessment.[66] The close interrelationship of physical activity with obesity and diet, two factors associated with many cancers, also makes its role in relation to cancer risk more difficult to assess.

Increased physical activity consistently has been found to be protective for colon cancer[67–69] and precancerous colon polyps.[70] Mounting evidence suggests that increased physical activity is protective for breast cancer.[71,72] Intense physical activity at the age of usual menarche may be especially important, since it can cause a delay in onset of menarche. Late onset of menarche is known to be protective against breast cancer.[73] Increased physical activity is known to be protective against heart disease, and a general increase in physical activity throughout the population would be beneficial for health.

### Occupational exposures

It is estimated that 4%–9% of cancer deaths can be attributed to exposure to occupational carcinogens. The lung is the most commonly affected site.[10]

Reasons for conducting epidemiological studies of industrial populations include surveillance of groups for the following:

- to identify unusual disease patterns that might indicate exposure to previously unidentified hazards

- to monitor and reevaluate "safe" levels of identified hazards

- to monitor human exposure to complex mixtures of different chemicals or materials that probably have not been tested in animal experiments in the laboratory

A summary of substances that are thought to cause cancer, and occupations in which they are used, is found in Table 4-5.[74]

### Pollution

Pollution accounts for less than 1%–5% of cancer deaths in the United States.[10] It can affect the air we breathe, the water we drink, and the food we eat. Epidemiological studies of pollution present a difficult methodological problem, that is, the assessment of exposure, specifically assessment of both how long a subject has been exposed and the level of exposure.

Air pollution has been studied primarily in relation to risk for lung cancer. It seems probable that in heavily polluted areas air pollution may contribute to lung cancer mortality; however, insufficient data are available to quantify the risk.[75] Evidence is much stronger for the association of air pollution and increased mortality from respiratory diseases, showing the importance of air pollution as a health risk.

Associations between water pollution and site-specific cancer risk are also unproved. Arsenic in drinking water appeared to be associated with an increase of skin cancer in Taiwan[76] but not in the United States.[77] This observed difference may be due to a higher intensity of exposure in Taiwan. Another more common pollutant of drinking water, trihalomethanes may be linked to rectal and bladder cancer.[78] These compounds are produced by the action of chlorine on organic waste.

**TABLE 4-5**  Known and Suspected Occupational Carcinogens

| Carcinogen | Occupation | Cancer |
|---|---|---|
| Polynuclear aromatic compounds in soots, tars, some mineral oils | Various, including sweeps, tar workers, cotton spinners, roofers, boat-builders and repairers, fishermen, tool setters | Scrotum, other skin |
| 2-naphthylamine, 4-aminobiphenyl | Chemicals, rubber, cable-making | Bladder |
| Benzidine | Chemicals, dyestuffs, laboratory reagent | Bladder |
| ? Michler's ketone | Auramine manufacture | Bladder |
| Mustard gas | Chemicals, warfare | Lung, larynx |
| *bis*(Chloromethyl)ether, technical chloromethyl methyl ether | Chemicals | Lung |
| ? Diisopropyl sulphate | Isopropanol manufacture by strong acid process | Nasal sinuses |
| ? Benzotrichloride | Manufacture of benzoyl chloride, etc. | Lung |
| Vinyl chloride (monomer) | Polyvinyl chloride manufacture | Liver angiosarcoma, ? other sites |
| Benzene | Chemicals, solvent | Leukemia |
| Unknown ? via immunosuppression | Professional chemists | Lymphoma, ? brain |
| Arsenic compounds | Manufacture, use of arsenical pesticides, mining, smelting of various metals | Lung, skin |
| Nickel subsulfide, oxide, etc. | Nickel refining | Nasal sinuses, lung |
| Zinc chromate, other Cr(VI) compounds | Production and use of chromates | Lung |
| Beryllium compounds | Mining and various uses | Lung |
| Cadmium oxide, etc. | Battery manufacture, alloying, plating, etc. | ? Prostate, ? lung |
| Radon + ? | Underground mining of hematite and other ores | Lung |
| Asbestos dust | Mining, multiple uses | Lung (synergism with smoking), mesothelioma of pleura, peritoneum |
| Wood dusts | Furniture manufacture | Nasal sinuses |
| Leather dusts | Shoe-making | Nasal sinuses |

Reprinted with permission from Searle and Teale.[74]

A type of pollution that may indirectly increase cancer risk is that of chlorofluorocarbons (CFCs), which are destroying the ozone layer in the stratosphere.[79] It is predicted that this destruction will increase the amount of ultraviolet light reaching the earth's surface, thereby increasing the risk for nonmelanoma and melanoma skin cancer. The Environmental Protection Agency (EPA) reports that for every 1% decrease in stratospheric ozone, there is a 2% increase in ultraviolet-B intensity, potentially increasing the incidence of skin cancer by 1%–3% each year that the condition of the deteriorating ozone exists.[80]

### Reproductive factors and sexual behavior

Risk factors related to reproduction and sexual behavior have been identified only for cancers in women; these are summarized in Table 4-6. The risk factor patterns are similar for breast, endometrial, and ovarian cancers. Pike[81] discusses the reasons for these observed similarities, such as exposure to unopposed estrogen. In contrast, cervical cancer has a very different risk factor pattern, with only multiple sexual partners being identified as a sexual behavioral risk factor. The number of sexual partners is a measure of the likelihood that an individual has been exposed to the human papilloma virus, which has been implicated as a cause of cervical dysplasia.[82]

In general, the reproductive risk factors associated with breast, endometrial, and ovarian cancers are unavoidable. Furthermore, there are no other proven risk factors for these cancers that can be avoided. Thus, early detection of these cancers is very important. Unfortunately, only breast cancer screening is available, although screening methods for ovarian cancer are being investigated. Nurses can play a strong role in encouraging all women to obtain mammography and in educating women regarding early signs of endometrial and ovarian cancer. For further information on screening refer to chapter 7.

**TABLE 4-6**    Reproductive and Sexual Factors Associated with Female Cancers

| Risk Factor | Breast | Cervical | Endometrial | Ovarian |
|---|---|---|---|---|
| Early menarche | X | | X | X |
| Late menopause | X | | X | X |
| Nulliparity | X | | X | X |
| Late first pregnancy, > 35 years old | X | | | |
| Obesity | X* | | X | |
| Multiple sexual partners | | X | | |

*Postmenopausal women only.

### Viruses and other biological agents

Zur Hausen[83] suggests that 15% of worldwide cancer incidence is due to viruses. Table 4-7 lists several putative human cancer viruses and their associated cancers. Epidemiological evidence for their role in cancer causation is relatively strong. Hepatitis B virus and human T-cell lymphotrophic virus type 1 may be sufficient alone to cause cancer, whereas Epstein-Barr virus alone is insufficient, and requires the host to be immunodeficient.[84] Burkitt's lymphoma, which is associated with the Epstein-Barr virus, is seen primarily in Africa, where malarial infection causes the required immunodeficiency state.

A very strong body of evidence exists supporting a role for human papillomavirus (HPV) in the development of cervical cancer,[85] with subtypes HPV16 and HPV18 being most strongly associated with the disease.

Both cohort and case-control studies suggest that gastric cancer may be linked to infection with *Helicobacter pylori*.[86] However, intervention studies that eradicate infection with *Helicobacter pylori* will be required to prove causality between infection and gastric cancer.

*Schistosoma haematobium*, a parasitic flatworm, is common in Iraq, Egypt, and southeast Africa; there is strong epidemiological evidence of its causative role in bladder cancer in these regions.[87]

### Radiation

Doll and Peto[10] estimate that 3% of cancer deaths are due to natural sources of radiation, excluding occupational exposure.

***Ionizing radiation***    For most of the earth's population, over 80% of exposure to ionizing radiation is from natural sources, such as the food chain, air, water, minerals on or near the earth's crust, and cosmic rays. Man-made sources are x-rays (80% of exposure to man-made sources in the United States),[88] fallout from nuclear explosions, and emissions and waste from nuclear power stations.

Several populations have been studied to assess the cancer risk of ionizing radiation. These include survivors from Nagasaki and Hiroshima, people who received radiation therapy for medical reasons, and underground miners who were exposed to radon gas and decay products. There is no doubt that ionizing radiation causes many different cancer types, with the breast, thyroid, and bone marrow being particularly sensitive sites.[89,90] However, determining the effect of low-dose exposure, the level at which most such exposure occurs, is difficult. Dose extrapolation poses many problems. For example, attempting to extrapolate from the cancer risk of the high radon dose that miners receive to the relatively low dose that individuals living in a radon-contaminated house receive requires many assumptions regarding exposure to both the miners and the householders.[91] Using extrapolated risk estimates, Lubin et al[91] calculated that in the United States 10% of all lung cancer deaths annually may be due to exposure to radon in the home, thus making radon exposure a great public health concern.

Occupational exposure to ionizing radiation is highest among underground uranium miners, commercial nuclear power plant workers, fuel fabricators, physicians, flight crews and attendants, industrial radiographers, and well loggers.[92]

**TABLE 4-7**    Cancer Types Associated with a Virus or Other Biological Agent

| Virus or Biological Agent | Cancer |
|---|---|
| Hepatitis B virus | Hepatocellular carcinoma |
| Human papillomavirus (types 16 and 18) | Cervical cancer |
| Epstein-Barr virus | Burkitt's lymphoma |
| Human T-cell lymphotrophic virus type 1 | Adult T-cell leukemia/ lymphoma (ATLL) |
| Human immunodeficiency virus* | Kaposi's sarcoma; non-Hodgkin's lymphoma |
| *Schistosoma* | Bladder cancer |
| *Helicobacter pylori* | Gastric cancer |

*The association may be due to immunosuppression caused by HIV, which places the individual at increased risk. But even HIV-seropositive patients with no measurable immunosuppression appear at higher risk.

***Ultraviolet radiation*** Ultraviolet radiation (UVR) is the major cause of nonmelanoma skin cancer, with cumulative exposure and number of lifetime sunburns being predictive of risk.[93,94] The relationship of UVR to melanoma skin cancer is not as clear, because the site of melanoma does not mimic the site of exposure, as happens in nonmelanoma skin cancer. However, it is thought that intense intermittent exposure to UVR, especially in childhood, is a risk factor for melanoma.[95] UVR also has been shown to act synergistically with pipe smoking as a risk factor for lip cancer.[10]

Individual exposure to UVR is dependent on latitude, altitude, humidity, and personal behaviors, such as wearing protective clothing, using sunscreens, and staying out of the sun as much as possible.

***Nonionizing radiation*** Nonionizing electromagnetic fields (EMF) are generated from a variety of electrical power, radar, and microwave sources[96] and have only recently been suspected of increasing cancer risk. Both occupational and residential exposures have been studied, and the results from some studies suggest that exposure to EMF is associated with increased cancer risk.[97] Early studies suggested that residential exposure is associated with an increased risk of leukemia and brain tumors in children and that occupational exposure is associated with increased leukemia risk in adults.[98] However, two recently published large case-control studies found no detectable effect of residential magnetic field exposure on the development of brain tumors in children.[99,100]

The ubiquitous nature of EMF exposure makes its measurement difficult.[101] In addition, measurement of quantitative exposure to EMF is generally based on assumptions regarding the relationship of EMFs to the electrical wiring configuration of the home, which may not always be correct.

## Drugs

The mechanism of action of many antineoplastic drugs is to damage cellular DNA, thereby killing the cell. However, since these drugs currently cannot be targeted to act specifically on tumor cells, normal cells also are damaged. A late effect of this damage can be the development of a second malignancy. Second tumors most frequently involve hematopoietic and lymphatic systems, but solid tumors also can occur. Single or combinations of antineoplastic drugs that have been implicated in the cause of second malignancies are listed in Table 4-8.[102]

Other drugs that have been associated with malignancies include the following:

- phenacetin: associated with lower urinary tract cancers

- the immunosuppressive drugs azathioprine and cyclosporine: the former associated with an increase in non-Hodgkin's lymphoma and squamous cell cancer of the skin, the latter with an increased risk of lymphoma[102]

**TABLE 4-8**   Antineoplastic Agents That Have Been Evaluated by IARC* Working Groups as Carcinogenic, Probably Carcinogenic, or Possibly Carcinogenic to Humans

| Agent | Status |
|---|---|
| Adriamycin | Probably carcinogenic |
| Azacitidine | Probably carcinogenic |
| Azaserine | Possibly carcinogenic |
| N,N-Bis(2-chloro-ethyl)-2-naphthylamine (chlornaphthazine) | Carcinogenic |
| Bischloroethyl nitrosourea (BCNU) | Probably carcinogenic |
| 1,4-Butanediol dimethylsulphonate (Myleran) | Carcinogenic |
| Chlorambucil | Carcinogenic |
| 1-(2-Chloroethyl)-3-cyclohexyl-1-nitrosourea (CCNU) | Probably carcinogenic |
| 1-(2-Chloroethyl)-3-(4-methylcyclohexyl)-1-nitrosourea (Methyl-CCNU) | Carcinogenic |
| Chlorozotocin | Probably carcinogenic |
| Cisplatin | Probably carcinogenic |
| Cyclophosphamide | Carcinogenic |
| Dacarbazine | Possibly carcinogenic |
| Daunomycin | Possibly carcinogenic |
| Melphalan | Carcinogenic |
| Merphalan | Possibly carcinogenic |
| Mitomycin C | Possibly carcinogenic |
| MOPP and other combined chemotherapy, including alkylating agents | Carcinogenic |
| Nitrogen mustard | Probably carcinogenic |
| Nitrogen mustard N-oxide | Possibly carcinogenic |
| Procarbazine hydrochloride | Probably carcinogenic |
| Streptozotocin | Possibly carcinogenic |
| Tris(1-aziridinyl) phosphine sulphate (Thiotepa) | Carcinogenic |
| Treosulphan | Carcinogenic |
| Trichlormethine | Possibly carcinogenic |
| Uracil mustard | Possibly carcinogenic |

*International Agency for Research on Cancer.
Reprinted with permission from Tomatis.[75]

- 8-methoxypsoralen combined with UVR, used for the treatment of psoriasis and vitiligo: associated with an increased risk of squamous cell cancer of the skin[103]

### Exogenous hormones

Exogenous hormones are prescribed most commonly for women, either as a contraceptive or as replacement therapy following natural or induced menopause. They are also utilized for disorders of the menstrual cycle and to control abnormal uterine bleeding. Progestins have been used in obstetrics to prevent premature labor and in the management of threatened abortions.

Diethylstilbestrol, a synthetic estrogen used in the past for the treatment of threatened abortions, has been associated with vaginal and cervical cancers in the daughters of treated women.[104] This is the only known carcinogen to act transplacentally.[102] The cancers occur 10–30 years after treatment.

In contrast, use of combined oral contraceptives has been associated with a decreased risk of endometrial and ovarian cancer. Five years of usage is associated with a 55% reduction of endometrial cancer and a 40% reduction of ovarian cancer, compared with nonusers.[105]

An increased risk of liver cancer in young women also has been associated with oral contraceptive use; because this is a rare tumor, however, the absolute number of cases is low.[106] Oral contraceptive use has been associated with an increased risk of breast cancer in women diagnosed at young ages.[107,108] The effect, if any, of oral contraceptive use on breast cancer risk in women diagnosed when older is still unclear.

Estrogen replacement therapy (ERT) in postmenopausal women has been shown to increase the risk of endometrial cancer. However, when estrogen is combined with progestin, the increased risk is eliminated.[109] A small increase in breast cancer risk has been associated with long-term ERT. Key and Pike[110] estimate that five years of ERT is associated with a 10% increase in breast cancer when users are compared with nonusers. In contrast, there is evidence that ERT is associated with a reduced risk of large bowel cancer.[111]

## HOST CHARACTERISTICS INFLUENCING CANCER SUSCEPTIBILITY

### Age

Although cancer can occur at any age, it is very much a disease of the elderly, with those over age 65 being ten times more likely (incidence rate 1983.3 per 100,000) than those under 65 (incidence rate 189.8 per 100,000) to develop cancer.[112] Cancer is most common in the elderly because with time the chance of prolonged exposure to cancer-inducing agents increases, and the ability of the immune system to prevent cancer declines.[113]

Increasing cancer incidence is not, however, uniform with advancing age for all cancer sites (Figure 4-1),[112] and the leading cause of cancer deaths changes with age (Table 4-9).[114] Leukemia is the leading cause of death for children under 15 years of age but is no longer among the five leading causes of cancer death after the age of 35; in contrast, lung cancer is rarely a cause of death under the age of 30 but is the leading cause of death over the age of 35.

Because age is such an important determinant of cancer risk, it is important in epidemiological studies to make adjustments for age in the statistical analysis unless comparison groups have the same age distribution.

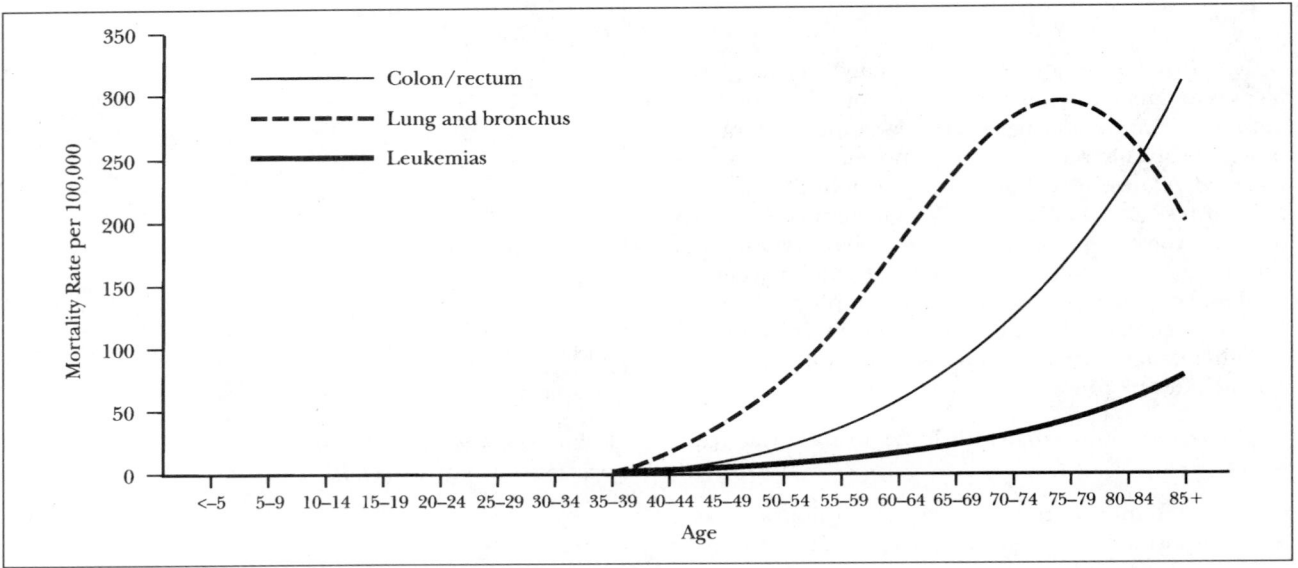

**FIGURE 4-1**   Changing cancer mortality with age for three cancer sites. (Data from Ries et al.[112])

**TABLE 4-9**   Mortality for the Five Leading Cancer Sites by Age, United States, 1992

| MALES | | | | | |
|---|---|---|---|---|---|
| **All Ages** | **Under 15** | **15–34** | **35–54** | **55–74** | **75 +** |
| All Cancer 274,838 | All Cancer 937 | All Cancer 3,655 | All Cancer 28,127 | All Cancer 141,171 | All Cancer 100,931 |
| Lung 91,405 | Leukemia 375 | Leukemia 676 | Lung 8,882 | Lung 54,973 | Lung 27,394 |
| Prostate 34,240 | Brain and CNS 218 | Non-Hodgkin's lymphomas 524 | Colon and rectum 2,490 | Colon and rectum 13,823 | Prostate 21,486 |
| Colon and rectum 28,434 | Endocrine 93 | Brain and CNS 454 | Non-Hodgkin's lymphomas 1,749 | Prostate 12,407 | Colon and rectum 11,922 |
| Pancreas 12,672 | Non-Hodgkin's lymphomas 53 | Skin 241 | Brain and CNS 1,550 | Pancreas 6,904 | Pancreas 4,390 |
| Leukemia 10,609 | Connective tissue 49 | Hodgkin's disease 232 | Pancreas 1,330 | Non-Hodgkin's lymphomas 4,684 | Leukemia 3,959 |

| FEMALES | | | | | |
|---|---|---|---|---|---|
| **All Ages** | **Under 15** | **15–34** | **35–54** | **55–74** | **75 +** |
| All Cancer 245,740 | All Cancer 742 | All Cancer 3,457 | All Cancer 29,961 | All Cancer 111,663 | All Cancer 99,904 |
| Lung 54,538 | Leukemia 257 | Breast 615 | Breast 9,239 | Lung 31,399 | Lung 17,510 |
| Breast 43,068 | Brain and CNS 218 | Leukemia 460 | Lung 5,491 | Breast 19,395 | Colon and rectum 15,956 |
| Colon and rectum 28,942 | Endocrine 80 | Cervix uteri 347 | Colon and rectum 2,060 | Colon and rectum 10,774 | Breast 13,811 |
| Pancreas 13,399 | Bone 35 | Brain and CNS 301 | Ovary 1,844 | Ovary 6,679 | Pancreas 6,767 |
| Ovary 13,393 | Connective tissue 31 | Non-Hodgkin's lymphomas 218 | Cervix uteri 1,629 | Pancreas 5,763 | Ovary 4,742 |

Reprinted with permission from Parker SL, Tong T, Bolden S, Wingo PA: Cancer statistics, 1996. *CA* 65:5-27, 1996.[114]

## Sex

The incidence of cancers that are not sex-specific (e.g., prostate and cervix) is generally lower in females (Table 4-10).[112] The distributions of cancer types in each sex are shown in Figure 4-2.[114] In part this is due to the differences in lifestyles between the sexes that are associated with cancer; for example, smoking prevalence historically has been lower in females, and therefore smoking-related cancers are less common in females.

## Genetic Predisposition

Epidemiological investigation of genetic predisposition to cancer is growing as developments in molecular biol-ogy make it possible to study genetic markers in large populations. The ongoing Human Genome Project[115] is almost certain to accelerate this work by the discovery of new genes or gene markers associated with increased genetic predisposition for cancer.

Two genes have recently been discovered that are associated with susceptibility to breast cancer, *BRCA1*[116] and *BRCA2*.[117] The *BRCA1* gene is associated with increased susceptibility to both breast and ovarian cancer, whereas *BRCA2* is associated only with an increase in breast cancer. The genes are estimated to be involved in 5% of breast cancer cases and appear to be more strongly associated with breast cancer diagnosed at an early age. Much work remains to be done to further investigate the

**TABLE 4-10** Age-Adjusted Cancer Incidence for Males and Females, 1973–1987 (per 100,000)

| Site | Males |  | Females |  |
|---|---|---|---|---|
|  | <65 | 65+ | <65 | 65+ |
| Oral and pharynx | 10.7 | 77.6 | 4.1 | 28.9 |
| Esophagus | 3.2 | 34.1 | 0.9 | 10.8 |
| Stomach | 4.7 | 79.6 | 2.1 | 35.9 |
| Colon/rectum | 22.1 | 417.5 | 16.6 | 288.0 |
| Liver and intrahepatic | 1.9 | 22.2 | 0.8 | 8.5 |
| Pancreas | 4.5 | 72.8 | 3.1 | 55.8 |
| Larynx | 4.9 | 40.7 | 1.1 | 6.2 |
| Lung and bronchus | 38.4 | 502.2 | 20.5 | 173.7 |
| Melanoma of skin | 8.5 | 39.8 | 7.7 | 19.5 |
| Urinary bladder | 11.1 | 197.4 | 3.0 | 47.5 |
| Kidney and renal pelvis | 6.2 | 57.8 | 3.0 | 26.0 |
| Brain and nervous system | 5.4 | 22.8 | 3.8 | 16.5 |
| Thyroid gland | 2.0 | 6.5 | 5.7 | 8.8 |
| Hodgkin's disease | 3.1 | 5.1 | 2.2 | 3.0 |
| Non-Hodgkin's lymphoma | 8.9 | 73.1 | 5.5 | 55.0 |
| Multiple myeloma | 2.0 | 33.8 | 1.4 | 22.3 |
| Leukemia | 6.6 | 72.0 | 4.4 | 37.4 |

Reprinted from Ries et al.[112]

effects of these genes, including how other known risk factors for breast cancer modulate the risk conferred by the breast cancer genes.

Familial polyposis of the colon is an example of an autosomal dominant syndrome, where those with the syndrome develop colon cancer at a young age, in their 30s or 40s, and have a high number of adenomatous polyps in the colon. The genetic steps required for the development of colon cancer have been studied in subjects with familial polyposis as well as in unaffected individuals who have adenomas or colon cancer. Vogelstein and colleagues[118] reported that the steps include mutational activation of an oncogene, coupled with the loss of several genes that normally suppress tumorigenesis. The mutation affecting individuals with familial polyposis, located on chromosome 5, represents one of these steps.

It has been observed for many years that cancer aggregates in some families. Such familial aggregation could be due to an inherited susceptibility or to common familial exposure(s), for example, diet. The majority of studies of this phenomenon have identified cancer familial aggregation for one cancer type, for example, colon cancer in relatives of individuals with colon cancer. However, Li and Fraumeni have identified an autosomal dominant syndrome from studying the kindred of children with

rhabdomyosarcoma[119] in which the kindred have increased risk of developing cancers other than rhabdomyosarcoma. The genetic defect in these families may be a mutation in the suppressor gene $p53$.[120]

Some gene defects may increase a person's risk for cancer because they have an impact on carcinogen metabolism. It has been found that subjects who have slow acetylator status (i.e., the metabolism of aromatic amines by acetyltransferase is comparatively slow) are at higher risk for bladder cancer in certain occupational settings.[121] Acetylator status is genetically determined. Similarly, subjects who are slow metabolizers of the probe drug debrisoquine, due to a recessive Mendelian trait, appear to be at lower risk for lung cancer.[122]

## Ethnicity and Race

Ethnicity and race can be important issues to assess in epidemiological research. However, several factors must be borne in mind when considering these points. First, ethnicity and race are both prone to misclassification. There is no accepted scientific definition for race. An individual may have grandparents from two or more ethnic or racial backgrounds, and could be classified in many ways. Frost and Shy, in a study of childhood deaths,[123] found that race at birth and race at death were different for 12% of African-Americans and 34% of Native Americans, indicating the complexity of this problem.

Second, ethnicity and race are often highly correlated with SES. African-Americans, American Hispanics, and Native Americans generally have a lower SES than white non-Hispanics. Distinguishing an ethnic or racial effect from a socioeconomic effect may be difficult.

However, assessing biological or genetic differences, along with cultural differences, that may make an ethnic or racial group at increased or decreased risk of a specific cancer is important so that special attention can be given to high-risk groups. Racial or ethnic groups may also differ in attitudes to illness, care seeking, and prevention. It is important to identify such differences so that approaches can be tailored to each group to increase preventive health behavior.

There are four main racial/ethnic groups in the United States: African-Americans (blacks), Hispanic Americans, Asian/Pacific Islanders, and Native Americans. For most cancer sites, African-Americans have higher incidence rates than non-Hispanic Caucasians; in contrast, Hispanics and Native Americans have, overall, lower incidence rates.[124] A comparison of cancer incidence and mortality rates for African-Americans and non-Hispanic whites is shown in Figure 4-3.[125]

## Socioeconomic Factors

Socioeconomic status is usually assessed by data on income, education, or percent below the poverty level,

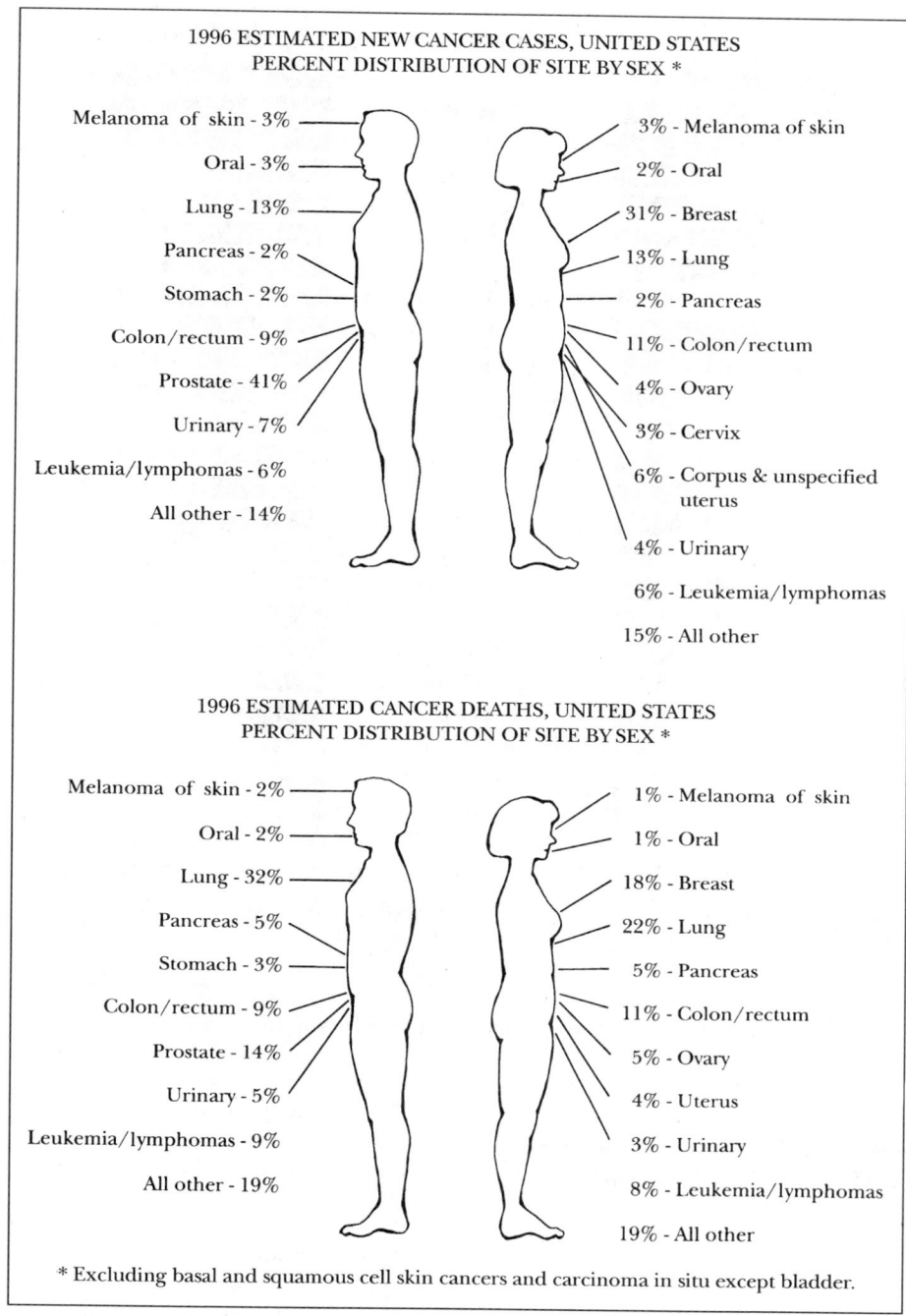

**FIGURE 4-2** Estimated cancer incidence and deaths by site and sex for 1996. (Reprinted with permission from Parker et al.[114])

and has been found to be associated with some cancers, independent of race.[126] Clearly, SES is not a cause of cancer but is a proxy measure for lifestyle characteristics that differ for cancer type and the particular situation under study. For example, cervical cancer has been associated with lower SES. In this case SES may be a proxy for the number of partners the individual or her

male spouse or partners have had; the larger the number, the greater the chance of the female partner's being HPV-positive. Alternatively, SES may be a proxy for Pap test frequency.

SES is now strongly associated with smoking prevalence, with low-income earners being more likely to smoke cigarettes.[127] Therefore, higher lung cancer rates

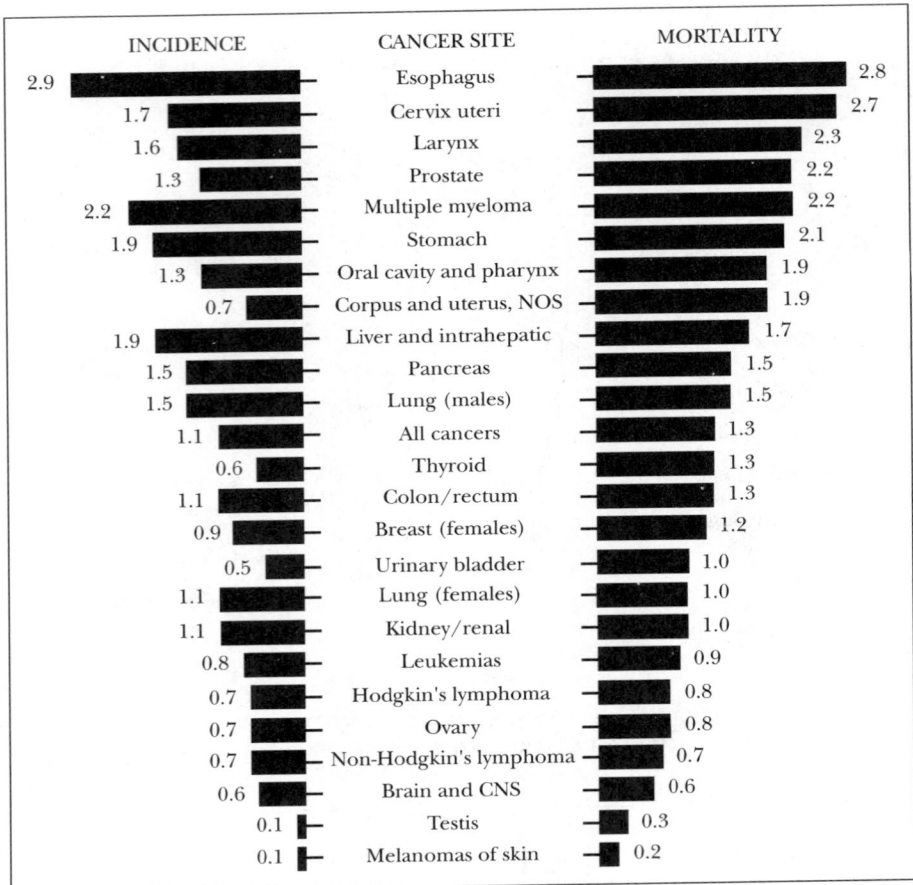

**FIGURE 4-3** SEER cancer incidence and U.S. mortality rates, 1988–1992: Ratio of black rate to white rate for all ages. (Reprinted from Kosary et al.[125])

in the lower SES group are likely to be due to this association.

## OTHER APPLICATIONS OF EPIDEMIOLOGY IN ONCOLOGY

### Survival

Survival analysis is the calculation of the probability that an individual with a specific disease will be alive at a particular time point after diagnosis; five years is commonly used as this time point. For most cancers the survival rate is greatly affected by the stage of cancer at diagnosis. For example, the five-year survival rate for melanoma diagnosed as local disease is 87%; in comparison, the equivalent survival rate for metastatic melanoma is 11%. The histology of the cancer also affects survival time. For example, men with oat cell lung cancer have a five-year survival rate of 4%, in comparison to other lung histologies, where the five-year survival is 13%. African-Americans have a lower survival rate for most cancer sites as compared with whites (Figure 4-4),[125] due in part to the distribution of stage at diagnosis for the two groups. In turn, stage at diagnosis may be influenced by knowledge or attitudes about cancer (e.g., the importance of early diagnosis). Lack of access to care may also cause a delay in diagnosis.

Survival analysis is also used to assess the effectiveness of new treatment modalities for cancer, where survival following the new treatment is compared with survival following the standard treatment.

## CANCER CONTROL

*Cancer control* has been defined as "the reduction of cancer incidence, morbidity, and mortality through an orderly sequence, from research on interventions and their impact in defined populations to the broad, systematic application of the research results."[128] In this definition the term *cancer control* encompasses both cancer preven-

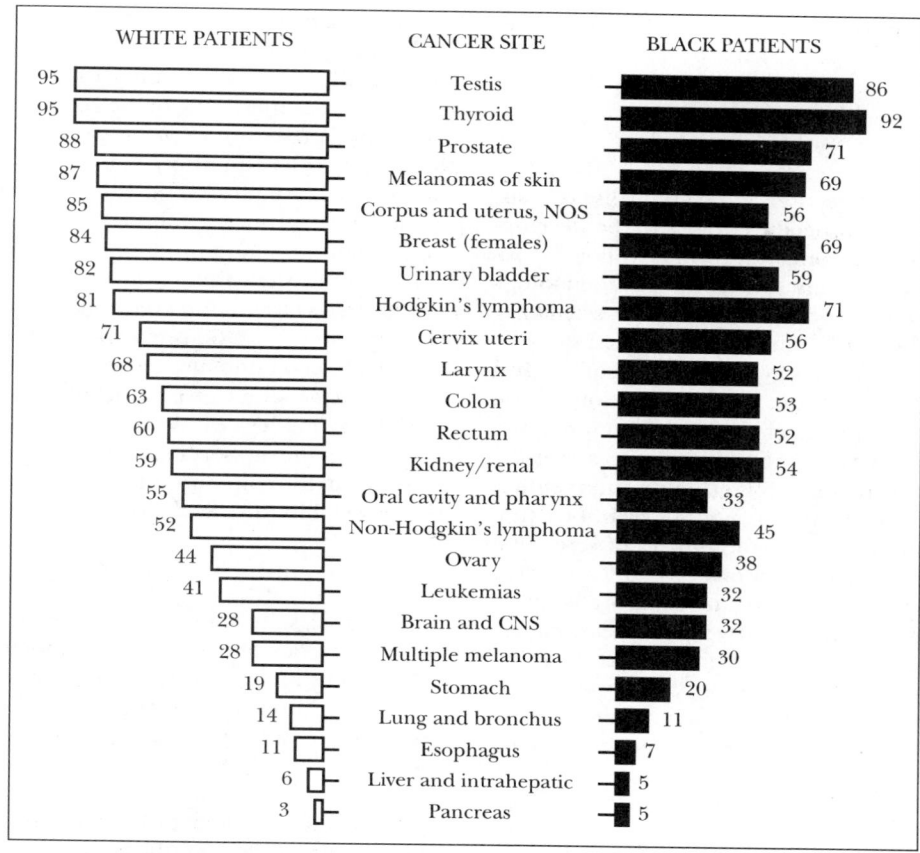

**FIGURE 4-4** Five-year relative survival rates for black and white patients: SEER Program, 1983–1991. (Reprinted from Kosary et al.[125])

tion and control. The term will be used similarly in this chapter.

In 1985 Greenwald and Cullen[128] pointed out the need for a national strategy for cancer control so that the results of research efforts of the National Cancer Program could be translated into a nationwide reduction in cancer incidence and mortality. To help improve cancer control, a model for cancer control research was developed, the phases of which are shown in Figure 4-5.[128] In phase I, hypotheses are developed from basic biomedical research, for example, from the results of epidemiological research. In phase II the necessary methods are then developed, for example, the feasibility of an intervention is examined. In phase III the efficacy of the intervention is being determined in a group of subjects. In phase IV the impact of the intervention is tested using a sample representative of a large target population. In phase V an intervention that has been proven effective in phase IV is applied to a larger population, and the effect of the intervention in the population is evaluated.

In the Healthy People 2000 Study,[129] high-priority research needs for cancer control science in the United States were identified. These needs reflect the numerous disciplines and areas of research involved in the field of

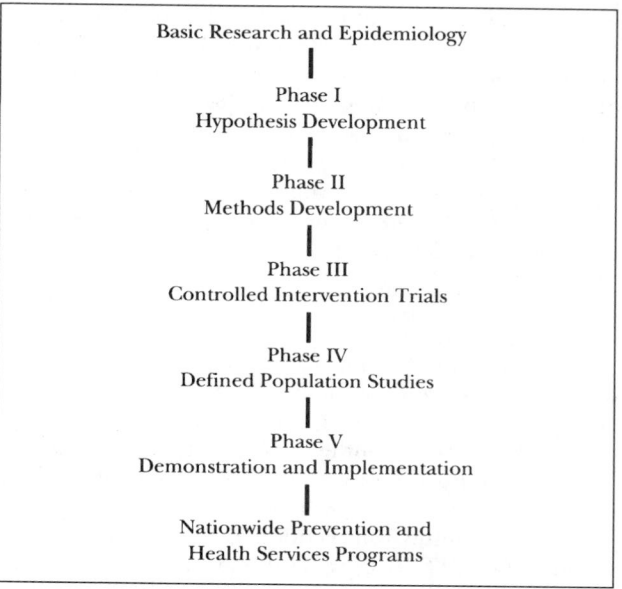

**FIGURE 4-5** Phases of cancer control research. (Reprinted with permission from Greenwald and Cullen.[128])

cancer control. Some of the main areas of research involved in cancer control are discussed next.

## Screening

*Screening* refers to the detection of disease by use of tests, examinations, or other procedures prior to the development of symptoms. Additional test(s) must follow a positive screening test to diagnose the disease. Epidemiology is an important aspect of developing and evaluating screening programs. During development, data must be available on the incidence, prevalence, distribution, and natural history of the disease. The distribution of the disease may influence the target population for screening and so improve the cost-benefit ratio of the screening program. Evaluation requires following an intervention (screened) population and a nonintervention (unscreened) population to assess the impact of screening on mortality. An implicit assumption regarding screening is that early detection will lead to a more favorable prognosis because treatment begun early in the disease course will be more effective than later treatment. This has shown to be the case for mammography and breast cancer mortality;[130] however, early detection of lung cancer using cytology or x-rays has proved to have no effect in reducing lung cancer mortality.[131]

## Barriers to Participation in Screening Programs

General barriers to participation in screening programs have been reviewed by Melnyk[132] and include cost, availability, discrimination, time, and patient characteristics such as culture and knowledge. These factors can prevent individuals from benefiting from early detection of cancer. Several studies show that females from minority groups or of low SES are less likely to seek mammography or Pap tests for screening.[133,134] In the study of Stein and colleagues,[134] specific barriers to receiving mammography included lack of knowledge, cost, embarrassment, and fear of radiation. Interventions to increase screening compliance, especially among low-utilizer groups, must continue to be developed.

### Behavioral change

Increasing public knowledge regarding a risk factor for cancer does not automatically result in a behavioral change within the at-risk group. Groups with differing characteristics, for example, demographics or risk behaviors, may require differing interventions to achieve behavioral change.

The Community Intervention Trial for Smoking Cessation (COMMIT)[135] is an example of a program that incorporated several intervention strategies, the goal of which was to increase smoking cessation. COMMIT incorporated many interventions that had been shown to be individually successful. Within the target communities, several task forces were formed, each of which had several goals. For example, some of the goals of the Public Education Task Force were to promote social action that leads to a smoke-free community, to maintain quality and quantity of tobacco education in local schools, and to reduce adolescent exposure to tobacco products by encouraging endorsement of approved restrictions. In this trial, 22 communities were randomized to receive the intervention or to receive no intervention. The results of the trial showed that the multifaceted approach used in COMMIT had no effect on smoking cessation rates in heavy smokers (the primary target group) but had a significant effect in light to moderate smokers.[136] Such divergent results emphasize the importance of testing intervention approaches at the community level and measuring the effectiveness within different groups.

### Government policy

National, state, and local government have an impact on cancer control through legislation. Such legislation may directly affect cancer control. For example, in 1990 legislative action made screening mammography a covered benefit under Medicare.[137] Legislation may also indirectly affect cancer control. An example is recent legislation to mandate food labeling and to address the issue of health claims made by food companies.[138] This legislation will provide the public with information with which to select a healthier diet. Many state and local governments have restricted smoking in public places, effectively reducing the public's exposure to sidestream smoke.

Cancer control efforts are affected by the monies specifically appropriated to cancer control in the National Institutes of Health budget by the government. The government can influence advancement in this area by setting national goals for cancer control, such as those in the Healthy People 2000 document.

## THE APPLICATION OF EPIDEMIOLOGY TO NURSING PRACTICE

Nursing professionals play integral roles in all aspects of cancer prevention and cancer control. These involve the planning and implementation of cancer screening and educational programs, the design and coordination of cancer-related research projects, and clinical application of cancer control treatments. These roles involve much more than data collection: nurses function as principal investigators, as program directors, as educators, and as patient managers.

Within their roles in cancer prevention and control, nurses apply epidemiological data and research principles to three main phases of their work:[139]

1. *The development phase.* The epidemiological statistics of cancer incidence and mortality assist nursing professionals in identifying high-risk groups and individuals within their patient community. Changes in incidence and mortality rates over time, demographic characteristics of cancer patients, health-related behaviors, and environmental conditions associated with cancer promotion can be obtained through epidemiological data. These data can provide a basis for the development of research hypotheses and the theoretical foundation for program planning.

2. *The planning phases of research and prevention programs.* By using appropriate epidemiological research principles, nurses can design studies that are focused, valid, and ultimately important in the scientific and clinical communities. Program development and short- and long-term goals for cancer prevention and control can be based on epidemiological evidence from previous projects and new surveys that highlight changing cancer trends.

3. *The evaluation phase.* Via appropriate statistical methods, changes in cancer incidence and mortality rates, in stage of disease at diagnosis, in behavioral changes, and in survival time can be used to evaluate program effectiveness.

In all of these areas in which nurses are full participants, epidemiology supplies important information and the methodological foundation for the development, planning, and evaluation of cancer prevention and control programs.

## REFERENCES

1. MacMahon B, Pugh TF: *Epidemiology: Principles and Methods.* Boston, Little, Brown, 1970

2. Rothman K: *Modern Epidemiology.* Boston, Little, Brown, 1986, pp 92–94

3. Hennekens CH, Buring JE: *Epidemiology in Medicine.* Boston, Little, Brown, 1987

4. Walter SD, Marrett LD, From L, et al: The association of cutaneous malignant melanoma with the use of sunbeds and sunlamps. *Am J Epidemiol* 131:232–243, 1990

5. Horowitz RL, Feinstein AR: Alternative analytic methods for case-control studies of estrogens and endometrial cancer. *N Engl J Med* 299:1089–1094, 1978

6. Dawber TR: *The Framingham Study: The Epidemiology of Atherosclerotic Disease.* Cambridge, MA, Harvard University Press, 1980

7. Postservice mortality among Vietnam veterans: The Centers for Disease Control Vietnam Experience Study. *JAMA* 257:790–795, 1987

8. The Steering Committee of the Physicians' Health Study Research Group. Preliminary Report: Findings from the aspirin component of the ongoing physicians' health study. *N Engl J Med* 318:262–263, 1988

9. Hennekens CH, Buring JE, Manson JE, et al: Lack of effect of long-term supplementation with beta carotene on the incidence of malignant neoplasms and cardiovascular disease. *N Engl J Med* 334:1145–1149, 1996

10. Doll R, Peto R: The causes of cancer: Quantitative estimates of avoidable risks of cancer in the United States today. *J Natl Cancer Inst* 66:1193–1308, 1981

11. *Tobacco Smoking,* IARC Monographs on the Evaluation of Carcinogenic Risks of Chemicals to Humans, vol 38. Lyon, France, International Agency for Research on Cancer, 1986

12. Wynder EL, Hoffman D: Tobacco, in Schottenfeld D, Fraumeni JF Jr (eds): *Cancer Epidemiology and Prevention.* Philadelphia, Saunders, 1982, pp 277–292

13. U.S. Department of Health and Human Services, Office on Smoking and Health: *The Health Consequences of Smoking: Cancer.* A Report of the Surgeon General. DHHS[PHS] 82-50179. Washington, DC: U.S. Government Printing Office, 1982

14. Rogot E: Smoking and mortality among U.S. veterans. *J Chronic Dis* 27:189–203, 1974

15. Janerich DT, Thompson WD, Varela LR, et al: Lung cancer and exposure to tobacco smoke in the household. *N Engl J Med* 323:632–636, 1990

16. Fielding JE, Phenow KJ: Health effects of involuntary smoking. *N Engl J Med* 319:1452–1460, 1988

17. Ives, JC, Buffler PA, Selwyn BJ, et al: Lung cancer mortality among women employed in high-risk industries and occupations in Harris County, Texas, 1977–1980, *Am J Epidemiol* 127:65–74, 1988

18. Blot WJ, Fraumeni JF: Passive smoking and lung cancer. *J Natl Cancer Inst* 77:993–1000, 1986

19. Blot WJ, Fraumeni JF: Passive smoking and cancer, in DeVita VT Jr, Hellman S, Rosenberg SA (eds): *Cancer Prevention.* Philadelphia, Lippincott, 1989, pp 1–10

20. Tredaniel J, Boffetta P, Saracci R, et al: Exposure to environmental tobacco smoke and risk of lung cancer: The epidemiological evidence. *Eur Respir J* 7:1877–1888, 1994

21. Rouse BA: Epidemiology of smokeless tobacco use: A national study. *NCI Monogr* 8:29–33, 1989

22. Mattson ME, Winn DM: Smokeless tobacco: Association with increased cancer risk. *NCI Monogr* 8:13–16, 1989

23. Fiore MC, Novotny TE, Pierce JP: Trends in cigarette smoking in the United States: The changing influence of gender and race. *JAMA* 261:49–55, 1989

24. Devasa SS, Blot WJ, Fraumeni JF: Declining lung cancer rates among young men and women in the United States: A cohort analysis. *J Natl Cancer Inst* 81:1568–1571, 1989

25. Nelson DE, Giovino GA, Shopland DR, et al: Trends in cigarette smoking among US adolescents, 1974 through 1991. *JAMA* 85:34–40, 1995

26. Brown CC, Kessler LG: Projections of lung cancer mortality in the U.S. 1985–2025. *J Natl Cancer Inst* 80:43–51, 1988

27. Mahaney FX Jr: Lung cancer rates in white males leveling off. *J Natl Cancer Inst* 84:83–84, 1992

28. Novotny TE, Fiore MC, Hatziandreu EJ, et al: Trends in smoking by age and sex, United States, 1974–1987: The implications for disease impact. *Prev Med* 19:552–561, 1990

29. Centers for Disease Control (CDC): Smoking-attributable mortality and years of potential life lost—United States, 1988. *MMWR* 40:62–63, 69–71, 1991

30. Armstrong B, Doll R: Environmental factors and cancer incidence and mortality in different countries, with special reference to dietary practices. *Int J Cancer* 15:617–631, 1975

31. Willett WC (ed): *Nutritional Epidemiology.* New York, Oxford University Press, 1990

32. Willett WC: Implications of total energy intake for epidemiologic analyses, in Willett W (ed): *Nutritional Epidemiology.* New York, Oxford University Press, 1990, pp 245–271

33. Willett WC, Stampfer MJ, Colditz GA, et al: Dietary fat and the risk of breast cancer. *N Engl J Med* 316:22–28, 1987

34. Hunter D: Biochemical indicators of dietary intake, in Willett W (ed): *Nutritional Epidemiology.* New York, Oxford University Press, 1990, pp 143–216

35. Doll R: Lifestyle: An overview. *Cancer Detect Prev* 14:589–594, 1990

36. Wynder EL, Shigermatsu T: Environmental factors of cancer of the colon and rectum. *Cancer* 20:1520–1561, 1967

37. Whittemore AS, Wu-Williams AH, Lee M, et al: Diet, physical activity and colorectal cancer among Chinese in North America and China. *J Natl Cancer Inst* 82:915–926, 1990

38. Jain M, Cook GM, Davis FG, et al: A case-control study of diet and colo-rectal cancer. *Int J Cancer* 26:757–768, 1980

39. Lyon JL, Mahoney AW, West DW, et al: Energy intake: Its relationship to colon cancer risk. *J Natl Cancer Inst* 78:853–861, 1987

40. Potter JD, McMichael AJ: Diet and cancer of the colon and rectum: A case-control study. *J Natl Cancer Inst* 76:557–569, 1986

41. Trock B, Lanza E, Greenwald P: Dietary fiber, vegetables, and colon cancer: Critical review and meta-analyses of the epidemiologic evidence. *J Natl Cancer Inst* 82:650–651, 1990

42. Slattery ML, Sorenson AW, Ford MH: Dietary calcium intake as a mitigating factor in colon cancer. *Am J Epidemiol* 128:504–514, 1988

43. Garland C, Shekell RB, Barrett-Connor E, et al: Dietary vitamin D and calcium, and risk of colorectal cancer: A 19-year prospective study in men. *Lancet* 1:307–309, 1985

44. Sorenson AW, Slattery ML, Ford MH: Calcium and colon cancer: A review. *Nutr Cancer* 11:135–145, 1988

45. Kune S, Kune GA, Watson LF: Case-control study of dietary etiological factors: The Melbourne Colorectal Cancer Study. *Nutr Cancer* 9:21–42, 1987

46. Newmark HL, Lipkin M: Calcium, vitamin D and colon cancer. *Cancer Res* 52:2067s–2070s, 1992

47. Howe GR, Hirohata T, Hislop TG, et al: Dietary factors and risk of breast cancer: Combined analysis of 12 case-control studies. *J Natl Cancer Inst* 82:561–569, 1990

48. Willett W, Hunter D, Stampfer MJ, et al: Dietary fat and breast cancer: Eight-year follow-up. Program and abstracts of the 15th Annual Meeting of the American Society of Preventive Oncology, 1991

49. Kushi L, Potter J, Drinkard C, et al: Dietary fat and risk of breast cancer according to hormone receptor status. *Cancer Epidemiol Biomarkers Prev* 4:9–11, 1995

50. Steinmetz KA, Potter JD: Vegetables, fruit and cancer: I. Epidemiology. *Cancer Causes Control* 2:325–327, 1991

51. Wattenberg LW: Inhibition of carcinogenesis by minor dietary constituents. *Cancer Res* 52:2085s–2091s, 1992

52. Moon TE, Micozzi MS: *Nutrition and Cancer Prevention: Investigating the Role of Micronutrients.* New York, Marcel Dekker, 1989

53. The Alpha-Tocopherol, Beta-Carotene Cancer Prevention Study Group: The effect of vitamin E and beta-carotene on the incidence of lung cancer and other cancers in male smokers. *N Engl J Med* 330:1029–1035, 1994

54. Omenn GS, Foodman GE, Thornquist MD, et al: Effects of a combination of beta carotene and vitamin A on lung cancer and cardiovascular disease. *N Engl J Med* 334:1150–1155, 1996

55. Freedman LS, Prentice RL, Clifford C, et al: Dietary fat and breast cancer: Where are we? *J Natl Cancer Inst* 85:764–765, 1993

56. Alberts D, Ritenbaugh C, Story J, et al: Randomized, double-blinded, placebo-controlled study of effect of wheat bran fiber and calcium on fecal bile acids in patients with resected adenomatous colon polyps. *J Natl Cancer Inst* 88:81–92, 1996

57. Greenwald P, Kelloff G, Burch-Whitman C, et al: Chemoprevention. *CA Cancer J Clin* 45:31–49, 1995

58. *The Executive Summary in Diet and Health: Implications for Reducing Chronic Disease.* Washington, DC, National Academy Press, 1989, pp 3–22

59. Longnecker MP: Alcohol consumption in relation to risk of breast cancer: Meta-analysis and review. *Cancer Causes Control* 5:73–82, 1994

60. *Alcohol Drinking.* IARC Monographs on the Evaluation of Carcinogenic Risks of Chemicals to Humans, vol 44. Lyon, France, International Agency for Research on Cancer, 1988

61. Seitz HK, Simanowski UA: Alcohol and colorectal carcinogenesis, in Watson RR (ed): *Alcohol and Cancer.* Boca Raton, FL, CRC Press, 1992, pp 167–177

62. Spiegelhalder B, Eisenbrand G, Preussmann R: Contamination of beer with trace quantities of N-nitrosodimethylamine. *Food Cosmet Toxicol* 17:29–31, 1979

63. Longnecker MP, Newcomb PA, Mittendorf R, et al: Risk of breast cancer in relation to lifetime alcohol consumption. *J Natl Cancer Inst* 87:923–929, 1995

64. Byers T: Nutritional risk factors for breast cancer. *Cancer* 74:288–295, 1994

65. Colditz GA: A prospective assessment of moderate alcohol intake and major chronic diseases. *Ann Epidemiol* 1:167–177, 1990

66. Washburn RA, Montoye HJ: The assessment of physical activity by questionnaire. *Am J Epidemiol* 123:563–576, 1986

67. Slattery ML, Abd-Elghany N, Derber R, et al: Physical activity and colon cancer: A comparison of various indicators of physical activity to evaluate the association. *Epidemiology* 1:481–485, 1990

68. Gerhardsson De Verdier M, Steinbeck G, Hagman U, et al: Physical activity and colon cancer: A case-referent study in Stockholm. *Int J Cancer* 46:985–989, 1990

69. Albanes D, Blair A, Taylor PR: Physical activity and risk of cancer in NHANES 1 population. *Am J Public Health* 79:744–750, 1989

70. Kono S, Shinchi K, Ikeda N, et al: Physical activity, dietary habits and adenomatous polyps of the sigmoid colon: A study of self-defense officials in Japan. *J Clin Epidemiol* 44:1255–1261, 1991

71. Bernstein L, Ross RK, Henderson B: Prospects for the primary prevention of breast cancer. *Am J Epidemiol* 135:142–152, 1992

72. Bernstein L, Henderson BE, Hanisch R, et al: Physical exercise and reduced risk of breast cancer in young women. *J Natl Cancer Inst* 86:1403–1408, 1994

73. Merzenick H, Boeing H, Wahrendorf J: Dietary fat and sports activity as determinants for age at menarche. *Am J Epidemiol* 138:217–224, 1993

74. Searle CE, Teale OJ: Occupational carcinogens, in Born GV, Cooper CS, Grover PL (eds): *Chemical Carcinogenesis and Mutagenesis 1: Handbook of Experimental Pharmacology,* vol 94/1. Berlin, Springer-Verlag, 1990 pp 103–151

75. Tomatis L (ed): Pollution, in *Cancer: Causes, Occurrence and Control.* Lyon, France, International Agency for Research on Cancer Scientific Publications, 1990, pp 229–239

76. Tseng WP: Effects and dose-response relationships of skin

cancer and blackfoot disease with arsenic. *Environ Health Perspect* 19:109–119, 1977

77. Morton W, Starr G, Pohl D, et al: Skin cancer and water arsenic in Lane County, Oregon. *Cancer* 37:2523–2532, 1976

78. Morris RD, Audet A, Angelillo IF, et al: Chlorination, chlorination by-products and cancer: A meta analysis. *Am J Public Health* 82:955–963, 1992

79. McFarland M, Kaye J: Chlorofluorocarbons and ozone. *Photochem Photobiol* 55:911–929, 1992

80. National Institutes of Health Consensus Development Conference Statement: *Sunlight, Ultraviolet Radiation, and the Skin.* Bethesda, MD, U.S. Department of Health and Human Services, Public Health Service, National Institutes of Health, Office of Medical Applications of Research, 1989

81. Pike M: The prevention of breast, endometrial and ovarian cancer, in Fortner JG, Rhoads JE (eds): *Accomplishments in Cancer Research.* Philadelphia, Lippincott, 1989, pp 327–356

82. Ley C, Bauer HM, Reingold A, et al: Determinants of genital human papillomavirus infection in young women. *J Natl Cancer Inst* 83:997–1003, 1991

83. Zur Hausen H: Viruses in human cancers. *Science* 254:1167–1173, 1991

84. Henderson BE: Establishment of an association between a virus and a human cancer. *J Natl Cancer Inst* 81:320–321, 1989

85. Schiffman MH, Bauer HM, Hoover RN, et al: Epidemiologic evidence showing that human papillomavirus infection causes most cervical intraepithelial neoplasia. *J Natl Cancer Inst* 85:958–964, 1993

86. Munoz N: Is *Helicobacter pylori* a cause of gastric cancer? An appraisal of the seroepidemiological evidence. *Epidemiol Biomarkers Prev* 3:445–451, 1994

87. Gentile JM: Schistosome-related cancers: A possible role for genotoxins. *Environ Mutagen* 7:775–785, 1985

88. Henderson BE, Ross RK, Pike MC: Toward the primary prevention of cancer. *Science* 254:1131–1138, 1991

89. Shigematsu I, Kagan A (eds): *Cancer in Atomic Bomb Survivors.* Japanese Cancer Association. GANN Monograph on Cancer Research 32. Tokyo, Scientific Societies Press; New York, Plenum Press, 1986

90. BEIR III, Committee on the Biological Effects of Ionizing Radiation: *The Effects on Populations of Exposure to Low Levels of Ionizing Radiation.* Washington, DC, National Academy Press, 1980

91. Lubin JH, Boice JD, Edling C, et al: Lung cancer in radon-exposed miners and estimation of risk from indoor exposure. *J Natl Cancer Inst* 87:817–826, 1995

92. *Exposure of the U.S. Population to Occupational Radiation.* NCRP report No. 101. Bethesda, MD, National Council on Radiation Protection and Measurements, 1989

93. Strickland PT, Vitasa BC, West SK, et al: Quantitative carcinogenesis in man: Solar ultraviolet B dose dependence of skin cancer in Maryland watermen. *J Natl Cancer Inst* 81:1910–1913, 1989

94. Grodstein F, Speizer FE, Hunter DJ: A prospective study of incident squamous cell carcinoma of the skin in the Nurses' Health Study. *J Natl Cancer Inst* 87:1061–1066, 1995

95. Armstrong BK, English DR: Epidemiologic studies, in Balch CM, Houghton AN, Milton GW, et al (eds): *Cutaneous Melanoma* (ed 2). Philadelphia, Lippincott, 1992, pp 12–20

96. Adey WR: Joint actions of environmental nonionizing electromagnetic fields and chemical pollution in cancer promotion. *Environ Health Perspect* 86:297–305, 1990

97. Savitz DA, Pearce NE, Poole C: Methodological issues in the epidemiology of electromagnetic fields and cancer. *Epidemiol Rev* 131:763–773, 1990

98. London SJ, Bowman JD, Sobel E, et al: Exposure to magnetic fields among electrical workers in relationship to leukemia risk in Los Angeles County. *Am J Indust Med* 26:47–60, 1994

99. Preston-Martin S, Navidi W, Thomas D, et al: Los Angeles study of residential magnetic fields and childhood brain tumors. *Am J Epidemiol* 143:105–119, 1996

100. Gurney JG, Mueller BA, Davis S, et al: Childhood brain tumor occurrence in relation to residential power line configurations, electric heating sources, and electric appliance use. *Am J Epidemiol* 143:120–128, 1996

101. Poole C: Invited commentary: Evolution of epidemiologic evidence on magnetic fields and childhood cancers. *Am J Epidemiol* 143:120–128, 1996

102. Tomatis L: Drugs and exogenous sex hormones, in *Cancer: Causes, Occurrence and Control.* Lyon, France, International Association for Research on Cancer Scientific Publications, 1990, pp 148–154

103. Stern RS, Thibodeau LA, Kleinerman RA, et al: Risk of cutaneous carcinoma in patients treated with oral methoxsalen photochemotherapy for psoriasis. *N Engl J Med* 300:809–813, 1979

104. Herbst AL, Ulfelder H, Poskanzer DC: Adenocarcinoma of the vagina: Association of maternal stilbestrol therapy with tumor appearance in young women. *N Engl J Med* 284:878–881, 1971

105. The WHO collaborative study of neoplasia and steroid contraceptives: Endometrial cancer and combined oral contraceptives: *Int J Epidemiol* 17:263–269, 1988

106. Henderson BE, Preston-Martin S, Edmonson HA, et al: Hepatocellular carcinoma and oral contraceptives. *Br J Cancer* 48:437–440, 1983

107. Briton LA, Daling JR, Liff JM, et al: Oral contraceptives and breast cancer risk among younger women. *J Natl Cancer Inst* 87:827–835, 1995

108. Rosenberg L, Palmer JR, Rao RS, et al: Case-control study of oral contraceptive use and risk of breast cancer. *Am J Epidemiol* 143:25–37, 1996

109. Lobo RO: Benefits and risks of estrogen replacement therapy. *Am J Obstet Gynecol* 173:982–989, 1995

110. Key TJA, Pike MC: The role of oestrogens and progestagens in the epidemiology and prevention of breast cancer. *Eur J Cancer Clin Oncol* 24:29–43, 1988

111. Newcomb PA, Storer BE: Postmenopausal hormone use and risk of large-bowel cancer. *J Natl Cancer Inst* 87:1067–1071, 1995

112. Ries LAG, Hankey BF, Edwards BK (eds): *Cancer Statistics Review 1973–1987.* U.S. Department of Health and Human Services, NIH publication No. 90-2789, Bethesda, MD, 1991

113. Holmes FF: *Aging and Cancer.* New York, Springer-Verlag, 1983

114. Parker SL, Tong T, Bolden S, et al: *Cancer Statistics, 1996. CA Cancer J Clin* 46:5–27, 1996

115. The Human Genome Project: Implications for human genetics. *Am J Hum Genet* 49:687–691, 1991

116. Futreal PA, Liu Q, Shattuck-Eidens De, et al: *BRCA1* mutations in primary breast and ovarian carcinomas. *Science* 266:120–122, 1994

117. Wooster R, Neuhausen SL, Mangion J, et al: Localization of a breast cancer susceptibility gene *BRCA2*, to chromosome 13q12–13. *Science* 265:2088–2090, 1994

118. Vogelstein B, Fearon ER, Hamilton SR, et al: Genetic alterations during colorectal-tumor development. *N Engl J Med* 319:525–532, 1988

119. Li FP, Fraumeni JF Jr: Rhabdomyosarcoma in children: Epidemiologic study and identification of a familial cancer syndrome. *J Natl Cancer Inst* 43:1365–1373, 1969

120. Li FP, Fraumeni JF Jr, Mulvihill JJ, et al: A cancer family syndrome in twenty-four kindreds. *Cancer Res* 48:5358–5362, 1988

121. Cartwright RA, Glashan RW, Rogers HJ, et al: Role of N-acetyltransferase phenotypes in bladder carcinogenesis: A pharmacogenetic epidemiological approach to bladder cancer. *Lancet* 2:842–845, 1982

122. Ayesh R, Idle JR, Ritchie JC, et al: Metabolic oxidation phenotypes as markers for susceptibility to lung cancer. *Nature* 312:169–172, 1984

123. Frost F, Shy KK: Racial differences between linked birth and infant deaths records in Washington State. *Am J Public Health* 70:974–976, 1980

124. Jones LA, Newell GR: Introduction to section 1, in Jones LA (ed): *Minorities and Cancer.* New York, Springer-Verlag, 1989, pp 3–4

125. Kosary CL, Ries LAG, Miller BA, Hankey BF, et al (eds): *SEER Cancer Statistics Review, 1973–1992: Tables and Graphs.* National Cancer Institute, NIH publication No. 96-2789. Bethesda, MD, 1995

126. Baquet CR, Horm JW, Gibbs T, et al: Socioeconomic factors and cancer incidence among blacks and whites. *J Natl Cancer Inst* 83:551–557, 1991

127. Centers for Disease Control, Center for Chronic Disease Prevention and Health Promotion, Office on Smoking and Health: *Tobacco Use in 1986: Methods and Basic Tabulations from Adult Use of Tobacco Survey.* DHHS publication No. OM-90-2004. Rockville, MD, Centers for Disease Control, 1990

128. Greenwald P, Cullen JW: The new emphasis in cancer control. *J Natl Cancer Inst* 74:543–551, 1985

129. *Healthy People 2000: National Health Promotion and Disease Prevention Objectives.* DHHS publication No. (PHS) 91-50212. Washington, DC, U.S. Government Printing Office, 1991

130. Feig SA: Follow-up studies of the Health Insurance Plan Study and the Breast Cancer Detection Demonstration Project Screening Trials in the U.S.A. *Recent Results Cancer Res* 119:39–52, 1988

131. Fontana RS, Sanderson DR, Woolner LB, et al: Screening for lung cancer: A critique of the Mayo Lung Project. *Cancer 67:* 1155–1164, 1991

132. Melnyk KAM: Barriers: A critical review of recent literature. *Nurs Res* 37:196–201, 1988

133. Peters RK, Moraye BB, Thomas D: Barriers to screening for cancer of the cervix. *Prev Med* 18:133–146, 1989

134. Stein JA, Fox SA, Murata PJ: The influence of ethnicity, socioeconomic status, and psychological barriers on use of mammography. *J Health Soc Behav* 32:101–113, 1991

135. COMMIT Research Group: Community Intervention Trial for Smoking Cessation (COMMIT): Summary of design and intervention. *J Natl Cancer Inst* 83:1620–1628, 1991

136. Community Intervention Trial for Smoking Cessation (COMMIT): I. Cohort results from a four-year community intervention. *Am J Public Health* 85:183–192, 1995

137. Oakar MR: Legislative effect of the 102nd Congress: Cancer prevention, detection, treatment, and research. *Cancer* 69:154–156, 1992

138. McNamara S: The brave new world of FDA nutrition regulation: Some thoughts about current trends and long-term effects. *Crit Rev Food Sci Nutr* 34:215–221, 1994

139. Rempusheski VF: Ask an expert. *Appl Nurs Res* 4:96–98, 1991

# PART II

# Prevention, Detection, and Diagnosis

# Chapter 5

# Factors Affecting Health Behavior

Jayne I. Fernsler, RN, DSN, AOCN

Mary Ann Miller, RN, PhD

## INTRODUCTION

Promotion of positive health behavior has become a national initiative. The knowledge that unhealthful personal lifestyle choices account for a large proportion of both morbidity and mortality in the United States and the subsequent cost of these choices to society have been the impetus for major policy and program development.

The health behavior initiative is an important component of cancer care. Personal choices with regard to diet, tobacco use, alcohol consumption, and sun exposure can have a powerful impact on cancer prevention. In addition, personal decisions about learning and performing routine self-examinations, participating in cancer screening activities, and seeking appropriate help when cancer signs and symptoms are noted are pivotal to the early detection and potential cure of cancer. Also, behavior with regard to following a recommended treatment regimen and maintaining a healthful lifestyle while experiencing cancer may enhance both quantity and quality of life. Consequently, individual health behavior is a concern of health care professionals who interact with people at any phase of the cancer continuum.

The purpose of this chapter is to define *health behavior* and related terms, to identify national initiatives, and to describe factors that influence health behavior. Selected models and theories of health behavior are explained, and their applications in research on cancer care are described. Nursing practice implications of health behavior theory and research are discussed in the conclusion of the chapter.

## NATIONAL INITIATIVES

The evolving body of knowledge about the association between personal behavior and cancer control has spurred activity in both the public and the private sectors. Major initiatives are the National Cancer Institute (NCI) objectives for 1985–2000,[1] the American Cancer Society's (ACS) priorities for the 1990s,[2] and the U.S. Department of Health and Human Services (DHHS) objectives for health promotion and disease prevention.[3] The NCI's goal of reducing cancer mortality by 50% by the year 2000, as well as the ACS's stated priority on cancer prevention and detection, and the DHHS objectives for cancer control all focus strongly on efforts to influence people's health behavior. The behaviors of people who are disadvantaged and/or at high risk for cancer are a major target of these efforts.

## DEFINITIONS

### Health Behavior

Generally, *behavior* involves something that people do or refrain from doing, consciously or unconsciously, voluntarily or involuntarily.[4] A number of definitions of health behavior have been advanced by experts in the field. Gochman defines *health behavior* as "those personal attributes, such as beliefs, expectations, motives, values, perceptions, and other cognitive elements; personality characteristics, including affective and emotional states and traits; and overt behavior patterns, actions and habits that relate to health maintenance, to health restoration and to health improvement." Such "personal attributes are influenced by, and otherwise reflect family structure and processes, peer group and social factors, and societal, institutional, and cultural determinants."[5,p.169]

Health behavior involves actions taken by persons who believe they are healthy, and who have not been experiencing any signs or symptoms of illness, in order to remain disease free.[6,7] According to this definition, health behavior is confined to preventive actions. In 1979 Harris and Guten[8] introduced the broader term *health protective behavior* to include both preventive and health-promoting activities. They define it as "any behavior performed by a person, regardless of his or her perceived or actual health status, in order to protect, promote or maintain his or her health, whether or not such behavior is objectively effective toward that end."[8,p.18]

Pender[9] differentiates between the concepts of *health promotion* and *disease prevention*. She defines *health promotion activities* as those directed toward increasing the level of well-being that already exists, thus actualizing the health potential of individuals. Primary prevention activities decrease the probability of specific illnesses; secondary prevention activities focus on early diagnosis and intervention; tertiary prevention activities involve rehabilitation and restoration to optimal level of functioning. Whereas prevention is disease specific, health promotion is not. Prevention represents avoidance behavior, whereas health promotion activities aim to increase one's positive potential for health.

### Illness Behavior

Kasl and Cobb define *illness behavior* as "any activity, undertaken by a person who feels ill, to define the state of his health and to discover a suitable remedy."[6,p.246] Thus, illness behavior refers to a person's perceptions and actions resulting from the recognition of bodily signs or symptoms, recognition of the need for advice, the decision whether to seek it, and the choice of advisor, whether it be relatives, friends, and/or lay or professional health care practitioners.[10–12] Illness behaviors are undertaken to clarify the meaning of certain signs and symptoms. This may mean waiting to see if the symptoms will disappear without therapy.

## Sick Role Behavior

*Sick role behavior* is the activity taken by individuals who believe themselves (or whom others believe) to be ill in order to get well. It usually involves a range of dependent behaviors, includes accepting treatment, and leads to some neglect of one's usual duties.[6]

The distinctions made among these various types of health behaviors (Figure 5-1) and their determinants should not be minimized.[4] Although their apparently common relationship to "health" unites them, more research is needed to confirm underlying commonalities among the categories or to uncover the variety of determinants to which each category is specifically related.[4]

## MODELS AND THEORIES OF HEALTH BEHAVIOR

A number of theories and models to explain health behavior have been developed during the past 20 years. Their evolution has emphasized the complexities of health behavior and its determinants.

To determine similarities and differences among the explanatory approaches to health and illness behavior, Cummings, Becker, and Maile[13] reviewed 14 such models, all drawn from a variety of theoretical constructs and chosen because of their predictive ability and frequency of citation. The authors found the general classes of explanatory variables to be quite similar. A set of six categories emerged from the original 109 variables described in the models. These include attitudes toward health care

benefits and health care quality, perception of symptoms and beliefs about susceptibility to illness, accessibility of health services, knowledge about the disease/condition, social support characteristics, and demographic variables (particularly social status, income, and education). Because there is not a single unifying theory on which the models are based, health care practitioners have had to choose the model that best fits a specific health behavior in order to determine appropriate interventions to stimulate behavior change. Some of the predominant theories and models used to explain health behavior and their application to cancer care are presented in the following sections.

## Social Learning Theory

Bandura's social cognitive theory currently represents one of the most formally developed theories of behavior.[14] It provides an umbrella framework for analyzing health behavior in terms of a continuous, mutual interaction among cognitive, behavioral, and environmental determinants (reciprocal determinism). According to Bandura, "the primary determinants of adoptive behavior are the influences closely tied to it—the stimulus inducements, the anticipated satisfactions, the observed benefits, the experienced functional value, the perceived risks, the self-evaluative derivatives, and the various social barriers and economic constraints."[15,p.54]

The environment is the source of social supports that provide cues for reinforcement of behavior. The environment also provides the social and physical situation within which a person must function. In so doing, it provides the incentives and disincentives for the performance of behavior (expectancies). People have the potential for self-control over their actions. In order to do this, they must have a certain amount of knowledge and skill. They can anticipate certain events and outcomes and respond to them, based on their own past experiences or the

| Behavior | Health | Illness | | Sick role | |
|---|---|---|---|---|---|
| Identity | Healthy | Feel sick | | Am sick | |
| Role performance | Usual social roles | Diminished function | Preparing to enter sick role | Being in sick role | Leaving sick role |
| Health | Health | Asymptomatic disease | Symptoms | Diagnosis | Treatment | Outcome |

**FIGURE 5-1**   Continuum from health to disease, related to behavior, identity, and role performance. (Kasl S, Cobb S: Health behavior, illness behavior, and sick role behavior: I. Health and illness behavior. *Arch Environ Health* 12:246–266, 1966. Reprinted with permission of the Helen Dwight Reid Educational Foundation. Published by Heldref Publications, 1319 Eighteenth St., N.W., Washington, D.C. 20036-1802. Copyright © 1966.)

experiences of others whom they have observed. If all other things are equal, people will choose to perform an activity that maximizes a positive outcome or minimizes a negative one (principle of maximization).[14]

### Sources of influence

Bandura[15] views human behavior in terms of three interdependent sources of influence: antecedent determinants, consequent outcomes, and cognitive determinants of behavior. Antecedent determinants stem from objects or events that precede behavior change. Cognitive factors partly determine which external events will be observed, how they will be perceived, and how information they convey will be organized for future use. In order to function effectively, individuals must anticipate the probable consequences of these different events and courses of action. They then regulate their behavior on the basis of such predictive antecedent events.

The more individuals believe that influences of past events remain viable, and the more severe the outcome they expect (e.g., their perceived susceptibility to ill effects due to a particular behavior), the stronger their anticipatory reaction will be. The failure of anticipated risks to materialize reinforces the expectation that the subsequent behaviors prevented their occurrence. Thus, most behavior is maintained by anticipated rather than by immediate consequences.[15]

Rewarding experiences are repeatedly associated with expressions of the interest and approval of others (their social support) and unrewarding experiences with their disapproval. These social reactions themselves become influential predictors of consequences and become incentives. Thus, the impact of rewards or punishments can be explained in terms of motivation. By representing foreseeable outcomes symbolically, individuals can convert future consequences into current motivations of behavior.[15]

### Efficacy and outcome expectations

Bandura[15] proposes that behavioral changes are generated from the common mechanisms of personal efficacy and outcome expectations. An *outcome expectation* is defined as a personal belief that a given behavior will lead to certain outcomes.[16] An *efficacy expectation* is the conviction that one can successfully execute a specific behavior required to produce a specific outcome.[17,18] Outcome and efficacy expectations are differentiated because individuals can believe that a certain course of action will produce certain outcomes but question whether they can perform those actions. Both outcome and efficacy expectations reflect individuals' beliefs about their capabilities and behavior-outcome links. Although self-efficacy and outcome expectations are conceptually distinct, the types of outcomes that people anticipate are strongly influenced by efficacy expectations, the most important prerequisite for behavior change.[14,19]

The strength of people's convictions in their own ef-

fectiveness determines whether they will even try to cope with difficult situations. Bandura[16] speculates that perceived efficacy forms a mediating link between knowledge and behavior. Efficacy expectations determine how much effort people will expend and how long they will persist in the face of barriers and aversive experiences. In general, stronger efficacy expectations will produce more active and sustained efforts.[18]

Perceptions of efficacy usually are acquired through direct environmental interaction or through social experiences.[18] The most dependable and powerful source of efficacy expectations is personal experience.[15] Another source is vicarious experience, i.e., live or symbolic modeling or seeing what happens to others who perform activities with certain consequences. Of the numerous cues that influence behavior, none is more common than the actions of others.[15,16,20]

A third source of information about efficacy expectations is verbal persuasion. The efficacy expectations that it generates, however, are likely to be weak, and short in duration. The fourth source is one's own physiological state or emotional arousal (anxiety, agitation, fatigue) in threatening situations.[20]

Efficacy expectations vary greatly, depending on a particular task that confronts the person. Individuals with low self-efficacy about a particular task may concentrate on personal deficiencies rather than thinking about accomplishing the task at hand. This can impede successful performance of the task.[21]

### Application of beliefs about self-efficacy to cancer care

In the application of social learning theory to analysis of health behavior, a major task becomes trying to learn what beliefs a person has developed about targeted health problems or behaviors. Taking the theoretical application one step further, one might conclude that, when strong beliefs about health risks are combined with a strong sense of efficacy for avoiding them and a belief in the value of the avoidance behaviors, healthier outcomes can result.

The influence of self-efficacy has been studied in relation to general cancer prevention practices,[22] dietary cancer prevention practices,[23] smoking cessation,[24-27] testicular self-examination (TSE),[28,29] breast self-examination (BSE),[30-34] and compliance with screening for fecal occult blood.[35] Generally, a strong belief in one's ability to carry out a required activity was a powerful influence in the decision to engage in healthy behavior. Self-efficacy has been shown to be particularly influential in promoting positive action among smokers who have contemplated quitting.[25-27] In a study on general health promotion, subjects who smoked had the lowest self-efficacy scores.[36]

### Summary

Social learning theory as an umbrella framework addresses many of the constructs that will be discussed in the models and theories that follow. Along with the Health Belief Model (HBM) and the Theory of Reasoned Action, it contains constructs that can be viewed as belonging to the larger family of expectancy-value theories. Outcome value has been a traditional component of these theories. While the HBM explicitly sets forth outcome benefits/barriers as a variable, Bandura[15] suggests the construct of outcome value by emphasizing the role of rewarding outcomes in determining behavior. The Theory of Reasoned Action includes evaluation of outcomes as a specific determinant of attitude toward behavior. This is another variable that is made explicit in the HBM. There is already a body of research to support the utility of both the concept of self-efficacy, as explained by Bandura,[15] and the variables of the HBM in studies of preventive health behavior.[37,38]

Another influential variable, social support, is alluded to in the reciprocal determinism of social learning theory, the environmental influence proposed by the HBM, and the variable of social norms in the Theory of Reasoned Action. Janis[39] asserts that social support is especially important for individuals who find it difficult to sustain a high level of motivation when pursuing a stressful course of action, such as trying to abstain from smoking. A high level of motivation is often contingent on the presence of "personal assets" or resources, including the presence of "important others" for emotional support.

Early social learning theory also provided the foundation for current behavioral theories that include the variable of personal control. These include locus of control and health locus of control. Control also appears as a variable in attribution theory.

## Health Belief Model

The Health Belief Model (HBM) was originally developed in the 1950s by Rosenstock and Hochbaum to explain preventive health behavior using psychosocial variables and psychological theories of decision making.[40] It evolved from a central tenet of Lewin's theory of goal setting: that behavior depends on the value that individuals attach to a given outcome and their expectation that a particular action will result in that outcome.[41] Translated to health behavior, the value becomes the desire to avoid illness or to get well, and the expectancy is the belief that a particular personal action will prevent or lessen the threat of illness. People will usually choose the behavior that they think will produce the maximum number of good outcomes and the minimum number of bad ones (principle of maximization).[14]

The HBM is based on the assumption that an individual's subjective perception of the environment determines behavior.[42] Variables tested in current applications of the model are susceptibility, severity, benefits, barriers, and self-efficacy. See Table 5-1. Research has shown that the variable *perceived barriers* is the most powerful single predictor of behavior, although *perceived susceptibility* and *benefits* are strong also. *Perceived severity* is the weakest

**TABLE 5-1** Health Belief Model

| Variable | Definition |
|---|---|
| Perceived susceptibility | Perception of vulnerability to a condition |
| Perceived severity | Perception of the seriousness of the consequences of developing a condition |

Together the two variables above constitute a perceived **Threat** and provide the individual with a psychological readiness to take action.

| | |
|---|---|
| Benefits | Effectiveness of the action in reducing threat |
| Barriers | Psychological and other costs or negative aspects associated with the proposed action |
| Cue to action | Stimulus to behave in a certain manner |
| Self-efficacy | Conviction that one can successfully behave in the manner required to achieve a specific outcome |
| **Modifying variables** | |
| Demographic | Age, gender, etc. |
| Structural | Access |
| Attitudinal | Satisfaction |
| Interactional | Patient/practitioner relationship |
| Enabling | Social pressure |

Compiled from Strecher, DeVellis, Becker, et al;[37] Rosenstock;[42,43] Becker, Maiman.[44]

predictor, but appears to be strongly related to sick role behaviors.[38,43]

The stimulus or cue to action may be internal, such as the perception of a symptom, or external, such as interaction with others or mass media communications.[40] Many researchers have found health care providers' recommendations to be a primary cue to action regarding cancer prevention and early detection.[45–50] The true role of such stimuli has been difficult to study because they may be only barely perceptible in the individual's consciousness.[43] If perceived susceptibility and severity are high, relatively insignificant stimuli may result in behavior change but stronger stimuli may be required to effect change in the face of low perceptions of susceptibility and severity.[43]

A 1992 meta-analysis of published research using the HBM as a framework resulted in only 16 studies that met minimal criteria for valid representation of all HBM dimensions.[51] Relatively weak relationships were found between the HBM variables and health behaviors in much of the literature. However, as long as research indicates that the dimensions of the HBM interact systematically in predicting health behavior, the model will continue to guide attempts to understand why people do what they do with regard to their health.

It is believed that self-efficacy must be added to the HBM in order to increase its explanatory power.[37] Efficacy expectations, or the belief that one can successfully execute the behavior required to produce the outcome, are crucial in lifestyle behaviors requiring long-term changes, such as smoking. They affect how much effort a person puts into a given task and what levels of performance are attained. Repetition builds self-efficacy, which affects task persistence and endurance, and thus promotes behavior change.[43]

### Application of the Health Belief Model to health behavior

The HBM has been applied to all preventive health actions, illness behaviors, and sick role behaviors. The model has been one of the most influential and widely used psychosocial approaches to explaining health-related behavior, and, in fact, is one of the few psychosocial models developed expressly to promote understanding of health behavior.[43]

Underlying the ability of the model to explain health behavior is the assumption that people can accept the possibility that they may have a serious illness in the complete absence of symptoms. This may provide the rationale for many decisions to seek screening for health-related reasons. For example, the failure to believe in the possibility of asymptomatic illness may help to explain less-than-desirable responses to cancer screening programs.[43,52]

The HBM is based on the premise that health is a valued goal for most individuals. As such, it can only account for as much of the variation in individuals' health-related behaviors as can be explained by attitudes and beliefs.[38] Other forces also influence behavior. There is a habitual component to some behavior (e.g., smoking); some behaviors occur for nonhealth reasons (e.g., dieting to appear more attractive); and, in some cases, economic or environmental factors prevent an individual from taking a preferred mode of action (e.g., residing in a city with high air pollution).[22,43]

Another limitation of the HBM is its lack of quantification beyond an ordinal scale. One of the advantages of the model, its ability to measure beliefs specific to a given condition, is also one of its limitations. There is not a generic instrument with proven reliability and validity that can be used by all researchers. Instead, a multitude of measures exist, each with different behaviors as targets.

### Application of the Health Belief Model to cancer care

The Health Belief Model has been used extensively as a framework for the identification of individuals who engage in behaviors relevant to primary and secondary cancer prevention. The HBM has been used to identify health beliefs of individuals who practice BSE,[31,34,53–61]

TSE,[62–64] skin cancer prevention,[65–67] cancer risk reduction and early detection,[68] and general health promotion.[36] In addition, health beliefs have been studied in relation to participation in a diet intervention program,[69] mammographic screening for breast cancer,[45,47,50,70–73] Pap smear screening for cervical cancer,[74,75] and fecal occult blood screening for colorectal cancer.[35]

In general, health motivation and/or perceived barriers are strong predictors of people's intentions and behaviors related to cancer prevention and screening activities.[31,36,45,47,50,52,55,60,61,65,67,69,71] Perceived susceptibility was found to be associated positively with BSE,[58,61] having a mammogram,[50] and having a Pap test when perceived benefits were high.[75] The relationship between beliefs about severity of a potential illness and health behavior has both been supported[47] and not supported[45,71,76] in some cancer literature. In fact, a strong belief in severity could inhibit participation in screening.[77,78]

The influence of health beliefs alone on people's behaviors with regard to cancer prevention and screening activities is equivocal and may be modified by other factors. Consequently, several researchers have used the HBM in conjunction with other concepts and theories in an attempt to predict health behaviors, as discussed later in the chapter.

## Theory of Reasoned Action

Ajzen and Fishbein's Theory of Reasoned Action,[79] like the HBM, is also a value-expectancy theory. It has been used to predict a person's intention to perform a behavior in a specific situation. The model is based on the assumption that intention to perform (or not to perform) a specific behavior is the immediate determinant of that behavior. For intention to predict behavior, the behavior must be under voluntary control, and the intention must be assessed close to the time of the behavior. The longer the time interval between statement of intention and the behavior, the more likely events will occur that may change the intention.

Two factors contribute to the strength of the intention to perform a specific behavior: attitude toward the behavior, and the influence of the social environment or general subjective norms on the behavior. See Figure 5-2. Attitude is determined by an individual's belief that a specific outcome will occur if he or she performs the behavior (similar to outcome expectation) and by an evaluation of the outcome (cost/benefit analysis). The influence of norms stems from a person's belief about what significant others believe that he/she should do, weighted by the individual's motivation to comply with their wishes (social pressure to perform).[80] The model also emphasizes normative influences that might affect intention for *any* reason, health-related or otherwise, thus adding a cultural component to the prediction of behavior.[21]

Variables other than attitude or subjective norm can influence intention and behavior indirectly. For example,

1. *Behavior* is determined by *behavioral intention.*
2. Strength of *behavioral intention* depends on *attitude toward the behavior* and influence of the social environment or social norms.
   A. Attitude toward the behavior is determined by:
      1. Belief that a specific outcome will occur if the behavior is performed
      2. Evaluation of the outcome as positive or negative
   B. Social norm is determined by:
      1. The person's belief about what significant others think should be done
      2. The person's motivation to do what others wish

**FIGURE 5-2**   Theory of Reasoned Action. (Compiled from Ajzen, Fishbein.[79])

variables such as personality traits and demographic characteristics can affect intention and behavior through their influence on the attitudinal or subjective normative components.[81]

When this theory is used to explain health behavior, the effectiveness of interventions to encourage people to change behavior is greatly determined by the professional's ability to identify major concerns and barriers that the person confronts in making the decision to change. Data generated through interviews and open-ended questions with selected individuals ultimately result in the development of a questionnaire that can be used to identify beliefs that can be changed. Although this method provides for a systematic identification of those issues that are most salient to the person's decisions about performing a specific behavior, it is possible that not all important variables will be discovered in the interview process. The method also involves a measurement technique that can be complicated, cumbersome, and time-consuming. Although the model is very well developed theoretically, there is not yet a large body of data on which to judge its predictive validity.[80]

### Application of the Theory of Reasoned Action to cancer care

The Theory of Reasoned Action has been used in research on perceptions about cancer detection in general,[82] BSE,[83] mammography screening,[84] women's beliefs, attitudes, and behaviors regarding Pap tests,[74,83] seeking care for symptoms of breast cancer,[81] and adolescents' intention to chew tobacco.[85] In a study of medically underserved African-American women, Burnett et al[83] supported the propositions of the Theory of Reasoned Action in relation to breast and cervical cancer screening and found no relationship between intentions and demographic variables.

Timko[81] found that in women with a breast cancer symptom, intention to delay seeking medical care was associated with having a positive attitude toward delay and perceiving social pressure to delay. Women who delayed did not foresee a negative health outcome.

## Theory of Planned Behavior

The Theory of Reasoned Action was designed to apply to behaviors that are under complete volitional control. Its ability to predict behavior decreases when the behavior in question is one over which the individual has only limited control, such as access to health services. The Theory of Planned Behavior takes this phenomenon into consideration by extending the Theory of Reasoned Action to include a dimension of perceived control. Perceived control reflects past experience as well as perceived ease or difficulty in achieving a behavioral goal. It focuses on the person's control over factors that may influence a successful behavioral outcome, such as information, skills, willpower, time, opportunity, etc. Perceived control can affect behavior in several ways. It may facilitate intention to behave in a certain way by providing motivation; it may directly affect behavior to the extent that it realistically represents actual control over the behavior; or it may interact with intention to predict behavior. The addition of this construct to the Theory of Reasoned Action has been shown to increase the explanatory power of the model.[86–88]

### Application of the Theory of Planned Behavior to cancer care

The Theory of Planned Behavior has been used to support research in the area of colorectal cancer when the variable of perceived control not only enhanced prediction of intention to complete screening in low- and high-risk groups, but also had a direct effect on screening behavior in the high-risk group.[89] Perceived behavioral control was also shown to be significantly related to BSE frequency,[90] and adherence to a program of BSE or TSE in young adults.[91]

## Social Support

The field of relationships that individuals have with others in daily living has been called their social or personal network. It depends on the existence of people on whom individuals can rely, who will let them know that they care about, value, or love them.[92] Conceptual definitions of social support abound. The definition proposed by Kahn is "interpersonal transactions that include one or more of the following: the expression of positive affect of one person toward another, the affirmation or endorsement of another person's behaviors, perceptions, or expressed views; the giving of symbolic or material aid to another."[93,p.85] Thus Kahn proposes affect, affirmation, and aid as the three components of supportive transactions.

The precise mechanism of action linking social support and health is not known. Researchers have advanced three hypotheses.[94] The first is that social ties provide a buffer against the effects of high stress. The second is that social ties increase the development of coping strategies, thereby facilitating adaptation to change. The third hypothesis is that a perceived sense of support from others leads to a person's more generalized sense of control and responsibility.

Langlie[95] points to two other considerations in how social support may influence health status. One is that social groups differ in terms of both their norms regarding preventive health behavior and their ability to exert pressure to conform to those norms. The other is that interaction with others may provide specific practical information, such as how to prevent disease and where to go for health services.

### Relevance of social support to health behavior

Becker and Maiman[96] found increasing evidence that social support, particularly that provided by the patient's family, has a positive influence on compliance with medical advice. They emphasize that the patient's family remains a largely untapped means for reminding, assisting, encouraging, and reinforcing the patient with regard to following therapeutic directions.

Gottlieb[97] and McKinlay[98] elaborate on this association. They state that members of the help seeker's social network perform two functions prior to their mobilization as a support system. Initially they engage in formal and informal diagnostic functions. Through the former, they help to shape the definition of the help seeker's problem and judge its significance for well-being. Through the latter, they control the direction of help seeking and condition expectations about how help will be given. For example, a woman in a new town seeking health care will consult other women she has met either at work or in the community, trying to identify medical resources that are best suited to her health beliefs and special needs.

The lay network controls flow of clients to practitioners. By conditioning accurate expectations about the type of help given by health professionals, the lay network can decrease the likelihood of the help seeker's dropping out of treatment. It can speed or delay use of professional services by involving the help seeker in long or short periods of informal referral. It can contradict or concur with professionals' diagnoses of problems and attributions about their causes and improve or interfere with the patient's ability to follow the prescribed regimen.

### Application of social support to cancer care

Applications of the theory of social support in the area of cancer-related health behavior are found in the study of smoking behavior.[99,100] Support and/or smoking behavior of either family members or close associates was related to the smoking behavior of the subjects. Those subjects whose close social contacts were either nonsmokers or former smokers were likely to be nonsmokers or successful abstainers also. Social support also has been found to be influential in women's participation in screening for breast cancer.[101,102]

## Locus of Control/Health Locus of Control

### Locus of control

When Rotter[103] applied early social learning principles to clinical psychology in 1954, he developed the concepts of *internal* and *external locus of control*. They refer to the degree to which individuals perceive events in their lives as being a consequence of their own actions, and thereby controllable (internal control), or as being unrelated to their own behavior, and therefore beyond personal control (external control). Rotter proposed that people who were more internally controlled were more likely to self-initiate change. Those who were externally controlled were more likely to be influenced by others.[104]

### Health locus of control

In 1978 Wallston and Wallston[105] developed a new construct, the *health locus of control*, a generalized expectation about whether health is controllable by one's own behavior or by forces external to oneself. The Wallstons saw this construct as more useful in health-related research because an individual's sense of control often varies according to health-related experiences. Their model includes the concepts of internal and external locus of control. External locus of control is represented by two constructs, that of *chance* (health determined by fate) and *powerful others* (health determined by externals such as health professionals).

The conviction that outcomes (good health) are determined by one's own actions can have a number of effects on behavior. People who view health as personally determined but who believe they lack the skills needed to carry out the behaviors that would result in good health (low self-efficacy) would approach those activities with a sense of futility.[21]

Beliefs about internal locus of control, in combination with a high value placed on health, should predict preventive health behaviors. However, there is no theoretical reason for people with such beliefs who do *not* value health highly to perform health-relevant behaviors. Thus, if these constructs are used to study health behavior, the interaction between health value and health locus of control should be examined. The fact that many investigators have not done this may explain why beliefs about health locus of control have not been linked consistently to the performance of a variety of preventive health behaviors.[106]

In general, Oberle[107] found that nursing studies related to locus of control have yielded little information that is useful for nursing practice. However, use of recently developed disease specific locus of control scales, including one for cancer, may provide more helpful data.[108,109]

### Application of health locus of control to cancer care

The influence of beliefs about health locus of control has been examined in relation to BSE behavior,[58,110,111] seeking medical care for breast symptoms,[81] and adjustment to cancer.[112,113] Among a sample of southern African-American hospital employees, BSE was practiced less frequently by women who believed that powerful others (health professionals) had control over their health.[111] In young Caucasian women[58] and elderly Hispanic women,[110] BSE was practiced more frequently by women who perceived an internal locus of control. Internal locus of control has also been associated with more positive adjustment to cancer.[112,113]

## Attribution Theory

Attribution Theory involves the explanations that individuals use to make sense of their world and the behavioral and emotional consequences of those explanations. The assumption is made that people are motivated to engage spontaneously in attributional activities; they ask "why?" or "why me?" This search for information is ultimately connected to the broader concept of personal or cognitive control.[114]

Ascribing causes can be especially relevant when one's health is threatened, when symptoms or tensions are heightened, or when a catastrophic event takes place. If one can assign a cause, one can manage the situation more effectively and can plan future action.

Attributions can be used to predict behavior, feelings, and expectancies, and can serve to maintain self-esteem and reduce anxiety.[114] Attributions may be conscious and deliberate, or preconscious. There are four dimensions of causal attributions. Each of them is associated with certain consequences. See Table 5-2.

Attributions that people generate have significant implications for their subsequent thoughts, feelings, and actions. Lewis and Daltroy[114] speculate that there is some optimal set of attributions that best predict a person's exercise of health behaviors. Attributions of success are usually related to stable, global, and internal causes. In general, the goal of the health professional is to encourage attribution of failure (e.g., failure to stop smoking) to unstable, specific, uncontrollable, and external causes. The person can then act on the belief that the health behavior in question was not potentially achievable at that time, and that it was not a personal deficiency that resulted in the failure. It becomes possible, therefore, for the individual to try again in the future. By obtaining information on the individual's attributions, the health professional can begin to understand the motivations behind the behaviors and can tailor health behavior interventions appropriately.[114] Research in the area of causal attributions is still limited, and much more needs to be done in order to determine whether the dimensions of attributions can be manipulated, in what manner, and by what method.

### Application of Attribution Theory to cancer care

The influence of beliefs about attribution has been examined in relation to adjustment or response to can-

**TABLE 5-2**  Attribution Theory

| Dimensions of Attributions (Causes) | Consequences |
|---|---|
| **Locus of Cause** | |
| Internal to the person (*Example:* innate ability) | Can be associated with low self-esteem or depression or taking responsibility for one's treatment |
| External to the person (*Example:* chance, luck, environmental pollutants) | Can be associated with poorer long-term morbidity or better coping and adjustment |
| **Controllability** | |
| Controllable (*Example:* level of effort) | Usually results in increased effort, enhanced performance |
| Uncontrollable (*Example:* innate ability, task difficulty) | Offers little hope of influencing future outcomes |
| **Stability** | |
| Stable (*Example:* personal ability) Unstable (*Example:* attention span, mood) | Both stability and instability are important determinants of goal expectations and can be used to predict cognitive and motivational deficits |
| **Globality** | |
| Global (*Example:* innate intelligence) | Affects a wide variety of outcomes; can result in extensive performance deficits |
| Specific (*Example:* test anxiety) | Affects a limited set of outcomes in a given situation |

Compiled from Lewis, Daltroy;[114] Weiner.[115,116]

cer.[117–127] Lewis et al[124] found that patients with late-stage cancer used several processes, such as monitoring progress to maintain control over their lives, despite their terminal illness. Other researchers have attempted to relate patients' attributions of the cause of their cancer to adjustment behaviors.[117,118,120–123,125–127] Timko and Janoff-Bulman[127] found that adjustment of women with non-metastatic breast cancer was associated positively with attributions to an individual's own behavior and negatively with attributions to other people or to the individual's personality. Berckman and Austin[118] found negative relationships between causal attributions and aspects of adjustment. Although no clear association has been validated consistently,[120,125] Gotay[121] has suggested that not making strong causal attributions may be a positive factor in patients' adjustment. A recent study showed that making a causal attribution had no significant effect on women's adjustment to breast cancer, although attributing the cancer to an uncontrollable cause was associated with information-seeking behavior.[123]

## Transtheoretical Model of Change

A more recent theoretical approach to understanding health behavior was developed by Prochaska and DiClemente.[128,129] The Transtheoretical Model of Change is based on the assumption that a continuum of readiness to change applies to behavior. There are five stages in this process: precontemplation (not considering change and resistant to outside pressures to change); contemplation (starting to think about changing behavior within the next six months; more open to feedback and information; ambivalent about costs/benefits—can remain in this stage for years); preparation (taking some steps toward action and planning to change within the next month); action (initiating the new behavior and maintaining it for a minimal time); and maintenance (sustaining the change for more than six months). The process of behavioral change is not a linear one, but allows for cyclical relapses to an earlier point in the change process along the way to adoption of the new behavior.

The model also includes ten basic processes of change, overt and covert cognitive and behavioral strategies that individuals use to move through the five stages of change described above. These are consciousness-raising (increased awareness and more accurate information processing), self-liberation (belief in one's ability to change), social liberation (notice of social changes that support personal changes), self-reevaluation (affective and cognitive reexperiencing of one's self), environmental reevaluation (affective and cognitive reexperiencing of one's self), counter-conditioning (substituting more positive behaviors for negative ones), stimulus control (restructuring one's environment so that problem stimuli are less likely to occur), reinforcement management (reinforcement of positive behaviors and punishment of negative ones), dramatic relief (experiencing and releasing feelings), and helping relationships (involving openness, caring, trust, and empathy). In general, the processes of consciousness-raising and dramatic relief are used most frequently by individuals in the early stages of behavioral change, and helping relationships and reinforcement management in the later stages.[129,130] Individuals in different stages of adopting a new behavior tend to use different processes of change.[131] Thus interventions for behavioral change can emphasize processes that promote movement to the next behavioral stage.[132]

In addition to the stage and process variables, the model also highlights elements of decision making. Decisional balance is achieved by a comparison of the perceived strengths of the new behavior (pros) with the perceived negative aspects of the behavior (cons). This variable has been operationalized in the Decisional Balance Scale.[133,134] The stages of behavioral adoption have been found to correspond to differences in the pros and cons separately and to the more general measure of decisional balance.[135] The model hypothesizes that individuals in the later stages of behavior adoption should have a decisional balance favoring the positive (pro) aspects of the target behavior, in the precontemplation stage, a balance favoring the negative (con) aspects of the behavior, and in the contemplation stage, a decisional balance somewhere in-between.

While the Transtheoretical Model does not focus directly on a particular psychological variable, its constructs draw heavily on those proposed by the Health Belief Model, the Theory of Reasoned Action, and Social Learning Theory among others and are integrated in a different and, perhaps, more comprehensive manner.

### Application of the Transtheoretical Model of Change to cancer care

The Transtheoretical Model of Change has been applied extensively to smoking.[124,129–131,136] Work by Rakowski et al[135,137] has demonstrated the usefulness of stage of adoption and decisional balance as guides for designing specific interventions to increase mammography rates. Smoking cessation and mammography screening interventions that have been tailored to individuals' stages of behavioral change have been more successful than more traditional programs.[138,139]

## Combined Theoretical Approaches to Health Behavior

In an attempt to enhance the explanatory power of the models described previously, many researchers have combined models or selected variables from the models. To explain behavior related to cancer screening, the Health Belief Model has been combined with Social Learning Theory constructs,[57,140–144] Theory of Reasoned Action and Social Learning Theory,[146,147] Locus of Control,[111,148–150] the Transtheoretical Model of Change,[70] and Transtheoretical Model of Change and Theory of Reasoned Action.[151] When self-efficacy was added to the Theory of Planned Behavior to predict BSE or TSE, perceived control was a better predictor than self-efficacy.[91] The addition of facilitating conditions and perceived normative belief[152] or habit[153] to the constructs of the Theory of Reasoned Action increased the variance accounted for by the theory components alone in adherence to BSE in older women[152] and mammography participation.[153]

## RELATED FACTORS

### Sociodemographics

The influence of sociodemographics on health behavior is variable. In a relatively homogeneous sample of rural women, Gray[55] found that practicing BSE was not significantly related to sociodemographic variables. Reno[62] found similar results with regard to TSE practice among college males.

### Knowledge and educational level

Because knowledge is often related to educational level, both factors are discussed in this section. Being knowledgeable about a specific cancer or cancer detection or screening measure has been found to relate positively to health behaviors such as skin protective behavior,[46,65] having a mammogram,[142,145,154] having a Pap test,[155,156] practicing BSE,[48,53,147,157] and practicing TSE.[63] Likewise, educational level has been found to relate positively to having a mammogram,[49,145,154,158] practicing BSE,[48,59,147] and having a Pap test.[155,156]

On the other hand, being knowledgeable and/or having a high level of education is not associated consistently with positive health behaviors.[52,60,67] Gould[159] found that education was associated negatively with monitoring one's own health and that consciousness about health in general was unrelated to demographic variables. In relation to cancer detection, women at high risk for breast cancer were found to be more knowledgeable about BSE than low-risk women but did not practice it more frequently.[77] Similarly, women who had personal knowledge about breast cancer did not necessarily report their symptoms of breast cancer promptly.[160]

In one study, an educational intervention was found to increase men's knowledge about TSE, but other factors such as attitude and perceived self-efficacy were better predictors of TSE behavior.[29] In another study of TSE behavior, the educational intervention did not increase men's knowledge about testicular cancer, but did increase their practice of TSE.[63] With regard to mammography screening for breast cancer, an educational intervention was found to increase levels of knowledge and perceived benefits among women, but did not increase their use of mammography.[73]

Knowledge and educational level apparently influence health behavior both positively and negatively. Other factors, such as fear,[155] may override the positive influence of knowledge on behavior. On the other hand, fear messages can have a positive effect if they are used with a person whose fear level about a disease is not already overwhelming, and who believes that certain health behaviors would be helpful. If fear messages are used, they are likely to be most influential if they are given in the initial attempt to change behavior and if they contain advice that can be quickly and easily followed.[21]

### Socioeconomic status

Educational level is sometimes used as an indicator of socioeconomic status (SES), another factor that has a strong association with health behavior. People of low SES have been found to be less likely than people of high SES to report symptoms of colorectal cancer,[161] participate in screening for cervical cancer,[155] and participate in screening for breast cancer.[162] In addition, individuals of low SES are less likely to be successful with smoking cessation,[27] and more fearful of getting cancer.[64]

### Age

Like educational level and SES, age is an important influence on health behavior. For example, perceived barriers to performing BSE vary among different age groups of women, although frequency of practice is no different.[60] Age modifies the influence of health beliefs, and confidence in one's ability to carry out a task is influential regardless of age.[35] Although several researchers found that older women were more likely than younger women to practice BSE,[111] others have found the reverse, especially in regard to the Pap test[74,75,163,164] and mammography.[142] Older women tend to believe that they no longer require Pap tests because they are no longer sexually active or bearing children.[75] Also, they tend to have fewer close associates, such as spouses and friends, who would encourage them to have the test.[74] Older women have been found to delay seeing a health care provider for evaluation of symptoms of breast cancer.[160] In one study, older adults (over age 65) were found to be significantly less compliant than younger people (ages 20–35) with skin protective measures, after an educational intervention.[165] In another study, older adults were found to be more compliant.[148]

### Race

Differences in cancer incidence, mortality, and survival rates among people of different races have stimulated researchers to examine the health behaviors of these groups. The influence of race, exclusive of SES and educational level, is not evaluated easily. In Bloom and colleagues'[163] study of African-Americans, most of the women had had breast examinations and Pap tests, and knew the warning signs of cancer but not the predisposing factors. Many believed that cancer was spread by air, and women were more likely than men to harbor cancer myths. Vaz and associates[64] found no difference between African-American and white adolescent males' knowledge about TSE or testicular cancer, although the African-American adolescents were more afraid of getting testicular cancer, less likely to consult a physician, and less optimistic about the prognosis. McCoy et al[166] found that African-American and Hispanic men were twice as likely to have never had a digital rectal exam for prostate cancer. In a worksite study[167] on skin cancer prevention, African-Americans and Hispanics reported that they would be less likely than Caucasians to seek care for suspicious skin lesions.

Secondary analysis of data from the 1987 National Health Interview Survey[168] revealed that race was not a predictor of health behavior when knowledge was considered as a factor. One exception to this finding was that African-American women were found to smoke less than white women. Nevertheless, Guillory[169] cautioned that African-Americans are not a homogeneous group with regard to health behavior, and health care professionals should avoid stereotyping them.

The causal attributions, values, and traditional remedies of Native Americans can influence their health behaviors.[119,170] They may attribute cancer to exposure to lightning,[119] to witchcraft, or to breaking a taboo,[119,170] and may not seek prompt help in the health care system. Navajos are reluctant to address the potential fatality of an illness and are more interested in finding out why they contracted the disease.[119] Interestingly, Navajos have a low rate of cigarette smoking and a low rate of lung cancer.[119]

In a study of 600 elderly Hispanic women, Richardson and colleagues[157] found no differences in their breast cancer screening behaviors in comparison to the general population. However, 10% of the Hispanic women refused to touch the breast model. In another study, the fatalistic beliefs and lack of value in early diagnosis expressed by Mexican American subjects were attributed to lack of education rather than to cultural factors.[171] More recent research supports the interaction of acculturation and education in influencing the responses of Mexican American and other Hispanic/Latino women to cancer risk factors.

## Family Factors

Families in the childbearing years are likely to access the health system for obstetrical and child care services and may be more likely than older families to hear health-related messages directly from providers. These messages can influence health behaviors positively.[46,156,164] For example, in one study[46] parents who received information frequently from health care providers practiced more sun protective measures for themselves and their children.

Family ethnicity can be a powerful influence on health behavior. Some ethnic groups, such as Native Americans,[170] Japanese Americans, and Hispanic Americans,[173] place great value on family involvement in decisions and care and do not value individualism. In one study, Arab women with breast cancer were found to seek support from the matriarchal family rather than from their husbands.[174]

## Social Factors

Social support, social roles, and social stigma all influence health behavior of individuals with regard to cancer prevention, detection, and treatment. Social support has been found to have a positive influence on people's smoking cessation efforts.[99,100] Social roles may influence health behavior either positively or negatively. Being married has been positively associated with women's having a mammogram,[82] practicing monthly BSE, and having a yearly professional breast examination.[147] Also, having

support from a spouse has been associated with women's participation in a diet intervention program for breast cancer.[69] As alluded to previously, women in childbearing and child-rearing roles who may have more contact with the health care system are more likely than older women to practice BSE and participate in cancer screening programs. Older women, on the other hand, who are no longer wives and/or engaged in childbearing often perceive that they do not need Pap tests. In addition, fear of embarrassment at having to expose certain body parts may negatively influence a woman's participation in cancer screening.[155]

Cultural factors have been found to influence people's decisions both to participate in screening and to delay seeking help for symptoms of cancer. In Moslem culture, delay in seeking care is associated with the belief that disease is not present unless it is accompanied by noticeable signs.[174] Also, reluctance to talk about one's cancer is related to the belief that this disclosure inhibits recovery.[174] Egyptians are doubtful of the benefits of cancer prevention and early detection practices and believe that a diagnosis of cancer is God's will.[175] In Native American culture, delay in seeking care may be related to the use of Native American remedies rather than to denial of illness.[170]

Cancer is discussed relatively freely in the dominant culture of the United States. Media coverage of the diagnosis and treatment of cancer in both President[176] and Mrs. Reagan[177,178] had a positive influence on the information-seeking and cancer screening behaviors of the public.

## Institutional Factors

The organization of the health care delivery system influences people's health behavior. Services organized around care for the sick often include barriers for those people who seek prevention or screening services. Social priorities and, to some extent, the political system determine the allocation of resources to various health services. In the United States, women at high risk for cervical cancer often do not participate in screening, whereas in Sweden all women are screened.[179] The Swedish system eliminates barriers such as cost, and provides reminders to women as a cue to initiate healthy behavior. Cost and reminders are two areas that have been identified as a focus for interventions to increase women's participation in cervical screening[59,74,180] as well as breast cancer screening[49,181–183] in the United States. Current availability of at least some level of Medicaid reimbursement for Pap tests in most states, and mammography in many states[184] should reduce the cost barrier for many disadvantaged women.

Health care providers influence people's health behavior in a number of ways. Individuals have reported that a health care provider's recommendation or reminder to have a cancer screening test was important in their decision to do so.[45–50,74,156,164,185] In a sample of elderly women, frequency of the practice of BSE was associated with having been taught BSE by health care providers.[48,76] Nurses may not recognize the powerful influence they can exert on patients' health behaviors. The majority of nurses in one study rarely or only occasionally taught women about mammography.[187] Prompt, courteous, and competent examinations by health care providers were associated with women's continuation in a national breast screening study,[186] and with intention to engage in breast and cervical cancer screening.[83]

## IMPLICATIONS FOR NURSING PRACTICE

People's health behaviors are influenced by multiple interacting factors. Theories and models continue to evolve to identify and describe the interaction of these variables and to predict and prescribe health behavior. Nevertheless, human behavior is not totally predictable, and the totality of its complexity has not yet been described.

Nurses can apply some of the empirically validated concepts and propositions of health behavior by incorporating them into the nursing process. The models provide guidelines for assessment, nursing diagnosis, intervention, and evaluation. For example, health beliefs, self-efficacy, intentions, stages of readiness, and beliefs about control can be incorporated into all steps of the nursing process.

Considering the association between health behavior and demographics,[188] nurses need to examine this aspect of the community. A thorough assessment of people's cultural beliefs and practices[169] and the use of developmental and communication principles[189] are crucial to nurses' success in influencing people's health behaviors positively.

## REFERENCES

1. Greenwald P, Sondik EJ: Cancer control objectives for the nation: 1985–2000. *NCI Monographs* 2:3–11, 1986
2. American Cancer Society: *American Cancer Society Priorities for the 1990s.* Atlanta, Author, 1990
3. U.S. Department of Health and Human Services: *Healthy People 2000.* National Health Promotion and Disease Prevention Objectives (DHHS publication No. (PHS) 91-50212). Washington, DC, U.S. Government Printing Office, 1991
4. Gochman D: Health behavior: Plural perspectives, in Gochman D (ed): *Health Behavior: Emerging Research Perspectives.* New York, Plenum, 1988, pp 3–17
5. Gochman D: Labels, systems and motives: Some perspectives for future research. *Health Educ Q* 9:167–174, 1982
6. Kasl S, Cobb S: Health behavior, illness behavior, and sick role behavior: I. Health and illness behavior. *Arch Environ Health* 12:246–266, 1966
7. Rosenstock I: Why people use health services. *Milbank Mem Fund Q* 44:94–124, 1966
8. Harris D, Guten S: Health protective behavior: An exploratory study. *J Health Soc Behav* 20:17–29, 1979
9. Pender N: *Health Promotion in Nursing Practice* (ed 2). Norwalk, CT, Appleton and Lange, 1987
10. Mechanic D: *Medical Sociology* (ed 2). New York, Free Press, 1978
11. Steele J, McBroom W: Conceptual and empirical dimensions of health behavior. *J Health Soc Behav* 13:382–392, 1972
12. Mechanic D: Response factors in illness: The study of illness behavior, in Jaco E (ed): *Patients, Physicians and Illness: A Sourcebook in Behavioral Science and Health* (ed 2). New York, Free Press, 1972, pp 118–130
13. Cummings K, Becker M, Maile M: Bringing the models together: An empirical approach to combining variables used to explain health actions. *J Behav Med* 3:123–145, 1980
14. Perry C, Baranowski T, Parcel G: How individuals, environments, and health behavior interact: Social learning theory, in Glanz K, Lewis F, Rimer B (eds): *Health Behavior and Health Education.* San Francisco, Jossey-Bass, 1990, pp 161–186
15. Bandura A: *Social Learning Theory.* Englewood Cliffs, NJ, Prentice-Hall, 1977
16. Bandura A: Self-efficacy: Toward a unifying theory of behavioral change. *Psychol Rev* 84:191–215, 1977
17. Bandura A: The self system in reciprocal determinism. *Am Psychologist* 33:344–358, 1978
18. Bandura A: Self-referent thought: A developmental analysis of self-efficacy, in Flavell J, Ross L (eds): *Social Cognitive Development: Frontiers and Possible Futures.* Cambridge, Eng., Cambridge University Press, 1981, pp 200–239
19. Bandura A: Recycling misconceptions of perceived self-efficacy. *Cog Ther Res* 8:231–255, 1984
20. Bandura A: Self-efficacy mechanism in human agency. *Am Psychologist* 37:122–147, 1982
21. Becker M: Theoretical models of adherence and strategies for improving adherence, in Shumaker S, Schron E, Ockene J (eds): *The Handbook of Health Behavior Change.* New York, Springer-Verlag, 1990, pp 5–43
22. Seydel E, Taal E, Wiegman O: Risk-appraisal, outcome and self-efficacy expectancies: Cognitive factors in preventive behavior related to cancer. *Psychol Health* 4:99–109, 1990
23. Hertog JK, Finnegan JR, Rooney B, et al: Self-efficacy as a target population segmentation strategy in a diet and cancer risk reduction campaign. *Health Communication* 5: 21–40, 1993
24. DiClemente C, Prochaska J, Gibertini M: Self-efficacy and the stages of self-change of smoking. *Cog Ther Res* 9: 181–200, 1985
25. Godding P, Glasgow R: Self-efficacy and outcome expectations as predictors of controlled smoking status. *Cog Ther Res* 9:583–590, 1985
26. Strecher V, Becker M, Kirscht J, et al: Psychosocial aspects of changes in cigarette smoking behavior. *Patient Educ Counsel* 7:249–262, 1985
27. Wilcox NS, Prochaska JO, Velicer WF, et al: Subject characteristics as predictors of self-change in smoking. *Addict Behav* 10:407–412, 1985
28. Brubaker RG, Fowler C: Encouraging college males to perform testicular self-examination: Evaluation of a persuasive message based on the revised Theory of Reasoned Action. *J Appl Soc Psychol* 20:1411–1422, 1990
29. Brubaker RG, Wickersham D: Encouraging the practice

of testicular self-examination: A field application of the Theory of Reasoned Action. *Health Psychol* 9:154–163, 1990

30. Baker J: Breast self-examination among older women. *Health Educ Res* 3:181–189, 1988

31. Champion VL: Breast self-examination in women 35 and older: A prospective study. *J Behav Med* 13:523–538, 1990

32. Olson R, Mitchell E: Self-confidence as a critical factor in breast self-examination. *J Obstet Gynecol Neonatal Nurs* 18: 476–481, 1989

33. Rippetoe PA, Rogers RW: Effects of components of Protection-Motivation Theory on adaptive and maladaptive coping with a health threat. *J Pers Soc Psychol* 52:596–604, 1987

34. Rutledge DN, Davis GT: Breast self-examination compliance and the Health Belief Model. *Oncol Nurs Forum* 15: 175–179, 1988

35. Hoogewerf PE, Hislop G, Morrison BJ, et al: Health belief and compliance with screening for fecal occult blood. *Soc Sci Med* 30:721–726, 1990

36. Kelly RB, Zyzanski SJ, Alemagno SA: Prediction of motivation and behavior change following health promotion: Role of health beliefs, social support, and self-efficacy. *Soc Sci Med* 32:311–320, 1991

37. Strecher V, De Vellis B, Becker M, et al: The role of self-efficacy in achieving health behavior change. *Health Educ Q* 13:73–91, 1986

38. Janz N, Becker M: The Health Belief Model: A decade later. *Health Educ Q* 11:1–47, 1984

39. Janis I: The role of social support in adherence to stressful decisions. *Am Psychologist* 38:143–160, 1983

40. Maiman L, Becker M: The Health Belief Model: Origins and correlates in psychological theory, in Becker M (ed): *The Health Belief Model and Personal Health Behavior*. Thorofare, NJ, Slack, 1974, pp 9–26

41. Lewin K: *A Dynamic Theory of Personality: Selected Papers*. New York, McGraw-Hill, 1935

42. Rosenstock I: Historical origins of the Health Belief Model, in Becker M (ed): *The Health Belief Model and Personal Health Behavior*. Thorofare, NJ, Slack, 1974, pp 1–8

43. Rosenstock I: The Health Belief Model: Explaining health behavior through expectancies, in Glanz K, Lewis F, Rimer B (eds): *Health Behavior and Health Education*. San Francisco, Jossey-Bass, 1990, pp 39–61

44. Becker M, Maiman L: Sociobehavioral determinants of compliance with health and medical care recommendations. *Med Care* 13:10–24, 1975

45. Aiken LS, West SG, Woodward CK, et al: Health beliefs and compliance with mammography screening recommendations in asymptomatic women. *Health Psychol* 13: 122–129, 1994

46. Buller DB, Callister MA, Reichert T: Skin cancer prevention by parents of young children: Health information sources, skin cancer knowledge, and sun-protection practices. *Oncol Nurs Forum* 22:1559–1566, 1995

47. Johnson JD, Meischke, H: Factors associated with adoption of mammography screening: Results of a cross-sectional and longitudinal study. *J Women's Health* 3:97–105, 1994

48. Morrison C: Determining crucial correlates of breast self-examination in older women with low incomes. *Oncol Nurs Forum* 23:83–93, 1996

49. Rimer BK, Trock B, Engstrom PF, et al: Why do some women get regular mammograms? *Am J Prev Med* 7:69–74, 1991

50. Stein JA, Fox SA, Murata PJ, et al: Mammography usage and the Health Belief Model. *Health Educ Q* 19:447–462, 1992

51. Harrison JA, Mullen PD, Green LW: A meta-analysis of studies of the Health Belief Model with adults. *Health Educ Res* 7:107–116, 1992

52. Rimer B, Keintz M, Kessler H, et al: Why women resist screening mammography: Patient-related barriers. *Radiology* 172:243–246, 1989

53. Bottimore AH, Hailey BJ: Promotion of breast self-exam behavior: An attempt to modify health beliefs. *Int Q Community Health Educ* 9:273–282, 1988–89

54. Chrvala C, Iverson D: Predictive models for frequency and proficiency of BSE performance. *Prog Clin Biol Res* 293: 159–173, 1989

55. Gray ME: Factors related to practice of breast self-examination in rural women. *Cancer Nurs* 13:100–107, 1990

56. Hill D, Shugg D: Breast self-examination practices and attitudes among breast cancer, benign breast disease and general practice patients. *Health Educ Res* 4:193–203, 1989

57. Lu ZJ: Variables associated with breast self-examination among Chinese women. *Cancer Nurs* 18:29–34, 1995

58. Redeker N: Health beliefs, health locus of control, and the frequency of practice of breast self-examination in women. *J Obstet Gynecol Neonatal Nurs* 18:45–51, 1989

59. Ronis DL, Harel Y: Health beliefs and breast examination behaviors: Analyses of linear structural relations. *Psychol Health* 3:259–285, 1989

60. Sensiba ME, Stewart DS: Relationship of perceived barriers to breast self-examination in women of varying ages and levels of education. *Oncol Nurs Forum* 22:1265–1268, 1995

61. Wyper MA: Breast self-examination and the Health Belief Model: Variations on a theme. *Res Nurs Health* 13:421–428, 1990

62. Reno DR: Men's knowledge and health beliefs about testicular cancer and testicular self-examination. *Cancer Nurs* 11: 112–117, 1988

63. Rudolf VM, Quinn KL: The practice of TSE among college men: Effectiveness of an educational program. *Oncol Nurs Forum* 15:45–48, 1988

64. Vaz RM, Best DL, Davis SW: Testicular cancer. Adolescent knowledge and attitudes. *J Adolesc Health Care* 9:474–479, 1988

65. Cody R, Lee C: Behaviors, beliefs, and intentions in skin cancer prevention. *J Behav Med* 13:373–389, 1990

66. Cockburn J, Hennrikus D, Scott R, et al: Adolescent use of sun protection measures. *Med J Aust* 151:136–140, 1989

67. Marlenga B: The health beliefs and skin cancer prevention practices of Wisconsin dairy farmers. *Oncol Nurs Forum* 22: 681–686, 1995

68. Millon-Underwood S, Sanders E: Factors contributing to health promotion behaviors among African-American men. *Oncol Nurs Forum* 17:707–712, 1990

69. Naslund GK, Fredrikson M, Holm LE: Psychosocial factors associated with participation and nonparticipation in a diet intervention program. *J Psychosoc Oncol* 10(4):93–107, 1993

70. Champion VL: Beliefs about breast cancer and mammography by behavioral stage. *Oncol Nurs Forum* 21:1009–1014, 1994

71. Fischera SD, Frank DI: The Health Belief Model as a predictor of mammography screening. *Health Values* 18(4): 3–9, 1994

72. Hyman RB, Baker S, Ephraim R, et al: Health Belief Model variables as predictors of screening mammography utilization. *J Behav Med* 17:391–406, 1994

73. Reynolds K, West S, Aiken L: Increasing the use of mammography: A pilot program. *Health Educ Q* 17:429–441, 1990

74. Hennig P, Knowles A: Factors influencing women over 40 years to take precautions against cervical cancer. *J Appl Soc Psychol* 20:1612–1621, 1990

75. Lerman C, Caputo C, Brody D: Factors associated with inadequate cervical cancer screening among lower-income primary care patients. *J Am Board Fam Pract* 3:151–156, 1990

76. Williams RD: Factors affecting the practice of breast self-examination in older women. *Oncol Nurs Forum* 15:611–616, 1988

77. Alagna SW, Morokoff PJ, Bevett JM, et al: Performance of breast self-examination by women at high risk for breast cancer. *Women and Health* 12:29–46, 1987

78. Strauss L, Solomon L, Costanza M, et al: Breast self-examination practices and attitudes of women with and without a history of breast cancer. *J Behav Med* 10:337–350, 1987

79. Ajzen I, Fishbein M: *Understanding Attitudes and Predicting Social Behavior.* Englewood Cliffs, NJ, Prentice-Hall, 1980

80. Carter W: Health behavior as a rational process: Theory of Reasoned Action and Multiattribute Utility Theory, in Glanz K, Lewis F, Rimer B (eds): *Health Behavior and Health Education.* San Francisco, Jossey-Bass, 1990, pp 63–91

81. Timko C: Seeking medical care for a breast cancer symptom: Determinants of intentions to engage in prompt or delay behavior. *Health Psychol* 6:305–328, 1987

82. Nichols BS, Misra R, Alexy B: Cancer detection: How effective is public education? *Cancer Nurs* 19:98–103, 1996

83. Burnettt CB, Steakley CS, Tefft MC: Barriers to breast and cervical cancer screening in underserved women of the District of Columbia. *Oncol Nurs Forum* 22:1551–1557, 1995

84. Crooks CE, Neutens JJ: Prediction and verification of a woman's intention to participate in a mammography screening program. *J Health Educ* 24:369–374, 1993

85. Gerber RW, Newman IM, Martin GL: Applying the Theory of Reasoned Action to early adolescent tobacco chewing. *J Sch Health* 58:410–413, 1988

86. Ajzen I: From intentions to actions: A theory of planned behavior, in Kuhl J, Beckmann J (eds): *Action Control: From Cognition to Behavior.* Berlin, Springer-Verlag, 1985, pp 11–39

87. Ajzen I, Madden TJ: Prediction of goal-directed behavior: Attitudes, intentions, and perceived behavioral control. *J Exp Soc Psychol* 22:453–474, 1986

88. Madden TJ, Ellen PS, Ajzen I: A comparison of the Theory of Planned Behavior and the Theory of Reasoned Action. *Pers Soc Psychol Bull* 18:3–9, 1992

89. DeVellis BM, Blalock SJ, Sandler RS: Predicting participation in cancer screening: The role of perceived behavioral control. *J Appl Soc Psychol* 20:639–660, 1990

90. Lierman LM, Young HM, Powell-Cope G, et al: Effects of education and support on breast self-examination in older women. *Nurs Res* 43:158–163, 1994

91. McCaul KD, Sandgren AK, O'Neill HK, et al: The value of the Theory of Planned Behavior, perceived control, and self-efficacy expectations for predicting health-protective behaviors. *Basic Appl Soc Psychol* 14:231–252, 1993

92. Sarason I, Levine H, Basham R, et al: Assessing social support. *J Pers Soc Psychol* 44:127–139, 1983

93. Kahn R: Aging and social support, in Riley M (ed): *Aging from Birth to Death: Interdisciplinary Perspectives.* Boulder, CO, Westview Press, 1979, pp 77–91

94. Hamburg B, Killilea M: Relation of social support, stress, illness, and use of health services, in *Public Health Service: Healthy People: The Surgeon General's Report on Health Promotion and Disease Prevention—Background Papers* (DHEW pub-

lication No. (PHS) 79-55071A). Washington, DC, U.S. Government Printing Office, 1979, pp 253–256

95. Langlie J: Social networks, health beliefs, and preventive health behavior. *J Health Soc Behav* 18:244–260, 1977

96. Becker M, Maiman L: Strategies for enhancing patient compliance. *J Community Health* 6:113–135, 1980

97. Gottlieb B: *Social Support Strategies.* Beverly Hills, CA, Sage, 1983

98. McKinlay J: Social networks, lay consultation, and help-seeking behavior. *Soc Forces* 51:275–292, 1973

99. Lauer R, Akers R, Massey J, et al: Evaluation of cigarette smoking among adolescents: The Muscatine Study. *Prev Med* 11:417–428, 1982

100. Mermelstein R, Lichtenstein E, McIntyre K: Partner support and relapse in smoking cessation programs. *J Consult Clin Psychol* 51:465–466, 1983

101. Kang SH, Bloom JR, Romano PS: Cancer screening among African-American women: Their use of tests and social support. *Am J Public Health* 84:101–103, 1994

102. McCance KL, Mooney KH, Field R, et al: Influence of others in motivating women to obtain breast cancer screening. *Cancer Pract* 4:141–146, 1996

103. Rotter J: *Social Learning and Clinical Psychology.* Englewood Cliffs, N.J.: Prentice-Hall, 1954

104. Rotter J: Generalized expectancies for internal versus external control of reinforcement. *Psychol Med Monogr* 80:1–28, 1966

105. Wallston K, Wallston B: Locus of control and health. *Health Educ Monogr* 6:107–117, 1978

106. Lau R: Beliefs about control and health behavior, in Gochman D (ed): *Health Behavior: Emerging Research Perspectives.* New York, Plenum, 1988, pp 43–63

107. Oberle K: A decade of research in locus of control: What have we learned? *J Adv Nurs* 16:800–806, 1991

108. Dahnke GL, Garlick R, Kazoleas D: Testing a new disease-specific Health Locus of Control scale among cancer and aplastic anemia patients. *Health Communication* 6:37–53, 1994

109. Wallston KA, Stein MJ, Smith CA: Form C of the MHLC scales: A condition-specific measure of locus of control. *J Pers Assess* 63:534–553, 1994

110. Bundek NI, Marks G, Richardson JL: Role of Health Locus of Control beliefs in cancer screening of elderly Hispanic women. *Health Psychol* 12:193–199, 1993

111. Nemcek MA: Factors influencing black women's breast self-examination practice. *Cancer Nurs* 12:339–343, 1989

112. Blood GW, Kauffman SM, Dineen M, et al: Perceived control, adjustment, and communication problems in laryngeal cancer survivors. *Percept Mot Skills* 77:764–766, 1993

113. Watson M, Greer S, Pruyn J, et al: Locus of control and adjustment to cancer. *Psychol Rep* 66:39–48, 1990

114. Lewis F, Daltroy L: How causal explanations influence health behavior: Attribution Theory, in Glanz K, Lewis F, Rimer B (eds): *Health Behavior and Health Education.* San Francisco, Jossey-Bass, 1990, pp 92–114

115. Weiner B: A theory of motivation for some classroom experiences. *J Educ Psychol* 71:3–25, 1979

116. Weiner B: A theory of motivation for some classroom experiences, in Gorlitz D (ed): *Perspectives on Attribution Research and Theory, The Bielefeld Symposium.* Cambridge, MA, Ballinger, 1980, pp 39–74

117. Bearison DJ, Sadow AJ, Granowetter L, et al: Patients' and parents' causal attributions for childhood cancer. *J Psychosoc Oncol* 11(3):47–61, 1993

118. Berckman KL, Austin JK: Causal attributions, perceived

control, and adjustments in patients with lung cancer. *Oncol Nurs Forum* 20:23–30, 1993

119. Csordas TJ: The sore that does not heal: Cause and concept in the Navajo experience of cancer. *J Anthrop Res* 45:457–485, 1989

120. Eiser C, Havermans T, Eiser JR: Parents' attributions about childhood cancer: Implications for relationships with medical staff. *Child Care Health Dev* 21:31–42, 1994

121. Gotay CC: Why me? Attributions and adjustment by cancer patients and their mates at two stages in the disease process. *Soc Sci Med* 20:825–831, 1985

122. Kroode H, Oosterwijk M, Steverink N: Three conflicts as a result of causal attributions. *Soc Sci Med* 28:93–97, 1989

123. Lavery JF, Clarke VA: Causal attributions, coping strategies, and adjustment to breast cancer. *Cancer Nurs* 19:20–28, 1996

124. Lewis FM, Haberman MR, Wallhagen MI: How adults with late-stage cancer experience personal control. *J Psychosoc Oncol* 4:27–42, 1986

125. Lowery BJ, Jacobsen BS, DuCette J: Causal attribution, control, and adjustment to breast cancer. *J Psychosoc Oncol* 10(4):37–53, 1993

126. Taylor SE, Lichtman RR, Wood JV: Attributions, beliefs about control, and adjustment to breast cancer. *J Pers Soc Psychol* 46:489–502, 1984

127. Timko C, Janoff-Bulman R: Attributions, vulnerability, and psychological adjustment: The case of breast cancer. *Health Psychol* 4:521–544, 1985

128. Prochaska JO, DiClemente CC: Transtheoretical therapy: Toward a more integrative model of change. *Psychother: Theory Res Pract* 19:276–288, 1982

129. Prochaska JO, DiClemente CC: Stages and processes of self change of smoking: Toward an integrative model of change. *J Consult Clin Psychol* 51:390–395, 1983

130. Prochaska JO, Redding CA, Harlow LL, et al: The Transtheoretical Model of Change and HIV prevention. A review. *Health Educ Q* 21:471–486, 1994

131. Prochaska JO, Velicer WF, DiClemente CC, et al: Measuring the process of change: Applications to the cessation of smoking. *J Consult Clin Psychol* 56:520–528, 1988

132. Hecht JP, Emmons KM, Brown RA, et al: Smoking interventions for patients with cancer: Guidelines for nursing practice. *Oncol Nurs Forum* 21:1657–1666, 1994

133. Prochaska JO, Velicer WF, Rossi JS, et al: Stages of change and decisional balance for 12 problem behaviors. *Health Psychol* 13:39–46, 1994

134. Velicer WF, DiClemente CC, Prochaska JO, et al: A decisional balance measure for predicting smoking cessation. *J Pers Soc Psychol* 48:1279–1289, 1985

135. Rakowski W, Dube CE, Marcus BH, et al: Assessing elements of women's decisions about mammography. *Health Psychol* 11:111–118, 1992

136. DiClemente CC, Prochaska JO, Fairhurst S, et al: The process of smoking cessation: An analysis of precontemplation, contemplation and preparation stages of change. *J Consult Clin Psychol* 59:259–304, 1991

137. Rakowski W, Fulton JP, Feldman JP. Women's decision making about mammography: A replication of the relationship between stages of adoption and decisional balance. *Health Psychol* 12:209–214, 1993

138. Prochaska JO, DiClemente CC, Velicer WF, et al: Standardized, individualized, interactive and personalized self-help programs for smoking cessation. *Health Psychol* 12:399–405, 1993

139. Skinner CS, Strecher VJ, Hospers H: Physician recommendations for mammography: Do tailored messages make a difference? *Am J Public Health* 84:43–49, 1994

140. Duke SS, Gordon-Sosby K, Reynolds KD, et al: A study of breast cancer detection practices and beliefs in black women attending public health clinics. *Health Educ Res* 9:331–342, 1994

141. Friedman LC, Nelson DV, Webb JA, et al: Dispositional optimism, self-efficacy, and health beliefs as predictors of breast self examination. *Am J Prev Med* 10:130–135, 1994

142. Glanz K, Resch N, Lerman C, et al: Factors associated with adherence to breast cancer screening among working women. *J Occup Med* 34:1071–1078, 1992

143. Kurtz ME, Given B, Given CW, et al: Relationships of barriers and facilitators to breast self-examination, mammography, and a clinical breast examination in a worksite population. *Cancer Nurs* 16:251–259, 1993

144. Marshburn J, Bradham DD, Studnicki J, et al: Mass mammography screening. *Cancer Pract* 2:146–153, 1994

145. King E, Rimer BK, Balsheim A, et al: Mammography-related beliefs of older women. *J Aging Health* 5:82–100, 1993

146. Myers RE, Ross E, Jepson C, et al: Modeling adherence to colorectal cancer screening. *Prev Med* 23:142–151, 1994

147. Phillips JM, Wilbur J: Adherence to breast cancer screening guidelines among African-American women of differing employment status. *Cancer Nurs* 18:258–269, 1995

148. Carmel S, Shani E, Rosenberg L: The role of age and an expanded Health Belief Model in predicting skin cancer protective behavior. *Health Educ Res* 9:433–447, 1994

149. Funke BL, Nicholson ME: Factors affecting patient compliance among women with abnormal pap smears. *Patient Educ Counsel* 20:5–15, 1993

150. Murray M, McMillan C: Health beliefs, locus of control, emotional control and women's cancer screening behavior. *Br J Clin Psychol* 32:87–100, 1993

151. Beardall S, Edwards N: Social and cultural determinants of smoking behavior in selected immigrant groups: Results of key informant interviews. *Fam Community Health* 18:65–72, 1995

152. Lierman LM, Kasprzyk D, Benoliel JQ: Understanding adherence to breast self-examination in older women. *West J Nurs Res* 13:46–66, 1991

153. Montano DE, Taplin SH: A test of an expanded Theory of Reasoned Action to predict mammography participation. *Soc Sci Med* 32:733–741, 1991

154. Champion VL: The relationship of selected variables to breast cancer detection behaviors in women 35 and older. *Oncol Nurs Forum* 18:733–739, 1991

155. Peters RK, Bear MB, Thomas D: Barriers to screening for cancer of the cervix. *Prev Med* 18:133–146, 1989

156. Mamon JA, Shediac MC, Crosby CB, et al: Inner-city women at risk for cervical cancer: Behavioral and utilization factors related to inadequate screening. *Prev Med* 19:363–376, 1990

157. Richardson JL, Marks G, Solis JM, et al: Frequency and adequacy of breast cancer screening among elderly Hispanic women. *Prev Med* 16:761–774, 1987

158. Anda RF, Sienko DG, Remington PL, et al: Screening mammography for women 50 years of age and older: Practices and trends. *Am J Prev Med* 6:123–129, 1990

159. Gould SJ: Health consciousness and health behavior. The application of a new health consciousness scale. *Am J Prev Med* 6:228–237, 1990

160. Lierman LM: Discovery of breast changes. Women's re-

sponses and nursing implications. *Cancer Nurs* 11:352–361, 1988

161. Funch DP: Predictors and consequences of symptom-reporting behaviors in colorectal cancer patients. *Med Care* 26:1000–1008, 1988

162. Fink R, Shapiro S: Significance of increased efforts to gain participation in screening for breast cancer. *Am J Prev Med* 6:34–41, 1990

163. Bloom JR, Hayes WA, Saunders F, et al: Cancer awareness and secondary prevention practices in Black Americans: Implications for intervention. *Fam Community Health* 10: 19–30, 1987

164. Paskett ED, Carter WB, Chu J, et al: Compliance behavior in women with abnormal pap smears. *Med Care* 28:643–656, 1990

165. Robinson J: Behavior modification obtained by sun protection education coupled with removal of a skin cancer. *Arch Dermatol* 126:477–481, 1990

166. McCoy CB, Anwyl RS, Metsch LR, et al: Prostate cancer in Florida: Knowledge, attitudes, practices, and beliefs. *Cancer Pract* 3:88–93, 1995

167. Friedman LC, Bruce S, Weinberg AD, et al: Early detection of skin cancer: Racial/ethnic differences in behaviors and attitudes. *J Cancer Educ* 9:105–110, 1994

168. Jepson C, Kessler LG, Portnoy B, et al: Black-white differences in cancer prevention knowledge and behavior. *Am J Public Health* 81:501–504, 1991

169. Guillory J: Ethnic perspectives of cancer nursing: The black American. *Oncol Nurs Forum* 14:66–69, 1987

170. Antle A: Ethnic perspectives of cancer nursing: The American Indian. *Oncol Nurs Forum* 14:70–73, 1987

171. Sugarek NJ, Deyo RN, Holmes BC: Locus of control and beliefs about cancer in a multi-ethnic clinic population. *Oncol Nurs Forum* 15:481–486, 1988

172. Balcazar H, Castro FG, Krull JL: Cancer risk reduction in Mexican American women: The role of acculturation, education and health risk factors. *Health Educ Q* 22:61–84, 1995

173. Kagawa-Singer M: Ethnic perspectives of cancer nursing: Hispanics and Japanese Americans. *Oncol Nurs Forum* 14: 59–65, 1987

174. Baider L, De-Nour AK: The meaning of a disease: An exploratory study of Moslem Arab women after a mastectomy. *J Psychosoc Oncol* 4:1–13, 1986

175. Ali N, Khalil H: Cancer prevention and early detection among Egyptians. *Cancer Nurs* 19:104–111, 1996

176. Brown ML, Potosky AL: The presidential effect: The public health response to media coverage about Ronald Reagan's colon cancer episode. *Public Opin Q* 54:317–329, 1990

177. Lane DS, Polednak AP, Burg MA: The impact of media coverage of Nancy Reagan's experience on breast cancer screening. *Am J Public Health* 79:1551–1554, 1989

178. Stoddard A, Zapka J, Schoenfield S, et al: Effects of a news event on breast cancer screening survey responses. *Prog Clin Biol Res* 339:259–268, 1990

179. Howard J: "Avoidable mortality" from cervical cancer: Exploring the concept. *Soc Sci Med* 24:507–514, 1987

180. Lovejoy NC: Multinational approaches to cervical cancer screening: A review. *Cancer Nurs* 19:126–134, 1996

181. Baines CJ, Christen A, Simard A, et al: The National Breast Screening Study: Pre-recruitment sources of awareness in participants. *Can J Public Health* 80:221–225, 1989

182. Lane DS, Polednak AP, Burg MA: Breast cancer screening practices among users of county-funded health centers vs women in the entire community. *Am J Public Health* 82: 199–203, 1992

183. Mayer JA, Kellogg MC: Promoting mammography appointment making. *J Behav Med* 12:605–611, 1989

184. Boss LP, Guckes FH: Medicaid coverage of screening tests for breast and cervical cancer. *Am J Public Health* 82: 252–253, 1992

185. Vogel VS, Graves DS, Vernon SW, et al: Mammographic screening of women with increased risk of breast cancer. *Cancer* 66:1613–1620, 1990

186. Baines CJ, To T, Wall C: Women's attitudes to screening after participation in the National Breast Screening Study. *Cancer* 65:1663–1669, 1990

187. Fischera S, Frank DI: Attitudes, practices, and role of nurses in the use of mammography. *Cancer Nurs* 17:223–228, 1994

188. Fink D, Sheehan H: Cancer prevention and detection: An overview of variables influencing adoption and practice. *Cancer* 61:2391–2395, 1988

189. Buller DB, Buller MK: Approaches to communicating preventive behaviors. *Semin Oncol Nurs* 7:53–63, 1991

# Chapter 6

# Dynamics of Cancer Prevention

Lois J. Loescher, RN, MS

# INTRODUCTION

Many believe that the best way to control cancer is to prevent it, specifically by reducing the risk of cancer.[1,2] The focus on cancer treatment and "cure" by clinicians, researchers, and funding agencies is slowly beginning to shift to prevention. Since the passage of the National Cancer Act in 1971, cancer prevention and control activities gradually have been integrated into the National Cancer Program. Now, less than three years from the end of the twentieth century, scientists in many disciplines, including nursing, are faced with the challenges of translating the findings of behavioral, epidemiological, clinical, and basic science research into specific interventions for preventing cancer.[3] This chapter presents a conceptual overview of cancer prevention as a component of cancer control. For information about cancer risk, risk assessment, and specific screening activities, refer to chapters 7 and 8.

# DEFINITIONS OF CANCER PREVENTION

The definition of cancer prevention is evolving and is often unclear. In the past, nurses generally have used a stage-of-disease model[4] to define prevention as all measures that limit the progression of disease at any time during its course. These prevention measures can occur anywhere along the health continuum. Three levels of prevention traditionally have been defined in the nursing literature. *Primary prevention* decreases the vulnerability of a healthy individual or population to illness or dysfunction through health promotion strategies and specific protection recommendations. *Secondary prevention* defines and identifies high-risk individuals and populations, including those with precursor lesions or syndromes, and consists of early diagnosis, early detection, screening, and treatment of early stages of disease. *Tertiary prevention* minimizes morbidity resulting from permanent or irreversible disease by preventing complications.[5]

Although this traditional definition of prevention, which encompasses the entire health continuum, has guided nursing science and practice for years, it does not reflect the evolving science or sentiment concerning cancer prevention.[6] Generally, cancer prevention is achieved when modulation or modification of self-care behaviors or exogenous factors results in reduced cancer risk.[7,8] This definition broadly covers preventive measures such as avoidance or reduction of exposure to carcinogens, use of chemopreventive agents, or surgical removal of precancerous lesions.[7] Byar and Freedman[7] have suggested that primary prevention should relate to initiation, secondary prevention to promotion, and tertiary prevention to progression. Thus, *primary prevention* is the avoidance of exposure to carcinogens (e.g., viruses, radiation, pollutants, chemicals), tobacco use, changes in diet, and the administration of specific agents (e.g., chemopreventives) to limit exposure to the carcinogens that initiate carcinogenesis. *Secondary prevention* is the prevention of promotion by smoking cessation, changes in diet, and administration of chemopreventive agents presumed to act on promotion. Mechanisms might be inhibiting the activation of proto-oncogenes or by antagonizing the effects of oncogene expression.[9,10] Byar and Freedman[7,p.413] stated, "The term secondary prevention has often been used to describe screening activities. This usage should be discouraged because it is conceptually awkward to imagine preventing a lesion that is already present and that we wish to detect." *Tertiary prevention* consists of arresting, removing, or reversing a premalignant lesion (e.g., with chemoprevention or surgery) to prevent recurrence or progression to cancer.[9] Not all investigators have adopted the definitions of Byar and Freedman.

The traditional definition of cancer prevention used by nursing now more aptly falls under the broad umbrella of cancer control, rather than cancer prevention per se.[6] The Division of Cancer Prevention and Control (DCPC) at the National Cancer Institute (NCI) defines cancer control as "the reduction of cancer incidence, morbidity, and mortality through an orderly sequence from research on interventions and their impact in defined populations to the broad, systematic application of the research results."[11,p.9] Smart[12] further specified cancer control as prevention, screening and early detection, diagnosis and treatment, and rehabilitation and continuing care.

# MODERN APPROACHES TO CANCER PREVENTION

The multidisciplinary scientific community uses three main approaches to achieve primary, secondary, and tertiary prevention: (1) education and knowledge, (2) regulation, and (3) host modification.[13]

## Education and Knowledge

Lifestyle factors that have a known impact on cancer development are tobacco use, alcohol consumption, and diet.[14] Education focuses on changing lifestyle behaviors to reduce cancer incidence through translation of scientific findings into sensible and practical recommendations.[11,13] These recommendations may be based on objectives such as those proposed by the DCPC in its *Cancer Control Objectives for the Nation: 1985–2000.* These objectives target four areas of prevention (smoking, diet, sun exposure, counseling) that reflect an analysis and synthesis of current knowledge about cancer prevention

(Table 6-1).[11] In addition to messages aimed at tobacco cessation, sun avoidance, and dietary changes, cancer prevention education primarily consists of modifying sexual practices and decreasing exposure to environmental and occupational carcinogens.[13]

Prevention education has been carried out by the U.S. Public Health Service, the NCI, state and local health care agencies, cancer centers, and voluntary health organizations such as the American Cancer Society and the American Lung Association. A large part of public health education has been facilitated by the lay media, particularly by newspapers, magazines, and television programs that learned about scientific discoveries and reported the news in a reader-friendly fashion to the public.[15,16]

Education alone, however, does not effect lifestyle change, and bridging the gap between knowledge and actually adopting or modifying lifestyle cancer preventive behaviors remains a critical and problematic issue. Several variables, including knowledge of the principles underlying prevention, perceived susceptibility to developing cancer, and perceived consequences of prevention and lack of prevention influence a person's decision to put knowledge into practice.[17] These and other variables critical for lifestyle changes aimed at preventing cancer are illustrated in Figure 6-1.

Education efforts must be directed toward persuading people and populations to adopt preventive behaviors. Health care providers need to remember that persuasion is a nonlinear process and that lasting change is not achieved in a single encounter.[17] Persuasion depends on the following factors: (1) recipients of the information need to receive it from a source that is credible and is similar and attractive to the recipient; (2) the quality, quantity, and timing of messages are critical; (3) channels for communicating messages must maximize exposure or coverage of at-risk populations, speed of transmission, cost, and message function; and (4) the characteristics of the receiver (e.g., age, culture, ethnicity, developmental level, gender) must be considered.[17]

## Regulation

Regulation related to cancer prevention, much of which is a result of public demand, occurs in the form of legislation prohibiting the sale of alcohol and tobacco to minors and prohibiting smoking in public places. Imposing and increasing excise taxes on tobacco and alcohol products to reduce their accessibility also is an important form of regulation. Additionally, regulation decreases or eliminates man-made environmental carcinogens (e.g., 2-naphthylamine, benzene) and prohibits the addition of carcinogens to food. Regulatory efforts monitor homes for radon and limit exposure to occupational carcinogens (e.g., asbestos).[13]

Unfortunately, the etiology for most cancers is unknown, thereby limiting the application of exposure-based regulatory strategies.[10] Additionally, the impact of regulatory efforts concerned with cancer prevention are difficult to evaluate. For example, it is still too early to evaluate the long-term gains from tobacco regulation.[13]

## Host Modification

Host modification is the alteration of the body's internal environment to prevent initiation or progression of cancer. The principle methods are immunization and chemoprevention.[13]

### Immunization

Viruses may contribute to over 20% of human cancers.[18] Tumor-associated viruses probably are necessary but not sufficient for tumor causation. Generally, the cancer-causing virus is integrated into cellular DNA. A long latent period occurs between the initial infection and cancer.[19] Well-known viruses thought to cause human cancers are Epstein-Barr virus (EBV), associated with Burkitt's lymphoma and nasopharyngeal cancer; hepatitis B and C viruses (HBV and HCV), associated with liver cancer; human papillomavirus (HPV), linked with cervical, penile, and some anal cancers; human T-cell leukemia retrovirus types 1 and 2 (HTLV-1 and HTLV-2), associated with T-cell leukemia and lymphoma; and human immunodeficiency virus (HIV), associated with non-Hodgkin's lymphoma and Kaposi's sarcoma. Table 6-2 lists viral mechanisms and cofactors involved in cancer development. More information about these viruses and their

**TABLE 6-1** Cancer Control Healthy People 2000 Prevention Objectives

| Factor | Year 2000 Objectives |
|---|---|
| Smoking | Reduce percent of adults who smoke to 15% or less. |
| | Reduce percent of youths who smoke by age 20 to 15% or less |
| Diet | Reduce dietary fat to 30% of total calories or less. |
| | Reduce saturated fat to less than 10% of total calories (ages 2 and older). Increase complex carbohydrates and fiber in adult diets to 5 or more servings of fruit and 6 or more servings of grain products daily. |
| Sun exposure | Increase to 60% or more people who limit sun exposure, use sunscreens and protective clothing when exposed to sunlight, and avoid artificial sources of ultraviolet light. |
| Counseling | Increase to 75% or more primary care providers who routinely counsel patients about tobacco cessation, diet modification, and screening recommendations. |

Adapted from the Division of Cancer Prevention and Control: *'94 Annual Report.* Bethesda, MD, National Cancer Institute, 1994, p 13.

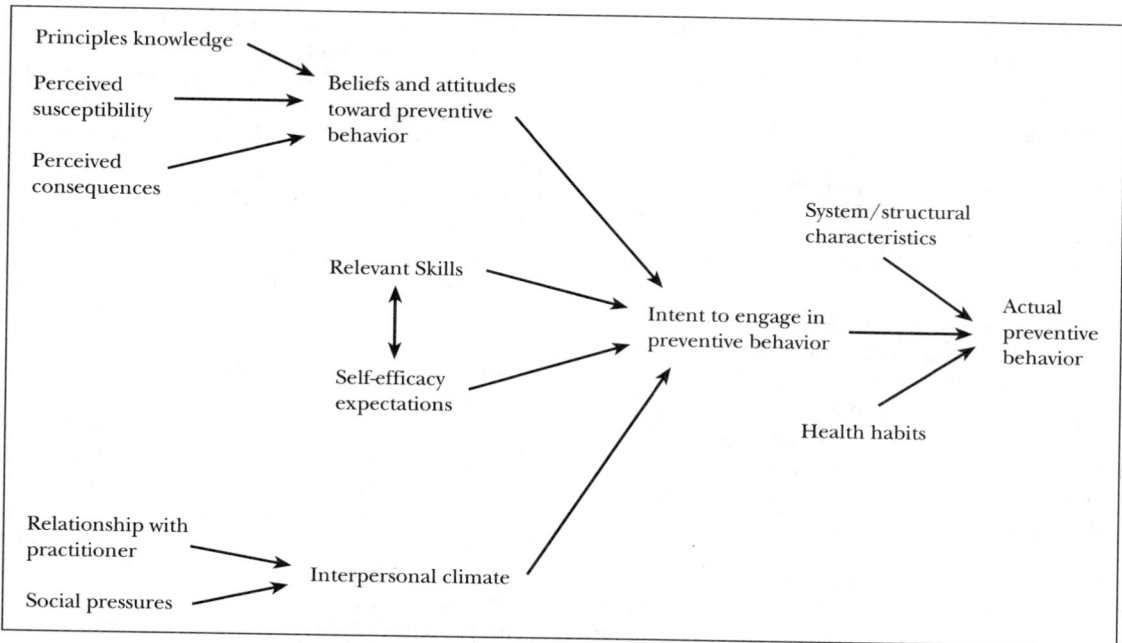

**FIGURE 6-1**   Factors affecting cancer prevention behavior. (Adapted with permission from Buller and Buller.[17])

**TABLE 6-2**   Viral Mechanisms and Cofactors Involved in Cancer Development

| Virus | Cancer-Causing Mechanisms | Probable Cofactors |
|---|---|---|
| Epstein-Barr virus | Affects B lymphocytes, activates *myc* oncogene, suppresses function of specific T lymphocytes | Malaria, eating salted fish in childhood, exposure to cigarette smoke |
| Hepatitis B virus | Integrates with viral DNA, causes cell proliferation, inactivates *p53* tumor-suppressor gene | Aflatoxins, alcohol, cigarette smoking |
| Human papillomavirus | Viral oncoproteins inactivate tumor-suppressor genes (retinoblastoma and *p53*) in premalignant conditions | Cigarette smoking, coinfections, exposure to solar radiation and x-rays, natural carcinogens |
| Human T-cell leukemia virus 1 | Oncogene-like action | None implicated |
| Human immuno-deficiency virus | Aberrant growth factor stimulation, loss of normal immune surveillance | Coinfections, lifestyle |

Adapted from Fischinger.[19]

relationship to human cancers is found in chapters 34, 41, 42, 44, and 46.

The discovery of cancer-causing viruses in humans shows some promise for cancer prevention in that similar viruses in animals have been eliminated by vaccines made from the attenuated (inactivated) viruses.[18] The current approach to vaccination in humans is to attenuate viruses and use them for immunostimulation.[20] Newer direct approaches to cancer vaccines currently are being explored or are in the planning stages. The direct approach uses two methods. In one, gene sequences of the desired antigen are delivered to the host by inserting the gene for the antigen via a nonreplicating plasmid vector. The gene coding for the desired protein is put into purified plasmid DNA, suspended in saline, and injected into the skin or muscle. The other method introduces the gene by bombarding the skin with particles containing the plasmid DNA with a "gene gun."[20,21]

Clinical trials of cancer vaccines are in various phases of testing. EBV vaccine trials currently are under way in England. At-risk populations who have received the existing HBV vaccine (a third-generation vaccine is in phase III testing) will need careful follow-up to determine its possible role in preventing cancer. HPV and HTLV vaccines are not ready for human trials. Two vaccines for HIV are safe for phase I or II trials. Tumor antigen vaccines against breast and pancreatic cancers are under development.[18,19] The Cancer Research Institute, a non-profit organization that supports cancer immunology research, is establishing a cancer vaccine trial registry that will serve as a centralized source of information about all ongoing cancer vaccine trials.[21]

## Chemoprevention

The most tested and promising form of host modification is chemoprevention, which is the use of defined, noncytotoxic nutrients and/or pharmacological agents to inhibit or reverse the process of carcinogenesis. Chemopreventive agents enhance the inactivation of carcinogens, modify the expression of oncogenes, or interfere with cell proliferation. Nutrient chemopreventives include dietary constituents (e.g., beta-carotene), vitamins (e.g., vitamins A, C, and E), and micronutrients (e.g., selenium). Examples of pharmacological chemopreventives are synthetic retinoids (e.g., isotretinoin), antiestrogens (e.g., tamoxifen), and nonsteroidal anti-inflammatory drugs (NSAIDs).[22,23]

***Chemoprevention and carcinogenesis*** Although chapters 2 and 3 explain carcinogenesis in detail, knowledge of certain aspects of the process is fundamental to understanding chemoprevention. Multiple changes in cellular genetics occurring together, rather than a single event, are thought to initiate cancer.[10] During initiation, the DNA of a normal cell undergoes somatic mutation. If the cell repairs the DNA damage, cancer may not develop. However, after initiation, a mutation may remain dormant in an extended latency period. During this period the multiple initiating events or promotion of a genetically altered cell required for tumor growth may begin.[10,23]

Proto-oncogenes, which code for proteins involved in normal cell growth and differentiation, most likely are involved in initiation and promotion of cancer.[24] The conversion of proto-oncogenes to oncogenes can occur through genetic mechanisms (e.g., translocation, gene amplification, point mutation) that may result from spontaneous somatic events or from exposure to carcinogens or mutagens.[10] Tumor-suppressor genes code for proteins that inhibit unregulated growth. Thus, within this genetic framework, the theoretical disruption of carcinogenesis at several points provides the rationale for use of chemopreventive agents.[10,23]

Agents that inhibit carcinogenesis generally are classified by the point in the process at which they are effective. For example, chemopreventive agents could be used to prevent or limit exposure to tumor initiators or promoters; stimulate inactivation and excretion of potential initiators or promoters; inhibit, modify, or block the activation of proto-oncogenes, thereby blocking the oncogene expression; or inactivate tumor-suppressor genes to regain control over cell replication and differentiation.[10,24]

Chemopreventive agents can affect carcinogenesis in many ways. Antioxidants (e.g., vitamins C and E, beta-carotene) have been well studied as potential chemopreventive agents. Antioxidants serve as "scavengers" to protect against cellular damage produced by active oxygen during the promotional phase of carcinogenesis.[9] Retinoids can control expression of certain oncogenes and growth factor receptors, thereby regulating cell differentiation and proliferation in most epithelia that are sites for cancer development.[24] Steroid hormones or analogues, such as tamoxifen (a synthetic antiestrogen) or finasteride (a synthetic antiandrogen), can bind to protein receptors in the cell nucleus and regulate translation. Anti-inflammatory agents may inhibit the synthesis of prostaglandins, which reduce the formation of colon polyps.[10] Chemoprevention, therefore, has the potential for primary, secondary, and tertiary prevention.[9]

***Biological end points of chemoprevention*** A major limitation of chemoprevention is identification of end points that measure efficacy of the agent. Although detection of cancer is the definitive end point, it is not feasible because the time to cancer occurrence may be long, or the incidence uncommon, even in persons at high risk.[25] Thus, the current approach for assessing efficacy of chemoprevention consists of using biological parameters, or biomarkers, as intermediate end points. *Biomarkers,* which have the capacity to reveal responses to chemopreventive agents within a shorter time,[26] can be defined as "measurable markers of cellular or molecular events associated with specific stages of the multistep evolution and progression of carcinogenesis."[27,p.556] For chemoprevention to be feasible and cost-effective, biomarkers must reveal earlier changes in carcinogenesis and more information about risk of transformation to cancer. Additionally, biomarkers need to be sensitive, specific, quantitative, and reproducible.[27] Validation of a biomarker requires that its biological or biochemical properties correlate with the definitive end point—cancer.[22]

Table 6-3 lists some biomarkers of end points of chemoprevention, specifically genetic, proliferation, and differentiation markers; markers of biochemical, immune, and micronutrient status; and tissue markers. Combinations of these markers may most accurately predict the response to a chemopreventive agent.[26]

With the discovery of proto-oncogenes, oncogenes, and tumor-suppressor genes, use of *genetic markers* in clinical chemoprevention studies will become feasible. For example, gene amplification or mutations in people at high risk for cancer and changes in expression during chemopreventive treatment may provide information on both treatment and the disease course.[26] Reports of DNA adducts (DNA damage following carcinogen exposure) and micronuclei (chromosomal fragments created in proliferating cells during carcinogenic damage to DNA) as sole intermediate end point markers remain inconclusive.[25-27]

As *proliferation markers,* precancerous lesions can show regression to a lower degree of precancer, progression to a higher degree, and the status of surrounding unaffected tissue and its relation to the precancer (field cancerization effect).[25,27] Measures of cellular proliferation using mitotic index, thymidine labeling, proliferating cell nuclear antigen (PCNA), and Ki 67 antigen have been impressive biomarkers of chemoprevention activity.[25,27]

**TABLE 6-3** Biomarkers of Intermediate End Points of Chemoprevention

| |
|---|
| Genetic markers |
|    Oncogenes and oncoproteins |
|    Nuclear aberrations (e.g., micronuclei) |
|    DNA adducts |
| Proliferation markers |
|    Precancerous lesions |
|    Cellular proliferation indexes (e.g., mitotic index, thymidine labeling, proliferating cell nuclear antigen, Ki 67 antigen) |
| Differentiation markers |
|    Growth factors and receptors |
|    Cytokeratins |
|    Involucrin |
|    Blood antigens |
| Biochemical and immunologic markers |
|    Ornithine decarboxylase |
|    Transglutaminase |
|    Altered cellular/humoral immunity |
| Micronutrient and tissue markers |
|    Vitamins and trace elements |
|    Intrinsic effect of chemopreventive agents in target tissue |

Adapted from Meyskens,[25] Pillai et al,[26] and Lippmann et al.[27]

*Differentiation markers* include growth factors and epithelial markers such as cytokeratins, involucrin, and certain blood-related antigens of epithelial cells. Growth factors are promising intermediate end-point markers of differentiation because of their postulated link to oncogenes.[26] Cytokeratins are epithelial intracellular filaments comprising keratin-like proteins that are expressed in different epithelia in different patterns. As epithelial cells undergo differentiation, the patterns change. Involucrin, a protein component synthesized by human epithelial cells, reflects epithelial differentiation. Expression of Lewis blood antigens has been correlated with histological type and degree of colonic epithelial cell dysplasia.[26]

Ornithine decarboxylase (ODC), the rate-limiting enzyme in polyamine synthesis (which has an essential role in cell proliferation), has been established as a *biochemical marker* for chemopreventive activity in people with Barrett's esophagus, familial polyposis of the colon, and adenomatous colon polyps. Epidermal transglutamase serves as a marker of squamous cell differentiation of epithelial tissue. *Immunologic markers* are not well understood but may reflect changes in cellular or hormonal immunity or identify cellular and molecular alterations in incipient tumor cells.[22]

Examples of *micronutrient markers* are serum levels of micronutrients, such as vitamins and trace elements that can serve as useful intermediate markers of intake and tissue distribution.[25,26] Effects of the chemopreventive agent directly on the target tissue also serve as an intermediate *tissue marker* of efficacy, but correlations with the definitive end point (e.g., changes in precancers, cancer occurrence) could take some time.[25]

## CHALLENGES OF CONDUCTING CANCER PREVENTION TRIALS

The overall goal of cancer prevention research is to identify the preventable causes of cancer and to reduce cancer incidence by effectively applying prevention strategies in specific populations.[28]

### Comparisons of Prevention and Treatment Trials

Although cancer prevention trials resemble cancer treatment trials in that they commonly use prospective design, random assignment of participants, control groups, blinding when feasible, and rigorous statistical analyses, cancer prevention trials do have some unique features.[29,30] Cancer prevention trials commonly involve more collaboration with biology, epidemiology, and behavioral sciences than do treatment trials.[31] The specific goals of cancer chemoprevention trials are safety and efficacy. Safety is important because cancer prevention trials usually involve an essentially healthy rather than an ailing population and therefore should not expose participants to undue risk. Efficacy of a selected agent establishes its cancer prevention effect.[32]

Similar to cancer treatment trials, clinical cancer chemoprevention trials have specific phases. Phase I trials develop pharmacokinetic safety and toxicity profiles on potential chemopreventive agents. Phase II trials demonstrate efficacy and develop biomarkers of efficacy. Phase III trials demonstrate modulation of surrogate end points of cancer or demonstrate cancer incidence reduction.[11,23] Table 6-4 further compares cancer prevention and cancer treatment trials.

### Design

Cancer prevention trials usually are randomized, single- or double-blinded studies. Generally a high-risk population selected for study is one with a risk for a particular cancer that exceeds the risk of the general population by a factor of at least two.[7] Usual eligibility criteria include age, family history of the same cancer or related cancers, abnormalities of specific laboratory tests, carcinogen exposure, and the presence of other risk factors identified in epidemiological studies.[7] Depending on the statistical power (the probability that the study will detect a statistically significant benefit), the recruitment pool can range from hundreds to thousands of people.

Selection of the intervention used in a cancer prevention trial, particularly a chemoprevention trial, may be influenced by the identification of human carcinogenic exposures to determine high-risk study participants, the availability of biomarkers to assess risk status of

**TABLE 6-4** Features of Cancer Prevention Trials versus Cancer Treatment Trials

| Variable | Prevention Trial | Treatment Trial |
|---|---|---|
| Goals | Decrease incidence/mortality | Increase cancer cure/remission rates |
| | Prevent/ameliorate precancerous lesions or markers of cancer risk | Decrease cancer morbidity/mortality |
| | Prevent second primary cancer | |
| Study population | People without cancer | People with confirmed diagnosis of cancer |
| | General population | |
| | High-risk population | |
| | People with precancerous lesions | |
| | Disease-free cancer survivors | |
| Toxicity of agent | None to moderate, acceptable | Moderate to severe, acceptable |
| Study protocol | Design | Design |
| | Simple (dichotomy) | Simple (dichotomy or multiagent) |
| | Intervention versus placebo | Therapy versus placebo |
| | Factorial | Therapy A versus therapy B |
| | Intervention A versus intervention B versus intervention AB versus placebo | Therapy A versus therapy B versus therapy C |
| | Multiple simultaneous interventions, including interactions | |
| | Large scale (thousands of subjects) | Small scale (hundreds of subjects) |
| | Pilot study usually required | Pilot study rarely needed |
| | Placebo run-in useful | Run-in inappropriate |
| | Study may require 5–10+ years of intervention and follow-up | Study length may be short for aggressive cancers, longer for slower-growing cancers or adjuvant studies |
| Adherence | Adherence to protocol may be difficult to maintain, i.e., subject-dependent | Adherence to protocol easier to maintain, i.e., physician-dependent |

Adapted with permission from Greenwald P, Nixon DW, Malone WF, et al: Concepts in cancer chemoprevention research. *Cancer* 65:1487, 1990.

participants or efficiently serve as intermediate end points, and the interest and ability of potential study participants to adopt and adhere to behaviors specified in the trial.[3] Prevention trial interventions usually contain many dimensions beyond the participant, such as family, social network, school, work site, health care system, and the mass media. Chemoprevention trials usually combine the chemopreventive agent or placebo with corresponding behavioral interventions (e.g., smoking cessation, dietary modification, avoidance of sun exposure).[3] Other factors considered in the design of a cancer prevention trial include the number of study groups, the unit of randomization, end points (e.g., death, cancer diagnosis, changes in a precancerous lesion, or targets of a biological marker), and the duration. Other independent variables may include behavioral changes and quality-of-life measures.[33] Analysis of the trials may be affected by factors such as nonadherence, delays in the effect of the intervention, and available statistical methods.

## Recruitment

Finding people at high risk for a certain cancer is much more difficult than finding people at ordinary risk.[7] Recruitment also is made more difficult by the fact that only 10%–25% of eligible subjects will choose to enroll in a chemoprevention trial.[9] Recruitment to chemoprevention trials, therefore, requires considerable cost, time, and effort on the part of study personnel.

The pool of potential subjects for cancer chemoprevention trials emanates from a variety of sources such as insurance company lists, referrals from physician specialists who would likely care for the population under study (e.g., people with premalignant conditions), and public relations campaigns.[9] Other recruitment sources include screening clinics, tumor registries, pathology databases, behavioral instruments that assess lifestyle, genetic and hereditary cancer screening, and cancer survivors who are at high risk for a second malignancy.[3]

Criteria for trial eligibility or ineligibility may pose some barriers to recruitment. These criteria vary according to the design of the trial, the cancer under study, and the agent being tested. To be eligible for a trial, potential participants may be asked to cease taking certain medications that they have been using for general health maintenance. For example, the Breast Cancer Prevention Trial (BCPT) requires women to discontinue estrogen they may have taken for years to control symptoms of menopause. In general, women who are pregnant or who intend to become pregnant are not candidates for chemoprevention studies because of actual or potential teratogenic effects of the intervention.

In most chemoprevention trials, participants are randomly assigned to either an intervention (treatment) arm using a chemopreventive agent or a placebo arm. Thus, potential participants need to be well informed about the short- and long-term toxicities of the chemopreventive agents under study before enrolling in a trial. Learning all the known potential side effects of the intervention may be sufficiently daunting to dampen the person's desire to enroll in the trial. Additionally, people who suspect they might be assigned to the placebo arm may choose not to enroll in the trial because they desire the chemopreventive agent. If a compound that is easily available over-the-counter, such as a vitamin or a mineral, is being used as a study agent, potential participants may choose not to enroll in the study and subsequently self-prescribe their own treatment. Thus, health care providers are responsible for educating potential participants and reinforcing teaching of the possible hazards involved in self-treatment.[34] The NCI has published a patient education booklet that discusses some of these issues and provides general information about chemoprevention trials for potential participants.[35]

## Enrollment

### Toxicity monitoring

Once a person provides written, informed consent to enroll in a trial and is randomly assigned to the intervention or control arm, study personnel are responsible for several important tasks to ensure the participant's safety. Early identification of toxicity is critical and entails carefully following the trial protocol and seeing that participants undergo proper testing (e.g., laboratory tests, radiographs) to evaluate toxicity. Maintaining a current record of concomitant prescription and over-the-counter medications is also important because some compounds interfere with chemopreventive agents.

### Adherence

Study personnel also monitor and promote short- and long-term adherence to the assigned regimen. This is a challenging task in that most chemoprevention trials last between five and ten years and ideally incorporate long-term follow-up after completion of the intervention. Several trials also involve lifestyle changes, and adherence to these changes is considerably more difficult than adherence to taking a medication.[7]

Some trials build a run-in period into the design to assess likely adherence. During this period, study personnel ask potential participants to adhere to similar tasks (e.g., taking a pill, eating a certain diet) that will be required of them following randomization. If their adherence is unacceptable during the run-in period, the potential participants are not enrolled in the trial.[7]

Enrolled participants who are assigned to the inter-vention group and fail to adhere to the regimen are called *dropouts*, whereas participants in the control group who adopt the intervention are called *drop-ins*.[7] These forms of nonadherence may be influenced by the media, advice from other health care providers not involved in or knowledgeable about the trial, health fads, alternative therapies, or family. Unfortunately, this information may not always be accurate or based on well-designed scientific research. Study personnel must therefore be continually aware of media and scientific developments in the area of cancer prevention and must educate subjects appropriately. Study personnel need to develop a relationship based on honesty and trust with each participant in order to facilitate exchange of accurate information and promote adherence.[32,34]

## CHEMOPREVENTION RESEARCH

Chemoprevention research at the NCI began in the late 1970s. In 1982 the NCI established the Chemoprevention Research Program, which is divided into two broad categories: chemoprevention, and diet and nutrition. These areas of research are pursued through extramural and intramural funding to identify and evaluate the efficacy of specific micronutrients, natural compounds, and drugs in reducing cancer incidence.[10,11]

## Chemoprevention Trials

Table 6-5 provides a summary of representative phase II and phase III chemoprevention trials funded by the NCI. High-priority trials designated by the NCI include the BCPT and the Prostate Cancer Prevention Trial (PCPT).

### Breast Cancer Prevention Trial

The BCPT began in 1992 as a ten-year study to test the ability of tamoxifen to prevent breast cancer in healthy women at high risk for the disease. This randomized, double-blind trial determines women's risk by age (women aged 35–39 must have a risk that is equal to that of a 60-year-old woman); number of first-degree relatives with a history of breast cancer; age at first live birth; number of benign breast biopsies, especially for atypical hyperplasia; and age at menarche. Women with a history of lobular carcinoma in situ also are eligible. Ineligible women include those with concurrent health conditions that may affect their ability to complete the trial. Women who are taking hormone replacements for menopausal symptoms and women who use oral contraceptives are eligible only if they cease taking the medication three months before considering enrollment. Approximately 16,000 women, aged 35 and older, are being randomly assigned to receive oral tamoxifen (20 mg daily) or pla-

**TABLE 6-5**   Phase II and III Clinical Cancer Chemoprevention Trials Funded by the National Cancer Institute, Division of Cancer Prevention and Control

| Study Site/Population | Institution | Study Title/Phase | Agent Dose and Schedule |
|---|---|---|---|
| Bladder/Resected superficial tumors | Instituto Nazionale per la Ricerca sul Cancre (Italy) | DNA content modulation by HPR in bladder tumors/phase II | 4-HPR 200 mg/day vs. control |
| Bladder/Transitional cell carcinoma | University of Wisconsin | Markers of bladder cancer and their modulation by DFMO/phase II | DFMO 0.5 or 1.0 g/day vs. placebo |
| Breast/Stage I/II within 1 year of adjuvant therapy, NED | American Health Foundation | Women's Intervention Nutrition Study (WINS)/phase III | Low fat diet (<15% calories) vs. standard diet |
| Breast/Status post–stage I breast cancer | Instituto Nazionale Tumori (Italy) | Breast cancer prevention with synthetic retinoid (4-HPR) | 4-HPR 200 mg/day |
| Breast/High risk | University of Pittsburgh | Breast Cancer Prevention Trial/phase III | Tamoxifen 20 mg/day vs. placebo |
| Breast/Proliferative breast disease | University of Utah | Effect of tamoxifen on proliferative breast disease/phase II | Tamoxifen 20 mg/day vs. placebo |
| Cervix/CIN I, II | Albert Einstein Medical Center | Beta-carotene clinical trial monitoring cervical dysplasia/phase II | Beta-carotene 30 mg/day vs. placebo |
| Cervix/CIN II, III | University of California, Irvine | Chemoprevention of cervical cancer with beta-carotene/phase III | Beta-carotene 30 mg/day vs. placebo |
| Colon | Dallas Veteran's Administration Medical Center | Aspirin, mucosal prostaglandins, and colon proliferation/phase II | Aspirin 325 mg/day and 81 mg/day vs. placebo |
| Colon/Previous cancerous polyp | Dartmouth College | Aspirin prevention of large bowel polyps/phase II | Aspirin 80 or 325 mg/day vs. folic acid vs. placebo |
| Colon/Previous colon cancer | Loyola University of Chicago | Effects of beta-carotene on colonic cell proliferation/phase II | Beta-carotene 30–180 mg/day |
| Colon/Status post–Dukes' A & B1 colon cancer | New England Deaconess Hospital | Mucosal proliferation and fish oil in colorectal cancer/phase II | Omega-3 fatty acids 10 mg/day vs. placebo |
| Colon/Previous colon adenoma | Tufts University | Folate: effects on intermediary markers of colon cancer/phase II | Folic acid 5 mg/day vs. placebo |
| Colon/Previous colon adenoma | University of Arizona | Colon cancer prevention program project: phase III trial of wheat bran fiber | Wheat bran 13.5 g/day vs. placebo |
| Colon/Previous colon adenoma | University of Arizona | Colon cancer prevention program project: phase II trial of piroxicam | Piroxicam 7.5 mg/day vs. placebo |
| Colon/Previous colon adenoma | University of California, Irvine | Polyamine depletion and chemoprevention of colon cancer/phase II | DFMO 0.0655 g/day, 0.125 g/day, 0.25 g/day |
| Colon/Previous colon adenoma | University of Utah | Sulindac therapy for sporadic colorectal adenomas/phase III | Sulindac 150 mg/bid vs. placebo |
| Colon/Previous colon adenoma; Prostate/status post–A/B prostate cancer, serum PSA 3-10 | University of Wisconsin | Modulating intermediate end points by DFMO/phase II | DFMO 0.5 g/day vs. placebo |
| Head and neck | Northern California Oncology Group | Double-blind phase III trial of effects of low-dose 13-cis retinoic acid on second primaries | 13-cis retinoic acid vs. placebo |
| Lung/Women, smokers | Brigham and Women's Hospital | Vitamin E and aspirin in women (Women's Health Study) | Aspirin 100 mg/qod, vitamin E 600 mg/qod vs. placebo |

**TABLE 6-5** Phase II and III Clinical Cancer Chemoprevention Trials Funded by the National Cancer Institute, Division of Cancer Prevention and Control (continued)

| Study Site/Population | Institution | Study Title/Phase | Agent Dose and Schedule |
|---|---|---|---|
| Lung/Men, asbestosis | University of Washington (multi-institutional) | Cancer prevention with retinol and beta-carotene in persons with asbestosis (CARET Study)/ phase III COMPLETED | Beta-carotene 30 mg/day, retinol 25,000 IU/day |
| Lung/Cigarette smokers | University of Washington (multi-institutional) | Chemoprevention of lung cancer with retinoids and beta-carotene (CARET Study)/phase III COMPLETED | Beta-carotene 30 mg/day, retinol 25,000 IU/day |
| Physicians | Harvard Medical School | Randomized trial of aspirin and beta-carotene in U.S. physicians (Physicians' Health Study) COMPLETED | Beta-carotene 50 mg/qod; aspirin 325 mg/qod vs. placebo |
| Prostate/Normal DRE, PSA ≤3.0 | Southwest Oncology Group | Prostate Cancer Prevention Trial (PCPT) | Finasteride 5 mg/day vs. placebo |
| Skin/Actinic keratoses | University of Arizona | Chemoprevention of skin cancer program project: topically administered chemopreventive agents/ phase II | Topical DFMO, vitamin E, epigallocatechin gallate vs. placebo |
| Skin/Actinic keratoses | University of Arizona | Chemoprevention of skin cancer program project: clinical pharmacology of dose-intensive vitamin A/phase II | Retinyl palmitate 25,000–100,000 IU/day vs. placebo |

CARET = Carotenoid and Retinoid Efficacy Trial; CIN = cervical intraepithelial neoplasia; DRE = digital rectal examination; DFMO = difluoromethylornithine; HPR = 4-hydroxyphenyl retinamide; NED = no evidence of disease; PSA = prostate-specific antigen.
Data from National Cancer Institute, Division of Cancer Prevention and Control, Chemoprevention Branch; David S. Alberts, MD, personal communication (December 1995).

cebo for an initial five-year period.[36] More than 12,000 women have been enrolled in the trial.

### Prostate Cancer Prevention Trial

Initiated in 1993, the PCPT is a double-blind, randomized, intergroup trial testing the ability of finasteride to prevent prostate cancer in healthy men aged 55 and older. Enrollment of the 18,000 men was completed in the fall of 1995. The men were randomly assigned to oral finasteride (5 mg) per day or placebo. Participants will be followed for seven years, and trial results can be expected sometime in 2003. The primary end point of the study is a prostate biopsy that is negative for cancer. Secondary objectives include evaluating side effects and toxicity, and determining grade and stage of prostate and other cancers, cancer mortality, incidence of benign prostatic hypertrophy, effectiveness of prostate-specific antigen screening and digital rectal examination, and quality of life.[37]

## Completed Phase III Chemoprevention Trials

Alberts and Garcia[23] critically reviewed results of several positive phase III chemoprevention studies reported in

the literature. In brief, patients with non–small cell lung cancer who received retinol developed fewer second primary lung cancers than controls. Synthetic retinoids (isotretinoin and 4-hydroxyphenyl retinamide) provide significant clinical improvement and reduction in relapse for oral leukoplakia. Patients with familial adenomatous polyposis who took a wheat bran fiber supplement had a significant inverse correlation between the number of polyps and amount of ingested prescribed fiber. Another study of familial polyposis showed that sulindac significantly decreased the number of polyps.

The Nutritional Intervention Studies of Esophageal Cancer Studies, conducted in Linxian, China, looked at the effects of dietary supplementation with four different vitamin-mineral combinations. Linxian served as the study site because the rural county has the highest rate of esophageal cancer in the world and because it is suspected that the population's chronic deficiencies of multiple nutrients may contribute to esophageal cancer etiology.[11] Approximately 30,000 participants were randomized to one of three treatment arms that enabled evaluation of four combinations of nutrients: retinol/zinc, riboflavin/niacin, vitamin C/molybdenum, and beta-carotene/vitamin E/selenium. Participants who received daily beta-carotene/vitamin

E/selenium had a lower incidence of cancer, particularly stomach cancer, and a significant reduction in mortality. No other combinations had apparent chemopreventive activity.[38]

The Alpha-Tocopherol, Beta-Carotene Lung Cancer Prevention Study (ATBC) investigated the efficacy of daily oral alpha-tocopherol and beta-carotene in preventing lung cancer among male cigarette smokers. Over 29,000 participants were enrolled in the trial. The ATBC found no reduction in lung cancer incidence among men who received alpha-tocopherol. Unexpectedly, men who took beta-carotene had an 18% higher incidence of lung cancer. These results raised the possibility that the chemopreventive agents may have harmful as well as beneficial effects.[39]

The Carotenoid and Retinoid Efficacy Trial (CARET), a randomized, double-blind trial testing the efficacy of beta-carotene and retinol in two high-risk groups for lung cancer (men and women current heavy smokers or former smokers, and men with extensive occupational asbestos exposure) was terminated by the investigators in early 1996. The primary end point of the trial was incidence of lung cancer. Over 18,000 participants received a placebo or a combination of oral beta-carotene (30 mg) and retinol (25,000) daily for an average of four years. The intervention was halted 21 months early because it did not reduce lung cancer and because, similar to the ATBC trial, participants in the intervention arm had more lung cancers and deaths from lung cancer than those in the placebo arm. Follow-up of the subjects will continue for another five years.[40]

The Physicians' Health Study was conducted among male physicians in the United States over a 12-year period. By the scheduled end of the study (December 31, 1995), over 22,000 subjects had received 50 mg of beta-carotene every other day or placebo. The end points of the study were incidence and mortality of cancer or cardiovascular disease. Results showed that beta-carotene produced neither benefit nor harm as far as incidence of cancer, cardiovascular disease, or death from all causes.[41]

## Diet and Nutrition Research

The NCI is sponsoring several studies targeting diet and nutrition in cancer prevention. These include (1) physiochemical effects of dietary fiber on transit time, stool weight, pH, bile acids, serum lipids, mineral absorption, and intestinal flora; (2) retinoids and carotenoids (identify mechanisms that control absorption of vitamin A and carotenoids, evaluate conversion of carotenoids to retinol, and evaluate storage in tissues); (3) nutritive and nonnutritive constituents of fruits and vegetables (develop analytic methods for identifying and quantifying these constituents and determine their biological activity, absorption, metabolism, and mechanisms of action); and (4) biomarkers for monitoring dietary changes.[11]

# CANCER PREVENTION CONTROVERSIES AND DILEMMAS

## Incomplete Knowledge

Epidemiological reports of cancer prevention and detection may use statistical analyses to group associated risk factors of certain cancers. Although these risk factors may be confounded either with each other or with their reputed effects, interventions aimed at reducing risks often are implemented before the relationship among the factors is known.[42] The controversy surrounding the role of diet and cancer illustrates this dilemma.

Diet can be considered a lifestyle factor or a carcinogenic risk factor. The current dietary recommendations for preventing cancer (Table 6-1) are based largely on epidemiological research. Although one author[43] stated that good dietary epidemiological data are scarce and inconsistent, overviews of epidemiological research do provide compelling evidence that dietary intake of naturally occurring chemopreventive agents (e.g., vitamin A, beta-carotene) is inversely associated with cancer incidence.[9,10] However, countless variables interfere with the interpretation of some epidemiological dietary studies. For example, participants' recall of dietary information (particularly long-term recall) is imprecise and incomplete; dietary patterns correlate with socioeconomic and political characteristics; the distribution of dietary components among individual foods varies greatly; the interactive roles of dietary components are not completely understood, particularly when several components are present in individual foods; and the period of life during which dietary intake most affects carcinogenesis is uncertain.[10,43] Publication bias may come into play if more "positive" dietary findings than "negative" findings are printed.[43] Proponents of dietary guidelines for cancer prevention argue that the recommended diet is healthful even if it does not reduce cancer incidence and mortality.[42]

Kottke[44] suggested that lack of evidence from randomized, controlled trials for an intervention's efficacy should not prevent us from recommending the intervention if other evidence is compelling, and that equal weight should not be assigned to all classes of evidence. He stated, "We should not be embarrassed to admit that a recommendation must be based on a 'best guess' because of inadequate information."[44,p.902] Kottke recommended using the consensus process to summarize and simplify knowledge that may be difficult to interpret. It also can facilitate action by minimizing the appearance of tentativeness and minimizing potential contradictory messages by individuals or organizations.

## Overselling Prevention

Goodman and Goodman[42] commented that in their enthusiasm to move from tentative hypotheses to implementing programs, health care organizations and industries, such as the food industry, acknowledge the caveats and qualifications of science but use more of a marketing approach than an educational approach to disseminating information. For example, when the ACS published its dietary guidelines a decade ago, it also mobilized millions of volunteers to promote them.[42]

The public education sponsored by many cancer organizations is a noble focus. However, these campaigns, which may cost thousands of dollars and be disseminated to thousands of people, often are not rigorously evaluated for their effectiveness in terms of efficacy, outcomes, economic impact, and benefit. If a campaign is not evaluated for its ability to change a certain behavior, for example, one could question the logic and underlying motivation for conducting the campaign. Is it being conducted purely to enhance knowledge? (Even though this outcome was not determined via evaluation.) To provide visibility for the sponsor? Many organizations keep statistics to document the number of people reached with a certain prevention message (e.g., numbers of brochures distributed). These numbers do not constitute an evaluation of a campaign. The earnestness and vigor of these organizations cannot be discounted, since in the minds of many, one life saved is worth the cost of the campaign. However, these groups need to take care not to eclipse hard information about cancer with notions of cancer prevention, particularly in this era of budget cutting and cost containment. Teutsch[4] recommended that prevention campaigns also be evaluated for their ability to determine the potential and practical consequences of prevention strategies, including social, legal, and ethical factors.

From the standpoint of the media's role in selling prevention, Brody[16,p.164] stated that health care professionals must provide the mass media with "sound scientific information and well-considered comments based on real evidence, not speculation or hysteria-mongering possibilities." She recommended that cancer prevention messages avoid a "quick-fix" mentality, emphasize that healthful living is not an all-or-nothing phenomenon, and encourage moderation of lifestyle behaviors.

## Attribution of Responsibility

The ongoing discoveries of carcinogens and cancer genes generate skepticism, making people indifferent to changing or adopting behaviors aimed at preventing cancer.[13] People also are reluctant to give up behaviors such as suntanning or cigarette smoking in order to gain health.[5] However, after developing cancer it is natural to seek meaning for why the event happened. In all human societies, morality may be a frame of reference for that meaning, that is, something was done incorrectly or not at all. When an illness such as cancer occurs, solace and exoneration are found in assigning blame for the disease to someone or something.[42]

Obversely, cancer prevention programs must take care not to impart a false sense of security. Even the person who faithfully adheres to prevention and screening guidelines could still develop cancer. Participants in prevention and screening campaigns need to be reminded that observance of guidelines does not guarantee a cancer-free existence, particularly when guidelines are based on incomplete knowledge.

The focus on the individual's role in preventing cancer may also serve to shift responsibility for health away from other bodies such as the federal government. Goodman and Goodman[42,p.36] stated that "recognizing the role of individual choice and discipline [in practicing preventive behaviors] is no substitute for health insurance, research, therapy, or exercising responsibility for the environment."

## CANCER PREVENTION AND CHANGES IN HEALTH CARE

The role of prevention has been overshadowed by more dramatic advances in medical science.[45] For cancer prevention to be successful, the health care community and policy makers need first to change the existing treatment-oriented model to one that is prevention-oriented.[15,46] They also must recognize the importance of intervening before carcinogenesis or during initiation or promotion, when the process may be halted, slowed, or reversed. This concept of early intervention parallels that used in cardiovascular disease, which is now accepted by the health care community and reimbursers alike. As with cardiovascular disease, the health care community must be aware of the biological significance of precancerous lesions and the importance of early detection of these lesions, so as to treat them with effective agents to prevent progression to cancer.[24]

Historically in the United States, cancer prevention services have not been reimbursed by payers at all levels. Most private health insurance plans do not pay for prevention counseling and testing. They may only pay for counseling that is incidental to the problem (e.g., reimbursing for tobacco cessation counseling of a patient with lung cancer but not reimbursing for identical counseling of a healthy individual).[47] The growth of managed care and capitation and the increasing use of primary health care providers as gatekeepers are driving the coverage of preventive services. Quality-control efforts by health plans carefully monitor whether patients received necessary preventive services.[46] However, funding for preventive services remains inadequate, even in prepaid health systems. These plans may need to earmark revenues (e.g., a percentage of capitation dues) to be devoted to prevention.[48]

Effective cancer prevention counseling and intervention often require additional time spent with the patient (e.g., to conduct a complete risk assessment, explain available clinical trials) and repeated visits or examinations that may be necessary to establish eligibility for clinical trials. Managed care groups generally will not reimburse health care providers for these efforts, a decision that could have two main effects: (1) health care providers will choose to spend less time counseling and educating patients about cancer prevention, and (2) the successful implementation of clinical cancer prevention trials may be compromised. However, cancer prevention guidelines and programs disseminated to even a portion of managed care groups can reach thousands of health care professionals who can serve as a conduit to millions of people.[46]

The health care community must recognize that no individual or single public or private agency can achieve the goal of prevention.[46] People will have to be actively involved in their own health care and in the management of their health.[48] Partnerships of public health agencies at all levels with professional, voluntary, and community organizations; health care organizations; academic institutions; philanthropic foundations; industry and labor; and schools, churches, and other local institutions will be needed for prevention to be achieved.[46,49]

## IMPLICATIONS FOR NURSING

Nurses play a key role in cancer prevention. They perform valuable, traditional services such as identifying people at high risk and counseling and educating patients about cancer prevention.[5] Additionally, nurses must strive to keep pace with the science of cancer prevention. For example, in the near future, individual risk profiles based on genetic factors, lifestyle behaviors, environmental exposure, history of precursor lesions, or any combination of these will define specific interventions, such as chemoprevention, for modulating cancer risk.[24] With sophisticated molecular biology techniques, it also may be possible to identify early damage to key proto-oncogenes in individuals at high risk.[22] Another future preventive strategy, gene transfer technology, may replace deficient genes prior to cancer development.[14]

To understand and participate in these advances in cancer prevention, nursing education, clinical practice, and research will need to have a stronger foundation in genetics, carcinogenesis, bioethics, behavioral change strategies, health policy, and environmental health.[5,50] Oncology nurse educators bear much of the responsibility for preparing nurses with knowledge and skills to participate in cancer prevention. Educators need to continually assess and update cancer prevention information in nursing program curricula at all levels.[8] This is no small task in light of the rapid changes in cancer prevention. Similarly, health care administrators should allow nurses time to plan and implement cancer prevention services. Given the opportunity, nurses can be instrumental in developing cancer prevention standards of care along with developing, supporting, and steering health policies related to cancer prevention. By being actively involved in collaborative, multidisciplinary research, nurses have a key opportunity to influence prevention interventions and outcomes. Oncology nurses are particularly well positioned to conduct cancer prevention research in socioeconomically disadvantaged populations. Engelking[51] succinctly stated the onus to oncology nurses: to meet the challenges of cancer prevention, nurses must prepare proactively, not reactively.

## ACKNOWLEDGMENTS

The author thanks David S. Alberts, MD, for scientific review of this chapter.

## REFERENCES

1. Garfinkel L: Perspectives on cancer prevention. *CA Cancer J Clin* 45:5–7, 1995 (editorial)
2. Meyskens FL Jr: Coming of age: The chemoprevention of cancer. *N Engl J Med* 323:825–827, 1990 (editorial)
3. Gritz ER, Moon TE: The new cancer prevention and control. *Cancer Epidemiol Biomarkers Prev* 1:163–165, 1992
4. Teutsch SM: A framework for assessing the effectiveness of disease and injury prevention. *MMWR* 41(RR-3):1–12, 1992
5. Frank-Stromborg M, Cohen R: Assessment and interventions for cancer prevention and detection, in Groenwald SL, Frogge MH, Goodman M, Yarbro CH (eds): *Cancer Nursing: Principles and Practice* (ed 3). Boston, Jones and Bartlett, 1993, pp 124–169
6. Loescher LJ: Commentary: Expanding our horizons with an alternative approach to cancer prevention and detection. *Semin Oncol Nurs* 9:147–149, 1993
7. Byar DP, Freedman LS: The importance and nature of cancer prevention trials. *Semin Oncol* 17:413–424, 1990
8. McMillan SC: Nurses' compliance with American Cancer Society Guidelines for Cancer Prevention and Detection. *Oncol Nurs Forum* 17:721–727, 1990
9. Bertram JS, Kolonel LN, Meyskens FL Jr: Rationale and strategies for chemoprevention of cancer in humans. *Cancer Res* 47:3012–3031, 1987
10. Greenwald P, Nixon DW, Malone W, et al: Concepts in chemoprevention research. *Cancer* 65:1483–1490, 1990
11. Division of Cancer Prevention and Control: *1994 Annual Report*. Bethesda, MD, National Institutes of Health/National Cancer Institute, 1994
12. Smart CR: Screening and early detection. *Semin Oncol* 17: 456–462, 1990
13. Cole P, Amoateng-Adjepong Y: Cancer prevention: Accomplishments and prospects. *Am J Public Health* 84:8–10, 1994 (editorial)
14. Greenwald P: Keynote address: Cancer prevention. *J Natl Cancer Inst Monogr* 12:9–14, 1992
15. Terris M: Healthy lifestyles: The perspective of epidemiology. *J Public Health Policy* 13:186–194, 1992
16. Brody JE: Communicating cancer-prevention information. *J Natl Cancer Inst Monogr* 12:163–164, 1992

17. Buller DB, Buller MK: Approaches to communicating preventive behaviors. *Semin Oncol Nurs* 7:53–63, 1991
18. Dalgleish AG: Viruses and cancer. *Br Med Bull* 47:21–46, 1991
19. Fischinger PJ: Prospects for reducing virus-associated human cancers by antiviral vaccines. *J Natl Cancer Inst Monogr* 12:109–114, 1992
20. Marwick C: Exciting potential of DNA vaccines explored. *JAMA* 273:1403–1404, 1995
21. Skolnick AA: Essential components now in place for clinical testing of cancer vaccine strategies, experts say. *JAMA* 273:528–530, 1995
22. Meyskens FL Jr: Chemoprevention of cancer in humans 1990: Where do we go from here? in Pastorino U, Hong WK (eds): *Chemoimmuno Prevention of Cancer: Proceedings of the First International Conference, Vienna, Austria.* New York, Thieme Medical Publishers, 1991, pp 245–252
23. Alberts DS, Garcia D: An overview of clinical cancer chemoprevention studies with emphasis on positive phase III studies. *J Nutr* 125:692S–697S, 1995
24. Greenwald P, Kelloff G, Burch-Whitman C, et al: Chemoprevention. *CA Cancer J Clin* 45:31–49, 1995
25. Meyskens FL Jr: Biomarkers as intermediate endpoints and cancer prevention. *J Natl Cancer Inst Monogr* 13:177–181, 1992
26. Pillai R, Garewal HS, Wood S, et al: Biological monitoring of cancer chemoprevention. *J Surg Oncol* 51:195–202, 1992
27. Lippman SM, Lee JS, Lotan R, et al: Biomarkers as intermediate end points in chemoprevention trials. *J Natl Cancer Inst* 82:555–560, 1990
28. Greenwald P, Sondik E, Lynch BS: Diet and chemoprevention in NCI's research strategy to achieve national cancer control objectives. *Annu Rev Public Health* 7:267–291, 1986
29. Hennekens CH: Issues in the design and conduct of clinical trials. *J Natl Cancer Inst* 73:1473–1476, 1984
30. Nixon DW: Special aspects of chemoprevention trials. *Cancer* 74:2683–2686, 1994 (suppl)
31. Meyskens FL Jr: Commentary: Thinking about cancer causality and chemoprevention. *J Natl Cancer Inst* 80:1278–1281, 1988
32. Padberg RM: Chemoprevention trials. *Cancer Pract* 2:154–156, 1994
33. Moon TE: Planning the analysis of a breast cancer prevention trial. *Prev Med* 20:109–118, 1991
34. Loescher LJ: Chemoprevention of human skin cancers. *Semin Oncol Nurs* 7:45–52, 1991
35. National Cancer Institute: *What Are Chemoprevention Clinical Trials?* NIH publication No. 93-3595. Bethesda, MD, National Cancer Institute, 1992
36. National Surgical Adjuvant Breast and Bowel Project. *Protocol P-1. A clinical trial to determine the worth of tamoxifen for preventing breast cancer.* Pittsburgh, NSABP, 1992
37. Thompson I, Brawer M, Crawford ED, et al: *Chemoprevention of prostate cancer with finasteride (Proscar). Protocol no. 9217.* San Antonio, Southwest Oncology Group, 1993
38. Blot WJ, Li J-Y, Taylor PR, et al: Nutrition intervention trials in Linxian, China: Supplementation with specific vitamin/mineral combinations, cancer incidence, and disease-specific mortality in the general population. *J Natl Cancer Inst* 85:1483–1492, 1993
39. The Alpha-Tocopherol, Beta Carotene Cancer Prevention Study Group: The effect of vitamin E and beta carotene on the incidence of lung cancer and other cancers in male smokers. *N Engl J Med* 330:1029–1035, 1994
40. Omenn GS, Goodman GE, Thornquist MD, et al: Effects of a combination of beta carotene and vitamin A on lung cancer and cardiovascular disease. *N Engl J Med* 334:1150–1155, 1996
41. Hennekens CH, Buring JE, Manson JE, et al: Lack of effect of long-term supplementation with beta carotene on the incidence of malignant neoplasms and cardiovascular disease. *N Engl J Med* 334:1145–1149, 1996
42. Goodman LE, Goodman MJ: Prevention: How misuse of a concept undercuts its worth. *Hastings Cent Rep* 16(2):26–38, 1986
43. Modan B: Diet and cancer: Causal relation or just wishful thinking? *Lancet* 340:162–164, 1992.
44. Kottke TE: Clinical preventive services: How should we define the indications? *Mayo Clin Proc* 65:899–902, 1990
45. Sutchfield FD, Hartman KT: Physicians and preventive medicine. *JAMA* 273:1150–1151, 1995
46. Satcher D, Hull F: The weight of an ounce. *JAMA* 273:1149–1159, 1995 (editorial)
47. Fogle S: Bench notes special report. Pitching prevention: Will doctors listen? *J NIH Res* 3:90–92, 1991
48. Thompson RS, Taplin SH, McAfee TA, et al: Primary and secondary prevention services in clinical practice: Twenty years' experience in development, implementation, and evaluation. *JAMA* 273:1130–1135, 1995
49. Baker EL, Melton RH, Stange PV, et al: Health reform and the health of the public: Forging community health partnerships. *JAMA* 272:1276–1282, 1994
50. Loescher LJ: Genetics in cancer prediction, screening and counseling: Part 1. Genetics in cancer prediction and screening. *Oncol Nurs Forum* 22:10–15, 1995 (suppl)
51. Engelking C: New approaches: Innovations in cancer prevention, diagnosis, treatment, and support. *Oncol Nurs Forum* 21:62–71, 1994

# Chapter 7

# Cancer Risk and Assessment

**Rebecca F. Cohen, RN, EdD, MPA, CPHQ**

**Marilyn Frank-Stromborg, EdD, JD, NP, FAAN**

## INTRODUCTION

Health risk appraisal has been credited to Dr. Lewis C. Robbins, who worked extensively on the prevention of cervical cancer and heart disease during the 1940s. He developed a "health hazard chart" to give the medical examination a more prospective orientation toward preventive efforts. By the end of the 1960s, life insurance actuarial principles were being applied to risk assessment, and risk multipliers were quantified for patient characteristics that affect mortality risk. The presence of these necessary elements thus led the way to quantitative risk appraisal. In 1970 Robbins and Hall[1] published a manual entitled *How to Practice Prospective Medicine*, which provided a complete health risk assessment (HRA) package, including questionnaire, risk computations, and feedback strategy.

When HRAs were first presented for use, the medical profession generally ignored their presence. However, the potential for computerization of the risk-estimation procedure, commercial interest, and the involvement of government agencies led to a proliferation of HRA programs. As of 1985, there were approximately 52 HRAs identified by the Office of Disease Prevention and Health Promotion in the U.S. Department of Health and Human Services. While questions have been raised concerning the validity of the databases and procedures used in HRA risk estimation, few empirical evaluations of the adequacy of the HRA procedures have been reported.[2]

Precise prediction of disease or mortality by any means currently is not an attainable goal because of incomplete knowledge of the total set of risk factors, their time-dose levels, and the true functional form of their contribution to risk. Similar risk models are successful in differentiating high-, medium-, and low-risk individuals and in estimating relative risk, but are much less successful in estimating absolute risk in individuals or across populations. In contrast, measurements applied to individuals should attain higher levels of accuracy than measurements used only in correlational studies, where there is opportunity for random errors to offset one another.[2]

HRA as a vehicle for what might be termed *prospective health assessment* potentially has a number of very desirable qualities for clinicians and health educators: preventive orientation, systematic approach, ability to emphasize modifiable factors, and a scientific knowledge base. However, a major concern is the value of quantitative estimates of absolute risk. Would the use of relative risk, risk scores, health scores, and other less quantitative measures, given the limitations in scientific knowledge and risk-estimation methods, be more helpful than the dependence on absolute risk assessment? Schoenbach[2] suggests that while HRAs may have valuable purposes, sophistication and precision in risk estimation are not necessarily the measure of their quality.

## DEFINITIONS OF RISK

*Risk* is the potential realization of unwanted consequences of an event. Both a probability of occurrence of an event and the magnitude of its consequences are involved.[3,4] According to Rowe,[5] *hazard* implies the existence of some threat, whereas *risk* implies both the existence of a threat and its potential for occurrence. Since a risk can occur only if a potential pathway for exposure exists, a hazard may exist without implying risk. For example, there are toxic chemicals that are hazardous, but until the chemical actually exists in some form with a potential pathway to humans or the environment there is no risk. A risk estimate in this case involves both potency of the substance and exposure to a population in terms of the number of individuals who might receive specified dose levels. This definition of risk does, however, imply that risk is always negative. A more general definition of risk, which would not be in conflict with other definitions, is that risk "is the downside of a gamble."[5] This definition implies that (1) living itself involves gambles, (2) some gambles are involuntary, (3) trade-offs are often required between quality and quantity of life, and (4) there is no such thing as zero risk, only involuntary and voluntary gambles for which minimum risk for acceptable gain is one criterion for decision making.[5]

A person's "cancer risk" would generally mean a factual estimate of the likelihood and severity of adverse effect, or the odds of incurring cancer. The estimation of health risks is an empirical problem filled with many uncertainties. After risks are estimated, decisions must be made about whether to bear the risks or to minimize them by reducing their source or taking protective actions. These decisions, often referred to as *risk evaluation,* are based on personal and social value judgments.[3,4] As Rowe[5] has stressed, the issue is really whether a particular risk is "acceptable" or is similar to risks already accepted or to the risks of alternatives.

Two approaches that can be used to calculate risk are relative risk and attributable risk. *Relative risk* is a ratio that compares the rate of the disease among exposed persons with the rate of the disease among unexposed persons. Although relative risk does not reveal the probability that the exposed person will have the disease, it does measure the strength of the association between a factor and the outcome.[6] The *attributable risk* is the difference in the disease rates between the group exposed to the factor and unexposed groups. Attributable risk is used to calculate the magnitude of change when a particular factor is added or subtracted.[6]

## CANCER RISK FACTORS

Cancer prevention strategies can be divided into two major areas: (1) identification of the contributors to the cause(s) of cancer, and (2) the action taken in response to this knowledge. Identification is the function of the researcher, and action is usually enacted by legislative control or preferably by voluntary actions taken on the part of concerned individuals. It is, according to Newell,[7] very possible that we could know the cause of every cancer and not be able to prevent any of them. Cancer prevention depends, therefore, on what individuals do with this knowledge and how they perceive, accept, and act on it. What really counts is behavior modification, or agent change, whether in the environment, the medical care system, or the individual.

Cancer risk factors are specific risk factors or individual characteristics that are associated with an increased cancer risk: personal behavior, genetic makeup or familial traits, and exposure to a known cancer-causing agent.[3–10] Breslow[9] divides the factors that cause cancer into two groups: those that are under a person's control (personal habits, such as cigarette smoking), and those outside a person's control (age; hereditary characteristics such as familial polyposis). Risk factors have also been divided according to whether they are unique to an individual or shared by a group of persons. Individual risk factors include the individual's lifestyle, nutritional habits, medical conditions, and exposure to radiation or drugs. Group risk factors are those shared by persons from the same geographic residence or the same occupation.[10] Eventually the role of such factors may be describable in terms of chemical or metabolic mechanisms that might relate to multistage or cocarcinogenesis in humans.[3]

One important function of categorizing risk factors is to provide a database from which to develop an individual's cancer risk profile, to make recommendations about risk factors, and to plan specific interventions for risk reduction. The two biggest challenges for the cancer research establishment are (1) the implementation of interventions to prevent cancers from known or proven causes, and (2) the verification of highly suspected causes of major types of cancer.[10]

Another function of categorization is to emphasize the many causative factors and the complex etiology of cancer. For example, some cancers, such as skin cancer, appear to have one factor that is especially important (i.e., ultraviolet radiation). For most types of cancer, however, it appears that an interaction of multiple factors is probably necessary.[3,11–15]

In general, the predominant carcinogenic risk factors believed to be responsible for 70%–90% of cancers in humans in Western industrial societies can be put into the following categories:

A. Environmental
   1. Nonoccupational
      a. Habits
         i. Smoking
         ii. Alcohol consumption
         iii. Sunbathing
         iv. Dietary factors
      b. Customs (e.g., noncircumcision)
      c. Air and water pollution
   2. Occupational
      a. Chemical (e.g., asbestos)
      b. Physical (e.g., radiation)
B. Sex differences (e.g., hormones)
C. Virus
D. Racial differences
E. Habitat: urban vs. rural environment
F. Genetic factors
G. Marital status
H. Socioeconomic class
I. Psychological
   1. Personality profile theory
   2. Stressful life events
J. Medical therapy–related cancers

## CANCER RISK FACTORS IN MINORITY POPULATIONS

### Racial/Multifactorial Aspects

The American Cancer Society estimates that about 1,359,150 cancers will be diagnosed in the United States in 1996. Approximately 136,380 of these cancers will be among black Americans and 38,000 among other minority Americans.[16] Blacks have a higher incidence and mortality for cancers of the esophagus, uterine cervix, stomach, liver, prostate, and larynx, and for multiple myeloma. Esophageal cancer rates are three times higher among blacks than whites.[16]

Data from 1986 through 1992 indicate that 42% of blacks with cancer survive five years, while the rate is 58% for whites. A part of this difference in survival is attributed to more advanced stage upon diagnosis among blacks, whereas many cancers in whites are more often diagnosed in a localized stage.

Native Americans, Asian and Pacific Islanders, and Hispanics have lower incidence and mortality rates for cancers of the lung, breast, prostate, colon, and rectum than do whites. However, these minority groups have higher incidence and mortality rates for other tumor types. The fact that cancer risk is associated with lifestyle and behavior can help researchers understand these differences in cancer rates among ethnic and cultural groups. High-incidence cancers for specific ethnic groups, by site, are identified in Table 7-1.[16–20]

These aggregate data may, however, mask the fact that subgroups within an ethnic minority may be at increased risk of cancer. These subgroups include immigrants, the elderly, the non–English speaker, the illiterate, and the economically disadvantaged. Members of these subgroups may not attend screening programs because of real or perceived barriers such as language difficulties, negative cancer beliefs, fear of cancer, and cost of services.[17]

**TABLE 7-1** High-Incidence Cancers, by Site, for Specific Ethnic Groups

| Ethnic Group | Cancers of Highest Incidence |
| --- | --- |
| **Hispanic** | |
| Men and women | Gallbladder, liver, stomach, pancreas |
| Men | Prostate |
| Women | Cervical |
| **Black** | |
| Men | Prostate, lung, bronchial, pancreas |
| Women | Cervical, breast |
| Men and women | Multiple myeloma |
| **Hawaiian** | |
| Men and women | Lung, stomach, rectal, esophageal |
| Women | Uterine, cervical, breast |
| Men | Liver, pancreas |
| **Alaskan Natives** | |
| Men | Lung, nasopharyngeal |
| Eskimo men | Liver |
| Women | Renal cell, gallbladder, thyroid, colorectal |
| Men and women | Gallbladder |
| **Navajo** | |
| Children | Retinoblastoma |
| Men and women | Melanoma, gallbladder |
| Men | Lung |
| **Pueblo** | |
| Men and women | Mesothelioma |
| **Other Tribes** | |
| Chippewa | Gallbladder |
| Sioux | |
| Arapaho | |
| Shoshone | |
| Pima | |
| Apache | |
| **Chinese** | Nasopharyngeal, liver, esophageal, lung, stomach |
| **Japanese** | Stomach, esophageal, liver, gallbladder |
| **Korean** | Liver, biliary, lymphoma, thyroid |
| **Philippino** | Liver, biliary, lymphoma, thyroid |

Adapted with permission from Frank-Stromborg and Olsen[20]

## Socioeconomic/Educational Factors

Studies considered income and education in relation to the incidence of cancer. For example, Devesa and Diamond[21] found a significant inverse trend between lung cancer incidence and both income and education among white and black males, and the effect of income exceeded that of education. Poor Americans, regardless of race, are at a disproportionate risk of dying of cancer. Americans living below the poverty level have a five-year cancer survival rate that is 10%–15% lower than that for other Americans.[22,23] In addition, by the time

a diagnosis is made among poor people, the disease is usually terminal.[23,24]

Several factors contribute to the increased mortality and morbidity from cancer among the poor.[22,24] These factors include the following:

1. inadequate education
2. lack of employment
3. substandard housing
4. lack of access to medical care
5. chronic malnutrition
6. fatalistic attitudes about cancer despite advances in both diagnosis and treatment

Jenks[23] noted that the following critical issues involving cancer and the poor must be considered in any analysis of cancer morbidity and mortality:

1. The poor face substantial obstacles in obtaining and using health insurance and often do not seek needed care if they cannot pay for it.
2. Poor people and their families must make personal sacrifices to obtain and pay for health care, and often have to choose between food or shelter and paying for care.
3. Cancer education and outreach efforts are insensitive and irrelevant to many poor people, whose primary concern is survival.

While a key element in the development of state-of-the-art prevention and treatment programs is the clinical trial, many obstacles have hindered recruitment efforts and entry of the economically disadvantaged to clinical trials. These obstacles include patient finances, perceptions of health, and attitudes toward clinical trials. Strategies to recruit the economically disadvantaged to clinical trials must consider the ethnic and cultural environment as well as the barriers faced by the target group.[25]

Finally, based on findings related to cancer rates and socioeconomic level, the American Cancer Society Special Report has presented a number of recommendations to reduce the disproportionate effect of cancer in the socioeconomically disadvantaged. The following are some examples of these recommendations related to cancer risk assessment:[22, pp. 22–23]

1. Efforts should be made to improve the cost-effectiveness of cancer screening, with the ultimate goal of providing all Americans at risk with this preventive measure, through advocacy and/or direct involvement.

2. Funding mechanisms, both direct and indirect, should be developed to screen indigent populations at high risk for specific cancer sites.

3. Emergency rooms and clinics should have outreach programs, including mobile vans, for screening people in high-risk categories presenting themselves for treatment of other illnesses at primary care clinics, and

emergency rooms should be encouraged to avail themselves of cancer screening.

4. Studies should be performed to evaluate factors that affect prognosis and survival for the socioeconomically disadvantaged, such as compliance, nutrition, and home environment.

5. Studies should be performed to determine the most effective strategies for smoking cessation among the socioeconomically disadvantaged.

6. Profiles of each community to be served should be developed, with the principles based on encouraging people to modify their behavior to help reduce the risk of cancer.

7. Emphasis should be placed on encouraging lifestyle and behavioral changes that might help reduce the risk of developing cancer.

8. A major effort should be made to educate health professionals about the important role of socioeconomic factors in the incidence and mortality of cancer, particularly cervical, prostate, lung, esophageal, laryngeal, and oral cancers, since many of these sites lend themselves to risk reduction through altering lifestyle factors such as smoking and drinking.

9. Strategies should be developed to enlist and train the socioeconomically disadvantaged to serve as volunteers in their own communities.

10. Innovative communication strategies should be devised to reach the socioeconomically disadvantaged with specific messages about cancer control.

11. Additional research is needed on the factors affecting the cancer incidence and survival of Hispanic, Asian, and other populations.

## Ethnic/Cultural Factors

Cancer morbidity and mortality are higher among African-Americans than Caucasians. In a study conducted by the University of Pittsburgh Cancer Institute, it was found that constant presence, cultural sensitivity, and repetition are necessary to overcome the barriers to increased awareness and behavioral changes in the African-American community.[26]

It has also been suggested that the greatest potential for reducing cancer mortality in high-risk populations may be realized through aggressive implementation of prevention, diagnostic, and state-of-the-art treatment programs and increasing participation in cancer trials. However, African-Americans are often underrepresented in such programs and/or trials. Various studies have provided evidence that multiple factors contribute to this situation, including the impact that perceptions, attitudes, and beliefs have on willingness to participate in investigational programs and/or trials. Millon-Underwood et al[27] found that the factor having the greatest influence on willingness to participate was the perceived efficacy of the investigational programs and/or trials. It was noted that when participants were given information on the opportunities for participation in prevention, diagnostic, and treatment programs, and on the benefits of participation, they were more willing to take part in the study. Jepson and Colleagues[28] also found that when knowledge variables were excluded in their study of factors affecting cancer prevention behaviors, race was not a significant predictor of behavior except among women, where African-Americans were found to smoke less than Anglo-Americans.

Overall, providing cancer prevention information and screening to the diverse minority subgroups of the United States is a challenge. In order to screen the African-American, Native American, Native Alaskan, and Native Hawaiian populations, cancer screening and prevention methods must be ethnically and culturally based.[29–31] For example, there is a high rate of cervical cancer among Native American Indian women,[32] and a high rate of smoking has increased the incidence of lung cancer.[33,34] Among African-American women, recent studies have found that breast cancer knowledge scores were uniformly low, and statistically significant associations were found between the frequency of breast self-examination and the variables age, prior experience with breast disease, "powerful other" locus of control, health values, and health beliefs.[35,36]

The need for understanding culturally based knowledge in order to provide screening, prevention, and treatment programs was strongly pointed out in a study that evaluated knowledge and attitudes about breast cancer risk factors among 28 Salvadoran and 39 Mexican immigrants, 27 Chicanas, 27 Anglo-American women, and 30 primary care physicians in Orange County, California. Results indicated that two cultural models of breast cancer risk factors emerged. The risk factors emphasized in a Latina model were breast trauma and "bad" behaviors, including drinking alcohol and using illegal drugs. A biomedical model, expressed by the physicians and Anglo-American women, emphasized risk factors identified in medical literature, such as family history and age.[37]

## Gender Differences

Devesa[38] points out that six cancers account for almost 70% of cases in women and more than 60% of deaths, namely, breast, lung, colorectal, cervix uteri, corpus uteri, and ovarian cancers. However, disparity exists between the scientific advances made for female Euro-Americans and for female African-Americans, Hispanics, Native Americans, and Asian/Pacific Islanders. The major variables in cancer morbidity and mortality in ethnic populations compared with Anglo-Americans appear to be physiological and biochemical differences, socioeconomic factors, structural barriers, and cultural factors.[39]

Numerous factors in the social environment may affect the incidence and mortality from cancer in women. Women's work roles, possible exposure to workplace hazards, social class, social roles, social stress, access to health care, and health care behaviors act together to help determine a woman's health.[40] Also, there are differences between the mortality rates for certain cancers in younger versus older women, most notably breast cancer. Part of this difference has been theorized to be due to biological processes such as increased immune suppression with aging, but most of the distinction between the courses of breast cancer in older and younger individuals has been related to decreased screening during advanced age.[41]

## RISK FACTORS FOR SPECIFIC CANCERS

When assessing risk factors for specific cancers, it is important to recognize that risk factors can replace each other. A very high blood pressure and normal serum cholesterol may have the same effect as a moderate blood pressure and hypercholesteremia. It appears that the actual risk from a single factor depends on (1) the number and intensity of other coexisting factors in a given individual, and (2) the intensity of the factor itself. It is possible for a person with only one risk factor to be placed in a "high-risk" level because of the potency of that factor. Also, as age advances, more factors accumulate and come into play, thus potentiating each other. This makes risk appraisal of the elderly an important nursing concern. Risk factors for specific cancers are summarized in Table 7-2. The risk factors presented are those for which there is strong evidence from laboratory, epidemiological, or clinical research of being linked to the development of cancer.[42,43]

### Bladder Cancer

The strongest risk factors for bladder cancer involve occupational exposures and lifestyle practices. In some cohorts of chemical workers exposed to aromatic amines, more than 80% have died of bladder cancer.[44] In developing countries, bladder infection with the parasite *Schistosoma haematobium* has been linked to the development of bladder cancer.[45] In the United States, however, risk factors for bladder cancer involve primarily occupational exposures and tobacco use. Workers exposed to aromatic amines (2-naphthylamine, benzidine) have a fourfold greater risk of bladder cancer.[44,46] People in high-risk occupations include apparel, textile, and leather workers, workers in the dye industry, rubber workers, metal workers, and painters.

Cigarette smoking is the most important known risk factor for bladder cancer. Smokers develop bladder cancer two to three times more often than nonsmokers.[47] It is estimated that as many as 60% of bladder cancers may result from smoking.[46] Drug use has also been found to increase the risk of bladder cancer. Cyclophosphamide

**TABLE 7-2**  **Risk Factors for Selected Cancers**

| BLADDER CANCER | |
| --- | --- |
| Personal risk factors | Male |
| | White |
| | Infection with schistosomiasis |
| Lifestyle | Cigarette smoking |
| | Coffee drinking? |
| | Drinking liquids with artificial sweeteners? |
| | Drinking water in rural areas with heavy pesticide use? |
| Occupation | Occupations working with benzidine, aniline dye, and 2-naphthylamine—apparel, textile, and leather workers, workers in dye industry, rubber workers, metal workers, painters, petroleum workers, hairdressers |
| Drugs | Cyclophosphamide (alkylating drug) |

| BREAST CANCER | |
| --- | --- |
| Personal risk factor | History of benign breast disease |
| | Jewish descent |
| | Single lifestyle |
| | Some researchers believe that all women should be treated as being at risk |
| Lifestyle | Alcohol consumption |
| | Higher socioeconomic status |
| | Diet high in fat |
| Reproductive history | Early menarche |
| | Nulliparity |
| | Late menopause |
| | Late age at birth of first child |
| Family history | Family history of breast cancer |

| CERVICAL CANCER | |
| --- | --- |
| Personal risk factors | Black women |
| | Dysplasia |
| | Infection with herpes genitalis and condyloma acuminatum |
| Reproductive history | Early age at first marriage or coitus |
| | Multiple marriages or sexual partners |
| | Use of nonbarrier contraceptives |

| COLORECTAL CANCER | |
| --- | --- |
| Personal risk factors | Increasing age |
| | Family history of colon cancer |
| | Disease with hereditary predisposition—Gardner's syndrome, Turcot syndrome, Peutz-Jeghers syndrome, familial polyposis of colon |
| | Ulcerative colitis |
| | Crohn's disease |
| | History of colon cancer, female genital cancer, bladder cancer, breast cancer |
| | Sporadic colorectal adenomas |

*(continued)*

**TABLE 7-2** Risk Factors for Selected Cancers (continued)

### COLORECTAL CANCER

| | |
|---|---|
| Lifestyle | A diet high in fat, low in fiber, and low in fruits and vegetables containing vitamins A and C<br>Obesity<br>Sedentary lifestyle |
| Geographic location | Living in highly developed countries |

### LIVER CANCER

| | |
|---|---|
| Personal risk factors | Men between the third and fifth decades of life<br>Cirrhosis<br>Infection with hepatitis B virus<br>Infection with hepatitis C virus |
| Lifestyle | Living in non-Western countries, e.g., China, Asia, Africa<br>Homosexual and bisexual men, who are at increased risk for hepatitis B virus |
| Medical treatments | Hemodialysis patients, who are at increased risk for hepatitis B virus |
| Chemicals | Vinyl chloride |

### LUNG CANCER

| | |
|---|---|
| Personal risk factors | Cigarette smoking<br>Family history of lung cancer |
| Lifestyle | Exposure to smokers over a period of time<br>Exposure to high levels of indoor radon |
| Occupation | Working with iron oxide, nickel, arsenic, chromium, asbestos, petroleum-related products, mustard gas, chloromethyl ether; occupations involved: iron ore miners, nickel smelters, miners, chromium producers, millers, textile workers, insulation workers, shipyard workers, mustard gas workers, chemical workers, diesel jet testers, iron foundry workers, oil refiners, vintners |
| Geographic location | Living in an urban area or coastal community |

### ORAL CANCER

| | |
|---|---|
| Personal risk factors | Tobacco use<br>Heavy alcohol use<br>Nutritional deficiencies<br>Poor dentition and oral hygiene<br>Plummer-Vinson syndrome |
| Occupation | Occupations resulting in long-term exposure to the sun (lip cancer) |

### OVARIAN CANCER

| | |
|---|---|
| Personal risk factors | White upper-income groups in the Western hemisphere |

**TABLE 7-2** (continued)

### OVARIAN CANCER

| | |
|---|---|
| Personal risk factors | Cancer of the breast<br>Family history of ovarian cancer |
| Reproductive history | Delayed age at first pregnancy<br>Nulliparity |
| Medical treatments | Radiation to the pelvic area |
| Occupation | Occupations involving asbestos |

### PROSTATE CANCER

| | |
|---|---|
| Personal risk factors | Increasing age<br>Black males—highest incidence in the world |
| Lifestyle | Diet high in fats, oils, sugar, eggs, milk, animal protein (under investigation)<br>Sexual activity?<br>History of venereal disease? |
| Occupation | Occupations related to use of cadmium |

### SKIN CANCER

| | |
|---|---|
| Personal risk factors | Light-skinned, fair-haired, freckles, burns easily<br>History of severe sunburn under the age of 20<br>Increasing age<br>Presence of congenital moles<br>Personal history of dysplastic nevi, cutaneous melanoma<br>History of excessive sunbathing<br>Xeroderma pigmentosum (a progressive sun-sensitive disease that develops in early childhood)<br>Albinism<br>Epidermodysplasia verruciformis (multiple virus-induced warty lesions that develop in early childhood)<br>History of tropical ulcers, burns, and scars related to squamous cell carcinoma and increased incidence |
| Family history | History of melanoma in children, siblings, and parents |
| Occupation | Outdoor work—farming, ranching<br>Uranium miners, radiologists |
| Drugs | Treatment for psoriasis known as PUVA |
| Precursor lesions | Solar (actinic) keratosis<br>Bowen's disease |
| Chemicals | Polycyclic aromatic hydrocarbons |
| Immunologic factors | Organ transplant recipients |

### TESTICULAR CANCER

| | |
|---|---|
| Personal risk factors | White males<br>Family history<br>Younger men (ages 20–40)<br>Cryptorchidism<br>Higher socioeconomic status |

**TABLE 7-2** Risk Factors for Selected Cancers (continued)

| ENDOMETRIAL (UTERINE CORPUS) CANCER | |
|---|---|
| Personal risk factors | Obesity |
| | Hypertension |
| | Diabetes mellitus |
| Lifestyle | Higher socioeconomic status |
| Reproductive history | History of menstrual irregularities |
| | Nulliparity |
| | Infertility through anovulation |
| Drugs | Long-term use of conjugated estrogens |

| VAGINAL CANCER | |
|---|---|
| Personal risk factors | Mother's use of DES during pregnancy |
| | Radiation of cervix for cancer |
| | Elderly |

can cause bladder cancer.[48] It has been reported that there is a latency period of as much as 18 years before bladder tumors develop after exposure to carcinogens.[49]

There is conflicting information concerning the role of coffee drinking and the use of artificial sweeteners and the risk of bladder cancer. Further research is needed to determine the association between these two substances and the incidence of bladder cancer.[50] It has also been reported that drinking water in rural areas with high pesticide use is associated with increased risk of bladder cancer.[46]

## Breast Cancer

The primary risk factors for breast cancer are increasing age, family history of breast cancer, history of benign breast disease, late age at first live birth, nulliparity, early age at menarche, late age at menopause, higher socioeconomic status, being Jewish, estrogen replacement therapy, exposure of the female breast to ionizing radiation in infancy, mammographic parenchymal patterns that are dense (P2 and DY), having complex fibroadenomas, and being single.[51–55] However, some clinicians stress that all women 35 or older should be treated as being at risk for breast cancer.[56]

There are conflicting data on the relationship between alcohol consumption and risk of breast cancer. Some investigators have noted a dose-response relationship between alcohol and breast cancer.[57] One study found that all types of alcoholic beverages were associated with an increase in breast cancer risk. It has been suggested that alcohol may increase breast cancer risk by mediating the level of endogenous estrogen exposure in the breast.[58] Several other reports found no association between alcohol and breast cancer.[59]

In the past, the same type of debate revolved around the use of birth control pills and increased risk of breast

cancer.[60] A study by the Centers for Disease Control and the National Institute of Child Health and Human Development found that use of birth control pills did not increase the risk of breast cancer.[61] An extensive review by Malone et al concluded that oral contraceptives should not be associated with an increase in breast cancer risk.[62]

There is considerable debate about the influence of diet on the development of breast cancer. Since the worldwide distribution of breast cancer is very similar to that of colorectal cancer, it is believed by many researchers that a high fat intake is a causative factor in breast cancer, especially in older women.[63] Additional evidence of this association comes from clinical and laboratory animal studies.[63] How much reduction in fat intake is necessary to lower the risk of cancer is also unknown at this time. Willett et al[64] reported from their study of 85,538 U.S. nurses that a moderate reduction in fat intake by women is unlikely to result in a substantial reduction in the incidence of breast cancer.

A recent study conducted in Sweden found no association between fat intake and breast cancer risk.[65] It is believed that 5%–10% of all breast cancers are due to highly penetrant mutated tumor-suppressor genes, namely, *BRCA1* on chromosome 17q21 and *BRCA2* on chromosome 13q12-13.66. Weber[66] reports that "age-specific risks provide a clear picture of the contribution of breast susceptibility, suggesting that as many as 30% of women diagnosed with breast cancer under the age of 35 may have inherited susceptibility, while less than 1% of women diagnosed after age 75 have breast cancer associated with a dominant susceptibility gene."[66,p.12]

A woman with a strong family history of breast cancer is generally defined as having four or more genetically related women affected with the disease; about 40% of their cancers are caused by an inherited mutation in the gene *BRCA1* and another 40% by *BRCA2*.

A recent study by Madigan and colleagues reports that established risk factors account for only 41% of breast cancer cases in the United States.[67] The established risk factors were later age at first birth, nulliparity, family history of breast cancer, and higher socioeconomic status.

Table 7-3 shows the various known risk factors for breast cancer and the approximate degree of increased risk. This table compares the increased-risk group (e.g., women in North America) with a group known to be at low risk for breast cancer (e.g., women in Asia) and gives the approximate degree of increased risk.[68]

## Cervical Cancer

Race, personal factors, and venereal disease are the major risk factors associated with cervical cancer. Personal risk factors include early age at first coitus, multiple marriages or sexual partners, and use of nonbarrier contraceptives.[69,70] Venereal infections associated with increased risk are herpes genitalis and condyloma acuminatum caused by human papillomaviruses (HPV).[71] With the existence of major new sexually transmitted infectious diseases (i.e.,

**TABLE 7-3** Risk Factors in Human Breast Cancer

| Factors* | RISK GROUP | | |
| | Increased-Risk Group | Comparison Group | Approximate Degree of Increased Risk |
| --- | --- | --- | --- |
| Sex | Female | Male | High |
| Geography | North America | Asia | High |
| Age (years) | >50 | <35 | High |
| Personal history of cancer | Breast | Negative | High |
| | Endometrium, ovary | Negative | Moderate |
| Personal history of: | | | |
| Atypical hyperplasia (ductal, lobular) | Positive | Negative | Moderate |
| Carcinoma in situ | Positive | Negative | High |
| Mammographic parenchymal pattern | Extremely dense, dysplastic (Dy) | Negative | Moderate–high |
| Family history of breast cancer | Any first-degree relative | Negative | Mild–high |
| | Premenopausal bilateral breast cancer in first-degree relative | Negative | Moderate–high |
| Reproductive status: | | | |
| First full-term pregnancy at age (years) | >30 | <20 | Moderate |
| Parity | Nulliparous | Multiparous | Moderate |
| Menopause | Late | Early | Moderate |
| Menarche | Early | Late | Moderate |
| Alcohol | Consumers of >3 drinks/week | Abstainers | Mild–moderate |
| Radiation | Heavily exposed | None | Mild–moderate |

*Additional factors with risk ≤2 or not presently conclusively quantified include (high-risk group first): Jewish vs. gentile; high vs. low socioeconomic status; obesity vs. leanness (postmenopausal); high vs. low fat consumption; use of birth control pills or menopausal hormone vs. no use.

Reprinted with permission from Stefanek,[68] Table 1.

human immunodeficiency virus [HIV] infection, *Chlamydia trachomatis,* genital herpesvirus), health professionals anticipated that sexual practices would markedly change to reflect a desire on the part of women to avoid infection. A study of women who consulted gynecologists at a university student health service in 1975, 1986, and 1989 found that sexual practices among college women did not change markedly in 14 years.[72] Although the use of condoms increased, the majority of sexually active women reported that their partners do not use condoms regularly.

Incidence rates for black women are 66% higher than those for whites: 13.1 versus 7.9 per 100,000. The highest proportion of late-stage diagnoses of cervical cancer occurs among Native Americans (53.3%).[73] The rates for Orientals and whites are similar.[74] Certain religious groups in the United States have been noted to have low incidence rates of cervical cancer: Jews, Mormons, and Seventh-Day Adventists.[75]

Recent information supports an association between smoking and the incidence of cervical cancer. It has been reported that smokers' risk of developing cervical cancer is four times greater than that of nonsmokers. Researchers have confirmed that women smokers carry tobacco carcinogens in their cervical tissues, this strengthens a long-suspected hypothesis linking smoking and cervical cancer.[76,77]

## Colorectal Cancer

High rates of colorectal cancer are found in highly developed countries (e.g., North America, Northern and Western Europe, New Zealand), and low rates are found in Asia, Africa, and most countries of Latin America. There is substantial evidence that differences between nations in the incidence of colorectal cancer are due at least in part to environmental factors, such as diet.[78] Obesity, high fat intake, low fiber content, and a dearth of fruits and vegetables containing vitamins A and C have been identified as risk factors.[79–82] A sedentary lifestyle has also been implicated as a risk factor for colorectal cancer.

Age is considered a significant risk factor for colorectal cancer. Risk begins to increase at age 40, increases rapidly above age 55, and roughly doubles with each successive decade, reaching a peak at age 75.

Familial and hereditary factors are another significant risk.[83,84] The specific diseases with a hereditary predisposition are Gardner's syndrome, Turcot syndrome, Peutz-Jeghers syndrome, and familial polyposis of the colon.[85]

It is estimated that familial adenomatous polyposis accounts for 1% of all colon cancers; Lynch family syndromes and related syndromes about 10%; other inherited patterns 40%–90%, and noninherited cases 10%–50%.[86,87]

Adenomatous polyps are precursors of most colorectal cancers, and their prevalence increases with age. The practice of removing polyps at colonoscopy is based on the assumption that their removal prevents progression to cancer.[88] The National Polyp Study demonstrated that colonoscopic polypectomy resulted in an incidence of colorectal cancer that was 76%–90% lower than expected.[89] Müller and Sonnenberg also demonstrated that endoscopic procedures of the large intestine in conjunction with polyp removal reduced the risk for developing colorectal cancer by 50%.[90]

Having ulcerative colitis is another significant risk factor for colorectal cancer. The risk of carcinoma of the large intestine is 20 times greater than in the general population among individuals with extensive ulcerative colitis for ten years or more. Because of the strong association of ulcerative colitis and colorectal cancer, it has been recommended that in "patients with ulcerative colitis that is diagnosed before the age of 15 prophylactic proctocolectomy might be an alternative to close surveillance in reducing mortality from colorectal cancer."[91,p.1233] Crohn's disease also places individuals at higher risk of colorectal cancer. Persons with a past history of colon cancer and adenomatous intestinal polyps are also at increased risk.

## Liver Cancer

The incidence of hepatocellular carcinoma (HCC) increases with age, predominantly affects men, and occurs most often between the third and fifth decades of life.[92,93] There is a pronounced geographic variation in its incidence throughout the world. In the United States and Western countries, HCC is rare, ranking 25th among cancers in the United States and occurring at a rate of four to five per 100,000 population in North America, the United Kingdom, and Australia. In contrast, HCC is probably the most common cancer in the world among men. The risk factors for HCC include hepatitis B virus, cirrhosis, hepatitis C virus, and the chemical vinyl chloride.[94–98]

Groups at high risk for hepatitis B infection in the United States include institutionally developmentally disabled, intravenous drug users, homosexual and bisexual men, and hemodialysis patients.[99,100] It is generally believed that "chronic hepatitis B virus infection is probably the leading cause of HCC throughout the world, accounting for 75%–90% of the world's cases."[101, p.1956] Epidemiological evidence has shown that at least in some high-risk populations the chance of developing HCC is more than 160 times greater in hepatitis B virus (HBV) carriers than in HBV-free individuals.[101]

Although rare, oral contraceptives taken for more than eight to nine years have been associated with HCC.[102] The etiologic relationship between liver disease and subsequent HCC has long been debated and remains controversial.[103]

## Lung Cancer

The major risk factors for lung cancer are cigarette smoking, occupation, air pollution, environmental tobacco smoke, and radon exposure.[16,104,105] Cigarette smoking increases the risk of lung cancer to a greater degree than any other risk factor. Cigarette smoking in the United States contributes to 90% of lung cancers among men and 79% among women.[16] Black men have the highest risk for lung cancer of any group; the incidence of lung cancer in black men is 60% higher than that for white men.[106] Approximately 44.1 million adults were former smokers in 1990.[107]

In 1993 it was estimated that 46 million adults (25%) in the United States smoked—24 million men and 22 million women. Smoking prevalence is highest among some minority groups—in particular, black males, Native Americans, and Alaskan Natives—and among those with the least education and those living below the poverty level.[108] The World Health Organization estimates that 200 to 300 million children and adolescents under age 20 currently alive will eventually be killed by tobacco.[109]

Studies have also found an elevated risk of lung cancer as well as heart disease among individuals who have never smoked but are living with a spouse who smokes cigarettes.[110] There is a wide body of evidence that points to the likelihood that the involuntary inhalation of tobacco smoke increases the risk of lung cancer in nonsmokers. It is estimated that approximately 17% of lung cancers among nonsmokers can be attributed to high levels of exposure to cigarette smoke during childhood and adolescence.

Long-term exposure to environmental tobacco smoke increases the risk of lung cancer in women who have never personally smoked; this increased risk is more marked for women who have also been exposed to environmental tobacco smoke during childhood.[110,111]

Another environmental risk factor for lung cancer is indoor radon exposure. "Radon exposure may be the most significant risk factor for the nonsmoker that can be readily reduced."[112,p.274] Radon exposure may be responsible for about 10,000 lung cancer deaths per year, while smoking accounts for 85% of the lung cancer deaths annually. Much of the increased risk seems to occur in smokers. There has been some suggestion that radon acts synergistically with cigarette smoking to enhance the risk of lung cancer.

High-risk occupations are those in which persons work with asbestos, polycyclic hydrocarbons, chromium, mustard gas, chloromethyl ethers, radon, nickel, and inorganic arsenic. Included in this group are welders, gas workers, roofers, uranium miners, workers in the chrome pigment industry, nickel refinery workers, copper smelter workers, vineyard workers, and insulation workers.[113,114] The proportion of lung cancer in males due to occupational agents has been estimated to be from 5% to 36%.[114] Occupations among males with the highest rates of cigarette smoking include painters, construction laborers, auto mechanics, assemblers, and electricians. Thus, workers with the most opportunity for exposure to workplace respiratory toxins are also at the highest risk for cigarette smoking and its associated diseases. The deleterious effects of cigarette smoke and selected occupational agents are frequently additive and sometimes multiplicative in their interaction.[114]

International studies of geographic variation have shown that lung cancer is most common in urban and coastal communities.

## Oral Cancer

Tobacco is a major risk factor for oral cancer. The habitual smoking of cigarettes, cigars, and pipes and the use of chewing tobacco or snuff has long been associated with oral cancer.[115,116] In other countries, different tobacco-chewing habits place users at increased risk of oral cancer. In India, betel nut, or "pan," is chewed; in Bombay, "bidi" is chewed; "keeyo" is chewed in Thailand; and "nass" is chewed in central Asia. Mixing tobacco with these other products increases the risk of oral cancer.[117] Another significant risk factor for oral cancer is excessive alcohol intake. The risk of oral cancer among heavy drinkers and smokers is approximately 6 to 15 times greater than among nonsmokers and nondrinkers.[115,118] Alcohol appears to act chiefly by augmenting the effects of tobacco.

Other risk factors are nutritional deficiencies and poor dentition. Plummer-Vinson syndrome has a positive association with oral cancer. However, other nutritional deficiencies linked with an increased risk of oral cancer may be related to heavy use of alcohol, which influences dietary intake.[119] A relationship between infrequent vegetable intake and ingestion of hot infusions (maté) has been linked to cancer of the tongue in men in Uruguay.[120]

Evidence indicates that physical irritation (e.g., from dentures, irregular or sharp teeth, hot or spicy foods) plays little or no part in the natural history of oral carcinoma.[118] Occupations related to long-term exposure to the sun have been associated with cancer of the lip.

## Ovarian Cancer

The risk factors for ovarian cancer are less well known than those for the other major gynecologic cancers.[121] Women who have two or more first-degree relatives with a history of ovarian cancer have a significantly increased risk for this cancer.[122] Analysis of families with ovarian cancer suggests it has an autosomal dominant mode of inheritance with variable penetrance. A woman who has only one first-degree relative with ovarian cancer has an overall risk that is two to four times the average risk of 1.4% in the general population.[123] Ovarian cancer tends to be more common among white upper-income groups in highly industrialized countries.[124] Jewish women experience a 40% higher incidence rate than do African-American, Hispanic, and Native American women. The probable cause is delay or absence of childbearing.[123] The risk of ovarian cancer is associated with delayed age at first pregnancy and with a smaller number of pregnancies. These risk factors suggest an abnormality of endocrine secretion as an important component of ovarian carcinogenesis.[125] Present information suggests that oral contraceptive use might protect against ovarian cancer.[126] Other risk factors are radiation to the pelvic area, cancer of the breast, and occupations involving asbestos.

## Endometrial (Uterine Corpus) Cancer

The risk factors for cancer of the uterus are well known, with estrogen now considered the major risk factor. Obesity, high socioeconomic status, hypertension, and diabetes mellitus have been correlated with the development of endometrial cancer.[127] Women who have a history of menstrual irregularities and infertility through anovulation are also at increased risk. Long-term use of conjugated estrogens is an iatrogenic risk factor for endometrial cancer.[128] There is a national debate about whether postmenopausal women should be routinely given estrogen replacement. The Canadian and U.S. task forces advise against routine estrogen replacement therapy. Rather, they advocate hormone replacement therapy (HRT) for women who are at risk for osteoporosis and fracture.[129] Estrogens reduce the risk of coronary heart disease and fractures but greatly increase the risk of endometrial cancer and may increase the risk of breast cancer.[130] HRT is also believed to increase the risk for ovarian cancer. Concomitant use of progestins with estrogen eliminates the risk of endometrial cancer but has no effect on fracture, and its effect on breast cancer and coronary heart disease is unknown. The American College of Physicians recommends estrogen replacement in women who have had a hysterectomy and recommends combined HRT in women at high risk of heart disease. It makes no recommendation for other groups. The use of oral contraceptives (containing both estrogen and progesterone in each pill) for at least one year has a protective effect against endometrial cancer.[131,132]

## Prostate Cancer

Age and race are significant risk factors for prostate cancer. Black Americans have the highest prostate cancer incidence rate in the United States, and Japanese American men have the lowest incidence rate.[133,134] African-American men have an incidence rate that is nearly twice that of the general population and a death rate that is up to three times greater.[135] Prostate cancer affects the elderly more than the young to a greater extent than any other cancer.[136] Average age at diagnosis of prostate cancer is 70, and 80% of cases are found in men over 65.[137]

Other risk factors for prostate cancer are tentative at this time and require more research. A positive relationship has been found between the consumption of fats, oils, sugar, animal protein, eggs, and milk ("overnutrition") and mortality rates among men with prostate cancers.[138,139]

The results of a number of dietary intake surveys support the possibility that a high-fat diet may increase the risk of clinically significant prostate cancer. Dietary fat is presumably converted to androgens, leading to increased androgenic stimulation of the prostate. This may translate into an increased risk of hormonally induced tumors. Diets high in fat are associated with an increased production of sex hormones. Overall, a diet in which 40%–60% of calories come from fat appears to increase the relative risk of developing prostate cancer by a factor of 1.6 to 1.9.[140]

There may be a familial tendency toward the development of prostate cancer. If a man has a first-degree relative (i.e., father or brother) with prostate cancer, he has a 2.5 relative risk for developing prostate cancer.[141] However, whether it is due to environmental or genetic factors has not been determined. An increased risk of prostate cancer in association with an increasing number of sexual partners, prior history of venereal disease, frequency of sexual intercourse, and an early onset of sexual activity has been suggested.[136] Occupations that have been linked to increased risk of prostate cancer are those in which workers are exposed to cadmium (e.g., welding, electroplating, alkaline battery production). However, other studies have linked the development of prostate cancer with a multitude of other occupations that have no common carcinogenic exposure. At this time the evidence relating occupation and increased risk of prostate cancer is weak and needs further study.

## Skin Cancer

The chief risk factor for the development of basal cell and squamous cell carcinomas of the skin is exposure to ultraviolet radiation (UVR). Exposure to UVR in a tanning booth may also increase the risk of skin cancer.[142,143] Melanoma is also related to UVR, but there are several other influential risk factors: familial predisposition, hormonal factors, dysplastic nevus syndrome, and nearness to the equator.[144] The risk in the general population for developing malignant melanoma is approximately 0.53%, while the risk in a dysplastic nevus syndrome population is 10% (20 times greater), and even greater is the risk for a dysplastic nevus family member who has already developed malignant melanoma.[145]

Overall, those at greatest risk of skin cancer are fair-skinned white persons, particularly those with reddish or blond hair and blue or light eyes, those with a tendency to freckle or burn easily, and individuals who have spent considerable time in the sun.[146] Non-Europeans with various skin pigmentations have a substantial incidence of melanomas of the volar surface of the feet, but Africans seem to be notably less pigmented in that area and certainly have, for the same area of skin, particularly increased rates of occurrence of melanoma.[147] Other risk factors for skin cancer are occupation, personal risk factors, family history, drugs, precursor lesions, chemicals, and immunologic factors.[148]

## Testicular Cancer

A significant risk factor for testicular cancer involves race and age. This cancer occurs about 4.5 times more frequently in whites than in blacks and in men between the ages of 20 and 40 years and again in late adulthood over age 60.[149] Another significant risk factor is undescended testicles, especially in men who have a testicle that descended after the age of 6 or a testicle that never descended (cryptorchidism).[150] A history of cryptorchidism is found in nearly half the men with bilateral tumors and is consistent with observations that bilateral dysgenesis occurs frequently even in patients with unilateral maldescent.[149] About 5%–10% of patients with a history of cryptorchidism develop malignancy in the contralateral normally descended gonad. During the past few decades, several case reports and series of familial testicular cancers have been described in the literature, supporting the possibility of familial testicular cancer.[151] Other possible risk factors are trauma, hormonal drugs, and socioeconomic status.

The possibility that intrascrotal temperature is involved in the etiology of testicular cancer was investigated by Karagas et al.[152] They interviewed 323 men with germ cell tumors of the testis diagnosed between 1977 and 1984, and 658 randomly selected controls were interviewed with regard to type of shorts worn, use of long underwear, heat-resistant clothing, and hot tubs or saunas, and a history of varicocele. Their results provided little or no support for the hypothesis that intermittent intrascrotal temperature elevation plays a role in the etiology of germ cell testicular cancer.

## Vaginal Cancer

A risk factor for vaginal cancer that has received much attention is diethylstilbestrol (DES). Adenosis of the vagina has been identified in the offspring of women who received DES during pregnancy. This agent is no longer given to women to prevent threatened miscarriages. Another risk factor is radiation of the cervix for cancer of this organ. Postradiation carcinoma in situ of the vagina is of the epidermoid type and may occur one or more years after apparently successful treatment of cancer of the cervix.[153] Brinton et al[153] conducted a study of 41 patients with carcinoma in situ or invasive cancer of the vagina and compared them with 97 community controls in an effort to identify potential risk factors for vaginal cancer. They report that some risk factors for vaginal cancer are similar to those for cervical cancer and include low education and family income, history of genital warts, history of previous abnormal Pap smear, and vaginal discharge or irritation.

## CANCER RISK ASSESSMENT

The purposes of a cancer risk assessment include the following:

1. providing an individual with information about his or her health-related behavior that may increase cancer risk
2. serving as an effective aid for educating patients about the relationship between risk factors and the likelihood of cancer
3. stimulating a person to participate in activities aimed at changing lifestyle and improving health[9,154]

In addition, analysis of cancer risk may help individuals identify their options so that they can make realistic decisions about their health care. Physicians have also found that risk analyses help in the development of health regimens that are tailored to each individual's risk and tolerance for living with that risk.[155–160]

Before information is provided about an individual's specific risks, however, it is important that there be an understanding of the risk to an average person in the population.[154] This average risk serves as a baseline against which individuals can measure the magnitude of their increased risk, if any. Also, tables that show risks to various ages are useful because they indicate that cancer risk in the general population usually increases with certain activities (i.e., smoking) and with age.

One of the problems that exists in assessment of cancer risks is that some persons are unwilling to seriously consider what their risks might be. If a relative has had cancer, they may assume that their risk is "high" but fear that an examination of this assumption might in some way further increase their risk. They may also be dealing with various emotions, such as low self-esteem, denial, fear, anger, guilt, embarrassment, and insecurity, which are often seen in persons who come from families with a history of cancer. These emotions act as barriers to effective communication and can result in an inability to

face a risk analysis. Other individuals may believe that as long as they suffer by worrying about their high risk, their worry will act as a shield, and they will be spared the suffering of cancer itself. Finally, there often is the belief that if one worries about risks, one is engaging in "negative thinking that can cause cancer." Through the process of learning to understand one's fears, learning that such ideas are perfectly normal, and taking positive action to reduce the risks, an individual can be helped to understand the importance of risk assessment. Those who have received information about risk are more likely to schedule regular checkups and undergo necessary diagnostic procedures than are those who hold unrealistic health beliefs.[161]

It is also extremely important that a clear definition of the meaning of risk be provided when a health risk analysis is conducted. Many believe that when one's cancer risk is considered to be "high," it means that one's risk of dying is high. This, of course, is inaccurate because risk implies occurrence of disease and complications, not just mortality rate. Therefore, health professionals need to make sure that health care consumers understand such concepts as "carcinogen," "risk," "cancer risk," "carcinogenic risk factors," and "cancer risk assessment" so that they will know exactly what the assessment can and cannot do for them and how to use the data obtained.

According to the American Cancer Society,[16] *risk assessment* is a two-step process: identifying the toxic properties of potential oncogenic hazards and measuring the extent of human exposure. The first step, *hazard identification*, evaluates the chemical or physical nature of hazards and their oncogenicity in observed clinical and epidemiological studies and in laboratory tests using animals or cell systems. Special attention is given to any evidence suggesting that cancer risk may increase with dose.[16] The second step, *exposure measurement*, determines the levels of hazards in the environment (air, water, food, etc.) and the extent to which people are actually exposed.[16,155] Since assessment is only one aspect of a complete risk analysis, a comprehensive risk analysis should include (1) the identification of risks and the estimation of the likelihood and magnitude of risk occurring, and (2) an evaluation that measures *risk acceptance* (the acceptable levels of societal risk) and *risk management* (the control of risks, including methods of reducing and avoiding risk).[155]

Constanza et al[156] point out that risk assessment not only is a part of cancer prevention but also must be included in detection procedures to maximize the chance that one can discover cancer at its smallest or earliest possible stage. Achievement of National Institutes of Health and American Cancer Society goals for reduction in cancer mortality will require increased efforts directed at risk reduction and early detection in the general population. To accomplish these goals, it is vital that a quantifiable cancer risk appraisal tool be utilized to promote cancer prevention and screening and to enhance the ability of the health care provider to identify risk and carry out patient counseling.[157]

# Evaluation

The assessment of every individual should start with the history. The history format should include information on the following factors:[4]

- demographic data
- current past medical problems
- family medical history
- surgical and (if appropriate) obstetric history
- childhood illnesses

- allergies
- current medications
- psychological status
- social history
- environmental background
- review of systems

In most cases this information, excluding the review of systems, can be supplied by the individual on one of the many questionnaire forms available (see Table 7-4).

**TABLE 7-4**   Health Risk Assessment Instruments

| Instrument | Description | Source |
|---|---|---|
| COMPUTER-SCORED HRAs | | |
| CANCER RISK ASSESSMENT TOOL | Completed by the patient in approximately 10–15 minutes. IBM-compatible format permits easy quantification by laser scanning and computer analysis. Program quantitates risk arising from interacting independent factors and estimates the effects of primary prevention interventions. Program output includes age- and sex-specific ACS screening guidelines and discussion of intensified screening measures in high-risk subjects. | Lippman SM, Bassford TL, Meyskens FL: A quantitatively scored cancer-risk assessment tool: Its development and use. *J Cancer Educ* 7:15–36, 1992 |
| COSTPREDICT AND HEALTHPREDICT | Calculates costs and savings related to 51 health-related conditions and 44 risk factors. Reports give predicted costs and savings related to risks, absenteeism, and hospitalization. (200-item questionnaire re: habits, stress, medical history, and women's health) | CompuHealth Associates (also available for IBM-PC) |
| HEALTH AND LIFESTYLE QUESTIONNAIRE | Emphasizes current quality of life over long-term risks. Report assigns scores ranging from "excellent" to "immediate attention" and discusses the individual's risks. (54-item questionnaire re: health habits, psychological and job attitudes, and social relationships) | Health Enhancement Systems |
| HEALTH HAZARD APPRAISAL | Computer analysis provides a 4- to 5-page report that is a combination of bar graph, narrative, and tabulated data, including summaries of health age, projected health cost, and stress. (80-item questionnaire re: medical history, family history, lifestyle, stress, and women's health) | Prospective Medicine Center |
| HEALTHLINE | A 4-page report discusses leading probable causes of death and alterable risk factors. A 15-page report shows specific risks such as frustrations, satisfactions, and stresses. (44-item questionnaire re: medical history, lifestyle, women's health, stress, social and psychological factors, exercise, and nutrition) | Health Logics |

*(continued)*

**TABLE 7-4**  Health Risk Assessment Instruments (continued)

| Instrument | Description | Source |
|---|---|---|
| COMPUTER-SCORED HRAs | | |
| HEALTHLOGIC | 20-page report focuses on impact of lifestyle changes on health, fitness, and risk of chronic disease. (17-page booklet with questions on health history, men's and women's health, stress, and motor vehicle safety) | HMC Software Inc. |
| HEALTHPATH | 14-page report scores participants in 11 health habit areas. Helps to serve cost-containment objectives of a corporation. (72-item questionnaire covers 13 risk/lifestyle areas; physical measurements and laboratory data are optional) | Control Data Corp. |
| HEALTHPLAN AND HEALTHPLAN PLUS | 12-page booklet provides narrative and graphic information on 8 health areas, current risk as compared with average and achievable risk, and specific recommendations for behavior change. Individual's 5 leading health problems in order of importance are included. HealthPlan Plus has a longer and more detailed profile. (111-item questionnaire re: personal and family medical history, behavior habits, socioeconomic status, and women's health) | General Health, Inc. |
| HEALTH RISK APPRAISAL | 4-page report tabulates risks for 5 leading causes of death, recommends ways to reduce risks, and gives a 20-year future projection. (50-item questionnaire re: health habits and medical status; a wider-ranging Lifestyle Development Questionnaire is available) | University of Michigan (also available for IBM-PC) |
| HEALTH RISK APPRAISAL QUESTIONNAIRE | 2-page report explains patient's risk factors for the 12 leading causes of death as percentages by which he or she deviates from the average; appraisal and achievable ages are given as behavioral changes that could reduce risks. (39-item questionnaire re: personal and family medical history, health habits, and women's health) | St. Louis County Health Department |
| HEALTH RISK ASSESSMENT | Report recommends ways to reduce risks and compares the client's risk factors with those of others of the same age, sex, and race. (85-item questionnaire re: personal and family medical history, alcohol, smoking, and driving habits, and women's health) | University of California |
| HEALTH RISK ASSESSMENT QUESTIONNAIRE | 3-page report describes risks and gives information on health age, achievable age, and top 10 mortality causes and risk factors sorted into 4 categories: ideal, average, risky, and nonmodifiable. (96-item questionnaire re: medical history, physical examination, family history, women's health, and personal health habits) | Wisconsin Center for Health Risk Research |
| HEALTH RISK QUESTIONNAIRE | Report discusses risk factors for 15 major diseases with an emphasis on cancer. (39- | Health Enhancement Systems (also available for IBM-PC) |

**TABLE 7-4** Health Risk Assessment Instruments (continued)

| Instrument | Description | Source |
|---|---|---|
| COMPUTER-SCORED HRAs | | |
| HEALTH RISK QUESTIONNAIRE (continued) | item questionnaire re: lifestyle, medical history, and physical and laboratory measurements) | |
| HEALTH WRAP | Both a standard risk profile and a "wellness index" are provided. (93-item questionnaire) | Lifestyle and Health Promotion |
| LIFE | Report lists 20 major risk indicators (mostly physical measurements), patient's values for these, and recommended values. Also lists 20 leading causes of death for patient's age and sex, making recommendations to reduce risks where appropriate. A nutrition profile, stress profile and appraisal, and achievable ages are included. (16-page questionnaire re: personal and family medical histories, habits, and lifestyle, attitudes about health, physical measurements, diet, exercise, and other health habits) | Wellsource |
| LIFESCORE PLUS | Report projects life span and identifies risks. Booklet suggests guidelines to reduce or eliminate health risks. (62-item questionnaire: biomedical measurements, lifestyle habits, health history) | Center for Corporate Health Promotion |
| LIFESTYLE ASSESSMENT QUESTIONNAIRE (LAQ) | Printout suggests specific resources on topics selected and compares level of wellness with average of others who have taken the LAQ. The top 10 risk factors are listed, as well as ways to reduce them. (270-item questionnaire re: "Wellness Inventory" section with six dimensions of wellness and "Personal Growth" section to identify preferred topics for further information) | National Wellness Institute |
| LIFESTYLE DIRECTIONS | Short, 30-question instrument, which covers diet, exercise, and health. Report presents graphic information on risks for five major diseases. | Lifestyle Directions, Inc. |
| PERSONAL STRESS PROFILE | 12-page booklet aimed at employees in a workplace environment contains explanations on stress and specific recommendations for behavior change. (167-item questionnaire re: personal and family medical history, lifestyle behaviors, socioeconomic status, and stress) | General Health, Inc. |
| RHRC HEALTH RISK APPRAISAL | In addition to assessing individual risks, this instrument estimates the impact of workplace wellness programs. 5-page report includes 10-year mortality estimates for the 12 leading causes of death, estimated annual hospital days, and advice on reducing risks. A group profile includes the estimated reduction in workforce mortality and hospitalization | Regional Health Resource Center (also available for IBM-PC) |

*(continued)*

**TABLE 7-4**  Health Risk Assessment Instruments (continued)

| Instrument | Description | Source |
|---|---|---|
| **COMPUTER-SCORED HRAs** | | |
| RHRC HEALTH RISK APPRAISAL (continued) | achievable through specific wellness programs. (39-item questionnaire re: lifestyle, medical history, frequency of medical screening, optional laboratory data, and women's health; an additional "General Well-Being Questionnaire" measures stress) | |
| WELL AWARE HEALTH RISK APPRAISAL | Emphasis is on quality of life and current risks. 16-page report includes mortality predictions and stresses practical measures to improve health. (Questionnaire includes health habits, lifestyle, health knowledge, stress, women's health, diet, motor vehicle safety, alcohol use, sociability, and physical and laboratory data) | Well Aware About Health |
| **MICROCOMPUTER-BASED HRAs** | | |
| AVIVA | Provides an overall risk score adjusted for age and sex, the contribution of each risk factor to the score, and suggestions for modifying risks. This instrument assesses hospitalization risks but concerns only those risks that an individual can modify. (5- to 10-minute or 15- to 20-minute versions available; screens users to ensure that the interview is appropriate; questions cover alcohol use, driving habits, weight, blood pressure, cholesterol levels, depression, and smoking; user can ask why certain information is requested and receive explanations) | Center for Research in Medical Education and Health Care, Jefferson Medical College |
| HEALTH AWARENESS GAMES | This is a set of 5 microcomputer programs that draw on statistics about lifestyle and health as they relate to life expectancy. Appropriate for junior high school through college and is suitable for home use. (5 programs include Coronary Risk, Why Do You Smoke? Exercise and Weight, Life Expectancy, and Life-Style) | Queue Inc. |
| HEALTH RISK APPRAISAL | Profile displays the user's risks for 10 leading causes of death and provides a 1-page summary printout. (40-item questionnaire re: lifestyle and physiological indicators. For Apple II, II+, IIe, and IBM-PC) | University of Minnesota Media Distribution |
| LIFESCAN | Each individual receives a printout listing his or her top 10 risk factors and suggested methods to reduce those risks. Special feature is a listing of the individual's positive lifestyle behaviors. (40-item questionnaire re: physical activity, drug usage, driving habits, cholesterol level, medical history, and women's health issues. For IBM-PC) | National Wellness Institute |

**TABLE 7-4**   Health Risk Assessment Instruments (continued)

| Instrument | Description | Source |
|---|---|---|
| MICROCOMPUTER-BASED HRAs | | |
| PERSONAL HEALTH APPRAISAL | There are two versions: The personal version is interactive, and the professional version can be used in either an interactive or a batch-processing mode and can store and update profiles. The user's life expectancy is calculated at the end, and it includes an analysis of the user's "Cancer Early Warning Signs" and preventive health practices. (84-item questionnaire re: medical history, occupational health information, lifestyle, and women's health. For IBM-PC) | MedMicro |
| SPHERE | The 25-item questionnaire covers medical and lifestyle characteristics. Reports explain each user's risks and appraisal and achievable ages. Available in English and French. (For IBM-PC) | University of British Columbia |
| SELF-SCORED QUESTIONNAIRES | | |
| HEALTHSTYLE: A SELF-TEST | 2-page, 24-item questionnaire published by the U.S. Public Health Service. Gives specific suggestions for reducing risks. Topics covered include nutrition, alcohol and drug use, smoking, fitness, stress, and safety. | ODPHP National Health Information Center (1-800-336-4797) |
| HOPE HEALTH APPRAISAL | A complete health kit designed to help an individual manage his or her health risk and improve lifestyle. | International Health Awareness Center |
| HOW DO YOU RATE AS A HEALTH RISK? | Booklet includes 40 questions on smoking, alcohol and other drugs, nutrition, weight control, exercise, stress, and safety. Provides suggestions to improve the individual's present condition. | Channing L. Bete Co., Inc. |
| LIFESCORE-C | Designed for employee health programs. Results yield an individual score and can be batch-processed to yield a group profile. Questions cover lifestyle, environmental factors, family medical history, and utilization of health care. Scores are given for general health and life expectancy. | Center for Corporate Health Promotion (also available as LIFESCORE-M FOR IBM-PC) |
| OTHER INSTRUMENTS | | |
| CANCER RISK ASSESSMENT | Check-off questions for men and women related to cancer risks. Specific areas include skin, head and neck, lung, breast, colon-rectum, cervix, endometrium, vulva, vagina, prostate, testes. | White LN: Cancer risk assessment. *Semin Oncol Nurs* 2:184–190, 1986 |
| C.A.R.E.S. (CANCER AWARENESS RISK EDUCATION SERVICE) | C.A.R.E.S. was designed to assist health educators in providing cancer risk reduction information to the general public. It is used on a Compaq 386 with 1024K of memory and an EGA board. User | H. Lee Moffitt Cancer Center and Research Institute, Inc. P.O. Box 280179, Tampa, FL 33682-0179 |

*(continued)*

**TABLE 7-4** Health Risk Assessment Instruments (continued)

| Instrument | Description | Source |
|---|---|---|
| OTHER INSTRUMENTS | | |
| C.A.R.E.S. (CANCER AWARENESS RISK EDUCATION SERVICE) (continued) | responds to questions about personal health history, family history, personal habits related to skin, lung, colorectal, breast, gynecologic, prostate, testicular, stomach, head and neck, and esophageal cancers. A comprehensive component on dietary habits, stress, and exercise is also included. The user receives a printed analysis of his or her personal risk for developing the cancers listed. | |
| INCREASED RISK ASSESSMENT | Check-off list related to carcinogenic exposure, genetic predisposition, personal history of cancer, and certain associated diseases. Next to each item is the associated cancer for which the person is at increased risk. | Costanza et al: Cancer prevention and detection: Strategies for practice, in *Cancer Manual* (ed 7). Boston, American Cancer Society, 1986 |
| RISK APPRAISAL FORM | A Risk Appraisal Form that is practical and useful for office or clinic setting was developed. Questions are presented related to risk for cardiovascular disease, malignant diseases, auto accidents, suicide, diabetes. Scores are summarized to provide total number of risk factors for which the patient is in the highest risk level, and this is then converted to a percentage. Form indicates factors that provide low, medium, and high risk for patient. | Pender N (ed): Health promotion, in *Nursing Practice*. New York, Appleton-Century Crofts, 1982 |

### RESOURCES FOR HEALTH RISK ASSESSMENT INSTRUMENTS

Center for Corporate Health Promotion
1850 Centennial Park Dr.
Suite 520
Reston, VA 22091

Center for Research in Medical Education and Health Care
Jefferson Medical College
Philadelphia, PA 19107

Channing L. Bete Co., Inc.
200 State Rd.
South Deerfield, MA 01373

CompuHealth Associates
13795 Rider Trail
Earth City, MO 63045

Control Data Corp.
StayWell/EAR Division
901 East 78th St.
Minneapolis, MN 55420

General Health, Inc.
3299 K. St., NW
Washington, DC 20007

Health Enhancement Systems
9 Mercer St.
Princeton, NJ 08540

Health Logics
111 Deerwood Pl
San Ramon, CA 94583

HMC Software Inc.
4200 North MacArthur Blvd.
Irving, TX 75038

International Health Awareness Center
157 South Kalamazoo Mall
Suite 482
Kalamazoo, MI 49007-4895

Lifestyle and Health Promotion
59 Monterrey Ave.
Kenner, LA 70065

Lifestyle Directions, Inc.
300 Ninth St.
Conway, PA 15027-1696

MedMicro
6701 Seybold Rd.
Suite 220A
Madison, WI 53719

National Wellness Institute
University of Wisconsin–Stevens Point
South Hall
Stevens Point, WI 54481

ODPHP National Health Information Center
P.O. Box 1133
Washington, DC 20013

Prospective Medicine Center
Suite 219
3901 North Meridian
Indianapolis, IN 46208

Queue Inc.
562 Boston Ave.
Bridgeport, CT 06610

Regional Health Resource Center
Medical Information Laboratory
1408 West University Ave.
Urbana, IL 61801

St. Louis County Health Department
1001 East First St.
Duluth, MN 55805

University of British Columbia
Health Care and Epidemiology
5804 Fairview Crescent
Mather Building
Vancouver, BC V6T W5
Canada

**TABLE 7-4**  Health Risk Assessment Instruments (continued)

| Instrument | Description | Source |
|---|---|---|
| RESOURCES FOR HEALTH RISK ASSESSMENT INSTRUMENTS | | |

University of California
Epidemiology and International Health
1699 HSW
San Francisco, CA 94143

University of Michigan
Fitness Research Center
401 Washtenaw Ave.
Ann Arbor, MI 48109-2214

University of Minnesota
Media Distribution
Box 734, Mayo Building
420 Delaware St., SE
Minneapolis, MN 55455

Well Aware About Health
P.O. Box 43338
Tucson, AZ 85733

Wellsource
15431 Southeast 82nd Dr.
Suite E
P.O. Box 569
Clackamas, OR 97015

Wisconsin Center for Health Risk Research
University of Wisconsin Center for Health Sciences
600 Highland Ave., Room J5/224
Madison, WI 53792

National Health Information Center, Washington, DC.

It is important to remember that there is an element of fear of the diagnostic implications of admitting to certain symptoms that can create problems in cancer prevention/detection. The history, therefore, is helpful not only in detecting early, vague symptoms but also in identifying signs and symptoms that the patient might deny if asked outright. In addition, the history helps to identify factors, such as a family history of genetic susceptibility, that may increase an individual's risk of specific cancers. In such situations the physician may order special tests that are not included in the guidelines for the public in general.[156] A complete physical examination should follow the health history to provide objective data that can complement and verify the health history's subjective data.

For individuals identified as having a high risk of cancer, advice should be given about avoiding additional exposure to carcinogens, and rigorous intervention may be indicated (e.g., excision of the colon in a patient with chronic ulcerative colitis before the appearance of cancer or removal of a dysplastic nevus to prevent progression to melanoma). In high-risk individuals, screening might also be carried out more frequently and in greater detail than in those at low risk. Women at high risk of breast cancer may need to have mammography and periodic physical examinations performed more frequently and started at an earlier age than women who are at low risk. The recommended schedule of prevention and detection procedures for the general population, as suggested by the American Cancer Society, is shown in Table 7-5.[43,130]

## EDUCATION

Education of individuals at high risk of cancer cannot be treated as something separate and distinct from general education of the public about cancer, although it has certain features. The aims of public education are

- to inform and educate about treatable forms of cancer and to reassure people that treatment is advantageous

- to persuade people, particularly those at special risk, to undertake preventive action, to undergo tests so that cancer can be detected at an earlier stage, or to seek medical advice quickly when recognizable signs of ill health occur[162]

Consequently, organized cancer education attempts to maintain positive health behavior or to interrupt a behavior pattern that is linked to increased risks of cancer. The behavior usually is that of the persons whose health is in question, but often it includes the behavior of others who control resources or rewards for behavior, such as community leaders, parents, employers, peers, teachers, and health professionals. Whether it is at the primary, secondary, or tertiary stage of prevention, a cancer education program is an intervention to prevent disability, illness, or death or to enhance quality of life through voluntary change of cancer-related behavior.[163]

Areas that should be covered in educational programs include tobacco, alcohol, occupations and cancer, environmental pollutants, sexual activity, radiation, infective and genetic factors, and diet.[164] Each of these areas should be discussed in terms of the risks they impose for certain types of cancer, actions to reduce risks, signs and symptoms of specific cancers, screening and detection methods, and personal responsibility in prevention. To reduce fears that may prevent compliance, reassurance must be given that some forms of cancer respond well to treatment. These deep-seated fears influence behavior and often create situations in which the person knows what ought to be done but does not do it.

## CONCLUSION

From experience to date, we know that more than 80% of the causes of cancer are theoretically avoidable. This tells us that cancer is not inevitable and that cancer prevention is feasible and practical. As LeMaistre[15] points out, "If we are willing to use the knowledge we now have

**TABLE 7-5**   Summary of American Cancer Society Recommendations for the Early Detection of Cancer in Asymptomatic Persons at Average Risk

| Examination | Sex | Age | Frequency |
| --- | --- | --- | --- |
| Sigmoidoscopy | M and F | 50 and over | One exam every 3–5 years |
| Stool guaiac slide test | M and F | Over 50 | Every year |
| Digital rectal examination | M and F | Over 40 | Every year |
| Digital rectal examination | M | Over 50 | Check for prostate cancer every year. |
| Prostate-specific antigen blood test | M | Over 50 | Every year |
| Pap test and pelvic examination | F | All women who have been sexually active or have reached age 18 | Every year. After 3 or more satisfactory consecutive, normal annual examinations, the Pap test may be performed less frequently, at the discretion of the physician. |
| Endometrial tissue sample | F | At menopause Women at high risk* | At menopause |
| Breast self-examination | F | 20 and older | Every month |
| Clinical breast examination | F | 20–39 40 and older | Every 3 years Every year |
| Mammography | F | 35–39 40–49 50 and over | Baseline Every 1–2 years Every year |
| Health counseling† | M and F | Over 20 | Every 3 years |
| Cancer checkup‡ | M and F | Over 40 | Every year |

*History of infertility, obesity, failure to ovulate, abnormal uterine bleeding, or estrogen therapy.

†To include counseling about tobacco control, sun exposure, diet and nutrition, risk factors, sexual practices, and environmental and other occupational exposures.

‡To include examination for cancers of the thyroid, testicles, prostate, ovaries, lymph nodes, oral cavity, and skin.

Reprinted with permission from the American Cancer Society.[43,130]

about how to prevent cancer as effectively as we do the knowledge about how to cure cancer, then and only then will we be on the road to eliminating cancer." The concept of prevention is sound, but successful application will require that we move forward aggressively in two directions: (1) basic research in cancer prevention, and (2) understanding more about motivating human behavioral change. A first step in refocusing our cancer prevention efforts occurred when a consensus was achieved that cancers are caused by specific risk factors in our environment and in our lifestyle. However, efforts at developing effective cancer prevention strategies have been hampered by the fact that the knowledge base and understanding of each risk factor varies. We must, therefore, acquire additional knowledge about each individual risk factor and determine how it affects the body. This information, combined with strong public education, will prove to be the cornerstone of cancer prevention.

# REFERENCES

1. Robbins LC, Hall JH: *How to Practice Prospective Medicine.* Indianapolis, Methodist Hospital of Indiana, 1970
2. Schoenbach V: Appraising health risk appraisal. *Am J Public Health* 77:409–411, 1987

3. Higginson J: Existing risks for cancer, in Deisler P (ed): *Reducing the Carcinogenic Risks in Industry.* New York, Marcel Dekker, 1984, pp 1–19

4. Bodnar B, Pedersen S: The nursing process, in Edelman C, Mandel C (eds): *Health Promotion throughout the Lifespan.* St. Louis, Mosby, 1986, pp 44–71

5. Rowe W: Identification of risk, in *Risk and Reasons: Risk Assessment in Relation to Environmental Mutagens and Carcinogens.* New York, Alan R. Liss, 1986, pp 3–22

6. Cartmel B, Reid M: Cancer control and epidemiology, in Groenwald SL, Frogge MH, Goodman M, Yarbro, CH (eds): *Cancer Nursing: Principles and Practice* (ed 3). Boston, Jones and Bartlett, 1993, pp 3–27

7. Newell G: Lifestyles and cancer prevention, in *Progress in Cancer Control IV: Research in the Cancer Center.* New York, Alan R. Liss, 1983, pp 55–66

8. Yarbro, JW: Milestones in our understanding of the causes of cancer, in Groenwald SL, Frogge MH, Goodman M, Yarbro, CH (eds): *Cancer Nursing: Principles and Practices* (ed 3). Boston, Jones and Bartlett, 1993, pp. 28–46

9. Breslow L: Review and future perspectives of cancer screening programs, in Nieburgs H (ed): *Prevention and Detection of Cancer. Part II. Detection.* New York, Marcel Dekker, 1978, pp 1177–1212

10. White L: Cancer risk assessment. *Semin Oncol Nurs* 2: 184–190, 1986

11. Boyd NF: The epidemiology of cancer: Principles and methods, in Tannock IF, Hill RP (eds): *The Basic Science of Oncology.* New York, Pergamon Press, 1987

12. Meili L: Epidemiology, in Otto SE (ed): *Oncology Nursing.* St. Louis, Mosby Year Book, 1991, pp 19–27

13. Lin R, Kesseler I: A multifactorial model for pancreatic cancer in man. *JAMA* 245:147–152, 1981

14. Woods NH, Woods J: Epidemiology and the study of cancer, in Marino L (ed): *Cancer Nursing.* St. Louis, Mosby, 1981, pp 139–175

15. LeMaistre C: Reflections on disease prevention. *Cancer* 62:1673–1675, 1988 (suppl)

16. American Cancer Society: *Cancer Facts and Figures, 1996.* Atlanta, American Cancer Society, 1996

17. Lovejoy N, Jenkins C, Wu T, et al: Developing a breast cancer screening program for Chinese-American women. *Oncol Nurs Forum* 16:181–187, 1989

18. Millon-Underwood S, Sanders E: Factors contributing to health promotion behaviors among African-American men. *Oncol Nurs Forum* 17:707–720, 1990

19. Baquet CR, Ringen K: *Cancer Among Blacks and Other Minorities.* Publication No. 86-2785. Washington, DC, U.S. Department of Health and Human Services, Public Health Service, National Institutes of Health, March 1986

20. Frank-Stromborg M, Olsen S (eds): *Cancer Prevention in Minority Populations: Cultural Implications for Health Care Professionals.* St. Louis, Mosby, 1993

21. Devesa S, Diamond E: Socioeconomic and racial differences in lung cancer incidence. *Am J Epidemiol* 118: 818–829, 1983

22. Freeman H: Cancer in the socioeconomically disadvantaged, in *Cancer and the Socioeconomically Disadvantaged.* Atlanta, American Cancer Society, 1990

23. Jenks S: War on cancer confronts poverty. *Med World News,* August 14, 1989, p 31

24. Wilkes G, Freeman H, Prout M: Cancer and poverty: Breaking the cycle. *Semin Oncol Nurs* 10:79–88, 1994

25. McCabe MS, Varricchio CG, Padberg RM: Efforts to recruit the economically disadvantaged to national clinical trials. *Semin Oncol Nurs* 10:123–129, 1994

26. Robinson KD, Kimmel EA, Yasko JM: Reaching out to the African-American community through innovative strategies. *Oncol Nurs Forum* 22:1383–1391, 1995

27. Millon-Underwood S, Sanders E, Davis M: Determinants of participation in state-of-the-art cancer prevention, early detection/screening and treatment trials among African-Americans. *Cancer Nurs* 16:25–33, 1993

28. Jepson C, Kessler LG, Portnoy B, et al: Black-white differences in cancer prevention knowledge and behavior. *Am J Public Health* 81:501–504, 1991

29. Boehm S, Coleman-Burns P, Schlenk EA, et al: Prostate cancer in African American men: Increasing knowledge and self-efficacy. *J Community Health Nurs* 12:161–169, 1995

30. Allen ME, Edwards K: Cancer prevention: Implications for ethnic and racial minorities. *Fam Community Health* 10: 62–66, 1987

31. Olsen SJ, Frank-Stromborg M: Cancer prevention and early detection in ethnically diverse populations. *Semin Oncol Nurs* 9:198–209, 1993

32. Thiemann Kay MB: Native women at risk: Addressing cancer prevention. *Winds of Change* 9:30–33, 1994

33. Hampton JW: Cancer prevention and control in American Indian/Alaska Natives. *Am Indian Culture Res J* 16:41–49, 1992

34. Welty TK: Cancer and cancer prevention and control programs in the Aberdeen Area Indian Health Services. *Am Indian Culture Res J* 16:117–137, 1992

35. Nemcek MA: Factors influencing black women's breast self-examination practice. *Cancer Nurs* 12:339–343, 1989

36. Nemcek MA: Health beliefs and breast self-examination among black women. *Health Values* 14:41–52, 1990

37. Chavez LR, Hubbell FA, McMullin JM, et al: Understanding knowledge and attitudes about breast cancer: A cultural analysis. *Arch Fam Med* 4:145–152, 1995

38. Devesa SS: Cancer patterns among women in the United States. *Semin Oncol Nurs* 11:78–87, 1995

39. Kagawa-Singer M: Socioeconomic and cultural influences on cancer care of women. *Semin Oncol Nurs* 11:109–119, 1995

40. Stellman JM, Stellman SD: Social factors: Women and cancer. *Semin Oncol Nurs* 11:103–108, 1995

41. McCool WF: Barriers to breast cancer screening in older women: A review. *J Nurse Midwifery* 39:283–299, 1994

42. Fink D: *Guidelines for the Cancer-Related Checkup: Recommendations and Rationale.* Atlanta, American Cancer Society, 1991

43. Update January 1992: The American Cancer Society Guidelines for the Cancer-Related Checkup. *CA Cancer J Clin* 42:44–45, 1992

44. Landrigan P: The prevention of occupational cancer. *CA Cancer J Clin* 46:67–69

45. Gray N: Cancer risks and cancer prevention in the third world, in Vessey M, Gray M (eds): *Cancer Risks and Prevention.* Oxford, Oxford University Press, 1985, pp 269–299

46. Lamm D, Torti F: Bladder cancer, 1996. *CA Cancer J Clin* 46:93–112, 1996

47. Brownson RC, Chang JC, Davis JR: Occupation, smoking, and alcohol in the epidemiology of bladder cancer. *Am J Public Health* 77:1298–1300, 1987

48. Hossan E, Striegel A: Carcinoma of the bladder. *Semin Oncol Nurs* 9:252–256, 1993

49. Skegg D: Other drugs, in Vessey M, Gray M (eds): *Cancer*

*Risks and Prevention.* Oxford: Oxford University Press, 1985, pp 211–230

50. Whitmore W: Bladder cancer: An overview. *CA Cancer J Clin* 38:213–221, 1988

51. American Cancer Society: *Breast Cancer Facts and Figures 1996.* Atlanta, American Cancer Society, 1996

52. Kelsey JL, Gammon MD: The epidemiology of breast cancer. *CA Cancer J Clin* 41:146–165, 1991

53. Henderson D, Ross R, Bernstein L: Estrogens as a cause of human cancer: The Richard and Hinda Rosenthal Foundation Award Lecture. *Cancer Res* 48:246–253, 1988

54. DuPont W, Page D, Parl F, et al: Long-term risk of breast cancer in women with fibroadenoma. *N Engl J Med* 331:10–15, 1994

55. King S, Schottenfeld D: The "epidemic" of breast cancer in the U.S.: Determining the factors. *Oncology* 10:453–464, 1996

56. Seidman H, Stellman S, Hushinski M: A different perspective on breast cancer risk factors: Some implications of the non-attributable risk. *CA Cancer J Clin* 32:301–313, 1982

57. Schatzkin A, Longnecker M: Alcohol and breast cancer: Where are we now and where do we go from here? *Cancer* 74:1101–1110, 1994 (suppl)

58. Harris RE, Wynder EL: Breast cancer and alcohol consumption: A study in weak associations. *JAMA* 259:2867–2871, 1988

59. Schatzkin A, Jones Y, Hoover RN, et al: Alcohol consumption and breast cancer in the epidemiologic follow-up study of the first national health and nutrition survey. *N Engl J Med* 316:1169–1173, 1987

60. Petrakis N, Ernster V, King M: Breast, in Schottenfeld D, Fraumeni J (eds): *Cancer Epidemiology and Prevention.* Philadelphia, Saunders, 1982, pp 855–870

61. The Cancer and Steroid Hormone Study of the Centers for Disease Control and the National Institute of Child Health and Human Development: Oral-contraceptive use and the risk of breast cancer. *N Engl J Med* 315:405–411, 1986

62. Malone K, Daling J, Weiss N: Oral contraceptives in relation to breast cancer. *Epidemiology Review* 15:80–97, 1993

63. Wynder E, Rose D, Cohen L: Diet and breast cancer in causation and therapy. *Cancer* 58:1804–1813, 1986

64. Willett WC, Stampfer MJ, Colditz GA, et al: Dietary fat and the risk of breast cancer. *N Engl J Med* 316:22–28, 1987

65. Holmberg L, Ohlander E, Byers T: Diet and breast cancer risk. *Arch Intern Med* 154:1805–1811, 1994

66. Weber B: Genetic testing for breast cancer. *Sci Am Med* 3:12–21, 1996

67. Madigan M, Ziegler R, Benichou J, et al: Proportion of breast cancer cases in the United States explained by well-established risk factors. *J Natl Cancer Inst* 87:1681–1685, 1995

68. Stefanek ME: Counseling women at high risk for breast cancer. *Oncology* 4:27–38, 1990

69. Herrero R, Brinton L, Reeves W, et al: Sexual behavior, venereal disease, hygiene practices, and invasive cervical cancer in a high-risk population. *Cancer* 65:380–386, 1990

70. Villa L, Franco E: Ludwig Institute for Cancer Research Human Papillomavirus Study Group: Epidemiologic correlates of cervical neoplasia and risk of human papilloma virus infection in asymptomatic women in Brazil. *J Natl Cancer Inst* 81:332–340, 1989

71. Maiman M, Fruchter R, Guy L, et al: Human immunodefi-

ciency virus infection and invasive cervical carcinoma. *Cancer* 71:402–406, 1993

72. DeBuono B, Zinner S, Daamen M, et al: Sexual behavior of college women in 1975, 1986, and 1989. *N Engl J Med* 322:821–825, 1990

73. Martin L, Parker S, Wingo P, et al: Cervical cancer incidence and screening. *Cancer Pract* 4:130–134, 1996

74. Eddy D: Screening for cervical cancer. *Ann Intern Med* 113:214–226, 1990

75. Hendershot GE: Coitus-related cervical cancer risk factors: Trends and differentials in racial and religious groups. *Am J Public Health* 73:299–301, 1983

76. Brinton LA, Schairer C, Hasenszel W: Smoking and invasive cervical cancer. *JAMA* 255:3265–3269, 1986

77. More bad news for women smokers. *Cope* 12:7, 1996

78. Carroll KK, Lipkin M, Weisburger JH: Diet's key role in preventing cancer. *Patient Care* 23:54–63, 1989

79. National Research Council: *Diet and Health Report.* Washington, DC: National Academy of Sciences, 1990

80. Council on Scientific Affairs: Dietary fiber and health. *JAMA* 262:542–546, 1989

81. Willett WC, Stampfer MJ, Colditz GA, et al: Relation of meat, fat, and fiber intake to the risk of colon cancer in a prospective study among women. *N Engl J Med* 323:1664–1672, 1990

82. Kritchevsky D: Diet and cancer. *CA Cancer J Clin* 41:328–333, 1991

83. Colon cancer gene offers new target for drug designers. *J NIH Res* 3:37, 1991

84. Bufill JA: Colorectal cancer: Evidence for distinct genetic categories based on proximal or distal tumor location. *Ann Intern Med* 113:779–788, 1990

85. Fleischer DE, Goldberg SB, Browning TH, et al: Detection and surveillance of colorectal cancer. *JAMA* 261:580–585, 1989

86. Smigel K: Group defines directions for colorectal cancer screening. *J Natl Cancer Inst* 86:958–960, 1994

87. DeCosse J, Tsioulias G, Jacobson J: Colorectal cancer: Detection, treatment, and rehabilitation. *CA Cancer J Clin* 44:27–42, 1994

88. Atkin W, Cuzick J, Northover J et al: Prevention of colorectal cancer by once-only sigmoidoscopy. *Lancet* 341:736–740, 1993

89. Winawer S, Zauber A, Ho M, et al: Prevention of colorectal cancer by colonoscopic polypectomy. *N Engl J Med* 329:1977–1981, 1993

90. Müller A, Sonnenberg A: Protection by endoscopy against death from colorectal cancer. *Arch Intern Med* 155:1741–1748, 1995

91. Ekbom A, Helmick C, Zack M, et al: Ulcerative colitis and colorectal cancer. *N Engl J Med* 323:1228–1233, 1990

92. Di Bisceglie A: Hepatocellular carcinoma: Molecular biology of its growth and relationship to hepatitis B virus infection. *Med Clin North Am* 73:985–995, 1989

93. Prevention of liver cancer. *World Health Organ Tech Rep Ser* 691:1–30, 1983

94. Kaklamai E, Trichopoulos D, Tzonou A, et al: Hepatitis B and C viruses and their interaction in the origin of hepatocellular carcinoma. *JAMA* 265:1974–1976, 1991

95. Simonetti RG, Camma C, Fiorello F, et al: Hepatitis C virus infection as risk factor for hepatocellular carcinoma in patients with cirrhosis. *Ann Intern Med* 116:97–102, 1992

96. Falk H: Vinyl chloride–induced hepatic angiosarcoma, in

Miller RW (ed): *Unusual Occurrences as Clues to Cancer Etiology.* Tokyo, Japan Scientific Societies Press, 1988, pp 39–46

97. Fleisher JM: Occupational and non-occupational risk factors in relation to an excess of primary liver cancer observed among residents of Brooklyn, New York. *Cancer* 65:180–185, 1990

98. Rustigi VK: Epidemiology of hepatocellular carcinoma. *Gastroenterol Clin North Am* 16:545–551, 1987

99. Regan LS: Screening for hepatocellular carcinoma in high-risk individuals. *Arch Intern Med* 149:1741–1744, 1989

100. Rosenblum L, Darrow W, Witte J, et al: Sexual practices in the transmission of hepatitis B virus and prevalence of hepatitis delta virus infection in female prostitutes in the United States. *JAMA* 267:2477–2481, 1992

101. Beasley RP: Hepatitis B virus: The major etiology of hepatocellular carcinoma. *Cancer* 61:1942–1956, 1988

102. Hsing A, Hoover R, McLaughlin J: Oral contraceptives and primary liver cancer among young women. *Cancer Causes Control* 3:43–48, 1992

103. Lisker-Melman M, Martin P, Hoofnagle JH: Conditions associated with hepatocellular carcinoma. *Med Clin North Am* 73:999–1009, 1989

104. Boyle P, Maisonneuve P: Lung cancer and tobacco smoking. *Lung Cancer* 12:167–181, 1995

105. Oleske D: The epidemiology of lung cancer: An overview. *Semin Oncol Nurs* 3:165–173, 1987

106. Cresanta J: Epidemiology of cancer in the United States. *Primary Cancer* 19:419–441, 1992

107. Cigarette smoking among adults: United States, 1990. *JAMA* 267:3133, 1992

108. Bartecchi C, MacKenzie T, Schrier R: The global tobacco epidemic. *Sci Am* 273:44–51, 1995

109. Voelker R: Young people may face huge tobacco toll. *JAMA* 274:203, 1995

110. Jonthan ET, Correa P, Reynolds P, et al: Environmental tobacco smoke and lung cancer in nonsmoking women. *JAMA* 271:1752–1759, 1994

111. Wang F, Love E, Liu N, et al: Childhood and adolescent passive smoking and the risk of female lung cancer. *Int J Epidemiol* 23:223–230, 1994

112. Harley NH, Harley JH: Potential lung cancer risk from indoor radon exposure. *CA Cancer J Clin* 40:265–275, 1990

113. Jöckel K, Ahrens W, Wichmann H, et al: Occupational and environmental hazards associated with lung cancer. *Int J Epidemiol* 21:202–213, 1992

114. Markowitz S: Primary prevention of occupational lung disease: A view from the United States. *Isr J Med Sci* 28:513–519, 1992

115. Mahboubi E, Sayed G: Oral cavity and pharynx, in Schottenfeld D, Fraumeni J (eds): *Cancer Epidemiology and Prevention.* Philadelphia, Saunders, 1982, pp 583–595

116. Holmstrup P, Pindborg J: Oral mucosal lesions in smokeless tobacco users. *CA Cancer J Clin* 38:230–235, 1988

117. Sankaranarayanan R, Duffy SW, Day NF, et al: A case-control investigation of cancer of the oral tongue and the floor of the mouth in southern India. *Int J Cancer* 44:617–621, 1989

118. Mashberg A, Samit AM: Early detection, diagnosis, and management of oral and oropharyngeal cancer. *CA Cancer J Clin* 39:67–87, 1989

119. Peto R: The preventability of cancer, in Vessey M, Gray M (eds): *Cancer Risks and Prevention.* Oxford, Oxford University Press, 1985, pp 1–14

120. Oreggia F, DeStefani E, Correa P, et al: Risk factors for cancer of the tongue in Uruguay. *Cancer* 67:180–183, 1991

121. Weiss N: Ovary, in Schottenfeld D, Fraumeni J (eds): *Cancer Epidemiology and Prevention.* Philadelphia, Saunders, 1982, pp 871–880

122. Ozols RF: The current status of the treatment of ovarian cancer. *Mediguide to Oncology* 11:1–5, 1991

123. Ovarian cancer: Risk factors and how best to screen patients. *Primary Care & Cancer* 14:9–10, 1994

124. White L: The nurse's role in cancer prevention, in Newell G (ed): *Cancer Prevention in Clinical Medicine.* New York, Raven Press, 1983, pp 91–112

125. Henderson B, Gerkins V, Pike M: Sexual factors and pregnancy, in Fraumeni J (ed): *Persons at High Risk of Cancer: An Approach to Cancer Etiology and Control.* New York, Academic Press, 1975, pp 267–284

126. The Cancer and Steroid Hormone Study of the Centers for Disease Control and the National Institute of Child Health and Human Development: The reduction in risk of ovarian cancer associated with oral-contraceptive use. *N Engl J Med* 316:650–655, 1987

127. Pritchard KI: Screening for endometrial cancer: Is it effective? *Ann Intern Med* 110:177–179, 1989

128. Gambrell RD: Estrogen-progesterone replacement and cancer risk. *Hosp Pract* 25:81–100, 1990

129. Sox H: Preventive health services in adults. *N Engl J Med* 330:1589–1595, 1994

130. American Cancer Society: *Guidelines for the Cancer-Related Checkup.* Atlanta, American Cancer Society, 1992

131. Michell D: Contraception. *N Engl J Med* 320:777–787, 1989

132. Persky V, Davis F, Barrett R, et al: Recent time trends in uterine cancer. *Am J Public Health* 80:935–939, 1990

133. Crawford ED, Nabors WL: Diagnosing prostate cancer: Role of the primary care physician. *Primary Care & Cancer* 10:19–24, 1990

134. Littrup PJ, Lee F, Mettlin C: Prostate cancer screening: Current trends and future implications. *CA Cancer J Clin* 142:198–211, 1992

135. Littrup P, Goodman A, Mettlin C, et al: The benefit and cost of prostate cancer early detection. *CA Cancer J Clin* 43:134–149, 1993

136. Greenwald P: Prostate, in Schottenfeld D, Fraumeni J (eds): *Cancer Epidemiology and Prevention.* Philadelphia, Saunders, 1982, pp 938–967

137. Diagnosis and treatment of prostate cancer. *Senior Medical Review. AARP* 3:1–8, 1989

138. Doll R, Peto R: *The Causes of Cancer: Quantitative Estimates of Avoidable Risks of Cancer in the United States Today.* New York, Oxford University Press, 1981

139. Rose D, Boyar A, Wynder E: International comparisons of mortality rates for cancer of the breast, ovary, prostate, and colon, and per capita food consumption. *Cancer* 58:2363–2371, 1986

140. Brawley O, Thompson I: Chemoprevention of prostate cancer. *Urology* 43:594–599, 1994

141. Willson PC: Prostate cancer II: The nurse's role in screening and early diagnosis for primary disease and recurrence. *Nursing Interventions in Oncology.* (M.D. Anderson Cancer Center, Houston, TX) 4:4–5, 1992

142. Council on Scientific Affairs: Harmful effects of ultraviolet radiation. *JAMA* 262:380–384, 1989

143. Stewart DS: Indoor tanning: The nurse's role in preventing skin damage, in Reed-Ash C, Jenkins JF (eds): *Enhancing*

*the Role of Cancer Nursing.* New York, Raven Press, 1990, pp 79–94

144. Lawler PE, Schreiber S: Cutaneous malignant melanoma: Nursing's role in prevention and early detection. *Oncol Nurs Forum* 16:345–352, 1989

145. Devereux DF: Diagnosis and management of dysplastic nevus syndrome and early melanoma. *Oncology* 4:73–83, 1990

146. Koh HK, Lew RA, Prout MN: Screening for melanoma/ skin cancer: Theoretic and practical considerations. *J Am Acad Dermatol* 20:159–172, 1989

147. Lee JAH: The melanoma epidemic thus far. *Mayo Clin Proc* 65:1368–1371, 1990

148. Campbell EM, Redman S, Sanson-Fisher WS: Screening for melanoma: A community survey of prevalence and predictors. *Med J Aust* 154:338–343, 1991

149. Richie J: Detection and treatment of testicular cancer. *CA Cancer J Clin* 43:151–175, 1993

150. Schottenfeld D, Warshauer M: Testis, in Schottenfeld D, Fraumeni J (eds): *Cancer Epidemiology and Prevention.* Philadelphia, Saunders, 1982, pp 947–957

151. Shreyaskumar PR, Kvols LK, Richardson RL: Familial testicular cancer: Report of six cases and review of the literature. *Mayo Clin Proc* 65:804–808, 1990

152. Karagas MR, Weiss NS, Strader CH, et al: Elevated intrascrotal temperature and the incidence of testicular cancer in noncryptorchid men. *Am J Epidemiol* 129:1104–1109, 1989

153. Brinton LA, Nasca PC, Mallin K, et al: Case-control study of in situ and invasive carcinoma of the vagina. *Gynecol Oncol* 38:49–54, 1990

154. Kelly P: Counseling persons who have family histories of cancer, in Newell G (ed): *Cancer Prevention in Clinical Medicine.* New York, Raven Press, 1983, pp 147–164

155. Baeck M, Eisenberg M: Carcinogenic risk assessment: Concepts and issues. *Md Med J* 34:672–674, 1985

156. Constanza M, Li F, Green H, et al: Cancer prevention and detection: Strategies for practice, in *American Cancer Society. Cancer Manual* (ed 7). Boston, American Cancer Society, 1986, pp 14–35

157. Lippman SM, Bassford TL, Meyskens FL: A quantitatively scored cancer risk assessment tool: Its development and use. *J Cancer Educ* 7:15-36, 1992

158. Koss L: Counseling persons who have family histories of cancer, in Fraumeni J (ed) *Persons at High Risk of Cancer: An Approach to Cancer Etiology and Control.* New York, Academic Press, 1975, pp 85–102

159. White LN: Cancer risk and early detection assessment. *Semin Oncol Nurs* 9:188–197, 1993

160. Wamstad K: Commentary on a quantitatively scored cancer risk assessment tool: Its development and use. *Oncol Nurs Scan* 1:2, 1992

161. Cohen J, Jaffe D: Holistic health: The future, in Edelman C, Mandle C (eds): *Health Promotion throughout the Life-Span.* St. Louis, Mosby, 1986, pp 643–666

162. Wakefield J: Education of the public, in Fraumeni J (ed): *Persons at High Risk of Cancer: An Approach to Cancer Etiology and Control.* New York, Academic Press, 1975, pp 415–434

163. Green L, Rimer B, Elwood T: Public education, in Schottenfeld D, Fraumeni J (eds). *Cancer Epidemiology and Prevention.* Philadelphia, Saunders, 1982, pp 1100–1110

164. Peto R: The preventability of cancer, in Vessey M, Gray M (eds). *Cancer Risks and Prevention.* Oxford: Oxford University Press, 1985, pp 1–14

# Chapter 8

# Assessment and Interventions for Cancer Detection

**Marilyn Frank-Stromborg, EdD, JD, NP, FAAN**

**Rebecca F. Cohen, RN, EdD, MPA, CPHQ**

## INTRODUCTION

Despite its long history, cancer became a relatively important health problem only during the twentieth century. It was among the first chronic diseases recognized as potentially "controllable," that is, amenable to public health strategies consistent with its magnitude and social impact. In 1937 the Congress of the United States took its first significant action on the problem of cancer by passing the National Cancer Institute Act. This law established the National Cancer Institute for purposes of conducting research relating to the cause, diagnosis, and treatment of cancer and the application of research results, with a view to the development and prompt widespread use of the most effective methods of prevention, diagnosis, and treatment of cancer.[1] Congressional intent toward the cancer problem was reaffirmed by the passage of the National Cancer Act of 1971. This act expanded activities

> to develop, through research and development efforts, the means to significantly reduce the morbidity and mortality from cancer by: preventing as many cancers as possible, curing patients who develop cancer, providing maximum palliation to patients not cured, rehabilitating treated patients to as nearly normal a state as possible.[2]

Although a clear expression of congressional intent existed regarding cancer control, results of the 1971 legislation tended to be in the direction of research. It had been hoped that the legislation would result in the following cancer control efforts: (1) improved identification of techniques or methods with a potential for combating the disease, (2) improved community testing of these technological methods for safety and efficacy, (3) provision for evaluation of the results of the testing, and (4) enhanced promotion of the appropriate general use of technological techniques in the community through professional and public education. Obstacles existed, however, that made it much more difficult to initiate cancer control efforts than it had been to control communicable diseases. One of the obstacles included the fact that physicians generally did not view cancer as epidemic in nature. It was believed that governmental action to establish public services for cancer diagnosis or treatment was an intrusion into physicians' freedom to practice. In addition, economic resistance to control measures, for example, by the tobacco industry, was assisted by the fact that the long latency period of cancer helped to make etiologic factors less identifiable. Finally, cancer's multiple etiology engendered an extensive research effort when an additional attack on the disease was mounted. Money for research and training of personnel was held onto tightly by special interest groups that resisted public expenditures for cancer control as a threat to their own existence.[3,4]

Thus organized cancer control in the United States has had three strong adversaries: the private medical world, the private industrial world, and the biomedical research establishment that emerged after the passage of the National Cancer Institute Act of 1937 and the subsequent creation of the National Institutes of Health (NIH) in 1948. In some situations these forces, feeling threatened by cancer control, have developed strong lobbies against cancer control.

## Can We Prevent Cancer?

The arguments that cancer can be prevented are familiar to almost everyone. Different populations throughout the world suffer from different kinds of cancer, but those who migrate tend to acquire the pattern of cancers characteristic of their new home. It is therefore concluded by scientists that the incidence of cancers is determined by environment.[5,6] Research indicates that Americans could cut their incidence of cancer to little more than half the national average simply by adopting the lifestyle of the Seventh-Day Adventists and moving to the Rocky Mountain states or becoming Mormons and migrating to Utah.[7]

Evidence clearly illustrates that people resist changes in lifestyle.[8-12] Such attitudes as "there is not much a person can do to prevent cancer" and "scientists say everything causes cancer" create further resistance to altering lifestyle to prevent cancer.[13] Everyone knows about the link between cigarettes and lung cancer, and people expect to be exposed to lectures about the dangers of smoking. However, it has become customary to brush this aside and concentrate attention on modern industry as the supposed cause of most of our ills. It is attractive to distrust science and technology because they lay the blame on the imagined avarice of others rather than on one's own self-indulgence.[7]

In fact, some scientists[7,12] believe that there is really no evidence that any of the products of modern technology (except cigarettes) contribute to the common cancers. Thus most of the major cancers, except lung cancer, are not any more common today than they were 50 years ago.[7,12] It is suggested, however, that new industrial products be monitored for mutagenicity and carcinogenicity and that industries are deterred from adding hazardous ingredients or waste to our environment. However, cancer cannot be conquered simply by the surveillance and control of industry. To effectively conquer the common cancers, preventive measures must reach the individual and seek to modify personal habits and lifestyles.[7,12] For example, cancer of the lung is due to a highly addictive habit; cancer of the head and neck is associated with tobacco and excessive alcohol use; cancer of the large intestine and breast are most common in affluent countries and are thought to be related to diet; cancer of the skin is linked to ultraviolet rays and for some individuals is connected with increased leisure time.[10,20] The strategies for preventing these cancers may conflict with the immediate desires of individuals.[11] Apart from giving up smoking, sunbathing, and alcohol, the most recent change that we have been asked to make is in diet—the consumption of less fat, less cholesterol, and more fruits, vegetables, and cereals.[14-20]

Whether people will be willing to give up certain immediate desires for health and prolonged life remains to be seen. However, the National Cancer Institute (NCI) has established as its "Year 2000 Cancer Control Objective" a 50% reduction in the cancer mortality rate.[10] About 90% of the 800,000 skin cancers that were expected to be diagnosed in 1996 could have been prevented by protection from the sun. All cancers caused by cigarette smoking and heavy use of alcohol could be prevented completely. It was estimated that in 1996 about 170,000 lives would be lost to cancer because of tobacco use, and that about 19,000 cancer deaths would be related to excessive alcohol use. Diets high in fruits, vegetables, and fiber may reduce the incidence of some types of cancers. Regular screening and self-exams can detect cancers of the breast, tongue, mouth, colon, rectum, cervix, prostate, testis, and melanoma at an early stage when treatment is more likely to be successful. These sites include over half of all new cases and about two-thirds of all of these patients currently survive five years. With early detection, about 95% would survive. This means that of those individuals diagnosed with these cancers in 1996, about 115,000 more would survive if their cancers had been detected in a localized stage and treated promptly.[20]

It is apparent, therefore, that the best treatment of cancer is its prevention. Advances in understanding cancer formation, the development of effective screening modalities, the identification of major avoidable risk factors for cancer development, and chemoprevention suggest that the contribution of cancer prevention to decreasing the overall morbidity and mortality from cancer will increase rapidly in the next few years. Meyskens[21] urges specialists in cancer care to incorporate the strategies of cancer prevention into their activities to ensure maximal benefit and to provide continuity of care for patients and their families.

Of all the approaches to cancer control that can reduce mortality, screening holds the greatest promise for a rapid and major impact and is an important prevention strategy. Screening is defined as looking for disease in asymptomatic populations while early detection is looking for disease in asymptomatic and symptomatic patients (case finding). The boundary between screening and early detection is becoming increasingly blurred as we are able to identify "disease" at earlier stages.[21,22] Early detection is not useful for all cancers, such as cancer of the pancreas, which has no early detection tests available, and leukemia, which has no apparent localized phase.[22,23] Also, in only two modalities are the data sufficiently impressive for their widespread general use to be recommended. These include mammography in women between the ages of 40 and 69 and Papanicolaou cytology in sexually active women. Evidence of the efficacy of other screening tests, such as the Hemoccult screening in colon cancer and routine flexible sigmoidoscopy in individuals over age 50 have increased, but there is no definitive

information that supports the use of screening tools for lung, bladder, stomach, prostate, or ovarian cancers.[21,23] However, the investigation into using screening and early detection to help discover cancers that may never have surfaced in life is becoming increasingly important for cancers such as prostate cancer. The discovery of occult prostate carcinomas upon autopsy in elderly men has suggested that an increase in detection rates could increase survival and decrease mortality.[22]

In order for early detection to be useful, there must be a test or procedure that will detect cancers earlier, and there must be evidence that earlier treatment will result in an improved outcome. The majority of all detectable cancers can be discovered on a routine physical examination. Observation and palpation are valuable detection procedures for finding external cancers. Internal cancers require an extension of observation through the use of x-rays, ultrasound, laboratory tests, and scopes. Concerns regarding effectiveness, yield, and cost of these tests play an important role in decisions to detect internal cancers in asymptomatic individuals. Effectiveness of tests is measured in terms of sensitivity, specificity, and positive predictive values.[22]

There are several benefits and disadvantages to the increased use of screening measures for cancer. The greatest benefit includes improved prognoses for some patients whose disease is detected by screening. Those who benefit are primarily those who would have died from their disease without screening. In addition, less radical treatment may be needed to cure some patients of their disease because it is detected at an early stage. Reassurance for those with negative test results can be beneficial as well as resource savings and lower treatment cost if less radical treatment is instituted.[23]

Several disadvantages to screening exist. For example, earlier detection can create a longer period of morbidity for patients whose prognosis is unaltered. Overtreatment of borderline abnormalities that might never have been recognized without a positive screening test and false reassurance for those with false-negative screening results are negative aspects of screening. In situations where a false-negative occurred, the development of symptoms may be ignored with consequent postponement of the diagnosis and a poorer prognosis. Another disadvantage of screening may be unnecessary morbidity for those with false-positive screening results that may cause the individual to undergo multiple and varied diagnostic tests. Finally, there are resource costs of administering the screening test and from the overtreatment of borderline abnormalities.

It is important to evaluate not only the screening test itself but also the screening program to determine effectiveness of early identification of cancer. The process of evaluating the effectiveness of the screening test should begin with determining whether it has adequate sensitivity and specificity. The test should be acceptable to those who are to be screened. The screening program should be evaluated to determine if it is free of biases that may interfere with determining its effectiveness. If screening has been judged to be effective, the programs should be monitored to ensure that they achieve the expected benefits and that changes are not required in their organization.

Several obstacles also exist that may prevent screening from making a major contribution to cancer control: (1) an unfavorable natural history of some cancers (e.g., lung cancer), (2) poor organization of screening programs, and (3) poor compliance of those at risk (e.g., cancer of the cervix).[23] Also, the issue of poor compliance in following American Cancer Society (ACS) guidelines on mammography screening for breast cancer may be exacerbated by economic barriers that prevent the person from having the test or the physician from ordering it. Thus, there is some feeling that screening is a less productive approach to the control of cancer than prevention. However, the reality is that it may take many years for prevention strategies to achieve their full potential. Screening, which offers more return from appropriate investment, should, therefore, remain a major aspect of cancer control.

# DETECTION OF MAJOR CANCER SITES

Physical assessment has become a vital part of the nursing role, regardless of the nurse's setting. The use of physical assessment techniques is not limited to nurses who have completed a nurse practitioner program. Rather, it is now routinely taught in all undergraduate nursing programs, and the expectation is that nursing students will incorporate the four cardinal techniques (inspection, palpation, percussion, and auscultation) into their daily clinical practice. Physical assessment techniques enable the nurse to assume an active role in the early detection of cancer.

Cancers of the lung, breast, cervix, colon/rectum, and prostate are among the cancers that result in the highest morbidity and mortality rates in the United States.[24] The nursing interventions for these five cancers and for skin, testicular, head and neck, and other gynecologic cancers will be discussed. Each of the following sections presents the nursing role in terms of obtaining the health history, conducting the physical examination, using screening tests for asymptomatic individuals, and initiating patient education for primary and secondary prevention of the cancer.

## Lung Cancer

It was estimated that in 1996 177,000 Americans would be diagnosed with lung cancer.[25] It is the leading cause of death from cancer in men and women over 35 years of age. Once considered a male disease, since the late 1980s lung cancer has replaced breast cancer as the chief cause of cancer deaths among women. Of all the known risk factors for lung cancer, the most important environmental carcinogen related to the increased incidence of lung cancer is cigarette smoking. Cigarette smoking is the largest single preventable cause of premature death and disability and the major single cause of cancer mortality.[26]

### History assessment

When obtaining the history, the nurse should inquire into smoking habits, including marijuana use, occupational history, and the general respiratory environment in both the workplace and the home. Individuals at high risk for lung cancer are those exposed to high levels of respiratory carcinogens in their workplace, in their general environment, and in their homes. Because of the risks of passive smoking, a detailed history should be taken of the number of smokers in the home and the length of time the individual has been exposed to the smoke environment.[27,28]

Although obtaining a detailed, lifetime occupational history is time-consuming, it is strongly recommended for anyone who has worked in shipyards or who is believed to have been exposed to asbestos; significant exposures may have been as brief as one month and may have occurred many years ago, even during World War II. Because the World War II work force was composed of women as well as men, the female patient should not be overlooked. The same type of detailed, lifetime occupational history should be obtained if exposure to other known carcinogenic respiratory agents, such as those found in the following occupations, is suspected: clothing and textile workers, laundry workers, meat wrappers and cutters, hairdressers, agricultural workers, chemical workers, electrical machinery manufacturers, and health care workers.[29] In the assessment of elderly individuals, prior employment in settings unregulated by the National Institute of Occupational Safety and Health, the Occupational Safety and Health Act of 1970, or the Toxic Substances Control Act of 1976 must be considered because of possible exposure to toxic chemical or carcinogens that are no longer manufactured or permitted in unsupervised occupational settings.

An occupational history includes dates of employment, a list of current and longest-held jobs, average hours worked per week, exposure to potential hazards in the workplace, common illness in coworkers, and personal protective equipment worn on the job. Figure 8-1 presents a systematic approach to the occupational and environmental health history.[30]

Questions that should be included in the history and review of systems for lung cancer are the following:

1. When was your last chest x-ray film?
2. When was your last tuberculin skin test? If positive, what was the treatment?
3. Do you presently smoke? How many packs a day and for how many years? (*Pack-years* equal packs per day times years of smoking.) What do you smoke? Are they filtered? What's your style of smoking? Have you ever tried to stop smoking? What happened? Do you

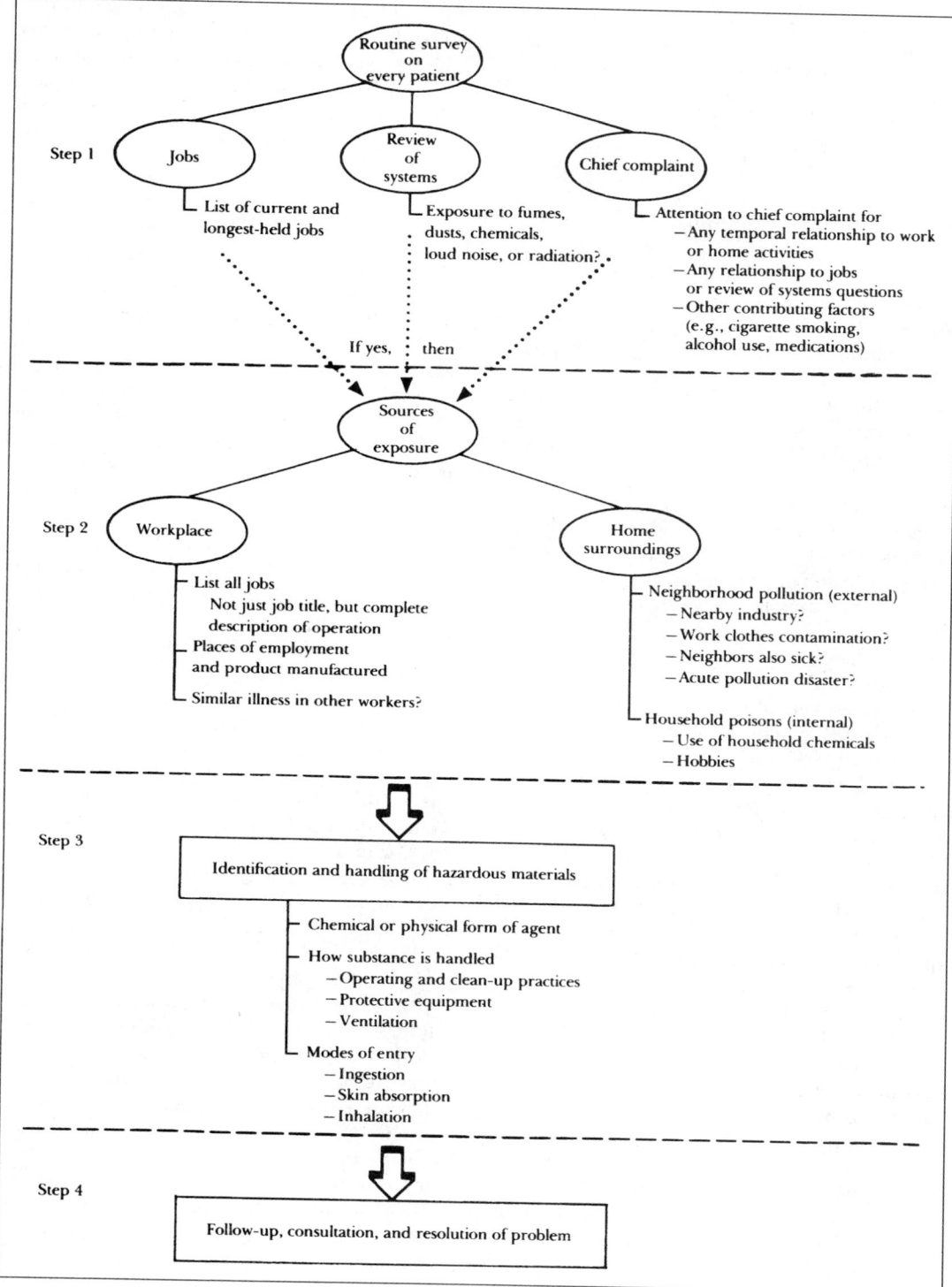

**FIGURE 8-1**   Systematic approach to the occupational and environmental health history. (Goldman R, Peters J: The occupational and environmental health history. *JAMA* 246:2832–2836, 1981.)

have a "smoker's" cough? Who else in the home smokes, and how much do they tend to smoke a day? Are you exposed to smoking in your work setting?

4. Has your home ever been tested for radon? Have homes around you been tested for radon and found to have high levels? If you tested your home for radon, was it high or low? If high, what did you do to remedy the situation?
5. Do you have bronchitis or asthma?
6. Have you ever had pneumonia?
7. Do you get short of breath when walking? climbing stairs? while resting? exercise?
8. Have you ever been told you have emphysema?
9. How many pillows do you sleep on? What happens if you don't use pillows?
10. Do you ever spit or cough up blood?
11. *Smokers:* What color is the sputum you cough up? Does it have a smell? How much is routinely coughed up in the morning?
12. What occupations have you had?
13. *Chronic obstructive pulmonary disease:* How often do you get flu shots? Have you been taught ways to drain the secretions from your lungs?
14. Have you ever had a pulmonary function test? What were the results?
15. Do you ever wheeze?
16. Do you cough a lot?
17. Do you have any skeletal deformities? Or were you born with any skeletal conditions?
18. Have you had any broken ribs?
19. Do you have to purse your lips to breathe?
20. Are you aware of any sounds when you breathe?
21. Have you noticed any color changes of your lips or nails?
22. Are you now (or have you been at some time in the past) exposed to fumes, chemicals, dust, or radiation?

The majority of patients have no profound early symptoms, but most have some combination of cough, chest pain, weight loss, dyspnea, fever, fatigue, and transient hemoptysis. Because these symptoms are general in nature, they usually cause no alarm and delay diagnosis. The most frequently reported symptom of lung cancer is a cough that is productive and often associated with hemoptysis or chest pain. Cough may be the primary or only complaint in such varied diseases as congestive heart failure, asthma, upper respiratory infection, pneumonia, and bronchitis. The irritative cough may occur at night accompanied by mucoid expectoration. However, if the lung cancer is centrally located or if only the main carina is involved, the cough is nonproductive.

Later symptoms are increased frequency of early symptoms and some combination of wheezes, pleuritic pain, hoarseness, nerve disorders from local invasion, edema of head, neck, or arms, and dysphagia. There is a high index of suspicion in anyone with a history of smoking or exposure to carcinogenic agents who complains of pneumonitis that persists longer than two weeks despite antibiotic therapy. Unfortunately, the first symptoms of lung cancer are usually not alarming and therefore tend to be considered lightly by health professionals. Because elderly individuals experience changes in respiratory structure and function, their initial vague respiratory complaints go unnoticed or are attributed to the aging process or chronic illnesses (e.g., congestive heart failure).

## Physical examination

**Inspection** On inspection there may be many systemic, as well as localized signs that will alert the practitioner to the possibility of lung cancer.

*Finger clubbing* This may be either an early or a late sign of thoracic disease, and it may be absent even in the presence of advanced disease. Approximately 5%–12% of patients with carcinoma of the lung will have clubbing of the fingers. It also may be seen in other diseases such as industrial lung disease (e.g., asbestosis).[31] It is important to inspect the nails closely and to palpate them for sponginess. With clubbing, the nail bed becomes thickened and boggy, which is first observed by palpating the nail bed to elicit fluctuation. Clubbing usually occurs first in the thumb and the index finger and then spreads to the other fingers.

The changes associated with clubbing usually occur gradually over many weeks, months, and years. However, they have been noted to appear within a week of the onset of lung cancer. Clubbing is best assessed by viewing the finger from the side. A normal finger viewed from this direction has an angle of about 160° between the base of the nail and the skin next to the cuticle (Figure 8-2). In clubbing, this base angle is obliterated and becomes 180° or more.[32]

*Barrel chest* This is characterized by prominence of the sternum and a barrel-shaped configuration of the chest that appears to be held in a state of full inspiration. This finding is associated with pulmonary emphysema or normal aging. Emphysema can be inherited, but the vast majority of individuals with this disease have acquired it from a lifetime of smoking. Those with emphysema are at high risk for lung cancer. Typical physical findings of emphysema are pursed lips during breathing, retraction of the intercostal spaces during inspiration, use of accessory muscles during quiet respirations, and audible wheezes.

*Abnormal breathing* With obstructive types of pulmonary disease, expiration is prolonged and inspiration is gasping and may require the use of the accessory muscles of respiration in the neck and about the shoulder girdle.[33] Figure 8-3 shows the stance taken by individuals with pulmonary obstruction. This stance is called the "professorial attitude" because it resembles a professor lecturing.

*Bulges on the thorax* With the use of indirect lighting, the practitioner may observe a bulge on the chest. Neoplasm of the ribs may protrude and will be visible on inspection.

*Breathlessness* The patient's breathlessness during the history taking may indicate obstruction of the lungs.

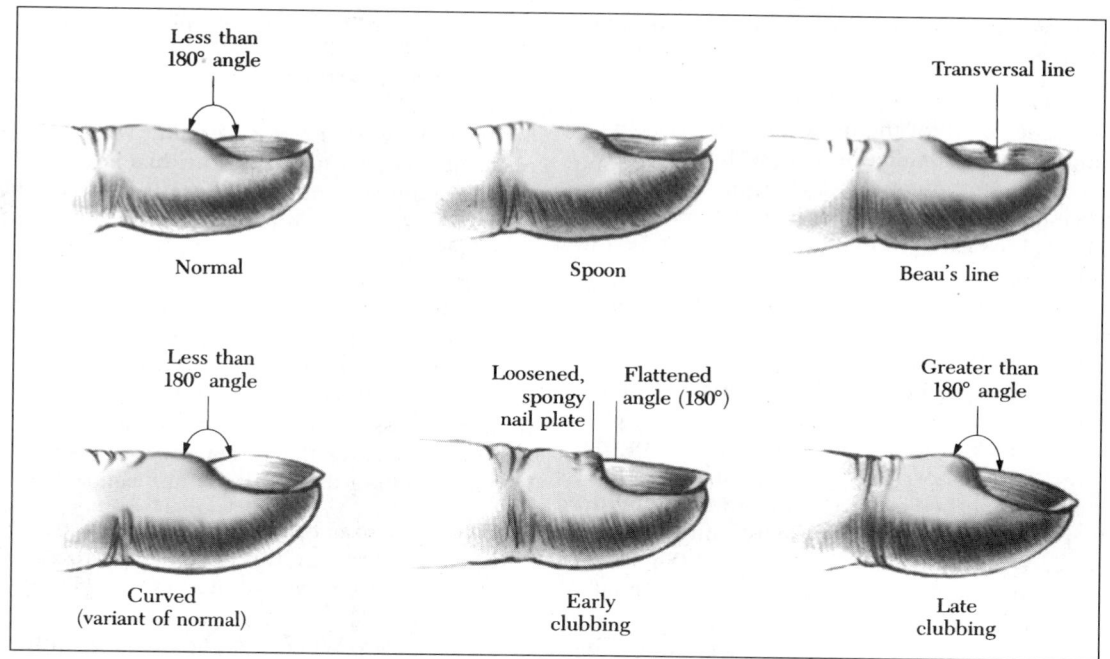

**FIGURE 8-2**   Normal and abnormal nails. (Grimes J, Burns E (eds): *Health Assessment in Nursing Practice* (ed 2). Boston, Jones and Bartlett, 1987.)

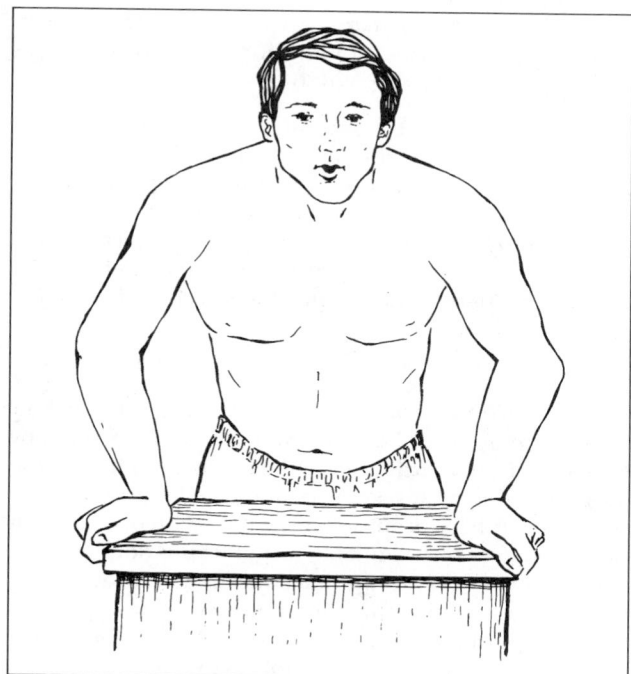

**FIGURE 8-3**   Patient fixes the arms and leans forward to use pectoral muscles as accessory inspiratory muscles for obstructed breathing.

*Skin*   Inspection of the skin of a heavy smoker may reveal premature wrinkling. Heavy cigarette smokers (>50 pack-years) are 4.7 times more likely to be wrinkled than nonsmokers.[34]

*Superior vena cava obstruction*   Obstruction of the superior vena cava is a common complication of lung cancer; approximately 80% of these cases are caused by undifferentiated neoplasms arising in proximal right bronchi.[35] The clinical picture is described by Buckingham:

Edema of both eyelids, arms, and hands develops and will "pit" on pressure; . . . the face is a dusky blue color, the lips are deeply cyanotic; and the swollen, blue head sits on a thick "bull neck" which is distended by many large tense collateral veins. The shoulders, chest, and upper abdomen are covered with a lacy collateral venous pattern.[33]

*Palpation*   Palpation of the thorax includes testing for vocal fremitus, respiratory excursion and compression, and ascertaining the position and movability of the trachea. The following discussion presents physical signs on palpation that may indicate lung cancer.

*Deviation and fixed trachea*   Normally the trachea is located in the midline and is freely movable. Localized disease may produce tracheal shift, or the trachea may be fixed by disease in the surrounding structures. Carcinoma of the lung rarely causes displacement except by producing atelectasis.[36]

*Thoracic wall*   Palpation of the thoracic wall reveals masses.

*Vocal fremitus*   Decreased or absent vocal fremitus indicates local bronchial obstruction from bronchial carcinomas, adenomas, or foreign bodies. Sound transmission through the bronchus is interrupted, causing the change in fremitus. Absent vocal fremitus also may indicate pleural effusions. Lung tumors immediately adjacent to the visceral pleura often cause early, insidious formation of pleural effusion that is responsible for the initial complaint of dyspnea.

***Percussion and auscultation***    These may provide the final clues to assessment of the individual who is at high risk for lung cancer. Auscultation is best done with the diaphragm of the stethoscope in a slow, methodical sequence of upper, middle, and lower zones and front, sides, and back. Physical signs that would require referral to a physician are discussed next.

*Dullness*    In the normal chest the sound on auscultatory percussion is resonance. If any pathological condition exists between the sound source (manubrium) and the reception point (stethoscope), the sound produced is a duller tone than normal.

An excellent technique for assessing dullness in the thorax is the auscultatory-percussion technique. This technique is accomplished by having the examiner lightly percuss the patient's manubrium while listening with the diaphragm piece on the posterior chest wall[37] (Figure 8-4). This technique enables the examiner to detect small, deep areas of pathological disease.

Dullness on percussion indicates either pleural effusion or a consolidated lung. Lung cancer is the most common cause of hemorrhagic pleural effusion in middle-aged and elderly male smokers. The early production of pleural fluid by most tumors produces the classic signs of pleural effusion: flatness, absence of fremitus, and breath sounds.[36]

*Decreased or absent breath sounds*    Breath sounds are decreased or absent when air flow is decreased or when

fluid or tissue separates the air passages from the stethoscope.

*Unilateral wheezing and the bagpipe sign*    Tumors in the main bronchus may cause a localized expiratory and/or inspiratory wheeze, or "honk," which sometimes is reproduced only when the individual lies on the affected side. When a continuous wheeze is heard at the end of expiration as air continues to whistle out past a partial obstruction, this is known as the *bagpipe sign*.

*Presence of whispered pectoriloquy, bronchophony, and egophony*    When the lungs are normal, whispered test words are faint and their syllables are not distinct when the examiner listens with a stethoscope over the lungs. When a lung is consolidated or compressed by a pleural effusion, transmission of voice sounds is altered. The sounds are louder, clearer than usual, and sometimes changed in quality. These three criteria are assessed as follows:

1. *Whispered pectoriloquy.* The patient whispers numerals (e.g., one, two, and three). Normally these sounds are muffled; in consolidation they are clearly transmitted.[38]
2. *Bronchophony.* When the patient says a number (e.g., 99), the sound normally is muffled. When the sound transmitted is a clear sound of the vocalized numerals, it is created by mucus- or fluid-filled alveoli or by cellular mass replacing alveolar tissue.[39]
3. *Egophony.* The patient says *e*, which normally results in a muffled, indistinct sound. In pleural effusion the *e* sound is heard as a nasal-sounding *a*.

Figure 8-5 presents a synopsis of the physical findings commonly seen with tumors of different anatomic sites in the lungs. The majority of physical signs discussed previously are found in late or advanced lung cancer. The *only early* physical finding that most strongly suggests lung cancer is wheezing localized to a single lobe of the lung in an elderly person with a long history of smoking.

### Screening tests for asymptomatic individuals

There are no recommended screening programs or tests for lung cancer because studies have not shown any evidence of a significant reduction in mortality from these programs. Recent research has indicated that molecular genetics may hold promise for the detection of early lung cancer. Mao et al[40] were able to follow the development of clinical lesions after sputum collection, indicating that these gene mutations may be detected with significant lead time prior to clinical diagnosis.[40] The ACS focuses on primary prevention: helping smokers to stop and keeping nonsmokers from starting.

### Smoking cessation

The greatest reduction in mortality can be achieved by cessation of smoking. Between 80% and 85% of deaths from lung cancer are directly attributable to smoking, thus making smoking the leading cause of cancer mortality in the United States.[41] Smoking in the United States is

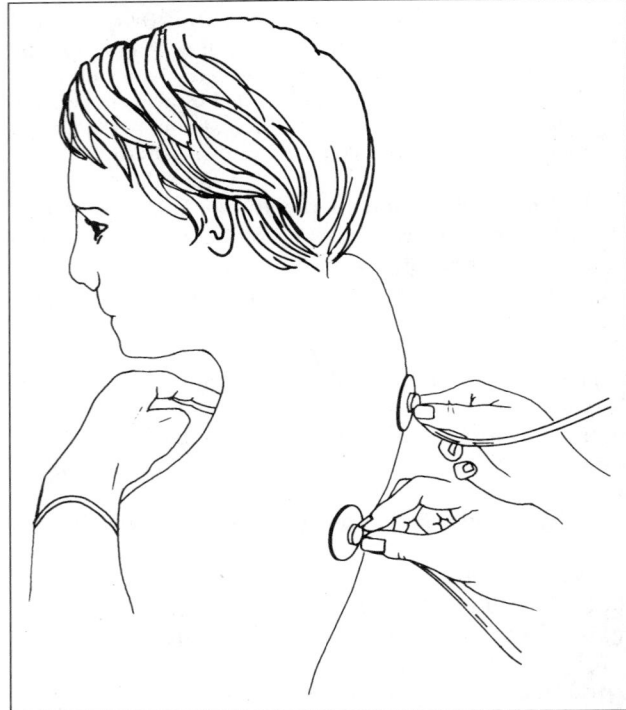

**FIGURE 8-4**    Auscultatory-percussion technique.

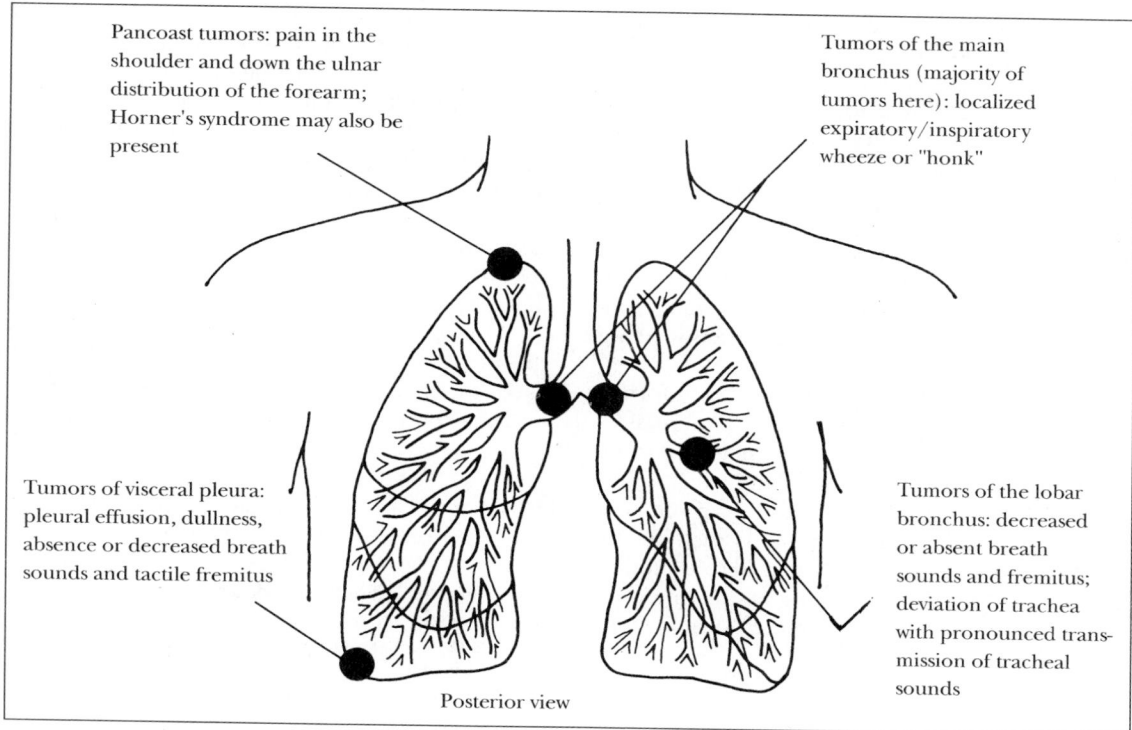

Pancoast tumors: pain in the shoulder and down the ulnar distribution of the forearm; Horner's syndrome may also be present

Tumors of the main bronchus (majority of tumors here): localized expiratory/inspiratory wheeze or "honk"

Tumors of visceral pleura: pleural effusion, dullness, absence or decreased breath sounds and tactile fremitus

Tumors of the lobar bronchus: decreased or absent breath sounds and fremitus; deviation of trachea with pronounced transmission of tracheal sounds

Posterior view

**FIGURE 8-5**   Synopsis of physical findings of lung cancer.

on the decline. Per capita cigarette consumption among adults fell from 4141 in 1974 to 3196 in 1987, and this is the lowest per capita consumption since 1944.[42] In general, smoking prevalence is decreasing across all race-gender groups, although at a slower rate for women than men.[43] However, smoking prevalence has increased among American teens.[44] The latest data collected by the National Health Interview Surveys indicate that educational level is the major demographic predictor of whether an individual will smoke cigarettes. Regardless of gender, a person who does not attend college is more than twice as likely to start smoking than the person who does. In addition, smoking cessation occurs more frequently in groups with higher levels of education than in groups with less education, and the gap is widening over time.[45]

Cigarette advertising campaigns have been directed to groups that tend to smoke (youth, women, minorities, and blue-collar workers) in order to recruit new smokers or to increase cigarette consumption among smokers.[46] Knowing the groups that tend to smoke and that are being targeted by the tobacco industry should assist health professionals in identifying and predicting patterns of cigarette use and in developing health promotion materials specifically designed for these high-risk groups.[47] Chapter 66 of this text provides a list of smoking cessation materials specifically written for blue-collar workers, minorities, and women.

Obviously, the nurse wants to monitor most aggressively those who smoke, who have had a history of heavy smoking, or who were employed in high-risk occupations. These individuals should have (1) a complete baseline respiratory assessment, (2) a thorough assessment of respiratory symptoms, and (3) physical assessment of their respiratory system at periodic intervals. Deviations from normal merit referral for chest x-ray studies and/or sputum cytological findings. In this high-risk population a cold that lingers or "smoker's cough" that is accompanied by fatigue and weight loss should not be ignored.

One fallacy commonly heard about individuals who smoke is that because they have smoked for years, "what harm is there in letting them continue?" Nothing could be further from the truth or more detrimental to their health. Continual smoking damages not only their already compromised respiratory system but their cardiovascular system as well. Research clearly documents that smoking cessation results in improved sensory, respiratory, and cardiovascular status.[48] Fielding[41] noted that a British physician study reported that ex-smokers who had not smoked for five years had a lung cancer mortality rate approximately 40% that of a current smoker. After 15 years without smoking the mortality rate of ex-smokers was only slightly greater than that of nonsmokers. No one is ever too old nor has smoked too long to *stop* smoking.

The nurse should take a nonjudgmental approach with those who refuse or are unable to stop smoking. The 1988 surgeon general's report stated that "an extensive body of research has shown that nicotine is the drug in tobacco that causes addiction. However, the processes that determine tobacco addiction are similar to those that determine addiction to drugs such as heroin and cocaine."[49] Because of the addicting qualities of nicotine, many ex-smokers are not able to give up the habit on the first attempt but must try three or more times before finally succeeding.[43] In the hope of reducing the adverse health consequences of smoking, health professionals frequently advise individuals who cannot quit to smoke fewer cigarettes, to smoke cigarettes with less than 10 mg of tar, to smoke filtered cigarettes, and to smoke only half of each cigarette. However, habitual smokers may compensate for the reduced number of cigarettes by taking in more smoke per cigarette ("oversmoking").[50]

It is the nurse's responsibility to disseminate information actively and assertively on the disease potential of smoking whenever possible. Every assistance should be afforded to those who want to stop smoking. Nurses who smoke are less likely to discuss the need to stop smoking or the various smoking cessation methods that can be employed. It is essential that nurses act as role models by not smoking and by actively working at creating nonsmoking environments in both their employment and their home settings.

Nurses have frequent opportunities to advise smokers to quit either in health care settings or in the community. The importance of counseling smokers to quit is underscored by the research of Anda et al.[51] In their study of 5875 Michigan adults who smoked, of those who had seen a physician in the previous year, only 44% reported being told to quit smoking by a physician. In general, most smokers did not perceive physicians to be even minimally involved in their efforts to quit. In fairness to physicians, there may be a tendency for smokers to hear only what they want to hear.[52] For this reason, the U.S. Preventive Services Task Force recommends that smokers be exposed to a variety of intervention techniques on multiple occasions delivered by *both* physicians and nonphysicians to improve smoking cessation rates.[53] Kottke et al[54] also found that the best result for helping smokers quit was to use a team of physicians and nonphysicians that employed multiple intervention modalities to deliver individualized advice on multiple occasions. The U.S. Agency for Health Care Policy and Research's *Smoking Cessation Clinical Practice Guidelines* provides recommendations for primary care clinicians, smoking cessation specialists, and health care administrators, insurers and purchasers on the treatment of tobacco addiction.[55] The multiple smoking cessation interventions suggested by all authorities include the following:

1. direct, face-to-face advice and suggestions on smoking cessation
2. smoking cessation self-help materials that are culturally and educationally relevant to the individual person
3. referral to community smoking cessation programs
4. drug therapy when appropriate (e.g., nicotine gum, nicotine patch)
5. scheduled reinforcement with the smoker

Table 8-1 presents the process the nurse should follow to successfully assist the smoker in quitting, and Table 8-2 lists the factors associated with successful smoking cessation.[57] When individuals are referred to smoking cessation programs, it is advised that cost effectiveness be considered in the selection. Altman et al[58] found that self-help programs not only had the lowest total cost and lowest time requirement for participants, but their quit rate percentage was also the lowest. In contrast, smoking cessation classes were expensive but had the most success in getting individuals to stop smoking.

A new development to assist smokers in quitting is the nicotine patch (e.g., Habitrol, Nicoderm, Prostep, Nicotrol, Nicolan, Nicotinell). These can be purchased over-the-counter and don't require a physician's prescrip-

**TABLE 8-1  Smoking Cessation Strategies**

1. Ask
   - Identify patient's smoking behavior
   - Review smoking history
   - Provide risk–benefit information, personalizing when possible
   - Assess health beliefs about smoking

2. Advise
   - Urge smokers to quit

3. Assess
   - Determine interest in smoking cessation
   - Determine patient's readiness to quit in terms of motivation, intention, and self-efficacy

4. Assist
   - Aid patient in quitting
   - Set the target quit-date
   - Pick a realistic calendar quit-date
   - Stop smoking "cold turkey"
   - Encourage nicotine replacement therapy as appropriate
   - Provide materials and referral sources
   - Describe preparatory techniques
     - List reasons for quitting; review previous quit attempts
     - Become aware of smoking-related situations
     - Seek social support
     - Reduce number of cigarettes and/or amount of nicotine
     - Replace cigarettes with gum or food (preferably low-fat, low-calorie)
     - Eliminate environmental cues, alcohol
     - Avoid, distract, delay
   - Discuss withdrawal symptoms
   - Review cognitive and behavioral strategies to use in high-risk situations—social, relaxation, work, and upsetting situations

5. Follow-up
   - Contact during the first week and again within first month
   - Congratulate success
   - Encourage the maintenance of successful abstinence and discuss "slips"
   - Review relapse and refer to more specialized program
   - Assess nicotine replacement therapy use and problems

Data from Fiore et al[55] and Gritz.[56]

**TABLE 8-2** Factors Associated with Successful Smoking Cessation

**Motivational Factors**

Desire to overcome minor smoking-related symptoms (coughing, wheezing, shortness of breath)
Expectation of improved future health
Sense of personal vulnerability to risk
Desire to increase self-mastery and self-esteem
Expectation of many benefits of quitting—health, freedom, social, and economic
Expectation of success
Expectation that benefits will outweigh difficulties
Support and encouragement from family (especially spouse), friends, work associates

**Effective Quitting Skills**

Quitting abruptly instead of tapering off
Using a variety of coping methods for withdrawal symptoms, such as deep breathing, positive thinking, and specific cigarette substitutes
Using a variety of methods to remain off cigarettes, such as avoiding temptations to smoke, finding alternative ways to relax and to cope with stress (such as hobbies or exercise), using substitute self-rewards to counteract sense of loss and prevent relapse
Taking a long-range, problem-solving approach

**Social Supports/Psychosocial Assets**

Personalized and medical quit-smoking advice and support
Encouragement, inspiration, and advice from ex-smokers
Good psychosocial resources (such as education and income)

**Smoking Habit Factors**

Lower smoking rate and nicotine intake/dependence
Less reliance on cigarettes for regulation of negative effect
Past success in quitting for 6 months or more
Good stress management skills

Orleans CT: Understanding and promoting smoking cessation: Overview and guidelines for physician intervention. *Annu Rev Med* 36:51–61, 1985.

tion. These patches are available in three sizes that deliver 21 mg, 14 mg, or 7 mg of nicotine over 16–24 hours. The nicotine is either directly released through the skin or through a membrane system in contact with the skin. Side effects are minimal and include: mild-to-moderate sleep disturbances; skin reactions including transient itching, burning, and erythema; poorly defined body aches; and increased cough.

Significant changes in the social and work-related environments have occurred in this country that have resulted in less tolerance of smoking and that have made smokers more receptive to the antismoking messages of health professionals. The 1987 Bureau of National Affairs survey of 623 large corporations found that 54% had adopted some type of plan to restrict employee smoking. This was a 36% increase from a similar survey the previous year.[59] In the health care field the Joint Commission on Accreditation of Healthcare Organizations, which accredits about 80% of all U.S. Hospitals, has mandated a ban on smoking in hospitals.[60] In addition, many states have passed laws that place limitations on smoking. These anti-smoking policies appear to have a dramatic effect on the nation's smoking habits. Theoretically, they will encourage people to quit smoking by increasing the social pressure against it and by restricting the time available for it.

## Gastrointestinal Cancer

Colorectal cancer incidence and mortality in the United States are second only to those of lung cancer. It is estimated that in 1996, 133,500 new colorectal cases will be diagnosed, and 54,900 people will die of this cancer. In both men and women 35 years of age and older, colorectal cancer is one of the leading causes of deaths from cancer.[25]

### History assessment

Several conditions and health practices must be questioned to obtain a realistic picture of the patient's gastrointestinal system. For example, after the age of 50 years, approximately 25% of the population has demonstrable diverticulosis, and by age 80 years the proportion is 70%.[61] Slight rectal bleeding commonly is found with this disorder. Another condition that causes symptoms that mimic gastrointestinal cancer is depression. Depression is more common in the elderly than in the young because of increasing losses and limitations that accompany the aging process.[61] Some of the cardinal manifestations of depression are anorexia, constipation, and somatic pains. In addition, weight loss in the elderly may be due to nutritional disturbances rather than a malignancy. Loss of income, depression, decreased sensation of taste, loss of teeth, and difficulty swallowing all contribute to decreased food intake. Another important part of the nursing assessment is a thorough history of drug intake. The elderly tend to use aspirin frequently for the pain of arthritis and to abuse laxatives. Considering these factors, the history and review of systems should include the following questions:

1. Do you have a history of cancer of the bowel or ulcerative colitis?
2. Have you ever been told you have polyps of the bowel? Gardner's syndrome? Have you had any polyps removed?
3. Do any of your relatives have (or have any had) bowel cancer?
4. Would you characterize your diet as consisting of more red meat than fish, veal, and poultry? Has your diet usually consisted of more starches and sweets than vegetables and fruits? Would you characterize your diet as being high in fats?
5. Do you take laxatives? If so, what kind, how often, what amount? How long have you taken laxatives?
6. Have you noticed a difference in your bowel habits?

Do you have more constipation, more diarrhea? Do these two conditions seem to alternate?

7. What is your usual bowel habit? Has this changed in the last few years? Has the shape of your bowel movements changed recently?

8. Have you ever been told you have diverticulosis? ulcers? nervous stomach?

9. Have you had gastrointestinal x-ray studies within the last two to three years? Have you had a barium enema, proctoscopy, or related procedure to examine your rectum and colon in the last two to three years? If you did, why was the test done and what were the results?

10. Do you take aspirin? How often and how much? What other medications (antacids, stool softeners, antispasmodics) are you now taking?

11. Are you familiar with at-home stool guaiac testing? Have you ever used this?

12. Do you have hemorrhoids or anal fissures?

13. Have you noticed any change in appetite? Are you experiencing nausea or vomiting?

14. Have you experienced any weight loss recently?

15. Do you have excessive gas? feelings of being bloated? abdominal pain?

16. Do you have the feeling after you have a bowel movement that you still have to go to the bathroom and expel more stool? Do you experience pain before, with, or after defecation?

The signs and symptoms of cancers of the colon and rectum often are related to the portion of intestine involved. Figure 8-6 identifies the most frequent presenting signs and symptoms of each area of the intestinal tract affected by cancer.

Physical examination

*Inspection*   The assessment of the gastrointestinal system begins with inspection. The findings that may suggest cancer of the gastrointestinal system include the following:

1. Nodular umbilicus. Abdominal carcinoma, especially gastric, may metastasize to the navel. This is called Sister Joseph's nodule.

2. Masses that distort the abdominal profile and indicate organomegaly.

3. Subcutaneous nodules under the skin that are visible with tangential lighting.

4. Distention. The abdominal profile should be inspected because neoplasms can distort the profile. The examiner may see distention of the lower half, lower third, or upper half of the abdomen.

5. Venous distention caused by blockage of the inferior vena cava, which can occur from spread of cancer. In this condition there is edema of the eyelids, a bluish face and lips, prominent neck veins, and pitting edema

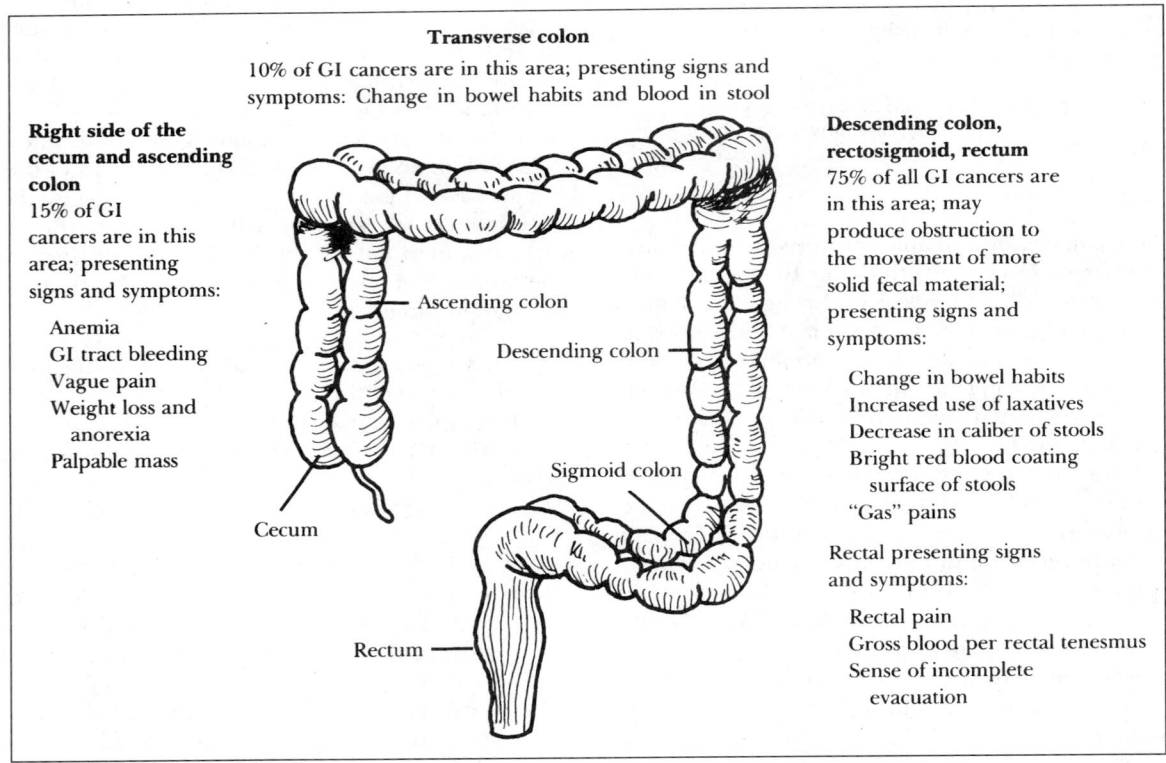

**Transverse colon**

10% of GI cancers are in this area; presenting signs and symptoms: Change in bowel habits and blood in stool

**Right side of the cecum and ascending colon**
15% of GI cancers are in this area; presenting signs and symptoms:

Anemia
GI tract bleeding
Vague pain
Weight loss and anorexia
Palpable mass

Ascending colon

Descending colon

Sigmoid colon

Cecum

Rectum

**Descending colon, rectosigmoid, rectum**
75% of all GI cancers are in this area; may produce obstruction to the movement of more solid fecal material; presenting signs and symptoms:

Change in bowel habits
Increased use of laxatives
Decrease in caliber of stools
Bright red blood coating surface of stools
"Gas" pains

Rectal presenting signs and symptoms:

Rectal pain
Gross blood per rectal tenesmus
Sense of incomplete evacuation

**FIGURE 8-6**   Presenting signs and symptoms of colorectal cancers based on location in the intestinal tract.

of the arms and large veins over the upper portions of the chest and shoulders.

6. Visible peristaltic waves, which may appear in normal individuals with thin abdomens and may be accentuated in patients with obstruction to the forward passage of gastrointestinal contents. Small-bowel obstruction gives rise to a condition resembling a "bag of worms" or a "step ladder." Numerous segments of small bowel contract and relax in an irregular manner, and the peristalsis has no recognizable pattern.

7. Bulging of the flanks may signal intraabdominal fluid.

*Auscultation*   After a thorough inspection of the abdomen is performed with the use of tangential lighting, the abdomen should be auscultated. Bowel sounds that are heard without the use of a stethoscope are called *borborygmi.* Bowel sounds heard with the stethoscope bell range from absent to frequent. Significant types of bowel sounds include the following:

- High-pitched, long, intense peristaltic rushes occur with any hypermotile state such as partial obstruction.

- High-pitched "tingling" sounds indicate a more complete mechanical intestinal obstruction.

- Extremely weak or infrequent sounds may also indicate bowel immobility.

- Absent bowel sounds, determined by listening to the bowel for at least *five minutes,* may indicate advanced intestinal obstruction.

Another sound that may signal obstruction of the small intestines is a *succussion splash.* Succussion splash is produced by a combination of air and fluid in the gut when the examiner shakes the stomach or vigorously moves the abdomen. The sound resembles very loud splashes.

Some abdominal circulatory sounds also signal cancer (Figure 8-7). A bruit heard over the liver with the bell of the stethoscope when the patient takes a deep breath may indicate a hepatoma with arteriovenous shunting. In addition, a hepatic friction rub heard with the bell of the stethoscope may also indicate a hepatoma. A bruit heard over the pancreas may indicate pancreatic carcinoma. A murmur over the left hypochondrium is one of the rare physical signs that suggests an early carcinoma of the body of the pancreas. Thus auscultation of the abdomen may indicate a bowel obstruction, a hepatoma, or pancreatic carcinoma.

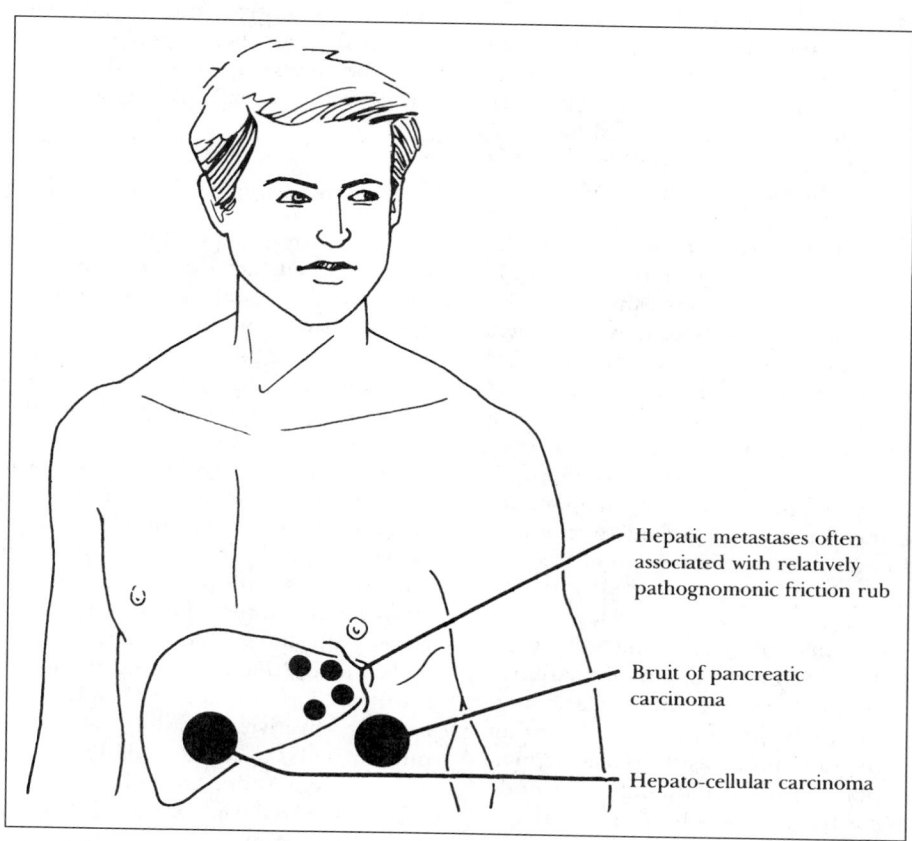

Hepatic metastases often associated with relatively pathognomonic friction rub

Bruit of pancreatic carcinoma

Hepato-cellular carcinoma

**FIGURE 8-7**   Abdominal sounds that indicate cancer.

***Palpation and percussion***   The information obtained from inspection and auscultation should alert the examiner to expected findings during palpation and percussion of the abdomen. On palpation of the abdomen the organs that are normally palpated are the abdominal aorta, the edge of the liver, the lower pole of the right kidney, the descending colon and the sigmoid, and the ascending colon. The following findings on palpation and percussion merit further attention, and may signal colorectal cancer.

*Hepatomegaly*   Total liver span is the best estimate of liver size because liver height cannot be determined by feeling only the edge. Palpation alone detects the inferior portion as it descends below the costal margin. A normal liver at the midclavicular line is 10–12 cm in span. Nodules on the liver or an irregular edge suggest malignancy.

*Splenomegaly*   Because the normal spleen is rarely palpable, a spleen that descends below the left costal margin on deep inspiration is enlarged. Cancer conditions that enlarge the spleen are leukemias and lymphomas.

*Enlargement of the colon*   Carcinoma of the colon may produce a palpable mass anywhere along the course of the colon.

*Fluid*   Several tests can be used to determine if there is free fluid in the abdomen. The presence of intraperitoneal fluid is suspected when there is abdominal distention with bulging flanks and possibly an everted umbilicus. *Shifting dullness* and *fluid wave* are two tests frequently used to detect fluid in the abdomen. The *puddle sign* has the advantage of detecting small amounts of intraabdominal fluid. After the patient has been on hands and knees for several minutes, the examiner percusses the periumbilical area to detect a line between fluid and air, as in the determination of shifting dullness. As little as several hundred milliliters of ascitic fluid can be detected by this method.[36]

*Rectal examination*   Half the cancers that occur in the rectum and colon are within reach of the examining finger. Lesions high in the rectum are sometimes felt more readily when the patient bears down as if having a bowel movement. On palpation the examiner may feel a *rectal shelf*, which, in men, is a stony hard mass above the prostate on the anterior rectal wall. In women it is felt as a stony hard mass in the cul-de-sac. The shelf indicates a carcinoma that has metastasized to the pelvic floor and therefore is a sign of advanced malignancy. Carcinoma of the rectum causes plateaulike, nodular, annular, and cauliflower masses in the rectum.[33]

• • •

Several physical findings in other parts of the body, which are not revealed in the abdominal examination, are typical in abdominal carcinoma. For instance, enlargement of a single node, usually in the left supraclavicular group, is a sign of carcinomatous metastasis from a primary lesion in the upper portion of the abdomen. This node, called *Virchow's node,* is frequently behind the clavicular head of the left supraclavicular group. The Valsalva maneuver causes the node to rise, which enables the nurse to palpate the node.

Another physical finding associated with abdominal carcinoma is *acanthosis nigricans,* a skin lesion. Acanthosis nigricans is probably the most well-known cutaneous syndrome of intestinal malignancy. It is a velvety, brownish skin eruption that strongly suggests an intestinal malignancy when it occurs in patients older than 40 years of age.[62]

Another systemic finding related to pathology of the gastrointestinal system is jaundice. Jaundice and accompanying steady pain may indicate hepatic or pancreatic lesions. Although painless obstructive jaundice is said to be a feature of carcinoma of the head of the pancreas, the majority of individuals with pancreatic cancer have some degree of anterior abdominal or back pain. By means of daylight or fluorescent light the sclerae, the undersurface of the tongue, and the frenulum of the tongue should be examined for jaundice.

Although there are many physical findings that suggest cancer of the gastrointestinal system, the findings that *most strongly* suggest cancer of the colorectal area are (1) a mass palpated in the rectum, (2) a palpable mass in the abdomen, and (3) evidence of blood in the feces. Nurses who work with the elderly or high-risk individuals in nursing homes, residential settings, acute-care institutions, and physicians' offices are encouraged to take the time to thoroughly assess an individual's gastrointestinal complaints. Often the elderly will share their complaints with the nurse rather than the physician because they hesitate to bother the doctor with "trivial" problems.

### Screening tests for asymptomatic individuals

The two most important screening tests for asymptomatic individuals are examination of the feces for occult blood and the digital rectal examination.[63] There is professional debate about the use of fecal occult blood tests as a mass screening tool. The results from the only true randomized controlled study in this country that assessed the effect of occult blood screening on colorectal cancer mortality has thus far shown a 33% decrease in the 13-year cumulative mortality from colorectal cancer.[64] This study made extensive use of rehydration of Hemoccult slides, a process that makes detection of blood more likely.[65] There are researchers who argue against the use of rehydrated slides because of the possibility of more positive test results. However, researchers in Italy who have been rehydrating Hemoccult slides since 1982 recommend this procedure and conclude that rehydrated Hemoccult slides should be introduced as the standard test for screening in order to increase sensitivity for colorectal cancer and adenomas. A randomized trial conducted in Sweden using rehydration of Hemoccult slides[66] found that the cancers detected in this randomized trial were at a less advanced stage than in the control group. However, the researchers commented that it was too early to show any effect of screening on mortality from colorectal cancer.

One problem with occult blood tests is the number of false-positive results that necessitate additional tests. It is argued that although the test itself is inexpensive, the recommended follow-up diagnostic procedure is expensive. For instance, if one million people were screened, about 100,000 of them (10%) would show positive findings and the costs of the follow-up tests would be $50 million for the detection of 2300 colorectal cancers. Table 8-3 presents the causes of false-positive and false-negative test results when Hemoccult slides are used.[67]

The American Cancer Society, the National Cancer Institute, and the American College of Surgeons recommend that asymptomatic individuals have a sigmoidoscopic (preferably flexible) examination every three to five years in conjunction with an annual fecal occult blood test beginning at age 50.[68] The American Cancer Society further advocates an annual digital rectal examination starting at age 40. In contrast, the Canadian Task Force on the Periodic Health Examination concluded that the evidence in favor of colorectal cancer screening was still insufficient to recommend it.

A small benefit from annual screening for colorectal cancer with the Hemoccult test was found in patients >40 years of age. Encouraging results were shown with sigmoidoscopy, but the evidence was subject to study design biases. Insufficient evidence exists to support screening with colonoscopy. Hemoccult testing and sigmoidoscopy were neither included nor excluded from the periodic health examination and colonoscopy was not recommended.[69]

Although the role of fecal occult blood tests in the early detection of colorectal cancer is still being evaluated, the nurse should be aware of the following specific recommendations that will increase the accuracy of the test:

1. Duplicate samples should be taken from different parts of the feces each day for three consecutive days while the patient follows a meat-free diet.[70] It is important for the nurse to encourage the patient to collect stool for three consecutive days because not all bowel cancers bleed, and occult blood is not always uniformly distributed in feces. Increasing the number of tests may therefore address these two causes of false-negative tests.[71] Presently no scientific validation exists for a high-residue diet during the three days of stool specimen collection.[71]

2. During the three days of stool collection, patients should avoid:
   a. aspirin-containing compounds (cause false-positive reaction)
   b. antibiotics (cause false-positive reaction)
   c. anti-inflammatory drugs (cause false-positive reaction)
   d. ascorbic acid (cause false-negative reaction)
   e. foods high in peroxidase—broccoli, cabbage, potatoes, cantaloupe, turnips, apricots, apples, pears, horseradish (cause false-positive reaction)
   f. oral iron compounds (cause false-positive reactions)[72]

3. The stool specimens should be read within six days of collection because delay contributes to false-negative results.

Because of the false-positive and false-negative results frequently obtained with the current tests for occult stool by means of guaiac-impregnated cards, alternate methods to detect colorectal cancer are being sought. Several researchers have published preliminary data on immunochemical tests that do not rely on blood loss to detect gastrointestinal changes caused by cancer.[73] Nakama and Kamijo conducted a mass screening for colorectal cancer using immunological fecal occult blood testing.[73] The sensitivity and specificity of the immunological fecal occult blood tests were 91% and 96% respectively. These values indicate an accuracy higher than that achieved by chemical occult testing. Dietary restrictions have been reported to decrease compliance and self-administered fecal occult blood tests have not been found to increase compliance either.[74] Those who are most likely to be helped by screening (e.g., the elderly) are less likely to cooperate. Those studies that report good compliance usually deal with a highly motivated or selected group of volunteers.

The carcinoembryonic antigen (CEA) assay is not conclusive in the diagnosing of colorectal cancer.[63] A normal

**TABLE 8-3**   Causes of False-Positive and False-Negative Tests Using the Hemoccult Method

| False-Positive Tests | False-Negative Tests |
| --- | --- |
| Meat in diet | Failure to employ high-residue diet |
| Medications; antibiotics, aspirin, anti-inflammatories, oral iron compounds | Vitamin C in diet |
| Diverticulosis | Time lag between specimen collection and specimen examination |
| Minor anorectal problems   Hemorrhoids   Fissures   Proctitis | Failure to prepare slides properly or complete all six slides |
| Peroxidases in skins of vegetables and fruits (tomatoes and cherries) | Follow-up examinations that failed to detect lesion |
| Upper gastrointestinal pathology   Gastritis from ASA   ingestion   Ulcer | Lesion not bleeding at the time of stool collection |
| Hiatus hernia | Outdated Hemoccult slides or reagent |
| Gastric malignancy | |

Sugarbaker P, Gunderson L, Wittes R: Colorectal cancer, in DeVita VT, Hellman S, Rosenberg SA (eds): *Cancer: Principles and Practice of Oncology* (ed 2). Philadelphia, Lippincott, 1986, pp. 795–884.

level does not rule out colon cancer, and elevated levels have been found in cancer of the pancreas as well as in nonmalignant diseases of the colon, lung, and liver. Because it is nonspecific, it is not considered a good screening test for colorectal cancer.

The American Cancer Society recommendations for screening asymptomatic patients for colorectal cancer are shown in Figure 8-8.

### Additional nursing interventions

Nurses have a variety of roles in colorectal cancer detection. Not only are they practitioners, they also are educators, coordinators, counselors, and researchers. One of the most important roles the nurse assumes is that of educator. Two surveys conducted by the Gallup Organization for the American Cancer Society have found that

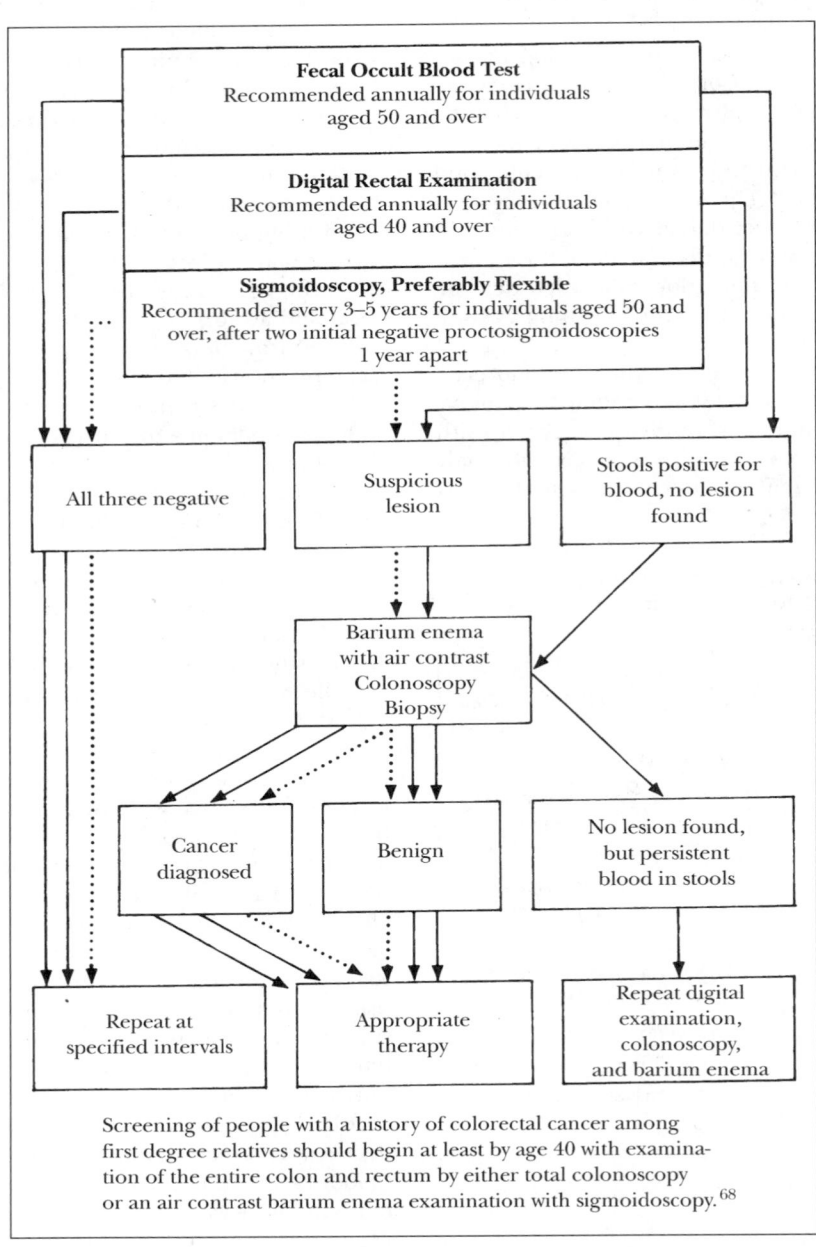

**FIGURE 8-8** Diagnostic guide for asymptomatic patients. (Leffall L: *Early Diagnosis of Colorectal Cancer.* New York, American Cancer Society [Professional Educational Publication 81-50M-No. 3311-PE], 1981. Adapted to reflect most recent ACS recommendations.)

only a small percentage of the public has taken the necessary steps to detect colorectal cancer at its earliest stages.[75] The surveys also revealed that few people were asking their physicians for the tests during regular physical examinations. There was little knowledge about this type of cancer, and attitudes toward its early detection were pessimistic. A little more than one-third of Americans in the 40-plus age group knew that colorectal cancer was one of the most common forms of cancer. More than 40% believed that surgery for colorectal cancer would result in a permanent colostomy, and more than 50% had little faith that anything could be done to cure colorectal cancer. In addition, there were general misconceptions about the recommended early detection tests. Twenty-five percent believed that if no blood is found in a stool blood test, the digital rectal and proctoscopic examinations are not needed.

As educators, nurses can play an important role in colorectal cancer detection by (1) informing the general public about colon and rectum cancer, as well as by making a special effort to inform the elderly and other high-risk groups, and (2) encouraging the participation of the general public and high-risk groups in early detection of the disease through the use of a stool guaiac slide test, digital rectal examination, and, after 50 years of age, proctosigmoidoscopic examination. The most effective public education approach to general screening for colorectal cancer is (1) to emphasize the effectiveness of the stool guaiac test, (2) to stress that it is painless and convenient (it can be administered in the privacy of one's home), and (3) to indicate the value of early detection of colorectal cancer (e.g., President Reagan's successful bout with a malignant tumor of the colon).[76]

Nurses who work in community organizations, clinics, nursing homes, retirement centers, geriatric day care centers, and hospitals are in ideal settings to provide education and to plan and participate in colorectal screening programs. These screening programs could be conducted by community organizations such as the American Cancer Society, local service groups, and community religious groups, with the nurse coordinating the efforts.

Another role for the nurse as educator is to promote the following dietary recommendations of the American Cancer Society and the National Cancer Institutes to lower overall cancer risk including colorectal cancer:

1. Avoid obesity.
2. Decrease total fat intake. It is recommended that fat be only 30% of total calories. The year 2000 cancer control objective is to reduce average consumption of fat from 40% to 25% or less of total calories.[77] There are many simple methods to reduce dietary fat in the diet: for example, (1) use low-fat cottage cheese instead of sour cream for dips, (2) use baked potatoes instead of French fries, (3) use nonstick pans or a cooking spray for grilling sandwiches instead of grilling them in oil, and (4) select bagels or whole wheat bread for breakfast instead of doughnuts, rolls, or croissants.
3. Consume more high-fiber foods, such as whole grain cereals, fruits, and vegetables. The year 2000 cancer control objective is to increase the average consumption of fiber from 8–12 g/day to 20–30 g/day.
4. Include foods rich in vitamins A and C in the daily diet. Foods rich in carotene, a form in vitamin A, are carrots, tomatoes, spinach, apricots, peaches, cantaloupes. In general, dark green and deep yellow vegetables are rich in vitamin A.
5. Be moderate in the consumption of alcoholic beverages.
6. Be moderate in the consumption of salt-cured, smoked, and nitrite-cured foods.
7. Include cruciferous vegetables in the diet, such as cabbage, broccoli, brussels sprouts, kohlrabi, and cauliflower.[78–80]

Research supports the assumption that Americans will change their diet in an effort to be healthier. A survey in Illinois, conducted in 1982 and in 1986, found that 42% of the 46,830 subjects reported a major change in their diet since the first survey. Subjects reported eating less meat and pork and more fish and chicken, and there was a shift toward whole grains from refined grains and an increase in the number of times per week that subjects ate cruciferous vegetables.[81]

In the role of researcher, it is extremely important that a nurse be knowledgeable about emerging information on the relationship between diet and colorectal cancer. Future research may establish definitive relationships, as well as additional relationships not presently known. Nurses also should be able to evaluate research findings. Those reports that are based on sound, ethical research principles may be judged appropriate for inclusion in patient education. Because of debate about the use of stool guaiac tests in screening programs in terms of lowering mortality from colorectal cancer, nurses need to remain alert to new research that either supports or refutes the use of this early detection test. Nurses also can plan or participate in the wide range of research projects related to colorectal cancer such as health behaviors, dietary habits, motives that facilitate early detection and dietary changes, and effective educational approaches for changing dietary patterns. Results certainly would benefit existing nursing practice as it relates to the prevention and early detection of colorectal cancer.

As practitioners, nurses are urged to use their physical assessment skills when they deal with individuals who have gastrointestinal complaints. Geriatric patients often share their symptoms first with a sympathetic nurse. Thus the nurse is in the ideal position to detect colorectal cancer in its *initial stages*. Physical assessment of the abdomen may reveal subtle clues of a pathological condition that merits referral, one that otherwise might be overlooked by an elderly patient. Hospital-based nurses are cautioned not to assume that elderly patients must have had a thorough physical examination because they are in the hospital. If the complaints are not related to the gastrointestinal system, that system may not have been thoroughly assessed.

## Prostate Cancer

Prostate cancer is currently the second most common cancer in American men. In men older than 75 years of age, it is estimated that the prevalence of prostate cancer is 500/100,000. The American Cancer Society estimates that in 1996 there will be 317,100 new cases of prostate cancer and 41,400 deaths caused by this cancer.[25] A large percentage of men have advanced disease at the time of diagnosis; approximately 35% have metastases to the bones or lymph nodes, and another 40% have extracapsular invasion.[82] African-American men have the highest incidence of prostate cancer in the world. Between 1937 and 1985 the incidence of prostate cancer increased 53.5% among white men and more than 100% in black men.[83] Prostate cancer increases in incidence with age more rapidly than any other cancer.

### History assessment

There are *no* real symptoms of early, probably curable, disease. Most symptoms are related to late complications of stage III or IV prostate cancer. Because many of the initial symptoms may be related to carcinomatous obstruction of the prostatic urethra, the inquiries made during the history should be about nonspecific urinary symptoms. The following questions are recommended:

1. Do you have to wait for your stream to begin?
2. Does your stream stop while you still have the urge to void?
3. Do you have to strain to urinate?
4. Does your stream seem very weak to you?
5. Do you have the urge to urinate but find you can't?
6. Have you noticed blood in your urine? Has your urine changed in color or smell at all?
7. Does the blood seem to come at the beginning or end of your stream?
8. Do you dribble after urinating?
9. Do you find you have to urinate more than you used to?
10. Do you have pain on urination?
11. Do you ever wet your pants?
12. How often do you urinate during the day? Do you get up at night to urinate? How often?
13. When was your last rectal examination? Why was this done? What was found?

Symptoms that suggest prostatic cancer are urinary difficulty manifested by a decrease in urinary stream and a frequency and urgency to urinate, often associated with pain. These symptoms also are found with prostatic enlargement (benign prostatic hypertrophy) that is very common in older men. The most frequent initial symptoms of prostate cancer are frequency of urination, difficult or painful urination, pain, complete urinary retention, and hematuria.

### Physical examination

An early diagnosis of prostate cancer can be done only by rectal palpation of the prostate (Figure 8-9). It is recommended that the examiner flex the distal finger joint 2–3 mm into the gland substance rather than keep the finger straight (Figure 8-10). Having the patient perform the Valsalva maneuver during the rectal examination will bring the prostate gland closer to the examining finger. Early prostatic carcinoma is a nodule *within,* not *on,* the gland. Simply rubbing the gland is not effective for early detection of prostate cancer.[84]

The normal prostate on palpation is usually a rounded structure about 4 cm in diameter, feels firm rather than boggy, soft, or rock hard, and usually is not tender. Some examiners describe the consistency of the normal prostate as that of a pencil eraser. Cancer of the prostate typically appears as a stony-hard nodule, whereas benign prostatic hypertrophy usually results in a diffuse enlargement of the prostate without masses.

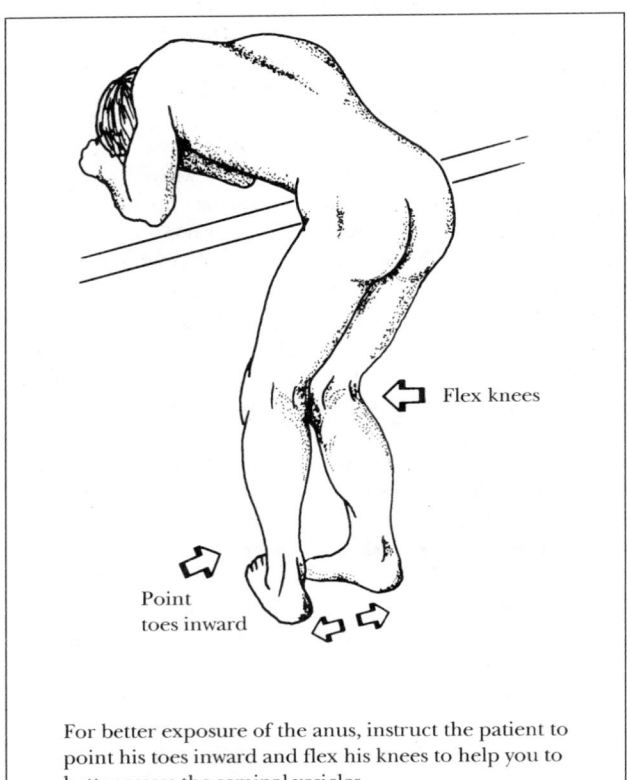

Flex knees

Point toes inward

For better exposure of the anus, instruct the patient to point his toes inward and flex his knees to help you to better assess the seminal vesicles.

**FIGURE 8-9** Recommended position for digital rectal examination. (Adapted from Guinan P, Sharifi R, Bush I: Prostate cancer: Tips toward earlier detection. *Your Patient & Cancer* 4:37–42, 1984.)

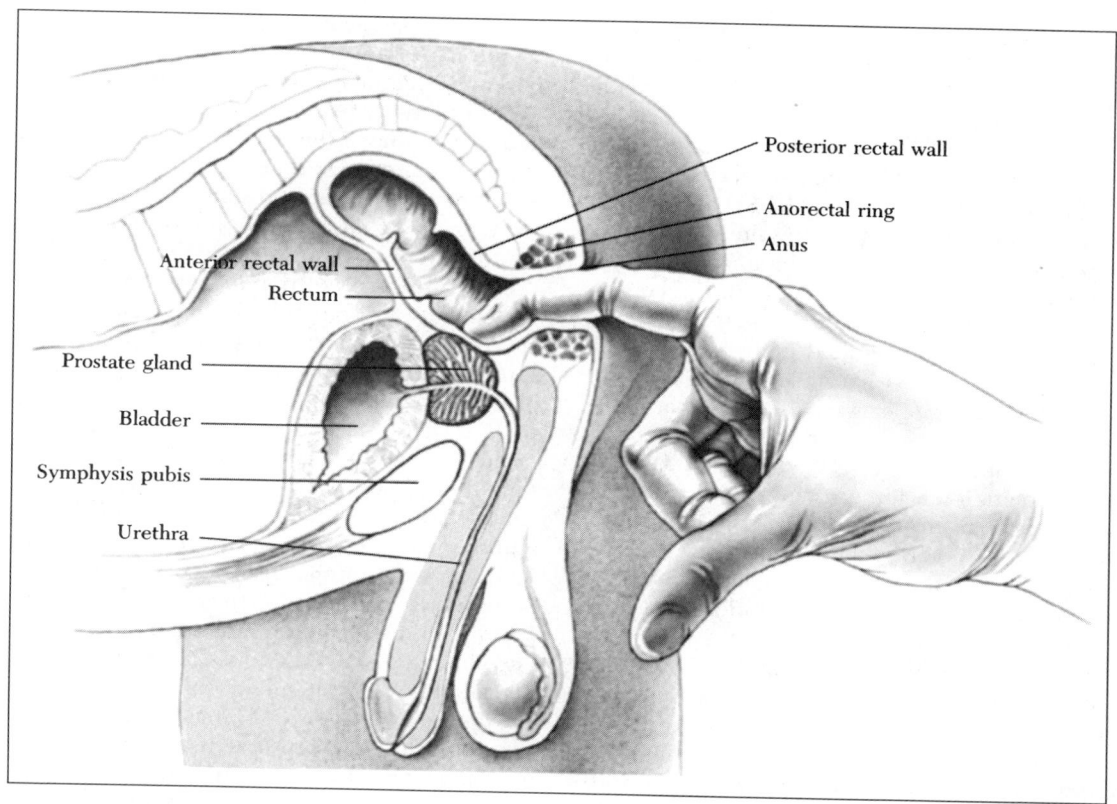

**FIGURE 8-10** Technique for palpation of the prostate gland. (Grimes J, Burns E (eds): *Health Assessment in Nursing Practice* (ed 2). Boston, Jones and Bartlett, 1987.)

It is common to find in older men a diffusely enlarged prostate gland without masses (benign prostatic hypertrophy). Carcinoma of the prostate is manifested by a palpable hard nodule near the posterior surface of the prostate. As the carcinoma grows, the entire gland may become stony hard, or there may be several hard nodules.[36]

### Screening tests for asymptomatic individuals

There is national and international debate over the issue of screening asymptomatic men for prostate cancer.[85–87] The debate involves multiple factors including the low percentage of localized cancers diagnosed by conventional methods, lack of evidence that early treatment reduces the probability of dying of prostate cancer, and the development of serum prostate-specific antigen (PSA) assay, which improves the early detection of prostate cancer. Because of these factors, the Canadian Task Force on the Periodic Health Examination concluded that there is insufficient evidence to promote screening for prostate cancer among asymptomatic men.[87] The U.S. Preventive Services Task Force also does not recommend screening for prostate cancer among asymptomatic men.[86] In contrast, the American Cancer Society and the American Urological Association recommend that men older than 50 years be tested annually using digital rectal examination and PSA. The major argument against screening for prostate cancer revolves around the absence of any randomized clinical trials documenting that screening reduces mortality or increases life expectancy. Two such studies, the Prostate Cancer Intervention Versus Observation Trial (PIVOT) and the National Cancer Institute Prostate, Lung, Colon, Ovarian Cancer (PLCO) screening project, have been launched in the United States and should answer many questions and doubts about screening for prostate cancer.[88] Unfortunately, it will take about 10 to 15 years before these trials are completed. Until mortality and morbidity benefits are known, it is recommended that screening be limited to men with life expectancies greater than 10 years.

While morbidity and mortality issues affect the practicality of screening for prostate cancer, cost considerations are also a significant barrier to the use of PSA and transrectal ultrasound in screening for this cancer. Handley and Stuart[89] investigated the routine use of PSA as a screening test in a managed care HMO organization. They concluded that use of PSA to screen for prostate cancer did not meet the criteria for an effective screening program and if PSA screening had continued, there would have been $4,800,000 in increased costs (400,000 patients). While there has been enthusiasm for the use of PSA screening and aggressive treatment of localized disease, there is no evidence that PSA can distinguish between indolent and aggressive cancer, that aggressive treatment of localized cancer decreases disease-specific mortality, or that PSA screening decreases disease-specific mortality for a population.

Krahn et al[90] used a cost-utility analysis to compare three screening strategies (PSA, digital rectal examination (DRE), transrectal ultrasound (TRUS)) with a strategy of not screening. Transrectal ultrasound consists of a probe that is inserted into the rectum and ultrasound images of the prostate are recorded on film. It is considered by most men to be less uncomfortable than a digital examination. Two questions guided their research: (1) Given the available evidence, what is the net clinical benefit of screening for prostate cancer, and (2) What is the economic burden of screening for this cancer? Their analysis did not support using PSA, TRUS, or DRE to screen asymptomatic men for prostate cancer. Furthermore, they do not advocate selecting high-prevalence populations since to do so would not improve the benefit of screening. The recommendation to not screen for prostate cancer centered on cost considerations and poor health outcomes of treatment.

A *tumor marker* is a biochemical indicator for the presence of a tumor. In clinical use the term refers to a molecule that can be detected in plasma or other body fluids.[91] PSA is a tumor marker that the Food and Drug Administration in 1994 approved for use with digital rectal examination for early detection of prostate cancer. As discussed earlier, the use of this tumor marker has resulted in unnecessary biopsies (low specificity) due to the test's lack of discrimination between prostate cancer and benign conditions that elevate PSA. However, two recent developments have dramatically improved the specificity of the test. In a recent refinement of the test for serum PSA values, the relative percentage of free PSA and PSA that binds to serum proteins (bound PSA) is determined. Men with a higher ratio of bound to free PSA are more likely to have prostate cancer seen on examination of biopsy specimens regardless of total serum PSA level.[91] The other recent refinement is the development of age-specific reference ranges. The ultimate value of this approach is that it decreases the number of biopsies in older patients with PSA values greater than 4 ng/ml and that it may increase the rate of cancer detection in younger men with PSA values less than 4 ng/ml.[91] It is suggested that normal ranges of PSA for men aged 50–59 is 0.0–3.5, 60–69 years of age is 0.0–4.5, and men aged 70–79 is 0.0–6.5 ng/ml. These two recent refinements of PSA address the recommendation of the American Cancer Society-National Prostate Cancer Detection Project that "more specific PSA assay needs to be highly encouraged" to lower net detection costs.[92]

What has added further to the debate over the screening of prostate cancer is the Gann study of U.S. male physicians who participated in the Physicians' Health Study, which started in 1982.[93] Before the physicians were randomized in the double-blind trial, they sent blood samples (n = 14,916). Gann et al examined and con-ducted PSA analysis on a smaller sample of the blood samples. The researchers found a single PSA level would have detected nearly 80% of all aggressive cancers diagnosed within five years and about 5% of aggressive cancers as much as nine or ten years later. Specificity of the single PSA measurement was also high—only 96 of 1098 men who remained free of a prostate cancer diagnosis through ten years had a false-positive test result. The final recommendation of this study echoed that of the ACS-National Prostate Cancer Detection Project. These results support the conclusion that PSA has the highest validity of any circulating cancer screening marker discovered thus far. Intensive efforts to identify cost-effective screening strategies incorporating PSA testing is warranted.

One of the most important roles the nurse can assume in the detection of early prostate cancer is that of educator. All men older than 40 years of age, especially African-American men, should be informed of the importance and rationale for yearly or biannual rectal examinations. Men with strong family histories of prostate cancer should be urged to *request and expect* rectal examinations and a PSA blood test at their annual physical. Men need to be encouraged to discuss the risk-benefits of early detection of prostate cancer with their primary health care provider. In some managed care settings, the man may be asked to pay for the PSA blood test if the health care plan does not follow the ACS recommendations.

In some communities it may be necessary for the nurse to conduct the physical examination that includes the rectal examination for prostate as well as colorectal cancer. Female nurses who conduct physical examinations but omit the rectal assessment because of their embarrassment or the patient's discomfort must request a male physician or nurse practitioner to complete this portion of the examination rather than omitting it. In other settings it may be possible to develop a once-a-year volunteer transportation program that will enable infirm or geographically isolated elderly men to have the recommended yearly examination. The development of a prostate screening program for each isolated, poor, or infirm elderly man is a problem all nurses should attempt to solve. At the very least the nurse should question all hospitalized elderly men about their last rectal examination and contact the physician about those men who have not had one within the last year (or who have "deferred" written on their chart next to "rectal examination").

## Breast Cancer

Breast cancer is the most common cancer in women in the western world.[94] It is the leading cause of cancer deaths in American women aged 40 to 55 and the second cause of cancer deaths in women older than 55 years of age.[25] It was estimated that in 1996, 185,700 women would be diagnosed with invasive breast cancer and 44,560 would die of the disease.[25] The probability that breast cancer will develop in a woman's lifetime is 12.6% or one in eight.[95]

### History assessment

Questions that may be asked during the history include the following:

1. Do you practice breast self-examination (BSE)?
   a. *"Yes" response:* How often do you do BSE? Where did you learn to do this? Do you feel comfortable doing BSE, or would you like me to go over it with you?
   b. *"No" response:* Have you ever been shown BSE? Would you be interested in learning BSE? Some women don't examine their breasts because they feel unsure, embarrassed, or frightened about doing it. Do you feel this way about BSE?
2. Have you ever been advised to have a mammogram? If you have had a mammogram, what were the results?
3. Do you experience sore breasts?
4. Have you ever been told you had "lumpy" or "cystic breasts"?
5. Have you noticed any color or temperature change on your breasts? Do you have trouble with scaly, itching nipples?
6. Have you ever had breast infections?
7. Have you ever had breast surgery or cosmetic surgery on your breasts? Tell me about the surgery that was done.
8. Do you have any sores or open wounds on your breasts?
9. Have you noticed any "dimpling" of your breasts?
10. Have you noticed any change in your nipples or discharge?
11. Have you ever been told that you had cancer of the breast?
12. Do you have or have you discovered any breast lumps?
13. Is there anyone in your family—grandparents, siblings, cousins, parents, aunts, and uncles—who have or had cancer? Breast cancer? Can you remember how old your _____ was when she first was diagnosed as having breast cancer?
14. At what age (or grade in school) did you start menstruating? At what age did you stop menstruating?

The *most common* presenting complaint of women with breast cancer is a painless lump or mass in the breast. It is estimated that 90% of all palpable breast tumors are discovered by women themselves either accidentally or through planned self-examination.[96]

### Physical examination

***Inspection***    The physical examination begins with inspection of the breast with the woman sitting relaxed with arms at side, then sitting with arms at side pressed against body, hands on waist pressed against body, and then sitting with arms overhead (Figure 8-11).[97] Visible signs of cancer of the breast include the following:

1. *Dimpling of the breast* results from a shortening of Cooper's ligaments as the tumor spreads in the breast.
2. *Unilateral flattening of the nipple* is caused by fibrosis and contraction of this fibrotic tissue, thus producing retraction signs, including flattening or deviation of the nipple.[38]
3. *Abnormal contours or flattening* becomes apparent as the woman changes positions. It is important to compare one breast with the other. An excellent position for observing this is when the woman leans forward.
4. *Peau d'orange,* orange peel skin, is caused by interference with the lymphatic drainage of the skin (Figure 8-12).
5. *Increased venous prominence* usually is unilateral. Carci-

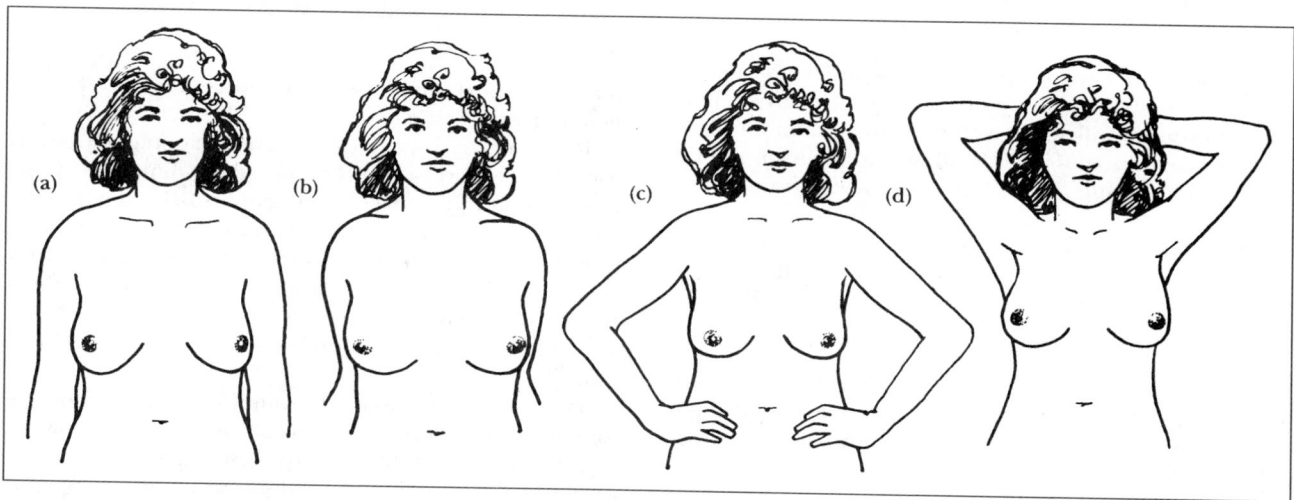

**FIGURE 8-11**    Positions for inspection of the breast. (a) Arms at side with woman relaxed; (b) arms at side pressed against body; (c) hands on waist pressed against body; (d) arms over head. (Adapted from Olsen S: *Examinations for Detecting Breast Cancer.* Cancer Prevention Program, Wisconsin Clinical Cancer Center, 1300 University Ave.-7C, Medical Science Center, Madison, WI 53706.)

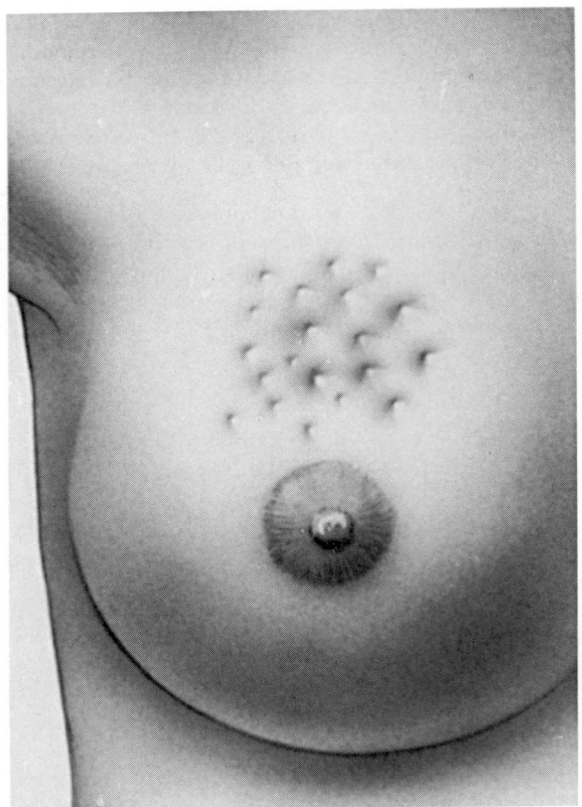

**FIGURE 8-12** Peau d'orange. Note the rough, pitted appearance. (Grimes J, Burns E (eds): *Health Assessment in Nursing Practice* (ed 2). Boston, Jones and Bartlett, 1987.)

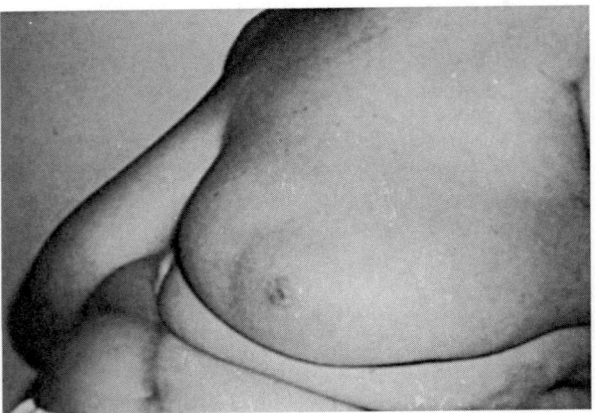

**FIGURE 8-13** Woman sitting. Note that breasts appear normal. (Rosemond G, Maier W: *Breast Cancer.* New York, Famous Teachings in Modern Medicine, Medcom, 1974.)

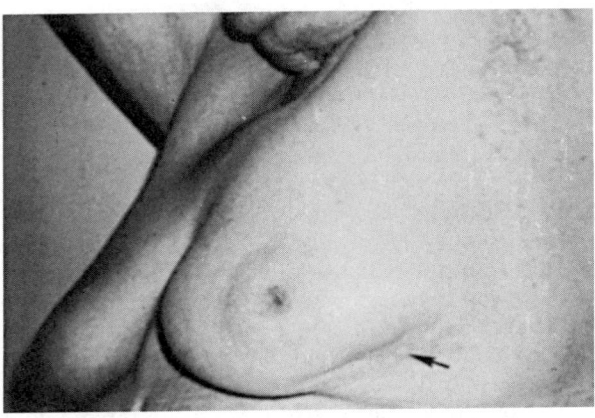

**FIGURE 8-14** Woman raising her hands during breast inspection. Note dimpling, which becomes evident with this maneuver. (Rosemond G, Maier W: *Breast Cancer.* New York, Famous Teachings in Modern Medicine, Medcom, 1974.)

nomas demand an increased blood flow; thus the dilated venous channels will be obvious on inspection.

6. *Scaling or eczematoid lesions* of the nipple indicate Paget's disease, a slow-growing intraductal carcinoma.

It is essential that good lighting (e.g., use of gooseneck lamp) be used for examination of the woman so that subtle contours will be detected by the examiner. The initial inspection *must* include all positions shown in Figure 8-11 and having the woman lean forward to observe abnormal contours; omitting a position may cause the nurse to miss important pathological findings. The photographs in Figures 8-13 and 8-14 show the differences when the woman has her hands at her sides and when she raises her arms.

*Palpation* After inspection, the entire breast should be lightly palpated for thickening. This is accomplished by using the pads of your fingers. Palpation for thickening is done very lightly and slowly toward the nipple enabling the nurse to detect subtle differences in consistency in the breasts. It should be viewed as a "scouting expedition" before palpation for masses is begun. If the woman complains of a lump, she should find it for the examiner. It is best to first palpate the normal breast. Cancer occurs

as a hard, poorly circumscribed nodule, fixed to the skin or underlying tissue.

If cancer is suspected, the breast should be gently moved or compressed and observed for dimpling. A malignant tumor that may be attached to the deep fascia will limit the mobility of the breast on the chest wall. The examiner checks for such a lump by having the patient place her hands on her hip; then the examiner moves the breast medially and laterally with the muscles relaxed and then with the muscles under tension by forced adduction.

The breasts need to be thoroughly palpated while the woman is supine with her arms above her head. Powder on the breasts may be useful to establish a frictionless surface. Palpation should be done with the flat part of the tips of three fingers. Using a spiral motion, rotate the fingers in small circles. It is recommended that the nurse start at the areolar margin and examine the breast by palpation in ever-widening concentric circles. Any mass that is felt should be charted as to its location, size, shape, consistency, discreteness, mobility, tenderness, erythema, and dimpling over the mass. Location of a nodule should be charted in terms of the quadrant, that is, right upper, left outer, and so forth. Special attention should be paid to the breast tissue along the inframammary crease. In its early stage cancer in this area may be hidden under the overlying breast tissue, and the normal induration of the inframammary crease can be confusing.[98] A device called a "sensorpad" may be used to conduct physical palpation of the breasts. The sensorpad consists of two thin round sheets of plastic that have liquid silicone sealed between them, allowing the two sheets of plastic to slide easily over each other. The sensorpad increases the ability to detect breast lesions because it reduces friction between the woman's fingers and her breast during BSE. The device, made by Inventive Products, Inc. (Decatur, IL), has received FDA clearance for marketing by prescription only.

Heymann[99] recommends that physical examination of a woman's breasts include right and left semilateral decubitus positions (Figure 8-15). The rationale for this is as follows: lesions deep within the medial aspects, upper outer quadrants, or axillary tail, especially in large breasts, may be hidden within dense parenchyma or a thick layer of fat or may sink between ribs onto intercostal muscles when they are examined in the usual erect and supine positions (Figure 8-15a). By means of the right and left semilateral decubitus positions with both of the patient's arms elevated (Figure 8-15b), both breasts will fall dependently, thereby thinning the lateral aspects, upper outer quadrant, and axillary tail of the upper portion of the breasts and the medial aspect of the lower portion of the breast[99] (Figure 8-15c).

Next, the examiner needs to check for nipple discharge. Because the ducts are like spokes of a wheel, a discharge from the ten o'clock position indicates trouble in the upper inner quadrant, and so forth. The nipple should be gently compressed in *all* directions for the presence of discharge. Smears should be taken for cytological examination of any suspicious discharge.

Because carcinoma of the breast may metastasize to regional lymph nodes, a careful palpation of the axillae and the supraclavicular regions is necessary. Most clinicians believe that the axilla is best palpated with the patient sitting erect and at a higher level than the examiner. Hard, fixed nodes palpated in the axillae or the supraclavicular region raise the suspicion of cancer. Normally, lymph nodes are felt as soft, movable structures.

When the clinician examines the breasts of an older woman, it should be kept in mind that the physiological changes that normally occur with aging may simulate cancer of the breast. As a woman ages, there is atrophy of glandular elements that accentuates anatomic landmarks and reduces the amount of palpable tissue. Shrinkage and fibrotic changes of the breast may cause retraction of the nipple, and the terminal ducts are more visible. Both these changes may cause the examiner to suspect cancer. Because of the high incidence of breast cancer in elderly women, it is best to refer all suspicious findings rather than assume they are due to aging.

In conclusion, the physical signs that most *strongly* suggest cancer of the breast are dimpling, peau d'orange, abnormal contours of the breast, flattening of the nipple, palpable hard, poorly circumscribed nodules that are fixed to the skin or underlying tissue, and palpable hard, fixed nodes in the axillae or supraclavicular region.

## Screening tests for asymptomatic individuals

Three methods used in screening for breast cancer are physical examination of the breast by the health professional, teaching the woman BSE, and mammography.

The American Cancer Society's revised recommendations for screening for breast cancer are as follows:

1. All women from age 20 years should perform BSE monthly.
2. Women 20–40 years of age should have a breast physical examination every three years, and women older than 40 years should have a breast physical examination every year.

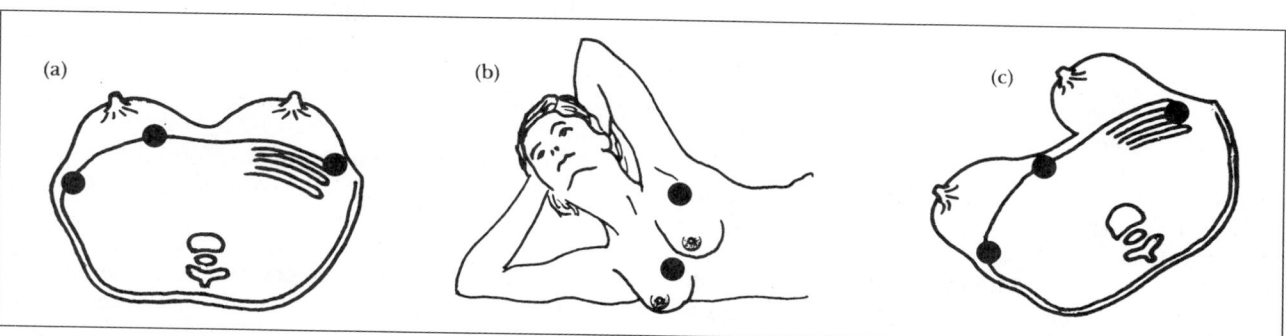

**FIGURE 8-15** Semilateral decubitus breast examination. (a) Small masses obscured by breast parenchyma or ribs when breast is examined in upright or supine position; (b) semilateral decubitus position; (c) thinning of parenchyma with clarification of obscured masses when patient is in semilateral decubitus position. (Adapted from Heymann A: Semilateral decubitus breast examination. *JAMA* 243:1713, 1980.)

**3.** Screening mammography should begin by age 40; women 40–49 years of age should have a mammogram every one to two years; and women older than 50 years of age should have a mammogram every year.[100,101]

The National Cancer Institute's cancer control objective for the year 2000 is to increase from 45% to 80% the percentage of women from ages 50–70 years who have an annual breast examination and mammogram.[102] A study conducted by the Health Insurance Plan of New York (HIP) demonstrated that the mortality rate of carcinoma of the breast can be reduced by a combination of physical examination and mammography.[103]

The Breast Cancer Detection Demonstration Project (BCDDP) showed that mammography alone was responsible for the detection of 41.6% of 3557 cancers diagnosed in 280,000 women. In women 40–49 years of age, mammography alone detected 35.4% of 762 cancers. These percentages are better than the mass screening study of 160,000 women developed by HIP a decade earlier, which showed that mammography alone detected 33.3% of all cancers and 19.4% of the cancers in women 40–49 years of age. At ten years, mortality is reduced 30% in women older than 50 years of age who are screened for breast cancer by mammography and physical examination. A study in Sweden duplicates the 30% mortality reduction found in the HIP study.[104] The BCDDP study also showed results consistent with the reduction in mortality from breast cancer found in the HIP and the Swedish study.[102] In all the studies, there is unequivocal benefit for those older than 50 years of age. However, the benefits for those 40–50 years of age have been widely debated in the literature.[103] In the HIP study women in the 40–49 age group exhibited only a 5% decrease in mortality.

A new analysis of the HIP data has indicated significant reductions in breast cancer mortality for women younger than 50 years of age which may help settle the under-50 screening debate.[105] The investigators attribute the new finding to longer follow-up and more efficient statistical methods. At the same time, recent analysis of the BCDDP data supports the new HIP findings that mammographic screening lowers mortality for the 40–49 age group. The National Cancer Institute, the American Cancer Society, and the American College of Radiology now recommend that women between 40 and 49 years of age have a mammogram every one to two years.[101,105]

***Breast self-examination***   The importance of BSE is based on the fact that approximately 95% of breast cancers are self-discovered either accidentally or through planned examination. Because approximately 10% of cancers termed *interim cancers* will become apparent within a year of an examination with negative results, reliance has been placed on BSE to find these lesions. There has been considerable debate about the value of BSE in reducing mortality and increasing survival rates.[106–109] The problem is that to date there have been no prospective randomized studies testing the benefits of BSE. The World Health Organization is sponsoring a prospective trial of BSE in Russia, and there is also a British randomized trial of breast cancer screening under way, but any data from these trials are several years away.[107] Because BSE has not been studied in a prospective, controlled trial with mortality as an outcome, the U.S. Preventive Services Task Force does not make a recommendation about the inclusion or exclusion of teaching BSE during the periodic health examination.[108] In addition, the World Health Organization does not recommend BSE screening programs as public health policy, although there is insufficient evidence to change them where they already exist.[108]

Although there probably is not sufficient evidence to justify BSE as a large-scale, community-based intervention, many authorities believe it should be encouraged as part of a woman's regular medical care.[102,110] A study by Huguley et al[111] of 2093 women with breast cancer found that self-examiners tended to seek medical care more rapidly and to have earlier stages of disease at diagnosis than nonself-examiners. Five years after diagnosis the cumulative observed survival rates in breast cancer were 76.7% among self-examiners and 60.9% among nonexaminers ($p < 0.0001$). The researchers acknowledge that the observed survival advantage may be due to characteristics of the self-examiners other than BSE per se; however, they encourage BSE as an adjunctive technique for the early detection of breast cancer.[111]

In any discussion of BSE it must be remembered that the majority of American women do not practice monthly BSE. Although nearly all women (90%–99%) are aware of this early detection practice, only 15%–40% perform BSE monthly.[109] Bennett et al[112] interviewed 616 women and found that women who were more likely to practice BSE on a frequent basis were living with their sexual partner, had a maternal history of breast disease, had been shown how to perform BSE, and were confident in their examination technique. They found no association between monthly BSE practice and formal education. Studies consistently have shown that lack of knowledge and low confidence are related to low rates of practice or no practice at all. In a review article on BSE, Kegeles[113] noted that knowledge of how it should be done and confidence in one's ability were the characteristics that consistently differentiated frequent from less frequent practitioners of BSE. Table 8-4 provides several educational approaches to help women detect breast cancer early.

Many researchers, including those of the Gallup poll, found that personal instruction results in more frequent BSE than do films, pamphlets, or lectures. It also has been shown that individual contact is successful in bringing both low users of health services and women at high risk for cancer into cancer screening programs.[113] Self-instruction includes teaching a woman to do BSE by *using her own hand on her breast under the direct guidance of a professional.* Because women can be taught to detect lesions of 1 cm or less in their own breasts, those who

**TABLE 8-4** Educational Efforts to Help Women Detect Breast Cancer Early

1. Increase competence of women in doing BSE
   a. Cognitive component—Educate women about importance of becoming familiar with their breasts in order to identify changes if they occur.
   b. Tactile-skill competence—Women are shown BSE and then *return* the demonstration. Women should be seen 6 months later to again demonstrate their technique and findings.
2. Increase frequency and retain persistence of BSE
   a. Habit component of BSE—Provide calendar or other stimulus memory aid noting date on which BSE should be performed.
   b. Memory component of BSE—Provide woman with a record form to be filled out each month; form should enable woman to chart findings.
   c. Reinforcement component of BSE—Offer praise whenever possible either verbally or through tangible rewards (i.e., buttons, stickers).
3. Reduce delay in reporting findings and increase access to physicians
   a. Share the fact that BSE is not enough if something different is discovered. Need to have suspicious findings followed up by mammography and biopsy if necessary.
   b. Educate women about the favorable outcome of breast cancer that is found at stage I and the substantial risk in delay.
   c. Encourage woman to have physician who will welcome her if she finds differences in any monthly findings. Woman should change physicians if her present physician is not supportive of her early detection efforts.

Kegeles S: Education for breast self-examination: Why, who, what, and how? *Prev Med* 14:702–720, 1985.

practice regular BSE will detect tumors within a size range that will maximize chances for survival and minimize chances for axillary node involvement.[114] When teaching BSE, the nurse should also review the American Cancer Society guidelines, stressing the importance of a yearly physical examination by a health professional and mammographic examination at intervals determined by the woman's age.

Because a high percentage of cancerous lesions are potentially palpable, it is important for nurses to include one-on-one instruction in BSE techniques whenever possible. Research documents the effectiveness of registered nurses teaching BSE to women in their place of employment.[96,115,116] In the BSE program reported by Styrd,[117] more than 60% of the eligible female employees participated in the program, and one year later 80% reported performing BSE some time during the three months before being surveyed. In addition, the proportion of employees who indicated they had performed BSE on a monthly basis increased significantly after the program ($p < 0.001$).

Primary nursing, as well as public health and occupational health nursing, afford the nurse excellent opportunities for BSE education. To date, there is some empirical evidence that supports nurses' ability to promote the practice of BSE in the acute care setting. Shamian and Edgar[118] studied the knowledge and the frequency pattern of 223 women taught BSE by nurse clinicians. They concluded that nurses influence positively the factual and proficiency knowledge base and the frequency of BSE practice. To reinforce personal instruction in BSE there could be posters, multimedia events such as slide-tape and films, and educational panels portraying the techniques of BSE. These methods, however, should reinforce, *not* replace, personal instruction.

## Testicular Cancer

Although testicular cancer is relatively rare (1% of all cancers), it is the most common solid tumor in young men between 20 and 34 years of age.[119] A lesser peak occurs in early childhood. Testicular cancer, which is uncommon after 40 years of age, affects white men more than black men. It is estimated that in 1996, 7400 men will be diagnosed with this cancer and 370 will die from it.[25]

### History assessment

When obtaining the health history, the nurse should inquire about the following:

1. Do you have a history of undescended testicles? Was this surgically corrected? At what age?
2. Is there a history of mumps, orchitis, or testicular cancer in the family? History of inguinal hernia?
3. Did your mother take any type of hormones while she was pregnant with you?
4. Are you aware of any lumps in your scrotum?
5. Were there signs of early puberty as a child?
6. Have you noticed any changes in your genital organs or interest in sex?
7. Are you aware of any scrotal heaviness or heavy discomfort in the scrotum or lower portion of the abdomen and groin?
8. Are you aware of any breast swelling or nipple tenderness?
9. Do you practice testicular self-examination (TSE)? If not, have you ever been shown?
10. Are you aware of any recent trauma to the genital organs?

Although there is no direct proof that trauma causes testicular cancer, many men link swelling or a lump to a recent trauma. The most common presenting complaint is a painless enlargement of the testis, or "heaviness," which is noticed by about two-thirds of men.[120] Nodules in the testes are typically small, hard, and usually painless, and they are slightly more common in the right testis (52.3%) than in the left (47.7%).[121]

The major obstacle to early detection of testicular cancer is the delay that commonly occurs between initial detection of the lesion in the testis to the time of treatment. Approximately six months will elapse before treatment is either sought by the patient or begun by the physician.[120] The uninformed young man may ignore the unilateral enlargement for quite some time for the following reasons: (1) the man may hope that the testis will spontaneously revert to normal; (2) he may feel a certain pride in his enlarging sexual organ; (3) he may perceive the tumor as punishment for past sexual sins; (4) he may perceive the lack of pain as an indication that the lump is innocent; and (5) he may fear it is cancer.[120]

In 1978 Conklin et al[122] explored the need for and the interest in a health education program about TSE at the University of Vermont. Although 58% of the 90 students interviewed had taken a health-related course in the previous two years, 75% had never heard of testicular cancer. None knew how to examine their testes correctly, and only one knew what to palpate for. In 1986 Blesch[123] surveyed a random sample of 233 professional men about their knowledge and perceptions of testicular cancer and TSE and found the same lack of knowledge about TSE as Conklin et al. Of 129 responses, only 31.1% of the sample subjects were aware of TSE and only 9.5% practiced TSE. Although more than half the sample (61.2%) were aware of testicular cancer, four out of nine men with a personal history of undescended testis (a significant risk factor) had not heard of testicular cancer.[123] Because the effectiveness of TSE in lowering mortality has not been documented, there is debate about recommending this practice for men in screening programs.[102]

### Physical examination

The examination begins with inspection of the scrotum. Cancer of the testes may be manifested by asymmetry of the scrotum. In most men the left side of the scrotal sac descends lower than the right because of the greater length of the left spermatic cord.[124] Another clue to the presence of a tumor in the scrotum is scrotal skin that appears stretched and thin over the tumor.

Palpation of the scrotal contents can be done with the man standing or in a recumbent position; however, the examination should be thorough and gentle because the testes are exquisitely tender to physical pressure.[125] The examiner must conduct the palpation as gently as possible to avoid eliciting the cremasteric reflex. Stimulation of the scrotum or inner thigh may elicit this reflex and cause the testes to be retracted into the inguinal canal (migratory testis). Several procedures are recommended

for palpating the testes. Some authors advocate that the examiner palpate the scrotal contents with both hands to help differentiate the testicles from the other scrotal structures—epididymis, vas deferens, and spermatic cord. Palpating bimanually also improves the chances of detecting any weight differential between the testicles, an important clue to malignancy.[126] The bimanual procedure of using index and middle fingers to separate testes and scrotum so that the right testis and epididymis can be examined with left hand and vice versa is illustrated in Figure 8-16. DeGowin and DeGowin[36] recommend comparing both testes simultaneously by grasping one with each hand, using the thumb and forefinger. As is true with breast lesions, if the man has symptoms, the uninvolved testis should be examined first to provide a baseline comparison.[127]

A normal testicle has a somewhat rubbery, spongy consistency, and the consistency is uniform throughout with a surface free of lumps or indurations. Diffuse induration of the testis in the absence of discrete nodularity also may be the initial abnormality.[128] The most common sites for tumors are on the testicular anterior and lateral surfaces.[129] In the young male, the testis is apt to feel firm and smooth, whereas in the elderly male it may be very soft, almost mushy.[124] Even though the testes feel normal, each should be transilluminated. One may be atrophied and the normal size attained by a hydrocele.[36] Transillumination is helpful in distinguishing cystic from solid masses. Transillumination can be accomplished by aiming a small flashlight behind or on the side of the scrotum in a darkened room. It should be remembered that hydroceles may develop as a result of a tumor.[130] Testicular tumors tend to remain ovoid, being limited by the tough tunica albuginea. Spread to the epididymis may occur in 10%–15% of men.[125] Typically, a testicular tumor occurs as a painless scrotal mass that does not transilluminate. The size may range from less than 1 cm to 10 cm in diameter. The examiner needs to be aware that the scrotal skin overlying the tumor is rarely attached, although attachment may exist in lymphomatous involvement of the testis.[124]

Other areas should be checked to ascertain if there has been metastasis; for example, a mass in the epigastrium or an enlarged left supraclavicular node (Virchow's node) may be palpable. The examiner also should palpate the abdomen for retroperitoneal lymph node involvement. To feel any metastatic nodes the examiner will have to palpate the abdomen fairly deeply. Metastatic nodes usually lie at the level of, or slightly caudal to, the umbilicus. Ultrasonographic examination is often useful in further defining an abnormality of the testicular parenchyma.[128]

### Education: testicular self-examination

There is a need for nurses to educate themselves, their colleagues, and their patients about testicular cancer and TSE. The major deterrent to early detection and treatment is young men's lack of knowledge of the great danger of testicular cancer and the lack of awareness of the

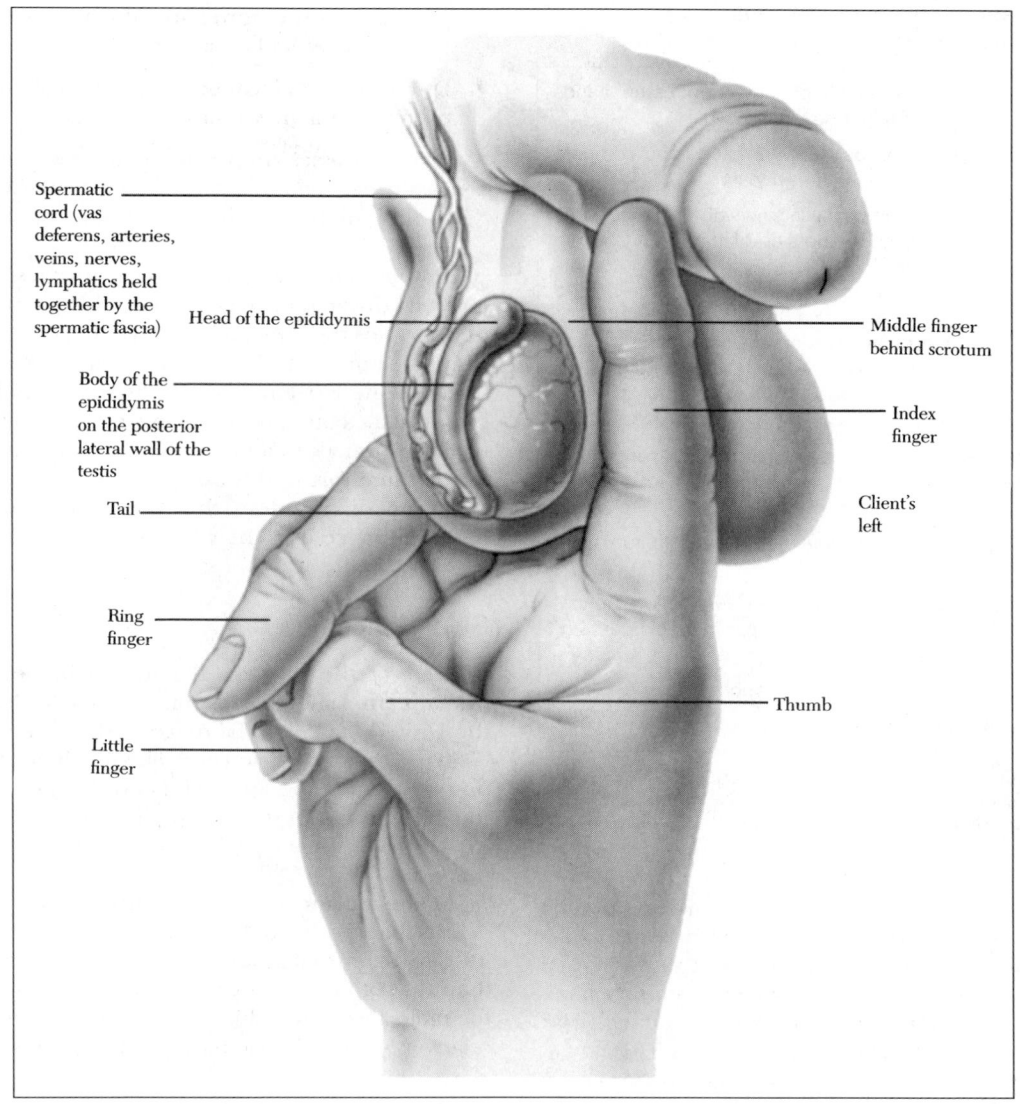

Spermatic cord (vas deferens, arteries, veins, nerves, lymphatics held together by the spermatic fascia)

Head of the epididymis

Body of the epididymis on the posterior lateral wall of the testis

Tail

Ring finger

Little finger

Middle finger behind scrotum

Index finger

Client's left

Thumb

**FIGURE 8-16**   Palpation of the scrotum. Bimanual procedure of using the index and middle fingers to separate the testes and scrotum so that the right testes and epididymus can be examined with the left hand and vice versa. (Grimes J, Burns E (eds): *Health Assessment in Nursing Practice* (ed 2). Boston, Jones and Bartlett, 1987.)

need for regular self-examination.[123] Because the prognosis is good when the tumor is treated early, there is a vital need to educate the public about early detection and treatment. The majority of men discover the changes in the testes while bathing or showering, or it is found by their sexual partners. Only 4% of tumors are detected by clinicians doing a work-up for infertility.[121]

Pediatric hospital and office-based nurses, pediatric nurse practitioners, and school nurses must instruct the parents of high-risk boys and adolescents—those who have or have had undescended testes—how to correctly palpate the scrotum and what physical findings are significant. These same children should be instructed in TSE as they mature. TSE techniques should be included in

health education classes just as breast self-examinations are now routinely included in these classes. Education should emphasize the importance of reporting abnormal findings immediately because delay in reporting testicular lesions is common. Table 8-5 summarizes what should be taught during TSE.[131]

Nurses who work in the military, in occupational health settings, in physicians' offices, and in educational settings are in ideal clinical settings for teaching TSE and providing education that will dispel the myths that contribute to delay once a testicular lump is found.

Teaching TSE should be incorporated into routine physical examinations by the examining health professional. A nursing assessment of any male younger than

**TABLE 8-5** Summary Chart: Testicular Self-Examination (TSE)

- Perform monthly while bathing or showering. Lather hands with soap to increase finger sensitivity.

- Hold the scrotum in the palm of the hands and compare each half of the sac for equal heaviness.

- Examine the side of the scrotal sac individually. Place index and middle fingers on the underside of the testis and the thumb on top. Palpate the ovoid-shaped testis for lumps. Locate the epididymis and palpate. It is a comma-shaped structure on top of and extending down behind the testicle. It is usually soft and slightly tender. Position the thumb and fingers into the deep groove between the anterior oval testis and the posterior epididymis. The testis is firmer than the epididymis.

- Identify the spermatic cord (vas deferens) that ascends from the epididymis. It is a smooth, firm, movable, tubular structure.

- During TSE, apply gentle pressure. If there is pain, too much pressure is being applied.

- Examination of the testis should be done with a slow, gentle, rolling action. Check for any small lump, slight enlargement, or change in consistency.

- Repeat the same procedure for the opposite testicle.

- Report any changes to a physician for immediate evaluation.

White L: The nurse's role in cancer prevention, in Newell G (ed): *Cancer Prevention in Clinical Medicine*. New York, Raven Press, 1983, pp. 91–112.

40 years of age should include a health history to elicit any subjective symptoms and established risk factors for testicular cancer. A man who complains of vague scrotal symptoms should be referred for a careful genital examination, and those men identified as being at high risk for testicular cancer should be instructed in TSE.

The following methods to disseminate information about testicular cancer and TSE have been proposed by Carlin.[121]

- Teach male patients in clinics for sexually transmitted disease.

- Publish articles on TSE and early detection in local papers, radio, and television.

- Include discussions of TSE in all health education classes at the junior high and high school levels.

- Distribute TSE pamphlets to physicians' offices (especially offices of urologists), hospitals, pediatric clinics, clinics for women, infants, and children, immunization clinics, and other health care settings.

- Teach personnel in public health departments the importance of including discussions of testicular cancer and how to perform TSE when they work with parents of young boys and with men who attend the health clinic.

- Publish articles in college newspapers and offer health

programs at the university infirmary on the early detection of testicular cancer.

- Discuss testicular cancer and TSE in all health-related programs for new military recruits.

- Provide classes and written materials to male employees in occupational settings, particularly young men in the "high-tech" occupations.

In summary, the best defense against testicular cancer is a well-educated male population that practices TSE and understands the importance of seeking medical attention when a "lump" is discovered. Much progress has been made in the last ten years in discussing and promoting breast self-examination among women. The time has come for nurses to address the issue of testicular cancer in the same forthright, open manner that breast cancer has been discussed so that men will incorporate this health practice into their lives.

## Skin Cancer

Cancers of the skin are the most common cancers in humans. In 1996, it is estimated that 38,300 people in the United States will be diagnosed with melanoma and 7300 will die of skin cancer.[25] The incidence rate of melanoma is increasing approximately 4% per year.[20] Today the lifetime risk of developing invasive melanoma is 1 in 87. However, this is projected to increase to 1 in 75 by the year 2000.[132]

Malignant melanoma accounts for about 74% of all deaths that result from cutaneous cancers.[133] The mortality rate from malignant melanoma is increasing faster than that of any other cancer except lung cancer. Today the majority of individuals with malignant melanoma are relatively young: the median age at diagnosis is 45 years.[134]

### History assessment

When obtaining the health history, the nurse should inquire about the following:

1. Have you noticed any changes in any of your moles in terms of color, size, surface characteristics, sensation, areas around the mole, and elevation of the mole?
2. Are you aware of any skin lesions on your body that are new or don't seem to "go away"?
3. Are you aware of the development of any new moles?
4. Have you ever been told you should have a mole removed? Why were you told this?
5. Have you (or any members of your family) ever been told you have dysplastic nevi? Have you (or any members of your family) ever had skin cancer? melanoma? If yes, where was the cancer?
6. Do you feel you have a lot of moles? Where are the majority of these moles?
7. Do you sunbathe? How often? Do you use sunscreen?
8. Do you go to a tanning salon or use a tanning bed? How often?

9. Does your skin generally burn when in the sun or tan?
10. What is your occupation? Have you ever worked in a position in which you were outside for long periods of time? How long did you hold that job?
11. Have you ever worked in occupations in which you were exposed to tar and pitch, oils, paraffins, arsenic, x-rays, or radium?
12. Were you ever burned, or do you have scarring from corrosive or thermal damage?
13. Do you have any outdoor recreational habits or hobbies that you consistently engage in?

When obtaining a health history, the nurse must inquire whether any of the aforementioned changes in moles have occurred. A history of change, often extending over a period of weeks or months, in a preexisting mole or the development of a new mole in an adult is of great importance and requires inspection. The nurse needs to be aware that almost half the melanomas arise in moles or pigmented areas; thus there should be a high index of suspicion in any mole that is changing or enlarging.[135]

## Physical examination

It is essential that the entire integument be inspected during the examination of a patient. Skin assessment includes inspection of the inner lip mucosa, the axillae, the nail beds, the external genitalia, the webs between the toes, the soles of the feet, and the areas in skin folds.[136] This is best accomplished in a setting with good lighting (e.g., a gooseneck lamp) that enables the nurse to project the light obliquely across the body surface. A pen light can be used instead of a gooseneck lamp. A magnifying glass also allows closer inspection of minute details.[137]

All areas that are chronically exposed to the sun should be meticulously assessed, including the neck, ears, shoulders, face, scalp, arms, and hands. Areas that have been chronically exposed to sunlight are common sites for basal cell and squamous cell carcinomas. However, melanomas are found on head, neck, and trunk, which may or may not be exposed to sun, and on the legs in women; occurrence of malignant melanoma is infrequent in rarely exposed or unexposed areas (breasts and bathing suit area of women and bathing trunk area of men).[138] The surface distribution of melanomas in African-Americans differs from that in Caucasians; the relatively depigmented palms, soles, nail beds, and mucous membranes are primary sites in almost all African-American patients.[139]

It is recommended that the entire posterior and anterior aspect of the body be viewed and the location of moles be mapped to serve as baseline data for future skin assessments. If a skin lesion is detected, the nurse has three responsibilities: accurate documentation (size, location, description of the lesion), referral of the patient to a physician for diagnosis, and follow-up for recurrent disease.[136]

There are three types of skin cancer: basal cell carcinoma, squamous cell carcinoma, and melanoma. The nurse should be aware of the following precancerous skin lesions: leukoplakia (found in the oral mucosa), senile and actinic keratoses, and dysplastic nevi. Table 8-6[133,140,141] lists the incidence, clinical characteristics, and common sites of actinic keratoses and basal cell and squamous cell skin cancer. Table 8-7 compares the clinical features of a normal mole, dysplastic mole, and malignant melanoma.

## Education

Of all the known risk factors, ultraviolet radiation from the sun is the leading cause of skin cancer. Fortunately, the most carcinogenic of the ultraviolet wavelengths can be blocked by sunscreening agents. Sunscreens are rated according to *sun protection factor* (SPF), on a scale currently ranging from 2 to 35. An SPF of 2 in a sunscreen means that proper application allows users to stay in the sun twice as long as they could without any protection at all. Sunbathing should be avoided during the 2-hour period around noon, because two-thirds of the day's ultraviolet light comes through during that time. Skin types are similarly rated from 1 to 6 according to intensity of sunburn in the first 30–45 minutes of unprotected exposure to the sun after a period of no exposure. Skin type 1 burns easily and never tans, whereas skin types 5 and 6 rarely burn and tan well.

The following information about decreasing or eliminating skin cancer risks should be discussed with each patient:

1. Ultraviolet rays can penetrate thin clothing like cotton T-shirts; those who desire protective clothing should select hats, long-sleeved shirts, and beach robes rather than rely on T-shirts.
2. Individuals with skin types 1 and 2 should avoid sunbathing.
3. People who live or vacation in areas of higher altitudes need to be aware that there is less atmosphere to filter out ultraviolet rays so that the sun's effects are more intense.
4. Individuals need to be informed that the sun's rays are reflected off snow, sand, and water and that significant sun exposure can result from activities on these surfaces.
5. As the ozone layer of the earth changes, people need to be aware that this significantly alters the amount of ultraviolet radiation that reaches the earth.

Routine self-examination of the skin is the best defense against skin cancer, especially malignant melanoma. It is inexpensive, noninvasive, and totally free of danger. Periodic self-examination for melanoma and examination by others may result in improved survival.[142] It is recommended that individuals older than 30 years of age who have fair skin and are subject to heavy sun exposures be taught skin self-assessment. Those with dysplastic nevus syndrome or a history of melanoma in a first-degree relative also should have regular medical examinations that

**TABLE 8-6** Incidence, Clinical Characteristics, and Common Sites of Premalignant Skin Cancers and Skin Cancer

| Skin Carcinoma | Incidence | Clinical Characteristics | Common Sites |
|---|---|---|---|
| Actinic keratoses (senile keratoses, solar keratoses) | Most common premalignant keratoses; develop in persons with fair complexions as result of excessive exposure to light; located on sun-exposed areas | Appear as circumscribed dry patches with adherent scales on slightly red, inflamed skin | Most commonly found on the face and the backs of hands. 20% of cases lead to squamous cell carcinoma |
| Basal cell carcinoma | Most common form of skin cancer; occurs primarily in persons exposed to intense sunlight, especially fair-complexioned white persons with light eyes and hair | *Nodular basal cell carcinoma:* elevated papule to lesions with an ulcerated center, raised margin, and waxy or "pearly" border; firm | Commonly found on the nose, eyelids, cheeks, and neck |
| | | *Superficial basal cell carcinoma:* plaque, usually with a crusted and erythematous center, flat, and defined margins | Commonly found on trunk and extremities |
| Squamous cell carcinoma | Less common than basal cell carcinoma: occurs primarily on areas exposed to actinic or ultraviolet (UV) radiation | Appearance varies from an elevated nodular mass to a punched-out ulcerated lesion or a large fungating mass. Unlike basal cell carcinoma, squamous cell tumors are opaque and aggressive | Commonly found on head and hands |

Adapted from Friedman et al,[133] Helm and Helm,[140] Epstein.[141]

**TABLE 8-7** Comparison of Common Nevi, Dysplastic Nevi, and Malignant Melanoma

| Characteristic | Common Nevi | Dysplastic Nevi | Malignant Melanoma |
|---|---|---|---|
| Color | Uniformly tan or brown | Variable mixtures of tan, brown, black, or red/pink within a single nevus; nevi may look very different from each other | Variegated colors ranging from various hues of tan and brown to black and sometimes intermingled with red and white |
| Shape | Round; sharp, clear-cut borders between the nevus and the surrounding skin; may be flat or elevated | Irregular borders; pigment may fade off into surrounding skin; always have a flat portion level with the skin, which often occurs at the edge of the nevus | Borders of early malignant melanomas usually irregular, notched or angular |
| Size | Usually <6 mm in diameter like this: ● | Usually >6 mm; may be >10 mm; occasionally <6 mm | Diameters of macular malignant melanomas often >5 mm (it is not unusual to see 1.0 to 1.5 cm); 98.5% have a diameter ≥ 5 mm |
| Number | In a typical adult: 10 to 40 are scattered over the body | Often very many (>100), but some people may not have an unusual number of nevi | |
| Location | Generally on the sun-exposed surfaces of the skin above the waist; the scalp, breasts, and buttocks rarely are involved | Sun-exposed areas: the back is the most common site, but also may be seen on the scalp, breasts, and buttocks | Relatively uncommon body areas that are always covered, especially the breast and pelvic area in women; sharp increase in incidence in the head, neck, trunk of men, and arms and lower legs of women |

Adapted from Friedman R, Rigel D, Kopf A: Early detection of malignant melanoma: The role of physician, examination and self-examination of the skin. *CA Cancer J Clin* 35:130–151, 1985.

include measurement and charting of location of unusual pigmented lesions.[133] It also is recommended that patients be given copies of blank body charts so that they can chart lesions found during self-skin assessment. Figure 8-17 illustrates the correct procedure for self-assessment of skin.

Along with self-assessment of the skin, patients should be instructed about the changes in moles that merit immediate medical attention: size, color, elevation, surface characteristics, and sensation. Melanoma is more likely to develop in individuals and families with a history of dysplastic nevus syndrome (DNS) than it is in most people.[143] The initial diagnosis is based on a physical examination and confirmed by the removal and biopsy of several moles. Individuals with familial DNS should visit their clinician or dermatologist twice a year for assessment and follow-up. They also should conduct self-assessments of the skin on a monthly basis. Assistance usually is necessary because many of the nevi are present in areas such as the scalp or back that are difficult for the individual to inspect.

The elderly constitute the highest-risk group for skin cancer because of the number of years of exposure to the sun. It is estimated that 40%–50% of all those who live to be 65 years of age will have at least one skin cancer during their lifetime.[144] Changes normally occur in the skin with age, which increase the risk of skin cancer. Keratoses, lentigines, and pigmented alterations develop with aging and in areas of chronic solar exposure. Elderly persons should be taught skin self-assessment and the importance of having a health professional examine any new lesions or changing lesions. Any setting where older adults congregate offers the nurse an excellent opportunity to provide an educational program on skin self-examination and early detection for skin cancer. Any areas that have been chronically exposed to the sun should be meticulously screened.

## Oral Cancer

It is estimated that in 1996 there will be 29,490 new cases of oral cancer in the United States. The majority of these cancers (11,300) will be cancers of the mouth. There will be 8260 deaths from oral cancer.[25] These figures indicate that oral cancer incidence is not declining nationally and that we have not made significant headway in treatment during the last decade.[145] Approximately 95% of all oral malignancies begin in the surface mucosa. Although the surface of the oral mucosa is easily inspected and palpated, by the time of diagnosis more than 60% of oral cancers have spread to the lymph nodes.[145]

### History assessment

When the nurse obtains the health history, it is important to ask the following questions:

1. Do you smoke? How much do you smoke, and how many years have you smoked (pack-years)?

2. Do you chew tobacco or dip snuff? How long have you done this? How much tobacco do you use in a day? Can you describe where you place the tobacco in your mouth?

3. Do you smoke a pipe? How long have you smoked a pipe? Do you smoke cigars?

4. Do you drink alcohol? Approximately how much alcohol do you drink in a day? What type of alcohol do you consume?

5. *For the patient from Southeast Asia or Central Asia:* Do you chew *betel quid*? Do you use betel quid with any form of tobacco (chewing or smoking)?[146]

6. Do you wear dentures? Do you have any sore spots in your mouth from your dentures? Do you inspect under your dentures at least weekly?

7. When was your last dental examination?

8. How often do you brush your teeth? floss your teeth?

9. Have you ever been in an occupation in which you spent a lot of time outside? Do you have any hobbies or sports interests that involve spending a great deal of time outdoors? Do you wear lip balm when outdoors to protect your lips?

10. Have you noticed any white or red sores in your mouth for longer than a month? any lumps, swelling, or rough spots?

11. Have you been aware of any limitation of tongue or jaw movement?

12. Have you noticed taste changes, dry mouth, speech changes, hoarseness, or chronic cough?

13. Are you aware of any sore or crusts on your lips?

14. Are you aware of any lumps or growing "bumps" in your neck or face?

15. Do you have problems with persistent halitosis that does not seem to respond to any home remedies?

### Physical examination

The majority of oral cancers cause no symptoms in their early stages. Most individuals who notice a white or bright red spot, "sore," or a swelling in their mouth attribute it to their teeth or dentures and thus seek the consultation of a dentist.

Physical examination of the mouth includes inspection, digital palpation, and olfaction of the oral cavity. The following maneuvers should be performed during the oral examination:

1. Have the patient extend the tongue and move it from side to side. The patient also should be asked to move the jaw from side to side and up and down. Limitation of normal movement could indicate that a tumor is interfering with muscle action.

2. Palpate the tongue with a gloved hand. Palpation may reveal a lesion not otherwise visible. Palpation of a hard lesion should be referred for biopsy to establish the diagnosis.[147]

3. Inspect the anterior two-thirds of the tongue by grasping the tip of the tongue with a piece of gauze and gently pulling the tongue forward and to each side.

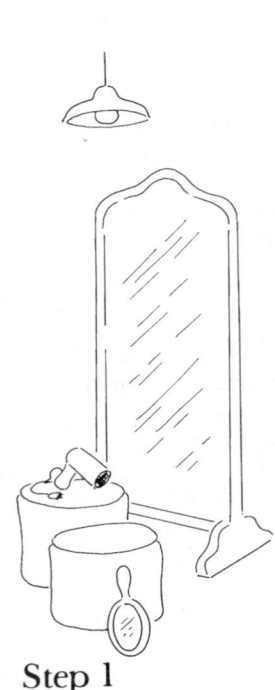

## Step 1

Make sure the room is well-lighted and that you have nearby a full-length mirror, a hand-held dryer, and two chairs or stools. Undress completely.

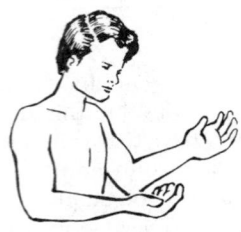

## Step 2

Hold your hands with the palms face up, as shown in the drawing. Look at your palms, fingers, spaces between the fingers, and forearms. Then turn your hands over and examine the backs of your hands, fingers, spaces between the fingers, fingernails, and forearms.

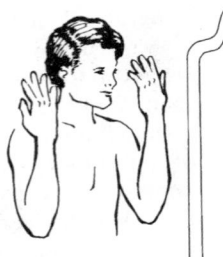

## Step 3

Now position yourself in front of the full-length mirror. Hold up your arms, bent at the elbows, with your palms facing you. In the mirror, look at the backs of your forearms and elbows.

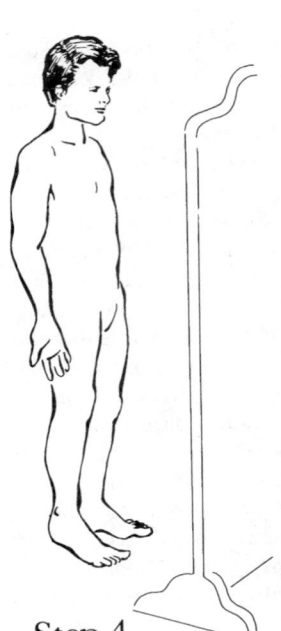

## Step 4

Again using the full-length mirror, observe the entire front of your body. In turn, look at your face, neck, and arms. Turn your palms to face the mirror and look at your upper arms. Then look at your chest and abdomen, pubic area, thighs and lower legs.

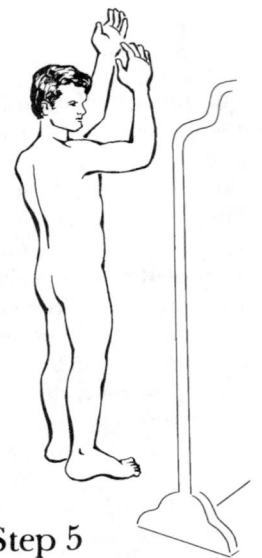

## Step 5

Still standing in front of the mirror, lift your arms over your head with the palms facing each other. Turn so that your right side is facing the mirror and look at the entire side of your body—your hands and arms, underarms, sides of your trunk, thighs, and lower legs. Then turn, and repeat the process with your left side.

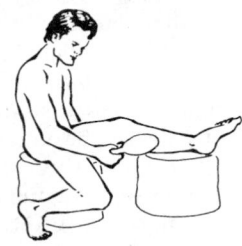

## Step 9

Sit down and prop up one leg on a chair or stool in front of you as shown. Using the hand-held mirror, examine the inside of the propped-up leg, beginning at the groin area and moving the mirror down the leg to your foot. Repeat the procedure for your other leg.

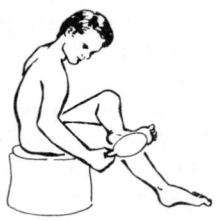

## Step 10

Still sitting, cross one leg over the other. Use the hand-held mirror to examine the top of your foot, the toes, toenails, and spaces between the toes. Then look at the sole or bottom of your foot. Repeat the procedure for the other foot.

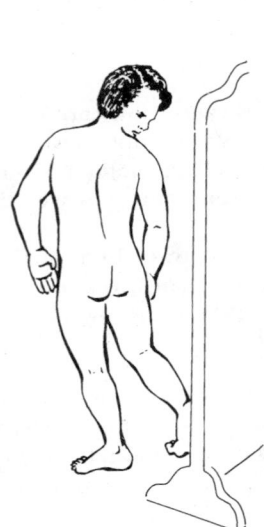

## Step 6

With your back toward the full-length mirror, look at your buttocks and the backs of your thighs and lower legs.

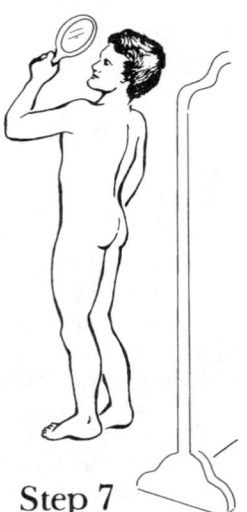

## Step 7

Now pick up the hand-held mirror. With your back still to the full-length mirror, examine the back of your neck, and your back and buttocks. Also examine the backs of your arms in this way. Some areas are hard to see, and you may find it helpful to ask your spouse or a friend to assist you.

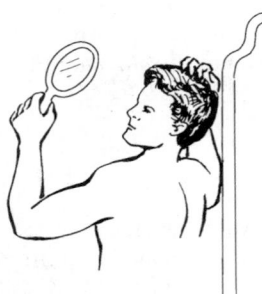

## Step 8

Use the hand-held mirror and the full-length mirror to look at your scalp. Because the scalp is difficult to examine, we suggest you also use a hand-held blow dryer turned to a cool setting to lift the hair from the scalp. While some people find it easy to hold the mirror in one hand and the dryer in the other while looking in the full-length mirror, many do not. For the scalp examination in particular, then, you might ask your spouse or a friend to assist you.

**FIGURE 8-17** Self-examination of the skin. (Friedman R, Rigel D, Kopf A: Early detection of malignant melanoma: The role of physician examination and self-examination of the skin. *CA Cancer J Clin* 35:130-151, 1985.)

Lesions of the base of the tongue are most often overlooked and must be both inspected and palpated. The nurse should be aware that most tongue cancers appear on the lateral surfaces.

4. The floor of the mouth should be inspected by having the patient place the tongue on the hard palate. Squamous cell carcinomas frequently are found on the floor of the mouth. The floor of the mouth should be palpated bimanually, with the fingers of one hand in the floor of the mouth and the fingers of the other hand placed on the skin under the right side of the jaw.

5. Inspection of the mouth may reveal snuff keratosis from the use of snuff in one spot in the mouth and nicotine stomatitis from cigar or pipe smoking. Nicotine stomatitis is a diffuse white condition that contains numerous red dots. This lesion usually covers the entire hard palate and is almost always associated with pipe smoking and has minimal or no malignant potential. Complete resolution should occur with cessation of smoking.

Individuals who use smokeless tobacco may develop leukoplakias in the exact region where they hold the quid. The leukoplakia may vary from a very mild whiteness, which may be difficult to see, to a very obvious white lesion.[148,149] When a white oral lesion is found, the area should be rubbed to see if it can be removed. White lesions that adhere to the surface are classified as keratotic and have a greater probability of malignancy. Leukoplakia occurs in men more commonly than in women, and the vast majority are seen in individuals older than 40 years of age.

In erythroplakia, also considered premalignant, a red plaque or well-defined red patches have a velvety consistency and often have tiny areas of ulceration. Erythroplakia lesions usually have a more malignant histological component than does leukoplakia.[147] Erythroplakia patches are characteristically painless and occur with about equal frequency in men and women who usually are older than 50 years of age.

Mashberg and Samit recommend using Toluidine blue as a rinse to spotlight suspicious lesions.[148] The topical application of this dye to suspicious lesions serves as a diagnostic "control" over the clinician's subjective impression. Lesions not detected during a visual examination may therefore be revealed by the stain. If an entire lesion or portion of a lesion stains dark blue in a solid or strippled pattern, malignancy must be considered. Normal tissue does not absorb stain, but small areas of intense, mechanically retained stain may be observed. (See Mashberg and Samit[148] article for specific details on this procedure and follow-up questions and answers on this article in *CA-Cancer Journal for Clinicians* 46:126–128, 1996.)

6. While inspecting the lips, observe them for any skin changes, such as keratosis of the lips from excessive sun exposure and pipe smoking. Solar keratoses occur on sun-exposed surfaces and are flat, reddish-to-tan plaques that are usually scaly. In the earliest stages a cancerous lesion may appear as a small swelling or induration that may be difficult to see but that can be palpated. An area of roughness, induration, or granularity often is the best clue to the diagnosis of early carcinoma. The upper lip should be grasped between the index finger and the thumb and bidigitally palpated along its complete length to discover masses that may be located deep under the surface.[147]

7. Olfaction of the breath. An odor of sourness may indicate obstruction and fermentation, whereas fetid and foul odors may signal necrotic neoplasms indicative of advanced disease. All large, fungating oral cancers produce a marked halitosis; however, small oral cancers are not particularly associated with mouth odor.[148] Referral to a dentist may be necessary if the breath odors indicate advanced dental decay and poor oral hygiene.

8. Palpate the parotid, submandibular, and submental areas and the cervical lymph nodes.

## Screening

Because alcoholics who smoke constitute the largest risk group for oral cancers, screening programs should be geared to this population. Any screening programs would have to be conducted in settings in which alcoholics could be approached as a group, such as in reform organizations, Salvation Army facilities for this population, shelters for the homeless, or alcoholic rehabilitation units. Although primary prevention by limiting alcohol intake and cessation of smoking is a more desirable goal, many alcoholics cannot be reached by these types of programs. Thus the more realistic approach with this group is to encourage periodic oral examinations so that cancer can be detected in the early stages.

It is important for the nurse to explain to individuals 40 years of age and older that it is necessary to have a complete oral and dental examination on a periodic basis to detect serious lesions. Individuals with complete dentures frequently believe they no longer require periodic oral examinations because of their loss of natural teeth.[150]

The use of smokeless tobacco (e.g., snuff and chewing tobacco) has risen dramatically in the last ten years. The increase in the sales of smokeless tobacco, predominantly snuff, since the early 1970s has been estimated at 11% per year, representing an estimated 7–12 million users.[151] In the early 1970s a majority of users were men 50 years of age and older; now most are young men between 16 and 29 years of age. Nurses need to stress that smokeless tobacco is *not* a safe substitute for smoking. Long-term use of smokeless tobacco increases the risk of gingival and buccal carcinomas nearly 50-fold.[148] Many young people are not aware that smokeless tobacco is as addicting as cigarette smoking.[152] Information about the health hazards of smokeless tobacco should be shared with young people. Because so many users are very young children, it is advocated that education on the dangers of smokeless tobacco should begin with children as young as 6 and 7 years of age.[153] School nurses and nurses who work in settings with young people need to actively initiate educational programs on this subject or make sure that whenever smoking is discussed in health and science classes that the issue of smokeless tobacco also is addressed. In addition, parents, teachers, and athletic coaches should not neglect the powerful influence they can have as positive role models. Youngsters perceive the use of smokeless tobacco as "macho," and athletic coaches can have a tremendous influence in dispelling this myth. Chapter 66 provides a list of sources for obtaining patient education materials on smokeless tobacco.

In summary, education first begins with the identification of individuals at high risk for oral cancer. Depending on the risk factors identified, the individual could be referred to a physician or a dentist or taught oral self-examination for the early signs of cancer, or the nurse could conduct the oral examination at predetermined intervals. Grabau[154] found that about half those taught self-examinations for early signs of cancer continued these examinations at regular intervals. It is advocated that oral self-examination techniques need to be popularized in the same manner as breast self-examination techniques.

## Gynecologic Cancer

It is estimated that in 1996 there will be 34,000 cases of endometrial cancers and 15,700 cases of cervical cancers in the United States. The anticipated mortality rates in this same period are expected to be 4900 deaths from cervical cancer and 6000 deaths from endometrial cancer.[25] The risk of endometrial cancer is age-related; the disease usually occurs in women 50–60 years old.

In stark contrast are the incidence and mortality rates for ovarian cancer. It was estimated that in 1996, 26,700 U.S. women would be diagnosed with this cancer and 14,800 would die of the disease. Ovarian cancer accounts for about 26% of all gynecologic cancer and about 52% of all genital cancer deaths. The greatest number of cases of ovarian cancer are found in the age group of 55- to 74-year-old women.

### History assessment

The health history should include questions that will elicit an accurate menstrual, obstetric, gynecologic, and sexual history. The majority of women at risk for cancer of the reproductive organs can be identified only after a thorough and complete gynecologic history has been obtained. The following questions will help identify high-risk women:

1. When was your last Pap smear? Do you remember the results? Was any follow-up done or recommended?
2. Have you ever been told that you have herpes? genital warts? Were the genital warts treated? What type of treatment was done for the genital warts? Have you been treated for pelvic inflammatory disease or any other sexually transmitted diseases?
3. Do you have any vaginal bleeding or discharge not connected with menses?
4. Do you have spotting between menstrual periods?
5. Do you have bleeding or spotting although you no longer have menstrual periods?
6. Do you have bleeding after intercourse or douching?
7. At what age did you start sexual activity?
8. Have you had a consistent sexual partner since beginning sexual activity, or have you had different partners?
9. What is the approximate number of sexual partners you have had?
10. What age did you start menstruation?
11. What age did you start menopause? When was your last period?
12. How many pregnancies have you had? How many live births? miscarriages? elective abortions?
13. Have you ever taken birth control pills? How long did you take birth control pills? Do you remember the name of the pill that you took?
14. Have you ever taken estrogens? How long did you take these? What was the dose that you were given? What follow-up tests were recommended for you while taking estrogens?
15. Have you ever had infertility problems? Have you ever had endometriosis? polycystic ovaries? Stein-Leventhal syndrome? uterine fibroids?
16. Are you aware of abdominal distention or vague abdominal discomfort?
17. Are you aware if your mother received diethylstilbestrol (DES) when she was pregnant with you?
18. Have you had any gynecologic surgery—hysterectomy, tubal pregnancy, sterilization, ovarian cysts, cancer?
19. Have you ever had office procedures for a gynecologic problem, such as cervical cautery and colposcopic examination?
20. Has your present sexual partner ever had a sexual partner who had cervical cancer?
21. Have any women in your family had ovarian cancer? Who?

### Physical examination

The early signs and symptoms of gynecologic cancer are as follows. Ovarian cancer usually has no early manifestations. There may be vague abdominal discomfort, dyspepsia, indigestion, gas with constant distention, flatulence, eructation, a feeling of fullness after a light meal, or slight loss of appetite.[155] The majority of patients with endometrial cancer have unexplained bleeding. In postmenopausal women, abnormal bleeding takes the form of intermittent spotting or bleeding that the patient describes as a "very light period." A malodorous watery discharge may be noticed as an early sign. The symptoms of cervical cancer typically are abnormal vaginal discharge, irregular bleeding, elongation of menstrual period, or bleeding that may occur after douching or intercourse.[156]

The gynecologic examination includes *inspection* and *palpation*. The nurse should be aware of the following maneuvers performed during the gynecologic examination and related signs that indicate cancer.

**Abdomen**  The abdomen must be thoroughly and slowly palpated to detect any masses, areas of tenderness, or inguinal adenopathy. A mass in the upper portion of the abdomen may suggest the presence of omental cake, the solid mass formed when the omentum is infiltrated with cancer, which is a sign of advanced ovarian disease. It may be palpated or detected by ballottement during the abdominal examination. Other signs of advanced ovarian cancer are abdominal distention and ascites.[155]

**Vulva**  The vulva should be inspected and palpated for signs of cancer of the vulva: excoriation of skin because of pruritis, ulcers, lumps, leukoplakia, bleeding, atrophy of the labia, and narrowing of the introitus.[157]

Infection with human papillomavirus (HPV) may produce the typically raised exophytic tumors (warts) that can be seen with simple inspection of the vulva. There is, however, a variety of anogenital warts known as "flat" or "noncondylomatous" warts that may be invisible before the application of acetic acid. Several gauze pads (4-in. diameter) that are soaked in 3%–5% acetic acid should be compressed on the vulva and left in place for 10 minutes. After the compress is removed, the area should be inspected with a high-quality magnification lens for the *acetowhite reaction*. Acetic acid will cause the surface of both flat and exophytic warts to turn white.[158] Colposcopic examination also can be used to inspect lesions after acetic acid application. Further, carcinoma in situ also may appear as a hyperpigmented lesion. In addition, HPV can infect the entire lower female genital tract—the vagina and cervix. Patients with vulvar HPV lesions should have a thorough examination of the vagina, cervix, and perirectal epithelium with the use of an acetic acid compress application and a colposcopic examination.[158] In 1989 a minimum of 10% of the population, and probably much higher, was infected with HPV.[159] About half the individuals infected with HPV are carriers of the high-risk types of HPV virus.[16,18,25–27]

**Vagina**  The vagina should be inspected and palpated for cancer—masses, vaginal bands, texture changes, ulcers, erosions, leukoplakia, pink blush, induration, telangiectasis, and erythematosus. Induration and nodulation may indicate submucosal vaginal lesions. Most squamous cell carcinomas are found in the posterior vaginal wall, but 25% involve the anterior wall and at least 15% arise from the lateral walls.[160] The majority of lesions occur in the upper third of the vagina.

The nurse may elect to do a Schiller's test on any suspicious area of the vagina or cervix. The mucosa is painted with an iodine solution (Lugol's solution), and the normal mucosa becomes brown whereas areas of abnormal epithelium remain uncolored. This test is merely an adjunctive aid to colposcopic examination or used when colposcopy is not available. It indicates a glycogen-free area and delineates biopsy sites.[157]

**Cervix**  The cervix should be inspected and palpated, and a Pap smear should be taken for cytological examination. To avoid contamination of the cell sample with foreign material, vaginal jelly should not be used before Pap smears are obtained. The cervical sample should contain cells from the squamous epithelium of the vaginal portion of the cervix, from the squamo-columnar junction (also known as the transformation zone), and from the endocervical epithelium.[159,161] With aging the transformation zone becomes increasingly invisible as it moves into the endocervical canal. In women during and after menopause, a sample of the vaginal pool cells is obtained, in addition to the cervical smear, to identify cancer cells from the endometrium, tubes, and ovaries.

The nurse should inspect and palpate the cervix for position, shape, consistency, regularity, mobility, friability, and tenderness. The cervix is freely movable, firm, and smooth, and if it has been invaded by cancer, it becomes hard and immobile. In addition to rendering the cervix much harder than normal, malignancy produces a rough, granular surface and is likened to both the feel and appearance of a cauliflower.[124] However, the nurse needs to be cognizant of the fact that early carcinoma has an appearance that cannot be well differentiated visually from erosion. Cancer arising within the cervical canal may cause no abnormal appearance of the cervix.

Several physical changes may be apparent in the cervix that indicate possible patient exposure to DES in utero. Cervical ectropion, or cervical bumps or ridges ("cockscombs," "hoods," or "collars"), and other non-neoplastic changes are immediate clues to DES exposure. These physical signs merit referral to a physician.

The conventional Pap smear, taken in the usual manner for cervix cancer screening, is inaccurate for a diagnosis of endometrial lesions.[162] For this reason an annual suction curettage is recommended for menopausal women and women who have taken estrogen without progestational modification for a prolonged period after menopause. Suction curettage can provide an excellent sample and in most cases can be done in the office without need for anesthesia. Monitoring of women who have received long-term estrogen therapy will detect those whose endometrium is overstimulated (adenomatous hyperplasia), and appropriate referrals can be made.

**Uterus and adnexa**  A bimanual examination of the uterus and adnexa should be done. The nurse should note the size, shape, mobility, position, tenderness, and consistency of the uterus. Uterine tenderness, immobility, or enlargement merits further investigation and appropriate referrals. An enlarged boggy uterus is an indication of advanced disease.

**Ovaries**  Palpation of the ovaries in prepubertal girls or postmenopausal women also merits investigation because (1) normal ovaries and tubes are usually not palpable, (2) ovaries in these two groups of women are smaller than the usual ovarian size of 4 cm in its largest dimension, and (3) three to five years after menopause the ovaries usually have atrophied and are no longer palpable. In actively menstruating women, any ovarian enlargement that persists or increases more than 5 or 6 cm requires prompt referral.[155] In general the findings on the pelvic examination that can alert the nurse to a possible ovarian cancer are adnexal enlargement, fixation or immobility, bilateral irregularity or nodulation and masses, relative insensitivity of the mass, and bilaterality of the mass.

***Rectovaginal palpation*** *Rectovaginal* palpation, as well as rectal palpation, should be done. It is extremely important that the anterior rectal wall in the region of the peritoneal rectovaginal pouch, or Douglas' cul-de-sac, be palpated. Thickening of this area occurs from spread of cervical carcinoma, whereas spread from ovarian cancer may be felt as a shelf, nodule, or handful-of-knuckles on rectal palpation.

## Screening of asymptomatic individuals

The American Cancer Society recommends that all women who are, or who have been, sexually active or have reached 18 years of age have an annual Pap test and pelvic examination. After a woman has had three or more consecutive satisfactory normal annual examinations, the Pap test may be performed less frequently at the discretion of her physician.[163] Numerous other professional health organizations also have approved a similar or identical recommendation.

***Cervical smears*** Because of the Pap test, the death rate from invasive cervical cancer has decreased by at least 70% over the last 40 years.[77] However, 15%–20% of American women do not have regular Pap testing.[163] The majority of women in whom cervical cancer develops have not had the test on a regular basis.

The importance of regular Pap smears was documented by Stenkvist et al.[164] They studied 207,455 women for ten years and found that when women were screened at least once, the incidence of cervical cancer dropped from 32/100,000 to 10/100,000 (a 75% decrease in invasive cervical cancer incidence among women who had smears taken at least once during the ten-year period). Among women with at least one normal smear, the incidence drops still lower, to 7/100,000. Because elderly women will constitute 17.3% of the adult population by the year 2020, screening programs for older, high-risk women will be needed.

In the past 20 years, the screening rate in older women has been low, with up to 62% of women older than the age of 65 reporting that they never had a Pap smear. This is of concern because older women comprise 25% of patients with carcinoma of the cervix but 40% of the deaths. A disproportionate number of older women present with locally advanced massive cancer of the cervix, which explains the poor survival of these women.[165]

Mandelblatt and Fahs[166] conducted a study of the cost-effectiveness of a cervical cancer screening program for infrequently screened elderly women. The results of the Pap smears were abnormal in 11/816 women screened. This early detection of cervical neoplasia saved $5907 and 3.7 years of life per 100 Pap tests. The average medical costs per year of life extended by screening were included, and the program cost $2874 per year of life saved. The researchers concluded that the benefits from cervical cancer screening for elderly women can offset the costs of these programs.

Several factors contribute to false-negative results from Pap smears and other errors:

*Patient error* Patient error consists of women failing to have follow-up annual examinations, delay in seeing a physician while symptoms are present, and refusal to undergo diagnostic measures.

*Physician error* Physician error consists of failure to act on reports of abnormal cytological findings, failure to perform a pelvic examination with a Pap smear, reading of Pap smears by untrained physicians, and diagnosis of "dysplasia," which is considered inconsequential by uninformed physicians.

*Laboratory error* Koss[159] reports in his excellent review article that studies have found a false-negative laboratory rate for invasive cancer of approximately 50%. The rate of screening errors for precancerous lesions was at least 28%.

Although nurses generally do not have control over laboratory errors, they can play a significant role in decreasing patient and physician error (1) by educating women about the early symptoms of gynecologic cancer and the necessity of seeking medical advice with these early symptoms; (2) by educating women about the recommended intervals for Pap smears; (3) by educating women, particularly older women, to the necessity of asking for a Pap smear when they have a physical examination; (4) by educating women to request information about the mechanism used by the health care setting to inform them about the results of their Pap smears: women with a history of abnormal or questionable Pap smear results should be encouraged to personally call about their results rather than rely on the health professional to alert them; (5) by educating women about the importance of receiving additional medical care with an abnormal or a questionable Pap smear finding; and (6) by performing Pap smears only after they are thoroughly versed in the proper procedures for obtaining a smear. Improperly done smears probably contribute to at least half of the 10%–35% false-negative rate generally reported for Pap smears.[167] Errors made by cytotechnologists may be minimized in the future by new experimental technological techniques that measure the DNA content of standard Pap smears. Several groups of researchers are investigating the feasibility of automating the procedure of reading Pap smears on the basis of optical density of the specimens or DNA content of cell nuclei.[168,169] Studies are being conducted to determine the feasibility of these approaches.

Two classification methods are used to identify abnormal changes in the Pap smear. One method is the classification system accepted by the World Health Organization. This system identified two types of lesions, dysplasia and carcinoma in situ. The dysplasias are subdivided into very mild, mild, moderate, and severe grades, depending on the extent of involvement of the epithelium.[170] Another classification method is the cervical intraepithelial neoplasia (CIN) nomenclature. CIN is a continuum of change and generally begins as a well-differentiated lesion (CIN 1, or mild dysplasia), passes through a less well-differentiated phase (CIN 2, or moderate dysplasia), and leads to an undifferentiated intraepithelial lesion (CIN 3).[161] CIN 3 is the severe dysplasia/carcinoma in situ in the World Health Organization system. Table 8-8 compares the commonly used Papanicolaou terminology and relationship to the CIN classification method, and Figure 8-18 is a schematic representation of precancerous cervical lesions.[171]

Colposcopic examination is an accurate and reliable method for evaluating the cervix and vagina of a woman with an abnormality revealed by Pap smear. This modality (a well-illuminated binocular microscope) not only provides visualization of the cervical transformation zone but also allows directed biopsy of specific areas of the epithelium, removing only small amounts of tissue.

### Additional nursing interventions

Reaching those women who are at high risk for gynecologic cancer is one of the most challenging roles for nurses. Patient acceptance and increasing the availability of screening are areas that will require major effort on the part of nurses if the entire population at greatest risk

is to be reached. Because cytological screening is closely tied to obstetric care and contraceptive services, a higher proportion of women are screened among the groups that require such attention than among those that do not. This is effective for screening for cervical and vaginal cancer in the reproductive years but does not reach the postmenopausal women who are at risk for ovarian and endometrial malignancies. Nurses who work in retirement centers, extended care facilities, physicians' offices, factories, public health agencies, and ambulatory care settings are urged to provide health education programs that include the early signs and symptoms of ovarian, cervical, and endometrial cancer and to stress the need for gynecologic examinations after menopause as well as during the reproductive years. Female patients being followed routinely for chronic problems (such as hypertension, diabetes, heart condition, or chronic lung disease) should be asked when they had their last pelvic examination.

When appropriate, nurses should discuss the myths about menopause with women who are in their late 30s and early 40s. There are several significant barriers to early detection of gynecologic cancer in older women. Many women have the mistaken belief that once they are past childbearing years and/or are sexually inactive, they no longer need pelvic examinations. There are also physical changes that occur that make the gynecologic examination difficult for older women. There is decreased mobility of the femoropelvic structure, which leads to pain when the woman is put in the lithotomy position for a gynecologic examination. Nurses need to be aware of this physical barrier and suggest the use of the left lateral Sims' position instead of the traditional lithotomy position. Because the vaginal orifice may have narrowed with age, the insertion of the traditional speculum may cause discomfort or admit only the passage of one finger.

Nurses must conduct educational programs in community settings that dispel these myths that surround menopause and aging and provide factual information on the early signs and symptoms of the common gynecologic cancers in older women, as well as discuss methods to make the gynecologic examination more comfortable for the woman. Women taking estrogens should be advised that they should be routinely monitored by their physician in terms of an examination to detect endometrial cancer.[172,173]

Nurses need to be aware that older women are at high risk for endometrial, vulvar, vaginal, and ovarian cancer. Several premalignant conditions commonly found in elderly women predispose them to gynecologic cancers. These premalignant conditions are leukoplakic vulvitis, which precedes epidermoid carcinoma; lichen sclerosus et atrophicus, which precedes epidermoid carcinoma; and endometrial adenoma, which precedes hyperplastic lesions. Normal changes that occur with aging frequently obscure the early symptoms of cancer. The vaginal mucosa thins with aging, and there is a decrease in vaginal/cervical lubrication. Bleeding that results from endometrial or vaginal cancer is shrugged off as normal

**TABLE 8-8**   Classification and Comparative Nomenclature of Cervical Smears

| |
|---|
| **Class I**<br>Normal smear<br>No abnormal cells |
| **Class II**<br>Atypical cells present below the level of cervical neoplasia |
| **Class III**<br>Smear contains abnormal cells consistent with dysplasia<br>　Mild dysplasia　　　= CIN 1<br>　Moderate dysplasia = CIN 2 |
| **Class IV**<br>Smear contains abnormal cells consistent with carcinoma in situ<br>　Severe dysplasia and carcinoma in situ = CIN 3 |
| **Class V**<br>Smear contains abnormal cells consistent with invasive carcinoma of squamous cell origin |

*CIN,* cervical intraepithelial neoplasia.

Nelson J, Averette H, Richart R: Dysplasia, carcinoma in situ, and early invasive cervical carcinoma. *CA Cancer J Clin* 34:307, 1984. Courtesy of James H. Nelson Jr.

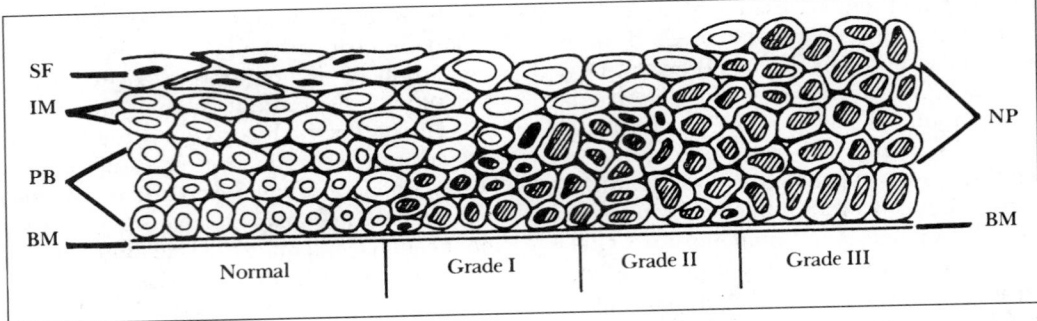

**FIGURE 8-18**   Cervical intraepithelial neoplasia *(CIN)*, showing infiltrating normal epithelium. CIN is dysplasia that occurs in the transformation zone. When CIN is suspected from abnormalities seen on a Pap smear of cervical secretions, a colposcopic examination should be done. (*SF* = superficial cells; *IM* = intermediate cells; *PB* = parabasal cells; *BM* = basement membrane; *NP* = neoplastic cells). *Grades* refer to degree of epithelium involved by dysplasia. *Grade I* = ¼ in thickness; *grade II* = ¼–¾ thickness; and *grade III* = ¾ to full thickness of epithelium. (McCauley K, Oi R: Evaluating the Papanicolaou smear: Part I. *Consultant* 28(12):31–40, 1988.)

"postmenopausal bleeding" or attributed by health professionals to atrophic vaginitis and often is not followed up.[162]

Young women who have had venereal disease (syphilis, gonorrhea, genital herpes, or HPV infection) must be alert to the necessity of having regular Pap smears. Women with vulvar condyloma acuminatum should be referred for a thorough examination of the vagina, cervix, and perirectal epithelium with the use of acetic acid compress application, a colposcopic examination, and a Pap smear. It also is recommended that these women (and infected male partners) have frequent follow-up examinations to detect precancerous conditions caused by a latent virus in clinically and histologically normal tissue.[158] Infection of the genital tract by HPV is a common disease and often encountered in clinics for family planning, prenatal care, and sexually transmitted diseases. Women whose Pap smears indicate the presence of warty infections such as koilocytotic cells or who show cells consistent with squamous papilloma or warty atypia also should be referred to a physician for further evaluation.[174]

Nurses are urged to acquire physical assessment skills that will enable them to perform pelvic examinations. It has been documented that nurses who perform pelvic examinations can detect gynecologic malignancies, that patient acceptance and satisfaction are high, and that pelvic examinations done by nurses are cost-effective.[162,175]

Nurses trained to conduct gynecologic examinations are in an ideal position to reach those women who are at highest risk for the development of various types of gynecologic cancers but who are least likely to use conventional screening programs or have routine health examinations, such as older women in residential settings or older poor women in the community. Nurses actively involved in conducting pelvic examinations would increase the availability of screening programs and thus reach more women.[175]

## REFERENCES

1. The National Cancer Institute Act, Aug. 5, 1937. PL 244, 75th Congress, 1st Session. Chapter 565 (S. 2067)
2. The National Cancer Act of 1971. *J Natl Cancer Inst* 48: 577–584, 1972
3. Schottenfeld D, Fraumeni JF: *Cancer Epidemiology and Prevention.* Philadelphia, Saunders, 1982
4. Vessey MP, Gray M: *Cancer Risks and Prevention.* Oxford, Engl., Oxford University Press, 1985
5. Enstrom J, Austin D: Interpreting cancer survival rates, in Kruse L, Reese J, Hart L (eds): *Cancer: Pathophysiology, Etiology and Management.* St. Louis, Mosby, 1979, pp 28–37
6. Bailar JC, Smith EM: Progress against cancer. *N Engl J Med* 314:1226–1232, 1986
7. Hamburg D: Healthy people: The surgeon general's report on health promotion and disease prevention, background papers. Washington, DC, DHEW publication No. (PHS) 79-55071A, 1979, p 162
8. Schottenfeld D: *Cancer Epidemiology and Prevention: Current Concepts.* Springfield, IL, Thomas, 1975
9. Pollner F: Debate over cancer survival rate is heating up. *Medical World News* 72:Apr. 25, 1988
10. McGinnis JM, Richmond JB, Brandt EN, et al: Health progress in the United States: Results of the 1990 objectives for the nation. *JAMA* 268:2545–2552, 1992
11. Fisher S: Cancer: Prevention, screening and early diagnosis. *Aust Fam Physician* 6:269–277, 1977
12. Van Parifs LG, Eckhardt S: Public education in primary and secondary cancer prevention. *Hygiene* 111:16–28, 1984
13. Slenker S, Spreitzer EA: Public perceptions and behaviors regarding cancer control. *J Cancer Educ* 3:171–180, 1988
14. Bal DG, Nixon DW, Foerster SB, et al: Cancer prevention, in Murphy GP, Lawrence W, Lenhard RE (eds): *American Cancer Society Textbook of Oncology* (ed 2). Atlanta, GA, American Cancer Society, 1995, pp 40–63
15. Block G, Patterson B, Subar A: Fruit, vegetables, and cancer prevention: A review of the epidemiological evidence. *Nutr Cancer* 18:1–29, 1992

16. Bright MA: Public health initiatives in cancer prevention and control. *Semin Oncol Nurs* 9:139–146, 1993

17. Samuels SE: Project LEAN: A national campaign to reduce dietary fate consumption. *Am J Health Promotion* 4:435–440, 1990

18. Bal DG, Foerster SB: Dietary strategies for cancer prevention. *Cancer* 72:1005–1010, 1993 (suppl 3)

19. Weinhouse S, Bal DG, Adamson R, et al: American Cancer Society Guidelines on diet, nutrition, and cancer. *CA Cancer J Clin* 41:334–338, 1991

20. American Cancer Society: *Cancer Facts and Figures: 1996.* New York, American Cancer Society, 1996

21. Meyskens FL: Principles of cancer prevention, in Haskell CM (ed): *Cancer Treatment* (ed 4). Philadelphia, Saunders, 1995, pp 10–13

22. Smart CR, Chu KC, Conley VL, et al: Cancer screening and early detection, in Holland JF, Frei E, Bast RC, Kufe DU, Morton DL, Weichselbaum RR (eds): *Cancer Medicine* (ed 3). Philadelphia, Lea and Febiger, 1993, pp 408–431

23. Miller AB: Cancer screening, in DeVita VT, Hellman S, Rosenberg SA (eds): *Cancer: Principles and Practice of Oncology* (ed 4). Philadelphia, Lippincott, 1993, pp 564–573

24. Hospital discharge rates for four major cancers—United States, 1970–1986. *JAMA* 260:3412–3416, 1988

25. Parker SL, Tong T, Bolden S, Wingo P: Cancer statistics 1996. *CA Cancer J Clin* 46:5–27, 1996

26. Bartecchi C, MacKenzie T, Schrier R: The human costs of tobacco use. *N Engl J Med* 330:907–912, 1994

27. Fielding J, Phenow J: Health effects of involuntary smoking. *N Engl J Med* 319:1452–1460, 1988

28. Humble C, Samet J, Pathak D: Marriage to a smoker and lung cancer risk. *Am J Public Health* 77:598–601, 1987

29. Stellman J, Stellman S: Occupational lung disease and cancer risk in women. *Occup Health Nurs* 31:40–46, 1983

30. Goldman R, Peters J: The occupational and environmental health history. *JAMA* 246:2832–2836, 1981

31. National Cancer Institute: *Asbestos Exposure.* DHEW publication No. 78-1622. Washington, DC, National Cancer Institute, 1978

32. Grimes J, Burns E (eds): *Health Assessment in Nursing Practice* (ed 2). Boston, Jones and Bartlett, 1987

33. Buckingham W: *A Primer of Clinical Diagnosis* (ed 2). New York, Harper & Row, 1979

34. Kadunce D, Burr R, Gress R, et al: Cigarette smoking: Risk factor for premature facial wrinkling. *Ann Intern Med* 114:840–844, 1991

35. Rohwedder J: Neoplastic disease, in Guenter C, Welch M (eds): *Pulmonary Medicine.* Philadelphia, Lippincott, 1977, pp 300–320

36. DeGowin E, DeGowin R: *Bedside Diagnostic Examination* (ed 5). New York, Macmillan, 1987

37. Guarino J: Auscultatory-percussion, a technique for detecting unsuspected lung disease. *Diagnosis* January: 20–26, 1981

38. Bates B: *A Guide to Physical Examination* (ed 3). Philadelphia, Lippincott, 1983

39. Burns K, Johnson P: *Health Assessment in Clinical Practice* (ed 2). Englewood Cliffs, NJ, Prentice-Hall, 1980

40. Mao L, Hruban R, Boyle J, et al: Detection of oncogene mutations in sputum precedes diagnosis of lung cancer. *Cancer Res* 54:1634–1637, 1994

41. Fielding J: Smoking: Health effects and control. *N Engl J Med* 313:491–498, 1985

42. Fiore M, Novotny T, Pierce J, et al: Trends in cigarette smoking in the United States. The changing influence of gender and race. *JAMA* 261:49–55, 1989

43. Novello AC, Davis RM, Giovino GA: The slowing of the lung cancer epidemic and the need for continued vigilance. *CA Cancer J Clin* 41:133–136, 1991

44. Davis RM: The ledger of tobacco control. Is the cup half empty or half full? *JAMA* 275:1261–1284, 1996 (editorial)

45. Pierce J, Fiore M, Novotny T, et al: Trends in cigarette smoking in the United States. Educational differences are increasing. *JAMA* 261:56–60, 1989

46. Davis R: Current trends in cigarette advertising and marketing. *N Engl J Med* 316:725–732, 1987

47. Ernster V: Trends in smoking, cancer risk, and cigarette promotion: Current priorities for reducing tobacco exposure. *Cancer* 62:1702–1712, 1988

48. Hermanson B, Omenn G, Kronmal R, et al: Participants in the Coronary Artery Surgery Study: Beneficial six-year outcome of smoking cessation in older men and women with coronary artery disease. *N Engl J Med* 319:1365–1369, 1988

49. Koop report equates nicotine with narcotic addiction. *Oncology & Biotechnology News* 2(6):3, 1988

50. Benowitz N, Jacob P, Kozlowski L, et al: Influence of smoking fewer cigarettes on exposure to tar, nicotine, and carbon monoxide. *N Engl J Med* 315:1310–1313, 1986

51. Anda R, Remington P, Sienko D, et al: Are physicians advising smokers to quit? The patient's perspective. *JAMA* 257:1916–1919, 1987

52. Smith J: Letter to the editor. *JAMA* 258:472, 1987

53. U.S. Preventive Services Task Force: Recommendations for smoking cessation counseling. *JAMA* 259:2882, 1988

54. Kottke T, Battista R, Defriese G, et al: Attributes of successful smoking cessation interventions in medical practice. A meta-analysis of 39 controlled trials. *JAMA* 259:2883–2889, 1988

55. Fiore MC, Wetter DW, Bailey WC, et al: *Smoking Cessation Clinical Practice Guideline.* Rockville, MD: Agency for Health Care Policy and Research, Public Health Service, U.S. Dept. of Health and Human Services, 1996

56. Gritz E: Cigarette smoking: The need for action by health professionals, *CA Cancer J Clin* 38:194–212, 1988

57. Orleans CT: Understanding and promoting smoking cessation: Overview and guidelines for physician intervention. *Annu Rev Med* 36:51–61, 1985

58. Altman D, Flora J, Fortmann S, et al: The cost-effectiveness of three smoking cessation programs. *Am J Public Health* 77:162–165, 1987

59. New rules extinguish "smoking lamp" in growing number of public places. *JAMA* 259:2809, 1988

60. Longo DR, Brownson RC, Johnson JC, et al: Hospital smoking bans and employee smoking behavior. Results of a national survey. *JAMA* 275:1252–1257, 1996

61. Schuster M: Disorders of the aging GI system, in Reichel W (ed): *The Geriatric Patient.* New York, HP Publishers, 1978, pp 73–81

62. Bunn PA, Ridgway EC: Paraneoplastic syndromes, in DeVita VT, Hellman S, Rosenberg SA (eds): *Cancer: Principles and Practice of Oncology* (ed 4). Philadelphia, Lippincott, 1993, pp 2026–2071

63. Leffall L: *Early Diagnosis of Colorectal Cancer.* New York, American Cancer Society [Professional Education Publication 81-50M-No. 3311-PE], 1981

64. Mandel J, Bond J, Church T, et al: Reducing mortality from colorectal cancer by screening for fecal occult blood. *N*

*Engl J Med* 328:1365–1371, 1993 [Erranum *N Engl J Med* 329:329; 672, 1993]

65. Castiglione G, Biangini M, Barchielli A, et al: Effect of rehydration on guaiac-based fecal occult blood testing in colorectal cancer screening. *Br J Cancer* 67:1142–1144, 1993

66. Reiventer J, Brevinge H, Engarás B, et al: Results of screening, rescreening, and follow-up in a prospective randomized study of colorectal cancer by fecal occult blood test. *Scand J Gastroenterol* 29:468–473, 1994

67. Sugarbaker P, Gunderson L, Wittes R: Colorectal cancer, in DeVita VT, Hellman S, Rosenberg SA (eds): *Cancer: Principles and Practice of Oncology* (ed 2). Philadelphia, Lippincott, 1986, pp 795–884

68. De Cosse J, Tsioulias G, Jacobson J: Colorectal cancer: Detection, treatment, and rehabilitation. *CA Cancer J Clin* 44:27–42, 1994

69. Solomon M, McLeod R: Canadian Task Force on the Periodic Health Examination: Periodic health examination, 1994 update: 2. Screening strategies for colorectal cancer. *Can Med Assoc J* 15:150:1961–1970, 1994

70. Rakel R: A clinician's guide: Tips on fecal occult blood testing. *Your Patient & Cancer* 3:33–38, 1983

71. Simon J: Occult blood screening for colorectal carcinoma. A critical review. *Gastroenterology* 88:820–837, 1985

72. Winawer S: Introduction to position papers from the Third International Symposium on Colorectal Cancer. *CA Cancer J Clin* 35:130–133, 1985

73. Nakama H, Kamijo N: Accuracy of immunological fecal occult blood testing for colorectal cancer screening. *Prev Med* 23:309–313, 1994

74. Robinson M, Pye G, Thomas J, et al: Haemoccult screening for colorectal cancer: The effect of dietary restriction on compliance. *Eur J Surg Oncol* 20:545–548, 1994

75. Poll finds public misconceptions re colorectal cancer detection. *Oncology Times*, September 9, 1986, p 25

76. Callahan L: Colorectal cancer: Clinical trial/community outreach. Proceedings of the Fourth National Cancer Communications Conference. DHEW publication No. (PHS) 78-1463. Washington, DC, National Institutes of Health, 1977

77. Greenwald P, Sondik E, Lynch B: Diet and chemoprevention in NCI's research strategy to achieve national cancer control objectives. *Annu Rev Public Health* 7:267–291, 1986

78. American Cancer Society Special Report: *Nutrition and Cancer: Cause and Prevention.* New York, American Cancer Society [Professional Education Publication 84-50M-No. 3389-PE], 1984

79. Kritchevsky D: Diet and cancer. *CA Cancer J Clin* 41:328–333, 1991

80. The Work Study Group on Diet, Nutrition, and Cancer: American Cancer Society Guidelines on diet, nutrition, and cancer. *CA* 41:334–338, 1991

81. The changing diet: Illinois 1982–1986. *American Cancer Society Cancer Prevention Study II Newsletter* 5(2):3, Fall 1987

82. Chodak G, Schoenberg H: Early detection of prostate cancer by routine screening. *JAMA* 252:3261–3264, 1984

83. National Cancer Institute: *Cancer Among Blacks and Other Minorities: Statistical Profiles.* NIH publication No. 86-2785. Washington, DC, National Cancer Institute, 1986

84. Guinan P, Sharifi R, Bush I: Prostate cancer: Tips toward earlier detection. *Your Patient & Cancer* 4:37–42, 1984

85. Chodak G: Screening for prostate cancer, the debate continues. *JAMA* 272:813–814, 1994

86. Sox H: Preventative health services in adults. *N Engl J Med* 330:1589–1595, 1994

87. Feightner J: The early detection and treatment of prostate cancer: The perspective of the Canadian Task Force on the Periodic Health Examination. *J Urol* 152:1682–1684, 1994

88. Lange P: New information about prostate-specific antigen and the paradoxes of prostate cancer. *JAMA* 273:336–337, 1995

89. Handley M, Stuart M: The use of prostate-specific antigen for prostate cancer screening: A managed care perspective. *J Urol* 152:1689–1692, 1994

90. Krahn M, Mahoney J, Eckman M, Trachtenberg J, et al: Screening for prostate cancer: A decision analytic view. *JAMA* 272:773–780, 1994

91. Garnick M, Fair W: Prostate cancer: Emerging concepts. Part I. *Ann Intern Med* 125:118–125, 1996

92. Littrup P, Goodman A, Mettlin C: The Investigators of the American Cancer Society-National Prostate Cancer Detection Project: the benefit and cost of prostate cancer early detection. *CA Cancer J Clin* 43:134–149, 1993

93. Gann P, Hennekens C, Stampfer M: A prospective evaluation of plasma prostate-specific antigen for detection of prostate cancer. *JAMA* 273:289–294, 1995

94. Henderson IC: Breast cancer, in Murphy GP, Lawrence W, Lenhard RE (eds): *American Cancer Society Textbook of Oncology.* Atlanta, GA, American Cancer Society, 1995, pp 198–219

95. American Cancer Society: *Breast Cancer Facts and Figures 1996.* Atlanta, GA, American Cancer Society, 1996

96. Wilkes B: The development of a two-tier BSE educational program, in *Progress in Cancer Control III: A Regional Approach.* New York, Alan R. Liss, 1983, pp 127–131

97. Olsen S: *Examinations for Detecting Breast Cancer.* Cancer Prevention Program, Wisconsin Clinical Cancer Center, 1300 University Ave-7C, Medical Science Center, Madison, WI 53706

98. Scanlon E: A photo checklist for a better breast palpation. *Primary Care & Cancer* 7:13–20, 1987

99. Heymann A: Semilateral decubitus breast examination. *JAMA* 243:1713, 1980

100. Feig S: Mammography screening: Published guidelines and actual practice. *Recent Results Cancer Res* 105:78–88, 1987

101. Update January 1992: The American Cancer Society guidelines for the cancer-related checkup. *CA Cancer J Clin* 42:44–45, 1992

102. Greenwald P, Sondik E: *Cancer Control Objectives for the Nation: 1985–2000.* NIH publication No. 86-2880, no. 8. Washington, DC, National Institutes of Health, 1986

103. Dodd G: Screening for the early detection of breast cancer. *Cancer* 62:1781–1783, 1988

104. Tabar L, Fagerberg C, Gad A, et al: Reduction in mortality from breast cancer after mass screening with mammography. *Lancet* 1:829–832, 1984

105. Boyd J (ed): New analysis of HIP study supports mammographic screening age 40–49. *Cancer Lett* 14(37):4–6, 1988

106. Frank J, Mai V: Breast self-examination in young women: More harm than good? *Lancet* 2:654–657, 1985

107. Foster R, Costanza M, Worden J: The current status of research in breast self-examination. *NY State J Med* 85:480–482, 1985

108. U.S. Preventive Services Task Force: Recommendations for breast cancer screening. *JAMA* 257:2196, 1987

109. O'Malley M, Fletcher S: Screening for breast cancer with breast self-examination. A critical review. *JAMA* 257: 2197–2203, 1987

110. Feldman J: Breast self-examination—A practice whose time has come? *NY State J Med* 85:482–483, 1985

111. Huguley C, Brown R, Greenberg R, et al: Breast self-examination and survival from breast cancer. *Cancer* 62: 1389–1396, 1988

112. Bennett S, Lawrence R, Fleischmann K, et al: Profile of women practicing breast self-examination. *JAMA* 249: 488–491, 1983

113. Kegeles S: Education for breast self-examination: Why, who, what, and how? *Prev Med* 14:702–720, 1985

114. Study shows survival advantage for women who examine their breasts. *Medical World News* 25:31, 1984

115. Boyle M, Michalek A, Bersani G, et al: Effectiveness of a community program to promote early breast cancer detection. *J Surg Oncol* 18:183–188, 1981

116. Diem G, Rose D: Has breast self-examination had a fair trial? *NY State J Med* 85:479–480, 1985

117. Styrd A: A breast self-examination program in an occupational health setting. *Occup Health Nurs* 30:33–35, 1982

118. Shamian J, Edgar L: Nurses as agents for change in teaching breast self-examination. *Public Health Nurs* 4:29–34, 1987

119. Kassabian VS, Graham SD: Urologic and male genital cancers, in Murphy GP, Lawrence W, Lenhard RE (eds): *American Cancer Society Textbook of Oncology.* Atlanta, GA, American Cancer Society, 1995, pp 311–329

120. Swanson D: Why you should conscientiously promote self-examination. *Consultant* 27(4):142–147, 1987

121. Carlin P: Testicular self-examination: A public awareness program. *Public Health Rep* 101(1):98–102, 1986

122. Conklin M, Klint K, Morway A, et al: Should health teaching include self-examination of the testis? *Am J Nurs* 78: 2073–2074, 1978

123. Blesch K: Health beliefs about testicular cancer and self-examination among professional men. *Oncol Nurs Forum* 13(1):29–33, 1986

124. Smith J, Hollenbeck Z: Genitalia, in Prior J, Silberstein J, Stang J (eds): *Physical Diagnosis. The History and Examination of the Patient.* St. Louis, Mosby, 1981, pp 330–364

125. Richie J: Detection and treatment of testicular cancer. *CA Cancer J Clin* 43:151–175, 1993

126. Boyd J (ed): Office urology: When your patient fears testicular cancer. *Patient Care* 9:102, 1975

127. Frank-Stromborg M: The role of the nurse in cancer detection and screening. *Semin Oncol Nurs* 2:191–199, 1986

128. Garnick M: Urologic cancer, in Rubenstein E, Federman D (eds): *Oncology,* vol. 9. New York, Scientific American Medicine, 1988, pp 1–17

129. Murray B, Wilcox L: Testicular self-examination. *Am J Nurs* 78:2074–2075, 1978

130. Malasanos L, Barkauskas V, Moss M, et al: *Health Assessment.* St. Louis, Mosby, 1986, pp 401–414

131. White L: The nurse's role in cancer prevention, in Newell G (ed): *Cancer Prevention in Clinical Medicine.* New York, Raven Press, 1983, pp 91–112

132. Rigel DS: Malignant melanoma: Perspectives on incidence and its effects on awareness, diagnosis, and treatment. *CA Cancer J Clin* 46:195–198, 1996

133. Friedman RJ, Rigel DS, Silverman MK, et al: Malignant melanoma in the 1990s: The continued importance of early detection and the role of physician examination and

self-examination of the skin. *CA Cancer J Clin* 41:201–226, 1991

134. Legha S: Malignant melanoma. Pitfalls and controversies in diagnosis and treatment. *Consultant* 28(6):111–124, 1988

135. Schleper J: Cancer prevention and detection: Skin cancer. *Cancer Nurs* 7:67–84, 1984

136. White L, Patterson J, Cornelius J, et al: *Cancer Screening and Detection Manual for Nurses.* New York, McGraw-Hill, 1979, pp 9–16

137. Finley C: Malignant melanoma: A primary care perspective. *Nurse Pract* 11(4):18–38, 1986

138. Fitzpatrick T, Rhodes A, Sober A: Prevention of melanoma by recognition of its precursors. *N Engl J Med* 312:115–116, 1985

139. Smith T, Mihm M, Sober A: Malignant melanoma, in *Cancer Manual* (ed 7). New York, American Cancer Society, Massachusetts Division, 1986, pp 106–113

140. Helm F, Helm J: On guard against skin cancer, in Murphy G (ed): *Cancer. Signals and Safeguards.* Littleton, MA: PSG Publishing, 1981, pp 67–80

141. Epstein E: *Common Skin Disorders. A Manual for Physicians and Patients.* Oradell, NJ: Medical Economics, 1979

142. Rhodes A, Weinstock M, Fitzpatrick T, et al: Risk factors for cutaneous melanoma. A practical method of recognizing predisposed individuals. *JAMA* 258:3146–3154, 1987

143. Ketcham M, Loescher LJ: Skin cancers, in Groenwald SL, Frogge MH, Goodman M, Yarbro CH (eds): *Cancer Nursing: Principles and Practice* (ed 3). Boston, Jones and Bartlett, 1993, pp 1238–1257

144. Diekmann J: Cancer in the elderly: Systems overview. *Semin Oncol Nurs* 4:169–177, 1988

145. Wood N: Oral cancer: An overview. *Ill Dental J* 57:323, 1988

146. Winn D: Smokeless tobacco and cancer: The epidemiologic evidence. *CA Cancer J Clin* 38:236–243, 1988

147. Sawyer D, Wood N, Lehnert J: Examination, detection, diagnosis and referral. *Ill Dental J* 57:326–329, 1988

148. Mashberg A, Samit A: Early detection of asymptomatic oral and oropharyngeal squamous cancers. *CA Cancer J Clin* 45: 328–351, 1995

149. Holmstrup P, Pindborg J: Oral mucosal lesions in smokeless tobacco users. *CA Cancer J Clin* 38:230–235, 1988

150. Kabot T, Heffez L, Bergschneider J: Prevention, detection and referral. Responsibility of the dental team: Prevention and patient education. *Ill Dental J* 57:324–325, 1988

151. Squier C: The nature of smokeless tobacco and patterns of use. *CA Cancer J Clin* 38:226–229, 1988

152. Benowitz N: Nicotine and smokeless tobacco. *CA Cancer J Clin* 38:244–247, 1988

153. Schroeder K, Iaderosa G, Chen M, et al: Bimodal initiation of smokeless tobacco usage: Implications for cancer education. *Cancer Education* 2:15–21, 1987

154. Grabau J: Oral/facial self-examination, in Nieburgs H (ed): *Prevention and Detection of Cancer. Part I* (vol 2), Prevention. New York, Marcel Dekker, 1978, pp 2263–2274

155. Williams T: Ovarian cancer. Fewest signs, greatest challenge. *Diagnosis* 3(5):53–60, 1981

156. White L: Cancer prevention and detection: Cervical cancer. *Cancer Nurs* 7:335–345, 1984

157. Beecham J, Helmkamp BF, Rubin P: Tumors of the female genital tract, in Rubin P (ed): *Clinical Oncology for Medical Students and Physicians* (ed 6). New York, American Cancer Society, 1983, pp 428–481

158. Mitchell MF, Sandella JA, White LN: Cervical cancer: The role of the human papillomavirus, in Hubbard SM, Greene

PE, Knobf MT (eds): *Current Issues in Cancer Nursing Practice Updates*. Philadelphia, Lippincott, 1992, pp 1–9

159. Koss L: The Papanicolaou test for cervical cancer detection. A triumph and a tragedy. *JAMA* 261:737–743, 1989

160. Jones H: Vaginal cancer. Common signs, uncommon cause. *Diagnosis* 3(5):71–85, 1981

161. Nelson J, Averette H, Richart R: Dysplasia, carcinoma in situ, and early invasive cervical carcinoma. *CA Cancer J Clin* 34:306–327, 1984

162. Persky V, Davis F, Barrett R, et al: Recent time trends in uterine cancer. *Am J Pub Health* 80:935–939, 1990

163. Fink D: Change in American Cancer Society checkup guidelines for detection of cervical cancer. *CA Cancer J Clin* 38:127–128, 1988

164. Stenkvist B, Bergstrom R, Eklund G, et al: Papanicolaou smear screening and cervical cancer. What can you expect? *JAMA* 252:1423–1426, 1984

165. Brooks S: Cervical cancer screening and the older woman. *Cancer Pract* 4:125–129, 1996

166. Mandelblatt J, Fahs M: The cost-effectiveness of cervical cancer screening for low-income elderly women. *JAMA* 259:2409–2413, 1988

167. Eddy DM: Screening for cervical cancer. *Ann Int Med* 113:214–226, 1990

168. Diagnosing cervical cancer by measuring DNA content. *Primary Care & Cancer* 8:13, 1988

169. Jones G: Densitometric screening found accurate for detecting cervical cancer. *Oncology & Biotechnology News* 2(2):3, 1988

170. Lovejoy N: Precancerous lesions of the cervix. Personal risk factors. *Cancer Nurs* 10:2–14, 1987

171. McCauley K, Oi R: Evaluating the Papanicolaou smear: Part I. *Consultant* 29(12):31–40, 1988

172. Braunstein G: The benefits of estrogen to the menopausal woman outweigh the risks of developing endometrial cancer [Opinion: Pro]. *CA Cancer J Clin* 34:210–219, 1984

173. Morrow C: The benefits of estrogen to the menopausal woman outweigh the risks of developing endometrial cancer [Opinion: Con]. *CA Cancer J Clin* 34:220–231, 1984

174. Jones W, Saigo P: The "atypical" Papanicolaou smear. *CA Cancer J Clin* 36:237–242, 1986

175. Stromborg M, Nord S: A cancer detection clinic: Patient motivation and satisfaction. *Nurse Pract* 4:10–14, 1979

# Chapter 9

# Diagnostic Evaluation, Classification, and Staging

Sharon Saldin O'Mary, RN, MN, OCN®

## DIAGNOSTIC EVALUATION

### Factors That Affect the Diagnostic Approach

Cancer is a significant health care problem in this country. The etiology of most cancers remains unknown and cancer prevention measures are complicated by multiple economic, behavioral, social, and cultural factors. Early detection efforts and comprehensive diagnostic evaluations hold the most promise for controlling the associated morbidity and cost of the cancer illness. This chapter focuses on the process of diagnostic evaluation, classification, and staging when a suspicion of cancer exists for an individual.

The major goals of the diagnostic evaluation for a suspected cancer are to determine the tissue type of the malignancy, the primary site of the malignancy, the extent of disease within the body, and the tumor's potential to recur in the future. This information is the critical first step in planning the therapeutic management. The approach to the diagnostic evaluation depends on the following factors: the person's presenting signs and symptoms, the person's clinical status and ability to tolerate invasive procedures, the anticipated goal of treatment when the diagnosis is made, the biological characteristics of the suspected malignancy, the diagnostic equipment available in the community, and the third-party payer approval of diagnostic procedures.

The diagnosis and staging of cancer have been affected by rapidly changing technology in imaging modalities and biochemical analysis. Historically there has been a progression from the gross evaluation of a tumor mass at surgery to the assessment of genetic expression and structure of tumor cells to diagnose and predict the natural history of the disease.

Even with the sophisticated armamentarium presently available for cancer diagnosis, the key to survival continues to be early detection of disease. The discovery of a precancerous lesion or a malignant neoplasm at its earliest stage affords the very best opportunity for cure, extended survival, and less extensive treatment. For example, the nonpalpable breast mass found on a screening mammogram or the isolated tumor found incidentally on a chest film is more likely to be diagnosed as localized disease amenable to treatment and cure. More typically, the tumor goes undetected until specific signs or symptoms become apparent and prompt the person to consult a health professional.

Frequently, these symptoms include the complaints of weight loss, persistent pain, unexplained fever, fatigue, or one of the seven warning signals that have brought the early detection of cancer into public awareness.[1] Unfortunately, many of the people at greatest risk for developing cancer have an inadequate understanding of the importance of early attention to symptoms. A study of cancer knowledge among the elderly revealed an inability to recall more than one or two of the seven warning signals of cancer and a lack of awareness that elderly individuals have an increased cancer risk.[2] Table 9-1 identifies the most common warning signals of cancer, the significance of each signal or symptom, and the persons at greatest risk for developing an associated malignancy.[1,3]

The worst prognosis can be expected in those people who delay seeking medical evaluation at the onset of their symptoms, in those cancers for which technological methods are unavailable to make an early diagnosis, and in people for whom the primary lesion cannot be found. For the person who presents with widespread extensive disease, the palliative goal of treatment may direct and abbreviate an otherwise exhaustive and expensive diagnostic workup.

An effective clinical evaluation of the person with a suspected malignancy includes a comprehensive history with the identification of known risk factors, a thorough physical examination, laboratory and imaging tests, and perhaps most importantly, the histological verification of the malignancy. Known biological characteristics of the suspected malignancy and the typical routes of regional and distant metastases will direct the approach of further diagnostic and staging procedures. In some situations, extensive laboratory and imaging examinations precede tissue biopsy in the attempt to locate the primary tumor or an accessible tumor. In other patients, results of a biopsy specimen that confirm the presence of malignancy direct further testing that will be done to accurately stage the extent of disease. Those tests that are the least taxing to the individual, that are cost effective, and that yield the information necessary for treatment planning are considered.

In the present era of cost containment in health care, the judicious selection and sequencing of diagnostic studies are stressed. The proper test is one that yields information on the suspicious site of malignancy and complements rather than merely confirms known information. The relative benefits of competing imaging technologies such as computed tomography and magnetic resonance imaging are being evaluated for several organ sites by the Radiology Diagnostic Oncology Group, a cooperative group funded by the National Cancer Institute.[4–6] The increased availability of sophisticated equipment, the fear of litigation, and pressure from patients and families are all factors that influence the physician to overinvestigate. At least one study has indicated that patients believed extensive test ordering correlated with physician quality.[7]

It is apparent that third-party payers, prospective payment systems, and managed care networks also play an important role as gatekeepers in the diagnostic evaluation. Blue Cross of California is an example of a health insurance provider with published practice guidelines for breast cancer screening, diagnosis, staging, and treatment.[8] It is also likely that diagnostic evaluations will be completed in the ambulatory setting unless patients are acutely ill, requiring hospitalization.

### Nursing Implications in Diagnostic Evaluation

Many opportunities exist for nurses to promote the early detection and diagnosis of cancer. Serving as role models

**TABLE 9-1** Seven Warning Signals of Cancer and Their Significance

| Warning Signals | Significance of Warning Signal | Persons at Greatest Risk |
|---|---|---|
| Change in bowel or bladder habits | Changes in stool caliber and regular bowel function are frequent signs of colorectal cancer; dependent on the area of intestine involved. A change in bladder function, frequency, dysuria, retention, or hematuria may indicate prostate or bladder cancer. | *Colorectal cancer:* over age 40, personal or family history of polyps or colorectal cancer, family history of polyposis syndromes, inflammatory bowel disease<br>*Prostate cancer:* over age 65, black males<br>*Bladder cancer:* smokers, males, chemical exposure |
| Unusual bleeding or discharge | Any unusual bleeding or discharge can signify malignancy. Occult or bright red blood may be seen with colorectal cancer. Abnormal vaginal bleeding is the most frequent sign of endometrial or cervical cancer. A clear, milky, or bloody discharge from the nipple is the second-most common symptom of breast cancer. Hemoptysis is a sign of lung cancer. Hematuria is the most frequent sign of bladder cancer and is also seen in renal and prostate cancer. | *Endometrial cancer:* postmenopausal women over age 50, family history of endometrial cancer, obesity, diabetes, hypertension, prolonged estrogen administration<br>*Cervix cancer:* first vaginal intercourse at early age, multiple sexual partners, genital human papillomavirus, smokers |
| A sore that does not heal | Delayed healing of a sore or a change in a skin lesion's size, color, or shape, particularly on a surface exposed to ultraviolet light, can represent basal cell or squamous cell cancer. Oral lesions and leukoplakia, particularly in tobacco or alcohol users, need careful follow-up. Persistent sores or itching of the vulva can indicate a preinvasive or malignant lesion. | *Skin cancer (nonmelanoma):* exposure to UV radiation, psoralens, and UV light, or chemical carcinogens; fair-skinned Caucasians<br>*Oral cancer:* males, over age 40, tobacco users (chewed or smoked), pipe smokers, combined tobacco and alcohol use |
| Obvious change in wart or mole | A change in a mole's color and pigmentation pattern, irregularities in border or surface topography, or increasing size causes suspicion of malignancy. Occurs in areas protected from or exposed to the sun. | *Melanoma:* fair-skinned Caucasians with history of sun exposure, family or personal history of melanoma or dysplastic nevi, large congenital moles |
| Thickening or lump in breast or elsewhere | A painless lump or mass is most common presenting sign in cancer of the breast, testis, and soft-tissue sarcoma. Persistent enlarged lymph nodes can signify lymphoma or metastatic nodal disease. | *Breast cancer:* all women, particularly over age 50, personal or family history of breast cancer, nulliparity or first child after age 30<br>*Testis cancer:* males aged 20–35, undescended testes |
| Nagging cough or hoarseness | Persistent, productive cough is the most frequently reported symptom of lung cancer. Hoarseness may indicate lung, laryngeal, or thyroid cancer. | *Lung cancer:* all smokers, black males, history of asbestos exposure<br>*Larynx cancer:* males over age 50, combined tobacco and alcohol use |
| Indigestion or difficulty in swallowing | Indigestion, gastroesophageal reflux, painful "spasms" after eating, or difficulty swallowing can be symptoms of cancer of the esophagus, stomach, or pharynx. | *Stomach cancer:* males over age 50, Japanese emigrants, history of pernicious anemia<br>*Esophagus cancer:* males over age 60, history of Barrett's esophagus, achalasia, caustic injury to esophagus |

by incorporating early detection practices into their personal health care is a beginning point. As respected members of the health profession, nurses are consulted formally and informally about perceived signs or symptoms of cancer. It is imperative not only that nurses be able to recognize and understand the meaning of a clinical sign, but that they assess the individual's risk for cancer and then take responsibility for encouraging investigation and intervention.[9] Nurses can facilitate entry into the health care system by encouraging appropriate follow-up without delay, providing accurate information on cancer detection and diagnostic procedures, clarifying misconceptions, and referring to trusted health care providers or community programs. Frank-Stromborg and Rohan provide an extensive review of nursing involvement in cancer prevention and early detection and point out that efforts have been concentrated in the areas of breast, cervical, and lung cancer.[10]

Table 9-1 presents information on the significance of early warning signals of cancer and can be used by nurses to design education programs for the community that target individuals who are at the highest risk for developing a malignancy and are most likely to delay seeking medical attention. The program content should stress the importance of recognizing symptoms early to improve survival. The rationale should be given for participating in screening or annual physical examinations that include rectal and pelvic examinations. Nurses proficient in physical assessment and screening techniques can perform early detection and diagnostic procedures, including digital rectal examinations, sigmoidoscopy, pelvic examinations and Papanicolaou tests, and testicular and breast examinations.[11–13] Integrating instruction on breast self-examination or testicular self-examination can be done by nurses in most practice settings. Displaying posters and pamphlets from the American Cancer Society that identify warning signals and recommendations for a cancer-related checkup is a free and effective way to reach many people. Educational programs will be most accessible and acceptable if they are community based in the local church, work site, shopping center, health fair, senior center, or wherever participation can be maximized. Successful examples of this include a testicular and prostate cancer awareness program presented to 3000 men at their work site, a breast cancer screening and awareness program for Chinese American women at a Chinese YWCA, and a colorectal screening and education program in community black churches.[14–16]

Nurses are integral members of the professional team providing support to individuals facing the potential threat of cancer. The time elapsed between the discovery of a suspicious symptom, such as a breast lump, and the seeking of medical attention and the completion of diagnostic evaluation will vary in every situation, and for many reasons. However, the potential for stress, disruption, anxiety, and fear exists for every person and family member. Marino and Kooser separate the prediagnostic period from the diagnostic period to identify specific patient concerns and behaviors.[17] During the prediagnostic period, any delay in seeking attention depends on the perceived threat or importance attached to the symptom, the severity of the symptom, personal beliefs about cancer and treatment, and personal and financial resources. Once the individual acts on her or his concerns and seeks medical attention, the diagnostic period begins. Anxiety about the results of examinations and fear and curiosity regarding the technology of procedures are common.[18] The emotional impact of the cancer diagnosis, once confirmed, ranges from relief, disbelief, anger, depression, and hopelessness to intellectualization.[19,20] Guilt feelings from not seeking attention earlier or from lifestyles that may have contributed to the cancer are not uncommon.[17] Professional nurses in diverse settings are able to intervene by taking time to listen to concerns, respond to questions, and provide support. Being able to project optimism and hope in a serious situation helps to counter the "worst possible" assumptions often made by the patient and family.

Oncology nurses play a key role in providing information and support to reduce the stress of going through a diagnostic evaluation for a suspected malignancy. An accurate assessment of the individual's and family's desire to know, in addition to their ability to understand, is the first step in providing this much-needed support. Educational preparation for an examination should include an explanation of the procedure to be followed, as well as a description of any physical sensations that might be expected, such as pain, discomfort, and facial flushing. The purpose of the examination, what information can and cannot be gleaned from the examination, when the results can be expected, and from whom to expect them should be identified. Reinforcing verbal information with written materials targeted for the individual has proven to be helpful.[21,22]

Nurses also must be cognizant of any potential for complications during or after a procedure, including reactions to contrast agents, bleeding, vasovagal response, and the need for intravenous analgesia or conscious sedation. Nurses may be assisting with the procedure, performing the procedure, or providing postprocedure care.

Including the family members in all aspects of the diagnostic evaluation is helpful to the individual and family and to the health care team. Families are able to reinforce instructions and information, assist with examination preparation, observe for untoward effects from procedures as well as provide emotional support for the patient. An assessment of the entire family's adjustment to the cancer diagnosis may lead to referrals for more extensive support.

Other specific nursing interventions depend on identified nursing diagnoses. These might include[23]:

1. knowledge deficits related to lack of exposure to or misconceptions about cancer
2. anticipatory grieving related to the stigma of cancer or probable prognosis
3. ineffective coping related to the meaning of the diagnosis, financial stress, inadequate support, and the demands of decision making
4. spiritual distress related to challenged belief because of diagnosis
5. fear of death, treatment, and body image changes related to inability to control events and knowledge deficit
6. self-care deficit related to effects of the malignancy

## Laboratory Techniques

Laboratory studies are performed to help formulate or confirm a clinical diagnosis and to monitor the patient's response to or relapse from a specific therapy. The data provide information on the functioning of specific organs and metabolic processes that may be altered by disease or a malignant process.

Biochemical analysis of blood, serum, urine, and other body fluids identifies chemical and hematologic values outside the narrow, homeostatic range. Specific malignancies characteristically alter chemical composition of the blood, but no single value is diagnostic for a malignancy. For example, elevated serum levels of bilirubin, alkaline phosphatase, and glutamic-oxaloacetic transaminase are seen in approximately 50% of individuals presenting with liver cancer, and the abnormalities are significant in their correlation with shorter survival. Nonspecific changes such as anemia, leukocytosis or leukopenia, and thrombocytosis or thrombocytopenia also may contribute to the diagnostic evaluation.

Tumor markers are proteins, antigens, genes, ectopically produced hormones, and enzymes that are expressed by the tumor (tumor derived) or produced by normal tissue in response to the tumor (tumor associated). Markers have been recognized in serum and body fluids, in tissue, and, with recent technologies like flow cytometry, at the cellular and genetic levels.

The accuracy of a particular laboratory study or imaging technique often is reported in terms of sensitivity or specificity. *Sensitivity* establishes the percentage of people with cancer who will have positive (abnormal) test results, known as *true-positive* results. Test results of people with cancer that are negative (normal) are *false-negative* findings. *Specificity* establishes the percentage of people without cancer who will have negative (normal) test results, known as *true-negative* results. People who are free of disease and show positive (abnormal) results are considered to have *false-positive* results. A clinically useful test will detect a malignant abnormality early in its development (sensitivity) and exclude nonmalignant sources for the abnormality (specificity). In reality, many tests are highly sensitive but not very specific. The *predictive value* of a test establishes the probability that a test result correctly predicts the actual disease status.

Ideally, a tumor marker is produced exclusively by the tumor cell and not in other conditions (highly specific), is present and detectable in early, occult disease (highly sensitive), is detectable in levels directly reflecting tumor mass (proportional), predicts disease response and recurrence (predictive), and is cost effective and commercially available (feasible).[24] The only marker that approaches this ideal is human chorionic gonadotrophin in gestational trophoblastic tumors.[25] Several other markers are clinically useful in monitoring tumor activity during treatment and in detecting recurrent cancer but lack the specificity to be good screening tools. The assay for carcinoembryonic antigen is highly sensitive and correlates well with tumor burden and prognosis in gastrointestinal neoplasms.[26,27] It lacks specificity, however, because the antigen is expressed by benign as well as many different malignant cells. Table 9-2 identifies several tumor markers and their clinical significance in the diagnosis and monitoring of cancer.[28–32]

Recent technological advances in monoclonal antibody production, radioimmunoassay, and flow cytometry have provided diagnostic and prognostic information in a variety of cancers. Techniques to produce monoclonal antibodies that detect specific tumor antigens have been important to the diagnosis, classification, localization, and treatment of several solid tumors, T- and B-cell lymphomas, and leukemia. Identified tumor antigens include surface immunoglobulins (cytoplasmic membranes), surface epitopes (antigen sites), antigens in various stages of cell differentiation, and enzymes.[33]

Radioimmunoassay, an important technique in the measurement of tumor markers, determines the amount of tumor antigen in a serum sample. A known amount of radio-labeled antigen combined with antibody is added to a serum sample. The individual's unlabeled antigen displaces the radio-labeled antigen, which permits quantification.

Flow cytometry rapidly measures and identifies DNA characteristics and cell surface markers that correlate with patient prognosis and are useful to diagnose a malignancy and monitor response to therapy. A cell sorter measures fluorescence and light scatter as cells flow past an excitation source. In hematologic and lymphoid malignancies, fluorescent-marked antibodies directed against specific cell surface antigens (T-cell antigens, common acute lymphocytic leukemia antigen) help to differentiate hematopoetic cell lines. The primary application of flow cytometry analysis in solid tumors has been to determine DNA content (ploidy) and the percentage of cells synthesizing DNA (the S-phase fraction). Normal DNA is characterized as diploid and contrasts with abnormal, disorganized DNA, which is aneuploid. The proliferative potential of a tumor is measured by the percentage of cells in the synthesis phase of the cell cycle. Both of these factors—aneuploidy and high S-phase fraction—correlate with the biological aggressiveness of several tumors.[34,35] Breast cancer is a tumor in which DNA aneuploidy and high S-phase appear to be predictors of poor prognosis for women regardless of their node-negative or node-positive status. Although no standard for treatment has been established, some physicians and research protocols are incorporating this information into adjuvant treatment decisions.[36]

## Tumor Imaging

Many diagnostic procedures are available to ascertain the presence of a tumor mass, localize the mass for biopsy, provide tissue characterization, and further assess or stage the anatomical extent of disease. Although diagnostic imaging has benefited from the technology that produced computerized tomography (CT) and magnetic resonance imaging (MRI), an important role remains for the conventional diagnostic procedures. Examinations are selected that are efficient in detecting suspicious lesions and that also result in the least risk, discomfort, and expense for the individual. Table 9-3 identifies preferred imaging procedures for tumor definition and staging in several organ sites.[37–51] Table 9-4 elaborates on the patient preparation and education for select examinations.[52,53] The following section discusses imaging techniques available for diagnosis and staging.

### Radiographic techniques

Radiographic studies, or x-ray films, allow visualization of internal structures of the body. Distinction is made between normal and abnormal structure and function. X-rays or gamma rays are passed through the body, are absorbed variably by tissues of differing densities, and react on specially sensitized film or fluoroscopic screens.

**TABLE 9-2**  Selected Markers in the Diagnosis and Monitoring of Malignant Disease

| Laboratory Test | Associated Malignancy | Comments |
|---|---|---|
| **ENZYMES** | | |
| Lactic dehydrogenase (LDH) | Lymphoma, seminoma, acute leukemia, metastatic carcinoma | Elevated in 50% of patients with advanced disease; also in hepatitis and myocardial infarction |
| Prostatic acid phosphatase (PAP) | Metastatic cancer of prostate, myeloma, lung cancer, osteogenic sarcoma | Elevated in 80% of patients with bone metastases from prostate cancer; also in prostatitis, nodular prostatic hypertrophy |
| Placental alkaline phosphatase (PLAP) | Seminoma, lung, ovary, uterus | Elevated in pregnancy |
| Neuron-specific enolase (NSE) | Small-cell lung cancer, neuroendocrine tumors, neuroblastoma, medullary thyroid cancer | |
| Creatine kinase-BB | Breast, colon, ovary, prostate cancers | Elevated in bowel infarction, renal failure, stroke |
| Terminal deoxynucleotidal transferase (TdT) | Lymphoblastic malignancy | |
| **HORMONES** | | |
| Parathyroid hormone | Ectopic hyperparathyroidism from cancer of the kidney, lung (squamous cell), pancreas, ovary, myeloma | Elevated in primary hyperparathyroidism |
| Calcitonin | Medullary thyroid, small-cell lung, breast cancer, and carcinoid | |
| Antidiuretic hormone (ADH) | Small-cell lung cancer, adenocarcinomas | Inappropriate secretion associated with pneumonia, porphyria |
| Adrenocorticotropic hormone (ACTH) | Lung, prostate, gastrointestinal cancers, neuroendocrine tumors | Elevated in Cushing's disease |
| Human chorionic gonadotrophin, beta subunit (B-HCG) | Choriocarcinoma, germ cell testicular cancer, ectopic production in cancer of stomach, pancreas, lung, colon, liver | Elevated in almost all choriocarcinoma, 60% of testicular cancer; also in pregnancy |
| **METABOLIC PRODUCTS** | | |
| 5 Hydroxyindoleacetic acid (5 HIAA) | Carcinoid, lung | Drugs and diet interfere with test |
| Vanillylmandelic acid (VMA) | Neuroblastoma | Drugs and diet interfere with test |
| **PROTEINS** | | |
| Protein electrophoresis (urine—Bence Jones) (serum—immunoglobulins) | Myeloma, lymphoma | Elevated in connective tissue disease, benign monoclonal gammopathy, chronic renal failure |
|   IgG | IgG myeloma | |
|   IgA | IgA myeloma | |
|   IgM | Waldenström's macroglobulinemia | |
|   IgD | IgD myeloma | |
|   IgE | IgE myeloma | |
| | advanced neoplasms | |
| Beta-2 microglobulin | Myeloma, lymphoma | |
| **ANTIGENS** | | |
| Alpha-fetoprotein (AFP) | Nonseminomatous germ cell testicular cancer, choriocarcinoma, gonadal teratoblastoma in children, cancer of the pancreas, colon, lung, stomach, biliary system, liver | Elevated in 80% of hepatocellular cancer, 60% of nonseminomatous germ cell cancer; also in cirrhosis, hepatitis, toxic liver injury |

(continued)

**TABLE 9-2**  Selected Markers in the Diagnosis and Monitoring of Malignant Disease (continued)

| Laboratory Test | Associated Malignancy | Comments |
|---|---|---|
| **ANTIGENS** | | |
| Carcinoembryonic antigen (CEA) | Cancer of the colon-rectum, stomach, pancreas, prostate, lungs, breast | Elevated in smokers, chronic obstructive pulmonary disease, pancreatitis, hepatitis, inflammatory bowel disease |
| Prostate-specific antigen (PSA) | Prostate cancer | Elevated in prostatitis, nodular prostatic hyperplasia |
| Tissue polypeptide antigen (TPA) | Breast, colon, lung, pancreas cancer | Marker for cell proliferation in benign or malignant disease |
| CA—125 | Ovary (epithelial), pancreas, breast, colon cancer | Elevated in >85% of ovarian cancer; also in endometriosis, pelvic inflammatory disease, peritonitis |
| CA—19-9 | Pancreas, colon, gastric cancer | Differentiates benign from malignant pancreatobiliary disease |
| CA—15-3 | Breast cancer | |
| CA—72-4 | Gastric cancer | |
| **OTHER** | | |
| Lipid-associated sialic acid (LSA) | Leukemia, lymphoma, melanoma, most solid tumors | |
| Chromosome rearrangements (deletion, translocation, inversion) | Melanoma, small-cell lung, renal, testicular cancers, liposarcoma, neuroblastoma, lymphoma, leukemia, and others | |
| Amplified oncogenes | | |
| *myc* | Neuroblastoma, small-cell lung cancer | |
| *c-erbB* | Glioblastoma, squamous cell carcinomas | |
| *c-erbB₂* | Breast, adenocarcinomas | |

Radiographs may be site specific, such as the standard chest film (Figure 9-1) or mammogram, or they may view the dynamic function of an entire organ system. For example, in a gastrointestinal series a continuous flow of x-rays passes through the digestive tract to assess the action of peristalsis, to detect displacement of structures, and to visualize mucosal abnormalities.

Mammographic examination is performed primarily in x-ray units dedicated solely to this procedure. These units are distinguished by the incorporation of a tissue compression device or cone that improves the quality of the image and reduces the amount of primary and scatter radiation. Assuring women that this examination offers a low dose of radiation and a high-quality mammographic image that is sensitive to abnormalities has been necessary to promote participation in screening efforts. Since 1987 the American College of Radiology (ACR) has provided accreditation of mammography facilities that has resulted in a standard of quality assurance.[54] Additionally, many states have passed legislation or regulation to monitor the quality of mammography. In an attempt to establish national uniform quality standards, Congress enacted the Mammography Quality Standards Act in 1992. Effective in October 1994, every mammography facility, except those in the Department of Veteran's Affairs, must be certified by the Food and Drug Administration, accredited by an approved accrediting body, undergo annual inspection, and meet standards for personnel, equipment, equipment performance, and quality control practices.[55] A list of qualified facilities can be obtained from a local American Cancer Society office, the ACR, or the National Cancer Institute.

Diagnostic mammography is indicated when symptoms or clinical findings exist that suggest an abnormality. The examination requires that more views be taken than for the standard two-view screening mammogram, as well as spot compression and magnification views of suspicious spots. Frequently, mammography is used to guide the placement of a wire, needle, dye, or catheter near a suspicious lesion in preparation for biopsy or surgery. Figure 9-2 shows a mammographically guided needle localization of a nonpalpable breast lesion. The localizer penetrates and extends beyond the lesion for more reliable surgical excision.

Thermography, which images variations in radiant heat produced by blood flow through the breast, now is

**TABLE 9-3** Preferred Imaging Procedures for Tumor Definition and Staging

| Site | Imaging Techniques | Comments |
|------|-------------------|----------|
| Central nervous system | MRI with contrast | MRI with contrast is superior to CT due to exquisite sensitivity of lesions <1 cm and lack of bone artifact in posterior fossa imaging |
| Head and neck | CT<br>MRI | CT best for osseous change<br>MRI superior for soft-tissue lesions, tumor–tissue interface, parapharyngeal spaces |
| Lung | CXR<br>CT<br>MRI | CXR good for detection of peripheral lesions<br>CT preferred for parenchyma and mediastinal nodes<br>MRI's advantage over CT is in chest wall, hilum, and mediastinal vascular invasion |
| Esophagus | Esophagram with contrast<br><br>Endoscopic ultrasound (EUS)<br>CT | Esophagram preferred for measuring lesion length, necessary for staging<br>EUS superior to CT (except with severe stenosis) for depth of tumor invasion and lymph node assessment |
| Stomach | Barium studies with double contrast<br>Endoscopic ultrasound | Barium studies good for detection<br>EUS preferred over CT for staging due to better detection of small nodes |
| Colon | Barium enema with double contrast<br><br>CT<br>Endoscopic ultrasound | Most tumors originate in mucosa, where barium studies will detect 70%–90% of lesions<br>CT assesses liver or distant node metastasis<br>EUS is accurate in determining depth of tumor invasion and regional lymph nodes |
| Liver | Ultrasound (US)<br><br>CT or MRI with contrast | US preferred for differentiating biliary obstruction from hepatic parenchymal disease<br>CT has been preferred for imaging, but MRI with contrast may be equivalent |
| Bladder | Intravenous pyelogram (IVP)<br>MRI or CT | IVP detects lesions >1.5–2 cm<br>MRI preferred for bladder wall invasion, identifying large nodes, and separating them from vessels |
| Kidney | Intravenous pyelogram<br>CT | IVP preferred for detection<br>CT with contrast provides 90% accuracy for staging |
| Musculoskeletal | X-ray<br>Bone scan<br><br>CT or MRI | X-ray for initial detection<br>Bone scan more sensitive than x-ray in identifying metastatic bone lesions (except multiple myeloma)<br>CT preferred for intraosseous lesion; MRI preferred for extraosseous lesion or intraosseous lesion extending into bone |
| Breast | Mammogram | Mammography provides the standard for breast imaging; detects the 50% of breast lesions that are nonpalpable |
| Prostate | Transrectal ultrasound (TRUS)<br><br>MRI or CT | TRUS is being evaluated as detection tool; detects extracapsular extension of lesion with 90% accuracy<br>MRI preferred for staging seminal vesicle invasion |
| Endometrium | MRI | Primary staging is by surgery; MRI assists with staging of local and nodal disease |
| Ovary | Ultrasound or CT | Tumor mass >1 cm can be defined by US or CT; primary staging is by surgery |
| Lymphoma and Hodgkin's disease | CXR<br>CT of chest and abdomen<br><br><br>Lymphangiogram (LAG) | CRX required<br>CT replacing need for LAG in non-Hodgkin's lymphoma; CT of abdomen images upper retroperitoneal and mesenteric nodes, liver, and spleen<br>LAG has 95% sensitivity for imaging nodes in Hodgkin's disease and defines characteristic, abnormal, foamy lymph node architecture; doesn't visualize high celiac, splenic, hilar, or mesenteric nodes, requiring CT of abdomen |

**TABLE 9-4**   Several Tumor Imaging Techniques with Instructions for Preparing the Patient

| Tumor Imaging Examination | Patient Instructions | Comments |
|---|---|---|
| Barium studies | • Restriction of diet, smoking, and most medication before examination<br><br>• Laxatives and enemas to cleanse bowel before colon examination<br><br>• Will lie on tilting x-ray table, secured<br><br>• Barium will taste chalky, milkshake consistency<br><br>• Barium enema (BE) will feel cool, may cause cramping<br><br>• Laxatives to clear barium after UGI<br><br>• *Time: 30–60 min* | Bowel cleansing and procedure are exhausting for elderly patients. BE must precede UGI and small-bowel series. BE should follow other imaging examinations.<br>Average cost for BE = $325. |
| Computerized tomography | • Diet restrictions before examination<br><br>• Will lie still on adjustable table; x-ray tube rotates around patient to take many pictures<br><br>• Machinery noisy<br><br>• Test painless<br><br>• May receive intravenous contrast dye; may feel burning sensation as injected<br><br>• May report feelings of nausea, vomiting, flushing, itching, bitter taste<br><br>• Drink fluids after examination to eliminate dye<br><br>• *Time: 30–90 min* | Careful history required to determine prior adverse reaction to contrast.<br>Average cost for CT of abdomen and pelvis = $1600. |
| Angiogram | • Diet restriction before examination<br><br>• May receive sedative just before examination<br><br>• Will lie still on x-ray table<br><br>• Skin over selected artery site cleansed and anesthetized<br><br>• Cannula passed into artery or vein<br><br>• Contrast die rapidly injected, may feel burning sensation as injected<br><br>• Several x-ray films taken<br><br>• May report feelings of nausea, vomiting, flushing, itching, bitter or salty taste<br><br>• Cannula removed after examination, pressure applied, limb immobilized<br><br>• *Time: 1–3 hr* | Decreased use as diagnostic procedure. Being replaced by percutaneous procedures. Useful in preoperative planning and therapeutic embolization. |
| Lymphangiogram | • No diet restrictions<br><br>• Blue dye injected into interdigital webs of feet; some discomfort<br><br>• May discolor urine, stool, skin for 48 hr<br><br>• Skin over lymphatic vessel on foot anesthetized<br><br>• Small incision made on each foot, and cannula inserted<br><br>• Contrast dye infused for 1–2 hr<br><br>• May be uncomfortable during beginning of infusion, but must lie still | Decreased use, but still has a role in staging Hodgkin's disease and lymphoma.<br>Average cost = $1000. |

*(continued)*

**TABLE 9-4**  Several Tumor Imaging Techniques with Instructions for Preparing the Patient (continued)

| Tumor Imaging Examination | Patient Instructions | Comments |
|---|---|---|
| | • X-ray films taken after dye infused<br>• *Time:* 2–3 hr<br>• Must return following day for more x-ray films<br>• *Time:* 30 min | |
| Magnetic resonance imaging | • No diet restriction<br>• Remove anything affected by a magnet<br>• Lie still on table, secured with Velcro straps<br>• Table will move into narrow magnet opening<br>• Knocking or beating sound in machinery is normal<br>• Painless<br>• May receive intravenous contrast dye<br>• May report nausea, vomiting, itching if given contrast dye<br>• *Time:* 45–60 min | Difficult to titrate medication for comfort and sedation during lengthy procedures.<br>Average cost for MRI of abdomen = $1425. |
| Ultrasonogram | • Diet restriction before examination<br>• Full bladder for pelvic ultrasound<br>• Will lie on exam table<br>• Ultrasound gel applied over skin of area to be examined<br>• Transducer passes over skin<br>• May feel pressure; no pain<br>• *Time:* 30 min | Increased use of probes introduced into the body (transrectal, transvaginal) for detection of cancer. Also has intraoperative use for intracranial and intra-abdominal tumor localization.<br>Average cost for abdominal ultrasound = $300. |
| Nuclear medicine imaging | • No diet restriction<br>• Radioisotope injected before exam (15 min to 2 hr)<br>• Will lie on scanner table, may have to vary positions<br>• Scanner moves back and forth, taking several pictures<br>• Procedure painless<br>• Radioisotope harmless<br>• *Time:* 30–60 min | Increased use of radioimmunoimaging using radio-labeled monoclonal antibodies.<br>Average cost of liver and spleen scan = $620.<br>Average cost of single-photon emission computer tomography = $730. |
| Endoscopy | • Diet restriction before examination<br>• Mild sedation before procedure, but patient remains conscious<br>• Intravenous infusion for medications and hydration<br><br>*Oral:*<br>• Local anesthetic sprayed in mouth<br>• Flexible tube passed through mouth to level to be examined<br>• Tongue and throat feel swollen; difficult to swallow<br>• May feel pressure and fullness if scope in stomach | Screening sigmoidoscopy is recommended every 3–5 yr, beginning at age 50.<br>Average cost = $100. Medicare does not pay for screening procedure. Colonoscopy requires more extensive preparation.<br>Average cost = $350. |

(continued)

**TABLE 9-4**   Several Tumor Imaging Techniques with Instructions for Preparing the Patient (continued)

| Tumor Imaging Examination | Patient Instructions | Comments |
|---|---|---|
| | *Rectal:* <br>• Prepared for exam with laxatives, enemas <br>• Lubricated endoscope inserted anally <br>• Feels cold, urge to defecate <br>• May need to change positions during examination as scope is advanced <br>• *Time:* 30–60 min | |
| Mammogram | • Breast is compressed between 2 plates on x-ray cassette <br>• Compression may feel tight, but not painful <br>• Radiation exposure is minimal and safe <br><br>*Screening:* <br>• Two views are taken of each breast: one view from head to foot (craniocaudal), the other lateral <br>• *Time:* 15 min <br><br>*Diagnostic:* <br>• Three views taken of breast; craniocaudal, lateral, oblique <br>• Spot compression and magnification films <br>• *Time:* 30 min | Clinical breast exam and instruction on breast self-examination should be included. <br>Average cost for screening mammogram = $100. Covered by Medicare. <br>Average cost for diagnostic mammogram = $175. |

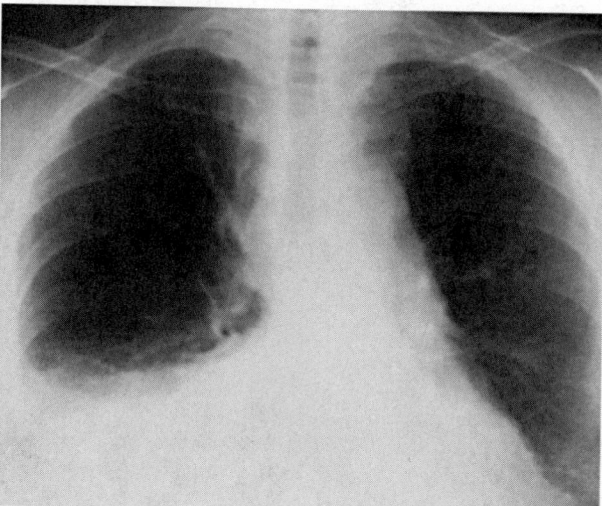

**FIGURE 9-1**   Initial chest x-ray film taken of a patient with small-cell lung cancer presenting with mediastinal adenopathy and right pleural effusion. (Courtesy of Scripps Memorial Hospital, Department of Radiology, La Jolla, CA.)

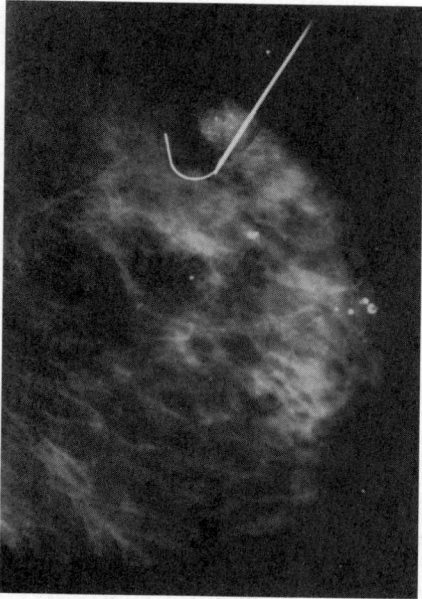

**FIGURE 9-2**   Mammographically guided hook-wire needle localization of nonpalpable breast lesion with multiple pathologic microcalcifications. (Courtesy of Scripps Memorial Hospital, Department of Radiology, La Jolla, CA.)

considered to be an ineffective modality for breast cancer screening.[56]

Tomography provides a radiographic image of a selected layer or plane of the body that would otherwise be obscured by shadows of other structures. Tomograms are particularly helpful in evaluating small calcified or cavitated lesions in the chest, hilar adenopathy, and mediastinal abnormalities.

Computerized axial tomography (CT or CAT) also provides sectional (axial, coronal, or sagittal) views of structures in the body. After serial x-ray exposures are taken through different angles of the body, a computer analyzes the information and provides a three-dimensional, reconstructed picture of the area studied. Computerized tomography is one of the most useful, informative, and available tests in the diagnosis and staging of malignancies. It is able to detect minor differences between tissue densities in any area of the body. The major drawback is its production of artifact in areas of cortical bone content. Tissues surrounded by bone (such as the posterior fossa), the base of the skull, and the spine are most affected.[57] CT may be completed with or without radioiodinated contrast agents. Figure 9-3 demonstrates two different tumors imaged by CT with intravenous contrast. CT frequently is used to direct a needle to a tumor site for percutaneous biopsy.

Several radiographic examinations rely on contrast materials to enhance or outline the structures to be visualized. Angiography, venography, cholangiography, and urography, in addition to computerized tomography, all rely on the intravascular administration of iodinated contrast agents for optimal visualization of body structure and function. An example is the excretory radiograph, also known as the intravenous pyelogram (IVP), which is used in the initial diagnostic evaluation of renal masses.

Approximately 5% of the patients who undergo examinations with iodinated contrast material experience an adverse reaction to the contrast medium.[58] Most commonly this reaction includes nausea, localized pain at the injection site, a metallic or bitter taste, and a sensation of warmth and flushing, lasting from one to three minutes. Urticaria and facial edema may last 30–60 minutes.[59] These symptoms do not require treatment and will not progress to life-threatening reactions. The incidence of a severe reaction such as cardiopulmonary arrest is extremely uncommon, occurring in only 0.1% of patients.[58] There is not a good predictor for severe reactions; however, patients with any history of allergic response should be closely monitored. People considered at risk for reaction may receive a test dose of the contrast agent and be given premedication with diphenhydramine, adrenocorticotropic hormone, or epinephrine. At least one study refutes this practice, stating that even a test dose may be life-threatening and that premedication does not minimize or prevent adverse reactions.[59] Nonionic contrast agents are available at considerable expense for use with patients who have had serious reactions in the past.

An oily iodinated contrast material is employed in lymphangiography (LAG). The lymphatic vessels in each foot, or, less commonly, each hand, are injected to allow visualization of the lymphatic vessels and nodes. This is indicated in the diagnosis and staging of Hodgkin's and non-Hodgkin's lymphomas and in some pelvic cancers. In addition to the risk of a reaction to the iodine in the contrast medium, as described previously, there is a

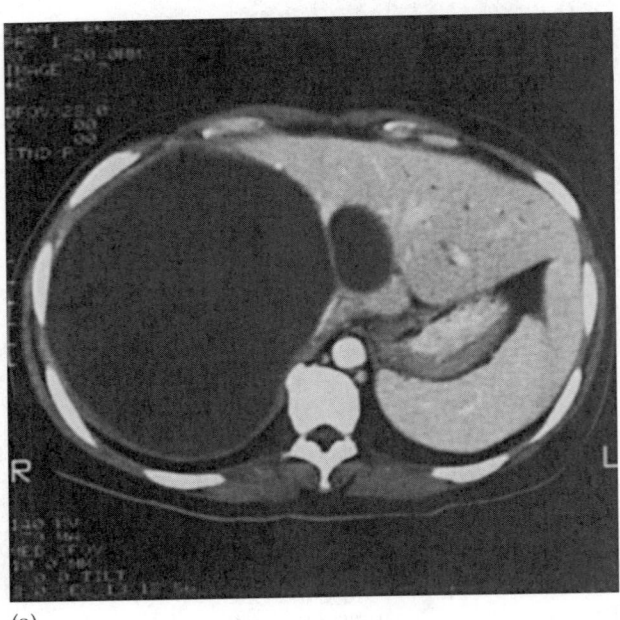

(a)

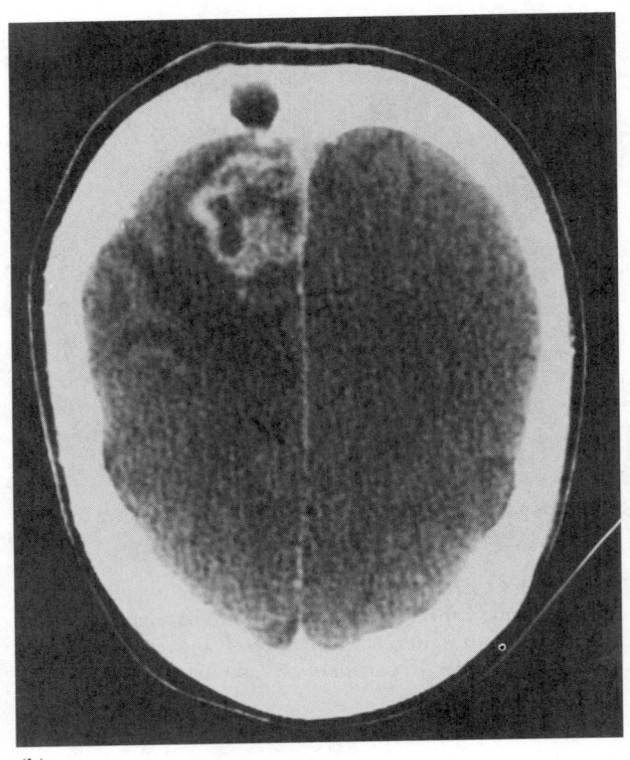

(b)

**FIGURE 9-3**   Examples of contrast-enhanced CT: CT abdominal scan revealing huge cystadenocarcinoma involving most of the liver (a), and CT head scan demonstrating lobular glioblastoma with peripheral rim enhancement (b). (Courtesy of Scripps Memorial Hospital, Department of Radiology, La Jolla, CA.)

potential reaction of pulmonary microembolization. This is of greatest concern if the lymph channels of the upper portion of the body are imaged. The thoracic duct empties into the lungs, and a degree of embolization is likely to occur. Patients with compromised pulmonary reserve are at highest risk, since a significant decrease in lung diffusing capacity may occur. Symptoms to be observed for are shortness of breath, chest pain, hypotension, and cyanosis, which should last only a few hours. Nursing actions after lymphangiogram include instruction in deep breathing and coughing to keep the lungs expanded.

Intrathecal contrast agents are used in myelography and in computerized tomography. Radiographs of the subarachnoid space are taken after the injection of either an oily or a water-soluble contrast agent. The contrast agent will flow only to the point of obstruction, and more than one injection may be required. This is one reason why magnetic resonance imaging has become the superior examination for detection of spinal cord compression as well as for skeletal metastatic deposits. A water-soluble myelographic contrast agent often is used with computerized tomography if a single disease site within the spinal canal is suspected.[52]

Barium sulfate is a nonabsorbable, radiopaque agent used to enhance the contrast between the lumen of the gastrointestinal tract and adjacent soft tissues. Studies that use barium include esophagraphy, upper gastrointestinal (UGI) series, small-bowel series, barium enema, and hypotonic duodenography. Barium is ingested or introduced into the gastrointestinal tract and allowed to coat the intraluminal surfaces. Radiographs are taken that can detect primary malignancies of the gastrointestinal organs or extrinsic compression from other tumor sites. Figure 9-4 presents a classic annular lesion of the colon imaged with radiopaque contrast. By combining barium and air, a double-contrast study is performed that is more sensitive than barium alone in detecting primary gastrointestinal tumors.[60] There are seldom complications to this examination unless there is an obstruction or a perforation of the digestive tract. Retention of the barium may cause fecal impaction and discomfort in some patients. The administration of a laxative or an enema may be necessary to assist with bowel evacuation.

Meglumine diatrizoate, a contrast agent containing water-soluble iodine, can be used instead of barium.

### Nuclear medicine techniques

Nuclear medicine imaging involves the intravenous injection or the ingestion of radioisotope compounds (technetium-99m methylene diphosphate, technetium-99m diethylenetriaminepentaacetic acid, technetium-99 sulfur colloid, iodine-123/131, or gallium-67 citrate), followed by camera imaging of those organs or tissues that have concentrated the radioisotopes. Nuclear medicine studies are extremely sensitive and often will detect sites of abnormal metabolism or early malignancy several months

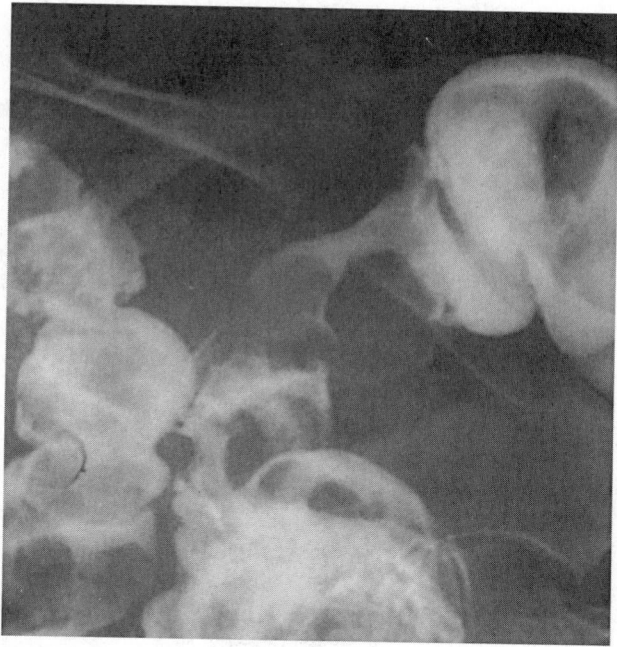

**FIGURE 9-4** Barium enema visualizes annular, "apple core" lesion that is constricting the colon. (Courtesy of Scripps Memorial Hospital, Department of Radiology, La Jolla, CA.)

before changes are seen on a radiograph. Scans of the bones, liver and spleen, brain, thyroid, and kidneys are useful in the detection of malignancy. Figure 9-5 shows an abnormal bone scan suggestive of widespread metastasis from prostate cancer. Gallium scans are particularly sensitive in detecting bronchogenic carcinomas and lymphomas. However, the increased use and the sensitivity of computerized tomography have replaced many radioisotope examinations.

Positron emission tomography (PET) is an imaging modality that provides information based on the biochemical and metabolic activity of tissue. Infused biochemical compounds such as glucose are tagged with radioactive particles that emit positrons detectable by gamma camera tomography. F-18 fluorodeoxyglucose (FDG) is the most widely used radiopharmaceutical. The most extensive application in clinical oncology has been in brain imaging. PET-FDG is particularly useful in differentiating low-grade tumors from high-grade tumors and in distinguishing treatment-induced tissue necrosis from recurrent tumor. Many insurers have accepted this technology for imaging brain tumors and are offering reimbursement. The accuracy of PET imaging has also been demonstrated in other neoplasms (e.g., breast). Practical limitations of this modality are its expense and the need for a cyclotron to produce the isotopes.[61,62] Single-photon emission computed tomography (SPECT) uses commercially available radioisotopes and has much broader application.

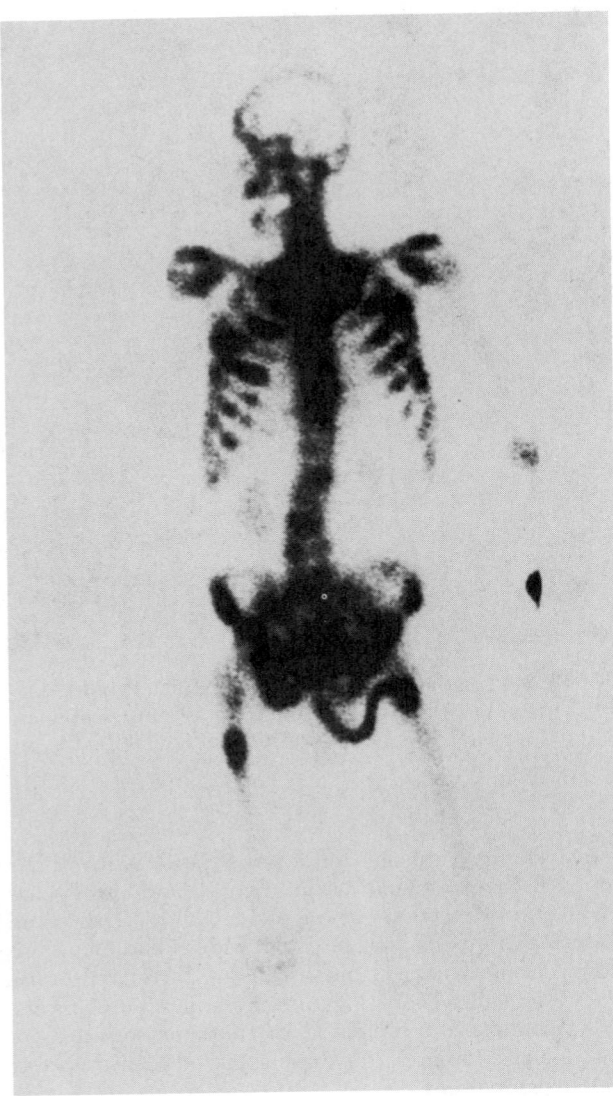

**FIGURE 9-5** Abnormal bone scan suggesting widespread bony metastasis in central axial skeleton, pelvis, hips, and right proximal femur. (Courtesy of Scripps Memorial Hospital, Department of Radiology, La Jolla, CA.)

Nuclear imaging with radio-labeled monoclonal antibodies visualizes microscopic sites of metastasis or suspected malignancy. This technique requires that a monoclonal antibody targeted against a specific tumor antigen be combined with tracer amounts of radioactivity. After intravenous injection, the antibody binds to antigen on the tumor. Tumor sites then "light up" with imaging scanners. CYT-103 (OncoScint OV/CR) is the first FDA-approved radiolabeled monoclonal antibody for diagnostic use in cancer. The Indium-111–labeled antibody targets the tumor-associated glycoprotein (TAG-72) found in mucin-producing adenocarcinomas.[63] In clinical trials, imaging has been successful in several disease sites, including the colon,[64] the breast and the ovaries,[65] and in melanoma[66] and T-cell lymphomas.[67]

## Ultrasonography

Ultrasonography (US) is a nonradiographic and noninvasive technique of imaging deep soft-tissue structures within the body. The reflecting echoes of high-frequency sound waves directed into specific tissues are recorded on an imaging screen. The echoes are variable, depending on the tissue density, and can be used to discriminate masses. A limitation of the examination is its inability to visualize through bone or air. Ultrasonography is most applicable in detecting tumors within the pelvis, the retroperitoneum, and the peritoneum of patients with cancer.[52] Masses greater than 2 cm in diameter can be detected and localized for possible percutaneous biopsy. Transrectal ultrasound is useful in guiding a needle biopsy of suspicious prostate lesions, but has not proven an effective screening tool. In the diagnosis of breast cancer, ultrasound is an important adjunct to mammography for distinguishing cysts from solid lesions with 98%–100% accuracy.

## Magnetic resonance imaging

Magnetic resonance imaging creates sectional images of the body, similar to computerized tomography, but does not expose the patient to ionizing radiation. Images are created by placing the individual within a powerful magnetic field that aligns the body's hydrogen nuclei in one direction. Radio-frequency pulses are used to excite the magnetized nuclei and change their alignment. Between radio-frequency pulses the nuclei return to a state of relaxation, and variable signals are transmitted on the basis of tissue characteristics. These signals are analyzed by the computer, and multiplaner (sagittal, coronal, and axial) images are produced with exquisite clarity. Magnetic resonance imaging can be enhanced with the intravenous paramagnetic contrast agents gadolinium diethylenetriaminepentaacetic acid (DTPA) and gadotetrate meglumine (DOTA).[68] These agents work by reducing tissue relaxation time, thus increasing signal intensity and image production. Adverse reactions to gadolinium DTPA, which are rare, include nausea, pain localized to the injection site, and headache occurring several hours after the examination. Anaphylactoid reactions to the contrast agent have been reported.[69]

Magnetic resonance imaging is most applicable in the detection, localization, and staging of malignant disease in the central nervous system, spine, head and neck, and musculoskeletal system. Contrast-enhanced MRI is the superior imaging modality in brain tumors (Figure 9-6).[70] MRI examination of the spinal cord essentially has eliminated the use of myelography in patients with cancer.[37]

Significant limitations do exist in the use of MRI. Persons with aneurysm or surgical clips, pacemakers, im-

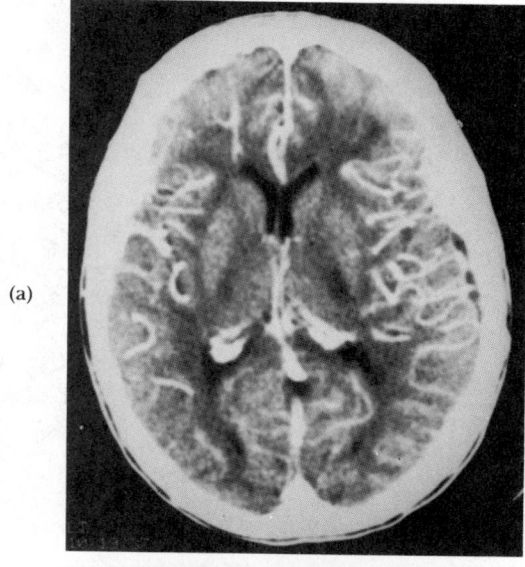

(a)

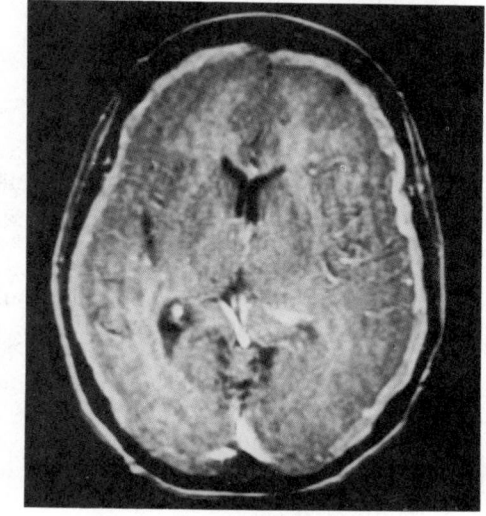

(b)

**FIGURE 9-6** Contrast-enhanced CT (a) and contrast-enhanced MRI (b) of metastatic intracranial tumor. MRI shows "rind" of metastatic deposit around brain that was invisible on CT due to bone artifact. (Courtesy of Scripps Memorial Hospital, Department of Radiology, La Jolla, CA.)

planted pumps, tattooed eyeliner, or any ferromagnetic metallic implant cannot undergo MRI examination. The magnetic pull of the MRI is capable of dislodging the implant or interfering with its operation, or may actually remove the object from the person's body. This excludes the MRI examination for acutely ill patients with life-support or monitoring devices. Nonferrous metallic implants may produce artifacts that distort the MRI image, but are generally safe for the patient. Implanted ports, frequently used in cancer patients to provide vascular, peritoneal, and epidural access, are made from many different materials. Shellock provides a list of ports that do not move or deflect during exposure to magnetic

scanning.[71] Camp-Sorrell identifies ports causing the least artifact, but concludes that attention must be paid to the manufacturer's recommendations as materials change and new ports are developed.[72] High-grade titanium and nonmetal ports produce the least or no artifact.

Claustrophobic individuals may require sedation if they are to undergo an MRI scan, but they also benefit from explanations prior to the procedure, a support person nearby, verbal contact, MRI-compatible headphones, prisms or mirrors to allow a view outside of the tube, and relaxation techniques.[71] The cost of the MRI, length of the examination (one to two hours for a total scan of the spine), and somewhat limited availability of this diagnostic tool are additional disadvantages.

## Invasive Diagnostic Techniques

### Endoscopy

Endoscopy is a method of directly visualizing the interior of a hollow viscus by the insertion of an endoscope into a body cavity or opening. The endoscope contains fiberoptic glass bundles that transmit light and then return an image to the optical head of the endoscope. The instrument may be rigid or flexible. Visual inspection, tissue biopsy, cytological aspiration, staging the extent of disease, and the excision of pathological processes are possible through the endoscope.

By passing a flexible scope through the mouth, endoscopic examinations can visualize directly the larynx, the upper airway passages and the bronchial tree, the esophagus, the stomach, and the upper duodenum. Visualization of the distal sigmoid colon, the rectum, and the anal canal is performed by means of a rigid scope. The entire large intestine can be viewed with a flexible colonoscope that is inserted anally.

Endoscopic retrograde cholangiopancreatography combines the diagnostic procedures of endoscopy and contrast-enhanced radiography to evaluate biliary tract obstruction and pancreatic masses.

The endoscopic ultrasound (EUS) may prove superior to other imaging modalities for assessing direct depth of tumor invasion and local lymph node status for esophageal, gastric, and colon malignancy. EUS, where available, is indicated to distinguish benign from malignant lesions, to stage neoplasms, to establish operability and surgical approach, and to determine response or recurrence.[73]

The cervix and vagina are visualized with the use of the magnification lens of the colposcope. Peritoneoscopy or laparoscopy permits assessment of surfaces within the peritoneal cavity by the insertion of a peritoneoscope through a small incision below the umbilicus. Thoracoscopy allows visualization of the visceral and parietal pleura, the mediastinum, and the diaphragm by means of a thoracoscope passed through an incision in the mid-axillary line of the sixth to the eighth intercostal space. The direct visualization of the tissues and organs of the mediastinum is performed by passing an endoscope into the mediastinum through a small incision above the manubrium.

## Biopsy

The importance of obtaining histological or cytological proof of malignancy cannot be overstated. Treatment decisions for cancers arising within the same organ differ on the basis of the histopathology report. An example is the very different treatment regimens for small-cell cancer of the lung and adenocarcinoma of the lung. Exactly what tissue is to be biopsied depends on several factors: the clinical status of the person, the person's willingness to undergo invasive procedures, the size and location of the identified tumor, and the amount of tissue needed by the pathologist for analysis.[74]

The cytological examination of aspirated fluid, secretions, scrapings, or washings of body cavities may reveal malignant cells that have exfoliated from a primary or metastatic tumor. Tissue will not be obtained by this method, and the pathologist's ability to establish the primary site of the malignancy may be limited. Cancer of the cervix is one example of a malignancy that is successfully detected by the cytological examination of cells acquired from a Papanicolaou smear.

The fine-needle aspiration biopsy, guided by palpation or an imaging technique, is extensively used and is available in the ambulatory setting. It provides not only cytological information but also microhistologic information if adequate tissue fragments are obtained. Table 9-5 provides general instructions for preparing the patient for an image-guided fine-needle aspiration biopsy.[75] Figure 9-7 shows a patient undergoing a CT-guided needle biopsy of an abdominal mass.

Stereotactic localization is another diagnostic tool utilizing CT or MRI to establish the coordinates of a lesion and accurately position a needle for the tissue biopsy. Stereotactic breast biopsy of nonpalpable lesions is comparable to conventional needle-localization surgical biopsy with a sensitivity of 90%–95% for breast cancer

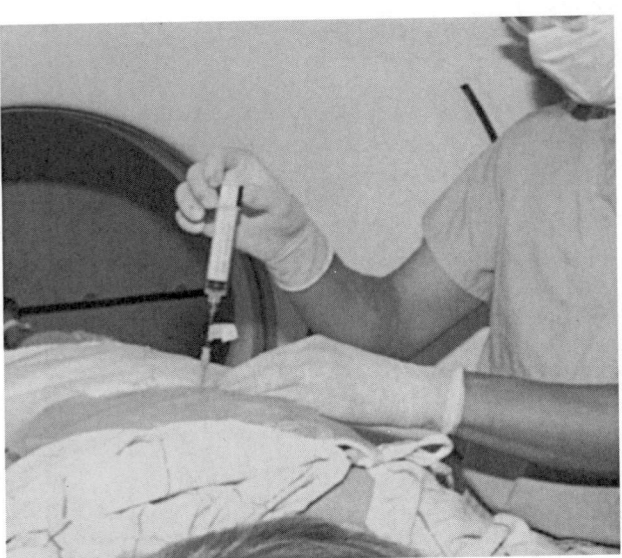

**FIGURE 9-7**   Patient undergoing CT-guided needle biopsy of retroperitoneal lymph node. (Courtesy of Scripps Memorial Hospital, Department of Radiology, La Jolla, CA.)

**TABLE 9-5**   Instructions for Preparing the Patient for Image-Guided Fine-Needle Aspiration Biopsy

- Contrast agent may be required—intravenous or oral.
- Sedatives may be offered.
- Vital signs and oximetry will be monitored if intravenous sedation is used.
- Some pain may be experienced; local anesthetic is used.
- Skin at biopsy site is cleansed, and the needle inserted.
- Needle position is established by an imaging technique, (e.g., CT, ultrasound, or chest fluoroscopy).
- Syringe is attached to the needle, and the fluid and tissue are aspirated.
- Patient is observed for infection, bleeding, or increase in pain.

detection.[76] Figure 9-8 demonstrates stereotactic images of a breast nodule and the accurate placement of a needle for biopsy. Stereotactic brain biopsy of suspicious lesions is a relatively safe and quick procedure. A stereotactic head frame is fixed to the skull under local anesthetic, the lesion is scanned for localizing landmarks, including the location of arteries and vessels, a small hole is made in the skull, and the biopsy is then directed by an instrument attached to the frame.

The biopsy provides tissue for histological examination. The following are commonly recognized techniques for obtaining a biopsy: needle biopsy, incisional biopsy, excisional biopsy, punch biopsy, and bone marrow aspiration. These procedures and their nursing implications are discussed in chapter 12. For a definitive diagnosis of malignancy it is imperative that the pathologist receive an adequate, representative, and well-preserved tissue specimen. A cytological or histological report that is negative for malignancy may only signify a specimen that is inadequate for diagnostic evaluation, thus necessitating repeat biopsy. Only a complete excisional biopsy can exclude malignancy with certainty. When the results of a biopsy are equivocal the specimen should be sent to an outside source for a second evaluation. The Armed Forces Institute of Pathology in Washington, DC is used by pathologists worldwide as a reference and for review.

Not infrequently, the biopsied tissue will confirm malignancy but the primary site or tissue of origin cannot be established by the pathologist or the clinician. An example is the individual who undergoes biopsy of a cervical node and is diagnosed with squamous cell carcinoma but for whom a thorough examination of the chest

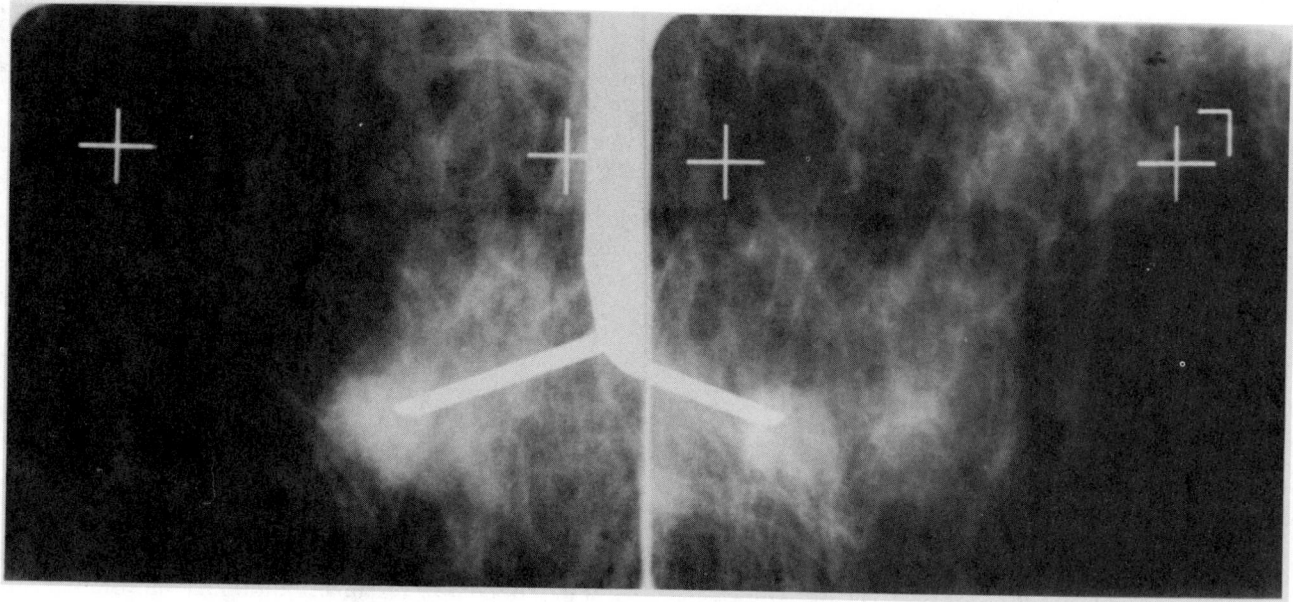

**FIGURE 9-8**   Pair of images confirming accurate placement of needle at the margin of a breast nodule for stereotactic core biopsy. (Courtesy of Scripps Memorial Hospital, Department of Radiology, La Jolla, CA.)

and head and neck area fails to yield the source of the malignancy. The goals for pursuing the primary site in this situation are discussed later in this chapter in the section on "Tumors of Unknown Origin."

## CLASSIFICATION AND NOMENCLATURE

### Basic Terminology

The terms *cancer* and *tumor* often are used interchangeably and inappropriately and can be misleading for patients, families, and professionals. A *tumor* is a swelling or mass of tissue that may be benign or malignant. *Cancer,* synonymous with *malignant neoplasm,* is an uncontrolled "new growth" capable of metastasis and invasion that threatens host survival.

The term *primary tumor* is used to describe the original histological site of tumorigenesis. A *secondary,* or *metastatic tumor* resembles the primary tumor histologically but sometimes may be so anaplastic as to obscure the cell of origin. A *second primary lesion* refers to an additional, histologically separate malignant neoplasm in the same patient. Although this is a relatively unusual occurrence, it must be excluded at the time of an apparent recurrence. Tables of probability for recurrence exist to guide the clinician in these determinations. A general rule is always to biopsy the first recurrence, because it may actually represent a new, curable or treatable malignancy. An example is the person with a history of breast cancer who presents with suspicious lymph nodes and is found on biopsy to have lymphoma. Unfortunately, some recur-

rences present in sites where the morbidity from biopsy is so significant that the lesion is treated without tissue confirmation. The woman with breast cancer presenting with a vertebral pedicle lesion is an example of this situation.

### Benign and Malignant Tumor Characteristics

Certain biological, histological, and cytological characteristics distinguish a benign tumor from a malignant tumor. However, with the exception of the properties of invasion and metastasis, which are found only in cancer, the differences between a benign process and a malignant process are relative. In some circumstances a definitive diagnosis of benign tumor versus malignant tumor cannot be made. For example, a well-differentiated follicular carcinoma of the thyroid may be solitary and encapsulated and may mimic a benign adenoma of the thyroid. Occasionally a benign tumor will transform into a malignant tumor over time. An adenomatous polyp of the colon is an example of a relatively benign process that can transform into cancer of the colon if left untreated.

In general, the following features distinguish benign tumors from those that are malignant. The *benign* tumor is relatively slow-growing. Tumor stasis or regression may occur. Growth occurs as the tumor expands locally within a capsule of fibrous tissue. Benign tumors do not invade adjacent tissues, destroy normal tissue, or metastasize elsewhere in the body. Although death from a benign tumor is rare, distressing symptoms may result from a tumor's pressure on vital organs or from ectopic hormone production. Cytological examination reveals uniform, well-differentiated cells that resemble those of the adult tissue of origin and demonstrate little or no anaplasia and rare mitoses.

In contrast, the *malignant* tumor is characterized by its generally high mitotic rate, rapid growth, and disregard for normal growth limitations. Malignant tumors are almost never encapsulated. The malignant cells invade surrounding tissue, lymphatic vessels, and blood vessels and metastasize to distant sites. Malignant tumor cells are anaplastic, vary in morphological characteristics within the same tumor, are poorly differentiated, and have abnormal and inconstant numbers of chromosomes.

## Tumor Classification System

The most relevant classification systems will universally communicate clinical and prognostic information. Tumors may be classified not only by their biological behavior (benign versus malignant) but also by their tissue of origin.

To understand the nomenclature of tumors it is useful to review normal cell differentiation in the embryonic state. An early occurrence in the life of the embryo is the development of three primary germ layers: the ectoderm, the mesoderm, and the endoderm. The cells within these layers divide, specialize, and give rise to all cells, tissues, and organs within the body. The ectoderm differentiates into the skin and nervous system. The mesoderm differentiates into several organs and connective tissue: bones, blood, cartilage, fat, fibrous tissue, muscle, and blood and lymph vessels. The endoderm differentiates into the lining of the digestive and respiratory tracts, the bladder, and the urethra.

Virtually every cell type in the body is capable of transforming into a malignant cell. Chapter 3 provides a complete discussion of carcinogenic transformation. It is fairly well accepted that the malignant cell derives from a postembryonic cell that is arrested in the process of differentiation.

Most tumors will retain sufficient characteristics of the normal, differentiated cell to allow recognition of the type of tissue from which they were derived, which is the basis of distinguishing tumors in the histogenetic classification system (Table 9-6).[77,78] Specific nomenclature provides information on characteristics of the neoplasm. A suffix is added to the name of the tissue or cell type under pathological study to designate its benign or malignant nature. Benign tumors usually end in the suffix *-oma,* the Greek root for "tumor." Most malignant tumors end in either the suffix *-sarcoma* or the suffix *-carcinoma,* depending on the tissues from which they arise. For example, lipoma is a benign tumor of fat tissue, and liposarcoma is a malignancy of fat tissue. *Sarcoma* specifies a malignant tumor of the connective tissues, that is, those tissues originating from the mesodermal embryonic layer. *Carcinoma* specifies a malignant tumor arising from epithelial tissues. Epithelium covers or lines surfaces in the body and arises from the ectodermal, mesodermal, or endodermal embryonic layers.

Carcinomas are further delineated by the prefixes *adeno-,* for tumors that arise from glandular epithelial tissue, and *squamous,* for tumors that originate from squamous epithelial tissues. Descriptive terms such as *cystic, follicular, papillary, medullary, exophytic,* and *polypoid* are added to further define histological characteristics.

The suffix that refers to malignant tumors that resemble the primitive blastula phase in embryonic development is *-blastoma.* Examples are neuroblastoma and retinoblastoma.

Mixed tumors, such as adenosquamous carcinoma of the bronchi, represent tumors with mixed squamous and glandular elements but that arise from the same germ layer and tissue. Some tumors, although rare and highly malignant, have such primitive differentiation that characteristics of a carcinoma and sarcoma may be evident.[77,79]

Teratoma and its malignant counterpart, teratocarcinoma, arise from tissue of all three germ layers and have no relationship to the site of origin.[77]

Several exceptions exist to the classification system just described. For instance, lymphoma, melanoma, and hepatoma are malignant tumors with the *-oma* suffix. In addition, some malignancies are named after the person who characterized them. Hodgkin's disease, Ewing's sarcoma, and Wilms' tumor are examples. The hematopoietic malignancies are classified separately by predominant cell type and their acute versus chronic nature.

## Tumors of Unknown Origin

Five to ten percent of patients diagnosed with cancer each year are found to have a malignancy from an unknown primary site.[80] Most frequently the histological classification will be adenocarcinoma, but the site of origin may never be determined, even on autopsy. The prognosis is poor, with an overall median survival of five months.[81] The goal of proceeding with a diagnostic investigation in this situation is to identify those malignancies, even if they are disseminated, that are potentially curable or palliated with known, effective treatment. For example, lymphomas and germ cell tumors are potentially curable with systemic chemotherapy. Lesions in the nasopharynx may be cured with radiation. Local complications such as bowel obstruction, spinal cord compression, and pathological fractures can be palliated with surgery or radiation treatment even when the primary site of malignancy is unknown. Hormonal therapy may be recommended if the presumptive diagnosis, based on tumor markers or hormone receptor analysis, is breast, prostate, or endometrial malignancy.

Patients and their families who are facing cancer from an unknown source present unique challenges for the nurse. Not only do they need information and preparation for extensive imaging and laboratory testing, but they also need support when these tests fail to yield a definitive diagnosis. It is often hoped, though not necessarily true, that a known primary source of malignancy will

**TABLE 9-6**  Select Benign and Malignant Neoplasms Listed by Histogenetic Classification

| Tissue of Origin | Benign Neoplasm | Malignant Neoplasm |
|---|---|---|
| **Epithelial (Endodermal)** | | |
| Squamous | Squamous cell papilloma | Squamous cell or epidermoid carcinoma |
| Glandular | Adenoma | Adenocarcinoma |
| | Papilloma | Papillary carcinoma |
| | Cystadenoma | Cystadenocarcinoma |
| Respiratory tract | | Bronchogenic carcinoma |
| Renal epithelium | Renal tubular adenoma | Renal cell carcinoma (hypernephroma) |
| Urinary tract | Transitional cell papilloma | Transitional cell carcinoma |
| Placental epithelium | Hydatidiform mole | Choriocarcinoma |
| Testicular epithelium | | Seminoma |
| | | Embryonal carcinoma |
| Liver | Liver cell adenoma | Hepatocellular carcinoma (hepatoma) |
| Biliary tree | Cholangioma | Cholangiocarcinoma |
| Stomach | Gastric polyp | Gastric carcinoma |
| Colon | Colonic polyp | Adenocarcinoma of the colon |
| **Mesenchymal (Mesodermal)** | | |
| *Connective* | | |
| Fibrous tissue | Fibroma | Fibrosarcoma |
| Adipose tissue | Lipoma | Liposarcoma |
| Cartilage | Chondroma | Chondrosarcoma |
| Bone | Osteoma | Osteosarcoma |
| *Muscle* | | |
| Smooth muscle | Leiomyoma | Leiomyosarcoma |
| Striated muscle | Rhabdomyoma | Rhabdomyosarcoma |
| *Endothelial* | | |
| Blood vessels | Hemangioma | Hemangiosarcoma |
| Lymphatic vessels | Lymphangioma | Lymphangiosarcoma |
| *Hematopoietic and lymphoreticular* | | |
| Hematopoietic cells | | Leukemias |
| Lymphoid tissue | | Lymphomas |
| | | Hodgkin's disease |
| Plasma cells | | Plasmacytoma (multiple myeloma) |
| **Neural (Ectodermal)** | | |
| Meninges | Meningioma | Meningeal sarcoma |
| Glia | Astrocytoma | Glioblastoma multiforme |
| Nerve cells | Ganglioneuroma | Neuroblastoma |
| | | Medulloblastoma |
| Melanocytes | Nevus | Malignant melanoma |
| **Mixed Tissues** | | |
| Kidney | | Wilms' tumor |
| Salivary gland | Mixed tumor of salivary gland (pleomorphic adenoma) | Malignant mixed tumor of salivary gland |

be more treatable or curable than an unknown primary. Coping with any cancer diagnosis is difficult. Coping with an "unknown" cancer accentuates the feelings of loss of control, anxiety, and frustration. The involved nurse can be most helpful by identifying psychosocial concerns and available support systems early in the diagnostic period, clarifying and reinforcing known information and the rationale for extensive testing, and providing hope and reassurance that treatment is offered for the most probable and most treatable source of malignancy.[82]

# STAGING AND GRADING CLASSIFICATIONS

## Staging the Extent of the Disease

The staging process is a method of classifying a malignancy by the extent of its spread within the body. It is a clinical and histological determination that depends on the natural course of each particular type of cancer. Staging is based on the premise that cancers of similar histological features and site of origin will extend and metastasize in a predictable manner. Although most staging classifications are based on the anatomic extent of disease, other criteria are included for specific malignancies. For thyroid cancer, the age of the patient and the histological diagnosis (papillary, follicular, medullary, or anaplastic) are included in the staging system. In the staging of prostate cancer, soft-tissue sarcomas, primary malignant tumors of the bone, and brain tumors the histopathological grade of the tumor is significant.

There are multiple objectives of solid-tumor staging but the most important is to provide the necessary information for individual treatment planning. Other reasons for using a uniform staging system are the following: to give prognostic information, to assist in treatment evaluation, to facilitate the exchange of information and comparative statistics among treatment centers, and to stratify individuals who may be eligible for clinical trials.[83]

With the goal of developing an internationally consistent system of staging solid-tumor malignancy, the TNM committee of the International Union Against Cancer (UICC) and the American Joint Committee on Cancer (AJCC) have agreed on the TNM staging system. The TNM staging system classifies solid tumors by the anatomic extent of disease, as determined clinically and histologically. Three categories are quantified, with gradations representing progressive tumor size or involvement. The extent of the primary tumor (T) is evaluated on the basis of depth of invasion, surface spread, and tumor size. Secondly, the absence or presence and extent of regional lymph node (N) metastasis are considered, with attention to the size and location of the nodes. Thirdly, the absence or presence of distant metastasis (M) is assessed. A subscript may specify the site of metastasis. For example, M1PUL denotes pulmonary metastasis. The TNM system is further classified by whether the assessment is obtained clinically (cTNM or TNM), after pathological review (pTNM), at the time of retreatment (rTNM), or on autopsy (aTNM). For reporting purposes, the TNM stage classification remains constant throughout the disease process. Progression of disease does not change the initial stage of disease. Table 9-7 presents the nomenclature of the TNM system for classification.[83]

It is important to distinguish the cTNM, based on a clinical exam, from the pTNM, which is determined after surgery when the true extent of the disease is known and treatment decisions can be made. This is particularly true in breast cancer, where the lymph node status (pN) is the most precise prognostic indicator and directs adjuvant therapy decisions. Surgical nurses are well aware of the support needed by the woman with breast cancer in the first 24–48 hours after lymphadenectomy while she is awaiting the pathologist's review of lymph nodes. Another example occurs in the treatment of prostate cancer when the discovery of tumor in the pelvic lymph nodes (pN) at the time of surgery precludes the anticipated radical prostatectomy.

After numerical values are assigned to the T, N, and

**TABLE 9-7**   TNM Classification System for Describing the Anatomic Extent of Disease

**TNM Definitions**

(T)   Primary tumor

| | |
|---|---|
| TX | Primary tumor cannot be assessed |
| T0 | No evidence of primary tumor |
| Tis | Carcinoma in situ |
| T1, T2, T3, T4 | Increasing size and/or local extent of the primary tumor |

(N)   Regional lymph nodes

| | |
|---|---|
| NX | Regional lymph nodes cannot be assessed |
| N0 | No regional lymph node metastasis |
| N1, N2, N3 | Increasing involvement of regional lymph nodes |

(M)   Distant metastasis

| | |
|---|---|
| MX | Presence of distant metastasis cannot be assessed |
| M0 | No distant metastasis |
| M1 | Distant metastasis |

**TNM Classifications**

| | |
|---|---|
| cTNM or TNM | *Clinical Classification:* Based on information obtained from the physical examination, laboratory and imaging studies, endoscopy, biopsy, and surgical exploration. Clinical staging uses all information available before the initiation of definitive treatment. |
| pTNM | *Pathologic Classification:* Based on information acquired before treatment, supplemented or modified by information from surgery and the pathologic examination of a resected specimen. This includes resected tumor (pT), lymph nodes (pN), and distant metastasis (pM). |
| rTNM | *Retreatment Classification:* Based on all information available after a disease-free interval or at the time of a second-look surgery. The extent or absence of disease recurrence is documented before retreatment planning is begun. |
| aTNM | *Autopsy Classification:* Based on all information available at the time of a postmortem examination. It is helpful in answering questions about the tumor's response to treatment, recurrence patterns, and the extent of disease at the time of death. |

Adapted from Beahrs OH, Henson DE, Hutter RVP, et al: *American Joint Committee on Cancer: Manual for Staging of Cancer* (ed 4). Philadelphia, Lippincott, 1995

M categories, they are clustered into one of four stages (I through IV), or stage O for carcinoma in situ. Stage IV consistently includes distant metastases (M1) and predicts the worst prognosis. All tumor sites are grouped differently on the basis of characteristics of the disease. A typical TNM grouping is depicted in Table 9-8.[84]

Several established and accepted staging classifications other than TNM exist for particular malignancies. Melanomas are staged histologically by the level of invasion of the primary lesion, since this is the major determinant of prognosis. The Clark levels of invasion are widely

**TABLE 9-8** A Typical Stage Grouping Based on TNM Classification

- *Stage I, T1, N0, M0:* Clinical examination reveals a mass limited to the organ of origin. The lesion is operable and resectable, with only local involvement, and there is no nodal and vascular spread. This stage affords the best chance for survival.

- *Stage II, T2, N1, M0:* Clinical examination shows evidence of local spread into surrounding tissue and first-station lymph nodes. The lesion is operable and resectable, but because of greater local extent there is uncertainty as to completeness of removal. The specimen shows evidence of microinvasion into capsule and lymphatics. This stage affords a good chance of survival.

- *Stage III, T3, N2, M0:* Clinical examination reveals an extensive primary tumor with fixation to a deeper structure, bone invasion, and lymph nodes of a similar nature. The lesion is operable but not resectable, and gross disease is left behind. This stage affords some chance of survival.

- *Stage IV, T4, N3, M+:* There is evidence of distant metastases beyond the site of origin. The lesion is inoperable. There is little to no chance of survival.

Rubin P: Statement of the clinical oncologic problem, in Rubin P (ed): *Clinical Oncology for Medical Students and Physicians: A Multidisciplinary Approach* (ed 6). New York, American Cancer Society, 1983, p 10

accepted. The TNM stages for melanoma incorporate Clark's classification into primary tumor (T) assessment. The Duke's staging system for colorectal cancer, with its many subsequent modifications, classifies colorectal tumors by their depth of invasion and presence of nodal metastasis. The International Federation of Gynecology and Obstetrics has an accepted staging system for cervical and endometrial cancers. Hodgkin's disease and non-Hodgkin's lymphoma are standardly described by the Ann Arbor classification, which recognizes disease distribution and symptoms. Cancers of the brain are not entirely suited to the TNM system because there are no lymphatic structures to categorize nodal (N) involvement.

The nonsolid tumors do not conform to solid-tumor staging principles because of their disseminated nature. Leukemias are best classified according to their predominant cell types (i.e., lymphocytic or nonlymphocytic), cell maturation, and acute or chronic nature. Clinical, morphological, histochemical, and immunologic findings help to define favorable or unfavorable prognostic categories in acute lymphoblastic leukemia. The French-American-British classification, has clinical and prognostic significance in acute myeloblastic leukemia but is not a staging system. In chronic lymphocytic leukemia, more than one staging system exists: the Rai classification, the Binet classification, and a relatively new system prepared by the International Workshop on chronic lymphocytic leukemia.[85] For patients with myeloma there is a staging classification that correlates M proteins with myeloma cell mass to provide prognostic information.[86]

The AJCC, with the UICC, is currently developing staging systems for malignancies not yet classified by the TNM system. These include cancers of the small intestine, mesothelioma, spinal cord, carcinoid, and Kaposi's sarcoma. Additionally, they are likely to incorporate tumor markers into the present anatomic staging to produce a system with better prognostic indexes.[87] This has important implications for patients with early-stage disease (based on anatomic staging) but who are actually at risk for recurrence based on other measurements of malignant potential and who will need further treatment. The 30% of women with node-negative breast cancer who eventually experience a recurrence are a subset of people with early stage disease with a less favorable prognosis. The staging system of the future will be an estimation of risk (of local extension and distant metastases) based on the sum of risks associated with anatomic stage, morphological grade, biological grade, and genetic potential.[88] In breast cancer this could include the TNM stage, degree of morphological anaplasia, estrogen and progesterone receptor status, S-phase fraction and aneuploidy, epidermal growth factor receptors, and *Her-2/neu, c-erB-2,* or *c-myc* oncogene expression.[88]

## Patient Performance Classification

An individual's physical performance status at the time of diagnosis and staging often will influence the type of treatment selected and provide prognostic information.[89] Bedridden patients are much less likely to respond to any treatment than those who are asymptomatic and able to maintain the activities of daily living. Performance scales that measure a person's functional status are used frequently in the eligibility criteria for cooperative group clinical trials and also periodically to evaluate the effects of treatment and disease. It is important to assess whether aggressive, toxic treatment protocols actually will permit people to feel better and to maintain their optimum functional status. The most prevalent performance scales are the Karnofsky Performance Status scale, the Eastern Cooperative Oncology Group (ECOG) scale, and the World Health Organization (WHO) scale.[90–92] In an attempt to standardize this classification, the American Joint Committee on Cancer (AJCC) developed a simplified performance scale.[83] The four scales are compared in Table 9-9. Nurses need to be familiar with the scoring systems, for they may be able to contribute the most accurate information to a primarily subjective rating. Moderate interobserver reliability and weak correlation between the functional status score and the patient's self-assessment have been concerns with established scales.[93,94]

## Grading

Grading a malignant neoplasm is a method of classification based on histopathological characteristics of the tis-

**TABLE 9-9**  Comparison of Frequently Used Performance Status Scales

| Karnofsky Scale | | ECOG Scale | | WHO Scale | | AJCC Scale | |
|---|---|---|---|---|---|---|---|
| % Score | Status | Score | Status | Score | Status | Score | Status |
| 100% | Normal; no complaints; no evidence of disease | 0 | Asymptomatic | 0 | Fully active, able to carry out all predisease activities without restriction | H0 | Normal activity |
| 90 | Able to carry on normal activity; minor signs or symptoms of disease | 1 | Symptomatic; fully ambulatory | 1 | Restricted in strenuous activity but ambulatory and able to carry out light work or pursue sedentary occupation | H1 | Symptomatic and ambulatory; cares for self |
| 80 | Normal activity with effort; some signs or symptoms of disease | | | | | | |
| 70 | Cares for self; unable to carry on normal activity or to do active work | 2 | Symptomatic; in bed less than 50% of day | 2 | Ambulatory and capable of all self-care but unable to do any light work; up and about more than 50% of waking hours | H2 | Ambulatory more than 50% of time; occasionally needs assistance |
| 60 | Requires occasional assistance, but able to care for most needs | | | | | | |
| 50 | Requires considerable assistance and frequent medical care | 3 | Symptomatic; in bed more than 50% of day but not bedridden | 3 | Capable of only limited self-care; confined to bed or chair more than 50% of waking hours | H3 | Ambulatory 50% or less of time; nursing care needed |
| 40 | Disabled; requires special care and assistance | | | | | | |
| 30 | Severely disabled; hospitalization indicated, although death not imminent | 4 | Bedridden | 4 | Completely disabled; unable to carry out any self-care and confined totally to bed or chair | H4 | Bedridden; may need hospitalization |
| 20 | Very sick; hospitalization necessary; active supportive treatment necessary | | | | | | |
| 10 | Moribund; fatal processes progressing rapidly | | | | | | |
| 0 | Dead | | | | | | |

sue. The pathologist assesses the aggressiveness or degree of malignancy of tumor cells by comparing the cellular anaplasia, differentiation, and mitotic activity with normal counterparts. Specific characteristics vary with each type of cancer.

The objective of grading a tumor is to quantify information to assist with treatment planning and prognostic determinations. For selected tumors the grade is considered more significant than anatomic staging in terms of prognostic value and treatment. In cancer of the prostate, a well-differentiated T1a tumor requires no specific ther-

apy other than close observation; however, a poorly differentiated T1 tumor needs to be treated aggressively with radiation or radical prostatectomy if the lymph nodes are negative for disease.[95] In soft-tissue sarcomas the grade is the primary determinant of stage of disease and of prognosis. Cure rates for grade 1 sarcoma are 80%, whereas cure rates for grades 2 and 3 drop dramatically to 60% and 40%, respectively.[96] In other tumors, such as melanoma of the skin, testicular and thyroid cancer, and neuroblastoma, histological grading has no useful application.

Two grading systems are commonly seen. One descriptively identifies the tumor as well differentiated (i.e., retaining most of the morphological features and behavior of the normal cell of the tissue of origin), moderately well differentiated, poorly differentiated, or undifferentiated. The other system numerically grades from 1 to 3 or 4, with 1 being the most differentiated and 3 and 4 being the least well differentiated. Grade 4 applies to tumors with no specific differentiation. It is important to remember that the grade 1, well differentiated tumor implies the best prognosis for the patient. The AJCC recommends the following grading classification[83]:

GX  grade cannot be assessed

G1  well differentiated

G2  moderately well differentiated

G3  poorly differentiated

G4  undifferentiated

Certain problems exist with grading classifications: A tumor's level of differentiation may vary with time. Several grades of malignancy may exist within one tumor, in which situation the tumor should be labeled as the least favorable level of differentiation. It is essential that an adequate and representative biopsy specimen has been obtained for a valid interpretation by the pathologist. Nurses aware of the significance of a malignant tumor's grade and stage, as well as new prognostic, molecular markers, will be able to respond realistically to the person's questions about treatment and prognosis.

## CONCLUSION

The diagnostic phase of a cancer illness is a time of adjustment, learning, anxiety, and uncertainty for the individual and family members. With adequate knowledge of the symptoms of disease and of the diagnostic process required for evaluation, nurses can help prepare patients, thereby easing the anxiety associated with the unknown. During this time nurses will interact with the individual in several health care settings—primary clinics, inpatient and outpatient units, and extended care units—as well as in the community. Oncology nurses have used their expertise to (1) facilitate early diagnosis of cancer by promoting awareness of "warning signals" of cancer and conducting screening programs, (2) educate and prepare individuals for a diagnostic evaluation of suspicious signs or symptoms, (3) perform or assist with diagnostic procedures and interpret or clarify results, (4) counsel and support the individual and family in a therapeutic relationship, and (5) prepare the individual for the possible treatment options once a definitive diagnosis is made. Nurses are in pivotal positions to promote the detection of cancer at the earliest possible stage and to assist the individual and family to regain hope, control, and quality of life once the diagnosis of cancer has been determined.

## REFERENCES

1. *Cancer Facts and Figures.* Atlanta, American Cancer Society, 1991
2. Weinrich SP, Weinrich MC: Cancer knowledge among elderly individuals, in Ash CR, Jenkins JF (eds): *Enhancing the Role of Cancer Nursing.* New York, Raven Press, 1990, pp 217–233
3. Fink DJ, Mettlin CJ: Cancer detection: The cancer-related checkup guidelines, in Murphy GP, Lawrence W, Lenhard RE (eds): *American Cancer Society Textbook of Clinical Oncology* (ed 2). Atlanta, American Cancer Society, 1995, pp 178–193
4. Gatsonis C, McNeil BJ: Collaborative evaluations of diagnostic tests: Experience of the RDOG. *Radiology* 175:571–575, 1990
5. Tempany CM, Zhou X, Zerhoundi EA, et al: Staging of prostate cancer: Results of Radiology Diagnostic Oncology Group project comparison of three MRI imaging techniques. *Radiology* 192:47–54, 1994
6. Webb WR, Gatsonis C, Zerhoundi EA, et al: CT and MRI imaging in staging non-small cell bronchogenic carcinoma: report of the Radiology Oncology Diagnostic Oncology Group. *Radiology* 178:705–713, 1991
7. Marton KI, Sox HC, Alexander J, et al: Attitudes of patients toward diagnostic tests: The case of the upper gastrointestinal series roentgenogram. *Med Decis Making* 2:439–448, 1982
8. Blue Cross of California Presents: Breast Cancer Practice Guidelines. Woodland Hills, Blue Cross of California, 1995
9. Rovinski CA: Nurses and cancer's seven warning signals. *Cancer Nurs* 3:53–55, 1980
10. Frank-Stromborg M, Rohan K: Nursing's involvement in the primary and secondary prevention of cancer. *Cancer Nurs* 15:79–108, 1992
11. Melillo KD: Who needs health maintenance? *J Gerontol Nurs* 11:18–21, 1985
12. Rosevelt J, Frankl H: Colorectal cancer screening by nurse practitioners using 60-cm flexible fiberoptic sigmoidoscope. *Dig Dis Sci* 29:161–163, 1984
13. White L, Cornelius J, Judkins A, et al: Screening of cancer by nurses. *Cancer Nurs* 1:15–20, 1978
14. Martin J: Male cancer awareness: Impact of an employee education program. *Oncol Nurs Forum* 17(1):59–64, 1990
15. Lovejoy NC, Jenkins C, Wu T, et al: Developing a breast cancer screening program for Chinese-American women. *Oncol Nurs Forum* 16(2):181–187, 1989
16. Mitchell-Breen ME, Dodds ME, Choi KL, et al: A colorectal cancer prevention, screening and evaluation program in community black churches. *CA* 39:115–118, 1989
17. Marino LB, Kooser J: The psychosocial care of cancer clients and their families: Periods of high risk, in Marino LB (ed): *Cancer Nursing.* St. Louis: Mosby, 1981, pp 53–66
18. Peteet JR, Stomper PC, Ross DM, et al: Emotional support for patients with cancer who are undergoing CT: Semistructured interviews of patients at a cancer institute. *Radiology* 182:99–102, 1992

19. Frank-Stromborg M, Wright P, Segulla M, et al: Psychological impact of the cancer diagnosis. *Oncol Nurs Forum* 11(3): 16–22, 1984

20. Vettese T: Problems of the patient confronting a diagnosis of cancer, in Cullen JW, Fox BH, Isom RN (eds): *Cancer: The Behavioral Dimensions.* New York, Raven Press, 1975, pp 275–281

21. Mahon SM, Casperson D: Teaching women about mammography through use of a brochure. *Oncol Nurs Forum* 18(8): 1375–1378, 1991

22. Habegger D, Ellerhorst-Ryan JM: Needle localization for nonpalpable breast lesions. *Oncol Nurs Forum* 15(2):192–194, 1988

23. Herberth L, Gosnell DJ: Nursing diagnosis for oncology nursing practice. *Cancer Nurs* 10:41–51, 1987

24. Lovejoy NC, Thomas ML, Halliburton P, et al: Tumor markers: Relevance to clinical practice. *Oncol Nurs Forum* 14(5): 75–82, 1987

25. Braunstein GD, Vaitukaitis JL, Carbone PP, et al: Ectopic production of human chorionic gonadotropin by neoplasm. *Ann Intern Med* 78:39–45, 1973

26. Wolmark N, Fisher B, Wieand HS, et al: The prognostic significance of preoperative carcinoembryonic antigen levels in colorectal cancer. Results from NSABP clinical trials. *Ann Surg* 199:375–381, 1984

27. Zamcheck N: The present status of carcinoembryonic antigen (CEA) in diagnosis, detection of recurrence, prognosis and evaluation of therapy of colonic and pancreatic cancer. *Clin Gastroenterol* 5:625–638, 1976

28. Tietz NW: *Clinical Guide to Laboratory Tests* (ed. 3). Philadelphia, Saunders, 1995

29. Byrne CJ, Saxton DF, Pelikan PK: *Laboratory Tests: Implications for Nursing Care* (ed 2). Menlo Park, CA, Addison-Wesley, 1986

30. Perkins AS, Vande Woude GF: Principles of molecular cell biology of cancer: Oncogenes, in DeVita VT, Hellman S, Rosenberg SA (eds): *Cancer Principles and Practice of Oncology* (ed 4). Philadelphia, Lippincott, 1993, pp 35–59

31. Ghosh BC, Ghosh L: *Tumor Markers and Tumor Associated Antigens.* New York, McGraw-Hill, 1987, pp 1–10

32. Bates SE, Longo DL: Use of serum markers in cancer diagnosis and management. *Semin Oncol* 14:102–138, 1987

33. Ravel R: *Clinical Laboratory Medicine* (ed 6). St. Louis, Mosby, 1995, pp 63–84

34. Madeya ML, Pfab-Tokarsky JM: Flow cytometry: An overview. *Oncol Nurs Forum* 19:459–463, 1992

35. Williams NN, Daly JM: Flow cytometry and prognostic implications in patients with solid tumors. *Surg Gynecol Obstet* 171: 257–266, 1990

36. Collins-Hattery AM, Blumberg BD: S phase index and ploidy prognostic markers in node negative breast cancer: Information for nurses. *Oncol Nurs Forum* 18(1):59–62, 1991

37. Bragg DG: State-of-the-art assessment: Diagnostic oncologic imaging. *Cancer* 64:261–265, 1989 (suppl)

38. Dillon WP, Harnsberger HR: The impact of radiologic imaging on staging of cancer of the head and neck. *Semin Oncol* 18(2):64–79, 1991

39. Bragg DG: The application of imaging in lung cancer. *Cancer* 67:1150–1154, 1991 (suppl)

40. McClennan BL: Oncologic imaging, staging, and follow-up of renal and adrenal carcinoma. *Cancer* 67:1199–1208, 1991 (suppl)

41. Hricak H: Role of imaging in the evaluation of pelvic cancer, in DeVita VT, Hellman S, Rosenberg SA (eds): *Important*

*Advances in Oncology 1991.* Philadelphia, Lippincott, 1991, pp 103–131

42. Castellino RA: Diagnostic imaging evaluation of Hodgkin's disease and non-Hodgkin's lymphoma. *Cancer* 67:1177–1180, 1991 (suppl)

43. Tio TL, Cohen P, Coene PP, et al: Endosonography and computed tomography of esophageal carcinoma: Preoperative classification compared to new (1987) TNM system. *Gastroenterology* 96:1478–1486, 1989

44. Shaha AR, Strong EW: Cancer of the head and neck, in Murphy GP, Lawrence W, Lenhard RE (eds): *American Cancer Society Textbook of Oncology* (ed 2). Atlanta, American Cancer Society, 1995, pp 355–377

45. Sussman SK, Halvorsen RA, Illescas FF, et al: Gastric adenocarcinoma: CT vs. surgical staging. *Radiology* 167:335–349, 1988

46. Hatch TR, Barry JM: The value of excretory urography in staging bladder cancer. *J Urol* 135:49, 1986

47. Johnson CD, Dunnick NR, Cohan RM, et al: Renal adenocarcinoma: CT staging of 100 tumors. *Am J Radiology* 148:59–63, 1987

48. Pettersson H, Gillespy T, Hamlin D, et al: Primary musculoskeletal tumors: Examination with the MR imaging compared with conventional modality. *Radiology* 164:237–241, 1987

49. Rubin P, Bragg DG, O'Mara RE: Principles of oncologic imaging and tumor imaging strategies, in Rubin P (ed): *Clinical Oncology: A Multidisciplinary Approach for Physicians and Students* (ed 7). Philadelphia, Saunders, 1993, pp 169–176

50. Salo JO, Kivisaari L, Rannikko S, et al: Computerized tomography and transrectal ultrasound in the assessment of local extension of prostatic cancer before retropubic prostatectomy. *J Urol* 137:435–438, 1987

51. Clouse ME, Harrison DA, Grassi CJ, et al: Lymphangiography, ultrasonography, and computed tomography in Hodgkin's disease and non-Hodgkin's lymphomas. *J Comput Assist Tomography* 9:1–8, 1985

52. Borg SA, Rosenthal S: *Handbook of Cancer Diagnosis and Staging: A Clinical Atlas.* New York, Wiley, 1984

53. *Diagnostics: The Nurse's Reference Library.* Nursing 81 Books. Springhouse, PA, Intermed Communications, 1981

54. McLelland R, Hendrick RE, Zinninger MD, et al: The American College of Radiology Mammography Accreditation Program. *Am J Radiology* 157:473–479, 1991

55. Mammography Quality Control Standards Act of 1992. U.S. Congress, Senate. 102nd Congress, 2nd session, October 1, 1992. Senate Report 102–448.

56. Paulus DD: Imaging in breast cancer. *CA Cancer J Clin* 37: 133–150, 1987

57. Castellino RA, Delapaz RL, Larson SM: Imaging techniques in cancer, in DeVita VT, Hellman S, Rosenberg SA (eds): *Cancer Principles and Practice of Oncology* (ed 4). Philadelphia, Lippincott, 1993, pp 507–530

58. Ehrlich RA, McCloskey ED: *Patient Care in Radiography.* St. Louis, Mosby, 1989, pp 139–167

59. Shehadi WH: Contrast media reactions: Occurrence, recurrence, distribution patterns. *Radiology* 143:11–17, 1982

60. Thompson WM: Imaging strategies for tumors of the gastrointestinal system. *CA Cancer J Clin* 37:165–185, 1987

61. Gupta NC, Frick MP: Clinical applications of positron-emission tomography in cancer. *CA Cancer J Clin* 43:235–254, 1993

62. Wahl RD, Hawkins RA, Larson SM, et al: Proceedings of a

National Cancer Institute workshop: PET in oncology—a clinical research agenda. *Radiology* 193:604–606, 1994

63. Harrison KA, Tempero MA: Diagnostic use of radiolabeled antibodies for cancer. *Oncology* 9:625–631, 1995

64. Petersen BM, Bass BL, Bates HR, et al: Use of the radiolabeled murine monoclonal antibody 111-In-CYT-103 in the management of colon cancer. *Am J Surg* 165:137–142, 1993

65. Epenetos A, Britton KE, Mather S, et al: Targeting of 1-123 tumor-associated antibodies to ovarian, breast, and gastrointestinal tumors. *Lancet* 2:999–1005, 1982

66. Siccardi AG, Buraggi GL, Callegaro L, et al: Multicenter study of immunoscintigraphy with radiolabeled monoclonal antibodies in patients with melanoma. *Cancer Res* 46:4817–4822, 1986

67. Carrasquillo JA, Bunn PA, Keenan AM, et al: Radioimmunodetection of cutaneous T-cell lymphoma with 111In-labeled T101 monoclonal antibody. *N Engl J Med* 315:673–680, 1986

68. Watson AD, Rocklage SM: Theory and mechanisms of contrast enhancing agents, in Higgins CB, Hricak H, Helms CA (eds): *Magnetic Resonance Imaging of the Body*. New York, Raven Press, 1992, pp 1257–1287

69. Lufkin RB: Severe anaphylactoid reaction to GD-DTPA. *Radiology* 176:879, 1990

70. Stack JP, Antoun NM, Jenkins JPR, et al: Gadolinium-DPTA as a contrast agent in magnetic resonance imaging of the brain. *Neuroradiology* 30:145–154, 1988

71. Shellock FG: MRI biologic effects and safety considerations, in Higgins CB, Hricak H, Helms CA (eds): *Magnetic Resonance Imaging of the Body*. New York: Raven Press, 1992, pp 233–265

72. Camp-Sorrell D: Magnetic resonance imaging and the implantable port. *Oncol Nurs Forum* 17(2):197–199, 1990

73. Nickl NJ, Cotton PB: Clinical application of endoscopic ultrasonography. *Am J Gastroenterol* 85:675–682, 1990

74. Neiman RS, Smith TJ: Biopsy principles, pathologic evaluation of specimens and staging, in *Cancer Manual* (ed 8). Boston, American Cancer Society, Massachusetts Division, 1990, pp 70–77

75. Ell SR: Imaging techniques: Fine-needle aspiration of various organs and body sites, in Bibbo M (ed): *Comprehensive Cytopathology*. Philadelphia, Saunders, 1991, pp 615–620

76. Schmidt RA: Stereotactic breast biopsy. *CA* 44:172–191, 1994

77. Pitot HC: *Fundamentals of Oncology* (ed 3). New York, Marcel Dekker, 1986, pp 21–33

78. Cotran RS, Kumar V, Robbins SL: Neoplasia, in *Robbins Pathologic Basis of Disease* (ed 4). Philadelphia, Saunders, 1989, pp 239–305

79. Sirica AE: Classification of neoplasms, in Sirica AE (ed): *The Pathobiology of Neoplasia*. New York, Plenum Press, 1989, pp 25–39

80. Greco FA, Hainsworth JD: Cancer of unknown primary site, in DeVita VT, Hellman S, Rosenberg SA (eds): *Cancer Principles and Practice in Oncology* (ed 4). Philadelphia, Lippincott, 1993, pp 2072–2092

81. Altman E, Cadman E: An analysis of 1,539 patients with cancer of unknown primary site. *Cancer* 57(1):120–124, 1986

82. Yeomans AC, Washington JB: Occult primary malignancies. *Oncol Nurs Forum* 18(3):539–544, 1991

83. Beahrs OH, Henson DE, Hutter RVP, et al: *American Joint Committee on Cancer: Manual for Staging of Cancer* (ed 4). Philadelphia, Lippincott, 1992

84. Rubin P: Statement of the clinical oncologic problem, in Rubin P (ed): *Clinical Oncology for Medical Students and Physicians: A Multidisciplinary Approach* (ed 6). New York, American Cancer Society, 1983, pp 2–19

85. Santoro A: Chronic leukemias, in Bonadonna G, Robustelli della Cuna G (eds): *Handbook of Medical Oncology*. Milan, Italy, Masson, 1988, pp 756–777

86. Durie BGM, Salmon SE: A clinical staging system for multiple myeloma correlation of measured myeloma cell mass with presenting clinical features, response to treatment and survival. *Cancer* 36:842–854, 1975

87. Henson DE: Future directions for the American Joint Committee on Cancer. *Cancer* 69:1639–1644, 1992 (suppl)

88. Preisler HD, Raza A: The role of emerging technologies in the diagnosis and staging of neoplastic diseases. *Cancer* 69:1520–1526, 1992 (suppl)

89. Stanley KE: Prognostic factors for survival in patients with inoperable lung cancer. *J Nat Cancer Institute* 65:25–32, 1980

90. Karnofsky DA, Abelmann WH, Craver LF, et al: The use of the nitrogen mustards in the palliative treatment of carcinoma. *Cancer* 1:634–656, 1948

91. Zubrod CG, Schneiderman M, Frei E, et al: Appraisal of methods for the study of chemotherapy in man: Comparative therapeutic trial of nitrogen mustard and triethylene thiophosphoramide. *J Chron Dis* 11:7–33, 1960

92. World Health Organization: *World Handbook for Reporting Results of Cancer Treatment*. Geneva, WHO, 1979

93. Poelhuis EHK, Hart AAM, Burgers JMV, et al: Assessment of quality of life: Scoring performance status in cancer patients, in Aaronson NK, Beckmann J (eds): *The Quality of Life of Cancer Patients*. New York, Raven Press, 1987, pp 93–99

94. Hutchinson TA, Boyd NF, Feinstein AR: Scientific problems in clinical scales, as demonstrated in the Karnofsky index of performance status. *J Chron Dis* 32:661–666, 1979

95. Shipley WU, Meares EM, Schwartz JH, et al: Cancer of the prostate, in *Cancer Manual* (ed 8). Boston, American Cancer Society, Massachusetts Division, 1990, pp 284–294

96. Suit HD, Mankin JH, Antman KH, et al: Sarcomas of bone and soft tissue, in *Cancer Manual* (ed 8). Boston, American Cancer Society, Massachusetts Division, 1990, pp 315–326

# PART III

# Treatment

# Chapter 10

# Quality of Life as an Outcome of Cancer Treatment

**David Cella, PhD**

## INTRODUCTION

The term *quality of life* (QL or QOL) or *health-related quality of life (HQL)* has emerged to organize and galvanize a collection of outcome evaluation activities in cancer treatment research over the past two decades. Prior to this, length of survival, regardless of its quality, was considered to be the only primary outcome in oncology treatment research. It is now widely accepted that in most circumstances *quality* of survival is as important as *quantity* of survival. This implies that a severely toxic treatment must be evaluated for its detrimental impact as well as its survival benefit. It also raises a less obvious point: that treatments can be considered efficacious if the quality of life is improved even in the absence of survival benefit. Thus, investigating the impact of cancer treatments on HQL is a two-tailed enterprise in which treatment toxicity is traded not only with survival time but also with posttreatment function and well-being.

HQL evaluation entails a multidimensional quantification of patient functional status, usually as perceived by the patient.[1-13] In the decades to come, treatment intensification strategies that increase toxicity are likely to continue, given the advent of hematopoietic growth factors and improved antiemetic regimens. This further increases the importance of evaluating toxicity, patient function, and patient preferences for treatment. HQL evaluation differs from classic toxicity ratings in two important ways: (1) it incorporates more aspects of function (e.g., mood, affect, social well-being) than those that typically have been attributed to treatment, and (2) it focuses on the patient's perspective.

## THE ROLE OF NURSING

Nursing has always played a central role in the clinical appreciation and treatment of quality of life, as evidenced by interest in managing disease symptoms and treatment side effects. Symptoms and side effects represent a major component of HQL as it is understood today. Managing these problems has for centuries been the primary domain of nurses caring for people with cancer. Nurses play a leadership role in HQL evaluation of cancer clinical trials, including a detailed analysis of the relative impact of symptoms and side effects on the patient's HQL.

Since the early 1950s, most of the important large-scale oncology clinical trials have been conducted by one of the cooperative clinical trials organizations within the United States, Canada, Europe, and Australia. One cannot help noticing the rapid growth of interest shown by cooperative groups to include HQL evaluation in selected trials. For the first time since their inception, *every* large cooperative clinical trials organization in Europe and North America is actively examining quality of life in some of its trials. In many groups (e.g., Southwest Oncology Group, Radiation Therapy Oncology Group, Gynecologic Oncology Group, Eastern Cooperative Oncology Group) nursing has played a leadership role in these initiatives. This chapter presents background information to help the nurse-investigator understand and evaluate quality-of-life studies in oncology clinical trials, and a selected review of measures available to the investigator aspiring to participate in the broad-based evaluation of experimental cancer treatments.

## EVALUATING METHODS OF ASSESSMENT

Along with the evolution of interest in HQL, many efforts to measure the construct have been created and promoted. A number of validated HQL measures have become accepted for use in oncology in particular[14-20] and chronic illness in general,[21-27] so it is increasingly unlikely that a single "gold standard" measure will ever emerge. The diversity of available measures is potentially valuable in that it provides the user with choices based on specific characteristics of a given disease site, clinical trial, or HQL domain of interest. This chapter provides the reader with some understanding of criteria to evaluate whether an HQL measure is likely to accomplish its stated purpose. Such an understanding can guide the reader who wishes to critically evaluate the development, initial testing, and field performance of a given measure.

### Construct Definition as a Frame for Measurement

Any construct must be defined before it can be measured. There are many different definitions of HQL in the literature,[28-32] but disagreement about its definition or its dimensions does not mean that it cannot be measured. It does, however, suggest that all measures are not equivalent, so one must therefore be clear on the definition of HQL as put forth by the group that developed a particular measure. Definitions of HQL may differ across study groups and still be measured reliably and validly within the parameters of a definition. For example, most agree that important HQL domains include physical, mental, and social dimensions. Whereas virtually all currently accepted HQL measures provide some ability to separate physical and psychological dimensions, social functioning is much less evenly represented. Some measures cover social well-being and function more than others. For example, deHaes et al[33] do not measure social functioning as a component, and yet their scale can be evaluated for reliability and validity within their range of item content. Regarding the social dimension of HQL, there may well be a distinction between social *well-being* (perceived social support, satisfaction with relationships, etc.) and social *functioning* (ability to see friends, leisure activity). Clearly, the most empirically substantiated distinction has been between the correlated, but distinct, dimensions of physical well-being and mental well-being.[33–35]

# APPROACHES TO MEASURING HEALTH-RELATED QUALITY OF LIFE

Over time, two approaches to measuring HQL have evolved: psychometric and utility. These approaches have evolved independent of one another, largely because they were developed within different scientific disciplines. Psychometric approaches derive from psychology, whereas utility approaches derive from economics. Only recently have investigators considered integrating these two approaches. This remains a critical challenge in HQL measurement.

## Psychometric Approach

The psychometric approach includes generic health profile measurement (e.g., Sickness Impact Profile[27]) and specific instruments intended to measure the multidimensional impact of a specific disease, treatment, or condition (e.g., Functional Living Index—Cancer[17]). The psychometric approach places heavy emphasis on an individual's response and response variability across individuals. An important contribution of the psychometric approach is that it measures subjective or perceived well-being. Psychometric measures may or may not include a summary or total score. When available, only rarely have these summary scores been connected to patients' values for their current health status. This poses a problem, because without a rating of patient preference, one cannot appropriately make a decision about the value of a given treatment to a given patient. Very often, one of two patients with identical disease and treatment options declines therapy while the other accepts it enthusiastically. Because psychometric measures typically neither incorporate patient-specific weights for individual domains nor anchor states of health to a common standard, evaluating trade-offs between quality of life and length of life, or between one dimension of HQL and another, is difficult. This presents a challenge in a clinical trial where the primary purpose for integrating HQL measurement is to incorporate data on the impact of treatment on both length of life and quality of life into conclusions about treatment efficacy. The collection of patient preferences in clinical trials would allow evaluation of the effect of treatment on quality-adjusted survival as well as on conventional outcome measures. Further, the addition of patient preference assessments to clinical trial outcome evaluation can make it possible to distinguish patients who favor one treatment over another when both may have equivalent survival outcomes. A strategy for doing this has been described by Till and colleagues.[36]

## Utility Approach

In contrast to the psychometric approach, the utility approach is explicitly concerned with treatment decision making, usually at a policy level. In this approach, treatments typically are evaluated as to their benefit compared in some way to their cost. The utility approach to health status measurement evolved from a tradition of cost-benefit analysis, into cost-effectiveness approaches and, most recently, cost-utility approaches.[37] The cost-utility approach extends the cost-effectiveness approach conceptually by evaluating the HQL benefit produced by the clinical effects of a treatment, thereby including the patient's (presumed) perspective. To be used this way, HQL must be measured as a utility since, by definition, utilities can be multiplied by time to yield a meaningful quantity. Two general cost-utility methods are the standard gamble approach and the time trade-off approach.[38] In the *standard gamble* approach, people are asked to choose between their current state of health and a "gamble" in which they have various probabilities for death or perfect health. The *time trade-off* method is easier to perform and involves asking people how much time they would be willing to give up in order to live out their remaining life expectancy in perfect health. All utility approaches share in common the use of 0–1 scale in which $0 = $ death and $1 = $ perfect health. In practice, most cost-utility analyses employ expert estimates of utility weights, or, in some cases, weights provided by healthy members of the general public. It is often assumed that these weights are reasonable approximations of patient preferences. However, several studies have demonstrated that utilities obtained from patients are generally higher than those provided by physicians, which are, in turn, higher than utilities for the same health states obtained from healthy individuals.[39] There are practical impediments to collection of utilities directly from patients, including the complexity of the concepts involved and the requirement for an interviewer-administered questionnaire (often unfeasible in the cooperative group setting). In addition, utility assessments provide little information on important disease and treatment-specific problems and are probably less sensitive to changes in health status over time than psychometric data.[40,41] Finally, the few studies that have been done involving simultaneous measurement of utilities and health status have found them at best to be moderately correlated, with measures of mood and depression correlating more highly than other measures with utilities.[42]

A modified utility approach was developed to evaluate the effectiveness of adjuvant chemotherapy for early-stage breast cancer.[43] This approach, the Quality-adjusted Time Without Symptoms and Toxicity (Q-TWiST), has been extended to other diseases and treatments. The Q-TWiST approach discounts survival time by subtracting from observed survival a utility-weighted estimate of the quality of time spent in various partitioned health states, such as treatment toxicity and recurrent disease. Most often, utilities are estimated, not actually gathered, or data are presented in a way that allows one to judge the value of therapy based on different utilities. In this approach, thresholds for decision making are determined by modeling actual survival data using judgments made by investigators regarding where patient preferences are likely to fall relative to these threshold values. There is no theoretical reason that actual patient preference data could not be used in Q-TWiST analyses or other studies of quality-adjusted survival. If the relationship between psychometric data and utilities can be established, it will become possible to collect psychometric data and base utility estimates on the reports of patients rather than the best guesses of others.

In summary, the existing science of HQL measurement is organized around a presumed (but theoretically unsubstantiated) dichotomy between psychometric and utility approaches. Neither approach alone is sufficient to understand clinical trial outcome data. The psychometric approach provides the detailed perspective of the patient, but it does not tell us how important a given problem or set of problems is to a group of patients. The utility approach informs us about the relative value of various health states; however, because of its emphasis on a single summary score, it fails to reflect the specific problems that might emerge. To date, it has also usually relied on surrogates rather than on patients to provide the utility weights. The psychometric approach can uncover specific areas of difficulty or dysfunction, yet patients may not consider these areas to be worthy of provider attention or a change in treatment. On the other hand, the utility approach does not generally reveal the nature of specific problems or dysfunctions, which clearly hampers the provider's efforts in planning interventions or treatment changes. In fact, identification of health dimensions uniquely important to an individual and quantifying patient status within those dimensions has been proposed.[44] These approaches can and must be integrated in order to continue to advance the field. Previous efforts to combine psychometric and utility approaches have been rare and, where present, poorly integrated.[45] An integrative approach could be applied in which a well-validated HQL scale can be administered to a patient in a clinical trial (or in clinical practice, for that matter). This patient's total score can be converted to a standardized score that allows for both ease of communication and possible utility analysis.

# EVALUATING PSYCHOMETRIC MEASURES

Asking a psychometric consultant if a given HQL measure is valid is like asking a bacteriologist if a given antibiotic is effective. Unless the measure is clearly invalid, the answer will always begin with a question such as: "Under what circumstances, and with which patients?" Just as there is no antibiotic for every infection, there is no HQL measure for every investigation. Similarly, when

the question is: "Which HQL measure should I use for evaluating (X) treatment for (Y) disease," the answer has necessary contingencies: "At which phase of treatment?" "What differences do you expect?" In short, the investigator's task is to select the measure most likely to be effective for a given purpose. This is best accomplished by careful consideration of the purpose of the investigation, critical evaluation of the psychometric properties and known performance of available measures, and review of item content for relevance and appropriateness. This last activity is not trivial inasmuch as it can prevent selection of an otherwise-valid measure that will be insensitive for the application selected. For example, the short forms (e.g., SF-36) derived from the Medical Outcomes Study[22,23] have a long history of development and demonstrate good psychometric properties, but may be inappropriate at the high end of HQL (e.g., adjuvant chemotherapy) because they emphasize mobility and physical function over social well-being, sexuality, and body image. The issue of disease severity cuts across virtually all self-report measures of HQL, in that it becomes difficult if not impossible to obtain self-report HQL data from very weak, cognitively impaired, or emotionally upset patients. This is an unfortunate irony given that these patients are often the very ones for whom quality-of-life concerns take first priority in treatment decision making. Efforts to use surrogate ratings have been disappointing, showing that health providers and, to a lesser extent, family members cannot be considered as reliable surrogate raters.[46]

## Reliability

Two synonyms for *reliability* are repeatability and consistency. *Repeatability* refers to the extent to which a measure, applied two different times (test-retest) or in two different ways (alternate form and interrater), produces the same score. Consistency refers to the homogeneity of the items of a scale. A measure's internal consistency is usually expressed in terms of Cronbach's coefficient α, because it is the most comprehensive strategy among those available, and can be easily done with most computer statistical packages.

A ruler is a perfectly reliable measure because it will always produce the same score when applied to the same object, whether done by the same person or two different people. No HQL measure can ever expect to achieve such perfection, expressed as a correlation coefficient of 1.0, but close approximations (e.g., correlations above .70) are important.[47]

### Reliability is a matter of degree

Reliability is not a fixed property of a measure but rather a property of a measure used with certain people under certain conditions. Because it is not a fixed property, reported reliability cannot be assumed to be generalizable and therefore should be reevaluated in later applications. Reevaluation may be unreasonable to expect of test-retest reliability, but certainly not of internal consistency or interrater reliability (when appropriate).

### Reliability depends on the number of items

As the number of items goes up, so too does the reliability coefficient. It is this observation that led to the Spearman-Brown correction of the split-half reliability technique, which evaluates the internal consistency of a test by splitting it in half and correlating the two halves (Cronbach's α is the average of all split halves). In our effort to reduce the number of items in a scale so as to lower patient and staff burden, we cannot allow ourselves to go so far as to drop reliability below an acceptable level. Another important corollary to this basic principle is that subtests will usually have lower reliability than the total score, because they have fewer items. It would be acceptable, for example, to implement a measure that has Cronbach α coefficients ranging from, say, .65 to .80, for the subtests, and to .85 for the total score. One might be more cautious about interpreting data from the least internally consistent subtest, especially if it were the only one with significant results.

### Reliability is increased by heterogeneous samples

This increase in reliability occurs because heterogeneous samples produce a greater spread of scores, which inflate the reliability coefficient. Therefore, a coefficient of .70 for a group of patients with advanced pancreatic cancer may reflect superior reliability compared to a coefficient of .80 obtained with a sample combining healthy and very ill people.

## Validity

*Validity* refers to a scale's ability to measure what it purports to measure. A scale must be reliable in order to be valid, but it needn't be valid in order to be reliable. The ruler described earlier, for example, is certainly reliable; however, its validity must be clarified. As a measure of length, it can be demonstrated to be valid; in fact, it is a "gold standard" against which other measures of length could be compared. However, it has limited validity as a measure of weight. Length and weight are two different physical constructs, one that is perfectly measured by a ruler, the other that can be estimated by a ruler (assuming constant density). If we had no better measure of weight than a ruler, it could arguably be used as a reasonably valid approximation, but certainly not as a gold standard. In some sense, this is where we find ourselves today in HQL measurement: without a gold standard, trying to approximate a construct we agree is important and measurable. Data collected to substantiate this effort are validity data.

Validity generally has been subdivided into three types: content, criterion, and construct. *Content validity* is further divided into *face validity* (the degree to which the scale superficially appears to measure the construct in

question), and *true content validity* (the degree to which the items accurately represent the range of attributes covered by the construct). Two things are important to understand about content validity. First, since content validity does not include statistical evidence to support inferences made from tests (the central feature of validity), some[48] do not consider content of items to be a true measure of a scale's validity. Second, with a multidimensional construct such as HQL, content coverage should cut across at least three broad domains (i.e., physical, psychological, and social) in order to be considered valid from the perspective of item content. The scale reviewer can evaluate this by examination of the development strategy for the scale as well as the actual content of the items themselves, which may or may not be reflected by subtest scores.

*Criterion validity* is also subdivided into two types, *concurrent validity* and *predictive validity*. The distinction between the two is a function of when the criterion data are collected. Criterion data that are collected simultaneously with the scale data provide evidence of concurrent validity. Data that are collected some time after the scale data provide evidence for predictive validity. It is common to see scores on the self-report measure of HQL in question correlated to another "standard" that has been completed at the same time, provided as evidence of concurrent validity. Generally, when the method of completion is the same and the timing is concurrent, one would seek coefficients only slightly below the internal consistency coefficients for the reference and comparison scales. Similarly, test-retest reliability coefficients can be considered as upper bounds of predictive validity.

*Construct validity* extends criterion-related validity into a broader arena in which the scale in question is tested against a theoretical model and adjusted according to results that can, in turn, help refine theory. There are many different approaches to construct validation. One is to examine a matrix of correlations between the scale in question and the following: other measures of the same construct; measures of related constructs; measures of unrelated constructs; and different methods of data collection (e.g., self-report versus observer rating). This multitrait-multimethod matrix permits one to test for the presence of hypothesized high correlations (convergent validity) and hypothesized low correlations (discriminant validity).

Other contributions to construct validity can be derived from multidimensional scaling and factor analytic approaches that can confirm the presumed multidimensional nature of HQL. It might seem contradictory, but it may also help to conduct item analyses based on a unidimensional scaling model for the overall measure as well as the component subtests, given the fact that HQL dimensions are intercorrelated.

The ability of an instrument to differentiate groups of patients expected to differ in HQL is also an important validation of its sensitivity. A "known groups technique"[49] can be employed in which patients with, for example, advanced disease are compared to those with limited disease to determine whether the HQL measure detects the known clinical differences between groups. The same could be done by comparing HQL scores of inpatients to those of outpatients, scores of patients receiving adjuvant therapy to those of a clinically comparable group receiving no therapy, scores of homebound patients to those of ambulatory patients, and so forth. Finally, the demonstration of an instrument's sensitivity or responsiveness to change over time, parallel to changes in clinical status[50] is an important example of its validity that can easily be neglected in early psychometric evaluations.

### Validity is not absolute

Like reliability, validity should not be considered to be an absolutely achieved status of a measure. Validity data are cumulative, requiring ongoing updates and refinements. Validity is relative, in that a given measure might be valid (i.e., sensitive) in one setting and not in another. Consider a measure that emphasizes activities of daily living skills and physical sensations. Such a measure may be valid in the context of metastatic breast cancer, but insensitive in early-stage disease, where virtually all patients will score at the top of the scale. The potential for sample-dependent ceiling effects such as this (and for floor effects in the reverse case) warrants caution when selecting the best instrument for a given population.

### An HQL measure should assess well-being in addition to impairment

A criterion of content validity is that a scale measure the full range of HQL. Given that the concept of HQL includes positive aspects of health status (well-being), it is important that a measure of HQL address well-being in addition to functional ability/limitations.

### Statistical significance is not always clinically meaningful

Related to validity is the issue of meaningfulness of the data obtained. A comparison of treatment arms might indeed result in differences in HQL. But how much of a difference is clinically meaningful, as opposed to statistically significant? For a seven-point Likert scaling of symptoms, Jaeschke et al[51] suggested a difference of approximately 0.5 units as a minimal clinically important difference. For other types of scaling (e.g., linear analog), Jacobson and Truax[52] recommend a Reliable Change Index that estimates whether a change measured is real or just a consequence of imprecise measurement.

## Acceptability of Measures

In addition to reliability and validity, the acceptability of an instrument to patients and staff is also very important. Intrusiveness or inappropriateness of items can damage the integrity of an HQL measure that might otherwise be quite sound. Also, while reliability and validity are certainly important, they are not static standards. Just as our understanding of HQL is evolving, so also should our measurement approaches.

## QUALITY-OF-LIFE MEASURES FOR USE IN ONCOLOGY

The fact that there are now many available measures of HQL is both a blessing and a curse. On the one hand, having many questionnaires available provides the user with choices based on specific characteristics of a given disease site or clinical trial. On the other hand, the choices potentially fragment the field of HQL measurement, thereby impeding our ability to make comparisons across studies and measures. This section presents some of the more commonly used and adequately validated measures of HQL that have been designated as cancer-specific. The designation of cancer-specific is rather arbitrary in that some measures considered to be cancer-specific could be (and have been) applied to other diseases. Examination of item content of some of these measures reveals that indeed many of the concepts measured are generic rather than cancer-specific.

### Psychometric Measures

#### Quality-of-Life Index (QLI)[21]

This scale is perhaps the best example of a "cancer-specific" scale that in reality measures generic health concepts. Although not the first cancer-specific quality-of-life measure to appear in the literature,[53] the QLI was certainly an early entry. Intended by its authors as conceptually equivalent to a neonatal Apgar score,[54] it was developed originally as a 10-point physician rating of five areas of functioning (activity, daily living, health, support, outlook). Since then, many have used this observer rating scale as a patient-rated scale, with reasonable success.[46] The QLI was constructed using expert advisory panels comprised of patients and professionals, and has been subjected to study in at least 28 empirical investigations. In their thorough review, Wood-Dauphinee and Williams[55] conclude that the QLI is a well-validated global measure of HQL. Proxy ratings and interrater agreement data for subscales of activity, daily living, and health are more robust than those for support and outlook. As a five-item index, its internal consistency is often quite low (below .60), raising concern about the wisdom of combining these five items. The QLI has demonstrated the ability to distinguish cancer patients with terminal disease from either patients with recent disease or ones who were engaged in active treatment.[56] The QLI has also been positively related to the Uniscale and Multiscale Measures of Quality of Life and self- and physician ratings of HQL in cancer patients,[57] although the relationship with the Karnofsky Performance Status (KPS) scale has been variable.

### European Organization for Research and Treatment of Cancer Quality-of-Life Questionnaire—Core (EORTC-QLQ)[14,15]

This measure is a 36-item instrument consisting of both dichotomous responses (yes/no) and responses that utilize a 4-point rating scale ranging from "not at all" to "very much." The core instrument was developed from a conceptual model and measures physical, role, emotional, and social functioning, along with disease symptoms, financial impact, and global quality of life across different cultural contexts. Aaronson et al[14] report α's for individual scales ranging from a low of .59 for a three-item subset of the physical functioning dimension to a high of .85 for the two-item global quality-of-life dimension. Multitrait scaling techniques using 156 tests of item discriminant validity yielded only one definite and three probable scaling errors and interscale correlations supported the notion of nonorthogonal dimensions ($p <$ .001) in quality of life. Finally, Aaronson et al demonstrated that the seven scales significantly predicted differences in patient clinical status.[14] The 36-item QLQ has been replaced with a 30-item version that reduces the number of physical- and emotional-functioning items and replaces the single concentration and memory item with two separate items.[15] Three new items have been added, creating a QLQ-C33 version in current use.

### Functional Living Index—Cancer (FLIC)[17]

This is a 22-item scale on which patients indicate the impact of cancer on "day-to-day living issues that represent the global construct of functional quality of life,"[17] using a 7-point Likert-type rating. The scale provides a total HQL score only. Although only a total score is available, factor analyses have consistently revealed two primary factors (physical and psychological) with other smaller factors also present. It might therefore be appropriate to create at least two subtest scores from this instrument. Convergent validity studies on the FLIC suggest that the emotional factor is more highly correlated with other well-validated measures assessing depression and anxiety than with measures of physical functioning. Conversely, the physical factor of the FLIC is more highly correlated with measures of physical functioning than with measures of emotional distress. The FLIC has been used extensively in oncology, with predominantly positive results.

### Functional Assessment of Cancer Therapy (FACT) scales[16,18]

This instrument is a 29–49-item compilation of a generic core (29 items) and over 20 specific subscales, which reflect symptoms or problems associated with different diseases (e.g., breast, bladder, colorectal, head and neck, and lung cancers, and HIV infection), treatments (e.g., bone marrow transplantation, neurotoxicity), symptoms (e.g., fatigue, anorexia/cachexia), or other concerns (e.g., spirituality).[16,18] The scale was originally developed

from a model similar to that of the EORTC, using 135 patients with advanced cancer and 15 oncology specialists. It was validated on a second sample of 630 patients with a variety of cancers at different stages. The measure yields a total HQL score and subtest scores for physical well-being, social/family well-being, relationship with doctor, emotional well-being, functional well-being, and disease-specific concerns. Six additional experimental items request information regarding how much each dimension affects HQL, using a rating scale that ranges from 0 ("not at all") to 10 ("very much so").

The FACT-G (general core) is able to distinguish metastatic ($M = 79.6$) from nonmetastatic disease ($M = 83.7$), $F(1,334) = 5.38$, $p < .05$. It also distinguishes between stage I, II, III, and IV disease, $F(3,308) = 2.94$, $p < .05$, and between inpatients and outpatients from different centers, $F(2,411) = 17.0$, $p < .001$. Concurrent validity is supported by Pearson correlations with the Functional Living Index—Cancer (.80) and a patient-completed version of the QL Index (.74). A unique feature of the FACT scales is that they provide supplemental valuative ratings that allow patients to provide domain-specific utility weights. These scales were developed primarily out of the psychometric tradition; however, there was an early eye toward movement into a utility approach.

### Ferrans and Powers Quality of Life Index (QLI)[58]

The QLI is a 68-item index of overall quality of life, which provides a summary score of four health domains: health and physical functioning; social and economic; psychological/spiritual; and family. A unique feature of the instrument is its two-part response format, which allows people to rate satisfaction with 34 areas and then second has them rate their perceived importance of those same areas, thus producing 68 items. Scores are obtained by summing weighted satisfaction and importance scores.[58] The "cancer-specific" version was a modification of an earlier general population version of the QLI, and was developed based upon a review of the oncology literature. Initial testing was in breast cancer patients; however, considerably more testing and applications have been published. Internal consistency and reliability for the subscales ranged in the initial studies from .65 (family) to .93 (psychological/spiritual). The total QLI score correlates highly with the measure of life satisfaction, and on review of content appears to be more "general" than other commonly used cancer-specific quality-of-life questionnaires.[58]

### Cancer Rehabilitation Evaluation System—Short Form (CARES—SF)[19,20]

This is a 59-item self-administered rehabilitation and HQL instrument composed of a list of statements reflecting problems encountered by cancer patients. Patients complete a minimum of 38 to a maximum of 57 items, depending on their treatments as well as on other medical and demographic factors. Statements are rated in terms of how applicable each is to them using a 5-

point rating scale ranging from "not at all" to "very much." The measure yields a global score (summed ratings) reflecting overall HQL, five summary scores reflecting physical, psychosocial, medical interaction, marital and sexual dimensions, and 31 subscales. Adequate test-retest reliability (10 days, $r = .92$ for global score, and ranges from .69 to .87 for subscales), internal consistency ($\alpha$'s for five subscales range from .67 to .83), and concurrent validity with other HQL measures ($r$'s range from $-.50$ to .74, $p < .0001$) are reported,[19] and the shortened form is correlated with the longer, 139-item version at $r = .98$. The global CARES score is sensitive to extent of disease in patients with colorectal, lung, and prostate cancer, and to improvement in HQL in patients with breast cancer over a 13-month period.[20] Summary scales, in part, have replicated global CARES scores, particularly in colorectal and lung disease.[20]

### Linear Analogue Self-Assessment (LASA) scales

LASA scales use a 100-mm line with descriptors at each extreme. Respondents are required to mark their current state somewhere along that line, which is then measured as a score in centimeters or millimeters from the 0 point. There are three noteworthy LASA scales for cancer patients. The original LASA scale of Priestman and Baum[53] was a 10-item scale for studying HQL in advanced breast cancer. This was later extended to 25 items in a study comparing chemotherapy and hormone therapy for advanced breast cancer.[57] These items included ten on symptoms and side effects, five on physical functioning, five on mood, and five on social relationships.

Two other LASA scales are the 31-item measure of Selby et al,[59] which subsequently was reduced to 29 items,[60] and the 14-item LASA of Padilla and colleagues.[61,62] Much of the Selby measure[59,60] was derived from the 12 Sickness Impact Profile (SIP) categories,[27] and supplemented with items to measure pain, mouth sores, concern with appearance, and other breast cancer-specific concerns. Test-retest reliability and internal consistency coefficients are above .70.[57,59] Concurrent validity coefficients with the appropriate SIP scales ranged from .28 to .98, with most above .60. Reliability coefficients on the Padilla et al scale are acceptably high, with a factor analysis of 130 cancer patients revealing three factors (physical well-being, psychological well-being, symptom control) accounting for 73% of the total variance.[61] Padilla et al have also developed a longer (23-item) measure for patients with colostomies.[62]

Linear analogue scales are appealing because they are easy to administer and are usually presumed to have robust sensitivity due to interval scaling and a wide range of scores. They have also been criticized on the grounds that their sensitivity may be illusory and that it is difficult to know the minimal clinically significant difference. They also cannot be administered over the telephone, which can be limiting. However, they have performed rather well in studying individuals with metastatic breast cancer. For example, women receiving cytotoxic therapy were found to suffer more adverse physical reactions with a subsequent improvement in well-being on Priestman and Baum's scale, as long as there was an objective clinical response.[53] Later that decade, the much-quoted, counterintuitive results of Coates et al[63] were reported in which women with metastatic cancer did better on continuous chemotherapy than those on intermittent chemotherapy. They used a very simple five-item linear analogue scale along with the Spitzer QLI. Finally, Tannock et al,[64] using the Selby LASA, demonstrated trends toward better HQL in women receiving higher dosages of cytotoxic chemotherapy as opposed to lower doses, presumably because of the increased tumor response and survival advantage gained from the increased dosage. All of these studies point to the same general conclusion about management of metastatic breast cancer: that the advantages of continuous cytotoxic chemotherapy outweigh the costs, assuming sufficient dosing and assuming the presence of measurable response to therapy. Taken together, these findings can provide valuable guidance in patient counseling and management with respect to the costs and benefits of cytotoxic chemotherapy in advanced breast cancer. In fact, Tannock has put forth a set of guidelines for managing metastatic breast cancer based on available treatment and HQL data.[65]

### Medical Outcomes Study—Short-Form Health Status Survey (MOS SF-36)[22,23]

The Medical Outcomes Study—Short-Form Health Status Survey (MOS SF-36) is a self-administered 36-item measure of eight health concepts: physical functioning, limitations in role functioning due to physical health problems, social functioning, bodily pain, general mental health, limitations in role functioning due to emotional problems, vitality, and general health perceptions.[22] It was developed to reproduce the previously well-validated, full-length scales, but in a shorter format. Responses vary as a function of the attribute measured, and range from dichotomous to a maximum of five possible choices. Its standardized scoring system yields a profile of eight health scores, which are summed scores of individual scale items (some of which have been reverse-scored) as well as summary indices. The SF-36 is reported to have satisfactory reliability (coefficients ranging from .73 to .94). Validity studies have demonstrated the ability to distinguish between patients with and without a chronic condition, discriminate levels of severity within a medical diagnosis, and reflect changes in health-related quality of life associated with changes in disease severity.[23]

## Utility Measures

### Quality of Well-Being (QWB) Scale[24–26]

The QWB is a utility-based measure of HQL. Kaplan and Anderson[24] focus on the qualitative dimension of functioning rather than exclusively on the psychological and social attributes of health outcomes, and use the term *health-related QL* to refer to the impact of health conditions on function. The Quality of Well-Being (QWB) scale is a 25-item list of symptom/problem complexes (CPX) covering the domains of mobility, physical activity, and social activity, each representing related but distinct aspects of daily functioning.[24] There are community weights for each CPX control for relative desirability, with higher weights reflecting more desirable states. The QWB is administered in a standardized interview and yields information about both specific states (CPX) and a total quality of well-being score (range = 0–1), expressed as the average of relative desirability scores. It is reported to demonstrate good test-retest reliability ($r$'s ranging from .78 to .99, with most correlation coefficients being above .90) over a 1-day period across different populations and health problems,[26] and adequate content, convergent, and discriminant validity.[25]

### Quality-adjusted Time Without Symptoms and Toxicity (Q-TWiST)[43]

The only utility approach developed specifically for assessing cancer patients, the Quality-adjusted Time Without Symptoms and Toxicity (Q-TWiST) approach, attempts to evaluate the effectiveness of treatments relative to one another by partitioning posttreatment time into distinct health states.[43] (See discussion earlier in this chapter.) The Q-TWiST approach discounts survival time by reducing it according to a predetermined utility weight (0–1 range), which accounts for the impact of disease symptoms and treatment side effects. The Q-TWiST approach does not clearly account for the effect of the time trade-off of most patients, who are usually quite willing to trade acute treatment toxicity for extended survival benefit. Given that it typically infers rather than measures patient preferences, the Q-TWiST approach may be regarded as related to but conceptually distinct from patient-rated HQL. It carries some advantages over patient-rated approaches in that it is inexpensive to derive and allows for adjustment of survival time with the (presumed) HQL of that time. It may be possible to integrate the Q-TWiST approach with a psychometric scale or a patient preference scaling approach that increases sensitivity of measurement by adding the perspective of the patient.

## OTHER APPLICATIONS OF HQL DATA

Although this chapter has focused on HQL as an outcome of cancer therapy, there are other important applications of HQL data. These include rehabilitation planning, predicting survival and treatment response, and predicting treatment preferences. Nursing efforts at patient rehabilitation are helped by systematic, structured assessment of HQL concerns. The CARES[20] was developed to fill exactly

this demand for structured, comprehensive assessment of rehabilitation needs.

Survival prediction is a feature common to virtually every HQL assessment tool that has tested this component of prediction validity. Knowledge of survival probability in a cohort of patients can be useful in planning long-term care and placing patients into treatment protocols.

There are other predictive capabilities of HQL instruments that are not as obvious but provide opportunity for further clinical insight. For example, Yellen and Cella[66] found that aggressive treatment preferences in advanced cancer were predicted by social well-being and not the patient's physical or emotional state. It appears that the strongest predictor of aggressive treatment preference is the positivity of one's social milieu and not, as clinicians have tended to think, the physical or mental well-being of the patient. Findings such as this provide food for thought to the nurse who must counsel patients about current and future treatment options.

## CONCLUSION

This chapter provides a brief update of a sampling of cancer-specific health-related quality-of-life measures and approaches that have shown promise. Examination of sample measures is possible elsewhere.[4] Some of the measures described here have already contributed to an understanding of the diverse costs and benefits of cancer therapies. Most of the progress has been in the study of breast cancer and, to a lesser extent, lung, colorectal, and prostate cancers. Further attention must be directed to less common (e.g., hematologic) malignancies as well as to intensive experimental therapies with severe toxicity and uncertain benefit (e.g., bone marrow transplantation with solid tumors). The issues in these areas may be sufficiently distinct to require new or appropriately adapted measurement. Because of their clinical experience and expertise, and because of their position at the forefront of cancer practice settings, nurses are in a unique position to assume leadership in evaluating the broad spectrum of costs and benefits associated with today's cancer therapies.

## REFERENCES

1. Aaronson NK, Beckman J: *The Quality of Life of Cancer Patients.* Monograph Series of the European Organization for Research on Treatment of Cancer (EORTC), vol. 17. New York, Raven Press, 1987
2. Spilker B (ed): *Quality of Life Pharmacoeconomics in Clinical Trials* (ed 2). New York, Raven Press, 1996

3. Osoba D (ed): *Effect of Cancer on Quality of Life.* Boca Raton, FL, CRC Press, 1991

4. Tchekmedyian NS, Cella DF, Winn P (eds): Economical quality of life outcomes in oncology. *Oncology* 9(11), 1995 (suppl)

5. U.S. Department of Health and Human Services (DHHS), Public Health Service, National Institutes of Health: *Quality of Life Assessment in Cancer Clinical Trials: Report of the Workshop on Quality of Life Research in Cancer Clinical Trials.* Bethesda, MD, National Cancer Institute, 1990

6. Moinpour CM, Feigl P, Metch B, et al: Quality of life end points in cancer clinical trials: Review and recommendations. *J Natl Cancer Inst* 81:485–495, 1989

7. Cella DF, Tulsky DS: Measuring quality of life today: Methodological aspects. *Oncology* 4:29–38, 1990

8. Gotay CC, Korn EL, McCabe MS, et al: Quality-of-life assessment in cancer treatment protocols: Research issues in protocol development. *J Natl Cancer Inst* 84:575–579, 1992

9. Donovan K, Sanson-Fisher RW, Redman S: Measuring quality of life in cancer patients. *J Clin Oncol* 7:959–968, 1989

10. Fayers PM, Jones DR: Measuring and analyzing quality of life in cancer clinical trials: A review. *Stat Med* 2:429–446, 1983

11. Fetting JH: Evaluating quality and quantity of life in breast cancer adjuvant trials. *J Clin Oncol* 6:1795–1797, 1988

12. Skeel RT: Quality of life assessment in cancer clinical trials—It's time to catch up. *J Natl Cancer Inst* 81:472–473, 1989

13. Cella DF, Cherin EA: Quality of life during and after cancer treatment. *Compr Ther* 14:69–75, 1988

14. Aaronson NK, Ahmedzai S, Bullinger M, et al: The EORTC Core Quality-of-Life Questionnaire: Interim results of an international field study, in Osoba D (ed): *Effect of Cancer on Quality of Life.* Boca Raton, FL, CRC Press, 1991

15. Aaronson NK, Ahmedzai S, Bergman B, et al: The European Organization for the Research and Treatment of Cancer QLQ-C30: A quality of life instrument for use in international clinical trials in oncology. *J Natl Cancer Inst* 85:365–376, 1993

16. Cella DF, Bonomi AE: The Functional Assessment of Cancer Therapy (FACT) and Functional Assessment of HIV Infection (FAHI) quality of life measurement system, in Spilker B (ed): *Quality of Life and Pharmacoeconomics in Clinical Trials* (ed 2). New York, Raven Press, 1996, pp 203–214

17. Schipper H, Clinch J, McMurray A, Levitt M: Measuring the quality of life of cancer patients: The Functional Living Index—Cancer: Development and validation. *J Clin Oncol* 2:472–483, 1984

18. Cella DF, Tulsky DS, Gray G, et al: The Functional Assessment of Cancer Therapy (FACT) scale: Development and validation of the general version. *J Clin Oncol* 11:570–579, 1993

19. Schag CAC, Ganz P, Heinrich RL: Cancer Rehabilitation Evaluation System—Short Form: A cancer-specific rehabilitation and quality of life instrument. *Cancer* 68:1406–1413, 1991

20. Ganz PA, Schag CAC, Lee JJ, Sim MS: The CARES: A generic measure of health-related quality of life for patients with cancer. *Qual Life Res* 1:19–29, 1992

21. Spitzer WO, Dobson AJ, Hall J, et al: Measuring the quality of life of cancer patients: A concise QL index for use by physicians. *J Chron Dis* 34:585–597, 1981

22. Ware JE, Sherbourne CD: The MOS 36-Item short-form health survey (SF-36): I. Conceptual framework and item selection. *Med Care* 30:473–83, 1992

23. McHorney CA, Ware JE, Rogers W, et al: The validity and relative precision of MOS Short- and Long-Form Health Status Scales and Dartmouth COOP Charts: Results from the Medical Outcomes Study. *Med Care* 30:253–265, 1992, (suppl 5)

24. Kaplan RM, Anderson JP: The general health policy model: An integrated approach, in Spilker B (ed): *Quality of Life Assessment in Clinical Trials.* New York, Raven Press, 1990

25. Kaplan RM, Bush JW, Berry CC: Health status: Types of validity and the Index of Well-Being: *Health Serv Res* 11:478–507, 1976

26. Anderson JP, Kaplan RM, Berry CC, et al: Interday reliability of function assessment for a health status measure: The Quality of Well-Being Scale. *Med Care* 27:1076–1084, 1989

27. Bergner J, Bobbitt RA, Carter WB, Gilson BS: The Sickness Impact Profile: Development and final revision of a health status measure. *Med Care* 19:787–806, 1981

28. Campbell A, Converse PE, Rodgers WL: *The Quality of American Life.* New York, Sage, 1976

29. Till JE, McNeil BJ, Bush RS: Measurement of multiple components of quality of life. *Cancer Treatment Symposium* 1:177–181, 1984

30. Calman KC: The quality of life in cancer patients—An hypothesis. *J Med Ethics* 10:124–125, 1984

31. Schipper H, Levitt M: Measuring quality of life: Risks and benefits. *Cancer Treat Rep* 69:1115–1123, 1985

32. George L, Bearon L: *Quality of Life in Older Persons: Meaning and Measurement.* New York, Human Sciences Press, 1980

33. deHaes JCJM, vanKnippenberg FCE, Neijt JP: Measuring psychological and physical distress in cancer patients: Structure and application of the Rotterdam Symptom Checklist. *Br J Cancer* 62:1034–1038, 1990

34. Hays RD, Stewart AL: The structure of self-reported health in chronic disease patients. *Psychol Assess* 2:22–30, 1990

35. Ware J: Measuring functioning, well-being and other generic health concepts, in Osoba D (ed): *Effect of Cancer on Quality of Life.* Boca Raton, FL, CRC Press, 1991, pp 7–23

36. Till JE, Sutherland HJ, Meslin EM: Is there a role for preference assessments in research on quality of life in oncology. *Qual Life Res* 1:31–40, 1992

37. Drummond MF, Stoddart GL, Torrance GW: *Methods for Economic Evaluation of Health Care Programmes.* Oxford, Eng., Oxford University Press, 1987

38. Torrance GW: Measurement of health state utilities for economic appraisal: A review article. *J Health Econ* 5:1–30, 1986

39. Boyd NF, Sutherland HJ, Heasman KZ, et al: Whose utilities for decision analysis? *Med Decis Making* 10:58–67, 1990

40. Tsevat J, Goldman L, Soukup JR, Lee TH: Stability of utilities in survivors of myocardial infarction. *Med Decis Making* 10:323, 1990

41. Canadian Erythropoietin Study Group: Association between recombinant human erythropoietin and quality of life and exercise capacity of patients receiving hemodialysis. *Br Med J* 300:573–578, 1990

42. Tsevat J, Cook EF, Soukop JR, et al: Utilities of the seriously ill (abst). *Clin Res* 39:589A, 1991

43. Gelber RD, Goldhirsch A, Cavalli F: Quality-of-life-adjusted evaluation of adjuvant therapies for operable breast cancer. *Ann Intern Med* 114:621–628, 1991

44. Llewellyn-Thomas HA, Sutherland HJ, Tritchler DL, et al: Benign and malignant breast disease: The relationship between women's health status and health values. *Med Decis Making* 11:180–188, 1991

45. Feeny D, LaBelle R, Torrance GW: Integrating economic

evaluations and assessments, in Spilker B (ed): *Quality of Life Assessments in Clinical Trials.* New York, Raven Press, 1990, pp 71–83

46. Slevin ML, Plant H, Lynch D, et al: Who should measure quality of life, the doctor or the patient? *Br J Cancer* 57:109, 1988

47. Nunnally JC: *Psychometric Theory.* New York, McGraw-Hill, 1967

48. Messick S: The once and future issues of validity: Assessing the meaning and consequences of measurement, in Wainer H, Braun HI (eds): *Test Validity.* Hillside, NJ, Lawrence Erlbaum Associates, 1988

49. Bohrnstedt GW: Measurement, in Rossi PH, Wright JD, Anderson AB (eds): *Handbook of Survey Research.* New York, Academic Press, 1983

50. Guyatt G, Walter S, Normal G: Measuring change over time: Assessing the usefulness of evaluative instruments. *J Chron Dis* 40:171, 1987

51. Jaeschke R, Singer J, Guyatt GH: Measurement of health status: Ascertaining the minimal clinically important difference. *Controlled Clin Trials* 10:407–415, 1989

52. Jacobson NS, Truax P: Clinical significance: A statistical approach to defining meaningful change in psychotherapy research. *J Consul Clin Psychol* 59:12–19, 1991

53. Priestman TJ, Baum M: Evaluation of quality of life in patients receiving treatment for advanced breast cancer. *Lancet* April 24:899–901, 1976

54. Apgar V: Proposal for new methods of evaluation of newborn infants. *Anesth Analg* 32:260, 1953

55. Wood-Dauphinee S, Williams JI: The Spitzer Quality-of-Life Index: Its performance as a measure, in Osoba D (ed): *Effect of Cancer on Quality of Life.* Boca Raton, FL, CRC Press, 1991, pp 169–184

56. Mor V: Cancer patients' quality of life over the disease course: Lessons from the real world. *J Chron Dis* 40:535, 1987

57. Baum M, Priestman T, West RR, Jones EM: A comparison of subjective responses in a trial comparing endocrine with cytotoxic treatment in advanced carcinoma of the breast. *Eur J Cancer* 16:223–226, 1980 (suppl 1)

58. Ferrans, CE: Development of a Quality of Life Index for patients with cancer. *Oncol Nurs Forum* 17:15–21, 1990, (suppl)

59. Selby PJ, Chapman JAW, Etazadi-Amoli J, et al: The development of a method for assessing the quality of life of cancer patients. *Br J Cancer* 50:13–22, 1984

60. Boyd NF, Selby PJ, Sutherland HJ, Hogg S: Measurement of the clinical status of patients with breast cancer: Evidence for the validity of self assessment with linear analogue scales. *J Clin Epidemiol* 41:243–250, 1988

61. Padilla GV, Presant C, Grant MM, et al: Quality of life index for patients with cancer. *Res Nurs Health* 6:117–126, 1983

62. Padilla GV, Grant MM: Quality of life as a cancer nursing outcome variable. *Am Nurs Sci* 8:45–60, 1985

63. Coates A, Gebski V, Stat M (for the Australian-New Zealand Breast Cancer Trials Group): Improving the quality of life during chemotherapy for advanced breast cancer. *N Engl J Med* 317:1490, 1987

64. Tannock IF, Boyd NF, DeBoer G, et al: A randomized trial of two dose levels of cyclophosphamide, methotrexate and fluorouracil chemotherapy for patients with metastatic breast cancer. *J Clin Oncol* 6:1377, 1988

65. Tannock IF: Management of breast and prostate cancer: How does quality of life enter the equation?, in Tchekmedyian NS, Cella CF (eds): *Quality of Life in Oncology Practice and Research.* Williston Park, NY, Dominus (PRR), 1991

66. Yellen SB, Cella DF: Someone to live for: Social well-being, parenthood and decision-making in oncology. *J Clin Oncol* 13:1255–1264, 1995

# Chapter 11

# Principles of Treatment Planning

**Mary B. Maxwell, RN, C, PhD**

## INTRODUCTION

Because "cancer" includes more than 101 different disease entities involving virtually every organ system in the body, choosing among the therapeutic alternatives is a complex task. Fundamentally, treatment decisions in oncology are based on the location, cell type, and extent of the malignancy, with established modes of therapy (surgery, radiation, chemotherapy) directed toward the particular disease presentation. The aim of treatment is to cure if possible, causing minimal structural or functional impairment. If cure is not possible, then the aim is to control or palliate the disease. The sequence and intellectual considerations in cancer treatment planning are the same as in any problem-solving activity: gathering information, planning, executing the plan, and evaluating. In this chapter the factors involved in problem solving for cancer treatment are examined in detail. The material is organized temporally, following the usual sequence in planning treatment for a patient. An initial, brief historical look at treatment will set the stage for understanding the basis of contemporary therapy, from which projections can be made for the future.

The recipient of cancer treatment is a unique human being, and every aspect of the design and evaluation of therapeutic activities must take this into consideration. A therapeutic plan that seems indicated by abstract scientific analysis may have to be modified or changed by human events in the real world. Cancer treatment and care should be a humanistic application of established modes of therapy to a unique individual. Optimal treatment for both cure and palliation requires not only individualization of treatment but an approach that uses all therapeutic disciplines capable of improving results.

## HISTORICAL PERSPECTIVES ON CANCER TREATMENT

In the haste to find more effective ways to treat cancer, new methods were and are continually being devised. Treatment assumptions that can seem so logical are often not borne out with time or by the application of rigorous scientific research methods. A hundred years from now, current treatments may seem as bizarre to clinicians as bloodletting and purging seem to us today. Understanding cancer involves unraveling the mysteries of the basis of life itself, and we are still far from this understanding. Until cancer can be prevented, therapeutic interventions will continue to evolve and change. Every year new discoveries are made and old methods modified or discarded. From the earliest times, the treatment of cancer has been based on the prevailing ideas about the etiology of the disease.[1] In any era, such ideas stem from theories of the structure and function of the human body, the philosophical view of nature, and the available technology.[2]

### Ancient Times

The Egyptians used arsenical ointment in 1500 B.C. to attack cancer's external manifestations, which were believed to be most important. Hippocrates cauterized cancer in the neck in the fourth century B.C. Celsus (30 B.C. to A.D. 38) excised breast cancer, leaving the pectoral muscles intact. Cato administered charcoal, and many therapists employed metallic salts, particularly copper and lead, treatments that persisted for centuries.

### Dark Ages/Medieval Period

Galen (A.D. 131–20) classified tumors, and considered cancer a systemic disease caused by an excess of black bile humor, being thereby beyond the cure of operation. He advocated vegetable diets and purging, cautioning against eating walnuts. The theory of humors came from ancient Greek beliefs that universal elements (fire, air, wind, earth) and qualities (hot, cold, moist, dry) were assigned to four humors: blood, phlegm, yellow bile, and black bile.[2] Treatment for cancer in this era was mostly surgical, including lancing and bloodletting, aimed at releasing the offending collection of humor causing the cancer. The basic principle was first to purge the black humors and then to excise the affected area. These ideas predominated until the dawn of the eighteenth century.

### The Enlightenment

As discoveries were made about anatomy and the lymphatic and circulatory systems, the humoral theories and the idea that cancer was a constitutional disease gave way to more scientific notions. In 1704 Valsalva advanced the theory that cancer was first a local lesion capable of cure by surgery, which then spread via the lymphatics to regional nodes, thus tending to recur as secondary lesions. The principles of modern cancer surgery are based on this theory.

### The Nineteenth Century

John Hunter, father of scientific surgery, thought coagulated lymph was a cause of cancer and that tumors were nourished by lymph vessels. This led to a more chemical orientation in which corrosive acids or ferments of lymph were seen as culprits. Hunter removed local lymph nodes when possible and ligated vessels supplying the tumor.

With the aid of the microscope and advances in chemistry and science in general, it later became accepted that the body was composed of fibers and tissues. The new tissue theories, coupled with findings from embryonic studies, led to a better understanding of cancer metastasis. This was followed by the cellular theory, which recognized cells as the basic structural units of tissues, including tumors. Toward the end of this era, the only available treatment, surgery, progressed in a dramatic manner due to the development of anesthesia and antiseptic techniques.

## The Twentieth Century

An anatomical basis for cancer surgery arose about 100 years ago. *En bloc* resections (radical mastectomy, radical prostatectomy), in which the primary tumor as well as adjacent lymphatics and lymph nodes were removed in one continuous section, were deemed the proper cancer operation. Cancer surgery based on these considerations has persisted, with the goal being the surgical removal of every cancer cell. By the 1970s, however, the superradical procedures, such as hemicorporectomy and hindquarter operations, were seldom performed; patient survival had not been improved.

As a consequence of conceptual changes arising from new information about tumor biology, a biological basis for cancer treatment emerged.[3] It became generally accepted that even the smallest solid tumor that could be diagnosed with contemporary methods was already systemic at the time of presentation. Since cancer is a systemic disease involving a complex spectrum of host-tumor interrelations, variations in local-regional therapy are unlikely to affect survival substantially. The primary aim of oncological surgery became to reduce the tumor burden to a number of viable cells that could be destroyed by host immunologic factors, chemotherapy, or immunotherapy. If surgery was followed by one or more of these treatments, it was called *adjuvant* (aiding or assisting) *therapy*.

The goal of adjuvant chemotherapy is to significantly prolong the patient's survival while maintaining quality of life. Disease-free survival (time from diagnosis until first relapse) and overall survival (time from diagnosis until death) are end points evaluated in any adjuvant clinical trial. Quality of life assessment is used to evaluate the therapeutic ratio (benefit versus risk) of a treatment.[4]

More recently, *neoadjuvant therapy* (the use of drugs at the earliest possible time for induction) has been used for some tumors.[5,6] This involves giving a short course of chemotherapy prior to a surgical procedure, in an attempt to eliminate micrometastasis up front. These are examples of *multimodal therapy*, the integration of more than one antineoplastic therapy into a treatment program in order to improve therapeutic results, reduce toxicities (as compared to single modality treatment), or both.[7] The objective to eradicate every malignant cell remained the same, but the method for its accomplishment changed from exclusively surgical as other cancer treatment modalities became available.

## Radiation Discovered

The discovery of x-rays, radioactivity, and radium before the turn of the century was soon followed by the therapeutic application of the new agents. By 1899, a basal cell carcinoma had been cured by radiation.[8] It was thought that a miraculous new cure for cancer had been discovered because of the dramatic initial responses seen in the treatment of skin and superficial lesions. Then followed a period of disillusionment and pessimism as recurrence and serious injuries to normal tissues were realized. These first 25 years were the "dark ages" of radiotherapy. The physical nature and biological effects of the new agents were not understood, and equipment was primitive. There was no reliable way to measure dose. Many scientists lost their lives through their work with radiation during this time. Because most of the earliest practitioners were surgeons, they used treatment methods involving single, massive exposures aimed at eradicating a tumor in a single treatment. As might be expected, those individuals who lived through the immediate postirradiation period, although they had impressive initial regressions of their lesions, usually developed serious complications as well as early recurrences. Starting in 1919, the technique of successive fractionated daily doses of radiotherapy evolved from clinical research. Impressive results became evident in the treatment of head and neck and cervical lesions. In the early 1950s, the emergence of megavoltage equipment greatly improved delivery. Recent technological innovations such as beam-modifying devices, radiation sensitizers, and radioprotectors have enhanced the tumoricidal effect of radiation therapy. Where previously radiation was used only for palliation, it began to be used for cure in some situations.

## Chemotherapy Introduced

Cancer chemotherapy has its origins in observations made of chemical warfare during World War I. Soldiers who breathed mustard gas suffered severe bone marrow suppression, aplasia, and death. It was hypothesized that these effects could be exploited in the treatment of cancer. Nitrogen mustard subsequently became the first chemotherapeutic agent to undergo clinical trials.

In the 1940s, the laborious task of ascertaining which of some 200,000 known chemicals possessed cancericidal properties was begun. Effective chemotherapeutic agents were produced by the synthesis of toxic radicals with chemical substances required by the malignant cell for division and multiplication. In the 1950s antibiotics (Adriamycin, bleomycin) began to be used as antineoplastics. Thioguanine, mercaptopurine, and folic antagonists were introduced. The prospective, randomized clinical trial was introduced into clinical medicine as a mechanism for hypothesis testing, obtaining natural history information about the cancer, and for evaluating the worth of a particular treatment. The advent of clinical trials allowed cancer treatment to be based on rational choice rather than on anecdote and trial and error.[9]

Where at first single drugs were given continuously or daily over a period of time, the use of systemic chemotherapy has evolved to *pulse dosing* (high doses given intermittently), with multiple drugs being given concurrently (*combination chemotherapy*).[10] Because agents used in combination are chosen for their overlapping toxicities as well as their sensitivity to a particular tumor, higher tumor cell kill can theoretically be achieved with each treatment, resulting in fewer side effects. *Biological response modifiers*, agents meant to modulate biological or immune responses that affect cancer, were introduced in the 1980s.[11] These agents are described in chapter 17. Biological response modifiers may be considered a noncytotoxic type of chemotherapy. There are currently over 50 antineoplastic agents available (plus investigational drugs in testing stages) for treating cancers. Pharmacological considerations, variables, and patient factors make for an infinite variety of combinations and sequences that have been, are, and will be tried for treatment.[12] *First-line drugs*, those used during initial treatment, are also those known to be most effective against the tumor and most likely to lead to remission, or "cure." If the tumor recurs, *second-line drugs* may be in order, because the drugs used initially failed (probably due to resistance). Second-line drugs are those with less activity against the tumor, but for which a response or a second remission may be possible if the tumor is sensitive to them. In some cases, such as hematologic malignancies, third- and fourth-line drugs may be capable of eliciting a tumor response.

## The Cancer Team

Traditionally, surgeons had managed the treatment of most people with cancer. During the 1960s, medical oncology, an offshoot of internal medicine, became a specialty. Radiotherapy is a consultative discipline, and radiation oncologists see patients only on referral by other physicians. Whereas up to 30 years ago the primary qualifications for an oncology nurse were a kind heart and the ability to improvise,[13] the current variety and complexity of care opportunities has called forth a new breed of professional nurse. Advanced formal education, oncology nursing certification, research skills, and clinical sophistication are mandatory as nursing roles have expanded and nurses have assumed increased responsibility for all aspects of patient management. Even with the prevalence of managed care and hospital downsizing, the certified oncology nurse (OCN® and AOCN) is highly valued in all care settings. Modern cancer treatment and care is a team effort involving the expertise of specialists from a variety of disciplines.

## Treatment Centers

Because treatment approaches are not always clearly defined, the consultative assistance of qualified oncological specialists is available to patients throughout the United States through tumor boards in hospitals with accredited cancer programs. Tumor boards enable a group of physicians and clinicians specializing in cancer to meet, discuss particular cases, and give their opinions about the advantages and disadvantages of treatment alternatives. In many larger centers, there are even specialty tumor boards that review cases in one particular field (e.g., breast, urology, pediatrics).

Patients can now usually be treated in their own communities, avoiding the long periods away from home and family that used to be necessary. The care provided by the major cancer centers has become highly technological, palliative, or research oriented. Many community cancer centers have been established, as well as special oncology units in local hospitals, and hospices for the terminally ill. These cancer programs offer not only the latest treatment with state-of-the-art national protocols, but also rehabilitation and support programs for patients and families. Due to cost-containment efforts, most cancer treatment is now given in ambulatory settings, and patients are receiving home care instead of hospital care more frequently.

But the care of the person with cancer has not always been so enlightened. The first cancer hospital opened in Rheims in 1740 under the supervision of the Hotel Dieu (in Paris, the oldest hospital in Europe). In 1770, because of the superstition that cancer was contagious, the hospital was moved outside the city. The first cancer service in a general hospital was established in Middlesex Hospital in England. It consisted of 12 beds for patients who were permitted to remain until they either improved or succumbed. In the United States, the present Memorial Sloan-Kettering Cancer Center in New York City was established by J. Marion Sims, who was ridiculed and threatened for his efforts to treat cancer.

Because primary therapy has improved and combined methods of treatment offer a wide variety of interventions to manage the disease after recurrence, people with cancer are living longer. This often means additional therapeutic planning sessions and visits to the tumor board or cancer team as new problems arise. Figure 11-1 charts the usual sequence of events in planning cancer treatment.

## FACTORS INVOLVED IN TREATMENT PLANNING

### The Patient Presents

Any person with a physical complaint who seeks health care may have cancer. Any complaints of weight loss,

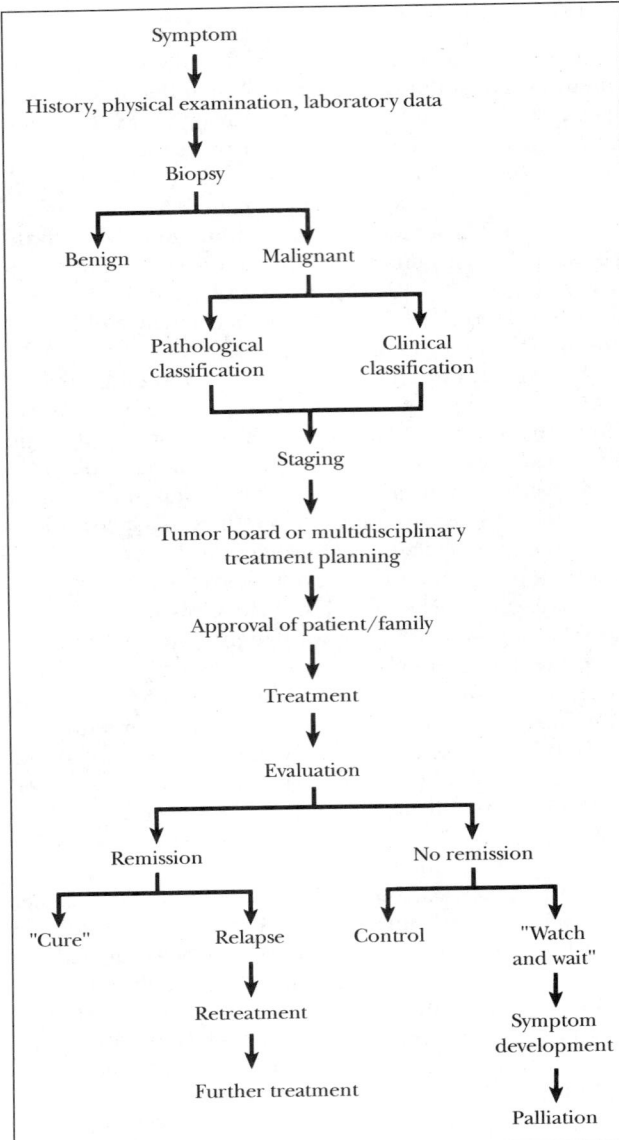

**FIGURE 11-1** Usual sequence of events in planning cancer treatment.

unexplained pain, unexplained loss of energy, or irregularities of the alimentary, respiratory, genital, urinary, or neurologic system, or concerns about lumps or bumps should alert the primary clinician to the possibility of cancer.

## A Diagnostic Workup Is Begun

When neoplastic disease is suspected, a detailed history (including family and occupational information), physical examination, and hematological, biochemical, and radiological studies must be performed to establish the likelihood of cancer as the diagnosis and the necessity for obtaining histological proof. When the clinical evidence points to the presence of malignancy, the next step is to establish by biopsy the nature of the lesion.

## A Biopsy Is Done

Histological proof of malignancy is the cornerstone of diagnosis and treatment. It is crucial because neoplasms can masquerade as benign or inflammatory conditions, and vice versa. A biopsy is also a useful guide to prognosis, and a definitive diagnosis fosters the economical, orderly, and planned use of all available resources. It prevents hasty local treatment measures that might jeopardize later interventions. No matter how difficult it may be to obtain tissue (e.g., a suspected pancreatic tumor), proceeding to treat without a tissue diagnosis could lead to disaster if the lesion were later found to be benign. The site that is least risky to disrupt and most likely to provide the necessary information is biopsied. Chapter 9 describes methods for performing biopsies.

Any biopsy report that is equivocal or inconsistent with the clinical findings should be reviewed by an outside source (such as the Armed Forces Institute of Pathology) or a new biopsy should be obtained. Recurrent or metastatic disease requires the same critical diagnosis as the primary lesion.

## The Biopsy Establishes the Diagnosis

The pathologist's report is crucial in oncology because it conveys the significance of a given neoplasm. The information is expressed in a kind of shorthand, condensing abundant information into a few terms. The language used must be understood by all involved and it must be simple enough to be practical for use in the clinical setting. It has been standardized so that cross-comparisons of different cancers in different individuals in different geographic locations can be made.

The two major agencies involved in the standardization of the language of malignant disease are the International Union Against Cancer (UICC) and the American Joint Committee on Cancer (AJCC). Not only does a common language assist the individual clinician in planning treatment and determining the patient's prognosis, but it assists oncology specialists around the world to share results of research and treatment outcomes.

## Classifying the Tumor

Cancers are classified, or staged, via two main approaches: *pathological*, based on information about the tumor, and *clinical*, based upon information concerning the host. Table 11-1 compares these two systems, and chapter 9 discusses classification in greater detail.

### Pathological classification

The current and best pathological classification system is a combination of approaches: anticipated biologi-

**TABLE 11-1**   Tumor Classification Approaches: Pathological and Clinical

| Approach | Describes | Based On | Performed By | When Performed | Information Provided | Useful For | Standardization |
|---|---|---|---|---|---|---|---|
| Pathological staging | Tumor | Microscopic examination of biopsy | Pathologist | Before first treatment | | 1. Diagnosis<br>2. Prognosis<br>3. Selection of treatment<br>4. Prevention of complications<br>5. Exchange of information<br>6. Research | Guidelines for reporting developed by College of American Pathologists and Joint Commission on Accreditation Health Care Organizations |
| a. Biological behavior<br>b. Histological type<br>c. Grade | | | | | a. Benign or malignant<br>b. Cell tissue of origin<br>c. Degree of malignancy | | |
| d. Special studies, flow cytometry, cytogenetic, DNA probe analysis, electron microscopy, tumor markers | | | | | d. Differential diagnosis, quantification of cellular subpopulations | | |
| e. Tumor size, margins, nodes, invasion | | Microscopic examination of resected specimen | | After surgical resection | e. Anatomic extent of disease | | |
| Clinical staging<br>a. Initial | Host | Physical exam, labs, x-rays, imaging, etc. | Clinician | a. Before first treatment | Extent of disease and organs involved | Same as for pathological staging | TNM staging system developed by International Union Against Cancer and American Joint Committee on Cancer |
| b. Retreatment | | | | b. After recurrence when further treatment needed | | | |
| c. Autopsy | | | | c. At death | | | |

cal behavior, histogenesis (tissue of origin), and grade.[14,15] In terms of *biological behavior,* tumors can be divided into benign or malignant groups. A benign tumor is well circumscribed or encapsulated: microscopically, it appears orderly and is made up of cells similar to those of its parent tissue. A malignant tumor invades the organs from which it originated and eventually the surrounding tissues; it is made up of cells that vary greatly in size and shape and contain large, hyperchromic nuclei and prominent nucleoli. Many mitotic figures are present in cancerous tissue, some of which are atypical, and lymph and blood vessels are often permeated with malignant cells.

Various suffixes are used to complete the nomenclature of tumors. The suffix *oma* implies, simply, tumor,

and benign tumors are named by adding this suffix to the name of the cell type of tissue (such as fibroma or lipoma). Malignant tumors arising in epithelial tissues are known as *carcinoma. Sarcoma* refers to malignant tumors involving mesenchymal tissues. Because epithelial tissue contains three germ layers, neoplasms of the squamous epithelium are called *squamous cell carcinomas,* neoplasms of transitional epithelium are called *transitional cell carcinomas,* and those involving glandular epithelium are called *adenocarcinomas.*

*Histopathological type* is a qualitative assessment whereby a neoplasm is categorized in terms of the tissue or cell type from which it has originated (e.g., lobular carcinoma, osteosarcoma, squamous cell carcinoma).

Knowing the organ of origin does not provide much information, because tumors arising from different tissues in the same organ behave differently. Conversely, tumors of the same tissue from different organs behave in a similar fashion. For example, adenocarcinoma of the lung and adenocarcinoma of the rectum behave similarly, whereas adenocarcinoma of the lung and squamous cell carcinoma of the lung have different natural histories. The tissue of origin determines the behavior of the tumor, and the cell type can be relied on not to change. The general region of the tumor (e.g., lung, testicle) is primarily descriptive. A lesion with the same cell type but at a site other than the original site would indicate a *metastatic* tumor. A different cell type originating from another lesion anywhere in the body would indicate a *second primary* cancer. An important factor in cancer management is determining whether the tumor is in situ, microinvasive, or frankly invasive.

*Histopathological grade* is a quantitative assessment of the extent to which the tumor resembles the tissue of origin. Grade is expressed in both numerical and descriptive terms. The language of grading refers to the appearance of the malignant cells and their degree of anaplasia or differentiation. Grading is done numerically from I to IV. Grade I indicates that the cells are so well differentiated that they closely resemble the normal parent cells. Grade IV tumor cells are so anaplastic that it is often difficult for the pathologist to determine their cell of origin. Grades II and III are intermediate designations. Grading can also be expressed by the terms well differentiated (grade I), moderately differentiated (grade II), poorly differentiated (grade III), or undifferentiated (grade IV).

Reports of the degree of cell differentiation are particularly important in deciding treatment approaches for tumors such as lymphomas. The prognostic value of grading varies with different types of tumors. For some, such as bladder cancers, the tumor grade is directly related to the ultimate prognosis of the patient, with the prognosis worsening as the cells become less differentiated. For other tumors, such as melanoma, grading has little or no prognostic value.

Sometimes the routinely assessed microscopic features of a cancer are not sufficiently conclusive for a firm diagnosis to be made. New technologies have provided the means for additional sophisticated studies to be performed on cells or tissues. For instance, electron microscopy, immunohistochemistry, in situ hybridization, and DNA probe analysis help distinguish between microscopic "look alikes." Nuclear DNA measurements may be useful for predicting distant metastasis and response to chemotherapy.[17] Flow cytometry permits rapid quantitative measurements of cellular characteristics.[16] Along with tumor markers and cytogenetics, all these special procedures are performed by the pathologist and may provide further information for critical diagnosis, prognosis, and treatment decisions.

Cytogenetic analysis plays an important part in the diagnostic workup of many individual patients, particularly in hematological neoplasms where the knowledge of chromosomal abnormalities is more complete than with solid tumors. Such information can assist in the subclassification of the malignant disease and thus the definitive selection of the most appropriate treatment.[18,19]

In parallel with cytogenetic data implicating specific genetic changes in carcinogenesis, molecular genetic techniques have enlarged the understanding of the molecular mechanics in the development of cancer. Researchers can now study tumor cells at the level of individual genes, even single base pairs.[20] The cytogenetic and molecular genetic techniques assess two quite different organizational levels of the genome and the two approaches provide complimentary and equally important clinical information.

Before these analytic techniques can have widespread application in clinical settings other than research institutions, however, certain problems must be solved. These include standardization and simplification of the technologies, selection of those that provide the most clinically meaningful information, and the conduct of large-scale clinical trials allowing multivariate statistical analysis to evaluate whether the new procedures actually improve the present ability to diagnose and stage cancer patients.[21]

Quality assurance guidelines for information to be included in routine pathology reports for different types of primary cancers have been developed by the Cancer Committee of the College of American Pathologists (CAP) and Joint Commission on Accreditation of Health Care Organizations (JCAHO).[15]

Years of accumulated experience have shown that a tumor with a particular appearance of cells, with a certain level of differentiation, arranged in a certain way, and originating in a particular organ will behave in a predictable way. This knowledge permits the medical team to plan therapy based on collective information about what happened to numerous individuals with the same tumors in the past. For instance, a pathology report revealing a "seminoma" carcinoma of the testes means that metastasis to the nearby lymph nodes is likely. It also means that this type of tumor has a fairly good prognosis, because the primary lesion is usually resectable and lymph node metastasis is radiosensitive. High cure rates are expected. On the other hand, a report of an embryonal cell carcinoma of the testis is ominous. This type of tumor tends to metastasize early to the lung, liver, bone marrow, and brain. It is radioresistant, with a 50% mortality rate.

### Clinical classification

Once the diagnosis is established, further testing is needed to assess the clinical extent of the disease. This process is called *staging*. There is no routine set of evaluations to be obtained on all patients. A knowledge of the natural history and patterns of spread of the particular neoplasm serve to focus and expedite the staging workup. Whole-lung tomography, magnetic resonance imaging, abdominal scans, bone marrow biopsies, or more routine procedures such as cystoscopy or chest x-ray are meant to focus on areas of possible hidden metastasis. Staging procedures are expensive and should be ordered in a cost-effective manner.

When all the essential information is at hand, the patient's disease can be staged. This process has been standardized using the TNM classification system.[22,23] By following the TNM system, the extent of disease is evaluated separately with respect to the primary tumor site (T), the regional lymph nodes (N), and the presence or absence of metastasis (M). The basic TNM model is expanded by using subcategories to describe how far the disease has progressed and the extent of metastasis if any. Tis indicates tumor in situ or tumor with all the histological characteristics of malignancy except invasion. T, with the possible numbers, 1, 2, 3, and 4, denotes increasing primary tumor extension. Increments of progressive lymph node involvement are indicated by N0, N1, N2, and N3. In like manner, M0, M1, M2, and M3 mean an advancing metastatic involvement and degree of organ impairment. On the basis of information about each of the TNM components, a stage designation can be assigned. Stage designations differ for each anatomic site, depending on the knowledge of spread and clinical behavior of the specific cancer. Stage designations have been developed for more than 40 primary tumor types. *Stage groupings* involve combining the various classification elements of defined T, N, and M. Table 11-2 illustrates the staging of breast cancer.

Once a cancer is staged at a certain period of time, the stage of the tumor at that time is not subject to change. There are two main staging periods. The first, *pretreatment staging*, is based on tests and evidence gathered before the first treatment is begun. There are two aspects to pretreatment staging of a previously undiagnosed cancer: *clinical-diagnostic* staging, for patients who have had a biopsy but are otherwise in the preoperative phase of study, and *postsurgical resection-pathological* staging, which includes a complete evaluation of the surgical specimen by a pathologist. Restaging, or reevaluation, may be done after a prescribed course of treatment to document remission. The second main staging period occurs if the patient has a recurrence following a disease-free interval and needs further treatment. This is termed *retreatment staging*. In addition, *autopsy staging* may occur to assess the extent of disease at death.

Previously, many other staging systems had been developed and modified, such as the Duke's classification for colorectal cancer and the Ann Arbor classification system for lymphomas. Consequently, data related to the management and prognosis of many cancers were not comparable. An attempt has been made to make the now-universally accepted TNM system consistent with several of these well-known classification systems already in use. The UICC published its pamphlet on the staging of cancer in 1987 and the fourth and latest edition of the AJCC's manual on cancer staging became available in 1992.[24] TNM information data forms, and "pocket stagers" are readily available from any hospital's tumor registry. Since January 1991, TNM staging for all cancer patients is required for approval of cancer programs by the Com-

mission on Cancer. To maintain approval status, implementation of this universal staging system for all tumor sites must have been completed by 1995. Future plans of the AJCC include improving uniformity in staging, expansion of the TNM system to include new prognostic markers (development of a prognostic index), the testing of prognostic indices using national and regional tumor registries, and development of staging systems for anatomic sites of types of cancer not yet classified by TNM (mesothelioma, carcinoid tumors). The goal of the AJCC is that all patients with cancer should be staged (universal staging).[25]

Although the TNM system gives an excellent description of a tumor's size and extent of anatomic spread, it does not take into account the cancer's physiological function. In 1992, a committee was established by the AJCC to develop more advanced classification systems based on multiple prognostic factors, including TNM. These factors include information on a patient's symptoms (which reflect some of the tumor's biological behavior), and patient comorbidity apart from the cancer itself. The purpose of this highly complex effort will be to improve treatment selection and accuracy of outcome prediction.[26,27]

During the time of staging, additional factors that might influence the treatment plan must be considered. It is important to assess the patient's general clinical condition in terms of age, general debility, previous treatment for the same or other cancers, and the presence of other major illness. Table 11-3 lists the many factors to evaluate and consider in the cancer treatment process.[28] Psychosocial status and family support can be evaluated in terms of discharge planning and home care needs during the course of treatment. The patient's educational background and medical sophistication have implications for the level and extent of patient education that will be needed.

## DETERMINING THE TREATMENT PLAN

A series of crucial decisions concerning management are now ready to be made. Careful integration of the extent of disease and the individual's condition with an extensive body of knowledge relating to treatment, anticipated complication rates, survival statistics, and other relevant clinical considerations will determine whether and when surgery, chemotherapy, radiation, biotherapy, hormone therapy, bone marrow transplant, or "watch and wait" will be offered to the patient. The most effective, most definitive treatment aimed at cure for a given cancer is called *primary therapy.*

### Should Treatment Be Aimed at Cure?

This is the vital question. In general, the oncologist tends to think of tumors with five-year survival probabilities in

**TABLE 11-2** Staging for Breast Cancer

### PRIMARY TUMOR (T)

| | |
|---|---|
| TX | Primary tumor cannot be assessed |
| T0 | No evidence of primary tumor |
| Tis | Carcinoma in situ: Intraductal carcinoma, lobular carcinoma in situ, or Paget's disease of the nipple with no tumor |
| T1 | Tumor 2 cm or less in greatest dimension |
| T1a | 0.5 cm or less in greatest dimension |
| T1b | More than 0.5 cm but not more than 1 cm in greatest dimension |
| T1c | More than 1 cm but not more than 2 cm in greatest dimension |
| T2 | Tumor more than 2 cm but not more than 5 cm in greatest dimension |
| T3 | Tumor more than 5 cm in greatest dimension |
| T4 | Tumor of any size with direct extension to chest wall or skin |
| T4a | Extension to chest wall |
| T4b | Edema (including peau d'orange) or ulceration of the skin of breast or satellite skin nodules confined to same breast |
| T4c | Both T4a and T4b |
| T4d | Inflammatory carcinoma |

### LYMPH NODE (N)

| | |
|---|---|
| NX | Regional lymph nodes cannot be assessed (e.g., previously removed) |
| N0 | No regional lymph node metastasis |
| N1 | Metastasis to movable ipsilateral axillary lymph node(s) |
| N2 | Metastasis to ipsilateral axillary lymph node(s) fixed to one another or to other structures |
| N3 | Metastasis to ipsilateral internal mammary lymph node(s) |

### PATHOLOGIC CLASSIFICATION (pN)

| | |
|---|---|
| pNX | Regional lymph nodes cannot be assessed (e.g., previously removed, or not removed for pathologic study) |
| pN0 | No regional lymph node metastasis |
| pN1 | Metastasis to movable ipsilateral axillary lymph node(s) |
| pN1a | Only micrometastasis (none larger than 0.2 cm) |
| pN1b | Metastasis to lymph nodes, any larger than 0.2 cm |
| pN1bi | Metastasis in 1–3 lymph nodes, any more than 0.2 cm and all less than 2 cm in greatest dimension |
| pN1bii | Metastasis to 4 or more lymph nodes, any more than 0.2 cm and all less than 2 cm in greatest dimension |
| pN1biii | Extension of tumor beyond the capsule of a lymph node metastasis less than 2 cm in greatest dimension |
| pN1biv | Metastasis to a lymph node 2 cm or more in greatest dimension |
| pN2 | Metastasis to ipsilateral axillary lymph nodes that are fixed to one another or to other structures |
| pN3 | Metastasis to ipsilateral internal mammary lymph node(s) |

### DISTANT METASTASIS (M)

| | |
|---|---|
| MX | Presence of distant metastasis cannot be assessed |
| M0 | No distant metastasis |
| M1 | Distant metastasis (includes metastasis to ipsilateral supraclavicular lymph node(s)) |

### STAGE GROUPING

| | | | |
|---|---|---|---|
| 0 | Tis | N0 | M0 |
| I | T1 | N0 | M0 |
| IIA | T0 | N1 | M0 |
| | T1 | N1 | M0 |
| | T2 | N0 | M0 |
| IIB | T2 | N1 | M0 |
| | T3 | N0 | M0 |
| IIIA | T0 | N2 | M0 |
| | T1 | N2 | M0 |
| | T2 | N2 | M0 |
| | T3 | N1 | M0 |
| | T3 | N2 | M0 |
| IIIB | T4 | Any N | M0 |
| | Any T | N3 | M0 |
| IV | Any T | Any N | M1 |

Reprinted with permission from American Joint Committee on Cancer: *Manual of Staging for Cancer* (ed 4). Philadelphia, Lippincott, 1992.

**TABLE 11-3** Factors Influencing Cancer Treatment Choices

---

**Tumor Factors**
- Size
- Anatomic location
- Histology/aggressiveness
- Sensitivity to chemotherapy or radiation
- Natural history
- Survival statistics

**Treatment Factors**
- Availability of treatment modalities
- Availability of research protocols/clinical trials
- Experience of the treatment team
- Potential morbidity/mortality
- Prior cancer treatment

**Patient Factors**
- Age
- Sex
- General health
- Patient/family values and preferences
- Physical performance status
- Quality of life
- Cardiac, renal, liver, bone marrow, and respiratory status
- Immune system function
- Psychological status
- Life expectancy

**Treatment Goals**
- Cure
- Control
- Palliation

**Environmental Factors**
- Geographic distance from treatment center
- Financial
- Social network

**Ethical Factors**
- Patient autonomy in decision making
- Informed consent
- Justice: individual rights to scarce and expensive resources vs. the public good

---

the range of 1%–5% as having no or only minimal chance for cure. The oncologist will therefore ask whether any method can offer the person even such a small chance for cure. The risks involved must then be related to the person's age and condition. An intensive treatment program that offers a small chance for permanent cure may be justified for a young, vigorous adult but inappropriate for a frail, elderly person, even though their cancers may be of the same type and extent. A correct decision on whether to treat for cure is one of the most important decisions that the oncologist must make. Overly aggressive attempts can expose individuals who are incurable to needless morbidity, prolonged and expensive treatment, and distressing complications. On the other hand, therapeutic decisions that are too pessimistic may deprive the person who has a small but significant opportunity for cure of the chance to live out the rest of life. The patient's feelings and values are crucial to the decision. Some

people, even knowing they have only a small chance for cure, will prefer an aggressive plan of action. Others will make it clear that they prefer to maximize quality of life.

## Which Modality Should Be Used?

After it has been decided that treatment will be aimed at cure, the next decision involves choosing the optimal treatment modality or combination thereof. In the past, cancer was treated only by surgery *or* radiation *or* chemotherapy, depending on the stage of the disease. Two or three therapies may have been used, but they would have been used only one at a time in the above order. First, surgery if the tumor was localized, then radiation if there was actual or potential recurrence, and last, chemotherapy if the cancer involved vital organs or had spread to such an extent that more surgery and radiation were impossible. Today, this treatment strategy has been replaced by multimodality therapy. There is not universal agreement yet on what the optimal combination or best sequence of therapies is for many malignancies, but the following broad principles have evolved.

1. When tumors are large, locally aggressive, and contiguous to adjacent structures (e.g., head and neck tumors), radiotherapy might be given prior to surgery. This would cause tumor shrinkage and thus make the surgical resection easier. Intraoperative radiation also may be given during a surgical procedure[29] such as surgery for cancer of the pancreas.

2. Both radiation and chemotherapy may be given after surgery.
   a. Radiation will usually be indicated if the tumor is found to be invading nearby tissues that cannot be surgically resected. Chemotherapy would be used to eliminate micrometastasis.
   b. Radiation and chemotherapy have been combined in an attempt to produce a more powerful antitumor effect than either treatment can produce alone. Chemotherapy is sometimes used prior to radiotherapy to shrink a lesion, since radiation has a more effective tumoricidal action against smaller lesions.

3. The new biological therapies are being blended with standard radiotherapy and chemotherapy, and research on these combinations is ongoing. For instance, monoclonal antibodies once thought of as the "magic bullet," have now been used for over a decade in a variety of ways to treat cancer patients. Although major responses have been seen in patients with various lymphomas, monoclonal antibodies have not yet gained a role in standard therapy.[11]

A broad body of knowledge about all aspects of clinical oncology must be used by those planning cancer treatment, including an understanding of tumor growth and cell kinetics[30] as well as the anticipated results of surgery, chemotherapy, and radiotherapy, either alone or in combination with other procedures. Since cancer therapy is always evolving, cancer specialists must keep abreast of the most recent literature and attend professional meetings where research findings and other cancer information are presented. Each major modality has its advantages and its disadvantages, as illustrated in Table 11-4. Current treatment programs are designed to enable the greatest curative potential of each modality by using each to exploit the different biological characteristics of a variety of cancers.

The best approach for treatment planning and evaluation is for an interdisciplinary group to share in the decision-making process. The surgeon specifies the therapeutic potential and resectability of the patient's tumor. The radiation oncologist shares the expectation of curability by primary radiotherapy or the augmentation effect that radiotherapy might have prior to or following surgery and/or chemotherapy. The medical oncologist specifies the contribution that chemotherapy could make to cure the tumor and the potential for chemotherapeutic or hormonal palliation if surgical or radiotherapeutic cure are impossible. The pathologist explains the details of the biopsy and microscopic appearance of the tumor. The radiologist reviews the various radiographs and scans.

Nurses may be involved in any number of ways: as enterostomal therapists, clinical specialists or nurse practitioners providing case management, or discharge planners, to name a few. The nurse can participate in cancer treatment planning by providing a broad perspective on what impact a proposed treatment program will have on the particular patient and family. Aspects of the nurse's role include patient education, particularly in symptom management, self care, assessing the benefits and toxicities of therapy, and coordination of participation in clinical trials. Nurses may also be involved in conducting and collecting data on companion studies aimed at quality of life assessment and symptom management.

Because the basic principle of cancer therapy is to cure the person with the least functional and structural impairment, the interdisciplinary planning team considers how aggressive and radical a treatment should be based on the following factors: the aggressiveness of the cancer, the predictability of spread, the morbidity and mortality that can be expected from the treatment, the cure rate, and the patient's desires. These are hard decisions, and the choice is often relative. What percentage of survival is acceptable for a debilitating surgical, radio-

**TABLE 11-4** Advantages and Disadvantages of Treatment Modalities

| Treatment Modality | Advantages | Disadvantages |
|---|---|---|
| Surgery | <ul><li>No biological resistance by tumors</li><li>No carcinogenic effects</li><li>May cure localized cancers</li><li>Gives the most accurate estimate of extent of disease and definition of histological features of tumor</li></ul> | <ul><li>No specificity for malignant tissues</li><li>Acute threat to life, possible morbidity</li><li>May result in deformity or loss of function</li><li>If cancer is disseminated, cannot cure: local/regional treatment only</li><li>May leave behind viable malignant cells</li></ul> |
| Radiation | <ul><li>May be curative if disease is localized</li><li>Delivers large tumoricidal dose to a specific area</li><li>Minimal residual deformity or loss of function*</li><li>Palliative</li></ul> | <ul><li>May develop side effects over a period of time</li><li>May leave behind viable malignant cells</li><li>Time-consuming</li><li>Has carcinogenic effect</li><li>If cancer is disseminated, cannot cure: local/regional only</li><li>Some tumors not radiosensitive</li></ul> |
| Chemotherapy | <ul><li>Systemic</li><li>Specificity for rapidly dividing (cancer) cells</li><li>Can cure some disseminated cancers</li><li>Potential for eliminating micrometastasis</li><li>Minimal residual deformity or loss of function</li><li>Potential to cure hematologic malignancies</li></ul> | <ul><li>Biological resistance by tumor often develops</li><li>Affects rapidly dividing normal cells resulting in side effects over a period of time</li><li>Has carcinogenic effect</li><li>Less effective with large, bulky tumors</li><li>Some tumors not chemosensitive</li></ul> |
| Biologicals | <ul><li>Not cytotoxic</li><li>Enhance immune system function</li></ul> | <ul><li>Still primarily experimental</li><li>Often major side effects</li></ul> |

*Exception: pediatrics, gonadal exposure

therapeutic, or chemotherapeutic maneuver? Is the tendency to be more radical justified as the chance for cure diminishes? Will a more conservative approach only lead to recurrence? The final decision must ultimately be personal judgment based on clinical experience and the experiences of others published in the literature. It is clearly in the patient's best interest to have the highly individualized prescription afforded by a multidisciplinary approach. The therapeutic aggressiveness of one member of the team is often tempered by the more conservative therapeutic bend of a colleague, and each member present brings a fresh approach. Although, in the majority of instances, the indications for one discipline or the other are clear-cut and noncompetitive, the decisions made by an interdisciplinary team are not easy. The construction of an overall treatment plan for the patient should provide for both immediate management and anticipated future developments.

## The Benefit of Clinical Trials

Oncology clinicians, realizing the limitations of their own experience and of haphazard observations in general, turn for guidance to organized clinical trials. At present and for the future, these constitute the only sure foundation for therapeutic progress. Clinical trials involve objectivity, rigor, and the use of empirical data in a systematic manner. A randomized clinical trial can be defined as a carefully and ethically designed experiment that aims to answer a specifically framed question, such as determining which intervention is superior among alternatives. The study design is prospective in nature so the entire study group can be followed over time for the outcomes of interest. An absolute necessity is a valid protocol that covers all foreseeable eventualities and ambiguities. Clinical trials for chemotherapy drug testing proceed through several phases that are described in chapter 14. The publication of the results of clinical trials allows clinicians around the world to evaluate outcomes and build on treatment successes. Replication of the experiments at other institutions ensures that treatment outcomes are not serendipitous.

Incidental advantages of clinical trials include the freedom from having to make individual choices of treatment for each patient, and that the actual conduct of the trial can provide opportunities for a valuable exchange of ideas among the physicians involved. Clinical trials are not perfect. No trial can determine absolutely the best treatment for an individual. Also, it is hard to control the confounding variables that are possible with a human subject. Any type of therapy or combination thereof can be made the objective of a clinical trial. Most clinical trials are planned and organized under the auspices of a federally funded cooperative study group such as the Southwest Oncology Group (SWOG) or the Gynecology Oncology Group (GOG). Such cooperative groups achieve the goal of obtaining adequate numbers of study patients so that meaningful answers can be derived to improve therapeutic regimens for specific categories of malignant disease.

## Selecting a Treatment Plan

Although in many instances the therapeutic decision is straightforward and clearly follows an established treatment pattern, there are often a variety of approaches that might be used. The optimal treatment plan from the physician's point of view would have the patient entered into an existing clinical trial (see Table 11-5). However, this is not always possible, for a number of reasons. The facility where treatment is to occur may not participate in a cooperative study group. There may not be a protocol available that fits the patient's stage of disease. If a protocol exists, the patient might be ineligible. The patient may refuse to be in a study for one reason or another.

An alternate approach is to use a conventional treatment program. Conventional or standard regimens are those that have been studied extensively, used for a long time, and are widely accepted for common cancers. For instance, the MOPP regimen (nitrogen mustard, oncovin, procarbazine, prednisone) has been a standard treatment choice for stage III or IV Hodgkin's disease, while CMF chemotherapy (cyclophosphamide, methotrexate, 5-fluorouracil) is a commonly used treatment for breast cancer. Conventional treatment programs involve drugs that are commercially available; clinical trials usually test recently developed investigational drugs that are available only to patients entered into a study. These newest drugs may provide a breakthrough not available with the older drugs, another reason why a clinical trial could offer the patient an advantage. On the other hand, the newest drugs may be less effective than those "tried and true."

If a patient is not eligible for a clinical trial and there is no conventional treatment program suitable for the case, the physician usually tries to find a study in the literature that documents a successful treatment program for the situation. Publications in journals usually involve larger numbers of patients and a longer post-treatment period for evaluating the effectiveness of the therapy. More details are provided in a journal article about side effects and dose modification than are provided in an abstract. If a journal article is unavailable, an abstracts publication could be used. Abstracts, that is, published synopses of oral presentations at professional meetings, offer few protocol details but often provide information about the latest drug combinations and doses being tried.

**TABLE 11-5**  Types of Treatment Plans (in order of preference by physician)

1. Clinical trial
2. Conventional treatment plan
3. Protocol published as journal article
4. Published abstract
5. Individualized treatment plan

Finally, if no existing treatment programs are available, the physician develops a protocol specific to the situation. Agents that are active against the tumor are specified for a regimen unique to that patient, the disease state, and any coexisting medical problems.

## ASSESSING RESPONSE TO TREATMENT

Responses to treatment may be classified as *objective* or *subjective* (Table 11-6). Objective parameters of the disease are measured before initiating therapy to give a baseline for evaluating treatment success or failure. Types of objective response parameters are listed in Table 11-7.[10] When the treatment course is completed, these indicators of response are measured again. This reevaluation, often called *restaging*, focuses particular attention on the disease parameters that were positive at diagnosis to signal a search for any remaining evidence that treatment should continue. Restaging does not imply that if a remission is obtained the patient reverts to a lesser disease stage. The stage ascribed at the time of diagnosis is the one referenced throughout the illness.

**TABLE 11-6** Response Criteria for Assessing Treatment Outcomes

| OBJECTIVE RESPONSE | |
|---|---|
| Complete response (CR) | Complete disappearance of signs and symptoms (for at least 1 month) |
| Partial response (PR) | 50% or more reduction in sum of products of greater and lesser diameters of all measured lesions (for at least 1 month), with no new lesions appearing |
| Minimal response (MR) | Same as for PR but less than 50% reduction |
| Progression | 25% or more increase in sum of products of greater and lesser diameters of all measured lesions, or appearance of new lesions |
| Stable disease | Measurable tumor does not meet criteria for CR, PR, MR, or progression |

| SUBJECTIVE RESPONSE |
|---|
| • Patient feels better |
| • Increased strength, decreased fatigue |
| • Appetite improved, gains weight |
| • Decrease in pain |

**TABLE 11-7** Common Parameters for Assessing Objective Response to Treatment

| | |
|---|---|
| Tumor size | Measured by palpation, x-ray films, radioisotope scans |
| Serum and urinary paraproteins, carcinoembryonic antigen | Decrease or increase |
| Peripheral white blood count | Decrease, increase, or blasts |
| Bone marrow biopsy | Types and condition of precursor cells |
| Gonadotropin titer | Decrease or increase |
| Pleural effusion status | Improves or worsens |
| Retroperitoneal nodes on abdominal CT scan | Larger, decreased in size, or not enlarged |
| Organ function | Improved or worse |

## Survival Statistics

In oncology, it is difficult to evaluate the comparative efficacy of therapeutic interventions. If a person succumbs after being treated, therapy has clearly failed. On the other hand, normal recovery—with the return to health, weight gain, and the resumption of normal activity—is not conclusive evidence that a cure has been achieved. The nature of cancer is such that even after a long time interval of apparent health, the disease may reappear and the person may die.

If at autopsy there is no evidence of tumor, a cancer can be said to have been cured. This is the only precise definition of "cure," but it is of little practical value. Freedom from clinical evidence of recurrent metastatic disease during the patient's lifetime is accepted by most clinicians as a reasonably reliable estimate of cure in a personal sense. In oncology, "cure" is a statistical term that applies to groups of cancer patients rather than to individuals.

The observation over time of individuals with cancer and the calculation of their probability of dying over several time periods is called *survival analysis*. A time interval is selected that must elapse without evidence of recurrence. The time at which survival can be called "cure" varies according to how soon after the primary treatment residual disease usually becomes evident. It is best understood as the time after treatment at which the annual death rate, given the age and sex of the treated person, is no longer greater than that of the normal population. Because this does not occur for 15–20 years after primary treatment in many tumors, five-year survival rates, which have been customary to report the results of treatment, are important only in the more aggressive tumors (lung, pancreas). Since statistical cure is unlikely for the majority of cancer patients, it is apparent that despite our best treatment efforts, only palliation is usually achieved.

## Patient Follow-up

Continued follow-up of patients is extremely important for the compilation of conclusive data. An integral part of a hospital's cancer program is a tumor registry or cancer data center. Information is compiled over time on each person diagnosed with cancer at that institution. These data not only aid in systematic follow-up of individuals with cancer but facilitate the hospital's evaluation of the effectiveness of different modes of therapy. Larger state, regional, and national cancer databases help in examining trends in cancer therapy and patient survival. The now widely used standardized methods of reporting the results of therapy are important to making such evaluation possible.

## WHEN A CURE IS NOT ACHIEVED

Should the disease recur, there may be a long period during which treatment is aimed at control. Cancer can thus be viewed as a chronic disease, similar to diabetes or heart disease, where cure is impossible and control is the objective. With some tumors, such as myeloma, cure is not yet an option and therapy is aimed at control from the beginning. When relapse has occurred, survival can often be prolonged and improved with proper treatment.

Does the person have recurrent disease symptoms that require palliation? Radiation or even chemotherapy may be effective in relieving pain, bleeding, and compression or obstruction of vital organs. A palliative surgical procedure may provide relief from a bulky tumor mass impinging on other organs. Palliative treatment should be used with discretion, based on sound clinical indications, and have a specific objective. It should minimize cost, inconvenience, discomfort, and risks, as well as be completed in the shortest possible time. Palliative measures may sometimes need to be used for people who are asymptomatic in whom the impending development of a catastrophic problem can be predicted, such as obstruction of the superior vena cava or a major bronchus, or a collapsing vertebral body. However, palliative treatment of most patients who are asymptomatic and incurable is usually deferred until the appearance of specific problems. Such persons should be followed closely to offer emotional support and for reassurance that appropriate palliative therapy will be initiated should the need arise.

## FUTURE PROSPECTS

The evolution in cancer therapy over the years has been the result of technological advances and increasingly sophisticated knowledge about the structure and function of the human body and of cancer biology. As reviewed in this chapter, the current era of cancer treatment features rather crude interventions based on our understanding of the disease: that cancer is usually systemic at presentation and that it involves a complex spectrum of host-tumor interrelations. Future efforts are being directed toward an increased understanding of these host-tumor interrelationships.[31] The rate of progress will depend on developments in molecular biology, immunology, and genetics as scientists delve deeper and deeper into the mysteries of both normal and abnormal microcellular function.

Postmodern strategies for cancer treatment may feature gene therapy, antineoplastic agents and delivery systems that exploit the differences between normal and malignant cells, the use of new and improved biologicals to prevent toxicity and extend the effectiveness of chemotherapy, and biological response modifiers to boost, direct, and restore the body's normal immune defenses.[32] As more is learned about the role of each biological substance, more effective manipulation of the immune system will be possible. Chemoprevention, the use of agents to impede the carcinogenic process, may lower the rate of cancer incidence. Vaccines to prevent some cancers are in development. Ultimately, the only permanent solution to the cancer treatment problem is prevention.

## REFERENCES

1. Yarbro JW: Milestones in our understanding of the causes of cancer, in Groenwald SL, Frogge MH, Goodman M, Yarbro CH (eds): *Cancer Nursing, Principles and Practices* (3rd ed). Boston, Jones and Bartlett, 1993, pp 28–46
2. Gallucci BB: Selected concepts of cancer as a disease: From Greeks to 1990. *Oncol Nurs Forum* 12:67–71, 1995
3. Fisher B: A biological perspective of breast cancer: Contributions of the National Surgical Adjuvant Breast and Bowel Project clinical trials. *CA* 41:97–111, 1991
4. Lydon J: Metastasis: Biology and Prevention. *Oncol Nurs Forum* 2(5):1–13, 1995
5. Goldie JH: Scientific basis for adjuvant and primary (neoadjuvant) chemotherapy. *Semin Oncol* 14:1–7, 1987
6. Harris DT, Mastrangelo MJ: Theory and application of early systemic therapy. *Semin Oncol* 18:493–503, 1991
7. Scofield RP, Liebman MC, Popkin JD: Multimodality therapy, in Baird SB, McCorkle R, Grant M (eds): *Cancer Nursing: A Comprehensive Text*. Philadelphia, Saunders, 1991, pp 334–354
8. Ahiya RK, Milligan AJ, Dobelbower RR: Radiation therapy in cancer management: Principles and complications, in Moossa AR, Martin C, Schimpff SC (eds): *Comprehensive Textbook of Oncology*. Baltimore, Williams & Wilkins, 1986, pp 257–268
9. Kennedy BJ: Evolution of chemotherapy. *CA* 41:261–263, 1991
10. Haskell CM: Principles of cancer chemotherapy, in Haskell CM (ed): *Cancer Treatment* (ed 3). Philadelphia, Saunders, 1990, pp 21–39

11. Goldenberg DM: New developments in monoclonal antibodies for cancer detection and therapy. *CA Cancer J Clin* 44:43–64, 1994

12. Krakoff IH: Cancer chemotherapy and biologic agents. *CA Cancer J Clin* 41:265–277, 1991

13. Yarbro CH: The history of cancer nursing, in Baird SB, McCorkle R, Grant M (eds): *Cancer Nursing: A Comprehensive Text.* Philadelphia, Saunders, 1991, pp 10–20

14. Pfeifer JD, Wick MR: The pathologic evaluation of neoplastic disease, in Holleb AI, Fink DJ, Murphy GP (eds): *Clinical Oncology.* Atlanta, American Cancer Society, 1991, pp 7–24

15. Hutter RV: The role of the pathologist in the management of breast cancer. *CA Cancer J Clin* 41:283–299, 1991

16. Madeya ML, Pfab-Tokarsky JM: Flow cytometry. *Oncol Nurs Forum* 19:459–463, 1992

17. Kimura T, Sato T, Onodera K: Clinical significance of DNA measurements in small cell lung cancer. *Cancer* 72(11): 3216–3222, 1993

18. Sandberg AA: Cancer cytogenetics for clinicians. *CA Cancer J Clin* 44(3):136–159, 1994

19. Mitelman, F: Chromosones, genes, and cancer. *CA Cancer J Clin* 44(3):133–135, 1994

20. Weinberg, RA: Oncogenes and tumor suppressor genes. *CA Cancer J Clin* 44(3):160–171, 1994

21. Preisler HD, Raza A: The role of emerging technologies in the diagnosis and staging of neoplastic disease. *Cancer* 69: 1520–1526, 1992 (suppl)

22. Beahrs OH: Staging of cancer. *CA Cancer J Clin* 41:121–125, 1991

23. Scott-Conner CE, Christie DW: Cancer staging using the American Joint Committee on Cancer TNM system. *J Am College of Surgeons* 81:182–188, 1995

24. American Joint Committee on Cancer: *Manual for Staging of Cancer* (ed 4). Philadelphia, Lippincott, 1992

25. Henson DE: Future directions for the American Joint Committee on Cancer. *Cancer* 69:1639–1644, 1992 (suppl)

26. Peccirillo JF, Feinstein AR: Clinical symptoms and comorbidity significance for the prognostic classification of cancer. *Cancer* 77(7):834–841, 1996

27. Hermanek P, Sobin LH, Fleming ID: What do we need beyond TNM? *Cancer* 77(5):815–817, 1996

28. Haskell CM: Introduction, in Haskell CM (ed): *Cancer Treatment.* Philadelphia, Saunders, 1990, pp 1–9

29. Haibeck SV: Intraoperative radiation therapy. *Oncol Nurs Forum* 15:143–147, 1988

30. Lind J: Tumor cell growth and cell kinetics. *Semin Oncol Nurs* 8:3–9, 1992

31. Yarbro JW: Future potential of adjuvant and neoadjuvant therapy. *Semin Oncol* 18:613–619, 1991

32. Jenkins J: Biology of cancer: Current issues and future prospects. *Semin Oncol Nurs* 8:63–69, 1992

# Chapter 12

# Surgical Therapy

**Margaret Hansen Frogge, RN, MS**

**Barbara Hansen Kalinowski, RN, MSN, OCN®**

## INTRODUCTION

Greater understanding of the biology of cancer has dramatically altered the place surgery has in the treatment plan for individuals with cancer. The natural history of cancer is such that the initial treatment plan, whether single approach or combination therapy, is the critical opportunity to cure a patient with cancer. Once disease recurs, cure is unlikely. Surgery is the treatment of choice for many tumors, but current understanding of tumor biology and advances in interdisciplinary cancer management have changed the reliance on surgery and have caused practitioners to reevaluate the magnitude of surgical resections. Approximately 55% of all individuals with cancer are treated with surgical intervention. Surgery and radiation therapy are the most successful methods available today to treat localized and regionally localized primary cancers.[1] By using combinations of surgery, chemotherapy, radiotherapy, or biotherapy, disease-free intervals have been significantly lengthened and survival advantages have been realized.[2] Surgery can be used for prevention, diagnosis, definitive treatment, rehabilitation, or palliation.

This chapter will review the role surgery plays in the many aspects of cancer treatment. It also will highlight some areas of nursing care specific to caring for individuals with cancer who will be having surgery.

## FACTORS INFLUENCING SURGICAL ONCOLOGY

### Ambulatory Surgery

Over 50% of the surgical procedures performed in the United States today occur within the ambulatory setting.[3] Ambulatory surgical services are provided in hospitals, freestanding ambulatory surgery centers, or in mobile units. Technological and scientific advances in surgery and anesthesia have enabled this change in venue for the delivery of surgical care. Economic pressures have had a significant influence on the rapidity of change to ambulatory surgery.

Most often, an ambulatory surgical procedure is performed and the patient is discharged to home care or to family care in less than 23 hours following surgery. Educating the patient and his or her family in self-care is a significant challenge to surgical nurses, office staff, and family members providing supportive care. Educational materials are needed to supplement the verbal teaching that is done in the perioperative period. Since the average reading level of Americans is about eighth grade, and it is estimated that 20% of the population has a serious literacy problem, educational materials must be carefully selected if maximum benefit is to be derived.[4] Visuals and videos can be useful adjuncts to written materials.

Individuals with cancer who have an ambulatory procedure for treatment or diagnosis, such as breast lumpectomy or prostate biopsy, are usually in need of additional support and education beyond what can be provided in such a brief period. Support groups, follow-up phone checks, individual consultation, and educational sessions can be used to help the patients and families understand the disease and the necessary follow-up care.

### Technological Advances

Lasers, laparoscopes, endoscopes, conscious sedation, and new anesthetic agents are among the leading approaches in ambulatory surgical care. Patients are quite accepting of less invasive ambulatory surgical procedures because there are fewer surgical risks, less pain, and a less extensive recovery period.[5]

For example, laparoscopes are used to perform splenectomy, adrenelectomy, pancreatectomy, colon resection, and pelvic lymphadenectomy.[6-9] Cancer staging and a variety of palliative procedures also can be done via laparoscope. Before a laparoscopic approach is selected, the surgeon must be reasonably certain that the disease can be resected with adequate margins using the laparoscope. Though laparoscopic procedures are generally less costly and easier for the patient to tolerate, if an open surgical approach becomes necessary during a laparoscopic procedure, then the overall cost and the patient variables change significantly.[10]

Surgical techniques of microvascular surgery, laser surgery, and cryosurgery result in less blood loss, which has reduced operative mortality. Laser vaporization with a variety of laser beam sources is used in the treatment of small, early lesions. Cryosurgery, or thermal surgery through extreme cooling, is used for certain gynecologic and neurological surgeries. The extreme temperatures result in cryogenic necrosis of the surrounding tissues, capillaries, and venules.[11] Surgical anesthesia, intraoperative monitoring, and postoperative management techniques continue to be refined.

### Economic Forces

Economic forces and managed care have precipitated development of aggressive measures to reduce lengthy and costly hospital stays. Preoperative preparation, surgical management, and postoperative care are all scrutinized closely for ways to decrease utilization of diagnostic tests and reduce the costs of surgical care. Ambulatory surgery, increased efficiency, clinical pathways, algorithms, and changes in medical education are a few of the measures that have been taken to reduce the cost of surgical care.[12] The individual with cancer who is approaching a surgical procedure may need help navigating the health care course in the least traumatic way possible. In many settings, nurses act as case managers to assist the patient and family in the complex negotiations that are often necessary in the continuum of cancer care.

# FACTORS INFLUENCING TREATMENT DECISIONS

## Tumor Cell Kinetics

An understanding of the biology and natural history of individual tumors is fundamental to the surgical treatment of cancer.[13] Tumor cell characteristics such as growth rate, differentiation, metastatic potential, and metastatic pattern affect the treatment decision. It was once thought that cancer was essentially a mass of uncontrolled, rapidly proliferating cells that extended into surrounding tissues and lymph nodes and inevitably reached the circulatory system. With this in mind, surgeons felt that time was of the essence in curing cancer and that the lymph nodes had to be included in any resection because metastatic extensions would rest there. With these ideas guiding surgeons to extend the surgical margin and resect more tissue, extensive radical procedures such as hemicorporectomies and radical mastectomies were performed with better, but still disappointing, results. Such radical procedures have failed to significantly increase cure rates.[14–16]

An explosion of knowledge in the field of tumor biology has led clinicians to recognize that interdisciplinary collaboration and treatment planning are necessary to select the most effective treatment method for cancer.[13,17] Oncology practitioners must understand the potential of surgery, chemotherapy, radiation, and biotherapy in order to select the most effective course of therapy. The factors that affect the decision of whether an individual with cancer should be treated by surgery will be discussed in the following sections.

### Growth rate

The rate of growth of a tumor is expressed in terms of volume-doubling time. The time it takes for a tumor mass to double in size depends on the cell cycle activity of proliferating cells comprising the tumor; the growth fraction, or number of cells proliferating in the tumor; and the rate of cell loss from the tumor. In general, tumors that are slow growing and that consist of cells with prolonged cell cycles lend themselves best to surgical treatment, because these types of tumors are more likely to be confined locally.[18]

### Invasiveness

Any cancer cell remaining after treatment constitutes a potential risk for recurrence or metastasis if that cell is capable of proliferating. Therefore, a surgical procedure intended to be curative must involve resection of the entire tumor mass and normal tissue surrounding the tumor to ensure a margin of safety for removal of all cancer cells. Some cancers (e.g., melanomas) invade deeply into adjacent tissues, either requiring extensive surgical procedures to remove the tumor mass or making surgery an impractical treatment option. Other tumors, such as basal cell carcinoma and chrondrosarcoma, are highly cohesive and are more amenable to complete surgical excision. Local, less radical procedures are performed for those particular tumors where research has demonstrated an equally effective result compared with radical surgery.[19–22]

### Metastatic potential

The initial operation performed for removal of a cancer has a better chance for success than a subsequent operation performed for a recurrence; thus, knowledge of metastatic patterns of individual tumors is crucial for planning the most effective therapy.

Some tumors metastasize late or not at all, and, even if advanced, may be cured by aggressive therapy. Other tumors predictably metastasize to local or regional sites, and cure may be achieved by a procedure that involves removal of the primary tumor-bearing organ and the involved adjacent tumor sites or lymph nodes. Some tumors are known to metastasize early. In such cases surgery may not be warranted (e.g., lung cancer), or surgery may be used to remove all visible tumor in preparation for adjuvant system therapy or after a number of courses of chemotherapy to resect remaining disease (e.g., testicular cancer).[19–22]

Subclinical metastasis or occult disease is responsible for most recurrences when surgery has been the only treatment used. It is thought that micrometastases are present in 60% of individuals by the time a tumor is large enough to be detected clinically.[23] Interdisciplinary planning and selection of the most appropriate treatment methods are important to improve survival and to lower an individual's risk of systemic metastasis.

## Tumor Location

Once the location and extent of the tumor are determined through diagnostic and staging procedures, the clinician assesses the structural and functional changes that can be expected as a result of the surgical procedure. This assessment will assist the clinician and patient and family in weighing the benefits and risks involved in treatment. In some cases, the decision to treat an individual's cancer with surgery may rest solely on whether the tumor involves vital structures. Superficial and encapsulated tumors are more easily resected than those that are embedded in inaccessible or delicate tissues or those that have invaded tissues in multiple directions.

## Physical Status

Careful preoperative assessment is critical for evaluating the significant factors that would potentially increase the risk of surgical morbidity and mortality. Evaluation of respiratory, cardiovascular, nutritional, immunologic, renal, and central nervous system (CNS) status are important.[24] The severity of the underlying illness and co-morbid conditions are considered in the decision regarding surgical therapy. The health care team assesses the patient's rehabilitation potential, particularly if the intended surgery will significantly alter normal physiological function. In some cases the intended surgical procedure may produce physiological alterations that are beyond that particular individual's capabilities. Since cancer incidence is much greater in elderly patients, age can be a factor to weigh in the treatment decision. In general, elderly individuals have a higher surgical risk than younger individuals. However, the elderly individual should also be treated as aggressively as possible but may require additional preoperative support (e.g., hyperalimentation and/or blood products). Elderly individuals with cancer do not appear to have a higher risk or complication rate than their age-matched cohorts.[25,26]

## Quality of Life

The goal of therapy for the patient with cancer varies according to the stage of disease. Selection of the treatment approach includes consideration of the quality of the individual's life when treatment is complete. Research has shown that some radical surgical procedures are not warranted, either because they do not improve the end result or because they interfere unduly with the individual's functional or psychological well-being. Multidisciplinary planning that includes the individual with cancer and significant others will facilitate the selection of a treatment plan tailored to that individual's unique needs and desires.

## PREVENTING CANCER USING SURGICAL PROCEDURES

Certain conditions, diseases, and genetic or congenital traits are known to be associated with a higher risk of developing cancer. In some instances, surgical removal of nonvital benign tissue or an organ that is responsible for predisposing the individual to higher risk can lower incidence and possibly prevent occurrence of cancer. Polyposis is a clear example of a condition that increases the individual's risk for developing colon cancer. Surgical excision of colon polyps is a relatively simple preventive procedure to reduce the risk of developing colon cancer.[27] Another, more complex situation is that of women who have a high risk for breast cancer. After careful review and thorough explanation, some women may elect to undergo prophylactic bilateral mastectomy to lower the risk of breast cancer.[28,29] At this time, prophylactic mastectomy is highly controversial. The role of surgery in cancer prevention is somewhat limited; however, epidemiological and etiologic findings may indicate a more definitive role for surgery in the future. Genetic testing and chemoprevention will undoubtedly influence the use of surgery in the prevention of cancer.

## DIAGNOSING CANCER USING SURGICAL TECHNIQUES

Each type of cancer responds differently to therapy; therefore, a histological diagnosis is crucial to selecting effective treatment. Surgical diagnostic techniques such as endoscopy, needle aspiration, incisional biopsy, excisional biopsy, and core needle biopsy are commonly used to procure cells or tissue specimens for histopathologic examination.

An adequate biopsy requires careful planning by the physician. The biopsy specimen should contain both normal cells and tumor cells for comparison; it should be intact and not crushed or contaminated; and it should be labeled and preserved properly for complete evaluation. An important principle to note in the diagnosis of cancer is that only positive biopsy findings are definitive. A negative biopsy finding can mean no cancer, but it can also mean that the biopsy specimen was not representative of the tumor. If a high index of suspicion for cancer exists, another biopsy technique may be in order.

Before selecting the most appropriate biopsy technique, the surgeon will consider the possible treatment approaches to be used if cancer is diagnosed. The placement and orientation of the biopsy incision should facilitate any further surgical resections deemed necessary. Because tumor cells can contaminate the biopsy site, the biopsy incision should be located so it will be removed during definitive surgery, or the biopsy itself should contain the tumor in toto.[30] Minimum disruption or disturbance to the bulk of the tumor, while achieving an adequate specimen, requires careful consideration prior to biopsy. Aesthetic results are also considered, so that incision lines and subsequent incisions will be located in cosmetically acceptable areas or folds, if possible.

Important principles of biopsy include minimizing dissection as much as possible and maintaining adequate hemostasis to avoid iatrogenic tumor spread. Use of incisional, excisional, aspiration, or core biopsy depends on tumor size, location, and growth characteristics. Figure 12-1 illustrates these four techniques.[31] Possible complications following any biopsy are pain, bleeding, hematoma, infection, dehiscence, and tumor cell seeding.

Individuals should be instructed about biopsy site care and possible complications. Individuals should know in advance when the biopsy results will be available and how the physician will give the results (e.g., by phone call

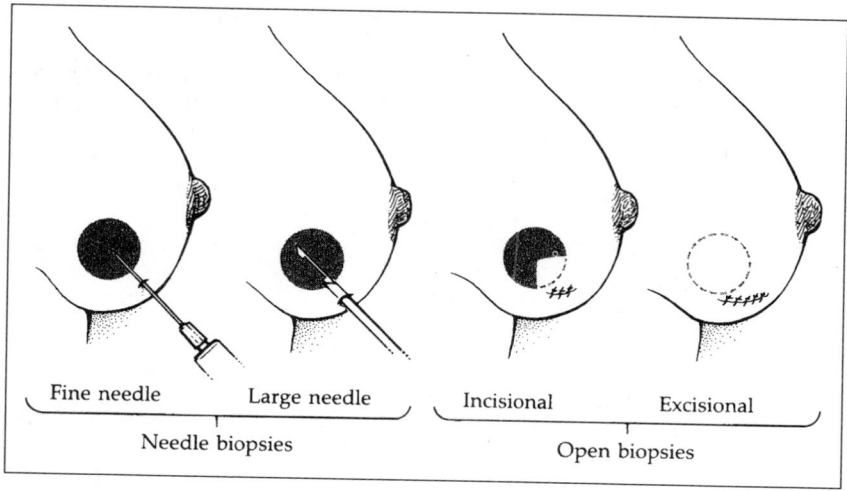

**FIGURE 12-1**   Possible approaches for breast biopsy. (Love S: *Dr. Susan Love's Breast Book*. Reading, MA, Addison-Wesley, 1990. Reprinted with permission.)

or in person). The individual should be informed as to whether the result will be known immediately (frozen section result) or whether the physician prefers to wait until the permanent sections have been prepared and interpreted, usually between two and five days later.

## Needle Biopsy: Fine Needle and Core Needle

Needle biopsies are usually performed in an outpatient or office setting, since they do not require extensive surgical support and are simple and safe for the patient. Cooperation and skill are required of the surgeon, pathologist, and the affiliated pathology lab to assure that an accurate diagnosis is made. Local or topical anesthesia is commonly used. Table 12-1 lists specific details of each type of needle biopsy: (1) aspiration needles, (2) cutting or core needles, (3) large cutting needles, and (4) automated biopsy systems (biopsy guns). Some needles have carriers that shield and guide the actual biopsy needle, cup, or punch used to obtain the specimen. The carrier reduces the possibility of contaminating the needle tract with tumor cells from the specimen as the needle is withdrawn. An unfortunate limitation of either needle aspiration or core biopsy is the possibility that the tumor will be missed; therefore only a positive finding of malignancy is diagnostically significant.[1,30,32,33]

Fine-needle aspiration or biopsy is the procedure of choice when there is a high index of suspicion for malignancy and the lesion is both accessible and solid. The biopsy needles are small bore, usually 20- to 23-gauge. Fine-needle biopsies are well tolerated by the patient, result in a small amount of trauma to tissue, and cause minimal manipulation of the tumor. Hematoma and infection are potential complications.

Core biopsies, which include percutaneous biopsies, are usually indicated when there is a need to confirm malignancy, yet there is clinical and diagnostic evidence

that the disease will be treated with nonsurgical approaches. If surgery is likely, the biopsy approach selected is often the fine needle rather than the core biopsy. Fluoroscopy, ultrasound, or computed tomography (CT) is often used to guide the clinician during core biopsy procedures. Local anesthesia is used. Hematoma, infection, and pain are postbiopsy considerations.

Regional biopsy is performed using a variety of approaches and needles. Regional biopsy involves obtaining several samples of tissue from different locations within a tumor or within a diseased organ. Regional biopsies are used to diagnose metastatic disease in a defined, but not localized, region of the body. Regional biopsies are also used to sample diffuse disease within an organ or to sample multiple nodes within a region. Examples include: transthoracic, pancreatic, adrenal gland, liver, pelvic mass, prostate, renal, breast, thyroid, and bone regional biopsies.[34]

## Surgical Biopsy: Excisional, Incisional, Endoscopic

Surgical biopsies are careful and delicate procedures performed to secure a piece of tumor tissue larger than that possible with a needle. The types of biopsy techniques are excisional, incisional, and endoscopic.

*Excisional biopsy* is performed on small, discrete, accessible tumors to remove the entire suspected mass with little or no margin of surrounding normal tissue included in the biopsy specimen. In some cases, such as tumors of the lip, nose, ear, or breast, excisional biopsy alone will be definitive therapy. The pathologist and the surgeon will determine whether the extent of the excisional biopsy is sufficient to eliminate the possibility of residual disease or whether more extensive surgery is indicated. Figure 12-2 illustrates a technique used to prepare tissue to allow visualization of the specimen margin.[31] The tissue is covered with ink, sliced, and then put on the slide for microscopic evaluation.

*Incisional biopsies* are generally selected for the diagnosis of large tumors that will require major surgery for complete removal. A portion of the mass is removed by incisional biopsy for pathological examination. Incisional biopsy should be positioned in such a way that the biopsy site will be totally excised with subsequent definitive surgery.

*Endoscopy* is a surgical technique used to obtain biopsy specimens for diagnosis of tumors in accessible lumens.[35] Tumors of the gastrointestinal, genitourinary, or pulmonary system, and more recently the ductal system of the breast, can be diagnosed by inserting an

**TABLE 12-1**   Approaches for Biopsy

| Type | What Used For | Where Done | Rationale |
|---|---|---|---|
| **Needle Biopsy** | | | |
| *Fine-Needle Aspiration:* (21–22 g needle 5-cc syringe) local anesthesia | Solid, palpable lesion (i.e., breast mass, thyroid nodule) | Outpatient setting Operating room | Involves only small amount of trauma to tissue, so if positive then surgical procedure is avoided. Used when there is a high level of suspicion of malignancy. |
| *Steriotaxic Fine-Needle Aspiration:* (21–22 g needle, steriotaxic equipment) local anesthesia | Solid, nonpalpable lesion (i.e., mammographic abnormality) | Outpatient setting Radiology center | Same as for fine-needle aspiration, but able to sample small, *nonpalpable* lesions |
| *Core Needle Biopsy:* (special cutting needle) local anesthesia; can use ultrasound to help guide | Solid, accessible tumor | Outpatient setting | Removes larger amount of tissue than fine-needle aspiration; may allow for more information (i.e., hormone receptor tests) |
| **Surgical Biopsy** | | | |
| *Excisional Biopsy:* usually local anesthesia | Solid, palpable mass (i.e., melanoma, breast mass) | Day surgery | Attempt is made to remove the whole mass only, without regard to clear margin. Result should be cosmetically acceptable. |
| *Incisional Biopsy:* usually local anesthesia | Solid, palpable large mass (i.e., large, ulcerating or bleeding mass) | Day surgery | Biopsy is for diagnosis; mass is too large to remove without major surgery. May bleed profusely. |
| *Endoscopy:* (special endoscope) may use sedation | Solid mass in an accessible lumen (i.e., colon, esophagus) | Outpatient setting Day surgery | May be for diagnosis or treatment. Avoids surgical trauma. |

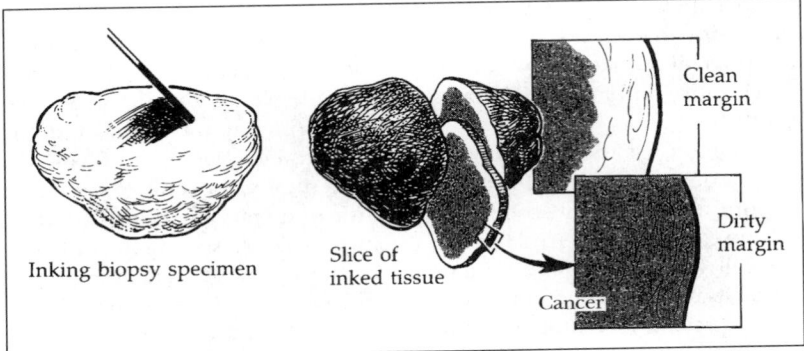

Inking biopsy specimen

Slice of inked tissue

Cancer

Clean margin

Dirty margin

**FIGURE 12-2**   Technique for obtaining inked surgical margins. (Love S: *Dr. Susan Love's Breast Book.* Reading, MA, Addison-Wesley, 1990. Reprinted with permission.)

optical instrument into the lumen to examine the area and to secure a biopsy for analysis or secretions for cytological examination. Flexible instruments have made endoscopy more tolerable for the patient and more functional for the clinician. Bleeding and infection are potential problems.

## STAGING CANCER USING SURGICAL PROCEDURES

Surgical procedures are selected for the precise diagnosis of cancer and for defining the stage of the disease. For example, staging laparotomy is an important diagnostic measure for the pathological staging of Hodgkin's disease. Exploratory surgical procedures can be done to diagnose most intracavitary tumors or to define the extent of tumor growth, size, nodal involvement, implants, or multiorgan involvement.

The American Joint Committee on Cancer Staging has developed a system for staging most solid tumors. The TNM classification defines the extent of the solid tumor based on size and local extension (T), the presence or absence of nodal involvement (N), and the presence or absence of distant metastasis (M) and degree of organ dysfunction. (See chapter 9 for more details on the TNM system.) Descriptions of staging and classification of each tumor type are included throughout this text.

Before recommending a surgical resection of the tumor for cure, the physician will undertake a search for evidence of distant metastasis. This metastatic workup is important for accurate staging of disease. If distant metastases are present, radical or body-altering surgery is usually not indicated, and the focus of treatment quickly shifts from local control to systemic treatment or palliation.

During the diagnostic phase, including the biopsy and staging tests, the patient with cancer and his or her family will probably experience profound anxiety, which can be alleviated or reduced to some extent. It is important to assess the factors that could contribute to anxiety, such as previous hospitalizations, experience with other individuals with cancer, influence of the mass media, formal and informal sources of information, and the patient's developmental stage. The nurse should carefully assess the patient's understanding of the diagnostic procedures and the significance of the findings.

Although seeking information is considered a healthy coping behavior, only the patient can cue the nurse on how much information is adequate. During the diagnostic period, many individuals become quite aggressive seeking information from a myriad of sources. The Internet, magazines, neighbors, friends, and television are common sources of both information and misinformation. It is important to help the individual quickly and completely understand the variability of approaches used to treat cancer and the biological basis on which the treatment decision will be made. This can help the individual with

cancer and their family to have a better understanding of the disease and to have more control of their own information-seeking process.

## SURGERY FOR TREATMENT OF CANCER

After diagnosis, staging, and classification of the tumor, the interdisciplinary oncology team will propose the most appropriate plan and sequence of therapy. The goal of therapy is based on the patient's desires, general condition, and tumor stage and classification. The sequence and methods of treatment used will be guided by the most effective treatment protocols available for that particular tumor type. Surgical intervention may be the definitive treatment or may be part of a sequence of combined treatment modalities.

Preoperative considerations include a thorough patient and family history and physical examination. Assessments are made of lifestyle, concomitant disease, general physical condition, nutritional status, hematologic status, and pulmonary status. Measures to improve the patient's overall status are initiated before surgery whenever possible.[24] In addition, an assessment of the patient's understanding of the surgery and rehabilitation should be completed. Involving the individual's significant others in preoperative teaching can often facilitate understanding and reduce anxiety (see Table 12-2).

### Surgery Aimed at Cure

Advances in our understanding of cancer biology have changed the surgical approach for cure from "more is better" to an approach that focuses on tissue and functional preservation and relies on effective use of radiotherapy, chemotherapy, and biotherapy. Tumors that are solid, accessible, have relatively well-defined margins, and are without evidence of spread can generally be surgically excised with a goal of eradicating the tumor.

#### Resection—local and radical

The type of surgical procedure selected for curative treatment of a primary tumor depends on the specific tumor cell characteristics, site, and extent of involvement. In the preoperative period, the surgeon is challenged to identify those patients who will best be treated by limited or extensive surgery and to select the adjuvant therapies that will control local and distant disease.[1]

The magnitude of the surgical excision for many tumors has been greatly modified in recent years. There is a limit beyond which larger excisions fail to yield improved long-term outcomes. A better understanding of the biology and natural history of specific cancers, combined with advances in adjuvant treatment, has led to less radical surgery for some cancers. Breast cancer is probably the

**TABLE 12-2** Preoperative Assessment/Teaching Guide

| What to Assess | Teaching Strategies |
| --- | --- |
| Understanding of procedure | *Visual:* books, diagrams, models of equipment<br>*Verbal:* Q & A session with patient and significant other, in person or on telephone; arrange network with patient who has had similar procedure |
| Understanding of process | Facility tour to include room and waiting area; explanation of expected sequence of events and the individual's anticipated participation |
| Preoperative physical condition<br>• history and physical<br>• special tests<br>• hospital-specific requirements<br>• previous therapy—especially chemotherapy or radiation<br>• venous access devices | Discuss donating autologous blood<br>Routine preoperative teaching (respiratory and circulatory exercises, wound care, catheter care, IVs, intensive care stay, etc.) |
| Anxiety about procedure | Teach relaxation exercises<br>Encourage use of techniques already helpful to patient (e.g., music, meditation)<br>Discuss expectations of pain management<br>Offer and discuss patient-controlled analgesia if available |

best example of a tumor that is approached much differently now because of our understanding of tumor biology.[16,36]

Local resection is used for small lesions if the entire tumor and an adequate margin of tumor-free tissue can be encompassed in the excision. Tumors of the ear, skin, or lip are typical lesions where local excision can be used as definitive therapy for cure. Hemostasis and infection are the major postoperative concerns.

Radical surgical resections are performed when the tumor is surgically accessible and there is hope that the tumor can be resected en bloc along with the necessary local or regional tissues and lymphatics. If possible, it is desirable to include a wide margin of normal tissue to assure complete resection of the tumor.

Depending on the characteristic pattern of spread of the tumor involved, a radical resection may include the primary tumor and the regional lymph nodes surrounding the area. The surgeon must carefully identify the collecting nodes and lymphatic channels to include in this type of resection. The en bloc regional lymph node dissection is critical to preventing local tumor recurrence.[1] Extensive surgery may be needed if the disease is to be eradicated and the patient is to be given the chance to live a normal life span. Surgical resections can greatly alter an individual's body image as well as the structure and function of his or her body. There are obvious tradeoffs and concessions that the individual with cancer must consider. Striking a balance between length of life and quality of life is a major challenge in surgical oncology.

Extensive radical resections or supraradical procedures are not used often, but they can provide a chance for cure for a limited set of individuals with cancer. Indica-

tions for extensive radical surgery include primary tumors that grow slowly, have wide local infiltration, and are large. The entire spectrum of care for an extended radical procedure is best handled by a highly experienced team of clinicians. Examples of these procedures are hemipelvectomy, forequarter amputation, and pelvic exenteration. The emotional and adaptive challenges to the patient receiving this type of surgery must be carefully assessed and evaluated before electing to proceed with the procedure.

During the preoperative period, the nurse instructs the individual on what to expect throughout the surgical course. It is important that the individual understand the anticipated outcomes of surgical therapy, as well as how surgery fits in the overall plan of therapy. Very often, the patient and significant others have many questions and need information repeated and validated. Encouraging dialogue and allowing adequate time for instruction and verbalization of feelings and fears during the preoperative period can enhance adjustment and acceptance of the surgery and its effects. Discussion of specific nursing management and rehabilitation of the patient following various surgical procedures is included in Part V on the management of malignancies.

### Surgery and adjuvant therapies

Surgery is local therapy and thus is limited in what it can achieve as a treatment modality for cancer. Surgery was once the sole therapy for many solid tumors, such as carcinoma of the breast, colon, and head and neck. Survival rates for these cancers and others have not been satisfactory with surgery alone.[2] For this reason, combination or adjuvant therapies are used to improve the rates of cure and disease-free survival. Adjuvant therapy can be initiated preoperatively, intraoperatively, or postoperatively. Surgery may be combined with radiotherapy for local and regional tumor control. Chemotherapy is given to provide systemic control of micrometastases and distant metastases.

In some situations, surgery, called cytoreductive surgery, is used to debulk or reduce the tumor mass to a size where combination therapy can be most effective.[37] Ovarian cancer is usually spread throughout the peritoneum by the time of diagnosis, and clinicians have found that cytoreductive surgery followed by aggressive chemotherapy has resulted in significantly improved survival rates.[37] The individual may undergo definitive therapy for months or even years. Other examples of tumors in which debulking procedures have been used are Burkitt's lymphoma, rhabdomyosarcoma, chordoma, glioblastoma multiforme, and some neoplastic syndromes. This adjuvant approach to the treatment of the person with cancer requires a multidisciplinary team effort.

### Excision of metastatic lesions

Surgery also may be used to resect a metastatic lesion if the primary tumor is believed to be eradicated, if the metastatic site is solitary, and if the patient can undergo surgery without significant morbidity. Resection of the metastatic lesion is not indicated if there is evidence of additional metastatic disease or if the metastatic lesion is particularly aggressive or inaccessible. A solitary pulmonary lesion, a liver lesion, and a cerebral mass are examples of metastatic sites that may be amenable to resection with a curative intent, with approximately 25% of patients achieving cure.[1,38]

## Surgery Aimed at Palliation

Surgical procedures are commonly performed for the palliation of the debilitating manifestations of cancer. These procedures are aimed at controlling the cancer and improving the quality of life for the individual with cancer, even when all the cancer cannot be removed. If the quality of the individual's life cannot be improved as a result of the surgery, then surgery is not warranted. If the surgery carries an unnecessary risk of morbidity or mortality, it is also not indicated. Issues such as biological pace of the disease, the patient's life expectancy, and expected outcome of the palliative procedure all require careful consideration if the patient is to benefit from the procedure. Open communication among the patient, the family, and the physician is of paramount importance. The patient must know the goals of the procedure and realistically understand the expected outcome. If the patient's hope is unrealistic, the potential disappointment experienced postoperatively can be devastating. For instance, consider the individual experiencing chronic pain who is offered a surgical procedure that can possibly alleviate suffering. It is more compassionate to ensure that the individual understands and accepts that the pain may be relieved only temporarily rather than indefinitely. The patient who lives with cancer knows well the meaning of palliation. Clinicians should always respect the courage and will of the individual with uncontrolled cancer and promote his or her active participation in the plan of care.

The goal of palliative surgery is to relieve suffering and minimize the symptoms of the disease. For example, palliative surgery may involve removal of a tumor that has become ulcerative and a likely source of infection or may involve the amputation of a nonfunctioning, painful limb with sarcoma. Some tumors are slow growing, and although metastatic sites are evident and the patient is technically incurable, resection of the primary tumor is warranted to prevent future complications such as bleeding or obstruction. Several surgical techniques are used for palliation of cancer: fulgeration, electrocoagulation, lasers, photodynamic therapy, shunts, and bone stabilization procedures.[25,39,40]

Palliative procedures are not undertaken unless the clinician is reasonably confident that the wound will heal. For example, surgery is contraindicated for the patient who has a local recurrence and lung metastasis following radiotherapy to an oropharyngeal lesion. In this case a surgical wound would probably not heal without extensive skin flap reconstruction, which would not be warranted in view of the distant metastasis.

Palliative surgery is particularly useful in relieving suffering caused by an obstructive process. Obstruction occurs in the respiratory, gastrointestinal, or urinary system. Surgical intervention such as a tracheostomy will restore airway patency, and a gastrostomy tube will facilitate adequate nutrition. Through palliative procedures, the individual can be supported while therapy is initiated to control the primary disease. Surgery may also be used to decompress vital structures (i.e., laminectomy) or to help in the control of pain.

## Surgery for Rehabilitation

Although surgical procedures have long been used to treat cancer, their use in rehabilitation of individuals with cancer is underemphasized. Today, significant value is placed on the quality of life for the individual with cancer. With this emphasis has come an effort to develop techniques to restore an individual to as near a normal life as possible following surgery for cancer. Cosmetic and functional success have been achieved through procedures such as: breast reconstruction following mastectomy, facial reconstruction after head and neck surgery, and skin grafting following major resections for melanoma.[1] The development of various implants, microvascular surgery, allografts, and autogenous reconstructive techniques has enlarged the scope of reconstructive surgery.[30] Reconstructive procedures can be done immediately following resection or can be delayed several days or years.[41]

Rehabilitation potential is considered before initiation of primary therapy. Careful interdisciplinary planning will assist the clinician to prepare the patient emotionally and physically for both the primary treatment and subsequent rehabilitation. In preparing an individual for rehabilitation, the clinician strikes a fine balance between optimism and realism. Rehabilitative teaching and counseling generally are begun before primary surgical therapy is initiated. Some people fear that their desire for rehabilitative surgical procedures will be interpreted as valuing their physical appearance or function as more important than the length of their life. Nurses can assist the patient to see that rehabilitation is desirable and sometimes necessary for achieving the highest possible level of functioning.[42]

Success of surgery for rehabilitation purposes is measured not only by aesthetic improvement but also by improvements in function and self-esteem. As surgical techniques improve, more people with cancer will select and enjoy the benefits of surgical rehabilitation.

## SPECIAL CONSIDERATIONS FOR NURSING CARE

Nursing care of the patient with cancer who is undergoing surgery follows many of the same principles as care for an individual undergoing non-cancer-related surgery. The nurse's role in coordination, education, and communication within the health care team is of utmost importance since surgical procedures are complex, surgical stays are short, and patients receive several forms of cancer therapy in a short amount of time.

### Surgical Setting and Length of Stay

Historically, surgical procedures were performed in an inpatient hospital setting, with a generous amount of time for recuperation in the hospital before discharge. In recent years, the health care delivery system has been changed by the many advances in surgical and anesthetic technique, as well as the multiple measures to contain costs.[43] Since 1990, more surgical procedures are done on an ambulatory basis than on an inpatient basis.[3] This change in the method of delivery of surgical care presents challenges for both inpatient and ambulatory nurses who are striving to support patients in various stages of crisis and aiming to ensure that adequate information is given, surgical procedures are performed safely, and postoperative complications are minimized.

Patients identify that their most important concerns are the effectiveness of treatment, the options for treatment, the effects of therapy on life expectancy, and how to manage the effects of treatment.[44] Many educational strategies can be used to support patients; however, because the period of contact with health care professionals during surgical care is of such short duration, it is most important for patients and their families to know whom to contact and how to do so when they need help or further information.

### General Surgical Care and Oncological Emergencies

Surgical teams are well acquainted with typical surgical complications of pulmonary problems, sepsis, perforation, and hemorrhage. The nursing care issues and considerations for care are well summarized by Polomano et al in Table 12-3.[45] The current challenges in surgical care are rapidly changing as the technology of surgical instrumentation (lasers, laparoscopes, endoscopes) and the role of adjuvant therapies advance. Particularly challenging is the patient with concomitant diseases (cardiac, pulmonary, renal, endocrine) who will receive aggressive treatment for the cancer because of advances made in the management and supportive therapies available today. Antibiotic therapy, hematopoietic growth factors, implantable pumps, high-tech infusion equipment, and transplantation are a few of the overall advances that contribute to the challenging care of the surgical oncology patient today.

**TABLE 12-3**  General Nursing Care Issues in the Care of Surgical Oncology Patients

| Potential/Actual Complication | Contributing Factors | Nursing Considerations |
|---|---|---|
| ARDS | Hemorrhage<br>Aspiration<br>Prolonged atelectasis<br>Infection<br>Pulmonary edema<br>Deposition of platelets<br>Trauma to lung parenchyma<br>Cardiopulmonary bypass<br>Pulmonary emboli | 1. Maintain patent airway.<br>2. Optimize mechanical ventilation, avoid toxic levels of oxygen, use PEEP as tolerated.<br>3. Administer corticosteroids and/or anti-inflammatory agents such as indomethacin as ordered.<br>4. Use colloid if fluid replacement is necessary—invasive hemodynamic monitoring.<br>5. Optimize nutrition.<br>6. Add mucolytic agents via nebulizer.<br>7. Turn frequently.<br>8. Monitor chest x-ray. |

**TABLE 12-3**  General Nursing Care Issues in the Care of Surgical Oncology Patients (continued)

| Potential/Actual Complication | Contributing Factors | Nursing Considerations |
|---|---|---|
| Aspiration pneumonia | Difficulty in swallowing<br>Mechanical obstruction from cancer<br>Excessive sedation | 1. Keep head of the bed elevated 30°.<br>2. Maintain NPO status if gag reflex is not intact—Use NG tube.<br>3. Consult speech therapy for swallowing techniques.<br>4. Avoid excessive sedation in nonintubated patients.<br>5. Soft mechanical diet once taking PO.<br>6. Frequent suctioning when intubated.<br>7. Keep patient in lateral position.<br>8. Monitor chest x-rays.<br>9. Monitor daily CBC. |
| Infection | See Chapter 21 | 1. Assess vital signs frequently.<br>2. Check insertion sites, IV lines, suture lines, and wounds for signs of infection.<br>3. Isolation as indicated—no fresh flowers or fresh fruit for neutropenic patients.<br>4. Institute skin-care precautions.<br>5. Minimize invasive procedures.<br>6. Direct all visitors to use strict hand-washing techniques.<br>7. Check daily CBC (absolute neutrophil and lymphocyte counts).<br>8. Monitor chest x-ray.<br>9. Obtain blood culture for temperature >101 °F. |
| Bleeding | Hypothermia<br>Prolonged cardiopulmonary bypass<br>Medications | 1. Place bleeding precautions sign at bedside.<br>2. Observe for signs/symptoms of bleeding: purpura, oozing, pallor, hemoptysis, petechia, hemorrhage, and ecchymosis.<br>3. Test all excreta for blood.<br>4. Turn and reposition frequently.<br>5. Monitor CBC, PT, PTT.<br>6. Eliminate aspirin and aspirin-containing compounds and heparin from IV lines.<br>7. Avoid invasive procedures.<br>8. Secure peripheral arterial lines and observe site for bleeding. |
| Poor wound healing | Prior radiation therapy<br>Steroid therapy<br>Chemotherapy<br>Local tumor invasion<br>Malnutrition<br>Immune dysfunction<br>Neutropenia | 1. Assess wound for drainage and erythema.<br>2. Keep dressing dry and secure with a nonirritating tape.<br>3. Optimize nutrition.<br>4. Consider vitamin E cream. |
| Stomatitis | Antimetabolite chemotherapeutic agents<br>Bleomycin<br>Head and neck radiation<br>Dehydration | 1. Assess oral membranes for ulcerations.<br>2. Administer frequent oral care with a cleansing agent like chlorhexidine or hydrogen peroxide.<br>3. Moisten membranes and lips with a water-soluble gel or artificial saliva preparation.<br>4. Secure endotracheal tubes with tape, avoiding contact with lips.<br>5. Avoid mouth rinses containing alcohol.<br>6. Watch for oral candidiasis and administer topical or systemic antifungal agents. |

Abbreviations: NPO = nothing by mouth; NG = nasogastric; CBC = complete blood count; PO = by mouth; IV = intravenous.

Adapted with permission from Polomano R, Weintraub FN, Wurster A.: Surgical Critical Care for Cancer Patients. *Semin Oncol Nurs* 10:165–176, 1994

The effects of the disease and of the treatments can lead to clinical situations that are categorized as oncology emergencies. The surgical patient may experience a complex set of reactions and responses to therapy that may be precipitated by the concomitant therapies or the complications of the underlying disease process itself. Beyond classic surgical complications and emergencies, the surgical team should be aware of the most common oncology

**TABLE 12-4**   Oncological Emergencies and Treatment Complications

**Metabolic**
Hypercalcemia
Hypoglycemia
  Insulinoma
  Other tumors
Hyperuricemia
Tumor lysis syndrome
SIADH

**Respiratory**
Infectious
  Bacterial, fungal, viral
Iatrogenic
  Bleomycin/mitomycin-C, radiation therapy
Massive hemoptysis
Proximal lower airway obstruction
Tracheoesophageal fistula
Complications of tracheostomy
  Obstruction
  Sepsis
  Tube displacement
  Early hemorrhage
  Tracheoarterial fistula

**Gastrointestinal**
Acute abdomen
  Visceral perforation
    Due to tumor
    Due to treatment (radiation, chemotherapy)
    Other (peptic ulcer perforation, appendicitis)
  Obstruction
    Adhesions, hernias, other benign causes
    Neoplasm (intrinsic, extrinsic, transcoclomic)
    Radiation enteritis/proctitis
  Inflammatory
    Diverticulitis, appendicitis, other nonneoplastic
    Neutropenic enterocolitis
Perianal/perirectal sepsis
Jaundice
  Biliary obstruction
    Intrinsic/extrinsic neoplasia
    Intrahepatic/extrahepatic
  Hepatic metastases (massive replacement)
Transfusion-related
  Hemolytic reactions
  Hepatitis B or C
Complications from intraperitoneal catheters

**Genitourinary**
Obstructive uropathy
  Retroperitoneal/pelvic neoplasia
  Prostatism
Urosepsis
Priapism

**Neurological**
ALTERED MENTAL STATES AND SEIZURES
Metabolic
  Hypercalcemia
  Hypoglycemia
  Hepatic/uremic encephalopathy
  Hyponatremia
  Hypomagnesemia
Infectious
  Meningitis
    *Listeria*
    *Candida, Cryptococcus*
    Viral
  Brain abscess
    Anaerobes, Gram-positive aerobes, *Pseudomonas*
    *Aspergillus*
  Viral encephalitis
Cerebrovascular
  Embolic infarction
  Thrombotic infarction
  Intracranial hemorrhage
    Intracerebral neoplasm/metastasis
    Coagulopathy (e.g., DIC, IV heparin)
Iatrogenic
  Chemotherapeutic encephalopathy
    Nitrogen mustard, BCNU, VP-16, ifosfamide, interferons, methotrexate, procarbazine, cytosine arabinoside
  Brain irradiation
  Medications
    Corticosteroids, antiemetics, narcotics,
    Hypnotics/sedatives
Neoplastic
  Intracranial mass lesions
    Primary/metastatic tumor
    Hemorrhage into metastasis
  Leptomeningeal involvement
    Acute hydrocephalus
    Encephalopathy
SPINAL CORD COMPRESSION

**Cardiovascular**
CARDIAC
  Cardiac tamponade
  Arrhythmias
VASCULAR
  Arterial
    Hemorrhage
      Invasion/erosion by tumor
      Treatment-related
    Embolism
      Nonbacterial marantic endocarditis
  Venous
    Superior vena cava syndrome
    Thromboembolism
      Deep vein thrombosis
      Phlegmasia cerulea dolens
      Pulmonary embolism

**Hematologic**
Disseminated intravascular coagulation
  Chronic and acute
Venous thromboembolism
Hemorrhagic complications
  Thrombocytopenia
  Platelet function defects
  Thrombocytosis

**Related to Chemotherapy**
Extravasation injuries
Allergic/hypersensitivity reactions
  Anaphylaxis ± other allergic phenomena
    Actinomycin-D
    Bleomycin
    Cyclophosphamide
    DTIC
    Methotrexate
    VP-16
    L-asparaginase
    *cis*-Platinum
    Doxorubicin
    Melphalan
    Nitrogen mustard

SIADH = syndrome of inappropriate secretion of antidiuretic hormone; DIC = disseminated intravascular coagulation; IV = intravenous; BCNU = carmustine; VP-16 = etoposide; DTIC = dacarbazine.
Reprinted from Moffat and Ketcham.[30]

emergencies that can occur.[30] These clinical situations are listed in Table 12-4. The reader is referred to specific chapters in this book for detailed discussion of care for the emergencies.

## Autologous Blood Donation

Autologous blood donation is being considered more commonly in situations where the surgical procedure is not emergent and the patient is hemodynamically stable to donate. Some hospitals have their own autologous donation programs; others use the services of the American Red Cross Autologous Donor Program. It is important to schedule this donation well in advance of surgery. Nonanemic patients can donate up to 6 units of blood prior to surgery. Blood usually can be donated from 42 days to 72 hours prior to surgery. Because of the small, but real, risk from homologous blood transfusions, most individuals are eager to donate their own blood.[12,46]

## Anxiety and Pain Control

Anxiety and pain control should be addressed prior to the actual operation to allow patients to verbalize fears, to discuss previous experiences, and to be made aware of advances in pharmacological methods of pain relief as well as the advantages of behavioral methods of pain control and relaxation techniques. Carr et al[47] recommend discussions in the preoperative period of expectations of pain and its relief to include dosing of analgesic medicine, availability of patient-controlled analgesia (PCA) units, use of rating scales to measure pain, and nonpharmacological maneuvers to decrease pain and anxiety[48] (Table 12-5). The reader is also referred to chapter 20 for additional information.

Relaxation and hypnosis have been used in the pediatric setting to help decrease the trauma of painful procedures.[49] These same techniques can be applied to the adult surgical population with effective results in reducing both anxiety and pain.[50,51] Relaxation, deep breathing,

**TABLE 12-5**  Nonpharmacologic Interventions for Pain Control[48]

| | Intervention* | Type of Evidence† | Comments |
|---|---|---|---|
| Simple relaxation (begin preoperatively) | • Jaw relaxation<br>• Progressive muscle relaxation<br>• Simple imagery | Ia, IIa, IIb, IV | Effective in reducing mild to moderate pain and as an adjunct to analgesic drugs for severe pain. Use when patients express an interest in relaxation. Requires 3–5 minutes of staff time for instructions. |
| | Music | Ib, IIa, IV | Both patient-preferred and "easy listening" music are effective in reducing mild to moderate pain. |
| Complex relaxation (begin preoperatively) | Biofeedback | Ib, IIa, IIb, IV | Effective in reducing mild to moderate pain and operative site muscle tension. Requires skilled personnel and special equipment. |
| | Imagery | Ib, IIa, IV | Effective for reduction of mild to moderate pain. Requires skilled personnel. |
| Education/instruction (begin preoperatively) | | Ia, IIa, IIb, IV | Effective for reduction of pain. Should include sensory and procedural information and instruction aimed at reducing activity-related pain. Requires 5–15 minutes of staff time. |
| TENS | | Ia, IIa, III, IV | Effective in reducing pain and improving physical function. Requires skilled personnel and special equipment. May be useful as an adjunct to drug therapy. |

*Selected references are included in this Clinical Practice Guideline. For more complete references, see: Acute Pain Management Guideline Panel: *Acute Pain Management: Operative or Medical Procedures and Trauma. Guideline Report.* AHCPR Pub. No. 92-0022. Rockville, MD: Agency for Health Care Policy and Research, Public Health Service, U.S. Department of Health and Human Services, 1992.

†Insufficient scientific evidence is available to provide specific recommendations regarding the use of hypnosis, acupuncture, and other physical modalities for relief of postoperative pain.

Key to Type of Evidence
Ia  Evidence obtained from meta-analysis of randomized controlled trials
 b  Evidence obtained from at least one randomized controlled trial
IIa  Evidence obtained from at least one well-designed controlled study without randomization
 b  Evidence obtained from at least one other type of well-designed quasi-experimental study
III  Evidence obtained from well-designed nonexperimental studies, such as comparative studies, correlational studies, and case studies
IV  Evidence obtained from expert committee reports or opinions and/or clinical experiences of respected authorities

visualization, guided imagery, and self-hypnosis are techniques to help patients decrease anxiety and pain during painful procedures (i.e., bone marrow biopsy, needle localization, breast biopsy) as well as during the postoperative period. Specially trained nurses may be available in the health care setting to provide training for hypnosis, meditation, or relaxation, and they also may be able to coordinate referrals to other specialists in the institution or in the community for assistance in learning these techniques. Many people already incorporate these behavioral methods into their normal daily routine, so it may be a matter of reminding patients to use skills already at their disposal (e.g., using Lamaze breathing during a painful procedure). Health care professionals should make it a priority to encourage and teach methods of reducing anxiety and providing pain relief to individuals anticipating a surgical procedure. A team approach focused on communication and anticipation of needs is of the utmost importance and will benefit the patient greatly.[51]

In the preoperative period, nurses should be acutely aware of problems that can occur as a result of the cancer disease process itself, as well as anticipating possible postoperative complications. The patient with cancer should be cared for by professionals who have a keen eye for the complications that are common with this disease.[52]

## Nutritional Support

Protein-calorie malnutrition is a common occurrence among cancer patients, especially those with advanced disease. The nutritionally debilitated individual with cancer is a poor surgical candidate and will likely experience severe postoperative complications unless the nutritional status of the patient is fully assessed and an aggressive plan of support is developed and initiated. Complications of surgery associated with malnutrition include pneumonia, ileus, sepsis, wound dehiscence, and diminished tolerance of subsequent antineoplastic therapies. The individual with cancer undergoing surgery may be experiencing the advanced symptoms of cachexia: a syndrome of weight loss, anorexia, and wasting of lean body mass. Anorexia, a voluntary decrease in intake, can occur as a result of systemic effects of the tumor itself or the anorexia that can occur as a result of chemotherapy and radiation therapy.

When subjected to a major stress, such as surgical trauma or infection, the patient with cancer who is malnourished or has cachexia will not mount the usual defense of conserving lean body mass. The catabolism of body mass that accompanies cancer is persistent and somewhat refractory to nutritional therapy. The challenge of supporting the surgical patient with nutritional therapy requires a knowledgeable and comprehensive team approach because the simple approach of increased caloric intake by whatever route possible will likely not produce adequate results to avoid significant morbidity.[53–55]

An important first step in the management of the malnourished surgical cancer patient is to carefully assess the nutritional status through history, physical examination, and laboratory tests. The nutritional plan is based on the metabolic needs of the patient, which can vary from hypermetabolic to hypometabolic. The route of administration of nutritional support should be considered in the following sequence:[53]

1. Enteral nutrition—the preferred route when the gastrointestinal (GI) tract is functioning. There are significant benefits of enteral nutrition over the parenteral route, such as GI mucosal and enzyme function, immune status, and balanced microflora of the gut.
2. Total parenteral nutrition (TPN) for brief periods (7–10 days)—though not scientifically validated as an effective method of nutritional support, especially for mildly malnourished surgical patients or those with rapidly advancing disease, TPN may be indicated in a severely malnourished patient who cannot be fed via the enteral route.
3. Total parenteral nutrition for prolonged periods or home TPN—this approach is only indicated in situations where enteral feeding is not feasible because of advanced disease or severe toxicities of cancer therapies.

There are special indications for the use of TPN with surgical patients that do not fit the above pattern. Patients with enterocutaneous fistulas will not be able to use the enteral route for nutrition because oral intake stimulates fistula output and can lead to metabolic and electrolyte disturbances. The fistula may close more rapidly if the person is nutritionally well supported. Hepatic failure due to chemotherapy or major surgery, acute renal failure, prolonged ileus, and acute radiation enteritis are all clinical situations that may benefit from the addition of TPN to the treatment plan.

The nutrition plan should be as aggressive as the cancer treatment plan.[56] Specific nursing measures to improve the nutritional status of patients are discussed in chapter 24.

## Hemostasis

Another common manifestation of cancer that can significantly increase the risk of postoperative complications is altered hemostasis, particularly hypercoagulability and thrombosis.[57] Elevated clotting factors and shortened partial thromboplastin and prothrombin times have been noted to occur in individuals with cancer. The individual with cancer therefore is highly susceptible to minor changes in the hemostatic process. An individual with cancer is more likely to develop postoperative thrombophlebitis than is an individual without cancer.

The nursing management of the individual with cancer undergoing surgery is based on accurate assessment of hemodynamic parameters and an understanding of the implications of abnormalities in clotting factors that can result in bleeding tendencies and hemorrhage. The importance of early postoperative ambulation cannot be overemphasized. Because these individuals are at high risk for deep-vein thrombosis, the nurse observes the patient for signs and symptoms of this disorder. Bleeding abnormalities in individuals with cancer are discussed in more detail in chapter 22.

## Combined Modality Therapy

The combined modality treatment of cancer has introduced a new set of challenges for health care providers. Chemotherapy, radiation therapy, and biotherapy are being given for certain tumors in varied sequences according to the most effective protocol, including preoperative, intraoperative, and postoperative treatment. The synergistic and augmented effects of combined therapies can produce postoperative reactions and complications that may be difficult to manage.

Preoperative chemotherapy or radiotherapy, alone or in combination, is used with particular tumors that have better response rates when combination therapy is sequenced in this manner. The timing and extent of surgery may require modification following radiation or chemotherapy, depending on the type of treatment, the individual's response to therapy and the side effects experienced. Given the trend toward more aggressive chemotherapy and radiotherapy, wound healing may become a more significant problem in the future. These concerns point to the need for further research to determine the optimal doses and timing sequence for combination therapy.

Surgical procedures sometimes become necessary during active radiation or chemotherapy treatment cycles, such as inserting a vascular access device, relieving an obstruction, or repairing a perforation. Preoperative assessment of the patient who is actively receiving combination therapy is specifically focused on those body systems and organs that are being affected by the current therapy. For example, if a patient has been receiving anthracycline chemotherapy (adriamycin, bleomycin, mitomycin C, or mithramycin), there are known cardiac and pulmonary toxicities that will require special attention during any operative and postoperative period.[58]

Intraoperative radiotherapy and intraoperative chemotherapy are being researched for their potential to decrease recurrence and metastases. Radiotherapy or chemotherapy given intraoperatively involves the delivery of a single, high dose directly to the surgically exposed tumor or tumor bed. Intraoperative therapy requires extensive multidisciplinary collaboration. Patient and staff safety are carefully considered.[59] Potential side effects of intraoperative therapy are not yet fully known but appear to be similar to those of traditional delivery methods. Intraoperative treatments, used predominantly in major cancer centers, are administered for locally advanced abdominal and pelvic malignancies. Gastric, pancreatic, ovarian, bladder, and colorectal are a few of the tumor types being treated with intraoperative radiotherapy.[59,60]

A major challenge in caring for a patient who has received combination therapy is wound healing. If the patient was previously treated with radiation to the surgical site, there may be long-term damage to the underlying tissues, such as fibrosis and obliteration of lymphatic and vascular channels.[61] Once the integrity of the tissue is damaged by radiation, additional trauma is not tolerated well. Postoperative wound dehiscence, infection, tissue necrosis, and bone necrosis are potential complications of surgery performed on previously irradiated tissue. It is also known that radiation itself will interfere with healing if it is administered in the early postoperative period.

In some cases, it becomes necessary or highly desirable to initiate chemotherapy early in the postoperative period. There are many unanswered questions regarding the appropriate timing and effects of specific chemotherapeutic agents on wound healing. Table 12-6 outlines some of the potential postoperative complications as a result of intraoperative or early postoperative chemotherapy.[62]

Certain chemotherapeutic agents are toxic to specific organ systems, resulting in long-term side effects that can increase the individual's risk of surgical complications. Table 12-7 presents some of the agents that may have an effect on surgical outcome and wound healing.[63]

Critical phases of wound healing last for about 25 days following incision. During this time, inflammatory processes release growth factors and cytokines and stimulate production of platelets and acute inflammatory cells. During the proliferative phase of wound healing, which can last from 3 to 25 days following surgery, granulation tissue is formed and provides the characteristic strength of a wound.

Most chemotherapy agents act by interfering with protein synthesis. Because of this interference, it follows that wound healing could be disrupted by the administration of most chemotherapeutic agents in the early phases of wound healing. Research studies on humans to test this deduction are limited, but animal studies have been conducted that indicate that the immediate and early postoperative period is a time when wound healing could be adversely affected or delayed by the administration of chemotherapy. Typical patterns of care allow a period of recovery before combination therapy is initiated.

The nurse needs to be aware of these effects and focus assessments and nursing care toward early identification and measures to minimize complications. As new therapies become available and are used aggressively in an

**TABLE 12-6**   Effects of Chemotherapy on Wound Healing

Alteration of nitrogen balance (suppressed protein synthesis)
Impeded aggregation of platelets and deposition of fibrin
Inhibition of inflammatory cells
Inhibition of fibroplasia
Decreased production of hydroxyproline and collagen
Delayed vasodilatation and neovascularization
Impaired wound contraction
Slowed epithelialization
Impairment of collagen cross-linking
Promotion of wound infection

Reprinted from Schaffer and Barbal.[62]

**TABLE 12-7** Effects of Chemotherapy on Specific Organs[63]

| Organ | Chemotherapeutic Agent | Effects |
|-------|------------------------|---------|
| Respiratory system | Bleomycin | May predispose patient to postoperative acute adult respiratory distress syndrome |
| | Methotrexate Busulfan | May produce diffuse interstitial and alveolar pneumonitis |
| Renal system | Cis-platinum Streptozocin Methotrexate VP-16 | Can result in persistent decrease in glomerular filtration rate (GFR) |
| Cardiac system | Doxorubicin Daunorubicin | With cumulative dose of 500 mg/m² increased risk of intraoperative and postoperative congestive heart failure and pulmonary edema |

attempt to eradicate malignancies, the potential exists for different and more severe complications to occur.

## CONCLUSION

Surgery for cancer is the oldest form of cancer therapy still in use; however, there have been advances and changes in the scope and role of surgical therapy. Most individuals with cancer will have some sort of surgical procedure as part of their treatment plan. Current understanding of cancer biology and the natural history and progression of certain tumors has caused the role of surgery to be questioned and modified in many instances. Radical surgery is still a reasonable and valid approach for several tumor types, but not for others. Breast cancer is the most profound example of a less drastic surgical approach.

Adjuvant therapy can lengthen survival and disease-free intervals and improve the quality of life. The potential side effects of combination modality therapies present new challenges to health care practitioners.

Nurses who interact with individuals with cancer having surgery will find many useful practices and applicable concepts from other fields. Oncology nurses will find much satisfaction interacting with nurses in the operating room, the recovery room, and the various surgical settings to learn more about the patient's overall experience.

Prospective clinical research, both physiological and psychological, that includes active participation of surgical practitioners will continue to be needed.[64-66] Effective surgical cancer therapy depends on a solid integration of the biological and clinical sciences of cancer. In addition to important strides in the understanding of the biology of cancer, clinicians have learned a great deal about the educational, psychological, social, and rehabilitative needs of individuals who are undergoing surgical procedures for cancer therapy.[67]

## REFERENCES

1. Balch CM, Pellis NR, Morton DL, et al: Oncology, in Swartz SI, Shires GT, Spencer FC (eds) *Principles of Surgery* (ed 6). New York, McGraw-Hill, 1994, pp 305–385
2. Henderson IC: Adjuvant systemic therapy of breast cancer, in Harris JR, Hellman S, Henderson IC, Kinne D (eds): *Breast Diseases.* Philadelphia, Lippincott, 1991, pp 427–486
3. Stone MD, Doyle J: The influence of surgical training on the practice of surgery. *Surg Clin North Am* 76:1–10, 1996
4. Doak LG, Doak CC, Meade CD: Strategies to improve cancer educational materials. *Oncol Nurs Forum* 23:1305–1312, 1996
5. Rosenberg SA: Principles of surgical oncology, in DeVita VT, Hellman S, Rosenberg SA (eds): *Cancer: Principles and Practice of Oncology* (ed 4). Philadelphia, Lippincott, 1993, pp 238–247
6. Rege RV, Merriam LT, Joehl RJ: Laparoscopic splenectomy. *Surg Clin North Am* 76:459–468, 1996
7. Gagner M: Laparoscopic adrenelectomy. *Surg Clin North Am* 76:523–538, 1996
8. Salky BA, Edye M: Laparoscopic pancreatectomy. *Surg Clin North Am* 76:539–546, 1996
9. Schirmer BD: Laparoscopic colon resection. *Surg Clin North Am* 76:571–584, 1996
10. Traverso LW: The laparoscopic surgical value package and how surgeons can influence costs. *Surg Clin North Am* 76:631–640, 1996
11. Schwartz SI: Hemostasis, surgical bleeding, and transfusion, in Schwartz SI, Shires GT, Spencer FC (eds): *Principles of Surgery.* New York, McGraw Hill, 1996, 1806–1812
12. Campion FX, Rosenblatt MS: Quality assurance and medical outcomes in the era of cost containment. *Surg Clin North Am* 76:139–160, 1996
13. Preisler HD, Taza A: The role of emerging technologies in the diagnosis and staging of neoplastic diseases. *Cancer* 9:1520–1525, 1992 (suppl)
14. Herrera L, Luna P, Villarreal J: Perspectives in colorectal cancer. *J Surg Oncol* 2:92–103, 1991 (suppl)
15. Jeekel J: Can radical surgery improve survival in colorectal cancer? *World J Surg* 11:412–417, 1987
16. NIH Consensus Conference: Treatment of early-stage breast cancer. *JAMA* 265:391–394, 1991

17. Steele G, Cady B: The surgical oncologist as the patient manager, in Steele G, Cady B (eds): *General Surgical Oncology.* Philadelphia, Saunders, 1992, pp 18–21

18. Tannock IF: Principles of cell proliferation: Cell Kinetics, in DeVita VT, Hellman S, Rosenberg S (eds): *Cancer: Principles and Practice of Oncology* (ed 3). Philadelphia, Lippincott, 1989, pp 3–13

19. Douglass HO: Adjuvant treatment in colorectal cancer: An update. *World J Surg* 11:478–492, 1987

20. Schuller DE, Laramore G, Al-Sarraf M, et al: Combined therapy for resectable head and neck cancer. *Arch Otolaryngol Head Neck Surg* 115:364–368, 1989

21. Shepard FA, Ginsberg RJ, Patterson GA, et al: A prospective study of adjuvant surgical resection after chemotherapy for limited small cell lung cancer. *J Thorac Cardiovasc Surg* 97: 177–186, 1989

22. Siegel B, Mayzel K, Love S: Level I and II axillary dissection in the treatment of early-stage breast cancer. *Arch Surg* 25: 1144–1147, 1990

23. Liotta L, Stetler-Stevenson WG: Principles of molecular cell biology of cancer: Cancer Metastases, in DeVita VT, Hellman S, Rosenberg S (eds): *Cancer Principles and Practice of Oncology* (ed 4). Philadelphia, Lippincott, 1993, pp 134–149

24. Ewer M, Ali MK: Surgical treatment of the cancer patient: Preoperative assessment and perioperative medical management. *J Surg Oncol* 44:185–190, 1990

25. Patterson WB: Surgical issues in geriatric oncology. *Semin Oncol* 16:57–65, 1989

26. Law TM, Hesketh PJ, Porter KA, et al: Breast cancer in elderly women: Presentation, survival, and treatment options. *Surg Clin North Am* 76:289–308, 1996

27. Ravikumar TS, Steele G: Colon cancer, in Steele G, Cady B (eds): *General Surgical Oncology.* Philadelphia, Saunders, 1992, pp 149–169

28. Wapnir IL, Rabinowitz B: A reappraisal of prophylactic mastectomy. *Surg Gynecol Obstet* 171:171–181, 1990

29. Lopez MJ, Porter KA: The current role of prophylactic mastectomy. *Surg Clin North Am* 76:231–242, 1996

30. Moffat FL, Ketcham AS: Surgery for malignant neoplasia: The evolution of oncologic surgery and its role in the management of cancer patients, in McKenna RJ, Murphy GP (eds): *Cancer Surgery.* Philadelphia, Lippincott, 1994, pp 1–20

31. Love S: *Dr. Susan Love's Breast Book.* Reading, MA, Addison-Wesley, 1990

32. Bibbo M, Underhill S: Cytology of fine-needle aspiration, in Harris JR, Hellman S, Henderson IC, Kinne D (eds): *Breast Diseases.* Philadelphia, Lippincott, 1991, pp 297–300

33. Flynn MB, Wolfson SE, Thomas S, et al: Fine needle aspiration biopsy in clinical management of head and neck tumors. *J Surg Oncol* 44:214–217, 1990

34. Turner AF: Radiographically guided techniques of biopsy, in McKenna RJ, Murphy GP (eds): *Cancer Surgery.* Philadelphia, Lippincott, 1994, pp 21–34

35. Greene FL, Williams RB: Endoscopic management of gastrointestinal malignancy, in McKenna RT, Murphy GP (eds): *Cancer Surgery.* Philadelphia, Lippincott, 1994, pp 35–46

36. Kalinowski BH: Local therapy for breast cancer. Treatment choices and decision making. *Semin Oncol Nurs* 7:187–193, 1991

37. Young RC, Perez CA, Hoskins WJ: Cancer of the ovary, in DeVita VT, Hellman S, Rosenberg S (eds): *Cancer: Principles and Practice of Oncology.* Philadelphia, Lippincott, 1993, pp 1226–1263

38. Steele G, Ravikumar TS, Benotti PN: New surgical treatments for recurrent colorectal cancer. *Cancer* 65:723–730, 1990

39. Russin DJ, Kaplan SR, Goldberg RI, et al: Neodymium-YAG laser. *Arch Surg* 121:1399–1403, 1986

40. Dyck S: Surgical instrumentation as a palliative treatment for spinal cord compression. *Oncol Nurs Forum* 18:515–521, 1991

41. Corral CJ, Mustoe TA: Controversy in breast reconstruction. *Surg Clin North Am* 76:309–326, 1996

42. Schain WS, Wellisch DK, Pasnau RO, et al: The sooner the better. A study of psychological factors in women undergoing immediate versus delayed breast reconstruction. *Am J Psychiatry* 142:40–46, 1985

43. Sangermano CA: Practice and principles of ambulatory surgery, in Meeker MH, Rothrock JC (eds): *Alexander's Care of the Patient in Surgery* (ed 9). St. Louis, Mosby Yearbook, 1991, pp 964–979

44. Griffiths M, Leek C: Patient education needs: Opinions of oncology nurses and their patients. *Oncol Nurs Forum* 22: 139–144, 1995

45. Polomano R, Weintraub FN, Wurster A: Surgical critical care for cancer patients. *Semin Oncol Nurs* 10:165–176, 1994

46. Lichtiger B, Huh YO, Armintor M, et al: Autologous transfusions for cancer patients undergoing elective ablative surgery. *J Surg Oncol* 43:19–23, 1990

47. Carr DB, Jacox A, Chapman CR, et al: *Pain Control After Surgery: A Patient's Guide.* Agency for Health Care Policy and Research publication No. 92-0021. Rockville, MD, U.S. Department of Health and Human Services, 1992

48. Carr DB, Jacox A, Chapman CR, et al: *Acute Pain Management: Operative or Medical Procedures and Trauma.* Agency for Health Care Policy and Research, publication No. 92-0032. Rockville, MD, U.S. Department of Health and Human Services, 1992

49. Valante S: Using Hypnosis with children for pain management. *Oncol Nurs Forum* 18:699–704, 1991

50. Blankfield RP: Suggestion, relaxation, and hypnosis as adjuncts in the care of surgery patients: A review of the literature. *Am J Clin Hypn* 33:172–186, 1991

51. Alberts MS, Lyons JS, Moretti RJ: Psychological interventions in the pre-surgical period. *Int J Psychiatry Med* 19: 91–106, 1989

52. Paice JA, Mahon SM, Faut-Callahan M: Factors associated with adequate pain control in hospitalized postsurgical patients diagnosed with cancer. *Cancer Nurs* 14:298–305, 1991

53. Sarantos P, Copeland EM, Souba WW: Nutritional support of the surgical oncology patient, in McKenna RJ, Murphy GP (eds): *Cancer Surgery.* Philadelphia, Lippincott, 1994, pp 761–772

54. Falcone RE, Nappi JF: Chemotherapy and wound healing. *Surg Clin North Am* 64:779–794, 1984

55. Ehrlichman RJ, Seckel Br, Bryan DJ, et al: Common complications of wound healing. *Surg Clin North Am* 71:1323–1351, 1991

56. Daly JM, Redmond HP, Lieberman MD, et al: Nutritional support of patients with cancer of the gastrointestinal tract. *Surg Clin North Am* 71:523–536, 1991

57. Kemplin S, Gould-Rossback P, Houland WS: Disorders of hemostasis in the critically ill cancer patient, in Howland WS, Carlon GC (eds): *Critical Care of the Cancer Patient.* Chicago, Year Book 1985

58. Mathes DD, Bogdonoff DL: Preoperative evaluation of the cancer patient, in Lefor AT (ed): *Surgical Problems Affecting*

*the patient with Cancer: Interdisciplinary Management.* Philadelphia, Lippincott-Raven, 1996, pp 273–304

59. Smith R: Intraopertive radiation therapy, in Dow KH, Hilderley L (eds): *Nursing Care in Radiation Oncology.* Philadelphia, Saunders, 1992

60. Haibeck SV: Intraoperative radiation therapy. *Oncol Nurs Forum* 15:143–147, 1988

61. Chahbazian CM: The skin, in Moss WT, Cox JD (eds): *Radiation Oncology: Rationale, Techniques, Results* (ed 6). St. Louis, Mosby Year Book, 1989, pp 83–111

62. Schaffer M, Barbul A: Chemotherapy and wound healing, in Lefor AT (ed): *Surgical Problems Affecting the Patient with Cancer: Interdisciplinary Management.* Philadelphia, Lippincott-Raven, 1996, pp 305–320

63. Chabner BA, Myers CE: Clinical pharmacology of cancer chemotherapy, in DeVita VT, Hellman S, Rosenberg SA (eds): *Cancer: Principles and Practice of Oncology.* Philadelphia, Lippincott, 1989, pp 349–395

64. Avis FP, Ellenberg S, Friedman MA: Surgical oncology research. *Ann Surg* 207:262–266, 1988

65. Jacobs JR, Pajak TF, Snow JB, et al: Surgical quality control in head and neck cancer. *Arch Otolaryngol Head Neck Surg* 115:489–493, 1989

66. Thorne SE: Helpful and unhelpful communication in cancer care: The patient perspective. *Oncol Nurs Forum* 15: 167–172, 1988

67. Morra ME: Choices: Who's going to tell the patients what they need to know? *Oncol Nurs Forum* 15:421–425, 1988

# Chapter 13

# Radiotherapy

Laura J. Hilderley, RN, MS

## INTRODUCTION

Radiation therapy has been used in the treatment of cancer since the early 1900s. Roentgen's discovery of the x-ray in 1895 followed by Marie and Pierre Curie's investigation of radioactive sources led to recognition of the ionizing property of radiation and its effect on living matter. Through many years of trial and discovery, the science of radiation oncology has evolved to its current place as a primary cancer treatment modality.

## THE CURRENT APPLICATION OF RADIOTHERAPY IN THE MANAGEMENT OF THE PATIENT DIAGNOSED WITH CANCER

Radiotherapy often is combined with surgery or chemotherapy and immunotherapy, as well as being the sole treatment for cancer in some instances. For example, stage II B adenocarcinoma of the endometrium is treated with preoperative radiation followed by hysterectomy, whereas stage II B squamous cell carcinoma of the cervix is treated with radiation alone.

The goal or intent of radiotherapy may be curative, as in the treatment of skin cancer, carcinoma of the cervix, Hodgkin's disease, or seminoma. Treatment is vigorous and often lengthy, but the prognosis and probability of long-term survival make such an attempt worthwhile.

For certain other lesions, cure or eradication is not possible, and control of the cancer for periods ranging from months to years may be the goal. Recurrent breast cancer, some soft-tissue sarcomas, and lung cancer are examples of cancers controlled by radiotherapy in combination with surgery or chemotherapy.

Palliation may be another goal of radiotherapy. Relief of pain, prevention of pathological fractures, and return of mobility can be achieved with radiation to metastatic bone lesions from primary sites such as breast, lung, and prostate. Pain relief often is dramatic, and it is not uncommon for one individual to receive multiple palliative courses to different bony structures over the course of several years. Between such metastatic episodes the individual sometimes can live a near-normal life. Palliative radiotherapy also is given for the relief of central nervous system (CNS) symptoms caused by brain metastasis or spinal cord compression. Hemorrhage, ulceration, and fungating lesions effectively can be reduced and in some instances eliminated by palliative radiotherapy.

"Anticipatory" palliation is a useful application of radiotherapy in treating potentially symptomatic lesions before they become a problem. Examples of anticipatory palliation include treatment of a mediastinal mass that threatens to produce a superior vena caval syndrome and treatment to a vertebral lesion when spinal cord compression is impending.

Although treatment techniques and equipment may vary, the fundamental principles of radiobiology and radiation physics form the basis on which a course of treatment is selected and designed for each patient. Understanding these principles will enable the oncology nurse to support and care for the patient diagnosed with cancer receiving radiotherapy, meeting the emotional as well as the physical needs that result from the disease and the therapy.

## APPLIED RADIATION PHYSICS

The use of ionizing radiation in the treatment of cancer is based on the ability of radiation to interact with the atoms and molecules of the tumor cells to produce specific harmful biological effects. Ionization affects either the molecules of the cell or the cell environment.

An understanding of atomic structure is basic to understanding the ionizing effects of radiation. The atom, the basic unit of molecular structure, consists of two parts: the nucleus, containing positively charged protons and neutrons that have mass but no charge; and the shells (orbits), containing electrons (equivalent to the number of protons), each of which has a negative charge. Each shell can accommodate only a certain number of electrons; if this number is exceeded, a second or third shell is established more distant from the nucleus (Figure 13-1). The negatively charged electrons orbit the nucleus, held in place by the attractive force of the positive protons in the nucleus, thus maintaining a stable state. Certain

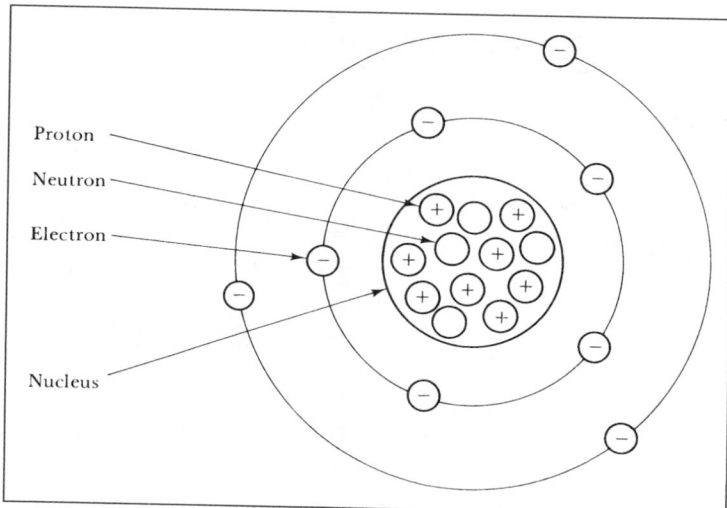

**FIGURE 13-1** Basic structure of an atom. Protons, which are positively charged, and neutrons, which have no electrical charge, are the major components of the nucleus of an atom. The number of protons is equal to the number of negatively charged electrons orbiting the nucleus. Atoms of any given element may have different numbers of neutrons in the nucleus, thus giving atoms of the same element different atomic weights. An atom of a given element that differs only in its atomic weight is called an isotope.

atoms are known to be unstable, however, and it is in this process of decay or breakdown into a more stable state that alpha, beta, or gamma rays may be emitted. Radium, radon, and uranium are examples of unstable atoms that produce ionizing radiation.

Stable atoms also may be made to produce ionizing radiation through excitation, ionization, and nuclear disintegration. Radiation produced by these processes can be classified into two groups: *electromagnetic radiation* and *particulate radiation*. The electromagnetic spectrum can be further divided into five levels of decreasing wavelength:

1. radio waves
2. infrared radiation
3. visible light
4. ultraviolet radiation
5. ionizing radiation

Ionizing radiation has the shortest wavelength and the greatest energy of the electromagnetic spectrum and is therefore the form of energy used in radiotherapy. A classification system for ionizing radiations is shown in Figure 13-2. As seen in the figure, the terms *x-ray* and *gamma ray* both describe ionizing electromagnetic radiation and differ only in their means of production. That is, x-rays are produced by specially designed equipment, and gamma rays are emitted by radioactive materials such as $^{60}$Co undergoing nuclear transition. Both x- and gamma rays have no mass, but rather are packets of available energy ready to be released on collision with a substance. Because they have no mass, x- and gamma rays can penetrate much deeper into tissue before releasing their energy.

Particulate radiation, on the other hand, is composed of alpha and beta particles, as well as electrons and neutrons, which have mass. The relatively large size of alpha particles allows them to penetrate only a short distance into tissue before collision and energy release take place; beta particles, which are smaller than alpha particles, will

penetrate deeper, but because of their mass do not have the ability to reach as deeply into tissues as do x- and gamma rays. The significance of these variations in ability to penetrate tissue will be obvious when treatment beams and equipment are discussed.

X-rays are produced when a stream of fast-moving electrons, accelerated by the application of high voltage (between the filament and the target), strikes the target, and the electrons give up their energy. This radiation loss occurs because the electron is attracted to and slowed down by the nucleus of the tungsten (target) atom. Figure 13-3 illustrates the basic structure of an x-ray tube.

In addition to x-rays, some treatment machines (betatron, linear accelerator) are equipped to produce particle irradiation in the form of electrons. Electron energy is produced in an x-ray tube by bypassing one of the steps used to produce x-rays (see Figure 13-3). Electrons from the heated tungsten filament are injected into the vacuum tube, are accelerated at a high velocity, and emerge from a window in the vacuum tube, thus bypassing the tungsten target and emerging as electron particles suitable for treating surface lesions and those located a few centimeters below the skin.

Electromagnetic and particulate radiations also are produced through the process of decay of radioactive elements and radioactive isotopes. This process, which produces radiation in the form of alpha, beta, or gamma rays, is illustrated as follows:

$$\text{atom} \xrightarrow{\text{radioactive decay}} \text{atom } y + \text{radiation}$$

The time required for half the radioactive atoms present at any time to decay is known as the *half-life* of that radioactive element or isotope.

Because most radioisotopes are produced by neutron bombardment of stable elements ($^{60}$Co, $^{32}$P, $^{182}$TA, $^{198}$Au) or nuclear fission of uranium in a nuclear reactor ($^{90}$SR, $^{137}$Cs), they are referred to as artificial isotopes to distinguish them from naturally occurring radioisotopes such

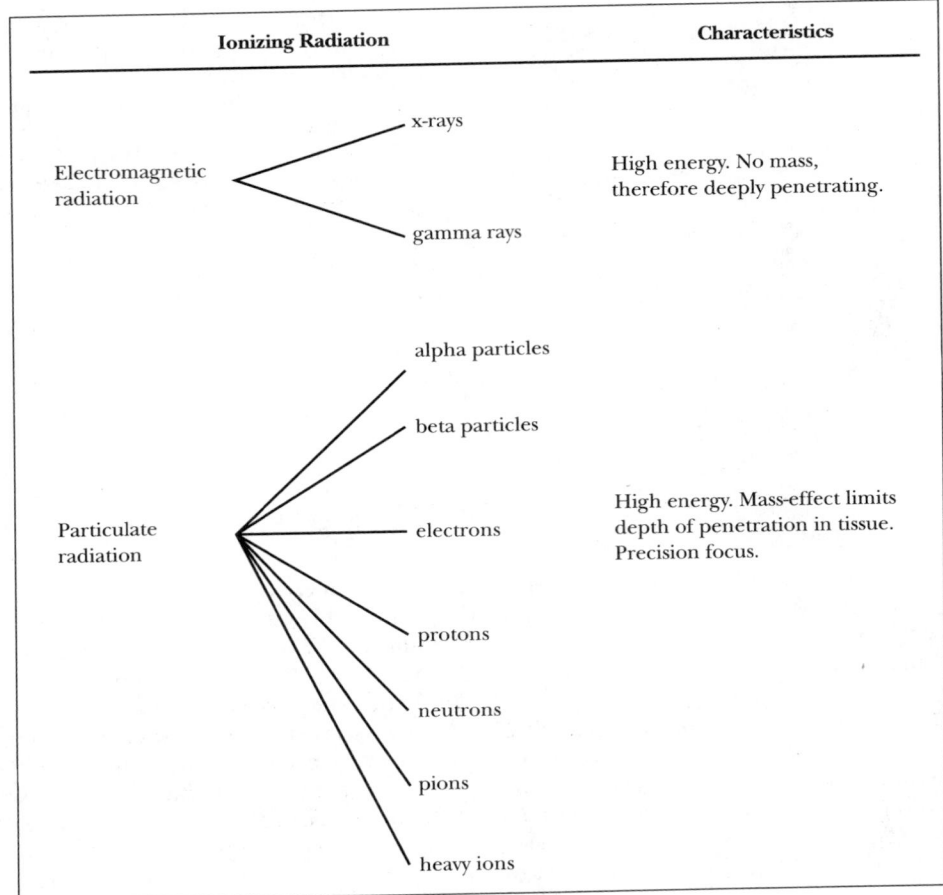

**FIGURE 13-2**  Characteristics of ionizing radiations.

as $^{226}$Ra and $^{222}$Rn. Radioisotopes are listed in Table 13-1.

## EQUIPMENT, BEAMS, AND MATERIALS USED IN RADIOTHERAPY

The types of equipment and beams used in radiotherapy are numerous and vary considerably in their application to clinical practice. A large radiotherapy center will have available a selection suitable for the treatment of almost any malignancy in any part of the body. On the other hand, the equipment available in a private office or small general hospital may be limited to whatever is easiest to use and maintain.

Equipment can be classified according to use: external radiation, or *teletherapy* (radiation from a source at a distance from the body), and internal application, or *brachytherapy* (radiation from a source placed within the body or a body cavity).

A useful classification system of various beams, equipment, and radioactive materials is given in Figures 13-4

and 13-5. In addition to teletherapy and brachytherapy, radiotherapy can be administered systemically using radioisotopes. *Contact therapy* using $^{90}$Sr isotopes for conjunctival lesions and *surface (mould) therapy* for superficial skin lesions are additional applications of brachytherapy.

### Teletherapy (External Radiation)

#### Conventional or orthovoltage equipment

Conventional or orthovoltage equipment produces x-rays of varying energies, depending on the voltage used. The higher the voltage, the greater the depth of penetration of the x-ray beam. In selecting the proper beam for treatment of a particular lesion, the percentage depth dose of the beam must be known, as well as the depth of the lesion within the body. *Percentage depth dose* is defined as the percentage of the intensity of any given beam at a given depth in tissue compared with the presumed 100% dose level. The maximum, or 100% level, occurs at varying depths depending mainly on the energy of the radiation being produced. Equipment in the range of 40–120 kV (1 kV = 1000 V) is suitable only for superficial

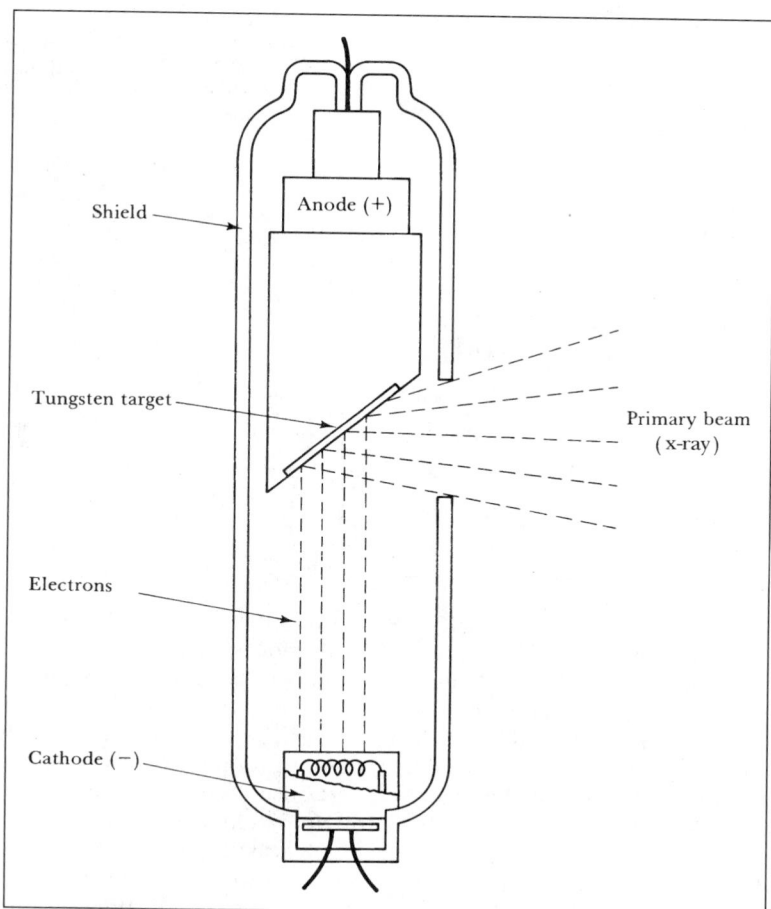

**FIGURE 13-3** Basic structure of an x-ray tube. Electrons emitted from a heated tungsten filament are accelerated across a high-voltage source. These high-speed electrons then strike a positively charged tungsten target, producing x-rays. The primary beam of radiation thus produced penetrates tissues. The greater the voltage, the greater the penetrating power of the beam.

skin lesions and those no deeper than 1 cm. Beams in the 250–400 kV range (orthovoltage) have greater penetration and have been in use for many years. There are, however, a number of disadvantages to orthovoltage beams in addition to the poor depth of penetration. The most important disadvantages are the severe skin reactions, due to the fact that most of the dose is at skin level, and bone necrosis, which can result because bone absorbs more orthovoltage radiation than does soft tissue. As a result of bone absorption, a tumor located distal to bone in the treatment field receives less than the desired dose of radiation.

## Megavoltage equipment

Megavoltage equipment, operating at 2–40 MeV (million electron volts), has distinct advantages over orthovoltage beams. The primary advantages of megavoltage therapy are (1) deeper beam penetration, (2) more ho-

mogeneous absorption of radiation (minimizing the excessive absorption by bone that occurs with orthovoltage treatment), and (3) greater skin sparing. Equipment used in megavoltage therapy includes the Van de Graaf generator, cobalt and cesium units, the betatron, and linear accelerators. Largely experimental units such as those producing heavy ions, neutron beams, and negative pi-meson particle beams will be briefly mentioned.

The Van de Graaf generator, operating at 2 million volts, was one of the forerunners in megavoltage equipment. Its use today is relegated primarily to the experimental laboratory, having been replaced in cancer therapy by more sophisticated equipment.

Cobalt-60 radiotherapy units were once the most common megavoltage equipment. The cobalt machine is easy to operate and maintain, not having the complicated electronics of linear accelerators. Because the radiation source is a radioactive isotope of cobalt, it is undergoing constant decay, at the rate of about a 10% per year de-

**TABLE 13-1** Radioactive Isotopes Used in Radiotherapy

| Isotope | Symbol | Half-Life | | Emissions | | |
|---------|--------|-----------|---|-------|------|-------|
| | | | | Alpha | Beta | Gamma |
| Cesium | $^{137}$Cs | 30 | years | | | X |
| Cobalt | $^{60}$Co | 5.3 | years | | X | X |
| Gold | $^{198}$Au | 2.69 | days | | X | X |
| Iodine | $^{131}$I | 8.0 | days | | X | X |
| Iridium | $^{192}$Ir | 74.5 | days | | X | X |
| Phosphorus | $^{32}$P | 14.3 | days | | X | |
| Radium | $^{226}$Ra | 1622 | years | X | X | X |
| Radon | $^{222}$Rn | 3.83 | days | X | X | X |
| Strontium | $^{90}$Sr | 28 | years | | X | |
| Tantalum | $^{182}$Ta | 118 | days | | X | X |
| Yttrium | $^{90}$Y | 64 | hours | | X | |

crease in output. Cobalt sources are measured in curies (Ci), and 3000–9000 Ci typically are needed in a teletherapy unit. Gamma rays are emitted as the $^{60}$Co atoms decay; with a half-life of 5.3 years, this means that the cobalt source would need to be replaced every 5–6 years to avoid lengthy treatment times. Cobalt units are also characterized by lower dose rates and a lower percentage depth dose compared with a linear accelerator of 10 MeV.

Cesium in the form of $^{137}$Cs also is used in teletherapy units, primarily those outside the United States. Because of the low specific activity of a $^{137}$Cs source, the source must be placed about 35 cm from the skin. This short source-to-skin distance (SSD) adds to surface skin dose by electron contamination, producing greater skin reactions. In comparison, $^{60}$Co usually is placed at 80 cm SSD.

Linear accelerators, although more complex in terms of operation and maintenance than cobalt units, are widely used in most hospital-based radiotherapy departments as well as in the private practice setting. Linear accelerators have distinct treatment advantages, includ-

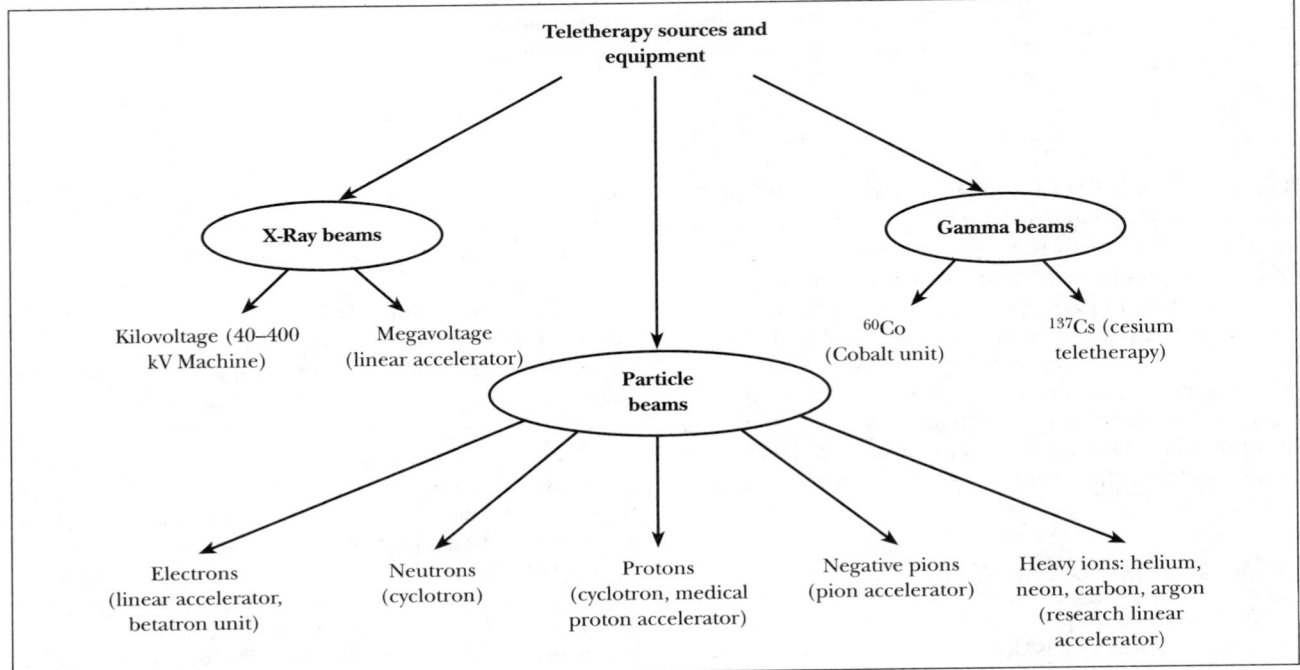

**FIGURE 13-4** Classification system for teletherapy sources and equipment.

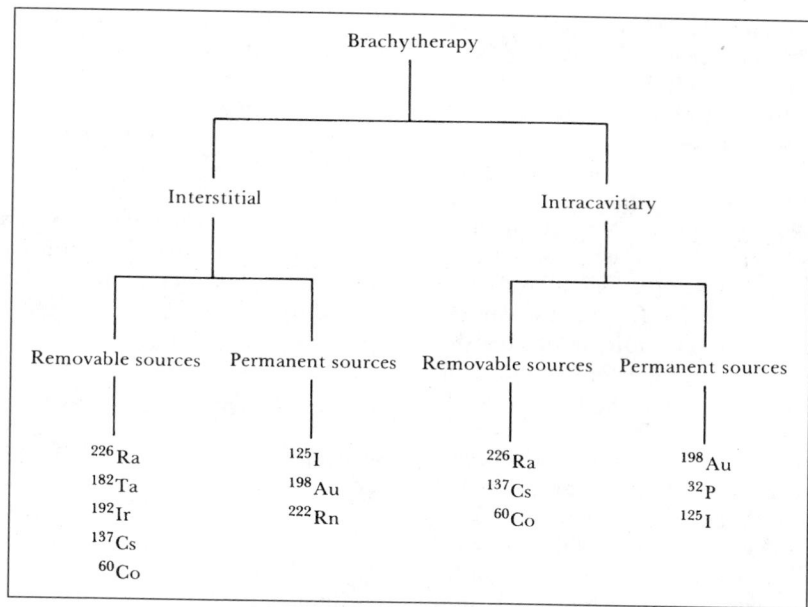

**FIGURE 13-5**   Radioactive sources used in brachytherapy.

ing the speed with which treatments can be given. Not only is this an advantage in terms of efficient use of time but, more important, it means that the person being treated spends less time in awkward, sometimes uncomfortable positions. In addition, a sharply defined field of irradiation can be obtained, thus treating only the desired tissue volume.

Linear accelerators are so named because of the method of x-ray production, which involves accelerating electrons along a radio frequency electromagnetic wave, achieving energies equivalent to those that could be obtained only in a conventional x-ray tube at excessively high voltage. Some linear accelerators are also equipped to allow use of the electron beam (particulate radiation) itself. Electron beam therapy is useful for relatively superficial lesions such as chest wall recurrence of breast cancer, skin cancer, and superficial nodes. It may be used to provide a booster dose to a limited site following treatment with megavoltage therapy. Electron particles are the equivalent of beta particles, differing only in their origin (beta particles are produced by radioactive decay) and their limited penetration into tissue. Limited penetration is a distinct advantage over x- or gamma radiation in that almost all the electron energy is expended at a particular tissue depth, thus sparing whatever structures lie beyond the tumor site.

The betatron is an electron and x-ray therapy machine that predates the development of the linear accelerator. Electrons produced from a heated tungsten filament are injected into a doughnut-shaped porcelain envelope and accelerated by a changing magnetic field. These high-velocity electrons range in energy from 10–30 MeV and are useful for deep-seated lesions. X-rays (18–40 MeV) also may be produced by the betatron when the electron beam is directed at a tungsten target.

## High LET and charged particle radiation therapy

There are two basic forms of radiation used in radiotherapy, those classified as low LET (linear energy transfer) radiation, such as x-rays, gamma rays, and electrons, and high LET radiation, such as neutron beams, heavy ions, and negative pi-mesons (pions). Basically, the difference between low and high LET radiation is in the rate of energy deposition in the tissue molecule. (See Figure 13-12.) Low LET radiation could conceivably pass through a molecule without damaging it. In contrast, the number of ionizing events produced in molecules by high LET radiation is much greater and damage is invariably produced.

High-energy radiation facilities are limited in the United States and elsewhere. Years of experimentation have shown that there are distinct advantages to this form of therapy, yet the cost of such facilities and the technological sophistication needed to operate the facilities have meant that they are usually only referral centers for carefully selected individuals with cancer.[1] High LET radiation has several advantages over low LET radiation:

1. greater relative biological effectiveness (RBE)
2. reduced relative radioresistance of hypoxic cells in tumors (low oxygen enhancement ratio (OER))
3. less intertreatment recovery of tumor cells in fractionated dosage

***Neutron beam therapy***   Fast neutrons are produced by a cyclotron, equipment in which high-energy neutrons bombard targets of either beryllium or tritium. Neutron therapy is less expensive than other high LET energy producers; however, technological problems and the low dose rate (5–6 cGy/min) are among the disadvantages to this form of therapy.

*Heavy charged particle therapy* Heavy ions, such as protons, helium, and nitrogen, are mainly useful for small tumors, because the dose distribution is best for treating a small volume. As the tumor size increases, treatment volume and OER will also increase.

Clinical trials with proton beam therapy are currently being conducted by the Proton Radiation Oncology Group, established in 1991. This cooperative group gathers data from 14 centers around the world, three of which are located in the United States. Approximately 16,000 patients were treated with protons by July 1994 in centers around the world. Current application of protons includes treatment of pituitary tumors, arteriovenous malformations, uveal melanomas, sarcomas and chondrosarcomas of the skull base and cervical spine. Recently several groups have taken advantage of the dose localization characteristics of the proton beam to treat carcinoma of the prostate, postsurgical rectal carcinoma, and paravertebral soft-tissue sarcomas. Favorable results have also been reported in proton treatment of such common tumors as lung, esophagus, digestive tract, gynecologic, and genitourinary sites.[2]

*Negative pi-meson therapy* Negative pi-mesons (pions) are small, negatively charged particles found in the nuclei of atoms that "cement" protons and neutrons together. Pions are produced when protons are accelerated at approximately 131,000 miles/sec before striking a carbon target. The pions are then collected by a system of magnets, and the beam of high LET energy is directed at the target tissue. The first application of this form of treatment for human subjects took place at the Los Alamos Meson Physics Facility in Los Alamos, New Mexico in 1974. The advantage of pion therapy, like other forms of high LET radiation, is that the beam can be shaped to fit the tumor precisely, thus minimizing the amount of radiation to surrounding normal structures. Pions can be aimed and stopped at a specific target site by adjusting the momentum of the particles.

At Los Alamos a number of tumor sites and histologies were treated with good local cure rates and minimal morbidity, particularly in cancers of the head and neck, lung, bladder, cervix, and prostate gland. Tumors of the large bowel, pancreas, or brain did not respond as well. The Los Alamos program was terminated in 1981, however, because overall results were not impressive and costs were prohibitive.

A second pion facility opened in 1979 in Vancouver, BC and a third in Villigen, Switzerland in 1980. Approximately 500 patients were treated at Villigen with a high incidence of long-term toxicities noted. The severity of late effects was attributed to the use of treatment volumes nearly three times that used by the Vancouver group. The program at Villigen was discontinued in 1993.

The Vancouver pion group completed two randomized trials in late 1995 comparing photon and pion irradiation for high-grade gliomas and advanced prostate cancers. The glioma study found no difference between the two treatment groups in overall survival, time to recurrence, toxicity, and quality of life. The prostate trial has a median follow-up of only two years, therefore outcome data are not yet definitive. Acute effects of pion therapy were increased over photon therapy; however, late toxicity was reduced in pion treatment.

Raju[2] concludes that clinical results with pions appear to be about equal to photons for all sites investigated except for the bladder. Because of the cost and complexity of building and operating pion facilities, Raju also concludes that pion radiation will not likely be pursued in the future.

## Brachytherapy (Internal Radiation)

*Brachytherapy,* the use of sealed sources of radioactive material placed within or near a tumor, is the treatment of choice for a variety of lesions. Brachytherapy frequently is combined with teletherapy and also may be used preoperatively and postoperatively.

Radioactive isotopes for brachytherapy application are contained in a variety of forms, such as wires ($^{182}$TA), ribbons or tubes ($^{192}$Ir), needles ($^{137}$Cs, $^{226}$Ra), grains or seeds ($^{198}$Au, $^{222}$Rn), and capsules ($^{137}$Cs, $^{226}$Ra). The source is selected by the radiotherapist according to the site to be treated, the size of the lesion, and whether the implant is to be temporary or permanent.[3]

Needles, wires, and ribbons (either preloaded or afterloaded) are particularly useful in treating head and neck lesions. Intra-abdominal and intrathoracic lesions can be implanted with gold or iodine seeds introduced either through hollow needles or tubes or through a "seed gun" that injects the radioactive sources into the tumor bed. Isotopes implanted in this manner usually are permanent, and radiation precautions may be needed after the individual is discharged.

Intracavitary radiotherapy most often is employed in the treatment of gynecologic lesions. A variety of techniques and types of equipment have been designed (Figure 13-6) to provide a desired dosage to the tissues around the radiation source.[4] Most gynecologic applicators are based on the "Manchester method."[5] According to this method, the radioactive source is contained in two vaginal ovoids separated by a spacer, and a central uterine tandem is added when both the corpus and cervix are to be treated. Many of these applicators are the afterloading type that can be positioned in the operating room and loaded with the radioactive source at a later time after the proper position has been checked by radiograph and the patient returned to her room. The afterloading method is most desirable because it prevents unnecessary radiation exposure for personnel.

Brachytherapy equipment and techniques have been a subject of intense interest and development in recent years. Standard applications and operative procedures as described earlier are still the most common method of treating with radioactive sources. However, the newer techniques involving high-dose rate, remote afterloading procedures, and equipment are being utilized through-

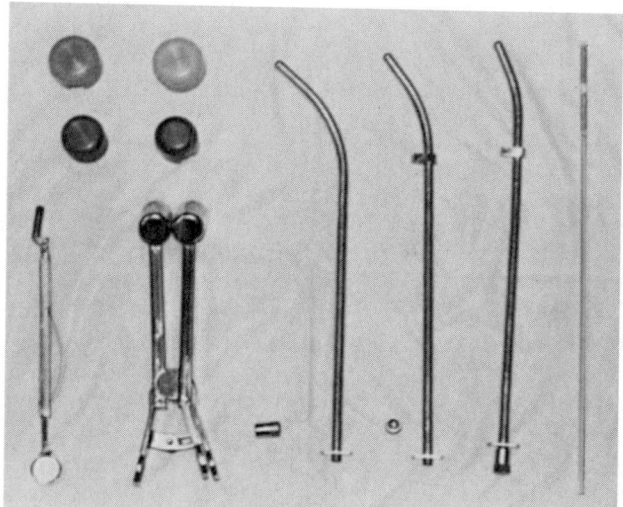

**FIGURE 13-6** Examples of gynecologic applicators. Left to right: carrier for radioactive source to be inserted in colpostat; afterloading vaginal colpostats with plastic caps used to increase the size; afterloading uterine tandems; plastic tube containing radioactive sources to be inserted into tandem.

out the world and with increasing frequency in the United States.[6]

Use of high-dose-rate (HDR) sources for brachytherapy has distinct advantages over low-dose-rate (LDR) sources in that HDR produces the same radiobiological effect in a shorter period of time. With standard brachytherapy techniques with LDR sources, the patient is hospitalized for up to 72 hours of continuous therapy. With HDR technique, 500–1000 cGy can be delivered in less than ten minutes. Number of fractions and total dose must be chosen carefully for each body site and tumor type in order to produce the desired tumor effect while minimizing the effect on both early-responding (acute effect) and late-responding (chronic effect) normal tissues.

HDR brachytherapy can be used for intralumenal (lung, esophagus, bile duct), interstitial, intracavitary, and surface lesions. Under appropriate sedation, hollow catheters are placed within or adjacent to the lesion, the catheters are connected to the delivery system, and the appropriate dose is administered by propelling the radioactive source via catheter to the target site for the prescribed length of time. If the patient should require care (i.e., suctioning) before the treatment is completed, the radioactive sources simply are returned to the storage system via the catheter until care is completed.

Major advantages of the remote afterloading HDR technique include reduced exposure of personnel, flexible techniques, shorter treatment time, and outpatient options. In addition to the specialized equipment that must be acquired in order to utilize this method of brachytherapy, computer planning systems and physics programs must be added. A multidisciplinary team (including radiation oncologists, radiation therapists, physicists, nurses, and operating room personnel) usually is involved when remote afterloading brachytherapy is implemented. The nursing role in HDR brachytherapy is significant in all phases of the procedure: pretreatment teaching and patient assessment, treatment-phase support and monitoring of patient condition, and posttreatment education and follow-up. Nursing care during HDR for endobronchial lesions is detailed by Jordan and Mantravadi.[7] An excellent patient education booklet has also been published by Jordan and Buck.[8]

## SIMULATION AND TREATMENT PLANNING

The decision to employ radiotherapy is made after consideration of a number of factors. Histological confirmation of the diagnosis and staging of the disease by appropriate clinical, surgical, and laboratory procedures are necessary before a treatment decision can be made. In addition, such factors as the patient's age and general condition, site of tumor, radio-responsiveness of the tumor, risk versus benefit, patient consent, and availability of treatment facilities must all be considered to select a plan of therapy. The radiation oncologist devises the treatment plan utilizing an array of sophisticated equipment and involving a team of personnel.

One of the first steps in planning is localizing the tumor and defining the volume to be treated. Some lesions are visible and their dimensions can be determined clinically. However, often it is necessary to employ a simulator to determine treatment volume accurately. A simulator may have several component parts (Figure 13-7). It contains a diagnostic x-ray unit for visualizing the proposed treatment site. Fluoroscopic examination also may be done. From radiographs taken on the simulator the physician can determine the field of treatment and draw in the proposed field outline on the radiograph. The radiation therapist (formerly called radiation technologist or radiographer) then duplicates these markings on the patient's skin using a marking pen to trace the field outline projected onto the patient's skin by the simulator. Treatment portals can be identified by several small tattoos placed at the corners of the field. Tattooing is a simple process in which a drop of India ink is placed on the skin and a needle is used to introduce the ink into the skin, leaving a tiny permanent black dot. This procedure, which produces only momentary discomfort, can be distressing to the patient if it is not explained carefully beforehand. For individuals receiving head and neck irradiation, where the field markings are particularly visible, tattoos may be substituted for inked lines once the reproducibility of the field has been ensured. Injection molding equipment also can be employed to form head holders of clear or mesh plastic. The holders are tailored to each patient to provide a form-fitted mold that the patient's head is repositioned within for each treatment

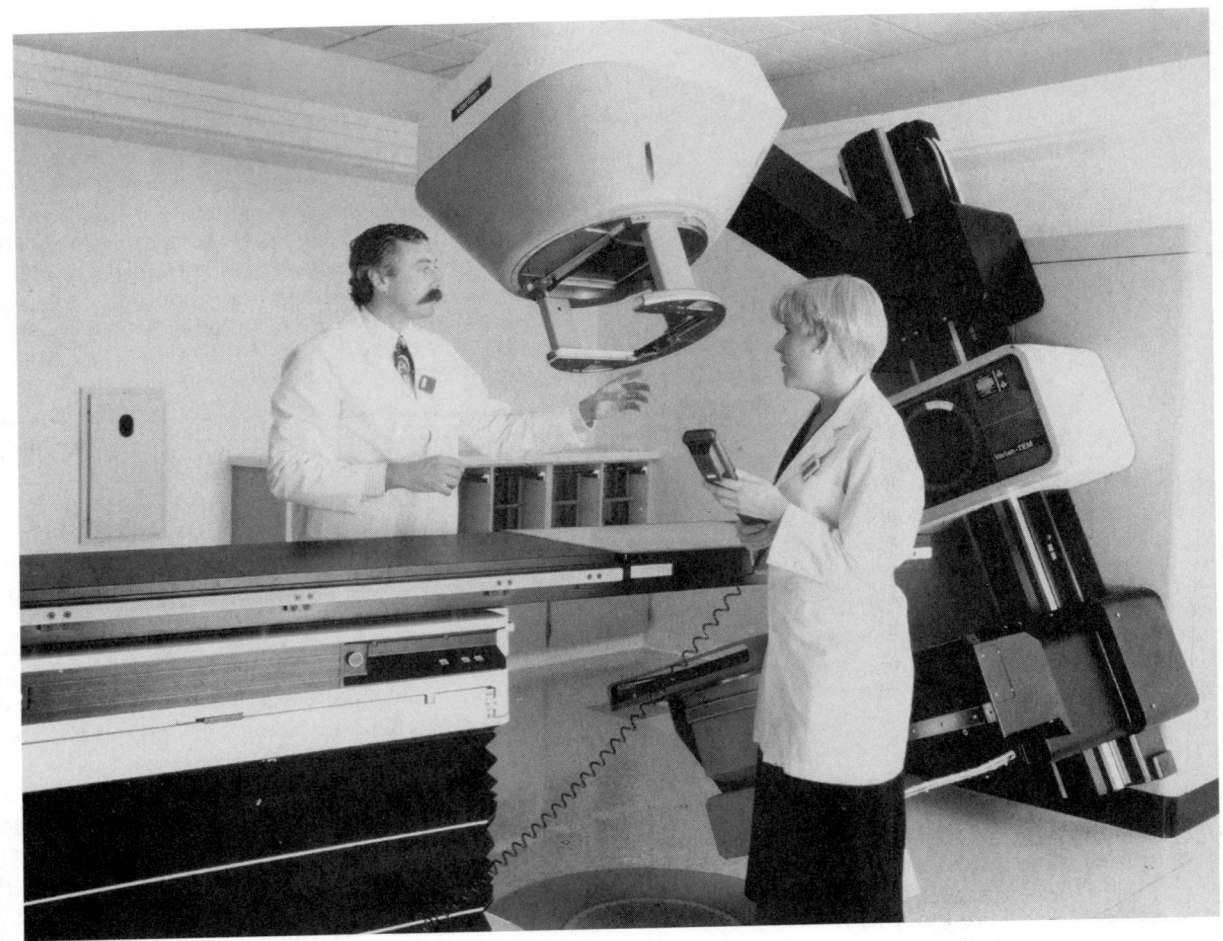

**FIGURE 13-7** A Varian Ximatron™ C-Series radiation therapy simulator. (Photo courtesy of © Varian Associates, Inc., Palo Alto, CA)

session. Field markings can be placed on these masks rather than on the skin, avoiding conspicuous facial marks. In some instances, however, tattoos are not placed until the end of the treatment course because a field may shrink or change as surface contours change and tumor volume shrinks. Tattoos are a useful means of identifying a previously treated area if a patient returns for further therapy.

Some simulators also are capable of transverse axial tomography. Tomography is a radiographic technique for showing detailed images of body structures at any given plane in the body. This technique obtains a three-dimensional view of the tumor and surrounding structures, allowing greater precision in planning and delivering treatment. Computerized tomography (CT scan) and magnetic resonance imaging (MRI) can provide the radiation oncologist with even finer detail for treatment planning.

Some simulators are also equipped with an ultrasound device that produces an image of internal structures. This technique employs ultrasound (inaudible sound with frequencies ranging from 16,000 to 10 billion cycles per second [cps]) that is reflected back as an echo from the tissues it strikes. Differences in density and elasticity of tissues and organs produce differences in the echo, which are recorded as an image of the target structures. Ultrasound is another means of defining tumor volume and relationship to nearby vital structures.

Various restraining or positioning devices may be designed at the time of simulation to aid in immobilizing the patient. Lying still in exactly the same position each day sometimes is difficult but is necessary to deliver the prescribed treatment to the prescribed volume. For children, especially, a custom-made body cast sometimes is used to ensure immobility. The adult also may be more accurately positioned by means of various headrests, armboards, handgrips, and the like.

An important part of simulation and treatment planning is shaping the field and determining what structures are to be blocked and protected from radiation. The therapy machine produces a rectangular field, which can be made larger or smaller. However, that rectangular field must then be trimmed and shaped, with portions eliminated in varying patterns to meet individual require-

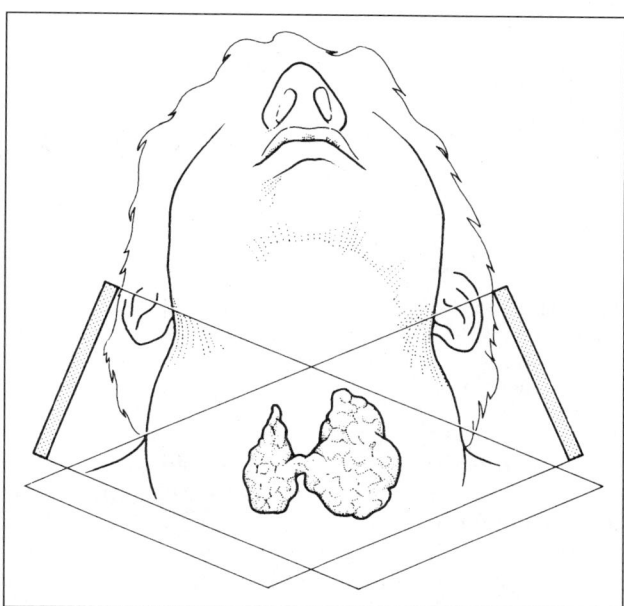

**FIGURE 13-8**   Two vertically wedged field arrangements for the treatment of thyroid carcinoma.

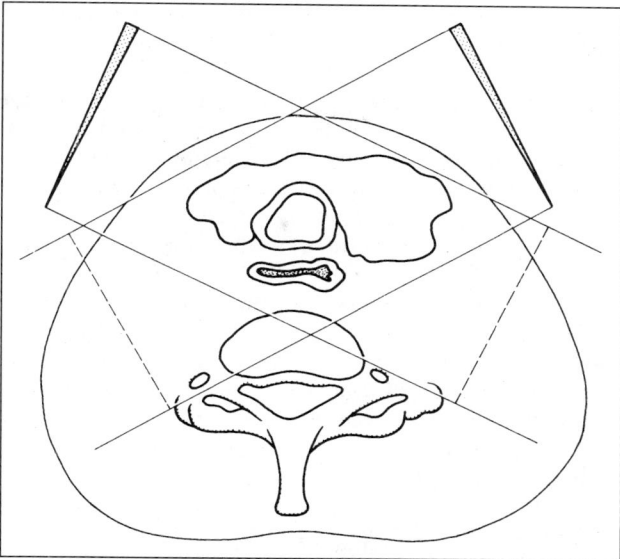

**FIGURE 13-9**   Cross section of the neck showing the zone of high-dose irradiation to a thyroid tumor; the dose to the spinal cord is low, although the skin dose is high.

ments. Blocks to protect vital body organs and tissues are secured to a plastic tray that is then placed on the head of the treatment machine between the beam and the patient. *Portal films* (sometimes called *beam films*) are radiographs taken through the treatment machine to confirm the treatment field and the placement of blocks in the desired position.

During simulation, contours of the patient's body may be obtained and then traced onto paper. Information from the tracings is fed into a computer, which then produces an isodose plot to guide the radiation oncologist and physicist in designing the best field arrangement possible. Some examples of various field arrangements for treating tumors in different locations are shown in Figures 13-8 and 13-9.

The physicist plays an important role in simulation and treatment planning. Working together, the physicist and radiation oncologist design the field arrangement, determine the dose calculations, monitor tumor response, and ensure accuracy of technical aspects. Physicists also are often involved in the maintenance and calibration of treatment machines.

For the patient with cancer, simulation and treatment planning usually are the first introduction to the equipment and methods used in a radiotherapy department. Thorough and careful explanation about the purpose of this preliminary phase of treatment is important in order to allay anxiety about the planning procedures and about the delay in getting treatment started. If the patient can be helped to understand the importance of careful planning, the steps necessary in simulation and treatment planning will be accepted or at least tolerated better.

## RADIOBIOLOGY

The biological effects of radiation on humans are the result of a sequence of events that follows the absorption of energy from ionizing radiation and the organism's attempts to compensate for this assault. Radiation effect takes place at the cellular level, with consequences in tissues, organs, and the entire body.

### Cellular Response to Radiation

Radiation effect at the cellular level may be either direct or indirect, according to the target theory.[9] *A direct hit* occurs when any of the key molecules within the cell, such as DNA or RNA, are damaged. After high-dose radiation of DNA molecules in vitro, the types of damage observed are (1) change or loss of a base (thymine, adenine, guanine, or cytosine), (2) breakage of the hydrogen bond between the two chains of the DNA molecule, (3) breaks in one or both chains of the DNA molecule, and (4) cross-linking of the chains after breakage. Such unrepaired breaks or alterations in the base lead to mutations resulting in impaired cellular function or cell death.

An *indirect hit*, according to target theory, occurs when ionization takes place in the medium (mostly water) surrounding the molecular structures within the cell. Radiation absorbed by the water molecules results in the formation of a free radical when an electron is literally knocked out of orbit surrounding the ion. These free radicals may trigger a variety of chemical reactions, producing new compounds that are toxic to the cell. Figure 13-10 illustrates the ionizing effect of radiation on the water contained within a cell.

It generally is agreed that a direct hit (i.e., DNA damage and chromosomal aberrations) accounts for the most effective and lethal injury produced by ionizing radiation.[9,10] However, because of the relative proportion of water to DNA in a single cell, the probability of indirect damage through ionization of intracellular water is much greater.

In addition to the damage produced by a direct or indirect hit, experimental evidence shows that radiation can cause damage to proteins, carbohydrates, and enzymes within the cell. Damage to these additional molecules, as well as alterations in the permeability of the cell membrane, may all contribute to the ultimate effect of radiation at the cellular level.

## Cell cycle and radiosensitivity

According to Hall and Cox,[11] radiosensitivity appears to be maximum during the M and $G_2$ phases of the cell cycle (Figure 13-11). Thus the maximum effect from radiation should occur just before and during actual cell division. In early research, Bergonie and Tribondeau[12]

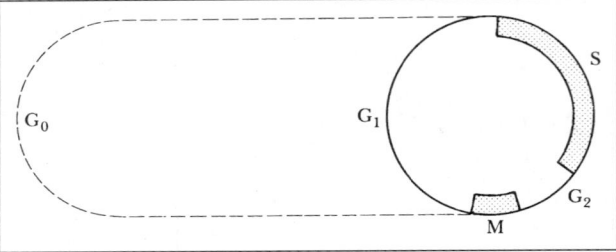

**FIGURE 13-11** Stages in cell replication cycle: $S$ = DNA synthesis; $G_2$ = the gap between DNA synthesis and mitosis; $M$ = mitosis; $G_1$ = the gap between the end of mitosis and the start of DNA synthesis.

formulated a law stating that the sensitivity of cells to irradiation is in direct proportion to their reproductive activity and inversely proportional to their degree of differentiation. A differentiated cell is one that is morphologically or functionally specialized (such as the erythrocyte) and does not undergo mitosis. An undifferentiated cell (such as the red blood cell stem cell or erythroblast) has few specialized morphological or functional characteristics, and its primary purpose is to divide and provide new cells to maintain its own population. Because the effect of radiation is known to be greatest during mitosis, undifferentiated cell populations generally are most sensitive to radiation. In contrast, well-differentiated cells are relatively radioresistant.

Changes in mitotic activity due to radiation can be classified as either *delayed onset* or *complete inhibition*. *Delayed onset* of mitosis indicates that although damage occurred at some point during prophase, repair was accomplished and division occurred. *Complete inhibition* of mitosis, or cell sterilization, renders the cell incapable of division, although it may continue to live in a nonreproducing state.

## Cell death

There are three types of cell death: mitotic (or genetic) death, interphase death, and instant death. *Mitotic death* occurs after one or more divisions and usually with much smaller radiation doses than those required to produce interphase death. *Interphase death* occurs many hours after irradiation and before the cell begins the mitotic process. *Instant death* occurs following extremely high doses of radiation and would take place only in the experimental laboratory or in the event of a nuclear accident.

## Contributory biological factors

A number of additional factors directly affect the biological response to radiation and ultimately the treatment outcome. Among these are the oxygen effect, linear energy transfer, relative biological effectiveness, dose rate, radiosensitivity, and fractionation.

***Oxygen effect*** Well-oxygenated tumors show a much greater response to radiation, that is, they are more radio-

---

The final products of the ionization of water molecules (HOH) by radiation are an ion pair (H$^+$, OH$^-$) and free radicals (H$^\cdot$, OH$^\cdot$), which are capable of damaging the cell. The ionization of water is shown in the following steps:

$$HOH \xrightarrow{\text{radiation}} HOH^+ + e^-$$

The free electron (e$^-$) is then captured by another available water molecule and, as shown in the next step, forms the second ion:

$$HOH + e^- \rightarrow HOH^-$$

Because the two ions (HOH$^+$, HOH$^-$) produced by these reactions are unstable, rapid breakdown occurs (in the presence of other, normal water molecules), forming yet another ion and a free radical as follows:

$$HOH^+ \rightarrow H^+ + OH^\cdot$$
$$HOH^- \rightarrow OH^- + H^\cdot$$

Although the resulting pair of ions (H$^+$, OH$^-$) have some potential for cellular damage through chemical reactions, they are more likely to recombine and form water (HOH). The free radicals (H$^\cdot$, OH$^\cdot$) are extremely reactive, and they too may simply recombine to form water. However, free radicals appear to be more likely to undergo chemical interactions with other free radicals, forming cytotoxic agents, as shown in this reaction:

$$OH^\cdot + OH^\cdot \rightarrow H_2O_2 \text{ (hydrogen peroxide)}$$

Free radicals that result from the interaction of radiation with water are capable of triggering a variety of chemical reactions within the cell and are therefore believed to be a major factor in the production of damage in the cell.

**FIGURE 13-10** The effect of ionizing radiation on water molecules.

sensitive than poorly oxygenated tumors. Extensive laboratory and clinical research[9,13] has shown that the existence of oxygen tension between 20–40 mm Hg at time of radiation greatly enhances the radiosensitivity of the cells. Theoretically, the mechanism of the oxygen effect is related to the ability of oxygen to combine with the free radicals formed during ionization, producing new and toxic combinations. A second theory holds that the presence of oxygen at time of irradiation prevents the reversal (and thus the repair) of some of the chemical changes that occur as the result of ionization. The clinical significance of the oxygen effect is that oxygen modifies the dose of radiation needed to produce a given degree of biological damage. The magnitude of the oxygen effect is expressed as the oxygen enhancement ratio (OER). The OER is the ratio of radiation dose in the absence of oxygen (or hypoxia) to the radiation dose in the presence of oxygen required for the same biological effect.

***Linear energy transfer***   Linear energy transfer (LET) describes the rate at which energy is lost from different types of radiation while traveling through matter. Its usefulness is seen in designating the quality of radiation emitted from various radiations, such as x-rays, neutrons, and alpha particles. Low-LET radiations (x- and gamma rays) are sparsely ionizing, having a random pathway that results in few direct hits within the cell nucleus. Radiation of higher LET (alpha particles, neutrons, and negative pi-mesons) has a greater probability of interacting with matter and producing more direct hits within the cell (Figure 13-12).[10]

***Relative biological effectiveness***   Because different radiations have varying rates of energy loss, the biological response likewise will be different. Therefore, the term relative biological effectiveness (RBE) is used to compare a dose of test radiation with a dose of standard radiation that produces the same biological response. The following formula is used to express RBE:

$$RBE = \frac{\textit{Dose of reference radiation to produce a given biological effect}}{\textit{Dose of test radiation to produce the same biological effect}}$$

***Dose rate***   Dose rate refers to the rate at which a given dose is delivered by a treatment machine or equipment. Studies have shown low dose rates to be much less effective in producing lethal cell damage than high dose rates, primarily because low dose rates permit cell repair to occur before the lethal dose has been reached.

***Radiosensitivity***   According to Bergonie and Tribondeau's law, ionizing radiation is most effective on cells that are undifferentiated and undergoing active mitosis.[12] Laboratory and clinical experience has shown this to be true in most tissues.

***Fractionation***   Fractionation, or the dividing of a total dose of radiation into a number of equal fractions, is based on four important factors: repair, redistribution, repopulation, and reoxygenation,[9,10,14] commonly referred to as the four Rs of radiobiology.[15]

*Repair*   Repair of intracellular sublethal damage by normal cells between daily dose fractions is one benefit of fractionation. The goal of fractionation is to deliver a dose sufficient to prevent tumor cells from being repaired while allowing normal cells to recover before the next dose is given. Although some tumor cells may be repaired between daily doses, they may also reoxygenate, rendering them more radiosensitive when the next dose is given. Thus although some degree of repair of tumor cells is possible between fractionated doses, repeated daily doses ultimately would lead to tumor control.

*Redistribution*   Redistribution of cell age (within the cell cycle) as a result of daily radiation is advantageous because more tumor cells are made radiosensitive. Theoretically, with succeeding daily doses of radiation, more and more tumor cells would be delayed in cycle and reach the mitotic phase as the next dose is given, thus increasing the cell kill. Certain chemotherapeutic agents, such as methotrexate and hydroxyurea, are being used in combination with radiation to take advantage of this synchronization in the cell cycle.

*Repopulation*   Repopulation of normal tissues takes place through cell division at some time during a multifraction treatment course. Fractionation of dose allows this repopulation in normal tissues, sparing them from some of the late consequences that might occur if repopulation (new growth) was inhibited. On the other hand, those tumor cells that do succeed in dividing while undergoing a fractionated course of radiotherapy usually are incapable of surviving because of the radiation effect.

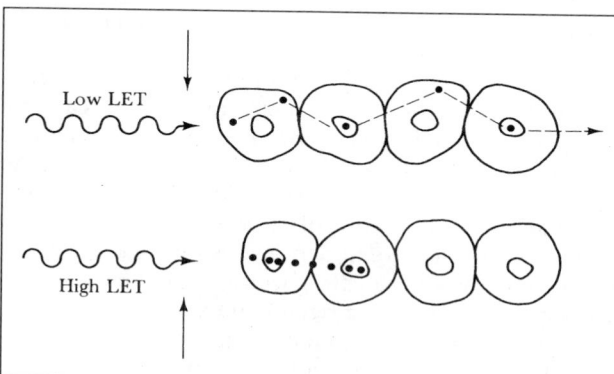

**FIGURE 13-12**   Comparison of the effects of low- and high-LET radiations on a population of cells. Notice the irregular path of the low-LET radiation, interacting with four cells, compared with the relatively straight path of the high-LET radiation, which is interacting with only two cells. However, the low-LET radiation produces only *one* hit in two nuclei, whereas the high-LET radiation produces *two* hits in two nuclei. (Travis EL: *Primer of Medical Radiobiology.* Chicago, Year Book Medical Publishers, 1975, p 71. © 1975 Year Book Medical Publishers. Reproduced with permission.)

Thus fractionation favors normal tissue while still eradicating tumor.

*Reoxygenation* Reoxygenation is the fourth consideration favoring fractionation of the radiation dose. Whereas normal tissues usually are well oxygenated, tumors characteristically range from normal to hypoxic to anoxic. As discussed earlier, radiosensitivity is closely related to oxygen tension in the tumor cell; hypoxic or anoxic cells generally are radioresistant, whereas oxygenated cells are radiosensitive. Fractionating the dose allows time between treatments for the tumor to reoxygenate.

Tissue and organ response to radiation is based on the sensitivity of cellular components. It is important to note that tissues and organs are composed of more than one cell category, each cell category having different degrees of radiosensitivity. A second factor in determining tissue response is related to the parenchymal versus stromal substance found in that tissue. The parenchyma is composed of cells characteristic of the tissue or organ, and if those cells are radiosensitive (e.g., the testis), ionizing radiation has its greatest impact on the parenchyma. However, if parenchymal tissue is relatively radioresistant (e.g., the spinal cord), radiation response in that organ is due to the indirect effects on the stromal components (especially the vasculature) that support the parenchyma. Table 13-2 lists various organs according to their degree of radiosensitivity as measured by parenchymal hypoplasia.

# CHEMICAL AND THERMAL MODIFIERS OF RADIATION

## Radiosensitizers and Radioprotectors

The goal of radiotherapy is to achieve maximum tumor cell kill while minimizing injury to normal tissues (therapeutic ratio). Efforts to improve the therapeutic ratio have resulted in the development of certain compounds that act to increase the radiosensitivity of tumor cells or to protect normal cells from radiation effect. Combined modality therapy with both radiation and certain cytotoxic agents also takes advantage of enhanced tumor cell kill. Drugs such as doxorubicin, actinomycin-D, cyclophosphamide, bleomycin, and cisplatin often are used along with radiation to achieve greater cell kill than either therapy could achieve if used independently. When used alone, chemical modifiers of radiation therapy (radiosensitizers), however, are not generally cytotoxic like the chemotherapeutic agents.

Phillips[16] proposed several definitions useful in describing the various interactions of radiation with other agents. *Enhancement* or *potentiation* describes any radiation effect that is greater in the presence of the chemical than in its absence. If the effect is less than that caused by the most active agent in the combination, then this is known as *interference*. *Antagonism* is the term used to describe an

**TABLE 13-2** Degree of Radiosensitivity of Various Organs Based on Parenchymal Hypoplasia

| Organ | Radiosensitivity |
|---|---|
| Lymphoid organs, bone marrow, blood, testes, ovaries, intestines | High |
| Skin, cornea, oral cavity, esophagus, rectum, bladder, vagina, cervix, ureters | Fairly high |
| Optic lens, stomach, growing cartilage, fine vasculature, growing bone | Medium |
| Mature cartilage or bone, salivary glands, respiratory organs, kidneys, liver, pancreas, thyroid, adrenals, pituitary gland | Fairly low |
| Muscle, brain, spinal cord | Low |

outcome less than that of the least effective agent in a given combination. In clinical radiotherapy, enhancement by noncytotoxic sensitizers is called *radiosensitization*. Antagonism by protective compounds is called *radioprotection*.

*Radiosensitizers* are compounds that apparently promote fixation of the free radicals produced by radiation damage at the molecular level. The mechanism of this action is similar to the oxygen effect described earlier, in which biochemical reactions in the damaged molecules prevent repair of the cellular radiation damage. Free radicals (such as $OH^\bullet$) are captured by the electron-affinic radiosensitizers, rendering the molecules incapable of repair.

The two most biologically active radiosensitizing compounds first tested in phase II and III studies were metronidazole (Flagyl) and misonidazole (RO-07-0582). Major side effects are neurotoxicity, including peripheral neuropathies, somnolence, confusion, and transient coma. Nausea and vomiting are also frequent side effects that seem to be dose-related.

Early clinical trials using misonidazole as a radiosensitizer indicated some degree of effectiveness in treatment of squamous carcinoma of the head and neck and of the uterine cervix. Overall results were disappointing, however, due to severe toxicity and only marginal improvement in tumor control.[17] Misonidazole is the only such substance to have undergone extensive clinical trial evaluation. Misonidazole has been shown to increase the cytotoxicity of alkylating agents, nitrosoureas, 5-fluorouracil (5-FU), cyclophosphamide, and melphalan. However, the side effects commonly experienced with these agents also are apparently enhanced by the addition of misonidazole. This nonselective enhancement significantly detracts from the potential benefits to be gained.

The compound SR-2508 (etanidazole) has been tested with encouraging results in phase II and III trials.[18] This member of the nitroimidazole group of compounds appears to be less toxic to the CNS tissue than misonidazole, and has also been shown to cross the blood-brain barrier in limited quantity.

Early studies[19] with nitroimidazoles used in vitro showed that these radiosensitizers are also capable of cytotoxic activity in hypoxic cells after periods of long exposure. The high doses required to achieve actual cell kill in vitro have, however, prohibited their use in vivo for this purpose.

The established basis for use of chemical radiosensitizers is based on extensive laboratory research.[20] However, clinical trials thus far have failed to establish the overall efficacy of radiosensitizers as adjuncts to radiation therapy in the clinical setting.

*Radioprotectors* are compounds that can protect oxygenated (nontumor) cells while having a limited effect on hypoxic (tumor) cells. This selective action serves to increase the therapeutic ratio by promoting the repair of irradiated normal tissues. Repair or return to a non-damaged state takes place through the chemical process of reduction. Free electrons are captured by the radioprotective substance and thus are unavailable to participate in further chemical reactions that lead to cellular damage. This process can be viewed as the opposite of what occurs when radiosensitizers are used.

The sulfhydryl groups contained in the nonprotein fraction of most cells aid in the reduction process following radiation damage. Thiophosphate compounds (such as cysteine and cysteamine) containing sulfhydryl and aminopropyl groups were among the earliest radioprotectors synthesized. The compound that appears to be most useful at present is designated WR-2721.[21]

The study of radiosensitizers and radioprotectors has extended to phase II and III clinical trials in the continued effort to achieve better results in cancer treatment with radiotherapy. With combined therapy, toxicity can be increased and patient comfort may be compromised. Some nursing responsibilities in the use of radiosensitizers and radioprotectors would include:

1. providing patient and family education
2. participating in obtaining informed consent
3. administering investigational agents
4. timing and coordinating drug administration with radiotherapy treatment
5. observing and documenting expected and previously unreported effects and side effects
6. managing side effects, including developing interventions for those newly observed

A thorough discussion of the nursing implications for patients receiving chemical modifiers of radiation can be found in Noll.[22]

## Combined Modality Therapy

Treatment of cancer with any single modality (surgery, chemotherapy, or radiation) does not always produce the desired effect of tumor eradication. Chemotherapy and radiation therapy produce dose-limiting side effects that govern the extent of single modality treatment. In order to increase or improve the therapeutic index (ratio of tumor control versus normal tissue damage), various combinations of chemotherapy and radiation have been studied.

Ideally, a chemotherapeutic agent (or combination of agents) will shrink a tumor when given *prior* to local radiation (neoadjuvant chemotherapy); enhance or increase radiation cell kill when given *during* radiation (concomitant therapy); or control micrometastases and subclinical disease *after* a course of radiation (adjuvant therapy). Radiation and chemotherapy sometimes are given on a planned, alternating schedule using the so-called *sandwich technique*. This approach utilizes a split course of radiation in which the patient is treated with chemotherapy during a planned break in the total course of radiation therapy.[23]

Combined modality therapy is being used in the treatment of a variety of cancer types, including squamous cell cancer of the cervix, anus, head and neck, and lung. Cancers of the bladder, esophagus, pancreas, and stomach frequently are treated with both modalities in varying schedules. Vigorous combined modality therapy has allowed organ preservation for some individuals with carcinoma of the larynx, bladder, or anus.[23,24]

Some of the chemotherapeutic agents in common use for their radiosensitizing effect include cisplatin, methotrexate, doxorubicin, vinblastin, VP-16, mitomycin C, 5-fluorouracil, actinomycin D, and bleomycin. As would be expected, combined-modality therapy has the potential for enhanced side effects as well as enhanced tumor effect. Organ systems at greatest risk for toxicity are the gastrointestinal, integumentary, and myeloproliferative systems.

Nursing implications for care of the patient receiving combined-modality therapy are based on the individual's treatment plan and an understanding of the principles of combined therapies. Enhanced side effects of both radiation and chemotherapy are common. Awareness of the drugs and radiation site and dose are essential elements in anticipating toxicities, monitoring acuity, and implementing appropriate care. Hirshfield-Bartek[25] and Held and Volpe[23] developed detailed nursing guidelines for assessment and management of the patient receiving combined-modality therapy.

## Hyperthermia

The use of hyperthermia to achieve a synergistic effect with radiotherapy has been studied and applied in clinical situations with considerable enthusiasm. Although it is technically arguable whether hyperthermia actually sensitizes tumor cells to radiation effect or simply combines to produce a greater effect than either modality can achieve on its own, it is generally agreed that this combined technique is warranted and research continues.[26–29]

The biological basis for combining hyperthermia with radiation involves several factors. Heat is cytotoxic to cancer cells but is also destructive to healthy tissue if applied in excess of tolerable ranges. Controlled hyperthermia combined with radiation achieves tumor cell kill without excess toxicity.

Tumor cells are *least* radiosensitive during S phase. Hyperthermia is most effective during S phase; therefore, the combined effect of radiation and hyperthermia on a tumor produces greater cell kill than either does alone. Similarly, hypoxic cells, which are generally radioresistant, have been found to be quite thermosensitive. Heat is also known to inhibit the repair of radiation damage, thus increasing the therapeutic ratio.

Valdagni et al[30] reviewed the important parameters that may influence tumor response to combined hyperthermia and radiation therapy. Pretreatment parameters include tumor size, histological findings, and disease site. Treatment parameters include total dose of radiation and dose per fraction, thermal dose, total and weekly number of hyperthermia sessions, and, finally, the sequencing of hyperthermia and radiation.

Hyperthermia is achieved in various ways, including immersion of the local area in a heated bath, ultrasound, microwaves, interstitial implants, and perfusion techniques. The choice of technique depends on whether local, regional, or whole-body hyperthermia is desired.[31-36]

Side effects of combined hyperthermia and radiation include local skin reaction, pain, fever, gastrointestinal effects, and cardiac arrhythmias. Late effects, such as necrosis and ulceration, can occur but do not seem to be significant enough to preclude continued use of this combined modality. Wojtas[37] details the nursing care of patients receiving hyperthermia treatments as well as the role nurses might take in administering the actual treatment. Table 13-3 provides an overview of the nursing care.

**TABLE 13-3** Potential Nursing Responsibilities in Hyperthermia Treatment

---

**Pretreatment evaluation phase**
1. Assess suitability for treatment.
2. Assess ability to tolerate treatment.
3. Assess cardiac and neurological status.
4. Assess for presence of metal objects.
5. Provide thorough patient and family education.

**Treatment phase**
1. Vital signs, gastrointestinal preparation, sedation.
2. Assist during surgical placement of thermometry probes.
3. Position for comfort and access to applicator probes.
4. Monitor patient throughout treatment.
5. Provide physical and emotional support.

**Posttreatment phase**
1. Clean and dress cannula sites.
2. Observe and document thermal changes at treatment site.
3. Provide discharge instructions.
4. Manage subsequent local reactions.

---

## TISSUE AND ORGAN RESPONSE TO RADIATION

When discussing the effect of radiation on tissues, one must consider both the acute (or immediate) effects, seen within the first six months following treatment, and the late effects, seen after six months. In general, acute effects are due to cell damage in which mitotic activity is altered in some way. If early effects are not reversible, late or permanent tissue changes occur. These late effects can be attributed to the organism's attempt to heal or repair the damage inflicted by ionizing radiation.

The unit of radiation dose is called a *gray* (Gy). This term was officially adopted in 1985, replacing the term *rad* (an acronym for *r*adiation *a*bsorbed *d*ose). One Gy equals 100 rad. One cGy equals 1 rad.

In the following sections, radiation changes in normal tissues are presented according to body systems. It is important to remember that treatment volume, *dose rate* (number of cGy in a given unit of time), and *dose-time* factor (total number of cGy in a total number of days), as well as beam quality, may alter the tissue reaction. Except for those systemic effects described, radiation response is seen only in the tissues and organs that are within or immediately adjacent to the treatment field. Thus, an individual being treated to an abdominal field will not lose scalp hair from radiation, nor will the patient being treated to the mediastinum develop radiation-induced diarrhea. Similarly, those patients undergoing brachytherapy will develop site-specific reactions to treatment, which vary with the site, dose, volume, and energy of the source. For example, cesium needle implants to the tongue will produce intraoral mucositis but usually no skin reaction. Application of a radioactive source intravaginally produces vaginal mucositis and often results in diarrhea due to the effect of radiation on the adjacent intestinal and rectal mucosa. The important point to remember is that side effects from radiation are specific, and therefore preparation, teaching, and care must be planned specifically for each individual.

### Integumentary System

The outer layer of skin (epidermis) is composed of several layers of cells, with mature, nondividing cells at the surface and immature, dividing cells at the base. Normal mature cells constantly are being shed from the skin surface and replaced by new cells from the basal layer. This continual state of reproductive activity accounts for the high radiosensitivity of skin. Although the skin may be the primary site of radiation (as in skin cancer), it is also irradiated when any other site within the body is treated because radiation must pass through whatever tissues it encounters before reaching the target site. Depending on the equipment used and the beam quality, skin of the exit portal also may be affected. Erythema may be the only manifestation, or the skin reaction may progress to dry and then moist desquamation. Healing may be slow, but is usually complete and leaves minimal evidence of the acute damage except for changes in pigmentation. Fibrosis and atrophy may occur after high doses, as may ulceration, necrosis, and skin cancer. Such changes are uncommon with modern equipment and techniques. It is important to note that skin in certain areas, such as the groin, gluteal fold, axilla, and under the breasts, usually exhibits a greater and often earlier reaction to radiation due to the natural warmth and moistness in these areas and to friction caused by apposition of skin surfaces.

Use of the term *burn* or *radiation burn* to describe skin reactions is no longer appropriate. The severe skin reactions of the past are uncommon because of the skin-sparing effect of modern equipment. Burn implies accidental or unexpected damage, neither of which should take place in a controlled therapeutic setting. There are specific instances in which the patient will experience a severe reaction, especially when receiving electron beam therapy in the range of 5500–6000 cGy.

Skin reactions of this nature progress from a brisk erythema to a florid state, followed by a moist desquamation and loss of the epidermis. This, however, is an *expected* reaction because of the particular beam quality (see the earlier section entitled "Equipment, Beams, and Materials Used in Radiotherapy"), and despite the severity of the acute reaction, the involved skin usually heals well.

Hair follicles and glands (sweat and sebaceous) are also radiosensitive. The radiosensitivity of the hair follicle is due to the relatively high rate of growth (mitotic activity) taking place; thus, these follicles are more susceptible to radiation damage. Under normal circumstances, hair grows and new hair is formed at a rate that keeps pace with the regular loss or shedding of the mature hair, with the net result being no obvious change in the amount of hair on the head. However, when the scalp is irradiated, the resulting inhibition of growth of new hair coupled with the accelerated hair loss due to damage to the follicle produces a net loss of hair, or *alopecia*. Epilation occurs in doses as low as a single dose of 500 cGy but is usually temporary. Regrowth may not begin for several months following the end of treatment, and the new hair may have a different quality or color. Higher doses (4500 cGy or greater) may produce permanent alopecia or delay regrowth for a year or more. Sebaceous and sweat glands usually will experience a decrease in activity during treatment and may cease functioning altogether at high doses (over 6000–7000 cGy). Return of function is proportional to the dose received.

## Hematopoietic System

Red bone marrow is responsible for producing mature functional cells for the circulating blood. The stem cells are highly radiosensitive, and when large areas of red bone marrow (in the adult) are irradiated, including ilia, vertebrae, ribs, metaphyses of the long bones, skull, and sternum, the number of circulating mature cells decreases because production is suppressed. More erythroblasts (red blood cell precursors) are damaged by moderate doses than myeloblasts, but they recover rapidly, and thus anemia is not a prominent or early feature. Myeloblasts (white blood cell precursors) are suppressed at the same rate as erythroblasts, but the rate of recovery is much slower. Megakaryocytes (platelet precursors) are affected one to two weeks after exposure and take the longest time to recover (two to six weeks).

Mature, nondividing blood cells in the circulating blood have a limited life span and are relatively insensitive to radiation. Peripheral blood does, however, reflect marrow activity. Thus, the patient receiving radiotherapy may have depressed blood counts if sufficient radiation was given to active red bone marrow, especially if prior or concomitant chemotherapy has been given. The usual pattern seen in individuals whose marrow has been affected is a decrease first in lymphocytes, then in neutrophils, and then in platelets and red blood cells. It sometimes is necessary to interrupt a course of radiotherapy for varying periods to allow the bone marrow to recover.

Radiation to the spleen alters its physiological functions of hemolysis, red blood cell and iron storage, and antibody production, as well as causing shrinkage of the spleen itself. Lymph nodes, like the spleen, are highly radiosensitive, whereas lymphatic vessels appear to be relatively radioresistant. Interference with lymphatic vessel function is thought to be caused by fibrotic changes and obstruction.

## Gastrointestinal System

The gastrointestinal tract, from mouth to rectum, is lined with mucous membrane that contains layers of cells. A large proportion of these cells are undifferentiated and highly mitotic and are thus extremely radiosensitive. In addition, glandular tissue, ranging from large distinct bodies such as the parotids to multiple small mucous glands, is embedded in much of the mucous membrane of the intestinal tract. The effect of radiation on glandular tissue can be summarized as follows:

1. Initial swelling and edema of the epithelial lining of the ducts results in partial obstruction.
2. Secretion is inhibited by damage to the acini.
3. Atrophy and fibrosis occur as healing takes place, with permanent reduction in secretion, the amount depending on the dose received and the volume of mucous tissue irradiated.

Oral mucous membrane may develop a confluent mucositis, especially on the soft palate and the floor of the mouth, during the third and fourth weeks of therapy at the usual dose rate. Salivary function is altered as damage to the serous and mucous acini occurs, and saliva becomes viscous after moderate doses. Higher doses of radiation lead to atrophy of the salivary glands, with greatly diminished saliva and increased acidity. Such changes in saliva production and acidity often are permanent and are a factor in the development of radiation caries and infection. Alterations in the sense of taste occur early in treatment but are rarely permanent, depending on the dose of radiation received.

The esophagus and stomach also develop dose-dependent reactions. Changes in the glandular tissues of the stomach brought about by radiation are even more complex than those that occur in the glands of the oral mucous membranes. Gastric secretions, in addition to mucus, include pepsin and hydrochloric acid. If 1600 cGy are delivered in approximately ten days to the stomach, all three secretions will be reduced; this may be accompanied by nausea, dyspepsia, and pyloric spasm. Inflammation of the mucosa (esophagitis and gastritis) occurs with moderate to high doses and produces dysphagia, anorexia, and sometimes nausea and vomiting. Late changes may include atrophy, ulcerations, and fibrosis.

The most sensitive area of the entire gastrointestinal tract is thought to be the small intestine. When one considers the length of the small intestine and also the fact that its loops overlap and fill a large portion of the abdomen, even a small radiation field of 5–8 cm on the abdomen will contain a large surface area of intestinal mucosa. Crypt cells (rapidly dividing, undifferentiated stem cells) arise from the base of the villi on a continuous basis to replace mature cells of the villi that are lost as part of the normal sloughing process. The high degree of radiosensitivity of these crypt cells and resultant changes in the intestinal villi account for the sometimes severe reactions that occur when abdominal or pelvic radiation is given.

Radiation reaction in the small intestine is characterized by shortening of the villi and loss of absorptive surface. Temporary reactions usually can be tolerated with minimal nutritional consequences. However, if reactions are prolonged and severe, as in some individuals receiving 5000–6000 cGy to the abdomen or pelvis, the nutritional consequences can be major. Shortening of the villi and denuding of the intestinal mucosa prevent adequate absorption of the end products of digestion, namely, amino acids (protein), simple sugars (carbohydrates), and glycerol and fatty acids (fats). Late changes following high doses of radiation include fibrosis, ulcerations, necrosis, and hemorrhage. Intestinal obstruction, although not common, can occur in a patient receiving abdominal or pelvic irradiation. This is more likely to happen postoperatively, when the trauma of surgical manipulation combined with the effects of radiation can result in paralytic ileus.

Such a reaction depends on many factors, including total dose, fractionation, volume, and site. Most individuals receiving pelvic irradiation experience only some degree of anorexia, nausea, diarrhea, or cramping, which can be managed readily with appropriate medication and diet.

The effect of radiation on the colon and rectum is similar to that seen in the small intestine, with the addition of the distressing symptom of tenesmus, which sometimes occurs when the anal sphincter is irradiated.

## Liver

The liver is considered an accessory digestive organ and has been shown to be moderately radiosensitive. Although the parenchymal cells do have a regenerative capacity and are therefore vulnerable, the greatest damage produced by radiation to the liver is due to vascular injury. Early changes may be detectable only by liver function tests. However, radiation hepatitis is a possible consequence of doses over 2500 cGy, and the severity will depend on the volume irradiated.

## Respiratory System

Mucous membrane lines the pharynx, trachea, and bronchi, and reactions that occur are due to the response of that sensitive tissue to irradiation. Hoarseness due to laryngeal mucous membrane congestion sometimes occurs. More significant in terms of radiation is the response of the bronchial tree and alveoli. Radiation pneumonitis, usually a transient response to moderate doses, is the result of changes in the alveolar wall plus the accumulation of exudate in the air sac, similar to pneumonia. Late changes are manifested by fibrosis in the lung tissue itself plus some thickening of the pleura. Such changes will compromise respiratory function in the area treated, but the degree of disability is related to the amount and condition of remaining untreated lung tissue.

## Reproductive System

The cervix and uterine body are quite radioresistant and usually present no problem for the patient being irradiated. However, vaginal mucous membrane responds to radiation much the same as the oral mucous membrane, with mucositis and inflammation. Following brachytherapy, vaginal stenosis due to permanent fibrotic changes is a potential problem. Radiation to the ovaries produces either temporary or permanent sterility, depending on the age of the individual being treated and the dose of radiation. Permanent sterilization will occur at doses of 600–1200 cGy, and older women are sterilized at lower doses than younger women.

Maturation of graafian follicles and release of ova are essential for fertility. Radiation is most damaging to the intermediate follicle, thus preventing its development into a mature form. Small follicles are most radioresistant, and fertility may return if these small follicles are able to undergo repair and release ova. Mature graafian follicles are only moderately radiosensitive, and an ovum can be released, which accounts for the period of fertility that sometimes occurs after moderate doses of radiation.

In addition to sterility, hormonal changes (especially loss of estrogen production) and early menopause may occur. Perhaps most significant in terms of late or long-term consequences of radiation to the gonads in both the male and female is the potential for genetic damage. Chromosomal aberrations are a possibility that must be considered, especially at low doses. (For further reading on the genetic effects of radiation, the reader is referred to Travis,[10] Beir V,[38] and Liber et al.[39])

Radiation to the male testes damages and prevents maturation of the immature spermatogonia. Sterility can be permanent even after a dose of 500–600 cGy, and temporary sterility usually is seen following doses as low as 250 cGy.

## Urinary System

Radiation-induced cystitis and urethritis are early and transient effects on the urinary tract that usually respond well to symptomatic treatment. Of major significance when considering the effect of radiation on the urinary system is damage to the kidneys in the form of nephritis. Early changes brought about by high doses of radiation lead to permanent fibrosis and atrophy, largely due to sclerosis of the vasculature. Renal failure and death can result. Protection of the kidneys is essential when the abdomen is irradiated.

## Cardiovascular System

Damage to the vasculature of an organ or tissue (i.e., to stroma) can be the primary reason for the radioresponsiveness of that organ or tissue. Blood vessels (lined with epithelium) may become occluded when excessive cell production takes place during repair and regeneration in response to radiation injury. Thrombosis may be induced by the thickening that occurs during regenerative activity, thus further occluding the vessels. Late changes can be seen in the form of telangiectasia, petechiae, and sclerosis. The heart muscle itself is thought to be relatively radioresistant. However, at doses above 4000 cGy, pericarditis may occur in addition to the damage to the vasculature of the heart muscle.

## Nervous System

The brain and spinal cord are considered to be relatively radioresistant, and peripheral nerves are even more so. However, therapeutic doses between 3000 and 6000 cGy have produced transient symptoms in the CNS, usually following a latent period in which no functional damage is seen. Especially noticeable is the response called *Lhermitte's syndrome,* which may occur following irradiation to the cervical cord. This syndrome is characterized by paresthesia in the form of shocklike sensations that radiate down the back and extremities when the neck is bent forward. Stretching of the cord in this manner compromises circulation, which may partially account for the sensations experienced. Myelopathy usually is transient, but at higher doses may lead to paralysis or paresis. When large volumes of the spinal cord (15 cm or more) are irradiated, doses of 4500–5000 cGy will produce transverse myelitis. The tissues of the nervous system are composed of a variety of cells, most sensitive of which are the neurons found in olfactory, gustatory, and retinal receptors. Radiation to these neurons can therefore alter or destroy the function of the particular sense organ. Because the nervous system is thought to be relatively radioresistant in itself, damage that does occur following radiation probably relates to vascular insufficiency. As described earlier, the vasculature of the body is radiosensitive. In addition, preexisting disorders such as diabetes, hypertension, and arteriosclerotic changes can enhance the effect of radiation on nervous tissue.

## Skeletal System

Mature bone and cartilage are radioresistant and seldom present a problem in planning radiotherapy. However, late avascular necrosis can occur after high doses, causing pain and possible pathological fracture. This is a relatively rare complication with supervoltage equipment.

Of much greater clinical significance is the effect of radiation on growing bone and cartilage. Children treated for spinal, thoracic, or abdominal tumors are susceptible to deformity as a result of radiation to the vertebrae. Failure to attain normal height due to spinal irradiation has occurred, as has shortening of a limb when the epiphyses are irradiated. Such orthopedic problems, although serious in themselves, may be considered a necessary compromise in terms of tumor eradication.

## Systemic Effects of Radiation

Aside from or in addition to the specific local effects of radiation to tissues and organs already presented, the patient receiving radiotherapy may experience certain subjective systemic effects, including nausea, anorexia, and malaise. Although the psychological component of these symptoms cannot be overlooked, these systemic effects theoretically can be linked to the release of toxic waste products into the bloodstream resulting from tumor destruction. The presence of these toxins may account for the nausea and anorexia, whereas the increased metabolic rate required to dispose of the waste products might be partially responsible for the frequent complaint of fatigue. The physical effort needed to make a daily trip to the radiotherapy department for four or five weeks also may account for the malaise experienced by many individuals.

It is important to note that the response of the whole body (nausea, anorexia, malaise) to radiation of a limited site depends on the volume of the irradiated area, the anatomic site, and the dose. Consequently, not all individuals experience these systemic symptoms, and the degree of disability due to the symptoms will vary from mild to severe. Most individuals receiving radiotherapy tolerate treatment remarkably well and experience only mild systemic symptoms.

### Total-body and hemibody radiation

Total body and hemibody irradiation are relatively infrequent therapeutic applications of radiation. The effect on the patient varies with the dose, dose rate, and dose-time factor. For example, total-body irradiation (TBI) of 150 cGy is being used in some centers in the treatment of chronic lymphocytic leukemia. This total dose is delivered at the rate of 5 cGy/day for ten days, followed by a two-week break, and then repeated for two more cycles to reach the total of 150 cGy. When TBI is delivered in this manner, which calls for small daily doses fractioned over a ten-week period, the side effects are negligible.

Total body irradiation for "conditioning" prior to bone marrow transplantation has three purposes: (1) myeloablation to create space for engraftment of donor marrow, (2) immunosuppression in the recipient to prevent graft rejection, and (3) clearing of any residual malignant cells.

Fractionation of the dose (120–400 cGy per day to a total of 1200–1600 cGy) appears to be more beneficial and less likely to produce tissue tolerance and late effects.[40] Acute effects of TBI include graft-versus-host disease, nausea, vomiting, diarrhea, mucositis, erythema, and alopecia. Chronic or late effects occurring up to three months after TBI include cataracts, growth disturbances, endocrine dysfunction, and nephrotoxicity. The single most significant chronic effect is interstitial pneumonitis which carries a 70% mortality rate.[40]

*Hemibody radiation* refers to treatment of the upper, middle, or lower body in a single large fraction of approximately 500–800 cGy. This approach is used primarily for the patient with widespread bone metastases to achieve rapid palliation of pain. Often, this individual has had one or several localized treatment courses, but no sooner achieves local pain relief than another site becomes problematic. Although individual sites can be treated sequentially, this is very time consuming as well as demoralizing for both patient and family. Treating a large volume in a single fraction is a viable alternative.[41]

Hemibody radiation, while generally effective in relieving pain, may produce significant side effects related to the site treated. Pretreatment medications such as antiemetics and steroids usually are administered for upper and mid-body treatment to alleviate nausea and possible radiation pneumonitis.

Lower hemibody radiation is better tolerated, although some patients experience brief periods of posttreatment nausea and occasional abdominal cramping or diarrhea. Bone marrow suppression is likely to occur because of the large volume treated. In addition, many patients who are candidates for hemibody treatment have had prior chemotherapy (and radiation) and are therefore already immunocompromised. Blood counts must be monitored pre- and posttreatment with hemibody radiation. If sequential hemibody treatment is required, there is usually a gap of several weeks between treatments to ensure marrow recovery.

### Altered fractionation schedules

Standard treatment with radiation therapy calls for single daily fractions, given five days per week in daily doses in the range of 180–300 cGy. Patient tolerance, convenience, staff availability, and (most important) tissue tolerance are the factors governing today's standard fractionation schedules.

In the evolution of today's standard approach, numerous variations in time-dose relationships were tried, with results ranging from cure to severe radiation injury. Modern clinical experience with hyperfractionation began in the 1970s, progressing to randomized trials during the 1980s,[42] continuing into the 1990s. The development of flow cytometry allowed rapid measurement of tumor doubling time, increasing scientists' awareness of the danger of rapid tumor cell proliferation. These findings spurred further attempts to explore fractionation schemes in order to increase the therapeutic ratio of tumor cell kill versus normal tissue tolerance.

Two approaches to altered fractionation currently being explored are pure hyperfractionation and accelerated fractionation. Advanced, nonresectable, squamous cell carcinomas of various head and neck sites are the most frequent subject of these studies. *Hyperfractionation* (HFX) involves an increased number of fractions delivered over the same total treatment time as in standard fractionation. Typical doses are 115–125 cGy per dose, twice daily. *Accelerated fractionation* (AFX), on the other hand, uses three fractions per day to achieve the same total dose as HFX while shortening overall treatment time by approximately two weeks.[43,44]

Horiot et al[44] report that one study of HFX using two fractions per day has shown improved local-regional control without increasing incidence and severity of normal tissue damage, compared to a single fraction per day. Early results from an AFX study show that delivering three fractions per day is feasible; however, there is evidence of significant increase in acute morbidity and a trend indicating increased severe late effects.

One other alteration in standard fractionation schedule is the *dynamic fractionation* approach, in which doses are escalated over the length of the treatment course. One study calls for two fractions per day increasing from 150–200 cGy per fraction over five weeks.[43] Another study, cited by Fowler,[43] utilizes twice-daily fractions of 120–160 cGy plus two to four 200-cGy doses, achieving a total dose of 7200–7600 cGy in five weeks' time. As with any research, large prospective clinical trials are needed in order to determine efficacy as well as practicality of altered fractionation schedules in radiation oncology.[45]

### Chronic low-dose exposure

Chronic low-dose radiation exposure occurs to all individuals, due to background radiation from naturally occurring radioactive substances and cosmic rays.[46] Such exposure is largely unavoidable and within the safe limits defined by federal regulations. Radiation workers are exposed to a somewhat higher level of ionizing radiation, but the allowable limit is well below that which is known to produce ill effects.

### Total-body radiation syndrome

*Total-body radiation syndrome* refers to the effects of the acute exposure of the organism to doses of radiation received in a matter of minutes rather than hours or days. Acute exposure of human beings has been studied through data obtained from industrial and laboratory accidents, individuals exposed at Hiroshima and Nagasaki, Pacific Testing Grounds fallout exposure, and medical treatment procedures.[47] Doses of 150–2000 cGy delivered to the whole body in a short time produce life-shortening or lethal damage through effects on the hematopoietic, gastrointestinal, and central nervous systems. The April 1986 nuclear accident in Chernobyl, Ukraine undoubtedly will produce additional significant information about the somatic and genetic effects of exposure to high levels of radioactivity. For greater detail and for information on the effects of radiation exposure to the embryo and fetus, the reader is referred to Travis.[10]

### Radiation-induced malignancies in humans

The carcinogenic effects of radiation, often called "late effects," from both chronic low-dose exposure and acute exposure to the whole body are of particular interest and concern to the nurse, especially in providing support to the individual who is hesitant about accepting treatment. The key to understanding lies in the fact that acute exposure and chronic low-dose exposure are the exceptions, occurring in radiation accidents, occupational exposure, and the early stages of the development of the science of radiotherapy. The usually prescribed therapeutic doses (in the range of 2500–6500 cGy) are believed to be less carcinogenic than lower doses given over a much longer time period. Theoretically, a cell that has survived in a damaged or altered state after low-dose irradiation may undergo carcinogenic mutation in the presence of other conditional factors. On the other hand, a cell that has been sterilized or destroyed by therapeutic doses of radiation should be incapable of malignant changes.

The most common malignancies associated with radiation exposure are skin carcinoma and leukemia, and evidence also implicates radiation in some sarcomas, thyroid carcinoma, and lung cancer.[48–50] Recent reports have suggested the possibility of inducing breast cancer in females by frequent radiographic exposure for screening for tuberculosis, other lung disease, and breast cancer itself.

Radiation carcinogenesis depends on a number of variables.[51] These include a latent period of from 1–30 years, radiation dose, concomitant factors in the radiated organism's environment, and the actual fate of the cell as it responds to radiation injury. For a more comprehensive review of radiation carcinogenesis, the reader is referred to Bucholtz.[52]

## NURSING CARE OF THE PATIENT RECEIVING RADIOTHERAPY

Caring for the patient receiving radiotherapy gives nurses an opportunity to put into practice all the theory and science acquired in their education and work experience. The patient receiving radiotherapy is first and foremost an individual with all the needs and problems generated by the diagnosis of cancer. Care cannot focus solely on the disease site (i.e., a "lung" patient, a "cervix" patient, a "Hodgkin's" patient, and so on). Nor can nursing care be based solely on meeting the immediate needs generated by treatment and its side effects without considering the individual's long-term needs. Nursing care must be individualized and holistic, intelligent and thoughtful, scientific and compassionate. All these qualities can be achieved in nursing care of the patient receiving radiotherapy. By applying the scientific background material provided in earlier sections of this chapter and using specific nursing care measures detailed in the following pages, the nurse will be able to devise a comprehensive plan of care for each individual receiving radiotherapy.

Assessing the individual's situation is the first step in planning care. A number of questions must be asked and answered:

1. What is the diagnosis? The prognosis?
2. What is the goal of treatment?
3. Does the patient know and understand the diagnosis?
4. Does the family (or significant others) know and understand the diagnosis?
5. What is the plan of treatment? Radiotherapy alone? Surgery? Chemotherapy? All three?
6. Will therapy be given on an inpatient or an outpatient basis?
7. What does the patient know and understand about radiotherapy?
8. Where can the correct information about the individual's treatment plan be obtained?

When the individual with cancer is an inpatient, the staff should begin this assessment on admission and build on the care plan as the diagnosis becomes available and treatment plans are formulated by the medical staff. Coping with the diagnosis may be the only crisis a particular patient can handle at this early stage; elaborate plans and explanations about treatment may go largely unheard as the individual struggles to resolve feelings about the diagnosis of cancer. In contrast, another individual moves quickly past the diagnosis and literally pleads to get treatment under way before a total care plan has been formulated. Each patient must be assessed and managed on an individual basis.

In seeking answers to some of the assessment questions posed previously, the hospital nurse can turn to the patient's physician, the patient, and the family. After the patient has been referred to a radiation oncologist and evaluated, the physician (and nursing staff from that department, if available) can provide further information that can be useful in devising the care plan.

What are some of the facts about radiotherapy the nurse must understand when caring for the individual in the pretreatment phase? How can these facts be incorporated into the nursing care plan? Most individuals newly diagnosed with cancer have a number of misconceptions about treatment stemming from the experiences of other people. The worst side effects are always the ones that are remembered and are often exaggerated in the retelling. Of course, side effects do occur, but their severity depends on such factors as treatment site, treatment volume, fractionation, total dose, and especially on the individual being treated. Knowing what side effects can be expected and, most important, knowing that measures are available to alleviate most symptoms can be reassuring to the individual. In general, most individuals respond best to a reassuring pretreatment discussion in which side effects specific to their treatment are discussed, stressing that symptomatic relief is available. Knowing what to expect usually helps prevent the patient from worrying that a treatment-related side effect represents a worsening or recurrence of disease. At this time the nurse can also mention briefly the reactions that will not occur. Some might argue that this only puts ideas into the anxious patient's mind, but most people are reassured to know, for example, that they will not lose their hair or be nauseated if this is the case.

Thus nurses should know the facts about treatment site and related potential side effects when they are caring for individuals before and during radiotherapy. Most people experience few or at least manageable side effects today. Many individuals are able to continue working, perhaps with some changes in schedule, or manage a home and family just as they did before diagnosis and treatment. Less common are those who are debilitated by the disease or treatment, making it impossible to continue in their former roles.

In planning nursing care for the patient receiving radiotherapy, another important consideration is the length of the treatment course. Specifically, it is important to determine the need for transportation and to help the individual and family obtain this transportation. Although some palliative treatment is given over a period of seven to ten days (often while the patient is hospitalized), most individuals receive radiotherapy as an outpatient for an average of five weeks, and some may be treated over seven or eight weeks. The patient with stage III Hodgkin's disease receiving total nodal irradiation will be making trips to the radiotherapy department for approximately three months, with several two-week breaks interspersed. Transportation for these lengthy periods can be a major challenge requiring assistance of professionals to mobilize many resources.

Some individuals are able and willing to drive themselves, and some have family and friends who can provide this service, but many, especially elderly persons, are without transportation on a steady basis and will need assistance. Sources of transportation vary, but some available services are as follows:

- senior citizens transportation (a federal or locally funded service in many parts of the United States)
- American Red Cross
- American Cancer Society
- religious groups
- service and civic organizations

In addition to meeting transportation needs, explaining potential side effects, and dispelling misconceptions, the staff nurse or community nurse can provide a great service to the individual undergoing radiotherapy by describing the treatment facilities and equipment. People are sometimes frightened by the size and complexity of the equipment and the fact that they must be alone in the room during treatments. Of course, no nurse can be familiar with every radiotherapy facility. However, nurses working in oncology settings or regularly caring for individuals with cancer should make it a part of their own education to visit and familiarize themselves with the radiotherapy departments and facilities where their patients are frequently referred. Individuals being treated and visitors are sometimes disturbed by the fact that a radiotherapy facility is in a basement or an underground location. Again, a factual explanation about the necessity for proper shielding and architectural support will help allay some of these fears.

The well-informed nurse who is familiar with local radiotherapy facilities can provide the support and reassurance needed during the pretreatment phase of an individual's illness. The confidence that familiarity brings can significantly increase the nurse's ability to meet some of the pretreatment needs of a patient about to begin radiotherapy.

The personnel an individual comes in contact with during radiotherapy can play an important role in alleviating anxiety. The radiation oncologist who prescribes, directs, and evaluates treatment is primarily responsible for the patient's care during treatment and for varying periods afterward. This often is done in conjunction with a family physician, oncologist, or surgeon. Nurses in a radiotherapy department can offer much of the supportive care needed to cope with the emotional and physical needs of the patient and his or her family. Symptomatic relief of side effects, nutritional support, and social and financial assistance are all nursing concerns. Coordination of complex treatment schedules and protocols also may be part of the nurse's role. Some departments employ one or more nurses to meet these patient needs, and in others an oncology nurse is shared by both medical and radiation oncology. The reality is that nurses are in short supply in radiotherapy departments and nursing care needs often go unmet, thus underscoring why the role of the staff nurse, office nurse, or community nurse is so important.

The individual with whom the patient has the most frequent contact and establishes the closest relationship is often the radiation therapist. The therapist is a highly skilled individual, certified by the American Society of Radiologic Technologists, and is responsible for giving the daily treatments under the direction of the radiation oncologist. Although the therapist's primary focus is the physics and mechanics of treatment, attention is also given to the patient as an individual with particular wants and needs. Nursing care sometimes is carried out by the therapist in departments where there are no nurses. However, it would be unfair to expect that a radiation therapist could or would be able to devote as much attention to nursing needs as to the technical responsibilities of the job. In recognition of this need for combined skills, some centers have employed, trained, and prepared nurses for certification as radiation therapists.

Regardless of who will be treating and caring for the patient in a radiotherapy department, it is important and comforting for the individual and family to know that caring individuals are available who will try to make the total treatment experience as untraumatic as possible. Most individuals experience few or no treatment-related problems, and those who do experience problems can usually be managed effectively. The patient should be encouraged to ask questions, report symptoms, and regard radiotherapy as part of a total plan for managing the cancer.

Assessment of individual needs and implementation of nursing interventions are ongoing processes in oncology nursing. For individuals receiving radiotherapy, this is especially true because needs change as treatment progresses. Initial nursing concerns focus on diagnosis and the individual's acceptance of treatment, preparation (both physical and psychological) for treatment, transportation arrangements, and so on. As treatment progresses, many of the initial fears and misconceptions disappear, and the patient settles into the somewhat routine process of coming for daily treatments. Expected side effects usually occur after 10–14 days, depending on dose, volume, and site. Individuals undergoing treatment frequently count the days and keep track of the number of treatments received. Although a plan has been made from the beginning prescribing the number of daily fractions, this plan is subject to change as the radiation oncologist deems appropriate. There are a number of reasons for adding to, subtracting from, or changing the plan, and if the patient understands this from the beginning, changes will not be interpreted as signs of recurrence or disease progression. Although most individuals want to

know how many treatments will be given so that they can adjust their activities accordingly, they should be helped to understand that this number may be subject to change.

Apathy or a sense of futility may develop as treatment progresses and the patient does not see any obvious changes in his or her disease. Visible lesions frequently can be observed to shrink or disappear with treatment, and this is encouraging. However, when a tumor is not visible or when treatment is an adjuvant treatment in cases where no measurable lesion exists, the patient sometimes finds it difficult to continue in the absence of obvious and immediate benefits. This is especially true if side effects produce symptoms that are more troublesome than those created by the disease. Regardless of the setting, the nurse plays a vital role in helping the patient to accept and continue treatment for its long-term potential despite the immediate discomforts. A telephone call to the physician, nurse, or therapist in the radiation department from the nurse caring for the individual in another setting can be helpful in such situations to assure continuity of care and consistency of support.

## SPECIFIC NURSING CARE MEASURES FOR PATIENTS RECEIVING RADIOTHERAPY

During a course of radiotherapy, certain treatment-related side effects can be expected to develop, most of which are site specific as well as dependent on volume, dose fractionation, total dose, and individual differences. Many symptoms do not develop until approximately 10–14 days into treatment, and some do not subside until two or more weeks after treatments have ended.

Nursing care measures and medical management described in the following sections reflect the patterns and practices that are most commonly used. It should be noted that alternative means do exist for medical management and nursing care, any of which may be suitable to a particular setting or individual patient situation.

### Fatigue

Fatigue or malaise is common among individuals with cancer, and may be even more pronounced during and after a course of radiation treatment. Although a number of theories exist that attempt to explain radiation-induced fatigue, the mechanism is still not well understood.[53,54]

Some of the potential contributors to the fatigue experienced with radiation treatment are relatively obvious and therefore may be amenable to interventions. Table 13-4 lists the more common factors contributing to fatigue.[55] Nursing assessment of the contributing factors is particularly important, since these factors often can be addressed. Pain management is especially important, because chronic and uncontrolled pain is one of the most wearisome challenges faced by some patients. Extra rest

**TABLE 13-4**  Factors Contributing to Fatigue in the Patient Receiving Radiation Treatment

- Recent surgery
- Prior or concurrent chemotherapy
- Pain
- Malnourishment
- Medications
- Frequency of treatment visits
- Maintaining usual lifestyle
- Tumor burden
- Anemia
- Respiratory compromise

and a reduction in the normal activity level may be necessary during treatment. Individuals receiving radiation treatments should be encouraged to nap, go to bed early, or alter their daily schedule to allow for rest periods rather than to "fight it," as some are prone to do. Some individuals report that taking a nap immediately after returning home from their treatment gives them enough energy for the rest of the day. Others prefer to retire earlier than usual at night. The patient who is bedridden at home or is hospitalized will need provisions for rest and quiet according to individual need.

Pretreatment patient education should include information about the potential for fatigue during treatment. With the knowledge that treatment-induced fatigue usually is self-limiting, most patients are better able to tolerate this common side effect.

## Anorexia

Anorexia may occur among individuals receiving radiotherapy, regardless of the treatment site. Anorexia, like fatigue, is probably related to the presence in the patient's system of the waste products of tissue destruction. Other possible causes for anorexia include anemia, inactivity, medications, alterations in the individual's ability to ingest and digest foods, and psychological factors. The cause often cannot be identified clearly, and therefore the symptom must be treated utilizing all the techniques known to encourage adequate nutritional intake. A self-perpetuating cycle of anorexia/weight loss/weakness/inactivity/anorexia can develop if the symptom is untreated. For detailed information on the management of anorexia and cachexia in the individual with cancer, see chapter 24 in this text, and Iwamoto.[56]

## Mucositis

The reaction induced by radiation within the mucous membranes of the body (gastrointestinal, genitourinary, and respiratory systems) is called mucositis. Mucositis can be described as a patchy, white membrane that becomes confluent and may bleed if disturbed. This reaction is most visible when radiation is given to the mouth and oropharynx, and severe reactions cause considerable dis-

comfort to the patient. A number of measures can be employed in treating mucositis in the oral cavity, but it is first important to enlist the patient's cooperation in avoiding irritants such as alcohol, tobacco, spicy or acidic foods, very hot or very cold foods and drinks, and commercial mouthwash products (they are too astringent even when diluted).

Although a 1:1 solution of hydrogen peroxide has been used for mouth care for many years, this solution can actually be very damaging to tissues if it is not diluted correctly. Normal saline is an acceptable solution, although it does little to refresh the mouth. One ounce of diphenhydramine hydrochloride (Benadryl) elixir diluted in one quart of water provides an ideal agent for mouth care in individuals with mucositis. The diphenhydramine hydrochloride solution provides a soothing, nontoxic, pleasant-tasting means for the patient to rinse and gargle as needed. Mouth care should be done as often as every three or four hours and is especially important before mealtime. One technique is to use an air-powered spray apparatus to deliver a fine mist of the diphenhydramine hydrochloride solution, which can be directed at all surfaces of the mouth and oral cavity. This irrigation technique is effective in loosening retained food particles, breaking up the usually tenacious mucus, and soothing the mucosa. Care should be taken not to dislodge the plaquelike formations of mucositis, because dislodgement will cause bleeding and denude the mucosal surface. Outpatients can receive this irrigation treatment daily, as can inpatients when they are brought to the radiotherapy department for their radiation treatment. In addition, inpatients can be given mouth care by a modified technique at their bedside several times daily. A disposable irrigation bag is hung from an intravenous pole, using gravity to deliver a spray of solution to the mouth and oropharynx.

In addition to diphenhydramine hydrochloride mouth care solution, agents that coat and soothe the oral mucosa, such as Maalox, are sometimes used. Lidocaine hydrochloride 2% viscous solution may provide some relief from discomfort. Among other oral anesthetic solutions now available are Orajel Mouth-Aid®, Zila Dent® Oral Analgesic, Zilactin® Medicated Gel, and Hurricaine® liquid or spray. Instituting an active approach to mouth care for radiation-induced mucositis enables most individuals to tolerate the effects of radiation better. Occasionally, a break from treatment will have to be given when reactions are excessive, but constant, daily nursing support appears to be a factor in promoting tolerance of treatment.

## Xerostomia

The dry mouth resulting from radiation to the salivary glands or portions of them is known as xerostomia. Alterations in taste frequently accompany xerostomia. Whether the condition is temporary or permanent depends on the dose received and the percentage of the total salivary tissues irradiated. During the course of radiation, little can be done to relieve this annoying symptom. The sensitivity of the mucous membranes precludes the use of saliva substitutes at this point, and frequent sips of water seem to be the best method of providing moisture. Saliva, though present, is thick and viscous, often causing the patient to gag and to expectorate with difficulty. Frequent mouth care, especially before meals, will provide some relief. When a course of therapy has ended and any intraoral reaction has subsided, some individuals will benefit from the use of a saliva substitute to provide moisture and lubrication for two to four hour periods. During the night, xerostomia causes the patient to awaken frequently with a dry, almost choking sensation that is relieved only by taking a drink of water. Some individuals find that using the saliva substitute allows them to sleep uninterrupted for several hours. A small container of this mixture can be carried easily in pocket or purse for use when he or she is away from home. One formula for saliva substitute is as follows:

| | |
|---|---|
| Cologel | 98.2 ml |
| Glycerin | 110.0 ml |
| Saline | 1000.0 ml |

The solution should be mixed well and refrigerated. It is stable for three months. The patient with xerostomia should use one to two teaspoons every three or four hours. The solution is swished in the mouth and swallowed. Several brands of saliva substitute are available for over-the-counter purchase including Xerolube®, Moi-stir®, and Orabalance®. Pilocarpine (Salagen®) is a parasympathomimetic agent shown to be effective in stimulating saliva flow after radiation-induced xerostomia.

Chapter 29 in this text provides detailed oral care guidelines for patients with treatment-induced alterations in oral mucosal integrity.

## Radiation Caries

Although it is a potential late effect of irradiation to the mouth and oropharynx, radiation caries can be greatly reduced or avoided by proper care before, during, and after a course of treatment. Absence or decrease in saliva and the altered pH produced by treatment promote decay. Before the start of therapy, a thorough dental examination and prophylaxis should be carried out. If extensive decay and generally poor dentition exist, full mouth extraction is usually the treatment of choice. However, if teeth are in good repair, a vigorous preventive program is begun to protect them from the late effects of radiation. This can include daily diphenhydramine hydrochloride mouth sprays for their cleansing effect, followed by a 5-minute application of fluoride gel. Brushing the teeth with a soft-bristled brush several times daily is also important. Such vigorous efforts to prevent decay in individuals receiving radiotherapy can be initiated by the nurse, and nursing support and encouragement are necessary in helping to ensure continuation of this preventive treatment when radiotherapy is completed.

A patient information sheet on oral and dental care is shown in Table 13-5.

## Esophagitis and Dysphagia

When radiation is directed to the mediastinum, as, for example, in treating patients with Hodgkin's disease or cancer of the lung or breast, areas of the esophagus may receive a sufficient dose to produce symptoms of esophagitis.[56] This is a transient effect in which the esophageal mucous membrane becomes somewhat edematous, and mucositis can develop. The patient will first notice some difficulty in swallowing solids (dysphagia), which is often described as "a lump in my throat, only deeper." This may then progress to a definite esophagitis, which makes swallowing painful and can be responsible for a decrease in intake of foods and fluids. Newer treatment techniques are available that minimize this effect, and a treatment technique or schedule can be adjusted to allow the reaction to subside. The following mixture provides temporary relief from radiation esophagitis:

Radiotherapy mixture
**Mylanta** (Stuart)—450 ml (three 5 oz bottles)
**Lidocaine** hydrochloride viscus 2%—100 ml
**Diphenhydramine** hydrochloride elixir—60 ml
Shake well and refrigerate
Dosage: 1–2 tablespoons 5 minutes
before meals and before bedtime

When esophagitis occurs, ensuring adequate nutrition becomes a major nursing concern. The patient receiving treatment should be encouraged to substitute high-calorie, high-protein, high-carbohydrate liquids and soft, bland foods for their regular meals. Eggnogs, milk shakes, "instant" liquid meals, and commercially prepared liquid supplements all may be used between meals as well as substituted for solids. Blenderized foods from the patient's regular diet are less expensive than commercial products, and the patient with esophagitis should be encouraged to try this method.

The individual and family need continual encouragement and support through this difficult period. Weight loss caused by decreased intake can be interpreted by the patient undergoing therapy as treatment failure and lead to a defeatist attitude. The temporary nature of the esophagitis and dysphagia should be emphasized.

## Nausea and Vomiting

Of the potential side effects from radiotherapy, nausea or vomiting are probably the most distressing to the patient being treated. Although nausea and vomiting are not common, the fear that they will occur causes great stress in many individuals. As with other side effects, treatment site and volume are the variables to be considered, along

**TABLE 13-5** Dental Care for Patients Receiving Radiation to the Mouth Area

**Before You Start Radiation Treatments:**

Make an appointment with your dentist for dental prophylaxis. This includes inspection, polishing, scaling of teeth (if indicated), flossing, and repair or restoration of existing teeth. Daily fluoride treatments are necessary to help prevent future dental problems. Ask your dentist to recommend either a fluoride rinse or gel and applicator tray.

**During a Course of Radiation Treatment:**

| Helpful Hints | Stay Away from These |
| --- | --- |
| • Use a soft toothbrush, brushing gently after meals and at bedtime. | • Do not use any commercial mouthwash. |
| • Use toothpaste if desired. Otherwise, just brush with lukewarm water. | • Avoid very hot foods and drinks. |
| • Use diphenhydramine mouthwash as a rinse and gargle 4–6 times daily or more often as needed. Directions for this mouthwash will be given to you. | • Do not drink alcoholic beverages. |
| • Eat a high-calorie, high-protein diet including plenty of liquids. Instant breakfast drinks and liquid nutritional supplements help add calories and protein. | • Do not smoke. |
| • Eat soft/bland foods if mouth is sore (eggs, custard, pudding, potato, cheese, milk and ice cream drinks). | • Avoid spicy, highly seasoned foods, and acidic foods such as oranges, grapefruit, and tomatoes. |
| • We will provide you with nutritional information and hints on food preparation. | |

**If You Wear Dentures:**

Dentures or partial plates may be cleaned in your usual manner. If your mouth becomes irritated, we may ask you to stop wearing dentures except at mealtime.

Courtesy of Philip G. Maddock, MD, and Laura J. Hilderley, RN, MS, Radiation Oncology Services of Rhode Island.

with preexisting conditions related to surgery, chemotherapy, and sites of disease. The patient's emotional state and apprehension about the disease and treatment are sometimes responsible for nausea when treatment is unlikely to be the cause.

Generally, the patient receiving radiotherapy can be expected to experience some degree of nausea when treatment is directed to any of the following sites: whole abdomen or portions of it, large pelvic fields, hypochondrium, epigastrium, or para-aortic areas.

Some patients report nausea with whole-brain irradiation or wide mediastinal fields. However, the majority of patients experience little or no difficulty with this side effect. When nausea does occur, it usually can be controlled by antiemetics administered on a regular schedule and by adjusting the eating pattern so that treatment is given when the stomach is relatively empty. Delaying intake of a full meal until three or four hours after treatment is also helpful because nausea, if it occurs, will usually appear from one to three hours after treatment.

## Diarrhea

Diarrhea, like nausea and vomiting, is not an expected side effect in most individuals receiving radiotherapy. However, it does occur if areas of the abdomen and pelvis are treated after about 2000 cGy have been given. Some individuals experience only an increase in their usual number of bowel movements, whereas others develop loose, watery stools and intestinal cramping. Occasionally, treatment must be interrupted to allow the bowel to recover from radiation effects, especially in elderly or debilitated individuals. When diarrhea and vomiting both occur, active intervention with intravenous fluids for short-term replacement may be needed, as well as a rest from treatment.

For most individuals with radiation-induced diarrhea, a low-residue diet and prescription of loperamide hydrochloride usually are sufficient. The low-residue diet may be all that is required in some instances. Many individuals are not sufficiently knowledgeable about foods and their composition to manage this on their own, and a low-residue diet sheet has been developed to supplement the teaching done by the nurse (Table 13-6). When reviewing the diet with the patient (and with the individual preparing meals at home), it is especially important to emphasize the "Foods Allowed" and to point out that a daily multiple vitamin should be included. Vitamin C is notably lacking from the diet, as well as those vitamins found in leafy green vegetables. A favorite food from the "Foods to Avoid" list may be added now and then, if it does not increase symptoms. Diets such as this one should be individually designed to meet the particular geographic and ethnic food patterns of the population, hence the inclusion of well-washed clams and pasta without sauces on the sample.

**TABLE 13-6** Low-Residue Diet for Control of Radiation-Induced Diarrhea

| Foods Allowed | | Foods to Avoid | |
|---|---|---|---|
| Beverages | Skim or low-fat milk, buttermilk, tea, soda (decaffeinated only), Gatorade | Beverages | Coffee, beer, liquor, fruit juice, chocolate milk, hot chocolate, cocoa |
| Breads and Cereals | White bread and rolls, plain muffins, saltines, melba toast, cream of wheat or rice, farina, corn and rice cereals, well-cooked oatmeal | Breads and Cereals | Dark, whole-grain breads, rolls, and cereals (ie: whole wheat, cracked wheat, bran, pumpernickel, rye, granola, wheat germ, shredded wheat, bran flakes, cereals with dried fruit/nuts) |
| Starchy Foods | White potatoes (no skin), plain spaghetti, macaroni, noodles, other pasta (no tomato sauce), white rice | Starchy Foods | Sweet potatoes, potato skins, wild or brown rice |
| Vegetables | Well-cooked carrots, squash, green beans | Vegetables | All other vegetables (cooked or raw) especially cabbage, broccoli, brussels sprouts, baked beans, peas, radishes, cucumbers, corn |
| Fruits | Bananas, apples in any form (baked, raw, applesauce, apple juice) | Fruits | All other fruits and juices |
| Proteins | Chicken (stewed, creamed, broiled or baked, all without skin), turkey, lean beef, veal, pork, lamb, ham, fish, canned or well-washed clams, cottage cheese, hard cheese, and eggs | Proteins | All fried, tough or spicy meats, hot dogs, sausage, poultry skins, gritty seafood, pork and beans, peanut butter |
| Miscellaneous | Broth, bouillion, consomme, creamed soups, salt, sugar, jelly, honey, plain jello, custard, tapioca pudding, other puddings (except chocolate), hard candies, low-fat ice cream, sherbet, low-fat yogurt (plain, vanilla, lemon) | Miscellaneous | All seasonings, jams, pickles, popcorn, olives, coconut, nuts, dried seeds, chocolate cake and chocolate cookies |

Courtesy Philip G. Maddock, MD, and Laura J. Hilderley, RN, MS, of Radiation Oncology Services of Rhode Island.

## Tenesmus, Cystitis, and Urethritis

Although infrequent, tenesmus, cystitis, and urethritis do occur in some individuals receiving pelvic irradiation. Tenesmus of the anal or urinary sphincter produces a persistent sensation of the need to evacuate the bowel or bladder. Relief sometimes can be obtained from gastrointestinal and urinary antispasmodics and anticholinergic preparations. The problem may persist, however, until after the course of treatment has ended.

Cystitis and urethritis resulting from radiation to the bladder area is distressing to the patient being treated and usually is brought to the physician's or nurse's attention soon after it develops. A clean-voided urine specimen for culture and sensitivity testing should be obtained, and appropriate antibiotic therapy instituted if indicated. Usually, no infection is found, and treatment consists of urinary antiseptics and antispasmodics for symptomatic relief. High fluid intake is encouraged. Sitz baths, which are commonly prescribed for tenesmus, cystitis, and urethritis, are contraindicated if the perineal area is being irradiated. The added moisture will only enhance any potential or actual skin reaction.

## Alopecia

The loss of hair is traumatic to most people, regardless of whether they are prepared for this change in body image. The needless fear of this loss is equally traumatic; thus if patients are being prepared for radiotherapy that does not include the scalp, they should be reassured that hair loss will not occur as a result of treatment.

During treatment of the whole brain, as in metastatic disease or for primary brain tumor, alopecia will occur and follows a typical pattern. At about 2500–3000 cGy fractionated over two or three weeks, the patient will notice excessive amounts of hair in the brush or comb and a gradual thinning of the hair. This continues for two or three weeks, and then quite suddenly most of the hair comes out, and the patient awakens to find the remainder of his or her hair on the pillow. The patient who is prepared for this with a wig or attractive scarves or caps will adjust to this change with less emotional trauma than one who is totally unprepared either emotionally or physically.

In some instances hair loss may occur regionally or in patches rather than over the entire scalp. Examples include the patient being treated for a pituitary lesion with a two- or three-field technique involving portals of approximately 6 × 6 cm or the person receiving mantle irradiation for Hodgkin's disease that includes the suboccipital lymph nodes. The latter patient will lose hair at the base of the scalp from the hairline to several centimeters above, with a strip remaining in the midline due to a block inserted to protect the spinal cord. Whenever possible, the patient with this or similar field arrangements in which patchy hair loss is expected should be advised to grow the hair longer. In some instances the long hair can be combed to cover areas of alopecia.

Care of the hair and scalp while receiving radiation to the scalp includes very gentle brushing or combing and infrequent shampooing. Permanent waves and hair coloring are contraindicated because of the potential harm to the irradiated skin of the scalp. Individuals being treated in the neck or facial areas should likewise avoid any procedures on the hair that involve the use of harsh chemicals, because such substances may run down onto treated skin. As in the case of irradiated skin in general, the scalp should be treated with care and caution for several months to a year or more after healing has taken place. The top of the head, especially in males (who have less of a protective layer of hair), should be protected from sunburn with a cap. The forehead, ears, and neck also may exhibit more sensitivity to the sun than before radiation treatment was given.

## Skin Reactions

The response of normal skin to radiation treatments varies from mild erythema to moist desquamation that leaves a raw surface similar to a second-degree burn. Because megavoltage and cobalt beams deliver the maximum dose beneath the skin, skin reactions have become less significant. Although an acute response may occur during the course of therapy in which brisk erythema progresses to dry and then moist desquamation, healing and cosmesis usually are satisfactory. Some individuals may exhibit a permanent tanning effect in the treatment area, with no change in the texture of the skin and subcutaneous tissues. Other individuals will have fibrosclerotic changes in the subcutaneous structures, and their skin will be smooth, taut, and shiny. Telangiectasia also may be evident.

Acute and chronic changes in irradiated skin depend on many factors that govern the severity and permanence of the radiation effect.[57,58] As in other treatment-related side effects, total dose, fractionation, and volume are important factors. Quality of the treatment beam and its percentage depth dose (see the section entitled "Applied Radiation Physics," earlier in the chapter) will determine the amount of skin sparing. Individuals treated with electron beams will exhibit considerable skin reaction when the electron beam is intended for lesions located on the skin or a few centimeters below the surface. Characteristics of the electron beam are such that maximum dose buildup occurs within 1 cm below the skin, especially at energies below 20 MeV. However, even more severe reactions that include areas of moist desquamation and peeling will heal well, leaving some patchy depigmentation and telangiectasis.

Skin in some areas of the body, such as the groin, perineum, buttocks, inframammary folds, and axillae, has a relatively poor tolerance to radiation. This is due to the normal warmth and moisture found in these areas rather than any characteristic of the skin itself. Reactions to radiation in these sites are likely to be more severe than in adjacent areas receiving identical treatment.

Because moisture enhances skin reactions, the patient should be advised to keep the skin in the treated area as dry as possible. Bathing or showering is permissible, but long periods of soaking are inadvisable. Treated skin should be bathed gently with tepid water and mild soap. The area should be rinsed thoroughly and gently patted (not rubbed) dry. Lines or markings placed on the skin at simulation should not be removed until the radiation therapist advises the patient to do so. It may therefore be necessary for the patient to take sponge baths rather than tub baths or a shower for some time to avoid washing off the markings.

General guidelines to follow for care of the skin within the treatment site include the following:

1. Keep the skin dry.
2. Avoid using powders, lotions, creams, alcohol, and deodorants.
3. Wear loose-fitting garments.
4. Do not apply tape to the treatment site when dressings are applied.
5. Shave with an electric razor only. Do not use preshaves or aftershaves.
6. Protect the skin from exposure to direct sunlight, chlorinated swimming pools, and temperature extremes (e.g., hot water bottle, heating pad).

Such precautions are necessary throughout the course of treatment and until any skin reaction has disappeared following cessation of therapy.

Specific measures useful in treating skin reactions include the use of a light dusting of cornstarch for pruritus from erythema and dry desquamation. If moist desquamation and denuded areas appear, a thin layer of A & D ointment may be applied, followed by a Telfa (nonstick) dressing to protect the clothing and the skin. The therapist or radiation oncology nurse should always be consulted regarding specific skin care measures appropriate to the individual.

When planning for skin care for the patient receiving radiotherapy, it should be remembered that individuals often are treated by parallel opposing portals and only one of these portals may be marked to indicate the field. This means that in addition to the clearly marked portal on the patient's abdomen or chest (for example), there may be a corresponding field on the posterior that needs the same careful attention. A telephone call to the nurse or therapist will provide the information needed to identify the treatment portal or portals. Tattoos that indicate the treatment site (as described in the earlier section entitled "Simulation and Treatment Planning") also may be present on the patient's skin and may be helpful in determining which areas of skin require special care.

Skin care in radiotherapy varies considerably from one treatment center to another.[58] The radiotherapy nurse or physician should always be consulted about skin care if there is any question concerning institutional or office policy. Outpatients should be given explicit directions for managing at home, and written directions are very helpful in addition to the verbal instructions (see Table 13-7).

One area of skin care about which there usually is some question is the matter of exposure to the sun. Any restrictions on exposure apply only to the treated area or areas. No special precautions are needed for sites that normally are covered by clothing when outdoors. (One exception is skin that exhibits a moderate or severe reaction to radiation, which may become sunburned when protected only by a sheer or light fabric covering.) During treatment and for a month or more afterward, treated skin should not be exposed to direct sunlight. Individuals whose treatment site is exposed usually can go from home to car or elsewhere for brief periods without difficulty. However, during seasons when the sun is most intense or in locales where the exposure is more intense, even a brief trip outdoors without protective garments may enhance the reaction on treated skin, depending on the dose of radiation received. Caution and common sense should prevail.

When a course of radiotherapy has ended and after any reaction has subsided and healed, a cautious approach to sun exposure may be resumed. Previously treated areas may be exposed gradually (15 min/day), using a number 15 sunblock. Each individual must determine his or her own tolerance to the sun and proceed accordingly.

Because of the skin-sparing effect of today's treatment machines, most individuals are able to enjoy outdoor activities without incident after their treatment course has ended. Again, it is important to emphasize caution and common sense. A patient information sheet for sense in the sun is shown in Table 13-8.

## TABLE 13-7  Skin Care During Radiation

Skin over the area where you are receiving radiation therapy needs to be treated with gentle care. During your course of radiation treatment, please follow these guidelines:

**Keep the treated area dry and free from irritation.**

- Do not wash the treated area until the therapist tells you to. This may not be until 2 or 3 days after the start of treatments.

- Do not remove the lines or ink marks that have been placed on your skin until your therapist or doctor tells you to.

- When permitted, wash the treated skin gently, using a mild soap, and rinse well before patting dry. Always use warm or cool water, *not* hot water.

- Do not apply any lotions, creams, alcohol, aftershave, perfume, deodorants, etc. to the treated area.

- Heating pads and hot water bottles should not be used on treated skin.

- Avoid friction; that is, avoid clothing that is tight or may rub over the treated skin, such as shirt collars, ties, undergarments, belts.

- Men should use an electric razor if they are receiving treatment to the face and/or neck area. Do not use aftershave.

- If treated skin becomes reddened or tender, you may apply a thin layer of Vitamin A&D ointment. Be sure to tell us when this happens. If further irritation develops, we will give you special instructions or medications for skin care.

- Protect the treatment area from exposure to direct sunlight. While you are receiving a course of therapy, do not sunbathe or spend more than a few minutes in the bright sun if the treated area is exposed. We will give you special instructions about future sun exposure when you finish your course of treatment.

Courtesy of Philip G. Maddock, MD, and Laura J. Hilderley, RN, MS, Radiation Oncology Services of Rhode Island.

## TABLE 13-8  Sense in the Sun After Radiation Treatment

Skin that has been treated with radiation will need special attention in the bright sunlight. When your course of radiation therapy is finished, you may have some dryness or raw areas in the treatment field. These will clear up in a few weeks with continuation of the special care instructions given to you during treatment.

Until the skin is completely healed, you should not expose the area to sunlight. When healing is complete, you may gradually begin to sunbathe, using a #15 sunscreen in the treated area, and increasing the exposure time very slowly and carefully. If the area becomes reddened or irritated—discontinue sun exposure. You may have to wait another season before trying again.

Wear a T-shirt, cover-up, broad-brimmed hat, or some other means of protecting the treated skin. Remember that a thin, gauzelike layer of fabric does not block the harmful ultraviolet light.

Remember that the beach is not the only place where sunburns can occur. Use caution when riding in the car with your arm, neck, and face near a sunny window, when working in the yard or garden, when at a ballgame or other summer outing, when in a boat, and even when skiing on a bright sunny day.

While these instructions for special care refer primarily to skin that has been treated with radiation, we urge you to use care and common sense in general whenever the sun is bright.

Courtesy of Philip G. Maddock, MD, and Laura J. Hilderley, RN, MS, Radiation Oncology Services of Rhode Island.

## Bone Marrow Suppression

When large volumes of active bone marrow are irradiated (especially the pelvis or spine in the adult), the effect on the marrow can be quite significant. Other areas of concern when large fields are treated include the sternum, ribs, metaphyses of the long bones, and skull. During simulation and treatment planning, provision is made for shielding as much of this active marrow as possible without compromising the treatment. Because of careful planning and trimming of fields to include only the necessary volume, the majority of people receiving radiotherapy are able to tolerate a course of treatment without experiencing bone marrow depression. Nonetheless, weekly blood counts should be done on all individuals receiving radiotherapy and two to three times weekly in some instances. The latter is necessary for individuals receiving concomitant chemotherapy or those who have had extensive chemotherapy before radiation. A notable example would be the patient with Hodgkin's disease or non-Hodgkin's lymphoma who has received several cycles of combination chemotherapy. Individuals receiving total-body irradiation or splenic irradiation for chronic lymphocytic leukemia will require daily blood counts before treatment to avoid (or at least anticipate) a precipitous drop in white blood cells or platelets.

For the individual whose bone marrow is affected by treatment or a combination of factors, a number of support measures can be employed. Transfusions of whole blood, platelets, or other blood components may be necessary for the patient who has dangerously low blood counts. Treatment may have to be adjusted or interrupted. Nursing care should include observation of the patient for signs and symptoms of bleeding, anemia, and infection. Patients and their families must be taught what to look for and to report to the physician, therapist, or nurse whenever symptoms occur.

## Radiation Side Effects: Special Considerations

As previously stated, most people are less anxious if told ahead of time what specific side effects they may expect from their treatment. Knowing that diarrhea is quite likely to result from pelvic irradiation will help the patient prepare for such an event, both in terms of dietary adjustments and in helping to avoid embarrassing accidents. There are, however, a number of side effects that do not occur with any predictability or regularity, and an individual being treated would not necessarily benefit from knowing about them ahead of time. The nurse, who is sometimes the first caregiver to whom a patient may report symptoms, should be aware of these less common but possible side effects of radiotherapy to specific sites.

### Transient myelitis

When lymph nodes in the cervical region are radiated, as in the mantle technique employed when treating patients with stage III Hodgkin's disease, the spinal cord is blocked to protect it from unnecessary radiation. However, a radiation effect on the spinal cord can still occur. Some individuals will experience paresthesia (a shocklike sensation radiating down the back and over the extremities) when flexing the neck. This is known as Lhermitte's syndrome and occurs after a latent period of two to three weeks after treatment to the site has ended. The symptoms usually improve gradually or spontaneously, leaving no permanent effect. The dose of radiation that can produce a transient myelopathy is well below the dose that results in a permanent injury to the spinal cord. A possible explanation for the symptoms found in Lhermitte's syndrome is the effect of radiation on the vasculature supplying the cervical spinal cord. If the blood vessels are compromised by radiation injury, stretching or bending the neck can cause a temporary occlusion and decrease in blood supply to the cord, resulting in paresthesia. Paresthesia can be frightening to a patient. However, the temporary nature of this effect should be stressed and the patient reassured that this is a known side effect that sometimes occurs.

### Parotitis

Parotitis is a painful swelling and inflammation of the parotid glands that sometimes occurs in individuals receiving radiation to the maxillomandibular area. It may occur with mantle irradiation for Hodgkin's disease, as well as with treatment to the area for other forms of cancer. The onset of symptoms is sudden and usually follows the first two or three treatments. Although uncomfortable, the symptoms subside almost as quickly as they arise, and no specific treatment is necessary.

### Visual and olfactory disturbances

During radiation to the pituitary area, some individuals occasionally experience visual or olfactory disturbances that can be distressing. Some have reported seeing lights or smelling something burning, among other things, after several treatments. The explanation for this phenomenon lies in the anatomic proximity of the optic and olfactory nerves to the hypophysis and the fact that ionization taking place in or near these structures can cause alterations in the sensations of sight and smell. A multiple-field technique usually is employed when treating patients with pituitary lesions to deliver a high dose to the tumor with a minimal dose to surrounding structures. However, the optic nerves, chiasma, and optic tract lie between the hypophysis and the bulk of the brain, and the olfactory bulb and tract lie superior and anterior to the hypophysis, which means that the olfactory and optic structures are likely to be included in the field arrangement. Again, reassurance and explanation tailored to the person's ability to understand are the best means of handling these disturbing but uncommon side effects.

### Radiation recall

Although not technically a radiation reaction, *radiation recall* can occur in a previously irradiated site that exhibited mucositis or erythema. Radiation recall occurs in response to the systemic administration of certain chemotherapeutic agents (for example, actinomycin) several months to a year or more after radiation was received. Typically, the person develops intraoral mucositis or a skin reaction in the exact pattern corresponding to the previously treated radiation portal. Treatment is symptomatic, and the drug dosage or choice of agent may be modified if necessary.

## NURSING CARE OF THE PATIENT WITH A RADIOACTIVE SOURCE

Nursing care of individuals being treated with implanted radioactive sources is a challenge that goes beyond basic medical-surgical theory and requires an understanding of radiation safety, biology, and physiological manifestations. Rather than fear, the nurse should develop a healthy respect for all that is implicit in working with radioactive isotopes and proceed to plan and deliver optimum care under the special conditions encountered in each situation.

Radioactive materials for therapeutic usage are listed in Table 13-1 and specific sources for brachytherapy are outlined in Figure 13-5. In addition to being implanted in tissues or inserted into body cavities, some radioactive isotopes may be administered orally, intravenously, or by instillation. These materials are absorbed or metabolized by the body, and specific safety precautions are required, depending on the particular source and mode of administration. Adsorbed or metabolized isotopes used most commonly include $^{131}$I, $^{32}$P, and $^{198}$Au, all of which are administered as colloids or solutions. Liquid sources such as these present a possibility of contamination of equipment, dressings, and linens, depending on the mode of administration and metabolism. In contrast, sealed sources such as $^{137}$Cs and $^{226}$Ra for implantation through a mechanical device are not metabolized and therefore are not excreted in body fluids.

The following information is necessary to provide safe and effective nursing care for individuals being treated with brachytherapy (sealed radioactive source placed within a body cavity or tissue) or with metabolized or adsorbed radiation:

1. What is the source being used?
2. What is the half-life of that source?
3. What is the type of emission (alpha, beta, gamma)?
4. How much radioisotope is being used (energy)?
5. What method of administration/application is being used?
6. Is the source metabolized? adsorbed? neither?

From this information, the nurse can plan and administer nursing care utilizing the appropriate precautions, including disposal of wastes and care of linens and equipment. This information will also help to determine what radiation safety precautions, if any, are necessary at home or after hospital discharge.

Radiation safety and radiation protection are the concerns of every caregiver involved with brachytherapy patients. This includes the radiation oncologist, other physicians, nurses, therapists, physicists, and allied health workers who may come in contact with the patient. Guiding this team is the radiation safety officer, who is responsible for implementing radiation safety procedures and monitoring all use of radioactive materials. Most institutions also will have a radiation safety committee composed of representatives from among the disciplines listed previously, whose responsibilities are the control and enforcement of the use of radioisotopes in the hospital as required by the Nuclear Regulatory Commission.

Three primary factors in radiation protection should be foremost in the minds of all personnel involved in care of the patient: time, distance, and shielding. Each factor can be used to minimize unnecessary radiation exposure for those around a patient with a radioactive source implanted, ingested, or applied.

### Time

The amount of exposure to radiation that personnel receive is directly proportional to the time spent within a specific distance from the source. Nursing care must be planned and organized so that the nurse spends as little time as possible in close contact with the individual being treated while still providing for his or her needs. A team of providers with a clearly defined plan for care is a common approach used to minimize a nurse's exposure yet adequately meet the patient's needs.

### Distance

As radiation is emitted from a point source, the amount of radiation reaching a given area decreases according to the law of inverse square. Figure 13-13 illustrates this principle. Nurses can use distance creatively when noncontact care is being given.

### Shielding

When a sheet of absorbing material is placed between a radiation source and a detector, the amount of radiation that reaches the detector decreases, depending on the energy of the radiation and the nature and thickness of the absorbing material (shield). The thickness of a shielding material that is required to reduce the radiation to half of its original quantity is referred to as the *half-value layer* (HVL). The HVL for $^{137}$Cs (a commonly used radioactive source) is approximately 6 mm of lead or 10 cm of concrete. The practical implications of this shielding approach are evident.

When planning nursing care for the patient with a

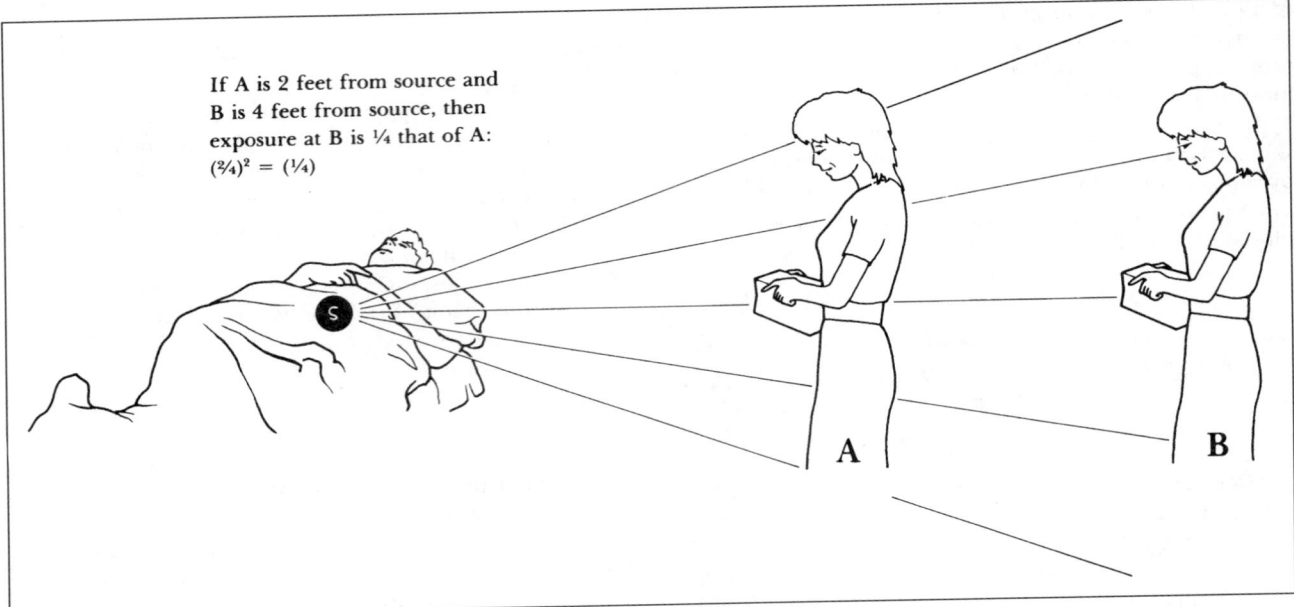

If A is 2 feet from source and B is 4 feet from source, then exposure at B is ¼ that of A: $(2/4)^2 = (1/4)$

**FIGURE 13-13**   The inverse square law. As distance from a radiation source increases, exposure decreases by the square of that distance.

radioactive source, time and distance are the two variables that can most readily be controlled. Because shielding from gamma radiation requires lead or concrete in the previously specified thicknesses, it is usually impractical to expect that much physical care can be given from behind such a shield. Portable radiation shields (similar in design to a moving blackboard on wheels) are available and do protect the caregiver who places it between himself or herself and the source. However, this is useful primarily in doing tasks within the patient's room other than direct care. The so-called lead aprons used in diagnostic radiology are not of sufficient thickness to stop gamma rays and cannot protect the caregiver from exposure when caring for individuals, for example, with radium or cesium sources.

Because shielding is not always possible or practical, time and distance are the two factors that nurses must incorporate into the care plan. Some of the ways in which exposure to personnel can be reduced are listed in Table 13-9.

## Patient Education and Support

With all the emphasis on haste and elimination of nonessential care, it is sometimes easy to eliminate that most important consideration of emotional and social support of the patient. Individuals who are isolated for radiation precautions often feel "unclean" or "contaminated." The fact that visitors are allowed only at the doorway and that housekeeping personnel are barred from the room adds to this sense of isolation. Because the nurse also must limit the time spent in giving direct care, the patient's sense of rejection often is heightened.

**TABLE 13-9   Some Ways to Reduce Exposure to Personnel Providing Care for the Individual with a Radioactive Source**

1. Use appropriate radiation precaution signs, wristbands, and tags.
2. Plan care to avoid delays at the person's bedside.
3. Eliminate the bedbath except for what the person can manage alone.
4. Change linens less frequently or only when soiled.
5. Prepare meal trays outside of the person's room instead of at the bedside (cut up meats, open containers, etc.).
6. Work quickly; concentrate on accomplishing the necessary tasks in as short a time as possible.
7. Position the bedside table, call bell, and television controls within easy reach of the person to avoid frequent return trips to the bedside.
8. Use appropriate monitoring devices and heed the information regarding total individual exposure.
9. Never care for more than two individuals at a time with radioactive sources.
10. Keep long-handled forceps and a shielded transport cart in the person's room at all times.
11. Use long-handled forceps to retrieve a radioactive source that has accidentally been dislodged.
12. Arrange the chair so that ambulatory individuals can be seated as far from the bed (and thus the caregiver) as possible while linens are being changed.

Planning and providing emotional support are major components of nursing care for all individuals, but especially for those with an implant or other form of radioactive material. Preparation for these procedures should include all the following points of information:

1. *Description of the procedure.* For example, although performed in the operating room under anesthesia, insertion of vaginal tandem and ovoids will not involve a surgical incision.

2. *Possible change in appearance.* For example, individuals with needle implants in the facial region often request a mirror and should be prepared for their sometimes grotesque appearance while needles are in place.

3. *Anticipated pain or discomfort and measures available for relief.* For example, the presence of gynecologic applicators (such as in Figure 13-6) combined with bed rest and restricted movement often produces a low backache. Appropriate analgesics are prescribed and should be administered as needed.

4. *Potential short-term and long-term side effects and complications.* An example of a short-term side effect: Needle implants to the tongue usually produce edema, causing the tongue to be noticeably swollen during the procedure and for several days afterward. A long-term complication, such as occurs with vaginal brachytherapy, may result in scarring and the formation of adhesions that cause dyspareunia.

5. *Restrictions on activity while the radioactive sources are in place.* For example, individuals with gynecologic applicators in place are confined to bed for the duration of the treatment, which may be as long as three to four days.

6. *Visiting restrictions.* For example, policy varies depending on the availability of appropriate shielding devices and the energy of the sources being used. However, visitors usually are restricted from the patient's room, and, when allowed, visits must be brief.

7. *Radiation precautions observed by hospital personnel.* For example, individuals should be reassured that their personal care needs will be met but that the nurse's time at the bedside and in the room will be restricted because of the presence of the radioactive sources.

The patient also should be helped to prepare for such procedures by planning for suitable activities such as reading, handwork, television, and so on. Boredom and isolation sometimes are the most difficult part of treatment with a radioactive source. The nurse has a primary responsibility to meet those treatment-induced needs, as well as those of a physical nature. With the proper application of the principles of radiation safety and careful attention to the special emotional needs of individuals being treated with brachytherapy, this challenge for nursing care can be met.

## ADVANCES IN RADIOTHERAPY

Radiation oncology in the 1990s can be characterized by continual refinement of treatment techniques and expanded application of multimodal therapy. Numerous cooperative group studies employ radiation as primary or adjuvant therapy. Variations such as hyperfractionation (more than one treatment per day) for particularly resistant tumors are being tested. Whole-body or hemibody irradiation for widespread metastases is providing rapid palliation for some individuals.[41]

Use of particle radiation such as fast neutrons, deuterons, helium ion beams, and negative pi-mesons will continue to be tested and refined for use in situations where conventional radiation is of little value. The expense and limited applicability of such treatment methods currently confine their use to a small proportion of cancer patients.

In February 1989, an announcement was made of the first proton beam accelerator built for hospital use. This device was moved out of the physics laboratory setting (Fermi Laboratory in Illinois, Harvard University, the University of California at Berkeley, as well as several sites abroad), where limited numbers of patients had been treated since the early 1970s. Loma Linda University Medical Center, Los Angeles, began using the $40 million treatment device in 1990.

*Radiolabeled antibody therapy* has been the subject of considerable interest and effort since the 1970s.[59] This treatment technique is based on the information acquired in recent years regarding immunobiology and the isolation of many tumor-specific monoclonal and polyclonal antibodies. Among the numerous radioactive isotopes that have been used therapeutically,[131]I and [90]Y, in particular, have been adopted for use in radiolabeled antibody therapy.

The underlying principle of radiolabeled antibody therapy involves attaching a radioactive isotope to the tumor-specific antibody to deliver therapeutic radiation directly to the target tumor. Theoretically, this avoids prolonged radiation exposure to healthy cells while delivering lethal or sublethal doses to the tumor. Among numerous phase I, II, and III clinical trials over the past two decades, some of the more significant results have been achieved in the treatment of hepatoma.[60] Studies involving treatment of intrahepatic biliary carcinoma, nonresectable, non-oat-cell carcinoma, and recurrent Hodgkin's disease are ongoing.[60]

*Intraoperative radiotherapy* (IOR) was developed in the United States during the late 1970s at Howard University and at Massachusetts General Hospital. Unresectable tumors had been the primary target of IOR before the 1980s. By 1985, however, IOR was used increasingly in a prophylactic approach combined with resection of primary tumors, such as locally advanced colorectal carcinoma; pancreatic, gastric, and bladder cancers; and soft-tissue sarcomas.

Compared with external beam therapy, intraoperative radiotherapy has the advantage of increasing tumor dose in relation to normal tissue dose. After surgically exposing the target volume, a single, large fraction of radiation is delivered directly to the tumor site by a specially built cone attached to the therapy machine. The surgical procedure is then completed, and a further postoperative course of conventional radiotherapy is given. Some institutions give a preoperative rather than postoperative course of conventional radiotherapy, but rarely is IOR the definitive treatment.

There are a number of differences in the exact IOR procedures at the various institutions in the United States now using IOR.[61-63] Although some have installed radiotherapy equipment in an operating room or built a special room to perform the combined therapy, others have worked out a detailed procedure for transporting the fully anesthetized and surgically opened patient through the hospital corridors to the radiotherapy department. Despite the technical difficulties in performing IOR, it appears to have potential for further development and application in cancer management.

*Conformal radiation therapy* is an outgrowth of computer technology and the continued search to more precisely target the tumor site while sparing surrounding healthy tissue. Computerized treatment planning has been in use since the late 1960s and has dramatically enhanced the speed of planning. Beam profiles were stored in the computer and could be quickly placed onto the patient contour. Cross-sectional anatomy, however, was based on a single cross-section through the center of the target volume. This single slice obviously could not represent the structure of the entire treatment volume and thus had significant limitations. Since then, with the advent of the computed tomography (CT) scanner in the late 1970s, three-dimensional planning became a reality. Advances in three-dimensional radiotherapy treatment planning included:

1. use of multiple cross-sectional slices
2. integration of all cross-sectional imaging modalities—magnetic resonance imaging (MRI), single photon emission computed tomography (SPECT), and positron emission tomography (PET)
3. full three-dimensional description of the target region[64]

From three-dimensional treatment planning, field shaping and blocking became more highly defined, and there soon emerged the concept of *conformal* radiation therapy delivery. By tightly conforming the zone of high-dose volume to the target volume, dose outside the target volume would be greatly reduced. Theoretically, if this precision could be reached, then tumor dose could be increased with greater cell-kill and normal tissue sparing.

Conformal therapy utilizes either a multifield technique or the newer multileaf collimator. Multifield technique can involve as many as six separate fields and sets of blocks which is very time-consuming both in the planning and block-making process as well as during treatment when the therapist must manually replace blocks for each field.[64] The multileaf collimator on a linear accelerator, however, changes both the field shape and blocking in a matter of seconds. A multileaf collimator located in the head of the treatment machine contains many pairs of thin lead leaves. Each leaf is motorized and computer controlled to respond to the individually designed field-shaping program. Thus, in a matter of seconds, each of the precision fields can be changed without removing and adding the standard lead blocks. Conformal therapy is being used in a number of centers, primarily for treatment of prostate, lung, and nasopharynx cancers.[65,66]

*Stereotactic radioneurosurgery* for the treatment of intracranial tumors is currently being studied and refined in the continuous effort to more effectively deliver a high single-radiation dose to a very small volume within the brain. Stereotactic radiosurgery uses multiple convergent beams via a coordinate system. A stereotactic frame is secured to the patient's skull, for use in pin-pointing the lesion, and for directing the placement of interstitial catheters if brachytherapy and/or hyperthermia is to be used.

Three high-energy radiation techniques currently are in use for radiosurgery in approximately 200 centers in the United States.[67] The most common technique employs a linear accelerator with a specially adapted collimator. Patients are usually treated supine. However, some facilities utilize a sitting arrangement in which the patient is rotated about a fixed or moving linac beam. When the patient is in a supine position, both treatment couch and linac gantry may move to create a series of arc-shaped beams.

The Gamma Knife is the second most common high-energy source for stereotactic radiosurgery. This unit utilizes 201 $^{60}$Co sources positioned in individual beam channels inside a large helmetlike structure. The patient, with stereotactic frame in place, is positioned with his or her head inside this helmet and the frame is locked into the device assuring stability and precision. Treatment to one or several isocenters is then delivered according to the carefully constructed treatment plan, which defines the target and directs the deployment of the appropriate number of $^{60}$Co sources radially toward the target.

The third technique for delivering stereotactic radiation utilizes charged particle beams (described earlier under Equipment, Beams, and Materials Used in Radiotherapy) produced by cyclotrons or synchrotrons. Charged particle beams deliver increased dose at depth in tissue and then stop at a fixed depth dependent on the beam energy.[67] An effective three-dimensional dose distribution can be obtained with only a few (two to six) intersecting stationary beams.

Stereotactic radioneurosurgery historically has been used primarily for treating arteriovenous malformation and other benign tumors. In recent years, however, this modality has been used effectively for treatment of small metastatic brain tumors, for treating brain metastases that progress or recur after external beam therapy, and for small, relatively spherical high-grade gliomas. Most patients treated with radiosurgery only have been followed for a short time, therefore firm conclusions about outcome have not been reached. Prospective randomized trials are currently underway.[68]

## CONCLUSION

Radiotherapy in the treatment of cancer has indeed come a long way from its exciting beginning in the late 1800s. Much has been learned about the beneficial as well as the harmful effects of ionizing radiation. As we move toward the year 2000, innovations in technology will help to further refine the applications of radiotherapy in cancer treatment. Special approaches such as intraoperative radiation, hyperthermia, and monoclonal antibody therapy will either be adopted or abandoned. At the same time, stereotactic radioneurosurgery, conformal therapy, and high dose-rate brachytherapy are becoming more widely used as the efficacy of these techniques becomes apparent.

Along with advances in therapy there has been increased recognition of the important role of the nurse as educator and care provider for individuals receiving radiation treatment and their families. As new radiation centers open and others are restructured, nurses increasingly are being added to the team of caregivers. Nurses now are taking a major role as collaborative caregivers with the radiation oncologist. Advances in nursing science and nursing care parallel advances in radiotherapy as a treatment modality. Advanced practice nurses have an important role in the multidisciplinary radiation oncology team.

## REFERENCES

1. Munzenrider JE, Crowell C: Charged particles, in Mauch PM, Loeffler JS (eds): *Radiation Oncology, Technology and Biology*. Philadelphia, Saunders, 1994, pp 34–55
2. Raju MR: Particle radiotherapy: Historical developments and current status. *Radiat Res* 145:391–407, 1996
3. Maddock PG: Brachytherapy sources and applicators. *Semin Oncol Nurs* 3:15–22, 1987
4. Schiff PB, Brenner DJ, Hall EJ: Brachytherapy: Low dose rate and its alternatives, in Mauch PM, Loeffler JS (eds): *Radiation Oncology, Technology and Biology*. Philadelphia, Saunders, 1994, pp 514–523
5. Crook J, Esche BA: The uterine cervix, in Cox JD (ed): *Moss' Radiation Oncology: Rationale, Technique, Results* (ed 7). St. Louis, Mosby, 1994, pp 617–682
6. International Brachytherapy. *Programme and Abstracts 7th International Brachytherapy Working Conference, Sept. 6–8, 1992, Baltimore/Washington*. Veenendaal, Netherlands, Nucletron International B.V., 1992
7. Jordan L, Mantravadi RVP: Nursing care of the patient receiving high-dose rate brachytherapy. *Oncol Nurs Forum* 18:1167–1171, 1991
8. Jordan L, Buck S: A teaching booklet for patients receiving high-dose rate brachytherapy. *Oncol Nurs Forum* 18:1235–1238, 1991
9. Hall EJ: *Radiobiology for the Radiologist* (ed 4). Philadelphia, Lippincott, 1994
10. Travis E: *Primer of Medical Radiobiology*. Chicago, Year Book Medical Publishers, 1975
11. Hall EJ, Cox JD: Physical and biologic basis of radiation therapy, in Cox JD (ed): *Moss' Radiation Oncology: Rationale, Technique, Results* (ed 7). St. Louis, Mosby-Yearbook, Inc., 1994, pp 3–66
12. Bergonie J, Tribondeau L: Interpretation of some results of radiotherapy and an attempt at determining a logical technique of treatment. *Radiat Res* II:587, 1959
13. Gray LH: Radiobiologic basis of oxygen as a modifying factor in radiation therapy. *Am J Roentgenol* 85:805, 1961
14. Ritter MA: Cell proliferation, in Mauch PM, Loeffler JS (eds): *Radiation Oncology, Technology and Biology*. Philadelphia, Saunders, 1994, pp 525–544
15. Withers HR: Biologic basis of radiation therapy, in Perez CA, Brady LW (eds): *Principles and Practice of Radiation Oncology* (ed 2). Philadelphia, Lippincott, 1992, pp 64–96
16. Phillips TL. Biochemical modifiers: Drug-radiation interactions, in Mauch PM, Loeffler JS (eds): *Radiation Oncology, Technology and Biology*. Philadelphia, Saunders, 1994, pp 113–151
17. Brown JM: Hypoxic cell radiosensitizers: Where next? *Int J Radiat Oncol Biol Phys* 16:987–993, 1989
18. Coleman CN, Beard CJ, Hlatky L, et al: Biochemical modifiers: Hypoxic cell sensitizers, in Mauch PM, Loeffler JS (eds): *Radiation Oncology, Technology and Biology*. Philadelphia, Saunders, 1994, pp 56–89
19. Hall EJ, Miller R, Astor M, et al: The nitroimidazoles as radiosensitizers and cytotoxic agents. *Br J Cancer* 37:120, 1978 (suppl 3)
20. Cox JD: Clinical applications of new modalities, in Cox JD (ed): *Moss' Radiation Oncology: Rationale, Technique, Results* (ed 7). St. Louis, Mosby-Yearbook, Inc., 1994, pp 971–986
21. Fowler JF: Chemical modifiers of radiosensitivity—theory and reality: A review. *Int J Radiat Oncol Biol Phys* 11:665–674, 1985
22. Noll L: Chemical modifiers of radiation therapy, in Hassey-Dow K, Hilderley L (eds): *Nursing Care in Radiation Oncology*. Philadelphia, Saunders, 1992, pp 264–274
23. Held J, Volpe H: Bladder preserving combined modality therapy for invasive bladder cancer. *Oncol Nurs Forum* 18:49–57, 1991
24. Cummings BJ, Keane TJ, O'Sullivan B, et al: Epidermoid anal cancer: Treatment by radiation alone or by radiation and 5-fluorouracil with and without Mitomycin-C. *Int J Radiat Oncol Biol Phys* 21:1115–1125, 1991
25. Hirshfield-Bartek J: Combined modality therapy, in Hassey-Dow K, Hilderley L (eds): *Nursing Care in Radiation Oncology*. Philadelphia, Saunders, 1992, pp 251–263
26. Coughlin CT, Wong TZ, Ryan TP, et al: Interstitial microwave-induced hyperthermia and iridium brachytherapy for the treatment of obstructing biliary carcinoma. *Int J Hyperthermia* 8:157–171, 1992
27. Kapp KS, Kapp DS, Stuecklschweiger G, et al: Interstitial hyperthermia and high-dose rate brachytherapy in the treatment of anal cancer: A phase I–II study (Review). *Int J Radiat Oncol Biol Phys* 28:189–199, 1994
28. Seegenschmiedt MH, Martus P, Fietkau R, et al: Multivariate analysis of prognostic parameters using interstitial thermoradiotherapy (IHT-IRT): Tumor and treatment variables predict outcome. *Int J Radiat Oncol Biol Phys* 29:1049–1063, 1994
29. Moros EG, Straube WL, Klein EE, et al: Clinical system for simultaneous external superficial microwave hyperthermia and cobalt-60 radiation. *Int J Hyperthermia* 11:11–26, 1995
30. Valdagni R, Fei-Fei L, Kapp D: Important prognostic factors

influencing outcome of combined radiation and hyperthermia. *Int J Radiat Oncol Biol Phys* 15:959–972, 1988

31. Sneed PK, Stauffer PR, Gutin PH, et al: Interstitial irradiation and hyperthermia for the treatment of recurrent malignant brain tumors. *Neurosurgery* 28:206–215, 1991

32. Robins HI: Combined modality clinical trials for favorable B-cell neoplasms: Lonidamine plus whole body hyperthermia and/or total-body irradiation (Review). *Semin Oncol* 18:23–27, 1991 (suppl 4)

33. Kapp DS, Cox RS, Fessenden P, et al: Parameters predictive for complications of treatment with combined hyperthermia and radiation therapy. *Int J Radiat Oncol Biol Phys* 22:999–1008, 1992

34. Zimmerman M, Schorcht J, Andree W: Theoretical and experimental investigations of a newly developed intracavitary applicator system for the radiothermotherapy of gynecological tumours. *Int J Hyperthermia* 9:463–477, 1993

35. Prionas SD, Kapp DS, Goffinet DR, et al: Thermometry of interstitial hyperthermia given as an adjuvant to brachytherapy for the treatment of carcinoma of the prostate. *Int J Radiat Oncol Biol Phys* 28:151–162, 1994

36. Montes H, Hynynen K: A system for the simultaneous delivery of intraoperative radiation and ultrasound hyperthermia. *Int J Hyperthermia* 11:109–119, 1995

37. Wojtas F: Hyperthermia and radiation therapy, in Hassey-Dow K, Hilderley L (eds): *Nursing Care in Radiation Oncology*. Philadelphia, Saunders, 1992, pp 307–319

38. Beir V: Health effects of exposure to low levels of ionizing radiation, Committee on the Biological Effects of Ionizing Radiation. Washington, DC, National Academy Press, 1990

39. Liber HL, Kelsey KT, Little JB: Radiation mutagenesis and carcinogenesis, in Mauch PM, Loeffler JS (eds): *Radiation Oncology, Technology and Biology*. Philadelphia, Saunders, 1994, pp 470–486

40. Tarbell NJ, Chin LM, Mauch PM, in Mauch PM, Loeffler JS (eds): *Radiation Oncology, Technology and Biology*. Philadelphia, Saunders, 1994, pp 387–404

41. Dudjak L: Alternatives in dose fractionation and treatment volume, in Hassey-Dow K, Hilderley L (eds): *Nursing Care in Radiation Oncology*. Philadelphia, Saunders, 1992, pp 285–294

42. Thames HD: On the origin of dose fractionation regimens in radiotherapy. *Semin Radiat Oncol* 2:3–9, 1992

43. Fowler JF: Intercomparisons of new and old schedules in fractionated radiotherapy. *Semin Radiat Oncol* 2:67–72, 1992

44. Horiot JC, LeFur R, Schraub S, et al: Status of the experience of the EORTC Cooperative Group of radiotherapy with hyperfractionated and accelerated radiotherapy regimes. *Semin Radiat Oncol* 2:34–37, 1992

45. Peters LK, Ang KK: Altered fractionation schemes, in Mauch PM, Loeffler JS (eds): *Radiation Oncology, Technology and Biology*. Philadelphia, Saunders, 1994, pp 545–565

46. Mettler FA and Upton AC: *Medical Effects of Ionizing Radiation* (ed 2). Philadelphia, Saunders, 1995, pp 73–112

47. Kato H, Schull WJ: Studies of the mortality of A-bomb survivors. Mortality, 1950-78. I. Cancer mortality. *Radiat Res* 90:395–432, 1982

48. March HC: Leukemia in radiologists in a twenty-year period. *Am J Med Sci* 220:282, 1950

49. Pack GT, Davis J: Radiation cancer of the skin. *Radiology* 84:436, 1965

50. Conrad RA, Hicking A: Medical findings in Marshallese people exposed to fallout radiation: Results from a ten-year study. *JAMA* 214:316, 1970

51. Rubin P, Costine L, Fajardo LF: Overview: Late effects of normal tissue (LENT) scoring system. *Int J Radiat Oncol Biol Phys* 31:1041–1042, 1995

52. Bucholtz J: Radiation carcinogenesis, in Hassey-Dow K, Hilderley L (eds): *Nursing Care in Radiation Oncology*. Philadelphia, Saunders, 1992, pp 342–357

53. Winningham ML, Nail LM, Burke MB, et al: Fatigue and the cancer experience: The state of the knowledge. *Oncol Nurs Forum* 21:23–36, 1994

54. Nail LM, Winningham ML: Fatigue and weakness in cancer patients: The symptom experience. *Semin Oncol Nurs* 11:272–278, 1995

55. Hilderley L: Pain and fatigue, in Hassey-Dow K, Hilderley L (eds): *Nursing Care in Radiation Oncology*. Philadelphia, Saunders, 1992, pp 57–68

56. Iwamoto R: Altered nutrition, in Hassey-Dow K, Hilderley L (eds): *Nursing Care in Radiation Oncology*. Philadelphia, Saunders, 1992, pp 69–95

57. Sitton E: Early and late radiation-induced skin alterations, Part I: Mechanisms of skin changes. *Oncol Nurs Forum* 19:801–807, 1992

58. Sitton E: Early and late radiation-induced skin alterations, Part II: Nursing care of irradiated skin. *Oncol Nurs Forum* 19:907–912, 1992

59. Bucholtz J: Radiolabeled antibody therapy, in Hassey-Dow K, Hilderley L (eds): *Nursing Care in Radiation Oncology*. Philadelphia, Saunders, 1992, pp 275–284

60. Macklis R: Radioimmunoconjugates and other target-selective therapeutic radiopharmaceuticals, in Mauch PM, Loeffler JS (eds). *Radiation Oncology, Technology and Biology*. Philadelphia, Saunders, 1994, pp 357–381

61. Liming PR: IORT perioperative nursing challenges. One hospital's experience. *Todays OR Nurse* 15:35–38, 1993

62. Stelzer KJ, Koh WJ, Greer B, et al: Intraoperative radiotherapy in soft tissue sarcomas. *Radiother Oncol* 34:160–163, 1995

63. Smith R: Intraoperative radiation therapy, in Hassey-Dow K, Hilderley L (eds): *Nursing Care in Radiation Oncology*. Philadelphia, Saunders, 1992, pp 295–306

64. Lichter AS, Ten Haken RK: Three-dimensional treatment planning and conformal radiation dose delivery, in De Vita VT, Hellman S, Rosenberg SA (eds): *Important Advances in Oncology 1995*. Philadelphia, Lippincott, 1995, pp 95–109

65. Armstrong JG: Three-dimensional conformal radiotherapy. Precision treatment of lung cancer (Review). *Chest Surg Clin North Am* 4:29–43, 1994

66. LoSasso T, Chui CS, Kutcher GJ, et al: The use of a multileaf collimator for conformal radiotherapy of carcinomas of the prostate and nasopharynx. *Int J Radiat Oncol Biol Phys* 25:161–170, 1993

67. Loeffler JS, Larson DA, Shrieve DC: Radiosurgery for intracranial lesions, in De Vita VT, Hellman S, Rosenberg SA (eds): *Important Advances in Oncology 1995*. Philadelphia, Lippincott, 1995, pp 141–156

68. Flickinger JC, Loeffler JS, Larson DA: Stereotactic radiosurgery for intracranial malignancies (Review). *Oncology* 8:81–86, 1994

# Chapter 14

# Chemotherapy: Principles of Therapy

Peter V. Tortorice, PharmD, BCPS

# HISTORICAL PERSPECTIVE

The term *chemotherapy* was first coined to describe the use of chemicals or drugs to treat microbial and later neoplastic diseases.[1] In the 1940s nitrogen mustard, the first cytotoxic drug, was introduced for cancer chemotherapy. Nitrogen mustard, a derivative of mustard gas used as a chemical deterrent in the two world wars, was developed as an antineoplastic agent after it was learned that soldiers exposed to this drug developed reversible leukopenia. Following soon after the introduction of nitrogen mustard, methotrexate, cyclophosphamide, and fluorouracil were made available for treatment of advanced cancers. Two significant developments occurred in the 1960s and late 1970s that opened the door for modern-day cancer chemotherapy; the first was the introduction of platinum-coordinated complexes as cytotoxic therapy, and later was the introduction of combination chemotherapy to improve response rates and survival without significantly affecting toxicity.[2]

The screening, synthesis, and clinical testing of new compounds or analogues of currently active agents continued through the 1970s and 1980s. Among the most useful agents discovered during this period were the semisynthetic podophyllotoxin etoposide, and the natural product paclitaxel isolated from the western yew tree. The development of the anthracycline analogue doxorubicin also had a significant impact on the treatment of breast cancer and sarcomas. The biologic response modifiers were first recognized as having antineoplastic activity in the 1980s. The search for new agents to treat cancer continues into the 21st century.

Currently strategies being emphasized for drug development in the 1990s include drugs with novel mechanisms of action, drugs that avoid or reverse drug resistance, and drugs used for supportive care of the cancer patient. Supportive therapies that have made administering and managing chemotherapy easier and safer include simple and effective antiemetic therapy and hematopoietic growth factors.

Historically the goals of early chemotherapy were primarily limited to palliation of symptoms. An increase in available agents and more experience with cytotoxic therapy produced significant tumor regression and control of cancer. The development and acceptance of combination chemotherapy greatly improved the outcome of otherwise incurable neoplastic diseases. This approach to cancer treatment incorporated the theoretical point that targeting multiple biochemical processes would have a greater overall effect on tumor regression and remission. The goals of chemotherapy shifted to a curative approach for those cancers in which complete responses to chemotherapy were seen. Table 14-1 lists those cancers for which cures and increases in survival have been accomplished using chemotherapy alone or in combination with other modalities of treatment such as surgery and radiation therapy.[2] Although chemotherapy has produced cures in a subset of patients with some cancers such as acute leukemia,

**TABLE 14-1**  Chemotherapy Outcomes of Specific Cancers

| Curable Cancers |
| --- |
| *Type of Cancer (cure rate)* |
| Acute lymphoblastic leukemia in children (75%) |
| Acute lymphoblastic leukemia in adults (40%) |
| Acute myeloblastic leukemia (15%) |
| Burkitt's lymphoma (50%) |
| Diffuse histiocytic lymphoma (50%) |
| Gestational trophoblastic tumors (60%–90%) |
| Hodgkin's disease (80%) |
| Osteogenic sarcoma (65%) |
| Rhabdomyosarcoma (70%) |
| Testicular carcinoma (90%) |
| Wilms' tumor (65%) |

| Cancers with Complete Remission and Potentially Increased Survival |
| --- |
| *Type of Cancer* |
| Breast cancer |
| Chronic granulocytic leukemia |
| Multiple myeloma |
| Neuroblastoma |
| Ovarian cancer |
| Prostate cancer |
| Small-cell lung cancer |

Hodgkin's disease, and testicular tumors, significant cure rates for the most common cancers such as breast cancer, lung cancer, and colon cancer have not been achieved.

The use of drugs to control or eradicate cancer has developed into the specialization of medical oncology. The treatment of individuals with cancer is probably one of the most rapidly expanding and dynamic fields in medicine and demands continuous reevaluation and reappraisal of new as well as established therapies. To continue to develop and improve cancer treatment, more patients need to participate in controlled clinical trials. It is estimated that less than 10% of eligible patients actively being treated for cancer are enrolled in clinical trials. The clinician is a key figure in encouraging cooperation not only from the patient and his or her family but also from the health care community, including providers and sponsors (third-party payers). Increased survival and, more important, the maintenance or improvement of quality of life for patients with cancer can be achieved with the appropriate use of chemotherapy.

# CANCER CHEMOTHERAPY DRUG DEVELOPMENT

Drug discovery and the eventual development of cancer treatment compounds involve numerous strategies. The most successful methods seek to combine current knowledge of the biology of cancer and the pharmacological properties of potentially therapeutic compounds. Synthesis and testing of analogues of compounds with known antineoplastic activity is one of the approaches that has had some success. Synthesis of chemically or mechanistically similar compounds with different pharmacokinetic or toxic properties has yielded clinically useful new agents. An example of this approach may be found with the introduction of the new camptothecins topotecan and irinotecan. Both agents are effective topoisomerase I inhibitors but lack the unpredictable urotoxicity seen with earlier camptothecin derivatives. Another approach to developing new antineoplastic agents is further identifying the proposed mechanism of action for previously identified active compounds. The elucidation of the specific effects of paclitaxel on tubulin formation and the identification of etoposide as a topoisomerase inhibitor are examples of this approach to drug development.

The oncology research community is composed of national and local study groups, university-based research programs, and pharmaceutical manufacturers. The National Cancer Institute (NCI) assists in coordinating the massive efforts of researchers and clinicians in screening and developing drugs for use in cancer treatment. A significant amount of research and development is also conducted outside the NCI primarily by pharmaceutical manufacturers.

The drug approval process in the United States is very rigorous and comprehensive. New compounds undergo extensive testing in animals and then in humans before becoming commercially available for general medical practice. Because of the unique and potentially life-threatening toxicities associated with antineoplastic drugs, this approval process may become both lengthy and expensive. The average time and cost to bring a drug to market may be 10–12 years and $40–$80 million, respectively.

## Preclinical Evaluation

The National Cancer Institute coordinates the screening of over 10,000 compounds each year in an attempt to find new and potentially useful drugs for treating cancer.[3] Less than 1% of screened compounds proceed to clinical trials. Compounds with known or suspected antineoplastic activity are screened by a number of methods, including transplantable rodent tumor models. Positive compounds are further evaluated against a panel of human tumor cell lines grown in defined media.[4] Cell lines in use include lung, ovarian, and renal cell cancer; malignant melanoma; brain tumors; and leukemias. Because of the interest in the impact drug resistance may have on chemotherapy effectiveness, a multidrug resistant (MDR) variant of a human breast cancer and murine leukemia cell lines are also available for testing.[5]

Compounds having demonstrated significant antineoplastic activity then undergo preclinical toxicology studies. The purpose of these studies is to determine a safe starting dose for use in humans. The lethal dose in 10% of animals tested ($LD_{10}$) is then used to calculate a starting

dose for clinical trials. Although mice are the primary toxicology test animal, the dose determined for clinical trials is first tested in dogs to avoid excessive risk to humans. Body surface area (BSA) is the preferred reference point used for making interspecies dose comparisons.

## Phase I Trials

The primary objective of the first phase of clinical testing is to determine a maximum tolerated dose (MTD) for one or more schedules of drug administration. Although normal volunteers are usually recruited for phase I testing, because of the potential for significant toxicity with antineoplastic drugs, patients with advanced cancer are instead enrolled in these trials. These patients may also benefit from these new therapies. Dosing starts at 10% of the $LD_{10}$ determined in mice and is escalated until significant toxicity is seen in 50% or more of the patients treated. This dose is the MTD, and one step below the MTD is used for phase II testing. Another approach to dose escalation uses a concentration-time curve and is based on achieving a systemic exposure similar to what was seen in preclinical animal studies. This method may be more efficient in conducting a dose escalation study and is being tested in NCI phase I trials.

Pharmacological and pharmacokinetic studies are also done in this phase. Data from these trials will help determine the most effective dose and administration schedule for subsequent trials.[6] Prohibitive and excessive toxicity is often cause to discontinue further clinical testing.

## Phase II Trials

Identifying activity of a new drug in a specified tumor type is the primary objective of phase II clinical trials. The ideal patients for phase II testing are previously untreated; however, most tend to be patients who have shown little or no response to previous chemotherapy. Other information about the drug is gathered, such as administration techniques, identifying and managing acute toxicity, and supportive care.

A drug may be dropped from further testing for a number of reasons, including lack of sufficient responsiveness or excessive or intolerable toxicity. Usually response rates of higher than 20% indicate the agent may have therapeutic usefulness and warrant further clinical testing. Sufficient testing is also done on a number of possible doses and administration schedules before a compound is eliminated. Drugs found to be effective when given at certain doses and schedules in specific tumors then enter phase III testing before Food and Drug Administration (FDA) approval for marketing.

## Phase III Trials

In phase III testing new drugs are tested as single agents or combined with other drugs and compared with the standard treatment for a specific tumor. Traditionally response rates, duration of response, survival, and toxicity are measured; however, quality of life has also become the focus of clinical trials. Phase III trials typically require a large number of patients to be treated and observed over a prolonged time period before final results are available. At the conclusion of phase III testing it should be known if the new treatment is better than the standard therapy in terms of response, survival, toxicity, and what impact it has on the patient's quality of life. The actual role the new drug or drug combination will have in treatment may be further determined in postmarketing evaluations.

### Phase IV Trials

Clinical trials carried out following the FDA approval of a drug are referred to as *postmarketing* or *phase IV studies*. Trials are usually designed to answer questions regarding other uses, doses, and schedules of commercially available drugs, as well as new information regarding risks and toxicity of a new treatment. Phase IV studies generally involve the use of drugs in combination with other therapies where cure is the goal of treatment.

## SCIENTIFIC BASIS OF CHEMOTHERAPY

Researchers have only recently begun to identify what is thought to be the primary pharmacological activity for many antineoplastic agents.[7,8] The actual mechanism or combination of mechanisms responsible for killing tumor cells remain elusive. This disparity is in part a function of the lack of a clear understanding of how cancer cells originate, grow, and regress. The following section will address tumor cell biology and how chemotherapeutic drugs may selectively exert their cytotoxicity.

### The Cell Cycle

Much of what is known regarding the effects of cytotoxic chemotherapy relies on understanding the cell cycle. The cycle is made of five phases: $G_1$, S, $G_2$, M, and $G_0$. The phases describe periods of time for different cellular processes that ultimately result in a cell's reproduction or death (Figure 14-1). In any population, only some cells are actively proliferating. The *growth fraction* is the portion of cells actively cycling compared to the entire population. Following mitosis, a cell can do any one of the following: leave the cycle, differentiate, and eventually die; enter a resting state ($G_0$) and reenter the cycle at some later time (stem cells); or enter the $G_1$ phase and continue to cycle. Synthesis of RNA and proteins occurs predominantly in the $G_1$ phase. *Synthesis*, or *S phase*, is

when DNA is being replicated and is a relatively short period compared with the overall time a cell is cycling. The $G_2$ *phase* is typically brief, occurring after DNA synthesis and just before cell division. *Mitosis*, or *cell division*, ensues during the *M phase*, resulting in two identical daughter cells. The time from mitosis to mitosis is described as the *cycling time*. Cells that have left the cycle to enter $G_0$ are considered in a *resting* or *dormant phase*. These cells can actively synthesize RNA and proteins and differentiate; however, they are typically resistant to the cytotoxic effects of chemotherapy.

### Tumor Cell Kinetics

Tumor cells may be distinguished from cells of normal tissues by their loss of controlled cell division, lack of differentiation, and ability to invade surrounding tissues and establish new growth at distant sites in the body. Theoretically, most antineoplastic agents utilize the rapid proliferation rate of tumor cells as a target for their cytotoxic effects. This is also the mechanism of many of the toxicities seen in cells of normal tissues since they are also going through the cell cycle and dividing, but at a much slower rate. A kinetic model has been developed to explain the selective effects of antineoplastic drugs on both normal and tumor cells.[9] The model states that tumor growth is often exponential, doubling times vary widely between tumors, and chemotherapy-sensitive tumors tend to grow faster than slow-growing tumors that are less responsive to chemotherapy.

Doubling time of both malignant and normal tissues is widely variable. The factors that affect doubling time are cell cycle time; growth fraction; cell loss by either cell death (apoptosis) or differentiation or metastasis.[10] Cells with a rapid cycling time and a tumor with a large growth fraction should be the most responsive to cytotoxic therapy.[11] Table 14-2 classifies some normal tissues and tumors by their doubling time. Although tumor cells may exhibit rapid cycling, the rate is not higher than what is seen with normal renewal tissues such as the bone marrow and gastrointestinal mucosa. Therefore, uncontrolled cell division is not the primary distinguishing trait of tumor cells. Loss of homeostatic mechanisms such as contact inhibition and cell differentiation and maturation leads to an increased proliferative rate, which exceeds cell death.[12] This leads to the accumulation of tumor cells.

### The Effects of Chemotherapy on Tumor Cells

#### Cell kill hypothesis

The cell kill hypothesis is a basic principle often used to describe the effects of cancer chemotherapy on normal and tumor cells. The hypothesis describes a first-order kinetic process that predicts the number of cells killed

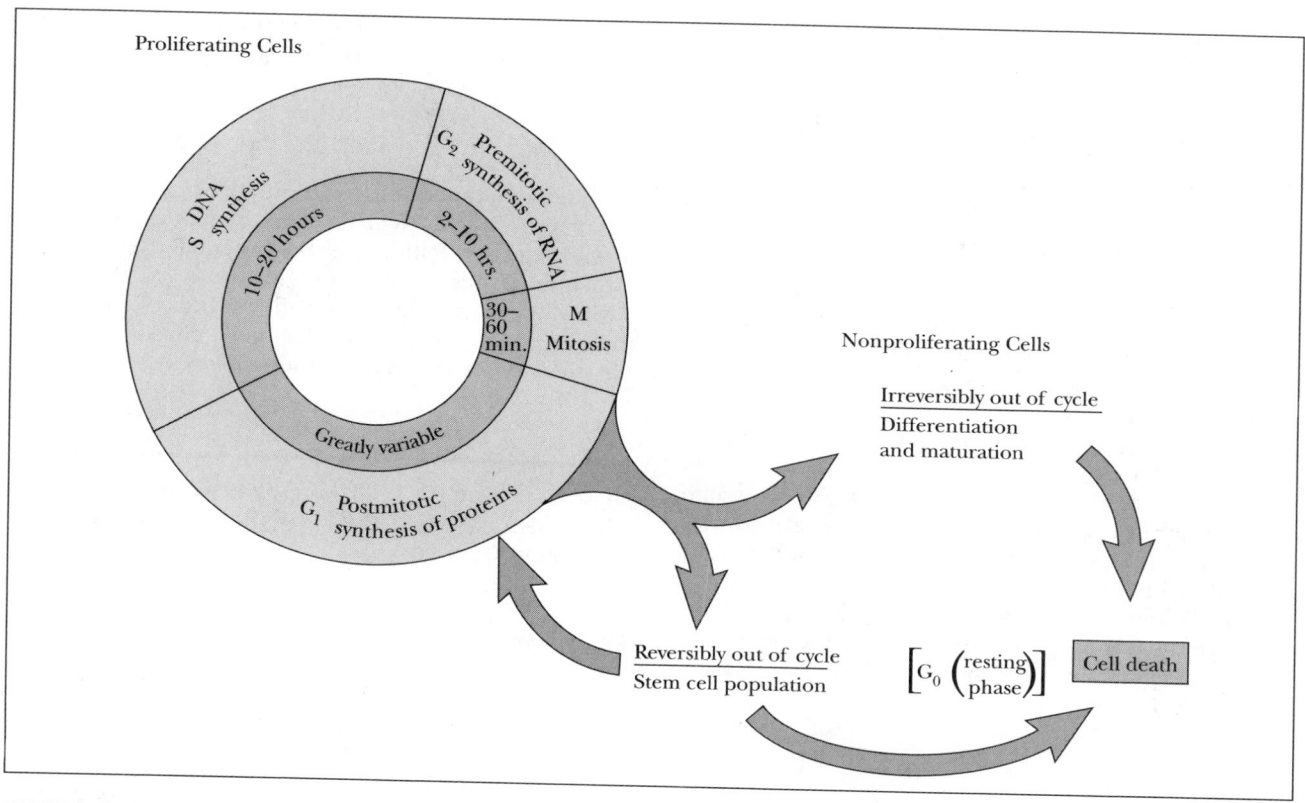

**FIGURE 14-1** Diagrammatic representation of the life of a cell emphasizing the relationships between the cell cycle and proliferating and nonproliferating cells.

**TABLE 14-2**   A Comparison of Doubling Time for Some Normal Tissue and Common Tumors

| Doubling Time | Normal Tissues | Malignant Tumors |
|---|---|---|
| Short (3–4 weeks) | Gastrointestinal mucosa<br>Bone marrow<br>Ovary<br>Testis | Burkitt's lymphoma<br>Testicular germ cell tumors<br>Acute myelogenous leukemia |
| Intermediate (4–6 weeks) | Skin<br>Hair follicles<br>Endocrine glands | Small-cell lung cancer<br>Hodgkin's disease<br>Malignant lymphomas |
| Long (8–12 weeks) | Liver<br>Kidney<br>Lung | Breast cancer<br>Non–small-cell lung cancer<br>Colon cancer |

Data from Steel GG: *Growth Kinetics of Tumours: Cell Population Kinetics in Relation to the Growth and Treatment of Cancer.* Oxford, Clarendon Press, 1977; and Charbit A, Malaise EP, Tubiana M: Relation between the pathological nature and the growth rate of human tumors. *Eur J Cancer,* 7:307–315, 1971.

based on the dose of chemotherapy given. The hypothesis applies only to cells that are actively proliferating and assumes treatment sensitivity does not change and growth rate is constant. A model of this concept was originally described by Skipper and Schabel in the early 1960s[13,14] using a leukemia L1210 tumor in mice. The cell kill model is based on a log-kill relationship for dose of chemotherapy and a constant proportion of cells killed per treatment. If a given drug at a given dose produces a 1-log kill or a 90% reduction, then a tumor of $1 \times 10^5$ will be decreased to $1 \times 10^4$. A treatment with a 3-log kill is necessary to produce a tumor reduction of 99.9%. Essentially, no treatment can completely reduce the number of tumor cells to zero. Although the number of cells is reduced by a 1-log, the net effect on viable tumor cells is surviving cells plus regrowth before the next treatment. Because of these limitations, Skipper's model is not applicable to most human tumors. Malignancies that do follow this model include Burkitt's lymphoma and germ cell tumors. The cell kill hypothesis is still used today in determining tumor cell growth inhibition of newly derived cancer treatment compounds.

## Gompertzian curve

The effect of antineoplastic drugs on human tumors cannot be fully explained by the cell kill model since not all tumor cells are in a proliferative state. A Gompertzian growth curve (Figure 14-2) probably best describes the growth of human tumors and the responses observed with the administration of antineoplastic drugs.[5] Tumor growth fraction and proliferative rate are not constant but instead decrease with time as a tumor goes from a small, undetectable clump of cells to a large mass. The doubling time of a tumor increases as the mass increases in size. Eventually the tumor reaches a growth plateau phase where further increase in size becomes minimal because of the slower doubling time.

The Gompertzian curve is also useful in describing the observed tumor response to chemotherapy.[15] If cytotoxic chemotherapy is given in the growth phase of the tumor, the portion of cells actively proliferating (growth fraction) is large; therefore, a high percentage of cells will be susceptible to the effects of the drugs. However, in a more advanced stage of the disease, when growth has reached a plateau, fewer cells will be dividing and thereby less susceptible to chemotherapy.

When surgery or radiation therapy has been utilized to reduce the tumor mass, chemotherapy may be useful in eradicating remaining residual and micrometastatic disease.[16,17] However, since metastatic cells are often the result of numerous prior divisions, the possibility that either primary or secondary drug resistance has developed is significant.

### Mechanisms and sites of action of chemotherapy

Chemotherapeutic drugs induce their cytotoxicity on tumor cells and normal tissue by one or more mechanisms. Figure 14-3 illustrates the potential sites and proposed mechanisms of action for many of the drugs currently available for cancer chemotherapy. Central to the diagram is the genetic machinery, considered to be the focus for most effective cytotoxic drugs.

## CHEMOTHERAPY DRUG SELECTION AND FACTORS AFFECTING RESPONSE TO CHEMOTHERAPY

There is wide interpatient variability in both therapeutic response and unacceptable toxicity observed in patients receiving chemotherapy. This variability may be explained by differences in factors involving the patient with cancer, the chemotherapy being given, and the type of tumor being treated.

### Patient Factors

Patient factors include toxicity response, organ dysfunction, previous treatment, and age. The occurrence and severity of toxicity are widely variable between patients and often necessitate chemotherapy dose reduction or treatment delay. Preexisting organ dysfunction such as renal or hepatic insufficiency may also require dose or schedule alteration or preclude using known effective antineoplastic drugs. Patients who have received previous chemotherapy may not be candidates to receive the same drug again or a drug with similar toxicity. Drug toxicity may influence the choice of chemotherapy. For example, receiving more than the recommended maximum lifetime dose of the anthracycline drug doxorubicin greatly increases the patient's risk for developing severe cardiomyopathy. Drugs with similar toxicities such as neurotoxicity must be avoided in patients with preexisting neurological defects. Previous bone marrow transplant or the use of severely marrow-toxic drugs may preclude the use of full doses of myelosuppressive drugs. All these factors may have an adverse effect on the patient's antineoplastic response and the overall potential to cure or control the cancer.

### Drug Factors

Antineoplastic activity, pharmacokinetics, dose, and schedule are important drug factors that can influence

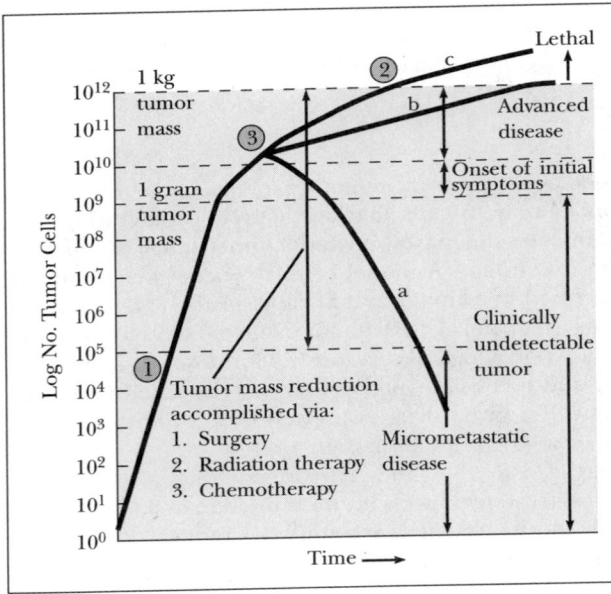

**FIGURE 14-2** Gompertzian Tumor Growth Curve: relationship of tumor mass, diagnosis, symptoms, and potential treatment regimens. Growth phases and chemotherapy response: 1) log phase (high growth fraction, short doubling time); 2) plateau phase (low growth fraction, longer doubling time); 3) initiation of chemotherapy treatments: a. tumor cells responsive to drugs; b. tumor exhibits initial response to treatment but develops resistance (secondary or somatic resistance); c. tumor unresponsive to drug regimen (primary resistance). Data adapted with permission from Buick RN: Cellular basis of chemotherapy, in Dorr RT, Von Hoff DD (eds): *Cancer Chemotherapy Handbook* (ed 2). Norwalk, CT, Appleton & Lange, 1994, pp 3–14.

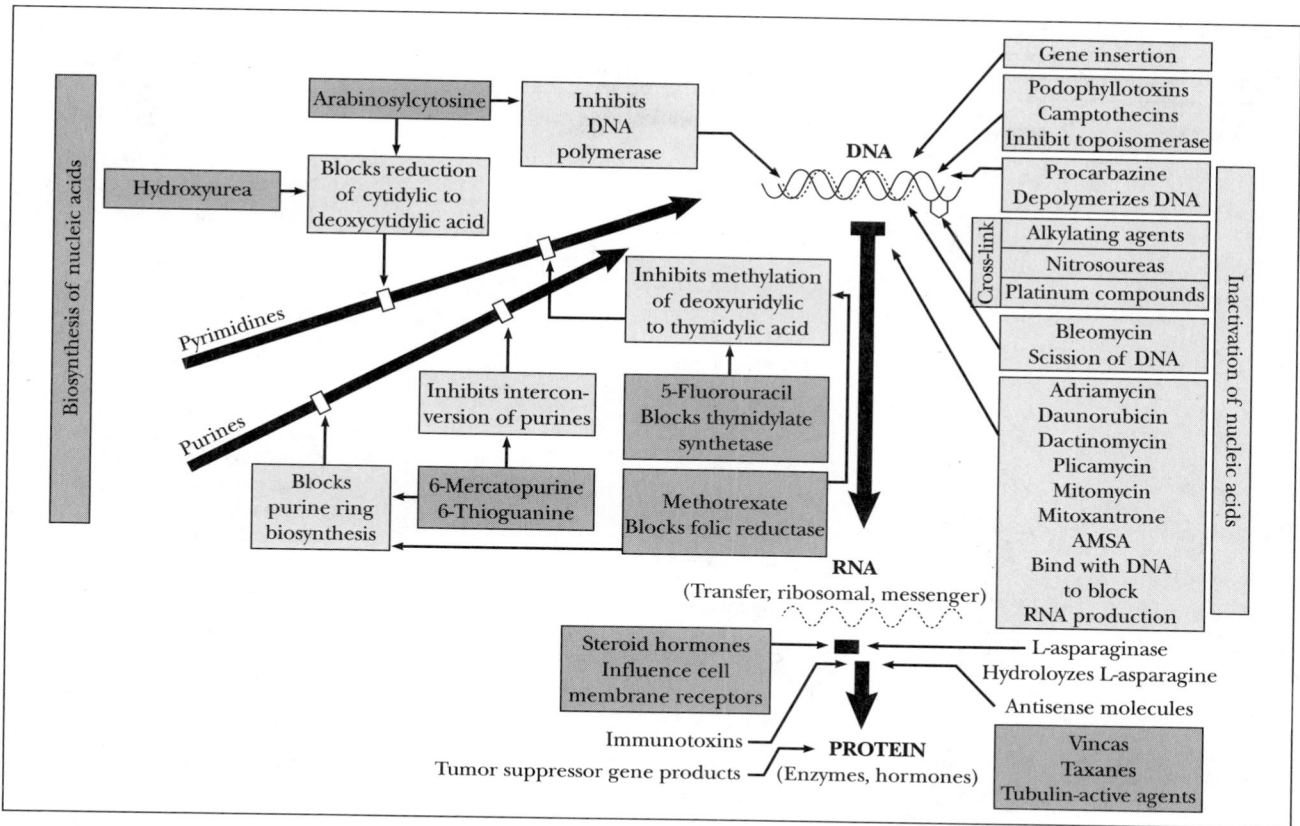

**FIGURE 14-3** Proposed mechanisms of action for chemotherapeutic drugs. From Krakoff IH: Systemic treatment of cancer. *CA Cancer J Clin* 46: 134–141, 1996. Printed with permission.

chemotherapy response and toxicity. The relative cytotoxicity of any antineoplastic drug is dependent on the origin of the tumor and the presence of intrinsic drug resistance.[5] Intrinsic resistance is probably a type of generic defense mechanism present in cells of certain histological type. Pharmacokinetic factors determine the ability of chemotherapeutic drugs to reach their cellular targets. Changes in these factors such as decreased metabolic activation or increased drug clearance from the body may decrease antitumor response. Similarly, alterations in protein binding of certain drugs such as etoposide or teniposide may enhance clinical toxicity. Poorly lipophilic drugs administered systemically are ineffective for tumors found in lipophilic tissues such as the central nervous system. Administration of drugs such as methotrexate or cytarabine directly into the intrathecal space will circumvent this obstacle. The ability to deliver the optimal dose of chemotherapy for a specific cancer is often limited by the maximally tolerated dose. The clinical use of hematopoietic growth factors such as granulocyte colony-stimulating factor (G-CSF) and granulocyte-macrophage colony-stimulating factor (GM-CSF) has allowed the dose of severely myelotoxic drugs to be escalated in an attempt to improve response.

## Tumor Factors

Tumor growth and size significantly influence the response to chemotherapy. As previously discussed, larger tumors have small growth fractions and are therefore less responsive to the cytotoxic effects of antineoplastic drugs. The ability of chemotherapy to reach large solid tumors may be hindered by inadequate blood flow. Surgical excision or debulking of tumors can increase the responsiveness of these tumors by recruiting more cells into the proliferative phase.

Chemotherapy response is also influenced by tumor cell histology. Table 14-3 differentiates tumor types by their sensitivity to chemotherapy and what outcomes may be expected in patients successfully treated with chemotherapy. Selectivity of certain types of malignancies for specific chemotherapeutic agents is also seen. Fluorouracil is most active in cancers of endodermal tissue such as gastrointestinal and breast neoplasms. Epithelial tumors such as squamous cell cancers are especially sensitive to the cytotoxic effects of bleomycin. As discussed previously, tumor location may present a dilemma for optimal chemotherapy administration, and special administration techniques must be utilized to achieve significant chemotherapy responses.

**TABLE 14-3**   Chemotherapy-Sensitive Tumors

| Relative Chemosensitivity | Expected Survival Outcome | Type of Cancer |
| --- | --- | --- |
| Highly | Normal survival, possible cure | Acute leukemia in children<br>Hodgkin's disease<br>Diffuse large-cell lymphoma<br>Burkitt's lymphoma<br>Testicular carcinoma<br>Embryonal carcinoma<br>Ewing's sarcoma<br>Wilms' tumor<br>Skin cancer |
| Moderately | Increase in survival | Ovarian carcinoma<br>Breast carcinoma<br>Endometrial carcinoma<br>Acute leukemia in adults<br>Small-cell lung cancer<br>Prostate cancer<br>Stomach cancer<br>Cervical cancer<br>Neuroblastoma |
| Minimally | Some increase in survival | Head and neck cancers<br>Gastrointestinal cancers<br>Endocrine gland tumors<br>Malignant melanoma<br>Osteogenic sarcoma<br>Soft-tissue sarcoma |
| Marginally | No documented increase in survival | Bladder cancer<br>Esophageal cancer<br>Non–small-cell lung cancer<br>Pancreatic carcinoma<br>Hepatocellular carcinoma |

DeVita VT, Young RC, Canellos GP: Combination versus single agent chemotherapy: A review of the basis for selection of drug treatment of cancer. *Cancer,* 35:98–110, 1975. Copyright © 1975 American Cancer Society. Reprinted by permission of Wiley-Liss, Inc., a subsidiary of John Wiley & Sons, Inc.

## LACK OF RESPONSE TO CHEMOTHERAPY AND STRATEGIES TO OVERCOME TREATMENT FAILURE

### Theoretical Basis for Chemotherapy Resistance

The failure of chemotherapy to control tumor growth and induce a remission is one of the most important problems facing the oncology clinician today. Several theories and models have been developed to explain this phenomenon. The previously described cell kill model served as an early attempt to explain neoplastic cell growth and lack of response to cytotoxic chemotherapy. According to the model, increasing the dose of a cytotoxic drug or adding other drugs results in an increase in cell kill. Therefore, failure of chemotherapy to eradicate a tumor is the result of inadequate dose intensity or the presence of biochemically resistant tumor cells. Although this theory is applicable to tumor regression, clinical data do not necessarily support this concept.[15] Another possible explanation for treatment failures is the stem cell concept. Stem cells continually produce progeny that go on to become mature cells but themselves do not differentiate. Stem cells constitute a small portion of the total population of cells. Therefore, eradicating the stem cell population would theoretically eliminate the source of malignant cells and induce tumor regression. However, this must be accomplished without greatly increasing the rate of genetic mutation and producing other biochemically resistant stem cell lines.

Currently the most popular explanation for chemotherapy treatment failures is the development of drug resistance. The genetic instability of tumor cells with high mitotic rates is possibly responsible for the emergence of resistant clones within a population of tumor cells. A quantitative explanation of this process was first described by Goldie and Coldman in 1979.[18,19] Treatment failure could be explained by the existence of drug-resistant cells that resulted from random genetic mutations occurring before or during cytotoxic chemotherapy. The best chance for curing cancer would be to apply effective drugs early to reduce the total number of cancer cells while preventing resistant cells from developing, thus supporting the established concepts of combination chemotherapy.[20]

Tumors that recur following effective initial treatment often present a treatment dilemma. Disease that recurs within six months usually is considered resistant to initial chemotherapy, and an alternative drug regimen is used. However, recurrence more than six months following treatment may be successfully treated with the same or similar chemotherapy regimen. This phenomenon may be explained by either the reversion of resistant cells to drug-sensitive cells, or the predominance of initially sensitive cells in the relapsed tumor.[15] Although the Goldie-Coldman model presents an important concept of quantitative drug resistance, the assumptions are not always applicable to human tumors. Continued diligence in exploring the mechanisms behind chemotherapy treatment failure is a goal of modern chemotherapy.

## Cytotoxic Drug Resistance

Although patient and drug factors play an important role in response to chemotherapy, genetic instability of the tumor cell and emergence of resistance are currently considered the most significant determinants of response.[21] Since it is unlikely the biology of the disease or genetic composition of the tumor can be altered, strategies for overcoming resistance need to be developed and implemented. However, without a clear concept of how resistance develops or how to prevent it, strategies for overcoming drug resistance are slow to be applied in clinical practice.

Cytotoxic drug resistance may be expressed as a temporary or permanent insensitivity to one or more antineoplastic drugs. Temporary resistance is usually observed only in vivo with drugs known to be active against a specific cancer. Tumor location and adequate blood supply may adversely affect chemotherapy outcomes. Large tumors are usually poorly vascularized and thereby less accessible to systemically administered cytotoxic therapy. Tumors located in anatomic sanctuary sites such as the central nervous system or testes are poorly reached with standard chemotherapy. Altered pharmacokinetic parameters such as decreased metabolic activation or increased clearance from the body will affect therapeutic outcome. As yet undefined host defense mechanisms may also have a negative impact on treatment success. In some conditions temporary resistance may be reversed by altering drug delivery, dose, or scheduling of drug administration.

Permanent or phenotypic drug resistance, an inheritable resistance mechanism, is the result of a genetic mutation or preexisting trait.[22] This form of resistance may be present prior to treatment (primary resistance) or may develop after exposure to antineoplastic drugs (secondary resistance). Cytotoxic drug resistance may develop from genetic changes such as point mutations or gene amplification. Point mutations usually occur in a single cell and are independent of drug concentration. Gene amplification is influenced by drug concentration and occurs with repeated exposure over an extended period of time. Expression of the *mdr-1* gene is thought to be responsible for the development of multidrug resistance (MDR).[23,24]

### Biological basis of phenotypic drug resistance

Phenotypic drug resistance is probably a major factor contributing to chemotherapy failure.[25] Goldie and Coldman proposed that drug resistance arises from spontaneous genetic mutations that regularly occur in a population of tumor cells.[22,26,27] Their model was based on Luria and Delbruck's observations of the development of acquired resistance in bacteria.[28] A mutational origin appears responsible for the development of antibiotic resistance in bacterial cells, which is analogous to cytotoxic drug resistance observed in tumor cells. Antibiotics or cytotoxic drugs selectively kill sensitive cells and leave behind phenotypically resistant cells that reproduce and expand the tumor volume. This process has been demonstrated in mouse lymphoma cells, which exhibited resistance to folic acid antagonist after exposure to methotrexate.[29]

The development of drug resistance is dependent on the spontaneous mutation rate of tumor cells, the timing of a significant mutation relative to the tumor's growth, and overall tumor burden. All biological systems have an inherent probability of undergoing genetic variation from random changes. These random changes may result in minor effects, no effect, or a mutation that alters the cell's characteristics and sensitivity to cytotoxic drugs. Neoplastic cells are genetically unstable and exhibit a high rate of mutation. If mutations occur early in the growth of a population of tumor cells, a high fraction of resistant cells would result. A mutation occurring later would produce only a small fraction of resistant clones. If no resistant cells develop prior to treatment, then a cure would be probable with the appropriate chemotherapy. Cytotoxic therapy directed at minimal tumor burden has a much greater likelihood of being successful.

The Goldie and Coldman model provides a strong argument for the use of adjuvant and combination chemotherapy. Adjuvant chemotherapy is used in an attempt to eradicate undetectable or micrometastatic tumor cells. If the probability of cure decreases as the number of tumor cells or the mutation rate increases, then eliminating all possible cells or clones should induce a cure or a complete response. The model also supports the use of combination chemotherapy with non–cross-resistant drugs to potentially eliminate subpopulations of resistant tumor cells. The chance of a cell being resistant to two or more antineoplastic drugs simultaneously is less than that of being resistant to single agents when used alone.

### Mechanisms of drug resistance

Tumor cells exposed to antineoplastic drugs sometimes develop mechanisms to protect themselves against the drug's cytotoxic effect. Table 14-4 lists known mechanisms of resistance and the drugs most often affected. Resistance may result from alterations in cytotoxic drug metabolism, including decreased activation of pro-drugs such as cyclophosphamide and increased breakdown of active compounds such as the deamination of purine and pyrimidine analogues.[32] Decreased intracellular availability of a biochemical cofactor will significantly reduce the cytotoxicity of certain antineoplastic drugs. An example of this mechanism is seen with the lack of reduced folates and resistance to fluorouracil seen in colon and rectal tumor cells. Alterations in cytotoxic targets are other ways cells become resistant to antineoplastic drugs. Cancer cells can overcome the effects of cytotoxic drugs either by increasing the amount of target enzymes or by modifying the enzyme so as to interfere with binding to antagonistic drugs. Enzyme systems that exhibit this type of resistance include dihydrofolate reductase, thymidylate synthase, and topoisomerase II.[33–35] The ability of cells to repair DNA lesions such as strand breaks, errors in base pairing, and premature chain termination is an important resistance mechanism seen with alkylating agents and cisplatin.[36] Intracellular drug concentrations may be significantly reduced as a result of decreased influx carrier proteins, enhanced efflux pump functioning, or both. The most familiar example of this mechanism of cytotoxic drug resistance is the P-glycoprotein (P-gp) efflux pump associated with overexpression of the MDR gene.[23]

**TABLE 14-4** Possible Mechanisms of Cytotoxic Drug Resistance

| Type of Resistance | Mechanism of Resistance | Drugs Involved |
|---|---|---|
| Drug metabolism | Reduced drug activation | Cytarabine Fluorouracil 6-Mercaptopurine Methotrexate |
| | Increased drug deactivation | Alkylating agents Cytarabine Doxorubicin |
| Cytotoxic targets | Increased enzyme levels | Fluorouracil Methotrexate |
| | Alteration in enzyme-substrate binding | Doxorubicin Etoposide Fluorouracil 6-Mercaptopurine Methotrexate |
| Biochemical modification | Use of alternative (salvage) pathways | Cytarabine Fluorouracil 6-Mercaptopurine Methotrexate |
| | Decreased cofactor concentrations (reduced folate pool) | Fluorouracil |
| DNA repair systems | Increased DNA repair | Alkylating agents Cisplatin Mitomycin |
| Intracellular drug concentration | Decreased cellular uptake | Mechlorethamine Methotrexate |
| | Increased efflux (P-glycoprotein mediated) | Anthracycline antibiotics Etoposide Paclitaxel Vinca alkaloids |

Data from Yarbro JW: The scientific basis of cancer chemotherapy, in Perry MC (ed): *Chemotherapy Source Book*, Baltimore, Williams & Wilkins, 1992, pp 2–14; and Buick RN: Cellular basis of chemotherapy, in Dorr RT and Von Hoff DD (eds): *Cancer Chemotherapy Handbook* (ed 2). Norwalk, CT, Appleton & Lange, 1994, pp 3–14.

## Multidrug-resistance phenotype

Tumor cells that exhibit resistance to a group of drugs that are structurally dissimilar, with unrelated cytotoxic mechanisms, or both are expressing a MDR phenotype. Resistance usually develops intrinsically or is acquired following exposure to a particular drug in the group.[37] MDR may occur as a result of overexpression of P-gp membrane efflux pump, enhancements of the glutathione detoxification pathway, or alterations in topoisomerase enzyme systems. The identification and further investigation of this type of resistance and strategies to prevent MDR will have broad clinical implications for the use of chemotherapy as a form of cancer treatment.

The classic form of MDR is associated with overexpression of *mdr-1* gene, which encodes for an energy-dependent cell membrane efflux pump, P-gp. This phenomenon was first described in tumor cells selected for resistance to dactinomycin that also exhibited resistance to vinca alkaloids, daunorubicin, and mitomycin.[37] Figure 14-4 is a model of P-gp structure. The pump naturally functions to transport toxic molecules from inside the cell to the external environment and is found in low concentrations in normal tissues, including the renal tubules, colon, small intestine, bile canaliculi, and vascular epithelia of the brain and spinal cord.[38–40] Cytotoxic drugs that have entered the cell probably bind to a carrier protein before reaching their cellular targets, and are transported out of the cell via the pump.[41] The actual process of drug binding and extruding from the cell is unknown. Currently the list of drugs exhibiting P-gp-associated cross-resistance include several natural products and an antimetabolite (Table 14-5).

Levels of P-gp have been found in many human tumors, including acute and chronic leukemias, ovarian cancer, multiple myeloma, breast cancer, soft-tissue sarcomas, renal cell carcinoma, and small-cell lung cancer.[42–45] Their presence has typically been associated with prior cytotoxic therapy, intrinsically resistant tumors, and inferior treatment outcomes. The detection of the *mdr-1* gene product from cells of tumors typically resistant to chemotherapy, such as colon, kidney, liver, and pancreas, further supports the importance of P-

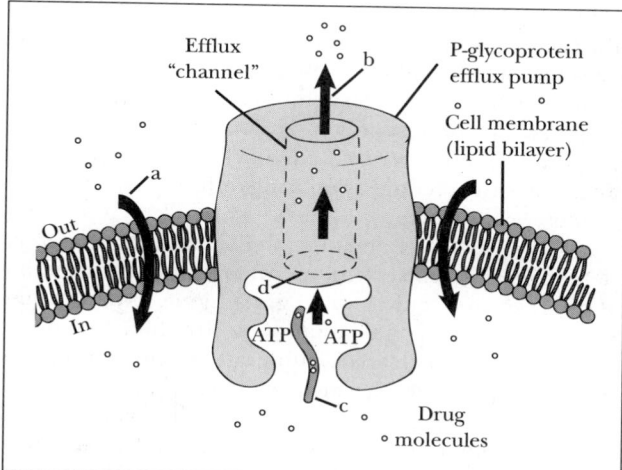

**FIGURE 14-4**  Model of P-glycoprotein as an energy-dependent (ATP) drug efflux pump.
Key: a. drug influx; b. drug efflux via p-glycoprotein "channel"; c. possible carrier protein-assisted efflux; d. possible site for binding of pump inhibitors.
In this model, drugs enter the cell by diffusing across the lipid bilayer (a), drugs bind directly to P-glycoprotein and are transported out of cell (b), drugs bind to a carrier protein and are transported out of cell (c), and efflux may be inhibited by the binding of chemosensitizers (d). Adapted from Dalton WS: Overcoming the Multidrug-Resistant Phenotype, in DeVita VT, Hellman S, Rosenberg SA (eds): *Cancer: Principles and Practice of Oncology* (ed 4). J.B. Lippincott Co., 1993, pp 2655–2666. Adapted with permission.

**TABLE 14-5**  Chemotherapeutic Drugs Exhibiting Cross-Resistance in P-Glycoprotein Associated Multidrug Resistance

| |
|---|
| Dactinomycin |
| Daunorubicin |
| Doxorubicin |
| Etoposide |
| Mitomycin |
| Mitoxantrone |
| Paclitaxel |
| Trimetrexate |
| Vinblastine |
| Vincristine |

Data from Dalton WS: Overcoming the multidrug-resistant phenotype, in DeVita VT, Hellman S, Rosenberg SA (eds): *Cancer: Principles and Practice of Oncology* (ed 4). Philadelphia, J. B. Lippincott Co., 1993, pp 2655–2666.

gp and chemotherapy failure.[45] Therefore, further understanding and elucidating the structure and function of P-gp will contribute to the strategies to overcome this type of resistance. A second mechanism of MDR also associated with increased drug efflux but not P-gp mediated has been described.[46] Some cell lines have increased expression of a protein that likely functions as a drug transporter similar to P-gp. This multidrug resistance-associated protein (MRP) gene confers resistance to structurally unrelated natural products. MDR cells may coexpress P-gp, MRP, and other transport proteins. Therefore, as strategies are applied for reversing resistance, tumor samples may need to be analyzed for the presence of P-gp or other transport proteins.

***Strategies for reversing MDR***   Approaches to overcoming MDR are receiving much attention. Strategies being investigated include the use of high-dose chemotherapy to increase intracellular cytotoxic drug concentrations; the use of non–cross-resistant drug regimens to prevent the emergence of resistant clones; and using modulators to inhibit or reverse the effects of specialized resistance mechanisms such as P-gp associated drug efflux. Several pharmaceutical agents currently available for treatment of nonmalignant conditions have been identified in vitro as modulators of P-gp MDR, including calcium channel blockers, calmodulin inhibitors (phenothiazines), cyclosporine, and steroid hormones (Table 14-6).[47] The two most widely investigated modulators are verapamil and cyclosporine A. These drugs are believed to act directly by binding to special sites on the P-gp molecule and inhibiting the efflux of cytotoxic drugs. The specific binding sites and mechanism of interaction are not known; however, the outcome is decreased efflux and higher intracellular concentrations of the antineoplastic drug. Only a few clinical trials using these agents have been performed to date.[48] Responses were most often observed in patients with hematologic malignancies and some solid tumors such as breast cancer.

Clinical trials have identified several problems associated with the use of modulators to overcome P-gp–associated MDR.[49–52] Obtaining adequate blood levels of modulators is only achievable for half of the agents tested; however, plasma levels do not necessarily reflect concentration of the modulator at the active site. Another concern is the potential for these drugs to inhibit efflux pumps in normal cells, thereby increasing the toxicity observed in these tissues. This observation has not yet been seen in clinical trials to date. Modulators may reverse resistance by altering the pharmacokinetics

**TABLE 14-6**  Drugs Demonstrating Potential to Reverse P-glycoprotein Associated MDR

| Pharmacological Class | Drug Name |
|---|---|
| Calcium channel blocker | Verapamil |
| Calmodulin inhibitor | |
|   Phenothiazine | Trifluoperazine |
| Cyclosporine | Cyclosporine A |
| Hormonal agent | Tamoxifen |

Data from Ford JM and Hait WN: Pharmacology of drugs that alter multidrug resistance in cancer. *Pharmacol Rev* 42:155–199, 1990.

of the antineoplastic drug in addition to or as the sole mechanism of MDR reversal.[48] Verapamil is known to inhibit hepatic microsomal enzymes responsible for the metabolism of many antineoplastic drugs, and prolonged clearance of etoposide was reported when a combination of etoposide and cyclosporine was administered.[51] Pharmacokinetics of both the modulator and the chemotherapeutic drug should be studied to evaluate this potential mechanism.

Drugs used as modulators of MDR are often given in doses at or above their therapeutic range, often producing significant toxicity. Cardiotoxicity, such as first-degree heart block, hypotension, sinus bradycardia, and junctional rhythms, has been reported with verapamil given to patients for MDR modulation.[53] Dose-limiting extrapyramidal side effects were commonly seen in patients receiving trifluoperazine for reversal of doxorubicin resistance.[54] Cyclosporine A is frequently associated with dose-limiting renal, hepatic, and neurological toxicity. The toxicities observed in these clinical trials have been attributed to the resistance modulators and not to the chemotherapeutic drugs.

Laboratory and clinical research is ongoing to identify compounds that may be used to reverse or prevent MDR. Ideal agents would be easy to administer, would not hinder the pharmacology or pharmacokinetics of the chemotherapy, and would have minimal toxicity of their own. Clinical trials have recently begun using a stereoisomer of verapamil, which is equally effective in reversing MDR but is associated with much less cardiotoxicity.[55] Another approach to modulation of MDR involves the inhibition of protein kinases, which are enzymes that control the phosphorylation of P-gp and thereby regulate its function.[56] Therapies aimed at suppressing *mdr-1* gene expression may also be considered as alternative approaches to modulating resistance. Yet another strategy focuses on sequencing non–cross-resistant chemotherapy regimens to prevent the survival of resistant clones.[57]

P-glycoprotein–mediated MDR may be an important factor contributing to the failure of cytotoxic drugs to eradicate otherwise sensitive tumors. Although the exact mechanism of resistance is not known, important factors include overexpression of the *mdr-1* gene and the functioning of an energy-dependent efflux pump. Although much has been learned about MDR and drugs that may reverse it, the clinical use of modulators is not routinely practiced. Prospective, randomized, controlled clinical trials are needed to define the role of modulators and their safe and effective use.

### Other mechanisms of MDR

Another type of MDR has been described in cells cross-resistant to topoisomerase poisons such as etoposide, doxorubicin, daunorubicin, and topotecan. Although most of the drugs associated with this type of MDR are also associated with P-gp–mediated MDR, the pattern of resistance is different and cells retain sensitivity to vinca alkaloids.[58] Resistance may be conferred by the tumor cell's ability to decrease the activity of or change the binding properties of topoisomerase enzymes. Tumor cells that have developed resistance to one type of topoisomerase II poisons such as intercalators (e.g., doxorubicin) may not be resistant to an alternative type such as epipodophyllotoxins (e.g., etoposide). Therefore, resistance may be overcome by utilizing different types of topoisomerase II poisons.

MDR may also be demonstrated in cells with increased detoxifying systems such as glutathione S-transferase (GST) enzymes and elevated glutathione levels.[59] These enzymes catalyze conjugation of electrophilic hydrophobic compounds such as alkylating agents and their metabolites with glutathione, which facilitates elimination from the tumor cell. Alkylating agents, their metabolites, and platinum compounds are among the most frequent substrates of these enzymes.[60] Strategies being investigated for reversing this type of resistance include administering inhibitors of GST and glutathione synthesis such as buthionine sulfoxaminde (BSO).[61]

## Chemotherapy as a Treatment for Cancer

### Primary and adjuvant chemotherapy

Chemotherapy given with curative intent may be either primary therapy or adjuvant therapy. Chemotherapy is considered primary treatment for patients with cancers for which no effective alternative treatment is available or the alternative treatment is less than optimal.[62] *Induction* is a common term used to describe chemotherapy given to patients with leukemia or other advanced disease that is highly sensitive to drugs. *Neoadjuvant chemotherapy* describes chemotherapy given prior to alternative treatments in patients who present with primarily local disease.[63] This approach has had some success in preserving organ structure and function in cancers of the lung and larynx.[64–65] However, there is some concern that neoadjuvant treatment may delay the administration of definitive local therapy such as surgery or radiotherapy. Chemotherapy given concurrently instead of sequentially with radiotherapy is becoming a popular approach, especially for cancers of the head and neck.

Adjuvant chemotherapy is a well-established and routine part of treatment for cancers of the breast and bowel. Systemic therapy is usually given following surgical resection of the primary tumor with the intent of improving the potential for cure.[25] Although effective chemotherapy would theoretically eradicate clinically undetected and micrometastatic disease, the overall effect on tumor recurrence has been less than dramatic.

### Therapeutic strategies

***Combination chemotherapy***   Administering a combination of clinically effective anticancer drugs is the standard chemotherapeutic approach for most malignancies. Although individually the drugs are biochemically and clinically active, they are rarely used alone as single agents.

Combination chemotherapy was first applied with success in the treatment of leukemias and lymphomas and is now employed routinely for most other malignancies. The work of Goldie and Coldman supports the use of combination chemotherapy as a mechanism to prevent the survival or emergence of resistant cell lines.[18] The objectives of combination chemotherapy are achieving maximal tumor cell kill without excessive toxicity; providing cytotoxic drugs that are active against potentially resistant heterogeneous tumor populations; and avoiding selection of resistant cell lines. Table 14-7 delineates the principles by which antineoplastic drugs are usually chosen for combination regimens. When overlapping toxicities are unavoidable, as is often the case with bone marrow–suppressive drugs, administration of less than full doses or longer intervals between treatments may be necessary. Recovery time for normal tissues is typically used to determine the retreatment or cycle time. The time for the bone marrow to reach its nadir (lowest counts) and recover is different depending on the drugs administered. Nadir and recovery periods are critical for determining the length of a treatment cycle. Therefore, chemotherapy cycles for drugs with significant myelosuppression are approximately three to four weeks. The duration of treatment is usually based on the response rate or a number determined from clinical trials.

### Dose intensity

Delivering a sufficient amount of drug over a specified period of time is of great importance in curing drug-sensitive malignancies. However, many situations often prevent the proper dose from being delivered, such as the necessity for a dose reduction or a delay in treatment because of unacceptable toxicity. Dose reductions as small as 20% often translate into a loss of cure without affecting clinical response rates for most drug-sensitive tumors. Decreasing the dose or adjusting the schedule of treatment may explain the failure of chemotherapy to cure drug-sensitive tumors.

The concept of dose intensity has been developed to assist the researcher and clinician in evaluating the impact these changes in doses have on treatment outcomes.[66] Dose intensity is expressed as the amount of drug delivered per unit of time, or simply $mg/m^2/week$. The effect of a new regimen on treatment outcome can be expressed as the relative dose intensity (RDI), which is calculated by dividing the dose intensity of a test regimen by that of a standard regimen. This calculation can be done for a single drug or for an average of all the drugs in a combination regimen.[67] The impact of dose reductions or treatment delays is best evaluated when dose intensity is based on actual or received doses instead of intended or protocol doses.

The concept of dose intensity has been applied to a number of diseases to improve response rates. Increasing the dose has improved outcomes in lymphomas and advanced tumors of the ovary, breast, and colon.[68–70] High-dose chemotherapy regimens with hematopoietic support are quickly becoming an acceptable treatment alternative for refractory lymphomas, breast cancer, childhood sarcomas, and neuroblastomas.

### Chemoprotective agents

Antineoplastic drugs are among the most toxic drugs administered to humans. Most toxicity, such as nausea, vomiting, mucositis, alopecia, and lethargy, is not life-threatening. Bone marrow suppression is both common and potentially life-threatening; however, it is dose-dependent and can be managed by reducing doses, delaying therapy, or administering hematopoietic growth factors. Several drugs are known to induce life-threatening and permanent cellular injury. Chemoprotective and rescue agents have been developed and are under investigation for use in preventing or reversing drug-induced toxicity for some anticancer agents including cisplatin, doxorubicin, ifosfamide, and methotrexate. Availability of these compounds has permitted expanded clinical development and usefulness of the anticancer drugs whose toxicity they ameliorate. Table 14-8 lists currently available chemoprotective and rescue agents, along with their clinical indications, proposed mechanism of action, and toxicities.[71–73]

### High-dose chemotherapy with peripheral blood stem cell transplant

High-dose chemotherapy with autologous rescue is being used more frequently in cancers that respond to increasing doses of marrow-ablative therapy such as leukemias, lymphomas, breast cancer, and ovarian cancer. This form of therapy, once available only at select treatment centers, is now being offered at most major medical centers and many large community hospitals. Reasons for the expansion of this form of cancer treatment include the curative potential, more experience with administering and managing these therapies, and advancements in supportive care available to these patients. The introduction of the hematopoietic growth factors (HGFs) such as G-CSF and GM-CSF has been among the major advancements in supportive care measures. Their availability has allowed the procedure of harvesting hematopoietic stem cells from peripheral blood and in most situations avoiding costly and painful bone marrow harvesting. Peripheral blood stem cells (PBSCs) are committed progenitor cells existing in peripheral blood, which have the capacity of restoring hematopoiesis.[74]

Before receiving marrow-ablative chemotherapy, patients are given HGFs with or without chemotherapy, typically cyclophosphamide, to mobilize stem cells into the peripheral blood from the bone marrow.[75,76] Patients then undergo leukopheresis to remove mobilized stem

**TABLE 14-7**   Principles for Selection of Antineoplastic Drugs for Combination Chemotherapy Regimens

1. Choose drugs with single-agent activity. Drugs producing complete responses are preferred.
2. Avoid drugs with overlapping toxicities.
3. Administer drugs at their optimal dose and schedule as previously determined by clinical trials.
4. Give chemotherapy at regular intervals (cycles) and minimize the time between cycles.

**TABLE 14-8** Drugs Used as Chemoprotective and Rescue Agents for Cancer Chemotherapy[71-73]

| Chemoprotective Drug | Anticancer Drug | Mechanism of Action | Target Organ | Side Effects |
|---|---|---|---|---|
| Amifostine (Ethyol®) | Cisplatin | Reduces DNA damage | Kidney | Hypotension, vomiting |
| Dexrazoxane (Zinacard®) | Doxorubicin | Inhibits free radical formation | Heart | Myelosuppression, nausea and vomiting |
| Leucovorin (folinic acid) | Methotrexate | Circumvents enzyme inhibition | Bone marrow GI Kidney | Hypersensitivity, rash |
| Mesna (Mesnex®) | Ifosfamide Cyclophosphamide | Binds toxic metabolites in bladder | Kidney Bladder | Nausea, vomiting, hypersensitivity |

cells from the peripheral blood.[77] Leukopheresis may be performed two to six times to collect an adequate number of cells. Following high-dose chemotherapy, radiation therapy, or both, which is intended to eradicate the cancer cells and by consequence the bone marrow stem cells, the patient's PBSCs are reinfused. As with other forms of hematopoietic cell transplantation, infused stem cells migrate to the bone marrow and engraft. Compared with patients receiving autologous bone marrow alone, patients who receive PBSCs either alone or with bone marrow transplantation typically have fewer days of neutropenia and thrombocytopenia. A major disadvantage of PBSC transplantation is nausea, vomiting, and hypertension associated with infusion of the large amounts of the cryopreservative DSMO along with the large volume of cells needed to be infused. Another concern is the potential to reinfuse mobilized tumor cells, as well as hematopoietic stem cells. The significance of this contamination for relapse rates is yet to be determined.[78] The use of monoclonal antibodies to manufacture a product devoid of tumor cells is currently under investigation.

***Chemotherapy as a radiation sensitizer*** The concomitant use of chemotherapy and radiation therapy has received significant attention in the literature.[79-82] The primary goal of this type of combined-modality treatment is to overcome radiation resistance and improve locoregional control of disease. A number of theoretical considerations may explain the improved results seen when chemotherapy and radiation are given concomitantly to specific tumors. The modalities affect different tumor cell subpopulations; therefore, their combined use may better eradicate cells resistant to the other modality. Tumor cell regrowth following radiation therapy is slowed by the addition of chemotherapy, and cells undergoing growth are more vulnerable to the cytotoxic effects of chemotherapy. The cytoreductive effects of chemotherapy improve tumor oxygen supply, resulting in an increased susceptibility to radiation effects. In addition, direct interaction of the combined modalities, as yet undefined, may explain the improved response seen especially at a locoregional level. A positive interaction is defined as enhanced radiation effects in tumor cells and

less toxicity observed.[83] Significant improvement in quality of life may be achieved by utilizing combined-modality regimens to preserve organs affected by cancer such as the larynx, anal canal, bladder, and esophagus.[84,85]

Chemoradiotherapy with fluorouracil has demonstrated improved overall survival for individuals with cancers of the head and neck, rectum, pancreas, and lung.[79] Cisplatin has also been investigated as a radiation enhancer, with the greatest activity seen in tumors sensitive to cisplatin.[86] Cisplatin combined with other antineoplastic drugs such as paclitaxel, fluorouracil, or etoposide for radiation enhancement have also been studied.[87,88] The results of clinical trials combining cisplatin and radiation with or without fluorouracil for head and neck cancer have shown improved disease-free survival over radiation alone.[89,90] Although chemoradiotherapy may improve survival rates and preserve organs, the optimal drugs, dosing, and scheduling need to be defined.

***Modulation of fluorouracil by leucovorin*** Leucovorin, or folinic acid, has been developed primarily as an antidote for antifolate therapy. Another emerging role of leucovorin is in the modulation of the cytotoxicity of fluorouracil. Although fluorouracil is the most active antineoplastic drug in cancers of the gastrointestinal tract, it is only modest in controlling progression of these cancers. Therefore, investigators have sought to enhance this efficacy in an attempt to better control and potentially cure these cancers. In the presence of increased folate pools the active form of fluorouracil binds more tightly to the target enzyme.[91]

The interaction of leucovorin and fluorouracil has been studied in over 650 patients, with significantly improved response rates being seen with the combination compared with fluorouracil alone.[92] Although the optimal dose and schedule of leucovorin have not been determined, a prolonged or five-day intermittent dosing schedule is preferred. The results of current trials suggest that a maximal benefit of combined therapy is seen in patients with less advanced disease.[92,93] Other drugs that have been tested as biochemical modulators of fluorouracil include methotrexate, PALA, and alfa-interferon.

***Chronopharmacology and cancer chemotherapy*** *Chronopharmacology* is described as the temporal variation in the handling of drugs by the body.[94] This new and emerging science examines the variance of chemical and physical processes of a biological system with respect to time. The antineoplastic and toxic effects of several anticancer drugs exhibit variable and predictable daily or circadian rhythms in murine and human trials.[95–97] Both normal and tumor cells exhibit circadian cytokinetic rhythms; however, most of the time these rhythms are asynchronic.[98] By exploiting these differences in chronobiology, the timing of cancer chemotherapy may be successful in maximizing therapeutic activity and minimizing toxicity.

Clinical trials to date have focused on minimizing the toxic effects of antineoplastic drugs; however, some information is available on improved efficacy with chronochemotherapy dosing regimens.[96,97,99,100] Floxuridine given by continuous infusion produced less toxicity with increasing dose intensity when the majority of the daily dose was given in the evening hours (3 P.M. to 9 P.M.).[96,101] The catabolism of fluorouracil follows a circadian variation that may be exploited to allow maximum dose delivery during a period of decreased catabolic activity.[102] When the dose of cisplatin was administered in evening hours, the risk of nephrotoxicity was lessened as a result of increased urinary platinum concentrations and increased urine output.[103] The combination chemotherapy regimen of cisplatin and doxorubicin has also demonstrated circadian variation with respect to myelosuppression. Several studies suggest the ideal timing is the early morning for doxorubicin, and late afternoon or early evening for cisplatin.[95] The vinca alkaloids vincristine and vinblastine are least toxic when administered in early and midday activity times, respectively.[104,105] Other drugs that have been investigated for chronochemotherapy variability include cytarabine and methotrexate.

# PHARMACOLOGY OF CHEMOTHERAPEUTIC DRUGS

## Pharmacokinetics of Antineoplastic Drugs

### Principles of pharmacokinetics

*Pharmacokinetics* is the study of the movement of drugs in the body. Several parameters have been utilized to describe the pharmacokinetics of drugs.[106] The half-life of a drug is the time required for the serum concentration of the drug to decrease by one-half. The drug's half-life determines the time required to reach steady-state concentrations in the serum and the appropriate dosing interval. The concept of steady-state serum concentration is less useful in chemotherapy since most antineoplastics are administered as single doses. However, knowing the half-life of a drug may be useful when evaluating the interval necessary for most of the drug to be removed from the body. This time period is equal to three half-lives of the drug. Clearance is the most important phar-

macokinetic parameter because it determines the steady-state concentration and is independent of half-life. Clearance is determined by blood flow to an organ, usually the kidney or liver, and the organ's efficacy in extracting the drug from the blood. If a drug is cleared from the body by more than one organ, then the total clearance is a sum of the individual clearance of each extracting organ. Clearance may be altered by changes in blood flow to an organ, by enzyme function, and by protein binding. Cyclophosphamide is highly dependent on metabolizing enzymes for activation and inactivation. Therefore, induction or inhibition of enzymes may cause a more rapid or slower clearance of the drug. Changes in protein binding caused by either hypoalbuminemia or interactions with other drugs may alter the removal of highly protein-bound drugs such as etoposide or teniposide. The volume of distribution ($V_D$) relates the amount of drug in the body to the serum concentration. This parameter is usually different among individuals and is a function of the drug's protein-binding capabilities and its ability to distribute to extravasular compartments (tissue binding). Half-life is dependent on clearance and $V_D$; therefore, variability in half-life may be the result of changes in clearance, $V_D$, or both. Variability in these parameters may help explain the differences in response and toxicity seen among patients treated with similar doses and schedules of chemotherapy.

The basic principles of clinical pharmacokinetics may be divided into four major areas: absorption, distribution, metabolism, and excretion.

*Absorption* Absorption from the gastrointestinal tract should be sufficient to ensure adequate bioavailability of the drug. Because the bioavailability of most anticancer drugs is poor and unpredictable, they are usually given parenterally to ensure accurate dosing and optimal systemic exposure. Drugs administered orally for cancer treatment include some alkylating agents (cyclophosphamide, chlorambucil, and melphalan), etoposide, lomustine, methothexate, and procarbazine. Although oral absorption is less than optimal for some of these drugs, the amount that reaches systemic circulation and, more important, the tumor is sufficient to produce a response.

*Distribution* Distribution of drugs in the body is determined primarily by their ability to penetrate different tissues and their affinity for binding to plasma proteins. Drugs that are highly lipophilic tend to be more readily taken up by lipophilic tissues such as bone marrow, fat, and the central nervous system. Nitrosoureas such as carmustine and lomustine are useful for brain and hematopoietic malignancies since they readily penetrate these tissues. Decreased levels of plasma proteins, especially albumin, often occur in patients with cancer. This may be the result of nutritional deficiencies or decreased hepatic synthesis of albumin. The cytotoxic activity of highly protein-bound chemotherapy drugs such as etoposide and teniposide may be enhanced in these patients because a greater percentage of the drug is unbound. An increase in the unbound fraction can also occur if two highly bound drugs are administered concurrently. Methotrexate abnormally distributes in ascites and pleural effusions, delaying clearance and enhancing hematologic and mucosal toxicity.[107]

*Metabolism* The metabolic activation and inactivation or catabolism of drugs is carried out primarily by the liver. Some of these enzymatic processes are also performed in normal and tumor cells. Many chemotherapy drugs require activation intracellularly or systemically before they are able to exert their cytotoxic effect (Table 14-9). Antimetabolites such as fluorouracil and cytarabine are phosphorylated to active nucleotides in tumor cells. Cisplatin undergoes a chemical aquation with water molecules intracellularly that generates a positively charged species that forms adducts with DNA molecules.[108] Cyclophosphamide and ifosfamide are transformed by hepatic microsomal enzymes into active alkylating species.[109] Many chemotherapeutic drugs are metabolized to inactive compounds, which are then excreted by the body. The rate of metabolic conversion may be affected by a number of factors, including hepatic dysfunction (either drug-induced or tumor-induced) or genetic differences in drug metabolism. Changes in liver function or metabolic enzymes may result in decreased cytotoxic activity, increased treatment-related toxicity, or both. Table 14-10 lists drugs known to alter microsomal enzymes and potentially affect antineoplastic drug disposition.

*Elimination* The kidneys are responsible for the majority of the elimination of drugs and drug metabolites from the body. A number of anticancer drugs are highly dependent on renal function for their elimination. Significant decreases in renal function can decrease the clearance of these compounds from the body and cause excessive toxicity (Table 14-11). Cisplatin and methotrexate are both eliminated primarily by the kidney and are nephrotoxic themselves; therefore, decreased renal function may produce enhanced toxicity and a further decline in renal function. The biliary tract is the primary route of elimination for vinca alkaloids, and urinary excretion is minimal.

## Pharmacokinetic principles applied to chemotherapeutic drugs

Chemotherapeutic drugs must reach their target site in order to exert their antineoplastic activity. Often their targets are intracellular structures and molecules such as DNA, enzymes, and microtubules. Adequate blood supply to tumor cells is necessary for optimal delivery of chemotherapy to their site of action. Then, once at the tumor cell, the drug must be transported intracellularly via passive, facilitated, or active transport mechanisms.[110] Transport mechanisms may either facilitate drug entry into the cell or hasten its removal. As mentioned previously, efflux from the cell is a major limitation of antineoplastic drug efficacy. Systemic drug exposure is also an important parameter in ensuring the optimal cytotoxic response and minimal toxicity. The area under the serum concentration-time curve (AUC) is a measure of systemic drug exposure. Since the AUC is dependent on drug administration and elimination, changes in these parameters may greatly affect the systemic exposure. Patients with a more rapid drug clearance may need larger doses than those with a slower clearance. Therefore, methods of dose prediction based on target AUCs and a measure of drug elimination may provide a more optimal treatment intensity.

Pharmacokinetic parameters should be routinely applied in clinical practice to assist in delivering the optimal dose with the least risk of serious toxicity. Interpatient variability should always be considered when evaluating therapeutic or toxic response to therapy.

**TABLE 14-9** Chemotherapy Drugs That Depend on Hepatic Metabolism for Activation and Elimination from the Body

| Chemotherapy Drug | Activation | Clearance |
|---|---|---|
| Anthracycline antibiotics | X | X |
| Daunorubicin | | |
| Doxorubicin | | |
| Cyclophosphamide | X | X |
| Dacarbazine | X | X |
| Hexamethylmelamine | | X |
| Ifosfamide | X | |
| Nitrosoureas | | X |
| Carmustine | | |
| Lomustine | | |
| Procarbazine | X | |

**TABLE 14-10** Drugs Known to Enhance or Inhibit Hepatic Microsomal Metabolism

| Enhance | Inhibit |
|---|---|
| Cyclophosphamide | Cimetidine |
| Phenobarbital | Alfa-interferon |
| Phenytoin | Ketoconazole |
| Rifampin | Verapamil |

**TABLE 14-11** Chemotherapeutic Agents Cleared by Kidneys that Cause Excessive Toxicity in Renal Insufficiency

| Drugs Requiring Dose Modification | |
|---|---|
| Bleomycin | Cyclophosphamide |
| Carboplatin | Etoposide |
| Cisplatin | Methotrexate |
| | Streptozotocin |

## Drug Interactions in the Patient Receiving Chemotherapy

A drug interaction occurs when the effects of one drug, therapeutic or toxic, are modified by the presence of another. Interactions may result in a beneficial effect such as improving therapeutic response or preventing or reducing toxicity. However, the majority produce undesirable outcomes such as a suboptimal therapeutic response or enhanced adverse effects. Tables 14-12[71,111-122] and 14-13[71,123,124] list numerous clinically significant drug interactions in patients receiving cancer chemotherapy.

Clinically significant drug interactions may be described as having a direct, indirect, or additive effect on the chemotherapy treatment. Direct interactions involve changes in the pharmacokinetics of the primary drug such as oral absorption, distribution, metabolism, and excretion. Drugs may also interact by indirectly altering the eliminating function of the organs of the body.

Drug-induced renal or hepatic dysfunction may cause chemotherapy drugs to be eliminated more slowly, thereby increasing the potential for and severity of adverse reactions. Chemotherapeutic drugs often share similar toxicities with other drugs. Therefore, additive toxicities may occur, such as myelosuppression and gastrointestinal disturbances.

Not all drug interactions result in clinically significant therapeutic or toxic outcomes. Most interactions occur only under specific pharmacological and physiological situations; therefore, drug interactions should be judged by their overall effect on therapeutic response and patient care. The potential for serious interaction increases with the number of drugs a patient receives. Since most patients with cancer are receiving chemotherapy drugs, supportive care drugs, and conceivably pain management drugs, the potential for drug interactions is relatively high. Many patients with advanced disease have significant organ dysfunction, are elderly, or have concomitant

**TABLE 14-12** Selected Clinically Significant Drug Interactions in Patients Receiving Cancer Chemotherapy[71, 111-122]

| Chemotherapy Drug | Interacting Drug | Pharmacokinetic/Pharmacodynamic Effect[a] | Management of Interaction |
|---|---|---|---|
| Asparaginase | Methotrexate | ↓ toxicity[b] | Give methotrexate 3–24 hours prior |
| Bleomycin | Cisplatin | ↓ renal elimination, ↑ pulmonary toxicity | Monitor renal function in patients previously treated with cisplatin |
| | Oxygen | ↑ risk of acute pulmonary inflammation | Avoid inspired oxygen above 25% |
| Busulfan | Phenytoin[c] | ↑ metabolic clearance, ↓ bone marrow cytotoxicity | Begin phenytoin therapy briefly before busulfan |
| Carmustine | Phenytoin | ↓ phenytoin blood level, ↓ anti-seizure effect | Monitor phenytoin level and adjust dose |
| Cisplatin | Anticonvulsant drugs (carbamazepine, phenytoin, valproic acid) | ↓ oral absorption of anticonvulsant drug, ↓ blood levels | Monitor levels and increase dose as needed |
| | Aminoglycoside antibiotics | Additive risk of renal toxicity | Monitor renal function and electrolytes |
| | Sodium thiosulfate Mesna | Chemical incompatibility, ↓ cytotoxic and toxic effects, Sodium thiosulfate may be used as an antidote for cisplatin toxicity | Do not administer in same infusion device |
| Cyclophosphamide | Allopurinol | ↓ renal elimination of alkylating metabolite, ↑ toxicity | Monitor bone marrow and urologic toxicity |
| | Digoxin | ↓ oral absorption of digoxin tablet | Monitor digoxin levels |
| | Succinylcholine | ↓ metabolic clearance of succinylcholine, Prolonged neuromuscular block | Use neuromuscular blocking drugs cautiously |
| Corticosteroids (Dexamethasone, hydrocortisone, methylprednisolone) | Aminoglutethimide Mitotane | ↑ metabolic clearance, ↓ therapeutic effect | Adjust corticosteroid dose to avoid adrenal crisis |
| | Streptozocin | Additive diabetogenic effect | Monitor blood glucose |

*(continued)*

**TABLE 14-12** Selected Clinically Significant Drug Interactions in Patients Receiving Cancer Chemotherapy[71, 111–122] (continued)

| Chemotherapy Drug | Interacting Drug | Pharmacokinetic/Pharmacodynamic Effect[a] | Management of Interaction |
|---|---|---|---|
| Etoposide | Phenobarbital Phenytoin | ↑ metabolic clearance, ↓ cytotoxicity | Avoid co-administration |
| | Highly protein-bound drugs | ↓ protein binding, ↑ myelotoxicity | Avoid co-administration |
| Fluorouracil | Alfa interferon | ↓ metabolic clearance, ↑ cytotoxicity | Monitor for severe gastrointestinal toxicity |
| | Methotrexate | Cytotoxic antagonism of both drugs | Give methotrexate before or with 5FU |
| | Metronidazole | ↓ metabolic clearance, ↑ toxicity | Co-administer with caution |
| Ifosfamide | Phenobarbital | ↑ metabolic activation, ↑ toxicity | Monitor bone marrow suppression and neurotoxicity |
| Alfa interferon | Theophylline | ↓ metabolic clearance of theophylline | Monitor theophylline blood levels |
| Interleukin-2 | Corticosteroids | Block antitumor effect, ↓ tumor response rate | Use corticosteroids only for IL-2 toxicity management |
| Levamisole | Alcohol | Blocked metabolic clearance of alcohol, Disulfiram-like reaction (flushing, headache, nausea, vomiting, hypotension) | Avoid co-administration |
| Melphalan (High dose) | Cyclosporine | ↑ risk of severe nephrotoxicity | Monitor renal function and cyclosporine blood levels |
| Mercaptopurine | Allopurinol | ↓ metabolic clearance, ↑ serum levels, Prolonged bone marrow suppression | Decrease dose of mercaptopurine by 75% |
| | Cotrimoxazole (trimethoprim, sulfamethoxazole) | ↑ oral absorption, ↓ metabolic activation | Monitor bone marrow suppression |
| Methotrexate | Cotrimoxazole | ↓ renal clearance, Additive antifolate activity, ↑ bone marrow toxicity | Monitor methotrexate levels and toxicity |
| | Ethanol (alcohol) | ↑ intrahepatic uptake of methotrexate, ↑ risk of hepatotoxicity | Limit alcohol intake |
| | NSAIDs salicylates | ↓ renal clearance, ↓ protein binding, ↑ bone marrow and gastrointestinal toxicity | Monitor methotrexate levels and toxicity (FATAL outcomes reported in cases of oral methotrexate and NSAID use) |
| | Probenecid Penicillin G | ↓ renal clearance, ↑ toxic effects | Monitor methotrexate levels and toxicity |
| Paclitaxel | Cisplatin | ↓ total body clearance, ↑ myelotoxicity | Give paclitaxel before cisplatin |
| Procarbazine | Ethanol | Blocks metabolism of alcohol, Disulfiram-like reaction | Avoid co-administration |
| | Sympathomimetic drugs (ephedrine, epinephrine) Tricyclic antidepressant drugs (amitriptyline, imipramine) | MAO inhibition,[d] Hypertensive crisis, tremor, excitation | Most interactions are not clinically important |
| | CNS depressant drugs (narcotics, phenothiazines, barbiturates) | Additive CNS depression and respiratory depression | Co-administer cautiously |
| Tamoxifen | Aminoglutethimide | ↑ metabolic clearance | Avoid concurrent use |

**TABLE 14-12** Selected Clinically Significant Drug Interactions in Patients Receiving Cancer Chemotherapy[71, 111-122] (continued)

| Chemotherapy Drug | Interacting Drug | Pharmacokinetic/Pharmacodynamic Effect[a] | Management of Interaction |
|---|---|---|---|
| Teniposide | Highly protein-bound drugs[e] | ↓ protein binding, ↑ in free (active) drug blood level | Avoid co-administration |
| Thiotepa | Succinylcholine | ↓ metabolic clearance of succinylcholine, Exaggerated skeletal muscle relaxation | Co-administer cautiously |
| Vinblastine | Phenytoin | ↓ phenytoin blood level | Monitor phenytoin level and adjust dose as needed |
| | Mitomycin C | Acute pulmonary reaction (dyspnea, bronchospasm) | Discontinue therapy and treat with oxygen and bronchodilators |
| Vincristine | Asparaginase | ↑ risk of peripheral neurotoxicity | Give vincristine first |
| | Teniposide | ↑ risk of peripheral neurotoxicity | Monitor for toxicity |

a. refers to chemotherapy drug unless otherwise specified

b. result of methotrexate-induced block of protein synthesis

c. for seizure prophylaxis for patients receiving high-dose busulfan for bone marrow transplant therapy

d. monoamine oxidase inhibition decreases the metabolism of sympathomimetic drugs, neurotransmitters released by tricyclic antidepressants and endogenous amines

e. specifically sodium salicylate, sulfonamide drugs and tolbutamide

**TABLE 14-13** Chemotherapy Drug Interactions with Warfarin[71,123,124]

| Chemotherapy Drug | Possible Mechanism of Interaction | Effect on Prothrombin Time |
|---|---|---|
| Aminoglutethimide | ↑ metabolic clearance | Shorten |
| Ifosfamide/mesna | Enzyme inhibition, protein-binding displacement | Prolong |
| Levamisole | Unknown | Prolong |
| Mercaptopurine | Antagonize anticoagulant effect | Shorten |
| Mitotane | ↑ metabolic clearance | Shorten |
| Tamoxifen | Unknown, enzyme inhibition and/or protein-binding displacement | Prolong |

illness, which all add to the seriousness of harmful drug interactions. The cancer patient's overall quality of life may be severely affected by toxic or subtherapeutic treatment that may result due to a significant drug interaction. Therefore, the clinician should always be aware of the potential for interactions to occur and make changes in therapy or monitor for undesirable outcomes.

## Antineoplastic Drugs

Cancer chemotherapeutic drugs have traditionally been classified by their mechanism of action, chemical struc-ture, or biological source. Grouping antineoplastic drugs into categories is done primarily for convenience. Although drugs within a class share some characteristics, there are often major differences in their indications, toxicities, and pharmaceutical properties. Tables 14-14 and 14-15 list the commonly used antineoplastic drugs and hormonal agents and their primary indications.[71] Figure 14-3 illustrates the proposed mechanisms and sites of action for most chemotherapeutic drugs. Information about dose, preparation, and administration, as well as more detailed descriptions of toxicity and management, are found in chapters 15 and 16.

### Alkylating and alkylating-like agents

***Classic alkylators*** Alkylating agents were among the first drugs used to treat malignancies in humans, and they continue to play a major role in chemotherapy. This group consists of a wide array of cytotoxic drugs that possess single-agent tumoricidal activity as well as a significant role in combination chemotherapy. Alkylating agents contribute electrophilic, alkyl groups ($R-CH_2-CH_2$) to attack electron-rich, nucleophilic sites on biological macromolecules such as DNA. The most common site of DNA alkylation is the N-7 position of guanine, with adducts at other positions on other bases being less frequent.[125] These DNA adducts may produce a variety of lesions, including strand breaks, nucleotide base deletions, and ring openings. Cytotoxicity and mutagenicity of alkylating agents usually result from these DNA adducts as well as interference with replication and transcription.[125,126,127] Many of the DNA lesions may be restored by repair enzymes; however, if the repair is only partial, additional DNA damage may result. Alkylators are non-

**TABLE 14-14** Classification of Commonly Used Antineoplastic Drugs and Their Primary Indications[71]

| Drug Name(s) | Primary Indications |
|---|---|
| **ALKYLATING AGENTS** | |
| *Classic Alkylators:* | |
| Busulfan (Myleran®) | CML |
| | AML[1] |
| Chlorambucil (Leukeran®) | CLL |
| | Multiple myeloma |
| Cyclophosphamide (Cytoxan®, Neosar®) | Breast cancer |
| | Lymphoma |
| | Ovarian cancer |
| | AML, ALL |
| Ifosfamide[2] (Ifex®) | Testicular cancer |
| | Sarcoma |
| | NCSLC |
| Mechlorethamine (Nitrogen mustard, Mustargen®) | Hodgkin's disease |
| | Lymphoma |
| | CML, CLL |
| Melphalan (L-PAM, Alkeran®) | Multiple myeloma |
| | Ovarian cancer |
| | Breast cancer |
| Thiotepa (TESPA) | Bladder cancer |
| | Breast cancer |
| *Nitrosoureas:* | |
| Carmustine (BCNU, BiCNU®) | Brain tumors |
| | Lymphomas |
| Lomustine (CCNU, CeeNU®) | Hodgkin's disease |
| Streptozocin (Zanosar®) | Pancreatic cancer |
| **ALKYLATING-LIKE AGENTS** | |
| *Platinum-containing Compounds:* | |
| Cisplatin (Platinol®) | Testicular cancer |
| | Ovarian cancer |
| | NSCLC, SCLC |
| Carboplatin (Paraplatin®) | Ovarian cancer |
| | AML |
| | NSCLC, SCLC |
| *Other Alkylating-like Drugs:* | |
| Dacarbazine (DTIC®) | Hodgkin's disease |
| | Malignant melanoma |
| Procarbazine (Matulane®) | Hodgkin's disease |
| | Brain tumors |
| Altretamine (Hexalen®) | Ovarian cancer |
| **ANTITUMOR ANTIBIOTICS** | |
| *Anthracycline Antibiotics:* | |
| Daunorubicin (Daunomycin®) | AML, ALL |
| Liposomal daunorubicin (DaunoXome®) | Kaposi's sarcoma |
| Doxorubicin (Adriamycin®) | Breast cancer |
| | Sarcomas |
| | Lymphomas |
| | Gastric cancer |
| | Ovarian cancer |

**TABLE 14-14** Classification of Commonly Used Antineoplastic Drugs and Their Primary Indications[71] (continued)

| Drug Name(s) | Primary Indications |
|---|---|
| Liposomal doxorubicin (Doxil®) | Kaposi's sarcoma |
| Idarubicin (Idamycin®) | AML |
| Mitoxantrone (Novantrone®) | AML |
| | Lymphomas |
| | Breast cancer |
| *Other Antitumor Antibiotics* | |
| Bleomycin (Blenoxane®) | Lymphomas |
| | Head/Neck cancer |
| | Germ cell tumors |
| Dactinomycin (Actinomycin D, Cosmegen®) | Wilms' tumor |
| | Ewing's sarcoma |
| | Kaposi's sarcoma |
| Mitomycin C (Mutamycin®) | Gastrointestinal cancer |
| | NSCLC |
| | Breast cancer |
| Plicamycin (Mithramycin, Mithracin®) | Malignant hypercalcemia |
| **ANTIMETABOLITES** | |
| *Antifolates:* | |
| Methotrexate (Folex®) | Breast cancer |
| | AML, ALL |
| | Squamous cell cancer |
| | Trophoblastic neoplasms |
| Trimetrexate Neutrexin®) | Pneumocystis carinii pneumonia |
| | Breast cancer[3] |
| | Esophageal cancer[9] |
| *Pyrimidine Analogs:* | |
| Fluorouracil (5FU) | Colorectal cancer |
| | Breast cancer |
| | Pancreatic cancer |
| | Head/neck cancer |
| Floxuridine (FUDR®) | Colorectal cancer[4] |
| | Liver tumors |
| | Brain tumors |
| Cytarabine (Ara-C, Cytosar®) | AML |
| 5-Azacytidine (5-AC) | AML |
| Gemcitabine (Gemsar®) | Pancreatic cancer |
| *Purine Analogs:* | |
| Mercaptopurine (Purinethol®) | ALL, AML |
| | CML |
| 6-Thioguanine (Tabloid®) | ALL, AML |
| | CML |
| Fludarabine (Fludara®) | CLL |
| Cladrabine (Leustatin®) | Hairy cell leukemia |
| | Lymphocytic lymphomas |

**TABLE 14-14** Classification of Commonly Used Antineoplastic Drugs and Their Primary Indications[71] (continued)

| Drug Name(s) | Primary Indications |
|---|---|
| **PLANT DERIVATIVES** | |
| *Vinca Alkaloids:* | |
| Vinblastine (Velban®) | Hodgkin's disease<br>Testicular cancer<br>Kaposi's sarcoma<br>Breast cancer |
| Vincristine (Oncovin®) | AML, ALL<br>Lymphomas<br>SCLC<br>Breast cancer<br>Multiple myeloma |
| Vinorelbine (Navelbine®) | NSCLC<br>Breast cancer |
| *Taxanes:* | |
| Paclitaxel (Taxol®) | Ovarian cancer<br>Breast cancer<br>NSCLC |
| Docetaxel (Taxotere®) | Ovarian cancer<br>Breast cancer<br>NSCLC |
| *Epipodophyllotoxins:* | |
| Etoposide (VP-16, VePesid®) | Testicular cancer<br>SCLC, NSCLC<br>Lymphomas |
| Teniposide (Vumon®) | AML<br>Lymphomas |
| *Camptothecin Analogs:* | |
| Topotecan (Hycamtin®) | Ovarian cancer<br>SCLC |
| Irinotecan (Camptosar®) | Colon cancer |
| **MISCELLANEOUS ANTINEOPLASTIC DRUGS** | |
| L-asparaginase (Elspar®) | ALL |
| Pegaspargase (Oncaspar®) | ALL[5] |
| Hydroxyurea (Hydrea®) | CML<br>Ovarian cancer<br>Malignant melanoma |
| Amsacrine [IND] (m-AMSA) | AML |

Key: ALL, acute lymphocytic leukemia; AML, acute myelocytic leukemia; CLL, chronic lymphocytic leukemia; CML, chronic lymphocytic leukemia; H.d., high dose; IND, Investigational New Drug; NSCLC, non-small cell lung cancer; SCLC, small cell lung cancer.

1. High-dose with bone marrow transplant support.
2. Administered concurrently with Mesna (Mesnex).
3. Investigational use only.
4. Regional therapy.
5. For use in patients hypersensitive to L-asparaginase.

**TABLE 14-15** Commonly Used Hormonal Agents, Their Pharmacological Effects and Their Primary Indications[71]

| Pharmacological Class | Drugs | Primary Indication |
|---|---|---|
| Androgens | Fluoxymesterone<br>Testosterone | Breast cancer |
| Estrogens | Conjugated estrogens<br>Diethylstilbestrol<br>Estradiol | Prostate cancer<br>Breast cancer |
| Progestins | Medroxyprogesterone<br>Megestrol[1] | Endometrial cancer<br>Breast cancer |
| Antiestrogens | Tamoxifen | Breast cancer |
| Antiandrogens | Flutamide | Prostate cancer |
| LH-RH antagonists | Gosereline<br>Leuprolide | Prostate cancer<br>Breast cancer |
| Estrogen-mustard conjugate | Estramustine phosphate | Prostate cancer |
| Aromatase inhibitors[2] | Arimidex<br>Aminoglutethimide<br>Mitotane | Breast cancer<br>Adrenal cancer |
| Corticosteroids | Dexamethasone<br>Hydrocortisone<br>Methylprednisolone<br>Prednisone | Acute and chronic leukemias<br>Hodgkin's disease<br>Malignant lymphomas<br>Breast cancer<br>Multiple myeloma |

1. Also used as an appetite stimulant and weight gain agent for breast cancer and AIDS-related cachexia.
2. Inhibits the synthesis of all classes of steroids including corticosteroids and sex steroids.

cell cycle phase-specific and are most active in the resting cell ($G_0$). Most alkylating agents are considered mutagens and potentially carcinogenic; therefore, the health care professional should be especially careful to avoid exposure when working with these compounds.

Mechlorethamine (nitrogen mustard) was the first alkylating agent introduced for cancer therapy. The drug spontaneously undergoes molecular rearrangement in aqueous solution to form a reactive species with two chloroethyl groups available for formation of cross-links of DNA strands.[125] Nitrogen mustard has a very short half-life and is usually undetectable in the blood within a few minutes of administration. It is a severe vesicant that must be handled with caution to prevent exposure of the clinician and to prevent extravasation during administration. Dose-limiting toxicities are myelosuppression, which may be severe, and rapid-onset nausea and vomiting. The major therapeutic role of mechlorethamine is in the MOPP chemotherapy regimen for Hodgkin's disease. Other uses include topical application for mycosis fungoides or skin cancer, and intracavitary instillation for malignant pleural or pericardial effusions.

Melphalan, busulfan, and chlorambucil are usually given orally. Melphalan and busulfan are currently available as injectable products for specific indications. Melphalan was developed as a targeted agent for selective uptake in tumors actively using phenylalanine and tyrosine, such as melanin-producing malignant cells. The drug is transported into cells via two amino acid transport systems, a highly active l-amino acid system and a second, less active, amino acid system.[128] Absorption from the gastrointestinal tract is variable and is slowed when the drug is taken with food; therefore, it should be taken on an empty stomach. Melphalan may be given parenterally when the oral route is not appropriate; however, a 50% dose reduction should be considered in patients with a significant decrease in renal function. Chlorambucil is completely absorbed from the gastrointestinal tract. It has a predictable myelotoxicity profile and is well established in the treatment of chronic lymphocytic leukemia. Busulfan is a bifunctional alkylating agent with two reactive groups on opposite ends of the molecule, which form DNA adducts resulting in cross-linked strands.[125] Besides its use in chronic lymphocytic leukemia (CML), busulfan is also used in high-dose chemotherapy conditioning regimens along with allogeneic or autologous bone marrow transplantation.

Cyclophosphamide and ifosfamide undergo a multistep activation process in vivo involving both hepatic microsomal and cellular enzyme systems to generate reactive chemical species. The two active metabolites of cyclophosphamide responsible for the majority of the drug's cytotoxicity are phosphoramide mustard and acrolein.[129] Acrolein is also primarily responsible for inducing hemorrhagic cystitis in approximately 10% of patients. This complication may be avoided by ensuring the patient is adequately hydrated and encouraging frequent urination within 24 hours of cyclophosphamide administration. Ifosfamide administration is associated with a much higher incidence of urotoxicity than cyclophosphamide. This is the result of an altered pharmacokinetic profile, which generates more urotoxic metabolite precursors than is found with cyclophosphamide.[130] Cystitis can be prevented by the co-administration of mesna, a compound that inactivates urotoxic metabolites in the bladder. Because cyclophosphamide and ifosfamide rely on both the kidneys and the liver for elimination, their toxicity may be prolonged in patients with compromised renal or hepatic failure.

Thiotepa is a polyfunctional alkylating agent that induces multiple types of DNA damage, including interstrand cross-links. Thiotepa may be administered by various routes: intravenous for breast cancer, intravesical for superficial bladder cancer, intrapleural for malignant pleural effusions, and intraperitoneal for refractory ovarian cancer.[131] Thiotepa has some unique skin toxicities, including an acute erythroderma and dry desquamation of the palms and soles; and chronic darkening or bronzing of the skin when used in high-dose regimens.

Nitrosoureas decompose in aqueous solutions to form two reactive intermediates, a chloroethyldiazohydroxide and an isocyanate group.[132] The chloroethyldiazohydroxide form undergoes further decomposition to yield chloroethyl carbonium ions, which form adducts with DNA and induce interstrand cross-links. Isocyanate groups react with amine groups and produce carbamoylation reactions and thereby deplete glutathione and inhibit DNA repair. The interaction of chloroethyl carbonium ions with DNA is most likely the major cytotoxic effect. Nitrosoureas are distinct from other alkylators in that they are highly lipid-soluble and readily cross the blood-brain barrier, lending themselves highly active in intracranial tumors. Other uses include Hodgkin's and non-Hodgkin's lymphoma and malignant melanoma.

***Platinum-containing compounds*** Drugs in this group constitute a highly active group of antineoplastic agents widely used for cancer treatment. Platinum compounds undergo an aquation reaction that enables them to react with macromolecules with strong binding sites such as DNA.[133] Cisplatin-induced DNA adducts and formation of intrastrand DNA cross-links correlate well with the drug's cytotoxicity and antitumor activity.[134,135] Although cisplatin and other platinum analogues behave similarly to alkylators, their cytotoxicity is probably the result of a combination of mechanisms of action, including inhibition of DNA and protein synthesis, alteration in cell membrane transport, and suppression of mitochondrial function.[136]

Cisplatin and carboplatin are both highly dependent on renal elimination as their primary route of excretion. Cisplatin is removed from the blood in both its free and protein-bound forms following a triphasic elimination model. In the first two phases primarily the unbound or free form of cisplatin is eliminated. Since 90% of the drug is excreted by the kidneys, adequate renal function is important in preventing drug accumulation and excessive toxicity.[137] Cisplatin given intraperitoneally produces peak levels that are as much as 21 times higher than peak plasma levels using similar doses.[138] Sodium thiosulfate may be administered systemically to decrease severe toxicities experienced with intraperitoneally administered cisplatin. Carboplatin elimination follows a triphasic pattern similar to that of cisplatin.[139] The dose of carboplatin should be reduced in the patient with compromised renal function. Patients who previously received cisplatin may be at increased risk for toxicity with carboplatin and should be evaluated for decreased renal function.

Although both platinum analogues possess similar antitumor activity, there are significant differences in their dosing, administration, and side effect profiles. The dose-limiting toxicity of cisplatin is nephrotoxicity. Acute renal failure may occur within 24 hours of drug administration.[131] Patients most at risk are those who receive inadequate hydration. Nephrotoxicity may usually be avoided by adequately hydrating the patient and administering diuretics such as furosemide, mannitol, or both. Carboplatin, although dependent on good renal function for elimination, is not necessarily nephrotoxic and rarely requires concomitant hydration and diuresis. Nausea and vomiting are common in patients receiving either platinum compound. However, emesis is often more severe and prolonged with cisplatin. Combination antiemetic regimens are usually necessary to prevent and treat this side effect, which is often most feared by the patient. Dose-limiting myelosuppression is much more of an issue with carboplatin than with cisplatin. Neurotoxicity and ototoxicity are more commonly associated with cisplatin.

***Other alkylating-like drugs***  Other drugs with alkylating-like activity include dacarbazine, procarbazine, and altretamine (hexamethylmelamine). These drugs, like most other alkylating agents, are dependent on metabolic activation for the formation of reactive species. Dacarbazine functions primarily as an alkylating agent but may also act as an antimetabolite by inhibiting purine nucleoside incorporation into DNA.[140,141]

Dacarbazine does not appear to be cell cycle-phase specific and kills cells in all phases of the cycle. The drug is extremely sensitive to light and will undergo spontaneous decomposition to both active and inactive compounds. The most significant adverse events are nausea and vomiting, which may decrease with repeated courses. Other toxicities include a flulike syndrome, myelosuppression, and photosensitivity. Dacarbazine is also associated with hepatic veno-occlusive disease characterized by fever and acute hepatic necrosis.[142] Procarbazine is administered orally and is a major therapeutic agent in the treatment of Hodgkin's disease and brain tumors. Two significant drug interactions are possible in patients taking procarbazine.[143] The first is the drug's ability to inhibit the enzyme monoamine oxidase, which is responsible for metabolism of amines. Inhibition of vasoactive amine metabolism may lead to hypertensive crisis, severe headache, sweating, and coma. Patients should avoid eating foods high in tyramine such as wine, ripe cheese, chocolate, and liver to prevent this drug interaction. The second interaction is seen when patients on procarbazine consume alcohol. They experience a disulfiram reaction, which is characterized by nausea, vomiting, palpitations, and sweating. Hexamethylmelamine is an orally administered agent whose mechanism of action is uncertain but probably of an alkylating type.

## Antitumor antibiotics

***Anthracycline antibiotics***  The antitumor antibiotics constitute a large and diverse group of antineoplastic drugs originally derived from natural sources. Anthracyclines are a group of highly colored compounds known as *rhodomycins,* with both antineoplastic and antimicrobial activity. Anthracyclines (daunorubicin, doxorubicin, and idarubicin) and the chemically related anthracenedione (mitoxantrone) have multiple mechanisms of cytotoxicity, including intercalation, covalent DNA binding, free radical formation, and topoisomerase II enzyme inhibition. The two mechanisms now thought responsible for

the majority of the cytotoxicity are free radical formation and inhibition of topoisomerase II enzyme. Anthracyclines can also interfere with the DNA unwinding process catalyzed by the nuclear enzyme topoisomerase II.[144,145] A "cleavable complex" is produced by inhibiting the enzyme's re-ligation function, thereby creating double-strand breaks in the DNA structure. Anthracyclines generate oxygen radicals by at least two mechanisms. The quinone structure common to all anthracyclines can donate an electron to an oxygen molecule and generate a superoxide. The superoxide is converted to hydrogen peroxide by superoxide dismutase and finally to a hydroxyl radical. Hydroxyl radical, the most reactive compound known, rapidly attacks DNA and cell membrane lipids.[146,147] An iron-anthracycline complex may also produce hydroxyl radical from hydrogen peroxide. Most normal tissues and tumor cells possess enzymes capable of detoxifying hydrogen peroxide. Both catalase and glutathione peroxidase convert hydrogen peroxide to water. Heart muscle cells lack the enzyme catalase, and anthracycline compounds destroy glutathione peroxidase.[148] This leaves cardiac tissue unable to detoxify hydrogen peroxide, which may then give rise to a reactive hydroxyl radical. There is now substantial evidence that the drug-iron complex plays an important role in the cytotoxicity of anthracylines. Hydroxyl radical formation in cardiac tissue may be significantly decreased by the use of an edetate analogue dexrazoxane, that effectively chelates iron.

Anthracyclines are metabolized to both active and inactive compounds by the liver. The major metabolites of most anthracyclines are their alcohols, such as doxorubinicinol, which have antitumor activity but not as significant as do the parent compounds. The anthracycline dose should be reduced in patients with hepatic dysfunction, especially if the bilirubin is elevated. Dose adjustment is not necessary in renal failure since renal clearance of anthracyclines is minimal.

Cardiac toxicity of anthracyclines may manifest as acute changes in ECG and arrhythmias, which is more significant in patients with preexisting heart disease. However, the more common and often therapy-limiting cardiotoxicity is the development of cardiomyopathy leading to congestive heart failure.[146] Up to 10% of patients receiving a cumulative dose of doxorubicin greater than 550 mg/m$^2$ will develop this toxicity. Cardiac function is usually monitored with serial measurements of left ventricular function (MUGA scan) and ECG. Potential strategies to prevent or lessen cardiotoxicity include prolonged infusions of doxorubicin and cardioprotectant drugs such as dexrazoxane (Zinacard).

Mitoxantrone may be associated with less nausea, vomiting, and alopecia. Cardiac toxicity in patients treated with mitoxantrone appears to be less than that seen with doxorubicin.[149] However, there may be no difference in the incidence of cardiomyopathy at doses equipotent to doxorubicin. Daunorubicin, doxorubicin, and idarubicin are vesicants and can induce a severe extravasation injury characterized by pain, erythema, and tissue necrosis. Mitoxantrone is considered an irritant, and extravasation injury is much less common. Other toxicities of anthracyclines include mucositis, nausea, vomiting, and alopecia.

Liposomal encapsulation of doxorubicin and daunorubicin have provided two new anticancer agents with therapeutic and toxicity profiles different from the free form of these drugs. The mechanism of action is believed to be unchanged; however, the liposomal formulation changes the pharmacokinetics, allowing for a longer half-life and increased uptake by tumor cells.[150] Liposomal daunorubicin and liposomal doxorubicin are currently established treatments for Kaposi's sarcoma in patients with acquired immunodeficiency syndrome (AIDS). There are also significant data suggesting activity in breast cancer. Less alopecia, nausea, vomiting, and neurotoxicity is seen with these agents compared with their nonliposomal or free drug formulations. Cardiac toxicity appears to be less dose-limiting with the liposomal encapsulated drugs. Doses greater than 1000 mg/m² have been given without significant changes in left ventricular function. An infusion reaction consisting of back pain, chest tightness, and flushing has been seen in approximately 7% of patients receiving their first dose of liposomal doxorubicin.[151] This rarely requires discontinuing treatment and is usually managed with administration of diphenhydramine and restarting the infusion at a slower rate. Palmarplantar skin eruptions with swelling, pain, erythema, and desquamation of skin have also been seen in some patients receiving liposomal doxorubicin.

***Other antitumor antibiotics*** Bleomycin is a polypeptide composed of many low-molecular-weight proteins, isolated from the fungus *Streptomyces verticullus*. A drug-iron-oxygen complex binds to DNA by intercalation and generates oxygen radicals, which attack the nucleotide bases.[152] This results in single- and double-strand DNA breaks. Tumor cells are most sensitive to bleomycin in the premitotic, or $G_2$, phase, or in the mitotic phase of the cell cycle. Bleomycin has been used to synchronize cells into the $G_2$ and S phases so that other antineoplastic agents that act in those phases may have an increased cell kill potential. Bleomycin is also useful in combination chemotherapy regimens because of its lack of significant myelosuppressive effects.

Bleomycin is highly dependent on renal clearance for elimination from the body. Significant renal failure necessitates decreasing the dose by 50%–75% of full dose.[131] Renal function of patients previously treated with renal toxic drugs or those who are currently receiving cisplatin should be monitored closely. Pulmonary toxicity of bleomycin may initially present as cough, dyspnea, and pleuritic chest pain. Patients at higher risk for developing bleomycin-related pulmonary fibrosis include older patients ($\geq$70 years), those with preexisting pulmonary disease, and those who have received mediastinal radiation therapy. Although a cumulative dose greater than 450 units is associated with a higher incidence of fibrosis, clinically significant pulmonary toxicity has been documented at lower doses.

Dactinomycin (actinomycin D) also binds to DNA by intercalation and induces single-strand breaks similar to those seen with doxorubicin.[153] The drug is currently limited to use in pediatric tumors and gestational trophoblastic neoplasms. Dactinomycin is not metabolized to a significant amount but instead is excreted unchanged in the urine and bile.

Mitomycin C is activated to an alkylating agent and its cytotoxicity is the result of cross-links with DNA leading to inhibition of DNA synthesis and cell death. The drug is preferentially activated in hypoxic tissues such as the environment common to solid tumors.[154] Metabolism of mitomycin by the liver is poorly defined, and renal clearance plays only a minor role in total elimination. Mitomycin degrades at pHs lower than 6; therefore, when the drug is used intravesicularly for bladder cancer a pH higher than 6 should by maintained in the bladder to ensure potency. A delayed and cumulative myelosuppression is seen with mitomycin. However, the development of a hemolytic-uremic syndrome resulting in renal failure, which is rarely reversible, is of more concern.

### Antimetabolites

***Antifolates*** Antimetabolites used in cancer chemotherapy are structural analogues of nucleotide bases, which are the building blocks of DNA and RNA. The antineoplastic effect of this group of drugs is related to their ability to inhibit nucleic acid synthesis or to falsely be incorporated into the DNA double helix. Antifolate drugs methotrexate and trimetrexate inhibit the enzyme dihydrofolate reductase (DHFR), which catalyzes the reduction of dihydrofolate (folic acid) to tetrohydrofolate (folinic acid). Reduced folates act as 1-carbon donors necessary for the synthesis of purine and pyrimidine bases. Inhibition of DHFR by methotrexate depletes the intracellular reduced folate pool, thereby blocking de novo synthesis of nucleotide bases. These compounds also inhibit other folate-dependent enzymes such as thymidylate synthase, which catalyzes uracil to thymidine. Cytotoxicity is the result of an arrest of folate-dependent enzymatic reactions, including DNA, RNA, and protein synthesis.[155]

Rapidly proliferating cells in S phase are most susceptible to methotrexate-induced depletion of reduced folates.[129] Therefore, longer exposure of tumor cells to methotrexate will allow more cells to enter the DNA synthesis phase of the cell cycle and result in enhanced cell kill. Most cells can function with relatively small amounts of DHFR to maintain sufficient reduced folate pools. Therefore, a high intracellular concentration of antifolate drugs should be maintained to ensure complete enzyme inhibition. This may be accomplished by administering large amounts of methotrexate such as that seen in treatment for malignant lymphomas and sarcomas. The ability to administer such high doses is possible only with the timely administration of leucovorin (folinic acid). Leucovorin circumvents methotrexateinduced enzyme blockade and "rescues" normal cells by providing them with the reduced folates they need for nucleic acid and protein synthesis.[156]

Methotrexate is one of the most extensively studied antineoplastic drugs for its pharmacokinetics, in part because there is a simple and readily available assay to measure the blood concentration of methotrexate. This assay is frequently used to monitor for potential toxicity when administering moderate to high doses of methotrexate. The drug is well absorbed orally at moderate to low doses. Elimination occurs primarily through renal excretion via glomerular filtration and active secretion in the proximal tubule.[157] Excretion is highly dependent on adequate renal function and may be inhibited by a number of compounds (see Drug Interactions in this chapter). Doses should be reduced in patients with decreased renal function, and blood levels should be monitored following each dose. Patients with blood levels greater than $1 \times 10^{-6}$ M at 48 hours post dose are at increased risk for severe myelosuppression and mucositis.[158,159] Leucovorin therapy should be continued in these patients until methotrexate blood levels are below $5 \times 10^{-8}$ micromolar. Dose reductions vary and should be proportionate with reductions in creatinine clearance. Patients with a creatinine clearance of 10–50 ml/minute should receive 30%–50% of the original dose, and those with creatinine clearance less than 10 ml/minute only 15% of original dose.[160] The pharmacokinetics of methotrexate are altered by distribution into third-space fluid collections such as ascitic accumulation in the peritoneal cavity. Elimination is prolonged and toxicity is increased because of the slow redistribution of the drug from the peritoneum back into the blood.[161]

Methotrexate-associated toxicities, besides myelosuppression and mucositis, include nephrotoxicity, hepatotoxicity, and pulmonary fibrosis. Hepatotoxicity may result from high-dose therapy and result in acute and reversible elevations in liver function enzymes. Methotrexate is useful as treatment or prophylaxis for meningeal leukemia; however, the drug poorly distributes into the cerebrospinal fluid (CSF). Therefore, methotrexate may be injected directly into the CSF by lumbar puncture or intraventricular device (Ommaya reservoir). Toxicities seen with intrathecal administration include severe headache, nuchal rigidity, vomiting, and fever; in severe cases a demyelinating encephalopathy may develop.

*Pyrimidine analogues* The fluoropyrimidine 5-fluorouracil (5-FU) undergoes extensive metabolism intracellularly to an active metabolite fluoro-deoxyuridine monophosphate (FdUMP). FdUMP covalently binds with thymidylate synthase (TS) and inhibits the enzyme's ability to synthesize deoxythymidine triphosphate (dTTP), a precursor of DNA synthesis. Other metabolic pathways are conversion of 5-FU to fluorouradine triphosphate (FUTP), which may be incorporated into RNA, and conversion of FdUMP to the triphosphate form, which may be incorporated into DNA. Cytotoxicity of 5-FU by these metabolic pathways results in depletion of dTTP or false incorporation of other metabolites into DNA and RNA.[162–164] The administration of 5-FU and leucovorin concurrently enhances this reaction and increases the cytotoxic effect of 5-FU (see Modulation of 5-Fluorouracil by Leucovorin).

5-FU is rapidly cleared by the liver and has a plasma half-life of 6–20 minutes. There may be considerable variation in half-life time among patients. 5-FU is metabolized to dihydrofluorouracil by the enzyme dihydropyrimidine dehydrogenase in the liver and other tissues. Patients who are deficient in this enzyme experience greatly increased 5-FU levels and resultant toxicity.[165] When 5-FU or floxuridine is administered directly into the hepatic artery or portal vein, hepatic metastases are directly exposed to the drug with minimal systemic exposure because of the drug's significant first-pass clearance.

The major dose-limiting toxicity of 5-FU is dependent on the schedule of administration. Myelosuppression is more prominent when the drug is given by rapid bolus injection, whereas mucositis and gastrointestinal toxicity are more common with prolonged infusions over four to five days. Cholestatic jaundice and biliary sclerosis are complications of intrahepatic adminstration of fluoropyrimidines. 5-FU therapy has sometimes caused chest pain, elevation in cardiac enzymes, and ECG changes similar to those seen with myocardial ischemia. This syndrome may be associated with 5-FU–induced coronary vasospasm.[166]

Cytarabine was originally isolated from the sponge *Cryptothethya crypta*. The parent drug is phosphorylated to ara-CTP, which competes with the normal substrate deoxycytidine triphosphate (dCTP) to inhibit DNA polymerase-alpha.[167] DNA polymerases are critical enzymes in the synthesis and repair of DNA. The metabolite ara-CTP may also incorporate into DNA and interfere with chain polymerization and repair of damaged DNA strands.[168] As seen with other antimetabolites, tumor cells and normal tissues are most sensitive to cytarabine in the S phase of the cell cycle.

Cytarabine is rapidly converted to the inactive metabolite ara-U by the enzyme cytidine deaminase, which is present in many tissues, including the gastrointestinal epithelium and liver. The half-life is 7–20 minutes, with more than 70% of the dose appearing in the urine as ara-U. Cytarabine is usually administered by continuous infusion following a bolus dose. This regimen is used to maintain cytotoxic levels despite the drug's rapid inactivation and to maximally expose all cycling cells to the cytotoxic effects during the S phase of the cell cycle. Cytarabine may be used alone or in addition to methotrexate for meningeal leukemia; however, direct intrathecal administration is necessary to obtain sufficient drug concentrations in the CSF. Only small amounts of cytarabine are needed intrathecally because deamination is minimal in the CSF. Toxicity of cytarabine includes myelosuppression and gastrointestinal epithelial injury. When high-dose cytarabine is used for refractory acute myelogenous leukemia (AML), 20% of patients may experience a cerebral and cerebellar dysfunction. This syndrome is more often seen in individuals older than 50 and is characterized by slurred speech, ataxia, confusion, and coma.[170] High-dose cytarabine is also associated with conjunctivitis, which can usually be prevented by giving the patient steroid ophthalmic drops.

***Purine analogues*** Thiopurines 6-mercaptopurine (6-MP) and 6-thioguanine (6-TG) are converted to their respective monophosphates, which inhibit purine synthesis and cause an accumulation of nucleic acid precursors. These precursors in turn facilitate the conversion of 6-MP and 6-TG to their active nucleotide forms. The triphosphate nucleotides of these drugs incorporate into DNA and induce strand breaks, which are correlated with cytotoxicity.[171] Methotrexate, an inhibitor of de novo purine biosynthesis, is synergistic with the 6-thiopurines by blocking purine synthesis and enhancing thiopurine activation. The cytotoxicity of fludarabine and cladrabine (2-chlorodeoxyadenosine) is associated with their ability to inhibit DNA polymerase and other enzymes utilized in the synthesis of DNA and RNA.[172,173]

## Plant derivatives

Antineoplastic drugs derived from plant sources represent a large and diverse group of chemotherapeutic drugs. Many of the drugs in this group (plant alkaloids, paclitaxel) are naturally occurring alkaloids that were isolated from plant material. Others are the result of synthetic and semisynthetic processes used to manufacture analogues of compounds originally extracted from plants. Examples include etoposide, docetaxel, and topotecan. The discovery of new plant-derived compounds with antitumor activity is ongoing and will continue to provide important and novel agents for the treatment of cancer.

***Vinca alkaloids*** Natural alkaloids present in small quantities in the periwinkle plant, play a major role in cancer chemotherapy. Although the drugs in this group are dramatically similar in chemical structure, their antitumor activity and toxicity differ greatly.[129] Vincristine has a broad spectrum of activity, including leukemia, lymphoma, breast cancer, lung cancer, and multiple myeloma, while vinblastine is used primarily in germ cell tumors and advanced Hodgkin's disease. Vinblastine is myelotoxic and neurotoxic; vincristine is also neurotoxic but has amazingly minimal myelotoxicity. Vinorelbine is the newest vinca alkaloid to become available in the United States. It is active in breast cancer and non–small-cell lung cancer and is both myelotoxic and neurotoxic. Vindesine is widely available in Europe but currently not available in the United States except in clinical trials.

Vinca alkaloids belong to a group of compounds now known as the *tubulin interactive agents*. They exert their cytotoxic effects primarily by interfering with normal microtubule formation and function, which is critical for the mitosis phase of the cell cycle and ultimately cell division. Microtubules have other important cellular functions that are affected by the vinca alkaloids, including maintenance of cell shape and intracellular transport. Vinca alkaloids bind to specific sites on tubulin, preventing formation of tubulin dimers and inhibiting the formation of microtubule structures. Although mitotic arrest is the primary mechanism of cell death, vinca alkaloids may have a cytolytic effect on resting cells in $G_0$ phase and other cells in $G_1$ or S phase.[174] Cells are sensitive to low concentrations of vincristine, and duration of exposure is critical in cytotoxic effect.

Despite the wide range of clinical uses of the vinca alkaloids, there is surprisingly little information available to describe their pharmacological and pharmacokinetic profiles. This may be primarily the result of lack of a sensitive drug assay for quantitating the low concentration found in patients receiving vincas. Vincristine is highly bound to serum proteins, blood cells, and especially platelets. Vincristine is metabolized primarily by the liver and concentrates in the bile. Seventy percent of a dose is excreted in the feces, and approximately 10% is excreted in the urine.[175] Dose modification should be considered in patients with hepatic dysfunction, particularly patients with biliary obstructions. Vinblastine and vinorelbine have similar pharmacokinetic profiles with excretion occurring primarily through the biliary tract. All the vinca alkaloids have a prolonged terminal elimination phase half-life of one to four days.

Vinca alkaloids are known for their peripheral neurotoxicity, which is frequently a cumulative dose-limiting toxicity. Peripheral neurotoxicity initially presents as sensory impairment (stocking-and-glove distribution) and paresthesias. Patients may later develop neuritic pain and motor dysfunction. Loss of deep tendon reflexes, foot and wrist drop, ataxia, and paralysis may occur with continued vinca alkaloid therapy. The only effective management is discontinuation of therapy. Accidental intrathecal administration of vincristine induces an ascending paralysis resulting in death. Constipation and abdominal pain are frequent complaints of older patients while on vincristine. Myelosuppression is also a dose-limiting toxicity of vinblastine and navelbine, but not vincristine. The vinca alkaloids are vesicants, and extravasation should be avoided.

***Taxanes*** The taxanes are emerging as an extremely important group of antitumor compounds with activity in a wide range of cancers. Extracted and isolated from the bark of the Pacific yew tree *Taxus brevifolia*, paclitaxel has demonstrated antitumor activity in preclinical studies in a broad range of tumor models.[176] Taxanes are complex chemical structures and difficult to synthesize in the laboratory; therefore, extraction and isolation from plant material was the only source for paclitaxel until recently, when a semisynthetic process using a taxane precursor was introduced. Because of the drug's poor water solubility, the injectable formulation must contain 50% Cremophor EL vehicle to maintain aqueous solubility. This creates problems with administration since Cremophor

EL can leach hepatotoxic plasticizer from PVC plastic infusion devices and is also associated with severe hypersensitivity reactions.

Initially, the mechanism of action of paclitaxel was thought to be inhibition of microtubule formation similar to that of the vinca alkaloids. Interest in the drug's development was renewed when it was discovered that stabilization of microtubules was identified as the primary mechanism of activity. Paclitaxel preferentially binds to microtubules over tubulin dimers, and inhibits microtubule disassembly, which is necessary for normal functioning of microtubule structures.[177] Cells exposed to paclitaxel display many arrays of disorganized microtubules during all phases of the cell cycle.[178] Although taxanes have these distinct antimicrotubule effects on cells, the actual mechanism of cell death is unclear. The mechanism of action and cytotoxic effect of docetaxel are similar to those of paclitaxel.[179]

Hepatic metabolism and biliary excretion probably constitute the major routes of elimination for paclitaxel and docetaxel.[180,181] Urinary excretion accounts for less than 5% of total body clearance of the drug. Paclitaxel clearance is reduced by as much as 30% when given following cisplatin.[182] This interaction results in increased peak plasma concentrations of paclitaxel and more severe myelotoxicity than is seen with the reverse administration schedule. For routine use of paclitaxel with cisplatin or carboplatin, the paclitaxel should be given first, followed by cisplatin or carboplatin. The taxanes also exhibit a high degree of protein binding (90%–95%). Among the most significant toxicities associated with taxanes are myelosuppression, neurotoxicity, hypersensitivity, total-body alopecia, and transient myalgias and arthralgias. Hypersensitivity reactions were seen in 10% of patients receiving paclitaxel during early clinical trials.[183] Hypersensitivity reactions usually occur within the first ten minutes of the initial infusion and may be characterized by hypotension, bronchospasm, dyspnea, abdominal and leg pain, and severe facial flushing. Major hypersensitivity reactions may be prevented in most patients by the preinfusion administration of a corticosteroid (dexamethasone), an antihistamine (diphenhydramine), and a H₂-blocking drug (cimetidine). Paclitaxel may be safely given parenterally with infusions lasting 24, 3, or 1 hours. The 3-hour infusion rate has been associated with less neutropenia than the 24-hour infusion.

The toxicity profile of docetaxel is different from that of paclitaxel.[184] The incidence of hypersensitivity reactions is lower with docetaxel, with severe reactions experienced in fewer than 1% of patients treated. Skin reactions, including pruritus, macular or papular lesions, erythema, and desquamation, are seen in 50%–70% of patients treated with docetaxel. Nail changes, consisting of an orange discoloration and thickening of the nails, were also observed in many patients in clinical trials. A more significant complication is fluid retention and weight gain, which can occur in 6% of patients. Characteristics of this side effect include peripheral edema, generalized edema, pleural effusion, and cardiac tamponade. A five-day regimen of corticosteroid is useful in preventing and lessening the fluid retention, and is also useful for prevention of hypersensitivity reactions.

***Epipodophyllotoxins*** Podophyllotoxin, an extract of the mandrake plant, is an antimitotic drug that binds to tubulin and inhibits microtubulin formation. This compound was not further developed as an antitumor agent because of its unacceptable toxicity in humans. Etoposide and teniposide are glycosidic derivatives of podophyllotoxin that possess significant activity in many human tumors such as germ cell tumors and lung cancer, with a more predictable and mild toxicity profile. Initially, these drugs were thought to work as antimicrotubule agents similar to podophyllotoxin and vinca alkaloids. However, these agents produced no effect on microtubule assembly.[185] Cell cycle studies demonstrated epipodophyllotoxins induced arrest of cells in late S or early G phase instead of the expected M-phase arrest common with antimitotic drugs. Along with the observation of drug-induced DNA strand breaks, scientists have suggested the primary cytotoxic mechanism of these compounds is inhibition of topoisomerase II.[186] Epipodophyllotoxins stabilize the enzyme-DNA formation, thereby inhibiting the reunion of the two DNA strands originally cleaved by the enzyme. Additionally, the synergy of the etoposides with antimetabolite drugs may be the result of inhibition of nucleoside transport into the cell.[131]

Etoposide and teniposide are highly protein-bound (94% and 99%, respectively) to the albumin. Drugs that interfere with the protein binding of teniposide may induce greater toxicity in patients receiving both drugs (see Drug Interactions in Oncology Patients). Renal clearance is the major route of elimination for etoposide, with approximately 40%–60% of the drug excreted unchanged in the urine. Biliary excretion and hepatic metabolism are responsible for elimination to a lesser extent.[187] Teniposide is more extensively metabolized, with only 5%–20% excreted unchanged in the urine. The cytotoxic effects of etoposide exhibit a schedule dependency in the treatment of extensive small-cell lung cancer.[188] Etoposide is available as an oral formulation, which has a bioavailability of approximately 50%.

The toxicities of both agents are similar, with myelosuppression, hypersensitivity, and infusion-related blood pressure changes being the most significant. Both agents are also poorly water-soluble, necessitating the addition of tween 80 or Cremophor EL and other excipients to maintain the drugs in aqueous solution. The manufacturer of teniposide recommends avoiding the use of PVC plastic infusion devices to prevent exposing the patient to potentially hepatotoxic plasticizers leached from the plastic by the Cremophor vehicle.

***Camptothecin derivatives*** Camptothecin sodium was originally tested in the early 1970s as an antitumor compound. Despite the drug's significant activity in both preclinical and clinical trials, it was abandoned because of unpredictable and often severe hemorrhagic cystitis.

Later interest in this group of drugs was renewed with the introduction of semisynthetic analogues of camptothecin. Topotecan and irinotecan have undergone extensive clinical evaluation and were recently approved by the FDA as single-agent therapy for refractory ovarian cancer and relapsed colon cancer, respectively. Their proposed mechanism of action is inhibition of topoisomerase I, an enzyme responsible for maintaining the three-dimensional structure of DNA. Topoisomerase inhibitors bind with the DNA-enzyme complex, thereby inducing DNA strand breaks and cell death.[189]

Camptothecins appear to exist in two species in aqueous solutions, a closed lactone ring, which possesses cytotoxic activity, and an open carboxylate form, which does not. The conversion is pH-dependent, with the open form predominating in an alkaline environment and the closed, or active, form predominating in an acidic solution. Much of the unpredictable urotoxicity seen in early trials of camptothecin sodium may be explained by the lack of knowledge of the pH-dependent conversion and the shift of the equilibrium toward the active species in the acidic environment of the bladder. Irinotecan is a pro-drug and must be converted to its active form via carboxylesterase in the body.[190] Myelosuppression is the major dose-limiting toxicity of topotecan, while diarrhea is the primary dose-limiting toxicity for irinotecan when administered on a once-weekly schedule. To effectively manage the diarrhea associated with irinotecan, patients should be instructed to start a high-dose loperamide regimen (2 mg of loperamide every two hours) until they are diarrhea-free for 12 hours.

### Miscellaneous agents

L-asparaginase induces a rapid and complete depletion from the blood of the amino acid L-asparagine. This biochemical process is cytotoxic to tumor cells highly dependent on exogenous sources of the amino acid. The major cytotoxic effect is the inhibition of protein synthesis, with a secondary effect of inhibition of nucleic acid synthesis also observed in sensitive cells.[131] L-asparaginase is considered cell cycle phase nonspecific despite the drug's ability to block cells in $G_1$ and S phases of the cell cycle. The drug's only antineoplastic use is as part of the induction and consolidation therapy for acute lymphocytic leukemia in both children and adults. L-asparaginase is extracted from *Escherichia coli* bacteria and is associated with a high incidence of anaphylaxis. Patients who develop severe hypersensitivity reactions to the bacterial source product may receive pegaspargase, which is chemically altered to be less immunogenic. Other toxicities seen with L-asparaginase include hyperglycemia, hypoprothrombinemia, and neurotoxicity.

Hydroxyurea is a DNA-selective antimetabolite that inhibits ribonucleotide reductase and has minimal inhibitory effect on RNA and protein synthesis. Its major indication is in rapidly controlling blood counts in acute leukemia and other myeloproliferative diseases such as polycythemia vera and essential thrombocytosis. Allopurinol should be used in conjuction with hydroxyurea to prevent tumor lysis syndrome.

## Hormonal Therapy

Hormonal manipulations were among the first treatments used to control cancer. Initially they had limited potential to induce significant response in sensitive tumors; currently, however, they are critical components in the treatment for many different neoplasms. Table 14-15[69] lists the commonly used hormonal agents and their primary indications. Steroids and steroid analogues constitute the majority of drugs used for hormonal therapy.[191] Their mechanism of action is incompletely understood but probably involves the inhibition of steroid-specific receptors located on the surface of cells. Luteinizing hormone releasing hormone agonists are synthetic analogues of the naturally occurring hormone. Initially these drugs induce an increase in testosterone levels secondary to their stimulation of luteinizing hormone release. However, with continued use, the pituitary gland becomes desensitized, resulting in a dramatic decrease in the production of estrogens and androgens. Blocking these receptors prevents the cell from receiving normal hormonal growth stimulation, thereby decreasing the growth fraction of the tumor. This mechanism of action is seen with the antiestrogen drug tamoxifen, which is used for breast cancer. Another approach is to administer steroids with opposite or antagonistic effects, such as estrogens in prostate cancer or androgens in breast cancer. Estramustine is a unique compound made up of a molecule of estradiol phosphate combined with nitrogen mustard. Originally thought to have alkylating properties, the drug's mechanism of action is now thought to be related to antimicrotubule activity.[192]

## Retinoids

Retinoids, a class of compounds structurally related to vitamin A (retinol), have been found to influence proliferation and differentiation of normal and tumor cells.[193] The two compounds most studied for their effect on controlling or preventing tumor growth are 13-*cis* retinoic acid (isotretinoin) and all-trans retinoic acid (tretinoin). Isotretinoin is currently marketed as the antiacne product Accutane®, however, it is under extensive evaluation, often in combination with alfa-interferon, for the prevention of new and recurrent squamous cell tumors.[194,195] Other potential uses for isotretinoin include myelodysplastic syndromes and acute and chronic leukemias.[196–198] Tretinoin (Vesanoid®) has recently been approved for use in induction and maintenance regimens for acute promyelocytic leukemia. Toxicity of these compounds is similar to the pharmacological effects of hypervitaminosis A, which include dry lips and mucous membranes, skin fragility, brittle nails, photosensitivity, and conjunctivitis.[199] Other side effects are headache, nausea and vomiting, transaminase and triglyceride elevations, and arthralgia and bone pain. Tretinoin is also associated with a severe leukocytosis, which may induce fevers, respiratory distress, pulmonary and pericardial effusions, and hypotension.[200] All retinoids are teratogens and therefore should never be given to pregnant female patients.

## CONCLUSION

Drug therapy for the control and cure of cancer has come a long way from early experimentation with mustard gas derivatives. Currently a multitude of drugs with a variety of treatment schedules are among the oncologist's armamentarium. Research efforts must continue to focus on improving the oncology patient's life by evaluating new drugs and therapies, as well as reevaluating old ones. Biological therapies are also being actively investigated for their ability to control tumor growth and generation. The development of gene therapy approaches may hold the key to more effective and better-tolerated treatment for cancer. New knowledge of this type is expanding exponentially as technology enhances our ability to peer into the genetic workings of the tumor cell. Future directions for research in oncology should include combining chemotherapy and biological therapy, gene therapy or all of these to achieve optimal patient outcomes.

## REFERENCES

1. Kennedy BJ: Evolution of chemotherapy. *CA Cancer J Clin* 41:261–263, 1991 (editorial)
2. Einhorn LH, Donohue J: Cis-Diamminedichloroplatinum, vinblastine and bleomycin: Combination chemotherapy in disseminated testicular cancer. *Am Intern Med* 87:293–298, 1977
3. Zubrod CG, Schepartz S, Leiter J, et al: The chemotherapy program of the National Cancer Institute: History, analysis and plans. *Cancer Chemother Rep* 50:349–540, 1966
4. Shoemaker RH, Wolpert-DeFilippes MK, Kern DH, et al: Application of a human tumor colony-forming assay to new drug screening. *Cancer Res* 45:2145–2153, 1985
5. DeVita VT: Principles of chemotherapy, in DeVita VT, Hellman S, Rosenberg SA (eds): *Cancer: Principles and Practice of Oncology* (ed 4). Philadelphia, Lippincott, 1993, pp 276–292
6. VonHoff DD, Kuhn J, Clark GM: Design and conduct of phase I trials, in Buyse ME, Staquet MJ, Sylvester RJ (eds): *Cancer Clinical Trials, Methods and Practice*. New York, Oxford University Press, 1984, pp 210–220
7. Heidelberger C, Chaudhuri N, Weston E: The metabolism of 5-fluorouracil-2-C14 in humans. *Proc Am Assoc Cancer Res* 2:306, 1958
8. Riggs CE: Antitumor antibiotics and related compounds, in Perry MC (ed): *Chemotherapy Source Book*. Baltimore, Williams and Wilkins, 1992, pp 318–358
9. DeVita VT: Cell kinetics and chemotherapy of cancer. *Cancer Chemother Rep* 2:22–23, 1971
10. Steel GG: Cell loss as a factor in the growth rate of human tumors. *Eur J Cancer* 3:381–387, 1967
11. Charbit A, Malaise EP, Tubiana M: Relation between the pathological nature and the growth rate of human tumors. *Eur J Cancer* 7:307–315, 1971
12. Pierce GB, Shike R, Fink LM: *Cancer: A Problem of Developmental Biology*. Englewood Cliffs, NJ, Prentice-Hall, 1978
13. Skipper HE, Schabel FM, Wilcox WS: Experimental evaluation of potential anticancer agents XII: On the criteria and kinetics associated with "curability" of experimental leukemia. *Cancer Chemother Rep* 35:1–111, 1964
14. Skipper HE, Schabel FM, Mellet LB, et al: Implications of biochemical cytokinetic, pharmacologic, and toxicologic relationships in the design of optimal therapeutic schedules. *Cancer Chemother Rep* 54:431–450, 1950
15. Norton L: The Norton-Simon hypothesis, in Perry MC (ed): *Chemotherapy Source Book*. Baltimore, Williams and Wilkins, 1992, pp 36–53
16. Norton L, Day R: Potential innovations in scheduling in cancer chemotherapy, in DeVita VT, Hellman S, Rosenberg SA (eds): *Important Advances in Oncology*. Philadelphia, Lippincott, 1991, pp 57–73
17. Norton LA: A Gompertzian model of human breast cancer growth. *Cancer Res* 48:7067–7071, 1988
18. Goldie JH, Coldman AJ: A mathematic model for relating the drug sensitivity of tumors to their spontaneous mutation rate. *Cancer Treat Rep* 63:1727–1733, 1979
19. Goldie JH: Scientific basis for adjuvant and primary (neoadjuvant) chemotherapy. *Semin Oncol* 14:1–7, 1987
20. DeVita VT, Young RC, Canellos GP: Combination versus single agent chemotherapy: A review of the basis for selection of drug treatment of cancer. *Cancer* 35:98–110, 1975
21. Skipper HE, Simpson-Herren L: Relationship between tumor cell heterogeneity and responsiveness to chemotherapy, in DeVita VT, Hellman S, Rosenberg SA (eds): *Important Advances in Oncology*. Philadelphia, Lippincott, 1985, pp 63–77
22. Goldie JH, Coldman AJ: The genetic origin of drug resistance in neoplasms: Implications for systemic therapy. *Cancer Res* 44:3643–3653, 1984
23. Endicott JA, Ling V: The biochemistry of P-glycoprotein–mediated multidrug resistance. *Annu Rev Biochem* 58:137–171, 1989
24. Riordan JR, Ling V: Genetic and biochemical characterization of multidrug resistance. *Pharmacol Ther* 28:51–78, 1985
25. DeVita, VT: The relationship between tumor mass and resistance to chemotherapy. *Cancer* 51:1209–1220, 1983
26. Goldie JH: Relevance of drug resistance in cancer treatment strategy, in Muggia FM (ed): *Cancer Chemotherapy*. New York, Martinus Nijhoff, 1983, pp 1–30
27. Goldie JH: Drug resistance and cancer chemotherapy strategy in breast cancer. *Breast Cancer Res Treat* 3:129–136, 1983
28. Luria SE, Delbruck M: Mutations of bacteria from virus sensitivity to virus resistance. *Genetics* 28:491–511, 1943
29. Law LW: Origin of the resistance of leukemic cells to folic acid antagonists. *Nature* 169:628–629, 1952
30. Yarbro JW: The scientific basis of cancer chemotherapy, in Perry MC (ed): *Chemotherapy Source Book*. Baltimore, Williams and Wilkins, 1992, pp 2–14
31. Buick RN: Cellular basis of chemotherapy, in Dorr RT, Von Hoff DD (eds): *Cancer Chemotherapy Handbook* (ed 2). Norwalk, CT, Appleton and Lange, 1994, pp 3–14
32. Stewart CD, Burke PJ: Cytidine deaminase and the develop-

ment of resistance to cytosine arabinoside. *Nature* 233: 109–117, 1971

33. Armstrong RA: Fluoropyrimidine activity and resistance at the cellular level, in Kessel D (ed): *Resistance to Antineoplastic Drugs*. Boca Raton, FL, CRC Press, 1989, pp 317–332

34. Haber DA, Beverly SM, Kiely ML, et al: Properties of altered dehydrofolate reductase encoded by amplified genes in cultured mouse fibroblasts. *J Biol Chem* 256:9501–9510, 1981

35. Pommier Y, Kerrigan D, Schwartz JA, et al: Altered DNA topoisomerase II activity in Chinese hamster cells resistant to topoisomerase II inhibitors. *Cancer Res* 46:3075–3079, 1988

36. Chao CCK, Lee YL, Cheng PW, et al: Enhanced host cell reactivation of damaged plasmid DNA in HeLa cells resistant to cis-diamminedichlorplatinum (II). *Cancer Res* 51: 601–605, 1991

37. Biedler J, Riehm H: Cellular resistance to actinomycin D in Chinese hamster cells in vitro: Cross-resistance, radioautographic, and cytogenetic studies. *Cancer Res* 30: 1174–1182, 1970

38. Gill DR, Hyde SC, Higgins CF, et al: Separation of drug transport and chloride channel functions of the human multidrug resistance P-glycoprotein. *Cell* 71:23–32, 1992

39. Cordon-Carlo C, O'Brien JP, Boccia J, et al: Expression of the multidrug resistance gene product (p-glycoprotein) in human normal and tumor tissues. *J Histochem Cytochem* 38: 1277–1287, 1990

40. Sugawara I, Hamada H, Tsuruo T, et al: Specialized localization of P-glycoprotein recognized by MRK 16 monoclonal antibody in endothelial cells of the brain and the spinal cord. *Jpn J Cancer Res* 81:727–730, 1990

41. Dalton WS: Overcoming the multidrug-resistant phenotype, in DeVita VT, Hellman S, Rosenberg SA (eds): *Cancer: Principles and Practice of Oncology* (ed 4). Philadelphia, Lippincott, 1993, pp 2655–2666

42. Marie J, Zittoun R, Sikic B: Multidrug resistance (*MDR-1*) gene expression in adult acute leukemias: Correlations with treatment and in vitro drug sensitivity. *Blood* 78: 586–592, 1991

43. Bell DR, Gerlach JH, Kartner N, et al: Detection of P-glycoprotein in ovarian cancer: A molecular marker associated with multidrug resistance. *J Clin Oncol* 3:311–315, 1985

44. Schneider J, Bak M, Efferth TH, et al: P-glycoprotein expression in treated and untreated breast cancer. *Br J Cancer* 60:815–818, 1989

45. Goldstein LJ, Galski H, Fojo A, et al: Expression of a multidrug resistance in human cancers. *J Natl Cancer Inst* 81: 116–176, 1989

46. Cole SPC, Sparks KE, Fraser K, et al: Pharmacological characterization of multidrug resistant MRP-transfected human cells. *Cancer Res* 54:5902–5910, 1994

47. Ford JM, Hait WN: Pharmacology of drugs that alter multidrug resistance in cancer. *Pharmacol Rev* 42:155–199, 1990

48. Murren JR, DeVita VT: Another look at multidrug resistance. *PPO Updates* 9:1–12, 1995

49. Miller TP, Grogan TM, Dalton WS, et al: P-glycoprotein expression in malignant lymphoma and reversal of clinical drug resistance with chemotherapy plus high-dose verapamil. *J Clin Oncol* 9:17–26, 1991

50. Sonneveld P, Durie BGM, Lonkhorst HM, et al: Modulation of multidrug resistant myeloma by cyclosporin: The Leukemia Group of the EORTC and the HOVON. *Lancet* 340: 225–229, 1992

51. Yahanda AM, Adler KM, Fisher GA, et al: Phase I trial of etoposide with cyclosporine as a modulator of multidrug resistance. *J Clin Oncol* 10:1624–1634, 1992

52. Linn SC, van Kalken C, van Tellingen O, et al: Clinical and pharmacologic study of multidrug resistance reversal with vinblastine and bepridil. *J Clin Oncol* 12:812–819, 1994

53. Pennock GD, Dalton WS, Roeske WR, et al: Systemic toxic effects associated with high-dose verapamil infusion and chemotherapy administration. *J Natl Cancer Inst* 83: 105–110, 1991

54. Miller RL, Bukowski RM, Budd GT, et al: Clinical modulation of doxorubicin resistance by the calmodulin inhibitor trifluoperazin: A phase I trial. *J Clin Oncol* 6:880–888, 1988

55. Keilhauer C, Emling F, Raschack M, et al: The use of R-verapamil (R-VPM) is superior to racemic verapamil (VPM) in breaking multidrug resistance (MDR) of malignant cells. *Proc Am Assoc Cancer Res* 30:503, 1989 (abstr)

56. Fan D, Regenass U, Bettran P, et al: Protein kinase C inhibitor staurosporin derivative CGP 41251 reverses MDR in murine and human cancer cell lines. *Anticancer Drugs* 5:29, 1994 (suppl 1)

57. Bonadonna G, Zambetti M, Valagussa P: Sequential or alternating doxorubicin and CMF regimens in breast cancer with more than three positive nodes: Ten-year results. *JAMA* 273:542–547, 1995

58. Glisson BS: Multidrug resistance mediated through alterations in topoisomerase II. *Cancer Bull* 41:37, 1989

59. Mannervik B, Danielson UH: Glutathione transferases: Structure and catalytic activity. *Crit Rev Biochem* 23:283–337, 1988

60. Lazo JS, Basu A: Metallothionein expression and transient resistance to electrophilic antineoplastic drugs. *Cancer Biol* 2:267–271, 1991

61. Ozols RF, O'Dwyer PJ, Hamilton TC, et al: The role of glutathione in drug resistance. *Cancer Treat Rev* 17:45–50, 1990 (suppl A)

62. Holland JF: Induction chemotherapy: An old term for an old concept, in *Neoadjuvant Chemotherapy*. Philadelphia, Colloque INSERM, 1986, pp. 45–47.

63. Frei A III, Clark JR, Miller D: The concept of neoadjuvant chemotherapy, in Salmon SE (ed): *Adjuvant Therapy of Cancer V*. Orlando, FL, Grune and Stratton, 1987, p 67–72

64. Jacobs C, Pinto H: Adjuvant and neoadjuvant treatment of head and neck cancers: The next chapter. *Semin Oncol* 22:540–552, 1995

65. Friedland DM, Comis RL: Perioperative therapy of non–small cell lung cancer: A review of adjuvant and neoadjuvant approaches. *Semin Oncol* 22:571–581, 1995

66. Hryniuk WM: The importance of dose intensity in the outcome of chemotherapy, in DeVita VT, Hellman S, Rosenberg SA (eds): *Important Advances in Oncology 1988*. Philadelphia, Lippincott, 1988, pp 121–142

67. Hryniuk WM: Average relative dose intensity and the impact on design of clinical trials. *Semin Oncol* 14:65–74, 1987

68. Hryniuk WM, Levine MN: Analysis of dose intensity for adjuvant chemotherapy trials in stage II breast cancer. *J Clin Oncol* 4:1162–1170, 1986

69. Bonadonna G, Valagussa R: Dose-response effect of adjuvant chemotherapy in breast cancer. *N Engl J Med* 304: 10–15, 1981

70. Canellos GP, Pocock SJ, Taylor SG III, et al: Combination chemotherapy for metastatic breast cancer: Prospective comparison of multiple drug therapy with L-phenylalanine mustard. *Cancer* 38:1882–1886, 1976

71. Dorr RT, Von Hoff DD (eds): *Cancer Chemotherapy Handbook* (ed 2). Norwalk, CT, Appleton and Lange, 1994

72. Product information: Etyol. Palo Alto, CA, Alza Pharmaceuticals, 1986

73. Seifert CF, Nesser ME, Thompson DF: Dexrazoxane in the prevention of doxorubicin-induced cardiotoxicity. *Ann Pharmacother* 28:1063–1072, 1994

74. Rice A, Reiffers J: Peripheral blood stem cells contain pluripotent stem cells. *Int J Cell Cloning* 10:101, 1992 (suppl 1)

75. Bregni M, Sierna S, Magni M, et al: Circulating hemopoietic progenitors mobilized by cancer chemotherapy and by rhGM-CSF in the treatment of high-grade non-Hodgkin's lymphoma. *Leukemia* 5:123, 1991 (suppl 1)

76. Haas R, Ho AD, Bredthauer U, et al: Successful autologous transplantation of blood stem cells mobilized with recombinant human granulocyte-macrophage colony-stimulating factor. *Exp Hematol* 18:94–98, 1990

77. Kessinger A: Autologous transplantation with peripheral blood stem cells: A review of clinical results. *J Clin Apheresis* 5:97, 1990

78. Brugger W, Bross KJ, Blatt M, et al: Mobilization of tumor cells and hematopoietic progenitor cells into peripheral blood of patients with solid tumors. *Blood* 83:636–640, 1994

79. Vokes EE, Weichselbaum RR: Concomitant chemoradiotherapy: Rational and clinical experience in patients with solid tumors. *J Clin Oncol* 8:911–934, 1990

80. Rotman M, Aziz H: Concomitant continuous infusion chemotherapy and radiation. *Cancer* 65:823–835, 1990

81. Third International Conference on the Interaction of Radiation Therapy and Systemic Therapy. *Int J Radiat Oncol Biol Phys* 20:195–386, 1991

82. Rotman M, Rosenthal CJ: *Concomitant Continuous Infusion Chemotherapy and Radiation.* New York, Springer-Verlag, 1991

83. Tannock IF, Rotin D: Keynote address: Mechanisms of interaction between radiation and drugs with potential for improvements in therapy. *Monogr Natl Cancer Inst* 6:77–83, 1988

84. McNeil BJ, Weichselbaum RR, Pauker S: Speech and survival: Tradeoffs between quality and quantity of life in laryngeal cancer. *N Engl J Med* 305:982–987, 1981

85. Wolf GT, Hong WK, Gross-Fischer S, et al: Induction chemotherapy plus radiation compared with surgery plus radiation in patients with advanced laryngeal cancer: The Department of Veterans Affairs Laryngeal Cancer Study Group. *N Engl J Med* 324:1685–1690, 1991

86. Begg AC, Van der Kolk PJ, Dewit L, et al: Radiosensitization by cisplatin of R1F1 tumor cells in vitro. *Int J Radiat Biol* 50:871–884, 1986

87. Kallman RF, Rapachhietta D, Zaghloul MS: Schedule-dependent therapeutic gain from the combination of fractionated irradiation plus c-DDP and 5-FU or plus C-DDP and cyclophosphamide in C3H/Km mouse model systems. *Int J Radiat Oncol Biol Phys* 20:227–232, 1991

88. Pfeffer MR, Teicher BA, Holden SA, et al: The interaction of cisplatin plus etoposide with radiation ± hyperthermia. *Int J Radiat Oncol Biol Phys* 19:1439–1447, 1990

89. Bachaud J-M, David J-M, Boussin G, et al: Combined postoperative radiotherapy and weekly cisplatin infusion for locally advanced squamous cell carcinoma of the head and neck: Preliminary report of a randomization trial. *Int J Radiat Oncol Biol Phys* 20:243–246, 1991

90. Merlano M, Rosso R, Benasso M, et al: Alternating chemotherapy and radiotherapy vs radiotherapy in advanced inoperable SCC-HN: A cooperative randomized trial. *Proc Am Soc Clin Oncol* 10:198, 1991 (abstr)

91. Santi DV, McHenry CS, Sommer H: Interaction of thymidylate synthetase with 5-fluorouridylate. *Biochemistry* 13: 471–480, 1974

92. Piedbois P, Buyse M, Rustum Y, et al: Modulation of fluorouracil by leucovorin in advanced colorectal cancer: Evidence in terms of response rate. *J Clin Oncol* 10:896–903, 1992

93. Gerstner J, O'Connell MJ, Wieand HS, et al: A prospectively randomized clinical trial comparing 5FU combined with either high or low dose leucovorin for the treatment of advanced colorectal cancer. *Proc Am Soc Clin Oncol* 10:134, 1991 (abstr)

94. Reinberg A, Smolensky MH: Circadian changes of drug disposition in man. *Clin Pharmacokinet* 7:401–420, 1982

95. Levi F, Boughattas NA, Blazsek I: Comparative murine chronotoxicity of anticancer agents and related mechanisms, in Reinberg A, Smolensky M, Labrecque G (eds): *Annual Review of Chronopharmacology,* vol 4. Oxford, Pergamon Press, 1987, pp 283–331

96. von Roemeling R, Hrushesky WJM: Circadian patterning of continuous floxuridine infusion reduces toxicity and allows higher dose intensity in patients with widespread cancer. *J Clin Oncol* 7:1710–1719, 1989

97. Hrushesky WJM: Circadian timing of cancer chemotherapy. *Science* 228:73–75, 1985

98. Garcia-Sainz M, Halberg F: Mitotic rhythms in human cancer reevaluated by electronic computer programs: Evidence for chronopathology. *J Natl Cancer Inst* 37:279–292, 1966

99. Caussanel JP, Levi F, Brienza S, et al: Phase I trial of 5-day continuous venous infusion of oxaliplatin at circadian rhythm-modulated rate compared with constant rate. *J Natl Cancer Inst* 82:1046–1050, 1990

100. Bjarnason GA, Hrushesky WJM: Circadian cancer chemotherapy: Clinical trials. *J Infus Chemother* 2:79–88, 1992

101. Valvassori L, Bellegotti L, Marchiano A, et al: Continuous circadian-shaped infusion FUDR effectively reduces toxicity. *Proc Am Soc Clin Oncol* 8:427, 1989 (abstr)

102. Harris BE, Song R, Song S, et al: Circadian variation of 5-fluorouracil catabolism in isolated perfused rat liver. *Cancer Res* 49:6610–6614, 1989

103. Hrushesky WJM, Borch R, Levi F: Circadian time dependence of cisplatin urinary kinetics. *Clin Pharmacol Ther* 32: 330–339, 1982

104. Halberg F, Gupta B, Haus E, et al: Steps toward a chronopolychemotherapy, in *Proceedings of the 14th International Congress of Therapeutics.* Paris: L' Expansion Scientifique Française, 1977, pp 151–196

105. Mormont MC, Berstka J, Mushiya T, et al: Circadian dependence of vinblastine toxicity, in Reinberg A, Smolensky M, Labrecque G (eds): *Annual Review of Chronopharmacology,* vol 3. Oxford, Pergamon Press, 1986, pp 187–190

106. Baur LA: Individualization of drug therapy: Clinical pharmacokinetics and pharmacodynamics, in DiPiro JT, Talbert RL, Hayes PE, et al (eds): *Pharmacotherapy* (ed 2). Norwalk, CT, Appleton and Lange, 1993, pp 15–31

107. Chabner BA, Stoller RG, Hande K, et al: Methotrexate disposition in human case studies in ovarian cancer and following high-dose infusion. *Drug Metab Rev* 1:107–117, 1978

108. Lippard SJ: New chemistry of an old molecule: cis(Pt NH$_3$)$_2$ Cl$_2$). *Science* 218:1075–1082, 1982

109. Moore MJ: Clinical pharmacokinetics of cyclophosphamide. *Clin Pharmacokinet* 20:194–208, 1991

110. Goldman ID: Pharmacokinetics of antineoplastic agents at the cellular level, in Chabner BA (ed): *Pharmacologic Principles of Cancer Treatment*. Philadelphia, Saunders, 1982, pp 15–44

111. Hansten PD, Horn JR (eds): *Drug Interactions and Updates*. Vancouver, WA, Applied Therapeutics, 1995

112. Balis FM: Pharmacokinetic drug interactions of commonly used anticancer drugs. *Clin Pharmacokinet* 11:223–235, 1986

113. Finley RS: Drug interactions in the oncology patient. *Semin Oncol Nurs* 8:95–101, 1992

114. Loadman PM, Bibby MC: Pharmacokinetic drug interactions with anticancer drugs. *Clin Pharmacokinet* 26:486–500, 1994

115. Ignoffo RJ: Drug interactions with antineoplastic agents. *Highlights on Antineoplastic Drugs*, Feb/Mar:2–7, 1989

116. Grossman SA, Sheidler VR, Gilbert MR: Decreased phenytoin levels in patients receiving chemotherapy. *Am J Med* 87:505–510, 1989

117. Evans WE, Christensen ML: *Drug Interactions with Methotrexate*. Wayne, NJ: Lederle Laboratories, 1985

118. Thyss A, Milano G, Kubar J, et al: Clinical and pharmacokinetic evidence of a life-threatening interaction between methotrexate and ketoprofen. *Lancet* 1:256–258, 1986

119. Ellison NM, Servi RJ: Acute renal failure and death following sequential intermediate-dose methotrexate and 5-FU: A possible adverse effect due to concomitant indomethacin administration. *Cancer Treat Rep* 69:342–343, 1985

120. Fitzsimmons WE, Ghalie R, Kaizer H: The effect of hepatic enzyme inducers on busulfan neurotoxicity and myelotoxicity. *Cancer Chemother Pharmacol* 27:27–32, 1990

121. Cerny T, Pedrazzini A, Joss RA, et al: Unexpected high toxicity in a phase II study of teniposide in elderly patients with untreated small-cell lung cancer. *Lung Cancer* 4:A102, 1988 (abstr)

122. Konits PH, Aisner J, Sutherland JC, et al: Possible pulmonary toxicity secondary to vinblastine. *Cancer* 50:2771–2774, 1982

123. Hall G, Lind MJ, Huang M, et al: Intravenous infusions of ifosfamide/mesna and perturbation of warfarin anticoagulant control. *Postgrad Med J* 66:860–861, 1990

124. Lodwick R, McConkey B, Brown AM: Life-threatening interaction between tamoxifen and warfarin. *BMJ* 295:1141, 1987 (letter)

125. Ludlum DB: Alkylating agents and the nitrosoureas, in Becker FF (ed): *Cancer: A Comprehensive Treatise*, vol 5. New York, Plenum Press, 1977, pp 285–307

126. Hanawalt PC, Cooper PK, Ganesan AK, et al: DNA repair in bacteria and mammalian cells. *Annu Rev Biochem* 48:783–836, 1979

127. Bohr VA, Phillips DH, Hanawalt PC: Heterogeneous DNA damage and repair in the mammalian genome. *Cancer Res* 47:6426–6436, 1987

128. Vistica DT: Cytotoxicity as an indicator for transport mechanism: Evidence that melphalan is transported by two leucine-preferring carrier systems in the L1210 murine leukemia cell. *Biochim Biophys Acta* 550:309–317, 1979

129. Colvin M: A review of the pharmacology and clinical use of cyclophosphamide, in Pinedo HM (ed): *Clinical Pharmacology of Antineoplastic Drugs*. Amsterdam, Elsevier-North Holland, 1978, pp 245–261

130. Colvin M: The comparative pharmacology of cyclophosphamide and ifosfamide. *Semin Oncol* 9:2–7, 1982 (suppl 1)

131. Chabner BA: Anticancer drugs, in DeVita VT, Hellman S, Rosenberg SA (eds): *Cancer: Principles and Practice of Oncology* (ed 4). Philadelphia, Lippincott, 1993, pp 325–417

132. Montgomery JA: Chemistry and structure: Activity studies of the nitrosoureas. *Cancer Treat Rep* 60:651–664, 1976

133. Pascoe JM, Roberts JJ: Interaction between mammalian cell DNA and inorganic platinum compounds: I. DNA interstrand cross-linking and cytotoxic properties of platinum (II) compounds. *Biochem Pharmacol* 23:1345–1357, 1974

134. Zwelling LA, Anderson T, Kohn KW: DNA-protein and DNA interstrand cross-linking by cis- and trans-platinum (II) diamminedichloride in L1210 mouse leukemia cells and its relation to cytotoxity. *Cancer Res* 39:365–369, 1979

135. Rosenberg B: Possible mechanisms for the antitumor activity of platinum coordination complexes. *Cancer Chemother Rep* 59:589–598, 1975

136. Reed E: Platinum analogs, in DeVita VT, Hellman S, Rosenberg SA (eds): *Cancer: Principles and Practice of Oncology* (ed 4). Philadelphia, Lippincott, 1993, pp 390–400

137. Gormley PE, Bull JM, LeRoy AF, et al: Kinetics of cis-dichloro-diammineplatinum. *Clin Pharmcol Ther* 25:351–357, 1979

138. Howell SB, Pfeifle CE, Wung W, et al: Intraperitoneal cisplatin with systemic thiosulfate protection. *Ann Intern Med* 97:845–851, 1982

139. Oguri S, Sakakibara T, Mase H, et al: Clinical pharmacokinetics of carboplatin. *J Clin Pharmacol* 28:208–215, 1988

140. Montgomery JA: Experimental studies at Southern Research Institute with DTIC (NSC-45388). *Cancer Treat Rep* 60:125–134, 1976

141. Hayward IP, Parson PG: Epigenetic effects of the methylating agent 5-(3-methyl-1-triazeno) imidazole-4-carboxamide in human melanoma cells. *Aust J Exp Biol Med Sci* 62:597–606, 1984

142. Sutherland CM, Krementz ET: Hepatic toxicity of DTIC. *Cancer Treat Rep* 65:321–322, 1981

143. Holt GA (ed): *Food and Drug Interactions: A Health Care Professional's Guide*. Chicago, Precept Press, 1992

144. Zhang H, D'Arpe P, Liu LF: A model for tumor cell killing by topoisomerase poisons. *Cancer Cells* 2:23–27, 1990

145. Zwelling LA: Topoisomerase II as a target of antileukemia drugs: A review of controversial areas. *Hematol Pathol* 3:101–112, 1989

146. Myers CE: Anthracyclines, in Chabner B (ed): *Pharmacologic Principles of Cancer Treatment*. Philadelphia, Saunders, 1982, pp 416–434

147. Goodman J, Hochstein P: Generation of free radicals and lipid peroxidation by redox cycling of Adriamycin and daunomycin. *Biochem Biophys Res Commun* 77:797, 1977

148. Myers CE, McGuire WP, Liss RH, et al: Adriamycin: The role of lipid peroxidation in cardiac toxicity and tumor response. *Science* 197:165–167, 1977

149. Henderson IC, Allegra JC, Woodcock T, et al: Randomized clinical trials comparing mitoxantrone with doxorubicin in previously treated patients with metastatic breast cancer. *J Clin Oncol* 7:560–571, 1989

150. Forssen EA, Coulter DM, Proffitt RT: Selective in vivo localization of daunorubicin small unilamellar vesicles in solid tumors. *Cancer Res* 56:2066–2075, 1996

151. Product information: Doxil. Menlo Park, CA, Sequoia Pharmaceuticals, 1995

152. Kozarich JW, Worth L, Frank BL, et al: Sequence-specific isotope effects on the cleavage of DNA by bleomycin. *Science* 245:1396–1399, 1989

153. Ross WE, Glaubiger DL, Kohn KW: Quantitative and qualitative aspects of intercalator-induced DNA damage. *Biochim Biophys Acta* 562:41–50, 1979

154. Crooke ST, Bradner WT: Mitomycin C: A review. *Cancer Treat Rev* 3:121–139, 1976

155. Goldman ID: Analysis of the cytotoxic determinants for methotrexate (NSC-740): Role of "free" intracellular drug. *Cancer Chemother Rep* 6:51–61, 1975

156. Pinedo HM, Zaharko DS, Bull JM, et al: The reversal of methotrexate cytotoxicity to mouse bone marrow cells by leucovorin and nucleosides. *Cancer Res* 36:4418–4424, 1976

157. Evans WE, Crom WR, Yalowich J: Methotrexate, in Evans WE, Schentag J.J, Juskow, J (eds): *Applied Pharmacokinetics: Principles of Therapeutic Drug Monitoring* (ed 2). Spokane, WA, San Francisco, Applied Therapeutics, 1986, pp 1009–1056

158. Isacoff WH, Morrison PF, Aroesty J, et al: Pharmacokinetics of high-dose methotrexate with citrovorum factor rescue. *Cancer Treat Rep* 61:1665–1674, 1977

159. Stoller RG, Hande KR, Jacobs SA, et al: Use of plasma pharmacokinetics to predict and prevent methotrexate toxicity. *N Engl J Med* 297:630–634, 1977

160. Campbell MA, Perrier DG, Dorr RT, et al: Methotrexate: Bioavailability and pharmacokinetics. *Cancer Treat Rep* 69: 833–838, 1985

161. Chabner BA, Stoller RG, Hande KR, et al: Methotrexate disposition in humans: Case studies of ovarian cancer and following high-dose infusion. *Drug Metab Rev* 8:107–117, 1978

162. Heidelberger C, Chandhari NK, Dannenberg P, et al: Fluorinated pyrimidines: A new class of tumor inhibitory compounds. *Nature* 179:663–666, 1957

163. Mandel HG: Incorporation of 5-fluorouracil into RNA and its molecular consequences. *Prog Mol Subcell Biol* 1:82–135, 1969

164. Schuetz JD, Collins JM, Wallace HJ, et al: Alteration of secondary structure of newly synthesized DNA from murine bone marrow cells by 5-fluorouracil. *Cancer Res* 46: 119–123, 1986

165. Diasio RB, Schuetz JD, Wallace HJ, et al: Dihydrofluorouracil, a fluorouracil catabolite with antitumor activity in murine and human cells. *Cancer Res* 45:4900–4903, 1985

166. Burger AJ, Mannino S: 5-fluorouracil-induced coronary vasospasm. *Am Heart J* 114:433–436, 1987

167. Chu MY, Fischer GA: A proposed mechanism of action of 1-beta-arabinofuranosyl-cytosine as an inhibitor of the growth of leukemia cells. *Biochem Pharmacol* 11:423–430, 1962

168. Fram RJ, Egan EM, Kufe DW: Accumulation of leukemic cell DNA strand breaks with Adrimycin and cytosine arabinoside. *Leuk Res* 7:243–249, 1983

169. Kufe DW, Munroe D, Herrick D, et al: Effects of 1-beta-D-arabinosuranosyl-cytosine incorporation on eukaryotic DNA template function. *Mol Pharmacol* 26:128–134, 1984

170. Herzig RH, Hines JD, Herzig GP, et al: Cerebellar toxicity with high-dose cytosine arabinoside. *J Clin Oncol* 5: 927–932, 1987

171. Christie NT, Drake S, Meyn RE, et al: 6-Thiopurine-induced DNA damage as a determinant of cytotoxicity in cultured Chinese hamster ovary cells. *Cancer Res* 44:3665–3672, 1984

172. Tseng W-C, Derse D, Cheng Y-C, et al: In vitro biological activity of 9-beta-D-arabinofuranosyl-2-fluoroadenine and the biochemical actions of its triphosphate on DNA polymerase and ribonucleotide reductase from HeLa cells. *Mol Pharmacol* 21:474–477, 1982

173. Seto S, Carrera CJ, Kubota M, et al: Mechanism of deoxyadenosine and 2-chlorodoxyadenosine toxicity to nondividing human lymphocytes. *J Clin Invest* 75:377–383, 1985

174. Madoc-Jones H, Mauro F: Interphase action of vinblastine and vincristine: Differences in their lethal action through the mitotic cycle of cultured mammalian cells. *J Cell Physiol* 72:185–196, 1968

175. Nelson RL: The comparative clinical pharmacology and pharmacokinetics of vindisine, vincristine, and vinblastine in human patients with cancer. *Med Pediatr Oncol* 10: 115–127, 1982

176. Wani MC, Taylor HL, Wall ME, et al: Plant antitumor agents: IV. The isolation and structure of taxol, a novel antileukemic and antitumor agent from *Taxus brevifolia. J Am Chem Soc* 93:2325–2327, 1971

177. Schiff PB, Fant J, Horowitz SB: Promotion of microtubule assembly in vitro by taxol. *Nature* 22:665–667, 1979

178. Rowinsky EK, Donehower RC, Jones RJ, et al: Microtubule changes and cytotoxicity in leukemic cell lines treated with taxol. *Cancer Res* 48:4093–4100, 1988

179. Bissery MC, Guenard D, Gueritte-Voegelein F, et al: Experimental antitumor activity of taxotere (RP 56976, NSC 628503), a taxol analogue. *Cancer Res* 51:4845–4852, 1991

180. Rowisnky EK, Burke PJ, Karp JE, et al: Phase I clinical and pharmacokinetic study of taxol. *Cancer Res* 49:4640–4647, 1989

181. Extra JM, Rousseau F, Bruno R, et al: Phase I and pharmacokinetic study of taxotere (NSC 628503) given as a short intravenous infusion. *Cancer Res* 53:1037–1042, 1993

182. Citardi M, Rowinsky EK, Schaefer KL, et al: Sequence-dependent cytotoxicity between cisplatin and the antimicrotubule agents taxol and vincristine. *Proc Am Assoc Cancer Res* 31:2431, 1990

183. Weiss RB, Donehower RC, Wiernik PH, et al: Hypersensitivity reactions from taxol. *J Clin Oncol* 8:1263–1268, 1990

184. Chevallier B, Fumoleau P, Kerbrat P, et al: Docetaxel is a major cytotoxic drug for the treatment of advanced breast cancer. *J Clin Oncol* 13:314–322, 1995

185. Loike D, Horwitz SB: Effects of podophyllotoxin and VP-6 on microtubule assembly in vitro and nucleotide transport in HeLa cells. *Biochemistry* 15:5435–5442, 1976

186. Yang L, Rowe RC, Liu LF: Identification of DNA topoisomerase II as an intracellular target of antitumor epipodophyllotoxins in Simian virus 40–infected monkey cells. *Cancer Res* 45:5872–5876, 1985

187. Creaven PJ: The clinical pharmacology of VM-26 and VP-16-213: A brief overview. *Cancer Chemother Pharmacol* 7: 133–140, 1982

188. Slevin ML, Clark PL, Joel SP, et al: A randomized trial to evaluate the effects of schedule on the activity of etoposide in small-cell lung cancer. *J Clin Oncol* 7:1333–1340, 1989

189. Jones SF, Burris HA: Topoisomerase I Inhibitors: Topotecan and irinotecan. *Cancer Pract* 4:51–53, 1996

190. Rothenberg ML, Kuhn JG, Burris HA, et al: Phase I and pharmacokinetic trial of weekly CPT-11. *J Clin Oncol* 11: 2194–2204, 1993

191. Sutherland DJ: Hormones and cancer, in Tannock IF, Hill RP (eds): *The Basic Science of Oncology.* New York, Pergamon Press, 1987, pp 204–222

192. Stearns ME, Tew KD: Antimicrotubule effects of estramustine, an antiprostatic tumor drug. *Cancer Res* 45:3891–3897, 1985

193. Sporn MB, Roberts AB: Interactions of retinoids and transforming growth factor–beta in regulation of cell differentiation and proliferation. *Mol Endocrinol* 5:3–7, 1991

194. Lippman S, Kessler J, Al-Sarraf M, et al: Treatment of advanced squamous cell carcinoma of the head and neck with isotretinoin: A phase II randomized trial. *Invest New Drugs* 6:51–56, 1988

195. Lippman S, Parkinson D, Itri L, et al: 13-*cis*-Retinoic acid and interferon alpha-2a: Effective combination therapy for advanced squamous cell carcinoma of the skin. *J Natl Cancer Inst* 84:235–241, 1992

196. Clark R, Ismail S, Jacobs A, et al: A randomized trial of 13-*cis*-Retinoic acid with or without cytosine arabinoside in patients with myelodysplastic syndrome. *Br J Haematol* 66:77–83, 1987

197. Fontana J, Rogers J, Durham J: The role of 13-*cis*-Retinoic acid in the remission induction of a patient with acute promyelocytic leukemia. *Cancer* 57:209–217, 1986

198. Kramer Z, Boros L, Wiernik P, et al: 13-*cis*-Retinoic acid in the treatment of elderly patients with acute myeloid leukemia. *Cancer* 67:1484–1486, 1991

199. Kamm J, Ashenfelter K, Ehmann C: Preclinical and clinical toxicology of selected retinoids, in Sporn M, Roberts A, Goodman D (eds): *The Retinoids*. Orlando, FL, Academic Press, 1984, pp 287–326

200. Warrell RR: All-trans-Retinoic acid, in *American Society of Clinical Oncology Educational Book, 28th Annual Meeting, San Diego, California, May 17–19, 1992,* pp 107–112

**Chapter 15**

# Chemotherapy: Principles of Administration

**Michelle Goodman, RN, MS, OCN®**

**Mary Beth Riley, RN, MS**

# CHEMOTHERAPY ADMINISTRATION

Dramatic changes in health care delivery systems have occurred over the past ten years have an impact on the practice of medical oncology. In the past chemotherapy was primarily administered in a hospital setting. Today the practice of medical oncology involves delivery of care to patients in a variety of care settings. The majority of cancer patients receive systemic chemotherapy in an ambulatory care setting that may be adjacent to a university hospital, or a 23-hour unit designed to care for patients requiring lengthy infusions. Others may receive their chemotherapy in a freestanding clinic or in their homes. Few actually require hospitalization for chemotherapy despite the fact that treatment regimens are frequently more aggressive and dose-intensive in nature. Admissions are therefore reserved for patients who require intensive monitoring or those who are acutely ill. Even bone marrow transplant and peripheral blood stem cell transplant programs are moving to the outpatient setting.[1]

This shift to outpatient ambulatory care services has grown out of the need for more efficient and economical health care delivery systems as hospitals prepare for increases in managed care and capitation. Managed care is rapidly replacing fee-for-service in all aspects of the health care delivery system.[2] Oncology nurses are challenged with the increased responsibility for coordinating quality patient care with limited resources and support. Through team building and working across settings and disciplines, the nurse must effectively assess and develop a plan of care that ensures continuity of care regardless of the care setting. The real challenge lies in finding ways to promote self-care in an aging population with limited personal and social resources. This chapter deals with both basic and advanced principles in chemotherapy administration. It focuses on clinical practice, methods of drug delivery, and vascular access devices (VADs).

## Professional Qualifications

Educational guidelines for nurses administering chemotherapy are almost universally implemented in a variety of practice settings.[3] The *Oncology Nursing Society's Cancer Chemotherapy Guidelines* contain a section entitled "Recommendations for Cancer Chemotherapy Course Content and Clinical Practicum." State boards of nursing have also recognized the need for specialized chemotherapy training and have enacted rules that require adherence to national standards.[4] Both the Intravenous Nurses' Society and the Oncology Nursing Society have published position statements regarding the administration of antineoplastic agents and the preparation of the nurse.[5,6]

Basic qualifications for nurses administering antineoplastic agents include:

1. current licensure as a registered nurse
2. certification in CPR
3. intravenous therapy skills
4. educational preparation and demonstration of knowledge in all areas related to antineoplastic drugs (pharmacology, kinetics, handling, administration, side-effect management, laboratory-value monitoring, patient education, and resources)
5. demonstration of the skill of drug administration
6. ongoing acquisition of updated information and verification of continuing knowledge and skills
7. policies and procedures to govern specific actions (see Table 15-1)

Formal chemotherapy certification programs developed by and for oncology nurses use a variety of teaching strategies. Program lengths vary from several days to several weeks. The most common approach involves organized lectures in a classroom setting, but some courses are designed independently, using videotapes, programmed instruction modules, and self-study materials. Programs should include a pre- and a posttest to verify learning and a supervised clinical demonstration of the skill. Structured chemotherapy training has eliminated much of the fear and uncertainty for new oncology nurses and helps to ensure quality patient care and maintain high safety standards.[7,8] Chemotherapy certification also provides proof of formalized training and skill demonstration, which is extremely important from a professional liability perspective. Antineoplastic agents have serious, even life-threatening side effects, and it is in the best interests of both the patient and the nurse that educational preparation be obtained and documented. Additionally, clinically oriented policies and procedures that are part of ongoing quality improvement help to provide a firm practical and legal foundation for this aspect of oncology nursing practice.

**TABLE 15-1** Institutional Policies and Procedures That Should Be Established to Guide Oncology Nursing Practice in the Area of Chemotherapy Administration

- Staff education for chemotherapy and other specialty procedures (i.e., VADs, Ommaya reservoirs)
- Chemotherapy administration (all routes)
- Vesicant management
- Allergic reactions
- Safe drug handling and disposal
- Patient and family education
- Management of vascular access devices
- Documentation methods (extravasation record)
- Coordination of home care
- Outcome standards
- Oncology quality-improvement process

## Handling Cytotoxic Drugs

Scientific articles regarding potential or actual hazards of cytotoxic drug exposure have been appearing in medical, pharmaceutical, and nursing literature for many years.[9-11] Direct exposure to these cytotoxic agents can occur during admixture, administration, or handling, and involve inhalation, ingestion, or absorption.[12,13] The drugs are known to be mutagenic, teratogenic, and carcinogenic. Additionally, exposure has been reported to result in rashes, skin discolorations, scarring, blurred vision, and dizziness. Guidelines containing recommendations to prevent cytotoxic drug exposure to personnel and the environment have been established by the Occupational Safety and Health Administration (OSHA), Oncology Nursing Society, and American Society of Hospital Pharmacists.[10,13] Detailed drug handling guidelines are outlined in Table 15-2. These guidelines are to be used by those determining the specific institutional policies and procedures of cytotoxic drug handling.

A major area of controversy during drug administration is the need for protective clothing, which could be uniforms, lab coats, scrubs, or disposable gowns. Some institutions mandate specific garb according to risk of exposure; others leave it to the discretion of the individual or supervisor to determine if spills or splashes are likely to occur.

It is well known that the drugs and their metabolites are excreted in the urine and stool beyond 48 hours after drug administration. The OSHA guidelines recommend gowning and gloving to handle excreta during this time frame; however, most nurses wear only regular exam gloves. Double gloving was a common practice at one time, but is now usually seen only when cleaning up large spills.

Personnel policies regarding pregnancy are quite varied, despite OSHA's suggestion that appropriate protective practices should reduce any potential reproductive hazards.[13] While OSHA recommends that employees be informed of potential risks and, if necessary, reassigned to other duties, it is not uncommon to find institutional policies that prohibit pregnant or lactating women from working with cytotoxic drugs. Another personnel issue is medical surveillance, which usually includes a preemployment health assessment, a baseline CBC, and thorough documentation of any risk factors in the health history.[14] It's becoming less common to require more extensive testing, for there are no data to support a cause-and-effect relationship between precautionary cytotoxic drug handling and abnormal physical or laboratory findings.

Patient education regarding cytotoxic drug handling is important so that patients and family members understand why gloves and/or gowns are being worn and do not feel alienated by the practice. Education is a crucial element if chemotherapy is being provided in the home setting, since family members need to be instructed in drug containment practices. The health care professional should provide the patient with written instructions which specify that gloves be worn when working with the medications, used materials be placed in the provided containers, care be taken to avoid direct exposure, spills be cleaned up with the spill kit provided, and direct external exposure be managed with copious flushing and washing.[15] Despite proof that exposure to cytotoxic drugs can be harmful, a large percentage of health professionals continue to disregard personal protective measures.[16,17] There appears to be a perception that low-level exposure is not harmful, since no absolute scientific quantification of exposure has been defined. It is not known if a little exposure is harmless or how much is too much or even if some drugs are more harmful than others. Given the fact that stiff financial penalties can be incurred if OSHA ascertains noncompliance with established guidelines, the minimum standards to be met include: (1) knowledge of the latest scientific information; (2) established policies and procedures; and (3) ongoing monitoring to ensure compliance and continuous quality improvement.

## Patient and Family Education

Educating patients and their family members about cancer is usually initiated by the physician, who explains the diagnosis of cancer, treatment options, risks and benefits, alternatives, and prognosis. The nurse's role usually begins with clarifying information and disabusing misconceptions, especially the old wives' tales that exist about cancer and cancer treatment. Nurses are responsible for informing the patient and family of specific information about treatment side effects and measures to recognize and minimize their consequences. Teaching self-care measures is critically important given the often limited resources and support services available. Self-care guides such as those detailed by Groenwald, Frogge, Goodman, and Yarbro in *Cancer Symptom Management*[18] are ideal because they can be copied and given to the patient to reinforce teaching. Details regarding mouth care, skin care, wig shops, over-the-counter medications, food intake, and many other aspects of daily life are frequently addressed by the nurse. Identifying problems or side effects a patient might experience due to the chemotherapy as a whole rather than addressing each drug separately is most efficient, due to the wide range of side effects encountered. Some basic steps to follow when planning and implementing patient education are included in Table 15-3.

It is very important in the preparation and planning stages to ensure adequate knowledge of the drugs, their side effects, and the treatment goal. Assessment of the patient should include the individual's response to the diagnosis, communication style, ability to read/comprehend information, family status, lifestyle, and treatment outcome expectations.

The patient and nurse should both be relaxed, with time to discuss the treatment and its side effects. Asking the patient if there are any questions helps to address

**TABLE 15-2**  Cytotoxic Drug Handling Guidelines[3,9,10,13]

**Preparation**

- Verify current drug order with patient profile.
- Ensure accuracy of dose and drug.
- Don a disposable gown that is lint-free, low- or nonpermeable, long-sleeved, cuffed, and solid-fronted.
- Don a pair of powder-free, thick, surgical-quality latex gloves, ensuring that the cuffs of the gloves overlap the cuffs of the gown.
- Admix all cytotoxic drugs in a class II biologic safety cabinet (vertical air flow) that meets national standards and is inspected appropriately.
- Use a disposable, plastic-backed liner for the preparation area and appropriate equipment such as Luer-Lok syringes.
- Clean the cabinet daily with 70% alcohol, and decontaminate it weekly or if spills occur.
- Use aseptic technique.
- Take care to avoid drug dispersement by venting vials, handling ampules carefully, avoiding overfilling of containers, and adding diluents slowly.
- Attach and prime IV tubing before adding the cytotoxic drug to the IV solution.
- Wipe all syringes and containers, and label them appropriately, including a warning label indicating that the contents are cytotoxic.
- When dispensing vincristine affix a label that indicates that the drug can be lethal if injected intrathecally.
- Do not clip or recap needles; discard all sharps in a convenient and appropriately labeled, puncture-proof container.
- Discard protective clothing and used materials in a separate trash bag labeled as cytotoxic.
- Wash hands.
- Verify with a colleague/pharmacist that the drug order is identical to the drug prepared and that the dose is customary and reasonable.

**Administration**

- Receive appropriately labeled cytotoxic drugs in clean, dry syringes or bags of IV fluids. Syringes may be inside zip-close plastic bags. Inspect bags before opening to ensure no spillage within the bag.
- Wash hands and don protective clothing. If dripping or splashing can occur, this should include a disposable gown that is lint-free, low- or nonpermeable, long-sleeved, cuffed, and solid-fronted.
- Don a pair of powder-free, thick, surgical-quality latex gloves, ensuring that the cuffs of the gloves overlap the cuffs of the gown, if a gown is being worn.
- Place a plastic-backed absorbent pad over the work area to absorb any drips.
- Use intravenous administration sets and syringes with Luer-Lok fittings.
- If the administration set is not attached to the intravenous fluids and primed by the pharmacist, it should be attached and primed with caution to prevent exposure of the drug to the environment. It may be primed into a gauze pad inside a zip-close bag, or it may be piggybacked to plain fluids and primed by retrograde flow ("back-primed").

- Secure all connections and Y-sites with tape.
- Keep a gauze pad at hand to wipe droplets off Y-sites or connecting points.
- Do not expel air from syringes. If air is in a syringe, hold it in such a way that the air is up near the plunger and simply stop pushing on the plunger when all of the drug is injected.
- Do not use intravenous bottles with venting tubes.
- Monitor administration sets and connection sites for leakage.
- Do not clip or recap needles. Discard the needle-syringe unit into a convenient and appropriately labeled, puncture-proof container.
- Discard all gauze, tubing, bags, bottles, etc., in appropriately labeled bags, and seal. Remove gown and gloves and discard in a similar manner.
- Wash hands.

**General Handling and Disposal**

- Dispose of all sharps, containers, and cytotoxic waste according to appropriate state and federal guidelines (usually, incineration or burial in a hazardous waste landfill).
- Contain all grossly contaminated linen of treated patients within 48 hours in labeled double bags, and wash twice (same procedure as for infectious wastes).
- Obtain spill kits, and place them in the admixture and administration areas.
- Clean up spills using available kits and disposable towels or sponges. For large spills, double gloving is recommended.
- If direct exposure occurs, immediately rinse the area with running water. For eye exposure, rinse with an eye wash solution or sterile saline.
- Report all episodes of exposure to employee health or the equivalent resource.

**Personnel**

- Identify all personnel who handle cytotoxic drugs.
- Educate and train personnel in proper drug handling.
- Establish a mechanism to monitor cytotoxic drug handling practices, from receipt through disposal.
- Provide ready access to information regarding cytotoxic drugs.
- Address pregnancy and medical surveillance issues.
- Monitor all spills and occurrences of direct exposure through a quality-improvement program.
- Develop patient education materials as needed, particularly for use in the home.

**TABLE 15-3  Chemotherapy Patient Education Guidelines**

**Preparation**

- Accompany the physician when the treatment plan is explained to the patient and family to better reinforce what they have been told.
- Identify learning needs and specific written instructions for prevention and management of side effects.
- Emphasize the importance of self-care strategies and provide the patient and family with self-care guidelines that are clearly written at an eighth-grade level of understanding.
- Determine whether audiovisuals are appropriate teaching aids. Test equipment and establish a time for patient/family to view.
- Review policies, procedures, and documentation forms.

**Planning**

- Know the basics about the patient to be taught and the goal of the treatment plan. Review the chart. It is especially important to know if the patient speaks and reads English, if that is the language being used.
- If possible, separate the teaching session from the actual drug administration procedure.
- Encourage the patient to have a family member present during instruction sessions.
- Assemble all teaching materials including calendar, prescriptions, drug information sheets, and other teaching materials before you begin, to avoid interruptions.

**Presentation**

- Introduce self and purpose.
- Determine if the patient has any specific questions or concerns to address before proceeding.
- Discuss the treatment process (i.e., starting intravenous infusion, administering drugs, length of time, immediate events, expected follow-up, monitoring side effects, and home care). Describe any sensations the patient might have during the infusion/injection (e.g., coolness, perirectal burning, light-headedness, nasal stuffiness).
- Describe the potential side effects and interventions in order to minimize their consequences. Include specific information about what to look for, what's normal, how to take a temperature, where to buy a wig, which mouth care regimen to use, and other appropriate recommendations. Provide written information regarding when to call the physician or nurse.
- Avoid overloading the patient with information about rare or unusual risks of chemotherapy. Give written information regarding this aspect of his or her treatment and elaborate where appropriate.
- Ensure that informed consent has been obtained.
- Maintain a responsive atmosphere that is open to questioning.
- Give written instructions regarding activity, diet, hygiene, medications, and other self-care behaviors for the patient to follow for the next few days or weeks.

**Follow-Up**

- Document the encounter and the patient's response. (See Patient Teaching and Documentation Tool, chapter 16.)
- Question the patient to assess his or her understanding of the information imparted.
- When possible, observe the patient to determine if his or her actions indicate an understanding of the information (e.g., hydration, mouth care, medications).
- It is optimal to contact the patient within 24 hours of drug administration to determine if there are any questions or problems to be resolved, especially if the patient and nurse are no longer together in the same setting (i.e., hospital or home).

concerns immediately and establishes an open exchange of information. Anxiety during the presentation is unavoidable, but the nurse should observe the patient's facial expression and body language to help measure the impact of the information on the patient, for it is sometimes necessary to allow time for the facts to be assimilated. More complex instruction is required when a patient is entering a research protocol, since there is a written informed consent, usually several pages in length, that is read to the patient or reviewed in great detail. Participation in a research study is usually the only circumstance under which the patient's signature on a written consent form is required by law. While some health care agencies require signed consent forms for all chemotherapy, many others consider that consent is granted when the patient allows the drug to be given.

Follow-up includes assessment of the patient's understanding of the information imparted and determination that the outcome has been achieved. Observation of the patient and questioning regarding actions and activities are usually sufficient to ensure comprehension. Documentation of the entire process is very important and can involve a detailed written note or a checklist-type form[19–23] (see chapter 16).

## Professional Issues

The delivery of chemotherapy, as well as the education of the patient and family is primarily the responsibility of the registered professional nurse. The nurse must be properly educated in the pharmacology of the drugs including distribution and elimination patterns, the proper techniques of drug preparation and administration, and especially drug interactions. Table 15-4 and Appendix A describe the dosing, metabolism, preparation, administration precautions, and special considerations regarding the administration of the more common oral and intravenous antineoplastic agents.

Because the administration of chemotherapy is pri-

**TABLE 15-4**  Oral Antineoplastic Agents

| Drug and Disease Indications | Dose and Schedule | Side Effects: Acute or Delayed | Pharmacokinetics | Comments |
|---|---|---|---|---|
| Cyclophosphamide (Cytoxan, Endoxan)<br>Breast cancer<br>Multiple myeloma<br>Small-cell lung cancer<br>Malignant lymphomas<br>Leukemias | *Tab:* 25–50 mg<br>*Dose:* 1–5 mg/kg/day<br>60–120 mg/m$^2$<br>Adjust dose in presence of renal dysfunction | *Nadir:* 7–14 days<br>Bone marrow suppression (BMS)<br>Anorexia, nausea, and vomiting<br>Alopecia<br>Hemorrhagic cystitis with gross or microscopic hematuria<br>Amenorrhea<br>Sterility | Activated in the liver<br>Oral absorption in 1 hr<br>30% of drug excreted unchanged in urine | Vigorous hydration (3 liter/day). Encourage frequent voiding to prevent hemorrhagic cystitis (a sterile inflammation of the urinary bladder). If patient complains of burning on urination or bladder incontinence, urinalysis may reveal occult blood. Control by withdrawal of the drug and hydration. May take pills in divided doses early in the day and with meals or all at one time. Better tolerated with cold foods. Barbiturates and other inducers of hepatic microsomal enzymes may enhance toxicity, e.g., cimetidine. Allopurinol may enhance BMS. |
| Chlorambucil (Leukeran)<br>Leukemia<br>Hodgkin's disease | *Tab:* 2 mg white<br>*Dose:* 4–8 mg/m$^2$/day ×<br>3–6 wk<br>16 mg/m$^2$/wk every 4 wk | *Nadir:* 7–10 days<br>Severe BMS<br>Slight nausea and vomiting<br>Occasional dermatitis<br>Abnormal liver function<br>Pulmonary fibrosis with prolonged use<br>Second malignancy<br>Sterility | Hepatic metabolism to active compound<br>Renal excretion of 50% of unchanged drug | Good oral absorption. Concomitant barbiturate administration may enhance toxicity. Marrow suppression may be prolonged. |
| Busulfan (Myleran)<br>Leukemia | *Tab:* 2 mg white<br>*Dose:* 4–12 mg/day; for several weeks | *Nadir:* 10–30 days delayed marrow recovery<br>Potentially teratogenic<br>Pulmonary fibrosis with long-term use<br>Dermatologic hyperpigmentation<br>Gynecomastia<br>Amenorrhea | Well absorbed<br>Extensive hepatic metabolism to inactive compounds<br>Renal excretion | Bone marrow recovery may be delayed; therefore caution is advised with long-term use. Hydration and allopurinol may be indicated to prevent hyperuricemia. Total cumulative dose: 600 mg. Long-term daily administration is not recommended due to the risk of second malignancies with chronic alkylating agents. |
| 6-Thioguanine<br>Leukemia | *Tab:* 40 mg green/yellow<br>*Dose:* 80–100 mg/m$^2$<br>Reduce dose if stomatitis occurs | *Nadir:* 7–28 days<br>Stomatitis<br>Diarrhea<br>Hepatotoxicity | Variable, incomplete absorption<br>Hepatic metabolism<br>Renal excretion | Administer on an empty stomach.<br>Does not require dose reduction when used in conjunction with allopurinol. |
| 6-Mercaptopurine (6 MP)<br>Leukemia | *Tab:* 50 mg off-white<br>*Dose:* 80–100 mg/m$^2$/day<br>Titrate dose based on blood counts<br>Reduce dose in presence of hepatic or renal dysfunction | *Nadir:* 10–14 days<br>Nausea, vomiting<br>Mucositis<br>Diarrhea<br>Drug fever<br>Intrahepatic cholestasis<br>Pulmonary toxicity with prolonged use | Incomplete oral absorption<br>Hepatic inactivation<br>Renal excretion 10% unchanged in 24 hr | Protect pills from light. Administer as single dose on an empty stomach. Increased toxicity with allopurinol (reduce dose by one-third to one-fourth of the original dose). Administer with caution to patients on sodium warfarin (Coumadin). Monitor liver function tests. |
| Hexamethylmelamine (Altretamine hexalene)<br>Ovarian cancer | *Cap:* 50 mg clear<br>*Dose:* 240–320 mg/m$^2$/day | *Nadir:* 21–28 days<br>Acute liver toxicity is dose-limiting; nausea and vomiting are dose-related<br>Mild BMS<br>Abdominal cramping<br>Diarrhea<br>Peripheral neuropathies<br>Agitation, confusion | Variable absorption<br>Rapid metabolism<br>Urine excretion 90% in 72 hr | Pyridoxine 50 mg/day may decrease neuropathy.<br>Take with food, prophylactic antiemetics.<br>May worsen vincristine-related peripheral neuropathy. |

**TABLE 15-4** Oral Antineoplastic Agents (continued)

| Drug and Disease Indications | Dose and Schedule | Side Effects: Acute or Delayed | Pharmacokinetics | Comments |
|---|---|---|---|---|
| L-phenylanine mustard (melphalan, alkeran)<br><br>Multiple myeloma<br>Ovarian cancer | *Tab:* 2 mg white<br>*Dose:* 0.1–0.15 mg/kg/day × 2–3 wk<br>Reduce dose with hepatic or renal impairment | *Nadir:* 10–18 days<br>Nausea and vomiting usually mild<br>Dermatitis<br>Pulmonary fibrosis<br>Long-term therapy can result in acute leukemia | Hepatic metabolism<br>Renal excretion 20%–35% (10% unchanged)<br>20%–50% excreted in feces within 6 days | Protect pills from sunlight.<br>Take on an empty stomach.<br>BMS may be cumulative in older patients.<br>Leukemogenic. |
| Lomustine (CCNU)<br>Brain cancer<br>Lymphomas | *Cap:* 100 mg green/green, 40 mg green/white, 10 mg white<br>*Dose:* 100–130 mg/m² q 6–8 wk | *Nadir:* 28–42 days<br>Severe cumulative BMS<br>Nausea and vomiting 4–6 hr after dosing<br>Anorexia<br>Alopecia<br>Stomatitis<br>Hepatotoxicity | Absorbed rapidly (<60 min)<br>Hepatic metabolism<br>Renal excretion of 50% in 24 hr and 75% in 96 hr<br>Crosses into CSF | Dispense one dose at a time to prevent accidental overdose.<br>Take on an empty stomach just before bedtime.<br>Pretreat with aggressive antiemetics.<br>Protect pills from heat and humidity. |
| Hydroxyurea (Hydrea)<br>Chronic myelocytic leukemia<br>Melanoma<br>Head and neck cancer | *Cap:* 500 mg<br>*Dose:* 80 mg/kg/day every third day<br>750–1000 mg/m²/day × 5<br>Decrease dose in presence of renal dysfunction<br>Store in tight container in a cool environment | *Nadir:* 13–17 days<br>Acute nausea and vomiting<br>Chronic and severe anemia<br>Neurological seizures and hallucinations<br>Dermatitis<br>Dysuria<br>Azotemia | Well absorbed<br>Hepatic metabolism<br>Renal excretion of 80% of compound in 12 hr<br>Crosses into CSF | Concomitant radiation and/or 5-FU may enhance neurotoxicity.<br>Dysuria and renal impairment may occur.<br>Consider pretreatment with allopurinol. |
| VP-16-213 (etoposide, VePesid)<br>Lung cancer<br>Testicular cancer | *Cap:* 50 mg pink<br>*Dose:* 2 × the intravenous dose or 100–200 mg/m²/day over 3–5 days every 3–4 wk | *Nadir:* 7–14 days (white blood cell count)<br>Nausea and vomiting: 9–16 days (platelets)<br>Alopecia<br>BMS is dose limiting | Renal and hepatic metabolism<br>Incomplete and variable absorption | Nausea is mild though can be more severe with oral route than with intravenous route. |
| Procarbazine (Matulane)<br>Hodgkin's disease | *Cap:* 50 mg<br>*Dose:* 100 mg/m²/day × 14 days every 4 wk; reduce dose in presence of hepatic or renal dysfunction | *Nadir:* 4 wk<br>BMS, nausea, vomiting, and diarrhea gradually subside; flulike syndrome, paresthesias, neuropathies, dizziness, and ataxia | Well absorbed from the gastrointestinal tract<br>Metabolized in the liver with a biological half-life of about 1 hr<br>70% of the drug is eliminated by 24 hr in the urine, 5% appears as unchanged drug | Drug and food interactions can occur.<br>Central nervous system (CNS) depression can occur with concomitant administration of procarbazine and CNS depressants.<br>Hypertensive crisis can occur when procarbazine is administered with certain antidepressants (tricyclics and monoamine oxidase inhibitors) and tyramine-rich foods.<br>Severe nausea and vomiting can occur if taken with ethanol, mixed drinks, and beer. |
| Methotrexate<br>Squamous cell carcinoma<br>Lung cancer | *Tab:* 2.5 mg yellow<br>*Dose:* 2.5–10 mg/day PO or 15–30 mg/day PO × 5 days every 1–3 wk | *Nadir:* 7–10 days<br>Nausea and anorexia can occur; stomatitis and ulcerations can occur and are dose-limiting. | Serum half-life is 2–4 hr<br>Excreted by the kidneys | Dose is reduced with renal impairment; dosing on an empty stomach may enhance bioavailability. Excretion may be impaired in patients with simultaneous administration or weak acids such as salicylates or vitamin C; oral dosing is generally well tolerated. Avoid administration of methotrexate with keto-protein or probenecid because toxicity of methotrexate may be enhanced. |

Adapted from Goodman M: Delivery of cancer chemotherapy, in Baird S, McCorkle R, Grant M (eds): *Cancer Nursing: A Comprehensive Textbook.* Philadelphia, Saunders, 1991, p 311. Used with permission.

marily the nurse's responsibility, the nurse must be skilled in venipuncture, accessing, and management of numerous types of vascular access devices and drug administration systems. The nurse is also responsible for the prevention, early detection, and management of acute reactions associated with chemotherapy, including hypersensitivity, anaphylaxis, hypotension, extravasation, and nausea and vomiting. Through instructions, both oral and written, the nurse prepares the patient to manage the anticipated side effects of chemotherapy and to report their symptoms to the health care team early to avoid more serious toxic reactions.

One of the primary responsibilities of the nurse in the delivery of chemotherapy is to ensure that the correct dose of the appropriate drug is given to the appropriate individual. Despite the fact that safeguards are in place, serious errors in drug dosing do occur.[24,25] Such tragic events are regrettable but not so remarkable when one considers the number of chemotherapy doses given and the number of patients treated. Such significant drug errors occur at a rate of less than 1 percent.

As practitioners it is important to consider the potential origins and the settings in which drug errors are likely to occur. Combinations of complicated regimens of potentially lethal drugs are currently being given in high doses in a variety of settings, not just the research institutions where procedures intended to guard against drug errors are usually in place. Consequently, even though the caregiver may recognize a cumulative dose as higher than the usual dose they may still fail to question the order. In addition, institutions are being pressured to dramatically scale back, so that as resources diminish and individuals are required to do more with less the risk of error increases. Nurses are being required to be more efficient and to deliver the same quality of care with fewer support services. In some settings, in an effort to reduce expenditures, highly trained and experienced nurse practitioners are being replaced by individuals who are less experienced, less knowledgeable, and therefore less qualified, which increases the possibility of error.

In an effort to reduce the risk for drug error the following safeguards should be instituted wherever chemotherapy is admixed and administered.

1. Only the most senior physician responsible for the care of the patient and most familiar with the drug regimen and dosing schedule should write the chemotherapy orders.
2. The drug name should be written clearly and in full. Abbreviations are to be avoided, especially where drugs with similar sounding names are concerned (e.g., cisplatin and carboplatin, taxol and taxotere, mitomycin and mitoxantrone, vinblastine and vinorelbine, 5-Fudr and 5-Fu).
3. When the drug order is written (usually in triplicate) the drug name, dose in $mg/m^2$, total daily dose, and cumulative dose should be written. The original order that is sent to the pharmacy or individual preparing the drug should not be transcribed again before it reaches the pharmacy.
4. Once the order reaches the pharmacy the order is checked by the pharmacist against previous orders for that patient. If the drug or dose varies from the previous order, the order should be verified. If the patient is on a research protocol, the pharmacy staff should have a copy of the protocol to verify the order.
5. The person writing the order for the drug should avoid the use of extraneous ".0" because this allows the false interpretation of "100.0" as "1000." Probability of error could be further reduced by spelling out the amount as "one hundred" which will rarely, if ever, be read as "one thousand."
6. In most settings computer-generated labels are used. Ideally, the computer should be programmed to fail to print the label if the dose/cumulative dose are out of the ordinary and customary range. To override the computer and print the label would then require verification and authorization.
7. Drugs should be dispensed on large trays or in plastic ziplock bags large enough to hold all the drugs to be given to one patient. In a busy clinic, syringes of chemotherapy and bags of drugs to be given are often placed on a counter with the drug orders. Drugs intended for one patient may be confused with another patient's order if they are not contained properly in a bag or on a tray.
8. Once the pharmacist signs off on the drug, verifying that it is the right dose of the right drug for the right patient, the complete order is given to the nurse. The nurse then checks the drugs against the original written order to again confirm the accuracy of the order prior to treating the patient. If at all possible the person preparing the drug should not be the same person double-checking the order to make certain that what was ordered was prepared. If a nurse is working alone in a clinic the physician should be available to double-check the drugs prior to administration.
9. Everyone responsible for drug preparation and administration (pharmacist, pharmacy technicians, and nurses) needs to be properly trained in the specialty of chemotherapy drugs, and regularly reviewed according to institutional policy and procedure. In the rare situation where the patient is receiving chemotherapy at home, the nurse must have proof of certification to administer chemotherapy by an approved chemotherapy administration program.
10. Policies and procedures for drug preparation and administration should be reviewed by committee on a yearly basis.
11. Everyone responsible for chemotherapy drug preparation and administration should be empowered with the ability to question the order. If there is any question related to the drug, the dose, or the route or schedule, the individual must clarify the order, and be further encouraged to do so.

12. Any protocol involving unusual dosing patterns or dose intensive regimens should be reviewed carefully by all. No one should be expected to prepare or administer a drug with a dose-intensive schedule without the opportunity to review the protocol at least 24 hours in advance, especially if the study involves an investigational agent.

It is not uncommon in a busy outpatient clinic for a nurse to have no prior knowledge that a patient is beginning a new chemotherapy protocol before the patient appears in the clinic ready to be treated. This is not optimal because the nurse has no time to review the protocol and to prepare the patient's learning packet. Errors can be made whenever drugs are given in a hurried and unprepared manner. Communication between the physician, pharmacist, and nurse is critical to providing a safe level of care.

It is further recommended that all licensed registered nurses should have malpractice insurance regardless of their practice setting, but especially if their practice involves intravenous therapy.[26,27] To infiltrate a vesicant chemotherapeutic agent is not an act of negligence or malpractice. The issue is how much fluid infiltrated the tissues, over what length of time, the nurse's specific actions, and the completeness of the documentation and follow-up. At issue will also be the nurse's level of preparation and skill in IV drug administration and whether or not she has been certified to administer certain drugs, specifically vesicant chemotherapy. General certification in oncology nursing does not qualify the nurse to administer chemotherapy. Specific guidelines for certification and training to safely administer chemotherapy have been suggested by the Oncology Nursing Society Cancer Chemotherapy Guidelines.[3] Critical to these guidelines is the supervised training and experience of administering vesicant agents.

Specific policies and procedures that reflect standards of practice for IV drug administration should be readily available, reviewed frequently, and updated as necessary. If the nurse does not have knowledge of a specific procedure or does not follow it, he or she is not practicing according to the hospital's policy, and his or her actions are therefore indefensible in court. If the supervisor failed to inform the nurse of the policy and procedure, the supervisor (physician, nurse manager, hospital administration) may also be found at fault.

When a drug error occurs or an extravasation of a vesicant is suspected or certain, the nurse must document the event as thoroughly as possible to verify exactly what actions were taken to ensure optimal patient care. When the event involves infiltration of a vesicant agent an extravasation record (Figure 15-1) is useful to prompt the nurse to document the event as thoroughly as possible. When called upon to testify in a legal case one cannot be expected to recall events that occurred five years ago. If the nurse does not document what she did and what the patient reported at the time, it is as if she did nothing,

and what the patient currently says is true, no matter what the nurse says she did or what she recalls the patient reporting. It is important to document, if possible, the amount of fluid infiltrated and the size of the involved area. The site should be drawn on the extravasation record to identify the location and a color photograph should be attached to the extravasation record to compare to serial photographs to be taken on a weekly basis until the degree of damage can be determined. The format of an extravasation record should identify what the patient reported (subjective data), what the nurse observed (objective data), what the nurse did in detail (action), and the immediate plan of care including instructions for the patient and follow-up site care (plan). The nurse must document that the physician was notified and that instructions for care were explained and given to the patient including future plans for care such as a return appointment for evaluation and possible referral to a plastic surgeon and/or physical therapist.

Another issue that needs to be addressed is the patient's risk for extravasation. Often patients have been offered a vascular access device because of the nature of their treatment or their poor venous access and then refuse the device. This should be documented in the medical record. Ten years ago, before access devices were so readily available, it may have been acceptable to stick a patient three and four times with an angiocath or a scalp vein needle to secure an adequate, but likely suboptimal, venous access. Today, venous access devices are not only available but in many settings are the logical solution for any patient who requires chemotherapy for an indefinite period of time.

Chemotherapy is never (with rare exception) an emergency treatment in which a delay of two or three days to place an access device would be detrimental to the patient's condition. On the other hand an extravasation is associated with extreme morbidity, and an access device is inevitable under these circumstances. It is far better for the patient that the nurse refuse to attempt another venipuncture rather than to forge ahead with even more risk of extravasation. Unfortunately the pressure to complete the task at hand and the fact that refusing to try one more time might mean the drug will be wasted, often leads to poor judgment. As nurses we need to give each other permission to make the appropriate choice and provide the support to one another that is needed once that choice is made.

## ROUTES OF DRUG ADMINISTRATION

### Dose Calculation

The dose of drug to be administered is generally based on the individual's body surface area, usually expressed in milligrams per square meter or milligrams per kilo-

Patient _____ Date infiltration occurred _____

Drug _____ Dilution mg/ml _____ vesicant _____ irritant _____

**Amount of drug infiltrated:** < 1ml _____ 1–3 ml _____ 3–5 ml _____ 5–ml _____ > 10 ml _____

**Method of drug administration:**

_____ Two syringe technique IV push

_____ Side-arm with IV freely running

_____ Continuous infusion: rate _____ ml/hour

peristaltic pump _____ yes _____ no

_____ VAD: _____ port _____ tunneled catheter

type of needle _____

_____ Other _____

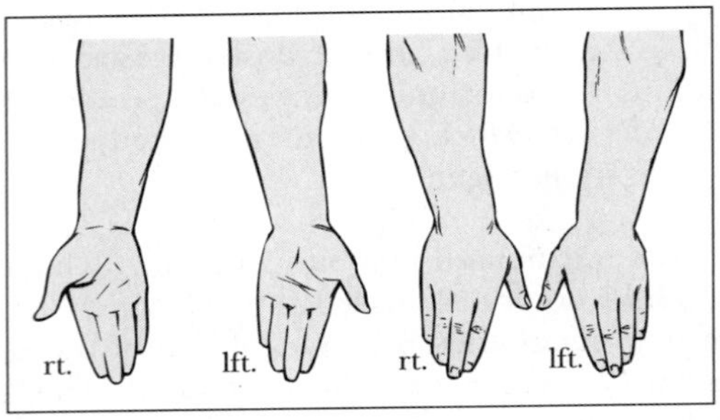

right arm          left arm
(attach photograph)

**Description of site:**

Size _____ Color _____ Texture _____
(Indicate location on diagram)

**Process Documentation:** Describe the events that occurred during the drug administration

S: (Patient's Symptoms) _____

_____

_____

O: (Clinical Symptoms) _____

_____

_____

A: (Assessment) _____ suspected extravasation _____ definite extravasation _____

_____

P: (Plan of care) Initial actions: _____

_____

Physician notified: _____ Instruction _____

_____

**Follow-up Instructions:** _____

_____

**Additional Comments:** _____

Consultations: _____ Plastic Surgery _____ Physical Therapy _____ Other _____

Date of referral: _____ Follow-up _____

Return appointment: _____ Written instructions for site care reviewed with patient _____

(RN Signature _____ )

Follow-up visit #1 (date _____) Describe site and care instructions: attach photo _____

_____

Follow-up visit #2 (date _____) Describe site and care instructions: attach photo _____

_____

Follow-up visit #3 (date _____) Describe site and care instructions: attach photo _____

_____

**FIGURE 15-1** Documentation record for suspected or actual chemotherapy drug extravasation.
Reprinted with permission from Goodman M: Rush Cancer Institute Chicago, IL

gram. The patient's body surface area is usually determined by a height and weight nomogram. There is controversy regarding the accuracy and safety of this method since some patients may have been heavily pretreated and therefore unable to tolerate higher doses of drugs or dose-intensive regimens. In addition many patients are clinically obese, which is defined as weighing 30% or more over ideal body weight. Empiric decreases in the doses of anticancer agents given to obese patients based on ideal body weight are not supported by available data.[28] Georgiadis et al[29] found no significant association between obesity and toxicity measured primarily as white blood cell nadir. It is important to bear in mind that inappropriate dose reduction may compromise efficacy, which is particularly meaningful when the intent of treatment is cure. However, in situations where a dose reduction is necessary and the patient's weight is significantly greater than their ideal, a simple method of calculating their dose is to take the average of the ideal and actual weight. If an ideal weight table is not available, start with 100 pounds for 5 feet and add five pounds for each additional inch. So, someone who is 5'5" would ideally weigh 125 pounds. That weight plus their actual weight divided by two would give the weight upon which to calculate dose per square meter.

Attempts are often made to individualize the dose of a drug so that optimal therapeutic response is achieved without toxic effects. However, the outcome is generally less than ideal and patients, especially the elderly, are frequently underdosed because of the potential for severe toxicity. It is often proposed that individual doses be calculated based on a person's physiological age rather than their chronological age. One example of this approach involves the application of the Calvert formula for carboplatin dosing.[30] The Calvert formula makes it possible to individualize the carboplatin dose in order to obtain a maximally effective dose with tolerable side effects.

Carboplatin is excreted by the kidneys, in particular glomerular filtration with little excretion or reabsorption by the renal tubules. Therefore pretreatment assessment of renal function or glomerula filtration rate (GFR) can be used to individualize carboplatin dose in adults. The GFR is essentially equivalent to the creatinine clearance which can be estimated from the patient's age, serum creatinine, and weight. Another factor in the Calvert formula involves the area under the curve (AUC), or target drug concentration for carboplatin. The AUC dosing correlates more closely with drug toxicity than do doses based on body surface area.[31] In the presence of impaired renal function the delayed clearance of carboplatin would result in prolonged drug exposure (increased AUC): in patients with high renal clearance decreased AUC could result in subtherapeutic dosing. Since AUC or carboplatin exposure, rather than toxicity, is the measurement, it is not influenced by concurrent myelosuppressive therapy or supportive treatment. The following formula is applicable in single-agent, combination therapy, or high-dose studies:

$$\text{CARBOPLATIN DOSE (MG)} = \text{TARGET AUC} \times (\text{GFR} + 25)$$

AUC: Area under the curve
GFR: Glomerular filtration rate

The AUC ranges from 4 to 11 and is selected for appropriate clinical situations. For example if the patient has had prior treatment or is receiving carboplatin in combination with another myelosuppressive agent, an AUC of 4–5 might be selected. If the patient is receiving carboplatin alone and has not been previously treated with ablative chemotherapy, an AUC of 7–11 might be selected.

The GFR is equivalent to the creatinine clearance, which can be measured or estimated from the patient's age, weight, and serum creatinine. It is important to note that the dose calculation for carboplatin using this formula is the total dose, not $mg/m^2$.

## Pretreatment Considerations

Table 15-5 includes specific tasks involved in antineoplastic drug administration that are applicable in all practice settings. Of special note would be any procedure that would address patient safety such as anaphylaxis or extravasation. All emergency equipment should be available and in good working order. Standing orders for emergency care should be readily available as well as appropriate personnel in the event that an emergency situation should arise. In the current practice environment, it is not uncommon for one or two nurses to be the sole providers of care in an ambulatory care setting with a clinic full of patients who have seen the physician and are receiving their medicines or waiting to begin their treatment. The physicians often see their patients and leave to do rounds in the hospital or to go to another freestanding oncology facility. Standards of practice dictate that a physician be physically available where chemotherapy is administered. This applies to all settings where drugs of an experimental nature are given, but in fact reactions and emergency situations can arise when more commonly used drugs like etoposide are given. The first consideration is the safety of the patient, and the policies and procedures governing the setting in which chemotherapy is given should specifically indicate that a physician should be present physically, not just available by phone.

There are other specific factors to be considered for individual drugs (e.g., test dosing prior to administering bleomycin). While not a common practice, it is still considered appropriate to administer a test dose of bleomycin prior to administering the full dose because the first dose of bleomycin has been known to cause rare but severe allergic reactions, especially in patients with lymphoma.[31] Test dosing involves giving 0.5–1.0 unit of bleomycin IV, IM, or subcutaneously prior to the first dose of the drug.

## TABLE 15-5  Chemotherapy Administration Guidelines

**Professional Preparation**

- Maintain appropriate knowledge and skills regarding chemotherapy drug protocols and administration procedures.

- Review applicable policies and procedures.

- Review drug protocol and research guidelines.

**Patient Preparation**

- Verify patient identity (arm band, driver's license, verbalization of name).

- Ensure appropriate patient education.

- Confirm that appropriate laboratory tests have been completed and are within normal limits.

- Measure and record baseline vital signs.

- Verify patient's allergy history.

- Assess venous access status (i.e., need for VAD).

- Initiate pretreatment therapies, if ordered (e.g., hydration, test dosing).

**Drug Preparation**

- Verify drug order (including body surface area and dosage calculations).

- Obtain prepared drug, and double-check label for the correct drug, dose, route, and patient. If admixing, follow appropriate guidelines for cytotoxic drug admixture.

- Ensure rapid access to extravasation kit and medications necessary if allergic reaction occurs (parenteral diphenhydramine hydrochloride, epinephrine, and hydrocortisone should be immediately available).

- Obtain necessary supplies and equipment for safe drug administration.

- Wash hands, and don gloves and appropriate protective clothing.

**Venipuncture Guidelines**

- Establish work area with plastic-backed pad.

- Organize materials, needle box, syringes, flush, IV start materials, and IV fluids.

- Select needle size and type according to setting, patient's veins, and treatment to be administered.

- Determine appropriate site for venous access, avoiding:
  - limbs with recent (i.e., 30 min) venipunctures
  - limbs with axillary node dissections, extensive radiation therapy, or obstructive process
  - antecubital fossa (for peripheral sticks)
  - ecchymotic or sclerosed areas
  - bony prominences and joints

- Ensure adequate lighting and visualization of area to be accessed.

- Remove jewelry near access site.

- Select a large vein if administering drugs known to be irritating (mechlorethamine, BCNU, streptozotocin, paclitaxel, docetaxel, vinorelbine).

- Administer vesicants only at sites designated by established policies and procedures, specifically in areas with underlying subcutaneous tissue. Areas to be avoided when administering vesicants include veins over joints, bony prominences, neurovascular bundles, tendons, and areas of existing soft-tissue damage.

- For peripheral sites, begin at the most distal areas.

- Utilize an appropriate sterile technique for access.

- Achieve a "clean" venipuncture and determine patency. The needle should not puncture through the back of the vein and then be resettled within the vein. There should be a brisk, immediate blood return and no swelling at the needle site.

- Secure needle with tape, but ensure visualization of the site.

- Flush needle with sterile NS or D5W to clear the line and establish patency. Observe the site at this time to ensure that swelling is not occurring at the needle site.

- Use Luer-Lok fittings for intravenous (IV) sets and syringes; use sterile gauze or alcohol pad for priming IV sets.

**Drug Administration Guidelines**

- Check patient's condition periodically during drug administration, and explain actions being taken, when appropriate.

- Monitor the status of the venous access site periodically during the process.

- If administering a vesicant, observe the site continuously throughout the injection.

- Administer antiemetics (if not already given).

- Ensure drug containment at all times. Wipe any droplets at the connector or Y-site with a gauze pad.

- Administer chemotherapy drugs as ordered, using slow, steady pressure.

- Check for a blood return every few mls and before and after each drug.

- Flush between each drug with sterile NS or D5W to avoid drug admixture and potential precipitation.

- When administering short-term drips or infusions, establish the infusion, taping all connections securely, and set the appropriate flow rate.

- Generally, place long-term infusions on an infusion pump.

- Flush after last drug with sterile NS or D5W.

- If appropriate, discontinue the IV needle. For peripheral sites, hold pressure manually over the site for a few minutes, then apply small, sterile dressing.

- Do not clip or recap needles.

**Postadministration Guidelines**

- Discard all materials (needles, syringes, bags, tubing, gown, gloves, etc.) appropriately.

- Assess patient's status and provide for follow-up:
  - *Inpatient:* Call button within reach; fluids available, etc.
  - *Outpatient:* Transportation ready; return appointment and prescriptions obtained; telephone number of physician or nurse available
  - *Home care:* Caregiver available; telephone number of nurse-on-call available

- Document all actions (flow sheets or specialized forms are recommended). (See chapter 16.)

It is preferable to test dose 24 hours prior to administration, but it is commonly done one or two hours before the full dose, followed by very close observation. Diphenhydramine 50 mg and acetaminophen 1000 mg may be given with the bleomycin and again four hours later. The hypersensitity reactions including hypotension, rash, facial flushing, and bronchospasm can progress to anaphylaxis; but in general most patients experience only a relatively high fever, chills, and a flu-like syndrome. These symptoms are usually preventable if the patient is given the diphenhydramine and the acetaminophen and remembers to take it again four hours later.

Another issue involves prevention of hypersensitivity reactions (HSR) with paclitaxel or docetaxel. When paclitaxel is given, patients must remember to begin taking dexamethasone 20 mg by mouth 13 and 7 hours prior to dosing with taxol. In addition, patients are given diphenhydramine 50 mg IV and an H2 blocker (ranitidine 50 mg or cimetidine 300 mg) 30 minutes prior to taxol. Most reactions, if they are going to occur with taxol, occur within the first three courses and are thought to be due to Cremophor EL, the formulation vehicle.

In the case of etoposide, the primary reaction is hypotension. Severe hypotension can occur if the drug is infused in less than 45 minutes. Etoposide is formulated in benzyl alcohol and Tween 80. Caution should be taken when giving etoposide for the first and second time. The infusion is started slowly at a 60-minute rate and all nursing personnel are informed that the patient is receiving the drug for the first or second time. The patient is instructed to report any light-headedness, dizziness, rash, or difficulty breathing. Bronchospasm with severe wheezing can occur and responds to antihistamines and glucocorticosteroids. It is advisable, especially if the individual is atopic or has a prior history of reaction to paclitaxel or cisplatin, to have diphenhydramine 50 mg available if needed. If the patient is receiving both paclitaxel and etoposide, special pretreatment and monitoring for hypersensitivity reactions may be needed.[32] Inhaled bronchodilators, epinephrine and diphenhydramine 50 mg, should be readily available in the treatment area.

Docetaxel is a drug similar to paclitaxel, but is associated with less risk of HSR and initially in phase I studies was given without premedication. Currently most patients are given dexamethasone 8 mg twice a day for five days beginning one day prior to docetaxel. This precaution appears to delay the onset and decrease the severity of fluid retention characterized by peripheral edema, pleural effusions, and ascites.

The last pretreatment consideration involves the sequencing of various drugs to either enhance cytotoxicity or minimize toxicity to normal tissues. For example the administration of slightly higher doses of intravenous methotrexate one hour prior to 5-fluorouracil with leucovorin rescue 24 hours later appears to enhance the cell kill effect of both the methotrexate and the 5-FU. Similarly the sequence of cisplatin before paclitaxel induces more profound neutropenia than the alternate sequence. The incidence of neutropenia is felt to be due to the lower paclitaxel clearance rates when cisplatin precedes paclitaxel.[33] In addition the cytotoxic effects of paclitaxel preceding platinol were additive, whereas the reverse sequence resulted in pronounced antagonism.[34]

A study by Clark et al[35] demonstrated that administering paclitaxel before carboplatin resulted in significantly greater cytotoxicity than when administering the drugs in the reverse sequence. The toxicity profile was not effected by sequence of drug administration. Therefore to achieve the greatest efficacy with no increase in toxicity the paclitaxel is routinely administered prior to carboplatin.

Another example of the importance of sequencing in chemotherapy administration involves the administration of doxorubicin and paclitaxel. A moderate to severe mucositis can occur when paclitaxel is given prior to doxorubicin, but not when it was given in the reverse sequence. The paclitaxel-related mucosal damage concomitant with neutropenia has been thought to contribute to the development of typhlitis, which can be life threatening. Pharmacokinetic data indicate that when paclitaxel is given immediately prior to doxorubicin there is a 31.6% average decrease in the clearance of doxorubicin, which contributes greatly to profound neutropenia.[36] Based on this, the sequence of doxorubicin followed by paclitaxel is recommended.

Chemotherapy was designed as a systemic treatment for cancer, having the ability to travel throughout the body via the bloodstream and to damage or kill dividing cells. It is now possible to direct drugs systemically as well as to almost every anatomic region in the body: to specific organs, inside body cavities, and to body spaces. Intravenous chemotherapy remains the most common route of drug delivery, but other systemic routes include oral, intramuscular, and subcutaneous. Regional drug delivery utilizes the following routes: topical, intra-arterial, intraperitoneal, intrapleural, intravesical, intrathecal, and intraventricular. It is even possible to use these techniques to administer the drugs directly into the center of a tumor (intratumoral).

## Topical

Cutaneous malignant lesions can be treated in a variety of ways, including the topical application of antineoplastic agents. This is most commonly done for cutaneous T-cell lymphoma, basal cell carcinoma, Kaposi's sarcoma, and squamous cell carcinoma. The agents used include nitrogen mustard for cutaneous T-cell lymphoma and fluorouracil for the two mentioned carcinomas.[37] The topical agent is usually applied once or twice daily until the lesions progress to the necrosis phase, which may take one to three weeks. The affected area is not washed vigorously during the treatment period. The expected result of topical antineoplastic administration is local sloughing of the affected area and eventual regranulation of normal tissue, so it is normal for the treated area to become red and tender, then to form a lesion that becomes necrotic, followed by superficial sloughing of the dead tissue and regrowth of healthy skin. It is unusual for the patient to experience any systemic side effects of the drugs unless the majority of the skin is being treated; but incidences of mild, delayed side effects such as nausea have been reported.

Special nursing considerations for these patients include:

1. patient education, with special consideration for body image issues
2. application of the drug using cotton swabs or non-metal applicators
3. close attention to application only in the prescribed (affected) area
4. careful avoidance of the eyes, nares, mouth, or other areas very close to mucous membranes
5. utilization of safe drug handling practices (e.g., gloves and strict attention to drug containment)
6. when using nitrogen mustard, having sodium thiosulfate available (to neutralize the nitrogen mustard) and applying it to areas of the skin that may be inadvertently exposed (after removal of the drug)
7. application of dressings, if prescribed
8. observation for untoward sequelae (e.g., severe burning or rashes, which may require discontinuation of therapy or subsequent dose reduction)
9. monitoring disease response

## Oral

A variety of antineoplastic agents are administered orally to treat numerous types of cancer (Table 15-4).[38] The oral route is convenient, economical, noninvasive, and often less toxic. Most oral drugs are well absorbed as long as the gastrointestinal tract is functioning normally.

The nursing responsibilities for oral drug administration include safe handling (gloves are considered acceptable if physical contact with the tablet or capsule is required) and monitoring for drug absorption and compliance with the prescribed therapy. If the patient experiences emesis immediately after drug ingestion and the pills or capsules cannot be visualized, the drug is usually not repeated. Several oral antineoplastic agents are also available in parenteral forms, providing an option for patients intolerant of or noncompliant with oral regimens. Other recommendations include:

1. Prescribe one "course" at a time, to avoid inadvertent overdosing that could be life threatening.
2. Instruct the patient to take the medication on an empty stomach with water to enhance absorption, unless the drug is tolerated better with food, as is the case with prednisone, cyclophosphamide, and tamoxifen.
3. Familiarize the patient with both generic and brand names of the drug, to avoid confusion or double dosing (many physicians prefer to prescribe brand name

antineoplastic agents to avoid the possibility of the generics not being bioequivalent).
4. Instruct the patient to maintain a record of drugs being taken.
5. Obtain a list of any drugs currently being taken by the patient to ensure compatibility.
6. Advise the patient to avoid any over-the-counter drugs unless first checking with the physician or nurse.
7. Question the patient at each visit regarding the medication (i.e., how much was taken, whether any doses were omitted, and why).

It is important that the patient comply with the treatment regimen to maximize the goal of therapy (i.e., remission or cure). Oral agents give the patient control over administration, and noncompliance is not common. However, tamoxifen can cause hot flashes and mood swings, cyclophosphamide and etoposide can cause emesis, and levamisole can cause neurotoxicity. A patient might decide to omit a dose in order to feel better temporarily. The patient needs to understand the importance of dosing and scheduling and how critical it is that the prescribed regimen be followed exactly. With therapy such as leucovorin following methotrexate, noncompliance could be fatal. It is common for patients receiving oral antineoplastic agents to be given a calendar with the doses indicated and space to record each dose. The nurse checks the previous treatment calendar and questions the patient about any omitted doses during each encounter. The regimen can often be modified to enhance the patient's tolerance of the side effects (e.g., administering an antiemetic to minimize nausea or changing the time of dose administration).

## Intramuscular and Subcutaneous

Utilization of intramuscular (IM) or subcutaneous (SQ) antineoplastic drug delivery was uncommon in the past, since only a few drugs were indicated by this route. The development of the biological agents (such as interferon, colony-stimulating factors) has increased the number of drugs given IM or SQ. These convenient and quick routes are handled according to standard injection methods. Since some of the drugs can sting or burn, IM injections are usually given into large muscles, with the Z-track method being optional. Subcutaneous injections of small volumes (up to 3 ml) are in the usual sites and should be rotated if being given daily. Many drug manufacturers have distributed videos, charts, or posters that clearly outline the steps to follow for patients self-administering SQ medications. One drug that is administered subcutaneously in a rather unique way is goserelin acetate (Zoladex®; ICI Pharma), a hormonal agent used in the treatment of breast cancer and prostate cancer. It is actually a dry drug pellet that is implanted in the soft tissue of the abdomen, where it gradually is absorbed over a 28-day period. A local anesthetic such as Emla Cream®

or a lidocaine injection is usually used to minimize discomfort, since the needle is large (16-gauge).

## Intravenous

The intravenous (IV) route of drug delivery is the most common and most reliable method of drug delivery. Detailed nursing actions concerning IV drug administration are included in Table 15-5. Selection of a venous access device, an angiocath, or a butterfly will be determined by the type of therapy the patient is to receive and the condition of the patient's veins. For most patients a 21-gauge needle is adequate for extended infusions for hydration and for three- and four-hour infusions of chemotherapy. If an IV needs to stay in over one hour it is best to place an angiocath that will be less likely to infiltrate and will be less traumatic to the veins. If the patient is to receive only an injection of chemotherapy and IV antiemetics without hydration, a 23- or 21-gauge butterfly needle is preferred because it is easy to insert into small veins and is less traumatic because it is not left in for an extended period of time. The problem with small butterfly needles (25-gauge) is that the blood return is often lost because the needle is so small. When giving a vesicant it is always better to have a blood return throughout the injection so a smaller-gauge needle is not preferable in that situation. Unfortunately, patients often have such small veins that the smaller needles are needed. In this situation choosing an angiocath like the Intima®, that is thin-walled with an over-the-needle cannula, permits a large internal diameter once the stylet is removed without overly traumatizing the vein. Choosing the appropriate device is important but taking the time to find the most appropriate vein is even more important. Staying focused on finding the vein can be difficult considering the numerous distractions that exist in a busy ambulatory care center. The initial and careful assessment of both arms (if appropriate) is critical to vein selection. Too often the nurse fails to assess the veins properly, fails to distend the veins sufficiently prior to attempting venipuncture, and fails to apply adequate traction on the vein to prevent the vein from rolling. If a vein is not obvious it is advisable to apply moist heat to the arms for five to ten minutes and have the patient drink warm liquids prior to attempting venipuncture. If the patient is known to have small, hard-to-find veins the patient should drink four to six glasses of fluid the morning of treatment, dress warmly, and practice vein distention by squeezing a handball for ten minutes prior to the nurse attempting venipuncture. If the nurse has difficulty accessing an appropriate vein after one or two attempts, she should seek the assistance of a colleague. If a patient repeatedly requires more than three sticks and the plan is to have chemotherapy indefinitely, or at least for an extended period of time, a vascular access device is appropriate. The longer the patient has the device the longer he or she benefits from having it placed. Even if a person has great veins, if he or she has metastatic disease and will require an access device at some point, it is appropriate to propose it early on in the course of treatment.

When selecting a vein the general rule is to start distally and gradually proceed proximal. Another rule might be to select the best vein, provided that vein is not the antecubital vein. Some nurses might prefer the antecubital area for venous access because it contains large veins to facilitate rapid drug delivery. However, this area should be avoided, especially if the patient is receiving a vesicant agent. Placing a needle in the antecubital area restricts patient mobility and increases the risk of dislodgment. Any extravasation that occurs is difficult to detect because the area is dense and a lot of fluid can infiltrate before it is detected.

Another issue involves the order in which chemotherapeutic agents are given. Except where sequencing is important pharmacologically the order of drug delivery is probably not critical. However, when administering a vesicant agent, it is wiser to administer the antiemetic and any antianxiolytic agent after the vesicant. No agent, except perhaps nitrogen mustard causes emesis in the first hour, so giving the vesicant before the antiemetic is sound practice. It is important that the patient be alert and able to communicate how they are feeling throughout the injection of the vesicant. The reasons to give the vesicant before any other agent is (1) the venous integrity is greatest earlier on in the procedure, and (2) the nurse's assessment skills and the patient's level of awareness and sensitivity are most acute at the initiation of the infusion. The possibility that the vein will be irritated by other drugs (decadron) or by movement is eliminated. The idea that if the vein takes the nonvesicants without any problem then the vesicant will infuse without difficulty is faulty reasoning. The risk of infiltration of any IV increases over time. Often other drugs can cause venous irritation and even spasm that can result in a loss of blood return, a major assessment criteria for safe administration of chemotherapy.

Another factor in the intravenous administration of chemotherapy is the pain associated with the needle stick. Patients seldom become accustomed to the discomfort and often grow to dread the event more as time goes on. The pain of venipuncture can be dealt with in a number of ways: first needle phobia is a major reason for insertion of a vascular access device. However, while the placement of an access device does diminish the discomfort of a needle stick, it by no means eliminates it. Ethyl chloride spray has been used to numb the site prior to needle stick, but it does not work well. Ice has been used over ports to ease the discomfort, but again patients will still feel the needle stick and it is messy. There is one approach to pain prevention with a needle stick that works remarkably well and is especially indicated for anyone with a needle phobia and with children. Emla Cream® (ASTRA Inc., Westborough, MA) is a mixture of lidocaine 2.5% and prilocaine 2.5%. A dollop of cream is placed over the vein, port, or selected site for IM or SQ injection approximately one to four hours prior to treatment. An occlusive dressing (provided with the 5 g tubes) is applied over the Emla Cream without spreading out the cream. When the time comes to begin the procedure the dressing is removed and the site is cleansed thoroughly prior to the needle stick. Having patients turn their heads away or close their eyes guarantees elimination of the psychological component of fear of needle sticks, although it does not totally eliminate the anticipation of the pain—until the patient sees how well the approach works to prevent pain and discomfort. Patients who in the past have experienced severe anxiety and pain with venipuncture claim they feel nothing when the needle goes in, not even pressure, especially when the Emla is in place for at least two hours. One word of caution—Emla should not be used in patients who are also receiving a vesicant agent peripherally because they will not be able to feel the pain if the vesicant should infiltrate. Using Emla cream means that the nurse needs to take a little time to help the patient select the vein that will be used at the next treatment and the nurse must try to access a vein in that area. In patients with few veins it is a good idea to select two sites to prepare with the Emla cream. Patients should be cautioned that it is not always possible to access a vein in a previously selected site. When it does work out, however, the patient is extremely appreciative. For the nurse it is especially rewarding to be able to eliminate what is surely the most dreaded aspect of the patient's treatment. Even patients with ports become devoted users of Emla cream.

## Vesicant Extravasation Issues

Several of the most commonly administered chemotherapy drugs are vesicants, meaning that they cause tissue necrosis if they infiltrate or extravasate out of the blood vessel and into the soft tissue. While a few nonantineoplastic drugs are vesicants (e.g., Levophed and Dilantin), the number of antineoplastic vesicants is significant; they are listed in Table 15-6 along with the agents known to be irritating to the vein during drug administration. It is critical that the nurse administering chemotherapy both be aware of those drugs that are vesicants and employ a number of safety measures to try to prevent extravasation.

When infiltration of a vesicant occurs, underlying tissue is damaged. The damage can be severe enough to result in physical deformity or a functional deficit, such as loss of joint mobility, loss of vascularity, or loss of tendon function. If a sufficient amount of an irritant infiltrates, it too can cause significant damage beyond discoloration and pain. The following guidelines are suggested to minimize the risk of extravasation.

1. Be aware of certain patients at increased risk for extravasation:
   a. patients unable to communicate to the nurse about the pain of extravasation
   b. elderly, debilitated, or confused patients with diabetes or general vascular disease

**TABLE 15-6    Antineoplastic Vesicants and Irritants***

**Vesicants**
Dactinomycin (Cosmegen)
Daunomycin (Cerubidine)
Doxorubicin (Adriamycin)
Estramustin (Estracyte)
Idarubicin (Idamycin)
Mitomycin C (Mutamycin)
Nitrogen mustard (Mustargen)
Teniposide
Vinblastine (Velban)
Vincristine (Oncovin)

**Irritants**
Carmustine (BCNU)
Dacarbazine (DTIC)
Etoposide (VP-16)
Liposomal doxorubicin (Doxil)
Mithramycin (Plicamycin)
Mitoxantrone (Novantrone)
Paclitaxel (Taxol)
Streptozocin (Zanosar)
Docetaxel (Taxotere)
Vinorelbine (Navelbine)

*There is some controversy regarding these lists. The practitioner is urged to remain up to date with current research and literature reports regarding these drugs as well as any new agents becoming available.

   c. any patient with very fragile veins
2. Generally, avoid infusing vesicants over joints, bony prominences, tendons, neurovascular bundles, or the antecubital fossa.
3. Never give vesicants intramuscularly or subcutaneously.
4. Avoid giving vesicant drugs in areas where venous or lymphatic circulation is poor (e.g., operative side for a mastectomy patient, patient with superior vena cava syndrome) or in sites that have been previously irradiated.
5. Make sure the peripheral IV site is adequate and less than 24 hours old. A brisk blood return and easy flow of fluids are to be determined before administering vesicants in any IV needle or catheter (peripheral or central).
6. Visualize the needle or catheter insertion site and observe the site continuously. (Never leave the patient unattended when administering a vesicant peripherally.)
7. When giving more than one chemotherapy agent, give the vesicant agent first.
8. Give vesicants in a steady, even flow, checking frequently (every 1–2 ml) for a blood return. When checking for a blood return, do so gently so as to avoid excessive pressure in the vein.
9. If a vesicant is ordered as an *infusion,* it is given through a central line only and checked every 1–2 hours in health care facilities and every 2–4 hours

when the patient is receiving vesicant infusions in the home.

10. An extravasation kit containing all materials necessary to manage an extravasation should be available wherever vesicant agents are administered. Include in the kit a copy of the extravasation policy and procedure.

Despite these precautions, vesicant extravasation does occur, although the incidence is low among experienced oncology nurses in cancer specialty settings (0.1%) and somewhat higher in general hospital settings (2%–5%).[39]

Detection of a vesicant extravasation in its earliest stage is most likely to result in the least possible soft-tissue damage. The nurse should be aware of the following symptoms that could indicate extravasation. It is important to note that an extravasation can occur without any symptoms.

- swelling (most common)

- stinging, burning, or pain at the injection site (not *always* present)

- redness (not often seen initially)

- lack of blood return (if this is *only* occurrence, the IV should be reevaluated; if still no blood return, consider other options); lack of a blood return *alone* is not always indicative of an extravasation. An extravasation can occur even if a blood return is present.

If an extravasation is suspected, the infusion is to be stopped immediately and the needle site inspected.

Chemotherapy drug extravasation is a known complication of cancer treatment. The occurrence of extravasation of vesicant chemotherapeutic agents is probably underreported, but according to the literature the incidence ranges from 0.5% to 5% of patients receiving peripheral intravenous chemotherapeutic agents[40,41] and 6.4% of patients ($n = 300$) receiving vesicant chemotherapy via implanted vascular access ports.[42]

The most benign, inconsequential local reaction to chemotherapy is venous flare (see Figure 15-2—Plate 1). This reaction occurs most commonly in patients receiving doxorubicin and is characterized by a localized erythema, venous streaking, and pruritis along the injected vein. This localized allergic reaction is distinguishable from an extravasation by the absence of pain or swelling and the presence of a blood return. Once this important distinction is made, it is safe to continue injecting the agent. Flushing the vein with saline and slowing the injection rate appear to ease the symptoms, which dissipate without treatment within 20–30 minutes of the injection.

Another local tissue reaction characterized by pain, venous irritation, and chemical phlebitis can occur with certain nonvesicant chemotherapy agents. These agents are called *irritants* and are listed in Table 15-6. While any drug given in concentrated form in sufficient amount can cause tissue damage if infiltrated, these agents are not associated with ulceration if infiltrated. Irritants cause intravascular irritation often accompanied by pain (described as achiness or as tightness) only during the infusion and may, as is the case with carmustine, be a function of the diluent.

Vinorelbine can cause venous irritation. Infusing 250 ml of fluid and injecting the drug over six to ten minutes followed by a 250 ml infusion of saline or dextrose in water will minimize discomfort when infusing vinorelbine into a peripheral vein. When administering vinorelbine into a central line the flush is probably not important but it is generally done as a precaution. Liposomal doxorubicin (Doxil) is an irritant that is given as an infusion over 30–60 minutes. If infiltrated there may be redness and edema but no ulceration. A cold compress is appropriate to ease discomfort. With some irritants like dacarbazine or streptozocin increasing the dilution, applying a cold pack, or slowing the drip rate will ease the pain associated with infusion.

The most devastating skin reactions caused by chemotherapy occur when a vesicant agent is infiltrated causing an extravasation injury. The degree of injury to local tissues is related to the vesicant properties of the drug infiltrated, the concentration of the drug, and the amount of the drug infiltrated. For example, in the animal model 0.2 ml of doxorubicin at a concentration of 2 mg/ml produces a 1 cm-diameter lesion taking seven or eight weeks to heal.[40]

By definition, an *extravasation* is the infiltration of a vesicant chemotherapeutic agent. A *vesicant* is a drug that, if infiltrated, is capable of causing pain, ulceration, necrosis, and sloughing of damaged tissue. While all vesicants are capable of causing significant ulceration and morbidity due to pain, tissue necrosis, and potential loss of function of the affected area, this rarely occurs when these drugs are given by professional nurses who are trained in the proper techniques of chemotherapy drug administration. Although infiltration of vesicant agents can occur even when these drugs are given by properly trained individuals, the sequelae are usually inconsequential and the wound usually heals spontaneously over time.

To infiltrate a vesicant agent is traumatic for patient and nurse, but it is not an act of negligence. In many situations the patient is elderly with small frail veins, or obese with deep and difficult-to-access veins. In such cases the occurrence of an extravasation is more a function of venous integrity than the administration technique. Patients should be thoroughly informed regarding the vesicant potential of the drugs they are receiving and the importance of reporting any pain, burning, or stinging during the injection.

To ensure the best outcome possible in the event of an extravasation, the nurse must be able to recognize that an infiltration has occurred and act appropriately. When vesicant agents are administered by nurses and physicians who are not trained in the skills of chemotherapy administration, the subtle early signs and symptoms of an extravasation may go unnoticed, resulting in extensive tissue damage and possible loss of function, even amputation (see Figures 15-3 and 15-4—Plates 2 and 3).

## Prevention and assessment

Because there are no universally effective, optimal means of treating vesicant extravasation, the best approach is prevention. The Cancer Chemotherapy Guidelines and Recommendations for the Management of Vesicant Extravasation is an excellent resource for nurses and physicians to implement preventive care and for the design of appropriate policies and procedures in individual practice settings. The official position of the Oncology Nursing Society is that all personnel who administer chemotherapy should receive training in chemotherapy drug administration and management of toxicities including drug extravasation. Institutionally approved guidelines for extravasation management should be readily available, reviewed, and revised regularly as appropriate. The physician's guidelines or institutional protocol for the management of a presumed or proven extravasation should be readily available wherever vesicant drugs are administered and instituted immediately in the event of an extravasation. The procedure for documenting and reporting an actual or suspected extravasation should be clearly defined.

The signs and symptoms of an extravasation may be very obvious or extremely subtle. The one obvious sign of drug infiltration is a bleb formation at the injection site that is readily apparent in a superficial vein, or swelling that occurs in more deeply accessed veins. In the absence of pain, swelling, or diffuse induration, an extravasation may go unnoticed, especially when the vein lies deeply in an obese limb. In this situation a large amount of drug can infiltrate, especially if the drug is injected very slowly.

Pain can be an early or late symptom depending upon the patient's ability to report this sensation. If a patient is elderly and confused or heavily sedated, symptoms may go unreported. Any antiemetics, sedatives, or analgesics that may affect the patient's ability to readily report any change in sensation at the injection site should be withheld until after the vesicant has been safely administered. The report of any change in sensation such as pain, stinging, or burning at the injection site warrants further investigation to ensure an intact vein. The vesicant injection is stopped immediately and the vein is aspirated to ensure a blood return. In the absence of any swelling, pain, or evidence of infiltration, the injection of the vesicant may continue following a copious (30–40 ml) saline flush. If the patient again complains of discomfort despite the presence of a blood return and absence of swelling, the site should be flushed with saline once more and the intravenous discontinued. Drug administration is resumed at another appropriate site despite the absence of any evidence of extravasation. Mitomycin has been associated with subtle extravasation; therefore, in the presence of any discomfort, the nurse is cautioned to immediately stop the injection, flush copiously with saline, and restart the IV despite the absence of any objective signs of extravasation.

A blood return should be assessed every 1–2 ml of drug administration. The presence of a blood return is valuable to determine venous access but does not always ensure an intact vein. A blood return can be obtained in the presence of an extravasation as the needle may extend partially through the vein, allowing for a subtle leakage of the vesicant into the subcutaneous tissues. In this situation the blood return will be weak instead of full and brisk. On the other hand, the absence of a blood return in no way confirms an extravasation. The needle bevel or cannula tip may upon aspiration become positioned against the vein wall, preventing appropriate and obvious blood return. In this situation the clinician may choose to restart the intravenous or rely on other measures of assessing venous integrity. Often the patient does not have numerous venous access sites from which to choose. While one would always want to spare the patient another needle stick, it is often better to restart the intravenous elsewhere, especially when, after flushing with saline, there remains any doubt of an intact vein.

Rarely, if ever, is the administration of chemotherapy an emergency situation, meaning that if the nurse determines that the patient has no optimal means of safely receiving the vesicant agent, then the nurse should confer with the physician regarding placement of a vascular access device, after which the drug may be administered. In the current milieu of cancer treatment and the variety of short-and long-term vascular access devices available, the nurse should not feel compelled to administer vesicant agents in less than optimally safe circumstances. These devices have become a common method of drug delivery and, depending on the patient's individual treatment plan, may be recommended prior to beginning chemotherapy.

While generally considered a reliable and safe means of drug delivery, implanted ports and, less commonly, tunneled catheters do sometimes result in extravasations of vesicant agents. In the case of implanted ports, the cause of drug extravasation is usually a misplaced or displaced needle. In this situation the drug extravasates into the port pocket or area surrounding the port. Another mechanism for drug extravasation from ports involves retrograde subcutaneous leakage from percutaneously inserted catheters obstructed by a fibrin sheath.[43,44] Extravasation may also occur into the subcutaneous tunnel either from thrombosis and backtracking or from a damaged or fractured central venous catheter. Extravasation may also occur into the intrathoracic cavity as a complication of catheter placement.

Prior to injecting or infusing a vesicant into a tunneled central venous catheter or a nontunneled centrally or peripherally placed central venous catheter (e.g., PICC), examine the exit site for leaks and the insertion site for evidence of swelling or venous thrombosis. Catheter displacement may be evidenced by the appearance of the cuff extruding from the exit site or of the obviously more white segment of catheter at the exit site indicating that the catheter has been pulled or slipped out of place. Observe the insertion site (usually the ipsilateral supraclavicular area) for evidence of swelling during fluid bolus. Any evidence of swelling or subjective complaints by the patient of pain or discomfort during fluid bolus warrants investigation.

The presence of a blood return from an implanted port or a tunneled catheter usually confirms catheter tip placement. However, it is not uncommon for a catheter to be properly placed without evidence of catheter damage, and still have an absent or intermittent blood return. The catheter or port is still safe to use provided it flushes easily without subjective complaints. If, however, the patient complains of discomfort with fluid injection or if the flow demonstrates resistance, becomes sluggish, or does not flow freely with gravity, it is possible that the catheter tip is somehow intermittently obstructed, the catheter has drifted or migrated into a smaller ancillary vein, or it has otherwise become bent or coiled preventing back flow of blood (Figures 15-5 and 15-6). It is important in these situations to determine catheter placement by radiological means. The injection of fluid or chemotherapy should be withheld pending physician examination.

When giving vesicant agents through a port, whether

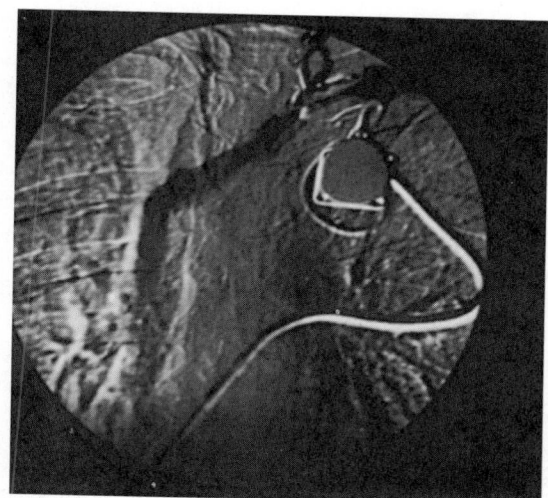

**FIGURE 15-6**   Catheter coiled around port as demonstrated by digital subtraction venogram.

by simple injection or long-term infusion, it is important to use a 90-degree bent huber point needle rather than a straight needle. Straight needles can easily become dislodged because there is no way to stabilize them regardless of how brief the injection time. Patients are instructed to report any pain, burning, tightness, stinging, or discomfort over the chest area during the injection or infusion. When injecting a vesicant, the blood return is assessed before the injection and at the conclusion of the injection. During the short-term or long-term infusion of a vesicant, assessment of blood return is variable depending upon the status of the patient. In some situations where the patient is confused or uncooperative, it is reasonable to question whether it is safe to use a port for long-term vesicant infusions because these needles can become dislodged even under the best of conditions.

It is difficult to determine how frequently a catheter should be aspirated during the infusion of a vesicant in the hospitalized individual to determine the presence or absence of a blood return. If the catheter or port never had a blood return prior to instituting the vesicant infusion, then assessment of the site every hour as one would any intravenous infusion seems appropriate. If a blood return is known to exist, then assessment of blood return will vary from institution to institution, but the beginning of each shift seems appropriate, with hourly visual examination of the infusion/insertion site. More frequent catheter aspiration such as at the beginning and end of each shift or every four hours would appear excessive and could significantly increase risk for infection.

The ideal catheter for infusion of vesicant agents in the outpatient/home environment is the tunneled externally based catheter or PICC line. In some situations where a port is already in place, this device can safely be employed for vesicant infusions provided the patient is capable of regularly assessing the site for proper needle placement.

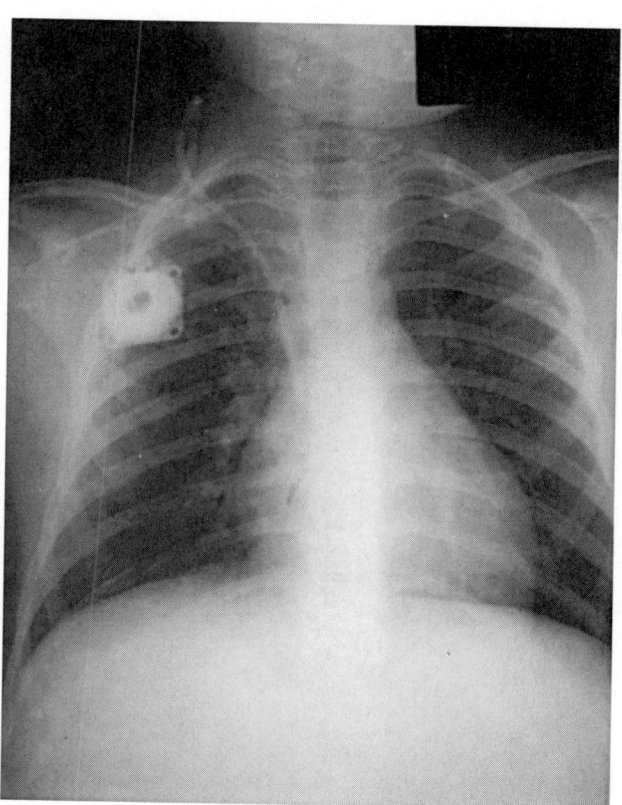

**FIGURE 15-5**   Catheter bent causing resistance during infusion and lack of blood return.

## Management

If a frank extravasation has occurred, it will usually be obvious to patient and nurse at the time it occurs. In some situations, however, the actual symptoms are delayed for 24–48 hours. The patient may report a redness over the injection site that is warm to touch. Most often these delayed symptoms indicate that only a small amount of drug actually infiltrated. Figure 15-7 (Plate 4) depicts a doxorubicin extravasation 12 days after drug administration. There was no pain with movement of the area, which healed spontaneously without local treatment. Figure 15-8 (Plate 5) demonstrates erythema and edema at the injection site one week after doxorubicin administration. At the time of administration, blood return was lost and the patient complained of slight pain at the site. The drug was stopped. After flushing with saline, slight swelling was noted over the area. Ice was applied. This area progressed to blister formation in three weeks with clear demarcation of the damaged area (see Figure 15-9—Plate 6), which was surgically excised (see Figure 15-10—Plate 7).

When there is cause to believe that an extravasation of a vesicant agent has occurred during drug administration, prompt nursing action will, in general, minimize tissue damage. The nurse is responsible for ensuring that all antidotes and diluents are readily available and accessible. The following outlines appropriate steps to be taken if an extravasation is suspected.

1. Stop the administration of the chemotherapeutic agent. If injecting through the side arm of a free-flowing intravenous, stop the fluid flow immediately. Failure to do so further disperses the infiltrated drug into the tissues.
2. Disconnect the intravenous tubing or syringe and attach an empty 10-ml syringe. Attempt to aspirate any residual drug in the tubing and at the site. Stabilize the extremity and tape the syringe in place.
3. If unable to aspirate any blood or residual drug from the tubing, remove the needle. Gentle apply a sterile 2 × 2 gauze pad over the needle entrance site.
4. Prepare the antidote according to institutional policy and procedure (see Table 15-7).[45–47]
5. Replace syringe with antidote-filled syringe and inject the antidote.
6. If the needle has been removed, inject the antidote subcutaneously into the extravasation site using a single injection of a 25-g needle.
7. Remove the needle.
8. Avoid applying direct manual pressure to the site.
9. Photograph the extravasation site prior to applying a loose sterile dressing.
10. Apply a warm compress in the event of a plant alkyloid extravasation 15 minutes or more q.i.d. for 24 hours.
11. Apply ice for 15 minutes or more every three to four hours for 24–48 hours as tolerated in the event of an anthracycline extravasation.
12. Notify the attending physician that an extravasation has occurred or is suspected.
13. Instruct the patient on local care, systemic analgesics, and plan for follow-up.
    a. Elevate the extremity for 48 hours.
    b. After the first 48 hours the patient should be encouraged to use the extremity normally. Failure to do so may result in stiffness, neuropathy, and causalgia.[46]
    c. Arrange for a return appointment once or twice weekly depending on the amount of drug suspected to have extravasated and the patient's individual concerns.

**TABLE 15-7**   Management of Selected Vesicant Extravasations

| Chemotherapeutic Agent | Mechanism of Tissue Damage and Clinical Course | Pharmacologic Antidote | Local Management | Comments |
|---|---|---|---|---|
| Doxorubicin (Adriamycin) | Binds to nucleic acids leading to prolonged tissue damage | None | Apply ice for 15 min every 3–4 hr as tolerated for 24–48 hr | Less extensive (1–2 ml/2 mg/ml) extravasations tend to heal spontaneously |
| | Drug is steadily released from dead or dying cells, thereby causing damage to neighboring cells | | Elevate the extremity for 48 hr Resume normal activities after 48 hr | More extensive (>3 ml) extravasations follow an indolent course, usually causing ulceration, eschar formation, and pain |
| | | | Physical therapy may be appropriate to prevent stiffness and neuralgia | Surgical intervention with skin grafting may be required |
| | | | Topical (1–2 ml) dimethylsulfoxide (99%) applied to the site every 6 hr may be beneficial | |

**TABLE 15-7** Management of Selected Vesicant Extravasations (continued)

| Chemotherapeutic Agent | Mechanism of Tissue Damage and Clinical Course | Pharmacologic Antidote | Local Management | Comments |
|---|---|---|---|---|
| Daunorubicin (Cerubidine, daunomycin) | Binds to nucleic acids leading to prolonged tissue damage. (See doxorubicin.)<br><br>Severe pain may be noted during infusion of the drug<br><br>Cellulitis may occur without extravasation | None | Ice or local cooling has not been beneficial, but may be used to increase comfort<br><br>Heat increases ulceration<br><br>Surgical excision is usually needed to remove necrotic tissue and locally entrapped drug<br><br>Little information is currently available. Extravasations may be managed like doxorubicin extravasation | Topical DMSO 99% may help to minimize ulceration |
| Epirubicin Idarubicin (Idamycin) | Both drugs have vesicant properties similar to doxorubicin | None | Little information is currently available. Extravasations may be managed like doxorubicin extravasation | |
| Mechlorethamine (nitrogen mustard, Mustargen) | Drug rapidly fixes to tissues, causing immediate tissue damage<br><br>Drug is probably not recycled locally<br><br>Immediate, often intense pain is noted if extravasated<br><br>Thrombophlebitis of the injected vein is common<br><br>Perivenous hyperpigmentation may occur following a single injection | Isotonic sodium thiosulfate<br><br>Mix 4 ml 10% sodium thiosulfate with 6 ml sterile $H_2O$<br><br>or<br><br>1.6 ml 25% sodium thiosulfate with 8.4 ml sterile $H_2O$<br><br>Yield 10 ml 1/6 molar solution sodium thiosulfate | Inject 1–4 ml 1/6 molar solution of sodium thiosulfate through existing IV line or subcutaneously if IV has been removed<br><br>Inject 1 ml for each mg extravasated<br><br>Topical cooling may promote comfort but does not appear to minimize ulceration | Sodium thiosulfate neutralizes nitrogen mustard<br><br>Initiate local treatment immediately<br><br>Ensure availability of sodium thiosulfate and sterile water for injection in extravasation kit prior to initiating injection of nitrogen mustard |
| Vincristine (Oncovin) | These agents do not bind to DNA, but inhibit mitosis. | Hyaluronidase (Wydase) (refrigerate) | Inject 1.4 ml through existing IV line or subcutaneously if IV has been removed | Both hyaluronidase and heat act to enhance the systemic absorption from subcutaneous spaces |
| Vinblastine (Velban) | Tissue damage tends to follow a more indolent course | Mix 150 u/ml hyaluronidase with 1 ml of sodium chloride | | |
| Teniposide (Vumon) | | | Administer 1 ml for each ml extravasated | |
| Vindesine (Eldisine) | Pain, localized swelling, and erythema typically occur if these drugs are extravasated | | Apply warm compress 15 min four times a day for 48 hr | Local cooling, vitamin A cream, and hydrocortisone injection significantly increase vinca alkaloid skin ulcers |

(continued)

**TABLE 15-7** Management of Selected Vesicant Extravasations *(continued)*

| Chemotherapeutic Agent | Mechanism of Tissue Damage and Clinical Course | Pharmacologic Antidote | Local Management | Comments |
|---|---|---|---|---|
| Vindesine *(continued)* | | | | Symptoms of vindesine extravasation may be delayed. Ulceration and delayed healing (6 mo) have been noted |
| Vinorelbine (Navelbine) | | | | Vinorelbine may be associated with an intense aching along the injected vein 12–24 hr after the injection, persisting for 3–4 days. Systemic analgesics may be necessary. |
| | | | | To reduce incidence of phlebitis administer vinorelbine over 6–10 minutes into the side-port or a free flowing IV most distant from the patient. |
| Etoposide (Vepesid) | Blister formation may occur within a week of extravasation and gradually resolve without frank ulceration | | | |
| | If ulceration does occur, healing is often prolonged, taking 5–6 mo | | | |
| Mitomycin C (Mutamycin) | Frank and obvious mitomycin C extravasation is associated with intense pain gradually resulting in painful ulceration, necrosis, and eschar formation | None | DMSO may provide some benefit in the treatment of mitomycin C extravasation, but further research is needed | Mitomycin C may cause dermal ulceration at sites distant from injection site |
| | Surgical debridement is usually necessary where significant extravasation has occurred | | Protect from sunlight | Glucocorticoids appear to offer no therapeutic benefit in the treatment of immediate or delayed mitomycin C extravasations, and may even worsen ulceration |
| | Delayed skin ulceration may appear at a previous injection site | | | Neither heating nor cooling has proven therapeutic |
| | Extravasation may occur without any evidence of pain or swelling at the site with delay of ulceration occurring weeks to months later | | | |
| Dactinomycin (Actinomycin D, Cosmegen) | Dactinomycin is a potent intercalating agent that causes intense pain and ulceration if extravasated | None | Ice may be applied to the site to increase comfort | Neither topical cooling nor DMSO is effective local treatment for extravasation of dactinomycin |
| | | | Elevate area for 48 hr Resume normal activities after 48 hr | Heat may significantly enhance tissue damage |
| | | | Consult plastic surgeon if pain persists for >7–10 days | |

d. Photograph the site weekly as appropriate. Document degree of erythema, induration, pain, and whether there is evidence of ulceration or necrosis.

e. If pain persists beyond 7–10 days, confer with physician regarding a plastic surgery consultation, especially if there is evidence of ulcer demarcation.

f. Consider physical therapy consultation to encourage normal use of the extremity during healing.

14. Complete extravasation documentation record (Figure 15-1), paying special attention to subjective complaints and objective observations of the details immediately surrounding the extravasation event.

Paclitaxel and docetaxel are similar antineoplastic agents that are considered to be moderate irritants with the potential to cause ulceration if large amounts of the drug infiltrate. These drugs are routinely infused via peripheral veins, some with the assistance of an infusion pump. In most health care settings vesicants are not administered with the force of a peristaltic infusion pump into a peripheral vein. In the case of these drugs it is important to use caution in the manner in which they are given. There is evidence clinically that both paclitaxel and docetaxel cause a moderate degree of tissue damage when infiltrated and most clinicians consider them to be irritants. Once infiltrated, the amount of tissue damage appears to be related to the amount of concentration of the drug infiltrated.[47] The injection of hyaluronidase (300 units) into the area of infiltration has been recommended.[3] Currently the application of heat to the site of infiltration of either paclitaxel or taxotere is not recommended. Figure 15-11 (Plate 8) depicts a taxotere infiltration. At four weeks the area is peeling and somewhat tender. No ulceration occurred. The clear line of demarcation is the outline of the warm cloth that appeared to aggravate the condition more than help.[48]

Extravasation from a central venous catheter (tunneled, nontunneled, implanted port, or PICC line) may be substantial before detected since infusions are not monitored constantly and the vesicant may be more diluted than when given by intravenous injection. Therefore, pain at the site may not be noted early. Dressings over the port site may mask swelling. Because infusions tend to be given very slowly, a considerable amount of drug can extravasate without obvious evidence of leakage. In the case of an implanted port, the cause is usually needle dislodgment from the port septum, where the needle is found lying in the subcutaneous tissue. The degree of tissue damage will depend on the concentration of the drug and the amount infiltrated. In some cases there may be no tissue breakdown; in others, wide excision including mastectomy may be required for the wound to heal.

If an extravasation is suspected from a central venous catheter, the infusion is immediately stopped and the physician is notified. An attempt should be made to estimate the amount of drug extravasated. It may be possible to aspirate residual drug from the site. An antidote can be administered if available. Otherwise, the needle should be removed. Efforts to manually express fluid from the site should be avoided. Instead, a sterile dressing should be applied over the needle entrance site and changed frequently. Ice or warm packs should be applied per institutional policy and procedure. Appropriate documentation (extravasation documentation record) should be completed, and plans for careful follow-up and additional consultation with a surgeon may be appropriate.

## Intra-arterial

Intra-arterial drug administration, a drug delivery practice that gained popularity in the early 1980s, involves cannulation of the artery that provides a tumor's blood supply and subsequent administration of the drug directly through the arterial catheter to the tumor bed.[53] This practice increases the concentration of the drug to known areas of tumor and decreases the systemic drug concentration and thus the side effects. The primary utilization of this route is the hepatic artery for the management of potential or actual metastasis of colon cancer to the liver. It has also been used for hepatocellular carcinoma. The antineoplastic drugs used include fluorouracil, floxuridine, doxorubicin, and mytomycin C, among others.

The most common method of intra-arterial drug delivery involves placement of a silastic catheter into the main artery supplying the tumor. This catheter is then attached either to an implanted port or a pump (Medtronics or Infusaid pump). The Infusaid pump (Infusaid, Inc., Norwood, MA) and the Synchromed Infusion System (Medtronics, Inc., Minneapolis, MN) are examples of subcutaneously implanted pumps, (see Figures 15-12–15-14). The catheter is inserted into the appropriate artery and then attached to the pump located in a surgically created subcutaneous pocket, usually in the lower abdomen or upper chest. The pump chamber is accessed via a noncoring needle and filled with either chemotherapy or heparinized sterile saline. The flow rates are dependent on pump design and are either preset prior to implantation or adjustable via an external electronic wand that communicates with the internal pump. Obviously,

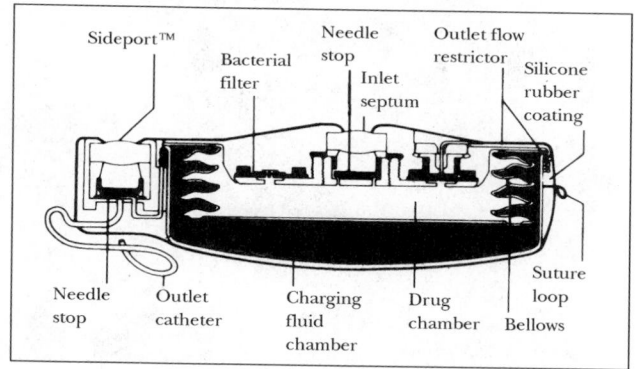

**FIGURE 15-12**  Schematic drawing of Infusaid pump, model 400. (Courtesy of Infusaid, Inc., Norwood, MA)

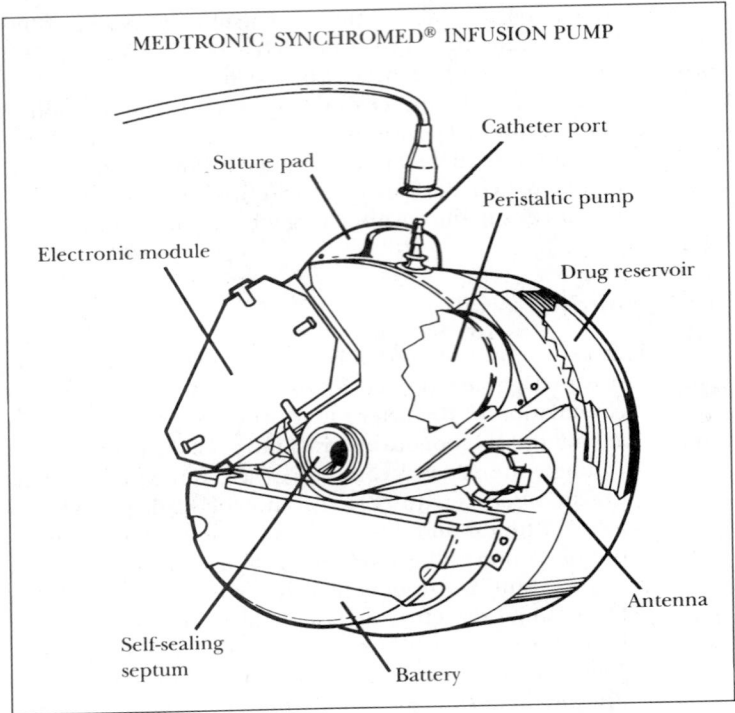

MEDTRONIC SYNCHROMED® INFUSION PUMP

Catheter port
Suture pad
Peristaltic pump
Electronic module
Drug reservoir
Antenna
Self-sealing septum
Battery

**FIGURE 15-13**  Schematic drawing of Synchromed infusion pump. (Courtesy of Medtronic, Inc., Minneapolis, MN)

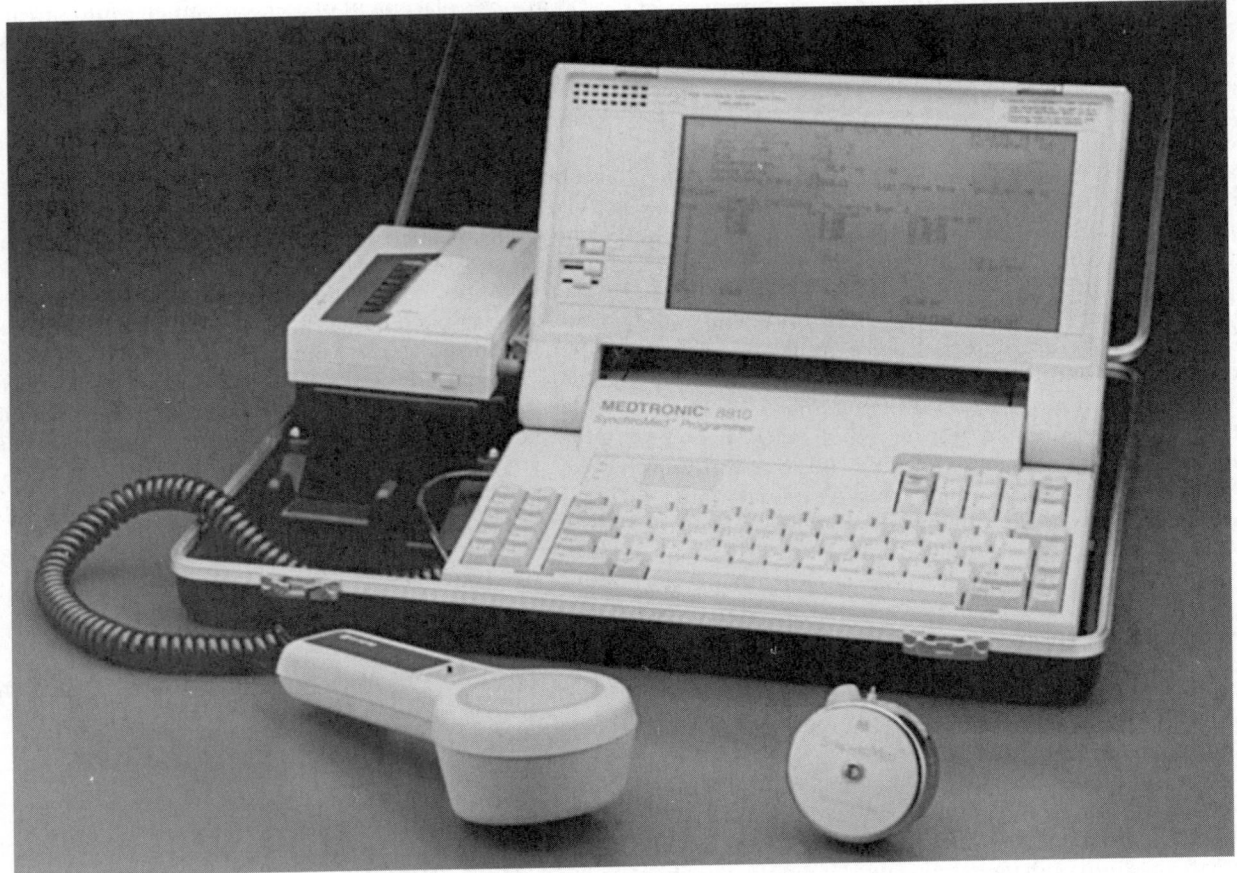

**FIGURE 15-14**  Synchromed infusion system. (Courtesy of Medtronic, Inc., Minneapolis, MN)

care and maintenance of these devices by the nurse requires a formalized educational program and ongoing monitoring of pump functioning.

The implantable pump offers the patient the greatest level of freedom when receiving intra-arterial chemotherapy, and the pumps have lower complication rates than the external methods. One potential disadvantage is the cost; the pump plus the implantation can be very costly and insurance companies under managed care may not agree to pay. When compared to intermittent hospitalization, an ambulatory pump is usually felt to be cost-effective if therapy is anticipated for a minimum of three to six months or longer. In fact, long-term therapy with an external pump can eventually cost more due to the cost of disposable supplies.

Nursing considerations involve monitoring for drug side effects and potential pump complications, such as infection, occlusion, extravasation, and malfunction. Some unique nursing actions are necessary when dealing with implantable pumps, such as not aspirating the center septum, monitoring or establishing pump flow rate, and detecting malfunctions. The oncology nurse is referred to the manufacturers' instructions and guidelines regarding the management of these innovative and advanced nursing responsibilities.

## Intraperitoneal

Regional delivery of chemotherapy into the peritoneal space has been found to be a safe and effective treatment for locally recurrent ovarian and colon cancers. The antineoplastic agents used include cisplatin, carboplatin, etoposide, doxorubicin, and cytarabine, among others.

The semipermeable nature of the peritoneal space allows high concentrations of the drugs to be achieved at the tumor sites throughout the peritoneal space, but with lower concentrations entering the bloodstream. The procedure causes local side effects due to the large volume of fluid filling the space, and the drugs cause systemic side effects that are mild or delayed when compared to intravenous administration of the same drugs. It is possible with some of the drugs to minimize the systemic side effects by simultaneously infusing an agent intravenously to counteract drug side effects through the venous system. This is most commonly achieved during the intraperitoneal instillation of cisplatin by infusing intravenous sodium thiosulfate, which appears to decrease the renal toxicities of the cisplatin.[49]

There are three methods of accessing the peritoneal space: (1) intermittent placement of temporary indwelling catheters; (2) placement of a Tenckhoff external catheter; and (3) placement of an implantable peritoneal port.[50,51] Intermittent placement might be used if the therapy is planned for a short time, such as for symptom relief or palliation. Tenckhoff catheters or ports are placed when several months of therapy are planned, especially when the treatment goal is cure of minimal or microscopic residual disease. Tenckhoff catheters have the advantages of a rapid flow rate (10–15 minutes for 2 liters) and the allowance of catheter manipulation to dislodge fibrin deposits, if necessary. The disadvantages are that they are external, thus requiring care and maintenance by the patient, and possibly resulting in an increased incidence of infection or leakage around the catheter. The advantages of the implanted port are that it is internal and requires no care when not accessed, and has a potentially lower rate of infection. Disadvantages include a slower flow rate (30–45 minutes for 2 liters), a needle stick is required for access, and a surgical procedure is necessary for removal.

Nursing considerations include patient education, assessing the catheter or port patency, establishing access, administering systemic therapies as ordered, instilling the infusate, monitoring patient response to the procedure, draining the infusate (if ordered), side effect management, and documentation as outlined in Table 15-8.

Side effects of the drugs used for intraperitoneal chemotherapy are variable and depend on the agents being administered. Regardless of the drugs administered, complications specific to the intraperitoneal route include respiratory distress, abdominal pain, discomfort, and diarrhea, which are due to increased intra-abdominal pressure. Appropriate interventions to manage these problems include elevation of the head of the bed, instructing the patient to roll from side to side, and administering analgesics. Mechanical difficulties can occur, and include inflow or outflow occlusions caused by fibrin sheath formation over the catheter, other outflow occlusions, and catheter migration. Other complications include infection, chemical irritation of the peritoneal space, electrolyte imbalances, and (with an implantable port) drug extravasation.

In general, intraperitoneal chemotherapy is well tolerated by patients and provides a safe, effective treatment for the management of peritoneal disease, particularly ovarian carcinoma. Patients are frequently able to maintain a normal lifestyle, for this route is successfully utilized in inpatient, ambulatory, and home care settings, with fewer side effects than traditional intravenous therapy.

## Intrapleural

Care of the patient with a pleural effusion traditionally involves insertion of chest tubes, drainage of the fluid, and sclerosis of the pleural space to prevent recurrence of the effusion. When the effusion is caused by malignant cells, the preferred treatment is sclerosis with an antineoplastic agent such as nitrogen mustard or bleomycin.[52] This is accomplished in the usual sterile manner by injecting the drug directly into the chest tube and clamping it for a specified time (e.g., 24 hours). The procedure can be repeated daily for several days if necessary. Nursing management of intrapleural chemotherapy includes

**TABLE 15-8**   Nursing Considerations in Intraperitoneal Drug Administration

| | |
|---|---|
| **Patient Education** | ● Open the clamp on the tubing, and infuse the warmed IP chemotherapy at the prescribed rate (usually over 30 min to several hours). |
| ● Instruct the patient in the care of the catheter or port prior to its insertion. | ● Stop infusion immediately if severe pain is experienced and check for catheter migration (usually with x-ray verification). |

**Patient Education**

● Instruct the patient in the care of the catheter or port prior to its insertion.

● Immediately prior to initiating therapy, explain the drug administration process, side effects of the drugs, side effects of the route, and measures to manage/minimize the side effects.

● Teach the patient and/or family how to care for the catheter at home, if appropriate.

**Pretreatment and Site Access**

● Verify the drug order and normal serum electrolyte levels.

● Insert a urinary catheter to straight drainage, if ordered, and initiate intake and output measurements.

● Ensure that intravenous therapy is proceeding as ordered. (IP cisplatin infusions usually include prehydration for 12–24 hr with IV fluids containing potassium and magnesium supplements. A few moments before initiating the IP cisplatin, IV sodium thiosulfate is begun to neutralize the systemic cisplatin and to prevent renal toxicities and severe nausea and vomiting.)

● Gather appropriate supplies and materials, and wash hands.

● Assess the area around the catheter or port for redness, edema, warmth, or tenderness.

● Organize materials, don gloves (and gown if desired).

● Access external catheter directly after a thorough povidone-iodine scrub of the external hub using aseptic technique, *or*

● Access implanted port using aseptic technique and a large-gauge, noncoring, 90° needle of appropriate length (usually 1–1.5 in.); anesthetize the skin surface prior to access, if desired, with 2% xylocaine, Emla Cream®, or ice.

● Flush the catheter with 10–20 ml of nonbacteriostatic sterile saline; catheter should flush easily.

● Administer antiemetics, if ordered.

**Drug Administration**

● Initiate IV sodium thiosulfate, if ordered.

● Position patient comfortably in a semi-Fowler's position (elevate head of bed).

● Open the clamp on the tubing, and infuse the warmed IP chemotherapy at the prescribed rate (usually over 30 min to several hours).

● Stop infusion immediately if severe pain is experienced and check for catheter migration (usually with x-ray verification).

● Slow the rate of infusion if the patient experiences shortness of breath or discomfort.

● Administer analgesics as prescribed, if necessary.

● Apply blankets if patient feels chilled.

● Close the clamp on the tubing when the infusion is complete, and encourage repositioning from side to side every 15 min during the dwell time (usually 2–4 hr).

● Monitor patient's comfort levels and observe for shortness of breath, abdominal discomfort, or diarrhea.

● After the prescribed dwell time, open the clamp to the drainage bag and allow the solution to drain. If flow is sluggish, check tubing for kinks, help patient roll from side to side, have patient use the Valsalva maneuver, apply manual pressure to the abdomen, or irrigate the catheter with normal saline.

● Recognize that the volume of drained fluid may be less than that infused, and reassure patient that the fluid will be reabsorbed and metabolized.

● Clamp tubing on drainage bag after fluid has drained (usually 30 min to 2 hr), and send specimen, properly labeled as cytotoxic, to cytology or dispose of in proper hazardous waste container.

**Postadministration Care**

● Flush catheter or port with nonbacteriostatic sterile saline; if using a port, follow with heparinized saline.

● Secure site using standard technique (i.e., cap and secure catheter or remove needle from port, and cover site with a small dressing, if necessary).

● Establish IV fluids as prescribed, or discontinue IV needle.

● Assess patient's status; ensure ability to perform self-care, if appropriate.

● Document procedure in medical record.

patient education, safe drug handling, and side effect management. Nitrogen mustard is well known for its emetogenic properties, and treatment with adequate antiemetics is necessary. Also, severe pleural pain can accompany intrapleural nitrogen mustard, and a strong narcotic such as morphine sulfate is frequently ordered as a premedication and for 24–48 hours afterward. Use of a patient-controlled anesthesia (PCA) pump is ideal for patient control of the analgesic agent to ensuring adequate pain control. Bleomycin is not known to cause these symptoms but instead may cause mild nausea or fever and chills, similar to its intravenous side effect profile. In general, nursing care focuses on emesis control, pain control, respiratory status, chest tube secu-

rity, and other comfort measures, depending on the drug utilized.

The process just described is a standard procedure that has been moderately successful for many years. The quest for newer and better forms of sclerosing therapy has led to a variety of alternatives that appear equal to or better than traditional therapy. These include:

1. use of other agents, including methylprednisolone,[53] doxorubicin hydrochloride-containing poly (L-lactic acid) microspheres (ADR-MS),[54] and cisplatin plus cytarabine[55] (all agents being used investigationally by some physicians)

2. insertion of small-bore percutaneously placed cathe-

ters or implantable ports with drainage and subsequent sclerosing instead of large-bore closed-tube thoracostomy.[56,57] (see chapter 30)

3. implantation of pleuroperitoneal shunts[58]

The most noteworthy of these advances is small-bore catheter placement, which is easily accomplished with only mild discomfort and without the major trauma of regular chest tube insertion. Also, for recurrent pleural effusion, thoracentesis can be performed repeatedly via an implantable port, with the catheter portion in the pleural space and the portal on the lower rib cage. Acceptance and clinical utilization of these techniques are variable, and the oncology nurse is encouraged to be aware of the specific procedures used and the established policies describing the nurse's role in administering intrapleural chemotherapy.

## Intravesical

Direct instillation of chemotherapy into the bladder has been proven to be a very effective and simple method of controlling superficial bladder cancer and carcinoma in situ. Agents such as thiotepa, doxorubicin, mitomycin C, and bacillus Calmette-Guerin (BCG) have all been shown to be effective, especially BCG. Instillation is usually weekly for 4–12 weeks and involves insertion of a urinary catheter, instillation of the drug (usually in 50–60 ml of sterile solution), and retention of the drug for one to two hours (with frequent movement to disperse the drug throughout the bladder) prior to unclamping the catheter or voiding. Some physicians prefer to have the urinary catheter remain clamped and in place for the dwell time. In this case, the fluid that drains from the catheter when it is unclamped should be contained and disposed of properly (i.e., sealed, then labeled as cytotoxic waste). If the physician prefers to withdraw the catheter after drug instillation and instructs the patient to void in one to two hours, the patient should flush the toilet twice after voiding. Local side effects such as bladder irritation or, with mitomycin C, dermatitis of the external genitalia can be experienced. A unique side effect of BCG is a "creepy-crawling" feeling sometimes referred to as "BCG-osis."[59,60] Patients report feeling as if their skin is creeping or little things are crawling on them. Administration of a mild sedative can be considered if this side effect occurs.

While initial studies demonstrated an apparent decrease in incidence of recurrence of bladder tumors, this finding has not been corroborated by longer-term studies. Therefore, it appears that the role of intravesical chemotherapy will be as a single postoperative instillation rather than as long-term maintenance therapy.[61]

Nursing considerations for patients receiving intravesical chemotherapy include patient education (stressing hand washing and personal hygiene), drug administration, side effect monitoring, and safe drug handling. For most oncology nurses it is unusual to have experience with this method of drug delivery, since it is commonly performed in urologists' offices as part of a postoperative office visit.

## Intrathecal or Intraventricular

Cancer cells can cross the blood-brain barrier and appear in the cerebrospinal fluid (CSF), resulting in central nervous system involvement of the malignancy. This phenomenon is seen most commonly in leukemia (meningeal leukemia) and to a lesser extent in other malignancies, such as breast cancer, lymphoma, and rhabdomyosarcoma (meningeal carcinomatosis). Unfortunately, available antineoplastic agents are unable to enter the CSF in sufficient concentrations to kill the cancer cells effectively, so chemotherapy is injected directly into the CSF as prophylaxis or to manage existing disease. The antineoplastic drugs used include methotrexate, cytarabine, thiotepa, and interferon. When prepared for use by this route, the preservative-free drug is always admixed under strictly sterile conditions with a preservative-free diluent such as sodium chloride USP (unpreserved) or Ringer's injection USP (unpreserved). Methotrexate is available in an unpreserved lyophilized form for intrathecal use. Cytarabine is supplied with a diluent that contains benzyl alcohol and should be replaced with an appropriate unpreserved diluent (sodium chloride or Ringer's solution).

The two primary methods of instillation are intrathecal and intraventricular. The intrathecal route is achieved by performing a standard lumbar puncture, using established techniques to ascertain placement, and injecting 10–12 ml of drug, followed by withdrawal of the needle. This procedure usually is performed by a physician or a nurse practitioner on a daily to weekly basis, depending on the protocol being followed. This method is quick and easy to perform but is disadvantageous because the drug may reach only epidural or subdural spaces. Even when it reaches the subarachnoid space, therapeutic levels of the drug usually are not achieved in the ventricles. For this reason, many physicians prefer intraventricular drug administration.

Central instillation of the drug into the ventricle can be achieved via an Ommaya reservoir (see Figure 15-15), which is surgically implanted through the cranium. A skin flap is created, and the Ommaya reservoir is placed underneath the skin, with the catheter extending from the reservoir to the ventricle. Once the surgical site has healed, the only visible evidence of the device is a small bump on the head. Placement of this reservoir obviously involves greater risk than performance of a lumbar puncture, but it provides permanent intraventricular access for those patients in whom repeated translumbar puncture is impractical. Ommaya reservoirs are usually accessed by specially trained nurses. The patient is usually in a supine position but can be sitting if that is more comfortable. The site is assessed for tenderness, redness, or warmth. The area above the Ommaya reservoir is prepped in a sterile manner with betadine in a standard circular mo-

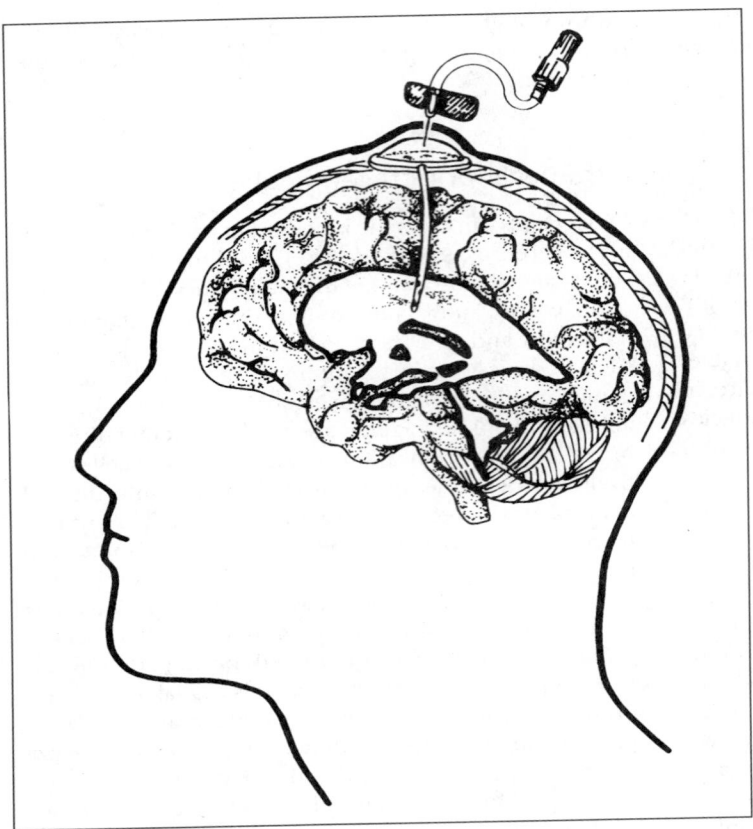

**FIGURE 15-15**    Ommaya reservoir placement.

tion, using three swabs (shaving a small area is desirable). Access is achieved using a small-gauge, noncoring needle (see Figure 15-16). Cerebrospinal fluid, in a volume equal to the amount of drug to be injected, is gently aspirated, and if necessary can be sent for cytology or laboratory studies. The drug is administered slowly, and resistance should not be felt. The reservoir volume is approximately 1.5–2 ml, and the needle usually is flushed with a small volume of nonbacteriostatic saline to clear the drug from the needle prior to its removal. After needle withdrawal, it is common to gently "pump" the reservoir to aid in adequate drug dispersement. The patient frequently will hear a slight whooshing or squishing sound when the reservoir is depressed and then refills. No heparinization or intermittent flushing is necessary, as CSF flows freely through the device. Patients are instructed to rest in a supine position for approximately 30 minutes following the procedure.

Regardless of the specific delivery method, nursing considerations include patient education, assessment of the access site, administration (or assistance with administration) of the drug, safe drug handling, and side effect management. Even though intravenous drugs do not cross the blood-brain barrier in sufficient concentration to treat meningeal disease, the intraventricular drugs are capable of entering the systemic bloodstream. Side effects of the drugs, such as nausea, stomatitis, and mild myelo-

suppression, are to be anticipated. Special care should be taken with methotrexate especially if it is given with another drug such as cytarabine or in conjunction with radiation therapy. Leucovorin may be given orally to prevent unnecessarily severe systemic toxicities. The expected side effects related to intraventricular drug administration include headache, nausea, vomiting, ataxia, blurred vision, and transient paresthesias. The most serious complication for which to observe is infection, which is manifested by tenderness, redness, drainage, warmth or fever, stiff neck, and headache (with or without vomiting). Acute chemical arachnoiditis characterized by headache, back pain, vomiting, fever, and nuchal rigidity has been reported. This reaction appears to be more common in the elderly and in the presence of reduced cerebral glucose and protein metabolism accompanied by altered blood-brain barrier permeability.[62]

## VASCULAR ACCESS DEVICES

The development of central venous catheters (CVCs) and other types of long-term vascular access devices (VADs) has enhanced the lives of oncology patients but added a new series of concerns and challenges for their caregivers.

---

*Description:* The Ommaya reservoir has a catheter that rests in the lateral ventricle. The general uses of the reservoir include:

1. Sample CSF
2. Monitor CSF pressure
3. Administer analgesics into the CSF
4. Administer antibiotics into the CSF
5. Administer chemotherapy into the CSF

*Equipment:* Accessing the Ommaya reservoir is a sterile procedure; assemble all equipment before you begin:

Sterile gloves

Betadine swabs #3

Alcohol wipes #3

Shave/prep kit (optional)

Noncoring (huber point) needle with attached tubing (23-gauge)

Premixed drugs (preservative-free)

Equipment for specimen collection: 3 ml syringes, collection tubes, requisitions

Small dressing or bandaid

Procedure: NOTE: shave area if needed prior to establishing a sterile field

1. Assemble equipment: prepare a sterile field.
2. Position patient in a semi-recumbent position. Support head with pillow.
3. Examine reservoir for any signs of infection. Palpate disc to locate center.
4. Cleanse area over disc in a circular motion with Betadine swabs (x3).
5. Repeat using alcohol.
6. Using a sterile procedure puncture the disc perpendicularly with the needle. Normally, CSF is clear and colorless as it rises into the tubing. Aspirate slightly to collect 2–3 ml of CSF. Set aside to flush the reservoir after drug instillation. Aspirating the CSF from the reservoir is not contraindicated, but should be done gently as it may cause the reservoir catheter to become obstructed. If this occurs, flush to clear and continue collection.
7. Obtain CSF specimens for cytology/microbiology with separate syringes and set aside.
8. Attach syringe of medicine and inject drug slowly over 5–10 minutes. The fluid being injected should be amply diluted to prevent irritation to the meninges (e.g., methotrexate is usually mixed in 12 ml of preservative-free solvent).
9. Follow medicine with 2–3 ml of CSF flush.
10. Remove needle, and apply a small dressing.

**FIGURE 15-16**  Intraventricular Chemotherapy: Use of the Ommaya Reservoir

Device selection, patient selection, use, maintenance, complication management, and product development continue to be refined by practice and research. Use of VADs is not restricted to the cancer population and the oncology nurse often serves as an expert resource to other users of the devices.

There are many different kinds of catheters, needles, and implantable ports used for cancer chemotherapy delivery. Some of the major VAD types and features are outlined in Table 15-9. The nurse has an important role in assessing the patient's vascular access needs and selecting or recommending placement of the proper device. Intermittent peripheral venous access is preferred for patients with good veins, on limited intermittent therapies not involving vesicant infusions. Even multiday infusional therapy can easily be administered through peripheral veins when vascular integrity is good. A VAD should be considered in patients with poor veins, requiring multi-infusional therapy (e.g., the patient with acute leukemia receiving chemotherapy, blood products, antibiotics, and TPN), long-term therapy, or continuous infusion of vesicants.

As with other aspects of chemotherapy administration, education of both the nurse and the patient and family is essential when dealing with vascular access devices. The oncology nurse should be knowledgeable in all aspects of VAD care: selection, placement, postinsertion care, accessing, flushing, site care, troubleshooting, repairing, and removing. There is no universal standard of care for these devices. There is a need for randomized prospective clinical trials to help define the standards of care for VADs. The nurse is urged to be familiar with the particular brands of devices, the manufacturers' recommendations, existing clinical practice trends, and the established policies and procedures of the employing institution.[63,64] Patient and family education is critical, since many devices have self-care aspects that must be considered when selecting the VAD. Any patient having an external device must be able to flush, clean, and care for the device. Consideration should be given to the patient's ability to understand instructions, physical ability to manipulate the catheter, financial ability to purchase supplies, access to a clean area in the home, willingness to perform self-care activities, and compliance in reporting problems. Many excellent booklets and videotapes have been developed by VAD manufacturers and also by hospitals and health care agencies, but their usefulness depends on the nurse's assessment of the patient's ability to understand and comply with the actions described.[65]

## General Management

The selection, care, and maintenance of the long-term devices varies with the type of VAD, and will be addressed separately for nontunneled CVCs, tunneled central venous catheters (TCVCs), and implantable ports. Many of the major complications are handled in similar ways, so the management of complications will be addressed together for all the devices, immediately following this discussion of general management. Most CVCs will be inserted so the catheter tip ends in the superior vena cava, but for those patients for whom this is not possible, a femoral approach with the catheter tip in the inferior vena cava may be an option.

**TABLE 15-9**  Overview of Available Vascular Access Devices

| Type | Description | Longevity | Comments |
|---|---|---|---|
| Peripheral needle<br>  Scalp vein<br>  Butterfly | • Stainless steel<br>• Single lumen<br>• 27–19-gauge | Minutes to days | • Excellent for short-term access, especially outpatient<br>• Increased risk of infiltration with long-term use |
| Peripheral catheter | • Catheter over needle<br>• Teflon or polyurethane<br>• Elastomeric hydrogel, which softens and expands one lumen size after insertion<br>• Single and double lumen<br>• 26–14-gauge | Hours to days | • Excellent for multiday infusional therapy<br>• Provides greater patient mobility since less likely to infiltrate<br>• Elastomeric hydrogel catheter has been known to remain patent and functioning for 1–2 weeks, due to its softer composition |
| Nontunneled central venous catheter | • Polyurethane or silicone catheter<br>• Single, double, and triple lumen | Hours to months | • Excellent for emergency need for CVC<br>• Can augment existing VAD for acute care needs or longer-term use<br>• Inserted by physician at bedside or in procedure room |
| Peripherally inserted central catheters (PICCs) | • Silicone elastomer or other polymers<br>• Single and double lumen<br>• 24–16-gauge | Weeks to months | • Excellent for continuous infusion over several weeks or months<br>• Can be inserted at bedside by specially trained nurse<br>• Quick, easy central access without surgical procedure<br>• Requires external site care and routine flushing |
| Tunneled central venous catheter | • Silicone catheter with Dacron cuff<br>• Single, double, and triple lumen<br>• 4.2–19.2 Fr; 40–90-cm length<br>• Groshong has slit valve, requiring less flushing | Months to years | • Excellent for long-term, continuous, or intermittent therapy<br>• Preferred for long-term TPN administration<br>• Preferred by many for vesicant infusional therapy<br>• Requires external site care and routine flushing |
| Implantable port | • Titanium, stainless steel, silastic, or plastic portal attached to catheter<br>• Single and double lumen<br>• Access with noncoring needle | Months to years | • Excellent for long-term, intermittent infusional therapy<br>• No site care required when not in use so excellent for patients unable to perform site care<br>• Surgical procedure required for removal |
| Peripheral port | • Titanium portal attached to silastic catheter<br>• Single lumen<br>• Access with noncoring needle | Months to years | • Excellent for frequent, intermittent access, particularly for those patients with active lifestyles or body image concerns<br>• No external site care when not in use |

## Nontunneled central venous catheters

Short-term use of a nontunneled CVC, such as a standard subclavian line, is common practice in urgent situations. When an immediate need for a central line arises, it commonly is placed by a physician at the bedside, in the intensive care unit, or in the emergency room. For oncology patients, it is primarily intended to provide immediate access until the emergency can be resolved, or in some practices silastic catheters may be used for months with low infection rates.[66] These devices are also used in oncology patients with the need for multi-infusional therapy beyond the capabilities of an existing tunneled CVC or implantable port. A multilumen subclavian catheter might be placed in a patient with acute leukemia who is on chemotherapy, hydration, antibiotics, TPN, blood products, and other medications or in a patient on a complex investigational drug protocol. The triple-lumen central catheter can augment the long-term device during the hospitalization and be removed prior to discharge, or left in place for outpatient care. The oncology patient may have a CVC in place for apheresis or dialysis. These catheters are usually dedicated to those procedures and care is directed by those departments.

For long-term use, the gap that exists between the trauma of subclavian lines and the investment in a long-term tunneled catheter or port has been narrowed with the use of peripherally inserted central catheters (PICCs).[67] From the patient's viewpoint, the PICC is the least expensive and most easily inserted long-term CVC, but it requires self-care capabilities and often a caregiver, since it is located at the antecubital fossa and self-care has to be one-handed. These small-gauge, thin-walled catheters are inserted at the antecubital fossa into the basilic or cephalic vein (Figure 15-17). The procedure is performed by a physician or a specially trained nurse at the patient's bedside, and the catheter can be advanced into the superior vena cava, in which case x-ray verification of placement is required. A few state boards of nursing consider the placement of a CVC to be outside the role of a professional nurse, so it is important for the nurse to verify that placement of a PICC is within the scope of nursing as defined by the state. Some states allow PICC insertion by a nurse if it is considered a long-line catheter and is only advanced into the axillary or subclavian veins, in which case x-ray verification of placement is not necessarily required but is preferred, especially for vesicant administration. Formal training in the intricacies of PICC insertion is required since the insertion techniques vary greatly among the specific devices and success is usually technique-dependent and due to repeated practice.[66–68]

PICCs are ideal for short-term access (one week to several months) in patients with adequate antecubital veins, self-care capabilities, and the need for a wide variety of intravenous therapies, including antibiotics, chemotherapy, TPN, and analgesics. The thin, flexible nature of the catheter does not lend itself well to blood with-

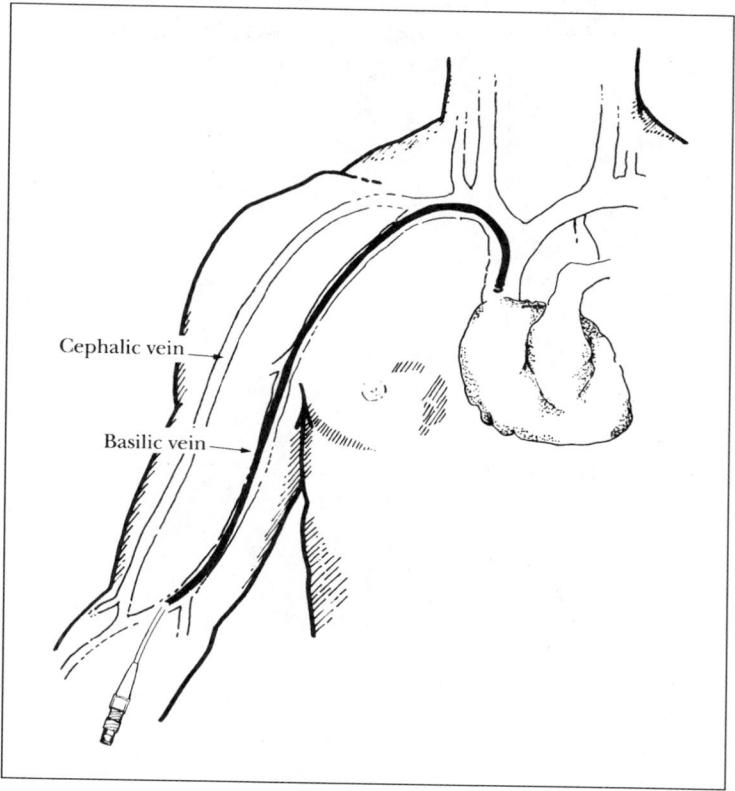

**FIGURE 15-17**   Peripherally inserted central catheter (PICC) placement.

Cephalic vein

Basilic vein

**TABLE 15-10** PICC Overview

**Catheter Features**

- Multiple manufacturers and insertion techniques are available.
- Composed of silicone elastomer or other polymers.
- Available in single- and dual-lumen styles.
- Sizes range from 16–24 gauge and 20–60 cm in length.
- Insertion kits with introducers are available from some manufacturers.
- Cost effective compared to all other VADs.

**Placement**

- Successful placement is highly technique dependent; requires formal training.

- A sterile procedure; at bedside; performed by registered nurse or physician.
- Requires adequate antecubital veins and x-ray verification.

**Use**

- Is excellent for central access for one week to several months.
- Blood withdrawal can be difficult; may be dependent on catheter gauge.
- Requires regular flushing/heparinization.
- Requires sterile dressing.
- Easily removed by registered nurse at bedside.
- Over time, multiple insertions can cause venous scarring and decrease the ability to reuse the site.

drawal, but it is not contraindicated and may be successfully achieved with gentle application of pressure via the syringe used for blood withdrawal. The complication rate is similar to that for other VADs in terms of infection, clotting, and malfunction.[69] Some studies suggest a higher rate of phlebitis, which may be technique-dependent or caused by powdered gloves. Meticulous attention to sterile technique during insertion and rinsing the powder off the gloves prior to handling the PICC seem to decrease these complications. An overview of PICC features is given in Table 15-10.[68]

### Tunneled central venous catheters

The tunneled CVC provides safe and reliable long-term access (months to years) with a low incidence of infection, suitable for almost all hematology/oncology patients and many others as well. TCVCs continue to be well accepted and have been modified by the various manufacturers who now market similar devices. The unique features of the TCVC (see Figure 15-18) include a Dacron cuff around which granulation tissue forms, actually helping to hold the catheter in place. The 4–10-

**FIGURE 15-18** Tunneled central venous catheter placement.

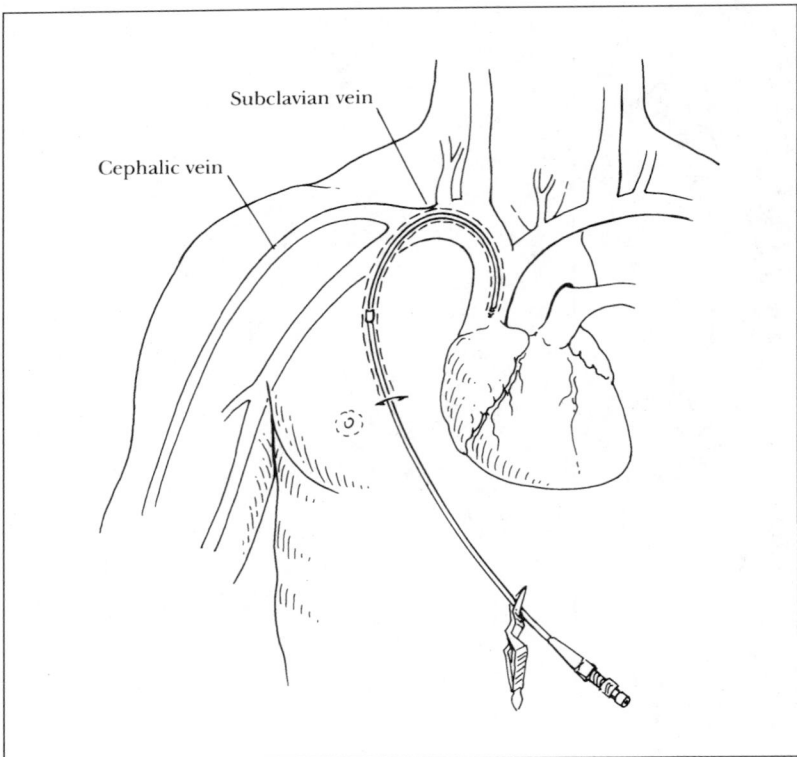

Subclavian vein

Cephalic vein

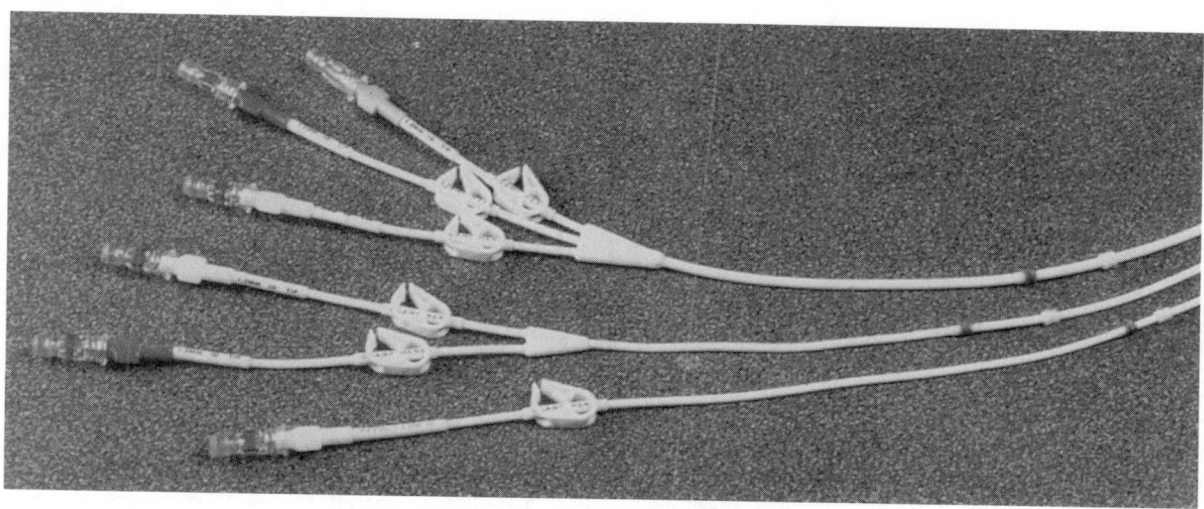

**FIGURE 15-19**  Hickman catheters—single, double, and triple lumen. (Courtesy of Bard Access Systems, Salt Lake City, UT)

inch tunnel through which the catheter is channeled serves to prevent the easy passage of bacteria from the skin into the vein. Also, the cuff is thought to help stop bacteria traveling along the subcutaneous portion of the catheter. A second cuff (VitaCuff) impregnated with silver ions can be attached to any catheter to help decrease the infection rate (see Figure 15-19). The catheter material is usually radiopaque silicone to aid insertion and subsequent placement verification. The external portion of the TCVC has a Luer-Lok hub (to allow direct access with an intravenous infusion set) or placement of a prn/heparin lock adapter (to allow access via a needle or

needleless system). Single-, double-, and triple-lumen TCVCs are available in various gauges and lengths. Areas of development include newer materials and antibiotic bonded catheters.[70]

One unique variation of a TCVC is the Groshong catheter (see Figure 15-20), which features a closed-end radiopaque tip. Flow through the catheter is achieved via a patented slit valve, which opens out into the bloodstream when fluid is infusing into the catheter, opens inward into the catheter lumen when blood is being withdrawn from the catheter, and remains closed when no pressure is being applied. Groshong catheter technology

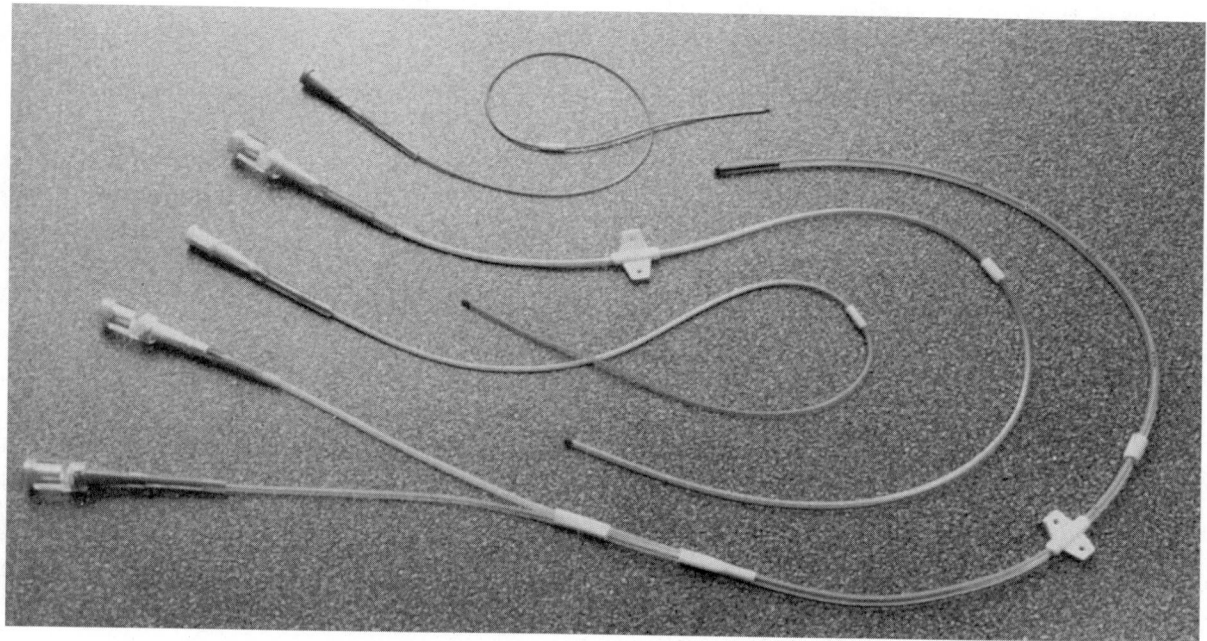

**FIGURE 15-20**  Various Groshong catheters (pediatric, CVC, TCVC, dual-lumen TCVC). (Courtesy of Bard Access Systems, Salt Lake City, UT)

has been applied to the other VADs, and Groshong ports and PICCs are available, as well as the tunneled and nontunneled CVCs. This design prevents the need for regular heparinization of the catheter, which usually is flushed with sterile normal saline (NS) once a week when not in use, making it advantageous in those patients for whom heparin is contraindicated.

Patient selection is a key issue with the TCVC because it requires regular care and maintenance. The patient or significant other must be willing and physically able to clean the exit site, flush the catheter, change the cap, and assess and report complications. The patient must be able to afford the equipment (needles, syringes, heparin or saline, and dressing materials) and must have access to a clean area in the home in which to perform self-care. Body image and patient lifestyle can be issues because of the catheter exit through the chest wall, which can be distressing or embarrassing to some patients, particularly adolescents. Also, whereas swimming in chlorinated pools is allowed by some practitioners, swimming in ponds, rivers, or the ocean usually is not recommended.

There are several major advantages of the TCVC, including its elimination of needle sticks for those people who have a needle phobia, and the ease with which it is removed when no longer needed for care. It also allows for a great deal of flexibility in terms of use, being a preferred device for long-term TPN, vesicant infusion therapy, and continuous infusions. It also is the only long-term device that offers a triple-access option. Finally, it is less expensive in terms of both the device and the insertion costs than an implantable port; however, there is some debate as to the long-term cost effectiveness, since supplies are needed for care and their cost depends on the regimen of care and frequency and type of flushing. An overview of TCVC features is given in Table 15-11.

Despite the common use of TCVCs for over two decades, there is very little standardization of their insertion and care. Insertion is not without risks, and complications include pneumothorax and arterial puncture.[71] A variety of techniques is used for placement, and experienced oncology nurses are beginning to work with physicians and patients prior to insertion to help select a site that is convenient when considering clothing and body contours. Adequate instruction of the patient and family both before and after placement is critical to a successful experience with a TCVC.

When developing policies and procedures governing the use of TCVCs, it is recommended that the following aspects of care be included:

1. Requires sterile site care with dressings until the formation of granulation tissue and verification of normal absolute neutrophil counts, at which time site care involves bathing the chest wall and securing the catheter with tape to prevent dislodgment.
2. When not in use, requires daily, every other day, or even weekly flushing with 3–5 ml of heparinized saline (10 u/ml).

## TABLE 15-11 Tunneled Central Venous Catheter Overview

**Catheter Features**
- Multiple manufacturers.
- Composed of silicone or polyurethane with Dacron cuff.
- Available as single-, double-, and triple-lumen catheters.
- Sizes range from 4.2–19.2 Fr and 40–90 cm in length.
- Inner diameter ranges from 0.7–1.6 mm, with a priming volume of 0.3–2.5 ml.
- Insertion kits with introducers are available from all manufacturers.
- Cost-effective, especially with percutaneous insertion (eliminates operating room cost).

**Placement**
- Technique-dependent; training or observation of the technique is strongly encouraged.
- A sterile procedure, performed by physician, usually in operating room, although some can be inserted percutaneously at the bedside or in a radiology suite.
- Exit site on the nondominant side should be preselected by the nurse, with the patient erect and clothed to prevent placement at an inappropriate site (e.g., under the breast).
- Groshong catheters require a reverse tunneling technique and cannot be trimmed at the proximal end.
- Can be placed through numerous veins, including the jugular, cephalic, and subclavian veins for catheter tip placement in superior vena cava. Occasionally inguinal approach for tip placement in inferior vena cava is necessary.
- Frequently placed under fluoroscopy; x-ray verification of placement is required.
- Suture should be placed at exit site to retain proper catheter placement until granulation occurs around the cuff (usually within 2 wk), and then the suture should be removed.

**Use**
- Excellent for long-term access for several months to years.
- Preferred for TPN, vesicants, and continuous infusions.
- Requires regular flushing/heparinization (daily to weekly).
- Groshong requires weekly flushing with sterile NS when not in use.
- Requires exit site care.
- Blood withdrawal is easy; can use vacutainer technique.
- Usually removed by physician.

**Differences with nontunneled CVCs**
- Do not have Dacron cuffs.
- Insertion may take place at bedside or in procedure room.
- Nylon sutures remain in place for duration of catheter life.
- May be used for days to months.
- Easily removed by nurse or physician at bedside.

3. Allows blood withdrawal for all laboratory tests (except coagulation studies), which can be achieved via vacutainer technique, if desired; vacutainer technique is preferred, since it minimizes the risk of accidental needle sticks.

4. Whenever blood has been aspirated into the catheter, it is flushed with 20 ml of saline prior to hep-locking or resuming an infusion.

5. Must avoid intraluminal mixing of potentially incompatible drugs, which can be achieved by flushing with plain fluid between each drug.

6. Must avoid scissors, sharp objects, and needles longer than 1 inch.

7. Access is either direct or via prn/heparin lock adaptor cap; all connections must be Luer-Loked.

8. Continuous infusions should be directly connected to the catheter hub.

Perhaps one reason there is so much variation in technique among states, settings, and facilities is because it may not really matter that much which type of dressing is used or how often and with what the catheter is flushed. Several small studies regarding dressings have suggested equivocal results. One study showed a slight increased risk of infection with transparent vs. gauze dressings, while the other showed no statistically significant difference between transparent, gauze, or no dressing.[72,73] Similarly, Kelley et al[74] analyzed existing data regarding flushing regimens, conducted a three-year study, and concluded that weekly flushing with 100 units heparin/ml was safe and effective for 86.5% of study participants. Another group, routinely flushing with sterile saline weekly in pediatric patients, reported that the most striking finding of the study was the fact that the majority of infections occurred during the summer months, when children might be expected to be outside playing and swimming and are perhaps at high risk for infection.[75] Interpretation of these findings and resolution of some of these issues will continue to require assessment, documentation, and reporting of research study results.

One unique care issue related to TCVCs is fracture, puncture, or cutting of the external portion of the catheter. Puncture can be prevented by not using scissors or sharp objects near the catheter and limiting needles used for access to 1 inch in length or by using needleless systems. It is also advisable to avoid clamping the catheter continuously or, if a clamp is used, padding and rotating the clamp site. As long as at least 2 inches of undamaged catheter exits the skin, it can be repaired using a repair kit available from the manufacturer. Most repair kits are designed only for a specific catheter, especially the double- and triple-lumen repair kits when the break is in the main portion of the catheter. Emergency repairs to a single-lumen can be conducted via the following steps:

1. Clamp catheter close to chest wall.
2. Clean catheter with alcohol at the most distal undamaged point.
3. Using sterile scissors, cut the catheter.
4. Remove the inner metal stylus from a 14-g or 16-g peripheral IV catheter, and insert the IV catheter into the TCVC until the cut edge touches the hub.
5. Secure with tape or suture.
6. Apply heparin lock adapter cap, unclamp, and gently flush catheter; heparinize or use in the normal manner.
7. Obtain a repair kit as soon as possible for permanent repair.

One major advantage of the TCVC is the ease with which it is removed by the physician when no longer needed or desired by the patient. Prior to withdrawal of the catheter, some catheter manufacturers suggest a very short surgical incision, under local anesthesia, to mechanically release the Dacron cuff from the subcutaneous tissue. If the cuff is not removed with the catheter it may become infected later. Catheter removal is achieved by cleaning the exit site and manually pulling on the catheter until it loosens in the tunnel. Pressure is then applied manually over the entrance site into the vein and maintained for several minutes after catheter removal. Steady, slow pressure is applied while pulling on the catheter until the entire catheter is removed and inspected to ensure that it is intact, since breakage or splintering can occur. The exit site is dressed with a small dressing, if necessary.

## Implantable ports

The implantable port has proven to be a unique development in vascular access devices because when it is not in use, it requires almost no care or maintenance (see Figures 15-21 and 15-22). A *port* is a hollow housing of

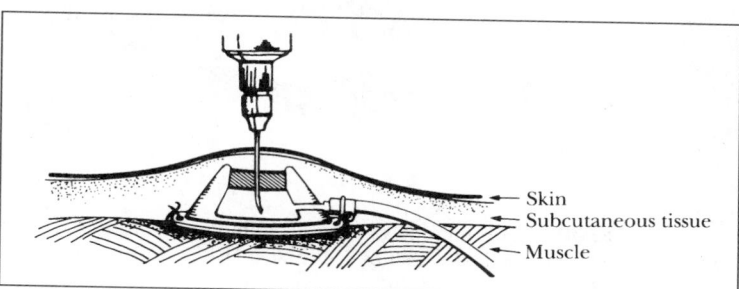

Skin
Subcutaneous tissue
Muscle

**FIGURE 15-21** Schematic drawing of an implantable port.

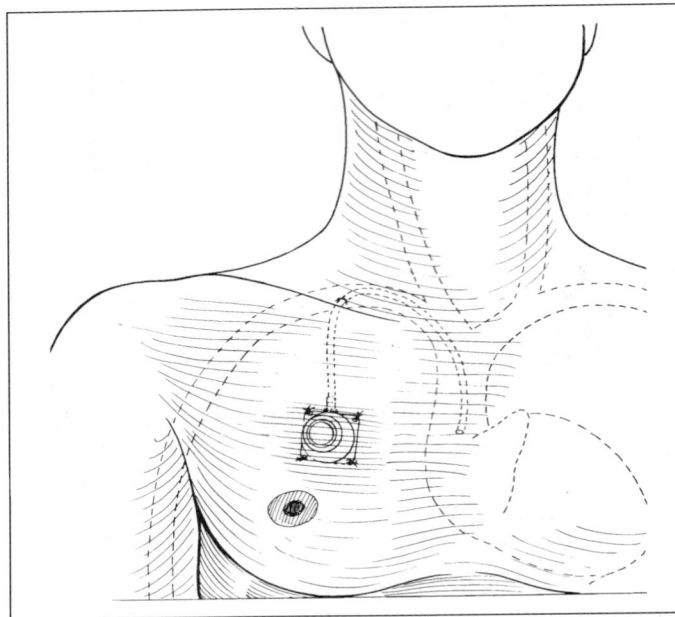

**FIGURE 15-22**  Venous port placement. (© 1990 Pharmacia Deltec, Inc. Courtesy of Pharmacia Deltec, Inc., St. Paul, MN)

stainless steel, titanium, or plastic containing a compressed latex septum over a portal chamber connected via a small tube to a silicone or polyurethane catheter that is inserted into a blood vessel (see Figures 15-23 and 15-24). It is placed subcutaneously and accessed percutaneously using a special noncoring needle. The needle has an offset bevel, which prevents coring the septum and allows 1000–3600 punctures per port, depending on manufacturer and needle size. The plastic and titanium ports are advantageous because they cause little if any disturbance on x-ray film during imaging procedures. Ports are available with: (1) the catheter permanently

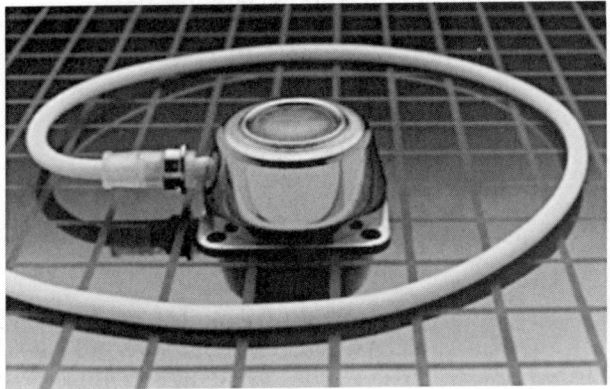

(a)

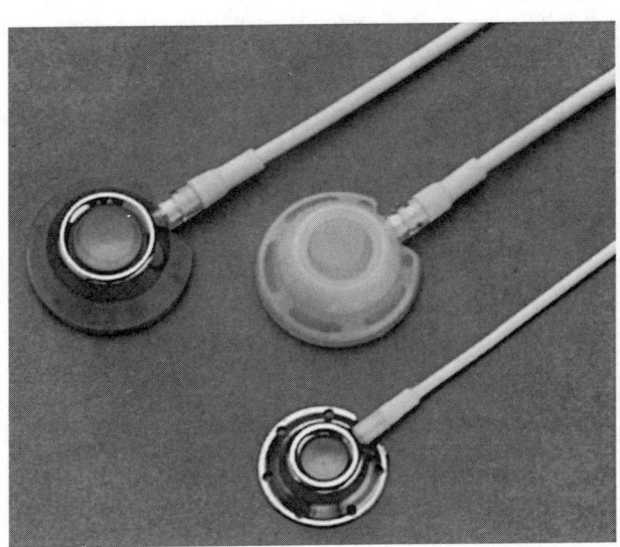

**FIGURE 15-23**  Various implantable port designs. (Courtesy of Bard Access Systems, Salt Lake City, UT)

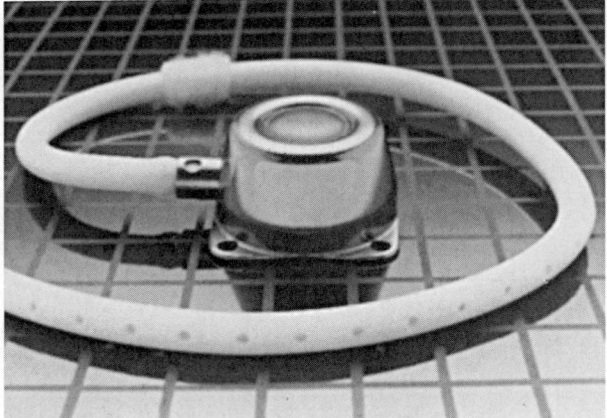

(b)

**FIGURE 15-24**  Port-a-Cath implantable ports. (a) venous; (b) peritoneal. (© 1990 by Pharmacia Deltec, Inc. Courtesy of Pharmacia Deltec, Inc., St. Paul, MN)

attached to the portal housing, in which case the surgeon adjusts the length by trimming the distal portion of the catheter prior to insertion, or (2) the catheter separate from the portal housing, in which case the surgeon trims the proximal end prior to attaching and securing it to the portal during the implantation procedure. They are available in single and double designs, with the double port having two distinct portal chambers to allow simultaneous administration of separate solutions. Most ports are accessed through the top. A portal design that provides access via the side, allowing the needle to be positioned parallel to the skin, is available but is not commonly used by practitioners today. An overview of port features is given in Table 15-12.

*Port routes* There are five major types of ports: venous, arterial, peritoneal, intrapleural, and epidural. The unique portal design allows access to more than just the vascular system. While the portal housings are all essentially the same, the catheters are designed, located, and cared for differently. The arterial and epidural ports have specially designed catheters with very small lumens, since the flow rate through these devices is often as low as 2–3 ml per day. At the opposite end of the spectrum is the peritoneal catheter, which has a very large lumen and multiple fluid outlet holes in the catheter to allow rapid infusion of fluids. The venous ports have varying-sized lumens and flow rates. Placement of these ports, illustrated in Figure 15-25, is usually over a bony structure in the left or right upper chest, lower chest, or lower abdomen. Usually, venous ports are placed in the upper chest area. Arterial ports can be placed in any of the sites. Peritoneal ports are consistently placed on the lower rib cage, but could be on the lower abdomen. Epidural ports could be at either of the lower positions. Unfortunately, there is no standardized placement of the different types of ports, which creates major problems for the nurse unfamiliar with a new patient. It is imperative that the type of device and its purpose be determined prior to access of the port. It is not common, but it is important to remember that ports can be located in other areas of the body. Most patients are given an identifying wallet card and information regarding their ports. If that information is unavailable and the patient is unsure of the device type, then the health care professional must seek the operative note in the hospital chart to confirm device type and catheter route.

Nursing issues related to arterial, peritoneal, epidural, and intrapleural ports are summarized in Table 15-13 and have been discussed in some detail in the previous portion of this chapter dealing with routes of drug administration.

*Port usage* The routine care of the venous port when not being used is to flush it once every three to four months with sterile heparinized saline (usually 5 ml of 100 unit/ml solution). It is an ideal choice for patients who are unable or unwilling to care properly for an external device, receiving intermittent therapies, concerned

## TABLE 15-12 Port Overview

### Port Features

- Multiple manufacturers available.
- Composed of stainless steel, titanium, or plastic, with catheter of silicone or polyurethane.
- Available with preattached or attachable catheters in single and double designs.
- Can be accessed with a noncoring needle, usually through the top; side-access model is available.
- Types include: venous, arterial, peritoneal, intrapleural, and epidural.
- Venous variations include central and peripheral insertion techniques.
- Available in pediatric and low-profile styles.
- Insertion kits with introducers are available from all manufacturers.
- Expensive, both in terms of port cost and implantation procedure.
- Possibly the least expensive of all VADs for routine care and maintenance.

### Placement

- Technique-dependent; training or observation of the technique is required.
- A sterile procedure, performed by surgeon in operating room.
- Exit site on the nondominant side should be preselected by the nurse, with the patient erect and clothed to prevent placement at an inappropriate site (e.g., under the breast, in the breast, or under the arm).
- Groshong port catheters cannot be trimmed at the proximal end.
- Frequently placed with fluoroscopy; x-ray verification of placement required.
- Suture line should not be over the top of the port.
- Port should be accessed with an infusion set and a dressing applied prior to leaving the operating room if it is to be used immediately; some practitioners prefer to wait 14 days prior to use to allow postoperative edema to resolve and wound to heal.

### Use

- Can remain in place and functional for many years.
- Ideal for intermittent therapies.
- Must be accessed using noncoring needle.
- Ice or a local anesthetic can be used to decrease discomfort prior to accessing.
- When not in use, must be flushed every 4–6 weeks (usually with 3–5 ml of sterile 100 u/ml heparinized saline).
- For continuous access, site care is provided and needle is changed per established policy (usually every 7 days or prn).
- Blood withdrawal is easy; can use vacutainer technique.
- Removal requires surgical procedure.

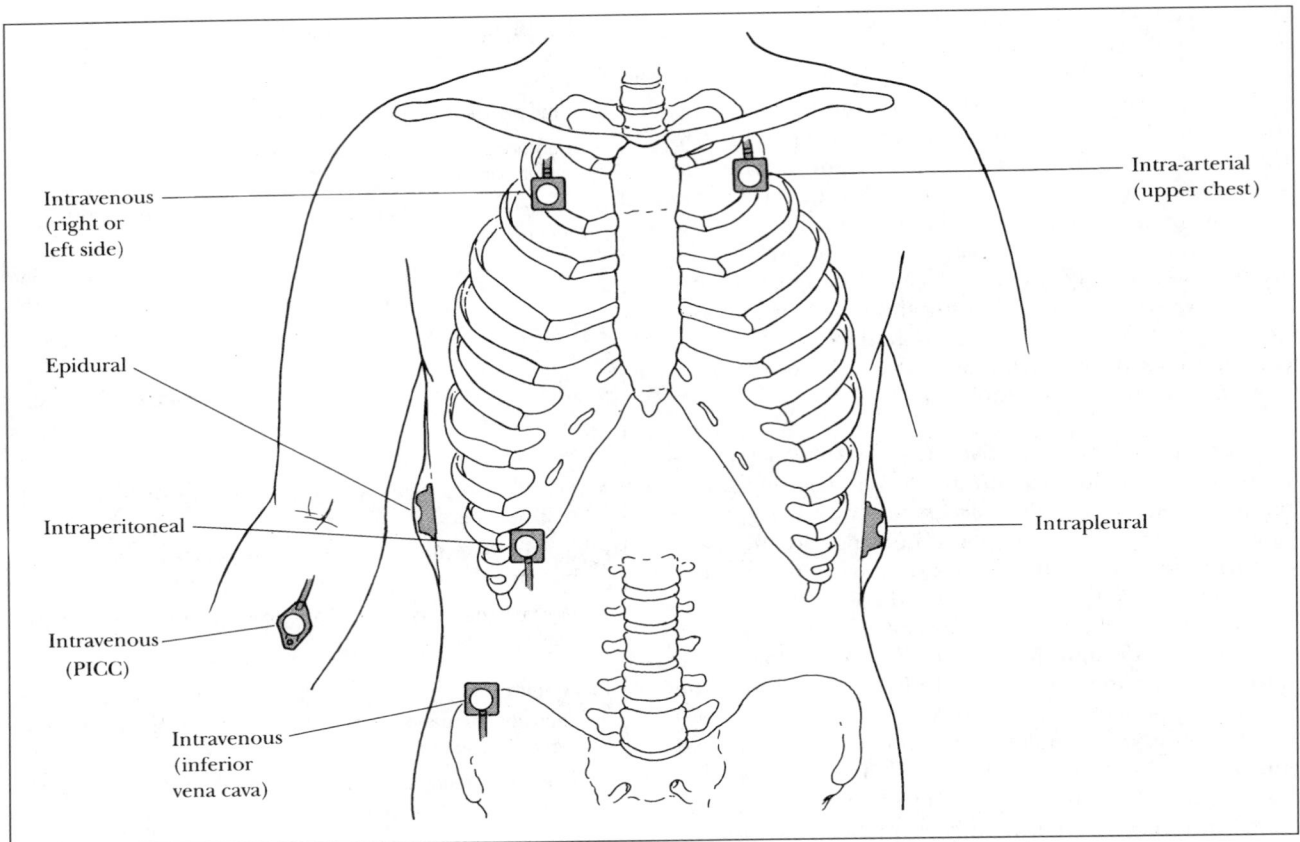

**FIGURE 15-25** Implantable port placement sites.

about body image, or physically active (especially if swimming in unchlorinated bodies of water). Its major disadvantage is that it requires a needle to pass through the skin and into the port for usage. The procedure of accessing the port could introduce infective organisms, cause a hematoma in a thrombocytopenic patient, cause anxiety in a patient with a needle phobia, or result in extravasation of fluid around the port if performed incorrectly or if the needle subsequently becomes dislodged. There is also a very remote chance that the device could extrude through the skin.

Nursing management of ports involves assessing the site, accessing the device, infusing or withdrawing fluids, and flushing. The nurse should help select the portal site prior to implantation. With the patient erect and clothed, the nondominant side should be examined for a convenient location. Ideally, the port can be located over a rib in an area easy for the patient to visualize for care but not visible when clothed. Consideration should be given to clothing, brassiere straps, lifestyle (e.g., frequent holding of a telephone receiver between the head and chest), and physical activities (e.g., swimming). Thin patients may need low-profile ports; obese patients may need large ports. Also, in obese patients or large-breasted women, placement of the port near the sternum provides better needle stability and ease of access. Care should be taken

to avoid placement of the port under the arm, under the breast, in the breast, or in the soft tissue of the abdomen (for nonvenous ports). The preferred site and an alternate should be marked on the skin as a reference for the surgeon. It is also helpful if the surgeon offsets the port pocket so that the suture line is 1–2 inches away from the top of the port.

Port access usually is achieved under sterile or aseptic technique after a betadine scrub using noncoring needles that can be either straight or bent at a 90° angle. The needle penetrates the septum and is advanced until it touches the bottom of the portal chamber. The most popular access needles are actually infusion sets consisting of needle, tubing, Luer-Lok hub, and containing a Y-site and a clamp. These infusion sets allow great flexibility and multiple access sites and can be left in place for up to seven days. For long-term access, a sterile dressing (usually transparent) is placed over the site and assessed on a daily basis. Redness, rash, or blistering of the skin around the port could be indicative of an allergic reaction to the tape or dressing, and is resolved by using an alternative type of tape, dressing, or skin disinfecting agent.

There are several other aspects of port accessing that are especially important to the patient. The area is tender and edematous for a week or so after implantation, causing manipulation of the device to be uncomfortable or

**TABLE 15-13**  Unique Types of Implantable Ports

**Arterial**

- Used to administer continuous or intermittent intra-arterial chemotherapy.

- Catheter is placed into an artery, and port is usually placed on the lower rib cage.

- Accessed and managed in the usual manner, except heparinization procedure may be different, with increased frequency (i.e., weekly) or higher concentrations of heparin (100–1000 u/ml).

- Catheter has a small lumen and seems to form clots more easily than venous catheters; hence the need for at least weekly flushing.

**Peritoneal**

- Used to administer intermittent intraperitoneal chemotherapy for ovarian or colon cancer.

- Catheter is placed in the peritoneal space, and port is usually placed on the lower rib cage but can be in the lower abdominal area.

- Accessed and managed in the usual sterile manner except 19-gauge noncoring needles are used to facilitate large-volume infusions; the portal is flushed after use with sterile saline, and heparinization usually is not required.

- Catheter has a very large lumen with several ridges or cuffs to secure placement and multiple exit holes in the distal portion for rapid fluid infusion.

**Epidural**

- Used to administer intrathecal or epidural medications, including chemotherapy and analgesics.

- Catheter is placed into the intrathecal or epidural space and tunneled through a long subcutaneous passage from the spinal area to the side of the abdomen, where the port is placed on the lower rib cage or the abdominal area. The portal is designed with a 60-micron screen filter to remove particulate matter.

- Accessed using special 24-gauge noncoring needles, *always* with meticulous sterile technique, including sterile gloves, prep drape, and procedure tray.

- **Never to be flushed with heparin.**

- Preservative-free chemotherapy or morphine is instilled or infused into the port.

- After usage, 1–2 ml of sterile, preservative-free saline may be used to flush the line.

- Catheter has a small lumen (0.5-mm inner diameter), which is suitable for this type of drug delivery.

**Intrapleural**

- Used to drain pleural effusions periodically in patients who are unresponsive to sclerosing.

- Accessed with noncoring needle only.

- Patient's position is changed frequently during "tap."

- Flushed with 3 ml of saline. (See chapter 30.)

even painful. Some practitioners prefer to wait until the site has healed and the edema is gone before using the port. When immediate use is indicated, the port should be accessed and dressed securely in the operating room. For routine use once the site is healed, the needle stick usually is not a concern to most patients and causes little discomfort. An occasional patient will have a needle phobia or experience pain during insertion. Effective options to increase patient comfort include application of a small ice pack to the area for a few minutes or application of a topical anesthetic agent to numb the area before accessing. Most patients prefer to have the site anesthetized prior to access with application of a topical anesthetic such as ethyl chloride or Emla Cream®.

All types of medications and fluids can be administered through venous ports, but some problems have been noted with TPN, which can cause drug crystals or sludge to build up inside the portal housing and occlude the device. As with TCVCs, blood withdrawal can be accomplished for all laboratory studies except those involving coagulation, and the vacutainer technique can be utilized. There is a concern when administering continuous-infusion vesicants because the needle could become dislodged from the septum and remain under the skin, causing a port pocket extravasation. For this reason, vesicant infusions are monitored frequently (every 1–2 hours), and some practitioners prefer that PICCs or TCVCs be placed instead of ports if it is known in advance that this type of therapy may be necessary.

As with other VADs, the nurse must know and assess for the signs and symptoms of complications with utilization of the device. The port should have a brisk blood return, easy flow of fluids, and there should be no edema, redness, or pain in the surrounding tissues. If any problems are noted, measures should be taken to resolve them; if necessary, verification of the patency of the port should be ascertained using x-ray film, venogram, or contrast study (cathetergram).

***Peripheral implantable port***  A variation of the venous port that combines the properties of a PICC and a port is the peripherally inserted port.[76] The P.A.S.-Port (Peripheral Access System, Pharmacia Deltec, Inc., Minneapolis, MN) allows the peripheral insertion of a port near the antecubital fossa. Insertion and proper placement are achieved using an electronic device that enables insertion at the bedside or in the physician's office. The P.A.S.-Port is about half the size of a regular port and allows patients to experience the advantages of port placement (unobtrusive, long-term access, intermittent use) without having to expose the chest area to achieve access. Access is achieved through a very short (0.5-inch) noncoring needle or infusion set. In all other aspects except placement, it is managed like other implantable venous ports.

## Complication Management

Occlusions, infections, and other complications can occur with all of the long-term vascular access devices.

The incidence and type of complication depend on the device, insertion technique, care regimen, and to a great extent physiological factors inherent in the introduction of a long-term catheter into the venous system.[77–80]

## Intraluminal catheter occlusion

The complete inability to withdraw blood or infuse fluid in a VAD is most commonly the result of a blood clot within the catheter. It can also be caused by incompatible drugs or lipids that have crystallized or precipitated and have obstructed the catheter. The nurse is instrumental in assessing the catheter and its most recent usage to determine which of these causes are most likely to have occurred. Blood clots can build up over time (i.e., sluggish catheter) but can also appear suddenly. Drug precipitates tend to be more directly related to a recent infusion and are seen more often with TPN and lipids.[81] Measures to prevent either occurrence include the following:[71,82–84]

1. Maintain positive pressure within the catheter and vigorously flush the catheter provided there is no resistance. If there is intermittent resistance it may mean that the catheter is being pinched off at the level of the clavicle and first rib. Vigorously flushing in this situation can cause an aneurysm in the catheter.
2. Advise patient to avoid excessive manipulation (i.e., pinching or bending) of external catheters.
3. Vigorously flush with at least 20 ml of sterile NS after any blood has gotten into the catheter. This helps to prevent sludge build-up within the ports.
4. Document each patient's VAD experience, and adjust concentration, volume, and frequency of heparinized flush, as needed.
5. Question patient and family regarding actual catheter maintenance activities to assess compliance with recommended care and usage.
6. Flush between each drug with at least 10 ml of plain IV fluid to avoid incompatible drug admixture.
7. Vigorously flush catheter every 8–12 hours when administering TPN or lipids.
8. Do not administer IV fluid or TPN containing visible precipitates (which is more likely to occur if the solution is more than 24 hours old).

In the case of ports, the inability to infuse or aspirate usually is due to the needles being improperly placed in the septum rather than the portal. Advancing the needle into the portal usually will solve the problem.

Management of an occluded catheter when a blood clot is suspected involves the instillation of urokinase which is almost universally successful. A dose of urokinase 5000 units in 1–3 ml is instilled using a 3-ml or larger syringe and a gentle to-and-fro motion. The catheter is then clamped for 30 minutes or longer after which an attempt is made to aspirate the catheter contents. If successful, the catheter is flushed and used; if unsuccessful the procedure is repeated. If a second instillation of urokinase is unsuccessful, a variety of options exist. Some success has been obtained with a 24 "lock" of urokinase,

while continuous infusions of urokinase for 4–24 hours have also been reported to clear occluded catheters successfully.[85] Certain drug precipitates can be cleared using 0.1N hydrochloric acid for some crystals or ethanol 70% for lipid deposits.[86–89] The process is similar to that used for urokinase, with the gentle instillation of 0.2–1 ml of drug. After a dwell time of 30–60 minutes, an attempt is made to aspirate the catheter contents. If TPN is not involved and a specific drug is known or suspected, a pharmacist should be consulted about possible agents that might dissolve the precipitate and enable it to be aspirated from the catheter. Figure 15-26 describes a possible decision-making matrix to consider when dealing with a completely occluded catheter.

## Extraluminal catheter occlusion

Catheter sluggishness or partial occlusion can be due to two extraluminal phenomena: fibrin sheath formation and thrombosis. The catheter position can also affect flow, so a partial occlusion, in the absence of pain or discomfort, should first be managed by instructing the patient to change positions, raise the arms, deep breathe, and/or cough (Figure 15-27). Each of these might release the open lumen of the catheter from the vein wall and allow easy flushing and blood withdrawal. If a withdrawal occlusion exists (flushes easily but backflow is very sluggish or nonexistent), fibrin sheath formation or thrombosis should be considered. Fibrin sheaths can form at the catheter insertion site and float, like a sleeve, around the outside of the catheter. If the sheath extends beyond the lumen, it can cause withdrawal occlusions. Lysis of the sheath may be achieved by instilling urokinase 5000–10,000 units into the catheter with an extended dwell time of 1–24 hours.[83]

Venous thrombosis can be caused by a variety of factors, including endothelial injury, hypercoagulability, multiple catheters, catheter stiffness (i.e., polyvinyl chloride), catheter size (i.e., larger bore), and catheter placement (i.e., left side or in a smaller vein). The incidence of catheter thrombosis with clinical symptoms appears to be as high as 10%. Actual incidence in the absence of clinical symptoms could be as high as 50%.[90] Signs and symptoms are related to impaired blood flow and include: edema of the neck, face, shoulder, or arm; prominent superficial veins; neck pain; tingling of the neck, shoulder, or arm; and skin color or temperature changes. A variety of radiographic studies can be used to diagnose and define the extent of the thrombosis accurately.

Management of venous thrombosis usually involves anticoagulants or thrombolytic agents. Several authors report success with the continuous infusion, centrally and/or peripherally, of urokinase for 4–24 hours.[91] It is recommended that all lumens of a multilumenal device be treated. The serum fibrinogen level should be maintained at 80–100 mg/dl by titration of the urokinase.[91] The success of this treatment may be related to a short period of symptoms prior to the infusion. Prophylactic administration of low-dose warfarin (1 mg/day) appears

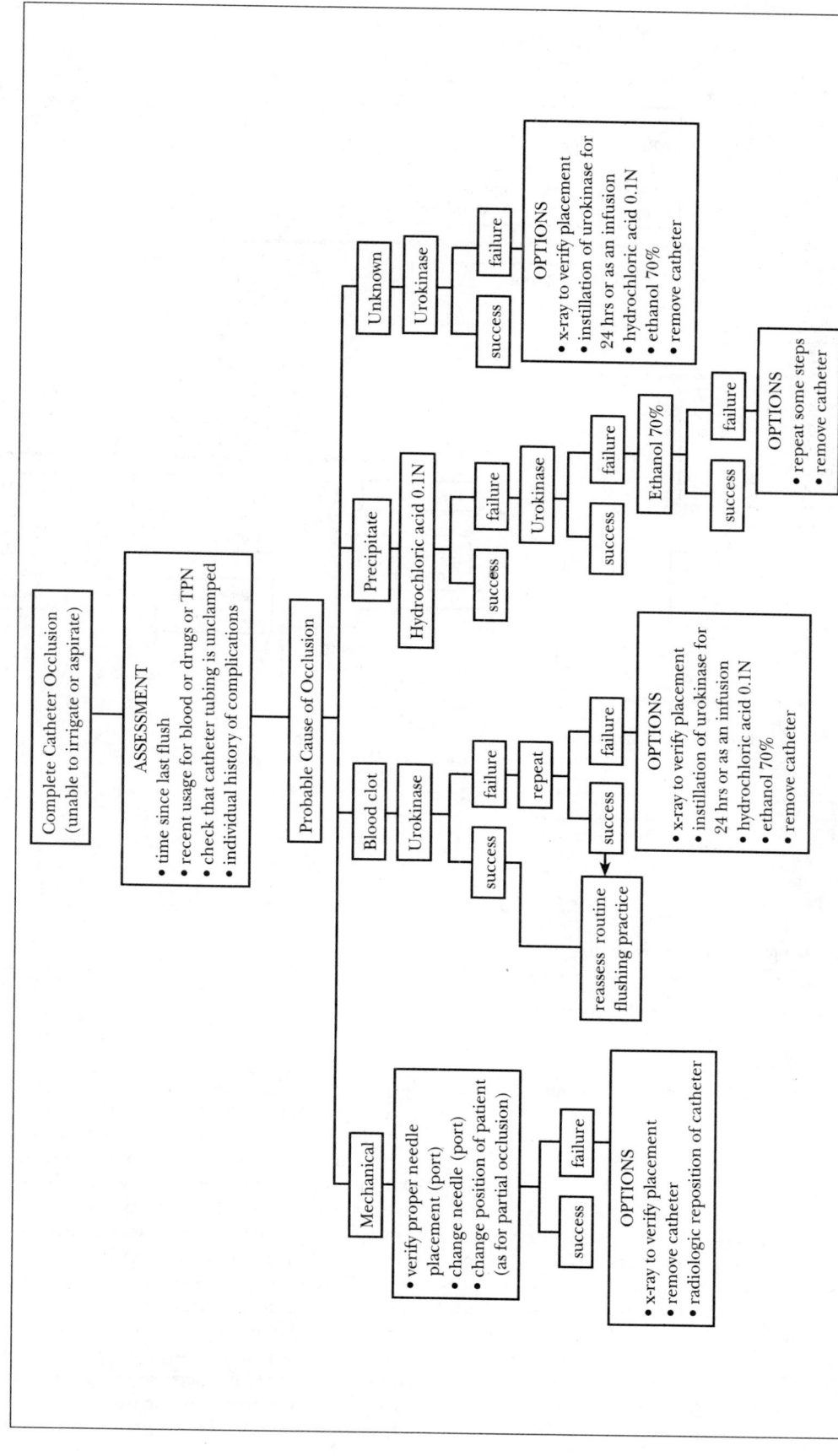

**FIGURE 15-26**   Managing complete catheter occlusion.

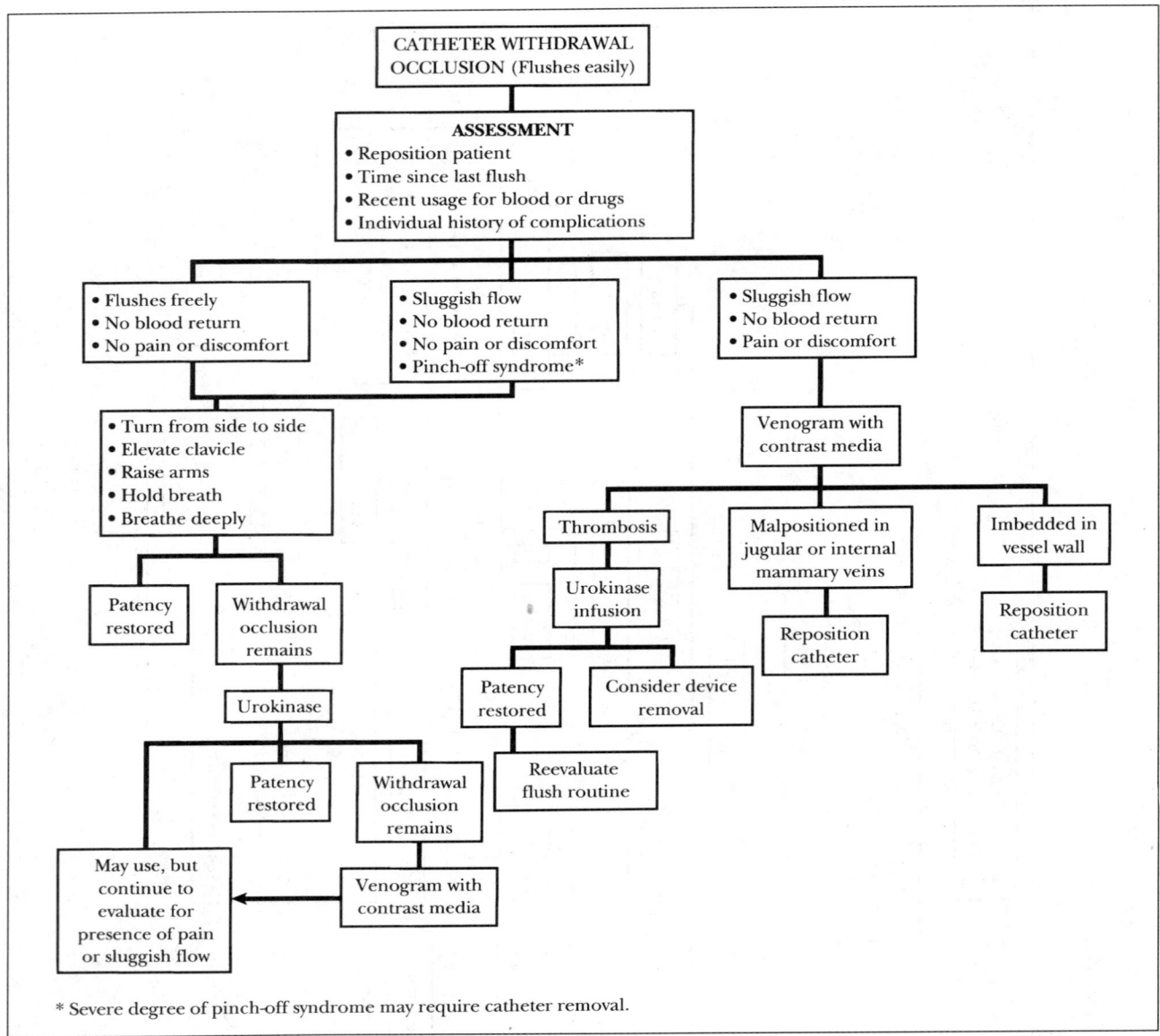

**FIGURE 15-27** Managing catheter withdrawal occlusion.

to prevent or decrease the incidence of thrombus formation.[68,92]

## Infection

Long-term central venous catheters are designed to minimize the risk of infection compared to regular venous catheters, but infection still occurs in 2.7%–60% of devices.[77,79] This wide range is probably dependent on the techniques used to insert and care for the VADs as well as the diagnoses and physical conditions of the patients involved. Infections can occur locally (on the skin), in the catheter tunnel/port pocket, or systemically. Infections are more common in patients with neutropenia (<500 granulocytes/mm³), those with multilumen cathe-

ters, and those receiving TPN or chemotherapy. A study by Howell et al[79] indicated that neutropenia was the only independent risk factor for catheter-related infections.

Local infections at the catheter exit site or over the skin around the port needle insertion site usually are due to organisms on the skin such as *S. aureus* and *S. epidermis*. Symptoms can include redness, warmth, discomfort, and exudate. Management includes culture of the area, increased frequency of dressing changes with meticulous site care, and administration of appropriate oral or IV antibiotics.[77,85] The needle should be removed from an implantable port if a skin infection occurs over the port, and it should not be reaccessed until the infection clears.

Infections in the catheter tunnel or port pocket usually involve a variety of different organisms and are manifested by redness, edema, tenderness or discomfort, exudate, skin warmth, and/or fever. After cultures have been taken, including aspiration of any port pocket exudate, appropriate IV antibiotic therapy is initiated. If the causative organism is identified and appropriate anti-infective therapy fails to resolve the infection, consideration should be given to removal of the device.

Systemic infections can be thrombus-related or caused by intraluminal catheter colonization with a wide variety of infective organisms. Signs and symptoms include fever and chills. Blood cultures are taken through each lumen of the device as well as peripherally and can be positive either in the device only or via both routes. Administration of appropriate antibacterial or antifungal therapy is initiated, and blood cultures are repeated. Failure to resolve the infection is cause to consider removal of the device.

Preventing infection is a primary concern when caring for all types of VADs. Attention should be focused on the techniques used in routine maintenance, and care should be taken to employ measures to decrease the risk of infection such as decreasing the catheter manipulations and aseptic handling of the hubs. The VitaCuff (Vitaphore, San Carlos, CA), is impregnated with silver ions, and can be attached to any catheter before insertion to provide an antimicrobial barrier within the catheter tunnel. It has been reported to decrease the incidence of catheter infections.[93] Another preventive measure successful in decreasing catheter infection rates is the "locking" of the device with a heparinized vancomycin solution (instead of only heparinized saline).[94] No toxicities or complications have been noted, and no patients have experienced bacteremia due to intraluminal colonization of vancomycin-susceptible organisms, although infection due to other organisms has occurred. Another approach has been to investigate the use of antibiotic bonded catheters and the possible impact of these catheters on infection rates.[70]

### Other complications

Occlusions and device malfunctions can occur for a variety of other reasons, and careful assessment of the device when occlusion occurs should always include consideration of malpositioning or breakage. Catheters can be kinked, compressed by tumor, compressed between the rib and clavicle ("pinch-off sign"), malpositioned due to patient manipulation ("twiddler's syndrome"), malpositioned for other reasons, severed, punctured, split, or separated. The port access needle can be embedded in the septum; be inaccurately placed into the side of the port or catheter, instead of the portal housing; or become dislodged from the port and remain under the skin.

Thrombus formation can result in a retrograde flow of blood or fluid along the catheter tract, with subsequent extravasation into the subcutaneous tissues. Infusion of drugs into a severed, punctured, or separated catheter can also result in extravasation. Prevention of vesicant extravasation is discussed elsewhere in this chapter, but it is prudent to reiterate that all vascular access devices should be patent and functioning appropriately before initiating vesicant therapy. Extravasation of vesicants into the chest wall or thorax can result in severe deformity, loss of function, or death.

All of the vascular access devices are popular, and manufacturers are continually developing new designs with innovative features every year. Oncology nurses frequently review these new devices and are called on to evaluate their effectiveness. Table 15-14 contains product selection guidelines that might be useful in determining the product to be utilized by an individual health care institution. Cost containment is a growing concern, and the best price usually can be achieved if all of the devices selected come from a limited number of vendors, thus consolidating buying power. The oncology nurse contributes greatly to this interdisciplinary team by his or her clinical experience with the product and evaluation of specific outcome measures.

## REPORTING DEFECTS

The Safe Medical Devices Act of 1995 requires health care facilities and manufacturers to report device-related events that did or could have caused serious injury or death. The MEDWatch system through the FDA makes the reporting process simple and confidential. Forms can be obtained by calling 1-800-FDA-1088.[95]

## CONCLUSION

Cancer chemotherapy administration is a rapidly evolving area of oncology nursing practice that offers exciting opportunities for both beginning and seasoned oncology nurses. The level of responsibility for monitoring patients receiving chemotherapy and managing many aspects of their care continues to increase. Expanded outpatient and home care settings, where the majority of chemotherapy is given, offer opportunities for triage assessment and nursing intervention at an increasingly autonomous level. The technical explosions in drug delivery systems are a constant informational challenge, as is maintaining the personal and rewarding relationships with patients for whom these advanced technologies are utilized.

Health care will continue to move toward more and more ambulatory and home care, with hospitals becoming virtually intensive care buildings. Reimbursement, lobbying, litigation, and legislation are predominant issues for the 1990s, and they will continue into the twenty-first century. The oncology nurse has a vital role in establishing effective policies and procedures by serving on institutional practice or policy committees. An oncology

**TABLE 15-14**   Vascular Access Devices: Product Selection Guidelines

**VAD Selection Team Members**

- Vascular or general surgeon or interventional radiologist
- Oncology nurse
- Purchasing representative
- Medical oncologist (optional or consultant to team)
- Others, as appropriate (i.e., nutritional support nurse, IV therapy nurse)

**Manufacturer Considerations**

- Length of time in business
- Manufacturer vs. distributor
- Distribution system and supply turnaround
- Availability of representative (i.e., locally or regionally)
- Reputation of reliability or quality
- Commitment to product (e.g., R & D department)
- List of all customers using device
- Return policy
- Purchasing plan (e.g., group discount)
- Price
- Training and in-service capabilities
- Availability of professional and patient education material

**Device Selection**

- Material (silastic vs. polyurethane; titanium vs. plastic)
- Ease of access; simplicity of use
- Design advantages (i.e., preattached vs. attachable catheters)

- Lumen size and flow requirements
- Choice and size/type variations
- Supplies necessary for use and their cost
- Standardization of design (to minimize errors)
- History of malfunctions and manufacturer's response
- Frequency of major design changes

**VAD Selection Team Actions**

- Examine VAD needs (i.e., type, flow rate, infusion usage, patient population, and surgical preferences).
- Establish specifications, including points of view of all members.
- Contact manufacturers for written material.
- Research subject matter (e.g., infection rates, pros, cons, etc.).
- Select 2–4 manufacturers to make individual presentations.
- Contact current users of devices from list provided by manufacturer.
- Use devices from 1–2 manufacturers on a trial basis, if necessary.
- Select most advantageous device(s).
- Implement educational plan and device usage.
- Evaluate device using preestablished expectations (specifications). Include patient responses.
- Maintain records on usage, function, and complications.
- Publish process and utilization results.
- Consider specialized clinic/insertion service area.

clinical practice committee with responsibility for reviewing and recommending procedures can also serve to evaluate new technologies. Methods for assuring competency also are being developed and documented.[96] Patient care evaluation and quality improvement are key responsibilities recognized by the Joint Commission on the Accreditation of Healthcare Organizations, which initiated clinical indicators for oncology to more closely monitor quality in the health care setting.

# REFERENCES

1. Buchsel PC: Ambulatory care for the bone marrow transplant patient, in Buchsel PC, Yarbro CH (eds): *Oncology Nursing in the Ambulatory Setting*. Boston, Jones and Bartlett, 1993, pp 185–216
2. Baird S: The impact of changing health care delivery on oncology practice. *Oncol Nurs Forum* 2:1–13, 1995
3. Oncology Nursing Society: *ONS Cancer Chemotherapy Guidelines and Recommendations for Practice*. Pittsburgh, Oncology Nursing Society, 1996
4. Alabama Board of Nursing: *Alabama Board of Nursing Administrative Code*. Montgomery, AL, Alabama Board of Nursing, 1990
5. Rutherford C: Position Paper—Administration of antineoplastic agents. *J Intraven Nurs* 15:8–9, 1992
6. Oncology Nursing Society: *Position Statement—Preparations of the professional registered nurse who administers and cares for the individual receiving chemotherapy*. Pittsburgh, Oncology Nursing Society, 1991
7. Krohner KM, Spitak AF: Cancer nursing education in the community hospital: Principles and practice. *Oncol Nurs Forum* 19:783–786, 1992
8. Creaton EM, Leonard ED, Day AL: A hospital-based chemotherapy education and training program. *Cancer Nurs* 14:79–90, 1991
9. American Society of Hospital Pharmacists: ASHP technical assistance bulletin on handling cytotoxic drugs in hospitals. *Am J Hosp Pharm* 42:131–137, 1985
10. American Society of Hospital Pharmacists: *Safe Handling of Cytotoxic and Hazardous Drugs Study Guide*. Bethesda, MD, American Society of Hospital Pharmacists, 1990
11. Anderson RW, Puckett W, Dana W, et al: Risk of handling

injectable antineoplastic agents. *Am J Hosp Pharm* 39: 1881–1887, 1982

12. Stellman JM, Aufiero BM, Taub RN: Assessment of potential exposure to antineoplastic agents in the health care setting. *Prev Med* 13:245–255, 1984

13. Occupational Safety and Health Administration: *Work Practice Guidelines for Personnel Dealing with Cytotoxic (antineoplastic) Drugs* (OSHA Instruction CPL 2-2.20B) Washington, DC, US Department of Labor Publication, 1995

14. Parillo VL: Documentation forms for monitoring occupational surveillance of health care workers who handle cytotoxic drugs. *Oncol Nurs Forum* 21:115–118, 1994

15. Blecke C: Home chemotherapy safety procedures. *Oncol Nurs Forum* 16:719–724, 1989

16. Valanis B, McNeil V, Driscoll K: Staff members' compliance with their facility's antineoplastic drug handling policy. *Oncol Nurs Forum* 18:571–576, 1991

17. Stajich GV, Barnett CW, Turner SV, et al: Protective measures used by oncologic office nurses handling parenteral antineoplastic agents. *Oncol Nurs Forum* 13:47–49, 1986

18. Groenwald SL, Frogge MH, Goodman M, Yarbro CH, (eds): *Cancer Symptom Management*. Boston, Jones and Bartlett, 1996

19. Lynch M, Yanes L: *Flowsheet documentation of chemotherapy administration and patient teaching.* Pittsburgh, Oncology Nursing Society, 1989

20. Cushman KE: A tool for documenting chemotherapy administration quickly and completely. *Oncol Nurs Forum* 18: 599–600, 1991

21. Moore JM, Knobf MT: A nursing flow sheet for documentation of ambulatory oncology. *Oncol Nurs Forum* 18:933–939, 1991

22. Coker M, Lampert A: Teaching checklist for home infusion therapy. *Oncol Nurs Forum* 17:923–926, 1990

23. Pickett RR: Outpatient oncology chemotherapy documentation tool. *Oncol Nurs Forum* 19:515–517, 1992

24. Cancer Letter, Goldberg KB (ed): 21 pp 1–5, June 1995

25. Lippman H: Malpractice protection, how much is enough? *RN* 56:61–67, 1993

26. Senders JW: Detecting, correcting and interrupting errors. *J Intraven Nurs* 18:23–32, 1995

27. Masoorlis S: Infusion therapy lawsuits: An occupational hazard. *J Intraven Nurs* 18:88–91, 1995

28. Baker K, Grochow LB, Donehower R: Should anticancer drug doses be adjusted in the obese patient? *J Natl Cancer Inst* 87:333–335, 1995

29. Georgiadis MS, Steinberg SM, Hankins LA, et al: Obesity and therapy-related toxicity in patients treated for small cell lung cancer. *J Natl Cancer Inst* 87:361–366, 1995

30. Calvert AH, Newell DR, Gumbrell LA, et al: Carboplatin dosage: Prospective evaluation of a simple formula based on renal function. *J Clin Onc* 7:1748–1756, 1989

31. Riggs CE: Anti-tumor antibiotics and related compounds, in Perry MC (ed): *The Chemotherapy Source Book*. Baltimore, Williams & Wilkins, 1992, pp 318–358

32. Friedland D, Gorman G, Treat T: Hypersensitivity reaction from taxol and etoposide. *J Natl Cancer Inst* 85:2036, 1993

33. Rowinsky EK, Gilbert MR, McGuire WP, et al: Serious hypersensitivity reactions related to its Cremophor EL formulation vehicle. *J Clin Oncol* 9:1692–1703, 1991

34. Van Hoefer U, Harstrick A, Wilke H, et al: Schedule dependent antagonism of paclitaxel and cisplatin in human gastric and ovarian carcinoma cell lines in vitro. *Eur J Cancer* 31A:92–97, 1995

35. Clark JW, Santos-Moore AS, Choy H: Sequencing of taxol and carboplatinum therapy. *Proc Am Assoc Cancer Res* 36: 298, 1995 (abstr 1772)

36. Holmes FA, Newman RA, Madden T, et al: Schedule dependent pharmacokinetics (pk) in a phase I trial of taxol and doxorubicin as initial therapy for metastatic breast cancer. A489, NCI-EORTC, 1994

37. Gilyon K, Kuzel T: Cutaneous T-cell lymphoma. *Oncol Nurs Forum* 18:901–908, 1991

38. Martin V, Walker FE, Goodman M: Delivery of cancer chemotherapy, in Stromberg M, McCorkle R, Grant M (eds): *Cancer Nursing: A Comprehensive Textbook*. Philadelphia, Saunders, 1996, pp 397–399

39. Rudolph R, Larson DL: Etiology and treatment of chemotherapeutic agent extravasation injuries: A review. *J Clin Oncol* 5:1116–1126, 1987

40. Laughlin RA, Landeen JM, Habal MB: The management of inadvertent subcutaneous adriamycin infiltration. *Am J Surg* 137:408–412, 1979

41. Ignoffo RJ, Friedman MA: Therapy of local toxicities caused by extravasation of cancer chemotherapeutic drugs. *Cancer Treat Rev* 7:17–27, 1980

42. Brothers TE, Niederhuber JE, Roberts JA, Ensminger WD: Experience with subcutaneous infusion ports in three hundred patients. *Surg Gynecol Obstet* 66:295–301, 1988

43. Gemlo BT, Rayner AA, Swanson RJ, et al: Extravasation: A serious complication of the split-sheath introducer technique for venous access. *Arch Surg* 123:490–492, 1988

44. Mayo DJ, Pearson DC: Chemotherapy extravasation: A consequence of fibrin sheath formation around venous access devices. *Oncol Nurs Forum* 22:675–680, 1995

45. Bertelli G, Gozza GB, Vidili S, et al: Topical DMSO Dimethylsulfoxide for the prevention of soft tissue injury after extravasation of vesicant cytotoxic drugs: Prospective Clinical Study. *J Clin Oncol* 13:2851–2855, 1996

46. Rudolph R, Larson DL: Etiology and treatment of chemotherapeutic agent extravasation injuries: A review. *J Clin Oncol* 5:1116–1126, 1987

47. Ajani J, Dodd LG, Daugherty K, et al: Taxol induced soft-tissue injury secondary to extravasation: Characterized by histopathology and clinical course. *J Natl Cancer Inst* 86: 51–53, 1994

48. Goodman M: Taxol and Taxotere Infiltrations: Special considerations in management. *Oncol Nurs Forum* 23:87, 1996

49. Howell SB, Pfeifle CL, Wung WE, et al: Intraperitoneal cisplatin with systemic thiosulfate protection. *Ann Intern Med* 97:845–851, 1982

50. Zook-Enck D: Intraperitoneal therapy via the Tenckhoff catheter. *J Intrav Nurs* 13:375–382, 1990

51. Malloy J: Administering intraperitoneal chemotherapy: A new approach. *Nursing* 1:58–62, 1991

52. Moores D: Malignant pleural effusions. *Semin Oncol* 18: 59–61, 1991 (suppl 2)

53. Bartal AH, Gazitt Y, Zidan G, et al: Clinical and flow cytometry characteristics of malignant pleural effusion in patients after intracavitary administration of methyl-prednisolone acetate. *Cancer* 67:3136–3140, 1991

54. Ike O, Shimizu Y, Hitomi S, et al: Treatment of malignant pleural effusions with doxorubicin hydrochloride containing poly (L-lactic acid) microspheres. *Chest* 99:911–915, 1991

55. Rusch VW, Figlin R, Godwin D, et al: Intrapleural cisplatin and cytarabine in the management of pleural effusions: A Lung Cancer Study Group trial. *J Clin Oncol* 9:313–319, 1991

56. Parker LA, Charnock GC, Delany DJ: Small-bore catheter drainage and sclerotherapy for malignant pleural effusions. *Cancer* 64:1218–1221, 1989

57. Walsh FW, Alberts WM, Soloman DA, et al: Malignant pleural effusions: Pleurodesis using a small-bore percutaneous catheter. *South Med J* 92:963–965, 1989

58. Tsang V, Fernando HC, Goldstraw P: Pleuroperitoneal shunt for recurrent malignant pleural effusion. *Thorax* 45:369–372, 1990

59. Herr HW, Badalament RA, Amato DA, et al: Superficial bladder cancer treated with bacillus Calmette-Guerin: A multivariate analysis of factors affecting tumor progression. *J Urol* 141:22–29, 1989

60. Brosman SA, Lamm DL: The preparation, handling and use of intravesical bacillus Calmette-Guerin for the management of stage Ta, T1, carcinoma in situ and transitional cell cancer. *J Urol* 144:313–315, 1990

61. Lamm DL, Riggs DR, Traynelis CI: Apparent failure of current intravesical chemotherapy prophylaxis to influence the long-term course of superficial transitional cell carcinoma of the bladder. *J Urol* 153:1444–1450, 1995

62. Phillips PC: Methotrexate Neurotoxicity, in Rottenberg DA (ed): *Neurologic Complications of Cancer Treatment.* Boston, Butterworth-Heinemann, 1991, pp 155–123

63. Oncology Nursing Society: *Access Device Guidelines: Recommendations for Nursing Education and Practice.* Pittsburgh, Oncology Nursing Society, 1996, pp 2–86

64. ACS Nursing Subcommittee: *Venous Access Devices Standards of Care.* Salt Lake City, American Cancer Society, 1990, p 8

65. Lucas AB: A critical review of venous access devices: The nursing perspective, in Hubbard SM, Greene PE, Knobf MT (eds): *Current Issues in Cancer Nursing Practice.* Philadelphia, Lippincott, 1991, pp 1–10

66. Raad I, Davis S, Becker M, et al: Low infection rate and long durability of nontunneled silastic catheters. *Arch Intern Med* 153:1791–1796, 1993

67. Alexander HR, Lucas A: New technologies in long-term venous access and peripherally inserted central venous catheters, in Alexander HR (ed): *Vascular Access in the Cancer Patient: Devices, Insertion Techniques, Maintenance, and Prevention of Complications.* Philadelphia, Lippincott, 1995, pp 130–146

68. Ryder M: Peripherally inserted central venous catheters. *Nurs Clin North Am* 28:937–971, 1994

69. Alexander HR: Infectious complications associated with long-term vascular access devices: Etiology, diagnosis, treatment, and prophylaxis, in Alexander HR (ed): *Vascular Access in the Cancer Patient: Devices, Insertion Techniques, Maintenance, and Prevention of Complications.* Philadelphia, Lippincott, 1995, pp 112–128

70. Maki DG, Wheeler SJ, Stoltz SM, et al: Clinical trial of a novel antiseptic-coated central venous catheter. *ICAAC, American Society of Microbiology*, 1991 (abstr)

71. Lucas A: Routine maintenance and care of long-term vascular access devices, in Alexander HR (ed): *Vascular Access in the Cancer Patient: Devices, Insertion Techniques, Maintenance, and Prevention of Complications.* Philadelphia, Lippincott, 1995, pp 148–164

72. Hoffman KK, Weber DJ, Samsa GP, et al: Transparent polyurethane film as an intravenous catheter dressing: A meta-analysis of the infection rates. *JAMA* 267:2072–2076, 1992

73. Hutchinson SK, Waskerwitz M, Martin K, et al: Non-occlusive, clean permanent right atrial dressing change procedures compared with occlusive, sterile permanent right atrial catheter dressing change procedures in children with cancer. *J Pediatr Oncol Nurs* 7:71, 1990

74. Kelly C, Dumenko L, McGregor SE, et al: A change in flushing protocols of central venous catheters. *Oncol Nurs Forum* 19:599–605, 1992

75. Wiernikowski JT, Elder-Thornley D, Dawson S, et al: Bacterial colonization of tunnelled right atrial catheters in pediatric oncology: A comparison of sterile saline and bacteriostatic saline flush solutions. *Am J Pediatr Hemotol Oncol* 13:137–140, 1991

76. Winters V, Peters B, Coila S, et al: A trial with a new peripheral implanted vascular access device. *Oncol Nurs Forum* 17:891–896, 1990

77. Groeger S, Lucas A, Thaler H, et al: Infectious morbidity associated with long-term use of vascular access devices in patients with cancer. *Ann Intern Med* 153:1167–1174, 1993

78. Danzig L, Shat L, Collins K, et al: Bloodstream infections associated with a needleless system in patients receiving home infusion therapy. *JAMA* 23:1862–1864, 1995

79. Howell P, Walters P, Donowitz G, et al: Risk factors for infection of adult patients with cancer who have tunneled central venous access devices. *Cancer* 75:1367–1375, 1995

80. Keung Y, Watkins D, Chen S, et al: Comparative study of infectious complications of different types of chronic vascular access devices. *Cancer* 73:2832–2837, 1994

81. Kupensky D: Use of hydrochloric acid to restore patency in an occluded implantable port. *J Intraven Nurs* 18:198–201, 1995

82. Breaux CW, Duke D, Georgeson KE, et al: Calcium phosphate crystal occlusion of central venous catheters used for total parenteral nutrition in infants and children: Prevention and treatment. *J Pediatr Surg* 22:829–832, 1987

83. Wickham R, Purl S, Welker D: Long-term central venous catheters: Issues for care. *Semin Oncol Nurs* 8:133–147, 1992

84. Wickham R, Purl S, McHale M: Long-term central venous catheters, in Kitt S, Selfridge-Thomas J, Proehl J, Kaiser J (eds): *Emergency Nursing. A Physiologic and Clinical Perspective.* Philadelphia, Saunders, 1995, pp 640–664

85. Holcombe BJ, Forloines-Lynn S, Garmhausen LW: Restoring patency of long-term central venous access devices. *J Intraven Nurs* 15:36–41, 1992

86. Duffy LF, Kerzner B, Gevus V, et al: Treatment of central venous catheter occlusions with hydrochloric acid. *J Pediatr* 114:1002–1104, 1989

87. Pennington CR, Pithie AD: Ethanol lock in the management of catheter occlusion. *J Parent Enter Nutrit* 11:507–508, 1987

88. Thompson B, Veal D: Pharmacologic treatment of pediatric catheter occlusion. *Hospital Pharmacy* 27:137–141, 1992

89. Shulman RJ, Reed T, Pitre D, et al: Use of hydrochloric acid to clear obstructed central venous catheters. *J Paren Enter Nutrit* 12:509–510, 1988

90. Gray WJ, Bell WR: Fibrinolytic agents in the treatment of thrombotic disorders. *Semin Oncol* 17:228–237, 1990

91. Fraschini G, Jadeja J, Lawson M, et al: Local infusion of urokinase for the lysis of thrombosis associated with permanent central venous catheters in cancer patients. *J Clin Oncol* 5:672–678, 1990

92. Bern MM, Lokich JL, Wallach SR, et al: Very low doses of warfarin can prevent thrombosis in central venous catheters: A randomized perspective trial. *Ann Intern Med* 112:423–428, 1990

93. Flowers RH, Schwenzer KJ, Kopel RF, et al: Efficacy of an

attachable subcutaneous cuff for the prevention of intravascular catheter-related sepsis. *JAMA* 261:878–883, 1989

94. Schwartz C, Hendrickson KJ, Roghmann K, et al: Prevention of bacteremia attributed to luminal colonization of tunneled central venous catheters with vancomycin-susceptible organisms. *J Clin Oncol* 8:1591–1597, 1990

95. Dessler DA: Introducing MEDWatch, a new approach to reporting medication and device adverse effects and product problems. *JAMA* 269:2765–2768, 1995

96. Dool J, Rodehaver CB, Fulton JS: Central venous access devices, issues for staff education and clinical competence. *Nurs Clin North Am* 28:973–984, 1993

97. Chabner B, Longo D (eds): *Cancer Chemotherapy and Biotherapy: Principles and Practice* (ed 2). Philadelphia, Lippincott-Raven, 1996, pp 600–824

98. Barton-Burke M (ed): *Cancer Chemotherapy: A Nursing Process Approach.* Sudbury, MA, Jones and Bartlett, 1996, pp 187–495

99. Dorr R, VanHoff DD (eds): *Cancer Chemotherapy Handbook* (ed 2). CT, Appleton and Lange, pp 112–935, 1993

100. Fischer DS, Knobf MT, Durivage HJ (eds): *Cancer Chemotherapy Handbook* (ed 4). St. Louis, Mosby, pp 58–215, 1993

## APPENDIX A  Intravenous Antineoplastic Agents

| Efficacy | Dosage | Mechanism of Action | Metabolism | Administration Precautions | Side Effects and Special Precautions |
|---|---|---|---|---|---|
| ALDESLEUKIN (IL-2, Proleukin) | | | | | |
| Renal cell carcinoma Malignant lymphoma Chronic lymphocytic leukemia | Proleukin 600,000 IU/kg per dose as a 15 min. infusion every 8 hours for 14 doses Continuous infusion over several days may reduce toxicity. | Stimulates production of cytokines. | t1/2 = variable depending on route; range 5–45 min. Renal elimination | Administered IV, SQ, and IM. Store under refrigeration. May be given over 15–30 min. or 24-hour infusion. Dosage: 600,000 IU/kg over 15 min as an IV infusion. Acetaminophen and indomethacin may be useful to prevent flu-like syndrome. SQ injections can cause local inflammation. | High-dose therapy can cause severe hypotension. Cardiac monitoring may be recommended. MI can be fatal. Renal dysfunction and capillary leak syndrome can occur. Corticosteroids may interfere with IL-2 activity. Flu-like syndrome: malaise, fever, chills, nausea, vomiting, and diarrhea. H2 antagonist may be given to prevent ulcer formation. DLT: Capillary leak syndrome: hypotension, pulmonary edema, weight gain, reduced cardiac output, azotemia, oliguria, and sodium retention. Anemia occurs with high-dose therapy. CNS toxicity: Somnolence, confusion. |
| AMSACRINE (AMSA, M-AMSA) (investigational) | | | | | |
| Acute nonlymphocytic leukemia Advanced ovarian cancer Lymphomas | 70 mg/m² q 14 days or 120 mg/m² q 3 weeks. In poor risk patients: 50 mg/m² q 14 days or 90 mg/m² every 3 weeks. | Cell-cycle phase specific S-phase; arrests cells in $G_2$ | Broken down in the liver, excreted in the bile and urine t1/2 = 12 min. | Precipitates in sodium chloride solutions. Dilute in D5W. Infuse over 2 hours via central line (if possible). Drug has vesicant potential. | DLT: Leukopenia, nadir occurs 7–14 days, recovery by day 21–25 Platelet-sparing |

*(continued)*

**APPENDIX A** Intravenous Antineoplastic Agents (continued)

| Efficacy | Dosage | Mechanism of Action | Metabolism | Administration Precautions | Side Effects and Special Precautions |
|---|---|---|---|---|---|
| | | | | Pain and phlebitis can occur. Reconstitute using glass syringe. Stable for 48 hours but use within 8 hours. Monitor cardiac status. Acute ventricular fibrillation can occur with hypokalemia. Dose reduction is recommended for patients with renal/hepatic dysfunction: BUN 20 mg/dl Serum creatinine 1.5 mg/dl: Bilirubin 2 mg/dl. Observe for HSR. Skin rash can occur. | Monitor liver functions. Skin discoloration can occur. Urine is orange following treatment. Transient paresthesias, hearing loss, and seizure activity have been reported. Nausea and vomiting occur but tend to be mild. Monitor cardiac ejection fraction. CHF can occur. Mucositis is dose-related. Hair loss occurs. |

BLEOMYCIN (Blenoxane)

| Efficacy | Dosage | Mechanism of Action | Metabolism | Administration Precautions | Side Effects and Special Precautions |
|---|---|---|---|---|---|
| Cervical cancer Head and neck cancer Penis, skin, and testicular cancer Hodgkin's lymphoma, Non-Hodgkin's lymphoma Kaposi's sarcoma | May be given IM, SQ, IV, intratumoral, intra-arterial. 10–20 U/m$^2$ once or twice a week Intrapleural/pericardial sclerosing dose: 50–60 U/m$^2$ in 50–100 ml NS or D5W: not to exceed 40 U/m$^2$ in geriatric population | Cell-cycle phase specific for G$_2$ and M phase. Binds to DNA. Inhibits cell progression out of G$_2$ resulting in cellular synchronization for subsequent drug therapy. | t1/2 = 20 min. Renal elimination | Administer with caution to patients with significant pulmonary or renal disease. Prior cisplatin therapy may reduce bleomycin clearance increasing plasma half-life and toxicity. Test dose: Bleomycin is associated with HSR and a test dose of 2 u IV in 50 ml D5W over 15 min. followed by observation. Observe for anaphylactic reaction for 1–2 hours posttest dose. Lymphoma patients are more at risk for HSR and should be tested for the first two doses. | Lifetime cumulative dose is 400 U. 25% dose reduction for creatinine clearance of 30–50 ml/min. 50% dose reduction for creatinine clearance of 20–30 ml/min. Fever occurs in approximately 50% of patients. Premedicate with acetaminophen 1 gram and diphenhydramine 50 mg. (Repeat 6 hours later.) Dermatologic reactions such as hyperpigmentation, hyperkeratosis, and erythema on palms and fingers; urticaria, rash, mucositis, and alopecia. Anorexia and mild nausea. Interstitial pneumonitis and pulmonary fibrosis occurs more commonly in patients who also have mediastinal radiation, are elderly, and receive higher cumulative doses. |

**APPENDIX A** Intravenous Antineoplastic Agents (continued)

| Efficacy | Dosage | Mechanism of Action | Metabolism | Administration Precautions | Side Effects and Special Precautions |
|---|---|---|---|---|---|
| | | | | | Assess for dyspnea, cough, fine rales, and altered pulmonary functions. |

### CARBOPLATIN (Paraplatin)

| Efficacy | Dosage | Mechanism of Action | Metabolism | Administration Precautions | Side Effects and Special Precautions |
|---|---|---|---|---|---|
| Ovarian carcinoma Testicular cancer Head and neck cancer Cervical cancer Lung cancer | IV: 360 mg/m² q 4 weeks Higher doses are given in pretransplant protocols and intraperitoneally or intra-arterially. Dose calculations are most therapeutically based on the desired serum concentration (AUC), renal status, and whether or not the patient has been previously treated with chemotherapy (Calvert Method). Note that doses calculated according to the Calvert formula are total mg, not mg/m² (see text). | Maximal cytotoxicity occurs when cells are in the S-phase although cell kill by intrastrand DNA cross-linkage occurs throughout $G_1$, S, and $G_2$ phases of the cell cycle. | t1/2 = 2.5 hours 60% eliminated unchanged in the urine Major route of elimination is glomerular filtration and tubular secretion. | Available as lyophilized (powdered) form to distinguish it from cisplatin, which is only available in aqueous solution. Usually administered over 15–30 min. in 500 cc of saline or D5W, without further hydration. May also be administered as a continuous 24-hour infusion or longer. Forms a precipitate when in contact with aluminum causing loss of antitumor potency. Injection site irritation and erythema can occur with infiltration but no ulceration or necrosis. Physically compatible with ondansetron. | DLT: myelosuppression, particularly thrombocytopenia Nadir occurs at 2–3 weeks. Nausea and vomiting are mild and rarely last beyond 24 hours. Ototoxicity and neurotoxicity (paresthesias) are uncommon. Alopecia, mucositis, and abnormal liver functions have been reported. Nephrotoxicity occurs, but is less common than with cisplatin. |

### CARMUSTINE (BiCNU)

| Efficacy | Dosage | Mechanism of Action | Metabolism | Administration Precautions | Side Effects and Special Precautions |
|---|---|---|---|---|---|
| Brain tumors Multiple myeloma Hodgkin's disease Non-Hodgkin's lymphoma Melanoma | IV: 150–200 mg/m² q 6 weeks Higher doses have been used in pretransplant protocols. | Inhibits enzymatic reactions involved in DNA synthesis. Inhibits DNA repair. Acts predominantly during late G and early S phase. Readily crosses the blood-brain barrier. | Metabolized by the liver. 80% eliminated via the kidneys t1/2 = 15–20 min. | Soluble in water and absolute alcohol. Protect from light. Administer in 100–500 cc of D5W or normal saline as a 1–2 hour infusion. Infusion may burn as it goes in and should be monitored closely. Heat provides symptomatic relief. Slowing the infusion rate also eases vein discomfort. Hypotension can occur if the infusion is given rapidly. Facial flushing and dizziness occur infrequently. Compatible with ondansetron. Incompatible with polyvinylchloride infusion bags and with sodium bicarbonate. Avoid contact with skin. A brown stain may result. | DLT: Leukopenia and thrombocytopenia occur 3–5 weeks after treatment, recovery at 8 weeks. Myelosuppression may be cumulative. Nausea and vomiting are common and require aggressive antiemetic therapy. Pulmonary fibrosis has been reported and generally presents as a dry cough and dyspnea. Alopecia is common. Elevation of LFTs and azotemia can occur with higher doses. Cimetidine has been shown to potentiate carmustine toxicity. |

*(continued)*

**APPENDIX A**   Intravenous Antineoplastic Agents (continued)

| Efficacy | Dosage | Mechanism of Action | Metabolism | Administration Precautions | Side Effects and Special Precautions |
|---|---|---|---|---|---|
| | | CISPLATIN (Platinol; CDDP) AQUEOUS SOLUTION | | | |
| Bladder<br>Ovarian<br>Testicular carcinoma<br>Nonsmall cell lung cancer<br>Head and neck cancer | IV: 20–40 mg/m² day for 3–5 days q 3–4 weeks<br>20–120 mg/m² single dose q 3–4 weeks<br>IP: 100–270 mg/m² in 2 liters of warmed NS Infuse via gravity over 10 min. Allow 4 hours dwell time. | Binds to DNA affecting DNA replication.<br>Forms DNA protein cross-links.<br>Interacts with cellular glutathione. | 90% bound to plasma proteins<br>20–45% eliminated unchanged via kidney<br>t1/2 = 60–90 hours<br>10% eliminated in bile | Dose reductions: 25% dose reduction for patients with creatinine clearance of 30–50 ml/min and a 50% dose reduction for patients with creatinine clearance < 30 ml/min.<br>Administer after appropriate hydration (1–2 liters with mannitol).<br>Maintain urinary output (125ml/hour). Mixing cisplatin in 0.9% NaCl maintains drug stability.<br>Cisplatin may react with aluminum resulting in loss of cisplatin potency.<br>Physically compatible with ondansetron. Sodium thiosulfate and MESNA directly inactivate cisplatin.<br>Administer with caution in patients receiving other potentially nephrotoxic drugs (aminoglycosides). | Concomitant administration of probenecid enhances cisplatin renal toxicity.<br><br>Monitor patient for HSR: tachycardia, wheezing, hypotension, and facial edema.<br><br>Acute and delayed nausea and vomiting are preventable with aggressive antiemetics including 5 HT3 receptor antagonists, dexamethasone, and metoclopramide.<br><br>High frequency hearing loss may occur in up to 30% of patients.<br><br>Tinnitis, vestibular dysfunction, and ototoxicity occur infrequently and are preventable with adequate hydration and mannitol diuresis.<br><br>Peripheral neuropathy including numbness, tingling, and sensory loss occurs in arms and legs with long-term administration.<br><br>Hypomagnesemia is seen with high dose (>200 mg/m²) and is preventable with oral and IV supplements.<br><br>Hemolytic anemia is seen with higher doses and responds to recombinant erythropoietin. |
| | | CYCLOPHOSPHAMIDE (Cytoxan) | | | |
| Breast<br>Ovary<br>Leukemias<br>Lymphomas<br>Multiple myeloma<br>Lung cancer | PO: 50–200 mg/m² orally each day for 14 days q 28 days IV: 500 mg–1.5g/m² IV q 3 weeks or 60 mg/kg IV for 2 days prior to BMT | Activated by hepatic microsomal enzymes; prevents cell division by cross-linking DNA strands.<br><br>Noncell-cycle phase specific. | t1/2 = 3–10 hours<br>Metabolized in the liver<br>Excreted in the kidney (15% unchanged) 33% of drug is excreted unchanged in the stool | When doses >1000mg are given, patients should receive hydration of 500–1000ml of normal saline.<br>Administer IV dose slowly to prevent nasal congestion, headache, and dizziness. | Hemorrhagic cystitis occurs rarely with conventional doses. Hydration and MESNA are indicated with high dose and pretransplant therapy. |

## APPENDIX A Intravenous Antineoplastic Agents (continued)

| Efficacy | Dosage | Mechanism of Action | Metabolism | Administration Precautions | Side Effects and Special Precautions |
|---|---|---|---|---|---|
| | | | | Encourage fluid intake of 3 liters per day while taking cytoxan. When taking oral doses encourage patient to take all pills before 5 P.M. to minimize bladder contact with toxic metabolites. Phenytoin and chloral hydrate may enhance the conversion of cytoxan to toxic metabolites, thereby increasing toxicity. | SIADH can occur with high-dose cytoxan. Nausea and vomiting are preventable with aggressive antiemetic therapy. Alopecia is common. Metallic taste occurs during injection and when taken orally. Encourage the patient to chew gum, peppermint or lemon candy. Myelosuppression (leukopenia) is dose-limiting. Amenorrhea and reversible oligo-spermia occur and are dose-dependent. Cytoxan 1mg/ml is compatible with doxorubicin, cisplatin, MESNA, and other drugs. Blurring of vision has been reported. Cardiac toxicity can occur with high-dose therapy, especially if given with radiation to the chest area. |
| | | **CYTARABINE (Cytosar; ARA-C, Cytosine Arabinoside)** | | | |
| Acute leukemia Myeloid leukemia Acute nonlymphocytic leukemia Meningeal leukemia | IV: 5–10 day CI of 100–200 mg/m² Intrathecal: 5–70 mg/m² 1–3×/week Subcutaneous: 1 mg/kg 1–2×/week or 100 mg 2x/day for 5 days every 28 days | Inhibits DNA polymerase causing DNA chain elongation and arrest. Cell-cycle phase specific for the S phase. Antimetabolite | Metabolized in the liver At 24 hours, 90% of the drug is eliminated in the urine t1/2 = 2–3 hours | Given IV push or IV infusion over 30 min. 5–10 day continuous infusions may be optimal for antitumor cytotoxicity because of the S-phase specificity. For intrathecal use mix drug with lactated Ringer's solution or NS without preservatives. Rotate sites for SQ and IM injections. | Myelosuppression is the DLT. Nadir at 5–7 days, recovery in 2–3 weeks Anemia is common. Nausea, vomiting, anorexia, metallic taste, stomatitis, and diarrhea are reported. Minimal alopecia Skin erythema can occur. Arthralgias and myalgias occur. After intrathecal use patients may experience nausea, vomiting, fever, and headache. Ocular toxicity: excessive tearing, photophobia, and blurred vision. |

*(continued)*

## APPENDIX A    Intravenous Antineoplastic Agents (continued)

| Efficacy | Dosage | Mechanism of Action | Metabolism | Administration Precautions | Side Effects and Special Precautions |
|---|---|---|---|---|---|
| | | | | | High-dose therapy can lead to CNS toxicity: lethargy, confusion, ataxia. |
| | | | | | ARA-C may decrease the cellular uptake of methotrexate. |
| | | | | | Compatible with vincristine, prednisolone, sodium phosphate, and ondansetron. |
| | | | | | Physical changes are noted with methotrexate and 5-FU and heparin. |
| | | | | | Compatible with vancomycin for 4–8 hours. |

### DACARBAZINE (DTIC)

| Efficacy | Dosage | Mechanism of Action | Metabolism | Administration Precautions | Side Effects and Special Precautions |
|---|---|---|---|---|---|
| Malignant melanoma Soft tissue sarcomas Hodgkin's disease | 375 mg/m² q 3–4 weeks or 150–250 mg/m² q day × 5 days q 3–4 weeks or 850 mg/m² on day 1 q 3–4 weeks | Causes cross-linkage and breaks in DNA strands. Inhibits RNA and DNA synthesis. Cell-cycle phase nonspecific, but has more activity in late $G_2$. | Activated by liver microsomes. Excreted renally; t1/2 = 35 min. | Reconstitute with D5W or saline. Solution can be painful and should be administered slowly in 250–500 cc of solution over 30–60 min. Moist heat along the vein eases pain. Stable for 8 hours at room temperature, 72 hours if refrigerated. Drug should be protected from light. May turn to a pinkish color if exposed to light. HSR can occur, hypotension occurs with high-dose therapy. | DLT: moderate degree of myelosuppression Nadir occurs at 21–25 days. Anemia can occur. Severe nausea and vomiting can occur. Aggressive pretreatment with antiemetic therapy is needed. Nausea and vomiting lessen by day 3–4 of treatment. Hepatotoxic; monitor liver functions Flu-like syndrome may occur with fever, myalgia, and malaise at about 7 days, lasting 1–3 weeks. Photosensitivity can occur; protect skin from sunlight. |

### DACTINOMYCIN (Actinomycin D; ACT-D, Cosmegen)

| Efficacy | Dosage | Mechanism of Action | Metabolism | Administration Precautions | Side Effects and Special Precautions |
|---|---|---|---|---|---|
| Wilms' tumor Embryonal rhabdomyosarcoma Choriocarcinoma Malignant melanoma Hodgkin's and non-Hodgkin's lymphoma | 10–15 μ/kg/day × 5 days q 3–4 weeks or 2.4 mg/m² in divided doses over 1 week or 2 mg/m² IV q 3–4 weeks | Binds between purine-pyrimidine base pairs in DNA. Inhibiting the synthesis of DNA-dependent RNA and messenger RNA. Action is cell-cycle nonspecific but is more active during $G_1$ and in cells that are cycling. | Excreted unchanged in bile and urine | Reconstitute with preservative-free sterile water for injection. Preserved diluent may cause precipitation. Use drug as soon as possible. Monitor liver functions: dose reductions may be necessary. | DLT: myelosuppression occurs within 7–10 days of dosing. Nadir may be delayed, occurring at 3 weeks. Due to its immuno-suppressive effects avoid administering Act-D to patients who have an active viral infection. |

**APPENDIX A**  Intravenous Antineoplastic Agents (continued)

| Efficacy | Dosage | Mechanism of Action | Metabolism | Administration Precautions | Side Effects and Special Precautions |
|---|---|---|---|---|---|
| | | | | Use extreme caution during administration. Act-D is a severe vesicant. Act-D is compatible with ondansetron. When calculating dose, double-check the order since the drug is ordered both as micrograms per kg and mg/m². | Nausea and vomiting can be severe. Aggressive pretreatment with antiemetics is appropriate.<br><br>Mucositis and diarrhea can be severe; institute preventive oral hygiene regimen.<br><br>Alopecia occurs commonly.<br><br>Erythema, hyperpigmentation, and an acne-like rash occur commonly.<br><br>Act-D can cause a radiation recall reaction.<br><br>Hepatic-veno-occlusive toxicity manifested as elevated SGOT and bilirubin can occur. |

### DAUNORUBICIN (daunomycin, Cerubidine)

| Efficacy | Dosage | Mechanism of Action | Metabolism | Administration Precautions | Side Effects and Special Precautions |
|---|---|---|---|---|---|
| ALL<br>AML<br>Acute monocytic leukemia<br>Acute nonlymphocytic leukemia | 30–60 mg/m² daily for 3–5 days q 3–4 weeks | Intercalates DNA, thereby blocking DNA, RNA and protein synthesis. It is an anthracycline antitumor antibiotic. | Metabolized in the liver. About 40% of the drug is eliminated via the bile. 20%–25% is eliminated via the urine. t1/2 = 20–25 hours | 20 mg vial is reconstituted with 4 ml of sterile water = 5 mg/ml. QS to 15–20 ml of NS<br><br>Stable for 24 hours at room temperature and 48 hours under refrigeration.<br><br>Incompatible with heparin, 5-fluorouracil, and dexamethasone<br><br>Compatible with ondansetron.<br><br>CAUTION: Because the solution is red, as is doxorubicin and with a similar sounding name, the vial should be double-checked against the order.<br><br>Urine will be pink to red for 12–24 hours after administration.<br><br>Daunorubicin is a severe vesicant. Extreme caution should be used in administration of this drug. Administer via the side arm of a freely running IV or by the two-syringe technique. | DLT: myelosuppression.<br><br>WBC nadir occurs at 7–14 days; recovery at 3 weeks. Thrombocytopenia and anemia occur.<br><br>Stomatitis occurs, but is mild.<br><br>Diarrhea occurs infrequently.<br><br>Nausea and vomiting occur 1–5 hours after dosing but are prevented with aggressive antiemetic therapy.<br><br>Alopecia is abrupt and involves all body hair.<br><br>Hyperpigmentation of the nails occurs. Urticaria and a generalized rash have been reported.<br><br>Monitor liver functions. If elevated LFTs are noted, dose reduction is indicated.<br><br>Cardiac toxicity can occur. Dose is limited to 500–600 mg/m². |

(continued)

**APPENDIX A** Intravenous Antineoplastic Agents (continued)

| Efficacy | Dosage | Mechanism of Action | Metabolism | Administration Precautions | Side Effects and Special Precautions |
|---|---|---|---|---|---|
| | | | | | Manifestation of CHF is characterized by dyspnea on exertion, fatigue, and arrhythmias. |

DOCETAXEL (Taxotere)

| Efficacy | Dosage | Mechanism of Action | Metabolism | Administration Precautions | Side Effects and Special Precautions |
|---|---|---|---|---|---|
| Ovarian cancer Breast cancer Non-small cell lung cancer | 80–100 mg/m² every 3 weeks as a one-hour infusion | Antimicrotubule agent–a mitotic spindle poison. Enhances microtubule assembly and inhibits the depolymerization of tubulin. This process leads to increased bundles of microtubules in the cell. The cell is then unable to divide. | Metabolized in the liver, excreted in the feces and minimally excreted in the urine. t1/2 = 11 hours | Taxotere solution contains 2 mg (40 mg/ml) of Taxotere in polysorbate/tween 80. Refrigerated vial sits at room temperature for 5 min. Once mixed with solvent the solution contains 10 mg/ml. The appropriate amount of taxotere is mixed with D5W in a concentration <1 mg/ml. Once diluted, taxotere is stable for 8 hours at room temperature. Avoid infiltration: the drug is an irritant, but can cause tissue damage depending on the concentration. Hyaluronidase SQ injections (maximum volume of 3 ml) have been recommended for treatment of infiltration. Apply cold to the site—NOT HEAT. Monitor liver functions carefully; dose adjustments are appropriate if LFTs are elevated 2.5× normal. | The DLT for taxotere is neutropenia and thrombocytopenia. All patients receive dexamethasone 8 mg po b.i.d. for 5 days starting one day prior to taxotere. Diphenhydramine 50 mg is also given 30 min. prior to prevent hypersensitivity reactions. If mild HSR occurs with flushing, skin reactions, or pruritus, the infusion rate is slowed with observation. If the patient experiences rash, flushing, mild dyspnea, or chest discomfort the infusion is stopped and the patient is treated with IV diphenhydramine and dexamethasone. The infusion may be resumed after symptoms abate. If severe symptoms such as generalized urticaria, angioedema, or hypotension occur the infusion is stopped and the patient is treated with antihistamine, steroid, and if necessary epinephrine or bronchodilators. The patient may still receive the taxotere depending on the severity of the response. If the patient reacts a second time the patient probably should not receive the drug again. Nausea and vomiting are minimal. Alopecia occurs within 3 weeks of the first treatment. |

**APPENDIX A** Intravenous Antineoplastic Agents (continued)

| Efficacy | Dosage | Mechanism of Action | Metabolism | Administration Precautions | Side Effects and Special Precautions |
|---|---|---|---|---|---|
| | | | | | Nail separation may occur. |
| | | | | | Drug-associated fluid retention or edema including pleural effusions, ascites, and peripheral edema occur and may be managed with a diuretic, which may or may not be helpful. |
| DOXORUBICIN (Adriamycin, Rubex) | | | | | |
| Acute nonlymphocytic leukemia<br>Acute lymphocytic leukemia<br>Wilms' tumor<br>Neuroblastoma<br>Soft-tissue sarcoma<br>Breast cancer<br>Hepatocellular carcinoma<br>Ovarian carcinoma | 60–75 mg/m² as bolus or as a continuous infusion over 3–4 days q 3–4 weeks. Higher doses are used in dose-intensive regimens.<br><br>Doxorubicin may also be given intra-arterially, intrapleu-rally, and by bladder in-stillation. | Binds directly to DNA base pairs and inhibits DNA, RNA, and protein synthesis. Antitumor antibiotic. Cell-cycle specific for the S-phase. | Extensively metabolized by the liver. 40%–50% of the drug is eliminated in the bile. 5% is eliminated in the urine.<br>t1/2 = 18–30 hours. | Available in liquid and lyophilized form.<br><br>Reconstitute with sterile water for injection, D5W, normal saline to form a solution of 2 mg/ml.<br><br>Stable for 35 days at room temperature.<br><br>Incompatible with hep-arin, dexamethasone, 5-fluorouracil, furose-mide, aminophylline.<br><br>Compatible with cyclo-phosphamide, cis-platin, dacarbazine, droperidol, vinblastine, vincristine, and on-dansetron.<br><br>Adriamycin turns the urine a reddish orange for 8–10 hours after ad-ministration.<br><br>Since adriamycin is me-tabolized and elimi-nated by the liver, liver function tests are moni-tored frequently. Eleva-tion in bilirubin to 1.2–3 mg/dL warrants a 50% dose reduction; biliru-bin of 3 mg/dL calls for a 75% dose reduction.<br><br>Administer with ex-treme caution. Adria-mycin is a severe vesicant. It will cause tissue damage, ulcer-ation, and necrosis if in-filtrated. Inject through the side arm of a freely running and well-estab-lished IV or by using the two syringe technique.<br><br>CAUTION: Because it has a similar name and color to daunorubicin it is important to check | DLT: Myelosuppres-sion, especially leuko-penia. Nadir occurs at 10–14 days. Recov-ery is swift at 3 weeks.<br><br>Cardiac toxicity can occur. Dose is limited to 450–550 mg/m². Adriamycin causes damage to the myo-cyte of the heart caus-ing various degrees of damage, but mani-fests as CHF as the heart begins to func-tion less efficiently as a pump.<br><br>MUGA scans are done periodically to monitor left ventricu-lar function. Early symptoms of CHF in-clude tachycardia, dyspnea on exertion, arrhythmias, and EKG changes.<br><br>Alopecia occurs pre-dictably and is dose dependent. Doses greater than 50 mg are associated with moderate to severe loss. Doses of 90–100 mg cause hair loss in 2.5 weeks.<br><br>Stomatitis is dose-limiting and can be more severe with continuous infusions. Continuous infusions are only given through central lines, never through peripheral lines.<br><br>Nail bed changes occur and include hy-perpigmentation es-pecially in African-Americans and in indi- |

(continued)

**APPENDIX A**   Intravenous Antineoplastic **Agents** (continued)

| Efficacy | Dosage | Mechanism of Action | Metabolism | Administration Precautions | Side Effects and Special Precautions |
|---|---|---|---|---|---|
| | | | | the drug order against the vial to ensure the right dose of the right drug. | viduals of Mediterranean descent. |

| | | ETOPOSIDE (VePesid, VP-16) | | | |
|---|---|---|---|---|---|
| Small-cell lung cancer Testicular cancer | 50–100 mg/m² IV qd × 5 (testicular) q 3–4 weeks<br><br>75–200 mg/m² IV qd × 3 (small-cell lung cancer) q 3–4 weeks Oral dose is twice the intravenous dose.<br><br>400 mg/m²/day for 3 days prior to bone marrow transplant. | Inhibits DNA synthesis in S and $G_2$. Causes single-strand breaks in DNA.<br>Cell-cycle phase specific for S and $G_2$ phase. | Extensively protein bound. Metabolized in the liver. Excreted in the bile and urine<br>t1/2 = 8–14 hours | Following dilution in normal saline or 5% dextrose the drug is stable for 72–96 hours at room temperature. At room temperature, stability is dependent on concentration:<br>  .6 mg/ml = 24 hour<br>  1 mg/ml = 4 hour<br>  2 mg/ml = 2 hour<br><br>Etoposide is administered slowly over at least 30–45 min.<br><br>Hypotension can occur, monitor patients for drug sensitivity. | DLT: Leukopenia, dose-related. Nadir occurs 7–14 days, recovery by day 21.<br><br>Nausea and vomiting are uncommon. Anorexia occurs, especially with oral dosing.<br><br>Alopecia occurs more commonly with IV dosing. Radiation recall and pruritus can occur.<br><br>HSR reactions are rare. |

| | | 5-FLUOROURACIL (5-FU, Adrucil) | | | |
|---|---|---|---|---|---|
| Cancer of the breast, colon, rectum, pancreas, stomach, head and neck | Doses vary: 300–600 mg/m² IV for 5 days every 3–4 weeks; 450–600 mg/m² IV weekly; 800–1200 mg/m² continuous infusion for 14–21 days to toxicity | Inhibits the formation of thymidine which is necessary for DNA synthesis. Causes abnormal RNA synthesis. Acts synergistically with methotrexate.<br><br>Cell-cycle phase specific for the S-phase. | Poorly absorbed by mouth. After IV administration the drug is metabolized to active metabolites. Approximately 45% of the drug is metabolized by the liver. 15% is eliminated unchanged in the urine. t1/2 = 10–20 min. | May be given a variety of ways: IV as a continuous infusion, IV push, arterial infusion, intracavitary, or intraperitoneally.<br><br>Store at room temperature and protect from light.<br><br>Incompatible with daunorubicin, doxorubicin, idarubicin, cisplatin, cytarabine, and diazepam.<br><br>Compatible with vincristine, methotrexate, potassium chloride, and magnesium sulfate. | Mylosuppression may be dose-limiting, but less common with continuous infusion.<br><br>Mucositis is most common DLT with continuous infusions. Symptoms of erythema, soreness, and ulceration may begin within 5–8 days of therapy. Sucking on ice chips as tolerated may decrease oral stomatitis. Diarrhea can be severe, even life threatening, especially when 5-FU is given in higher doses with leucovorin.<br><br>Nausea, vomiting, and anorexia occur less frequently, but are more common when 5-FU is given simultaneously with radiation to the abdomen.<br><br>Skin and nail bed changes occur especially with continuous infusion. Partial nail loss can occur as well as banding. Palmarplantar erythrodysethesias can be severe, necessitating |

**APPENDIX A**    Intravenous Antineoplastic Agents (continued)

| Efficacy | Dosage | Mechanism of Action | Metabolism | Administration Precautions | Side Effects and Special Precautions |
|---|---|---|---|---|---|
| | | | | | dose reduction and treatment delays. Hyperpigmentation and photosensitivity are common. Patients are cautioned to protect themselves from the sun. Excessive lacrimation due to tear duct stenosis and blurred vision occur in about 25% of patients. |
| | | | | | Headache, cerebellar ataxia, nystagmus, and confusion occur with higher doses. |
| | | | | | Administering 5-FU based on the patient's circadian rhythm may lessen toxicity in general. |
| | | | | | Alopecia is dose-dependent. |
| | | | | | Ataxia occurs in elderly patients. Other CNS changes include headache, drowsiness, and blurred vision. |

FLOXURIDINE (FUDR, 5-FUDR)

| Efficacy | Dosage | Mechanism of Action | Metabolism | Administration Precautions | Side Effects and Special Precautions |
|---|---|---|---|---|---|
| Adenocarcinoma metastatic to the liver | 0.1–0.6 mg/kg/day by intrahepatic infusion Therapy is continued to toxicity, usually 7–14 days.<br><br>Circadian infusion protocols have been used.<br><br>Intravenous doses range from 0.5–1.0 mg/kg/day for up to two weeks by continuous infusion. | Antimetabolite, similar to 5-FU, interrupts DNA synthesis causing cell death. Cell-cycle phase specific for the S-phase. | Metabolized to 5-FU when given IV. 70%–90% of the drug is metabolized by the liver and metabolites are excreted by the kidneys and lungs. When given intrahepatic FUDR has a much higher first pass extraction rate compared to 5-FU and therefore the cytotoxic effect is more localized to the liver.<br><br>t1/2 = 0.3–3.6 hours | Caution should be exercised since both 5-FU and floxuridine (also called 5-FUDR) are supplied in 500 mg vials and the doses of each are dramatically different. With such similar names it is important to note that mistaking 500 mg of FUDR for 500 mg of 5-FU could be lethal. FUDR 500 mg vial of lyophilized powder is reconstituted with sterile water.<br><br>Generally given via an intra-arterial infusion pump.<br><br>Heparin is added to the FUDR to prevent clotting of the catheter due to the slow infusion rate. | When given as an intra-arterial infusion an H2 antihistamine such as ranitidine may be recommended (150 mg b.i.d.) to prevent peptic ulcer disease.<br><br>The intra-arterial route is usually associated with less systemic toxicity.<br><br>Bone marrow suppression is more common with IV bolus injections.<br><br>Nausea, vomiting, and anorexia are common. Abdominal cramps with severe diarrhea are indications to interrupt therapy.<br><br>Mucositis does not occur often and if it occurs is an indication to |

(continued)

**APPENDIX A** Intravenous Antineoplastic Agents (continued)

| Efficacy | Dosage | Mechanism of Action | Metabolism | Administration Precautions | Side Effects and Special Precautions |
|---|---|---|---|---|---|
| | | | | | interrupt the treatment and to reduce the dose. |
| | | | | | Skin changes can occur and include edema, dermatitis, rashes, and pruritus as well as hyperpigmentation. |
| | | | | | Alopecia can occur but is usually mild. |

| GEMCITABINE (Gemsar) | | | | | |
|---|---|---|---|---|---|
| Pancreas cancer Non-small cell lung cancer Breast cancer | 800–1000 mg/m² weekly for 3 weeks every 4 weeks | An antimetabolite. Inhibits DNA synthesis. Cell-cycle specific for the S-phase. | Eliminated by the kidneys. t1/2 = 20 min. | Reconstitute with sodium chloride to a solution containing 10 mg/ml. Dilute in 100–1000 ml of saline and infuse over 30 min. to 3 hours. | Myleosuppression, especially thrombocytopenia can be dose-limiting.

Flu-like syndrome with fever, mild nausea, and vomiting can occur. Fever generally occurs within 8 hours of dosing. Acetaminophen generally relieves symptoms.

Rash may occur within 2–3 days of the infusion. Topical steroids may be helpful.

Peripheral edema may occur. |

| IDARUBICIN (Idamycin) | | | | | |
|---|---|---|---|---|---|
| Acute nonlymphocytic leukemia | 12 mg/m²/day for 3 days Doses vary Generally given in combination with other drugs. | Cell-cycle phase specific for S-phase. Analog of daunorubicin. Inhibits RNA synthesis. | Excreted primarily in the bile and urine. 25% of the drug is eliminated over approximately 5 days.

t1/2 = 13–26 hours

Metabolized in the liver to active form | Reconstituted with normal saline.

Protect from light.

Caution is used during administration because drug is a vesicant.

Incompatible with 5-fluorouracil, etoposide, dexamethasone, heparin, hydrocortisone, methotrexate, and vincristine. | DLT: Leukopenia and thrombocytopenia are expected.

Urine can be pink to red for 48 hours after administration.

Nausea can be mild to moderate and preventable with standard antiemetic.

Diarrhea and mucositis can occur.

Alopecia occurs gradually. Cumulative cardio-myopathy and congestive heart failure can occur with large cumulative doses. |

**APPENDIX A**   Intravenous Antineoplastic Agents (continued)

| Efficacy | Dosage | Mechanism of Action | Metabolism | Administration Precautions | Side Effects and Special Precautions |
|---|---|---|---|---|---|
| IFOSFAMIDE (Ifex) | | | | | |
| Testicular cancer Soft-tissue sarcoma Hodgkin's and non-Hodgkin's lymphoma Acute leukemias Ewing's sarcoma Osteosarcoma | IV: 1–1.2 g/m² day over a 5 day period every 3–4 weeks. Higher doses of 2.5–3.7 g/m²/day over a 2–3 day period. MESNA at a dose of 20% of the ifosfamide dose is given just prior to the ifosfamide and every 4 hours for 2 more doses. MESNA may be given IV or orally. | Ifosfamide is an alkylating agent. It is a prodrug and requires activation in the liver by microsomal enzymes. | Metabolized by the liver to inactive metabolites. 15%–56% of the drug is excreted unchanged in the urine. t1/2 = 7–15 hours Drug elimination may be hindered by renal dysfunction. | Ifosfamide is administered over at least 30 minutes with aggressive hydration to reduce the incidence of hemorrhagic cystitis. The uroprotectant MESNA is also given either as a continuous infusion or in divided doses every 4 hours × 3 doses. Ifosfamide and MESNA are compatible and can be infused concurrently when high dose ifosfamide is given. | Myelosuppression is the DLT. WBC nadir usually occurs 7–10 days posttreatment. Urinary tract toxicity is the dose-limiting toxicity and is manifested as hemorrhagic cystitis. Patients may complain of dysuria and frequency 2–3 days after the infusion. Encourage oral intake of 2–3 liters per day prior to and after dosing. Encourage patients to empty their bladders every 2–3 hours. Nausea and vomiting are common with higher doses. Symptoms are preventable with serotonin antagonist therapy. Avoid sedation with neurotoxic drugs that can exacerbate the lethargy and confusion that can occur due to the accumulation of chloracetylaldehyde, a metabolite with neurotoxic properties. Alopecia is more common with higher doses and occurs usually within 3 weeks of therapy. |
| L-ASPARAGINASE (Elspar) Erwinia Asparaginase (investigational) | | | | | |
| Acute lymphocytic leukemia | Used in combination with other drugs active in ALL 200 IU/day for 28 days 1000 IU/kg × 10 days or 20,000 IU/m² per week | Inhibits protein synthesis | Biphasic elimination t1/2 = 4–9 hours and 1.4–1.8 days Binds to vascular binding sites. May be eliminated by the liver. | Dilute in nonpreserved sterile saline or water. Use within 8 hours. Refrigerate before and after reconstitution. Do not infuse through a filter. IV slow push over 30 min., or IM. Do not use if solution is cloudy. Skin test with 2 IU | Anaphylactic reactions can occur in 20%–35% of patients. Monitor closely with appropriate support. IM use is associated with delayed allergic response. If HSR occurs, the Erwinia preparation |

(continued)

**APPENDIX A**   Intravenous Antineoplastic Agents (continued)

| Efficacy | Dosage | Mechanism of Action | Metabolism | Administration Precautions | Side Effects and Special Precautions |
|---|---|---|---|---|---|
| | | | | intradermal at least 1 hour prior to dosing. Administer subsequent doses with caution despite negative skin test. | may be used with prophylactic premedication. Urticarial eruptions are common. Incidence of reactions increases with each subsequent dosing. Slight anemia can occur, leukopenia is rare. Malaise, anorexia, nausea, and vomiting occur frequently. Hepatic toxicity is uncommon. Lethargy, somnolence, disorientation, and loss of recent memory occur with higher doses. |

### MECHLORETHAMINE HYDROCHLORIDE (nitrogen mustard, Mustargen)

| Efficacy | Dosage | Mechanism of Action | Metabolism | Administration Precautions | Side Effects and Special Precautions |
|---|---|---|---|---|---|
| Hodgkin's disease Chronic myelogenous leukemia Lymphosarcoma | IV: 6 mg/m² on days 1 and 8 Topically: 10 mg/ 60ml ointment | Alkylating agent results in abnormal base pairing causing DNA miscoding, cross-linking of DNA, and strand breakage. Cell-cycle nonspecific | Rapidly deactivated in the blood t1/2 = 15 min. | Once reconstituted with sterile water or normal saline the drug should be used within 60 min. because of its instability. Nitrogen mustard should be administered by intravenous push via a freely running IV line. Administering nitrogen mustard via direct IV push technique can cause venous thrombosis and pain. Nitrogen mustard is a severe vesicant and must be given with extreme caution. Assess for a blood return every 1 ml of injection. If extravasation occurs inject a solution of sodium thiosulfate (1/ 6 M) into the area to neutralize the drug. For 1 mg of nitrogen mustard infiltrated inject 2 ml of the 10% thiosulfate solution. Preparation: 4 ml sodium thiosulfate Injection (10%) diluted with 6 ml of sterile water for injection. | Myelosuppression is the DLT. Leukopenia occurs 8–14 days following treatment. Severe thrombocytopenia may occur. Severe nausea and vomiting within 1 hour of IV administration. Patients should be premedicated with aggressive antiemetic therapy. Alopecia is common. A metallic taste is common during the injection and can be masked by encouraging the patient to chew gum or bite on a lemon rind. Amenorrhea and impaired spermatogenesis occurs and is dose dependent. |

## APPENDIX A   Intravenous Antineoplastic Agents (continued)

| Efficacy | Dosage | Mechanism of Action | Metabolism | Administration Precautions | Side Effects and Special Precautions |
|---|---|---|---|---|---|
| MELPHALAN (Alkeran, L-PAM, L-Phenylalanine Mustard) | | | | | |
| Multiple myeloma Epithelial carcinoma of the ovary Bone marrow transplant | IV: 16 mg/m² every 3 weeks for 4 doses then every 4 weeks ORAL: 2 mg/kg/day for 5 days every 4–6 weeks BMT: 50–60 mg/m² IV | Alkylating agent; cycle specific Forms DNA cross-links | 80%–90% of the drug is bound to plasma proteins 10%–15% of the drug is eliminated unchanged in the urine. t1/2 = 1.5–4 hours | Reconstitute with 10 ml of supplied diluent for a concentration = 5 mg/ml. Dilute in NS to a concentration of 0.45 mg/ml and use within 60 min. Do not refrigerate reconstituted product. When taken orally peak plasma levels are reached within 2 hours. The drug is poorly absorbed when taken with food. | Myelosuppression is the DLT. GI: mild anorexia, nausea and vomiting when taken orally. Nausea and vomiting can be severe with higher IV doses. Mucositis, diarrhea, and oral ulceration occur infrequently. Leukopenia and thrombocytopenia peak at 2–3 weeks and may be cumulative with a prolonged recovery period of 6 or more weeks. Pruritus, dermatitis, and rash may occur. Alopecia is not common with oral dosing. Amenorrhea and oligospermia are common. Second malignancies (leukemias) have been reported. |
| METHOTREXATE (MTX, Mexate, amethopterin) | | | | | |
| Trophoblastic neoplasms Acute leukemias Meningeal leukemias Carcinoma of the breast Osteogenic sarcoma Burkitt's lymphoma | 15–30 mg/day for 5 days or 20–30 mg/m² twice weekly. Single doses of 1.5–20 gm/m² with leucovorin rescue. Intrathecal dosing 10–15 mg in 7–15 ml of preservative-free saline. | MTX tightly binds to dihydrofolate reductase thereby blocking the reduction of dihydrofolate to tetrahydrofolic acid, the active form of folic acid. This process effectively arrests DNA, RNA, and protein synthesis. Antimetabolite; cell-cycle specific for the S-phase of the cell cycle. | MTX is distributed freely in water, which means that it will circulate in third space fluid increasing the toxicity of the drug since it is not being metabolized. Patients with effusions or ascites should be monitored carefully to avoid severe toxicity. MTX is highly protein bound and should not be given with acids that may compete for binding (elimination) sites which would increase the AUC of the MTX, resulting in extreme toxicity. 90% of MTX is eliminated from the kidneys in the urine as unchanged drug. BUN and creatinine levels should be | Lower doses (<100mg) are usually given IVP without leucovorin rescue. When given with 5-FU for breast cancer the methotrexate dose is followed in one hour by the 5-FU. The drugs are synergistic when given this way. Leucovorin rescue is needed because the dose of MTX is generally > 100 mg. Preservative-free MTX used for intrathecal injection should be prepared just prior to use. Protect infusions from light. | Myelosuppression is the DLT. Leukopenia is dose-dependent and is more likely to occur with prolonged exposure. Nausea and vomiting are common with higher doses. Diarrhea can be dose limiting. Stomatitis is more common with higher doses and more lengthy infusions. Skin erythema, hyperpigmentation, photosensitivity, rash, folliculitis, and pruritus may occur. MTX can cause enhanced radiation side effects if given simultaneously. Renal dysfunction is dose-related and |

(continued)

**APPENDIX A**   Intravenous Antineoplastic Agents (continued)

| Efficacy | Dosage | Mechanism of Action | Metabolism | Administration Precautions | Side Effects and Special Precautions |
|---|---|---|---|---|---|
| | | | monitored regularly. If there is evidence of renal impairment lower doses should be given with leucovorin rescue. | | more common in patients who are dehydrated. When given in higher doses the patients urine pH must be > 7 to prevent precipitation of the MTX in the renal tubules with subsequent renal damage. Administer bicarb as directed. The BUN and creatinine are monitored prior to high-dose therapy. Neurological dysfunction can occur with intrathecal administration, especially if cranial radiation has also been given. Photophobia, excessive lacrimation, and conjunctivitis have been noted. |

MITOMYCIN (Mutamycin, mitomycin C)

| Efficacy | Dosage | Mechanism of Action | Metabolism | Administration Precautions | Side Effects and Special Precautions |
|---|---|---|---|---|---|
| Adenocarcinoma of the stomach, pancreas Cancer of the bladder, breast | 20 mg/m² as a single dose repeated every 6–8 weeks For bladder instillation: 20–40 mg is mixed with 20–40 ml of water or saline and is given every 1–2 weeks | Antitumor antibiotic Active during the G₁ and S-phase of the cell cycle. Disrupts DNA synthesis secondary to alkylation. | Mitomycin is inactivated by microsomal enzymes in the liver and is metabolized in the spleen and kidneys. 10%–30% of the drug is eliminated unchanged in the urine. t1/2 = .5–1 hour | Reconstitute in sterile water. 10 ml in 5 mg vial = 0.5 mg/ml. Use within 3 hours. Mitomycin is a severe vesicant. Administer with caution. Give IV push through the side arm of a freely running IV to minimize venous irritation. Assess for a blood return every 1 ml of drug. Discontinue the injection immediately if the patient complains of pain or burning. Mitomycin can cause tissue damage without evidence of drug infiltration. Skin ulceration may occur at sites distant from the site of drug administration. | Myelosuppression is the DLT. Leukopenia and thrombocytopenia occur late at 4–5 weeks with recovery at 7–8 weeks. Both are cumulative. Anemia and hemolytic–uremic syndrome have been reported. Nausea and vomiting are mild. Alopecia is mild, photosensitivity, skin rash, and pruritus are uncommon. Veno-occlusive disease of the liver with abdominal pain, hepatomegaly, and liver failure occur in patients receiving mitomycin and BMT. Pulmonary fibrosis has been reported. |

MITOXANTRONE (Novantrone)

| Efficacy | Dosage | Mechanism of Action | Metabolism | Administration Precautions | Side Effects and Special Precautions |
|---|---|---|---|---|---|
| Acute monocytic leukemia AML | 10–12 mg/m²/day for 5 days for induction of acute nonlymphocytic | Antitumor antibiotic Intercalates into DNA; disrupts cell division | Metabolized in the liver and excreted in the bile and urine | Dark blue solution in vials; Dilute in at least 50 ml D5W or NS. | Leukopenia is the DLT. Nausea and vomiting are mild and |

**APPENDIX A** Intravenous Antineoplastic Agents (continued)

| Efficacy | Dosage | Mechanism of Action | Metabolism | Administration Precautions | Side Effects and Special Precautions |
|---|---|---|---|---|---|
| Acute promyelocytic leukemia<br>Breast cancer<br>Primary hepatocellular carcinoma | leukemia; 12 mg/m² every 3–4 weeks | | t1/2 = 24–37 hours | Stable for 7 days at room temperature.<br><br>Administer IV over at least 5 minutes as an infusion. | preventable. Alopecia is common. Diarrhea and stomatitis may occur.<br><br>Cumulative cardiomyopathy can occur. Monitoring the left ventricular ejection fraction is indicated, especially in patients who are at risk for heart disease or who have received adriamycin in the past.<br><br>Blue discoloration of the sclera may occur. The urine may remain blue-green for 48 hours following treatment. |

PACLITAXEL (Taxol)

| Efficacy | Dosage | Mechanism of Action | Metabolism | Administration Precautions | Side Effects and Special Precautions |
|---|---|---|---|---|---|
| Ovarian carcinoma<br>Breast cancer<br>Non-small cell lung cancer | 200–250 mg/m² every 3 weeks or in heavily pretreated patients 135–170 mg/m² every 3 weeks. | Promotes assembly of microtubules and stabilizes them, thereby blocking mitosis. Taxol also prevents transition of the cell from $G_0$-phase to S-phase by blocking cellular response to growth factors. | The majority of Taxol is protein bound. Elimination is primarily hepatic. Minimal renal excretion<br>t1/2 = 1.3–8 hours | Formulated in 50% polyoxyethylated castor oil (Cremophor EL) and 50% dehydrated alcohol.<br><br>Administer only in glass bottles or non-PVC containers (polyolefin containers using polyethylene-lined nitroglycerin tubing sets). Cremophor containing solutions will leach the plasticizer DEHP from polyvinyl chloride containers. DEHP can cause liver toxicity.<br><br>Inline filtration is needed (.02micron) due to the natural origins of the drug.<br><br>Administration rate varies from 1–3 hours to 24–96 hours. In general the longer the infusion, the more likely the patient will experience myelosuppression that is dose-limiting.<br><br>Hypersensitivity reactions can occur with Taxol infusion and are thought to be related to the Cremophor EL. Patients are premedicated with | Hypersensitivity reactions occur infrequently with proper premedication. Most HSR occur within the first or second dosing. Symptoms include dyspnea, urticaria, flushing, and hypotension. Dose-limiting toxicity is myelosuppression. Leukopenic nadir occurs 7–10 days after dosing with recovery at 15 days. Anemia and thrombocytopenia occur less frequently.<br><br>Peripheral neuropathy occurs more commonly in patients who are also receiving cisplatin. Hyperesthesias and burning pain in the feet may also occur. Myalgias and arthralgias occur usually 3–4 days after dosing.<br><br>Alopecia is complete at 3 weeks.<br><br>Mucositis occurs more commonly with prolonged infusions. Nausea and vomiting are mild. Diarrhea occurs infrequently. |

*(continued)*

**APPENDIX A**    Intravenous Antineoplastic Agents (continued)

| Efficacy | Dosage | Mechanism of Action | Metabolism | Administration Precautions | Side Effects and Special Precautions |
|---|---|---|---|---|---|
| | | | | dexamethasone 20 mg at 13 and 7 hours prior to treatment; Diphenhydramine 50 mg IV 30 min. prior and an H2 blocker (cimetidine 300 mg or pepcid 20 mg) 30 min. prior. | Taxol is an irritant but can cause blistering and skin breakdown if large amounts of more concentrated drug are infiltrated. |
| | | | | When administering Taxol with doxorubicin the doxorubicin is given first; likewise when Taxol is given with cisplatin or carboplatin the Taxol is given first to avoid disruption in the elimination of the platinum compound and enhanced toxicity. | |

TENIPOSIDE (Vumon, VM-26)

| Efficacy | Dosage | Mechanism of Action | Metabolism | Administration Precautions | Side Effects and Special Precautions |
|---|---|---|---|---|---|
| Relapsed or refractory acute lymphoblastic leukemia Small-cell lung cancer | 100 mg/m² 1–2 times weekly and 20–60 mg/m² for 5 days or 90 mg/m²/day for 5 days for lung cancer | Plant alkaloid, topoisomerase II inhibitor Phase specific, acts in late S-phase and early $G_2$ phase | Bound to plasma protein, metabolized in the liver with less than 10% of the unchanged drug in feces. Eliminated in the urine. t1/2 = 20 hours | Dosage is diluted in sodium chloride and is physically stable for approximately 24 hours at room temperature in glass containers. Drug may precipitate in plastic containers. Administer over at least a 45 min. period to avoid severe hypotension. Avoid extravasation. Local phlebitis may occur. HSR occur and include blood pressure changes, bronchospasm, tachycardia, urticaria, facial flushing, diaphoresis, periorbital edema, vomiting, and/or fever. | Leukopenia is the DLT occurring at 10–14 days. Nausea and vomiting are rare. Alopecia occurs gradually; skin rash is rare. With high-dose therapy severe skin rashes can occur. Hemolytic anemia with renal failure has occurred. HSR may be related to the Cremophor EL vehicle. Secondary malignancies occur infrequently. Hyperbilirubinemia, SGOT, and SGPT elevations can occur. |

THIOTEPA

| Efficacy | Dosage | Mechanism of Action | Metabolism | Administration Precautions | Side Effects and Special Precautions |
|---|---|---|---|---|---|
| Breast cancer Ovarian cancer Superficial bladder cancer Lymphoma Hodgkin's disease | 12–16 mg/m² every 1–4 weeks 900 mg/m² (transplant dose) 30–60 mg every week for 4 weeks for intravesicular 1–10 mg/m² 1–2 times per week for intrathecal use. | An alkylating agent similiar to nitrogen mustard | Variably absorbed through the bladder mucosa following intravesical injection. Metabolized in the liver. t1/2 = 2–3 hours | 15 mg vial is reconstituted with 1.5 ml of sterile water and further diluted with saline for intrathecal use (preservative free). Intravenous and intravesical solutions may be diluted with saline, D5W, or lactated Ringer's solution and are chemically stable for at | Myelosuppression is the DLT and may be cumulative. Leukopenia occurs 7–10 days postinjection. Thrombocytopenia may be delayed. Nausea and vomiting are not common in nontransplant doses. |

**APPENDIX A** Intravenous Antineoplastic Agents (continued)

| Efficacy | Dosage | Mechanism of Action | Metabolism | Administration Precautions | Side Effects and Special Precautions |
|---|---|---|---|---|---|
| | | | | least 5 days in the refrigerator and 24 hours at room temperature.<br><br>Intravesical instillation involves placement of a catheter in the bladder and instillation of the drug with retention of the liquid for up to 2 hours. The patient is repositioned every 15 min. to maximize exposure to the tissues of the bladder.<br><br>Intrathecal doses are mixed in up to 20 ml of Ringer's lactate to maximize CNS distribution.<br><br>Intravenous administration may be given IVP or as an infusion. Thiotepa is not a vesicant. | Stomatitis may be severe in transplant doses.<br><br>Abdominal pain, hematuria, dysuria, frequency, and urgency occur with intravesical instillation.<br><br>Second malignancies have been reported. |

### TOPOTECAN (Hycamtin)

| Efficacy | Dosage | Mechanism of Action | Metabolism | Administration Precautions | Side Effects and Special Precautions |
|---|---|---|---|---|---|
| Small-cell lung cancer<br>Ovarian cancer<br>Esophageal cancer | 1.3–1.6 mg/m² IV infusion over 30 min., 2 hours, or 24 hours; or 1.5–2 mg/m² daily as a 30 min. infusion daily for 5 days. | Topoisomerase I inihibitor causing single strand breaks in DNA causing the cell to die during DNA replication | Up to 48% of the drug is eliminated unchanged in the urine.<br>t1/2 = 3 hours | 5 mg vial is reconstituted with 2 ml of sterile water and diluted in D5W. Stable for up to 48 hours at room temperature. Given intravenously as an infusion. | Leukopenia is the DLT and the nadir occurs at day 10–12 with recovery at 3 weeks.<br><br>Thrombocytopenia and anemia occur but are not usually dose-limiting.<br><br>Mild to moderate nausea and vomiting may occur. Diarrhea has been reported to occur during or shortly after the infusion.<br><br>Fever and mild flu-like symptoms are reported.<br><br>Alopecia and skin rash may occur.<br><br>Elevated LFTs are common. Headache, dizziness, lightheadedness, and peripheral neuropathy have been reported. |

(continued)

## APPENDIX A   Intravenous Antineoplastic Agents (continued)

| Efficacy | Dosage | Mechanism of Action | Metabolism | Administration Precautions | Side Effects and Special Precautions |
|---|---|---|---|---|---|
| VINBLASTINE (Velban) | | | | | |
| Hodgkin's disease<br>Non-Hodgkin's lymphoma<br>Testis cancer<br>Kaposi's sarcoma<br>Breast cancer<br>Melanoma<br>Cancers of the kidney, bladder, and cervix<br>Head and neck cancers<br>Lung cancer<br>Ovarian cancer | 6–10 mg/m$^2$ every 2–4 weeks; 1.7–2 mg/m$^2$/day weekly as a continuous infusion or over a period of 96 hours | Cell-cycle phase specific for the M phase—a plant alkaloid that binds to tubulin causing inhibition of the microtubule assembly which inhibits mitotic spindle formation. | Metabolized by the liver. Less than 1% is eliminated unchanged in the urine.<br>t1/2 = 20 hours | Reconstituted with 10 ml of bacteriostatic normal saline to yield a concentration of 1 mg/ml. Dose may be further diluted with D5W or normal saline for continuous infusion.<br><br>Continuous infusions may only be given through central lines because vinblastine is a severe vesicant if infiltrated.<br><br>Store in the refrigerator. Stable for 14 days at room temperature and 30 days under refrigeration. | Leukopenia is the DLT. Thrombocytopenia and anemia are less common.<br><br>Nausea and vomiting, anorexia, diarrhea, and mucositis are rare.<br><br>Peripheral neuropathy, constipation, paralytic ileus, and urinary retention may occur.<br><br>Alopecia occurs with higher doses.<br><br>Rash and photosensitivity may occur.<br><br>Infiltration may cause ulceration depending on the amount of drug extravasated.<br><br>Treatment with hyaluronidase and heat may minimize ulceration.<br><br>Incompatible with heparin and furosemide.<br><br>Compatible in solution with doxorubicin, metoclopramide, dacarbazine, and bleomycin. |
| VINCRISTINE (Oncovin) | | | | | |
| Acute leukemia<br>Hodgkin's disease<br>Non-Hodgkin's lymphoma<br>Rhabdomyosarcoma<br>Neuroblastoma<br>Wilms' tumor<br>Ewing's sarcoma<br>Melanoma<br>Multiple myeloma<br>Breast cancer<br>Lung cancer | .5–1.4 mg/m$^2$ every 1–4 weeks<br>Continuous infusion regimens of 0.5 mg/day–0.5 mg/m$^2$/d for 4 days may be used. | Plant alkaloid. Binds to tubulin causing inhibition of microtubule assembly which inhibits mitotic spindle formation. M phase specific. | Metabolized by the liver. 40%–70% excreted in the bile.<br>t1/2 = 70–100 hours | Store in the refrigerator. Stable for at least 30 days at room temperature. Doses for continuous infusion are further diluted with normal saline or D5W. Compatible with doxorubicin, bleomycin, cytarabine, fluorouracil, methotrexate, and metoclopramide.<br><br>Vincristine is a vesicant that should be given with caution and through a central line | Myelosuppression is mild. Nausea, vomiting, anorexia, and diarrhea are rare.<br><br>Constipation and abdominal pain may occur due to the neurological toxicity of the drug.<br><br>Prophylactic stool softeners and laxatives may be indicated in patients at high risk for constipation.<br><br>Alopecia is minimal. Paresthesias, ataxia, hoarseness, |

**APPENDIX A**  Intravenous Antineoplastic Agents (continued)

| Efficacy | Dosage | Mechanism of Action | Metabolism | Administration Precautions | Side Effects and Special Precautions |
|---|---|---|---|---|---|
| | | | | when given as a continuous infusion.<br><br>Hyaluronidase plus heat to disperse the antidote are indicated if the drug should infiltrate.<br><br>Greater than 2 mg total dose is usually contraindicated due to the toxicity of the drug.<br><br>Vincristine is lethal if given intrathecally and should be labeled as such when dispensed by the pharmacist.<br><br>Administer with caution in patients with obvious liver dysfunction. | myalgias, headache, and seizures may occur.<br><br>Severe pain in the jaw may occur. |

VINORELBINE TARTRATE (Navelbine)

| Efficacy | Dosage | Mechanism of Action | Metabolism | Administration Precautions | Side Effects and Special Precautions |
|---|---|---|---|---|---|
| Breast cancer<br>Ovarian cancer<br>Head and neck cancer<br>Esophageal cancer<br>Nonsmall cell lung cancer<br>Lung cancer<br>Germ cell cancers<br>Hodgkin's disease | Oral: 40 mg capsule for oral use (investigational)<br>IV: 30–40mg/m² weekly | Cell-cycle specific produces cell blockade in $G_2$ and M phase.<br>Blocks polymerization of microtubules.<br>Impairs mitotic spindle. | Hepatic elimination<br>Binds to plasma proteins<br>Nonrenal elimination | Venous irritation occurs in about 25% of patients. Symptoms include erythema and pain at the site, vein discoloration and tenderness along the vein.<br>Administer drug over 6–10 minutes through the side arm of a freely running IV. Inject through the port furthest from the IV site.<br>Follow injection with 75–125 cc of IV fluid to flush the line (peripheral IV sites only). Local tissue damage/necrosis, phlebitis may occur if the drug infiltrates.<br>Dose reduction may be appropriate for patients with impaired liver function: If bilirubin is >2.1 the dose of navelbine is reduced 50%–75% (i.e., 15–7.5 mg/m²).<br>Pain at the tumor site can occur during administration.<br>Navelbine is compatible with metoclopramide, ondansetron, chlorpromazine, promethazine, and dexamethasone.<br>Navelbine is | DLT: Noncumulative neutropenia<br><br>Alopecia/hair thinning after several treatments<br><br>Anorexia<br><br>Asthenia<br><br>Peripheral neuropathy<br><br>Constipation occurs in about ⅓ of patients and increases after several treatments.<br><br>Fatigue can be cumulative.<br><br>Arthralgias and myalgias<br><br>Rash (rare)<br><br>Typhlitis with abdominal pain and fever occur 3–4 days after treatment in heavily pretreated patients.<br><br>Jaw pain is rare. |

*(continued)*

**APPENDIX A**   Intravenous Antineoplastic Agents (continued)

| Efficacy | Dosage | Mechanism of Action | Metabolism | Administration Precautions | Side Effects and Special Precautions |
|----------|--------|---------------------|------------|----------------------------|--------------------------------------|
|          |        |                     |            | incompatible with 5-fluorouracil, thiotepa, furosemide, amphotericin, ampicillin, piperacillin, aminophyllin, and sodium bicarbonate. |  |

Key: HSR: hypersensitivity reaction; DTL: dose-limiting toxicity; CHF: congestive heart failure; MI: myocardial infarction; AUC: area under the curve; SIADH: syndrome of inappropriate antidiuretic hormone; q: every; IP: intraperitoneal; IT: intrathecal; LFT: liver function test; t1/2: half-life; CI: continuous infusion

Data from Chabner B and Longo D (eds);[97] Barton-Burke M (ed);[98] Dorr R and VonHoff DD (eds);[99] and Fischer DS, Knobf MT, and Durivage HJ (eds).[99]

# Chapter 16

# Chemotherapy: Toxicity Management

**Dawn Camp-Sorrell, RN, MSN, AOCN, FNP**

# INTRODUCTION

Chemotherapy is administered based on a dose-response relationship (i.e., the more drug administered, the more cancer cells killed). Characteristically, these agents have a narrow therapeutic index, with anticipated acute toxicities expressed in rapidly dividing normal tissues, such as the bone marrow, the gastrointestinal (GI) tract, the gonads, and the hair follicles. Acute and long-term toxicities from chemotherapy may also be a function of the drug's effect on specific cells of a given organ. The incidence and severity of toxicities are related to the drug's dosage, administration schedule, specific mechanism of action, concomitant illness, and specific measures employed to prevent or minimize toxicities. Chemotherapeutic agents cause side effects that can appear immediately or after a few days (acute), within a few weeks (intermediate), or months to years after chemotherapy administration (long term).[1]

Since virtually every organ is affected by chemotherapy, the toxicities of the drug will commonly determine the maximum amount of drug that can be administered safely. Side effects such as stomatitis, alopecia, myelosuppression, nausea, vomiting, anorexia, and diarrhea are common, depending on the agent administered.[2] These are expected side effects that can be managed effectively, and generally do not warrant reducing the dose or discontinuing the drug. *Toxic* effects refer to life-threatening, often dose-limiting effects characteristic of high dosages. Cumulative and irreversible damage to certain vital organs, such as the heart, limits the total dosage of chemotherapy.[3]

Providing nursing care to the patient receiving chemotherapy presents many challenges. Interventions focus on preventing or minimizing side effects caused by the chemotherapeutic agent. The key is to assess accurately the patient's status and to complete a health history to detect risk factors before initiating therapy that provides baseline data.[2] After the patient begins treatment, it is important to assess any changes from the baseline and to evaluate the effectiveness of interventions implemented.

# PRETREATMENT EVALUATION: RISK ANALYSIS

Individuals with an overall weak physical condition and poor nutritional status are not likely to tolerate a vigorous treatment course.[3] Patients previously treated with multiple chemotherapy agents, radiation, or immunotherapy may lack marrow reserve, placing them at a higher risk for infection, bleeding, or anemia. The inability or unwillingness of an individual to perform self-care may increase the severity of a side effect and also delay the seeking of appropriate care from health care professionals.

Preexisting disorders such as hepatic or renal dysfunction can alter the absorption, distribution, metabolism, and excretion of chemotherapy, causing abnormal accumulations of the drug and its metabolites. Hypovolemia due to nausea/vomiting, diarrhea, inadequate dietary intake, third spacing, or hypoalbuminemia may increase the risk of acute renal failure.[4] Thus the patient could be placed at a higher risk for organ toxicities.

Since the incidence of cancer increases with age, nurses must be aware of possible additional risks for the elderly. Age-related changes in physical stature, body composition, kidneys, liver, and other organs influence the pharmacokinetic and pharmacodynamic properties of drug therapy, possibly prolonging the agent's half-life.[5] Many elderly people, especially those over age 85, are physically frail secondary to chronic and debilitating illness or poor nutrition or as a result of aging. Chronic illnesses such as arthritis, heart disease, diabetes, glaucoma, high blood pressure, cognitive deficits, and hearing and vision loss are common in the elderly. These conditions may interfere with the ability to perform basic activities of daily living and, consequently, elderly patients may be unable to perform preventive measures to minimize side effects.

Gradual but substantial changes occur in body composition with age. The percentage of body fat increases, with a corresponding decrease in muscle mass and percentage of body water. Decreases occur in cardiac output, kidney function, hepatic blood flow, the ability to conjugate drugs, and the effectiveness of the immune system.[5,6] Cardiovascular changes occur including thickening of blood vessel walls, atherosclerotic plaque formation, and loss of elastin fibers which can lead to cardiac hypertrophy, diastolic dysfunction, and myocardia ischemia.[7] With advancing age the kidneys atrophy, bringing subsequent decrease in renal function. Vasoconstriction of the renal vasculature decreases renal blood flow, glomerular filtration rate, and the ability to concentrate/dilute urine, resulting in a decreased creatinine clearance.[4] Bone marrow reserves decrease and the ability to replicate myeloid and erythroid progenitor cells decrease. In addition, the functional ability of peripheral mononuclear cells are impaired.[7,8]

Historically, elderly patients with cancer have not been treated as aggressively as their younger counterparts because it was speculated that the elderly would not be able to tolerate the stresses imposed by chemotherapy. This trend is changing, however, and many elderly patients now receive aggressive treatment for their cancer.[7–17] Numerous studies have looked at the consequences of treating older patients with chemotherapy. Although the study results are often variable and contradictory, the degree of tolerance to chemotherapy has depended on the type of malignancy and dose intensity.

In general, for many solid tumors, geriatric patients tolerate chemotherapy, used either for adjuvant or palliation therapy, as well as young patients.[12] Cisplatin in moderate doses (60 to 100 mg/m²) have been found to be safe in patients >80 years old.[18] Geriatric patients with a systemic malignancy such as lymphoma or acute leukemia usually develop more treatment-related toxicity than younger patients. Leukemia in the elderly is frequently associated with poor prognostic features such as prior preleukemia, myelodysplastic syndrome, and chromosome abnormalities that may place them at an increased risk for toxicities such as infection.[11,13] However, geriatric patients can achieve complete response from chemotherapy if they survive the intensive initial therapy.[12]

A retrospective analysis was conducted on six Eastern Cooperative Oncology Group (ECOG) clinical trials for breast, lung, and colon cancers. Elderly patients were defined as 70 years or older in the lung and colon studies and 60–65 years of age in the breast studies. All patients had normal renal, hepatic, and cardiac function. When compared to nonelderly controls, the incidence of severe toxic reactions in the two groups was comparable.[15]

While it is critical to be knowledgeable regarding the potential problems the elderly may encounter as a consequence of physiological aging, age alone has not been shown to be a significant factor in the incidence and severity of toxicity to chemotherapy.[9,15–17] Chronic illness that often accompanies longevity is a better predictor for tolerance than age alone.[9] The one exception has been hematologic toxicity, probably related to decreased marrow reserve and/or renal function. Health care professionals therefore should monitor hematologic values closely to minimize potential ill effects. Patients older than 70 years of age with normal renal and hepatic function and without serious medical conditions have been found to tolerate chemotherapy as well as individuals in younger populations.[12]

## QUALITY OF LIFE AND CHEMOTHERAPY TOXICITY

Treatment considerations include the patient's quality of life, the impact chemotherapy will have on the patient's quality of life, and the patient's physical as well as mental well-being.[19] Complications or side effects of chemotherapy are weighed against its potential benefits. If tumor control or palliation is the goal, the side effects are weighed against such benefits of chemotherapy as pain control and prolonged survival time.

In the past, cancer treatment was evaluated by tumor response and survival rates rather than by functional ability or quality of life.[20] Quality of life is difficult to measure. It should be based on the physical, psychological, social, and spiritual characteristics of what gives life value to the individual.[21] Currently, there is a movement to recognize and include quality of life as an acceptable end point in clinical trials, which has been influenced by viewing cancer as a chronic condition instead of as an acute event. Groups of cancer survivors have indicated to the health care community that quality of life is as important to the patient as is the overall therapeutic effect.[22]

Physical symptoms can result in significant distress that has a marked impact on the patient's quality of life.[21,23] It is important to realize that the patient's perception of cancer and chemotherapy treatment will influence how the patient reacts and ultimately adapts.[24] Side effects can impair a patient's abilities to function at work or at home, maintain sexual relationships, and engage in social activities. The degree of self-reported symptoms relates to the individual's perceived quality of life such as when an increase in symptoms correlates with a decrease in quality of life.[21] Feelings of helplessness are heightened, since patients are dependent on health care professionals to deliver their treatment. Anxiety can develop at key decision points, such as diagnosis, beginning of treatment, while awaiting test results, when the treatment plan is altered, or when the chemotherapy treatment plan has been successfully completed.[25] Chemotherapy-related changes in physical appearance are often described as a distressing aspect of cancer treatment. Weight changes and alopecia commonly occur and can be especially devastating because they can be viewed as public manifestations of having cancer.[24]

To help the patient cope with potential side effects, a trusting relationship between patient and nurse must be developed so that sufficient information can be provided for the patient to retain control over his or her care. An important aspect of establishing a partnership with the patient and family in the pretreatment phase is knowing what concerns about the treatment need to be explored and what information needs to be provided. Such information helps patients formulate questions about available options when making difficult decisions about their care. Feelings of control are enhanced, resulting in an improved functional status, sense of well-being, and performance of effective self-care.[26] Nurses must focus on developing practical interventions to reduce the psychological distress of treatment and to provide needed information, thereby increasing the patient's quality of life.

## SELF-CARE

There is undeniable evidence that cost factors are dictating health care. Institutional, state, and federal regulatory bodies have assumed increasing jurisdiction over how and where patients will be treated. Diagnostic related groups (DRGs) and prospective payment, cost-control measures by other insurers, and increased out-of-pocket medical expenses by consumers have all combined to create a shift from hospital-based care to outpatient and home care settings.[27] The change from inpatient to outpatient administration of chemotherapy necessitates a shift in responsibility for managing treatment of side effects from health care providers to patients and their families. To facilitate self-care, nurses must understand the nature, incidence, and relative severity of each side effect, as well as being aware of effective self-care activities for reducing the severity of side effects.

Dodd assessed self-care behaviors used for side effects from chemotherapy.[28] Via a self-care behavior questionnaire, 48 patients were asked to indicate how severe the side effects were and what actions were taken to alleviate those side effects. The side effects with the greatest frequency were nausea and vomiting (83%), loss of hair (75%), taste and smell changes (71%), and decreased appetite (69%). Patients initiated self-care most frequently for nausea and vomiting, constipation, and loss of hair.

In an attempt to test patients' self-care behavior, Dodd gave information on side effect management techniques to one of two groups of patients with cancer who were undergoing chemotherapy. Patients who received the information on side effect management reported initiating self-care behaviors with a higher degree of perceived effectiveness than those who did not receive this information. The informed patients also initiated self-care behaviors before side effects became persistent and severe.[29]

In another study, patients and family members were asked to describe self-care behaviors initiated by patients and their family members and to determine the relationship between patients and family members' affective states.[30] Data were collected over three cycles of chemotherapy from 42 patients and 40 family members. The independent variables were affective states (measured by the Profile of Mood Status), family functioning (measured by the Family Crises–Oriented Personal Scales), and self-care behavior (recorded in a Self-Care Behavior Log). Self-care behavior was defined as any activity initiated by patient, family, or friends to alleviate a side effect from chemotherapy.

Side effects reported most frequently were nausea (90%), fatigue (65%), vomiting (62%), mouth sores (31%), and weakness (31%). Patients did not delay in initiating self-care behaviors more than 24 hours, especially if a family member was present to help. However, with increasing severity of the side effect, patients became more immobilized, and delayed initiating self-care behaviors up to several days. The patients' mood disturbances were greater than the family members' during all three cycles, but the differences were more marked at the initiation of chemotherapy and decreased over time. These studies recommend that follow-up from the nurse be initiated at least one to three days postchemotherapy to assess the patients and to determine if side effects were being managed adequately. In addition, the studies concluded that patient education is essential to ensure that the patient and family understand what self-care measures need to be taken for side effects experienced.

Two other studies[31,32] evaluated the relationship between individual side effects and distress from chemotherapy using standard scales. Nausea, hair loss, and tiredness were reported by more than 80% of patients as the most distressing symptoms. Vomiting was reported by 54%. The degree of distress reported by individuals correlated with the number of side effects experienced. Thus, a cumulative effect from experiencing several side effects had a greater impact on the patients' daily activities and quality of life.

Nail et al studied the incidence of side effects from chemotherapy and the use of self-care activities, using a closed-ended approach provided by a self-care diary.[33] A total of 49 patients receiving chemotherapy on an outpatient basis were asked to complete the self-care diary on the second and fifth days after treatment. The self-care diary included a list of side effects that the patient might experience from chemotherapy, and self-care activities that the patient might initiate to minimize individual side effects. Although there were 24 different drug combinations used, the most common regimens included 5-fluorouracil, cyclophosphamide, methotrexate, and doxorubicin.

Fatigue was the most frequently reported side effect (81%). Sleeping difficulty, nausea, and decreased appetite each were reported by approximately 50% of the subjects. The majority of side effects were rated as moderately severe, with the highest severity rating being for hair loss, followed closely by fatigue. Self-care activities used to gauge fatigue included obtaining extra sleep by napping, going to bed earlier, or sleeping later. The most effective activity for dealing with nausea was taking antinausea medication. The majority of patients' self-care activities were rated as slightly to moderately helpful. The authors recommend that nurses prepare patients for the occurrence of fatigue and review self-care activities directed to combating fatigue. Also, patients should be encouraged to use prescribed antiemetics.

This study also found that some patients believed that side effects from chemotherapy had to be endured. This was reinforced by health care professionals who did not tell patients what actions could be taken to alleviate the side effects. Several patients believed that if the interventions suggested did not alleviate the side effects, there were no other alternatives. These authors concluded that health care professionals either are not providing adequate information or are providing information in a form that the patient cannot absorb, retain, and recall when needed.[33]

Self-care activities are initiated pretreatment and are used throughout the treatment phase. Self-care activities are intended to manage or minimize chemotherapy side effects. In situations where patients are unable to participate or are unwilling, efforts must be made to include family members or visiting nurses to ensure compliance. Without compliance, the side effects could be severe and lead to further complications. Hospitalization and death may be the consequences of side effects that are not managed effectively.[30] From the studies just described it appears that the side effects that seem to be the most distressing to patients include fatigue, nausea, vomiting, alopecia, anorexia, and mouth sores. Nurses must continue to develop effective strategies to assist patients in minimizing these effects. Documenting effective strategies that have been successful, including those suggested by the patients, can serve as a useful resource for future teachings.

## PATIENT EDUCATION AND FOLLOW-UP

Although teaching may be initiated while the patient is still hospitalized, most teaching regarding chemotherapy takes place in the outpatient setting and is provided by the nurse who will administer the drugs. The intent of teaching is more than to give information; it provides support and knowledge to empower the patient to manage self-care effectively.[34,35] For patient education to be most effective, it should begin early in the diagnostic phase and serve as a guide throughout treatments and follow-up care. Teaching patients about their treatment reduces fear, increases self-confidence, improves compliance, and enhances their participation in self-care.[34] The nurse is in a valuable position to identify what the patient needs to know about managing chemotherapy side effects and what resources are available to augment those teachings.

One approach to identifying the informational needs of the patients and family members is to focus on the various phases of cancer care: diagnosis, treatment, rehabilitation, survivorship, and recurrent disease. Goals of chemotherapy teaching include:

1. helping the patient adjust to the treatment
2. explaining how the treatment will affect the cancer
3. imparting the sequence of administration
4. recognizing and controlling side effects
5. encouraging self-care behaviors that minimize the side effects
6. listing side effects pertinent to report to the health care professional

All information offered to the patient must be documented in the patient's record (see Figure 16-1), for future reference as well as to comply with professional regulations.

An earlier study by Dodd indicated that despite the efforts of health care professionals, patients are not absorbing and retaining the information they need.[34] It was not uncommon for patients to attribute the majority of their symptoms to chemotherapy regardless of other medical conditions or medicines used. The symptoms most frequently attributed incorrectly to chemotherapy were nervousness, irritability, insomnia, and numbness/tingling of hands and feet. In conclusion the author stressed the importance of reinforcing teachings periodically, since retention without reinforcement is short-lived.

In the outpatient setting the nurse very frequently screens phone calls and triages the patient to assist in evaluating symptomatology and initiating the appropriate treatment measures. Most patient problems can be managed without the patient's needing to be seen on an emergency basis. It is important, however, for the nurse to be able to gather sufficient data to determine whether the patient needs medical intervention, and if so whether the patient will be cared for most appropriately in the outpatient setting or whether the patient needs emergency care. Figure 16-2 is a phone triage flow sheet listing basic steps that might be appropriate in managing patient problems over the phone. Obviously, the nurse needs to be highly knowledgeable about the patient's history, the last chemotherapy treatment, and whether this complaint is related to the treatment, and/or the disease, or is unrelated.

Objective and subjective data must be gathered methodically in order to formulate an opinion regarding the patient's deposition. After consulting with the physician, the nurse once again speaks to the patient, either to gather more information or to relay instructions to the patient and/or family regarding care. Examples of specific phone triage flow sheets are included in the discussion of various chemotherapy side effects later in the chapter.

## CHEMOTHERAPY TOXICITIES

### Grading of Toxicities

Standardization of assessment and documentation of side effects are crucial in evaluating the therapeutic use of chemotherapy.[36] Specific therapies can be assessed by comparing their benefits with toxicity occurrence. To assess toxicity, the following information should be included in relation to chemotherapy administration:[37]

1. which toxicities occurred
2. toxicity severity
3. time of onset
4. duration of the effect
5. interventions incorporated to minimize the effect

It is important in the recognition and evaluation of toxicities to be able to discriminate between an expected versus a toxic reaction from chemotherapy and to distinguish these from the complications related to the cancer. For example, if a patient with lymphoma presents to the clinic with a complaint of paresthesias, numbness, and tingling, the patient must be evaluated for possible spinal cord compression from tumor progression versus peripheral toxicity from vincristine administration.

Using specific parameters and operational definitions to define the degree of a given toxicity ensures consistency in documenting observed reactions (see Table 16-1). Toxicity grading scales have been developed by the World Health Organization and various cooperative study groups to provide consistency in reporting. Adequate assessment and documentation of the side effect experienced, the patient's overall response to the regimen, and

CHEMOTHERAPY TEACHING CHECKLIST

Assessment Summary: _____

_____

_____

_____

_____

_____

Patient
name: _____
Primary
nurse: _____

Drugs: _____

_____

_____

| LEARNING NEED | TEACHING INITIATED (DATE & INITIALS) | KNOWLEDGE CONFIRMED (DATE & INITIALS) | COMMENTS |
|---|---|---|---|
| 1. Patient education booklets/drug cards | | | |
| 2. Viewed chemotherapy video<br>Other: | | | |
| 3. Common side effects and treatment | | | |
| a. Nausea and vomiting—antiemetics | | | |
| b. Stomatitis—mouth care | | | |
| c. Alopecia—wigs/scarves | | | |
| d. Decreased white blood cells—infection precaution | | | |
| e. Decreased red blood cells—fatigue | | | |
| f. Decreased platelets—bleeding precaution | | | |
| g. Skin changes—hygienic needs | | | |
| h. Loss of appetite—nutrition | | | |
| i. Diarrhea—medication/diet | | | |
| j. Constipation—diet/medication | | | |
| k. Flu-like symptoms | | | |
| l. Urine discoloration | | | |
| m. Hemorrhagic cystitis | | | |
| n. Other | | | |
| 4. Specific teaching | | | |
| a. Subcutaneous injections | | | |
| b. Maintaining adequate nutrition | | | |
| c. Precautions to report during drug administration: | | | |
| (1) Stinging, burning pain | | | |
| (2) Flushing of face | | | |
| (3) Metallic taste | | | |
| (4) Feeling of numbness | | | |
| (5) Itching at site (or generalized itching) | | | |
| (6) Allergic reactions | | | |

**FIGURE 16-1** Chemotherapy teaching checklist.

| LEARNING NEED | TEACHING INITIATED (DATE & INITIALS) | KNOWLEDGE CONFIRMED (DATE & INITIALS) | COMMENTS |
|---|---|---|---|
| d. Reproductive changes<br>   *Dyspareunia<br>   *Menopausal symptoms | | | |
| e. Activity | | | |
| f. Interaction with other drugs/food | | | |
| g. Vascular access device | | | |
| h. Perineal burning (Decadron) | | | |
| 5. Symptoms to report to physician: | | | |
| a. Bleeding | | | |
| b. Prolonged nausea or vomiting | | | |
| c. Fever/chills | | | |
| d. Stomatitis | | | |
| e. Diarrhea/constipation | | | |
| f. Numbness or tingling of extremities | | | |
| g. Difficulty breathing or shortness of breath | | | |
| h. Other | | | |
| 6. Prescriptions given to patient with<br>Instructions: □ Antiemetics _____<br>□ Wig □ Blood counts □ Other | | | |
| 7. Schedule of drug treatment | | | |
| 8. Instructions to obtain blood counts | | | |
| 9. Follow-up or referral to community<br>resources | | | |

Comments: _____

_____

_____

_____

Patient signature: _____

RN signature: _____

RN signature: _____

**FIGURE 16-1** Chemotherapy teaching checklist (continued).

subsequent quality of life can be essential for evaluating the impact of treatment. Decisions regarding the need for appropriate adjustments in the treatment plan can be determined on the basis of sound, objective data documented by the nurse.[38]

Specific guidelines need to be taught and to be given in written form to the patient and caregiver to ensure they report any type of toxicity. Misinterpretation of the patient's report can make a significant difference in changes made in the treatment protocol. Nurses will continue to be challenged to design effective assessment and documentation systems that ensure accurate patient ob-

servation and reporting of toxicities, especially in the home setting.

## Systemic Toxicities

### Bone marrow suppression

Myelosuppression is not only the most common dose-limiting side effect of chemotherapy but also potentially the most lethal.[39–42] All hematopoietic cells divide rapidly, regardless of their developmental stage, and are therefore

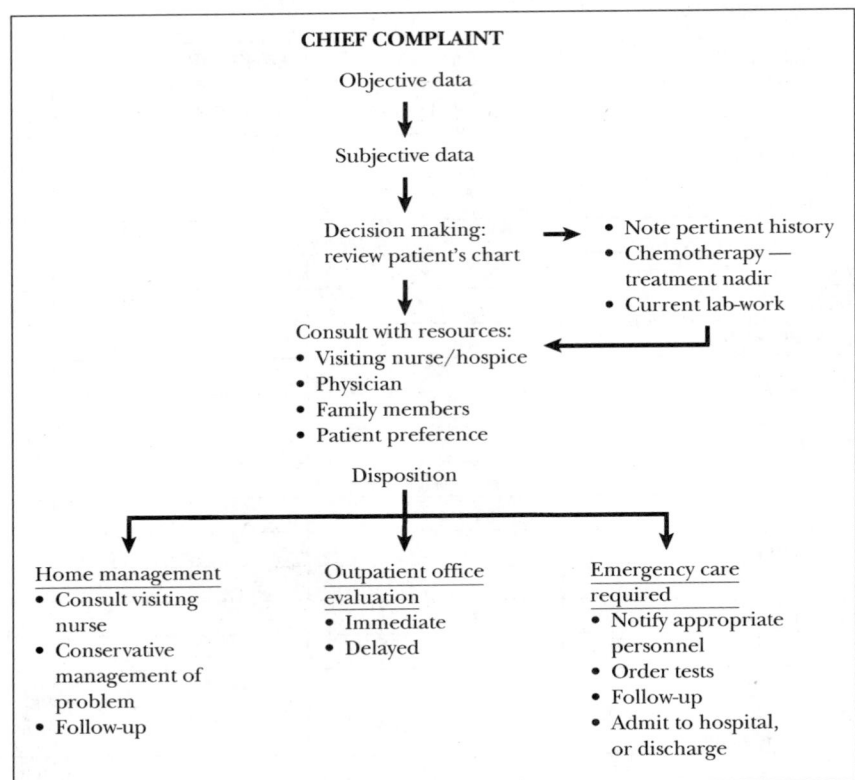

**FIGURE 16-2** Phone triage flow sheet.

vulnerable to chemotherapy. Proliferating progenitor cells that produce the mature granulocytes, erythrocytes, and thrombocytes in the peripheral circulation are commonly destroyed. As immature cells in the marrow and preexisting mature cells are destroyed, the nadir becomes apparent, usually 7–14 days after chemotherapy. At the same time, cells in the bone marrow are maturing and are ready to be released into the peripheral blood. Within a short period of time (three to four weeks) the nadir will resolve.[42] However, when high doses are administered, the stem cell population may fail to repopulate quickly enough, resulting in a prolonged nadir period.

The majority of chemotherapy drugs cause some degree of myelosuppression.[40] Agents most active against cells that are cycling or those active during a specific phase of the cell cycle can produce rapid cytopenia. Because alkylating agents and nitrosoureas affect cycling cells as well as noncycling cells, these drugs are more likely to destroy the marrow stem cells. Antimetabolites, vinca alkaloids, and antitumor antibiotics are most damaging to cells that are in a specific phase of the cell cycle; thus, myelosuppression is less severe with these agents.[43] However, dose intensification and drug combinations can produce severe and prolonged neutropenia. For many drugs myelosuppression can be the dose-limiting toxicity, especially for newer agents such as paclitaxel, docetaxel, vinorelbine, and gemcitabine.[44–50] Paclitaxel can cause neutropenia with the severity dependent on the adminis-

tration schedule, dose, extent of previous treatment, and pharmacological exposure to the drug. Although preliminary data reveal that three-hour infusion induces less neutropenia, the neutropenic effect is not cumulative and permanent toxicity does not occur to the bone marrow. Gemcitibine can cause myelosuppression, especially thrombocytopenia. The hematologic toxicity has been found to be cumulative with the maximum tolerated dose of 1500 mg/m²/week over a 30 minute infusion. Docetaxel results in an early short-lasting type of neutropenia at a dose of 100 mg/m² or greater when infused over one hour every three weeks. The nadir usually occurs at the eighth day and resolves in one to two weeks, which has not been found to be a cumulative effect.

Younger patients are more tolerant of chemotherapy, due to their more cellular marrow and a decreased percentage of fat. Risk factors such as tumor cells in the bone marrow, prior treatment with chemotherapy or radiation, and a high negative nitrogen balance will compromise the marrow and increase the degree and duration of cytopenia.[43] It has been recognized that an increased risk of infection occurs among individuals suffering from protein-calorie malnutrition, causing lymphopenia, diminished levels of the complement system and a decrease of certain immunoglobulins.[51] In addition, myelotoxicity caused by chemotherapy and radiotherapy is enhanced by protein deprivation resulting from cancer cachexia.[52]

Differences in the lengths and kinetics of the life

**TABLE 16-1** Grading Toxicities from Chemotherapeutic Agents

| Toxicity | Grade 0 | Grade 1 | Grade 2 | Grade 3 | Grade 4 |
|---|---|---|---|---|---|
| | | | HEMATOLOGIC | | |
| WBC (1000/mm$^3$) | >4.0 | 3.0–3.9 | 2.0–2.9 | 1.0–1.9 | <1.0 |
| Granulocytes (1000/mm$^3$) | >2.0 | 1.5–1.9 | 1.0–1.4 | 0.5–0.9 | <0.5 |
| Platelets (1000/mm$^3$) | >100 | 75–99 | 50–74 | 25–49 | <25 |
| Hemoglobin (g/100 ml) | >11 | 9.5–10.9 | 8.0–9.4 | 6.5–7.9 | <6.5 |
| Hemorrhage | None | Slight, no transfusion | Mild, 1–2 transfusions/ episode | Gross, 3–4 transfusions/ episode | Massive, >4 transfusions/ episode |
| Infection/fever | None | Temp; <38°C No antibiotics | Temp: 38°–40°C Broad-spectrum antibiotics | Temp: >40°C Antifungal coverage | Signs of sepsis: reevaluate medication |
| | | | GASTROINTESTINAL | | |
| Nausea/vomiting | None | Slight nausea, 1 episode of vomiting Maintains intake | Occasional nausea, 2–5 episodes of vomiting Maintains intake | Frequent nausea, 6–10 episodes of vomiting Intake decreased | Constant nausea, >10 episodes of vomiting No intake |
| Diarrhea | None | 2–3 stools | 4–6 stools Moderate cramps | 7–9 stools Severe cramps | >10 stools; needs rehydration |
| Constipation | None | Dry, hard passage of painful stool Stool softener | No stool >2 days Laxatives | No stool >4 days Rule out obstruction or cause | — |
| Anorexia | None | Mild | Moderate, with weight loss | Severe Needs supplements | Life-threatening |

cycles of particular blood cells account for the frequency of neutropenia, thrombocytopenia, and anemia.[42] Maturation of cells in the bone marrow takes eight to ten days. The life span of platelets is seven to ten days. Thrombocytopenia usually occurs 8–14 days after chemotherapy and in most cases concomitantly with neutropenia. Chemotherapy may be held if the count drops below 100,000/mm$^3$. Manifestations of thrombocytopenia are easy bruising, bleeding from gums, nose, or other orifices, and petechiae on the upper and lower extremities, pressure points, elbows, and palate (see Figure 16-3).

Red blood cells (RBCs) have a life span of 120 days. Chemotherapy-induced anemia occurs rarely, because the bone marrow begins to recover before the number of circulating RBCs decreases significantly. Although low hemoglobin and hematocrit levels will not prevent administering chemotherapy, low levels affect how the patient feels and functions. Anemia is manifested by pallor, hypotension, headaches, irritability, and fatigue. Tachycardia and tachypnea may be present due to the hypoxic effects on the heart. Secondary problems include skin or mucous membrane breakdown arising from decreased tissue oxygenation, and cardiopulmonary stress. The incapacitating symptoms of anemia have a profound impact on quality of life.[53]

Anemia of chronic disease is associated with erythroid hypoplasia of the bone marrow.[54] This results in a slight decrease in reticulocytosis, hypoferremia, and a decrease in serum erythropoietin. Actions of certain chemotherapeutic agents such as cisplatin may inhibit the maturation of the erythroid lineage cells in the bone marrow.[55]

Erythropoietin can be administered in an attempt to correct anemia induced by chemotherapy. This is a growth factor for erythroid progenitor cells that promotes proliferation and maintains their survival.[56] The usual dose is 150 u/kg subcutaneously three times a week until the target hematocrit is reached. The target range is 36%–40% which is monitored weekly.[56] Once the patient reaches the target range, a maintenance dose is administered. Although a response from erythropoietin may take two to eight weeks, the maintenance dose is the dose the patient was receiving when the target hematocrit was reached.

Patients with iron deficiency require iron supplementation since adequate iron stores are necessary to support erythropoiesis. The most common side effect from erythropoietin is hypertension, therefore the patient's blood pressure should be monitored biweekly.[57]

Currently the standard of practice is to administer platelets prophylactically if the platelet count falls below 20,000 ul. In a recent study of 182 patients with gynecologic cancers, no intracranial or life-threatening bleeding

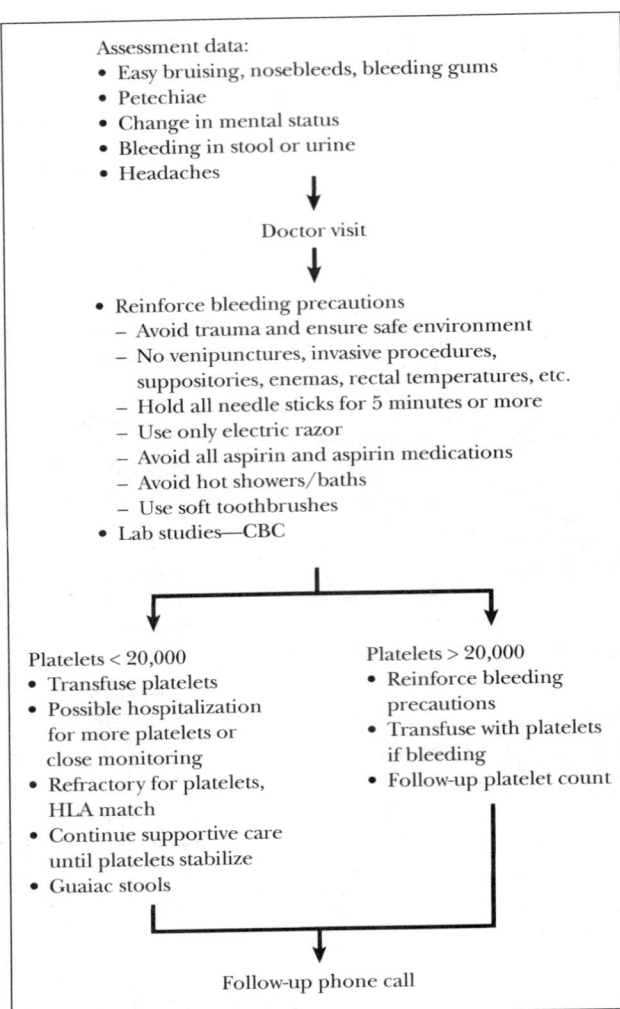

Assessment data:
- Easy bruising, nosebleeds, bleeding gums
- Petechiae
- Change in mental status
- Bleeding in stool or urine
- Headaches

↓

Doctor visit

↓

- Reinforce bleeding precautions
  - Avoid trauma and ensure safe environment
  - No venipunctures, invasive procedures, suppositories, enemas, rectal temperatures, etc.
  - Hold all needle sticks for 5 minutes or more
  - Use only electric razor
  - Avoid all aspirin and aspirin medications
  - Avoid hot showers/baths
  - Use soft toothbrushes
- Lab studies—CBC

Platelets < 20,000
- Transfuse platelets
- Possible hospitalization for more platelets or close monitoring
- Refractory for platelets, HLA match
- Continue supportive care until platelets stabilize
- Guaiac stools

Platelets > 20,000
- Reinforce bleeding precautions
- Transfuse with platelets if bleeding
- Follow-up platelet count

Follow-up phone call

**FIGURE 16-3** Thrombocytopenia phone triage flow sheet.

was evident when platelet levels decreased below 10,000 ul. These researchers recommend prophylactic platelet transfusions when levels decrease below 10,000 ul or if bleeding occurs.[58] Anemia and thrombocytopenia can usually be corrected with blood component transfusions.[40]

The life span of the granulocyte is six to eight hours after release from the marrow. Neutropenia typically develops 8–12 days after chemotherapy, with recovery in three to four weeks. Chemotherapy is usually withheld if the patient's white blood cell (WBC) count is between 1000 and 3000/mm³ or if the absolute neutrophil count (ANC) is below 1500/mm³. Neutropenia generally is defined as an ANC below 1500 cells/mm³. In normal individuals, neutrophils, including both the segmented and slightly less mature band forms, are found in concentrations ranging from 1830 to 7250 cells/mm³.[40] Profound neutropenia (grade 4) usually is defined as an ANC <500 cells/mm.[59]

It is important to note that neutropenia can occur when total WBC count is within a normal range (4000–10,000/mm³). Consequently, quantitating the ANC is essential to achieving a correct assessment of neutrophil status. An ANC is calculated by multiplying the total WBC count by the differential proportion of combined band and segmented neutrophils in a blood sample. Thus, in a patient with a WBC count of 4000 cells/mm³, a differential of 34% segmented neutrophils plus 3% band neutrophils yields an ANC of

$$4000 \text{ cells/mm}^3 \times 37\% = 1480 \text{ cells/mm}^3$$

Monocyte count should also be monitored since an increase in monocytes precedes and predicts resolution of neutropenia.[60]

Since the prime function of neutrophils is phagocytosis, neutropenia eliminates one of the body's prime defenses against bacterial infection.[60] Infections, due to invasion and overgrowth of pathogenic microbes, increase in frequency and severity as the ANC decreases. In addition, risk for severe infections increase when the nadir persists for more than seven to ten days.

Signs of an infection may not be apparent with the inhibition of phagocytic cells. The only response may be fever, and this at times may not be present. It is estimated that 80% of the infections that occur arise from endogenous microbial flora (GI or respiratory tract).[42] When the neutrophil count is less than 500, approximately 20% or more of febrile episodes will have an associated bacteriemia caused principally by aerobic gram-negative bacilli (*Escherichia coli*, *Klebsiella pneumoinis*, and *Pseudomonas aeruginosa*) and gram-positive cocci (coagulase-negative staphylocci, streptococci species, and *Staphylococcus aureus*).[60]

Chemotherapy-induced damage to the alimentary canal and respiratory tract mucosa facilitates the entry of infecting organisms; therefore pneumonia and sinusitis are commonly seen. The nurse must assess for inflammation at the sites most commonly infected, including the periodontium, pharynx, lower esophagus, lung, perineum, anus, skin, and venous access exit sites. Prevention, early detection, good hand-washing technique, and prompt management of infections in patients with neutropenia are essential if sepsis and septic shock are to be avoided.[40,60–62] (see Figure 16-4).

Once appropriate cultures are obtained, antibiotics are used to treat chemotherapy-induced infections: (1) until cultures indicate eradication of the causative organism, (2) for a minimum of seven days, or (3) until the neutrophil count is greater than 500/mm³.[62] In a recent study of children and adolescents, discontinuing antibiotics after 48 hours was found to be safe in the absence of documented infection and the patients remained afebrile for 24 hours.[63] To achieve a broad coverage, therapy with a broad-spectrum cephalosporin or penicillin in combination with an aminoglycoside has been the mainstay of empiric treatment in neutropenic patients for the past decade.[64] Ceftazidine alone has been found to be as effective as a combination of piperacillin and tobramycin for

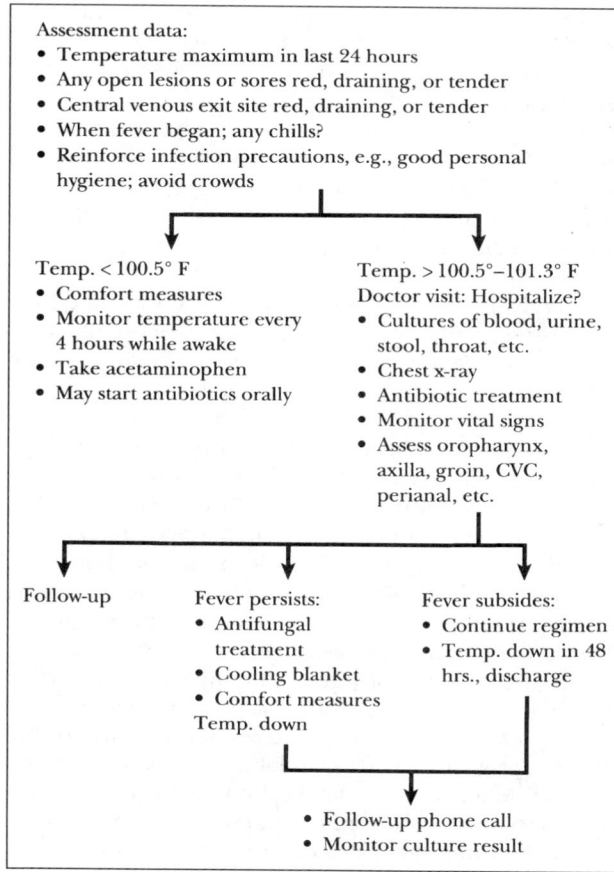

**FIGURE 16-4** Fever phone triage flow sheet.

empiric treatment of febrile neutropenia without evidence of anaerobic or staphylococcal infections.[65] Fever persisting for over three days without identification of an infected site or organism suggests: (1) a nonbacterial cause, (2) resistance to the antibiotic, (3) emergence of a second bacterial infection, (4) inadequate antibiotic serum and tissue levels, (5) drug fever, or (6) infection at avascular sites (abscess).[66] At this point, antifungal therapy is started.[41,67] Antiviral drugs are usually counterrecommended unless mucosal lesions or viral disease is suspected. Risk for recurrent fever and infection is significant for neutropenic patients or those with poor marrow recovery such as disease-related bone marrow dysfunction.[63]

Among all the problems identified with myelosuppression, infection is the most serious associated with significant morbidity and mortality.[68] For this reason, much attention has been focused on the therapeutic application of recombinant colony-stimulating factors (CSFs) to augment neutrophil counts. Hematopoietic growth factors are a family of glycoprotein hormones that act as natural regulators of hematopoiesis to promote the proliferation and differentiation of hematopoietic progenitor cells along multiple pathways.[69] While hematopoietic stimulants have not changed the decline rate of granulocytes,

they have shortened the duration of neutropenia, thereby dramatically reducing the morbidity and mortality from infections. The discovery of CSFs offers hope that the myelosuppression associated with chemotherapy can be ameliorated and full dosages of chemotherapy can be used in cancer therapy.

The American Society of Clinical Oncologists have developed clinical practice guidelines for appropriate use of CSFs.[68] After reviewing available literature, the following guidelines were developed to assist the practitioner in use of CSFs:

1. CSFs are appropriate to initiate if subsequent chemotherapy regimens are delayed from prolonged neutropenia and dose reduction is not possible.
2. CSFs are appropriate in febrile neutropenia in conjunction with antibiotics only in clinical deterioration such as multiorgan failure.
3. CSFs are appropriate when febrile neutropenia is expected in >40% of patients such as result from high-dose chemotherapy.
4. CSFs are appropriate with autologous bone marrow transplants to shorten neutropenia and infectious complications.
5. CSFs are effective in mobilizing peripheral blood progenitor cells for transplantation.

Inconclusive data exist on the use of CSFs with other conditions, especially febrile neutropenia. One study attempted to determine the usefulness of G-CSF in 218 febrile neutropenic patients. These patients were randomly assigned G-CSF or placebo. The researchers concluded that G-CSF accelerated neutrophil recovery and shortened the duration of febrile neutropenia, however the number of days with fever and duration of hospitalization was not decreased.[70]

### Fatigue

Fatigue is a common adverse effect of cancer and its therapy; however, it is underdescribed in the literature as related to chemotherapy administration. When fatigue begins to have an adverse effect on the patient's well-being and interferes with activities of daily living, relationships, and compliance with medical therapy, interventions must be incorporated.[71]

Specific causative mechanisms underlying fatigue are unclear. Changes in skeletal muscle protein stores or metabolite concentration may be one physiological mechanism.[72] Fatigue may result from the body's response to the accumulation of various metabolites and the metabolism of end products from cell destruction by chemotherapy. Other contributing factors could include other side effects, changes in energy usage, disease patterns, anemia, and psychological patterns.

Fatigue manifests as weariness, weakness, and lack of energy. The nurse must assess the onset, the duration, the intensity, the impact on lifestyle, and aggravating and alleviating factors.[73] Acute fatigue protects the individual from exhaustion, which usually dissipates with a good night's sleep. Chronic fatigue is described as a totally overwhelming experience. Chronic fatigue is not easily resolved, and a combination of approaches may be needed. Interventions to overcome fatigue include energy conservation, rest, setting priorities for activities, and delegating tasks.

### Gastrointestinal tract

**Anorexia** Anorexia is a frequent complaint of patients with cancer and contributes to decreased caloric intake with subsequent weight loss. Weight loss often leads to cachexia and is indicative of a poor prognosis.[74] Anorexia or declining food intake implies alterations in food perception, taste, and smell that result from the effects of chemotherapy.[75] Abnormalities of carbohydrate, protein, and fat metabolism are central features of anorexia. Visceral and lean body mass depletion are common, along with muscle atrophy, visceral organ atrophy, and hypoalbuminemia.[76,77] Anorexia can lead to compromised immune status as manifested by decreased macrophage mobilization, depressed lymphocyte function, and impaired phagocytosis.[78]

Nutritional assessment is the first step in meeting the nutritional needs. This includes a physical assessment, a health history, and the obtaining of specific nutritional parameters (albumin, transferrin, nitrogen balance, and oxygen consumption). Other information to obtain during the initial interview include: financial resources for the purchase of food or supplements; individuals responsible for purchasing, storing, and preparing food; and community resources available for food preparation and purchase. The interview and physical assessment can identify the usual nutritional patterns, the physiological and psychological deficits affecting nutritional intake, and those individuals who are at high risk for the development of protein-calorie malnutrition.[79–81] A loss of more than 10% of body weight within the previous six months or an unintentional weight loss of more than 1 kilogram a week is considered a significant risk factor.

The success of maintaining nutritional status depends on a number of factors, including patient motivation, nutritional status at the time of diagnosis, site of the cancer, type of treatment, and severity of side effects. The patient must be taught that adequate nutrition is required for protein synthesis, cellular repair, and tissue growth. For patients receiving chemotherapy, an increase of 4.4 cal/kg and 2 g/kg of protein per body weight must be incorporated when developing a nutritional plan.[82] One strategy could be for the nurse to contract with the patient to increase the intake of calories and protein each day. Hyperalimentation, nutritional supplements, or enteral nutrition can be alternatives for sufficient nutritional intake. Short walks before meals and smaller more frequent meals may be helpful for the patient. Nutrition is an important aspect in providing care to the patient with cancer. Planning nutritious diets gives patients as well as families the ability to actively participate in their care.

**Diarrhea** Diarrhea is an increase in stool volume and liquidity resulting in three or more bowel movements per day. Diarrhea results from the destruction of the actively dividing epithelial cells of the GI tract. When these cells are destroyed, atrophy of the intestinal mucosa and shortening or denuding of the intestinal villa occur. The villi and microvilli become flattened, reducing the absorptive surface area and resulting in a "slick gut." Thus the intestinal contents move rapidly through the gut, reducing absorption of nutrients.[83]

The degree and duration of diarrhea depend on the agent, dose, nadir, and frequency of chemotherapy administration. Patients may experience abdominal cramps and rectal urgency with 5-fluorouracil-leucovorin therapy, which can evolve into nocturnal diarrhea or fecal incontinence leading to lethargy, weakness, orthostatic hypotension, and fluid/electrolyte imbalance. Without adequate management, prolonged diarrhea will cause dehydration, nutritional malabsorption, and circulatory collapse.[84]

Although 5-fluorouracil is the most common drug to cause diarrhea, other agents include methotrexate, docetaxel, actinomycin D, doxorubicin, and irinotecan. Recent manipulations of 5-fluorouracil metabolism with agents such as leucovorin have potentiated its antitumor effect as well as increased diarrhea occurrence.[84]

Thorough evaluation to determine the cause of the diarrhea provides a firm foundation for planning interventions. Management may be limited to dietary measures, such as a low-residue, high-caloric, and protein diet, or pharmacological measures. Stool cultures need to be obtained initially, to rule out an infectious process so appropriate therapy can be implemented. *Clostridium difficile* has been reported in patients receiving chemotherapy who have had prior antibiotic exposure. Antidiarrheal agents should never be given to counteract diarrhea resulting from an infection, since these agents slow the passage of stool through the intestines, prolonging the mucosa's exposure to the organism's toxins. Usually when the diarrhea is a result of an organism, it will resolve in a few days with the use of vancomycin or metronidazole.[85]

Pharmacological intervention for diarrhea is varied. Anticholinergic drugs such as atropine sulfate and scopolamine reduce gastric secretions and decrease intestinal peristalsis. Opiate therapy binds to receptors on the smooth muscle of bowel, slowing down the intestinal motility and increasing fluid absorption. Loperamide is a long-acting opioid agonist, without central opioid activity.[84] Octreotide acetate, a synthetic analog of the hormone octapeptide, inhibits the release of gut hormones, including serotonin and gastrin from the GI tract. It affects the GI tract by prolonging intestinal transit time, increasing intestinal water and electrolyte transport, and decreasing GI blood flow.[86,87] Octreotide acetate is indicated for patients who have excessive diarrhea as a result of GI resections or when other pharmacological treatments have proven ineffective to manage chemotherapy-induced diarrhea.

Chemotherapy usually is administered despite the occurrence of diarrhea. However, diarrhea can be severe enough to be a dose-limiting toxicity of some chemotherapeutic agent combinations, specifically 5-fluorouracil and leucovorin. The nurse must carefully monitor the patient's status to provide appropriate therapy, such as antidiarrheal medications, fluid/electrolyte replacements, and perirectal care to prevent further complications (see Figure 16-5).

***Constipation***   Constipation is defined as infrequent, excessively hard and dry bowel movements resulting from a decrease in rectal filling or emptying.[41] Risk factors that contribute to constipation include narcotic analgesics, a decrease in physical activity, a low-fiber diet, a decrease in fluid intake, and bed rest. Vincristine, vinblastine, and navelbine are the most common chemotherapy agents to cause constipation, as a result of autonomic nerve dysfunction manifested as colicky abdominal pain and ileus. Rectal emptying is specifically diminished because nonfunctional afferent and efferent pathways from the sacral cord are interrupted. Symptoms occur within three to seven days of drug administration and may be accompanied by evidence of peripheral nerve dysfunction.[84,86]

Patients are instructed to be aware of bowel movements. If a bowel movement does not occur every other day, a laxative must be taken. If there are no results, the physician should be asked for further instructions. Laxative therapy or prophylactic stool softener is recom-

mended prior to the administration of drugs known to contribute to constipation, especially if the patient has a history of or is at risk for constipation. The patient should be encouraged to increase the amount of high-fiber foods in the daily diet as well as to increase fluid intake. The patient also should be encouraged to increase physical activity, if that is tolerated. It should be stressed to the patient never to wait more than three days without a bowel movement before calling the physician, since a complication such as impaction or ileus can arise (see Figure 16-6).

***Nausea/vomiting***   During the past decade, the management of chemotherapy-related nausea and vomiting has vastly improved. Understanding the pathophysiology of the symptoms, the efficacy and limitations of pharmacological interventions, and the use of nonpharmacological techniques is essential in minimizing nausea and vomiting. Emesis is a complicated process that requires coordination by the vomiting center (VC) in the lateral reticular formation of the medulla (see Figure 16-7). The VC lies close to the respiratory center on the floor of the fourth ventricle and is directly activated by the visceral and vagal afferent pathways from the GI tract, chemoreceptor trigger zone (CTZ), vestibular apparatus, and the cerebral cortex. When the VC is stimulated, emesis is

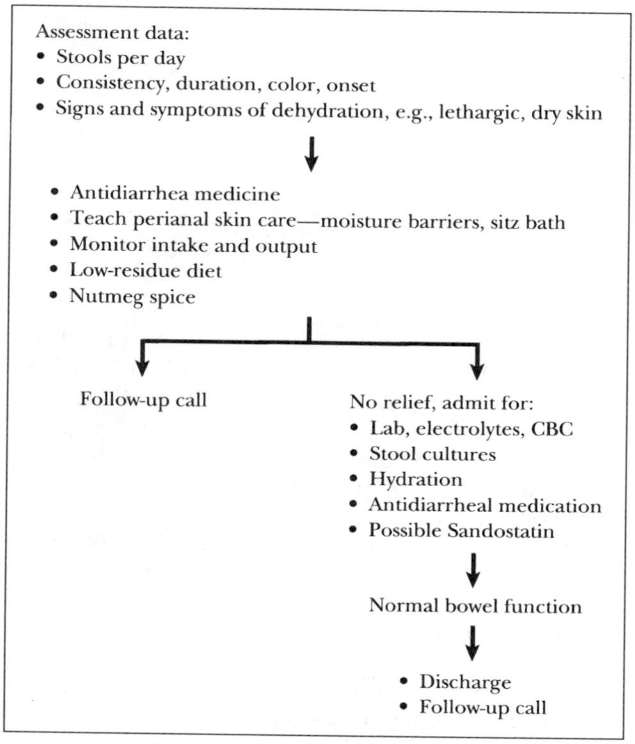

**FIGURE 16-5**  Diarrhea phone triage flow sheet.

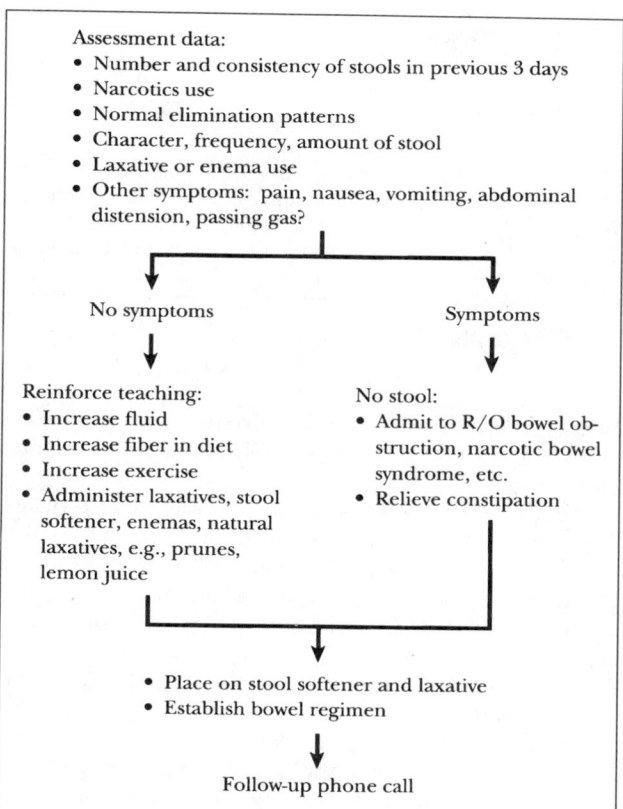

**FIGURE 16-6**  Constipation phone triage flow sheet.

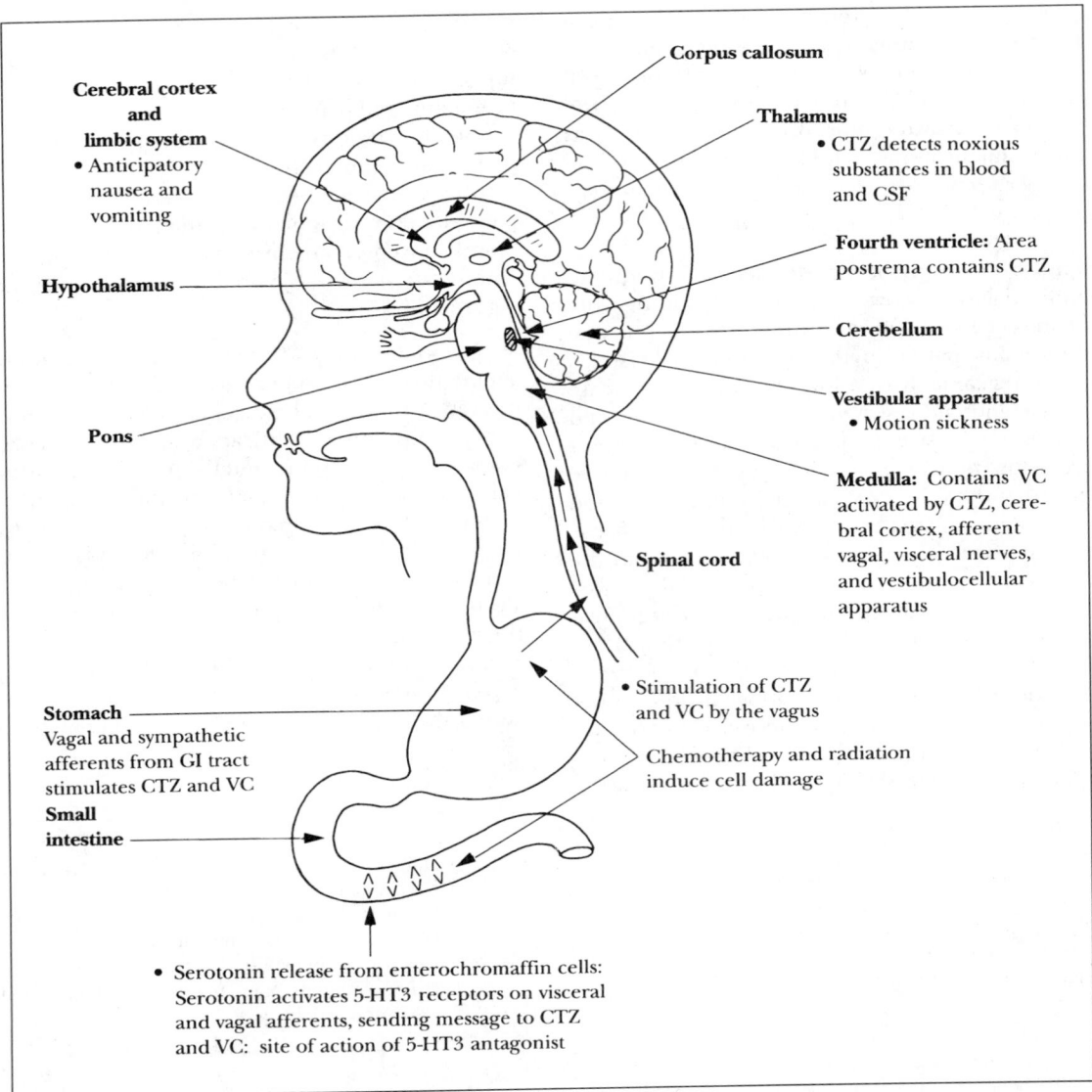

Corpus callosum

Cerebral cortex
and
limbic system
• Anticipatory
nausea and
vomiting

Thalamus
• CTZ detects noxious
substances in blood
and CSF

Fourth ventricle: Area
postrema contains CTZ

Hypothalamus

Cerebellum

Vestibular apparatus
• Motion sickness

Pons

Medulla: Contains VC
activated by CTZ, cere-
bral cortex, afferent
vagal, visceral nerves,
and vestibulocellular
apparatus

Spinal cord

Stomach
Vagal and sympathetic
afferents from GI tract
stimulates CTZ and VC
Small
intestine

• Stimulation of CTZ
and VC by the vagus

Chemotherapy and radiation
induce cell damage

• Serotonin release from enterochromaffin cells:
Serotonin activates 5-HT3 receptors on visceral
and vagal afferents, sending message to CTZ
and VC: site of action of 5-HT3 antagonist

**FIGURE 16-7** Pathways of nausea and vomiting.

induced via impulses to the salivation and respiratory centers and to the pharyngeal, GI, and abdominal muscles.[88,89]

Vestibular-cerebellar afferent pathway areas transmit impulses to the cerebellum and then to the VC, which is experienced as motion sickness. When rapid motion change occurs, the receptors of the labyrinth in the inner ear are stimulated, which is associated with nausea.[90] Obstruction, irritation, inflammation, or delayed gastric emptying may stimulate the GI tract through vagal visceral afferent pathways.[91] Conditioned and anticipatory response are controlled by the cerebral cortex and limbic system, which can be stimulated by sights, sounds, or odors that the patient associates with chemotherapy, thereby making the patient nauseated.[88]

The VC is rich in neurotransmitter receptors sensitive to chemical toxins in the blood and cerebrospinal fluid.[92]

The major receptors are: dopamine, serotonin ($5\text{-HT}_3$), and muscarinic cholinergic in the CTZ; muscarinic in the VC, vestibular apparatus, and the efferent vagal motor nuclei; and histamine in the VC and the vestibular apparatus.[89] A summary of the numerous factors involved in emesis, neurotransmitters, and pharmacological management are summarized in Figure 16-8.

Although nausea, retching, and vomiting commonly occur together, they are considered separate conditions.[93,94] *Nausea* is described as a subjective conscious recognition of the desire to vomit and is manifested by an unpleasant wavelike sensation in the epigastric area, at the back of the throat, or throughout the abdomen. Nausea is mediated by the autonomic nervous system and accompanied by symptoms such as tachycardia, perspiration, light-headedness, dizziness, pallor, excess salivation, and weakness.

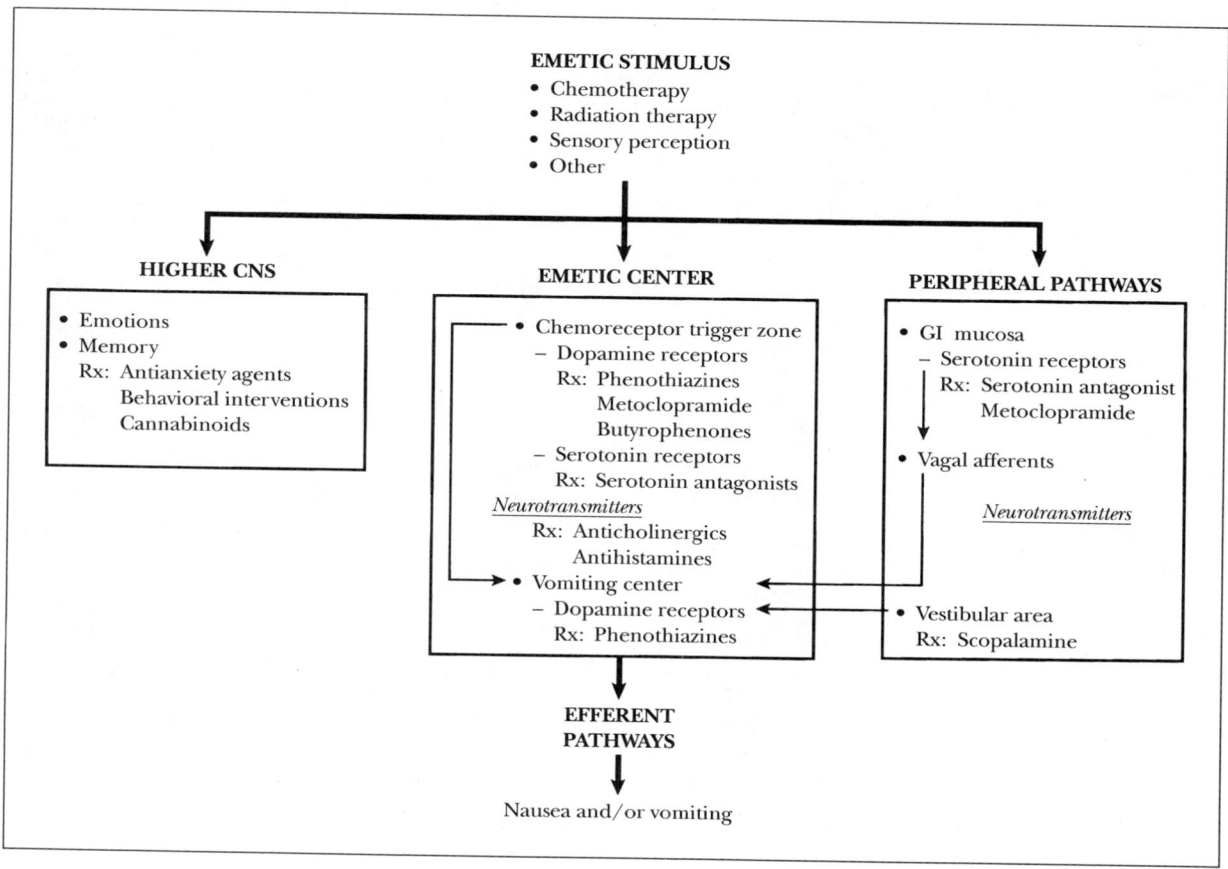

**FIGURE 16-8**   Physiology of chemotherapy-induced nausea/vomiting with proposed sites of action for interventions. (Published with permission of Wujcik, D: Current research in side-effects of high-dose chemotherapy. *Semin Oncol Nurs* 8:102–112, 1992.)

*Retching* is a rhythmic and spasmodic movement involving the diaphragm and abdominal muscles controlled by the respiratory center in the brainstem near the VC. Negative intrathoracic pressure and positive abdominal pressure result in unproductive retching. When the negative pressure becomes positive, vomiting occurs. *Vomiting* is a somatic process performed by the respiratory muscles causing the forceful oral expulsion of gastric, duodenal, or jejunal contents through the mouth.[89,90]

Nausea and vomiting can be classified as acute, delayed, and anticipatory. *Acute* nausea and vomiting occurs a few minutes to one to two hours after treatment, resolving within 24 hours. The pattern is determined by the emetogenicity of the chemotherapy and pretreatment with an antiemetic agent. *Delayed* nausea and vomiting persist or develop 24 hours after chemotherapy, perhaps due to the ongoing effect that the metabolites of chemotherapy continue to exert on the CNS or GI tract. Although cisplatin is thought to be the culprit, cyclosphamide, doxorubicin, and ifosfamide can cause delayed nausea. If nausea was controlled within the first 24 hours after therapy, delayed patterns are less likely to occur. However, despite effective antiemetic regimens, 93% of patients receiving a high dose of cisplatin experience delayed nausea and vomiting up to six to seven days.[95,96] Oral ondansetron has been found to control delayed nausea and vomiting 48–72 hours after cisplatin.[97] *Anticipatory* nausea and vomiting occur in 25% of patients as a result of classic operant conditioning from stimuli associated with chemotherapy usually 12 hours prior to administration. Such conditioned responses are experienced after a few sessions of chemotherapy and occur most commonly when efforts to control emesis are unsuccessful.[97–99] Lorazepam has been found to relieve anticipatory effects as well as delayed nausea.[100]

It is possible to predict the degree and severity of nausea and vomiting as well as the onset and duration (see Table 16-2). Mechlorethamine, for example, induces emesis within 30 minutes of intravenous administration, whereas other highly emetic agents cause emesis at least one hour after infusion. With moderate to highly emetic drugs, emesis develops within six hours of administration. Drugs with low emetic potential usually cause emesis 12–48 hours after administration. Variability in occurrence and onset suggests that each drug may cause emesis via different mechanisms or by stimulating different pathways.[98,99] Rate and route of chemotherapy administration also affect emetic onset, intensity, and duration. For ex-

**TABLE 16-2**  Emetogenic Potential of Chemotherapeutic Agents

| Incidence | Agent | Onset (hours) | Duration (hours) |
|---|---|---|---|
| Very High (>90%) | Cisplatin | 1–6 | 24–48+ |
| | Dacarbazine | 1–3 | 1–12 |
| | Mechlorethamine | 0.5–2 | 8–24 |
| | Melphalan—high dose | 0.3–6 | 6–12 |
| | Streptozocin | 1–6 | 12–24 |
| | Cytarabine—high dose | 2–4 | 12–24 |
| High (60%–90%) | Carmustine | 2–4 | 4–24 |
| | Cyclophosphamide | 4–12 | 12–24 |
| | Procarbazine | 24–27 | variable |
| | Etoposide—high dose | 4–6 | 24+ |
| | Semustine | 1–5 | 12–24 |
| | Lomustine | 4–6 | 12–24 |
| | Dactinomycin | 2–5 | 24 |
| | Plicamycin | 1–6 | 12–24 |
| | Methotrexate—high dose | 1–12 | 24–72 |
| Moderate (30%–60%) | Doxorubicin | 4–6 | 6+ |
| | Mitoxantrone | 4–6 | 6+ |
| | 5-Fluorouracil | 3–6 | 24+ |
| | Mitomycin C | 1–4 | 48–72 |
| | Carboplatin | 4–6 | 12–24 |
| | Daunorubicin | 2–6 | 24 |
| | L-Asparaginase | 1–4 | 2–12 |
| | Topotecan | 6–12 | 24–72 |
| | Ifosfamide | 3–6 | 24–72 |
| Low (10%–30%) | Bleomycin | 3–6 | — |
| | Cytarabine | 6–12 | 3–12 |
| | Etoposide | 3–8 | — |
| | Melphalan | 6–12 | — |
| | 6-Mercaptopurine | 4–8 | — |
| | Methotrexate | 4–12 | 3–12 |
| | Vinblastine | 4–8 | — |
| | Hydroxyurea | — | — |
| | Teniposide | — | — |
| | Gemcitabine | — | — |
| | Vinorelbine | — | — |
| Very low <10% | Vincristine | 4–8 | — |
| | Chlorambucil | 48–72 | — |
| | Busulfan | — | — |
| | Thioguinine | — | — |
| | Hormones | — | — |
| | Paclitaxel | 4–8 | — |
| | Docetaxel | — | — |

ample, rapid infusion of cytarabine is more often associated with an earlier onset of severe emesis than is slower infusion.[92]

Management begins with obtaining an in-depth emetic history and developing a preventive action plan with antiemetics (see Table 16-3). Characteristics that affect the occurrence of nausea and vomiting include susceptibility to motion sickness, poor previous emetic control, and being young. Individuals with a heavy alcohol intake seem to have a decreased occurrence of nausea and vomiting.[99]

Successful antiemetic regimens interrupt the stimulation of the VC. Combination regimens must be individual-ized and developed according to the emetic potential of the chemotherapy regimen, expected duration of the nausea and vomiting, and current pattern of symptoms. Numerous combinations are being investigated extensively to eliminate the stimulation of the VC. These regimens use drugs with proven single-agent antiemetic activity, optimum doses, routes, and minimum overlapping toxicities (see Table 16-4).[101–105] For example, combinations of dopamine antagonists with steroids have been found to provide complete control of nausea and vomiting in up to 100% of patients undergoing high-dose cisplatin-base regimens. The combination of on-dansetron and dexamethasone have been found more

**TABLE 16-3**   Antiemetic Therapy

| Classification | Drugs | Availability/Dose | Schedule | Duration/ Half-Life | Comments |
|---|---|---|---|---|---|
| **Benzodiazepines**<br><br>*Mechanism of action:* CNS depressant; interferes with afferent nerves from cerebral cortex; sedative<br>*Common side effects:* Sedation, amnesia, confusion | Lorazepam (Ativan)<br><br>Diazepam (Valium) | *Tablet:* 1–3 mg po or sublingual<br>*IV:* 0.5–2.5 mg<br>*Tablet:* 2–4 mg<br>*IV:* 2–10 mg | q3–4 hr<br><br><br>q4–6 hr | 4–8 hr<br>*Half-life:* 10–15 hr<br><br>4–8 hr<br>*Half-life:* 30–40 hr | Reduces anticipatory nausea and vomiting. May aggravate CNS effects of ifosfamide. Use with caution in patients with hepatic and renal dysfunction. |
| **Butyrophenones**<br><br>*Mechanism of action:* Dopamine antagonist in the CTZ, esophagus, and stomach<br>*Common side effects:* Sedation, hypotension, tachycardia, EPS | Droperidol (Inapsine)<br><br>Haloperidol (Haldol) | *IM:* 2.5–10 mg<br>*IV:* 0.5–2.5 mg<br>*Tablet:* 3–5 mg<br>*IM:* 1–2 mg<br>*IV:* 1–3 mg | q3–4 hr<br><br>q4 hr<br>q2–6 hr | 2–4 hr<br>*Half-life:* 10 hr<br>2–6 hr<br>*Half-life:* 12–18 hr | Diphenhydramine 25–50 mg po or IV will prevent EPS. EPS more common in young patients. May have additive effects. Use caution in patients with cardiac disorders. |
| **Cannabinoids**<br><br>*Mechanism of action:* Suppresses pathways to VC (speculated)<br>*Common side effects:* Sedation, dizziness, dysphoria, dry mouth, disorientation, impaired concentration, orthostatic hypotension, tachycardia | Dronabinol (Marinol) | *Tablet:* 5–10 mg | q4 hr | 4–6 hr | May be difficult to obtain in outpatient setting. Elderly patients generally do not tolerate side effects. Generally used for second-line antiemetic therapy. |
| **Phenothiazines**<br><br>*Mechanism of action:* Blocks dopamine receptor in the CTZ; inhibits VC by blocking autonomic afferent impulses via vagus nerve<br>*Common side effects:* Sedation, orthostatic hypotension, EPS, dizziness, drowsiness | Prochlorperazine (Compazine)<br><br><br><br><br>Promethazine (Phenergan)<br><br>Thiethylperazine (Torecan)<br><br>Chlorpromazine (Thorazine)<br><br>Perphenazine (Trilafon) | *Tablet:* 5–25 mg<br>*Sustained release:* 10–30 mg po<br>*IM/IV:* 5–20 mg<br>*Rectal:* 25 mg q4 hr<br>*Tablet:* 12.5–25 mg<br>*IM/IV:* 10–25 mg<br>*Rectal:* 25 mg<br>*Tablet:* 10 mg<br>*IM:* 10 mg<br>*Rectal:* 10 mg<br>*Tablet:* 25–50 mg<br>*IM/IV:* 25–50 mg<br>*Rectal:* 25–100 mg<br>*Tablet:* 4 mg<br>*IM/IV:* 5 mg | q4–6 hr<br>q10–12 hr<br><br>q3–4 hr<br>q4–6 hr<br><br>q4–6 hr<br><br><br>q4–6 hr<br><br><br>q4–6 hr<br><br><br>q4–6 hr | 3–4 hr<br>10–12 hr<br><br>3–4 hr<br>3–4 hr<br><br>3–4 hr<br><br><br>3–4 hr<br><br><br>3–4 hr<br><br><br>3–4 hr | Administer IV dose over 15–30 min. EPS more common in person <30. Side effects can be cumulative in the elderly. Do not exceed 5 mg/min with IV dose Dystonia can occur with chlorpromazine, especially with IM. Chlorpromazine generally second-line antiemetic therapy. Diphenhydramine can prevent EPS and dystonia. Sustained-release form can prevent delayed nausea and vomiting. |
| **Substituted Benzamide**<br><br>*Mechanism of action:* Dopamine antagonist; accelerates gastric emptying and small-bowel transit; CTZ<br>*Common side effects:* Sedation, diarrhea, anxiety, EPS, fatigue, headache | Metoclopramide (Reglan) | *Tablet:* 5–10 mg<br>*IV:* 1–3 mg/kg | q2–3 h × 3–5 doses | 2–3 hr<br>*Half-life:* 4–6 hr | EPS more common in young patients. Administer over 15 min to prevent intense anxiety. Use with caution in patients with renal dysfunction. |

*(continued)*

**TABLE 16-3** Antiemetic Therapy (continued)

| Classification | Drugs | Availability/Dose | Schedule | Duration/ Half-Life | Comments |
|---|---|---|---|---|---|
| **Steroids** <br> *Mechanism of action:* Antiprostaglandin synthesis activity? <br> *Common side effects:* Insomnia, euphoria, anxiety, hypertension, edema | Dexamethasone (Decadron) <br> Solu Medrol | *Tablet:* 4 mg <br> *IV:* 10–20 mg <br> *IV:* 125–250 mg | q4 hr <br><br> q3 hr | *Half-life:* 2–3 hr | Rapid infusion causes perineal itching. |
| **Antihistamines** <br> *Mechanism of action:* Histamine H-1; receptor antagonist <br> *Common side effects:* Sedation, hypotension | Diphenhydramine (Benadryl) | *Tablet:* 25–50 mg <br> *IM/IV:* 12.5–50 mg | q3–4 hr | *Half-life:* 5–8 hr | Prevents acute dystonic reactions. <br> Use with caution in patients with hepatic dysfunction. |
| **Serotonin Inhibitors** <br> *Mechanism of action:* Serotonin receptor; (5-HT3) antagonist <br> *Common side effects:* Hypotension, headache, constipation, sedation minimal | Ondansetron (Zofran) | *IV:* 32 mg × 1 or 0.15 mg/kg × 3 <br> *po:* 4-mg and 8-mg tablets | q4 hr | *Half-life:* 3–4 hr | Transient elevations of LFTs may occur with cisplatin and ondansetron administration. |
| | Granisetron (Kytril) | *IV:* 10 mcg/kg <br> *po:* 1 mg every 12 hours | 30 min prior to chemo | *Half-life:* 8–10 hr | Single dose of Kytril may be sufficient for a 12-hr time period. <br> Neither granisetron nor ondanestron are recommended for delayed or anticipatory nausea/vomiting. |
| | Tropisetron (investigational Navoban) | *IV:* 5 mg <br> *po:* 5 mg everyday × 5d | 30 min prior to chemo | | |
| **Anticholinergic** <br> *Common side effects:* Dry mouth, sedation, blurred vision, restlessness | Scopolamine (Transderm Scop) | *Patch:* 0.5 mg/24° every 3d | | Duration 72° | May irritate skin. <br> May be difficult to obtain. |

*VC*, vomiting center; *CTZ*, chemoreceptor trigger zone; *EPS*, extrapyramidal symptoms; *LFTs*, liver function tests

efficacious than ondansetron alone in controlling emesis.[104]

With the addition of the serotonin inhibitors, the management of chemotherapy-induced nausea and vomiting has improved. After extensive review of studies using serotonin inhibitors, several findings were supported: (1) no greater efficacy is found among ondansetron, granisetron, or tropisetron; (2) efficacy appears more pronounced for cisplatin-containing regimens; (3) less effectiveness is found for delayed nausea and vomiting; (4) dexamethasone increases the efficacy of all three; (5) efficacy seems to diminish over repeated days or repeated chemotherapy cycles.[101–105]

Behavioral interventions such as progressive muscle relaxation, hypnosis, and systematic desensitization can be taught to the patient to help interrupt the association of nausea and vomiting with chemotherapy. The nurse can try to minimize in the environment any aversive sounds or smells that could stimulate the VC. Distraction with audiotapes, radios, or television programs should be provided in the treatment area to help minimize nausea. Each of these techniques has been found effective in decreasing the frequency and duration of vomiting as well as in decreasing anxiety.[106,107]

It is important to teach the patient about the potential side effects of antiemetic therapy, such as drowsiness and diarrhea. If the patient is returning home after an emetogenic chemotherapy treatment, ensure that someone can provide transportation and care in the immediate hours following therapy. Phone follow-up 24–48 hours after treatment is essential to ensure that appropriate antiemetic management is being followed (see Figure 16-9).

**TABLE 16-4**  Combination Antiemetic Regimens

- When possible, antiemetics should be started 30 minutes prior to chemotherapy.
- When giving vesicant chemotherapeutic agents via a peripheral vein do not sedate patient until safe administration of the vesicant.
- All regimens designed for outpatient unless specified otherwise.

I. Low Emetic Potential

   A. Prochlorperazine 15 mg SR
     Lorazepam 1 mg po prn

   B. Thiethylperazine 10 mg po
     Dexamethasone 10 mg IV

   C. Droperidol 2–2.5 mg IV
     Dexamethasone 10 mg IV

II. Moderate–Severe Emetic Potential

   A. A • B • C • D (low dose)
     Lorazepam: 1 mg po or IV
     Diphenhydramine: 25–50 mg IV over 30 min
     Prochlorperazine: 15–20 mg IV over 30 min
     Dexamethasone: 10 mg IV

     *At Hour of Sleep:*
     Lorazepam: 1 mg po
     Diphenhydramine: 25 mg po
     Prochlorperazine: 15 mg SR po

   B. A • B • C • D (high dose)
     Lorazepam: 1–2 mg po q6 hr beginning 24 hr before morning of treatment
     Lorazepam: 1–2.5 mg IV
     Diphenhydramine: 50 mg IV
     Prochlorperazine: 20 mg IV infusion over 30 min q3 hr × 2
     Dexamethasone: 20 mg IV

     *At Hour of Sleep:*
     Lorazepam: 2 mg po or SL
     Diphenhydramine: 50 mg po
     Prochlorperazine: 15 mg SR in morning and q12 hr prn

   C. Metoclopramide: 1–2 mg/kg 30 min prior and q2 hr for 2 additional doses
     Diphenhydramine: 50 mg IV
     Lorazepam: 1–2 mg po or IV
     Dexamethasone: 20 mg IV

   D. Metoclopramide: 1 mg/kg prior and q2 hr for 2 additional doses
     Diphenhydramine: 50 mg IV
     Dexamethasone: 20 mg IV
     Diazepam: 5 mg IV
     Thiethylperazine: 10 mg supp q4–6 hr for 24 hr

   E. Metoclopramide: 1–2 mg IV 30 min prior and q2 hr for 2 additional doses
     Diphenhydramine: 50 mg IV
     Lorazepam: 1–2 mg po or IV
     Decadron: 20 mg IV
     *continue*
     Metoclopramide: 0.5 mg/kg po 4 × a day 1–4 days postchemotherapy
     Dexamethasone: 8 mg po bid days 1 & 2, 4 mg po bid days 3 & 4

**TABLE 16-4**  (continued)

   F. For inpatient receiving cisplatin daily for 5 days with 5-FU or VP-16.
     Prochlorperazine: 12 mg IV q8 hr with
     Diphenhydramine: 25 mg IV q8 hr
     Lorazepam: 1–2 mg po q4–6 hr prn
     *or*
     Ondansetron: 0.15 mg/kg IV infusion over 15 min q8 hr × 5 days or granisetron 1 mg IV q12 hr
     Lorazepam: 1 mg sublingually q4–6 hr
     Dexamethasone: 10 mg IV daily × 5, or 8 mg po bid days 1, 2, and 3 and 4 mg po bid days 4 and 5

   G. Ondansetron: 0.15 mg/kg IV infusion over 15 min, 30 min prior to chemotherapy and again in 8 hr
     Dexamethasone: 10–20 mg IV
     Lorazepam: 1–2 mg po

     *At Hour of Sleep:*
     Prochlorperazine: 15–30 mg SR
     Lorazepam: 1–2 mg po
     Diphenhydramine: 25–50 mg po

     This regimen works well for outpatient high-dose doxorubicin and cyclophosphamide or cisplatin and etoposide.

   H. Ondansetron: 32 mg IV infusion over 45 min, 30 min prior to chemotherapy (one dose only) or granisetron 1 mg IV every 12 hrs
     Dexamethasone: 20 mg IV

     *At Hour of Sleep:*
     Prochlorperazine: 15–30 mg SR
     Lorazepam: 1–2 mg po
     Diphenhydramine: 25–50 mg po

## Organ Toxicities

Certain chemotherapy drugs may cause direct damage to specific cells of a given organ or cause indirect damage by the effects of cellular breakdown by-products. In general, organ toxicities are predictable based on the cumulative dose, the presence of concomitant organ dysfunction, the age of the patient, and the manner in which the drug is given. Of interest is the fact that the toxicity profile may be changing as a result of the more widespread use of dose-intensive regimens and CSFs. These approaches to managing the disease are likely to result in more organ toxicities as myelosuppression becomes less prominent. Each of the major organ toxicities will be discussed. Tables 16-5 through 16-10 provide a review of major toxicities in terms of risk factors, signs of toxicity, preventive measures, grading, and management.

### Cardiotoxicity

Cardiotoxicity is described as an acute or chronic process. The acute form consists of transient electrocardiogram (ECG) changes, occurring in approximately 10% of patients receiving chemotherapy. Acute effects are im-

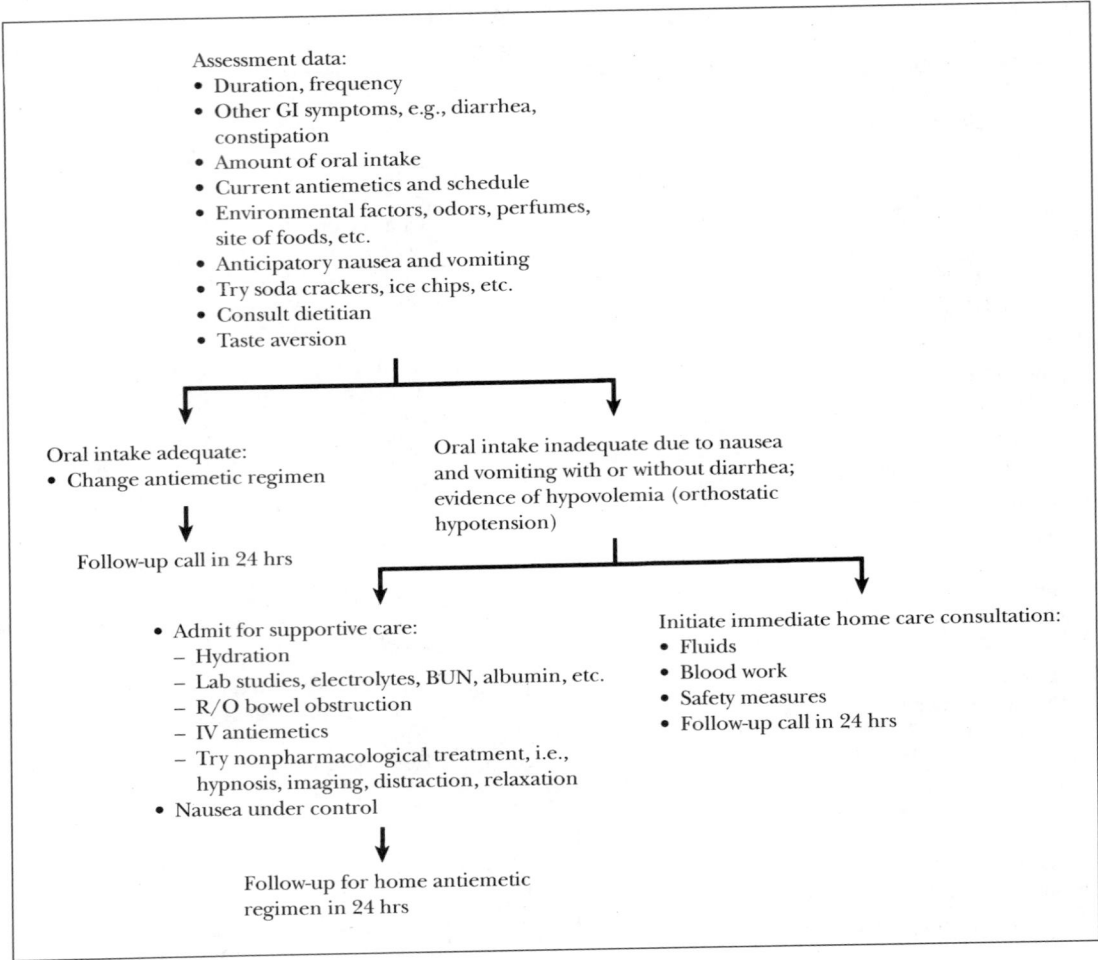

Assessment data:
- Duration, frequency
- Other GI symptoms, e.g., diarrhea, constipation
- Amount of oral intake
- Current antiemetics and schedule
- Environmental factors, odors, perfumes, site of foods, etc.
- Anticipatory nausea and vomiting
- Try soda crackers, ice chips, etc.
- Consult dietitian
- Taste aversion

Oral intake adequate:
- Change antiemetic regimen

Follow-up call in 24 hrs

Oral intake inadequate due to nausea and vomiting with or without diarrhea; evidence of hypovolemia (orthostatic hypotension)

- Admit for supportive care:
  - Hydration
  - Lab studies, electrolytes, BUN, albumin, etc.
  - R/O bowel obstruction
  - IV antiemetics
  - Try nonpharmacological treatment, i.e., hypnosis, imaging, distraction, relaxation
- Nausea under control

Follow-up for home antiemetic regimen in 24 hrs

Initiate immediate home care consultation:
- Fluids
- Blood work
- Safety measures
- Follow-up call in 24 hrs

**FIGURE 16-9**    Nausea and vomiting phone triage flow sheet.

mediate in onset and resolve quickly without serious complications. These effects are not dose related and are not an indication to stop the drug. Less than 5% of patients develop chronic cardiotoxicity from a cumulative drug effect requiring immediate discontinuation of the drug.[108,109] Chronic effects occur weeks or months after administration, involving nonreversible cardiomyopathy presenting as a classic biventricular congestive heart failure (CHF) with a characteristic low-voltage QRS complex. Signs and symptoms are classical for CHF, including complaints of a nonproductive cough, dyspnea, and pedal edema. Generally, it is poorly responsive to diuretics or digitalis, becoming progressively worse, with a 60% mortality.

Anthracyclines are known to cause cardiotoxicity by directly damaging the cardiac myocyte cells. The incidence of cardiotoxicity is 2%–3% after cumulative doses are administered.[109] Total cumulative dosages have been established at 550 mg/m² for doxorubicin and 600 mg/m² for daunomycin, with a decrease in dose to 450 mg/m² if mediastinal radiation has been administered.[110]

The mechanism of action occurs in the presence of oxygen, where the anthracyclines form a bond or union with iron or copper. These complexes inhibit lipid peroxidation, allowing a free oxygen radical to damage the myocytes directly. This results in a loss of myocardial fibrils, mitochrondrial changes, and cellular destruction.[110,111] As a result, the myocyte has limited contractility, leading to hypertrophy of the cardiac muscle, which increases the demand for oxygen.

In an attempt to decrease cardiotoxicity occurrence, altering the dose scheduling of doxorubicin to frequent lower doses has resulted in reduction of cardiotoxicity without compromise of antitumor effects.[111] Chemoprotectants are being evaluated to protect the cardiac tissue by blocking the anthracycline's damage to the myocytes.[112] Razoxane (ICRF-159), an investigational drug, has been shown to have chemoprotectant activity against daunomycin and doxorubicin in studies with mice. It appears that ICRF-159 competes with specific metals, such as iron, that are required for the anthracycline-induced cardiotoxicity.

ICRF-187 (Dexrazoxane, Zinecard) is a similar compound currently being investigated that is more water soluble and easier to administer. This compound has permitted doses of doxorubicin up to 700 mg/m² to be administered without cardiotoxicity occurring.[113] It appears to interfere with the intracellular process responsible for anthracycline-induced cardiomyopathy.[114] Zinecard has been FDA-approved as a cardioprotective agent for patients with metastatic breast cancer who have received cumulative doses of 300 mg/m² and continuing treatment with doxorubicin (not for initial treatment). Patients have been able to tolerate greater cumulative doses of doxorubicin with a decreased risk of cardiac events. The agent is administered 30 minutes prior to doxorubicin, calculated on a 10:1 ratio. Thus with a 50 mg dose of doxorubicin, 500 mg of dexrazoxane would be administered.[114]

In an attempt to reduce further the cardiotoxicity from the anthracyclines, analogs that have greater antitumor activity and may have reduced cardiotoxicity have been developed. Epirubicin appears to be similar to doxorubicin, but the cardiotoxicity is significantly less. Patients can receive twice the cumulative dose of 1000 mg/m² before the risk of clinical cardiotoxicity begins to rise significantly.[115] Idarubicin, esorubicin, and aclarubicin also show less cardiotoxicity occurrence than doxorubicin. Although mitoxantrone has been associated with rare cardiac events, it is considered less cardiotoxic.[116,117]

Acute pericarditis has been reported with high-dose cyclophosphamide therapy (90–270 mg/kg) used in the bone marrow transplant (BMT) population with subsequent pericardial effusion and cardiac tamponade.[118] Cyclophosphamide damages the myocytes, similar to anthracyclines, where swelling and decreased contractility lead to less effective pumping of the heart. Hemorrhagic myocardial necrosis has been reported, with leakage of blood through capillaries. Transient complete heart block requiring temporary pacemaker support has been reported. Myocardial edema results from the induced injury to the capillary endothelium.[119] Toxicity ranges from minor, transient ECG changes and asymptomatic elevation of cardiac enzymes to fatal myopericarditis and myocardial necrosis.[120]

Myocardial ischemia has been reported with 5-fluorouracil infusion in patients with or without preexisting heart disease. Coronary vasospasm with resulting angina pectoris, myocardial infarction, S-T segment elevations, and ventricular ectopy has been described. The pathophysiology is unclear, although a direct cardiomyopathic effect from the release of vasoactive substances in the presence of 5-fluorouracil has been suggested.[121] It has been speculated that angina is a coronary artery spasm of the Prinzmetal's type, and it does respond to nitrates.[122] Cessation of therapy does not appear to be absolutely necessary, since patients who have such a syndrome can be pretreated with calcium antagonists known to prevent coronary artery spasm.

Asymptomatic bradycardia has been reported in about 30% of patients with ovarian cancer who have received Taxol.[123] Other cardiac disturbances that have been reported in 5% of patients included atrioventricular conduction blocks, left bundle branch blocks, ventricular tachycardia, and symptoms of cardiac ischemia. In five patients who received both cisplatin and Taxol, episodes of ventricular tachycardia occurred. The majority of Taxol-related cardiac disturbances were not associated with clinical symptoms and were noted incidentally during continuous cardiac monitoring. Taxol infusion is not discontinued unless associated with progressive atrioventricular conduction disturbances. The mechanism is unclear; however, it is speculated to be the result of the administration vehicle cremophor EL causing activation of selected cardiac-histamine receptors. Stimulation of these receptors in the cardiac tissue increases myocardial oxygen demand and produces coronary vasoconstriction. Although cardiac disturbances are usually benign, a case report documents the occurrence of myocardial ischemia during Taxol administration which resulted in death.[124]

Cardiac function should be evaluated throughout therapy for patients at high risk for cardiotoxicity or those who will be receiving high dosages of an anthracycline. Methods to evaluate cardiac function include noninvasive monitoring with ECG, echocardiography, and radionuclide cardiography. An ejection fraction less tha 55% of resting or a decrease of 5% or more from the resting value with exercise is considered abnormal. Further doses of chemotherapy are not recommended if the ejection fraction drops to 45% or less at rest or deteriorates to greater than 5% from baseline.[108] Although an endomyocardial biopsy can reveal damage to the myocytes prior to clinical detection, the procedure is costly and technically difficult and requires considerable expertise.

It has been recommended to obtain an ECG at three months and also at one year after the last anthraccline dose to determine cardiac status and risk for late abnormality. A radionuclide cardiac scan should be obtained with one of these tests to confirm cardiac status and to serve as a posttreatment baseline.[125,126] Low-risk patients have been defined as those receiving less than 200 mg/m² of an anthracycline and ano mediastinal radiation or exhibiting no cardiac abnormality. Long-term follow-up has been recommended to include an ECG every two to three years, with a radionuclinde cardiac scan with exercise stress every five years. High-risk patients are considered to have received more than 500 mg/m² of an anthracycline, to have received mediastinal radiation, or to have abnormal cardiac function. For long-term follow-up it has been recommended to include a minimum of an echocardiography yearly and a cardiac scan every five years if the patient remains asymptomatic.

Accurate documentation and monitoring of total cumulative dosages is essential. Cardiac assessment is imperative to evaluate for a third heart sound or gallop, which could indicate cardiac insufficiency. Cardiac monitoring may be necessary for administering high dosages of chemotherapy, such as with cyclophosphamide. Once the patient develops chronic cardiotoxicity, nursing interventions include teaching the patient about conservation of energy, managing fluid retention, and minimizing sodium in the diet. Supportive care with digitalis to enhance the cardiac output and with diuretics to manage fluid should also be instituted. Eventually the patient may need supplemental oxygen to relieve dyspnea. Heart transplantation has become an accepted procedure to treat end-stage heart disease for anthracycline cardiomyopathy. Early preparation for possible cardiac transplant is imperative to ensure success.[127] The degree of cardiac injury determines the limitations on activities of daily living the individual will experience. Few are prepared for this debilitating effect, and nurses must initiate interventions that will assist the patient and family in coping. Patients are also taught the importance of close cardiac follow-up, once the treatment is complete, to monitor for late cardiac effects (see Table 16-5).

### Neurotoxicity

The clinical picture of chemotherapy-induced neurotoxicity can arise as a direct or an indirect damage to the central nervous system (CNS), peripheral nervous system, cranial nerves, or any combination of the three. The majority of patients experience temporary neurotoxicity; however, some will have permanent neurological deficits. Significant neurotoxicity usually requires holding the treatment until the symptom resolves and reinstituting with a 50% dose reduction or discontinuing the drug.[128]

The central and peripheral nervous systems are protected against potentially neurotoxic effects by the blood-brain barrier and blood-nerve barriers. If intact, these barriers exclude most chemotherapeutic agents that are water soluble and also exclude relatively large molecules. Biopsies of damaged nerves from chemotherapy have demonstrated a mild decrease in the number of large diameter myelinated nerve fibers, and ultrastructural studies have shown scattered degenerating nerve fibers both in the axon and in the myelin sheaths. Severity of neurotoxicity is usually dose-related, with symptoms exhibited in a variable and unpredictable fashion.

The CNS is made up of collections of neurons and their connections organized into the brain and spinal cord areas. CNS damage primarily involves the cerebellum, which produces altered reflexes, unsteady gait, ataxia, and confusion. The peripheral nervous system is basically a set of communication channels located outside the CNS and consisting of the cranial and spinal nerves. Damage to the peripheral nervous system produces paralysis or loss of movement and sensation to those areas affected by the particular nerve. The autonomic nervous system (ANS) includes those peripheral nerves that regulate functions occurring automatically in the body, such as the cardiovascular, respiratory, and endocrine systems. Damage to the ANS causes ileus, impotence, or urinary retention.

Vincristine is well known for potential peripheral neuropathy characterized by myalgias, loss of the deep tendon reflex at the ankle, progressing to complete areflexia, distal symmetric sensory loss, motor weakness, foot drop, and muscle atrophy.[128] Autonomic neuropathy is characterized by ileus, constipation, impotence, urinary reten-

tion, or postural hypotension. The mechanism of damage is thought to involve disruption of the microtubules in the neural tissues, which thereby inhibits the mitotic spindle movements necessary for the mitosis phase of cellular reproduction.[129] Vincristine doses greater than 2 mg increase the risk of neurotoxicity.

Neuropathy related to cisplatin is reversible, although cases of persistent progression after the discontinuation of the drug have been reported.[130] Cisplatin affects the large-diameter fibers of the neural tissues, resulting in sensory changes. The earliest sign of peripheral neuropathy is decreased vibratory sense described as hand and feet paresthesias with the classic stocking glove distribution. Sensory loss occurs initially; and without dose modification, loss of the Achilles reflex, muscle weakness, and loss of the deep tendon reflex occurs. Symptoms of neuropathy are seen at cumulative doses of 300 mg/m$^2$ to 500 mg/m$^2$. As the neuropathy progresses, position sense is impaired, and a marked sensory ataxia develops. Peripheral neuropathy has been reported from combined Taxol and cisplatin. Sensory-motor neuropathy occurs 1–21 weeks after initiation of therapy. Neuropathy appears to be progressive with additional courses and more pronounced with higher doses of Taxol (cumulative $\geq$ 1500 mg/m$^3$).[131]

High tone loss is speculated to be related to the loss of hairs in the organ of Corti from cisplatin. Rapid drug delivery, simultaneous administration of aminoglycosides, and dehydration seem to increase the potential for ototoxicity. The loss can be reversed with discontinuation of the drug; however, permanent damage has been reported, resulting in the need for a hearing aid.[132] Carboplatin has minimal neurotoxicity at normal doses, exhibited as peripheral neuropathy and ototoxicity.[128]

Neurotoxicity characterized by metabolic encephalopathy manifested as blurred vision, subclinical electroencephalographic changes, urinary incontinence, motor system dysfunction, cranial nerve dysfunction, seizures, or irreversible coma has been reported in 5%–30% of patients treated with ifosfamide.[133] Signs have occurred within two hours of bolus administration and up to 28 days after therapy. Within 48–72 hours of cessation of ifosfamide, most abnormalities clear spontaneously.[134] Risk factors associated with neurotoxicity include duration of administration, hepatic insufficiency, previous cisplatin, presence of bulky disease, low serum albumin, and high serum creatinine.[135] Although the cause is not completely understood, the encephalopathy is thought to result from an accumulation of drug metabolites (chloracetaldehyde) causing direct CNS damage.

High-dose methotrexate (>1 g/m$^2$) occasionally causes encephalopathy after several courses, which usually is transient and reversible.[128] Intrathecal methotrexate may cause a chemical meningitis, with fever, headache, muscle rigidity, and cerebrospinal fluid leukocytosis. This is rare, but it occurs within hours of the intrathecal injection and resolves spontaneously.

5-FU may cause an acute cerebellar dysfunction, usually more common in the elderly. It is characterized by the

**TABLE 16-5**   Organ Toxicity of Chemotherapy Agents: Cardiotoxicity

| Toxicity/ Symptoms | Grade | General Risk Factors | Chemotherapy Agent/Risk Factors | Mechanism of Damage | Protective/ Management Measures |
|---|---|---|---|---|---|
| • Tachycardia<br>• Dyspnea<br>• Nonproductive cough<br>• Neck vein distention<br>• Gallop rhythm<br>• Rales<br>• Pedal edema<br>• Cardiomegaly<br>• Dull or sharp precordial pain, may radiate to neck and shoulder<br>• Cardiac friction rub<br>• ST-T wave changes<br>• Supraventricular<br>• Tachyarrhythmias<br>• T-wave flattening | *Cardiac Dysrhythmias:*<br>0 = None<br>1 = Asymptomatic, transient, requires no therapy<br>2 = Recurrent or persistent, no therapy required<br>3 = Requires treatment<br>4 = Requires monitoring. Hypotension, ventricular tachycardia, or fibrillation<br>*Cardiac Function:*<br>0 = None<br>1 = Asymptomatic decline of resting ejection by less than 20% of baseline<br>2 = Asymptomatic, decline of resting ejection fraction by more than 20% of baseline<br>3 = Mild CHF, responsive to therapy<br>4 = Severe or refractory CHF | • Age<br>• Cumulative dose<br>• Schedule of drug administration<br>• History of cardiac disease (i.e., atherosclerosis, mitral valve prolapse, hypertension)<br>• Use of combination drugs<br>• Hepatic dysfunction<br>• Prior mediastinum radiation<br>• History of CHF<br>• Prior anthracycline exposure | *Anthracyclines*<br>• Doxorubicin ($>550$ mg/m$^2$)<br>• Daunorubicin ($>600$ mg/m$^2$)<br>• Dactinomycin<br>• Doxorubicin-enhanced effect with: actinomycin, mitomycin, vincristine, melphalan, bleomycin cyclophosphamide<br>• *Mitoxantrone* ($>160$ mg/m$^2$)<br>• *Cyclophosphamide* High dose ($>144$ mg/kg $\times$ 4 days)<br>• *5-fluorouracil*<br><br>• *Taxol* | *Acute Changes:*<br>• Hypereosinophilia of myocytes<br>*Chronic Changes:*<br>• Loss of contractile elements<br>• Mitochondrial changes<br>• Myocyte damage<br><br><br>• Hemorrhagic myocardial necrosis<br><br>• Fibrin deposition in interstitium<br><br>• Coronary spasm of the Prinzmetal's type<br>• Speculated to be related to Cremaphor EL, the administration vehicle that causes activation of selected cardiac histamine receptors | • Limit cumulative dose of doxorubicin to $<550$ mg/m$^2$<br>• Administer doxorubicin at lower doses more frequently<br>• ECG before treatment<br>• Radionuclide cardiac scan<br>• Administer Zinecard (ICRF-159) before anthracycline dose<br>• Administer calcium channel blockers before anthracycline dose<br>• Limit cumulative dose of daunorubicin to $<600$ mg/m$^2$<br>• Avoid alcohol, smoking, and cocaine use<br>• Moderate exercise and low-fat, low-salt diet<br>• Prevent thrombus with daily aspirin or Coumadin |

rapid onset of gait ataxia, limb incoordination, dysarthria, nystagmus, and diplopia. Effects are reversible with drug withdrawal or dose reduction. Multifocal cerebral demyelination has been described to occur as the result of 5-FU and levamisole or leucovorin administration.[136] Symptoms that have been exhibited include acute confusion, ataxia, slurred speech, and restlessness. With the use of steroids and discontinuing chemotherapy the patient's symptoms improve.

High-dose cytarabine can cause encephalopathy, leukoencephalopathy, and sometimes peripheral neuropathy with doses over 18 g/m$^2$. High doses increase the transport rate over the cell membranes, enhancing the intracellular drug concentrations and prolonging the cellular exposure to the drugs' metabolites. CNS toxicity usually occurs 5–7 days after the start of therapy.[137] Ocular toxicity (conjunctivitis, photophobia, burning, and decreased acuity), cerebellar, and cerebral dysfunction can also occur. Once the drug is stopped, the neurological symptoms may resolve partially or completely.

Arthralgia and myalgia have been reported to occur infrequently with Taxotere administration. If symptoms occur, they are usually experienced a few days after administration lasting up to four days. Severity of discomfort can be reduced by the use of prophylactic analgesics such as ibuprofen.[45] Transient myalgia and arthralgia are common after moderate to high doses of Taxol administration. Symptoms usually occur two to three days after treatment and resolve in approximately six days. The shoulder and paraspinal muscles seem to be the most common area of occurrence, however other muscle groups can be effected.[44] Reports indicate the use of seldane has been found to reduce the discomfort.

One of the principal nonhematologic toxicities of Taxol is sensory neuropathy which is experienced at doses 250 mg/m² or greater. Symptoms consist of numbness, tingling, or burning pain of the lower extremities. Perioral numbness has been reported that may be asymmetrical at onset and progress in a symmetrical pattern. Neurotoxicity is typically cumulative with large-fiber modalities (vibration, proprioception) more frequently affected than loss of small-fiber modalities (pain and temperature).[44] Mild symptoms improve or resolve within several months after the discontinuation of Taxol. Amitriptyline has been found to be beneficial in relieving discomfort of the symptoms. Autonomic neuropathy has been reported with high doses of Taxol (250 mg/m² or greater) exhibited as paralytic ileus and orthostatic hypotension. Patients with diabetes mellitus experience this neuropathy more frequently.

Taxotere administration can produce mild sensory neuropathy. At a cumulative dose of 600 mg/m² severe and disabling neuropathy can develop. Symptoms include paresthesia, numbness, loss of sensory qualities and decrease in deep tendon reflexes.[138]

Astute neurological assessment is critical in patients receiving potentially neurotoxic agents. Baseline assessment should include sensory function, motor function, gait, range-of-motion, cranial nerves, and reflexes. Renal and hepatic functions should be monitored closely.[128] Chemotherapy agents such as ifosfamide and cytarabine will have increased neurotoxicity with renal dysfunction.[4] Sedatives, tranquilizers, and antiemetics, which are CNS depressants, must be used with caution since their usage may increase toxicity. In addition, other causes of these symptoms, such as electrolyte imbalances, metastasis, or other medical diseases, can cause similar effects. Neurotoxicity will affect patients by decreasing their mobility, ability for self-care, and ability to perform fine motor skills such as writing and buttoning a shirt. An occupational therapist may need to be consulted to help the patient adapt to loss of motor skills. Patients must be taught the importance of reporting any change in status, such as numbing and tingling of extremities. If neurological deficits become severe, safety measures must be initiated to protect the patient from harm (see Table 16-6).

### Pulmonary toxicity

Pulmonary toxicity usually is irreversible and progressive as a result of chemotherapy administration. The initial site of damage seems to be the endothelial cells, with an inflammatory-type reaction resulting in drug-induced pneumonitis. Another type of damage occurs as a result of an immunologic mechanism. Either the lung or the drug may act as the antigen in an allergic-type reaction.[139] Chronic exposure to chemotherapy causes an extensive alteration of the pulmonary parenchyma, with changes in the connective tissue, obliteration of alveoli, and dilatation of airspaces, known as "honeycombing."[140] Continuous injury and repair result in restrictive lung disease, with a thickened, still interstitium, increased work of breathing, and a functionally reduced lung volume leading to impaired gas exchange. Hypoxemia results because oxygen does not diffuse in the damaged areas while perfusion continues.

Pulmonary toxicity usually presents clinically as dyspnea, unproductive cough, bilateral basilar rales, and tachypnea. The chest x-ray may be within normal limits, but can show a pattern of diffuse interstitial markings. Arterial blood gases reveal hypoxia with hypocapnia and respiratory alkalosis. The most sensitive pulmonary function test is the carbon monoxide diffusion capacity measurement that becomes abnormal before the onset of clinical symptoms.[141] Other pulmonary function tests can show a restrictive pattern when pulmonary fibrosis has occurred. The best method to establish a histopathological diagnosis is to obtain involved tissues by means of an open lung biopsy or a fiberoptic bronchoscopy. As a result, bacterial or fungal infections and metastasis can be ruled out.

Bleomycin is known to cause pulmonary toxicity. The incidence is 5% for a total cumulative dose of 450 units and 15% for higher dosages. Bleomycin is concentrated preferentially in the lung and is inactivated by a hydrolase enzyme. This enzyme is relatively deficient in lung tissue as compared with other tissues, such as liver. These findings may explain the relative sensitivity of bleomycin to lung tissue causing: (1) early endothelial cell damage, (2) decrease in type I pneumocytes, with subsequent proliferation, and (3) migration of type II pneumocytes into alveolar spaces, inducing interstitial changes.[140] Following destruction of type I cells, repair is characterized by hyperplasia and dysplasia of the type II pneumocytes. Fibroblast proliferation, with subsequent pulmonary fibrosis, is probably the basis for irreversible changes induced by bleomycin.[141]

Cytarabine exerts a direct toxic effect on the pneumocytes and capillary endothelial cells to diminish the integrity of cell membranes and increase capillary permeability. A capillary leak syndrome, involving primarily the lung, occurs 2–21 days after the first dose, resulting in pulmonary edema and respiratory failure with features of adult respiratory disease (ARD). It appears to be related to high doses and continuous administration.[139]

Mitomycin C damage to the lung presents as diffuse alveolar damage with capillary leak and pulmonary edema. Incidence ranges from 3%–36%, occurring 6–12 months after therapy; however, occurrence may be after a brief exposure. If dyspnea occurs with a normal chest

**TABLE 16-6**   Organ Toxicity of Chemotherapy Agents: Neurotoxicity

| Toxicity/Symptoms | Grade | General Risk Factors | Chemotherapy Agent/Risk Factors/ Symptoms | Mechanism of Damage | Protective/ Management Measures |
|---|---|---|---|---|---|
| *Cerebellar:*<br>• Unsteady gait<br>• Nystagmus<br>• Ataxia<br>• Dizziness<br>• Seizures<br>• Hemiparesis<br>• Confusion<br>• Coma<br><br>*Autonomic:*<br>• Ileus<br>• Constipation<br>• Impotence<br>• Urinary retention<br>• Postural hypotension<br><br>*Peripheral/Cranial:*<br>• Facial palsies<br>• Diplopia<br>• Paresthesia of hands and feet<br>• Muscle atrophy<br>• Foot drop<br>• Loss of deep tendon reflexes<br>• Areflexia<br>• Sensory loss<br>• Sensory perception loss<br>• Hoarseness | *Neurocerebellar:*<br>0 = None<br>1 = Slight incoordination dysdiadokinesis<br>2 = Intention tremor dysmetria, slurred speech<br>3 = Locomotor ataxia<br>4 = Cerebellar necrosis<br><br>*Neurocortical:*<br>0 = None<br>1 = Mild somnolence or agitation<br>2 = Moderate somnolence or agitation<br>3 = Severe somnolence or agitation, confusion, disorientation, hallucination, aphasia<br>4 = Coma, seizures, psychosis<br><br>*Neurosensory:*<br>0 = None<br>1 = Mild paresthesias, loss of deep tendon reflexes<br>2 = Mild or moderate objective sensory loss, moderate paresthesias<br>3 = Severe objective loss, or paresthesias that interfere with function<br><br>*Neuromotor:*<br>0 = None<br>1 = Subjective weakness<br>2 = Mild objective weakness<br>3 = Objective weakness with impairment of function<br>4 = Paralysis | • Dosage<br>• Cranial radiation<br>• Intrathecal administration<br>• Age<br>• CNS depressants, i.e., antiemetics, tranquilizers, and sedatives | *Ifosfamide:*<br>• High doses<br>• Cerebellar and cranial dysfunction<br><br>*Vincristine:*<br>• Dose related >2 mg/m² of unit dose<br>• Hepatic dysfunction<br>• Autonomic, peripheral dysfunction<br><br>*Cisplatin:*<br>• Dose related<br>• Renal dysfunction<br>• Dehydration<br>• Autonomic, peripheral dysfunction<br>• Concurrent treatment with vincristine or etoposide<br><br>*Methotrexate:*<br>• High dose (>1 g/m²)<br>• Cerebellar dysfunction<br>• Concurrent cranial radiotherapy<br>• Intrathecal dose<br>• Increases effect with cytarabine, daunorubicin, salicylates, sulfonamides, vinblastine, vincristine<br><br>*Cytarabine:*<br>• High doses (>2 g/m²)<br>• Cerebellar and peripheral effects<br><br>*5-fluorouracil:*<br>• Cerebellar dysfunction<br>• Dose and schedule related<br><br>*Taxanes:*<br>• peripheral neuropathies<br>• Myalgias/arthralgia | • Accumulation of drug metabolite (chloracetaldehyde) with direct CNS effect<br><br>• Disrupts microtubules in the neural tissues<br><br>• Damages large fibers, resulting in sensory change<br>• Damage/loss of inner hair cells in the organ of Corti<br><br>• Demyelination of nerve fibers | • Place on bowel regimen<br>• Oral diazepam 5 mg every 6 hr at the time of treatment, to manage muscle spasms<br>• Eliminate furosemide<br>• Avoid concurrent administration of aminoglycosides<br>• Audiometric testing for high risk<br>• Ethyol (amifostine)<br>• Withhold therapy for severe toxicity, i.e., muscle weakness or pain<br>• Neurological recovery, start drug at 50% dose reduction<br>• Monitor neurological signs and symptoms<br>• Monitor electrolytes<br>• Institute safety measures |

radiograph, it may be necessary to discontinue mitomycin from the treatment plan.[142]

Cyclophosphamide causes pulmonary toxicity in less than 1% of patients and is associated with high doses (120 mg/kg/day for four days). Histological findings include endothelial swelling, pneumocyte dysplasia, edema, fibrosis, and fibroblast proliferation. The result of damage is alveolar hemorrhage and fibrin deposition.[139]

Carmustine inhibits lung glutathione disulfide reductase, which mediates the resultant cellular injury. Damage occurs after a long latency period, averaging three years, but may occur after only six weeks of therapy. High-dose carmustine has an incidence of 20%–30% when a cumulative dose of 1500 mg/m² is given. An insidious cough with dyspnea or sudden respiratory failure occurs. It has been suggested that this reaction may be more common when cyclophosphamide is given simultaneously.[143] Glucocorticoid administration has improved symptoms; however, mortality still occurs in a small percentage of patients.

Methotrexate can also produce an acute or a chronic process related to endothelial injury.[144] Diffuse alveolar damage is characterized by the disappearance of type I pneumocytes, hyaline membrane formation, and the presence of inflammatory cells in the alveoli and interstitium. The incidence is less than 1%, with an acute onset of pulmonary edema producing ARDs or more gradual systemic toxicity, such as fever, chills, and malaise being present before the appearance of pulmonary symptoms. Radiographic features may be unique, with pleural effusion occurring alone or in conjunction with pulmonary infiltrates, peripheral consolidations, or chronic eosinophilic pneumonia. Discontinuation of the drug is not always required for recovery, and reinstitution of the drug may not result in recurring symptoms.[145]

An uncommon side effect of Taxotere is fluid retention. The incidence is related to the cumulative dose which can be disabling, worsening with higher doses. Fluid retention is exhibited peripherally, as abdominal ascites, as a pleural effusion, or as a combination. The fluid retention is reversible and can be controlled with diuretics.[45]

Because lung damage usually is irreversible and progressive, it is imperative to detect evidence of pulmonary toxicity as early as possible. The causative agent may be discontinued or dose-reduced to prevent further damage to lung tissue. High concentrations of inspired oxygen are toxic to the lungs, and the simultaneous administration of various chemotherapy drugs may induce lung damage. Nurses need to be aware of this phenomenon and need to monitor the patient's oxygen saturation and breath sounds closely for early signs and symptoms of pulmonary toxicity.

When oxygen saturation is compromised due to restrictive lung damage, the patient experiences dyspnea on exertion or at rest. As a result, the patient will have an increased effort to perform simple activities of daily living. Nursing care is centered on teaching the patient to prioritize daily activities and to use breathing techniques such as pursed lips to lessen the effects of dyspnea. Supplemental oxygen therapy may be necessary to relieve the dyspnea. The family and patient must be taught how to administer the oxygen and what safety precautions to institute for oxygen therapy. Steroids are usually administered to lessen the pulmonary symptoms. Single lung transplantation may be an option for drug-induced pulmonary toxicity.[146] To prevent further complications, the nurse must also teach the patient how to mobilize secretions by maintaining an adequate fluid intake and performing effective cough and deep breathing techniques (see Table 16-7).

### Hepatotoxicity

Chemotherapy agents can cause a variety of hepatotoxic reactions. The initial site of damage seems to be the parenchymal cells. Obstruction to hepatic blood flow results in fatty changes, hepatocellular necrosis, cholestasis, hepatitis, and veno-occlusive disease (VOD). Hepatotoxicity usually is diagnosed initially by transient elevations of the hepatic enzymes during treatment that can progress to hepatomegaly, jaundice, and abdominal pain. Unless extensive fibrosis or necrosis has occurred, hepatotoxicity is reversible. For patients with hepatic dysfunction, the drug dose may need to be reduced or eliminated from the treatment plan.[147]

The incidence of VOD following high-dose chemotherapy in preparation for BMT is 20%, with a 50% mortality rate. Risk factors include increased age, hepatitis, and elevated SGOT before BMT. Clinical signs of VOD include insidious weight gain and jaundice that precede the development of abdominal pain, hepatomegaly, ascites, encephalopathy, and elevated bilirubin and SGOT laboratory values. VOD has also been documented after exposure to conventional or extremely high doses of a wide variety of chemotherapeutic agents, such as 6-mercaptopurine, cytarabine, thioguanine, dacarbazine, cyclophosphamide, carmustine, lomustine, busulfan, and mitomycin.[148]

Chemotherapy-induced VOD is sporadic manifesting with variable severity. Signs of chemotherapy-induced VOD have been described as (1) unexplained thrombocytopenia refractory to platelets, (2) sudden weight gain, (3) sudden decrease in hemoglobin, (4) increase in liver enzymes, (5) intractable ascites, and (6) associated with dactinomycin. Spontaneous recovery usually occurs from chemotherapy-induced VOD.[149]

VOD involves the partial or complete occlusion of the branches of the hepatic veins by endophlebitis and thrombosis. Normal hepatic circulation allows sinusoids to empty into the terminal hepatic venule through the small pores that penetrate the endothelial lining. When these pores are obstructed, the fluid and cellular debris become trapped, and eventually fibrosis of the venous walls occurs. Central hepatocellular necrosis occurs as well. Vascular engorgement results in hepatomegaly and

**TABLE 16-7** Organ Toxicity of Chemotherapy Agents: Pulmonary Toxicity

| Toxicity/Symptoms | Grade | General Risk Factors | Chemotherapy Agent/Risk Factors | Mechanism of Damage | Protective/Management Measures |
|---|---|---|---|---|---|
| • Low-grade fever<br>• Nonproductive cough<br>• Dyspnea<br>• Tachycardia<br>• Diffuse basilar crackles<br>• Wheezing<br>• Pleural rub<br>• Fatigue<br>• Malaise<br>• Chest pain<br>• Night sweats<br>• Tachypnea<br>• Cyanosis | *Dyspnea:*<br>0 = None<br>1 = Asymptomatic with abnormal PFTs<br>2 = Dyspnea on exertion<br>3 = Dyspnea at normal activity<br>4 = Dyspnea at rest<br><br>*Pulmonary Fibrosis:*<br>0 = Normal<br>1 = Radiographic changes, no symptoms<br>2 = N/A<br>3 = Changes with symptoms<br><br>*Pulmonary Edema:*<br>0–2 = None<br>3 = Radiographic changes and diuretics required<br>4 = Requires intubation<br><br>*Pneumonitis (Noninfectious):*<br>0 = Normal<br>1 = Radiographic change, symptoms do not require steroids<br>2 = Steroids required<br>3 = Oxygen required<br>4 = Requires assisted ventilation<br><br>*Pleural Effusion:*<br>0 = None<br>1–4 = Present<br><br>*ARDs:*<br>0 = None<br>1 = Mild<br>2 = Moderate<br>3 = Severe<br>4 = Life threatening | • Age<br>• Preexisting lung disease, i.e., COPD, TB<br>• History of smoking<br>• Cumulative dose<br>• Long-term therapy<br>• Mediastinal radiation<br>• High inspired concentration of oxygen | *Bleomycin:*<br>• Synergistic with vincristine<br>• Cumulative dose >450 mg/m$^2$<br>• Oxygen exposure >50%<br><br>*Mitomycin:*<br>• History of cyclophosphamide and/or methotrexate administration<br>• Oxygen concentrations >50%<br><br>*Carmustine:*<br>• Dose related (>1500 mg/m$^2$)<br>• Concurrent administration with cyclophosphamide<br><br>*Busulfan*<br><br>*Cyclophosphamide:*<br>• High dose >120 mg/kg/day × 4 days<br><br>*Methotrexate*<br><br>*Cytarabine:*<br>• High doses (5 g/m$^2$) | • Initial injury to capillary endothelium cells<br>• Necrosis of type I epithelial cells<br>• Hypertrophy of type II alveolar pneumocytes<br>• Pulmonary fibrosis<br><br>• Hypersensitivity reaction or immune complex related<br>• Damage similar to bleomycin<br>• Increased effect with VM-26, vincristine<br><br>• Inhibition of glutathione reductase in alveolar macrophages<br><br>• Hyperplasia and dysplasia of the type II pneumocytes<br><br>• Alveolar hemorrhage and fibrin deposition<br>• Increased effect with cisplatin, VM-26, vincristine<br><br>• Capillary leak syndrome, pulmonary edema<br>• Interstitial pneumonitis<br><br>• Capillary leak syndrome | • Assess for risk factors<br>• Obtain baseline pulmonary function tests<br>• Monitor cumulative dose<br>• Limit cumulative dose<br>• Limit oxygen to keep arterial PO$_2$ >60 mm Hg<br>• Discontinue drug if dyspnea occurs<br>• Assess for pulmonary symptoms<br>• Administer steroids and oxygen<br>• Monitor activities to minimize energy<br>• Stop or reduce dose of drug<br>• Fluid restriction<br>• Administer diuretics<br>• Follow-up with pulmonary function tests |

ascites. As the hepatocytes degenerate and necrose, liver serum enzyme levels become elevated, which can lead to liver necrosis, fibrosis, and portal hypertension.[150,151]

In clinical studies pentoxifylline (PTX) has been shown to have a marked effect on cell mediators of inflammation and tissue injury. The therapeutic effect of PTX is to stimulate vascular endothelial production of noninflammatory prostaglandins (E and I series), enhancing regional blood flow and promoting thrombolysis. These prostaglandins are responsible for the autoregulation of blood flow in several organs, including the liver, promoting diuresis and maintenance of blood flow. Studies suggest that PTX might preserve hepatic function and prevent VOD in the BMT population.[151]

Liver toxicity induced by high-dose methotrexate is transient and usually does not result in chronic liver disease. Elevation of hepatic enzyme levels is common, rising with successive courses and tending to be higher in patients treated on a daily schedule than those treated on intermittent schedules. All abnormalities usually resolve within one month following cessation of methotrexate therapy.[152]

High-dose cytarabine may induce intrahepatic cholestasis, possibly as a result of injury to the hepatocyte transport system. Changes are reversible; therefore they do not appear to limit cytarabine use.[153] 5-FU with combination levamisole has resulted in an increase in alkaline phosphatase, increase in transaminases, and increase in bilirubin. These changes resolve with the discontinuation of therapy without the need for medical intervention.[154] Gemcitabine can cause a transient increase of hepatic enzymes which resolve after discontinuing the drug.[47]

Fluorodeoxyuridine, usually administered as a continuous arterial dose, can cause chemical hepatitis, with rises in transaminases, alkaline phosphatase, and serum bilirubin levels. Stricture of intrahepatic or extrahepatic bile ducts can also occur. Toxicity appears to be both time and dose dependent. Liver function usually normalizes when the drug is discontinued. However, the development of biliary sclerosis is irreversible.[155]

Hepatocellular or cholestatic liver disease occurs with the administration of 6-mercaptopurine in daily doses exceeding 2 mg/kg. Histological pattern includes features of intrahepatic cholestasis and parenchymal cell necrosis. Moderate elevations occur in transaminases, alkaline phosphatase, and serum bilirubin, with episodes of jaundice occurring 30 days after initiation of therapy.[147]

Amsacrine is concentrated in the liver, where it undergoes conjugation to glutathione and is excreted in the bile. Its half-life is prolonged in patients with hepatic dysfunction manifested as elevations in bilirubin and alkaline phosphatase values. A 40% dose reduction in patients with bilirubin greater than 2 mg/100 ml is recommended.[156]

Few guidelines exist for the use of drugs when hepatic dysfunction is present. Known hepatotoxic drugs must be avoided when liver test results are abnormal. Impaired liver function delays excretion and results in increased accumulation in the plasma and tissues, especially for drugs such as doxorubicin Taxotere, vincristine, and vinblastine, which are excreted primarily by the liver into the bile. It has been recommended to reduce or not to administer the dose of these agents if the serum bilirubin is between 1.5 and 3 mg/dl. If the SGOT is between 60 and 180 international units, the drug should be reduced by 50%.[147]

Hepatic toxicity is uncommon, but it can be a serious consequence of chemotherapy administration, ranging from transient enzyme elevations to permanent cirrhosis. Because there are many disease- and treatment-related factors that can be hepatotoxic, it is difficult to attribute hepatic toxicity definitely to specific agents. During chemotherapy administration, the nurse monitors liver function tests closely, since enzymatic changes may be the first clinical evidence of hepatotoxicity. Third spacing (the shift of fluid from the vascular space to the interstitial space) can occur as a result of hepatotoxicity. Signs of fluid shift are decreased blood pressure, increased pulse rate, low central venous pressure, decreased urine output, increased specific gravity, low levels of serum albumin, and hemoconcentration.[150] Albumin is administered to replace the plasma protein and hopefully assist with absorption of the fluid. Fluid restriction minimizes third spacing, which enhances renal blood flow, decreases systemic congestion, and improves patient comfort. Other supportive care measures include diuretics, decreased protein intake, lactulose, and emotional support (see Table 16-8).

### Hemorrhagic cystitis

Hemorrhagic cystitis is a bladder toxicity resulting from cyclophosphamide and ifosfamide therapy. Hemorrhagic cystitis ranges from microscopic hematuria to frank bleeding, necessitating invasive local intervention with instillation of sclerosing agents. Symptoms range from transient irritative urination, dysuria, suprapubic pain to life-threatening hemorrhage. Transient cystitis has an early onset and short duration due to the direct effect of the deposition of acrolein, a by-product of metabolism, on the urothelium.[157]

After oral or intravenous administration, cyclophosphamide is metabolized by hepatic microsomal enzymes to hydroxycyclophosphamide and later by target cells to phosphamide mustard (active) and acrolein (urinary metabolite). The binding of acrolein to the bladder mucosa results in inflammation and ulceration. Approximately 10% of people receiving cyclophosphamide experience microscopic hematuria.[148] Early diagnosis is accomplished by urine dipstick or visual observation of red-tinged urine. If necessary, a confirmed diagnosis can be accomplished by cystoscopy, which shows discrete bleeding capillaries or diffuse mucosal ulceration, hemorrhage, and necrosis.

When hemorrhagic cystitis develops, drug therapy probably should be discontinued. In many patients discontinuation will lead to amelioration of the symptoms

**TABLE 16-8** Organ Toxicity of Chemotherapy Agents: Hepatotoxicity

| Toxicity/ Symptoms | Grade | General Risk Factors | Chemotherapy Agent | Mechanism of Damage | Protective/ Management Measures |
|---|---|---|---|---|---|
| • Elevated bilirubin, LDH, SGOT, alkaline phosphatase, SGPT<br>• Chemical hepatitis<br>• Jaundice<br>• Ascites<br>• Decreased albumin<br>• Cirrhosis<br>• Hepatomegaly<br>• Right upper quadrant pain<br>• Fatigue<br>• Anorexia<br>• Nausea<br>• Decreased clotting factor synthesis<br>• Hyperpigmentation of skin | Bilirubin:<br>0–1 = Normal<br>2 = <1.5<br>3 = 1.5–3.0<br>4 = >3.0<br><br>SGOT/SGPT:<br>0 = Normal<br>1 = <2.5<br>2 = 2.6–5.0<br>3 = 5.1–20<br>4 = >20<br><br>Alkaline Phosphatase:<br>0 = Normal<br>1 = 2.5<br>2 = 2.6–5.0<br>3 = 5.1–20<br>4 = >20<br><br>Liver Clinical:<br>0–2 = No change<br>3 = Precoma<br>4 = Hepatic coma | • Prior liver damage, e.g., hepatitis<br>• Dose<br>• Diabetes mellitus<br>• Tumor involvement<br>• Irradiation of liver<br>• Alcoholism<br>• Liver infections<br>• Concurrent administration of hepatotoxic drugs, e.g., phenothiazines<br>• Age<br>• Hepatic dysfunction<br>• Total bilirubin >2 mg/100 ml | • Methotrexate<br>• 6-Mercaptopurine<br>• Cytarabine<br>• Fluorodoxyuridine<br>• Nitrosoureas<br>• Etoposide, high dose<br>• Cisplatin, high dose<br>• L-Asparaginase<br>• Amsacrine<br>• Cyclophosphamide, high dose<br>• Doxorubicin<br>• Vincristine<br>• Vinblastine<br>• Docetaxel | Direct Toxic Effects:<br>• Parenchymal cell damage<br>• Intrahepatic cholestasis<br>• Hepatic fibrosis<br>• Fatty changes | • Pentoxifylline<br>• Reduce dose in presence of liver dysfunction for drugs metabolized in liver, e.g., vinca alkaloids or doxorubicin<br>• Avoid alcohol intake<br>• Monitor liver function tests<br>• If bilirubin >1.5 mg, reduce dose by 50%<br>• If bilirubin >3.0 mg, reduce dose by 75% |

without sequelae; however, microhematuria can continue long after discontinuing cyclophosphamide.[157] When therapy is not stopped, up to 55% of patients have persistent symptoms. Extensive chronic bleeding and mucosal inflammation can produce long-term cystitis, irreversible bladder fibrosis, bladder contraction, and an increased risk for bladder cancer.[158]

In an attempt to prevent cyclophosphamide-induced hemorrhagic cystitis, several drugs have been investigated to decrease this toxicity by inactivating acrolein within the bladder. Intravesical instillation of N-acetylcysteine, a thiol compound, may produce sulfhydryl complexes and subsequent detoxification of acrolein. Prostaglandin E2 and sucralfate may have therapeutic roles as intravesical agents for acrolein inactivation. In high doses, MESNA has been successful in protecting the bladder from the harmful effects of acrolein.[158]

Ifosfamide has a slower rate of metabolic activation into acrolein, allowing larger dosages to be administered as compared to cyclophosphamide. MESNA, a uroprotectant, contains a sulfhydryl group believed to bind acrolein within the urinary collecting system and detoxifies ifosfamide. MESNA is administered before ifosfamide and then intermittently up to 24 hours afterward to protect the bladder.[158]

In clinical trials gemcitabine caused microscopic hematuria and proteinuria, especially with repeated cycles. The occurrence was not found to be correlated with a cumulative dose or treatment duration.[47]

Protection of the bladder from either drug focuses on hyperhydration, frequent voiding, and diuresis. If cystitis occurs, the treatment includes bladder irrigations through a three-way Foley catheter to clear developing clots. The various solutions that cause a protein precipitate to form over the bleeding surfaces include saline, potassium aluminum sulfate, silver nitrate, and formalin. Vasopressins such as amino caproic acid may be administered intravenously or orally to decrease clotting. Cystoscopy may be necessary to cauterize bleeders, if the bladder irrigations were ineffective in controlling the bleeding. As a last resort, a cystectomy may be necessary.

During administration of chemotherapy agents, the nurse should monitor the urine for blood, through dip-sticking or observation. Strict intake and output measures are imperative to ensure minimal contact of acrolein with the bladder mucosa. The patient must be taught to maintain adequate hydration and to void frequently. If feasible, cyclophosphamide should be administered early in the day so the patient can drink fluids and void frequently without interruption of sleep. Insertion of a Foley catheter may be necessary when high doses of cyclophosphamide are administered, to ensure that the agent is being cleared from the bladder continuously (see Table 16-9).

### Nephrotoxicity

Nephrotoxicity is a dose-limiting side effect of some chemotherapeutic agents. Serious fluid and electrolyte imbalances that can progress to renal failure are the result of the direct and indirect effects of these agents on the kidney. Prevention of nephrotoxicity primarily involves aggressive hydration, urinary alkalization, diuresis, and careful monitoring of laboratory values. The hospitalized patient receiving other potentially nephrotoxic drugs, such as aminoglycosides, should be assessed prior to administering the agent. For patients with preexisting renal disease or who exhibit early signs of renal toxicity, the dosage may need to be reduced or the agent eliminated from the treatment plan.

Many chemotherapy agents are both metabolized and excreted by the kidneys; others are merely excreted as metabolites or as unchanged drugs. The manner in which chemotherapy damages the kidney varies from direct renal cell damage to an obstructive nephropathy as a result of precipitate formation. Renal failure, acid/base disorders, or electrolyte abnormalities may also occur as a result of tumor lysis syndrome or uric acid nephropathy.[159] When renal clearance of a specific drug with linear pharmakinetics is 35%–40% and the patient has moderate-to-severe renal function, a significant increase of the drug in the area under the plasma concentration curve (AUC) can occur.[4] (See acute tumor lysis syndrome.)

Cisplatin can cause mild-to-severe nephrotoxicity, with specific damage to the proximal and distal tubules. Platinum metal chelates in the renal tubules cause direct damage to the proximal tubular cells, damaging the tubular basement membranes, and can cause focal tubular necrosis.[160] Acute damage can occur within 3–21 hours after cisplatin administration, as evidenced by renal enzyme changes when precautions are not taken.[161,162] Renal dysfunction can persist for several years following cisplatin administration and may be irreversible.[4] Damage is characterized by degeneration of renal tubular epithelium, thickening of tubular basement membrane, and mild interstitial fibrosis. To avoid toxicity, patients should receive vigorous saline hydration of 1–2 liters as well as diuresis during therapy.

The use of mannitol in facilitating and inducing diuresis is a means of ensuring adequate urine flow. Mannitol possibly prevents immediate binding of cisplatin onto the renal tubules. Loop diuretics such as furosemide must be used with caution, since an increase in cisplatin toxicity has been reported.[163] Frequent determinations of renal function should be obtained, and if the creatinine clearance falls to less than 50 mg/ml, the drug should be withheld until renal function improves. Daily magnesium supplementation is indicated during cisplatin therapy, and electrolyte levels should be monitored frequently.[163]

Amifostine is an organic thiophosphate that has recently received FDA approval to reduce the cumulative renal toxicity associated with repeated administration of cisplatin in patients with advanced ovarian or nonsmall cell lung cancer. Although limited data exist, amifostine does not appear to decrease the effectiveness of cisplatin because of the differences in the normal cells' and cancer

**TABLE 16-9** Organ Toxicity of Chemotherapy Agents: Hemorrhagic Cystitis

| Toxicity/ Symptoms | Grade | General Risk Factors | Chemotherapy Agent/Risk Factors | Mechanism of Damage | Protective/ Management Measures |
|---|---|---|---|---|---|
| • Gross hematuria<br>• Dysuria, urgency<br>• Suprapubic pain | 0 = None<br>1 = Micro only<br>2 = Gross, no clots<br>3 = Gross, with clots<br>4 = Requires transfusion | • Dose-related<br>• Pelvic radiation | *Cyclophosphamide:*<br>• High dose (>2.5 g)<br><br>*Synergistic Effect:*<br>• Cisplatin<br>• VM-26<br>• Vincristine | • Drug metabolite acrolein damages bladder mucosa | • Vigorous hydration<br>• Frequent emptying of bladder, especially at night<br>• Monitor urine for blood<br>• 3-way Foley irrigation with saline, alum, or formaldehyde<br>• Administer amino caproic acid IV or po |
| | | | *Ifosfamide:*<br>• Single high dose vs multiple dose | | • MESNA given in a dose of 20%–30% of ifosfamide q 4hr × 3 |

cells' physiology and transport between the two tissue types. Other benefits seen with amifostine administration include: (1) reduced occurrence of hypomagnesemia, (2) protected effect of the kidneys from nephrotoxic antibiotics, and (3) reduced cumulative nephrotoxicity associated with cisplatin.[164,165]

Amifostine is dephosphorylated at the tissue site by alkaline phosphatase to form free thiol. Within the cell, thiol neutralizes reactive components of cisplatin before damage occurs to the DNA and RNA of the normal cell. Thiol acts as a potent scavenger of oxygen-free radicals and superoxide anions. This phenomenon is important because free radicals can damage cell membranes, DNA, and other vital cell components.[164,165]

A dose of 910 mg/m² is administered to the patient over 15 minutes intravenously after the patient has been adequately hydrated. Fifteen minutes afterwards cisplatin is administered. The most common side effect has been transient systolic hypotension, therefore it is recommended to administer amifostine with the patient in a supine position. The blood pressure is monitored every five minutes throughout the infusion and five minutes after the infusion. If the blood pressure drops below threshold from the baseline, the infusion is interrupted. The infusion can be restarted if the blood pressure returns to threshold within five minutes and if the patient is asymptomatic. If the blood pressure does not return, the infusion is discontinued and the next dose is reduced to 740 mg/m².[164,165]

| Baseline | <100 | 100–119 | 120–139 | 140–179 | >180 |
|---|---|---|---|---|---|
| Drop of 20 mm Hg of B/P interrupt infusion | 20 | 25 | 30 | 40 | 50 |

Transient systolic hypotension is short term, reversible, and treated with fluid administration and placing the patient in Trendelenburg position. Increased nausea and vomiting have occurred which could be a potentiating effect with cisplatin. Antiemetics must be given prior to amifostine administration and continued with cisplatin. Other side effects that have been observed include flushing, feeling of warmth or coldness, chills, syncope, somnolence, hiccups, and sneezing.[164,165]

Another compound being used as a cisplatin chemoprotectant agent is diethyldithiocarbamate (DDTC). This compound reportedly removes tissue-bound platinum through chelation, without reversing cisplatin's antitumor activity. Protection is provided against nephrotoxicity, bone marrow suppression, and GI toxicity. DDTC is administered intravenously and can cause flushing, diaphoresis, chest discomfort, and uneasiness if given rapidly.[165]

Standard doses of methotrexate are not associated with renal toxicity unless the patient has preexisting renal dysfunction. High doses (>1 g/m²) can cause an obstructive nephropathy from precipitation of methotrexate or its metabolites (7-OH mtx) in the renal tubules. Risk factors associated with drug-induced nephrotoxicity include: (1) low urine pH, (2) dehydration, (3) low methotrexate clearance, (4) decreased urine output, and (5) concurrent intrathecal treatment.[166] In general, urinary alkalization to maintain a urine pH greater than 7 with simultaneous administration of sodium bicarbonate or diamox prevents precipitate formation, permitting high-dose therapy.

Streptozocin in doses over 1.5 g/m² is associated with renal dysfunction in more than 65% of patients. Characteristically, streptozocin causes a tubulointerstitial nephritis and tubular atrophy due to direct damage of the tubules. This toxicity is manifested by hypokalemia, proteinuria, increased BUN, and increased creatinine levels.[161] Renal function tests and creatinine clearance tests should be obtained before beginning streptozocin therapy. Patients who develop an elevation of serum creatinine, even if it subsequently returns to normal, are cautioned against receiving further streptozocin, since severe toxicity may occur.

Lomustine and carmustine can cause a delayed renal failure months or years following therapy. Azotemia and proteinuria are manifested, followed by progressive renal failure, often requiring dialysis. It appears that the incidence of renal failure increases dramatically after a total dose of 1500 mg/m².[167]

Mitomycin C has been associated with a syndrome of renal failure and microangiopathic hemolytic anemia. This toxicity occurs in approximately 20% of patients who have received a cumulative dose of 100 mg or more after approximately six months of therapy and is characterized by an abrupt onset of microangiopathic hemolytic anemia, thrombocytopenia, azotemia, proteinuria, and hematuria. It generally is reversible.[168]

Nurses play a vital role in preventing nephrotoxicity. Preventive management includes aggressive hydration with hyper-tonic saline, diuresis, urinary alkalinization, and careful monitoring of urine output. Renal function tests, especially creatinine clearance, should be monitored before administering nephrotoxic drugs. Patients that must receive other nephrotoxic drugs, such as aminoglycosides, should be monitored closely for early signs and symptoms of toxicity. Assessment of renal function should continue throughout treatment and periodically after the completion of therapy (see Table 16-10).

*Acute tumor lysis syndrome* (ATLS) is a complication of cancer therapy that occurs most commonly in patients with tumors that have a high proliferation index and are highly sensitive to chemotherapy. ATLS is most commonly seen in patients with high-grade lymphoma, acute myelogenous leukemia, chronic myelogenous leukemia in blastic transformation, and non-Hodgkin's lymphoma.

ATLS is characterized by the development of acute hyperuricemia, hyperkalemia, hyperphosphatemia, and hypocalcemia with or without acute renal failure.[169] Patients with large tumor burdens in combination with high white blood cell count, lymphadenopathy, splenomegaly, and elevated lactate dehydrogenase are at particularly high risk. They will require close monitoring of metabolic parameters, including potassium, phosphorus, calcium,

**TABLE 16-10  Organ Toxicity of Chemotherapy Agents: Nephrotoxicity**

| Toxicity/ Symptoms | Grade | General Risk Factors | Chemotherapy Agent/Risk Factors | Mechanism of Damage | Protective/ Preventive Measures | General Management |
|---|---|---|---|---|---|---|
| • Increased BUN, creatinine<br>• Oliguria<br>• Azotemia<br>• Proteinuria<br>• Decreased creatinine clearance<br>• Hyperuricemia<br>• Hypomagnesemia<br>• Hypocalcemia | *Creatinine:*<br>0 = WNL<br>1 = <1.5<br>2 = 1.5–3.0<br>3 = 3.1–6.0<br>4 = >6.0<br><br>*Proteinuria:*<br>0 = No change<br>1 = 1+ or <3 g/liter<br>2 = 2–3+ or 3–10 g/liter<br>3 = 4+ or >10 g/liter<br>4 = Nephrotic syndrome<br><br>*Hematuria:*<br>0 = None<br>1 = Micro<br>2 = Gross, no clots<br>3 = Gross, with clots<br>4 = Requires transfusion<br><br>*BUN mg%:*<br>0 = WNL <20<br>1 = 21–30<br>2 = 31–50<br>3 = >50 | • Age<br>• Dose of agent<br>• Preexisting disease of kidneys<br>• Nutritional status<br>• Duration of cancer therapy<br>• Concurrent: Aminoglycoside therapy Amphotericin-B<br>• Renal damage<br>• Dehydration<br>• Large tumor mass<br>• Ileal conduits | *Nitrosoureas:*<br>• Cumulative dose of 1200 mg/m² for carmustine and lomustine<br><br>*Mitomycin C:*<br>• Increased effect with vincristine and VM-26<br><br>*Anthracyclines:*<br>• High dose (1.5 g/m²/wk)<br><br>*Streptozotocin:*<br>• Dose (>1.5 g/m²/wk)<br><br>*Cisplatin:*<br>• Multiple doses (>50 mg/m²)<br>• High dose<br>• Increased effect with cyclophosphamide<br><br><br>*Methotrexate:*<br>• High dose (>1 g/m²)<br>• Enhanced effect with cisplatin | • Direct cell damage in glomerulus<br>• Chronic interstitial nephritis<br>• Tubular atrophy<br>• Direct cell damage in glomerulus<br>• Microangiopathic hemolytic anemia<br>• Tubular atrophy<br><br>• Diffuse tubulointerstitial nephritis<br>• Tubulointerstitial nephritis<br>• Tubular atrophy<br>• Direct cell damage in tubules<br>• Necrosis of proximal and distal renal tubules<br><br><br>• Precipitation of metabolites in the acid environment of the urine<br>• Obstructive nephropathy | These following four measures apply to all drugs<br>• Monitor renal function tests<br>• Saline diuresis<br>• Hydrate patient (3000 ml/day)<br>• Decrease uric acid production with allopurinol<br><br><br>• Stop drug if creatinine does not return to baseline<br>• Diuresis with mannitol<br>• Administer WR-2721 15 min before administration<br>• Administer DDTC<br><br>• Maintain alkalinization of urine pH >7<br>• Administer leucovorin<br>• Administer bicarbonate<br>• Avoid vitamin C<br><br>Acids (ASA, vitamin C) compete for drug elimination sites that increases serum concentration of methotrexate | • Substitute analogue drug<br>• Reduce dose for creatinine clearance (normal 125 ml/min)<br><br>*30–60 ml/min:*<br>Cisplatin—50%<br>Methotrexate—50%<br>Mitomycin—75%<br>Nitrosoureas—hold dose<br><br>*10–30 ml/min:*<br>Cisplatin—hold dose<br>Mitomycin—75%<br><br>*<10 ml/min:*<br>Cyclophosphamide—50%<br>Mitomycin—50% |

Note: Pharmacokinetics of the following drugs suggest dose reduction when the patient has renal impairment:
fludarabine
carboplatin (increased thrombocytopenia with renal dysfunction)
ifosfamide (increased CNS toxicity)
melphalan IV

pentostatin (increased serious toxicity)
etoposide (increased bone marrow toxicity)
topotecan (increased neutropenia)
bleomycin (increased pulmonary toxicity)
dacarbazine
hydroxyurea (increased bone marrow toxicity)

uric acid, blood urea nitrogen, and creatinine levels. For high-risk patients, baseline renal function is assessed before the initiation of aggressive antineoplastic therapy.[170] Electrolytes and serum phosphorus, calcium, magne-sium, uric acid, creatinine and blood urea nitrogen levels are measured daily.

Uric acid crystallization in the renal tubules causing obstruction, decreased glomerular filtration, and/or acute renal failure is a major complication that can be prevented by prophylactic alkalinization of urine, thus increasing the solubility of uric acid (Table 16-11). This is accomplished by maintaining the urine pH at a level greater than 7, with the use of sodium bicarbonate and vigorous intravenous hydration to decrease the uric acid concentration in the urine. A recommended fluid regimen is D5W/0.45NS with sodium bicarbonate, 60 mEq/l, at 150 ml/hr. Sodium bicarbonate administration should be discontinued once serum uric acid has normalized since overly vigorous alkalinization may accelerate phosphate precipitation in the renal tubules. Also, alkalosis may predispose the patient to neuromuscular irritability by further lowering the calcium level.[169]

Potassium and magnesium may need to be replaced if deficits in these electrolytes appear. Simultaneous hydration and diuresis promote the excretion of phosphorus

**TABLE 16-11**   Prevention and Management of the Metabolic Complications of Acute Tumor Lysis

| |
|---|
| Control of hyperuricemia<br>　Begin allopurinol administration at a dose of 600–900 mg/day and reduce to half after 3–4 days. |
| Urinary alkalinization<br>　Maintain urine pH ≥ 7 by addition of 50–100 mEq of $NaHCO_3$ to each liter of IV fluid<br>　Acetazolamide 250–500 mg IV daily if above measure is ineffective or serum $HCO_3$ >27 mEq/l<br>　Discontinue urinary alkalinization once hyperuricemia is corrected (serum uric acid <10 mg/dl) |
| Forced diuresis<br>　Maintain urine flow at >150–200 ml/hr with infusion of 5% dextrose 0.5NS at 200 ml/hr<br>　Initiate low-dose dopamine and diuretics in patients with preexisting evidence of fluid retention (marked edema or ascites) or oliguria<br>　Do not insert Foley catheter unless patient has altered mental status or evidence of urinary retention |
| Maintain fluid balance<br>　Avoid fluid overload: administer IV furosemide (20–100 mg q 4–8hr) if urine output falls below fluid intake<br>　Obtain daily weights<br>　Maintain scrupulous records of intake and output |
| Monitoring of blood chemistries<br>　Serum electrolytes, BUN, creatinine, uric acid, calcium, phosphorous, magnesium q 6–8hr during the first 72 hr following chemotherapy |
| Acute hyperkalemia<br>　Initiate hypertonic glucose and insulin infusion, Kayexalate and furosemide |
| Hyperphosphatemia<br>　Initiate hypertonic glucose and insulin infusion, and oral antacids |

Dietz K, Flaherty AM: Oncologic emergencies, in Groenwald S, Frogge MH, Goodman M, Yarbro CH (eds): *Cancer Nursing: Principles and Practice* (ed 3). Boston, Jones and Bartlett, 1993, pp 801–839.

and potassium. Urine output should be maintained at a minimum of 100 ml/hr. Diuretics may be administered as adjunctive therapy, particularly when the person has a co-existing condition (e.g., impaired cardiac function) that could potentiate the risk of fluid overload. If adequate urine output is not achieved, furosemide 40–80 mg intravenously, or mannitol 12.5 g intravenously, may be given to promote diuresis.[169] Fluid balance is assessed by monitoring of intake, output, and weight and observation for edema of lower extremities or sacrum. Distended neck veins or shortness of breath should be noted and the lungs should be auscultated for adventitious sounds (rales). Decreased urine output, hematuria, and urine pH < 7 are reported immediately. Meticulous records of intake and output are necessary to monitor effectiveness of therapy.

If a patient is at high risk for ATLS with chemotherapy, allopurinol is generally given as a prophylactic measure. Allopurinol decreases uric acid levels by interfering with purine metabolism. If tumor lysis syndrome develops, allopurinol 600–900 mg/day is given and then reduced to 300–450 mg/day after three to four days. It may cause a skin rash within seven days of initial dosage, requiring palliative relief measures with lotion or diphenhydramine hydrochloride. If adequate renal function is maintained and metabolic parameters have been corrected, ATLS will usually resolve within seven to ten days of treatment (see Figure 16-10.)

### Gonadal toxicity

From the beginning of the use of chemotherapy in the treatment of cancer, gonadal failure, infertility, and premature menopause have been reported as consequences of chemotherapy. The likelihood that chemotherapy will affect a patient's fertility depends in part on the patient's gender, age, and the specific drugs. In contrast to males, the age of female patients is an important predictor of treatment-induced sterility. The aging ovary has progressively fewer germ cells, which are not replaced. Therefore, women over the age of 30 are less likely to regain ovarian function because they have fewer oocytes.[171-173] Treatment-induced gonadal function is quantified by elevation in the gonadotropins, follicle-stimulating hormone (FSH), and luteinizing hormone (LH), which reflects the efforts of the hypothalamic-pituitary axis to stimulate the injured gonads to function normally.[173,174]

Cycle-nonspecific drugs such as alkylating agents are the most detrimental to fertility.[171] Effects on fertility are presumably due to the constant mitotic cycles essential for spermatogenesis, compared with the relative inactivity of oocyte formation. Therefore the testes are more susceptible to injury from alkylating agents than the ovaries. Alkylating agents are most commonly associated with compromised fertility, and combination regimens have a greater effect than single agents. Busulfan causes amenorrhea, atrophic endometrium, and symptoms associated with menopause. Nitrogen mustard, chlorambucil, mel-

**FIGURE 16-10** Clinical pathway for tumor lysis syndrome. (Dietz K, Flaherty AM: Oncologic emergencies, in Groenwald SL, Frogge MH, Goodman M, Yarbro CH (eds): *Cancer Nursing: Principles and Practice* (ed 3). Boston, Jones and Bartlett, 1993, pp 801–839.)

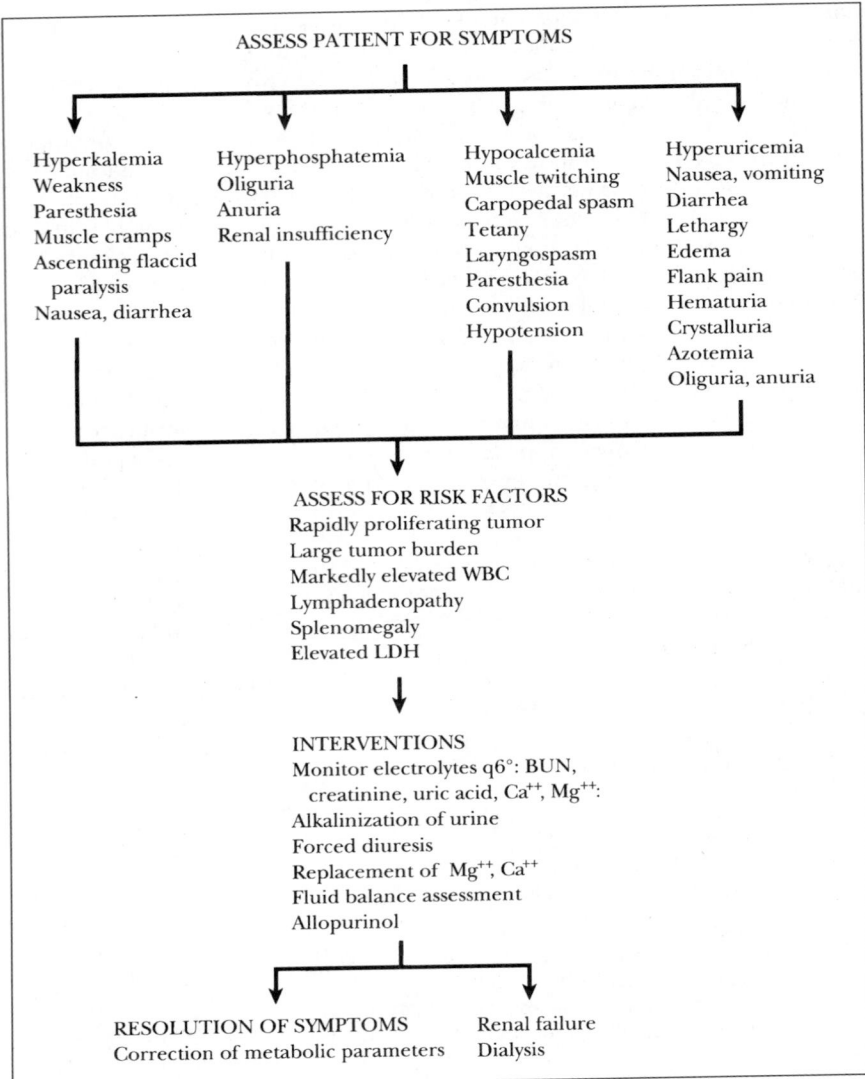

ASSESS PATIENT FOR SYMPTOMS

Hyperkalemia
Weakness
Paresthesia
Muscle cramps
Ascending flaccid
  paralysis
Nausea, diarrhea

Hyperphosphatemia
Oliguria
Anuria
Renal insufficiency

Hypocalcemia
Muscle twitching
Carpopedal spasm
Tetany
Laryngospasm
Paresthesia
Convulsion
Hypotension

Hyperuricemia
Nausea, vomiting
Diarrhea
Lethargy
Edema
Flank pain
Hematuria
Crystalluria
Azotemia
Oliguria, anuria

ASSESS FOR RISK FACTORS
Rapidly proliferating tumor
Large tumor burden
Markedly elevated WBC
Lymphadenopathy
Splenomegaly
Elevated LDH

INTERVENTIONS
Monitor electrolytes q6°: BUN,
  creatinine, uric acid, $Ca^{++}$, $Mg^{++}$:
Alkalinization of urine
Forced diuresis
Replacement of $Mg^{++}$, $Ca^{++}$
Fluid balance assessment
Allopurinol

RESOLUTION OF SYMPTOMS
Correction of metabolic parameters

Renal failure
Dialysis

phalan, and procarbazine cause ovarian atrophy. Cyclophosphamide elevates FSH levels, pointing to a direct toxic effect on the ovaries.[175]

It is difficult to define the effects of chemotherapy on gonadal function in children. Frequently, childhood cancers are treated with multimodality therapy combining chemotherapy and radiation therapy. In addition, children are in various stages of sexual and growth development. Presently, long-term follow-up is being conducted but has not been conclusive on long-term gonadal functions.

The testes of adult men are particularly vulnerable to chemotherapeutic agents. A progressive dose-related depletion of the germinal epithelial lining of the seminiferous tubule results in the disappearance of the spermatocytes and spermatogonia, leaving only Sertoli cells. Drug-induced testicular damage results in azoospermia, oligospermia, and abnormalities of semen volume, motility, and sperm forms in postpubertal men. Assessment of

male gonadal function includes: (1) semen analysis, (2) presence of testicular atrophy, (3) FSH levels, and (4) testosterone levels.[176] The incidence and length of time for recovery of spermatogenesis depend on the patient's age and the total drug dose. For example, cyclophosphamide produces azoospermia at a total dose of 9 grams, with a recovery of normal spermatogenesis in 100% within 31 months of treatment.[171,174] Male patients who desire to preserve childbearing ability may elect to utilize semen preservation, along with subsequent artificial insemination or in vitro fertilization.[177]

Chemotherapy affects fertility by injuring the germinal epithelium of the gonad. It is clear that prepubertal ovaries are profoundly affected histologically after chemotherapy. Ova become nonfunctional by direct injury or indirect injury resulting from loss of supporting follicular cells. These changes include focal stromal fibrosis, follicular maturation arrest, and reduction in numbers of ova despite exposure to lower total doses of drugs.[178–180]

Women who develop amenorrhea after cytotoxic therapy often experience hot flashes, with menopausal blood levels of FSH, LH, and estradiol. Menopausal symptoms may be treated with hormonal replacement, low-dose clonidine, or progesterone.[176,181]

Over time, the more serious consequences of premature estrogen deprivation, such as osteoporosis and vaginal atrophy, can develop, but if not contraindicated can be effectively treated with hormonal replacement.[174] With failing ovary syndrome, there is a period of months or years of erratic ovarian function, with many months of amenorrhea interspersed with occasional normal menstrual periods.[173] Depending on the woman's age as well as the type and total dose of chemotherapy, ovarian function may resume after a period of time. Because the onset of chemotherapy-related ovarian failure is age-related and progressive, a young woman might remain amenorrheic for several years and then begin to menstruate sporadically and even conceive during these cycles.[175,178] Ovarian function can be evaluated by menstrual history, reproductive history, FSH/LH/estradiol levels, presence of vaginal atrophy, and menopausal symptoms.[181] Attempts have been made to preserve ovarian function during chemotherapy through the use of oral estrogens, which produce negative feedback to the hypothalamic-pituitary axis, thereby decreasing gonadotropic stimulation of the ovaries.

For women who have conceived and must receive chemotherapy, few complications have been reported, provided the drugs are given in the second and third trimester.[179,182] The antimetabolites and alkylating agents administered during the first trimester cause teratogenesis. Even though chemotherapy agents are known to cross the placental barrier, second- or third-trimester chemotherapy exposure may result in low birth weight or prematurity.

In general, patients surviving cancer may be advised to wait at least two years after completion of therapy before attempting parenthood. This allows plenty of time for the elimination of chromosome breaks and damaged germ cells.[183,184] In women who conceive after receiving chemotherapy, the incidence of spontaneous abortion and fetal abnormality is not increased.[182,185] Currently no firm evidence exists that progeny of former cancer patients have an increase frequency of spontaneous abortions, genetic diseases, or congenital anomalies.[176]

Although many patients experience reproductive dysfunction during chemotherapy, information is still needed regarding the possibility of conception and the effects that could occur during chemotherapy administration. Birth control pills can be used if the patient does not have a cancer that is hormonally sensitive and the risk of cardiovascular side effects is not a concern. Intrauterine devices are not recommended when the patient is experiencing myelosuppression, since bleeding or infection could occur. Diaphragms, sponges, vaginal inserts, and condoms require careful attention to the insertion technique and personal hygiene after usage. A water-soluble lubricant may be needed if vaginal dryness is being experienced prior to intercourse.

Accurate information can make a significant difference in the patient's ability to deal with sexual concerns regarding chemotherapy. In general, most chemotherapy agents are excreted from the body in the first 72 hours following administration. Patients need to be instructed to use condoms and to avoid oral sex during this period in the event that the semen or vaginal secretions contain chemotherapy metabolites.

Female patients may need instruction on coping with ovarian dysfunction and guidance on managing hot flashes and vaginal dryness. Although high-dose chemotherapy may affect the male's ability to achieve or maintain an erection, usually this is not a problem. However, all patients may need to be counseled about decreased libido due to fatigue or the lack of sexual desire. Providing information that chemotherapy will not be transferred by kissing, hugging, or cuddling is reassuring and helps patients come to terms with feelings about cancer and sexuality.

## SECONDARY/THERAPY-RELATED CANCERS

One of the most serious long-term consequences of cancer is that the treatment intended to cure the patient may contribute to the occurrence of a second malignancy.[186] *Second malignancy* refers to a new neoplasm that has developed after treatment of the initial or primary cancer.[187,188] It implies that the new neoplasm is related in some way to treatment that was not only cytotoxic but also carcinogenic. Although the risk for a secondary cancer is small, treatment for the primary cancer usually outweighs that risk.[186,189]

Therapy-related malignancies generally have a poor prognosis, and treatment is often unsuccessful. The mechanism of oncogenesis after treatment remains unclear but could relate to interactions between immunosuppressive factors, direct cellular damage produced by fibrotic tissue changes, or carcinogenic effects from other environmental carcinogens. Lethal damage to the neoplastic cell is the obvious intent of chemotherapy; yet if cellular damage is not repaired in the normal cell, malignant transformation and/or mutation can occur.[190] Long-term survivors of Hodgkin's disease who have received both chemotherapy and radiation have the highest incidence of secondary malignancies.[191,192] Other risk factors include the primary neoplasm, the natural history of the disease, the type of chemotherapy, the cumulative dose of the agent, the age of the patient during chemotherapy administration, the patient's immune status, and the patient's environment.[193,194]

The alkylating agents, nitrosoureas, and procarbazine are the agents most implicated in chemotherapy-related malignancies.[193–195] Although all alkylating agents have been implicated in producing a myelodysplastic disease or acute leukemia, melphalan is probably the most potent leukemogenic agent. Alkylating agents cause the two strands of DNA to become cross-linked so that DNA replication is inhibited. Due to a change in the structural configuration of guanine, miscoding of thymidine may occur, leading to abnormal base pairing.[186] Sister chromatid exchanges frequently occur after the use of alkylating agents and may be responsible for mutagenesis. Chromosomes 5 and 7 are involved in 90% of those with cytogenetic abnormalities. Observed deletions of all or part of those chromosomes strongly support the diagnosis of chemotherapy-associated acute leukemia. In addition, damage to the stem cells in the bone marrow by alkylating agents may result in the emergence of leukemic clones.[193]

After receiving alkylating agents, patients have a 1.6%–2.3% risk of developing acute nonlymphocytic leukemia (ANLL) within ten years, peaking at two to three years.[195] Older patients have been found to have shorter intervals between treatment and preleukemic changes. This may be related in part to a declining immune status associated with age combined with long-term immunosuppressive effects of alkylating agents.[186]

The schedule of chemotherapy administration may have some bearing on the development of leukemia.[187] Patients with multiple myeloma who received intravenous doses of melphalan, carmustine, and cyclophosphamide had a rate of 0.7% in developing leukemia as compared to 2.6% of patients who received daily oral doses of melphalan. Patients with multiple myeloma developed acute myelocytic or myelomonocytic leukemia at a risk of 2.5% at five years and 9.2% at ten years.[193] Women receiving melphalan for ovarian cancer are two or three times more likely to develop leukemic disorders than those receiving cyclophosphamide.[195] The interval between the onset of cyclophosphamide therapy and the occurrence of bladder, kidney, ureter, or urethra malignancy averaged more than five years, with a range of 1–12 years.[187]

Maintenance chemotherapy with chlorambucil and the use of mechlorethamine for induction seems to be a major contributor to the development of acute leukemia in patients with Hodgkin's disease. The ten-year actual risk of ANLL was 10.9% in a series of 172 patients with Hodgkin's disease given radiation and chemotherapy.[190–192] This risk was 5.6% for patients under 40 years of age and 30.9% for those over 40. Risk also increased in direct proportion to the cumulative dose of alkylating agents as well as combination regimens.

Relative risks for developing leukemia after treatment for breast cancer with cyclophosphamide was 1.3%–2.7% and up to 30% with the use of melphalan and radiotherapy.[196,197] Increased risk was confined to women older than 50 years of age. It has been reported that etoposide may induce a leukemia with the morphological and cytogenetic features of acute monoblastic leukemia rather than those seen with ANLL.[194] Patients with germ cell tumors treated with high-dose etoposide, cisplatin, and bleomycin are at an increased risk for developing myelodysplastic syndrome and acute myelocytic leukemia.[198]

Although the number of patients who develop a second malignancy is small, patients must be taught the importance of continual follow-up for the rest of their lives after treatment. The nurse may need to encourage patients to implement lifestyle changes to improve their health. The American Cancer Society warning signs of cancer should be taught to patients for their own follow-up. Patients who develop a second malignancy are a challenge to the nurse, especially when it involves a long-term survivor with whom there is a strong bonding relationship. It is imperative that the nurse assist the patient and family in coping with the diagnosis and impending treatment.

## CONCLUSION

Advances in cancer therapy are made by continual investigations, evaluation of treatment results, and their incorporation into the practice of oncology. Because of the amount of time spent directly with the patient receiving chemotherapy, the nurse is often the health care provider best able to recognize subtle changes in the patient's status that could be indicative of pending complications from chemotherapy. Nursing responsibilities are multifaceted, and include patient education, ongoing physical assessments, identification of risk factors, and prompt therapeutic interventions with ongoing evaluation for modification.

Occurrence of side effects does not necessarily preclude withholding of chemotherapy but instead alerts nurses to the need for careful assessment, management, and evaluation. The nurse's assessment of a patient's response to treatment and assistance in preventing or managing side effects can make the difference in the patient's overall perceived quality of life. Once the treatment is complete, nurses can be instrumental in encouraging patients to have a yearly comprehensive physical examination to detect cancer recurrence, second malignancies, and other long-term effects of chemotherapy.

## REFERENCES

1. Lilly LL: Side effects associated with pediatric chemotherapy: Management and patient education issues. *Ped Nurs* 16:252–255, 1990
2. Camp-Sorrell D: Controlling adverse effects of chemotherapy. *Nurs 91* 4:34–42, 1991
3. Goodman M: Managing the side effects of chemotherapy. *Semin Oncol Nurs* 5:29–52, 1989 (suppl 1)
4. Kintzel PE, Dorr RT: Anticancer drug renal toxicity and elimination: Dosing guidelines for altered renal function. *Cancer Treat Rev* 21:23–64, 1995
5. Montamat SC, Cusack BJ, Vestal RE: Management of drug therapy in the elderly. *N Engl J Med* 321:303–309, 1989
6. Annesley T: Pharmacokinetic changes in the elderly. *Clin Lab Sc* 3:100–102, 1990
7. Vose JM: Cytokine use in the older patient. *Semin Oncol* 22(1):6–8, 1995 (suppl 1)

8. Lipschitz DA: Age-related declines in hematopoietic reserve capacity. *Semin Oncol* 22(1):3–5, 1995 (suppl 1)

9. Boyle DM: Realities to guide novel and necessary nursing care in geriatric oncology. *Cancer Nurs* 17(2):125–136, 1994

10. Blesch KS: The normal physiological changes of aging and their impact on the response to cancer treatment. *Semin Oncol Nurs* 4:178–188, 1988

11. Leslie WT: Chemotherapy in older cancer patients. *Oncology* 6:74–80, 1992

12. Damon LE: Anemia of chronic disease in the aged: Diagnosis and treatment. *Geriatrics* 47:47–57, 1992

13. Yates J, Glidewell O, Wiernick P, et al: Cytosine arabinoside with daunorubicin or adriamycin for therapy of acute myelocytic leukemia. *Blood* 60:454–462, 1982

14. Begg CB, Cohen JL, Ellerton J: Are the elderly predisposed to toxicity from cancer chemotherapy? *Cancer Clin Trials* 3:369–374, 1980

15. Begg CB, Carbone PP: Clinical trials and drug toxicity in the elderly: The experience of the Eastern Cooperative Oncology Group. *Cancer* 52:1986–1992, 1983

16. Begg CB, Elson PG, Carbone PP: A study of excess hematologic toxicity in elderly patients treated on cancer chemotherapy protocols, in Yancik R (ed): *Cancer in the Elderly: Approaches to Early Detection and Treatment.* New York, Springer-Verlag, 1989

17. O'Reilly S, Klimo P, Conners J: Low-dose ACOP-B and VABE: Weekly chemotherapy for elderly patients with advanced stage diffuse large-cell lymphoma. *J Clin Oncol* 9:741–747, 1991

18. Thyss A, Saudes L, Otto J, et al: Renal tolerance of cisplatin in patients more than 80 years old. *J Clin Oncol* 12(10):2121–2125, 1994

19. Thomasma DC: Ethics and professional practice in oncology. *Semin Oncol Nurs* 5:89–94, 1989

20. Schipper H, Levitt M: Measuring quality of life: Risks and benefits. *Cancer Treat Rep* 69:1115–1123, 1985

21. Youngblood M, Williams PD, Eyles H, et al: A comparison of two methods of assessing cancer therapy-related symptoms. *Cancer Nurs* 17(1):37–44, 1994

22. Aaronson NK: Quality of life: What is it? How should it be measured? *Oncology* 2:69–74, 1988

23. Ferrans CE: Quality of life: Conceptual issues. *Semin Oncol Nurs* 6:248–254, 1990

24. McCabe MS: Psychological support for the patient on chemotherapy. *Oncology* 5:91–107, 1991

25. Cella DF, Cherin EA: Quality of life during and after cancer treatment. *Comp Ther* 14:69–75, 1988

26. Morra ME: Choices: Who's going to tell the patients what they need to know? *Oncol Nurs Forum* 15:421–425, 1988

27. Yasko JM, Verfurth M: Closing comment: Future trends. *Semin Oncol Nurs* 8:156–158, 1992

28. Dodd M: Assessing patient self-care for side effects of cancer chemotherapy. Part I. *Cancer Nurs* 5:447–451, 1982

29. Dodd M: Self-care for side effects in cancer chemotherapy: An assessment of nursing interventions. Part II. *Cancer Nurs* 6:63–66, 1983

30. Musci EC, Dodd MJ: Predicting self-care with patients' and family members' affective states and family functioning. *Oncol Nurs Forum* 17:394–400, 1990

31. Holland JC, Lesko LM: Chemotherapy, endocrine therapy and immunotherapy, in Holland JC, Rowland JH (eds): *Handbook of Psychooncology.* New York, Oxford University Press, 1989, pp 146–162

32. Love RR, Leventhal H, Douglas V, et al: Side effects and emotional distress during cancer chemotherapy. *Cancer* 63:604–611, 1989

33. Nail LM, Jones LS, Greene D, et al: Use and perceived efficacy of self-care activities in patients receiving chemotherapy. *Oncol Nurs Forum* 18:883–887, 1991

34. Dodd M: Cancer patients' knowledge of chemotherapy: Assessment and informational interventions. *Oncol Nurs Forum* 9:39–44, 1982

35. Fernsler JI, Cannon CA: The whys of patient education. *Semin Oncol Nurs* 7:79–86, 1991

36. Miller AB, Hoogstraten B, Staquet M, et al: Reporting results of cancer treatment. *Cancer* 47:207–214, 1981

37. Kisner DL: Reporting treatment toxicities, in Buyse ME, Staquet M, Sylvester RJ (eds): *Cancer Clinical Trials: Methods and Practice.* New York, Oxford University Press, 1984, pp 178–190

38. Mili L: The community hospital perspective of clinical trials and the role of the nurse educator. *Semin Oncol Nurs* 7:280–287, 1991

39. Link DL: Antibiotic therapy in the cancer patient: Focus on third generation cephalosporins. *Oncol Nurs Forum* 14:35–41, 1987

40. Rostad ME: Current strategies for managing myelosuppression in patients with cancer. *Oncol Nurs Forum* 18:7–15, 1991 (suppl)

41. Gootenberg JE, Pizzo PA: Optimal management of acute toxicities of therapy. *Pediatr Clin North Am* 38:269–297, 1991

42. Maxwell MB, Maher KE: Chemotherapy-induced myelosuppression. *Semin Oncol Nurs* 8:113–123, 1992

43. Hoagland HC: Hematologic complications of cancer chemotherapy, in Perry MC (ed): *The Chemotherapy Source Book.* Baltimore, Williams & Wilkins, 1992, pp 498–507

44. Rowinsky EK, Eisenhauer EA, Chaudhry V, et al: Clinical toxicities encountered with paclitaxel (Taxol). *Semin Oncol* 20:1–15, 1993, (suppl 3)

45. Pronk LC, Stoter G, Verweij J: Docetaxel (taxotere): Single agent activity, development of combination treatment and reducing side effects. *Cancer Treat Rev* 21:463–478, 1995

46. Guchelaar HJ, Richel DJ, van Knapen A: Clinical, toxicological and pharmacological aspects of gemcitabine. *Cancer Treat Rev* 22:15–31, 1996

47. Shepherd FA, Burkes R, Cormier Y, et al: Phase I dose-escalation trial of gemcitabine and cisplatin for advanced non-small cell lung cancer: Usefulness of mathematic modeling to determine maximum tolerable dose. *J Clin Oncol* 14:1656–1662, 1996

48. Hudis CA, Seidman AD, Crown JPA, et al: Phase II and pharmacologic study of docetaxel as initial chemotherapy for metastatic breast cancer. *J Clin Oncol* 14:58–65, 1996

49. Hohneker J: A summary of vinorelbine (Navelbine) safety data from North American clinical trials. *Semin Oncol* 21:42–47, 1994, (suppl 10)

50. Wargin WA, Lucas V: The clinical pharmacokinetics of vinorelbine (Navelbine). *Semin Oncol* 21:21–27, 1994, (suppl 10)

51. Corman LC: The relationship between nutrition, infection, and immunity. *Med Clin North Am* 69:519–531, 1985

52. Balducci L, Hardy C: Cancer and malnutrition: A critical interaction. *Am J Hematol* 18:91–103, 1985

53. Leitgeb C, Pecherstorfer M, Ludwig H: Quality of life in chronic anemia of cancer during treatment with recombinant human erythropoietin. *Cancer* 73(10):2535–2542, 1993

54. Krantz SB: Pathogenesis and treatment of anemia of chronic disease. *Am J Med Sci* 307:353–359, 1994

55. Vose JM, Armitage JO: Clinical applications of hematopoietic growth factors. *J Clin Oncol* 13, 1023–1035, 1995

56. Means RT: Clinical application of recombinant erythropoietin in the anemia of chronic disease. *Hematol Oncol Clin North Am* 8:933–944, 1994

57. Rieger PT, Haeuber D: A new approach to managing chemotherapy-related anemia: Nursing implications of Epoietin Alfa. *Oncol Nurs Forum* 22:71–86, 1995

58. Goldberg GL, Gibbon DG, Smith HO, et al: Clinical impact of chemotherapy-induced thrombocytopenia in patients with gynecologic cancer. *J Clin Oncol* 12:2317–2320, 1994

59. Wujcik D: A case management approach to patients receiving G-CSF. *Oncol Nurs So Monograph* May:8–13, 1992

60. Oniboni AC: Infection in the neutropenic patient. *Semin Oncol Nurs* 6:50–60, 1990

61. Nauseef WM, Maki DG: A study of the value of simple protective isolation in patients with granulocytopenia. *N Engl J Med* 304:448–453, 1981

62. Gucalp R: Management of the febrile neutropenic patient with cancer. *Oncology* 5:137–148, 1991

63. Jones GR, Konsler GK, Dunaway RP, et al: Risk factors for recurrent fever after the discontinuation of empiric antibiotic therapy for fever and neutropenia in pediatric patients with a malignancy or hematologic condition. *J Pediatr* 124:703–708, 1994

64. Koeppler H, Pflueger KH, Seitz R, et al: Three-step empiric treatment for severely neutropenic patients with fever: Ceftazidime, vancomycin, amphotericin B. *Infection* 17: 142–145, 1989

65. De Pauw BE, Deresinski SC, Feld R, et al: Ceftazidime compared with piperacillin and tobramycin for the empiric treatment of fever in neutropenic patients with cancer. *Ann Intern Med* 120:834–844, 1994

66. Hughes WT, Armstrong D, Bodey GP, et al: Guidelines for the use of antimicrobial agents in neutropenic patients with unexplained fever. *J Infect Dis* 161:381–396, 1991

67. Sugar AM: Empiric treatment of fungal infections in the neutropenic host. *Arch Intern Med* 150:2258–2264, 1990

68. Miller L, Ozer H, Anderson JR, et al: American Society of Oncology recommendations for the use of hematopoietic colony-stimulating factors: Evidence-based, clinical practice guidelines. *J Clin Oncol* 12:2471–2508, 1994

69. Sallerfors B, Olofsson T: Granulocyte-macrophage colony-stimulating factor (GM-CSF) and granulocyte colony-stimulating factor (G-CSF) in serum during induction treatment of acute leukaemia. *Br J Hematol* 78:343–351, 1991

70. Maher DW, Lieschke GJ, Green M, et al: Filgrastim in patients with chemotherapy-induced febrile neutropenia: A double-blind, placebo-controlled trial. *Ann Intern Med* 121:492–501, 1994

71. Winningham ML, Nail LM, Burke MB, et al: Fatigue and the cancer experience: The state of the knowledge. *Oncol Nurs Forum* 21:23–36, 1994

72. St. Pierre BS, Kasper CE, Lindsey AM: Fatigue mechanisms in patients with cancer: Effects of tumor necrosis factor and exercise on skeletal muscle. *Oncol Nurs Forum* 19:419–425, 1992

73. Piper BF, Lindsey AM, Dodd MJ: Fatigue mechanisms in cancer patients: Developing nursing theory. *Oncol Nurs Forum* 14:17–23, 1987

74. Tchekmedyian NS, Hickman MN, Siau J, et al: Megestrol acetate in cancer anorexia and weight loss. *Cancer* 69: 1268–1274, 1992

75. Langstein HN, Norton JA: Mechanisms of cancer cachexia. *Hematol Oncol Clin North Am* 5:103–123, 1991

76. Nelson K, Walsh D: Management of the anorexia cachexia syndrome. *Cancer Bul* 43:403–406, 1991

77. Lindsey AM, Piper BF, Stotts NA: The phenomenon of cancer cachexia: A review. *Oncol Nurs Forum* 9:38–42, 1982

78. Lin EM: Nutritional support: Making the difficult decisions. *Cancer Nurs* 14:261–269, 1991

79. Eng-Hen N, Lowry SF: Nutritional support and cancer cachexia. *Hematol Oncol Clin North Am* 5:161–184, 1991

80. Crosley MA: Watch out for nutritional complications of cancer. *RN* 48:22–27, 1985

81. Nunnally C, Donoghue M, Yasko JM: Nutritional needs of cancer patients. *Nurs Clin North Am* 17:557–578, 1982

82. Ramstack JL, Rosenbaum EH: *Nutrition for the Chemotherapy Patient.* Palo Alto, CA, Bull Publishing, 1990

83. Wujcik D: Current research in side effects of high-dose chemotherapy. *Semin Oncol Nurs* 8:102–112, 1992

84. Levy MH: Constipation and diarrhea in cancer patients. *Cancer Bul* 43:412–422, 1991

85. Suppaiah L: Pseudomembranous colitis induced by *Clostridium difficile. Crit Care Nurs* 8:65–68, 1988

86. Mitchell EP, Schein PS: Gastrointestinal toxicity of chemotherapeutic agents, in Perry MC (ed): *The Chemotherapy Source Book.* Baltimore, Williams & Wilkins, 1992, pp 620–634

87. Katz MD, Erstan BL, Rose C: Treatment of severe diarrhea with octreotide in a patient with AIDS. *Drug Intell Clin Pharm* 22:134–136, 1988

88. Borison HL: Anatomy and physiology of the chemoreceptor trigger zone and area postrema, in Davis CJ, Lake-Bakarr CV, Grahame-Smith DG (eds): *Nausea and Vomiting Mechanisms and Treatment.* New York, Springer-Verlag, 1986, pp 10–17

89. Borison JL, McCarthy LE: Neuropharmacology of chemotherapy induced emesis. *Drugs* 25:8–17, 1983

90. Morrow GR: The effects of susceptibility to motion sickness on the side effects of cancer chemotherapy. *Cancer* 55: 2670–2766, 1985

91. Akwar O: The gastrointestinal tract in chemotherapy-induced emesis. A final common pathway. *Drugs* 25:18–34, 1983

92. Tortorice PV, O'Connell MB: Management of chemotherapy-induced nausea and vomiting. *Pharmacotherapy* 10: 129–145, 1990

93. Hogan CA: Advances in the management of nausea and vomiting. *Nurs Clin North Am* 25:475–497, 1991

94. Ettinger DS: Preventing chemotherapy-induced nausea and vomiting: An update and review of emesis. *Semin Oncol* 22:6–18, 1995 (suppl 10)

95. Grunber SM: Advances in the management of nausea and vomiting induced by non-cisplatin containing chemotherapeutic regimens. *Blood Rev* 3:216–221, 1989

96. Goodman M: Management of nausea and vomiting induced by outpatient cisplatin (Platinol) therapy. *Semin Oncol Nurs* 3:23–35, 1987

97. Navari RM, Madajewicz S, Anderson N, et al: Oral ondansetron for the control of cisplatin-induced delayed emesis: A large, multicenter, double-blind, randomized comparative trial of ondansetron versus placebo. *J Clin Oncol* 13: 2408–2416, 1995

98. Gralla RJ: Progress in the development of antiemetics for chemotherapy-induced nausea and vomiting. *Cancer Bul* 43:407–411, 1991

99. Aapro MS: Controlling emesis related to cancer therapy. *Eur J Cancer* 27:356–361, 1991

100. Malik IA, Khan WA, Qazilbash M: Clinical efficacy of lorazepam in prophylaxis of anticipatory, acute, and delayed nausea and vomiting induced by high doses of cisplatin. *Am J Clin Oncol* 18:170–175, 1995

101. Bruntsch U, Drechsler S, Eggert J, et al: Prevention of chemotherapy-induced nausea and vomiting by tropisetron (Navoban) alone or in combination with other antiemetic agents. *Semin Oncol* 21:7–11, 1994 (suppl 9)

102. Hesketh PJ, Beck T, Uhlenhopp M, et al: Adjusting the dose of intravenous ondansetron plus dexamethasone to the emetogenic potential of the chemotherapy regimen. *J Clin Oncol* 13:2117–2122, 1995

103. Madej G, Krzakowski M, Pawinski A, et al: A report comparing the use of tropisetron (Navoban): a 5-HT3 antagonist, with a standard antiemetic regimen of dexamethasone and metoclopramide in cisplatin-treated patients under conditions of severe emesis. *Semin Oncol* 21:3–6, 1994 (suppl 9)

104. Morrow GR, Hickok JT, Rosenthal SN: Progress in reducing nausea and emesis: Comparisons of ondansetron (Zofran), granisetron (Kytril), and tropisetron (Navoban). *Cancer* 76:343–357, 1995

105. Navari RM, Kaplan HG, Gralla RJ, et al: Efficacy and safety of granisetron, a selective 5-hydroxytryptamine-3 receptor antagonist, in the prevention of nausea and vomiting induced by high-dose cisplatin. *J Clin Oncol* 12:2204–2210, 1994

106. Zeltzer LK, Dolgin MJ, LeBaron S, et al: A randomized, controlled study of behavioral intervention of chemotherapy distress in children with cancer. *Pediatrics* 88:34–42, 1991

107. Cotanch PH, Strum S: Progressive muscle relaxation as antiemetic therapy for cancer patients. *Oncol Nurs Forum* 14:33–37, 1987

108. Kantrowitz NE, Bristow MR: Cardiotoxicity of antitumor agents. *Prog Cardiovasc Dis* 27:195–200, 1984

109. Torti FM, Lum BL: Cardiac toxicity, in DeVita VT, Hellman S, Rosenberg SA (eds): *Cancer: Principles and Practice of Oncology* (ed 3). Philadelphia, Lippincott, 1989, pp 2153–2169

110. Bristow MR: Toxic cardiomyopathy due to doxorubicin. *Hosp Pract* 17:101–111, 1982

111. Kaszyk LK: Cardiac toxicity associated with cancer therapy. *Oncol Nurs Forum* 13:81–88, 1986

112. Dorr RT: Chemoprotectants for cancer chemotherapy. *Semin Oncol* 18:8–58, 1991 (suppl 2)

113. Speyer JL, Green MD, Zeleniuch-Jacquotte A: ICRF-86 permits longer treatment with doxorubicin in women with breast cancer. *J Clin Oncol* 10:117–127, 1992

114. Hochster H, Wasserheit C, Speyer J: Cardiotoxicity and cardioprotection during chemotherapy. *Curr Opin Oncol* 7:304–309, 1995

115. Hurteloup P, Ganzina F: Clinical studies with new anthracyclines: Epirubicin, idarubicin, esorubicin. *Drugs Exp Clin Res* 12:233–246, 1986

116. Crossley RJ: Clinical safety and tolerance of mitoxantrone. *Semin Oncol* 11:54–58, 1984 (suppl 1)

117. Shenkenber TD, Von Hoff DD: Mitoxantrone: A new anticancer drug with significant clinical activity. *Ann Intern Med* 105:67–81, 1986

118. Mill BA, Roberts RW: Cyclophosphamide-induced cardiomyopathy. A report of two cases and review of the English literature. *Cancer* 43:2223–2226, 1979

119. Ramireddy K, Kane KM, Adhar GC: Acquired episodic complete heart block after high-dose chemotherapy with cyclophosphamide and thiotepa. *Am Heart J* 127:701–704, 1994

120. Braverman AC, Antin JH, Plappert MT, et al: Cyclophosphamide cardiotoxicity in one marrow transplantation: A prospective evaluation of new dosing regimens. *J Clin Oncol* 9:1215–1223, 1991

121. Weidmann B, Teipel A, Niederie N: The syndrome of 5-fluorouracil cardiotoxicity: An elusive cardiopathy. *Cancer* 73:2001–2002, 1994

122. Kleiman NS, Lehane DE, Geyer CE, et al: Prinzmetal's angina during 5-fluorouracil chemotherapy. *Am J Med* 82:566–568, 1987

123. Rowinsky EK, McGuire WP, Guarnieri T, et al: Cardiac disturbances during the administration of taxol. *J Clin Oncol* 9:1704–1712, 1991

124. Soe MS, Berkman A, Mardelli, J: Case report: Paclitaxel-induced myocardial ischemia. *Med J* 45:41–43, 1996

125. Steinherz LJ, Steinherz PG, Tan CT, et al: Cardiac toxicity 4 to 20 years after completing anthracycline therapy. *JAMA* 266:1672–1677, 1991

126. Steinherz LJ, Steinherz PG, Tan C: Cardiac failure and dysrhythmias 6–19 years after anthracycline therapy: A series of 15 patients. *Med Pediatr Oncol* 24:352–361, 1995

127. Deng MC, Kececioglu D, Weyand M, et al: Successful long-term course after heart transplantation for anthracycline cardiomyopathy in a young boy despite neurological complications. *Thorac Cardiovasc Surg* 42:122–124, 1994

128. MacDonald DR: Neurotoxicity of chemotherapeutic agents, in Perry MC (ed): *The Chemotherapy Source Book.* Baltimore, Williams & Wilkins, 1992, pp 666–679

129. Forman A: Peripheral neuropathy in cancer patients: Clinical types, etiology, and presentation. *Oncology* 4:85–89, 1990

130. Mollman JE, Glover DJ, Hogan WM, et al: Cisplatin neuropathy: Risk factors, prognosis, and protection by WR-2721. *Cancer* 61:2192–2195, 1988

131. Chaudhry V, Rowinsky EK, Sartorius SE, et al: Peripheral neuropathy from taxol and cisplatin combination chemotherapy: Clinical and electrophysiological studies. *Ann Neurol* 35:304–311, 1994

132. Schaefer SD, Post JD, Close LG, et al: Ototoxicity of low and moderate dose cisplatin. *Cancer* 56:1934–1939, 1985

133. Miller LJ: Ifosfamide-induced neurotoxicity. *Cancer Bul* 43:456–457, 1991

134. Anderson RN, Tandon DS: Ifosamide extrapyramidal neurotoxicity. *Cancer* 69:72–75, 1991

135. Cain JW, Bender CM: Ifosfamide-induced neurotoxicity: Associated symptoms and nursing implications. *Oncol Nurs Forum* 22:659–666, 1995

136. Fassas ABT, Gattani AM, Morgello S: Cerebral demyelination with 5-fluorouracil and levamisole. *Cancer Invest* 12:379–383, 1994

137. Conrad KJ: Cerebellar toxicities associated with cytosine arabinoside: A nursing perspective. *Oncol Nurs Forum* 13:57–59, 1986

138. Hilkens PHE, Verweij J, Stoter G, et al: Peripheral neurotoxicity induced by docetaxel. *Am Academy of Neurol* 46:104–111, 1996

139. Twohig KJ, Matthay RA: Pulmonary effects of cytotoxic agents other than bleomycin. *Clin Chest Med* 11:31–54, 1990

140. Chandler DB: Possible mechanisms of bleomycin-induced fibrosis. *Clin Chest Med* 11:21–30, 1990

141. Sleijfer S, van der Mark TW, Koops S, Mulder NH: Decrease

in pulmonary function during bleomycin-containing combination chemotherapy for testicular cancer: Not only a bleomycin effect. *Br J Cancer* 71:120–123, 1995

142. Luedke D, McLaughlin TT, Daughaday C, et al: Mitomycin C and vindesine associated pulmonary toxicity with variable clinical expression. *Cancer* 55:542–545, 1985

143. Kalaycioglu M, Kavuru M, Tuason L, Bolwell B: Empiric prednisone therapy for pulmonary toxic reaction after high-dose chemotherapy containing carmustine (BCNU). *Chest* 107:482–487, 1995

144. White DA, Rankin JA, Stover DE, et al: Methotrexate pneumonitis. *Am Rev Respir Dis* 139:18–21, 1989

145. Sostman HD, Matthay RA, Putman CE, et al: Methotrexate-induced pneumonitis. *Medicine* 55:371–388, 1976

146. Santamauro JT, Stover DE, Jules-Elysee K, et al: Lung transplantation for chemotherapy-induced pulmonary fibrosis. *Chest* 105:310–312, 1994

147. Perry MC (ed): Hepatotoxicity of chemotherapeutic agents, in Perry MC: *The Chemotherapy Source Book.* Baltimore, Williams & Wilkins, 1992, pp 635–647

148. Wujcik D, Downs S: Bone marrow transplantation. *Crit Care Clin* 4:149–166, 1992

149. Kanwar VS, Luiza M, Albuquerque C, et al: Veno-occlusive disease of the liver after chemotherapy for rhabdomyosarcoma: Case report with a review of the literature. *Med Pediatr Oncol* 24:334–340, 1995

150. Keith JS: Hepatic failure: Etiologies, manifestations, and management. *Crit Care Nurs* 5:60–86, 1985

151. Blanco JA, Appelbaum FR, Nemunaitis J, et al: Phase I–II trial of pentoxifylline for the prevention of transplant-related toxicities following bone marrow transplant. *Blood* 78:1205–1211, 1991

152. Lewis JH, Schiff E: Methotrexate-induced chronic liver injury: Guidelines for detection and prevention. *Am J Gastroentrol* 88:1337–1345, 1988

153. George CB, Mansour RP, Redmond J: Hepatic dysfunction and jaundice following high-dose cytosine arabinoside. *Cancer* 54:2360–2362, 1984

154. Moertel CG, Fleming TR, Macdonald JS, et al: Hepatic toxicity associated with fluorouracil plus levamisole adjuvant toxicity. *J Clin Oncol* 11:2386–2390, 1993

155. Kemeny N, Daly J, Reichman B, et al: Intrahepatic or systemic infusion of fluorodeoxyruidine in patients with liver metastases from colorectal carcinoma. *Ann Intern Med* 107:459–475, 1987

156. Applebaum FR, Shulman HM: Fatal hepatotoxicity associated with AMSA therapy. *Cancer Treat Rep* 66:1863–1865, 1982

157. Stillwell TJ, Benson RC: Cyclophosphamide-induced hemorrhagic cystitis. *Cancer* 61:451–457, 1988

158. Shepherd JD, Pringle LE, Barnett M, et al: Mesna versus hyperhydration for the prevention of cyclophosphamide-induced hemorrhagic cystitis in bone marrow transplantation. *J Clin Oncol* 9:2016–2020, 1991

159. Patterson WP, Reams GP: Renal and electrolyte abnormalities due to chemotherapy, in Perry MC (ed): *The Chemotherapy Source Book.* Philadelphia, Williams & Wilkins, 1992, pp 648–665

160. Safirstein R, Winston J, Goldstein M, et al: Cisplatin nephrotoxicity. *Am J Kidney Dis* 8:356–357, 1986

161. Vogelzang NJ: Nephrotoxicity from chemotherapy: Prevention and management. *Oncology* 5:97–112, 1991

162. Daley-Yates PT, McBrien DC: A study of the protective effect of chloride salts on cisplatin nephrotoxicity. *Biochem Pharmacol* 34:2363–2369, 1985

163. Corden BJ, Fine RL, Ozols RF, et al: Chemical pharmacology of high-dose cisplatin. *Cancer Chemother Pharmacol* 14:38–41, 1985

164. Walker EM Jr, Fazekas-May MA, Bowen WR: Nephrotoxic and ototoxic agents. *Clin Lab Med* 10:323–354, 1990

165. Treskes M, Nijtmans LGJ, Fichtinger-Schepman AMJ, et al: Effects of the modulating agent WR-2721 and its main metabolites on the formation and stability of cisplatin-DNA adducts in vitro in comparison to the effects of thiosulphate and diethyldithiocarbamate. *Biochem Pharmacol* 43:1013–1019, 1992

166. Relling MV, Fairclough D, Ayers D, et al: Patient characteristics associated with high-risk methotrexate concentrations and toxicity. *J Clin Oncol* 12:1667–1672, 1994

167. Tuttle SE, Sharma HM, Bay WH, et al: Glomerular basement membrane splitting and microaneurysm formation associated with nitrosourea therapy. *Am J Nephrol* 5:388–394, 1985

168. Hrozencik SP, Connaughton MJ: Cancer-associated hemolytic uremic syndrome. *Oncol Nurs Forum* 15:755–759, 1988

169. Flombaum CD: Electrolyte and renal abnormalities, in Groeger JS (ed): *Critical Care of the Cancer Patient* (ed 2). St. Louis: Mosby, 1991, pp 140–164

170. Dietz KA, Flaherty AM: Oncologic Emergencies, in Groenwald SL, Frogge MH, Goodman M, Yarbro CH (eds): *Cancer Nursing: Principles and Practice* (ed 3). Boston, Jones and Bartlett, 1993, pp 801–837

171. Averette HE, Boike GM, Jarrell MA: Effects of cancer chemotherapy on gonadal function and reproductive capacity. *CA Cancer J Clin* 40:199–209, 1990

172. Yarbro CH, Perry MC: The effect of cancer therapy on gonadal function. *Semin Oncol Nurs* 1:3–8, 1985

173. Chapman RM: Gonadal toxicity and teratogenicity, in Perry MC (ed): *The Chemotherapy Source Book.* Baltimore, Williams & Wilkins, 1992, pp 710–753

174. Chapman RM: Gonadal injury resulting from chemotherapy. *Am J Int Med* 4:149–161, 1983

175. Shalet SM: Effects of cancer chemotherapy on gonadal function of patients. *Cancer Treat Rev* 7:141–152, 1980

176. Myers SE, Schilsky RL: Prospects for fertility after cancer chemotherapy. *Semin Oncol* 19:597–604, 1992

177. Sanger WG, Armitage JO, Schmidt MA: Feasibility of semen cryopreservation in patients with malignant disease. *JAMA* 244:789–790, 1980

178. Nicosia SV, Matus-Ridley M, Meadows AT: Gonadal effects of cancer therapy in girls. *Cancer* 55:2364–2372, 1985

179. Rustin GJS, Pektasides D, Bagshawe KD, et al: Fertility after chemotherapy for male and female germ cell tumors. *In J Androl* 10:389–392, 1987

180. Gulati SC, Vega R, Gee T, Kozner B, et al: Growth and development of children born to patients after cancer therapy. *Cancer Invest* 4:197–205, 1986

181. Lamb MA: Effects of cancer on the sexuality and fertility of women. *Semin Oncol Nurs* 11:120–127, 1995

182. Mulvihill JJ, McKeen A, Rosner F, et al: Pregnancy outcome in cancer patients. *Cancer* 60:1143–1150, 1987

183. Salooja N, Chatterjee R, McMillan AK, et al: Successful pregnancies in women following single autotransplant for acute myeloid leukemia with a chemotherapy ablation protocol. *Bone Marrow Transplant* 13:431–435, 1994

184. Samuelsson A, Fuchs T, Simonsson B, et al: Successful pregnancy in a 28-year-old patient autografted for acute lymphoblastic leukemia following myeloablative treatment including total body irradiation. *Bone Marrow Transplant* 12:659–660, 1993

185. Mustieles C, Munoz A, Alonso M, et al: Male gonadal func-

tion after chemotherapy in survivors of childhood malignancy. *Med Pediatr Oncol* 24:347–351, 1995

186. Uhlenhopp MB: An overview of the relationship between alkylating agents and therapy-related acute nonlymphocytic leukemia. *Cancer Nurs* 15:9–17, 1992

187. Hydzik CA: Late effects of chemotherapy: Implications for patient management and rehabilitation. *Nurs Clin North Am* 25:423–446, 1990

188. Heyne KH, Lippman SM, Lee J, et al: The incidence of second primary tumors in long-term survivors of small-cell lung cancer. *J Clin Oncol* 10:1519–1524, 1992

189. Green DM, Zevon MA, Reese, PA: Second malignant tumors following treatment during childhood and adolescence for cancer. *Med Pediatr Oncol* 22:1–10, 1994

190. Tucker MA, Coleman CN, Cox RS, et al: Risk of second cancers after treatment for Hodgkin's disease. *N Engl J Med* 318:76–81, 1988

191. Koletsky AJ, Bertino JR, Farber LR, et al: Second neoplasms in patients with Hodgkin's disease following combined modality therapy. *J Clin Oncol* 4:311–317, 1986

192. Beaty O, Hudson MM, Greenwald C, et al: Subsequent malignancies in children and adolescents after treatment for Hodgkin's disease. *J Clin Oncol* 13:603–609, 1995

193. Kyle RS, Genta MA: Second malignancies after chemotherapy, in Perry MC (ed): *The Chemotherapy Source Book.* Baltimore, Williams & Wilkins, 1992, pp 689–702

194. Ratain MJ, Kaminer LS, Bitran JD, et al: Acute nonlymphocytic leukemia following etoposide and cisplatin combination chemotherapy for advanced non-small cell carcinoma of the lung. *Blood* 70:1412–1417, 1987

195. Tucker MA, Fraumeni JF: Treatment-related cancers after gynecologic malignancy. *Cancer* 60:2117–2122, 1987

196. Valagussa P, Tancini G, Bonadonna G: Second malignancies after CMF for resectable breast cancer. *J Clin Oncol* 5: 1138–1142, 1987

197. Curtis RE, Boice JD, Stovall M, et al: Risk of leukemia after chemotherapy and radiation therapy for breast cancer. *N Engl J Med* 326:1745–1751, 1992

198. Pedersen-Bjergaard J, Caugaard G, et al: Increased risk of myelodysplasia and leukemia after etoposide, cisplatin, and bleomycin for germ-cell tumors. *Lancet* 338:359–363, 1991

# Chapter 17

# Biotherapy

Vera S. Wheeler, RN, MN, OCN®

Side Effects and Key Nursing Strategies
>  Flu-like syndromes (FLS)
>  Fatigue
>  Cardiovascular-respiratory changes
>  Capillary leak syndrome (CLS)
>  Dermatologic changes

>  Gastrointestinal symptoms
>  Neurological effects
>  Anaphylactic reactions

**The Patient's Experience with Biotherapy**

**THE FUTURE OF BIOTHERAPY**

**REFERENCES**

# INTRODUCTION

Biotherapy has been described as the fourth modality of cancer therapy, but unlike other therapies that are fully developed and mature, the biggest achievements in biotherapy are yet to come. However, there are present day successes that provide the basis for optimism about the future of biotherapy. For example, cytokines such as epoetin and filgrastim have become an integral part of cancer therapy. Also, patients have already been treated with gene-labeled cells in autologous bone marrow transplantation. How biotherapy will mature depends on the further development of scientific knowledge and biotechnology, and on the clinical experience with current cytokines, monoclonal antibodies, and other biological agents.

This chapter will describe the major current applications of biotherapy and those being investigated in clinical trials. It will review basic immunological principles for these therapies and major toxicities commonly experienced by patients.

# FOUNDATION CONCEPTS FOR BIOTHERAPY

## Immune Defense Against Malignancy: An Overview

### Immune surveillance

Immune surveillance is a theory first proposed in the 1950s to explain the role of the immune system in defending against neoplastic cells. Tumor cells express abnormal tumor antigens on their surfaces that can be recognized and subsequently destroyed by immune cells. The immune system is believed to destroy many circulating malignant cells before they can become established sites of tumor. Although the response of immune defense cells to specific tumors has been demonstrated, the theory fails to explain why some cancers elude immune detection and response. Abbas et al suggest that immuno-

surveillance may be most effective in a subset of virally-caused cancers.[1]

### Effector mechanisms of immune function

Defense against foreign antigens, either exogenous microbes or endogenous altered or virally-transformed cells, is accomplished through components of the immune response. Effector or cell killing mechanisms are initiated through a complicated recognition system of self/non-self surface molecules known as the major histocompatibility complex (MHC). The primary defense against transformed cells is cell-mediated immunity carried out by T-lymphocytes and aided by B cells and humoral immunity. The key components of the immune response are shown in Figure 17-1. Stimulated by the presence of an antigen, the macrophage activates a T helper ($T_H$) cell. The activated $T_H$ cell along with cytokines initiates a B cell response and the generation of antibody, an increase in cytotoxic T8 cells, activation of natural killer (NK) cells, and the stimulation of hematopoietic stem cells. The following is a further description of these cells that also are adapted to cancer therapy as biological agents.

*Monocyte/macrophage*  The macrophage is a versatile cell that is a primary initiator to an inflammatory immune response. It originates in the bone marrow and circulates as a monocyte. It becomes a macrophage when it enters tissue at a site of infection. The macrophage is first a phagocytic cell capable of engulfing microbes and altered cells, and processing them in lysosomes with cytolytic enzymes. The macrophage then presents a portion of the processed antigen along with the MHC class II surface molecules as an antigen-presenting cell (APC) to initiate both humoral- and cell-mediated immune functions.[2]

The macrophage is also a secretory cell, manufacturing key pyrogenic cytokines such as interleukin 1, tumor necrosis factor, and interleukin 6. These cytokines can have diverse pro-inflammatory actions throughout the body, including generating fever.

*T helper lymphocyte ($T_H$ or T4)*  The $T_H$ cell is the coordinator of the immune response and cell-mediated immunity. It is activated by binding to the APC's MHC

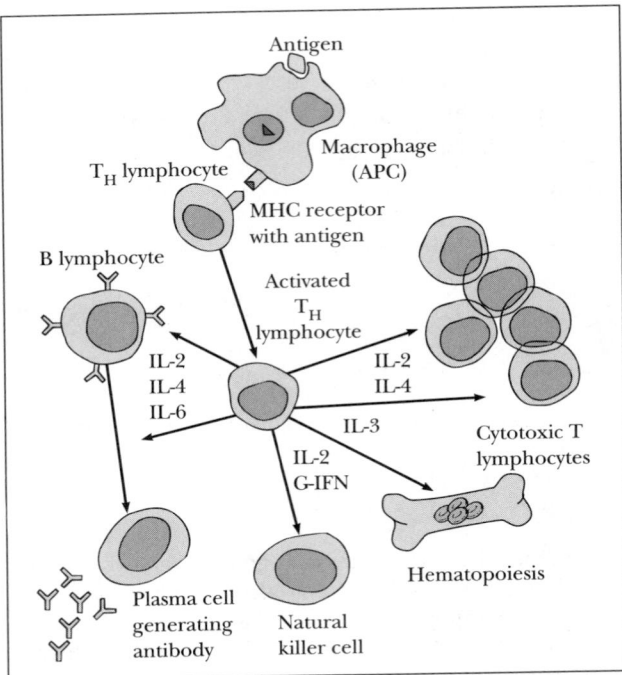

**FIGURE 17-1** Major Components of the Immune Response. (APC: antigen presenting cell; $T_H$ Cell: T helper lymphocyte; IL-2: interleukin 2; IL-3: interleukin 3; IL-4: interleukin 4; IL-6: interleukin 6; G-IFN: gamma-interferon)

class II receptor with antigen complex. When activated, the $T_H$ cell manufactures cytokines—primarily interleukin 2, 3, 4, 6, and alpha- and gamma-interferon. It also has surface receptors for IL-1 and IL-2, which participate in an autocrine, positive feedback loop.

***Cytotoxic T-lymphocytes (CTL)*** CTL or T8 cells are lymphocytes with MHC class I surface molecules. They are activated primarily by IL-2 and other cytokines, and rapidly increase clonally. They are MHC restricted; that is, they need to recognize MHC class I receptors on the surface of the target cell in order to initiate their cytotoxic response and are capable of linking to these cells. Through the use of cytolytic enzymes they damage the target cell wall and the cell dies.

***Natural killer (NK) cells*** These cells lack T and B cell surface markers and are able to function without MHC recognition. When activated primarily through cytokines, NK cells are capable of killing transformed cells. Lymphokine activated killer (LAK) cells are a special population of cytotoxic cells used in cancer therapy that are made up primarily of NK cells, capable of nonspecific tumor cell killing.

***B-lymphocyte*** This cell is identified by the surface immunoglobulin that it displays. It is a sedentary cell located in lymph nodes and the spleen. When it combines with antigen, it also can function as an antigen-presenting cell to $T_H$ lymphocytes. When activated with antigen and

cytokines—primarily IL-2, IL-4, and IL-6—the B lymphocyte differentiates into a plasma cell and manufactures immunoglobulin or antibody specific to the initiating antigen. Later, the plasma cell can evolve into a memory cell, capable of a more rapid response on future exposures with the same antigen.[3]

***Antibody (Ab)*** Ab is a specific protein product of plasma cells that is also known as immunoglobulin. There are five classes of immunoglobulin, with IgG and IgM being the most frequently generated classes of immunoglobulin. Ab is not a cytotoxic substance itself, but is essentially an adaptor that enhances the capability of immune effector cell functions. When antibody links to an antigenic target, the resulting Ab/Ag complex greatly increases the phagocytic capability of the macrophages and can initiate the serum complement protein cascade on the surface of a foreign cell, resulting in lysing of the cell.

***Antibody dependent cell-mediated cytotoxicity (ADCC)*** ADCC is the cell-killing process enabled by antibody. Ab attaches to foreign cells at the Fab or variable end and facilitates the attachment of an NK cell and other cytotoxic cells that attach to the Fc or constant end of the antibody.

***Cytokines*** These are glycoprotein products of immune cells such as lymphocytes and macrophages that coordinate and initiate effector defense functions. They are not cytotoxic agents themselves with the exception of tumor necrosis factor alpha (TNF-$\alpha$) and lymphotoxin. The characteristics of the primary host defense cytokines are shown in Table 17-1 and include interleukins 1, 2, 4, 6, 12; interferons alpha, beta, and gamma; TNF-$\alpha$; lymphotoxin; and transforming growth factor beta. Interleukins 3, 5, and 7 have a primary role in hematopoiesis and will be discussed in a later section.

Cytokines generally share certain properties despite the disparity of their names. These characteristics are[1,4]:

- They mediate and regulate immune defense functions of the body by providing communication and coordination among a variety of diverse immune cells. They have been called the hormones of the immune system.

- They have brief half-lives and usually function over short distances.

- They are produced by many different cell types and also act upon diverse cell targets both within the immune system and in other organ targets such as the liver.

- Their actions are overlapping, redundant, and sometimes contradictory. They can influence the stimulation of other cytokines to produce synergistic effects as in a cytokine network, or to antagonize the actions of other cytokines.

- They bind to surface receptors of target cells and act as regulators of cell growth or as mediators of defense functions.

**TABLE 17-1** Table of Cytokines

| Names/Alternative Names | Source | Biological Actions |
|---|---|---|
| INTERLEUKINS | | |
| Interleukin 1 alpha and beta<br>IL-1a, IL-1b; endogenous pyrogen; catabolin; lymphocyte activating factor; hematopoietin | Monocyte/macrophage; NK cells; dendritic cells | Activates T cells; induces cytokine release from T cells; induces fever, tissue catabolism, and release of $PGE_2$; co-stimulates proliferation of B cells |
| Interleukin 2<br>IL-2; T cell growth factor; aldesleukin | Activated T cells | Activates cytotoxic T cells; cofactor for activation and differentiation of B cells; increases monocyte and NK cell cytotoxicity; induces immune response cytokines. |
| Interleukin 3<br>IL-3; multi-CSF; hematopoietin 2 | Activated T cells | Stimulates hematopoietic progenitor cell growth; stimulates mast cell growth; activates eosinophils; promotes macrophage cytotoxicity and phagocytosis. |
| Interleukin 4<br>IL-4; B cell growth factor (BCGF); B cell stimulating factor (BSF); T cell growth factor II | Activated T cells | Growth factor for B cells; cofactor for T cell growth and differentiation; promotes LAK activity; cofactor for mast cell growth; inhibits IL-1, IL-8, and TNF-$\alpha$ secretion. |
| Interleukin 5<br>IL-5; B cell growth factor II; eosinophil CSF | Activated T cells | Induces proliferation and differentiation of eosinophils; induces proliferation of B cells; enhances actions of cytotoxic T cells. |
| Interleukin 6<br>IL-6; IFN-$\beta_2$; Hybridoma growth factor; B cell differentiation factor (BCDF) | Monocyte/macrophage; fibroblasts; T cells | Cofactor for T cell activity and IL-2 production; augments NK cell and LAK activity; induces B cell differentiation and Ig secretion; bone marrow stem cell proliferation. |
| Interleukin 7<br>IL-7; pre-B cell growth factor (pBCGF) | Bone marrow stromal cells | Induces pre-B cell and pre-T cell proliferation; stimulates generation of LAK cells. |
| Interleukin 8<br>IL-8; PF4 superfamily of molecules | Activated lymphocytes, monocytes, endothelial cells | Chemotactic and activation factor for neutrophils, eosinophils, T and B cells and monocytes; stimulates inflammatory actions of leukocytes. |
| Interleukin 9<br>IL-9; P40 | T helper cells | Enhances growth of bone marrow derived mast cells and response to IL-3. |
| Interleukin 10<br>IL-10; B derived T cell growth factor; mast cell growth factor III | T and B cells | Inhibitory factor for $T_H$ cell cytokine synthesis and macrophage activity; inhibits gamma-interferon production. |
| Interleukin 11<br>IL-11 | Bone marrow stromal cells | Stimulates megakaryopoiesis and platelet production; enhances macrophage development. |
| Interleukin 12<br>IL-12; NK cell stimulatory factor | B lymphoblastoid cell | Stimulates activated CD4 and CD8 T cells; synergizes with IL-2 for stimulation of cytotoxic T lymphocytes; augments NK activity. |
| OTHER CYTOKINES | | |
| Tumor necrosis factor, alpha<br>TNF-$\alpha$; cachectin | Activated monocyte/macrophage; NK cells | Promotes inflammatory reactions; mediates catabolic processes, septic shock, and inflammation; directly cytotoxic to tumor cells. |

*(continued)*

**TABLE 17-1** Table of Cytokines (continued)

| Names/Alternative Names | Source | Biological Actions |
|---|---|---|
| OTHER CYTOKINES | | |
| Tumor necrosis factor, beta<br>TNF-β, lymphotoxin | Activated T cells | Cytotoxic to malignant, transformed cells; endogenous pyrogen. |
| Transforming growth factor beta<br>TGF-β, inhibin | T cells; activated macrophages; platelets | Inhibits B and T cell growth and maturation; macrophage and NK cell activity; counteracts pro-inflammatory effects of cytokines; promotes healing. Acts as a negative regulator for immune response. |
| Granulocyte colony stimulating factor<br>G-CSF; filgrastim | Macrophage; fibroblast; endothelial cells | Stimulates differentiation of granulocytes. |
| Granulocyte-macrophage colony stimulating factor<br>GM-CSF; sargramostim | Activated T cells; monocyte; fibroblast | Stimulates growth and differentiation of myeloid progenitor cells and megakaryocytes; induces phagocytosis and neutrophil cytotoxicity; induces synthesis of IL-1, A-IFN, G-IFN. |
| Macrophage colony stimulating factor<br>M-CSF | Macrophage; fibroblast | Stimulates differentiation of monocytes. |

NK: natural killer cell; A-IFN: alpha-interferon; G-IFN: gamma-interferon; CSF: colony stimulating factor; LAK: lymphokine-activated killer cell

The cytokine network is an overlapping, interactive communication pattern within the immune system. The secretion of one cytokine (or the administration of a recombinant form) can initiate a large release of secondary cytokines. Figure 17-2 illustrates one aspect of this network. When a bolus of high-dose IL-2 is administered, it potentially stimulates three cell types: NK, macrophage, and CTL cells. These cells secrete a variety of cytokines responsible for both the flu-like symptoms that manifest, as well as potential tumor cell killing. Other administered cytokines will engage in their own unique interactions within the cytokine network.

## Origins of Biotherapy

### Coley's toxins

William Coley, a New York surgeon, observed in 1893 that a patient with metastatic sarcoma had a complete remission of his cancer after two episodes of erysipelas, a streptococcal infection. Coley continued to explore this relationship of acute infection and tumor regression by injecting live and later killed bacterial extracts into patients' tumors. These extracts, known as Coley's toxins, were administered in a highly variable manner, but are believed to have contained *streptococcus pyogenes* with *serratia marcesens* and *bacillus prodigiosus*. Patients received these injections for weeks, months, or even up to a year.

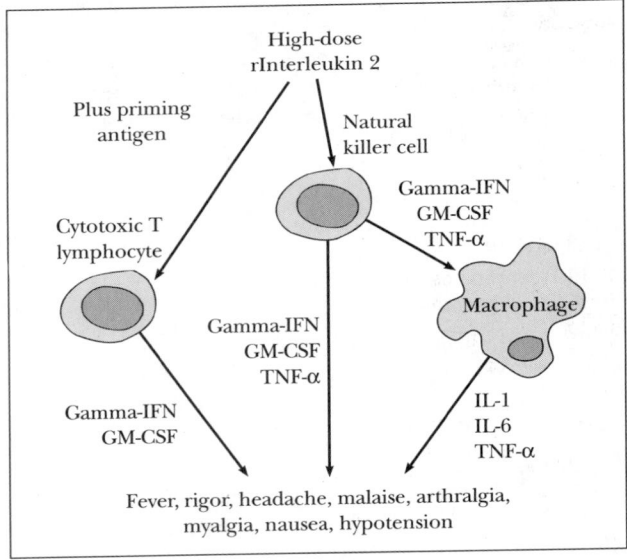

**FIGURE 17-2** High-dose rIL-2 cytokine cascade: rIL-2 given parenterally can result in a massive release of cytokines and symptoms of inflammation from the activation of peripheral blood mononuclear cells and their pyrogenic cytokines.[4] (GM-CSF: granulocyte-macrophage colony stimulating factor; IFN: interferon; IL-1: interleukin 1; IL-6: interleukin 6; TNF-α: tumor necrosis factor-alpha)

They reacted with fever, chills, and other systemic effects that Dr. Coley believed was an essential part of the treatment. Although approximately one-fourth of Coley's patients had a complete regression of their tumor, interest in these toxins waned with the onset of radiotherapy and chemotherapy.[4,5] It is now believed that the active ingredient in these toxins was endotoxin, a component in bacterial cell walls that generated TNF and other cytokines in the patient.

### BCG and modern immunotherapy

In the 1960s and 1970s, nonspecific immunopotentiators such as Bacillus Calmette-Guerin (BCG) were being tested in clinical trials. BCG was originally developed as a vaccine for tuberculosis. The use of BCG as adjuvant therapy after chemotherapy demonstrated increased survival of children with acute lymphoblastic leukemia and sparked interest in immunotherapy as a new fourth modality of cancer treatment.[5] However, many subsequent clinical studies showed little difference in the cancer recurrence rates using BCG, *C. parvum*, and other immunopotentiators. Interest in immunotherapy again faded.

### Biologic Response Modifiers (BRMs)

Advances in molecular biology and computerization, and the advent of genetic engineering in the early 1980s provided a large number of new substances from the mammalian genome that were capable of modulating immune functions. Oldham describes BRMs as a "medicine cabinet" of new biologicals that may directly or indirectly have antitumor activity.[6] Unlike previous immunotherapeutic agents, these were homogenous, pure substances that were capable of more specific effects in the immune system. BRMs are defined as "agents or approaches that will modify the relationship between tumor and host by modifying the host's biological response to tumor cells, with resultant therapeutic benefit."[7,p3] These agents can be classified as: (1) agents that restore, aug-ment, or modulate host antitumor immune mechanisms; (2) cells or cellular products that have direct antitumor effects such as tumor necrosis factor; and (3) biological agents that have other biological, antitumor effects, for example, interfering with the metastatic ability of tumor or differentiating agents.[8] BRMs are more broadly defined and encompass a greater number of substances than the earlier field of immunotherapy, even though the terms are sometimes used interchangeably. *Biotherapy* and *biologic therapy* have become the more prevalent terms. Biotherapy is defined as the use of agents derived from biological sources or that affect biological responses.[9] It now describes agents that are biological in origin that may not have antitumor effects.

## Recombinant DNA Technology

Recombinant DNA, or the combining of genes from different sources to produce an organism with new qualities, is an important basic principle to biotherapy. (See Table 17-2 for definitions of terms used in biotechnology.) This advance in molecular biology has enabled the current generation of biological agents to be available for use in cancer therapy. When the process of recombinant DNA was discovered in the 1970s, there was much controversy over how this new technology might be used or misused. However, recombinant DNA technology produces proteins that have created a new class of drugs called biopharmaceuticals. Table 17-3 identifies major classifications of biopharmaceuticals presently available or in clinical trial.

The process of recombinant DNA starts with the isolation of a specific segment of one strand of DNA (see Figure 17-3). This segment, a sequence of base pairs responsible for the manufacture of a particular protein, is cut from the DNA strand using a specific restriction enzyme. The remaining "sticky ends" enable the fragment to be joined to DNA in the plasmid by the binding of complementary base pairs, thymine to adenine and guanine to cytosine. The splice in the DNA strand is completed by another enzyme and the plasmid is inserted

**TABLE 17-2**  Common Terms for Biotechnology

| | |
|---|---|
| Biopharmaceuticals:<br>proteins, usually the product of recombinant DNA technology, that are used as drugs (e.g., interferon, human growth hormone). | Plasmid:<br>an autonomously replicating, circular molecule of DNA. It is used as a vector for the introduction of a gene. |
| Gene:<br>a unit of DNA that forms a discrete part of a chromosome of an organism. | Restriction enzymes:<br>enzymes that act like "molecular scissors" to cut strands of DNA at specific cleavage sites to make specific DNA fragments. |
| Genetic Engineering:<br>the formation of new combinations of genes that are placed into an organism in which these genes do not occur naturally. | Recombinant DNA:<br>a genome that contains genes from different sources that have been combined by genetic engineering methods. |
| Polymerase chain reaction (PCR):<br>a method of gene amplication that does not require use of bacterial vectors. | Vector:<br>a carrier for the DNA in genetic engineering. Typical vectors are plasmids and viruses. |

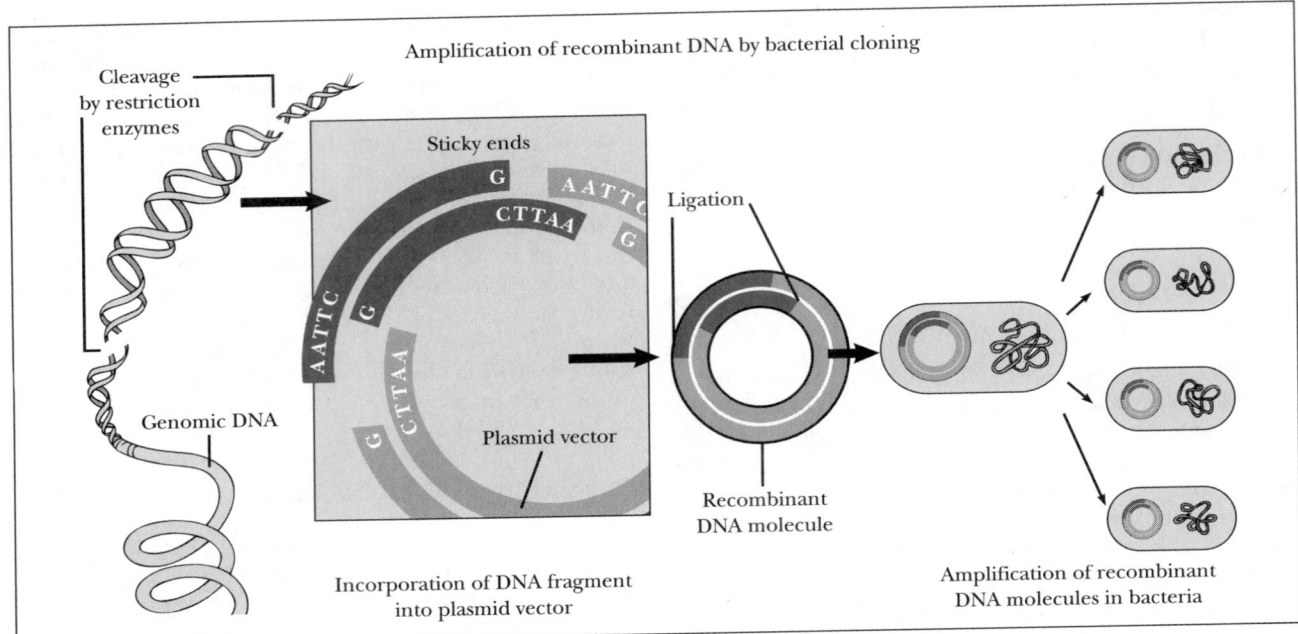

**FIGURE 17-3** Amplification of recombinant DNA by bacterial cloning. In the example shown, the DNA segment to be amplified is separated by cleavage with a restriction enzyme that produces "sticky ends." The restriction enzyme cuts each strand as well as the plasmid DNA at a single site generating "sticky ends" on the plasmid that are complementary to the ends of the DNA fragments. The cut ends of the DNA fragments and the plasmid form smooth joints with ligase enzyme. The new molecule is carried into bacteria that replicate the plasmid as they grow in culture. Data from Rosenthal[10]

**TABLE 17-3** Major Classifications of Biopharmaceuticals

| Category | Examples |
|---|---|
| 1. Enzymes and enzyme regulators | Alteplase; Tissue plasminogen activator or TPA (Activase®)<br>Ceredase-glucocerebrosidase for Gaucher's disease (Cerezyme®) |
| 2. Hormones and hormone-like growth factors | Human insulin (Humulin®)<br>Erythropoietin (Procrit®)<br>Platelet-derived growth factor (PDGF) |
| 3. Cytokines | Alfa-interferon (Intron A®)<br>Aldesleukin, Interleukin 2 (Proleukin®)<br>Filgrastim (Neupogen®) |
| 4. Vaccines | Hepatitis B Vaccine (Recombinvax®) |

into a bacterial cell and cultured to produce the desired protein.[10]

The process used currently is called polymerase chain reaction (PCR) and is used to create copies of a specific segment of DNA without using vectors and bacteria. Short-stranded DNA fragments, known as *primers,* correspond to the short segment of DNA to be amplified. The DNA and primers are separated by heating and by the addition of DNA polymerase that generates new additions to the strands, doubling the number of DNA fragments. These cycles are repeated within minutes and can generate millions of copies of the DNA fragments.[10]

The future of biotherapy is influenced by new developments in biotechnology. The first generation of biotechnology produced recombinant versions of immune cell proteins such as alfa interferon and interleukin 2. These were pure, homogenous, contaminant-free products used in clinical trials to modulate or initiate antitumor responses.

The second generation of biotechnological products is now being evaluated. They are genes for the naturally-occurring proteins that have been combined to make hybrid products.[11] The aim is to eliminate troublesome side effects and increase the effectiveness of the agents. These agents are called fusion proteins. Some examples currently in clinical trials include PIXY 321 combining GM-CSF and IL-3, and DAB$_{486}$-IL-2, an immunotoxin. Consensus interferon is another example of combining active portions of many separate subclasses of interferon into one molecule. It is unclear at present whether these molecules will be a significant improvement over the naturally-occurring proteins.

A third generation of biological products is close to entering clinical trial. These are chemical mimics of large molecules that refine the recombinant molecule to target specific molecular sites of activity to achieve the desired therapeutic effect. For example, a collagenase inhibitor molecule has been developed to decrease the joint destruction associated with rheumatoid arthritis. It also may have usefulness in interfering with metastatic tumor growth in bones of women with breast cancer.[11]

# HEMATOPOIETIC GROWTH FACTORS

One of the most successful applications for biotherapy has been hematopoietic growth factors (HGFs). Unlike other applications in which cytokines are administered as primary anticancer therapy, HGFs are used as supportive therapy to myelosuppressive chemotherapy or bone marrow transplantation (BMT). Some cytokines such as IL-1 and IL-6 have pleiotropic actions and may have application in both primary and supportive therapy.

HGFs are cytokines, hormones, colony stimulating factors, and other molecules that influence the development of bone marrow—derived cells to their mature form. These growth factors are usually synthesized by stromal cells in the bone marrow or rarely by non-hematopoietic cells (e.g., the synthesis of erythropoietin by kidney and liver cells).

## The Hematopoietic Microenvironment

The bone marrow is a dense organ with approximately $3–9 \times 10^8$ cell/ml. The marrow requires a high flow of plasma to supply nutrients to a large number of rapidly dividing cells, and to remove waste products. It receives directly approximately 5% of the cardiac output.[12] Approximately $6 \times 10^{11}$ cells (600 billion) are produced each day in the bone marrow.[13] In times of stress, the bone marrow is capable of increasing its output 3 to 20 fold depending on the particular cell type. Thus, the bone marrow is characterized by its stability and ability to produce a variety of cells over a long period of time under varied conditions.

The bone marrow is a complex organ composed of hematopoietic stem cells (HSC), progenitor and maturing cells of various lineages, as well as a supportive matrix for developing cells. HSCs reside in niches in the bone marrow. The stroma of the bone marrow consists of non-stem cell-derived endothelial cells, fibroblasts, fat cells, macrophages, and circulating cells such as lymphocytes and monocytes.[12] A close cell-to-cell contact of progenitor cells and stroma as required for hematopoiesis, is supported by matrix proteins, hemonectin, and fibronectin. These proteoglycans have adhesive surface molecules that help maintain close cell-to-cell contact and high levels of HGFs.[14]

From one originating stem cell, the bone marrow is capable of producing approximately 10 distinct cells that function in body defense (neutrophil, eosinophil, basophil, mast cell, monocyte/macrophage, B- and T-lymphocyte, natural killer cell), oxygen-carrying capability (erythrocyte), and clotting (platelet). As shown in Figure 17-4, these mature cells develop from cell lineages that gradually produce a more differentiated, specialized cell in the bone marrow under the influence of growth factors. The major cell lineages and related HGFs will now be discussed along with the status of these growth factors as biopharmaceutical agents for clinical use.

## Hematopoietic Progenitor Cells and HGFs

### Multipotential precursor cells

The hematopoietic stem cell (HSC), also called a totipotent stem cell, is a self-renewing, originating cell that divides asynchronously. In other words, one daughter cell replaces the parent stem cell and the other becomes a progenitor (HPC) cell, losing its capacity for self-renewal. The HSC is also a rare cell, believed to be 1 cell per 100,000 nucleated marrow cells, and usually resides in a noncycling or $G_0$ state. It is unclear what stimulates an HSC to enter the cell cycle as it is not believed to be responsive to any of the known growth factors.[14]

HPCs are multipotential precursor cells, also referred to as stem cells, that are responsive to growth factors. They are cells capable of repopulating the marrow after myelosuppressive therapy and maintaining hematopoiesis. These pluripotent cells have CD34 positive surface markers.[15]

***Stem cell factor*** The major HGF that influences the multipotential precursor cells, or CFU blast, to develop into myeloid or lymphoid lineages is stem cell factor (SCF). SCF is also known as steel factor or kit ligand, names derived from its discovery in Steel mutant mice and as the ligand for *c kit* proto-oncogenes. SCF is a molecule that stimulates undifferentiated multipotential progenitor cells and committed cell lineage precursors (e.g., colony forming unit-granulocyte erythrocyte monocyte megakaryocyte (CFU-GEMM)) to further develop into mature cells (see Figure 17-4). When administered alone, SCF has demonstrated little colony stimulating effect. However, in combination with other HGFs such as G-CSF, GM-CSF, IL-3, or EPO, it increases the number and size of cell colonies suggesting that it influences early progenitor activity.[16]

SCF may have clinical application in expanding the hematopoietic progenitor population that is responsive to a specific lineage factor such as EPO. It may also have a role in restoring chemotherapy-induced myelosuppression by accelerating bone marrow restoration in BMT or restoring bone marrow function in aplastic anemia or myelodysplastic syndrome.[16]

A phase I clinical trial of recombinant methionyl human SCF was completed in patients with advanced lung and breast cancer.[17] Patients were given daily subcutaneous (SQ) SCF doses for 14 days at 5 to 50 µg/kg/day. The most frequent side effects were injection site reactions and mild to severe symptoms of hypersensitivity reactions with urticaria, dyspnea, and throat tightness. These symptoms were believed to result from the mast cell stimulation. Patients were given $H_1$-receptor antagonist medication with future SCF doses.

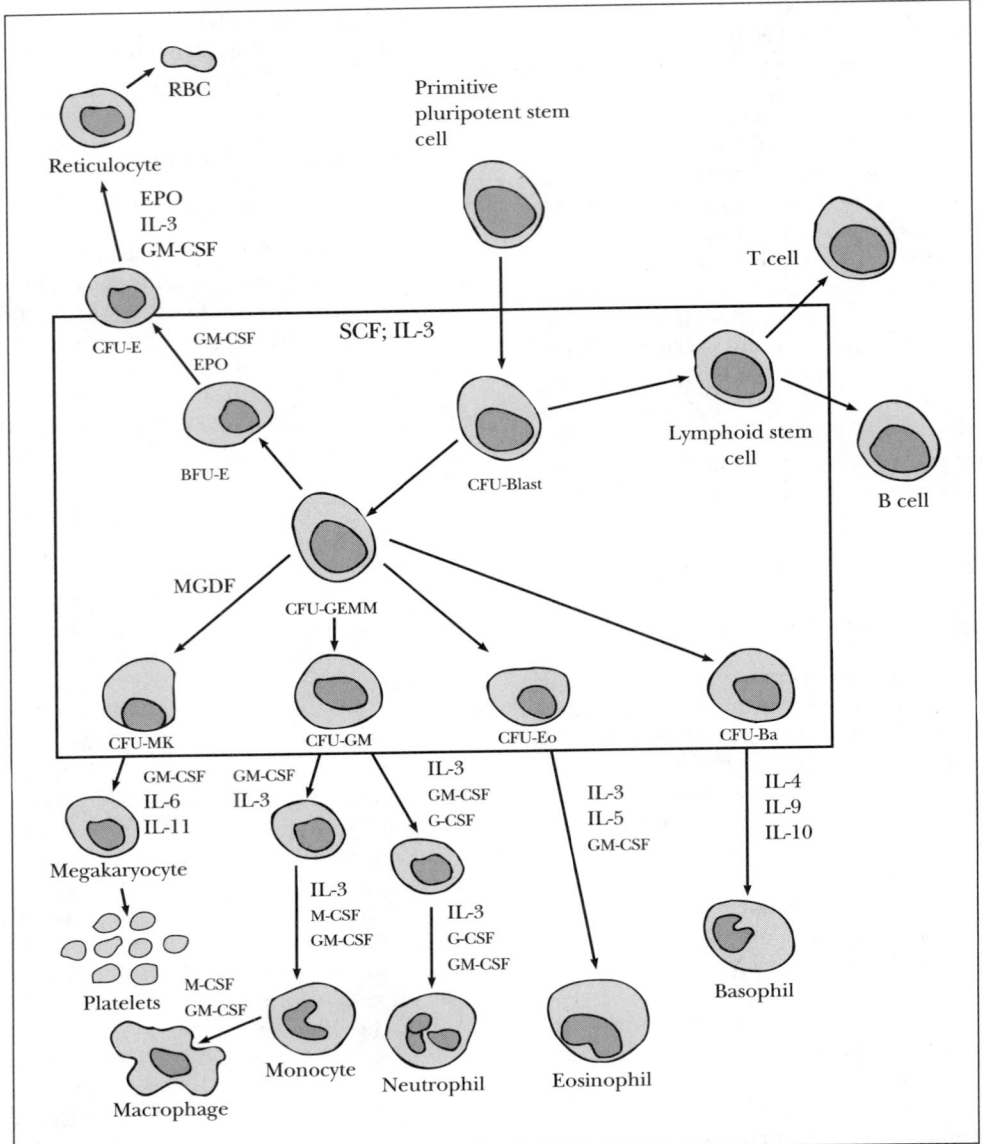

**FIGURE 17-4**   The Hematopoietic Cascade. CFU: colony-forming unit; BFU: burst-forming unit; GEMM: granulocyte/erythrocyte/monocyte/megakaryocyte; GM: granulocyte-monocyte; MK: megakaryocyte; Eo: eosinophil; Ba: basophil; SCF: stem cell factor

***Interleukin 3***   This cytokine is also known as multi-CSF or IL-3. As shown on Figure 17-4, its major role is to promote growth and differentiation of multipotential committed progenitor cells such as the CFU-GEMM for the myeloid cell lineages and the lymphoid progenitor cells.[18]

IL-3 has been tested in several phase I and II clinical trials to evaluate its potential to reverse the myelosuppressive effects of chemotherapy and to restore hematopoiesis in patients with aplastic anemia.[19–21] Doses of 30 to 1,000 $\mu g/m^2$ day of rIL-3 were administered either SQ or as a short intravenous infusion in various treatment regimens. Typical side effects included flu-like symptoms, headache,

bone pain, neck stiffness, and injection site redness. Modest increases in neutrophils, eosinophils, reticulocytes, and platelets were noted in these studies.

It is not clear at present what role IL-3 may have in providing hematopoietic support as a single agent. However, Hoffman[22] suggests that it may have a potential role in mobilization of blood progenitor cells for peripheral stem cell transplantation.

### Erythrocyte lineage

The RBC or erythrocyte is the mature cell of a specialized cell lineage that starts with the CFU-GEMM (see

Figure 17-4). The first committed progenitor cell for this lineage is the erythroid burst forming unit (BFU-E). Initially, these cells are stimulated by SCF, IL-3, and granulo-cyte-macrophage-colony stimulating factor (GM-CSF) and they develop erythropoietin receptors making them responsive to erythropoietin (EPO). They evolve into CFU-E and to the reticulocyte in the presence of the hormone EPO. As the cells mature to erythrocytes, they lose their surface receptors to EPO.[23]

***Erythropoietin*** EPO is a hormone normally synthesized by peritubular cells in the kidney and secondarily by hepatocytes. Its production and plasma levels are closely regulated by many factors, including tissue oxygenation. EPO production is increased by hypoxia and decreased by inflammatory cytokines such as interleukin-1, gamma interferon, and TNF.

There are two identical recombinant products of epoetin alfa or EPO available for use. Procrit® (Ortho Biotech) is licensed for use in anemia associated with cancer chemotherapy, and Epogen® (Amgen) is approved for anemia of chronic renal failure, AIDS, and nonmyeloid malignancies. Both products are given by SQ injection and cause a rise in the red blood cell count within a few days to weeks.

### Platelet cell lineage

The platelet cell is another highly-specialized cell of the bone marrow that develops from the multipotential myeloid progenitor cell (see Figure 17-4). The first committed cell is CFU-megakaryocyte (CFU-MK). It is stimulated by SCF, IL-3, and megakaryocyte growth and development factor (MGDF). The CFU-MK becomes more differentiated under the influence of several additional growth factors of GM-CSF, IL-6, and possibly IL-11 as the megakaryocyte cell fragments into platelets.

There are three growth factors under evaluation for use in platelet support during high-dose chemotherapy. They are IL-1, IL-6, and MGDF or thrombopoietin.

***Interleukin 1*** It is believed that IL-1 stimulates multipotential progenitor cells that later result in increased numbers of cells from multicell lineages including platelets. However, the exact mechanism is unclear. IL-1A is known to have a myeloprotective effect when given prior to radiation or high-dose chemotherapy.[24] Patients with ovarian cancer given IL-1A prior to carboplatinum therapy appear to demonstrate a lessening of myelosuppression with a moderate leukocytosis and significant reduction in the duration of postchemotherapy thrombocytopenia. Patients given IL-1B over five days also showed a rise in their platelet counts after cessation of IL-1B therapy, reaching a maximum 10 days after treatment.[25] In both studies, unlike treatment with CSFs, the cytokine was administered before rather than after chemotherapy, and the rise in platelets occurred after the therapy stopped.

***Interleukin 6*** IL-6 is a cytokine with many actions within the immune system and in hematopoiesis. It is believed to have a role in thrombopoiesis as a cofactor in stimulating the CFU-MK progenitor cell. It is synergistic to other growth factors such as IL-1 and IL-3 in increasing the number of CFU-MK colonies. IL-6 also promotes differentiation and maturation of megakaryocytes.[26]

In phase I clinical studies, IL-6 has been shown to increase platelet counts after the cytokine was stopped.[27] Typical side effects with SQ administration include fever, chills, malaise, and a rise in hepatic enzymes particularly in patients with hepatic disease. IL-6's role in thrombopoiesis appears to be as a cofactor with other growth factors.

***Thrombopoietin (TPO) or MGDF*** This growth factor was isolated and described as the factor that stimulates the proliferation of CFU-MK cells and the differentiation of megakaryocytes into platelets. It has several names—MGDF, TPO, *c-mpl* ligand—as it was characterized independently by four groups of researchers. However, it is believed to be the same molecule.[28] Clinical studies are currently underway to investigate its toxicity as well as its therapeutic effects for maintaining platelet counts during chemotherapy and BMT.

### Monocyte/macrophage and neutrophil cell lineages

Another series of differentiated cells is the monocyte/macrophage and neutrophil lineages (see Figure 17-4). They develop from the common multipotential progenitor cell, the CFU-GEMM, into the CFU-GM under the influence of SCF and IL-3. The CFU-GM differentiates into a monocyte with stimulation of IL-3, GM-CSF, and M-CSF. The latter CSFs may influence development of the macrophage from the monocyte.

The CFU-GM can also differentiate into the neutrophil under the influence of IL-3, GM-CSF, and G-CSF. G-CSF acts on committed granulocyte precursors to increase the number of progeny. Although G-CSF is considered to be a lineage-specific HGF, it has also been found to have some effect on multipotential precursor cells.[18]

***GM-CSF*** This colony stimulating factor or growth factor has effects on myeloid precursor cells as well as on maturing monocytes and macrophages. It also enhances the antibody-dependent cytotoxicity of mature cells.

Sargramostim (Leukine®, Immunex, Seattle) is a recombinant form of GM-CSF that is approved by the Food and Drug Administration (FDA) for use in decreasing myelosuppressive effects of allogeneic or autologous BMT. It can also be used for other neutropenia-associated diseases such as HIV and myelodysplastic syndrome.[29]

Side effects of Sargramostim include fever, lethargy, myalgia, bone pain, anorexia, injection site redness, and rash. There is a "first dose reaction" characterized by flushing, tachycardia, hypotension, dyspnea, nausea, and vomiting.[30]

***M-CSF***    M-CSF is a lineage-specific CSF that stimulates the differentiation and maturation of promonocytes into monocytes and macrophages. It also acts on mature cells to enhance their phagocytosis of bacteria, fungi, and potential tumor cells.

Phase I studies of *E. Coli* derived recombinant M-CSF have been conducted in cancer patients. M-CSF doses ranged from 10 to 100,000 µg/m²/day. Patients at the highest doses experienced malaise, nausea, headache, and various ocular symptoms such as iritis, periorbital edema, and photophobia. Significant increases in monocyte counts were observed in patients receiving greater than 1000 µg/m²/day.[31]

M-CSF may also play an important role as an antifungal agent in cancer patients. Nemunaitis et al[32] reported that 10 of 13 patients with fungal infections demonstrated improvement or complete resolution when given M-CSF infusions at 100–2000 µg/kg. A few responding patients had fungal infections refractory to other medications.

***G-CSF***    Another lineage specific CSF is G-CSF. It is the prime growth factor in the late development of neutrophils, stimulating the proliferation and activation of these cells. It increases the mature cell's infection-fighting capability.

Filgrastim (Neupogen®, Amgen) is a recombinant form of G-CSF that is currently approved by the FDA for use in decreasing neutropenia related to chemotherapy, HIV infection, myelodysplastic syndrome, or BMT. It also can be used to stimulate peripheral blood stem cells for autologous BMT.[13] The most frequent side effect of filgrastim is bone pain.

### Eosinophils and basophils/mast cell lineages

Another form of rare and specialized cell is the eosinophil. It also originates from the multipotential CFU-GEMM and develops into the first committed progenitor cell, CFU-EO, under the influence of IL-3 and SCF (see Figure 17-4). Further differentiation of the committed precursor cell to its mature form is influenced by IL-3, IL-5 (an eosinophil growth factor), and GM-CSF.

Basophils/mast cells also develop from the myeloid precursor cell, the CFU-GEMM. Under the influence of SCF and IL-3, they develop into the first committed cell CFU-BA. Further development into a basophil or mast cell is influenced by IL-4, IL-9, IL-10, and SCF.

## Second Generation HGFs: Fusion Proteins

A second generation of HGFs, the fusion protein called PIXY 321, has begun clinical evaluation. PIXY 321 is a synthetic molecule combining IL-3 and GM-CSF made by genetic engineering techniques. The coding regions of these cytokines are combined to make a product ten times more potent a stimulator of BFU-E and CFU-GEMM than either substance alone.[16]

Vadhan-Raj et al[33] administered PIXY 321 to individuals with sarcoma in a phase I-II clinical trial. PIXY 321 was first given before chemotherapy and then administered in a later cycle after combination chemotherapy. Doses ranged from 25–1000 µg/cm²/day administered SQ b.i.d. Side effects were typical for other growth factors: malaise, headache, fever, myalgia, bone pain, nausea, and injection site redness and induration. No capillary leak or weight gain was observed.

Patients showed increased levels of neutrophils, monocytes, eosinophils, reticulocytes, and platelets, suggesting stimulation of progenitor cells. The pattern of platelet rise was similar to what was observed with IL-3; however, the WBC count was less than has been seen when GM-CSF is given alone. Further study will be needed with this new class of growth factors to better understand its capabilities and limitations. PIXY 321 may be the first in a series of genetically-engineered molecules to combine several growth factors with the potential to maximize the desired therapeutic effects of growth factors while decreasing their toxic effects.

## ANTICANCER CYTOKINE THERAPY

### Interferon (IFN)

Interferon was the first cytokine to be explored as an anticancer biological agent. It was extensively studied both in natural and recombinant forms in a variety of doses and schedules. The early enthusiasm for interferon as a "magic bullet for cancer" did not become a reality, but now interferons are being used as part of biological therapy in low-dose regimens and in combination with other cytokines and chemotherapy regimens.[34]

Interferon was discovered in 1957 with the observation that cells infected with a virus produced a substance that prevented further viral infection to nearby cells.[35] In the 1970s and 1980s, interferon's anticancer qualities led to clinical trials using a natural product extracted from leukocytes and later recombinant varieties when they became available. Table 17-4 describes interferons presently approved by the FDA for clinical use.

#### Types

There are three major types of interferon (IFN) in the body: alpha, beta, and gamma. Alpha and beta are type I IFN and are located on chromosome 9. While beta IFN has only one form, there are 23 subtypes of alpha IFN. Alpha-IFN is primarily made by virally-stimulated leukocytes; beta-IFN is made by activated fibroblasts. Both of these IFNs primarily have antiviral and cell growth regulatory functions.

Gamma IFN is the only type II IFN and its gene is

**TABLE 17-4**   Types of Interferons: A Comparison of Characteristics

| Type/Subtype | Primary Function | Cell Source | Commercial Product | FDA Approved Uses |
|---|---|---|---|---|
| **Type I** Alpha-Interferon (A-IFN) | Antiviral; Antiproliferative | Leukocytes; host cells infected by virus | Leukocyte IFN IFN Alfa 2A Roferon® (Roche) | HCL; AIDS-related Kaposi's sarcoma |
| | | | IFN Alfa 2B Intron A® (Schering) | HCL; AIDS-related Kaposi's sarcoma; Chronic Hepatitis B; Hepatitis C |
| | | | Lymphoblastoid IFN IFN Alfa Wellferon® (Burroughs Wellcome) | |
| Beta-Interferon (B-IFN) | Antiviral; Antiproliferative | Fibroblast; endothelial cells | Interferon Beta 1b Betaseron® (Berlex/Chiron Labs) | Relapsing, Remitting multiple sclerosis |
| **Type II** Gamma-Interferon (G-IFN) | Immunomodulatory | Activated T cells; NK cell | IFN Gamma-1b Actimmune® (Genentech) | Chronic granulomatous disease |

located on chromosome 12. It is made by antigen-activated T cells and NK cells as part of an immune response. Gamma IFN's chief function is immunomodulation. It induces class II major histocompatibility (MHC) receptor molecules, activates macrophages, and increases the cytotoxicity of T cells and NK cells. Gamma IFN also induces other cytokines such as IL-2 and TNF-α.[36]

All three of these IFNs have recombinant forms and are approved for use in cancer and other diseases, primarily hepatitis (see Table 17-4). One commercial IFN, Wellferon®, is a natural product derived from lymphoblastoid cells.

There is also a second generation type of interferon called Consensus IFN (rIFN-con-1). It modifies the interferon to create a synthetic IFN that combines the amino acid sequences of the first eight known subtypes of alfa-IFN.[37] Toxicities are similar to those experienced with alfa-IFN. The efficacy of rIFN-con-1 over naturally occurring recombinant IFNs is currently being evaluated.

Another new class of IFN has also been identified. IFN Tau or trophoblastin has a structure similar to α-IFN. Preliminary laboratory studies suggest that it may have antiviral and antineoplastic activity.[35]

### Side effects

The effects a patient experiences when receiving IFN depends on the IFN type, dose level, and schedule. The higher the dose, the more severe the side effects. Table 17-5 lists the side effects that the patient typically experiences. Patients receiving alfa-interferon experience the worst flu-like symptoms on the first dose. With continued administration, they develop tachyphylaxis or the lessening of intensity and disappearance of symptoms. How-

**TABLE 17-5**   Common Toxicities Related to Interferon Administration

Acute:
Fever, chills, rigor
Malaise
Myalgia
Headache
Nausea, vomiting, diarrhea

Chronic:
Anorexia
Weight loss
Fatigue
Mental slowing
Confusion
Neutropenia, thrombocytopenia
Increased liver enzymes

ever, if the IFN is stopped and restarted, the acute symptoms recur. Patients receiving gamma IFN do not experience tachyphylaxis to acute symptoms.

### Clinical application of alfa-interferon

Alfa-interferon was the first agent to be approved for use in hairy cell leukemia (HCL). However, other more active drugs have generally replaced its use in HCL. It has also been approved for use in a high-dose regimen for AIDS-related Kaposi's sarcoma. Alfa IFN has shown activity in chronic myelogenous leukemia (CML) with low-dose regimens that prolong the chronic phase. Alfa IFN also has shown activity in malignant melanoma, renal cell carcinoma, non-Hodgkin's lymphoma, multiple myeloma, and squamous cell cancer of the skin.

## Interleukins (ILs)

Interleukins (ILs) are cytokines that act primarily between lymphocytes. The name *interleukin* literally means between white cells. However, since their discovery, ILs have been found to have broader activity, interacting with other immune cells and body organs that have a role in the inflammatory immune response.

ILs are referred to by several names as they were discovered by a variety of researchers and given functional names to describe their identified action. To reduce confusion, the International Congress of Immunology designates interleukins by number as soon as the interleukin gene is described.

Unlike other forms of cancer therapy such as chemotherapy, interleukins are not directly cytotoxic to tumor cells. They act as messengers to initiate, coordinate, and sometimes amplify potent immune defense activities. Thus, they require a functional, intact immune system to achieve their therapeutic effects. Immunosuppressive agents such as corticosteroids can block the therapeutic actions of these interleukins and other cytokines when they are used as an anticancer therapy. This has implications for health care professionals in the selection of medications for the management of symptoms commonly associated with cytokine therapy.

The following is a description of the recombinant interleukins currently being evaluated for their anticancer therapeutic potential.

### rInterleukin-2 (aldesleukin)

Recombinant interleukin-2, also known as aldesleukin (Proleukin®), is the first cytokine of the class of interleukins to be approved by the FDA as a cancer therapy. Although it has been studied extensively in many cancers, aldesleukin has demonstrated the best therapeutic effect in renal cell carcinoma (RCC). The approved method of administration is a high-dose regimen of 600,000 or 720,000 international units (IU)/kg by intravenous bolus every eight hours as tolerated up to 15 doses. This regimen is based on a multicenter study of 255 patients with RCC in which 14% of participants responded to the therapy. For those patients who responded, the remission was durable and averaged 20.3 months.[38]

In the years since the FDA's approval of aldesleukin, the high-dose regimen has not been widely accepted, primarily because of its toxic effects. Patients experience symptoms resembling acute sepsis with hypotension, tachycardia, oliguria, weight gain, pulmonary edema, and mental status changes. Many of these symptoms are due to a dose-related capillary leak syndrome. Although these symptoms are reversible when therapy is stopped, they often require intensive medical and nursing care. There is a reluctance to use costly resources for a minority of responders.[39]

Evaluation of lower doses of aldesleukin to treat RCC is currently underway to determine whether lower doses will have similar efficacy but fewer toxicities, and whether low-dose aldesleukin is appropriate to an ambulatory setting. Table 17-6 compares the efficacy and toxicity of two different interleukin regimens—one high-dose bolus rIL-2[40] and the second low-dose.[41] An advantage to the low-dose regimen is that patients with poorer functional status may be able to tolerate as well as benefit from the therapy.

### Interleukin 1

Interleukin 1 (IL-1) is one of the oldest known cytokines with broad, pleiotropic effects on the body. Only recently has it been evaluated for potential use as a cancer therapy. IL-1 is a primary coordinator of the body's inflammatory response to microbial invasion. It is described as having a major role in a variety of inflammatory and autoimmune diseases and is responsible for the harmful host effects of acute sepsis. In host defense, it stimulates both T- and B-lymphocytes and is a cofactor in the activation of NK cells. It also stimulates secondary cytokine production of IL-2, IL-3, colony stimulating factors, IL-6, and TNF. These actions frequently manifest in the side effects experienced by patients receiving rIL-1 in phase I clinical studies.

IL-1 has three molecular forms, all with potential application to patient care. IL-1A and IL-1B are structurally similar molecules, but IL-1B is produced at 10–50 fold greater amounts than IL-1a. Both molecules bind to the same cell surface receptor and have similar biological activity.

IL-1 receptor antagonist (IL-1RA) is the third member of the IL-1 group. It acts as a suppressor to block IL-1 effects stimulated by other interleukins. IL-1RA binds to the IL-1 receptor, preventing initiation of cellular activation. This blockage by IL-1RA may have a valuable role in decreasing the deleterious effects of inflammation without suppressing overall immune responsiveness.[43] It also may decrease unwanted side effects associated with rIL-2 administration without interfering with therapeutic effects.

Several phase I clinical studies have explored the potential side effects and dose-limiting toxicities associated with IL-1a and IL-1b administration. Table 17-7 summarizes the reported dose ranges, maximum tolerated dose (MTD), and toxicity noted in these studies. Both IL-1A and IL-1B promptly produced symptoms typical of acute sepsis (i.e., fever, rigor, hypotension, and nausea). Inflammation occurred at surgical wounds and phlebitis at intravenous sites. Pain was reported as headache, myalgia, and arthralgia. The severity of symptoms was dose related, higher at the MTD level with hypotension as the dose-limiting toxicity. No tumor responses were reported in these studies. Further studies are being conducted to determine the antitumor potential of rIL-1A and rIL-1B

**TABLE 17-6** A Comparison of Two Recombinant Interleukin-2 Treatment Regimens in Patients with Renal Cell Carcinoma Based on Dose Level

| Type of Therapy/ Care Setting | Dose and Schedule | Comparative Dose* | Response Rate** | Major Toxic Effects |
|---|---|---|---|---|
| **High Dose:** Inpatient care with ICU supports[40] | 600,000–720,000 IU/ kg q8h IV bolus for 15 doses and 2 cycles as tolerated | 139–167 MIU/day | 19% (53/283) | Fever, chills, malaise, hypotension, weight gain, oliguria, dyspnea, nausea, vomiting, diarrhea, CNS changes, cardiac arrhythmias |
| **Low Dose:** Ambulatory care[41] | 9–18 MIU SQ q day for 5 days/week over 6 weeks | 9–18 MIU/day | 23% (6/26) | Fever, chills, nausea, skin desquamation, SQ site inflammation |

(IU: international units; IV: intravenous; kg: kilograms; MIU: million international units; SQ: subcutaneous)

*Dose is based on a patient with the following dimensions: 77.3 kg (170 lbs), height 6 feet, BSA 2.0 meters. All doses have been translated into million international units.

**Response rate is the percentage of complete responders (CR) and partial responders (PR) of the total number of study patients. Data from references: Rosenberg, et al, 1994[40]; Sleijfer D, 1992[41]

Adapted from Wheeler V: Interleukins: The search for an anticancer therapy. *Semin Oncol Nurs* 12:106–114, 1996[42]

when given in combination with other cytokines such as rIL-2.

### Interleukin 4

Interleukin 4 or IL-4 is primarily a growth factor for B cells and cofactor for T cell development. It is capable of stimulating the growth and activation of mast cells and eosinophils. This action may be related to the incidence of an allergic inflammatory reaction with symptoms of sinusitis, periorbital edema, and headache in patients receiving IL-4.[47]

Another function of IL-4 is that it inhibits the produc-tion of secondary cytokines such as IL-1 and TNF-α from monocytes while increasing MHC class I and II surface molecules. Therefore, one possible use for recombinant IL-4 (rIL-4) might be to decrease the side effects of IL-2 without losing its therapeutic effects.

Truitt et al[47] reviewed over 10 phase I/II studies of rIL-4, starting in 1988, to evaluate the toxicity and potential efficacy of this agent. rIL-4 was administered subcutane-ously, as a parenteral bolus or continuous infusion and was scheduled three times daily or daily for several weeks. Table 17-7 describes one study using rIL-4.[44] The maxi-mum tolerated dose (MTD) was identified as 10 mcg/kg/dose given as a bolus three times daily. Similar MTDs

**TABLE 17-7** Phase I Studies of Anticancer Interleukins

| Type of Interleukin | Dose Range/Schedule | Major Toxicities |
|---|---|---|
| rInterleukin-1A[44] | 0.01 to 1.0 µg/kg IV bolus MTD 0.3 µg/Kg | Fever, chills, fatigue, headache, hypotension, somnolence, nausea, abdominal pain, dyspnea, confusion |
| rInterleukin-IB[45] | 0.002 to 0.1 µ/kg/day 30 minute infusion for two days MTD 0.1 µg/Kg/day | Fever, chills, headache, arthralgia, myalgia, phlebitis, hypotension, transient hypertension, abdominal pain |
| rInterleukin-4[46] | 10 to 15 µg/kg Q8 hr for 5 days MTD: 10–15 µg/Kg | Nasal congestion, fatigue, nausea & vomiting, diarrhea, headache, dyspnea, capillary leak syndrome, orthostatic hypotension |
| rInterleukin-6[27] | 3, 10, 30 µg/kg SQ q day for 7 days and 2 cycles MTD not defined | Fever, chills, fatigue, nausea, anemia, hyperglycemia, headache, hepatotoxicity |

(µg: micrograms; SQ: subcutaneous; MTD: maximum tolerated dose.) From Wheeler V: Interleukins: The search for an anticancer therapy. *Semin Oncol Nurs* 12:106–114, 1996, p 111.[42] Used with permission.

were reported in other studies. Major side effects included flu-like symptoms, fluid retention and significant nasal congestion, headache, and malaise. A few studies also noted that nausea, vomiting, gastritis, and ulceration with hemorrhage occurred. The severity of symptoms was dose-related; the greater the dose the more intense the symptom. None of the studies reported significant tumor response in patients receiving rIL-4; however, rIL-4 did not induce detectable levels of TNF in contrast to IL-2.

### Interleukin 6

Interleukin 6 (IL-6), like IL-1, has pleiotropic or wide-ranging action to promote host defense. The primary sources of IL-6 are the monocyte/macrophage and activated T helper cells. IL-6 also inhibits tumor growth and is a cofactor in thrombopoiesis and B cell differentiation.[36] Like IL-1, IL-6 is a pyrogenic cytokine capable of inducing fever.

IL-6 was first identified as IFN-α2 due to its similarity to alpha-and beta-interferons and antiviral activity. It is also known as a hybridoma growth factor in the production of monoclonal antibodies and the growth of myeloma.[47] IL-6 is being evaluated for its potential effects on platelet development; however, preclinical evaluations also suggest potential antitumor effects.

A phase I study of rIL-6 has been described in hematopoietic growth factors and is summarized in Table 17-7. No tumor responses were noted.

### Interleukin 12

Interleukin 12 (IL-12) is a recently described cytokine with immune activity involving NK and cytotoxic T cells. IL-2 and IL-12 act synergistically to facilitate maturation of cytotoxic T-lymphocytes, and to induce and prolong LAK cell activity. IL-12 is synergistic to IL-3 and steel factor in stimulating hematopoietic stem cells. Finally, IL-12 is a potent inducer of gamma-interferon by both resting and activated T cells.[47]

rIL-12 is now in clinical phase I trials and reports on its toxicities and clinical efficacy are pending.

## Combination Therapy

The next step in developing an effective anticancer regimen using cytokines is to evaluate them in combination. However, the major dilemma is how to combine them to their best advantage. The important variables of agent, dose, route, sequencing of agents, and duration of treatment are only a few that may influence significantly the therapeutic outcome for the patient.

Many combinations of cytokines have been evaluated such as rIL-2 and rIL-4, rIL-2 and rTNF-α. Two combinations with promising results are as follows:

1. rIL-2 and alfa-interferon—Preclinical studies of these agents in combination demonstrated significant anti-tumor synergy. However, the toxicities were also increased with greater hepatic, cardiac, and especially neurotoxicity. Studies are continuing to evaluate moderate- to low-dose rIL-2 and IFN-α in patients with renal cell cancer.[48,49]

2. rIL-2 and rIL-1—Although this combination has only been recently used, Triozzi et al[50] reported that of patients with colon cancer who received low doses of this combination in an outpatient setting, three patients responded at the lowest dose levels including one who continued to respond for 12 months. These preliminary results will need further study to determine if they are significant.

Another form of combination therapy is combining a cytokine or group of cytokines with chemotherapy. This is a complex therapy that attempts to preserve the immune function stimulated by the cytokines along with tumoricidal effects of chemotherapy. Numerous studies have evaluated rIL-2 or alfa-IFN in combination with 5-FU, cyclophosphamide, adriamycin, and other drugs. One of the most promising areas is in the treatment of melanoma using various combinations of dacarbazine, cisplatin, tamoxifen, carmustine, or vinblastine along with alfa-interferon and rIL-2. Response rates are variable among studies, but average approximately 25%.[51] Toxicities of fatigue, nausea, vomiting, fever, chills, and thrombocytopenia can be significant. Further clinical trials will be needed to determine if chemo-biotherapy combinations are superior to either therapy alone.

## Tumor Necrosis Factors (TNFs)

TNFs are a group of glycoproteins produced by immune cells in response to a pathogen. They are the active substances first seen in Coley's toxins. TNF-α, or cachectin, is produced primarily by macrophages, NK cells, and T cells. They elicit a variety of immune response actions including increased catabolism, enhanced phagocytosis, and tumor destruction.[36]

TNF-β or lymphotoxin, is also a cytokine produced by T cells in response to antigen. It is a cytotoxin that when released is capable of killing any nearby cells. TNF-β's cell killing is enhanced by IFN-g.[36]

TNF is one of the few cytokines that has direct, tumoricidal capability. Although the exact method of cell killing is yet unknown, TNF is capable of damaging tumor blood vessels leading to necrosis and loss of nutrients and oxygen.[52]

The recombinant form of TNF-α (rTNF-α) was evaluated in phase I clinical trials in 1987. The MTD was 250 μg/m²/d; however, the toxicities were severe constitutional symptoms and hypotension, resembling symptoms of septic shock.[53] While rTNF-α was shown to be effective in preclinical trials, in murine tumors, the MTD of TNF-α in clinical studies was substantially less than the effective dose in murine tumors.[54]

Researchers are now investigating the use of rTNF-α in a regional infusion as a way to limit systemic toxicity yet increase the dose to tumors. Patients with tumors isolated to a limb have received 90 minute perfusions of the arm or leg using rTNF-α along with gamma-interferon and melphalan. Significant and sometimes dramatic necrosis of melanoma or sarcoma tumors have been seen with this treatment. Side effects included fever and chills, skin rash, limb-swelling, and hypotension in the immediate postoperative period. Patients with leakage from the perfusion circuit experienced the most side effects.[54] This procedure is now being used to palliate necrotic tumors in patients without life-threatening metastasis to major organs.[55]

# ACTIVATED CELL THERAPY (ADOPTIVE IMMUNOTHERAPY)

The discovery and development of recombinant cytokines such as IL-2 has facilitated the development of activated cell therapy. These activated cells are immune cells that are removed from the patient and placed in culture with rIL-2, which greatly increases their numbers and enhances their cytolytic capacity. The cells are then administered to the patient as adoptive immunotherapy. Activated cells are capable of targeting cancer cells without killing normal cells.

There are two types of activated cells: lymphokine activated killer (LAK) cells and tumor-infiltrating lymphocytes (TIL). LAK is primarily made up of NK cells activated on exposure to high levels of IL-2. They are nonspecific killer cells that can lyse tumor cells without MHC recognition and specificity.[56]

## Lymphokine Activated Killer Cells (LAK)

LAK therapy was first initiated in 1984 at the National Institutes of Health (NIH) and later administered to patients at major cancer research centers. LAK therapy begins with the administration of high-dose rIL-2 to stimulate cell production. These cells are then removed by a series of plasmaphereses and are cultured in rIL-2 for several days. They are returned to the patient along with additional rIL-2 doses as tolerated.

The side effects of the therapy are caused by the rIL-2 administered with the cells: fever, chills, hypotension, oliguria, weight gain, mental status changes, and pruritis. Only pulmonary congestion and dyspnea are attributable to LAK cells themselves.

One of the first patients with melanoma to be given IL-2/LAK therapy had a durable complete remission. However, long-term evaluation of IL-2/LAK therapy has shown that only 5%–10% of patients with melanoma or renal cell carcinoma have responded to therapy. The addition of LAK cells has not demonstrated an advantage in response rates over patients receiving high-dose rIL-2 alone.[57]

## Tumor-Infiltrating Lymphocytes (TIL)

TIL are a second type of activated cell used in cell transfer therapy. TIL are derived from tumor sites and are cytotoxic to autologous (patient's own), but not allogeneic (others of the same type) tumors. They are also 50 to 100 times more potent than LAK. Although the TIL cell population may vary according to the type of cancer, in melanoma approximately 60% are CD4/CD8 cells and NK cell numbers are low. They also differ from LAK as they travel to tumor sites, recognize MHC and tumor antigens.[58]

TIL therapy begins with the isolation of these cells from fresh resected tumor that is enzymatically digested into single cell suspensions. TIL and tumor cells are then cultured in a medium containing antibiotics and rIL-2. Within 2 weeks, tumor cells disappear; over 30 days, the number of TIL rapidly increases and is allowed to grow to a size predicted from preclinical studies to be therapeutically effective. The cells are then removed from culture, washed, and prepared for reinfusion. They are administered intravenously in saline in divided doses depending on the total numbers of cells. High-dose rIL-2 is also administered as tolerated to keep the cells active.[59]

The toxicity of TIL therapy reflects the same side effects of high-dose rIL-2. Side effects directly related to TIL infusions are pulmonary symptoms such as dyspnea, pulmonary congestion, and hypoxia.

Rosenberg et al[60] reported the 5 year NIH experience with TIL therapy in malignant melanoma: 86 patients were treated with TIL and rIL-2 with or without cyclophosphamide (CTX). The objective response rate was 34% with more patients responding to TIL derived from subcutaneous metastatic tumor deposits than TIL derived from lymph nodes. No significant difference was reported for patients who also received CTX. There were patients who responded to TIL who previously had failed to respond to high-dose rIL-2 alone.

TIL therapy is being investigated in patients with renal cell cancer and ovarian cancer in which TIL are administered by intraperitoneal infusions. TIL has also been grown from colon, breast, and lung cancers.

As cancer therapy moves to a molecular-based level, a new generation of more effective TIL may be created. Early gene therapy trials utilized TIL transduced with genes for cytokines such as TNF and IL-2 that were designed to deliver high concentrations of TNF to tumor sites with decreased systemic effects.[61] Now TIL are being developed with more specific recognition ability using immunodominant peptides of tumor-associated antigens. These peptides can be used in ex vivo cultures to generate TIL with specific immunoreactiveness and greater potency than previous TIL.[62,63]

# MONOCLONAL ANTIBODIES

Monoclonal antibodies (Mab) are the product of a single clone of cells sensitized to a specific antigenic protein present on the surface of a target tumor. Mab therapy, also known as *serotherapy,* was one of the first forms of modern biotherapy using a highly specific cytotoxic agent directed against cancer cells and sparing normal tissue.

## Manufacture of Antibodies and the Hybridoma Technique

In the 1970s, the hybridoma technique established the ability to make highly specific antibodies in large quantities and made it possible to develop monoclonal antibodies into a potential cancer therapy. However, it also introduced one of this therapy's biggest problems—the use of foreign immunogenic protein.

As shown in Figure 17-5, the hybridoma process begins with immunizing a mouse with a selected antigen. B cells within the spleen of the mouse soon produce immunoglobulin directed against this injected antigen. These mouse spleen cells are then fused in polyethylene glycol with immortal B cells, myeloma cells, that are capable of continued antibody production in cell culture. Thus, B spleen cells with the desired genetic antibody information are combined with cells having continued antibody production potential. These hybrid daughter cells are separated using a medium that eliminates all nonhybrid cells, and then selected for those clones that produce the desired antibody against the immunizing antigen. The selected cell clones can then be stored or cultured for mass production.[65,66]

This classic method of Mab production has now been modified through the use of genetic engineering techniques. The use of recombinant DNA allows the reshaping of Mab structure to include portions made of human protein or to delete undesired sections of the antibody structure.[67] The newer methods currently being explored include the use of transgenic animals or the genetic engineering of a mouse to produce human instead of mouse antibodies. Some biotechnology companies are evaluating the use of bacteria such as *Escherichia coli* (*E. coli*) as antibody factories to mass produce a specific antibody.[68] It is unclear at present which of these genetic engineering methods will prove most economical and useful in Mab production.

## Mab in Cancer Therapy

Monoclonal antibodies have three essential roles in cancer therapy. The most successful role is in diagnostic and screening functions. Radioisotope-labeled Mab are capable of identifying sites of tumor in the patient that may not be detectable by other methods. A further discussion of this function can be found in chapter 9. A second

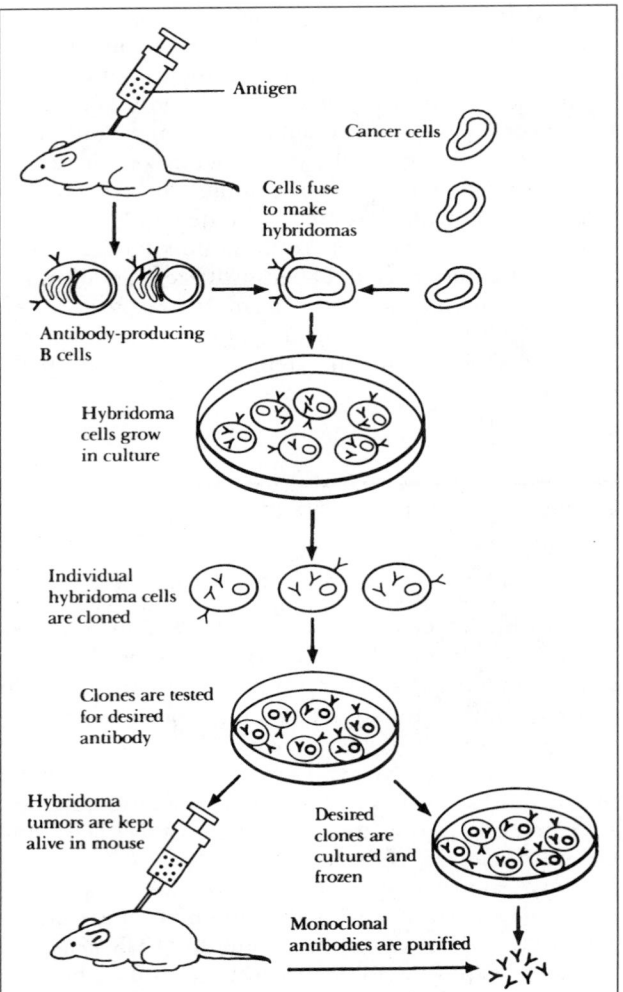

**FIGURE 17-5** A diagram of the Hybridoma Technology for Manufacturing Monoclonal Antibodies.[64]

role for Mab has been to purge autologous bone marrow of malignant cells ex vivo. This will be discussed further in chapter 19. The third role of Mab, as a cancer therapy capable of killing tumor cells with high specificity, is still evolving and will be the focus of this discussion.

The first generation of Mab was used in its native, unconjugated form, and functioned like human immunoglobulin. This form of unaltered antibody is dependent on host immune mechanisms for cell killing since the antibody itself is not a cytotoxic agent. Some of these immune mechanisms include activation of the complement cascade on the surface of tumor cells that can result in cell killing through enzymes; enabling phagocytic cells to attach to and ingest tumor cells; and enhancing NK cell tumor destruction by antibody-dependent cell-mediated cytotoxicity (ADCC).

The specificity of monoclonal antibodies is dependent on identifying antigenic proteins on the surface of tumors that are not present on normal tissues. Mabs have been developed and directed toward many tumor-associated antigens. Schlom[69] describes some of the categories of Mab antigen targets:

**1.** Oncofetal antigens—The most well-known is the carcinoembryonic antigen (CEA), one of the prominent tumor markers. Some Mabs can identify "pancarcinoma" antigens or antibodies developed against one tumor type that also react to many other cancers (e.g., B72.3, 17-1A, KS1/4).[65]

**2.** Differentiation antigens—Antibodies that are capable of binding to cells with surface proteins in a given state of differentiation (e.g., CALLA, Anti-CAA).

**3.** Tissue specific antigen—There are few antigen targets currently identified that are specific to one type of tissue. One example is D612, a gastrointestinal antigen.

**4.** Growth factor and oncogene products—An increasing number of growth factor molecules have been identified with tumors. Some are epidermal growth factor, transforming growth factor-β (TGF-β), or IL-2. C-erb/B-2 is an oncogene being evaluated as a potential Mab target.

**5.** Anti-idiotype—An idiotype is the specific binding region of an antibody. Anti-idiotype Mabs are directed to the antigen binding sites of antitumor antibodies, and have been used in clinical trials with B cell lymphoma and melanoma.

## Design of Monoclonal Antibodies

The repetitive use of antibodies containing foreign protein is strongly immunogenic in immunocompetent patients. It is estimated that 50% of patients develop human antimouse antibody (HAMA) on the first exposure and up to 90% of patients who receive three or more Mab doses develop HAMA.[69] HAMA can bind to the Mab, increasing its clearance from the body and potentially leading to increased toxicity.

In an attempt to decrease the incidence of HAMA, changes in the structure of Mabs have been made to include more human protein that would be less immunogenic. Figure 17-6 shows some of the major modifications currently being evaluated. Chimera antibodies combine the mouse Fab or variable portion with a humanized constant region or Fc. These Mab have a longer circulating half-life and are less immunogenic than murine antibodies.[67] Another Mab design is predominately human protein and is called "humanized antibody." Short segments of murine antibody have been inserted in the variable end on a human antibody structure. These antibodies are currently in clinical trials to evaluate their therapeutic effectiveness and immunogenicity.

Another approach to antibody design has been to decrease the size of the antibody and use the antibody fragments. These fragments—Fab, F(ab')2, or Fv—lack a constant Fc region and thus cannot attach to host cells. They are less immunogenic, are able to penetrate tissues more than an intact antibody, but are rapidly cleared

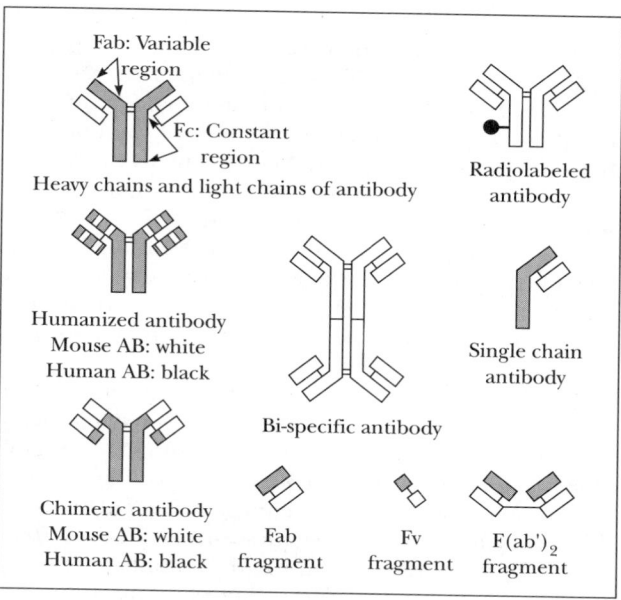

**FIGURE 17-6** Antibody anatomy: variations on the structure of murine, human, and chimeric antibodies.

from the circulation. Antibody fragments are also used as vehicles for toxins or radioisotopes.[70]

### Antibody conjugates

As previously mentioned, unaltered Mabs were the first Mabs to be tested in clinical trials. However, many of the early clinical trials of these unaltered Mabs were done in advanced cancer patients with large tumor burdens. The studies produced only occasional complete or partial responses that were not durable.[69,71]

Another strategy was developed to utilize the ability of a Mab to bind specifically to a target, spare normal tissues, and deliver a cell poison to the tumor cell. These carrier or conjugated Mabs are capable of cell killing and do not require the host's immune competence. Conjugated Mabs have three major divisions:

**1.** Immunotoxins—An immunotoxin (IT) is a Mab or growth factor that is joined to a plant or bacterial cell poison. Ricin is the most commonly used plant toxin; however, some studies have tried saporin or gelonin. These are potent cell poisons that require only minute amounts to be incorporated into the cell to inhibit protein synthesis and cause cell death. Pseudomonas exotoxin (PE) and diptheria toxin are the two most frequently used bacterial toxins.

First generation ITs used a toxin chemically coupled to an unaltered Mab. These bonds were sometimes unstable and could separate in vivo.[70] Unexpected toxicity occasionally occurred. One example was the Mab OVB3 coupled to pseudomonas exotoxin or OVB3-PE. When this agent was tested in phase I studies in patients with ovarian cancer, unexpected severe neurotoxicity occurred due to cross-reactivity and binding of the Mab to neural tissue.[72] Efforts were then directed to methods to decrease toxicity and increase efficacy.

Second generation ITs utilize recombinant DNA technology to reshape both the Mab carrier and toxin, splicing desired genes and removing sites of binding from the toxin to decrease toxicity. Mab fragments can be combined with altered PE to decrease binding to hepatocytes, which has resulted in hepatic necrosis.

Growth factors such as IL-2 and transforming growth factor-alpha (TGF-$\alpha$) also have the capability to bind to specific cell surface receptors that may be overexpressed by malignant cells. These growth factors have also been linked to bacterial toxins as fusion proteins. For example, DAB$_{486}$ IL-2 combines the A domain of diptheria toxin molecule with the gene for IL-2. It is currently being evaluated in phase I clinical trials in patients with non-Hodgkin's lymphoma and cutaneous T cell leukemia.[72] TP-40 is a fusion protein combining TGF-$\alpha$ and modified PE. It is being evaluated for intravesical use in the treatment of bladder cancer, and has the advantage of being a regional infusion and decreasing the opportunity for undesirable tissue binding. Table 17-8 lists other ITs in clinical trials.

**2.** Antibody-drug conjugates—Mabs have been linked to chemotherapeutic agents with the goal of increasing drug concentration at the tumor site. However, problems in getting sufficient concentrations of drug at the site of bulky, often necrotic, and poorly vascularized tumors has been a limiting factor.

**3.** Radioimmunoconjugates—Mab or Mab fragments have been used as carriers of radiation to tumor sites. Radiation has the advantage of killing tumor cells without requiring cell uptake. The most frequently used radionuclides are beta emitters such as I$^{131}$ and Y$^{90}$. They have a relatively short half-life and are capable of transmitting energy a distance of several cell diameters.[67] Table 17-8 lists a selection of the radioimmunoconjugates currently under investigation. Problems with radioimmunoconjugates include potential liver damage due to radiation effects during Mab clearance, stability of the conjugated Mab, and the ability of the Mab to reach its target.[66,67]

### Problems in Mab Therapy

A primary factor that diminishes the effectiveness of Mab therapy is the host's immune response to foreign protein. HAMA, as previously mentioned, can develop rapidly with repetitive doses of Mab. There is concern that patients with increased levels of HAMA can have a hypersensitivity reaction to Mab; however, few reports have documented this toxicity.[74] The greater concern with HAMA is that it alters the effectiveness of the antibody and increases its clearance from the body.

Other problems encountered in Mab therapy center on the characteristics of the tumor target. Unbound circulating antigen from the tumor can bind Mab and prevent them from reaching their target. Also, tumors modulate or change surface antigens, making it difficult for the Mab to link to the target. Often tumors are bulky, hypoxic, and poorly vascularized, making it difficult for circulating Mabs to gain access. For these reasons, Mabs can have low uptake rates, particularly in solid tumors.[75]

### Side Effects of Mab Therapy

Acute side effects that occur during Mab infusion are most commonly fever, chills, malaise, myalgia, nausea, and vomiting. Not all Mab therapy causes side effects and the intensity of the symptoms is variable. Dyspnea, cough, and chest pain can occur during a Mab infusion and may be related to the rate of infusion. The symptoms often resolve if the rate is slowed.

The primary potential toxicity with Mab therapy is an allergic reaction to the foreign protein. A small number of patients may experience symptoms such as bronchospasm, urticaria, pruritis, flushing, restlessness, and hypotension. Skin testing by the administration of small test doses does *not* always identify those patients who will react.[74]

Another potential reaction to Mab therapy is serum sickness. This may occur two to four weeks after therapy and results from circulating immune complexes. It is characterized by urticaria, pruritis, malaise and other flu-like symptoms, arthralgia, and generalized adenopathy.[76]

Side effects of conjugated Mabs vary with the agent used. Myelosuppression is common when radioimmunoconjugates are used. Patients receiving IT therapy occasionally experience vascular leak syndrome with pulmonary edema and weight gain, hypoalbuminemia, and increased liver enzymes. It is unclear what mechanism causes these symptoms.

## HUMAN GENE THERAPY (HGT)

HGT is the insertion of a functioning gene into the cells of a patient to correct a genetic disorder or introduce a new function to the cell.[77] Gene therapy is part of a larger technology known as gene transfer or the transfer of genetic material into human cells.

Gene transfer is a technique that has been performed in laboratories for a decade or more, but its first approved use in humans, in 1989, was to transfer a marker gene to TIL in patients with melanoma to determine TIL's long-term survival and persistence at tumor sites.[78] This trial and subsequent gene therapy trials have demonstrated the safety and feasibility of this developing new technology. HGT is still in its infancy with promising applications in cancer, HIV, and other diseases including cardiovascular and genetic disease. It has the potential to revolutionize biotherapy and cancer therapy in the

**TABLE 17-8** Monoclonal Antibodies Under Investigation*

| | Antibody | Source | Target/Antigen | Conjugate | Comments |
|---|---|---|---|---|---|
| Native/ Unmodified | 3F8 | Murine | Anti-GD$_2$ | | Neuroblastoma or melanoma trials |
| | 14.G$_2$a | Murine | Anti-GD$_2$ | | Neuroblastoma patients |
| | 14.18 | Chimeric (mouse/human) | Anti-GD$_2$ | | Neuroblastoma patient |
| | Shared anti-1D (SID) | Murine | Anti-B cell | | A percentage of lymphomas react to this panel of antibodies |
| | 17-1A | Chimeric (mouse/human) | Colorectal cancer | | Randomized trial showed survival benefit |
| | Campath 1-H | Chimeric (rat/ human) | Lymphocyte, monocyte | | Repeated injections did not result in antiglobulin response |
| | Campath 1-M | Chimeric (rat/ human) | Lymphocyte, monocyte | | Used to deplete T cells in bone marrow to prevent GVH |
| | 16.88 | Human | Colorectal cancer | Rhenium–186 | |
| | 88.BV59 | Human | Colorectal cancer | Rhenium–186 | |
| Immunotoxin conjugates | T-101 | Murine | Anti-CDS | Ricin A | |
| | B$_4$ | Murine | Anti-CD19 | Blocked ricin | NHL, CLL patients |
| | NRLU-10 | Murine | Adenocarcinomas | Pseudomonas exotoxin | Used ex vivo for marrow purging |
| Radioimmuno-conjugates | BC8 | Murine | Anti-CD5 | Iodine–131 | |
| | P67 | Murine | Anti-CD33 | Iodine–131 | AML transplant preparative regimen |
| | M195 | Murine | Anti-CD33 | Iodine–131 | Marrow ablation in relapsed or refractory myeloid leukemia |
| | B1 | Murine | Anti-CD29 | Iodine–131 (high dose and BMT) | B cell NHL |
| | B1 | Murine | Anti-CD29 | Iodine–131 (low dose) | B cell NHL |
| | Lym-1 | Murine | Anti-DR variant | Iodine–131 | NHL |
| | Lym-1 | Murine | Anti-DR variant | Copper–67 | NHL |

*Partial listing—Over 80 antibodies are in early clinical investigation.
Modified with permission from Wheeler V, Appelbaum J: Module 5, Biotechnologic Agents in Clinical Practice, NFSNO Biotechnology Nursing Core Curriculum, National Federation for Specialty Nursing Organizations (NFSNO), 1995, p. 64.

future as recombinant genetic engineering changed immunotherapy over two decades ago.

At this time, HGT is limited to somatic cell therapy; that is, a genetic change in an individual's cells is limited to the individual's lifetime. For example, the gene placed in the lymphocytes of a child with severe combined immunodeficiency syndrome (SCID) to correct an enzyme deficiency cannot be passed on to their offspring who may inherit SCID.

Germline therapy alters the human genome for future generations by placing the gene into the egg or sperm cells. This form of therapy, although feasible, is not presently used in clinical trials and is the subject of intense ethical, social, and legal debates.[79,80]

One method of classifying HGT clinical trials in cancer is by the method of gene transfer used. The following is a review of some of the primary methods being investigated.

## Retroviral Gene Transfer

Viruses have a special ability to enter a cell's genome and convert the cell's machinery to manufacture virions. In gene transfer techniques, the virus is used as a vector or carrier to deliver the desired gene to a target cell. The virus is disabled from replication by removing its reproductive genes. This process is usually done ex vivo, in culture. For example, the target cells, such as lymphocytes, are exposed to the retroviral vector carrying the desired gene, TNF. Transduced cells, those that incorporate the gene, are returned to the patient and evaluated for their desired effect. Safety monitoring ensures that the retroviruses are not capable of reproducing and that they are not present in the transduced cells being returned to the patient.[77]

An example of research in this method of gene transfer involves the multiple drug resistance (MDR) gene. The MDR gene is one mechanism whereby cancer cells become resistant to chemotherapy. The multiple drug resistance pump exists in the cell membrane and effectively acts as an "efflux pump" that pumps the chemotherapy out of the cancer cell before it has an opportunity to cause cellular damage and death. By employing the process of gene transfer, it may be feasible to transfer the MDR gene into a patient's hematopoietic stem cells as a means of preventing damage to the hematopoietic cells, thereby preventing myelosuppression from chemotherapy. A clinical trial of MDR gene transfer in patients receiving high-dose chemotherapy for ovarian or breast cancer is underway.[81]

A different technique of retroviral gene transfer is the insertion of the herpes simplex virus thymidine kinase (HSV-TK) gene into brain tumor cells to confer a sensitivity to the antiviral agent, gancyclovir. The retrovirus is picked up only by cells that are actively dividing. When the patient is given gancyclovir intravenously, the altered brain tumor cells are killed and normal noncycling brain tissue is spared. Another phenomenon, known as the "bystander effect," occurs when nearby tumor cells that were not transduced also are killed. One possible explanation is that toxic metabolites are transferred from cell to cell. This technique is also being evaluated in other cancers (e.g., ovarian cancer) and as adjuvant therapy.[82]

Finally, retroviral gene transfer has been used to answer questions about the cause of relapse in patients undergoing autologous bone marrow transplantation (AuBMT). Cells removed from the bone marrow were marked with a gene for neomycin resistance (Neo®) that confers resistance to the neomycin analog, G418. Cells that are transduced with Neo® are protected from the lethal effects of G418 while nontransduced cells are not. Brenner et al[83] found that patients who relapsed after AuBMT had Neo®-marked cells suggesting that the cause of relapse was ineffective purging of the marrow specimen.

The use of this permanent genetic marker that persists in cell lineages derived from the marked cell has provided valuable information about cancer therapy in BMT as well as in other non-cancer clinical situations.[84]

## Direct Gene Transfer

There is growing interest in developing methods of transfering genes to a target cell without the use and associated problems of a viral vector. One method being investigated is the use of liposomal carriers. Liposomes are nontoxic fat droplets in which drugs or gene-containing plasmids can be placed. Nabel et al[85] reported on a first trial using DNA-liposome complexes containing the gene for a foreign major histocompatibility molecule HLA-B7 and targeting melanoma cells. The objective was to increase the immunogenicity of tumors as well as test the safety and feasibility of this technique. Results were that the HLA-B7 molecule could be recovered by tumor biopsy and that one patient demonstrated regression of both the injected tumor nodules and other metastatic sites.

Additional studies are now underway using an improved cationic lipid and HLA-B7 DNA plasmid delivered by catheter to metastatic tumor sites in patients with renal cell or colon cancer. In other studies, tumor cells are transduced with genes expressing various cytokines, antigens, or foreign MHC molecules to increase their immunogenicity for use as a cancer vaccine.[86]

Other researchers are proposing to use direct injection of "naked DNA" into tissues with plasmid DNA encoding for peptide products of tumor specific proteins such as carcinoembryonic antigen (CEA). These peptide products act as immunizing agents. The genes are attached to particles that are delivered by a "gene gun," a technique borrowed from plant molecular biology that bombards a target tissue with the peptide particles and propels them into the cells.[61,87] The expression of these particles on cells results in their uptake by antigen presenting cells, stimulating an immune response.

## Safety Concerns

The primary concern with HGT involves the safety of using viral vectors. It is possible for the viruses to reacquire the ability to replicate through interaction with intact benign viruses, and infect the patient. Also, there is the potential for insertional mutagenesis; that is, the insertion of the virus into the genome could potentially disrupt a tumor suppressor gene controlling normal cellular growth. However, thus far, currently existing viral gene transfer methods have been evaluated and found to be safe.[88]

Other concerns about gene transfer center on the ability to control the expression of the transduced gene. Cells that are transduced with cytokines may express IL-2 or TNF and lack feedback controls of native cytokine expression. These are issues that are considered at the time approval for the clinical study is discussed. Some protocols may be required to build in methods of eliminating transduced cells when untoward effects occur.

## Nursing Considerations

It is unclear at present how gene therapy will change nursing practice. Patient and nursing considerations for these studies are largely identical to those for any phase I clinical research. Important priorities include ensuring informed consent of patients enrolling in clinical trials, and providing patient education with therapies that involve complex genetic and molecular biology techniques.

However, there are two concerns with gene therapy of particular interest to nurses. First, what symptoms or side effects will the patient experience from HGT? A review of initial gene therapy studies by the Recombinant DNA Advisory Committee showed that the initial gene therapy studies demonstrated little to no toxicity directly related to the gene-altered cells.[89] However, patients participating in these clinical trials may experience symptoms resulting from associated drug treatments. In other words, patients receiving AuBMT with Neo® cells experienced myelosuppression and other side effects of the transplantation procedure, but had no detectable side effects from the Neo® transduced cells.

Another issue of concern to nurses is safety for the health care provider when handling gene therapy agents, particularly when retroviruses are employed for cell transduction. For those gene therapy protocols that utilize retroviruses, the FDA requires that institutions manufacturing gene therapy vectors conduct stringent quality control testing before a product is utilized in the clinical setting.[90] Although there are no studies or reported incidents that suggest any dangers related to gene therapy, nurses are advised to use universal precautions or simple barriers such as gloves to guard against known viral hazards (e.g., hepatitis and HIV).[91]

## The Future of Gene Therapy

Gene therapy has caught the interest of the general public, and through the news media, the expectations for this technology have far exceeded its present capabilities.[92] An article in a weekly news magazine criticized that gene therapy protocols have not demonstrated the ability to cure anything after five years of study.[93] There is pressure to demonstrate immediate benefit to justify costs and to help patients, which could compromise the testing and development of this technology.

Problems that must be solved include improving the efficiency of gene delivery methods to the target cells and improving their expression. Friedman states, "What lies ahead now is the difficult process of implementation—of developing tools to make it all work."[94, p.271]

## OTHER IMMUNOMODULATING AGENTS

An immunomodulating agent can be broadly defined as a substance that stimulates host defense mechanisms or indirectly augments aspects of immunity that are beneficial in cancer therapy. Immunostimulants are often nonspecific agents that target key immune cells such as the monocyte/macrophage, provoking secondary responses involving increased cytokines, cytotoxic cell activation, and increased immunoglobulins.

Nonspecific immunostimulation is based on the theory that the host's responsiveness to a tumor can be increased through overall stimulation of host defense mechanisms using nontumor-related antigenic agents such as microorganisms.[95] In localized therapy, the tumor may be an "innocent bystander" but killed in the reaction to the provoking agent. This concept has been pursued in numerous clinical studies since the 1970s with occasional positive outcomes.[5] These results underscore the need to better understand the complexities of the host-tumor relationship in order to apply this theory to clinical practice.

Some immunomodulating agents, such as cancer vaccines, provide active specific immunotherapy directed to a specific tumor target. Immunomodulator agents also include those that target specific aspects of host defense to stimulate cell differentiation (e.g., thymic hormones acting on T cell differentiation); chemical substances that act as nonspecific immunostimulants (e.g., levamisole); vitamin preparations such as retinoids and even chemotherapeutic agents such as cyclophosphamide that may decrease suppressor T cell function or stimulate immune cells after initial immunosuppression.[95]

Nonspecific immunomodulating agents require that the host be capable of developing an immune response. Permanent damage to the immune system or persistent immunosuppression will interfere with the agent's effectiveness. In addition, the patient's tumor burden should be low. Large, bulky tumors are believed to significantly suppress host defense mechanisms. Therefore, immunomodulators frequently are used as adjunctive therapy with surgery or chemotherapy to reduce the patient's tumor burden.[95,96]

The following discussion will briefly describe immunomodulating agents that are approved for cancer therapy or for clinical trials.

## Bacillus Calmette-Guerin (BCG)

This is a nonspecific immunostimulant that was originally derived from attentuated *mycobacterium bovis* isolated in 1920. There are various BCG strains available (e.g., Glaxo, Pasteur, Tice); they vary according to the number of organisms per unit of dose administered. BCG has been administered intradermally, subcutaneously, by scarification, or via intracavitary infusion. It produces both localized side effects of swelling, pain, inflammation, and ulceration of the injection site as well as systemic flu-like symptoms of fever, chills, malaise, and arthralgia. Patients can have hypersensitivity reactions to BCG preparations if they have had previous exposure to BCG or a positive PPD. A small number of patients receiving BCG may develop a disseminated BCG infection.[95,97,98]

Special precautions are used with the patient receiving BCG, particularly intralesional therapy.[97] They include

- Assess the patient's potential for a hypersensitivity reaction to BCG before and during therapy. Patients with prior exposure to this agent will have a more rapid response that can be severe and can lead to anaphylaxis. Changes in the BCG dosage may be required.

- Premedication of patients with acetaminophen and diphenhydramine may decrease the severity of systemic flu-like symptoms.

- Patients are monitored for prolonged flu-like symptoms and organ dysfunction (liver, kidney, and pulmonary abnormalities) that suggest potential BCG infection.

- All BCG syringes and other materials that have come in contact with BCG should be disposed of as hazardous waste to prevent environmental contamination. Consult the health agency's epidemiology official for other BCG safety guidelines.

There are two accepted applications of BCG. It is used as an intralesional injection for superficial metastatic malignant melanoma lesions. Patients with melanoma receiving intralesional therapy achieved complete control of superficial lesions in about 60% of immunocompetent patients. Long-term survival occurred in approximately one-fourth of responding patients.[97]

A second application is the administration of BCG as a bladder instillation for maintenance therapy of superficial bladder tumors after transurethral resection. Patients receive repeated two-hour bladder instillations of BCG at weekly or monthly intervals. Patients who received BCG instillations had a greater disease-free interval after surgical resection than patients who did not receive BCG. BCG was also capable of creating an immunologic memory to future tumor recurrences that was not possible with instillations of chemotherapeutic agents.[98]

The side effects of intravesical BCG therapy include hematuria and dysuria from the inflammatory mucosal reaction to BCG, fever, and rarely, disseminated BCG infection. A long-term outcome of BCG bladder instillations can be a contracted bladder.

## Levamisole

This drug, also known as Ergamisol, is a nonspecific chemical immunomodulator that was originally developed in the 1960s as an agent for common intestinal parasites.[95,99] It was investigated in the 1970s as a stimulant of host defense to augment or restore deficient immune function through stimulation of T cells and macrophages after immunosuppression.[100] A large national study using an adjuvant regimen of oral levamisole with intravenous 5-fluorouracil found a significant survival advantage in a subset of patients with Dukes C colon carcinoma.[101]

Not all studies using levamisole in colon and other cancers have had positive results. Although it is still unclear how levamisole works, particularly in a subset of patients with Dukes C colon cancer, several factors may contribute to its success. Like with other immunomodula-

tors, the host must have an immune system capable of responding to an immunostimulant. The dose amount and timing also may influence therapeutic results. Levamisole appears most effective as adjuvant therapy administered with other cytoreductive therapies such as surgery or chemotherapy.[96,102]

Levamisole is usually given orally at 50 mg three times per day. The peak blood levels occur two to four hours after administration and the drug is metabolized in the liver. Side effects of levamisole therapy include mild nausea, liver dysfunction, leukopenia, skin rash, flu-like symptoms, and, rarely, neurological effects such as cerebellar dysfunction and mental confusion. Patients who consume alcohol during levamisole administration may experience increased side effects including flushing, throbbing headaches, and respiratory distress.[99]

## Retinoids

Retinoids are a group of compounds that are natural derivatives of retinol or vitamin A. They include all *trans* retinoic acid (ATRA), 13-*cis* retinoic acid (13-*cis* RA or isotretinoin), and 9-*cis* retinoic acid (9-*cis* RA).

Retinoids are essential in the physiological processes of vision, fertility, and embryonal growth. In cancer, retinoids act as immunomodulators by inducing cellular differentiation and suppressing proliferation.[103,104] Cancers that may be responsive to retinoids include leukemias, melanoma, neuroblastoma, and various epithelial cancers.

Retinol is absorbed from the gastrointestinal tract and is bound in the circulation to retinol-binding plasma proteins in minute amounts. Intracellularly, retinol is oxidized to form 13-*cis* RA, 9-*cis* RA, or other compounds. They target receptors in the nucleus capable of binding retinol as well as steroids, estrogen, and thyroid. Here they interact with DNA to affect cellular growth and functions. For example, retinol can suppress the synthesis of stromelysin by tumor cells, a compound that allows tumors to metastasize by degrading stromal tissue.

Clinically, dramatic effects have been seen using retinoids in acute promyelocytic leukemia (APL). ATRA acts on APL cells to increase their differentiation into mature granulocyte cells and induce clinical remission.[104,105] However, the remission often is not durable and APL reoccurs.

A serious side effect of retinol therapy in APL is the retinoic acid syndrome.[103,106] Patients receiving retinoids can exhibit fever, respiratory distress, interstitial pulmonary infiltrates, pleural effusions, and weight gain. Retinoic acid syndrome can be fatal if not promptly recognized and treated, usually with high-dose corticosteroids. It occurs in approximately 25% of patients and can appear within 2 to 21 days of onset of therapy. Symptoms do not abate or reverse when the drug is discontinued.[106]

Retinoids have been combined with alpha- and beta-interferons to enhance the antiproliferative actions of both compounds. This combination has been evaluated in squamous cell carcinoma of the skin with a 68% response rate. Major side effects of retinoids in this study included mucocutaneous dryness, flu-like symptoms, and dose-limiting fatigue.[107] Other studies are exploring the use of retinoids and alfa-interferon in head and neck, cervical, breast, esophageal, endometrial, vulval, and penile cancer.

## Cancer Vaccines

A vaccine is an immunostimulant that utilizes live, inactivated, killed, or portions of an organism. Vaccinations increase immunity to a specific disease prior to exposure. In cancer, the term vaccine is actually a misnomer as the patient already has the disease and the intent is to stimulate the patient's own immune system to recognize and destroy the tumor.

Cancer or tumor vaccines are also known as active specific immunotherapy (ASI). They differ from other immunomodulating therapies in that they stimulate an immune response directed to a specific target versus creating a generalized immune response. ASI requires, however, that the patient be immunocompetent and not have a large tumor burden that may interfere with immunity.[108]

Cancer vaccines have been a part of immunotherapy research for approximately 25 years or more. The studies are usually long-term requiring years to demonstrate survival differences.[109] First generation cancer vaccines were frequently made of tumor cells, either whole irradiated or an immunogenic portion of the tumor cell along with an adjuvant. Adjuvants are a variety of agents added to the tumor cell preparation to stimulate an immune response. Freund's incomplete adjuvant is a water-in-oil emulsion that forms a slow-release depot for the vaccine antigen.[36] Other frequently used adjuvants are bacterial preparations. BCG is a frequently used nonspecific immunostimulant. DETOX® (Ribi Immunochemicals) is an adjuvant composed of portions of *salmonella minnesota* and *mycobacterium phlei* combined with the tumor vaccine. In other studies, viral proteins called viral oncolysates, are added to tumor cell preparations to stimulate the immune system.

The source of tumor cells varies. Autologous vaccines are made from the patient's own tumor; allogeneic or polyvalent vaccines contain the same tumor-type cells from several patients.

Hoover et al[110] used a tumor cell/adjuvant preparation in a trial of adjuvant cancer vaccine in postsurgical patients with colorectal cancer. Postoperative patients received four injections of irradiated autologous tumor cells with BCG as an adjuvant or no additional treatment. Study patients showed a 70% delayed hypersensitivity reaction to the tumor cells. Patients receiving vaccinations had an increased disease-free survival time compared to those receiving no treatment.

Second generation vaccines are also being evaluated. They contain a more specific antigenic molecule to stimulate a cell-mediated and/or humoral reaction. One disadvantage to this method is that the material might not contain the right antigen. However, some researchers suggest that the product is more consistently reproducible among patients and studies.[111] In a study using this more purified material, melanoma cell antigen ganglioside GM$_2$ plus BCG and cyclophosphamide were administered to patients with melanoma in four to five treatments over six months. Patients who developed antibodies to GM$_2$had significantly improved survival rates versus patients who did not demonstrate antibody production.[112] Patients typically experience fever, chills, and injection site reactions. These site reactions resolve over several weeks. The interest in cancer vaccine studies has increased considerably in the last few years. These studies are conducted primarily in ambulatory care settings and create few side effects in participants compared with cytokine studies.[113] However, more time is needed to determine efficacy in clinical practice.

## NURSING MANAGEMENT OF THE PATIENT RECEIVING BIOTHERAPY

Biotherapy, like chemotherapy, has a distinctive constellation of common side effects. Patients frequently experience fever and chills, headache, malaise, and arthralgia. Some patients experience injection site redness, induration, and pain. A few patients may develop generalized swelling, rash, weight gain, hypotension, and, occasionally, respiratory changes.

Not all biological agents have the same profile of toxicities. High-dose cytokines, particularly high-dose IL-2 can result in a broad spectrum of toxicities affecting nearly all organ systems. On the other hand, CSFs, particularly G-CSF (Filgrastim), are well-tolerated. One possible explanation for this variability is that a few cytokines, particularly interleukins 1, 2, and 6, like native interleukins, are capable of initiating broad, inflammatory activities throughout the body either directly or mediated through secondary cytokines. Other agents have a narrow range of activity.

### Effects of Dose and Schedule

Biological agents differ from chemotherapy in the dose level required to achieve therapeutic effects. Often the best results from chemotherapy are obtained from high-dose, intensive regimens given at the maximum tolerated dose (MTD). Biological agents, on the other hand, may stimulate the desired biological activity at a dose level far less than the MTD. This dose is called the optimal biological dose (OBD).[113] Thus, the evaluation of a new biological agent is more complex than evaluation of a new drug. Different dose levels can initiate opposite immunological reactions. For example, for melanoma patients, the most effective results are obtained with high-dose rIL-2. In contrast, in renal cell cancer, patients respond to rIL-2 when it is given at much lower doses. At the lowest dose, approximately 180,000 U SQ, rIL-2 is an effective treatment for leprosy.[114]

Different symptoms predominate with variations in the method of administration (subcutaneous versus parenteral), dose level, and schedule. For example, Thompson et al[115] evaluated for toxicity four dose levels and schedules of IL-2 administration. They found that patients given 300,000 U/m²/day as a two-hour infusion experienced fever, chills, emesis, diarrhea, and occasionally rash. Patients receiving the same dose given over 24 hours also experienced hypotension, 5%–10% weight gain, and increased creatinine—all symptoms of a capillary leak syndrome. Patients given a higher IL-2 dose (3 million U/day) by either schedule experienced greater flu-like symptoms, more severe fluid retention, hemodynamic changes, oliguria, and gastrointestional symptoms.

## Preparation, Administration, and Safe Handling of Biological Agents

Many biological agents such as recombinant growth factors are reconstituted by nurses and patients. Therefore, it is important to be aware of some key differences between biopharmaceuticals and drugs. Biopharmaceuticals are protein-based agents that often require refrigerated storage. Patients who travel should be cautioned that these products cannot tolerate the extremes in temperature commonly found in car trunks and airplane baggage holds. When the lyophilized product is reconstituted the vial should not be shaken or the diluent directed into the dried powder. Excessive foaming that can denature the protein may occur. Finally, some biopharmaceuticals are not compatible with all plastic syringes and intravenous tubing. The package insert can provide valuable information on storage and compatibility of a particular product. Many pharmaceutical companies have toll-free numbers to answer questions and supply additional information regarding their products.

At present, there are no known safety hazards associated with exposure to cytokines, monoclonal antibodies, or cell therapies. However, the use of simple barriers is recommended to prevent inadvertent exposure to immunogenic substances. For products containing BCG, it is recommended that barriers be used with special disposal to prevent environmental contamination with mycobacterium. The Oncology Nursing Society has published a monograph on biotherapy that provides more specific instructions on safe handling.[116]

## Side Effects and Key Nursing Strategies

### Flu-Like Syndromes (FLS)

FLS is a constellation of nonspecific symptoms that typically occurs when one develops an influenza infection.

The major symptoms include chills and possible rigors, moderate to high fever (100–104° F), myalgias, arthralgias, and malaise. These symptoms may be associated with one or more related symptoms such as headache, anorexia, nausea, vomiting, diarrhea, sinusitis, and hyperalgesia.

Body temperature is controlled by preoptic anterior hypothalamic brain centers in a feedback mechanism with peripheral sensors (see Figure 17-7). According to the set-point theory of temperature control, the hypothalamic centers "sense" deviations from a set temperature range of 36.4 to 37.3° C (97.5–99.5° F) and regulate thermal balance with heat producing vasoconstriction and shivering or with heat loss actions such as vasodilation and sweating.[117,118] Pyrogenic pathogens, toxins, or drugs stimulate the release of endogenous pyrogenic cytokines such as IL-1, TNF, and IL-6 that act on thermal brain centers via prostaglandin release to create an upward reset of the body's temperature set-point. Feedback mechanisms now read the body temperature as cold and initiate heat producing actions such as involuntary muscular contractions or rigors. The hypothalamic temperature set-point can be returned to normal when blood levels of endogenous pyrogen at the brain centers fall or are blocked by antipyretics such as aspirin.[118] The excess heat is then released through diaphoresis.

Shivering or rigors requires a large energy expenditure and increased oxygen consumption three to five fold greater than normal.[117] This involuntary, vigorous exercise may put a strain on both the cardiovascular system as well as the large muscle groups of the body. Therefore, it is important to control rigors as soon as they occur to prevent undue cardiovascular stress.

FLS is most frequently a side effect of cytokine therapy

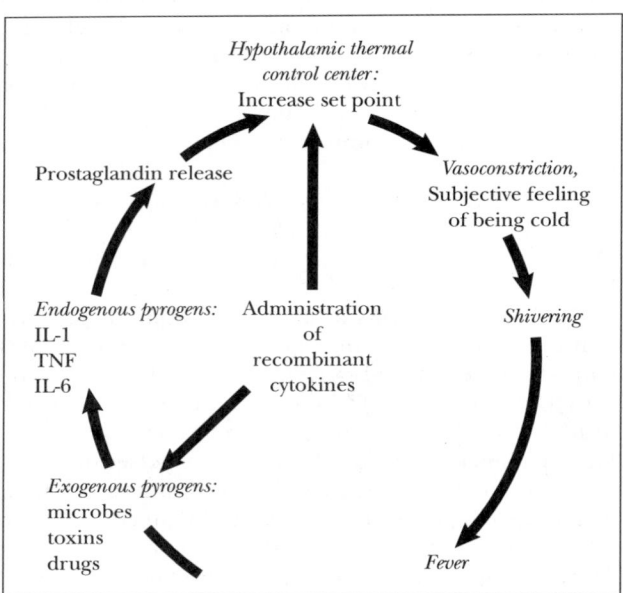

**FIGURE 17-7**  Pathogenesis of cytokine-related fever.

although not all cytokines produce the full spectrum of symptoms or at the same intensity. For example, headache is a typical symptom of IL-3 and sinusitis is typical of IL-4. *Tachyphylaxis,* or the development of tolerance to a symptom with repeated frequent doses, commonly occurs with interferon therapy. The FLS symptoms are most severe with the first doses and then lessen and disappear. The FLS symptoms return only when the therapy is stopped and restarted.

Monoclonal antibody (Mab) therapy has its own FLS pattern of symptoms. Some Mabs do not cause fever at all; others create a biphasic fever pattern with fever occurring at the onset of administration and then several hours after completion. Arthralgias, possibly due to circulating immune complexes, rather than myalgias may accompany the fever.[119]

Colony stimulating factors such as G-CSF and EPO generally do not cause fever. GM-CSF is an exception. Fever may accompany its administration probably through stimulation of endogenous pyrogen release from monocytes and macrophages.

*Nursing management*   Guidelines for the nursing management of FLS in a patient receiving biologic therapy are as follows:

- Evaluate the risk for FLS symptoms: Cytokine therapy, monoclonal antibody infusions, and the first dose of interferons are the highest risk.

- Premedicate the patient one hour prior to the first dose: Common medications are acetaminophen and indomethacin (optional).

- Keep the patient warm: Use warm blankets at the first sign of a chill.

- For rigors: Administer meperidine 25–50 mg parenterally as appropriate to the patient care setting.

- For arthralgia, myalgia, or headache: Continue the use of acetaminophen and indomethacin as appropriate.

- For uncontrolled, high fevers: Use cooling blanket or tepid bath.

- Consider alternate times of administration: Give biological agent at bedtime rather than in the morning.

- Consider other sources of fever: Infection may be a complication of cytokine therapy, particularly if the patient is receiving high-dose IL-2. If fever persists and is accompanied by hypotension, consider the following possible sources of infection: Pulmonary, urinary tract, IV site or central venous catheter, existing wound or skin lesion, or septicemia from unknown sources.

## Fatigue

Fatigue is a symptom commonly experienced by cancer patients and especially those receiving radiation therapy and chemotherapy. It is also a common side effect of many types of biotherapy and severe enough in certain high-dose, long-term cytokine regimens to be a dose-limiting factor.

Fatigue's subjective nature can make definition challenging. Aistairs[120] defines fatigue as subjective feelings of generalized weariness, weakness, exhaustion, and lack of energy resulting from prolonged stress that is directly or indirectly attributable to the disease process. Winningham[121] describes fatigue as a subjective feeling of tiredness that is multidimensional and multisensory. She distinguishes acute fatigue—that which is protective and disappears after a short rest—from chronic fatigue that is not relieved by rest, but that is constant and debilitating. All of these definitions help define the experience of biotherapy-related fatigue: A chronic fatigue characterized by generalized weariness, weakness, exhaustion, and feelings of tiredness. It can be accompanied by other symptoms such as fever, myalgia, and headache. Fatigue of biotherapy is a symptom that can disrupt physical, psychological, and spiritual well-being.[122]

*Interferon*   When alfa-interferon was first investigated in phase I/II clinical trials, the impact of severe fatigue on a patient's functional status was recognized for the first time. Quesada et al[123] note that daily schedules of interferon at doses of 20 million units or greater can result in profound toxicity including fatigue. Davis[124] describes the patient experience of fatigue while receiving escalating doses of alfa-interferon, as fatigue increasing over time and positively related to the dose level. Patients reported feeling tired all the time. They had increased leg weakness and the need to lie down. Maintenance of nutrition and fluid balance became a problem as patients were too tired to make the effort to eat, or even lift food to their mouths.

Davis[124] observes that patients experienced mood changes, increased irritability and impatience, and decreased sociability. They were too tired for conversation or to be interested in activities. Sleep patterns were disrupted by frequent daytime naps and patients experienced a restlessness and inability to get comfortable when lying down.

*Interleukins*   Fatigue is a common side effect with nearly all interleukins such as IL-1, IL-2, IL-4, and IL-6, particularly in long-term outpatient regimens. Only phase I studies of IL-3 do not list fatigue in their top five side effects. When interleukins are combined with interferons, fatigue appears to be additive. Nearly 100% of patients receiving combined therapy reported fatigue and in some patients, it was a dose-limiting symptom.[48,49]

*Monoclonal antibodies, colony stimulating factors*   Fatigue is not a common side effect of either Mabs or CSFs.

***Nursing management*** The following are nursing guidelines for the care of patients experiencing biotherapy-related fatigue. The reader is also referred to chapter 23 for additional information.

- Assessment: Evaluate the patient self-report of fatigue for perception of amount of fatigue, peak severity, patterns of activity and sleep, impact on self-care activities, and nutritional balance.

- Patient education: Teach patient and family the relationship of fatigue to therapy; methods of saving energy and value of activity in spite of fatigue.

- Maintain activity: Plan with patient how to maintain activity and prevent prolonged bedrest. Patients receiving interferon who maintained activity despite fatigue were observed to have improved functioning.[124]

## Cardiovascular-respiratory changes

Cardiovascular changes are associated most frequently with high-dose IL-2, and usually occur in association with the capillary leak syndrome (CLS). These changes include supraventricular arrhythmias such as atrial fibrillation and supraventricular tachycardia, symptoms of ischemia, and decreased cardiac contractility.[125] These symptoms occur in approximately 10% of patients undergoing treatment. Myocarditis and myocardial infarction have also occurred, possibly in patients who may have underlying coronary artery disease.

Cytokines such as rIL-1, rIL-2, and TNF typically cause hypotension, decrease in central venous pressure, and oliguria necessitating fluid administration. Mab and vaccine therapy are not associated with cardiovascular changes.

Respiratory changes may arise from two sources: First, hypersensitivity reactions may cause wheezing and bronchospasm. Secondly, respiratory changes may occur in high-dose IL-2 therapy with pulmonary edema, dyspnea, shortness of breath, and hypoxia. The administration of activated cell therapy can worsen these symptoms.[125]

***Nursing management***
- Monitor: Watch the patient's cardiovascular and respiratory status at frequent intervals during high-dose IL-2 therapy.

- Patient education: Teach patient to report chest pain, palpitations, or changes in respiration that occur during therapy.

## Capillary Leak Syndrome (CLS)

The capillary or vascular leak syndrome (CLS) is an important side effect that is unique to biological agents, most frequently described in patients receiving high-dose rIL-2. It is the extravasation of fluids and albumin into body tissues, associated with a decreased peripheral vascular resistance, hypotension, and intravascular volume.[125] Compensatory mechanisms of oliguria, increased creatinine levels, tachycardia, and weight gain also occur as fluids are administered to maintain the blood pressure. Major organ dysfunction such as mental status changes, nausea and diarrhea, and pulmonary edema occur with a rapid weight gain, sometimes up to 10% of pretreatment body weight.

CLS can occur rapidly or increase gradually over hours. Although it is a toxicity most frequently associated with high-dose IL-2 therapy, it has been reported in varying degrees with other cytokines and high-dose GM-CSF. It rarely occurs with Mab therapy, and has not been described with interferons and nonspecific immunomodulators.

***Nursing management***
- Monitor: Assess regularly the patient's blood pressure, pulse, respiratory status, urine output, and body weight during therapy. Have the patient remove all restrictive jewelry, particularly rings, before treatment begins.

- For hypotension and oliguria: Administer fluid boluses per physician order. Low-dose dopamine may be administered by peripheral vein to increase urine output. Intensive care monitoring may be required if patient does not respond to above measures.

- Patient education: Instruct patient to stand gradually and allow blood pressure to adjust to the upright position. Request patient to report symptoms of dizziness.

## Dermatologic changes

The skin is not generally considered a primary immune organ; however, it often exemplifies what is happening in the person's immune system. Administration of biological agents can stimulate immunoreactive cells such as Langerhans cells in the skin that function like macrophages and along with activated T cells, release cytokines and vasoactive substances contributing to the redness, swelling, and itching seen in patients receiving cytokine therapy.[126]

Allergic reactions, particularly to a foreign protein such as Mab, can occur. These symptoms include acute development of an erythematous rash on the face and upper body, swelling, hives, and pruritis.

IL-2 therapy, particularly high-dose IL-2, can create similar reactions, but over a longer period of time. Erythema starting on the face and upper body progresses to severe dryness and flaking; pruritis can be intense. In severe cases, skin erosions and the sloughing of the palms, soles, and nails can occur with gradual healing after therapy ends.[41,127] Hair thinning may occur, but alopecia is rare. Patients with preexisting psoriasis can experience a worsening of their disease with IL-2 therapy possibly due to T cell activation.

When cytokines such as IL-2 and GM-CSF are given

subcutaneously, inflammatory reactions at the injection site often occur. Swelling and pain resolve within days, but a firm nodule may remain at the site for months.[41]

***Nursing management***   Interventions that may aid healing, decrease discomfort, and prevent infectious complications are as follows (see chapter 29 for additional nursing measures):

- Apply hypoallergenic emollient lotions and creams on the skin frequently. Use bath oil and hypoallergenic soaps for bathing.

- For pruritis: For severe itching, administer antipruritic medications such as hydroxyzine HCL, or diphenhydramine. Use Lorazepan with severe itching as needed. Use colloidal oatmeal baths (Aveeno®).

- For subcutaneous site inflammation: Rotate sites and do not reuse until firmness resolves. Use local anesthetics and possibly cooling for inflammation.

## Gastrointestinal symptoms

Anorexia, nausea, vomiting, and diarrhea can occur primarily with cytokine therapy, but also with Mab therapy in association with flu-like symptoms. It can be sporadic and not require medication.

The most severe nausea, vomiting, and diarrhea occur with IL-2 therapy, particularly high-dose regimens. Figlin[49] reported that 93% of patients receiving low-dose IL-2 and alfa-IFN reported these gastrointestinal (GI) symptoms. In a few patients, it was a dose-limiting factor to treatment. Rosenberg et al[40] reported that approximately one-third of patients receiving high-dose IL-2 regimens experienced nausea, vomiting, and diarrhea at grade three or four toxicity. Although these GI complaints do not receive the same attention as IL-2-related cardiovascular and respiratory problems, they can have a major impact on the patient's quality of life.

There are few studies exploring the cause of GI problems with IL-2 therapy. The most likely possibility is the vascular leak syndrome or the leakage of fluid and albumin into the GI tract. Diarrhea can be severe with loss of fluid and electrolytes. Colon perforation and GI bleeding have been also reported, particularly in early studies with IL-2.[125]

***Nursing management***   The interventions for nausea, vomiting, and diarrhea previously used with chemotherapy may be applicable for use in IL-2 therapy. One exception is that steroids should not be used as an antiemetic because of their effects on immune function. The following interventions may be useful in managing IL-2 related gastrointestinal symptoms:

- *Evaluate:* Know the potential that the type of therapy has for moderate to severe nausea, vomiting, or diarrhea.

- *For nausea and vomiting:* Medicate patients either with antiemetics on an "as needed" basis, or administer on a regular schedule, depending on severity of symptoms.

- *For diarrhea:* Use antidiarrheal medications as needed, starting with the least potent. Observe patient for symptoms of bowel stasis, distension, and signs of an acute abdomen.

- *Monitor:* Assess patients for symptoms of fluid and electrolyte imbalance.

## Neurological effects

Patients receiving alfa-interferon or IL-2 can experience simple memory changes, increased anxiety, nightmares, and other sleep disturbances. One symptom frequently encountered but poorly described is the loss of concentration or inability to pay attention.[128] More severe symptoms of disorientation, somnolence, and even coma can occur. These symptoms are reversible with supportive care. However, unless therapy is stopped when early signs of neurotoxicity appear, symptoms may worsen and persist for days to weeks before improving.[129]

Neurological changes are infrequent in cytokine therapy and are rare in Mab or other biological therapy. Although rare, neurotoxicity can be severe, particularly in high-dose alfa-interferon or rIL-2 therapy. When these cytokines are combined, the incidence of neurotoxicity is significantly higher than with IL-2 or alfa-interferon alone.

Figlin[51] reported that 17% of patients receiving outpatient alfa-interferon and IL-2 experienced disorientation, somnolence, or paresthesias. Neurological symptomatology was a dose-limitation in this study.

Rosenberg et al[40] reported that in 283 patients receiving high-dose IL-2, 14% experienced disorientation, 5% somnolence, and 2% coma. Marincola et al[130] reviewed 189 patients who received varying dose combinations of alfa-interferon and high-dose IL-2. They found a greater incidence of neurotoxicity than previously reported for either agent alone.

***Nursing management***   The following are interventions to be used with patients receiving high-dose interleukin or alfa-interferon therapy:

- *Assessment:* Assess patient prior to start of therapy for baseline neurological functioning. Elderly patients are at increased risk.

- *Patient education:* Teach patient and his or her family members early signs of mental status changes that should be reported to the patient's health team.

- *Monitor:* Protect patient from harm and observe frequently when mental status changes occur.

- *Decrease stress:* Reduce environmental demands that increase attentional fatigue.[130]

### Anaphylactic reactions

Type I hypersensitivity reactions (anaphylaxis) are rarely seen with the administration of biological agents. However, anaphylaxis is always a concern when administering agents that are designed to stimulate or potentiate immune function.

Anaphylaxis results from the stimulation of mast or basophil cells when IgE antigen complexes bind to surface receptors. This results in the release of mediators such as histamine, leukotrienes and, prostaglandins.[131] Within minutes, the patient develops symptoms of redness, swelling, urticaria, nervousness, angioedema, respiratory distress, abdominal cramping, and hypotension.

Anaphylactoid reactions have most commonly occurred with Mab therapy. Most of these reactions occurred with Mab in their early development and in administration to patients with lymphoma or leukemia, or when Mabs were administered by rapid infusion.[66]

Although anaphylaxis is not described with interferons and most interleukins, high-dose IL-2 administration has been associated with the development of increased sensitivity to other agents. Patients on IL-2 therapy have experienced an increased incidence of contrast dye reactions and also allergic reactions to chemotherapeutic agents such as cisplatin when they are administered in combination with IL-2.[132] The mechanism of this increased sensitivity is unknown.

***Nursing management***

- *Review emergency procedures:* Have essential drugs, steroids, epinephrine, and antihistamines available when administering Mab or other biological agents to patients with a history of hypersensitivity reactions.

- *Patient education:* Instruct patient and family about the symptoms of hypersensitivity. Request that they call their physician if symptoms occur or seek immediate medical assistance if symptoms develop rapidly.

## The Patient's Experience with Biotherapy

A patient receiving biological agents such as high-dose cytokines usually experiences a constellation of symptoms. Many of these symptoms are largely subjective with fever, chills, malaise, and hard-to-describe pains in the head, on the skin, and in joints and muscles. The person looks unwell, feels crummy and his symptoms "are not terribly interesting from a medical point of view."[133,p.68]

A physician or nurse assessing a patient during therapy evaluates objective signs such as lab value changes, vital signs, and indications of organ dysfunction. In contrast, a patient judges his or her well-being on feeling well versus feeling miserable. As shown in Figure 17-8, many symptoms that are common to biological agents such as interferon can have a negative impact on the patient's sense of well-being despite the lack of objective changes in cardiac and lung function. Patients may stop treatment

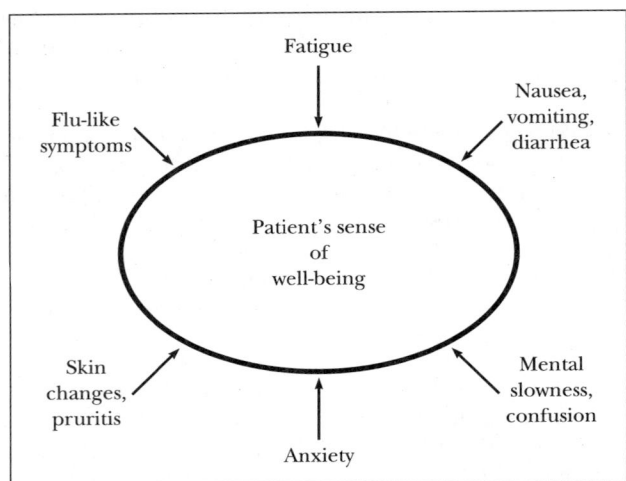

**FIGURE 17-8**   The impact of symptoms on a patient receiving high-dose cytokine therapy.

prematurely because their endurance for the burden of these symptoms runs out.

Nurses have always been interested in how patients feel. However, the nurse may not fully assess the amount of distress the patient is experiencing with the reported symptoms. The concept of symptom distress—the amount of suffering or burden endured by the patient for the duration of the symptom—has begun to be considered more in the description of the patient's symptoms. Symptom distress is the patient's interpretation of the importance of suffering endured as a result of symptoms.[134]

Patients receiving cancer therapy always carry a significant burden of symptoms and symptom distress. For biotherapy, however, many of these symptoms are ill-defined and have only recently received attention from nurse researchers. The studies on the symptom of acute and chronic fatigue and more recently, Cimprich's[128] description of attentional fatigue have brought greater understanding to the patient's experience and helped patients with suggestions on self-care regimens.

The subjective symptoms frequently experienced by patients receiving biotherapy offer great opportunities for nurse researchers to better define the symptom experience and interventions to decrease the burden experienced by the patient. Fever and chills, arthralgia and myalgia, fatigue, nonspecific neurological changes particularly in the elderly, nausea and vomiting with cytokines, and pruritis are typical symptoms for which significant improvements in understanding and intervention might occur.

## THE FUTURE OF BIOTHERAPY

From mid 1980 to the mid 1990s, there was a tremendous amount of growth in the field of biotherapy. Numerous studies of cytokines, activated cells, and hematopoietic growth factors have been published and human gene therapy has begun. The approval by the FDA of several growth factors and IL-2 has established biotherapy as a qualified yet still limited cancer therapy.

The next era, however, will also change biotherapy. Research and development support and reimbursement money will become increasingly scarce. Biotherapy may indirectly benefit as it may force prioritization and refocusing on biological agents that are practical, economically feasible, and the best possibilities for improving the treatment of cancer. Already there has been a reconsideration of cancer vaccine research that previously was only a minor aspect of biotherapy.[111] Finally, the incorporation of gene transfer technology into biotherapy provides promising new ventures that may bring a cure, effective treatment, or even the prevention of cancer into reality.

# REFERENCES

1. Abbas AK, Lichtman AH, Pober JS: *Cellular and Molecular Immunology.* Philadelphia, Saunders, 1991

2. Grey HM, Sette A, Buus S: How T cells see antigen. *Sci Am* 261:56–64, 1989

3. Male D: *Immunology, An Illustrated Outline* (ed 2). London, Gower Medical Publishing, 1991

4. Balkwill FR: *Cytokines in Cancer Therapy.* Oxford, Engl, Oxford University Press, 1989

5. Oettgen HF, Old LJ: The history of cancer, in DeVita V, Hellman S, Rosenberg SA (eds): *Biologic Therapy of Cancer.* Philadelphia, Saunders, 1991, pp 104–110

6. Oldham RK: Cancer biotherapy: General principles, in Oldham RK (ed): *Principles of Cancer Biotherapy* (ed 2). New York, Marcel Dekker, 1991, pp 1–22

7. Mihich E, Fefer A (eds): *National Cancer Institute Monograph, 63.* NIH publication No. 83-2606. Bethesda, MD, National Institutes of Health, 1983

8. Clark J, Longo D: Biological response modifiers. *Mediguide to Oncology* 6:1–4, 1986

9. Rieger PT: *Biotherapy, A Comprehensive Overview.* Boston, Jones and Bartlett, 1995

10. Rosenthal N: Tools of the trade—recombinant DNA. *New Eng J Med* 331:315–317, 1994

11. Richards B: New ways from biotechnology to detect and treat old and new diseases. *Biotechnol Educ* 3:2–8, 1992

12. Emerson SG, Taichman R: The hematopoietic microenvironment, in Armitage JO, Antman KH (eds): *High-Dose Cancer Therapy* (ed 2). Baltimore, Williams & Wilkins, 1995, pp 151–158

13. Lee ME, Crawford J: Delivery of high-dose chemotherapy with recombinant human granulocyte-stimulating factor support, in Armitage JO, Antman KH (eds): *High-Dose Cancer Therapy* (ed 2). Baltimore, Williams & Wilkins, 1995, pp 342–371

14. Ratajczak MZ, Gewirtz AM: The biology of hematopoietic stem cells. *Semin Oncol* 22:210–217, 1995

15. Golde DW: The stem cell. *Sci Am* 261:86–93, 1991

16. Bernstein SH, Kufe DW: Future of basic/clinical hematopoiesis research in the era of hematopoietic growth factor availability. *Semin Oncol* 19:441–448, 1992

17. Sheridan WP, McNiece I: Stem cell factor, in Armitage JO, Antman KH (eds): *High-Dose Cancer Therapy* (ed 2). Baltimore, Williams & Wilkins, 1995, pp 429–444

18. Guillaume T, Symann M: Interleukin 3: General biology, preclinical and clinical studies, in Armitage JO, Antman KH (eds): *High-Dose Cancer Therapy* (ed 2). Baltimore, Williams & Wilkins, 1995, pp 372–401

19. Kurzrock R, Talpaz M, Estrov Z, et al: Phase I study of recombinant human interleukin 3 in patients with bone marrow failure. *J Clin Oncol* 9:1241–1250, 1991

20. Lindemann A, Ganser A, Hermann F, et al: Biologic effects of recombinant human interleukin 3 in vivo. *J Clin Oncol* 9:2120–2127, 1991

21. Postmus PE, Gietema JA, Damsma O, et al: Effects of recombinant human interleukin 3 in patients with relapsed small cell lung cancer treated with chemotherapy: A dose-finding study. *J Clin Oncol* 10:1131–1140, 1992

22. Hoffman R: Interleukin 3: A potentially useful agent for treating chemotherapy-related thrombocytopenia. *J Clin Oncol* 11:2057–2060, 1993

23. Spivak JL: Cancer-related anemia: Its causes and characteristics. *Semin Oncol* 21:3–8, 1994 (suppl 3)

24. Vadhan-Raj S, Kudella AP, Garrison L, et al: Effects of interleukin 1 alpha on carboplatin-induced thrombocytopenia in patients with recurrent ovarian cancer. *J Clin Oncol* 12:707–714, 1994

25. Tewari A, Buhles WC, Starnes HF: Preliminary report: Effects of interleukin-1 on platelet counts. *Lancet* 336: 712–714, 1990

26. Weber J: Interleukin 6: Multi-functional cytokine. *Biol Ther of Cancer Updates* 3:1–9, 1993

27. Weber J, Yang JC, Topalian S, et al: Phase I trial of subcutaneous interleukin 6 in patients with advanced malignancies. *J Clin Oncol* 11:499–506, 1993

28. Steele FR: Research in their blood: Scientists find elusive thrombopoietin. *J NIH Res* 6:53–57, 1994

29. Lieschke GJ, Burgess AW: Granulocyte colony-stimulating factor and granulocyte-macrophage colony-stimulating factor, part II. *New Engl J Med* 327:99–106, 1992

30. Lieschke GJ, Burgess AW: Granulocyte colony-stimulating factor and granulocyte-macrophage colony-stimulating factor, part I. *New Engl J Med* 327:28–35, 1992

31. Sanda MG, Yang JC, Topalian SL, et al: Intravenous administration of recombinant human macrophage colony stimulating factor to patients with metastatic cancer: A phase I study. *J Clin Oncol* 10:1643–1649, 1992

32. Nemunaitis J, Meyers JD, Buckner CD, et al: Phase I/II trial of recombinant human macrophage-colony stimulating factor (M-CSF) in patients with invasive fungal infection. *Blood* 76:159a, 1993 (suppl)

33. Vadhan-Raj S, Papadopoulos NE, Burgess MA, et al: Effects of PIXY 321, a granulocyte-macrophage colony-stimulating factor/interleukin-3 fusion protein, on chemotherapy-induced multilineage myelosuppression in patients with sarcoma. *J Clin Oncol* 12:715–724, 1994

34. Jenks S: After the early hype, interferons spark interest. *J Natl Cancer Inst* 85:773–775, 1993

35. Johnson HM, Bazer FW, Fuller W, et al: How interferons fight disease. *Sci Am* 264:68–75, 1994

36. Tizard IR: *Immunology, An Introduction* (ed 3). Fort Worth, Texas, Saunders College Pub, 1992

37. Glaspy JA, Souza L, Scates S, et al: Treatment of hairy cell leukemia with granulocyte colony-stimulating factor and recombinant consensus interferon or recombinant interferon-alpha-2b. *J Immunother* 11:198–208, 1992

38. Fisher RI: Introduction: Interleukin-2—Advances in clinical research and treatment. *Semin Oncol* 20:1–2, 1993 (suppl 9)

39. Parkinson DR, Sznol M: High-dose interleukin-2 in the therapy of metastatic renal cell carcinoma. *Semin Oncol* 22:61–66, 1995

40. Rosenberg SA, Yang JC, Topalian SL, et al: Treatment of 283 consecutive patients with metastatic melanoma or renal cell cancer using high-dose bolus interleukin 2. *JAMA* 271:907–913, 1994

41. Sleijfer DT, Janssen RAJ, Buter J, et al: Phase II study of subcutaneous interleukin-2 in unselected patients with advanced renal cell cancer on an outpatient basis. *J Clin Oncol* 10:1119–1123, 1992

42. Wheeler V: Interleukins: The search for an anticancer therapy. *Semin Oncol Nurs* 12:106–114, 1996

43. Dinarello CA, Wolff S: The role of interleukin 1 in disease. *New Engl J Med* 328:106–113, 1993

44. Smith JW, Urba WJ, Curti BD, et al: The toxic and hematologic effects of interleukin-1 alpha administered in a phase I trial to patients with advanced malignancies. *J Clin Oncol* 10:1141–1152, 1992

45. Crown J, Jakublwski A, Kemeny N, et al: A phase I trial of recombinant human interleukin-1B alone and in combination with myelosuppressive doses of 5-fluorouracil in patients with gastrointestinal cancer. *Blood* 78:1420–1427, 1991

46. Atkins MB, Trehu EG, Mier JW: Combination cytokine therapy, in DeVita VT, Hellman S, Rosenberg SA (eds): *Biologic Therapy of Cancer: Principles and Practice* (ed 2). Philadelphia, Lippincott, 1995, pp 443–466

47. Truitt RL, Borden EC, Keever CA: Role of IL-4, IL-6, and IL-12 in cancer therapy, in DeVita VT, Hellman S, Rosenberg SA (eds): *Biologic Therapy of Cancer, Principles and Practice* (ed 2). Philadelphia Lippincott, 1995, pp 279–293

48. Hirsh M, Lipton A, Harvey H, et al: Phase I study of interleukin-2 and interferon alfa-2A as outpatient therapy for patients with advanced malignancy. *J Clin Oncol* 8:1657–1663, 1990

49. Figlin RA, Belldegrun A, Moldawer N, et al: Concomitant administration of recombinant human interleukin-2 and recombinant interferon alfa-2A: An active outpatient regimen in metastatic renal cell carcinoma. *J Clin Oncol* 10:414–421, 1992

50. Triozzi PL, Kim JA, Martin EW, et al: Phase I trial of escalating doses of interleukin-1B in combination with a fixed dose of interleukin-2. *J Clin Oncol* 13:482–489, 1995

51. Buzaid AC, Legha SS: Combination of chemotherapy with interleukin-2 and interferon-alfa for the treatment of advanced melanoma. *Semin Oncol* 21:23–28, 1994 (suppl 14)

52. Old LJ: Tumor necrosis factor. *Sci Am* 258:59–75, 1988

53. Feinberg B, Kurzrock M, Talpaz M, et al: A phase I trial of intravenously-administered recombinant tumor necrosis factor-alpha in cancer patients. *J Clin Oncol* 6:1328–1334, 1988

54. Fraker DL, Alexander HR: The use of tumor necrosis factor in isolated limb perfusions for melanoma and sarcoma. *Principles and Practice of Oncology Updates* 7:1–10, 1993

55. Fraker DL, Alexander HR, Andrich M, et al: Palliation of regional symptoms of advanced extremity melanoma by isolated limb perfusion with melphalan and high-dose tumor necrosis factor. *The Cancer Journal* 1:122–130, 1995

56. Rosenberg SA: Adoptive immunotherapy for cancer, in Paul WE (ed): *Immunology, Recognition and Response.* New York, Freeman, 1990, pp 109–121

57. Sznol M, Parkinson DR: Clinical applications of IL-2. *Oncology* 8:61–66, 1994

58. Platsoucas CD, Freedman RS: Tumor-infiltrating lymphocytes in gene therapy. *Cancer Bull* 45:118–124, 1993

59. Topalian SL, Solomon D, Avis FP, et al: Immunotherapy of patients with advanced cancer using tumor-infiltrating lymphocytes and recombinant interleukin-2: A pilot study. *J Clin Oncol* 6:839–853, 1988

60. Rosenberg SA, Yannelli Jr, Yang JC, et al: Treatment of patients with autologous tumor-infiltrating lymphocytes and interleukin 2. *J Natl Cancer Inst* 86:1159–1164, 1994

61. Rosenberg SA: Gene therapy for cancer. *JAMA* 268:2416–2419, 1992

62. Rosenberg SA: The development of new cancer therapies based on the molecular identification of cancer regression antigens. *The Cancer Journal* 1:89–100, 1995

63. Bronte V: Molecular genetics of cancer, gene therapy, and other novel therapeutic approaches. *Cancer* 76:1878–1881, 1995

64. Schindler LW: *Understanding the Immune System.* NIH publication No. 88-529. Bethesda, MD, U.S. Department of Health and Human Services, 1988

65. Goldenberg DM: Recent advances in cancer detection and therapy with radiolabeled antibodies. *Mediguide to Oncology* 10:1–10, 1990

66. DiJulio JE, Liles TM: Monoclonal antibodies, in Rieger PT (ed): *Biotherapy, A Comprehensive Overview.* Boston, Jones and Bartlett Publishers, 1995, pp 135–160

67. Lobuglio AF, Saleh MN: Monoclonal antibodies, in Niederheber JE (ed): *Current Therapy in Oncology.* New York, BC Decker, 1993, pp 41–49

68. Gibbs WW: Try, try again. *Sci Am* 263:101–103, 1993

69. Schlom J: Antibodies in cancer therapy: Basic principles of monoclonal antibodies, in DeVita VT, Hellman S, Rosenberg SA (eds): *Biologic Therapy of Cancer.* Philadelphia, Lippincott, 1991, pp 464–481

70. Vitteta ES, Thorpe PE: Immunotoxins, in DeVita V, Hellman S, Rosenberg SA (eds): *Biologic Therapy of Cancer.* Philadelphia, Lippincott, 1991, pp 482–495

71. Vaickus L, Foon KA: Overview of monoclonal antibodies in the diagnosis and therapy of cancer. *Cancer Invest* 9:195–209, 1991

72. Pai LH, Pastan I: Immunotoxins and recombinant toxins for cancer treatment, in DeVita VT, Hellman S, Rosenberg SA (eds): *Important Advances in Oncology 1994.* Philadelphia, Lippincott, 1994, pp 3–19

73. National Federation for Specialty Nursing Organizations (NFSNO): *Biotechnology Nursing Core Curriculum.* Pitman, NJ: Anthony J. Jannetti, 1995, p 64

74. Khazaeli MB, Conry RM, LoBuglio AF: Human immune response to monoclonal antibodies. *J Immunother* 15:42–52, 1994

75. Goldenberg DM: Challenges to the therapy of cancer with monoclonal antibodies. *J Natl Cancer Inst* 83:78–79, 1991

76. Dillman JB: Toxicity of monoclonal antibodies in the treatment of cancer. *Semin Oncol Nurs* 4:107–111, 1988

77. Rosenberg SA: Gene therapy for cancer, in DeVita V, Hellman S, Rosenberg SA (eds): *Important Advances in Oncology 1992.* Philadelphia, Lippincott, 1992, pp 17–38

78. Cournoyer D, Caskey CT: Gene transfer into humans, a first step. *New Engl J Med* 323:601–602, 1993

79. Fox JL: The ethical roar of germline gene therapy. *Biotechnology* 13:18–19, 1995

80. Jenkins J, Wheeler V, Albright L: Gene therapy for cancer. *Cancer Nurs* 17:447–456, 1994

81. Deisseroth AB, Kavanagh JJ, Hanania EG, et al: Gene therapy: Chemoprotection, immunoenhancement, and modification of tumor cells. *Cancer Bull* 45:139–145, 1993

82. Seachrist L: Successful gene therapy has researchers looking for the bystander effect. *J Natl Cancer Inst* 86:82–83, 1994

83. Brenner MK, Rill DR, Moen RC, et al: Gene-marking to trace origin of relapse after autologous bone marrow transplant. *Lancet* 341:85–87, 1993

84. Morgan RA, Anderson WF: Human gene therapy. *Annu Rev Biochem* 62:191–217, 1993

85. Nabel GJ, Nabel EG, Yang Z, et al: Direct gene transfer with DNA-liposome complexes in melanoma: Expression, biologic activity, and lack of toxicity in humans. *Proc Natl Acad Sci USA* 90:11307–11311, 1993

86. Vile R, Russell SJ: Gene transfer technologies for the gene therapy of cancer. *Gene Ther* 1:88–98, 1994

87. Spooner RA, Deonarian MP, Epenelos AA: DNA vaccination for cancer treatment. *Gene Ther* 2:173–180, 1995

88. Anderson WR, McGarrity GJ, Moen RC: Report to the NIH Recombinant DNA Advisory Committee on murine replication-competent retrovirus (RCR) assays. *Human Gene Therapy* 4:311–321, 1993

89. Jenks S: Gene therapy finds few complications. *J Natl Cancer Inst* 85:1188–1190, 1993b

90. Anderson WF: Making clinical grade gene therapy vectors. *Human Gene Ther* 5:925–926, 1994

91. Wheeler VS: Gene therapy: Current strategies and future applications. *Oncol Nurs Forum* 22:20–26, 1995 (suppl)

92. Jenks S: Panel says gene therapy "hype" should be toned down. *J Natl Cancer Inst* 88:9–10, 1996

93. Begley S: Promises, Promises. *Newsweek* 126:60–62, 1995

94. Friedmann T: The promise and overpromise of human gene therapy. *Gene Ther* 1:217–218, 1994

95. Hersh EM, Taylor CW: Immunotherapy by active immunization: Use of nonspecific stimulants and immunomodulators, in DeVita V, Hellman S, Rosenberg SA (eds): *Biologic Therapy of Cancer.* Philadelphia, Lippincott, 1991, pp 613–626

96. Spreafico F: The use of levamisole in cancer patients. *Drugs* 19:105–116, 1980

97. Morton DL, Hunt KK, Bauer RL, et al: Immunotherapy by active immunization of the host using nonspecific agents—clinical applications using intralesional therapy, in DeVita V, Hellman S, Rosenberg SA (eds): *Biologic Therapy of Cancer.* Philadelphia, Lippincott, 1991, pp 627–642

98. Herr H: Instillation therapy for bladder cancer, in DeVita V, Hellman S, Rosenberg SA (eds): *Biologic Therapy of Cancer.* Philadelphia, Lippincott, 1991, pp 643–650

99. Wilkes GM, Ingwersen K, Burke MB: *Oncology Nursing Drug Reference.* Boston, Jones and Bartlett, 1994

100. Miller M: The use of levamisole in parasitic infections. *Drugs* 19:122–130, 1980

101. Fuchs CS, Mayer RJ: Adjuvant chemotherapy for colon and rectal cancer. *Semin Oncol* 22:472–487, 1995

102. Renoux G: The general immunopharmacology of levamisole. *Drugs* 19:89–99, 1980

103. Parkinson DR, Smith MA, Cheson BD, et al: Trans-retinoic acid and related differentiation agents. *Semin Oncol* 19:734–741, 1992

104. Warrell RP: Applications for retinoids in cancer therapy. *Semin Hematol* 31:1–13, 1994 (suppl 5)

105. Miller WH, Dmitrovsky E: Retinoic acid and its rearranged receptor in the treatment of acute promyelocytic leukemia, in DeVita V, Hellman S, Rosenberg SA (eds): *Important Advances in Oncology 1993,* Philadelphia, Lippincott, 1993, pp 81–93

106. Gillis JC, Goa KL: Tretinoin. *Drugs* 50:897–923, 1995

107. Moore DM, Kalvakolano DV, Lippman SM, et al: Retinoic acid and interferon in human cancer: Mechanisms and clinical studies. *Semin Hematol* 31:31–37, 1994 (suppl 5)

108. Ruddon RW: *Cancer Biology* (ed 3). New York, Oxford University Press, 1995

109. Morton DL, Foshag LJ, Hoon DSB, et al: Prolongation of survival in metastatic melanoma after active specific immunotherapy with a new polyvalent melanoma vaccine. *Ann Surg* 216:463–482, 1992

110. Hoover HC, Brandhorst JS, Petus LC, et al: Adjuvant active specific immunotherapy for human colorectal cancer: 6.5-year medical follow-up of a phase III prospectively randomized trial. *J Clin Oncol* 11:390–399, 1993

111. Cohen J: Cancer vaccines get a shot in the arm. *Science* 262:841–843, 1993

112. Nathan FE, Mastrangelo MJ: Adjuvant therapy for cutaneous melanoma. *Semin Oncol* 22:647–661, 1995

113. Rieger PT: Dosing and scheduling biological response modifiers, in Rieger PT (ed): *Biotherapy, A Comprehensive Overview.* Boston, Jones and Bartlett, 1995, pp 43–66

114. Smith K: Lowest dose interleukin-2 immunotherapy. *Blood* 81:1414–1423, 1993

115. Thompson JA, Lee DJ, Lindgren CG, et al: Influence of dose and duration of infusion of interleukin 2 on toxicity and immunomodulation. *J Clin Oncol* 6:669–678, 1988

116. Conrad KJ, Horrell CJ (eds): *Biotherapy: Recommendations for Nursing Course Content and Clinical Practicum.* Pittsburgh, Oncology Nursing Press, 1995

117. Holtzclaw BJ: Shivering, a clinical nursing problem. *Nurs Clin North Am* 25:977–986, 1990

118. Dinarello CA, Cannon JG, Wolff S: New concepts on the pathogenesis of fever. *Rev Infectious Dis* 10:168–189, 1988

119. Haeuber D: Recent advances in the management of biotherapy-related side effects: Flu-like syndrome. *Oncol Nurs Forum* 16:35–40, 1989 (suppl)

120. Aistairs J: Fatigue in the cancer patient: A conceptual approach to a clinical problem. *Oncol Nurs Forum* 14:25–30, 1987

121. Winningham ML: Fatigue, in Groenwald SL, Frogge MH, Goodman M, Yarbro CH (eds): *Cancer Symptom Management.* Boston, Jones and Bartlett, 1996, pp 42–58

122. Skalla KA, Rieger PT: Fatigue, in Rieger PT (ed): *Biotherapy, a Comprehensive Overview.* Boston, Jones and Bartlett, 1995, pp 221–242

123. Quesada JR, Talpaz M, Rios A, et al: Clinical toxicity of interferons in cancer patients: A review. *J Clin Oncol* 4:234–243, 1986

124. Davis C: Interferon-induced fatigue. *Oncol Nurs Bull* 1:4–5, 1987

125. Siegel JP, Puri RK: Interleukin-2 toxicity. *J Clin Oncol* 9:694–704, 1991

126. Dummer R, Miller K, Eilles C: The skin: An immunoreactive target organ during interleukin 2 administration? *Dermatologica* 183:95–99, 1991

127. Gaspari AA, Lotze MT, Rosenberg SA: Dermatologic changes associated with interleukin 2 administration. *JAMA* 258:1624–1628, 1987

128. Cimprich B: Symptom management: Loss of concentration. *Semin Oncol Nurs* 11:279–288, 1995

129. Forman AD: Neurologic complications of cytokine therapy. *Oncology* 8:105–110, 1994

130. Marincola FM, White DE, Wise AP, et al: Combination therapy with interferon alfa-2a and interleukin-2 for the treatment of metastatic cancer. *J Clin Oncol* 13:110–112, 1995

131. Fox GW, Ream MA: Hypersensitivity reactions, in Yasko JM, Dudjak LA (eds): *Biological Response Modifier Therapy: Symptom Management.* Emeryville, CA, Park Row Publishers, 1990, pp 187–196

132. Weber JS, Heywood GR, Rosenberg SA: Allergic reactions to chemotherapy agents in patients receiving interleukin-2 (IL-2). *Proc Am Soc Clin Oncol* 13:297, 1994 (abstr)

133. Sapolsky RM: Why you feel crummy when you're sick. *Discover* 11:66–70, 1990

134. McDaniel RW, Rhodes VA: Symptom experience. *Semin Oncol Nurs* 11:232–233, 1995

# Chapter 18

# Allogeneic Bone Marrow Transplantation

**Patricia Corcoran Buchsel, RN, MSN**

## INTRODUCTION

Bone marrow transplantation (BMT) has evolved during the past 30 years from an experimental procedure to an established and effective treatment for increasing numbers of selected patients. The International Bone Marrow Transplant Registry (IBMTR), an organization dedicated to BMT scientific research, reports that more than 230 marrow transplant teams are currently reporting data on over 2000 allogeneic and syngeneic transplants worldwide[1] (Figure 18-1). Improvements in the management of graft-versus-host disease (GVHD) and cytomegalovirus pneumonia (CMV), advancement of enhanced supportive care measures, the increasing availability of unrelated volunteer donors, and wider treatment applications are responsible for much of this growth.[2] The number of autologous bone marrow transplants performed to date has surpassed that of allogeneic marrow transplantation and will continue to do so in the future. Chapter 19 offers a complete discussion of autologous marrow and blood cell transplantation (BCT). The advent of BCTs, although promising as a less expensive treatment for a number of diseases currently treated by marrow transplantation, may appear to be eclipsing marrow transplantation, but much research on sustained engraftment, tumor contamination, and disease-free long-term survival is needed before blood cell transplantation replaces marrow transplantation. Until such time, marrow transplantation as it is known today will continue to grow as a treatment option for many who would otherwise die of their disease. With the increase of BMT, oncology nurses working in the area will need to expand their knowledge and skills to encompass immunology, hematology, pediatrics, ambulatory care, home care, critical care, research, and nursing administration.[3]

## HISTORICAL PERSPECTIVES

The earliest marrow transplantation in humans was reported by Brown-Sequard in 1888. They described a procedure wherein an extract of marrow was given by mouth to patients with pernicious anemia and lymphadenoma.[4] In 1837, Schretzenmayr administered bone marrow intramuscularly. Although his studies were encouraging, they were not accepted by his peers. These early attempts were soon followed by unsuccessful attempts to use marrow given by the intramedullary and intravenous routes.[5]

After World War II, studies of radiation-induced bone marrow failure led to treatments using infusions of bone marrow in aplastic anemia and radiation-induced bone marrow failure patients.[6] In 1949 and 1951, research in murine and canine models showed that animals given lethal doses of irradiation survived after parenteral infusion of bone marrow.[5]

The first modern human marrow transplants were conducted without success in patients with end-stage diseases.[6] It was not until the mid-1960s that medical research focused on the importance of human tissue typing and applied these concepts to organ and marrow transplantation.[7] By the late 1960s, following the institution of histocompatible leukocyte antigen (HLA) typing to identify suitable sibling donors, successful human allogeneic transplants were carried out in increasing numbers. Simultaneously, the technology of platelet transfusions and methods of prophylaxis against infection were developed.[8,9] In the 1980s, changes in pretransplant conditioning regimens, prophylaxis, and treatment of infectious diseases decreased transplant-related morbidity and mortality. Only a modest increase in leukemia-free survival rates occurred after identical-sibling BMT. This remains a major research priority today.

Significant shifts in pretransplantation conditioning agents have occurred in recent years. Historically, total-body irradiation (TBI) plus cyclophosphamide has been the most common pretransplantation conditioning regimen. Currently, the use of fractionated (versus single dose) TBI and antileukemic drugs, such as high-dose etoposide and high-dose cytosine arabinoside, with TBI has increased markedly. The increased use of busulfan and cyclophosphamide without TBI for pretransplant conditioning is another important trend. This latter shift is an attempt to reduce the risk of leukemia relapse and to eliminate the late effects of irradiation, especially in the pediatric patient. Finally, the technique of T-cell marrow depletion has been effective in reducing the risk of graft-versus-host disease; however, it has been largely abandoned because of significantly high relapse rates and graft failure in recipients of T-cell-depleted marrow infusions.[10] Aggressive research continues in this area.[11]

In the early 1980s most allogeneic marrow recipients received methotrexate alone or in combination therapy. Cyclosporine; a newly discovered immunosuppressive drug, emerged as an important treatment and was used with corticosteroids to prevent GVHD.[12] By mid-decade, research demonstrated that cyclosporine with or without corticosteroids was a more effective treatment than other regimens. Thus, cyclosporine in combination with methotrexate was largely abandoned, and standard prophylaxis for GVHD currently is cyclosporine with corticosteroids.[12] Prophylaxis against viral infections, especially CMV infections, improved. Protective environments, including laminar airflow (LAF) rooms and high-efficiency particulate air filters, were developed. The use of protective isolation continues to be an important tenet in marrow transplantation medicine. Due to the cost and lack of convincing data on survival, new construction of LAF rooms has ceased, although the use of high-efficiency particulate air (HEPA) protective isolation and simple protective isolation remain an important deterrent to infection in the profoundly immunosuppressed recipient. As BMT technology moved into the 1990s, the role of recombinant colony stimulating factors (CSFs) dominated clinical research. These cytokines have clearly decreased posttransplant infections, decreased antibiotic use, and shortened hospitalization and hospital readmissions for thousands of recipients. To date the role of CSFs has been most dramatic in early engraftment in the autologous marrow and blood cell transplant recipient but clinical investigators are studying the efficacy of CSFs in allogeneic donors. Concomitant with these phenomena, the use of blood cells rather than marrow for allogeneic transplantation is becoming an important area of study and many researchers predict that blood cell transplantation may replace marrow transplantation in the next millennium. However, large cooperative randomized clinical trials are needed to determine sustained engraftment and long-term survival before this transition occurs.[13,14]

The number of older patients receiving BMT has increased, particularly in the treatment of chronic myelogenous leukemia, younger patients are undergoing transplantation for early acute leukemia. The availability of volunteer donors for unrelated donor transplantation has increased from 400,000 in 1988 to 1.7 million in 1996.[15] The 25th anniversary of the first three children transplanted for birth defects was recently reported. All three children are alive and largely or completely free of their underlying disease.[16] It is estimated that more than 2000 long-term survivors, defined as those patients who remain disease-free one year after BMT, and 10,000 recipients are alive at least five years following allogeneic marrow transplant.[17] These encouraging results are a direct consequence of advances in medical technology, improved support of the immunosuppressed patient, and improved communication between long-term follow-up teams and referring physicians.

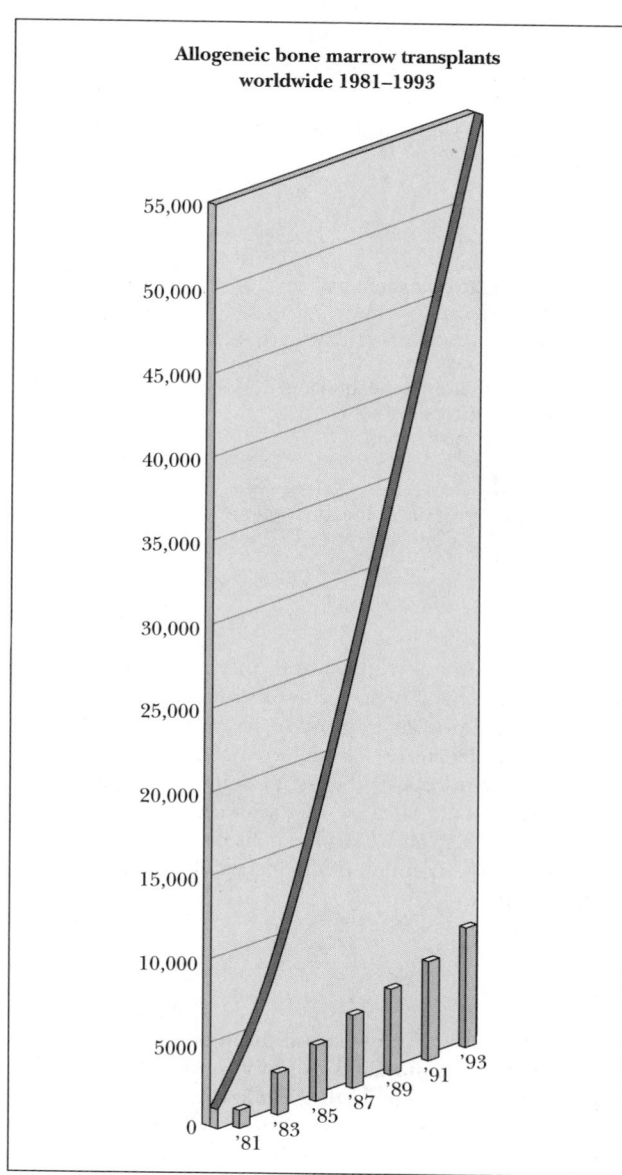

**FIGURE 18-1**   Current annual and cumulative number of patients receiving allogeneic bone marrow transplants worldwide.

## CONCEPTS OF BONE MARROW TRANSPLANTATION

Replacing diseased marrow with healthy donor marrow is simple in concept. However, the toxicities of high-dose chemotherapy and irradiation used in preparative regimens make the treatment hard to implement successfully.

Specialized medical and nursing care is required. The basic concepts of the BMT process are as follows.

- The dose of most chemotherapeutic agents administered to cure a patient's disease is limited by subsequent dose-related marrow toxicity.

- The availability of donor marrow for transplantation and engraftment make it possible to administer chemoradiotherapy in supralethal doses in an effort to kill malignant cells (preparative regimens for BMT).

- The patient is then rescued with donor marrow to prevent iatrogenic death (bone marrow transplantation).

- The infused marrow will reconstitute the patient's (host) hematopoietic and immunologic system, and the patient (host) will be rescued (engraftment).

- Complications that follow BMT are the result of the (1) high-dose chemotherapy and irradiation conditioning regimens used to prepare the patient to receive the donor marrow (acute and chronic complications); (2) graft-versus-host disease and its management; (3) adverse effects of medication; and (4) relapse.

Table 18-1 presents the sequence and time of events in the process of allogeneic BMT.

## TYPES OF BONE MARROW TRANSPLANTATION

Originally, only patients with leukemia refractory to conventional therapy were considered for marrow transplantation. Successful marrow grafts are now performed in patients with a variety of hematologic and nonhematologic malignant disorders. The selection of marrow transplantation to treat any such disease is highly contingent on an available and appropriate donor source. Allogeneic donor sources are related family members or unrelated matched volunteers. If the recipient's twin is the donor, the transplant is called a syngeneic (twin) transplant. Umbilical stem cell transplantation is emerging as a promising treatment for children with Fanconi's anemia and some leukemias and may soon be offered to selected adults as a treatment for their disease.[18] Numerous ethical issues surround umbilical stem cell transplantation. Questions of ownership, informed consent, the possibility of infectious disease, privacy and confidentiality, fair and equitable harvesting, and access to umbilical blood.[18] Other alternative donor sources currently being investigated for possible use are the use of fetal liver cells and cadavers.[19,20] Fetal liver cell transplants will not likely become an option in the near future because of ethical concerns. Cadaveric transplants present significant logistical difficulties making it unlikely as an alternative for allogeneic donors.

**TABLE 18-1** Process of Allogeneic Bone Marrow Transplantation: Sequence and Time of Events

| Event | Time |
|---|---|
| 1. Diagnosis of patient with disease treatable with BMT | Days (AA) to years (CML, CP) |
| 2. Identification of histocompatible donor | 2 wk |
| 3. Evaluation of patient and donor for BMT | 2 wk |
| 4. Placement of multilumen central catheter in patient | 1 day |
| 5. Admission to hospital for BMT | — |
| 6. Initiation of pretransplantation conditioning regimen with high-dose chemoirradiation given either alone or in combination therapy | 2–10 days |
| 7. Admission of donor for marrow harvest | Day of BMT |
| 8. Infusion of donor marrow into patient | Day of marrow harvest; several-hour infusion |
| 9. Engraftment | 2–4 wk |
|    Acute complications | Day 0 to 100 days after BMT |
| 10. Discharge to outpatient setting | 30–40 days after BMT |
| 11. Outpatient care | 30–100 days after BMT |
| 12. Late acute and early chronic complications | 30–100 days after BMT |
| 13. Return to referring health care team for continuing care | 100 days after BMT |
| 14. Chronic complications | 100 days—4–5 yr after BMT |

*AA*, Aplastic anemia; *CML*, chronic myelogenous leukemia; *CP*, chronic phase

### Syngeneic

A syngeneic marrow transplant is one in which the donor is an identical twin (who by definition is a perfect HLA match). Conditioning regimens are determined by the disease being treated.[7,12] A higher incidence of leukemic relapse has been reported in syngeneic than in allogeneic marrow recipients because of the demonstrated antileukemic effect of graft-versus-host disease.[9] This is known as graft-versus-leukemia effect, and will be discussed later in this chapter.

### Allogeneic

Allogeneic marrow transplantation depends on the availability of an HLA-matched donor (Figure 18-2). GVHD, a complication unique to allogeneic marrow transplantation and a major impediment to successful transplantation, is discussed later in this chapter. Intensive supportive care with protective environments, gut decontaminates, prophylactic and therapeutic antibiotics, red cell and platelet transfusions, and administration of CSFs are required and their use will differ among institutions. Granu-

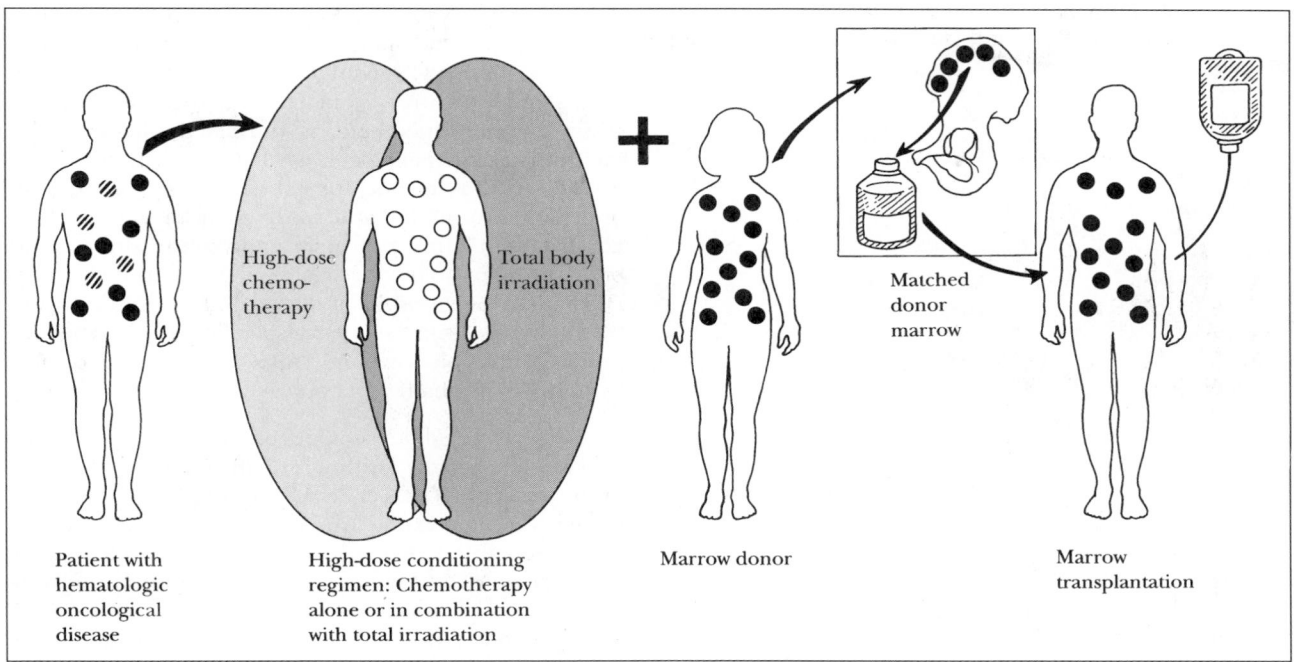

**FIGURE 18-2**  Schematic for allogeneic bone marrow transplantation.

locyte transfusions are rarely used because of consistently poor results. Specialized nursing care is essential to manage these patients.[21]

### Diseases treated with allogeneic BMT

Allogeneic transplantations are done most commonly for acute and chronic leukemia, lymphomas, multiple myeloma, severe aplastic anemia, genetic disease, immunologic deficiencies, and inborn errors of metabolism. Table 18-2 identifies the diseases treated with allogeneic BMT and disease-free survival statistics.[22]

***Genetic disease***   Children with aplastic anemia, thalassemia, or Fanconi's anemia have received successful allografts. BMT for sickle cell anemia is under investigation; however, considerable controversy still exists in this area. The risks intrinsic to BMT for sickle cell anemia must be balanced against the expected morbidity and mortality of the disease. Weighing these risks is difficult, since the clinical course of sickle cell disease is quite variable. The cost-effectiveness of using BMT for a disease with a 40-year life expectancy is also questionable.[23]

***Immunologic deficiencies***   Cures have been reported in patients with congenital immunodeficiency diseases, including severe combined immunodeficiency disease syndrome (SCIDS), Wiskott-Aldrich syndrome, and some rare inherited disorders. Currently, marrow transplantation is a treatment choice only in the presence of an HLA-matched sibling.[24] The first human gene therapy experiment for the treatment of adenosine deaminase deficiency, a form of SCIDS, has paved the way for treat-

ment of a wider variety of genetic diseases.[25] Considerable research is needed to understand the limitations and potential use of in vivo gene transfer therapy.

***Inborn errors of metabolism***   Allogeneic BMT has been utilized successfully to treat diseases of inborn errors of metabolism, such as Gaucher disease, chronic granulomatosis disease, osteoporosis, mucopolysaccharidosis (Hurler's syndrome), Sanfilipp B disease, and Maroteaux-Lamy syndrome. Lipidosis diseases include adrenoleukodystrophy (ADL) and metachromatic leukodystrophy (MLD). Treatment of these diseases has been limited to those patients with a histocompatible sibling. But as increasing numbers of volunteer donors become available, more unrelated donor searches may be initiated.[24,26]

## Donors

### Tissue typing

***Human leukocyte antigen/mixed lymphocyte culture***   Selecting the most appropriate donor for a patient begins with an understanding of the major histocompatibility complex in humans, which is composed of a series of closely linked genetic loci on chromosome 6. The antigens located at HLA-A and HLA-B are defined serologically, and those of the HLA-A locus are detected by the mixed leukocyte culture (MLC) test. A locus identical with or closely related to HLA-D, called HLA-DR, can be serologically typed using T lymphocytes. A chromosomal region is known as a *haplotype*. Every person inherits one haplotype from each parent, and within any given family

**TABLE 18-2** Diseases Treated with Allogeneic Bone Marrow Transplantation and Disease-Free Survival Statistics

| Disease | Disease-Free Survival | Range of Follow-Up (Median) |
|---|---|---|
| Aplastic anemia | 61%–94% | 6 months to 15 years |
| Chronic myelogen-ous leukemia (CML) | | |
| CML BC (twin) | 20% | 5 years |
| CML CP (twin) | 65% | 5 years |
| CML BC (HLA matched) | 10%–20% | 5 years |
| CML CP | 30%–45% | 5 years |
| CML AP | 50%–60% | 5 years |
| Acute myeloid leukemia (AML) | | |
| Relapse | 15%–20% | 2–14 years |
| 1st remission | 45%–65% | 12–14 years |
| Acute lympho-blastic leukemia | | |
| 1st CR | 22%–71% | 1–4.8 years |
| CR2nd | 10%–65% | 2–9 years |
| CR3rd | 10%–33% | 2–17 years |
| Acute lymphocytic leukemia (ALL) | | |
| children | 23%–84% | 2.5–10.4 years |
| Myelodysplastic and myeloproliferative disorders | 50%–67% | 7 years |
| Multiple myeloma | | |
| HLA matched siblings | 45%–50% | 6 years |
| Unrelated | 40%–50% | 6 years |
| Osteopetrosis | 50% | 13 years |
| Acquired immunodeficiency syndrome (AIDS) (8 patients) | 0% | weeks |
| Hodgkin's disease—HLA matched sibling | rarely reported | not known |
| Neuroblastoma | 30%–40% | 3–4 years |
| Thalassemia | 80% | 10 years |
| Wiskott-Aldrich syndrome | | |
| HLA matched | 50%–90% | 10 years |
| Unrelated | 30%–40% | 10 years |
| Severe combined immunodeficiency disease | 70%–80% | 12 years |
| Sickle cell disease (48 patients) | 90% | 3 years |
| Lymphoma | 12%–75% | 18–44 months |

AP = Accelerated Phase, BC = Blast Crisis, CP = Chronic Phase, CR = Complete Remission
Data from Forman SJ, Blume KG, Thomas CD (eds): *Bone Marrow Transplantation.* Boston, Blackwell Scientific Publications, 1994

there can be only four haplotypes. There is approximately a 25% chance for a person to be an HLA-match with a sibling[6] (Figure 18-3). Until recent years, most allogeneic transplantations were from HLA-identical siblings, but selected family members or unrelated phenotypically identical donors have been used successfully as marrow donors. As the demand for marrow transplantation donors increases, faster and more accurate methods are needed to identify the most appropriate donor. One breakthrough in this area allows the identification of HLA allelic polymorphism directed at the DNA level by hybridization with sequence-specific ologonucleotide probes ("HLA ologotyping") after identification of DNA by polymerase chain reaction.[27]

***ABO typing*** Major ABO-incompatible marrow grafting can be performed without significant hemolytic transfusion reactions. This is because effective techniques to remove red blood cells from donor marrow, and plasma exchange of patient marrow, have reduced the risk of such reactions.[28] Blood group typing, however, must be done on all patients and potential donors.[29] If unmanipulated incompatible ABO marrow is transfused, it, like any incompatible blood product transfusion, will cause a major hemolytic transfusion reaction, which can result in death. After transplantation, the patient's ABO type will become the same type as the marrow donor.

### Marrow collection

Donor marrow is harvested in the operating room under sterile conditions, with the donor anesthetized under general or spinal anesthesia. The marrow is obtained from the posterior iliac crests in 2-ml aspirates, up to a total of 10 to 15 mg/kg recipient body weight. If necessary, the anterior iliac crests and the sternum can be used. Although 150 to 200 aspirates are necessary to obtain sufficient marrow, only six to ten skin punctures are made, with the aspiration needles redirected to different sites under the skin.[9] The heparinized marrow is screened through a series of progressively finer mesh screens to filter out bone particles and fat. Marrow is then placed in blood administration bags and infused into the patient within two to four hours.[5,9,20] The steps of marrow collection and harvest are outlined in Figure 18-4.

***T-Cell depletion*** One of the major limiting factors of allogeneic marrow transplantation is GVHD. Ex vivo T-cell depletion of donor marrow has proven to be the most successful method to prevent life-threatening GVHD. As discussed earlier for patients with leukemia, the benefits of less GVHD and no posttransplant immunosuppression have been offset by increased incidence of graft failure in patients, especially those with chronic myelogenous leukemia. Because aggressive studies continue in this area, it is important for oncology nurses to have some understanding of the T-cell depletion process.

The purpose of T-cell depletion is to remove T-cells

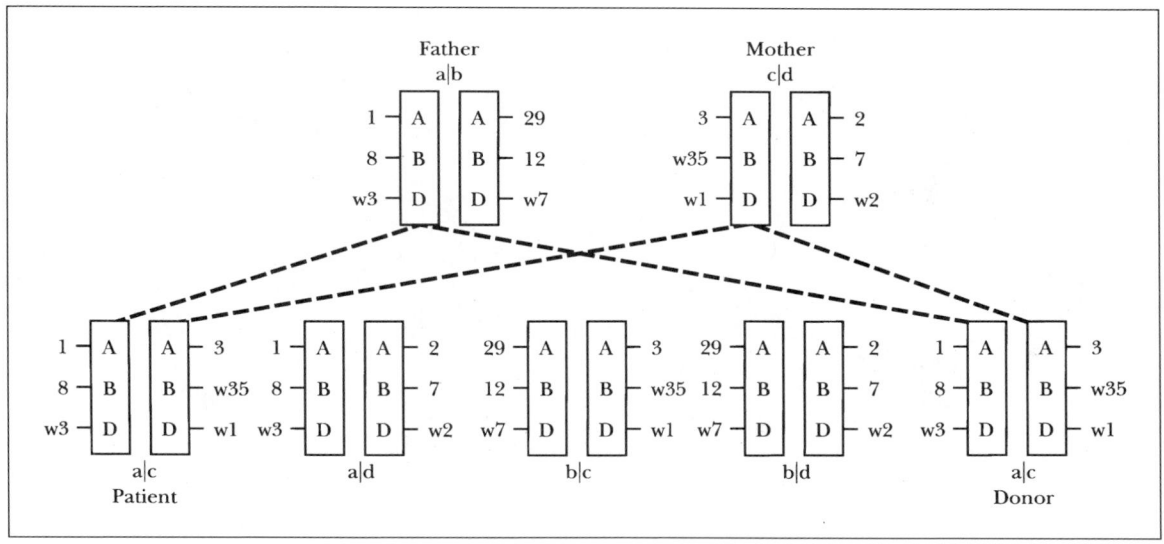

**FIGURE 18-3**   Diagram of possible combinations of human leukocyte antigen (HLA) region of chromosome 6 inherited by offspring from parents. The recipient and donor have inherited the same two haplotypes and are genotypically HLA identical.

thought to be responsible for GVHD before the donor marrow is reinfused. There are three methods of T-cell depletion: physical, immunologic, and pharmacological. Physical methods include soybean lectin separation plus E-rosette depletion; E-rosette alone; albumin gradient fractionation; and counterflow elutriation. Immunologic purging uses immunotoxins and murine or rat monoclonal anti-T-cell antibodies and complement alone or in combination with magnetic immunobeads to lyse the T-cells while preserving progenitor cells.[9] Finally combinations of physical and monoclonal antibody techniques or soybean agglutination plus monoclonal antibodies are used.

***Unrelated donors***   The use of unrelated volunteer donors has increased substantially. As of 1996, the National Marrow Donor Program (NMDP) has approved 76 centers to perform allogeneic BMT for unrelated donors. There are 105 donor centers with 11 recruiting groups and unrelated donor marrow harvests are performed at 111 approved collection centers. Since November 1988, the NMDP has facilitated over 4000 unrelated donor bone marrow transplantations and this number is increasing at more than 55 transplants per month.[29] However, the majority of donors are Caucasian and, consequently, transplants between unrelated individuals are primarily limited to the white middle class. Public education regarding the efficacy and benefits of unrelated donor marrow transplants, and the thrust to recruit African-American, Hispanic, Oriental, Jewish, and mixed European minority donors, makes possible marrow transplantation for thousands of patients without matched family donors. Improvements in genetic tissue typing with serological and restrictive fragment-length polymorphism techniques

hold promise for improving the reliability and speed of current screening methods. Scientific investigators working with unrelated donor transplants are striving to develop improved therapies to prevent the major complications of marrow rejection, GVHD, and infection.

## PROCESS OF BONE MARROW TRANSPLANT

The oncology nurse in the referring physician's office or clinic can contribute significantly to the continuity of care for the BMT candidate, donor, and family. Anxiety associated with the decision to physically relocate to participate in an expensive life-threatening treatment has been well documented.[30,31] Community-based nurses can prepare and support BMT candidates, donors, and families by providing literature specific to BMT. The National Institutes of Health (NIH) provides material that explains the BMT process. Long-term survivors of BMT in the candidate's community may be an additional source of inspiration and information. Good communication between BMT coordinator nurses and community nursing care managers will enhance continuity of care between the community and the BMT center.

### Pretransplant Evaluation and Preparation of the Patient

Marrow candidates require comprehensive evaluations to determine the patients' ability to sustain BMT. These evaluations, listed in Table 18-3, usually are done in the

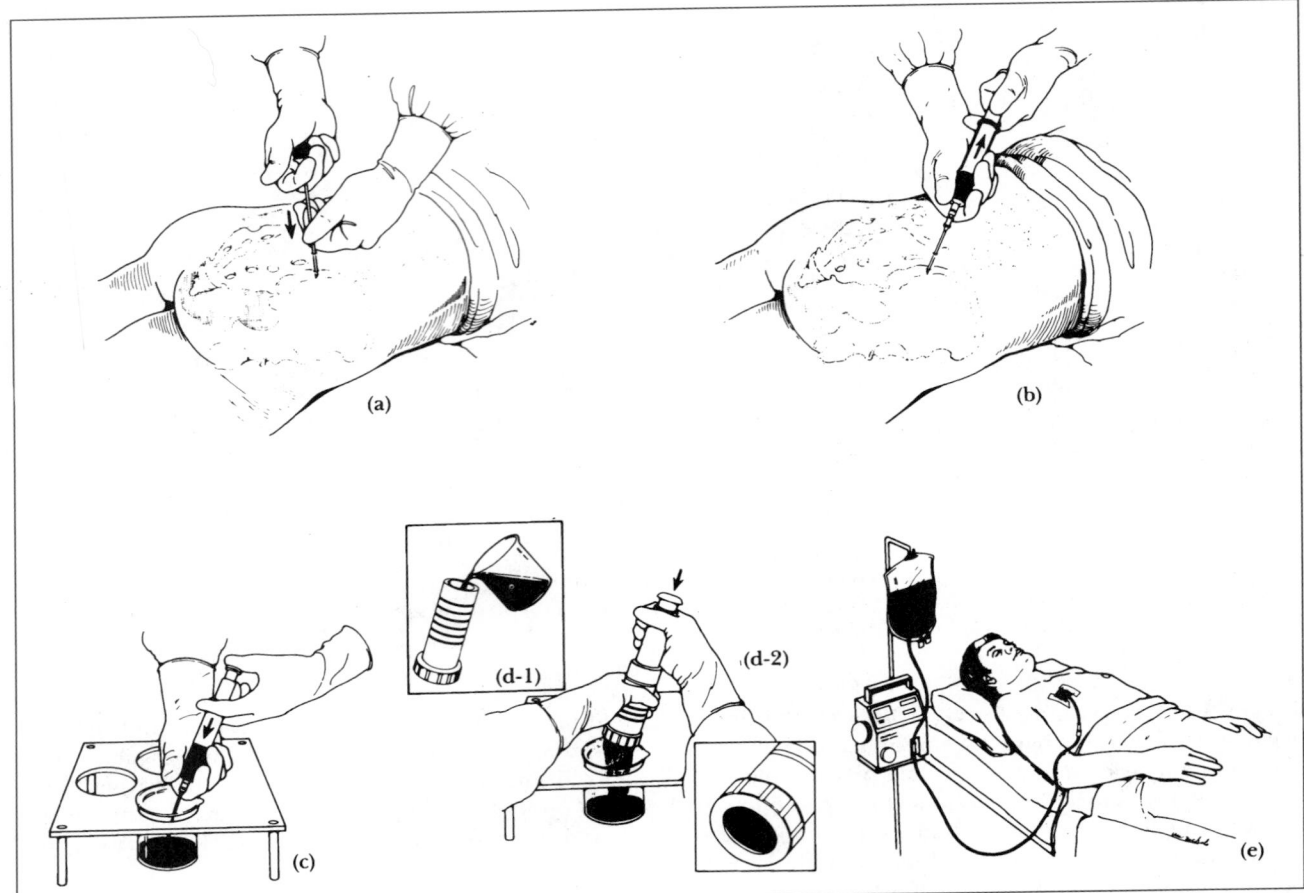

**FIGURE 18-4** Figure series of steps in donor marrow aspiration and harvest. (a) Large-bore needle placed in the posterior iliac crest. (b) Multiple aspirations. (c) Marrow drawn up in large syringe. (d-1) Marrow placed in collection beaker; (d-2) strained through metal grid. (e) Marrow placed in a blood administration bag and administered through multilumen central catheter.

BMT outpatient setting or even prior to the patient's arrival. A patient and family conference is held in the outpatient setting prior to the transplantation. The purposes of this conference are (1) to obtain informed consent, (2) to discuss expected risk and transplant-related morbidity and mortality, and (3) to discuss expected outcomes with the patient. A clear understanding of the BMT process is critical at this time. Often the patient discovers that actual survival statistics and other clinical data are very different from initial expectations. For example, a patient with acute myelogenous leukemia (AML) in second complete remission may have been told, prior to arrival at the center, that the statistical probability of a five-year, disease-free survival for the disease was 80%. In reality, the probability of disease-free survival is 50%.[32] Outpatient nurses can support the patient faced with the difficulties of accepting treatment realities and making critical treatment decisions. Patient and family preparation for hospitalization can be conducted during the wait for hospital admission. Familiarizing the patient with pro-

tective isolation and various complex treatment and research protocols can decrease the patient's anxiety concerning the procedures. Formalized instruction using videotapes and booklets is effective. Many BMT centers provide written information about their center, including maps, important telephone numbers, activities, and a glossary of BMT terms. All patients have multilumen indwelling central catheters inserted before admission. Atrial catheters are essential to accommodate large volumes of parenteral fluids that will be required. Peripheral inserted catheters (PICs), placed by certified nurses, are gaining attention but it is not clear if most of these catheters can withstand the duration of a transplant. Gonadal failure caused by the high-dose chemotherapy and total-body irradiation used in preparative regimens is a concern for BMT patients. The option of sperm banking should be discussed prior to hospitalization in patients with adequate sperm counts.[2] Fertilized ova storage may be an option for women; however, ethical issues may arise if the woman should die during BMT.

**TABLE 18-3** Pretransplantation Preparation and Evaluation of Candidate and Donor for BMT

| Evaluation | Candidate | Donor |
|---|---|---|
| **Clinical evaluation** | | |
| • Histocompatible tissue typing (HLA, MLC, HLA-DR-RFLP) DNA study | X | X |
| • ECG, possible cardiac-ejection fraction, appropriate scans | X | X |
| • Complete history and physical examination | X | X |
| • Immunization history | X | X |
| • Diagnostic procedures (bone marrow aspiration, biopsies) | X | |
| • Oral examination | X | |
| • Pulmonary function test, arterial blood gases | X | |
| • Chest films | X | X |
| • Informed consent | X | X |
| • Nutritional evaluation | X | |
| • Psychological evaluation, if recommended | X | X |
| • Gynecologic consultation for women of menstrual age | X | |
| • Appropriate consultations | X | X |
| • Sperm storage and ova storage if appropriate | X | |
| **Laboratory evaluation** | | |
| • Complete blood count with differential and platelet count | X | X |
| • Chemistry profile | X | X |
| • IgG, IgA, IgM levels | | |
| • Hepatitis screen | | |
| non-A | X | X |
| non-B | X | X |
| A | X | X |
| B | X | X |
| C | X | X |
| • HIV antibody status | X | X |
| • Serological test for syphilis | X | X |
| • ABO and Rh groups | X | X |
| • CMV antibody status | X | X |
| • HCG, FSH, LH, estradiol levels | X | X |
| **Preparation and intervention** | | |
| • Placement of right atrial catheter | X | |
| • Ferrous gluconate medication | | X |
| • Preoperative and postoperative teaching regarding marrow harvest | X | X (autologous) |
| • Postoperative care and evaluation of marrow aspiration sites | X | X |

*RFLP,* restriction fragment-length polymorphism; *HCG,* human chorionic gonadotropin; *DNA,* deoxyribonucleic acid; *FSH,* follicle stimulating hormone; *LH,* luteinizing hormone.

## Preparation of the Donor and Nursing Care

Selected allogeneic donors, in addition to being HLA matched, need to be relatively healthy, give informed consent, and be available for marrow harvest and platelet donation. Donors who are minors may present certain legal and ethical considerations. For example, in the state of Washington, parents do not have the legal prerogative to give consent for their childrens' marrow donation because the procedure is legally viewed as having no medical benefit for the child and could be potentially dangerous. To solve this problem, all minor donors in Washington are made wards of the court, limited legal guardians are appointed, and court approval obtained for marrow harvest. The rationale is that the child donor may experience psychological harm if not allowed to donate marrow.[32] In another incident the Illinois Supreme Court ruled that half-siblings cannot be required to undergo tissue-typing for a stepbrother requiring a BMT.[33]

Although risks are minimal, donors need to be comprehensively evaluated prior to surgery, especially for the ability to tolerate general or spinal anesthesia. To minimize the risks of blood transfusion, donors weighing more than 50 kilograms donate a unit of autologous whole blood to be reinfused intraoperatively at the time of marrow harvest. A small study (n = 10) showed that administration of erythropoietin to boost normal donor hematocrit levels to avoid postoperative transfusions showed a 16% increase in postharvest hematocrit count.[34] Further trials are necessary to define donor populations that will benefit from this approach and to determine possible long-term effects on donors. Several factors influence the amount of counseling and education a donor needs prior to donation. These include the relationship between the donor, the patient, and the family, as well as the donor's own life responsibilities.[35,36] For example, donors often need to provide platelet support for the patient up to three months after marrow transfusion. This demand can create hardships for the donor. Donors can experience long-term psychological effects when the patient has died after the BMT. Long-term sequelae, including mood changes, lack of self-esteem, altered relationships, and guilt, can occur depending on the donor's perception of the success or failure of the BMT.[37,38] These studies, however, are dated and new research is needed. As with the patient, donors and their families can be effectively supported through education and written information to minimize anxiety and to promote realistic expectations. In the case of unrelated volunteer donors few psychological pressures are involved and most individuals donate from altruism. Direct contact between unrelated marrow donors and recipient is prohibited by the National Marrow Donor Program in the United States. There is debate on this issue and some centers allow written contact prior to transplant and shortly thereafter. In time, some donors and marrow recipients have formed long-term relationships.[32] Several important and significant studies assessing the effects of unrelated marrow donation note that donors were generally positive about the donation process. Butterworth et al noted the psychosocial effects of 493 donors from the National Marrow Donor Program.[39] The majority (88%) reported that they would donate a second time. Stroncek et al studied the same group and found that, similar to related donors, they described fatigue (74.8%), pain at the collection site (67.8%), and low-back pain (51.6%).[40] These studies have implications for nurses working in community settings where unrelated marrow transplant harvest occurs.

Preparation of the donor may cause anxieties surrounding the coming events. The World Marrow Donor Association published recommendations and requirements for standard practices when BMT involves unrelated volunteer donors.[41] There is a trend toward outpatient marrow harvest. Bolwell et al[42] reported that outpatient marrow harvesting is feasible and that the need for red blood cell transfusions can be reduced by using red blood cells collected during the harvest. Brandwein and colleagues[43] assessed outpatient marrow harvesting for marrow recipients. Over a 13 month period, 39 patients underwent outpatient marrow harvest. Of these, 36 were discharged later the same day with oral iron supplements and no adverse postoperative sequelae. Two patients required hospital admission—one for hypotension and the other for fever. In another study,[42] researchers asked 211 marrow donors to describe the side effects of outpatient marrow donation. Of the 65% who responded, the most common side effects were pain at the donation site (90%), low-back pain (60%), nausea (43%), vomiting (31%), sore throat (43%), fever (18%), and bleeding at the donation site (6%). Similar complications are noted in marrow donors admitted for longer periods of time. Physical and psychological follow-up care for the donor is essential.[41]

Nursing care of the donor often is overshadowed by the attention given to the marrow recipient. Nurses can be instrumental in recognizing this phenomenon and making appropriate referrals to social workers or psychologists. Donors may be under stress due to separation from work and family, worries about lost income, and strained interpersonal relationships. Unrelated donors are typically harvested in a hospital away from the marrow recipient, for confidentiality and convenience. Unrelated donors are not asked to remain available for future platelet transfusions to the marrow recipient. Nurses caring for unrelated donors should be sensitive to the ethical issues of confidentiality, especially regarding the donor's motivations.[44]

The use of laminar air flow (LAF) rooms to decrease infection-related morbidity and mortality versus simple protective isolation is still under debate, and transplant centers differ in isolation techniques. Early studies showed that only patients with aplastic anemia admitted to LAF rooms survived longer when compared to patients not placed in LAF rooms.[45,46] There is no convincing evidence that patients cared for in LAF rooms have significantly higher survival rates than patients placed in conventional hospital rooms where reverse isolation, gloves, face masks, or filtered air are used.[47,48] Applicable research data on this topic in the past decade have been confounded by an accompanying increase in oral nonabsorbable antibiotic administration. Despite the uncertainty about the most effective protective isolation techniques, the use of LAF rooms and rooms with high-efficiency particulate air filters has increased during the past decade.

Patients transplanted in protective isolation require specialized nursing care. These patients undergo decontamination of their gastrointestinal tracts, skin, and body cavities. Decontamination techniques include ingestion of concentrated antibiotic solution, application of antibiotic powders or ointment in nostrils, ears, umbilicus, axillae, rectum, and groin areas, and bathing with sterile water and antibacterial soap. Nursing care includes supporting compliance with these medications as well as offering psychological support. The loss of human touch can induce psychological problems.[49,50] However, further nursing research is needed in this area.

Poe et al[51] surveyed 88 BMT programs in the United States and noted little standardization in infection prevention measures. Almost all units surveyed used some type of protected environment including skin contamination (69%), gut decontamination with oral nonabsorbable antibiotics (30%), antifungal therapy (73%), administration of colony stimulating factors (58%), and modified microbial diets (66%). A wide variety of mouth care regimens, visitor and patient precautions, and environmental maintenance were described. Anecdotal reports and clinical observations suggest that use of masks and garment covers is declining. Cost-benefit analysis does not convince that such methods eliminate or reduce infection. Handwashing, scrupulous hygiene, and protective isolation may be the most cost-effective and meaningful conventions for infection control.[51] Oncology nurses can play a key role in identifying the most beneficial environmental methods to reduce infection-related morbidity and mortality.

## THE BONE MARROW TRANSPLANT

### Admission to the Hospital

Once patients have been thoroughly evaluated for BMT, they are admitted to the hospital and placed in a protective isolation room. Several isolation methods exist.

## Pretransplant Conditioning Regimens

Recipients of marrow transplant usually are admitted to the hospital one day prior to the start of their conditioning regimen. The methods used to prepare patients for grafting differ according to the underlying disease. Patients receive high-dose chemotherapy alone or with supralethal doses of irradiation. This serves to eradicate malignant cells and to prevent graft rejection by the patient's own immune system.[52]

The array of drugs for high-dose chemotherapy in preparation for marrow transplantation is limited secondary to major organ toxicity. For example, doxorubicin can cause cardiac toxicity placing the patient at significant risk to succumb during or immediately after transplantation. Historically, cyclophosphamide in combination with total-body irradiation (TBI) has been the standard treatment used in BMT preparative regimens. Cyclophosphamide is the most common chemotherapeutic agent because it provides tumor cell kill as well as immune ablation. Other agents sometimes used in combination with TBI include cytosine arabinoside and etoposide. The use of busulfan and cyclophosphamide without TBI has increased markedly during the last decade in efforts to avoid the long-term effects of irradiation, especially for children.[1]

Total-body irradiation is delivered in varying doses from cobalt or linear accelerator units. TBI offers optimal tumor cell kill because of its ability to penetrate the central nervous system and other privileged sites.[52] Lung shielding sometimes is used in efforts to reduce life-threatening pulmonary complications. TBI can be delivered in single or fractionated doses, but prevailing practice favors fractionated doses to reduce toxicities.[52] Pretransplant "booster" radiotherapy to previous tumor sites may be used in patients with bulky disease to reduce the chances of relapse.[53]

## Marrow Infusion

The day of marrow infusion is "day 0," with subsequent days numbered from this time. The actual marrow infusion is a procedure similar to a blood transfusion. The marrow is infused through a central lumen catheter over the course of several hours. Marrow cells pass through the lung and home to the marrow cavity. Complications may include volume overload and pulmonary abnormalities from fat emboli. Symptoms similar to blood transfusion reactions can occur (i.e., chills, urticaria, and fever) and should be treated with antihistamines, antipyretics, or by decreasing the rate of infusion.[54] Within two to four weeks, the marrow graft becomes functional, and peripheral platelets, leukocytes, and red cells increase in number. Intensive nursing care is required to prevent complications until the recipient's marrow recovers.

## COMPLICATIONS OF BONE MARROW TRANSPLANTATION

Although BMT holds potential cure for a number of diseases, acute and chronic toxicities can complicate the posttransplantation course. Complications are the result of (1) high-dose chemotherapy and irradiation for conditioning regimens, (2) graft-versus-host disease, or (3) problems associated with the original disease and the adverse effects of medications used in the process.[55] The sequence of major complications following allogeneic BMT is presented in Figure 18-5. The major complications following autologous BMT are similar, except for GVHD.

## Interrelationships of BMT Complications

The major symptoms of marrow transplant-related complications overlap (Figure 18-6) and are interrelated as follows:

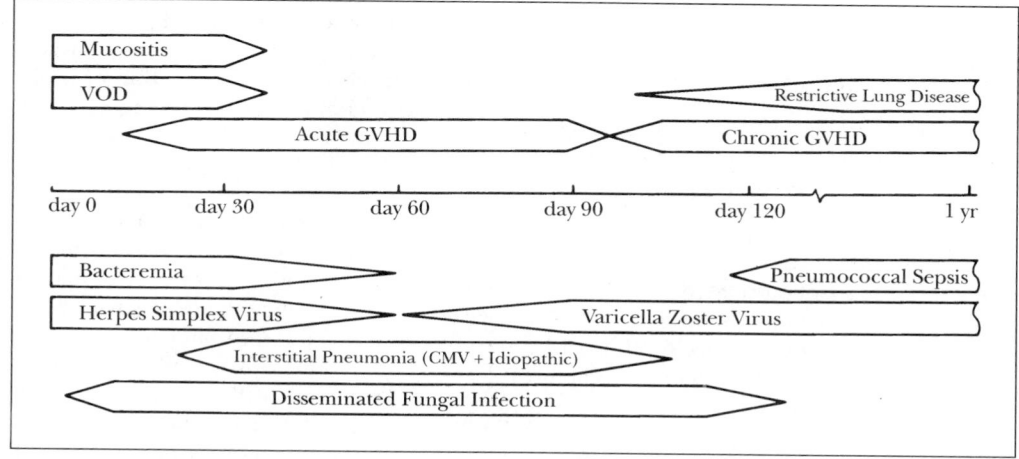

**FIGURE 18-5**   Temporal sequence of major complications after allogeneic bone marrow transplantation, from day 0 to one year after BMT. (Press OW, Schaller RT, Thomas ED: *Complications of Organ Transplantation.* New York, Marcel Dekker, 1987. Reprinted with permission of Marcel Dekker, Inc.)

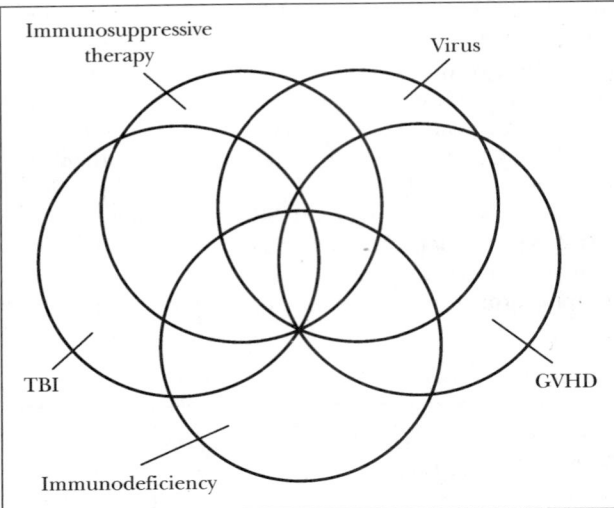

**FIGURE 18-6** The multifactorial nature of acute and chronic complications following marrow transplantation. (Degg JH: Delayed complications of marrow transplantation. *Marrow Transplant Reviews* 2:11, 1992 Reprinted with permission.)

- The chemoradiation therapy the patients receive would be fatal if the patients were not rescued with marrow infusion.

- Major complications after transplantation usually result from the chemoradiation used to prepare for transplantation or from the marrow transplantation, not from the original disease.

- Complications often occur simultaneously.

- Clinical manifestations of some complications may be sudden yet subtle.

- The clinical manifestations of different complications can be identical; one complication can cause or exacerbate another.

- The treatment of one complication can cause or exacerbate another complication.

- The prophylaxis or treatment for one complication may have to be modified or terminated because of the development of another complication.

Nursing care of marrow recipients requires an ability to organize procedures and therapies aimed at prevention and treatment of transplant-related toxicities.[21] Patients and families experience anxiety and stress associated with this treatment, and nurses require psychosocial nursing skills and the ability to interact with multidisciplinary teams to address patient needs.

## Acute Complications

Acute complications are seen several days after BMT and affect multiple organ systems. Because pretransplantation chemoradiotherapy ablates all cell lines, complications will be most severe until early engraftment. Table 18-4 presents a detailed summary of the cause, incidence, onset, manifestations, and interventions associated with acute complications of BMT.

### Gastrointestinal toxicity

***Mucositis*** The gastrointestinal tract is affected by TBI and chemotherapy preparative conditioning. Inflammation of the oral and pharyngeal tissues may occur two to three days after marrow infusion. Initially, oral tissues become hyperkeratotic; as mucositis continues, the cheeks, lips, and tongue become edematous. Patients often develop pharyngitis, complain of a sore throat, and have difficulty swallowing. Bleeding ulcerations and acute GVHD may occur on the buccal mucosa or sides of the tongue. Concomitant herpes simplex lesions and other local or systemic secondary infections can further damage the oral mucosa.[56] The major symptom in all oral infections is protracted pain, which usually is treated with intravenous morphine.[57] Mucositis is further complicated by severe thrombocytopenia and aspiration pneumonia can occur.[56] These problems resolve once engraftment occurs and serious long-term problems are rare. Nursing care includes supporting good oral hygiene measures and patient and family education in use of saline mouthwashes, toothettes, and flossing. Frequent use of saline can ease minor tissue irritation and drying and dissolve thick secretions. Applications of ice bags or packs can control facial swelling and throat discomfort. Topical anesthetics may be useful for mild to moderate pain. Most patients, however, will require parenteral analgesics. Patient-controlled analgesia (PCA) delivery systems have been used successfully. Patients using PCA systems reported better pain control and reduced nausea and vomiting when compared to marrow recipients receiving continuous infusion analgesics.[57] Mucosal coating agents such as antacids, sucrafate, sodium alginate, and cellulose film may increase comfort and promote healing. Epstein et al demonstrated the effectiveness of benzydamine hydrochloride rinse in the reduction of oral mucositis.[58] It is not clear if immunomodulators such as colony stimulating factors and cytokines reduce the incidence of mucositis.[59]

***Nausea and vomiting*** Nausea and vomiting following chemotherapy and TBI is a consistent problem.[60] Protracted nausea and vomiting also may be caused by GVHD, CMV esophagitis, or gastrointestinal infections. In these cases, a differential diagnosis must be made and may include endoscopy with duodenal biopsy.[60] Nursing care of the patient with nausea and vomiting includes administration of antiemetics, careful recording of fluid intake and output, monitoring of acid and electrolyte balances, and psychological support. Traditionally, the most frequently used antiemetic agents included high-dose metoclopramide, droperidol, metoclopramide, diphenhydramine, and lorazepam.[20,60] Most recently, the

**TABLE 18-4**   Possible Acute Complications of Bone Marrow Transplantation

| Complication | Cause | Incidence Rate (%) | Time of Onset after BMT (days) | Signs and Symptoms | Nursing Intervention | Medical Intervention |
|---|---|---|---|---|---|---|
| **Gastrointestinal** | | | | | | |
| Oral mucositis | High-dose conditioning regimen of chemotherapy; TBI (immuno-suppression) plus coexistent infection; HSV, methotrexate | 100 Universal to chemotherapy and irradiation | 0–28 | Profuse, watery to thick ropy mucus, severe pain, bleeding ulceration, infection, potential airway obstruction, xerostomia | Assess nasal and oral cavities for integrity of mucous membrane | Acyclovir for HSV infection; topical antibiotics; lidocaine, dyclonine, IV morphine sulfate |
| Esophageal mucositis | Same | 100 | Same | Esophageal dysphagia, bleeding, infection | Administer IV analgesic medication; provide frequent, vigorous oral care | IV morphine sulfate; daily chest film and CBC; viral cultures; parenteral support |
| Gastric mucositis | Same | 100 | Same | Anorexia, nausea, vomiting, bleeding, infection | Monitor with care, assess fluids and electrolytes I & O, fluids, and man-agement of pain | Parenteral nutrition, biopsy, appropriate antibiotic therapy |
| Intestinal mucositis | Same | 100 | Same | Watery diarrhea, cramping pain, ulcerations, infections | Monitor vital signs q 4 hr; accurately measure I & O; manage pain | Surgical intervention; gut biopsy; antibiotic therapy |
| Gastrointestinal lower bowel toxicity | High-dose TBI and chemotherapy; GVHD | 100 | 0–30 | Nausea, vomiting, diarrhea | Monitor with care fluids and electrolytes, assessment of I & O; administer antiemetics, TPN | Antiemetics, fluid management, gut biopsy |
| **Acute GVHD** | | | | | | |
| Skin | Reaction of im-munocompetent donor T-lymphocytes against immuno-incompetent host | 40–50 | 10–70; median onset day 25 after BMT | Maculopapular rash on trunk, palms, soles, ears; generalized erythroderma with desquamation | Assess integumentary system; understand side effects of drugs used in treatment; provide psychological support of patient | Immuno-suppressive therapy with methotrexate, cyclosporine; treated T-cell–depleted donor marrow before BMT; antithy-mocyte globulin; corticosteroids; skin biopsy; analgesics |
| Liver | Same | 40–50 | Same | Elevated liver enzymes, alkaline phosphatase, right upper quadrant pain, hepatomegaly, jaundice | Monitor liver function tests | Liver biopsy |
| Gastrointestinal tract | Same | 40–50 | 10–70 | Green watery diarrhea, abdominal cramping, anorexia, nausea, vomiting | Monitor guaiac stool test, weigh, accurate I & O, central venous pressure, CBC and electrolytes; administer antiemetics | Gut biopsy; differential diagnosis to rule out infection, VOD, gut rest, parenteral nutrition |
| Renal insufficiency | Nephrotoxins, amphotericin B, cyclosporine, methotrexate, | 25 | 1–50 | Decreased urine output, asymptomatic azotemia, | Monitor vital signs, with postural BP; careful fluid | Dialysis (5%–10% of BMT patients), removal or reduction of |

*(continued)*

**TABLE 18-4**  Possible Acute Complications of Bone Marrow Transplantation (continued)

| Complication | Cause | Incidence Rate (%) | Time of Onset after BMT (days) | Signs and Symptoms | Nursing Intervention | Medical Intervention |
|---|---|---|---|---|---|---|
| | aminoglycoside plus septic shock or cardiogenic shock or volume depletion because of diarrhea; hepatorenal syndrome of VOD | | | proteinuria, hypertension, renal failure, thrombocyto-penia purpura, thirst, dizziness; flat or distended neck veins, peripheral edema; doubling of baseline serum creatinine | management, accurate I & O; monitor serum creatinine, BUN, electrolyte levels; monitor urine electrolyte collections, specific gravity q 4 hr; measure daily abdominal girth, weight; assess for peripheral edema; monitor patient during dialysis | nephrotoxic drugs; correction of fluid electrolyte and acid-base imbalance; treatment of infections |
| Hemorrhagic cystitis | High-dose cyclo-phosphamide | 24 | Immediately | Hematuria, dysuria, frequency, blood clots | Assess fluid intake; force fluids | Three-way catheters, continuous bladder irrigation |
| Veno-occlusive disease | High-dose conditioning regimens; patients with previous liver disease; patients >15 yr old | 21 (6% mortality rate) aplastic anemia (rare) | 6–15 | Weight gain >12%, ascites, hepatic metabolism, bilirubin >20 mg/dl, SGOT >40 mU/ml; right upper quadrant pain; encephalopathy, hepato-megaly | Carefully and frequently assess fluid balance; monitor weight BID, vital signs with postural BP, accurate I & O; measure abdom-inal girth daily, restrict fluid, sodium; monitor narcotics and, if indicated, hemo-dynamics; assess neurological and mental changes | No known treatment; maintain intravascular volume and renal profusion; restrict sodium, maintain hematocrit >35%; albumin; low-dose dopamine; supportive care |
| Infection | | 100 | 0–30 | | | |
| Bacterial | | 10 | | Neutropenia, fever >38°C, sepsis, cough, lethargy | Provide LAF rooms; prevent infection; use good hand-washing techniques; wear mask in patient's room; provide surveillance, cultures, pan cultures; administer antibiotics; manage side effects of treatment drugs; regulate BP with pressor agents and hemodynamics monitoring; manage fluid and electrolyte acid-base balances; institute fever reduction measures | Prophylactic measures, i.e., protective isolation, LAF rooms, oral nonabsorbable antibiotics, low-bacteria diet, TMP-SMX for pneumocystis; acyclovir prophy-laxis for HSV; passive immuni-zation with CMV-Ig, IgG, CMV blood product screening; surveillance chest films; total-body skin cleaning; treatment with broad-spectrum prophylactic antibiotics; appropriate antibiotics for bacterial, viral, fungal, and protozoal infection |
| *Escherichia coli* | | 5.5 | | | | |
| *Staphylococcus epidermidis* | | 35.9 | | | | |
| *Staphylococcus aureus* | | 7.8 | | | | |
| *Streptococcus* species | | 6.3 | | | | |

**TABLE 18-4** Possible Acute Complications of Bone Marrow Transplantation (continued)

| Complication | Cause | Incidence Rate (%) | Time of Onset after BMT (days) | Signs and Symptoms | Nursing Intervention | Medical Intervention |
|---|---|---|---|---|---|---|
| **Viral** | | | | | | |
| Herpes simplex | Reactivation of latent virus | 70–80 | 0–30 | Pain, ulceration, bleeding, fever, infection | Provide vigorous mouth care; administer pain medication | Prophylaxis and treatment with IV acyclovir; analgesics |
| CMV pneumonia | Reactivation of latent virus | 70 in allogeneic 10 in autologous | 60–70 | Dyspnea, infiltrates on chest film; abnormal ABGs, PFTs; may be asymptomatic | Administer medication, chest auscultation | Diagnostic bronchoscopy, DHPG, CMV-Ig; bronchial washings |
| Fungal *Aspergillus (Candida)* | Immuno-suppression caused by TBI and chemotherapy | 10% unknown | 0–30 | Fever | Administer amphotericin B; monitor serum electrolytes, hydration status, side effects of amphotericin B; administer pre-medications to reduce drug reactions, (e.g., hydrocortisone, meperidine diphenhydramine | Amphotericin B; endoscopic examination with biopsy |
| Alopecia | High-dose chemotherapy, TBI | 100 | 7–10 | Loss of body hair | Help patient cope with body image changes; acquaint patient with cosmetic head coverings | Psychological support |

*ABG*, arterial blood gas; *BID*, twice daily; *BP*, blood pressure; *BUN*, blood urea nitrogen; *CBC*, complete blood count; *CMV*, cytomegalovirus; *DHPG*, dihydroxyproproxymethylguanine; *HSV*, herpes simplex virus; *HZV*, herpes zoster varicella; *Ig*, immunoglobulin; *IgG*, immunoglobulin G; *I & O*, intake and output; *IV*, intravenous; *LAF*, laminar air flow; *PFT*, pulmonary function test; *SGOT*, serum glutamic oxaloacetic transaminase; *TBI*, total-body irradiation; *TMP-SMX*, trimethoprim-sulfamethoxazole (Bactrim); *TPN*, total parenteral nutrition, VOD, veno-occlusive disease.

use of 5-HT3 antagonists (ondansetron) is playing an important role in relief of nausea and vomiting associated with TBI and high-dose chemotherapy in children.[61] A randomized controlled study of ondansetron administered to transplant recipients reported equal relief of nausea and vomiting episodes but fewer extrapyramidal reactions and sedation compared to chlorpromazine.[62] Granisetron hydrochloride, an antagonist of serotine-3, is the newest 5-HT3 blocker to be studied in the marrow transplant community for prevention of single and fractionated TBI.[63]

***Diarrhea*** Diarrhea is one of the most obsequious symptoms associated with BMT and can continue up to 100 days after BMT. It is difficult to differentiate clinically between infectious and noninfectious causes. A prospective study of 296 marrow transplant patients over age 10 years were studied to identify risk factors for diarrhea.[64] The incidence of diarrhea 20 days after transplant was not related to the cytoreductive therapy regimen. Protective environmental factors, such as laminar air flow rooms, nonabsorbable antibiotics, and low-bacterial content food, did not reduce the incidence of either GVHD or

infection. The cause of diarrhea was intestinal infection in 13%, GVHD in 48%, and unknown in 39%. Patients with diarrhea from any cause had similar clinical signs and symptoms, so identification of the cause required intestinal mucosal biopsy. This study confirmed clinical observation that diarrhea as a result of high-dose conditioning regimens seldom persists beyond day 15. Oral magnesium and nonabsorbable antibiotics (vancomycin, tobramycin, and nystatin) can cause mild diarrhea.[65] Diarrhea associated with acute GVHD and infections is seen as early as day 7 in mismatched BMT patients; this is discussed later in the chapter.

## Hematologic complications

Transplant recipients are at high risk for pancytopenia and must be supported with blood component therapy and in some cases with CSFs until the donor marrow becomes fully engrafted and functional. The use of CSF erythropoietin is being studied in clinical trials in the hopes that red cell transfusions can be decreased. If a cost-effective and efficacious CSF can increase hematopoietic recovery, the associated risks for transfusion-related infections and eco-

**TABLE 18-5** Prevention and Management of Hemorrhage in the Recipient of Bone Marrow Transplantation

| Complication | Cause | Nursing Intervention | Medical Intervention |
|---|---|---|---|
| Nosebleed | High-dose chemotherapy and TBI (immunosuppression of megakaryocyte/erythrocyte lines) | Apply pressure and ice packs to nasal area; administer platelets; avoid invasive procedures | Daily CBC, blood product support, topical adrenalin and cocaine, ENT consult |
| Mouthbleed | Same as above | Assess airway for patency; provide vigorous mouth care, use toothettes, discourage toothbrushes; provide oral airway at bedside | Same; dental medicine consult |
| Cranial | Same as above | Frequent neurological assessment for headache, seizure, confusion; lumbar puncture only with platelet count >50,000/mm³; avoid emesis and straining | Daily CBC; blood product support, neurological consult; MRI, CT scans |
| Gastrointestinal | High-dose chemotherapy and TBI, mucosal irritation, infection, stress | Observe emesis and stools; avoid nasogastric tubes, enemas, rectal temperatures | Daily CBC; blood product support; endoscopy with platelets >50,000/mm³; coagulation studies |
| Invasive procedures | High-dose chemotherapy and TBI (immunosuppression of megakaryocyte/erythrocyte lines) | Place sandbags to surgical site after insertion of atrial catheters; avoid intramuscular injections | Platelet count >50,000/mm³; avoid cutdowns; use percutaneous procedures for Swan-Ganz catheters |
| Hemorrhagic cystitis | Same as above | Assess for blood in urine; irrigate bladder during administration of cyclophosphamide; use care in insertion of urinary catheters | Bladder irrigation; daily CBCs; IV hydration; blood product support |
| Menstrual bleeding | Same as above | Observe bleeding carefully (count number of sanitary pads); administer medroxyprogesterone acetate | Medroxyprogesterone acetate; daily CBCs; blood product support |
| Petechiae, bruising | Same as above | Turn patient frequently; avoid pressure sores; use eggshell mattress, sheepskin, alternating pressure mattress | |

*CBC,* complete blood count; *CT,* computerized tomography; *ENT,* ear, nose, and throat; *IV,* intravenous; *MRI,* magnetic resonance imaging; *TBI,* total-body irradiation.

nomic costs may be avoided. Blood products must be irradiated to destroy T-lymphocytes that can cause GVHD in the marrow recipient. Patients whose platelets become refractory to random platelet transfusions can receive HLA-matched platelets from family or community donors, and platelets that have undergone plasmapheresis from marrow donors yield optimal increments. Alloimmunization and platelet refractoriness contribute to a 1% case fatality rate from hemorrhage complications. Bleeding can occur from all body orifices and requires immediate intervention. Table 18-5 outlines clinical manifestations and interventions for management of hemorrhages.[21]

***Hemorrhage cystitis*** Seventy percent of marrow recipients may develop hemorrhagic cystitis as a result of the urotoxic effect of acrolein metabolites in cyclophosphamide in conditioning regimens. Hemorrhagic cystitis can have a sudden onset, be delayed, or manifest itself months after BMT. Prevention of hemorrhagic cystitis involves continuous bladder irrigation and/or aggressive intravenous (IV) therapy to flush cyclophosphamide metabolites from the bladder. Continuous bladder infusion administered prophylactically has been shown to be well tolerated and significantly decreases the incidence of hemorrhagic cystitis.[66] Intravenous drug therapy with MESNA (2-mercaptoethane sulfonate sodium) has been shown to be of benefit in preventing hemorrhagic cystitis by combining MESNA with acrolein, but the drug must be administered prior to manifestation of the problem.[67–69]

### Acute graft-versus-host disease

GVHD is an immunologic disease that is a direct consequence of allogeneic marrow transplantation and occurs in an acute and chronic form. Despite prophylaxis with postgrafting in vivo immunosuppression, this disease remains a major impediment to successful marrow grafting and occurs in 30%–50% of HLA-identical recipients and up to 75% of unrelated donor transplants.[70] GVHD is thought to be a graft-host response in which the grafted donor T-lymphocytes recognize disparate non-HLA host cell antigens and initiate cytotoxic injury directed against host (patient) tissue.[65,70] Acute GVHD targets the skin, liver, and gut.[70] Symptoms range from mild to severe. The clinical states of acute graft-versus-host disease are outlined in Table 18-6. GVHD-related complications account for approximately 10% of all BMT deaths.[71] Risk factors for the development of acute GVHD from HLA-matched transplantation are (1) patient and donor age greater than 18 years of age, (2) donor alloimmunization through transfusion or pregnancy, (3) mismatched-gender BMTs, (4) diagnosis of CML, (5) CMV negativity in patient and donor, and (6) type of GVHD prophylaxis.[71] Marrow recipients receiving unrelated donor transplants experience significantly worse GVHD than those receiving HLA-identical sibling transplants.[72]

*Clinical manifestations* Clinical manifestations of acute GVHD typically begin with a maculopapular erythema that may be pruritic and may cover about 25% of the body. The disease can progress to a generalized erythroderma with frank desquamation and blistering similar to second-degree burns. Liver involvement may appear consistent with or subsequent to the onset of GVHD of the skin. On abdominal examination, patients may have pain in the right upper quadrant of the abdomen and hepatomegaly. In addition, increases in liver enzymes may be noted. Jaundice indicates progressive liver involvement. Gastrointestinal involvement of acute GVHD can result in nausea, vomiting, anorexia, abdominal cramping, and pain. A typical early symptom is green, watery diarrhea that may exceed 2 liters/day.

*Diagnosis* The diagnosis of GVHD may be difficult to distinguish from symptoms secondary to infection or the high-dose conditioning regimens. Skin and liver biopsy and clinical, laboratory, and x-ray data help establish the differential diagnosis imperative to treatment.

*Prophylaxis and treatment* One of the most important concepts in transplantation medicine is the prevention of GVHD and its related symptoms. Immunosuppressive medications are aimed at removing or inactivating T-lymphocytes that attack target organs. Cyclosporine and methotrexate inhibit T-lymphocytes that are believed to be responsible for acute GVHD and are the first line therapy. Used in combination, they are more effective than either agent alone. The use of T-cell depletion of donor marrow to decrease GVHD has been abandoned because of increased relapse rates and graft failure.[73] Because GVHD commonly manifests itself in the face of prophylactic measures, treatment approaches to contain GVHD are of paramount importance to patient survival. Cyclosporine and methotrexate continue to be the first line approach to treating GVHD, while adding corticosteroids (1–60 mg/kg) to the treatment regimen is the second line of therapy. Patients who fail treatments with combinations of these agents may show response with OKT3, a monoclonal antibody, but this therapy has been associated with toxicity and tumor necrosis factor. Polyvalent intravenous immunoglobulin (IVIg) has been found to reduce the frequency of acute GVHD but the expense of this therapy needs to be balanced against the likely gains and overall costs of alternative approaches. One of these alternatives includes the use of ultraviolet irradiation to suppress skin GVHD. Initially used to treat chronic skin GVHD, several studies demonstrate encouraging results for patients with acute GVHD using Psoralen and ultraviolet A irradiation (PUVA). This therapy also has application for chronic GVHD and will be discussed elsewhere in this chapter.[74] Other medications used to prevent and modify acute GVHD are antithymocyte globulin (ATG) and monoclonal antibodies. ATG, once thought to be an important treatment for GVHD, has been disappointing in randomized clinical trials.[75] Symptom management includes gut rest, hyperalimentation, pain control, antibiotic prophylaxis, and psychological support. Octreotide, a somatostatin analogue, prolongs gastrointestinal transit time, decreases endogenous fluid secretion in the jejunum, and stimulates intestinal absorption of water and electrolytes. This agent is currently being investigated for controlling secretory diarrhea resulting from acute GI GVHD.[76]

*Nursing implications* Nursing care of patients with acute GVHD requires a thorough understanding of its tempo and manifestations, and skillful assessment and

**TABLE 18-6** Clinical Stages of Acute Graft-Versus-Host Disease

| Stage | Skin | Liver | Gut |
|---|---|---|---|
| + (mild) | Maculopapular rash <25% body surface | Bilirubin 2–3 mg/dl | Diarrhea 500–1000 ml/day |
| + + (moderate) | Maculopapular rash 25%–50% body surface | Bilirubin 3–6 mg/dl | Diarrhea 1000–1500 ml/day |
| + + + (severe) | Generalized erythroderma | Bilirubin 6–15 mg/dl | Diarrhea >1500 ml/day |
| + + + + (life-threatening) | Desquamation and bullae | Bilirubin >15 mg/dl | Pain or ileus |

management of its early complications. Drugs given to treat or prevent GVHD may have adverse side effects and confound the clinical course (i.e., cyclosporine and steroids). Nursing care includes management of burnlike wounds, abdominal pain, and voluminous diarrhea. Frequent clinical reassessment is required to monitor fluid replacement, hyperalimentation, transfusions, and antibiotic therapy.[77] Large volumes of diarrhea mandate intensive nutritional assessment as well.

## Renal complications

Renal complications after BMT occur in over 50% of marrow recipients and can be the result of one event or a combination of events. Multiple nephrotoxic drugs used for prevention and treatment of transplantation-related problems (e.g., amphotericin B, cyclosporine, methotrexate, aminoglycosides) are implicated in renal toxicities. These toxicities, superimposed on patients with prerenal dysfunction, septic shock, volume depletion, veno-occlusive disease, or tumor necrosis syndrome act in concert to exacerbate renal hemodynamic complications further.[68,69]

*Clinical manifestations/monitoring* Clinical manifestations of renal complications include the abrupt onset of anuria,[67-69] which may be an early indication of acute tubular necrosis or acute renal failure. Acute tubular necrosis is defined as damage to the epithelial cells of the lining of the renal tubules from nephotoxic or ischemic injury. This insult leads to compromised renal flow with consequent impaired ability to eliminate fluid, electrolytes, and metabolic wastes.[78] Anuria results from postrenal obstruction arising from cyclophosphamide-related hemorrhagic cystitis. Renal failure, defined as a doubling of baseline creatinine, stems from tumor lysis resulting from high-dose chemotherapy. Early symptoms of renal failure include anuria and acid-based imbalances from the lack of elimination of nitrogenous wastes, water, electrolytes, and acids. Renal dysfunction in marrow transplant recipients usually is mild, and patients can be managed by dose adjustments of medications and careful fluid regulation. After allogeneic transplantation, however, 5% to 10% of patients will require renal dialysis; mortality is 85% in this group.

*Nursing implications* Nursing assessment for acute tubular necrosis focuses on early recognition of symptoms of either prerenal or intrarenal failure. It includes the monitoring of routine vital signs, with postural blood pressures, determination of urine specific gravity, measurement of urine electrolytes, and determination of accurate intake and output of bodily fluids. Complaints of thirst or dizziness or indications of mental confusion are also indicators of renal compromise. Distended neck veins or peripheral edema must be noted. Correct determination of abdominal girth and daily weight are important nursing assessments to distinguish between prerenal and intrarenal conditions. Knowledge of interactions and adverse effects of the pharmacological agents given to the recipient is also imperative.[68]

## Veno-occlusive disease of the liver

Veno-occlusive disease is almost exclusive to BMT, and is the most common nonrelapse life-threatening complication of preparative-regimen-related toxicity for bone marrow transplantation.[79-81] Peak onset is 21 weeks after transplant. The diagnosis of VOD often is clouded by overlapping BMT-related symptoms. Risk factors for developing VOD include: (1) patients with hepatitis and infections before BMT, (2) those who receive repeated doses of chemotherapy prior to transplant in addition to high-dose irradiation in pretransplant conditioning regimens, (3) the use of antimicrobial therapy with acyclovir, amphotericin, or vancomycin, (4) and mismatched or unrelated allogeneic marrow grafts.

*Clinical manifestations* Liver damage caused by chemoradiotherapy involves two histopathological processes: (1) venule occlusion and/or veno-occlusive process involving terminal hepatic venules and sublobular veins and (2) hepatocyte necrosis. Clinical symptoms, which occur in the first weeks after transplantation, include rapid fluid retention, sudden weight gain, abdominal distention, pain in the right upper quadrant of the abdomen, jaundice, hepatomegaly, icteric skin and sclerae, encephalopathy, possible bleeding, and elevated serum bilirubin levels. These symptoms are the result of significant obstruction and intrasinusoidal hypertension. Morbidity ranges from 21%–50%.

*Treatment* Currently, there is no prevention or treatment for VOD, although researchers are exploring the use of prostaglandins, tumor necrosis factor, and ursodexecholic acid. Treatment with recombinant tissue plasminogen activator holds some promise but prospective randomized trials should occur. Symptom management and supportive measures to maintain the patient until the VOD has run its course are the mainstay of care. Treatment consists of fluid management, with diuresis and restriction of water. Hematocrit levels should be kept above 35% to maintain intravascular volume and renal perfusion. Supportive care must include the respiratory system as well because of fluid overload.[82] An interesting note: Marrow recipients who require renal dialysis also have VOD because of liver-kidney hemodynamic interaction. As the number of unrelated marrow transplants increases concomitant with more toxic conditioning regimens, the greater the need to identify preventive treatment techniques for this illusive syndrome.

*Nursing implications* Continuous and careful monitoring of the fluid status of the patient is a nursing responsibility. This includes weighing the patient twice a day, obtaining daily abdominal girth measurements, monitoring for signs of bleeding, monitoring postural blood pressures, and administering and monitoring the effectiveness of diuretics and colloids.

## Pulmonary complications

Pulmonary complications are a major cause of morbidity and mortality occurring in up to 40%–60% of recipients appearing as early and late sequelae. They occur as a result of chemoradiotherapy toxicity or bacterial, viral, or fungal infection in severely immunosuppressed patients.[83,84] Complications include alveolar capillary injury characterized by increased pulmonary vascular permeability, leakage of plasma into the pulmonary interstitium, and reduced pulmonary compliance. Pulmonary VOD, however, is rare.[85] Pulmonary edema syndromes caused by sodium excess and cardiomyopathy, myocarditis, and volume overload from VOD can occur immediately after transplant. Early complications, caused by severe mucositis, can occur days after marrow transplantation, and aspiration of secretions and blood can lead to upper airway obstruction that requires intubation. Interstitial pneumonia presents symptoms similar to those of adult respiratory distress syndrome (ARDS) and occurs early (before day 100) or late (after day 100) of transplantation.

***Clinical manifestations***   Manifestations of pneumonia may include nonproductive cough, dyspnea, hypoxemia, and fever. A chest x-ray may demonstrate evidence of interstitial infiltrates and arterial blood gas levels may show hypoxia. These symptoms have rapid onset in the compromised host, and the patient's condition deteriorates quickly. Differential diagnosis must be made rapidly to ensure appropriate treatment. Bronchoalveolar lavage with centrifugation culture, rather than an open lung biopsy, has improved the care of the marrow recipient with pneumonia by eliminating surgery and hastening identification of causative organisms and treatment. CMV antigenemia assays consisting of direct staining of granulocyte-enriched peripheral blood leukocytes with monoclonal antibodies is currently under investigation for more rapid accurate detection of CMV pneumonia.[86] Practices for CMV diagnosis, prophylaxis, and treatment continue to be the subject of serious discussion worldwide.[87,88] Major aims are focused on reaching consensus in management of this major hurdle in transplant medicine.

***Interstitial pneumonia***   Interstitial pneumonia is a process that occurs in the interstitial spaces of the lungs. It occurs in approximately 35% of allogeneic marrow recipients and is the most frequent cause of death during the first 100 days after transplant. The overall mortality rate from interstitial pneumonia is approximately 20% in allogeneic recipients transplanted for advanced hematologic malignancy.[85]

***CMV pneumonia***   CMV pneumonia is the leading cause of infectious pneumonia after BMT. It occurs in 20% of patients who receive allogeneic marrow transplantation and has a fatality rate up to 85%. The incidence of CMV pneumonia may be higher in the allograft versus autograft recipients because of prolonged periods of immunosuppression caused by medication. Onset of early CMV is greatest between 5 and 13 weeks after transplanta-

tion. High-risk factors include: (1) patients older than 30 years of age, (2) severe GVHD, (3) TBI conditioning regimen, (4) CMV seropositivity in patients, and (5) advanced hematologic malignancies.[85] The most effective prophylaxis against CMV pneumonia is the avoidance of viral infection by infusing only CMV-negative blood products in cases in which both donor and patient demonstrated CMV seronegativity prior to BMT.[86-88] Patients who receive screened blood products must continue to do so through day 100 after BMT. The results of a five-year randomized study concluded that patients administered blood filtered through a mechanical device (experimental group) versus CMV blood screened at a blood bank (control) had a 2.4% probability of developing CMV infection compared to those who received screened products.[89] This percentage is within the acceptable rate of less than or equal to a 5% infection rate. This landmark study has wide implications. Marrow transplant recipients are the greatest users of blood products and the average patient receives approximately 23 units of RBCs and 120 units of platelets over the course of a treatment. The costs of processing blood products for CMV screening and the depletion of blood banks' stores of CMV negative blood for use in marrow and solid organ transplants have decreased.

Patients who are seropositive and whose donors are seropositive may benefit from the use of antiviral agents such as acyclovir, or from passive antibody prophylaxis with immunoglobulin. Recently over five studies using prophylactic ganciclovir have shown a reduction in CMV infection but without a reduction in transplant mortality.[90] Historically, treatment of CMV pneumonia has been largely unsuccessful, despite the use of various antiviral drugs and immunotherapeutic agents used alone or in combination therapy. However, treatment regimens that use combination ganciclovir and intravenous cytomegalovirus immunoglobulin have demonstrated a 40%–50% survival rate in marrow recipients whose diagnosis occurred during the initial episode of CMV pneumonia.

***Idiopathic pneumonia***   Idiopathic pneumonia accounts for 30% of all interstitial pneumonias in marrow recipients. It is believed to be a result of high-dose irradiation. Idiopathic pneumonia is diagnosed when no specific organism is recovered in bronchial lavage washings or lung biopsy tissue.[90]

***Other pneumonias***   Other pneumonias that occur may be caused by a virus (e.g., adenovirus, herpes simplex, or varicella zoster), bacteria, or fungus. These account for 15% of pneumonia in marrow recipients, and may be successfully treated. Respiratory syncytial virus (RSV) pneumonia has been identified in the BMT recipient.[91] RSV is a common cause of winter outbreaks of acute respiratory disease that causes a high death rate in the immunocompromised patient or neonate. Sources of acquired infection include infected patients, staff, visitors, or contaminated fomites. Strict attention to contact-isolation procedures must be reinforced once this virus is known to exist. Prophylaxis with intravenous RSV immunoglobulin for high-risk patients may become available during future RSV seasons and vaccines for RSV are being developed, but significant research is needed in this area before application to the transplant recipient can be assured.[92] Aerosolized ribavirin, successfully used in the neonate, has been used to manage BMT recipients with RSV, but research is needed to document treatment efficacy. *Pneumocystis carinii* pneumonia caused significant mortality in the early years of marrow transplantation, but has been successfully prevented by the use of prophylactic trimethoprim-sulfamethoxazole (TMP-SMX). Bacterial or fungal pneumonias are not a major cause of death in the marrow recipient.[70,93]

***Nursing implications***    The median time of onset for interstitial pneumonias is 60–70 days following BMT. Typically, patients have been discharged from the acute-care setting and are being followed up in a clinic or a physician's office. Classic symptoms are related to the patient's inability to engage in daily activities and may manifest as fatigue, malaise, and/or dyspnea. Patients must undergo routine chest x-rays and thorough physical examinations, including chest auscultation and determination of arterial blood gases in cases of suspected interstitial pneumonia. Readmission to the hospital is usually necessary, and patients may need respiratory support with mechanical ventilation.

## Neurological complications

Neurological and neuromuscular complications occur in 59%–70% of marrow recipients, with a resulting 6% fatality rate.[94] The peak time of onset is from pretransplantation to 21 days after transplantation. Neuropathy and somnolence occur earliest (−13 to −8 before BMT) while confusion or disorientation peak around 12 days after transplantation.[95] The underlying causes are pretransplant chemoradiotherapy, central nervous system infection, and immunosuppressive agents, such as cyclosporine, steroids, and intrathecal methotrexate. Neurological complications from hemorrhage are rare because of the administration of prophylactic platelet transfusions to prevent bleeding. Recurrence of malignancy after BMT may occur in the CNS in up to 38% of the recipients who receive no posttransplant intrathecal prophylaxis.[96]

Leukoencephalopathy has been reported in the 7% of marrow transplant recipients who have had prior cranial irradiation and intrathecal methotrexate. Symptoms include lethargy, somnolence, dementia, coma, and personality changes. Patients who receive cyclosporine for posttransplantation immunosuppression have documented hypomagnesemia, which can result in neurological sequelae, such as seizure activity.[94–99] Magnesium dosing differs among institutions. Oncology nurses are often the first to identify neurological alteration and neurological nursing assessments must be a part of the routine care of marrow recipients.

## Cardiac complications

Life-threatening cardiac complications can develop within several days following administration of high-dose cyclophosphamide and occur in approximately five to ten of recipients who receive cyclophosphamide-containing preparative regimens. Cardiomegaly, congestive heart failure, and fluid retention can develop, and can be managed with fluid balance to avoid iatrogenic pulmonary edema. These symptoms usually resolve during the first 100 days after BMT and have a fatality rate of less than 1%.[100] Assessment of patients includes obtaining a history of previous therapy with cardiotoxic drugs (e.g., doxorubicin) and monitoring cardiac function with routine electrocardiograms, cardiac ejection fractions, and exercise tolerance tests during the first 100 days after BMT.[101]

## Infection

Infections, as a result of profound immunosuppression caused by myeloablative therapy used in conditioning regimens and postBMT immunosuppression, remain a major impediment to successful marrow grafting. The duration of neutropenia differs relative to the number of stem cells used for marrow reconstitution, the occurrence of viral infections such as CMV, agents used in management of GVHD, and use of colony stimulating factors. The most common sites of infections are the gastrointestinal tract, oropharynx, lung, skin, and indwelling catheter sites.

Dramatic improvements during the past decade have reduced marrow-transplantation-related infection through the development of antimicrobial therapy, immunomodulators, new diagnostic techniques, and changes in blood transfusion therapy. The tempo and sequence of high-risk periods for bacterial, viral, fungal, and protozoal complications, which peak at predicted times after transplant, are well documented.[90]

The most common infections (90%) during the first month (preengraftment stage), are gram-negative and gram-positive bacterial infections, concomitant with fungal and herpes simplex virus. During the second and third months (early postengraftment stage), cytomegalovirus, fungi, gram-positive bacteria, and *Pneumocystis carinii* place marrow recipients at risk. After engraftment has been established, recipients are at risk for infection from encapsulated bacteria, varicella zoster, and *Pneumocystis carinii*.[90]

***Preengraftment (days 0–30)***    The herpes simplex virus (HSV) types I and II, Epstein-Barr virus, cytomegalovirus, and varicella zoster virus are the major viruses that occur in the first 30 days after BMT. Active HSV infection, which peaks at 17 days after the conditioning regimen is initiated, is caused almost exclusively by reactivation of HSV, and is seen in 70%–80% of seropositive patients. Oral ulceration is the common clinical manifestation of HSV type I infection, and genital ulcerations are caused by HSV type II reactivation. Mucocutaneous infections can contribute to decreased oral intake, severe pain, and serve as portals of entry for bacteria and fungi. Standard treatment for HSV is acyclovir. Considerable debate has existed about the prophylactic use of acyclovir for patients with histories of HSV because of the concern of the development of HSV resistance. Recent studies, however, have noted that the resistant virus can manifest itself during the treatment phase, but rarely during the prophylactic phase. Furthermore, debate continues about the economics of administering acyclovir versus the costs of suprainfection and patient discomfort. Treatment of acyclovir-resistant HSV is foscarnat and vivbrine. More research is needed in this area to test the possible toxic effects.[102]

Neutropenia with concomitant damage to mucosal surfaces contributes to gram-negative bacteremia immediately after transplantation. Classic approaches to management have been semisynthetic penicillin, plus an aminoglycoside administered empirically at the first sign of fever during neutropenia. The advantage of this strategy is potential synergy in treating the infection. The advent of the fluoroquinolones (e.g., norfloxacin, ciprofloxacin) and development of effective regimens that do not include aminoglycosides have improved the control and treatment of gram-negative infections. Aminoglycoside, a known nephrotoxic agent, further compromises renal toxicity in many allogeneic marrow recipients who are receiving nephrotoxic immunosuppressive therapy with cyclosporine.[90,103]

Profound immunosuppression with resulting neutropenia concomitant with denuding of the mucosa in the gastrointestinal tract places marrow recipients at risk for *Candida* infection. In addition, systemic *Candida* infections commonly occur during periods of neutropenia. The most common *Candida* species that cause infection are *C. tropicalis* and *C. albicans*. Amphotericin B is the agent of choice for the treatment of *Candida* infection. Newer strategies being explored include prophylaxis with imidazole. Intravenous miconazole has been shown to be an effective prophylactic agent, but its use is limited by its cost. Recently, fluconazole has shown to prevent colonization and infection with *Candida* species other than *C. krusei* and *Torulopsis glabrala*. Elevation of cyclosporine concentrations because of interaction between azoles and cyclosporine requires close monitoring of plasma drug levels. The advantages of fluconazole are that it can be administered either orally or intravenously and one daily dose may be sufficient.

*Aspergillus* is a major infectious problem during days 0–30. The portal of entry for *Aspergillus* infection is the respiratory tract, and the risk for *Aspergillus* infection increases with the duration and degree of neutropenia. Diagnosis from blood cultures is difficult, and percutaneous-needle, bronchoscopic, or open-lung biopsy may be used. Early diagnosis and aggressive treatment with high doses of amphotericin B in combination with flucytosine have improved survival outcomes in the marrow recipient. Less common fungal pathogens that have emerged in recent years include *Trichosporon* species, *C. lusitaniae*, *C. krusei*, and *Fusarium* species. Aggressive therapy with

high doses of amphotericin B and flucytosine is the recommended treatment.

***Early engraftment (days 30–90)***   Cytomegalovirus infection is the most significant infection during this phase and accounts for a 15%–20% mortality rate in marrow recipients. Risk factors are the presence of positive serological titers, GVHD, and the degree of HLA tissue-typing between patient and donor. The most severe CMV disease after BMT is interstitial pneumonitis, which is reviewed elsewhere in this chapter. CMV enteritis and retinitis occur less frequently in the marrow recipient.[104]

Bacterial infections are less frequent from day 30 to day 90 following marrow transplantation. Gram-positive infections associated with the central lumen catheter present a major risk for systemic infection. Gram-negative septicemia or infection related to flushing right atrial catheters has been documented in the outpatient setting.[105]

Fungal infections are problematic during this recovery phase, and marrow recipients with GVHD are at higher risk for infections than recipients without GVHD. *Pneumocystis carinii* pneumonia accounts for 10% of interstitial pneumonitis in marrow recipients.[70] Open-lung biopsy and bronchoscopic washings remain classic diagnostic measures, and trimethoprim-sulfamethoxazole (TMP-SMX) is effective as a preventive and therapeutic agent. Aerosolized pentamidine is an alternative therapy for those patients who report true allergies to TMP-SMX. Long-term effectiveness of aerosolized pentamidine has not been evaluated.

***Clinical manifestations***   Fever is the cardinal symptom of infection. The neutropenic condition of marrow recipients masks the classic infection-related symptoms of inflammation, pus formation, and elevated white blood cell counts. Consequently, cultures of blood, throat, urine, stool, and sputum are necessary to identify and treat pathogenic organisms. Risk factors associated with life-threatening infections and measures to treat and prevent infections are outlined in Table 18-7.

***Treatment***   Prevention and treatment of infection in the marrow recipient BMT patient is aimed at identifying the invasive organism and treating the accompanying infection with appropriate antibiotics. Antimicrobial therapy has proven to be successful, while granulocyte transfusions have been largely abandoned.[1] The role of immunoglobulin (Ig) therapy in marrow transplantation continues to be studied and potential uses of Ig include: (1) modifying or preventing CMV infections and CMV-related interstitial pneumonia, (2) decreasing GVHD, (3) preventing infections other than CMV, and (4) treating autoimmune complications of marrow grafting. Results of studies indicate that Ig given before and at 100 days posttransplant reduced the incidence of CMV pneumonia.[104,106] The expense of this therapy should be balanced against the likely gains and the overall costs of alternative approaches.

**TABLE 18-7** Nursing and Medical Management of Infection in the Bone Marrow Transplant Recipient

| Possible Infections | Incidence Rate | Cause | Nursing Management | Diagnostic Tools | Medical Management |
|---|---|---|---|---|---|
| PHASE I: DAYS 0–30 | | | | | |
| **Bacterial** Gram negative Gram positive | 100% | High-dose chemotherapy and TBI; immuno-suppressive drugs for TBI | Complete nursing assessments, with particular attention to mouth and central catheter site; vital signs q 2–4 hr; administration of antibiotics; pan cultures in presence of fever or chilling; surveillance cultures; ice packs and cooling blankets | Blood and tissue cultures, chest x-rays, CAT scan | Prophylactic treatment with antibiotics, (e.g., fluoroquinolones (nafloxacin, ciprofloxacin), aminoglycosides, antilipopoly-saccharide antibodies); LAF, HEPA filter rooms, masks, hand washing; colony stimulating factors |
| **Viral** Herpes simplex I and II, Epstein-Barr, CMV | 70%–80% | CMV reactivation; high-dose chemotherapy and TBI | Complete nursing assessments, with particular attention to mouth, genital areas | Blood and tissue cultures, chest x-rays, acid-fast cultures | Prophylactic treatment with acyclovir |
| Adenovirus | 5% | CMV reactivation; high-dose chemotherapy and TBI | Stool cultures | Stool cultures | Appropriate antibiotics |
| **Fungal** *Candida tropicalis, albicans* | 100% | CMV reactivation; high-dose chemotherapy and TBI; broad-spectrum antibiotics | Complete nursing assessments, with particular attention to mouth and central catheter site; vital signs q 2–4 hr; administration of antibiotics; pan cultures in presence of fever or chilling; surveillance cultures | Blood and tissue cultures, chest x-rays, CAT scan, needle biopsy | Amphotericin B, imidazole, miconazole, fluconazole, iatraconazole |
| *Aspergillus, Trichosporon* species, *C. lusitaniae, C. krusei, Fusarium* species | 100% | High-dose chemotherapy and TBI | Complete nursing assessments, with particular attention to mouth and central catheter site; vital signs q 2–4 hr; administration of antibiotics; pan cultures in presence of fever or chilling; surveillance cultures | Percutaneous needle biopsy, bronchoscopy, open lung biopsy | Prophylactic treatment with antifungals, amphotericin B, flucytosine |
| PHASE II: DAYS 30–90 | | | | | |
| Bacterial | 100% | High-dose chemotherapy and TBI; immuno-suppressive drugs, | Complete nursing assessments, with particular attention to mouth and | Blood and tissue cultures, chest x-rays, CAT scan | Prophylactic treatment with anti-biotics (e.g., |

**TABLE 18-7**  Nursing and Medical Management of Infection in the Bone Marrow Transplant Recipient (continued)

| Possible Infections | Incidence Rate | Cause | Nursing Management | Diagnostic Tools | Medical Management |
|---|---|---|---|---|---|
| | | central lumen catheter | central catheter site; vital signs q 2–4 hr; administration of antibiotics; pan cultures in presence of fever or chilling; surveillance cultures | | fluoroquinolones (nafloxacin, ciprofloxacin), aminoglycosides, antilipopoly-saccharide antibodies); colony stimulating factors |
| **Viral** CMV pneumonia | 20% allogeneic 2% autologous | CMV-positive recipient or donor; advanced hematologic malignancy; mismatched patients | Complete nursing assessment; assessment for cough, dyspnea, hypoxemia; vital signs q 2–4 hr; chest auscultation | Bronchial lavage and centrifugation culture, chest x-ray, arterial blood gases | Immunoglobulin, acyclovir, CMV-negative blood products, leukopoor, blood products |
| Respiratory syncytial virus (RSV) | Unknown | High-dose chemotherapy and TBI; RSV+ | Complete nursing assessment; assessment for cough, dyspnea, hypoxemia | Bronchial washings | Ribavirin |
| **Fungal** *Pneumocystis carinii* pneumonia | 80% or higher with GVHD | High-dose chemotherapy and TBI | Complete nursing assessment; determine patient compliance for TMP-SMX | Chest x-ray, CAT scans | Prophylactic treatment; aerosolized pentamidine treatments |
| **PHASE III: DAYS 100 TO 2 YEARS** | | | | | |
| **Bacterial** Pneumonia, encapsulated bacteria, *Streptococcus pneumoniae*, *Neisseria meningitidis*, *Haemophilus influenzae*, septicemia, sinusitis | Unknown | High-dose chemotherapy and TBI; chronic GVHD | Complete nursing assessment; monitoring of chest x-rays; assessment for sinusitis, sepsis; assessment for patient compliance for medications | Chest x-ray, sputum culture | TMP-SMX prophylactically, appropriate antibiotic therapy; wearing mask, hand washing, avoiding crowds; immunizations after 1 yr without GVHD; immune testing with GVHD |
| **Viral** Varicella zoster virus | 25%–40% | High-dose chemotherapy and TBI; reactivation of HZV | Complete nursing assessment, with attention to prodromal symptoms of pain, itching, burning | | Acyclovir 500 mg/kg IV q 8 hr for 7–10 days; HZV immunoglobulin for seropositive recipients exposed to HZV |

*TBI*, total-body irradiation; *CAT*, computerized axial tomography; *LAF*, laminar air flow room; *HEPA*, high-efficiency particulate air; *CMV*, cytomegalovirus; *RSV*, respiratory syncytial virus; *GVHD*, graft-versus-host disease; *TMP-SMX*, trimethoprim-sulfamethoxazole; *HZV*, herpes zoster varicella.

***Nursing implications*** Astute nursing assessments are important in determining the onset and course of infectious problems. Fever may be associated with GVHD and administration of blood and drug products. Steroid administration in immunosuppressed patients masks fever and nurses need to be alert to the subtle signs of infection. Current research continues to examine the effects of more palatable oral antibiotics for gastrointestinal decontamination. It is hoped that these drugs will provide optimal patient compliance while preventing bacterial and fungal infections.

## DISCHARGE FROM THE HOSPITAL

Hospital discharge after allogeneic BMT averages 20–25 days and will differ among institutions.[107] The use of CSFs has decreased the length of hospital stays for autologous recipients, but has not been as dramatic for the allogeneic recipients. Nonetheless the number of days that allogeneic patients remain hospitalized has become increasingly shorter in direct response to the current economic climate. Recipients are being discharged to outpatient settings supported with multiple antibiotics, blood component therapy, and hyperalimentation. Accordingly, the profile of the newly discharged patient is one of higher acuity and symptomatology. Paralleling these events are additional family caregiver responsibilities that can further complicate the outpatient course of numerous allogeneic recipients. Consequently institutions offering "outpatient transplants" or short hospitalizations are making enormous efforts to prepare caregivers for responsibilities for management of the marrow recipient outside of the hospital setting. Some institutions are offering outpatient TBI as well as dose-intensive chemotherapy.[108] Guidelines to prepare the patient/family for discharge are outlined in Table 18-8. Chielens and Herrick have described the discharge process and the role of the discharge planner.[109]

### Discharge Criteria

Established discharge criteria for marrow recipients are becoming more liberal because of new trends in outpatient care. Antimicrobial and biotechnological therapies have helped to diminish the effects of transplantation-related complications, and sophisticated infusion pump technology permits patients to receive numerous intravenous therapies in outpatient settings. In addition, economic pressures prompt earlier discharge for patients who, until recently, would have remained in the hospital for their care. Discharge criteria for marrow recipients differ among institutions and depend on the stability of the patient, the presence of skilled outpatient teams, and caregiver support at home.[107] The following are represen-

**TABLE 18-8** Patient and Caregiver Guidelines upon Discharge from the Hospital

**Report the following symptoms**
- Fever >38.4°C (101.4°F)
- Difficulty flushing the central or peripheral catheter
- Bleeding of any kind
- Frequent urination or pain and burning on urination
- Redness, swelling, itching of skin
- Pain in any part of the body
- Cough, sneezing, runny nose, shortness of breath, or discomfort in the chest
- Light sensitivity to the eyes; blurring of vision, burning, itching, or sense of "grittiness" in the eyes
- Inability to sweat or perspire
- Redness, swelling, or drainage from the central catheter site
- Blisters around the mouth or in the genital area
- Any beeping or alarming of pump if receiving home infusion therapy

**Further guidelines**
- Report any problem or concern.
- Report all tests, examinations, and procedures.
- Take and record your medications. Renew all prescriptions immediately.
- Do not receive immunizations until advised by the physician.
- Avoid children or other persons who have had live-virus vaccines (such as the Sabin oral polio vaccine, measles, mumps, rubella, yellow fever, or small pox).

**Personal health guidelines**
- Avoid crowds for 6 months after bone marrow transplantation.
- Avoid swimming in public swimming areas until the central lumen or peripheral catheter is removed.
- Take a daily shower or bath using a mild soap. Use skin lotions without alcohol.
- Avoid sharing personal care items with family members (e.g., towels, combs, washcloths).
- Daily, brush your teeth with a soft toothbrush and floss. Use saline rinses for a mouthwash, and avoid commercial mouthwashes.
- Practice safe sex; use condoms or dental dams.
- Keep your home environment clean. However, it is not necessary to sterilize personal items, such as dishes, and cooking areas.
- Avoid cleaning cat litter boxes, fish bowls, and bird cages.
- Houseplants may remain in the home environment, but avoid cut flowers in water, which harbor bacteria.

tative discharge criteria common among marrow transplantation centers:

- availability of 24-hour outpatient medical care provided by a multidisciplinary outpatient BMT team

- evidence of oral intake requirements

- nausea, vomiting, and pain controlled without IV medications

- diarrhea controlled at <500 ml/day

- a platelet count supportable at 5000–15,000 mm$^3$

- granulocytes >500 mm$^3$ for 24 hours

- hematocrit >25%

- tolerating PO medications for 24 hours (i.e., narcotics, antihypertensives, cyclosporine, and prednisone)

- family support at home

Ideally, patients and a strong support person need to reside near the transplant center until discharged home to the referring care physician. Comprehensive outpatient care of the BMT recipient patient consists of daily-to-weekly clinic visits to assess the patient's stability. Blood products, parenteral nutrition, intravenous medications, and procedures can be delivered effectively in ambulatory care settings. Clear, consistent patient/family teaching aimed at prevention and early recognition of transplant-related problems must be emphasized. Because a large portion of the care of the allogeneic recipient is being given in outpatient areas, family caregivers need to be taught their expanding roles and increased responsibilities throughout the transplant trajectory. Patients and families are taught to prevent infections by avoiding crowds, school, and work for one year after BMT. Currently, the readmission rate is 50% for treatment of fever and neutropenia.[110]

# CLINICAL MANAGEMENT OF THE BMT OUTPATIENT

The role of ambulatory care and home care for the marrow recipient has gained dramatic importance in the face of economic mandates for cost containment. A major bone marrow transplant center recently studied the effects of early discharge relative to morbidity, mortality, nursing management, caregiver burden, and psychological measures of care. One hundred and forty patients were randomized to early discharge with outpatient clinic and home care support or traditional discharge with outpatient support only. The investigators found that there was no greater morbidity and mortality, number of hospital days over 100 days after BMT, or out-of-pocket expenses in the early discharge group compared to the traditional group. An additional important finding was that there was no decrease in overall costs because of the additional expense of home care for the early discharge patients.[111] This study serves as an important model for changing clinical practices and scrutinizing costs and charges. The role of outpatient nursing was also under-

scored. Early identification and management of multi-symptomatic patients by outpatient and home care nurses contributed significantly to the success of outpatient management as evidenced by equal readmission rates in each group. Another study emphasized the importance of nursing support for marrow recipients in outpatient settings during the first four weeks following BMT.[112] By 30–34 days, BMT recipients were found to have an increase in positive thinking and physical activity, to want their families to be present, and to want physicians to be consistent and responsible in meeting their needs. They viewed nurses as the coordinators of their care and the ones to "keep things in order."[112] The importance of nursing in outpatient settings is further evidenced by the increase in nurse-managed outpatient clinics staffed with advance practice nurses working in concert with transplant physicians.

## Outpatient Home Care

Outpatient care requires keen clinical management as well as nursing care delivered by oncology nurses highly knowledgeable of the BMT process, possible complications, and appropriate medications. As more acutely ill patients are cared for in outpatient settings, management of early complications typically restricted to hospital care are now a common challenge. Home care for the marrow recipient and family caregiver has become an increasingly important service. Sophisticated ambulatory pump technology and the growing number of nurses experienced in care of the marrow transplant recipient allow patients to receive administration of large volumes of IV fluids, multiple antibiotics, and blood component therapy in their homes. Numerous corporate and hospital-based home care programs exist. Clinic and home care teams must outline communication pathways so that duplication of services is avoided, emergency care is efficient, continuity of care is established, and cost containment is monitored. If the BMT center contracts with outside home care providers, joint inservicing and cross training of home care staff will reassure patients and families of continuity of care.[113]

Chronic complications of BMT may appear around 80 days after BMT. The outpatient and home care staff must be able to distinguish the tempo, duration, signs, and symptoms of acute and chronic GVHD, herpes, varicella zoster, cytomegalovirus, *Pneumocystis carinii* pneumonia, sexually transmitted diseases, and other transplantation-related problems. Symptom management of the BMT outpatient is accomplished with a multidisciplinary team of physicians, nurses, dietitians, dentists, and social workers. Common marrow-transplant-related symptoms and their possible causes are shown in Table 18-9. The numerous tests and evaluations needed to assess, manage, and treat BMT recipients are presented in Table 18-10. Historically, marrow recipients remain under the care of the BMT team until approximately 100 days after BMT. Because of cost containment measures centers are

**TABLE 18-9** Common Outpatient Allogeneic Marrow-Transplant-Related Symptoms and Their Possible Causes

| Symptoms | Possible Causes |
|---|---|
| Fever | Bacterial (gram-negative, gram-positive sepsis), fungal infection (Candida, Aspergillus) Interstitial pneumonia (bacterial, viral, idiopathic) Herpes simplex virus, varicella zoster GVHD Hepatitis Granulocytopenia Blood product transfusions/drug toxicity Recurrent disease |
| Nausea, vomiting | GVHD Gastrointestinal infection (CMV, Salmonella, Shigella, C. difficile) |
| Diarrhea | Mucositis Leukoencephalopathy, encephalitis, subdural hematoma Septicemia Adrenal insufficiency Liver disease Cholecystitis, pancreatitis Hyperalimentation withdrawal Psychological Drug toxicity |
| Bleeding | Thrombocytopenia GVHD, gut Hemorrhagic cystitis Drug-related (prednisone) Herpes simplex virus infection |
| Pruritus | Acute and chronic GVHD Herpes varicella zoster Drug toxicity Blood product transfusions |
| Rash | GVHD, HSV, drug toxicity |
| Fatigue | Drug-related (interferon) Altered sleep patterns Premature menopause Psychological stress |
| Dyspnea | Sinopulmonary infection Restrictive, obstructive lung disease CMV pneumonia |
| Pain | Herpes zoster, relapse GVHD Peptic ulcer disease Mucositis Gastritis |
| Weight loss | Dehydration Relapse Mucositis GVHD Drug-related therapy Depression Malabsorption Body image |

**TABLE 18-9** Common Outpatient Allogeneic Marrow-Transplant-Related Symptoms and Their Possible Causes (continued)

| Symptoms | Possible Causes |
|---|---|
| Vasomotor instability: nervousness, anxiety, irritability, depression | Leukoencephalopathy Premature menopause, drug toxicity Hypomagnesemia |
| Jaundice | GVHD Infection Drug toxicity Hepatitis |
| Body image changes | Alopecia GVHD Wearing a mask Corticosteroids Drug-related (cyclosporine/prednisone) Hyperalimentation High-dose chemotherapy, TBI Presence of venous access catheter Early menopause/sterility Growth and development problems |
| Psychological: role changes, adaptation/integration into community | Issues of survival Feelings of taking advantage of donor Rehabilitation needs Rebirth or Lazarus syndrome Survival syndrome Role changes within family |

Adapted with permission from Corcoran PC: Ambulatory care of the bone marrow transplant patient. *Puget Sound Quarterly, Oncology Nursing Society* 12:4–7, 1989

forced to discharge patients to their home as soon as they are relatively stable. Most allogeneic recipients experience at least three months of severe immune deficiency. Consequently, they are at considerable risk for bacterial, viral, and fungal infections. Evidence of improvement and return of immune function generally is seen between six and nine months after BMT. Immune recovery is delayed in allogeneic patients with chronic GVHD. The consequence of the syndrome is discussed elsewhere in this chapter.[75]

## 100-Day Evaluation

An evaluation determining the allogeneic recipient's stability and risk factors for discharge home is usually initiated approximately 80 days after BMT (Table 18-11). If the patient remains at the BMT center during this time, the patient's BMT course is reviewed, and a final discharge conference is scheduled with the physician, the patient, and the family. A nurse from the continuing care team attending this meeting can ensure continuity of care and bridge the gap between outpatient care and the outpatient's referring care physician. If the patient has returned to the primary care physician, exquisite coordination between the BMT center and the primary care physician is

**TABLE 18-10**  Typical Assessments, Procedures, and Tests for Allogeneic Bone Marrow Transplantation Outpatients

- One to two clinic visits a week for full medical and nursing assessment to monitor for BMT-related problems
- Weekly assessments with the nutrition team for evaluation for parenteral support and nutritional counseling
- Once-a-month examination with the medical dental department to determine infection status of mouth for fungal, viral, and bacterial overgrowth
- Once-a-week consultations with social worker to assess ongoing psychological/social needs
- Consultation with gynecologists for all postpubertal women for evaluation of possible early menopause and sexual dysfunction
- Consultation visits with ophthalmologist, cardiologist, renal pulmonary physician, gynecologist, infectious disease physician as needed
- Weekly evaluation of medication schedules and refills of medications

**Procedures routinely required for BMT outpatient**
- Daily to twice weekly blood draws to monitor blood chemistries, and engraftment and immune recovery status
- Once or twice weekly urine tests for infection surveillance
- Weekly throat cultures for infection surveillance
- Periodic bone marrow aspirations and biopsies for evaluation of engraftment and disease status
- Intrathecal methotrexate for prophylaxis against central nervous system disease
- Skin biopsies for evaluation of graft-versus-host disease and diagnosis of other possible skin ailments
- Pulmonary function test and arterial blood gases for assessment of potential interstitial pneumonia
- Weekly surveillance chest x-rays for assessment of ongoing pulmonary complications

**TABLE 18-11**  Evaluation of Allogeneic Marrow Transplant Recipients Prior to Their Return Home

**All marrow transplantation recipients**
- Pulmonary function test and arterial blood gases for possible infection and obstructive/restrictive lung disease
- Bone marrow aspiration and biopsy to establish engraftment and disease state (remission or relapse)
- Complete blood counts and serum alkaline phosphatase, SGOT, bilirubin to evaluate hepatic function
- Follicle-stimulating hormone and testosterone levels to evaluate gonadal function
- Serological indicators for return of immune function: ANA, AMA, ASMA, RA, IgA, IgM, IgE; C3, C4 (complement studies); immunoglobulin subclasses, immunoglobulin titer; direct Coombs test
- Repeated CAT scans and x-rays performed at pretransplant evaluation for comparison to determine possible underlying disease
- Medical-dental examination for dental caries, xerostomia
- Gynecologic examination for postpubertal women for sexual counseling and prescribing of appropriate gonadal hormones
- Physical assessment of the skin and skin biopsy to determine possible skin graft-versus-host disease
- Physical assessment of the eye to determine ocular GVHD
- Schirmer's tear test to determine "dry" eye
- Physical assessment of the mouth to assess for chronic graft-versus-host disease

*GVHD,* graft-versus-host disease.

required to orchestrate numerous tests, blood sampling, and procedures to determine risks of future problems.

GVHD is only one of the many potential long-term sequelae of BMT. Other potential transplantation-related problems are assessed before a marrow recipient's return to the care of the primary physician. These tests are critical to the quality of patients' long-term recovery and the data amassed contribute to the research determining factors affecting patients after BMT and their disease-free long-term survival. Marrow recipients view this "final" process with a mixture of anxiety and excitement. Relapse or treatment failure remains a limiting factor in BMT, and it may be at this critical time that a patient is found to have relapsed. In this case, the patient and his or her significant others are given the diagnosis, prognosis, and alternate plans of care. Options may include chemotherapy, irradiation, a second BMT, or hospice care. Outpatient nurses need to act as essential coordinators to orchestrate procedures and tests and to support the pa-

tient through this final phase of care. The importance of the referring care oncology team has risen to new levels in supporting the recipient after return from the transplant center because of earlier discharge.

Community-based physicians and nurses can expect to see a patient at least weekly for the first month alone. If no new medical problems develop and the patient is stable, these intervals can be lengthened to two weeks for the next two months, and eventually to three-week or monthly intervals depending on the patient's clinical status. Monitoring of liver function tests, chest x-rays, complete blood counts, food intake, and weekly weights (on the same scale) is considered routine care during this period. Nurses caring for BMT recipients spend a large part of their nursing time teaching and reassuring patients and their families, assessing for infection and potential long-term complications, and interacting with long-term follow-up teams at the BMT center. Communication between community-based oncologists and long-term follow-up teams is essential to care for the growing number of long-term survivors of BMT. Nurses working in long-term follow-up settings triage and serve as liaison between BMT physicians and referring oncologists. Historically, all communication has been done by telephone. Facsimile machines now facilitate the exchange of information and aid in early diagnosis of transplant-related problems.

As economic constraints in health care systems continue, more allogeneic marrow recipients will be sent home prior to the traditional 100th day after BMT. This will increase the demand for keen nursing assessment skills as well as for sophisticated long-term follow-up systems. Copel and Smith[114] studied a select group of inpatient BMT nurses' knowledge of GVHD and found that nurses who participated in journal reading and who attended conferences relevant to GVHD scored higher than BMT nurses who did not. Like BMT nurses, community-based nurses will benefit from active participation in educational activities. Administrative managers are encouraged to budget time and money for nurses to pursue these opportunities.

## Annual Assessments

Patients typically return to the BMT center for annual evaluations for up to three years following BMT, to identify current or impending problems associated with the BMT. Outpatient nurses are extensively involved in annual assessments and procedures. Sensitive nursing support is needed because patients and their families revisiting the facility will recall the emotional experiences associated with the BMT. The marrow recipient usually wants to visit with clinical staff. Patients may not understand when staff are too busy to stop and make hall visits. Solutions to this dilemma include providing continuity of care through nurse practitioners, or a social event scheduled by clinic staff at which patients, their families, and staff can renew acquaintances.

## LATE COMPLICATIONS OF BMT

The number of marrow recipients living disease-free for years after BMT increases annually. It is estimated that more than 10,000 allogeneic marrow recipients survive five years after transplantation; some have survived more than 20 years.[115] Many recipients, however, will encounter late complications. Late complications, like the acute complications, are a direct result of high-dose conditioning regimens, GVHD and its long-term immunosuppressive management, and other transplant-related insults. Late complications are defined as those developing 100 days or more after transplant.[107,115] The incidence, time period, manifestations, and interventions of these late effects are outlined in Tables 18-12[116] and 18–13.

## Chronic Graft-Versus-Host Disease (Allogeneic BMT)

Allogeneic marrow recipients remain at considerable risk for chronic GVHD despite extensive research. Risk factors include mismatched donors/recipients, female to male transplants, positive herpes simplex and CMV virus, over 18 years of age, prior grade 2–3 acute GVHD, and CML recipients who received methotrexate and cyclosporine as chronic GVHD prophylaxis. Risk factors are cumulative and those recipients who have more complications have a higher probability of extensive chronic GVHD. Chronic GVHD typically develops more than three months after transplantation and differs from acute GVHD in both clinical presentation and target organs affected.[117–120] Figure 18-7 identifies the organ system involvement of chronic GVHD.

Chronic GVHD is a major cause of morbidity after allogeneic BMT and occurs in 33% of HLA-identical transplants, 49% of HLA-mismatched family members, and 65% of unrelated donor marrow transplantations. In addition, the time to onset of chronic GVHD is shortened with greater allogeneic mismatch transplants. For example, onset for HLA-identical siblings is 201 days versus 159 days for mismatched family members versus 133 days for unrelated donors.[115] Chronic GVHD is a multisystem disorder of the skin, mouth, eyes, sinuses, liver, gut, vaginal mucosa, serosal surfaces, and pulmonary, nervous, urologic, hematopoietic, lymphoid, and endocrine systems.[116–119] Figure 18-8 depicts chronic GVHD of the skin. Clinical and pathological findings resemble several naturally occurring autoimmune diseases, such as scleroderma, lupus erythematosus, lichen planus, rheumatoid arthritis, and Sorgen's syndrome (sicca syndrome).

### Onset and classification

The onset of chronic GVHD may be progressive, quiescent, or de novo. *Progressive* onset, a direct extension of acute GVHD, has the poorest prognosis. *Quiescent* onset develops after clinical resolution of acute GVHD, and these patients have a fair prognosis. Patients with *de novo* onset have had no prior acute disease and have the best prognosis. Chronic GVHD may be limited or extensive. Limited disease targets only the skin and liver and has a favorable course if untreated, whereas extensive disease affects numerous organ systems and can be fatal if not treated.

### Clinical manifestations of chronic GVHD

**Skin** The skin is affected in more than 70%–80% of patients diagnosed with chronic GVHD. Some patients have a sudden onset of erythema that can be activated by exposure to the sun. Other involvement can include the entire integument and produce alopecia and nail ridging. Initially, patients will complain of itching and burning of the skin. Patchy hyperpigmentation, mottled-appearing skin, or dyspigmentation may occur. In the extreme, fibrosis can result in joint contracture, skin ulcerations, and poor wound healing requiring extensive multidisciplinary collaboration that includes medical, nursing, dietary, and physical and occupational therapy (Figure 18–9—plate 9). Sweat gland function can be de-

**TABLE 18-12** Nursing and Medical Management of Possible Late Effects of Allogeneic Bone Marrow Transplantation Caused by High-Dose Chemotherapy and/or Irradiation in Conditioning Regimens

| Late Effect | Incidence Rate | Time PostBMT | Signs and Symptoms | Nursing Management | Diagnostic Tools | Medical Management |
|---|---|---|---|---|---|---|
| **Pulmonary complications** | | | | | | |
| Interstitial pneumonia Bronchiolitis obliterans | 10% | 3 mo to 2 yr | Cough, wheezing, dyspnea; decreased ability to perform daily living activities due to pulmonary insufficiency | Anticipatory teaching of pulmonary toilet; routine vital signs; chest x-ray; monitor PFT and ABG | Bronchial lavage washings, decreased midexpiratory flow, open lung biopsy | Prophylactic— TMP-SMX; Appropriate antibiotic therapy; ganciclovir; acyclovir; immuno-globulin |
| | | | | | | Antimicrobial therapy; high-dose steroids; cyclosporine; pred-nisone; colony stimulating factors; corticosteroids; pentami-dine, IV or aerosolized |
| Restrictive disease | 20% | | May be asymptomatic or cough | | Total lung capacity, diffusion capacity | Respiratory therapy; bronchodilation |
| Obstructive disease | 10% | | | | Pulmonary function test; IgG, IgA levels | Immuno-suppressive therapy |
| **Neurological complications** | | | | | | |
| Leukoencephalo-pathy | 7% | 1–5 mo | Lethargy, somnolence, dementia, seizures, spastic quadriplegia, coma, personality changes | Early intervention; multidisciplinary approach with special education program; routine neurological assessments | Periodic head computer-assisted tomography (CAT) scans of the head and psychometric evaluation | Symptomatic and supportive management |
| Impaired memory Learning disorders | Reported | Months to years | Loss of concentration, memory lapses, poor school/work performance | | | Rehabilitative consultation |
| Hypomagnesemia | Common occurrence | | Tremors, seizures | Monitor magnesium serum levels | | Magnesium replacement |
| **Cataracts** | | | | | | |
| Total-body irradiation, fractionated | 86% | 1.5–6 yr | Poor vision | Anticipatory teaching of BMT risk factors; ophthalmologist recommendation | Examination with slit-lamp microscopy | Intraocular lens replacement |
| Total-body irradiation, single dose | 100% | 1.5–6 yr | | | | |
| **Psychological complications** | 5%–10% | Months to years | Depression; weight change; altered body image; survival syndrome; sibling rivalry; altered concentration; decreased IQ levels in children | Allow patient/family to verbalize feelings; identify coping mechanisms, personal strengths; refer to mental health resources | Psychological testing | Mental health evaluation and treatment from appropriate source |

*(continued)*

**TABLE 18-12** Nursing and Medical Management of Possible Late Effects of Bone Marrow Transplantation Caused by High-Dose Chemotherapy and/or Irradiation in Conditioning Regimens (continued)

| Late Effect | Incidence Rate | Time PostBMT | Signs and Symptoms | Nursing Management | Diagnostic Tools | Medical Management |
|---|---|---|---|---|---|---|
| **Impaired growth in children** | | | | | | |
| Irradiation only | 100% | Months to years | Subnormal growth and development | Anticipatory teaching to patients/parents; annual evaluation of growth pattern; serial height/weight | Adrenocortical function; growth hormone; thyroid hormone | Possible appropriate hormone replacement; long-term follow-up |
| **Late infectious complications** | | | | | | |
| Bacterial Encapsulated bacteria *Haemophilus influenzae Streptococcus pneumoniae Neisseria meningitidis* | >50% | 3 mo to 1 yr | Fever, wheezing, rales, postnasal drip, signs of infection, unexplained fever, otitis media, sinusitis, bronchopulmonary infection, septicemia | Preventive teaching; mask-wearing until 6 mo postBMT; good hand-washing techniques; avoid infectious persons (measles, chicken-pox, mumps); avoid school/work, until 6 mo postBMT; avoid hot tubs, public swimming pools until 6–9 mo postBMT; limit number of sexual partners; avoid live-virus vaccines | Positive blood culture for bacteria, fungus, virus; abnormal chest x-ray studies, pulmonary function tests (PFT); pulmonary infiltrates; open lung biopsy; changes in CBC; decreased serum levels of IgG; impaired splenic reticuloendothelia function | Appropriate antibiotic support |
| Cytomegalovirus *Pneumocystis carinii* | 80%–100% 10% | 3 mo to 1 yr | Fever, sepsis, hypotension, lethargy; cough, dyspnea may be asymptomatic | Anticipatory preventive teaching; routine vital signs; chest auscultation and percussion (A&P); monitor PFT, arterial blood gases (ABG) | Chest x-ray studies, CBC, ABG, PFT; positive cultures for bacterial, fungal, and viral microorganisms; bronchoscopy; IgA, IgG levels | Prophylactic— TMP-SMX; appropriate antibiotic therapy; ganciclovir; acyclovir, immunoglobulin |
| Varicella zoster virus | | | | | | |
| Without chronic GVHD | <50% | 3 mo to 1 yr | Lesions, pain, malaise, tenderness, neurologic manifestation | Relieve pruritus with calamine lotion; cool compresses; prevent secondary infection | Positive herpes zoster varicella (HZV) cultures | Strict isolation until lesions are crusting; IV acyclovir 500 mg/m² q 8hr × 7 days |
| With chronic GVHD | >75% | | | | | |
| **Dental** Tooth decay | Known in children | 3 mo to 1 yr | Oral sicca syndrome; abnormal tooth development | Oral assessments, preventive teaching | Panorex | Dental medicine consults |
| **Avascular necrosis of the bone** | Reported | 3 mo to 1 yr | Limited range of motion in legs/hips, joint contractures; pain, swelling in areas of head of femur | Assess for history of steroid therapy | Computer-assisted tomography | Antimicrobial therapy, femur head replacement |
| **Genitourinary effects** | | | | | | |
| Bladder shrinkage Chronic urinary disorder | Reported | 4.5–26 mo | *Adenoviral*, CMV, *Viral,* polyomaviruses, bladder | Monitor urinary analyses, creatinine levels, assessment of urologic | Urinary analyses; culture and sensitivities; cystoscopy; | Appropriate antimicrobial therapy; urologic consultation |

**TABLE 18-12** Nursing and Medical Management of Possible Late Effects of Bone Marrow Transplantation Caused by High-Dose Chemotherapy and/or Irradiation in Conditioning Regimens (continued)

| Late Effect | Incidence Rate | Time PostBMT | Signs and Symptoms | Nursing Management | Diagnostic Tools | Medical Management |
|---|---|---|---|---|---|---|
| Radiation nephritis Hemolytic uremic syndrome Delayed-onset nephrotic syndrome | | | infections, hematuria, dysuria, vague abdominal pain | complaints, drug history for cyclo-sporine | increased serum creatinine levels | |
| Graft failure—marrow dysfunction | HLA-matched marrow—rare HLA-mis-matched—20% T-cell depleted—50% Autologous—20% | | Profound immuno-suppression, infection, bleeding, hypoxemia, relapse | Assessment for pancytopenia | CBC, bone marrow aspiration and biopsy; determine engraftment with cytogenetic analysis, ABO blood type, red cell antigen, enzyme markers | Supportive therapy |
| Second malignancy | 6%–22% | 1–14 yr | Fever, fatigue, swollen glands, abnormal bleeding, pain, night sweats | Complete nursing assessments; knowledge of treatment prescription; promote routine cancer screening | CBC, diagnostic CAT scans, x-rays, needle biopsy | Traditional cancer therapy, chemotherapy, irradiation |
| **GONADAL DYSFUNCTION** Effects of high-dose chemotherapy (single agent) | | | | | | |
| Females, prepubertal | Usually 0% | | Usually no abnormalities; menarche onset 12–13 yr | Careful monitoring of development | Tanner sexual maturity scales | |
| Males, prepubertal | Usually 0% | | Usually no abnormalities | Careful monitoring of development | | |
| Females <26 yr | 100% | | Usually no abnormalities; return of menstrual period, median = 6 mo | Menstrual history; fertility counseling | Normal luteinizing hormone (LH); normal follicle-stimulating hormone (FSH) | |
| Females >26 yr | 66% | Immediate | Premature menopause; sterility | Anticipatory teaching/counseling | LH levels; FSH levels | Cyclic hormone therapy |
| Males | 33% | Immediate | Sterility | Anticipatory teaching/counseling; semen analysis; sperm storage prior to BMT | Testosterone levels | Testosterone therapy, if appropriate |
| Effects of high-dose chemotherapy (high-dose cyclophospha-mide and busulfan without TBI) | | | | | | |
| Females | Unknown | Immediate | Sterility; premature menopause | Anticipatory teaching/counseling; menstrual history; fertility counseling | LH levels; FSH levels | Ova storage; cyclic hormone therapy |

*(continued)*

**TABLE 18-12** Nursing and Medical Management of Possible Late Effects of Bone Marrow Transplantation Caused by High-Dose Chemotherapy and/or Irradiation in Conditioning Regimens (continued)

| Late Effect | Incidence Rate | Time PostBMT | Signs and Symptoms | Nursing Management | Diagnostic Tools | Medical Management |
|---|---|---|---|---|---|---|
| Males | Unknown | Immediate | Sterility | Anticipatory teaching; sexual counseling | Gonadotropin; low sperm counts | Sperm storage prior to BMT; testosterone therapy, if appropriate |
| **Effects of high-dose irradiation** | | | | | | |
| Females, prepubertal | 100% | Immediate | Delayed onset of puberty; failure to reach menarche | Anticipatory teaching/ counseling | Tanner development scores; LH levels; FSH levels | Neuroendocrine evaluation; appropriate hormone therapy |
| Males, prepubertal | 100% | Immediate | Delayed onset of puberty | Anticipatory teaching/ counseling | Tanner development scores; testosterone levels | Neuroendocrine evaluation; testosterone therapy may be helpful |
| Males, adolescent | 100% | Immediate | Sterility | Sperm storage prior to BMT | Tanner development scores; gonadotropin; sperm counts | Testosterone therapy |
| Females | 95%–100% | Immediate | Premature menopause | Anticipatory teaching; sexual counseling | LH levels; FSH levels | Cyclic hormone therapy |
| Males | 95%–100% | Immediate | Sterility | Sperm storage prior to BMT; anticipatory teaching/ counseling | Gonadotropin; low sperm counts | Testosterone therapy |

Adapted from the *Oncology Nursing Forum* with permission from the Oncology Nursing Press, Inc. Corcoran-Buchsel P: Long-term complications of allogeneic bone marrow transplantation: Nursing implications. *Oncol Nurs Forum* 13:61–70, 1986.

creased, thereby impairing the body's ability to hydrate and cool itself leading to hyperthermia.

Skin biopsies may be required for differential diagnosis of chronic GVHD. Nurses and physicians need to ensure that platelet counts are adequate (approximately 20,000 mm³) before a skin biopsy is performed. Infection and bleeding may be a potential problem following skin biopsy. For recipients with severe dermal chronic GVHD, manifestations are similar to burn patients. Closure of portals of entry for infection may require skin allografting. The classic features of untreated chronic skin GVHD characterized by generalized bronze-colored hide-bound skin and pressure point ulceration accompanied by joint contractures are rare today. Nursing care of the patient with chronic skin GVHD requires thorough assessment of the integument and education of patient and family of prevention and/or palliative care of the many skin manifestations.

*Liver*   Liver disorders are observed in about 50% of patients with chronic GVHD. Pathological findings are characterized by damaged or absent small bile ducts with concomitant severe cholestasis similar to that seen in primary biliary cirrhosis. Alkaline phosphatase, serum glutamic oxaloacetic transaminase (SGOT), and bilirubin levels are elevated. With treatment, bilirubin values return to normal within several weeks, but elevated alkaline phosphatase and SGOT may persist for months. Drug metabolism may be altered and levels of blood clotting factors and albumin may be abnormal. Chronic liver GVHD manifests symptoms that mimic those of viral infection, heptotoxic drug reactions, gallstones, and infiltrative hepatic abnormalities.[21] Symptoms may include right upper quadrant pain, heptamomegaly, and jaundice. Bile acid displacement therapy with ursodexcholic acid has shown limited success as treatments for this problem but more research is needed in this area. Other patient management strategies include alteration of medications to maintain normal, therapeutic drug levels, and monitoring of liver function tests (LFTs), coagulation factors, fluid status, and albumin levels. Nursing management includes monitoring liver function laboratory values and an awareness that jaundice in a patient 3–12 months after BMT may indicate liver involvement in chronic GVHD (see Table 18-13).

**TABLE 18-13** Nursing and Medical Management of Late Effects of Allogeneic Bone Marrow Transplantation: Chronic Graft-Versus-Host Disease (GVHD)

| Late Effect | Incidence Rate | Time Post-BMT (days) | Signs and Symptoms | Nursing Management | Diagnostic Tools | Medical Management |
|---|---|---|---|---|---|---|
| Skin | 95% | 100–400 | Rough, scaly skin; malar erythema; generalized rash; hypo/hyper-pigmentation; dyspigmentation; premature graying; alopecia; joint contractures; scleroderma; loss of perspiration | Use of nonabrasive soaps, lotions, sunscreen; cosmetic support, makeup, wigs; range-of-motion activities; patient/family education; monitor compliance to treatment protocols | Skin biopsy positive for GVHD; Karnofsky score | Lanolin-based creams; possible systemic immunosuppressive therapy with cyclosporine, prednisone, Imuran |
| Liver | 30% | 100–400 | Jaundice | Infection precautions until differential diagnosis is made; monitor LFTs; low-fat diet | Alkaline phosphatase; SGOT; bilirubin | Possible systemic immunosuppressive therapy with cyclosporine, prednisone, Imuran |
| Oral | 80% | 100–400 | Pain, burning, dryness, irritation, soreness, loss of taste; lichenoid changes, atrophy, erythema in oral cavity; *Candida* infection; stomatitis; dental caries; xerostomia | Encourage soft, bland diet; dental hygiene education, soft toothbrush, flossing; saline rinses; dental medicine referral/recommendation; salivary gland stimulants, sugarless mints, artificial saliva | Labial mucosa biopsy positive for GVHD; secretory IgA levels; mouth culture positive for yeast organisms; mouth culture positive for bacterial and viral etiologies; radiographs | Possible systemic immunosuppressive therapy with cyclosporine, prednisone, Imuran; artificial saliva; clotrimazole troches or Nystatin, swish and swallow; appropriate topical medication; topical fluoride treatment; appropriate dental therapy |
| Ocular | 80% | 100–400 | Grittiness, burning of eyes; dry eyes; sicca syndrome | Artificial tears; Schirmer's tear test; if <10 mm of wetting, refer to ophthalmologist | Keratoconjunctivitis; corneal ulceration; slit-lamp microscopy | Lacriset plugs; soft contact lens; punctal ligation for obliteration of tear duct outflow; keratoplasty; tarsorrhaphies |
| GI tract, esophagus | 36% | 100–400 | Anorexia; difficulty eating; painful swallowing; retrosternal pain; weight loss; vomiting | Serial weights; high-calorie food supplements; recommend nutritional counseling | Barium swallow of esophagus and small bowel follow-through | Esophageal dilatation; possible systemic immunosuppressive therapy with cyclosporine, prednisone, Imuran; parenteral nutrition |
| Vagina | 20% | 100–400 | Inflammation; stricture formation causing obstruction of menstrual flow; adhesions; dry vagina; painful intercourse; marital problems | Water-soluble lubricants; recommend sexual counseling and therapy | Papanicolaou smear | Vaginal stents; estrogen cream; surgical intervention |

***Oral*** Oral mucosal involvement will develop in approximately 70% of patients with extensive chronic GVHD. Xerostomia, in combination with decreased or absent salivary lubrication, and IgA secretion may be present. Stomatitis may be a common symptom. Lichenoid lesions can be confused with candidiasis.[120] Labial mucosa biopsy is a major diagnostic tool to screen for the presence of chronic GVHD. Salivary changes occur, and xerostomia may cause rampant tooth decay. Early subtle signs are complaints of changes in food tastes and burning after

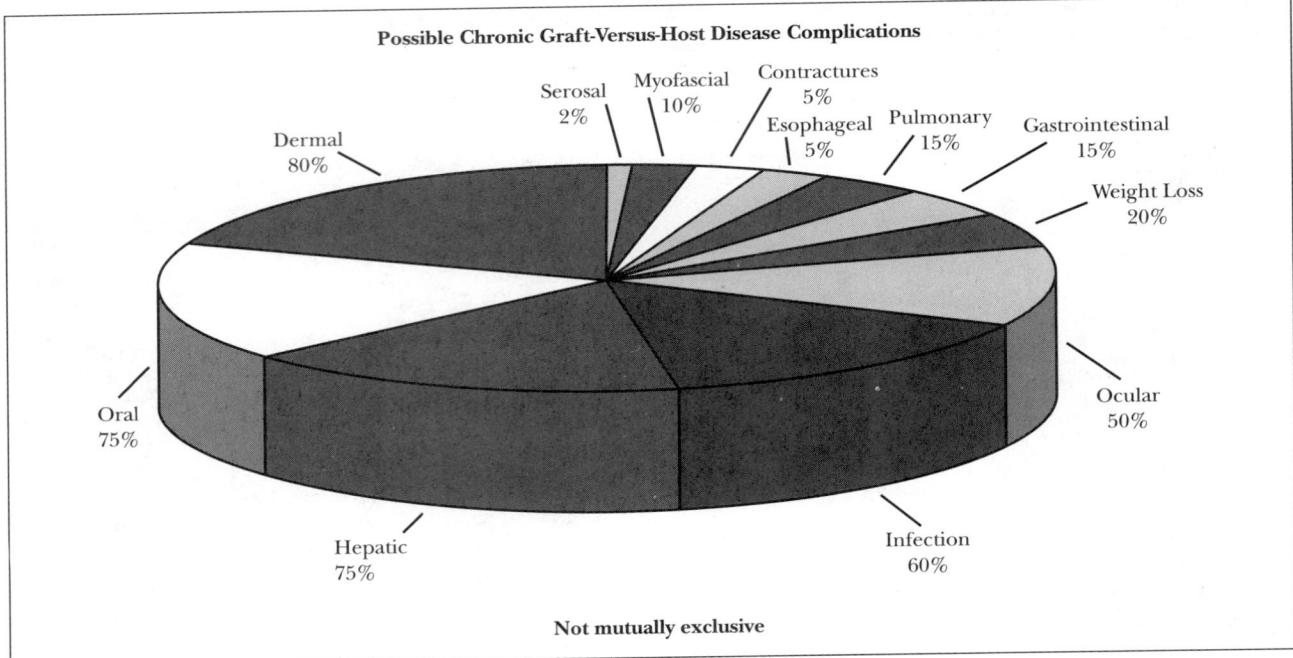

**FIGURE 18-7**   Organ System Involvement in Chronic Graft-Versus-Host Disease.
Data from Sullivan K: Graft-vs-Host Disease, in Forman SJ, Blume KG, Thomas ED (eds): *Bone Marrow Transplantation*. Boston, Blackwell Scientific Publications, 1994, pp 339–362

brushing of the teeth. Herpes simplex virus often accompanies chronic GVHD and serial viral cultures may be needed to make a differential diagnosis of chronic GVHD. The complete nursing assessment of the patient after transplantation must include examination of the oral cavity at each clinic visit.

***Ocular***   Ocular involvement occurs in 50% of patients with extensive chronic GVHD. Major symptoms include burning, itching, and complaints of a "gritty" feeling in the eye. Patients sometimes experience inability to close the eyelid and may lack the ability to form tears. Unfortunately, these symptoms usually appear after corneal stippling has already occurred from lachrymal insufficiency. Schirmer's tear test may be employed four times a year to measure the tearing capacity of the eye. Supportive measures with artificial tear replacement and wearing glasses shielded to prevent entry of dust particles will prevent keratitis sicca, which can lead to corneal erosion, perforation, or scarring.[115,116,119,121,122] Nurses must assess for the early symptoms of ocular chronic GVHD to prevent permanent damage.

***Sinuses***   Sinusitis is common in patients with chronic GVHD and is caused by a combination of sicca syndrome involving the sinuses and the predisposition to gram-positive bacterial infections. The most common causative organisms are *Streptococcus pneumoniae* and *Haemophilus influenzae*. Typical symptoms are fever and headache.[115–119,122]

***Gastrointestinal tract***   Esophageal abnormalities, once a common complication in advanced cases of chronic GVHD, occur less frequently because of advances made in management of this disorder.[115–120] Symptoms include dysphagia, painful swallowing, and retrosternal pain caused by esophageal thinning. Patients may need to be readmitted to inpatient care for management of nutritional problems and pain. Upper and lower intestinal involvement can occur in chronic GVHD. Symptoms include diarrhea and abdominal pain. Malabsorption and submucosal fibrosis also have been documented in ad-

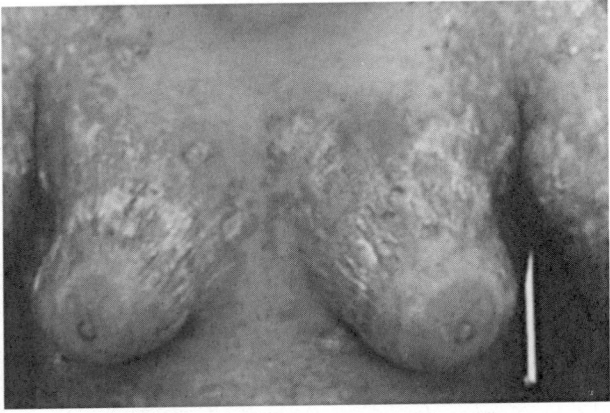

**FIGURE 18-8**   Chronic graft-versus-host disease of the skin.

vanced cases.[115–119,121,122] Responsible nursing management requires early detection of nutritional deficiencies.

*Vaginal* Significant vaginal problems have been documented in women with chronic GVHD. Vaginal inflammation, stricture formation, and adhesions have occurred one to three years after transplantation. Stricture formation severe enough to require surgery to relieve menstrual obstruction with abdominal distention and pain is now rare. Vaginal atrophy may cause painful intercourse leading to sexual dysfunction.[123] The use of a water-soluble, nonperfumed lubricating jelly during sexual intercourse helps women overcome pain associated with the thinning of the vaginal mucosa and loss of natural lubrication. Treatment measures include vaginal dilation in conjunction with immunosuppressive therapies for chronic GVHD. A routine gynecologic examination should be incorporated into the care of female recipients of BMT. Female recipients who are experiencing symptoms associated with high-dose conditioning transplant-related menopause will have confounding and exacerbated symptoms.[116] Nurses interacting with affected women can contribute significantly to their quality-of-life issues and offer intervention promoting emotional and physical healing.

*Other* Problems in other organ systems will develop in 20% of patients with extensive chronic GVHD. The musculoskeletal system can be affected in a manner similar to rheumatoid arthritis, with arthralgia, serosal effusions, joint contracture, and polymyositis. Tendinitis and arthritis accompanied by muscle aches, cramping, and carpal spasms have also been identified as well as peripheral neuropathy and myasthenia gravis resulting from neuropathy associated with subcutaneous fibrosis. Some cases of renal involvement presenting clinically as a nephrotic syndrome or severe cystitis have been reported.[124] Dyspnea may be a manifestation of bronchiolitis obliterans.

### Treatment

Most often, chronic GVHD does not manifest itself until after the patients return to their communities. A dangerous scenario could occur if chronic GVHD remained undetected by an oncology team unfamiliar with its clinical manifestations, diagnosis, and treatment. Consequently, allogeneic recipients have a battery of tests specific for diagnosing the presence of chronic GVHD; these were discussed earlier in the chapter (see Table 18-11). If chronic GVHD is present, appropriate treatment protocols are begun. Nurses involved in preparing allogeneic marrow recipients to return home may be coordinators of this "work-up," clinical assessments, and required tests. As more third-party payers mandate that marrow recipients return to their communities prior to 100 days postBMT, referring physicians and the BMT center will need to cooperate in establishing the type and time of these evaluations.

Early detection and monitoring to detect subclinical chronic GVHD have proven key in preventing and treating chronic GVHD. Classic treatment of chronic GVHD is long-term administration of cyclosporine using a slow taper of 5%/week starting at week 7 following the transplant, followed by an abrupt taper. If acute GVHD flare-up occurs, the initial treatment is to reinstitute full-dose cyclosporine therapy. If resolution does not occur after several weeks, prednisone may be added and followed by a rapid taper. Sullivan et al, in a prospective randomized study, found prednisone alone to be superior to prednisone with azathioprine in preventing GVHD. Although immunosuppressive agents have been the underpinnings of chronic GVHD management, long-term immunosuppressive treatment, particularly steroids, presents a host of problems that include emotional lability, avascular necrosis, secondary malignancies, and increased susceptibility to infections.[75,125] The use of psoralen ultraviolet (PUVA) therapy has been effective for some cases of resistant chronic GVHD of the mouth and skin.[126] Clinical trials using thalidomide for prevention and treatment of chronic GVHD are under way.[127] Etrelenate, a retinoid often used in the treatment of psoriatric patients, is being tested for efficacy and safety in the transplant recipient with chronic skin GVHD. Major adverse effects include teratogenetic effects, corneal erosion, hypertriglyceridemia, and hypercholesterolemia. Other new treatment strategies under review are cytokine antagonists and oxpentifylline.[115] Current and future studies will continue to evaluate agents to control chronic GVHD while allowing a sufficient degree of chronic GVHD to preserve the graft-versus-leukemic effect (explained next). Nurses working within ambulatory settings will need to keep abreast of new treatment therapies for early detection, prevention, and treatment of chronic GVHD (see Table 18-12 and Table 18-13).

*Graft-versus-leukemic effect* The graft-versus-leukemic (GVL) effect is a curious phenomenon that has been demonstrated in vitro since the early 1950s. The GVL effect was first observed in twins receiving syngeneic marrow transplantations who had a twofold higher relapse rate than allogeneic marrow patients who developed graft-versus-host disease. Studies of marrow recipients transplanted for leukemia suggest that GVHD is accompanied by a graft-versus-leukemic effect noted by a lower rate of relapse in patients with GVHD. Although not well understood, there is a significant interest in maintaining some GVHD in allogeneic recipients and inducing GVHD in the autologous recipient in attempts to decrease relapse rates. Intense interest and investigation continues to identify techniques to remove T-cells, the cause of graft-versus-host disease, from donor marrow through T-cell depletion techniques to prevent graft failure yet preserve the antileukemic effect of GVHD. Recently, selected depletion of the T-cell, CD-8, from marrow transplant recipients reduced the incidence of acute GVHD from 50% to 20%, and graft failure to 10% without high relapse rates.[121,122] Preliminary research is beginning to identify vaccines and in vitro expansion of leukemia reactive lymphocytes.[75]

## Late Infectious Complications

As the immune system recovers, infectious complications generally decline. Marrow recipients with persistent acute GVHD or those who develop chronic GVHD, however, remain at considerable risk for infection due to immune dysfunction.[90] Long-term survivors without chronic GVHD are remarkably free of infections after one year. In contrast, patients in whom chronic GVHD develops remain at high risk for bacterial pneumonia, septicemia, and sinusitis, for their donor-derived immune systems have not yet matured and cannot adequately protect against invasive organisms.[115] Figure 18-10 shows the effects of chronic GVHD on the returning immune system.[128] The tempo and type of microbial infections follow a predicted path.

### Varicella zoster virus (VZV)

Seropositive marrow recipients are at substantial risk for VZV infection and nearly one-third to one-half of long-term allogeneic BMT survivors develop recurrent

VZV. Peak time of onset is six to nine months after BMT. Reactivation occurs most often in marrow recipients with chronic GVHD; however, autologous BMT patients also are at risk. Patients may report the prodromal symptoms of burning, pain, and pruritus that may be accompanied by fever and chills. Dermatomal zoster represents 50%–70% of postBMT VZV with significant infectious complications in 20%–30% of cases. As the infection progresses, vesicular lesions erupt and can be localized or disseminated over several dermatomes. Bacterial superinfection with subsequent scarring can be an additional problem if VZV is not treated promptly. Cutaneous infection can predispose BMT recipients to visceral VZV dissemination. The lung, liver, and central nervous system are other common sites for VZV visceral dissemination resulting in pneumonia, hepatitis, intravascular coagulopathy (DIC), and encephalitis. Aggressive antiviral therapy with intravenous acyclovir at 500 mg/kg every eight hours for seven to ten days is the standard therapy. Caution must be used in administering high-dose oral acyclovir (800 mg, five times daily) because peak serum concentrations often are lower than the concentrations required to inhibit many VZV in vitro. For seronegative marrow recipients exposed to VZV, early administration of VZV immunoglobulin may reduce the risk for infection. Patients with nonspecific suppressor cells and chronic GVHD may be at greater risk for VZV as a result of prolonged immunosuppression.

### Encapsulated bacteria

All marrow recipients with chronic GVHD are at risk for infection from encapsulated bacteria. The common cause is sinopulmonary infection caused by *Streptococcus pneumoniae, Neisseria meningitidis,* and *Hemophilus influenzae.* Resulting occult sinusitis and overwhelming sepsis can occur. All patients with chronic GVHD should receive antibiotic prophylaxis with penicillin or trimethoprim-sulfamethoxazole. Marrow recipients with IgG subclass 2 deficiency and recurrent sinopulmonary infection may benefit from intravenous immunoglobulin supplementation. Current research is focusing on the cost-benefit ratio of this therapy.[102]

A major concern after a BMT patient is discharged home is infection. Historically, transplantation teams recommended that patients wear surgical masks for at least six months after transplant to reduce the risk of infections due to microorganisms, fungal spores, and pollen. Due to lack of convincing evidence that masks prevent infection in combination with cost issues, mask wearing has been largely abandoned. Scrupulous handwashing, personal hygiene, and antibiotic and immunosuppressive agents are the mainstay for prevention and treatment of infectious complications. Immunizations against a number of infectious diseases play an important role in these patients. Practices may differ among institutions. Some allogeneic recipients, free of GVHD, develop sufficient amounts of tetanus, diphtheria, and measles antibody virus from their donor marrow; however, standard prac-

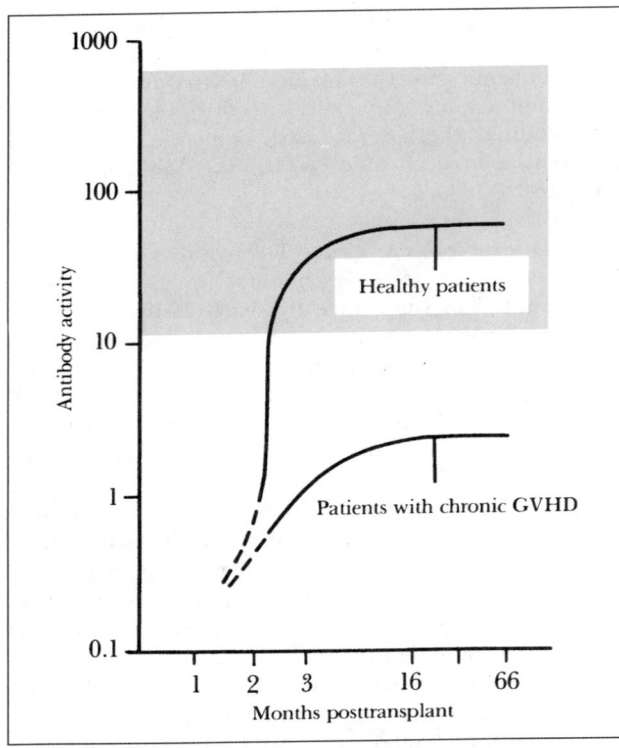

**FIGURE 18-10**  Effects of chronic graft-versus-host disease on the return of the immune system. (Adapted from Witherspoon RP, Lum LG, Storb R: *Semin Hematol* 21:2-10, 1984. Reprinted with permission.)

tice is to reimmunize recipients so that antibody titers reflect normal laboratory values. For those patients free of chronic GVHD, booster immunizations with diphtheria, pertussis tetanus (DPT), *H. influenza* (Hib) conjungate, inactivated Salk poliovirus, influenza, and pneumococcal vaccines are advised. Live attenuated vaccines, such as mumps, measles, and rubella should be given in the second year after BMT but only to those patients without chronic GVHD. Family members of BMT recipients should not be given the Sabin oral polio vaccine during the first years following BMT because of possible virus shedding with subsequent infection in the recipient. If the vaccine is given, the patient needs to be isolated from that family member for 8 to 12 weeks.[129]

## Pulmonary Complications

Restrictive pulmonary abnormalities are rarely observed in long-term survivors and are associated with chemoirradiation and recurrent pneumonia.[75,90] The incidence of restrictive disease peaks at one year. Obstructive pulmonary disease, which occurs in approximately 15% of long-term survivors with chronic GVHD, presents clinical and pathological features of obliterative bronchiolitis. Late interstitial pneumonia occurs in 10%–20% of long-term survivors with chronic GVHD and carries a 50% mortality rate. Studies have identified specific pneumonias as idiopathic: CMV, varicella zoster, and *Pneumocystis carinii*. Twenty percent of patients with chronic GVHD will have restrictive lung disease, 10% will have obstructive lung disease, and 10% will be at risk for bronchiolitis obliterans. Complete nursing assessments of long-term survivors require careful histories and physical examinations. Specifically, inquire about changes in activities of daily living, perform chest auscultation and percussion, and monitor pulmonary capacities and volumes.[130]

## Gonadal Dysfunction

Most transplant patients conditioned with TBI will demonstrate gonadal dysfunction. Some recipients prepared with chemotherapy alone will retain or recover gonadal function and successfully have children. Table 18-12 describes possible gonadal dysfunction and related management in BMT recipients. The adverse effects of single agent high-dose chemotherapy on gonadal function depends on the patient's age at the time of BMT. Girls and boys who are prepubertal at the time of BMT develop normally. Younger women (under 26 years of age) can expect return of menstrual periods, but only a few have borne children. Women over the age of 26 develop early menopause. Men usually return to normal gonadotropin levels and low to normal sperm counts, and can father children.[131] Initial data reviewing high-dose chemotherapy regimens containing combination therapy using cyclophosphamide and busulfan suggest that gonadal dysfunction is similar to that of regimens containing TBI.

These studies await further data collection and analyses as children and adults receiving this therapy advance through their reproductive years.

### TBI

**Women** Almost all female recipients conditioned with TBI have gonadal dysfunction, including sterility and early menopause. A few accounts exist about live births from women receiving such conditioning. Cyclic oral or transdermal hormone replacement therapy commonly is used to reduce symptoms of premature menopause and to prevent long-term disorders, such as osteoporosis or vulvar and vaginal atrophic changes. Vasomotor symptoms, such as hot flashes, sweating, palpitation, irritability, headache, sleep disturbances, and genitourinary tract symptoms, are common. Dysuria, vaginal dryness, dyspareunia, and vulva vaginitis are reported and are often the underlying cause of sexual dysfunction. Successful in vitro fertilization plus artificial insemination has been reported. Rio et al reported a full-term pregnancy from a donated oocyte in a 36-year-old woman six years after receiving an allogeneic BMT after TBI and cyclophosphamide.[132] This approach cannot routinely be advised until further research is done. These fertility techniques raise new ethical issues as an increasing number of BMT candidates inquire about the possibilities of such treatment.

Gonadal dysfunction, although it occurs immediately after BMT, is historically classified as a long-term effect. The ideal time, however, to prepare the patient and significant others is prior to BMT with sensitive counseling by gynecologists, nurse practitioners, or staff nurses working in ambulatory and home care. Several centers offer the expertise of advanced nurse practitioners to help women understand and cope with issues of sexuality, premature menopause, and child-bearing concerns. Information for understanding and managing sexual issues exists for the oncology patient and can be useful for the marrow transplant recipient.

**Men** Most men conditioned with TBI preserve Leydig cell function and testosterone and luteinizing hormone production, but spermatogenesis usually is absent. A few men have fathered children. Young males and men having viable sperm prior to BMT and who wish to father children in future years should be directed to store sperm for future use. Most literature studies of sexual dysfunction after BMT have been limited to men. A recent study of gonadal function and psychosexual adjustment in male patients receiving autologous and allogeneic BMT noted that 50% (n = 29) were dissatisfied with their sexual life. None of these patients had a history of GVHD and there was no difference in sexual concerns between men who had received TBI and those who received chemotherapy only. The predominant problems reported were impotence/erectile difficulties (37.9%), low sexual desire (37.9%), and altered body image (20.7%).[133] Little attention has focused on male sexual dysfunction issues, however, this important quality of life issue should not go unattended because of embarrassment. Nurses who are comfortable with sexuality issues may prepare men for this condition. Those nurses who are not comfortable may suggest sexual counseling.

***Children*** Most prepubertal girls who receive TBI have primary ovarian failure, do not achieve menarche, and do not develop secondary sexual characteristics. A few prepubertal boys conditioned with TBI develop secondary sexual characteristics, but most have delayed onset of puberty. The children most profoundly affected are prepubertal boys who receive testicular irradiation prior to marrow conditioning. Testosterone therapy may be effective, but longer follow-up is needed.

Sexual counseling prior to BMT is important for all marrow transplant candidates. Pediatric long-term survivors require special consideration in assessing possible gonadal dysfunction. Children who fail to reach puberty require neuroendocrine evaluation, and young adolescents reaching puberty will need information about possible sterility. Oncology nurses who work with these families can be instrumental in assessing and teaching both parents and children. New pretransplantation conditioning regimens, aimed at decreasing toxicities, use high-dose busulfan and cyclophosphamide with TBI. Preliminary results demonstrate that the combination of these two agents induces gonadal impairment, as measured by decreased levels of estradiol and elevated levels of luteinizing hormone and follicle-stimulating hormone. In males, testosterone and luteinizing hormone levels have remained normal while FSH is only slightly elevated.

***Growth in children*** Children who undergo conditioning with high-dose cyclophosphamide alone have normal growth and development.[123,131] In contrast, children receiving cyclophosphamide and busulfan face the possibility of growth and development problems. Children transplanted at less than 9 years of age have normal growth velocity curves but older children demonstrate decreased growth velocity curves with no pubescent growth spurt. Careful research monitoring larger numbers of children is needed to make a more definite determination of growth and development problems in this group. Glucocorticoid treatment can suppress growth hormone; thus it is not surprising that decreased growth and development have been noted in children treated with these agents for GVHD. TBI used in conditioning regimens causes abnormalities of growth and development in children. All children have decreased growth rates after TBI, and those who have chronic GVHD are the most significantly affected. Bone age does not seem to be as affected and often is consistent with chronological age, but adrenocortical function, growth hormone levels, and thyroid function have been subnormal in some children, especially those given prior prophylactic with cranial irradiation.[123,131] Radiation can interfere with dental and facial bone development and is particularly harmful to the pediatric patient. TBI results in significantly reduced lengths of both the maxilla and the mandible, and reduction in vertical growth of the upper face, especially in children less than 6 years of age. Facial and dental bone development is compromised resulting in poor calcification, root blunting, apical closure, and mandibular hypoplasia.[131] Correction of these problems may require years of dental surgery and orthodontist care.

Establishing parental awareness of the potential late effects of irradiation is an important nursing function and should be addressed prior to and at regular intervals after transplant. Growth patterns should be evaluated annually, and those who demonstrate a decreased growth rate should be referred to a pediatric endocrinologist. A pubertal developmental staging tool (Tanner Staging) should be used and serum luteinizing hormone (LH) and estradiol levels should be obtained in females at age 12 if the development of secondary sexual characteristics is not apparent. In addition to staging, assessment parameters for testicular dysfunction in adolescent males should include testicular volume, semen analysis, serum LH and FSH if secondary sexual characteristics are not apparent by age 14. Education and counseling are key management and nursing considerations. It is essential that oncology nurses assess and evaluate growth and development patterns in children and young adults. Complete health history and physical examination, head circumference, height and weight, as well as growth hormone levels should be documented in the medical record. Nurses need to be mindful of pretransplant cranial radiation or TBI, and a history of chronic GVHD. The administration of hormones may be necessary to ensure appropriate sexual maturity. As the pediatric BMT survivor approaches adolescence and young adulthood, sexual and reproductive counseling needs to be part of routine long-term follow-up care. Adversely affected children need to be referred to endocrinologists for evaluation. Intervention and careful long-term follow-up through puberty will be necessary.[131] Growth hormone and appropriate sex hormone therapy may be indicated.

## Thyroid Dysfunction

Thyroid dysfunction occurs in 30%–60% of patients prepared for BMT with a regimen that includes single-dose TBI.[123,131] 40% to 55% of children given high-dose TBI show a deficiency of growth hormone; in children with previous cranial irradiation, the incidence may be as high as 90%. As indicated earlier, sexual development may be severely impaired in both boys and girls receiving single-dose TBI.

## Ophthalmologic Effects

Ophthalmologic effects include chronic GVHD and posterior capsular cataracts.[121] Cataract formation peak onset is three years after BMT with a range of 1.5 to 5 years postBMT and is caused by TBI and long-term steroid therapy for GVHD. Historically, it was thought that those patients receiving single-dose TBI were at greatest risk for cataract formation while those receiving fractionated radiation were spared. New information suggests that little difference exists between these two groups. Cataract formation was evaluated in 197 patients treated at a major international transplant center. Thirty-six percent of patients studied (n = 197) developed cataracts with 23% needing surgical repair. All recipients receiving single-dose TBI developed cataracts while 86% of those treated with fractionated TBI had the probability of developing cataracts six years after BMT.[134]

Lens shielding during TBI should be considered as a preventative measure. The treatment of cataracts with surgical extraction is highly successful. Glucocorticoid therapy for treatment of GVHD increases the risk of cataract formation by 25% in patients who have had fractionated TBI or high-dose chemotherapy only. Patients may report poor vision and complain of grittiness, burning, or dryness of the eyes. Keratoconjunctivitis sicca or dry eye syndrome also is noted as an ocular complication. Sicca syndrome usually is associated with GVHD; however, it has been observed in patients without GVHD. Artificial tears can alleviate discomfort. An important nursing function is to educate and prepare patients for the possibility of cataract development and treatment, and to encourage annual eye examinations[116] (see Tables 18-12 and 18-13).

## Graft Failure

Graft failure occurs rarely in an HLA-matched marrow transplantation. However, graft failure in patients who have had transplantation with HLA-mismatched or T-cell-depleted marrow typically occurs early, or months after transplantation. Graft failure differentiates into either primary graft failure or transient engraftment. *Primary graft failure* is the absence of hematologic recovery in patients surviving more than 21 days postBMT. *Transient engraftment* is defined as complete or partial recovery of hematopoiesis, in the absence of moderate to severe GVHD, followed by recurrent pancytopenia. The causes for graft failure include immunologic rejection of the donor, minor histocompatible antigens, and inhibition of hematopoiesis by infection. Disease status at the time of transplantation, the degree of HLA compatibility, pretransplant treatment, preconditioning regimens, T-cell marrow depletion, and immunosuppressive therapy for GVHD can also influence engraftment and outcome. Diagnosis is difficult because pancytopenia can result from other causes such as drug toxicities (ganciclovir [DHPG], TMX-SMX, alfa interferon), viral infections (CMV), or GVHD. Final diagnosis is usually determined by the presence of host T-cells in the presence of graft failure. Graft failure and marrow dysfunction can be life-threatening for BMT recipients. Patients usually die from overwhelming infection, or if a second BMT is done, from multiorgan drug toxicities. Risk factors associated with the development of graft failure differ in allogeneic and autologous transplant.

## Avascular Necrosis

Avascular or aseptic necrosis of the bone, particularly of the humerus or femur head, has been observed in the allogeneic long-term BMT survivor.[135] This syndrome is a direct result of bone softening associated with steroid therapy given for GVHD management. The incidence rate is thought to be as high as 10% and has a median onset of 545 (range 249–731) days posttransplant. Patients can present with complaints of pain and limited range of motion. Treatment often includes an interdisciplinary approach to provide symptom management for pain, physical therapy to maintain mobility, antimicrobial therapy, and femur head replacement. Nurses caring for marrow recipients need to examine closely the patient's medical history for prior or current steroid therapy.

## Dental Effects

Dental effects related to pretransplant conditioning or to chronic GVHD can lead to dental decay. Oral sicca, or dry mouth syndrome, is a common late effect causing oral caries, infection such as *Candida*, HSV, CMV, and other dental health problems. Brush-on fluoride gels or rinses should be prescribed to reduce the risk of tooth decay associated with long-term xerostomia. Taste dysfunction is a common complaint that can affect the patient's nutritional oral intake and overall sense of well-being. Patients often report an increased sensitivity to the taste of sweet foods and complain that many foods taste salty. Saline and water mouth rinses before and after meals may help alleviate these symptoms. Transient dermal hypersensitivity to cold can affect a few or all of the teeth and can be relieved by topical fluoride therapy and desensitizing dentifrice. Temporomandibular dysfunction or myofascial pain dysfunction may also be a problem. Symptoms include toothache, facial pain, ear problems, and headache. The use of hot or cold packs, physical therapy, and tricyclic antidepressants or muscle relaxants may reduce symptomatology. Radiation can directly affect dental and facial bone development, resulting in poor calcification and root blunting. Defects usually are more severe in the pediatric marrow recipient and have been discussed elsewhere in this chapter. These dental effects are often overlooked in relation to the overall long-term assessment of transplant recipients. Nurses can encourage routine head and neck examinations to prevent and manage these emerging long-term complications[120] (see Table 18-12).

## Genitourinary Effects

Until recently, genitourinary toxicity has not been reported as a long-term sequela of BMT. BMT recipients may develop chronic renal failure resulting from radiation injury, the chemotherapeutic process, or drug toxicity secondary to antimicrobial or immunosuppressive therapy (i.e., cyclosporine). Total-body irradiation, drug toxicity related to antimicrobial therapy, and cyclosporine are causative factors. The median time of onset is nine months, with a range of 4.5–26 months. Renal insufficiency is characterized by increased serum creatinine, decreased glomerular filtration rate, anemia, hypertension, and proteinuria. Urinary effects caused by scarring from early onset of hemorrhagic cystitis can lead to bladder shrinkage and chronic urinary disorders. Abdominal pain, microscopic or gross hematuria, and anemia are common clinical findings in late hemorrhagic cystitis.[136]

## Radiation Nephritis

Radiation Nephritis from radiation damage has recently been described and occurs approximately five months postBMT. It is thought that multiagent preparative regimens are the underlying cause.[139]

Hemolytic uremic syndrome (HUS) associated with renal failure is also a delayed and fatal complication after BMT. The etiology is unclear and some studies suggest HUS is related to high-dose conditioning regimens, infection, and cyclosporine.[137] Patients present with the triad of microangiopathic hemolytic anemia, renal insufficiency, and thrombocytopenia 30 to 875 days after BMT. Treatment consists of supportive care with administration of packed red blood cells and platelets until HUS resolution. Prevention is the primary intervention for these infrequent late urologic complications. Vigorous hydration, bladder irrigations, and the administration of MESNA during the preconditioning phase of BMT can minimize hemorrhagic cystitis. The delayed effects of urologic complications are influenced by many factors throughout the transplant process. Nurses must now recognize that these urologic sequelae of conditioning regimens can declare themselves months to years after BMT as well as in the acute stage.

## Neurological Complications

Neurological complications in the BMT recipient are associated with intrathecal methotrexate, central nervous system (CNS) irradiation, and immunosuppressive agents. The incidence of neurological sequelae has been reported to be as high as 60%–70% at various intervals along the transplantation continuum. Many complications are reversible upon drug withdrawal or dose reduction. However leukoencephalopathy, with irreversible CNS toxicity, occurs between one to five months after BMT in about 7% of patients transplanted for leukemia. Symptoms include subsequent impaired memory, shortened attention span, and impaired verbal skills and may not appear for months or even years after transplantation. Learning disabilities in children have been reported, including abnormal motor, perceptual, behavioral, and language performance. Clinical signs and symptoms may be subtle and may require careful observation of the behavior of the pediatric patient. Meyers and colleagues studied 61 marrow recipients to evaluate cognitive and emotional functioning prior to BMT, at two weeks after BMT, at hospital discharge, and at eight months after BMT. Baseline scores prior to BMT showed that 20% of the patients had mild cognitive dysfunction, and nearly 40% had significant anxiety. Although few patients developed problems with cognition or mood during the study, short-term memory deficits nearly doubled at follow-up compared with baseline. Anxiety decreased significantly during hospitalization and remained unchanged at follow-up evaluations. Oncology nurses assessing BMT survivors must be mindful of possible neurological and developmental dysfunction and perform CNS assessments as part of follow-up care. Referral to rehabilitative programs is important[95] (see Table 18-12).

## Second Malignancy

Second malignancies are being reported with increasing frequency and occur at the rate of up to almost four times the normal population. An analysis at a major transplant center of 1,926 combined allogeneic and autologous marrow recipients transplanted for hematologic malignancies reported 35 secondary malignancies. This phenomenon is similar to secondary malignancies experienced by solid organ transplant recipients and may be the result of lengthy immunosuppressive periods and the use of corticosteroids.[138] TBI, viral infection, immunosuppression, chronic immune stimulation, and genetic predisposition are possible etiologies. The onset of de novo malignancy ranges from two to four years after BMT. Common secondary malignancies after BMT encompass a wide range of lymphoproliferative disorders as well as solid tumors. Types of secondary cancers include ALL, ANL, granulocytic sarcomas, non-Hodgkin's lymphoma, carcinomas, malignant melanomas, glioblastoma multiform, and invasive vulvar carcinoma.[139]

## RELAPSE

The success rate of BMT has increased during the past 30 years, but relapse remains a major problem. Most patients in whom relapse occurs have disease in host cells, which indicates that the conditioning regimen for transplantation was not sufficient to eradicate residual leukemic cells that found sanctuary in the marrow recipient. Late relapse in cells of donor origin has been detected by molecular analysis of donor and host DNA.[139] Patients in whom relapse occurs after BMT need intensive supportive care, because families and patients feel they have exhausted not only their medical options but also their psychological and economic strengths. Options for these patients may include a standard oncological treatment of chemotherapy, irradiation, surgery, second transplant, or possibly hospice care. Nurses who work with the families of patients who ultimately will die of their original disease or of transplantation-related problems will be challenged to support patients and families on death and dying issues.

Although marrow transplantation holds the promise of cure for many patients who would otherwise die of their disease, many problems exist and are the subject of ongoing research. Relapse of malignancy after marrow transplantation remains a significant impediment to successful transplantation. Conditioning protocols with new regimens of chemotherapeutic agents and hyperfractionated irradiation hold promise of obtaining optimal conditioning for BMT.

Involved-field irradiation given in addition to TBI to patients with lymphoma may reduce relapse rates and irradiation toxicity. The extra irradiation may be given before or after BMT, and is being investigated in the hope of increasing tumor cell kill and lessening irradiation toxicities.[140] Monoclonal antibodies targeted to tumor or immunotoxins show encouraging early results.[141] Bone-seeking isotopes designed to ablate tumor cells in the marrow without creating additional toxicities to otherwise healthy organs show significant application to BMT.[140,141] Earlier transplantation for younger patients with CML and ALL are improving relapse rates.

## PSYCHOSOCIAL ISSUES

### Patients

Research on the psychosocial issues unique to the BMT recipient is appearing with increasing regularity. Haberman[30] in a seminal article, noted that patients have consistently identified specific stresses associated with each phase of the BMT process. Each phase is eclipsed by particular concerns and provides a framework for nurses who care for these patients to offer appropriate support through patient preparation and teaching. More recently, Andrykowski[142] has advanced areas of psychosocial concerns of the marrow recipient into more succinct compartments with research recommendations for each phase.

Despite the continued research in psychological complications in the BMT recipient, few long-term problems have been identified. Once discharged from the hospital, marrow recipients often experience a normal reactive depression because of neuropsychological deficits, body image changes, malaise, sexual dysfunction, and a slower than anticipated return to normal activities.[143,144] These symptoms might progress to clinical depression if not recognized and treated promptly. Recently, a small study of 20 families with children who underwent BMT docu-

mented that parents may develop posttraumatic stress disorder. Parents considered the BMT process a traumatic occurrence and reexperienced the event through intrusive thoughts and a variety of emotional and cognitive responses. The investigators concluded that family preparation prior to BMT may decrease anxiety related to relocation to a BMT center and the BMT process.[145]

Unusual psychological reactions include suicidal ideation, depression greater than expected from the normal grief reaction, disruptive anxiety, pathological regression, and organic delirium. These cases represent a small but significant percentage of BMT recipients. Individual psychological counseling and antidepressant therapy may be required. Important considerations are early psychiatric intervention, ruling out organic factors, and identifying a consistent team to interact with these patients.[146] Nurses can anticipate these normal reactions and direct patients and their families to supportive resources that include hospital or community-based support groups, national survivorship organizations, and programs offered by the American Cancer Society. An Internet support group for BMT recipients meets weekly on America Online. As the cyberspace technology advances, survivors will have rapid access to support systems in their own home.[147]

### Donors

Donors experience a variety of psychological reactions before and after their marrow donation. Donor-related stresses have been identified; they were reviewed earlier in this chapter.

### Family/Caregivers

Families may experience considerable psychological, emotional, and social problems before and after marrow transplantation. For example, transplant centers often are located far from familiar support systems, and relocation requires dramatic changes in every aspect of family dynamics. These changes include significant economic issues and medical consequences of marrow transplant. Families need to confront the long-term issues of caring for a recovering family member until the physical sequelae of treatment have vanished. Strong social work teams are beneficial in transplant settings to prepare families for this experience and to identify community resources. This intervention lessens the likelihood of developing family-related dysfunctions. Studies examining the burden on the caregivers of BMT patients are needed to identify the nature and timing of stressors and which caregiver burdens can be alleviated through nursing interventions.

### Staff

Provision of psychological support for staff members who care for patients undergoing marrow transplantation is essential to the quality of nursing care provided to marrow recipients and their families. Inherent to BMT nursing is chronic stress related to caring for patients whose condition may change rapidly. These nurses are challenged by family interactions as well as patient concerns, and they become part of a psychosocial team caring for acutely ill patients who may die. Winters et al[148] recently characterized the nature of patient-nurse psychosocial interactions in the BMT milieu. Five core concepts were identified and include: (1) discovering the patient and family's interpretation of the BMT experience, (2) intuitive awareness of the group relationships, (3) undocumented and informal interactions between the nurse and patient, (4) direct and indirect interactions, and (5) monitoring family interactions vis-a-vis the patient. The findings of this study raise important issues related to clinical practice, education, and to defining the role of the psychosocial nurse practicing with patients and families.

Excellence in patient care, staff retention, and emotionally healthy nurses can be the result of programs designed to support staff nurses. Implementation of successful programs has been described in the literature and requires a nursing administration committed to assisting nurses in coping with the stresses of their environment.[149–151] As the economics of health care increasingly influence practice by soaring workloads, former successful efforts to effect retention are rapidly disappearing. Perhaps one of the major impediments to staff satisfaction and subsequent retention of experienced nursing staff are administrative budgetary constraints reducing or eliminating professional education, travel, and subscription to professional nursing journals.

## Quality of Life

Early quality of life (QOL) studies focused mainly on morbidity based on physical disabilities measured by Karnofsky Performance Scales. More recently, researchers have attempted to measure quality of life in four domains: physical, social, psychological, and spiritual.[152] Although the number of BMT QOL studies are increasing, most are retrospective studies or studies that did not collect baseline data immediately prior to transplant. Two notable studies are exceptions. Andrykowski et al[153] studied the physical and psychosocial status of 28 adult BMT recipients prior to BMT and at 12–16 months after BMT. Analysis of group mean showed few significant differences between pre- and postBMT assessments but residual change scores suggested that physical and psychosocial status improved following BMT for women and younger recipients while men and older recipients did less well. The investigators emphasize the need for baseline physical and psychosocial status assessments prior to BMT so that those problems reported after BMT are not seen as direct transplant-related sequelae. The second study done at a major BMT center surveyed patients before and after BMT. Results showed that severe chronic GVHD coupled with pretransplant family conflict predicted subsequent impaired physical and emotional recovery. In addition unmarried males did less well than married males or single or married women.[144]

Haberman et al[154] surveyed, retrospectively, 125 adult survivors of allogeneic (87%) and syngeneic/autologous (13%) transplants and found that 80% of those surveyed reported their QOL to be good or excellent, while only 5% rated it as poor. The most frequently cited problem of recovery was a perceived lack of social support. Baker et al[155] studied 135 patients 6 to 149 months after transplant. Survivors showed a high degree of general satisfaction with life but were least satisfied with their bodies, level of physical strength, and ability to attain sexual satisfaction. Similar to the Syrjala[144] study, patients with previous GVHD were least satisfied with major life domains. Another significant study evaluated health, functional ability, and employment status of 171 adults living six months or longer after BMT.[156] Most patients (80%) reported return of normal function with few physical problems. Global health was noted to be good to excellent (67%) and most (80%) reported that social activities were unimpaired or only slightly affected. Three-fourths of the patients had returned to work or school. A quality-of-life instrument specifically for long-term follow-up of BMT recipients measures physical symptoms (e.g., weight loss, frequent colds, skin changes, cataracts, sexual problems), psychological symptoms (e.g., worry about recurrence of disease, adjustment to illness, social concerns, relationship adjustment, return to work), and spiritual well-being (e.g., sense of control, future goals).[156]

Many sophisticated qualitative research studies in BMT are emerging. Studies of hope, meaning, and quality of life provide physical, psychological, and social findings to help oncology nurses perform thorough and meaningful psychosocial assessments.[154–157]

Few studies exist on pediatric QOL issues, but anecdotal evidence from patients often praise the improved family life of disease-free survivors. A recent prospective, longitudinal study evaluated 65 pediatric BMT recipients with standardized measures of global intelligence and academic achievement and selected tests of neuropsychological function. Tests were administered preBMT and 12–16 months after BMT. Cognitive and neuropsychological function remained stable during the study periods. Declines were noted in social competence, self-esteem, and general emotional well-being. Surprisingly, and in contrast to other studies, BMT conditioning regimens were not associated with significant neuropsychological impairment. More prospective studies following pediatric recipients over longer periods of time are needed. Nurses can guide long-term survivors and their families to necessary community support groups to help patients reintegrate successfully into their communities.

As medical costs soar and health care resources diminish, only those procedures that balance successful long-term outcome with the cost of treatment will remain available. BMT QOL studies that use meaningful and reliable instruments specific to the recovering BMT recipients are necessary to help justify the benefits of this treatment to third-party payers. Instruments need to be easy to use and not burdensome to a fatigued or compromised recipient. New studies should define the ultimate success of BMT as a return to a productive life not compromised with expensive long-term treatment. Family functioning and caregiver burden also need to be measured. Nurses practicing in alternate care and home care milieus are a rich resource for collaborative research concerning this important issue.

## Ethical Issues

Marrow transplantation can involve complex moral and ethical considerations. Informed consent for experimental procedures is standard, but the effectiveness of these explanations is poorly understood. The rights of children and their welfare continue to challenge medical and legal systems.[158] Broader social issues, such as allocation of resources, prolonged life support in the face of irreversible organ failure, and the competitive selection of marrow recipients, are being examined.[159,160] As new technologies and stem cell sources evolve, even greater moral issues emerge. Concerns relative to the possible long-term effects of colony stimulating factors used in normal marrow donors haunt researchers involved in such investigations. Worldwide banking of placental blood for transplant raises questions of (1) tissue ownership, (2) informed consent, (3) infectious disease and genetic information, (4) privacy and confidentiality, and (5) the need for fair and equitable access to placental blood. These and other complex questions provide opportunities for multidisciplinary studies of some of the major biopsychosocial issues of our time.

## FUTURE APPLICATIONS

A new era of clinical research on treatment of autoimmune diseases with marrow or blood transplantation is under discussion. Disorders such as systemic lupus erythematosus, cerebral palsy, multiple sclerosis, sickle cell anemia, cystic fibrosis, and rheumatoid arthritis affects millions of people who may benefit from this therapy.[161] Before this treatment becomes accepted for these disease entities, the costs and long-term disease-free survival must be assured through cooperative trials.

## Stem Cell Technology

Treatment failure or relapse remains one of the major impediments to successful allografting. Research on techniques for separation of hematopoietic stem cells includes studies of sedimentation techniques, monoclonal antibodies, and immunoabsorption columns. Alternate donor sources are emerging rapidly and numerous inves-

tigators predict that marrow transplantation as it is known today will not exist by the next millennium. Allogeneic stem cell transplants are the subject of intense research. Fetal liver stem cell transplants have been reported in the treatment of selected patients with severe combined immunodeficiency disease syndrome (SCIDS).[162] Successful allogeneic stem cell transplants for children and adults using umbilical cord blood are now being reported. Early fears that GVHD would be an insurmountable problem have not materialized. The ability to use cord blood has generated cord blood banks to store this tissue for possible autologous use and for unrelated genetically diverse transplants. Cord blood may be an optimal vehicle for gene therapy and treatment of metabolic diseases such as thalassemia and Fanconi's anemia.[163]

## Gene Transfer

Gene transfer holds dramatic promise for future applications of BMT and other genetic diseases. This involves replacement of defective genetic material with healthy genes in marrow transplantation candidates with genetic diseases.[164,165] Adenosine deaminase deficiency is the first disease to be treated with gene transfer therapy but other genetic disorders of lymphohematopoietic cells including hemoglobinopathies, immune deficiencies, and storage diseases are being studied in preclinical trials. Substantial preclinical improvements in transfer efficiency are required before wider clinical studies can be conducted.

## CONCLUSION

The number of bone marrow transplantations will continue to increase to unanticipated numbers until blood cell transplantation is perfected as an appropriate substitute. Most of the treatment, including TBI, will occur in outpatient settings. Expert training programs for physicians and advanced nurse clinicians at large transplant centers will generate new transplantation teams to provide treatment to more patients. Nurses will interact more with third-party payers. BMT coordinators will assume more comprehensive roles in establishing safe and cost-effective care. Nurse-managed clinics will be established benefiting the large number of recipients requiring intensive outpatient monitoring. The number of third-party-payer corporate case managers will increase and will influence the management of the patient. BMT education of these and other professionals will be crucial.

Growth of the unrelated donor pool will continue to increase the allogeneic marrow and stem cell population to unprecedented levels. Existing transplantation resources, including physicians and nurses, blood banking capabilities, and other supportive services, will require expansion. New models of care for stable BMT recipients will incorporate 24-hour clinics, day hospitals, infusion suites, and high-tech home health services. Research studies, in addition to safety and efficacy of treatment, will identify cost-benefit ratios, cost-effectiveness measures, and QOL issues.[166-171] Centers of excellence are being identified by third-party payers who may limit reimbursement to BMTs received at an approved site.

The roles and responsibilities of oncology and bone marrow transplant nurses are rapidly changing. Nurses greatly influence the success of transplantation by the care given to marrow recipients before and after the procedure. BMT outpatients are more acutely ill than in the past and require new treatments and therapies. Nurses require in-depth, complex treatment protocols and the ability to continually assimilate new technologies. Unifying the goals of medical research and nursing care will continue to challenge multidisciplinary teams. Nursing management will be challenged to create an environment that promotes staff education and retention. As the number of patients undergoing marrow transplantation increases, the demand for BMT nurses of the highest professional caliber will continue to increase.

## REFERENCES

1. Bortin MM, Horowitz MM, Rowlings PA, et al: 1993 progress report from the International Bone Marrow Transplant Registry. *Bone Marrow Transplant* 12:97–104, 1993
2. Rimm AA: Increasing utilization of allogeneic bone marrow transplantation. *Ann Intern Med* 116:505–512, 1992
3. Corcoran-Buchsel PB, Ford RC: Introduction. *Semin Oncol Nurs* 4:1–2, 1988
4. Quine WE: The remedial application of bone marrow. *JAMA* 26:1012–1013, 1896
5. Santos GW: History of bone marrow transplantation. *Clin Haematol* 12:611–639, 1983
6. Thomas ED, Storb R, Clift RA, et al: Bone-marrow transplantation. *N Engl J Med* 292:832–843, 895–902, 1975
7. Weiden PL, Flournoy N, Thomas ED, et al: Antileukemic effect of graft-versus-host disease in human recipients of allogeneic-marrow grafts. *N Engl J Med* 300:1068–1073, 1979
8. Doney KC, Buckner CD: Bone marrow transplantation: An overview. *Plasma Ther Transfus Technol* 6:149–161, 1985
9. Thomas ED, Sargur M: Bone marrow transplantation, in Cerilli J (ed): *Organ Transplantation and Replacement*. Philadelphia, Lippincott, 1988, pp 608–616
10. Goldman JM, Gale RP, Horowitz MM, et al: Bone marrow transplantation for chronic myelogenous leukemia in chronic phase: Increased risk of relapse associated with T-cell depletion. *Ann Intern Med* 108:806–814, 1988
11. Barrett J, Jiang S, Dermime S, et al: Mechanisms of graft versus leukemia: Blood cell and bone marrow transplants. *Proceedings of Advances and Controversies in Bone Marrow Transplantation*, 1996, p 27 (abstr 12)
12. Storb R, Thomas ED: Allogeneic bone marrow transplantation. *Immunol Rev* 71:78–102, 1983
13. Korbling M, Juttner CA, Henon P, et al: Blood research in bone marrow transplants, in Gale P, Juttner CA, Henon P

(eds): *Blood Cell Transplants*. New York, Cambridge University Press, 1994, pp 87–98
14. Buchsel P, Kapustay P: Peripheral stem cell transplantation. *Oncology Nursing: Patient Treatment and Support* 2(2):1–14, 1995
15. O'Reilly RJ, Hansen J, Kurtzberg J, et al: Allogeneic marrow transplantation for patients lacking a donor. *Hematol:* 4:132–146, 1996
16. Bortin MM, Bach FH, van Bekkumm DW, et al: 25th anniversary of the first successful allogeneic bone marrow transplants. *Bone Marrow Transplant* 14:211–212, 1994
17. Deeg JH: Delayed complications of marrow transplantation. *Marrow Transplant Reviews: Issues in Hematology, Oncology and Immunology* 2:10–16, 1992
18. Sugarman J, Reisner EG, Kurtzberg J: Ethical aspects of banking placental blood for transplantation. *JAMA* 274:1783–1785, 1995
19. Blazer BR, Lasky LC, Perentesis JP, et al: Successful donor cell engraftment in a recipient of bone marrow from a cadaveric donor. *Blood* 67:1655–1660, 1986
20. Zanjani EM, Harrison MR, Tavassoli M: In utero transplantation of fetal hematopoietic stem cells (HSC). *J Cell Biochem Suppl* 16a:179, 1992 (abst D 030)
21. Ford R, Ballard B: Acute complications after bone marrow transplantation. *Semin Oncol Nurs* 4:15–24, 1988
22. Forman SJ, Thomas ED, Blume K (eds): *Bone Marrow Transplantation*. Cambridge, MA, Blackwell Scientific Publishers, 1994
23. Beutler E, Sullivan K: Marrow transplantation in sickle cell disease, in Forman SJ, Thomas ED, Blume K (eds): *Bone Marrow Transplantation*. Cambridge, MA, Blackwell Scientific Publishers, 1994, pp 840–848
24. Parkman R: Bone marrow transplantation for genetic diseases. *Pediatr Ann* 20:677–681, 1988
25. Blaese RM, Culver KW: Progress toward the application of gene therapy, in Nance SJ (ed): *Clinical and Basic Science Aspects of Immunohematology*. Arlington, VA, American Association of Blood Banks, 1988, pp 1–11
26. Armitage J: Bone marrow transplantation. *N Engl J Med* 330:827–838, 1994
27. Tiercy JM, Morel C, Freidel AC, et al: Selection of unrelated donors for bone marrow transplantation is improved by HLA class II genotyping with oligonucleotide hybridization. *Proc Natl Acad Sci USA* 88:7121–7125, 1988
28. Bensinger WI, Buckner CD, Thomas ED, et al: ABO-incompatible marrow transplants. *Transplant* 33:427–429, 1982
29. Hansen JA, Anasett C, Petersdorf E, et al: Marrow transplants from unrelated donors. *Transplant Proc* 26:1710–1712, 1994
30. Haberman MR: Psychosocial aspects of bone marrow transplantation. *Semin Oncol Nurs* 4:55–59, 1988
31. Durbin M: Bone marrow transplantation: Economic, ethical, and social issues. *Pediatrics* 82:774–778, 1988
32. Buckner CD, Peterson FB, Bolonesi B: Bone marrow donors, in Forman SJ, Blume K, Thomas ED (eds): *Bone Marrow Transplantation*. Cambridge MA, Blackwell Scientific Publishers, 1994, pp 259–268
33. Curran WJ, Hyg SM: Beyond the best interests of a child: Bone marrow transplantation among half-siblings. *N Engl J Med* 324:1818–1819, 1992
34. York A, Cliff R, Sander J, et al: Recombinant human erythropoietin (Rh-Epo) administration to normal donors. *Bone Marrow Transplant* 10:415–417, 1992
35. Dudjak LA: HLA typing: Implications for nurses. *Oncol Nurs Forum* 11:1130–1135, 1984

36. Ruggiero MR: The donor in bone marrow transplantation. *Semin Oncol Nurs* 4:9–14, 1988

37. Lesko LM, Hawkins DR: Psychological aspects of transplantation medicine, in Akhtat S (ed): *New Psychiatric Syndromes: DSM-III and Beyond.* New York, Aronson, 1983, pp 265–309

38. Patenaude AF, Rappeport H: Psychological costs of bone marrow transplantation in children. *Am J Orthopsychiatry* 49:409–422, 1979

39. Butterworth VA, Simmons RG, Bartsch G, et al: Psychosocial effects of unrelated bone marrow donation: Experiences of the national marrow donor program. *Blood* 81:1947–1959, 1993

40. Stroncek DF, Holland PV, Bartsch G, et al: Experiences of the first 493 unrelated marrow donors in the national marrow donor program. *Blood* 81:1940–1946, 1993

41. Goldman JM: A special report: Bone marrow transplantation using volunteer donors—recommendations and requirement for a standardized practice throughout the world—1994 update. *Blood* 84:2833–2838, 1996

42. Bolwell B, Lichtin A, Sands K, et al: An analysis of complications of outpatient bone marrow harvesting. *Proc of Keystone Symposia on Molecular and Cellular Biology,* p 200, 1992 (abstr) (suppl)

43. Brandwein JM, Callum J, Rubinger M, et al: An evaluation of outpatient bone marrow harvesting. *J Clin Oncol* 7:648–650, 1989

44. Weinberg P: The human leukocyte antigen (HLA) system, the search for a matching donor, national marrow donor program development, and marrow donor issues, in Whedon M (ed): *Bone Marrow Transplantation: Principles, Practice, and Nursing Insights.* Boston, Jones and Bartlett, 1988, pp 105–132

45. Storb R, Prentice RL, Buckner CD, et al: Graft-versus-host disease and survival in patients with aplastic anemia treated with marrow graft from HLA-identical siblings: Beneficial effect of a protective environment. *N Engl J Med* 308:302–307, 1983

46. Storb R, Deeg HJ, Whitehead J, et al: Methotrexate and cyclosporine compared with cyclosporine alone for prophylaxis of acute graft-versus-host disease after marrow transplantation for leukemia. *N Engl J Med* 314:729–735, 1986

47. Russell JA, Poon MC, Jones AR, et al: Allogeneic bone-marrow transplantation without protective isolation in adults with malignant disease. *Lancet* 339:38–40, 1992

48. Buckner CD, Clift RA, Sander JE, et al: Protective environment for marrow transplant patients: A prospective study. *Ann Intern Med* 89:893–901, 1978

49. Whedon M (ed): *Bone Marrow Transplantation: Principles, Practice, and Nursing Insights.* Boston, Jones and Bartlett, 1988

50. Thomas ED: Bone marrow transplantation: A lifesaving applied art. *JAMA* 249:2528–2536, 1983

51. Poe SS, Larson E, McGuire D, et al: A national survey of infection prevention practices on bone marrow transplantation units. *Oncol Nurs Forum* 21:1687–1694, 1994

52. Thomas ED, Fefer A: Bone marrow transplantation, in De Vita VT, Hellman S, Rosenberg SA (eds): *Cancer: Principles and Practice of Oncology* (ed 2). Philadelphia, Lippincott, 1989, pp 2320–2325

53. Phillips G, Wolff S, Herzig G: Local radiotherapy followed by cyclophosphamide, fractionated total body irradiation and autologous marrow transplantation for refractory malignant lymphoma. *Blood* 62:228, 1983 (suppl 1)

54. Freedman S, Hainsfield ME, McQuire DB, et al: Nursing considerations in the administration of blood component therapy. *Semin Oncol Nurs* 6:155–162, 1990

55. Sullivan KM, Storb R: Allogeneic marrow transplantation. *Cancer Invest* 2:27–38, 1984

56. Schubert MM, Sullivan KM, Truelove EL: Head and neck complications of bone marrow transplantation, in Peterson ED, Sonis ST, Elias EG (eds): *Head and Neck Management of the Cancer Patient.* Boston, Martinus Nijhoff, 1986, pp 401–427

57. Hill HH, Chapman RC, Kornell JA, et al: Self-administration of morphine in bone marrow transplant patients reduces drug requirement. *Pain* 40:121–129, 1990

58. Epstein JB, Stevenson-Moor P, Jackson S: Prevention of oral mucositis in radiation therapy: A controlled study with benzamine hydrochloride rinse. *Int J Radiat Oncol Biol Physics* 16:1571–1575, 1989

59. Brandt SJ, Peters WP, Atwater SK, et al: Effect of recombinant human granulocyte-macrophage colony stimulating factor on hematopoietic reconstitution after high-dose chemotherapy and autologous bone marrow transplantation. *N Engl J Med* 318:869–876, 1988

60. Wolford JL, McDonald GB: A problem-oriented approach to intestinal and liver disease after marrow transplantation. *J Clin Gastroenterol* 10:419–433, 1988

61. Hewitt M, Cornish D, Pamphilon D, et al: Effective emetic control during conditioning of children for bone marrow transplantation using ondansetron, a 5-HT3 antagonist. *Bone Marrow Transplant* 7:431–433, 1988

62. Bosi A, Guide S, Messori A, et al: Ondansetron versus chlorpomizine for preventing emesis in bone marrow transplant recipients: A double-blind randomized study. *J Chemother* 5:188–196, 1993

63. Feuvret L, Jammet P, Campana F, et al: Value of granisetron in the prevention of digestive disorders in total body irradiation. *Bull Cancer Radiother* 81:41–44, 1994

64. Cox GJ, Matsui SM, Lo RS, et al: Etiology and outcome of diarrhea after marrow transplantation: A prospective study. *Gastroenterology* 107:1398–1407, 1994

65. Press OW, Schaller RT, Thomas ED: Bone marrow transplant complications, in Toledo-Pereyra LH (ed): *Complications of Organ Transplantation.* New York, Marcel Dekker, 1986, pp 399–424

66. Turkeri LN, Lum LG, Uberti JP, et al: Prevention of hemorrhagic cystitis following allogeneic bone marrow transplant preparative regimens with cyclophosphamide and busulfan: Role of continuous bladder irrigation. *J Urol* 153:637–640, 1995

67. Brady HR, Brenner BM: Acute renal failure in Isselbacher KJ, Braunwald E, Wilson JD, Martin JB, Falici AS, Kasper DL (eds): *Harrison's Principles of Internal Medicine.* New York, McGraw-Hill, 1994, pp 1265–1274

68. Ballard B: Renal and hepatic complications, in Whedon MB (ed): *Bone Marrow Transplantation: Principles, Practice, and Nursing Insights.* Boston, Jones and Bartlett, 1988, pp 240–261

69. Klingemann H-G: Urinary tract, in Deeg HJ, Klingemann H-G, Phillips GL (eds): *A Guide to Marrow Transplantation.* New York, Springer-Verlag, 1988, pp 135–139

70. Sullivan KM: Acute and chronic graft-versus-host disease in man. *Int J Cell Clon* 4:42–93, 1986 (suppl 1)

71. Meyers JD: Infection in bone marrow transplant recipients. *Am J Med* 81:27–38, 1986 (suppl 1A)

72. Weisdorf D, Hakke R, Blazar B, et al: Risk factors for acute graft-versus-host disease in histocompatible donor bone

marrow transplantation. *Transplantation* 51:1197–1203, 1988

73. Butturina A, Gale RP: T-cell depletion in bone marrow transplantation for leukemia: Current results and future directions. *Bone Marrow Transplant* 3:185–192, 1988

74. Reinauer S, Lehmann P, Plewig G, et al: Photochemotherapy (PUVA) of acute graft-versus-host disease. *Hautarzt* 44:708–712, 1993

75. Sullivan KM. Graft-versus-host disease, in Forman SJ, Blume KG, Thomas ED (eds): *Bone Marrow Transplantation.* Cambridge, MA, Blackwell Scientific Publishers, 1994, pp 339–375

76. Lamberts SWJ, Van Der Lely AJ, DeHerder WW, et al: Drug therapy: Octreotide. *N Engl J Med* 334:246–253, 1996

77. Ford R, Eisenberg S: Bone marrow transplant: Recent advances and nursing implications. *Nurs Clin North Am* 25:405–422, 1990

78. Oncology Nursing Society: *Manual for Bone Marrow Transplantation: Recommendations for Practice and Education.* Pittsburgh, Oncology Nursing Press, 1994

79. McDonald GB, Sharma P, Matthews DE, et al: The clinical course of 53 patients with veno-occlusive disease of the liver after marrow transplantation. *Transplant* 39:603–608, 1985

80. Dulley FL, Kanfer EF, Appelbaum FR, et al: Veno-occlusive disease of the liver after chemoradiotherapy and autologous bone marrow transplantation. *Transplant* 43:870–873, 1987

81. Shulman HM, Hinterberger W: Hepatic veno-occlusive disease-liver toxicity syndrome after bone marrow transplantation. *Bone Marrow Transplant* 10:197–214, 1992

82. Bearman SI: The syndrome of hepatic veno-occlusive disease after marrow transplantation. *Blood* 85:3005–3020, 1995

83. Buckner CD, Meyers JD, Springmeyer SC, et al: Pulmonary complications of marrow transplantation: Review of the Seattle experience. *Exp Hematol* 12:1–5, 1984 (suppl 15)

84. Sullivan KM, Meyers JD, Flournoy N, et al: Early and late interstitial pneumonia following human bone marrow transplantation. *Int J Cell Cloning* 4:107–121, 1986 (suppl 1)

85. Crawford SW, Bowden RA, Hackman RC, et al: Rapid detection of cytomegalovirus pulmonary infection by bronchoalveolar lavage and centrifugation culture. *Ann Intern Med* 108:180–185, 1988

86. Rowe JM, Ciobanu N, Ascensao J, et al: Recommended guidelines for the management of autologous and allogeneic bone marrow transplantation: A report from the Eastern Cooperative Oncology Group. *Ann Intern Med* 120:143–158, 1994

87. Ljungman P, DeBock R, Cordonnier C, et al: Practices for cytomegalovirus diagnosis, prophylaxis and treatment in allogeneic bone marrow recipients: A report from the working party for infectious diseases of the EBMT. *Bone Marrow Transplant* 12:393–403, 1993

88. Goodridge JM, Boeckh M, Bowden R: Strategies for the prevention of cytomegalovirus disease after marrow transplantation. *Clin Infect Dis* 19:287–289, 1994

89. Bowden RA, Slichter S, Sayers M, et al: A comparison of filtered leukocyte-reduced and cytomegalovirus (CMV) seronegative blood products for the prevention of transfusion-associated CMV infection after marrow transplant. *Blood* 86:3599–3603, 1995

90. Wingard JR: Management of infectious complications of bone marrow transplantations. *Oncology* 4:69–76, 1990

91. Harrington RD, Hooten T, Hackman RC, et al: An outbreak of respiratory syncytial virus in a bone marrow transplant center. *J Infect Dis* 165:987–993, 1992

92. Update: Respiratory syncytial virus activity—United States, 1995–1996 season. *JAMA* 275:29, 1995

93. Gucalp R: Management of the febrile neutropenic patient with cancer. *Oncology* 5:137–144, 1988

94. Davis D, Patchell RA: Neurologic complications of bone marrow transplantation. *Neurol Clin* 6:377–378, 1988

95. Meyers CA, Weitzner M, Byrne K, et al: Evaluation of the neurobehavioral functioning of patients before, during, and after bone marrow transplantation. *J Clin Oncol* 12:820–826, 1994

96. Furlong T: Neurologic complications of immunosuppressive cancer therapy. *Oncol Nurs Forum* 20:1337–1352, 1993

97. Thompson CB, June CH, Sullivan KM, et al: Association between cyclosporine neurotoxicity and hypomagnesemia. *Lancet* 2:1116–1120, 1984

98. Klingemann H-G: Central nervous system (CNS), in Deeg HJ, Klingemann H-G, Phillips GL (eds): *A Guide to Marrow Transplantation.* New York, Springer-Verlag, 1988, pp 135–139

99. Meriney DK: Neurologic and neuromuscular complications of bone marrow transplantation, in Whedon MB (ed): *Bone Marrow Transplantation: Principles, Practice, and Nursing Insights.* Boston, Jones and Bartlett, 1988, pp 262–279

100. Peterson FB, Bearman, SI: Preparative regimens and their toxicity, in Forman SJ, Blume K, Thomas ED (eds): *Bone Marrow Transplantation.* Cambridge, MA, Blackwell Scientific Publishers, 1994, pp 79–95

101. Larsen RL, Barber Heise CT, et al: Exercise assessment of cardiac function in children and young adults before and after bone marrow transplantation. *Pediatrics* 89:722–729, 1992

102. Schulman KA, Glick HA, Rubine H, et al: Cost-effectiveness of HA-1A monoclonal antibody for gram-negative sepsis: Economic assessment of a new therapeutic agent. *JAMA* 266:3466–3471, 1992

103. Momin F, Chandrasekar PH: Antimicrobial prophylaxis in bone marrow transplantation. *Ann Intern Med* 123:205–215, 1995

104. Guglielom JB, Wong-Beringer A, Lonker CA: Immune globulin therapy in allogeneic bone marrow transplant: A critical review. *Bone Marrow Transplant* 13:499–510, 1994

105. Buchsel P, Benson A, Counts G, et al: Etiology and prevention of gram-negative septicemias (GNS) in bone marrow transplant (BMT) outpatients: Relation to nursing care of right atrial catheters (RAC). *Proc American Cancer Society First National Conference on Cancer Nursing Research.* Atlanta, American Cancer Society, 1989 (abstr 15)

106. Sullivan KM, Kopecky KJ, Jocom J, et al: Immunomodulatory and antimicrobial efficacy of intravenous immunoglobulin in bone marrow transplantation. *N Engl J Med* 323:705–712, 1990

107. Buchsel PC: From hospital to home: Making the transition, in Whedon MB (ed): *Bone Marrow Transplantation: Principles, Practice, and Nursing Insights.* Boston, Jones and Bartlett, 1988, pp 240–261

108. Algara M, Valls A, Vivancos P, et al: Outpatient total body irradiation for bone marrow transplanation. *Bone Marrow Transplant* 14:381–382, 1994

109. Chielens D, Herrick E: Recipients of bone marrow transplants: Making a smooth transition to an ambulatory care setting. *Oncol Nurs Forum* 17:857–862, 1990

110. Buchsel P: Bone marrow transplants: Managing BMT patients in alternate site health care settings with infusion therapy. *Continuing Care* 11:27–36, 1992

111. Sullivan KM, Moinpouir C, Chapko M, et al: Reducing the costs of blood and marrow transplantation: A randomized study of early hospital discharge and the results of revised standard practice guidelines. *Blood* 84:1994 (abstr)

112. Larson PJ: Patients' perception of needs in the first four weeks after bone marrow transplant. *Oncol Nurs Forum* 19: 313, 1992 (abstr 271)

113. Buchsel P: Patterns of symptoms experienced by bone marrow transplant recipients during an early discharge trial. *Oncol Nurs Forum* 21:355, 1994 (abstr)

114. Copel LC, Smith ME: Oncology nursing knowledge of graft-versus-host disease in bone marrow transplant patients. *Cancer Nurs* 10:243–249, 1989

115. Sullivan KM, Mori M, Sander J: Late complications of allogeneic and autologous marrow transplantation. *Bone Marrow Transplant* 10:127–134, 1992

116. Corcoran-Buchsel P: Long-term complications of allogeneic bone marrow transplantation: Nursing implications. *Oncol Nurs Forum* 13:61–70, 1986

117. Atkinson K, Horowitz MM, Gale RP, et al: Risk factors for chronic graft-versus-host disease after HLA identical sibling bone marrow transplantation. *Blood* 75:2459–2465, 1990

118. Sullivan KM: Graft-versus-host disease, in Blume KG, Petz LD (eds): *Clinical Bone Marrow Transplantation*. New York, Churchill-Livingstone 1983, pp 88–129

119. Atkinson K: Chronic graft-versus-host disease following marrow transplantation. *Marrow Transplantation Reviews: Issues in Hematology, Oncology and Immunology* 2:10–16, 1992

120. Lloid M: Oral medicine concerns of the BMT patient, in Buchsel PC, Whedon MB (eds): *Bone Marrow Transplantation: Administrative and Clinical Strategies*. Boston, Jones and Bartlett, 1995 pp 257–276

121. Sullivan KM, Agura E, Anasett C, et al: Chronic graft-versus-host disease and other late complications of bone marrow transplantation. *Semin Hematol* 28:250–259, 1988

122. Ferrara JLM, Deeg HJ: Graft-versus-host disease. *N Engl J Med* 324:667–674, 1991

123. Sanders JE, Seattle Marrow Transplant Team: Effect of bone marrow transplantation on reproductive function, in *Late Effects of Childhood Cancer*. New York: Wiley, Liss, 1992, pp 95–101

124. Spencer, S, Haake J, Weisdorf D: Hemorrhagic cystitis after bone marrow transplantation. *Transplantation* 56:875–879, 1993

125. Russell JA, Blahey WA, Stuart TA, et al: Avascular necrosis of bone in bone marrow transplant patients. *Med Pediatr Oncol* 17:1140–1143, 1989

126. Jampel RM, Farmer ER, Vogelsang GB, et al: PUVA therapy for chronic cutaneous graft-vs-host disease. *Arch Dermatol* 127:1673–1678, 1988

127. Vogelsang GB, Hess AD, Santos GW: Thalidomide for treatment of graft-versus-host disease. *Bone Marrow Transplant* 3:392–398, 1988

128. Witherspoon RP, Lum LG, Storb R: Effects of chronic graft-versus-host disease on the return of the immune system. *Semin Hematol* 21:2–10, 1984

129. Somani J, Larson, RA: Reimmunization after allogeneic bone marrow transplantation. *Am J Med* 98:389–398, 1995

130. Nims JW, Strom S: Late complications of bone marrow transplant recipients: Nursing care issues. *Semin Oncol Nurs* 4:47–54, 1988

131. Sanders J: Growth and development after bone marrow transplantation, in Forman SJ, Blume KG, Thomas ED (eds): *Bone Marrow Transplantation*. Cambridge, MA, Blackwell Scientific Publishers, 1994, pp 3527–3537

132. Rio B, Letur-Konirsch H, Ajchenbaum-Cymbalista, et al: Full-term pregnancy with embryos from donated oocytes in a 36-year old woman allografted for chronic myeloid leukemia. *Bone Marrow Transplant,* 13:487–488, 1994

133. Molassiotis A, van den Akkekr OBA, Milligan DW, et al: Gonadal function and psychosexual adjustment in male long-term survivors of bone marrow transplantation. *Bone Marrow Transplant* 16:253–259, 1995

134. Tichelli A: Late ocular complications after bone marrow transplantation. *Nouv-Rev Fr Hematol* 36:S79–82, 1994 (suppl)

135. Atkinson K, Cohen M, Biggs J: Avascular necrosis of the femoral head secondary to corticosteroid therapy for graft-versus-host disease after marrow transplantation: Effective therapy with hip arthroplasty. *Bone Marrow Transplant* 2: 421–426, 1987

136. Wujcik D, Ballard B, Camp-Sorrell D: Selected complications of allogeneic bone marrow transplantation. *Semin Oncol Nurs* 10:28–41, 1994

137. Jackett M, Perry EH, Daniels BS, et al: Hemolytic uremic syndrome following bone marrow transplantation. *Bone Marrow Transplant* 7:405–409, 1988

138. Giralt SA, Champlin R: Leukemia relapse after allogeneic bone marrow transplantation: A review. *Blood* 84:3603–3612, 1994

139. Witherspoon RP, Fisher LD, Schoch G, et al: Secondary cancers after bone marrow transplantation for leukemia or aplastic anemia. *N Engl J Med* 321:784–789, 1989

140. Appelbaum FR, Matthew DC, Eary JF, et al: The use of radiolabeled anti-CD33 antibody to augment marrow irradiation prior to marrow transplantation for acute myelogenous leukemia. *Transplantation* 54:829–833, 1992

141. McNeil C: A new generation of monoclonal antibodies arrives at the clinic. *J Natl Cancer Inst* 87:1658–1660, 1995

142. Andrykowski, MA: Psychosocial factors in bone marrow transplantation: A review and recommendations for research. *Bone Marrow Transplant* 13:357–375, 1994

143. Syrjala KL, Chapko MK, Vitaliano PP, et al: Recovery after allogeneic marrow transplantation: Prospective study of predictors of long-term physical and psychosocial functioning. *Bone Marrow Transplant* 11:319–327, 1993

144. Syrjala K: Meeting the psychological needs of recipients and families, in Buchsel PC, Whedon MB (eds): *Bone Marrow Transplantation: Administrative and Clinical Strategies*. Boston, Jones and Bartlett, 1995, pp 283–302

145. Heiney SP, Neurberg RW, Myers D, et al: The aftermath of bone marrow transplant for parents of pediatric patients: A post-traumatic stress disorder. *Oncol Nurs Forum,* 21: 843–847, 1994

146. Wellisch DK, Wolcott, DL: Psychological issues after bone marrow transplantation, in Forman SJ, Blume KG, Thomas ED (eds): *Bone Marrow Transplantation*. Cambridge, MA, Blackwell Scientific Publishers, 1994, pp 3527–3537

147. New bits. *BMT Newsletter.* 6(5):8, 1995

148. Winters G, Miller C, Marachich L, et al: Provisional practice; the nature of psychological bone marrow transplant nursing. *Oncol Nurs Forum* 21:1147–1154, 1994

149. Sarantos S: Innovations in psychosocial staff support: A model program for the marrow transplant nurse. *Semin Oncol Nurs* 4:69–73, 1988

150. Kelleher J, Jennings M: Nursing management of a marrow transplantation unit: A framework for practice. *Semin Oncol Nurs* 4:60–68, 1988

151. Buchsel P, Kapustay P: New models of care for blood and marrow transplantation, in Whedon MB, Wujcik D (eds): *Blood and Marrow Transplantation: Principles, Practices, and Nursing Insights,* Boston, Jones and Bartlett (in press)

152. Whedon MB, Ferrell BR: Quality of life in adult bone marrow transplant patients: Beyond the first year. *Semin Oncol Nurs* 10:42–57, 1994

153. Andrykowski MA, Henslee PJ, Barmett RL: Longitudinal assessment of psychosocial functioning of adult survivors of allogeneic bone marrow transplantation. *Bone Marrow Transplant* 6:505–508, 1989

154. Haberman M, Bush N, Young K, et al: Quality of life of adult bone marrow transplantation survivors. *Oncol Nurs Forum* 20:1545–1553, 1993

155. Baker, F, Wingard J, Curbow B, et al: Quality of life of bone marrow transplant long-term survivors. *Bone Marrow Transplant* 13:589–596, 1994

156. Ferrell B, Grant M, Schmidt G, et al: The meaning of quality of life for bone marrow transplant survivors: Part 2. Improving quality of life for bone marrow transplant survivors. *Cancer Nurs* 15:247–253, 1992

157. Coxon VJ: Subjective perceptions of the demands of hospitalization and anxiety in bone marrow transplant patients. *Proc American Cancer Society Second National Conference on Cancer Nursing Research.* Atlanta, American Cancer Society, 1992, p 27–B (abstr)

158. Serota FT, O'Shea AT, Woodward WT Jr, et al: Role of a child advocate in the selection of donors for pediatric bone marrow transplantation. *J Pediatr* 98:847–850, 1981

159. Crawford W: Decision making in critically ill patients with hematologic malignancy. *West J Med* 115:488–493, 1988

160. Vaughan WP, Purtileo RB, Butler CD, et al: Ethical and financial issues in autologous marrow transplantation: A symposium sponsored by the University of Nebraska Medical Center. *Ann Intern Med* 105:134–135, 1986

161. Tyndall AG: Options for bone marrow transplantation in severe arthritis. *Blood Cell and Bone Marrow Transplants.* Proceedings of Keystone, 1996, p 28 (abstr 15)

162. Gale RP: Fetal liver transplants. *Bone Marrow Transplant* 9:11, 1992 (suppl 1)

163. Gluckman E, Wagner J: Workshop on umbilical cord blood stem cells and transplantation. *Bone Marrow Transplant* 15:146–150, 1994 (suppl)

164. Kohn DB, Krall W, Chalita H, et al: Gene therapy for congenital hematologic and immune disorders. *Bone Marrow Transplant* 15:288–296, 1994 (suppl)

165. Thomas ED: The future of marrow transplantation. *Semin Oncol Nurs* 4:74–78, 1988

166. Chapman JR, Atkinson K, Lapsely H: Cost of bone marrow transplants using unrelated donors. *Blood Rev* 5:112–116, 1988

167. Hillner RE, Smith TJ, Christopher ED: Estimating the cost-effectiveness of autologous bone marrow transplantation for metastatic breast cancer. *Proc Am Soc Clin Oncol* 10:A60, 1988 (abstr)

168. Boros L, Asbury RF, Chang AY, et al: Cost controls in autologous bone marrow transplantation. *Proc Am Soc Clin Oncol* 9:A388, 1990 (abstr)

169. Sullivan KM, Appelbaum FR: Comparative trials of chemotherapy and bone marrow transplantation in acute non-lymphocytic leukemia. *Rinsho Ketsueki* 31:527–533, 1990

170. Welch HG, Larson EB: Cost-effectiveness of bone marrow transplantation in acute nonlymphoblastic leukemia. *N Engl J Med* 321:807–812, 1988

171. Wingard JR: Health, functional status, and employment of long-term survivors after bone marrow transplantation. *Ann Intern Med* 114:114–118, 1988

# Chapter 19

# Autologous Bone Marrow and Blood Cell Transplantation

Debra Wujcik, RN, MSN, AOCN

# OVERVIEW OF BONE MARROW TRANSPLANTATION

## Allogeneic Bone Marrow Transplantation

Allogeneic bone marrow transplantation (BMT) has been a treatment for some diseases for more than 30 years. The primary purpose of allogeneic BMT is to treat patients with defective bone marrow in nonmalignant disease such as aplastic anemia or diseased marrow such as leukemia. The replacement marrow is obtained from a related or unrelated human leukocyte antigen (HLA)-matched donor. The cells harvested from the bone marrow are pluripotent stem cells (PPSCs). These are cells that have the capacity for both myeloid and lymphoid (multilineage) differentiation, proliferation, and self-renewal.[1,2] The exact number of PPSCs needed to repopulate a marrow destroyed by chemotherapy and/or radiation has not been determined; however, 5% of the nucleated cells found in adult human marrow contain sufficient PPSCs for transplant.[3]

There are many limitations to allogeneic BMT. The biggest drawback is the availability of an appropriate marrow donor. Only one in four persons needing a BMT has a related match. The National Marrow Donor Program provides a pool of nearly 2 million potential donors, but the registry is hindered by the numbers of donors from different races. The best opportunity to find a match is within one's own race, and the largest race in the registry is white. Histocompatibility is another limitation of allogeneic BMT. The greater the histoincompatibility between patient and donor, the greater the risk of graft failure, graft rejection, and graft-versus-host disease (GVHD).[4]

## Autologous Bone Marrow Transplantation

There is a steep dose-response relationship in some malignancies, with response rates improving with dose escalation of chemotherapy and radiation therapy. The limiting toxicity, myelosuppression, can be overcome by "rescue" with the patient's own PPSCs that have been harvested and stored prior to therapy. The first use of autologous bone marrow transplantation (ABMT) to regenerate the bone marrow was reported in 1958 by Kurnick et al.[5] In the early days, failure was due to inadequate treatment after transplant. The lessons of supportive care learned from allogeneic BMT were applied to ABMT with enhanced infection control and transfusion support. Improvements in the technology for cell storage, harvesting, and purging have contributed to increased survival. In turn, ABMT is increasingly used as a treatment option.

## Blood Cell Transplantation

Concern regarding the potential for minimal disease remaining in the bone marrow of autologous donors led researchers to look for new sources of PPSCs. It was learned that cells for autologous transplant could also be obtained from the peripheral blood. Some PPSCs circulate in the peripheral blood in small numbers, and committed progenitors circulate in greater numbers.[6] Progenitors are cells that have limited ability to divide and are irreversibly committed to one or more lines of differentiation.[7] The colony-forming unit–granulocyte, erythrocyte, macrophage, megakaryocyte (CFU-GEMM) and colony-forming unit–lymphocyte (CFU-L) are committed stem cells. Although they are irreversibly committed to the separate lineages, they remain capable of differentiating to one of several cell lines[8] (Figure 19-1).

The peripheral blood progenitor cells represent 1%–10% of the marrow progenitors. Once it was proved that these cells could be reinfused into animals (mice, dogs, and baboons) and restore hematopoiesis, the process was applied to humans.[9] The first transplant using cells obtained from peripheral blood was reported in 1985, with several more the following year.[10]

This process has historically been referred to as peripheral blood stem cell transplant (PBSCT) or peripheral blood progenitor cell transplant (PBPCT). The process involves obtaining and infusing an unspecified number of true PPSCs with or without committed progenitor and precursor cells.[2,11] The current terminology for this process is *blood cell transplant* (BCT). BCT is considered to be more precise and is preferred to other terms to differentiate the PPSCs obtained from the bone marrow for allogeneic BMT and ABMT from the combined PPSCs and committed progenitors obtained from the peripheral blood for BCT.[2]

The cells needed for successful engraftment after high-dose chemotherapy and irradiation are difficult to isolate by current techniques. The CD34 antigen is expressed on the surface of early progenitor cells. The antigen does not appear on the PPSCs but is present on the committed progenitors. Currently the CD34 assay is the best technique available to identify the cells that have been proved to be correlated with successful engraftment.[12–14]

There are advantages to using peripheral PPSCs and progenitor cells obtained from peripheral blood. One advantage is the more rapid recovery of neutrophils and platelets when progenitor cells are used.[15,16] This is because the committed progenitors collected for BCT are farther along the differentiation pathway than the PPSCs harvested from the bone marrow. Another advantage is that no anesthesia is required for BCT so there is less risk of complications and fewer medical contraindications than with bone marrow harvest. Also, individuals who cannot have bone marrow harvested because of marrow involvement or prior radiation therapy to large areas of bone marrow may be able to undergo BCT.

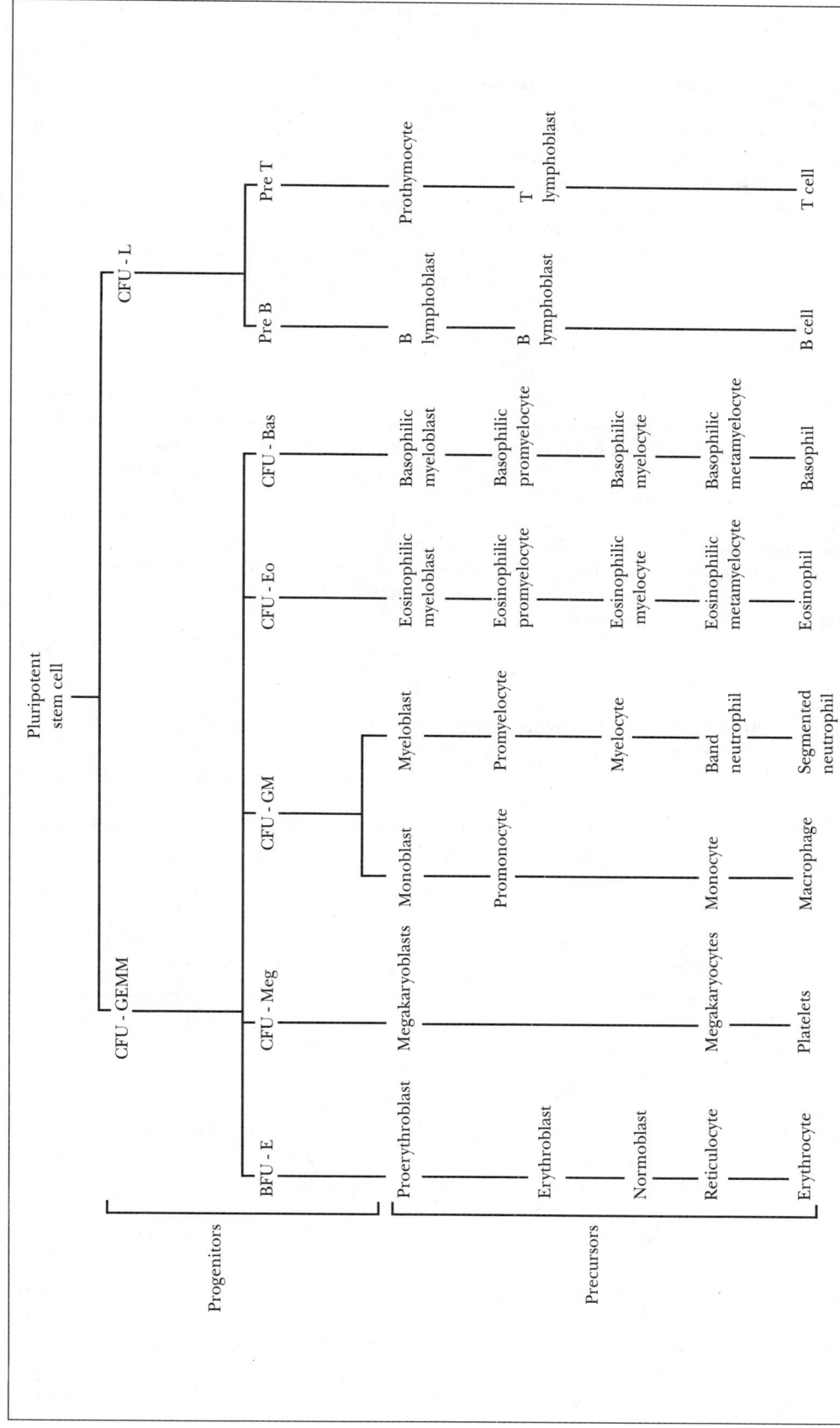

**FIGURE 19-1**   Hematopoietic cascade. Pluripotent stem cells (PPSCs) are harvested from bone marrow for bone marrow transplantation. PPSCs and progenitor cells are collected from peripheral blood for blood cell transplantation. CFU = colony-forming unit; GEMM = granulocyte, erythrocyte, megakaryocyte, macrophage; L = lymphocyte; BFU = burst-forming unit; Meg = megakaryocyte; GM = granulocyte, macrophage; Eo = eosinophil; Bas = basophil. (Reprinted with permission from Wujcik D: *Hematopoiesis,* adapted from Figure 1, Whedon MB, Wujcik D: *Stem Cell and Marrow Transplantation: Principles, Practice, and Nursing Insights.* (ed 2). Boston, Jones & Bartlett, 1997.)

## Standards Development

Two organizations are collecting and organizing data to evaluate the trends and outcomes of transplantation. The International Bone Marrow Transplant Registry, formed in 1970, collects all data on allogeneic and syngeneic BMT patients. The Autologous Blood and Marrow Transplant Registry, formed in 1990, records similar data on ABMT patients.[17] These organizations report annually on the number and types of transplants being performed worldwide and on the outcomes for patients with various diseases.

The standards for transplantation are being set by a number of organizations (Table 19-1). The American Society for Blood and Marrow Transplantation published guidelines for clinical centers and training of transplant staff in 1995.[18,19] The American Society of Clinical Oncology, the American Society of Hematology, and the Eastern Cooperative Oncology Group have published guidelines as well.[20–22]

Centers of excellence for BMT and BCT are being developed and mandated by insurers. This approach is a form of managed care that usually involves a financial contract between the transplant center and the third-party payer.[23] There is shared risk by both parties that allows discount pricing and agreement of selection criteria. A successful partnership should increase the volume of patients for the transplant center as well as decrease the cost for the insurance company. It is hoped that the centers of excellence are built upon the standards set by the professional organizations.

The idea of transplants being performed only in large, usually academic, centers was first challenged by those performing ABMT. The care of ABMT patients is similar to care for those undergoing induction and consolidation therapy for acute myelogenous leukemia (AML). Therefore, physicians with expertise in the care of AML patients in community hospitals have developed successful ABMT programs. Today, patients and those performing BCT are developing successful BCT programs in the community. BCT apheresis can be performed safely in hospital outpatient clinics as well as in for-profit outpatient settings. The availability of the technology in the community setting, along with the knowledge of lay people about this availability, has increased the demand for community BCT programs. There are increasing numbers of joint ventures with hospitals and for-profit apheresis centers as well as networks of community hospitals under the umbrella of university transplant programs. The challenge is to continue to conduct clinical trials to evaluate this treatment while providing accessible, reimbursable care.

**TABLE 19-1**    Standards for Autologous Bone Marrow and Blood Cell Transplantation Programs

| PERSONNEL | |
| --- | --- |
| Director | Licensed and board-certified<br>One year specific clinical training or 2 years as attending for patients undergoing transplantation |
| Other physicians | Trained under the director with demonstrated competency in the managment of myelosuppressed patients |
| Surgeon | Skilled in catheter placement |
| Consultants | Consultants available who are board-certified in pulmonary, gastroenterology, nephrology, infectious disease, cardiology, psychiatry, and radiation oncology |
| Nurses | Formally trained and experienced in care of BCT and ABMT patients; skills in administration of chemotherapy and blood components and management of infections |
| Technologist | Trained for handling of stem cells |
| CLINICAL PRACTICE | |
| Marrow and blood stem cells | Established method for procurement and cryopreservation of stem cells |
| Transfusion support | Policies to maintain hemoglobin > 9.0 g/dl and platelets > 20,000/mm$^3$; all blood products are irradiated and leukocyte depleted; blood bank support available 24 hours per day |
| Infection prophylaxis | Infection prophylaxis includes trimethoprim and sulfamethoxazole for pneumocystis, empirical amphotericin B for fungal infection, and acyclovir for patients with history of oral or genital herpes simplex |
| Vascular access | Multilumen, indwelling catheters used for administration of chemotherapy, antibiotics, and blood products |
| Nutrition management | Criteria and administration policies for total parenteral nutrition |
| Patient care areas | Designated inpatient beds with high-efficiency particulate air filtration recommended |

# INDICATIONS

There are very few randomized trials comparing high-dose chemotherapy plus ABMT or BCT rescue with conventional therapy. There is considerable variation in professional opinion about the value of the high-dose approach because of higher toxicity and lack of proven efficacy. Managed-care considerations of cost and public demand for any potentially lifesaving treatment have led to a high level of controversy that has made recruitment to randomized trials difficult. Therefore, most conclusions are derived from uncontrolled clinical trials.

## Indications for ABMT

The use of ABMT is well established in patients with leukemia, lymphoma, and some solid tumors. The advantages for ABMT over allogeneic BMT are the absence of GVHD and fewer toxicities. The advantages of BCT over ABMT are yet to be proved.

### Leukemia

ABMT is indicated for patients with AML who do not have an allogeneic donor. There is a 40%–50% remission rate in patients transplanted during first remission.[24] Purging of the marrow increases the disease-free survival (DFS).[25,26] The advantage of ABMT over allogeneic BMT in leukemia is less toxicity since there is no veno-occlusive disease or GVHD. However, there is a potential risk of tumor contamination in the autologous marrow, and there is no benefit of the graft-versus-leukemia (GVL) effect, which is thought to be due to the T lymphocytes of the graft identifying and destroying the malignant cells of the host. The presence of GVL is associated with lower relapse rates.[27]

One study analyzed data from the European Bone Marrow Transplantation Registry Group for patients with AML receiving transplant in first remission. The study reviewed data from patients who received ABMT, ABMT with purging, and BCT. Survival was the same for all three groups, but the period of white blood cell counts < 1000/mm³ was significantly shorter for the BCT group. Platelet recovery was the same.[28]

ABMT is used in individuals with acute lymphocytic leukemia who have relapsed or are at high risk for recurrence of disease.[29] The results are improved with the use of purged marrow. There are no randomized trials to determine which type of transplant produces the best survival in this group.

Allogeneic BMT is the treatment of choice for cure in individuals with chronic myelogenous leukemia (CML). Patients in the chronic phase of CML do not benefit from ABMT. Patients in the acute phase may receive ABMT to reestablish the chronic phase 80% of the time. Although this may allow time to continue the search for a matched unrelated donor, the remissions are of short duration.[30,31]

### Lymphoma

Individuals with early or relapsed Hodgkin's disease may be treated with ABMT. The prognosis is better for those previously treated with one or two courses of therapy rather than extensive prior treatment.[32] ABMT is curative for low-grade non-Hodgkin's lymphoma.[33] Individuals with intermediate- to high-grade lymphoma who do not achieve remission with first-line therapy are generally referred for transplant as well.[34,35]

### Solid tumors

The overall disease-free survival of patients with advanced breast cancer receiving ABMT is similar to those receiving standard therapy. However, those who respond to ABMT have a longer duration of response than those who respond to chemotherapy.[36,37] Since the early studies of ABMT in breast cancer were conducted with women with metastatic disease, the trend is now to recommend ABMT before there is a large tumor burden.[38]

Individuals with germ cell tumors generally respond well to chemotherapy. However, a small percentage who are refractory to treatment or who relapse quickly respond well to ABMT, with a 15%–20% DFS after ABMT.[39,40]

Women with ovarian cancer are usually diagnosed with advanced disease. The standard treatment is chemotherapy and debulking surgery. Those women with residual disease are candidates for ABMT. The results are 50% complete response, with 30%–50% DFS at three years.[41]

## Indications for BCT

Most studies demonstrate decreased hematopoietic toxicity with BCT, but none yet say that BCT is better than ABMT for these individuals.[7,42]

### Leukemia

The rationale for BCT in patients with AML is that there would be less malignant cell contamination than in ABMT and faster hematopoietic recovery using committed progenitors. Juttner[43] analyzed the published results of three studies of AML patients who received BCT, which clearly demonstrate hematopoietic repopulation that is earlier after BCT than after either purged or unpurged ABMT. Platelet recovery is more rapid with BCT as well, although it seems to be more directly related to the dose of cells collected. There is no conclusive evidence yet of relapse rates with BCT versus ABMT for patients with AML. Juttner suggests that because BCT apheresis is easier to accomplish, the patient may be able to proceed to transplant more quickly. In addition, one group suggests BCT, having less morbidity, may be more beneficial for treating older individuals, since 25% of patients were greater than 60 years old and 42% were greater than 50 years.[44]

BCT is considered only for those patients with CML who have no options for related or unrelated allogeneic BMT. It is known that ABMT using marrow harvested during the chronic phase and performed during the accelerated or blastic phase can restore the patient to the chronic phase. However, the likelihood of cure is minimal. A few patients who received BCT in the chronic phase reportedly have achieved a complete response as indicated by Philadelphia chromosome negativity.[45] The use of BCT in CML remains investigational.

### Lymphoma

Poor-risk lymphoma patients who received either ABMT or conventional chemotherapy may benefit from BCT. BCT recipients showed an improved complete response rate, freedom from relapse, and increased disease-free survival, although the overall survival was no different.[46]

### Multiple myeloma

BCT has been used to treat small numbers of individuals with multiple myeloma. Fernand et al,[43] in a study with 48 patients, reported a 92% response.[47] Although 32% later relapsed, 66% remained in a state of remission for a median of 35 months. Others have shown similar results.[48]

### Solid tumors

The use of BCT in women with breast cancer is highly controversial due to the high number of women with breast cancer and the large number of breast cancer advocacy groups. Lay people and women with breast cancer are well aware of the potential option of BCT and many have concluded it is appropriate therapy even without published results from clinical trials. In one study of women with poor-prognosis breast cancer, myeloid recovery was decreased from 23 days to 10 days in patients receiving BCT versus ABMT. There was decreased tumor contamination as indicated by recurrence of disease.[14]

BCT can provide effective consolidation for early metastatic breast cancer.[49] Blue Cross and Blue Shield is supporting a large randomized study of standard chemotherapy versus high-dose chemotherapy and BCT to help answer the question of appropriate use of BCT.[50]

Small numbers of individuals with sarcoma, small cell lung cancer, ovarian cancer, neuroblastoma, and Wilms' tumor have also been treated with BCT. The results are encouraging, although the numbers are few and the follow-up is short.[51]

## PROCESS OF AUTOLOGOUS TRANSPLANTATION

The process of autologous transplantation is the same for ABMT and BCT except for the procedure for obtaining the cells used to recover hematopoiesis. Both groups of patients undergo the same evaluation, conditioning, reinfusion, and supportive care procedures. Figures 19-2 and 19-3 show the timelines for ABMT and BCT.

### Patient Evaluation

The first step in patient evaluation for transplant is to determine whether the patient is a candidate for transplantation and which type of transplant is most appropriate. The disease, stage of disease, performance status of the patient, and availability of an appropriate protocol are considered. The type of transplant the patient will receive is decided early in the process since the preauthorization, timing, and scheduling are influenced by this information.

The clinical evaluation, which occurs simultaneously with an insurance preauthorization process, includes determining whether there is any organ dysfunction—specifically in the lungs or heart—secondary to disease or prior therapy. Other screening tests include viral studies to rule out human immunodeficiency virus (HIV) or hepatitis, among others[52,53] (Table 19-2).

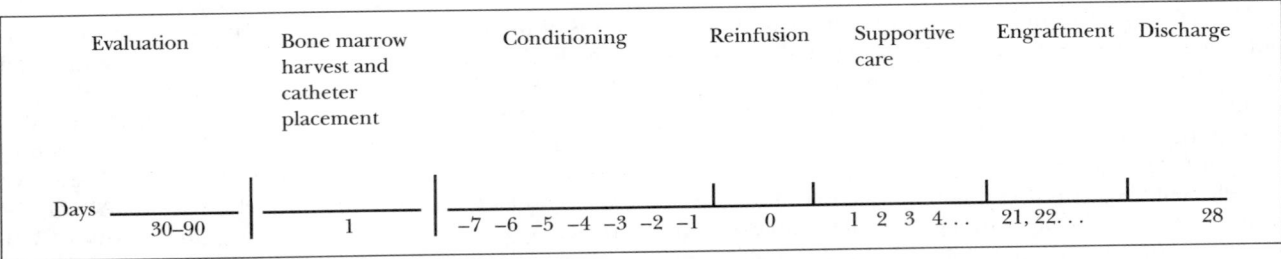

**FIGURE 19-2** Timeline for autologous bone marrow transplantation (ABMT). The number of days for evaluation are variable. Bone marrow harvesting requires one day. The process can be interrupted after evaluation or after harvest if necessary. The days of conditioning are referred to as minus days. Once conditioning begins, the process of BMT cannot be interrupted.

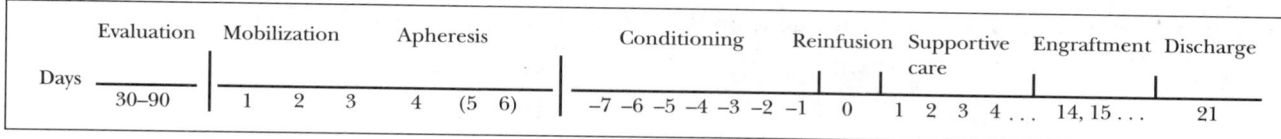

| Days | Evaluation | Mobilization | | | Apheresis | | | Conditioning | | | | | | | Reinfusion | Supportive care | | | Engraftment | Discharge |
|---|---|---|---|---|---|---|---|---|---|---|---|---|---|---|---|---|---|---|---|---|
| | 30–90 | 1 | 2 | 3 | 4 | (5 | 6) | −7 −6 −5 −4 −3 −2 −1 | | | | | | | 0 | 1  2  3  4 . . . | | | 14, 15 . . . | 21 |

**FIGURE 19-3**  Timeline for blood cell transplantation (BCT). The number of days for evaluation is variable. Mobilization and apheresis require four to six days depending on the patient response to the mobilization method (chemotherapy or hematopoietic growth factor). The process can be interrupted after evaluation or after apheresis if necessary. The days of conditioning are referred to as *minus days*. Once conditioning begins, the process of BCT cannot be interrupted.

**TABLE 19-2**  Baseline Evaluation for Patients Undergoing Autologous Bone Marrow or Blood Cell Transplantation

Complete blood count, including differential and reticulocyte
Complete blood chemistry profile
Prothrombin time
Partial thromboplastin time
Thyroid function tests
Urinalysis
Chest x-ray (PA-Lat)
Cardiac ejection fraction by (resting) MUGA scan
Pulmonary function tests (including DLCO)
12-lead ECG
Type and screen
HSV serology
EBV serology
HIV antibody
HTLV-1 antibody
Varicella zoster serology
Hepatitis A, B, C battery
VDRL

Key:
PA-Lat = posterior anterior-lateral
MUGA = multigated angiogram
DLCO = diffusion capacity of carbon monoxide
ECG = electrocardiogram
HSV = herpes simplex virus
EBV = Epstein Barr virus
HIV = human immunodeficiency virus
HTLV = human T-cell lymphocytic virus
VDRL = venereal disease research laboratory

The insurance appraisal must occur early in the evaluation process because of the expense and the frequent investigational nature of the studies. An insurance counselor or transplant coordinator works closely with the transplant team and advises them of potential reimbursement obstacles. Preauthorization is usually required. Sometimes during this process, it is learned that the patient must go to a different transplant center where the insurance company has an existing contract. Successful preauthorization generally requires knowledge of the patient's history and the transplant process along with experience in negotiations with the insurers.[54]

In general allogeneic BMT and ABMT for acute leukemia in remission, resistant non-Hodgkin's lymphoma, advanced Hodgkin's lymphoma, recurrent neuroblastoma, and medulloblastoma are covered by insurers. However, autologous transplant for patients with solid tumors remains controversial.[55] Some patients have to sue for coverage.[56] Some payers such as Blue Cross and Blue Shield have agreed to support patients enrolled in clinical trials until the results are known.[50] Often patients without insurance coverage must raise their own funds and have a certain amount raised before the transplant.

Beginning with this period of evaluation and continuing throughout the process of transplantation, the patient and family receive extensive education (Table 19-3). It is useful to provide both written and oral instructions and to allow sufficient time for patients and family members to synthesize information and ask questions.[57] Use of critical pathways may allow the teaching to be presented in a consistent, sequential manner with reinforcement at the appropriate time.[54]

## Cells for Autologous Transplant

The process of obtaining PPSCs and progenitor cells for autologous transplantation differs according to the type of transplant. With ABMT the cells are obtained through a bone marrow harvest. In BCT the number of PPSCs and progenitors in the peripheral blood must first be enhanced, then collected in an apheresis procedure.

### Harvest for autologous BMT

The process of obtaining bone marrow for ABMT is the same as for allogeneic BMT, but the volume harvested may be greater if there is a need for purging or other manipulation. The bone marrow is harvested when the patient is in remission and recovered from other treatment. The harvest is usually done in the operating room with the patient anesthetized.

Multiple aspirations are obtained from each posterior ileac crest to obtain the necessary volume. The dose of bone marrow CD34+ cells needed for engraftment is $1 \times 10^6$/kg body weight.[58] The marrow is placed in a heparinized tissue culture medium, filtered for removal of fat and bone particles, then sent to the laboratory for processing and cryopreservation.

Postoperatively, pressure dressings are applied to the puncture sites. The nurse assesses the patient for bleeding, pain, and fluid balance. Because 400–600 ml of whole blood are aspirated during the harvest, the patient may

**Table 19-3** Topics for Education of Autologous Bone Marrow or Blood Cell Transplant Patients

| Phase | ABMT | Both | BCT |
|---|---|---|---|
| Evaluation | | Overview<br>Tests<br>Laboratory specimens<br>Local housing | |
| Catheter | | Placement<br>Catheter care<br>Complications | |
| Procurement of cells | Harvest procedure<br>Complications | | Mobilization<br>Pheresis<br>Complications |
| Conditioning | Specific drugs<br>± TBI | | Specific drugs<br>TBI rare |
| Reinfusion | | Preparation<br>Procedure<br>Complications | |
| Supportive care | | Antibiotics<br>HGFs<br>Blood products<br>TPN | |
| Discharge | | Criteria for discharge<br>Continued care at<br>home | |

ABMT = autologous bone marrow transplantation; BCT = blood cell transplantation; TBI = total body irradiation; TPN = total parenteral nutrition; HGF = hematopoietic growth factor.

receive an autologous unit of blood that was collected before the procedure. The complication rate for bone marrow harvest is low, and the patient is usually discharged the next day.[59]

A double- or triple-lumen silicone catheter is placed centrally to use for reinfusion of bone marrow cells, administration of conditioning chemotherapy and hydration, and supportive therapy such as antibiotics and transfusions of blood products. The catheter is placed at the time of harvest or at the first day of conditioning therapy unless the patient has a preexisting catheter from prior therapy. Catheter care includes insertion site care, dressing changes, and flushing procedures. Patients are taught signs and symptoms of infection and management of complications such as occlusion or accidental puncture of the catheter. The timing of catheter placement determines the extent and timing of the education for the patient and caregiver.

### BCT mobilization

The purpose of mobilization for BCT is to release an increased number of PPSCs and progenitor cells into the peripheral bloodstream. The number of progenitor cells in the bloodstream in the steady state is only 1%–10% of the marrow progenitors.[16] The number of PPSCs and progenitors can be increased up to 100–500-fold through the use of hematopoietic growth factors (HGFs), chemo-

therapy, or both.[16,60,61] Without mobilization, it would take 10 to 14 procedures to obtain the required number of cells needed for BCT.[7,58] The number of cells required for BCT is $\geq$5–7 $\times$ $10^8$ mononuclear cells/kg and/or $\geq$ 1–5 $\times$ $10^6$ CD34 cells/kg.[62] With appropriate mobilization this usually requires two to three apheresis procedures. However, the optimal process for mobilization is not yet defined.

Chemotherapy is used for mobilization either alone or in combination with HGFs. The results using chemotherapy are variable and less predictable than with HGFs. Rebound leukocytosis occurs after single-agent chemotherapy with high-dose cyclophosphamide or with multiple drug regimens using etoposide, cyclophosphamide, and cisplatin.[63,64] It is important not to use drugs that induce thrombocytopenia at the time of maximum progenitor output or to use drugs, such as carmustine or melphalan, that are damaging to progenitor cells.[7]

Chemotherapy alone for mobilization is useful in patients with residual malignancy, but there are disadvantages as well. Fever and pancytopenia that occur as side effects of the drugs can interfere with the schedule for apheresis. In addition, since rebound leukocytosis occurs 10 to 14 days after chemotherapy, it is often difficult to plan ahead for collection of cells.[65] Finally, if an adequate volume of cells is not harvested, the patient must undergo further chemotherapy that is not related to the BCT process itself.

If there is no malignancy in the bone marrow, if the patient received minor pretreatment with chemotherapy, and appropriate mobilization is used, a single apheresis can obtain the desired number of cells.[65] Although two to three procedures usually are needed, investigations continue to find strategies to decrease the number to one.[66] This would benefit the patient by decreasing both the volume of bone marrow withdrawn and the amount of dimethyl sulfoxide (DMSO) reinfused into the patient.[58]

HGFs provide a much more controlled response for mobilization. HGFs stimulate enhanced proliferation and maturation of neutrophils. Granulocyte colony-stimulating factor (G-CSF) is indicated for mobilization at 10 μg/kg/day given subcutaneously for four to five days. This administration usually allows pheresing to begin on the fourth day.[67,68] Two other HGFs have been used for mobilization as well: granulocyte-macrophage colony-stimulating factor (GM-CSF)[69] and interleukin-3.[70,71]

Ex vivo expansion of the number of cells with stem cell factor, interleukin-1, interleukin-6, gamma-interferon, and erythropoietin is being explored.[72] If successful, this process would allow the pheresing of a small amount of cells that would then be grown and expanded in the laboratory until the desired number of cells were produced.

### BCT apheresis

Blood cell separators have been used since the 1980s for various clinical indications. Third-generation machines are now being used for plasma apheresis and leukapheresis.[60,73] Blood cell separators collect the PPSCs and progenitor cells since each cell type has a different density. The machines work by using a centrifuge to separate and collect mononuclear cells, which include the progenitor cells, and other blood components.[16] The Fenwal CS3000 (Fenwal Laboratories, Deerfield, IL) and Cobe Spectra (Cobe Laboratories, Lakewood, CO) are the most commonly used machines.[74] Both use a continuous flow mode. The Spectra relies on the operator to position the buffy coat correctly and has little RBC and platelet contamination. The Fenwal has been improved to provide a comparable product, but it is not as useful for high-volume pheresis. These machines extract the mononuclear cell layer from the buffy coat. One goal is to develop machines that will draw off only CD34 + cells.

Patients are prepared for apheresis through extensive education, placement of the central venous catheter, and being started on specific medications. Teaching at this time covers catheter care, the process of pheresis, mobilization, and potential complications.[57]

The patient undergoing BCT requires a catheter that is stiffer than the traditional CVC used for ABMT because of the need for high volume and pressure during pheresis (about 60–70 ml/minute versus 30 ml/minute). Subclavian silicone catheters placed centrally and used in ABMT are not stiff enough to withstand the rapid withdrawal of blood. In the past, a more rigid catheter used for dialysis was frequently used for BCT apheresis. This catheter was replaced by another after apheresis for extended use during BCT. Currently, the PermCath (Quinton®, Boothal, WA) is a double-lumen catheter suitable for use during pheresis, conditioning chemotherapy, and supportive care. The catheter is placed in an outpatient setting usually at the beginning or during the period of mobilization and is used throughout BCT.

The mobilization process is initiated at the appropriate time (see Figure 19-3). If growth factor is being used, the patient must learn subcutaneous administration. It is usually administered daily for five to six days, with the collection of cells beginning on the fourth day. If chemotherapy is used for mobilization, the drugs are given and the individual returns home. Blood counts are monitored daily, and apheresis begins when the desired white blood cell (WBC) count is achieved. To prevent platelet clumping during apheresis, ibuprofen 200 mg is given daily starting several days before apheresis begins. Oscal-D 500 mg orally three times daily also begins to minimize hypocalcemia during apheresis.

Collection of cells begins once the WBC count is adequate. When chemotherapy is used for mobilization, adequate WBC count is >10,000 cells/mm³ and there is clear evidence of rising counts. If growth factor is used to stimulate neutrophil production, a count of 20,000 cells/mm³ indicates that the patient is ready to be pheresed. Baseline blood specimens, including red blood cell, platelet, and calcium, are drawn. Next the patient is connected to the machine using the central venous catheter. About 7–15 liters of blood are processed through the machine in a four- to eight-hour period. The mononuclear cell layer is drawn off and the rest is returned to the patient. Chilling can occur due to the large volume of blood leaving the body and cooling to room temperature before being returned to the patient. However, the patient is generally comfortable during the procedure and can watch television or use other diversions.

Several potential procedural complications can be avoided or minimized by early intervention.[75] A large volume of the anticoagulant sodium citrate is used to keep the blood from clotting.[60] The citrate binds to ionized serum calcium, causing hypocalcemia, in which the patient experiences tingling in the extremities and around the mouth. Nurses routinely give TUMS® (SmithKline Beecham) at the beginning of apheresis and as needed throughout the procedure. Intravenous (IV) calcium gluconate may be needed if the hypocalcemia becomes severe. Hypovolemia may also be a problem, especially for patients with a history of cardiac problems. The patient may complain of light-headedness, chilling, dizziness, and shaking, and may experience dysrhythmia. Thrombocytopenia is problematic with some types of equipment because platelets are destroyed by the process. Because platelet counts may even drop by one-half during the apheresis, the patient should have an adequate platelet count (> 150,000/mm³) before the procedure. Occasionally the blood flow rate may be altered or decreased. Usually a position change by the patient quickly remedies the problem.

## Cell Processing/Storage

The cells obtained from either the bone marrow or the peripheral blood for autologous transplant are processed and cryopreserved in the same way. The American Association of Blood Banking (AABB) has strict standards for processing and storing the cells.[76] Processing begins with the identification of the cells needed for engraftment. Previously, the colony-forming unit-granulocyte macrophage (CFU-GM) assay was used to identify the adequate dose. This technique requires 14 days, which is problematic when trying to determine whether additional cells should be collected. More recently, the CFU-GM assay has been replaced by the CD34 assay, an easier, standardized method that provides a real number of circulating progenitor cells, not a number predicted after growth in culture.[77] At present, CD34+ selection is the most reproducible and standardizable technique available. However, most agree that further development of techniques to identify the number and type of cells essential for engraftment needs to continue.[7,78]

Quality assurance is monitored with bacterial and fungal cultures of the collected cells. DMSO is added so that cells will not lyse when thawed. Freezing of the cells begins at $-1°$/minute down to $-40°$, and $-2°$/minute from $-40°C$ to $-80°C$. The cells are stored in liquid nitrogen between $-100°C$ and $-196°C$.[79]

One of the main reasons to use cells derived from blood rather than from bone marrow was to avoid tumor contamination from bone marrow. CD34 assays are also useful to separate the malignant cells in a positive selection process. CD34 antigens are not present on breast tumors, neuroblastoma, lymphoma, and multiple myeloma cells.[14] Therefore, stem cell isolates should be free from tumor contamination. That is, in theory, selecting only CD34+ cells should produce a product that is free from malignant cells for those diseases.[80] However, the purity is incomplete because of the limitations of current techniques, so the process is not yet perfected.[12] In addition, lack of randomized trials and relative short-term follow-up of BCT recipients has not yet allowed the issue of tumor contamination in BCT to be answered.[81]

Minimal residual disease is especially important for patients with hematologic malignancy. The outcome after either ABMT or BCT in individuals with AML is similar. Therefore, the shortened nadir period produced by BCT may be the only advantage of one procedure over the other. In patients with solid tumors, there are not enough data to evaluate the significance of minimal residual disease.[82] There is also some evidence that although CD34+ selection does not eliminate leukemia cells, current technology using polymerase chain reaction assays indicate that if bone marrow cells are contaminated, so are peripheral progenitor cells.[83]

Purging of autologous bone marrow and peripheral blood cells is another strategy to decrease the risk of tumor contamination. Purging is done after the harvest or apheresis and before cryopreservation. A number of procedures are used to remove the malignant cells, all of which have the potential to harm the PPSCs and progenitor cells.[84,85] This manipulation often results in delayed or failed engraftment. Pharmacological methods use chemotherapeutic agents such as 4-hydroperoxycyclophosphamide (4HC) or mafosfamide. Immunologic methods use monoclonal antibodies and toxins. Physical methods are used to mark the malignant cells, then separate them from the isolate.[86] To date, there are no randomized trials to identify the best purging methods.

## Conditioning Therapy

Conditioning therapy is given to remove any remaining malignant cells. In the process, the bone marrow is depleted and the immune response is altered. Protocols vary in length from four to seven days. The days of chemotherapy and irradiation before transplant are referred to as *minus days*, and the day of bone marrow or blood cell reinfusion is *day 0*[52] (see Figures 19-2 and 19-3). A commonly used protocol for patients with leukemia or lymphoma includes cyclophosphamide and total-body irradiation. The use of busulfan and cyclophosphamide without total-body irradiation has been proved to be effective as well. Patients receiving BCT for breast cancer may receive cyclophosphamide, cisplatin, and carmustine.

Cyclophosphamide, an alkylating agent that provides tumor cell kill and immunosuppression, is the most commonly used agent in ABMT and BCT. The side effects of cyclophosphamide are dose-related and include bone marrow depression, nausea and vomiting, hemorrhagic cystitis, and cardiotoxicity.

Hemorrhagic cystitis is a significant urologic toxicity that is often a deterrent to outpatient conditioning therapy. Hemorrhagic cystitis ranges from transient, difficult voiding to a life-threatening process. The incidence is up to 68% in all BMT patients, with significant hemorrhage in 8%–27%.[87] Transient cystitis, which has an early onset and a duration of less than seven days, is believed to be due to the direct effect of acrolein, a by-product of cyclophosphamide metabolism, on the urothelium. Long-lasting cystitis or cystitis that develops after completion of cyclophosphamide administration may be associated with viuria. This pathology results in sloughing, inflammatory response, regeneration of thinner epithelium, and formation of new blood vessels.[88]

Prevention of hemorrhagic cystitis is the key to success with aggressive use of hydration, Foley catheter, and administration of the uroprotectant mesna. Because there is no good treatment of hemorrhagic cystitis, prevention is paramount. Protocols vary but may include continuous bladder irrigation during and for 24 hours after cyclophosphamide administration, continuous mesna infusion, and hydration at 200 ml/hour. Protocols are being developed for outpatient administration of high-dose cyclophosphamide.[89]

Cardiomyopathy may result from use of high-dose cyclophosphamide as well.[90] This can be fatal, and patients with a previous history of receiving cardiotoxic drugs such as daunomycin or doxorubicin are at higher risk. The baseline assessment includes a multigated angiogram (MUGA) scan to establish any potential risk. Daily assessment includes cardiac and fluid assessment, with cardiac monitoring as indicated. Signs and symptoms such as dull or sharp precordial pain radiating to the neck or shoulder, dyspnea, friction rub, fever, or ST-T wave changes on electrocardiogram are reported to the physician.[91] Congestive heart failure is treated with fluid and sodium restrictions, digoxin, and diuretics. Pericardial effusion may also occur. Early dysrhythmia can signal risk for later problems.

Busulfan is an oral alkylating agent that causes bone marrow depression and pulmonary interstitial fibrosis. The nurse should be aware of signs and symptoms such as dyspnea, nonproductive cough, fever, and rales in the first weeks to months after transplant.[91]

Carmustine is a nitrosourea agent that crosses the blood-brain barrier. It also causes pulmonary fibrosis and hepatic toxicity as evidenced by abnormal liver function tests. Because carmustine is reconstituted in ethanol, a cool or pressure sensation in the chest and a drunken feeling can occur.

Etoposide, a topoisomerase inhibitor, is cell cycle-specific in the synthesis phase. To minimize risk of bronchospasm and hypotension, the drug is administered in a large amount of fluid (1 mg/1 ml fluid). This requires aggressive monitoring of the patient by the nurse to avoid fluid overload. Side effects include nausea, vomiting, bone marrow depression, and possible hepatic injury.

Total-body irradiation is given to provide maximum tumor cell kill. Total-body irradiation penetrates the sanctuary sites where cells may be hidden, such as the central nervous system and gonads. In the earlier days of transplant, total-body irradiation was delivered in a single dose, which often produced lethal organ toxicity. The current standard is for several days of fractionated dosing to provide maximum effect with minimal toxicity. Common side effects of total-body irradiation include nausea, vomiting, diarrhea, fever, and skin erythema and tenderness. Patients are advised that parotid tenderness, decreased salivation, and loss of taste are temporary side effects that may interfere with eating.[92]

## Reinfusion

The preparation of the patient for reinfusion of autologous cells includes psychological and physical aspects. Patient teaching includes a description of the steps in the reinfusion procedure, potential side effects, and measures to ensure patient comfort. The entire procedure usually takes less than an hour. The nurse ensures the patient is in a comfortable position and the catheter is patent. Preservative-free normal saline is used to flush the IV line and maintain patency.

Because the patient may experience sudden onset of nausea and vomiting, antiemetic prophylaxis is recommended. IV hydration for two hours prior to reinfusion is recommended to ensure optimal renal function.[60] Hemoglobulinuria develops due to red blood cell lysis. Patients are advised that reddish urine is expected for 12 to 24 hours after reinfusion.[52]

The cells are brought to the patient care unit or bedside in liquid nitrogen. A supply basket of needed items is at the bedside. The bags of frozen cells are thawed quickly in warm water. The cells can be given by rapid IV drip but it is preferable to give them by IV push to maintain maximum cell viability. A connector is inserted to break the vacuum on the bag and provide a needle puncture site. The cells are withdrawn from the bag using a large syringe and are handed to the nurse, who administers them by IV push. The bag is emptied, then rinsed with saline. The preservative DMSO is about 10% of the volume of the bag of cells. The maximum daily amount of DMSO tolerated by the patient is 1 ml/kg body weight. Therefore, the volume may be too great to administer at one time. The reinfusion may be divided into two procedures given eight hours apart.

Several complications can occur during and immediately after infusion. Nausea, due to the DMSO, is often acute but brief. The patient also experiences nausea and vomiting, chilling, cramping, and a bad taste from the DMSO. The characteristic odor of DMSO is present in the room and is excreted through the patient's breath and excretions for up to 12 hours after the infusion. Cough, dyspnea, chest tightness, decreased or increased blood pressure, and tachypnea may indicate pulmonary emboli or pulmonary overload. The nurse should monitor vital signs and oxygenation throughout the procedure. Anaphylaxis is rare, but if it does occur the procedure is stopped and treatment with epinephrine and hydrocortisone is instituted immediately.[52,54]

## POSTTRANSPLANT CARE

Posttransplant care for patients receiving ABMT and BCT requires a multidisciplinary team skilled in the management of severely myelosuppressed patients.[18,19,21,22] All patients undergoing transplantation experience common toxicities. The degree and duration depend upon a combination of variables that includes the conditioning protocol, disease and stage, and other patient variables such as age, concurrent medical conditions, and performance status. Table 19-4 provides a comparison of complications after BMT or BCT.[93]

### Infection

A predictable period of myelosuppression follows BMT[94] (Figure 19-4). Engraftment after ABMT for hematologic malignancy occurs beginning at day 21, with full recovery by day 30. This nadir period can be decreased with use of HGFs, especially for patients with solid tumor receiving ABMT.[95] Patients receiving BCT have a shorter period of

**TABLE 19-4**  Comparison of Frequency of Complications after Bone Marrow or Blood Cell Transplantion

| Toxicity/Complication | Related Allogeneic | Unrelated Allogeneic | Autologous | Blood Cell Transplantation |
|---|---|---|---|---|
| GVHD | + + | + + + | rare | − |
| Infection | + + | + + + | + | + |
| Gastrointestinal | | | | |
| Nausea/vomiting | + + | + + | + + | + |
| Diarrhea | + + | + + + | + | + |
| Stomatitis | + + | + + | + + | + + |
| Pulmonary | + + | + + | + + | + + |
| Genitourinary | | | | |
| Cystitis | + + | + + | + | + |
| Renal | + + | + + | + | + |
| Hepatic | | | | |
| Veno-occlusive disease | + + | + + | rare | rare |
| Neurotoxicity | + + | + + | + | + |
| Failure to engraft | + | + + | + | + |

− = absent; + = infrequent; + + = common; + + + = frequent; GVHD = graft-versus-host disease.

Reprinted with permission from Viele.[93]

neutropenia lasting 7 to 10 days with recovery by day 18 to 21 following transplant.[94] Platelet recovery is less predictable and immune recovery about the same or slightly increased since some CFU-Ls are infused in BCT. Typically the patient undergoing transplant has significant risk for infection before engraftment, with bacterial infection first, followed by viral infections and fungal infections. By decreasing the length of the nadir and with aggressive use of prophylaxis, there is less risk of infection with ABMT and BCT than with allogeneic BMT.

Recipients of allogeneic BMT remain immunosuppressed for six months to two years, depending upon the presence and degree of GVHD.[96] The immunosuppression predisposes them to opportunistic infections such as cytomegalovirus or aspergillus. Patients with ABMT and BCT do not have extended immunosuppression; therefore, there is less risk for late infections. Patients undergoing ABMT for hematologic malignancy receive aggressive prophylaxis with antivirals, trimethoprim-sulfamethoxazole, and broad-spectrum antibiotics. Those with

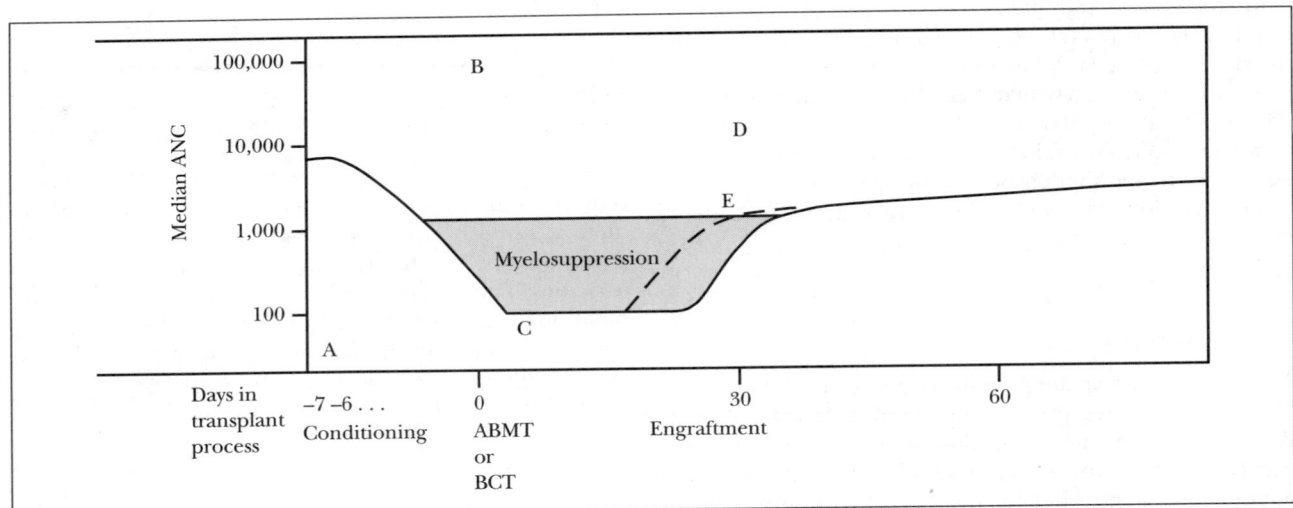

**FIGURE 19-4**  Infection risk and prophylaxis in patients undergoing autologous bone marrow transplantation (ABMT) and blood cell transplantation (BCT). A. Conditioning chemotherapy with or without total body irradiation is administered to prepare the patient for transplantation. B. Prophylactic antibiotics are given to decrease colonization. C. During the period of myelosuppression, empirical antibiotic therapy is initiated with the first fever. D. As the stem cells engraft and peripheral counts recover, prophylaxis for *Pneumocystis carinii* is added. E. The solid line indicates hematopoietic recovery after ABMT. The broken line indicates hematopoietic recovery after BCT. Recovery after BCT is more rapid due to the presence of the committed progenitor cells in the collected cells.

ABMT for solid tumor or BCT may require less aggressive prophylaxis.

Standard prophylaxis and empiric therapy are used to manage infection in patients undergoing ABMT and BCT. Infection prophylaxis includes administration of trimethoprim-sulfamethoxazole to prevent pneumocystis and acyclovir for patients with a history of oral or genital herpes simplex.[20] Some physicians use oral fluoroquinolones to minimize infections with gram-negative organisms.[97] Another strategy to decrease the risk of infection is to use HGFs to shorten the duration of neutropenia and enhance engraftment of the bone marrow and blood stem cells. G-CSF or GM-CSF, usually started on the day of reinfusion of the cells, is administered daily until the neutrophil count is >10,000 cells/mm$^3$.[15,98,99]

Empiric antibiotic therapy is initiated at the onset of fever in the presence of neutropenia. Although a complete daily assessment is performed on the patient, a source of infection is rarely documented. Common management of infection includes the combination of an aminoglycoside plus an extended-spectrum cephalosporin or a broad-spectrum penicillin.[100] If fever persists after several days of broad-spectrum therapy, antifungal therapy is added, usually amphotericin B.[101] A complete discussion of infection management is found in chapter 21.

## Bleeding

Bleeding may occur secondary to thrombocytopenia during the preengraftment period. Patients may require platelet transfusions to prevent life-threatening bleeding until the bone marrow begins producing sufficient megakaryocytes. The nose and mouth are the most common sites of bleeding, requiring diligence by the nurse to keep the airway patent. Intracranial bleeding is a threat when platelets are <20,000/mm$^3$. Signs and symptoms such as headache, blurred vision, and pupil changes are reported immediately. Platelets are usually administered to keep counts >20,000/mm$^3$ and >50,000/mm$^3$ if an invasive procedure is to be performed[52,54] (see chapter 22).

## Anemia

Fatigue and decreased oxygenation occur due to anemia. Red blood cell infusions are given to keep the hematocrit above 25%. Leukocyte-removing filters are used at the bedside to decrease risk of transfusion reactions. All products should be irradiated to decrease the risk of acute GVHD from transfused lymphocytes[102,103] (see chapter 26).

## Gastrointestinal Toxicity

Gastrointestinal toxicity is common with the chemotherapeutic drugs used for all types of transplant. Stomatitis, nausea, vomiting, and diarrhea can be severe enough to require hospitalization and aggressive supportive care. Numerous strategies are being evaluated to decrease the need for hospitalization. Outpatient protocols are being developed using continuous infusions of antiemetic cocktails. Aggressive oral care regimens are taught to the patient and family to decrease the infection and discomfort associated with mucositis. Selected conditioning protocols such as the combination of cyclophosphamide, cisplatin, and carmustine are being used for outpatient treatment. This combination is effective in patients with breast cancer or lymphoma and produces no stomatitis.[104] Some centers are seeing patients daily in the outpatient clinic for assessment and changes in the plan of care. Again, a smooth admission process must be available 24 hours a day to ensure timely inpatient care when needed.

## Urinary System Toxicity

Hemorrhagic cystitis can be a severe side effect of high-dose cyclophosphamide. One successful protocol, reported from a group with an aggressive outpatient program for ABMT and BCT,[89] allows the patient to be discharged 24 hours after the completion of chemotherapy. Hydration is accomplished with IV fluids at 200 ml/m$^2$/hour during chemotherapy. Standing orders allow an automatic increase if urine output falls below 200 ml/hour. Bladder irrigation with a Foley catheter is administered at 1 liter/hour during administration of cyclophosphamide and for the next 24 hours after cyclophosphamide, cisplatin, and carmustine. No visible or symptomatic hematuria was reported for the 303 patients reviewed. This report is an example of the many strategies being evaluated to determine how effective transplant therapy can be administered in a cost-effective manner.

In summary, many patients undergoing ABMT and BCT suffer significant toxicity from therapy. In addition, many patients remain hospitalized throughout their transplant process. Severe infections with opportunistic organisms can require weeks of multiple IV antibiotics. Many antibiotics can compromise renal function, especially in the setting of sepsis. Pulmonary, cardiac, and neurological toxicities may occur as well but with significantly less frequency than in patients undergoing allogeneic BMT (see chapter 18). However, the transplant team must remember that the care of these patients should never be considered routine.

## Outpatient Care

The trend of treatment is to move as much patient care to the outpatient setting as possible. Figure 19-5 provides an example of a care delivery model in which most of the care for individuals with breast cancer receiving ABMT is delivered in the outpatient setting.[104] Safe and effective care for ABMT and BCT requires significant allocation of resources and elimination of some typical administrative

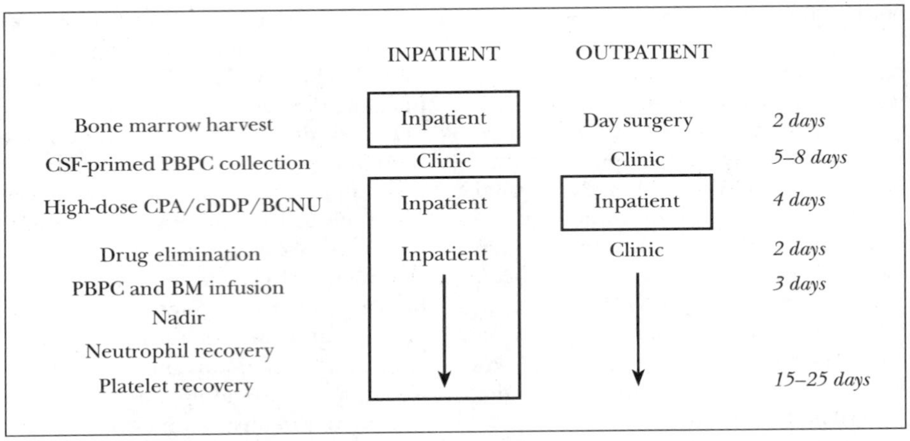

**FIGURE 19-5** Schematic comparison of traditional inpatient and outpatient ABMT management for breast cancer. CSF = colony-stimulating factor; PBPC = peripheral blood progenitor cells; CPA/cDDP/BCNU = cyclophosphamide/cisplatin/carmustine; BM = bone marrow. (Reprinted with permission from Anderson and Weinstein.[103])

obstacles. The neutropenic patient must be seen and evaluated daily. This can be accomplished in an outpatient clinic area or a designated space in the BMT unit for walk-in outpatient care. Having a bed exclusively designated for outpatient use ensures availability when needed without delays in the emergency room or admitting department.

Treatment and supportive care protocols must be reevaluated in order to facilitate outpatient care. For example, the use of HGFs and BCT can shorten the nadir period and subsequently decrease the risk of infection. Development of megakaryocyte growth factor may decrease the need for platelet transfusions.[105]

Outpatient protocols for the prevention of infection are being developed and tested. Gilbert et al used a specific protocol with 70 patients receiving both ABMT and BCT.[106] The prevention protocol was oral ciprofloxacin 500 mg every 8 hours and rifampin 300 mg every 12 hours. If fever developed during the neutropenic period, 30 mg/kg vancomycin and 5 mg/kg tobramycin were administered intravenously daily. Of the 70 patients, 43% remained afebrile, compared with less than 2% in the control group. For those who required IV antibiotics, the median duration of IV therapy was 4 days, compared with 11 days in the control group. The ciprofloxacin and rifampin were generally well tolerated. The original dose of rifampin every 6 hours produced nausea and vomiting, but decreasing the dose to every 12 hours alleviated the problem.

Another study evaluated the effectiveness of prophylactic antibiotics and the use of protective isolation in patients receiving ABMT. The patients were given oral ciprofloxacin 500 mg b.i.d. and either amphotericin B suspension and tablets (200 mg q.i.d.) or fluconazole 50 mg plus amphotericin tablets for fungal prophylaxis. To prevent alpha-hemolytic streptococcal infection, patients received either raxithromycin 150 mg b.i.d. or IV cephalothin 1000 mg every four hours for ten days following ABMT. In addition, isolation procedures were decreased from full isolation (high energy particulate air (HEPA) filtration, gowns, gloves, and masks by all entering the room, and low-microbial, sterilized foods) to minimal isolation (private room with no visitor restriction, hand washing, and low-microbial foods). There was no difference in incidence and outcome of infections.[107] The authors concluded that the use of expensive protective isolation may not be warranted in these patients. As studies continue to indicate that prophylaxis with oral and daily IV antibiotics is effective, outpatient therapy may become the standard for this group of patients.

## INFLUENCE OF HEALTH CARE REFORM

The influence of health care reform is felt in all settings across the health care continuum. In order to support the movement toward outpatient care, administrators and clinicians must work together closely to provide resources necessary for safe and effective care. Care must be available 24 hours a day, seven days per week, in order to provide for patients whose condition can deteriorate rapidly. Housing for out-of-town patients and families must be close to the health care facility, must be convenient, and must have facilities such as wheelchair ramps, handrails, and cooking equipment. Twenty-four-hour transportation to the facility must be available for those who cannot drive or are too weak to tolerate sitting in a car. Some patients have successfully contracted with third-party payers to pay for these accommodations since they significantly decrease the cost of inpatient care.[104]

## PRICE CAPITATION

Reports of the price of BCT range from $70,000 to $150,000 and ABMT from $80,000 to $120,000.[54] These amounts usually reflect the charges for the transplant process, including evaluation, transplant, and one year of follow-up care. What is not included are the aspects of care that are difficult to quantify: housing and meals for family members to stay nearby; travel; loss of income of the patient or caregiver during the lengthy period away from home; caregiver burden; and impact on quality of life.

Insurance carriers are inconsistent in the criteria used to approve and disapprove transplant.[108,109] One review examined the consistency of insurance preapprovals for 533 patients who received ABMT for breast cancer. All patients were enrolled in clinical trials supported by grants. The results showed significant variability in the frequency of approval both by different insurers and by individual insurers for different patients participating in the same investigational protocol. It was noted that of the 33% of patients who were initially denied authorization, about half went on to transplant after appealing the decision, a process that requires additional time and money.[108] Most health care providers recommend correlating insurance approval with protocol-based, medical decision making.

Analysis of the cost of care must consider many issues. One evaluation of the comparative cost of treatments for AML in first remission in 40 patients less than 50 years old reported that the average cost of allogeneic BMT and ABMT was significantly higher than the cost of chemotherapy when looking at the procedure and two years of follow-up.[110] The average cost of treatment for relapse was about the same regardless of the treatment group. Total cost including relapse was highest for ABMT and lowest for chemotherapy. The final analysis was the total cost per number of saved life years. The cost was again similar for allogeneic BMT and chemotherapy, and higher for autologous BMT. The authors concluded that allogeneic BMT was the best therapeutic and cost-effective approach for this group of patients.

Still others are evaluating transplant therapy as a way of decreasing the costs of high-dose therapy. A study of 26 patients who received high-dose chemotherapy with and without BCT showed decreased nadir and earlier platelet recovery, which translate to decreased hospital days, total parenteral nutrition, and transfusions. This study showed that use of BCT to support high-dose chemotherapy decreased costs by 44%.[111]

## FUTURE APPLICATIONS

It is well established in BMT that PPSCs from the bone marrow support long-term engraftment. It is also well documented that blood-derived cells provide short-term hematopoiesis.[112-114] However, it remains uncertain how effective peripheral progenitor and stem cells are in sustaining long-term hematopoiesis. It is believed that some residual hematopoietic function remains even after high-dose therapy. Therefore, the issue of long-term engraftment of the transfused cells may not be relevant. Others question the usefulness of the peripheral stem cells obtained from a matched related or unrelated donor for allogeneic transplantation if marrow ablation is not complete. If the short-term goal is only rapid recovery of bone marrow function, then BCT certainly achieves that goal.[115,116] Current data suggest that engraftment endures at least five years after BCT.[117] The type and number of cells needed for successful engraftment remain controversial, in spite of the apparent clinical success.[62,118]

Allogeneic BCT may be used in the future to increase recovery for the patient and decrease risk and discomfort for the donor. The first allogeneic BCT was performed in 1989.[119] Ten collections were needed to obtain sufficient cells, which were T lymphocyte–depleted to minimize GVHD. Although the patient died of infection one month after BCT, hematopoiesis had been reestablished. Since pheresis of cells for BCT is an easier process than bone marrow harvest, this option for allogeneic donation may increase public interest in donating for nonrelatives. Strategies to avoid the placement of a central venous catheter and improved techniques for mobilization such as ex vivo expansion would also need to be developed.[120]

Treatment with a combination of ABMT and BCT is also being evaluated. In addition to a shorter nadir period with the addition of the progenitor cells, the benefit may be to decrease thrombocytopenia, which thus far has not been reduced by the use of HGFs such as G-CSF or GM-CSF.[51,121]

Finally, strategies for ex vivo expansion of PPSCs and progenitor cells are being developed. Ex vivo stimulation would serve to increase the number of cells for transplant and to decrease the number of apheresis procedures required.[7,122,123]

## CONCLUSION

The field of transplantation continues to expand in response to technological developments and economic pressure. ABMT remains a therapeutic option for patients with leukemia, lymphoma, and some solid tumors. BCT is being evaluated as an alternative to BMT for some patients and as a new option for bone marrow recovery in patients with solid tumors receiving high-dose therapy. The process for ABMT and BCT is similar except for stem cell collection. Patient care for both patient populations is similar, with toxicities related to the specific conditioning regimen. Because bone marrow recovery after BCT is more rapid, many institutions have developed comprehensive outpatient programs. However, the issues of cost of care and the location where care should be delivered remain controversial.

## REFERENCES

1. Wujcik D: Hematopoietic growth factors, in Rieger PT (ed): *Biotherapy: A Comprehensive Overview.* Boston, Jones and Bartlett, 1995, pp 113–133
2. Coiffier B, Philip T, Burnett AK, et al: Consensus conference on intensive chemotherapy plus hematopoietic stem cell transplantation in malignancies, Lyon, June 4–6, 1993. *Ann Oncol* 5:19–23, 1994 (review)
3. Spangrude GJ: Biological and clinical aspects of hematopoietic stem cells. *Annu Rev Med* 45:93–104, 1994 (review)
4. Hegland J: Transplant immunology: HLA and issues of stem cell donation, in Whedon MB, Wujcik D (eds): *Stem Cell and Marrow Transplantation: Principles, Practice, and Nursing Insights* (ed 2). Boston, Jones and Bartlett, 1997
5. Kurnick NB, Montano A, Gerdes JC, et al: Preliminary observations on the treatment of post-irradiation hemopoietic depression in man by the infusion of stored autologous bone marrow. *Ann Intern Med* 49:973–975, 1958
6. Eaves CJ, Eaves AC: Stem and progenitor cells in the blood, in Gale RP, Juttner CA, Henon P (eds): *Blood Stem Cell Transplant.* New York, Cambridge University Press, 1994, pp 20–31
7. Juttner CA, Henon P, Gale RP: Blood stem cell transplants: Current state; future directions, in Gale RP, Juttner CA, Henon P (eds): *Blood Stem Cell Transplant.* New York, Cambridge University Press, 1994, pp 167–180
8. Wujcik D: Hematopoiesis, in Whedon MB, Wujcik D (eds): *Stem Cell and Marrow Transplantation: Principles, Practice, and Nursing Insights,* (ed 2). Boston, Jones and Bartlett, 1997
9. McCarthy DM, Goldman JM: Transfusion of circulating stem cells. *Crit Rev Clin Lab Sci* 20:1–24, 1984
10. Korbling M, Fliedner TM: History of blood stem cell transplants, in Gale RP, Juttner CA, Henon P (eds): *Blood Stem Cell Transplant.* New York, Cambridge University Press, 1994, pp 9–19
11. Craig JI, Turner ML, Parker AC: Peripheral blood stem cell transplantation. *Blood Rev* 6:59–67, 1995
12. Bensinger W: Isolating stem and progenitor cells, in Gale RP, Juttner CA, Henon P (eds): *Blood Stem Cell Transplant.* New York, Cambridge University Press, 1994, pp 32–42
13. Hogge DE, Sutherland HJ, Lansdrop PM, et al: The elusive peripheral blood hemopoietic stem cell. *Semin Hematol* 30:82–91, 1993
14. Shpall EJ, Jones RB, Bearman SI, et al: Transplantation of enriched CD34-positive autologous marrow into breast cancer patients following high-dose chemotherapy: Influence of CD34-positive peripheral-blood progenitors and growth factors on engraftment. *J Clin Oncol* 12:28–36, 1994
15. Sheridan W, Juttner C, Szer J, et al: Granulocyte-colony-stimulating factor (G-CSF) in peripheral blood stem cell (PBSC) and bone marrow (BM) transplantation. *Blood* 76:565–571, 1990
16. Sacher RA: Bone marrow and stem cell transplantation: Where are we going? *Semin Hematol* 30:130–133, 1993
17. Ezzone SA, Fliedner M: Transplant networks and standards of care: International perspectives, in Whedon MB, Wujcik D (eds): *Stem Cell and Marrow Transplantation: Principles, Practice, and Nursing Insights,* (ed 2). Boston, Jones and Bartlett, 1997 (in press)
18. Appelbaum FR, Fay J, Herzig G, et al: American Society for Blood and Marrow Transplantation guidelines for training. *Biol Blood Marrow Transplant* 1:1–2, 1995
19. Phillips G, Armitage JO, Bearman S, et al: American Society for Blood and Marrow Transplantation guidelines for clinical centers. *Biol Blood Marrow Transplant:* 1:3–4, 1995
20. Rowe JM, Ciobanu N, Ascensao J, et al: Recommended guidelines for the management of autologous and allogeneic bone marrow transplantation. *Ann Intern Med* 120:143–158, 1994
21. ASCO/ASH: The American Society of Clinical Oncology and American Society of Hematology recommended criteria for the performance of bone marrow transplantation. *J Clin Oncol* 8:563–564, 1990
22. ASCO/ASH: ASCO/ASH recommended criteria for the performance of bone marrow transplantation. *Blood* 75:1209–1212, 1990
23. Nelson JP: Centers of excellence for marrow transplantation, in Buchsel PC, Whedon MB (eds): *Bone Marrow Transplantation: Administrative and Clinical Issues.* Boston, Jones and Bartlett, 1995, pp 448–462
24. Rowlings PA, Gale RP, Horowitz MM, et al: Bone marrow transplantation in leukemia. *J Hematother* 3:235–238, 1994
25. Cassileth PA, Anderson J, Lazarus HM: An ECOG trial of autologous bone marrow transplantation in first remission of acute myeloid leukemia. *Blood* 76:352a, 1990
26. McMillan AK, Goldstone AH, Linch DC, et al: High-dose chemotherapy and autologous bone marrow transplantation in acute myeloid leukemia. *Blood* 76:480–488, 1990
27. Horowitz MM, Gale RP, Sondel PM, et al: Graft-versus-leukemia reactions after bone marrow transplantation. *Blood* 75:555–562, 1990
28. Reiffers J, Korbling M, Labopin M, et al: Autologous blood stem cell transplantation versus autologous bone marrow transplantation for acute myeloid leukemia in first complete remission. *Int J Cell Cloning* 10:111–113, 1992
29. Ramsay NKC, Kersey JH: Indications for marrow transplantation in acute lymphoblastic leukemia. *Blood* 75:815–818, 1990
30. Snyder DS, McGlave PB: Treatment of chronic myelogenous leukemia with bone marrow transplantation. *Hematol Oncol Clin North Am* 4:535–557, 1990
31. Gale RP, Butturini A: Intensive therapy of chronic myelogenous leukemia, in Armitage JO, Antman KH (eds): *High-Dose Cancer Therapy: Pharmacology, Hematopoietins, Stem Cells.* Baltimore, Williams and Wilkins, 1992, pp 619–625
32. Vose JM, Phillips GL, Armitage JO: Autologous bone marrow transplantation for Hodgkin's disease, in Armitage JO, Antman KH (eds): *High-Dose Cancer Therapy: Pharmacology, Hematopoietins, Stem Cells.* Baltimore, Williams and Wilkins, 1992, pp 651–661
33. Kessinger A, Nademanee A, Forman SJ, et al: Autologous bone marrow transplantation for Hodgkin's and non-Hodgkin's lymphoma. *Hematol Oncol Clin North Am* 4:577–587, 1990
34. Appelbaum FR: Treatment of aggressive non-Hodgkin's lymphoma with marrow transplantation. *Marrow Transplant Rev* 3:1–6, 1993
35. Armitage JO: Bone marrow transplantation in the treatment of patients with lymphoma. *Blood* 73:1749–1758, 1989

36. Peters WP: Autologous bone marrow transplantation for breast cancer. *Curr Sci* 4:279–282, 1992

37. Antman KH: Dose-intensive therapy in breast cancer, in Armitage JO, Antman KJ (eds): *High-Dose Cancer Therapy: Pharmacology, Hematopoietins, Stem Cells.* Baltimore, Williams and Wilkins, 1992, pp 701–718

38. Herzig RH: The role of autologous bone marrow transplantation in the treatment of solid tumors. *Semin Oncol* 19:7–12, 1992

39. Nichols CR, Tricot G, Williams SD, et al: Dose-intensive chemotherapy in refractory germ cell cancer: A phase I/II trial of high-dose carboplatin and etoposide with autologous bone marrow transplantation. *J Clin Oncol* 7:932–939, 1989

40. Nichols C, Tricot G, Williams SD: High-dose carboplatin and VP-16 with autologous bone marrow transplantation in patients with recurrent and refractory germ cell cancer: An Eastern Cooperative Oncology Group study. *J Clin Oncol* 10:558–563, 1992

41. Spitzer G, Spencer V, Dunphy FR: High-dose chemotherapy with autologous bone marrow support for ovarian cancer, in Armitage JO, Antman KH (eds): *High-Dose Cancer Therapy: Pharmacology, Hematopoietins, Stem Cells.* Baltimore, Williams and Wilkins, 1992, pp 719–728

42. Henon PR: Peripheral blood stem cell transplantation: Critical review. *Int J Artif Organs* 16:64–70, 1993

43. Juttner CA: Blood stem cell transplants in acute leukemia, in Gale RP, Juttner CA, Henon P (eds): *Blood Stem Cell Transplant.* New York, Cambridge University Press, 1994, pp 101–116

44. Szer J, Juttner CA, To LB, et al: Post-remission therapy for acute myeloid leukaemia with blood-derived stem cell transplantation: Results of a collaborative phase II trial. *Int J Cell Cloning* 10:114–117, 1992

45. Hoyle C, Goldman JM: Blood stem cell transplants in chronic myelogenous leukemia, in Gale RP, Juttner CA, Henon P (eds): *Blood Stem Cell Transplant.* New York, Cambridge University Press, 1994, pp 117–127

46. Kessinger A, Armitage JO: Peripheral stem cell transplantation for patients with non-Hodgkin lymphoma. *Int J Cell Cloning* 10:127–130, 1992

47. Fermand JP, Cheveret S, Hennequin M, et al: High-dose chemoradiotherapy and autologous blood stem cell transplantation for patients with multiple myeloma. *Int J Cell Cloning* 10:141–144, 1992

48. Ventura GJ, Barlogie B, Hester JP, et al: High-dose cyclophosphamide, BCNU and VP-16 with autologous blood stem cell support for refractory multiple myeloma. *Bone Marrow Transplant* 5:265–268, 1990

49. Vaughan WP, Reed EC, Edwards B, et al: High-dose cyclophosphamide, thiotepa and hydroxyurea with autologous hematopoietic stem cell rescue: An effective consolidation chemotherapy regimen for early metastatic breast cancer. *Bone Marrow Transplant* 13:619–624, 1994

50. Hillner BE, Smith TJ, Desch CE: Efficacy and cost-effectiveness of autologous bone marrow transplantation in metastatic breast cancer: Estimates using decision analysis while awaiting clinical trial results. *JAMA* 267:2055–2061, 1992

51. Kessinger A: Utilization of peripheral blood stem cells in autotransplantation. *Hematol Oncol Clin North Am* 7:535–545, 1993

52. Wujcik D, Downs S: Bone marrow transplantation. *Crit Care Nurs Clin North Am* 4:149–166, 1992

53. Jassak PF, Riley MB: Autologous stem cell transplant. *Cancer Pract* 2:141–145, 1994

54. King CR: Peripheral stem cell transplantation: Past, present, and future, in Buchsel PC, Whedon MB (eds): *Bone Marrow Transplantation: Administrative and Clinical Issues.* Boston, Jones and Bartlett, 1995, pp 187–211

55. Wodinsky HB, Dillman RO, MacDonald SA: Assessing peripheral blood stem cell transplant technology. *J Oncol Management* July/August 22–27, 1994

56. Wieseman T: Suing insurers: Litigation over autologous bone marrow transplants and breast cancer. *Oncology Issues* 6:7–12, 1991

57. Walker FE, Roethke SK, Sandman V, et al: Guiding patients and their families through peripheral stem cell transplantation with the help of a teaching booklet. *Oncol Nurs Forum* 21:585–591, 1994

58. Korbling M, Juttner CA, Henon P, et al: Blood versus bone marrow transplants, in Gale RP, Juttner CA, Henon P (eds): *Blood Stem Cell Transplant.* New York, Cambridge University Press, 1994, pp 87–98

59. Buckner CD, Clift RA, Sanders JE, et al: Marrow harvesting from normal donors. *Blood* 64:630–634, 1984

60. To LB: Mobilizing and collecting blood stem cells, in Gale RP, Juttner CA, Henon P (eds): *Blood Stem Cell Transplants.* New York, Cambridge University Press, 1994, pp 56–74

61. Bernstein ID, Andrews RG, Zsebo KM: Recombinant human stem cell factor enhances the formation of colonies by CD34+ and CD34+lin− cells, and the generation of colony-forming progeny from CD34+lin− cells cultured with interleukin-3, granulocyte-colony stimulating factor, or granulocyte-macrophage colony-stimulating factor. *Blood* 77:2316–2321, 1991

62. Bender JG, To LB, Williams S, et al: Defining a therapeutic dose of peripheral blood stem cells. *J Hematother* 1:329–341, 1992 (review)

63. To LB, Shepperd KM, Haylock DN: Single high doses of cyclophosphamide enable the collection of high numbers of hemopoietic stem cells from the peripheral blood. *Exp Hematol* 18:442–447, 1990

64. To LB, Haylock DN, Dyson PG, et al: A comparison between 4 g/m² and 7 g/m² cyclophosphamide for peripheral blood stem cell mobilization. *Int J Cell Cloning* 10:33–35, 1992

65. Korbling M, Fliedner TM, Holle R, et al: Autologous blood stem cell (ABSCT) versus purged bone marrow transplantation (pABMT) in standard risk AML: Influence of source and cell composition of the autograft on hemopoietic reconstitution and disease-free survival. *Bone Marrow Transplant* 7:343–349, 1991

66. Jones HM, Jones SA, Watts MJ, et al: Development of a simplified single-apheresis approach for peripheral-blood progenitor-cell transplantation in previously treated patients with lymphoma. *J Clin Oncol* 12:1693–1702, 1994

67. Sheridan WP, Begley CG, Juttner CA, et al: Effect of peripheral-blood progenitor cells mobilized by filgrastim (G-CSF) on platelet recovery after high-dose chemotherapy. *Lancet* 339:640–644, 1992

68. Henon P, Becker M: Cytokine enhancement of peripheral blood stem cells. *Stem Cells* 11:65–71, 1993

69. Socinski MA, Cannistra SA, Elias A, et al: Granulocyte-macrophage colony stimulating factor expands the circulating haemopoietic progenitor cell compartment in man. *Lancet* 1:1194–1198, 1988

70. Vose JM, Kessinger A, Bierman PJ, et al: The use of rhIL-3 for mobilization of peripheral blood stem cells in previously treated patients with lymphoid malignancies. *Int J Cell Cloning* 10:62–65, 1992

71. Guillaume T, D'Hondt V, Symann M: IL-3 and peripheral

blood stem cell harvesting. *Stem Cells* 11:173–181, 1993 (review)

72. Brugger W, Mocklin W, Heimfeld S, et al: Ex vivo expansion of enriched peripheral blood CD34+ progenitor cells by stem cell factor, interleukin-1 beta (IL-1beta), IL-6, IL-3, interferon-gamma, and erythropoietin. *Blood* 81:2579–2584, 1993

73. Valbonesi M: Hemopoietic stem cells: Technical and methodological considerations. *Stem Cells* 11:58–63, 1993 (review)

74. Padley D, Strauss RG, Wieland M, et al: Concurrent comparison of the Cobe Spectra and Fenwal CS3000 for the collection of peripheral blood mononuclear cells for autologous peripheral stem cell transplantation. *J Clin Apheresis* 6:77–80, 1991

75. Walker F, Roethke SK, Martin G: An overview of the rationale, process, and nursing implications of peripheral blood stem cell transplantation. *Cancer Nurs* 17:141–148, 1994

76. Bone marrow and peripheral blood progenitor cells, in Klein HG (ed): *16th Edition Standards for Blood Banks and Transfusion Services* (ed 16). Bethesda, MD, American Association of Blood Banks, 1994, pp 47–51

77. Di Nicola M, Siena S, Bregni M, et al: Quantization of CD34+ peripheral blood hematopoietic progenitors for autografting in cancer patients. *Int J Artif Organs* 16:80–82, 1993

78. Bender JG, Unverzagt K, Walker DE, et al: Phenotypic analysis and characterization of CD34+ cells from normal human bone marrow, cord blood, peripheral blood, and mobilized peripheral blood from patients undergoing autologous stem cell transplantation. *Clin Immunol Immunopathol* 70:10–18, 1994

79. Meagher RC, Herzig RH: Techniques of harvesting and cryopreservation of stem cells. *Hematol Oncol Clin North Am* 7:501–533, 1993

80. Berenson R: Human stem cell transplantation. *Leuk Lymphoma* 11:137–139, 1993 (review)

81. Henon PR: Peripheral blood stem cell transplantations: Past, present and future. *Stem Cells* 11:154–172, 1993 (review)

82. Sharp JG, Kessinger A: Minimal residual disease and blood stem cell transplants, in Gale RP, Juttner CA, Henon P (eds): *Blood Stem Cell Transplants*. New York, Cambridge University Press, 1994, pp 75–86

83. Nagafuji K, Harada M, Takamatsu Y, et al: Evaluation of leukaemic contamination in peripheral blood stem cell harvests by reverse transcriptase polymerase chain reaction. *Br J Haematol* 85:578–583, 1993

84. Freedman AS, Nadler LM: Developments in purging in autotransplantation. *Hematol Oncol Clin North Am* 7:687–715, 1993

85. Gulati SC, Duensing S: Evaluating the benefit of purging in stem cell transplantation. *Cancer Invest* 12:447–449, 1994 (review)

86. Shpall E, Cognoni P, Gehling U, et al: Bone marrow purging, in Armitage JO, Antman KH (eds): *High-Dose Cancer Therapy: Pharmacology, Hematopoietins, Stem Cells*. Baltimore, Williams and Wilkins, 1995, pp 609–619

87. Levine LA, Richie JP: Urological complications of cyclophosphamide. *J Urol* 141:1063–1069, 1989

88. Brugieres L, Hartmann O, Travagli JP, et al: Hemorrhagic cystitis following high-dose chemotherapy and bone marrow transplantation in children with malignancies: Incidence, clinical course, and outcome. *J Clin Oncol* 7:194–199, 1989

89. Meisenberg B, Lassiter M, Hussein A, et al: Prevention of hemorrhagic cystitis after high-dose alkylating agent chemotherapy and autologous bone marrow support. *Bone Marrow Transplant* 14:287–291, 1994

90. Braverman AC, Antin JH, Plappert MT, et al: Cyclophosphamide cardiotoxicity in bone marrow transplantation: A prospective evaluation of new dosing regimens. *J Clin Oncol* 9:1215–1223, 1991

91. Shapiro TW: Pulmonary and cardiac complications of blood cell and marrow transplantation, in Whedon MB, Wujcik D (eds): *Stem Cell and Marrow Transplantation: Principles, Practice, and Nursing Insights*. Boston, Jones and Bartlett, 1997

92. Dreifke L, DeMeyer E: Information guide for patients receiving total body irradiation before bone marrow transplantation. *Cancer Nurs* 15:206–210, 1992

93. Viele CS: Chronic myelogenous and acute promyelocytic leukemia: New bone marrow transplantation options. *Oncol Nurs Forum* 23:488–493, 1996

94. Henon PR, Liang H, Beck-Wirth G, et al: Comparison of hematopoietic and immune recovery after autologous bone marrow or blood stem cell transplants. *Bone Marrow Transplant* 9:285–291, 1992

95. Sheridan W, Morstyn G, Wolf M, et al: Granulocyte colony-stimulating factor and neutrophil recovery after high-dose chemotherapy and bone marrow transplantation. *Lancet* 2:891–895, 1989

96. Lum LG: Immune recovery after bone marrow transplantation. *Hematol Oncol Clin North Am* 4:659–675, 1990

97. Hooper DC, Wolfson JC: Fluoroquinolone antimicrobial agents. *N Engl J Med* 324:384–394, 1991

98. Brandt ST, Peter WP, Atwater SK, et al: Effect of recombinant human granulocyte-macrophage colony-stimulating factor on hematopoietic reconstitution after high-dose chemotherapy and autologous bone marrow transplantation. *N Engl J Med* 318:869–876, 1988

99. Brugger W, Clause JF, Lindemann A, et al: Role of hematopoietic growth factor combinations in experimental and clinical oncology. *Semin Oncol* 19:8–15, 1992

100. Armstrong D: Empiric therapy for the immunocompromised host. *Rev Infect Dis* 13:S763–S769, 1991

101. Wujcik D: Infection, in Groenwald SL, Frogge MH, Goodman M, Yarbro CH (eds): *Cancer Symptom Management*. Boston, Jones and Bartlett, 1996, 289–307

102. Hood AF, Vogelsang GB, Black LP, et al: Acute graft-versus-host disease: Development following autologous and syngeneic bone marrow transplantation. *Arch Dermatol* 123: 745–750, 1987

103. Anderson KC, Weinstein HJ: Transfusion-associated graft-versus-host disease. *N Engl J Med* 323:315–321, 1990

104. Peters WP, Ross M, Vredenburgh JJ, et al: The use of intensive clinic support to permit outpatient autologous bone marrow transplantation for breast cancer. *Semin Oncol* 21: 25–31, 1994

105. deSauvage RJ, Hass PE, Spencer SD, et al: Stimulation of megakaryocytopoiesis and thrombopoiesis by the c-Mpl ligand. *Nature* 369:533–538, 1994

106. Gilbert C, Meisenberg B, Vredenburgh J, et al: Sequential prophylactic oral and empiric once-daily parenteral antibiotics for neutropenia and fever after high-dose chemotherapy and autologous bone marrow support. *J Clin Oncol* 12: 1005–1011, 1994

107. Dekker AW, Verdonck LF, Rozenberg-Arska M: Infection prevention in autologous bone marrow transplantation and the role of protective isolation. *Bone Marrow Transplant* 14:89–93, 1994

108. Peters WP, Rodgers M: Variation in approval by insurance companies of coverage for autologous bone marrow transplantation for breast cancer. *N Engl J Med* 330:473–477, 1994

109. Mahaney FX: Bone marrow transplants for breast cancer: Some insurers pay, some insurers don't. *J Natl Cancer Inst* 86:420–421, 1994

110. Dufoir T, Saux MC, Terraza B, et al: Comparative cost of allogeneic or autologous bone marrow transplantation and chemotherapy in patients with acute myeloid leukemia in first remission. *Bone Marrow Transplant* 10:323–329, 1992

111. Uyl-de Groot CA, Ossenkoppele GJ, van Riet AA, et al: The costs of peripheral blood progenitor cell reinfusion mobilized by granulocyte colony-stimulating factor following high-dose melphalan as compared with conventional therapy in multiple myeloma. *Eur J Cancer* 30 A:457–459, 1994

112. Charbord P: Hemopoietic stem cells: Analysis of some parameters critical for engraftment. *Stem Cells* 12:545–562, 1994

113. Henon PR: Peripheral blood stem cell transplantation: Critical review. *Int J Artif Organs* 16:64–70, 1993

114. Orlic D, Bodine DM: What defines a pluripotent hematopoietic stem cell (PHSC): Will the real PHSC please stand up! *Blood* 84:3991–3994, 1994

115. Gale RP, Reiffers J, Juttner CA: What's new in blood progenitor cell autotransplants? *Bone Marrow Transplant* 14:343–346, 1994 (editorial)

116. Brugger W, Henschler R, Heimfeld S, et al: Positively selected autologous blood CD34+ cells and unseparated peripheral blood progenitor cells mediate identical hematopoietic engraftment after high-dose VP16, ifosfamide, carboplatin, and epirubicin. *Blood* 84:1421–1426, 1994

117. Gale RP, Henon P, Juttner CA (eds): Overview of blood stem cell transplants. *Blood Stem Cell Transplants.* New York, Cambridge University Press, 1994, pp 1–5

118. Kessinger A: Is blood or bone marrow better? *Stem Cells* 11:290–295, 1993 (review)

119. Kessinger A, Smith D, Strandjord S, et al: Allogeneic transplantation of blood derived, T cell-depleted hemopoietic stem cells after myeloablative treatment in a patient with acute lymphoblastic leukemia. *Bone Marrow Transplant* 4:643–646, 1989

120. Russell NH, Hunter AE: Peripheral blood stem cells for allogeneic transplantation. *Bone Marrow Transplant* 13:353–355, 1994

121. Mitchell PL, Shepherd VB, Proctor HM, et al: Peripheral blood stem cells used to augment autologous bone marrow transplantation. *Arch Dis Child* 70:237–240, 1994

122. Thomas ED: Stem cell transplantation: Past, present and future. *Stem Cells* 12:539–544, 1994

123. Murray L, Chen B, Galy A, et al: Enrichment of human hematopoietic stem cell activity in the CD34+ Thy−1 + Lin subpopulation from mobilized peripheral blood. *Blood* 85:368–378, 1995

# P A R T   I V

# Symptom Management

# Chapter 20

# Pain

Deborah B. McGuire, RN, PhD, FAAN

Vivian R. Sheidler, RN, MS

## INTRODUCTION AND BACKGROUND

### Definitions of Pain

Historically, pain has been a phenomenon not easy to define. During the seventeenth century, pain was viewed as a signal of bodily injury, with scant attention paid to its nonphysical aspects. This notion persisted until the twentieth century, when researchers began to formulate concepts of pain that recognized and included not only the physical "alarm" aspect but other neurological activities, cultural factors, and individual personality and experiential variables as well. Despite these broader concepts, a precise definition of pain eluded workers in the field, for as Livingston wrote, "The chief difficulty encountered in a search for a satisfactory definition of pain is the fact that it can be considered from either a physiologic or psychologic approach. Any consideration of pain, by one approach alone, without due regard to the other, is incomplete."[1,p.62]

Reconciliation of these two disparate approaches proved very difficult, since a single definition seemed unable to satisfy everyone. Melzack and Wall highlighted this problem when they wrote that "pain is such a common experience that we rarely pause to define it in ordinary conversation. Yet no one who has worked on the problem of pain has ever been able to give it a definition which is satisfactory to all of his colleagues."[2,p.9] In their view, pain was a "*category* of experiences, signifying a multitude of different, unique experiences having different causes, and characterized by different qualities varying along a number of sensory and affective dimensions."[2,p.71]

The need for a standard definition of pain, however, prompted the International Association for the Study of Pain (IASP) to form a subcommittee charged with developing a definition acceptable to both clinicians and researchers. The major result of their labors, published in 1979, was the following: "Pain is an unpleasant sensory and emotional experience associated with actual or potential tissue damage, or described in terms of such damage."[3] This definition accounted for both sensory and emotional aspects of pain as well as for pain of pathophysiological and psychological origin. It incorporated the essential elements of subjectivity and individual uniqueness in the pain experience.

In addition to this definition of pain, the IASP published a list of pain terms, with their definitions (e.g., *allodynia* and *causalgia*), which it viewed as a "minimum standard vocabulary for members of different disciplines who work in the field of pain."[3] Bouckoms wrote that the IASP definitions of pain and related terms provided a nontheoretical, relatively complete, valid taxonomy that was extremely useful to clinicians and researchers alike.[4] It is probably safe to say that since the IASP definition of pain was published, it has become commonly accepted and used by most pain specialists.

Since 1979 the IASP has continued its work on a taxonomy, or classification system, for pain. In 1986 it published additional pain terms with definitions, descriptions of chronic pain syndromes, and a classification and coding schema for these different syndromes.[5] A more recent publication lists a full taxonomy of chronic pain,[6] which includes many different types of cancer-related pain. One study[7] supports the clinical utility of the IASP coding schema as a means for deriving, coding, storing, and retrieving basic classification characteristics of pain.

Although the IASP publications just cited do not present a specific definition of acute pain, it is commonly accepted that chronic pain and acute pain are distinctly different phenomena. Bonica defined acute pain as "a complex constellation of unpleasant sensory, perceptual, and emotional experiences and certain associated autonomic, psychologic, emotional, and behavioral responses."[8,p.19] He emphasized that noxious stimulation from injury or disease to either cutaneous or deep tissues and the abnormal function of musculoskeletal or visceral tissues were the two major causes of acute pain. Furthermore, acute pain rarely has a strong psychopathological or environmental component, as does chronic pain, and it may recur periodically when an individual has recurrent acute pathophysiological processes, such as those commonly seen in persons with cancer.

### Theories and Mechanisms of Pain

Closely related to definitions of pain are theories of what pain is and how it occurs. Various theories have been proposed over the years and, as with definitions of pain, began with one or two simple anatomic or clinical aspects of pain and then expanded to include a multitude of anatomic, neural, physiological, clinical, and psychological variables. Until the mid–twentieth century, several traditional but opposing theories of pain were prominent. Price[9] reviewed and discussed these "classical" theories. In addition to the classical theories that have been described, there are several current theories of pain.[9] Most notable of these is the *gate control theory of pain,* proposed by Melzack and Wall in 1965[10] and discussed recently.[11] Although the gate control theory is not perfect, it is the most comprehensive theory of pain yet proposed and serves an extremely useful purpose in explaining pain mechanisms for most health care givers. It is now abundantly clear that pain has a sensory component as well as a reactive (emotional) component. Much research is being conducted to elucidate the specific processes and phenomena responsible for producing the sensory and emotional puzzle called pain. While it is not possible to describe these efforts in any detail in this chapter, a brief overview of general mechanisms of pain is provided next.

When considered strictly from the pathophysiological and biochemical processes that cause it, pain experienced by patients with cancer is no different than pain experienced by other individuals. Etiologic, clinical, and psychosocial characteristics of both tumor- and treatment-related cancer pain, however, distinguish it from other types of pain. These differences will be elaborated later in the chapter; in this section the basic mechanisms of pain in general are considered.

The perception of and response to pain are due to four distinct processes that operate simultaneously and are all required for pain to occur (Table 20–1).[12] The first of these processes, *transduction*, begins when a noxious (painful or tissue-damaging) stimulus affects a peripheral sensory nerve ending, depolarizing it and setting off electrical activity that initiates the whole phenomenon of pain perception. *Transmission*, the next process, consists of the series of subsequent neural events that carry the electrical impulses throughout the nervous system, from peripheral to central. *Modulation*, the third process, is a neural activity that controls pain transmission neurons, those originating in the periphery and/or the central nervous system (CNS). The fourth process, *perception*, is less an actual physiological/anatomic process than it is the vague subjective correlate of pain (how it feels) that encompasses complex behavioral, psychological, and emotional factors that are little understood. The reader interested in more detail is referred to Price,[9] Fields,[12] Wilkie,[13] and Wall and Melzack.[14] Figure 20–1 shows schematically where transmission and modulation occur.

## Cancer Pain as a Multidimensional Phenomenon

The notion of sensory and affective, or physiological and psychological, aspects of pain—developed and nurtured through the gate control theory of pain and its related model—has been used by researchers to develop a conceptual framework for cancer pain. Ahles and his colleagues[15] hypothesized five dimensions of the cancer pain experience: (1) *physiological* (organic etiology of pain), (2) *sensory* (intensity, location, quality), (3) *affective* (depression, anxiety), (4) *cognitive* (manner in which pain influences an individual's thought processes, how the individual views her- or himself, or the meaning of pain), and (5) *behavioral* (pain-related behaviors such as medication intake and activity level). Since these investigators found little in the literature to support their multidimensional conceptualization, they conducted a systematic study in a group of 40 cancer patients with tumor-related pain to assess each of the five dimensions in their model. They used a variety of reliable and valid tools to assess the dimensions and found support for their conceptual model. When compared with cancer patients without pain, the subjects in the study had more depression, were more irritable, engaged in less physical activity, and took more medications. Those who believed that pain indicated progression of cancer had elevated depression and anxiety scores. Ahles et al[15] suggested as a result of their findings that treatment for cancer pain consists of specific therapeutic modalities targeted to each of the five dimensions.

McGuire[16] adapted Ahles's conceptual framework to conduct a descriptive study of 40 cancer patients with pain and 40 without pain. In general, support was found for the five dimensions of the model. Patients with pain had more depression, poorer physical function, and more psychosocial and other problems than the pain-free patients. Another finding was that individuals with cancer

**TABLE 20-1**   Mechanisms of Pain

| Process | Anatomic and Physiological Components | Description |
|---|---|---|
| Transduction | • Peripheral nerve fibers<br>• Chemical substances | Noxious stimulus depolarizes peripheral nerve and sets off electrical activity |
| Transmission | • Afferent nerve fibers<br>• Dorsal horn of spinal cord<br>• Spinothalamic pathways<br>• Thalamus and cortex | Neural events that occur subsequent to transduction and carry electrical impulses throughout nervous system, from peripheral to central |
| Modulation | • Periacqueductal gray<br>• Descending neurons<br>• Dorsal horn of spinal cord<br>• Opiate receptors<br>• Opioid peptides<br>• Neurotransmitters | A central neural activity that controls transmission of pain impulses and contributes to variability of pain |
| Perception | • Transmission system<br>• Modulation system<br>• Cortical processes | Neural activities involved in transmission and modulation result in a subjective correlate of pain that encompasses complex behavioral, psychological, and emotional factors |

Data from Price[9] and Fields.[12]

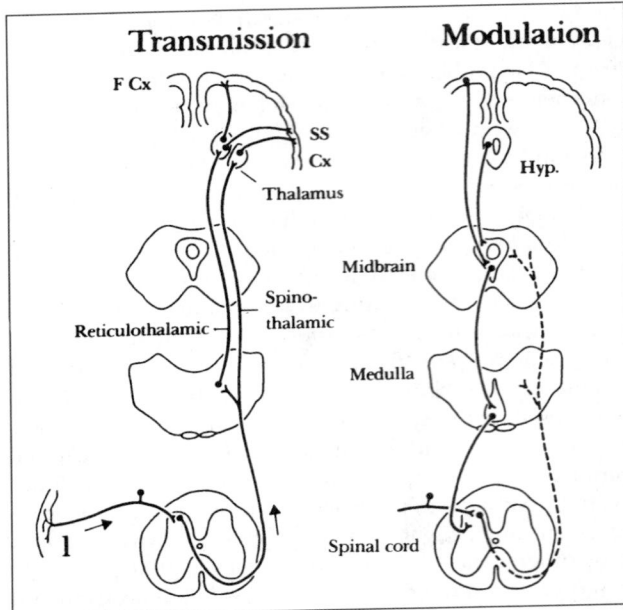

**FIGURE 20-1**  Pain transmission and modulation. **Left:** Transmission system for nociceptive messages. Noxious stimuli activate the sensitive peripheral ending of the primary afferent nociceptor by the process of transduction (*l*). The message is then transmitted over the peripheral nerve to the spinal cord, where it synapses with cells of origin of the two major ascending pain pathways, the spinothalamic and spinoreticulothalamic. The message is relayed in the thalamus to both the frontal (*F Cx*) and the somatosensory cortex (*SS Cx*). **Right:** Pain modulation network. Inputs from frontal cortex and hypothalamus (*Hyp.*) activate cells in the midbrain, which control spinal pain transmission cells via cells in the medulla. (Reprinted with permission from Fields HL: *Pain.* New York: McGraw-Hill, 1987.)

tion was based on earlier work by researchers at Memorial Sloan-Kettering Cancer Center in New York. In 1979 Foley[20] described three types of pain observed in patients with cancer, each with a different etiology: (1) pain associated with direct tumor involvement, (2) pain associated with cancer therapy, and (3) pain unrelated to either the tumor or its treatment. From this initial schema, she and a number of colleagues developed a comprehensive listing of more specific causes of pain that fit within the first two categories.[21]

Additional work on characterizing pain related to cancer therapy has been done.[22,23] The sources of pain associated with cancer treatment are many, ranging from initial diagnostic procedures causing acute, short-term pain, to standard therapeutic modalities (surgery, radiotherapy, chemotherapy) causing acute, short-term and/or chronic long-term pain. An example of acute, short-term pain is that associated with mucositis in patients receiving bone marrow transplantation.[24,25] Additional work is aimed at describing more fully treatment-related pain syndromes in specific populations, such as marrow transplant patients.[26] Additionally, literature from pediatric oncology strongly suggests that these pain etiologies and syndromes are also common in children with cancer pain.[27,28] Table 20–2 lists the major causes of tumor- and treatment-related cancer pain.

The third type of pain described by Foley[20] was pain unrelated to either cancer or its treatment. She estimated that it accounted for 3%–10% of the pain seen in cancer patients. Individuals with cancer pain are just as likely as the average individual to have pain from migraine headache, osteoarthritis, or degenerative disk disease. The presence of such pain, however, is important, and should be carefully assessed to be sure that it is *not* cancer related.

pain practiced a number of cognitive and behavioral coping strategies that they reported as moderately effective at reducing and controlling their pain.[17]

In addition to these five dimensions of the multidimensional model of cancer-related pain, there is a sixth important area—the *sociocultural dimension*.[18] This involves various demographic, social, and cultural characteristics that are related to the experience of pain. The six dimensions contribute to the individual's perception of and response to pain and are complex and interrelated.[18] Recent reviews of research literature indicate substantial support for this conceptualization of pain, for both cancer pain and other types of pain.[18,19] Further discussion of each dimension follows.

### Physiological dimension

Ahles et al[15] originally described the physiological dimension as consisting of the organic etiology of pain, specifying such causes as tumor that has metastasized to bone or infiltrated nerves or a hollow viscus. This defini-

**TABLE 20-2**  Causes of Cancer-Related Pain

| Tumor-Related | Treatment-Related |
|---|---|
| **Infiltration of bone** | **Diagnostic** |
| Base of skull | Mechanical injury |
| Vertebral bodies | Chemical irritation |
| Long bones | Inflammation |
| **Infiltration of nerves** | **Therapeutic (acute)** |
| Peripheral | Surgery |
| Plexus | Chemotherapy |
| Root | Radiotherapy |
| Epidural | |
| | **Posttherapeutic (chronic)** |
| **Infiltration of hollow viscus** | Surgery |
| Intestinal tract | Chemotherapy |
| Viscera | Radiotherapy |
| | **Complications** |
| | Tumor embolization |
| | Infections |

Data from Coyle and Foley,[21] Chapman et al,[22] Portenoy,[29] Payne,[30] and Kelly and Payne.[31]

The work of Foley, Chapman, their colleagues, and others on etiology of cancer pain has led to a greater understanding of the epidemiology and pathophysiology of cancer pain, including three specific pain syndromes that occur in patients with cancer and are caused by tumor.[29] These syndromes of somatic, visceral, and neuropathic pain are characterized by pain of different qualities, located in different anatomic parts of the body, and caused by different mechanisms (Figure 20–2). All three syndromes are usually discussed in reference to tumor-related pain, but they may apply equally as well to treatment-related pain.[30,31] It is important to note that many cancer patients with pain will have one or more of these three syndromes simultaneously,[32] and that each syndrome responds differently to therapeutic modalities.[33]

Related to etiology of pain are two other characteristics. *Duration* of pain refers to whether pain is acute or chronic. Acute pain generally is due to tissue damage, is self-limited, and resolves when the tissue damage heals. There is a clear pattern of onset and resolution. When acute pain occurs, there may be hyperactivity of the autonomic nervous system, although this is not diagnostic of the presence of pain. Chronic pain is also usually due to tissue damage, but not always. It may last three months or more[5] and is usually accompanied by adaptation, rather than hyperactivity, of the autonomic nervous system. There is not always a clear pattern of onset and resolution. Cancer pain, whether caused by tumor or treatment, can be subdivided into acute and chronic pain; sometimes both types occur simultaneously.

The second characteristic related to etiology of pain is the *pattern* that pain displays. Melzack first described patterns of pain in a quantifiable way in his McGill Pain Questionnaire,[34] where he identified three separate patterns: (1) brief, momentary, or transient, (2) rhythmic, periodic, or intermittent, and (3) continuous, steady, or constant. The few researchers who have studied patterns of pain in cancer patients have found that about half of individuals experience pain that is constant, with just fewer than half experiencing intermittent pain and a very small number reporting brief or transient pain.[16,35–37] Arathuzik noted that in her sample of 80 breast cancer patients with pain, most had pain lasting for one to several hours at a time, and many had pain lasting all day.[38] Most cancer patients experience two or more patterns simultaneously.

In summary, the physiological dimension of cancer pain includes organic etiology of the pain, which encompasses the specific anatomic sites affected. Additionally, duration and pattern of pain are inherent in this dimension. Finally, endogenous opioids and numerous psychophysiological variables have recently been proposed as components of the physiological dimension of pain.[18]

### Sensory dimension

The sensory dimension of cancer-related pain is related to where the pain is located and what it feels like. Three specific components of this dimension are location, intensity, and quality.

The first component, *location* of pain, is important. Many cancer patients have been reported to have pain at two or more locations.[38–40] Given the patterns of metastasis or sites of involvement seen in many solid tumors

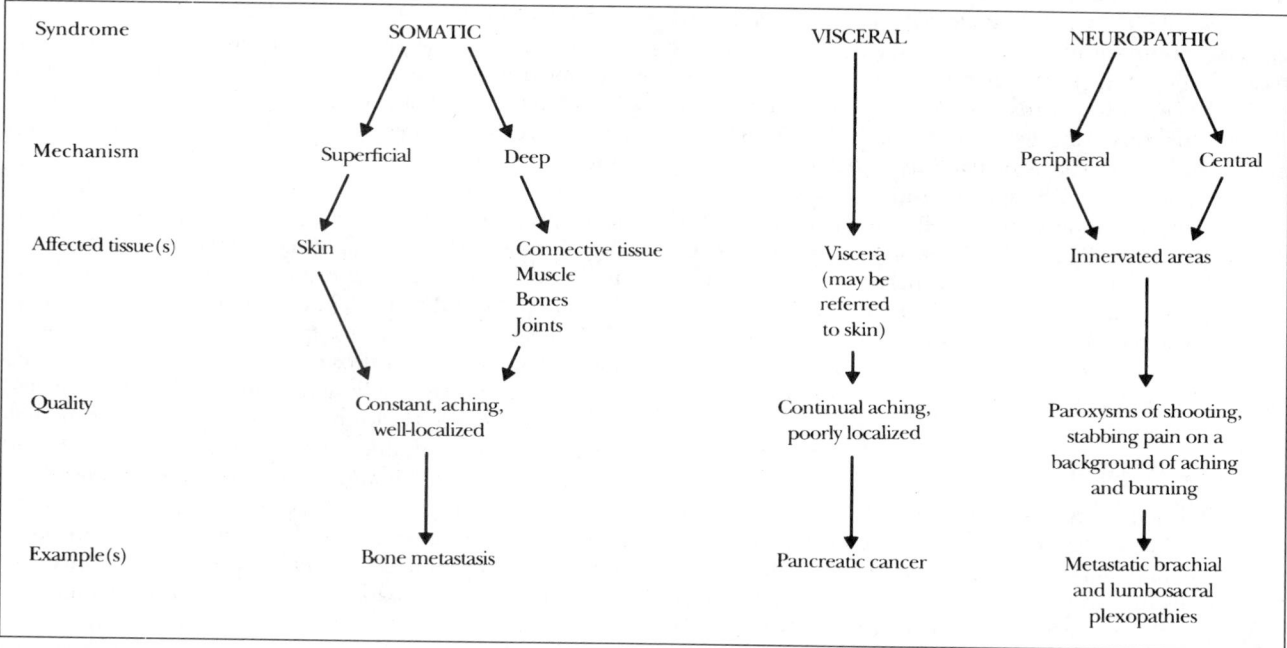

**FIGURE 20-2**   Pain syndromes in cancer.

and some hematologic malignancies, this finding is not surprising. The number of separate locations of pain has clear implications for the sensory dimension as well as for the entire pain experience.

*Intensity* of pain, or how strong it feels, is the second important component of the sensory dimension. Intensity is a perceived, and therefore a subjective, phenomenon, subject to individual sensation threshold (the least stimulus at which a person perceives a sensation, according to Twycross).[41] Although intensity depends primarily on etiology of pain, individual threshold may be affected by a variety of factors, such as physical comfort, mood, medications, and social environment, thus causing perceived intensity of pain to increase or decrease. Intensity is the most commonly assessed aspect of pain, and is characterized by words such as *none, mild, moderate, severe, intolerable, excruciating, bad,* and *intense.*

The third component of the sensory dimension is the *quality* of pain, which refers to how it actually feels. Melzack and Torgerson[42] were among the first to systematically study words that people used to describe pain. They composed a list of 102 words from the clinical literature on pain and organized them into classes that described sensory, affective, and evaluative properties of pain. Words placed in the sensory category referred to temporal, spatial, pressure, thermal, and other such aspects of pain. Examples of these sensory words are, respectively, *pulsing, radiating, penetrating, burning,* and *aching.* This initial work provided the foundation for the McGill Pain Questionnaire,[34] the first multidimensional measure of pain.

Some studies have revealed that patients with cancer pain use certain words more commonly than others to describe sensory aspects of their pain.[35-37,43-46] Words commonly used by patients in these studies included *sharp, tender, aching, throbbing, sore, stabbing, heavy, shooting,* and *gnawing.* Some authors distinguished between tumor- and treatment-related pain, but others did not, so it is not entirely clear which words describe which etiology. Nevertheless, the recurring word patterns found across time and in different groups of patients indicate that cancer pain is characterized by specific sensory qualities.

The sensory dimension of pain, as conceptualized by Ahles et al,[13] consists of location, intensity, and quality. The nature of and relationships among these three components are unique to each individual and undoubtedly have a strong impact not only on the entire experience of pain but on the affective, cognitive, behavioral, and sociocultural dimensions as well.

### Affective dimension

As defined by Ahles et al,[15] the affective dimension consists of depression, anxiety, or other psychological factors or personality traits associated with pain. Of the five dimensions proposed by Ahles, this one had the most support in the literature. In 1988 Dalton and Feuerstein[47] reviewed literature relating to biobehavioral factors in pain as well as affective, behavioral, and cognitive re-

sponses to pain. Although their review included both anecdotal and research reports relevant to the affective dimension of pain, it was clear that little research existed. A previous edition of this chapter identified 21 studies related to the affective dimension of cancer pain[48] and, in tabular format, indicated what psychological parameters were measured and what their relationships were to pain. Recent research and review articles[18,19,24,38,46,49-51] also support the importance of the affective dimension in cancer pain.

It is evident that parameters relevant to the affective dimension of pain range from specific personality traits (e.g., neuroticism) to affective disorders (e.g., depression) to vague general concepts such as psychological well-being. Taking into account the strong and weak points of studies in this area, it is possible to conclude the following: (1) specific personality factors probably are not related to the experience of cancer pain, (2) there is little evidence that affective disorders such as depression and anxiety are *strongly* related to pain, and (3) much more research on the relationships among these many psychological parameters and the experience of cancer pain is needed.

It is quite clear from the clinical perspective that there is an affective component to the pain experience and that it influences the individual's response to pain. The critical issue here is that psychological variables important to a particular patient's pain experience must be identified and dealt with to effectively manage pain.

### Cognitive dimension

The cognitive dimension of cancer pain, as conceived by Ahles et al,[15] encompassed the manner in which the pain influences a person's thought processes or the manner in which the person views her- or himself. In their study they found support for this dimension by assessing the meaning of each patient's pain. Almost two-thirds believed their pain was an indicator of progressive disease, and these individuals had significantly elevated anxiety and depression scores.

Spiegel and Bloom[52] found that in patients with metastatic breast cancer, the belief that pain indicated worsening disease was significantly correlated with reports of more pain, more anxiety, and more depression. Similarly, McGuire[16] found that 40% of patients considered pain an indicator of disease progression, and while they were more depressed than those without this view, the difference was not statistically significant. Barkwell[53] reported that cancer patients with pain ascribed meanings of challenge, punishment, and enemy to their pain. She found that patients who viewed pain as a challenge reported less pain and had lower depression and higher coping scores than those who viewed pain as punishment or an enemy. Ferrell and Dean[54] emphasized the importance of helping cancer patients determine the meaning of their pain so that they could better cope with it.

Several recent studies have examined the effects of opioid analgesics on cognitive function of patients with pain. They found that cognitive deficits occurred as opioids were first prescribed or when doses were adjusted upward but that the deficits were transient and that functioning returned to baseline when drug doses were stabilized for approximately two weeks.[55,56] Level and quality of cognition in relation to pharmacological therapy appear to be part of the cognitive dimension of pain, since they may influence the ability of individuals to report pain.

Another aspect of the cognitive dimension is knowledge about pain and its management. Such knowledge can affect responses both to pain and to interventions. Rimer and colleagues[57] demonstrated that an educational intervention of nurse counseling and printed materials resulted in a higher likelihood of cancer patients with pain taking the proper dose of analgesic on the proper schedule.

Finally, several researchers have examined cognitive strategies used by cancer patients to cope with pain. Such strategies clearly fall within the cognitive dimension of pain since they result from cognitive processes. Specific strategies include various forms of distraction (e.g., reading, watching television), use of coping self-statements, reinterpretation of painful sensations, selective inattention, withdrawal, suppression of pain, and trying to accept pain.[17,55,58,59]

### Behavioral dimension

The behavioral dimension of pain includes a variety of observable behaviors related to pain. Until recently, there was little research supporting this dimension of the cancer pain experience. Ahles et al[15] focused on level of activity and intake of analgesics as manifestations of this dimension in their study. They found that cancer patients with pain spent significantly less time walking or standing than those who did not have pain. Furthermore, 77% of the patients with pain reported that people in their immediate environment could tell when they were in pain because of their facial expressions, changes in mood or activity, or verbal complaints.

Communication of pain to others was examined systematically in a class study by Bond and Pilowsky,[60] who studied the relationships among advanced cancer patients' subjective reports of pain, their communication of pain, and reactions of nurses caring for them. About one-quarter of their patients with pain did not communicate it to nursing staff, and their self-reported pain scores were lower than those of patients who had pain and reported it or who were offered analgesics by staff. In another study, Francke and Theeuwen learned that patients who had undergone breast cancer surgery did not readily report their pain and expressed concern about "annoying" the staff.[61]

Keefe and his colleagues[62] conducted a study of the behavioral manifestations of pain in patients with head and neck cancer who were undergoing treatment for their disease. Guarded movements and grimacing were found to be the major behavioral indicators of pain, with grimacing correlating significantly with patients' reports of pain intensity. In addition, the amount of time patients spent walking or standing tended to decrease over the treatment period and time spent reclining increased. Finally, as treatment progressed, the number of simple daily activities that caused pain increased significantly.

Another component of the behavioral dimension of pain consists of simple strategies or activities that patients engage in to control pain. Several studies have examined these activities. McGuire[35] noted that inpatients most frequently used analgesics, but one-third also reported lying still, restricting movement, or positioning and moving of affected body parts. In a survey of 351 hospitalized patients, some of whom had cancer, researchers noted that the most commonly cited ($\geq$33%) pain reduction methods involved medications, rest or lying down, heat, and distraction.[63] Several studies found that cancer patients used an array of nonanalgesic, behaviorally oriented pain control methods, including heat, distraction, position change, massage, nonnarcotic drugs, exercise, positioning, pressure/manipulation, immobilization, guarding, and use of analgesics.[49,58,59,64,65] McGuire[17] noted the use of a variety of behavioral and cognitive coping strategies by both inpatients and outpatients, who reported moderate effectiveness of these methods of relieving pain.

It is clear that the studies just described support the behavioral dimension of the cancer pain experience as conceptualized by Ahles et al.[15] The findings offer directions for therapeutic approaches as well, which will be examined in a subsequent section.

### Sociocultural dimension

The sociocultural dimension of cancer pain consists of a variety of demographic, ethnic, cultural, spiritual, and related factors that influence a person's perception of and response to pain. There have been very few studies examining the relationships of any of these factors to cancer pain specifically, but research conducted on sociocultural aspects of clinical pain is reviewed briefly next, since some of the findings may pertain to the individual with cancer pain.

A number of studies used experimentally induced laboratory pain to examine racial, age, religious, and ethnic differences in pain.[66] Although none of the studies reviewed in this paper allowed definitive conclusions about differences in pain response due to the factors studied, a strong role of culturally determined attitudinal factors in pain perception and response was clearly supported. Wolff[67] lamented that little progress had been made in studying and understanding the important role ethnocultural factors played in pain. He maintained, however, that cultural factors such as majority/minority group status seemed to be the most likely causes of differences in pain perception and response.

Lipton and Marbach[68] corroborated this idea in their study of interethnic differences and similarities in reported pain experiences of black, Irish, Italian, Jewish, and Puerto Rican patients with facial pain. All five groups were similar in their reported responses to pain; however, the factors that *influenced* their responses were quite different. For example, Italians were most influenced by duration of pain, while Jews and Puerto Ricans were most influenced by level of psychological distress. These researchers suggested viewing the relationship between ethnicity and the pain experience as a subtle continuum of behaviors, attitudes, and feelings.

A descriptive study of Arab Americans' perceptions of and responses to pain emphasized that cultural characteristics heavily influenced individual behaviors.[69] For example, vehement, persistent, and perhaps exaggerated verbal messages were the norm for this group, and reporting of pain was included. Endurance of pain was not a priority, since modern technology was available; endurance was easier if Arab Americans understood that the consequences of pain would be more positive. Pain generally was perceived as unpleasant, to be avoided, and to be controlled by all means. Individuals with pain often displayed more behavioral manifestations of pain and were more vocal about it to family members rather than to health care providers. Family members assumed a major role in trying to manage pain, primarily through usurping the decision making related to care.

Age, sex, and race have been examined in relation to expression and management of pain. Females and older individuals were found to have increased verbal expressions of pain.[70,71] One study revealed that blacks used more moderate words than whites in describing pain.[70] Another study demonstrated no significant differences.[72]

Only a few studies have focused on cancer patients with pain. The sociocultural variables studied have been mixed but have included sex, race, age, and cultural background. In a study of cancer inpatients, McGuire[35] noted that females and nonwhites had significantly lower scores on the McGill Pain Questionnaire than males or whites. In a subsequent study of inpatients and outpatients, she found that blacks and older patients had less pain (as measured by the McGill Pain Questionnaire) and depression.[16] A study by Greenwald[75] indicated that despite few differences between ethnic identity and pain report, the ways in which people described affective aspects of pain using the McGill Pain Questionnaire varied across ethnic groups. He concluded that specific ethnic identities still condition the individual expression of pain even though assimilation into the American population has occurred.

McMillan[74] found that cancer patients with pain who were older (over age 55) reported less pain intensity than those who were younger. On the other hand, another study[75] found that the pain intensity of patients who were over 65 years of age was similar to that of those under 65.

Cleeland and associates,[76] using the Brief Pain Inventory (BPI), reported in their landmark study that female patients with metastatic cancer were significantly more likely to experience inadequate management of their pain, manifested by less and shorter pain relief and more pain-related functional impairment. These results suggest that gender may be linked in as yet unclear ways to efficacy of pain management in patients with cancer.

The research literature supporting the sociocultural dimension of cancer is just beginning to emerge. Fink and Gates recently reviewed relationships among culture, pain, and cancer.[77] Both the literature in noncancer populations and the slowly growing cancer literature make it clear that sociocultural factors are important in patients' perceptions of and responses to pain.

### Implications of the multidimensional model

The multidimensional conceptualization of cancer pain has been described as consisting of six interrelated dimensions,[18] a proposition that has begun to receive confirmation in recent research. Glajchen et al[78] studied 191 outpatients with cancer and found that pain disrupted their mood, activities, and enjoyment of life. They demonstrated relationships among pain intensity, family communication related to pain, and patients' educational level. These investigators concluded that psychological factors (affective and behavioral dimensions), demographics (sociocultural dimension), and medical factors (physiological, sensory, and behavioral dimensions) could interfere with assessment and management of cancer pain. In another study, Lancee and colleagues[79] tested a model for determinants of distress in cancer patients in 1309 individuals with cancer. Among their most striking findings was that pain (and other symptoms) had a direct effect on distress (affective dimension), and that pain was the single most significant factor related to distress. Additionally, pain exerted an indirect effect on distress through its effects on functional impairment (behavioral dimension) and cancer-related fears (cognitive dimension). Finally, Williamson and Schulz[80] demonstrated in 268 younger (aged 30–64) and older (65–90) cancer patients that the effects of pain on depression (affective dimension) are mediated by functional disability (behavioral dimension). This impairment was more distressing to the younger patients than to the older ones. These investigators also noted that patients' overall levels of depression were below those considered at risk for clinical depression.

The multidimensional conceptualization of cancer pain, as initially defined by Ahles et al;[15] expanded by McGuire,[18] and supported by the research of many investigators, provides the conceptual foundation for this chapter. The six dimensions are highly appropriate for assessment and management of cancer pain; each contributes in its own way to various aspects of these two critical processes. Additionally, the multidimensional framework allows the experience of cancer pain to be viewed as the complete, interrelated, interactive, and dynamic phenomenon that it is. Nursing assessment and management that are performed in a holistic, competent, and multidisciplinary manner will ensure that individuals with cancer pain achieve optimal quality of life regardless of the status of their disease.

# SCOPE OF THE CANCER PAIN PROBLEM

Pain in the cancer patient has long been recognized as a challenging clinical problem. The Oncology Nursing Society's (ONS) position paper on cancer pain[81] emphasized the fact that cancer pain often is managed inadequately. Similarly, the National Institutes of Health (NIH) consensus statement on an integrated approach to the management of pain[82] highlighted the inadequacies of current approaches to pain. A comprehensive understanding of the scope of the cancer pain problem requires knowledge of its prevalence, significance, and professional issues involved in its management.

## Prevalence

The incidence of cancer pain for all cancer diagnoses during all stages of the disease has been difficult to quantify. Most studies report prevalence data rather than incidence data. Coyle and Foley[21] identified several problems affecting the accuracy of prevalence data: (1) lack of systematic data collection and pain measurement techniques, (2) lack of documentation regarding the extent of patients' disease, (3) lack of identification of pain's etiology, and (4) inclusion of multiple cancer diagnoses as a single group. In spite of these problems, however, researchers have examined the prevalence of cancer pain, with the majority of reports appearing during the last 15 years.

The chapter on pain in a previous edition of this text[48] reviewed and discussed at length the literature on prevalence of cancer pain, presenting overviews in tabular format. In brief, prevalence of pain by clinical setting, regardless of cancer diagnosis, indicates that patients in hospice and specialty units report a higher prevalence of pain than patients in other settings. This observation can be understood by recognizing that patients with advanced, metastatic disease are often referred to these settings for terminal care. Patients with advanced disease report more severe pain than those who are in the early stages of their illness.

The severity of cancer pain, as opposed to the presence of pain, has been used as a means of reporting not only prevalence of pain but also its characteristics. Several studies cited in the chapter on pain in a previous edition of this text[48] revealed that patients with cancer-related pain described it as ranging from mild or moderate to severe or excruciating. Most patients, however, reported pain in the mild to moderate rather than the severe range.

Examination of pain prevalence data by cancer diagnosis shows the likelihood of pain becoming a significant problem with the progression of disease, particularly in common solid tumors such as lung and breast cancer. Several cancers, notably pancreatic and primary bone, exhibit relatively high prevalence rates of pain across all stages of disease.

Literature has addressed pain in children with cancer,[27,28] including prevalence and etiology. Very few studies of pain incidence or prevalence have been conducted in the pediatric oncology population, but the few data available suggest that between 25% and 78% of children may experience pain at some point during their cancer experience.

Taken together, the published studies on the prevalence of cancer pain indicate several important things. First, knowledge of cancer pain comes only from prevalence studies, since there are almost no published reports on the *incidence* of cancer pain. Second, pain clearly is more prevalent in those patients with advanced stages of disease and those being treated in hospice or specialty units. Third, certain common malignancies are more often associated with cancer pain, and it is these malignancies in which pain is better studied and understood. Finally, much of the available data are derived from patients with tumor- and/or treatment-related pain, rendering accurate rates for any specific type of pain difficult to ascertain.

Because of the complicated nature of cancer pain, with its different etiologies,[31] varied presentations,[32] multiple dimensions,[18] and variety of treatments, and the previously mentioned problems with studying the incidence and prevalence of the problem, one can speculate that the true prevalence is much greater than existing reports indicate.

## Significance

Although cancer pain clearly is a multidimensional phenomenon, the impact on patients who have it, or their families and friends, is only beginning to be understood. Cancer pain is a significant problem for a variety of reasons. It is already well known that individuals with cancer-related pain exhibit a variety of pain-related behaviors,[65] and experience many physical and psychosocial problems.[15,16,44,83–85] Additionally, the last eight to ten years have witnessed an explosion of clinical research, sociocultural, political, regulatory/legal, health policy, and professional activities that have increased knowledge about pain and have influenced in both positive and negative ways how it is managed. These developments encompass quality of life, family and home care issues, suicide risk, ethical concerns related to use of advanced technologies, financial costs associated with cancer pain, regulatory influences on use of controlled substances, legal impediments to adequate management of pain, health policy initiatives in pain, increased emphasis on cancer pain by national and international agencies, and increased federal and private research funding opportunities. The brief discussion that follows provides a cursory overview of these developments and demonstrates the far-reaching significance of the cancer pain problem.

Quality of life is a construct that has been examined in people with cancer pain as a domain of concern[46] as well as a potential outcome variable in treatment. Research has included refining the psychometric properties of a quality-of-life assessment tool[50] and using a quality-of-life tool in the clinical arena to evaluate pharmacological interventions with respect to impact on pain intensity as well as on the total person.[86] Additional research has documented the scope and extent of pain's influence on quality of life. For example, Strang and Qvarner[87] demonstrated in 84 patients with cancer-related pain that there was not only significant physical suffering but also negative influences on daily functional activities and concentration. Ferrell and colleagues[88] validated a conceptual model of quality of life in patients with cancer pain that included four domains: physical well-being and symptoms, social concerns, psychological well-being, and spiritual well-being. Research focused on this model has demonstrated quite clearly that quality of life is significantly affected by cancer pain, and that its assessment is important in evaluating both patients' responses to pain interventions and their overall status.[89]

Quality of life also serves as a foundation for reexamining the current issue of suicidal ideation or actual suicide in persons with progressive cancer accompanied by severe pain. Foley[90] recently reviewed the issues surrounding patients' requests for physician-assisted suicide as an option in the face of uncontrolled pain and multiple other adverse symptoms. She commented that physicians are not adequately trained to care for dying patients and, furthermore, are deterred from appropriate terminal care by economic considerations. She urged improved physician-patient communication, patient-centered care, better judgments about when to withhold or withdraw care, and familiarity with concepts of palliative care as ways to reduce physician-assisted suicide and euthanasia. Breitbart described specific factors that may make patients more likely to engage in suicidal ideation: pain and suffering, advanced disease with poor prognosis, depression and hopelessness, delirium, loss of control, preexisting psychopathology, prior family or personal history of suicide, and exhaustion or fatigue.[91]

Coyle has addressed the role of nursing in relation to current debates about euthanasia and physician-assisted suicide in patients with terminal cancer.[92] She emphasized the need for nurses to understand the issues surrounding these debates, including specific definitions, ethical principles underlying positions for or against euthanasia, and the positions of professional and global health organizations. She indicated that nurses also needed to understand the factors just cited that may make patients more vulnerable to considering suicide as an option, and to use all resources at their disposal to derive appropriate and individualized management plans for such individuals.

The impact of pain on family caregivers, particularly in the home environment, is an area that has been studied in some depth. A study of 85 family caregivers of patients with cancer pain[93] revealed that pain caused a significant burden for families. Their descriptions of pain centered on four themes: anatomic descriptions of pain, hidden pain (patient hides it), family fear and suffering, and overwhelming or unendurable pain. Families' experience of pain included three themes: helplessness, coping by denial of their own feelings (i.e., pretending to "be strong"), and a wish for the patient's death (a "welcome relief" from the suffering).

A second part of this same study[94] documented that family members played a major caregiving role in managing their loved one's pain. With respect to pharmacological interventions, they decided what medications to give and when, monitored them around the clock, kept records, dealt with fears of addiction, and assumed total responsibility for pain medications. In the realm of nonpharmacological interventions, they provided a number of physical interventions (e.g., positioning and/or mobility, massage, application of cold and heat) as well as cognitive interventions (e.g., being there, touch, talk). This research also revealed the questions and concerns family caregivers had about pain and its management, including their advice to professional caregivers (i.e., be there, offer hope, explain, be honest, listen, educate, give enough medicine) and their own personal perspectives (the future, understanding why, death, and fears about medications and handling pain at home).

Data from this same study, conducted in a community hospital, a national cancer center, and a home-based community hospice, were examined in relation to caregiver burden and family factors influencing pain management.[95] Areas of burden included physical dimensions, psychological responses, and interference with normal activities. Families of patients cared for in all three sites rated patients' pain and distress as severe, but caregivers in the home hospice setting reported lower burden, better mood, less distress, and more feelings of being supported in their attempts to care for their loved one. Recent research[96] suggests that patients and their family caregivers do not always agree on the presence and severity of pain and other symptoms. This assessment issue and other areas described above, document the significant impact pain has on the family system of cancer patients, and provide many directions for nursing practice.

Ethical concerns related to the use of high technology in medicine[97] are important issues, particularly with respect to costs, access, social justice, informed consent, and autonomy. In the management of cancer pain, the potential for violations of accepted principles of biomedical ethics (autonomy, beneficence, nonmaleficence, and justice) has been clearly explicated.[98] Examples include decision making by health caregivers who as experts feel they can decide for patients, lack of respect for patients' values, inadequate concern for the vulnerability of people in pain, conflicts of interest when caregivers have ownership in companies manufacturing or distributing high-technology equipment, selection of therapies that may not provide the best benefits for patients, implementation of therapies that increase risk of harm, denial of access to needed therapy because of reimbursement issues, and use of inappropriate interventions to increase reimbursement. Whedon and Ferrell[99] provided an excellent discussion of considerations in using high-technology management in cancer patients with pain. They emphasized the *appropriate* use of such technology, delineating the need for specific guidelines in clinical practice and for use of pain management principles in deciding on, selecting, and implementing various advanced technologies.

The costs associated with caring for patients with cancer-related pain have been explored empirically. Data from admissions records over a 12-month period in a national cancer center revealed that 26% of 5772 patients studied had at least one hospital admission for inadequately controlled pain, and that 54% of admissions for uncontrolled pain occurred within two weeks of the patient's most recent discharge.[100] The 255 readmissions for uncontrolled pain observed in this study were estimated to cost approximately $5 million over a one-year period. The investigators suggested that predischarge education related to pain management and potential barriers to effective pain management in the home and/or community needs careful exploration. Because reimbursement for unplanned readmissions for pain control may be limited, tremendous costs to both patients and health care facilities may result.

A different twist on costs is provided by a landmark legal case that involved the inadequate management of pain in a terminally ill cancer patient admitted to a nursing home in North Carolina.[101] In this case, opioid analgesics were withheld from the patient by the nurse because of concerns about addiction, and other medications were substituted. The family of the patient proved that failure of the nurse and her employer to fulfill their obligations and responsibilities resulted in increased pain and suffering and in "emotional and mental anguish." This "inhuman treatment" resulted initially in a $15 million jury award for compensatory and punitive damages. Although the award was later set aside and a confidential settlement figure agreed on,[102] the case underscored the importance of ethical and professional obligations to relieve pain and suffering and of individualized plans of care for patients with pain.

Regulatory and legal developments also have come to the forefront in the cancer pain issue. Because fear of regulatory scrutiny has been identified as a barrier in cancer pain management, state and national laws and regulations are also problematic.[103,104] Pain management advocates throughout the country have helped to defeat legislation that potentially limits patient access to opioids. For example, state-run multiple-prescription programs, which are intended to decrease substance abuse fraud and drug abuse, result in rapid decreases in the number of appropriate prescriptions written for controlled substances. Several states are considering repealing their triplicate prescription laws.[105] Other positive efforts in the legislative arena include the passing of intractable pain treatment laws, pain summit meetings, and, more recently, the establishment of state pain commissions.[106]

This brief review has highlighted several areas that demonstrate the far-reaching significance of the cancer pain problem. In addition, health policy initiatives and professional organizational efforts to reduce pain and improve its management are another recent and critically

important development.[106,107] Such initiatives have occurred both within the United States and internationally. Increased funding opportunities for basic and applied research on pain are more available than in past years, with some agencies specifically targeting pain.[19,108]

Finally, another area of enormous significance to the cancer pain problem is the extensive evidence suggesting that cancer pain is poorly managed worldwide by health professionals from a number of disciplines. Nurses in particular suffer from a lack of research-based knowledge about the prevalence of pain, the impact it has on patients and others, and effective ways of managing it. The next section explores a number of professional issues that influence management of pain.

## Professional Issues

### Organizational efforts

Organizations and agencies involved with cancer treatment and pain management have directed their efforts toward improving pain management. The ONS position paper[181] highlighted the fact that control of cancer pain is largely inadequate. Further, the paper pointed out that individuals with cancer pain have the right to have pain recognized as a problem and dealt with expediently. Similarly, the World Health Organization (WHO) has designated the relief of cancer pain as one of the goals of its cancer control program.[109] Additionally, the NIH consensus statement[82] recommended using multiple treatment modalities to help control cancer pain. At a national level, the American Pain Society (APS) recently published revised performance improvement standards on pain management[110] as well as having published the third edition of its principles for using analgesics to treat acute and cancer pain.[111] The American Society of Clinical Oncology (ASCO) issued a formal statement on the rights of patients to receive adequate pain management and published an educational curriculum for oncologists and oncologists in training.[112] The Agency for Health Care Policy and Research (AHCPR) has clinical practice guidelines for the management of cancer-related pain.[113] Finally, the International Association for the Study of Pain (IASP) published a pain curriculum for use in basic nursing education,[114] predicated on the notion that since nurses have frequent contact with patients receiving care in many settings, they need comprehensive knowledge about pain. The position papers, guidelines, recommendations, and curricula from these various groups have developed in part because of the compelling evidence documented over at least two decades that unrelieved cancer pain is a significant clinical problem.

### Obstacles to successful management

A number of obstacles to pain management can be attributed to health care professionals, patients and family, and the health care system (Table 20–3). Inaccurate knowledge about pharmacological principles represents a major problem area, as documented by many studies. Questionnaires administered to nurses, physicians, and students, as well as reviews of patients' records, indicate that in those with cancer pain, there are problems such as prolonged dosing intervals (i.e., not commensurate with the duration of action of the drug), lack of knowledge about equal analgesic doses, misconceptions about morphine's effectiveness as an oral analgesic, and use of doses too low to provide relief of pain.[76,115–120]

A related pharmacological problem stems from nurses' decision making in administering opioids. Sheidler and colleagues[116] found that when nurses were given hypothetical patient vignettes in which changes were made in drug, dose, route, or interval, very few nurses were able to select the appropriate "new" order.

Issues surrounding addiction and potential toxicities of potent opioids also have been cited as reasons for suboptimal pain control.[121–126] Although some evidence strongly suggests that addiction is not a problem for individuals who require opioids,[127] nurses, physicians, and medical students fear iatrogenically induced addiction and certainly overestimate its risk when opioids are prescribed.[128–130]

Ferrell et al[131] reviewed 14 pharmacology or medical-surgical nursing textbooks published since 1985 and found that only 1 out of 14 defined *opioid addiction* correctly and described accurately the likelihood of addiction developing with legitimate opioid use. This finding underscores the reason why there is so much confusion about addiction.

A more fundamental problem that nurses have demonstrated is a deficiency in the assessment of pain. A lack of basic assessment skills, failure to acknowledge and document the existence of pain, and inaccurate or nonexistent documentation when the problem is known to exist prohibit patients from receiving reasonable pain control.[39,132–134] Although there is strong evidence suggesting that systematic pain assessment and documentation can improve pain management,[135] these very basic nursing actions are not performed consistently.

**TABLE 20-3** Obstacles to Successful Pain Management

- Lack of understanding about pain
- Expectation that pain should be present
- Relief of pain not viewed as a goal of treatment
- Inadequate or nonexistent assessment
- Undertreatment with analgesics
- Inadequate knowledge of analgesics and other drugs
- Fears of addiction, sedation, and respiratory depression
- Inadequate knowledge of other interventions for pain
- Perceptual differences between patients and health care providers
- Legal impediments

Several other problems have been identified as obstacles to successful management of pain. Patients' reluctance to report pain to their health care providers and concerns about analgesics are major problems.[136] Perceptual differences between patients and professionals about severity of existing pain have been documented by several investigators.[125,135,137] Complete relief of pain traditionally has not been viewed as a treatment objective.[117,138] And finally, the role of government agencies, such as the Drug Enforcement Agency, and existing legal statutes have contributed to inadequate prescribing by physicians because of fear of regulatory scrutiny.[103,139,140]

### Improvements in management

Nurses and physicians have acknowledged their educational deficiencies related to cancer pain and its management.[124,141,142] The need for structured educational content in basic health professions' educational programs has been encouraged.[81,82,114,143–145] In nursing, Spross and colleagues[81] delineated positions involving not only basic and graduate nursing school education but also continuing education. ASCO recommends education about cancer pain management for all fellowship training programs,[112] and, as noted earlier, the IASP[114] has recommendations on pain curriculum in basic nursing education.

Initial efforts at improving pain management consisted of integrating both patients and caregivers into quality assurance efforts[146,147] and using a multidisciplinary team to get current pain knowledge into practice.[148] More recently, clinicians have reported a variety of creative programs in clinical and institutional settings that have improved pain management outcomes.[149–152] A structure common to several of these programs is teams or clinical partners who participate jointly in the educational activities, thus supporting the interdisciplinary nature of cancer pain practice.

In addition to such institutional programs, improvement of pain management can be accomplished through formal performance improvement programs.[147,153–155] The newly revised APS quality improvement guidelines for acute and cancer pain are applicable to both inpatient and outpatient settings.[110] Finally, major programmatic efforts, such as the state cancer pain initiatives and the WHO Cancer Control Program, have made the cancer pain problem much more visible, leading to heightened efforts to improve the care of patients with cancer pain.

### Delivery of pain management services

The delivery of pain management services is a controversial issue.[156] Individual practitioners who take care of oncology patients should possess basic skills in assessment and management. Recognizing the significant educational needs mentioned previously, some practitioners may feel more comfortable in referring a patient to a "specialist" for pain management, if one is available. A specialist may be an anesthesiologist, a medical or radiation oncologist, a neurologist, a neurosurgeon, a nurse, a pharmacist, a psychologist, a psychiatrist, or a social worker. Instead of an individual specialist, there may be a multidisciplinary pain team that can provide services.[157] When a referral is made to a specialist or to a pain team, several questions must be answered: (1) What is the level of responsibility of the consultant for the individual patient? (2) What role does the primary provider have after the consultation? (3) Does the patient incur significant additional costs by receiving care from a specialist or a multidisciplinary team? (4) If there are several options for a patient's pain management plan, how are decisions made, and who helps the patient and family with those decisions?

Gonzales et al[158] reported that in 64% of 276 patients referred for a pain consultation, the outcome of the evaluation (which usually required further diagnostic tests and analgesic changes) led to identifying the etiology of the pain problem. Metastatic disease was the most common cause of the pain. In addition, 22% of the patients received treatment for their pain problem with radiation, surgery, or chemotherapy. Walsh[159] described a palliative care service that saw approximately 400 patients per year. This consultant and management service was part of a hematology/medical oncology department, and was involved in research activities as well as providing full clinical services. Sheidler and Krumm[160] surveyed over 100 nurses involved in pain management activities and found that of the 42 nurses who indicated they were from settings that had a formal pain team, 55% of the 38 physician-led "pain management teams" were under departments of anesthesiology. When clinical settings had a formal service, only 40% of the nurses associated with the group spent more than 50% of the day in pain-related activities, indicating that most were involved in activities other than pain management. Although the multidisciplinary approach to managing cancer patients' pain may be optimal, utilization of resources, costs, and outcomes in today's health care climate needs careful consideration.

# PRINCIPLES OF ASSESSMENT AND MANAGEMENT

Effective clinical assessment and management of cancer pain rests on recognition and use of a number of critical principles. First is the importance of the nursing role in assessment and management.[161] The ONS position paper[81] delineated the nurse's role as (1) describing pain, (2) identifying aggravating and relieving factors, (3) determining the meaning of pain, (4) determining its cause, (5) determining individuals' definitions of optimal pain relief, (6) deriving nursing diagnoses, (7) assisting in selecting interventions, and (8) evaluating efficacy of interventions. Although nurses certainly contribute to the goals of the physician establishing and treating the cause

of pain, their emphasis is on the individual as a whole person, and on his or her response to pain. Thus, their focus is on individual definitions of optimal pain relief, psychosocial and physical problems amenable to nursing interventions, and evaluation of the overall response to treatment. Nurses are also interested in how pain affects an individual's significant others and support systems.

In addition to the critical importance of the nurse's role, there are other principles of assessment and management that are implicit in successful nursing management of cancer pain. These principles consist of the use of a multidisciplinary approach in the delivery of pain management services, a well-conceived scope of practice for nurses, a thorough assessment and diagnosis, incorporation of guidelines and standards into clinical practice, and approaches to managing pain in special populations of individuals. Each of these areas is explored in the following sections.

## Multidisciplinary Approach

The multidimensional conceptualization of cancer pain requires the involvement of multiple health care disciplines in assessment and management.[18,113] Treatment approaches, delineated later in this chapter, consist of chemotherapy, radiotherapy, surgery, anesthetic techniques, pharmacological agents, cognitive/behavioral methods, physical techniques, and many more. Clearly, there is no one best way to treat cancer pain, and no one best discipline or person prepared for managing cancer pain. Thus, input is required from specific health care professionals, including nurses, pharmacists, social workers, occupational therapists, physical therapists, psychologists, and physicians from many specialties and subspecialties (e.g., internal medicine, anesthesiology, surgery, radiation oncology, psychiatry).

## Nursing's Scope of Practice and Responsibilities

Nurses are an integral part of the multidisciplinary team approach to managing cancer pain. The ONS position paper[31] delineated a number of positions related to the management of cancer pain and suggested strategies to achieve the positions. Important components of the paper included the nurse's scope of practice relevant to pain and specific nursing responsibilities. Both of these key areas will be briefly summarized next; the interested reader is encouraged to read the original source.

Oncology nurses, by virtue of their prolonged contact with cancer patients in a variety of settings, and by virtue of their relationships with these individuals and their families, are best prepared to assume a leadership role in the assessment and management of cancer pain. Assumption of such a role is consistent with the ONS's mission of improving the care of persons with cancer. The NIH consensus statement[82] described and endorsed a pivotal role for professional nurses in the management of pain.

The ONS position paper[81] delineated a scope of practice for nurses with different levels of expertise (e.g., nurses and oncology clinical nurse specialists). These levels of expertise were made operational with specific knowledge and skills associated with each level. With the publication of the new scope and standards of oncology nursing practice,[162] the idea of levels of expertise can be easily translated into the general oncology nursing practice and advanced oncology nursing practice that are described in this publication. At the generalist level, the nurse needs a cancer pain–specific knowledge base that enables appropriate assessment, development of a care plan based on the nursing process, evaluation of the plan, and consultation with others when needed. At the advanced level, the nurse (an individual with a master's degree) should have substantially more theoretical knowledge and clinical expertise in cancer pain that allows assessment, diagnosis, analysis of complex problems, and the use of relevant research and theory to problem-solve.

Two positions set forth in the ONS position paper[81] dealt with the ethical and practice responsibilities of nurses in managing pain (Table 20–4). These positions,

**TABLE 20-4**  Oncology Nursing Society Position Paper on Cancer Pain

### POSITION STATEMENTS ON CANCER PAIN

**Ethics**

Individuals with cancer pain have a right to obtain optimal pain relief. Nurses caring for them have an ethical obligation to ensure exploration of everything possible within the scope of nursing practice to provide this relief.

**Practice**

Nurses caring for individuals with cancer pain must exercise leadership in identifying and assessing cancer pain and in planning, implementing, coordinating, and evaluating the interdisciplinary management of cancer pain.

- *Problem identification.* Nurses are responsible for identifying the problem of inadequate pain management in patients with cancer and for intervening responsibly to achieve optimal pain relief.

- *Assessment.* Nurses caring for individuals with cancer pain should perform initial and ongoing assessments of pain and communicate assessment data to colleagues.

- *Planning.* After assessing the individual experiencing cancer pain, the nurse develops a plan of care with the individual/significant other that includes specific measurable goals and effective pain management interventions; incorporates specific pain management techniques based on mutual goal setting; specifies a schedule for the timing of interventions and of ongoing assessment of pain, pain relief, and side effects associated with pain therapy, as well as overall effectiveness of the regimen; and addresses nursing responsibilities as well as communication and other collaborative interventions with other health care providers involved in the individual's care.

- *Implementation and coordination.* Nurses are responsible and accountable for implementation and coordination of the plan for management of cancer pain.

- *Evaluation.* Nurses are responsible for evaluating patient responses to interventions for cancer pain control and for using evaluation data to revise the care plan. Nurses use all available clinical and administrative resources to ensure progress toward achieving relief or control of cancer pain.

**Basic Nursing Education**

Basic nursing education programs should have theoretical and clinical curriculum content related to cancer pain and its management.

**Graduate Nursing Education**

Graduate nursing education programs preparing advanced practitioners should provide advanced theoretical, research, and clinical curriculum content on cancer pain and management.

**Responsibilities for Continuing Education**

Nurses are responsible for regularly updating their knowledge of cancer pain assessment and management. Opportunities should exist to develop competence in areas of cancer pain assessment, management, and evaluation.

**Patient and Public Education**

Patient education is an essential element of cancer pain management and is a primary responsibility of nurses. Nurses have a responsibility to educate the public, patients, and significant others about the right to relief from cancer pain and the resources available for assessment and treatment of cancer pain.

**Research**

Cancer pain and pain management are research priorities for oncology nurses and the Oncology Nursing Society (ONS).

**Research Utilization**

Nurses have a responsibility to use research findings relevant to assessment and management of cancer pain in their practice and to facilitate the dissemination and use of these findings by others.

**Nursing Administration**

Effective cancer pain management should be an organizational priority for nurse administrators, including establishment of nurses' lines of accountability and responsibility.

**Social Policy**

ONS is committed to initiating legislative and health policy activities that will overcome sociopolitical obstacles to cancer pain management and to evaluating legislative and health policy actions that can influence cancer pain management.

**Pediatric Cancer Pain**

Children experiencing pain because of cancer have a right to optimal pain relief. The nursing process, as outlined in previous position statements in this paper, should include the use of developmentally appropriate assessments and interventions. Effective management of pediatric cancer pain should reflect an understanding of particular pediatric pain issues (e.g., the role of the parents, procedural pain).

Reprinted from the *Oncology Nursing Forum* with permission from the Oncology Nursing Press, Inc. Spross JA, McGuire DB, Schmitt, RM: Oncology Nursing Society Position Paper on Cancer Pain Part I. *Oncol Nurs Forum* 17(4):595–603, 1990.

as well as all others, were based on several assumptions: (1) Patients have a right to relief of pain. (2) Unrelieved pain causes significant and unnecessary suffering for patients, families, friends, and health professionals. (3) Nurses and patients (i.e., society) have a social contract in which alleviation of pain and suffering is a tenet. (4) Nurses are often prevented from meeting this obligation because of inadequate education and a variety of sociocultural variables. (5) Nurses have sustained contact with patients and their significant others over the course of a cancer illness that make them key providers of care. (6) Cancer pain is an "orphan" problem with accountability for its relief unclear. (7) Cancer pain is a sociopolitical as well as a clinical problem.

It is clear that assumption of a leadership role in effective management of cancer patients' pain is a nursing responsibility. The scope of nursing practice delineated in the ONS paper provides the foundation for all positions relevant to nurses' roles and responsibilities in caring for persons with cancer-related pain.

## Assessment and Diagnosis

Literature documenting nurses' problems with assessing cancer pain has been discussed previously. This section presents the rationale for and basic principles of assessment, assessment parameters, tools for assessing pain, nursing diagnoses resulting from pain assessments, and strategies for incorporating assessment into institutional practice.

### Rationale and basic principles

Systematic nursing assessment of pain is important for several reasons.[163] First, it establishes a baseline from which to plan and begin interventions. Second, it assists in the selection of interventions. Third, it makes possible evaluation of the interventions. Assessment of pain is a critical process that aids in the clinical management of pain and, indeed, goes hand in hand with successful management. It is different from measurement of pain, which is used to quantify pain in a bias-free manner, and is generally carried out for research purposes.[163]

The timing of assessments is critical as well. Any cancer patient with pain who enters any health care setting should have an initial or baseline assessment. After the initiation of interventions, continuous or ongoing assessment is necessary for evaluation and revision of treatment plans. This approach to assessment is modeled on the nursing process. Collection of pain assessment data should be systematic and organized, just as the collection of general nursing data is.

The need for a complete nursing assessment of pain and documentation of the assessment was highlighted in several studies.[132,133] In addition, there are some "pitfalls" in assessment of pain. They include (1) the belief that patients with pain will demonstrate changes in vital signs or display overt behavioral manifestations of pain, (2)

the belief that all pain should have a documented organic cause, (3) the belief that pain in cancer patients may be of psychogenic origin ("all in the head"), (4) ascription of all pain in cancer patients to the tumor rather than to such "normal" problems as migraine headache or arthritis, and (5) feelings of being overwhelmed with clinical responsibilities and thus becoming insensitive to patients' pain and their related needs. Awareness and avoidance of these "pitfalls" should help nurses perform good pain assessments.

### Assessment parameters

The multidimensional conceptualization of pain described previously provides guidance in assessing pain.[18] The range of assessment parameters is quite wide and represents each of the multiple dimensions of cancer pain.[18] Key clinical parameters that require assessment in each dimension are highlighted in Table 20–5. Basic techniques for assessing pain, including the very important pain history, are discussed in a previous edition of this chapter[18] and in other sources.[161,163,164]

### Assessment tools

There is extensive literature on instruments to measure clinical pain, but a lengthy discussion is impossible here. The reader is referred to several recent publications in which this literature is reviewed and discussed, in adult and pediatric populations.[27,28,165] There is also literature on the assessment of cancer pain that focuses on generic issues of assessment and/or reviews available tools.[166,167] Table 20–6 presents clinical, psychometric, and practical information about tools most commonly used for assessing cancer pain in adult populations. Complete information can be found in a recent review chapter.[165] Additionally, categories of tools for assessing pain in children are illustrated, and the interested reader is urged to consult appropriate sources. The general discussion presented next about types of tools, their appropriate uses, and considerations in selecting them should help readers select the best tool for a given situation.

Pain assessment tools can be classified by the number of dimensions of pain they assess.[165] Unidimensional tools focus on one dimension of the pain experience, such as the sensory dimension, and within that dimension may focus on a specific parameter, such as pain intensity (see Table 20–6). Ten-centimeter visual analogue scales (VAS) (anchors of *no pain* and *worst possible pain*) or verbal descriptor scales (VDS) (words such as *none, mild, moderate,* and *severe*) measuring pain intensity are examples of commonly used unidimensional tools. Although most VASs and VDSs are of the paper-and-pencil variety, a new format consisting of a $5 \times 20$-cm plastic device with a sliding marker moving within a groove that measures 10 cm recently was tested and found to be reliable and valid at assessing pain intensity in cancer patients.[168] Pain relief can also be measured with VASs and VDSs simply by changing anchor and descriptor words. Although these

**TABLE 20-5** Assessment Parameters Using the Multidimensional Conceptualization of Cancer Pain

| Physiological | Sensory | Affective |
|---|---|---|
| • Onset | • Location | • Distress |
| • Associated factors | • Intensity | • Anxiety |
| • Duration | • Quality | • Depression |
| • Type of pain (acute or chronic) | • Pattern | • Mental state |
| • Syndrome | | • Perception of suffering |
| • Anatomy | | • Irritability/agitation |
| • Physiology | | • Pain relief |

| Cognitive | Behavioral | Sociocultural |
|---|---|---|
| • Meaning of pain | • Communication with others | • Ethnocultural/background |
| • Thought processes | • Interpersonal relationships | • Family/social life |
| • Coping strategies | • Activities of daily living | • Work/home responsibilities |
| • Knowledge | • Behaviors (pain-related, preventive, or controlling) | • Environment |
| • Attitudes/beliefs | | • Familial attitudes/beliefs/behaviors |
| • Previous treatments | • Use of medications | • Personal attitudes/beliefs |
| • Influencing factors (positive and negative) | • Sleep/rest patterns | |
| | • Fatigue | |

scales have documented reliability and validity in measuring cancer-related pain,[165] they measure only one parameter of one dimension of pain and thus are limited in their representation of the total pain experience. However, because pain intensity is such a salient aspect of pain, these scales are an excellent means to evaluate the success of specific interventions for pain. Indeed, the APS quality improvement guidelines[110] recommended regular use of pain intensity and relief scales, as did the AHCPR guidelines for both cancer pain and acute pain management.[113,169] Other unidimensional tools consist of body diagrams to assess location of pain and rating scales to assess behavioral indicators of pain[165] (see Tables 20–5 and 20–6).

Multidimensional tools focus on two or more dimensions of the pain experience (see Tables 20–5 and 20–6). The McGill Pain Questionnaire (MPQ)[34] is perhaps the most well-known example. The MPQ was originally developed to measure multidimensional aspects of pain in many diseases but has been shown to be reliable and valid in a number of different cancer patient populations.[34–37,43,45,165] Another comprehensive multidimensional (sensory, affective, cognitive, behavioral, sociocultural) tool is the Brief Pain Inventory (BPI), developed initially for assessing pain in general but used fairly extensively for cancer pain.[113,165,170–172] Recent research suggests that the BPI is a good tool for use in low-income African-Americans.[172] There are also several multidimensional tools that are short and easy to administer. For example, Melzack developed the short-form version of the MPQ[173] to assess sensory (including intensity and quality) and affective dimensions of pain. The Memorial Pain Assessment Card (MPAC) is another example.[174] It assesses pain intensity, pain relief, and mood (general psychological

**TABLE 20-6** Tools for Assessing Pain

| Tools | Dimension(s) Measured* | Patient Population(s) | Psychometric Properties | Advantages | Disadvantages |
|---|---|---|---|---|---|
| | | | ADULTS | | |
| Brief Pain Inventory[113,165,170–172] | P, S, A, C, B, So | Cancer, rheumatoid arthritis, orthopedic | Test-retest reliability; construct, predictive validity | Brief, simple, self-administered, comprehensive | Provides fairly superficial information |
| McGill Pain Questionnaire (long form)[34–37,42,43,45,165] | P, S, A, C, B | Acute, chronic, cancer, experimental | Test-retest reliability; content, concurrent, construct, predictive validity | Comprehensive, versatile | Time-consuming (5–20 min), may be difficult for some individuals to understand or complete |

**TABLE 20-6** Tools for Assessing Pain (continued)

| Tools | Dimension(s) Measured* | Patient Population(s) | Psychometric Properties | Advantages | Disadvantages |
|---|---|---|---|---|---|
| McGill Pain Questionnaire (short form)[165,173] | S, A | Acute postoperative, obstetric, dental, musculoskeletal | Reliability not reported; concurrent validity | Brief, simple, self-administered | Reliability is unclear; needs further psychometric evaluation in other groups with acute and chronic pain |
| Memorial Pain Assessment Card[165,174] | S, A | Cancer | Reliability not reported; construct, concurrent validity | Brief, simple | Reliability is unclear; requires further psychometric evaluation and extension to additional acute and chronic pain populations |
| Pain Affect Faces Scale[113,172] | S, A | Cancer | Reliability not reported; construct, concurrent validity | Brief, simple, combines affective and sensory, popular with low income patients | Needs more psychometric evaluation |
| Numerical Rating Scale[165,172] | S | Acute, chronic (also used in children) | Reliability not reported; construct, concurrent validity | Brief, simple, more sensitive than verbal descriptor scale, less confusing than Visual Analogue Scale, can be administered in written or verbal form | Unidimensional, sensitivity to pain treatment is unknown |
| Pain Assessment Tool (PAT)/Pain Flowsheet (PFS)[136,175] | P, S, A, C, B, So | Cancer | Interrater reliability (PAT); content validity (PAT); construct validity (PFS) | Both PAT and PFS are comprehensive, PFS helpful in managing pain | PAT time-consuming to complete |
| Verbal Descriptor Scale[161,164,165] | S (pain intensity, relief) | Acute, cancer, chronic, experimental (also used in children) | Test-retest reliability; construct, concurrent validity | Brief, simple, easy to score | Lacks sensitivity, forces selection of only one word, even if no word satisfactorily describes pain intensity; can be difficult for persons with limited vocabulary |
| Visual Analogue Scale[27,161,164–166] | S (pain intensity, relief), A (depression, mood) | Acute, chronic, cancer (also used in children) | Test-retest reliability; construct, concurrent validity | Brief, provides a sensitive measure, scores can be analyzed as interval data | May be difficult for some individuals; scoring is awkward in the clinical setting and may be a source of error |
| **CHILDREN†** | | | | | |
| Behavioral measures[178] | P, B | Postoperative, prolonged acute pain, during injections, cancer | Must read article(s) on specific tool(s) selected | Useful when self-report cannot be given or patient is preverbal | Does not allow for self-report |
| Self-report measures | S, A, C | Preschool, school-age, adolescent, injections, acute pain, chronic musculoskeletal pain, cancer | Must read article(s) on specific tool(s) selected | Allows self-report of various characteristics of pain, allows multidimensional assessment | May be difficult for preschoolers or for acutely ill youngsters |

*P, physiological; S, sensory; A, affective; C, cognitive; B, behavioral; So, sociocultural.

†Data from Ross DM, Ross SA: Assessment of pediatric pain: An overview, *ISS Compr Pediatr Nurs* 11:73–91, 1988; Beyer JE, Wells N: The assessment of pain in children. *Pediatr Clin North Am* 36:837–854, 1989.

distress) with VASs, and intensity with a series of verbal descriptors. Additional multidimensional methods for assessing pain have been developed to assist nurses in making both baseline and ongoing assessments, taking the form of comprehensive questionnaires and flow sheets.[135,175]

Clinicians and researchers have recently begun to recognize the importance of interactions between pain and other symptoms such as fatigue, sleep, and psychological distress.[176-178] Some symptoms, such as pain, fatigue, emotional distress, and sleep alterations appear to be associated with one another in cancer patients with pain.[176] Recent studies indicate that patients with cancer often suffer not only from pain but from numerous other symptoms. Those most commonly observed are pain, fatigue, weakness, lack of energy, worrying or feeling sad, and feeling drowsy or having difficulty sleeping.[177,178] These clinical observations have resulted in attempts to construct multidimensional tools to assess common cancer-related symptoms simultaneously, including pain. The Memorial Symptom Assessment Scale (MSAS), for example, is designed to collect information about the prevalence, characteristics, and distress of 32 common symptoms, including pain.[179] The MSAS has good preliminary evidence of reliability and validity, and may be useful to nurses wishing to perform a comprehensive symptom assessment.

Children with cancer pain represent a unique challenge to the nurse who wishes to assess pain. Because of their developmental characteristics, many of the assessment parameters already discussed are inappropriate. For example, infants and very young children lack verbal skills and therefore cannot tell others what their pain feels like, where it is located, and what makes it better or worse. Categories of measures include both behavioral and self-report.

Several instruments for measuring pain in children ages 3 years and older have been developed and tested[180] (see Table 20–6). These tools include the Oucher Scale[180] and the Children's Hospital of Eastern Ontario Pain Scale (CHEOPS), a behavioral scale for rating postoperative pain developed by McGrath and colleagues.[181] Additional tools recommended by McCaffery and Beebe[164] for assessing pain intensity in children include numerical scales (for ages 10 and older), the Wong/Baker Faces Rating Scale, the Eland Color Scale, and the Hester Poker Chip Scale. A discussion of each of these tools is beyond the scope of this chapter, but the reader who needs more information is referred to other sources.[27,28,182]

McCaffery and Beebe[164] urged nurses to use a multidimensional approach in assessing children's pain that included discussing pain with both child and family, obtaining the child's self-report if possible, identifying the presence of pathology with the potential to cause pain, observing behavioral manifestations of pain such as vocalizations or facial expressions, and considering a trial of analgesics with careful attention paid to the child's responses.

The choice of tools for assessing pain in both adults and children depends on several considerations.[161] Of foremost concern are the dimensions of pain that are most relevant in a given situation. For example, the behavioral dimension assumes primary importance in a preverbal child or in an adult cancer patient experiencing acute confusion or cognitive failure,[183,184] whereas the sensory and affective dimensions may predominate in an alert and oriented postoperative patient. The tool selected should be able to assess the relevant parameters of the dimension(s) of interest. The purpose of the assessment (i.e., baseline versus ongoing) is a second major consideration. In general, baseline assessments will require a more detailed and comprehensive tool, while ongoing assessments can use brief, simple tools.

A third consideration is related to the pain interventions being used. Effects of treatments aimed at the physiological and sensory dimensions (e.g., analgesics) should be evaluated by assessing parameters such as location, intensity, and quality. Treatments aimed at the cognitive, affective, and behavioral dimensions (e.g., distraction and relaxation) should be evaluated using tools assessing parameters of those dimensions (see Tables 20–5 and 20–6). A fourth important area relates to specific patient and setting factors, such as age, cognitive abilities, type of pain, level of acuity, physical function, literacy and language issues, personal preference, and type of clinical setting (inpatient, outpatient, home, hospice). Some of these patient-related factors may influence whether the tools selected are subjective (patient self-report) or objective (observational) in nature.

Finally, issues related to time, feasibility, and relevance to the clinical setting are a major consideration. Important considerations include the amount of time required to complete tools, format and amount of writing, overlap with existing documentation, relevance of parameters to setting and to clinicians, personal comfort and preference, and lines of responsibility and accountability.

## Nursing diagnoses and documentation

The outcome of a thorough baseline assessment of the cancer patient with pain should be identification of problems or nursing diagnoses that structure the design and implementation of the management plan. The North American Nursing Diagnosis Association (NANDA) included the diagnosis "Alteration in Comfort: Pain" in its 1988 taxonomy,[185] with two categories (pain and chronic pain). This diagnosis provided the framework for nursing management of patients with cancer pain in the ONS *Guidelines for Oncology Nursing Practice*.[186]

McCaffery and Beebe[164] cited 18 other nursing diagnoses that the nurse should consider as part of the assessment process: anxiety, constipation, ineffective individual coping, diversional activity deficit, fatigue, fear, knowledge deficit (specify), impaired physical mobility, powerlessness, feeding self-care deficit, bathing/hygiene self-care deficit, dressing/grooming self-care deficit, toileting self-care deficit, sexual dysfunction, sleep pattern disturbance, social isolation, spiritual distress (distress of the human spirit), and altered thought processes. In Carpenito's text[187] examples of NANDA-approved diagnoses that may be relevant are activity intolerance, anxiety, constipation, family coping, fatigue, and fear, among many others. The inclusion of *all* relevant nursing diagnoses will focus management efforts on the need for multiple disciplines to be involved in using multiple interventions for pain.

Of critical importance is the need for nurses to document their assessments and diagnoses in a manner appropriate for their clinical settings. The APS quality improvement standards[110] recommended the documentation of pain intensity and pain relief on standard patient records, such as the vital sign sheet or patient flow sheet. Similarly, the AHCPR guidelines on cancer pain management[113] suggested incorporation of assessment data into routine institutional records. The use of standardized pain assessment and documentation appears to have a positive impact on pain intensity and to facilitate management of pain.[135,154]

## Incorporation into Practice

Successful management of cancer pain will ultimately depend on the extent to which systematic processes, tools, documentation procedures, and lines of formal accountability and responsibility for pain management are incorporated into institutional settings. The ONS position paper,[81] as mentioned previously, places the *coordination* of pain management squarely on the oncology nurse. Several creative programs for helping oncology nurses assume this role were noted earlier.[150–153] The AHCPR cancer pain guidelines[113] provide a useful framework for incorporating sound pain assessment and management principles into clinical practice. Similarly, the use of components of the APS performance improvement standards,[110] such as assessment of patient satisfaction with pain management, can give clues to approaches that are working or that need improvement.[188] Strong institutionally supported programs for incorporating pain management into ongoing quality improvement mechanisms, such as the one described by Bookbinder et al,[154] have been successful in decreasing pain problems. Implementation of any effort to positively affect pain management must of necessity include evaluation of outcomes.[189,190]

## Special Populations

Because cancer is a group of diseases that affects individuals across the life span, the pain associated with it likewise occurs in groups of varying age, background, and clinical characteristics. Several populations—children, the elderly, individuals with substance abuse history, individuals with diverse sociocultural backgrounds, and the termi-

nally ill—require special consideration in the areas of pain assessment and management.

### Children

Assessment and management of pain in children with cancer have traditionally received little attention in the research arena.[191] The reasons for the paucity of published research are not entirely clear, but Stevens et al[192] proposed that they included theories of pain that are inadequate to explain children's pain, methodological and measurement difficulties, and clinical dilemmas brought about by differences in interpretation of children's behaviors coupled with nurses' and children's personal beliefs, values, fears, and pain experiences. The majority of existing research in children with cancer deals with the pain and distress of treatment-related procedures, such as bone marrow aspiration.[27,180,193]

Hester[194] reviewed research related to children's pain, covering the topics of prevalence of pain, children's perspectives on pain, assessment of pain, and management of pain. She concluded that although the volume of research in children's pain had increased dramatically over the past 20 years, much of it focused on measurement rather than on management of pain. She highlighted the need for studies of nonpharmacological and pharmacological interventions, and urged that the disparity between development of knowledge (i.e., research) and clinical practice be minimized, with the incorporation of research-based knowledge into practice as a major means for improving the care of children with pain.

The developmental level of children is directly related to how they perceive, interpret, and respond to pain, regardless of etiology.[195] Children's developmental stages have a number of implications for the assessment and management of their pain, and in fact can be used to help clarify a number of misconceptions that are held by health professionals and others about children with pain.

Generally speaking, the facts about children's pain can be represented by the following statements: There is significant evidence to indicate that neonates, including premature ones, do feel pain. Children who are verbally fluent may deny they have pain when in fact they *do* have it; this occurs when they have certain fears about pain or when they have adapted to it and do not realize it is worsening. Children's lack of willingness or ability to express pain or request treatment for it does *not* mean they do not have it. The child who sleeps, plays, or is otherwise distracted may still have a good deal of pain; such distractions are a common coping method used by children with pain. Children do *not* tolerate pain better than adults do. Opioids may be used safely in children provided there is an understanding of the pharmacokinetics and the children are properly observed; their use in all age-groups, including teenagers, generally is safe. Pain is *not* a harmless entity in children, without side effects or life-threatening potential; it has been documented that presence of pain in neonates may be harmful because of stressful reactions that can include prolonged crying leading to hypoxemia, and increased heart rate and blood pressure.[196] There is also the possibility of long-term psychological consequences from repeated episodes of acute pain or prolonged periods of unrelieved pain.[180]

The issue of undertreatment of children with pain is an important one. Although the evidence is not as massive as that documenting undertreatment of adults, there clearly is a problem in the pediatric arena. It was demonstrated that children who were hospitalized for surgery received very little of the analgesics ordered for them, and that, as compared with adults with the same diagnoses, they received 26 times *less* the amount.[197] Similarly, Schechter et al[198] demonstrated that hospitalized children and adults with the same diagnoses were treated differently with respect to administration of opioids. Children were likely to have less opioids than adults. One of the reasons suggested for these findings included the possibility that beliefs and attitudes of nursing and medical staff affected administration of drugs. A recent survey indicated that nurses caring for children with cancer had a poor understanding of pain management principles.[199]

A landmark document in the field of pediatric oncology was the report of the consensus conference on the management of pain in childhood cancer in 1990.[182] Key components of this report included assessment and methodological issues in managing pain, disease-related pain, management of pain associated with procedures and research priorities.

The subcommittee on assessment and methodological issues recommended the development and use of a pain problem list for children with cancer. This list resulted from the assessment process, including pain history, and characterization and key features that may influence decisions regarding therapy, particularly with respect to the multiple dimensions of pain and the multiple disciplines involved in its management.

Interventions for pain in children with cancer should be tailored to the type of pain they are experiencing.[28,182,191] Pain that is acute and related to operative procedures may be treated in the same manner as adult postoperative pain (i.e., with opioids, including patient-controlled analgesia if the patient is old enough). The AHCPR guidelines for cancer pain management explicitly addressed the management of pain in children.[113] It is important to note that children metabolize opioids more quickly than adults do, so their doses may need to be scheduled more frequently.[191] Since needles and shots are uniformly hated by children, the intravenous route immediately postoperatively followed by the oral route when possible is the preferred strategy. Management of other types of treatment-related pain, such as that caused by esophagitis or oral mucositis, can be successfully implemented through the use of continuous intravenous and even epidural and subarachnoid morphine infusions.[200]

The treatment of acute, procedure-related pain (e.g., bone marrow aspiration) is somewhat different. This type of pain usually is transient, though accompanied by a good deal of anxiety and fear. Interventions range from pharmacological approaches (e.g., sedatives) to cognitive and behavioral techniques (e.g., distraction and imagery).[201] Sedatives, particularly the combination of meperidine, promethazine, and chlorpromazine ("DPT") should be used with caution, for they do not decrease pain and anxiety[191] and they may even bring on respiratory depression.[202] A number of authors[28,191] recommend the combined use of premedications and cognitive/behavioral techniques for procedures such as bone marrow aspiration. The efficacy of several techniques has been documented.[203,204] Recent research suggests that use of ethyl chloride as a topical anesthetic reduces the pain of procedures and is well received by both children and parents.[205]

A newer agent, EMLA (eutectic mixture of local anesthetics), is also effective at providing local anesthesia during painful procedures.[206] The management of disease-related pain in children with cancer is a challenge. In the consensus conference report mentioned earlier,[182] the subcommittee on disease-related pain recommended the use of an algorithm for managing pediatric cancer pain. Guiding principles included (1) tailoring the route of administration to patients' conditions, (2) using simpler rather than complex technological approaches, (3) providing a level of comfort the patients find satisfactory, (4) treating side effects aggressively, (5) titrating analgesic doses to clinical effect without adherence to "standard doses," and (6) trying the oral route of administration first. An analgesic ladder was described that began with nonopioids for mild pain and progressed to combinations of these drugs, with strong opioids for severe pain. The use of nonpharmacological techniques was also recommended. Concurrent management of side effects and other symptoms, such as constipation, nausea, vomiting, urinary retention, and depression, was highlighted, with specific recommendations made regarding adjuvant analgesics. Finally, anesthetic and neurosurgical approaches were briefly discussed. This report offered a comprehensive and useful overview of managing pain in the pediatric cancer patient.

Finally, the management of pain due to terminal cancer is a challenging area, since the goal is pain relief without undue sedation. Oral analgesics administered around the clock often are helpful. Since children metabolize narcotics more quickly than adults, drugs with a longer duration of action, such as methadone, are advisable and have been shown to provide adequate pain relief.[207] Oral controlled-release morphine has been shown to be effective and safe when used in terminally ill children.[208] When pain is intractable, however, the parenteral route should be considered. And as noted, research clearly demonstrates that continuous intravenous or spinal infusions of morphine are safe and effective ways of relieving the pain of terminal cancer in children.[200,209]

In summary, assessment and management of cancer pain in children has been a significant clinical problem. Dispelling the misconceptions and misinformation that surround the assessment and management of pain in children is essential to achieving success. Although the research base of knowledge in this area is still limited, good assessment tools are continually being developed, and adequate interventions exist. The nurse caring for the pediatric cancer patient with pain plays a key role in managing this challenging problem, functioning within the scope of practice described by the ONS position paper.[81]

## The elderly

The elderly population in the United States (individuals aged 65 and older) more than doubled between 1950 and 1980 (from 12.3 million to 25.5 million), and one projection for the year 2030 is that the elderly population will increase to 64.3 million people.[210] As this population increases in number, one would expect to see a corresponding increase in the incidence of cancer and cancer-related deaths. Current American Cancer Society statistics indicate that for the five leading cancer sites, 51% of cancer deaths are in individuals between ages 55 and 74, and 37% are in individuals aged 75 or older.[211]

The problem of cancer pain in elderly cancer patients has been grossly neglected,[212,213] and prevalence surveys of pain are lacking. Ferrell[214] reviewed 11 geriatric medicine textbooks and found only 2 with chapters on pain in the elderly, with negligible content about cancer-related pain.

A misconception that lay individuals have about pain among the elderly is that pain is a normal sequela of aging. As a result of this belief, elderly patients may not report pain as a problem since it is considered "normal." In one study of "younger" elderly versus "older" elderly, there was a trend for the older elderly to report pain less often.[215] Similarly, if health care professionals are told about pain from elderly patients, they may dismiss the complaint as insignificant since pain becomes a manifestation of the aging process. While it may be true that people develop more chronic diseases as they age[216] the experience of pain does not need to be an expectation.

The normal process of aging creates unique problems in the management of cancer pain, especially as related to assessment. Ferrell et al[217] found that 71% of patients in a long-term care facility had pain, with an average of five chronic medical conditions. With the prevalence of more chronic diseases, there potentially will exist multiple causes of the same complaint. The elderly experience greater alterations in the musculoskeletal system and are more vulnerable to acute and soft-tissue pain.[218] Chronic problems such as arthritis, degenerative disk disease, osteoporosis, and peripheral neuropathy may confuse the pain problem for individuals who also have cancer-related pain.

Another unique problem is that the elderly may experience significant sensory and cognitive impairment.[164,213,218–220] The symptoms associated with these potential impairments alert the health care professional to be especially astute in obtaining a careful, detailed pain history.[164,213,218] The risk of historical inadequacies through the underreporting of symptoms, memory deficits, and concomitant depression-related symptomatology may lead to an inaccurate pain diagnosis and inappropriate treatment. A very important piece of assessment data to obtain in the elderly is any change from baseline behaviors, usual routines, and social interactions. A gradual loss of physical health, changes in family structure, limited economic resources, and a loss of social status can greatly influence a patient's quality of life and, therefore, the problem of pain.[164,221,222]

A third major unique problem is the issue of the sensitivity of elderly patients to both perception of pain and sensitivity to pharmacological interventions. The literature about perceptual sensitivity reveals contradictions. Bayer et al[223] reviewed symptoms of acute myocardial infarction in elderly patients and found that chest pain was reported less frequently than other symptoms, especially by patients over 85 years old. They proposed several explanations to account for this finding: higher pain threshold, autonomic dysfunction, or cortical failure from neurological disease. Conversely, McMillan[74] found that younger cancer patients (under 55 years of age) reported significantly more intense pain than older patients (over 55). In a review of the relationship between age and experimentally induced pain, Harkins et al[221] found no major age differences in pain sensitivity but noted that interindividual changes in pain sensitivity may have accounted for some differences. Similarly, Bressler et al[44] found no statistically significant differences in reports of pain intensity in cancer outpatients under versus over 60 years of age.

Issues related to sensitivity and response to pharmacological interventions have been examined by several investigators. Physiological responses to medication in light of changes in absorption, distribution, metabolism, and excretion of drugs are a major concern in the elderly population.[164,210,219,224–226] The changes reflect the contribution of the gastrointestinal system, nutritional composites, and hepatic and renal function, and relate to studies demonstrating that with increasing age, the elderly reported an increase in pain relief when given the same opioid and dose as younger patients.[227] If increasing age is associated with a decrease in morphine clearance, then the toxicities from opioids and other drugs potentially are much greater.

An issue related to toxicity is whether the elderly are at greater risk for adverse drug reactions. Problems with study design and definitions of adverse reactions have contributed to the conflicting evidence in this area.[228] Since the elderly have more chronic diseases and take more medications for these illnesses, the risk of adverse drug reactions may be higher solely because of increased drug intake. Ferrell et al[217] found that the average number of prescribed medications for the elderly in a long-term care facility was eight. Conn et al[229] reported that the average number of prescribed medications for patients either recently discharged from a hospital or who were at home was five. The interactions of multiple drug therapies are also an important issue related to toxicities.

A fourth and final issue relevant to pain in the elderly follows naturally from the issues already discussed. If assessment of cancer pain in the elderly is complicated by the possibility of multiple causative factors, sensory and cognitive impairment, differences in sensitivity, and pain relief because of normal physiological aging, does this population of patients receive adequate analgesic management? Several reports indicate that the elderly have fewer opioids prescribed for them than younger patients.[213,214,230,231] Portenoy[212] raised a very important issue in this regard: If the elderly perceive pain less often, indicating a lower prevalence of pain, then less frequent prescribing of analgesics is appropriate. If, however, the elderly experience pain similar to the younger population of patients, and choose not to report the pain, or respond more slowly to painful stimuli, indicating a higher prevalence of pain, then underprescribing creates needless suffering. As in other areas related to cancer pain, more well-controlled, epidemiological studies of the prevalence of pain in the elderly are needed to help delineate the scope of the problem in this vulnerable population and to assist in answering questions about appropriate management.

In summary, the problem of cancer pain in the elderly population is an important one. As individuals enter the later stages of life, the risk of developing cancer increases, and thus the risk of cancer pain increases. Specific attention to the unique physiological, pharmacological, psychological and sociological issues for these individuals is crucial for appropriate, successful management of cancer pain. Here are some general recommendations for management of pain in the elderly.[225,232,233]

1. Evaluate carefully for treatable, underlying conditions.
2. Differentiate new acute pains from chronic pains.
3. Avoid interactions among drugs.
4. Begin with smallest doses of specific drugs; use one-half to two-thirds of "younger" dose.
5. Adjust dose to accommodate for hepatic and renal abnormalities.
6. Individualize and simplify regimens; use analgesics one at a time.
7. Consider visual and auditory abilities/disabilities when giving instructions and when labeling medications.
8. Address the adherence issue by ensuring that patients can afford prescribed medications, can obtain them from a pharmacy, and can open the containers.
9. Monitor for toxicity, efficacy, and compliance.
10. Use drugs with short half-lives.
11. Look for additive effects from multiple drugs, especially adjuvant analgesics.
12. Maximize drug dosages before changing to another drug prematurely.
13. Use transdermal route with caution in elderly debilitated patients.
14. Incorporate nondrug interventions in the management plan.

### Substance abuse history

The national problem of drug abuse creates unique and different management challenges for health care professionals when pain and substance abuse occur simultaneously. Coyle and Foley[234] identified three patient groups in this special population: (1) those currently in a methadone maintenance program, (2) those actively using illicit drugs, and (3) those who used illicit drugs previously, many years ago.

For the patient in a methadone maintenance program or with a long-standing prior history, health care providers need to be concerned about recidivism, especially during a time of stress associated with a cancer diagnosis and pain.[234] McCaffery and Beebe[164] suggested that the patient be asked whether using opioids will be detrimental to continued or sustained recovery from illicit drug use. Similarly, the patient should be asked to share any concerns about using opioids for pain relief. The use of aggressive nonopioid approaches should be maximized in this population.[164]

For the patient who is actively using illicit drugs, there may be a fear of being punished or treated unfairly by health care providers. In addition, fear of withdrawal symptoms and not having those symptoms treated properly are legitimate concerns.[235] The active substance abuser may be more of a concern to physicians and nurses. Twycross[41] discussed potential errors with this population: (1) pain is discounted so that no matter what the patient says, it is unlikely that adequate medication will be provided; or (2) the patient is treated as a nonaddict so higher doses are given than are actually needed.

With all patients having any previous or current substance abuse history, it is important that an adversarial relationship not begin or escalate between patient and staff. As with any other patient, the substance abuse patient's report of pain should not be questioned or doubted.[164] Appropriate medications should not be withheld as a form of punishment[164] and pain relief should not become a bargaining tool.[235] Communication among all members of the health team, including the patient, about how pain will be managed should be instituted early in the course of contact with the patient. Sometimes a contract may be useful for establishing realistic goals between the health care provider and the patient. Regularly scheduled meetings to review the goals of care may avoid unnecessary conflict. In order to provide a consistent approach to management, several authors recommend having only one physician assume responsibility for writing all opioid orders and one nurse assume responsibility for coordinating nursing care.[234–236] The assistance of professionals experienced in substance abuse, analgesic management, and cognitive-behavioral approaches to pain may be helpful in developing a successful plan of care.

Individuals with a substance abuse history may require much higher doses of opioids for pain because of tolerance.[234] When a patient reports increasing pain that requires higher doses of opioids, the clinician should focus on the changing pain pattern as the reason for the need for more opioids and *not* on "drug seeking behavior." Twycross[41] recommended changing a patient from parenteral analgesics to oral or rectal routes so that the association between street drugs and pain relief is not present. Regardless of any history of substance abuse, the patient is entitled to receive reasonable, adequate care for a concomitant cancer pain problem. Obstacles to achieving this goal need to be discussed, examined, and resolved to ensure pain relief.

### Critical care

Patients who receive aggressive treatment for their malignancy or patients who experience serious symptoms from their disease may require intensive critical care monitoring. Management of pain in the midst of problems such as sepsis, acute respiratory distress syndrome, cerebral edema and increasing intracranial pressure, and severe graft-versus-host disease is an enormous challenge. When patients are unable to speak because of endotracheal intubation or are unable to communicate because of central nervous system dysfunction, the health care provider must rely on other means of communication to assess and manage pain. A detailed review of this topic is beyond the scope of this chapter, but excellent sources of information about pain assessment and management in the critically ill patient are available.[237,238]

### Culturally diverse populations

Nurses' assessment and management of individuals with cancer pain can be influenced by a number of factors, ranging from attitudes, beliefs, and personal history of pain to stereotypical notions about how people of specific ethnocultural backgrounds respond to pain.[48] As the racial and cultural diversity of the United States increases, more and more nurses find themselves caring for patients of ethnocultural backgrounds different from their own. In this section, approaches for dealing with culturally diverse patient populations are discussed.

"The American health care system, its philosophies, and its practices have their roots in white, middle-class values and beliefs."[239] That is, in the American system of health care, provision frequently is not made for even acknowledging the individual's ethnocultural perspective, let alone understanding or using it in planning health care interventions. There is a tendency on the part of nurses and other health care providers to become ethnocentric—that is, to believe that their own health practices are superior to those of others.[240] Since nurses

espouse the notion of holistic care, tailored to individuals' unique and specific needs, the idea of not only accepting but incorporating cultural diversity into plans for care is essential to achieving truly holistic care.

Different ethnic groups express pain and suffering differently.[77,241] The nurse's interpretation of individuals' behaviors and verbalizations related to pain should be based on knowledge of how the patient's culture views responses to pain.[77,240] Respect for cultures other than one's own, and for the fact that people have specific beliefs and behaviors that emanate from their cultural background, is known as cultural sensitivity.

Although providing nursing care for people who are culturally diverse can be extremely challenging, the nurse's commitment to delivering total care and supporting an individual's integrity and dignity can be exemplified by learning as much as possible about the individual's ethnocultural background and its influences on health and illness beliefs and behaviors.[242] Several authors have made recommendations that should be useful to nurses caring for individuals of culturally diverse backgrounds. Fong[240] discussed the importance of developing rapport as the foundation of successful nursing interventions. She urged the use of good manners, maintaining a broad and open attitude, and maintaining flexibility. Kagawa-Singer[242] highlighted the importance of developing good communication with patients and their family, followed by facilitation of their integrating the disease process and its treatment into their lives. A key principle is the use of negotiation to achieve feasible treatment plans and to enlist the patient's and family's participation in reaching treatment goals. These recommendations are generically useful and include identification and achievement of mutual goals, compromise and integration of different health care practices into the care plan, identification and discussion of nursing interventions with patient and family, stressing the importance of health education, use of vital teaching materials if language is a problem, and seeking additional information and assistance from cultural organizations and resources when necessary.

Although very little has been written specifically on dealing with cancer pain, or even with pain in general, in individuals of different cultural backgrounds, Fink and Gates[77] provide an excellent review. In their chapter, they discuss variables related to culture and pain, for example, the meaning of pain, gender, age, living and working environments, social class, religion, language, and level of assimilation and acculturation. Building on Fong's recommendations,[240] they list resources for nurses caring for diverse cultural groups, and use a case study to illustrate specific strategies for pain assessment and management.

Finally, in patients who are culturally different from their caregivers, as well as those who are similar, the area of spirituality is important. This construct is beginning to receive more attention, particularly as it relates to cultural differences, the nursing process, chronic illness, and dying.[243] Of special note are Jacik's chapter on the spiritual care of the dying adult[244] and Johnston Taylor and Ersek's chapter on the ethical and spiritual dimensions of cancer pain management.[245]

### Palliative and terminal care

Twycross wrote in 1987 that "the aim of terminal care is to help the patient, despite the cancer and increasing physical limitations, to go on having a good quality of life until he dies."[246,p.173] Wanzer and colleagues described the physician's responsibility toward dying individuals, emphasizing the "art of deliberately creating a medical environment that allows a peaceful death."[247,p.846] The parallel for nursing is obvious—the nurse must practice the art of creating a nursing environment that allows a peaceful death.

In recent years this approach has evolved into the multidisciplinary specialty of palliative care. Philosophical, organizational, and practical aspects of providing palliative care to terminally ill individuals with cancer pain have been described for inpatient and home hospice settings,[244,248–251] the home care setting,[41,252] extended care facilities,[253] general inpatient and cancer settings,[159,254–256] and the special situation of children and adolescents.[257] Several key aspects of caring for these individuals exist, regardless of setting, and need to be considered by nurses who are involved in palliative care.

The focus of terminal care is on relief of pain and other symptoms and on psychological support of both the patient and the family. Teamwork is requisite to the success of these efforts. Death often is accompanied by great fear, a normal human response that is part of the survival instinct.[245] In the care of terminal illness, not only are the dying afraid of death, but the living are as well. Withdrawal from those who are dying is a common reaction, yet remaining with the individual is one of the most important aspects of terminal care. Jacik wrote: "Human presence is a priceless source of comfort to dying persons."[244,p.267] For those dying with pain the knowledge that health care providers and others are not only present but continually focusing on relieving the pain serves as a great comfort.

Related to continual efforts at relieving pain are the issues of assessment and treatment, particularly when pain worsens or new pain appears. The goal of minimizing pain and increasing comfort in the terminally ill individual must not obstruct the normal response to complaints of pain or restrict the range of interventions that might be considered or attempted. There is no reason why terminally ill people with worsening or new symptoms of pain should be evaluated, diagnosed, and treated any differently than nonterminally ill individuals with cancer pain. For example, the development of new and painful metastatic lesions of the bone in a home hospice patient should not preclude use of radiotherapy if appropriate, even if it means that the patient must be moved. The goal is increased comfort, and all possible means to achieve it should be considered.

A flexible and adjustable care plan to meet the patient's changing needs as the disease progresses is essential.[247] Research indicates that pain and other symptoms during the last four weeks of life assume tremendous variability.[258] Tailoring of palliative care to meet these diverse needs involves the use of multiple interventions, including pharmacological therapies, and the expertise to use these interventions properly. Often there is inadequate knowledge of pharmacokinetics, neurology, and medical oncology.[259] Similarly, underutilization of opioids and adjuvant drugs can erode patients' confidence in the medical system and bring their dying into sharper focus. The WHO guidelines for cancer pain relief have been applied successfully to terminal cancer patients with pain.[260] Nonpharmacological, noninvasive interventions for pain are also appropriate in the terminal cancer patient.

In some clinical settings, such as hospice and home care, adjustments or modifications of interventions need to be made to accommodate the setting,[41,248,261] for example, the formulation of rectal diazepam, and systems such as reminder cards and special containers for home administration of opioids. Considerable creativity may go into devising methods for patients and their families to manage interventions on their own. Recent research has indicated the importance of addressing family factors that influence pain management, as well as the burdens home caregivers must deal with.[93–95] These activities, the ongoing need for assessment of pain, and coordination of pain management are well within the scope of practice for oncology nurses engaged in palliative care.

### Summary

When caring for special populations with cancer pain, a number of basic principles and special considerations need to be employed by nurses. Foremost is the need for a multidisciplinary approach. Exceedingly important as well, however, are a thorough understanding of the scope of nursing practice; accurate assessment and diagnosis; appropriate attention to developmental, clinical, and cultural issues; and knowledge about palliative care. Awareness and use of the information just presented will help nurses to identify and assess cancer pain and to plan, implement, coordinate, and evaluate its interdisciplinary management.[81] Specific approaches to the management of cancer pain are presented next.

## INTERVENTIONS

Methods for managing cancer pain can be categorized into three major approaches (Figure 20–3). In the first approach, treatment is aimed at the underlying pathology or organic etiology of the pain. In most cases this approach consists of attempts to reduce or eradicate tumor. The second approach aims at changing the individual's

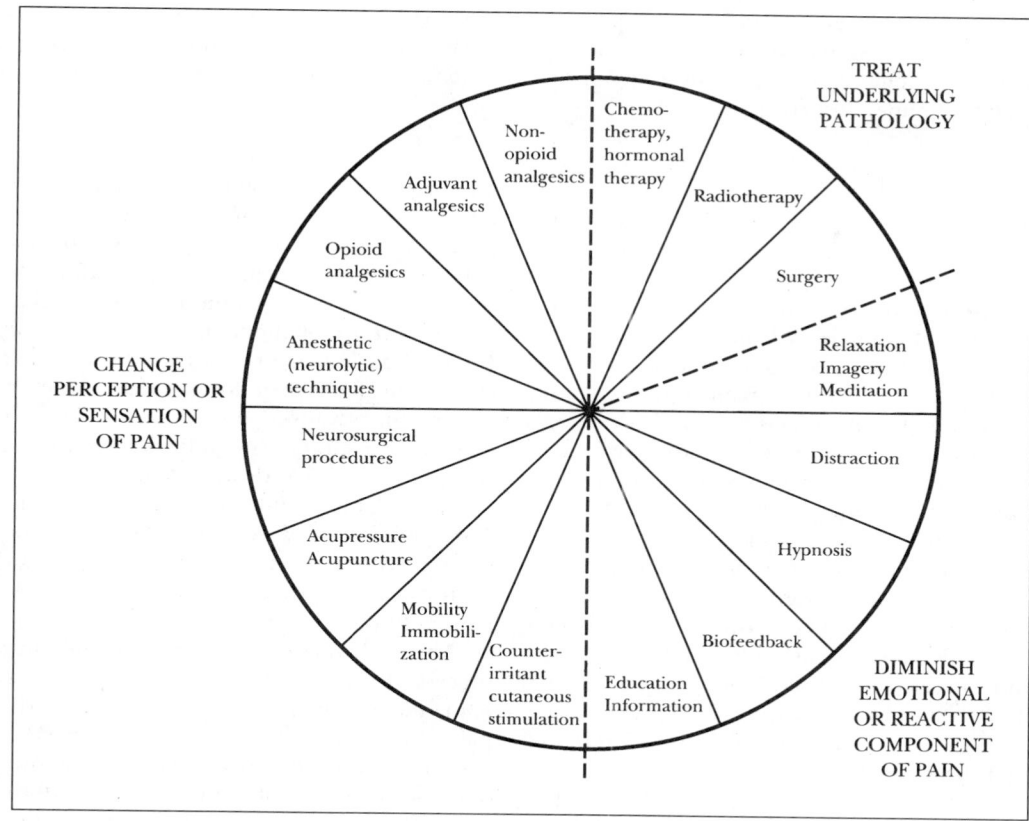

**FIGURE 20-3** Three major approaches to interventions for cancer pain.

perception or sensation of pain. A wide variety of techniques is available to help achieve this goal. The third approach consists of a number of interventions aimed at diminishing the emotional or reactive component of pain. Interventions from each of these three approaches may be, and commonly are, used simultaneously in a given individual.

With the wide variety of specific interventions available, a multidisciplinary treatment strategy clearly is the optimal approach to effective management of pain. In the following sections, specific interventions within each of the three major treatment approaches are discussed. Particular emphasis is put on the role of the nurse in relation to the intervention; some interventions will demand much more nursing knowledge and involvement than others.

## Treatment of Underlying Pathology

Chemotherapy, radiotherapy, and surgery are the major modalities used to treat cancer when cure is the intent, but they can also be useful when palliation is the goal. Hormonal therapy, a fourth treatment modality used for palliative treatment of certain tumors, is considered as chemotherapy. Each of the three modalities has specific

indications in the individual with cancer pain, which are reviewed in a recent cancer pain text[262] and discussed briefly in the following.

### Chemotherapy

The effect of chemotherapy on pain relief has not been well documented.[263–265] Relief of pain has not generally been an outcome measure for evaluating responses to chemotherapy. Patients with metastatic disease from breast and prostate cancer who respond to chemotherapy may report relief of pain, as will those receiving initial therapy for leukemia and lymphoma. Although common disease-related criteria are used to gauge responses to chemotherapy, standard assessment and evaluation of pain in treatment-related chemotherapy trials are not usually performed. With the increase in use of quality-of-life measures as outcomes in clinical trials, data on relief of pain can perhaps be extracted. Additionally, a staging system for cancer pain, such as that described by Bruera and colleagues,[266] may be useful in evaluating effects of chemotherapy.

Hormonal therapy has been used for many years to treat breast and prostate cancers. It provides palliation with fewer side effects and may afford significant relief of pain, sometimes even for prolonged periods of time.[267]

Investigators have reported good responses in painful bone metastases from breast and prostate cancers using a variety of therapies, including estrogen, androgen, progestin, aminoglutethimide, and corticosteroids.[268,269]

### Radiotherapy

Radiation has long been used to treat painful bone metastases, most often in cancers of the breast, lung, and prostate.[267,270,271] In addition, it is standard treatment for relieving pain from epidural cord compression, and it may be helpful in relieving pain from headaches and increased intracranial pressure due to brain metastases.[272] Radiotherapy also may be useful for pain resulting from nerve root infiltration, hepatic metastases, and advanced gynecologic, gastrointestinal, or upper aerodigestive cancers.[267] Relief of pain can begin to occur within 24–48 hours of initiation of radiotherapy.[267]

The evidence of the efficacy of radiotherapy in relieving cancer pain caused by bone metastases is quite convincing. One of the more recent radiotherapy approaches for palliation of pain is the use of strontium-89, a beta-emitter radionuclide that has been shown to decrease bone pain and decrease analgesic requirements in patients with prostate and breast cancer.[273–276] Given to patients intravenously in the outpatient setting no less than every three months, it localizes in the bone, especially in sites of active osteogenesis. Toxicities include myelosuppression and a temporary painful flare reaction within a few days after administration. Safety precautions with the administration of strontium-89 include universal precautions with blood and excretions, double-flushing toilets after use for one week, and washing clothes separately from other clothing if they get stained with blood and urine.[277]

### Surgery

Surgery as a modality for treating cancer pain can take many forms, but the primary goal is palliative. Direct palliative surgery either helps resolve oncological emergencies or other serious clinical situations such as bowel obstruction,[278] or helps improve the therapeutic effects of the previous two modalities by reducing tumor burden. Indirect palliative surgery involves surgical ablation of endocrine glands in endocrine-related tumors, e.g., ovariectomy for advanced breast cancer. Three other forms of palliative surgery for individuals with pain consist of procedures to provide direct access to areas of tumor (e.g., implants of infusion pumps or radiation seeds), orthopedic procedures to prevent or repair fractures from metastatic disease,[279] and neurosurgical procedures performed on various areas of the CNS to interrupt the pain pathway (discussed separately later).

Although very few data are available to indicate the success of these various surgical approaches at relieving pain, many clinical situations show anecdotal relief of pain. Chalmers,[280] for example, described a number of orthopedic procedures useful in dealing with skeletal metastases. Table 20–7 shows clinical conditions and tumors that may benefit from various types of palliative surgery; relief of pain from these conditions is obviously an outcome of the surgical procedures.

**TABLE 20-7**    Major Clinical Conditions Requiring Palliative Surgery for Pain

| Clinical Condition | Tumor | Type of Palliative Surgery |
|---|---|---|
| Breast tumor | Ulcerating<br>Fungating | Simple mastectomy |
| Abdominal cancer | | |
|   Intestinal occlusion | Colorectal carcinoma, ovarian, peritoneal carcinomatosis | Colostomy<br>GI bypass |
|   Intractable pelvic pain | Colorectal carcinomas | Intraarterial infusion (5-FU, nitrogen mustard) |
|   Serious ascites | Breast, ovarian cancer | Peritoneovenous shunt |
|   Acute urinary tract occlusion | *Upper tract:* flank and retroperitoneal tumor | Nephrostomy |
| | *Pelvic tract:* cancer of cervix, prostate, rectum | Cutaneous ureterostomy, cystotomy |
|   Rectovesical fistula | | Colostomy |
|   Rectovaginal fistula | | Colostomy |
| Tumors of the extremities | | |
|   Large lesions | Sarcomas, epithelial tumors, metastatic visceral tumors | Reductive surgery (amputation)<br>Disarticulation |
|   Pathological fracture | Metastases from lung, breast, prostate, renal, thyroid carcinomas | Amputation<br>Prostheses |
| | Primary advanced bone and soft-tissue tumors | Pins |
| Axial nervous system involvement | | |
|   Spinal cord compression | Metastases from lung, breast, prostate, renal, thyroid carcinomas<br>Lymphomas, sarcomas | Decompressive laminectomy |

Reprinted with permission from Azzarelli A, Crispino S: Palliative surgery in cancer pain treatment, in Swerdlow M, Ventafridda V (eds): *Cancer Pain.* Lancaster, England, MTP Press, 1987, pp 97–103.

The treatment modalities just described offer one approach to relieving cancer pain—treatment of the underlying pathology. Nursing responsibilities in relation to these methods are fairly standard, and quite similar to those when the same methods are used as first-line, curative therapies. In the second major approach to treating cancer pain, changing the perception and/or sensation of pain, the role and responsibilities of the nurse assume greater proportions.

## Change in Perception/Sensation of Pain

As can be seen in Figure 20–3, the number of interventions in this approach is quite extensive. The most effective and commonly used techniques are discussed in some detail next. Techniques used less frequently, and with a lesser nursing role, are discussed only briefly. Pharmacological therapy—consisting of nonopioids, opioids, and adjuvant drugs—is a major responsibility of nurses, and, as discussed previously, is an area about which much more knowledge and skill is needed.

### Pharmacological therapy

The pharmacological management of cancer pain accounts for the major source of pain treatment. Regardless of *when* a patient presents with a pain problem as a result of cancer or its treatment, the use of various pharmacological strategies must be incorporated into the plan of care.

During the past 17 years there have been a number of publications from physicians, nurses, and concerned health care professionals addressing the overall issue of pharmacological management of cancer pain.[41,164] This noninclusive, selected list of resources provides health care professionals with comprehensive information about pharmacological management of cancer-related pain.

In order to understand pharmacological management, one must be familiar with the terminology used to describe analgesics and their effects[164,284,285] (Table 20–8). These terms are especially important in understanding the actions of opioid drugs.

*Nonopioids* Although nonopioid drugs differ in their chemical structure and classification, they often are presented as two distinct categories—nonsteroidal anti-inflammatory drugs (NSAIDs) (which include aspirin), and acetaminophen. The similarities between categories are that they both have antipyretic and analgesic properties. Their site of action is primarily the peripheral nervous system. In addition, the nonopioids do not produce physical dependence, tolerance, or addiction, and they have a maximum ceiling effect for analgesic potential. Except for acetaminophen and choline magnesium trisalicylate, the NSAIDs have antiplatelet properties as well. This potential hematologic problem is caused by irreversible acetylation of platelet cyclooxygenase, which inhibits platelet aggregation.[12]

The mechanism of action for these drugs has been well described. The NSAIDs inhibit cyclooxygenase in peripheral tissues, which prevents arachidonic acid from converting to prostaglandin.[12,286] This action alters transduction in primary afferent nociceptors. Prostaglandins are associated with pain that results from injury or inflammation, and they can sensitize pain receptors to mechanical and chemical stimulation.

The indication for using nonopioids in patients with cancer pain is when pain is mild to moderate in intensity. Non–cancer-related pain, such as that caused by arthritis, primary dysmenorrhea, muscle sprains, orthopedic injuries, and dental pain, commonly is treated with nonopioids. In cancer-related pain, NSAIDs can be useful for (1) metastatic bone pain, (2) pain from mechanical compression of tendons, muscles, pleura, and peritoneum, and (3) nonobstructive visceral pain.[287]

Studies using NSAIDs in individuals with cancer pain indicate that the drugs are efficacious in providing pain relief.[288–292] The combination of nonopioids and opioids

**TABLE 20-8** Terminology in Analgesics

| | |
|---|---|
| Efficacy | Degree of analgesia provided by a given dose of an analgesic administered under a particular set of conditions |
| Dose response | Increase in dose accompanied by increase in effectiveness |
| Relative analgesic potency | Ratio of doses of two drugs |
| Relative analgesic potential | Relationship between efficacy and adverse effects |
| Half-life | Time it takes a drug to fall to half its original concentration in the blood |
| Opiate receptors | Specific recognition sites on which opioids produce their actions |
| Tolerance | A pharmacological phenomenon that develops when a given dose of a drug produces a decreased effect or when larger doses must be given to obtain the effects observed from the original dose |
| Physical dependence | An altered physiological state produced by the repeated administration of a drug, and which necessitates the continued administration of the drug to prevent the appearance of withdrawal |
| Addiction | A behavioral pattern of drug use characterized by overwhelming involvement with its use; also known as *psychological dependence* |

Data from McCaffery and Beebe,[164] Pasternak,[284] and Jaffe and Martin.[285]

administered simultaneously is designed to enhance analgesia.[293] One of the earliest studies with cancer patients demonstrated the beneficial effect of aspirin and morphine over morphine alone.[294] Another nonopioid, ibuprofen, was the drug of choice in two studies, the first involving two different doses of methadone.[295] and the second involving a variety of scheduled opioids.[296] Both studies showed increased analgesic efficacy with the ibuprofen/opioid combination compared with the opioid alone. Recently, however, Eisenberg et al's[297] meta-analysis of 25 studies using 16 NSAIDs in 1545 patients showed that the addition of NSAIDs to single or multiple doses of weak opioids provided no greater analgesia. In addition, they reported that there was a lack of studies to support the practice of using NSAIDs in patients with pain from bone metastases.

The major potential toxicities from NSAIDs are gastrointestinal disorders (nausea, vomiting, epigastric pain, ulcers, bleeding, diarrhea, constipation).[286,298] The loss of the cytoprotective effect of prostaglandin on the gastrointestinal epithelium contributes to these problems.[299] The elderly may have a significantly increased risk for developing peptic ulcer disease, especially with high doses.[300] Other potential toxicities include renal dysfunction, sodium and water retention, skin rashes, headaches, and cognitive dysfunction.[286,299,301]

The selection of a nonopioid for an individual patient often is based on individual preference and experience. Table 20–9 indicates many of the common drugs and doses. Portenoy[302] recommended a maximum ceiling of 1.5–2 times the recommended starting dose and continuing the drug for two to three weeks. Aspirin is considered by some to be a first-line nonopioid because it is relatively inexpensive and very efficacious,[41,109] Mannix and Rawlins[299] selected naproxen as their initial drug of choice because it is reasonably effective, comes in three formula-

tions (tablet, suspension, and suppository), and can be given on a twice-a-day schedule so as to simplify drug administration. Table 20–10 lists considerations in the use of nonopioids.

The benefits of nonopioids in patients who have pain of severe intensity and who require high doses of opioids has not been established. In designing analgesic regimens for these individuals, however, nonopioids need to be considered either alone or in conjunction with an opioid. In summary, nonopioids are useful in the management of cancer-related pain. Optimal use of this group of drugs requires a careful medical and analgesic history.

**Opioids** Opioids, which interfere with pain perception in the CNS, are the most important category of drugs for use in the pharmacological management of cancer pain. They are classified into three groups:

1. *Morphinelike opioid agonists.* These bind with mu and kappa receptors (mu receptors affect supraspinal analgesia, respiratory depression, euphoria, and physical dependence; kappa receptors affect spinal analgesia, miosis, and sedation); this group includes drugs such as codeine, fentanyl, hydromorphone, morphine, methadone, and oxycodone.
2. *Opioid antagonists.* These have no agonist receptor activity (naloxone is a pure opioid antagonist).
3. *Opioid agonist-antagonists.* These include partial agonists and mixed agonist-antagonists. Mixed agonist-antagonists, for example, pentazocine, butorphanol, and nalbuphine, act competitively at different receptor sites, and the partial agonists, which include buprenorphine, act at only one receptor site (mu).[285] It is generally accepted by cancer pain experts that opioid agonist-antagonist drugs have very limited usefulness in cancer pain management because of their propen-

**TABLE 20-9**  Nonopioids Commonly Used in Analgesic Treatments of Cancer Pain

| Name | Half-Life (hr) | Dosing Interval | Starting Dose (mg/day) | Maximum Dose (mg/day) |
|---|---|---|---|---|
| Acetaminophen | 2–3 | q 4 hr | 2000 | 6000 |
| Acetylsalicylic acid | 2–3 | q 4 hr | 2000 | 6000 |
| Choline magnesium trisalicylate | 9–17 | q 12 hr | 2000 | 4000 |
| Diclofenac | 1–2 | q 8–12 hr | 75–100 | 200 |
| Diflunisal | 8–12 | q 8–12 hr after loading dose | 500–1000 | 1500 |
| Ibuprofen | 3–4 | q 4–6 hr | 1600 | 3200 |
| Indomethacin | 4–5 | q 8–12 hr | 50–75 | 150–200 |
| Ketorolac | 4–9 | q 6 hr after loading dose | 60–120 | 150 |
| Naproxen | 10–20 | q 6–8 hr | 750 | 1250 |

Data from Insel PA: Analgesic-antipyretic and anti-inflammatory agents: Drugs employed in the treatment of rheumatoid arthritis and gout, in Gilman AG, Rall TW, Nies AS, et al (eds): *Goodman and Gilman's The Pharmacological Basis of Therapeutics* (ed 8). New York, Pergammon Press, 1990; *Physician's Desk Reference* (ed 46). Montvale, NJ, Medical Economics Data, 1992; *Drug Evaluations Annual 1991.* Milwaukee, American Medical Association, 1990; *American Hospital Formulary Service Drug Information.* Bethesda, MD, American Society of Hospital Pharmacists, 1992.

**TABLE 20-10**   Considerations in the Use of Nonopioid Analgesics

| Problem | Suggested Nonopioids |
|---|---|
| Need for strong anti-inflammatory activity | All drugs except acetaminophen |
| Need for parenteral route | Ketorolac |
| Risk of thrombocytopenia or other hematologic disorder | Acetaminophen, choline magnesium trisalicylate |
| Impaired renal function | Acetaminophen, diflunisal, sulindac |
| Altered gastrointestinal function | Acetaminophen, choline magnesium trisalicylate, salsalate |
| Compliance | Diflunisal, naproxen, piroxicam, choline magnesium trisalicylate |
| Risk of significant adverse side effects | Avoid indomethacin, phenylbutazone, oxyphenbutazone |
| Need for chronic use | Avoid mefenamic acid, meclofenamate |
| Cost | Aspirin, acetaminophen |

sity to induce opioid withdrawal. As a result, these drugs will not be discussed in this chapter.

There is certain information that is critical for physicians and nurses to know before prescribing and administering opioids. The specifics include the mechanism of action, purpose and category, common starting doses, equivalences of other analgesics when needed, duration of effect, half-life, available routes, and unique side effects.[303] Table 20–11 contains information about the relative potencies of commonly used analgesics for mild to moderate pain and for severe pain.

**TABLE 20-11**   Relative Potencies of Commonly Used Analgesics

| Mild to Moderate Pain | | Oral Dose (mg)* |
|---|---|---|
| | Codeine | 30 |
| | Meperidine | 50 |
| | Propoxyphene | 65 |
| | Acetaminophen | 650 |
| | Sodium salicylate | 1000 |

| Severe Pain | IM (mg)† | PO (mg)† | Plasma Half-Life (hr) | Average Duration of Action (hr) |
|---|---|---|---|---|
| Codeine | 130 | 200 | 2.5–3 | 3–5 |
| Meperidine | 75 | 300 | 3–5 | 2–4 |
| Oxycodone | 15 | 30 | 2–3 | 3–5‖ |
| Hydromorphone | 1.5 | 7.5 | 2–3 | 3–6 |
| Morphine | 10 | 60§ | 2–3.5 | 4–5‖¶ |
| Fentanyl‡ | 0.1 | — | 3–4 | 1–2 |
| Levorphanol | 2 | 4 | 11–16 | 4–5 |
| Methadone | 10 | 20 | 15–30 | 4–6 |
| Oxymorphone | 1 | — | 2–3 | 4–5 |

*Approximately equal to aspirin 650 mg.

†Approximately equivalent to morphine 10 mg IM. These values were determined from and based on clinical experience and single-dose studies of patients in acute pain.

‡Available as a transdermal patch, with a 72-hour duration of action.

§For chronic dosing, some pain experts believe that the oral morphine dose is approximately 20–30 mg, but this has not been demonstrated in any controlled trial.

‖Refers to immediate-release short-acting preparations; also available in q 12-hour preparations.

¶Available in a q 24-hour preparation.

Data from Houde,[277] Inturrisi,[283] Jaffe and Martin,[285] Foley,[303] Walsh,[325] and Houde.[331]

All opioid analgesics share common effects as a result of their action. CNS, respiratory, cardiovascular, gastrointestinal, genitourinary, and dermatologic effects of these drugs are included in Table 20–12. The four most common side effects, however, are sedation, respiratory depression, nausea and vomiting, and constipation. The problem of sedation is addressed in the discussion about psychostimulants in a subsequent section.

Respiratory depression rarely occurs if opioids are given based on commonly accepted principles. If it does occur, it can be treated easily and successfully with naloxone or with nalmefene, which has a longer duration of action than naloxone. The amount of naloxone a patient receives should be titrated to changes in respiratory rate. Rapid bolus injections of naloxone should be avoided in opioid-tolerant patients so as not to precipitate an abstinence syndrome response (nausea, vomiting, agitation, diaphoresis, intense pain). Respiratory depression is a concern when patients who have been maintained on opioid agonist drugs receive an anesthetic procedure that may totally eliminate their pain. The stimulus of pain on respiratory function is eliminated, which places the patient at risk for respiratory depression.

The chemoreceptor trigger zone (CTZ) in the brain is sensitive to chemical stimuli such as opioids. Similar to the effect of chemotherapy-related nausea and vomiting, the CTZ and the vomiting center can be stimulated to produce nausea and vomiting. In a retrospective review of 260 patients receiving opioids, Campora et al[304] found that in patients who received morphine ($n = 71$), 18.3% had moderate/severe nausea and 28% had vomiting.

If a patient experiences opioid-related nausea and vomiting, there are many options available. Portenoy and Coyle[156] recommended the following: (1) Treat aggressively on initial presentation. (2) Use antiemetics that act at the CTZ, such as prochlorperazine and thiethylperazine. (3) Use metoclopramide if gastroparesis is a possible etiology of the nausea and vomiting. (4) Use an antivertigo drug such as cyclizine or scopolamine if symptoms worsen with movement. (5) Consider drug combinations. (6) Maximize dose response, especially if symptoms partially improve. (7) Prescribe antiemetics on an around-the-clock basis for one to two weeks.

Constipation can become a significant clinical problem for patients taking opioid analgesics if preventive measures are not instituted. The simplest dietary measures include encouraging patients to increase their fluid intake and dietary fiber consumption. The use of laxative preparations generally is necessary when patients must take opioids. Table 20–13 lists six categories of laxatives, their mechanisms of action, and commonly available preparations. Patients frequently require laxatives from more than one category, such as a stimulant laxative and a detergent laxative. More detailed guidelines regarding constipation management are available.[41,164,305,306]

There are inherent properties in opioids that can create potential problems for patients if health care professionals do not understand the distinctions among them. Table 20–8 includes definitions of *tolerance, physical dependence,* and *addiction.* Tolerance requires that doses of specific analgesics be adjusted to accommodate the pharmacological phenomenon. Physical dependence is an issue when patients no longer require opioids for pain control and they must be tapered slowly off of them. It is also an issue if a patient inadvertently receives an agonist-antagonist drug causing acute withdrawal or if naloxone is required to reverse opioid-induced respiratory depression slowly. The problem of addiction was addressed earlier in this chapter, but to reiterate, addiction is not a problem for patients who require opioids for justifiable medical indications.

There has been considerable controversy over the last few years regarding the use of opioids for neuropathic pain.[156,307] Historically, neuropathic pain was thought not to be responsive to opioids. Portenoy et al[307] suggested that patients may, in fact, just require higher doses of opioids to relieve neuropathic pain and that opioids should not be excluded as a viable option for patients who have neuropathic pain.

*Specific drug selection* A wide variety of opioids and combination opioids are available. Various factors contribute to a specific opioid selection for an individual patient. These factors include pain intensity, patient age, concomitant medical illnesses, and specific drug characteristics. Opioid administration guidelines are described in Table 20–14.[308] In the sections that follow, the selected drugs discussed need special considerations when used to manage cancer pain.

**TABLE 20-12** Common Side Effects of Opioid Analgesics

| System | Side Effect |
|---|---|
| Central nervous | Sedation, drowsiness, mental clouding, euphoria, analgesia, nausea, vomiting, ↓ physical activity, lethargy, mood changes |
| Respiratory | ↓ Respiratory rate, ↓ ventilatory minute volume, ↓ tidal exchange, ↓ $Po_2$, ↑ $Pco_2$ |
| Cardiovascular | Hypotension from peripheral vasodilation or histamine release |
| Gastrointestinal | *Stomach:* ↓ motility; *small intestine:* ↓ propulsive contractions, delayed digestion from ↓ biliary and pancreatic secretions; *large intestine:* ↓ or absent propulsive peristaltic waves, causing delay in passage of contents; *biliary tract:* ↑ pressure from morphinelike drugs, causing epigastric distress to biliary colic |
| Genitourinary | ↑ Tone and amplitude of ureter contractions, ↑ tone of bladder muscles→urgency, ↑ tone of vesical sphincter |
| Dermatologic | Vasodilation of cutaneous blood vessels→ ↑ warmth and flushing of skin on face, neck, and upper thorax, sweating, pruritus |

Data from Jaffe and Martin.[285]

**TABLE 20-13** Laxatives for Opiate-Induced Constipation

| Category | Action | Common Preparations |
| --- | --- | --- |
| Bulk | Increases size, weight, and frequency of stool; requires high fluid intake | Metamucil, Maltsupex |
| Saline | Draws water into intestinal lumen and distends bowel, changes stool consistency | Milk of magnesia, magnesium citrate |
| Stimulant | Increases motor activity by direct action on the bowel | Bisacodyl, senna, Ex-Lax, Cascara |
| Lubricant | Reduces friction and coats the stool | Mineral oil |
| Osmotic | Increases volume in colon; promotes water retention | Lactulose, sorbitol |
| Detergent | Reduces surface tension | Docusate; available in combination with stimulant laxatives |

Data from Portenoy[306] and Levy.[308]

*Meperidine* Although used significantly less now than in recent years, meperidine is still not recommended for long-term analgesic management.[111,113] It is a drug that can produce serious CNS toxicities (agitation, tremors, myoclonus, and seizures),[309] and it has poor oral efficacy.[277]

*Morphine* Morphine is the most frequently used opioid analgesic for moderate to severe pain. It is used in the United States as well as in many foreign countries.[310–312] It is available as an oral, parenteral, rectal, and intraspinal preparation. The availability of long-acting morphine, which provides patients with 8–12-hour dosing schedules as opposed to 4-hour dosing, has contributed to improvements in patients' quality of life.[50] There can be considerable flexibility in dosing, since long-acting morphine comes in 15-, 30-, 60-, 100-, and 200-mg tablet sizes. Numerous studies, both controlled and uncontrolled, have demonstrated the efficacy and safety of long-acting morphine.[310,313–319] The design of these studies was similar: Patients were converted from their prestudy analgesic to

**TABLE 20-14** Guidelines for the Use of Opioids in Chronic Cancer Pain

1. Consider the role of this treatment in a multimodal approach.
2. Drug selection
   a. Consider pain intensity, age, whether major organ failure is present (especially renal, hepatic, or respiratory), and presence of coexisting disease.
   b. Consider pharmacological issues (e.g., accumulation of metabolites and effects of concurrent drugs and possible interactions).
   c. Consider individual differences (note prior treatment outcomes) and patient preference.
   d. Be aware of available routes of administration (e.g., oral, intravenous, subcutaneous) and formulation (e.g., controlled release or immediate release).
   e. Be aware of cost differences.
3. Route selection
   a. Use least invasive route possible.
   b. Consider patient compliance and convenience.
4. Dosing and dose titration
   a. Consider previous dosing requirement and relative analgesic potencies when initiating therapy.
   b. Start with low dose and increase until adequate analgesia is achieved or dose-limiting side effects are encountered.
   c. Consider dosing schedule (e.g., around-the-clock or as needed).
   d. Consider "rescue" doses for breakthrough pain.
   e. Recognize that tolerance is rarely the "driving force" for dose escalation; consider disease progression or psychological factors when increasing dose requirements occur.
5. Trials of alternative opioids
   Given individual differences in the response to various opioids, consider a trial of another opioid following treatment failure; be aware of incomplete cross-tolerance.
6. Treatment of side effects
   a. Be aware of the prevalence and impact of opioid side effects.
   b. Consider a preventative approach in the management of constipation.
7. Monitoring
   a. Monitor pain intensity and pain relief on an ongoing basis.
   b. Make necessary modifications to treatment plan.
   c. Be aware of potential for withdrawal if considering cessation of opioid therapy and need for tapering schedule.

Reprinted with permission from Coyle N, Cherny N, Portenoy RK: Pharmacologic management of cancer pain, in McGuire DB, Yarbro CH, Ferrell BR (eds): *Cancer Pain Management* (ed 2). Boston: Jones and Bartlett, 1995, p 99.

short-acting morphine, the dose was titrated to achieve adequate pain relief for 24–48 hours, and then the short-acting morphine was converted to long-acting morphine. Recently, a new once-a-day morphine preparation (Kadian, Zeneca, PA) was approved by the FDA.

Even though morphine is considered an effective oral analgesic,[320–322] its oral absorption rate is variable. Sawe et al[323] demonstrated that oral morphine's bioavailability was 15%–64%. A related issue is the oral-to-parenteral ratio of morphine. The study that showed the oral: parenteral ratio of 6:1 (60 mg PO = 10 mg intramuscular [IM] of morphine) was determined from a single-dose, postoperative study.[324] This number has been challenged by clinicians[41,325] who believe that based on clinical experience, the ratio is 2–3:1 (20–30 mg PO = 10 mg IM) in chronic dosing. This issue will be resolved best by a well-controlled clinical trial.[326]

One possible explanation for this analgesic effect of oral morphine in chronic dosing relates to a by-product of morphine metabolism, morphine-6-glucuronide. In patients with altered renal function, as well as in patients with normal renal function, morphine-6-glucuronide may be responsible not only for analgesia but also for the development of adverse side effects to morphine.[327–330]

*Methadone and levorphanol*  Both of these opioid analgesics have prolonged plasma half-lives (see Table 20–11) that do not correspond to the average duration of action. When patients are initially placed on fixed schedules of these drugs, they are at risk of developing significant sedation and respiratory depression as the level in their plasma rises.[331,332] Houde[331] has continued to recommend that patients initially receive methadone on an as-needed basis to determine their optimal dose and schedule. Clinicians must be aware of the potential toxicities associated with analgesics that have long plasma half-lives.

*Oxycodone*  Historically, oxycodone has been used in relatively low doses (e.g., 10 mg every four hours) either alone or in combination with aspirin or acetaminophen. Glare and Walsh[333] demonstrated the efficacy of high-dose oxycodone (e.g., 360 mg/day) in patients with cancer pain. Current thinking is that oxycodone does not have an upper limit or a ceiling effect. Oxycodone is now available as a twice-a-day controlled-release preparation in 10-, 20-, and 40-mg strengths, which allow for flexibility in low and high doses.[334–336]

*Tramadol*  Tramadol is a new centrally acting binary analgesic, which binds weakly to mu opioid receptors.[337] It has opioid agonists and monaminergic agonist actions. It can be considered as a weak opioid similar to codeine. The normal dose range is 50–100 mg every four to six hours, and side effects include dizziness, nausea, sedation, dry mouth, and diaphoresis. To date, there have been limited studies with cancer patients.[338]

**Adjuvant analgesics**  Adjuvant analgesics are defined as those medications that enhance the action of pain-modulating systems.[12] In general, adjuvant analgesics are indicated primarily for uses other than pain manage-

ment. There are at least ten types of adjuvant analgesics. The most common ones are discussed briefly in the following.

*Antidepressants*  Antidepressants are useful for patients with a neuropathic component to their pain. These drugs act by inhibiting the uptake of neurotransmitters into nerve terminals.[339] They have been used in many chronic nonmalignant pain problems, such as postherpetic neuralgia, diabetic neuropathy, and migraine headaches.[340–342] In cancer pain, their use has been for pain due to tumor infiltration of nerves or from treatment-related injury such as postmastectomy pain syndrome.[343,344] This type of pain can be described as having a continuous, dysesthetic, burning quality.

Walsh[345] reviewed nine studies involving antidepressants and cancer pain. He found they often were prescribed in an attempt to decrease opioid use. Although these studies were beset with significant design and methodological problems, he concluded that the drugs were useful in an opioid-potentiating role in cancer pain.

A partial list of antidepressants with starting and usual doses for cancer-related pain is given in Table 20–15. Dose changes at one- to two-day intervals in increments of 25 mg are recommended for these drugs.[346] The pain-relieving doses for antidepressants often are lower than those needed for treatment of depression. These drugs should not be used in patients with cardiac conduction disorders. Lower doses are used in elderly patients. If patients do not achieve a therapeutic benefit within a few weeks of initiating the drug, then another drug should be considered.

The major side effects from antidepressants are anticholinergic. Sedation, dry mouth, constipation, postural hypotension, and urinary retention can be troublesome, especially if a patient is already receiving opioid analgesics and is experiencing similar problems.

*Anticonvulsants*  The site and mechanism of the effectiveness of anticonvulsants for cancer-related pain are not well understood. They are a primary treatment for the pain caused by trigeminal neuralgia and have also been

**TABLE 20-15**  Antidepressants for Cancer-Related Pain

| Tricyclics | Usual Starting Dose (mg) | Usual Daily Dose (mg) |
|---|---|---|
| Amitriptyline | 10–25 | 75–150 |
| Nortriptyline | 25–50 | 75–100 |
| Imipramine | 10–25 | 50–200 |
| Desipramine | 10–25 | 75–200 |
| Doxepin | 25–50 | 75–150 |
| Second-generation | | |
| Trazadone | 50 t.i.d. | 150–250 |
| Maprotiline | 25 | 75–100 |

Data from Baldessarini[339] and Massie and Holland.[346]

used for diabetic neuropathy and postherpetic neuralgia as well.[347] Their effectiveness in chronic malignant pain has been supported by clinical observations and anecdotal experiences.

For patients who have neurogenic or neuropathic pain described as having a lancinating, stabbing quality, anticonvulsants may be beneficial.[347] Swerdlow and Cundill[348] studied 170 patients who had lancinating-type pain from a variety of etiologies. Each patient received four anticonvulsants (carbamazepine, clonazepam, phenytoin, valproate), proceeding from one to another after toxicity on each or lack of efficacy was demonstrated. Based on this study, the authors suggested that clinicians use carbamazepine or clonazepam as their first choice in treating lancinating-type pain.

Carbamazepine was used for six weeks in 13 patients for neurogenic pain caused by brachial plexus injury peripheral nerve injury, and postherpetic neuralgia.[349] Toxicities from ataxia and rash caused six patients to withdraw from the study early, but five of seven reported pain relief at a maximum dose of 1200 mg/day. The patients in this study had pain for a duration of six months to eight years.

Table 20–16 lists common doses and toxicities of four common anticonvulsants.[12,350–352] In addition to these four common drugs, a new one, gabapentin, is now being used for neuropathic pain. The drug is given in divided doses at a range of 900–1800 mg/day, but data are still limited with respect to its effectiveness.[353,354]

*Psychostimulants* Psychostimulants are useful in counteracting the sedation that accompanies opioid analgesics. If the sedation is present without any other CNS problems, such as delirium and confusion, and if pain occurs when the opioid dose is lowered, then psychostimulants may be indicated. In addition, they can potentiate opioid analgesia and can allow patients with difficult pain problems to receive higher doses.

Two psychostimulants used most often for opioid-related sedation are amphetamines and methylphenidate. Amphetamines are a more powerful CNS stimulant than methylphenidate. They both decrease the central depression caused by other drugs. Their effects may be from cortical stimulation and/or reticular activating system stimulation.[355] The starting doses for the two common psychostimulants are methylphenidate 10 mg and dextroamphetamine 2.5 mg. The first dose is given in the morning, and an early afternoon dose can be given if the morning dose is well tolerated. The dose can be titrated to response, with an expected benefit within two days.[356] Methylphenidate is particularly effective at treating opiate-induced sedation.[357]

The more desirable side effects are increased alertness, increased ability to concentrate, mood elevation, euphoria, and an increase in motor and speech activity. The more unpleasant side effects include confusion, agitation, dysphoria, apprehension, and fatigue.[355]

It has been only in the past decade that methylphenidate has been studied in cancer patients. In a controlled trial, Bruera et al[358] demonstrated an increased analgesic effect and decreased sedation when methylphenidate (15 mg/day) was compared with a placebo. In a subsequent study, Bruera and his colleagues[359] found that 91% of patients reported improvement in somnolence 48 hours after treatment. They also found that patients became tolerant to the methylphenidate with an initial dose of 15 mg/day and a mean maximal daily dose of 42 mg ± 6 after 39 ± 20 days. In a double-blind, placebo-controlled trial with methylphenidate, Wilwerding et al[357] reported an improvement in opioid-induced drowsiness and an increase in nighttime sleep.

*Phenothiazines/antihistamines* According to Dundee and Moore, the origin of the myth for the potentiation of analgesics with promethazine came from "observations after its [promethazine's] use with large doses of pethidine [meperidine] or other analgesics, and erroneously attributing reductions in barbiturate dosage and side effects during anaesthesia to the promethazine."[360,p.96] Even though promethazine was reported to be antianalgesic to meperidine almost 30 years ago,[360] the potentiation myth is still widely believed today. Similarly, Keats et al,[361] found that promethazine did not increase analgesic efficacy or meperidine-induced respiratory depression or prevent meperidine-induced nausea and vomiting, but that it *did* increase the sedative effects of meperidine. Methotrimeprazine is the only phenothiazine with demonstrated analgesic properties.[362,363]

Hanks et al[364] dispelled the myth about haloperidol potentiation from a retrospective review of 424 patients

**TABLE 20-16** Anticonvulsants for Pain Management

| Drug | Dose | Therapeutic Level | Toxicities |
|------|------|-------------------|------------|
| Phenytoin | 150–200 mg b.i.d. | 15–25 µg/ml | Drowsiness, dizziness, diplopia, ataxia |
| Carbamazepine | 100–200 mg b.i.d. increase q.o.d. until pain-free or side effects, total daily dose 600–1200 mg/day | 5–10 µg/ml | Drowsiness, dizziness, unsteadiness, gastric distress, anorexia, nausea |
| Clonazepam | 0.5–1.5 mg/day, maximum 3–4 mg/day | 20–80 ng/ml | Sedation, ataxia, behavioral disturbances |
| Valproic acid | 15 mg/kg, maximum 3000 mg/day | 50–100 µg/ml | Nausea, vomiting, indigestion, sedation |

Data from Fields,[12] McEvoy,[351] and Rall and Schleifer.[352]

who received different doses of haloperidol and found no opioid-sparing effect.

Perhaps one of the best examples of erroneously applying research to clinical practice is with hydroxyzine. Beaver and Feise[365] compared 100 mg IM hydroxyzine alone, morphine 8 mg IM alone, the combination of both drugs, and placebo in postoperative patients. In this *single-dose* study, the combination of morphine and hydroxyzine was superior to the other three groups. Hydroxyzine by itself was superior to placebo but less efficacious than morphine alone. Hydroxyzine seems to have analgesic properties, but it is not a potentiator of opioids, nor has it been shown to be less efficacious at a lower dose nor as an oral substitute (i.e., 25 mg PO q.i.d.).

*Steroids* Steroids are essential for managing the pain from epidural cord compressions, but their use as an adjuvant analgesic is based on limited data. Bruera et al[366] compared methylprednisolone 32 mg/day with placebo in a 14-day randomized double-blind study to evaluate pain relief and other associated symptoms. Pain improved significantly with the methylprednisolone as opposed to with the placebo. The researchers found an improvement in appetite (77%) and in daily activity (68%) and a decrease in depression (71%) and in analgesic consumption (57%). Walsh[367] suggested that steroids could be used for problems such as bone metastases, lymphedema, mass effects from solid tumors, and brachial and lumbosacral plexopathies.

The known toxicities from steroids, particularly an increase in appetite and elevation of mood, may be desirable in some patients, especially those with advanced disease. The morbidity from other toxicities, such as proximal myopathy, steroid-induced hyperglycemia, and cushingoid side effects, needs to be considered seriously if steroids are used early in the treatment of a patient's pain problem.

*Biphosphonates* These powerful inhibitors of bone resorption are used for treating disorders such as Paget's disease and hypercalcemia of malignancy. Preliminary evidence indicates these drugs may be useful for treating bone pain from metastatic disease. Ernst et al[368] found a statistically significant decrease in pain scores and an increase in activity level with clodronate 600 mg when compared with placebo in 24 patients with metastatic bone pain. In an open trial, Adami and Mian[369] gave intravenously (IV) clodronate 300 mg for ten days to men with metastatic prostate cancer and reported notable improvement in bone pain. In a more recent double-blind, placebo-controlled trial with pamidronate 90 mg given as a four-hour infusion for nine cycles to patients with multiple myeloma, patients who received pamidronate had significant decreases in bone pain.[370]

### Routes of opioid administration

The flexibility provided by many different routes of opioid administration allows the clinician to individualize a patient's analgesic regimen based on changing needs. There are five overall categories of routes of opioid administration: (1) oral, (2) parenteral (includes IM, subcutaneous, [SQ], and IV) by intermittent bolus or infusion), (3) transdermal, (4) rectal, and (5) intraspinal (includes epidural, subarachnoid, and intraventricular by intermittent bolus, continuous infusion via external or implanted pumps). Each route is discussed briefly next.

*Oral* The oral route is an effective, comparatively inexpensive, and safe way for patients to receive opioids. This route should be maximized for as long as possible. If a patient has an intact gastrointestinal system and can swallow the requisite number of pills or amount of liquid to achieve pain relief, then the oral route is the most appropriate route of administration.

Changing a patient to another route should be considered if high doses of oral opioids are ineffective or if toxicities occur that cannot be successfully treated.[371] For example, if a patient has nausea with morphine, an aggressive trial of antiemetics should be tried before switching to another oral opioid or *any* parenteral route. Similarly, if a patient has received excellent pain relief with hydromorphone 12 mg PO every four hours and now reports increasing pain, the dose of hydromorphone should be increased as needed to achieve relief while efforts to determine the cause of the increased pain are under way. High doses of oral and parenteral opioids are common. The scheduling of oral medications should be on a fixed-interval basis[41,109] except in a few circumstances. These exceptions are (1) initial dose titration for methadone and levorphanol,[324] (2) concomitant therapies, such as radiation and chemotherapy that may relieve pain, thus reducing the need for scheduled opioid analgesics, (3) simultaneous scheduling with around-the-clock administration to provide for incident or breakthrough pain (this also applies to continuous infusions), and (4) pain that is intermittent.

A variation on the use of the oral route is a new delivery system for fentanyl. Oral transmucosal fentanyl citrate (OTFC) is FDA-approved as an anesthetic premedicant and is currently in clinical trials as a treatment for breakthrough pain in cancer patients.[372,373] The fentanyl from the lozenge-like dosage form is rapidly absorbed through the oral mucosa, with relief in less than 15 minutes.[373]

*Parenteral* Patients with acute pain, such as postoperative pain, often are the recipients of intermittent IM or SQ injections. For cancer-related pain, if a patient requires immediate pain relief and does not have peripheral or central venous access then an occasional IM or SQ injection might be indicated. Prolonged analgesic administration with multiple injections per day should be replaced with other routes that do not produce pain when drugs are administered.

Intravenous bolus is a common alternative to IM or SQ injections. If scheduled bolus doses of IV opioids produce significant peak-and-trough effects, or if doses need to be given every two hours or less, then continuous parenteral infusion may be considered. Additional indications for infusional therapy are gastrointestinal problems such as uncontrollable vomiting or obstruction, inability to take the quantity of oral analgesic liquids or pills needed for pain relief, inadequate pain relief or unacceptable toxicities from intermittent bolus injections, and impracticality of frequent, repeated injections.[371]

The safety and efficacy of continuous intravenous infusions have been demonstrated.[371,374–376] Stuart et al[375] reported in a retrospective review of 79 patients that all patients had baseline control of their pain, but 54% needed additional analgesics. The median duration of the infusion was 7 days (range 24–162 days), and the morphine dose range was 0.5–300 mg/hour. Fourteen patients experienced toxicities, which included hallucinations, sedation, respiratory depression, and diaphoresis. Ferris et al[376] studied 135 patients receiving continuous infusions and found that 86% of the patients had good pain control without undue toxicity.

Continuous infusions provide the patient with steady blood levels of the opioid, and can avoid the potential side effects and the return of pain associated with intermittent dosing. Guidelines for initiating and managing continuous infusions have been based on clinical experience rather than on controlled studies.[371,377] These guidelines are highly useful, especially since infusional parenteral therapy has become a common mode of drug delivery. A summary of these suggested guidelines is given in Table 20–17.

*Continuous subcutaneous* Continuous SQ infusions are alternatives to continuous or bolus IV infusions if venous access is unavailable. With the availability of ambu-latory, computerized infusion devices, continuous SQ infusions have become a common analgesic delivery system.[378–385]

Morphine and hydromorphone have been the most commonly used opioids for SQ administration. Small-gauge needles (25 or 27) are placed in the SQ tissue, predominantly in the abdomen and anterior chest, but other sites can be used as well. Frequency of needle site changes has been quite variable. Reports have ranged from every six hours to every 21 days.[386] Brenneis et al[384] studied 45 patients receiving SQ infusions and found that the average duration of a needle remaining in place without toxicities was 7.3 days ± 5.2 (range 1–29).

For patients who are unable to use the oral route as a result of vomiting or obstruction, lack of control with the oral route, and no venous access, this delivery system is a reasonable alternative. The system has been shown to be efficacious and safe. Toxicities have included local skin irritation, leakage, swelling, and discomfort at the needle site. Teflon catheters appear to last longer than metal needles.[387] Bruera et al[383] reported that patients preferred this system for analgesic administration because they achieved better pain control and increased mobility and found it easy to administer. Moulin et al[388] used a randomized, double-blind crossover design to compare SQ and IV hydromorphone infusions. They concluded that there were no significant differences between the two routes with regard to pain intensity, pain relief, mood, and sedation. In fact, they strongly recommended abandoning the IV route for management. In another prospective trial, Lang et al[389] compared intermittent oral or SQ with continuous SQ and found statistically significant differences in pain relief and toxicities for the SQ route.

An important clinical issue for SQ infusions is the volume and concentration of the drug infused. How do differences in volume and concentration contribute to pain relief and the occurrence of toxicities? Morphine and hydromorphone can be reconstituted to make concentrations as high as 60 mg/cc and 100 mg/cc, respectively.[390] Bruera et al[391] demonstrated that with a mean hydromorphone concentration of 30 ± 15 mg/ml, hydromorphone can be safely given in concentrations higher than those commercially available. The volume per 24 hours without the addition of substances like hyaluronidase has been reported at 24–48 cc/day.[378,383] Bruera et al[381] reported on the successful use of hyaluronidase with a dextrose/saline solution to deliver SQ hydration and opioid analgesics. The rate of infusion was 20–100 ml/hour. A new continuous SQ delivery system using implantable hydromorphone polymers providing analgesia for four weeks has been developed.[392] Tested only in animals, this delivery system will be studied in clinical trials in the United States and India.

*Intermittent subcutaneous* An alternative to a continuous SQ infusion is scheduled, intermittent SQ injections.[393] With this system, an SQ needle is placed in a similar fashion as in continuous infusions. The same needle and administration set are used for multiple, sched-

**TABLE 20-17** Suggestions for the Management of Continuous Intravenous Infusion of Opioid Drugs

1. All infusions should be administered with a flow-calibrated infusion pump.
2. Convert the patient's current opioid drugs to an equal-analgesic parenteral dose of the drug that will be used for the infusion.
3. If the drug to be used for the infusion is the same one the patient is currently receiving, divide the parenteral dose by 24 to determine the hourly infusion rate.
4. If the drug to be used for the infusion is a different drug, use only half of the parenteral dose, and then divide by 24 to determine the hourly infusion rate.
5. Administer a loading dose at the beginning of the infusion and with each increase in the infusion rate. The amount of the loading dose depends on the patient's current opioid requirements.
6. Titrate the infusion until the patient reports pain relief or unacceptable side effects. Titration may occur the following ways:
   a. Increase the infusion rate by 10%–20% every few hours if the patient is receiving close monitoring.
   b. Administer additional doses of a short-acting opioid (preferably the same drug as the infusion) every 1–2 hr as needed. Give 25%–50% of the hourly dose for PRN dosing. Increase the infusion rate every 12–24 hr by the amount equal to the total number of milligrams during the preceding period divided by the number of hours in that period. Use this method if the patient is not receiving close monitoring.

Adapted from Portenoy RK: Continuous infusion of opioid drugs. *Med Clin North Am* 71:233–241, 1987.

uled injections throughout the day. This approach can also be used on an intermittent p.r.n. basis for breakthrough pain in patients who are using transdermal fentanyl and are unable to take medications orally.

*Transdermal* One of the newest opioid delivery systems is transdermal administration. Fentanyl, which is 75–100 times more potent than morphine, is the only opioid available via this route. It has been used in postoperative and cancer patients.[394–396] Calis et al[397] have written an excellent review of the pharmacology, efficacy, and clinical issues related to transdermal fentanyl. Although randomized, well-controlled clinical trials using transdermal fentanyl are lacking, many open-labeled studies indicate that this delivery system provides effective pain relief.[398–401] The toxicities from transdermal fentanyl are similar to those from other opioid agonist analgesics.

There are several unique features of this delivery system that have important clinical implications. First, after removing a patch, it takes approximately 16 hours for the serum concentrations to fall 50%.[402] If patients experience significant sedation or respiratory depression, simply removing the patch does not eliminate the risk of further problems from drug toxicity. Second, variability in body temperature of 3°C can increase the serum concentrations by 25%.[403] Finally, variability in skin thickness can significantly affect serum concentrations. Thin skin can produce 1.5 times, broken skin 5 times, the normal serum value. Thus, an individual with thick skin may have less drug absorbed.[403] Payne[404] presented important clinical guidelines for using transdermal fentanyl, including the following: (1) follow similar principles for chronic opioid use; (2) use in patients with stable baseline pain and minimal incident pain; (3) provide liberal rescue analgesia, especially during the first 24 hours; (4) use rescue doses to calculate dose increases; (5) rotate skin sites; (6) clarify patient and family expectations; and (7) allow several weeks for therapeutic trial. Advantages and disadvantages of transdermal fentanyl are highlighted in Table 20–18.

*Rectal* With the advent of transdermal fentanyl and sophisticated pump technology, the use of the rectal route may not be as common an alternative to orally administered analgesics. There are rectal preparations available for nonopioids (e.g., acetaminophen, aspirin, indomethacin) and opioids (e.g., morphine, hydromorphone, oxymorphone).

Controlled trials using the rectal route of administration in opioid-tolerant patients are lacking. A recent well-controlled randomized trial comparing a solution of morphine 10 mg orally versus rectally in opioid-naive patients showed significant differences in pain intensity. Reduction in pain relief for the rectal route took 10 minutes, compared with 60 minutes with the oral route.[405] Bioavailability of rectally administered morphine has been reported to be 31%–53.3%.[406–408] Exactly when the rectal route should be selected for patient use from all the available routes is unclear. Although there are three opioid agonist products commercially available, they do

**TABLE 20-18** Advantages and Disadvantages of Transdermal Fentanyl

| Advantages | Disadvantages |
|---|---|
| **FENTANYL TO ORAL** | |
| • Convenient | • More expensive |
| • Continuous delivery | • Slower onset |
| • Long duration | • Slower titration |
| | • Difficult to reverse side effects immediately |
| **FENTANYL TO IV/SQ** | |
| • Less invasive | • Slower onset |
| • No needles or pumps | • Slower titration |
| • Less expensive | • Difficult to reverse side effects immediately |
| • Easy for caregiver | • More experience with pump delivery systems |
| • Requires less technical nursing time | |

Data from Calis et al[397] and Payne.[404]

not allow flexibility in titration. For example, hydromorphone comes in 3-mg strengths, so patients who require high doses of hydromorphone would potentially need more suppositories per dose. Similarly, even though morphine is available in 10-, 20-, and 30-mg strengths, the same problem for patients who require high doses occurs with morphine. Controlled-release morphine designed for rectal administration has been studied,[409] but it is not FDA-approved for rectal use. Cole and Hanning[410] described the advantages and disadvantages of the rectal route of opioid administration, which are summarized in Table 20–19.

*Intraspinal* The identification of opiate receptors in the brain and spinal cord[411] and the results of early animal work involving spinal opioids[412] provided the bases for the use of intraspinal opioid administration for cancer pain. One of the earliest studies demonstrated complete pain relief for a mean of 15 hours after a single 0.5-mg injection of morphine,[413] indicating that epidural opioids could provide analgesia without sensory, motor, or sympathetic involvement. Subsequent work revealed similar findings for low-dose administration and prolonged pain relief. Many later studies have demonstrated that patients require higher doses of opioid to achieve pain relief.[414–417] Plummet et al[417] reported that in 284 cancer patients receiving intraspinal morphine, the minimum starting doses were 0.5–200 mg/day, the maximum doses were 1–3072 mg/day; not all patients responded to intraspinal administration.[414,418,419]

Max et al[419] gave possible explanations for patients receiving pain relief of brief duration: (1) the patients had been on high doses of systemic analgesics prior to intraspinal administration; and (2) the patients also had

**TABLE 20-19**  Advantages and Disadvantages of Rectal Opioid Administration

| Advantages | Disadvantages |
|---|---|
| • Absorption is not delayed by alterations in GI tract, such as vomiting | • Wide variation in systemic availability |
| • Useful if patients have difficulty swallowing, are unconscious, or NPO | • Delayed or limited absorption due to small surface area |
| • Drug can be removed if an adverse drug reaction develops | • Defecation or constipation may impair absorption |
| • Digestive enzymes do not affect drug breakdown | • Rectal-wall enzymes or microorganisms may degrade drug |
| • No unpleasant taste | • Invasive |
| • Significant first-pass effect from the liver may be avoided | • Self-medication may be difficult or impossible |
| • Easier to learn than sophisticated pump technology | |
| • Low cost | |

Data from Cole and Hanning.[410]

neuropathic pain problems that did not respond well to opioids.

Arner and Arner[416] presented a hierarchy of response to intraspinal analgesic from different pain problems. From best response to least response these are (1) somatic continuous pain, (2) visceral continuous pain, (3) somatic intermittent pain, (4) visceral intermittent pain, (5) neuropathic pain, either intermittent or continuous, and (6) cutaneous pain.

Morphine and fentanyl have been the most common agents used for intraspinal opioid administration. The combination of anesthetic agents such as bupivacaine and opioids is often used, especially in patients who have not been treated successfully with opioids alone.[420–422] Anesthetic agents, which act in part by reducing cell membrane permeability to sodium ions, act directly on the nerve roots.[423] Although there are added risks of motor, sensory, and sympathetic complications, the use of anesthetic agents can provide patients with effective pain relief. Nonopioids such as clonidine, an alpha-adrenergic agonist, have also been studied and are more effective than placebo in patients with neuropathic pain.[424]

Criteria for determining the appropriateness of a patient for intraspinal opioids include the following:[423,425–428]

1. opioid-responsive pain, but unacceptable toxicities from systemic opioids
2. pain below the midcervical dermatome
3. neuroablative or anesthetic procedures unsuccessful or not indicated
4. life expectancy of more than three months
5. satisfactory home and family support
6. successful response to trial of opioids or anesthetic agent through temporary catheter

Penn and Paice[427] evaluated response to temporary catheter placement by assessing (1) decrease in systemic opioids, (2) degree of pain relief, and (3) improvement in activity level. Responses were categorized as excellent, good, poor, or failure.

Intraspinal opioids can be administered by an externally placed epidural or intrathecal catheter, SQ catheter with a reservoir or a port for injection (either as a bolus injection or continuous infusion), and a totally implantable pump as a continuous infusion.[429,430] Factors that determine which type of system is used include life expectancy, clinician expertise, opioid and anesthetic needs, home care needs, and cost. Advantages and disadvantages of intraspinal drug delivery systems are highlighted in Table 20–20.[431]

Toxicities from these different techniques may include equipment-related problems, such as dislodgement, obstruction or occlusion, breakage, leakage from the catheter, and leakage of cerebrospinal fluid. They may also include drug-related problems, such as urinary retention, pruritus, nausea, vomiting, and respiratory depression.[429] The risk of infection is possible with all types of delivery systems. DuPen et al[432] reported a 5.4% incidence of infection (1 per 1702 catheter-days). The majority of the reported infections were exit-site or superficial epidural track infections. Catheters were removed only if a patient had a positive culture or an infection was present in the epidural space.

The basic knowledge nurses need to take care of patients receiving intraspinal opioids has been described.[433,434] This knowledge should include anatomy and physiology related to the neuroaxis, pharmacology of all agents, and potential complications related to type of procedure and agents used. Guidelines for patient monitoring, drug administration, and protocols involving potential complications and emergency situations need to be in place.

The nursing care of patients receiving intraspinal opioids can be divided into three major steps. The first step occurs before temporary catheter placement. The appropriateness of the therapy is determined, as discussed earlier. The patient and family have significant informational

**TABLE 20-20** Advantages and Disadvantages of Intraspinal Drug Administration

| System | Advantages | Disadvantages |
|---|---|---|
| Percutaneous temporary catheter | Used extensively both intraoperatively and postoperatively. Useful when prognosis is limited (< 1 month). | Mechanical problems include catheter dislodgment, kinking, or migration. |
| Permanent silicone-rubber epidural | Catheter implantation is a minor procedure. Dislodgment and infection less common than with temporary catheters. Can deliver bolus injections, continuous infusions, or PCA (with or without continuous delivery). | |
| Subcutaneous implanted injection port | Increased stability, less risk of dislodgment. Can deliver bolus injections or continuous infusions (with or without PCA). | Implantation more invasive than external catheters. Approved only for epidural catheter in U.S. Potential for infection increases with frequent injections. |
| Subcutaneous reservoir | Potentially, reduced infection in comparison to external system. | Difficult to access, and fibrosis may occur after repeated injection. |
| Implanted pumps (continuous and programmable) | Potentially, decreased risk of infection. | Need for more extensive operative procedure. Need for specialized, costly equipment with programmable systems. |

Jacox A, Carr DB, Payne R, et al: *Management of Cancer Pain: Adults Quick Reference Guide No. 9.* AHCPR publication No. 94-0593. Rockville, MD, Agency for Health Care Policy and Research, U.S. Department of Health and Human Services, Public Health Service, 1994, p 14.

needs about the procedure, required diagnostic tests, costs, possible expected outcomes, alternatives, and home care requirements. Assessment, documentation, and evaluation of interventions at this time is important, since the patient is experiencing unrelieved pain or unacceptable toxicities or both.

The second step occurs after temporary catheter placement. During this time attempts to determine the effectiveness of the opioid or anesthetic agent occur. Olsson et al[435] and Paice[436] have described care plans for patients receiving intraspinal opioids that include nursing diagnoses, patient outcomes, and nursing interventions. The nursing diagnoses include (1) potential alteration in respiratory function; (2) potential alteration in comfort related to pruritus, nausea, vomiting, pain on injection, and inadequate pain relief; (3) potential alteration in elimination (urinary); (4) knowledge deficit regarding epidural analgesia; and (5) potential infection at the catheter site. At the end of this step a decision about inserting a permanent catheter or an implantable pump is made.

The final step occurs after a permanent device has been placed. In addition to the nursing care described in step 2, significant attention is given to optimizing the patient's dose in anticipation of discharge from the hospital. Plans for follow-up, outpatient management and coordination of home care activities are critically important for the patient, who now has new equipment.

*Patient-controlled analgesia* Patient-controlled analgesia (PCA) has been used in patients who receive analgesics via the parenteral route and the epidural route. PCA has been used in postoperative patients since 1968,[437] but its use in cancer patients has been limited primarily to the last 15 years. PCA is designed to allow the patient to self-administer analgesics within preset programming parameters from special infusion pumps. Originally developed as a response to inadequate analgesic management in postoperative patients, PCA gives patients some independence in their care, allows individual response to analgesics to determine the amount of drug a patient will receive, and eliminates the usual lag time inherent in nurse-administered analgesics.

PCA is designed to avoid the peaks and troughs of conventional PRN parenteral administration.[438] PCA can be used in either of two ways: (1) bolus dosing only, or (2) bolus dosing with continuous infusion. Most pumps provide continuous infusion as an option, which would be similar to standard infusion pumps.

The routes for PCA can be IV, SQ, and epidural. Citron et al[439] used IV PCA and SQ PCA in 12 patients and found it to be safe and effective in both inpatients and outpatients. Bauman et al[440] used PCA requirements to change patients to oral analgesic regimens. They also found PCA to be safe and efficacious. Even though patients used PCA more in the first four hours of administration than at any other time period, Citron et al[439] reported no significant respiratory depression and sedation during the initial four hours.

PCA has also been successfully used in adolescents and adults to treat severe mucositis pain from the preparative regimen for a bone marrow transplantation.[441,442] Bruera et al[443] reported similar efficacy and toxicity with SQ PCA and SQ continuous infusions in 22 patients. Each PCA bolus dose was equivalent to four hours of the infusion. Kerr et al[444] reported that patients had improvement in pain control using PCA with SQ and IV opioid infusions. Maximum hourly doses for the opioids in the study were hydromorphone 60 mg, morphine 80 mg, and meperidine 50 mg. Grochow et al[445] used PCA to examine an unrelated research question concerning the duration of analgesia between IV methadone and morphine. The time between a patient's request and a nurse's administering the analgesic needed to be eliminated as a variable in the study. In a single-blind randomized study comparing PCA with and without continuous infusion in postoperative cancer patients, Hansen et al[446] reported no significant differences between the two groups with regard to pain relief and sedation.

Sophisticated computer technology and demonstrated efficacy and safety have contributed to clinicians more commonly using PCA pumps in inpatient and outpatient settings. Ferrell et al[447] identified some appropriate uses of PCA: (1) when the oral route is not available; (2) when the patient may benefit from increased self-control; and (3) as a useful modality for breakthrough pain. They also identified several inappropriate uses of PCA: (1) contraindicated in the sedated and confused patient; (2) when the oral route is inadequately tested; (3) potential conflict of interest if the owners of the equipment and the prescribers of the therapy are the same; (4) use only if it saves time; and (5) when there is inadequate training of staff.

The issues of appropriate use of PCA are only one aspect of a broader dilemma involving the use of technology in pain management. An ONS resolution addressing the appropriate use of technology in pain management included the use of intraspinal, IV, and SQ infusions.[448] The resolution addressed the significant financial, physical, and psychological burden that the use of high-tech therapies have on the patient and family. Although no one would argue that all patients are unequivocally entitled to receive pain relief, the process of selecting the methods to provide such relief is the issue. Ferrell and Rhiner[98] have used a biomedical ethical perspective in approaching this problem. The principles of autonomy, beneficence, nonmaleficence, and justice are relevant to the decisions whether to use high-tech therapies. Whedon and Ferrell[99] presented seven cases that involved the use of sophisticated therapies. These cases addressed the issues of patient selection, the need for a thorough assessment in determining the appropriateness of a treatment, informed consent, cost, family burden, conflict of interests, and morbidity. Indiscriminate use of therapies without clear indications and criteria is a major concern.

Nurses do not make the ultimate decision about whether a patient receives a specific high-tech therapy, but they are in a position to know what the benefits, risks, costs, and suitability are for an individual patient. Nurses can also take a leading role in developing standards for the use of pain technology as there is evidence to suggest clinicians are generally inconsistent in how they use such therapies.[449]

Regardless of the analgesic a patient receives or the route through which it is administered, nurses have a pivotal role in assuring adequate management. The obstacles to successful cancer pain management are entrenched in issues related to analgesics. Nurses must have a solid foundation in the pharmacology of analgesics in order to assess the effectiveness of an individual regimen. This content includes knowing the commonly used analgesics and understanding duration of action, dosing schedules, equal analgesic doses and drugs, and side effects. Nurses need effective communication skills to convey appropriate information about a patient's pain to physicians, other nurses, and other health care providers.

### Anesthetic and neurosurgical modalities

Anesthetic, or nerve-block, procedures for cancer-related pain help modulate a patient's neural responses to noxious stimuli.[450] According to Swerdlow,[451] proper use of analgesic drugs should necessitate the use of nerve blocks in 20% of patients with cancer pain. Local anesthetic agents prevent generation and conduction of nerve impulses.[452] The use of these agents, in addition to agents used for neurolytic blocks, makes up the major focus of anesthetic interventions.

Nondestructive nerve blocks serve two functions: (1) they are used for treatment of intractable pain such as neuropathic pain caused by invasion or compression of intraspinal nerve roots; and (2) they are used for prognostic/diagnostic purposes in which they help differentiate between visceral and somatic pain, demonstrate neural pathways for individual problems, and help predict the efficacy of more permanent neuroablative procedures.[450]

Neurolytic (destructive) nerve blocks can lead to more prolonged pain relief than nondestructive nerve blocks. They are used in conjunction with other therapies, for they often do not provide complete pain relief.[451]

Three categorical criteria can be used for determining the appropriateness of a patient for a neurolytic block:[453]

- *Physiological*—evaluate the extent of disease, know the pathophysiology of the pain syndrome.

- *Cognitive*—explain risks, benefits to both the patient and the family.

- *Functional*—the benefit of loss of function in performing the procedure.

The choices of neuroablative procedures are based on anatomy and type of pain (nociceptive versus deafferentation). For example, patients with nociceptive or deafferentation pain arising from the abdominal viscera, as with pancreatic cancer, may benefit from a celiac plexus block.[453]

Destructive neurosurgical procedures most often are used when standard pharmacological and nonpharmacological strategies are no longer effective. Patients are carefully selected for these procedures due to the potential motor and sensory losses associated with their use. Common neurosurgical procedures are as follows:

- *Peripheral neurotomy*—destroys sensory modalities from peripheral nerve; not recommended for pain in extremities.

- *Rhizotomy*—eliminates all sensation entering dorsal spinal cord; preserves motor function; percutaneous procedure an option for debilitated patients.

- *Cordotomy*—involves interruption of ascending pain and temperature fibers in anterolateral spinal cord; preserves major sensory function; good for unilateral pain.

- *Myelotomy*—interrupts pain and temperature fibers as they cross before reaching opposite spinothalamic tract; used for bilateral pain.[454]

The nursing responsibilities for patients undergoing anesthetic and neurodestructive procedures include (1) knowledge about the purpose of the procedure and how it is performed; (2) potential complications based on type of block, agent, and location; and (3) potential benefit of the procedure. An efficient way of obtaining some of this information is to participate in the explanation of the procedure to the patient and to talk with the anesthesiologist or neurosurgeon. Since this requisite information is based on the patient's individual pain problem, standard reference materials may provide incomplete information. The Core Curriculum for Neuroscience Nursing is a useful resource for patients undergoing neurodestructive procedures.[455]

## Diminishing the Emotional and Reactive Components of Pain

Interventions included in this approach to management of cancer pain are those that do not affect the underlying pathology or alter the perception or sensation of pain but, rather, help in a variety of ways to decrease emotional reactions to pain. The nonpsychiatric, nonpharmacological strategies encompassed in this major treatment approach are those that help individuals cope with their pain in a positive and proactive way.

It has long been known that both physicians and nurses have little information about nonpsychiatric, nonpharmacological interventions; in fact, one survey[456] revealed that individuals with cancer had a greater awareness of them than did their health care providers. This same survey also indicated that respondents found the techniques helpful at reducing pain.

Aside from being underutilized, the efficacy of these interventions has rarely been studied in a controlled way in the clinical environment.[457] The majority of evidence for their usefulness in treating cancer pain comes from anecdotal reports. Although there are a number of methodological and logistical difficulties inherent in conducting nonpharmacological intervention studies with cancer patients,[458] there is still a need to describe and evaluate in a systematic way their usefulness in management of cancer pain. In particular, information is lacking about how they are best used in conjunction with pharmacological approaches to therapy.

The role of these techniques is clearly that of an adjuvant to standard pharmacological therapy.[459] Drugs are used to treat the somatic (physiological and sensory) dimensions of pain, while nondrug methods are aimed at treating the affective, cognitive, behavioral, and sociocultural dimensions of pain. The benefits of many of the techniques are that they may increase sense of personal control, reduce feelings of helplessness, provide opportunities to become actively involved in care, reduce stress and anxiety, elevate mood, raise pain threshold, and thereby reduce pain.

Spross and Burke[460] recently published an excellent and comprehensive chapter on the use of nonpharmacological noninvasive interventions for patients with cancer pain. They used the multidimensional conceptualization of pain presented earlier to describe the numerous strategies available for managing pain, review research and anecdotal evidence for the efficacy of the strategies, and discuss the knowledge and skills nurses needed to implement them in clinical settings.

Spross and Burke[460] grouped noninvasive measures into the categories of interpersonal/spiritual, cognitive, behavioral, physical, and environmental. Each technique described in the chapter was included because it met one or more of the following criteria: easy to learn, easy to use in the clinical setting, not completely discussed in other resources readily available to nurses, important or efficacious in relieving cancer pain, potentially effective for relieving pain despite little scientific support, or documented efficacy in patients with noncancer pain. These interventions form the foundation of at least two classic nursing pain texts[164,461] and constitute the major interventional role that nurses can assume in the care of patients with cancer pain. Interested readers are enthusiastically referred to Spross and Burke for an in-depth discussion of noninvasive techniques for managing cancer pain.

Some of the treatment strategies aimed at diminishing the emotional and reactive components of pain are classified as cognitive, behavioral, or cognitive *and* behavioral techniques. *Cognitive* methods are those that attempt directly to modify thought processes in order to attenuate or relieve pain; they can be applied to thoughts, images, and attitudes. Examples include information, distraction, imagery, calming self-statements, identification of detrimental responses to pain, and informational or educational programs about pain and its management. *Behavioral* methods are those that modify physiological reactions to pain or behavioral manifestations of pain. Examples include relaxation, meditation, music therapy, biofeedback, hypnosis, and various desensitization strategies. Sometimes both cognitive and behavioral techniques are used simultaneously. Relaxation with guided imagery is one example.

Another group of interventions that diminish the emotional and reactive components of pain are those that provide counterirritant cutaneous stimulation; examples include menthol ointments, heat, cold, and massage. Although these methods fall within the major treatment approach of changing perception or sensation of pain, they are included here because they are behavioral interventions that clearly are within the scope of nursing practice.

Another category of interventions that change perception or sensation of pain but also diminish affective reactions and are considered behavioral in nature uses mobility and/or immobilization as the basis of nursing actions. Most of these interventions are simple and can be initiated when ongoing assessment of pain suggests a need for them. In each of the following sections, selected interventions are briefly discussed. The most recent research evidence supporting their efficacy in cancer pain, and additional information on implementing them, can be found in Spross and Burke.[460]

### Counterirritant cutaneous stimulation

This group of methods is thought to help relieve pain by somehow physiologically altering the transmission of nociceptive stimuli; these methods are based on the gate control theory of pain. Mentholated ointments are rubbed onto the skin in a painful area; heat is applied with hot packs, a heating pad, a hot water bottle, or a shower or bath; cold is applied with cold packs, cold cloths, ice, gel packs, or cold water; massage is applied with fingers, hands, or various devices; transcutaneous electrical nerve stimulation is administered by placing electrodes on selected areas of the body, depending on location of pain. Some of these methods are home remedies used very frequently by many people with pain, and combinations are common (e.g., massage with mentholated ointment). The relief achieved may outlast the actual application of the counterirritant. Most of the research that used these methods is descriptive in nature,[58,63,64] although one experimental study suggested that massage was an effective short-term intervention in male cancer patients with pain.[462] The use of transcutaneous electrical nerve stimulation (TENS) in cancer pain has been studied infrequently. Two studies reported beneficial effects from TENS upon initial use, but then responses dropped off.[463,464] Some patients taking opiates do derive benefit from TENS.[460]

### Immobilization/mobilization

Even when good pharmacological therapy has been instituted, some individuals may still experience pain on movement. Methods such as complete or partial immobilization of the body or parts of the body and positioning of specific body parts may be quite helpful. In other circumstances, mild exercise may help decrease pain, taking forms such as joint range of motion and stretching. Finally, rest or lying down may help in some instances, perhaps partly because of the relaxation that occurs. Again, the existing research is primarily descriptive[58,64] but does indicate benefit from these methods. One study examined the use of clinitron therapy and found it effective in promoting comfort in selected cancer patients.[465]

Spross and Burke thoroughly review other physically oriented interventions.[460]

### Distraction

Distraction is "directing one's attention away from the sensations or emotional reactions produced by a noxious stimulus; block[ing] awareness of the pain stimulus or its effects."[466] Distraction can be significantly helpful in reducing pain. A classic example is the focusing exercises (accompanied by relaxation techniques) taught in childbirth education classes. There are many individual distraction techniques and strategies; examples include conversation, verbalization to self or others, deep thinking, visualization and imagery, mind-body separation, routines/rituals, breathing exercises, counting, reading, and watching television. Caregivers do not always realize the broad scope and variety of distractive strategies; some may work for one individual and not for another.

The research that examines the methods just described falls into two categories—studies that asked patients to report what they used to help control cancer pain, and studies that used structured scales or questionnaires to collect this information. In the first group, several studies of both cancer inpatients and outpatients with pain[16,39,63–65,456] revealed that strategies such as heat, cold, distraction (including reading and television), relaxation, position change, exercise, inactivity, and massage helped to reduce pain to some degree. In one study that used a structured questionnaire to ascertain coping strategies,[17] patients with cancer pain employed a variety of cognitive and behavioral coping techniques (ignoring pain, reinterpreting the sensation, increasing physical activity, etc.) and rated them as moderately effective at reducing pain. Several other recent studies reported similar findings.[53,58,59]

### Relaxation and guided imagery

Relaxation training helps produce physiological and mental relaxation. The two most common methods are progressive muscle relaxation, which is the systematic tensing/relaxing of 16 muscle groups, and autogenic relaxation, which is the passive, quiet, and still use of autogenic phrases such as "my arms are warm and heavy." Training usually occurs in six to ten sessions with a therapist. Audiotapes can be used at home afterward, and individuals are encouraged to practice and use their new skills. Guided imagery, in which an individual visualizes pleasant places or things, is frequently used in conjunction with relaxation.

The literature on these techniques in the cancer patient population is scanty. Bayuk[467] provided anecdotal evidence of the helpfulness of relaxation in a group of bone marrow transplant patients. Additionally, she emphasized the importance of establishing rapport prior to using the technique, educating patients, involving friends and family, and advising practice and use of skills. One study of relaxation as an intervention[85] found that patients who used relaxation or relaxation in combination with distraction reported mild to quite good or complete relief of pain. Another study[468] found that taped transcripts using guided imagery or progressive muscle relaxation were equally effective in reducing pain and distress. Spross and Burke review additional research, but there is still a need to investigate the efficacy of these methods at reducing cancer pain, particularly when used with opioid analgesics.

### Biofeedback

Biofeedback is "a process in which a person learns to reliably influence physiological responses of two kinds: either responses that are not ordinarily under voluntary control or responses that ordinarily are easy to regulate but regulation has broken down because of trauma or disease.[469] There are several biofeedback techniques, electromyography being the most common. It is taught in six to ten sessions and often combined with relaxation. The purpose of the technique is to decrease muscle tension and/or sympathetically mediated responses, such as vasoconstriction, that might produce or worsen pain. A decrease in variables that amplify pain (e.g., anxiety) may occur as well. Only a few studies have examined systematically the effects of biofeedback, one of them with relaxation as well.[470–472]

### Hypnosis

Hypnosis is "a state of aroused, attentive focal concentration with a relative suspension of peripheral awareness."[473] It has been used for many years to relieve pain, relax muscles, and facilitate healing. When employed as a psychotherapeutic tool it can help alleviate symptoms, uncover forgotten memories, and facilitate behavioral changes. While an individual is under hypnosis, there are perceptual, motor, and cognitive alterations. With the help of a therapist or on one's own, several hypnotic strategies can be used for cancer pain: (1) block the pain from awareness; (2) substitute another sensation; (3) move pain to a smaller/less important area; (4) change the meaning of pain; (5) increase pain tolerance; or (6) dissociate part of the body from awareness.[474]

Although hypnosis has been in use for many years, the studies supporting its efficacy are fairly old, and are hindered by small sample sizes and nonexperimental designs. In a review of these studies, Twycross[41] concluded that most patients showed reduced pain using hypnosis. In an early prospective, controlled study of women with pain from metastatic breast cancer,[475] self-hypnosis training used in conjunction with a psychological support group decreased pain and improved mood. This study was fraught with attrition problems and variable pain experiences (e.g., 41% of patients had no pain at the start of the study but developed it later), but it did provide beginning evidence for the helpfulness of hypnosis. A recent study using hypnosis and cognitive behavioral training in bone marrow transplantation patients suggested that hypnosis was effective in reducing reported oral pain due to mucositis.[476] More research on these techniques, however, is clearly needed.

### Comprehensive cognitive/behavioral methods

Several individuals have proposed comprehensive cognitive and behavioral "treatment" packages for cancer pain. These proposals are based on cognitive and social learning models in which pain can be described in terms of objective qualities (e.g., location and intensity) and psychological significance. In Turk and Rennert's cognitive-social learning approach,[477] the goal is to help individuals modify thoughts, beliefs, or actions/behaviors that may exacerbate pain, depression, and anxiety, and to provide them with specific skills to cope with pain. In Fishman and Loscalzo's cognitive-behavior "specialized psychological approach,"[478] therapists provide short-term therapeutic interventions that are adaptable to the individual, with goals similar to those of Turk and Rennert.[477] Fishman and Loscalzo stated that their approach "can be very useful for both short-term and prolonged supportive care of cancer patients with pain" but provided only one case study as evidence. Another small body of work suggests that cognitive, educational treatment approaches are successful in helping patients better understand and adhere to pharmacological treatment regimens.[57]

### Miscellaneous methods

Other methods exist that diminish the emotional and reactive components of pain; these include music, humor, therapeutic touch, and interpersonal/spiritual interventions. Spross and Burke[460] reviewed existing research on these techniques, and additional research is clearly needed to document the efficacy of these interventions and their role in relation to pharmacological therapy.

### Summary and nursing implications

In summary, the evidence available from primarily descriptive research indicates that many of the nonpharmacological, independent nursing techniques just described may be useful in alleviating cancer pain. The majority of these techniques are familiar to nurses or may be easily learned and are conducive to use in a variety of settings. References are available to help nurses learn and understand these methods.[164,460,461] Many of these techniques require patient and family education, and a willingness to try them as adjuncts to pharmacological therapy. Finally, interventions such as hypnosis and biofeedback require specialized training and/or specific equipment and are best left to individuals who have or can obtain such training and equipment.

Table 20–21 presents the most commonly used nursing interventions for decreasing the emotional and reactive components of pain, along with advantages,

**TABLE 20-21** Common Nursing Interventions for Pain

| Intervention | Advantages/Disadvantages | Techniques |
|---|---|---|
| Cutaneous stimulation | *Adv:* Many methods available; eliminates or decreases pain sometimes after stimulation has stopped; produces relaxation and distraction<br>*Disadv:* May be viewed as curative; effects underestimated; tissue damage could occur; mild stimulation yields only mild pain relief | Superficial massage, pressure massage, vibration, superficial heat and cold, ice application and massage, menthol application to skin, transcutaneous electrical nerve stimulation (TENS) |
| Distraction | *Adv:* Increases pain tolerance; makes quality of pain more acceptable; improves mood and allows focusing on other things; gives sense of control<br>*Disadv:* Effective use can cause others to doubt presence of pain; pain may recur or increase when distraction ceases, along with more fatigue and irritability; patient needs pain relief measure that allows rest (e.g., analgesic) and that staff may be reluctant to give | Reading, watching TV, talking, singing/humming, rhyming, counting, word games, tactile/touch, rhythm, music, coping self-statements; try for auditory, visual, tactile, kinesthetic methods to stimulate all sensory modalities |
| Relaxation | *Adv:* Decreases oxygen consumption, respiratory rate, heart rate, and muscle tension; helps maintain normal blood pressure; increases alpha waves; aids sleep; helps decrease stress; improves problem solving; increases confidence and self-control; decreases fatigue; distracts from pain; increases effects of other pain treatments; elevates mood; decreases distress<br>*Disadv:* People think they are relaxed when they are not; some have trouble accepting it or connect it with "psychologic" pain; it is *not* a substitute for drugs; it may not help with very severe pain; must be highly individualized for patient; and sometimes will not work at all | Deep-breathe/tense, exhale/relax; yawn; humor for relaxation; heartbeat breathing; jaw relaxation; slow, rhythmic breathing; peaceful past experiences; meditative relaxation script; progressive relaxation script; simple touch, massage, or warmth |
| Imagery | *Adv:* Forms and strengthens nurse-patient relationship; assists expressions about pain, exploration/understanding of pain and illness beliefs; increases confidence in ability to control pain; increases effects of other measures; decreases intensity of pain or changes sensation to more acceptable one<br>*Disadv:* May connect it with "psychological" pain; not a substitute for standard measures; not well accepted by all health care givers; unwanted side effects can occur; trial and error; does not work for all; time-consuming; emotionally exhausting | Subtle conversation; simple, brief symptom substitution; standardized imagery techniques; systematically individualized imagery techniques |

Adapted with permission from McCaffery M, Beebe A: *Pain: Clinical Manual for Nursing Practice.* St. Louis, Mosby, 1989.

disadvantages, and information on specific techniques. For more detail and clinical examples, the reader is referred to McCaffery and Beebe's excellent clinical manual on pain, especially chapters 5–8.[164]

### Education and information

Accurate and appropriate education and information for patients with cancer-related pain and their caregivers are an essential aspect of comprehensive pain management. The importance of education was highlighted in the Agency for Health Care Policy guidelines on cancer pain,[113] which explicitly stated: "Because of the many misconceptions regarding pain and its treatment, education about the ability to control pain effectively and correction of myths about the use of opioids should be included as part of the treatment plan."[113,p.83] These guidelines included a patient guide specifically designed to help patients learn why pain control is important and how to work most effectively with their health care providers.[479]

Barriers, challenges, and solutions to the problem of pain education for patients, families, and nurses were recently reviewed by Grant and Rivera.[480] They provided a comprehensive list of resources for pain that included professional and volunteer organizations, publications, and information on patient service programs. This list should be extremely helpful to nurses who are developing educational plans for their patients with cancer pain.

Although an in-depth discussion of patient and family education is beyond the scope of this chapter, two key areas are emphasized. The first is the need to select appropriate content for pain education. Table 20–22 displays content originally developed for a home-based educational program in elderly individuals with cancer pain,[481]

**TABLE 20-22** Content Outline for Pain Education

---

**Part I: General Overview of Pain**

A. Defining pain
B. Understanding the cause of pain
C. Assessing pain intensity
D. Use of pain rating scales to document and communicate information about pain
E. The importance of taking a preventive approach to pain management
F. Participation of family caregivers in pain management
G. The relation between pain and other physical and psychological symptoms
H. Use of the self-care log to document pain and distress

   The patients are given an audiotaped reinforcement of this information and a Walkman cassette player.

**Part II: Pharmacological Management of Pain**

A. Overview of drug management of pain (ATC vs. PRN)
B. Principles of addiction
C. Drug dependence
D. Drug tolerance
E. Respiratory depression
F. Use of analgesics, including opioids, nonnarcotics, and other adjunct medications (WHO ladder, anti-inflammatory drugs, antidepressants, and antiseizure medications)
G. Talking to the physician about pain medications
H. Control of related symptoms; that is, anxiety, nausea, and constipation (aggressive treatment of the side effects for maximum comfort)

   The patients are also given an audiotaped reinforcement of this information.

**Part III: Nondrug Management of Pain**

A. The importance of nondrug interventions for pain
B. Use of nondrug interventions as an adjunct to medications
C. Review of previous use of nondrug comfort measures
D. Demonstrations of various nondrug pain relief methods
   1. Heat
   2. Cold
   3. Massage/vibration
   4. Relaxation/imagery
   5. Distraction
E. Participation of family members in nondrug pain management
F. Hands-on use of the nondrug methods chosen and the selection of appropriate sites for pain relief
G. Review of the handouts specific to the nondrug method selected.

---

Reprinted with permission from Ferrell BR, Rhiner M, and Ferrell BA: Development and implementation of a pain education program. *Cancer* 72:3426–3432, 1993. Copyright © 1993 American Cancer Society. Reprinted by permission of Wiley-Liss, Inc., a subsidiary of John Wiley & Sons, Inc.

and adapted by Rhiner and Coluzzi.[482] The second is the importance of incorporating sound teaching principles into the plan. Table 20–23 delineates specific guidelines for providing education to patients and families.[480,481] It is clear that pain education is a critical nursing role in helping patients and families cope with pain, and in improving their overall quality of life.

## CONCLUSIONS AND FUTURE DIRECTIONS

In this chapter the multidimensional phenomenon of cancer pain was presented, with special reference to the physiological sensory, affective, cognitive, behavioral, and sociocultural aspects of the experience. The importance of a multidisciplinary approach to management has been emphasized, with particular attention to the pivotal role of the nurse in this process. Various strategies for managing cancer pain have been presented, some of which call for more nursing involvement than others. Clearly, a great deal of information is readily available for nurses and other health professionals to use in achieving the best possible care for individuals with cancer pain. The challenge for the future is to utilize this knowledge to its fullest, to continue experimenting with new ways to treat pain, and to share the information gained with colleagues.

## REFERENCES

1. Livingston WK: *Pain Mechanisms: A Physiologic Interpretation of Causalgia and Its Related States.* New York, Macmillan, 1943

**TABLE 20-23**  Teaching Principles for Pain Education

Provide information that is accurate and current. Content should be reviewed by experts in the area and pilot tested in a sample of patients.

Precede teaching session by establishing what the patient already knows about his condition and pain management regimen.

Establish goals and objectives with the patient/family to enhance cooperation and compliance with the recommended plan of treatment. Information should be that which is immediately useful when teaching adults.

Teach the smallest amount possible rather than overload patient who may already be overburdened by illness and pain. The patient must know enough about his condition to understand the rationale behind the regimen and be able to carry out the desired behaviors.

Use a combination of educational methods such as written materials, lecture, discussion, and audiovisual tools.

Keep the teaching session brief with breaks as needed by the patient.

Present the most important material first. For example, it may be necessary to first overcome the patient's overwhelming fear of addiction before he will be at all open to using analgesics for pain management.

Use appropriate materials that convey the message/information to be taught. Can existing materials be used or is it necessary to produce new materials?

Evaluate the readability of written materials so that they are appropriate for the cognitive level of the patient. Generally speaking, no higher than a sixth-grade reading level is recommended. A readability index should be performed on all written information.

Use written materials in a larger print for elderly patients.

Reinforce written information with an audiocassette tape that can be replayed as often as necessary.

Use illustrations and written materials that are clear and concise. Avoid medical jargon.

Use repetition. Encourage questions. Ask questions. Have the patient/family state what they have learned in their own words.

Include family and supportive friends in the educational program whenever possible.

Choose an environment that is quiet with a temperature that is comfortable for the patient and family. The patient must be physically comfortable to learn.

Individualize education with consideration for cultural influences.

Reprinted with permission from Ferrell BR, Rhiner M, and Ferrell, BA: Development and implementation of a pain education program. *Cancer* 72:3426–3432, 1993. Copyright © 1993 American Cancer Society. Reprinted by permission of Wiley-Liss, Inc., a subsidiary of John Wiley & Sons, Inc.

2. Melzack R, Wall PD: *The Challenge of Pain.* New York, Basic Books, 1982

3. International Association for the Study of Pain Subcommittee on Taxonomy: Pain terms: A list with definitions and usage. *Pain* 6:249–252, 1979

4. Bouckoms AJ: Recent developments in the classification of pain. *Psychosom* 26:637–642, 645, 1985

5. International Association for the Study of Pain: Pain terms: A current list with definitions and notes on usage. *Pain* 3: S216–S221, 1986 (suppl)

6. Task Force on Taxonomy: *Classification of Chronic Pain: Descriptions of Chronic Pain Syndromes and Definitions of Terms* (ed 2). Seattle, International Association for the Study of Pain (IASP) Press, 1994

7. Brose WG, Cherry DA, Plummer J, et al: IASP taxonomy: Questions and controversies, in Bond MR, Charlton JE, Woolf CJ (eds): *Proceedings of the VIth World Congress on Pain.* Amsterdam, Elsevier, 1991, pp 503–507

8. Bonica JJ: Definitions and taxonomy of pain, in Bonica JJ (ed): *The Management of Pain,* vol 1, (ed 2). Philadelphia, Lea and Febiger, 1990, pp 18–27

9. Price DD: *Psychological and Neural Mechanisms of Pain.* New York, Raven Press, 1988

10. Melzack R, Wall PD: Pain mechanisms: A new theory. *Science* 150:971–979, 1965

11. Melzack R: Pain: Past, present, and future. *Can J Exp Psychol* 47:615–629, 1993

12. Fields HL: *Pain.* New York, McGraw-Hill, 1987

13. Wilkie DJ: Neural mechanisms of pain: A foundation for cancer pain assessment and management, in McGuire DB, Yarbro CH, Ferrell BR (eds): *Cancer Pain Management* (ed 2). Boston, Jones and Bartlett, 1995, pp 61–87

14. Wall PD, Melzack R: *Textbook of Pain* (ed 3). New York, Churchill Livingstone, 1994

15. Ahles TA, Blanchard EB, Ruckdeschel JC: The multidimensional nature of cancer-related pain. *Pain* 17:277–288, 1983

16. McGuire DB: Cancer-related pain: A multidimensional approach. *Dissert Abstr Internatl* 48(03), Sec B:705, 1987

17. McGuire DB: Coping strategies used by cancer patients with pain. *Oncol Nurs Forum* 14:123, 1987 (abstr)

18. McGuire DB: The multiple dimensions of cancer pain: A framework for assessment and management, in McGuire DB, Yarbro CH, Ferrell BR (eds): *Cancer Pain Management,* (ed 2). Boston, Jones and Bartlett, 1995, pp 1–17

19. NINR Priority Expert Panel on Symptom Management: Acute Pain: *Symptom Management: Acute Pain,* vol 6. NIH publication No. 94-2421. Bethesda, MD, National Institute of Nursing Research, U.S. Department of Health and Human Services, U.S. Public Health Service, National Institutes of Health, 1994

20. Foley KN: Pain syndromes in patients with cancer, in Bonica JJ, Ventafridda V (eds): *Advances in Pain Research and Therapy,* vol 2. New York, Raven Press, 1979, pp 59–75

21. Coyle N, Foley K: Prevalence and profile of pain syndromes

in cancer patients, in McGuire DB, Yarbro CH (eds): *Cancer Pain Management*. Philadelphia, Saunders, 1987, pp 21–46

22. Chapman CR, Kornell J, Syrjala K: Painful complications of cancer diagnosis and therapy, in McGuire DB, Yarbro CH (eds): *Cancer Pain Management*. Philadelphia, Saunders, 1987, pp 47–67

23. Schreml W: Pain in the cancer patient as a consequence of therapy (surgery, radiotherapy, chemotherapy). *Recent Results Cancer Res* 89:85–99, 1984

24. Gaston-Johansson F, Franco T, Zimmerman L: Pain and psychological distress in patients undergoing autologous bone marrow transplantation. *Oncol Nurs Forum* 19:41–48, 1992

25. McGuire DB, Altomonte V, Peterson DE, et al: Patterns of mucositis and pain in patients receiving preparative chemotherapy and bone marrow transplantation. *Oncol Nurs Forum* 20:1493–1502, 1993

26. Shivnan JC, Sheidler VR: Pain associated with bone marrow transplantation: Unique features and treatments. *Oncol Nurs Forum* 19:319, 1992 (abstr)

27. Sutters KA, Miaskowski C: The problem of pain in children with cancer: A research review. *Oncol Nurs Forum* 19:465–171, 1992

28. Patterson KL: Pain in the pediatric oncology patient. *J Pediatr Oncol Nurs* 9:119–130, 1992

29. Portenoy RK: Cancer pain: Epidemiology and syndromes. *Cancer* 63:2298–2307, 1989

30. Payne R: Cancer pain: Anatomy, physiology, and pharmacology. *Cancer* 63:2266–2274, 1989

31. Kelly JB, Payne R: Pain syndromes in the cancer patient. *Neurol Clin* 9:937–953, 1991

32. Banning A, Sjogren P, Henriksen H: Pain causes in 200 patients referred to a multidisciplinary cancer pain clinic. *Pain* 45:45–48, 1991

33. Samuelsson H, Hedner T: Pain characterization in cancer patients and the analgetic response to epidural morphine. *Pain* 46:3–8, 1991

34. Melzack R: The McGill Pain Questionnaire: Major properties and scoring methods. *Pain* 1:277–299, 1975

35. McGuire DB: Assessment of pain in cancer inpatients using the McGill Pain Questionnaire. *Oncol Nurs Forum* 11:32–37, 1984

36. Nicholson B, McGuire DB, Maurer VE: Assessment of pain in head and neck cancer patients using the McGill Pain Questionnaire. *The Journal* (official journal of the Society of Otorhinolaryngology and Head-Neck Nurses) 6:8–12, 1988

37. Graham C, Bond SS, Gerkovich MM, et al: Use of the McGill Pain Questionnaire in the assessment of cancer pain: Replicability and consistency. *Pain* 8:377–387, 1980

38. Arathuzik D: Pain experience for metastatic breast cancer patients. *Cancer Nurs* 14:41–48, 1991

39. Donovan MI, Dillon P: Incidence and characteristics of pain in a sample of hospitalized cancer patients. *Cancer Nurs* 10:85–92, 1987

40. Twycross RG, Fairfield S: Pain in far-advanced cancer. *Pain* 14:303–310, 1982

41. Twycross R: *Pain Relief in Advanced Cancer*. Edinburgh, Churchill Livingstone, 1994

42. Melzack R, Torgerson WS: On the language of pain. *Anesthesiology* 34:50–59, 1971

43. Dubuisson D, Melzack R: Classification of clinical pain descriptions by multiple group discriminant analysis. *Exp Neurol* 51:480–487, 1976

44. Bressler LR, Hange PA, McGuire DB: Characterization of the pain experience in a sample of cancer outpatients. *Oncol Nurs Forum* 13:51–55, 1986

45. Zimmerman L, Duncan K, Pozehl B, et al: Pain descriptors used by patients with cancer. *Oncol Nurs Forum* 14:67–71, 1987

46. Padilla GV, Ferrell B, Grant MM, et al: Defining the content domain of quality of life for cancer patients with pain. *Cancer Nurs* 13:108–115, 1990

47. Dalton JA, Feuerstein M: Biobehavioral factors in cancer pain. *Pain* 33:137–147, 1988

48. McGuire DB, Sheidler VR: Pain, in Groenwald S, Frogge MH, Goodman M, Yarbro CH (eds): *Cancer Nursing: Principles and Practice* (ed 2). Boston, Jones and Bartlett, 1990, pp 385–441

49. Dorrepaal KL, Aaronsen NK, van Dam FSAM: Pain experience and pain management among hospitalized cancer patients: A clinical study. *Cancer* 63:593–598, 1989

50. Ferrell BR, Wisdom C, Wenzl C: Quality of life as an outcome variable in the management of cancer pain. *Cancer* 63:2321–2327, 1989

51. Spiegel D, Sands S, Koopman C: Pain and depression in patients with cancer. *Cancer* 74:2570–2578, 1994

52. Spiegel D, Bloom J: Pain in metastatic breast cancer. *Cancer* 52:341–345, 1983

53. Barkwell DP: Ascribed meaning: A critical factor in coping and pain attenuation in patients with cancer-related pain. *J Palliat Care* 7:5–14, 1991

54. Ferrell BR, Dean G: The meaning of cancer pain. *Semin Oncol Nurs* 11:17–22, 1995

55. Bruera E, Macmillan K, Hanson J, et al: The cognitive effects of the administration of narcotic analgesics in patients with cancer pain. *Pain* 39:13–16, 1989

56. Sjogren P, Banning A: Pain, sedation and reaction time during long-term treatment of cancer patients with oral and epidural opioids. *Pain* 39:5–11, 1989

57. Rimer B, Levy MH, Keintz MK, et al: Enhancing cancer pain control regimens through patient education. *Patient Educ Counsel* 10:267–277, 1987

58. Wilkie DJ, Keefe FJ: Coping strategies of patients with lung cancer–related pain. *Clin J Pain* 7:292–299, 1991

59. Arathuzik D: The appraisal of pain and coping in cancer patients. *West J Nurs Res* 13:714–731, 1991

60. Bond MR, Pilowsky I: Subjective assessment of pain and its relationship to the administration of analgesics in patients with advanced cancer. *J Psychosom Res* 10:203–208, 1966

61. Francke AL, Theeuwen I: Inhibition in expressing pain: A qualitative study among Dutch breast cancer patients. *Cancer Nurs* 17:193–199, 1994

62. Keefe FJ, Brantley A, Manuel G, et al: Behavioral assessment of head and neck cancer pain. *Pain* 23:327–336, 1985

63. Donovan MI: Nursing assessment of cancer pain. *Semin Oncol Nurs* 1:109–115, 1985

64. Barbour LA, McGuire DB, Kirchhoff KT: Non-analgesic methods of pain control used by cancer outpatients. *Oncol Nurs Forum* 13:56–60, 1986

65. Wilkie D, Lovejoy N, Dodd M, et al: Cancer pain control behaviors: Description and correlation with pain intensity. *Oncol Nurs Forum* 15:723–731, 1988

66. Wolff BB, Langley L: Cultural factors and the response to pain: A review, in Weisenberg E (ed): *Pain: Clinical and Experimental Perspectives*. St. Louis, Mosby, 1975, pp 144–151

67. Wolff BB: Ethnocultural factors influencing pain and illness behavior. *Clin J Pain* 1:23–30, 1985

68. Lipton JA, Marbach JJ: Ethnicity and the pain experience. *Soc Sci Med* 19:1279–1298, 1984

69. Reizien A, Meleis AI: Arab-Americans' perceptions of and responses to pain. *Crit Care Nurs* 6:30–37, 1986

70. Miller JF, Shuter R: Age, sex, race affect pain expression. *Am J Nurs* 84:891, 1984

71. Swanson DW, Maruta T: Patients complaining of extreme pain. *Mayo Clin Proc* 55:563–566, 1980

72. Flannery RB, Sos J, McGovern P: Ethnicity as a factor in the expression of pain. *Psychosom* 22:39–40, 1981

73. Greenwald HP: Interethnic differences in pain perception. *Pain* 44:157–163, 1991

74. McMillan S: The relationship between age and intensity of cancer-related symptoms. *Oncol Nurs Forum* 16:237–241, 1989

75. Ferrell BA, Ferrell BR: The experience of pain and quality of life in elderly patients. *Gerontol* 28:76A, 1988 (suppl)

76. Cleeland CS, Gonin R, Hatfield AK, et al: Pain and its treatment in outpatients with metastatic cancer. *New Engl J Med* 330:592–596, 1994

77. Fink RS, Gates R: Cultural diversity and cancer pain, in McGuire DB, Yarbro CH, Ferrell BR (eds): *Cancer Pain Management* (ed 2). Boston, Jones and Bartlett, 1995, pp 19–39

78. Glajchen M, Fitzmartin RD, Blum D, Swanton R: Psychosocial barriers to cancer pain relief. *Cancer Pract* 3:76–82, 1995

79. Lancee WJ, Vachon MLS, Ghadirian P, et al: The impact of pain and impaired role performance on distress in persons with cancer. *Can J Psychiatry* 39:617–622, 1994

80. Williamson GM, Schulz R: Activity restriction mediates the association between pain and depressed affect: A study of younger and older adult cancer patients. *Psychol Aging* 10:369–378, 1995

81. Spross JA, McGuire DB, Schmitt R: Oncology Nursing Society position paper on cancer pain. *Oncol Nurs Forum* 17:595–614, 751–760, 825, 944–955, 1990

82. National Institutes of Health: The integrated approach to the management of pain. *NIH Consensus Development Conference Statement* 6(3). Bethesda, MD, NIH, 1986

83. Cleeland CS: The impact of pain on the patient with cancer. *Cancer* 54:2635–2641, 1984

84. Ferrell BR, Schneider C: Experience and management of cancer pain at home. *Cancer Nurs* 11:84–90, 1988

85. Norvell K, Zimmerman L: Psychological variables, and cancer pain. *Oncol Nurs Forum* 16:160, 1989 (suppl)

86. Ferrell B, Wisdom C, Wenzl C, et al: Effects of controlled release morphine on QOL for cancer pain. *Oncol Nurs Forum* 16:521–526, 1989

87. Strang P, Qvarner H: Cancer-related pain and its influence on quality of life. *Anticancer Res* 10:109–112, 1990

88. Ferrell BR, Grant M, Padilla G, et al: The experience of pain and perceptions of quality of life: Validation of a conceptual model. *Hosp J* 7:9–24, 1991

89. Ferrell BR: The quality of lives: 1,525 voices of cancer. *Oncol Nurs Forum* 23:907–916, 1996

90. Foley KM: Pain, physician-assisted suicide, and euthanasia. *Pain Forum* 4:163–178, 1995

91. Breitbart W: Cancer pain and suicide, in Foley KM, Bonica JJ, Ventafridda V (eds): *Advances in Pain Research and Therapy.* New York, Raven Press, 1990, pp 399–412

92. Coyle N: The euthanasia and physician-assisted suicide debate: Issues for nursing. *Oncol Nurs Forum* 19:41–46, 1992 (suppl)

93. Ferrell BR, Rhiner M, Cohen MZ, et al: Pain as a metaphor for illness: Part I. Impact of cancer pain on family caregivers. *Oncol Nurs Forum* 18:1303–1309, 1991

94. Ferrell BR, Cohen MZ, Rhiner M, et al: Pain as a metaphor for illness: Part II. Family caregivers' management of pain. *Oncol Nurs Forum* 18:1315–1321, 1991

95. Ferrell BR, Ferrell BA, Rhiner M, et al: Family factors influencing cancer pain management. *Postgrad Med J* 67: S64–S69, 1991 (suppl)

96. Kurtz ME, Kurtz JC, Given CC, et al: Concordance of cancer patient and caregiver symptom reports. *Cancer Pract* 4: 185–190, 1996

97. Ishay R: High technology in medicine: Ethical aspects. *Isr J Med Sci* 25:274–278, 1989

98. Ferrell BR, Rhiner M: High-tech comfort: Ethical issues in cancer pain management for the 1990s. *J Clin Ethics* 2: 108–112, 1991

99. Whedon M, Ferrell BR: Professional and ethical considerations in the use of high-tech pain management. *Oncol Nurs Forum* 18:1135–1143, 1991

100. Ropchan R, Ferrell BR, Grant M, et al: Pain management as a nursing administration concern. *Oncol Nurs Forum* 19: 317, 1992 (abstr)

101. Angarola RT, Donato BJ: Inappropriate pain management results in high jury award. *J Pain Symptom Manage* 6:407, 1991

102. Cushing M: The legal side: Pain management on trial. *Am J Nurs* 92:21–22, 1992

103. Angarola RT, Wray SD: Legal impediments to cancer pain treatment, in Hill CS, Fields WS (eds): *Advances in Pain Research and Therapy,* vol 11. New York, Raven Press, 1989, pp 213–231

104. Portenoy RK: The effect of drug regulation on the management of cancer pain. *NY State Med J* 91:13s–18s, 1991

105. Angarola RT, Bormel FG: Proposed legislative changes and access to pain medications. *APS Bull* 6:8–9, 1996

106. Joranson DE: State pain commissions: new vehicle for progress? *APS Bull* 6:7–9, 1996

107. Spross JA: Cancer pain relief: An international perspective. *Oncol Nurs Forum* 19:5–11, 1992 (suppl)

108. National Institute of Nursing Research: Symptom Management: Acute Pain RFA: NR-94-003. *NIH Guide* 23(1), 1994

109. World Health Organization: *Cancer Pain Relief* (ed 2). Geneva, WHO, 1996

110. Quality improvement guidelines for the treatment of acute pain and cancer pain. *JAMA* 274:1874–1880, 1995

111. American Pain Society: *Principles of Analgesic Use in the Treatment of Acute Pain and Cancer Pain* (ed 3). Skokie, IL, APS, 1992

112. Ad Hoc Committee on Cancer Pain of the American Society of Clinical Oncology: Cancer pain assessment and treatment curriculum guidelines. *J Clin Oncol* 10:1976–1982, 1992

113. Jacox A, Carr DB, Payne R, et al: *Management of cancer pain: Clinical practice guideline No. 9.* AHCPR publication No. 94-0592. Rockville, MD, Agency for Health Care Policy and Research, U.S. Department of Health and Human Services, Public Health Service, 1994

114. *Ad hoc* Committee: Pain curriculum for basic nursing education. *IASP Newsletter* Sept/Oct:4–6, 1993

115. Grossman SA, Sheidler VR: Skills of medical students and house officers in prescribing narcotic medications. *J Med Educ* 60:552–557, 1985

116. Sheidler VR, McGuire DB, Grossman SA, et al: Analgesic

decision-making skills of nurses. *Oncol Nurs Forum* 19: 1531–1534, 1992

117. Watt-Watson JH: Nurses' knowledge of pain issues: A survey. *J Pain Symptom Manage* 2:207–211, 1987

118. Charap AD: The knowledge, attitudes, and experience of medical personnel treating pain in the terminally ill. *Mt Sinai J Med* 45:561–580, 1978

119. Schauer PK, Wetterman TL, Schauer AR: Physicians' attitudes and knowledge about the management of cancer-related pain. *Conn Med* 52:705–707, 1988

120. McCaffery M, Ferrell BR: Nurses' knowledge about cancer pain: A survey of five countries. *J Pain Symptom Manage* 10: 356–369, 1995

121. Morgan JP: American opiophobia: Customary underutilization of opioid analgesics, in Hill CS, Fields WS (eds): *Advances in Pain Research and Therapy*, vol 11. New York, Raven Press, 1989, pp 181–195

122. Marks R, Sachar E: Undertreatment of medical inpatients with narcotic analgesics. *Ann Intern Med* 78:173–181, 1973

123. Hauck SL: Pain: Problem for the person with cancer. *Cancer Nurs* 9:66–76, 1986

124. Myers JS: Cancer pain: Assessment of nurses' knowledge and attitudes. *Oncol Nurs Forum* 12:62–66, 1985

125. Weis OF, Sriwatanakul K, Alloza JL, et al: Attitudes of patients, housestaff, and nurses toward post-operative analgesic care. *Anesth Analg* 62:70–74, 1983

126. Elliott TE, Elliott BA: Physician attitudes and beliefs about use of morphine for cancer pain. *J Pain Symptom Manage* 7:141–148, 1992

127. Porter J, Jick H: Addiction rare in patients treated with narcotics. *N Engl J Med* 302:123, 1980

128. Weissman DE, Dahl JL: Attitudes about cancer pain: A survey of Wisconsin's first-year medical students. *J Pain Symptom Manage* 5:345–349, 1990

129. Edgar L, Hamilton J: A survey examining nurses' knowledge of pain control. *J Pain Symptom Manage* 7:18–26, 1992

130. McCaffery M, Ferrell BR, O'Neil-Page E, et al: Nurses' knowledge of opioid analgesic drugs and psychological dependence. *Cancer Nurs* 13:21–27, 1990

131. Ferrell BR, McCaffery M, Rhiner M: Pain addiction: An urgent need for change in nursing education. *J Pain Symptom Manage* 7:117–124, 1992

132. Camp LD: Comparison of medical, surgical and oncology patients' descriptions of pain and nurses' documentation of pain assessments. *J Adv Nurs* 12:593–598, 1987

133. Dalton JA: Nurses' perceptions of their pain assessment skills, pain management practices, and attitudes toward pain. *Oncol Nurs Forum* 16:225–231, 1989

134. Paice JA, Mahon SM, Faut-Callahan M: Factors associated with adequate pain control in hospitalized patients diagnosed with cancer. *Cancer Nurs* 14:298–305, 1991

135. Faries JE, Mills DS, Goldsmith KW, et al: Systematic pain records and their impact on pain control: A pilot study. *Cancer Nurs* 14:306–313, 1991

136. Ward SE, Goldberg N, Miller-McCauley V, et al: Patient-related barriers to management of cancer pain. *Pain* 52: 319–324, 1993

137. Grossman SA, Sheidler VR, Swedeen K, et al: Correlation of patient and caregiver ratings of cancer pain. *J Pain Symptom Manage* 6:53–57, 1991

138. Rankin MA, Snider B: Nurses' perceptions of cancer patients' pain. *Cancer Nurs* 7:149–155, 1984

139. Weissman DE, Joranson DE, Hopwood MB: Wisconsin physicians' knowledge and attitudes about opioid analgesic regulations. *Wis Med J* 90:671–675, 1991

140. Hill CS: Pain management in a drug-oriented society. *Cancer* 63:2382–2386, 1989

141. Pritchard AP: Management of pain and nursing attitudes. *Cancer Nurs* 11:203–209, 1988

142. Von Roenn JH, Cleeland CS, Gonin R, et al: Physician attitudes and practice in cancer pain management: A survey from the Eastern Cooperative Oncology Group. *Ann Intern Med* 119:121–126, 1993

143. Pilowsky I: An outline curriculum on pain for medical school. *Pain* 33:1–2, 1988

144. Ferrell BR, McGuire DB, Donovan MI: Knowledge and beliefs regarding pain in a sample of nursing faculty. *J Prof Nurs* 9:79–88, 1993

145. Wisconsin Cancer Pain Initiative Nursing Education Committee: *Competency Guidelines for Cancer Pain Management in Nursing Education and Practice*. Madison, WI, Wisconsin Cancer Pain Initiative, 1995

146. Max MB: Improving outcomes of analgesic treatment: Is education enough? *Ann Intern Med* 113:885–889, 1990

147. Miaskowski C, Donovan M: Implementation of the American Pain Society Quality Assurance Standards for Relief of Acute Pain and Cancer Pain in oncology nursing practice. *Oncol Nurs Forum* 19:411–415, 1992

148. Weissman DE, Abram SE, Haddox AD, et al: Educational role of cancer pain rounds. *J Cancer Educ* 4:113–116, 1989

149. Weissman DE, Dahl JL: Update on the cancer pain role model education program. *J Pain Symptom Manage* 10: 292–297, 1995

150. Ferrell BR, Dean GE, Grant M, et al: An institutional commitment to pain management. *J Clin Oncol* 13:2158–2165, 1995

151. Ferrell BR, Grant M, Ritchey KL, et al: The pain resource nurse training program: a unique approach to pain management. *J Pain Symptom Manage* 8:545–556, 1993

152. McMenamin E, McCorkle E, Barg F, et al: Implementing a multidisciplinary cancer pain education program. *Cancer Pract* 3:303–309, 1995

153. Ward SE, Gordon D: Application of the American Pain Society quality assurance standards. *Pain* 56:299–306, 1994

154. Bookbinder M, Kiss M, Coyle N, et al: Improving pain management practices, in McGuire DB, Yarbro CH, Ferrell BR (eds): *Cancer Pain Management* (ed 2). Boston, Jones and Bartlett, 1995, pp 321–361

155. Ferrell B, Whedon M, Rollins B: Pain and quality assessment/improvement. *J Nurs Care Qual* 9:69–85, 1995

156. Portenoy RK, Coyle N: Controversies in the long-term management of analgesic therapy in patients with advanced cancer. *J Pain Symptom Manage* 5:307–319, 1991

157. Williams A, Kedziera P, Osterlund H, et al: Models of healthcare delivery in cancer pain management. *Oncol Nurs Forum* 19:20–26, 1992 (suppl)

158. Gonzales GR, Elliott KJ, Portenoy RK, et al: The impact of a comprehensive evaluation in the management of cancer pain. *Pain* 47:141–144, 1991

159. Walsh TD: Continuing care in a medical center: The Cleveland Clinic Foundation Palliative Care Service. *J Pain Sympt Manag* 5:273–278, 1990

160. Sheidler VR, Krumm SK: Pain management teams. Presentation at Oncology Nursing Society Congress, San Diego, May 1992

161. McGuire DB: Comprehensive and multidimensional assess-

ment and measurement of pain. *J Pain Symptom Manage* 7: 312–319, 1992

162. American Nurses Association and Oncology Nursing Society: *Statement on the Scope and Standards of Oncology Nursing Practice.* Washington, DC, 1996

163. Donovan MI: Clinical assessment of cancer pain, in McGuire DB, Yarbro CH (eds): *Cancer Pain Management.* Philadelphia, Saunders, 1987, pp 105–131

164. McCaffery M, Beebe A: *Pain: Clinical Manual for Nursing Practice.* St. Louis, Mosby, 1989

165. McGuire DB: Measuring pain, in Frank-Stromborg M, Olsen S. (eds): *Instruments for Clinical Nursing Research.* (ed 2). Boston, Jones and Bartlett, in press

166. Syrjala KL: The measurement of pain, in McGuire DB, Yarbro CH (eds): *Cancer Pain Management.* Philadelphia, Saunders, 1987, pp 133–150

167. Deschamps M, Band PR, Coldman AJ: Assessment of adult cancer pain: Shortcomings of current methods. *Pain* 32: 133–139, 1988

168. Grossman SA, Sheidler VR, McGuire DB, et al: A comparison of the Hopkins Pain Rating Instrument with standard visual analogue and verbal descriptor scales in patients with cancer pain. *J Pain Symptom Manage* 7:196–203, 1992

169. Acute Pain Management Guideline Panel: *Acute Pain Management: Operative or Medical Procedures and Trauma. Clinical Practice Guideline.* AHCPR publication No. 92-0032. Rockville, MD: Agency for Health Care Policy and Research. Public Health Service, U.S. Department of Health and Human Services, 1992

170. Daut RL, Cleeland CS, Flanery RC: Development of the Wisconsin brief pain questionnaire to assess pain in cancer and other diseases. *Pain* 17:197–210, 1983

171. Cleeland CS: Measurement and prevalence of pain in cancer. *Semin Oncol Nurs* 1:87–92, 1985

172. McGuire DB, Strickland OL: Assessment of cancer-related pain in low-income African Americans: Reliability, validity, and clinical utility of the Brief Pain Inventory and three pain intensity scales. *Abstracts: 8th World Congress on Pain,* 174, Aug. 1996, Vancouver, BC, Canada

173. Melzack R: The short-form McGill Pain Questionnaire. *Pain* 30:191–197, 1987

174. Fishman B, Pasternak S, Wallenstein SL, et al: The Memorial Pain Assessment Card: A valid instrument for the evaluation of cancer pain. *Cancer* 60:1151–1158, 1987

175. McMillan SC, Williams FA, Chatfield R, et al: A validity and reliability study of two tools for assessing and managing cancer pain. *Oncol Nurs Forum* 15:735–741, 1988

176. McGuire DB, Grimm PM, Baxendale-Cox L, et al: Pain, fatigue, and sleep alterations in cancer: A multidimensional perspective. Symposium presentation, American Pain Society Annual Meeting, Nov. 1994, Miami, FL.

177. Portenoy RK, Thaler HT, Kornblith AB, et al: Symptom prevalence, characteristics and distress in a cancer population. *Qual Life Res* 3:183–189, 1994

178. Donnelly S, Walsh D: The symptoms of advanced cancer. *Semin Oncol* 22:67–72, 1995

179. Portenoy RK, Thaler HT, Kornblith AB, et al: The Memorial Symptom Assessment Scale: An instrument for the evaluation of symptom prevalence, characteristics and distress. *Eur J Cancer* 30A:1326–1336, 1994

180. Beyer JE, Levin CR: Issues and advances in pain control in children. *Nurs Clin North Am* 22:661–676, 1987

181. McGrath PJ, Johnson G, Goodman J, et al: The Children's Hospital of Eastern Ontario Pain Scale (CHEOPS): A be-

havioral scale for rating postoperative pain in children, in Fields HL, Dubner R, Cervero F (eds): *Advances in Pain Research and Therapy,* vol. 9. New York, Raven Press, 1985, pp 395–402

182. Schechter NL, Altman A, Weisman S (eds): Report of the consensus conference on the management of pain in childhood cancer. *Pediatr* 86:5, 1990 (suppl)

183. Stiefel F, Fainsinger R, Bruera E: Acute confusional states in patients with advanced cancer. *J Pain Symptom Manage* 7:94–98, 1992

184. Bruera E, Fainsinger RL, Miller MJ, et al: The assessment of pain intensity in patients with cognitive failure: A preliminary report. *J Pain Symptom Manage* 7:267–270, 1992

185. North American Nursing Diagnosis Association: *Proc 8th Natl Conf NANDA.* St. Louis, 1988

186. McNally JC, Somerville ET, Miaskowski C, et al: *Guidelines for Oncology Nursing Practice* (ed 2). Philadelphia, Saunders, 1991, pp 125–142

187. Carpenito LJ: *Nursing Diagnosis: Application to Clinical Practice* (ed 4). Philadelphia, Lippincott, 1992, pp 211–248

188. Miaskowski C, Nichols R, Brody R, et al: Assessment of patient satisfaction utilizing the American Pain Society's Quality Assurance Standards on acute and cancer-related pain. *J Pain Symptom Manage* 9:5–11, 1994

189. Grant M, Ferrell BR, Rivera LM, et al: Unscheduled readmissions for uncontrolled symptoms: A health care challenge for nurses. *Nurs Clin North Am* 30:673–682, 1995

190. Dalton JA: Outcomes that provide evidence of change in cancer pain management. *Nurs Clin North Am* 30:683–695, 1995

191. Patterson KL, Klopovich PM: Pain in the pediatric oncology patient, in McGuire DB, Yarbro CH (eds): *Cancer Pain Management.* Philadelphia, Saunders, 1987, pp 259–272

192. Stevens B, Hunsberger M, Browne G: Pain in children: Theoretical, research, and practice dilemmas. *J Pediatr Nurs* 2:154–166, 1987

193. Broome ME, Lillis PP: A descriptive analysis of the pediatric pain management research. *Appl Nurs Res* 2:744–781, 1989

194. Hester NO: Integrating pain assessment and management into the care of children with cancer, in McGuire DB, Yarbro CH, Ferrell BR (eds): *Cancer Pain Management* (ed 2). Boston, Jones and Bartlett, 1995, pp 231–271

195. Katz ER, Kellerman J, Siegel SE: Behavioral distress in children with cancer undergoing medical procedures: Developmental considerations. *J Consult Clin Psychol* 48: 356–365, 1980

196. Beaver PK: Premature infants' response to touch and pain: Can nurses make a difference? *Neonatal Network* 6:13–17, 1987

197. Eland JM, Anderson JE: The experience of pain in children, in Jacox AK (ed): *Pain: A Sourcebook for Nurses and Other Health Professionals.* Boston, Little, Brown, 1977, pp 453–476

198. Schechter NL, Allen DA, Hanson K: Status of pediatric pain control: A comparison of hospital analgesic usage in children and adults. *Pediatr* 77:11–15, 1986

199. Schmidt K, Eland J, Weiler K: Pediatric cancer pain management: A survey of nurses' knowledge. *J Pediatr Oncol Nurs* 11:4–12, 1994

200. Collins JJ, Grier HE, Kinney HC, et al: Control of severe pain in children with terminal malignancy. *J Pediatr* 126: 653–657, 1995

201. Broome ME, Lillis PP, McGahee TW, et al: The use of

distraction and imagery with children during painful procedures. *Oncol Nurs Forum* 19:499–502, 1992

202. Nahata MC, Clotz MA, Krogg EA: Adverse effects of meperidine, promethazine, and chlorpromazine for sedation in pediatric patients. *Clin Pediatr* 24:558–560, 1985

203. Kuttner, L: *A Child in Pain: How to Help, What to Do*. USA: Hartley and Marks, 1996

204. Kuttner L, Bowman M, Teasdale M: Psychological treatment of distress, pain, and anxiety for young children with cancer. *J Dev Behav Pediatr* 9:374–381, 1988

205. Zappa SC, Nabors SB: Use of ethyl chloride topical anesthetic to reduce procedural pain in pediatric oncology patients. *Cancer Nurs* 15:130–136, 1992

206. Lander J, Nazarali S, Hodgins M, et al: Evaluation of a new topical anesthetic agent: A pilot study. *Nurs Res* 45:50–53, 1996

207. Miser AW, Miser JS: The use of oral methadone to control moderate and severe pain in children and young adults with malignancy. *Clin J Pain* 1:243–248, 1986

208. Goldman A: The role of oral controlled-release morphine for pain relief in children with cancer. *Palliat Med* 4:279–285, 1990

209. Dothage JA, Arndt C, Miser AW: Use of a continuous intravenous morphine infusion for pain control in an infant with terminal malignancy. *J Assoc Pediatr Oncol Nurs* 3(4):22–24, 1986

210. Gilford DM (ed): *The Aging Population in the Twenty-First Century: Statistics for Health Policy*. Washington, DC, National Academy Press, 1988

211. Parker SL, Tong T, Bolden S, et al: Cancer statistics, 1996. *CA Cancer J Clin* 46:5–27, 1996

212. Portenoy RK: Optimal pain control in elderly cancer patients. *Geriatr* 42:33–44, 1987

213. Ferrell BA, Ferrell BR: Assessment of chronic pain in the elderly. *Geriatr Med Today* 8:123–134, 1989

214. Ferrell BA: Pain in the elderly, in Watt-Watson JH, Donovan MI (eds): *Pain Management: Nursing Perspective*. St. Louis, Mosby Year Book, 1992, pp 349–369

215. Thomas MR, Roy R: Age and pain: A comparative study of the "younger and older" elderly. *Pain Manage* 1:174–179, 1988

216. Office of Technology Assessment: *Technology and Aging in America*. Publication No. OTA-BA-264. Washington, DC, Office of Technology Assessment, 1985

217. Ferrell BA, Ferrell BR, Osterweil D: Pain in the nursing home. *J Am Geriatr Soc* 38:409–414, 1990

218. Newton PA: Chronic pain, in Cassel KY, Walsh JR (eds): *Geriatric Medicine*, vol 2. *Fundamentals of Geriatric Care*. New York, Springer-Verlag, 1984, pp 236–274

219. Lamy PP: Pain management, drugs, and the elderly. *J Am Health Care Assoc* 10:32–36, 1984

220. Ferrell BA, Ferrell BR, Rivera L: Pain in cognitively impaired nursing home patients. *J Pain Symptom Manage* 10:591–598, 1995

221. Harkins SW, Kwentus J, Price DD: Pain in the elderly, in Bendetti C, Chapman CR, Morrica G (eds): *Advances in Pain Research and Therapy*, vol 7. New York, Raven Press, 1984, pp 103–121

222. Ferrell BR, Grant MM, Riner M, et al: Home care: Maintaining quality of life for patient and family. *Oncology* 6:136–140, 1992 (suppl)

223. Bayer AJ, Chadha JS, Farag RR, et al: Changing presentations of myocardial infarction with increasing old age. *J Am Geriatr Soc* 34:263–266, 1986

224. Schmucker DL: Drug disposition in the elderly: A review of the critical factors. *J Am Geriatr Soc* 32:144–149, 1984

225. Ouslander JG: Drug therapy in the elderly. *Ann Intern Med* 95:711–722, 1981

226. Amadio P, Cummings DM, Amadio PB: Pain in the elderly: Management techniques. *Pain Manage* 1:33–41, 1987

227. Kaiko RF, Wallenstein SL, Rogers AG, et al: Narcotics in the elderly. *Med Clin North Am* 66:1079–1089, 1982

228. Nolan L, O'Mallev K: Prescribing for the elderly: Part 1. Sensitivity of the elderly to adverse drug reactions. *J Am Geriatr Soc* 36:142–149, 1988

229. Conn VS, Taylor SG, Kelley S: Medication regimen complexity and adherence among older adults. *Image: J Nurs Schol* 23:231–235, 1991

230. Faherty BS, Grier MR: Analgesic medication for elderly people post-surgery. *Nurs Res* 33:369–372, 1984

231. Portenoy RK, Kanner RM: Patterns of analgesic prescription and consumption in a university-affiliated community hospital. *Arch Intern Med* 145:439–441, 1985

232. Portenoy R: Pain management in the older cancer patient. *Oncology* 6:86–98, 1992

233. Ferrell BR, Grant M, Chan J, et al: The impact of cancer pain education on family caregivers of elderly patients. *Oncol Nurs Forum* 22:1211–1218, 1995

234. Coyle N, Foley KM: Alteration in comfort: Pain, in Baird SB, McCorkle R, Grant M (eds): *Cancer Nursing: A Comprehensive Textbook*. Philadelphia, Saunders, 1991, pp 782–805

235. McCaffery M, Vourakis C: Assessment and relief of pain in chemically dependent patients. *Orthop Nurs* 11:13–27, 1992

236. Hoffman M, Provatas A, Lyver A, et al: Pain management in the opioid-addicted patient with cancer. *Cancer* 68:121–122, 1991

237. Puntillo KA (ed): *Pain in the Critically Ill: Assessment and Management*. Gaithersburg, VA, Aspen, 1991

238. Shelton BK: Pain, in Wright JE, Shelton BK (eds): *Desk Reference for Critical Care Nursing*. Boston, Jones and Bartlett, 1993, pp 1341–1357

239. Donnelly GF, Sutterley DC: From the editors (editorial). *Top Clin Nurs* 7: v, 1985 (entire issue on cultural diversity and nursing practice)

240. Fong CM: Ethnicity and nursing practice. *Top Clin Nurs* 7:1–10, 1985

241. Douglas MK: Cultural diversity in the response to pain, in Puntillo KA (ed): *Pain in the Critically Ill: Assessment and Management*. Gaithersburg, VA, Aspen, 1991, pp 65–76

242. Kagawa-Singer M: Ethnic perspectives of cancer nursing: Hispanics and Japanese-Americans. *Oncol Nurs Forum* 14:59–65, 1987

243. Carson VB (ed): *Spiritual Dimensions of Nursing Practice*. Philadelphia, Saunders, 1989

244. Jacik M: Spiritual care of the dying adult, in Carson VB (ed): *Spiritual Dimensions of Nursing Practice*. Philadelphia, Saunders, 1989, pp 254–288

245. Johnston Taylor E, Ersek M: Ethical and spiritual dimensions of cancer pain management, in McGuire DB, Yarbro CH, Ferrell BR (eds): *Cancer Pain Management* (ed 2). Boston, Jones and Bartlett, 1995, pp 41–60

246. Twycross RD: Terminal care: Organization and technical aspects, in Swerdlow M. Ventafridda V (eds): *Cancer Pain*. Lancaster, England, MTP Press, 1987, pp 173–184

247. Wanzer SH, Federman DD, Adelstein SJ, et al: The physician's responsibility toward hopelessly ill patients. *N Engl J Med* 320:844–849, 1989

248. Burchman SL: Hospice care of the cancer pain patient, in Abram SE (ed): *Cancer Pain*. Boston, Kluwer, 1989, pp 153–169

249. Kane RL, Bernstein L, Wales J, et al: Hospice effectiveness in controlling pain. *JAMA* 253:2683–2686, 1985

250. Austin C, Cody OP, Eyres PJ, et al: Hospice home care pain management: Four critical variables. *Cancer Nurs* 9:38–65, 1986

251. Fainsinger R, Miller MJ, Bruera E: Symptom control during the last week of life on a palliative care unit. *J Palliat Care* 7:5–11, 1991

252. Ventafridda V, Ripamonti C, DeConno F, et al: Symptom prevalence and control during cancer patients' last days of life. *J Palliat Care* 6:7–11, 1990

253. Degner LF, Fujii SH, Levitt M: Implementing a program to control chronic pain of malignant disease for patients in an extended care facility. *Cancer Nurs* 5:263–258, 1982

254. Bruera E, MacMillan K, Hanson J, et al: Palliative care in a cancer center: Results in 1984 versus 1987. *J Pain Symptom Manage* 5:1–5, 1990

255. Miller RD, Walsh TD: Psychosocial aspects of palliative care in advanced cancer. *J Pain Symptom Manage* 6:24–29, 1991

256. Chan H, Woodruff RK: Palliative care in a general teaching hospital: Assessment of needs. *Med J Aust* 155:597–599, 1991

257. Milch RA, Freeman A, Clark E: *Palliative Pain and Symptom Management for Children and Adolescents*. Alexandria, VA, Children's Hospice International, 1985

258. Coyle N, Adelhardt J, Foley KM, et al: Character of terminal illness in the advanced cancer patient: Pain and other symptoms during the last four weeks of life. *J Pain Symptom Manage* 5:83–93, 1990

259. Mount B. Challenges in palliative care (keynote address). *Am J Hosp Care* 2:22–29, 1985

260. Grond S, Zech D, Schug SA, et al: Validation of World Health Organization Guidelines for cancer pain relief during the last days and hours of life. *J Pain Symptom Manage* 6:411–422, 1991

261. Magrum LC, Bentzen C, Landmark S: Pain management in home care. *Semin Oncol Nurs* 12:202–218, 1996

262. Patt RB: *Cancer Pain*. Philadelphia, Lippincott, 1993

263. Bonadonna F, Molinari R: Role and limits of anticancer drugs in the treatment of advanced cancer pain, in Bonica JJ, Ventafridda V (eds): *Advances in Pain Research and Therapy*, vol 2. New York, Raven Press, 1979, pp 131–138

264. Russell JA: Cytotoxic therapy: Pain relief and recalcification, in Stoll BA, Parbhoo S (eds): *Bone Metastasis: Monitoring and Treatment*. New York, Raven Press, 1983, pp 354–368

265. MacDonald N: The role of medical oncology in cancer pain control, in Hill CS, Fields WS (eds): *Advances in Pain Research and Therapy*, vol 11. New York, Raven Press, 1989, pp 123–130

266. Bruera E, Schoeller T, Wenk R, et al: A prospective multicenter assessment of the Edmonton Staging System for Cancer Pain. *J Pain Symptom Manage* 10:348–355, 1995

267. Abrams RA, Hansen RM: Radiotherapy, chemotherapy and hormonal therapy in the management of cancer pain: Putting patient, prognosis, and oncologic options in perspective, in Abram SE (ed): *Cancer Pain*. Boston, Kluwer, 1989, pp 49–66

268. Pannuti F, Martoni A, Rossi AP, et al: The role of endocrine therapy for relief of pain due to advanced cancer, in Bonica JJ, Ventafridda V (eds): *Advances in Pain Research and Therapy*, vol 2. New York, Raven Press, 1979, pp 145–165

269. Stoll BA: Hormonal therapy: Pain relief and recalcification, in Stoll BA, Parbhoo S (eds): *Bone Metastasis: Monitoring and Treatment*. New York, Raven Press, 1983, pp 321–342

270. Needham PR, Hoskin PJ: Radiotherapy for painful bone metastases. *Palliat Med* 8:95–104, 1994

271. Hoskin PJ: Radiotherapy for bone pain. *Pain* 63:137–139, 1995

272. Ashby M: The role of radiotherapy in palliative care. *J Pain Symptom Manage* 6:380–388, 1991

273. Porter AT: Use of strontium-89 in metastatic cancer: US and UK experience. *Oncology* 8:25–29, 1994 (Suppl)

274. Ackery D, Yardley J: Radionuclide-targeted therapy for the management of metastatic bone pain. *Semin Oncol* 20:227–231, 1993 (suppl 2)

275. Robinson RG, Preston DF, Baxter KG, et al: Clinical experience with strontium-89 in prostatic and breast cancer patients. *Semin Oncol* 20:44–48, 1993 (suppl 2)

276. Kan MK: Palliation of bone pain in patients with metastatic cancer using strontium-89 (Metastron). *Cancer Nurs* 18:286–291, 1995

277. Bucholtz J: *Patient Information, Strontium-89*. Baltimore, The Johns Hopkins Oncology Center Division of Radiation Oncology, 1993

278. Azzarelli A, Crispino S: Palliative surgery in cancer pain treatment, in Swerdlow M, Ventafridda V (eds): *Cancer Pain*. Lancaster, England, MTP Press, 1987, pp 97–103

279. MacDonald N: The role of medical and surgical oncology in the management of cancer pain, in Foley KM, Bonica JJ, Ventafridda V (eds): *Advances in Pain Research and Therapy*, vol 16. New York, Raven Press, 1990, pp 27–44

280. Chalmers J: The management of bone metastases: Orthopaedic procedures. *Palliat Med* 1:121–127, 1987

281. Hanks GW: Opioid analgesics in the management of pain in patients with cancer: A review. *Palliat Med* 1:1–25, 1987

282. Twycross RG: Opioid analgesics in cancer pain: Current practice and controversies. *Cancer Surv* 7:29–53, 1988

283. Inturrisi CE: Management of cancer pain: Pharmacology and principles of management. *Cancer* 63:2308–2320, 1989

284. Pasternak GW: Biochemistry and pharmacology of multiple mu opioid receptors, in Foley KM, Inturrisi CE (eds): *Advances in Pain Research and Therapy*, vol 8. New York, Raven Press, 1986, pp 337–344

285. Jaffe JH, Martin WR: Opioid analgesics and antagonists, in Gilman AG, Rall TW, Nies AL, et al (eds): *Goodman and Gilman's The Pharmacological Basis of Therapeutics* (ed 8). New York, Pergamon Press, 1990, pp 485–521

286. Insel PA: Analgesic-antipyretic and anti-inflammatory agents: Drugs employed in the treatment of rheumatoid arthritis and gout, in Gilman AG, Rall TW, Nies AL, et al (eds): *Goodman and Gilman's The Pharmacological Basis of Therapeutics* (ed 8). New York, Pergamon Press, 1990, pp 638–681

287. Ventafridda V, Fochi V, DeConno D, et al: Use of nonsteroidal anti-inflammatory drugs in the treatment of pain in cancer. *Br J Clin Pharmacol* 10:3435–3465, 1980

288. Moertel CG: Treatment of cancer pain with orally administered medications. *JAMA* 244:2448–2450, 1980

289. Turnbull R, Hills LJ: Naproxen versus aspirin as analgesics in advanced malignant disease. *J Palliat Care* 1:25–28, 1986

290. Levich S, Jacobs C, Loukas DF: Naproxen sodium in treatment of bone pain due to metastatic cancer. *Pain* 35:253–258, 1988

291. Staquet MJ: Double-blind study with placebo control of

intramuscular ketorolac tromethamine in the treatment of cancer pain. *J Clin Pharmacol* 29:1031–1036, 1989

292. Ventafridda V, De Conno F, Panerai AE, et al: Nonsteroidal anti-inflammatory drugs as the first step in cancer pain therapy: Double blind, within-patient study comparing nine drugs. *J Int Med Res* 18:21–29, 1990

293. Beaver WT: Aspirin and acetaminophen as constituents of analgesic combinations, *Arch Intern Med* 141:292–300, 1981

294. Houde RW, Wallenstein SL, Rogers A: Clinical pharmacology of analgesics: A method of assaying analgesic effect. *Clin Pharmacol Ther* 1:163–174, 1960

295. Ferrer-Brechner T, Ganz P: Combination therapy with ibuprofen and methadone for chronic cancer pain. *Am J Med* 77:78–83, 1984

296. Weingart WA, Sorkness CA, Earhart RH: Analgesia with oral narcotics and added ibuprofen in cancer patients. *Clin Pharm* 4:53–58, 1985

297. Eisenberg E, Berley CS, Carr DB, et al: Efficacy and safety of nonsteroidal inflammatory drugs for cancer pain: A meta-analysis. *J Clin Oncol* 12:2756–2765, 1994

298. Allison MC, Howatson AG, Torrance CJ, et al: Gastrointestinal damage associated with the use of nonsteroidal anti-inflammatory drugs. *N Engl J Med* 327:749–754, 1992

299. Mannix KA, Rawlins MD: The management of bone metastases: Nonsteroidal anti-inflammatory drugs. *Palliat Med* 1:128–131, 1987

300. Griffin MR, Piper JM, Daughterty JR, et al: Nonsteroidal anti-inflammatory drug use and increased risk for peptic ulcer disease in elderly persons. *Ann Intern Med* 114:257–263, 1991

301. Kantor TG: Control of pain by nonsteroidal anti-inflammatory drugs. *Med Clin North Am* 66:1053–1059, 1982

302. Portenoy RK: Drug treatment of pain syndromes. *Semin Neurol* 7:139–149, 1987

303. Foley KM: The treatment of cancer pain. *N Engl J Med* 313:84–95, 1985

304. Campora E, Merlini L, Pace M, et al: The incidence of narcotic-induced emesis. *J Pain Symptom Manage* 6:428–430, 1991

305. Portenoy RK: Constipation in the cancer patient: Causes and management. *Med Clin North Am* 71:303–311, 1987

306. Levy MH: Constipation and diarrhea in cancer patients. *Cancer Bull* 43:312–422, 1991

307. Portenoy RK, Foley KM, Inturrisi CE: The nature of opioid responsiveness and its implications for neuropathic pain: New hypotheses derived from studies of opioid infusions. *Pain* 43:273–286, 1991

308. Coyle N, Cherny N, Portenoy RK: Pharmacologic management of cancer pain, in McGuire DB, Yarbro CH, Ferrell BR (eds): *Cancer Pain Management* (ed 2). Boston, Jones and Bartlett, 1995, pp 131–158

309. Kaiko RF, Foley KM, Grabinski PY, et al: Central nervous system excitatory effects of meperidine in cancer patients. *Ann Neurol* 13:180–185, 1983

310. Ventafridda V, Saita L, Barletta L, et al: Clinical observations on controlled-release morphine in cancer pain. *J Pain Symptom Manage* 4:124–129, 1989

311. Tsuneto S, Havashi A, Miyazaki M, et al: Clinical survey of controlled release morphine for cancer pain relief in a Japanese hospice. *Postgrad Med J* 67:79–81, 1991 (suppl)

312. Vijayaram S, Ramamani PV, Chandrashekhar NS, et al: Continuing care for cancer pain relief with oral morphine solution: One year experience in a regional cancer center. *Cancer* 66:1590–1595, 1990

313. Homesley HD, Welander CE, Muss HB, et al: Dosage range study of morphine sulfate controlled release. *Am J Clin Oncol* 9:449–453, 1986

314. Meed SD, Kleinman PM, Kantor TG, et al: Management of cancer pain with oral controlled-release morphine sulfate. *J Clin Pharmacol* 27:155–161, 1987

315. Savarese JJ, Shepherd L, Krant MJ: Long-acting oral morphine in cancer pain analgesia. *Clin J Pain* 3:177–181, 1987

316. Brescia FJ, Walsh M, Savarese JJ, et al: A study of controlled-release oral morphine (MS Contin) in an advanced cancer hospital. *J Pain Symptom Manage* 2:193–198, 1987

317. Khojasteh A, Evans W, Reynolds RD, et al: Controlled-release oral morphine sulfate in the treatment of cancer pain with pharmacokinetic correlation. *J Clin Oncol* 5:956–961, 1987

318. Thirwell MP, Sloan PA, Maroun JA, et al: Pharmacokinetics and clinical efficacy of oral morphine solution and controlled-release morphine tablets in cancer patients. *Cancer* 63:2275–2283, 1989

319. Goughnour BR, Arkinstall WW, Stewart JH: Analgesic response to single and multiple doses of controlled-release morphine tablets and morphine oral solution in cancer patients. *Cancer* 63:2294–2297, 1989

320. Walsh TD, Kadam BV: Morphine steady-state levels during repeated oral administration. *Br J Clin Pharmacol* 17:232, 1984

321. Walsh TD, Grabinski PY, Kaiko RF: Clinical implications of morphine plasma levels in advanced cancer, in Foley RM, Inturrisi CE (eds): *Advances in Pain Research and Therapy*, vol 8. New York, Raven Press, 1986, pp 31–35

322. Ventafridda V, Oliveri E, Caraceni A, et al: A retrospective study on the use of oral morphine in cancer pain. *J Pain Symptom Manage* 2:77–81, 1987

323. Sawe J, Dahlstrom B, Rase A: Morphine kinetics in cancer patients. *Clin Pharmacol Ther* 30:629–635, 1981

324. Houde RW, Wallenstein SL, Beaver WT: Clinical measurement of pain, in de Stevens G (eds): *Analgesics*. New York, Academic Press, 1965, pp 75–122

325. Walsh TD: Oral morphine in chronic cancer pain. *Pain* 18:1–11, 1984

326. Kaiko R: Controversy in the management of chronic cancer pain: Therapeutic equivalents of im and po morphine. *J Pain Symptom Manage* 1:42–45, 1986

327. Peterson GM, Randall CTC, Paterson J: Plasma levels of morphine glucuronide in the treatment of cancer pain: Relationship to renal function and route of administration. *Eur J Clin Pharmacol* 38:121–124, 1990

328. Portenoy RK, Thaler HT, Inturrisi CE, et al: The metabolite morphine-6-glucuronide contributes to the analgesia produced by morphine infusion in patients with pain and normal renal function. *Clin Pharmacol Ther* 51:422–431, 1992

329. Portenoy RK, Foley KM, Stulman, et al: Plasma morphine and morphine-6-glucuronide during chronic morphine therapy for cancer pain: Plasma profiles, steady state concentrations, and the consequences of renal failure. *Pain* 47:13–19, 1991

330. Faura CC, Moore RA, Horga JF, et al: Morphine and morphine-6-glucuronide plasma concentrations and effect in cancer pain. *J Pain Symptom Manage* 11:95–102, 1996

331. Houde RW: Misinformation: Side effects and drug interactions, in Hill CS, Fields WS (eds): *Advances in Pain Research and Therapy*, vol 11. New York, Raven Press, 1989, pp 145–161

332. Ettinger DS, Vitale PJ, Trump DC: Important clinical considerations in the use of methadone in cancer patients. *Cancer Treat Rep* 63:457–459, 1979

333. Glare PA, Walsh TD: Dose-ranging study of oxycodone for chronic pain in advanced cancer. *J Clin Oncol* 11:973–978, 1993

334. Benzinger DP, Levy SA, Fitzman RD, et al: Dose porportionality of 10, 20, and 40 mg controlled-release oxycodone hydrochloride tablets. *Pharmacotherapy* 15:391, 1995 (abstr)

335. Grandy R, Reder R, Fitzmartin R, et al: Steady-state pharmacokinetic comparison of controlled-release oxycodone tablets vs oxycodone oral liquid. *J Clin Pharmacol* 34:1015, 1994

336. OxyContin product information. Purdue Pharma L.P., 1995

337. Dayer P, Collart L, Desmeules J: The pharmacology of tramadol. *Drugs* 47:3–7, 1994 (suppl 1)

338. Wilder-Smith CH, Schimke J, Osterwalder B, et al: Oral tramadol, a mu-opioid agonist and monamine reuptake blocker, and morphine for strong cancer-related pain. *Ann Oncol* 5:141–146, 1994

339. Baldessarini RJ: Drugs and the treatment of psychiatric disorders, in Gilman AG, Rall TW, Nies AL, et al (eds): *Goodman and Gilman's The Pharmacological Bases of Therapeutics* (ed 8). New York, Pergamon Press, 1990, pp 383–435

340. Max MB, Lynch SA, Muir J, et al: Effects of desipiramine, amitriptyline, and fluoxethine on pain in diabetic neuropathy. *N Engl J Med* 326:1250–1256, 1992

341. Watson CPN, Chipman M, Reed K, et al: Amitriptyline versus maprotiline in postherpetic neuralgia: A randomized, double-blind crossover trial. *Pain* 48:29–36, 1992

342. Max MB: Thirteen consecutive well-designed randomized trials show that antidepressants reduce pain in diabetic neuropathy and postherpetic neuralgia. *Pain Forum* 4: 248–253, 1995

343. Portenoy RK: Practical aspects of pain control in the patient with cancer. *CA Cancer J Clin* 38:327–352, 1988

344. Eija K, Tasmuth T, Pertti J: Amitriptyline effectively relieves neuropathic pain following treatment of breast cancer. *Pain* 64:293–302, 1995

345. Walsh TD: Antidepressants for chronic pain. *Clin Neuropharmacol* 6:271–295, 1983

346. Massie MJ, Holland J: The cancer patient with pain: Psychiatric complications and their management. *Med Clin North Am* 71:243–258, 1987

347. McQuay H, Carroll D, Jadad AK, et al: Anticonvulsant drugs for management of pain: A systematic review. *Br Med J* 311:1047–1052, 1995

348. Swerdlow M, Cundill JG: Anti-convulsant drugs used in the treatment of lancinating pain: A comparison. *Anaesthesiol* 36: 1129–1132, 1981

349. Rapoport WG, Rogers KM, McCubbin TD, et al: Treatment of intractable neurogenic pain with carbamazepine. *Scott Med J* 29:162–165, 1984

350. Fromm GF: Trigeminal neuralgia and related disorders. *Neurol Clin* 7:305–320, 1989

351. McEvoy G (ed): *American Hospital Formulary Service*. Bethesda, MD, Amer. Soc. Hosp. Pharm., 1992

352. Rall TW, Schleifer LS: Drugs effective in the therapies of the epilepsies, in Gilman AG, Rall TW, Nies AL, et al (eds): *Goodman and Gilman's The Pharmacologic Basis of Therapeutics* (ed 8). New York, Pergamon Press, 1990, pp 436–462

353. Rosner H, Rubin L, Kestenbaum A: Gabapentin adjunctive therapy in neuropathic states. *Clin J Pain* 12:56–58, 1996

354. Beydoun A, Uthman BM, Sackellares JC: Gabapentin: Pharmacokinetics, efficacy, and safety. *Clin Neuropharmacol* 18: 469–481, 1995

355. Hoffman BB, Lefkowitz RJ: Catecholamines and sympathomimetic drugs, in Gilman AG, Rall TW, Nies AS, et al (eds): *Goodman and Gilman's The Pharmacological Basis of Therapeutics* (ed 8). New York, Pergamon Press, 1990, pp 187–220

356. Bruera E, Watanabe S: Psychostimulants as adjuvant analgesics. *J Pain Symptom Manage* 9:412–415, 1994

357. Wilwerding MB, Loprinzi CL, Mailliard JA, et al: A randomized, crossover evaluation of methylphenidate in cancer patients receiving strong narcotics. *Support Care Cancer* 3: 135–138, 1995

358. Bruera E, Chadwick S, Brenneis C, et al: Methylphenidate associated with narcotics for the treatment of cancer pain. *Cancer Treat Rep* 71:67–70, 1987

359. Bruera E, Brenneis C, Patterson AH, et al: Use of methylphenidate as an adjuvant to narcotic analgesics in patients with advanced cancer. *J Pain Symptom Manage* 4:3–6, 1989

360. Dundee JW, Moore J: The myth of phenothiazine potentiation. *Anaesth* 16:95–96, 1961

361. Keats AS, Telford J, Kurosu Y: "Potentiation" of meperidine by promethazine. *Anesthesiology* 22:34–41, 1961

362. Beaver WT, Wallenstein SL, Houde RW, et al: A comparison of the analgesic effect of methotrimeprazine and morphine in patients with cancer. *Clin Pharmacol Ther* 7: 436–446, 1966

363. Bloomfield S, Simard-Savoie S, Bernier J, et al: Comparative analgesic activity of levomepromazine and morphine in patients with chronic pain. *Can Med Assoc J* 90: 1156–1159, 1964

364. Hanks GW, Thomas PJ, Trueman T, et al: The myth of haloperidol potentiation. *Lancet* 2:523–524, 1983

365. Beaver WT, Feise G: Combination of analgesic effects of morphine sulfate, hydroxyzine and their combinations in patients with postoperative pain, in Bonica JJ, Albe-Fessard D (eds): *Advances in Pain Research and Therapy*, vol 1. New York, Raven Press, 1976, pp 553–557

366. Bruera E, Roca E, Cedaro L, et al: Action of oral methylprednisolone in terminal cancer patients: A prospective randomized double blind study. *Cancer Treat Rep* 69: 751–754, 1985

367. Walsh TD: Adjuvant analgesic therapy in cancer pain, in Foley KM, Bonica JJ, Ventafridda V (eds): *Advances in Pain Research and Therapy*, vol 16. New York, Raven Press, 1990, pp 155–169

368. Ernst DS, MacDonald N, Paterson AHG, et al: A double-blind, crossover trial of intravenous clodronate in metastatic bone pain. *J Pain Symptom Manage* 7:4–11, 1992

369. Adami S, Mian M: Clodronate therapy of metastatic bone disease in patients with prostatic carcinoma. *Recent Result Cancer Res* 116:67–72, 1989

370. Berenson JR, Lichtenstein A, Porter L, et al: Efficacy of pamidronate in reducing skeletal events in patients with advanced multiple myeloma. *N Engl J Med* 334:488–493, 1996

371. Portenoy RK, Moulin DE, Rogers A, et al: IV infusions of opioids for cancer pain: Clinical review and guidelines for use. *Cancer Treat Rep* 70:575–582, 1986

372. Ashburn MA, Streisand JB, Tarver SD, et al: Oral transmucosal fentanyl citrate for premedication in paediatric outpatients. *Can J Anaesth* 37:857–866, 1990

373. Fine PG, Marcus M, De Boer JA, et al: An open label

study of oral transmucosal fentanyl citrate (OTFC) for the treatment of breakthrough cancer pain. *Pain* 445:149–153, 1991

374. Citron M, Johnston-Early A, Fossieck B, et al: Safety and efficacy of continuous intravenous morphine for severe cancer pain. *Am J Med* 77:199–204, 1984

375. Stuart GJ, Davey EB, Wight SE: Continuous intravenous morphine infusions for terminal pain control: A retrospective review. *Drug Intell Clin Pharmacol* 20:968–972, 1986

376. Ferris FD, Kerr IG, DeAngelis C, et al: Inpatient narcotic infusions for patients with cancer pain. *J Palliat Care* 6:51–59, 1990

377. Portenoy RK: Continuous infusion of opioid drugs. *Med Clin North Am* 71:233–241, 1987

378. Coyle N, Mauskop A, Maggard J, et al: Continuous infusions of opiates in cancer patients with pain. *Oncol Nurs Forum* 13:53–57, 1986

379. Dickson RJ, Howard B, Campbell J: The relief of pain by subcutaneous infusion of morphine, in Wilkes E (ed): *Advances in Morphine Therapy: The 1983 International Symposium on Pain Control.* Royal Society of Medicine International Congress and Symposium Series #64. London, Royal Society of Medicine, 1983, pp 107–110

380. Miser AW, David DM, Hughes CS, et al: Continuous subcutaneous infusions of morphine in children with cancer. *Am J Dis Child* 137:383–385, 1983

381. Bruera E, Legris MA, Kuehn N, et al: Hypodermoclysis for the administration of fluids and narcotic analgesics in patients with advanced cancer. *J Natl Cancer Inst* 81:1108–1109, 1989

382. Drexel H, Dzien A, Spiegel RW: Treatment of severe cancer pain by low dose continuous subcutaneous morphine. *Pain* 36:169–176, 1989

383. Bruera E, Brenneis C, Michaud M, et al: Patient-controlled subcutaneous hydromorphone versus continuous subcutaneous infusion for the treatment of cancer pain. *J Natl Cancer Inst* 80:1152–1154, 1988

384. Brenneis C, Michaud M, Bruera E, et al: Local toxicity during subcutaneous infusion of narcotics: A prospective study. *Cancer Nurs* 10:172–176, 1987

385. Bruera E, Brenneis C, Michaud M, et al: Continuous sc infusion of narcotics using a portable disposable device in patients with advanced cancer. *Cancer Treat Rep* 71:635–637, 1987

386. Sheidler VR: New methods in analgesic delivery, in McGuire DB, Yarbro CH (eds): *Cancer Pain Management.* Philadelphia, Saunders, 1987, pp 203–222

387. Macmillan K, Bruera E, Kuehn N, et al: A prospective comparison study between a butterfly needle and a teflon cannula for subcutaneous narcotic administration. *J Pain Symptom Manage* 9:82–84, 1994

388. Moulin DE, Kreeft JH, Murray-Parsons N, et al: Comparison of continuous subcutaneous and intravenous hydromorphone for management of cancer pain. *Lancet* 337:465–468, 1991

389. Lang AH, Abbrederis K, Dzien A, et al: Treatment of severe cancer pain by continuous infusion of subcutaneous opioids. *Recent Results Cancer Res* 121:51–57, 1991

390. *The United States Pharmacopeia,* 21st rev., The United States Pharmacopeial Convention, Rockville, MD, 1984

391. Bruera E, MacEachern T, MacMillan K, et al: Local tolerance to subcutaneous infusions of high concentrations of hydromorphone: A prospective study. *J Pain Symptom Manage* 8:201–204, 1993

392. Lesser GL, Grossman SA, Leong KW, et al: In vitro and in vivo studies of subcutaneous hydromorphone implants designed for treatment of cancer pain. *Pain* 65:265–272, 1996

393. Crane RA: Intermittent subcutaneous infusion of opioids in hospice home care: An effective, economical, manageable option. *Am J Hosp Care* 11:8–12, 1994

394. Caplan RA, Ready LB, Oden RV, et al: Transdermal fentanyl for postoperative pain management. *JAMA* 261:1036–1039, 1989

395. Gourlay GK, Kowalski SR, Plummer JL, et al: The efficacy of transdermal fentanyl in the treatment of postoperative pain: A double-blind comparison of fentanyl and placebo systems. *Pain* 40:21–28, 1990

396. Simmonds MA, Richenbacher J: Transdermal fentanyl: Long-term analgesic studies. *J Pain Symptom Manage* 7:S36–S39, 1992

397. Calis KA, Kohler DR, Corso DM: Transdermally administered fentanyl for pain management. *Clin Pharm* 11:22–36, 1992

398. Miser AW, Narang PK, Dothage JA, et al: Transdermal fentanyl for pain control in patients with cancer. *Pain* 37:15–21, 1989

399. Herbst LH, Strause LG: Transdermal fentanyl use in hospice home-care patients with chronic cancer pain. *J Pain Symptom Manage* 7:S54–S57, 1992

400. Levy MH, Rosen SM, Kedziera P: Transdermal fentanyl: Seeding trial in patients with chronic cancer pain. *J Pain Symptom Manage* 7:S48–S50, 1992

401. Maves TJ, Barcellos WA: Management of cancer pain with transdermal fentanyl: Phase IV trial, University of Iowa. *J Pain Symptom Manage* 7:S58–S62, 1991

402. Varvel JR, Shafer SL, Hwang SS, et al: Absorption characteristics of transdermally administered fentanyl. *Anesthesiology* 70:928–934, 1989

403. Gupta SK, Southam M, Gale R, et al: System functionality and physiochemical model of fentanyl transdermal system. *J Pain Symptom Manage* 7:S17–S26, 1992

404. Payne R: Transdermal fentanyl: Suggested recommendations for clinical use. *J Pain Symptom Manage* 7:S40–S44, 1992

405. De Conno F, Ripamonti C, Saita L, et al: Role of rectal route in treating cancer pain: A randomized crossover clinical trial of oral versus rectal morphine administration in opioid-naïve cancer patients with pain. *J Clin Oncol* 13:1004–1008, 1995

406. Westerling D, Lindahl S, Anderson KE, et al: Absorption and bioavailability of rectally administered morphine in women. *Eur J Clin Pharmacol* 23:59–64, 1982

407. Johsson T, Christensen CB, Jordening H, et al: The bioavailability of rectally administered morphine *Pharmacol Toxicol* 62:203–205, 1988

408. Moolenaar F, Yska JP, Visser J, et al: Drastic improvement in the rectal absorbtion profile of morphine in man. *Eur J Clin Pharmacol* 29:119–121, 1985

409. Hanning CD, Vickers AP, Smith G, et al: The morphine hydrogel suppository: A new sustained release rectal preparation. *Br J Anaesth* 61:221–227, 1988

410. Cole L, Hanning CD: Review of the rectal use of opioids. *J Pain Symptom Manage* 5:118–126, 1990

411. Pert CB, Snyder SH: Opiate receptor demonstration in nervous tissue. *Science* 179:1011, 1973

412. Yaksh TL, Rudy TA: Analgesia mediated by a direct spinal action of narcotics. *Science* 192:1357–1358, 1976

413. Wang JK, Nauss CA, Thomas JE: Pain relief by intrathecally applied morphine in man. *Anesthesiology* 50:149–151, 1979

414. Zenz M, Schappler-Scheele B, Neuhaus R, et al: Long-term peridural morphine analgesia in cancer pain. *Lancet* 1:91, 1981

415. Coombs DW, Maurer LH, Saunders RL, et al: Outcomes and complications for continuous intraspinal narcotic analgesia for cancer pain control. *J Clin Oncol* 2:1414–1420, 1984

416. Arner S, Arner B: Differential effects of epidural morphine in the treatment of cancer-related pain. *Acta Anaesthesiol Scand* 29:32–36, 1985

417. Plummer JL, Cherry DA, Cousins MJ, et al: Long-term spinal administration of morphine in cancer and non-cancer pain: A retrospective study. *Pain* 44:215–220, 1991

418. Wang JK: Intrathecal morphine for intractable pain secondary to cancer of pelvic organs. *Pain* 21:99–102, 1985

419. Max MB, Inturrisi CE, Kaiko RF, et al: Epidural and intrathecal opiates: Cerebrospinal fluid and plasma profiles in patients with chronic cancer pain. *Clin Pharmacol Ther* 38:631–641, 1985

420. Sjoberg M, Appelgren L, Einarsson S, et al: Long-term intrathecal morphine and bupivacaine in "refractory" cancer patients: I. Results from the first series of 52 patients. *Acta Anaesthesiol Scand* 35:30–43, 1992

421. DuPen SL, Kharasch ED, Williams A, et al: Chronic epidural bupivacaine-opioid infusion in intractable cancer pain. *Pain* 49:293–300, 1992

422. Nitescu P, Appelgren L, Linder LE, et al: Epidural versus intrathecal morphine bupivacaine: Assessments of consecutive treatments in advanced cancer patients. *J Pain Symptom Manage* 5:18–26, 1990

423. Paice JA, Magolan JM: Intraspinal drug delivery. *Nurs Clin North Am* 26:477–498, 1991

424. Eisenach JC, DuPen S, Dubois M, et al: Epidural clonidine analgesia for intractable cancer pain. *Pain* 61:391–399, 1995

425. Krames ES, Gershow J, Glassberg A, et al: Continuous infusion of spinally administered narcotic for the relief of pain due to malignant disease. *Cancer* 56:696–702, 1985

426. Penn RD, Paice JA, Gottschalk W, et al: Cancer pain relief using chronic morphine infusion: Early experience with a programmable implanted drug pump. *J Neurosurg* 61:302–306, 1984

427. Penn RD, Paice JA: Chronic intrathecal morphine for intractable pain. *J Neurosurg* 67:182–186, 1987

428. Onofrio BM, Yaksh TL: Long-term pain relief produced by intrathecal morphine infusion in 53 patients. *J Neurosurg* 72:200–209, 1990

429. Krames ES: Intrathecal infusional therapies for intractable pain: Patient management guidelines. *J Pain Symptom Manage* 8:36–46, 1993

430. Nitescu P, Sjoberg M, Appelgran L, et al: Complications of intrathecal opioids and bupivacaine in the treatment of "refractory" cancer pain. *Clin J Pain* 11:45–62, 1995

431. Jacox A, Carr DB, Payne R, et al: *Management of Cancer Pain: Adults Quick Reference Guide No. 9.* AHCPR publication No. 94-0593. Rockville, MD, Agency for Health Care Policy and Research, U.S. Department of Health and Human Services, Public Health Service, 1994

432. DuPen SL, Peterson DG, Williams A, et al: Infection during chronic epidural catherization: Diagnosis and treatment. *Anesthesiology* 73:905–909, 1990

433. American Association of Nurse Anesthetists Position Statement: Provision of pain relief by medication administered via continuous epidural, intrathecal, intrapleural, peripheral nerve catheters, or other pain relief devices, June 1990

434. Paice JA, Williams AR: Intraspinal drugs for pain, in McGuire DB, Yarbro CH, Ferrell BR (eds): *Cancer Pain Management* (ed 2). Boston, Jones and Bartlett, 1995, pp 131–158

435. Olsson GL, Leddo CC, Wild L: Nursing management of patients receiving epidural narcotics. *Heart Lung* 18:130–138, 1989

436. Paice JA: Intrathecal morphine infusion for intractable cancer pain: A new use for implanted pumps. *Oncol Nurs Forum* 13:33–39, 1986

437. Sechzer PH: Objective measurement of pain. *Anesthesiology* 29:209–210, 1968

438. Sheidler VR: Patient-controlled analgesia. *Curr Conc Nurs* 1:13–16, 1987

439. Citron ML, Johnston-Early A, Boyer M, et al: Patient-controlled analgesia for severe cancer pain. *Arch Intern Med* 146:734–736, 1986

440. Bauman TJ, Batenhorst RL, Graves DA, et al: Patient-controlled analgesia in the terminally ill cancer patient. *Drug Intell Clin Pharmacol* 20:297–301, 1986

441. Hill HF, Saeger IC, Chapman CR: Patient-controlled analgesia after bone marrow transplantation for cancer. *Postgrad Med* 28:33–40, 1986

442. Mackie AM, Coda BC, Hill HH: Adolescents use patient-controlled analgesia effectively for relief from prolonged oropharyngeal mucositis pain. *Pain* 46:265–269, 1991

443. Bruera E, Brenneis C, Michaud M, et al: Patient-controlled subcutaneous hydromorphone versus continuous subcutaneous infusion for the treatment of cancer pain. *J Natl Cancer Inst* 80:1152–1154, 1988

444. Kerr IG, Sone M, DeAngelis C, et al: Continuous narcotic infusion with patient controlled analgesia for chronic cancer pain in outpatients. *Ann Intern Med* 108:554–557, 1988

445. Grochow LB, Sheidler VR, Grossman SA, et al: Does methadone provide longer-lasting analgesia than morphine? A randomized, double-blind study. *Pain* 38:151–157, 1989

446. Hansen LA, Noyes MA, Lehman ME: Evaluation of patient-controlled analgesia (PCA) versus PCA plus continuous infusion in post-operative cancer patients. *J Pain Symptom Manage* 6:4–14, 1991

447. Ferrell BR, Nash CC, Warfield C: The role of patient-controlled analgesia in the management of cancer pain. *J Pain Symptom Manage* 7:149–154, 1992

448. Oncology Nursing Society: Resolution: Use of technology in pain management. 1991 Congress Oncology Nursing Society, San Antonio, TX, May 8–11, 1991

449. Ferrell BR, Rhiner M: Use of technology in the management of cancer pain. *J Pharma Care Pain Symptom Control* 2:17–35, 1994

450. Abram SE: The role of non-neurolytic blocks in the management of cancer pain, in Abram SE (ed): *Cancer Pain.* Boston, Kluwer, 1989, pp 67–76

451. Swerdlow M: Role of chemical neurolysis and local anesthetic infiltration, in Swerdlow M, Ventafridda V (eds): *Cancer Pain.* Lancaster, England, MTP Press, 1987, pp 105–128

452. Ritchie JM, Greene NM: Local anesthetics, in Gilman AG, Rall TW, Nies AS, et al (eds): *Goodman and Gilman's The Pharmacological Basis of Therapeutics* (ed 8). New York, Pergamon Press, 1990, pp 311–331

453. Ferrer-Brechner T: Neurolytic blocks for cancer pain, in Abram SE (ed): *Cancer Pain.* Boston, Kluwer, 1989, pp 111–124

454. Carson B: Neurologic and neurosurgical approaches to cancer pain, in McGuire DB, Yarbro CH (eds): *Cancer Pain Management.* Philadelphia, Saunders, 1987, pp 111–124

455. Amidei CS: Pain and pain syndromes, in Cammermeyer M, Appeldorn C (eds): *Core Curriculum for Neuroscience Nursing* (ed 3). Chicago, American Association of Neuroscience Nurses, 1990

456. Peteet J, Tay V, Cohen G, et al: Pain characteristics and treatment in an outpatient cancer population. *Cancer* 57: 1259–1265, 1986

457. Ahles TA: Psychological techniques for the management of cancer-related pain, in McGuire DB, Yarbro CH (eds): *Cancer Pain Management*. Philadelphia, Saunders, 1987, pp 245–258

458. Ahles TA, Cohen RE, Blanchard ED: Difficulties inherent in conducting behavioral research with cancer patients. *Behav Ther* 7:69–70, 1984

459. Breitbart W: Psychiatric management of cancer pain. *Cancer* 63:2336–2342, 1989

460. Spross JA, Burke MW: Nonpharmacological management of cancer pain, in McGuire DB, Yarbro CH, Ferrell BR (eds): *Cancer Pain Management* (ed 2). Boston, Jones and Bartlett, 1995, pp 159–205

461. Watt-Watson J, Donovan MI: *Pain Management: Nursing Perspective*. St. Louis, Mosby Year Book, 1992

462. Weinrich SP, Weinrich MC: The effect of massage on pain in cancer patients. *Appl Nurs Res* 3:140–145, 1990

463. Avellanosa AM, West CR: Experience with transcutaneous electrical nerve stimulation for relief of intractable pain in cancer patients. *J Med* 13:203–213, 1982

464. Ventafridda V, Sganzerla EP, Fochi C, et al: Transcutaneous nerve stimulation in cancer pain, in Bonica JJ, Ventafridda V (eds): *Advances in Pain Research and Therapy*, vol 2. New York, Raven Press, 1979, pp 509–515

465. Walsh M Sr, Brescia FJ: Clinitron therapy and pain management in advanced cancer patients. *J Pain Symptom Manage* 5:46–50, 1990

466. McCaul KD, Malott JM: Distraction and coping with pain. *Psychol Bull* 95:516–533, 1984

467. Bayuk L: Relaxation techniques: An adjunct therapy for cancer patients. *Semin Oncol Nurs* 1:147–150, 1985

468. Graffam S, Johnson A: A comparison of two relaxation strategies for the relief of pain and its distress. *J Pain Symptom Manage* 2:229–231, 1987

469. Blanchard EB, Epstein LH: *A Biofeedback Primer*. Reading, MA, Addison-Wesley, 1978

470. Fotopoulos SS, Graham C, Cook MR: Psychophysiologic control of cancer pain, in Bonica JJ, Ventafridda V (eds): *Advances in Pain Research and Therapy*, vol 2. New York, Raven Press, 1979, pp 231–243

471. Fleming U: Relaxation therapy for far-advanced cancer. *Practitioner* 229:471–475, 1985

472. Fotopoulos SS, Cook MR, Graham C, et al: Cancer pain: Evaluation of electromyographic and electrodermal feedback. *Prog Clin Biol Res* 132D:33–53, 1983

473. Spiegel D: The use of hypnosis in controlling cancer pain. *CA Cancer J Clin* 35:4–14, 1985

474. Barber J, Gitelson J: Cancer pain: Psychological management using hypnosis. *CA Cancer J Clin* 30:130–136, 1980

475. Spiegel D, Bloom J: Group therapy and hypnosis reduce metastatic breast carcinoma pain. *Psychosom Med* 45: 333–339, 1983

476. Syrjala KL, Cummings C, Donaldson GW: Hypnosis or cognitive behavioral training for the reduction of pain and nausea during cancer treatment: A controlled clinical trial. *Pain* 48:137–146, 1992

477. Turk DC, Rennert K: Pain and the terminally ill cancer patient: A cognitive-social learning perspective, in Sobel HJ (ed): *Behavior Therapy in Terminal Care: A Humanistic Approach*. Cambridge, MA, Ballinger, 1981, pp 95–123

478. Fishman B, Loscalzo M: Cognitive behavioral interventions in management of cancer pain: Principles and applications. *Med Clin North Am* 71:271–287, 1987

479. Agency for Health Care Policy and Research: *Managing Cancer Pain: Consumer Version, Clinical Practice Guideline No. 9*. AHCPR publication No. 94-0595. Rockville, MD, U.S. Department of Health and Human Services, Public Health Service, 1994

480. Grant MM, Rivera LM: Pain education for nurses, patients, and families, in McGuire DB, Yarbro CH, Ferrell BR (eds): *Cancer Pain Management* (ed 2). Boston, Jones and Bartlett, 1995, pp 289–319

481. Ferrell BR, Rhiner M, Ferrell BA: Development and implementation of a pain education program. *Cancer* 72: 3426–3432, 1993

482. Rhiner M, Coluzzi PH: Family issues influencing management of cancer pain, in McGuire DB, Yarbro CH, Ferrell BR (eds): *Cancer Pain Management* (ed 2). Boston, Jones and Bartlett, 1995, pp 207–230

# Chapter 21

# Infection

Jan M. Ellerhorst-Ryan, RN, MSN, CS

## SCOPE OF THE PROBLEM

Infection in patients with cancer is a problem of great concern to health care providers. The types of infections presenting the greatest problems for cancer patients have changed over the years as a result of emerging resistant and opportunistic organisms. Effective antibiotic therapy has decreased much unnecessary mortality, but more aggressive cancer treatments have also created physiologic and immunologic challenges that are yet to be resolved.

### Incidence

Infection is a major cause of increased morbidity and mortality in individuals diagnosed with cancer. To understand why individuals with cancer are susceptible to infection, it is necessary to understand normal host defenses and the mechanisms by which they are impaired by cancer and cancer therapy.

### Etiology and Risk Factors

Infectious processes may be the result of the underlying malignancy, intensive treatment modalities, prolonged hospitalization, or a combination of these factors. The term *immunocompromised host* refers to a person who has one or more defects in natural defense mechanisms significant enough to predispose to severe, sometimes life-threatening infection.[1] Examples of defective protective mechanisms and factors contributing to infection in people with cancer are listed in Table 21-1.[2]

**TABLE 21-1** Factors Contributing to Infection in Cancer Patients

Disruption of natural physical barriers
  Skin and mucosal damage due to cytotoxic therapy
  Indwelling catheters, hyperalimentation lines, or
    hemodynamic monitoring devices
  Mechanical obstruction of natural drainage pathways and
    physiological disturbance due to the tumor
  Colonization by new pathogens due to antibiotics

Decrease of phagocytic capacity
  Qualitative and quantitative defects of granulocytes and
    monocytes due to cytotoxic therapy
  Qualitative defects in phagocytic function due to the disease

Disturbances in cellular immune function
  Defects related to specific neoplasms (e.g., Hodgkin's
    disease) or advanced malignancy
  Prolonged corticosteroid therapy
  Prolonged cytotoxic therapy

Disturbances in humoral immune function
  Defects related to specific neoplasms (e.g, multiple myeloma
    or chronic lymphocytic leukemia)
  Prolonged cytotoxic therapy

Disturbances in the reticuloendothelial system
  Defects in macrophage function
  Splenectomy

Malnutrition
  Defects in phagocytic capacity, B- and T-cell function (e.g.,
    cachexia)
  Bone marrow defects (for example, severe vitamin and iron
    deficiency)
  Poor integrity of integumental and mucosal barriers

Reprinted from Schwartsmann et al,[2] by permission of Oxford University Press.

## PHYSIOLOGICAL ALTERATIONS

### Normal Anatomy, Physiology, and Scientific Principles

#### Integumentary, mucosal, and chemical barriers

Intact skin constitutes the most important physical barrier against invasion by both exogenous and endogenous organisms. The skin is made up of cornified layers of epithelial cells that cover the body and protect tissues against dehydration and invasion by harmful bacteria. When a break in the skin occurs, environmental microbes and those that normally inhabit hair follicles and sebaceous glands may enter the body and cause infection.

A second major defense against infection is the mucociliary activity found in the mucous membranes. The cilia of the epithelial cells that line the respiratory tract beat rhythmically to propel mucus and its entrapped foreign particles toward the nose and throat. In the gastrointestinal tract the cilia propel bacteria and waste products to be removed in the feces. Microorganisms constitute up to 60% of the weight of the stool; therefore, an intact gastrointestinal mucous membrane is essential to prevention of infection.

A variety of other mechanisms serve to protect the body from microbial invasion. Acid pH inhibits or prevents bacterial growth on the skin and in the stomach, bladder, and vagina. Microbicidal elements found in prostatic fluid and in tears also provide a protective effect.

#### Leukocytes

Leukocytes, particularly polymorphonuclear neutrophils (PMNs), represent a significant defense against infection. PMNs, which are also referred to as *polys* or *segmented neutrophils (segs)* are short-lived white blood cells (WBCs) that respond quickly to bacterial invasion. PMNs are the most numerous of the leukocytes, constituting 55%–70% of circulating WBCs. The primary function of PMNs is the destruction and elimination of microorganisms through phagocytosis, the process of engulfing and ingesting foreign matter. In addition, PMNs secrete chemotactants, chemical substances that alert the body to the presence of an invader. Chemotactants stimulate increased production of PMNs and macrophages and direct them to the site of invasion. Without sufficient numbers of PMNs, the body's ability to mount an inflammatory response is compromised.

### Monocytes and macrophages

Monocytes and macrophages constitute what was previously referred to as the *reticuloendothelial system.* Monocytes are released from the bone marrow before they complete the maturation process; thus they are initially only capable of limited phagocytosis. After migrating into the tissues, full maturation occurs and the cells are then referred to as *macrophages.* Under normal conditions more than 95% of these cells are mature tissue macrophages, while less than 2% are circulating monocytes.[3]

Macrophages can survive several months to several years.[4] They are highly phagocytic and play important roles in the inflammatory, cellular, and humoral responses. Following initial contact with a foreign protein, macrophages process and present antigens to lymphocytes, which stimulate the immune response and cytokine production. Monocytes also produce specific components required for the complement cascade.[5]

### Lymphocytes

Lymphocytes, the cells responsible for cellular and humoral immunity, provide long-term protection against a variety of microorganisms. They usually constitute 25%–30% of the total WBC count. B lymphocytes, responsible for humoral immunity, produce antibodies, which neutralize, destroy, or facilitate phagocytosis of foreign proteins. T lymphocytes, providers of cellular immunity, initiate a variety of activities that, directly or indirectly, result in elimination of microorganisms or other foreign substances. T-helper cells are the most numerous of T-lymphocyte subsets, normally constituting over 75% of total T-lymphocyte counts. T-helper cells serve as the principal regulators of immune function through secretion of protein mediators (cytokines) that act on other cells involved in the immune and inflammatory responses.[6] Cytokines produced by T-helper cells include interleukin-2 through interleukin-6, gamma-interferon, and granulocyte-macrophage colony-stimulating factor (GM-CSF). The immune response is discussed in greater detail in chapter 17.

### Cytokines

Cytokines are small protein hormones synthesized by a variety of leukocytes. Cytokines produced by mononuclear phagocytes (monocytes, macrophages, PMNs, and eosinophils) are referred to as *monokines,* whereas cytokines secreted by T and B lymphocytes are called *lymphokines.*

Cytokines initiate and/or regulate a number of inflammatory and immune responses. They include interferons, interleukins, growth factors, and colony-stimulating factors. Specific information about cytokines and cytokine activity is detailed in chapter 17.

## Pathophysiology

### Alterations in nonspecific defenses

***Disruptions in protective barriers*** Skin and mucous membrane integrity is frequently impaired by cancer and cancer therapy. Primary and metastatic tumor growth invades healthy tissue and disrupts normal circulation, resulting in ulceration and necrosis. Chemotherapy and radiation may further alter the integrity of skin and mucosal surfaces, particularly in the gastrointestinal (GI) tract.

Diagnostic and treatment strategies typically include a variety of invasive procedures, including surgery, venipuncture, peripheral intravenous (IV) infusions, bone marrow biopsies and aspirations, vascular access catheters, "fingersticks," and bronchoscopy. Infection rates associated with diagnostic and therapeutic interventions are high, depending on the type of tumor or treatment.

Host defenses are further compromised by neurological consequences of primary or metastatic disease involving the central nervous system (CNS). Examples include aspiration pneumonia due to loss of gag reflex and urinary tract infections associated with inability to empty the bladder.

***Changes in normal flora*** Undisturbed, endogenous microbial flora exist as a carefully balanced synergistic microenvironment within the host. Alterations in normal flora predispose individuals with cancer to serious opportunistic or nosocomial infection.

Over 80% of infections developing in individuals with cancer arise from endogenous organisms, nearly half of which are acquired during hospitalization.[7–9] Institutional sources of potential infection include personnel, food, air, water, equipment, and procedures. The most significant factor contributing to transmission of infectious agents during hospitalization is poor hand washing by health care personnel.[8,10,11] Antibiotic use commonly alters normal flora, allowing overgrowth of pathogenic organisms.

***Obstruction*** Obstruction, usually associated with solid tumors or lymphoma, may contribute to risk of infection by interfering with normal clearing and drainage mechanisms. Sites most often involved include the pulmonary system, biliary tree, gastrointestinal system, and urinary tract.

### Granulocytopenia

There is a direct relationship between the number of circulating PMNs (segs) and incidence of infection. Individuals whose granulocyte count is lower than 1000/mm[3] are considered to be granulocytopenic and at increased risk of infection (Figure 21-1). When the granulocyte count is less than 500/mm³, risk of infection is significant. As the length of therapy and duration of granulocytopenia increase, so does the incidence of sepsis.[1,7]

Because of the short life span of circulating PMNs (segs), their absolute number must be determined on a daily basis for granulocytopenic individuals. The absolute neutrophil count (ANC) is calculated using data from the total WBC and the differential, which specifies the percentage of WBCs by cell type. The differential also notes the presence of abnormal or premature WBCs. The ANC is determined by multiplying the percentage of PMNs (segs) and bands times the total number of WBCs. For example, a patient has the following hematologic profile:

*Total WBC:* 2200 cells/mm³

33% PMNs (segs)*

18% bands

42% lymphocytes

1% eosinophils

1% basophils

5% monocytes
*Differential

To calculate the ANC, use the following formula:

$$ANC = \text{total WBC} \times (\% \text{ PMNs(segs)} + \% \text{ bands})$$
$$= 2200 \times (33\% + 18\%) = 1122$$

The individual in this example is not granulocytopenic, since the ANC is greater than 1000. The total WBC count may be approximately the same from one day to the next, but the percentage of PMNs and bands may vary significantly. The WBC count alone will not always provide enough information to determine the presence of granulocytopenia.

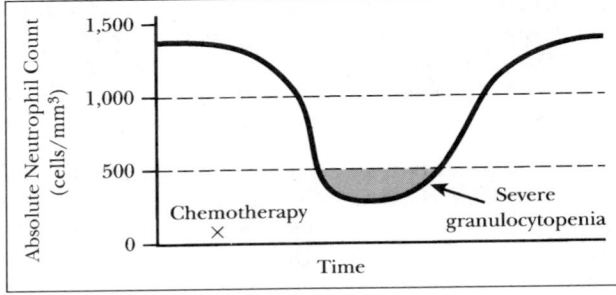

**FIGURE 21-1** Chemotherapy cycle. Days of risk for infection vary according to type of chemotherapy agent administered and individual response to treatment. The fall in the granulocyte count may begin a few days after chemotherapy or may be delayed for more than a week. Severe granulocytopenia occurs when absolute neutrophil counts are less than 500, and may persist for several days, a week, or sometimes longer.

***Implanted vascular access devices*** Surgically placed central venous catheters and ports provide long-term access for blood sampling and infusion therapy. These devices, however, are not without risk of complications, the most common being infection and thrombosis.

The incidence of catheter-related bacteremia is influenced by specific therapy, degree of use, patient population, catheter insertion technique, and care and maintenance procedures. However, neutropenia remains the primary risk factor for infection in vascular access catheters.[12]

Thrombus and fibrin sleeve formation have also been associated with catheter-related infection.[13] Thrombotic complications have been observed more frequently in patients with triple-lumen catheters when compared with double-lumen catheters, and in patients with catheter tips placed above the T3 level.[14] Urokinase is used in combination with antibiotic therapy to improve treatment outcome for catheter-related infections. It is thought that urokinase enhances antimicrobial therapy by removing sites of bacterial and fungal colonization in the lumen of the catheter.[15]

## Immunosuppression

***Infection*** Although infection is commonly viewed as a result of compromised immunity, certain infections actually contribute to impairment of immune function. Depression of lymphocyte function in vitro has been associated with a variety of viral infections, including cytomegalovirus (CMV), herpes simplex virus (HSV), and Epstein-Barr virus (EBV);[16,17] live vaccine (e.g., measles, mumps, and rubella); bacterial and mycobacterial infections, such as tuberculosis, leprosy, syphilis, and bacterial pneumonia; and fungal infections, such as candidiasis and coccidioidomycosis. It appears that both lymphocyte and macrophage functions may be abnormally depressed during and after acute infections, thereby extending susceptibility beyond the acute episode.[7]

***Acquired immunodeficiency syndrome*** Acquired immunodeficiency syndrome (AIDS) is characterized by loss of T-helper cells, resulting in progressive loss of immunocompetence, development of opportunistic infections and chronic wasting, impairment of the CNS, and emergence of unusual malignancies. The virus that causes AIDS, human immunodeficiency virus (HIV), has been isolated in blood, saliva, tears, urine, cerebrospinal fluid, semen, vaginal secretions, and breast milk. However, only blood, semen, and vaginal secretions are proven vectors, with limited evidence to suggest that transmission via breast milk is possible.[18]

Common opportunistic infections associated with AIDS include CMV, HSV, herpes zoster, *Candida albicans, Cryptococcus, Pneumocystis carinii, Toxoplasma gondii, Cryptosporidium, Mycobacterium avium* complex (MAC), and tuberculosis.

Infection with HIV is not synonymous with AIDS. AIDS is part of a continuum of illnesses related to infection with HIV. Many persons with primary HIV infection are asymptomatic even though they demonstrate seropositivity for antibodies to HIV. Others may have symptoms that can develop two to six weeks after primary infection, including lymphadenopathy, fever, rigors, arthralgia, rash, abdominal cramping, and diarrhea. These symptoms are often accompanied by mild immunologic deficiencies, including lymphopenia and thrombocytopenia, and transient elevations in hepatic enzymes.[19]

### Tumor-associated abnormalities

The types of infections that occur in persons diagnosed with cancer are somewhat predictable. Abnormal cell-mediated immunity in Hodgkin's disease and acute leukemia is associated with increased incidence of intracellular pathogens, including herpes zoster, *Cryptococcus neoformans*, *Brucella* species, *Mycobacterium tuberculosis*, *Listeria monocytogenes*, *Salmonella* species, and *T gondii*. Other malignancies such as advanced lung cancer and intracranial tumors are associated with a decreased sensitivity and an impaired ability to respond to a challenging antigen.[7,8]

The spleen has two major roles in infection management. The spleen serves as a mechanical filter, removing bacteria from the bloodstream, and it also participates in antibody production.[1,7] Individuals who are asplenic as a result of trauma, staging laparotomy for malignant lymphoma, hypersplenism, or sickle-cell disease have impaired opsonization that can increase susceptibility to infection.[1,16] The risk of overwhelming sepsis and death in persons with asplenia, especially those with Hodgkin's disease, is at least 50 times greater than in the normal population. It has been noted, however, that individuals with Hodgkin's disease in complete remission have a 2.30% cumulative risk of overwhelming postsplenectomy infection, whereas the rate of infection increases to 15.25% for those in whom relapse has occurred.[20]

Febrile episodes occur frequently in individuals diagnosed with cancer. Although fever may be caused by the underlying cancer, 55%–70% of fevers result from infection, especially during periods of granulocytopenia.[4,21] Lymphomas, hypernephromas, and hepatomas may cause fever unrelated to infection. In addition, tumor masses that cause local obstruction or compromise blood supply to normal tissue can predispose tissue to necrosis, local infection, and fever. Fever caused by an underlying cancer cannot be distinguished, on the basis of duration or the degree of temperature elevation, from fever caused by infection. Excluding febrile episodes related to the administration of blood products and chemotherapeutic agents, which resolve spontaneously, fevers in the individual with cancer warrant thorough and prompt evaluation to rule out infection as the cause.

### Nutrition

Cancer can affect nutritional status in several ways. The tumor can interfere with the functional capacity of GI structures or organs and may cause inlet or outlet obstruction. Chronic obstruction can compromise the blood supply to surrounding tissue, especially if vascular impairment is severe or prolonged. The resulting necrosis and ulceration will predispose the affected areas to hemorrhage and infection.

Cachexia is a complex metabolic syndrome characterized by significant involuntary weight loss. The exact mechanisms responsible for cachexia are not completely understood, but it is believed that faulty metabolism of nutrients is a major factor. Nutritional research suggests that the failure of certain cachectic cancer patients to increase lean body mass despite adequate nutritional support results from the tumor effects on the host's metabolism.[22]

There is substantial evidence to support the existence of a relationship between malnutrition and a variety of immune deficiencies. Cell-mediated immunity is most often affected, with decreased lymphocyte numbers and diminished response to antigen. Phagocytosis and the complement system are also impaired.[7,23] Immune defects related to nutritional deficiencies can be corrected by oral supplementation or parenteral nutritional support.

### Cancer therapy

***Surgery*** Surgery is commonly employed in diagnosis, staging, and treatment of individuals diagnosed with cancer. Various factors can increase the incidence of infectious complications in the individual undergoing surgery, including the duration of preoperative hospitalization, extent of surgery, length of the procedure, presence and degree of hemorrhage and tissue ischemia, nutritional status of the patient, prior chemotherapy or corticosteroid administration, and, most importantly, presence of infection or wound contamination during surgery. Preoperative prophylactic antibiotics may be given to provide protection during the perioperative risk period. The choice of antibiotic is based on the operative site, potential pathogens, presence of prior infection, or heavy colonization with particular microorganisms.[24]

The surgical wound is the most common site of infection during the postoperative period. Wound infections range in severity from minor inflammatory responses to major infections that can be life-threatening. Distinctive patterns of microorganisms are usually seen in different hospital environments. Each institution's infection-control team monitors patterns, trends, and incidence of specific microorganisms resulting in infection. Special concern must be directed toward the detection of resistant organisms, which can develop with astonishing rapidity within the hospital environment, causing significant morbidity.

A greater risk of sepsis accompanies certain surgical procedures. Surgical instrumentation of the genitourinary (GU) and GI tracts is associated with higher incidence of morbidity and mortality.

***Radiation therapy and chemotherapy*** Radiation therapy and chemotherapy interfere with essential metabolic functions of the cell and can cause inflammation and ulceration of normal tissues, predisposing the host to infection. Doses of chemotherapy and/or radiation that can be safely administered are determined by toxicity to normal tissues. Fractionation of radiation doses and administration of chemotherapy in intermittent cycles have been effective in enhancing therapeutic benefit while limiting toxicity. The major risks associated with therapeutic radiation and cytotoxic chemotherapy relate to the induction of granulocytopenia and immunosuppression.

Chemotherapy can induce immunologic defects that lead to bacterial, fungal, parasitic, or viral infection. Not all chemotherapeutic agents, however, produce immunologic compromise. The potential effects and side effects of each agent should be reviewed and incorporated into the patient's plan of care and assessment (see chapter 16 for specific information concerning management of chemotherapy toxicity).

Hematologic competency can be adversely affected by radiation therapy. During radiation therapy leukocytes are the first to decrease, followed by platelets and erythrocytes. Blood counts are monitored during radiation, especially if a large area is treated or if significant areas of bone marrow are included in the radiation field. Intensive radiation therapy results in a substantial reduction in cellular immune function that may persist for more than one year following treatment.[17]

Depending on the total dose and type of radiation, skin and mucous membrane integrity may be impaired, thereby predisposing to infection. Radiation reactions include epilation, erythema, dry and moist desquamation, mucositis, and necrosis. Nursing care for the patient receiving radiation therapy is discussed in chapter 13.

## CLINICAL MANIFESTATIONS

### Bacterial Infections

Changing patterns in bacterial infections are primarily the result of improvements in antibiotic therapy. During the 1950s and 1960s, *Staphylococcus aureus* was the most commonly identified organism in immunocompromised persons. Development of beta-lactamase–resistant penicillins provided highly effective therapy against *S aureus* and led to the subsequent emergence of gram-negative organisms as the predominant pathogen. Empirical use of combination antibiotic therapy, incorporating third-generation cephalosporins, has greatly reduced the number of documented gram-negative infections. However, a recent resurgence of gram-positive infections is believed to be the result of increased use of central venous access catheters and the prevalence of methicillin-resistant strains of *Staphylococcus*.[7,25,26]

#### Gram-negative organisms

Despite current shifts in the patterns of infection, the primary cause of infection in granulocytopenic patients continues to be gram-negative organisms, especially *Escherichia coli, Klebsiella pneumoniae,* and *Pseudomonas aeruginosa.*[1,7,26] The most significant consequence of gram-negative infection is the potential for endotoxic or systemic shock. Endotoxins are lipopolysaccharide protein complexes found on the outer membrane of gram-negative organisms. The release of endotoxin by these organisms initiates a cascade of events that, unless interrupted, will rapidly lead to death for the neutropenic patient. The actions of endotoxins include release of endogenous pyrogens, resulting in a febrile response; alteration of the vascular endothelium, causing formation of microthrombi; activation of the complement, coagulation, and fibrinolytic systems; and release of bradykinin, histamine, and serotonin, producing vasodilation and increased capillary permeability.[27] Without early detection and prompt initiation of treatment, endotoxic shock leads to hypotension, tissue ischemia, multisystem failure, and death.

#### Gram-positive organisms

*S aureus* and *Staphylococcus epidermidis* are responsible for most gram-positive infections occurring during periods of granulocytopenia; however, certain species of *Streptococcus* may also be encountered.[8] Although less common, infection with gram-positive organisms may result in shock produced by secretion of noxious proteins called *exotoxins*. The most well known exotoxin, produced by *S aureus,* is associated with toxic shock syndrome.

#### Treatment

Empirical antibiotic therapy is treatment initiated before infecting organisms have been identified. To date, a standardized regimen for treatment of bacterial infections in individuals with granulocytopenia has not been defined. Selection of antibiotic agents must be individualized to consider the probable cause of infection and likely site of origin, as well as institutional patterns of infection and antibiotic resistance. In general the empirical antibiotic regimen should cover a broad spectrum of pathogens without significant risk for emergence of resistant organisms or drug-related toxicity. Common combination therapies include a β-lactam antibiotic and an aminoglycoside.[26] Third-generation cephalosporins and carbapenems, which have a very broad range of activity and high bactericidal levels, may be effective when used as single agents.[7,26,28,29] Vancomycin may be added if gram-positive organisms are involved or suspected.

### Mycobacterial Infections

Although mycobacterial infections are uncommon in individuals with cancer, they tend to be associated with defects in cellular immunity. Latent infections with *M tuberculosis* may be reactivated. MAC, common in individuals with AIDS, has also been observed in those with hairy-cell leukemia and in those undergoing intensive chemotherapy for non-Hodgkin's lymphoma.[1]

### Treatment

While isoniazid is the treatment of choice for tuberculosis, it is not effective therapy for MAC. Combination therapy has been more successful in treating MAC, including amikacin, rifampin, ciprofloxacin, ethambutol, clofazamine, and clarithromycin.[30]

## Fungal Infections

In humans, fungi can exist in harmony with other endogenous flora in a carefully balanced synergistic microenvironment. Alterations in this environment, such as disrupted integumentary and mucosal barriers, treatment-induced granulocytopenia, immunosuppression, and alterations in normal flora can lead to invasive fungal infection. Fungal infections have become an increasingly important cause of morbidity and mortality in individuals with cancer, particularly hematologic and lymphoreticular neoplasms.

Factors predisposing to fungal infection include severe prolonged granulocytopenia, implanted vascular access catheters, administration of parenteral nutrition or corticosteroids, prolonged use of broad-spectrum antibiotics, and damage to oropharyngeal or GI mucosa due to disease or treatment. Immunosuppressed individuals who develop new or progressive pulmonary infiltrates while receiving broad-spectrum antibiotics present a major challenge for differential diagnosis. The possibility of fungal infection must be considered.

### Candida

*Candida* is the most common cause of invasive fungal infection. The presence of *Candida* in the sputum, mouth, or throat cannot be definitively correlated with infection because *Candida* can reside harmlessly in the healthy host. However, the immunosuppressed person is at risk when granulocytopenia occurs and/or when cellular immunity is impaired. Broad-spectrum antibiotics alter the function of normal bacterial flora and therefore are associated with increased risk of fungal overgrowth and infection.

Dermatologic infections with *Candida* occur most frequently in skin folds, such as the groin, perineum and perianal areas, and under the breasts. Oral candidiasis (thrush) is a common yeast infection that can disseminate throughout the GI tract. Disseminated candidiasis often involves the lungs, kidneys, bones, joints, and CNS.

### Aspergillus

*Aspergillus* is another common fungus that causes serious infections in individuals with cancer, particularly those who are granulocytopenic and/or are receiving immunosuppressive therapy. The fungus enters the host through the upper airway and typically causes pneumonia or sinus infection. Nosocomial transmission of *Aspergillus* has occurred in hospitals where spores contained in construction materials were disseminated through the ventilation system.

Aspergillosis is characterized by blood vessel invasion, which can lead to thrombosis and infarction of pulmonary arteries and veins. Blood cultures are rarely positive, even in disseminated aspergillosis. The infection is difficult to diagnose, often necessitating aggressive treatment before the diagnosis is confirmed. Without prompt and aggressive therapy with amphotericin, *Aspergillus* pneumonia is almost always fatal in granulocytopenic patients.[31,32]

### Cryptococcus

*Cryptococcus neoformans,* a yeast found in soil and in pigeon excreta, is generally acquired by inhalation. The infection appears most often in individuals with advanced Hodgkin's disease and other lymphomas. It commonly occurs as an insidious meningoencephalitis. Headache, vomiting, and diplopia without fever are typical symptoms. Cerebrospinal fluid examination reveals mononuclear pleocytosis and a low glucose level. Intrathecal administration of antifungal agents may be required for individuals whose cerebrospinal fluid does not clear with IV therapy. As with other fungi, cryptococcal infection can also occur in the lungs and disseminate to visceral organs.

### Histoplasma

Histoplasmosis generally occurs as a pulmonary infection, usually in individuals with lymphoreticular neoplasms. The infection commonly disseminates, causing adenopathy and hepatosplenomegaly, which may be confused with the underlying neoplasm. Disseminated histoplasmosis can occur in individuals whose cancer is in remission, as well as in those with active disease; therefore, histological examination of biopsy material for *Histoplasma* is necessary if this organism is suspected as a cause of infection.

### Phycomycetes

The Phycomycetes (*Mucor, Rhizopus,* and *Absidia*) are opportunistic fungi widespread in dust and air. The lungs, nasal sinuses, and GI tract are the three major sites of infection. After the fungi are inhaled into the lungs, the disease may disseminate to other body sites. Person-to-person transmission is rare.

### Coccidioides

*Coccidioides* is found in the soil of the southwestern United States and typically enters the body by inhalation. The organism is rapidly phagocytized in individuals who have a competent immune system and may cause no symptoms. Immunocompromised individuals, however, are susceptible to the development of serious pulmonary infection.[33]

### Treatment

Two major problems in treatment of fungal infections are the difficulty associated with culturing organisms from infected tissues and the limited number of effective agents available to manage severe fungal infections.

Amphotericin B is the drug of choice for treatment of systemic fungal infections. However, it is associated with significant side effects and toxicities, including fever, chills, rigors, nausea, vomiting, hypotension, bronchospasm, and occasionally seizures.

Premedication with acetaminophen and the addition of hydrocortisone sodium succinate to the IV solution generally reduce the reactions associated with the drug. IV meperidine (1 mg/kg) can be used to ameliorate fever and chills that frequently accompany the initial administration of amphotericin.[34]

The major toxicity of amphotericin is nephrotoxicity. With continued administration, elevated levels of creatinine and blood urea nitrogen can occur. Electrolyte imbalances, particularly hypokalemia, are common and warrant careful monitoring of fluid and treatment.

Flucytosine (5-FC) is another antifungal agent used for treatment of *Candida* and *Cryptococcus* infections. The major limitation to its use is the rapid onset of drug resistance. 5-FC is well absorbed orally, with side effects that include nausea, vomiting, diarrhea, myelosuppression, skin rash, nephrotoxicity, and hepatotoxicity.[34] 5-FC is commonly used in combination with amphotericin.

The antifungal agent fluconazole is well absorbed and is able to penetrate into cerebrospinal fluid, the eye, and peritoneal fluid. It is available in oral and parenteral form. Fluconazole is most often used to treat cryptococcal meningitis and oropharyngeal, esophageal, and systemic *Candida* infections. Side effects include exfoliative skin disorders (blistering, peeling, etc.), hepatotoxicity, and, less frequently, GI disturbances and headaches.[34]

Ketoconazole, another oral antifungal agent, is used to treat disseminated and pulmonary coccidioidomycosis, candidiasis, and histoplasmosis. The most frequent side effects are nausea, vomiting, and diarrhea. Rare instances of hepatotoxicity have been reported. High-dose ketoconazole therapy has been shown to suppress corticosteroid secretion, resulting in menstrual irregularities and decreased male libido.[34]

The oral agent itraconazole may be used in the treatment of aspergillosis in persons who are intolerant of or resistant to amphotericin. It may also be prescribed for treatment of histoplasmosis. Itraconazole should be taken with food to increase absorption. Patients with achlorhydria may require dosage elevations to compensate for decreased drug absorption.[34]

Miconazole is a parenteral antifungal agent primarily considered to be second-line therapy. It may be prescribed for treatment of candidiasis, coccidioidomycosis, and cryptococcosis. For treatment of fungal meningitis, IV miconazole must be supplemented with intrathecal administration to achieve therapeutic drug levels. Side effects include hypersensitivity reactions, phlebitis, GI disturbances, and, less frequently, anemia and thrombocytopenia. Infusions should be administered over a period of about two hours per 200-mg dose to prevent cardiac arrhythmias.[34]

## Viral Infections

Viruses, the smallest known infectious microorganisms, are visible only with the aid of an electron microscope. Viruses have no intrinsic energy system and consist only of a deoxyribonucleic acid (DNA) or ribonucleic acid (RNA) nucleus surrounded by a protein coat. Viruses are replicated by host cell mechanisms after invasion by a single virus. The primary virus invades the cell and initiates the formation of similar viruses by the host cell. Common viruses cause measles, mumps, rubella, respiratory infections, colds, and bronchitis. Most viral infections in granulocytopenic patients are caused by herpes viruses: HSV, varicella zoster virus (VZV), and CMV.

### Herpes simplex

HSV can cause serious infection in persons with cancer, from either primary exposure to or reactivation of a latent virus. Major sites of infection are the oropharynx, esophagus, eyes, skin, urogenital tract, and perianal area. In rare cases of HSV dissemination, pulmonary, CNS, and hepatic involvement may be seen.

Individuals with impaired cell-mediated immunity are at increased risk for recurrent HSV infections resulting in extensive mucocutaneous ulceration. Progression of the ulcers occurs as the virus, unimpeded by T-cell response, spreads across the squamous epithelium.[35]

### Varicella zoster

Infection with VZV ("chickenpox") can cause serious vesicular eruption in individuals with cancer, especially children, and results in a mortality rate of up to 18%.[36] Following primary VZV infection, reactivation ("shingles") can occur because the virus remains dormant in the spinal ganglia. Incidence of reactivation approaches 30% in those with Hodgkin's disease or following bone marrow transplant (BMT).[37,38] Radiotherapy can also increase the risk of developing VZV infection. Usually, dermatomes that are involved with VZV lesions have previously been encompassed in a radiation field.

Diagnosis of zoster is based on a history of chickenpox, characteristic dermatomal distribution of vesicular lesions, and positive culture results. Since skin lesions (vesicles) can become confluent, meticulous skin care is required to prevent secondary bacterial infection.

The major complication of VZV infection is visceral dissemination, resulting in pneumonitis, hepatitis, and meningoencephalitis. However, even in the immunocompromised patient, disseminated VZV is rarely fatal.[36] The risk of visceral dissemination is increased in individuals receiving chemotherapy during the time of infection, especially if lymphopenia occurs (<500 lymphocytes/mm³). Disseminated VZV is frequently complicated by secondary bacterial infections.

Varicella is highly contagious, and the risk of spread to other seronegative immunocompromised individuals is substantial, especially in adults with Hodgkin's disease and children with leukemia. Because of the severity of VZV infection in persons with cancer, infected individuals have been treated with varicella zoster-immune globulin (VZIG). When administered within 72 hours of exposure to VZV, VZIG generally modifies the infection to a subclinical or mild form. Management of individuals with cancer who are seronegative and who have been exposed to VZV includes interruption of therapy and administration of VZIG. Whenever possible, cancer therapy should not be reinstituted until the end of the incubation period, approximately 21 days. When clinical evidence of VZV infection occurs in individuals with cancer, immunosuppressive agents should be withheld until all skin lesions have dried and scabbed.

## Cytomegalovirus

CMV infection is usually a result of viral reactivation, particularly in association with immunosuppression. CMV is a common cause of interstitial pneumonitis in individuals with impaired cellular immunity or following BMT. CMV pneumonia characteristically occurs within three months of transplant and is often fatal.[39]

CMV retinitis is the most common opportunistic ocular infection noted in immunocompromised persons, especially those with AIDS. Direct viral invasion of retinal cells results in tissue damage, necrosis, and high risk of retinal detachment. Less commonly, CMV will infect the GI tract, resulting in esophagitis, gastritis, or colitis.

## Hepatitis virus

Hepatitis in individuals with cancer can occur as a primary infection with one of the hepatitis viruses (A, B [HBV], or C [HCV]) or as a secondary infection with other viruses. HBV and HCV are the major causative organisms in transfusion-related hepatitis.

Viral hepatitis occurs as an acute or chronic infection. Asymptomatic carriers may exhibit mild hepatic dysfunction. Although transfusions of blood products constitute the primary route of transmission, nonparenteral transmission occurs through sexual intercourse and contact with contaminated saliva, urine, and feces. Risk of infection to health care providers is high and warrants strict adherence to universal precautions outlined by the Centers for Disease Control (Table 21-2).[40] The CDC guidelines have been incorporated into the rules regarding occupational exposure to blood-borne pathogens released by the Occupational Safety and Health Administration (OSHA).[41]

## Treatment

Acyclovir is an antiviral agent preferentially taken up by cells infected with HSV and VZV. Treatment with acyclovir decreases viral shedding from infected cells, accelerates healing of lesions, and decreases pain and itching. Acyclovir offers significant prophylaxis against recurrent infection for immunocompromised individuals, especially those who have had allogeneic BMT. It is available in parenteral, oral, and topical forms; however, it is not well absorbed from the GI tract. Side effects are minimal and consist primarily of nausea, vomiting, diarrhea, and anorexia. Phlebitis is common with IV administration. Acute renal failure may occur if acyclovir is given by rapid injection, especially in patients with other risk factors for renal insufficiency.[34]

Vidarabine is an IV antiviral agent primarily used as second-line therapy for VZV and HSV infections. Due to poor solubility, the drug commonly requires 1.5–2 liters of

**TABLE 21-2**  Universal Precautions for Prevention of Transmission of Human Immunodeficiency Virus, Hepatitis B Virus, and Other Blood-Borne Pathogens

1. Never recap, bend, break, or clip needles.
2. Place needles and sharps promptly in an approved puncture-resistant container designated for needle disposal.
3. Use approved disposal containers in all areas.
4. Do not overfill containers.
5. Close container securely when three-quarters full.
6. Bag closed containers in red bags.
7. Protect open wounds from coming in contact with potentially infected materials.
8. Be sure to cover properly any broken skin surfaces.
9. Gloves are necessary when:
   a. drawing blood
   b. handling specimens that have obvious blood in them
   c. starting intravenous infusions (IVs)
   d. cleaning blood spills
   e. during cardiopulmonary resuscitation (CPR)
   f. suctioning (especially a new tracheostomy)
   g. changing dressings
10. Wear mask, gloves, and protective eyewear when:
   a. blood splattering may occur
   b. inserting or maintaining arterial lines
   c. doing oral care
   d. doing emergency procedures
   e. doing invasive procedures
   f. doing hemodialysis or hemapheresis
   g. doing peritoneal dialysis
11. Change gloves between patients.
12. Wash hands thoroughly before leaving the patient's room.

Adapted from Centers for Disease Control.[39]

fluid volume for administration. Toxicities include bone marrow suppression, GI disturbances, and neurological effects such as tremor, confusion, alterations in mentation and behavior, and ataxia.[42]

Ganciclovir is used in treatment of CMV infection. It is a virostatic agent and therefore does not eliminate existing CMV but suppresses viral replication. Ganciclovir is currently available in parenteral and oral forms. It has recently received FDA approval for administration via an intraocular implant for individuals with CMV retinitis who are intolerant of other forms of the drug. The most significant toxicities of ganciclovir are neutropenia and thrombocytopenia.[34]

Foscarnet is another virostatic agent that suppresses CMV replication. It also may be prescribed for acyclovir-resistant HSV infection. Oral absorption is poor; IV administration is required to achieve therapeutic serum levels. Primary side effects include anemia, nephrotoxicity, and hypocalcemia. Less common effects are CNS disturbances, including paresthesia, irritability, tremor, and headache.[34]

## Protozoa and Parasites

Protozoal infections are associated with defects in cell-mediated immunity. These organisms are ubiquitous, causing few problems, if any, in individuals who are immunocompetent. In the immunocompromised host, however, protozoal infections are often difficult to treat and quickly become life-threatening.

### Pneumocystis carinii

*Pneumocystis carinii* is most often classified as a protozoan based on its appearance, growth characteristics, and susceptibility to antiprotozoal agents. However, molecular and genetic analysis indicates that it is more closely related to fungi.[43] *P carinii* causes infection in malnourished infants, children with primary immunodeficiency disorders, persons with AIDS, and those with cancer undergoing immunosuppressive therapy. Clinical manifestations of infection include fever, nonproductive cough, tachypnea with intercostal retraction, and potentially life-threatening respiratory compromise. Rales are absent. Chest radiographs reveal hazy bilateral infiltrates, although some cases may present with unremarkable findings. Open lung biopsy is sometimes necessary to confirm the diagnosis.

### Toxoplasma

*T gondii* is an obligate intracellular parasite found in soil, cat excreta, and undercooked meats. It can remain encapsulated in host tissues, with reactivation of latent organisms causing infection. Persons at greatest risk include those with AIDS and those receiving immunosuppressive therapy for hematologic malignancies or prevention of organ transplant rejection. CNS involvement occurs in over 50% of infected individuals; however, in immunocompromised individuals the infection may be disseminated at the time of diagnosis.[39]

### Cryptosporidium

Although a common cause of enteritis in individuals with AIDS, cryptosporidiosis has only occasionally been observed in other immunocompromised patients. Routes of transmission include person-to-person, animal-to-person, and environmental particularly via contaminated water.[44] When severe immune deficiencies are present, cryptosporidiosis results in voluminous watery diarrhea and secondary malnutrition, dehydration, and electrolyte imbalance.

### Treatment

Untreated *P carinii* is fatal. Even with therapy, mortality is high. The treatment of choice for *P carinii* is trimethoprim-sulfamethoxazole. Side effects include rash, nausea, vomiting, hepatotoxicity, and myelosuppression.

In individuals with known history of sulfonamide sensitivity, dapsone-trimethoprim or atovaquone may be prescribed. GI absorption of atovaquone is low and variable. Absorption is significantly improved when the drug is administered with a high-fat meal. Atovaquone is usually well tolerated, with fever and skin rash the most common side effects. Side effects of dapsone may be more problematic, including hemolytic anemia, hypersensitivity reactions, blood dyscrasias, hepatic toxicity, and peripheral neuropathy.[34]

Pentamidine is effective in treating *P carinii* unresponsive to trimethoprim-sulfamethoxazole. Side effects, however, are troublesome and include azotemia, hypocalcemia, and hepatotoxicity. Rapid IV infusion may result in a precipitous fall in blood pressure. Severe, prolonged hypoglycemia has also been reported, usually associated with higher doses, longer duration of therapy, and retreatment within three months.[34]

Prophylactic treatment of high-risk patients is most often accomplished with trimethoprim-sulfamethoxazole. Alternative agents include aerosolized pentamidine, dapsone, pyrimethamine plus sulfamethoxazole, clindamycin, and atovaquone.[44]

Treatment with pyrimethamine plus sulfamethoxazole has been effective against *T gondii* in immunocompromised patients. Clindamycin can be substituted in patients with known allergies to sulfonamides.[45]

To date, there is no known treatment for cryptosporidiosis other than supportive therapy with antidiarrheal agents and replacement of fluid and electrolytes. Spiramycin is currently under investigation as an anticryptosporidial agent.[34]

# THERAPEUTIC APPROACHES AND NURSING CARE

## Prevention

Since most cancer care is delivered in the outpatient or home setting, nursing care focuses on prevention of infection, measures to optimize the person's health status, and aggressive therapeutic interventions when infection occurs. The individual with cancer and his or her family need to be well informed about protective self-care measures and symptoms of infection to report to the health care team. When an infection develops, prompt initiation of medical and nursing interventions is imperative to prevent life-threatening complications. Nursing care strategies for patients at risk for infection, including assessment parameters, interventions, and instructions for patients and caregivers, are summarized in Table 21-3.

### Reducing environmental pathogens

The single most important intervention to prevent infection is meticulous hand washing by every person who enters the room or comes in contact with the individual at risk for infection. Neutropenic patients are advised of their risk and are encouraged to remind staff, family, and visitors about hand-washing precautions.

When hospitalized, the patient is given a private room. Nursing assignments include consideration for whether a staff member has had a recent immunization or transmissible infection. Ideally, staff members caring for a patient with an active infection are not also assigned to a neutropenic patient. However, this precaution is probably unnecessary if thorough and meticulous hand washing is consistently performed. Visitors are also screened for recent immunization or transmissible infection.

When the ANC is less than 1000, live plants, cut flowers, and fresh fruit should not be brought into the patient's room. During times when granulocytes are adequate, bacterial content can be decreased by adding one teaspoon of chlorine bleach to each quart of water used in flower vases. Water in pitchers, denture cups, and nebulizers is changed at least once a day.

During granulocytopenic episodes, invasive procedures are kept to a minimum, with adherence to strict aseptic technique when they are performed. Indwelling urinary catheters are also avoided whenever possible. If any type of catheter placement is necessary, the smallest lumen size available is selected and the duration of use is kept as brief as possible. Communicating with laboratory staff to coordinate blood sampling can prevent unnecessary venipuncture.

### Optimizing health status

Adequate nutritional intake during periods of increased risk requires a high-calorie, high-protein diet. If severe neutropenia is anticipated, a low-bacteria cooked-food diet may be prescribed to minimize pathogenic colonization of the gut. A low-bacteria diet excludes fresh fruit, raw vegetables, fresh eggs, cold cuts, and many dairy products.[46]

Fluid intake is monitored to assure adequate hydration, especially during periods of nausea, vomiting, and diarrhea, and when therapy includes agents with bladder and renal toxicity. Supplemental IV fluid administration may be needed periodically.

Activities are organized to allow for periods of rest. Certain individuals may become frustrated or discouraged by their lack of stamina or endurance. Assisting them with realistic goal setting and planning may enable them to accomplish desired tasks without further compromising their health status.

Strategies to maintain skin and mucous membrane integrity are implemented. Meticulous personal hygiene is imperative, with strict attention to skin folds, including the axillae, perineum, groin, buttocks, and under the breasts. Mild soap and a water-soluble lubricant can help prevent drying of the skin. Shaving with an electric razor will reduce the occurrence of accidental cuts. Fingernails and toenails should be kept short; toenails that are difficult to trim should be brought to the attention of a podiatrist.

The optimal plan for oral hygiene includes use of a soft to medium toothbrush, toothpaste, and dental floss. However, periods of thrombocytopenia and oral stomatitis may require substitution of Toothettes® and normal saline. Oral care is performed after meals, at bedtime, and as indicated while the patient is awake.

Enemas, rectal temperatures, and suppositories are likely to traumatize fragile rectal mucosa and are avoided as much as possible in the high-risk patient. Prophylactic stool softeners are often recommended, particularly if hemorrhoids are present.

Activity consistent with current health status is encouraged to maintain optimal circulatory and pulmonary function. The patient is instructed and assisted in performing coughing and deep breathing exercises.

Although impaired cellular immunity and neutropenia are the primary causes of immunosuppression in individuals with cancer, humoral immunity can also be affected by either disease or treatment. Impaired humoral immunity compromises the efficacy of immunization, especially if chemotherapy is administered at the same time. Persons with cancer, especially those with acute leukemia, should receive pneumococcal and other vaccines only while in remission, since antibody response is limited during chemotherapy.[11]

## Management

### Early detection

In spite of strict adherence to protective measures, prolonged or severe neutropenia will allow rapid progres-

**TABLE 21-3** Nursing Care of Patient at Risk for Infection

| Problem | Assessment | Nursing Intervention | Patient/Significant Other Teaching |
|---------|-----------|---------------------|-----------------------------------|
| Potential for systemic infection | a. *Patient history:* factors that compromise immune function (e.g., cancer treatment, steroid use, nutritional status, chronic infections, HIV+)<br>b. Absolute neutrophil count<br>c. Vital signs<br>d. Comprehensive physical assessment<br>e. Response to antimicrobial, colony-stimulating factor therapy | a. Strict hand-washing measures<br>b. Appropriate protective measures (e.g., private room, protective isolation, dietary restrictions)<br>c. Adequate fluid/dietary intake<br>d. Adequate periods of rest<br>e. Aseptic technique for invasive procedures, dressing changes, etc. | a. Importance of hand washing<br>b. Rationale for protective measures<br>c. Importance of optimizing health status (e.g., diet, rest, personal hygiene)<br>d. Signs/symptoms of infection to report to health care team<br>e. Ability to read thermometer |
| Potential/actual disruption of skin integrity | a. *Patient history:* recent trauma to skin or conditions that predispose to disrupted skin integrity<br>b. *Physical assessment:* special attention to skin folds, wound sites; lesions suspicious for primary, recurrent malignancy<br>c. Characteristics of open areas (e.g., size, depth, discharge) | a. Meticulous personal hygiene, particularly to high-risk areas<br>b. Electric razors, dressing supplies less likely to traumatize skin<br>c. Moisturizing lotions, mild soaps to prevent drying, chapping, cracking of skin<br>d. Adequate fluid, dietary intake<br>e. Caution when moving bedfast patient<br>f. Activity consistent with health status<br>g. Special mattress to minimize pressure areas<br>h. Cultures of suspicious areas<br>i. Aseptic technique for dressing changes<br>j. Referral to home care agency for postdischarge follow-up | a. Self-care information regarding maintenance of skin integrity (e.g., avoiding exposure to sun, use of skin care products)<br>b. Rationale for precautions<br>c. Signs/symptoms to report to health care team<br>d. Proper techniques for wound care, dressing changes |
| Potential/actual pulmonary infection | a. *Patient history:* dysphagia, diminished gag reflex, tobacco use, asbestos exposure, COPD, HIV+, radiation therapy to chest, pulmonary toxicity due to chemotherapy<br>b. Respiratory rate, effort, use of accessory muscles<br>c. Chest auscultation<br>d. Recent changes in pulmonary status (cough, sputum) | a. Cough/deep breathing exercises<br>b. Activity appropriate for health status<br>c. Adequate hydration<br>d. Staff/visitors with respiratory infection restricted<br>e. TB testing<br>f. Review of x-ray, lab test results<br>g. Sputum specimen for culture<br>h. Aseptic technique when suctioning<br>i. Supplemental $O_2$ | a. Proper performance of cough/deep breathing exercises<br>b. Strategies for smoking cessation<br>c. Signs/symptoms to be reported to health care team<br>d. Home safety precautions when using $O_2$<br>e. Information about community resources |
| Potential/actual disruption of oral mucosa | a. *Patient history:* chemotherapy, radiation therapy to head/neck, HIV+, tobacco/alcohol use, periodontal disease, hydration/nutritional status<br>b. *Physical assessment of oral cavity:* color, moisture, lesions, ulcerations, amount and character of saliva<br>c. Patient's routine for oral hygiene, presence of oral pain | a. Oral hygiene plan—toothbrush, toothpaste, dental floss; cotton swab or Toothettes® if pain, bleeding preclude use of toothbrush<br>b. Normal saline, ¼ str. hydrogen peroxide, or sodium bicarbonate mouth rinses<br>c. Bacterial, fungal, and viral cultures if oral pain present<br>d. Adequate fluid intake<br>e. Topical or systemic analgesia for oral or esophageal pain<br>f. Water-soluble lubricant | a. Dietary modifications to reduce trauma to oral mucosa (avoiding spicy foods, temperature extremes, high acid content)<br>b. Consistent, thorough oral assessment and hygiene<br>c. Avoidance of tobacco, alcohol<br>d. Signs/symptoms to be reported to health care team<br>e. Use of dentures for meals only if oral mucous membrane integrity disrupted |

**TABLE 21-3**  Nursing Care of Patient at Risk for Infection (continued)

| Problem | Assessment | Nursing Intervention | Patient/Significant Other Teaching |
|---|---|---|---|
| Potential/actual disruption of rectal mucosa | a. *Patient history:* diet, sexual practices, medications, chemotherapy, HIV+, change in bowel habits<br>b. *Physical assessment of rectal area:* erythema, ulceration, hemorrhoids, bleeding<br>c. Character, frequency of bowel movements | a. Dietary modifications to reduce rectal trauma (increase fiber for constipation; low residue for diarrhea)<br>b. Avoid invasive procedures (e.g., rectal temperatures, suppositories, enemas)<br>c. Hygiene plan to prevent/ minimize anorectal excoriation, promote comfort (e.g., sitz baths, cotton balls or soft wipes instead of toilet tissue)<br>d. Stool softeners or antidiarrheal agents | a. Factors that increase risk of infection and strategies to reduce risk; dietary modification, alternative sexual practices, etc.<br>b. Signs/symptoms to be reported to health care team |
| Potential/actual genitourinary (GU) infection | a. *Patient history:* benign prostatic hypertrophy, HIV+, bladder-toxic chemotherapy; symptoms of GU infection (dysuria, urinary frequency, urgency, hematuria, pruritis, vaginal/penile discharge)<br>b. *Physical assessment of genitalia:* lesions, ulcerations, discharge<br>c. Characteristics of urine—color, turbidity, odor | a. Adequate hydration<br>b. Urine specimen (straight catheterization or clean catch) for culture and routine analysis<br>c. Culture genital discharge, lesions<br>d. Avoid indwelling urinary catheters<br>e. Antispasmodic; analgesic agents as indicated | a. Rationale, importance of adequate hydration<br>b. Signs/symptoms to be reported to health care team |

Reprinted with permission from Ellerhorst-Ryan JM: Nursing care plan for the immunocompromised patients. In Workman ML, Ellerhorst-Ryan JM, Koertge VH (eds.): *Nursing Care of the Immunocompromised Patient.* Philadelphia, Saunders, 1993.

sion of a localized infection to potentially life-threatening sepsis. When the inflammatory response is diminished or absent, classic signs and symptoms of infection—fever, erythema, edema, pain, and purulence—may not be present, making early identification difficult.

During neutropenic periods, patients need nurses with diligent physical assessment skills, including the ability to listen carefully to information provided by the patient and significant others and to identify subtle clues indicative of infection. The most reliable indicator of infection is a low-grade fever. A temperature elevation of 1° that persists for 24 hours may be the only early evidence of infection.

***Respiratory system***  The high incidence of pneumonia in immunocompromised patients mandates thorough assessment of the respiratory system. During hospitalization, chest auscultation is performed every two to four hours, depending on extent of risk, and with each nursing visit when at home. Neutropenic individuals may experience only slight temperature elevation and mild dyspnea if pneumonia is present. Assessment findings for upper respiratory infection range from pain, swelling, erythema, and discharge in nonneutropenic individuals to vague discomfort and possibly mild erythema in neutropenic individuals.

***Oropharynx***  The oral mucosa is often traumatized by chemotherapeutic agents, especially the antimetabolites and antibiotics. Local infections can occur if inflamed or injured mucosal surfaces become colonized with bacteria, predisposing to systemic infection. Teeth and gums in poor condition can become a source of sepsis during periods of granulocytopenia. Stomatitis can compromise nutritional status and fluid intake; when severe, it can necessitate interruption of chemotherapy.

The oral cavity is regularly inspected for white plaques, gingival edema, erythema, bleeding, and ulceration. Complaints of oral pain and dysphagia should be followed up with bacterial, fungal, and viral cultures.

***Gastrointestinal system***  Disruption of intestinal mucosa by anticancer therapy facilitates bacterial invasion and increases the potential for sepsis. If a granulocytopenic patient receiving broad-spectrum antibiotics complains of dysphagia and/or retrosternal burning, *Candida* or HSV esophagitis must be considered. Gastritis, enteritis, and colitis typically present with nausea, vomiting, diarrhea, and abdominal pain or tenderness. Hepatitis results in fatigue, anorexia, early satiety, and clay-colored stools. The perirectal area should be routinely inspected for signs of inflammation, infection, hemorrhoids, and fissures. Complaints of perineal itching, tenderness, co stipation, or pain with defecation can indicate early stages of perirectal cellulitis.

***Central nervous system***  Subtle changes in neurological function may signify either the onset of an infection or progression of malignancy. The development of any neurological abnormality warrants immediate attention.

CNS infections present with a variety of symptoms, depending upon the type and extent of infection. Typical complaints include headache, fever, visual impairment, personality changes, focal neurological signs, nuchal rigidity, altered mental status, and seizures.

***Urinary tract***  Urinary tract infections (UTIs) are common, especially in those cancer patients who have fever and granulocytopenia. Classic symptoms of UTI are typically absent in neutropenic patients. Observation of the clinical characteristics of the urine, specifically if cloudy and foul-smelling, is usually more helpful. *Candida* infection can result in erythema and pruritus in the perineal area.

***Skin***  Skin integrity should be regularly assessed, with special attention given to known areas of disruption at increased risk of breakdown.

***Cardiovascular system***  Symptoms of cardiovascular infection are generally nonspecific: fever, chills, malaise, and night sweats. Indications of possible cardiac infection include new or changing murmurs, thromboemboli, unexplained heart failure, and arrhythmias.[39]

## Nursing care during episodes of infection

Infection in the neutropenic patient is always considered a potentially life-threatening emergency. Fatality rates in untreated individuals during the first 48 hours of infection can exceed 50%.[9]

Cultures are obtained from all potential sites of infection, including urine, sputum, wound, stool, and blood. If vascular access catheters are present, culture specimens are obtained both from peripheral veins and through the catheter.

After culture specimens have been obtained, empirical broad-spectrum antibiotic therapy is promptly initiated and the patient's response closely observed. Monitoring for efficacy of antimicrobial treatment includes assessing vital signs every two to four hours; reviewing reports of chest x-rays and laboratory data, including arterial blood gases, blood counts, chemistry profiles, culture results, and serum antibiotic levels; and observing for signs of septic shock. If little or no improvement is apparent following three to five days of antibiotic treatment, cultures are repeated and the physician consulted about modifying the prescribed antimicrobial regimen.

Other supportive nursing care strategies include restoring circulatory fluid volume by administering IV fluids, blood or blood products, and vasopressors; maintaining adequate oxygenation through the use of supple-mental oxygen and, if necessary, mechanical ventilation. Additional measures are taken to promote optimal nutritional status by monitoring dietary intake, consulting with the dietitian, and conferring with the physician if enteral or parenteral nutrition is indicated.

## Treatment of infection

Persons with cancer who are not immunocompromised or granulocytopenic can be treated with appropriate antibiotic therapy for the specific infectious agent identified. Cultures are performed before the initiation of therapy and antibiotics are changed, if necessary, when the results of sensitivity testing are known. However, empirical treatment with a broad-spectrum antibiotic is initiated if a serious infection develops rapidly.

Patients who have fever during periods of granulocytopenia will have a thorough physical examination, chest radiograph, and appropriate laboratory studies. After cultures of all potential sources of infection have been obtained, empirical broad-spectrum antibiotic therapy is initiated.

Granulocytopenic patients may not manifest clinical evidence of infection because granulocytopenia prevents the mounting of an inflammatory response. Progression to systemic infection and septic shock is usually rapid. Therefore, individuals with granulocytopenia must be evaluated at frequent intervals for signs and symptoms of infection. Common sites of infection identified in patients with granulocytopenia and fever are listed in Table 21-4.

***Empirical antibiotics***  Empirical antibiotic therapy in the patient with fever and granulocytopenia reduces the number of infections that could become severe enough to be demonstrated by microbiological culture or clinical documentation. The decreasing incidence of septic shock in this high-risk population suggests that prompt aggressive antibiotic therapy is effective in reducing the serious

**TABLE 21-4**  Common Sites of Infections Identified in Febrile, Granulocytopenic Patients

| Site | Percentage |
| --- | --- |
| Mouth and pharynx | 25 |
| Respiratory tract | 25 |
| Skin, soft tissue, and intravascular catheters | 15 |
| Perineal region | 10 |
| Urinary tract | 5–10 |
| Nose and sinuses | 5 |
| Gastrointestinal tract | 5 |
| Others | 5–10 |

Reprinted from Meunier F: Infections in patients with acute leukemia and lymphoma, in Mandell GL, Bennett JE, Dolin R (eds): *Principles and Practice of Infectious Diseases* (ed 4). New York, Churchill Livingstone, 1995.

morbidity associated with gram-negative sepsis.[7,8] The particular empirical antibiotic regimen selected should meet the following criteria: provide broad-spectrum coverage for major pathogenic organisms; be synergistic and contain one bactericidal agent; and have minimal organ toxicity, satisfactory absorption by the route administered, consistent distribution to infected tissues, and adequate excretion.[47] Drug levels may be monitored periodically while the patient is receiving nephrotoxic antibiotics, and dosage adjustments made when indicated to maintain safe therapeutic levels.

*Isolation precautions and protected environments*  People with cancer receiving intensive therapeutic regimens are significantly more susceptible to infection than those receiving less intensive therapy. These severely immunocompromised persons are often placed on "protective" regimens intended to reduce the risk of infection. One such regimen, routine protective isolation, does not appear to reduce the risk of infection any more than consistent and frequent hand washing during patient care. Routine protective isolation fails to reduce the risk of infection from endogenous microorganisms or from colonization by contaminated hands of health care personnel.[48]

Efforts to exclude all microorganisms through use of patient isolator units (usually laminar air flow rooms), nonabsorbable prophylactic antibiotics, and sterilization of the patient's food and water may prevent or delay the onset of some infection. Therefore, these procedures have been recommended by some investigators for immunocompromised patients who have a predictable period of significant risk.[49,50] This is typically the period of greatest compromise associated with bone marrow transplants or high-dose chemotherapy.

Laminar air flow rooms are protected environments developed to protect the compromised host from exogenous and endogenous sources of infection. In this sophisticated isolation system, air is circulated through high-efficiency particulate air filters capable of removing from the air particles that are larger than 0.3 μm with a greater than 99.7% efficiency. The unidirectional (laminar) air flow significantly reduces air turbulence, which decreases the potential for microbial contamination in the consistently clean, protected environment. Semiportable units with horizontal air flow can be installed in regular hospital rooms.

To create an environment as free of microorganisms as possible, patients undergo cutaneous and GI decontamination with oral nonabsorbable antibiotics before entry into the room. All objects brought into the room are sterilized by steam or gas, and food is semisterile. Anyone who has physical contact with the patient wears gloves, mask, and gown.

The disadvantages of laminar air flow rooms are that the protective environment is elaborate, cumbersome, and expensive. In addition, the patient may experience depression due to social isolation and possibly psychotic episodes because of sensory deprivation. Although laminar air flow rooms reduce incidence of infection and improve short-term survival, they have not affected long-term survival.

*Granulocyte replacement*  Initial attempts at granulocyte replacement were in the form of granulocyte transfusions. However, limited efficacy, high cost, and serious complications, including development of lymphotoxic antibodies, made the procedure impractical.

Granulocyte colony-stimulating factor (G-CSF) and GM-CSF are hormonelike glycoproteins that promote the proliferation and maturation of phagocytes. Studies have shown that the duration of granulocytopenia following chemotherapy administration is markedly decreased when G-CSF or GM-CSF is used. In addition, mean recovery time for neutrophils following BMT is significantly shorter with the addition of CSFs.

## Approach to the patient with gram-negative sepsis

Shock develops in approximately 27%–46% of patients with gram-negative bacteremia,[10] resulting in inadequate tissue perfusion and circulatory collapse. Mortality approaches 80% unless vigorous treatment is begun promptly. The clinical syndrome is a result of a number of interrelated factors that include the direct effect of bacterial endotoxin on the cardiovascular system, activation of the coagulation and complement cascade systems, nutritional status of the patient, and the nature of the underlying disease. Signs and symptoms depend on the stage of shock, the causative organism, and the age of the patient. The first sign of impending shock in the immunocompromised host may be limited to a low-grade fever, shaking chills, and/or mild hypotension. Early recognition of sepsis and aggressive intervention are essential if irreversible damage to vital organs and subsequent death are to be averted (Table 21-5).

*Early (warm) shock*  Septic shock evolves through two phases that, although not always distinct, are characterized by different hemodynamic patterns. The early phase consists of vasodilation, decreased peripheral vascular resistance, normal to increased cardiac output, and mild hypotension. The signs of overt shock are not present in this phase. The patient may appear flushed with warm extremities and adequate urinary output. Central venous pressures are low, as are left ventricular and diastolic pressures, and respiratory alkalosis is present. During the early phase, peripheral vasodilation results in loss of fluid to the interstitial spaces. If myocardial function and fluid replacement are adequate, the syndrome may not progress provided immediate and appropriate antibiotic therapy is instituted. The duration of this early phase may vary from 30 minutes to 16 hours. However, if myocardial function is poor and volume replacement is inadequate, or if there is delay in initiating appropriate antibiotic therapy, severe life-threatening (late-phase) shock will develop.

**TABLE 21-5** Assessment of Patients with Septic Shock

| Assessment Parameter | Early Shock | Late Shock |
|---|---|---|
| Temperature | Low-grade fever, possible shaking chill | Febrile |
| Cutaneous | Flushed, warm | Cold, clammy; acrocyanosis |
| Cardiovascular | Tachycardia, normal to slightly low blood pressure | Hypotension, moderate to severe; decreased cardiac output; peripheral edema |
| Renal | Transient decrease in urine output | Oliguria, anuria |
| Pulmonary | Hyperventilation | Pulmonary edema |
| Central nervous system | Alert, possible mild confusion, apprehension | Restlessness, anxiety, confusion, lethargy, coma |
| Gastrointestinal | Nausea, vomiting, diarrhea | Hematemesis, melena, bright red bleeding from rectum |

*Late (cold) shock* The late phase of septic shock is characterized by a profound reduction in cardiac output, increased peripheral vascular resistance, oliguria, and metabolic acidosis. These factors create a cycle of vasoconstriction, ischemia, and vasodilation that result in irreversible damage to the heart, vascular system, kidneys, liver, and vasomotor center of the brain.

*Treatment of septic shock* The treatment of septic shock is based on two objectives: reversing the shock and treating the underlying sepsis. Individuals in shock require adequate oxygenation, effective circulation and tissue perfusion, nutritional support, and immediate, appropriate broad-spectrum antibiotic therapy (Figures 21-2 and 21-3).

Persistent hypotension despite fluid replacement may be managed through administration of vasoactive agents. In low to moderate doses, dopamine, the vasoactive agent of choice, increases arterial pressure without causing significant vasoconstriction and selectively increases renal, coronary, cerebral, and mesenteric flow.[34]

Any change in blood pressure, mental status, or urinary output in high-risk patients alerts the nurse to the probability of early shock. Once treatment has been initiated, nurses closely monitor for complications of shock, including disseminated intravascular coagulation, renal failure, GI bleeding, and hepatic abnormalities.

Finally, care is taken to meet the psychosocial needs of patients with septic shock and their significant others. The critical nature of septic shock, coupled with the inten-

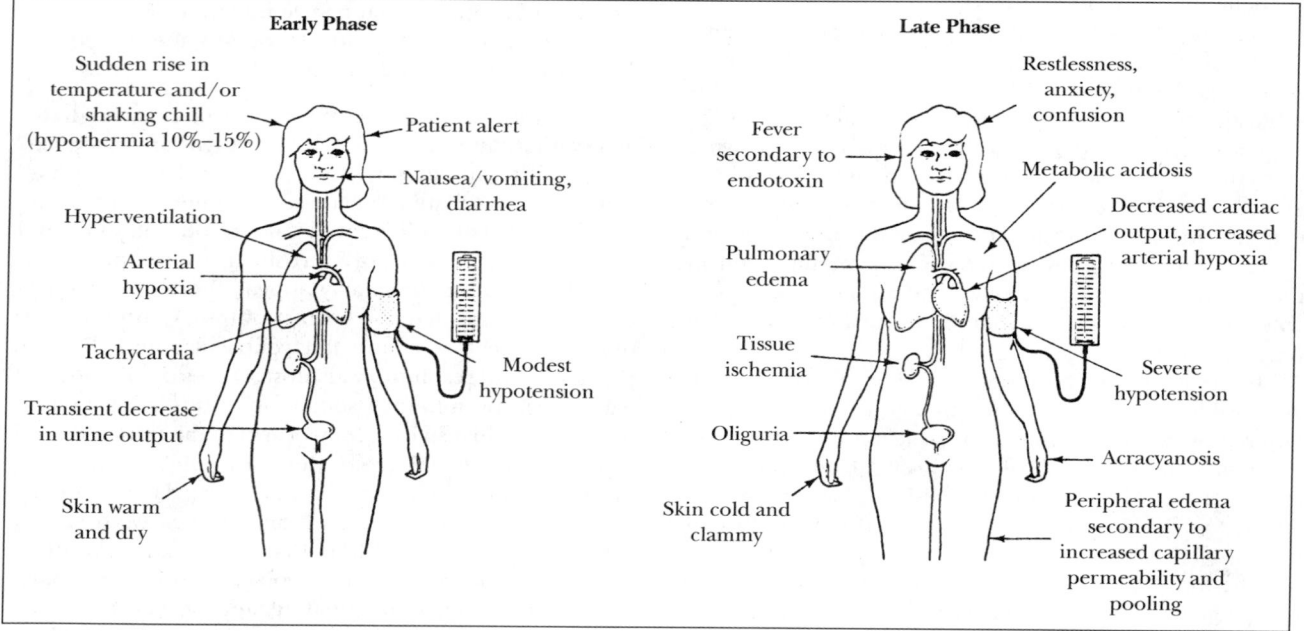

**FIGURE 21-2** Sepsis and septic shock.

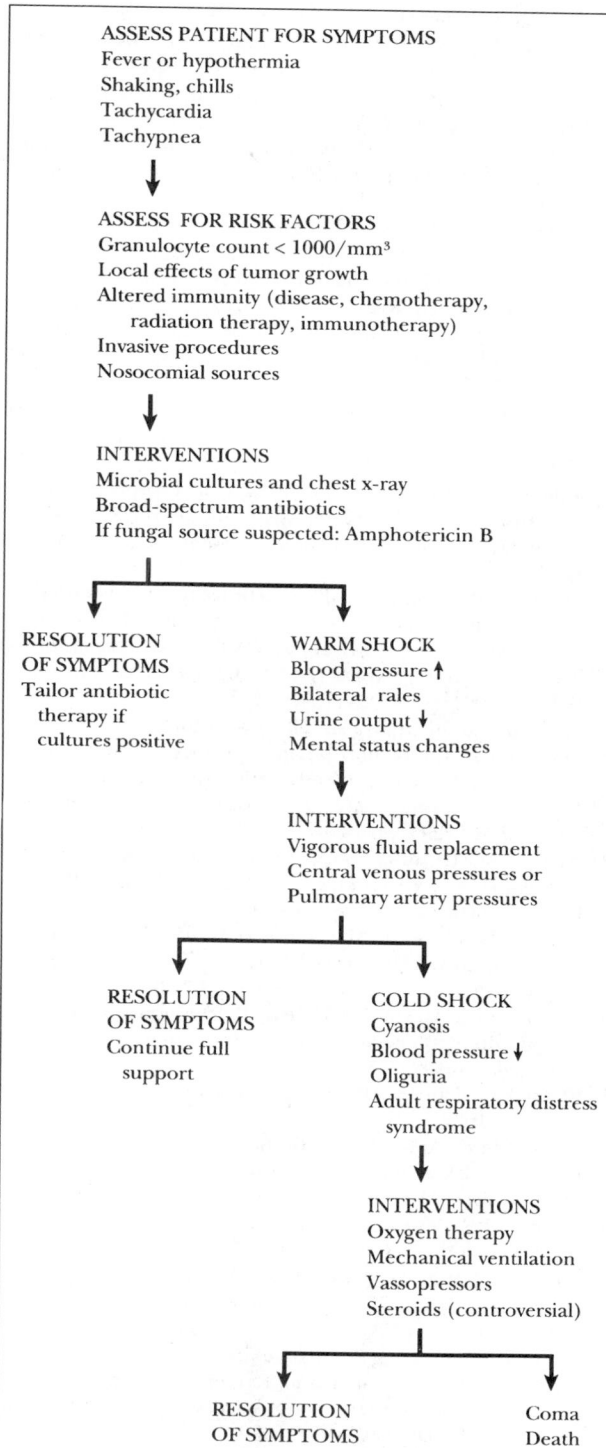

**FIGURE 21-3** Clinical pathway for septic shock.

sive treatment regimen, can be overwhelming. Patients may face not only fear of death but also loss of control and feelings of dependence. Nursing responsibilities include providing honest information, education, and assurance to both patients and family members.

### Approach to the HIV-infected patient with cancer

Nursing care of persons with AIDS, with or without malignancy, presents a unique challenge. These individuals are at increased risk for opportunistic infection not only because of HIV-related impairment of cellular immunity but also because of granulocytopenia secondary to cancer treatment and/or antimicrobial therapy (e.g., ganciclovir). Most opportunistic infections are the consequence of T-helper cell depletion and are caused by mycobacterial, viral, fungal, and protozoal organisms. Antimicrobial therapy is usually continued indefinitely, since discontinuing treatment commonly results in recurrent symptoms of infection. Side effects of therapy and progression of AIDS typically result in anorexia, nausea and vomiting, diarrhea, and malabsorption, which further compromise immune function.

## Continuity of Care

Education about risk of infection begins at the time of diagnosis. The patient and family are instructed about the impact of cancer and cancer treatment on the inflammatory and immune responses. They are also taught about blood counts, anticipated time until the nadir is reached, and self-care activities to minimize risk of infection. Information provided about prescribed dietary restrictions to prevent pathogenic colonization of the gut also includes the importance of thoroughly cleaning kitchen equipment, such as blenders and food processors, between uses.

The patient and caregiver must understand the necessity of communicating to the health care team any deviations from normal health status. Instructions include specific signs and symptoms of infection that are to be reported promptly. Temperatures are to be checked at least daily and at the same time of day. If the patient or caregiver is visually impaired or has difficulty reading a thermometer, a digital thermometer should be obtained.

If antibiotic therapy will be administered at home, patients and family members are informed of potential side effects, particularly those that are to be reported promptly to the health care team. Instructions include the dosing interval, dietary considerations that affect drug absorption, and the importance of compliance with the prescribed antibiotic therapy. If G-CSF/GM-CSF therapy is initiated, preparation and administration techniques are observed until safe and accurate performance of procedures has been adequately demonstrated. Referral to a home health agency should always be considered for an individual who is at risk for infection, especially if caregiver support is inadequate, if home environmental concerns are present (e.g., no indoor plumbing, possible insect or rodent infestation), or if reinforcement of instruction is indicated.

## CONCLUSION

Individuals with cancer are especially prone to develop infections as a result of impaired host defense mechanisms. Compromised immunity may be due to infection, nutritional deficiencies, tumor-associated factors, and/or cancer treatment. Most infections in this population are opportunistic and involve gram-negative and gram-positive microorganisms, although viruses, fungi, and protozoa are also involved in the spectrum of causative agents.

Infection in the immunocompromised person with cancer can quickly progress to life-threatening sepsis. Diligent nursing care directed toward prevention, early detection, and aggressive treatment is of primary importance for patient survival during high-risk periods.

## REFERENCES

1. Schimpff SC: Infections in the cancer patient: Diagnosis, prevention, and treatment, in Mandell GL, Bennett JE, Dolin R (eds): *Principles and Practice of Infectious Diseases* (ed 4). New York, Churchill Livingstone, 1995, pp 2666–2675
2. Schwartsmann G, Dekker AW, Verhoef J: Complications of cytotoxic therapy, in Peckham M, Pinedo HM, Veronisi U (eds): *Oxford Textbook of Oncology.* New York, Oxford University Press, 1995, pp 2307–2327
3. Locksley RM, Wilson CB: Cell mediated immunity and its role in host defense, in Mandell GL, Bennett JE, Dolin R (eds): *Principles and Practice of Infectious Diseases* (ed 4). New York, Churchill Livingstone, 1995, pp 102–149
4. Workman ML: Inflammatory responses, in Workman ML, Ellerhorst-Ryan JM, Koertqe VH: *Nursing Care of the Immunocompromised Patient.* Philadelphia, Saunders, 1993, pp 14–31
5. Phair JP: Laboratory assessment of immunocompetence, in Shulman ST, Phair JP, Sommers HM (eds): *Biologic and Clinical Basis of Infectious Diseases.* Philadelphia, Saunders, 1992, pp 87–93
6. Andre-Schwartz J, Schwartz R: Structure and function of the immune system, in Hoffman R, Benz EJ, Shatil SJ, Furie B, Cohen HJ, Silberstein LE (eds): *Hematology: Basic Principles and Practice* (ed 2). New York, Churchill Livingstone, 1995, pp 86–102
7. Pizzo PA, Meyers J, Friefeld AG, et al: Infections in the cancer patient, in Devita VT, Hellman S, Rosenberg SA (eds): *Cancer: Principles and Practice of Oncology* (ed 4). New York, Lippincott, 1993, pp 2292–2377
8. Schimpff SC: Infections in patients with cancer: Overview and epidemiology, in Moosa AR, Schimpff SC, Robson MC (eds): *Comprehensive Textbook of Oncology,* vol 2 (ed 2). Baltimore, Williams and Wilkins, 1991, pp. 1720–1732

9. Zimmer SH, Klatersky J: Infectious considerations in cancer, in Calabrisi P, Schein PS (eds): *Medical Oncology* (ed 2). New York, McGraw-Hill, 1993, pp 1073–1100
10. Martin MA: Epidemiology and clinical impact of gram-negative sepsis. *Infect Dis Clin North Am* 5:739–752, 1991
11. Klatersky J: Infections in patients with cancer: Prevention, in Moosa AR, Schimpff SC, Robson MC (eds): *Comprehensive Textbook of Oncology,* vol 2 (ed 2). Baltimore, Williams and Wilkins, 1991 pp 1749–1753
12. Howell PB, Walters PE, Donowitz GR, et al: Risk factors for infection of adult patients with cancer who have tunnelled central venous catheters. *Cancer* 75:1367–1375, 1995
13. Raad II, Luna M, Khalil SA, et al: The relationship between the thrombotic and infectious complications of central venous catheters. *JAMA* 271:1014–1016, 1994
14. Eastridge BJ, Lefor AT: Complications of indwelling venous access devices in cancer patients. *J Clin Oncol* 13:233–238, 1995
15. Jones GR, Konsler GK, Dunaway RP, et al: Prospective analysis of urokinase in the treatment of catheter sepsis in pediatric hematology-oncology patients. *J Pediatr Surg* 28:350–355, 1993
16. Robinson BE, Donowitz GR: Infections in patients with cancer: Host defenses and the immune-compromised state, in Moosa AR, Schimpff SC, Robson MC (eds): *Comprehensive Textbook of Oncology,* vol 2 (ed 2). Baltimore, Williams and Wilkins, 1991, pp 1733–1739
17. Sloas M. Rubin M, Walsh TJ, et al: Clinical approach to infections in the compromised host, in Hoffman R, Benz EJ, Shatil SJ, Furie B, Cohen HJ, Silberstein LE (eds): *Hematology: Basic Principles and Practice* (ed 2). New York, Churchill Livingstone, 1995, pp 1414–1972
18. Worth LA: HIV infection in women, in Cohen PT, Sande MA, Volberding PA (eds): *The AIDS Knowledge Base.* Boston, Little, Brown, 1994, pp 4.9/1–4.9/21
19. Crowe SM, McGrath MS: Acute HIV infection, in Cohen PT, Sande MA, Volberding PA, (eds): *The AIDS Knowledge Base.* Boston, Little, Brown, 1994, pp 4.2/1–4.2/7
20. Baccarani M, Fiacchini M, Galiene P: Meningitis and septicemia in adults splenectomized for Hodgkin's disease. *Scand J Haematol* 36:492–498, 1986
21. Klatersky J: Febrile neutropenia. *Supportive Care in Cancer* 1: 233–239, 1993
22. Blackburn G, Apovian CM, Bothe A: Nutritional factors in cancer, in Calabrisi P, Schein PS (eds): *Medical Oncology* (ed 2). New York, McGraw-Hill, 1993, pp 1149–1172
23. Chandra RK: Basic immunology and its application to nutritional problems, in Forse RA (ed): *Diet, Nutrition, and Immunity.* Boca Raton, FL, CRC Press, 1994, pp 1–8
24. Sawyer RG, Pruett TL: Wound infections. *Surg Clin North Am* 74:519–536, 1994
25. Kiehn TE, Armstrong D: Changes in the spectrum of organisms causing bacteremia and fungemia in immunocompromised patients due to venous access devices. *Eur J Clin Microbiol Infect Dis* 9:869–872, 1990
26. Meunier F: Infections in patients with acute leukemia and lymphoma, in Mandell GL, Bennett JE, Dolin R (eds): *Principles and Practice of Infectious Diseases* (ed 4). New York, Churchill Livingstone, 1995, pp 2674–2686
27. Warren J: Sepsis, in Shulman ST, Phair JP, Sommers HM (eds): *Biologic and Clinical Basis of Infectious Diseases.* Philadelphia, Saunders, 1992, pp 475–490
28. Bow EJ, Loewen R, Vaughn D: Reduced requirement for antibiotic therapy targeting gram-negative organisms in febrile, neutropenic patients with cancer who are receiving

antibacterial chemoprophylaxis with oral quinolones. *Clin Infect Dis* 20:907–912, 1995

29. Freifeld AG, Walsh T, Marshall D: Monotherapy for fever and neutropenia in cancer patients: A randomized comparison of ceftazidime versus imipenem. *J Clin Oncol* 13:165–176, 1995

30. Eccles E, Ptak J: Mycobacterium avium complex infection in AIDS: Clinical features, treatment and prevention. *J Assoc Nurses AIDS Care* 6:37–47, 1995

31. Walsh TJ: Invasive pulmonary aspergillosis in patients with neoplastic disease. *Semin Respir Infect* 5:111–122, 1990

32. Brown AE: Overview of fungal infections in cancer patients. *Semin Oncol* 17:2–5, 1990 (suppl 6)

33. Phair JP: Fungal infections of the respiratory tract, in Shulman ST, Phair JP, Sommers HM (eds): *Biologic and Clinical Basis of Infectious Diseases.* Philadelphia, Saunders, 1992, pp 208–220

34. United States Pharmacopeial Convention, Inc.: *Drug Information for the Health Care Professional* (ed 15). Rockville, MD, USPC, 1995

35. Yungbluth M: Infectious mononucleosis and viral infections of the upper respiratory tract, in Shulman ST, Phair JP, Sommers HM (eds): *Biologic and Clinical Basis of Infectious Diseases.* Philadelphia, Saunders, 1992, pp 120–137

36. Whitley RJ: Varicella-zoster virus, in Mandell GL, Bennett JE, Dolin R (eds): *Principles and Practice of Infectious Diseases* (ed 4). New York, Churchill Livingstone, 1995, pp 1345–1351

37. Finberg RW: Infection in the patient with neoplastic disease, in MacDonald JS, Haller DG, Mayer RJ (eds): *Manual of Oncologic Therapeutics* (ed 3). Philadelphia, Lippincott, 1995, pp 415–429

38. Rosenberg SA: Hodgkin's disease, in Calabrisi P, Schein PS (eds): *Medical Oncology* (ed 2). New York, McGraw-Hill, 1993, pp 401–415

39. Ellerhorst-Ryan JM: Infections in the immunocompromised host, in Workman ML, Ellerhorst-Ryan JM, Koertge VH, (eds): *Nursing Care of the Immunocompromised Patient.* Philadelphia, Saunders, 1993, pp 229–262

40. Centers for Disease Control: Universal precautions for prevention of transmission of human immunodeficiency virus, hepatitis B virus and other blood-borne pathogens. *MMWR* 37:377–387, 1988

41. Occupational Safety and Health Administration, United States Department of Labor: Occupational exposure to bloodborne pathogens. *Federal Register* 56:64175–64182, 1992

42. Hayden FG: Antiviral agents, in Mandell GL, Bennett JE, Dolin R (eds): *Principles and Practice of Infectious Diseases* (ed 4). New York, Churchill Livingstone, 1995, pp 441–450

43. Walzer PD: *Pneumocystis carinii,* in Mandell GL, Bennett JE, Dolin R (eds): *Principles and Practice of Infectious Diseases* (ed 4). New York, Churchill Livingstone, 1995, pp 2475–2487

44. Beaman MH, McCabe RE, Wong S, et al: *Toxoplasma gondii,* in Mandell GL, Bennett JE, Dolin R (eds): *Principles and Practice of Infectious Diseases* (ed 4). New York, Churchill Livingstone, 1995, pp 2455–2475

45. Remington JS, McLeod R: Toxoplasmosis, in Gorbach SL, Bartlett JG, Blacklow NR (eds): *Infectious Diseases.* Philadelphia, Saunders, 1992, pp 1329–1343

46. Carter LW: Bacterial translocation: Nursing implications in the care of patients with neutropenia. *Oncol Nurs Forum* 21:857–865, 1994

47. Wade JC: Infections in patients with cancer: Treatment, in Moosa AR, Schimpff SC, Robson MC (eds): *Comprehensive Textbook of Oncology,* vol 2 (ed 2). Baltimore, Williams and Wilkins, 1991, pp 1740–1748

48. Lynch P, Jackson MM, Cummings JM, et al: Rethinking the role of isolation practices in the prevention of nosocomial infections. *Ann Intern Med* 107:243–245, 1987

49. Poe SS, Larson E, McGuire D, et al: A national survey of infection prevention practices on bone marrow transplant units. *Oncol Nurs Forum* 21:1687–1694, 1994

50. Lynch LS: Infection in cancer patients, in Haskell CM (ed): *Cancer Treatment* (ed 4), Philadelphia, Saunders, 1995, pp 206–216

# Chapter 22

# Bleeding Disorders

Barbara Holmes Gobel, RN, MS

## SCOPE OF THE PROBLEM

Bleeding represents one of the most complex clinical challenges in the supportive care of the individual with cancer. The numerous and unique complications of each neoplasm, combined with the often toxic effects of various cancer treatments, create a difficult problem in the diagnosis and management of the individual with a bleeding disorder. Appropriate supportive measures are a vital aspect of the total care of these individuals. Supportive care may actually represent the difference between survival and death in an individual with a bleeding disorder. An exciting advancement in the supportive care of patients with cancer is the clinical availability of recombinant human growth factors. These factors are capable of stimulating the proliferation and maturation of bone marrow cells and promise to improve the results of chemotherapy. Growth factors may decrease the morbidity of current chemotherapy regimens, allowing drugs to be safely administered at higher doses or by a dose-intensity program.

Multiple hemostatic abnormalities may be involved in bleeding associated with cancer. Considerable differences exist in the presentation, proper management, and implications of these clinical problems. Minor bleeding may be the initial symptom that leads to the diagnosis of cancer. More severe bleeding may indicate the onset of a progressive or terminal disease. Because the morbidity and mortality of many bleeding problems are significant, prevention of the problem is clearly the best management plan. Rapid recognition, assessment, and knowledgeable treatment of the hemorrhagic complications of cancer will significantly improve quality of life, and possibly survival, for the individual with cancer.

This chapter includes a review of normal platelet and erythrocyte physiology, hemostasis, and coagulation, the etiology of bleeding associated with cancer, and patient assessment. Care of the individual with cancer who is experiencing bleeding, including both nursing and medical support, is reviewed. Blood component therapy and its use in cancer therapy are covered, as is home transfusion therapy. Finally, future perspectives on the issue of bleeding associated with cancer are discussed.

## PHYSIOLOGICAL ALTERATIONS

### Normal Hematopoiesis

Normal hematopoiesis is the process by which blood cells are formed. During fetal development the blood-forming organs include the spleen, the liver, and the bone marrow. The bone marrow is the primary site of hematopoiesis at the time of birth. During childhood this function takes place in the long bones, ribs, sternum, skull, pelvis, vertebrae, spleen, and liver. The major sites of blood cell development in adulthood include the vertebrae, ribs, sternum, skull, proximal epiphyses of long bones, pelvis, and spleen. The proportion of fatty marrow increases with age, so that only half of the ribs and sternum are sites of hematopoiesis in the elderly.[1] The marrow provides a differentiating inducing environment, known as the *hematopoietic inductive microenvironment* (HIM).[2] Within the HIM various elements interact to either enhance or inhibit hematopoiesis, depending on the type and balances of influences present at any time. These elements include the structural or stromal elements (fibroblasts, endothelial cells, fat cells) and the accessory cells (macrophages and lymphocytes) of the marrow. These elements can have a direct effect on early marrow cells through contact adherence or an indirect effect through release of substances known as *hematopoietic growth factors.*[3]

All of the blood cell lines derive from a pluripotent stem cell, or common progenitor cell. These pluripotent stem cells are capable of extensive, possibly lifelong, self-renewal and of differentiation to all cell lineages.[2] The stem cell normally is not in an active cell cycle.[4] When the cell is required to undergo division, as following injury or marrow depletion, a daughter cell leaves the stem cell pool and passes through a series of divisions and maturational changes. These changes culminate in the formation of the mature blood cells found in circulating blood. The processes of proliferation, differentiation, and maturation are mediated by various humoral factors. These factors are known to be predominantly an expanding set of hematopoietic growth factors, or *colony-stimulating factors* (CSFs). Refer to Figure 22-1 for an outline of blood cell development and the factors that mediate this process.

Early on in blood cell development the progeny of the pluripotent stem cell forms a population of *multipotent progenitor cells*. These cells are uncommitted to any one cell line and have a limited self-renewing capacity. The colony-forming unit (CFU-GEMM) is an example of the multipotent stem cell for granulocytes, erythroid, monocyte, and megakaryocyte lines. This stem cell can develop into any one of these cell lines. The lymphoid cell line follows a separate course of differentiation and maturation.[5]

As cells continue to differentiate they become committed to specific cell lines. At this level progenitor cells are called *unipotent* or *bipotent*, depicting their ability to follow, respectively, one or two cell lines. These cells include CFU-GM (granulocyte, monocyte, and macrophage), CFU-EO (eosinophil), burst-forming unit–erythroid (BFU-E) and CFU-E (erythroid), and CFU-Mega (megakaryocyte), and are considered committed stem cells.[3,5] Committed stem cells become increasingly differentiated and morphologically recognizable as belonging to a specific cell line. Ultimately the cell undergoes further division and becomes a mature component of the circulating blood.

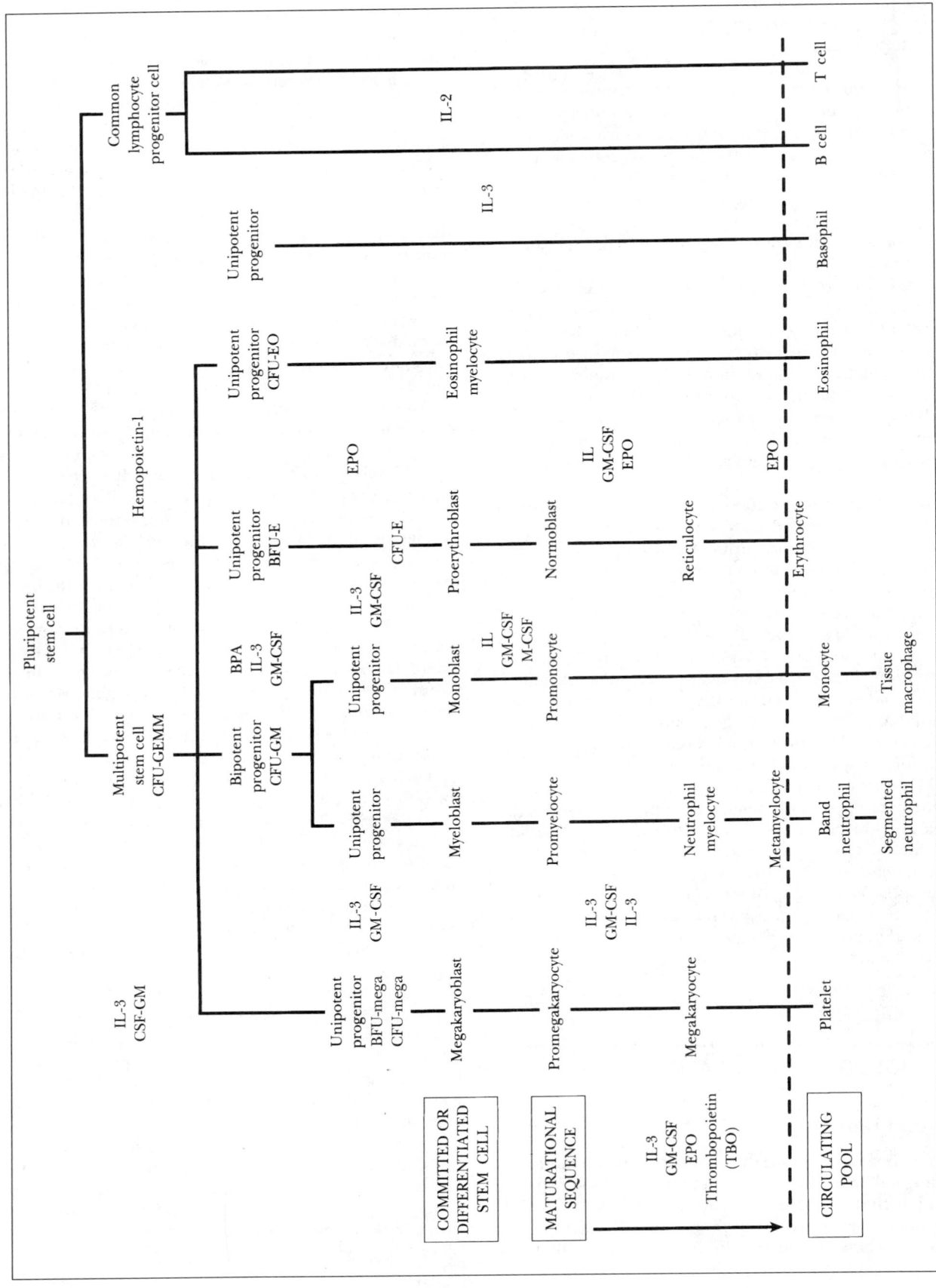

**FIGURE 22-1** Hematopoiesis.

## Colony-stimulating factors

CSFs are a set of hormonelike glycoproteins or cytokines that mediate hematopoiesis for all of the blood cell lines. These proteins govern the production of blood cells at every level of cell development, including the pluripotent stem cells.[6] CSFs appear to act on target cells via receptors on cell membranes. Different distribution of specific receptors may explain responsiveness to various CSFs.

Some of the CSFs appear to have their effect on more than one blood cell line. Interleukin-3 (IL-3), also called multi-CSF, is a growth factor for a variety of progenitor cells, as is the granulocyte-macrophage colony-stimulating factor (GM-CSF) (see Figure 22-1). These CSFs stimulate the growth of multipotential hematopoietic progenitor cells and of cells already committed to myeloid, erythroid, or megakaryocytic lines.[5] Other CSFs stimulate production of cells along single blood cell lines. Granulocyte-CSF (G-CSF), macrophage-CSF (M-CSF), and erythropoietin (EPO) stimulate the growth of predominantly granulocytes, monocytes, and red blood cells, respectively.[7] It is hypothesized that an overlap of the effects of one factor on another probably occurs, and that the CSFs are not truly lineage-specific.[8] CSFs appear to act on specific cells because of receptors that sit on the target cell membrane. It is the different distribution of these specific receptors that may help explain why these cells are responsive to certain CSFs and not to others.

CSFs are produced in the bone marrow, in the circulating blood, and by parenchymal cells in organs such as the kidney and liver. The stromal cells of the bone marrow and accessory cells (T lymphocytes and macrophages) in the marrow, and the peripheral circulation are primarily responsible for the production of the CSFs.[4]

## Erythrocyte physiology and function

The red blood cell (RBC) is a thin, biconcave disk-shaped cell with a thin membrane. The shape of the cell allows for oxygen transport and easy movement throughout the body. The normal RBC count in men is approximately 5.2 million cells/mm³, and in women 4.7 million cells/mm³.

RBCs are produced in the bone marrow from the pluripotent stem cell. Early stage of development is influenced by the following CSFs: burst-promoting activity (BPA), GM-CSF, and IL-3. The unipotent stem cell derived from the pluripotent stem cell is called the *BFU-E*, followed by a more differentiated progenitor cell called the *CFU-E*.[9] The reticulocyte is the immediate precursor of the RBC. The reticulocyte count is a useful indicator of bone marrow function with regard to RBC production. Once the cell becomes committed to the erythroid line, its development is induced by erythropoietin (EPO), one of the earliest identified of the hematopoietic growth factors. EPO is produced primarily in the kidneys in response to hypoxia or hyperoxia.[10,11] A small percentage of EPO is produced in the liver. Prostaglandin E and prostacyclin are also thought to induce renal EPO. The average life span of a red blood cell is 120 days. The cell becomes fragile as it ages, and it eventually ruptures, spilling its contents into the bloodstream. These by-products are then phagocytized by macrophages in the spleen.[12] The contents of the cell, including the membrane, are recycled in the body.

The major function of the RBC is the transport of hemoglobin, which carries oxygen to all tissues. The RBC also eliminates carbon dioxide, provides for hemoglobin synthesis and maintenance, and acts as a buffering agent in the blood.

## Platelet physiology and function

Platelets, also known as *thrombocytes*, are anuclear, disk-shaped fragments of large marrow cells, or *megakaryocytes*. Platelets are formed when the mature, granular megakaryocyte sheds its cytoplasm. The cytoplasmic fragments are released in the marrow and subsequently into the bloodstream. The normal platelet count in men and women is approximately 150,000–400,000 cells/mm³.

Platelets are derived from the pluripotent stem cell, which gives rise to a committed megakaryocytic progenitor cell (burst-forming unit–megakaryocyte [BFU-Mega]). Early-stage development is influenced by IL-3, GM-CSF, and EPO. Once a cell becomes committed to the megakaryocytic cell line, its production is also controlled by a growth factor called *thrombopoietin*, which is produced in the kidneys[13] (see Figure 22-1). Under normal circumstances, any reduction in the platelet count causes an increased production of megakaryocytes and platelets in the bone marrow.

Platelets remain in the vascular system and are not found in extravascular fluid. Normally about two-thirds of the platelet mass circulates in the bloodstream, and the rest is concentrated in the spleen. The life span of the platelet is about ten days. Most platelets die in repairing minor vascular injuries of daily life. Under normal conditions approximately 30,000 platelets are formed each day for each cubic millimeter of blood.

Circulating platelets perform several functions. First and most important is that of *hemostasis*, or the formation of a mechanical hemostatic plug. A second platelet function is to furnish a phospholipid surface, thereby facilitating the action of the clotting factors of the intrinsic system, which is an important component of hemostasis. Finally, platelets are necessary for *fibrinolysis*, or lysis of the fibrin clot, and vessel repair.

## Hemostasis

Hemostasis is the process by which the fluid component of blood becomes a solid clot. This process is initiated by vascular or tissue injury and culminates in the formation of a firm mechanical barrier, or a clot (made up of platelets and fibrin). The sequence of events after injury includes local constriction, platelet adherence to structures in the vessel wall, aggregation of platelets to form a hemostatic plug, and coagulation or solid clot formation.

When blood vessel injury occurs, vasoconstriction initially provides a minimal degree of control of the bleeding. Within seconds, platelets are attracted to and adhere to the underlying layer of collagen of the exposed subendothelial tissue.[14] Platelets then release a number of components, including calcium, serotonin, proteolytic enzymes, cationic proteins, thromboxane A, and nucleotide adenosine diphosphate (ADP).[14] ADP causes platelets to swell and become "sticky," thus increasing the adherence of platelets to one another. Increasing levels of ADP lead to clot contraction, degranulation, and ultimate fusion of the platelets. The end result of ADP-mediated platelet accumulation is the formation of a large platelet aggregate, or a hemostatic plug. Activated platelets also provide an anionic phospholipid surface for the clotting reactions that lead to thrombin generation, an essential precursor to fibrin. (See Figure 22-2 for the pathways to the formation of fibrin.[15]) This mass of platelets fills the gap in the vessel wall and arrests the bleeding, usually within five minutes. This primary hemostatic mechanism produces only a temporary cessation of bleeding.

## Coagulation

Blood coagulation may be considered a mechanism for rapid replacement of an unstable platelet plug with a stable fibrin clot. A series of interdependent, enzyme-mediated reactions ultimately act to activate fibrin. The fibrin clot is the final product of hemostasis.[16] When these enzymes or coagulation factors are stimulated, they become active in a sequential manner, not in numerical order (Table 22-1). This process often is referred to as the *coagulation cascade* (see Figure 22-2). Multiple inhibitors and control mechanisms keep these reactions localized to the site of the injury.

This process of the coagulation cascade has been an ever-evolving area of understanding over the years and recently has undergone substantial modification. Until recently the process of coagulation was interpreted as involving two separate pathways of factor activation: one initiated by tissue factor and the other initiated by contact activation and the activation of factor XII and factor XI. It is now known that people lacking factor XII (Hageman factor) do not experience significant hemorrhagic symptoms. Thus, it is generally accepted that factor XII is not involved in normal hemostasis.[17]

Coagulation is initiated by tissue factor, a transmembrane glycoprotein present on the surface of many cell types that is not normally in contact with the circulation. This factor is exposed to blood upon vascular damage. (It may also play a significant role in inflammation.)[15] Upon activation, tissue factor binds to factor VII as a cofactor and forms a complex; this complex is the plasma precursor (zymogen) to factor VIIa.[16] In the presence of calcium and anionic phospholipid, two natural substrates are activated—factors IX and X. The activation of factor X can apparently bypass any requirement for factor IX. The kinetics of this part of coagulation are not well understood, but it appears the factor IX–dependent route involves two enzyme-catalyzed reactions in sequence and can potentially promote extra amplification over the direct activation of factor X.[15]

The activation of prothrombin is catalyzed by factor Xa along with cofactor Va. Prothrombin is then converted to thrombin, the most powerful of the coagulation enzymes, which acts on fibrinogen to form fibrin.[16] This fibrin network is an essential portion of a clot. The clot is soluble until it becomes polymerized by factor XIIIa (fibrin-stabilizing factor), which converts it into a stable (insoluble) clot. Hemostasis is complete when the fibrin network alone is able to resist the hydrostatic pressure in the vessel.

Fibrin formation is an essential component of hemostasis, inflammation, and tissue repair, but it is a temporary reaction to an inciting stimulus. The fibrin clot must be remodeled and removed to restore normal tissue structure and function, as well as to restore normal blood flow. This is done by the fibrinolytic system that controls the enzymatic degradation of fibrin.

## Fibrinolysis

Fibrinolysis, or clot breakdown, is initiated by enzymes that are present in most body fluids and tissues (Figure 22-3). These enzymes, known as *plasminogen activators*, are present in most normal and neoplastic tissues as one

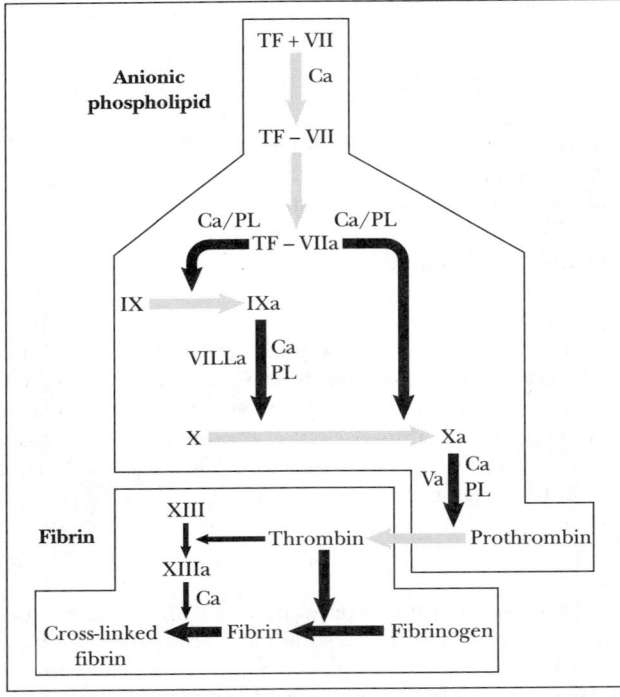

**FIGURE 22-2**   Blood coagulation. (Reprinted with permission from Jesty and Nemerson.[15])

**TABLE 22-1**  Normal Coagulation Factors

| Factor | Factor Name | Normal Range |
|---|---|---|
| I | Fibrinogen | 142–366 mg/dl |
| II | Prothrombin | 80%–120% |
| III | Tissue factor, tissue thromboplastin (extrinsic prothrombin activator) | 80%–120% |
| IV | Calcium | 8.5–10.5 mg/dl |
| V | Proaccelerin, accelerator globulin | 50%–150% |
| VI | Not assigned | |
| VII | Proconvertin, serum prothrombin conversion accelerator (SPCA) | 60%–140% |
| VIII | Antihemophilic globulin (AHG), antihemophilic factor (AHF) | 60%–150% |
| IX | Plasma thromboplastin component (PTC), Christmas factor | 60%–150% |
| X | Stuart-Prower factor | 60%–150% |
| XI | Plasma thromboplastin antecedent (PTA) | 60%–135% |
| XII | Hageman factor | 50%–150% |
| XIII | Fibrin stabilizing factor (FSF) | Present |

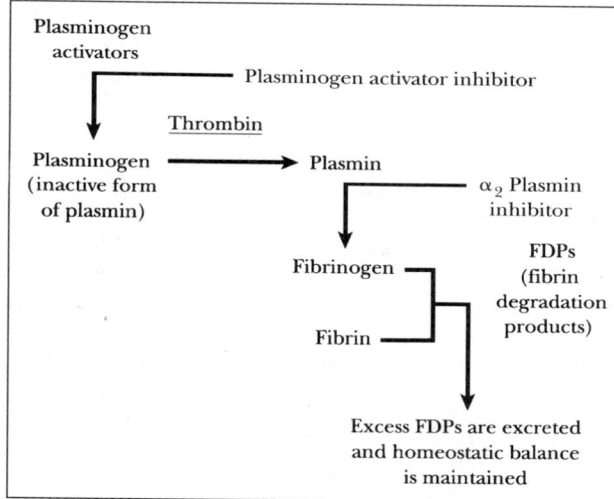

**FIGURE 22-3**  Fibrinolysis.

of two types: tissue-type plasminogen activator (t-PA) and urokinase-type plasminogen activator (u-PA).[18] Plasminogen activators activate plasminogen (an inactive precursor of plasmin) to plasmin in the presence of thrombin. It is plasmin that is responsible for the lysis of fibrin clots. The breakdown of fibrinogen and fibrin results in polypeptides called *fibrin degradation products* (FDPs), which are powerful anticoagulant substances that have a destructive effect on fibrin in the platelet plug. They also are able to impair platelet aggregation, reduce prothrombin, and interfere with polymerization of fibrin. When these products are increased in the circulation there is a predisposition to bleeding.[19]

Under usual conditions of homeostasis the processes of coagulation and fibrinolysis are localized to the sites of injury. These processes constitute a threat to the organism if they extend beyond the site of injury to the general circulation. This delicate balance of intermittent and localized fibrinolysis requires the coordinated interaction of plasminogen activators and naturally occurring inhibitors of fibrinolysis. The principal physiological inhibitor of plasmin is alfa$_2$-antiplasmin. Other inhibitors include alfa$_2$-macroglobulin, plasminogen activator inhibitor–1 (PAI–1), and plasminogen activator inhibitor–2 (PAI-2).[18]

# CLINICAL MANIFESTATIONS

## Causes of Bleeding in Cancer

### Tumor effects

Bleeding is a common presenting symptom of cancer, generally occurring as a result of tumor extension and local tissue invasion. Blood loss and the resultant iron-deficiency anemia are frequently the initial signs of lung, gynecologic, genitourinary, or colorectal carcinomas.[20–23] Bleeding may present as excessive pinkish, viscous sputum, which is typical of bronchoalveolar cell carcinoma, or as frank blood in the stool as a result of invasive left-sided colon cancer.

Frequently the most dramatic cause of bleeding in the individual with cancer is the invasion, erosion, and subsequent rupture of blood vessels. Any tumor involvement of vascular tissue or any tumor lying in close proximity to major vessels is seen as a threat of bleeding. Cancers of the large bronchi or lung may erode into the bronchial artery or branches of the pulmonary artery. Hemoptysis from tumor erosion into pulmonary blood vessels may appear as streaks of blood to gross blood loss. Head and neck tumors may also be associated with serious hemorrhage. Invasive neoplasms, particularly at the base of the tongue, can erode branches of the external carotid artery. Massive vaginal bleeding in individuals with pelvic tumor masses that invade major pelvic vessels is commonly seen in cervical carcinoma. Vaginal bleeding may also occasionally be seen with endometrial or ovarian carcinoma.

Other structural causes of bleeding that frequently occur in the individual with cancer include cavitational and ulcerative effects of local infections at sites of vessels; destructive effects of radiotherapy on normal structures in the radiation field; and denuded remains of vessels at the site of radical cancer surgery. One example of a surgical cause of bleeding is the potential of a carotid artery rupture after a radical neck dissection. This can occur more frequently when the patient has received prior radiotherapy.

Minor incidents of vascular bleeding that are eventually expressed as chronic occult blood loss occur in individuals whose neoplasms produce abnormal proteins of high viscosity. These paraproteins are common in individuals with multiple myeloma and Waldenström's macroglobulinemia. The hemostatic defects in patients with dysproteinemia are generally mild, although occasional patients have developed fatal hemorrhage.[24] Waldenström's macroglobulinemia is characterized by a malignant proliferation of lymphoplasmocytic cells and an overproduction of immunoglobulin M (IgM). The clinical manifestations of macroglobulinemia (bleeding, hyperviscosity, and neurological symptoms) are directly related to the overproduction of IgM.[25] The hyperviscosity associated with macroglobulinemia creates a circulating backflow in small vessels, thereby causing a vascular rupture with resultant microscopic hemorrhage.[26] A similar phenomenon is seen in individuals with acute leukemia with high white blood cell counts. Leukostasis, a potential complication of leukocytosis, results in aggregation and clotting of white blood cells in the microvasculature. This condition may mechanically stimulate obstruction, degeneration, and eventual disruption of small vessels, which results in bleeding.

In individuals with multiple myeloma, hemorrhage has been noted to be more common in those individuals with markedly increased serum proteins or viscosity, in patients who produce kappa rather than lambda light chains, and when abnormal platelet function was present.[27,24] A qualitative defect in platelet function can occur as a result of the M protein (myeloma protein or malignant protein of myeloma) coating the platelet and interfering with its function.[28,29] The thrombocytopenia associated with multiple myeloma is usually associated with chemotherapy and/or radiotherapy, or when the myeloma expands within the marrow compartment, further contributing to the risk of bleeding.

Invasion and replacement of bone marrow by tumor may affect hematopoiesis. This process, called *myelophthisis,* can result in anemia, thrombocytopenia, granulocytopenia, and impaired natural killer (NK) cell activity.[30] The decrease in production of normal marrow elements is thought to be a response to the physical "crowding out" of normal cells, competition for cellular nutrients, and the production by the invading cells' metabolic end products that are toxic to normal cells. Marrow infiltration may represent metastatic disease or a primary disease process such as acute leukemia in which the leukemia cells "pack" the marrow.

Clinically the individual may present with symptoms ranging from minor incidents of vaginal bleeding to gross blood loss. Direct injury to major blood vessels can lead to acute bleeding and a true oncological emergency. Specific symptoms depend on the site and extent of damage. Internal bleeding may present as massive hemoptysis, severe hematemesis, vaginal hemorrhage, loss of consciousness, or hypovolemic shock.

More gradual bleeding involving smaller circulatory structures is usually less obvious and therefore more difficult to diagnose. Melena due to colorectal carcinoma or the microscopic bleeding of macroglobulinemia can persist undetected until manifested by iron deficiency anemia. A continual loss of 6–8 ml of blood per day eventually will precipitate classic iron deficiency because the compensatory need for cell production exceeds the iron-producing capacity of the normal adult diet.

The most definitive diagnostic test for iron deficiency anemia is a bone marrow biopsy, which demonstrates absent stainable iron stores.[31] Other laboratory tests for diagnosing iron deficiency include studies to examine the RBCs and measurement of iron stores. Upon examination, the RBCs are small (microcytic) and irregularly shaped, with decreased amounts of hemoglobin (hypochromic). The serum ferritin level is decreased, which reflects a depletion in total body iron stores. The serum iron assay is often low but may be normal, and the iron-binding capacity is increased. The reticulocyte count is usually normal.[32,33]

The homeostatic mechanisms in the body provide such remarkable compensatory adaptation that iron deficiency anemia may be quite serious before the person actually develops significant symptoms. It is important to remember, therefore, that the onset of symptoms may reflect the rate of progression of the anemia better than does the severity. Fatigue, weakness, irritability, dyspnea, and tachycardia are typical clinical symptoms experienced by individuals with anemia.

Tumors lying near or on major vessels generally are treated aggressively to avoid complications. Surgery, radiotherapy, and/or chemotherapy are used to reduce or completely eliminate the neoplasm. If wound breakdown is in the neck area and carotid exposure occurs, wound debridement followed by a skin or skin-muscle flap carrying its own blood supply generally is done.[34] Prophylactic arterial ligation may be performed to minimize the risk of carotid hemorrhage. The patient who undergoes a bilateral ligation of the external carotid arteries runs the risk of a stroke. Small transient bleeding usually occurs before vessel ruptures. Careful observation can assist the caregiver in predicting and controlling such a complication. If vascular integrity is threatened by infection, antibiotic therapy is initiated. Preventing and treating infection is crucial in minimizing the potential for bleeding in the patient with cancer.

If acute bleeding occurs, direct methods to halt the hemorrhage are instituted immediately. Direct, steady pressure is applied at the site of bleeding. Mechanical pressure—such as insertion of an occlusion balloon catheter into the bronchus or the use of nasal packing during epistaxis—can be used if the site of bleeding is not directly exposed. Iced saline gastric lavages or enemas may help control gastrointestinal (GI) bleeding. Hypovolemic shock is to be avoided in situations of acute hemorrhage. Control of life-threatening hemorrhage is generally achieved by a combination of packed red cells with crystalloids or albumin, as opposed to whole blood, in correcting a volume deficit.[35]

Minor vascular bleeding due to capillary destruction is best controlled by treating the underlying malignancy. If iron deficiency anemia has occurred, oral or parenteral iron supplements are indicated. Oral iron preparations are often recommended since they are safe and usually correct the anemia within six weeks, but therapy generally continues for four to six months to adequately replace the iron stores.[32,33] Parenteral iron replacement may be given if the patient is not able to tolerate oral therapy or has a malabsorption problem. Iron dextran, generally given intravenously, requires a test dose because it is associated with a small risk of anaphylaxis.[32] If the hemoglobin level drops below 8 g/dl, blood replacement may be considered. Generally, blood replacement therapy is based on concurrent cardiac, pulmonary, or other conditions that can impair an individual's tolerance to anemia.

## Platelet abnormalities

Abnormalities of platelet production, function, survival, and metabolism frequently occur in individuals with cancer. These abnormalities may be due to a variety of causes. Generally, they are due to mechanical or humoral effects of the tumor itself or to abnormalities in the host induced by the tumor.

### Quantitative abnormalities

*Thrombocythemia* Thrombocythemia, also known as *essential* or *primary thrombocythemia,* is a clonal disorder of the multipotential hematopoietic stem cell. Thrombocythemia is characterized by abnormal expansion of the megakaryocytic progenitor cell part of the marrow. It is one of a group of related chronic myeloproliferative disorders, which includes chronic myelogenous leukemia, polycythemia vera, and ideopathic myelofibrosis.[36]

The major complications related to thrombocythemia are bleeding and thrombotic complications.[37,38] The most common sites of bleeding and potential hemorrhage associated with thrombocythemia are the mucosa and the GI tract, although bleeding at other sites such as the genitourinary tract and the skin can occur.[38] Thrombotic complications related to thrombocythemia are most frequently arterial in nature. The most common sites of arterial thrombosis involve the cerebrovascular, peripheral vascular, and coronary arterial circulation.[36] Deep vein thrombosis of the lower extremities can accompany thrombocythemia.

Care of patients with thrombocythemia may include no treatment for asymptomatic patients to a variety of platelet-reducing modalities. Platelet pheresis may be used for patients with acute and life-threatening hemostatic problems.[36] This treatment rapidly removes large numbers of circulating platelets. The platelet count can be reduced by 50% or more within a few hours. Unfortunately, the reduction in platelet count is transient and may have a rebound effect.

Other platelet-reducing modalities that are used with thrombocythemia include hydroxyurea, recombinant alfa-interferon, anagrelide, and antiplatelet agents. Hydroxyurea is a nonalkylating myelosuppressive agent that is considered an effective initial treatment for thrombocythemia and generally has not been considered leukemogenic. Anagrelide is another promising agent used in the platelet cytoreduction of thrombocythemia, as it is nonmutagenic.[39] Drugs considered for the prevention of thrombotic complications include aspirin and dipyridamole, due to their ability to interfere with platelet aggregation. They are used with caution because they can cause marked prolongation of the bleeding time with resultant bleeding in some patients with thrombocythemia.

*Thrombocytosis* Thrombocytosis, also known as *secondary* or *reactive thrombocytosis,* is used to describe the platelet count elevation in patients with a variety of other diseases. Thrombocytosis occurs in about 30%–40% of patients with malignant neoplasms. It is seen in lung, ovarian, pancreatic, breast, kidney, and GI carcinomas, in Hodgkin's disease, in splenectomized patients, and in individuals with widespread cancer.[40] Generally the platelet count is only mildly elevated when thrombocytosis is due to cancer (400,000–600,000 cells/mm$^3$).[41]

The patient with secondary thrombocytosis is usually asymptomatic, but thrombocytosis may cause thrombosis in a small proportion of cases. The risk of thrombosis increases in elderly patients or those with accompanying atherosclerosis, thrombotic complications, or immobility.[40] Thrombosis may result in symptoms associated with venous thrombosis, pulmonary embolism, transient cerebral ischemia, peripheral vascular ischemia, myocardial infarction and angina, or portal mesenteric vein occlusion.[42]

Patients with thrombocytosis who are asymptomatic do not require treatment. Symptomatic thrombocytosis can be treated with platelet pheresis. Aspirin and dipyridamole can be used, as in primary thrombocythemia, to prevent thrombotic complications or thrombocytosis.[41]

*Thrombocytopenia* Thrombocytopenia, a reduction in the number of circulating platelets, is the most frequent platelet abnormality associated with cancer. This disorder may be caused by a decrease in platelet production, a change in platelet distribution, platelet destruction, or vascular dilution.

*Platelet production*   The most common cause of thrombocytopenia in patients with cancer is a disorder of production involving decreased megakaryocytopoiesis. This may be due to tumor invasion of the bone marrow or to an acute or delayed effect of chemotherapy or radiation therapy. When tumor invasion is the cause of the decrease in platelet production, the resulting thrombocytopenia is generally part of the total picture of pancytopenia. A low platelet count is directly proportional to the degree of bone marrow infiltration by tumor cells. Bone marrow metastases are commonly seen in breast cancer, prostate cancer, and the hematologic malignancies but can occur in a variety of tumor types. An elevated serum alkaline phosphatase and lactic dehydrogenase often accompany diffuse marrow involvement.[43]

Chemotherapy is the treatment most often associated with hematologic toxicity and bone marrow suppression. The effects of chemotherapy are due in large part to the particular drugs used, dosages, schedules, routes of administration, previous cancer treatments, and concomitant therapy, and the individual's age, nutritional status, and tumor type. Acute chemotherapy-induced platelet toxicity usually is caused by the destruction of the proliferating cells of the platelet line, CFU-Mega. As these cells are destroyed, the circulatory platelets are cleared at the end of their life span and the nadir of a patient's blood cell count occurs. Considering that the average life span of a platelet is only seven days, this accounts in part for the high incidence of thrombocytopenia related to chemotherapy.[44]

The degree and duration of platelet toxicity related to various antineoplastic agents are the result of a number of factors, including the natural nadir of the drug, its potential for suppression, and cellular recovery time after the nadir. The major classification of these drugs also plays a part in how this toxicity is demonstrated. For example, cell-cycle phase nonspecific (CCNS) drugs, such as carmustine and lomustine, destroy cells in the resting phase of the cell cycle, damaging nonproliferating stem cells. These drugs can then have a delayed, prolonged, and cumulative suppressive effect.[1,45] The patient treated with carmustine will experience a platelet nadir approximately three weeks following treatment, and it may take as long as eight weeks for platelet recovery to occur. Cell-cycle phase specific (CCS) drugs, such as bleomycin, cytarabine, and vincristine, have their impact on proliferating progenitor cells and do not destroy cells in the resting phase of the cell cycle. These agents have an earlier nadir and a shorter recovery time and tend to be less toxic. See Table 22-2 for a list of chemotherapeutic agents associated with moderate to severe thrombocytopenia.

Radiation therapy can also cause hematologic toxicity, particularly when large areas of bone marrow are treated. The most significant factor that determines the risk of bone marrow depression related to radiation therapy is the volume of productive bone marrow in the radiation field. This risk factor is even more important than the therapeutic dose or the fractionation schedule.[46] Radiation-induced hematologic toxicity usually is caused by damage to the nonproliferating stem cells or to the cells in the resting phase of the cell cycle. Megakaryocytes are affected one to two weeks after exposure to the radiation, and take about two to six weeks for recovery. Radiation therapy is local treatment, except for total-nodal or total-body irradiation, and does not usually cause the nadirs in blood counts seen with chemotherapy. The localized nature of this treatment generally allows for the untreated marrow to compensate for the damage to the treated marrow.

*Platelet distribution*   Thrombocytopenia due to an abnormal distribution of platelets can occur in cancer patients with hypersplenism. An enlarged spleen may sequester up to 90% of the platelet population, making them unavailable in the circulation. Tumor metastasis to the spleen, particularly due to lymphomas and lung, breast, prostate, colon, and stomach cancers, are known to cause hypersplenism and subsequent platelet sequestration. Thrombocytopenia can also be due to congestive splenomegaly related to splenic vein obstruction in pancreatic cancer.[43] The thrombocytopenia related to hypersplenism is generally mild (platelet count 40,000–100,000 cells/mm³). The absence of a palpable spleen rules out this type of thrombocytopenic disorder. Areas denuded from surgery, mucositis resulting from chemotherapy and/or microbial toxins, and necrotic tumor can also cause platelet aggregation and a decrease in circulating platelets.

If the primary cause of thrombocytopenia is platelet sequestration, the bone marrow will contain normal to increased numbers of megakaryocytes. This is due to the attempt of the bone marrow to compensate for the decreased number of circulating platelets. When splenomegaly is accompanied by marrow infiltration by tumor, the degree of thrombocytopenia is compounded, for the compensatory production of platelets will be inadequate.

*Platelet destruction*   Thrombocytopenia can also be due to rapid platelet destruction, characterized by a dramatically shortened platelet life span and an abundance of megakaryocytes in the bone marrow. Although the platelet normally survives eight to ten days, it may live as little as a few hours.

This type of thrombocytopenia is seen in two situations. The first situation in which rapid platelet destruction occurs is immune thrombocytopenia, or idiopathic thrombocytopenic purpura (ITP). Signs and symptoms of ITP are similar to the bleeding disorders that accompany platelet disorders. Patients may be classified as having ITP that is mild (platelet counts > 80,000 cells/mm³), moderate (platelet counts > 50,000 cells/mm³), or severe (platelet counts < 30,000 cells/mm³).[47] This disorder occurs most frequently in individuals with lymphoproliferative diseases, such as chronic lymphocytic leukemia, acute lymphocytic leukemia, and non-Hodgkin's lymphoma.[24] ITP is rarely described with

**TABLE 22-2**  Chemotherapeutic Agents Associated with Significant Thrombocytopenia

| Chemotherapeutic Agent | Degree of Suppression | Nadir (days) | Recovery (days) | Comments |
|---|---|---|---|---|
| Busulfan (Myleran) | Moderate | 21–28 | 42–56 | CCNS, cumulative |
| Carmustine (BCNU) | Marked | 28–42 | 35–42 | Cell-cycle phase nonspecific (CCNS), cumulative toxicity |
| Chlorambucil (Leukeran) | Moderate | 21–28 | 42–56 | CCNS, cumulative |
| Cladribine (2-Cda) (Leustatin®) | Moderate | 14 | 60 | CCS |
| Cyclophosphamide (Cytoxan) | Moderate (dose related—100 mg/m²) | 7–14 | 21 | CCNS, cumulative |
| Cytarabine (Cytosar-U, ARA-C) | Marked | 10 | 21 | CCS |
| Dacarbazine (DTIC) | Marked (dose-related—200 mg/m² IV daily × 5 days) | 10–14 | 21–28 | CCNS |
| Dactinomycin (Actinomycin D) | Marked | 14 | 21–28 | CCNS |
| Daunorubicin hydrochloride (Cerubidine) | Marked | 10 | 21–28 | CCNS |
| Docetaxel (Taxotere) | Moderate to marked | 8 | 14 | CCS |
| Doxorubicin (Adriamycin) | Moderate to marked (dose-related) | 10–14 | 21 | CCNS |
| Epirubicin hydrochloride (Pharmorubicin) | Moderate | 10–14 | 21 | CCNS |
| 5-Fluorouracil (5-FU) | Moderate (dose-related—12–15 mg/kg) | 9–21 | 21 | Cell-cycle phase specific (CCS) |
| Hydroxyurea (Hydrea) | Moderate | 7 | 14 | |
| Lomustine (CCNU) | Marked | 21–28 | 42 | CCNS, cumulative |
| Mechlorethamine (nitrogen mustard) | Moderate | 10–14 | 21–28 | CCNS, cumulative |
| Methotrexate (Mexate) | Moderate (dose-related—100 mg/m²) | 10 | 14 | CCS |
| Mitomycin C (Mutamycin) | Marked | 21–28 | 42–56 | CCNS, cumulative |
| Paclitaxel (Taxol) | Marked | 8–15 | 21 | CCS |
| L-phenylalanine (L-PAM, Melphalan) | Moderate | 14–21 | 21–28 | CCNS, cumulative |
| Plicamycin (Mithracin) | Moderate | 14 | 21 | CCNS |
| Procarbazine (Matulane) | Moderate | 14 | 21–28 | |
| Streptozocin (Zanosar) | | | | CCNS, cumulative |
| 6-Thioguanine (6-TG) | Moderate to marked | 14–28 | 28–35 | CCS |
| Triethylenethiphosphoramide (Thiotepa) | Moderate | 14–21 | 40–50 | CCNS |
| Vinblastine (Velban) | Moderate to marked | 10 | 21 | CCS |
| Vinorelbine (Navelbine) | Mild to moderate | 14 | 21 | CCS |

solid tumors.[42] The rapid destruction of platelets is due to an autoimmune process in which antibodies are formed against the individual's own platelets. This process results in normal or increased numbers of megakaryocytes in the absence of any other cause of peripheral platelet destruction, such as sepsis or disseminated intravascular coagulation.[24]

The second type of rapid platelet destruction is seen in conditions of increased platelet consumption. This can be observed in various clinical syndromes with intravascular coagulation. Disseminated intravascular coagulation (DIC) is discussed in depth later in this chapter. In any condition involving increased platelet destruction, increased numbers of megakaryocytes will be present in the marrow as the body attempts to compensate for this abnormal state.

*Platelet dilution*  Dilution is another cause of thrombocytopenia. It is thought that rapid reconstitution of the intravascular volume by the use of stored platelet-poor blood dilutes thrombocytes that are already present. Whole blood can be stored up to 21 days with minimal decrease in erythrocyte survival. The platelets in the whole blood, however, lose considerable effectiveness after 24 hours at usual storage temperatures of 4 °C. This dilutional effect of platelets occurs in direct proportion to the amount of blood transfused. Stored blood is also deficient in factors V, VIII, and XI.[35,48]

The platelet count is considered the single most significant factor for predicting bleeding in the individual with cancer. Gaydos et al first reported an association between thrombocytopenia and an increased risk of bleeding in 1962.[49] The risk of spontaneous hemorrhage is considered to be greater than 50% when the platelet count is less than 20,000 cells/mm³. Manifestations of thrombocytopenia include easy bruising; bleeding from the mouth, gums, nose, or other orifices; petechiae; ecchymosis; melena; hematuria; and frank bleeding.

The platelet count is not the only determinant of a person's risk of bleeding. Concomitant infection, potential sources of bleeding, and a rapid decline in the platelet count commonly increase the risk of bleeding in an individual with cancer who is thrombocytopenic. Release of bacterial endotoxins from infection may stimulate a leukocyte response, which can enhance platelet consumption. Infection in the individual with thrombocytopenia increases the risk of bleeding. Potential sites of bleeding are numerous in the thrombocytopenic individual. They may be part of the disease process (e.g., necrotic tumor masses or intracranial bleeding) or may be related to treatment (e.g., mucositis or sites of injections). Risk for bleeding is greater in an individual with a rapidly falling platelet count compared with one that is rising, even if the absolute platelet count is the same. When the count is returning to normal, the platelets in circulation tend to be younger and larger and are able to clot more effectively.[50]

Although thrombocytopenia may be the immediate cause of bleeding in individuals with platelet disorders, therapy must address the underlying cause of the decreased platelet level. When decreased platelet production is the result of tumor infiltration of marrow, the best therapy is treatment of the tumor itself. The hematologic complications will remain or worsen as long as the marrow involvement persists. Platelet transfusions are often given to maintain a safe level of circulating thrombocytes until tumor regression occurs and marrow function returns. If platelet production has been depressed by chemotherapy or radiotherapy, in addition to platelet support if necessary, the dosage or administration schedule can be altered to maintain safe levels of platelet production.[51] (See Table 22-3 for a plan of care for the patient experiencing thrombocytopenia/bleeding.)

The use of recombinant colony-stimulating growth factors in accelerating hematologic recovery following ablative chemoradiotherapy continues to be an area of intensive investigation. Studies in both animals and humans have clearly shown that the administration of growth factors for granulocytes (rhG-CSF) and granulocytes-macrophages (rhGM-CSF) can reduce the hematopoietic toxicity that follows exposure to chemotherapy and radiation therapy.[52,53] GM-CSF possesses stimulating activities for granulocyte-macrophage, eosinophilic, and megakaryocytic progenitor cells in vitro. Different effects of GM-CSF on platelet levels have been reported. Gianni et al[54] reported that patients treated with continuous GM-CSF infusion (5.5 mg/kg/day) for 14 days after high-dose cyclophosphamide required fewer prophylactic platelet transfusions. A lack of platelet stimulation has been reported by other investigators.[55] According to Gianni et al, the lack of stimulation reported by these investigators might reflect differences in the myelotoxic damage underlying the conditions being treated with the growth factor.[54]

In addition to the intravascular (IV) route of administration, rhGM-CSF can effectively be administered by the subcutaneous (SQ) route. The recommended dose of GM-CSF is 250 mg/m²/day for up to 21 days.[56] When the drug is administered subcutaneously, local reactions, ranging from redness to infiltrates, may lead to cessation of rhGM-CSF.[57] deVries et al[57] reported that local reactions disappeared in most patients during the subsequent courses of treatment with GM-CSF. Reported side effects include a temporary generalized rash and pruritis, mild to moderate bone pain (sternum, ribs, shoulders, lower back, and hip areas), and muscle pain.[57,58] Discontinuation of treatment, rest, and analgesics have been used effectively to relieve these symptoms. Other mild side effects include fever, chills, myalgia, headaches, decreased appetite, nausea, and flushing. More serious reported toxicities include capillary leak syndrome and thrombosis.[56]

IL-3, currently under clinical investigation, is another multilineage growth factor that promotes growth and differentiation of various progenitor cells. In vitro IL-3 has been shown to stimulate growth of the neutrophil, monocyte, basophil, and thrombopoietic cell lines.[8,59] In a study in which patients with advanced malignancy with or without bone marrow hypoplasia were treated with recombinant IL-3, results revealed a dose-dependent increase in platelet counts as well as reticulocyte counts in most patients. Treatment with combinations of IL-3, interleukin-6, and interleukin–11 can increase the platelet count to a limited extent, but these hormones do not act specifically on megakaryocytes.[60] Side effects related to IL-3 include fever, flushing, headache, local irritation of the injection site, bone pain, lethargy, and nausea and vomiting.[61] Discontinuation of the IL-3 generally relieves these symptoms.

Investigational agents such as PIXY321 (a GM-CSF/IL-3 fusion protein) and the recently cloned thrombopoietin have shown promise in promoting maturation of the megakaryocyte.[52,62] PIXY321 holds promise of offering a substantial clinical benefit over either GM-CSF or IL-3.[62] The purification and cloning of thrombopoietin has led to phase I and II trials to study the effect of this cytokine on thrombopoiesis.[60,63]

**TABLE 22-3**  Plan of Care for the Patient Experiencing Thrombocytopenia/Bleeding

| Patient Problem | Expected Outcomes | Nursing Interventions |
|---|---|---|
| Potential for bleeding related to thrombocytopenia | The patient will be free of bleeding.<br><br>The patient/significant other will be able to state four signs/symptoms indicative of bleeding.<br><br>The patient/significant other will be able to demonstrate knowledge of their understanding of bleeding precautions. | 1. Monitor platelet count and other coagulation tests and report abnormal values.<br>2. Assess vital signs q 4° as indicated.<br>3. Hold myelosuppressive agents as indicated.<br>4. Test all excreta for occult blood and report positive results.<br>5. Assess patient for any signs/symptoms of bleeding (see Table 22-6).<br>6. Maintain and reinforce bleeding precautions.<br>7. Avoid trauma and provide for physical safety of the client:<br>　a. Use only electric razor.<br>　b. Use soft toothbrush or toothpaste.<br>　c. Use only alcohol-free mouthwash.<br>　d. Avoid use of dental floss and toothpicks.<br>　e. Avoid venipuncture, invasive procedures, rectal thermometers or suppositories.<br>　f. Apply pressure to puncture sites for at least 5 min.<br>　g. Avoid forceful coughing, sneezing, or nose blowing.<br>　h. Avoid constipation; may require stool softeners.<br>　i. Avoid cutting toenails and fingernails.<br>　j. During menses, monitor pad count.<br>　k. Avoid aspirin or any medications that may cause/aggravate thrombocytopenia.<br>　m. Avoid tight-fitting or constrictive clothing.<br>8. Administer platelet transfusion if ordered:<br>　a. Premedicate client as indicated.<br>　b. Use leukocyte-poor filter on platelet transfusion as indicated.<br>　c. Use HLA-matched platelets, if refractory platelets.<br>　d. Monitor, document, and notify physician if any allergic reaction (fever, chills, rash, hives, skin flushing).<br>　e. Obtain posttransfusion platelet count. |

Platelet sequestration within a spleen enlarged due to malignancy is treated most effectively by aggressive tumor therapy. Chemotherapy and radiotherapy usually are most effective. Sequestration of platelets is at times reversible with epinephrine, which causes a release of trapped platelets from an enlarged spleen. Transient control of platelet sequestration has also been achieved with corticosteroid therapy. Steroids have a capillary-stabilizing effect, which is important in minimizing the bleeding potential of thrombocytopenia. Splenectomy may be considered if other methods fail to control the sequestration of platelets.

Individuals who are found to have asymptomatic, mild or moderate ITP may be followed closely with no treatment. Individuals who experience severe thrombocytopenia are generally treated with prednisone therapy (1 mg/kg body weight).[64] This low-dose prednisone therapy may need to be maintained to keep the platelet count > 50,000 cells/mm³. If the platelet count drops during tapering of the prednisone, a high dose of prednisone may be required.[65]

Platelet transfusions are seldom indicated for patients with ITP because the survival time of transfused platelets is shortened. Platelet transfusions may be used for controlling severe hemorrhage.[64] Intravenous immune globulin therapy plays an important role in managing acute bleeding. The efficacy of platelets has been found to be improved immediately after an infusion of IV immune globulin. The recommended dosage of immune globulin is 1 g/kg/day for two days.[66]

Splenectomy for the management of ITP was used for many years before glucocorticoids were introduced. The decision to undergo a splenectomy for ITP is determined by the course and severity of the disease. Splenectomy may be done early on in the course of severe thrombocytopenia that is unresponsive to prednisone, or it may be done after several months if a remission from the disease cannot be attained.[64] If patients fail prednisone therapy or lack a response to a splenectomy, other treatments include splenic radiation or partial splenic embolization, vincristine, vinblastine, bleomycin, danazol, colchicine, anti-D antibody, and interferon-alfa$_{2b}$.[67-72]

### Qualitative abnormalities

*Platelet malfunction* At times patients with cancer may bleed despite normal platelet counts and/or coagulation factors. Alterations in platelet function may be responsible for the bleeding seen in these situations. A variety of hematologic diseases are associated with abnormal platelet function. Hemostatic abnormalities associated with abnormal platelet function include chronic myelogenous leukemia, acute myelogenous leukemia, acute lymphocytic leukemia in children, multiple myeloma, and Waldenström's macroglobulinemia.[26,73] The major abnormality noted in these diseases is a decrease in the procoagulant activity of the platelets, which is a measure of platelet factor III. Also noted in these diseases are platelets that are larger or smaller than normal, abnormally shaped platelets, and a variation in the number of storage pool granules. In multiple myeloma the qualitative defect in platelet function can occur as a result of the M protein coating the platelet and interfering with platelet aggregation.[25] Abnormal platelet function has also been described in patients with thrombocytosis, associated with the myeloproliferative disorders. This may help to explain the increased incidence of hemorrhage in patients with an increased platelet concentration.

Numerous drugs are known to affect platelet function. At times some of these drugs are administered deliberately for their antithrombotic effect, with diminished platelet function being the therapeutic goal (e.g., heparin). For many of the other drugs, the decreased platelet function is an unwanted side effect. For all of the drugs known to affect platelet function, the effect of the drug is measured by an abnormality of platelet function or bleeding time. Although these drugs are known to affect platelet aggregation or bleeding time, only aspirin has been demonstrated to cause a significant increased risk of bleeding. (See Table 22-4 for a discussion of commonly used drugs in cancer care that inhibit platelet function.) When aspirin is ingested, there is a predictable abnormality of impaired platelet aggregation with epinephrine, ADP, arachidonic acid, and low concentrations of collagen and thrombin. This is due to aspirin's ability to inactivate the enzyme cyclooxygenase.[73] This platelet aggregation abnormality associated with aspirin is so characteristic that abnormal platelet aggregation patterns of any etiology are often designated as "aspirin-like." The decreased platelet aggregation can lead to bleeding. Aspirin also prolongs bleeding time, although this is less consistent than the platelet aggregation abnormality. Daily ingestion of 30 mg or more of aspirin can produce an increased bleeding time.[74] It has also been demonstrated that the bleeding time can be prolonged for up to four days after a single dose of aspirin and that platelet aggregation tests may remain abnormal for up to a week, until normal platelet turnover results in a significant number of new platelets with normal function.[73]

The mechanism of action of nonsteroidal anti-inflammatory drugs appears to be similar to that for aspirin—that of inhibition of platelet cyclooxygenase. These drugs have only a temporary effect, causing inhibition only as long as the active drug is present in the circulation. Most of these drugs affect platelet function for only a few hours. One exception is piroxicam, which has a plasma half-life of more than 2 days. The short half-life of these drugs

**TABLE 22-4** Commonly Used Drugs in Cancer Care That Inhibit Platelet Function

| Drug | Effect | Comments |
|---|---|---|
| NONSTEROIDAL ANTI-INFLAMMATORY AGENTS | | |
| Aspirin | Impaired platelet aggregation Prolongs bleeding time | Has been demonstrated to cause a significant increased risk for bleeding, especially when patients have conditions predisposing to hemorrhage. |
| Others<br>Indomethacin (Indocin)<br>Ibuprofen (Advil, Motrin, Nuprin, Rufen)<br>Sulindac (Clinoril)<br>Naproxen (Naprosyn)<br>Phenylbutazone (Butazolidin)<br>Mechlofenamic acid (Meclomen)<br>Mefenamic acid (Ponstel)<br>Diflusinal (Dolobid)<br>Tolmetin (Tolectin)<br>Piroxicam (Feldene) | Impaired platelet aggregation Prolongs bleeding time, minimally and transiently | Cause less risk of increased bleeding than does aspirin. These drugs should be discontinued the day before surgery or an invasive procedure.<br><br>Has a half-life of more than 2 days; may increase the risk of bleeding slightly. |

**TABLE 22-4**   Commonly Used Drugs in Cancer Care That Inhibit Platelet Function (continued)

| Drug | Effect | Comments |
|---|---|---|
| **BETA-LACTAM ANTIBIOTICS** | | |
| **Penicillins**<br>Penicillin G<br>Carbenicillin (Geopen)<br>Ticarcillin (Ticar, Timentin)<br>Methicillin (Staphcillin)<br>Ampicillin (Polycillin, Omnipen)<br>Nafcillin (Nafcil, Unipen)<br>Piperacillin (Pipracil)<br>Azocillin (Azlin)<br>Mezlocillin (Mezlin)<br>Temocillin<br>Sulbenicillin<br>Apalcillin | Prolongs bleeding time<br>Impaired platelet aggregation and secretion | Effect on bleeding time occurs only in patients receiving large parenteral doses of antibiotics. Abnormalities do not subside for several days after these antibiotics are discontinued.<br><br>The frequency of clinically significant hemorrhage due *only* to the effects of antibiotics on platelet function is rare.[58] |
| **Cephalosporins**<br>Cephalothin (Keflin, Seffin)<br>Cefoxitin (Mefoxin)<br>Cefotaxime (Claforan)<br>Cefazolin (Ancef, Kefzol)<br>Cefoperazone (Cefobid)<br>Moxalactam (Moxam) | | |
| **PSYCHOTROPIC DRUGS** | | |
| **Phenothiazines**<br>Chlorpromazine (Thorazine)<br>Promethazine (Phenergan)<br>Trifluoperazine (Stelazine) | Impaired platelet aggregation and secretion response | Effect on platelets has not been associated with an increased risk of bleeding. |
| **Antidepressants**<br>Amitriptyline<br>Imipramine (Tofranil)<br>Nortriptyline (Pamelor) | | |
| **CHEMOTHERAPY AGENTS** | | |
| Mithramycin | Impaired platelet aggregation<br>Prolonged bleeding time<br>Mucocutaneous bleeding | Occurs with total dose of 6–21 mg. |
| BCNU (carmustine)<br>Daunorubicin (daunomycin)<br>Vinblastine<br>Vincristine | Impaired platelet aggregation and secretion when added to platelet-rich plasma | Effect on platelets has not been found to cause clinically significant bleeding. |
| **OTHER** | | |
| Aminophylline<br>Diphenhydramine (Benadryl)<br>Furosemide (Lasix)<br>Hydrocortisone<br>Methylprednisolone<br>Verapamil<br>Cyclosporin A | Impaired platelet aggregation through unknown mechanisms | |

suggests that they cause less risk of increased bleeding than does aspirin.[75]

Beta-lactam antibiotics, including the penicillins and cephalosporins, frequently are used in the cancer patient population. These antibiotics characteristically cause a prolonged bleeding time and abnormal platelet aggregation. These changes are most pronounced one to three days after administration of the antibiotic and may remain apparent for several days after the antibiotic has been stopped.[76] The mechanism by which certain antibiotics cause prolonged bleeding times is not entirely clear. It is thought that penicillins probably inhibit platelet function by binding to membrane components, which are necessary for platelet adhesiveness interactions (such as blocking ADP receptor activity on platelet membranes).[73] The frequency of clinically significant hemorrhage due solely to the effect of antibiotics on platelet function is rare, but risk of bleeding may be increased in patients with coexisting hemostatic defects such as thrombocytopenia or vitamin K deficiency.[73] The cephalosporins are another group of antibiotics that may cause a similar pattern of platelet dysfunction. Moxalactam is associated with a higher frequency of clinically significant hemorrhagic complications as compared with the other antibiotics. Although its effect on bleeding time and platelet aggregation is no different than that of the other antibiotics, it has been implicated in the inhibition of synthesis of vitamin K–dependent proteins. This process results in deficiencies of coagulation factors II, VII, IX, and X and impaired platelet function.[77]

Patients taking psychotropic drugs, such as tricyclic antidepressants and phenothiazines, may have impaired platelet aggregation and secretion responses to ADP, epinephrine, and collagen. This effect has not been found to be associated with an increased risk of bleeding.[73]

Administration of a few chemotherapeutic drugs has been found to be associated with abnormal platelet aggregation. Mithramycin, when administered to a total dose of 6–21 mg, has been associated with decreased platelet aggregation, increased bleeding time, and mucocutaneous bleeding. BCNU and carmustine are both known to inhibit platelet aggregation and secretion but are not linked to clinically significant bleeding caused by abnormal platelet function. Also, as single-agent therapy, they have not been shown to cause clinically significant platelet dysfunction.[78]

Management of hemorrhagic disorders due to platelet malfunction, such as when patients have a platelet factor III deficiency, frequently is aimed at the underlying cause. The patient will likely be treated with aggressive antineoplastic therapy.

Drug-induced platelet abnormalities must be assessed carefully in respect to the patient's total clinical picture. Aspirin has been demonstrated to cause an increased risk of bleeding. Because of this risk, the patient with cancer should avoid taking this drug or any compounds containing aspirin. A prolonged bleeding time due to aspirin may be corrected by infusion of desmopressin (1–deamino-8–D-arginine vasopressin, DDAVP).[79] (See the next section for a more thorough discussion of DDAVP.) The clinical risk for bleeding associated with nonsteroidal anti-inflammatory drugs is much less than that for aspirin. However, they should be used cautiously in patients with already-low platelet counts. The potential for beta-lactam–induced bleeding in patients with cancer generally does not prohibit patients from being treated with appropriate antibiotic coverage. These patients need to be monitored closely for any signs or symptoms of bleeding. Bleeding studies, including the bleeding time, are monitored closely as well. Platelet transfusions can be used during periods of thrombocytopenia to avoid hemorrhage, as well as during periods of acute bleeding.

### Hypocoagulation

Malignancy or the metabolic alterations that frequently accompany it may precipitate an imbalance in the coagulation factors, leading to an increased risk of bleeding. In 1974 Slichter and Harker[80] showed that these imbalances were related directly to tumor burden. Successful tumor therapy brought about a normalization of coagulation values. The most significant factor leading to a state of hypocoagulability is liver disease, which may be due to tumor invasion, chemotherapy, infection, or surgical resection. Regardless of the etiology, liver disease has been reported to cause a prolonged bleeding time, reduced platelet aggregation, and procoagulant activity.[81] Liver disease interferes with the synthesis of plasma coagulation factors I, II, V, VII, IX, and X. In addition to decreasing the production of these factors, liver disease may also interfere with their functioning. Decreased liver function allows for diminished liver clearance of fibrin degradation products and activated clotting factors, which further inhibits the coagulation mechanism.

A deficiency of vitamin K may also cause a hypocoagulation syndrome. This may be seen in patients with neoplastic disease in which there is dietary lack of vitamin K, biliary obstruction, malabsorptive states, with intestinal sterilization due to antibiotic administration, or to impaired clotting factor synthesis due to liver disease.[82] A deficiency of vitamin K results in a greatly reduced chemical activation of vitamin K–dependent proteins: factors II, VII, IX, and X. The result is a state of decreased hemostasis.

Individuals who undergo extensive surgical procedures and receive large amounts of frozen plasma may demonstrate a prolonged prothrombin time and a prolonged partial thromboplastin time. These individuals are prone to postsurgical bleeding. Frozen plasma has deficient levels of factors V and VIII, which can lead to an altered state of coagulation.

A nonspecific plasma antagonist of several coagulation proteins has been described in various disease states, including neoplastic disease. These anticoagulants have been identified in the acute leukemias, lymphocytic lymphomas, and other disease states in which white blood cell turnover is rapid. These inhibitors have also been found to be highest at the onset of chemotherapy when there is lysis of white blood cells, and in disease relapse when there is a large tumor burden.

Isolated factor deficiencies are also reported in neoplastic disease. Acquired Willebrand's syndrome has been demonstrated to occur in solid tumors, hematologic malignancies, myeloproliferative disorders, macroglobulinemia, and lymphoproliferative disorders. A small number of patients with malignant B-cell disease and Wilms' tumor have been reported to develop acquired Willebrand's syndrome.[83] Patients with this syndrome demonstrate mucosal bleeding, bruising, and GI hemorrhage. Coagulation studies show a prolonged bleeding time and diminished or absent factor VIII procoagulant activity (factor VIII:C), von Willebrand factor antigen (VWF:Ag), and ristocetin cofactor activity.[81] The factor VIII deficiency may be attributed to acquired inhibitors of coagulation proteins, which have been demonstrated in monoclonal immunoglobulin G (IgG) gammopathies, lymphoma, and macroglobulinemia.[24] The exact mechanism connecting the specific inhibitors and the underlying neoplastic disease is unclear. Factor XIII deficiency is also commonly affected by malignancy and liver disease.

Conditions of decreased coagulability are less common than the other types of hemostatic alterations discussed in this chapter. Although any type of coagulation abnormality can lead to bleeding, they less frequently cause serious bleeding when they do occur. Hemorrhages tend to develop in the deeper areas of the body, such as the subcutaneous or intramuscular tissue. Bleeding into the joints, especially of the distal extremities, may be seen in the hypocoagulability states. A deficiency of any factor will lead to abnormal fibrin formation, which provides an ineffective matrix for normal fibroblastic proliferation and wound healing.

Effective tumor therapy generally is the best means of controlling hypocoagulability abnormalities. Plasma and plasma derivative therapy may be used discriminately in specific clinical situations. Specific replacement of diminished factors is difficult because of the complex nature of these abnormalities. Generally, the treatment of specific inhibitors of coagulation factors depends on the severity of the abnormality. Life-threatening bleeding requires therapy, but lesser symptoms may require observation only.[84]

At times, liver disease associated with hemorrhagic diathesis and a decrease in the production of the vitamin K–dependent coagulation factors is treated by infusion of fresh-frozen plasma or prothrombin complex concentrates, when rapid correction of abnormalities is required. The therapeutic effectiveness of this therapy, however, is debated. Alternatively, albumin can be used as a volume expander when the patient is actively bleeding. Albumin is safer than plasma, since it carries no risk of hepatitis transmission. It may, however, precipitate congestive heart failure in patients with compromised cardiovascular function. The patient's cardiac and renal status must be monitored closely. When there is an attempt to shorten a prolonged prothrombin time, as before a needle biopsy of the liver, prothrombin complex (containing prothrombin and factors VII, IX, and X) may be given. The usual initial dose of prothrombin complex per kilogram of body weight is 40 units. Maintenance doses of 10–20 units are given daily until the patient's coagulation parameters normalize.[85] Infusion of DDAVP may be used when the patient with liver disease has a prolonged bleeding time with mild to moderate bleeding.[73] The usual dosage of DDAVP is 0.3–0.4 µg/kg body weight. The dose does not

usually exceed 20 g because of increased side effects, which include mild cutaneous vasodilation (the patient complains of feeling warm), facial flushing, tingling, and headache.[81] Episodes of acute thrombosis have occurred in a small number of patients treated with DDAVP.[86]

Generally, SQ vitamin K (Menaphthone, AquaMEPHYTON) is administered to correct the protein defects when this vitamin is deficient. The usual dose of vitamin K is a single SQ injection of 5–10 mg or less, which usually produces a complete correction of the prothrombin time within 12–24 hours.[87] Prothrombin complex concentrates or fresh-frozen plasma can be used in situations of vitamin K deficiency with concomitant severe bleeding.[84] The patient is also instructed on the dietary sources of vitamin K if absorption of the vitamin is not a problem. The major sources of dietary vitamin K are liver (92 g/100 gm), broccoli (175 µg/100 gm), and spinach (415 g/100 gm).[82]

Isolated factor deficiencies are generally treated by specific plasma components. When factors V and VIII are deficient because the patient has received large amounts of frozen plasma, the infusion of several units of fresh plasma may correct the disorder. Patients with acquired Willebrand's syndrome are generally treated when they experience bleeding or when they require an invasive procedure. The severity of the bleeding dictates the type and amount of therapy that will be used. Treatment for bleeding due to acquired Willebrand's syndrome includes fresh-frozen plasma and cryoprecipitate along with packed red cells and platelet concentrates, high-dose corticosteroid, factor VIII concentrates, DDAVP infusions, epsilon-aminocaproic acid (Amicar), IV gamma globulin, and extracorporeal immunoabsorption.[88,89]

Successful tumor therapy, including surgery, chemotherapy, or radiotherapy, may bring about the most significant response in the normalization of factor VIII-VWF complex parameters. Factor XIII deficiency (or fibrin-stabilizing factor deficiency) is readily treated by replacement therapy with plasma or cryoprecipitate.

## Hypercoagulation

Disseminated intravascular coagulation (DIC) is the most common serious hypercoagulable state in individuals with cancer. It represents an inappropriate and exaggerated overstimulation of normal coagulation, in which both thrombosis and thus hemorrhage may occur simultaneously. This seemingly paradoxical situation results in hypercoagulation, in which multiple small clots are formed in the microcirculation of many organs, and fibrinolysis, in which there is consumption of clots and clotting factors. Ultimately the body becomes unable to respond to vascular or tissue injury through stable clot formation, and thus hemorrhage ensues. This syndrome is always secondary to an underlying disease process, such as malignancy, septicemia, obstetric complications, or similar systemic stressors.

Although DIC is considered a common problem associated with malignancy, its incidence is difficult to estimate. The syndrome often remains undetected until severe hemorrhage occurs and frequently is discovered only at the time of autopsy. Currently, the overall incidence of DIC in patients with cancer is estimated to be approximately 10%.[90] DIC contributes strongly to morbidity and mortality in persons with cancer, particularly when there is thrombosis or bleeding into the lungs, central nervous system, or the GI tract.[40]

The most common cause of DIC is infection. It is believed that bacterial endotoxins, which are released from gram-negative bacteremia, activate the Hageman factor (factor XII). This factor can initiate coagulation as well as stimulate fibrinolysis. DIC is also seen in the presence of gram-positive bacteremia and with viremias. See Table 22-5 for a list of common causes of DIC in cancer.

Tumors themselves have been identified as stimulators of intravascular coagulation. The cancers most commonly associated with DIC include acute promyelocytic leukemia (APL) and the adenocarcinomas. APL has a high correlation with DIC. DIC associated with APL can occur before and in conjunction with chemotherapy administration.[40] A procoagulant substance has been identified on the promyelocytic blast cells that is similar to thromboplastin. This substance is believed to be released from granules on the promyelocytes, which subsequently initiate the clotting response.[91] The solid tumors most often associated with DIC are the mucin-producing adenocarcinomas, such as gastric, lung, pancreatic, and prostate tumors. Solid tumors develop new blood vessels that have an abnormal endothelial lining that is thought to activate the procoagulant system.[92] Tumors may also release necrotic tissue into the circulation or tissue enzymes, which could activate the coagulation mechanism.

Disseminated intravascular coagulation is always secondary to an underlying disease process. The pathophysiology of DIC involves an extensive triggering of the coagulation system by the underlying disease, which results in abnormal activation of thrombin formation. Excess circulating thrombin may abnormally activate both coagulation and fibrinolysis, which upsets the balance of hemostasis.

Thrombin cleaves fibrinogen, which combines easily with circulating fibrin degradation products to form a soluble form of fibrin. At times this combination forms insoluble clots that deposit in the microvasculature of various organs. These fibrin thrombi are considered the hallmark of DIC. The lodged clots further trap circulating platelets, which results in the thrombocytopenia associated with DIC.[93] This entrapment of platelets impedes blood flow, leading to tissue ischemia, hypoxia, and necrosis of multiple organs, along with consumption of clots and clotting factors.[94]

The abnormal activation of thrombin also results in increased fibrinolysis. Thrombin not only acts to convert fibrinogen to fibrin but also assists in the conversion of plasminogen to plasmin. Plasmin is responsible for the breakdown of fibrinogen and fibrin, which causes increased circulating fibrin degradation products that have strong anticoagulant properties. These then interfere with fibrin clot formation, as well as aiding in the consumption of clotting factors and platelets. The bleeding manifestations of DIC are caused by the combination of the consumption of platelets and certain clotting factors, plasmin's fibrinolytic properties, and the anticoagulant properties of the fibrin degradation products.

DIC can present as a chronic coagulation disorder or an acute hemorrhagic diathesis, or it can merely be detected through various laboratory studies. Clinical symptoms may be similar to those of other thrombocytopenic conditions.

The patient generally is not critically ill from chronic DIC. Chronic DIC may produce minimal or no clinical manifestations. Easy and spontaneous bruisability may be present. Mild petechiae, ecchymosis, gingival bleeding, and minor GI bleeding may be noted. Chronic DIC is more likely to cause thrombosis than bleeding. Venous thrombosis and endocarditis represent thrombotic complications of chronic DIC.[47] Laboratory tests may vary in chronic DIC but generally show minor coagulation abnormalities. Neurological dysfunction occasionally can occur in chronic DIC as a result of small episodic cerebral bleeding; however, it is often mistaken for metabolic encephalopathy or metastasis.

Acute DIC (also called *uncompensated*) occurs rapidly over hours to days. This condition rapidly depletes coagulation factors and inhibitors. Signs of acute DIC include petechiae; hematuria; acral cyanosis; bleeding or oozing from the gums, nose, or venipuncture sites; or oozing from surgical wounds.[94] Widespread thrombosis (purpura

---

**TABLE 22-5   Common Causes of Disseminated Intravascular Coagulation in Cancer**

**Neoplasms**
- Solid tumors (colon, lung, prostate, stomach, breast, gallbladder, ovary, melanoma, pancreas, gastric)
- Leukemia (acute promyelocytic, acute myelogenous, chronic myelogenous, acute lymphoblastic)

**Infections**
- Gram-negative bacteria (*pseudomonas, meningococcus, enterobacteriacae, salmonella, haemophilus*)
- Gram-positive bacteria (*Pneumococcus, Staphylococcus*)
- Viremias (hepatitis, varicella, cytomegalovirus)
- Septic shock
- Human immunodeficiency virus

**Liver disease**
- Obstructive jaundice
- Fulminant hepatic failure

**Intravascular hemorrhage**
- Multiple transfusions of whole blood
- Hemolytic transfusion reaction
- Minor hemolysis

fulminans—irregular hemorrhagic skin lesions) and significant bleeding can occur.[95] Overt hemorrhage involving multiple unrelated sites is not uncommon. The individual may display signs of shock and associated organ hypoxia. Hemoptysis, intraperitoneal hemorrhage, and intracranial bleeding all may pose life-threatening situations for the patient with DIC.

Thrombus formation often occurs simultaneously with bleeding in DIC. Thrombi generally form in the superficial and smaller veins, and may be clinically undetectable. Subtle signs and symptoms of thrombi include red, indurated tender areas found in multiple organ sites. When thrombosis occurs, the signs and symptoms include focal ischemia, acral cyanosis, superficial gangrene, altered sensorium, ulceration of the GI tract, and dyspnea, which can lead to acute respiratory distress syndrome.

There is no specific laboratory finding that is absolutely diagnostic of DIC. A battery of lab tests in conjunction with clinical evidence must be used to confirm the diagnosis, as well as to monitor response to treatment. A number of clinical conditions will affect these tests, which makes their interpretation difficult. For example, multiple blood product transfusions will dilute clotting factors or platelets, and liver disease with portal hypertension can lead to thrombocytopenia and the activation of the fibrinolytic system.

A classic triad of tests is generally done to help support the diagnosis of DIC: prothrombin time (PT), platelet count, and the plasma fibrinogen level (see Table 22-6). In DIC the PT is usually prolonged, which reflects decreased levels of clotting factors II and V and of fibrinogen. The platelet count drops below 150,000/mm³. A low platelet count is considered a cardinal diagnostic finding in DIC. In patients with acute leukemia and DIC, thrombocytopenia is more severe because of decreased thrombopoiesis. A low plasma fibrinogen level (< 150 mg/dl) results from the consumption of fibrinogen due to thrombin-induced clotting and from fibrinolysis in DIC. Other laboratory tests frequently used to detect DIC include FDP assays (increased in DIC), factor assays (decreased),

activated partial thromboplastin time (APTT) (prolonged), antithrombin III assay (decreased), and protamine paracoagulant test (negative in DIC with severe hypofibrinogenemia). The diagnosis of chronic DIC is supported by the appearance of red cell fragments, called *schistocytes*, on peripheral blood smears. This is seen in all patients with chronic DIC, and in only 50% of patients with acute DIC. FDPs are usually elevated and induce platelet dysfunction.[95,96]

Treatment of the underlying malignancy is vital in the patient with a hypercoagulability abnormality, for the tumor is the ultimate stimulus. All other therapy, although effective on a short-term basis, will provide only an interval of symptomatic relief. Identification of and early treatment for other precipitating factors must also be done (e.g., sepsis, volume deficit, transfusion reactions).

Early detection of the signs and symptoms of DIC may allow for prompt diagnosis and treatment. Major complications related to DIC include bleeding, with the potential of hemorrhage, altered fluid balance, decreased oxygenation, and thrombus formation. Close monitoring of the patient for any signs or symptoms of bleeding is essential to minimize blood loss. (See Table 22-7 for the physical examination of the patient with actual or potential bleeding.) Quantifying the amount of actual blood loss whenever possible is important in regard to replacement fluids and blood component therapy.

The fluid status of the patient with DIC is often tenuous. With significant blood loss the patient can quickly become hypovolemic. Replacement fluids may include red blood cells, platelets, fresh-frozen plasma, and albumin, in addition to IV solutions.[91] Caution must be used in treating the bleeding patient to avoid fluid overload and complications such as congestive heart failure.

Platelets can be given if the platelet count drops below 30,000/mm³. Packed red cells can be given if the patient is hemorrhaging. Fresh-frozen plasma also can be given for hemorrhage since it contains all of the clotting factors, including antithrombin III. It also can be given for vol-

**TABLE 22-6**  Clotting Studies of Disseminated Intravascular Coagulation

| Test | Abnormality | Cause |
|------|-------------|-------|
| Prothrombin time (PT)* | Prolonged | Elevated fibrin split products; decreased plasma clotting factor levels |
| Activated partial thromboplastin time (aPTT) | Prolonged | Elevated fibrin split products; decreased plasma clotting factor levels |
| Platelet count* | Decreased | Platelet consumption |
| Plasma fibrinogen* | Low | Consumption of fibrinogen by the clotting cascade and by fibrinolysis |
| FDP assays | Increased | Fibrinogen destruction by plasmin |
| Factor assays | Decreased | Consumption of clotting factors |
| Antithrombin III assay | Decreased | Consumption of clotting factors |
| Protamine paracoagulant | Negative | Severe hypofibrinogenemia |

*Classic triad of tests.

**TABLE 22-7   Physical Examination of the Patient with Actual or Potential Bleeding**

**Integumentary system** (assess entire skin surface, including intertrigonous areas)
Bruising, petechiae, purpura, ecchymoses, acrocyanosis (irregularly shaped cyanotic patches on the periphery of arms and legs associated with bleeding due to DIC); oozing from venipuncture sites or injections, biopsy sites, central lines, catheters, or nasogastric tubes; color and condition of gingival tissues

**Eyes\* and ears**
Visual disturbances, increased injection on the sclera, periorbital edema, subconjunctival hemorrhage (homogeneous red color that is sharply outlined on the sclera), headache, ear or eye pain

**Nose, mouth, and throat**
Petechiae on nasal/oral mucosa, epistaxis, tenderness or bleeding from gums or oral mucosa

**Cardiopulmonary system**
Crackles, wheezes, stridor, dyspnea, tachypnea, orthopnea, cyanosis, and hemoptysis (all possible signs of bleeding in the lungs); vital sign changes, color and temperature of all extremities, peripheral pulses, tachycardia; observe for angina

**Gastrointestinal system†**
Pain, bleeding, blood around rectum, tarry stools, frank or occult blood in stools, hemoptysis; observe for bleeding hemorrhoids (may respond to local measures)

**Genitourinary system**
Bleeding, character and amount of menses; monitor intake and output (if urine drops below 30 ml/hr it may be due to acute tubular necrosis secondary to thrombi, bleeding, or hypovolemia)

**Musculoskeletal system**
Check for complaint of painful joints while performing active or passive range of motion, which may indicate bleeding into the joints

**Central nervous system**
Mental status changes, including restlessness, confusion, lethargy, dizziness, obtundation, seizures, or coma (may indicate intracranial hemorrhage or impaired tissue perfusion)

\*Bleeding in the optic fundus could lead to permanent visual impairment.

†Guaiac all excreta for blood.

ume expansion. Albumin may be the component of choice for volume expansion for the reasons previously described. Specific coagulation factors may be given if laboratory data are able to identify the specific deficient factors. Antithrombin III is a coagulation factor that may be given to neutralize thrombin, plasmin, and activated forms of factors XII, XI, X, and VII, which may slow the process of DIC. Cryoprecipitate (a concentrated source of fibrinogen and factor VIII) may be used to treat the hypofibrinogenemia that often occurs in DIC. Usually two to four bags per 10 kg are given initially, with each bag containing 10–12 ml of given factors. Depending on individual laboratory data, the patient may be given one or more bags per 15 kg of body weight per day.[85]

A compromised respiratory status might result from bleeding. Inadequate oxygenation due to bleeding may be manifested as tachypnea, dyspnea, tachycardia, or orthopnea. Oxygen therapy and red blood cell transfusions may be required for inadequate oxygenation. Assisting patients to conserve energy and oxygen by helping them with any activities of daily living may also be necessary.[90]

Heparin therapy for DIC associated with malignancy is controversial.[40,93,97] The controversy stems primarily from the lack of randomized trials of heparin therapy use in patients with DIC due to malignancy. There is also a controversy as to whether high-risk patients (e.g., a promyelocytic leukemia patient undergoing chemotherapy) should be treated prophylactically with heparin therapy. The problem lies in the potential for unnecessarily exposing the patient to a risk of bleeding. Heparin therapy is used more frequently in the chronic DIC of malignancy associated with thrombotic, thromboembolic, or necrotizing complications.[40] The use of Coumadin has been studied in the treatment of chronic DIC, but it has not proved to be as effective as heparin.[95]

Heparin inhibits the formation of new clots by inhibiting factors IX and X, and may decrease the consumption of clotting factors. Heparin therapy for DIC is generally maintained until the symptoms disappear and laboratory values normalize. Large doses of heparin often are required to overcome intravascular clotting. A bolus of 10,000 units or more may be given, followed by a continuous or intermittent IV infusion. A continuous infusion is generally maintained if the heparin requirements (to maintain the PTT at 1.5 to 2 times normal) exceed 40,000/day. Intermittent SQ or IV infusions (every 6–8 hours) are used when the daily heparin requirement is lower.[40] Heparin use is contraindicated in patients with any signs of intracranial bleeding (e.g., headache), open wounds, or recent surgery.

Another drug that may be used with DIC is EACA, Amicar, a fibrinolytic inhibitor, although its use is also controversial. EACA can be used when the fibrinolysis of DIC has been resolved but uncontrolled bleeding persists. It is given to maintain platelet and fibrinogen levels, and only after intramuscular clotting has been brought under control, because it can lead to widespread fibrin deposition in the microcirculation and result in ischemic organ dysfunction.[94,95]

Prevention of further complications of DIC includes removal of any tight or restrictive clothing. If edema is present, it is measured daily. Elastic support stockings may help to minimize stasis and promote venous return. Other measures to decrease stasis and promote venous return include assisting the patient with leg lifts and/or elevating the legs to 15°–20° at intervals, and teaching the patient to wiggle his or her toes and perform ankle circles frequently while in bed. Compression to the knee vessels is minimized by avoiding placing anything under the knees while in bed (pillows, knee gatches), avoiding crossing of the knees or legs, and avoiding dangling the patient's legs over the side of the bed.

Education is a necessary component of care when a patient is at risk for DIC. Patients and families are taught to report any bleeding or unusual or abnormal symptoms. They are taught to save all excreta for the nurse to examine for blood. Finally, the patient and family will need excellent psychosocial support should the patient develop the paradoxical hemorrhage and thrombus formation of DIC.

## ASSESSMENT

Assessment begins with a thorough history and physical examination. Either component of the assessment may be comprehensive, as when interviewing a person suspected of having a malignancy, or cursory, as when caring for an individual with acute blood loss due to the malignancy. The information gathered in the assessment is instrumental in preparing an appropriate plan of care.

### Patient/Family History

The patient/family history is a vital component of the complete assessment. Because bleeding is a common problem in many malignancies, one must remain alert to findings that suggest hemostatic disorders. Patients may respond more openly and with greater ease if questions are focused toward activities of daily living, e.g., excessive bleeding while shaving, or prolonged bleeding after receiving minor cuts and scrapes while cooking or cleaning. Key aspects of a comprehensive history for the individual at risk for bleeding include the following:

1. bleeding tendencies, including easy bruising, excessive nosebleeds, gingival bleeding, presence of petechiae, change in color of stools or urine, stomach discomfort, vision problems, and painful joints
2. family history of any bleeding abnormalities
3. drugs and chemicals taken that might interfere with the coagulation mechanism or that might uncover an important symptom for which the person is taking medication
4. general performance status that helps to identify the effects of the disease or the presence of complications
5. current blood component therapy, including reason for and response to therapy
6. nutritional status, to identify vitamin K or C deficiency or generalized malnutrition that will affect the person's hematologic system
7. presence of any signs or symptoms of anemia, which may signify undetected long-term bleeding

### Physical Examination

Observation is perhaps the most important measure in early detection of bleeding. Diagnostic signals can be subtle, including skin petechiae noticed while bathing the person, traces of blood as the person brushes her or his teeth, and oozing from venipuncture sites or sites of injections. These are examples of the types of information that can lead to early diagnosis of hemostatic problems, and might prevent an incident of spontaneous hemorrhage.

The major problem associated with active bleeding is hemorrhage. Although bleeding can occur from any part of the body, common sites of hemorrhage include the gums, nose, bladder, GI tract, and brain. An examination of all body systems is done on a routine basis for any patient known to have a bleeding disorder (see Table 22-7).

### Screening Tests

Several screening tests provide information regarding hemostatic function. These groups of tests give information about both phases of hemostasis and fibrinolysis. The hematologic alterations leading to bleeding are complex, and test results will vary depending on the degree of original coagulation dysfunction and the cascading effect of related hemostatic mechanisms. A brief discussion regarding some of the most common screening tests of hemostatic function follows. A more comprehensive list is given in Table 22-8.

#### Bleeding time

This test measures the time it takes for a small skin incision to stop bleeding. The results depend on the platelet number and function and the ability of the capillary wall to constrict. The time varies from one to nine minutes. The bleeding time is prolonged when there is a lack of platelets or in diseases affecting the blood vessel walls. Examples of disease states in which a prolonged bleeding time may be found include thrombocytopenia, Willebrand's syndrome, infiltration of the marrow by tumor, and consumption of platelets in disseminated intravascular coagulation. Prolonged bleeding time is also found with drugs that affect platelet function, such as aspirin.

#### Platelet count

This test measures the actual number of circulating platelets per cubic millimeter of blood. Normal counts are considered to be 150,000–400,000/mm$^3$. Counts below 100,000/mm$^3$ are considered indicative of thrombocytopenia. Spontaneous hemorrhage generally is not a concern until the platelet count drops below 15,000/mm$^3$. Thrombocytosis occurs when the count rises above 400,000/mm$^3$.

#### Whole blood clot retraction test

This test, which measures the speed and extent of blood clot retraction in a test tube, is done to determine the degree of platelet adequacy. A normal clot shrinks to one-half its normal size in 1–2 hours and shrinks completely in 24 hours. Clot retraction is slower and the clot

**TABLE 22-8**  Tests of Hemostasis

| Test | Measures | Normal Value |
|---|---|---|
| **PLATELET FUNCTION** | | |
| Bleeding time | Platelet plug formation; response of small vessels | 1–9 min |
| Platelet count | Number of circulating platelets | 150,000–400,000/mm³ |
| Clot retraction | Ability of platelets to support retraction of a clot | 50% retraction within 1 hr; compare with normal value |
| Platelet aggregation | Ability of platelets to aggregate | Compare with normal control |
| Platelet phospholipid (factor 3) availability | Availability of platelet factor 3 for coagulation | Compare with normal control |
| **COAGULATION** | | |
| Partial thromboplastin time (aPTT) | Diminished or absent coagulation factors | Varies; compare with normal control (usually 30–40 sec) |
| Prothrombin time (PT) | Diminished or absent coagulation factors | Varies; compare with normal control |
| Thrombin time | Fibrinogen concentration; structure of fibrinogen; presence of inhibitors | Varies; compare with normal value |
| Specific factor assays | Concentration of functional factor in plasma | 50%–150% activity in pooled normal plasma |
| **FIBRINOLYSIS** | | |
| Assay of fibrinogen or fibrin degradation products (FDP) | Presence of FDP in serum | 1:8; 10 µg/ml<br>1:4; 0–8 µg/ml<br>10 µg/ml |

will stay soft and watery with thrombocytopenia or with abnormally functioning platelets.

### Prothrombin time

In this test, tissue thromboplastin and ionized calcium are added to citrated plasma, and the time required for clotting is recorded. The test is measured against the time needed for a normal sample of blood to clot. Test results are usually given as the actual time, in seconds, and are also compared with a normal or control value. When the clotting factors exist in diminished quantity, the PT is prolonged. Prolonged PT values are also seen in liver disease (hepatitis and tumor involvement), in obstructive biliary disease (e.g., bile duct obstruction secondary to tumor), and with coumarin ingestion.[98]

### Partial thromboplastin time (activated)

The aPTT is determined by adding phospholipid reagents to plasma in the presence of calcium chloride. Normal aPTT is 30–40 seconds. A prolonged aPTT is evidenced when clotting factors exist in inadequate quantities, as with consumptive coagulopathy, liver disease, and biliary obstruction, and with circulating anticoagulants such as heparin. There is a risk of spontaneous hemorrhage if the aPTT is greater than 100.[99]

The PT and PTT taken together can give a fair indication of the nature of the clotting defect. If both the PT and the PTT are normal, the vessels or platelets are probably defective. The defect is likely to be in the clotting mechanism if either the PT or the PTT is prolonged.

### Fibrin degradation products test

This test is determined by adding peripheral venous blood to serum containing antifibrinogen degradation fragments. The measurement of FDPs provides an indication of the activity of the fibrinolytic system. Agglutination is demonstrated if the patient's blood contains the degradation fragments. FDP levels greater than 10 g/ml indicate increased fibrinolysis, as seen in DIC and primary fibrinolytic disorders. No agglutination occurs if degradation products are absent in the patient's blood.

## THERAPEUTIC APPROACHES AND NURSING CARE

The physical safety of the patient is always ensured to prevent trauma in the individuals experiencing thrombocytopenia. Potential threats of injury in the environment are identified and then reduced or eliminated. Bumps or falls can be dangerous or even fatal in the individual with a low platelet count. (See Table 22-3 for a review of the plan of care of a patient experiencing thrombocytopenia/bleeding.)

Diligent measures to maintain skin integrity are instituted. Electric razors are used to prevent cuts while shaving. The mouth and gums are easily damaged when the platelet count drops, and they become an excellent potential source of infection. A systematic mouth care regimen should be used to minimize this problem. Soft-bristled toothbrushes help to avoid trauma to sensitive gums. When the platelet count drops below 20,000–30,000/mm,³ bristled toothbrushes are avoided and mouth swabs or Toothettes® are used. A nonirritating (alcohol-free) mouthwash is recommended. When the mouth and gums are irritated, dentures should not be replaced, particularly if they fit poorly. Patients requiring oxygen therapy via nasal cannula or endotracheal tube are assessed for irritation to the mucosa.

All unnecessary procedures are avoided in the thrombocytopenic patient, including intramuscular or SQ injections, rectal temperatures or suppositories, and indwelling catheters. If the patient requires parenteral administration of medication, the IV route is used whenever possible. Intramuscular and SQ injections place the patient at risk for the development of hematomas, which can become sites of infection when granulocytopenia is present. Injections, if unavoidable, are administered with the smallest possible gauge of needle. Pressure to the injection site is applied for several minutes, followed by the application of a pressure bandage to avoid hematomas. Similar care is taken at venipuncture sites.

Severe uterine hemorrhage can be a complication in thrombocytopenic women who are menstruating. Menses can be suppressed by pharmacological agents, generally progestational medications. In women whose menses are not suppressed, yet who have menstrual bleeding, careful napkin counts are done to help determine the volume of blood loss.

Forceful coughing, sneezing, or nose blowing can lead to bleeding. Epistaxis can be life-threatening in an individual with thrombocytopenia. The patient with epistaxis is placed in high Fowler's position. Ice packs, nasal packing, or topical adrenaline may also be used to decrease bleeding caused by small-vessel constriction within the nasal mucosa. Bowel strain caused by constipation can initiate rectal bleeding. Prescribed stool softeners may be necessary to avoid constipation. Instruction regarding proper diet and exercise to avoid constipation are also appropriate.

Hygiene is a problem in the patient who has active bleeding. The bleeding patient may require frequent baths and linen changes in order to feel and smell better. A room deodorizer may be needed, since blood exposed to air is malodorous.

Physical and emotional rest are essential when the patient is actively bleeding. Rest helps to decrease pulse rate and blood pressure, allowing for clot formation. A state of active bleeding is frightening and anxiety-producing for the patient and family. A calm approach and reassurance are in order in managing an individual who is actively bleeding. Sedation can also be used to decrease anxiety and the metabolic rate.

## Blood Component Therapy

Blood banking in the United States is a standardized industry that is heavily regulated by the federal government and some states. The blood-banking industry is regulated by the federal government under Title 21 of the Code of Regulations. These regulations place stringent requirements on collection, testing, storage, and distribution of blood and blood components.[100]

The technological advances in blood transfusion therapy, which allow for aggressive transfusion support for patients with cancer who receive highly toxic treatment regimens, have led to a decrease in the morbidity and mortality of cancer and its treatment. Except in situations of extreme emergency, transfusion therapy is provided to correct deficiencies in a specific component of whole blood. Whole blood is removed from a donor and is then "fractionated" into the various components, i.e., red blood cells, platelets, plasma, and plasma proteins. This fractionation process is accomplished via refrigerated centrifugation or automated equipment using continuous-flow cell separations.

The entire collection system is sterile, disposable, and never reused. It is therefore impossible for a donor to contract a transfusion-transmitted disease. The collection system is considered a closed system, being open only at the tip of the needle.

### Red blood cell therapy

In any patient the clinical concern for the adverse physiological effects of anemia is usually the basis for considering red blood cell replacement. The decision to transfuse generally is based on an overall clinical picture, including any underlying cardiac or pulmonary condition or any concurrent conditions that might impair the patient's tolerance for anemia.[50] Among the causes of anemia frequently seen in cancer patients, the two most common are decreased red cell production secondary to myelosuppressive therapy and the primary disease process.

An attempt is generally made to keep the patient's hemoglobin level higher than 8 g/100 ml. It is customary in most centers to delay transfusions until the hemoglobin is lower than 8 g/100 ml or until the patient is symptomatic. A patient is transfused with a sufficient quantity of red cells to raise the hemoglobin level to at least 10 or 11 g/100 ml, and to even higher levels if the patient has a concomitant infection.[101] Physiological signs of anemia (hyperventilation, rapid pulse, shortness of breath on exertion, rapid pulse, pallor, fatigue) should be relieved when the hemoglobin is raised to 10 or 11 g/100 ml.[35] If the patient is not actively bleeding, 1 unit of packed red cells should increase the peripheral hematocrit level by 3% and the hemoglobin by 1 g/dl.[102]

Packed erythrocytes usually are the therapy of choice. The advantage of packed red blood cells is that they provide more than 70% of the hematocrit of whole blood with only one-third of the plasma. This prevents unnecessary volume, electrolyte load, and anticoagulants that may otherwise be transfused.

Leukocytes in red blood cell transfusions can cause reactions if the recipient has antileukocyte antibodies, which can develop from previous transfusions or pregnancies. Transfusion of packed red cells in these patients can cause fever and chills. The patient can become alloimmunized, or refractory to transfusions. This condition is demonstrated when a transfusion of a unit of red cells fails to achieve an expected increase in the hemoglobin level. The use of leukocyte-poor blood component therapy is indicated for these patients. Another major indication for leukocyte-poor blood products is with patients who have had prior febrile nonhemolytic transfusion reactions or allergic reactions to packed erythrocytes.[35] (See leukocyte-depleted blood products in this chapter.)

Packed red blood cells are preserved at liquid storage 4–6 °C for a shelf life of 35 days. The shelf life can be extended to 42 days with the addition of certain solutions. The unit may also be frozen at −80° to −150° for storage for seven to ten years.[103]

### Platelet therapy

The use of platelet transfusions has proved to have tremendous therapeutic value in controlling and preventing hemorrhage in individuals with cancer. Generally the decision to transfuse is indicated when there is actual bleeding associated with thrombocytopenia, when the platelet count is > 20,000/mm³ yet bleeding is present, and in patients with abnormally functioning platelets who are bleeding. Prophylactic platelet transfusions can be given in the absence of clinical hemorrhage but during periods of intense chemotherapy, to prevent spontaneous hemorrhage into the brain. Other factors that determine appropriateness of transfusion therapy are determined on an individual basis. The presence of infection and a rapid decrease in circulating platelets may suggest a decreased tolerance to thrombocytopenia.

Theoretically, one unit of platelets should increase the recipient's peripheral blood platelet level by 10,000–12,000 cells/mm³. Traditionally, the attempt is made to maintain the patient's platelet count above 20,000/mm³ to minimize the potential for spontaneous hemorrhage. More recent experience indicates that platelet counts in the range of 10,000–20,000/mm³ can be monitored safely without the use of prophylactic transfusions.[104] Close observation of these patients to detect bleeding is essential. In the absence of normal platelet production, platelet transfusions generally are required every three days. Concomitant infection, with fever, or active bleeding will increase platelet transfusion requirements.

Platelets can be given in fresh whole blood, platelet-rich plasma, or platelet concentrates (see Table 22-9). The concentrated method is most widely used today. Platelets can be obtained from differential centrifugation of donated whole blood or from platelet pheresis of single donors. A donor can be pheresed frequently (up to every other day) if the donor's platelets provide the patient with good platelet count increases. One unit of platelets is routinely obtained from 500 ml of fresh whole blood. Platelets are stored at room temperature and are stored up to 5 days. Contaminating microorganisms may reach unacceptably high titers beyond 5 days. Platelet concentrates can be administered rapidly over 10–20 minutes.[50]

Several factors have been identified as important in determining posttransfusion platelet survival in an individual. Failure to achieve adequate increments in the circulating platelet count is often due to infection, fever, disseminated intravascular coagulation, or splenomegaly. Infection can enhance the consumption of platelets and increase the occurrence of hemorrhage. Patients with fever or sepsis require frequent transfusions to maintain an adequate platelet count. Patients with splenomegaly who are receiving platelet transfusions will have a reduced recovery of circulating platelets generally proportionate to the size of their spleen. If platelets are being transfused while the person is actively bleeding, increased increments will not be detected by laboratory data. However, their effectiveness can be measured by clinical improvement and control of bleeding.

Patients with fever due to infection can be premedicated with antipyretics prior to platelet transfusion in an attempt to minimize platelet destruction. When a fever is caused by the platelet transfusion, i.e., febrile reaction to the transfusion, premedication can consist of antipyretics, corticosteroids, and/or antihistamines. Demerol may be given if the patient is having shaking chills. Certain antimicrobial drugs occasionally have also been found to cause platelet refractoriness due to drug-induced antibodies. Drug-induced antibodies have been demonstrated against cotrimoxazole, amphotericin B, and certain semisynthetic penicillins.[105]

Platelet survival is greatly decreased when alloimmunization to the platelet transfusion develops. The patient is then considered to be refractory to platelet transfusions. In most cases alloimmunization is due to formation of antibodies to human leukocyte antigens (HLA) on the platelet cell surface, and from contamination of white cells in the platelet concentrate.[50,106] Because of repeated exposure of patient/recipient platelets to the HLA antigens on the donor's platelets, patients eventually may become refractory to random donor platelets. The patient may then respond to HLA-matched platelets. Leukocyte-poor transfusions may also be used to sustain an adequate platelet count and prevent bleeding (see Table 22-9). A one-hour postplatelet transfusion count is important in deciding if the patient is becoming refractory to platelets. A poor increment (< 10,000/mm³ rise in

**TABLE 22-9**  Platelet Transfusion Therapy

| Specific Component | Content and Volume | General Indications | Complications | Nursing Considerations |
|---|---|---|---|---|
| **Random donor (RD)**<br>• Fresh—best<br>• Frozen and cryopreserved (limited application because of poor recovery) | • Multiple donors (4+) approximately 200 ml<br>• Plasma, WBCs, few RBCs | • Bleeding and bleeding prophylaxis<br>• Prophylactic for platelet count <20,000/mm³ | • Exposure of patients to multiple tissue antigens, which initiates antigen-antibody formation, leading to refractoriness<br>• Hepatitis (increased risk with pooled products)<br>• Allergic reactions may be seen more often if leukocyte-poor filter is not used | • Gently agitate bag occasionally to prevent platelet clumping.<br>• Rapid infusion (per patient tolerance).<br>• Tubing should include a 170–220-mm in-line blood filter. Leukocyte-poor blood filter may be required.<br>• Less expensive than single donor of HLA-matched platelet concentrates |
| **Single donor (SD)**<br>• Fresh (maximum effectiveness up to 6 hr) | • One donor<br>• 1 unit—300 ml<br>• Plasma, WBCs, RBCs<br>• Number of platelets in a SD unit equals approximately the number of platelets in 5 RD units | • Bleeding and bleeding prophylaxis<br>• Severe febrile reactions<br>• Often used once a patient is refractory to random donor platelets<br>• Patients who require long-term platelet therapy<br>• Minimizes the transmission of viral disease | • Refractoriness to platelet may occur over time (see section on leukocyte-depleted blood products) | • Rapid infusion (generally 30 min +).<br>• Tubing as above. Leukocyte-poor blood filter may be required. |
| **Human-leukocyte antigen (HLA) matched concentrate** | • One donor compatible at the HLA complex<br>• 1 U—300 ml<br>• Plasma, WBCs, RBCs | • When patients become refractory to RD and SD platelets<br>• Minimizes transmission of viral disease | • Minimal | • HLA-matched platelets minimize patient exposure to multiple tissue antigens (HLA complex found on all blood cells—acts as a genetic monogram).<br>• Rapid infusion (30 min +).<br>• Tubing as above. Generally see more effective increases in the platelet count than with RD or SD. |

the platelet count) is seen with alloimmunization and splenomegaly. A 24-hour postplatelet transfusion count helps to determine if other factors are responsible for a poor platelet recovery, such as infection, fever, or another cause for accelerated platelet consumption.[107] An investigational method of preventing alloimmunization to platelets is the irradiation of platelet concentrates with ultraviolet light.[108]

Platelet increments may be negatively affected by leukoagglutinin reactions directed at non-HLA leukocyte antigens. In this situation donor platelets are contaminated with leukocytes. Once transfused there is subsequent antibody formation, causing allergic symptoms, which include hives, skin flush, fever, and chills. These reactions can be avoided by leukocyte depletion from the platelet concentrate during preparation.[109] Patients can also be premedicated with antipyretics, corticosteroids, and antihistamines to minimize this reaction.

The preparation and storage of platelets are also important factors in determining the quality of the platelet transfusion. To be most effective, platelets must be fresh and metabolically active. Maximum effectiveness remains for up to six hours after being obtained. Storage longer than 24 hours at 22 °C causes significant loss of platelet function due to release of ADP and alterations in platelet membrane permeability. Platelets can, however, be stored for up to five days. Platelets should be agitated gently during storage.

A therapy that continues to be investigated for the support of individuals refractory to all types of available transfusions is the use of IV gamma globulin (IVIgG). Some investigators have found that high-dose IVIgG (400 mg/kg/day for five days) improves the response to platelet concentrates in platelet-refractory patients.[110,111] This therapy is expensive but may be justified in the refractory patient with uncontrolled bleeding.

### Plasma therapy

Plasma, like the other blood components, can be separated from whole blood via centrifugation. As blood is withdrawn from a donor, the red blood cells are packed by centrifugation, leaving about 70% of the platelets suspended in plasma. This platelet-rich plasma is then spun again to yield a platelet concentrate in approximately 50 ml of plasma. The remaining plasma is then removed and rapidly frozen at less than 18 °C. The frozen plasma, called *fresh-frozen plasma*, contains all of the labile clotting factors and the plasma proteins. The plasma proteins such as albumin and cryoprecipitate, can be isolated and removed from plasma. Plasma and other blood components can also be obtained via apheresis.

The most common use of plasma and plasma components in cancer is with coagulation disorders associated with this disease. Plasma component therapy is also administered for severe bleeding, shock, bleeding associated with infections, and management of acute DIC. Plasma can be used to treat deficiences of factors II, V, VIII, X, XI, and XIII. Specific factor concentrates are available for factors VIII and IX. Factor concentrates for factors VII, XI, and XIII are under development. All patients who receive or are to receive clotting factor concentrates are advised to be vaccinated against hepatitis B.[85]

A number of variables are used to determine the optimal dosage of plasma and plasma components as replacement therapy in coagulation disorders. The primary considerations include severity of the deficiency, specific factor deficiency, severity of bleeding, possible danger of bleeding to the patient, and duration of therapy.[85] Replacement plasma is usually calculated in units, with 1 unit of plasma equaling the activity present in 1 ml of normal human male plasma.

Another consideration in plasma therapy is the metabolic half-life of plasma and plasma derivatives. Replacement therapy is given in doses high enough to compensate for the decrease in the plasma level as it is metabolized.[84] The metabolic half-life varies for each of the factors. Plasma and plasma factors usually are infused rapidly, so the maximum plasma level is reached before metabolic changes or degradation occurs. Plasma component therapy is generally given intravenously. (See Table 22-10 for further discussion of plasma therapy.)

## Transfusion Complications

There are many hazards associated with the administration of blood component therapy. These hazards may cause immediate or delayed reactions. The major hazards include hemolytic and nonhemolytic transfusion reactions, transmission of diseases, and complications associated with IV therapy and transfusions. (See Table 22-11 for a complete list of transfusion reactions and Table 22-12 for the nursing management of transfusion reactions.)

**TABLE 22-10** Commonly Used Plasma Components

| Component | Content Volume and Route | Shelf Life | Indications | Complications | Nursing Considerations |
|---|---|---|---|---|---|
| Normal human plasma (fresh or frozen) | Plasma; all plasma proteins and clotting factors; 200 ml, IV route | 1 yr frozen; 24 hr thawed | Severe blood loss; clotting factor deficiency (II, V, VII, X, XI, and XIII); plasma volume expander without increasing the hematocrit | Volume overload; hepatitis and other viruses; allergic reactions; hypernatremia, hypocalcemia | Requires ABO compatibility. Average adult dose is 3–5 units (12–15 ml/kg) given over 1 hr to several hrs (depending on the client's cardiovascular status); smaller doses may need to be given at periodic intervals; administer fresh-frozen plasma immediately after thawing to minimize deterioration of factors V and VIII; infusion should be slowed or stopped if patient demonstrates signs of citrate toxicity. |

**TABLE 22-10** Commonly Used Plasma Components (continued)

| Component | Content Volume and Route | Shelf Life | Indications | Complications | Nursing Considerations |
|---|---|---|---|---|---|
| Normal human serum albumin | Aqueous fraction of pooled plasma 5%: 250 ml and 500 ml; 25%: 25 ml and 50 ml, IV route | 3–5 yr | Rapid volume expansion | No hepatitis risk | Monitor cardiac and renal function closely; congestive heart failure may be precipitated by compromised function; each unit must be used immediately after opening as albumin does not contain preservatives; rate of administration of 5% solution should not be >2–4 ml/min; rate of administration of 25% solution should not be >1 ml/min. |
| Cryoprecipitate | Fibrinogen, factors VIII (100 U) and XIII, von Willebrand factor, fibronectin; 10–20 ml, IV route | 1 yr frozen; 6 hr thawed | Severe von Willebrand's disease; hypofibrinogenemia (DIC); fibronectin may have a role in wound healing | Hepatitis and other viruses | Best to be ABO-compatible; should be kept at room temperature until infused; administer within 3 min; infusion of cryoprecipitate will increase circulating plasma fibrinogen to pre-bleeding levels; a "fibrin sealant" can be made by adding bovine thrombin to cryoprecipitate; it may stop bleeding when applied topically. |
| Fibrinogen | Fibrinogen; 10 ml, IV route | 1 yr frozen | Clotting disorders; hemophilia A or B | | Monitor cardiac and renal function closely; administer rapidly; 1 U should raise level 10 U. |
| Purified AHF concentrate | Factor VIII (lyophilized); IV route | Per pharmacy label | Severe von Willebrand's disease; hemophilia A | High hepatitis risk (C) | Rate of administration is 2 ml/min, can be up to 10 ml/min; if patient's pulse increases significantly, rate of administration should be decreased. |
| Immune Globulin | Immunoglobulin from large pools of human plasma, IV and IM route | Per pharmacy label | Bleeding disorders, hypogammaglobulinemia, ITP | | May be given to clients who are refractory to a variety of platelet transfusions (Random donor, single donor, HLA matched platelets) |
| Antithrombin III (AT-III) Concentrates | Antithrombin III (lyophilized) | Per pharmacy label | Antithrombin III deficiency | | |
| Recombinant factor VIII | Factor VIII, IV route | Per pharmacy label | Hemophilia, especially for those patients who have never been exposed to blood products or have no evidence of transfusion-transmitted viruses | | |
| Heat-treated lyophilized prothrombin complex concentrates (PCC) | Prothrombin factors VII, IX, X; IV route | Per pharmacy label | Bleeding disorders; hemophilia B; factor VIII inhibitor | High hepatitis risk (C); thrombosis; no HIV with currently available products | Monitor patient for signs/symptoms of thrombosis (no lab test measures PCC effectiveness). |

Adapted with permission from Gobel.[84]

**TABLE 22-11** Complications of Transfusions

**Immediate**
Acute hemolytic transfusion reaction
Febrile reactions, chills
Allergy—urticaria, anaphylaxis
Bacterial contamination—shock, sepsis
Circulatory overload
Air embolism
Citrate toxicity
Hypocalcemia
Hyperkalemia
Hypothermia
Iron overload
Respiratory distress

**Delayed**
Delayed hemolytic transfusion reaction
Infection—hepatitis (A, B, or C), retrovirus, cytomegalovirus, human immunodeficiency virus, human T-cell lymphotrophic virus type 1, parasites
Graft-vs-host disease
Posttransfusion purpura
Alloimmunization
Bacterial contamination

Platelets generally can be transfused across incompatibilities of the major red blood cell antigens (ABO) unless there is gross red blood cell contamination into the transfusion pack. If significant spillage has occurred, the donor and recipient are matched by A,B,O antigens. If matching is not done when spillage occurs, hemolytic reactions are likely.

A serious transfusion complication in patients who are significantly immunosuppressed (e.g., bone marrow transplant recipients, patients undergoing combined treatment for Hodgkin's and non-Hodgkin's lymphoma, and leukemia patients undergoing induction chemotherapy) is the risk of developing graft-versus-host (GVH) disease. This complication can occur following the transfusion of blood products containing viable lymphocytes. The donor-competent T lymphocyte immunologically attacks the immunocompromised host tissue after transfusion. This disease, generally manifested in the skin, liver, and GI tract, can be fatal.[112] Pancytopenia can also occur as the hematopoietic cells are foreign to the attacking lymphocytes. The mortality rate is 85%–90% after a median of 21 days.[50]

It is generally recommended that all blood products given to the severely immunocompromised host be exposed to pretransfusion irradiation with 15 cGy.[113] Irradiation of blood is done to inhibit proliferation of lymphocytes without impairment of platelets, red cells, or granulocytes. There is additional cost with irradiation of blood component therapy. The current cost of the irradiator and the radiation source is approximately $50,000. Because of the additional cost, it is generally recommended that irradiated blood products be used only for specific indications.[50] Leukocyte-poor blood filters, which are capable of removing nearly all leukocytes, can serve as an alternate approach to preventing GVH disease.[114]

### Leukocyte-depleted blood products

Leukocytes remaining in donor blood collected for transfusion are responsible for many of the complications related to transfusion therapy, including immunologic effects, nonhemolytic febrile reactions, and transmission of viral infections.[114–117] (see Table 22-13). The removal of leukocytes, more specifically the microaggregates of leukocytes that form in a spontaneous and progressive manner in stored blood products, is done extensively to prevent febrile nonhemolytic reactions and other complications.[114] It has been demonstrated for decades that the likelihood of adverse reactions to blood component therapy is correlated with the absolute number of leukocytes transfused.[118]

The removal of leukocytes from stored blood products, by conventional filtration methods, can generally decrease the number of leukocytes to a point below the threshold for febrile reactions in a sensitized patient. (The pore size of a standard blood administration set in-line filter is 170 μm and effectively removes gross fibrin clots.) The number of remaining leukocytes, however, may be sufficient to enhance or cause alloimmunization to blood products.[114] The remaining leukocytes are also known to transmit viral infections. Some transfusion-induced infections are caused exclusively by white blood cells. Cytomegalovirus (CMV) infection caused by blood transfusion is caused by remaining leukocytes in the transfused blood. The use of CMV-seronegative blood products is currently the standard of care for severely immunosuppressed patients or for bone marrow transplant patients who are seronegative and who have seronegative bone marrow donors.[116] The demand for CMV-negative blood products may, however, exceed the supply at many blood centers, as the number of transplants has increased, and in areas where CMV-negative blood cannot be obtained (e.g., Washington, DC). Studies have shown that leukocyte reduction of blood products may significantly reduce the risk of CMV transmission.[115,119] A recent study demonstrated the relative safety and efficacy of leukocyte reduction of blood products versus CMV-seronegative blood products for the prevention of CMV infection and disease after allogeneic or autologous bone marrow transplant.[116]

In addition to the traditional methods of leukocyte depletion of blood products (sedimentation, centrifugation, cell washing, and freeze-thaw deglycerolization), two methods of leukocyte depletion that currently are being extensively investigated include laboratory filtration and bedside filtration of blood components.[120] The filters trap leukocytes by selective adsorption, with the most efficient medium being a nonwoven fiber mesh with a diameter less than 3 mm.[121] Most laboratory filters are capable of depleting 99% of the leukocytes present in a unit of

**TABLE 22-12**  Nursing Management of Selected Transfusion Reactions

| Type | Signs/Symptoms | Nursing Actions |
|---|---|---|
| Acute hemolytic transfusion reaction<br><br>● ABO incompatibility | Fever, chills, hypotension, increased pulse rate, nausea/vomiting, flushing, low back pain, decreased urine output, hematuria, dyspnea, bleeding, anaphylaxis | 1. Stop transfusion.<br>2. Maintain patent IV line.<br>3. Verify client and the blood unit with another nurse (the majority of reported fatalities with an acute hemolytic transfusion reaction involve human error).<br>4. Place in supine position.<br>5. Maintain open airway; provide CPR if necessary.<br>6. Obtain vital signs and record.<br>7. Notify physician.<br>8. Monitor intake and output.<br>9. Administer fluids and medications per physician order.<br>10. Vital signs.<br>11. Obtain blood and urine specimens.<br>12. Notify blood bank and return remainder of blood to blood bank.<br>13. Document event.<br>14. Admit patient to hospital if outpatient. |
| Febrile nonhemolytic transfusion reaction (FNHTRS)<br><br>● Antileukocyte antibodies in the recipient directed against the donor blood | Fever ± chills, headache, hypotension, increased pulse rate, dyspnea, chest pain, nausea/vomiting | 1. Stop transfusion.<br>2. Maintain patent IV line.<br>3. Obtain and monitor vital signs and record.<br>4. Assist in ruling out infection.<br>5. Notify physician.<br>6. Administer medications and fluids per physician order: acetaminophen for fever, meperidine for chills, antihistamine for dyspnea.<br>7. Continue transfusion if symptoms not severe.<br>8. Notify blood bank.<br>9. Document event.<br>10. For clients who are known to have FNHTRS or for clients who are at high risk for FNHTRS (multiply transfused clients) acetaminophen and antihistamines/steroids may be given before the transfusion to minimize or eliminate the transfusion reaction. The use of a leukocyte-poor filter may be indicated. |
| Allergic (usually mild)<br><br>● Recipient antibodies against immunoglobulin components or other soluble proteins in the plasma | Urticaria and hives; may develop severe allergic or even fatal anaphylaxis | 1. Obtain and monitor vital signs and record.<br>2. Slow or stop transfusion rate, depending on symptoms.<br>3. Measures to correct shock, maintain renal circulation, and to correct the bleeding depending on symptoms.<br>4. Notify physician.<br>5. Administer medications per physician order: antihistamines if reaction is mild.<br>6. Notify blood bank.<br>7. Document event. |
| Bacterial contamination<br><br>● Cold growing organisms | Fever, chills; may result in endotoxin shock | 1. Stop transfusion.<br>2. Maintain patent IV line.<br>3. Measures to correct shock and to maintain renal circulation.<br>4. Obtain vital signs and record.<br>5. Notify physician.<br>6. Notify blood bank and return remainder of blood to blood bank.<br>7. Obtain blood cultures of the client and the unit of blood.<br>8. Administer antibiotics per physician order.<br>9. Document event.<br>10. Admit client to hospital if outpatient. |
| Delayed hemolytic<br><br>● Development of alloantibodies to transfused blood | Delayed (7–10 days to weeks) decreased hemoglobin, low-grade fever, jaundice (increase in bilirubin and LDH) | Notify blood bank. |

**TABLE 22-13**  Immunologic and Infectious Complications of Blood Transfusion Attributed to the Infusion of Donor Leukocytes

---

**Immunologic consequences**
Alloimmunization to human leukocyte antigens
Febrile transfusion reactions due to granulocytes
Transient immunosuppression/immune tolerance
Graft-versus-host reaction/disease
Transfusion-related acute lung injury (TRALI)

**Transmission of blood-borne viruses (BBV)**
Cytomegalovirus (CMV)
Human immunodeficiency viruses (HIV-1/2)
Human T-cell lymphotrophic viruses (HTLV-III)
Hepatitis B virus (HBV)
Human herpesvirus type 6 (HSV-6)
Epstein-Barr virus (EBV)

---

Rawal BD, Davis E, Busch MP, et al: Dual reduction in the immunologic and infectious complications of transfusion by filtration/removal of leukocytes from donor blood soon after collection. *Trans Med Rev* 4:36–41, 1990. Reprinted with permission.

blood, whereas the bedside filters deplete 99.9% (3 logs 10) of the white blood cells.[122] Bedside filters require no special processing of the unit of blood. Currently, the leukocyte-depleting filters available for use in the United States are the Pall RC-100 for red cells, the Pall PL-50 for platelets (Pall Biomedical Products Corporation, Glen Cove, NY), and the Sepacell (Asahi Medical Co., Ltd., Tokyo, Japan).

## Home Transfusion Therapy for the Cancer Patient

The home care industry has grown tremendously during the past decade. Services that are now provided in the home include complex IV therapy, including blood transfusion therapy. These services that are provided in the home are motivated by many changes in the health care environment and third-party reimbursement policies.

Prior to 1986, home care agencies, hospitals, and blood banks were reluctant to provide home transfusion services because of liability issues and the potential of losing accreditation by the American Association of Blood Banks (AABB). The AABB published a book in 1986 that addressed issues regarding patient safety, liability, and reimbursement for home transfusion therapy.[123] Since that time many home care agencies have initiated home transfusion programs based on the standards of the AABB and the Joint Commission on the Accreditation of Healthcare Organizations.

Safety of the patient receiving blood transfusions in the home is of primary concern to all health care providers. Efforts to ensure safety of home transfusion services include establishing adequate standards of care upon which policies and procedures are developed, knowledge of marketing regulations and legal and ethical concerns, early hospital discharge planning, careful selection criteria of patients, and effective patient and caregiver education.[124]

There are a number of benefits to home transfusion therapy for the cancer patient, including the potential for decreased cost (compared with receiving transfusions in the hospital), convenience for the patient and family of being able to stay home for needed blood transfusion, psychological benefits, and the ability to be treated in a familiar environment with family available.[124,125] There are no specific legal constraints against transfusing patients at home, as long as the procedure is performed by licensed and qualified medical personnel.[126] However, regardless of precautions taken, the patient is at greater risk for complications than would be the case in a hospital setting (lack of sophisticated emergency equipment). Thus patients must be carefully selected for home transfusion using appropriate criteria, and medical personnel administering the blood must be trained properly. The recommendations made for home tranfusion follow those for out-of-hospital transfusion of the Transfusion Practices Committee of the American Association of Blood Banks.[127]

### Selection criteria

The seven basic criteria for inclusion in a home transfusion therapy program include the following:[125]

1. physical limitations of the patient that make transportation difficult
2. stable cardiopulmonary status
3. patients who do not have an acute need for blood or who do not require more than 2 units in a 24-hour period
4. absence of reactions to the most recent transfusion
5. a cooperative patient
6. presence of a responsible adult during and after transfusion
7. a telephone available for medical needs or the need to call an ambulance
8. a diagnosis supporting the need for transfusion therapy

The person administering the transfusion should be a registered nurse with current venipuncture and IV therapy skills. The nurse should have completed a competency-based educational program on transfusion therapy. Finally, the nurse's transfusion therapy skills should be supervised prior to independently transfusing a patient in the home.

### Preadministration considerations

Once the patient has been accepted as a candidate for home transfusion therapy, a number of appointments must be made and documents established. Appointments are made with the patient for pretransfusion blood samples and for the transfusions. Ideally, the pretransfusion blood sample collection is done the day before the scheduled transfusion (but may be done 48 hours prior to the tranfusion), and by the nurse who will administer the blood. The samples are placed in an insulated container with appropriate request forms and are returned to the blood bank for processing. Once the informed consent has been signed by the patient, a means of identification is placed on the patient and must remain in place until after the transfusion. It is recommended that a commercial wristband system that uses preprinted numbers be used to increase patient safety. Documentation records, established for each new patient, include physician's written orders for the blood transfusion, a signed informed consent, laboratory results, nursing progress records, and a "Home Transfusion Flow Sheet." This form provides for complete documentation of the blood transfusion process (see Figure 22-4). Much of the information on the flow sheet can be filled out prior to the blood administration: patient's name and address, physician's name and phone number, and emergency information. All of this information needs to be verified on the day of the transfusion.

Nurses who administer blood in the home setting take on a great deal of responsibility. Institutional policies and procedures must be adhered to closely in order to maximize patient safety. The home transfusion protocol outlined in Table 22-14 covers general administration considerations.

Once the transfusion is complete, the nurse will discontinue the transfusion bag yet maintain a patent IV

---

Date of transfusion: _____

Patient's name: _____    Patient's I.D. #: _____

Patient's address: _____

Patient's diagnosis: _____

Patient's blood type:    ABO _____    Rh _____    CMV Neg. _____    CMV Pos. _____

Physician's name: _____    Physician's phone #: _____

Order verified: _____ (Initials)

Name and location of emergency treatment facility: _____

_____

Name and phone # of emergency/ambulance service: _____

Patient identity verified:    Yes _____    No _____

Unique identifying number of the blood bag
same as cross-matched unit recorded:    Yes _____    No _____

Cross-matched units compatible:    Yes _____    No _____

Patient's name and I.D. # on
cross-match record verified with
patient identification:    Yes _____    No _____

Allergies: _____

Current medications: _____

IV solution: _____

  Time started: _____    By: _____ (initials)
  Amount infused: _____
  Site of infusion: _____
  Device (type and gauge): _____

**FIGURE 22-4**   Home transfusion flow sheet. (Adapted with permission from the American Association of Blood Banks.[102])

*(continued)*

Premedications:

    Acetaminophen _____     (dosae, route, time—initials)
    Benadryl _____
    Other _____

Filter type:

    In-line _____     Leukocyte-poor _____

Restrictions:

    Irradiation of products _____     Other _____

| Blood component | Whole Blood #/ Pool # | Time Started | Time Completed | Volume Infused |
|---|---|---|---|---|
| Single-donor platelets _____ | _____ | _____ | _____ | _____ |
| Random-donor platelets _____ | _____ | _____ | _____ | _____ |
| HLA-matched platelets _____ | _____ | _____ | _____ | _____ |
| Red blood cells _____ | _____ | _____ | _____ | _____ |
| Whole blood _____ | _____ | _____ | _____ | _____ |

| Nurses notes: | Time | BP | T | P | R | Lung Sounds (when indicated) |
|---|---|---|---|---|---|---|
| Baseline | _____ | _____ | _____ | _____ | _____ | _____ |
| 15 min | _____ | _____ | _____ | _____ | _____ | _____ |
| 30 min | _____ | _____ | _____ | _____ | _____ | _____ |
| 1 hr | _____ | _____ | _____ | _____ | _____ | _____ |
| 1-1/2 hr | _____ | _____ | _____ | _____ | _____ | _____ |
| 2 hr | _____ | _____ | _____ | _____ | _____ | _____ |
| 2-1/2 hr | _____ | _____ | _____ | _____ | _____ | _____ |
| 3 hr | _____ | _____ | _____ | _____ | _____ | _____ |
| 3-1/2 hr | _____ | _____ | _____ | _____ | _____ | _____ |
| 4 hr | _____ | _____ | _____ | _____ | _____ | _____ |
| Final | _____ | _____ | _____ | _____ | _____ | _____ |

Suspected reaction:          Yes _____     No _____

Symptoms: _____

Amount infused: _____

If yes, collect the following:     Blood sample _____     Urine sample _____

Physican notified _____ (initials)

*Return any blood bag to the blood bank when there is a suspicion of a blood transfusion reaction.

I have checked all information and find it to be correct. _____ R.N.
                                                        Signature

**FIGURE 22-4**   Home transfusion flow sheet. *(continued)*

line. The nurse remains with the patient for at least 30 minutes after transfusion to observe the patient and to monitor vital signs. If the patient is stable at this time, the IV line can be discontinued. All transfusion supplies are collected in a biohazard bag for disposal. If ordered, a posttransfusion blood sample can be obtained. Documentation of the entire blood transfusion process must be detailed and complete. Follow-up of the transfused patient should be done within 24 hours of the transfusion. Clinical indicators of the effectiveness of a transfusion include the hemoglobin level, the hematocrit, and the platelet count. Other measures to establish effectiveness of the tranfusion are the patient's energy/fatigue level and respiratory status.[128]

**TABLE 22-14** Home Transfusion Protocol

| Nursing Actions | Rationale |
|---|---|
| 1. Gather supplies:<br>• IV pole and pump (if required)<br>• Blood filter (if required)<br>• Saline<br>• Appropriate blood tubing<br>• Blood filters per institutional policies and procedures<br>• Needles, syringes, appropriate for type of vascular access device to be used<br>• Transfusion flow sheet<br>• Emergency drug kit (including epinephrine 1:10,000 and 1:1000 and diphenhydramine hydrochloride 50 mg), extra saline bag<br>• Transfusion reaction protocol<br>• Emergency plan to transport patient (physician's phone #, hospital and ambulance phone number | Most electromechanical pumps can safely administer RBC transfusions (see section on leukocyte-depleted blood products). Combining other solutions (including glucose) with RBCs can cause agglutination or hemolysis of the RBCs. All blood components require an in-line blood filter of 170 mm, at minimum. Some centers require all blood component therapy to be transfused through leukocyte-depleting blood filters or similar device. |
| 2. a. Check the physician's order to confirm the product type, dose, and rate of infusion.<br>b. Review client medical history/allergies, etc.<br>c. Obtain blood component from blood bank, on departure to client's home.<br>  • Check unit for client's full name, client's identification number, unique identifying numbers of the unit, the ABO and Rh type of the donor(s) and client, expiration date. Cross-check with blood bank employee and sign off.<br>  • Secure client's record and interpretation of compatibility test to the blood container.<br>  • Examine unit for unusual color, clots, or excessive air. | All blood components must be administered with a physician's written order.<br><br>Some medical conditions (e.g., congestive heart failure may make it necessary to modify usual administration practices i.e., administer blood over the longest, most appropriate length of time.<br><br>The primary cause of acute fatal transfusion reactions is major ABO incompatibility related to clerical errors.<br><br><br>Abnormalities may be an indication of contamination and/or improper collection or storage techniques. |
| 3. Transport the blood at a temperature between 1 °C and 10 °C (cool but not frozen).<br>• Best achieved by transporting RBCs in an insulated container with wet ice.<br>• Transport platelets at room temperature (between 20° and 24°); *do not* transport with wet ice.<br>• Blood components are not to be placed in the client's refrigerator at home. | RBCs cannot be returned to storage if the temperature exceeds 10 °C.<br><br><br>Platelets have best biological activity if stored at room temperature.<br>Temperatures in home refrigerators are not regulated. |
| 4. Confirm client identity:<br>• Verbally against the client record.<br>• Confirm client identification using the medical bracelet or other identification means and identify RBC compatibility on the tag attached to the unit and on all forms. | As above. |
| 5. Initiate blood component therapy:<br>• Explain procedure to client/family.<br>• Review with client and caregiver the signs/symptoms of adverse reactions; provide them with emergency phone numbers.<br>• Premedicate client as ordered.<br>• Establish baseline vital signs/record.<br>• Start RBC transfusion slowly.<br>• Vital signs per home transfusion flow sheet<br>• Observe for transfusion reaction.<br>• Adjust flow rate per order.<br>• Infuse RBCs within 4 hr.<br>• Observe and monitor vital signs 30 min after completion. | Transfusion reactions may be immediate or delayed.<br><br>May be required to alleviate allergic reactions.<br><br>Symptoms of a transfusion reaction (especially RBCs) are usually evident during infusion of first 50 ml of blood.<br><br>Minimize the risk of bacterial contamination. |
| 6. Documentation:<br>• Client identification procedure<br>• General condition of client and vital signs throughout procedure<br>• Record medication on flow sheet, etc.<br>• Record time of arrival/departure. | All to be part of the legal record. |

## CONCLUSION

Patients with cancer are at risk for the development of bleeding due to multiple factors. Bleeding can occur as the result of the cancer itself or as a result of the treatment of the cancer. Bleeding associated with cancer may be occult and chronic, or acute and life-threatening, as seen in the clotting and hemorrhage of DIC.

Treatment regimens for patients with cancer often are aggressive and place the patient at risk for complications, including bleeding. The use of blood component therapy and the newer colony-stimulating growth factors facilitates these aggressive treatment regimens. These sophisticated supportive care measures improve the prognosis of a number of malignancies. Care can be rendered in an acute care setting, an outpatient office or clinic, or the patient's home. With this increasing technology it is more crucial than ever before that nurses be educationally prepared to meet the complex needs of these patients. Early detection of the signs and symptoms of bleeding can allow for prompt diagnosis and treatment of the disorder.

## REFERENCES

1. Haeuber D, Spross JA: Alterations in protective mechanisms: Hematopoiesis and bone marrow depression, in Baird SB, McCorkle R, Grant M (eds): *Cancer Nursing: A Comprehensive Textbook.* Philadelphia, Saunders, 1991, pp 759–781

2. Haeuber D, DiJulio JE: Hematopoietic colony stimulating factors: An overview. *Oncol Nurs Forum* 16:247–255, 1989

3. Haeuber D, Spross JA: Bone marrow, in Gross J, Johnson BL (eds): *Handbook of Oncology Nursing* (ed 2). Boston, Jones and Bartlett, 1994, pp 373–399

4. Emerson SG: The stem cell model of hematopoiesis, in Hoffman R, Benz EJ, Shattil SJ, Furie B, Cohen HJ, Silberstein LE (eds): *Hematology: Basic Principles and Practice.* New York, Churchill Livingstone, 1991, pp 72–81

5. Quesenberry PJ: Hematopoietic stem cells, progenitor cells, and cytokines, in Beutler E, Lichtman MA, Coller BS, Kipps TJ (eds): *Williams Hematology* (ed 5). New York, McGraw-Hill, 1995, pp 211–228

6. Bagby GC, Segal GM: Growth factors and the control of hematopoiesis, In Hoffman R, Benz EJ, Shattil SJ, Furie B, Cohen HJ, Silberstein LE (eds): *Hematology: Basic Principles and Practice.* New York, Churchill Livingstone 1991, pp 91–121

7. Mayan H, Guilbert LJ, Janowska-Wieczorek A: Biology of the hematopoietic environment. *Eur J Haematol* 49: 225–233, 1992

8. Grosh WW, Quesenberry PJ: Recombinant human hematopoietic growth factors in the treatment of cytopenias. *Clin Immunol Immunopathol* 62:525–538, 1992

9. Mendelsohn J, Lippman ME: Principles of molecular cell biology of cancer: Growth factors, in DeVita VT, Hellman S, Rosenberg SA (eds): *Cancer: Principles and Practice of Oncology* (ed 4). Philadelphia, Lippincott., 1993, pp 114–133

10. Erslev AJ: Erythropoietin. *N Engl J Med* 324:1339–1344, 1991

11. Koury ST, Bondurant MC, Koury MJ, et al: Localization of cells producing erythropoietin in murine liver by in situ hybridization. *Blood* 77:2497–2503, 1991

12. Tabarra IA: Hemolytic anemia: Differential diagnosis and management of iron deficiency anemia. *Med Clin North Am* 76:549–566, 1992

13. Burnstein SA, Breton-Gorius J: Megakaryopoiesis and platelet formation, in Beutler E, Lichtman MA, Coller BS, Kipps TJ (eds): *Williams Hematology* (ed 5). New York, McGraw-Hill, 1995, pp 1149–1161

14. Jobe MI: Mechanisms of coagulation and fibrinolysis, in Lotspeich-Steininger CA, Stein-Martin EA, Koepke JA (eds): *Clinical Hematology: Principles, Procedures, Correlations.* Philadelphia, Lippincott, 1992, pp 579–598

15. Jesty J, Nemerson Y: The pathways of coagulation, in Beutler E, Lichtman MA, Coller BS, Kipps TJ (eds): *Williams Hematology* (ed 5). New York, McGraw-Hill, 1995, pp 1227–1238

16. Furie B, Furie BC: The molecular basis of blood coagulation, in Hoffman R, Benz EJ, Shattil SJ, Furie B, Cohen HJ, Silberstein LE (eds.): *Hematology: Basic Principles and Practice.* New York, Churchill Livingstone, 1991, pp 1213–1231

17. Neuenschwander PF, Morrissey JH: Deletion of the membrane anchoring region of tissue factor abolishes autoactivation of factor VII but not cofactor function: Analysis of a mutant with a selective deficiency in activity. *J Biol Chem* 266:21911, 1991

18. Francis CW, Marder VJ: Mechanisms of fibrinolysis, in Beutler E, Lichtman MA, Coller BS, Kipps TJ (eds): *Williams Hematology* (ed 5). New York, McGraw-Hill, 1995, pp 1252–1260

19. Pruett J: Bleeding, in Groenwald SL, Frogge MH, Goodman M, Yarbro CH (eds): *Cancer Symptom Management.* Boston, Jones and Bartlett, 1996, pp 269–288

20. Elpern EH: Lung cancer, in Groenwald SL, Frogge MH, Goodman M, Yarbro CH (eds): *Cancer Nursing: Principles and Practice* (ed 3). Boston, Jones and Bartlett, 1993, pp 1174–1199

21. Walczak JR, Klemm PR: Gynecologic cancers, in Groenwald SL, Frogge MH, Goodman M, Yarbro CH (eds): *Cancer Nursing: Principles and Practices* (ed 3). Boston, Jones and Bartlett, 1993, pp 1065–1113

22. Lind J, Krantz K, Grieg B: Urologic and male genital malignancies, in Groenwald SL, Frogge MH, Goodman M, Yarbro CH (eds). *Cancer Nursing: Principles and Practices* (ed 3). Boston, Jones and Bartlett, 1993, pp 1258–1316

23. Hampton B: Gastrointestinal cancer: Colon, rectum, and anus, in Groenwald SL, Frogge MH, Goodman M, Yarbro CH (eds): *Cancer Nursing: Principles and Practices* (ed 3). Boston, Jones and Bartlett, 1993, pp 1044–1064

24. Ey FS, Goodnight SH: Bleeding disorders in cancer. *Semin Oncol* 17:187–197, 1990

25. Sheridan CA: Multiple myeloma. *Semin Oncol Nurs* 12:59–69, 1996

26. Gobel BH: Bleeding disorders, in Groenwald SL, Frogge MH, Goodman M, Yarbro CH (eds): *Cancer Nursing: Principles and Practice* (ed 3). Boston, Jones and Bartlett, 1993, pp 575–607, 1993

27. Perkins HA, MacKenzie MR, Fudenberg HH: Hemostatic defects in dysproteinemias. *Blood* 35:695, 1970

28. Kyle RA: Diagnostic criteria of multiple myeloma. *Hematol Oncol Clin North Am* 6:347–358, 1992

29. Patterson WP, Caldwell CW, Doll DC: Hyperviscosity syndromes and coagulopathies. *Semin Oncol* 17:210–216, 1990

30. Sarzotti H, Baron S, Klingboll GR: El-4 metastases in spleen and bone marrow suppress the NK activity generated in the organs. *Int J Cancer* 39:117–125, 1978

31. Erickson JM: Anemia. *Semin Oncol Nurs* 12:2–14, 1996

32. Massey AC: Microcytic anemias: Differential diagnosis and management of iron deficiency anemia. *Med Clin North Am* 76:549–566, 1992

33. Fairbanks VF, Beutler E: Iron deficiency, in Beutler E, Lichtman MA, Coller BS, Kipps, TJ (eds): *Williams Hematology* (ed 5). New York, McGraw-Hill, 1995, pp 490–511

34. Swartz SS, Yuska CM: Common patient care issues following surgery for head and neck cancer. *Semin Oncol Nurs* 15: 191–194, 1989

35. Beutler E, Masouredis SP: Preservation and clinical use of erythrocytes and whole blood, in Beutler E, Lichtman MA, Coller BS, Kipps TJ (eds): *Williams Hematology* (ed 5). New York, McGraw-Hill, 1995, pp 1622–1635

36. Shafer AI: Essential (primary) thrombocythemia, in Beutler E, Lichtman MA, Coller BS, Kipps TJ (eds). *Williams Hematology* (ed 5). New York, McGraw-Hill, 1995, pp 1622–1635

37. Shafer AI: Essential thrombocythemia. *Prog Hemost Thromb* 10:69, 1991

38. Ravdi ML, Stocco F, Rossi C, et al: Thrombosis and hemorrhage in thombocytosis: Evaluation of a large cohort of patients (357 cases). *J Med* 22:213–217, 1991

39. Anagrelide Study Group: "Anagrelide," a therapy for thrombocytopenia states: Experience in 577 patients. *Am J Med* 92:69–76, 1992

40. Bunn PA, Ridgeway EC: Paraneoplastic syndromes, in DeVita VT, Hellman S, Rosenberg SA (eds): *Cancer: Principles and Practice of Oncology* (ed 4). Philadelphia, Lippincott, 1993, pp 2026–2071

41. Williams WJ: Secondary thrombocytosis, in Beutler E, Lichtman MA, Coller BS, Kipps TJ (eds): *Williams Hematology* (ed 5). New York, McGraw-Hill, 1995, pp 1361–1363

42. Schwartz CL, Cohen HJ: Myeloproliferative and myelodysplastic syndromes, in Pizzo PA, Poplack DG (eds): *Principles and Practice of Pediatric Oncology* (ed 2). Philadelphia, Lippincott, 1993, pp 519–536

43. Rosen PJ: Bleeding problems in the cancer patient. *Hematol Oncol Clin North Am* 6:1315–1328, 1992

44. Maxwell MB, Maher KE: Chemotherapy-induced myelosuppression. *Semin Oncol Nurs* 8:113–123, 1992

45. Hoagland HC: Hematologic complications of cancer chemotherapy, in Perry MC (ed): *The Chemotherapy Source Book*. Baltimore, Williams and Wilkins, 1992, pp 498–507

46. Hilderley L: Radiotherapy, in Groenwald SL, Frogge MH, Goodman M, Yarbro CH (eds): *Cancer Nursing: Principles and Practices* (ed 3). Boston, Jones and Bartlett, 1993, pp 235–269

47. Shuey KM: Platelet-associated bleeding disorders. *Semin Oncol Nurs* 12:15–27, 1996

48. Bick, RL: Platelet function defects associated with hemorrhage or thrombosis. *Med Clin North Am* 78:577–607, 1994

49. Gaydos LA, Frierich EJ, Mantel N: The quantitative relation between platelet count and hemorrhage in patients with acute leukemia. *N Engl J Med* 266:905–909, 1962

50. Wallerstein RO, Deisseroth AB: Bone marrow dysfunction in the cancer patient: Use of blood and blood products, in DeVita VT, Hellman S, Rosenberg SA (eds): *Cancer:*

*Principles and Practice of Oncology* (ed 4). Philadelphia, Lippincott, 1993, pp 2262–2275

51. Camp-Sorrell D: Chemotherapy: Toxicity management, in Groenwald SL, Frogge MH, Goodman M, Yarbro CH (eds): *Cancer Nursing: Principles and Practice* (ed 3). Boston, Jones and Bartlett, 1993, pp 235–269

52. Kanz L, Lindemann A, Oster W, et al: Hematopoietins in clinical oncology. *Am J Clin Oncol* 14:527–533, 1991

53. Wujcik D: Overview of colony-stimulating factors: Focus on the neutrophil, in Carrol-Johnson R (ed): *A Case Management Approach to Patients Receiving G-CSF*. Pittsburg, Oncology Nursing Society, 1992, pp 8–11

54. Gianni AM, Bregni M, Siena S, et al: Recombinant human granulocyte-macrophage colony-stimulating factor reduces hematologic toxicity and widens clinical applicability of high-dose cyclophosphamide treatment of breast cancer and non-Hodgkin's lymphoma. *J Clin Oncol* 8:768–778, 1990

55. Herrman F, Schulz G, Weiser M, et al: Effect of granulocyte-macrophage colony-stimulating factor on neutropenia and related morbidity induced by myelotoxic chemotherapy. *Hematol Blood Transfus* 33:717–723, 1990

56. Jassak PF: Biotherapy, in Groenwald SL, Frogge MH, Goodman M, Yarbro CH (eds). *Cancer Nursing: Principles and Practice* (ed 3). Boston, Jones and Bartlett, 1993, pp 366–392

57. deVries EGE, Biesma B, Willemse PHB, et al: A double-blind placebo-controlled study with granulocyte-macrophage colony-stimulating factor for chemotherapy for ovarian carcinoma. *Cancer Res* 51:116–122, 1991

58. Moore MAS: The clinical use of colony-stimulating factors. *Annu Rev Immunol* 9:159–191, 1991

59. Oster W, Frish J, Nicolay U, et al: Interleukin-3. Biologic effects and clinical impact. *Cancer* 67:2712–2717, 1991

60. Schick B: Hope for treatment of thrombocytopenia. *N Engl J Med* 331:875–876, 1994

61. Kurzrock R, Talpaz M, Estrov Z, et al: Phase I study of recombinant human interleukin-3 in patients with bone marrow failure. *J Clin Oncol* 1 9:1241–1250, 1991

62. Williams DE, Park LS: Hematopoietic effects of granulocyte-macrophage colony-stimulating factor/interleukin-3 fusion protein. *Cancer* 67:2705–2707, 1991

63. Lok S, Kaushansky K, Holly RD, et al: Promotion of megakaryocyte progenitor expansion and differentiation by the c-Mpl ligand thrombopoietin. *Nature* 369:565–568, 1994

64. George JN, El-Harake MA, Raskob G: Chronic idiopathic thrombocytopenic purpura. *N Engl J Med* 331:1207–1211, 1994

65. Tardio DJ, McFarland JA, Gonzalez MF: Immune thrombocytopenia purpura: Current concepts. *J Gen Intern Med* 8: 60–63, 1993

66. Blanchette VS, Kirby MA, Turner C: Role of intravenous immunoglobulin G in autoimmune hematologic disorders. *Semin Hematol* 29:72–82, 1992 (suppl 2)

67. Kirchner JT: Acute and chronic immune thrombocytopenic purpura. *Postgrad Med* 92:112–126, 1992

68. Calverly BC, Jones GW, Kelton JG: Splenic radiation for corticosteroid-resistant immune thrombocytopenia. *Ann Intern Med* 116:977–981, 1992.

69. Naouri A, Feghati B, Chabal J, et al: Results of splenectomy for idiopathic thrombocytopenic purpura. *Acta Haematol*, 89:200–203, 1993.

70. Figueroa M, Gehlsen J, Hammond D, et al: Combination chemotherapy in refractory immune thrombocytopenic purpura. *N Engl J Med* 328:1226–1235, 1993

71. Miyazaki M, Itoh H, Kaiho T, et al: Partial splenic embolization for the treatment of chronic idiopathic thrombocytopenic purpura. *Am J Roentgenol,* 163:123–126, 1994

72. Najean Y, Dufour V, Rain JD, et al: The site of platelet destruction in thrombocytopenic purpura as a predictive index of the efficacy of splenectomy. *Br J Haematol,* 79: 271–276, 1991

73. Shattil SJ, Bennett JS: Acquired qualitative platelet disorders due to diseases, drugs, and foods, in Beutler E, Lichtman MA, Coller BS, Kipps TJ (eds): *Williams Hematology* (ed 5). New York, McGraw Hill, 1995, pp 1386–1400

74. Kaullman R, Nieuwenhuis HK, de Groot PG, et al: Effects of low dose aspirin, 10 mg and 30 mg daily, on bleeding time, thromboxane production, and 6–keto-PGF$_{1_a}$ excretion in healthy subjects. *Thromb Res* 45:355, 1987.

75. George JN, Shattil SJ: Acquired disorders of platelet function, in Hoffman R, Berz EJ, Shattil SJ, Furie B, Cohen HJ, Silberstein LE (eds): *Hematology: Basic Principles and Practice.* New York, Churchill Livingstone, 1991, pp 1528–1546

76. Burroughs SF, Johnson GJ: B-Lactam antibiotic–induced platelet dysfunction: Evidence for irreversible inhibition of platelet activation in vitro and in vivo after prolonged exposure to penicillin. *Blood:* 75:1473–1480, 1990

77. Brown RB, Klar J, Lemenshow S: Enhanced bleeding with cefoxitin or moxolactam: Statistical analysis within a defined population. *Arch Intern Med* 146:2159, 1986

78. Karolak L, Chandra A, Kahn W, et al: High-dose chemotherapy-induced platelet defect: Inhibition of platelet signal transduction pathways. *Mol Pharmacol* 43:31, 1993

79. Lethagen S, Rugarn P: The effect of DDAVP and placebo on platelet function and prolonged bleeding time induced by oral acetyl salicylic acid intake in healthy volunteers. *Thromb Haemost* 67:185, 1992

80. Slichter SS, Harker LA: Hemostasis in malignancy. *Ann N Y Acad Sci* 230:252–261, 1974

81. Gralnick A, Ginsberg D: Von Willebrand's disease, in Beutler E, Lichtman MA, Coller BS, Kipps TJ (eds): *Williams Hematology* (ed 5). New York, McGraw-Hill, 1995, pp 1458–1480

82. Green D: Disorders of vitamin K–dependent coagulation factors, in Beutler E, Lichtman MA, Coller BS, Kipps TJ (eds): *Williams Hematology* (ed 5). New York, McGraw-Hill, 1995, pp 1481–1485

83. Murakawa M, Okamura T, Tsutsumi K, et al: Acquired von Willebrand's disease in association with essential thrombocythemia: Regression following treatment. *Acta Haematol* 87:83, 1992

84. Gobel BH: Plasma and plasma derivative therapy for coagulation disorders. *Semin Oncol Nurs* 6:129–135, 1990

85. Menitove JE, Gill JG, Montgomery RR: Preparation and clinical use of plasma and plasma fractions, in Beutler E, Lichtman MA, Coller BS, Kipps TJ (eds): *Williams Hematology* (ed 5). New York, McGraw-Hill, 1995, pp 1649–1663

86. Mannucci PM: Desmopressin and thrombosis. *Lancet 2:* 675, 1991

87. Shetty HGM, Backhouse G, Bentley DP, et al: Effective reversal of warfarin-induced excessive anticoagulation with low-dose vitamin K. *Thromb Haemost* 67:13, 1992

88. Jakaway JL: Acquired von Willebrand's disease. *Hematol Oncol Clin North Am* 6:1409, 1992

89. Eikenboom JCJ, VanderMeer FJM, Briet E: Acquired von Willebrand's disease due to excessive fibrinolysis. *Br J Hematol* 81:618, 1992

90. Bavier AR: Coagulopathies, in Gross J, Johnson BL (eds): *Handbook of Oncology Nursing* (ed 2). Boston, Jones and Bartlett, 1994, pp 729–794

91. Goodnough LT: Management of disseminated intravascular coagulation, in Rossi EC, Simon TL, Moss GS (eds): *Principles of Transfusion Medicine.* Baltimore, Williams and Wilkins, 1991, pp 373–382

92. Dietz KA, Flaherty AM: Oncologic emergencies, in Groenwald SL, Frogge MH, Goodman M, Yarbro CH (eds): *Cancer Nursing: Principles and Practice* (ed 3). Boston, Jones and Bartlett, 1995, pp 800–839

93. Young L: DIC: The insidious killer. *Crit Care Nurs* 10:26–33, 1990.

94. Bick RL: Disseminated intravascular coagulation: Objective criteria for diagnosis and management. *Med Clin North Am* 78:511–543, 1994

95. Marder JV, Martin SE, Colman RW: Clinical aspects of consumptive thrombohemorrhagic disorders, in Colman RW, Hirsh J, Marder JV, Salzman EW (eds): *Hemostasis and Thrombosis* (ed 3). Philadelphia, Lippincott, 1993, pp 665–693

96. Rutherford CJ, Frenkel EP: Thrombocytopenia: Issues in diagnosis and therapy. *Med Clin North Am,* 78:555–575, 1994

97. Gray WW, Bell WR: Fibrinolytic agents in the treatment of thrombotic disorders. *Semin Oncol* 17:228–237, 1990

98. Kee JL: *Handbook of Laboratory and Diagnostic Tests with Nursing Implications* (ed 2). Norwalk, CT, Appleton and Lange, 1994, pp 203–204

99. McFarland MB, Gant MM: *Nursing Implications of Laboratory Tests* (ed 3). Albany, NY, Delmar Publishing, 1994, pp 64–91

100. Food and Drug Administration: Title 21, Code of Federal Regulations. Washington, DC, U.S. Department of Health and Human Services, parts 600 and 601, 1989

101. Pavel JN: Red blood cell transfusions for anemia. *Semin Oncol Nurs* 6:117–122, 1990

102. American Association of Blood Banks: *Blood Transfusion Therapy: A Physician's Handbook* (ed 3). Bethesda, MD, American Association of Blood Bank Publications. 1993

103. Jassak PF, Godwin J: Blood component therapy, in Baird SB, McCorkle R, Grant M (eds): *Cancer Nursing: A Comprehensive Textbook.* Philadelphia, Saunders, 1991, pp 370–384

104. National Institutes of Health: *Transfusion Alert: Indications for Use of Red Blood Cells, Platelets, and Fresh Frozen Plasma.* Publication No. 89–2974a. Washington, DC, National Institutes of Health, 1989

105. Brand A, Claas FHJ, Falkenburg JHF, et al: Blood component therapy in bone marrow transplantation. *Semin Hematol* 21:141–153, 1984

106. Murphy S: Preservation and clinical use of platelets, in Beutler E, Lichtman MA, Coller BS, Kipps TJ (eds): *Williams Hematology* (ed 5). New York, McGraw-Hill, 1995, pp 1361–1363

107. Schiffer CA: Prevention of alloimmunization against platelets. *Blood* 77:1–4, 1991 (editorial)

108. Pamphilon DH, Blendell EL: Ultraviolet-B irradiation of platelet concentrates: A strategy to reduce transfusion recipient allosensitization. *Semin Hematol* 29:18, 1992

109. Hogman CF, Gong J, Eriksson L, et al: White cells protect donor blood against bacteria contamination. *Transfusion* 31:620–626, 1991

110. Berkman SA, Lee ML, Gale RP: Clinical uses of intravenous immunoglobulins. *Ann Intern Med* 27:245–247, 1990

111. Kickler T, Brain HG, Piantadosi S, et al: A randomized,

placebo-controlled trial of intravenous gammaglobulin in alloimmunized thrombocytopenic patients. *Blood* 75:313, 1990

112. Wedon MB: *Bone Marrow Transplantation: Principles, Practice, and Nursing Insights.* Boston, Jones and Bartlett, 1991

113. Vogelsang GB: Transfusion-associated graft-versus-host disease in nonimmunocompromised hosts. *Transfusion* 30: 101–103, 1990

114. Rawal BD, Davis E, Busch MP, et al: Dual reduction in the immunologic and infectious complications of transfusion by filtration/removal of leukocytes from donor blood soon after collection. *Transfus Med Rev* 4:36–41, 1990

115. Bowden RA, Slichter SJ, Sayers MH, et al: Use of leukocyte-depleted platelets and cytomegalovirus seronegative red blood cells for prevention of primary cytomegalovirus infection after marrow transplant. *Blood* 78:246–250, 1991

116. Bowden RA, Slichter SJ, Sayers MH et al: A comparison of filtered leukocyte-reduced and cytomegalovirus (CMV) seronegative blood products for the prevention of transfusion-associated CMV infection after marrow transplant. *Blood* 86:3598–3603, 1995

117. Williamson LM, Wimperis JZ, Williamson P, et al: Bedside filtration of blood products in the prevention of HLA-alloimmunization: A prospective randomized study. *Blood* 83:3028, 1994

118. Perkins HA, Payne R, Ferguson J, et al: Non-hemolytic febrile reactions: Quantitative effects of blood components with emphasis on isoantigenic incompatibility in leukocytes, *Vox Sang* II:578–600, 1966

119. Gilbert GL, Hayes K, Hudson IL, et al: Prevention of transfusion-acquired cytomegalovirus infection in infants by blood filtration to remove leukocytes. *Lancet* 1:1228, 1989

120. Pietersz RN, Steneker I, Reesink HW, et al: Comparison of five different filters for the removal of leukocytes from red cell concentrates. *Vox Sang* 62:76, 1992

121. Wenz B, Burns ER: Phenotypic characterization of white cells in white cell–reduced red cell concentrate using flow cytometry. *Transfusion* 31:829, 1991

122. Sirchia G, Wenz B, Rebulla P, et al: Removal of leukocytes from red blood cells by transfusion through a new filter. *Transfusion* 30:30–33, 1990

123. Snyder E, Menitove E (eds). *Home Transfusion Therapy.* Arlington, VA, American Association of Blood Banks, 1986

124. McAbee RR, Grupp K, Horn B: Home intravenous therapy: Part 1—Issues. *Home Health Care Serv Quart* 12:59–107, 1991

125. Rutman R, Kakaiya P, Miller WV: Home Transfusion for the Cancer Patient. *Semin Oncol Nurs* 6:163–167, 1990

126. Guilday TJ: Legal considerations of home blood transfusions, in Snyder EL, Menitove E (eds): *Home Transfusion Therapy.* Arlington, VA, American Association of Blood Banks, 1988, pp 41–52

127. Fridey JL, Issit LA, Kasprisin C: *Out-of-Hospital Transfusions.* Bethesda, MD, American Association of Blood Banks, 1994

128. Santiago DL: Establishing a community-based home transfusion program. *J Home Health Care Pract* 2:21–28, 1990

# Chapter 23

# Fatigue

**Lillian M. Nail, RN, PhD, FAAN**

## SCOPE OF THE PROBLEM

Fatigue is the most common side effect of cancer treatment.[1-6] People with cancer may also experience fatigue as a symptom of the disease or as a result of physical deconditioning. Bedrest, impaired mobility due to skeletal involvement, pain, or neurological problems, and muscle wasting caused by drugs or nutritional problems all contribute to physical deconditioning. Patients report that fatigue interferes with their ability to work, to maintain their roles within their homes and families, to concentrate, and to engage in their usual level of physical activity. Despite the high incidence of fatigue among individuals with cancer, widespread recognition of the need for preventing and treating cancer treatment–related fatigue (CRF) is relatively recent. Major impediments to addressing CRF in clinical practice include a misconception on the part of health care providers that CRF is transient and relieved by rest like the acute fatigue experienced in day-to-day life; confusion about the difference between fatigue and depression; lack of appreciation of the negative impact of fatigue on quality of life; use of ratings of treatment side effects and toxicities based upon the perceptions of health care providers rather than using data collected from patients prospectively; and lack of information about causal mechanisms needed to guide the development of interventions.

*Acute fatigue* is a relatively temporary state that is relieved by rest, although one night of undisturbed sleep may not provide complete relief. The popular view of the function of acute fatigue is that it protects individuals from harm by keeping them from engaging in excessive amounts of physical or mental activity. Feelings of fatigue usually are attributed to physical exertion, psychological stress, and inadequate sleep and rest. The advice given to people who complain of fatigue is often "Get some rest" or "Don't try to do so much." When fatigue persists over time, it is known as *chronic fatigue.*[7] Chronic fatigue is not readily relieved by rest, is often viewed by the person experiencing it as an "exaggerated" response to activity compared with their previous experience, and is extremely debilitating. Chronic fatigue is often seen in association with illnesses such as chronic obstructive lung disease, renal failure, heart disease, arthritis, multiple sclerosis, and fibromyalgia. The diagnosis of chronic fatigue syndrome is applied to those who present with a chronic fatigue pattern with no known physical or psychological etiology.[8,9]

Individuals with cancer may experience both acute and chronic fatigue as a result of the disease because of side effects of treatment, from sleep disruption produced by the psychological distress likely to accompany diagnosis of a potentially life-threatening condition or side effects of treatment, and as a response to increased demands imposed by adding cancer treatment to day-to-day activities.[1-5,10] The incidence of fatigue reported by cancer patients treated with surgery, radiation therapy, chemotherapy, or biologic response modifiers exceeds 90% in selected studies.[11-15] Despite the prevalence of fatigue in cancer patients and the extent to which it can interfere with daily activities, there is limited research describing the time of onset, duration, pattern, and severity of fatigue; identifying factors that contribute to fatigue; or testing interventions designed to prevent or ameliorate fatigue.

## DEFINITION OF FATIGUE

Fatigue is a complex concept that has been associated with many other terms such as tiredness, exhaustion, weariness, drowsiness, malaise, weakness, asthenia, somnolence, lack of energy, and feeling "bushed" or "beat." Fatigue has been defined in terms of both objective performance and subjective experience. Early fatigue research focused on individuals' jobs or athletic performances. The aim of this research was to identify the causes of fatigue and find ways to improve performance. In this approach to understanding fatigue, an objective indicator of the point at which performance declines, such as exercise endurance or accuracy of completion of a mental task, is used to define fatigue. Weakness is related to the objective view of fatigue, since it also represents a muscular performance deficit demonstrated on objective testing.

In the subjective experience approach, fatigue is conceptualized as a feeling state.[1,4,16] In contrast to weakness, defined as the *inability* either to initiate or to maintain specific muscular activities, subjectively defined fatigue has a voluntary component.[17] Individuals with CRF may push themselves to engage in a highly valued activity. This ability to overcome fatigue is not possible when muscle weakness is a problem. The subjective view of fatigue is analogous to the approach to pain: it is what the person experiencing it says it is.

The subjective view of fatigue is the most relevant to cancer care.[1] The actions individuals take in response to fatigue will be based on their perceptions rather than on the results of a performance test or an evaluation of their level of fatigue made by another person. Some will define their fatigue in terms of sensations, while others will define it in terms of their perceptions of their ability to engage in usual activities. However, level of activity or capacity to complete specific activities should be viewed as a response to fatigue rather than a measure of fatigue. This distinction is important because individuals experiencing CRF will choose to maintain specific activities, and some may purposefully increase activity in spite of fatigue. When assessment focuses on responses to CRF rather than the perceived severity of the sensation of CRF, it is possible to underestimate or overestimate the severity of fatigue and make inappropriate decisions about care needs.

# PATHOPHYSIOLOGY OF FATIGUE

## Theories of Causation

Although causes of fatigue have been explored in numerous studies, no clear support has emerged for any of the major hypotheses. The majority of the research was conducted before 1970 using normal human subjects in performance test situations. Specific hypotheses about fatigue in cancer patients remain untested. The extent to which findings from research on fatigue in healthy normal subjects or trained athletes apply to individuals with cancer is not known. A significant limitation of the research on CRF is that variables such as performance status or quality of life tend to be substituted for measures of subjective fatigue. In addition, most studies do not include measures of proposed physiological mechanisms.

### Accumulation hypothesis

Early research on fatigue led to the accumulation hypothesis, which proposed that a buildup of waste products in the body produces fatigue. This hypothesis was supported when rapid accumulation of lactic acid, pyruvic acid, and other metabolic products was found during strenuous exercise, although subsequent research failed to relate the accumulation of waste products to the occurrence of fatigue.[1,5,16] Although it is common for fatigue in cancer patients receiving radiation treatment or chemotherapy to be attributed to the presence of by-products of cell death, to date no research has been conducted to test this hypothesis.

### Depletion hypothesis

The depletion hypothesis was based on the idea that muscular activity is impaired when certain substances, such as carbohydrates, fats, proteins, adenosine triphosphate (ATP), and adrenal hormones, are not readily available.[18] The relationship between nutrition and muscular activity is complex, involving both the availability and the use of nutrients. When carbohydrates or fats are available for conversion into glycogen, protein is spared. With sustained muscle activity, glycogen is depleted, leading to fatigue.

The nutrition problems experienced by many cancer patients may lead to inadequate intake of nutrients; the way the body uses nutrients may change in the presence of cancer; and the tumor may successfully compete with normal tissues for available nutrients.[16,19,20] Therefore, indicators of changes in nutritional status, such as weight loss or changes in the nutrients available at the cellular level, should be associated with fatigue if the depletion hypothesis explains fatigue. The limited research in this area does not provide adequate support for this line of reasoning. For example, although weight loss was positively correlated with subjective postoperative fatigue in a group of general surgery patients, including some cancer patients, there was no association between fatigue and changes in specific muscle or plasma amino acids.[21] Tumor necrosis factor and cachectin are associated with muscle wasting that will contribute to fatigue; however, the relationship of these substances to subjective fatigue has not been examined.[22]

The fatigue produced by anemia can also be thought of as an example of the depletion mechanism. Anemia decreases the oxygen-carrying capacity of the blood, inhibiting the delivery of essential nutrients to the cells and decreasing the energy available to the organism. Cancer patients may experience a variety of conditions that could produce anemia.[23,24] When individuals who have experienced anemia and fatigue are treated with transfusions and subsequently demonstrate improvement in their hematocrit or hemoglobin values, they generally report a concurrent decrease in the severity of fatigue. Three published studies address the relationship of hematocrit to quality of life in cancer patients. Improving hematocrit was associated with improved performance status in two studies of anemic cancer patients receiving erythropoietin.[25,26] Subjective fatigue was not measured in either study. In the third study, hematocrit level was not associated with any of the outcome variables, but no data on hematocrit are reported.[27] It is important to note that studies of the adequacy of red blood cells in clinical populations utilize a dichotomous view of anemia (present or absent) based upon varying definitions of what constitutes anemia. Relatively few cancer patients exhibit bone marrow suppression during treatment that reaches the level of classic anemia, so studies focused on reversing anemia caused by bone marrow suppression may not generalize to most patients receiving cancer treatment. Anecdotal reports from patients under treatment suggest that some experience increased subjective fatigue with relatively small declines in hematocrit. Research on the relationship of level of hematocrit or hemoglobin to subjective level of fatigue is needed to begin addressing the relationship between depressed levels of red blood cells and severity of CRF.

### Biochemical and physiochemical phenomena

Changes in the production, distribution, use, balance, and movement of substances such as muscle proteins, glucose, electrolytes, and hormones may be important factors influencing the experience of fatigue.[18,28,29] Changes in the production and balance of hormones are central components of the Selye syndrome of stress response and may contribute to the fatigue experienced by individuals with cancer during physical or psychological stress.[30] Many of the drugs used to treat cancer or to manage side effects of treatment also can produce biochemical and physiochemical changes related to those believed to produce fatigue.[31] For example, the use of catabolic steroids as part of a treatment regimen is likely to produce muscle wasting and lead to increased CRF.

Endogenous cytokines, exogenous growth factors, and most medications that act on the central nervous system (CNS) have the potential to contribute to CRF.[16,32–34]

## Central nervous system control

In a 1970 review of the research on fatigue in animals and healthy human subjects, Grandjean concluded that central control of fatigue is vested in the brain's reticular formation.[35] In Grandjean's neurophysiological model of fatigue, the level of fatigue is determined by the balance between two opposing systems: the activating system and the inhibiting system. The *reticular activating system*, located in the reticular formation in the brain, controls alertness or wakefulness by stimulating the cerebral cortex and responding to both sensory stimulation and feedback from the cerebral cortex. The *inhibitory system*, believed to involve the cerebral cortex and the brain stem, depresses the activity of the reticular activating system. In Grandjean's model, both internal stimuli, such as thoughts and perceptions, as well as external stimuli (e.g., noise and light) stimulate the reticular activating system and promote wakefulness or alertness. The sustained arousal or wakefulness that occurs after environmental stimulation may be produced by release of adrenergic substances from the adrenal glands. Feelings of sleepiness or tiredness occur when the level of cortical stimulation of the reticular activating system is low, when there is little or no sensory input, or when the level of activity of the inhibitory system is high. Specific aspects of brain function have been explored as explanations of the etiology of chronic fatigue syndrome without definitive results.[36]

The neurophysiological model of fatigue may explain the occurrence of fatigue in conditions of low stimulation, such as immobility produced by bedrest, even when there is little expenditure of energy. It also accounts for rapid decreases in feelings of fatigue when danger or excitement is perceived or a sudden increase in intensity or change in the nature of environmental stimuli occurs. Reports of declines in the ability to concentrate and to process information are consistent with the neurophysiological model of fatigue.[37] The findings of studies in this area suggest that there are specific cognitive aspects of CRF. The cognitive changes seen in CRF may differ from the experience of acute fatigue in healthy individuals.[38,39] The exploration of attentional fatigue in people with cancer has important implications for the delivery of informational interventions, the process of making decisions about treatment, and the patient's ability to manage day-to-day responsibilities.

## Adaptation and energy reserves

Selye's approach to fatigue is that every individual has a certain amount of superficial energy available for adaptation and that fatigue occurs when that energy supply is depleted. Rest allows time for energy to be replenished from the individual's deep reserves so adaptation can continue.[30] As the reserves of adaptation energy are consumed, fatigue eventually leads to exhaustion and then to death. Selye's ideas incorporate accumulation, depletion, biochemical-physiochemical changes, and CNS control, since all these processes may be involved in the individual's response to stressors. The idea that fatigue is relieved by sufficient rest is consistent with the experience of healthy people experiencing acute fatigue but does not fit the chronic fatigue model applied to CRF. For example, patients receiving chemotherapy rate sleep and rest as partially rather than completely effective in relieving fatigue.[40,41] The possibility that too much rest may exacerbate fatigue is based in research on the effects of immobility and is a very real concern for individuals receiving cancer treatment.[1]

The quality of sleep and rest may also be important. Research on sleep patterns during illness tends to focus on environmental disruptions such as hospital noise and contact for the delivery of care.[42–45] The role of side effects and symptoms as well as illness management activities in sleep disruption has not been addressed. Examples of symptoms and side effects that disrupt sleep include hot flashes, urinary frequency, nausea, vomiting, pain, diarrhea, and coughing. Illness management activities that disrupt sleep include around-the-clock medications, alarms from pumps used for delivering medication, forcing fluids (and the inevitable consequence of frequent voiding), replacing hot or cold packs that have cooled or warmed, dressing changes, and supplemental feedings.

## Energy balance hypotheses

The relationship between activity or inactivity and energy is addressed by the psychobiological-entropy hypothesis and related research on immobility and deconditioning. According to the psychobiological-entropy hypothesis, decreased activity decreases the production of energy needed to support activity.[46,47] A trajectory that can be viewed as a downward spiral is then established in which the response to lower energy resources is to further decrease activity, which again decreases energy resources. The psychobiological-entropy hypothesis includes propositions that address the importance of achieving a balance between activity and rest.

Similarly, the deconditioning model, which served as the basis for most of the early work on immobility, proposes that muscle loss occurs rapidly in the face of immobility. As a result, the amount of energy expended in completing simple activities, such as getting out of bed, increases while capacity for work decreases. The work on deconditioning and immobility is based in the objective model of fatigue and has not been linked to subjective fatigue. The deconditioning model shares elements of the conceptual base of the psychobiological-entropy hypothesis and the depletion hypothesis.

Energy storage is another element drawn from the energy balance perspective and is typified by advice to save or conserve energy. The assumption behind this advice is that the individual has a finite amount of energy to invest in activity and that conservation will allow the saved energy to be devoted to another activity. In this conceptualization, energy is replenished through a variety of approaches, such as eating food to provide fuel and resting. This model has not been tested, although the concept of energy conservation frequently is presented in clinical guidelines for preventing or managing fatigue. It is clear that changes in the way specific activities are performed that result in decreased energy expenditure are perceived as helpful by cancer patients, suggesting that the conservation approach holds promise for further development.

# CANCER AND FATIGUE: PATHOPHYSIOLOGY AND PATHOPSYCHOLOGY

Fatigue is an important negative experience for cancer patients during and following treatment. For example, 37% of patients treated for Hodgkin's disease were dissatisfied with the return of their energy many years posttreatment.[48] Weakness and fatigue were among the sources of greatest suffering reported by patients with lung cancer receiving various forms of treatment.[49] Somnolence syndrome, often viewed as synonymous with fatigue, was reported by all of the patients participating in a study of experiences following cranial radiation treatment.[50] Researchers and clinicians acknowledge the problems inherent in isolating causes of fatigue among patients with cancer diagnoses receiving multiple treatments, measuring a variable that does not have one widely accepted operational definition, and facing the reality that very few interventions have been identified to prevent or ameliorate fatigue.[6,51,52]

## Treatment Effects

### Surgery

Patients undergoing surgery experience direct tissue damage as well as the effects of anesthetics and analgesics. Fatigue is a consistent finding in patients who are recovering from surgery and is generally assumed to have multiple causes.[53–57] A variety of preoperative, intraoperative, and postoperative factors have been examined in relation to postoperative fatigue with mixed results. Fatigue may persist up to six months following surgery. Since it is not unusual for patients to undergo several surgical procedures for diagnosis and initial treatment of cancer, the possible cumulative effects of multiple surgical procedures on fatigue are of concern to those who care for oncology patients. The effects of multiple surgical procedures on the severity and duration of postoperative fatigue have not been examined, and the effects of postoperative fatigue on the severity of fatigue associated

with subsequent cancer treatment have not been investigated.

### Radiation treatment

The majority of the side effects of radiation treatment are local and can be predicted based on the site of the treatment field. For example, individuals receiving radiation treatment to a pelvic field experience diarrhea, while those receiving treatment to the neck experience a sore throat. Fatigue is the only common *systemic* side effect of local radiation treatment and has been reported to be the most severe side effect of radiation during the last week of treatment. In a sample of 30 patients who received radiation therapy and completed the Pearson Byars Fatigue Feeling Checklist daily throughout the course of their treatment, the mean level of fatigue increased over the course of treatment, with decreases in the level of fatigue over the weekends (when patients were not treated).[58] A subgroup of the sample, consisting of patients with lung cancer, entered treatment with higher levels of fatigue than the other subjects and reported declines in fatigue before the end of treatment.

Weekly interviews of 96 patients undergoing radiation treatment revealed that fatigue was reported by 93% of the patients receiving treatment for lung cancer, 68% of the patients treated for head and neck cancer, 65% of the men treated for genitourinary cancer, and 72% of the women treated for gynecologic cancer. Among the patients with lung cancer, 60% reported fatigue at the first week of treatment compared with 5%–35% of the patients in the other three groups. In all four groups, fatigue declined gradually over the three months following treatment. Subjects reported that fatigue was intermittent early in treatment but became continuous by the end of treatment, that fatigue was worse in the afternoon or evening, and that resting or sleeping in the afternoon was helpful.[59] Several other studies of patients receiving radiation treatment document various levels of prevalence of fatigue and suggest that factors such as age, diagnosis, and pretreatment condition may influence the severity of fatigue experienced during treatment.[60–65]

The difference between the pattern of fatigue before and during radiation treatment reported by patients with lung cancer when compared with patients with other cancer diagnoses may be related to the characteristics of the disease. The high incidence of fatigue at the beginning of radiation treatment in patients with lung cancer may be explained by the increased energy expenditure required for breathing through partially obstructed airways. In research with healthy volunteers, decreases in airway diameter were associated with increased work of breathing.[66] If radiation treatment is successful in decreasing tumor size, individuals who enter treatment with some degree of airway obstruction are likely to experience some relief of fatigue as a result of the treatment.

The research on cancer patients' perceptions of fatigue as a side effect of radiation treatment is limited to patients receiving local radiation treatment. The experience of patients who receive total-body irradiation in preparation for bone marrow transplantation has not been examined. Since patients who receive total-body irradiation also receive a variety of drugs and undergo multiple medical procedures, their fatigue cannot be attributed to a single treatment modality and may be much different from that experienced by patients receiving local radiation treatment. In general, patients receiving local external radiation treatment alone experience increasing fatigue over the course of treatment. Following treatment, their fatigue declines over a period of weeks or months.[59,67] However, some patients report feeling that their energy level is lower than expected years after completing treatment.

### Chemotherapy

In general, the nature and severity of the side effects of cancer chemotherapy vary according to the type of drug(s) prescribed and the dose of the drug(s) (see chapter 16). Despite variation among treatment regimens, fatigue is the most frequently reported side effect of chemotherapy.[14,27,39,40,68–70] In a prospective study of 66 patients with advanced colon or rectal cancer receiving either intravenous or intraperitoneal 5-fluorouracil (5-FU), 90% of the patients receiving intravenous 5-FU and 85% of the patients receiving intraperitoneal 5-FU reported on a questionnaire completed at home that they experienced fatigue following each cycle of chemotherapy.[68] For patients with lung cancer receiving combination treatment with radiation plus either one of two drug regimens, fatigue increased compared with pretreatment levels in 68% of the patients in one group and 76% in the other group at the completion of treatment.[71] Seventy-five percent of 61 patients with malignant lymphoma, 90% of whom were receiving treatment at the time of the interview, reported fatigue as a side effect of chemotherapy.[72] In addition, fatigue was positively related to emotional distress. When individuals beginning chemotherapy and individuals who had already started treatment were interviewed at the beginning and end of a single cycle of chemotherapy, 63% of those just starting treatment reported worsening fatigue, with nearly 90% of all study participants reporting fatigue during the treatment cycle.[70] This finding is consistent in magnitude with the findings of other prospective studies of patients receiving chemotherapy.[40,73,74]

Women receiving adjuvant chemotherapy for breast cancer have provided much information about side effects of treatment and quality of life during cancer chemotherapy. Forty-eight (96%) of 50 women receiving adjuvant chemotherapy for stage II breast cancer reported fatigue as a side effect of treatment, and many reported fluctuations in the level of fatigue depending on the phase of the treatment cycle.[75] These subjects characterized their fatigue as a lack of ambition, a feeling of slowness, and a continuous feeling of tiredness.[75,76] Among 50 women receiving adjuvant chemotherapy for breast cancer and 28 women who had completed this treatment, fatigue received the highest physical distress

rating among women currently receiving treatment and the second-highest rating among those who had completed treatment.[77] Although fatigue produced the most distress of any of the physical symptoms reported by the women under treatment, the mean level of distress fell between 2 and 3 on a scale of 1 (no distress) to 5 (great distress). The finding of a low to moderate level of physical distress among women with breast cancer was replicated in a sample of 107 women who completed a self-administered questionnaire, with the mean level of distress from fatigue, insomnia, nausea, and pain falling between 2 and 3 on the same five-point scale.[78] When side effects reported by patients were compared by type of adjuvant chemotherapy regimen for breast cancer in a sample of 81 women, fatigue was the most frequently reported side effect regardless of drug regimen.[79]

Among 128 women beginning a course of daily aminoglutethimide and medroxyprogesterone acetate for advanced metastatic breast cancer, fatigue appeared in 50% of the women and gradually disappeared during the first six weeks of treatment.[78] In a group of 56 patients with a variety of types of cancer beginning their first cycle of chemotherapy, 46 (82%) of the patients reported experiencing fatigue by the completion of the second treatment cycle.[80] Fatigue was the second-most distressing symptom, after pain, reported by 26 patients with a variety of solid tumors who participated in a phase I clinical trial, with the level of distress produced by fatigue similar to that reported by patients receiving adjuvant chemotherapy for breast cancer.[81]

These studies indicate that fatigue is the most prevalent side effect experienced by patients receiving chemotherapy for cancer. Fatigue is an important problem regardless of cancer diagnosis and type of drug treatment, although the time of onset, duration, pattern, and severity of fatigue associated with chemotherapy and differences in the pattern of fatigue specific to individual drug regimens are not well documented.

### Biologic response modifiers

Fatigue is described as the most important dose-limiting side effect of interferons.[82–84] In a small sample of patients with leukemia ($n = 11$) given two different types of interferon, 50% of the patients who received beta-interferon and 60% of the patients who received gamma-interferon experienced fatigue.[85] Findings of a phase I study of beta-interferon demonstrated a positive relationship between dose and fatigue, with the incidence of fatigue reaching 100% at the highest dosage level administered in the protocol.[86] Findings of this study also suggest that patients may develop tolerance to some of the side effects of beta-interferon, including fatigue. Alfa-interferon produced fatigue similar to that produced by the other interferons.[87] Interleukin-2 produces multiple systemic toxicities such as fatigue, chills, fever, and headaches that resemble those produced by the interferons.[88]

Based on the limited information available on the incidence and characteristics of fatigue associated with the use of biologic response modifiers, it appears that this cancer treatment modality is likely to produce fatigue that is more severe than that associated with surgery, radiation treatment, and the most commonly used chemotherapy regimens. The severity of the fatigue may exceed the individual's level of tolerance, in terms of either the sensation of fatigue or the impact of fatigue on day-to-day activities, causing the patient to terminate treatment. Since fatigue is a dose-limiting side effect of biologic response modifiers, a high priority for nursing care of individuals receiving this form of treatment is preventing and ameliorating fatigue.

### Combined-modality treatment

The majority of cancer patients who present for adjuvant chemotherapy or radiation treatment already have undergone a surgical procedure. Some patients receive concurrent radiation treatment and chemotherapy, while others receive radiation and biologic response modifiers. Patients may receive three or four different types of treatment simultaneously or in a variety of sequences. Research to determine whether fatigue produced by sequential or combined-modality treatment exceeds that produced by the most toxic treatment alone is needed to determine the extent to which fatigue will be a problem for patients on these regimens and to design approaches to preventing and managing fatigue in patients receiving multiple forms of cancer treatment.

## Other Etiologic Factors

In addition to the direct effects of treatment, cancer patients experience a variety of problems that may produce fatigue.[1,4,5,10,89,90]

### Physical factors

Physical problems such as pain, pruritus, urinary frequency, diarrhea, nausea, and vomiting may interfere with patients' ability to rest or sleep. Nutritional deficits, changes in nutrient metabolism, and alteration in fluid and electrolyte balance are produced by anorexia, taste changes, nausea, vomiting, stomatitis, esophagitis, mucositis, xerostomia, diarrhea, use of a restricted diet as part of an unproven method of cancer treatment, inappropriate use of a weight-reduction diet, hepatic and renal damage, side effects of medications, changes in absorption due to surgery, or diabetes. Bone marrow depression can produce anemia, bleeding, and increased susceptibility to infection, all of which are believed to produce fatigue. Some physical conditions increase energy expenditure, such as amputation of a limb or a neurological deficit, weakness due to prolonged bedrest, a sensory deficit producing a need for increased vigilance, dyspnea, and decreased cardiac reserve. Alcohol and the use of prescription or nonprescription drugs also can contribute to feelings of fatigue, especially when the individual is using narcotics, sedatives, hypnotics, or antihistamines.

### Psychosocial factors

Fatigue is often viewed as a symptom of anxiety and depression. Anxiety is associated with feelings of panic or tension and can produce agitation that may be followed by intense feelings of fatigue. Depression is a state of sadness that results in low energy and low levels of activity,[91] but it is important to differentiate between fatigue and depression in patients who are undergoing cancer treatment as the approaches to dealing with depression and CRF are different. Assessment of depression in cancer patients should focus on the feeling of sadness that persists over time and is constant, rather than on symptoms like constipation and anorexia or sleep problems that are all potential side effects of treatment.[92] Receiving a diagnosis of cancer is certainly a frightening and stressful experience, and confronting a life-threatening disease can lead to depression. Conversely, feelings of anxiety and depression can result from the disruption in lifestyle produced by fatigue. When severe fatigue experienced as a side effect of cancer treatment forces the individual to decrease participation in social activities, transfer family responsibilities to others, and limit work activities, the person's response may include anxiety or depression as a result of the loss of usual social roles or the inability to reach desired goals. The impact of the severity of fatigue and associated changes in activity depends upon the individual's perception of what limitations are acceptable to the self and the family as well as the expected duration of the limitations. These value judgments will differ substantially from person to person, with some individuals finding a week of fatigue following chemotherapy to be unacceptable and others regarding it as a perfectly acceptable experience.

For those who strive to maintain all their usual activities in addition to dealing with the demands of cancer treatment, fatigue may be the result of expending too much energy. For example, a person who maintains a full-time work commitment while commuting one or two hours a day for radiation treatment may experience fatigue as the daily commute is added to an already full schedule. Individuals who deny the effects of their illness and its treatment may find it difficult to set priorities for their activities and consequently may experience more fatigue than those who curtail some activities. The relationship between level of daily activities and fatigue in individuals undergoing cancer treatment has not been examined systematically.

Responses to the provision of care may also influence level of fatigue. Patients who are concerned about the professional care they receive may become hypervigilant in health care settings as a self-protective measure. This hypervigilance state represents an investment of energy and may interfere with sleep and rest. In contrast, when care providers are effective in anticipating the needs of the patient and establishing a trust relationship, patients appear to accept the provider as the person who will maintain vigilance. Studies of the extent to which vigilance is practiced by cancer patients and the effect on fatigue of having a care provider take over the vigilance or remove the need for vigilance are needed.

# NURSING CARE OF THE CANCER PATIENT AT RISK FOR FATIGUE

The goal of nursing care for the patient with cancer is to minimize the negative impact of fatigue on quality of life. In order to reach this goal, the prevention and treatment of fatigue must be addressed in the plan of care. Understanding the possible causes of fatigue, the patient's values, coping resources, usual activities, and perception of fatigue is essential to providing care.

## Assessment

Systematic fatigue assessment was one of eight research-based practices assessed in a survey of oncology nurses.[93] Only 53% of the 1100 staff nurse respondents were aware of the need for systematic assessment of fatigue, and only 27% of those who were aware of it consistently assessed their patients' level of fatigue. The level of awareness for systematic assessment of fatigue was the lowest of the eight practices addressed in the survey. Among those who were assessing patients' level of fatigue, the average frequency of assessment was "sometimes." At the organizational level, a survey of supportive care programs in National Cancer Institute–designated cancer centers revealed that none of the responding centers had clinical programs that addressed fatigue.[94] These findings support the need for systematic education of health care providers, patients, family members, and the public about the need to address fatigue and the impact of fatigue on cancer patients.

### Level of fatigue

Since the patient's perception of fatigue will influence decisions about activities, participation in treatment, and overall quality of life, so-called objective ratings of fatigue made by health care professionals are much less relevant to the patient's situation than assessments made by the patient. Fernsler found that when the problems reported by cancer patients receiving chemotherapy were compared with nurses' reports of the problems they perceived the patients to be experiencing, patients reported three times more problems related to activity and rest than did their nurses.[95] Similar findings were reported for a sample of patients with advanced cancer.[96,97] In research on side effects of cancer treatment, various self-report measures have been used to obtain patients' ratings of the severity of fatigue or the distress produced by fatigue.[98] The measurement approaches used in these studies range from a single yes-no question to multiple-adjective checklists. Although the multiple-item instruments are more likely than the single-item measures to be subjected to psychometric testing to assess their reliability and validity, the longer instruments are not readily incorporated in clinical interviews. Clinicians often find it useful to ask patients to rate their fatigue on a scale of 0 to 10 or 1 to 10, with the lowest point representing no fatigue and the highest point representing extreme fatigue. This approach is analogous to pain ratings used in most practice settings and can be tailored to match the approach to rating pain for ease of use by patients and providers.

The definition of fatigue shifts as the person with cancer experiences it. This change takes the form of a new definition of the level at which one is fatigued, which is higher than that used prior to experiencing CRF.[99] The definition of what constitutes extreme fatigue also shifts upward. This shift in the standard of comparison is one reason why comparisons of healthy people with persons undergoing cancer treatment may yield comparable fatigue ratings. The healthy people are using a different—and lower—standard for fatigue than cancer patients who have experienced CRF.

The measures of fatigue based on health care providers' judgments or observations depend on observations of the individual's appearance, level of consciousness, activity level while in the hospital or during an outpatient visit, or patient reports of activity level. Using any measure of activity level as an indicator of fatigue is difficult conceptually because activity may represent a response to a variety of problems, such as nausea and pain, rather than a report of the sensation of fatigue. Measures of level of consciousness and appearance also are likely to capture multiple phenomena other than fatigue. In addition, this type of measure may not be very sensitive, since it is unlikely that the majority of patients experiencing fatigue will demonstrate marked changes in level of consciousness. At this time the use of motor or mental task performance tests such as those used in research with healthy individuals has limited relevance to the routine clinical assessment of individuals with cancer. The exception to this is in testing to determine ability to perform specific tasks that may be carried out in a work setting or as part of a rehabilitation assessment procedure.

Level of fatigue should be assessed at multiple points in time. Individuals who do not have fatigue when they begin treatment are likely to experience it at some point during treatment, and those whose fatigue does not gradually decrease once treatment is completed may require evaluation to determine if their fatigue is something other than an expected side effect of treatment. To assist patients in planning ways to deal with fatigue, the nurse must obtain information about both the daily pattern of fatigue and variations in fatigue in relation to the treatment cycle.

### Usual activities

Information about the type and intensity of the individual's usual activities can be obtained by asking the patient to describe a typical day. The description should include the time the patient arises and retires, the number of times the patient awakens during the night and the circumstances surrounding the awakening, physical and mental activities performed during the day, the extent to which naps or rests are taken during the day and the extent to which they relieve fatigue, and a comparison of the current level of activity to the individual's level of activity before this episode of illness or the beginning of the present course of treatment. Individuals who report fatigue should be asked to describe what they do about it and to indicate the extent to which their self-care activities are effective in relieving their fatigue.

To assist the person in planning ways of modifying daily activities, the nurse determines who might be available to assume some of the individual's usual responsibilities and gains an understanding of the meaning and value of each of the individual's activities. For example, a person who highly values maintaining his or her usual work role and places a lower value on recreation and entertainment will probably find it acceptable to suspend participation in sports and social events temporarily rather than take a leave of absence from work when experiencing fatigue as a side effect of cancer treatment. Individuals experiencing fatigue over time may gradually downgrade their perception of the level of activity that is "usual." They may not become aware of the impact of fatigue on their usual activities until months after treatment ends and it becomes apparent that routine seasonal household maintenance was not done or that their level of social activity is much lower than it was before treatment. Information about level of activity during treatment in relation to activity prior to treatment may also be obtained from family members or friends who have consistent, frequent contact with the patient.

### Additional assessment data

The assessment includes information about potential causes of fatigue. Chronic diseases such as diabetes, congestive heart failure, chronic obstructive pulmonary disease, Addison's disease, hyperthyroidism, hypopituitarism, renal or liver failure, anemia, and a variety of neurological disorders as well as infection, pain, acute CNS changes, sleep disruption, overexertion, dehydration, electrolyte imbalances, malnutrition, anxiety, and depression may contribute to fatigue. A careful review of the patient's medical and social history, including previous and current cancer treatment, laboratory data, and a thorough physical assessment, are essential in obtaining information about potential causes of fatigue.

## Interventions

Despite the prevalence of fatigue as a side effect of cancer treatment, little attention has been given to determining the efficacy of the self-care activities patients use to deal with fatigue or to developing and testing new approaches to the problem. It is important to be aware of the assumptions underlying most of the conventional advice provided to people experiencing fatigue about ways to manage or prevent fatigue. The most common suggestions are to rest or sleep more and do less. The advice to get more rest or sleep is based in the assumption, drawn from work on acute fatigue, that rest or sleep will eventually relieve the sensation of fatigue. Advice focused on decreasing activity assumes that fatigue is a response to activity. Both of these assumptions are questionable in CRF. However, they may address important responses to the reality of CRF in that they provide patients with permission to accept the natural response to overwhelming fatigue: decreasing activity.

Once treatable physiological problems such as anemia, electrolyte imbalance, or medication side effects have been eliminated as causes of fatigue in patients undergoing treatment, other forms of intervention become important. The interventions suggested for CRF include providing preparatory information, energy conservation and activity management, increasing sleep or rest, and exercise[1,2,3,5] (Table 23-1).

### Preparatory information

Preparatory information is used to structure the person's expectations about receiving chemotherapy or radiation therapy. In one type of preparatory information, individuals are told about the pattern of fatigue expected as a side effect of treatment based on data collected from patients who have had the same treatment. Preparatory information, combined with suggestions about planning for rest periods, has had positive effects on patients' maintenance of usual activities when combined with similar information about various aspects of the experience of receiving radiation treatment for prostate cancer.[100,101] Although there are reports of research on the effects of providing other types of preparatory informational interventions in samples of patients receiving cancer treatment, none of them include dependent variables relevant to level of performance of usual activities or fatigue. The rationale for providing preparatory information is that it provides patients with an accurate mental image of the impending experience. The importance of having accurate expectations or images should not be ignored, for this is the standard used by patients in processing information and assigning meaning. Patients who do not realize that fatigue is an expected side effect of treatment may believe that it means the treatment is not working, that information provided about a good prognosis was a lie, that they are not tolerating treatment well and that they should not tell their health care providers for fear the treatment will be stopped, and that fatigue that persists beyond the end of treatment is a sign of cancer progression or recurrence. Accurate information about impending experiences does not increase the num-

**TABLE 23-1** Intervention Guide for Cancer Treatment–Related Fatigue

| Intervention | Content | Rationale |
|---|---|---|
| **Preparatory information**<br>(for all patients beginning treatment) | 1. Introduce the idea that fatigue is a common side effect of treatment.<br>2. Describe the pattern of fatigue in neutral, objective (not evaluative) terms based upon information provided by other patients who have had the same treatment. | To set up accurate expectations about the experience so the patient can interpret the experience appropriately and make plans based upon accurate information. |
| **Sleep and rest**<br>(for patients experiencing CRF without an identified treatable cause) | 1. Address usual pattern of sleep and rest in assessment.<br>2. Identify sensations, thoughts, activities, etc., that interfere with sleep.<br>3. Anticipate and prevent sleep disruption caused by suggested illness management regimen.<br>4. Attend to noise, light, and people issues in institutional and home care setting.<br>5. Consider pharmacological management when initiating sleep is a problem.<br>6. Remember that sleep and rest are not likely to completely relieve fatigue but that most cancer patients find them to be helpful. | Try to tailor care to fit usual pattern (e.g., avoid suggesting naps to someone who reports that naps have never helped in the past, but do allow time for active rest for those who report being refreshed by reading) and develop awareness of interruptions of sleep and rest time. Timing of medication, meals, and other care activities should be considered in relation to sleep and rest. |
| **Energy conservation and activity management**<br>(for patients experiencing CRF without an identified treatable cause) | 1. Identify values, priorities, and recent changes in demand for activity during assessment.<br>2. Look for ways to conserve energy in the performance of usual activities like using a mobility aid, rearranging work area, sitting rather than standing, etc.<br>3. Consider physical therapy or occupational therapy referral for home evaluation and recommendation.<br>4. Identify other resources available to take over some activities.<br>5. Assist patient in developing an activity plan and evaluating the effectiveness of the plan.<br>6. Work with family and friends to aid with work without adding demands. | This intervention requires detailed evaluation of the environment and of the patient's usual level of activity, value systems, resources, and priorities. At times, having someone else take over an activity may create additional work for the patient rather than decreasing activity, so orientation for the helper is important. Mobility aids, work aids, referrals for evaluation and intervention, and coordination with occupational health personnel at the patient's employment site may be needed to establish an effective energy conservation plan. |
| **Exercise**<br>(some patients will use as a preventive or general health promotion measure, others may initiate when experiencing CRF in the absence of an identified treatable cause) | 1. Address usual level of physical activity in initial assessment.<br>2. Evaluate patient for contraindications for physical activity according to established guidelines (consider referral to physical therapy or cardiac rehabilitation).<br>3. If patient is interested in exercise prescription and there are no contraindications, refer for exercise prescription.<br>4. If patient has an established program that will continue, review special considerations such as signs of dehydration, infection, etc., that indicate the patient should not exercise; note special precautions in relation to laboratory tests, time since treatment, etc. | Safety is a key issue here. Consider weather-related risks as well as disease factors and individual level of fitness. Remember that commercial exercise facilities and programs vary in level of training of program staff. Follow established guidelines for staff qualifications in making referrals for fitness testing or exercise prescriptions. Unusual physical findings following the initiation of an exercise program should be investigated in relation to the exercise program (e.g., bruised skin in a radiation treatment field may be due to positioning during weight training rather than disease recurrence; localized pain may be a result of exercise rather than a metastatic process). |

*(continued)*

**TABLE 23-1**    Intervention Guide for Cancer Treatment–Related Fatigue (continued)

| Intervention | Content | Rationale |
|---|---|---|
| | 5. If the exercise program requires modification, refer patient to an appropriate resource with expertise in exercise and cancer.<br>6. Avoid unnecessary restrictions on physical exercise. | |

ber of patients who report specific side effects of treatment.

### Rest and sleep

Rest is the most frequently recommended intervention for cancer patients who experience fatigue. Rest may take the form of a nap, a period of inactivity, a lower level of activity than usual, or a momentary respite from contact with others. Increasing the length of nighttime sleep may be considered a form of rest. However, increased sleep or rest may not improve fatigue for all individuals. Some have reported that sleep helps with fatigue only because they do not notice the fatigue while they are asleep, while others find sleep and rest to be extremely effective in relieving fatigue.[40,41] Symptoms or treatment side effects that interfere with sleep and rest should be controlled to the extent possible. Nausea, vomiting, diarrhea, hot flashes, pain, urinary frequency, dry mouth, and urinary burning are examples of physical problems that can disrupt sleep. Assessment and aggressive management of these problems will address the component of CRF that results from sleep disruption. Establishing a schedule for medication administration, fluid administration, and self-monitoring activities that does not interfere with the individual's desired rest time may also be helpful in maintaining sleep. The use of medication to induce sleep or relieve anxiety that interferes with sleep or rest may be appropriate for some individuals.

### Energy conservation and activity management

Rearranging activities to allow for rest periods or to shorten the time that high-energy output is required is another approach to dealing with limitations imposed by fatigue. Individuals may rearrange their weekly errands so they are spread throughout the week or schedule strenuous or high-priority activities at the time of day or week when they have the most energy. Some activities will be abandoned, performed in a different way, or shifted to another person. Rhodes et al[102] provided a rich description of these changes in patients' lives as part of their research on self-care for the side effects of chemotherapy. Tiredness and weakness were the side effects that most interfered with self-care. The subjects limited energy expenditure through careful planning and scheduling, decreasing activities, and depending on others to complete some activities.

Even though energy conservation and activity management are widely accepted interventions, there are no specific protocols published for the use of these intervention strategies with cancer patients and there are no systematic tests of them to determine if they influence fatigue. Specific suggestions for energy conservation and activity management are used in the management of other chronic illnesses, such as multiple sclerosis, postpolio syndrome, and fibromyalgia, but research on these patient populations is also extremely limited and does not address the effect of the intervention on fatigue. Environmental modifications, such as sitting to prepare food or using a toilet seat that is elevated and has grab rails attached, are specific examples of the way in which changing how an activity is performed can reduce the energy demand of the activity.

### Exercise

Research involving women receiving adjuvant chemotherapy for breast cancer indicates that exercise may relieve fatigue. Patients who participated in a supervised, aerobic, interval training exercise program showed an improvement in fatigue measured as a component of mood, nausea, and functional capacity.[103,104] Women assigned to a combined structured walking and support group intervention had less fatigue, higher levels of psychosocial adjustment, and better physical performance than a control group.[105] The results of the research on exercise in women receiving adjuvant chemotherapy for breast cancer is encouraging. Further research is needed to determine the effects of different kinds of exercise on perceived fatigue in cancer patients with other diagnoses, stages of disease, and treatment regimens. Although exercise has the potential to be a powerful intervention, it is not without risk. Considerations in recommending exercise should include adherence to published recommendations for safety.[106,107] Medications such as catabolic steroids, mobility problems, neurological deficits, and dizziness are examples of factors that increase risk of injury in the use of exercise for cancer patients. Individuals for whom exercise is not contraindicated can be encouraged to try short walks or their usual exercise to see if the activity relieves their fatigue. One unstudied issue in cancer care is the extent to which cancer patients who exercised regularly prior to beginning treatment maintain their exercise program. There are no established practice standards that address this issue, and anecdotes from patients and providers suggest wide variation in recommendations provided to patients. Some practitioners suggest that patients continue their usual program of exercise, others suggest that the patient decrease the intensity and/or frequency of exercise, and some encourage patients to maintain their program of exercise based upon how they are feeling. Given the high level of acceptance of exercise by individuals who did not exercise regularly prior to joining the study, advice to decrease or terminate usual physical exercise in the absence of specific contraindications may be counterproductive.

### Posttreatment fatigue

When fatigue is experienced as a side effect of treatment, it does not disappear immediately once treatment ends. Individuals who have experienced fatigue during cancer treatment should be warned to expect a gradual lessening of fatigue over the months following treatment. The interventions that helped with fatigue during treatment may need to be continued, and activities that were decreased during treatment should be resumed gradually. Individuals with advanced cancer may complete treatment and subsequently experience worsening of their fatigue. For these individuals, the side effects of pain medications and immobility may contribute to the fatigue. The use of assistive devices such as wheelchairs and grab rails, systematic planning of activities to include those most valued by the individual, and careful conservation of energy to ensure that adequate energy is available for highly valued activities are important in enabling the individual to maintain the best possible quality of life.

## CONCLUSION

Although a number of hypotheses have been proposed to explain the causes of fatigue experienced as a symptom of cancer or as a side effect of cancer treatment, none has been adequately tested. Among the many side effects of cancer treatment, fatigue is the most prevalent but may be the most poorly understood.

The existing research on fatigue documents the incidence of fatigue among individuals receiving varying forms of cancer treatment. However, the measures of fatigue used in these studies represent a mix of patients' perceptions and those of physicians and nurses. Since the subjective view of fatigue is most relevant to patient care, both clinical assessment and further research should focus on the patient's assessment of fatigue. To plan nursing care for the patient who is experiencing fatigue, the patient's pattern of usual activities and the relative importance or value of each activity must also be understood. In addition, data also should be obtained on a variety of physical and psychosocial factors that may influence or produce fatigue.

The interventions routinely suggested to patients to lessen fatigue focus on increasing rest and decreasing the expenditure of energy. The specific activities suggested include naps, lengthening periods of sleep, rearranging schedules to spread strenuous activities over longer periods, and eliminating those activities that are unnecessary or are judged to be too taxing. Although some patients report using exercise to relieve fatigue, this intervention is not usually included in the clinical literature but is a subject of current research. Providing individuals with cancer with information about expected side effects of treatment, including fatigue, and assisting those who experience fatigue to plan alterations in their daily activities are important in helping individuals with cancer deal with their experience.

## REFERENCES

1. Winningham ML, Nail LM, Burke MB, et al: Fatigue and the cancer experience: The state of the knowledge. *Oncol Nurs Forum* 21:23–34, 1994
2. Richardson A: Fatigue in cancer patients: A review of the literature. *Eur J Cancer Care* 4:20–32, 1995
3. Smets E, Garssen B, Schuster-Uitterhoeve A, et al: Fatigue in cancer patients. *Br J Cancer* 68:220–224, 1993
4. Nail LM, King KB: Fatigue. *Semin Oncol Nurs* 3:257–262, 1987
5. Piper BF: Fatigue, in Carrieri VK, Lindsey AM, West CM (eds): *Pathophysiological Phenomena in Nursing: Human Responses to Illness* (ed 2). Philadelphia, Saunders, 1993, pp 279–302
6. Irvine DM, Vincent L, Bubela N, et al: A critical appraisal of the research literature investigating fatigue in the individual with cancer. *Cancer Nurs* 14(4):188–199, 1991
7. Potempa K, Lopez M, Reid C, et al: Chronic fatigue. *Image* 18:165–169, 1986
8. Farrar DJ, Locke SE, Kantrowitz FG: Chronic fatigue syndrome: 1. Etiology and pathogenesis. *Behav Med* 21:5–16, 1994
9. Kantrowitz FG, Farrar DJ, Locke SE: Chronic fatigue syndrome: 2. Treatment and future research. *Behav Med* 21:17–24, 1994
10. Aistars J: Fatigue in the cancer patient: A conceptual approach to a clinical problem. *Oncol Nurs Forum* 14:25–30, 1987
11. Copp G, Dunn V: Frequent and difficult problems perceived by nurses caring for the dying in community, hospice, and acute care settings. *Palliat Med* 7:19–25, 1993
12. Dean GE, Ferrell BH: Impact of fatigue on quality of life in cancer survivors. *Quality of Life: A Nurs Challenge* 4:25–28, 1995
13. Dean GE, Spears L, Ferrell BR, et al: Fatigue in patients with cancer receiving interferon alfa. *Cancer Pract* 3:164–172, 1995
14. Ferrell BR, Grant M, Dean GE, et al: "Bone tired": The experience of fatigue and impact on quality of life. *Oncol Nurs Forum* 23:1539–1547, 1996
15. Nail LM, Jones LS: Fatigue as a side effect of cancer treatment: Impact on quality of life. *Quality of Life: A Nurs Challenge* 4:8–13, 1995

16. Piper BF, Lindsay AM, Dodd MJ: Fatigue mechanisms in cancer patients: Developing nursing theory. *Oncol Nurs Forum* 14:17–23, 1987

17. Nail LM, Winningham ML: Fatigue and weakness in cancer patients: The symptom experience. *Semin Oncol Nurs* 11:272–278, 1995

18. Simonson E: *Physiology of Work Capacity and Fatigue.* Springfield, IL, Thomas, 1971

19. Brown JK: Gender, age, usual weight, and tobacco use as predictors of weight loss in patients with lung cancer. *Oncol Nurs Forum* 20:466–472, 1993

20. Langstein HN, Norton JA: Mechanisms of cancer cachexia. *Hematol Oncol Clin North Am* 5:103–123, 1991

21. Christensen T, Kehlet H, Vesterberg V, et al: Fatigue and muscle amino acids during surgical convalescence. *Acta Chir Scand* 153:567–570, 1987

22. St. Pierre B, Kasper CE, Lindsey AM: Fatigue mechanisms in patients with cancer: Effects of tumor necrosis factor and exercise on skeletal muscle. *Oncol Nurs Forum* 19:419–425, 1992

23. Diehl LF, Bolan CD, Weiss RB: Hemolytic anemia and cancer treatment. *Cancer Treat Rev* 22:33–73, 1996

24. Erickson JM: Anemia. *Semin Oncol Nurs* 12:2–14, 1996

25. Ludwig H, Fritz E, Leitgeb C, et al: Prediction of response to erythropoietin treatment in chronic anemia of cancer. *Blood* 84:1056–1063, 1994

26. Ludwig H, Sunday E, Percherstorfer M, et al: Recombinant human erythropoietin for the correction of cancer associated anemia with and without concomitant cytotoxic chemotherapy. *Cancer* 76:2319–2329, 1995

27. Blesch KS, Paice JA, Wickham R, et al: Correlates of fatigue in people with breast or lung cancer. *Oncol Nurs Forum* 18:81–87, 1991

28. Taylor LA, Rachman SJ: The effects of blood sugar level changes on cognitive function, affective state, and somatic symptoms. *J Behav Med* 11:279–291, 1988

29. Newsholme EA, Blomstrand E: The plasma level of some amino acids and physical and mental fatigue. *Experientia* 52:413–415, 1996

30. Selye H: *Stress without Distress.* Philadelphia, Lippincott, 1974

31. Dekhuijzen PN, Gayan-Ramirez G, Bisschop A, et al: Recovery of corticosteroid-induced changes in contractile properties of rat diaphragm. *Am J Respir Crit Care Med* 153:769–775, 1996

32. Gozdasoglu S, Unal E, Yavuz G, et al: Granulocyte-macrophage colony stimulating factor (rh-GM-CSF) in the treatment of chemotherapy-induced neutropenia. *J Chemother* 7:467–469, 1995

33. Harada M, Nagafuji K, Fujisaki T: G-CSF-induced mobilization of peripheral blood stem cells from healthy adults for allogeneic transplantation. *J Hematother* 5:63–71, 1996

34. Rapp SE, Egan KJ, Ross BK, et al: A multidimensional comparison of morphine and hydromorphone patient-controlled analgesia. *Anesth Analg* 82:1043–1048, 1996

35. Grandjean EP: Fatigue. *Am Ind Hyg Assoc J* 31:401–411, 1970

36. Cleare AJ, Bearn J, Allain T, et al: Contrasting neuroendocrine responses in depression and chronic fatigue syndrome. *J Affect Disord* 34:283–289, 1995

37. Cimprich B: Symptom management: Loss of concentration. *Semin Oncol Nurs* 11:279–288, 1995

38. Cimprich B: Attentional fatigue following breast cancer surgery. *Res Nurs Health* 15:199–207, 1992

39. Glaus A, Crow R, Hammond S: A qualitative study to explore the concept of fatigue/tiredness in cancer patients and in healthy individuals. *Eur J Cancer Care* 5:8–23, 1996 (suppl 2)

40. Nail LM, Jones LS, Greene D, et al: Use and perceived efficacy of self-care activities in patients receiving chemotherapy. *Oncol Nurs Forum* 18:883–887, 1991

41. Graydon JE, Bubela N, Irvine D, et al: Fatigue reducing strategies used by patients receiving treatment for cancer. *Cancer Nurs* 18:23–28, 1995

42. Jensen DP, Herr KA: Sleeplessness. *Adv Clin Nurs Res* 28:385–405, 1993

43. Sheely LC: Sleep disturbances in hospitalized patients with cancer. *Oncol Nurs Forum* 23:109–111, 1996

44. Lamb MA: The sleeping patterns of patients with malignant and nonmalignant diseases. *Cancer Nurs* 5:389–396, 1982

45. Silberfarb PM, Hauri PJ, Oxman TE: Assessment of sleep in patients with lung cancer and breast cancer. *J Clin Oncol* 11:997–1004, 1993

46. Winningham ML: How exercise mitigates fatigue: Implications for people receiving cancer therapy, in Johnson RM (ed): *The Biotherapy of Cancer V.* Pittsburgh, Oncology Nursing Press, 1992, pp 16–21

47. Winningham ML: The energetics of activity, fatigue, symptom management and functional status: A conceptual model. Presented at the First International Symposium on Symptom Management, San Francisco, March 12, 1992

48. Fobair P, Hoppe RT, Bloom J, et al: Psychosocial problems among survivors of Hodgkin's disease. *J Clin Oncol* 4:805–814, 1986

49. Benedict S: The suffering associated with lung cancer. *Cancer Nurs* 12(1):34–40, 1989

50. Faithfull S: Patients' experiences following cranial radiotherapy: A study of the somnolence syndrome. *J Adv Nurs* 16:939–946, 1991

51. Piper BF, Rieger PT, Brophy L, et al: Recent advances in the management of biotherapy-related side effects: Fatigue. *Oncol Nurs Forum* 16(6):27–34, 1989 (suppl)

52. Yarbro CH: Interventions for fatigue. *Eur J Cancer Care* 5:35–38, 1996 (suppl 2)

53. Christensen T, Kehlet H: Postoperative fatigue. *World J Surg* 17:220–225, 1993

54. Vara-Thorbeck R, Guerrero JA, Ruiz-Requena E, et al: Can the use of growth hormone reduce the postoperative fatigue syndrome? *World J Surg* 20:81–86, 1996

55. Watt-Watson J, Graydon J: Impact of surgery on head and neck cancer patients and their caregivers. *Nurs Clin North Am* 30:659–671, 1995

56. Schroeder D, Hill GH: Predicting postoperative fatigue: Importance of preoperative factors. *World J Surg* 17:226–231, 1993

57. Schulze S, Thorup J: Pulmonary function, pain, and fatigue after laparoscopic cholecystectomy. *Eur J Surg* 159:361–364, 1993

58. Haylock PJ, Hart LK: Fatigue in patients receiving localized radiation. *Cancer Nurs* 2:461–467, 1979

59. King KB, Nail LM, Kreamer K, et al: Patients' descriptions of the experience of receiving radiation treatment. *Oncol Nurs Forum* 12(5):55–61, 1985

60. Greenberg DW, Sawicka J, Eisenthal S, et al: Fatigue syndrome due to localized radiation treatment. *J Pain Symptom Manage* 7:38–45, 1992

61. Irvine DM, Vincent L, Graydon JE, et al: The prevalence and correlates of fatigue in patients receiving treatment with chemotherapy and radiotherapy. *Cancer Nurs* 17:367–378, 1994

62. Kubricht DW: Therapeutic self-care demands expressed by outpatients receiving external radiation therapy. *Cancer Nurs* 7:43–52, 1984

63. Larson PJ, Lindsey AM, Dodd MJ, et al: Influence of age on problems experienced by patients with lung cancer undergoing radiation therapy. *Oncol Nurs Forum* 20:473–480, 1993

64. Nail LM: Coping with intracavitary radiation treatment for gynecologic cancer. *Cancer Pract* 1:218–224, 1993

65. Oberst MT, Hughes SH, Chang AS, et al: Self-care burden, stress appraisal, and mood among persons receiving radiotherapy. *Cancer Nurs* 14:71–78, 1991

66. Shapiro M, Wilson K, Casar G, et al: Work of breathing through different sized endotracheal tubes. *Crit Care Med* 14:1028–1031, 1986

67. Walker BL, Nail LM, Larsen L, et al: Concerns, affect, and cognitive disruption following completion of radiation treatment for localized breast or prostate cancer. *Oncol Nurs Forum* 23:1181–1187, 1996

68. Gianola FJ, Sugarbaker PH, Barofsky I, et al: Toxicity studies of adjuvant versus intraperitoneal 5-FU in patients with advanced primary colon or rectal cancer. *Am J Clin Oncol* 9:403–410, 1986

69. Richardson A: The pattern of fatigue in patients receiving chemotherapy, in Richardson A, Wilson-Barnett J (eds): *Nursing Research in Cancer Care*. London, Scutari, 1995, pp 225–245

70. Richardson A, Ream E: The experience of fatigue and other symptoms in patients receiving chemotherapy. *Eur J Cancer Care* 5:24–30, 1996 (suppl 2)

71. Silberfarb PM, Holland JCB, Anbar D, et al: Psychological responses of patients receiving two drug regimens for lung carcinoma. *Am J Psychiatry* 140:110–111, 1983

72. Nerenz DR, Leventhal H, Love RR: Factors contributing to emotional distress during cancer chemotherapy. *Cancer* 50:1020–1027, 1982

73. Nail LM: Pattern of fatigue associated with cancer treatment. Paper presented at the Oncology Nursing Society Congress, Philadelphia, May, 1996

74. Foltz AT, Gaines G, Gullatte M: Recalled side effects and self-care actions of patients receiving inpatient chemotherapy. *Oncol Nurs Forum* 23:679–683, 1996

75. Meyerowitz BE, Sparks FC, Spears IK: Adjuvant chemotherapy for breast carcinoma: Psychosocial implications. *Cancer* 43:1613–1618, 1979

76. Meyerowitz BE, Watkins IK, Sparks FC: Quality of life for breast cancer patients receiving adjuvant chemotherapy. *Am J Nurs* 83:232–235, 1983

77. Knopf MT: Physical and psychological distress associated with adjuvant chemotherapy in women with breast cancer. *J Clin Oncol* 4:678–684, 1986

78. Ehlke G: Symptom distress in breast cancer patients receiving chemotherapy in the outpatient setting. *Oncol Nurs Forum* 15:343–346, 1988

79. Greene D, Nail LM, Fieler VK, et al: A comparison of patient-reported side effects among three chemotherapy regimens for breast cancer. *Cancer Pract* 2:57–62, 1994

80. Cassileth BR, Farber JM, Lusk EJ, et al: Chemotherapeutic toxicity: The relationship between patients' pretreatment expectations and post-treatment results. *Am J Clin Oncol* 8:419–425, 1985

81. Strauman JJ: Symptom distress in patients receiving phase I chemotherapy with Taxol. *Oncol Nurs Forum* 13(5):40–43, 1986

82. Piper BF, Rieger PT, Brophy L, et al: Recent advances in the management of biotherapy-related side effects: Fatigue. *Oncol Nurs Forum* 16(6):27–34, 1989 (suppl)

83. Quesada JR, Talpaz M, Rios A, et al: Clinical toxicity of interferons in cancer patients: A review. *J Clin Oncol* 4:234–243, 1986

84. Krown SE: Interferons and interferon inducers in cancer treatment. *Semin Oncol* 13:207–217, 1986

85. Tamura K, Makino S, Araki Y, et al: Recombinant interferon beta and gamma in the treatment of adult T-cell leukemia. *Cancer* 59:1059–1062, 1987

86. Grunberg SM, Kempf RA, Venturi CL, et al: Phase I study of recombinant beta interferon given by four-hour infusion. *Cancer Res* 47:1174–1178, 1987

87. Dean GE, Spears L, Ferrell BR, et al: Fatigue in patients with cancer receiving interferon alfa. *Cancer Pract* 3:164–172, 1995

88. Jassak PF, Stricklin LA: Interleukin-2: An overview. *Oncol Nurs Forum* 13:17–22, 1986

89. Chen MK: The epidemiology of self-perceived fatigue among adults. *Prev Med* 15:74–81, 1986

90. Silberfarb PM, Hauri PJ, Oxman TE, et al: Insomnia in cancer patients. *Soc Sci Med* 20:849–850, 1985

91. American Psychiatric Association: *Diagnostic and Statistical Manual of Mental Disorders* (ed 4). Washington, DC, American Psychiatric Association, 1994

92. Nail LM: Differentiating fatigue and depression in cancer patients, in Hogan C and Wickham R (eds): *Issues in Managing the Oncology Patient*. New York, Phillips Healthcare Communications, 1996, pp 36–41

93. Rutledge DN, Greene P, Mooney K, et al: Use of research-based practices by oncology staff nurses. *Oncol Nurs Forum* 23:1235–1244, 1996

94. Coluzzi PH, Grant M, Doroshow JH, et al: Survey of the provision of supportive care services at National Cancer Institute–designated cancer centers. *J Clin Oncol* 13:756–764, 1995

95. Fernsler J: A comparison of patient and nurse perceptions of patients' self-care deficits associated with cancer chemotherapy. *Cancer Nurs* 9:50–57, 1986

96. Morant R, Stiefel F, Radziwill A: Preliminary results of a study assessing asthenia and related phenomena in patients with advanced cancer. *J Supp Care* 1:101–107, 1993

97. Fernsler J: A comparison of patient and nurse perceptions of patients' self-care deficits associated with cancer chemotherapy. *Cancer Nurs* 9:50–57, 1986

98. Varricchio CG: Measurement issues in fatigue. *Qual of Life: A Nurs Challenge* 4:20–24, 1995

99. Breetvelt IS, Van Dam FSAM: Underreporting by cancer patients: The case of the response-shift. *Soc Sci Med* 32:981–987, 1991

100. Johnson JE, Nail LM, Lauver D, et al: Reducing the negative impact of radiation therapy on functional status. *Cancer* 61:46–51, 1988

101. Johnson JE: Coping with radiation therapy: Optimism and the effect of preparatory interventions. *Res Nurs Health* 19:3–12, 1996

102. Rhodes VA, Watson PM, Hanson BM: Patients' descriptions of the influence of tiredness and weakness on self-care activities. *Cancer Nurs* 11:186–194, 1988

103. MacVicar MG, Winningham ML: Promoting the functional capacity of cancer patients. *Cancer Bull* 38:235–239, 1986

104. Winningham ML, MacVicar MG: The effect of aerobic exercise on patient reports of nausea. *Oncol Nurs Forum* 15:447–450, 1988

105. Mock V, Burke MB, Sheehan P, et al: A nursing rehabilita-

tion program for women with breast cancer receiving adjuvant chemotherapy. *Oncol Nurs Forum* 15:447–450, 1994

106. Winningham ML, MacVicar MG, Burke CA: Exercise for cancer patients: Guidelines and precautions. *Physician and Sportsmedicine* 14(10):125–134, 1986

107. American College of Sports Medicine: *ACSM's Guidelines for Exercise Testing and Prescription* (ed 5). Baltimore, Williams and Wilkins, 1995

# Chapter 24

# Nutritional Disturbances

Ann T. Foltz, RN, DNS

## INTRODUCTION

Nutritional deficiencies in individuals with cancer occur along a continuum of nutritional adequacy ranging from optimal nutrition to malnutrition[1] (Figure 24-1). Malnutrition is a manifestation of both under- and overnutrition. In optimal nutrition nutrient intake provides adequate energy and protection from disease. When intake of nutrients is less than adequate or more than required, nutritional stores are reduced below or increased above normal. Nutritional lesions of varying magnitudes result, depending on the type and extent of the deficiency or excess.[2-4] The ability to prevent deficient or excessive intake and maintain optimal nutrition is influenced by the interaction among a number of external and internal factors (Table 24-1).

In the United States, recognition of the relationship between cancer and nutrition began in the 1930s[5] and became the subject of systematic research in the 1970s.[6-8] The research studies were of two main categories. One category, the relationship of nutrient intake to the development of cancer, has been discussed elsewhere in this text (see chapter 3). The second category, cancer-induced nutritional problems and their management, is considered in this chapter.

Because undernutrition is seen as the more common problem in both pediatric and adult cancer populations,[3,9-11] much of the chapter will deal with that form of malnutrition. However, the evidence that both under- and overnutrition negatively affect morbidity, survival, and quality of life[2,3,9-17] emphasizes the need for oncology nurses to evaluate the nutritional status of all individuals under their care.

## SCOPE OF THE PROBLEM

### Definitions

The two opposite end points of malnutrition in individuals with cancer are obesity and cancer cachexia. *Obesity* is defined as weighing more than 20% over ideal body weight. While obesity is most often thought of as increased

**TABLE 24-1**  Factors Influencing Individual Nutritional States

| External Factors | Internal Factors |
|---|---|
| Food supply | Inherited abnormalities, predispositions |
| Transportation | Individual demographics<br>  Age/development, education, income |
| Food enrichment programs |  |
| Food supplement programs | Family/cultural eating patterns<br>  Attitudes/beliefs about nutrition, "healthy foods," food as medicine, religious influences |
| Family/culture<br>  Cooking style, food choices, eating environment, family situation |  |
| Housing<br>  Living arrangement, cooking facilities | Psychological framework<br>  Mood, body image (importance of weight, history of bulimia, anorexia, obesity), concepts of food as reward, response to illness, stress |
| Geography<br>  Types of food available |  |
| Distribution of health, dental care | Disease/treatment<br>  Planned treatment, intactness of gastrointestinal tract, comorbid illness, presence of infection, fever, medications |

body fat, increased weight can be due to components other than fat. For example, bodybuilders often are overweight when compared with ideal body weight charts. Among individuals with cancer, increased weight may reflect tumor mass or fluid retention while masking loss of lean body mass. For example, children with abdominal masses are at risk for being considered at normal weight for height, despite loss of lean body mass.[11] Adults with ascites are at similar risk.

Terms used to describe nonmalignant nutritional deficiencies, and occasionally malignant starvation, are *kwashiorkor* (protein malnutrition with an adequate caloric intake) and *marasmus* (simple starvation with protein-calorie malnutrition). *Cachexia*, a general term meaning ill health, can occur in nonneoplastic diseases, such as sepsis, cardiac failure, and starvation. Although some in-

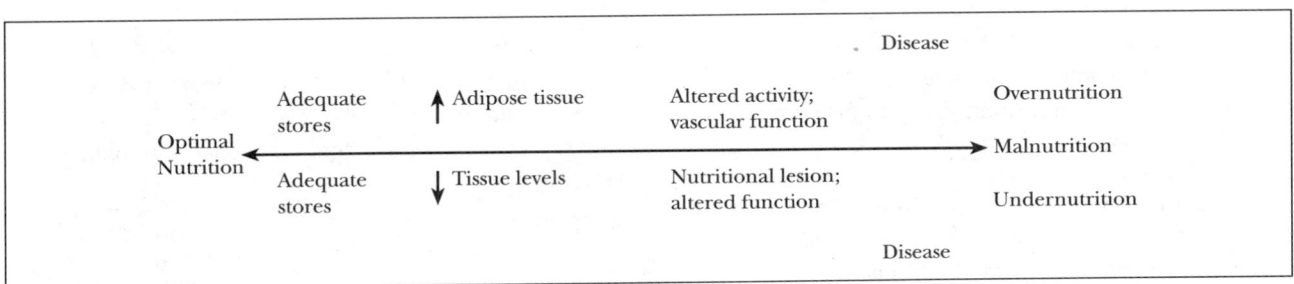

**FIGURE 24-1**  Nutritional continuum.

vestigators[12] suggest using the term *anorexia-cachexia cancer syndrome* (ACCS) to refer to the disorder in cancer populations, this distinction is rarely made. Cancer cachexia is characterized by anorexia, weight loss, skeletal muscle atrophy, and asthenia (loss of strength).[12,13,18] Other symptoms of cancer cachexia are early satiety, edema, anemia,[18] reduced attention span, organ dysfunction,[19] metabolic abnormalities,[19,20] and susceptibility to other diseases.[2,21]

Cancer-associated cachexia can be differentiated into primary and secondary types.[22] Primary cachexia results from tumor-produced metabolic abnormalities or host response. Secondary cachexia results from mechanical effects of the tumor or treatment. Primary cachexia resolves with successful cancer treatment. Secondary cachexia can be treated with a variety of approaches and is often more amenable to treatment than the primary form. *Repletion* describes the result of successful treatment of cachexia. Adequate nutritional status and normal body composition are reestablished.

Other terms are commonly used to describe conditions that result from cancer or its treatment. These include *hypogeusia* (decreased taste sensitivity), *dysgeusia* (perverted taste perception), *odynophagia* or *dysphagia* (painful swallowing), *hyposmia* (diminished ability to smell), and *inanition* (progressive deterioration with muscle wasting and energy loss).

## Incidence

Neither the incidence nor the prevalence of malnutrition is accurately documented in the cancer population.[23] The absence of these basic statistics arises from several factors. One problem is that nutritional status is not assessed when cancer is diagnosed, especially in the obese. Because assessment of nutritional status frequently is delayed, the opportunity to find minimal nutrient deficiencies in early stages is often lost. In addition, there is no consensus on what indicators of nutritional status should be used. Although weight is universally accepted as part of nutritional assessment, there is little agreement as to what other parameters must be included. Recommendations vary from a careful clinical exam[24] to the use of an array of laboratory tests.[11,25-28] There is also no agreement on how malnutrition should be graded. In clinical trials, study groups have developed toxicity scales for weight change and anorexia; however, these scales are better suited to determine side effect profiles rather than malnutrition levels.

Severe undernutrition was reported to be the single most common cause of death among individuals with cancer in the early twentieth century.[5] Incidence levels of significant protein-calorie malnutrition among hospitalized cancer patients ranged from 55% to 80% as late as the 1980s.[3,13,28,29] It is difficult to determine whether recent advances in cancer detection and nutritional interventions have decreased the rate of cancer-related malnutrition.

Overnutrition is most common in the breast cancer population. However, in a survey of the weight and nutritional status of 99 consecutive cancer patients admitted for treatment, Colletti et al found that 4% were underweight and 43% were overweight.[30] The incidence of obesity among women recently diagnosed with breast cancer ranges from 24% to 38%.[30,31] In addition, from 40% to 70% of women with breast cancer receiving adjuvant chemotherapy gain weight, and some become obese.[31-33] There is evidence that women who are obese may have poorer survival than women who are not.[16,34,35] Since breast cancer is a common cancer in women and adjuvant therapy is frequently employed, the incidence of this form of malnutrition is of major concern.

## Risk Factors

Identification of the risk factors for nutritional problems in cancer is based on assessment of the person's existing nutritional status and an appreciation of cancer malnutrition etiology. Both of these areas are complex and not yet completely understood.

Individuals who are nourished adequately at the time of diagnosis have fewer problems with both the cancer and its treatment. Adequate nourishment is the result of interaction among a number of external and internal factors.[4] Even with a satisfactory nutritional status, all individuals with cancer face two major risk factors for undernutrition: having the disease and being treated for it. The body's response to the tumor and the tumor-initiated metabolic changes are primary sources for undernutrition.[6-9,12,18,36-41] In addition, treatment imposes a burden by requiring repair of treatment-induced damage and by reducing the ability of the body to absorb nutrients.

The risk factors for overnutrition among cancer patients are even less well understood than the risks for undernutrition. There is some suggestion that treatment, especially chemotherapy, alters either the appetite-controlling hormones or the psychological restraints on nutritional intake.[31,33] There are external and internal cancer-related risk factors for under- and overnutrition in individuals with cancer.

### External and internal factors

External factors are the environmental and political climate surrounding an individual.[4] This climate encompasses the overall health of the country's economy, which has an impact on transportation, access to food shopping, availability of different nutrients, adequacy of housing and food preparation facilities, and programs that supplement food. These environmental factors influence the individual, who possesses cultural and attitudinal concepts about nutrition and eating behaviors. Other individual factors that influence a person's tendency to develop nutritional deficiencies include age, body image, past history of food fads or eating disorders, social support, educational level, alcohol or tobacco intake, and the presence of comorbid diseases. The effect of these factors on nutrition among individuals with cancer is an area of recent exploration.[42,43] Much more research in this area is needed before individuals at risk can be reliably identified.

## Cancer-related factors

The type of cancer affects the probability of malnutrition. Individuals with breast cancer or leukemia are at low risk, while those with cancers of the upper aerodigestive tract and gastrointestinal tract are at special risk for undernutrition.[10,44–46] These differences may arise from mechanical difficulties imposed by the location of tumors in the digestive area. Host responses to the cancer and the cancer itself cause changes in metabolism and energy needs.[36–41] Data about the variability in nutritional burden imposed by different cancer types come primarily from one study.[10] That study and other selected research findings are displayed in Table 24-2.[10,30,44–49]

## Treatment-related factors

All cancer therapies can cause nutritional deficiency. The magnitude of the treatment-related risk depends on the area of treatment, type of treatment, number of therapeutic modalities used, dosages of therapy used, and length of treatment.

*Surgery*  The effects of surgery on an individual's nutritional status depend on the extent of the procedure as well as the site of operation. Complications associated with surgery also are related to the nutritional status of the individual prior to the operation. Malnourished individuals have higher incidences of morbidity and mortality than do those who are adequately nourished.[9,10,50–52] This is of particular relevance to individuals with cancers of the aerodigestive or gastrointestinal tract. These patients may come to surgery with nutritional deficits because of cancer-related disruption of intake or absorption. In addition, they often are on restricted diets before surgery, with or without nonabsorbable antibiotics.

Surgery itself alters function. Major aerodigestive resections may produce hyposmia, dysgeusia, and reduced intake. Patients with abdominal and pelvic incisions will experience an ileus after surgery. Resections of large segments of the bowel can lead to malabsorption of fat, vitamin $B_{12}$ deficiency, anemia, and fluid-electrolyte imbalance.[46] These problems can become chronic, with reliance on tube feedings required by some patients.

For individuals with other cancer sites, nutritional problems resulting from surgical effects are often limited to the immediate perioperative period. Interruption of oral intake is usually minimal. The surgical procedure creates the same response to injury as does surgery for nonmalignant diseases. This stress is added to the psychological stress of dealing with a cancer diagnosis. Catecholamine, glucocorticoid, and glucagon outputs are increased, resulting in increased energy needs, loss of

**TABLE 24-2**  Percentages of Individuals with Weight Loss by Tumor Site

| Cancer Site | Percentage of Patients with Weight Loss > 5% | Comments |
|---|---|---|
| Breast | 14 | During clinical trials[11] |
|  | 5 | Stage I, II[11] |
| Colon | 28 | During clinical trials[11] |
| Head/neck | 37 | Preoperative[44] |
| Acute nonlymphocytic leukemia | 12 | Adults[11] |
| Acute lymphocytic leukemia | 0 | Children[45] |
| Non-Hodgkin's lymphoma | 18 | Favorable subtypes[11] |
| Non-Hodgkin's lymphoma | 28 | Unfavorable subtypes[11] |
| Small cell lung cancer | 34 | During clinical trials[11] |
| Non-small cell lung cancer | 36 | During clinical trials[11] |
| Non-small cell lung cancer | 30 | At diagnosis[47] |
| Pancreas | 54 | During clinical trials[11] |
| Prostate | 28 | During clinical trials[11] |
| Stomach | 67 | Measurable disease[11] |
| Stomach | 53 | Nonmeasurable disease[11] |
| Mixed | 4 | Sequential cancer patients[30] |
| Mixed | 37 | Advanced disease[48] |

nitrogen, and water and sodium retention. Surgery can increase energy requirements by 28 kcal/kg/day or 1.5 times normal dietary requirements.[53] For this reason, surgical candidates must be assessed carefully prior to treatment so that any nutritional deficiencies can be addressed proactively.

*Radiation*  Radiation therapy can alter nutritional status by both systemic and local effects. The percentage of individuals receiving radiation who experience nutritional side effects ranges from 32% to 83%.[54–56] The number varies with the area of the body being treated and the duration of treatment. Radiation alters function in the treatment area and poses particular problems for patients with aerodigestive or gastrointestinal cancers. Acute effects are transient and include anorexia, diarrhea, bleeding, nausea, vomiting, weight loss, mucositis, esophagitis, gastritis, xerostomia, and changes in taste.[55,56]

Local desquamation reactions can temporarily increase energy needs.

Indirect effects of radiation can also influence nutritional status. Fatigue and appetite changes commonly occur among individuals receiving radiation therapy.[55–57] These symptoms can alter the person's desire and ability to procure, prepare, and ingest food. Delayed effects of radiation, such as intestinal strictures, fibrosis or obstruction, fistulas, and pulmonary and hepatic fibrosis, cause mechanical problems in gut function and oxygenation. These in turn interrupt the person's ability to absorb and ingest food and may necessitate long-term management.[58]

***Chemotherapy*** Chemotherapy causes a number of direct and indirect effects on nutrition. Direct effects include alteration of the intestinal absorptive surface, excitation of the Chemoreceptor Trigger Zone and True Vomiting Center, and interference with specific metabolic and enzymatic reactions. The majority of chemotherapeutic agents, because of their damage to frequently reproducing cells, alter the length and surface area of intestinal villi. The ability of the gut to absorb nutrients and water can be negatively influenced. Diarrhea may also result.[46]

The direct excitation of the centers for nausea and vomiting occurs to varying degrees with the majority of chemotherapy drugs.[59–61] The variability is dependent on the drug, dosage, and individual response. In addition to these nonspecific changes in nutritional intake, some drugs cause specific nutritional lesions. For example, estrogen-containing compounds can cause hypercalcemia, and platinum-containing agents produce magnesium wasting. Both general and specific nutrient deficiencies can require treatment.

Indirect effects of chemotherapy on nutrition include interference with nutrient intake related to anorexia, fatigue, constipation, taste changes, and food aversions.[62–64] The number and magnitude of these various effects depend on the drugs chosen, their dosages, and the frequency and duration of drug administration. Although these side effects clearly alter nutrient intake, their clinical significance has not been adequately studied.

***Biotherapy/immunotherapy*** The effects of biotherapy on nutritional status are both direct and indirect. Biotherapy-induced fevers produce a direct increase in energy and fluid needs. Indirect influences, such as fatigue and flulike symptoms, can make food procurement and preparation difficult.[65,66] The magnitude and duration of these side effects are variable and may decrease over time. Their clinical effect on nutritional status is not well documented.

***Summary*** A variety of terms describe the effects of cancer and its treatment on nutrition. Nutritional problems vary in type and magnitude, depending on environmental and disease-related risk factors. Many individuals with cancer will develop nutritional problems. Late problems can arise from treatment-related damage to tissues involved in eating or digestion or from treatment failure.

However nutritional deficits do not always occur in individuals treated for cancer. Newer techniques in surgery and radiation produce less tissue destruction.[67,68] Improved medications for nausea and emesis control have reduced those side effects in radiation and chemotherapy.[59,60,69] Counseling can lessen the effect of changes such as food aversion; choice of a scapegoat food will spare pre-illness food preferences from treatment-induced aversions.[69] Moreover, the presence of symptoms like food aversion, taste change, and even nausea does not necessarily result in decreased nutrient intake.[31,69–71] The variability of the effect of treatment on nutrition implies the need to monitor all individuals receiving treatment and to recognize that some, but not all, will require some nutritional intervention.

## NORMAL NUTRITIONAL PHYSIOLOGY

Cioffi's model of nutrient intake[72] was modified for use in cancer (Figure 24-2). The model suggests that nutritional status is a function of an energy exchange system made up of four compartments: the *reference compartment, set point, controller,* and *body storage.*

The reference compartment is the repository of the standards governing nutrient intake. The standards have physiological (e.g., growth factors, insulin, glucose, thyroxine, taste transmitters), psychological (e.g., body image, self-esteem, meaning of food), and cultural (e.g., acceptable foods, eating patterns, social importance of food) determinants. These standards are monitored by the set point. The standards are maintained by the controller, largely through balancing energy intake and expenditure. Energy is obtained through the ingestion, digestion, and metabolism of macronutrients (carbohydrates, protein, lipids, and water) and micronutrients (minerals and vitamins). The controller requires an intact gastrointestinal tract and functioning taste and smell sensory mechanisms to work properly.

The result of the controller activity is the body storage, or body composition. The components of the body compartment include fat, protein (skeletal muscle, viscera,

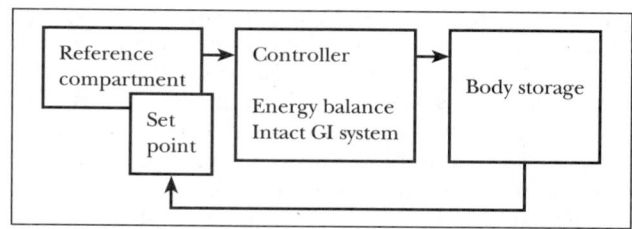

**FIGURE 24-2** Energy intake and expenditure model. (Modified from Cioffi L: General theory of critical periods and the development of obesity, in Smogyi J (ed): *Nutritional, Psychological and Social Aspects of Obesity,* Basel, Karger, 1968, p 20)

plasma, bone, cartilage, collagen), minerals and glycogen, and water (intracellular and extracellular).[9,73,74] The percentage of each of the components varies with genetics, gender, and age. The body storage provides feedback to the set point regarding its status via physiological, psychological, and cultural perceptions (serum glucose, perceived images, etc.). Under stress, feedback may be directed to the reference compartment, with the possibility that standard levels will be changed. The interplay among the compartments, in the setting of an adequate nutrient intake, results in sufficient body storage for energy needs and protection from illness.

## PATHOPHYSIOLOGY

Cancer, host response, and cancer treatment alter normal physiology. The alterations that affect nutritional status occur in the reference compartment, set point, and controller. These changes result in modified body storage, with the potential for development of obesity or cachexia.

### Cancer-Induced Changes in the Reference Compartment

#### Changes in appetite

There is some evidence that loss of appetite is related to circulating factors produced by the cancer and/or the host.[21,40,74–77] These factors may be produced peripherally but have a central effect on the reference standards for appetite. Cytokines have been proposed as one class of circulating anorectic agents. There is also support for an effect of serotonin and bombesin on appetite suppression, especially among individuals with carcinoid or lung cancers.[46] Animal studies support the importance of serotonin and ammonia as anorectics in cancer; studies in humans have been limited.[75] Increased circulating lipids and lactic acid caused by tumor metabolism can also decrease appetite.[46]

Loss of appetite also may be precipitated by cancer-induced psychological distress. Depression, anxiety, or situational factors (isolation, hospital food) may negatively influence food intake.[17,78] Cancer-induced pain and pain medication can also reduce intake.

Increased appetite has been reported among women with breast cancer. Grindel suggests that increased as well as decreased appetite may occur as a function of psychological distress.[33] Many women regularly limit their food intake. Following a breast cancer diagnosis, these women may lose their restraint, eat more, and gain weight. Additional study in this area is needed.

#### Changes in taste and smell

Altered taste and smell sensors, with loss of taste and olfactory cues, change the normal references that are part of appetite and intake.[79–81] Changes may be caused by direct tumor invasion; cancer-induced deficiencies in zinc, copper, nickel, vitamin A, and niacin;[82,83] or cancer-associated circulating factors.[75,76] Circulating factors are hypothesized sources of taste changes occurring early in the disease process.

Physiological increases in the recognition thresholds for sweet, sour, and salt and decreases in the recognition levels for bitter are common.[79–81] These threshold changes can lead to meat and other food aversions. Psychological factors may also contribute to food aversions. The hedonistic component of eating can be negatively influenced by alterations in taste or smell, leading to a reduced interest in eating and loss of appetite.[17,78]

#### Changes in electrolyte balance

Alterations in micronutrient availability occur in paraneoplastic syndromes. Cancer can cause hyper- and hypocalcemia, hyponatremia, and hypo- and hyperphosphatemia.[46,82,83] At least some of these abnormalities are caused by tumor-produced hormones and can be life-threatening. They also cause altered mental status, with associated problems in intake and adherence to treatment regimens.

### Cancer-Induced Changes in the Controller

#### Changes in energy expenditure

Patients with cancer can have increased energy needs initiated by cancer-induced sepsis, fistulas, or lesions. These energy demands can produce malnutrition in some patients, but they are not responsible for cachexia. The theory that cancer cachexia results from a tumor-driven increase in energy consumption has been suggested for more than 50 years.[84] Despite this long history, the studies of energy production have been inconsistent, with reports of increased, normal, and reduced resting energy expenditure.[84–88] Knox et al found all three energy states present in one study sample.[86]

Part of the inconsistency in findings may be due to differences in the definition of energy expenditure, difficulties in measurement, and the use of diverse patient populations with different diseases at different stages. Another factor may be the complexity of the mechanisms involved in energy use and distribution. Falconer et al reported on increased resting energy expenditure (REE) among patients with pancreatic cancer compared with controls.[87] In this study the subset of individuals with elevated REE also had increased levels of macrophage-produced tumor necrosis factor (TNF) and interleukin-6 (IL-6). However, total serum levels of TNF and IL-6 were not elevated. This suggests either that the macrophage reaction is localized in scope or that cytokine production does not explain the total picture regarding energy expenditure.

Other researchers have suggested that tumor-related

use of futile cycles for energy lead to increased metabolic rates. The Cori cycle has been the most frequently studied of these methods.[7,84,88,89] This process, in which tissue glucose is metabolized to lactate and then resynthesized as glucose in the liver, is energy-consuming. Unlike the normal situation in which the Cori cycle is utilized in response to specific needs, tumors may preferentially utilize this pathway, be forced to use this method because of poor oxygenation, or induce peripheral cells to increase Cori cycle activity for lactate production. This extremely wasteful process may cost as much as 300 kcal/day or 40% of the carbohydrates ingested.[38,87–90] However, investigators of Cori cycle activity note that Cori cycle abnormalities are not universal.[46,88,90]

Nixon et al[85] take another view and suggest that the problem is not one of increased expenditure but rather the failure to decrease expenditure in the face of an insufficient intake. This lack of accommodation results in an energy imbalance where energy expenditure exceeds energy intake. This situation is similar to other abnormal responses in which the individual with cancer responds to a decreased intake differently than an individual who has another disease. In any case, increased energy expenditure may be a problem for a subset of cancer patients, but it is not a factor in explaining cancer cachexia in all cancers.

## Changes in nutrient metabolism

Cancer is associated with abnormalities in carbohydrate, protein, and lipid metabolism. Changes in carbohydrate metabolism include increased Cori cycle activity, altered peripheral utilization of glucose, hepatic gluconeogenesis, increased glucose turnover, and glucose intolerance.[38,88–91] Cori cycle activity has been discussed. Glicksman and Rawson reported that over one-third of the cancer patients they studied demonstrated a diabetic glucose tolerance curve.[91] The abnormal curve was compatible with insulin resistance, similar to type II diabetes. Like diabetics, the individual with cancer has delayed glucose clearance, reduced glucose uptake in skeletal muscles, and an inability to produce glycogen in muscle. Unlike diabetics, individuals with cancer have normal plasma insulin levels. It is not known whether cancer patients also have normal insulin secretion. The origin of the glucose intolerance is unknown, but researchers have suggested that some cases may be the result of cytokines, produced by the host in response to the tumor.[76,91–93] Cheblowski and Heber point out that other influences, such as bedrest and sepsis, may also influence glucose metabolism.[92]

Increased hepatic glucose production has been reported in both undernourished and normal-weight cancer patients.[38,76,77] The elevated glucose level occurs as one of the features that differentiates cancer starvation/cachexia from normal starvation responses. In normal starvation, hepatic glucose production falls; this does not occur in cancer cachexia. The lack of a normal response

to a decreased intake may be related to the reliance of cancer on glucose and/or be the product of a cancer-associated abnormal growth hormone.[76,77]

Individuals with cancer may develop altered protein metabolism. Some studies indicate that the tumor preferentially takes up nitrogen-containing materials.[46,94] Glutamine, an abundant amino acid required for DNA synthesis, may be one of the substances taken up by cancers to the detriment of the host. In addition to the shunting of needed proteins to the cancer, there can be increased muscle breakdown and hepatic protein activity.[12,41,93–95] Despite the increased hepatic activity, protein synthesis does not match protein catabolism. The net result is increased whole-body protein turnover. Studies have reported whole-body protein turnover rates of 50% and 70% in patients with progressive disease and weight loss.[94,96] However, not all researchers find increased protein turnover, especially among cancer patients who are maintaining their weight.[96]

Abnormal lipid metabolism noted in cancer includes increased lipid mobilization and turnover, elevated triglyceride levels, decreased lipogenesis, altered glycerol transport, and decreased lipoprotein lipase activity.[12,46] To some degree the alteration in fat metabolism may be related to insulin resistance, with preferential oxidation of fat rather than carbohydrates.[97,98] In addition, lipolytic factors are produced by tumors in animal models and may play a part in human cancers as well.[99]

## Changes in the gastrointestinal tract

Controller function is heavily dependent on an intact gastrointestinal system. Cancer can produce direct negative effects on the digestive system. Cancers of the aerodigestive structures can cause primary reduction in food and nutrient intake associated with the following:

difficulty chewing or swallowing

partial or complete obstruction

dysmotility

inactivation of bile salts, pancreatic enzymes

blind loop syndrome

fistulas

interference associated with pain (ulceration, nerve compression, etc.)

bowel wall, mesenteric infiltration

protein-losing enteropathy

The type and magnitude of the nutritional deficit depend on the tumor site and size. Nongastrointestinal cancers can cause alterations in nutritional status by interfering with food intake or increasing energy demand. Examples of this type of direct and indirect interference with intake include pain, dyspnea, lymphatic blockages of mesentery or peritoneum, paraneoplastic syndromes that alter fluid or mineral balance, and altered cognitive function. Ulcerated lesions, both external and internal, are examples of cancer-associated increases in nutrient need.

### Changes in body storage

The degree of body storage alteration varies along the continuum of malnutrition. With small changes in nutrient intake or absorption, there may be no obvious change in body composition. In patients with weight gain, the compartment in which the change occurred should be determined. The most commonly affected compartments are the extracellular fluid and adipose tissue compartments. Unfortunately, lean body mass is less commonly improved.[100] The most striking change in body composition is seen in cachexia. The total body fat and skeletal muscle components can drop as much as 85% and 75%, respectively.[73] Reduction in intracellular water and mineral supplies also occurs, although not to the same degree. Feedback signals from the body storage compartment are deranged, reflecting the effect of cytokine activity and metabolic dysfunction. The altered feedback perpetuates the nutritional deficiencies.

## Treatment-Induced Changes in the Reference Compartment

### Changes in appetite

Just as cancer causes changes in appetite, so can therapy (See Table 24-3). Depressed appetite can be caused by some biotherapeutic agents, notably tumor necrosis factor.[65] Appetite loss can follow stimulation of the Chemoreceptor Trigger Zone and True Vomiting Center. Psychological responses to having and being treated for cancer can alter mood and change appetite. Medications prescribed for treatment also affect mood and appetite. Some of the drugs produce increased, rather than decreased, appetite or nutrient intake. Corticosteroids, prescribed in both pediatric and adult populations, can increase appetite. Foltz suggests that chemotherapy reduces production of estradiol, a regulatory hormone for appetite, leading to increased appetite.[31]

Chemotherapy and radiation produce indirect effects on appetite through the induction of nausea, vomiting, and food aversions.[59–61] Anticipatory nausea and vomiting become a conditioned response to chemotherapy. The clinical significance of these changes is unclear, since some patients alter choice and eating patterns but not their total intake when faced with these symptoms.[31,70,71]

Taste changes can follow head and neck surgery, radiation, and chemotherapy. These changes may be temporary and are sometimes related to zinc deficiency. However, radiation and surgical alterations in gustatory and olfactory structures can be permanent. This may result in an alteration of the normal references for food acceptability or a general reduction in the intake over time.

## Treatment-Induced Changes in the Controller

### Changes in energy expenditure

Treatment can affect energy needs both directly and indirectly. Some biotherapeutic agents elicit shaking chills and fever, which increase energy demands. Increased energy needs from fever and infection can also accompany bone marrow suppression. Moreover, antifungal agents administered to immunocompromised patients cause fever and chill responses. Nutritional needs increase as the body responds to repair damage induced by surgery, radiation, or chemotherapy. Energy requirements are related to the type and magnitude of the treatment.

### Changes in the gastrointestinal tract

Surgical resection removes or bypasses areas of the aerodigestive or gastrointestinal tract. Chemotherapy and

**TABLE 24-3**  Treatment-Associated Changes in the Gastrointestinal Tract

| Body Area | Surgical Changes | Radiation Changes | Chemotherapy Changes |
|---|---|---|---|
| Oropharynx | Dysphagia, inability to swallow | Xerostomia, dysphagia, taste loss, caries | Mucositis, glossitis, taste loss, pharyngitis |
| Esophagus | Gastric stasis, early satiety, hydrochlorhydria, regurgitation, diarrhea, steatorrhea | Esophagitis, fibrosis, stricture | Esophagitis |
| Stomach | Dumping syndrome, malabsorption, loss of intrinsic factor, early satiety, achlorhydria, hypoglycemia | Nausea, vomiting | Nausea, vomiting |
| Intestines | Decreased absorption; vitamin A, $B_{12}$, D, E deficit; dehydration; metabolic acidosis; calorie deficit; bile salt deficit; renal stones; calcium and magnesium deficit | Decreased absorption, diarrhea, stenosis, fibrosis, obstruction | Decreased absorption, diarrhea, constipation |

radiation cause direct injury to the intestinal villi, reducing the absorptive surface. These are major threats to the proper absorption of both macro- and micronutrients. Side effects of treatment include anorexia, nausea, vomiting, lactose intolerance, diarrhea, and constipation, all of which can create obstacles to normal gut function and intake. In addition, chronic changes can occur. Surgery, radiation, and bone marrow transplantation can produce significant alterations in gut function. Graft-versus-host disease, a complication of bone marrow transplantation, and radiation enteritis can lead to long-term patient dependence on parenteral nutritional support.

## CLINICAL MANIFESTATIONS

The most common clinical manifestation identified with cancer is cancer cachexia, which is characterized by skeletal muscle wasting, weight loss, and reduced function. The patient may complain of loss of appetite, inability to eat, or early satiety. However, because the nutrient deficiencies occur along a continuum, nutritional deficits can exist without these cardinal or extreme signs and symptoms. This is especially true of obese individuals, in whom weight loss can be overlooked. Fluid changes, such as edema or effusions, can mask protein and fat loss. The fact that nutritional disturbances can be subtle and are frequently nonspecific makes the need for assessment that much more important.

## ASSESSMENT AND GRADING

Nutritional assessment consists of four elements: anthropometrics, laboratory findings, clinical examination, and dietary evaluation. Recently there have been efforts to increase the accuracy of body composition determination and to add functional status evaluation.[27,101,102] In addition, a number of formulas and grading systems have been identified for quantifying nutritional status and risk.

### Anthropometrics

*Anthropometrics,* the measurement of the weight, size, and proportions of the body, commonly includes height, weight, and skinfold thickness. Weight is perhaps the single most important measure of nutritional status for the clinician, although its importance is often underemphasized. Standard weight measurement is inexpensive, quick, and practical. Serial measurements of weight can be used to identify trends in nutritional status. Underwater weighing has also been used in an effort to measure fat composition in relation to lean body mass.[27] The technique has been used with stable cancer patients but is primarily used in research studies.

Weight, in combination with height, is an indirect measure of body composition. It can be used to screen for both under- and overnutrition. The Metropolitan Life Insurance Company Height-Weight Table is a frequently used measure of nutritional status. The clinician must estimate whether the person has a small, medium, or large frame to establish the reference numbers. Estimation of frame size is accomplished by using a table derived from height and wrist circumference or by measuring elbow breadth. Anecdotal evidence suggests that many clinicians use clinical impression to estimate frame size, potentially leading to inaccurate interpretations. Also, the tables themselves are based largely on data from white, insured persons aged 25 to 59; the applicability to nonwhite, ill, or older populations is unclear.[101] Studies indicate that the Metropolitan tables are equivalent to nonwhite U.S. populations, but there have been few comparisons with African-American women and the majority of Asian Pacific populations.[103] Moreover, there continues to be considerable controversy over the range of age-related weight increases among older persons.[104,105] Thus, the Metropolitan tables should be used in conjunction with other measures to determine nutritional status. Frisancho has developed standards for height and weight for older adults, but these standards have not been used in the cancer population.[106]

Weight and height can also be used to calculate the body mass index (BMI). The BMI is considered a more accurate estimation of total body fat than the Metropolitan weight tables. The BMI has limited utility in individuals with increased lean muscle mass or with large frames. It is also more relevant for determining obesity than for assessing undernutrition. The formula for BMI calculation is as follows:

$$\text{Weight in kilograms/height in meters squared}$$

The result of the BMI calculation can then be plotted on a nomogram. It has been suggested that the acceptable BMI should increase with age to reflect the normal aging process, but standards have not been universally accepted.

Another important function of the anthropometric measures of height and weight is their use in calculating an individual's caloric needs. Resting metabolic rate nomograms have been developed for this purpose. Formulas are also commonly used. Caloric prescriptions for individuals with cancer are frequently based on the Harris-Benedict equation:

$$\text{For women: } = 655 + (9.6 \times \text{weight in kg}) + (1.7 \times \text{height in cm}) - (4.7 \times \text{age in years})$$

$$\text{For men: } 66 + (1.37 \times \text{weight in kg}) + (5 \times \text{height in cm}) - (6.8 \times \text{age in years})$$

or the ideal weight formula (Table 24-4). These equations indicate the number of calories expended while the indi-

**TABLE 24-4**  Ideal Body Weight Formula

|  | Ideal Weight Calculation | To Determine Caloric Need |
|---|---|---|
| Women | Add 100 pounds for first 60 inches, 5 pounds for each inch over 60 inches divided by 2.2 to obtain ideal weight in kilograms | Multiply ideal kilogram calculation × 24 hours × 0.9 calorie/kg = resting needs |
| Men | Add 106 pounds for first 60 inches, add 6 pounds for each inch over 60 inches, divide by 2.2 to calculate kilograms | Multiply ideal kilogram calculation × 24 × 1.0 calorie/kg = resting needs |
| Children | For children under the age of 12, energy needs are often set at 1000 calories plus 100 calories for each year of age. | |

vidual is at rest, or the *resting energy expenditure* (REE). This number is corrected for the level of required energy. The level varies according to activity, treatment, and morbid condition (Table 24-5). However, there have been no estimates of energy required by individuals with cancer; a correction factor is applied at the assessor's discretion. Souba suggests a correction of 1.10–1.45, depending on the extent of disease and treatment plans.[107]

Despite the overall importance, practicality, and clinical relevance of weight and height measures in nutritional assessment, the reliability of both measures is questionable. Measurement scales must be calibrated regularly. Self-calibrating scales also should be tested periodically. Staff members obtaining the data should follow a standard method of obtaining weight and height measures. (Table 24-6). Using patient-reported weight and height is often inaccurate and should be discouraged.[108] Training in accurate measurement and monitoring for quality assurance could improve the assessment process.

Anthropometric measures of skinfold thickness and various body part circumferences assess fat and muscle compartments. The basis for using skinfold measures lies in the fact that almost half of the body fat is located in subcutaneous tissue and is accessible for relatively straightforward measurement. The assumption is that total fat is fairly constant. However, fat deposition and relative percentage of fat do change over time, even among healthy individuals.

The necessity of routine use of skinfold measures is a subject of debate.[109] There are seven commonly identified skinfold measures. Thirty minutes or more may be neces-

**TABLE 24-6**  Measurement of Height and Weight

| Height | Weight |
|---|---|
| 1. Measure without shoes<br>2. Feet should be together, heel against the wall or measuring rod<br>3. Head should be erect, top of ear and corner of eye should be parallel to ground<br>4. The horizontal bar should be lowered to rest flat on the head<br>5. Measurement should be read to the nearest ¼ inch or 0.5 cm | 1. Measure in light clothing, without shoes<br>2. Measurement should be read to nearest 0.25 lb or 0.1 kg for children and 0.5 lb or 0.2 kg for adults |

sary to complete measurement of all seven sites. However, the accuracy of body composition estimates is lower when fewer than five sites are used. Nonetheless, the triceps skinfold (TSF) is often used alone or in combination with the midarm circumference (MAC).[25,27,101] The MAC and TSF determine the midarm muscle circumference (MAMC), a measure of lean arm mass and indicator of lean body mass. The calculation is as follows:

$$\text{Mid-arm muscle circumference (MAMC)}$$
$$= \text{arm circumference in cm} - [0.314$$
$$\times \text{ triceps skinfold in mm}]$$

This number can be compared with tables of standards. There are standards for older adults, making this one of a few measures applicable to adults of all ages. Measuring skinfold thickness requires adequate training, monitoring for interrater reliability, and consistency of measuring. The calipers used normally are insufficient for very large people. Use of skinfold thickness in people with a significant shift of fluid to the intracellular compartment will be misleading. These threats to accuracy must be considered when using skinfold measures for nutritional assessment.

A number of other techniques can be used to measure body composition. Ultrasound, computed tomography,

**TABLE 24-5**  Correction Factors for Caloric Needs Above REE

| Patient Situation | Energy Correction Factor |
|---|---|
| On bedrest | 1.2 |
| Out of bed | 1.3 |
| Fever | 1.0 + 0.13 per °C |
| Surgery | 1.0–1.2 |
| Sepsis | 1.4–1.8 |

infrared interactance, magnetic resonance imaging, dual-photon and dual-energy radiographic absorptiometry, neutron activation, total body potassium, total body water, and bioelectrical impedance have been used. These techniques vary in their invasiveness, availability, and expense. At this point the primary use of these types of measures is in nutritional research, not routine assessment.[27,101]

## Laboratory Tests

Table 24-7 lists the laboratory tests commonly used to evaluate nutritional status.[4,26,101] It is important to remember when using these tests in the nutritional assessment of individuals with cancer that the tests are not specific to malnutrition. There are a number of disease- and treatment-related variables that can cause abnormal values consistent with malnutrition. Examples include low blood count, decreased lymphocyte count, and delayed hypersensitivity testing, all of which can be affected by both cancer and cancer treatment. In addition, the tests are often not sensitive to nutritional deficiencies. For example, severe nutritional deficiencies may exist before albumin levels fall. Another consideration is cost. Some of the more sensitive measures, like prealbumin or retinol binding protein, are expensive and inadequately covered by insurance.[101]

## Physical Examination

Common physical changes caused by malnutrition are listed in Table 24-8. Individuals with cancer who are malnourished may display some of these manifestations. However, as Table 24-8 also indicates, cancer or its treatment can cause these same abnormalities, limiting the use of physical examination in distinguishing between the effects of cancer and those of nutritional deficiency. The fact that physical changes such as glossitis, muscle wasting, or diarrhea exist in many cancer patients secondary to their disease or treatment does not minimize their usefulness as indicators of problems in energy intake, absorption, or need. The nutritional problems resulting from cancer and its treatment differ from those caused by insufficient intake of nutrients. Management of symp-

**TABLE 24-7**   Laboratory Tests Used in Nutritional Assessment

| Test | Comments |
|---|---|
| Complete blood count: | Identifies macrocytosis (sign of possible folate or vitamin $B_{12}$ deficiency) and anemia (may identify iron-deficiency anemia). |
| Tests of immune function: | |
| Total lymphocyte count (TLC) | A quick but nonspecific measure of immune function; an indirect indicator of nutritional status. Levels below 1200 ccm suggest nutritional deficiency. Low TLC has been associated with increased morbidity and mortality in cancer patients. |
| Delayed hypersensitivity | This testing is based on the relationship between malnutrition and immune deficiency. The recall response to subcutaneous injections of antigens (usually *Candida*, tuberculin, mumps, streptokinase-streptodornase) is used as the measure. However, the test lacks both sensitivity and specificity for malnutrition. Nonetheless, anergic responses are related to increased infection and mortality rates and may be used to identify severely malnourished individuals in need of nutritional intervention prior to cancer treatment. |
| Mitogen function | T-cell response has been studied by incubating lymphocytes with mitogens like phytohemagglutinin. The magnitude of response has been used in research settings as a monitor of nutritional status. |
| Iron studies: | |
| Transferrin: | Can be used to identify iron deficiencies, which can be dietary or related to gastrointestinal blood loss. Transferrin can also be used as an indicator of protein status. (See section on protein studies for further info.) |
| Cholesterol: | Cholesterol below 160 mg/10dL indicates poor nutrition. Low cholesterol has been associated with increased mortality in nursing home residents. |
| Protein studies: | These measures indicate the state of protein catabolism, anabolism, and distribution. They are altered by a number of states and deficiencies. |
| Albumin | Albumin is a useful indicator because it is routinely obtained as part of a normal workup. It is not sensitive to minimal protein deficits and may be both insensitive and nonspecific to malnutrition in situations where major trauma exists. Levels are also affected by heart failure, sepsis, renal failure, bedrest, hepatic insufficiency, fluid problems, and surgery. When albumin levels are low, there is risk of increased surgical morbidity and mortality with longer hospital and intensive care stays. Because the half-life of albumin is 18–20 days, it is not useful for detecting rapid changes in nutritional status. |

*(continued)*

**TABLE 24-7** Laboratory Tests Used in Nutritional Assessment (continued)

| Test | Comments |
|------|----------|
| Transferrin | Transferrin is a major transport protein for iron and iron binding and may represent visceral protein stores to a greater extent than total protein or albumin measures. Transferrin has a half-life of 8–10 days and may be useful in monitoring changes in nutritional status. Levels of transferrin are increased with iron deficiency and decreased with age, fluid overload, and antibiotic therapy. Total iron-binding capacity can be used to derive transferrin levels when transferrin testing is not available. |
| Prealbumin | Prealbumin is a transport protein for thyroxine and retinol-binding protein with a serum half-life of 2–3 days. Prealbumin has potential advantages in monitoring changes in nutritional status. It has been used to measure the effectiveness of parenteral nutrition. |
| Retinol-binding protein | This small protein transports retinol. It has a shorter half-life than prealbumin and may be more sensitive to changes in nutritional status than other protein measures. It is increased in renal and hepatic disease and decreased in zinc and vitamin A deficiency and stress response. |
| Fibronectin | This glycoprotein is basic to many cellular structures and functions in immune responses. Fibronectin levels have increased in 1–4 days of nutritional intervention. However, the usefulness of fibronectin in assessment is not universally accepted. The test is also expensive and not routinely available. |
| Somatomedin (IGF-1) | Somatomedin C is an insulin-like growth factor that appears to be more specific and sensitive to changes in nutrient intake than albumin and prealbumin. The cost of the test and its limited availability restrict its use. |
| 3-Methyl-histidine | This component of myosin and actin is assessed by its presence in urine. It is a measure of skeletal mass. The test is limited by its expense and availability. Levels are influenced by age, stress, and recent diet. |
| Creatinine-height index (CHI) | Urinary creatinine excretion is a measure of muscle metabolism and lean body mass (protein stores). Holding weight constant, actual creatinine excretion is compared with ideal creatinine excretion rate. The CHI is more sensitive to malnutrition than the height-weight standards, especially among individuals with edema or obesity. However, its measurement requires stable dietary intake and normal renal function. |
| Nitrogen balance | Measures of nitrogen balance can be obtained by collecting 24-hour protein intake history and urinary urea nitrogen and using the following formula: Nitrogen balance = nitrogen intake − nitrogen output, where: Nitrogen intake = protein intake in g/24 hr (6.25 g protein/g of nitrogen) Nitrogen output = urinary urea nitrogen + 4 g nitrogen Nitrogen balance = (protein intake in g/6.25) − (24-hr urine urea nitrogen (g) + 4) |
| Electrolytes | Electrolyte levels are both insensitive and nonspecific assessments for malnutrition. However, decreases in serum sodium and calcium levels can reflect paraneoplastic syndromes, which have implications for nutritional care (e.g., fluid restriction and increased fluid intake, respectively). Other abnormalities, such as hypokalemia and hypomagnesemia, are deficiencies related to medications, while hypernatremia and elevated blood urea nitrogen or creatinine can be secondary to chemotherapy-related dehydration. |

toms of nutritional disturbances in cancer can include medication, oral care, and specific nutritional counseling as opposed to the simple dietary supplementation with vitamins and protein-rich foods used to treat symptoms caused by inadequate intake of nutrients.

Physical examination may identify other cancer-related changes that influence the intake or expenditure of energy. Examples include fever, fistulas, and external lesions. The importance of physical examination was reinforced by Baker et al,[24] who found that clinical identification of jaundice, cheilosis, glossitis, loss of subcutaneous fat, muscle wasting, and edema correlated well with anthropometric, body composition, and biochemical estimates of nutritional status. They suggested that careful clinical examination was as sensitive as more expensive and labor-intensive assessment methods.

## Dietary Information

### Diet history

Dietary intake information is used to identify potential nutritional excesses and deficits. In a full diet history, information that reflects both diet and general health is included. General questions alert the nurse to the need for the more in-depth study of dietary intakes. Dietary information is obtained using a number of approaches: 24-hour recall surveys, food frequency measures, diet diaries, calorie counts, or monthly purchase records. The last method is rarely used in clinical practice. Any of the types of food intake recordings provide information about energy, nutrient, vitamin, and mineral intakes. Obtaining this information requires variable amounts of time for data entry

**TABLE 24-8**  Physical Examination for Nutritional Deficiencies

| Organ/System | Signs of Deficiency | Nutritional Deficiency | Cancer-Related Source |
|---|---|---|---|
| Hair | Easy pluckability, dry, thin, lightening in color | Protein-calorie malnutrition | Chemotherapy- or cranial radiation–induced alopecia |
| Face | Nasolabial dyssebacea, moon face | Riboflavin, protein deficit | Cortisone treatment |
| Eyes | Pale conjunctiva | Iron deficit | Anemia secondary to bone marrow involvement, chemotherapy, radiation of active bone marrow |
| Lips | Fissures, cheilosis | B-complex deficits | Antimetabolite chemotherapy, retinoic acid |
| Gums | Spongy, bleeding | Vitamin C deficit | Chemotherapy |
| Tongue | Scarlet, glossitis | B-complex deficits | Chemotherapy, local radiation |
| Teeth | Caries, missing teeth | Fluoride deficit | Radiation effect |
| Skin | Dry, with desquamation, petechiae, pellagra | Vitamin A deficit Vitamin C Nicotinic acid | Radiation Chemotherapy, DIC |
| Nails | Spoon-shape, discoloration, ridged | Iron deficit | Doxorubicin |
| Musculoskeletal | Muscle wasting Rib, epiphyseal abnormalities | Protein-calorie deficit Vitamin D | Cachexia Radiation in children |
| Gastrointestinal system | Hepatomegaly Diarrhea | Protein-calorie deficit Thiamine deficit | Liver metastasis Chemotherapy, pelvic radiation |
| Cardiac system | Heart enlargement | Thiamine | Anthracyclines |
| Nervous system | Confusion, sensory loss, weakness | Thiamine, nicotinic acid deficit | Hypercalcemia, hyponatremia, brain metastasis, radiation, chemotherapy |

into nutrient analysis programs. The need for this depth of assessment will depend upon the setting.

Figure 24-3 lists items commonly included in a complete diet history. Questions about weight are extremely important. The usefulness of weight-height tables in establishing adequate nutrition, overnutrition, or undernutrition has already been discussed. Questions about changes in weight over time provide a basis for estimating the magnitude and rapidity of any changes. Weight change is calculated as follows:

$$\text{Percent usual weight} = \frac{\text{actual weight}}{\text{usual weight}} \times 100$$

$$\text{Percent weight change} = \frac{\text{usual weight} - \text{actual weight}}{\text{usual weight}} \times 100$$

Weight loss of 5% compared with usual weight is considered a sign of undernutrition. Greater than 25% percent loss reflects severe undernutrition.[11,25] These types of data are used in clinical trials to code toxicity during treatment. It is important to assess the length of time over which the weight loss occurred. A percent weight change of 2% in one week is much more ominous than the same degree of weight change over six months.[25]

A full diet history includes sociodemographic items, food preferences, religious restrictions, food allergies, past history of dieting, current drug therapy, activity, and measures of current intakes. The complete history can be extremely useful but is time-consuming.

---

Have you noticed any changes in your weight in the past two weeks?

How much do you think you weighed one month ago? Six months ago?

How much do you think you weighed this time last year? What would you say your usual weight is?

Are you having any problems eating?

Do you have: loss of appetite, nausea, vomiting, diarrhea, constipation, mouth sores, dry mouth, poorly fitting dentures, pain when eating or swallowing, other pain, taste change, fatigue, difficulty swallowing, indigestion, feeling full quickly, cramping, bloating?

Do you use tobacco?

How much alcohol do you drink a day?

Are there any food allergies?_____

Can you digest milk? _____ yes _____ no _____ don't know

Are you on a special diet? _____ yes _____ no

If yes, specify: _____

**FIGURE 24-3**  Common general health-related questions in diet history.

### 24-Hour recall

In a 24-hour dietary recall, the patient is asked to list all foods and beverages ingested, the time of consumption, preparation method, and an estimate of the amount consumed in the previous 24 hours. This method is useful since the patient can usually remember what was ingested and the interview time required is relatively short. The amount of detail depends on the skill of the interviewer. The reliability of the recall is also somewhat dependent on the interviewer's skill, as well as the patient's memory, accuracy of portion estimate, and willingness to list all foods and beverages ingested. However, the previous 24-hour intake may not be representative of usual intakes, especially among individuals who may be learning about or receiving care for cancer.

### Food frequency

A food frequency record usually consists of a checklist of common foods, a portion estimate, and a frequency estimate. This method provides a broader picture of consumption than does the 24-hour recall and can be completed relatively rapidly. It also can be designed to identify patterns of change, such as a trend to high fat or low calcium consumption. The accuracy of the data depends on the memory and truthfulness of the patient.

### Diet diary

A diet diary is a list of all foods and beverages consumed for from three to seven days. The patient typically is asked to list time, food or beverage, and a portion estimate. Some diaries also include information about the setting or emotional state of the person during the meal. These diaries can be extremely useful indicators of intake patterns. However, they rely on the honesty of the person reporting and continued cooperation during the period of collection. A variation of this method is the three-to-seven-day weighed intake record, which involves the reporting and actual weighing of foods. The technique can be burdensome to patients and may negatively influence adherence.

### Calorie count

A calorie count is a useful method of estimating intakes while the patient is hospitalized. This method has the advantage of providing reliable information about the weight and nutrient values of the food served. However, the accuracy of the count is dependent on the person observing and recording the intake. Often this is relegated to ancillary personnel or sometimes the patient, neither of whom may be cognizant of the importance of the information. In addition, the food choices and preparation may not reflect the patient's intake outside the hospital.

## Functional Assessment

Klidjian et al reported on the usefulness of including functional assessment as part of nutritional assessment.[110] Skeletal muscle strength is a sensitive indicator of both positive and negative changes in food intake. Muscle strength measures can be used to indicate both the degree of nutritional deficit and the effectiveness of nutritional intervention. Grip strength measurement is an uncomplicated way to measure function and has been used in a cancer population.[111]

## Nutritional Screening Methods

The need to assess nutritional status quickly and efficiently has led to the development of a number of screening assessment methods. The Nutritional Screening Initiative has developed a screening history.[112] This ten-question survey (Figure 24-4) provides a numerical score that is converted into categories of zero, moderate, and

*Read the following statements. Circle the number in the "yes" column for those that apply to you or someone you know. For each "yes" answer, score the number in the box. Total your nutritional score.*

| Statement | Yes |
|---|---|
| I have an illness or condition that made me change the kind and/or amount of food I eat. | 2 |
| I eat fewer than 2 meals a day. | 3 |
| I eat fewer fruits or vegetables or milk products. | 2 |
| I have 3 or more drinks of beer, liquor, or wine almost every day. | 2 |
| I have tooth or mouth problems that make it hard for me to eat. | 2 |
| I don't always have enough money to buy the food I need. | 4 |
| I eat alone most of the time. | 1 |
| I take 3 or more different prescribed or over-the-counter drugs a day. | 2 |
| Without wanting to, I have lost or gained 10 pounds in the last 6 months. | 2 |
| I am not always physically able to shop, cook, and/or feed myself. | 2 |
| **Total** | _____ |

If your score is:

| | |
|---|---|
| 0–2 | Good! Recheck in 6 months |
| 3–5 | You are at moderate nutritional risk |
| 6 or more | You are at high nutritional risk |

**FIGURE 24-4** Nutritional Screening Initiative Checklist. (Reprinted with permission of the Nutrition Screening Initiative, a project of the American Academy of Family Physicians, the American Dietetic Association, the National Council on the Aging, Inc., and funded in part by Ross Products Division, Abbott Laboratories.)

high nutritional risk. It is aimed primarily at older populations.

Detsky et al, using a similar approach, developed the Subjective Global Assessment of Nutritional Status (SGA).[113] The SGA evaluates weight change, dietary intake changes, gastrointestinal symptoms lasting more than two weeks, and activity levels. The patient's diagnosis and results from a focused physical examination are included. The clinician, considering all of the items, subjectively categorizes the patient as well nourished, having moderate or suspected malnutrition, or being severely malnourished. The SGA has been favorably compared with strictly objective measures in predicting infection susceptibility.[112] Ottery modified the original SGA for use in the cancer population.[18] The modified assessment includes more cancer-specific symptoms and a refinement of the activity level estimation. The patient is able to complete a portion of the assessment, thus decreasing clinician time in data collection.

There are also a number of formulas that integrate several objective measures into assessment of nutritional risk (see Table 24-9).[14] These include the Nutritional Index (NI),[114] the Prognostic Nutritional Index (PNI),[115] the Hospital Prognostic Index (HPI),[116] and the Nutrition Risk Index (NRI).[117] These indexes are especially helpful in identifying which individuals undergoing head and neck or gastrointestinal surgery might benefit from nutritional intervention prior to and following operation. The HPI and NRI utilize measures that are commonly used and readily available.

## Nutrition-Related Symptom Assessment

Assessment of symptoms that interfere with intake is part of an oncological nutritional assessment. These symptoms include anorexia, nausea, vomiting, diarrhea, constipation, mouth sores, dry mouth, pain when eating or swallowing, other pain, taste change, fatigue, difficulty in swallowing, indigestion, early satiety, cramping, and bloating. Linear analogue self-assessment, Likert scales, or objective grading scales are useful in identifying the severity of the problem and the effectiveness of intervention[18,48,56,62,63] (Figure 24-5). Although these techniques are reliable and valid, their utility as a part of routine clinical practice has not been studied.

## Summary

A number of methods for nutritional assessment are useful in cancer populations. The nurse is in the best position to determine the risk for malnutrition and to pursue further assessment. The nurse remains the most likely person to continue serial assessment, providing ongoing appraisal throughout the treatment trajectory.

## THERAPEUTIC APPROACHES AND NURSING CARE

### Introduction

Both deficiency and oversufficiency malnutrition have been associated with increased morbidity and mortality

---

**TABLE 24-9** Nutritional Assessment Formulas

**Nutritional Index (NI)**
$1.9579 - 0.0017 \times$ IgM $+ 0.0188 \times$ prealbumin $- 0.0075 \times$ complement factor C3 $- 0.0066 \times$ fibrinogen $+ 0.033 \times$ cholesterol $- 0.1858 \times$ vitamin A binding protein $+ 0.6636 \times$ thyroxine binding globubulin
*where:* IgM, complement factor, fibrinogen, cholesterol, vitamin A binding protein, and thyroxin binding globulin are measured in milligrams/deciliter.

**Prognostic Nutritional Index (PNI)**
PNI $= 158 - 16.6$ (albumin) $- 0.78$ (TSF) $- 0.2$ (transferrin) $- 5.8$ (DH)
*where:* PNI $= \%$ risk, albumin is measured in grams, TSF $=$ triceps skinfold in millimeters, transferrin is measured in milligrams per deciliter, and DH $=$ delayed hypersensitivity reaction, where 0 is nonreactive, 1 is less than 5 millimeters reactivity, 2 is equal to or more than 5 millimeters reactivity.

**Hospital Prognostic Index (HPI)**
HPI $= 0.91$ (albumin) $- 1.00$ DH $- 1.44$ (sepsis) $= .98$ (dx) $- 1.09$
*where:* albumin is measured in grams, DH $=$ delayed hypersensitivity, with 1 $=$ positive response to one or more antigens, and 2 $=$ no response; sepsis $= 1$ if present and 2 if no sepsis, and diagnosis $= 1$ if cancer present and 2 if the patient does not have cancer.

**Nutrition Risk Index**
NRI $= 15.19 \times$ albumin $+ 0.417 \times \%$UBW
*where:* albumin is measured in grams, and %UBW $= \dfrac{\text{actual weight}}{\text{usual weight}} \times 100$

---

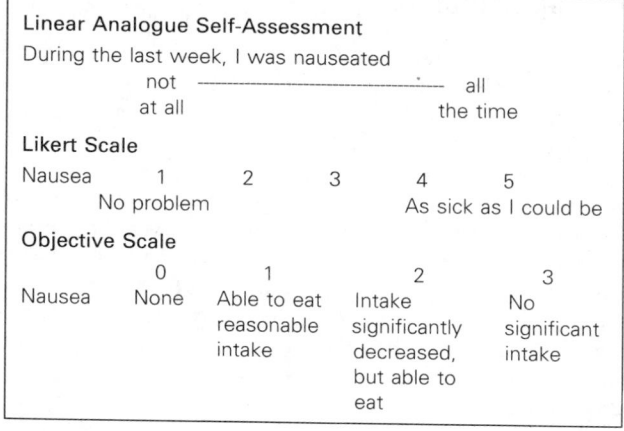

**FIGURE 24-5** Examples of nutritionally linked symptom measurement.

rates among individuals with cancer.[3,4,9–17] This finding suggests that nutritional intervention should reduce morbidity and mortality in the cancer population. While this is true for some people, it is not true for others. Positive outcomes can be expected for most individuals when the cancer is curative, the problems are due to treatment, or the deficit is mechanical. Use of specific food consistency, positioning, and swallowing techniques, for example, can be extremely effective for individuals with dysphagia.[118] But for other individuals, methods that reverse the nutritional deficits caused by the cancer and the host-cancer interaction are ineffective.[77,85,107,119,120] This reality makes the prescription of nutritional intervention complex. The prescription must be devised through cooperation among the patient and family and members of the health care team. The lack of understanding of the cancer-nutrient interaction means that for most patients, nutrition supports, and does not supplant, conventional treatment modalities.[18,22] However, there are clinical trials that evaluate nutrition as an intervention.[121–127] Individuals with cancer may also seek questionable methods that purport to treat cancer using nutritional manipulation.[128,129]

The nutritional prescription for any individual with cancer is best made with input from several disciplines. A nutritional team with expertise in cancer-associated malnutrition is optimal.[18] Nurses interested in such a team can contact the Society for Nutritional Oncology Adjuvant Therapy.[18] A general nutritional support team, responsible for identifying individuals in need of aggressive nutritional support, is a more commonly available group. When such specialization is not present, an approach to nutritional intervention can be determined with collaboration of nurses, physicians, dietitians, and, when needed, pharmacists, speech therapists, and social workers. The patient and family or significant others are an integral part of the effort. Without their participation in goal setting and method choice, it is unlikely that any intervention will be successful.

## Nutritional Interventions

The nutritional assessment, described previously and performed by members of the nutritional team, provides the basis for the nutritional prescription and development of intervention strategies. A range of available nutritional interventions exists, from general counseling about altering oral intakes and symptom management to combined use of total parenteral and enteral nutritional support. The level of intervention is dictated by the patient's baseline nutritional state, disease status, risks for malnutrition from treatment, anticipated response to therapy, and resources. Algorithms for individuals at normal weight and those who are undernourished are provided in Figures 24-6 and 24-7.

Intervention must also be based on realistic goals, which may target specific dietary components, caloric intake, morbidity, mortality, appetite, function, cost-bene-

fit ratio, or well-being. For patients in whom response to treatment is expected or for whom morbidity will be reduced, intervention is a sound practice. Goal determination can be more difficult in individuals with progressing disease, anorexia, and weight loss. Often, family members concentrate on the patient's lack of appetite and weight loss. This can put undue stress on the patient and the family relationship, especially since there is some evidence that increased intake may not increase survival.[53,70,121,122,126] Advising both the patient and the family that emphasis on eating does not improve survival may allow them to put their energies elsewhere. However, if eating is a major source of comfort or quality of life, then the use of medications that improve appetite and alter the metabolic abnormalities should be considered. Involving the patient and significant others in developing the nutritional prescription is imperative.

## Nutritional Prescription

### Alteration in single dietary components

The development of specific nutrient deficiencies is common across diseases. For example, low iron and serum potassium are not uncommon. In cancer patients these deficits arise from a combination of chemotherapy-related effects on bone marrow, anemia of chronic disease or from medications for comorbid conditions and/or antibiotic use. Other deficiencies that are more specific to cancer include hypomagnesemia related to platinum chemotherapy; hyponatremia and hypercalcemia, resulting from paraneoplastic syndromes; and zinc deficiency. Medication commonly is used to control these problems; however, dietary manipulation may be a supplemental treatment requiring education of the patient about foods high in potassium or zinc.

A target for specific intervention is dietary fat intake. There has been much emphasis on the reduction of the percentage of dietary fat consumed by patients with breast cancer.[34,35,121,122,125] Fat-intervention trials indicate that with verbal counseling, individuals can decrease fat intake to desired levels within three months. The altered intake pattern is sustained past the period of counseling with some follow-up. The usual approach employs individualized counseling over a variable number of sessions. These trials have not been in place long enough to determine the effect of fat reduction on mortality.

In another case study, a high-fat diet was utilized not as an adjunct but as salvage therapy.[127] Two children with advanced malignant astrocytoma who had exhausted other treatment measures were placed on a high-fat diet. The diet produced ketogenesis and reduced tumor uptake of glucose, producing disease stabilization in the children and improved cognitive function in one. This trial utilized what is known about the dependency of the nervous system on glucose and the alteration of carbohydrate metabolism in cancer. This approach requires much more study before its use can be expanded.

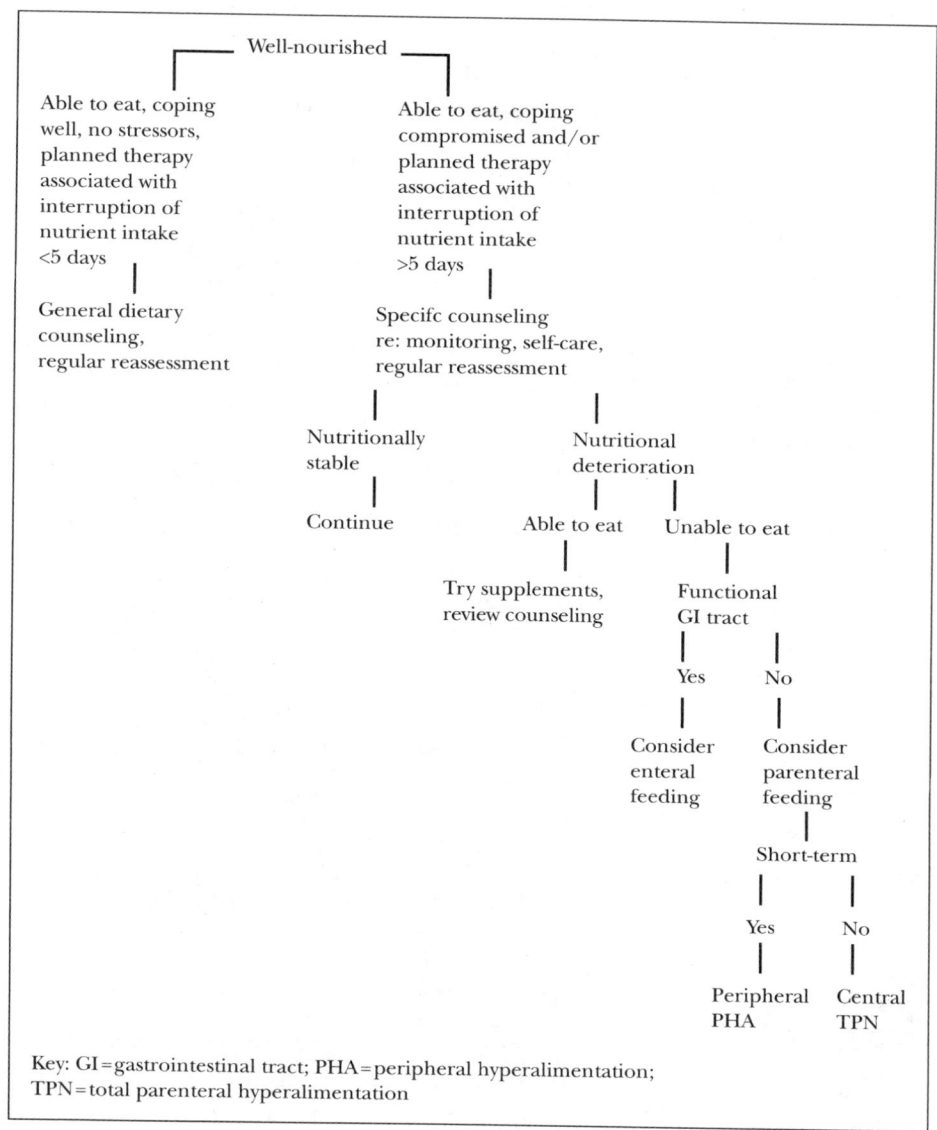

**FIGURE 24-6** Nutritional support algorithm for individuals well nourished at baseline.

Another investigational approach using nutrition as treatment includes the addition of arginine to improve cell-mediated immunity and numbers of circulating natural killer cells.[19] Glutamine has been used as a chemotherapy sensitizer and as a protecter for normal cells.[123] The success of these trials will depend on whether the nutritional lesions involved in the cancer-host relationship have been identified clearly enough.

A study targeting three specific nutrients has provided interesting data. The researchers found improved survival among patients with pancreatic and prostate cancers who were maintained on a low-fat, high-fiber, and lower-calorie diet following standard therapy.[126] The research was a retrospective case study and may not be generalizable. Nonetheless, it calls into question routine counseling for increased caloric intake in cancer patients.

### Alteration in total nutrient intake

***Nutrient interventions*** A more global approach to nutritional therapy has been taken in the attempt to alter the morbidity and mortality of cancer. A major emphasis has been on improving the patient's overall intake and nutritional status to minimize treatment side effects and maximize treatment delivery. Verbal counseling, use of supplements, enteral feedings, parenteral nutrition, and combinations of nutritional interventions have been used for this purpose. Results of selected research on the effect of each of these methods on the morbidity and mortality of individuals undergoing cancer treatment is summarized in Tables 24-10 through Table 24-13.[130–177] The interested reader is referred to Klein and Koretz for an extensive literature review.[178] The studies reviewed indi-

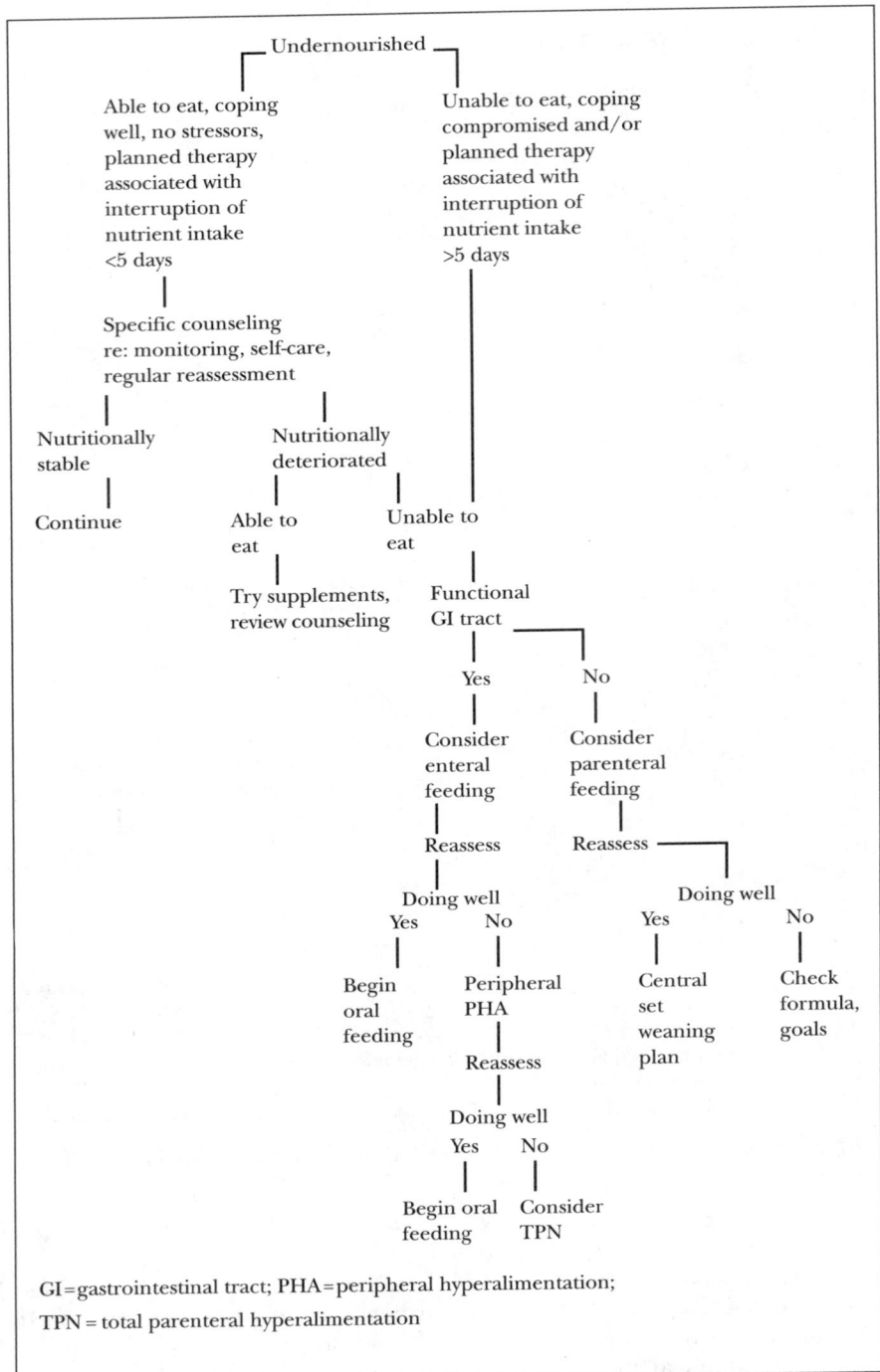

**FIGURE 24-7** Nutritional support algorithm for individuals undernourished at baseline.

cate that verbal counseling is a powerful tool in managing nutritional problems. More aggressive techniques are also of benefit. For example, enteral feeding is useful for individuals requiring protection of suture lines postoperatively or for those with gastrointestinal obstructions that can be bypassed by tube placement. Enteral feeding, especially in the upper gastrointestinal tract, maintains the normal stimulation of enzymatic and mucosal activity in the gut, which is not accomplished with parenteral nutrition. When oral intake is not sufficient or is contraindicated, and the gastrointestinal tract is functioning, enteral feeding is the intervention of choice. For individuals with-

**TABLE 24-10** Clinical Trials of Effect of Counseling Intervention on Morbidity and Mortality Associated with Cancer Treatment

| First Author | Intervention | N/Population | Findings/Comments |
|---|---|---|---|
| Evans[100] | Counseling vs. counseling with zinc, magnesium supplementation | 120 Lung, colon | ND morbidity, except mucositis worse with counseling than controls |
| Glimelius[124] | Verbal vs. control during CT | 58 Lung | ↑ mood, ↑ appetite; ND DFI, survival |
| Oveson[70] | Verbal vs. control | 29 ALL | ↑ intake and TSF; ND survival, weight, or QOL |
| Marcia[130] | Verbal vs. enteral | 93 H/N, GI, breast | Counseled lost weight; enteral stable |
| Kinsella[131] | Verbal vs. TPN during XRT | 32 GU | TPN had ↑ weight, ND survival |

↑ = increased or improved; TSF = triceps skinfold; ND = no difference; DFI = disease-free interval; QOL = quality of life; TPN = total parenteral nutrition; XRT = radiation; ALL = acute lymphocytic leukemia; H/N = head and neck cancer; GI = gastrointestinal; GU = genitourinary.

**TABLE 24-11** Clinical Trials of Effect of Dietary Supplement Use on Morbidity and Mortality Associated with Cancer Treatment

| First Author | Intervention | N/Population | Findings/Comments |
|---|---|---|---|
| Flynn[132] | Supplement vs. control 10 days preoperatively | 36 H/N | ND morbidity; supplement group had shorter LOS |

ND = no difference; LOS = length of stay; H/N = head and neck cancer.

**TABLE 24-12** Clinical Trials of Effects of Enteral Feeding Interventions on Morbidity and Mortality Associated with Cancer Treatment

| First Author | Intervention | N/Population | Findings/Comments |
|---|---|---|---|
| Besser[133] | Enteral vs. control during XRT | 18 Bladder | ND morbidity |
| Brown[134] | Enteral vs. control | 47 GYN | Morbidity reduced in blood count only |
| Elkort[135] | Enteral feeding vs. control during CT | 47 Breast | ND morbidity, response |
| Foschi[136] | Enteral vs. control 12 days preoperatively | 60 GI | ND morbidity |
| Jensen[137] | Enteral vs. TPN 8 days perioperatively | 20 Colon | ND morbidity |
| Lim[138] | Enteral feeding vs. TPN 4 weeks preoperatively | 19 GI | ↑ weight with TPN, ND mortality |
| Lipschitz[139] | Enteral feeding vs. control during CT | 14 Lung | Enteral group had less hematologic morbidity |
| Moloney[140] | Enteral vs. control during XRT | 84 Mixed | ND mortality |
| Nayel[141] | Enteral vs. control | 23 H/N | ND morbidity |
| Ryan[142] | Enteral vs. control 10 days postoperatively | 14 Colon | ND morbidity |
| Szeluga[143] | Enteral vs. TPN | 61 BMT, ALL | ↑ infection with TPN, ND mortality, some enteral also got TPN |
| Shukla[144] | Enteral vs. 10 days preoperatively | 110 H/N, GI, breast | Enteral group had ↓ morbidity, but 50% had problems with tube feedings |
| Smith[145] | Enteral vs. control 10 days postoperatively | 50 GI | Fed group had more problems |
| Tandon[146] | Enteral feeding vs. control during CT | 70 GI | ND in morbidity except stomatitis in enteral group, ND mortality |
| von Meyenfeldt[147] | Enteral feeding 10 days preoperatively | 100 GI | ND morbidity |
| Weintraub[148] | Enteral feeding vs. control | 40 GI | ND weight, QOL |
| Daly[149] | Enteral vs. enteral + arginine | 30 GI | ↓ infection, LOS in arginine group |

↑ = increased or improved; ↓ = decreased; ND = no difference; LOS = length of hospital stay; QOL = quality of life; TPN = total parenteral nutrition; XRT = radiation; CT = chemotherapy; BMT = bone marrow transplant; ALL acute lymphocytic leukemia; H/N = head and neck cancer; GI = gastrointestinal; GU = genitourinary; GYN = gynecologic cancer.

**TABLE 24-13**   Clinical Trials of Effects of Total Parenteral Nutrition Intervention on Morbidity and Mortality Associated with Cancer Treatment

| First Author | Intervention | N/Population | Findings/Comments |
|---|---|---|---|
| Bellantone[150] | TPN vs. control 7 days preoperatively | 100 GI | ND morbidity, mortality |
| Bonau[151] | TPN vs. control 7 days preoperatively | 20 GU | No complications either group |
| Brennan[152] | TPN vs. control | 117 GI | ↑ Infection in TPN group |
| Burt[153] | TPN vs. control 14 days preoperatively | 18 GI | ND morbidity, mortality |
| Buzby[154] | TPN vs. control > 10 days perioperatively | 395 GI, lung | ND morbidity, mortality; ↑ infection in subset TPN group; severely undernourished did better on TPN |
| Hansel[155] | TPN vs. control 4 days postoperatively | 20 Colon | ND morbidity, mortality |
| Muller[156] | TPN vs. control 10 days preoperatively | 125 GI | TPN ↓ morbidity, mortality |
| Sandstrom[157] | TPN vs. control postoperatively | 300 GI | ND morbidity, mortality; TPN group had more complications |
| Sclafani[158] | TPN vs. control 5–20 days postoperatively | 51 GI | ND morbidity, mortality |
| Sims[159] | TPN vs. control 10 days perioperatively | 30 GI | ND morbidity, mortality |
| Smith[160] | TPN vs. control 10 days preoperatively | 34 GI | ND morbidity, mortality |
| Thompson[161] | TPN vs. control 18 days perioperatively | 21 GI | ND morbidity, mortality |
| Woolfson[162] | TPN vs. control 6 days postoperatively | 122 GI | ND morbidity, mortality |
| Pearlstone[163] | TPN vs. TPN + insulin postoperatively | 11 Mixed | ↑ skeletal muscle synthesis in TPN + insulin group |
| Donaldson[164] | TPN vs. control during XRT | 25 Mixed pediatric | ↑ GI toxicity, ND mortality with TPN |
| Ghavimi[165] | TPN vs. control during XRT | 28 Mixed pediatric | ↑ morbidity, ND mortality with TPN |
| Coquin[166] | TPN vs. control during CT | 23 AL | More CR in TPN (191) group |
| Clamon[167] | TPN vs. control during CT | 119 Lung | ND response, ↑ infection, ↑ blood count return with TPN |
| DiCicco[168] | TPN vs. control during CT | 86 Mixed | ND morbidity |
| Drott[169] | TPN vs. control during CT | 23 Testicular | ND morbidity |
| Hays[170] | TPN vs. control during CT | 10 ANLL pediatric | ND morbidity |
| Jordan[171] | TPN vs. control during CT | 43 Lung | ↑ morbidity, ↓ mortality in TPN group |
| Nixon[172] | TPN vs. control | 45 Colon | ↓ survival time with TPN |
| Samuels[173] | TPN vs. control during CT | 30 Testicular | ↑ blood count, ↑ infection with TPN |
| Shamberger[174] | TPN vs. control during CT | 32 Sarcoma | ND morbidity, mortality |
| Valdivieso[175] | TPN vs. control | 65 Lung | ↓ response, ↑ morbidity with TPN |
| van Eys[176] | TPN vs. control during CT | 20 Mixed, pediatric | ↑ infection with TPN, ND mortality with TPN |
| Weisdorf[177] | Pre-transplant TPN vs. control | 137 BMT | ↑ infection, ↓ mortality with TPN |

↑ = increased; ↓ = decreased; ND = no difference; DFI = disease-free interval; QOL = quality of life; CR = complete response; TPN = total parenteral nutrition; XRT = radiation; CT = chemotherapy; ALL = acute lymphocytic leukemia; H/N = head and neck cancer, GI = gastrointestinal; GU = genitourinary.

out a functioning gastrointestinal tract or who need rapid repletion, total parenteral nutrition (TPN) may be the nutritional treatment of choice. TPN reduces morbidity in malnourished patients undergoing surgery. Patients with significant gastrointestinal malfunction, but otherwise with cured, controlled, or indolent disease, may also benefit from parenteral feeding. The largest group of cancer patients receiving home parenteral nutrition are those with severe enteritis following curative radiation treatment.[179]

Other uses of aggressive nutritional support are controversial, in part because of problems of design or methodology in the extant research. Many of the studies have small sample sizes. The studies frequently have different nutritional outcomes, differing patient populations, and different feeding formulas. They also reveal that, although subsets of patients benefit from nutritional repletion, aggressive nutritional intervention does not alter morbidity or mortality for the majority of individuals with cancer. A few studies, performed in animals or in in vitro tumor cell cultures, demonstrate an increase in cancer activity in the presence of TPN administration.[180,181] This area remains controversial. In addition, the risks associated with the various treatments must also be considered. The problems and common solutions associated with enteral and parenteral nutritional interventions are listed in Tables 24-14 and 24-15. The role of aggressive nutritional intervention in cancer treatment continues to require study. As the nutritional abnormalities created by cancer are better understood, better interventions will be developed.

***Pharmacological interventions***  Medications are used by patients to treat a number of nutrition-related problems. Taking medicine has been rated as one of the most effective self-care techniques in controlling constipation, diarrhea, nausea, vomiting, and mucosal irritation.[62,63,182] Medications also have been prescribed to improve appetite and increase nutrient intakes. The effectiveness of treatment depends in part on the origin of the symptom. For the most part, cancer-associated nutritional problems are best reversed by successful treatment of the malignancy. In treatment-induced changes, medication and self-care actions are usually helpful.

Medications commonly used to counter loss of appe-

**TABLE 24-14**  Enteral Feeding Considerations

**General Indications:**
Presence of protein-calorie malnutrition, oral intake compromised for more than 5 days, unable to take at least 50% of caloric needs for 7 or more days, severe dysphagia, head and neck surgery where suture area must be protected, low output fistulas, in combination with total parenteral nutrition (TPN) for bowel resections, continued anorexia in patient with otherwise acceptable quality of life

**Enteral Feeding Tube Sites:**
*Noninvasive placement:*
Nasogastric, nasoduodenal, nasojejunal
Comments: Nasal and esophageal irritation common; risk of regurgitation high with nasogastric tube, low with others, chance of removal high; long-term tolerance fair

*Invasive placement:*
Esophagostomy, gastrostomy, percutaneous endoscopic gastrostomy, jejunostomy
Comments: Esophagostomy and gastrostomy have some risk of regurgitation, chance for removal low, long-term tolerance good
Delivery methods: Bolus, intermittent, continuous, cycled

**TABLE 24-14**  (continued)

Common Enteral Feeding Problems and Solutions

| Problem | Solutions |
|---|---|
| Diarrhea | Give formula at room temperature, use lactose-free formula, add fiber, add antidiarrheal medicine, reduce rate of feeding, reduce volume or use continuous feeding schedule, reduce strength of formula, review other sources (medications, treatment) |
| Regurgitation | Check tube placement, check residuals and withhold feedings if more than 100 ml, keep in Fowler's position, use small-bore tube, place tube distally (jejunum, duodenum), consider drugs to increase motility |
| Nausea | Check tube placement, reduce rate, reduce anxiety, change formula, review other sources (infection, medications, treatment) |
| Distention | Use low-fat or hydrolyzed formula, encourage activity, review other sources (obstruction, constipation, organomegaly) |
| Dehydration | Increase water intake to ensure adequate amounts (usually 1 ml/kcal), control other sources (diarrhea, nausea), watch for glucosuria |
| Fluid overload | Reduce water intake |
| Constipation | Increase water, increase fiber, increase activity |
| Local | Clean area around tube, apply skin protecting agents, monitor for otitis media if using nasal tubes |
| Dry mouth | Frequent mouth rinsing, use xerostomia products, sugarless gum, or mints if medically allowed |
| Tube obstruction | Use room-temperature feedings, irrigate with water, use pump with high-density formulas (> 1.5 kcal/ml) or small-bore tubes, use liquid medicines rather than crushing pills whenever possible |
| Metabolic disturbances | Monitor carbon dioxide levels, reduce carbohydrate in formula, monitor glucose, monitor potassium and supplement if needed |

**TABLE 24-15**   Parenteral Feeding Considerations

**General Indications:**
Presence of protein-calorie malnutrition, nonfunctioning gastrointestinal tract, unable to begin enteral feedings 7 or more days, high output fistulas, in combination with enteral feedings for some bowel resections, severe radiation enteritis with or without malignant disease, temporary malabsorption secondary to aggressive therapy (example: bone marrow transplant), obstructed bowel but otherwise with acceptable quality of life

**Parenteral Catheter Sites:**
*Nonsurgically placed:* Percutaneously inserted central catheters
*Surgically placed:* Hickman®, Broviac®, Groshong®, implanted port
Comments: Choice depends on number of lines needed and expected duration of parenteral feeding
*Delivery Methods:* Continuous, cycled

**Common Parenteral Feeding Problems and Solutions**

| Problem | Solutions |
|---------|-----------|
| Pneumohemothorax | Put patient in Trendelenburg position for line placement, check x-ray postprocedure |
| Embolism | Follow flushing regimen, avoid use of small diameter syringes when flushing, avoid exposure to free air |
| Obstruction | Flush per protocol, check for flow per protocol, treat with antiembolics per institutional protocol |
| Dislodgment | Assess for patency. Be alert to patient complaints of pain or swelling in area of catheter insertion |
| Metabolic | Monitor levels of glucose, ammonia, phosphate; Abnormalities of liver enzymes, magnesium, potassium, hemoglobin/hematocrit |
| Infection | Perform careful site care and evaluation, monitor temperature, glucose levels, glucosuria |
| Trace element deficiency | Monitor vitamin and trace element orders |
| Bleeding | Monitor vitamin K administration |

tite include alcohol, corticosteroids, megestrol acetate, metoclopramide, and delta-9-tetrahydrocannabinol (THC). Other medications that have been investigated include cyproheptadine, insulin, hydrazine sulfate, fluoxymesterone, and pentoxifylline.[9,18,163,183-200] Psychotropic drugs also may assist those patients for whom depression is a factor in diminished appetite.

There have been no formal trials of alcohol as an appetite stimulant, although anecdotal evidence supports its benefit. Alcohol has the advantage of being readily available and inexpensive, although cultural, religious, and physical conditions may restrict its use. There are also relatively few trials of corticosteroids, although they have been used for over 20 years to treat anorexia.[185-187] The studies that are available report temporary, symptomatic improvement in appetite and function. The beneficial effect of corticosteroids is seen especially in individuals with asthenia and those with tumor-induced fever. Weight gain may not occur.[186] Nelson et al suggest beginning treatment with 4 mg of dexamethasone in the morning; dosages can be increased to twice daily.[12] The drug should be avoided in diabetics and in those who might be at added risk of infection. Measures to reduce gastrointestinal irritation also should be considered.

Megestrol acetate has been found to improve appetite, cause weight gain, control nausea, and improve quality of life among individuals with cancer.[188-191] Its mechanism of action may be related to its effect on cytokine activity and adipocytes. Dosages range from 160 to 800 mg/day. Factors to be considered in evaluating the use of the drug for an individual are the cost, the number of pills needed, and potential side effects. The drug now comes in a liquid form, reducing the mechanical problem of the patient having to swallow a number of tablets. Side effects include edema and hyperglycemia, with some increase in risk of an embolism. Because of this, megestrol acetate should be avoided in individuals with congestive heart failure, pericardial effusions, or a history of thrombotic problems. Diabetics should monitor themselves closely, especially during initiation of treatment.

Metoclopramide has been used to improve oral intake based on its effect on nausea and on gastric motility. The usual dose is 10 mg taken orally before meals and at bedtime. Very few trials have been performed to study the drug's effect on intake and weight. Metoclopramide does increase gastric motility and can reduce early satiety and minimize reflux.[192] The drug has also been used to reduce chemotherapy-related nausea.[59,69] More research is needed before the exact role of this drug in treatment of nutritional deficiencies is known.

THC, like metoclopramide, has been explored largely in terms of its effect on chemotherapy-induced nausea and vomiting. Increases in weight have been reported at doses ranging from 2.5 mg twice a day to 15 mg/day.[193,194] Changes in weight may be related to fluid retention rather than increased lean body mass. Effectiveness may be greater in individuals who have used the drug before. Side effects are more common in older persons, especially at higher doses, and may be reduced with timing administration of the drug after a meal. Nelson et al suggest taking THC after breakfast and lunch.[12] Cost and concern about the abuse of THC may limit its acceptance.

Several drugs have been tested for their appetite-stimulatory effect based upon their metabolic activity. Cyproheptadine was chosen because of its antiserotonin effects, since some tumors produce serotonin. It was shown to improve appetite in a study of 29 individuals with advanced cancer, but the benefit was minimal.[195] Insulin has been studied based on the carbohydrate abnormalities and insulin resistance found in some individuals with cancer. Although animal studies have been positive, use in humans is complicated by the difficulties of side effect management.[163,196]

Hydrazine sulfate, another drug associated with carbohydrate metabolism, initially showed promise in appetite stimulation.[197] Additional testing using randomized, double-blind, placebo-controlled designs revealed no benefit for individuals taking the hydrazine sulfate.[198,199] Pentoxifylline, an inhibitor of tumor necrosis factor (TNF), was similarly found to be helpful in initially increasing appetite; subsequent placebo-controlled trials have shown little benefit.[200] The appetite-stimulatory effect of anabolic steroids is being tested using fluoxymesterone, although prior study has not shown anabolic steroids to be effective appetite stimulants.[201] Despite the physiological rationale behind these drugs, their effectiveness and utility are still under study.

*Nonpharmacological interventions*  In addition to medication, a number of self-care actions have been proposed for treatment of cancer-induced nutritional problems. Patient education material commonly includes interventions for decreased appetite, nausea, vomiting, constipation, and taste changes. There has been little research exploring the effectiveness of most of these actions. Recent meta-analysis noted that of 423 nursing studies of symptom management interventions, only 28 utilized an experimental approach.[20] Of that 28, 26 utilized nonpharmacological interventions. This lack of rigor translates into the fact that much of what is suggested to patients for treatment of side effects is not based on scientific evidence or systematic review of patient experience. Moreover, some of the interventions are global in nature. For example, counseling and psychoeducational approaches have benefited patients having nausea, although the actual content of the counseling and psychoeducational interventions may not have been tested. Table 24-16 lists common nutritional interventions. Effectiveness ratings are noted when available. The ratings of effectiveness come essentially from the work of three groups of investigators.[56,62,63,182,203] The lack of effectiveness ratings demonstrates the need for more studies in the area of self-care actions for improving the nutritional status of cancer patients.

Patients and their families may self-prescribe self-care activities that are different from those commonly suggested in the cancer patient education literature. The oncology nurse must be aware of these actions and the beliefs underlying them. If the nurse determines

**TABLE 24-16**  Nonpharmacological Interventions Used to Treat Nutrition-Related Side Effects

| Side Effect | Interventions Suggested with Effectiveness Rating When Available† |
|---|---|
| Nausea | Relaxation (low effect size = 1.7),* mint candy (.28),** rest after meals (1.4, 3.5, 3.7),** avoid sight, smell of food (1.66),** eat cold food (.71),** eat room-temperature food (NR), alter diet (3.6),** increase oral hygiene (1.1, 2.8),** eat small, frequent meals (1.3, 1.4, 2.8),** eat slowly (1.1, 3.0),** chew food well (NR), get fresh air (.76, 2.8, 3.5),** drink clear liquids (1.6, 3.0),** drink between meals (NR), eat crackers, breathe through the mouth (NR), eat sour food (NR), eat low-fat food (NR), avoid spicy food (NR), eat sweet foods (NR) keep busy/distracted (1.0, 2.9, 3.5)** |
| Appetite change | Alter food choice (2.2, 2.9),** increase seasoning (NR), increase oral hygiene (2.0, 2.8),** avoid sight, smell of foods (1.5),** eat cold foods (.74),** eat sour foods (.90),** use straw (NR), use plastic utensils (NR), chew sugar-free gum (NR) |
| Constipation | Drink more liquid (2.1),** eat more fiber (1.6),** eat more fruit (1.5),** exercise (.74),** drink hot beverages (NR), add bran to foods (NR) |
| Diarrhea | Avoid gas-producing foods (.65),** drink clear liquids (.3),** rest (NR), eat small, frequent meals (NR), decrease fiber (NR), eat room-temperature foods (NR), avoid milk (NH), avoid fat (NR), increase potassium (NR), progress diet slowly (NR) |
| Dry mouth | None of the following interventions has been reported as being effective in research studies reviewed: increase liquids, suck on ice, chew sugarless gum, blend foods, use supplements, avoid acid, salty, or spicy foods, increase oral hygiene, apply lip balm, use extra gravies, soak dry food in liquids, humidify air |
| Sore mouth | Increase oral hygiene (4.0),** drink liquids (1.6, 2.6),** use soft toothbrush (1.6),** avoid spicy foods (1.36),** humidify air (.7),** use more gravy (.6),** use baking soda mouthwash (.4),** avoid alcohol, tobacco (NR), use straws (NR), use supplements (NR) |
| Taste change | Alter food choice (2.2, 2.9),** increase oral hygiene (2.0, 2.8),** avoid sight, smell of foods (1.48),* eat sour foods (.90),** eat cold foods (.74),** increase seasoning (NR), use straw (NR), avoid tart foods (NR), chew sugar-free gum (NR), eat less fat (NR), use plastic utensils (NR) |
| Vomiting | Relaxation, rest after meals (1.7, 1.8),** drink clear liquids (1.7),** avoid sight, smell of food (1.6),** chew slowly (1.4),** eat crackers (1.3),** eat cold foods (1.0),** get fresh air (.8),** mint candy (.57),** eat room-temperature food (NR), alter diet (NR), increase oral hygiene (NR), eat small, frequent meals (NR) |

*Numbers are percentages of individuals responding.

**Numbers are ratings of effectiveness on a scale of 1 to 5, with 1 having little effect and 5 being extremely effective.

**TABLE 24-17** Questionable Nutritional Interventions

| Intervention | Description | Potential Hazards |
|---|---|---|
| Metabolic diet | Attempts to excrete toxins, increase cell nutrition. Uses coffee enemas or colonics, high intake of vitamins C, E, A; laetrile, pangamic acid, zinc and selenium supplements | Bowel perforation, colitis, electrolyte imbalance |
| Macrobiotic diet | Although properly constructed diets are adequate, many practitioners do not provide balanced diets | Protein, calorie, iron, vitamin D, vitamin $B_{12}$ deficiencies |
| Megavitamin supplementation | Usually high doses of B complex, C, A, D, and E vitamins | Cardiac abnormalities, liver damage, kidney stones, soft-tissue calcification, coagulation abnormalities |

there is no potential harm, then ways to integrate the beliefs and more traditional activities must be devised. Discovery of such beliefs and folkways takes some perception and skill, and is basic to a full assessment of the patient.

### Questionable cancer nutritional interventions

An unknown number of individuals with cancer use questionable cancer therapies. These treatments are different from the cultural practices noted earlier, in that these methods offer cure outside standard treatment facilities. Research suggests that from 49% to 76% of individuals with cancer combine conventional and questionable therapies.[128,129] Nutritional approaches are the most commonly used questionable treatments and include metabolic, macrobiotic, and megavitamin therapy (Table 24-17). The oncology nurse must be alert to patient usage of these therapies since some have significant side effects. In addition, some medications should be avoided during therapy. There is some suggestion that antioxidant therapy should be avoided during radiation therapy and antimetabolite chemotherapy. The interested reader is encouraged to read the chapter on alternative cancer therapies in this text (chapter 58) and the excellent review articles that are available.[182,183]

## CONCLUSION

The link between nutrition and health was well recognized by Florence Nightingale. That link not only continues to exist today but is being given increasing scientific support. The connection is especially important in oncology, because nutrition influences carcinogenesis itself as well as the quantity and quality of life once the disease exists. The nurse's ability to take full advantage of nutritional interventions is hampered by the insufficient understanding of the pathophysiology of the tumor-host relationship. Without this knowledge, it is difficult to match a specific intervention with a specific nutritional problem.

This lack of knowledge emphasizes the importance of nursing care. Nurses are in the best position to detect undernutrition and overnutrition among individuals with cancer throughout the disease trajectory. The nurse can attend to basic nutritional information during the diagnostic process: height, weight, recent weight change, eating problems, unhealthy and healthful food choices, social situations that interfere with food procurement, and psychological responses that alter intake. Given this base, the nurse can work with other care providers to prioritize and define nutritional care. The nurse continues the assessment function throughout the patient's treatment and follow-up. Nutritional intervention can be devised in the overall context of the clinical situation and in accordance with the patient's beliefs and desires.

Although the scientific information is still far from complete, early nutritional intervention, when the tumor burden is relatively small, has the best chance to alter patient outcomes. This is particularly true for those undergoing surgery. Appropriate nutritional intervention reduces morbidity, length of hospital stay, and possibly mortality in these patients. For some patients the need for nutritional support will continue for a period following hospitalization. This group will need education and coordinated care, a function of nursing. The nurse must also be aware of the changing information regarding the effectiveness of nutritional support. At this time subsets of individuals, and not the whole population, benefit from aggressive refeeding. Understanding the limitations of nutritional interventions is important for both nurses and consumers. Assisting patients to make the best decisions for themselves within the confines of their understanding may reduce frustration and use of questionable methods.

Nurses also should be attuned to newer approaches in the use of nutrition as therapy. Whether these or other nutritional interventions will become part of the cancer armamentarium still needs to be determined by further study. Careful attention to side effects experienced by patients participating in such trials will be most helpful not only to those patients but also to patients who may follow.

Nurses also have an obligation to continue research into the self-care actions routinely prescribed in dealing with nutritional disturbances. Many of the actions commonly suggested have their basis in anecdotal evidence alone. Much more study is needed in this area so that the self-care actions that are most useful for a given patient can be prescribed. With the base of nursing research added to that of other disciplines, oncology nurses can truly influence the incidence and prevalence of nutritional deficiencies in cancer.

## REFERENCES

1. Beaton G, Bengoa J: *Nutrition and Preventive Medicine.* Geneva, World Health Organization, 1973
2. Chandra R: Nutrition and immunity: Lessons from the past and new insights into the future. *Am J Clin Nutr* 53:1087–1101, 1991
3. Nixon D, Heymsfield S, Cohen A, et al: Protein-calorie malnutrition in hospitalized cancer patients. *Am J Med* 68:683–690, 1980
4. Bender A, Bender D: *Nutrition for Medical Students.* New York, Wiley, 1982
5. Warren S: The immediate causes of death in cancer. *Am J Med Sci* 184:610–615, 1932
6. Gold J: Cancer cachexia and gluconeogenesis. *Ann N Y Acad Sci* 230:103–110, 1974
7. Holyrode C, Gabzuda T, Putnam R, et al: Altered glucose metabolism in metastatic carcinoma. *Cancer Res* 35:3710–3714, 1975
8. Lundholm K, Bylund A, Holm J, et al: Skeletal muscle metabolism in patients with malignant tumor. *Eur J Cancer* 12:465–473, 1976
9. Buzby G, Mullen J, Matthews D, et al: Prognostic nutritional index in gastrointestinal surgery. *Am J Surg* 139:160–167, 1980
10. DeWys W, Begg C, Lavin P, et al: Prognostic effect of weight loss prior to chemotherapy in cancer patients. *Am J Med* 69:491–497, 1980
11. Edelstein S: Nutritional assessment in cancer cachexia. *Pediatr Nurs* 17:237–240, 1991
12. Nelson K, Walsh D, Sheehan F: The cancer anorexia-cachexia syndrome. *J Clin Oncol* 12:213–225, 1994
13. Kern D, Norton J: Cancer cachexia. *J Parent Ent Nutr* 12:286–298, 1988
14. Norton J, Peacock J, Morrison S: Cancer cachexia. *Crit Rev Oncol Hematol* 7:289–293, 1987
15. Jain M, Cook G, Davis F, et al: A case control study: Nutrition and colorectal cancer. *Int J Cancer* 26:755–760, 1980
16. Bastarrachea J, Hortobagyi G, Smith T, et al: Obesity as an adverse prognostic factor for patients receiving adjuvant chemotherapy for breast cancer. *Ann Intern Med* 119:18–25, 1993
17. Grant M, Padilla G, Rhiner M: Patterns of anorexia in cancer patients. *First National Conference on Cancer Nursing Research,* American Cancer Society, Atlanta, November 30, 1989
18. Ottery F: Cancer cachexia. *Cancer Practice* 2:123–131, 1994
19. Heys S, Park G, Forlick P, et al: Nutrition and malignant disease: Implications for surgical practice. *Br J Surg* 79:614–623, 1992
20. Balducci L, Hardy C: Cancer and nutrition: A review. *Compr Ther* 13:59–63, 1987
21. Langstein H, Norton J: Mechanisms of cancer cachexia. *Hematol Oncol Clin North Am* 5:103–120, 1991
22. Ottery F: Supportive nutrition to prevent cachexia and improve quality of life. *Semin Oncol* 22:98–111, 1995
23. Knox L: Maintaining nutritional status in persons with cancer. *First National Conference on Cancer Nursing Research.* American Cancer Society, Atlanta, November 30, 1989
24. Baker J, Detsky A, Wesson D, et al: Nutritional assessment: A comparison of clinical judgment and objective measures. *N Engl J Med* 306:969–972, 1982
25. Blackburn G, Bistrian B, Maini B, et al: Nutrition and metabolic assessment of the hospitalized patient. *J Parent Ent Nutr* 1:11–23, 1977
26. Bozetti F, Migliavacca S, Gallus G, et al: Nutritional markers as prognostic indicators. *J Parent Ent Nutr* 9:462–467, 1985
27. Lipkin E, Bell S: Assessment of nutritional status. *Clin Lab Med* 13:329–352, 1993
28. Smale B, Mullen J, Buzby G, et al: The efficacy of nutritional assessment and support in cancer surgery. *Cancer* 47:2372–2377, 1981
29. Coates K, Morgan S, Barollucci A, et al: Hospitalized malnutrition: A reevaluation 12 years later. *J Am Diet Assoc* 93:27–33, 1993
30. Colletti R, Copeland K, Devlin J, et al: Effect of obesity on plasma insulin-like growth factor in cancer patients. *Int J Obes* 15:523–527, 1991
31. Foltz A: Weight gain among Stage II breast cancer patients: A study of five factors. *Oncol Nurs Forum* 12:21–26, 1985
32. Huntington M: Weight gain in patients receiving adjuvant chemotherapy for cancer of the breast. *Cancer* 56:472–474, 1985
33. Grindel C: Weight gain in breast cancer patients receiving adjuvant chemotherapy as a function of restraint and disinhibition. *Oncol Nurs Forum* 17:23–27, 1990
34. Boyd N, Campbell J, Germanson T, et al: Body weight and prognosis in breast cancer. *J Natl Cancer Inst* 67:785–789, 1981
35. Holm L, Nordevang E, Hjalmer M, et al: Treatment failure and dietary habits in women with breast cancer. *J Natl Cancer Inst* 85:32–36, 1993
36. Heber D, Byerly L, Chi J, et al: Pathology of malnutrition in the adult cancer patient. *Cancer* 58:1867–1873, 1983
37. Holyrode C, Reichard G: General metabolic abnormalities in cancer patients. *Surg Clin North Am* 66:940–950, 1986
38. Tayek J: Review of cancer cachexia and abnormal glucose metabolism in humans with cancer. *J Am Coll Nutr* 11:445–456, 1992
39. Heber D, Tchekmedyian N: Pathology of cancer. *Oncology* 49:28–31, 1992
40. Moldawer L, Rogy M, Lowry S: The role of cytokines in cancer cachexia. *J Parent Ent Nutr* 16:43S–49S, 1992
41. Heber D, Byerly L, Tchekmedyian N: Hormonal and metabolic abnormalities in the malnourished cancer patient. *J Parent Ent Nutr* 16:60S–64S, 1992
42. Larson P, Lindsey A, Dodd M, et al: Influence of age on problems experienced by patients with lung cancer undergoing radiation therapy. *Oncol Nurs Forum* 20:473–480, 1993
43. Waltman N, Bergstrom N, Armstrong N, et al: Nutritional status, pressure sores, and mortality in elderly patients with cancer. *Oncol Nurs Forum* 18:405–410, 1991
44. Guo C, Ma D, Zhang K: Applicability of the general nutritional status score to patients with oral and maxillofacial malignancies. *Int J Oral Maxillofac Surg* 23:167–169, 1994
45. Merritt R, Ashley J, Siegel S, et al: Calorie and protein

requirements of pediatric patients with acute nonlympho-cytic leukemia. *J Parent Ent Nutr* 9:303–306, 1987

46. Shils M: Nutrition and diet in cancer management, in Olson J, Shike M (eds): *Modern Nutrition in Health and Disease* (ed 8). Philadelphia, Lea and Febiger, 1994, pp 1319–1342

47. Staal-van den Brekel A, Schols A, ten Velde G, et al: Analysis of the energy balance in lung cancer patients. *Cancer Res* 54:6430–6433, 1994

48. Tchekmedyian N, Zahyra D, Halpert C, et al: Clinical aspects of nutrition in advanced cancer. *Oncology* 49(2):3–7, 1992

49. Bond S, Ham A, Wolton S, et al: Energy intake and basal metabolic rate during maintenance chemotherapy. *Arch Dis Child* 67:1318–1319, 1992

50. Ollenschlager G, Konkol K, Modder B: Implications for and results of nutritional therapy in cancer patients. *Recent Results Cancer Res* 108:172–184, 1988

51. Meguid M, Muhal M, Debonis D, et al: Influence of nutritional status on the resumption of adequate food intake in patients recovering from colorectal cancer operations. *Surg Clin North Am* 66:1167–1176, 1986

52. Daly J, Redmond H, Lieberman M, et al: Nutritional support of patients with cancer of the gastrointestinal tract. *Surg Clin North Am* 71:523–536, 1991

53. Williamson J: Physiologic stress: Trauma, sepsis, burns, and surgery, in Mahon L, Arliln M (eds): *Krause's Food, Nutrition and Diet Therapy* (ed 4). Philadelphia, Saunders, 1992, pp 503–504

54. Mood D: Radiation therapy effects. Presented at the Second National Conference on Cancer Nursing, Baltimore, MD, January 1992

55. Strohl R: The nursing role in radiation oncology. *Oncol Nurs Forum* 15:429–434, 1988

56. Dodd M: Radiation: Patterns of self-care of patients receiving radiation therapy. *Oncol Nurs Forum* 11(3):23–27, 1984

57. Grant M, Padilla G, Rhiner M: Patterns of anorexia in cancer patients. Presented at the First National Conference on Cancer Nursing, Atlanta, GA, November 1989

58. Rubin P: The Frank Buschke Lecture: Late effects of chemotherapy and radiation therapy: A new hypothesis. *Int J Radiat Oncol Biol Phys* 10(1):5–34, 1984

59. Wickham R: Managing chemotherapy-related nausea and vomiting: The state of the art. *Oncol Nurs Forum* 16:563–574, 1989

60. Jenns K: The importance of nausea. *Cancer Nurs* 17:488–493, 1994

61. Morrow G: Chemotherapy-related nausea and vomiting *CA: Cancer J Clin* 39:89–103, 1989

62. Dodd M: Patterns of self-care in patients with breast cancer. *West J Nurs Res* 10:7–24, 1988

63. Nail L, Jones L, Lauver D, et al: Use and perceived adequacy of self-care activities in patients receiving chemotherapy. *Oncol Nurs Forum* 18:883–887, 1991

64. Rhodes V, Watson P, Hanson B: Patients' descriptions of the influence of tiredness and weakness on self-care abilities. *Cancer Nurs* 11:186–194, 1988

65. Wujcik D: An odyssey into biologic therapy. *Oncol Nurs Forum* 20:879–887, 1993

66. Rosenberg S: Principles and applications of biologic therapy, in DeVita V, Hellman S, Rosenberg S (eds): *Cancer: Principles and Practice of Oncology* (ed 3). Philadelphia, Lippincott, 1993, pp 293–324

67. Antila H, Salo M, Nanto V, et al: The effect of postoperative radiotherapy on leukocytes, zinc, serum trace elements and nutritional status in breast cancer patients. *Acta Oncol* 31:569–572, 1992

68. Harrison L, Zclefsky M, Armstrong J, et al: Performance status after treatment for squamous cell cancer of the base of the tongue. *Int J Radiat Oncol Biol Phys* 30:953–957, 1994

69. Hawthorn J: *Understanding and Management of Nausea and Vomiting.* Cambridge, Blackwell Science, 1995

70. Ovesen L, Hannibal J, Allingstrup L: Dietary intake in patients with small cell lung cancer. *Eur J Clin Nutr* 46:435–437, 1992

71. Mattes R, Curran W Jr, Alavi J, et al: Clinical implications of learned food aversions in patients with cancer treated with chemotherapy or radiation therapy. *Cancer* 70:192–200, 1992

72. Cioffi L: General theory of critical periods and the development of obesity, in Smogyi J (ed): *Nutritional, Psychological and Social Aspects of Obesity.* Basel, Karger, 1968, pp 17–28

73. Fearnon K: The mechanisms and treatment of weight loss in cancer. *Proc Nutr Soc* 51:251–256, 1992

74. Goodwin W, Byers P: Nutritional management of the head and neck cancer patient. *Med Clin North Am* 77:597–610, 1993

75. Meguid M, Muscaritoli M, Beverly J, et al: The early cancer anorexia paradigm: Changes in plasma free tryptophan and feeding indexes. *J Parent Ent Nutr* 16:56S–59S, 1992

76. McNamara M, Alexander R, Norton J: Cytokines and their role in the pathophysiology of cancer cachexia. *J Parent Ent Nutr* 16:50S–55S, 1992

77. Tchekmedyian N, Heber D: Cancer and AIDS cachexia: Mechanisms and approaches to therapy. *Oncology* 7:55–59, 1993 (suppl)

78. Gormican A: Influencing food acceptance in anorexic cancer patients. *Postgrad Med* 68:145–162, 1980

79. Carson J, Gormican A: Taste acuity and food attitudes of selected patients with cancer. *J Am Diet Assoc* 70:361–365, 1977

80. Nielsen S, Theologides A, Vickers Z: Influence of food odors on food aversions and preferences in patients with cancer. *Am J Clin Nutr* 33:2253–2261, 1980

81. DeWys W, Walters K: Abnormalities in taste sensation in cancer patients. *Cancer* 36:1888–1896, 1975

82. Blackburn G, Bistrian B, Maini B, et al: The effect of cancer on nitrogen, electrolyte and mineral metabolism. *Cancer Res* 37:2345–2348, 1977

83. Hoffman F: Micronutrient requirements of cancer patients. *Cancer* 55:225–230, 1985

84. Cori C, Cori G: The carbohydrate metabolism of tumors. *J Biol Chem* 66:397–405, 1925

85. Nixon D, Kutner M, Heymsfield S, et al: Resting energy expenditure in lung and colon cancer. *Metabolism* 37:1059–1064, 1988

86. Knox L, Crosby L, Feurer I, et al: Energy expenditure in malnourished cancer patients. *Ann Surg* 197:152–162, 1983

87. Falconer J, Fearnon K, Plester C: Cytokines, the acute phase response and resting energy expenditure in cachectic patients with pancreatic cancer. *Ann Surg* 219:325–331, 1994

88. Eden E, Edstrom S, Bennegard K, et al: Glucose flux in relation to energy expenditure in malnourished patients with and without cancer during periods of fasting and feeding. *Cancer Res* 44:1718–1724, 1984

89. Shaw J, Wolfe R: Glucose and urea kinetics in patients with

early and advanced gastrointestinal cancer. *Surgery* 101: 181–185, 1986

90. Kokal W, McCulloch A, Wright P, et al: Glucose turnover and recycling in colorectal carcinoma. *Ann Surg* 198: 601–604, 1983

91. Glicksman A, Rawson R: Diabetes and altered carbohydrate metabolism in patients with cancer. *Cancer* 9:1127–1134, 1956

92. Cheblowski R, Heber D: Metabolic abnormalities in cancer patients. *Surg Clin North Am* 66:957–969, 1985

93. Heber D, Byerly L, Cheblowski R, et al: Medical abnormalities in the cancer patient. *Cancer* 55:225–229, 1985

94. Norton J, Stein T, Brennan M: Whole body protein synthesis and turnover in normal and malnourished patients with and without known cancer. *Ann Surg* 194:123–128, 1981

95. Istafan N, Wan J, Bistrian B: Nutrition and tumor promotion. *J Parent Ent Nutr* 16:76S–82S, 1991

96. Jeevanandam M, Lowry S, Horowitz G, et al: Cancer cachexia and protein metabolism. *Lancet* 1:1423–1426, 1984

97. Kitada S, McAndrew P, Hays E, et al: Lipid mobilizing factor in serum of cancer patients. *Proc Am Assoc Cancer Res* 25: 155, 1984 (abstr)

98. Vlassara H, Speigel R, Daval C, et al: Reduced plasma lipoprotein lipase activity in patients with malignancy associated weight loss. *Horm Metab Res* 18:698–703, 1986

99. Beck S, Tisdale M: Production of lipolytic and proteolytic factors by a murine tumor-producing cachexia in the host. *Cancer Res* 47:5919–5922, 1987

100. Evans W, Nixon D, Daly J, et al: A randomized study of oral nutritional support vs. ad lib nutritional intake during chemotherapy for advanced colorectal and non–small cell lung cancer. *J Clin Oncol* 5:113–124, 1987

101. Charney P: Nutrition assessment in the 1990s: Where are we now? *Nutr Clin Pract* 10:131–139, 1995

102. Lopes J, Russell D, Whitewell J, et al: Skeletal muscle function in malnutrition. *Am J Clin Nutr* 36:602–610, 1982

103. Robinett-Weiss N, Hixson M, Kier B, et al: The Metropolitan height-weight tables. *J Am Diet Assoc* 84:1480–1481, 1984

104. Andres R, Elahi D, Tobin J, et al: Impact of age on weight goals. *Ann Intern Med* 103(6, pt 2):1030–1033, 1985

105. Willett W, Stampfer J, VanItallie T: New weight guidelines for Americans: Justified or injudicious. *Am J Clin Nutr* 53: 1102–1103, 1991

106. Frisancho A: New standards of weight and body composition by frame size and height for assessment of nutritional status of adults and the elderly. *Am J Clin Nutr* 40:808–819, 1984

107. Souba J: Nutritional care of the individual with cancer. *Nutr Clin Pract* 3:173–176, 1988

108. Pirie P, Jacobs D, Jeffrey R, et al: Distortion in self-reported height and weight data. *J Am Diet Assoc* 78:601–606, 1981

109. Garn S, Sullivan T, Hawthorne V: Differential rates of fat change relative to body weight change at different body sites. *Int J Obes* 11:517–520, 1987

110. Klidjian A, Archer T, Foster K, et al: Detection of dangerous malnutrition. *J Parent Ent Nutr* 6:119–121, 1982

111. Kalfarentzos F, Spiliotis J, Velimezis G, et al: Comparison of forearm muscle dynamometry with nutritional prognostic index as a preoperative indicator in cancer patients. *J Parent Ent Nutr* 13:34–36, 1989

112. *Nutritional Screening Initiative Checklist.* Washington, DC, Nutrition Screening Initiative, 1992

113. Detsky A, McLaughlin J, Baker J, et al: What is subjective global assessment of nutritional status? *J Parent Ent Nutr* 11:8–13, 1987

114. Whitney E, Cataldo C, Rolfes S: *Understanding Normal and Clinical Nutrition* (ed 3). St. Paul, West Publishing, 1991

115. Buzby G, Mullen J, Matthews D, et al: Prognostic nutritional index in gastrointestinal surgery. *Am J Surg* 139:160–167, 1980

116. Harvey K, Moldwater L, Bistrian B, et al: Biological measure for the formulation of a hospital prognostic index. *Am J Clin Nutr* 34:2012–2015, 1981

117. Schlag P, Decker-Baumann C: Strategies and needs for nutritional support in cancer surgery. *Recent Results Cancer Res* 121:233–252, 1991

118. Bloch A: Nutritional management of patients with dysphagia. *Oncology* 7:127–138, 1993

119. Lundholm K, Hyltander A, Sandstrom R: Nutritional support in cancer treatment. *Curr Opin Oncol* 3:621–627, 1991

120. Goodman M, Kolonel L, Wilkens L, et al: Dietary factors in lung cancer diagnosis. *Eur J Cancer* 28:495–501, 1992

121. Holm L, Nordevang E, Hjalmar M, et al: Treatment failure and dietary habits of women with breast cancer. *J Natl Cancer Inst* 85:32–36, 1993

122. White E, Shattuck A, Dristal A, et al: Maintenance of a low-fat diet: Follow-up of the Women's Health Trial Cancer *Epidemiol Biomarkers Prev* 1:315–323, 1992

123. Klimberg V, Pappas A, Nwokedi E, et al: Effect of supplemental glutamine on methotrexate concentration in tumors. *Arch Surg* 127:1317–1320, 1992

124. Glimelius B, Birgegard G, Hoffman K, et al: Improved care of patients with small cell lung cancer. *Acta Oncol* 31: 823–831, 1992

125. de Waard F, Ramlau R, Mulders Y, et al: A feasibility study on weight reduction in obese postmenopausal breast cancer patients. *Eur J Cancer Prev* 2:233–238, 1993

126. Carter J, Saxe G, Newbold V, et al: Hypothesis: Dietary management may improve survival from nutritionally linked cancers based on analysis of representative cases. *J Am Coll Nutr* 12:209–226, 1993

127. Nebeling C, Miraldi F, Shurin S, et al: Effects of a ketogenic diet on tumor metabolism and nutritional status in pediatric oncology patients. *J Am Coll Nutr* 14:202–208, 1995

128. Cassileth B, Brown H: Questionable cancer medicine. *Cancer Invest* 4:591–598, 1986

129. Montbriand M: An overview of alternate therapies chosen by patients with cancer. *Oncol Nurs Forum* 21:1547–1554, 1994

130. Marcia E, Moran J, Santos J, et al: Nutritional evaluation and dietetic care in cancer patients treated with radiotherapy. *Nutrition* 7:205–209, 1991

131. Kinsella T, Malcolm A, Bothe A, et al: Prospective study of nutritional support during pelvic irradiation. *Int J Radiat Oncol Biol Phys* 7:543–548, 1981

132. Flynn M, Leight F: Preoperative outpatient nutritional support of patients with squamous cancer of the upper aerodigestive tract. *Am J Surg* 154:359–362, 1987

133. Besser P, Bonau R, Erlandson R, et al: Can enteral elemental diets (ED) protect the GI tract from acute radiation enteritis? *J Parent Ent Nutr* 10:4, 1986 (suppl)

134. Brown M, Buchanan R, Karran S: Clinical observations on the effects of elemental diet supplementation during irradiation. *Clin Radiol* 31:19–20, 1980

135. Elkort R, Baker F, Vitale J, et al: Long-term nutritional support as an adjunct to chemotherapy for breast cancer. *J Parent Ent Nutr* 5:385–390, 1981

136. Foschi D, Cavega G, Calloni F, et al: Hyperalimentation of jaundiced patients on percutaneous transhepatic biliary drainage. *Br J Surg* 73:716–719, 1986

137. Jensen S: Clinical effects of enteral and parenteral nutrition preceding cancer surgery. *Med Oncol Tumor Pharmacother* 2:225–229, 1985

138. Lim S, Choa R, Lam K, et al: Total parenteral nutrition versus gastrostomy in the preoperative preparation of patients with carcinoma of the oesophagus. *Br J Surg* 68:69–72, 1981

139. Lipschitz D, Mitchell C: Enteral hyperalimentation and hematopoietic toxicity caused by chemotherapy of small cell lung cancer. *J Parent Ent Nutr* 4:593, 1980 (abstr)

140. Moloney M, Moriarity M, Daly L: Controlled studies of nutritional intake in patients with malignant disease undergoing treatment. *Hum Nutr Appl Nutr* 37:30–35, 1983

141. Nayel H, El-Ghoneimy E, El-Haddad S: Impact of nutritional supplementation on treatment delay and morbidity in patients with head and neck tumors treated with irradiation. *Nutrition* 6:13–18, 1992

142. Ryan J, Page C, Babcock L: Early postoperative jejunal feeding of elemental diet in gastrointestinal surgery. *Am Surg* 47:393–403, 1981

143. Szeluga D, Stuart R, Brookmeyer R, et al: Nutritional support of bone marrow transplant recipients. *Cancer Res* 47:3309–3316, 1987

144. Shukla H, Rao R, Banu N, et al: Enteral hyperalimentation in malnourished surgical patients. *Indian J Med Res* 80:339–346, 1984

145. Smith R, Hartemink R, Hollinshead J, et al: Fine bore jejunostomy feeding following major abdominal surgery. *Br J Surg* 72:458–461, 1985

146. Tandon S, Gupta S, Sinha S, et al: Nutritional support as an adjunct therapy of advanced cancer patients. *Indian J Med Res* 80:180–188, 1984

147. von Meyenfeldt M, Meyerink W, Soeters P, et al: Perioperative nutritional support results in a reduction of major postoperative complications especially in high risk patients. *Gastroenterology* 100:A553, 1991 (abstr)

148. Weintraub F, Daly J, Polomano R, et al: The impact of home enteral nutrition on quality of life outcomes for postoperative patients with gastrointestinal (GI) malignancies. Presented at the Oncology Nursing Society, Cincinnati, May 4–7, 1994

149. Daly J, Weintraub F, Shou J, et al: Enteral nutrition during multimodal therapy in upper gastrointestinal cancer patients. *Ann Surg* 221:327–338, 1995

150. Bellantone R, Doglietto G, Bossola M, et al: Preoperative parenteral nutrition in the high risk surgical patient. *J Parent Ent Nutr* 12:195–197, 1988

151. Bonau A, Ang S, Jeevanandam M, et al: High-branched chain amino acid solutions. *J Parent Ent Nutr* 8:622–627, 1984

152. Brennan M, Pisters P, Posner M, et al: A prospective randomized trial of total parenteral nutrition after major pancreatic resection for malignancy. *Ann Surg* 220:436–441, 1994

153. Burt M, Stein T, Schwade J, et al: Whole-body protein metabolism I cancer-bearing patients. *Cancer* 53:1246–1252, 1984

154. Buzby G, Williford W, Peterson O, et al. Perioperative total parenteral nutrition in surgical patients: *N Engl J Med* 325:525–532, 1991

155. Hansel D, Davies J, Shenkin A, et al: The effects of an anabolic steroid and peripherally administered intravenous nutrition in the early postoperative period. *J Parent Ent Nutr* 13:349–358, 1989

156. Muller J, Brenner U, Dienst C, et al: Preoperative parenteral feeding in patients with gastrointestinal carcinoma. *Lancet* 1:68–71, 1982

157. Sandstrom R, Drott C, Hyltander A, et al: The effect of postoperative intravenous feeding (TPN) on outcome following major surgery evaluated in a randomized study. *Ann Surg* 217:185–195, 1993

158. Sclafani L, Shike M, Quesda E, et al: A randomized prospective trial of TPN following major pancreatic resection or radioactive implant for pancreatic cancer. Presented at the Society of Surgical Oncology, Orlando, FL, March 1991

159. Sims J, Oliver E, Smith J: A study of total parenteral nutrition (TPN) in major gastric and esophageal resection for neoplasia. *J Parent Ent Nutr* 4:42, 1980 (abstr)

160. Smith R, Hartemink R: Improvement of nutritional measures during preoperative parenteral nutrition in patients selected by the Prognostic nutritional index. *J Parent Ent Nutr* 12:587–591, 1988

161. Thompson B, Julian T, Stemple J: Perioperative total parenteral nutrition in patients with gastrointestinal cancer. *Surg Res* 30:497–500, 1981

162. Woolfson A, Smith J: Elective nutritional support after major surgery. *Clin Nutr* 8:15–21, 1989

163. Pearlstone D, Wolf R, Berman R, et al: Effect of systemic insulin on protein kinetics in postoperative cancer patients. *An Surg Oncology* 1:321–332, 1994

164. Donaldson S, Wesley M, Ghavimi F, et al: A prospective randomized clinical trial of total parenteral nutrition in children with cancer. *Med Pediatr Oncol* 10:129–139, 1982

165. Ghavimi F, Shils M, Scott B, et al: Comparison of morbidity in children requiring abdominal radiation and chemotherapy with and without total parenteral nutrition. *J Pediatr* 101:530–537, 1982

166. Coquin J, Maraninchi D, Gestaut J, et al: Influence of parenteral nutrition (PN) on chemotherapy and survival of acute leukemia. *J Parent Ent Nutr* 5:357, 1981 (abstr)

167. Clamon G, Feld R, Evans W, et al: Effect of adjuvant central IV hyperalimentation on the survival and response to treatment of patients with small cell lung cancer. *Cancer Treat Rep* 69:167–177, 1985

168. DiCicco M, Panarello G, Fantin D, et al: Parenteral nutrition in cancer patients receiving chemotherapy. *J Parent Ent Nutr* 17:513–518, 1993

169. Drott C, Unagaard B, Schersten T, et al: Total parenteral nutrition as an adjuvant to patients undergoing chemotherapy for testicular carcinoma. *Surgery* 103:499–506, 1988

170. Hays D, Merritt R, White R, et al: Effect of total parenteral nutrition on marrow recovery during induction therapy for acute nonlymphocytic leukemia in childhood. *Med Pediatr Oncol* 11:134–140, 1983

171. Jordan W, Valdivieso M, Frankman C, et al: Treatment of advanced adenocarcinoma of the lung with ftoraflur, doxorubicin, cyclophosphamide, and cisplatin (FACP) and intensive IV hyperalimentation. *Cancer Treat Rep* 65:197–205, 1981

172. Nixon D, Heymesfield S, Lawson D, et al: Effect of total parenteral nutrition on survival in advanced colon cancer. *Cancer Detect Prev* 4:421–427, 1981

173. Samuels M, Selig D, Ogden S, et al: IV hyperalimentation and chemotherapy for stage II testicular cancer. *Cancer Treat Rep* 65:617–625, 1981

174. Shamberger R, Brennan M, Goodgame J, et al: A prospec-

tive, randomized study of adjuvant parenteral nutrition in the treatment of sarcoma. *Surgery* 96:1–12, 1984

175. Valdivieso M, Frankmann C, Murphy W, et al: Long-term effects of intravenous hyperalimentation administered during intensive chemotherapy for small cell bronchogenic carcinoma. *Cancer* 59:362–369, 1987

176. Van Eys J, Copeland E, Cangir A, et al: A clinical trial of hyperalimentation in children with metastatic malignancies. *Med Pediatr Oncol* 8:63–73, 1980

177. Weisdorf S, Lysne J, Wind D, et al: Positive effect of prophylactic total parenteral nutrition on long-term outcome of bone marrow transplantation. *Transplantation* 43:833–838, 1987

178. Klein S, Koretz R: Nutrition support in patients with cancer: What do the data really show? *NCP* 9:91–100, 1994

179. Howard L: Home parenteral nutrition in patients with a cancer diagnosis. *J Parent Ent Nutr* 16:93S–99S, 1992

180. Torosian M: Stimulation of tumor growth by nutrition support. *J Parent Ent Nutr* 16:72S–75S, 1991

181. McNurian M, Heys S, Park K, et al: Tumour and host tissue responses to branched-chain amino acid supplementation of patients with cancer. *Clin Sci* 86:339–345, 1994

182. Foltz A, Gullatte M, Gaines G: Post-hospitalization self-care actions among medical oncology patients. *Oncol Nurs Forum* (in press)

183. Tchekmedyian N, Halpert C, Ashley J, et al: Nutrition in advanced cancer. *J Parent Ent Nutr* 16:88S–92S, 1991

184. Loprinzi C: Management of cancer anorexia/cachexia. *Support Care Cancer* 3:120–123, 1995

185. Moertel G, Schutt A, Reitemeier R, et al: Corticosteroid therapy of preterminal gastrointestinal cancer. *Cancer* 33:1607–1609, 1974

186. Popeila T, Lucchi R, Giongo F: Methylprednisolone as palliative therapy for female terminal cancer patients. *Eur J Cancer Clin Oncol* 25:1823–1829, 1989

187. Bruera E, Roca E, Cedaro L, et al: Action of oral methylprednisolone in terminal cancer patients. *Cancer Treat Rep* 69:751–754, 1992

188. Tchekmedyian N, Hickman M, Siau J, et al: Megestrol acetate in cancer anorexia and weight loss. *Cancer* 69:1268–1274, 1992

189. Breura E, Macmillasn K, Kuehn N, et al: A controlled trial of megestrol acetate on appetite, caloric intake, nutritional status, and other symptoms in patients with advanced cancer. *Cancer* 66:1279–1282, 1990

190. Kornblith A, Hollis D, Zuckerman E, et al: Effect of meges-trol acetate on quality of life in a dose-response trial in women with advanced breast cancer. *J Clin Oncol* 11:2081–2089, 1993

191. Loprinzi C, Michalek J, Scaid D, et al. Phase III evaluation of four doses of megestrol acetate as therapy for patients with cancer anorexia and/or cachexia. *J Clin Oncol* 11:762–767, 1993

192. Escott-Stump S: *Nutrition and Diagnosis Related Care* (ed 3). Philadelphia, Lea and Febiger, 1992

193. Plasse T, Gortner R, Krasnow S, et al: Recent clinical experience with dronabinol. *Pharmacol Biochem Behav* 40:695–700, 1991

194. Nelson K, Walsh D, Deeter P, et al: A phase II study of delta-9-tetrahydrocannabinol for appetite stimulation in cancer-associated anorexia. *J Palliat Care* 10:14–18, 1994

195. Kardinal C, Loprinzi C, Scaid D, et al: A controlled trial of cyproheptidine in cancer patients with anorexia and/or cachexia. *Cancer* 65:2657–2662, 1990

196. Cerosimo E, Pisters P, Pesola G, et al: The effect of graded doses of insulin on peripheral glucose uptake and lactate release in cancer cachexia. *Surgery* 109:459–467, 1991

197. Cheblowski R, Heber D, Richardson B, et al: Influence of hydrazine sulfate on abnormal carbohydrate metabolism in cancer patients with weight loss. *Cancer Res* 44:857–861, 1984

198. Cheblowski R, Bulcavage M, Grosvenor M, et al. Hydrazine sulfate in cancer patients with weight loss: A placebo controlled clinical experience. *Cancer* 59:406–410, 1987

199. Kosty M, Fleishman S, Herndon J, et al: Cisplatin, vinblastine and hydrazine sulfate in advanced non–small cell lung cancer. *Proc Am Soc Clin Oncol* 11:294, 1992

200. Goldberg R, Loprinzi C, Mailliard J, et al: A randomized placebo-controlled evaluation of pentoxifylline in patients with cancer anorexia and cachexia. *Proc Am Soc Clin Oncol* 13:459, 1994

201. Cheblowski R, Herrold J, Oktay E, et al: Influence of nandrolone decanoate on weight loss in cancer patients. *Cancer* 58:183–186, 1986

202. Smith M, Holcombe J, Stullenbarger E: A meta-analysis of intervention effectiveness for symptom management in oncology nursing research. *Oncol Nurs Forum* 21:1201–1209, 1994

203. Dodd M: Measuring informational intervention for chemotherapy knowledge and self-care behavior. *Res Nurs Health* 7:43–50, 1984

# Chapter 25

# Hypercalcemia

Jennifer Lang-Kummer, RN, MN, CS, FNP

# INTRODUCTION

## Incidence

Primary hyperparathyroidism and malignancy are responsible for 90% of all cases of hypercalcemia (Table 25-1). Overall, the incidence of primary hyperparathyroidism is twice that of malignancy-associated hypercalcemia and is most commonly described as a stable, asymptomatic disorder in an outpatient population of mostly elderly women. In hospitalized populations, hypercalcemia due to malignancy is much more common because of the more severe symptomatology and the progressive nature of the syndrome when associated with cancer. Since the hypercalcemia of malignancy is frequently associated with a high tumor burden and end-stage disease, hospitalizations for malignancy-associated hypercalcemia tend to be recurrent.

Hypercalcemia is a common complication of malignancy.[1] About 10%–20% of individuals with cancer will develop hypercalcemia at some point during the course of their disease. The incidence of hypercalcemia varies with the type of cancer, primarily due to the variability of the pathogenic mechanisms and circumstances responsible for the development of the condition. Patients with lung cancer account for 25%–35% of reported cases, while 20%–40% of cases occur in patients with breast cancer. Hypercalcemia is also seen frequently in patients with multiple myeloma and with head and neck cancer, while it is rare in cancers of the stomach, duodenum,

**TABLE 25-1** Causes of Hypercalcemia

Malignancy
   Humoral hypercalcemia of malignancy (HHM)
   Local osteolytic hypercalcemia (LOH)

Granulomatous disorders
   Sarcoidosis
   Tuberculosis
   Other granulomatous diseases

Immobilization
   Spinal cord injury
   Paget's disease
   Fractures
   Space travel

Endocrine
   Hyperparathyroidism
   Hyperthyroidism
   Adrenal insufficiency
   Pheochromocytoma

Drug-induced
   Thiazides
   Vitamin D intoxication
   Vitamin A
   Total parenteral nutrition
   Lithium

Renal dialysis and transplantation

colon, rectum, biliary tract, and prostate. The reported frequencies of malignancy-associated hypercalcemia by tumor type are summarized in Table 25-2.

Tumor histology is also a factor in the development of hypercalcemia in cancer patients. Although rare in patients with small-cell lung cancer, 23% of patients with squamous epidermoid cancer of the lung and 13% of those with large-cell anaplastic cancer of the lung will develop hypercalcemia.[6] Squamous histology also is the predominant feature for esophageal, head and neck, and many female reproductive system tumors, together making up 20% of cases.[7,8]

The high frequency of breast and lung cancer diagnoses among patients with hypercalcemia is related to the high overall incidence of these two types of cancers. Multiple myeloma, a relatively rare cancer, is the primary diagnosis in 10% of malignancy-associated cases. However, one-third of patients with multiple myeloma develop hypercalcemia.

Hypercalcemia of malignancy is usually progressive, causes unpleasant symptoms, can cause the patient to deteriorate rapidly, and may be the cause of death in some patients refractory to treatment. In the early stages, symptoms may be vague and nonspecific and can be confused with symptoms resulting from treatments such as radiation therapy, chemotherapy or biologic response modifiers, brain metastases, or progressive disease. The pathophysiology of hypercalcemia is complex, varies with tumor characteristics, and usually involves at least two basic mechanisms: increased bone resorption and decreased renal calcium clearance.

Uncorrected hypercalcemia leads to dehydration, renal failure, coma, and death. The availability of new generations of bisphosphonates and a growing understanding of the pathophysiology of malignancy-associated hypercalcemia (MAHC) has significantly expanded the options for prevention and management of hypercalcemia. Nurses play an important role in recognition of patients at risk, patient and family teaching, early recognition and monitoring of response to symptoms and response to treatment, and, when all else fails, assisting the patient and family in the terminal phases of the illness.

## Definition

The normal range of serum calcium in adults is 8.5–10.5 mg/dl (2.13–2.63 mmol/l). Hypercalcemia is considered to exist when the serum calcium level exceeds 11.0 mg/dl (2.75 mmol/l).

# PHYSIOLOGY OF CALCIUM HOMEOSTASIS

Calcium is essential for the maintenance of bones, teeth, clotting mechanisms, and intracellular metabolism. The majority of calcium (99%) is found in bone combined

**TABLE 25-2** Frequency of Malignancy-Associated Hypercalcemia

| Tumor Type | Fisken et al[2] (1980) | Fisken et al[3] (1981) | Mundy and Martin[4] (1982) | Blomqvist[5] (1986) | Combined Data No. | % |
|---|---|---|---|---|---|---|
| Lung | 54 | 24 | 25 | 24 | 127 | 27.3 |
| Breast | 44 | 20 | 18 | 33 | 115 | 25.7 |
| Multiple myeloma | 14 | 7 | 5 | 8 | 34 | 7.3 |
| Lymphoma/leukemia | 9 | 3 | 5 | 3 | 20 | 4.3 |
| Head and neck | 15 | 7 | 4 | 6 | 32 | 6.9 |
| Renal | 7 | 6 | 2 | 5 | 20 | 4.3 |
| Prostate | 3 | 1 | 2 | | 6 | 1.3 |
| Gastrointestinal | 9 | 4 | 4 | 2 | 19 | 4.1 |
| Esophagus | 13 | 4 | | 2 | 19 | 4.1 |
| Ureters, bladder, urethra | 15 | | | | 15 | 3.2 |
| Female genital | 14 | 2 | | | 16 | 3.4 |
| Others | 12 | 4 | 2 | 2 | 20 | 4.3 |
| Unknown primary | 10 | 7 | 5 | — | 22 | 4.7 |
| Total patients | 219 | 89 | 72 | 85 | 465 | |

Data have been combined from references 2–5 as follows: a 1-year prospective general hospital review,[2] a prospective general hospital review,[3] a 32-month retrospective general hospital review,[4] and a 1-year prospective oncology hospital review.[5]

with phosphate. The remaining 1% is divided evenly in the plasma between protein-bound (primarily albumin) and freely ionized forms. It is the freely ionized form that is biologically active. Maintenance of extracellular levels of ionized calcium within a narrow range is important for optimal function of numerous cellular and organ functions. Because of the important role extracellular calcium plays in influencing cell membrane permeability, alterations in extracellular calcium levels will affect nerve excitability and muscle contractility.

## Normal Calcium Homeostasis

Extracellular calcium levels are controlled tightly within a narrow range, primarily through the effects of three systemic hormones: parathyroid hormone (PTH), 1,25-dihydroxyvitamin D (the major biologically active metabolite of vitamin D), and calcitonin. Circulating levels of ionized calcium influence the secretion of each of these hormones through three negative-feedback loops. PTH and 1,25-dihydroxyvitamin D influence extracellular calcium levels by controlling calcium transport across three organs: bone, kidney, and small intestine.

Although 99% of the body's calcium is stored in the skeleton, bone makes little contribution to calcium homeostasis in the healthy adult. The ability to control extracellular calcium levels is influenced primarily by the rate of calcium absorption from the intestine and the kidney's threshold for calcium resorption. Renal regulation of

calcium is controlled by PTH and 1,25-dihydroxyvitamin D. Only when pathological states involving increased bone resorption (e.g., some malignancies, Paget's disease) occur do other homeostatic mechanisms come into play.

### Calcitonin

Secreted by thyroid parafollicular cells, calcitonin inhibits bone resorption and thus acts as a counterregulator to PTH. In healthy adults, calcitonin appears to play a minor role in calcium homeostasis, since abnormalities in calcium levels do not occur in the absence of the thyroid gland. However, calcitonin can be an important inhibitor of bone resorption in pathological states, although its effects are transient.

### Parathyroid hormone

Secreted by the parathyroid gland, PTH prevents serum calcium concentration from falling below the normal level directly by stimulating bone resorption and calcium liberation from the bony matrix and by calcium resorption in the renal tubules, and indirectly by influencing intestinal calcium absorption. The direct effect of PTH on the kidney is to rapidly regulate and fine-tune calcium balance. Normally, the kidneys filter approximately 10 g of calcium each day, 98% of which is resorbed by the tubules, resulting in a net excretion of 150–200 mg/day. A fall in plasma calcium concentration stimulates the release of PTH and increased renal absorption of calcium. The primary role of PTH on the kidney appears to be maintenance of extracellular calcium levels between 7.5 and 11.5 mg/dl. Outside of that range, the ability of PTH to regulate extracellular fluid calcium levels is quite limited.[9]

Sixty-five percent of calcium filtered by the glomerulus is resorbed in the proximal tubules, 20%–25% in the ascending limb of Henle's loop, and 10% in the distal convoluted tubules. In the proximal tubule, calcium resorption is closely linked with sodium and water resorption and is not influenced by PTH. Since phosphate resorption is inversely related to calcium resorption, PTH's actions in the proximal tubule are directed at inhibition of water, sodium, calcium, bicarbonate, and phosphate resorption.[10] When patients are dehydrated, renal blood flow is decreased and sodium resorption is enhanced. Calcium resorption accompanies sodium resorption, so dehydration can potentiate hypercalcemia by this mechanism.[9] PTH-mediated resorption of calcium occurs in the ascending limb of Henle's loop and in the distal tubule. In the distal convoluted tubule, about 1000 mg is resorbed daily and is under the effect of PTH enhanced by 1,25-dihydroxyvitamin D.[9–11] In healthy individuals the fractional excretion of calcium increases as the serum calcium increases to the point at which renal capability for calcium excretion is exceeded, usually 600 mg/day.[9,11]

In the skeleton, PTH plays a mediating role in bone resorption by stimulating the number and activity of bone osteoclasts, leading to the release of calcium and phosphate into the circulation. The exact mechanisms through which this occurs have not yet been identified.

## 1,25-dihydroxyvitamin D

Vitamin D is hydroxylated from 25-hydroxyvitamin D by enzymes found in the liver, gut, and kidney. 25-Hydroxyvitamin D is the major circulating and storage form of vitamin D. In the proximal tubules of the kidney, 25-hydroxyvitamin D is hydroxylated by 1-alpha-hydroxylase to 1,25-dihydroxyvitamin D, primarily under the influence of PTH.

In the gastrointestinal (GI) tract, 1,25-dihydroxyvitamin D stimulates the absorption of dietary calcium in response to low circulating levels of calcium. The net absorption of calcium from the gut is roughly equal to renal calcium excretion, about 150–200 mg/day. Calcium is absorbed from the gut through an active transport process and a passive diffusion process. While both of these processes are complex and imperfectly understood, the active transport process appears to occur through calcium binding with a protein regulated by 1,25-dihydroxyvitamin D. The passive diffusion process also appears to be mediated by 1,25-dihydroxyvitamin D.[9] Dietary intake of calcium influences the efficiency of calcium absorption from the gut. 1,25-Dihydroxyvitamin D acts to increase efficiency of calcium absorption when dietary calcium intake decreases. While the effect of PTH

on renal resorption of calcium occurs on a minute-to-minute basis, 1,25-dihydroxyvitamin D's effect on intestinal calcium absorption is less responsive to immediate changes in serum calcium levels and thus is responsible primarily for chronic calcium homeostasis.

A number of disease states influence circulating levels of 1,25-dihydroxyvitamin D and thus intestinal calcium absorption. In some types of hypercalcemia, 1,25-dihydroxyvitamin D levels may be increased, probably through extrarenal synthesis of 1,25-dihydroxyvitamin D, and include primary hyperparathyroidism, sarcoidosis, and T-cell or B-cell lymphomas.

In addition to its effect on calcium absorption in the gut, 1,25-dihydroxyvitamin D works in concert with PTH by acting directly on bone calcium mobilization by stimulating osteoclastic bone resorption and enhancing osteoblastic bone mineralization. In the bone marrow, 1,25-dihydroxyvitamin D plays an important role in the differentiation of cells of the monocyte-macrophage lineage and in enhancing the production of interleukin-1 by monocyte-macrophage cells.

In the kidney, 1,25-dihydroxyvitamin D works in concert with PTH to enhance calcium resorption and against PTH to enhance phosphate resorption.

## Homeostatic responses to increased calcium loads

With an increased extracellular fluid calcium load, the secretion of PTH is suppressed; this decreases physiological calcium release from bone and inhibits intestinal calcium resorption. This inhibitory effect occurs as a result of decreased renal synthesis of 1,25-dihydroxyvitamin D. In addition, decreased PTH results in increased urinary calcium excretion. The kidney is the principal route by which a calcium load can be cleared. To protect against an increased extracellular calcium level of hypercalcemic proportions, the kidney can increase calcium excretion approximately fivefold to a maximum of approximately 600 mg/day.[9] Mild hypercalcemia impairs glomerular filtration and urinary concentrating ability, creating a polyuric state. This predisposes a patient to dehydration and prerenal azotemia. Once the renal compensatory mechanisms are exceeded, further renal insufficiency enhances calcium resorption and phosphate wasting in the proximal tubule, further exacerbating the development of hypercalcemia and renal failure.

## The role of bone in calcium homeostasis

Skeletal bone serves as the body's calcium reservoir. In the healthy adult before middle life, bone resorption and formation are in balance and occur as a renewal process in response to the need for repair and to local mechanical factors such as weight bearing and fluid pressure. Only small amounts of skeletal calcium are exchanged daily with the extracellular fluid, and under most circumstances the exchange of calcium with extracellular fluid by the process of bone resorption and bone formation is in balance. However, in disease states skeletal calcium plays a larger role in extracellular calcium levels. There are two mechanisms through which skeletal calcium can enter extracellular fluid: bone remodeling and calcium exchange between the bone surface and extracellular fluid. This second mechanism is not well understood.

### Bone remodeling

The bone cells primarily concerned with the process of bone formation and resorption, known as *bone remodeling*, are the osteoclasts, osteocytes, and osteoblasts (Table 25-3). Incitement of bone remodeling is thought to be directed at the osteocyte, which prepares the bone surface for osteoclastic activity and liberates chemical messengers that not only attract osteoclasts but also initiate osteoblast precursor proliferation.[12] Thus, normal bone remodeling activity can be said to be "coupled" both geographically and chronologically; bone resorption is coupled with bone formation. "Uncoupling" refers to the failure of bone formation to follow the resorption process.[13]

The process of bone remodeling occurs in discrete units throughout the skeleton, and the location and frequency of bone remodeling activity appear to be influenced primarily by mechanical factors such as weight bearing; by the activity of the osteotropic hormones PTH, 1,25-dihydroxyvitamin D, and calcitonin; and by the presence of local factors such as cytokines, growth factors, prostaglandins, regulatory proteins, and constituents of the organic matrix.[9,12,14]

Local events lead to an increase in osteoclast activity that involves the formation of a mature multinucleated osteoclast from its precursor, differentiation of the committed progenitors, and then activation of the preformed cell. Bone is resorbed by the osteoclast through a process of extracellular degradation and proteolysis. The resorption phase of the remodeling process lasts for approximately ten days and is followed by a reversal process. In the reversal process, osteoclastic resorption ceases and the resorption bay is occupied by mononuclear cells.

Thereafter a team of osteoblasts aggregates at the resorption site, and repair of the defect and bone formation follow.[9] The repair and bone formation process is estimated to take three to five months. The action of PTH promotes the cellular differentiation of osteocytes, osteoblasts, and their precursors, while 1,25-dihydroxyvitamin D promotes the differentiation and fusion of osteoclasts (Table 25-4). At physiological levels of these hormones, bone remodeling takes place in an orderly and coupled manner (Figure 25-1). High levels of PTH and 1,25-dihydroxyvitamin D, on the other hand, stimulate large volumes of osteocytic and osteoclastic breakdown and resorption of calcified matrix.[10] Osteoclast growth factors and cytokines include the bone-resorbing cytokines interleukin-1 and interleukin-6 (IL-1 and IL-6), tumor necrosis factor (TNF), and transforming growth factors alpha and beta (TGF-alpha and TGF-beta).[9,15] An elevated serum acid phosphatase can indicate the presence of osteoclastic bone catabolism, as seen in metastatic skeletal involvement as well as in other disease states. An elevated serum alkaline phosphatase indicates osteoblastic activity, which can be seen in states of high bone turnover: Paget's disease, prostate cancer with blastic skeletal involvement, or healing of a bone fracture.

Since normal bone remodeling is a coupled process, skeletal calcium generally plays an insignificant role in calcium homeostasis. Although not important to the understanding of calcium homeostasis in the healthy adult, local and humoral factors that influence the liberation of calcium from bone in pathological states assume more significance.

## Pathophysiology

MAHC is a complex metabolic complication of hematologic malignancies, solid tumors with bone metastases, and solid tumors in the absence of bone metastases. Disruption of normal calcium homeostasis is caused by the action of tumor-produced factors on bone, kidney, and intestine. The two primary pathophysiological defects are

---

**TABLE 25-3** Cells Responsible for Bone Remodeling

| Cell | Origin | Function |
|------|--------|----------|
| Osteoblasts | Undifferentiated mesenchymatous cells | Bone-forming cells that secrete collagen; differentiation is promoted by PTH |
| Osteocytes | Osteoblasts buried within osteocytic lacunae in bone matrix | Responsive to PTH; liberate collagenase, which prepares bone surface for osteoclast resorption; communicate with osteoclasts through liberation of prostaglandin E |
| Osteoclasts | Mononuclear* bone marrow cells | Multinuclear bone cells that erode and resorb previously formed bone; chemotactic factors attract to osteocyte prepared bone; differentiation and fusion promoted by IL-1, 1,25-dihydroxyvitamin D; function inhibited by calcitonin |

*Osteoclast precursors are mononuclear cells that fuse to form large multinuclear units.
*PTH*, parathyroid hormone.
Adapted from Taylor BM, Weller LA: Hypercalcemia, in Groenwald SL (ed): *Cancer Nursing: Principles and Practice* (ed 1). 1987, p. 292.

**TABLE 25-4**  Hormonal Mediators of Calcium Homeostasis and Bone Remodeling

| Organ | Parathyroid Hormone | 1,25-dihydroxyvitamin D | Calcitonin |
|---|---|---|---|
| | Secreted by parathyroid gland in response to ↓ Ca++ | Synthesized in liver, kidney, and gut | Secreted by thyroid parafollicular cells in response to ↑ Ca++ |
| Bone | Promotes coupled bone remodeling through stimulation of osteocyte activity, number and activity of osteoclasts, differentiation of osteoblasts | Promotes differentiation and fusion of osteoclasts, differentiation of cells of monocyte lineage, stimulation of osteoclasts and osteoblast bone mineralization | Inhibits osteoclast bone resorption |
| Kidney | Maintains serum Ca++ levels between 7.5 and 11.5 mg/dl; mediates calcium resorption in Henle's loop and distal tubule; influences renal hydroxylation of 25-hydroxyvitamin D to 1,25-dihydroxyvitamin D | Enhances Ca++ resorption in concert with PTH in distal tubule; enhances PO4 resorption | |
| Small intestine | | Stimulates absorption of dietary Ca++ through active transport and passive diffusion | |

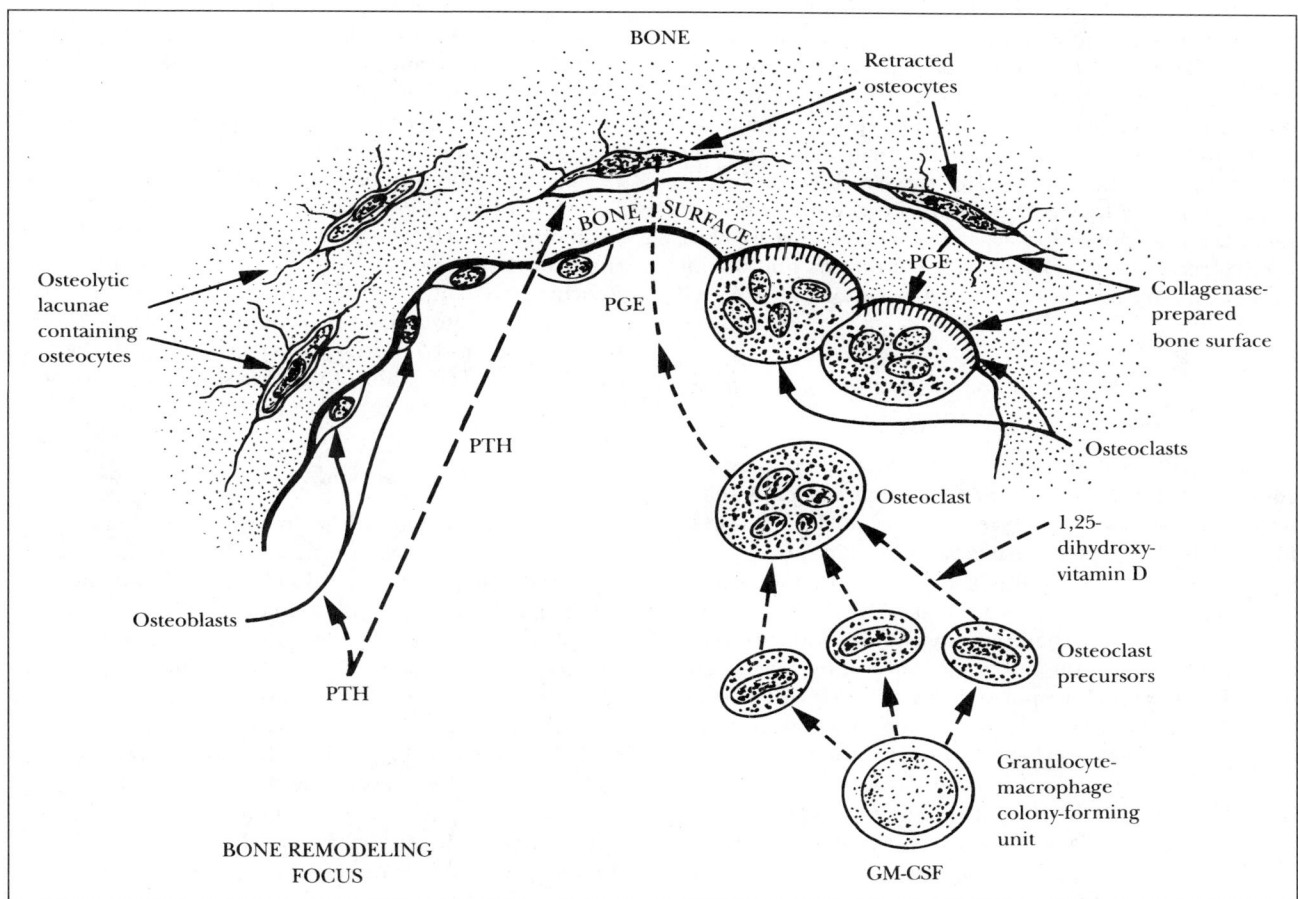

**FIGURE 25-1**  Coupled bone remodeling. *Bone Resorption:* Osteocytes retract within lacunae under the influence of PTH, liberating collagenase and messengers such as PGE. Collagenase prepares the bone surface for osteoclast resorption. The presence of PGE attracts osteoclasts to the bone surface. Osteoclast precursors, derived from granulocyte-macrophage colony-forming units, differentiate and fuse to form multinuclear osteoclasts under the influence of 1,25-dihydroxyvitamin D. *Bone Formation:* Osteoblasts differentiate under the influence of PTH, secreting collagen and mineralizing bone. Some osteoblasts become buried within osteocytic lacunae during the bone-forming process to become osteocytes. Osteoblasts recycle Ca++ liberated during the bone resorption process to mineralize new bone. (PTH, parathyroid hormone; PGE, prostaglandin E; GM-CSF, granulocyte-macrophage colony-stimulating factor.)

**TABLE 25-5**   Humoral Hypercalcemia of Malignancy

| Factor | Source | Action |
|---|---|---|
| PTHrP | Tumor cells | ↑ osteocyte and osteoclast activity; ↓ osteoblast activity (uncoupled bone resorption); ↑ renal calcium resorption and phosphate wasting; no stimulation of renal 1,25-dihydroxyvitamin D synthesis ≥ no ↑ intestinal Ca⁺⁺ transport |
| 1,25-dihydroxyvitamin D | Tumor-produced hydroxylase, which converts circulating substrates to 1,25-dihydroxyvitamin D; (?) synthesis by disease-activated macrophages | Enhanced intestinal Ca⁺⁺ transport; ↑ differentiation and fusion of osteoclast precursors; ↑ bone resorption |
| TGF-alpha | Most solid tumors | ↑ production of osteoclast progenitors, osteoclast activation; (?) stimulation of PGE |

enhanced osteoclastic bone resorption, which exceeds bone formation and the ability of the kidney to excrete extracellular calcium. Hypercalcemia impairs renal mechanisms that lead to calcium and sodium excretion. Our current understanding of MAHC is that there are two primary syndromes: humoral hypercalcemia of malignancy (HHM) and local osteolytic hypercalcemia (LOH), depending on whether a circulating hormone or local paracrine factors enhance bone resorption. While this delineation seems quite precise, the reality appears to be that both humoral and local factors are involved in the development of hypercalcemia in individuals with bone metastases. Tumors also release factors that increase renal tubular resorption of calcium. Rarely, tumors release vitamin D, which increases calcium absorption from the GI tract.

### Parathyroid hormone–related protein and humoral hypercalcemia of malignancy

HHM shares many factors with primary hyperparathyroidism, and it was this observation that led many scientists to believe that PTH played a role in MAHC. However, in the late 1980s, several investigators identified a previously unknown 141–amino acid peptide that was highly homologous to but not exactly like PTH.[16–19] Now it is generally accepted that parathyroid hormone–related protein (PTHrP) is the major mediator of hypercalcemia of malignancy and is responsible for 80%–90% of all cases of MAHC (Table 25-5). Since its identification in tumor tissue, PTHrP has also been found in normal keratinocytes, placenta, and fetal parathyroid glands, indicating that in addition to its role in mediating hypercalcemia in cancer it also plays an important endocrine role in the fetus and perhaps is implicated as a paracrine factor in a number of normal physiological processes.[19,20]

PTHrP stimulates adenylate cyclase in target tissues via PTH and PTHrP receptors, and while PTHrP stimulates some, it does not stimulate all PTH receptors, thus causing some but not all possible PTH effects. Individuals with HHM do not have elevated levels of 1,25-dihydroxyvitamin D and do not have increased levels of intestinal calcium absorption as is seen with elevated PTH levels

in primary hyperparathyroidism. Additionally, HHM is accompanied by an uncoupling of osteoblastic and osteoclastic activities such that bone resorption exceeds bone formation, and hypercalcemia and hypercalciuria occur to a greater degree than that which occurs with primary hyperparathyroidism. Considered the primary cause of hypercalcemia in solid tumors without bone metastases, the hypercalcemic effect of PTHrP is related to increased bone resorption, increased renal tubular calcium resorption, and phosphate wasting.

Several authors have suggested that PTHrP may be responsible for the hypercalcemic/hypophosphatemic renal effects of HHM, while another agent such as TGF-alpha works in concert with PTHrP to enhance bone-resorbing activity.[8,11,14,21–23] There is evidence that osteoclast-activating factors produced by both tumors and normal host immune cells act synergistically with PTHrP and TGF-alpha to increase bone resorption through osteoclast activation (Table 25-6).[14,15,23,24]

### 1,25-dihydroxyvitamin D

Several investigators have reported the presence of elevated levels of circulating 1,25-dihydroxyvitamin D in hypercalcemic patients with Hodgkin's disease and non-Hodgkin's lymphoma without bony metastases that resolved with effective treatment of the primary disease.[25–29] Proposed mechanisms of action are tumor production of 1-alpha-hydroxylase, which acts on the circulating substrate 25-hydroxyvitamin D to produce, independent of PTH, high circulating levels of 1,25-dihydroxyvitamin D that enhance bone resorption and increased intestinal transport,[28,30] monocyte-macrophage synthesis of 25-hydroxyvitamin D; and synthesis of 1,25-dihydroxyvitamin D or its precursor by disease-activated macrophages.[31]

### Other osteolytic factors

The cause of hypercalcemia in cancer patients with skeletal metastases such as breast cancer, multiple myeloma, and lymphoma is more heterogeneous, particularly in breast cancer. Many cancers invoke their hypercalcemic effect through a combination of humoral

**TABLE 25-6** Osteoclast-Activating Factors in Local Osteolytic Hypercalcemia

| Osteoclast-Activating Factor | Osteocytes | Osteoblasts | Sources Tumor Cells | Monocytes | Lymphocytes |
|---|---|---|---|---|---|
| Interleukin-1 (IL-1) | | X | X | X | |
| Interleukin-6 (IL-6) | | X | X | | |
| Prostaglandin E (PGE) | X | | X | X | |
| Tumor necrosis factor alpha (TNF-alpha) | | X | X | | |
| Tumor necrosis factor beta (TNF-beta) | | | X | X | |
| Interferon gamma (IFN-gamma) | | | | | X |
| Granulocyte-macrophage colony-stimulating factor (GM-CSF) | | | X | | X |
| Macrophage colony-stimulating factor (M-CSF) | | | X | X | X |
| Procathepsin D | | | X | | |
| Transforming growth factor alpha (TGF-alpha) | | | X | | |
| Transforming growth factor beta (TGF-beta) | | | X | | |

and local cell-mediated mechanisms. Three cellular mediators of osteolysis are proposed: osteoclasts, tumor-associated macrophages, and cancer cells.[14,15,17] The activities of these cellular mediators are influenced in a paracrine manner by the presence of one or more of the osteoclast-activating cytokines and growth factors: TGF-alpha and TGF-beta, IL-1 and IL-6, granulocyte-macrophage and granulocyte colony-stimulating factors (GM-CSF/G-CSF), and TNF-alpha and TNF-beta. Each of these factors has been found to be secreted by certain solid and hematologic tumors.[14,15,24,32,33]

## Local osteolytic hypercalcemia

The bone matrix contains growth factors and cytokines involved in the activation and differentiation of bone cells, while the bone marrow is rich in growth factors and cytokines normally involved in hematopoiesis. This environment, along with the presence of specific adherence molecules on tumor cell surfaces, makes the trabecular bone matrix particularly attractive to certain metastatic cancer cells.[15] Once adhered to bone, tumor cell–derived osteoclast-activating factors such as PTHrP, prostaglandin E (PGE), IL-1, IL-6, and TNF not only are capable of causing the development of HHM but also are thought to act as local osteoclast activators.[34] Recruitment and activation of osteoclasts appear to be essential to the development of bone metastases.[34] In animal models the development of bone metastases is associated with decreases in trabecular bone, increased numbers of osteoclasts, and virtual elimination of osteoblasts.[15]

***Breast cancer*** In breast cancer patients with hypercalcemia and bone metastases, 70%–80% will have elevated circulating levels of PTHrP and 50% will have raised urinary cyclic AMP levels, indicating an important role for PTHrP-induced hypercalcemia even when bone metastases are present.[14] Many cancers appear to invoke their hypercalcemic effect through a combination of humoral and local cellmediated mechanisms. In addition to TGF-alpha and the osteoclast-activating factors discussed earlier, other implicated factors include prostaglandins of the E series (PGE) and procathepsin D.[14] $PGE_2$ is a potent osteoclast stimulator that has been demonstrated to mediate hypercalcemia by stimulating bone resorption in several animal models. It is known that hormonally manipulated breast cancer cells do release prostaglandins.[11] Hypercalcemia in breast cancer patients is generally unresponsive to prostaglandin inhibitors, making understanding of the precise role of PGE in the pathogenesis of hypercalcemia difficult.

Hypercalcemia occurs in up to 40% of women with breast cancer.[35] Although the majority of individuals with hypercalcemia have widespread metastases, not all patients with metastases develop hypercalcemia.[35,36] Hypercalcemia and bone lesions are more common in estrogen receptor–positive tumors; in those patients in whom hypercalcemia occurs, extensive bone metastases are almost always present.[9]

While cultured breast cancer cells have been shown to resorb bone directly in vitro through tumor secretion of lysosomal enzymes and collagenase,[37] new evidence indicates that direct bone resorption by tumor cells is a minor component of the bone destruction that occurs with metastatic cancer.[22,33] The fact that hypercalcemia of breast cancer is generally responsive to osteoclast inhibitors indicates that osteoclast activation is the major mechanism associated with hypercalcemia.[9,33] Factors not produced by tumor cells also may be responsible for increased bone resorption at the metastatic site. The presence of breast cancer cells at the bone surface may be sufficient to stimulate a cell-mediated immune response and production of TNF-alpha or TNF-beta or IL-1, all of which are potent bone-resorbing factors. Some women with estrogen receptor–positive metastatic breast cancer treated with estrogens or antiestrogens suddenly develop hypercalcemia that may be associated with bone pain within one month of starting estrogens, androgens, or tamoxifen. Known as *tumor flare*, this response is associated with a temporary period of accelerated tumor growth shortly after beginning additive hormonal therapy. Tamoxifen-induced hypercalcemia occurs four to ten days after the initiation of hormonal therapy and has a rapid onset.[38] Tumor flare is generally self-limiting and is thought to indicate a hormonally responsive tumor. A decision to temporarily withdraw the hormone or to treat the patient with a bisphosphonate such as pamidronate without terminating the hormonal agent is usually influenced by the degree of hypercalcemia and its responsiveness to therapy.

***Hematologic malignancies*** Multiple myeloma is one of the malignancies most frequently associated with hypercalcemia, which occurs in 20%–40% of all individuals with myeloma at some time during the disease.[33,39] Hypercalcemia is more common in myeloma than in any other hematologic malignancy and can be either a presenting symptom or an indicator of terminal disease. Intractable bone pain is a prominent presenting symptom in 80% of patients.[40] Hypercalcemia in myeloma can be expected whenever patients become bedridden and may be caused by or contribute to renal failure.[41] While 50% of patients with multiple myeloma have elevated circulating PTHrP levels,[42] the pathophysiology of hypercalcemia in myeloma is different from that in most solid tumors. In most solid tumors, increased bone resorption and decreased urine calcium excretion are the cause. However, in myeloma the cause is increased bone resorption and decreased glomerular filtration.[43] Hypercalcemia in patients with myeloma is almost always accompanied by renal insufficiency due to impaired glomerular filtration caused by Bence Jones protein, uric acid nephropathy; pyelonephritis; or occasionally amyloidosis, which results in an inability to clear ultrafilterable calcium through the glomerulus.[11,39,43]

Hypercalcemia in myeloma always occurs in the presence of extensive bone destruction occurring adjacent to collections of myeloma cells.[33] In addition to PTHrP, other osteoclast-activating factors probably play a significant role. Whether these factors are produced by tumors or by normal immune cells in response to the presence of myeloma cells is not clear. In addition to the increased osteoclastic activity that takes place in myeloma, there is also evidence to support the presence of decreased osteoblastic activity as part of the pathological process.[33,40]

Hypercalcemia in patients with B-cell lymphomas is uncommon, occurring in up to 4% of cases.[41] However, HTLV-I and HTLV-II-associated adult T-cell lymphoma/leukemias (ATLL) are frequently associated with hypercalcemia, occurring in as many as 50% of patients.[9,44] In lymphomas, hypercalcemia is usually seen in patients with bone involvement, but humoral factors have also been found to play a part. As discussed previously, elevated levels of 1,25-dihydroxyvitamin D have been found in lymphoma patients without bone metastases. The presence of PTHrP has been demonstrated in more than half of patients with myeloma and ATLL, indicating that HHM is involved in some cases.[45–47] The osteoclast-activating factors IL-1, TNF-alpha, and TNF-beta have also been implicated as causes of hypercalcemia in these individuals. Most likely the cause of hypercalcemia will be found to be a combination of tumor-produced humoral and local osteoclast-activating factors. What differentiates the hypercalcemia found in myeloma from that found in lymphomas is the presence of renal insufficiency associated with myeloma.

***Other factors*** Immobilization, dehydration, poor nutrition, inappropriate use of diuretics, and generalized wasting all play important roles in the pathogenesis of malignancy-associated hypercalcemia.

Local mechanical forces such as weight bearing are important to stimulate osteoblast function and bone formation. Individuals with a preexisting state of high bone turnover are more likely to experience increased hypercalciuria and bone resorption when immobilized. Passive range-of-motion exercises may be useful in maintaining muscle and joint mobility but are not helpful in preventing hypercalcemia due to immobilization. Weight bearing is more important. Dehydration occurs as a result of diminished fluid intake (due to nausea, vomiting, or anorexia) as well as polyuria and inability to concentrate urine due to hypercalcemic interference with the effects of antidiuretic hormone (ADH) on the tubules.

Thiazide and potassium-sparing diuretics act on the distal tubule to enhance calcium but not sodium reabsorption. Thus, administration of such diuretics produces not only volume depletion but also a hypercalcemic effect.

## CLINICAL MANIFESTATIONS

The clinical presentation of hypercalcemia is variable, influenced not only by the degree of hypercalcemia, the rapidity of onset, and the patient's general physical and mental condition but also by the kidney's ability to maintain calcium homeostasis. Hypercalcemia that develops slowly and gradually is associated with few, if any, symptoms. Conversely, a rapidly expanding tumor burden associated with a progressively increasing rate of bone resorption may suddenly overwhelm renal compensatory mechanisms, producing a rapid and symptomatic rise in serum calcium levels. This is particularly true in HHM.

### Signs and Symptoms

Because of calcium's role in maintaining cell membrane permeability, hypercalcemia produces symptoms in almost all organ systems. Symptoms are numerous, vague, and nonspecific. Since many cancer patients with hypercalcemia have large tumor burdens and frequently die in less than six months (particularly those with HHM), symptoms of hypercalcemia may be confused with those of end-stage disease. Recognition of symptoms is important for early identification and treatment of the syndrome to reduce the risk of coma, irreversible renal failure, or a terminal cardiac event (Table 25-7). The symptomatology of hypercalcemia is potentially reversible

**TABLE 25-7**   Symptoms of Hypercalcemia

| System | Mechanism | Signs and Symptoms |
|---|---|---|
| Gastrointestinal | Depressed smooth muscle contractility causes delayed gastric emptying and decreased intestinal motility | Early: nausea, vomiting, anorexia, constipation<br>Late: obstipation and ileus; weight loss |
| Neuromuscular | Depressed excitability of neurons | Early: lethargy, drowsiness; restlessness, mood changes<br>Mid: mental status changes, poor calculation, decreased attention span, somnolence<br>Late: psychotic behavior, marked confusion, slurred speech, stupor, coma |
| | Impaired electrical conduction and cell membrane permeability in skeletal muscles | Early: muscle weakness, fatigue<br>Late: profound muscle weakness, hypotonia |
| | ? PGE-mediated bone resorption | Bone pain |
| Renal | Interference with action of ADH on renal collecting tubules → inability to concentrate urine and then volume contraction followed by ↓ GFR | Early: polyuria<br>Mid: polydipsia<br>Late: prerenal azotemia |
| Cardiovascular | Impaired electrical conduction and cell membrane permeability; altered intracellular metabolism; arterial vasoconstriction | Early: hypertension<br>Mid: sinus bradycardia, prolonged PR interval, shortened QT interval, dysrhythmias especially in digitalized patients<br>Late: prolonged QT interval due to widened T wave, coving of ST segment, AV block, asystole |

*ADH,* antidiuretic hormone; *GFR,* glomerular filtration rate; *PGE,* prostaglandin E; *Early,* mild hypercalcemia (<12 mg/dl); *Mid,* moderate hypercalcemia (12–15 mg/dl); Late, severe hypercalcemia (>15 mg/dl).

with treatment, and active treatment correlates with a better outlook and improved quality of life. However, it is most important to remember that the development of malignant hypercalcemia is usually associated with an extremely poor prognosis.[48] Common symptoms of hypercalcemia in order of reported frequency are fatigue, anorexia, weight loss, bone pain, constipation, polydipsia, muscle weakness, nausea and vomiting, mental changes, and polyuria.[1]

### Gastrointestinal

Elevated extracellular calcium levels depress smooth muscle contractility, leading to delayed gastric emptying and decreased GI motility. Anorexia, nausea, vomiting, abdominal pain, and constipation are early and common symptoms in hypercalcemic individuals. These symptoms may be exacerbated by the disease itself or by cytotoxic therapy. The development of obstipation and ileus are late findings associated with high serum calcium levels and are probably exacerbated by dehydration.

### Neuromuscular

Elevated extracellular calcium levels affect both the central nervous system (CNS) and neuromuscular function. Initial CNS dysfunction can present as personality changes, impaired concentration, mild confusion, drowsiness, and lethargy. Patients with rapidly advancing hypercalcemia may lapse into stupor or coma, usually at serum calcium levels > 15 mg/dl. Neurological manifestations are usually much more prominent in the elderly and

may persist for several days after normalization of serum calcium levels.

Personality changes occur subtly and often are unnoticed by the family or individual. Extreme restlessness, irritability, overt confusion, and progressive deterioration in cognitive function may develop. In a study of hospitalized patients with hypercalcemia, Mahon[49] reported increasing problems with memory span and attention span, inability to calculate, inappropriate conversation, slow mentation, and inappropriate behavior in patients with corrected serum calcium levels greater than 12.1 mg/dl.

Neuromuscular involvement is primarily neuropathic, involving decreased muscle strength and a decrease in respiratory muscular capacity. Impairment of skeletal muscle electrical conduction and cell membrane permeability leads to profound muscle weakness and hypotonia, usually with severe hypercalcemia.

### Renal

Hypercalcemia interferes with the action of ADH on the kidney's collecting tubules, causing an inability to concentrate urine and polyuria (a syndrome similar to nephrogenic diabetes insipidus). Subsequent volume contraction, which is exacerbated by nausea and vomiting, decreases the glomerular filtration rate (GFR). Decreased GFR stimulates sodium and water reabsorption in the proximal tubule. Since sodium and calcium are absorbed in parallel, hypercalcemia is exacerbated. In addition, evidence indicates that TGF-alpha also acts on the kidney's proximal tubule to enhance the resorption of calcium, while distal tubular calcium resorption is influenced by PTH and PTHrP. The downward spiral continues with the development of nitrogen retention, acidosis, and eventual renal failure. Renal failure is most common in patients with multiple myeloma.

### Cardiovascular

Calcium ions not only affect smooth, skeletal, and cardiac muscle contractility and cell membrane permeability but also influence conduction of electrical impulses within the heart. Hypertension may occur due to the direct effect of hypercalcemia on arterial smooth muscle. Hypercalcemia results in bradycardia, shortened QT intervals in moderate hypercalcemia, and prolonged QT intervals in moderate hypercalcemia, and prolonged QT intervals with calcium levels above 16 mg/dl. Prolonged QT intervals are due to widening of the T wave, with coving of the ST segment.[50] Prolonged PR intervals and significant dysrhythmias may also occur, particularly in patients taking digitalis.[51] Since the effects of digitalis are mediated partly by membrane-bound calcium, digitalis toxicity may be potentiated.[49] Atrioventricular block and asystole may occur when the serum calcium level reaches 18 mg/dl.[49,52]

### Laboratory Assessment

An elevated serum calcium level (corrected for abnormal protein values) is diagnostic. Calcium is found in the serum in three forms: 45% protein-bound (primarily to albumin), 45% freely ionized, and 10% complexed to ions such as sulfate, phosphate, or citrate. It is the freely ionized form that is biologically active. Normally, freely ionized calcium is in equilibrium with protein-bound calcium. When there is an abnormality in serum protein levels, serum calcium determinations may not represent true ionized calcium levels. Rarely, in multiple myeloma, a monoclonal protein may have an affinity for calcium and be associated with elevated protein-bound but normal ionized calcium levels, thus creating an illusion of an elevated serum calcium level. The more common finding in individuals with cancer is hypoalbuminemia, in which more calcium may be ionized due to low levels of serum albumin available for binding. Ionized serum calcium levels provide a more accurate means of measuring calcium when serum proteins are abnormal. A normal serum calcium is 8.5–10.5 mg/dl (2.13–2.63 mmol/l), while a normal serum ionized calcium level is 4.2–5.2 mg/dl (1.05–1.3 mmol/l). When ionized calcium levels are not available, total serum calcium levels can be corrected to more accurately reflect ionized serum calcium. A frequently used formula is

Corrected calcium (mg/dl) = Measured calcium +
[4 − albumin (g/dl)] × 0.8

or

Corrected calcium (mmol/l) = Measured calcium +
[40 − albumin (g/dl)] × 0.02

In the first example, 0.8 mg/dl of calcium is added (to the laboratory determination of serum calcium) for every 1 g/dl the serum albumin is less than 4.0, which is used as the midrange normal value for serum albumin.

## TREATMENT

Hypercalcemia results from a combination of excessive bone resorption and impaired renal calcium excretion. Treatment must therefore be directed at both causes. Most important initially is improving renal calcium excretion by correcting those factors impairing renal function, usually dehydration and diminished GFR. Second, bone resorption must be stopped either by eliminating the primary cause (treating the primary tumor) or by inhibiting osteoclast function to prevent recurrence of hypercalcemia. Unless the primary tumor or skeletal metastases can be controlled, all anti-hypercalcemia interventions tend to be palliative. If tumor ablation cannot be achieved, the median survival time after the initial episode of hypercalcemia is only one to three months.[14,53]

There are several nonspecific pharmacological approaches to the treatment of individuals with hypercalcemia (Table 25-8). Most pharmacological interventions are directed at osteoclast inhibition and thus do little to modify the increased renal tubular calcium resorption caused by PTHrP in HHM. It is this lack of effect on renal calcium resorption that is responsible for the partial or short-lived responses to osteoclast inhibitors in hypercalcemic individuals with solid tumors and no skeletal metastases. Currently calcitonin is the only drug available that blocks renal tubular calcium resorption.

The degree of urgency with which the hypercalcemia is treated depends on the serum calcium level and the patient's symptomatology. Patients with corrected serum calcium levels above 13.0 mg/dl or symptomatic patients with a calcium level <13.0 mg/dl should be treated aggressively, whereas asymptomatic individuals with lower calcium levels require more specific but less urgent treatment.

Despite new approaches to the treatment of hypercalcemia, MAHC continues to have a dismal prognosis with no survival advantage even when the hypercalcemia is successfully treated.[53] In patients with recurrent humoral hypercalcemia and end-stage disease where all cancer treatment options have been exhausted, physicians may, after discussion with the patient and family, elect not to treat further episodes of hypercalcemia, allowing the patient to lapse into a coma and, shortly thereafter, die. Since hypercalcemia can be associated with such unpleasant but manageable symptoms as mental status changes, nausea and vomiting, and abdominal pain, early dialogues among the physician, patient, and family are essential in order to determine what constitutes a "quality death" for the patient. Ralston et al reported that only

**TABLE 25-8**  Available Therapy for Malignant Hypercalcemia

| Therapy | Dosage | Comments |
|---|---|---|
| Tumor ablation | Tumor-specific | Only definitive approach to long-term resolution of hypercalcemia |
| Saline | 4 liters IV in first 24 hr, then 3 liters/day | Expands plasma volume, corrects dehydration and renal insufficiency, promotes calciuresis; may require cardiac and central venous pressure (CVP) monitoring with compromised cardiovascular or renal function. |
| Furosemide | Diuretic dose 20 mg q 4–6 hr; calciuretic dose 80–100 mg q 1–2 hr | Diuretic dose to control overhydration; calciuretic doses require ICU monitoring to replace electrolyte and fluid losses. |
| Bisphosphonates | | Prevent osteoclast recruitment and retention, attachment to bone matrix and bone resorption; given after rehydration; adverse effects include taste perversions and acute phase reactions (nausea, vomiting, and low-grade fever) |
|    Etidronate (Didronil) | 7.5 mg/kg/day IV over 2–3 hr × 3–7 days, or 30 mg/kg over 24 hr; then 5–10 mg/kg po for up to 3 months | Normalizes calcium level in 3–5 days; contraindicated in renal failure; osteomalacia with long-term use |
|    Pamidronate (Aredia) | 60–90 mg in 1000 ml IV fluid as single dose over 4–24 hr. Repeat q 2–3 weeks to maintain eucalcemia. | Higher doses for more severe hypercalcemia; onset of action within 24 hr; can be supplemented with calcitonin suppositories for more rapid effect; adverse effects include hypophosphatemia, hypokalemia, hypocalcemia, hypomagnesemia; infusion site reactions occur in 7%; ↓ risk of osteolytic sequelae: bone pain, pathological fractures with chronic use |
| Clodronate | 1.5 g/500 ml normal saline over 4 hr; 1600 mg po/day | Less effective than pamidronate, more effective than calcitonin; chronic oral dose ↓ risk of osteolytic sequelae in breast cancer and multiple myeloma |
| Calcitonin plus a glucocorticoid | 200 MRC units q 12hr IM/SQ + hydrocortisone 100 mg po q 6hr; calcitonin suppositories 300 mg q8h | Rapid onset of action; ↑ renal calcium excretion; safe in patients with cardiac or renal failure; most effective in hematologic malignancies |
| Plicamycin | 15–25 µg/kg (max. 1500 µg) as single dose IV over 4 hr. Can be repeated in 48 hr | Onset of action within 24–48 hr; variable duration of action; adverse effects ↑ with cumulative dosage include thrombocytopenia, hepatic and renal toxicity, nausea and vomiting. Cellulitis at injection site with extravasation. |
| Gallium nitrate | 200 mg/m²/day continuous IV infusion over 5–7 days | Inhibits osteoclast bone resorption. More effective than calcitonin or etidronate, less effective than pamidronate. |

28% of patients treated for hypercalcemia in his study actually died of uncontrolled hypercalcemia. The remainder died of other tumor-related complications after the hypercalcemic event.[54]

To correct the two major pathophysiological alterations of hypercalcemia, impaired renal calcium excretion and increased osteoclastic bone resorption, the cornerstones of therapy are hydration and saline diuresis followed by inhibition of osteoclast function.[55] The bisphosphonates, plicamycin, calcitonin, and gallium nitrate are all osteoclast inhibitors. Calcitonin acts most rapidly, but its duration of effectiveness is limited. Gallium nitrate is effective but inconvenient to administer, requiring five daily infusions. Plicamycin has cumulative toxicities.

Once rehydration has been established, initiation of bisphosphonate therapy is now considered the treatment of choice.[56,57] Bisphosphonates are effective when administered as a single four-hour infusion and in some cases when administered orally, making them quite useful in the outpatient setting for treatment of hypercalcemia, prevention of bone pain, skeletal fractures, and maintenance of normocalcemia.

## General Measures

Initial measures should involve correcting volume contraction and removing factors that may exacerbate hypercalcemia, such as thiazide diuretics, vitamins A and D, and, in some breast cancer patients, hormonal agents. Discontinuation of tamoxifen is not always indicated. Medications whose actions are potentiated by hypercalcemia, such as digoxin, should be adjusted.

Mobilization in an effort to promote weight bearing and osteoblast function should be encouraged whenever possible. Except in some patients with lymphoma in whom elevated levels of 1,25-dihydroxyvitamin D enhance intestinal calcium absorption, restriction of dietary calcium is without scientific basis. However, calcium supplementation in IV hyperalimentation formulas should be discontinued because of the IV route of administration.

## Hydration and Saline Diuresis

As a result of the polyuria that accompanies hypercalcemia, most patients are dehydrated. The initial step in hypercalcemic therapy is to expand volume, correct dehydration and renal insufficiency, and promote calciuresis. Since sodium and calcium are excreted in parallel, calciuresis and a small drop in serum calcium (<0.5 mmol/dl) can be promoted by administering 4 liters of normal saline.[14] Measurement of fluid intake and output and body weight, and frequent assessment for signs of fluid overload are important. Patients with compromised cardiovascular function or renal failure may need central venous pressure and cardiac monitoring during therapy. Hypokalemia, hypomagnesemia, and hypophosphatemia may occur with high fluid volumes.[4,58] Hyperosmolar states due to some patients' inability to excrete high sodium loads have been observed.[4]

## Loop Diuretics

Once rehydration has been established, loop diuretics such as furosemide may be used to enhance calcium excretion. Use of such diuretics, which block calcium and sodium reabsorption across the ascending limb of Henle's loop, is controversial. Mild to moderate hypercalcemia can usually be managed by saline diuresis alone, and the benefit of adding furosemide to saline diuresis has not been documented.[4,58]

There is a difference between the diuretic and calciuretic doses of furosemide.[4] Doses of 20 mg every four to six hours are usually sufficient to manage overhydration in patients with compromised cardiovascular or renal function. Patients treated with calciuretic doses of furosemide (80–100 mg every one to two hours) should be monitored in an intensive care setting to ensure that fluid and electrolyte losses are carefully replaced and that extracellular fluid volume is not depleted. Depletion of extracellular fluid volume in the hypercalcemic patient ensures reabsorption of calcium from the proximal tubule and further exacerbation of the hypercalcemia. Side effects of high-dose furosemide are severe potassium and magnesium loss.

Clinical improvement in mental status and relief of nausea often occur in younger patients within 24 hours of rehydration, but serum calcium levels may not normalize except in cases of mild hypercalcemia.[59] Once rehydration and improvement in renal function have been achieved, inhibition of osteoclastic bone resorption must be attained in order to achieve and maintain a normocalcemic state. Although antitumor therapy is the treatment of choice when available, pharmacological inhibition of bone resorption is usually indicated in order to prevent the movement of calcium from bone into extracellular fluid. Several treatment regimens are available.

## Bisphosphonates

The bisphosphonates (synonymous with diphosphonates or biphosphonates) are analogues of pyrophosphate, a naturally occurring substance that has an affinity for bone. They are effective inhibitors of osteoclast bone resorption, apparently by binding tightly to calcified bone matrix and preventing osteoclast bone resorption, preventing osteoclast attachment to bone matrix, and preventing osteoclast recruitment and retention.[14,60–62] Three generations of compounds have been described, each generation being more potent than the preceding generation, and include etidronate, clodronate, pamidronate, alendronate, risendronate, and tiludronate. A second-generation bisphosphonate, pamidronate, is widely used and is efficacious in inhibiting osteolysis-related sequelae of metastatic bone disease: bone pain, hypercalcemia, and pathological fractures.[15] The third-generation bisphosphonates show promise for prevention of development and progression of osteolytic metastases.[33] Alendronate, risendronate, and BM 21.0955 are as much as 500 times more potent than clodronate in inhibition of bone resorption.[33] Bisphosphonates are usually administered intravenously. Oral bisphosphonates tend to have low bioavailability and a high incidence of GI side effects with effective dose levels.

### Etidronate

Etidronate (Didronel,® MGI Pharma) is available in both IV and oral formulations. Etidronate has been shown to be more effective than either saline hydration alone[63] or calcitonin after saline hydration.[60] It has been demonstrated to be safe with few side effects. While the usual IV dose is 7.5 mg/kg/day administered over at least two hours for three to seven days followed by oral maintenance therapy at a dose of 5–10 mg/kg/day,[9] Flores et al report that etidronate is safe and more effective when 30 mg/kg is administered as a single infusion over 24 hours.[64] Side effects reported in fewer than 10% of patients included altered taste during etidronate infusion, nausea and vomiting, and low-grade fever following infusion. Elevated serum creatinine occurs rarely. Serum calcium nadirs usually occur by day 6 regardless of the infusion regimen, and the median duration of effect for IV etidronate in one study was reported to be 29 days.[60] Toxicities associated with long-term use (more than three months) include impaired mineralization of bone and increases in serum phosphate.[60]

### Pamidronate

Pamidronate (Aredia,® Ciba), a second-generation bisphosphonate approved for treatment of moderate to severe malignant hypercalcemia, has been demonstrated to be more effective than etidronate.[65] It inhibits bone resorption without preventing bone mineralization. Pamidronate has a rapid onset of action, with serum calcium levels responding within 24 hours and reaching nadir by seven days, and a longer duration of action than that seen with other therapies.[65–67] There appears to be a significant dose-response relationship, with more severe hypercalcemias requiring higher doses in order to achieve normocalcemia. Serum calcium responses are faster in patients receiving 4-hour infusions rather than the recommended 24-hour infusion.[68] A combination of IV pamidronate and calcitonin suppositories has been demonstrated to have a more rapid onset and better efficacy than IV pamidronate alone in a small study of 34 patients.[58] Recommended doses of pamidronate for moderate to severe hypercalcemia are 60–90 mg in 1000 ml of fluid (0.45% or 0.9% saline or 5% dextrose) administered as a single infusion over 4–24 hours in well-hydrated patients. The dose may be repeated after seven days if needed. Side effects are dose-related and include postinfusion temperature elevations (approximately 1 °C 24–48 hr postinfusion), nausea, anorexia, taste perversions, asymptomatic hypophosphatemia, hypokalemia, hypocalcemia, and hypomagnesemia. Seven percent of patients receiving pamidronate in one study were reported to experience infusion site reactions consisting of redness, swelling, induration, or pain at the intravenous catheter insertion site.[65]

The role of pamidronate in the prevention of osteolytic sequelae is a topic of scientific interest. In women with breast cancer and metastatic bone disease, pamidronate infusions of 60–90 mg over four hours every two to four weeks were associated with significant decreases in bone pain.[69] In an open randomized dosing study, oral pamidronate treatment in women with breast cancer and bone metastases led to reductions in the occurrence of hypercalcemia (65%), severe bone pain (30%), symptomatic impending fractures (50%), and need for radiotherapy (35%) compared with untreated controls. No survival advantage was demonstrated, and GI toxicity was associated with a 23% study dropout rate.[70] Clinical trials are now under way to evaluate the role of pamidronate in preventing the development of osteolytic metastases.

### Clodronate

Clodronate administered as a 1.5-g dose in 500 ml of normal saline over four hours has been reported to have an 80% complete response rate with onset of effect by day 3.[71] Oral clodronate as an adjunct to melphalan and prednisolone in patients with multiple myeloma showed a reduction in bone pain, episodes of hypercalcemia, and progression of osteolytic bone lesions.[72] In a double-blind placebo-controlled trial, Patterson et al demonstrated a reduction in the number of hypercalcemic episodes, incidence of vertebral fractures, and vertebral deformity with oral clodronate. There were no significant survival differences.[73]

### Third-generation bisphosphonates

Alendronate, neridronate, amifostine, tiludronate, YM175, and BM 21.0955 are all third-generation bisphosphonates with higher potency levels than first- and second-generation bisphosphonates. Dose-response studies have yet to identify their appropriate role in the prevention and management of hypercalcemia. Alendronate was approved by the FDA in 1995 for the prevention of postmenopausal osteoporosis.

## Calcitonin

Calcitonin, a 32–amino acid polypeptide normally produced by the parafollicular cells of the thyroid gland, produces transient (24–72 hours) inhibition of bone resorption through its direct effects on osteoclast formation. Calcitonin also acts directly on the kidney to promote urinary calcium excretion and can be used safely in patients with dehydration or renal failure. Onset of action is rapid, with declines in serum calcium within four to six hours of the first dose. Best responses are seen in persons with multiple myeloma and other hematologic neoplasms.[4] Unfortunately, inhibition of bone resorption is short, and tachyphylaxis or "escape" from therapeutic effect limits its usefulness. Use of calcitonin in severe hypercalcemia can buy time while waiting for a response to antineoplastic or other antihypercalcemic therapy with a longer onset of therapeutic effect. Administration in combination with glucocorticoids appears to be more effective because corticosteroids overcome the effect of renal tubular resistance to calcitonin, possibly through inhibition of PTHrP production.[55,74,75] Synthetic calcitonin can be administered subcutaneously at a starting dose of 4–12 units/kg body weight every 8–12 hours or as rectal suppositories at a dose of 300 mg three times daily for seven days. Side effects are mild and include nausea and vomiting, flushing, skin rashes, and occasionally allergic reactions. Skin testing is recommended before initiation of treatment.

## Glucocorticoids

Glucocorticoids (prednisone and hydrocortisone) are most effective in hypercalcemia associated with multiple myeloma, other hematologic diseases, and sometimes breast carcinoma. Hypercalcemia associated with other solid tumors is responsive only 30% of the time.[58] Glucocorticoids may be effective in hypercalcemia due to myeloma because they inhibit bone resorption mediated by osteoclast-activating factors or because they cause a decrease in calcium either by a direct tumor cytolytic effect or by inhibiting tumor-produced prostaglandins. Glucocorticoids also increase urinary calcium excretion and decrease intestinal calcium absorption. This latter effect may be important in those lymphomas that can hydroxylate 25-hydroxyvitamin D to produce high circulating 1,25-dihydroxyvitamin D levels, which stimulate intestinal calcium absorption. The benefits of long-term use of glucocorticoids outweigh potential side effects (Cushing's syndrome, osteomalacia), since side effects take longer to develop than the individual's anticipated survival time.

Glucocorticoids used alone are not as effective as when used with calcitonin. Both can be used in patients with renal or cardiac failure who are dehydrated, and they therefore are useful for treatment of hypercalcemia when saline diuresis is contraindicated. The advantages to combined use are a more rapid response and prevention of the escape phenomenon encountered with use of calcitonin alone. The usual dosage is prednisone 40–100 mg/dl in divided doses.

## Plicamycin

Plicamycin (mithramycin) is a cytotoxic drug with antihypercalcemic effects, probably through its toxic effects on osteoclasts and irreversible impairment of osteoclast bone resorption. Plicamycin has been associated with thrombocytopenia and with renal and hepatic toxicity. Nausea, vomiting, and toxic effects are related to cumulative dosage and rarely occur with the first or second dose. Since the drug is excreted through the kidneys, toxicity is more likely in patients with impaired renal function. Hypocalcemia and tetany also have been reported. Use of this agent is recommended only when other less toxic regimens have failed. Plicamycin's major disadvantages are cumulative myelotoxicity with thrombocytopenia, which may interfere with administration of myelotoxic anticancer therapy, and renal toxicity, which may further impair renal function in patients who already have renal insufficiency due to hypercalcemia.

Plicamycin is administered intravenously at a dose of 25 µg/kg (maximum dose 1500 mg) either as a slow bolus injection or as a four-hour infusion. Bolus injections are associated with a higher incidence of nausea and vomiting. Reduction in serum calcium occurs within 48 hours, and normocalcemia usually occurs after a single dose. The dose may be repeated if no detectable lowering of serum calcium occurs within 48 hours. Once the serum calcium is lowered, the duration of action is variable and unpredictable, lasting from three days to a week or more. Treatment is not repeated until hypercalcemia returns. Extravasation is associated with local irritation and cellulitis at the injection site. A change in the injection site and application of warm compresses are recommended by the manufacturer should extravasation occur (Miles Laboratories package insert).

## Phosphates

Phosphates prevent intestinal calcium absorption by forming poorly soluble Ca-PO$_4$ salts in the intestinal lumen, which makes less calcium available for absorption, and also by impairing conversion of 25-hydroxyvitamin D to 1,25-dihydroxyvitamin D (a major stimulator of intestinal calcium transport). In addition, phosphates inhibit mineral and bone matrix resorption. Oral phosphates are less toxic in patients with normal renal function and serum phosphorus levels under 4.0 mg/dl and are useful for chronic treatment of hypercalcemia once serum calcium levels have been reduced with other drugs. IV administration of inorganic phosphates rapidly decreases extracellular fluid calcium concentration by promoting skeletal calcification. Unfortunately, extraskeletal calcification also occurs and is associated with, among other things, impairment of renal function due to nephrocalcinosis. IV phosphates should not be employed except as a last resort. Soft-tissue and skeletal calcification also occurs to a lesser extent with oral than with IV phosphates, but lung and renal calcification has been documented with chronic administration. The most common and also most limiting side effect is diarrhea, since phosphates are administered in the form of sodium or potassium salts, Fleets Phospho Soda® being one of the preparations most commonly prescribed. The usual starting dosage is 1 g/dl in divided doses with titration of the dose upward to a maximum of 3 g/dl. Dose-limiting diarrhea usually occurs at 2 g/dl.[59] Despite an initial response, chronic administration is often accompanied by loss of effectiveness. No randomized prospective studies have evaluated the efficacy of oral phosphates. Phosphates are contraindicated in patients with renal failure and serum phosphorus levels greater than 3.8 mg/dl.

## Prostaglandin Inhibitors

Aspirin, indomethacin, and nonsteroidal anti-inflammatory drugs have been tried, but only on occasion is there an antihypercalcemic response.

## Gallium Nitrate

Gallium nitrate is a cytotoxic drug that has been found to inhibit bone resorption and restore normocalcemia with few side effects in 75%–85% of patients.[76] In a randomized double-blind trial comparing five-day infusions of gallium nitrate with salmon calcitonin intramuscularly every six hours for five days, 75% of the gallium nitrate patients compared with 31% of the calcitonin patients achieved normocalcemia. Median duration of normocalcemia before other cytotoxic or hypocalcemic therapy was six days with gallium nitrate and one day with calcitonin.[75] Gallium nitrate has also been found to be twice as effective as etidronate at usual doses.[77] Potential side effects in gallium-treated patients include asymptomatic hypophosphatemia and nephrotoxicity. It is contraindicated with serum creatinine levels >2.5 mg/dl. A major disadvantage to the use of gallium nitrate is the five-day continuous treatment regimen, which makes outpatient treatment inconvenient.

## CONCLUSION

Hypercalcemia is a common metabolic complication of malignancy with vague symptoms that can often be confused with those of other paraneoplastic syndromes as well as those of end-stage disease. Nurses caring for cancer patients must be cognizant both of patients at risk and of their associated risk factors. In an exploratory study

**TABLE 25-9**  What You Should Know About Hypercalcemia—A Patient Guide

Calcium is normally stored in the bones and a small amount is found circulating in the bloodstream. Proper levels of calcium in the bloodstream are needed to maintain body functions. Normally, the kidneys control the amount of calcium in the bloodstream. When this balance is offset by kidney disease, cancer in the bone, or another cause, hypercalcemia occurs.

Hypercalcemia occurs when the amount of calcium in the bloodstream is too high. Some types of cancer are more likely than others to cause hypercalcemia. Treatment of the disease process (cancer) is the best way to manage hypercalcemia.

### WHAT YOU CAN DO TO REDUCE YOUR RISK OF DEVELOPING HYPERCALCEMIA

Hypercalcemia cannot always be prevented. However, you may be able to reduce your risk of developing hypercalcemia by following these guidelines:

- Remain as active as possible. Walking, standing, or sitting is good because such activity stimulates new bone formation and keeps excess calcium in the bones, not in the bloodstream.

- Drink at least 3 quarts of fluid per day. Dehydration prevents the kidneys from excreting excess calcium. If nausea or vomiting prevent you from maintaining an adequate fluid intake, notify your doctor or nurse.

- If possible, avoid taking water pills such as hydrochlorthiazide (Diuril™), which can impair the kidney's ability to excrete calcium.

- Avoid taking vitamins A and D unless prescribed by your doctor.

- Unless your health care provider suggests otherwise, maintain a normal diet. The calcium in your diet will *not* increase your risk of hypercalcemia.

### SYMPTOMS OF HYPERCALCEMIA

The symptoms of hypercalcemia are due to the effects of excess calcium on the function of muscles and the nervous system. Early symptoms of hypercalcemia may be difficult for you or your family to identify because they are similar to the symptoms that you may already be experiencing due to your illness or your treatment. It is important that both you and your family report any change or worsening in the symptoms you experience. If you are developing hypercalcemia, the earlier that you get treatment, the less likely you are to experience severe symptoms. Treatment for high levels of calcium in the bloodstream usually requires hospitalization, while lower levels may be treated on an outpatient basis. Common early symptoms of hypercalcemia include the following:

- nausea, vomiting, or loss of appetite

- constipation and/or abdominal pain

- extreme fatigue or muscle weakness

- bone pain

- increased thirst or excessive urination

- sleepiness, difficulty thinking or concentrating

- inappropriate behavior or conversation

Physician's name and number _____

Nurse's name and number _____

---

of hospitalized and ambulatory hypercalcemic patients, 88% of the patients were not aware that hypercalcemia might occur, and 80%–95% were not aware of the various symptoms of hypercalcemia.[78] Counseling of patients and families regarding prevention and recognition of early symptoms enables therapy to commence before extreme debilitation develops (Table 25-9). Patient and family education regarding the purposes and goals of therapy promotes coping with yet another complication of cancer. Meticulous monitoring of fluid and electrolyte balance is essential for effective medical treatment. If hypercalcemia becomes refractory to treatment, nursing measures that facilitate coping with issues related to death and dying are essential.

Although theoretical knowledge regarding humoral and local factors associated with hypercalcemia is advancing, current therapies are nonspecific, aimed at osteoclast inhibition rather than at the mediating bone-resorbing factor itself. The development of specific antagonists to local and humoral hypercalcemic factors would theoretically improve treatment of malignant hypercalcemia.

## REFERENCES

1. Wysolmerski JJ, Broadus AE: Hypercalcemia of malignancy: The central role of parathyroid hormone–related protein. *Annu Rev Med* 45:189–200, 1994

2. Fisken RA, Heath DA, Bold AM: Hypercalcemia: A hospital survey. *Q J Med* 49:405–418, 1980

3. Fisken RA, Heath DA, Sommers S, et al: Hypercalcemia in hospital patients: Clinical and diagnostic aspects. *Lancet* 1:202–207, 1981

4. Mundy GR, Martin TJ: The hypercalcemia of malignancy: Pathogenesis and management. *Metabolism* 31:1247–1277, 1982

5. Blomqvist CP: Malignant hypercalcemia: A hospital survey. *Acta Med Scand* 220:455–463, 1986

6. Bender RA, Hansen H: Hypercalcemia in bronchogenic carcinoma: A prospective study of 200 patients. *Ann Intern Med* 80:205–208, 1974

7. Stewart AF, Romero R, Schwart PE, et al: Hypercalcemia associated with gynecologic malignancies: Biochemical characterization. *Cancer* 49:2389–2394, 1982

8. Strewler GJ, Nissenson RA: Nonparathyroid hypercalcemia. *Adv Intern Med* 32:235–258, 1987

9. Mundy GR: *Calcium Homeostasis: Hypercalcemia and Hypocalcemia*. London, Martin Dunitz, 1989, pp 1–126

10. Habener JF, Rosenblatt M, Potts JT: Parathyroid hormone: Biochemical aspects of biosynthesis, secretion, action, and metabolism. *Physiol Rev* 64:985–1040, 1984

11. Mundy GR: The hypercalcemia of malignancy. *Kidney Int* 31:142–155, 1987

12. Peck WA, Rifas L, Cheng SL, et al: The local regulation of bone remodeling. *Adv Exp Med Biol* 108:255–259, 1986

13. Meunier PJ: Cellular mechanisms of bone remodeling evaluated at the intermediary level of organization of bone. *Adv Exp Med Biol* 208:247–254, 1986

14. Walls J, Bundred N, Howell A: Hypercalcemia and bone resorption in malignancy. *Clin Orthop* 312:51–63, 1995

15. Orr WF, Sanchez-Sweatman OH, Kostenuik P, et al: Tumor-bone interactions in skeletal metastasis. *Clin Orthop* 312:19–33, 1995

16. Burtis WJ, Wu T, Bunch C, et al: Identification of a novel 17,000-dalton parathyroid hormone-like adenylate cyclase-stimulating protein from a tumor associated with humoral hypercalcemia of malignancy. *J Biol Chem* 262:7151–7156, 1987

17. Mangin M, Webb AC, Dreyer BE, et al: Identification of a cDNA encoding a parathyroid hormone-like peptide in messenger RNAs from a human tumor associated with humoral hypercalcemia of malignancy. *Proc Natl Acad Sci USA* 85:597–601, 1988

18. Ikeda K, Mangin M, Dreyer BE, et al: Identification of transcripts encoding a parathyroid hormone-like peptide in messenger RNAs from a variety of human and animal tumors associated with humoral hypercalcemia of malignancy. *J Clin Invest* 81:2010–2014, 1988

19. Martin JJ, Grill V: Hypercalcemia in cancer. *J Steroid Biochem Mol Biol* 43:123–129, 1992

20. Horwitz MJ, Bilezikian JP: Primary hyperparathyroidism and parathyroid hormone-related protein. *Curr Opin Rheumatol* 6(3):321–328, 1994

21. Guise TA, Yoneda T, Yates AJ, et al: The combined effect of tumor produced parathyroid hormone-related protein and transforming growth factor alpha enhance hypercalcemia in vivo and bone resorption in vitro. *J Clin Endocrinol Metab* 77(1):40–45, 1993

22. Mundy GR, Ibbotsen KJ, D'Souza SM: Tumor products and the hypercalcemia of malignancy. *J Clin Invest* 76:391–394, 1985

23. Sato K, Fujii Y, Kasono K, et al: Paraneoplastic syndrome of hypercalcemia and leukocytosis caused by squamous carcinoma cells (T3M1) producing parathyroid hormone-related protein, interleukin 1 alpha, and granulocyte colony stimulating factor. *Cancer Res* 49:4740–4746, 1989

24. Mundy GR: Pathophysiology of cancer-associated hypercalcemia. *Semin Oncol* 17:10–15, 1990

25. Mercier RJ, Thompson JM, Harman GS, et al: Recurrent hypercalcemia and elevated 1,25-dihydroxyvitamin D levels in Hodgkin's disease. *Am J Med* 84:165–168, 1988

26. Breslau NA, McGuire JL, Zerwekh JE, et al: Hypercalcemia associated with increased serum calcitriol levels in three patients with lymphoma. *Ann Intern Med* 100:1–7, 1984

27. Rosenthal N, Insogna KL, Godsall JW, et al: Elevations in circulating 1,25-dihydroxyvitamin D in three patients with lymphoma-associated hypercalcemia. *J Clin Endocrinol Metab* 60:29–33, 1985

28. Mudde AH, van den Berg H, Boshuis PG, et al: Ectopic production of 1,25-dihydroxyvitamin D by B-cell lymphoma as a cause of hypercalcemia. *Cancer* 59:1543–1546, 1987

29. Devogelaer JP, Lambert M, Boland B, et al: 1,25-dihydroxyvitamin D in lymphoma: Two case reports. *Clin Rheumatol* 9:404–410, 1990

30. Fetchik DA, Bertolini DR, Sarin PS, et al: Production of 1,25-dihydroxyvitamin $D_3$ by human T-cell lymphotrophic virus-l-transformed lymphocytes. *J Clin Invest* 78:592–596, 1986

31. Adams JS: Vitamin D metabolite-mediated hypercalcemia. *Endocrinol Metab Clin North Am* 18:765–778, 1989

32. Goni MH, Tolis G: Hypercalcemia of cancer: An update. *Anticancer Res* 13:1155–1160, 1993

33. Mundy GR, Yoneda T: Facilitation and suppression of bone metastasis. *Clin Orthop* 312:34–44, 1995

34. Kitazawa S, Maeda S: Development of skeletal metastases. *Clin Orthop* 312:45–50, 1995

35. Isales C, Carcangiu ML, Stewart AF: Hypercalcemia in breast cancer: Reassessment of the mechanism. *Am J Med* 82:1143–1147, 1987

36. Percival RC, Yates AJ, Gray RE, et al: Mechanism of malignant hypercalcemia in carcinoma of the breast. *Br Med J* 291:776–779, 1985

37. Eilon G, Mundy GR: Effects of inhibition of microtubule assembly on bone mineral release and enzyme release by human breast cancer cells. *J Clin Invest* 67:69–76, 1981

38. Legha S, Powell K, Budzan A, et al: Tamoxifen-induced hypercalcemia in breast cancer. *Cancer* 47:2803–2806, 1986

39. Mundy GR: Pathogenesis of hypercalcemia of malignancy. *Clin Endocrinol* 23:705–714, 1985

40. Mundy GR, Bertolini DR: Bone destruction and hypercalcemia in plasma cell myeloma. *Semin Oncol* 13:291–299, 1986

41. Muggia FM: Overview of cancer-related hypercalcemia: Epidemiology and etiology. *Semin Oncol* 17:3–9, 1990

42. Ratcliffe WA, Norbury S, Heath DA, et al: Development and validation of an immunoradiometric assay for parathyrin-related protein in unextracted plasma. *Clin Chem* 37:678–685, 1991

43. Mundy GR: Hypercalcemia factors other than parathyroid hormone–related protein. *Endocrinol Metab Clin North Am* 18:795–806, 1989

44. Kiyokawa T, Yamaguchi K, Takeya M, et al: Hypercalcemia and osteoclast proliferation in adult T-cell leukemia. *Cancer* 59:1187–1191, 1987

45. Fukumoto S, Matsumoto T, Watanabe T, et al: Secretion of parathyroid hormone–like activity from human T-cell lymphotropic virus type T–infected lymphocytes. *Cancer Res* 49:3849–3852, 1989

46. Moseley JM, Danks JA, Grill V, et al: Immunocytochemical demonstration of PTHrP in neoplastic tissue of HTLV-1 positive human adult T-cell leukemia/lymphoma: Implications for the mechanisms of hypercalcemia. *Br J Cancer* 64:745–748, 1991

47. Stewart AF, Horst R, Deftos LJ, et al: Biochemical evaluation of patients with cancer-associated hypercalcemia: Evidence for humoral and non-humoral groups. *N Engl J Med* 303:1377–1383, 1980

48. Pecherstorfer M, Schilling T, Blind E, et al: Parathyroid hormone–related protein and life expectancy in hypercalcemic patients. *J Clin Endocrinol Metab* 75:1268–1270, 1994

49. Mahon SM: Signs and symptoms associated with malignancy-induced hypercalcemia. *Cancer Nurs* 12:153–160, 1989

50. Poe CM, Radford AI: The challenge of hypercalcemia in cancer. *Oncol Nurs Forum* 12:29–34, 1985

51. Coward DD: Cancer-induced hypercalcemia. *Cancer Nurs* 9: 125–132, 1986

52. Bajorunas DR: Clinical manifestations of cancer-related hypercalcemia. *Semin Oncol* 17:16–25, 1990 (suppl 5)

53. Ling PJ, A'Hern RP, Hardy JR: Analysis of survival following treatment of tumor-induced hypercalcemia with intravenous pamidronate (APD). *Br J Cancer* 72:206–209, 1995

54. Ralston SH, Gallacher SJ, Patel U, et al: Cancer-associated hypercalcemia: Morbidity and mortality. Clinical experience in 126 treated patients. *Ann Intern Med* 112:499–504, 1990

55. Fetchik DA, Mundy GR: Hypercalcemia of malignancy: Diagnosis and therapy. *Compr Ther* 12:27–32, 1986

56. Warrell RP Jr: Etiology and current management of cancer-related hypercalcemia. *Oncology* 6(10):37–43, 1992

57. Fleisch H: Bisphosphonates: Pharmacology and use in treatment of tumor-induced hypercalcemia and metastatic bone disease. *Drugs* 42:919–944, 1991

58. Thiebaud D, Jacquet AF, Burckhardt P: Fast and effective treatment of malignant hypercalcemia: Combination of suppositories of calcitonin and a single infusion of 3-amino 1-hydroxypropylidene-1-bisphosphonate. *Arch Intern Med* 150: 2125–2128, 1990

59. Ritch PS: Treatment of cancer-related hypercalcemia. *Semin Oncol* 17:26–33, 1990

60. Singer FR: Role of the bisphosphonate etidronate in the therapy of cancer-related hypercalcemia. *Semin Oncol* 17: 34–39, 1990

61. Coleman RE: Bisphosphonate treatment of bone metastases and hypercalcemia of malignancy. *Oncology* 5:55–60, 1991

62. Houston SJ, Rubers RD: The systemic treatment of bone metastases. *Clin Orthop* 312:95–104, 1995

63. Singer FR, Ritch PS, Ringenberg QS, et al: Treatment of hypercalcemia of malignancy with intravenous etidronate: A controlled, multicenter study. The Hypercalcemia Study Group. *Arch Intern Med* 151:471–476, 1991

64. Flores JF, Singer FR, Rude RK: Effectiveness of a 24-hour infusion of etidronate disodium in the treatment of hypercalcemia of malignant disease: A dose ranging pilot study. *Miner Electrolyte Metab* 17:390–395, 1991

65. Gucalp R, Ritch P, Wiernik PH, et al: Comparative study of pamidronate and etidronate disodium in the treatment of cancer-related hypercalcemia. *J Clin Oncol* 10:134–142, 1992

66. Thiebaud D, Jaeger AF, Jacquet AF, et al: Dose-response in the treatment of hypercalcemia of malignancy by a single infusion of the bisphosphonate AHPrBP. *J Clin Oncol* 6: 762–768, 1988

67. Coleman RE, Rubens RD: 3(amino-1, 1-hydroxypropylidene) bisphosphonate (APD) for hypercalcemia of breast cancer. *Br J Cancer* 56:465–469, 1987

68. Gucalp R, Theriault R, Gill I, et al: Treatment of cancer-associated hypercalcemia. *Arch Intern Med* 154:1935–1944, 1994

69. Glover D, Lipton A, Keller A: Intravenous pamidronate disodium treatment of bone metastases in patients with breast cancer. *Cancer* 74:2950–2955, 1994

70. van Holten–Verzantvoort ATM, Kroon HM, Bijvoet OLM, et al: Palliative pamidronate treatment in patients with bone metastases from breast cancer. *J Clin Oncol* 11:491–498, 1993

71. O'Rourke NP, McCloskey EV, Vasikaran S, et al: Effective treatment of malignant hypercalcemia with a single intravenous dose of clodronate. *Br J Cancer* 67:560–563, 1993

72. Lahtinen R, Laasko M, Palva I, et al: Finnish Leukemia Group: Randomised, placebo-controlled multicentre trial of clodronate in multiple myeloma. *Lancet* 340:1049–1052, 1992

73. Patterson AH, Powles TJ, Kanis JA, et al: Double-blind controlled trial of oral clodronate in bone metastases from breast cancer. *J Clin Oncol* 11:59–65, 1993

74. Hosking DJ, Stone MD, Foote JW: Potentiation of calcitonin during the treatment of hypercalcemia of malignancy. *Eur J Clin Pharmacol* 38:37–41, 1990

75. Kasono K, Isozaki O, Sato K, et al: Effects of glucocorticoids and calcitonin on parathyroid hormone–related protein (PTHrP) gene expression and PTHrP release in human cancer cells causing humoral hypercalcemia. *Jpn J Cancer Res* 82:1008–1014, 1991

76. Warrell RP Jr, Israel R, Frisone M, et al: Gallium nitrate for acute treatment of cancer-related hypercalcemia: A randomized, double blind comparison to calcitonin. *Ann Intern Med* 108:669–674, 1988

77. Warrell RP Jr, Murphy WK, Shulman P, et al: A randomized double-blind study of gallium nitrate compared with etidronate for acute control of cancer-related hypercalcemia. *J Clin Oncol* 9:1467–1475, 1991

78. Coward D: Hypercalcemia knowledge assessment in patients at risk of developing cancer-induced hypercalcemia. *Oncol Nurs Forum* 15:471–476, 1988

# Chapter 26

# Paraneoplastic Syndromes

Irene Stewart Haapoja, RN, MS, OCN®

## INTRODUCTION

Paraneoplastic syndromes (PNSs), can be described as the "remote" or indirect effects of cancer. These rare diseases are the result of the secretion of substances, usually proteins, by the primary tumor or its metastases. These substances include hormones, growth factors, cytokines, antibodies, and other immune products, which indirectly result in a multitude of disorders of the endocrine, neurological, hematologic, cutaneous, renal, and gastrointestinal systems (see Figure 26-1). It is important for oncology nurses to understand these syndromes in order to recognize them as potential early warning signs of a malignancy, as a complication of malignancy, or as an indication of recurrent disease. Early detection and prompt effective treatment may minimize the morbidity associated with these syndromes.

It is estimated that PNSs occur in 10%–15% of all cancer patients.[1] While PNSs can occur with any malignancy, they most frequently occur with lung cancer, specifically small-cell lung carcinoma. The true incidence of PNSs is difficult to determine because they occur infrequently, they are associated with both benign and malignant disease, they are difficult to define in specific terms, and the diagnosis is often made by exclusion. Some general concepts exist concerning PNSs:[1]

1. PNSs may precede a diagnosis of malignancy or may occur concurrently; however, most appear in the later stages of the disease course.
2. PNSs rarely occur with childhood malignancies with the exception of Wilms' tumor and neuroblastoma.

3. The existence of a PNS frequently predicts a poor prognosis with regard to the malignancy; however, the severity of the PNS may not necessarily correlate with the extent of malignant disease.
4. A PNS may be useful as a monitoring tool to evaluate response of the malignancy to treatment and as an indication of recurrent disease.
5. The primary treatment of a PNS is treatment of the underlying malignancy. Response of the PNS to therapy frequently correlates with tumor response, especially in the case of the endocrine- or hormone-related PNSs. Unfortunately, the individual may be left with permanent deficits caused by the PNS even when the malignancy has been successfully eradicated, as is often seen with the neurological PNSs.

While oncology nurses are challenged every day by the more common PNSs, including anorexia-cachexia, hypercalcemia, and anemia of chronic disease, it is important to understand that many of these PNSs are extremely rare; in some instances only a few cases exist in the literature A review of the major PNSs affecting each body system is presented.

## ENDOCRINE PARANEOPLASTIC SYNDROMES

### Scope of the Problem

The endocrine PNSs are the most frequently occurring PNSs and the most well defined in terms of their etiology,

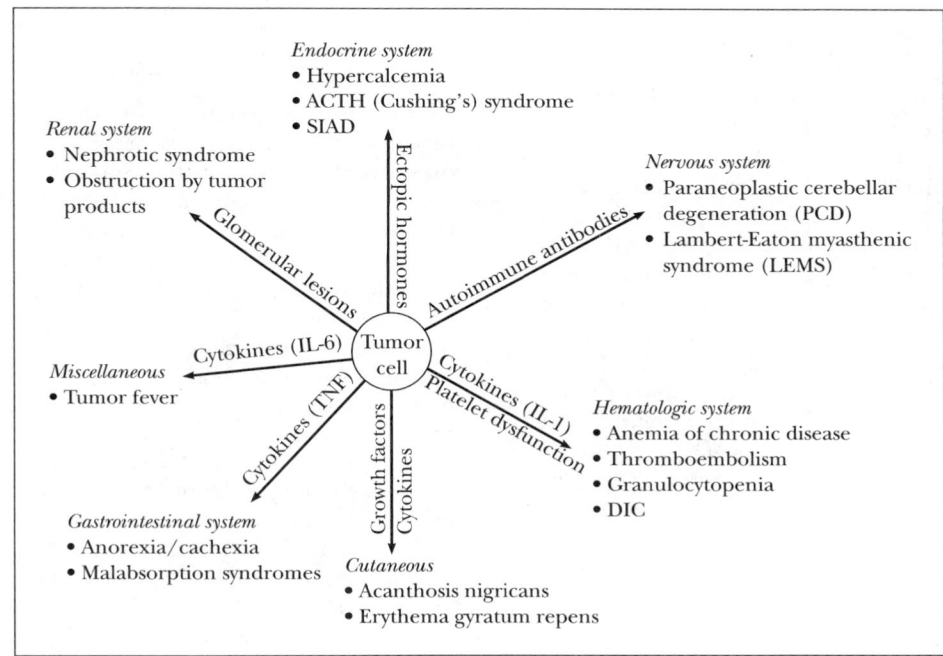

**FIGURE 26-1**  Paraneoplastic syndromes: Ectopic tumor effects.

clinical presentation, and disease course. These syndromes result from ectopic (tumor) synthesis of naturally occurring hormones or hormone precursors.[2] Definitive diagnosis depends on evidence that the tumor is synthesizing and secreting clinically significant amounts of the hormone, that the syndrome improves with successful treatment of the malignancy, and that it returns with recurrence of the malignancy. Confirmation that tumor tissue is synthesizing and secreting hormone can be done by in vitro testing; however, this extensive testing is not usually clinically useful and is rarely performed.[3]

Tumor cells have been shown to have the ability to produce almost every known hormone and hormone-releasing factor, resulting in the potential existence of multiple endocrine PNSs (Table 26-1).[4] The most common and well-known endocrine PNSs are hypercalcemia, paraneoplastic adrenocorticotropic hormone (ACTH) syndrome, and syndrome of inappropriate antidiuresis (SIAD).

## Definitions

Each endocrine PNS arises from tumor secretion of substances resulting in excessive amounts of circulating hormone that interrupt normal homeostatic mechanisms. Paraneoplastic or humoral hypercalcemia is defined as an elevated serum calcium level caused by tumor secretion of parathyroid hormone-related protein (PTHrP), and is usually distinguished from hypercalcemia arising from bony metastases. The normal range of serum calcium in adults is 8.5–10.5 mg/dl; hypercalcemia exists if the level exceeds 11.0 mg/dl.

Paraneoplastic ACTH syndrome is the development of pituitary-independent Cushing's disease caused by the secretion of ACTH by malignant cells, and must be distinguished from pituitary-dependent Cushing's disease produced by a pituitary neoplasm or hyperplasia.[4]

The syndrome of inappropriate secretion of antidiuretic hormone (SIADH) was initially described by Schwartz et al[5] in 1957 as the secretion of antidiuretic hormone (ADH) by the pituitary in response to a thoracic tumor. In 1963 Amatruda and colleagues[6] demonstrated that tumor production of ADH, not the pituitary, resulted in SIADH. SIADH is described as tumor production of ADH or arginine vasopressin (AVP) resulting in a syndrome of hyponatremia, urine inappropriately higher in osmolality than the plasma, and high urinary sodium in concentrations despite serum hyponatremia.[2] SIADH is more commonly referred to as SIAD or syndrome of inappropriate diuresis to reflect that vasopressin may not be the only agent to effect sodium excretion.[7]

## Incidence

Hypercalcemia is the most common metabolic complication of malignancy, occurring in approximately 10% of cancer patients, of which 10%–15% do not have metastatic bone disease. The malignancies most often associated with hypercalcemia are squamous cell carcinomas of the lung (15%), head and neck, and esophagus, followed by breast, uterine, cervical, lymphoma, multiple myeloma, and renal cell carcinomas.[2,4]

Although paraneoplastic ACTH syndrome occurs rarely, it is considered the second most frequent paraneoplastic syndrome. Bronchogenic carcinoma accounts for 60%–70% of the cases of paraneoplastic ACTH syndrome. Small-cell lung carcinoma represents the majority of these cases; approximately 5% of small-cell lung cancer patients will develop the syndrome during the course of their disease. Adenocarcinoma of the lung is less often associated (5%). Other malignancies associated with paraneoplastic ACTH syndrome include pancreatic carcinoma, carcinoid tumors, pheochromocytoma, colon carcinoma, and medullary thyroid cancer. Paraneoplastic ACTH syndrome occurs more often than the benign form of Cushing's disease.[8]

SIAD is primarily associated with small-cell lung cancer, which accounts for about 80% of cases. Most of these patients may have some aspects of SIAD without clinical evidence of the syndrome. Only about 9%–14% percent of patients with small-cell lung cancer have full-blown SIAD.[4] Other cancers associated with SIAD include non–small-cell lung cancer, carcinoid tumors, squamous cell cancer of the head and neck; carcinomas of the prostate, esophagus, pancreas, and colon; thymoma and Hodgkin's and non-Hodgkin's lymphomas. Central nervous system (CNS) metastases, such as meningeal carcinomatosis, have also been associated with SIAD. The incidence of SIAD with cancers other than small-cell lung cancer is extremely small; these cancers may actually have a small-cell component to their histology.[2]

## Etiology and Risk Factors

The etiology of paraneoplastic hypercalcemia involves tumor secretion of bone-resorbing cytokines, prostaglandins, transforming growth factors, 1,25-dihydroxyvitamin D, and parathyroid hormone related protein (PTHrP). Of these substances, PTHrP is the primary factor in the development of paraneoplastic hypercalcemia. Although this etiology has been distinguished from bone-related hypercalcemia in the past, there appears to be a paraneoplastic component to the development of hypercalcemia in patients with bone metastases. Many patients with bone metastases never develop hypercalcemia because their homeostatic mechanisms are able to compensate for the excess calcium. No relationship has been found between the incidence of hypercalcemia and the extent of bony disease.[9]

The etiology of paraneoplastic ACTH syndrome is ectopic secretion of ACTH by neoplastic cells, resulting in an excess of ACTH in the body. This leads to bilateral adrenal hyperplasia and the symptoms of Cushing's disease. ACTH syndrome has been widely reported, with more than 75% of the cases associated with tumors located in the chest and mediastinum.[4] The prognosis of the

**TABLE 26-1**  Endocrine Paraneoplastic Syndromes

| Syndrome | Hormone | Associated Malignancy | Clinical Presentation | Comments |
|---|---|---|---|---|
| Hypercalcemia | Parathyroid hormone-related protein (PTHrP) | *Solid Tumors:* Squamous cell <br>• Lung cancer<br>• Head and neck<br>• Esophagus<br>• Cervix<br>• Breast<br>• Ovarian<br>• Bladder<br>*Hematologic:* | • Confusion<br>• Weakness<br>• Lethargy | |
| | Osteoclast activating factors<br>1,25 hydroxyvitamin D | Multiple myeloma<br>Acute leukemia<br>Lymphoma | | |
| Paraneoplastic ACTH (Cushing's) syndrome | Adrenocorticotropic hormone (ACTH) | Small-cell lung carcinoma (6%)<br>Carcinoid<br>Pancreatic<br>Medullary thyroid<br>Pheochromocytoma | • Hypokalemia<br>• Muscle weakness/ atrophy<br>• Weight loss<br>• Hypertension | |
| Syndrome of inappropriate antidiuresis | Arginine vasopressin (AVP)<br>Atrial natriuretic hormone (ANP) | Small-cell lung carcinoma (80%)<br>Pancreatic<br>Thymus<br>Breast | • Water intoxication<br>• Hyponatremia | |
| Paraneoplastic growth hormone-releasing hormone syndrome (Acromegaly) | Growth hormone-releasing hormone (GHRH) | Bronchial carcinoid<br>Pancreatic carcinoma | • Acromegaly | Rapid onset |
| Paraneoplastic osteomalacia | 1,25 hydroxyvitamin D | "Strange tumors in strange places"<br>Soft tissue, bone tumors<br>• Hemangioma<br>• Angiosarcoma<br>• Osteoblastoma | • Skeletal pain<br>• Muscle weakness | Occurs in young adults |
| Paraneoplastic secretion of human chorionic gonadotropin | Human chorionic gonadotropin (HCG) | Ovarian<br>Testicular<br>Large-cell lung cancer<br>Gastric<br>Breast<br>Melanoma | Usually asymptomatic<br>• Dysfunctional bleeding<br>• Gynecomastia | |
| Hypoglycemia | Insulin-like growth factors | Mesothelioma<br>Fibrosarcoma<br>Neurofibrosarcoma<br>Hepatoma | • Diaphoresis<br>• Confusion— may progress to stupor/coma | Many patients asymptomatic unless fasting |
| Paraneoplastic erythrocytosis | Erythropoietin | Uterine fibroma<br>Cerebellar hemangioblastoma<br>Hepatocellular carcinoma | • ↑ RBC's<br>• ↑ Hgb/Hct<br>• ↑ Red blood cell mass | Remission achieved by surgical resection of tumor |

patient diagnosed with paraneoplastic ACTH syndrome is poor because ACTH may function as a growth factor for neoplastic cells, particularly small-cell lung cancer tissue, and excessive cortisol levels suppress immune function, leading to an increased risk of infection. ACTH syndrome patients are especially at risk for developing fungal infections.[10] They are also at risk for gastrointestinal ulceration and bleeding due to high cortisol levels.[11]

The etiology of SIAD as a PNS is related to ectopic production of vasopressin by malignant cells. The severity of SIAD usually correlates with the extent of malignant disease. Although structurally identical, ectopic AVP is not subject to normal physiological controls.[12] Small-cell carcinoma of the lung accounts for 80% of the malignancies associated with SIAD. Cyclophosphamide and vincristine, drugs frequently used in the treatment of small-cell lung cancer, have also been associated with the development of SIAD. Cyclophosphamide's direct effect on the renal tubule, combined with the vigorous hydration used to prevent hemorrhagic cystitis, can result in SIAD. SIAD in this instance represents a "secondary paraneoplastic syndrome."[2] Other factors contributing to the multifactorial etiology of SIAD in the small-cell lung cancer patient include smoking (nicotine), stress, pain, nausea, and the use of morphine, all of which can increase AVP production.[12]

## Pathophysiology

The pathophysiology of the endocrine PNSs is related to the effect of ectopic hormone production on the normal hormonal physiological pathways affecting the release and inhibition of various hormones.

Normal calcium homeostasis is maintained by the interactions of multiple factors that affect bone resorption and osteolysis. Prostaglandins ($PGE_1$, $PGE_2$), parathyroid hormone (PTH), osteoclast-activating factor, and thyroxine ($T_4$) stimulate bone resorption and osteolysis. Calcitonin and estrogen inhibit these mechanisms. Paraneoplastic or humoral hypercalcemia in solid tumors is most often caused by tumor secretion of parathyroid hormone-related peptide (PTHrP). This peptide is structurally similar to PTH and is present in small amounts in normal tissue. PTHrP binds to PTH receptors and mimics the effect of PTH, inducing bone resorption and phosphaturia.[13] In addition to inducing hypercalcemia, PTHrP may act as a growth factor for malignant cells.

Hypercalcemia associated with multiple myeloma and lymphomas results from local bone destruction rather than the effects of PTHrP. These tumors secrete osteoclast-activating factors that stimulate osteoclasts to resorb bone. Osteoclast-activating factors are made from one or several cytokines, such as interleukin-1-beta, released from malignant plasma cells.[8] Another cytokine, tumor necrosis factor (TNF)–beta, is secreted by multiple myeloma cells and stimulates bone resorption. Lymphoma, small-cell lung cancer, and malignant melanoma cells may produce active metabolites of vitamin D, which stimulates calcium absorbtion from the gut.[2]

Paraneoplastic ACTH syndrome is related to tumor secretion of ACTH, which stimulates the adrenal cortex to increase glucocorticoid production resulting in excessive amounts of corticosteroids and leading to the development of Cushing's disease. ACTH is actually part of a precursor molecule, which contains melanocyte-stimulating hormone (MSH) and immunologic forms of beta-endorphin. Due to the increased levels of MSH, patients with paraneoplastic ACTH syndrome may manifest marked hyperpigmentation. This precursor molecule contains many biologically inactive products; therefore, even though up to one-third of small-cell lung cancer patients have increased serum ACTH levels, only 1%–2% develop Cushing's syndrome.[8]

SIAD impacts the body's fluid and sodium balance. Normally, the body maintains fluid volume and concentration within a very narrow range regulated by the effect of the neurohypophyseal peptide arginine vasopressin (AVP) on the kidney. When AVP is present, the collecting duct is permeable to water resulting in water reabsorption and concentrated urine. Suppression of AVP leads to urine dilution. Malignant secretion of AVP overrides the normal negative feedback mechanism that suppresses AVP release when serum osmolality, blood volume, and sodium levels are homeostatic. The excess AVP stimulation leads to a scenario of water intoxication from an expanded extracellular volume, serum hypo-osmolality, hyponatremia, and hypertonic urine.[8]

## Clinical Manifestations

In many patients the gradual onset of hypercalcemia is asymptomatic and found only during routine electrolyte measurement. A rapid increase in calcium occurs with highly proliferative tumors causing accelerated bone resorption, which overwhelms the kidney's ability to excrete the excess calcium. The acute symptoms of hypercalcemia ensue and include polyuria, polydipsia, nausea, vomiting, anorexia, constipation, lethargy, weakness, and dehydration. Nausea, vomiting, and polyuria can exacerbate the dehydration, which then decreases the glomerular filtration rate and can worsen the hypercalcemia. Occasional complaints are headaches, irritability, anxiety, and insomnia. Confusion, disorientation, hallucinations, and coma are late signs of progressively elevated serum calcium.[14] Obviously these symptoms can arise from a multitude of oncological complications and/or therapies, making it difficult to detect the onset of hypercalcemia without frequent laboratory evaluation.

Excess calcium ions adversely affect cardiac muscle contractility, cell membrane permeability, and the conduction of electrical impulses through the heart. The resulting cardiovascular effects include heart block, bradycardia, ventricular arrhythmias, and asystole.[14]

Cushing's disease is a disorder of excess ACTH. Patients with paraneoplastic ACTH syndrome are most likely to exhibit hypokalemic alkalosis, glucose intolerance, and muscle weakness.[3,11] The classic features of Cushing's disease, such as fat distribution changes, hypertension, plethora, cutaneous hyperpigmentation, and edema, may be absent because these patients do not survive long enough to develop these characteristics.

Water intoxication accounts for the signs and symptoms seen with SIAD, although most patients are asymptomatic. Edema is rare since the retained water is distributed into cells and not interstitially. When the serum sodium level has fallen to 115–120 mEq/liter (normal range = 137–145 mEq/liter), symptoms may include nausea, weakness, anorexia, fatigue, and muscle cramps. These vague, nonspecific complaints can be easily attributed to the cancer, and often are not identified as early signs of hyponatremia. The symptomatology that a patient exhibits is dependent on both the severity of the hyponatremia and the rate at which it developed.[12]

As the hyponatremia worsens, symptoms may progress to include altered mental status, confusion, lethargy, combativeness, or psychotic behavior. When the hyponatremia is extremely severe (100–110 mEq/liter), seizures, coma, and death may occur.[2]

## Assessment

### Diagnostic studies

Diagnosis of hypercalcemia is based on combining the clinical picture with an elevated calcium level. The normal range for serum calcium is 8.5–10.5 g/dl. Hypercalcemia is defined as a serum calcium level >11.0 mg/dl. Measurement of ionized calcium levels is preferred to total serum calcium because it does not include protein-bound calcium and is considered more accurate.

Diagnosis of paraneoplastic ACTH (pACTH) syndrome is made primarily by lab testing. Plasma cortisol and 24-hour urinary free cortisol levels may be obtained. With ectopic ACTH, cortisol levels may be 140 times the normal level.[10] The simplest test to do is a dexamethasone suppression test. The patient receives 2 mg of dexamethasone every 6 hours for 48 hours, or a single 8-mg dose at midnight before obtaining a cortisol level at 8 A.M. the following morning. If the plasma cortisol levels do not suppress, the test is positive. A more recent development in the diagnosis of pACTH is the discovery that the malignancies most frequently associated with pACTH have somatostatin receptors.[4] These receptors are absent from pituitary adenomas, and these types of Cushing's disease do not respond to somatostatin analogues.

Most cases of SIAD are diagnosed inadvertently when hyponatremia is found through routine serum chemistry studies. The diagnosis of SIAD requires the presence of hyponatremia in addition to plasma hypo-osmolality and inappropriately concentrated urine. Plasma osmolality must be <280 mOsm/kg, and concurrent urinalysis must show increased levels of sodium (>20 mEq/liter). Serum chemistries frequently show a low BUN, creatinine, albumin, and uric acid as a result of the increased extracellular fluid volume. Measurement of serum AVP levels is possible by radioimmunoassay but is rarely done. The levels may be normal or elevated.[8] Other conditions that cause hyponatremia must be ruled out, such as dehydration, fluid retention or abnormal renal, adrenal, or thyroid function.

## Therapeutic Approaches and Nursing Care

Treatment of hypercalcemia involves vigorous hydration and the use of drug therapy. Intravenous pamidronate sodium has proved to be the most effective and least toxic therapy for hypercalcemia associated with solid tumors.[8]

Nursing care involves being able to recognize the subtle signs of early hypercalcemia and taking appropriate action (see chapter 25 on hypercalcemia).

Treatment of pACTH syndrome is primarily focused on treatment of the malignancy. Measures to control the effects of Cushing's disease while waiting for the malignancy to respond include the following:

- Aminoglutethimide: can be effective in lowering cortisol levels due to its effect on blocking hormone production from the adrenal gland. Glucocorticoid replacement may be necessary (dexamethasone)

- Ketoconazole: an imidazole derivative that impairs corticosteroid production

- Mitotane: an oral adrenal cytotoxic agent

- Bilateral adrenalectomy: used rarely in cases where the Cushing's syndrome is resistant to medical intervention, or the patient has an indolent tumor

The prognosis for patients with pACTH is poor. The reponse rates to combination chemotherapy are usually very low. The presence of Cushing's syndrome at the time of diagnosis is considered an adverse prognostic factor, worse than if it develops later at the time of recurrence. Patients with pACTH syndrome usually die of pneumonia or opportunistic fungal infections instead of progressive disease.[4] Achieving control of the Cushing's syndrome through normalization of the cortisol level prior to initiating chemotherapy may reduce the potential for infection.

The treatment of SIAD, as with all PNSs, is directed at the underlying malignancy. However, stabilization of the patient, and correction of the hyponatremia is essential. The severity of the hyponatremia and water intoxication determine the treatment of the SIAD. Fluid restriction of 800–1000 ml/day is the initial treatment of choice for mild hyponatremia (serum sodium between 125 and 134 mEq/liter), and may be the only treatment necessary.[12] Fluid restriction allows the plasma osmolality to gradually increase through the eventual loss of free water.

Severe hyponatremia (serum sodium <120 mEq/liter) requires more aggressive treatment, especially if the patient is experiencing seizures or coma. Hypertonic (3%) saline given intravenously at a rate of 0.1 ml/kg/minute over 24 hours should increase the serum sodium by 10 mmol/liter per day.[4] Intravenous (IV) furosemide (1 mg/kg) is often used to expedite water loss. Such therapeutic endeavors are instituted only in carefully controlled situations, such as an intensive care setting. The patient must be monitored carefully and the serum sodium and electrolytes checked frequently. An excessively rapid correction of the serum sodium may result in neurological damage. A thorough neurological assessment is documented daily. Restriction of oral and IV fluids should also be instituted.[12] The patient's fluid balance is monitored and the patient weighed daily.

Chronic mild to moderate hyponatremia may be managed with certain oral medications. Lithium carbonate stimulates diuresis by impairing the effect of AVP on the renal tubule. Because side effects include gastrointestinal toxicity, tremors, and muscle weakness, it is rarely used. Demeclocycline (900–1200 mg/day) is an antibiotic that is most frequently used to treat chronic SIAD. Its mechanism of action is the same as lithium, but it produces more reliable results. Demeclocycline allows a normal daily intake of water and other fluids. Superinfections and hematologic changes may occur. Another drug occasionally used to treat SIAD is urea, which produces an osmotic diuresis and also allows normal fluid intake.[2]

Outpatient oncology nurses, especially those caring for newly diagnosed lung cancer patients, should maintain a high index of suspicion for the development of SIAD. Obtaining a complete patient history, conducting careful nursing assessment, and reviewing serum chemistries assist with early diagnosis. Patients and their family members are instructed regarding the early symptoms of hyponatremia (nausea, weakness, muscle cramps, confusion, lethargy) and are encouraged to report these symptoms promptly.

# NEUROLOGICAL PARANEOPLASTIC SYNDROMES

## Scope of the Problem

Neurological PNSs are uncommon yet account for some of the most interesting and frustrating of the PNSs. As opposed to most of the other PNSs, the neurological syndromes do not always correlate with the status of the underlying malignancy, as nervous tissue is unable to repair certain types of damage. In some cases the malignancy may resolve and the patient is left to cope with the permanent neurological damage.[2]

Most neurological disorders in cancer patients are attributable to the effects of metastatic disease. However, the existence of paraneoplastic syndromes has been well established in some cases such as thymoma and myasthenia gravis. It is important to note that these neurological PNSs can also have a benign etiology. The possibility of cancer occurring simultaneously depends upon the type of PNS; for example, two-thirds of patients with Lambert-Eaton myasthenic syndrome (LEMS) have or will develop lung cancer, whereas malignancy is much less commonly associated with sensorimotor peripheral neuropathy. In general, the faster the onset of the neurological syndrome, the higher the odds that it is malignant in origin. Any segment of the nervous system, including the brain, spinal cord, and peripheral nervous system, may be affected by a PNS. In some cases more than one area may be affected at the same time.[15]

Unlike the endocrine PNSs, in which the tumor secretes excessive amounts of a naturally occurring hormone, the neurological PNSs are thought to occur from an autoimmune reaction to the tumor. Antibodies secreted by the immune system, in response to antigens shared by the tumor and nervous tissue, may attack nerve cells such as Purkinje cells, resulting in the neurological syndrome. This theory, which has evolved in the last 20 years, has increased the interest of the scientific community in PNSs. Identification of autoantibodies causing PNS

may lead to new diagnostic tests and the possibility of earlier diagnosis and treatment of both the malignancy and the PNS.[15]

Two major neurological PNSs are paraneoplastic cerebellar degeneration (PCD) and LEMS. Other neurological PNSs include sensory and motor neuropathies, limbic encephalitis, and retinal degeneration.

## Definitions

Subacute cerebellar degeneration is a group of paraneoplastic neurological disorders known to be caused by antineuronal antibodies that are characterized by progressive ataxia and severe vision changes. A number of antibodies have been identified in relation to PCD: Anti-Yo, Anti-Hu, Anti-Ri, Hodgkin's, and PCD/LEMS. In over 50% of patients the onset of PCD usually predates diagnosis of the cancer by several months. Occasionally, the malignancy is not detected for years and is discovered only upon autopsy.[16]

LEMS is a paraneoplastic antibody-mediated autoimmune disorder characterized by weakness and easy fatigability of muscles, that primarily affects patients with small-cell lung carcinoma.[17]

## Incidence

PCD is a rare disorder, with fewer than 300 cases having been reported in the literature. In some instances a PNS may go undetected and therefore unreported due to the subtle nature of the symptoms. This is not the case with PCD, where symptoms are severe and easily identifiable. The malignancy most often associated with PCD is ovarian cancer. Other cancers in which PCD may occur include small-cell lung cancer, Hodgkin's lymphoma, and to a lesser extent breast cancer. The autoantibody involved may differ depending upon the malignancy (Table 26-2).

LEMS occurs in approximately 6% of patients with small-cell lung cancer and has been incidentally reported in patients with breast, gastric, prostate, ovarian, and rectal cancers. An average of 40% of LEMS cases do not have a malignant etiology but result from a variety of autoimmune diseases, including rheumatoid arthritis, scleroderma, and multiple sclerosis.[17]

## Etiology and Risk Factors

Both paraneoplastic neurological syndromes result from the patient's immune system producing antibodies that mistake normal nerve cells for tumor cell antigens. The paraneoplastic cerebellar degeneration disorders arise from the presence of anti–Purkinje cell antibodies associated with specific neoplasms. The similarity between tumor cell antigens and onconeural antigens expressed by cerebellar Purkinje cells causes the immune system to

**TABLE 26-2**    Autoantibody-Associated Paraneoplastic Cerebellar Degeneration Syndromes

| Antibody | Malignancy | Syndrome | Clinical Features | Comments |
|---|---|---|---|---|
| Anti-Yo | • Ovarian carcinoma<br>• Breast carcinoma | Paraneoplastic cerebellar degeneration (PCD) | • Occurs only in women<br>• Occurs prior to malignant diagnosis in majority of patients<br>• Localized tumor<br>• Symptoms include severe dysarthria, oscillopsia, and diplopia | • Treatment with steroids or plasmapheresis is rarely effective<br>• PCD remains unchanged even if malignancy is cured<br>• 100 patients reported |
| Anti-Hu | • Small-cell lung cancer<br>• Prostate carcinoma<br>• Adenocarcinoma of lung<br>• Sarcoma | Paraneoplastic encephalomyelitis sensory neuropathy (PEM/SN) | • 60% of women<br>• Occurs prior to malignant diagnosis<br>• Sensory neuropathy may involve all 4 extremities | • 10% of SCLC patients have the Anti-Hu antibody but do *not* develop the syndrome<br>• Death usually occurs from autonomic nervous system failure, not progressive disease<br>• Treatment with steroids or plasmapheresis is rarely effective<br>• Presence of the antibody indicates an indolent disease course |
| Anti-Ri | Not associated with a particular malignancy seen in lung, breast cancer | Paraneoplastic opsoclonus-myoclonus (POM) | • Involuntary eye movement in all directions<br>• Truncal ataxia | • Clinical course is pattern of improvement and exacerbations independent of course of malignancy<br>• Extremely rare (< 20 patients studied) |
| Hodgkin's | • Hodgkin's lymphoma | PCD | • Male to female ratio is 6:1<br>• Younger age (20–40 years)<br>• Diagnosis usually made at time of malignant diagnosis<br>• Signs and symptoms similar to Anti-Yo PCD | • Only PCD syndrome in which remission occurs in conjunction with response of lymphoma to treatment |
| PCD/LEMS (antibody negative) | • Small-cell lung cancer | PCD combined with Lambert-Eaton myasthenic syndrome | • Subacute onset of PCD<br>• Lower extremity weakness<br>• Occurs prior to malignant diagnosis<br>• In some patients PCD is predominant; in others LEMS is predominant | • LEMS component may respond to plasmapheresis, steroids, or successful antineoplastic treatment; however, PCD component is usually unresponsive to therapy<br>• More common than other PCD syndromes except Anti-Yo (30 patients reported) |

mistakenly attack the Purkinje cells, with severe neurological consequences.[16]

LEMS as a PNS may be the result of autoantibodies attacking the neuromuscular structures involved in muscle nerve contraction. Small-cell lung carcinoma is thought to originate from neuroectodermal tissue; therefore, tumor cells may express neural antigens containing voltage-gated calcium channels (VGCCs) on their cell surface. The immune response to the presence of malignant cells produces IgG antibodies against these tumor antigens. These IgG antibodies mistakenly attack VGCCs in normal nerve tissue, leading to the development of LEMS.[17]

## Pathophysiology

PCD is a result of the loss or dysfunction of cerebellar Purkinje cells. The cerebellum is the area of the brain that assists in the coordination of movement. It processes sensory information to coordinate the activity of descending motor pathways. Coordinated gait, balance, head and eye movements, and muscle tone are the result of optimum cerebellar functioning. If cerebellar function is impaired, any or all of the following may occur: ataxia (staggered gait), intention tremors, loss of balance, loss of reflexes, or dysarthria (slow slurred speech). The cerebellum is only involved in the coordination of motor function; dysfunction does not produce sensory deficits.[18] However, sensory input from afferent fibers elicits action potentials in Purkinje cells, causing neuron discharge and transfer of electrical impulses to the cerebellar tissue.

### Antineural antibodies

The belief that PCD is an autoimmune disorder is based on the idea that the patient's immune response to the tumor produces antibodies that unfortunately recognize Purkinje cells as being similar to tumor cells, thereby attacking and destroying or disabling them.[16]

Several antibodies have been identified related to the development of PCD. These polyclonal IgG antibodies have been measured in the serum and cerebrospinal fluid (CSF) of patients with PCD. Not all patients with PCD have had antibodies present in their serum and CSF; however, the syndrome has been clinically identical to that in patients with antibodies. The presence of antibodies appears to have a positive prognostic significance as it is associated with a more indolent tumor course.

Western blot analysis allowed the antibodies to be first identified in the early 1980s. Initially designated "anti-Purkinje cell antibody," the first antibody identified has since been labeled *anti-Yo* (after the first two letters of the last name of the patient studied). Subsequent antibodies identified are *anti-Hu, anti-Ri, Hodgkin's,* and *pcd/LEMS.* Each antibody is associated with different malignancies, and PCD has since been categorized according to the autoantibody involved (see Table 26-2).

The pathophysiology involved in LEMS is a specific abnormality at the cholinergic presynaptic junction. In normal neural function nerve impulses are transmitted from one cell to another via electrical or chemical synapses. The structures involved with the transmission of a nerve impulse across a chemical synapse include the presynaptic neuron, a neurotransmitter substance, the synaptic cleft, and the postsynaptic cell. These structures are known as the *neuromuscular junction* (NMJ), which facilitates chemical impulses between motor neurons and skeletal muscle fibers. A nerve impulse or action potential is conducted from the motor neuron to the presynaptic neuron. Depolarization of the neuron plasma membrane opens calcium channels. Calcium influx stimulates the synaptic vesicles to fuse with the plasma membrane and

release acetylcholine (ACh) into the synaptic cleft. The synaptic vesicles are located in zones in the presynaptic nerve terminal that contain rows of large intramembrane particles. These particles are VGCCs that regulate ACh release. ACh is a neurotransmitter that crosses the synaptic cleft and combines with an ACh receptor protein (AChR) on the postsynaptic muscle cell. This ACh receptor complex increases conductance of $Na^+$ and $K^+$ currents, allowing depolarization of the postsynaptic muscle end plate. This end plate potential (EPP) triggers the action potential that results in muscle contraction.[17,18]

In LEMS, the presence of tumor cells stimulates an autoimmune response that produces IgG antibodies against calcium channels expressed by both the cancer and the neuromuscular junction. The IgG autoantibodies block the VGCCs in the presynaptic nerve terminal, resulting in insufficient ACh release into the synaptic cleft and therefore very low-amplitude muscle action potentials.[19]

## Clinical Manifestations

The onset of PCD usually occurs prior to the diagnosis of cancer. The cerebellar dysfunction is characterized by neurological signs and symptoms that are usually bilateral, symmetrical, and progressive. The initial symptoms are a slight difficulty in walking that rapidly progresses to severe ataxia. This deterioration may occur over days or weeks, with the movements of the arms, legs, and trunk becoming progressively uncoordinated. The patient may experience dysarthria, nystagmus, and oscillopsia, a subjective sensation that objects in the visual field are oscillating. Assistance may be needed to walk and sit, and eventually all activities of daily living are compromised. Communication may be difficult due to the dysarthria and the fact that most patients are unable to write due to hand tremors. Reading and watching television are challenging if not impossible due to the oscillopsia.[16]

Patients with PCD frequently have other mild neurological deficits. These include sensorineural hearing loss, dysphagia, diplopia, and peripheral neuropathy. Signs of mild dementia may occur, but this is difficult to assess due to the impaired ability to communicate. Vertigo is frequently present.[20]

Eventually the symptoms of PCD peak in their severity and stabilize. Unfortunately, even if the underlying malignancy is successfully treated the neurological symptoms rarely improve. However, there is a wide variety in the degree of severity of PCD. Some patients may experience only mild ataxia and impairment of writing and speaking abilities. A few patients may experience an improvement in neurological symptoms as their tumor responds to therapy.[16]

LEMS is characterized by muscle weakness and easy fatigability, with the muscle groups of the pelvic girdle and thighs primarily affected; the arms and shoulders to a lesser extent. Patients with LEMS complain of difficulty in climbing stairs, rising from a chair or toilet, walking, or running. Additional symptoms may include double or blurred vision, dysarthria, dysphagia, ptosis, parasthesias, and muscle pain.[2] The weakness associated with LEMS tends to amplify toward the end of the day. It may temporarily improve with voluntary effort from the patient. The autonomic nervous system may also be affected in LEMS due to antibody attack on smooth muscle resulting in complaints of constipation, urinary retention, and dry mouth.[17]

## Assessment

### Diagnostic studies

Routine neurological diagnostic studies include magnetic resonance imaging (MRI) and/or computed tomography (CT) scan of the brain, and lumbar puncture. Patients with PCD initially may have a normal MRI or CT brain scan. As the cerebellar failure progresses over a few months, these scans may exhibit diffuse cerebellar atrophy and a dilated fourth ventricle.[20] A positron emission tomography (PET) scan may show abnormal metabolism of the cerebral hemispheres. Initial analysis of CSF obtained via lumbar puncture may show elevated protein levels, an increased IgG, and increased lymphocytes. However, after the neurological symptoms have plateaued, the CSF frequently reverts to normal.[14]

The diagnosis of LEMS rests in part upon distinguishing it from another neurological disorder—myasthenia gravis (MG). LEMS is similar to MG but with some distinctions. In LEMS, in contrast to MG, muscle strength improves with exercise. The drug edrophonium (Tensilon), while very effective for the treatment of MG, has little effect in LEMS. The serum of MG patients contains ACh receptor antibodies that are not present in the serum of patients with LEMS.

Electromyography is used to assess muscle action potentials. Repeated nerve stimulation will cause an increase in muscle action potential, resulting in a temporary increase in muscle strength in LEMS. MG patients will experience a progressive decrease in muscle response.

## Therapeutic Approaches and Nursing Care

PCD rarely responds to treatment. The treatments that have been attempted include corticosteroids such as prednisone and dexamethasone. More recently, plasmapheresis has been used in an effort to remove the autoantibodies and antigen/antibody complexes, much as it is used to treat other autoimmune disorders. It has not proved to be successful. This may be due to the fact that the Purkinje cells may have been attacked and quickly destroyed early in the course of the syndrome long before treatment is initiated. The drug clonazepam has been

used to treat the ataxia associated with PCD; doses range from 0.5 mg to 1.5 mg daily.[16]

The most challenging issues for nurses caring for patients with PCD is helping them accept that the neurological symptoms may be permanent in spite of possible cure or improvement of their cancer. For most patients and families the symptoms occurred very rapidly, with little chance to adapt to the deterioration in abilities and the increasing dependence on others. Rehabilitation, psychological support, and counseling are essential to helping the patient and family adapt to changing roles and needs.

Treatment of LEMS, as with the previous PNSs, is based upon treatment of the underlying malignancy. Frequently the symptoms associated with LEMS improve with tumor response. If the neurological symptoms do not improve, a variety of medications and/or plasmapheresis may be implemented. The drugs used to treat LEMS are pharmacological agents that promote ACh release from the nerve terminal such as 3,4-diaminopyridine and guanidine. Guanidine is effective but has significant side effects such as seizures. 3,4-Diaminopyridine is the treatment of choice. It affects $K^+$ channels, thereby increasing the amount of ACh released into the synaptic cleft. Steroids, immune suppression, gamma globulin, and plasmapheresis have been utilized in the treatment of LEMS with mixed success. Plasmapheresis alone is associated with short-term clinical improvement. Weekly plasmapheresis, in combination with prednisone and azathioprine, has produced the most sustained clinical benefit.[21,22]

Patients with a neurological disorder such as LEMS require a great deal of emotional support. The initial phases of the illness can be frightening, as LEMS patients must learn to deal with a diagnosis of cancer as well as a potentially disabling neurological disease. The needs of the LEMS patient include ongoing assessment of the neurological status and comprehensive patient education regarding measures to cope with the chronic muscle weakness and fatigue.[23] Figure 26-2 depicts partial amputations of the fingertips and loss of the nails due to paraneoplastic sensory neuropathy, discussed in case study A (Table 26-3).

## HEMATOLOGIC PARANEOPLASTIC SYNDROMES

### Scope of the Problem

Hematologic abnormalities are frequent problems for oncology patients, often associated with tumor infiltration of the bone marrow or the effect of antineoplastic therapy. However, the most common hematologic problem is anemia of chronic disease or malignancy. Tumor secretion of cytokines, colony-stimulating factors, and factors that affect coagulation can produce a variety of hemato-

**TABLE 26-3**   Case Study A

*Subject:* Neurological paraneoplastic syndrome associated with large-cell lymphoma

*Summary:* A 38-year-old woman presenting with a profound ascending sensory neuropathy was subsequently diagnosed with a large-cell lymphoma of the lung. She later developed an autonomic neuropathy manifested by orthostatic hypotension and gastroparesis. She received 6 cycles of standard CHOP chemotherapy followed by radiation therapy for residual lung disease. She remains in complete remission three years following treatment.

*Clinical symptoms:* Initial complaints included fatigue, numbness and tingling of the arms and legs, right-sided facial numbness, difficulty ambulating, and dizziness when standing. Physical exam revealed severe orthostatic hypotension, the absence of fingernails, and sores on fingertips from patient biting. She also developed ulcerations of her lower extremities from trying to do housework.

*Clinical course and treatment:* The orthostatic hypotension has been successfully managed with Florinef, prednisone, and Sandostatin. She underwent three courses of plasmapheresis, which provided marked improvement of the fatigue but no change in the sensory neuropathy. However, in the past two years the sensory neuropathy has slightly improved. She currently ambulates with a wide-based gait using a single-prong cane. Following chemotherapy she developed osteomyelitis resulting in the partial amputation of several fingers (see Figure 26-2).

logic disorders, including anemia, granulocytopenia, eosinophilia, thrombocytosis, thromboembolism, thrombocytopenia, and coagulopathies such as disseminated intravascular coagulation (DIC). Blood coagulation abnormalities have been reported in over 90% of cancer patients.[24] Anemia of malignancy and thromboembolism will be discussed in more detail.

## Definitions

Anemia in the cancer patient may be due to the effects of chemotherapy or radiation, bleeding, bone marrow invasion by tumor, or a primary hematologic disorder. Anemia as a remote effect of neoplastic disease is much less common and is caused by tumor product impairment of bone marrow function and/or red cell metabolism.[2] When the cause of anemia in a cancer patient cannot be determined, the diagnosis of "anemia of chronic disease or chronic malignancy" is often made. This syndrome is characterized by a normocytic/normochromic anemia that is not associated with a particular malignancy.[2]

Cancer patients have a higher risk of thromboembolism (TE) or clot formation due to the hypercoagulable state induced by the malignancy. Paraneoplastic TE was first identified in 1865 by Trousseau, who noted an increased incidence of migratory venous thrombosis in patients with cancer. The definition of Trousseau's syndrome has been expanded over the years to reflect

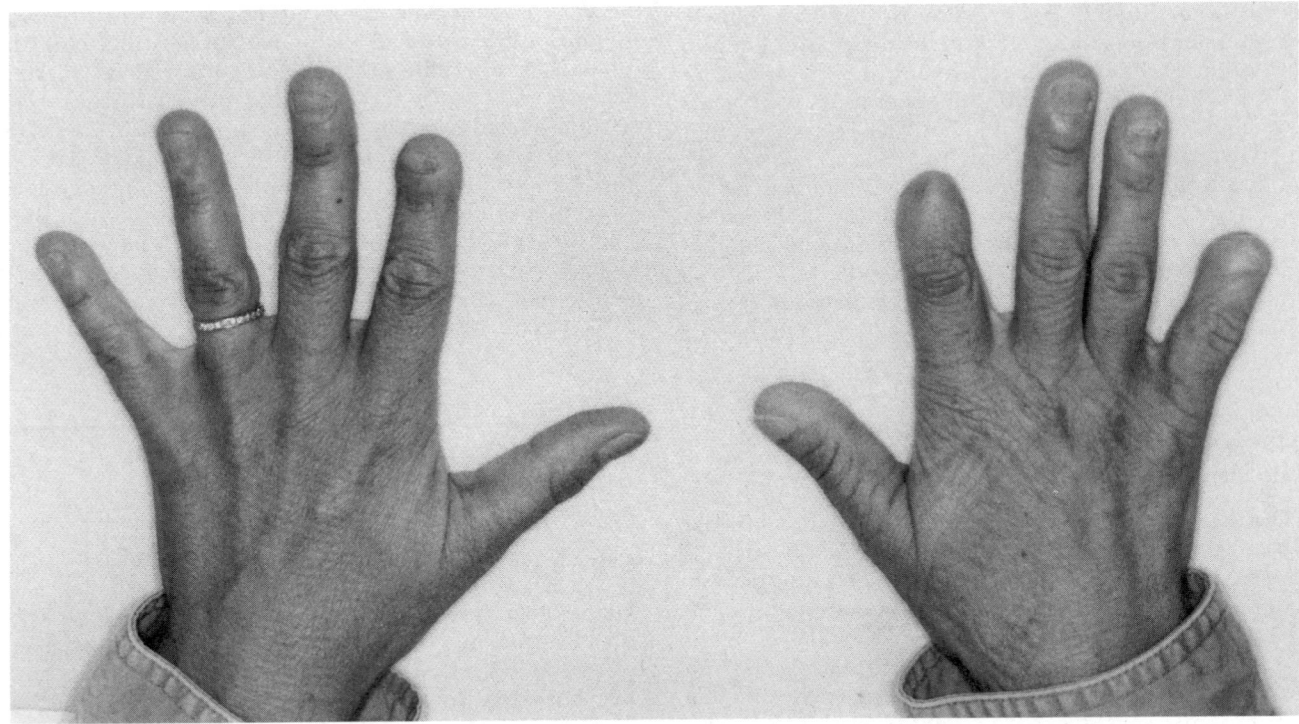

**FIGURE 26-2**   Hands of patient in Table 3 case study A, showing partial amputations of tips of fingers and lack of nails due to paraneoplastic sensory neuropathy.

a better understanding of the effect of cancer cells on vasculature and the coagulation pathways. Trousseau's syndrome now describes a variety of thromboembolic disorders affecting both veins and arteries, including specific types of peripheral vascular disease and ischemic heart disease.[25]

## Incidence

The incidence of anemia of malignancy is difficult if not impossible to determine because of the inability to separate treatment-related effects from a possible paraneoplastic etiology. Many oncology patients will experience some degree of anemia during their disease course, primarily related to treatment effects. Anemia of chronic malignancy is a diagnosis most commonly applied to patients with advanced disease.

The incidence of TE in cancer patients has been estimated to be between 1% and 11%. The thromboemboli are frequently found at the time of autopsy. The malignancies primarily associated with TE include small-cell lung cancer (SCLC) and non–small-cell lung cancer (NSCLC); and colon, pancreas, and—to a lesser extent—breast, prostate, ovarian, and bladder carcinomas. The type of cancer most often implicated is mucin-secreting adenocarcinoma of the gastrointestinal (GI) tract. The incidence of TE appears to rise during chemotherapy and hormonal therapy, possibly related to the thrombogenic effect of antineoplastic agents and hormones. The exact mechanism is unknown but may involve a reduction in antithrombin fibrin and fibrinolytic activity.[26,27]

## Etiology and Risk Factors

The etiology of anemia of malignancy is multifactorial. It involves the tumor secretion of cytokines, such as interleukin-1 (IL-1), affecting red cell metabolism; other factors include protein-calorie malnutrition, bone marrow failure, and chronic hemorrhage. Protein-calorie malnutrition will produce insufficiencies in iron and folic acid, and general hypoproteinemia. Heavily treated patients who have received multiple courses of chemotherapy and radiation are susceptible to bone marrow failure, which may be manifested by deficiencies in a single cell line such as red cells or platelets but more commonly presents as pancytopenia. Chronic microscopic bleeding usually results from the presence of primary or metastatic disease of the GI tract, genitourinary system, or upper and lower respiratory tract.[28]

The etiology of thromboembolism is the ability of tumor cells to affect systemic activation of coagulation and cause platelet dysfunction. Thromboembolic disease that is refractory to anticoagulation therapy is often indicative of underlying cancer. Several prospective studies have confirmed a relationship between recurrent, episodic idiopathic deep vein thrombosis (DVT), and the subsequent development of malignancy.[29,30] Idiopathic DVT (no identifiable risk factors) is associated with an estimated 10%–20% risk of malignancy. A significant proportion of these tumors are very small, presenting at an early stage, and are therefore potentially curable.[29]

## Pathophysiology

The multiple factors involved in the advent of anemia of malignancy include tumor secretion of cytokines that affect red cell metabolism and function. IL-1 has the ability to interfere in the transfer process of iron molecules from the reticuloendothelial system to red cell precursors in the bone marrow, resulting in an iron-rich bone marrow but iron-deficient erythrocytes.[28] Another function of IL-1 is stimulation of macrophages in the spleen, causing a decrease in red cell life span. Recently a protein called *anemia-inducing substance* has been identified in the plasma of patients with advanced malignancies that reduces the osmotic resistance of red blood cells, increasing their susceptibility to destruction.[31]

Tumor cells may remotely precipitate paraneoplastic TE by any one of three mechanisms: activation of the coagulation pathway, damage to the endothelial lining of blood vessels, or platelet activation.[25] (A review of the coagulation pathway and the association between clotting and cancer is discussed in chapter 22). Cancer cells are known to play a role in activation of the extrinsic clotting pathway. They may induce the cleavage of fibrinogen to fibrin and/or activate clotting factors such as factor VII or factor X, initiating the clotting cascade. This may be the combined result of direct and indirect effects of cancer cells. Stimulation of the patient's immune system by tumor cell antigens may activate monocyte-macrophages. These monocyte-macrophages in turn activate the clotting pathway through the expression of tissue factors. One theory describes the interaction of tumor cells, platelets, and inflammatory cells causing the formation of a "fibrin gel," a product essential to tumor growth and the development of metastases.[24]

Patients with cancer experience a variety of platelet disorders such as thrombocytopenia and platelet dysfunction. The exact mechanism by which tumor cells affect these disorders is unclear. One theory involves the production of thrombin.[25] Malignant cells may indirectly inflict damage to vascular endothelium via their activation of platelets. Platelets facilitate tumor cell adhesion to blood vessel walls through two mechanisms: the secretion of substances that promote further endothelial damage and the stimulation of increased platelet aggregation. This ability to affect platelet function is integral to the tumor's ability to invade, implant, and promote angiogenesis.[29]

## Clinical Manifestations

Anemia of malignancy is characterized by a low hemoglobin around 10 g/dl, and may be as low as 7.0–8.0

g/dl, which may or may not be symptomatic. Patients may complain of fatigue, dyspnea on exertion, reduced mental acuity, anorexia, and headaches. Physical signs include pallor, postural hypotension, edema, and splenomegaly. Paraneoplastic TE is characterized by venous or arterial thrombosis that may be recurrent and migratory, frequently occurring in veins in which DVTs are uncommon. Signs and symptoms are consistent with the presence of a DVT, including pain and edema of the extremity.

## Assessment

### Diagnostic studies

Anemia of malignancy is primarily a diagnosis of exclusion based on laboratory results combined with the clinical picture. It is characterized by a low serum iron and low iron-binding capacity. Other laboratory tests include hemoglobin, hematocrit, reticulocyte count, and serum ferritin. Bone marrow biopsy and aspirate may be performed. Trousseau's syndrome is diagnosed on the basis of the clinical presentation combined with ultrasound or radiographic confirmation of a thrombosis. Doppler ultrasound is most commonly performed.

## Therapeutic Approaches and Nursing Care

Anemia of malignancy is usually managed through the use of transfusions whenever the patient becomes symptomatic or the hemoglobin falls below 8.0 g/dl. Growth factors are employed conservatively due to the need for repeated injections and high cost. Iron, vitamin therapy, and steroids may be used but are generally not effective. Migratory TE is difficult to treat successfully. Anticoagulation therapy including heparin and warfarine is often instituted. Acute episodes of TE are managed with IV continuous-infusion heparin. Long-term management with coumadin therapy following the acute episode is usually unsuccessful. The advent of low-molecular-weight subcutaneous heparin has shown potential for the prevention of recurrent clot formation.

# RENAL PARANEOPLASTIC SYNDROMES

## Scope of the Problem

The majority of renal complications of malignancy are related to the effects of tumor infiltration of the kidneys, renal vein thrombosis, amyloidosis, urethral or ureteral obstruction, and complications of treatment, specifically chemotherapy. The only true renal PNSs are nephrotic syndrome produced by glomerular lesions and obstruction of the glomerulus by tumor products.[2] Obstruction by tumor products refers to the secretion of substances by malignant cells causing renal dysfunction. These are rare disorders such as mucoprotein secretion by pancreatic carcinoma cells resulting in intrarenal obstruction, and lysozyme secretion associated with acute leukemia resulting in renal potassium wasting and hypocalcemia. Nephrotic syndrome will be discussed in more detail.

## Definitions

The presence of paraneoplastic lesions in the renal glomerulus leads to a disease known as *nephrotic syndrome*, which is defined as impaired renal function resulting in massive proteinuria. Nephrotic syndrome fits the definition of a PNS in that it may precede the diagnosis of malignancy; a reduction in tumor burden by surgery or antineoplastic therapy is associated with a decrease in proteinuria; and increased proteinuria corresponds with tumor recurrence.[2]

## Incidence

The incidence of nephrotic syndrome as a PNS is difficult to determine. A review of 101 patients with nephrotic syndrome of unknown origin by Lee et al[32] in 1966 revealed 11 patients with evidence of malignancy. Hodgkin's lymphoma is the primary malignancy associated with nephrotic syndrome. To a lesser degree it is associated with non-Hodgkin's lymphomas such as Burkitt's lymphoma. Paraneoplastic nephrotic syndrome has also been reported in patients with lung, breast, colon, and prostate carcinomas as well as carcinoid tumors. Nephrotic syndrome precedes a diagnosis of cancer up to several months and possibly years in approximately 45% of cases; it follows a malignant diagnosis in 15%–20% of cases. The remaining 30%–40% of cases are diagnosed concurrently.[33]

## Etiology and Risk Factors

Nephrotic syndrome is most commonly known as a benign disorder either resulting from a primary glomerular disease or occurring secondary to infection, drugs, or systemic diseases such as diabetes mellitus, systemic lupus erythematosus, or rheumatoid arthritis.[34] The etiology of paraneoplastic nephrotic syndrome is the presence of glomerular lesions, with the type of lesion varying with the malignancy involved. In patients with carcinoma and nephrotic syndrome the etiology may involve products of the immune system, specifically antigen-antibody complexes, that become trapped within the glomerulus and impair glomerular function. The presence of nephrotic syndrome is considered a poor prognostic factor; however, death usually results from tumor progression and not from renal failure. Median survival following the diagnosis of nephrotic syndrome averages 12 months, and approximately 3 months from a malignant diagnosis.[35] However, successful eradication of the malignancy is associated with remission of the nephrotic syndrome.

## Pathophysiology

The glomerulus is the portion of the renal nephron, or functional unit of the kidney, responsible for the ultrafiltration of plasma and eventual urine formation. Ultrafiltration refers to the removal of plasma proteins and the passive flow of protein-free fluid from the glomerular capillaries into Bowman's space and the renal tubules.[18] The basement membrane of the glomerular capillaries is the main filtration barrier to plasma proteins and the location of most glomerular lesions. The glomerular lesions associated with the presence of a malignancy vary with the type of malignancy involved. The renal lesion present in 80% of patients with Hodgkin's lymphoma is known as *lipoid nephrosis*. Lipoid nephrosis is characterized by the presence of nephrotic syndrome and minimal glomerular changes on histological examination, also called *minimal change disease*.[36] Lipoid nephrosis may be linked to deficiencies in T-cell function, which are frequently seen in lymphomas. Membranous glomerulopathy and membranoproliferative glomerulonephritis represent the types of glomerular lesions seen in 20% of Hodgkin's lymphoma patients.[37]

Carcinomas are most often associated (80%–90%) with membranous glomerulonephritis, a type of glomerular lesion containing deposits of IgG and complement. Antigen-antibody complexes may become trapped in the glomerulus, resulting in lesions that adversely affect renal function. These types of complexes have been isolated from the kidneys of patients with lung and colon carcinomas and nephrotic syndrome. An example is the discovery of tumor-directed antibody and carcinoembryonic antigen present in the glomeruli of a patient with gastric carcinoma.[38]

The leakage of plasma proteins into the urine leads to the development of hypoalbuminemia, which in turn causes peripheral edema from the decrease in plasma oncotic pressure. The low plasma oncotic pressure instigates a series of homeostatic mechanisms, such as increased vasopressin secretion, in an effort to restore the plasma volume. The subsequent sodium and water retention further aggravate the peripheral edema, leading to anasarca. Another effect of insufficient plasma oncotic pressure is increased hepatic lipoprotein synthesis resulting in hyperlipidemia, specifically elevated cholesterol and low-density lipoprotein levels.[34]

## Clinical Manifestations

The clinical manifestations of nephrotic syndrome may precede a malignant diagnosis by 2–18 months. The cardinal sign of nephrotic syndrome is massive proteinuria, accompanied by hypoalbuminemia, hyperlipidemia, and edema. Signs and symptoms include brown, foamy urine and facial and peripheral edema, which may progress to anasarca or edema of all body tissues. The combined water and electrolyte retention may cause mild to moderate hypertension.

## Assessment and Grading

### Diagnostic studies

As with many PNSs, paraneoplastic nephrotic syndrome is a diagnosis of exclusion. Renal vein thrombosis, amyloidosis, and drug-related or benign disease etiologies must be ruled out. Nephrotic syndrome is diagnosed primarily by percutaneous renal biopsy combined with the clinical picture. On renal biopsy, minimal change disease is manifested by hyalinization of the glomeruli, narrowing or obliteration of the capillary walls, but completely normal capillary basement membranes, without evidence of immune deposits.[36] Renal biopsy results from patients with membranous glomerulonephritis related to carcinoma show fine holes in the glomerular basement membrane and focal capillary irregularities caused by granular deposits of IgG and possibly complement.[33]

Renal ultrasound may be utilized to eliminate renal vein thrombosis, or hydronephrosis as an etiology for the nephrotic syndrome. Findings usually reveal enlarged, occasionally asymmetrical kidneys and increased echogenicity consistent with parenchymal disease.

Laboratory studies include urinalysis, 24-hour urine collection, and serum chemistry profile. Urinalysis shows moderate heme, 2+ to 4+ protein, and 2+ granular casts. A 24-hour urine examination may contain protein levels of 3800–7000 mg. The chemistry profile may reveal an elevated creatinine, BUN, and cholesterol, with a decreased albumin.

Gallium scan may be performed and will show uptake by the kidneys. It can be utilized as a screening tool for patients with idiopathic nephrotic syndrome to screen for occult lymphoma.[39]

## Therapeutic Approaches and Nursing Care

The primary treatment of paraneoplastic nephrotic syndrome is focused on the underlying malignancy. The development of acute renal failure is a concern but rarely occurs. Resolution of the nephrotic syndrome is fairly rapid following tumor response to therapy. Sherman et al[40] report two cases of nephrotic syndrome associated with Hodgkin's lymphoma, characterized by anasarca, hypertension, hypoalbuminemia, and massive proteinuria. In both cases the patients received mantle radiation to the neck, axillae, supraclavicular areas, and mediastinum. Within one week of the radiation spontaneous diuresis occurred, the hypoalbuminemia resolved, and a significant decrease in the proteinuria was noted.

Another case of nephrotic syndrome associated with an adenocarcinoma of unknown primary was reported by

Robinson et al. In this situation the nephrotic syndrome preceded the malignant diagnosis by one year, and it waxed and waned with the malignancy. Recurrence of disease was heralded by symptoms of the nephrotic syndome.[39]

Management of the nephrotic syndrome itself includes the use of steroids and diuretics. The use of glucocorticoids is standard, i.e., prednisone 40–100 mg/day for four weeks followed by a reduced dose for an additional four weeks. A response to steroids is usually seen in 8–24 weeks. Side effects include muscle weakness, increased appetite, and the development of cushingoid symptoms. Loop diuretics are commonly used to relieve the edema. A high-protein diet may be recommended; however, most of the dietary protein will be excreted in the urine, and many cancer patients find this type of diet difficult to tolerate. Cytotoxic drugs such as cyclophosphamide and chlorambucil may be used but are usually reserved for patients who cannot tolerate steroids.[38]

# MISCELLANEOUS PARANEOPLASTIC SYNDROMES

## Cutaneous Paraneoplastic Syndromes

Malignant disease has always been associated with the development of a wide variety of cutaneous syndromes or dermatoses. In contrast to the previous PNSs, no one malignancy is predominantly associated with cutaneous PNSs in general, although some are pathognomonic for a certain malignancy. The etiology of most cutaneous PNSs is unknown. Possible theories include the secretion of transforming growth factor alpha resulting in abnormal stimulation of epidermal cells, peptide production by the tumor, or a type of autoimmune reaction involving dermal infiltration by neutrophils, lymphocytes, and eosinophils.[41,42]

Cutaneous PNSs are extremely rare; for example, only 50 reported cases of erythema gyratum repens exist[43] (Figure 26-3). These syndromes range from extremely rare but frequently associated with malignancy, to those that are equally associated with benign and malignant disease, to those that are infrequently associated with malignancy. Diagnosis of a cutaneous PNS is made on the basis of physical exam and skin biopsy. The presence of the syndrome should lead to a search for a malignant cause if not previously diagnosed or for recurrent disease in the patient with a history of malignancy.[41] A true cutaneous PNS must meet two criteria: (1) the appearance of the dermatosis must follow the development of the malignancy, and (2) the disease course of both the dermatosis and the malignancy must coincide.[42] The dermatoses considered to be true PNSs are described in Table 26-4.

The primary treatment of the cutaneous PNSs is treatment of the underlying malignancy. Topical and systemic corticosteroid therapy have been used with some success.[43] Other measures are strictly supportive, including nonsteroidal anti-inflammatory medications, lubricating lotions, and analgesics as needed. Nursing care depends upon the severity of the syndrome and may involve the use of wet dressings and the use of antihistamines to prevent scratching and the prevention of secondary infection. Patient education and emotional support are essential as the patient must cope with the effects of the syndrome while waiting for malignancy to respond to treatment.

## Anorexia-Cachexia Syndrome

The predominant and most well known PNSs affecting the GI system are anorexia and cachexia. Malabsorption syndromes are a rare phenomenon associated with histological abnormalities of the small bowel, characterized by a flattening of the mucosa and villous atrophy. The malignancies related to malabsorption syndromes include colon, lung, prostate, and pancreatic carcinomas, and lymphomas.[2] Anorexia refers to a loss of appetite and subsequent reduction in food intake. Cancer cachexia is a syndrome defined as progressive loss of body fat and lean body mass associated with anorexia, anemia, and profound weakness.[44] The incidence of anorexia and cachexia in the oncological population is difficult to determine but is estimated to occur in 60%–70% of patients with advanced malignant disease. It is considered a major contributing factor in the cause of death in 50% of patients with advanced disease.[45]

Anorexia-cachexia does not result from the nutritional demands of the malignancy. The reduced food intake resulting from anorexia is not sufficient to explain the cancer cachexia syndrome. The cancer cachexia syndrome is believed to be caused either by the effects of cytokines produced by malignant cells or by cytokines produced by the immune system in response to the malignancy. Anorexia-cachexia differs from other PNSs in that it is not associated with specific malignancies but can occur with any cancer. It is more commonly associated with end-stage disease but can occur at any time during the disease process and is usually related to the amount of tumor burden. The timing of the syndrome differs with the type of histology. Anorexia-cachexia is a dominant feature of lung cancer, occurring much earlier in the disease course than is seen in breast cancer patients. Anorexia-cachexia can severely impact a patient's ability to tolerate antineoplastic therapy and may potentiate adverse reactions.[45]

Several cytokines are believed to be responsible for the cancer cachexia syndrome. The major cytokine involved is tumor necrosis factor–alpha (TNF-alpha), also known as cachectin. IL-1 beta, IL-6, and gamma interferon may also play roles. The effect of TNF is alteration of metabolic controls affecting the mechanisms that regulate hunger, satiety, taste, and metabolism, specifically lipid metabolism.[2] TNF is a protein secreted by monocytes and macrophages that was initially named *cachectin* after

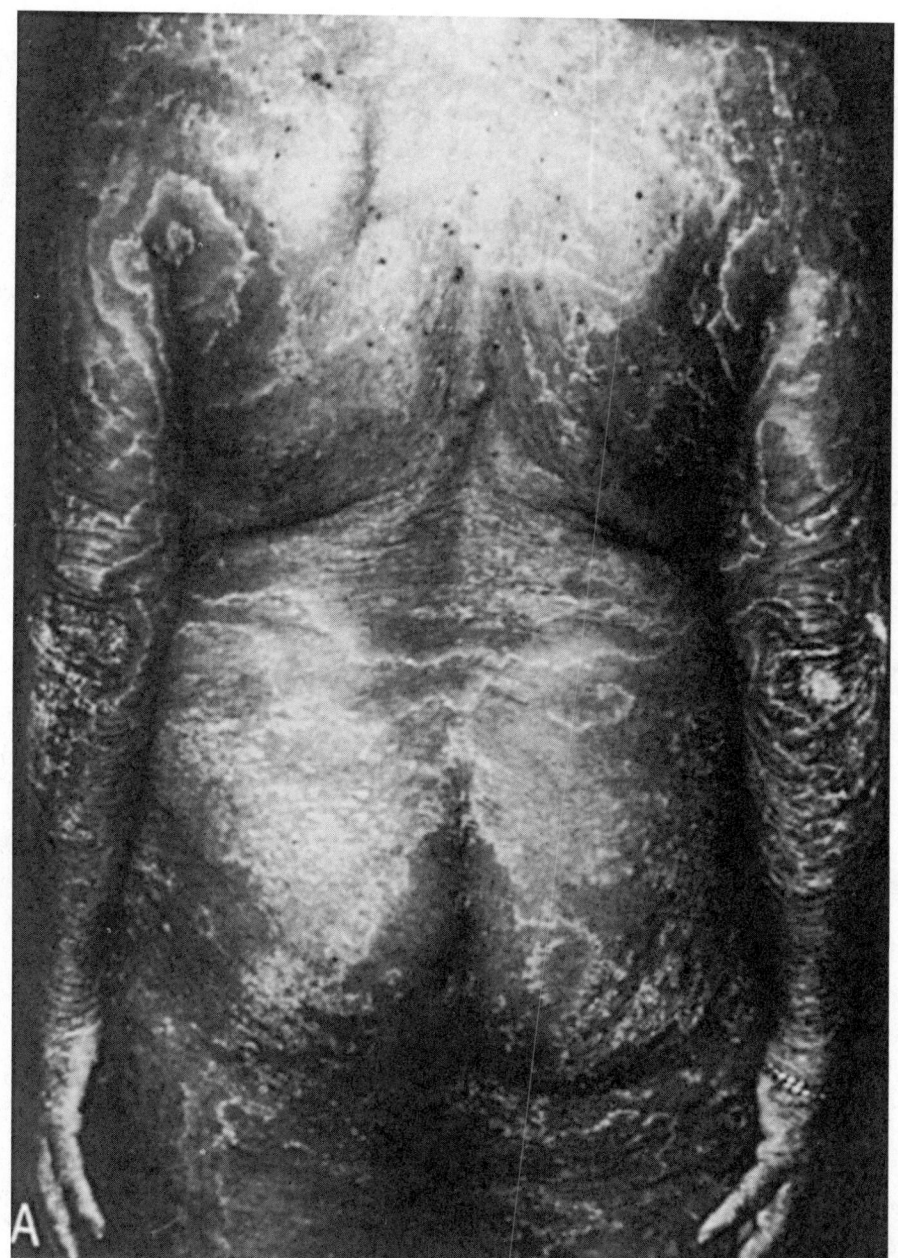

**FIGURE 26-3** Patient with erythema gyratum repens showing classic "wood grain" pattern most pronounced in the intertriginous areas (Photo reproduced with permission from Appell ML, Ward WQ, Tyring SK: Erythema gyratum repens—A cutaneous marker of malignancy. *Cancer* 62:548–550. Copyright © 1988 American Cancer Society. Reprinted by permission of Wiley-Liss, Inc., a subsidiary of John Wiley & Sons, Inc.)

its discovery in parasite-infected rabbits who developed anorexia and tissue wasting. Giving recombinant TNF to laboratory animals produces anorexia and weight loss but is dependent upon the method of administration. Intermittent bolus administration allowed the animals to become tolerant to the effects of the TNF and subsequently begin eating and gain weight. Continuous-infusion TNF produced more profound anorexia, weight loss, loss of muscle mass, and eventually death.[45]

TNF is also responsible for the systemic effects produced by the release of endotoxins in the body. Endotoxin stimulates the production of TNF, resulting in tissue inflammation, hypotension, anemia, fever, and hypoproteinemia. Patients who have received TNF in phase I clinical trials experienced fever, chills, hypotension, and anorexia but not weight loss. These infusions were bolus intermittent, and the TNF cleared from the body rapidly, which may have precluded the development of weight

**TABLE 26-4**    Paraneoplastic Cutaneous Syndromes

| Disorder | Clinical Presentation | Associated Malignancy | Comments |
|---|---|---|---|
| **Pigmented lesions**<br>• Acanthosis nigricans | • Velvety, brown, symmetrical lesions with hyperkeratosis that occur primarily in flexural areas—axilla, posterior neck, perineum, umbilicus | • 90% of cases associated with malignancy<br>• 60% gastric carcinoma<br>• 5% lung carcinoma | • Usually associated with advanced disease |
| • Sign of Leser-Trelat | • Multiple seborrheic (wart-like) lesions | • Adenocarcinomas<br>• Non-Hodgkin's lymphoma<br>• GI malignancies—43% | • Rapid development signals malignancy<br>• Pruritic |
| • Sweet's syndrome (acute, febrile neutrophilic dermatosis) | • Painful erythematous plaques covering arms, head, and neck | • 10–15% of cases associated with a malignancy, usually hematologic, leukemias (AML), myeloma<br>• GU, GI, breast—less common | |
| • Bazex's syndrome | • Scaly, pruritic psoriasiform rash affecting nails, nose, ears, elbows, knees, fingers, and toes | • Squamous cell carcinomas of head and neck, esophagus, lung<br>• Vulvar, esophageal, and uterine carcinomas | • Males primarily affected<br>• Females less common<br>• 100% association with malignancy |
| **Erythemas**<br>• Erythema gyratum repens (Repens is latin for "to crawl or creep") | • Expanding, scaly, concentric bands (gyri) with a "wood grain" pattern | • 32% lung carcinoma<br>• Breast<br>• Esophagus<br>• Uterine | • Pruritic<br>• Moves rapidly across skin surface—about 1 cm per day<br>• 2:1 male to female ratio<br>• 100% association with malignancy<br>• Tumor resection results in complete resolution within six weeks |
| • Glucagonoma syndrome (necrolytic migratory erythema) | • Erythematous patches<br>• Stomatitis | • Islet cell tumors of pancreas | • Tumor resection results in clearance of the eruption within 48 hours |
| • Flushing | • Intermittent episodes of facial flushing | • Carcinoid<br>• Medullary thyroid carcinoma | |
| **Endocrine/metabolic lesions**<br>• Porphyria cutanea tarda | • *Early* Photosensitive subepidermal vesicles, fragile skin, hyperpigmentation<br>• *Late* Alopecia, scarring, sclerodermoid changes | • Liver carcinoma | • Often painful, pruritic |
| • Systemic nodular panniculitis | • Fever, erythematous SQ nodules, fat necrosis of bone marrow, lungs, and other organs; abdominal pain | • Pancreatic adenocarcinoma | • Occurs rarely; also associated with benign pancreatic disease |
| **Miscellaneous**<br>• Pruritus | • Generalized itching with areas of excoriation from scratching<br>• Chronic, intensive itching of nostrils associated with advanced brain tumors | • Hodgkin's & T-cell lymphomas<br>• Polycythemia vera<br>• CNS malignancies | • 25% of Hodgkin's lymphoma patients experience generalized itching<br>• May be presenting symptom of malignancies<br>• Rapid onset |
| • Hypertrichosis lanuginosa (malignant down) | • Fine, silky hair occurring primarily on forehead and ears | • Lung, colon carcinomas, also bladder, uterine | • 90% association with malignancy |
| • Hypertrophic pulmonary osteoarthropathy (HPO) | • Painful, symmetric arthropathy involving fingers, wrists, elbows, and knees caused by periostitis | • Intrathoracic malignancies primarily lung carcinomas (88%)<br>• Histologies most common are large cell and adenocarcinoma of the lung | • Associated with clubbing of fingers and toes<br>• May resemble rheumatoid arthritis<br>• Usually precedes diagnosis of malignancy |

loss.[46] IL-1 and IL-6 appear to function synergistically with TNF. IL-1 alone can produce fever and anorexia.

## Tumor Fever

Tumor fever is a PNS primarily associated with lymphomas, as well as with leukemias, myelodysplastic syndromes, renal cell carcimona, hepatoma, and metastatic liver disease. It is produced by tumor secretion of cytokines, primarily IL-1, IL-6, interferon, and TNF. Fever may also result from an inflammatory reaction produced by the presence of tumor cells.[2]

The majority of patients with tumor fever do not follow a specific pattern. Fever patterns occur most commonly with lymphomas, specifically Hodgkin's lymphoma. A particular tumor fever known as Pel Ebstein fever occurs in Hodgkin's lymphoma, with a pattern of a three to ten day period of fever alternating with afebrile periods.[47]

The primary therapy for tumor fever is treatment of the underlying malignancy. However, because of the malaise that chronic fever may produce, symptomatic relief is important. Medications that may provide temporary relief include nonsteroidal anti-inflammatory drugs, naproxen, indomethacin, and steroids.

## CONCLUSION

The PNSs represent a fascinating group of diseases that may affect the endocrine, neurological, hematologic, renal, gastrointestinal, and cutaneous systems. These syndromes range in incidence from extremely rare, such as the paraneoplastic cerebellar disorders and cutaneous syndromes, to quite prevalent, such as anorexia-cachexia. As we gain a greater understanding of the substances that tumor cells secrete, the mechanisms involved, and their effect on normal tissue, we may be able to treat and possibly prevent the occurrence of PNSs. Oncology nurses need to understand these syndromes and the malignancies with which they are most commonly associated.

## REFERENCES

1. Eckhardt SL: Paraneoplastic syndromes. *Cancer Surv* 21: 197–209, 1994
2. Bunn PA, Ridgway EC: Paraneoplastic syndromes, in Devita VT, Hellman S, Rosenberg SA (eds): *Cancer: Principles and Practice of Oncology* (ed 4). Philadelphia, Lippincott, 1993, pp 2026–2071
3. Anderson KM: Paraneoplastic syndromes, in Bone R (ed): *Quick Reference to Internal Medicine.* New York, Igaku-Shoin Medical Publishers Inc., 1993, pp 1061–1065
4. Block JB: Paraneoplastic syndromes, in Haskell CM, Berek JS (eds): *Cancer Treatment* (ed 4). Philadelphia, Saunders, 1995, pp 245–264
5. Schwartz WB, Bennett W, Curelop S et al: A syndrome of renal sodium loss and hyponatremia probably resulting from inappropriate secretion of antidiuretic hormone. *Am J Med* 529–534, 1957
6. Amatruda TT, Mulrow PJ, Gallagher JC et al: Carcinoma of the lung with inappropriate antidiuresis. Demonstration of an antidiuretic–hormone-like activity in tumor extract. *N Engl J Med* 269:544–550, 1963
7. Moses AM, Scheinman SJ: Ectopic secretion of neurohypophyseal peptides in patients with malignancy. *Endocrinol Metab Clin North Am* 20:489–506, 1991
8. Becker KL, Silva OL: Paraneoplastic endocrine syndromes, in Becker KL (ed): *Principles and Practice of Endocrinology and Metabolism* (ed 2). Philadelphia, Lippincott, 1995, pp 1842–1852
9. Ralston SH: Pathogenesis and management of cancer-associated hypercalcemia. *Cancer Surv* 21:179–196, 1994
10. Pierce ST: Paraendocrine syndromes. *Curr Opin Oncol* 5: 639–645, 1993
11. Shepard FA, Laskey J, Evans WK, et al: Cushing's syndrome associated with ectopic corticotropin production and small cell lung cancer. *J Clin Oncol* 10:21–27, 1992
12. Poe CM, Taylor LM: Syndrome of inappropriate antidiuretic hormone: Assessment and nursing implications. *Oncol Nurs Forum* 16:373–381, 1989
13. Kaplan M: Hypercalcemia of malignancy: A review of advances in pathophysiology. *Oncol Nurs Forum* 21:1039–1046, 1994
14. Midthun DE, Jett JR: Clinical presentation of lung cancer, in Pass HI, Mitchell JB, Johnson DH, Turrisi AT (eds): *Lung Cancer: Principles and Practice.* Philadelphia, Lippincott-Raven, l996, pp 421–435
15. Posner JB, Furneaux HM: Paraneoplastic syndromes, in Waksman BH (ed): *Immunologic Mechanisms in Neurologic and Psychiatric Disease.* New York, Raven Press, 1990, pp 187–219
16. Posner JB: Paraneoplastic cerebellar degeneration. *PPO Updates* 5:1–13, 1991
17. Lang B, Newsom-Davis J: Immunopathology of the Lambert-Eaton myasthenic syndrome. *Springer Semin Immunopathol* 17:3–15, 1995
18. Berne RM, Levy MN: *Principles of Physiology.* St. Louis, Mosby, 1994, p 134
19. Lennon VA, Kryzer TJ, Griesmann GE, et al: Calcium-channel antibodies in the Lambert-Eaton syndrome and other paraneoplastic syndromes. *N Engl J Med* 332:1467–1474, 1995
20. Posner JB: Paraneoplastic syndromes. *Neurol Clin* 9:919–936, 1991
21. Newsom-Davis J, Murray N: Plasma exchange and immunosuppressive drug treatment in the Lambert-Eaton myasthenic syndrome. *Neurology* 34:480–485, 1984
22. Dau PC, Denys EH: Plasmapheresis and immunosuppressive drug therapy in the Lambert-Eaton syndrome. *Ann Neurol* 11:570–575, 1982
23. Struthers CS: Lambert-Eaton myasthenic syndrome in small cell lung cancer: Nursing implications. *Oncol Nurs Forum* 21: 677–683, 1994
24. Rickles FR, Edwards RL: Activation of blood coagulation in cancer: Trousseau's syndrome revisited. *Blood* 62:14–31, 1983
25. Naschitz JE, Yeshurun D, Lev LM: Thromboembolism in cancer. *Cancer* 71:1384–1390, 1993
26. Levine MN, Gent M, Hirsh J, et al: The thrombogenic effect

of anticancer drug therapy in women with stage II breast cancer. *N Engl J Med* 318:404–407, 1988

27. Bick RL, Strauss JF, Frenkel EP: Thrombosis and hemorrhage in oncology patients. *Hematol Oncol Clin North Am* 10:875–907, 1996

28. Turner AR: Haematological aspects of palliative medicine, in Doyle D, Hanks GWC, MacDonald N (eds): *Oxford Textbook of Palliative Medicine*. New York, Oxford University Press, 1994, pp 486–491

29. Silverstein RL, Nachman RL: Cancer and clotting: Trousseau's warning. *N Engl J Med* 327:1163–1164, 1992

30. Prandoni P, Lensing AWA, Buller HR, et al: Deep-vein thrombosis and the incidence of subsequent symptomatic cancer. *N Engl J Med* 327:1128–1133, 1992

31. Honda K, Ishiko O, Tatsuta I, et al: Anemia inducing substance from plasma of patients with advanced malignant neoplasms. *Cancer Res* 55:3623–3639, 1995

32. Lee JC, Yamaguchi H, Hopper J Jr: The association of cancer and the nephrotic syndrome. *Ann Intern Med* 64:41–51, 1966

33. Becker BN, Goldin G, Santos R, et al: Carcinoid tumor and the nephrotic syndrome: A novel association between neoplasia and glomerular disease. *South Med J* 89:240–242, 1996

34. Glassock RJ, Brenner BM: The major glomerulopathies, in Isselbacher KJ, Braunwald E, Wilson JD, Martin JB, Fauci AS, Kasper DL (eds): *Harrison's Principles of Internal Medicine*. New York, McGraw-Hill, 1994, pp 1295–1306

35. Eagen JW, Lewis EJ: Glomerulopathies of neoplasia. *Kidney Int* 11:297–306, 1977

36. Sherman RL, Susin M, Weksler ME, et al: Lipoid nephrosis in Hodgkin's disease. *Am J Med* 52:699–706, 1972

37. Gagliano RG, Costanzi JJ, Beathard GA, et al: The nephrotic syndrome associated with neoplasia: An unusual paraneoplastic syndrome. *Am J Med* 60:1026–1031, 1976

38. Juweid M, Kim CK, Heyman S: Nephrotic syndrome as an unusual paraneoplastic syndrome of Hodgkin's disease demonstrated on Gallium-67 scan. *Clin Nucl Med* 19:224–227, 1994

39. Robinson WL, Mitas JA, Haerr RW, et al: Remission and exacerbation of tumor-related nephrotic syndrome with treatment of the neoplasm. *Cancer* 54:1082–1084, 1984

40. Sherman RL, Susin M, Weksler ME et al: Lipoid nephrosis in Hodgkin's disease. *Amer Journal of Med* 52:699–706, 1972

41. Cohen PR: Cutaneous paraneoplastic syndromes. *Am Fam Physician* 50:1273–1282, 1994

42. McLean DI, Haynes HA: Cutaneous manifestations of internal malignant disease, in Fitzpatrick T (ed): *Fitzpatrick Dermatology and General Medicine* (ed 4). New York, McGraw-Hill, 1993, pp 2229–2248

43. Boyd AS, Neldner KH, Menter A: Erythema gyratum repens: A paraneoplastic eruption. *J Am Acad Dermatol* 26:757–762, 1992

44. Cotran RS, Kumar V, Robbins SL: *Robbins Pathologic Basis of Disease* (ed 5). Philadelphia, Saunders, 1994, pp 52–73

45. Alexander HR, Norton JA: Pathophysiology of cancer cachexia, in Doyle D, Hanks GWC, MacDonald N (eds): *Oxford Textbook of Palliative Medicine*. New York, Oxford University Press, 1994, pp 316–329

46. Vigano A, Watanabe S, Bruera E: Anorexia and cachexia in advanced cancer patients. *Cancer Surv* 21:99–115, 1994

47. Morant R, Hans-Jorg S: The management of infections in palliative care, in Doyle D, Hanks GWC, MacDonald N (eds): *Oxford Textbook of Palliative Medicine*. New York, Oxford University Press, 1994, pp 378–384

# Chapter 27

# Malignant Effusions and Edemas

Mary B. Maxwell, RN, C, PhD

## SCOPE OF THE PROBLEM

Fluid derangements are common in individuals with cancer. Abnormal leakage from blood and lymph vessels into tissues (edema) or cavities (effusions) occurs with many kinds of malignancy. Usually associated with advanced disease but sometimes occurring as the presenting symptom, effusions and edemas interfere with normal body function at the site where they develop and add new problems to those manifestations already present as a result of the underlying cancer and its treatment.

Although all cancers can metastasize to any of the body's serous cavities, *malignant effusions* occur most commonly in the pleural space of the lung (pleural effusion), the peritoneal cavity in the abdomen (ascites), or the space surrounding the heart (pericardial effusion). The brain and the extremities are frequent sites for *malignant edemas*. This chapter discusses normal fluid regulation in relation to fluid derangements seen in cancer patients and compares and contrasts the various edematous states. The pathophysiology, clinical manifestations, assessment, and interventions for the six most common fluid retention sites are presented.

## NORMAL FLUID REGULATION

The distribution pattern of body water is termed *fluid spacing*. *First spacing* describes a normal distribution of fluid in both the extracellular and intracellular compart-

ments. *Second spacing* refers to an excess accumulation of interstitial fluid (edema), while *third spacing* is fluid retention in areas that usually have no fluid or a minimum of fluid (effusion). Edema or effusion represents a disturbance in the normal distribution of extracellular fluid.

Extracellular fluids are separated into interstitial and intravascular compartments by the semipermeable membranes surrounding capillaries and cells. These membranes serve as the points where exchange takes place between each cell and its respective fluid environment (the interstitial fluid) and between the interstitial fluid and the plasma within the circulatory system. Various pressures as described by Starling's law influence fluid movement across the capillary membranes (Figure 27-1). More fluid moves out of the intravascular into the interstitial compartment than returns via the capillary membrane. The lymphatic capillaries take up the excess interstitial fluid and return it to the bloodstream via the lymphatic and thoracic ducts. Lymphatic drainage is particularly important for the removal of proteins that leak into the interstitial spaces, thereby keeping the interstitial osmotic pressure low. Edema results from any augmentation of the forces influencing movement of fluids from the intravascular compartment into the interstitial compartment.

## FLUID DISTURBANCES IN CANCER

### Effects of Cancer and Cancer Treatment

Cancer, either a primary tumor or a metastatic lesion, can affect fluid pressure dynamics in several negative ways: by

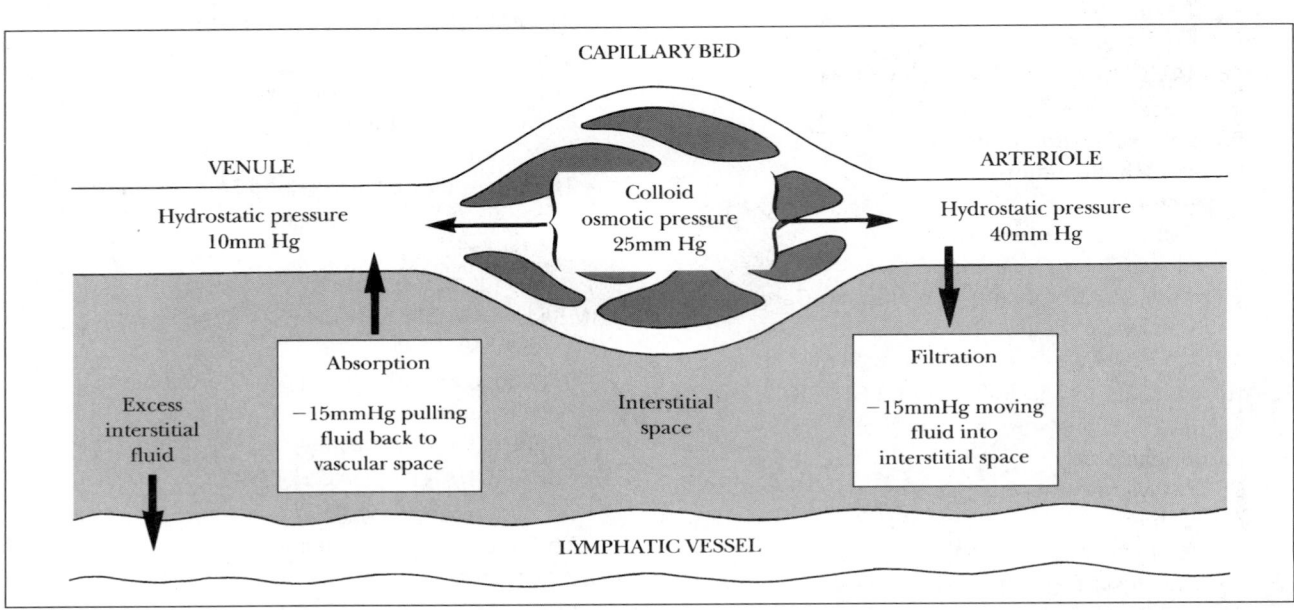

**FIGURE 27-1**   As described by Starling's law, the colloid osmotic pressure, hydrostatic pressure, capillary permeability, diffusion, and filtration pressure are all factors influencing fluid movement across the capillary membrane from the blood to the interstitial space.

direct extension of the tumor, by seeding of body cavities with malignant cells, by lymphatic or venous obstruction, and/or by causing severe hypoproteinemia (Table 27-1). Also, cancer treatments can affect or be altered by effusions/edemas. For instance, methotrexate given at routine doses can cause excessive myelosuppression in a patient who is experiencing third spacing. Edema can be a toxic side effect of growth factors given to a patient with a chronic inflammatory disease or an acute infection.[1] As a result of the syndrome of inappropriate antidiuretic hormone (SIADH), the severe fluid imbalance termed *water intoxication* can occur. It usually develops in patients with lung cancer or one receiving antineoplastic agents or analgesics (cyclophosphamide, vincristine, morphine).

## General Considerations: Similarities and Differences

### Benign versus malignant

Of the six fluid retention states discussed in this chapter, all except lymphedema are directly due to cancer.

**TABLE 27-1**   Causes of Malignant Edema (According to Underlying Physiological Mechanism)

---

### HYDROSTATIC PRESSURE ABNORMALITIES

Increased Capillary Fluid Pressure
  Increased venous pressure
    Vein obstruction
      Tumor
      Thrombophlebitis
    Increased total volume with decreased cardiac output
    Fluid overload
  Sodium and water retention, increased aldosterone from:
    Decreased renal blood flow
      Renal failure
    Increased aldosterone
      Corticosteroid therapy
    Inability to metabolize aldosterone
      Liver metastasis

### ONCOTIC PRESSURE ABNORMALITIES

Decreased Capillary Oncotic Pressure
  Loss of serum protein
    Anemia
    Bleeding
  Decreased protein intake
    Malnutrition
  Decreased albumin production
    Liver metastasis
Increased Interstitial Oncotic Pressure
  Increased capillary permeability to protein
    Inflammatory reactions
      Seeding of cavity surfaces with tumor cells
      Infection
  Obstructed lymphatics: decreased removal of tissue fluid and protein
      Malignant disease
      Surgical removal of lymph nodes

---

Lymphedema is a benign iatrogenic problem secondary to radical cancer surgery. Nonmalignant edema, always a possibility for a patient with cancer, should be considered in the differential diagnosis for any fluid accumulation.

### Incidence

Much of the data on incidence of effusion and edema are from autopsy reports in earlier years, when postmortem examinations were routinely carried out. Since autopsies are currently performed for only 10% of cancer deaths,[2] the actual incidence of metastasis and malignant fluid retention is less clear today. It is surmised that the incidence of these later complications is on the rise because longer survival after diagnosis is occurring as a result of improved treatments for primary disease.[3] The only fluid retention state that is decreasing in incidence is lymphedema, because fewer radical mastectomies are being performed for breast cancer. While pericardial effusion is usually seen only in end-stage disease, in contrast, pleural effusion, ascites, and cerebral edema may be the first indication of cancer.

### Rapid versus slow accumulation

Cavities and tissues can accommodate surprisingly large volumes of fluids if the abnormal liquid accumulates slowly over time. However, a rapid increase in volume, even a small amount, tends to overwhelm compensatory mechanisms, and life-threatening symptoms can occur. Malignant effusions and edemas usually begin slowly but then increase and expand exponentially.

### Assessment

Many more malignant pleural effusions than pericardial effusions are symptomatic. Thus, pericardial effusions are more difficult to diagnose. Often the individual's history and physical exam point to the likely etiology of the effusion/edema. The most helpful diagnostic tools for pleural effusion are the chest x-ray and examination of the pleural fluid, while the echocardiogram is the most important tool in pericardial effusions. The physical examination helps determine the diagnosis with ascites, lymphedema, and pedal edema. Brain lesions causing cerebral edema are usually diagnosed with computerized tomography (CT).

### Transudates versus exudates

Fluid accumulation at an effusion site can be classified as either a transudate or an exudate. Classification has diagnostic implications and can be a distinguishing characteristic between a malignant or a nonmalignant cause. A *transudate* is a low-protein fluid that has leaked from blood vessels due to mechanical factors, as in cirrhosis, congestive heart failure, or nephrotic syndrome. In contrast, an *exudate* is protein-rich fluid that has leaked from blood vessels with increased permeability. Most malignant effusions are exudates, caused by irritation of the serous membrane by sloughed cancer cells or solid tumor implants. The malignant exudate contains cells or cellular debris released by the resulting inflammation. Transudates and exudates can be distinguished by fluid protein to serum protein ratios and by fluid lactate dehydrogenase (LDH) to serum LDH ratios.[3]

## Treatment

For effusions, systemic treatment is usually employed first if the underlying cancer is responsive to chemotherapy. Otherwise, local therapy for malignant effusions is similar: drain the fluid, attempt to obliterate the third space, and prevent reaccumulation. No single clearly superior approach for local control of any of the effusions has been demonstrated by randomized clinical trial. A variety of treatment techniques have been advocated. Treatment for lymphedema and pedal edema involves application of local measures to the affected limb and possible administration of diuretics. Cerebral edema is treated quite differently, with steroids and radiation therapy. The main goals of treatment for malignant effusions and edemas are similar (see Table 27-2). Specific therapy depends upon the site where the fluid has accumulated and the individual patient and tumor-related factors (Table 27-3).

## Nursing Care

Although most patients will develop edemas or effusions when their cancer is advanced, ongoing *assessment* of each cancer patient for signs or symptoms of fluid retention is crucial so that interventions can be instituted early. When fluid accumulation occurs, the patient and family will need *emotional support* to counteract the stress and fears associated with advancing disease, cosmetic appearance changes, and the necessity for further medical intervention. With the treatment of effusions, the nurse will probably *assist* with potentially painful diagnostic and/or sclerosing procedures. Important nursing interventions include minimizing discomfort, providing reassurance, and *monitoring* the patient during and after these procedures for untoward reactions. *Patient education* will prepare the patient and family for tests and procedures as well as teaching them to recognize and report side

**TABLE 27-3** Factors Influencing Treatment Choices for Malignant Effusions/Edemas

| PATIENT-RELATED FACTORS |
| --- |
| Presence and degree of symptoms |
| Age |
| Performance status |
| Concomitant medical problems |
| Estimated life expectancy |
| Motivation |
| Quality of life |

| TUMOR-RELATED FACTORS |
| --- |
| Primary or metastatic cancer |
| Responsiveness to chemotherapy or radiation |
| Natural history of tumor type: histology, aggressiveness |
| Location and extent of tumor |
| Availability of therapies |
| Prior therapies |
| Concurrent therapies |

Reprinted from the *Oncology Nursing Forum* with permission from the Oncology Nursing Press. Gobel BH, Lawler PE: Malignant pleural effusions. *Oncol Nurs Forum* 12(4):49–54, 1985.

effects or complications. *Prevention* is important, particularly with lymphedema. Keeping records of fluid intake and output, evaluating the rate of fluid reaccumulation after cavity drainage, monitoring electrolytes and proteins, and helping the patient with a sodium-restricted diet may be important in some edemas. *Skin* care of the affected area is necessary with ascites, pedal edema, and lymphedema. *Pain evaluation and control* are often in order since the abnormal fluid accumulation can put pressure on nerve endings in surrounding structures. *Medications* (steroids, diuretics) may need to be administered and assessment for iatrogenic complications completed. If life-threatening cardiac tamponade or brain herniation occurs, *emergency care* is needed. Using the elements emphasized here, a complete plan of care for actual and potential problems specific to the fluid retention state should be developed for each patient. Additional detailed nursing care plans are available for selected aspects of fluid retention management (Table 27-4).

**TABLE 27-2** Goals of Treatment for Malignant Effusions or Edemas

| |
| --- |
| Short-term Goals |
|   Determine underlying cause |
|   Relieve discomfort |
|   Prevent fluid reaccumulation |
| Long-term Goals |
|   Prevent complications |
|   Prolong survival |
|   Enhance quality of life |

# LUNG: MALIGNANT PLEURAL EFFUSION

## Incidence

Although it is usually stated that approximately half of all newly diagnosed pleural effusions in adults are malignant,[4] there are no recent reports on the incidence of pleural effusion. Table 27-5 shows the tumor types associated with malignant pleural effusion and the incidence for each type.

**TABLE 27-4**   Nursing Care Plans for Patients with Malignant Effusions or Edemas

| Effusion or Edema Type | Plans | Reference |
|---|---|---|
| Pleural effusion | Nursing management during chest tube insertion and pleural sclerosing | Rossetti[9] |
| | Thoracostomy management in the home (patient education) | Hewitt and Jansen[15] |
| Pericardial effusion | Nursing plan of care for patients experiencing cardiac tamponade | Joiner and Kolodychuk[22] |
| | Nursing care plan for patients with pericardial window surgery for cardiac tamponade | Wojciechowicz[29] |
| | Nursing interventions for common complications of medical treatment for pericardial effusion | Mangan[25] |
| Peritoneal effusion | Patient care standards for patients with peritoneovenous shunt | Kehoe[38] |
| Lymphedema | Nursing interventions for patients with lymphedema | Getz[49] |
| | Guidelines for the care of the patient with altered tissue perfusion (lymphedema) | Kennelly and Yurkovic[54] |

Fifty percent of all cancer patients will develop pleural effusion at some time during their disease.[5] It may be the first sign of malignancy. Pleural effusion later in the disease progression is an ominous sign, but it does not necessarily mean the beginning of the terminal stage. Lung and breast cancer account for approximately 75% of malignant pleural effusions.[6,7] A median survival time of 14 months for breast cancer patients with effusions has been reported, compared with 6 months for patients with lung and other tumors and 16 months for patients with mesothelioma.[7] Most patients (90%) will have effusions of more than 500 ml, and approximately one-third will present with bilateral pleural effusions.[8]

## Physiological Alterations

Pleural fluid is a filtrate from the parietal pleura. It is formed and removed more slowly than formerly believed, with 100–200 ml being produced each 24 hours and then removed by the parietal pleural stomata.[6] The space between the parietal and visceral pleura contains a small amount of fluid (5–15 ml) that acts as a lubricant, allowing the two surfaces to move without friction. The parietal pleura contains nerve endings for pain, but the visceral pleura does not. In the presence of a massive effusion process, the interpleural space may contain as much as 1500 ml of fluid (Figure 27-2).

There are five ways that fluid equilibrium in the pleural space can be disturbed by cancer, either directly by origination in the pleura or indirectly via metastatic spread:

**1.** Most commonly, implantation with cancer cells on the pleural surface leads to increased capillary permeability and leakage from the intravascular to the interstitial compartment. This occurs with pleural effusions in patients with solid tumors such as lung cancer.

**2.** Obstruction of pleural or pulmonary lymphatic channels by malignant processes can prevent reabsorption of fluid. This is seen in pleural effusions related to lymphomas or breast cancer.

**3.** The pulmonary veins can be obstructed by tumor, leading to increased capillary hydrostatic pressure in the visceral pleura. This is another mechanism seen in lung cancer.

**4.** The pleural space colloid osmotic pressure may be increased by necrotic malignant cells being shed into the pleural space. This leads to a reduced absorption of fluid by the visceral pleural capillaries. It may be seen with lung and breast cancers.

**5.** The thoracic duct may be perforated, producing a chylous pleural effusion. This sometimes occurs with lymphoma.[3,6]

**TABLE 27-5**   Incidence of Pleural Effusion Related to Tumor Type

| Tumor Type | Incidence (%) |
|---|---|
| Lung cancer | 35 |
| Breast cancer | 23 |
| Adenocarcinoma, unknown primary | 12 |
| Leukemia/lymphoma | 10 |
| Reproductive tract | 6 |
| Gastrointestinal tract | 5 |
| Genitourinary tract | 3 |
| Primary unknown | 3 |
| Others | 5 |

Adapted with permission from *CA: Cancer J Clin* 41:165–179, 1991.

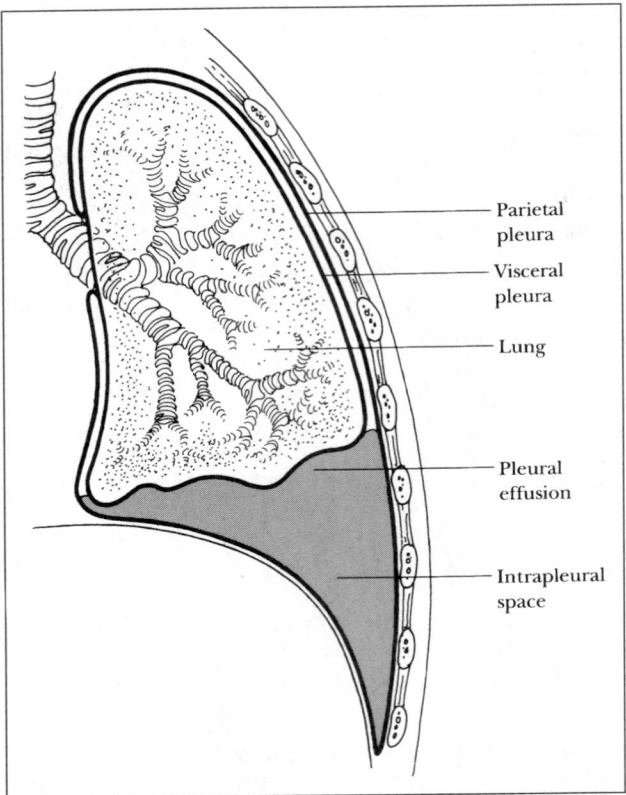

**FIGURE 27-2**  In the lung, fluid is constantly being filtered across the intrapleural space from the parietal pleural surface and reabsorbed through the visceral pleura. When obstruction by malignant processes prevents reabsorption, fluid accumulates in the intrapleural space and pleural effusion results.

In addition, tumor-related pathologies that can cause pleural effusion include superior vena cava syndrome (SVCS) (about 30% of patients with SVCS develop pleural effusions),[9] endobronchial obstruction with atelectasis, postobstructive pneumonitis, and pericardial constriction.

## Clinical Manifestations

The extent of alteration of respiratory function depends on the amount and rate of pleural fluid accumulation as well as the patient's underlying pulmonary status. The fluid accumulation restricts lung expansion, reduces lung volume, alters the ventilation and perfusion capacity, and results in abnormal gas exchange and hypoxia. Malignant pleural effusion may develop slowly over a period of several months. Pleural effusions due to noncancer causes usually have a more abrupt onset.

When pleural effusion develops in the patient with advanced cancer, it is often difficult to sort out the respiratory effects of the pleural fluid accumulation as opposed to shortness of breath due to thoracic muscle weakness and general debilitation. Breathing difficulties may also be aggravated by the side effects of chemotherapeutic agents (bleomycin and methotrexate) or prior lung irradiation.

Common presenting symptoms and signs are distressing to most patients (Table 27-6). Dyspnea is related to pulmonary compression. Cough is caused by compression of bronchial walls by fluid.[8] Dull, aching, continuous chest pain is the most common symptom and points to parietal pleural metastasis. Pleuritic chest wall pain is usually more intense and associated with parietal pleural inflammation.[8] The degree of subjective symptoms produced by a pleural effusion is not as dependent on the amount of fluid involved as on the rapidity with which it has accumulated. If the effusion has developed over a short time, the patient may be in extreme respiratory distress.[10] Although the majority of cancer patients with pleural effusions are symptomatic, 23% are not, with the effusion being found incidentally.[6]

## Assessment

### Radiographic examination

Chest x-rays are important in visualizing free fluid in the pleural cavity and relating accumulation to other structures. Most pleural effusions begin in the subpulmonic area between the lung and the diaphragm and appear as an elevated diaphragm on the affected side. The fluid casts an opaque shadow that has the same density as the heart. The larger the effusion, the more opaque it will appear. A pleural effusion will not be detected on a posterior-anterior chest film unless it contains at least 200–300 ml of fluid. A small effusion shows haziness at the base of the lung and obliterates the costophrenic angle. A lateral decubitus x-ray film is the

**TABLE 27-6**  Assessment of the Patient with Suspected Pleural Effusion

| SUBJECTIVE INDICATORS |
| --- |
| Dyspnea |
| Orthopnea |
| Dry, nonproductive cough |
| Chest pain, chest heaviness |

| OBJECTIVE INDICATORS |
| --- |
| Labored breathing |
| Tachypnea |
| Dullness to percussion |
| Restricted chest wall expansion |
| Impaired transmission of breath sounds |

| LABORATORY INDICATORS |
| --- |
| Fluid visualized on chest x-ray |
| Positive pleural fluid cytology |

Figure labels: Parietal pleura, Visceral pleura, Lung, Pleural effusion, Intrapleural space

best way to identify a small effusion, because gravity will cause the fluid to shift to a position along the dependent lateral rib cage where it is easier to visualize.[10]

Clues to the type of cancer causing the pleural effusion may be seen on x-ray. Mediastinum shift away from the effusion points to a disseminated nonthoracic tumor, such as breast or ovary. If the mediastinum is shifted toward the effusion, carcinoma of the lung, with some degree of bronchial obstruction, is probably involved. Mesothelioma or fixed central nodal metastasis is indicated if no mediastinal shift is seen.[4] If there is suspicion of pleural mesothelioma, CT can be useful.[3]

### Pleural fluid examination

Any new pleural effusion must be aspirated to confirm the presence of malignant cells and to rule out nonmalignant causes. Pleural fluid cytological analysis yields a definitive diagnosis in approximately 70% of patients with malignant pleural effusion.[7] Thoracoscopy with direct pleural biopsy leads to a diagnosis 100% of the time. If possible, the pleural fluid should be removed at the same time as the diagnostic thoracentesis, providing immediate relief for the distressing symptoms of large (1000–1500 ml) effusions.[3] Fluid should be removed slowly to avoid reexpansion pulmonary edema.

It is important to determine whether the fluid is an exudate or a transudate. Since malignant effusion is almost always an exudate, a transudative fluid would indicate a nonmalignant cause. The aspirated fluid is sent for cultures, gram and acid-fast stains, cell counts, and chemistry studies. Characteristics of the fluid that are helpful diagnostically are appearance (straw-colored, bloody, turbid, or milky) and levels of glucose amylase, protein, LDH, and lymphocytes.[3] A bloody effusion is the strongest indicator of malignancy.[8]

## Therapeutic Approaches and Nursing Care

How the malignant pleural effusion is treated depends on the type of tumor and previous therapy (Figure 27-3). Small, asymptotic effusions caused by lymphomas, leukemias, breast cancer, small cell lung cancer, and ovarian cancer are first treated with systemic chemotherapy or hormonal therapy. Unless the patient has been aggressively treated in the past and the tumor has become resistant to certain drugs, these types of tumors will usually respond and the effusion will disappear.[11] Patients with chemotherapy-resistant tumors (melanoma, non-small-cell lung cancer) will require alternative treatment approaches. If the underlying disease is unresponsive to therapy and the patient is symptomatic, palliative measures should be implemented.

### Removal of fluid

Relief of symptoms is a short-term treatment goal that is usually achieved when the pleural fluid is mechanically

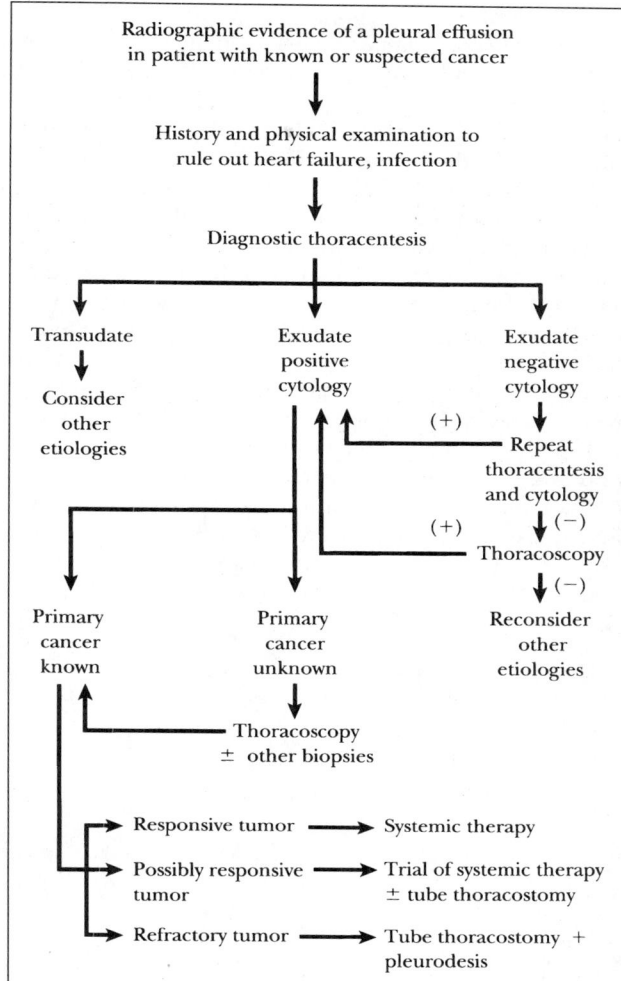

**FIGURE 27-3**   Algorithm for diagnosis and management of malignant pleural effusion. (Reprinted with permission of Ruckdeschel.[16])

drained. However, the fluid tends to reaccumulate when it is not possible to control the underlying cancer. Long-range treatment goals are directed toward the obliteration of the pleural space so that pleural fluid cannot reaccumulate.

*Thoracentesis*   In thoracentesis the pleural fluid is removed by needle aspiration through the chest wall. The patient is placed in an upright sitting position with arms and shoulders raised. This elevates and separates the ribs to make needle insertion easier. After the thoracentesis is completed and the pleural fluid has been drained, the patient is assessed for complications such as pneumothorax, pain, hypotension, or pulmonary edema. Patient education and support as well as medication and local anesthesia are important measures to prevent anxiety and discomfort during any of these therapeutic procedures.[12,13]

Although thoracocentesis alone is effective for diagnosis, palliation, or relief of acute respiratory distress, it is of little value for treating recurrent malignant effusions because the fluid usually reaccumulates quickly. In one study of 94 patients, the average reaccumulation time was four days and there was a 97% chance of recurrence within a month of the thoracentesis.[3] The risks of repeated thoracentesis include hypoalbuminemia, electrolyte imbalance, pneumothorax, fluid loculation, and infection.

Thoracentesis via an implanted port and intrapleural catheter is an alternative approach that can be advantageous for the patient whose cancer is refractory to treatment and thus will likely experience repeated pleural fluid reaccumulation.[14] Pleural fluid removal via an implanted port and interpleural catheter can be completed by the nurse in the ambulatory or home setting (Figure 27-4). Using the implanted port reduces the risk of pneumothorax and infection that can occur with repeated traditional percutaneous aspiration approaches. In addition, there can be significant reduction of health care resources consumed since nurses can evacuate the fluid accumulation before the symptoms of effusion become disabling. There is also a reduced need for repeat radiological examinations. Since a Huber point needle is used to access the implanted port, the patient experiences less pain than occurs with the large-gauge thoracentesis needle or a thoracostomy tube. Ease of performing the thoracentesis procedure, along with reduced pain and anxiety, significantly improves the patient's experience.

***Thoracostomy tube***   A thoracostomy tube may be inserted via video-guided thoracoscopy to facilitate fluid drainage and then left in place to assess the degree of fluid reaccumulation. However, chest tube drainage alone is only partially effective. Measures to prevent fluid reaccumulation are also needed. Nursing assessments while a thoracostomy tube is in place include observing for pneumothorax, pain, hypotension, and pulmonary edema as well as care of the closed-chest drainage system.[15] Care is taken to ensure that the chest tube remains patent since exudate fluid tends to clot. Thoracostomy tubes can also be used to instill sclerosing agents into the pleural space.

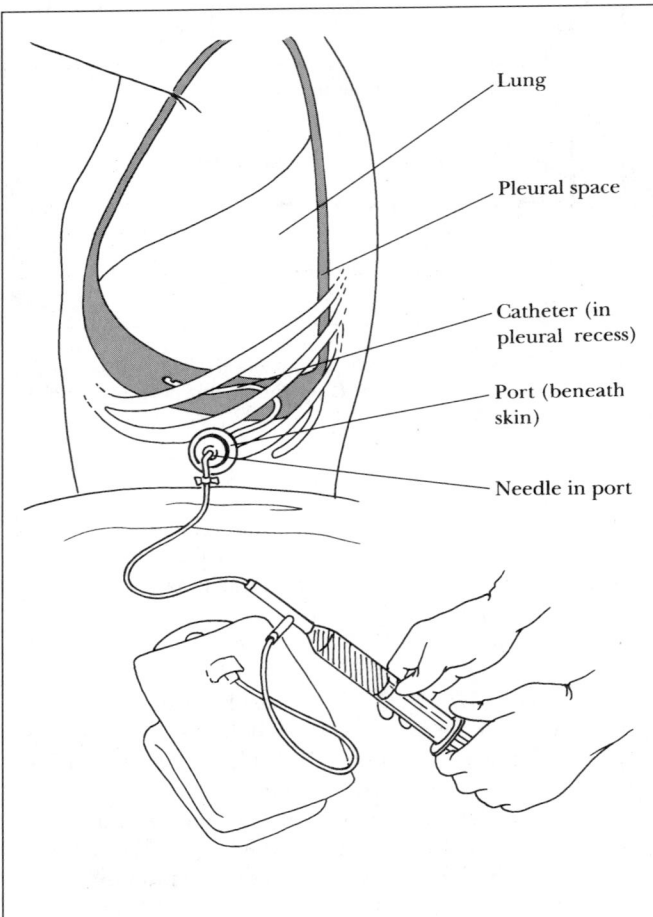

**Assemble equipment:**
1. Thoracentesis tray
2. Size 19g 90° Huber point needle with tubing and clamps
3. Heparin-saline solution (100 μ/ml 3 ml)
4. Betadine swabs
5. Sterile gloves (2 pairs)

**Procedure:**
1. Place patient in a comfortable position on side.
2. Open thoracentesis tray.
3. Place sterile Huber needle on sterile tray.
4. Don sterile gloves.
5. Connect 60-ml syringe to 2-way connector.
6. Connect one end of 2-way connector to the drainage bag and one end to sterile Huber needle (see illustration).
7. Prep site over port using sterile technique.
8. Change gloves.
9. Clamp Huber needle tubing.
10. Access port.
11. Tape needle securely.
12. Unclamp Huber needle tubing.
13. Draw back on plunger (fluid should be yellowish).
14. Fill syringe. Push on plunger to empty syringe into drainage bag. Repeat procedure until desired amount is obtained.
15. If the tube seems plugged, clamp the catheter, disconnect at 2-way valve and clear mucous plug.
16. If drainage seems to slow down or stop, have patient change position.
17. When tap is complete (1500 ml or so), clamp catheter. Disconnect drainage tube and flush with 3–5 cc of heparinized saline.
18. Withdraw needle from port.
19. Apply Band-Aid™.

Do not attempt to access port with thoracentesis needle. Must use Huber point needle. Procedure can be repeated as necessary.

Labels in figure: Lung · Pleural space · Catheter (in pleural recess) · Port (beneath skin) · Needle in port

**FIGURE 27-4**   Thoracentesis via an implanted port. (Procedure compliments of Michelle Goodman, RN, MS, Rush Presbyterian St. Luke's Medical Center.)

### Obliteration of the pleural space

If the pleural space can be obliterated, then the reaccumulation of pleural fluid may be prevented. Obliteration is achieved by instilling a chemical agent that causes the visceral and parietal pleura to become permanently adhered together. The chemical agent causes mesothelial fibrosis and the obliteration of small pleural blood vessels.[3]

***Chemical agents*** Many chemicals have been used over the years as sclerosing agents to prevent pleural effusion recurrence. Chemical sclerosing does not prolong the patient's life but may enhance quality of life by relieving symptoms and reducing the time a patient spends in the hospital. Agents used for pleural instillation in the past (nitrogen mustard, quinacrine, 5-fluorouracil, talc) have had side effects, such as nausea and vomiting, hypotension, pain, and bone marrow depression.

Until recently, bleomycin[15] and tetracycline were the two most common chemical agents used to control malignant pleural effusion in 70% or more of patients.[16] However, parenteral tetracycline is no longer available in the United States due to increasingly stringent manufacturing requirements.[17] An advantage of bleomycin is that it can be used without thoracostomy tube drainage for patients with smaller effusions.[4] The insufflation of talc has been popular for pleural effusion control in Great Britain and Europe.[18]

The selected sclerosing agent is instilled into the pleural space via the thoracentesis needle or the thoracostomy tube. Since the overall objective is to expose as much of the pleura as possible to the chemical, most of the pleural fluid will have to be removed and the lung reexpanded before the agent is instilled. The patient will be asked to move around and change position frequently to help distribute the agent. Nursing management during chest tube insertion and pleural sclerosing includes patient education and reassurance, pain control, positioning, and the management of the chest tube drainage as well as maintaining the drainage system.[9] Chest tube insertion and pleural sclerosing can be difficult and painful procedures for patients, who may already be debilitated due to their underlying disease.

Newer investigational methods for controlling malignant pleural effusion by pleural space obliteration include antibody-guided radiation using tumor-associated monoclonal antibodies radiolabeled with iodine 131. Biologicals such as interferons, interleukins, and *Cornebacterium parvum* are being tried as sclerosing agents to elicit a potent inflammatory and antitumor effect.[3] Recent reports from China describe good results with lymphokine-activated killer cells combined with recombinant interleukin 2.[8]

New technology using small-bore needles may permit management of malignant pleural effusions on an outpatient basis. At one institution, 28 outpatients were treated using radiologically placed small-bore catheters connected to a plastic bag with a one-way valve system for gravity drainage. Drainage was followed by intrapleural instillation of bleomycin. With palliation results comparable to in-hospital methods, greater patient comfort and lower health care costs can result from new approaches in outpatient management of effusion.[19]

***Surgical methods*** If a pleural effusion remains uncontrolled after other approaches have been tried, surgery is another option. If a patient has a good life expectancy and a good performance status, pleural stripping is advocated. Success rates approach 90%, but there can be serious complications such as air leak, bleeding, pneumonia, and empyema.[3]

Pleurectomy has been reported to be effective in some cases. Also, a pleuroperitoneal shunt has been developed for control of malignant effusion. The shunt is inserted into the subcutaneous tissue, and pleural fluid is diverted to the peritoneal cavity via manual compression of the shunt's main valve pump. The patient must be motivated, because he is required to conscientiously pump the valve intermittently (100 times five times a day) to prevent clogging. Failure of the shunt has plagued this procedure.[8,20]

***Radiation*** Although external beam radiation may be used as local treatment for mediastinal tumors (lymphoma and lung), hemithoracic radiation is not recommended as a first-line management of malignant pleural effusions due to the hazard of pulmonary fibrosis. Radiation is limited to treatment of the underlying disease, not the resultant effusion.

***Which treatment is best?*** Despite decades of experience with palliation of malignant pleural effusion, there is an urgent need for controlled studies using larger numbers of patients. Few studies have addressed such important factors as improvement, quality of life, performance status, or exercise tolerance. In summary, some general guidelines for treatment can be advanced:

1. Small, symptomless effusions often can be left alone.
2. If the underlying cancer will probably respond to treatment, specific treatment of larger effusions should wait (as long as the patient's symptoms are tolerable).
3. The patient's overall prognosis should be considered before embarking on an aggressive approach.
4. If pleurodesis is the option selected, it should be performed early.
5. If the effusion recurs or lung expansion is compromised due to pleural disease, pleuroperitoneal shunting may be attempted.[5]

## HEART: MALIGNANT PERICARDIAL EFFUSION

### Incidence

Autopsy series indicate metastasis to the heart and pericardium occurs in 8%–20% of cases.[3] However, only 30%

of affected patients are symptomatic. Since pericardial effusion is not easily detected by routine tests, it is often not discovered while the patient is alive. Lung (59%) and breast (11%) cancer are the most common tumor types associated with pericardial effusions (Table 27-7).[21]

## Pathophysiology

The pericardial sac or cavity that surrounds the heart is completely closed. Two layers make up the sac: a tough outer fibrous pericardium called the *parietal pericardium* and an inner layer of serous pericardium called the *visceral pericardium* (Figure 27-5). Malignant pericardial effusion collects within this cavity. The cavity ordinarily contains less than 50 ml of fluid, which serves as a lubricant.

Pericardial metastasis results from lymphatic or hematogenous spread or from direct invasion by an adjacent primary tumor. Tumor implants may stud the pericardial surface or completely encase the pericardium. Pericarditis secondary to prior radiation therapy can cause severe pericardial thickening. The majority of pericardial effusions result from obstruction of lymphatic and venous drainage of the heart. This obstruction disturbs the intrapericardial pressure and results in fluid buildup. The effects of pericardial fluid accumulation are largely dependent on the rate of exudation, the physical compliance capacity of the pericardial cavity, ventricular function, myocardial size, and blood volume. If the fluid accumulation is gradual, as is usually the case with metastatic spread, the pericardium can stretch to accommodate up to 4 liters of fluid. Rapid buildup of even 150–200 ml can trigger a cardiac oncological emergency.[8,22]

## Clinical Manifestations

Pericardial effusion interferes with cardiac function as the fluid burden occupies space and reduces the volume of the heart in diastole. Systemic circulatory effects of decreased cardiac output and impaired venous return lead to generalized congestion. The body tries to compensate in several ways: (1) a tachycardia is created by adrenergic stimulation to offset decreased stroke volume; (2) systemic and pulmonary venous pressure increase in an attempt to improve ventricular filling; and (3) the adrenergic stimulation increases the ejection fraction, leading to increased peripheral resistance that will support arterial blood pressure.[22]

Most persons with pericardial effusions are asymptomatic, so cardiac involvement may be overlooked. The individual may have only nonspecific symptoms at first: dyspnea, cough, and chest pain.[23] Often the patient is treated for right heart failure or complaints related to the underlying tumor. The clinician should have a high index of suspicion for pericardial involvement whenever cancer patients exhibit cardiovascular symptoms.[24] If not diagnosed early, pericardial effusion can lead to a life-threatening emergency.

Signs and symptoms of a developing pericardial effusion are often insidious (Table 27-8). These findings can be subdivided into three clinical stages, from mild effusion to tamponade.[25] Cardiac tamponade is characterized by impaired hemodynamic function due to increased intrapericardial pressure that overcomes normal compensa-

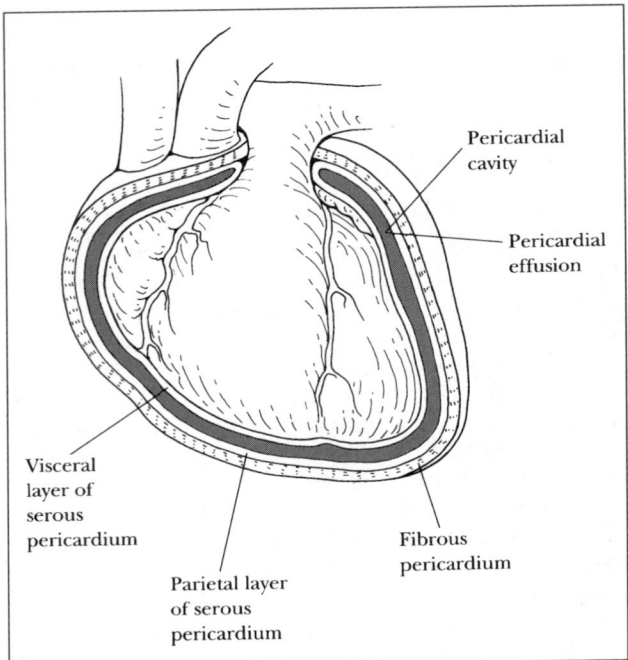

**FIGURE 27-5**  The pericardium is composed of two main compartments, the parietal pericardium and the visceral pericardium. Where the great vessels attach to the heart, these layers become continuous with each other to form the pericardial space. If venous or lymphatic drainage of the heart becomes obstructed by tumor-related processes, seepage of fluid through the visceral pericardium into the pericardial space leads to pericardial effusion. (Adapted from the *Oncology Nursing Forum* with permission from the Oncology Nursing Press. Mangan C: Malignant pericardial effusion, *Oncol Nurs Forum* 19(8):1216, 1992.)

**TABLE 27-7**  Incidence of Pericardial Effusion Related to Tumor Type

| Tumor | Incidence (%) |
| --- | --- |
| Lung cancer | 37 |
| Breast cancer | 22 |
| Leukemia and lymphoma | 17 |
| Sarcoma | 4 |
| Melanoma | 3 |
| Others | 19 |

Adapted with permission from *CA—Cancer J Clin* 41:165–179, 1991.

**TABLE 27-8**   Assessment of the Patient with Suspected Pericardial Effusion (in Order of Frequency Encountered)

| Signs and Symptoms | Frequency (%) |
|---|---|
| **SUBJECTIVE INDICATORS** | |
| Dyspnea | 79 |
| Cough | 47 |
| Chest pain | 27 |
| Orthopnea | 26 |
| Weakness | 20 |
| Dysphagia | 18 |
| Syncope | 4 |
| Palpitations | 3 |
| **OBJECTIVE INDICATORS** | |
| Pleural effusion | 51 |
| Tachycardia | 50 |
| Jugular venous distention | 45 |
| Hepatomegaly | 37 |
| Peripheral edema | 35 |
| Pulsus paradoxus | 31 |
| Hypotension | 31 |
| Distant heart sounds | 17 |
| Rales | 15 |
| Pericardial rub | 12 |
| **LABORATORY INDICATORS** | |
| Echocardiographic fluid | 100 |
| Abnormal ECG | 91 |
| Abnormal chest x-ray | 87 |
| Positive pericardial fluid cytology | 79 |
| Positive pericardial biopsy | 55 |

Adapted with permission from Press AW, Livingston R: Management of malignant pericardial effusion and tamponade. *JAMA* 257:1088–1092. Copyright 1987, American Medical Association.

tory mechanisms. Cardiac tamponade is the most severe symptom complex and is an oncological emergency.[19,21] It is seen in 16% of patients symptomatic for pericardial effusion and is more common in breast cancer than in lung cancer.[26] In one series, tamponade was the first manifestation of lung cancer in three patients.[27]

In addition to the symptoms listed in Table 27-8, the person with cardiac tamponade will position him- or herself in an upright, forward-leaning stance for maximum relief and will have anxiety, an ashen face with facial plethora, and vague gastrointestinal (GI) complaints due to visceral congestion.[8] When cardiovascular collapse is imminent, severe symptoms, profuse perspiration, and altered mental status can also occur.

Nursing management of patients in tamponade includes measures to minimize activity and promote adequate respiration, elevation of the head of the bed, and administration of oxygen and medications to relieve anxiety and pain. Intravascular volume maintenance with intravenous (IV) fluids, vasopressors, and other cardiac medications may be in order while preparation is made for pericardiocentesis or surgical intervention. Ongoing assessment for complications is imperative to prevent a fatality from occurring.[22]

## Assessment

### Radiography

Echocardiography is the fastest, least invasive, and most precise method for visualization and quantification of malignant pericardial effusion. It also allows for evaluation of ventricular function. However, it may take too much time to perform in a cardiac tamponade emergency. An upright anteroposterior (AP) x-ray view of the chest reveals cardiomegaly ("water bottle heart") but is not diagnostic. Bilateral pleural effusion, mediastinal widening, and hilar adenopathy can be observed. A small pericardial effusion may not be apparent on x-ray. Difficult-to-detect lesions may be better visualized by CT.

### Electrocardiography

Electrocardiograph (ECG) changes with neoplastic pericarditis or effusions include tachycardia, premature contractions, low QRS voltage, and nonspecific ST- and T-wave changes. Electrical alternans can occur with large effusions or with tamponade.[8,22]

### Pericardial fluid examination

Fluid withdrawn from the pericardial cavity by pericardiocentesis (needle aspiration using a subxiphoid approach) that has a bloody appearance is indicative of malignancy, especially with lung cancer. Such fluid is always exudative. Cytological examination can reveal tumor cells, but false-negatives are possible. The ability to make the diagnosis based on cytology can be difficult, particularly with effusions due to lymphoma or leukemia.[8]

## Therapeutic Approaches and Nursing Care

Medical and surgical treatment options for pericardial effusions have significant advantages and disadvantages.[21] Choice of treatment depends on the physiological impairment caused by the effusion and the degree of tamponade. If the individual is asymptomatic, it is usually expedient to simply watch and wait (Figure 27-6).

### Removal of fluid

***Pericardiocentesis alone***  Percutaneous pericardiocentesis (performed since 1840) guided by ECHO is an important diagnostic tool and is useful for initial drainage of fluid from the pericardium. This leads to dramatic relief of symptoms with minimal risk.[8] Using echocardiography to guide the procedure decreases the risk of puncturing the heart. Pericardial drainage alone as treatment for effusion has been equivocal, with most patients relapsing a short time after the tap. The complication rate ranges from 10% to 25%.[21] Pericardiocentesis is crucial with cardiac tamponade. Nursing care during the pericardiocentesis includes explaining the procedure to the patient and attempting to reduce anxiety and discomfort; positioning the patient in a semi-Fowler's position; maintaining asepsis; and having available a good light source, a defibrillator, and emergency medications. The nurse must continuously monitor the patient and the ECG during the pericardiocentesis, and afterward monitor for complications such as pneumothorax, myocardial laceration, and coronary artery laceration.[28] Other emergency

support measures may be needed first, such as IV fluids, oxygen, and drugs to increase cardiac output and blood pressure.[22,25,26]

***Subxiphoid pericardiotomy***  Under local anesthesia using a subxiphoid approach, subxiphoid pericardiotomy allows for a longer period of drainage and permits examination of the pericardial space as well as obtaining a pericardial biopsy. Complications are rare, and effusion usually does not recur.[29] Nursing care is the same as for pericardiocentesis.

***Balloon pericardiotomy***  After accessing the pericardial space by a conventional pericardiocentesis, a guide wire is threaded into the pericardium and a balloon dilating catheter inflated to create a window. Fluid then drains into the pleural space. Balloon pericardiotomy can be performed under local anesthesia, and in most cases allows for early hospital discharge.[30,31]

***Pericardioperitoneal shunt***  A Denver® pleuroperitoneal shunt has been used successfully to drain the pericardial effusion into the peritoneal cavity. The procedure is performed under local anesthesia and the patients are discharged two to four days later. In comparison, the more traditional methods of pericardial drainage led to higher postoperative morbidity and mortality and a much longer hospital stay.[32] This newer approach will need further study but could result in improved clinical outcomes.

### Obliteration of the pericardial space

***Pericardiocentesis with sclerosing agent instillation***  Sclerosing agents are instilled into the pericardial cavity via pericardiocentesis, but they are associated with significant toxicity. Sclerosing agents used in pericardial effusions include tetracycline, 5-fluorouracil, radioactive gold or phosphorus, quinacrine, and thiotepa. The degree of response varies with each agent. Effusions recur in approximately 50% of the patients thus treated.

***Surgery***  Surgical intervention, including pleuropericardial window via thoracotomy and pericardiectomy, is generally reserved for medically appropriate patients whose malignant effusion is unresponsive to other therapies or who have required repeated pericardiocentesis. General anesthesia and thoracotomy are required. Cardiac tamponade symptoms are usually present.

A nursing care plan for patients with tamponade undergoing pericardial window surgery includes preoperative measures to maintain blood pressure and heart rate, maintain urine output and mental status, provide sufficient oxygen, and decrease pain and anxiety. Nursing measures postoperatively include prevention of infection, atelectasis, pleural effusion, and pneumothorax, as well as ongoing assessment for cardiac arrhythmia due to surgical irritation or the presence of the pericardial catheter. Prevention of anxiety and pain and bleeding due to the catheter and maintaining free-flowing pericardial drainage are important.[29]

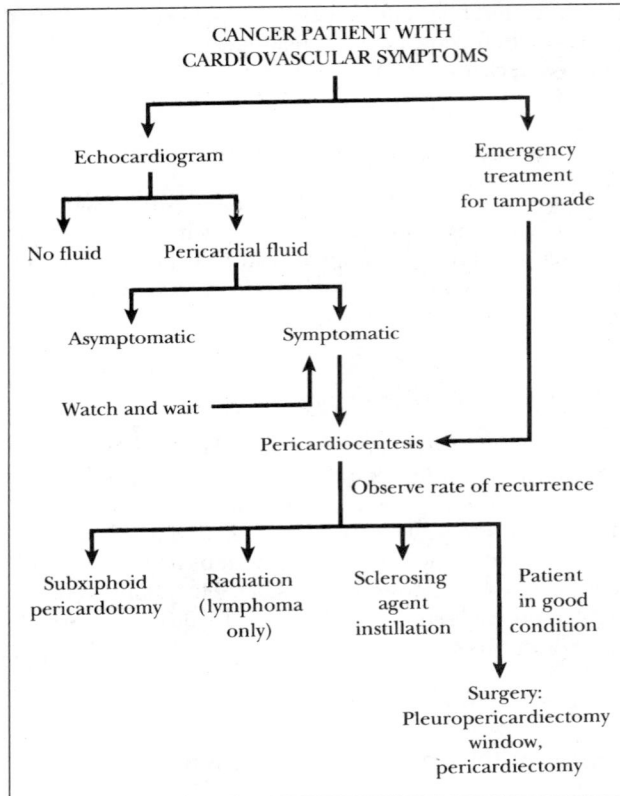

**FIGURE 27-6**  Algorithm for diagnosis and management of malignant pericardial effusion.

Recurrence following surgical intervention is rare. A reported experience with subxiphoid partial pericardiectomy, with or without a sclerosing agent, concluded that this procedure is a safe and effective treatment for malignant pericardial effusions. It was suggested that patients with symptomatic malignant pericardial effusions be treated first with subxiphoid partial pericardiectomy, thus reserving sclerosant instillation for those who have persistent drainage after surgery.[33]

***Radiation***   The use of external beam radiation is primarily reserved for pericardial effusion due to lymphomas, which are highly radiosensitive.[8] Approximately 50% of cases will respond. Carcinoma of the lung and breast are also sufficiently radiosensitive for radiation to be considered in the treatment plan.

## ABDOMEN: MALIGNANT PERITONEAL EFFUSION

### Incidence

Malignant peritoneal effusion (ascites) is most common in women with ovarian cancer (Table 27-9). Ascites will be found at presentation in 33% of these women, and over 60% will develop ascites at some time before death.[34] Ascites also develops in patients with GI malignancies, though it typically develops later in the course of the disease. The appearance of ascites in patients with advanced disease is prognostically grim, and palliation is usually all that can be offered. Life expectancy is a few months.

**TABLE 27-9**   Tumors Associated with Malignant Peritoneal Effusion

| | |
|---|---|
| Ovary | Gastric |
| Endometrial | Pancreatic |
| Breast | Lymphoma |
| Colon | Mesothelioma |

## Physiological Alterations

The peritoneal cavity is covered by a serous lining composed of the visceral peritoneum, which lines and supports the abdominal organs, and the parietal peritoneum. The parietal peritoneum covers the abdominal and pelvic walls and the undersurface of the diaphragm (Figure 27-7). As with the other third spaces, a small amount of fluid lubricates the cavity. Normally, the volume of peritoneal fluid is regulated by the pressure gradient balances described previously, with lymphatic channels draining 80% of all lymphatic peritoneal fluid.[12] When the production of peritoneal fluid exceeds the ability of the lymphatic channels to drain the cavity (the thoracic duct may be dilated to five to ten times the normal size), ascites develops.

The most common cause of ascitic fluid buildup is tumor seeding the peritoneum, resulting in obstruction of the diaphragmatic and/or abdominal lymphatics. This occurs primarily with gynecologic cancers. Excess intraperitoneal fluid production may also be a factor contributing to ascites. The tumor itself may elaborate humoral factors that cause increased capillary leakage of proteins and fluids into the peritoneum. In patients with diffuse liver metastasis and venous obstruction, hypoalbuminemia and low serum protein may play a part in the development of a transudative ascites.

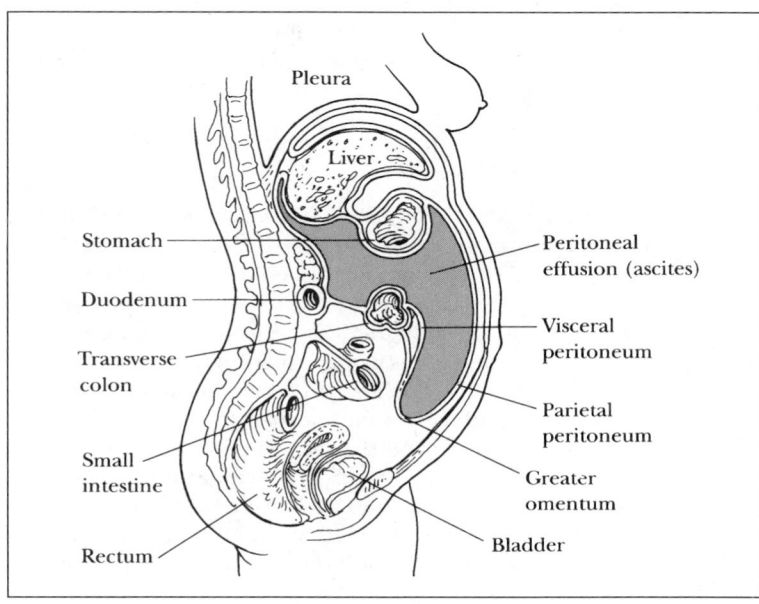

**FIGURE 27-7**   The peritoneal cavity is covered by the visceral peritoneum that lines and supports the abdominal organs, and the parietal peritoneum that covers the abdominal and pelvic walls and the undersurface of the diaphragm. If, due to malignant processes, the volume of fluid accumulating in the peritoneal space exceeds the capacity of lymphatic channels to drain the cavity, ascites develops. (Adapted from Pick TP, Howden R [eds]: *Gray's Anatomy* [rev. Am. ed from 15th Eng. ed]. New York: Bounty Books, 1977, p. 900.)

## Clinical Manifestations

The pressure of the ascitic fluid volume on nearby organs is uncomfortable and restrictive. Several liters of ascitic fluid can be accommodated in the abdomen. Some people report gaining 50–60 lb of body weight as a result of excess fluid. This massive accumulation of fluid leads to negative body image changes, anorexia, early satiety, and difficulty in breathing and walking. Subjective, objective, and laboratory findings illustrate the typical profile of a person with ascites (Table 27-10). Most physical signs appear after 1 liter or more of fluid is present.

## Assessment

Peritoneal effusion is diagnosed primarily by physical exam, with malignant characteristics confirmed by paracentesis. An abdomen filled with more than 500 ml of fluid appears as a single curve from the xiphoid process

**TABLE 27-10** Assessment of the Patient with a Peritoneal Effusion

| SUBJECTIVE INDICATORS |
| --- |
| Increasing abdominal girth—"clothes don't fit" |
| Indigestion and early satiety |
| Swollen ankles |
| Easily fatigued |
| Shortness of breath |
| Constipation |
| Reduced bladder capacity |

| OBJECTIVE INDICATORS |
| --- |
| Weight gain |
| Distended abdomen |
| Fluid wave |
| Shifting dullness |
| Bulging flanks |
| Everted umbilicus |
| Stretched skin |

| LABORATORY INDICATORS |
| --- |
| Abdominal flat plate: generalized ground-glass appearance, air-filled small-bowel loops occupy central position and are separated by fluid between loops |
| Ultrasound |
| Abdominal CT |
| Paracentesis |
|   Gross character on inspection: bloody, serous, milky, turbid |
|   Cell count and differential |
|   Chemistries: total protein, LDH, carcinoembryonic antigen (CEA), amylase levels |
|   Cytology |
|   Microbiology: Gram's stain and culture |

Adapted with permission from Baker AR, Treatment of malignant ascites, in DeVita VT, Hellman S, Rosenberg SA (eds): *Cancer: Principles and Practice of Oncology* (ed 3). Philadelphia, Lippincott, 1989.

to the pubis, with the umbilicus frequently everted. The following signs are characteristic of free fluid: bulging flanks, tympany at the top the abdominal curve, elicitation of a fluid wave, and shifting dullness. A small effusion is hard to detect. The "puddle sign" is said to detect as little as 120 ml of free fluid in the abdominal cavity. To elicit the puddle sign, the patient lies prone for five minutes, then rises on elbows and knees. A stethoscope is applied to the most dependent part of the abdomen, and the clinician repeatedly flicks the near flank with a finger. As the stethoscope is moved across the abdomen away from the examiner, the sound becomes louder. Small volumes of fluid in the abdomen can also be detected by ultrasonic examination. Detecting ascites in obese patients is difficult, even when it is marked.

## Therapeutic Approaches and Nursing Care

Many treatment approaches have been tried, but an optimal intervention has yet to be found.[34] No controlled trials comparing alternative therapies have been reported. It is difficult to carry out research in individuals whose longevity is limited to only a few months. An algorithm for the management of the patient with ascites includes the multiple factors influencing selection of treatment (Figure 27-8). Nursing care measures focus on maintaining fluid and electrolyte balance, comfort measures, and early recognition of complications.

### Diet and diuresis

Although diet and diuresis are important as therapy for individuals with ascites due to cirrhosis, sodium restriction and diuretics are usually ineffective in malignant ascites. Unless the underlying malignancy causing the ascites responds to antineoplastic therapy, the pathophysiology of ascites will remain unaltered and fluid accumulation will continue despite exogenous fluid restriction measures.

### Removal of fluid

*Paracentesis* Aside from its usefulness as a diagnostic tool, fluid removal by paracentesis alone is of little therapeutic benefit. It is usually reserved until a large volume of fluid has accumulated and the patient is profoundly symptomatic because the fluid reaccumulates rapidly. Of particular note, removal of 2–3 liters of fluid and repeated paracentesis taps can lead to severe protein depletion, postural hypotension, and electrolyte abnormalities. Injury to the viscera and the introduction of infection can occur. Although caution is urged regarding rapidly removing large volumes of ascitic fluid, there has been recent anecdotal evidence that rapid decompression via paracentesis is not harmful with malignant ascites, probably because the mechanism of its production differs from that of cirrhotic ascites.[35]

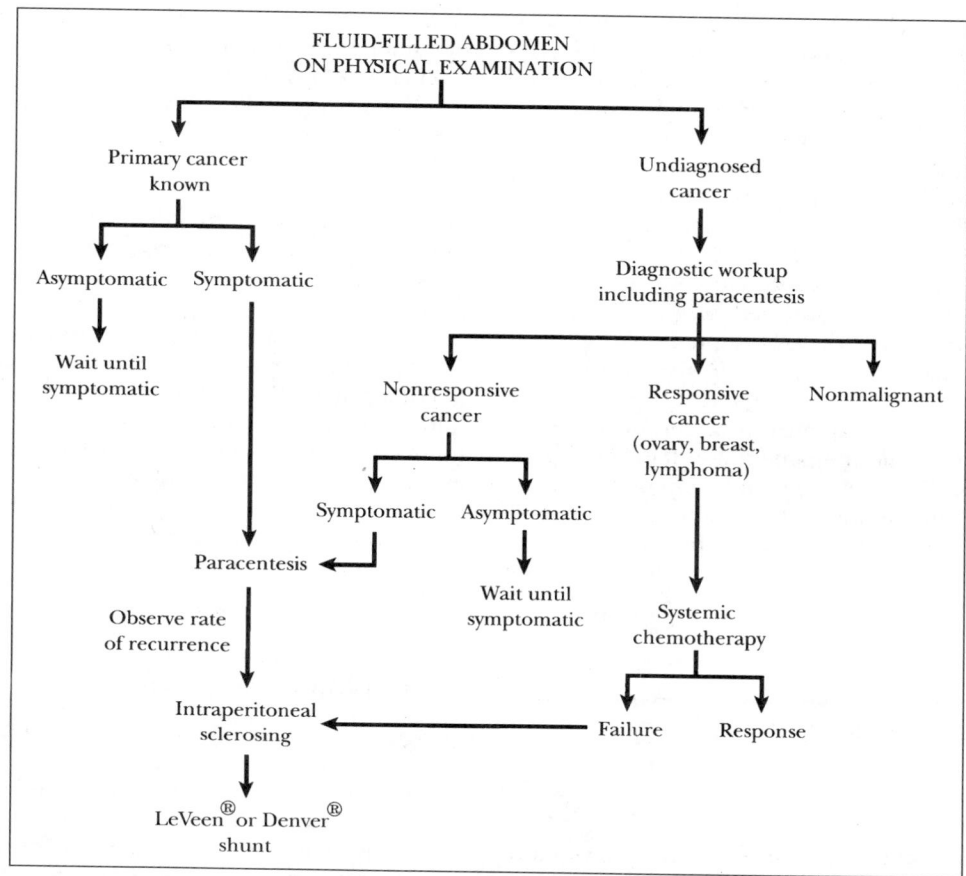

**FIGURE 27-8**  Algorithm for diagnosis and management of malignant peritoneal effusion.

***Obliteration of the intraperitoneal space***  In the past, intracavity therapy has consisted of instillation of a radioactive colloid suspension (no longer in favor) or a chemotherapeutic agent. The chemotherapy instillation is designed to provoke an inflammatory response leading to sclerosis of the peritoneal space linings. Although sclerosing therapy is effective in treating malignant pleural effusions, it is less successful with ascites.[26] Modest responses to bleomycin instillation for palliation have been reported with no significant side effects. Adriamycin, nitrogen mustard, and tetracycline instillations have been tried with small groups of individuals. Cisplatin has been administered intraperitoneally.

Access to the peritoneal cavity for drug administration is an important technical problem. The peritoneum can be entered on a temporary basis with various catheters, but repeated puncture of the abdominal wall and peritoneum is risky. Adhesions can occur, which increases the risk of bowel perforation and peritonitis. The Tenchoff® catheter is often used to provide repeated access to the peritoneum. It can remain in place indefinitely and allows peritoneal fluid sampling in addition to drug instillation. Problems with the Tenchoff® catheter have been poor return following drug and fluid instillation and abdominal pain or discomfort necessitating catheter removal.[12]

Using a Groshong® catheter for draining malignant ascites is an alternative to conventional paracentesis.[36] Use of the Groshong® catheter prevents needle access and does not require surgical removal upon completion of chemotherapy. Complex dressing changes like those required by the Tenchoff catheter are unnecessary.

***Peritoneovenous shunting***  Shunt devices (LeVeen® and Denver®) can be used to recirculate ascitic fluid continuously to the intravascular space. One end of a catheter is implanted in the peritoneal cavity and a tube is channeled through subcutaneous tissue to the superior vena cava, where the other end is implanted. A pressure differential between the abdominal cavity and the thoracic vein enables fluid to ascend from the peritoneal cavity into the superior vena cava. Since neoplastic ascites tends to contain more particulate matter than other fluid types (usually an exudate), a Denver® shunt may be preferred because it has a subcutaneous pump that can be manually compressed to prevent clogging of the tubing.[37] Despite this potential advantage, a functional superiority of one over the other of these devices has not been documented in the literature,[34] leaving the choice to the clinician's personal preference.

Peritoneovenous shunting is no panacea. It is usually

reserved for individuals in whom all other treatment options have failed. Median survival time after shunt placement is two to four months, so it is difficult to obtain objective evaluation criteria. When the shunt is functioning well, it provides good palliation. Complications can occur, with clotting occurring most frequently, but sometimes disseminated intravascular coagulation and pulmonary embolism develop. In some instances postoperative complications might be predicted by a preoperative procedure designed to assess patient tolerance to the proposed permanent shunt. Termed *peritoneovenous autotransfusion*, this preoperative evaluation can be accomplished by using an external shunting system trial over 48 hours.[38]

Nursing care of the patient with a peritoneovenous shunt includes teaching the patient and family the purpose and care of the shunt, signs and symptoms of problems with the shunt, and recognition and prevention of infection, as well as alleviating anxiety. In addition, nursing care includes measures related to the peritoneal effusion and advanced cancer.

## BRAIN: MALIGNANT CEREBRAL EDEMA

### Incidence

Cerebral edema results from an increase in brain volume caused by an increase in the fluid content of the brain.[39] There are three major types of cerebral edema: *vasogenic* edema (extracellular, the most common type); *cytotoxic* edema (intracellular, due to metabolic abnormalities); and *interstitial* edema (due to cerebrospinal fluid blockage). Malignant cerebral edema is the vasogenic type caused by increased permeability of the cerebral capillary endothelial cells. Although the edema can be iatrogenic, caused by radiotherapy or chemotherapy, most cerebral edema accompanies primary or metastatic brain tumors or carcinomatous meningitis. Any cancer can metastasize to the brain; brain metastasis occurs in 25%–35% of all persons with cancer. Lung cancer accounts for most of the metastatic lesions in the brain (40%–50%), followed by breast cancer (13%), melanoma, renal carcinoma, and others.[40]

### Physiological Alterations

Mechanisms thought to play a role in the formation of malignant cerebral edema are (1) direct injury to the vascular endothelium by the expanding tumor, (2) dysplastic vascular structures within tumor lesions, (3) biochemically mediated alterations of capillary permeability (including the excretion of a permeability factor by tumor cells),[41] and (4) a less stable blood-brain barrier. Capillary permeability varies depending on histology and tumor size. Within an individual brain tumor there are signifi-

cant variations in capillary permeability among regions of tumor necrosis and those of active tumor growth.[42] Edema develops as water and ions passively diffuse into the brain extracellular space to maintain isotonicity. The white matter of the brain is primarily affected (Figure 27-9). The progression of edema through brain tissue occurs as bulk fluid flow regulated by cerebral perfusion pressure. It is possible for edema fluid to travel along the longitudinal tracts of the white matter and thus increase local extracellular water content at a distance from the focal tumor.[43]

The tumor continuously produces edema fluid. There can be great differences in the volume of edema, depending on the level of productivity of that particular tumor.[44] How cerebral edema leads to neurological dysfunction is not clear, but it is probably related to ischemic effects of the mass itself and/or toxic inhibition of local neuron activity induced by metabolic abnormalities in the surrounding extravascular fluid. When the edema exceeds the limits of compensatory mechanisms, brain herniation can occur.

### Clinical Manifestations

Malignant cerebral edema produces diffuse signs and symptoms reflecting its more global effects on brain functioning, as opposed to the focal signs and symptoms caused by direct destruction of tissue by tumor.[43] Most patients with metastatic brain tumors have regional swelling of tissue, mostly in the cerebrum. In such patients the clinical deficits manifested are more often caused by

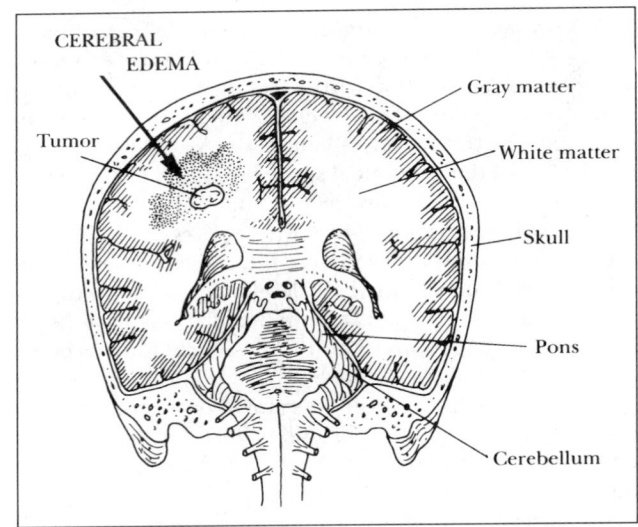

**FIGURE 27-9**  Vasogenic edema of the brain due to a primary tumor or metastatic lesion is characterized by increased permeability of brain capillary endothelial cells. The white matter of the brain is primarily affected. The progression of edema through the white matter of brain tissue occurs as bulk flow regulated by cerebral perfusion pressure.

peritumoral edema than by the tumor mass itself.[39] Subtle early changes in the patient's status are vague and usually observed only by someone who knows the patient well. Family members may notice the patient's lack of persistence in tasks, undue irritability, emotional lability, inertia, faulty insight, forgetfulness, reduced range of mental activity, indifference to common social practices, and lack of initiative and spontaneity. These early symptoms are often incorrectly attributed to worry, anxiety, or depression. Patients themselves often complain only of being weak, tired, or dizzy. As time progresses, the symptoms become more pronounced (Table 27-11).

Seizure is the most common symptom of acute onset. Headache, another common early symptom, is due to distortion and traction of pain-sensitive structures by the edema. Intermittent at first, headache usually is present in the morning and gradually increases in duration and frequency. Other indications of brain edema can be generalized or focal. Clinical signs may be observed that relate to specific parts of the brain, and these can be localized to the affected area by neurological assessment.[45]

**TABLE 27-11**   Assessment of the Patient with Cerebral Edema

| Signs and Symptoms | Frequency (%) |
| --- | --- |
| **SUBJECTIVE INDICATORS** | |
| Headache | 53 |
| Weakness, focal | 40 |
| Mental disturbance | 31 |
| Seizures | 15 |
| Gait disorder | 20 |
| Visual disturbance | 12 |
| Language disturbance | 10 |
| **OBJECTIVE INDICATORS** | |
| Hemiparesis | 66 |
| Impaired cognition | 77 |
| Sensory loss, unilateral | 27 |
| Papilledema | 26 |
| Ataxia | 24 |
| Aphasia | 19 |
| **LABORATORY INDICATORS** | |
| Computerized tomography (CT) brain | |
| Magnetic resonance imaging (MRI) | |

Adapted with permission from Wright DC, Delaney TF: Treatment of metastatic cancer to the brain, in DeVita VT, Hellman S, Rosenberg SA (eds): *Cancer: Principles and Practice of Oncology* (ed 3). Philadelphia, Lippincott, 1989.

## Assessment

Neurological examination, CT scanning, and magnetic resonance imaging (MRI) are the primary studies used for diagnosing a brain tumor mass. MRI is best for visualizing cerebral edema.[45] Surgery, such as stereotactic biopsy, is required for a definitive tissue diagnosis if a primary site is not in evidence elsewhere in the body.

## Therapeutic Approaches and Nursing Care

Aggressive therapy is warranted to sustain or restore neurological function. The principal treatment regimen is radiation therapy. In addition, patients receive supportive care and steroids to reduce edema. Patients with edema due to carcinomatous meningitis are aggressively treated with intrathecal chemotherapy. In most patients, neurological symptoms resolve or improve with treatment. Improvement is often maintained until the patient succumbs to systemic disease.

Nursing management of patients with cerebral edema focuses on assessment, administration of medication, management of side effects associated with these medications, the institution of safety and seizure precautions, and prevention of complications of immobility. Interventions may be targeted to the patient's specific neurological deficits. The nurse must be sensitive to changes in vital signs and be able to intervene rapidly. With advanced cerebral edema and the resultant intracranial hypertension, changes in vital signs such as bounding radial pulse, elevated temperature, and respiratory impairment may be seen. Early detection of brain herniation is essential to preserve brain function. Decreased level of consciousness, change in pupil size and reaction to light, and altered motor response, in addition to other vital sign changes, should alert the nurse to impending brain herniation, an oncological emergency.[45]

### Steroids and osmotherapy

The single most important adjunctive treatment to combat the effects of vasogenic cerebral edema is the use of glucocorticoids (dexamethasone, prednisone). These drugs rapidly reduce the rate of edema fluid formation by the tumor (by 30%) by inhibiting the capillary permeability factor produced by tumor cells.[44] The aim of steroid therapy is to reduce intracranial pressure and increase cerebral blood flow. The usual starting dose of dexamethasone is 16 mg/day in four divided doses. Dexamethasone is the preferred agent because of its minimal sodium-retaining properties and relative potency. Mannitol is an osmotherapy agent that can be used to reduce profound cerebral edema on a temporary basis.[43,46]

Once radiotherapy has relieved the neurological symptoms caused by the edema, steroids are slowly tapered to prevent addisonian crisis. Steroid withdrawal can result in headache, lethargy, postural dizziness, or nausea, even if there is no laboratory evidence of adrenal insufficiency. These symptoms can confuse the clinician, since they mirror symptoms associated with either adrenal suppression or progressive edema.[42]

Dexamethasone doses as high as 100 mg/day have been used for patients who are refractory at lower doses. Patients failing to improve after a seven-day trial at 100 mg/day are rapidly tapered to the lowest dose that will maintain stable neurological functioning. The continued long-term use of steroids can lead to serious toxic effects such as cataracts, hyperglycemia, peptic ulcer, and osteoporosis. The effects of long-term therapy should be considered in the nursing plan of care.[46]

### Radiation therapy

Ionizing radiation to the underlying tumor is the most effective way to decrease malignant edema as well as tumor bulk. Since it is assumed microscopic tumor is present in metastatic disease, the radiation port usually encompasses the whole brain. Treatment typically lasts two to three weeks. Interstitial brachytherapy (the implantation of seeds containing iodine 120 or iridium 192) can sometimes be used to achieve a high-dose "local" boost to the tumor while minimizing radiation exposure for normal brain tissue. Despite initial response rates of 80%, radiation accomplishes little in terms of survival. Median survival after treatment is three to six months.[43]

### Surgery

Surgical decompression may be in order in selected cases of resistant or relapsing cerebral metastasis. Surgical decompression or debulking can rapidly reduce the effect of the mass and remove the source of edema production. Neurosurgical procedures have significant associated risk, such as infection, hemorrhage, and operative mortality. Appropriate patient selection is a critical factor for successful surgical outcome. While surgery can sometimes remove a small, isolated metastasis identified early, individuals may not wish to sacrifice quality of remaining life for the hospitalization and recovery period required for a major neurosurgical procedure.

# ARMS/LEGS: IATROGENIC SECONDARY LYMPHEDEMA

## Incidence and Physiological Alterations

Unlike the other effusions and edemas, postsurgical lymphedema of the arm or leg is a benign condition. Arm lymphedema was the frequent postoperative sequela of the most common treatment for all types of breast cancer in the past: radical mastectomy with axillary node dissection followed by radiation. With the less invasive breast cancer treatments in use today, arm lymphedema occurs less frequently. Even so, lymphedema continues

to affect 5%–10% of women who have a modified radical mastectomy.[47]

Mechanical interruption (surgical technique) and radiation often produce lymphatic obstruction, the most common cause of lymphedema. Usually the more radical the surgery or radiation, the more severe the edema. Other factors contributing to the development of lymphedema are obesity,[48] insufficient muscle contraction, inflammation, trauma, formation of fibrosclerotic tissue within the lymph vessel, and scarring secondary to radiation therapy or infection. Narrower and fewer lymph channels remain, fluid transport is insufficient, and swelling occurs. Chronic lymphedema is a late postoperative complication that can occur anywhere from 6 weeks to 20 years after surgery. For most women the affected arm becomes enlarged within the first year after mastectomy.[49] The unpredictable and often delayed nature of lymphedema is postulated to be due to smoldering infection associated with subclinical lymphangitis.[50]

Lymphedema of the leg may develop after groin dissection, which is performed for the treatment of metastatic disease from primary tumors (melanoma, squamous cell carcinoma, or soft-tissue sarcomas) located in the anatomic area drained by the inguinal lymph nodes. The incidence of leg lymphedema after this type of surgery increases gradually over time, and by the fifth postoperative year is estimated to occur in 80% of patients.[51] Improved surgical technique and a preventive regimen of leg elevation and elastic stockings reduce the overall incidence of mild to moderate lymphedema to 20%, with no severe lymphedema occurring.[51]

The pathogenesis of lymphedema of the lower extremities (eventually including the genitalia) after groin dissection or radiation therapy is similar to that of the arm. Progressive interstitial fibrosis follows the mechanical interruption of lymph flow caused by the surgery, and scarring ensues. If the edema is severe, the result is the classic brawny, nonpitting, firm form of soft-tissue swelling. The edematous extremity is painful, can become contracted, and compromises the patient's ability to walk.

Rarely, a malignant lymphedema of the extremities occurs in a patient with an advanced, untreated lymphoma who has ignored earlier symptoms. Cancer cells obstruct lymph vessels or lymph nodes through intraluminal propagation or by external compression. This patient will usually respond to systemic treatment, and the edema will subside.

## Assessment

Assessment for extremity lymphedema includes monitoring the circumference of the limb, condition of the skin, mobility of the extremity, signs of infection, nutritional status, impairment of circulation, and constriction caused by clothing and other objects. Measurements of the arm circumference are taken prior to surgery and at each postoperative visit. The arm is measured 5.0 and 10.0 cm above and below the olecranon process. Measurement sites are documented and consistent for each patient. Leg measurements are done similarly at the level of the calf. Lymphedema is defined as present if there is a difference in measurement of 1.0 cm–1.5 cm compared with the unaffected extremity. It can be classified as mild (less than 3 cm), moderate (3.0–5.0 cm), or severe (more than 5 cm).[49]

## Therapeutic Approaches and Nursing Care

The goals of therapy are primarily aimed at prevention, to increase the flow of lymph away from the limb and minimize formation of new lymph fluid. Elevation, progressive mild exercise,[52] and massage[53] help mobilize fluid out of the limb. Use of an elastic sleeve is important to reduce the potential of stagnation of lymph fluid. Compliance and proper use are critical factors.[49] Prophylactic measures to prevent new fluid from forming include elastic support sleeves or stockings; sodium restriction; and avoidance of infection, excessive use of the limb, local heat, and trauma to the limb.[54] Mirolo et al describe a comprehensive lymphedema management program that stresses self-care.[54]

Nursing care is usually divided into primary, secondary, and tertiary interventions.[47,49] The primary nursing interventions for lymphedema involve measures to prevent complications. These begin preoperatively, with assessment of the patient's educational needs, nutritional status, and arm measurements. Instruction on postoperative hand and arm care and postoperative exercises should also occur at this time.

The secondary phase of nursing management is directed toward the early detection and initial treatment of lymphedema. The patient should be alerted to the signs and symptoms of lymphedema, the arms/legs should be measured at regular intervals, the affected limb should be elevated, massage therapy may be instituted, an elastic wrap or sleeve to the affected extremity may be needed, discomfort should be managed, and hand and arm care measures and exercise should be continued. The patient should be taught to recognize and prevent infection.

Tertiary care is associated with the long-term care of the patient with lymphedema and includes elevation of the arm, continued hand and arm care measures and exercises, massage therapy, elastic wrap or sleeve to the extremity, pain control, and assessment of the patient for general functioning and ability to perform activities of daily living.[53]

Diuretics are usually not helpful. Long-term use of diuretics is reserved for cases of generalized low-protein edemas in which the total body sodium content is elevated. In contrast, lymphedema is caused by the stagnation of proteins in the interstitium (a high-protein edema) and not by retention of sodium.

Although the condition is not life-threatening, breast cancer patients who developed lymphedema were found to have greater psychological morbidity, functional impairment, and disturbance in psychosocial adjustment.[55] Postmastectomy lymphedema therapy was found to have psychosocial benefit.[56]

## FEET: MALIGNANT PEDAL EDEMA

Peripheral, or dependent, edema is common in patients with far-advanced cancer. Among the multiple causes are the lack of normal muscular activity, which would ordinarily return fluids from the periphery to the central circulation; hypoalbuminemia; venous or lymphatic obstruction; compromised circulation; malnutrition; and hyperaldosteronism. As much as 10 lb of liquid can accumulate in the lower extremities before it is recognizable as pitting edema.[57] Many individuals will tolerate this fluid accumulation with no discomfort and will require no special therapy other than elastic stockings or elevation of the legs several times a day. However, patients and families are often disturbed by the cosmetic unsightliness of the swollen feet and ankles, especially when shoes no longer fit, and they may request more definitive intervention.

## Assessment

Measurement of the ankle is useful to record changes in circumference and note the effectiveness of treatment measures. Pitting can be assessed by pressing the thumb into the patient's skin over a bony surface.[57] The edema of advanced cancer is bilateral; a unilateral edema would lead to a search for a treatable cause such as thrombophlebitis. Serum albumin or serum total protein levels will indicate whether hypoalbuminemia is present, as will serum total proteins. The prealbumin level is a quick and accurate test that indicates malnutrition.[58]

## Therapeutic Approaches and Nursing Care

Three approaches can be taken in an attempt to relieve ankle edema.[58] First, the patient's nutritional status may be improved with concentrated dietary supplements. Protein is particularly important.[60] Overt sodium can be eliminated from the diet; however, most patients are eating little food at this point and have stopped eating salty foods at earlier stages of the illness. Water should be restricted if the patient is hyponatremic. Second, there is an effort to improve venous blood return by elevation of the legs while sitting, wearing of support stockings, eliminating clothing that constricts the lower legs, and gentle exercise. Third, diuretics may be helpful and can be tried on a short-term basis.[61] A typical diuretic regimen starts with low-dose hydrochlorothiazide and cautiously proceeds through progressively larger doses of spironolactone to furosemide until a diuretic response is achieved.[61] Serum electrolytes, blood urea nitrogen, and creatinine are monitored during such a trial.

## CONCLUSION

When fluid accumulates abnormally in the cancer patient, the consequences can range from life-threatening to merely irksome. A variety of interventions can be employed, mostly for palliation, depending on the amount of fluid present and the site where it is retained. Aggressive medical and nursing care can alleviate discomfort and may prolong life, or at least maintain its quality. The best hope for eliminating malignant effusions and edemas would be to discover a cure for cancer, or at least more effective therapies.

## REFERENCES

1. Maxwell MB, Maher KE: Chemotherapy-induced myelosuppression. *Semin Oncol Nurs* 8(2):113–123, 1992
2. Hill RB, Anderson RE: The autopsy in oncology. *CA Cancer J Clin* 42:47–56, 1992
3. Olopade OI, Ultmann JE: Malignant effusions. *CA Cancer J Clin* 41:166–179, 1991
4. Moores DW: Malignant pleural effusion. *Semin Oncol* 18:59–61, 1991 (suppl)
5. Miles DW, Kough RK: Diagnosis and management of malignant pleural effusion. *Cancer Treat Rev* 19:115–168, 1993
6. Lynch TJ: Management of malignant pleural effusions. *Chest* 103:3855–3895, 1993 (suppl)
7. Keller, SM: Current and future therapy for malignant pleural effusion. *Chest* 103:635–675, 1993 (suppl)
8. Pass HI: Treatment of malignant pleural and pericardial effusions, in DeVita VT, Hellman S, Rosenberg SA (eds): *Cancer: Principles and Practices of Oncology* (ed 4). Philadelphia, Lippincott, 1993, pp 2246–2255
9. Rossetti AC: Nursing care of patients treated with intrapleural tetracycline for control of malignant pleural effusion. *Cancer Nurs* 8:103–109, 1985
10. Wegmann JA, Forshee T: Malignant pleural effusion: Pertinent issues. *Heart Lung* 12:533–543, 1983
11. Hausheer FH, Yarbro JW: Diagnosis and treatment of malignant pleural effusion. *Semin Oncol* 12:54–75, 1985
12. Zehner LC, Hoogstraten B: Malignant effusions and their management. *Semin Oncol* 1:259–268, 1985
13. Gobel BH, Lawler PE: Malignant pleural effusion. *Oncol Nurs Forum* 12:49–54, 1985
14. Leff RS, Eisenberg B, Braisden CE, et al: Drainage of recurrent pleural effusion via an implanted port and intrapleural catheter. *Ann Intern Med* 104:308–309, 1986
15. Hewitt JB, Jansen WB: A management strategy for malignancy-induced pleural effusion: Long-term thoracostomy drainage: *Oncol Nurs Forum* 14:17–22, 1987
16. Ruckdeschel JC: Management of malignant pleural effusion: An overview. *Semin Oncol* 15:24–28, 1988 (suppl)
17. Petrou M, Kaplan D, Goldstraw P: Management of recurrent malignant pleural effusions. *Cancer* 75:801–805, 1995
18. Milanez RC, Vargas FS, Filomeno LB: Intrapleural talc for the treatment of malignant pleural effusion secondary to breast cancer: *Cancer* 75:2690–2692, 1995
19. Belani CP, Aisner J, Patz E, et al: Ambulatory sclerotherapy for malignant pleural effusion. *Proc Am Soc Clin Oncol* 14:524, 1995
20. Robinson RD, Fullerton DA, Alpert JD, et al: Use of pleural Tenckhoff catheter to palliate malignant pleural effusion. *Ann Thorac Surg* 57:286–288, 1994
21. Hawkins JW, Vacek JL: What constitutes definitive therapy of malignant pericardial effusion? Medical vs. surgical treatment. *Am Heart J* 118:428–432, 1989
22. Joiner GA, Kolodychuk GR: Neoplastic cardiac tamponade. *Crit Care Nurs* 11:50–58, 1991
23. Wilkes JD, Fideas P, Vaickus L, et al: Malignancy-related pericardial effusion. *Cancer* 76:1377–1387, 1995
24. Press OW, Livingston R: Management of malignant pericardial effusion and tamponade. *JAMA* 257:1088–1092, 1987
25. Mangan CM: Malignant pericardial effusions: Pathophysiology and clinical correlates. *Oncol Nurs Forum* 19:1215–1221, 1992
26. Okamoto H, Shinkai T, Yamakido M, et al: Cardiac tamponade caused by primary lung cancer and the management of pericardial effusion. *Cancer* 73:93–98, 1993
27. Fincher RM: Case report: Malignant pericardial effusion as the initial manifestation of malignancy. *Am J Med Sci* 305:106–110, 1993
28. Estes ME: Management of the cardiac tamponade patient: A nursing framework. *Crit Care Nurs* 5:17–26, 1985
29. Wojciechowicz V: Peripheral window surgery for cardiac tamponade. *Crit Care Nurs* 5:28–33, 1985
30. Vaikus PT, Herrmann HC, Le Winter MM: Treatment of malignant pericardial effusion. *JAMA* 272:59–64, 1994
31. Keane D, Jackson J: Managing recurrent malignant pericardial effusions: Percutaneous balloon pericardiotomy may have a role. *BMJ* 305:729–730, 1992
32. Wang N, Feikes JR, Morensen T, et al: Pericardioperitoneal shunt: An alternative treatment for malignant pericardial effusion. *Ann Thorac Surg* 57:289–292, 1994
33. Chan A, Rischin D, Clark CP, et al: Subxiphoid partial pericardiectomy with or without sclerosant instillation in the treatment of symptomatic pericardial effusions in patients with malignancy. *Cancer* 68:1021–1025, 1991
34. Baker AR, Weber JS: Treatment of malignant ascites, in DeVita VT, Hellman S, Rosenberg SA (eds): *Cancer: Principles and Practice of Oncology* (ed 4). Philadelphia, Lippincott, 1993, pp 2255–2261
35. Ratliff CR, Hutchinson M, Conner C: Rapid paracentesis of large volumes of ascitic fluid. *Oncol Nurs Forum* 18:1461, 1991
36. Hrozencik SP, Ness EA: Intraperitoneal chemotherapy via the Groshong catheter in the patient with gynecologic cancer. *Oncol Nurs Forum* 18:1245, 1991
37. Klopp A: Shunting malignant ascites. *Am J Nurs* 84:212–213, 1984
38. Kehoe C: Malignant ascites: Etiology, diagnosis, and treatment. *Oncol Nurs Forum* 18:523–530, 1991
39. Fishman RA: Brain edema. *N Engl J Med* 293:706–711, 1975
40. Ryan LS: Nursing assessment of the ambulatory patient with brain metastasis. *Cancer Nurs* 4:281–291, 1981
41. Ito U, Reulen HJ, Tomita H, et al: A computed tomography

study on formation, propagation, and resolution of edema fluid in metastatic brain tumors, in Long D (ed): *Advances in Neurology,* vol 52. New York, Raven Press, 1990

42. Weissman DE: Glucocorticoid treatment for brain metastases and epidural spinal cord compression: A review. *J Clin Oncol* 6:543–551, 1988

43. Wright DC, Delaney TF, Buckner JC: Treatment of metastatic cancer to the brain, in DeVita VT, Hellman S, Rosenberg SA (eds): *Cancer: Principles and Practice of Oncology* (ed 4). Philadelphia, Lippincott, 1993, pp 2170–2183

44. Reulen HJ, Huber P, Ito U, et al: Perihumoral brain edema, in Long D. (ed): *Advances in Neurology,* vol 52. New York, Raven Press, 1990

45. Saba MT, Magolan JM: Understanding cerebral edema: Implications for oncology nurses. *Oncol Nurs Forum* 18:499–505, 1991

46. Harper J: Use of steroids in cerebral edema: Therapeutic implications. *Heart Lung* 17:70–73, 1988

47. Getz DH: The primary, secondary, and tertiary nursing interventions of lymphedema. *Cancer Nurs* 8:177–184, 1985

48. Werner RS, McCormick B, Petrek J, et al: Arm edema in conservatively managed breast cancer: Obesity is a major predictive factor. *Radiology* 180:177–184, 1991

49. Knobf MK: Primary breast cancer: Physical consequences and rehabilitation. *Semin Oncol Nurs* 1:214–224, 1985

50. Witte CL, Witte MH, Dumont AE: Pathophysiology of chronic edema, lymphedema, and fibrosis, in Staub NC, Taylor AE (eds): *Edema.* New York, Raven Press, 1984, pp 521–542

51. Karakousis CP, Heiser MA, Moore RH: Lymphedema after groin dissection. *Am J Surg* 145:205–208, 1983

52. Granda, C: Nursing management of patients with lymphedema associated with cancer therapy. *Cancer Nurs* 17:229–235, 1994

53. Humble, CA: Lymphedema: Incidence, pathophysiology, management, and nursing care. *Oncol Nurs Forum* 22:1503–1509, 1995

54. Kennelly LF, Yurkovic CA: Altered tissue perfusion, peripheral, related to lymphedema, in McNally JC, Somerville ET, Miaskowski C (eds): *Guidelines for Oncology Nursing Practice.* Philadelphia, Saunders, 1991, pp 387–391

55. Tobin MB, Lacey HJ, Meyers L, et al: The psychological morbidity of breast cancer–related arm swelling. *Cancer* 72:3248–3252, 1993

56. Mirolo BR, Bunce IH, Chapman M, et al: Psychosocial benefits of postmastectomy lymphedema therapy. *Cancer Nurs* 18:197–205, 1995

57. Maxwell MB: Pedal edema in the cancer patient. *Am J Nurs* 82:1225–1228, 1982

58. Maxwell MB: Cancer, hypoalbuminemia, and nutrition. *Cancer Nurs* 4:451–458, 1981

59. Chlebowski RT: Nutritional support of the medical oncology patient. *Hematol Oncol Clin North Am* 5:147–159, 1991

60. Flombaum C, Isaacs M, Scheiner E, et al: Management of fluid retention in patients with advanced cancer. *JAMA* 245:611–614, 1981

61. Billings JA: Fluid accumulation: Edema and effusions, in Billings JA (ed): *Outpatient Management of Advanced Cancer.* Philadelphia, Lippincott, 1985, pp 106–110

# Chapter 28

# Sexual and Reproductive Dysfunction

Linda U. Krebs, RN, PhD, AOCN

## SCOPE OF THE PROBLEM

Although increasingly recognized as consequences of cancer or cancer therapy, sexual and reproduction dysfunctions often have been dismissed as normal side effects about which the caregiver can do little or nothing. Indeed, these dysfunctions often have gone underdiagnosed or underrated, or both, because of lack of concern, information, or knowledge on the part of the caregiver or because of fear, lack of knowledge, or embarrassment on the part of the patient or family. Often problems related to sexuality and reproduction are not addressed unless the patient is extremely assertive or presents to the health care provider in a crisis situation.[1]

Unfortunately, of all the complications associated with cancer, difficulties in the ability to be sexually intimate or to bear children have remained major problems that affect all aspects of the patient's and family's lives, sometimes influencing choices for therapy.[2,3] For some patients, sexual or reproductive dysfunctions may be temporary, with full recovery expected when therapy is completed. For many others, however, alterations in sexual or reproductive function are permanent, requiring adaptations in management of intimate relationships and lifelong plans to bear and raise children. Even short-term, temporary alterations can have long-term effects on the patient and family, influencing lifestyles and life choices.

Sexuality and reproductive ability are integral components of life, involving all aspects of our being.[4] Various factors may affect the cancer patient's sexuality and reproductive capacity, including the biological process of cancer, the effects of treatment, the alterations caused by cancer and treatment, and the psychological issues surrounding the patient and family.[5] Physiological problems of infertility and sterility, changes in body appearance, and the inability to have intercourse are exacerbated by the psychological and psychosexual issues of alteration in body image, fear of abandonment, loss of self-esteem, alterations in sexual identity, and concerns about self. Without appropriate education, counseling, and support, it may be difficult for the patient and family to adapt to the alterations that cancer can produce.

## PHYSIOLOGICAL ALTERATIONS

Gonadal function is regulated by the pituitary and the hypothalamus. The pituitary is divided into two distinct parts, the anterior and posterior portions. The pituitary is attached to the hypothalamus by the pituitary or hypophysial stalk, through which runs a minute blood vessel system, the hypothalamic-hypophysial portal vessels.[6,7]

The secretion of hormones by the anterior pituitary is controlled by hormones called *hypothalamic-releasing* or *hypothalamic-inhibiting hormones*. These are secreted within the hypothalamus and then spread via the portal vessel system to the anterior pituitary, where they act to influence glandular secretion. When produced in appropriate amounts, these hormones institute a feedback mechanism that shuts off hormonal secretion at the hypothalamus and/or pituitary level.[2,6-9]

In gonadal function, luteinizing hormone-releasing hormone (LHRH) or gonadotropin-releasing hormone (GnRH) is secreted by the hypothalamus and stimulates the anterior pituitary to produce luteinizing hormone (LH) and follicle-stimulating hormone (FSH). LH and FSH stimulate the testis or ovary to produce the appropriate hormones. When blood levels of these hormones are adequate, the hormones will exert a negative feedback on the pituitary, thus decreasing secretion.[2,6-9]

FSH and LH play major roles in the control of male sexual function. LH acts on the interstitial Leydig cells to produce testosterone; FSH, in conjunction with testosterone, is responsible for the conversion of spermatogonia into spermatocytes. A reciprocal inhibition of hypothalamic/anterior pituitary secretion of gonadotropic hormones by testicular hormones keeps the level of hormones stable. In this system the hypothalamus secretes GnRH, which causes the anterior pituitary to secrete LH. LH stimulates the Leydig cells to produce testosterone. The testosterone then negatively feeds back to the hypothalamus, inhibiting production of GnRH. Spermatogenesis is controlled in much the same manner, with FSH stimulating the Sertoli cells to convert spermatids into sperm. The Sertoli cells then secrete a hormone called *inhibin* that, through negative feedback, causes a decrease in FSH production, thus keeping spermatogenesis at a constant rate (Figure 28-1).[2,6-9]

The female hormonal system, like the male, consists of three levels of hormones: GnRH from the hypothalamus, LH and FSH from the anterior pituitary, and estrogen and progesterone from the ovary. In the nonpregnant female, monthly rhythmic changes in the rates of secretion of female hormones and responding changes in the sexual organs result in the female sexual (menstrual) cycle. As a result, a single mature ovum is released from an ovary and the endometrium of the uterus is prepared for implantation. FSH is responsible for growth of the ovarian follicle, which eventually will become the mature ovum. At the beginning of menstruation, FSH and LH increase, causing rapid cellular growth in about 20 follicles. Eventually one follicle begins to outgrow the others, causing atresia of the remaining follicles. During follicle growth, estrogen is secreted, probably causing a positive feedback that results in a surge of LH. This surge of LH, which occurs two days before ovulation, is necessary for follicular growth and ovulation. Around the time of ovulation the ruptured follicle, under the stimulation of LH, becomes the corpus luteum that secretes both estrogen and progesterone. After several days the estrogen and progesterone create a negative feedback to decrease secretion of FSH and LH. The corpus luteum,

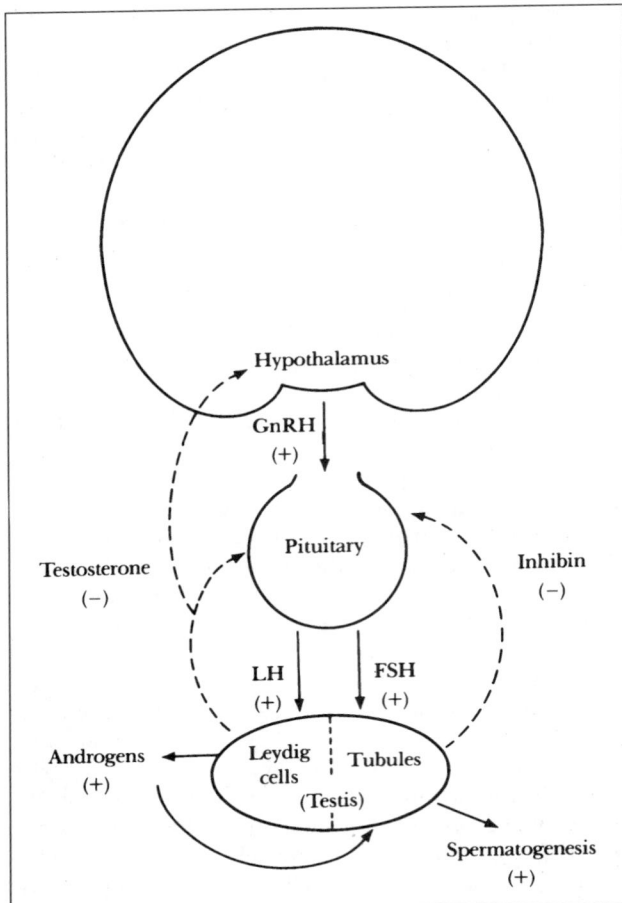

**FIGURE 28-1** Normal testicular function. FSH, follicle-stimulating hormone; GnRH, gonadotropin-releasing hormone; LH, luteinizing hormone. (Adapted from Yarbro and Perry,[2] Guyton,[6] and Gill.[7])

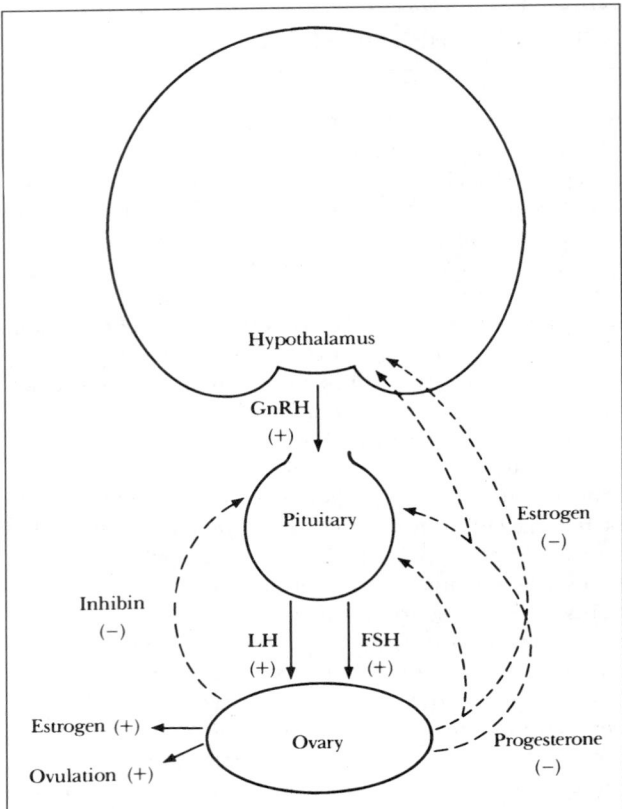

**FIGURE 28-2** Normal ovarian function. FSH, follicle-stimulating hormone; GnRH, gonadotropin-releasing hormone; LH, luteinizing hormone. (Adapted from Yarbro and Perry,[2] Guyton,[6] and Gill.[7])

which also secretes inhibin, slowly degenerates, creating a loss of the feedback mechanism and an associated rise in secretion of FSH and LH, beginning a new ovarian cycle and leading to menstruation[2,6–9] (Figure 28-2).

Ovarian failure and germinal aplasia can occur as a result of disease, therapy, nutritional status, psychological factors, or any combination of these. Ovarian failure also is related to age; as women near menopause, ovarian failure is more likely. In failure, damage to ovarian follicles causes decreased levels of estrogens and progesterones. This results in increased levels of LH and FSH with no compensating feedback mechanism. In addition, inhibin may be produced and react further to alter FSH production. Ovulation ceases, menstruation becomes erratic or ceases, and early menopause often results (Figure 28-3).[2,6–9] In the male, damage to the Leydig cells results in decreased testosterone production; LH and FSH will be elevated. Initially, Leydig cell activity may be compensated enough to produce adequate amounts of testosterone,

but continued damage results in temporary, but more often permanent, sterility (Figure 28-4).[2,6–10]

## CLINICAL MANIFESTATIONS: EFFECT OF CANCER THERAPY ON GONADAL FUNCTION

### Surgery

Some surgical procedures for cancer of the gastrointestinal and genitourinary tracts cause sexual dysfunction through the removal of sexual organs, through damage to nerves that enervate sexual organs, or through alteration in normal function. In addition, surgery on head and neck areas and the breast or amputations may alter body image and affect sexual identity. Organ dysfunction, either through loss of or alteration in normal function, is most common in cancers of the colon, rectum, bladder and associated urinary structures, and male and female genital tracts. Even when organs are not removed, normal function may be disrupted through the removal of tumor tissue surrounding an organ, through lymph node dissec-

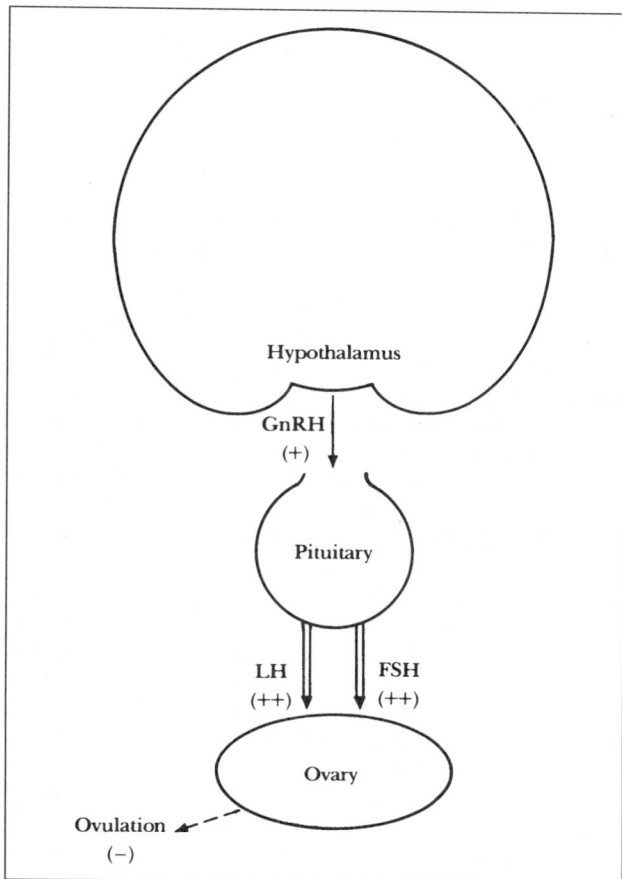

**FIGURE 28-3**  Ovarian failure. FSH, follicle-stimulating hormone; GnRH, gonadotropin-releasing hormone; LH, luteinizing hormone. (Adapted from Yarbro and Perry,[2] Guyton,[6] and Gill.[7])

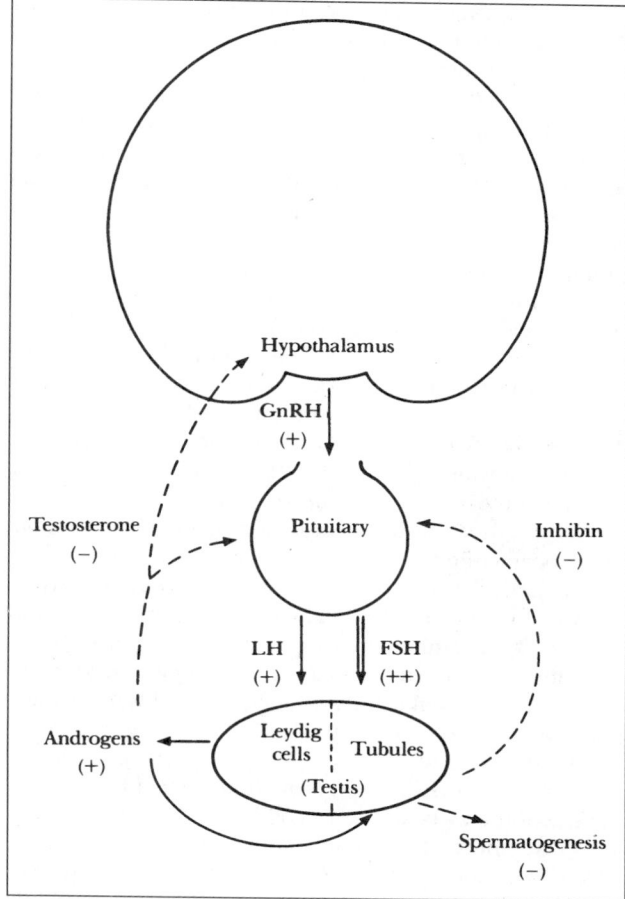

**FIGURE 28-4**  Germinal aplasia. FSH, follicle-stimulating hormone; GnRH, gonadotropin-releasing hormone; LH, luteinizing hormone. (Adapted from Yarbro and Perry,[2] Guyton,[6] and Gill.[7])

tion, or through associated physiological and psychological abnormalities related to the type of surgery.

### Cancer of the colon and rectum

Surgery for cancer of the colon or rectum may cause sexual dysfunction in both men and women. In general, sexual dysfunctions in women are more commonly related to psychosocial issues, whereas in men dysfunctions may be both organically and psychosocially caused. The most common surgery for colon cancer is some degree of colectomy with or without a colostomy. Whenever possible, primary anastomosis is performed. Cancer of the rectum and anus, however, may require anterior or abdominoperineal resection (APR). If possible, sphincter-preserving surgery without need for an ostomy may be done. Although such surgery is usually performed only for midrectal or high-rectal lesions, local excision of lesions in the distal third of the rectum may be possible if the lesion meets the criteria denoting minimal likelihood of metastases.[11] Excision is followed by radiotherapy and

chemotherapy. In addition, the use of the end-to-end anastomosis stapling device has allowed for more secure anastomoses at lower levels, minimizing the need for colostomy.[12] Because of this device, ultralow anastomoses are now more common. Although this saves the sphincter, the surgery is associated with increased bowel frequency, a sense of urgency, and fecal leakage in many patients.[13] The use of multimodality therapy has also minimized the size of surgical resections.[14] In general, the type of surgery will be associated with tumor location and available surgical techniques.[11,12]

For the patient who requires an APR, sexual dysfunction may be related to the placement of a colostomy, to removal of or interference with sexual organ function, or some combination of the two. A colostomy can be associated with sexual dysfunction because of the patient's negative changes in body image and self-esteem, as well as the responses of family and friends. In a study by MacDonald and Anderson[15] of 420 patients with rectal cancer, 265 had a permanent colostomy. Of these individuals, 16%

felt severely stigmatized because of the colostomy. Of those who were married or widowed since surgery, 48% of men and 27% of women younger than 65 years old (n = 116) felt that their married life had suffered as a result of the colostomy. In an extensive review of quality-of-life literature for patients with and without a stoma, Sprangers et al[13] found that the majority of patients with a stoma had some type of sexual dysfunction. The most common complaints were erectile dysfunction and ejaculatory impotence in men and dyspareunia and orgasmic dysfunction in women. As a group, those with a stoma were less sexually active and experienced more generalized distress than those without a stoma. Of additional importance was the finding that all patients with colorectal cancer experienced some degree of sexual dysfunction and decreased quality of life regardless of the type of therapy.

For the woman with an APR, the ovaries or uterus may be removed at the time of surgery in addition to colostomy, thus causing dysfunction from primary inability to bear children or from alterations in normal hormonal patterns. In addition, women may have part of the vagina removed, or healing of the perineal wound may result in vaginal scarring that causes painful or incomplete vaginal intercourse. A decreased incidence of orgasm and vaginal lubrication, reduced libido, and dyspareunia have also been noted.[12,16–19]

For the man who has an APR, sexual dysfunction is more severe, with a suggestion that permanent sexual dysfunction may be as high as 80%.[20] Although men may lose the ability to obtain or maintain an erection, 30%–35% maintain the ability to have an orgasm, and 25%–50% maintain the ability to ejaculate.[21,22] In a study by Andersen[19] it was reported that 30%–60% of men who have an APR will experience decreased desire, 30%–75% will have erectile dysfunctions, and 65%–85% will have ejaculatory dysfunctions. Age appears to be a factor, with the older patient more likely to suffer complete or incomplete erectile impotence.[23,24] This is most likely due to damage to parasympathetic and sympathetic nerves that control both erection and ejaculation. In addition to erectile dysfunction, decreased amount and/or force of ejaculation or retrograde ejaculation may occur. This occurrence, which may be temporary or permanent, adds to the trauma of surgery because of its unpredictable outcome. For all patients the removal of rectal tissue appears to be the most common denominator to organic sexual dysfunction. If the rectum remains intact, there rarely is an associated sexual dysfunction without direct tumor invasion.[25–27] Koukouras et al[28] reported sexual dysfunction, as denoted by cessation of sexual relationship, absence of erection, absence of ejaculation, or inability to penetrate, to occur in 15% of men who had a high anterior resection, whereas 54% of men with an APR experienced some type of dysfunction.

### Cancers of the genitourinary tract

***Bladder cancer***   The treatment of bladder cancer may alter sexual function in men and women. Repeated cystos-copy for local treatment of transitional cell cancer has been noted to cause pain with coitus for women, transient pain during erection and ejaculation in men, and temporary decrease in desire for both.[29,30] Transurethral resection or partial cystectomy may result in mild pain or dyspareunia; however, normal sexual function should not be altered.[30,31] For some patients, urinary incontinence may cause cessation of normal activities for fear of having an accident.[30] In addition, body image and self-esteem may be altered due to the need to use incontinence pads or other protective materials. Radical cystectomy results in sexual dysfunction for both men and women because of organ removal and/or enervation. In men, radical cystectomy consists of removal of the bladder, prostate, seminal vesicles, pelvic lymph nodes, and occasionally the urethra.[31] It has been noted that about 15% of men who undergo radical cystectomy will recover full erection potential and that men older than 60 are more likely to be negatively affected. Retrograde or no ejaculation may also result.[22] Orgasm may be experienced but is usually less intense and without ejaculate.[19] Sexual interest and penile sensation are not altered.[32,33] For these men the increasing availability and use of penile prostheses and the ability to perform revascularization of the penis have made erectile dysfunction a more manageable problem.[17,29] Boyd and Schiff[34] reported on 19 men who had inflatable penile prostheses implanted following surgery for transitional cell cancer. All were satisfied with appearance and function. For the woman who has radical cystectomy, the surgery usually includes removal of the bladder and urethra, the uterus, ovaries, fallopian tubes, and the anterior portion of the vagina. Although vaginal reconstruction usually is performed, the resulting vagina may be more narrow and shallow and provide less lubrication than before surgery, leading to difficulty with penetration. In addition, the removal of the ovaries, with associated estrogen loss, leads to dryness, inelasticity of the vagina, dyspareunia, and menopausal symptoms. Vaginal dilation and the liberal use of lubrication may provide relief.[19,24,35,36] For both sexes, urinary diversion is a necessity with radical cystectomy; it may result in alterations in self-esteem and body image and may lead to a decrease or cessation of all sexual activities.[30,37] In the past the ileal conduit, which necessitated the continuous use of an ostomy appliance, was the most common method for urinary diversions. Today the surgical development of a Kock pouch, or continent reservoir, has become more widely employed, resulting in overall improved sexual adjustment due to decreased odor and leakage.[30,31,38] Combined-modality therapies are being investigated that will allow for tumor reduction while maintaining the bladder. Success of these interventions should have direct effects on subsequent sexual function.[39]

***Penile cancer/cancer of the male urethra***   Cancer of the penis and male urethra are rare, with fewer than 1000 cases reported in the United States in 1996.[40] Treatment includes total or partial penectomy, radiation therapy, or topical chemotherapy, with radiation therapy or chemotherapy used for small, early lesions. The degree of limitation primarily relates to the amount of tissue removed.[32] Partial penectomy does not result in loss of erectile, ejaculative, or orgasmic abilities, whereas erectile ability obviously is absent with total penectomy.[19,29,31] Desire remains, and stimulation of the remaining genital tissue can produce orgasm.[41,42] Ejaculation, through the perineal urethrostomy, should continue. New techniques to create a penis have been used after a total penectomy. A semirigid or inflatable prosthesis restores the ability to have intercourse.[29,31,41–43] A Mayo Clinic study reported a successful placement rate of 90%–95% and an 8% mechanical failure rate in the three-year study period of men with penile implants. Eighty-nine percent of subjects and mates felt satisfied with function and appearance.[44] Opjordsmoen et al[45] reported on 30 men treated for penile cancer from 1 to 19 years prior to interview. Those treated with radiation therapy had significantly fewer concerns related to sexual dysfunction. Patients with partial or total penectomy had significantly increased complications, including decreased interest, enjoyment, frequency, and ability.

*Testicular cancer*  Testicular cancer, which represents about 1% of all cancers in men, is the leading cause of cancer in young men.[22] The treatment of testicular cancer includes an orchiectomy and usually retroperitoneal lymph node dissection and/or removal of a pelvic mass, usually followed by chemotherapy or radiation therapy. Unilateral orchiectomy will not result in infertility or sexual dysfunction providing that the contralateral testis is normal and the individual is fertile at diagnosis. Infertility before any definitive therapy is well documented and may be related to hormonal imbalance or the result of subacute chronic illness.[46–51] If bilateral orchiectomy is performed, sterility and decreased libido, related to loss of testosterone, will result. Retroperitoneal lymph node dissection (RPLND) done for staging or as treatment may result in temporary or permanent loss of ejaculation, whereas potency and the ability to have an orgasm remain.[29,31,46,48,51,52] Whenever possible, nerve-sparing RPLND should be done to preserve fertility.[51] Narayan et al[48] reported that 100% of 55 patients who underwent peritoneal lymphadenectomy reported loss of ejaculation, with 45% regaining function within three years following surgery. Nerve-sparing procedures with careful adherence to surgical boundaries and identification of sympathetic fibers have resulted in an almost 80%–99% preservation or return of ejaculation following lymphadenectomy.[46,49] Retrograde ejaculation has been noted in 25% of patients, whereas decreased libido, decreased pleasure at orgasm, and erectile dysfunction have occurred in 10%–38% of these men.[17,29,31,43,53] Gritz et al,[54] reported on the psychosexual status of 34 men and their partners a median of four years following treatment for testicular cancer. All men had a unilateral orchiectomy followed by additional surgery, chemotherapy, or radiation therapy. At the time of follow-up, 23% reported alterations in body image, 29% reported a decrease in sexual satisfaction, 20% an occasional problem with erection,

and 38% a decrease in frequency of intercourse. Of those who underwent retroperitoneal lymphadenectomy, 50% reported the inability to ejaculate and 54% experienced a decrease in the quality of orgasms. Forty-one percent of the couples desired children and expected to conceive, or adopt if necessary, in the future. Aass et al[55] reported on 76 patients treated for varying stages of testicular cancer. They noted that for more than 40% of all patients, discussions about sexuality before, during, and following treatment were considered crucial. Prior to therapy, an important aspect of discussion should be information about sperm banking.

*Prostate cancer*  Prostate cancer, because it generally occurs in men older than 50, often is not considered in terms of its potential to cause sexual dysfunctions. However, because sexual concerns are not necessarily related to age and because therapy for prostate cancer frequently causes sexual dysfunction, counseling and management of potential problems need to be addressed. Therapy for prostate cancer consists of various combinations of surgery, chemotherapy, radiation therapy, and hormonal manipulation, all of which have a potential to alter sexual function. Surgical treatment of prostate cancer includes prostatectomy (accomplished through transurethral, perineal, or transabdominal approaches) or bilateral orchiectomy. Transurethral resection of the prostate generally does not cause impotence or erectile dysfunction; however, retrograde ejaculation occurs in approximately 90% of all patients. Transabdominal resection of the prostate results in retrograde ejaculation in 75%–80% of patients and may cause erectile dysfunction. The perineal approach, or radical prostatectomy, includes removal of the prostate, seminal vesicles, and vas deferens and may result in permanent damage to erectile function with concomitant loss of emission and ejaculation.[25,31,32,56] Alterations in desire, penile sensation, and the ability to reach orgasm should not occur.[32] Nerve-sparing or potency-sparing surgery was developed by Walsh in the 1980s and, according to Church,[57] probably has been the most significant surgical development in the treatment of prostate cancer. Prior to the development of this procedure, 2%–15% of patients experienced urinary incontinence and 80%–90% experienced impotence. Eggleston and Walsh[58] evaluated 100 patients who had radical prostatectomies that incorporated nerve-sparing surgical techniques and reported that potency was maintained in approximately 86% of patients. Walsh and Schlegel[59] evaluated 320 men one to five years following surgery. Of the 259 who were potent prior to surgery and who had sexual partners, 192 (74%) were currently potent. Potency appeared to return gradually over a period of months to years. Bilateral orchiectomy causes sexual dysfunction through gradual diminution of libido, impotence, gynecomastia, penile atrophy, and body image changes.[17,31,33] Testicular implants filled with saline may be of benefit. Various methods, including the use of penile prostheses, suction or vacuum devices, intracorporeal injections of papaverine hydrochloride or prostaglandin E₁, or medications such as yohimbine hydrochloride, have been used to restore erectile potential. Fear of failure may also play a role. Since return of full erection potential may take as long as two years, it is suggested that the patient wait a minimum of six months after surgery to see if function will be restored.[29,31,60–62] With new techniques, sterility in individuals with retrograde ejaculation is not as frequent. Because of the ability to separate sperm from urine, artificial insemination of the mate may be possible.[63]

### Gynecologic malignancies

Surgical management of gynecologic malignancies includes surgery of the vulva, vagina, uterus and uterine cervix, ovary, and fallopian tube, and pelvic exenteration. Although the majority of gynecologic surgeries are invisible assaults to femininity, sexual identity and sexual functioning are often permanently affected. It is imperative that sexual and reproductive counseling be provided to the patient and family before surgical intervention because most surgeries permanently alter fertility and may alter sexuality.

***Vulvar cancer***  Vulvar cancer represents 1% of all cancers found in women, with approximately 85% of these cancers occurring in postmenopausal women.[64] However, it has been noted that the incidence appears to be increasing, particularly in younger women.[65] Treatment will not alter fertility but may affect sexuality, with 21%–90% of women reporting cessation of all sexual activities following radical vulvectomy.[66,67] Therapy for carcinoma in situ or preinvasive disease may include simple vulvectomy, wide local excision, skinning vulvectomy, topical 5-fluorouracil cream, or laser therapy. In general, good cosmetic results occur with treatment of early disease except for the simple vulvectomy, which removes the labia and subcutaneous tissue, with retention of the clitoris. Introital stenosis may result but may be easily managed through the use of lubrication and vaginal dilators. DiSaia[68] recommends conservative treatment with wide local excision and skin graft for the woman with early disease in order to maintain body image and minimally affect sexuality. Radical vulvectomy, which removes the labia minora and majora and the clitoris and usually includes a groin node dissection, frequently results in delayed wound healing, altered body image, abnormalities in sensory perception of the genital area, leg edema, decreased range of motion in lower extremities, altered orgasmic potential, and introital stenosis.[17,46,64,69] Evaluation of lymph nodes prior to radical surgery may allow for more limited surgeries with less compromise to sexuality.[65] Corney et al,[70] in a study of 105 women who underwent radical pelvic surgery, reported that generalized sexual dysfunction, including pain, anxiety, and decreased desire, was common, occurred earlier, and persisted unless appropriately treated. They further noted that, if there was a chance for cure, women were willing to live with sexual dysfunction and body image changes, provided adequate infor-

mation and discussion about causes of dysfunction and alternative methods of sexual satisfaction were given. All women need education on the effects of removal of tissue and on body image prior to surgery to promote self-esteem, function, and compliance with care.

***Vaginal cancer***  Vaginal cancer is rare. Surgery for the majority of gynecologic cancers results in some abnormality and/or need for reconstruction of the vagina. A shortened vagina can cause considerable sexual dysfunction because of decreased vaginal length and width, lack of lubrication, or pain on intercourse. Total vaginectomy without reconstruction precludes vaginal intercourse; however, there are multiple techniques for vaginal reconstruction.[43] Reconstruction can be accomplished using the large or small bowel. Because of its thicker wall, the large bowel is usually preferred.[71] It has been noted that in 30%–70% of patients who do have reconstruction there is a return of orgasmic sensations if they existed before surgery.[72] Despite this finding, reconstruction should not be considered a panacea for sexual dysfunction, with some women complaining that the new vagina is too large, too small, or has a persistent, annoying discharge.[73]

***Cervical cancer and endometrial cancer***  Invasive cancer of the uterine corpus and cervix are the first and second most common gynecologic malignancies, representing slightly less than 10% of all cancers in women.[39] Treatment for cervical intraepithelial neoplasia and carcinoma in situ includes conization, laser therapy, cryosurgery, loop electrosurgical excision (LEEP), or simple hysterectomy.[65,71,73] All but the last usually have no effect on fertility (conization may result in cervical stenosis or incompetence), nor should they cause any physiological sexual dysfunction. Simple hysterectomy precludes further childbearing but should not affect sexual functioning, although numerous authors have noted that altered sexual identity and/or body image may result in sexual dysfunction.[25,74–76] Treatment for invasive disease is usually radical hysterectomy, consisting of removal of the uterus and cervix, the supporting structures, and the upper third of the vagina and pelvic lymph nodes. For cancer of the endometrium, the ovaries and fallopian tubes also may be removed. If oophorectomy is included, menopausal symptoms with hot flashes and decrease in vaginal lubrication and elasticity may severely alter sexual functioning. Zussman et al[76] noted that 33%–46% of women who had a radical hysterectomy, including oophorectomy, reported decreased sexual desire, whereas Jenkins[77] and Schover et al[78] noted alterations in frequency of desire, orgasm, and frequency and enjoyment of intercourse in women who had abdominal hysterectomy and bilateral salpingo-oophorectomy and had received pelvic radiation for cervical or endometrial cancer. Schover et al[78] reported that 15% of these women became celibate within one year of treatment. One study[79] reported that 50% of patients treated for early-stage cervical cancer had a marked decrease in their sexual relationships and experienced extreme fatigue, lack of energy, depressed mood, weight gain, and anxiety. In women with endometrial cancer, effects of treatment and uncertainty about the future increased sexual difficulties.[80] Of those satisfied with their current sexual functioning, the majority noted that return to normalcy occurred gradually over a prolonged period. Although sexual feeling should not be altered after a radical hysterectomy, delayed bowel and bladder function may occur and necessitate discharge from the hospital with a urinary catheter. Long-term catheter placement may alter body image and affect sexuality. Intercourse can be accomplished through securing the catheter to the abdomen and making changes in coital position.[69,81] It also should be remembered that many women measure femininity by the ability to bear children. If this ability is removed, sexual dysfunctions may occur even in the absence of organic cause.[25]

***Ovarian cancer***   Ovarian cancer represents approximately 25% of gynecologic cancers and frequently is seen in the premenopausal female. Initial treatment is surgery, usually consisting of a radical hysterectomy with bilateral salpingo-oophorectomy and omentectomy. Fertility is lost and the associated menopausal symptoms occur. In the young woman with ovarian teratoma or borderline malignant epithelial neoplasia, it is possible to maintain fertility if disease is confined to one ovary and is of low grade; however, it is most common for radical surgery to be performed.[82-84] Treatment usually continues with combination chemotherapy, thus further compounding sexual and reproductive dysfunctions, including alterations in libido, frequency of intercourse, and desire for close physical contact.[85]

### Pelvic exenteration

Although pelvic exenteration may be performed in the man or woman with advanced colorectal or bladder cancer, the most common indication for pelvic exenteration is a locally advanced gynecologic malignancy. An anterior pelvic exenteration preserves the rectum, whereas a posterior exenteration preserves the bladder. A total pelvic exenteration involves removing the vagina, uterus, ovaries, fallopian tubes, bladder, and rectum (in the man, the prostate, seminal vesicles, and vas deferens are removed).[65,73,86,87] In patients with total pelvic exenteration a urinary conduit and colostomy also are created; a neovagina may be constructed.[65,71,86] In the woman, reproductive and sexual dysfunction are profound. Andersen and Hacker[87] reported that 80%–90% of women surveyed ceased all sexual activity except kissing. Dysfunction related to removal of all pelvic organs with resulting ostomies is obvious. In addition, body image, sexual identity, and self-esteem are disturbed, and appropriate interventions and education need to be provided. In the woman with vaginal reconstruction, intercourse will be possible; however, the physiological and psychological ramifications of this surgery may result in inability and/or lack of desire to participate in sexual activities.[88]

### Breast cancer

Although some surgeries may not be strictly related to sexual functioning, they may cause dysfunction as a result of the psychological issues related to the particular body part. The most likely assault to body image and sexual identity with resultant sexual dysfunction is surgical removal of all or part of the breast. Although fertility is not altered by mastectomy or lumpectomy, the inability or difficulty in breast-feeding should pregnancy be accomplished may be a major assault to the woman's femininity. In addition, removal or partial removal of a breast may result in sexual dysfunction because of fear of rejection, physical discomfort, anxiety about initiating sexual activities, feelings of being defective or different, or any combination of these factors.[89,90] Rutherford[91] noted that loss of even part of the breast can be seen as an alteration of self, with resultant alterations in body image and sexuality.

Although it has been previously reported that the use of breast-preserving surgery (lumpectomy) has been shown to cause significantly less alteration in body image, sexual desire, and frequency of intercourse,[73,89,90] recent studies[91-95] showed no difference between women receiving lumpectomy and radiotherapy and women undergoing mastectomy. Additionally, there appeared to be no difference between women who had or did not have reconstructive surgery following mastectomy.[95] What appears to be of significance is the opportunity or perceived opportunity to select the surgical technique employed. Thus, choices should be offered whenever possible. If breast-preserving surgery is not an option, breast reconstruction can be considered. The ability to have breast reconstruction has been shown to bolster sexual self-esteem and decrease reactions to body image alterations.[96] If such options are limited, sexual dysfunction, which should be temporary, may become permanent. Education and ongoing counseling should be available and may provide positive functional outcomes.

### Head and neck cancer

Although not generally considered an area responsible for sexual dysfunction, surgical treatment for cancers of the head and neck region are responsible for varying degrees of alteration in body image, leading to changes in sexuality and intimacy. Results of disease and treatment are readily apparent. Even with reconstructive surgery or the use of prostheses to ameliorate deformities, sexuality may be affected by the alterations in sensation, breathing, voice, the ability to use the mouth and tongue, or similar abnormalities. Presurgical counseling and long-term follow-up may be necessary for sexual rehabilitation.[81,97-99]

## Radiation Therapy

Radiation therapy can cause sexual and reproductive dysfunction through primary organ failure (e.g., ovarian failure and testicular aplasia), through alterations in organ function (e.g., decreased lubrication and impotence), and through the temporary or permanent effects of therapy not associated with reproduction (e.g., diarrhea and fatigue). Permanent effects most commonly are related to total dose, location, length of treatment, age, and prior fertility status.[63,100–102] In the woman, fertility depends on follicular maturation and ovum release. Radiation therapy to the ovaries has its most direct effect on the intermediate follicles. If these follicles are damaged by radiation and insufficient small follicles remain, permanent sterility results.[103] In the man, although the Leydig cell and mature sperm are relatively radioresistant, immature sperm and spermatogonia are extremely radiosensitive. Small doses of radiation will begin the process of infertility, which, depending on total dose, may be permanent.[7]

In women, temporary or permanent sterility is related to the dose of radiation, the volume of tissues radiated, the time period the ovaries are exposed to radiation, and the woman's age.[101–105] Because a woman has fewer oocytes as she nears menopause, radiation injury at that point in the life span is more likely to be permanent. Balducci et al,[63] and Hilderley[103] noted that a radiation dose of 600–1200 cGy is capable of inducing menopause; however, younger women appear to be more resistant to this effect. In addition, although age is an important factor, doses <400 cGy may result in temporary sterility whereas doses >400 cGy often result in permanent sterility. The number of oocytes is one of the most important factors in permanent sterility, with 95% of young women becoming sterile with a radiation dose >2000 cGy. In women older than 40, a dose of 600 cGy often is associated with subsequent menopause and the associated menopausal symptoms of hot flashes, amenorrhea, dyspareunia, loss of libido, and vaginal atrophy.[101,106] For some women the use of exogenous estrogens may alleviate these side effects.[78]

For women, movement of the ovaries out of the radiation field (oophoropexy), with appropriate shielding, has helped maintain fertility even when relatively high doses of radiation have been given. Ovaries can be moved to the midline of the uterus or to the iliac crests. In young women or those desiring to maintain both reproductive capacity and hormonal function, ovarian transposition, with the ovaries moved to the upper abdomen, can be undertaken.[101] In a study by Horning et al,[107] 8 of 19 patients treated with total lymphoid irradiation for Hodgkin's disease had reversible amenorrhea and seven eventually became pregnant. Even with oophoropexy and appropriate shielding, 30%–50% of all patients who receive >600–1000 cGy will have permanent menstrual cessation.[108,109]

In addition to sterility or transient infertility, radiation therapy can produce other sexual dysfunctions, which may be temporary or permanent. Decreases in sexual enjoyment, ability to attain orgasm, libido, and frequency of intercourse and sexual dreams, as well as vaginal stenosis or shortening, vaginal irritation, increased risk of infec-

tion, and decreased lubrication and sensation have been reported in women treated with radiation therapy. Painful intercourse and menstrual changes have also been reported.[105,110–115]

In men, temporary or permanent azoospermia also is a function of age, dose, tissue volume, and exposure time. When the testis is exposed to radiation, a reduction in sperm count begins within six to eight weeks and continues for up to one year after completion of therapy. Doses of <500 cGy usually are associated with temporary sterility, whereas doses of >500 cGy usually result in permanent sterility.[103] The return of normal spermatogenesis is related to total testicular dose, with a dose of <100 cGy taking 9 to 12 months for recovery, whereas 200–300 cGy may take two to three years and 400–600 cGy more than five years to infinity.[116] Kinsella et al[117] reported on 27 male adults with soft-tissue sarcoma who were treated with high-dose radiation therapy. The testes were not in the primary field and were shielded; however, significant scatter radiation still was received. In 11 of 27 patients who received <50 cGy, no abnormalities resulted, whereas in 6 patients with exposures of 50–150 cGy, FSH was elevated 200% and testosterone was decreased. In the ten patients who received >150 cGy, FSH was increased, whereas LH and testosterone were decreased; thus, testicular function was inadequate to support spermatogenesis. Fossa et al[118] evaluated the long-term morbidity of infradiaphragmatic radiotherapy in men with testicular cancer and noted that 23% of those previously thought to be fertile were found to be infertile following doses ranging from 36 to 50 GY. Gonadal dysfunction has been reported in survivors of childhood acute lymphoblastic leukemia who received at least 12 GY testicular irradiation.[119,120] In a follow-up of 60 long-term survivors, Sklar et al,[120] found that 50% of men exposed to craniospinal and extended abdominal field radiation experienced decreased testicular volume, abnormal germ cell function, and elevated FSH levels. Due to the morbidity of even low-level testicular radiation, Kinsella et al[121] suggest that those not requiring primary testicular irradiation receive additional testicular shielding to alleviate infertility sequelae.

The majority of men treated by external beam for prostate cancer have temporary or permanent impotence. Impotence is thought to be caused by fibrosis of pelvic vasculature or radiation damage of pelvic nerves. Van Heeringen et al[122] reported that 25% of men were impotent, 67% experienced decreased frequency, and more than 50% experienced decreased libido following radiation for localized cancer of the prostate. Herr[123] reported that 40 of 41 patients treated by lymphadenectomy remained potent if interstitial therapy was used, whereas Carlton et al[124] noted that only 25% of patients treated with internal and external therapy plus lymphadenectomy became impotent. This suggests that interstitial therapy may be less likely to cause impotence. In patients treated for testicular cancer, Schover and von Eschenbach[125] noted that 10% of 121 patients reported erectile dysfunction and 38% experienced a decrease in pleasure of orgasm. The inability to gain and maintain an erection may begin as early as two weeks into treatment and may last several weeks after treatment.[125] Occasionally impotence does not occur until after radiation therapy is completed. In these patients the effects usually are not reversible.[126] In addition to difficulty in gaining or maintaining erection, a decreased libido, inability to ejaculate, inability to lubricate, inability to achieve orgasm, and decreased sexual pleasure are common findings in men who receive radiation to the pelvis.

Along with direct assaults to sexual and reproductive function by radiation therapy, the general side effects and accompanying psychological effects frequently can alter sexual function. Severe fatigue can limit all activity. Nausea, vomiting, and diarrhea can decrease energy, sexual desire, and feelings of desirability and can interfere with a sense of general well-being. Inflammation, pain, and limited range of motion may make sexual activities difficult or impossible. In addition to physical limitations, fear, depression, anxiety, stress, body image alterations, and lowered self-esteem may be additional burdens.[127] The appropriate use of energy-conserving strategies, medications, lubricants, dilators, prostheses, time, and counseling may alleviate side effects, promote a sense of well-being, and improve sexual function.

## Chemotherapy

Chemotherapy-induced reproductive and sexual dysfunction is related to the type of drug, dose, length of treatment, age and sex of the individual receiving treatment, and length of time after therapy. In addition, the use of combination therapy with multiple agents and drugs given to combat side effects of chemotherapy also plays a role in infertility or sexual dysfunction.

Infertility and sterility after chemotherapy have been noted since the early 1970s, with reports of amenorrhea and azoospermia after single-agent or combination therapy.[128] Adult men are more likely to experience long-term side effects regardless of age, whereas women are more apt to have permanent cessation of menses as they near the age of 40.[129,130] The primary drugs that induce infertility are the alkylating agents, but others have been implicated, in particular, cytosine arabinoside, 5-fluorouracil, vinblastine, vincristine, cisplatin,[131] and procarbazine. Combinations of these drugs appear to prolong infertility[132–136] (Table 28-1).[129,130–136]

### Men

Infertility occurs in men primarily through depletion of the germinal epithelium that lines the seminiferous tubules. On testicular biopsy the interstitial Leydig cells appear normal, whereas the tubules are abnormal, contain Sertoli cells, and have depleted or absent germinal epithelium. Clinically, testicular volume decreases, oligospermia or azoospermia occurs, and infertility results.[137]

**TABLE 28-1   Chemotherapeutic Agents Affecting Sexual or Reproductive Function**

| Agent | Complication |
|---|---|
| **ALKYLATING** | |
| Busulfan | Amenorrhea, oligospermia, |
| Chlorambucil | azoospermia, decreased |
| Cyclophosphamide | libido, ovarian dysfunction, |
| Melphalan | erectile dysfunction |
| Nitrogen mustard | |
| **ANTIMETABOLITES** | |
| Cytosine arabinoside | As for alkylating agents |
| 5-fluorouracil | |
| Methotrexate | |
| **ANTITUMOR ANTIBIOTICS** | |
| Doxorubicin | As for alkylating agents |
| Plicamycin | |
| Dactinomycin | |
| **PLANT PRODUCTS** | |
| Vincristine | Retrograde ejaculation, erectile dysfunction |
| Vinblastine | Decreased libido, ovarian dysfunction, erectile dysfunction |
| **MISCELLANEOUS AGENTS** | |
| Procarbazine | As for alkylating agents |
| Androgens | Masculinization (women) |
| Antiandrogens | Gynecomastia, impotence |
| Estrogens | Gynecomastia, acne |
| Antiestrogens | Irregular menses |
| Progestins | Menstrual abnormalities, change in libido |
| Aminoglutethimide | Masculinization (women) |
| Corticosteroids | Irregular menses, acne |
| Interferons | Transient impotence, amenorrhea, pelvic pain |

Data from Yasko,[105] Dodd,[114] Schilsky and Erlichman,[129] Burke et al,[132] Otto,[133] Glasel,[134] Guy,[135] Goodman,[136] and Chapman.[138]

Chapman[138] reported that following drug-induced azoospermia, the process of spermatogenesis must start all over, as if the patient were going through puberty. Initially the germ stem cell must repopulate the testicle, then spermatogenesis should occur. This process may take several years.

Single-agent and combination chemotherapy have been reported to cause germinal aplasia, with alkylating agents the most extensively studied. Richter et al[139] reported that doses of chlorambucil <400 mg cause progressive oligospermia, whereas doses >400 mg have caused azoospermia and permanent germinal aplasia. They also studied cyclophosphamide and noted that doses as low as 50–100 mg/day for two months resulted in azoospermia. Recovery time was related to total dose and length of time since the completion of treatment. Nijman et al[53] studied the gonadal function of 54 men with testicular cancer who received chemotherapy with cisplatin (platinum), vinblastine, and bleomycin (PVB) after surgery. They noted, as have others,[140,141] that 72% of these men were infertile before treatment. Two years following therapy, 48% remained infertile, with increased levels of LH and FSH. Stoter et al[142] evaluated 48 men with testicular cancer who had been treated with PVB plus maintenance chemotherapy. With a minimum follow-up of seven years, 40% of participants reported a negative alteration in sexual life, with 21% experiencing decreased sexual desire, 8% experiencing erectile dysfunction, and 15% experiencing ejaculatory dysfunction. Drasga et al[141] reviewed 69 patients with disseminated testicular cancer treated with PVB with or without doxorubicin; 41 patients were part of a prospective study and 28 part of a retrospective study. In the prospective group only 6.6% of patients were able to meet sperm-banking requirements; the others had severe oligospermia or azoospermia. With a median of 17 months' follow-up, 100% of these men continue to be infertile. In the retrospective group, 46% had a normal sperm count at the time of evaluation. Thirty-two percent have successfully impregnated their wives. Male patients treated with cisplatin, doxorubicin, and dacarbazine (PADIC) for osteosarcoma were noted to be infertile during active treatment. However, within two years after completion of treatment, 70% had attained normal sperm counts. Those receiving more than 600 mg/m$^2$ cisplatin were more likely to remain infertile.[143] It appears that in some instances fertility may improve with time.

The most widely studied combination chemotherapy has been mechlorethamine, vincristine, procarbazine, and prednisone (MOPP), used in the treatment of Hodgkin's disease. Chapman[130] reported frequent sexual dysfunction and decreased fertility in men treated with MOPP. This is corroborated by Cunningham et al,[144] who noted that only one in ten men receiving MOPP and 1 in 13 receiving MOPP plus pelvic radiation were able to impregnate. Viviani et al[145] reported that azoospermia developed in only 54% of patients treated with doxorubicin, bleomycin, vinblastine, and dacarbazine (ABVD), whereas azoospermia occurred in 97% of patients treated with MOPP. In addition, 100% of those treated with ABVD had complete restoration of spermatogenesis, whereas only 14% of those treated with MOPP had return of spermatogenesis.

Hormonal manipulation and treatment with estrogens are well known as a cause of sexual dysfunction. The majority of patients who receive antiandrogen therapy experience a major reduction in interest in sexual intercourse and are unable to attain or maintain an erection.[146] Gynecomastia and decreases in libido, sexual excitement, and the ability to achieve sexual fulfillment are significant problems.[105,135,147]

## Women

Women experience sexual and reproductive dysfunction from chemotherapy as a result of hormonal alterations or direct effects that cause ovarian fibrosis and follicle destruction. Previous sexual health may also play a role. FSH and LH levels are elevated and estradiol is decreased, leading to amenorrhea, menopausal symptoms, dyspareunia, and vaginal atrophy and dryness.[132,137]

Like men, women experience reproductive dysfunction from both single-agent and combination chemotherapy; however, age appears to play a more significant role in infertility in women than in men, with women younger than 35 able to tolerate much higher doses of chemotherapy without resultant infertility. Amenorrhea has been noted in women with breast cancer who receive 40–120 mg/day of cyclophosphamide.[148] Busulfan, which may be used to treat chronic myelogenous leukemia, also induces amenorrhea.[149] Chapman et al[150] reported that amenorrhea developed in 49% of women treated with MOPP, while 34% experienced irregular menses, and 17% maintained normal menses. Of those with irregular or normal menses, 30% later experienced irreversible amenorrhea. Other investigators[141,151,152] have reported that permanent amenorrhea occurred in 26%–50% of women treated with MOPP combination chemotherapy and that permanent amenorrhea and early menopause were more common with advancing age. Indeed, in women under 25 years of age, 80% continued with normal menses. In women over 25, amenorrhea appeared to occur gradually after cessation of treatment. It was noted in a study of ABVD plus radiation therapy versus MOPP plus radiation therapy that 50% of women over 30 who received the latter therapy had prolonged amenorrhea.[153] In contrast, none of the women younger than 30 and none of the women receiving ABVD plus radiation therapy noted this side effect. Other combination therapy also has been reviewed, with similar results. In an analysis of nine studies, Chapman[138] concluded that amenorrhea occurred more commonly in women older than 40 and that ovarian failure correlated most closely to that seen in women treated solely with cyclophosphamide. Additionally, the author postulates that ovarian dysfunction occurs at all ages but is more reported and diagnosed in women closer to menopause.

It appears that any combination of drugs that contains an alkylating agent is apt to cause infertility, and as women near menopause, permanent cessation of menses is more likely. When hormonal manipulation includes androgens, not only sexual and reproductive function but also body image and feelings of sexual identity are affected. Chemotherapy contributed significantly to sexual dysfunction not only through menopausal symptoms but also through increased risk of urinary tract infections and monilial infections, vaginal irritation, exacerbations of genital herpes and human papillomavirus, and alterations in desire and arousal due to decreases in circulating androgens. In addition, the use of hormonal therapy, such as tamoxifen and aminoglutethimide, may be associated with menopausal symptoms and decreased desire.[154] Appropriate support and counseling should be provided.

### Children

The effect of chemotherapy on gonadal function in children has been extensively studied.[155–157] Primary effects include delayed sexual maturation and alterations in reproductive potential. Levy and Stillman[157] note that although the effects of chemotherapy are different in girls and boys, the primary effects appear to be age-related. Prepubescent boys seem to be minimally affected by chemotherapy and progress into and through puberty without major difficulty. Young men treated during puberty, however, appear to be more likely to have gonadal dysfunction with profound effects on both germ cell production and Leydig cell function, with a resultant increase in FSH and LH and a decrease in testosterone levels.[138,158,159] It should be noted, however, that since the reserve supply of spermatogonia in young males is much smaller than in adults, chemotherapy has the potential to significantly alter spermatogenesis. This cannot be easily assessed until puberty.[138] The majority of girls treated with combination therapy appear to have normal ovarian function; however, long-term follow-up is needed to assess whether these individuals will experience premature menopause.[2,138,160]

### Other issues

No discussion of gonadal dysfunction from chemotherapy is complete without acknowledgment that drugs used to manage chemotherapy side effects can alter sexual function. Impotence, decreased sexual desire, decreased sense of sexual fulfillment, and decreased ability to achieve orgasm all have been associated with these agents (Table 28-2).[105,128,134,147,161–163]

**TABLE 28-2  Cancer-Associated Drugs That Affect Sexual and Reproductive Function**

| Agent | Complication |
|---|---|
| **ANTIEMETICS/SEDATIVES/TRANQUILIZERS** | |
| Prochlorperazine Chlorpromazine Diazepam Lorazepam Metoclopramide Scopolamine | Sedation, orgasm without ejaculation, impotence, decreased sexual interest, decreased intensity of orgasm |
| **ANTIHISTAMINES** | |
| Diphenhydramine | Sedation, decreased sexual interest |
| **ANTIDEPRESSANTS** | |
| Amitriptyline Imipramine | Impotence, altered libido |
| **NARCOTICS** | |
| Morphine Hydromorphone Codeine | Decreased libido, sedation, impaired potency |
| **MISCELLANEOUS** | |
| Ketoconazole Cimetadine | Decreased libido Impotence |
| **STEROIDS** | |
| (see Table 28-1) | |

Data from Yasko,[105] Schilsky and Erlichman,[129] Glasel,[134] Kaempfer,[147,162] and Brager and Yasko.[163]

## Biologic Response Modifiers

Although now more frequently used in the adjuvant setting and for treatment of earlier stage disease, information is minimal about the sexual side effects associated with the biologic response modifiers (BRMs). Rieger[164] noted that most changes in sexuality are related to known BRM side effects, including fatigue, mucous membrane dryness, flulike symptoms, and body image changes. Some information is available on the use of the interferons, in particular alfa-interferon, alone or in combination with other agents. Decreased libido, amenorrhea, pelvic pain, uterine bleeding, and erectile dysfunction have been reported with alfa-interferon, and animals exposed to all interferons have demonstrated an increased rate of spontaneous abortions.[165] In addition to drug-induced dysfunction, the usual side effects of fatigue and flulike symptoms affect interest in and comfort with sexual activi-

ties. Nursing research on the subject of gonadal dysfunction related to BRMs is extremely important.

## Bone Marrow Transplantation

Until recently, few reports were available concerning the sexual and reproductive dysfunctions associated with bone marrow transplantation (BMT). Ostroff and Lesko[166] present a comprehensive review and note that late effects of BMT include chronic fatigue, body image alterations, gonadal dysfunction, and infertility. Women experienced decreased sexual desire and satisfaction, vaginal atrophy and decreased vaginal lubrication, and painful intercourse. Men frequently experienced premature ejaculation due to prolonged abstinence. They report that the standard germ-free environment and long hospitalization affect sexuality and intimacy; they further note that sexual interest and activity increase as health improves. Belec[167] evaluated 24 patients following BMT and noted that 50% experienced lack of energy and fatigue severe enough to impede normal activities. Cust et al[168] reported on 36 women who were treated for leukemia with BMT and total-body irradiation (TBI). Twenty experienced vaginal dryness, and 18 women reported dyspareunia. Forty percent complained of feelings of loss of femininity.

Sanders et al[169] evaluated patients following BMT with or without TBI and noted in those receiving BMT with TBI that all had primary gonadal dysfunction. Recovery of ovarian function occurred in less than 10% of the women, and 94% of men remained azoospermic. Milliken et al[170] reported three successful pregnancies in two women following BMT for acute leukemia. TBI was not used. The authors felt that the ability to conceive or father a child after BMT appeared to be related to age (older patients were less likely to reverse gonadal dysfunction) and treatment with TBI.

Numerous authors[171–174] have investigated quality of life in survivors of BMT. Decreased energy and moderate to severe fatigue were experienced by more than 50% of bone marrow transplant survivors up to ten years after transplant.[167,171,172] Other major concerns included infertility, inability to perform sexually, and alterations in sexual intimacy, pleasure, and the ability to achieve orgasm and/or an erection.[171,172] Sexual and reproductive implications of treatment should be discussed and counseling provided prior to, throughout, and following treatment.

# THERAPEUTIC APPROACHES AND NURSING CARE

## Sexual Counseling

All patients should receive information concerning the possible side effects of disease and treatment on sexuality and reproduction. Patients deserve the opportunity to have their sexual problems thoughtfully identified, and good communication among all parties is essential.[175] Potential side effects and possible methods for management should be discussed with the patient (and partner if available) at diagnosis, throughout treatment, and during follow-up visits.

Loescher et al[176] evaluated the impact of the cancer experience on 17 long-term survivors. Patients repeatedly listed problems and concerns related to sexuality and reproductive function, including concerns about alterations in physical function and libido, problems with erection and ejaculation, and infertility.

Auchincloss[177] suggests that in order to effectively assess a patient for alterations in sexuality, the nurse must understand the patient's medical, psychiatric, and psychosexual status, evaluate present relationships, and provide recommendations and encouragement. Nurses should include sexuality in their assessment of all patients and should provide hope, reassurance, and basic information.[24] Andersen and Lamb[73] described the ALARM model for assessment of sexual dysfunction. The model provides a structure for assessing information similar to that suggested by Auchincloss (see Table 28-3).

Once sexual functioning has been assessed, interventions are necessary to maintain optimal sexual functioning and to promote adaptation to the sexual and reproductive side effects of disease and treatment. Interventions should include the patient's partner whenever possible. The PLISSIT model is another method of intervention (see Table 28-4). This model can help the majority of patients without the need for intensive therapy.[178] In order to maintain integrity and to improve quality of life, it is essential that all patients receive counseling about sexual dysfunction, that open communication is encouraged, and that interventions are individualized and considered to be of value by the participants.

## Nursing Assessment and Management

Not every nurse can be a sexual counselor; however, listening to patient/family concerns, presenting factual information in a nonthreatening manner, managing noncomplex disease- and treatment-related symptoms, and providing appropriate referrals can be easily incorporated into routine care. Many health care providers rarely discuss issues related to sexual and reproductive concerns for a variety of personal and professional reasons. Primary reasons cited include personal discomfort, lack of training or knowledge, and fears of embarrassing themselves or their patients. Additional reasons include lack of time, concerns of inappropriateness of such discussions when dealing with a life-threatening illness, and the belief that

**TABLE 28-3**   Evaluation of Sexual Dysfunction

| ALARM Model | Auchincloss Model |
|---|---|
| A —Activity (sexual) | Evaluate sexual status: |
| L —Libido/desire | Present sexual function |
| A —Arousal and orgasm | Past experiences |
| R —Resolution/release | Relationships |
| M—Medical data | Evaluate medical, psychological, and cancer status |

Data from Andersen and Lamb[73] and Auchincloss.[24,177]

**TABLE 28-4**   PLISSIT Model for Intervention

| P —Permission |
|---|
| LI —Limited information |
| SS—Specific suggestions |
| IT —Intensive therapy |

Data from Annon.[178]

these subjects are not part of the nurse's job description.[179,180]

Although not always accurately portrayed, sexuality is more than the act of intercourse. It includes intimacy, touching, a multitude of activities to show affection, and a variety of methods to communicate with others. As Smith[179] notes, cancer and treatment may disrupt or permanently alter one's ability to perform in the previous sexual patterns or may cause infertility; however, cancer cannot alter the fact that one is a sexual being. This information needs to be reiterated and reinforced for the patient and family.

Many authors[30,80,115,179–184] have cited simple, easy-to-follow suggestions for nurses to assist patients and families with sexual alterations. All these authors emphasize the subject as congruent with and integral to the nurse's role in providing holistic care. They further assert that in order for nurses to provide assistance, they must understand their own sexual identity, what constitutes acceptable sexual patterns and practices, as well as the sociocultural, environmental and other beliefs that may have an impact on how the nurse interacts with others as sexual beings.

Asking about sexual practices early in the nurse's clinical assessment will legitimize and normalize the subject and give patients permission to discuss sexual issues. Current practices, cultural and religious beliefs, and general intimacy issues should be incorporated in the discussion. Additionally, whenever possible and appropriate, the patient's partner should be included. Medical jargon and value-oriented terminology should be avoided, and questions and responses should acknowledge the subject and related concerns as normal and important.[80,179–184]

Providing factual information about disease, treatment, and potential side effects is implicit in every nurse's role. Discussing potential alterations in sexual functioning, including fertility issues, prior to or early in treatment and continuing these discussions well into the follow-up phase is essential. Information is needed to dispel myths, decrease anxiety, minimize embarrassment, provide a basis for alternative strategies, and open lines of communication between the patient and others.[179,180,182]

Managing the side effects of cancer and treatment is also integral to the nurse's role. Offering simple suggestions and appropriately managing side effects may be sufficient for most patients to continue or reinstitute sexual activities and enhance intimacy. In addition to management of such traditional symptoms as pain, nausea, vomiting, and bone marrow depression, nurses should provide information and strategies about the importance of communication and openness; the need for exercise, rest, and adequate nutrition; the use of contraception; setting the stage for sexual activities (candles, music, sexy clothing); experimentation with alternative methods of intimacy and the liberal and adequate use of lubricants, foreplay, and more comfortable positions. Energy conservation techniques and information on the timing of medications and methods to maintain cleanliness and personal hygiene are also important.[30,80,115,179–184]

Finally, knowing when to make referrals and recognizing appropriate community resources is essential. Areas of referral include hormonal therapies, vacuum devices or medications to manage erectile dysfunction, sperm banking and other fertility-preserving options, and reconstructive surgery and/or prostheses. Some patients will require psychosexual counseling; others will not. Individualization of education and counseling is important for each patient. It is crucial that the nurse (or others) not invent sexual concerns for those who do not have them but rather anticipates, recognizes, advocates, and assists those who do.

## Fertility Considerations and Procreative Alternatives

Fertility and pregnancy following cancer diagnosis are fraught with a multitude of concerns, particularly the ability to conceive, carry to term, and deliver a healthy newborn with no congenital abnormalities and no increased risk for future malignancies because of either parent's previous diagnosis and treatment for cancer. Nicholson and Byrne,[185] who reviewed the current literature and reported on their own studies of subsequent fertility and pregnancy in children and adolescents treated for cancer, reiterated that radiation therapy and chemotherapy, alone or in combination, have the potential to induce infertility. They also note that proven fertility is measured by pregnancy rates and that even when fertility is preserved, conception may be delayed. The authors provide guidance for patients and health care providers, stressing that information about procreative alternatives, the potential for infertility, and issues related to genetic inheritance, mutagenicity, and timing of pregnancy be thoroughly discussed with potential parents prior to attempting conception.

### Mutagenicity

*Mutagenicity* is the ability to cause an abnormality in the genetic content of cells, resulting in cell death, alteration(s) in growth and replication, or no noticeable alteration in cell function. Mutagenicity following radiation therapy in mice has been documented; however, the mutagenic effects following radiation or chemotherapy in humans are less clear.[186] Possible germ cell mutations may not be evident for generations of offspring.[187–189]

Numerous researchers have investigated the offspring of individuals exposed to chemotherapy or radiotherapy as children or adolescents as a method to adequately assess mutagenicity following therapy.[190–194] Mulvihill et al[190] reviewed 12 retrospective case series of pregnancies in cancer survivors. There were 1573 pregnancies and 1240 live-born infants with 46 (4%) birth defects (which is comparable to the rate among the general population). The researchers noted only two instances of possible mutations. Hawkins[192] evaluated 2286 survivors of childhood cancer who were exposed to chemotherapy, radiotherapy, or both. In women who had received radiotherapy to the abdomen or gonads there was an increased rate of miscarriage (19%) for first pregnancies. No statistical difference for congenital anomalies was seen. Senturia and Peckham,[193] who evaluated children fathered by men treated with chemotherapy for metastatic testicular cancer, reported no statistical difference in congenital anomalies, although they did note a higher than expected rate of cardiac abnormalities. Green et al[194] examined the records of 306 men and women treated with chemotherapy for pediatric malignancies. No difference was noted in the rate of congenital anomalies; however, they did note that 10% of babies born to mothers who were given dactinomycin had structural congenital cardiac defects. In all studies it has been difficult to specifically implicate germ cell mutations as the cause of adverse outcomes to pregnancies. Chapman[138] reviewed the findings from 18 studies that included almost 1600 children born to 1078 mothers or fathers who had previously been treated for cancer. When compared with the general population, no increase in fetal wastage or in congenital defects could be noted in these offspring. Follow-up over several generations of patients and their offspring will be needed before definitive answers are obtained.

### Teratogenicity

*Teratogenicity* is the ability of a toxic compound to produce alterations in an exposed fetus. Both chemotherapy and radiotherapy are known to have teratogenetic effects on the fetus, causing spontaneous abortion, fetal malformation, or fetal death, especially during the first trimester. Low-dose radiation has also been implicated in fetal malignancy.[187,188,195–197] Mulvihill et al,[190] in their study of fetal exposure to radiotherapy or chemotherapy during gestation, noted a 28% abnormal outcome (spontaneous abortion or birth defects). Of five conceptions exposed only to radiotherapy, two were electively aborted, one was stillborn, and two were carried to term. All had some form of congenital malformation.

Fetal damage probably does not occur at doses <10 cGy and is only rarely reported at doses <50 cGy.[63] Radiation exposure during the first trimester represents the greatest risk to the fetus, with exposure ≥100 cGy resulting in fetal death, microcephaly, eye anomalies, and intrauterine growth retardation. In the second or third trimester, fetal death is unlikely, but growth retardation, sterility, and cataracts are common findings.[196]

Chemotherapy, particularly when received during the first trimester, has been related to congenital abnormalities, with approximately 10% of fetuses experiencing some type of anomaly. In general, the alkylating agents and antimetabolites have been most often associated with fetal malformations. Chemotherapy during the second or third trimester may cause premature birth or low birth weights, but congenital abnormalities are not increased over the normal pregnancy incidence.[195,198–200] Zemlickis et al[201] reported on 21 women treated with chemotherapy during pregnancy. Of those treated during the first tri-

mester (n = 13), five pregnancies were carried to term, four had spontaneous abortions, and four had therapeutic abortions. Of the five fetuses carried to term, two had major malformations and both infants died. In the women who received chemotherapy during the second and third trimesters (n = 8), there were six live births, none with major malformations. All infants were noted to have a lower mean birth weight and a shorter gestational period than matched controls. Doll et al[198] noted that the timing of chemotherapy is critical, with the period of teratogenicity limited to the time of embryonic organogenesis. They state that effects also are related to drug dose, length of exposure, frequency of administration, and type and number of drugs administered (Table 28-5).

## Reproductive Counseling

Discussions concerning fertility and reproduction issues need to be held prior to the onset of therapy and should continue well into posttreatment and follow-up. Current fertility status, desire for future childbearing, and contraception practices should be investigated during the initial assessment.[202] Potential alterations should be openly discussed and referrals made as appropriate. Counseling for possible risks of mutagenicity, increased cancer risk, and unknown sequelae of treatment for progeny should be included.[203] Birth control methods need to be implemented to minimize the possibility of an unplanned pregnancy during therapy. In addition, methods to maintain fertility during therapy should be investigated.

For those receiving radiotherapy, appropriate shield-

**TABLE 28-5  Teratogenetic Effects of Chemotherapy**

| Agent | Complication |
|---|---|
| **ALKYLATING** | |
| Busulfan | Spontaneous abortions |
| Chlorambucil | Skeletal malformations |
| Cyclophosphamide | |
| Nitrogen mustard | |
| **ANTIMETABOLITES** | |
| Cytosine arabinoside | Spontaneous abortions |
| 6-mercaptopurine | Skeletal malformations |
| 5-fluorouracil | |
| Methotrexate | |
| **MISCELLANEOUS AGENTS** | |
| Procarbazine | Atrial/septal defects |
| Glucocorticoids | Spontaneous abortions |
| Daunorubicin | Spontaneous abortions |
| Vinblastine | Spontaneous abortions |

Data from Balducci et al,[63] Glasel,[134] Green et al,[194] Robinson and Krebs,[195] Doll et al,[198] and Barnicle.[200]

ing of the testes or ovaries or oophoropexy to position the ovaries outside the radiation field may be of benefit. Birth control pills in women and Gn-RH analogues in men may protect the germ cells from damage by chemotherapeutic agents.[204,205] Studies in these areas continue, with results unclear.

Because it is often difficult to predict when an individual receiving chemotherapy is infertile, it is extremely important that methods to prevent pregnancy are discussed and appropriate drugs or devices provided. It has also been suggested that following cancer therapy an individual should wait a minimum of two years before attempting conception. This suggestion is made both to prevent pregnancy during the time recurrence is most likely and to allow for the recovery of spermatogenesis or ovarian function if it has been temporarily altered by therapy.[195,202,206] It should be noted, however, that this time frame may be too long for some women at risk for early menopause and that no benefit is known to be derived from a prolonged waiting time.[185,197]

## Sperm Banking

Semen storage for use in artificial insemination has been available for many years. Although initially used to establish pregnancy in infertile couples, sperm banking has more recently also been used to preserve procreation abilities in men undergoing cancer therapy. Unfortunately, the option to bank sperm will not be available to every man undergoing cancer therapy. As previously noted, many men will be subfertile or infertile at the time of diagnosis. In addition, since sperm banking needs to be completed prior to initiation of therapy, anyone with rapidly progressing disease frequently cannot delay the start of therapy to complete the cryopreservation process. Redman et al[207] investigated 79 men treated for Hodgkin's disease who had pretreatment semen analysis. Of these individuals, 28% were considered to be infertile at diagnosis. Of these men, 44 were followed posttherapy, and only 20% had normal sperm counts at a median of 27 months' follow-up. Eleven couples attempted pregnancy using the cryopreserved semen; thus far only three inseminations have been successful. Milligan et al[208] reported on semen cryopreservation in 2219 men treated for cancer. Only 133 of the men attempted conception, resulting in 27 pregnancies in 23 couples. Of the 27 pregnancies there were 21 live births and six miscarriages. Averette et al[152] reported on 157 patients among whom there were 22 inseminations resulting in six pregnancies. Of importance were sperm counts $>20 \times 10^6$/ml and postthaw counts >30%. Sweet et al[209] report that of the last 44 patients in their practice who used their banked semen, five pregnancies resulted. They noted the average time to conception was approximately three months, which is comparable to that seen in the general population.

Even if artificial insemination is never completed, the knowledge that semen has been banked and is available when needed can provide a significant psychological boost for the male undergoing cancer therapy.[209–211] All aspects of the sperm-banking process, from initial visit through the completion of insemination, should be fully discussed with the patient so that informed decisions can be made.

## In Vitro Fertilization/Embryo Transfer

In vitro fertilization, used for male infertility due to low sperm counts or for female infertility due to severe endometriosis, immunologic infertility, or absent or damaged fallopian tubes, has undergone remarkable technological advances, with more than 30,000 fertilization cycles undertaken each year.[212,213] In vitro fertilization requires ovarian stimulation followed by ova retrieval via ultrasound-guided needle aspiration of the preovulatory follicles. Laparoscopy also may be used. The retrieved oocytes are then incubated with sperm for 5–26 hours. Following incubation, these embryos are transferred to the uterus and released. The woman remains hospitalized and on bedrest for about six hours. Following discharge, she is encouraged to rest for 48–72 additional hours. Initial results of a single oocyte-retrieval procedure have resulted in a pregnancy rate of 10%–16%. It has been shown, however, that after four to six attempts, the rate of successful pregnancies may approach 50%–60%.[212,214] Fedele et al[215] reported on a woman with a tubal adenocarcinoma treated with salpingectomy. Following in vitro fertilization and embryo transfer, she delivered a normal male child. The mother remains alive and well. Other methods to attain fertility include the use of cryopreserved oocytes and zygotes, with pregnancy rates about 40%.[216,217]

# PREGNANCY AND CANCER

Although pregnancy complicated by a diagnosis of cancer is a rare event, it creates multiple problems for all concerned. Uncertainty about the prognosis of mother and fetus, the rigors of treatment, and the long-term sequelae of cancer for patient, infant, and family compound events that normally are surrounded by a myriad of conflicting emotions. Only with comprehensive care by many health care and ancillary individuals can a positive outcome for mother, fetus, and family be anticipated.

Cancer is the second-leading cause of death in the reproductive years. It is estimated that cancer complicates about 1 in 1000 pregnancies, and that approximately 1 in 118 women with cancer also have a concomitant pregnancy. The most commonly associated cancers are lymphoma, leukemia, malignant melanoma, and cancers of the breast, cervix, ovary, and colorectum—the cancers most commonly seen during the reproductive years.[83]

In general, most cancers do not adversely affect a pregnancy, nor does the pregnancy adversely affect the cancer outcome, although it is possible that the treatment necessary to manage the cancer may have an adverse effect on the pregnancy. Therapeutic abortion has not been shown to be of benefit in altering disease progression and should not be considered unless continued pregnancy will compromise treatment and thus prognosis. The wishes of the patient and family must be considered, with therapeutic options, including prognosis for mother and fetus, fully explained.

It was previously believed that cancer associated with pregnancy was more aggressive and the outcome for all patients dismal. It is now recognized that delay in diagnoses may be a more likely cause of advanced disease at the time of diagnosis. Diagnosing cancer during a pregnancy is difficult, and signs and symptoms of the disease may be misconstrued or underestimated. Treatment options should be evaluated as though the patient were not pregnant, and therapy instituted when appropriate.[83,195,206,218]

## Medical Management of Commonly Associated Cancers

### Breast cancer

Breast cancer is the cancer most commonly associated with pregnancy, representing 1 cancer for every 3000 pregnancies.[83,195,206] Parente et al[219] noted that collected series show a range from one to seven breast cancers per 10,000 pregnancies. Among all women with breast cancer who are still in their childbearing years, one in three will be pregnant at the time of diagnosis.[83,195]

Breast examination should be part of the initial prenatal visit. Although breast enlargement during pregnancy makes examination difficult, it is essential that all women have a thorough examination. If the woman does not practice breast self-examination (BSE), BSE education should be included. If a mass is felt, prompt evaluation is necessary. Although a mammogram is difficult to interpret because of the density of the breast, it may be safely undertaken if appropriate fetal shielding is used. Even if a mammogram shows negative results, a breast mass must be investigated until a definitive diagnosis is made.[83,195,220–223]

Treatment of breast cancer should be the same as in the nonpregnant woman. Biopsy with the patient under local anesthesia has not been shown to cause fetal harm and should be performed without delay.[220,221,224] Once a definitive diagnosis is made, further therapy can be tailored to time of gestation, physician recommendations, and patient wishes. In general, modified mastectomy with lymph node sampling is the standard treatment for early disease. Depending on gestational age, adjuvant chemotherapy can often be delayed until after delivery. For the woman desiring breast-conserving surgery, lumpectomy with lymph node sampling may be done if she is close to term, but radiation therapy and chemotherapy will be delayed until delivery. For advanced disease, surgery and chemotherapy should be undertaken without delay. Therapeutic abortion may be suggested during the first trimes-

ter in order to prevent chemotherapy exposure to the fetus.[83,198,220,221,224–226]

Chances for survival have been considered poor, with reports of 30%–57% survival rates.[223,227,228] Most authors note that when patients are matched stage for stage with nonpregnant control subjects, there appear to be no differences in survival rates.[223,227–229]

Pregnancy safety following cancer treatment has been extensively evaluated, particularly for women treated for breast cancer. Most authors[197,230–232] report no decrease in survival for women who become pregnant following breast cancer treatment. Some authors,[227,233] even suggest that a further pregnancy may actually protect against recurrence. Other authors[234,235] are concerned that there may be differences between those able to conceive and those unable to conceive. They also believe the number of reported pregnancies is small and thus most likely represents a select and nongeneralizable subset of women with breast cancer. Most authors suggest a wait of one to five years after treatment, depending on the stage of disease.[71,233,235]

Breast-feeding after breast cancer diagnosis also has been highly debated. Hassey[236] noted that breast-feeding should no longer be discouraged and, in fact, should be recommended if the woman desires. For the woman who has received primary breast radiation, it has been suggested that breast-feeding occur only on the nonirradiated side, primarily because of the possible increase in mastitis associated with breast-feeding in the irradiated breast but also due to diminished or absent lactation. Higgens and Haffty[230] reported breast asymmetry with little enlargement of the irradiated breast in women who became pregnant subsequent to breast radiation. Of their 11 patients, only four lactated from the radiated side, and only one woman successfully breast-fed her infant.

### Cancer of the cervix

The second most common cancer during pregnancy is cancer of the cervix, which occurs in 1 in 400 pregnancies. Approximately 1 in every 100 women diagnosed with cervical cancer will be pregnant at the time of diagnosis. Carcinoma in situ is most commonly found, with invasive disease seen in only 2%–5% of all cases. Signs and symptoms are similar to those found in the nonpregnant patient, with the majority of pregnant patients experiencing vaginal bleeding or discharge.[237] Diagnosis is most commonly made by Papanicolaou smear. If the smear is abnormal, colposcopy with appropriate biopsies should be undertaken. Cone biopsy is rarely indicated but may be undertaken to confirm a diagnosis of microinvasion. However, it is not without risks and is associated with a 30% complication rate, including hemorrhage, premature delivery, and infection.[65,84,195]

For carcinoma in situ the pregnancy may be allowed to continue. Biopsy should be repeated every six to eight weeks and, unless there is progression, definitive therapy delayed until after delivery. If frank invasion is found, treatment consistent with standard practice for nonpregnant women should not be delayed. During the first two trimesters, surgery or radiation therapy without therapeutic abortion usually is undertaken. Early stage disease (IA and IB) may be treated with radical hysterectomy and pelvic lymph node dissection, while in advanced disease, radiation therapy is the most common treatment. During the third trimester, fetal viability usually can be awaited and the baby can be delivered by cesarean section, after which the appropriate cancer therapy is given.[65,83,195,237–240]

Controversy exists over the safety of vaginal delivery. In reviewing the literature concerning vaginal delivery, Nevin et al[239] found that many authors believed vaginal delivery would disseminate the cancer or cause hemorrhage or infection; thus, cesarean section was recommended. Other authors have suggested that vaginal delivery actually may be associated with an improved overall survival and should be allowed if possible.[239,241] Gordon et al[242] reported the fourth case of recurrence in an episiotomy after vaginal delivery. They suggest that careful follow-up for recurrence is essential. The definitive answer remains unclear.

### Ovarian cancer

Ovarian masses are common during pregnancy, occurring once in every 81 pregnancies. In general, only 2%–5% of these are malignant, for an estimated 1 in 9000 to 1 in 25,000 case ratio. Most patients are asymptomatic, with an adnexal mass noted at the first prenatal visit.[195,214] There are a variety of ways to approach a pelvic mass during pregnancy. Orr and Shingleton[243] suggest that a mass >5 cm that lasts into the second trimester should be explored. Roberts[237] suggests that any mass that is symptomatic or >6 cm be immediately evaluated, whereas Barber[71] states that a unilateral, encapsulated, movable mass <10 cm can wait until the second trimester for evaluation.

If malignancy is diagnosed, treatment should proceed as in the nonpregnant woman. Early disease (stage IA) of low-grade histological findings can be managed by unilateral oophorectomy and biopsy of the other ovary. The pregnancy may be allowed to continue. For all other stages, standard therapy of radical hysterectomy, omentectomy, node biopsy, and peritoneal washings should be carried out. If the woman is near term, a cesarean section, followed by the appropriate therapy, may be performed. Unfortunately, 30%–50% of all women will be diagnosed with stage III or IV disease. Although recent management of stage III disease has resulted in improved survival, in general the prognosis for long-term survival is poor.[65,71,237,244] As in the treatment of all cancers, the wishes of the patient must be considered. It is not uncommon for a pregnant woman with advanced disease to delay treatment until the fetus is viable. Palliative treatment should be instituted at the earliest possible time.

### Malignant melanoma

Malignant melanoma is one of the most rapidly increasing cancers, with a predicted incidence of 1 in 100 whites by the year 2000. It occurs most often in a preexisting mole in fair-haired individuals with blue or green eyes and an inability to tan when exposed to the sun; the peak incidence is during the third and fourth decades.[243,245]

It has been suggested[246] that melanoma arising during pregnancy is associated with poor prognosis because it is hormonally influenced and thus exacerbated by pregnancy. At present this has yet to be definitely proved. What is known is that melanoma that occurs during pregnancy more often is found on the trunk, a site associated with a poor prognosis. In addition, all pigmented areas darken during pregnancy, making diagnosis of early changes more difficult. Biopsy and removal of questionable lesions are indicated. There appears to be no difference in survival between the pregnant and nonpregnant woman with melanoma.[246–250]

Treatment consists of wide excision with skin graft if necessary. Lymph node dissection remains controversial. Adjuvant therapy is being investigated, but no definite answers are available. The benefits of chemotherapy and biologic response modifiers remain unclear. For individuals with advanced disease, therapeutic abortion followed by palliative chemotherapy is advised. For the individual with brain metastasis, surgery or radiation therapy with appropriate fetal shielding may be undertaken.[243,248]

Malignant melanoma is known to metastasize to the placenta and fetus. The placenta should be carefully evaluated at delivery and the infant monitored for development of melanoma.[83,195,248,251–254] Further pregnancies should not be undertaken until at least two years after diagnosis and treatment.[255]

### Lymphomas

Both non-Hodgkin's lymphoma (NHL) and Hodgkin's disease (HD) occur with pregnancy, although the incidence is rare, with HD occurring in 1 in 6000 pregnancies and NHL rarely associated.[256,257] HD usually occurs as asymptomatic lymphadenopathy of the cervical, supraclavicular, or mediastinal regions. Disease confined to the neck or axilla usually can be treated with radiation therapy used with fetal shielding. Because more extensive disease requires combination chemotherapy, a therapeutic abortion is suggested during the first half of pregnancy. During the last half of pregnancy, therapy will be defined by the stage of the pregnancy. If viability is imminent, therapy may be delayed or single-drug treatment instituted and delivery awaited. For rapidly progressing disease, combination chemotherapy should be instituted immediately.[83,195,256,257]

Fewer than 50 cases of NHL and pregnancy have been reported in the literature. Steiner-Salz et al[258] reported on 6 cases of NHL that complicated pregnancy and reviewed an additional 22 cases. Therapy consisted of chemotherapy or radiation therapy, or both. Seventeen patients died within nine months of delivery, six infants died shortly after birth, and the remaining patients and offspring are believed to be alive and well. Although NHL is known to metastasize to the placenta and fetus and thus requires careful observations at delivery, NHL has not developed in these infants.[251,252]

### Leukemia

Leukemia occurs in 1 in 75,000 pregnancies. Diagnosis is often made on routine complete blood count. Treatment should be instituted immediately unless the fetus is viable or near viability. If the fetus is viable, delivery should not be delayed. If the fetus is near viability, leukapheresis may be utilized until delivery is possible. Therapeutic abortion is suggested in the first trimester to avoid fetal exposure to chemotherapy.[259,260] In a study of 20 children born of 18 women with acute leukemia, 1 was stillborn and 2 others died within 90 days of birth. Five of the 18 women remain alive; the other 13 died of recurrent leukemia. The 17 remaining children developed normally without apparent psychological or physiological abnormalities.[261] In another report[262] perinatal mortality was as high as 50%, with 75% of mothers dying within seven months of delivery. Leukemia also may spread to the placenta and fetus; thus, placental and fetal monitoring are important aspects of delivery and postpartum care.[251,252]

## Effects of Treatment and Malignancy on the Fetus

### Surgery

Maternal surgery can be safely accomplished with minimal risk to the fetus.[65,243] Pelvic surgery is more easily accomplished during the second trimester. There is little risk to the fetus from short exposure to anesthetic agents after the first trimester. Adequate ventilation and prevention of hypotension are of prime importance.[243] As long as competent surgeons and anesthesiologists with appropriate fetal monitoring equipment are available, no harm to the fetus should occur.[106]

### Radiation

Radiation doses of >250 cGY during pregnancy have been associated with fetal damage—for example, mental retardation, skin changes, and spontaneous abortions (depending on stage of gestation). Low doses of radiation associated with diagnostic x-ray studies (<0.5 cGY) are probably not harmful if adequate fetal shielding is provided. Radiation to the pelvis should be avoided.[263,264] Long-term effects of low-dose radiation remain unknown, but the concerns of chromosomal aberrations and an increase in childhood cancer in children exposed in utero remain. Follow-up over many generations may be necessary to determine the exact effects.[65,264]

### Chemotherapy

Chemotherapy has been administered prior to and concurrent with pregnancy.[265,266] As previously noted, chemotherapy during the first trimester has been associated with fetal wastage, malformations, and low birth weights. Many studies indicate that the incidence of fetal malformations is low (<10%) and may be minimized or avoided with careful selection of agents. Latent effects are still unknown, and offspring need continuous evaluation. It is important to note that pharmacokinetics of chemotherapeutic agents may be altered by the normal physiological changes of pregnancy. Monitoring for unexpected toxicities or altered response patterns is of extreme importance. Additionally, evaluation of the fetus for toxicities from administration of drugs immediately prior to delivery is paramount. Both neonatal metabolism and drug excretion may be suboptimal, and the placenta, which is the normal mechanism for excretion, has been eliminated.[266]

### Maternal-fetal spread

Only a few cancers spread from the mother to the fetus, with melanoma, NHL, and leukemia the most common. Because few series have been compiled, the exact incidence is unknown. Rothman et al[251] reviewed 11 cases and Potter and Schoeneman[252] 24 cases of maternal cancer that metastasized to the infant. Seventeen of the 35 women had metastatic melanoma. Fifteen infants died of cancer; an additional six died of events unrelated to cancer. Dildy et al[267] reviewed cases of maternal malignancy metastatic to products of conception and reported on 53 cases. The most common cancer was malignant melanoma. Metastasis to the placenta occurred in 12 cases and spread to the fetus in seven cases. The second most common were the hematological malignancies (leukemia and lymphoma), involving eight instances of placental spread and four cases of fetal spread. Breast and lung cancer were next; however, no cases of spread to the fetus have been reported. Because of the rare incidence of metastatic involvement to the infant, evaluation of the placenta and fetus is essential in women with disseminated cancers.

## Nursing Management of the Pregnant Patient

Nursing management of the pregnant patient with a concomitant diagnosis of cancer can be extremely complicated. Interventions including psychosocial, educational, and ethical considerations must be developed and implemented. It has been suggested that pregnancy and cancer be treated as a high-risk event with all the associated needs.[83] Careful explanations of all aspects of care, with special emphasis on support of the patient and her family, need to be included. Normal activities of pregnancy may be delayed or prevented by disease or treatment, and fears of fetal demise, cancer therapy, and death may prevent resolution of ambivalence toward pregnancy and establishment of emotional affiliation to the growing child. Ethical considerations become apparent as plans for pregnancy are contrasted with needs for therapy. In some instances therapeutic abortion may be necessary for optimal treatment; in other instances therapy delays may be requested to provide for the safety of the fetus. Nonjudgmental care by health care personnel is essential during these difficult times.

Nursing care of the woman with cancer and her baby is extremely complex and of utmost importance. With a focus on educational interventions, psychological support, and coordination of care, the nurse has an important role in the final outcome. Treatment plans; coordination of follow-up; education about cancer, pregnancy, and treatment; and emotional support of the patient and significant others are integral components of the comprehensive care needed by the pregnant woman with cancer. Without these essential elements, it may not be possible to provide the necessary care for a positive or improved maternal and fetal outcome.

## CONCLUSION

Sexual and reproductive dysfunction in cancer patients occurs much more frequently than previously recognized. Almost every patient exposed to cancer or cancer treatment may experience some form of sexual dysfunction at some point during the illness. With cancer survival rates improving and with the understanding that sexual and reproductive function are important to all individuals, it is essential that sexuality and sexual function be assessed and evaluated prior to therapy and that appropriate interventions be implemented throughout treatment and the follow-up period.

## REFERENCES

1. Ganz PA: Current issues in cancer rehabilitation. *Cancer* 65:742–751, 1990
2. Yarbro CH, Perry MC: The effect of cancer therapy on gonadal function. *Semin Oncol Nurs* 1:3–8, 1985
3. Yasko JM, Green P: Coping with problems related to cancer treatment. *CA Cancer J Clin* 37:107–125, 1987
4. Smith DB: Sexual rehabilitation of the cancer patient. *Cancer Nurs* 12:10–15, 1989
5. Fisher SG: The psychosexual effects of cancer and cancer treatment. *Oncol Nurs Forum* 10:63–68, 1983
6. Guyton AC: Endocrinology and reproduction, in Guyton AC (ed): *Human Physiology and Mechanism of Disease* (ed 4). Philadelphia, Saunders, 1987, pp 563–654
7. Gill GN: Endocrine, in West JB (ed): *Best and Taylor's Physiological Basis of Medical Practice* (ed 11). Baltimore, Williams and Wilkins, 1985, pp 844–933
8. Emslie-Smith D, Paterson CR, Schratcherd T, et al: Reproduction, in Emslie-Smith D, Paterson CR, Schratcherd T,
et al (eds): *Textbook of Physiology*. Edinburgh: Churchill Livingstone, 1988, pp 323–335
9. Marieb EN: Reproductive system, in Marieb EN (ed): *Essentials of Human Anatomy and Physiology*. Menlo Park, CA: Addison-Wesley, 1987, pp 311–333
10. Hobbie WL, Schwartz CL: Endocrine late effects among survivors of cancer. *Semin Oncol Nurs* 5:14–21, 1989
11. Jessup JM, Steele G: Rectal and anal carcinoma, in Steele G, Cady B (eds): *General Surgical Oncology*. Philadelphia, Saunders, 1992, pp 171–183
12. Wicks LJ: Treatment modalities for colorectal cancer. *Semin Oncol Nurs* 2:242–248, 1986
13. Sprangers MAG, Taal BG, Aaronson NK, et al: Quality of life in colorectal cancer: Stoma vs. nonstoma patients. *Dis Colon Rectum* 38:361–369, 1995
14. Cantril ST, Schoeppel P: Carcinoma of the anus: A review. *Semin Oncol Nurs* 4:203–299, 1988
15. MacDonald LD, Anderson HR: Stigma in patients with rectal cancer: A community study. *J Epidemiol Community Health* 38:284–290, 1984
16. Dobkin KA, Broadwell DC: Nursing considerations for the patient undergoing colostomy surgery. *Semin Oncol Nurs* 2: 249–255, 1986
17. Lamb MA, Woods NF: Sexuality and the cancer patient. *Cancer Nurs* 4:137–144, 1981
18. Donovan MI: Teaching the patient about sexuality, in Donovan MI (ed): *Cancer Care: A Guide for Patient Education*. New York, Appleton-Century-Crofts, 1981, pp 257–289
19. Andersen BL: How cancer affects sexual functioning. *Oncology* 4:81–88, 1990
20. De Bernardinis G, Tuscano D, Negro P, et al: Sexual dysfunction in males following extensive colorectal surgery. *Int Surg* 66:133–135, 1981
21. Hurney C, Holland J: Psychosocial sequelae of ostomies in cancer patients. *Cancer* 35:170–183, 1985
22. Shipes E, Lehr S: Sexuality and the male cancer patient. *Cancer Nurs* 5:375–381, 1982
23. Danzi M, Ferulano GP, Abate S, et al: Male sexual function after abdominoperineal resection for rectal cancer. *Dis Colon Rectum* 26:665–668, 1983
24. Auchincloss SS: Sexual dysfunction, in Holland JC, Rowland JH (eds): *Handbook of Psychooncology*. New York, Oxford University Press, 1989, pp 383–413
25. Glasgow M, Halfin V, Althausen AF: Sexual response and cancer. *CA Cancer J Clin* 37:322–333, 1987
26. Williams JJ, Slack WW: A prospective study of sexual function after major colorectal surgery. *Br J Surg* 67:772–774, 1980
27. Burnham WR, Leonard-Jones JE, Brooke BN: Sexual problems among married ileostomists. *Gut* 18:673–677, 1977
28. Koukouras D, Spiliotis J, Scopa CD, et al: Radical consequence in the sexuality of male patients operated for colorectal carcinoma. *Eur J Surg Oncol* 17:285–288, 1991
29. Schover LR, von Eschenbach AC, Smith DB, et al: Sexual rehabilitation of urologic cancer patients: A practical approach. *CA Cancer J Clin* 34:66–74, 1984
30. Ofman US: Preservation of function in genitourinary cancers: Psychosexual and psychosocial issues. *Cancer Invest* 13:125–131, 1995
31. Bachers ES: Sexual dysfunction after treatment for genitourinary cancer. *Semin Oncol Nurs* 1:18–24, 1985
32. Smith DB, Babaian RJ: The effects of treatment for cancer on male fertility and sexuality. *Cancer Nurs* 15:271–275, 1992

33. Ofman US: Psychosocial and sexual implications of genito-urinary cancers. *Semin Oncol Nurs* 9:286–292, 1993

34. Boyd SD, Schiff WM: Inflatable penile prostheses in patients undergoing cystoprostatectomy with urethrectomy. *J Urol* 141:60–62, 1989

35. Watt RC: Nursing management of a patient with a urinary diversion. *Semin Oncol Nurs* 2:265–269, 1986

36. Schover LR, Fife M: Sexual counseling of patients undergoing radical surgery for pelvic or genital cancer. *J Psychosoc Oncol* 3:21–41, 1986

37. Shipes E: Sexual functioning following ostomy surgery. *Nurs Clin North Am* 22:303–310, 1987

38. Mansson A, Johnson G, Mansson W: Quality of life after cystectomy: Comparison between patients with conduit and those with caeca reservoir diversion. *Br J Urol* 62:240–245, 1988

39. Held J, Volpe H: Bladder-preserving combined modality therapy for invasive bladder cancer. *Oncol Nurs Forum* 18:49–57, 1991

40. American Cancer Society: *Cancer Facts and Figures—1996*. Atlanta, American Cancer Society, 1996

41. Dobkin PL, Bradley I: Assessment of sexual dysfunction in oncology patients: Review, critique, and suggestions. *J Psychosoc Oncol* 9:43–74, 1991

42. Witkin MH, Kaplan HS: Sex therapy and penectomy. *J Sex Marital Ther* 8:209–221, 1982

43. Donovan MI, Girton SE: Self concept, in Donovan MI, Girton SE (eds): *Cancer Care Nursing* (ed 2). Norwalk, CT: Appleton-Century-Crofts, 1984, pp 506–556

44. Furlow WL: Sexual consequences of male genitourinary cancer: The role of sex prosthetics, in Vaeth JN (ed): *Frontiers of Radiation Therapy and Oncology*. Basel, Switzerland, Karger, 1980, pp 104–107

45. Opjordsmoen S, Waehre H, Aass N, et al: Sexuality in patients treated for penile cancer: Patients' experience and doctors' judgement. *Br J Urol* 73:554–560, 1994

46. Lange PH, Chang WY, Fraley EE: Fertility issues in the therapy of nonseminomatous testicular tumors. *Urol Clin North Am* 14:731–747, 1987

47. Blackmore C: The impact of orchiectomy upon the sexuality of the man with testicular cancer. *Cancer Nurs* 11:33–40, 1988

48. Narayan P, Lange PH, Fraley EE: Ejaculation and fertility after extended retroperitoneal lymph node dissection for testicular cancer. *J Urol* 127:685–688, 1982

49. Foster RS, McNulty A, Rubin LR, et al: The fertility of patients with clinical stage I testis cancer managed by nerve-sparing retroperitoneal lymph node dissection. *J Urol* 152:1139–1143, 1994

50. Donohue JP, Foster RS, Rowland RG, et al: Nerve-sparing retroperitoneal lymphadenectomy with preservation of ejaculation. *J Urol* 144:287–292, 1990

51. Brock D, Fox S, Gosling G, et al: Testicular cancer. *Semin Oncol Nurs* 9:224–236, 1993

52. Lamb MA: Alterations in sexuality and sexual functioning, in Baird SB, McCorkle R, Grant M (eds): *Cancer Nursing: A Comprehensive Textbook*. Philadelphia, Saunders, 1991, pp 831–849

53. Nijman JM, Koops HS, Kremer J, et al: Gonadal function after surgery and chemotherapy in men with stage II and III nonseminomatous testicular tumors. *J Clin Oncol* 5:651–656, 1987

54. Gritz ER, Wellisch DK, Wang H, et al: Long-term effects of testicular cancer on sexual functioning in married couples. *Cancer* 64:1560–1567, 1989

55. Aass N, Grunfeld B, Kaalhus O, et al: Pre- and post-treatment sexual life in testicular cancer patients: A descriptive investigation *Br J Cancer* 67:1113–1117, 1993

56. Heinrich-Rynning T: Prostatic cancer treatments and their effects on sexual functioning. *Oncol Nurs Forum* 14:37–41, 1987

57. Church PA: Prostate cancer, in Steele G, Cady B (eds): *General Surgical Oncology*. Philadelphia, Saunders, 1992, pp 275–285

58. Eggleston JC, Walsh PC: Radical prostatectomy with preservation of sexual function: Pathological findings in the first 100 cases. *J Urol* 134:1146–1148, 1985

59. Walsh PC, Schlegel PN: Radical pelvic surgery with preservation of sexual function. *Ann Surg* 208:391–400, 1988

60. Einhorn C: Helping the prostate surgery patient face sexual dysfunction. *Innovations Urol Nurs* 3:1, 9, 1992

61. Meredith CE: Treatment options for men with erectile dysfunction. *Innovations Urol Nurs* 3:2–4, 8, 11, 1992

62. Morales A, Condra MS, Owen JE, et al: Oral and transcutaneous pharmacologic agents in the treatment of impotence. *Urol Clin North Am* 15:87–93, 1988

63. Balducci L, Phillips DM, Gearhart JG, et al: Sexual complications of cancer treatment. *Am Fam Physician* 37:159–172, 1988

64. Lamb M: Vulvar cancer: Patient information booklet. *Oncol Nurs Forum* 13:79–82, 1986

65. DiSaia PJ, Creasman WT: *Clinical Gynecologic Oncology* (ed 4). St Louis, Mosby, 1993

66. Andersen BL, Turnquist D, LaPolla J, et al: Sexual function after treatment of in situ vulvar cancer: Preliminary report. *Obstet Gynecol* 71:15–19, 1988

67. Weijmar Schultz WCM, Van de Weil HBM, Bouma J, et al: Psychosexuality after cancer of the vulva. *Cancer* 66:402–407, 1990

68. DiSaia PJ: Conservative management of the patient with early gynecologic cancer. *CA Cancer J Clin* 39:135–154, 1989

69. Lamb MA: Psychosexual issues: The woman with gynecologic cancer. *Semin Oncol Nurs* 6:237–243, 1990

70. Corney RH, Crowther ME, Howells A: Psychosexual dysfunction in women with gynaecological cancer following radical pelvic surgery. *Br J Obstet Gynaecol* 100:73–78, 1993

71. Barber HRK: *Manual of Gynecologic Oncology* (ed 2). Philadelphia, Lippincott, 1989, pp 163–251

72. Hubbard JL, Shingleton HM: Sexual function of patients after cancer of the cervix treatment. *Clin Obstet Gynecol* 12:247–264, 1985

73. Andersen BL, Lamb M: Sexuality and cancer, in Murphy GP, Lawrence W, Lenhard RE (eds): *American Cancer Society Textbook of Clinical Oncology* (ed 2). Atlanta, American Cancer Society, 1995, pp 699–713

74. Morgan S: Sexuality after hysterectomy and castration. *Women Health* 3:5–10, 1978

75. Masters WH, Johnson VE (eds): *Human Sexual Response*. Boston, Little, Brown, 1966, pp 273–300

76. Zussman L, Zussman S, Sunley R, et al: Sexual response after hysterectomy-oophorectomy: Recent studies and reconsideration of psycho-genesis. *Am J Obstet Gynecol* 140:725–729, 1981

77. Jenkins B: Patients' reports of sexual changes after treatment for gynecologic cancer. *Oncol Nurs Forum* 15:349–354, 1988

78. Schover LR, Fife M, Gershenson DM: Sexual dysfunction and treatment for early stage cervical cancer. *Cancer* 63:204–212, 1989

79. Cull A, Cowie VJ, Farquarson DIM, et al: Early stage cervical

cancer: Psychosexual and sexual outcomes of treatment. *Br J Cancer* 68:1216–1220, 1993

80. Lamb MA, Sheldon TA: The sexual adaptation of women treated for endometrial cancer. *Cancer Pract* 2:103–113, 1994

81. Shell JA: Impact of cancer on sexuality, in Otto S (ed): *Oncology Nursing* (ed 2). St. Louis, Mosby Year Book, 1994, pp 737–760

82. Lamb MA, Bargman C, Brozovich K: Ovarian cancer: Patient information booklet. *Oncol Nurs Forum* 12:83–88, 1985

83. Krebs LU: Pregnancy and cancer. *Semin Oncol Nurs* 1:35–41, 1985

84. Martin LK, Braly PS: Gynecologic cancers, in Baird SB, McCorkle R, Grant M (eds): *Cancer Nursing: A Comprehensive Textbook.* Philadelphia, Saunders, 1991, pp 502–535

85. Thranov I, Klee M: Sexuality among gynecologic cancer patients: A cross-sectional study. *Gynecol Oncol* 52:14–19, 1994

86. Hampton BG: Nursing management of a patient following pelvic exenteration. *Semin Oncol Nurs* 2:281–286, 1986

87. Andersen BL, Hacker NF: Psychosexual adjustment following pelvic exenteration. *Obstet Gynecol* 61:331–338, 1983

88. McKenzie F: Sexuality after total pelvic exenteration. *Nurs Times* 84:27–29, 1988

89. Schain WS: The sexual and intimate consequences of breast cancer treatment. *CA Cancer J Clin* 38:154–161, 1988

90. Schain WS: Breast cancer surgeries and psychosexual sequelae: Implications for remediation. *Semin Oncol Nurs* 1:200–205, 1985

91. Rutherford DE: Assessing psychosocial needs of women experiencing lumpectomy. *Cancer Nurs* 11:244–249, 1988

92. Fallowfield LJ, Hall A: Psychosocial and sexual impact of diagnosis and treatment of breast cancer. *Br Med Bull* 47:388–399, 1991

93. Schover LR: The impact of breast cancer on sexuality, body image and intimate relationships. *CA Cancer J Clin* 41:112–120, 1991

94. Omne-Ponten M, Holmberg L, Burns T, et al: Determinants of the psycho-social outcome after operation for breast cancer: Results of a prospective comparative interview study following mastectomy and breast conservation. *Eur J Cancer* 28A:1062–1067, 1992

95. Wilmoth MC, Townsend J: A comparison of the effects of lumpectomy versus mastectomy on sexual behaviors. *Cancer Pract.* 3:297–285, 1995

96. Andersen BL: Sexual functioning morbidity among cancer survivors: Current status and future research directions. *Cancer* 55:1835–1842, 1985

97. Metcalf MC, Fishman SH: Factors affecting the sexuality of patients with head and neck cancer. *Oncol Nurs Forum* 12:21–25, 1985

98. Dropkin MJ: Coping with disfigurement and dysfunction after head and neck cancer surgery: A conceptual framework. *Semin Oncol Nurs* 5:213–219, 1989

99. Lamb MA: Effects of cancer on the sexuality and fertility of women. *Semin Oncol Nurs* 11:120–127, 1995

100. Witt ME, McDonald-Lynch A, Grimmer D: Adjuvant radiotherapy to the colorectum: Nursing implications. *Oncol Nurs Forum* 4:17–21, 1987

101. Granai CO, Amado PM, Goldstein AS, et al: The effects of cancer therapy on fertility. *Clin Adv Oncol Nurs* 3:1, 3, 7–9, 1991

102. Feldman JE: Ovarian failure and cancer treatment: Incidence and interventions for the premenopausal woman. *Oncol Nurs Forum* 16:651–657, 1989

103. Hilderley LJ: Radiotherapy, in Groenwald S, Frogge MH, Goodman M, Yarbro CH (eds): *Cancer Nursing: Principles and Practice* (ed 3). Boston, Jones and Bartlett, 1993, pp 235–269

104. Yasko JM: Sexual dysfunction, in Yasko JM (ed): *Care of the Client Receiving External Radiation Therapy.* Reston, VA, Reston, 1982, pp 192–231

105. Yasko JM: Sexual and reproductive dysfunction, in Yasko JM (ed): *Guidelines for Cancer Care: Symptom Management.* Reston, VA, Reston, 1983, pp 269–287

106. Stair J: Sexual dysfunction: Infertility, in McNally JC, Sommerville ET, Miaskowski C, Rostad M (eds), *Guidelines for Oncology Nursing Practice* (ed 2). Philadelphia, Saunders, 1991, pp 345–349

107. Horning SJ, Hoppe RT, Kaplan HS, et al: Female reproductive potential after treatment for Hodgkin's disease. *N Engl J Med* 304:1377–1382, 1981

108. Ray GR, Trueblood HW, Enright L, et al: Oophoropexy: A means of preserving ovarian function following pelvic megavoltage radiotherapy for Hodgkin's disease. *Radiology* 96:175–180, 1970

109. Baker JW, Peckham MJ, Morgan RL, et al: Preservation of ovarian function in patients requiring radiotherapy for paraaortic and pelvic Hodgkin's disease. *Lancet* 1:1307–1308, 1972

110. Seibel MM, Freeman MG, Graves WL: Carcinoma of the cervix and sexual function. *Obstet Gynecol* 55:484–487, 1980

111. Smith DB: Sexuality, in Gross J, Johnson BL (eds): *Handbook of Oncology Nursing.* Boston, Jones and Bartlett, 1994, pp 557–571

112. Jenkins B: Sexual healing after pelvic irradiation. *Am J Nurs* 86:920–922, 1986

113. Shell JA, Carter J: The gynecological implant patient. *Semin Oncol Nurs* 3:54–66, 1987

114. Dodd MJ: *Managing Side Effects of Chemotherapy and Radiation Therapy: A Guide for Nurses and Patients.* Norwalk, CT, Appleton and Lange, 1987, pp 139–189

115. Cartwright-Alcarese F: Addressing sexual dysfunction following radiation therapy for a gynecologic malignancy. *Oncol Nurs Forum* 22:1227–1232, 1995

116. Rowly MJ, Leach DR, Warner GA, et al: Effects of graded doses of ionizing radiation on human testes. *Radiat Res* 59:665–678, 1974

117. Kinsella TJ, Shapiro E, Fraass BA, et al: Testicular injury following high dose conventionally fractionated irradiation. *Int J Radiat Oncol Biol Phys* 9:136–137, 1983 (Suppl)

118. Fossa SD, Aass N, Kaalhus O: Long-term morbidity after infradiaphragmatic radiotherapy in young men with testicular cancer. *Cancer* 64:404–408, 1989

119. Costillo LA, Craft AW, Kernahan J, et al: Gonadal function after 12-Gy testicular irradiation in childhood acute lymphoblastic leukaemia. *Med Pediatr Oncol* 18:185–189, 1990

120. Sklar CA, Robison LL, Nesbit ME, et al: Effects of radiation on testicular function in long-term survivors of childhood acute lymphoblastic leukemia: A report from the Children's Cancer Study Group. *J Clin Oncol* 8:1981–1987, 1990

121. Kinsella TJ, Trivette G, Rowland J, et al: Long-term follow-up of testicular function following radiation therapy for early-stage Hodgkin's disease. *J Clin Oncol* 7:718–724, 1989

122. van Heeringen C, DeSchryver A, Verbeek E: Sexual function disorders after local radiotherapy for carcinoma of the prostate. *Radiother Oncol* 13:47–52, 1988

123. Herr HW: Preservation of sexual potency in prostatic cancer patients after iodine implantation. *J Am Geriatr Soc* 27:17–19, 1979

124. Carlton CE, Hudgins PT, Guerriero WG, et al: Radiotherapy in the management of stage C carcinoma of the prostate. *J Urol* 116:206–210, 1976

125. Schover LR, von Eschenbach AC: Sexual and marital counseling with men treated for testicular cancer. *J Sex Marital Ther* 10:29–40, 1984

126. Goldstein I, Feldman M, Deckers P, et al: Radiation-associated impotence. *JAMA* 251:903–910, 1984

127. Shell JA: Knowledge deficit related to radiation therapy, in McNally JC, Sommerville ET, Miaskowski C, Rostad M (eds): *Guidelines for Oncology Nursing Practice* (ed 2). Philadelphia, Saunders, 1991, pp 62–69

128. Longo DL, Fisher RI: Medical problems in long-term survivors of Hodgkin's disease. *Internal Med Spec* 4:165–171, 1983

129. Schilsky RL, Erlichman C: Late complications of chemotherapy: Infertility and carcinogenesis, in Chabner B (ed): *Pharmacologic Principles of Cancer Treatment*. Philadelphia, Saunders, 1982, pp 109–128

130. Chapman RM: Effect of cytotoxic therapy on sexuality and gonadal function. *Semin Oncol* 9:84–94, 1982

131. Wallace WHB, Shalet SM, Crowne EC, et al: Gonadal dysfunction due to cis-platinum. *Med Pediatr Oncol* 17:409–413, 1989

132. Burke MB, Wilkes GM, Berg D, et al: *Cancer Chemotherapy: A Nursing Process Approach*. Boston, Jones and Bartlett, 1991 pp 86–91, 139–372

133. Otto SE: Chemotherapy, in Otto S (ed): *Oncology Nursing* (ed 2). St. Louis, Mosby Year Book, 1994, pp 493–525

134. Glasel M: Effects on reproduction/sexual function, in Tenenbaum L (ed): *Cancer Chemotherapy and Biotherapy: A Reference Guide* (ed 2). Philadelphia, Saunders, 1994, pp 273–285

135. Guy JL: Medical oncology: The agents, in Baird SB, McCorkle R, Grant M (eds): *Cancer Nursing: A Comprehensive Textbook*. Philadelphia, Saunders, 1991, pp 266–290

136. Goodman M: Delivery of cancer chemotherapy, in Baird SB, McCorkle R, Grant M (eds): *Cancer Nursing: A Comprehensive Textbook*. Philadelphia, Saunders, 1991, pp 291–319

137. Schilsky RL, Lewis BJ, Sherins RJ, et al: Gonadal dysfunction in patients receiving chemotherapy for cancer. *Ann Intern Med* 93:109–114, 1980

138. Chapman RM: Gonadal toxicity and teratogenicity, in Perry MC (ed): *The Chemotherapy Sourcebook*. Baltimore, Williams and Wilkins, 1992, pp 710–753

139. Richter P, Calamera JC, Morgenfeld MC, et al: Effect of chlorambucil on spermatogenesis in the human with malignant lymphoma. *Cancer* 25:1026–1030, 1970

140. Viviani S, Ragni G, Santoro A, et al: Testicular dysfunction in Hodgkin's disease before and after treatment. *Eur J Cancer* 27:1389–1392, 1991

141. Drasga RE, Einhorn LH, Williams SD, et al: Fertility after chemotherapy for testicular cancer. *J Clin Oncol* 1:179–183, 1983

142. Stoter G, Koopman A, Vendrik CP, et al: Ten-year survival and late sequelae in testicular cancer patients treated with cisplatin, vinblastine and bleomycin. *J Clin Oncol* 7:1099–1104, 1989

143. Meistrich ML, Chawla SP, DaCunha MF, et al: Recovery of sperm after chemotherapy for osteosarcoma. *Cancer* 63:2115–2123, 1989

144. Cunningham J, Mauch P, Rosenthal DS, et al: Long-term complications of MOPP chemotherapy in patients with Hodgkin's disease. *Cancer Treat Rep* 66:1015–1022, 1982

145. Viviani S, Santoro A, Bon Pante V, et al: Gonadal toxicity after combination chemotherapy for Hodgkin's disease: Comparative results of MOPP vs ABVD. *Eur J Cancer Clin Oncol* 21:601–605, 1985

146. Rousseau L, Dupont A, Labrie F, et al: Sexuality changes in prostate cancer patients receiving antihormonal therapy combining the antiandrogen flutamide with medical (LHRH agonist) or surgical castration. *Arch Sex Behav* 17:87–98, 1988

147. Kaempfer SH: Male sexual dysfunction, in Baird SB (ed): *Decision Making in Oncology Nursing*. Toronto, Decker, 1988, pp 164–165

148. Warne GL, Fairley KF, Hobbs JB, et al: Cyclophosphamide-induced ovarian failure. *N Engl J Med* 289:1159–1162, 1973

149. Belohorsky B, Siracky YJ, Sandor L, et al: Comments on the development of amenorrhea caused by myleran in cases of chronic myelosis. *Neoplasma* 4:397–402, 1960

150. Chapman RM, Sutcliffe SB, Malpas JS: Cytotoxic-induced ovarian failure in women with Hodgkin's disease: II. Effects on sexual function. *JAMA* 242:1171–1181, 1979

151. Andrieu JM, Ochoa-Molina ME: Menstrual cycle, pregnancies and offspring before and after MOPP therapy for Hodgkin's disease. *Cancer* 52:435–438, 1983

152. Averette HE, Boike GM, Jarrell MA: Effects of chemotherapy on gonadal function and reproductive capacity. *CA Cancer J Clin* 40:199–209, 1990

153. Santoro A, Bonadonna G, Valagussa P, et al: Long-term results of combined chemotherapy-radiotherapy approach in Hodgkin's disease: Superiority of ABVD plus radiotherapy versus MOPP plus radiotherapy. *J Clin Oncol* 5:27–37, 1987

154. Schover LR: Sexuality and body image in younger women with breast cancer. *Monogr Natl Cancer Inst* 16:177–182, 1994

155. Meadows AT: Follow-up and care of childhood cancer survivors. *Hosp Pract* 15:99–108, 1991

156. Heiney SP: Adolescents with cancer: Sexual and reproductive issues. *Cancer Nurs* 12:95–101, 1989

157. Levy MJ, Stillman RJ: Reproductive potential in survivors of childhood malignancy. *Pediatrician* 18:61–70, 1991

158. Rivkees SA, Crawford JD: The relationship of gonadal activity and chemotherapy-induced gonadal damage. *JAMA* 259:2123–2125, 1988

159. Blatt J, Poplack DG, Sherins RJ: Testicular function in boys after chemotherapy for acute lymphoblastic leukemia. *JAMA* 304:1121–1124, 1981

160. Byrne J, Mulvihill JJ, Myers MH, et al: Effects of treatment on fertility in long-term survivors of childhood or adolescent cancer. *N Engl J Med* 317:1315–1321, 1987

161. Wilson B: The effects of drugs on male sexual function and fertility. *Nurse Pract* 16:12–24, 1991

162. Kaempfer SH: Female sexual dysfunction, in Baird SB (ed): *Decision Making in Oncology Nursing*. Toronto, Decker, 1988, pp 162–163

163. Brager BL, Yasko J: Sexual and reproductive dysfunction, in Brager BL, Yasko J (eds): *Care of the Client Receiving Chemotherapy*. Reston, VA, Reston, 1984, pp 287–297

164. Rieger PT: Patient management, in Rieger PT (ed): *Biotherapy: A Comprehensive Overview*. Boston, Jones and Bartlett, 1995, pp 195–219

165. Intron-A (package insert). Kenilworth, NJ, Schering Corporation, 1995

166. Ostroff JS, Lesko LM: Psychosexual adjustment and fertility issues, in Whedon MB (ed): *Bone Marrow Transplantation: Principles, Practice and Nursing Insights*. Boston, Jones and Bartlett, 1991, pp 312–333

167. Belec RH: Quality of life: Perceptions of long-term survi-

vors of bone marrow transplantation. *Oncol Nurs Forum* 19:
31–37, 1992

168. Cust MP, Whitehead MI, Powles R, et al: Consequences
and treatment of ovarian failure after total body irradiation
for leukaemia. *BMJ* 299:1494–1497, 1989

169. Sanders JE, Buckner CD, Amos D, et al: Ovarian function
following marrow transplantation for aplastic anemia or
leukemia. *J Clin Oncol* 6:813–818, 1988

170. Milliken S, Powles R, Parikh P: Successful pregnancy following bone marrow transplantation for leukaemia. *Bone Marrow Transplant* 5:135–137, 1990

171. Whedon M, Stearns D, Mills LE: Quality of life of long-
term adult survivors of autologous bone marrow transplantation. *Oncol Nurs Forum* 22:1527–1537, 1995

172. Haberman M, Bush N, Young K, et al: Quality of life of
adult long-term survivors of bone marrow transplantation:
A qualitative analysis of narrative data. *Oncol Nurs Forum*
20:1545–1553, 1993

173. Ferrell B, Grant M, Schmidt GM, et al: The meaning of
quality of life for bone marrow transplant survivors: Part
1. The impact of bone marrow transplant on quality of
life. *Cancer Nurs* 15:153–160, 1992

174. Ferrell B, Grant M, Schmidt GM, et al: The meaning of
quality of life for bone marrow transplant survivors: Part
2. Improving quality of life for bone marrow transplant
survivors. *Cancer Nurs* 15:247–253, 1992

175. Granai CO, Amado PM, Goldstein AS, et al: Female sexuality and cancer. *Clin Adv Oncol Nurs* 3(2):1–3, 7–9, 1990

176. Loescher LJ, Clark L, Atwood JR, et al: The impact of
the cancer experience on long-term survivors. *Oncol Nurs
Forum* 17:223–229, 1990

177. Auchincloss S: Sexual dysfunction after cancer treatment.
*J Psychosoc Oncol* 9:23–42, 1991

178. Annon JS: *The Behavioral Treatment of Sexual Problems.* Honolulu, Mercantile Printing, 1974, pp 43–47

179. Smith DB: Sexuality and the patient with cancer: What
nurses need to know. *Oncology Patient Care* 4(1):1–3, 15,
1994

180. Shell JA: The psychosocial impact of ostomy surgery. *Pro-
gressions* 4(1):3–6, 8–11, 14, 15, 1992

181. Ofman US: Psychosexual aspects of sexuality in the patient
with cancer. *Oncology Patient Care* 4(1):7, 8, 14, 15, 1994

182. Shell JA, Smith CK: Sexuality and the older person with
cancer. *Oncol Nurs Forum* 21:553–558, 1994

183. Small EC: Psycho-sexual issues. *Obstet Gynecol Clin North Am*
21:773–780, 1994

184. Baron RH: Dispelling the myths of pregnancy-associated
breast cancer. *Oncol Nurs Forum* 21:507–512, 1994

185. Nicholson HS, Byrne J: Fertility and pregnancy after treatment for cancer during childhood or adolescence. *Cancer*
71:3392–3399, 1993 (Suppl)

186. Mulvihill JJ, Byrne J: Genetic counseling of the cancer
survivor. *Semin Oncol Nurs* 5:29–35, 1989

187. Kaempfer SH: The effects of cancer chemotherapy on
reproduction: A review of the literature. *Oncol Nurs Forum*
8:11–18, 1981

188. Kaempfer SH, Wiley FM, Hoffman DJ, et al: Fertility considerations and procreative alternatives in cancer care. *Semin
Oncol Nurs* 1:25–34, 1985

189. Byrne J: Fertility and pregnancy after malignancy. *Semin
Perinatol* 14:423–429, 1990

190. Mulvihill JJ, McKeen EA, Rosner F, et al: Pregnancy outcome in cancer patients: Experience in a large cooperative
group. *Cancer* 60:1143–1150, 1987

191. Mulvihill JJ, Myers MH, Connelly RR, et al: Cancer in

offspring of long-time survivors of childhood and adolescent cancer. *Lancet* 2:813–817, 1987

192. Hawkins MM: Is there evidence of therapy-related increases
in germ cell mutation among childhood cancer survivors?
*J Natl Cancer Inst* 83:1643–1650, 1991

193. Senturia YD, Peckham CS: Children fathered by men
treated with chemotherapy for testicular cancer. *Eur J Cancer* 26:429–432, 1990

194. Green DM, Zevon MA, Lowrie G, et al: Congenital anomalies in children of patients who received chemotherapy for
cancer in childhood and adolescence. *N Engl J Med* 325:
141–146, 1991

195. Robinson WA, Krebs LU: Oncologic disease, in Abrams R,
Wexler P (eds): *Medical Care of the Pregnant Patient: Concepts
and Management.* Boston, Little, Brown, 1983, pp 307–319

196. Brent RL: The effect of embryonic and fetal exposure to
x-ray, microwaves and ultrasound: Counseling the pregnant and nonpregnant patient about these risks. *Semin
Oncol* 16:347–368, 1989

197. Reichman BS, Green KB: Breast cancer in young women:
Effect of chemotherapy on ovarian function, fertility, and
birth defects. *Monogr Natl Cancer Inst* 16:125–129, 1994

198. Doll DC, Ringenberg QS, Yarbro JW: Antineoplastic agents
and pregnancy. *Semin Oncol* 16:337–346, 1989

199. Garber JE: Long-term follow-up of children exposed in
utero to antineoplastic agents. *Semin Oncol* 16:437–444,
1989

200. Barnicle MM: Chemotherapy and pregnancy. *Semin Oncol
Nurs* 8:124–132, 1992

201. Zemlickis D, Lishner M, Degendorfer P, et al: Fetal outcome after in utero exposure to cancer chemotherapy.
*Arch Intern Med* 152:573–576, 1992

202. Kaempfer SH: Reproductive planning, in Baird SB (ed):
*Decision Making in Oncology Nursing.* Toronto, Decker, 1988,
pp 166–167

203. Hoskins IA: Genetic counseling for cancer patients and
their families. *Oncology* 3:84–92, 1981

204. Chapman RM, Sutcliffe SB: Protection of ovarian function
by oral contraceptives in women receiving chemotherapy
for Hodgkin's disease. *Blood* 58:849–851, 1981

205. Glode LM, Robinson W, Gould SF: Protection from cyclophosphamide-induced testicular damage with an analog
of gonadotropin releasing hormone. *Lancet* 1:1132–1134,
1981

206. Mott-Smith ME, Stolberg L: Sexual function and pregnancy, in Casciato DA, Lowitz BB (eds): *Manual of Clinical
Oncology* (ed 3). Boston, Little, Brown, 1995, pp 575–582

207. Redman JR, Bajoruna DR, Goldstein MC, et al: Semen
cryopreservation and artificial insemination for Hodgkin's
disease. *J Clin Oncol* 5:233–238, 1987

208. Milligan DW, Hughes R, Lindsay KS: Semen cryopreservation in men undergoing cancer chemotherapy: A UK survey. *Br J Cancer* 60:966–967, 1989

209. Sweet V, Servy EJ, Karow AM: Reproductive issues for men
with cancer: Technology and nursing management. *Oncol
Nurs Forum* 23:51–58, 1996

210. Kaempfer SH, Hoffman DJ, Wiley FM: Sperm banking: A
reproductive option in cancer therapy. *Cancer Nurs* 6:31–38,
1983

211. Koeppel KM: Sperm banking and patients with cancer:
Issues concerning patients and healthcare professionals.
*Cancer Nurs* 18:306–312, 1995

212. Speirs AL: The changing face of infertility. *Am J Obstet
Gynecol* 158:1390–1394, 1988

213. Meacham RB, Lipshultz LI: Assisted reproductive techno-

logies for male factor infertility. *Curr Opin Obstet Gynecol* 3: 656–661, 1991

214. Seibel MM: A new era in reproductive technology: In vitro fertilization, gamete intrafallopian transfer, and donated gametes and embryos. *N Engl J Med* 318:828–834, 1988

215. Fedele L, Cittadini E, Bortolozzi G, et al: Successful in vitro fertilization and embryo transfer after limited surgery for tubal adenocarcinoma. *Cancer* 64:1546–1547, 1989

216. Levran D, Dor J, Rudak E, et al: Pregnancy potential of human oocytes: The effect of cryopreservation. *N Engl J Med* 323:1153–1156, 1990

217. Abdalla HI, Barber RJ, Kirkland A, et al: Pregnancy in women with premature ovarian failure using tubal and intrauterine transfer of cryopreserved zygotes. *Br J Obstet Gynaecol* 96:1071–1075, 1989

218. Zemlickis D, Lishner M, Degendorfer P, et al: Maternal and fetal outcome after invasive cervical cancer in pregnancy. *J Clin Oncol* 9:1956–1961, 1991

219. Parente JT, Amsel M, Lerner R, et al: Breast cancer associated with pregnancy. *Obstet Gynecol* 71:861–864, 1988

220. Fiorica JV: Special problems: Breast cancer and pregnancy. *Obstet Gynecol Clin North Am* 21:721–732, 1994

221. Petrek JA: Breast cancer during pregnancy. *Cancer* 74: 518–527, 1994 (Suppl)

222. Zemlickis D, Lishner M, Degendorfer P, et al: Maternal and fetal outcome after breast cancer in pregnancy. *Am J Obstet Gynecol* 166:781–787, 1992

223. Shapiro CL, Mayer RJ: Breast cancer in pregnancy. *Adv Oncol* 8(3):25–29, 1992

224. Hoover HC: Breast cancer during pregnancy and lactation. *Surg Clin North Am* 70:1151–1163, 1990

225. Barnavon Y, Wallack K: Management of the pregnant patient with carcinoma of the breast. *Surg Gynecol Obstet* 171: 347–352, 1990

226. Van der Vange N, van Dongen JA: Breast cancer and pregnancy. *Eur J Surg Oncol* 17:1–8, 1991

227. Peters MV: The effect of pregnancy in breast cancer, in Forrest APM, Kunkler PB (eds): *Prognostic Factors in Breast Cancer.* Edinburgh, Livingstone, 1968, pp 65–89

228. Nugent P, O'Connell TX: Breast cancer and pregnancy. *Arch Surg* 120:1221–1224, 1985

229. Petrek JA, Dukoff R, Rogato A: Prognosis of pregnancy-associated breast cancer. *Cancer* 67:869–872, 1990

230. Higgins S, Haffty BG: Pregnancy and lactation after breast-conserving therapy for early stage breast cancer. *Cancer* 73: 2175–2180, 1994

231. von Schoultz E, Johansson H, Wilking N, et al: Influence of prior and subsequent pregnancy on breast cancer prognosis. *J Clin Oncol* 13:430–434, 1995

232. Dow KH, Harris JR, Roy C: Pregnancy after breast-conserving surgery and radiation therapy for breast cancer. *Monogr Natl Cancer Inst* 16:131–137, 1994

233. Danforth DN: How subsequent pregnancy affects outcome in women with a prior breast cancer. *Oncology* 5:23–35, 1991

234. Sankila R, Heinavaara S, Hakulinen T: Survival of breast cancer patients after subsequent term pregnancy: "Healthy mother effect." *Am J Obstet Gynecol* 170:818–823, 1994

235. Petrek JA: Pregnancy safety after breast cancer. *Cancer* 74: 528–531, 1994

236. Hassey KM: Pregnancy and parenthood after treatment for breast cancer. *Oncol Nurs Forum* 15:439–444, 1988

237. Roberts JA: Management of gynecologic tumors during pregnancy. *Clin Perinatol* 10:369–382, 1983

238. Duggan B, Muderspach LI, Roman LD, et al: Cervical

239. Nevin J, Soeters R, Dehaeek K, et al: Cervical carcinoma associated with pregnancy. *Obstet Gynecol Surv* 50:228–239, 1995

240. Sivanesaratnam V, Jayalakshmi P, Loo C: Surgical management of early invasive cancer of the cervix associated with pregnancy. *Gynecol Oncol* 48:68–75, 1993

241. Lee RB, Neglia W, Park RC: Cervical carcinoma in pregnancy. *Obstet Gynecol* 58:584–589, 1981

242. Gordon AN, Jensen R, Jones HW: Squamous carcinoma of the cervix complicating pregnancy: Recurrence in episiotomy after vaginal delivery. *Obstet Gynecol* 73:850–852, 1989

243. Orr JW, Shingleton HM: Cancer in pregnancy. *Curr Probl Cancer* 8:1–50, 1983

244. King LA, Nevin PC, Williams PP, et al: Treatment of advanced epithelial ovarian cancer in pregnancy with cisplatin-based chemotherapy. *Gynecol Oncol* 41:78–80, 1991

245. Rifkin RN, Thomas MR, Mughal TI, et al: Malignant melanoma: Profile of an epidemic. *West J Med* 149:43–46, 1988

246. Riberti C, Marola G, Bertani A: Malignant melanoma: The adverse effect of pregnancy. *Br J Plast Surg* 34:338–339, 1981

247. Shiu MH, Schohenfeld D, Maclean B, et al: Adverse effect of pregnancy on melanoma: A reappraisal. *Cancer* 37: 181–187, 1976

248. Houghton AN, Flannery J, Viola MV: Malignant melanoma of the skin occurring during pregnancy. *Cancer* 48:407–410, 1981

249. Slingluff CL, Reintgen DS, Vollmer RT, et al: Malignant melanoma arising during pregnancy: A study of 100 patients. *Ann Surg* 211:552–559, 1990

250. Wong JH, Sterns EE, Kopald KH, et al: Prognostic significance of pregnancy in stage I melanoma. *Arch Surg* 124: 1227–1231, 1989

251. Rothman LA, Cohen CJ, Astarloa J: Placental and fetal involvement by maternal malignancy: A report of rectal carcinoma and a review of the literature. *Am J Obstet Gynecol* 116:1023–1024, 1973

252. Potter JF, Schoeneman M: Metastasis of maternal cancer to the placenta and fetus. *Cancer* 25:380–388, 1970

253. Anderson JF, Kent S, Machin GA: Maternal malignant melanoma with placental metastasis: A case report with literature review. *Pediatr Pathol* 9:35–42, 1989

254. Brossard J, Abish S, Bernstein ML, et al: Maternal malignancy involving the products of conception: A report of malignant melanoma and medulloblastoma. *Am J Pediatr Hematol Oncol* 16:380–383, 1994

255. Mackie RM, Bufalino R, Morabito A, et al: Lack of effect of pregnancy on outcome of melanoma. *Lancet* 337:653–655, 1991

256. Ward FT, Weiss RB: Lymphoma in pregnancy. *Adv Oncol* 8(3):18–22, 1992

257. Kennedy BJ: Hodgkin's disease. *CA Cancer J Clin* 43: 325–346, 1993

258. Steiner-Salz D, Yahalom J, Samuelov A, et al: Non-Hodgkin's lymphoma associated with pregnancy: A report of six cases, with a review of the literature. *Cancer* 56:2087–2091, 1985

259. Henderson ES: A selected overview, in Gunz FW, Henderson ES (eds): *Leukemia* (ed 4). Orlando, FL, Grune and Stratton, 1983, pp 785–798

260. Caligiuri MA: Leukemia in pregnancy. *Adv Oncol* 8(3): 10–17, 1992

261. Aviles A, Niz J: Long-term follow-up of children born to

mothers with acute leukemia during pregnancy. *Med Pediatr Oncol* 16:3–6, 1988

262. Lilleyman JS, Hill AS, Anderkon KJ: Consequences of acute myelogenous leukemia in early pregnancy. *Cancer* 40:1300–1303, 1977

263. Dekaban AS: Abnormalities in children exposed to x-radiation during various stages of gestation: Tentative timetable of radiation injury to the human fetus. Part I. *J Nucl Med* 9:471–477, 1968

264. Jankowski CB: Radiation and pregnancy: Putting the risks in proportion. *Am J Nurs* 86:260–265, 1986

265. Schapira DV, Chudley AE: Successful pregnancy following continuous treatment with combination chemotherapy before conception and throughout pregnancy. *Cancer* 54:800–803, 1984

266. Doll DC: Chemotherapy in pregnancy, in Perry MC (ed): *The Chemotherapy Sourcebook*. Baltimore, Williams and Wilkins, 1992, pp 703–709

267. Dildy GA, Moise KJ, Carpenter RJ, et al: Maternal malignancy metastatic to the products of conception: A review. *Obstet Gynecol Surv* 44:535–540, 1989

# Chapter 29

# Integumentary and Mucous Membrane Alterations

Michelle Goodman, RN, MS, OCN®

Laura J. Hilderley, RN, MS

Sandra Purl, RN, MS, AOCN

# INTRODUCTION

The effects of radiation therapy and chemotherapy on the skin and mucous membranes can be profound. The oncology nurse is commonly faced with the challenge of deciding how to minimize and manage these complications of treatment. This chapter focuses on how and why these complications occur and creative management strategies.

# ANATOMY AND PHYSIOLOGY

## Integument

### Skin

The skin is the largest organ of the body, receiving approximately one-third of the heart's oxygenated blood. The skin is composed of three layers: the impermeable multilayered *epidermis;* a tough, durable but porous layer called the *dermis;* and a lipid, rich, deep layer called the *subcutaneous tissue* (Figure 29-1).

The epidermis is a stratified (multilayer) squamous epithelium that arises from the outer germ layer, the *ectoderm.* The epidermis forms a resistant surface cover and permeability barrier of varying thickness in different parts of the body. For example, the epidermis on the palms of the hands and the soles of the feet is usually thicker than the epidermis in other parts of the body. The epidermis renews itself continuously through cell division in its deepest layer (*basal layer*) and undergoes keratinization to produce scales that are shed from the outer layer (*stratum corneum*). It is avascular, receiving its nutrient support from the underlying dermis.

The epidermis is separated from the dermis by an anatomic dermal-epidermal junction that welds the two layers together. This interface, consisting primarily of dermal papilla, gives support to the basal cells of the epidermis and acts as a barrier to the movement of inflammatory and neoplastic cells between the dermis and epidermis.

The dermis lies between the epidermis and subcutaneous adipose tissue. It gives the skin its strength, elasticity, and softness. The dermis protects deeper structures from injury and contains blood vessels that regulate body temperature and provide nourishment to the epidermis. The dermis also interacts with the epidermis during wound repair.

The subcutaneous tissue lies beneath the dermis and is composed primarily of adipose tissue that serves as a cushion to physical trauma, an insulator to temperature change, and an energy reservoir. Nerves, blood vessels, and lymphatics that serve the skin course through this tissue.

The functions of the skin are many and include protection, regulation of body temperature, sensory perception, and vitamin D production, which is necessary for bone and teeth formation. In addition, the skin contains an interactive system of immunologic elements including dermal lymphocytes, mast cells, mononuclear phagocytes, and Langerhans cells, which provide an active system of immunologic defense.[1]

Intact skin is the first line of defense against bacteria and foreign substances, physical trauma, heat, or ultraviolet (UV) rays. If this barrier is weakened for any reason, permeability to bacteria, drugs, rays, and so on is increased. Protection against the environment is accomplished by (1) eccrine gland sweating, (2) insulation by the skin and the subcutaneous tissue, (3) regulation of cutaneous blood flow (vasoconstriction and vasodilation), and (4) muscle activity (e.g., shivering). Receptors for heat, cold, pain, and touch are present in the skin, making it possible for the skin to receive sensory stimuli. Another function of the skin is excretion. For example, loss of water and salt through excessive sweating is important for maintaining water balance in the body. Finally, because the skin is the part of the body visible to others, it is a way of communicating feelings and is involved in an individual's body image. The appendages of the skin are the hair, nails, apocrine and eccrine sweat glands, and sebaceous glands. The anatomy and physiology of each appendage will be discussed briefly.

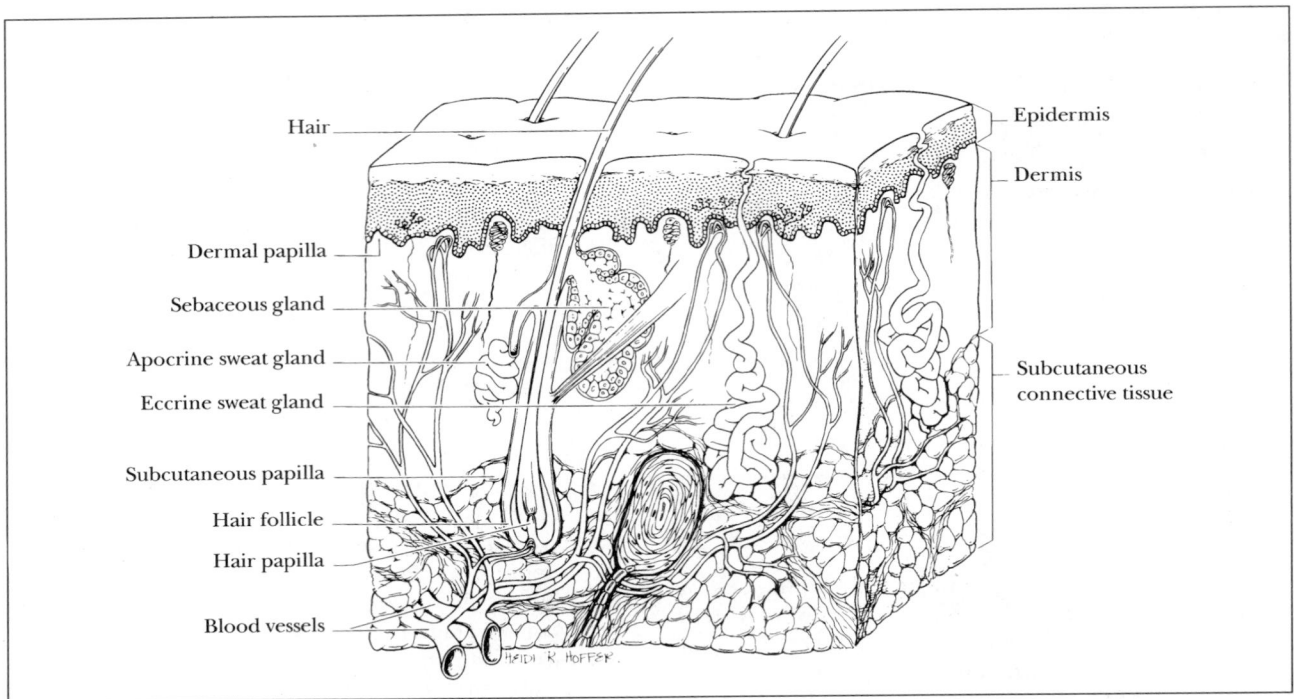

**FIGURE 29-1**   The structures of the skin.

## Hair

Hair, a product of the epidermis, is composed of tightly fused keratinized cells. Hairs are distributed widely over all body surfaces, being absent only on the lips, palms of the hands, soles of the feet, and nipples of the breast. Although the structure of hair is generally the same throughout the body, its thickness, length, and color vary not only in different body locations but also among different people and at different ages of life.

Each body hair develops from a *hair follicle* (a follicular involution of the epidermis). The full portion of the hair projecting from the surface of the skin is the *hair shaft;* the portion under the skin is the *hair root.* At the base of the root is the hair bulb, which is lodged in the hair follicle. At the hair bulb the dermis pushes up to form the dermal papilla, through which the blood and nerve supply reaches the hair. Over the surfaces of the dermal papilla lie the rapidly dividing stem cells (regeneration time of 24 hours) that give rise to the hair.

Human hair growth and loss occur in a continuous cyclic pattern, unlike in other mammals where hair growth and loss are seasonal. There are three phases in the hair growth cycle: anagen, catagen, and telogen.[2] Duration of each phase varies depending on body location of hair.

The *anagen* (growing) *phase* is the metabolically active period involving the growth of a hair from a follicle. The average hair root produces 0.35 mm of hair shaft daily, or 1 cm in 28 days. An average of 85%–90% of scalp hairs are in this anagen growth phase at any one time, but this

may vary from 35% to 100%. Scalp hair remains in anagen for two to six years, or an average of three years.

Generally, the anagen phase lasts longer in women than in men, explaining the existence of longer scalp hair in women. Once anagen has stopped, approximately 1%–2% of scalp hairs enter the *catagen* (transitional) *phase,* in which the follicle no longer produces hair and undergoes involution. Cell division stops, and the follicle shrinks toward the surface. This phase lasts two to three weeks. The *telogen* (resting) *phase* is normally the phase during which the hair is shed. About 10%–15% of scalp hairs are in this phase, which lasts approximately three months. Assuming the adult scalp averages 100,000 hair follicles, it is normal to shed about 100 telogen hairs each day and even more when the hair is washed.

In contrast to scalp hair, hairs located elsewhere on the body (legs, eyelashes, pubic area) have a shorter anagen phase and longer catagen and telogen phases, which explains why these hairs remain short. For example, the eyebrows actively grow for up to 30–60 days and then rest for approximately 105 days.

The function of hair is both physical and psychosocial in humans. Physically, the role of hair is to protect the surface of the skin, to enhance tactile senses, and to provide temperature regulation by conserving body heat. Specifically, scalp hair decreases exposure of the scalp to UV rays and minimizes loss of body heat from the head. Eyelashes and hairs lining the nose and ears act as filters to dust and other airborne contaminants.

Hair also contributes significantly to body image and is closely associated with secondary sexual characteristics.

For the most part, hair has cosmetic value as an adornment. Female or male, how the hair is groomed and styled makes an important statement about one's self-image and identity.

### Nails

The nail is a specialized epidermal structure made of keratinized cells cemented together. Specifically, nails are modifications of the stratum corneum and lucidum of the epidermis. Nails are found on the dorsal surfaces of the terminal phalanges of the fingers and toes. They rest on the nail bed, composed of the germinal layer of the epidermis and underlying dermis. The visible part of the nail, called the *body,* is highly vascular, resulting in the pink color seen through the semitransparent structure. The nail shapes the fingers and greatly enhances the coordinated fine motion of the finger.

### Glands

In humans there are two types of sweat glands: *apocrine* and *eccrine*. Apocrine glands have a duct that opens into a hair follicle, whereas eccrine glands have a duct that opens onto the skin surface independent of a hair follicle. Most of the apocrine sweat glands regress during embryonal life and are found only in limited areas in adults: axillae, nipples, periumbilical region, perineum, and genitalia. These glands become functional just before puberty and atrophy with age. Apocrine sweat glands are odiferous and increase evaporative heat loss.[3]

Some 1.6–4 million eccrine sweat glands are present over the entire body. These glands are especially plentiful in the palms, soles, and axillae and least abundant on the back. The main function of these glands is to cool the body through secretion and evaporation of water. Eccrine sweat glands secrete a thin, watery solution, primarily composed of sodium chloride and some sulfates, phosphates, and urea, known as *perspiration.*

The sebaceous glands are small, sacculated granular organs located in the dermis. Although not grossly visible, sebaceous glands are found in most parts of the skin, particularly on the face, scalp, upper chest, and back. They are not found on the palms or soles. The size and number of sebaceous glands vary from area to area. Each gland opens directly into a hair follicle and is lined by a cuboidal epithelium. Sebaceous glands continually secrete a mixture of fat, fatty acids, and cell remnants called *sebum* that is emptied into the hair shaft. Sebum keeps the skin and hair lubricated, pliable, and waterproof.

## Mucous Membranes

Epithelial membranes are formed in the body by epithelia combined with connective tissue. The major epithelial membranes are the *serous membranes, mucous membranes,* and the *cutaneous membrane* or skin. Serous membranes line the body cavities that do not open to the exterior, such as organs of the respiratory, digestive, excretory, and reproductive tracts. The skin is continuous with the mucous membranes. The function of the mucous membranes depends on their location in the body but may include absorption, transport, or secretion of mucus for lubrication of tissue surfaces. The rapidly proliferating cells of the epithelial layer of the mucous membranes make these membranes sensitive to the effects of both radiation and chemotherapy.

The oral mucosa is the body organ that forms a continuous lining of the oral cavity from the mucocutaneous junction of the lips to the oropharynx. The oral mucosa separates the interior of the oral cavity from the complex underlying organs. Because the oral mucosa is exposed to an aggressive environment in which injury and cell death are everyday occurrences, the epithelial lining of the mucosa constantly renews itself, with cell production meeting cell replacement needs. Maintenance of the integrity of the oral mucosa depends on continuous stem cell replication at the basement membrane. Epithelial cells produced at the basement membrane migrate upward to the mucosal surfaces to replace cells lost as a result of normal sloughing. Complete replacement of the epithelial layer occurs approximately every seven days.

The mucous membranes of the oral mucosa play a vital role in maintaining homeostasis. The primary function of the oral mucosa is to provide a first line of defense against infection. This is accomplished primarily by the epithelial lining of the mucosa. If, however, the integrity of the mucosa is altered and does not succeed in barring unwanted substances, the lamina propria of the connective tissue provides a second line of defense. Similar to the skin, the oral mucosa can both receive and transmit stimuli from the environment (e.g., heat, cold, pain, touch, and pressure). Sensory innervation of the oral mucosa is provided largely by the connective tissue component.

## ALTERATIONS TO THE INTEGUMENT

### Radiation Effects

The skin-sparing capabilities of newer megavoltage, high-energy equipment, and sophisticated treatment planning methods have reduced the incidence of severe tissue complications once associated with radiation therapy. However, certain acute and late side effects of radiation occur due to the effects of radiation on normal tissue and are, for the most part, expected and unavoidable.

The major effect of radiation on dividing cells is reproductive death, which leaves the cell unable to produce viable progeny capable of reproduction. The radiosensitivity of cells determines the degree to which they will be susceptible to injury from radiation as well as when that injury will manifest itself. Cells in a renewal system with rapid turnover and having little or no differentiation (e.g., skin cells, mucous membranes, hematopoietic stem cells) are radiosensitive. Cells that do not divide regularly or at all and are highly differentiated (e.g., muscle cells, nerve cells) are radioresistant. Damage from radiation is apparent early, within weeks to months of first exposure, in radiosensitive cells and is classified as an acute effect of radiation. In contrast, radioresistant cells may not manifest damage for months to years after exposure to radiation. These effects are classified as late effects of radiation.[4]

Acute effects of radiation are usually considered temporary, as the normal cells affected are often capable of repair. Late radiation effects are usually permanent and often become more severe as time goes on. The severity of acute and late effects is dependent upon dose-time-volume factors.[5] Higher doses given over shorter periods of time to larger volumes of tissue will result in more severe acute reactions. Acute damage results from the depletion of actively proliferating parenchymal or stromal cells and is characterized by vascular dilation, local edema, and inflammation. The severity of late effects is more dependent upon the total dose delivered and the volume of tissue irradiated. It appears that damage to endothelial or connective tissue results in late effects that occur as a result of narrowing or occlusion of small vasculature and fibrosis.[6]

It is important to note that the presence or severity of acute effects cannot be used to predict late effects of radiation. Late reactions such as tissue necrosis or dense tissue fibrosis can occur independently of acute reactions.

Side effects from radiation therapy, both acute and late, are local. That is, only those tissues within the irradiated area will be affected. The following discussion will focus on specific tissues of the integument and mucous membranes, their response to radiation, and symptom management.

## Acute radiation skin effects

Rarely can radiation treatments be delivered to a target without first penetrating the skin and its supporting connective tissue. The cells of the skin are highly radiosensitive due to their rapidly proliferating cell population. Maintenance of the skin's integrity depends on the consistent rate of mitotic reproduction in the basal cell layers. Radiation disrupts this balance, resulting in alterations in the skin's integrity.[7]

The acute skin reactions associated with radiation therapy include erythema, dry desquamation, pruritus, hyperpigmentation, and moist desquamation (Table 29-1).[4,7-11] Not all patients will experience all degrees of skin reaction, and many will have several occur simultaneously. For example, brisk erythema may surround patches of moist desquamation, or moist and dry desquamation may exist in adjacent areas being treated with photon and electron beams (see Figs. 29-2, 29-3, 29-4—Plates 10–12, respectively).

Several factors determine the degree, onset, and duration of radiation-induced skin reactions.[4,6,7]

1. *Dose-time-volume factors:* Higher doses given over shorter periods of time to larger volumes will result in more severe acute skin reactions.

2. *Equipment:* The energy or particular beam quality of a machine will influence the surface or skin dose. Electrons will produce greater skin reactions than photons. Electron therapy is often used to deliver high doses to superficial structures such as skin lesions, chest wall recurrence of breast cancer, and dermal lymphatics.

3. *Bolus material:* Placing tissue-equivalent material on the skin reduces the skin-sparing effect of radiation ther-

**TABLE 29-1** Acute Effects of Radiation on Skin

| Tissue Response | Onset/Duration | Clinical Presentation | Physiological Rationale |
|---|---|---|---|
| Erythema<br>Phase I (transient) | Within hours to days of first treatment<br>Resolves after several days but will recur if treatment continues | Faint, often unnoticed redness | Thought to be a vascular response to extracapillary cell injury |
| Phase 2 (erythema proper) | Following 2–3 wk of standard fractionated radiation therapy<br>Resolves 20–30 days following last treatment | Redness that outlines treatment field<br>Intensifies as treatment continues | Intensity greater with higher radiation doses and larger treatment fields (greater amount of vasculature) |
| | | Increased skin temperature | Increased blood flow through dermis from vasodilation |
| | | Edema | Capillary vasodilation with endothelial swelling and increased capillary permeability. Histamine and serotonin are released and microcirculation increases tissue perfusion allowing infiltration of the area by leukocytes. |

*(continued)*

**TABLE 29-1   Acute Effects of Radiation on Skin (continued)**

| Tissue Response | Onset/Duration | Clinical Presentation | Physiological Rationale |
| --- | --- | --- | --- |
| Dry desquamation | Following 3–4 wk of standard fractionated radiation therapy<br>Resolves 1–2 wk after completion of treatment | Dryness, flaking, and peeling often accompanied by itching | Each dose of radiation destroys a fixed percentage of basal cells. Surviving basal cells become cornified and are shed at an increased rate. Noncycling basal cells are stimulated and cell cycle time is shortened. |
| Pruritus | Occurs most commonly when exposure exceeds 20–28 Gy | Itching | Thinning of the epidermis with decreased sebaceous and sweat gland function results in dehydration of the stratum corneum, the water-retaining skin layer. |
| Hyperpigmentation | Following 2–3 wk of standard fractionated radiation therapy<br>Usually resolves 3 mo to 1 yr following completion of treatment, but may be chronic | Tanned appearance | Cornified basal cells carry more melanin into superficial layers of the epidermis and radiation stimulates tyrosinase to convert tyrosine to melanin.<br>Increased melanocyte activity causes cells to become darker. Darker-skinned people may have more hyperpigmentation because they traditionally have more melanin. |
| Perifollicular hyperpigmentation | | Brown dots at hair follicles | Hyperpigmentation of the epithelial cells surrounding hair follicles |
| Moist desquamation | Following 40 Gy or with trauma/excess friction<br>Recovery usually 2–4 wk after completion of treatment | Brilliant erythema<br>Sloughing skin<br>Exposed dermis<br>Serous exudate oozing from surface | Destruction of epithelium. All basal cells have been destroyed and no new cells are yet formed. |
| | | Pain | Nerve endings in the dermis are exposed. |
| Skin regrowth following moist desquamation | Dependent upon severity<br>Usually complete 2–3 mo following completion of treatment | Small areas of epithelium develop<br>New skin is smooth, pink, thin, and dryer | Epithelial cells migrate via proliferation from outside the treatment field and through peripheral migration. |
| | | Gradual thickening of skin over time, but skin does not regain former thickness | Migration occurs best over moist healthy tissue.<br>Fewer sweat and sebaceous glands result in chronic dryness. |

Data from Perez CA, Brady LW,[4] Dow KH, Hilderley LJ,[9] Margolin SG et al,[10] Sitton E,[7–8] and McDonald A.[11]

apy, allowing for maximum dose at the level of the skin. This approach is used to treat chest wall recurrence.

**4.** *Tangential fields:* This approach is used to deliver a more homogeneous dose to the treatment area, but it simultaneously increases the skin dose. This approach is used in the treatment of breast cancer.

**5.** *Concomitant chemotherapy:* The use of radiosensitizing chemotherapeutic agents such as doxorubicin, 5-fluoro-uracil, and actinomycin-D often results in increased severity of skin reactions.

**6.** *Anatomic location:* When treatment is targeted at areas of skin apposition (e.g., axilla, groin, skin folds), increased reaction secondary to warmth, moisture, and lack of aeration can be expected. Patients with ostomies, draining wounds, or tracheostomies in the treatment field are prone to more severe reactions as secretions may create a bolus effect. Treatment delivered over a bony prominence or surgical site may result in increased skin reactions due to alterations in vasculature and circulation.

**7.** *Patient-related considerations:* Normal age-related changes including thinning of the epidermis and dermis, diminished elasticity, and decreased dermal turgor result in delayed healing. Nutritional status must also be considered as appropriate nutrients are needed for cellular repair and wound healing.

### Late radiation skin effects

The late skin reactions associated with radiation therapy include photosensitivity, pigmentation changes, atrophy, fibrosis, telangiectasia, and, rarely, ulceration and necrosis (Table 29-2).[7,9,11]

Not all patients will have noticeable late effects, and those who do will experience them in varying degrees. Factors that may increase the risk and severity of late effects include dose and volume of irradiated tissue (higher total doses delivered to larger volumes) and altered physiological integrity of the tissue. For example, tissues with surgical changes such as fibrosis and those with severely depleted sweat and sebaceous gland functioning are more prone to late radiation skin effects. The potential for late effects limits the total dose that can be delivered to a particular target, which in turn may affect cure.

### Nursing considerations

Nurses play an important role in minimizing and managing the effects of radiation on skin. Nursing responsibilities include skin assessment, patient education, and management of skin reactions.

Initial assessment of the skin in the irradiated field including the exit site is necessary in order to determine the condition of the skin prior to treatment. Documentation should include the patient's present skin condition including surgical changes (edema, scars, unhealed wounds), preexisting skin disorders (skin cancers, psoriasis, maceration), medical conditions (especially those that may affect healing), medications (including past and present chemotherapeutic agents), age-related factors, and nutritional status. Knowledge of the individual's overall plan of treatment is necessary to identify treatment-related factors that may enhance skin reactions.

Skin assessment should be performed prior to initiation of treatment, at least weekly during treatment, one to two weeks following completion of treatment, and at each follow-up appointment thereafter. Consistency in assessment and documentation is imperative. Careful use of terminology related to radiation skin reactions will help prevent inconsistencies in reporting of toxicity. Grading scales are available and provide an objective system of categorizing impaired skin integrity. A commonly used system for grading acute radiation toxicity is one devised by the Radiation Therapy Oncology Group (RTOG) (Table 29-3).[12]

Patient education precedes initiation of radiation therapy and promotes self-care behaviors and optimal outcomes. Patients and their significant others require information regarding the anticipated skin reactions (both acute and late), probable time frame for each reaction including onset and duration, and skin care guidelines to be followed during and after radiation. Table 29-4 offers frequently recommended skin care guidelines. Written instructions are provided as an aid to patient learning. Patients should be informed that side effects usually do not occur for two to three weeks after beginning treatment, that they are usually gradual and become more severe as treatment progresses, and that most resolve two to three weeks after treatment is completed. It is also important to reassure patients that management of side effects and maintaining comfort are priorities. The importance of compliance with recommended skin care guidelines is reinforced frequently during the treatment course.

Management of basic skin care needs during and after radiation therapy is fairly standard, as are the approaches to management of reactions. Management of reactions such as severe dry desquamation with pruritus and moist desquamation is not well documented in the literature. Interventions are based on management goals and what is known about ideal wound-healing environments. Goals include promoting comfort and healing as well as prevention of infection and fluid loss. A clean, moist wound bed permits epithelial cells to migrate from healthy areas to areas of desquamation.[13] Table 29-5 reviews some of the commonly used interventions for severe acute skin reactions.[8,9,14,15] A team approach to managing side effects is most efficient and beneficial. Together, radiation oncologists, nurses, radiation therapists, and patients can often devise a plan that will meet the needs of the patient while ensuring optimal treatment outcomes.

Tissue fibrosis, ulceration, and necrosis are relatively infrequent late radiation skin effects and tend to be chronic in nature; therefore, they can significantly impact a patient's quality of life. Tissue fibrosis occurs in varying degrees from unnoticeable to severe. Moderate to severe fibrosis is occasionally seen in patients who have received surgery and radiation to the head and neck region and to the breast. Significant mobility restriction, pain, and lymphedema can result. Scar tissue integration therapy administered by registered physical or massage therapists is often extremely helpful in regaining mobility and pain reduction. Scar tissue integration therapy "breaks up" or loosens and redistributes scar tissue to increase mobility, decrease pain, and enhance lymphatic drainage. Qualified professionals are able to assess a patient's condition to determine appropriateness of this intervention. Following initiation of therapy, patients are usually instructed on exercises and techniques that can be done at home, which can make this therapy extremely cost-effective.[16,17]

In patients with fibrosis, ulcerations, and necrosis, pain may be a significant problem. A pain management program should be developed to ensure optimal relief of pain. Nonsteroidal anti-inflammatory agents are often effective in managing chronic pain of this nature; how-

**TABLE 29-2**   Late Effects of Radiation on Skin and Connective Tissue

| Tissue Response | Onset/Duration | Clinical Presentation | Physiological Rationale |
|---|---|---|---|
| Photosensitivity | Begins during treatment and is lifelong | Enhanced erythema over skin exposed to UV radiation from sun and tanning beds/booths | Destruction of melanocytes in the irradiated dermis and slower melanin production following irradiation reduce the skin's ability to protect itself from UV rays. |
| Pigmentation changes<br>  Hyperpigmentation | Refer to Table 29-1 | | |
|   Hypopigmentation | May begin anytime following resolution of hyperpigmentation<br><br>Permanent | Lack of skin color | Radiation doses necessary to eradicate cancer may permanently destroy melanocytes, which results in the skin's inability to form pigment. |
| Atrophy | Following epidermal regrowth<br><br>Permanent | Thin and fragile epidermis | Newly formed epidermis is thinner. The epidermis thickens over time, but never attains its preirradiation thickness. |
| Fibrosis | Usually begins 4–6 mo following completion of treatment<br><br>May worsen over time | Dense, hard, uneven skin texture<br><br>If extensive, may cause considerable induration | Fibroblasts, responsible for producing collagen, demonstrate uneven cellular division resulting in faulty collagen remodeling. Fibrotic tissue results, giving the skin an uneven texture. |
| Telangiectasia | Occurs up to 8 yr following radiation therapy<br><br>Permanent | Purple-red, spiderlike appearance of blood vessels in skin | Dose and fraction size–dependent. Basement membrane thickening results in a decreased permeability of material through capillary walls. With capillary occlusion, there are fewer functioning small vessels and a decreased capacity for capillary regeneration. This results in increased pressure of blood flow through remaining undamaged superficial structures. |
| Ulceration and necrosis | Infrequent<br><br>May occur up to 20 yr following treatment<br><br>Usually occurs as a result of inflammation and trauma to previously irradiated tissue | Painful ulcers with red, raised edges and a shaggy, necrotic base<br><br>Usually shows little or no tendency to epithelialize or contract<br><br>Despite local treatment, ulcers tend to deepen and become more painful | Although the mechanism is not clear, late ulceration and necrosis occur as a result of connective tissue damage.<br><br>Electron microscopic studies suggest that permanent damage to fibroblasts and their precursor cells prevents stem cell replication, angiogenesis, and wound contraction.<br><br>Occasionally, sustained vascular occlusion and tissue ischemia may be responsible for ulceration and necrosis. |

Data from Perez CA, Brady LW,[4] Dow KH, Hilderley LJ,[9] Margolin SG et al[10] Sitton E,[7–8] and McDonald A.[11]

ever, narcotic analgesia may become necessary. For basic principles of pain assessment and management in the oncology population, see chapter 20.

Management goals include promoting comfort and healing as well as prevention of infection and fluid loss. Radiation ulcers are often chronic and worsen over time; therefore, assessment of patient compliance and economic status should accompany wound assessment in

**TABLE 29-3** Acute Radiation Toxicities—Radiation Therapy Oncology Group Scale

| | 0 | I | II | III | IV |
|---|---|---|---|---|---|
| Skin | No change | Follicular erythema Dull redness Epilation Dry desquamation | Moderate edema Moist Bright erythema | Moist pitting edema | Necrotic Ulceration Hemorrhage |
| Mucous membranes | No change | Erythema | Patchy mucositis | Fibrinous mucositis Severe pain | Necrotic Ulceration Hemorrhage |
| Salivary glands | No change | Mild mouth dryness Thickened saliva Slightly altered taste | Moderate dryness Thickened saliva Markedly altered taste | Compete dryness | Acute salivary gland necrosis |
| Pharynx and esophagus | No change | Mild dysphagia or painful swallowing—may require anesthetic, nonnarcotic analgesia, soft diet | Moderate dysphagia or painful swallowing—may require narcotic analgesia, puree, or liquid diet | Severe dysphagia or painful swallowing Dehydration or weight loss requiring feeding tube, hyperalimentation, or IV fluids | Complete obstruction, ulceration, perforation, fistula |
| Upper gastrointestinal | No change | Anorexia with ≤5% weight loss from baseline Abdominal discomfort and nausea and/or vomiting not requiring medications | Anorexia with ≤15% weight loss Abdominal pain and nausea and/or vomiting requiring antiemetics and/or analgesics | Anorexia with ≥15% weight loss requiring nutritional support Severe abdominal pain despite medication Nausea and/or vomiting requiring NG or parenteral support | Ileus, subacute or acute obstruction, perforation, GI bleeding requiring transfusion, abdominal pain requiring tube decompression or bowel diversion |
| Lower gastrointestinal | No change | Increased frequency Change in quality Rectal discomfort No medications needed | Diarrhea requiring parasympatholytic drugs Minimal mucus discharge Rectal or abdominal pain requiring analgesics | Diarrhea requiring parenteral support Severe mucus or blood discharge requiring sanitary pads Abdominal distention | Acute or subacute obstruction, fistula, or perforation, GI bleeding requiring transfusion, pain requiring tube decompression or bowel diversion |

Data from Winchester D, Cox JD.[12]

order to develop an appropriate plan of care. A thorough nutritional assessment must also be performed. Successful wound healing requires adequate stores of protein, carbohydrates, fat, vitamins, and minerals.[10,13]

Wound care is individualized, based on the assessment and what is known about the optimal environment for wound healing. Wound beds should be moist, clean, free of debris and eschar, and without evidence of infection. Chronic radiation ulcers are heavily colonized with bacteria, which is responsible for the foul odor often associated with these wounds. Keeping the wound clean and managing infection helps to minimize odor while maintaining the integrity of the skin surrounding the wound. Table 29-6 lists various products used in managing wounds of this nature.

If conservative treatment is unsuccessful in providing wound closure, definitive debridement of the ulcer and underlying fibrotic bed with surgical closure of the wound may be attempted. Surgical wound closure is often unsuccessful for the following reasons: (1) irradiated tissue is fibrotic and unyielding, making it prone to dehiscence; (2) healthy tissue often cannot be reached surgically because the ulcers are so deep; and (3) radiation injury extends beyond the ulcer to surrounding tissues.[13,17] Myocutaneous flaps are the preferred method for surgical closure of radiation ulcers due to the rich vascular supply they provide to ischemic tissue and the greater resistance to infection. With modern radiotherapy techniques and equipment, such severe late tissue effects are uncommon.

**TABLE 29-4**  Skin Care Guidelines During and After Radiation Therapy

While receiving radiation therapy, the skin in the treatment area may become dry, reddened, tanned, and sensitive. Skin changes are usually gradual and become noticeable after 2 or 3 weeks of treatment, becoming more obvious as treatment continues. Care must be taken to protect the skin and prevent trauma. *The following guidelines pertain only to the skin within the radiation treatment field.*

| Guidelines | Rationale |
|---|---|
| **DURING TREATMENT** | |
| Shower or bathe using lukewarm water. Gently wash the area using fingertips. Rinse well and pat dry with soft cloth. | Extreme temperatures may further compromise vasculature. Mechanical irritation such as vigorous rubbing may cause trauma and an increased rate of superficial cell loss. |
| Avoid harsh soap. If it is necessary to use a cleaning solution, use baking soda and water (½ box to one tub of water) or a creamy mild soap made for sensitive skin (Basis,® Neutrogena,® Ivory®). | Perfumed soaps contain chemicals and heavy metal ions that irritate sensitive skin and may enhance skin reactions from radiation therapy. Mild soaps help to decrease the incidence of folliculitis and local skin infections. |
| Do not apply any ointment, cream, lotion, deodorant, perfume, cologne, powder, cosmetics, or home remedy to the skin unless specifically instructed to do so. Pure, unscented, kitchen cornstarch may be used in place of deodorant or to decrease itching. Apply lightly to *dry* skin using a powder puff or cotton ball. | Many products contain heavy metal ions and chemicals as described above. Cornstarch helps to reduce pruritus as well as moisture buildup, especially in the axilla, under the breast, and in skin folds. It must only be used on dry areas as its use on moist areas can promote fungal growth (by forming a glucose-rich environment), thereby increasing the risk of infection. |
| If instructed, apply a recommended mild, water-soluble lubricant to reduce itching and discomfort. Apply 2–3 times/day. Do not apply for at least 3 hr before treatment. | Use of water-soluble, mild aloe-based lubricant containing no heavy metal ions or perfumes is frequently recommended during radiation to prevent trauma from itching, promote comfort, and stimulate fibroblast formation. Examples include Natural Care Gel® (Bard Pharmaceuticals) and Skin Balm® (Carrington Laboratories). |
| Avoid shaving if possible. If it is necessary to shave, use an electric razor. | Shaving increases the rate of superficial cell loss resulting in earlier dry desquamation and can lacerate the skin thereby increasing the risk of infection. |
| Avoid extreme temperatures. Do not use water bottles, heating pads, sun lamps, ice bags, etc. | Irradiated skin has a decreased sensitivity to temperature, which can place the area at a higher risk for injury. Extreme temperatures may further compromise vascular reactions in the capillaries within the treatment area. |
| Avoid tight-fitting clothing made of irritating fabric. Clothes made of cotton or cotton blends are preferred over wool and polyester. If skin becomes irritated from clothing, change to a mild detergent such as Ivory Snow® or Dreft®. | Mechanical irritation caused by tight fitting clothes results in discomfort and trauma to fragile skin. Cotton clothing promotes air exchange and decreases moisture buildup. |
| Avoid exposing skin to sun. Use wide-brimmed hats, long sleeves, and gloves to prevent exposure. Always apply a sunscreen with an SPF of 15 or higher before sun exposure, even under lightweight clothing. | Destruction of melanocytes in the irradiated epidermis and a slower rate of melanin production in new epidermal cells render the skin at higher risk for sunburns. |
| Do not apply tape or adhesive bandages to skin in the radiation treatment field. | Removal can result in mechanical trauma to the already compromised epidermis. |
| Drink at least 3 qt of fluid each day. | Radiation to the skin and sweat and sebaceous glands causes dryness and itching. This is characterized by dehydration of the stratum corneum, the water-retaining layer of skin. |
| **AFTER TREATMENT** | |
| Continue following the above guidelines for 2–3 wk after the completion of treatment. | The acute effects of radiation are cumulative and may be at their peak 5–7 days after the last treatment. Great care must be taken to protect and preserve the fragile irradiated skin. |
| Apply an unscented hydrophilic emollient (lotion or cream) 2–3 times each day for 1–2 mo after treatment and then daily. Examples of moisturizers include Lubriderm®, Alpha Keri®, Nivea®, and Eucerin®. Application to damp (not wet) skin such as after bathing will help to seal in moisturizers. | Obliteration of sweat and sebaceous glands will cause permanent dryness to some degree. Lifetime use of a moisturizer should be encouraged to keep the skin lubricated and prevent fissuring. |
| Always avoid exposing previously irradiated skin to the sun. When this is not possible, use a sunscreen with an SPF of 15 or greater. | Melanocytes in the epidermis have been destroyed by radiation, and production of new cells and regeneration is slow and often not complete. Lifetime care must be taken to protect skin from injury. |

**TABLE 29-5** Management of Severe Acute Radiation Skin Reactions

| Agent | Application | Rationale | Comments |
|---|---|---|---|
| | DRY DESQUAMATION WITH PRURITUS | | |
| 1. Lubricants—water-soluble, aloe-based such as Natural Care Gel® (Bard Pharmaceuticals) and Skin Balm® (Carrington Laboratories) | Increase frequency to PRN Avoid application 3 hr prior to treatment | Decreases itching to increase comfort, stimulates epithelialization, and reduces the risk of skin cracking and fissure formation | Discontinue use if moist desquamation occurs |
| 2. Mild astringent soaks such as Domeboro® solution (Miles Laboratories) | Dissolve one tablet or packet in one quart of water (not one pint as suggested on package). Soak clean cloth in solution, lightly wring out, and apply to irritated area for 15 min 3–4 times a day. May be used in sitz bath for irritation from pelvic irradiation | Causes contraction of tissue and reduces inflammation by forming a protective film over the area, which aids in reducing or preventing fluid loss and infection. Anti-inflammatory response and cooling effect promote comfort. Provides gentle debridement of dead cells and exudate | Solution may be kept for 1 wk if refrigerated in a sealed glass container. May be used for dry and moist desquamation |
| 3. Topical steroids—mild | Apply as directed—usually 0.25% b.i.d. or t.i.d. Avoid application 3 hours prior to treatment. May be used in rectal preparations such as Anusol HC® (Parke-Davis), Preparation H® (Whitehall Laboratories), and Proctofoam® (Reed and Carnrick) | Anti-inflammatory and antipruritic actions. Often used when there is a risk for mechanical trauma from scratching or when sleep disruption occurs from pruritus | Use is controversial as topical steroids may result in further thinning of the epidermis causing the skin to be more susceptible to injury |
| | MOIST DESQUAMATION | | |
| 1. Mild astringent soaks (see above) | | | |
| 2. Hydrogel primary wound dressings such as Vigilon® (Bard Pharmaceuticals) and Spenco Second Skin® (Spenco Medical) | Remove film from one side and place hydrogel portion on the wound or skin. Cover with nonadherent dressing such as Telfa® and secure with paper tape placed outside of the radiation treatment field. May be used following mild astringent soaks | Composed of 98% water and 2% cellulose fiber. Maintains moist environment, protects newly formed epithelial cells from trauma, and increases comfort by covering exposed nerve endings. Mildly absorbent | Expensive. Difficult to secure. Must not be allowed to dry. Dressing can be removed and reapplied for routine soaks and cleaning. Must be removed during radiation treatment |
| 3. Wound cleansers such as Biolex Wound Cleanser (Bard Pharmaceuticals) and Caraklenz® (Carrington Laboratories), and epithelial stimulants such as Biolex Wound Gel® (Bard Pharmaceuticals) and Wound Dressing (Carrington Laboratories) | Cleanse wound with gentle spray b.i.d. or t.i.d. Apply liberal amount of gel to denuded area and cover with nonadherent dressing such as Telfa®. Secure with paper tape placed outside of the radiation treatment field, or flexible netting. | Cleanser aids in debridement and maintenance of wound bed pH. Does not harm proliferating fibroblasts. Wound gel maintains moist environment and stimulates epithelialization. Promotes comfort by covering exposed nerve endings | Expensive. Difficult to secure. Gel must be applied liberally to avoid drying between dressing changes. Must be removed during radiation treatment |
| 4. Occlusive hydrocolloid dressings such as DuoDerm® (Convatec), Restore® (Hollister), Cutinova hydro® (Beiersdorf, Inc.) | Cleanse wound. Choose dressing size that provides 1¼-in. margin around wound. Apply as directed on package. Dressing can remain in place for up to 7 days. Removal—use great care to prevent harm to new skin. If necessary, small amounts of sterile saline may be used to aid in removal. | Maintains moist environment. Promotes rapid epithelialization and aids in debridement. Isolates wound against bacterial contamination. Promotes comfort by covering exposed nerve endings and preventing friction. Absorbent | Cost-effective. Do not use if infection is present. May produce a malodorous yellow-brown fluid that may be mistaken as an infection. If this occurs, remove dressing, cleanse wound, and apply new dressing if needed. Should not be used during treatment as daily removal disturbs wound bed |

Data from Dangel, RB,[9] Lewis F, Levita M,[10] Dow KH, Hilderley LJ,[11] Ratliff C,[16] Hutchinson JJ, McGuckin M.[17]

**TABLE 29-6**  Agents Used in Wound Management

| Classification | Indication/Rationale | Product Examples |
|---|---|---|
| Absorption | Draining, noninfected wounds<br>Absorbs exudate, maintains moist environment<br>Some facilitate debridement | Wound filler products<br>  Debrisan Beads and Paste® (Johnson & Johnson)<br>  Bard Absorption Dressing® (Bard Pharmaceuticals)<br>  Comfeel Ulcus Powder and Paste® (Coloplast-Kendall)<br>  Duoderm Granules and Paste® (Convatec)<br>  Calcium Alginate Dressing-Kaltostat® (Calgon Vestal Labs)<br>  Sorbsan® (N.I. Medical) |
| | See above<br>Reduces pain<br>Prevents mechanical trauma | Occlusive hydrocolloid dressings<br>  Comfeel Ulcus® (Coloplast-Kendall)<br>  DuoDerm CGF and Extra Thin® (Convatec)<br>  Restore® (Hollister)<br>  Cutinova hydro® (Beiersdorf, Inc.) |
| | Absorbs exudate<br>Decreases frequency and number of dressing changes | Nonadherent dressings<br>  Lyo Foam® (Acme United Corp.)<br>  ExuDry® (Frastec Wound Care Products)<br>  Sanitary pads and disposable diapers with nonadherent lining |
| Antibiotics | Use in presence of known infection<br>Positive wound cultures of $>10^5$ bacteria | Topical or systemic<br>Agent dependent upon organism |
| Antiseptics | May be irritating to healthy skin surrounding wound | Hibiclens® (Stuart Pharmaceuticals)<br>Acetic acid 0.25%–5% |
| | Often caustic to wound | Hydrogen peroxide 1% |
| | Use with caution | Povidine iodine 1%<br>Sodium hypochlorite 0.5% (Dakins) |
| Cleansers | Aid in debridement<br>Soften eschar<br>Nontoxic to proliferating fibroblasts<br>pH-adjusted | Biolex Wound Cleanser® (Bard Pharmaceuticals)<br>Granulux® (Dow B. Hickman, Inc.)<br>Caraklenz® (Carrington Laboratories) |
| Debriding agents | Topical debridement of eschar and necrotic tissue | Granulex® (Dow B. Hickman, Inc.)<br>Elase® (Parke-Davis) |
| | May cause local irritation and disrupt granulation | Travase® (Sutilains)<br>Santyl® (Kaal)<br>Dakins solution |
| Deodorizers<br>  Sprays | Applied on dressing, act as odor antagonist—not to be applied directly to wound | Dignity® (Convatec)<br>Medi-Aire® (Bard Pharmaceuticals) |
|  Solutions and ointments | Applied directly to wound, act as odor antagonist and antibacterial agent to reduce odor and promote healing | Chloresium Ointment and Solution® (Rystan) |
|  Dressings | Applied over wound—charcoal absorbs odor | Lyofoam-C® (Acme United Corp.)<br>Carbonet® (Smith & Nephew, Inc.) |
| Epithelial stimulants | Create and maintain moist environment pH-adjusted | Biolex Wound Gel® (Bard Pharmaceuticals)<br>Carrington Wound Gel® and Carrington Hydrogel Wound Dressing®—(Carrington Laboratories) |
| Hemolytic agents | Arrest small vessel bleeds to provide hemostasis | Silver nitrate cauterizing stick<br>Surgical topical thrombin—Thrombogen® (Johnson & Johnson)<br>Absorbables—Gelfoam® and Xeroform® (Sherwood Medical) |
| Hydrogel dressings | Maintain moist environment<br>Reduce pain<br>Minimal absorption | Elasto Gel® (Southwest Technologies)<br>Spenco Second Skin® (Spenco Medical)<br>Vigilon® (Bard Pharmaceuticals) |

*(continued)*

**TABLE 29-6** Agents Used in Wound Management (continued)

| Classification | Indication/Rationale | Product Examples |
|---|---|---|
| Skin barriers | Protect healthy intact skin surrounding wound<br>Should not be applied directly to wound | Sween-A Peel® (Sween)<br>Bard Protective Spray® (Bard Pharmaceuticals)<br>Tincture of benzoin zinc oxide ointment<br>Moisture Barrier Ointment (Bard Pharmaceuticals)<br>Stomahesive |

## Chemotherapy Effects

### Hyperpigmentation

Numerous chemotherapeutic agents are associated with altered pigmentation of the skin. While the etiology of this purely cosmetic reaction is poorly understood, it is possible that the drug or a metabolic by-product of the drug stimulates melanocytes to produce increased quantities of melanin. It is unclear why some drugs are associated with widespread hyperpigmentation and others cause darkening confined to specific areas such as the nails, mucous membranes, or tongue.

Hyperpigmentation occurs more commonly in dark-skinned individuals and in persons receiving alkylating agents or antitumor antibiotics. Patients receiving busulfan often experience hyperpigmentation involving the neck, upper trunk, nipples, and abdomen. This complication occurs with increasing frequency in individuals also experiencing busulfan-induced pulmonary fibrosis.[18]

Hyperpigmentation associated with cyclophosphamide may be diffuse or confined to the palms, soles, nails, or gums. Skin contact with carmustine or nitrogen mustard can result in a contact dermatitis followed by postinflammatory hyperpigmentation.

Hyperpigmentation has been noted following 5-fluorouracil (5-FU) therapy, especially in those patients who receive high-dose weekly infusions with or without citrovorum factor (leucovorin). Hyperpigmentation occurs most readily in sun-exposed areas. Serpiginous hyperpigmented streaks overlying veins used repeatedly for infusions of 5-FU occur without any clinical evidence of cutaneous inflammation, phlebitis, or sclerosis (Figure 29-5).

Bleomycin also may cause a change in pigmentation over the veins into which the drug is given. However, bleomycin is more commonly associated with hyperpigmentation over pressure points (elbows) or with linear streaks occurring in areas of intense scratching, presumably due to a localized vasodilation that results in an increased concentration of the bleomycin in the skin (Figure 29-6).[19,20]

Doxorubicin, busulfan, cyclophosphamide, 5-FU, and etoposide have been associated with hyperpigmentation of the oral mucosa and tongue, especially in African-Americans (Figure 29-7). Doxorubicin and 5-FU also may cause skin darkening over the interphalangeal and meta-

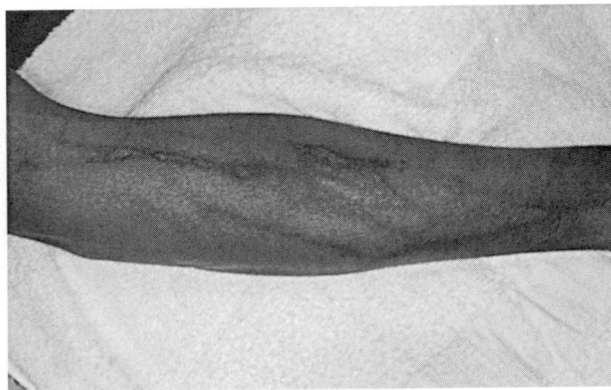

**FIGURE 29-5** Serpiginous hyperpigmentation following 5-fluorouracil infusion.

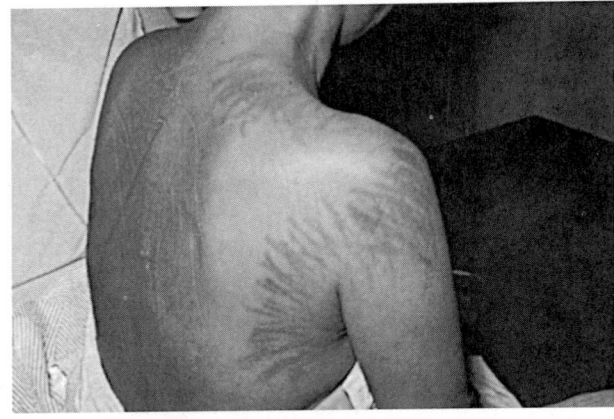

**FIGURE 29-6** Flagellate streaks of hyperpigmentation in an Asian woman occurring in areas of intense scratching following intracavitary (intrapleural) bleomycin.

carpophalangeal joints (Figure 29-8). The mechanism of this effect is not known, but the phalangeal darkening decreases once therapy is terminated.

### Hypersensitivity

Cutaneous hypersensitivity reactions (HSRs) to chemotherapy occur infrequently and tend not to be dose-

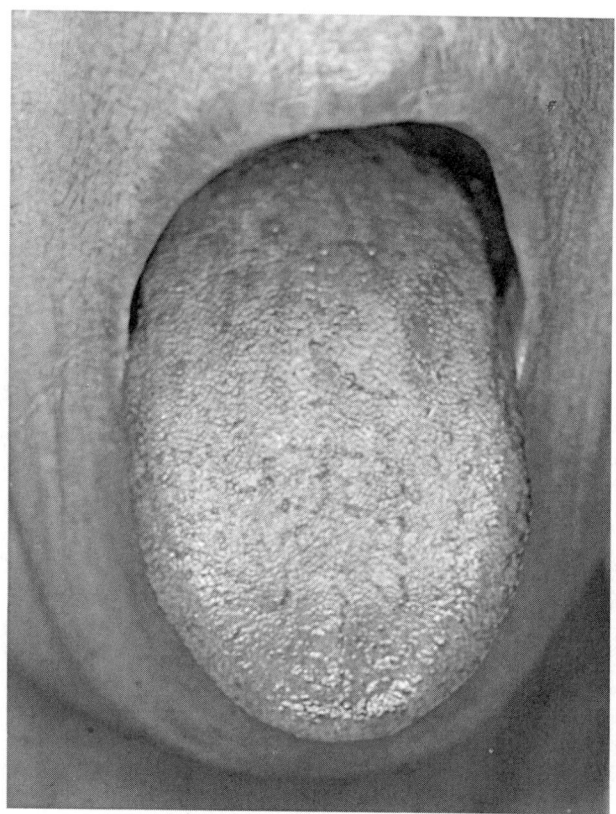

**FIGURE 29-7**  Black tongue following doxorubicin.

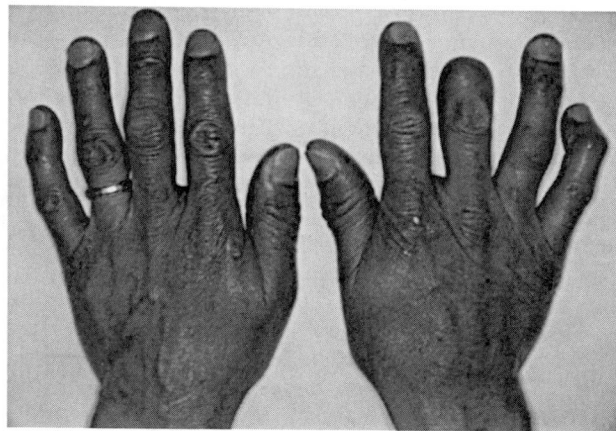

**FIGURE 29-8**  Skin darkening over the interphalangeal and metacarpophalangeal joints.

related. Cutaneous manifestations of immediate HSRs (type I reactions) generally present as urticaria angioedema or anaphylaxis. L-asparaginase, for example, is a polypeptide of bacterial origin that causes HSR in 10%–20% of patients receiving the drug.[21] Acute urticaria is the most frequent manifestation of L-asparaginase HSR,

with 10% of these patients progressing to life-threatening anaphylaxis.[18]

Paclitaxel has been observed to cause hypotension, rash, dyspnea, and bronchospasm within 10 minutes of initiating the drug, suggesting a nonimmunologic anaphylactoid reaction.[22] The cause of this HSR is felt to be due to the drug vehicle, Cremophor EL. Measures to minimize HSR with paclitaxel include prolonging drug infusion time (6–24 hours) and using a three-drug prophylactic regimen consisting of an antihistamine, a corticosteroid, and an H-2 receptor antagonist. Despite these precautions, approximately 2% of patients will experience HSRs.

Docetaxel, another taxane, is formulated in Tween 80 and is also associated with HSR, most notably skin rash, anaphylaxis, and fluid retention. Pretreatment with dexamethasone 8 mg twice daily starting one day prior to dosing and continuing for a total of five days has minimized these reactions.

Parenteral cisplatin, carboplatin, and nitrogen mustard can cause a type I HSR in approximately 5% of patients. The manifestations of this reaction include anxiety, pruritus, cough, dyspnea, angioedema, bronchospasm, rash, urticaria, and hypotension. These symptoms are generally relieved by prompt administration of antihistamines.[22]

Teniposide and parenteral etoposide can cause HSR with the initial dosing, manifesting as dyspnea, wheezing, hypotension, urticaria, pruritus, angioedema, facial flushing, and rash.[23] The incidence is higher with teniposide as it is formulated with Cremophor EL. Decreasing the infusion rate and premedicating with an antihistamine and a steroid generally permits further drug administration.

Other drugs producing rash, urticaria, pruritus, or angioedema include procarbazine, cytarabine, levamisole, alfa-interferon, interleukin, anthracycline antibiotics, melphalan, and methotrexate.

A common side effect of aminoglutethimide is a morbilliform maculopapular skin rash sometimes associated with fever. The rash usually disappears and does not necessitate cessation of therapy. Rarely it can progress and cause desquamation. Hydrocortisone may be given in higher than usual doses for the first two weeks of therapy in an attempt to decrease severity of the skin rash.

Dactinomycin folliculitis presents as diffuse erythematous papules over the face and trunk resembling acne, appearing approximately five days after therapy. The rash resolves in three to five days. Folliculitis has also been reported following administration of high-dose methotrexate.

Erythema multiforme has been infrequently associated with chemotherapeutic agents. Patients receiving high-dose combination chemotherapy are more at risk for erythema multiforme. This reaction is characterized by target lesions over the extremities, often involving the mucous membranes. Busulfan, etoposide, procarbazine, hydroxyurea, bleomycin, methotrexate, and cytarabine have been associated with such lesions, which occasionally develop into generalized blistering (toxic epidermal necrolysis).[18]

### Acral erythema

An intensely painful erythema, scaling, and epidermal sloughing from the palms and soles followed by desquamation and reepithelialization of the skin has been reported with continuous infusions of 5-FU,[24] doxorubicin, high-dose cytarabine,[25] and floxuridine (FUDR) (see Figure 29-9—Plate 13). This condition, also called *palmer-plantar erythrodysesthesia syndrome,* may represent a direct toxic effect on the epidermis and dermal vasculature or an accumulation of the chemotherapeutic agent in eccrine structures and sweat, causing erythema of the palms and soles, where there is a high concentration of eccrine glands.[20] Chemotherapy is usually suspended until symptoms subside and is then resumed at a lower dose. However, the symptoms may recur and may necessitate cessation of therapy.

### Pruritus

***Etiology*** Pruritus, or itching, may be localized or generalized and is associated with many medical conditions. Pruritus may occur in conjunction with thyroid disease, diabetes, anemia, polycythemia, leukemia, multiple myeloma, adenocarcinoma, Hodgkin's disease, non-Hodgkin's lymphoma, and acquired immunodeficiency syndrome (AIDS) and Kaposi's sarcoma. It may also occur as a consequence of obstructive biliary disease or a treatment side effect such as dry desquamation following radiation therapy, as a reaction to opiate analgesics, or an allergic dermatitis following chemotherapy. For example, aminoglutethimide has been associated with a pruritic rash that usually resolves spontaneously. Interleukin can cause a macular erythema most prominent on the head and neck region, with burning and pruritus. Pruritus may also occur as a result of acute or chronic graft-versus-host disease.

When pruritus is due primarily to systemic disease, toxic circulating substances such as peptides, histamine, bradykinin, and serotonin are thought to be the agents responsible for the itching.[26] Pruritus may also be a symptom of infection or a reaction to antibiotics. Whatever the cause, the urge to scratch can be overwhelming and distressing to the individual, as it commonly interferes with rest and sleep and can result in skin breakdown and infection.

***Assessment*** Assessment requires a thorough evaluation of the possible cause of the itching and any factors that might aggravate the condition. If the itching is due to a drug reaction, the condition is generally short-lived and subsides when the drug is stopped or gradually dissipates following antihistamine therapy despite continued administration of the offending agent. When the pruritus is due to Hodgkin's disease, it is often constant and presents as a burning sensation on the lower legs. The itching goes away with successful therapy. If relapse should occur, the pruritus is often the presenting symptom.

The characteristics of the pruritus and the patient's history will further assist in management and include the following: (1) localization, onset, duration, and intensity of the itching; (2) prior history of pruritus; (3) past or present cancer, cancer treatment, noncancer systemic disease, or use of analgesics or antibiotics; and (4) presence of infection. The nurse carefully examines all areas of the skin for any obvious signs of infection or drug reaction, as well as environmental conditions and level of hydration that may contribute to pruritus.

***Management*** Nursing care focuses on three areas: skin care, environmental control, and administration of therapeutics.[27,28]

Dry skin, whether caused by cancer therapy, dehydration, or aging, is subjectively uncomfortable and may lead to itching, skin cracking, and fissure formation. Adequate hydration promotes healthy skin. Drinking 3000 ml of fluid per day and eating a diet rich in iron, zinc, and protein promotes skin integrity. Medicated baths (Aveeno Colloidal Oatmeal Bath®) can be soothing, especially if antipruritic. Local anesthetic creams (e.g., Lanacaine®), emollient lotions (e.g., Lubriderm®, Alpha Keri®, Nivea®) may be useful. Soaps made especially for sensitive skin such as Aveeno Oatmeal Bar®, Neutrogena®, or Basis® should be used when skin cleansing is required. The patient is encouraged to employ alternate cutaneous stimulation methods to relieve the urge to scratch. These include massage, pressure, or rubbing the area with a soft cloth. The patient is instructed to avoid perfume, cosmetics, starch-based powders, and deodorants.

Environmental factors include keeping the room humidity at 30%–40% and the room temperature cool. Cotton clothing and sheets should be washed in hypoallergenic soaps. Distractions such as music, imagery, or relaxation may ease the itch sensation.

Medications may be recommended based on the etiology of the pruritus. If the itch is related to a drug reaction, an antihistamine and corticosteroid may be useful. If it is due to biliary obstruction, cholestyramine is often indicated. When itching is related to an infection, antibiotics or antifungal agents are indicated. Other measures include Aveeno® anti-itch cream, Periactin®, aspirin, Aquaphor, doxepin cream, and Atarax®. Dosages may be increased at the hour of sleep since pruritus generally worsens in the night.

### Photosensitivity

Photosensitivity is an enhanced skin response to UV radiation. This enhanced response may present like a sunburn with erythema, edema, blisters, hyperpigmentation, and desquamation or peeling. Rarely, photoallergy similar to a contact dermatitis with immediate wheal and flare reactions or delayed reactions may occur.

Photosensitivity is caused by a variety of topical or oral medications such as analgesics, antidepressants, antimicrobials, diuretics, antihistamines, nonsteroidal anti-inflammatory agents, and cytotoxic drugs. Photosensitivity has been reported following skin exposure to UV light following administration of 5-FU, dacarbazine, vinblastine, and high-dose methotrexate. In general, the exposed area becomes erythematous within a few hours and gradually subsides. Dacarbazine, however, has been associated with pruritus and erythematous edematous eruptions on the face, neck, and dorsal surfaces of both hands when sun exposure occurred within one to two hours following drug administration.[29]

Patients with cancer often are taking several different prescription and nonprescription medications, many of which can cause photosensitivity reactions. This fact highlights the importance of the oncology nurse obtaining a complete list of all medications that the patient has taken recently or is currently taking. In addition, patients commonly receive both radiation and chemotherapy, which further enhances the potential for photosensitivity.

Melanin commonly protects the skin by absorbing UV radiation from the sun. However, following radiation therapy the skin's ability to protect itself from UV rays is decreased as a result of destruction of melanocytes in the irradiated epidermis and the slower rate of melanin production in new epidermal cells in the radiation field. The newer and thinner epidermis after radiation is more easily damaged and is susceptible to all types of injuries: infectious, chemical, and physical.[7]

Nurses are responsible for educating patients on the dangers of exposure to UV radiation following treatment with radiation or certain chemotherapeutic agents. Verbal and written instructions concerning ways to reduce the risk of developing a photosensitivity reaction are given to the patient. Patients are instructed to avoid tanning booths and to limit their exposure to the sun, particularly between the hours of 10 A.M. and 3 P.M., when the harmful rays are most intense.

Because clouds allow 80% of the sun's UV light to reach the earth's surface, patients are still vulnerable to UV light on cloudy days. Therefore, protective clothing or a hat must be worn to protect areas of irradiated skin.

Most important, nurses provide instructions regarding the proper use of sunscreen based on the individual's skin type. Sunscreens contain a sun protection factor (SPF), which defines the ratio of the time it takes to develop erythema with the sunscreen applied compared with the time it takes to develop erythema without the sunscreen. For example, an individual who can only be in direct sunlight for 30 minutes without erythema may, by applying a sunscreen with an SPF of 8, remain outside for 240 minutes (30 × 8) without burning. The higher the SPF number, the more complete the sun protection. Products with an SPF higher than 15 are generally recommended for use in a tropical climate or for protection following chemotherapy or radiation therapy. Physical sun blocks with an SPF of 25 or more are available and recommended for children and fair-skinned individuals. In general, the greater the SPF, the greater the chance of skin irritation. Some sunscreens and blocks are water-resistant, but in general they should be applied frequently and directly to the skin. To maximize its effectiveness, sunscreen should be applied at least 15–30 minutes before sun exposure and as often as indicated by activities in which the individual is engaged. While some companies are developing products that are long-lasting and stay on until washed off with soap, most water-resistant products will provide protection for up to 40 minutes of continuous water exposure, while waterproof products will protect for up to 80 minutes of continuous water exposure.

## HAIR

### Radiation Effects

Hair follicles in the active growing phase (anagen) represent the most rapidly proliferating cell population in the human body. Rapid mitosis of epithelial cells in the hair root renders it quite radiosensitive; therefore, alopecia is a local effect of radiation therapy. While scalp hair is the most radiosensitive, other terminal hairs are also susceptible to the effects of radiation. In order of decreasing radiosensitivity are scalp, beard, eyebrow, eyelash, axillary, pubic, and fine hair of the body.

Radiation causes premature conversion of hair follicle cells from the anagen to the telogen or resting phase, which results in new hairs being shed at an increased rate. Radiation also affects hair growth and weakens the hair shaft, making it more susceptible to breakage.[14]

A number of factors determine the extent and duration of radiation-induced alopecia, including the total dose delivered to an area, the dose per fraction, the area being treated, and the individual's normal hair growth rate. Hair loss is either complete or partial depending on the treatment field. Complete scalp hair loss is usually seen in patients receiving whole-brain irradiation as treatment for primary or metastatic brain cancer, whereas patients who receive radiation to a portion of the brain will experience hair loss limited to the area treated.

Although hair loss patterns vary slightly, radiation-induced alopecia follows a somewhat predictable pattern. Hair thinning usually begins to occur after two to three weeks of treatment at a dose of 25–30 Gy and continues for an additional two to three weeks. Significant or complete hair loss occurs after a dose of 45–55 Gy has been delivered. While hair loss resulting from radiation to the scalp cannot be prevented, measures should be taken to reduce trauma to the remaining hair and the skin of the exposed scalp. General care of the hair and scalp is reviewed in Table 29-7. If hair regrowth occurs, it usually begins eight to nine weeks following completion of treatment. New hair usually has a slower growth rate, a finer texture, and may have

**TABLE 29-7** Nursing Diagnoses Related to Alopecia

| Diagnosis | Expected Outcome—Patient Will: | Nursing Interventions |
|---|---|---|
| I. Knowledge deficit regarding alopecia related to chemotherapy and/or radiation therapy | I. A. Verbalize understanding of the cause and expected sequelae of treatment-induced alopecia<br>B. Identify available resources related to alopecia | I. A. Assess patient's risk for hair loss related to treatment.<br>B. Inform patient of precise time of hair loss and how it will occur (complete, partial) if possible.<br>C. Explain rationale for alopecia specific to chemotherapy and/or radiation therapy. Discuss:<br>  1. Why hair falls out with specific therapy<br>  2. Variability of hair loss depending on therapy<br>  3. Possibility of hair regrowth—stress regrowth when appropriate<br>  4. Potential change in color and texture of new hair when regrowth occurs<br>D. Encourage verbalization of misconceptions regarding alopecia related to treatment.<br>E. Provide literature and resources related to alopecia. |
| II. Potential disturbance in body image and/or self-concept related to thinning or complete loss of hair | II. A. Verbalize feelings regarding hair loss and identify coping measures<br>B. Describe appropriate interventions to minimize degree and impact of alopecia | II. A. Assess the impact of hair loss on patient and significant other(s). Encourage verbalization of fears and concerns.<br>B. Identify ways to support patient's feelings in such areas as self-worth, masculinity and femininity, social contacts, and work activities.<br>C. Encourage patient to speak with others who have experienced and adjusted to hair loss.<br>D. Offer tips to minimize degree of alopecia:<br>  1. Shampoo gently one to two times/week with a mild protein-based shampoo. Check with radiation therapist before washing hair if marks have been placed on scalp.<br>  2. Rinse well with lukewarm water and gently pat dry with soft towel.<br>  3. Use a soft-bristled hairbrush or wide-toothed comb to reduce stress on the hair shaft.<br>  4. Use a satin pillowcase to minimize rubbing friction on scalp hair while lying down.<br>  5. Avoid use of hot rollers, hair dryers, curling irons, permanents, and hair dyes—all can dry the scalp and damage sensitive hair follicles.<br>  6. Avoid rollers in the hair while sleeping, braids, pony tails, or corn rows.<br>  7. Consider a short haircut—may reduce the weight on the hair shaft and make it easier to manage loose hairs.<br>  8. Utilize hair-preserving measures when appropriate and ordered by physician.<br>E. Provide information regarding wigs or hairpieces prior to hair loss. Include information on:<br>  1. Types of wigs (synthetic vs. human; machine-made vs. hand)<br>  2. Cost, fit, and style<br>  3. Area retailers or available wig banks such as a cancer organization<br>  4. Reimbursement—prosthetic coverage<br>    a. Health insurance companies (provide physician prescription; need invoice from retailer providing service)<br>    b. Tax deduction as medical expense<br>F. Identify wig alternatives.<br>  1. Scarves, turbans, bandannas, sports caps, hats |

**TABLE 29-7** Nursing Diagnoses Related to Alopecia (continued)

| Diagnosis | Expected Outcome—Patient Will: | Nursing Interventions |
|---|---|---|
| | | 2. Use of wardrobe, makeup, and jewelry to highlight other features and help to "feel good about oneself" <br> G. Encourage use of eyebrow pencil, false eyelashes, wide-brimmed eyeglasses to minimize loss. <br> H. Inform patient of "Look Good . . . Feel Better Program." Call 1-800-395-LOOK for information. |
| III. Alteration in protective mechanisms of hair: <br> A. Potential for impaired skin integrity related to scalp hair loss <br> B. Potential for eye injury related to loss of eyebrows and eyelashes | III. A. Verbalize knowledge of scalp care when hair loss is evident <br> B. Identify measures to minimize eye injury related to loss of eyebrows and eyelashes | III. A. Inform patient of the protective mechanisms of hair (scalp, eyebrows, eyelashes). <br> B. Instruct patient on scalp care: <br> 1. Wash scalp gently with mild shampoo 1–2 times/week. <br> 2. Use a head covering to protect scalp from wind, cold, and sun. <br> 3. Always apply a sunscreen with an SPF of 15 or more when sun exposure is expected. <br> 4. While receiving radiation therapy, apply a water-soluble, mild lubricant such as Natural Care Gel® (Catalin Corp), or Skin Balm® (Carrington Laboratories) 2–3 times daily. Do not apply 3 hours before receiving treatment. <br> 5. With chemotherapy cycles or after radiation treatments are completed, apply a hydrophilic lubricant containing no perfume 2–3 times daily. Examples include Lubriderm®, Eucerin®, and Special Care Cream®. Continue applying until hair regrowth begins. <br> 6. Ensure wig lining is comfortable and nonirritating. <br> C. Instruct patient on measures to protect eyes from injury (e.g., use of sunglasses, wide-brimmed hats, false eyelashes). |

a different color. Regrowth is unlikely if alopecia persists for greater than six months. The likelihood of hair regrowth also diminishes with age and higher doses of radiation.[9,14]

To minimize or delay hair loss and scalp irritation, basic hair and scalp care guidelines should be instituted at the onset of treatment. Although purely speculative, some clinicians theorize that the drug minoxidil may decrease the time needed for hair regrowth following radiation-induced alopecia. Even more uncertain is whether or not the drug would have any impact on what is considered to be permanent radiation-induced alopecia. This is clearly an area worthy of research.

Although controversial, hair transplantation by a punch or graft technique is the only reported treatment for permanent radiation-induced alopecia. Limited success for this procedure is thought to be a result of the compromised vascularity of irradiated skin. While it is reported that grafts take, the number of hairs that result per graft is poor. In cases where success has been reported, good technical cosmetic results have improved the patient's quality of life.[30]

## Chemotherapy Effects

### Alopecia

Alopecia is the most noticeable cutaneous side effect of chemotherapy and often one of the most distressing.[31] Although certainly not a life-threatening event, loss of hair has a profound social and psychological impact on individuals and their acceptance of treatment. Some may even refuse potentially curative therapy for fear of this side effect.

Cancer chemotherapeutic agents affect actively growing (anagen) hairs. Since anagen hair is the most rapidly proliferating cell population in the human body, alopecia is a common toxicity manifestation of these drugs. Extent of hair loss can range from thinning of scalp hair to total body hair loss.

With an average 85% of scalp hair follicles in the anagen phase at any given time, the most common location for hair loss is the scalp. The majority of other body hair follicles (e.g., eyebrows, axillae, pubic area) are in the catagen and telogen phases and therefore not initially affected. However, with multiple exposures from long-term therapy these hairs may also be lost as the percentage of hairs entering anagen increases.

Chemotherapy causes the hair shaft to be fragile or defective and thereby subject to breakage with minimal trauma. Mitotic activity is inhibited within the hair matrix such that hair shaft formation is impeded.

Higher doses of chemotherapy or more potent epilators cause complete mitotic arrest, resulting in atrophy of the root and loss of the hair root bulb. Hair falls out spontaneously or is lost easily when combed or washed. Drugs of less intensity temporarily inhibit or slow cellular activity, causing bulb deformity and narrowing of the hair shaft. When hair growth resumes again, narrow, weakened hair shafts are prone to breakage at the point of constriction. The hair root, however, remains intact and active, leaving a thinning pattern of hair loss.

Unlike natural hair loss, chemotherapy-induced alopecia occurs rapidly and usually starts two to three weeks following a dose of chemotherapy. It is most apparent after one to two months. Hair loss is diffuse and usually asymptomatic; however, some patients have described intense scalp discomfort one to two days prior to and during hair shedding. Mild pain relievers may be necessary.

The cytotoxic injury to hair follicles is essentially temporary and reversible. After discontinuation of the epilating drugs, regrowth is visible in four to six weeks, but complete regrowth may take one to two years. In situations involving very high doses of alkylating agents (bone marrow transplant), hair may not regrow.[32] Fortunately, this is an uncommon occurrence. In fact, regrowth may occur during active treatment because of developed drug resistance by cells of the hair matrix. As hair grows back, alterations in hair pigmentation (lighter or darker), hair texture (finer or coarser), and hair type (straight or curly) may be evident.

The severity and duration of chemotherapy-induced hair loss are related to several drug factors including the type of drug or combination of drugs, dose of drug (acute and cumulative), method of administration and pharmacokinetics, as well as patient-related factors. Contrary to public perceptions, all cytotoxic drugs do not cause hair loss. Rather, hair loss is a common side effect of a number of drugs that are used frequently in cancer treatment. Cytotoxic agents with the potential to cause alopecia when given alone or in combination include bleomycin, cyclophosphamide, dactinomycin, daunorubicin, doxorubicin, etoposide, 5-FU, hydroxyurea, idarubicin, docetaxel, ifosfamide, methotrexate, mitomycin, mitoxantrone, melphalan, paclitaxel, and vinblastine.

Bolus intravenous administration of chemotherapy results in immediate peak serum levels with subsequent exposure and damage of sensitive growing hairs resulting in hair loss. Infusions over several hours or longer are associated with a greater likelihood of alopecia. The risk of alopecia appears to be decreased with low-dose continuous infusion. This may be related to the fact that high peak serum levels are necessary to cause hair loss.

A patient-related factor that may influence the degree of scalp hair loss is the variability of scalp hair growth among individuals. Individuals who have relatively few hairs in the proliferative (anagen) phase will be less sensitive to the epilatory effects of chemotherapy. Another factor that must be considered is the condition of the patient's hair before treatment. Damaged hair (tinted, permed) may potentiate the risk for alopecia.

Other factors such as noncytotoxic drugs (e.g., heparin, propranolol, ibuprofen) and medical conditions (e.g., malnutrition, chronic stress, hypothyroidism) may also contribute to or cause alopecia in the cancer patient.[18]

### Prevention of alopecia

Since the 1960s through 1990 considerable efforts have been directed at reducing the incidence and severity of alopecia using empirical methods like scalp tourniquet[33,34] and scalp hypothermia.[35–38] The rationale is that each causes vasoconstriction of the superficial scalp veins, temporarily preventing drug uptake to the hair follicle and thereby preserving scalp hair.

Scalp hypothermia is thought to be more advantageous because it reduces cellular uptake of drugs that are temperature-dependent such as doxorubicin. Additionally, scalp hypothermia theoretically may lower the metabolic rate of cells, rendering hair follicles less susceptible to the epilatory effects of chemotherapeutic drugs.

Reviews of studies employing these methods report neither to be particularly useful in prevention of alopecia.[38,39] Although scalp cooling can sometimes be successful when an anthracycline (e.g., doxorubicin) is the sole alopecia-inducing drug, this method is less effective when doses exceed 50 mg/m$^2$ and when used in combination with cyclophosphamide.

Since the onset of hair preservation methods, several cases of scalp metastases have been reported following their use.[40,41] Therefore, these techniques are not recommended for all patients. In particular, they are contraindicated in patients with hematologic malignancies, with solid tumors that originate in the scalp, or with tumors that have a high incidence of scalp metastases. Risk of scalp micrometastasis must be considered especially when treating patients with curative intent.

Because of questions raised regarding the safety and efficacy of hypothermia devices in the prevention of chemotherapy-induced alopecia, manufacturers were requested by the Food and Drug Administration (FDA) to provide clinical data supporting their use. When no documentation was submitted, the FDA rescinded marketing approval effective January 1990 until proof is obtained.[42]

Even though commercial devices are unavailable for purchase, some institutions still provide scalp hypothermia for selected patients (e.g., the incurable patient, or the individual who would otherwise refuse potential curative treatment). For patients considering hair preservation techniques, discussion must include weighing the benefits (hair preservation) versus the risks (developing scalp metastases at a later date). Some institutions require the patient to sign an informed consent that becomes part of the patient's medical record.[43]

Protection from chemotherapy-induced alopecia has been preliminarily explored in animal models. In two separate but related studies using the biologic response modifiers Imu Ver® and interleukin-1 hair protection was demonstrated against cytosine arabinoside and doxorubicin (cell-cycle specific agents) but not against cyclophosphamide (cell-cycle nonspecific agent).[44,45] Additionally, the studies highlighted the different mechanisms by which hair loss is caused. The clinical relevance of these observations is as yet unknown.

The stigma associated with hair loss has also promoted research with products that have shown efficacy in male pattern baldness such as minoxidil. Although known to induce hair regrowth and prevent hair loss in male pattern baldness, minoxidil 2% topical solution has shown no benefit in prevention of chemotherapy-induced alopecia,[46] but may have a positive effect on regrowth.[47] Further research may be beneficial to evaluate minoxidil's role in accelerating regrowth of hair following treatment-related alopecia.

## Nursing Care

Hair contributes greatly to body image and is associated closely with one's sexuality. Consequently, the potential or actual loss of one's hair can have a devastating emotional impact on a patient and may represent a significant threat to self-image. In light of the absence of hair-preserving techniques, more emphasis needs to be placed on the psychological support of the patient experiencing hair loss from cancer treatment and creative measures to preserve self-image (Table 29-7).

It is essential that the nurse give the patient and family an adequate appraisal of the potential for treatment-related alopecia. The timing, extent, and duration of hair loss are addressed at the onset of therapy. While these are not always known, many times they are; for instance, when high-dose doxorubicin and cyclophosphamide are used, hair loss is nearly complete by three weeks. Patients should be encouraged to discuss their feelings regarding hair loss whether it is to be temporary or permanent. Great care must be taken not to minimize the potential impact on self-image.

It is often helpful for patients to prepare for probable alopecia by procuring a scalp prosthesis (wig or hairpiece) before it becomes necessary. This often reduces the anxiety associated with the uncertain timing of hair loss and makes it easier for a stylist to match color and style. Clinicians should encourage patients to question their insurance carriers regarding coverage for a "cranial therapeutic prosthesis for treatment-induced alopecia." Some insurance companies will reimburse with a physician's prescription and/or letter. Table 29-8 reviews suggestions for wig procurement and insurance reimbursement.

**TABLE 29-8   Tips for Wig Selection**

1. Select and purchase a wig prior to hair loss so hair color and style can be matched. If hair has thinned or complete loss has occurred, bring photographs to match.
2. Bring someone along whose opinion you trust.
3. If you need or want privacy, phone for an appointment or consultation.
4. Where to purchase: department stores, hair salons, and full-service wig stores. Ask your nurse or physician for area resources or contact your local cancer society.
5. Types of wigs: Wigs vary—human hair wigs are more costly and need more servicing; synthetic wigs are less expensive, easier to style, washable, and need less care. *Both look natural.*
6. Price: Ask what is included in the cost. Consider charges for fitting, altering, styling, accessories such as wigstand, shampoo, etc.
7. How to look natural: Consider *fit* (close on your head and feeling comfortable), *color* (choose one close to your own), *style* (handmade vs. machine-made). For men, hand-tied is best choice because of the need for close styling.
8. How many wigs: Life expectancy of a wig worn on a daily basis given proper care is 6 months; therefore, two wigs are preferred if hair loss is expected to be greater than 6 months.
9. Care of wig:

   Synthetic—wash with cold water using a capful of wig shampoo, do not brush when wet, and keep away from excess heat
   Human hair—as you care for normal hair
10. How to obtain insurance coverage for wig:
    - Get prescription from physician—"cranial therapeutic prosthesis for medical indication."
    - Obtain receipt from person servicing the wig.
    - Know your rights as the insured party and process claim.
    - If claim denied—appeal and ask for review by medical review board.
11. Alternative options to wigs: cap and hairpiece or scarf-type cap combinations
    - HEADLINER (Designs for Comfort, Inc., 1-800-443-9226)
    - Classicap™ (Susan's Special Needs, 1-800-497-7005)

Although alopecia is not preventable, certain measures may minimize or delay hair loss and scalp irritation. For example, some clinicians advise patients to cut long hair short in anticipation of hair loss. Short hair may make hair loss less noticeable, make remaining hair appear thicker, and possibly decrease the weight on the hair shaft. On the other hand, if hair is thinning or radiation therapy is given to a portion of the scalp, causing a balding area, longer hair may be a better style to camouflage thinning or lost hairs.

Once hair loss is significant, necessitating a wig or head covering, the patient may be advised to shave the remaining scalp hairs. This practice allows the hair to grow in at the same length, often permitting the patient to go without a wig sooner. In addition, shaving the head rids the patient of the problem of continuous shedding of hair.

Hair management to minimize hair loss should begin at the onset of therapy expected to cause alopecia. Recommendations should include using mild protein-based shampoos with conditioners, avoiding daily shampooing, allowing hair to dry naturally and grooming hair with wide-toothed combs.

The use or nonuse of hair care practices such as blow-drying, perming, or coloring hair is controversial and an area for further nursing research. Some claim these practices cause the hair to become brittle and fall out faster during chemotherapy, while others have not found these practices to be related to postchemotherapy hair loss.

The nurse is often the preferred person to assist patients in coping with personal image needs. Ehmann et al[48] describe an independent oncology nursing consultative service developed to intervene with patients at risk for alopecia. Other enterprising nurses have provided patients with an "alopecia packet" that includes a booklet describing hair loss and a cotton turban head covering[49] or have established the Scarf Bank, offering patients an alternative to wearing a wig.[50] A videotape demonstrating the best ways to wear the scarf is also available. Other motivational videotapes may facilitate nursing interventions for patients adapting to hair loss. One available resource is *The Beauty of Control: Overcoming the Cosmetic Side Effects of Cancer Treatment*, Medical Video Productions (800-822-3100).

Finally, guidelines are available for enhancing the appearance of patients undergoing chemotherapy and/or radiation therapy. The "Look Good . . . Feel Better" program is a national program developed by the American Cancer Society, the Cosmetology, Toiletry and Fragrance Association (CTFA) Foundation, and the National Cosmetology Association to offer women assistance and workable solutions for hair loss, skin care, and cosmetic concerns. Components of this program have been combined with a fashion show and one-to-one consultation as part of a rehabilitation program to restore self-image and self-esteem after cancer treatment.[51] Appearance mirrors positive attitude, and positive feelings enhance one's ability to cope.

## Hirsutism

Androgens are efficacious in the treatment of women with breast cancer, especially postmenopausal women with bone metastases. Troublesome side effects include loss of hair in the frontotemporal portion of the scalp (male pattern baldness) and hirsutism. *Hirsutism* is characterized by an excessive growth of hair in androgen-dependent areas of the body including the upper lip, chin, chest, abdomen, and anterior aspects of the thighs. The intensity of this side effect depends on the amount of drug taken, with distribution of hair returning to normal after the androgen is discontinued. Clinicians need to be aware that this excess hair growth may cause a great deal of distress and lead to refusal of treatment and non-compliance.

Nursing interventions are aimed at providing emotional support for body changes. Excess hair can be removed by tweezing or shaving. Electrolysis is not recommended unless approved by a physician because of the increased possibility of skin irritation and infection. If the hair is fine, bleaching may mask the condition.

## NAILS

While it is similar to that of a hair follicle by virtue of its rapidly proliferating cell population, the radiosensitivity of a fingernail or toenail is not usually of consequence in patients receiving radiation therapy. Rarely are these structures included in the radiation treatment field; however, there are exceptions. Patients receiving low-dose total-body irradiation (12–15 Gy) prior to bone marrow transplantation usually have minimal nail effects, while those patients whose nails receive higher doses (25–30 Gy), as seen in treatment for mycosis fungoides, may lose the nail(s). Radiation to the nail can result in decreased growth rates and the development of ridges when the nail attempts to grow. While nothing can be done to prevent nail changes when these structures are irradiated, patients need to be aware of the potential effects.[4,9]

Changes in the fingernails and toenails are commonly seen during chemotherapy. Pigmentation is seen most commonly and occurs with more regularity and intensity in African-Americans than in whites. The pigment generally is deposited at the base of the nail, causing transverse dark bands that correlate with the times the drug was administered. This reaction occurs most commonly with doxorubicin and cyclophosphamide but has been reported with melphalan, 5-FU, daunomycin, and bleomycin. If continuous infusion therapy of these drugs is given, the nails darken evenly.

Beau's lines (transverse white lines or grooves in the nail) indicate a reduction or cessation of nail growth in response to cytotoxic therapy. A partial separation of the nail plate (onycholysis) can be seen with 5-FU, doxorubicin, docetaxel, and bleomycin therapy.[18] (see Figure 29-10).

## GLANDS

Sebaceous glands are composed of cells that are destroyed and used in the production of sebum, which keeps the skin and hair lubricated and pliable. These cells undergo replacement through continuous cellular proliferation and, as a result, are radiosensitive. The loss of oil in the skin secondary to impairment or destruction of sebaceous glands is in large part responsible for the acute and late skin effects associated with irradiated skin such as pruritus and inelasticity.[4,26]

Irradiation of sweat glands can also contribute to the

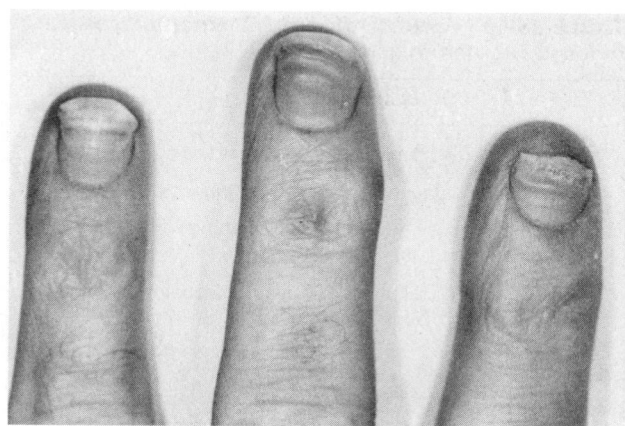

**FIGURE 29-10**   Nail separation following docetaxel therapy.

dryness of treated skin. The cells of sweat glands have long lives with a slower renewal system, making them only moderately radiosensitive. Complete and permanent destruction of sweat gland function occurs with a skin dose greater than 30 Gy delivered in three weeks, leaving the skin dry and itchy.

Great care must be taken to protect dry, irradiated skin as it is more susceptible to fissuring, subsequent infection, and late necrosis. Table 29-4 reviews basic post-irradiation skin care.

# ALTERATIONS OF THE GASTROINTESTINAL MUCOUS MEMBRANES

*Mucositis* is a general term that describes the inflammatory response of mucosal epithelial cells to the cytotoxic effects of chemotherapy as well as localized radiation therapy. Painful ulceration, hemorrhage, and secondary infection may develop when mucositis is not detected early or continues untreated. Since all mucous membrane–covered surfaces exhibit similar patterns of growth, replacement, and function, any mucous membrane–bearing site in the gastrointestinal (GI) tract from mouth to rectum or the vagina can be adversely affected by cancer treatment.

The epithelial cells lining the GI mucosa renew rapidly, which enables them to replace cells lost from general "wear and tear" that occurs when food is chewed, swallowed, digested, and eliminated from the body. Toxicity (mucositis) results when these mucosal cells damaged by cancer treatment are unable to adequately repair and replace normal cell loss. Manifestations of GI toxicity that will be discussed include mucositis in the oral cavity (stomatitis), in the esophagus (esophagitis), and in the intestines as diarrhea (enteritis).

## Stomatitis

The oral mucosa, with its rapid proliferation rate, is a prime target for complications secondary to cancer treatment, affecting approximately 400,000 patients annually.[52] The incidence is greatest for patients in high-risk categories such as those with leukemia, those receiving radiation therapy to the head and neck region, and those receiving more complex and intense treatment modalities such as bone marrow transplantation (BMT). Virtually all patients who receive radiation therapy to the head and neck region will experience oral mucositis, especially when the total dose exceeds 50 Gy.[53]

Oral complications resulting from treatment may be acute and/or chronic. Acute reactions include mucosal inflammation and ulceration, infection, and mucosal bleeding. Chronic complications occur as a result of changes in healthy tissue and include xerostomia, taste alterations, trismus, and soft-tissue and bone necrosis. In BMT patients, acute and chronic oral graft-versus-host disease (GVHD) is also observed.

The many factors contributing to the occurrence and severity of these complications are listed in Table 29-9. Recognition of these stressors and development of pretreatment and treatment strategies to minimize or prevent oral problems may result in decreased frequency, decreased morbidity, and an increase in patient well-being.

### Chemotherapy-induced stomatitis

Chemotherapy affects the oral mucosa either directly at the cellular level where the drug is destroying prolifer-

**TABLE 29-9**   Factors Contributing to Stomatitis in the Cancer Patient

Poor oral hygiene

Preexisting dental problems
  Dental caries
  Periodontal disease
  Partially erupted third molars

Exposure to irritants
  Chemical (citrus fruits, spicy foods)
  Physical (coarse food, ill-fitting dental prosthesis)
  Thermal (extremes in food temperatures)
  Tobacco and alcohol

Dehydration

Malnutrition

Drug therapy
  Antibiotics
  Chemotherapy
  Steroids

Radiation therapy
  Head and neck area

Surgical manipulation

Immunosuppression and myelosuppression
  Cancer
  Cancer therapy

ating cells (direct stomatotoxicity) or indirectly as a result of the drug's myelosuppressive action (indirect stomatotoxicity) (see Figure 29-11).[54]

**Risk factors**    The risk of developing chemotherapy-induced stomatitis is not the same for all patients, nor is it equal in similar drug regimens. Both patient-related and drug-related factors influence the incidence and severity (Table 29-10).

Diagnosis and aggressiveness of the chemotherapy regimen are predictors of oral complications. Breast cancer patients can have as low as a 12% risk and non-Hodgkin's lymphoma patients a 33% risk, compared with a 70% risk in leukemia patients.[53] The frequency of oral problems is two to three times higher in patients with hematologic malignancies than with solid tumors.[55] Stomatitis occurs more commonly in younger than older patients. The higher mitotic index of the oral mucosa and higher incidence of hematologic malignancies in the younger patient population may explain the age-related risk factor.

Preexisting oral disease (e.g., dental caries, periodontal disease, partially erupted third molars) as well as poor oral hygiene and local irritants (e.g., ill-fitting dental prostheses, tobacco, alcohol) will predispose chemotherapy patients to an increased risk of oral complications. Furthermore, research has substantiated that oral complications can be reduced or eliminated by meticulous oral assessment with interventions before, during, and between courses of chemotherapy.[56]

One of the most important variables influencing stomatotoxicity is the choice of cytotoxic agent. Nearly all chemotherapy drugs can cause some degree of stomato-

**TABLE 29-10**    Factors Affecting Chemotherapy-Induced Stomatotoxicity

| PATIENT-RELATED |
| --- |
| Type of disease (incidence higher in hematologic vs. solid tumor) |
| Age of patient (frequency greater in younger vs. older) |
| Condition of oral cavity pretreatment (preexisting oral or dental disease increases risk) |
| Level of oral care (risk decreases with adequate oral hygiene measures prior to, during, and between treatments) |

| DRUG-RELATED |
| --- |
| Drug (most frequently associated with antimetabolites and antitumor antibiotics) |
| Dose (more common with higher cumulative doses) |
| Administration schedule (eg, incidence increased with continuous infusion 5-FU vs. intravenous bolus 5-FU) |
| Drug metabolism (risk increases with impaired renal and hepatic function) |
| Concomitant therapy (increased risk with stomatotoxic drugs used concurrently with head and neck irradiation) |

toxicity. Those agents most associated with stomatitis are the antimetabolites and antitumor antibiotics, in particular bleomycin, doxorubicin, daunorubicin, 5-fluorouracil, and methotrexate (Table 29-11 and Figure 29-12—plate 14).

Although stomatotoxicity generally is dose-related and is more common with higher doses, patients differ in their ability to tolerate a given dose or combination. There is no way to predict which new patient will manifest oral mucositis and which will not, given the same dose of the same drug. However, those who develop stomatitis with one cycle of therapy will almost assuredly develop recurrence in subsequent courses unless the drugs or doses are changed.[57] This is especially the case when the body is unable to adequately eliminate a stomatotoxic drug. For example, in the presence of renal dysfunction or liver dysfunction, excretion of methotrexate and doxorubicin, respectively, may be compromised. Stomatotoxic drugs used in combination or combined with head and neck irradiation may also increase the degree of stomatitis. Mucositis is observed more often with 5-FU when combined with other mucositis-producing drugs such as methotrexate and doxorubicin and when 5-FU is given concurrently with leucovorin to augment its cytotoxicity.[58]

**Direct stomatotoxicity**    Direct stomatotoxicity results from the cytotoxic action of drugs on the cells of the oral basal epithelium causing a decrease in the rate of cell renewal. The sequelae are a thinned atrophic mucosa and initiation of an inflammatory response (stomatitis). Most often affected are the nonkeratinized mucosal areas including the buccal and labial mucosa, tongue, soft

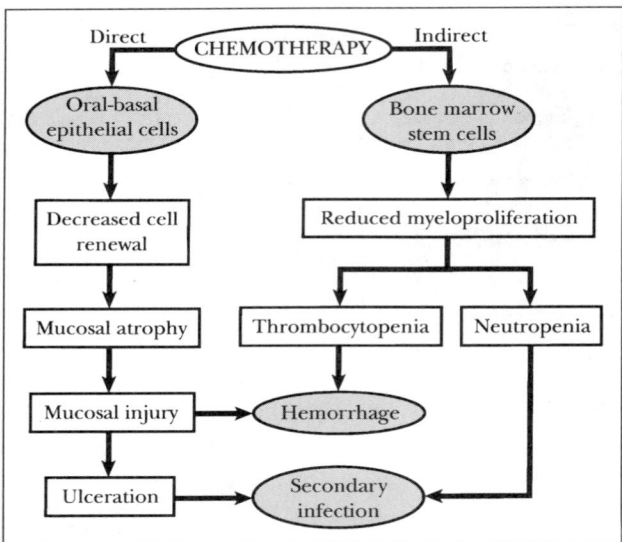

**FIGURE 29-11**    Stomatotoxic effects of chemotherapy. (Adapted with permission from Lockhart PB, Sonis ST: Relationship of oral complications to peripheral blood leukocyte and platelet counts in patients receiving cancer chemotherapy. *Oral Surg* 48:21–28, 1979.)

**TABLE 29-11**  Chemotherapeutic Drugs with Potential to Cause Stomatotoxicity

Antimetabolites
   Cytosine arabinoside
   Floxuridine
   5-Fluorouracil*
   6-Mercaptopurine
   Methotrexate*
   6-Thioguanine

Antibiotics
   Bleomycin*
   Dactinomycin*
   Daunorubicin
   Doxorubicin*
   Mitomycin

Alkylating agents
   Cyclophosphamide
   Nitrogen mustard

Plant alkaloids
   Vinblastine
   Vincristine
   Paclitaxel
   Docetaxel

Miscellaneous
   Hydroxyurea
   Procarbazine

*Frequently associated.

palate, and floor of the mouth. Rarely is the gingiva, or hard palate, involved.

Histologic changes can occur within five to seven days of initial drug exposure. A dry mucosa, tongue or lips; burning sensation in the oral cavity; and increased salivation result. Visible signs of inflammation and oral ulceration can be observed seven to ten days following therapy, just prior to the granulocyte nadir. Without complications and further insult from repeated drug administration, stomatitis is self-limiting and gradually reverses itself within two to three weeks in the nonmyelosuppressed patient. However, if a break in mucosal integrity occurs, secondary infection leading to sepsis can occur.

Oral pain is the major clinical problem associated with stomatitis. Pain results due to sloughing of the superficial epithelium, inflammation of the oral mucosa, and ulceration, making it difficult for patients to practice adequate oral hygiene, eat properly, and communicate. Treatment of drug-induced stomatitis is essentially palliative, involving topical anesthetics, analgesics, coating agents, and cleansing mouthwashes. In some situations (e.g., BMT) oral pain can be severe, necessitating intravenous analgesics by either intermittent or continuous infusion.

*Xerostomia*  Another potential direct effect on the oral mucosa following chemotherapy is salivary gland dysfunction, a decrease in the quality and quantity of saliva. Patients complain of dry mouth and accumulation of thick, ropy saliva that can interfere with nutrition, taste, and speech. Xerostomia is transient, with treatment aimed at lubricating the oral mucosa and alleviating pain. However, if prolonged, xerostomia may precipitate oral caries as well as candidal infections. Saliva substitutes, frequent rinses with ice water, chewing sugarless gum, or sucking hard sour candy may provide sufficient relief.

*Taste alterations*  Patients receiving chemotherapy may be susceptible to taste alterations in which there are actual or perceived changes in taste sensations. The drugs cause direct injury to taste cells composing the taste buds, resulting in taste changes that vary widely and are highly individualized. Commonly induced changes include lowered threshold for bitter taste, increase threshold for sweet taste, and complaints of a metallic taste. Chemotherapy drugs frequently associated with taste alterations are cyclophosphamide, dacarbazine, doxorubicin, 5-FU, levamisole, methotrexate, nitrogen mustard, and vincristine.

Some agents like doxorubicin and methotrexate may alter taste acuity, while others like cyclophosphamide and vincristine can be tasted while injected. Chemotherapy-induced taste alterations can further be influenced by poor oral hygiene, infection of the oral cavity, dentures (causing decreased taste sensations), and unpleasant odors.

Unless patients are specifically questioned, taste alterations are seldom reported spontaneously. When questioned, patients may report their taste changes as reasons for their loss of appetite or decreased weight. Nursing interventions are aimed at teaching patients self-care measures to maintain optimal nutrition. Eating hints should be customized in accordance with each patient's change in taste appreciation.

*Indirect stomatotoxicity*  Chemotherapeutic drugs can affect not only the cells of the oral mucosa but also other cell pools, especially those in the bone marrow. Reduced myeloproliferation is manifested by neutropenia and thrombocytopenia; infection and hemorrhage secondary to myelosuppression can then occur.

Since leukocytes and oral mucosal cells have similar cell renewal rates, changes in the oral status correlate with the timing of myelosuppression. Indirect stomatitis occurs most frequently near the nadir of the leukocytes (10–12 days following therapy). Oral healing occurs as the granulocyte count returns to normal, often preceding bone marrow recovery by two to three days.[54] Improvement in the status of the oral mucosa can therefore be predictive of a recovering white blood cell count.

The oral cavity is susceptible indirectly to infection because of chemotherapy-induced neutropenia. Patients with a granulocyte count less than 1000 mm³ have a greater than 50% chance of developing an opportunistic infection—bacterial viral, or fungal. Infections of the oral cavity will be discussed elsewhere in this chapter. It is important to remember that when a patient's granulocyte count is significantly reduced, classic signs of inflammation may be absent.

Oral bleeding and hemorrhage are indirect stomatotoxic sequelae from chemotherapy-induced thrombocytopenia. Bleeding results when the oral mucosa is traumatized or because of underlying periodontal disease and may occur anywhere in the mouth. The lips, tongue, and gingiva are the most common sites. The lower the platelet count, the greater the possibility of bleeding. As a general guideline, gingival bleeding may occur whenever the platelet count is less than 20,000/mm³ and generally is more severe in patients with preexisting periodontal disease or poor oral hygiene. For patients at risk, oral hygiene regimens should be modified to the less vigorous traumatic measures. Bleeding precautions should be exercised with oral hygiene measures for patients at risk. Management of bleeding with topical coagulants (thrombin-soaked gauze) and pressure is often helpful.

### Oral graft-versus-host disease

Acute and chronic GVHD is a significant complication of patients who undergo allogeneic BMT. Oral involvement has been reported in 33%–75% of patients with acute GVHD and nearly 80% of those with chronic GVHD.[59] Cultures are necessary to distinguish candidiasis and herpetic stomatitis from oral GVHD. Oral ulceration and pain are complications of acute GVHD and a scleroderma-like picture in chronic GVHD. Treatment strategies include systemic immunosuppressive therapy; topical steroids, which may or may not be beneficial; and fluoride therapy for patients at risk for caries secondary to xerostomia.

### Dental evaluation and prophylactic care

The pretreatment dental evaluation serves to establish a baseline, identify risk factors for developing complications, and allow development of a realistic preventive program. Regardless of dentition status, patients should have a comprehensive oral examination by the dentist at least two to three weeks before any therapy is initiated if possible. This will ensure adequate time for treatment of infections if present and for healing if invasive procedures are required. Using a mathematical model, Sonis et al[60] have analyzed the importance of a thorough pretreatment oral exam with regard to cost-efficiency.

Any preexisting oral problems, including decay, infection, and source of irritation, should be assessed. At minimum, radiographic examination should be panoramic for the edentulous patient and include appropriate bitewing for the dentulous patient. Teeth with caries and/or periodontal disease should be repaired or extracted if necessary. Dentures and prosthetic devices are evaluated and adjusted to ensure fit and prevent friction. A thorough cleaning to reduce bacteria that can result in local and systemic infection may include root planing, scaling, and curettage.

Emphasis on good oral hygiene techniques (flossing and brushing) must be continually reinforced to prevent accumulation of dental plaque. Guidelines regarding appropriate granulocyte and platelet counts when dental work is planned should be given to the patient.

Additionally, radiation-induced oral complications can significantly be reduced with daily fluoride treatments along with good oral hygiene. A custom-made fluoride carrier or tray is designed by the dentist to deliver topical fluoride. Patients should be instructed on proper brushing and flossing if not contraindicated. Fluoride gel (0.4% stannous fluoride and 1% sodium fluoride) is then placed in the carrier, which is inserted over the teeth and left in place for five to ten minutes daily. Bedtime is a preferred time of day as eating or drinking should be avoided for 30 minutes to one hour after use.

Oral care and status must be assessed frequently during and after the completion of treatment. Although recommendations vary, it is suggested that patients at risk for developing oral complications consult with a dentist before treatment, during treatment (if complications arise), and two months following completion of treatment or after acute effects have resolved. Routine dental evaluation is then every six months for two years and then annually.

### Radiation-induced stomatitis and oral complications

Oral mucosal side effects of radiation therapy can begin early in the treatment course and progressively worsen. Treatment to the oral cavity may result in stomatitis, hypogeusia (loss of taste), and xerostomia. If the esophagus is included in the treatment field, patients may experience esophagitis and/or dysphagia. While stomatitis, esophagitis, and dysphagia are usually temporary, taste alterations and xerostomia may be permanent in varying degrees. Other effects of radiation are less common and usually do not manifest for months to years after the completion of treatment. These effects include trismus, dental caries, tissue fibrosis, and tissue necrosis. Table 29-12 reviews potential radiation-induced GI toxicities.

The toxicities experienced as a result of radiation are directly related to the total dose delivered to a specific anatomic structure. Higher doses of radiation given to larger volumes over shorter time periods increase severity of oral complications, as does hyperfractionation. Methods of radiation delivery (external beam or interstitial brachytherapy) will influence incidence of stomatitis, as will multimodality therapy. Agents such as cyclophosphamide, 5-FU, and doxorubicin can have radiosensitizing effects and enhanced oral complications.

Poor nutritional status, use of irritants such as tobacco and alcohol, and large dental fillings and permanent prosthetic appliances have been found to significantly influence the onset, degree, and duration of stomatitis.[61,62] Dentures and appliances should be removed during treatment if possible. Nutritional deficiencies and smoking have both been shown to cause considerable delay in healing. Smoking cessation should be

**TABLE 29-12   Radiation-Induced Gastrointestinal Toxicities—Direct and Indirect**

| Tissue Response | Risk Factors: Onset/Duration | Clinical Presentation | Physiological Rationale |
|---|---|---|---|
| Stomatitis | 10 Gy | Mucosa appears white. Tenderness and increased sensitivity to extreme temperatures, acidic foods and fluids, and spicy or rough textured foods | Radiation results in a decrease in mitotic activity and subsequent retention of superficial cells, allowing cells to proceed to a higher degree of keratinization. Aggravated by alcohol and smoking. |
| | 20–25 Gy Progressively worsens Usually resolves 2–3 wk after treatment completion | Pain and burning first associated with eating and progressing to a continuous sensation Erythema | Increased sensitivity of nerve endings. Microvascular changes result in vascular congestion and increased capillary permeability. |
| | | Mucosal thinning and sloughing | As cells are lost, they are not sufficiently replaced by epithelial stem cells. |
| | | Edema Mucosal surface red | Mucosa becomes swollen as a result of vascular congestion and hyperemia. |
| | | White or tan, glistening membrane | Fibrinous exudate composed of serum and dead cells covers some areas. Mucosa is very thin and easily ulcerated. |
| | Trauma | Painful ulceration leaving bright red mucosa | Membrane is friable, fragile, and easily traumatized. |
| Esophagitis | | Refer to Stomatitis | Refer to Stomatitis. |
| | 20 Gy | Difficulty swallowing solids Mild to moderate dysphagia | Microvascular changes result in vascular congestion and increased capillary permeability. |
| | 20–30 Gy Usually resolves 2–3 wk after treatment completion | Substernal burning sensation Pain with swallowing May become progressively worse | Epithelial cells are destroyed without sufficient replacement cells being produced. |
| Taste alterations | 10 Gy exponential to 30 Gy | Diminished taste acuity Increased sensitivity to bitter and salty—appears first and lasts longest Decreased sensitivity to sweets | Indirectly, a function of changes in the oral mucosa and salivary glands (xerostomia). Directly, a result of damage of the microvilli of taste cells. |
| | >30 Gy Resolution:   Partial: 20–60 days after   treatment completion   Complete: 60–120 days after   treatment completion | May be unable to distinguish tastes | |
| | May have permanent alterations | Food may continue to taste bland, papery, or salty | Diminished salivary flow alters the electrolyte balance in the remaining saliva, creating altered taste perceptions. |
| Xerostomia | Dependent upon salivary glands within treatment field | | |
| | 10–20 Gy   50% decrease in saliva | Dry, smooth, shiny mucosa | Damage to salivary glands (major and/or minor) reduces amount of saliva produced. |

*(continued)*

**TABLE 29-12**  Radiation-Induced Gastrointestinal Toxicities—Direct and Indirect (continued)

| Tissue Response | Risk Factors: Onset/Duration | Clinical Presentation | Physiological Rationale |
|---|---|---|---|
| | >30 Gy 75% decrease in saliva | Thick, ropy saliva | Serous secretions are diminished first, leaving only mucin-type saliva. |
| | May be permanent | Difficulty chewing and swallowing | Progressive inflammation and degeneration of acinar and ductal cells result in replacement by fibrinous connective tissue infiltrated with lymphocyte and plasma cells. |
| Oral flora changes | Onset with xerostomia and stomatitis | Fungal and bacterial infection Erythema and burning sensation May have scattered irregular areas of white plaque that may or may not be easily removed—often difficult to distinguish from fibrinous exudate of stomatitis | An indirect function of radiation. Xerostomia results in a decrease in the volume of saliva and in the antimicrobial compounds responsible for chemical and mechanical debridement. Plaque and microorganisms accumulate. |
| | | Prime sites: tongue, buccal mucosa, and mucosal surfaces under dentures | Increase in cariogenic and decrease in noncariogenic bacteria. |
| Dental caries | Onset—variable | Decay—all teeth at risk | An indirect function of radiation. Xerostomia impairs the mechanical and chemical defenses against dental decay (refer to Oral flora changes). Decreased pH prevents saliva from acting as a buffer. |
| | Permanent risk | Begins as diffuse demineralization of teeth and can progress to rampant decay | |
| Mucosal atrophy | Following repair of acute mucosal injury Permanent | Thinned, shiny epithelium | Permanent decrease in keratinization and changes in microvasculature. |
| Fibrosis of subepithelial tissues | Several months following treatment completion Progressive and permanent | Severity/degree ranges from small induration to hard, stony fibrosis Contraction and shrinkage of tissue over time | Faulty collagen remodeling results in fibrotic tissue replacing submucosa. Perivascular and periglandular fibrosis. Increased susceptibility to chemical and mechanical trauma. |
| Soft tissue necrosis | Following repair of acute mucosal injury Permanent risk Induced by chemical or mechanical trauma | Pain and ulceration of epithelium and underlying tissue | Extracapillary fibrosis, inhibition of vascular remodeling, and vascular occlusion impairs the ability of tissue to respond to injury. |
| Bone necrosis (osteoradionecrosis) | Uncommon Progressive and irreversible Trauma-induced or spontaneous (rare) | Constant throbbing pain—most severe at night and during mastication Fistula formation Pathological fracture | Bone exposed by soft tissue damage is susceptible to infection by oral cavity bacteria. Radiation causes cellular and vascular injury within bone. Regional blood vessels thicken and result in bone hypoxia and disorganization of remodeling abilities. Destruction of osteocytes, absence of osteoblasts, and lack of new osteoid cells. |

**TABLE 29-12**   Radiation-Induced Gastrointestinal Toxicities—Direct and Indirect (continued)

| Tissue Response | Risk Factors: Onset/Duration | Clinical Presentation | Physiological Rationale |
|---|---|---|---|
| Trismus | May develop during treatment—usually 3–6 mo after treatment completion Permanent if untreated | Tonic muscle spasms Restriction in mouth opening Pain with swallowing | Fibrosis of the muscles of mastication and/or fibrotic changes in the capsule of the temporomandibular joint. |
| Nausea and vomiting | Dependent upon treatment field | Complaint of nausea with or without emesis | Direct response to mucosal irritation by radiation. |
|  | May occur within hours of receiving first treatment | Often accompanied by weight loss and dehydration | Indirect response to presence of toxic waste products of cellular destruction. |
|  | Usually resolves within 2–3 days following treatment completion |  | Stimulation of the vomiting center resulting from radiation-induced release of serotonin from enterochromaffin cells of the gastrointestinal tract. |
| Enteritis Acute | 20–30 Gy | Increased frequency | Transient mucosal atrophy and infiltration of the lamina propria with leukocytes and plasma cells. |
|  | Progressively worsens as total dose increases | Change in fecal consistency to loose or watery |  |
|  | Resolution usually begins 3 wk after treatment and is complete after 3 mo | Intestinal cramping (tenesmus) | Mucosal epithelial damage results in malabsorption of lactose, fat, bile acids, and vitamin $B_{12}$. |
|  |  |  | Fat malabsorption results in decreased bile salt reabsorption, which then acts as a cathartic in the colon by inhibiting water reabsorption and stimulating peristalsis. |
|  |  |  | Carbohydrate malabsorption results in unabsorbed sugars producing an osmotic effect that causes dilation and peristalsis. |
| Chronic | 6 mo–5 yr after treatment completion | Diarrhea, steatorrhea, abdominal cramping and pain, nausea and vomiting, malabsorption, and obstruction | Refer to malabsorption syndromes above. |
|  | Progressive |  | Progressive ischemia results in diffuse collagen deposition, mucosal atrophy, and tissue fibrosis. |
|  |  | Luminal narrowing, perforation, fistula formation | Mucosal ulceration and necrosis. |
|  |  | Partial or complete obstruction | Adhesions occur between the loops of the bowel. |

Data from Perez CA, Brady LW[4] Sutton E,[7,8] Dow KH, Hilderley LJ,[9] and Hall EJ, Cox JD.[5]

encouraged and facilitated if possible and nutritional deficiencies corrected.

As stomatitis and subsequent pain develop, patients are often unable to maintain an adequate intake of food and fluid. Early intervention and education can prevent or reduce the malnourishment that often accompanies stomatitis. It is not uncommon for patients to lose ten lb or more during a course of head and neck irradiation. Patients and their significant others need to understand the importance of nutrition and hydration and their impact on comfort, infection prevention, healing, and overall tolerance of treatment. Weight and hydration status must be closely monitored.

Patients may be reluctant to report pain and an inability to eat and should therefore be assessed frequently. Patients should be assured that measures can be taken to reduce the discomfort should it occur. Narcotic analgesia may be necessary. Appropriate management of pain will ensure that patients perform the oral care necessary to promote comfort and healing and prevent infection.

Few clinical trials evaluating various agents and methods of oral care have been conducted. One recent three-armed study comparing chlorhexidine mouthwash with antibiotic lozenges or placebo mouthwash concluded that chlorhexidine mouthwash was actually detrimental, producing taste changes, tooth discoloration, and local discomfort.[63] Makkonen et al[64] conducted a placebo-controlled, randomized study using sucralfate mouthwash for prevention of radiation-induced mucositis. All patients developed mucositis at approximately 30 Gy. Visual assessment and self-report of pain showed no degree of difference between the two groups. Measurement of salivary lactoferrin and albumin levels (suggested markers for degree of mucositis) did show, however, that while sucralfate did not prevent mucositis, it had a slight protective effect on the oral mucosa.

Radiation-induced stomatitis ranges in severity from tenderness to severe pain and ulceration. It is self-limiting and usually resolves two to three weeks after the completion of treatment if infection and further trauma are avoided. If severe, a break in treatment may be necessary in order to promote comfort, facilitate healing, and ensure willingness to complete treatment.

***Taste changes (hypogeusia)***    Alteration in taste sensation is a result of direct and indirect radiation changes in the oral mucosa, salivary function, and taste cells. Taste changes usually occur early in a course of therapy and increase with the cumulative dose. Complete taste loss may occur. Although usually not permanent, alterations in or loss of taste may take several months to resolve.

Hypogeusia can significantly impact nutritional status and quality of life as patients no longer find pleasure in eating. A positive correlation has been found between taste changes and weight loss in patients receiving radiation therapy.[61] Therefore, early intervention is necessary in order to reduce the potential for problems resulting from weight loss and malnourishment (see chapter 24).

***Xerostomia***    Xerostomia is one of the most common and can be one of the most devastating sequelae of radiation to the head and neck. It is a direct result of radiation damage and subsequent change in salivary function. Salivary glands are highly radiosensitive, with a drastic decrease in secretion evident after just 10 Gy that is usually permanent after 40 Gy.[61] Although some patients may report subjective improvement, this is more likely a result of adaptation than actual improvement in function. Unfortunately, doses used in an attempt to cure cancers of the head and neck exceed 40 Gy, making xerostomia a chronic problem with serious implications. Younger patients, such as those treated for Hodgkin's disease, may show some improvement in salivary function over time.

Adequate salivary gland function is essential for maintaining the integrity of the oral cavity. Saliva contains organic and inorganic compounds that provide significant protective capacity. Its buffering ability protects teeth, it serves to chemically and mechanically remove cellular and bacterial debris, and it acts as a barrier to irritants. In addition, saliva contains antibacterial agents, lysosomes, and immunoglobulin A, all of which influence the defense against bacterial and viral invasion.[61,62] Inadequate saliva creates difficulty in speaking, chewing, and swallowing, as well as altering the environment of the oral cavity, making it more prone to dental caries, mucosal lesions, pain, and infection.

Nursing assessment should include a review of medications that may contribute to xerostomia, including antihistamines, decongestants, anticholinergics, diuretics, tricyclic antidepressants, opioids, and phenothiazines. Avoiding these agents or using acceptable alternatives when possible will prevent a synergistic effect.

Nutrition is often a problem for patients with xerostomia. Thick, ropy saliva makes eating and swallowing difficult and unpleasant. Oral care before meals will help to freshen the mouth and stimulate appetite. Increasing fluid intake during meals and snacks will help to lubricate food and ease swallowing. Patients should be instructed to avoid dry, bulky, spicy, and acidic foods as they are more difficult to chew and swallow and can potentially damage friable mucosa. Softening or moistening food with milk or gravy may be helpful. Intake of at least eight glasses of fluid per day may help to prevent drying and cracking of the mucous membranes. The use of humidified air is often beneficial, especially at night, when frequent waking occurs from dryness. Many patients find it necessary to carry containers of water or other liquids for use throughout the day.

Irritants such as tobacco, alcohol, carbonated beverages, and caffeine should be avoided as they can dry and irritate the mucous membranes. Commercial mouthwashes contain astringent and antiseptic agents that may be drying and irritating and should be avoided. Commonly used in the past, lemon glycerin is also contraindicated as it dries and irritates the mucosa and can decalcify teeth.

Lubricating agents such as saliva substitutes are frequently used; however, they are expensive and have variable success. In the United States these products are primarily composed of carboxymethylcellulose solutions with a viscosity and electrolyte composition aimed at approximating normal saliva. They may help to temporarily decrease discomfort and buffer the hyperacidity associated with xerostomia. Lubricating agents may assist in protecting tissues under dental appliances and dentures by increasing the bond and reducing irritation. Vegetable or corn oil swished in the mouth may be a cost-effective alternative for artificial lubrication. Research aimed at identifying an effective lubricating agent should be a priority as this malady can greatly impact a patient's quality of life.

Use of proteolytic enzymes, papain and amylase, is

known to effectively dissolve and break up thick saliva in some patients. Papain is found naturally in papayas and papaya juice, is used in commercial meat tenderizers, and can be purchased over the counter. Eating or drinking papaya or swabbing the oral cavity with meat tenderizer before meals has been recommended. Pineapple contains amylase, an enzyme also helpful in cleansing the tongue and mouth. To avoid potential stinging in the mouth, eating frozen pineapple slices has been suggested.

Stimulating residual parenchyma to produce more saliva is often possible and useful. Sialagogues are agents that stimulate the secretion of endogenous saliva and include gustatory stimulants such as sugar-free lemon candy and masticatory stimulants such as sugar-free gum.

Systemic treatment with pilocarpine, a parasympatho-mimetic agent, has been shown to increase saliva production in patients with radiation-induced xerostomia. The cholinergic effect of pilocarpine stimulates any residual functional salivary gland tissue, bringing symptomatic relief.[65] Improvement in the sensation of dryness, in speaking ability, and in overall oral comfort has been noted. Side effects were considered minor, the most frequent of which was excessive sweating. Pilocarpine should be used with caution for those with cardiovascular disease due to the potential side effects of bradycardia, hypertension, and GI upset.

***Radiation-induced soft-tissue and bone necrosis*** Although less common, necrosis of soft tissue and bone following radiation to the head and neck is possible, and measures must be taken to prevent its occurrence. Necrosis can occur at any time after tissue has been irradiated and is usually precipitated by trauma.

Soft-tissue necrosis is a result of chemical, mechanical, or microbial insult. It is very painful, slow to heal, and enlarges rapidly unless treated. Prevention is best; however, if necrosis does occur, early irrigation with saline and baking soda rinses is usually employed. Antibiotics are given when necessary. The cause of trauma should be determined and corrected if possible.

Failure to effectively manage soft-tissue necrosis can result in exposure of underlying bone. This tends to occur most frequently in patients with chronic and advanced periodontal disease. Poor oral hygiene and exposure to irritants also contribute to exposure of bone.

Osteoradionecrosis is uncommon and can be a direct or indirect effect of radiation injury. It is usually precipitated by soft-tissue necrosis; however, pathological fractures can occur. Osteoradionecrosis results in severe pain, usually at night and during mastication, and can be accompanied by fistula formation.

Treatment begins with gentle debridement using saline irrigation. More aggressive debridement of dead or nonviable bone may become necessary. Antibiotic packs and systemic antibiotic therapy are used when infection is present.

***Radiation-induced trismus***   *Trismus* is the result of fibrosis of the muscles of mastication and/or fibrotic changes in the capsule of the temporomandibular joint. Restriction in mouth opening, tonic muscle spasms, and pain can limit access to the oral cavity and impair chewing. Treatment is best accomplished when initiated early. Repetition of jaw exercises should be used prophylactically in patients at high risk and should be initiated in others immediately after a problem develops. Patients are instructed to open their mouth as wide as possible 25 times. This is to be repeated three to four times each day. If trismus is severe, various appliances such as wedges, screws, springs, and elastics may be necessary. Surgical intervention to release fibrotic tissue is used only as a last resort.

### Nursing care

***Assessment***   Identification and treatment of oral complications secondary to chemotherapy and/or radiation therapy must be based on a comprehensive oral and dental assessment that includes examination of the physical condition of the oral mucosa, the patient's perception of any changes in oral sensations and function, and a dental evaluation with radiographic films as necessary. Assessment requires adequate knowledge of the anatomy and physiology of the oral cavity and the effects of radiation and chemotherapy on the structure and function of the oral mucosa.

Assessing the oral cavity requires adequate lighting, removal of all dental prostheses, and inspection and palpation of all mucosal surfaces. Use of a glove, tongue blade, and dental mirror facilitates a thorough exam.

Critical to assessment is the availability of an oral assessment tool that can describe and quantify the physical and functional condition of the oral cavity. A reliable and valid tool will ensure consistency in reporting, thereby facilitating initial and ongoing assessment. Additionally, a clinically useful tool enables stomatotoxic protocols to be identified and the efficacy of varied oral care regimens and interventions to be evaluated.

Eilers and associates[66] developed an oral assessment guide (OAG) based on clinical experience and nursing and dental literature (Table 29-13). The OAG utilizes three levels of descriptors to define oral health and function. Research validates the clinical usefulness of the OAG in BMT and hematologic patients receiving chemotherapy and/or radiation therapy.[67] Applicability in the clinical setting is strengthened because the OAG is understandable and requires only three to four minutes to complete.

A baseline assessment of the oral cavity should be done prior to the initiation of treatment. Dental prophylaxis, restoration, and repair should be completed before treatment begins, especially when radiation will be given to the oral cavity. When extraction rather than repair is necessary, 10–14 days should elapse to allow adequate healing before radiation is started.[61] Once treatment is initiated, an oral assessment should be repeated at regular intervals; outpatients should be instructed on self-assessment.

Nursing management of stomatitis will depend on its

**TABLE 29-13** Oral Assessment Guide (OAG)

| Category | Tools for Assessment | Methods of Measurement | Numerical and Descriptive Ratings | | |
| --- | --- | --- | --- | --- | --- |
| | | | 1 | 2 | 3 |
| Voice | Auditory | Converse with patient | Normal | Deeper or raspy | Difficulty talking or painful |
| Swallow | Observation | Ask patient to swallow To test gag reflex, gently place blade on back of tongue and depress | Normal swallow | Some pain on swallow | Unable to swallow |
| Lips | Visual/palpatory | Observe and feel tissue | Smooth and pink and moist | Dry or cracked | Ulcerated or bleeding |
| Tongue | Visual/palpatory | Feel and observe appearance of tissue | Pink and moist and papillae present | Coated or loss of papillae with a shiny appearance with or without redness | Blistered or cracked |
| Saliva | Tongue blade | Insert blade into mouth, touching the center of the tongue and the floor of the mouth | Watery | Thick or ropy | Absent |
| Mucous membranes | Visual | Observe appearance of tissue | Pink and moist | Reddened or coated (increased white-ness) without ulcerations | Ulcerations with or without bleeding |
| Gingiva | Tongue blade and visual | Gently press with tip of blade | Pink and stippled and firm | Edematous with or without redness | Spontaneous bleeding |
| Teeth or dentures (or denture-bearing area) | Visual | Observe appearance of teeth or denture-bearing area | Clean and no debris | Plaque or debris in localized areas (between teeth if present) | Plaque or debris generalized along gum line or denture-bearing area |

From Eilers J, Berger AM, Petersen MC: Development, testing, and application of the oral assessment guide, *Oncol Nurs Forum* 15:325–330, 1988. Reprinted with permission of June Eilers, University of Nebraska Medical Center, Omaha, NE.

severity, which is often described as mild, moderate, or severe. A grading system depicting degree of severity of mucosal damage includes the following:

Grade 1—erythema of oral mucosa

Grade 2—isolated small ulcerations (white patches)

Grade 3—confluent ulcerations (white patches) covering more than 25% of oral mucosa

Grade 4—hemorrhagic ulceration

***Management*** Systematic performance of oral care may be of greater significance in reducing the destructive effects of radiation and chemotherapy than the actual agents used.[64] Table 29-14 describes a protocol for oral care based on assessment and grade of stomatitis. Table 29-15 depicts various oral cleansing agents and devices, different means of lubricating and coating the oral cavity, and basic solutions and measures to manage oral discomfort.

Developing a plan of care that the patient finds acceptable may be more beneficial than employing complicated regimens. Because reinforcement promotes compliance, nurses should continually review with the patient the individual plan for oral care and assess its continued acceptability. Generally, the recommendation is that routine oral care be performed at least after meals and at bedtime, and that the frequency be increased as the severity of stomatitis increases.

Mouth rinses enhance removal of loosened debris and should be nonirritating and nondehydrating. Several solutions for rinsing have been studied and include normal saline, sodium bicarbonate, and hydrogen peroxide, as well as various combinations of these. Normal saline may be the least damaging; sodium bicarbonate is effective as a cleansing agent, but some patients complain of an unpleasant taste; hydrogen peroxide breaks down new tissues and should be avoided when fresh granulation surfaces are visible in the mouth.

A recent trial using chlorhexidine mouthwash to alleviate radiation-induced mucositis demonstrated an actual

**TABLE 29-14**  Stomatitis: Oral Care Protocol

I. Potential Stomatitis (Grade 0)
  A. Assess oral cavity daily
  B. Encourage routine oral hygiene regimen pc and hs
    1. Brush with soft toothbrush (e.g., Oral-B® 35 or 40) and nonastringent fluoride toothpaste using Bass technique
    2. Floss with unwaxed dental floss
    3. Rinse with mouthwash of patient preference—avoid mouthwashes with high alcohol content
    4. Remove, cleanse, and replace dental prostheses after oral care; store nightly in denture antiseptic solution (e.g., Efferdent®) (*Note:* Change solution daily to prevent growth of pathogens)
    5. Apply lip lubricant (e.g., Blistex, lipstick)
  C. Use oxidizing agent prn for mucolytic area
    1. 3% hydrogen peroxide and water (1:4 mixture)—swish, gargle, and expectorate (*Note:* Mix just prior to use to maintain oxidizing effect)
    2. Sodium bicarbonate solution (e.g., 1 tsp in 8 oz water)—swish, gargle, and expectorate
    3. Rinse with warm water or saline
    4. Remove thick, tenacious mucus with a swab as needed
  D. Provide daily fluoride treatment for patients with xerostomia and prophylactic use for patients receiving head and neck irradiation
  E. Use prophylactic chlorhexidine mouth rinse 15 ml—swish, gargle, and expectorate every 8 hrs for high-risk patients
  F. Consult dentist

II. Mild or Moderate Stomatitis (Grade 1 or Grade 2)
  A. Assess oral cavity twice daily
  B. Follow oral hygiene regimen (see IB above) every 2 hr while awake and every 6 hr during the night
    1. Use normal saline mouthwash if no crusts are present
    2. Alternate oxidizing agent with warm saline mouthwash if crusts are present
    3. Omit flossing if pain results or bleeding occurs with a low platelet count
    4. Remove, cleanse, and do not replace dental prostheses except for meals; store nightly in denture antiseptic solution (e.g., Efferdent®) (*Note:* Change solution daily to prevent growth of pathogens)
  C. Culture any suspicious oral lesions
    1. Culture for: viral, fungal, aerobic and anaerobic; send for Gram stain
    2. Use prophylactic oral antifungal, antiviral, and antibacterial agents per physician order as needed
  D. Apply topical anesthetics ac and prn for local pain control
    1. Lidocaine HCL viscous 2% or 5%
      a. apply directly on lesion(s) with cotton swab
      b. dilute 1 tablespoon with saline—"swish and spit" 10 min ac and hs; "swish and swallow" if throat is sore (*Note:* may cause decreased or absent gag reflex)
    2. Cetacaine or Hurricane® spray—1 to 2 sprays to mouth as needed
    3. "Stomatitis cocktail": mixture of equal parts lidocaine viscous, diphenhydramine HCl elixir (12.5 mg/5 ml)

and Maalox®—"swish and spit" 15–30 ml every 4 hr prn; "swish and swallow" if throat is sore (*Note:* May cause decreased or absent gag reflex)
    4. If xerostomia is not present: mixture of 50% Kaopectate® and 50% diphenhydramine HCI elixir (12.5 mg/5 ml)—"swish and spit" 15–30 ml every 4 hr prn
    5. Zilactin-hydroxypropyl cellulose or Oratect Gel® topical application—apply directly on lesion(s) with cotton swab prn
  E. Use oral analgesics for systemic pain control
    1. Take 1.5 hr ac and prn
    2. Schedule dose at regular intervals (e.g., every 3–4 hr) if pain is constant
    3. Titrate to pain control; may need alternate route of administration
  F. Provide oral lubricants (e.g., Moi-stir® swabs) or "artificial salivas" (e.g., Xero-Lube®) for patients with xerostomia
  G. Adapt diet to ensure maximum nutrition and fluid intake
    1. Encourage frequent small feedings with soft, bland foods; increase fluids to three liters/day
    2. Recommend diet high in protein and calories; add nutritional supplements (e.g., Ensure®, Sustacal®) as needed
    3. Avoid irritants
      a. chemical (citrus fruits, spicy foods)
      b. thermal (extremes in food temperatures)
      c. physical (coarse foods)
      d. tobacco and alcohol
    4. Consult dietician prn

III. Severe Stomatitis (Grade 3 or Grade 4)
  A. Assess oral cavity every 8 hr
  B. Assess for evidence of infection; culture any suspicious lesion(s) as in IIC
  C. Institute aggressive and timely antimicrobial therapy as ordered by physician
  D. Cleanse mouth every 2 hr while awake and every 4 hr at night
    1. Alternate warm saline mouthwash with antifungal or antibacterial oral suspension
    2. Use oxidizing agent (see IB) for mucolytic area every 4 hr followed by saline rinse
  E. Gently brush teeth every 4 hr avoiding trauma to gums; substitute soft foam toothettes if bleeding occurs or brushing is too painful
  F. Apply lip lubricant every 2 hr; if lips are bleeding or ulcerated, apply warm saline soaks every 4 hr for 20 min
  G. Remove, cleanse dental prostheses—do not replace; store in denture antiseptic solution (e.g., Efferdent®) (*Note:* Change solution daily to prevent growth of pathogens)
  H. Institute local pain control measures as in IID above
  I. Use systemic analgesics as needed, especially ac
  J. Provide adequate nutritional and fluid intake
    1. Liquid or pureed diet
    2. Intravenous fluids to prevent dehydration
    3. Enteral or total parenteral nutrition may be needed until healing occurs

Abbreviations: ac = before meals; pc = after meals; hs = at bedtime; prn = as required.

**TABLE 29-15** Prevention and Management of Perioral Complications of Cancer Treatment

| | | BASIC ORAL CLEANSING | | |
|---|---|---|---|---|
| Recommend routine oral cleansing after meals and at bedtime; increase frequency as stomatitis worsens; lip lubricant as needed | | | | |
| Avoid commercial mouthwashes and lemon glycerin swabs because they are drying and irritating to mucosal epithelia | | | | |

| Plan | Action | Active Ingredient | Schedule | Comments |
|---|---|---|---|---|
| *Cleansing Mouthrinses*<br>Normal saline | Mechanical plaque control—removes and washes away loose debris<br><br>Physical—moistens and soothes oral mucosa | Isotonic sodium chloride | Routine: 4 times daily (after meals and at bedtime) | Nonirritating<br>No unpleasant taste<br>Mixture preparation: 1 teaspoon salt in 1 quart warm water; use sterile saline if granulocytopenic or mouth ulcers present |
| Sodium bicarbonate solution | Mechanical plaque control—loosens hardened crusts and debris<br><br>Mucosolvent<br><br>Reduces acidity | Sodium bicarbonate | Routine: 4 times daily (after meals and at bedtime) | Decreases odor<br>Unpleasant taste reported<br>Mixture preparation: 1 tsp baking soda in 8 oz water for thick paste of sodium bicarbonate; water applied to gingival sulcus for use in mechanical plaque debridement |
| Hydrogen peroxide (3% solution) | Mechanical plaque control—loosens hardened crusts and debris<br><br>Mucosolvent<br><br>Germicidal | | Routine: 4 times daily (after meals and at bedtime) | Unpleasant taste<br>Use with caution on ulcers or fresh granulation surfaces—may break down tissue<br>Chronic use may alter normal oral flora and predispose to candidal infections<br>Mixture preparation: dilute 3% hydrogen peroxide to ¼ strength. *Note:* Mix just prior to usage to maintain oxidizing effect<br>Refrigerated solution may also provide local anesthetic effect |
| *Antimicrobial Mouthrinse*<br>Peridex | Broad-spectrum antimicrobial agent used to suppress oral microflora and prevent dental plaque formation<br><br>Decreases bacterial cloud in mouth<br><br>Prevents oral candidal infections | Chlorhexidine digluconate | 15 ml rinse for 30 sec three times daily<br><br>Do not swallow<br><br>Avoid eating or drinking 1 hr following use | Efficacy for the prophylaxis of therapy-induced mucositis is controversial<br><br>Most common local side effect from long-term use is staining of teeth and tongue. No systemic toxicity has been reported |

**TABLE 29-15** Prevention and Management of Perioral Complications of Cancer Treatment (continued)

### BASIC ORAL CLEANSING

| Plan | Action | Active Ingredient | Schedule | Comments |
|------|--------|-------------------|----------|----------|
| *Cleansing Devices* | | | | |
| Toothbrush | Mechanical cleansing and removal of debris | | Toothbrushing 4 times daily (after meals and at bedtime) | Cleansing instrument of choice Bass technique of brushing recommended |
| Toothette | Stimulate circulation to oral mucosa Removes debris more gently than toothbrush | | Every 4 hr and as needed | Recommended for cleansing when platelet count falls below 20,000 Use unflavored if stomatitis is present |

### MAINTENANCE OF MOISTURE

Cleanse cracked or ulcerated lips with gauze soaked in normal saline; encrusted lips with gauze soaked in sodium bicarbonate or $H_2O_2$ solution

A dry mouth (xerostomia) contributes to taste disturbances, which may affect appetite and nutritional status; radiation to the oral cavity is associated with xerostomia

Fluoride treatment recommended to prevent dental caries secondary to xerostomia

| Plan | Action | Active Ingredient | Schedule | Comments |
|------|--------|-------------------|----------|----------|
| *Lipcare* | | | | |
| K-Y Jelly® | Lubricates lips Prevents cracking and bleeding | Sodium carboxymethylcellulose Sodium alginate Glycerin | Apply as needed for moisture | Nonirritating Water-soluble Can be applied on oral mucosa also Safe for use in patients receiving oxygen |
| Petrolatum (e.g., Vaseline®, petroleum jelly) | Lubricates lips Prevents evaporation of moisture | Petrolatum | Apply as needed for moisture | Unpleasant taste Forms occlusive film on lips Harmful if aspirated |
| *Oral Cavity Care* | | | | |
| Orabalance® | Relief of dry mouth | | Use after rinsing mouth and after every brushing | A nondrying moisturizing gel May be applied around the teeth and along gum line |
| Saliva substitutes (e.g., Moi-Stir®) | Mouth-moistening salivary supplement | Sorbitol, sodium carboxymethyl-cellulose, and electrolytes present in saliva | Apply as needed for xerostomia | Available in oral swabsticks and spray |
| (e.g., Xerolube®) | Mouth moisturizer Caries inhibition | Carboxymethylcellulose | 5 ml orally as needed for xerostomia | Includes fluoride as an added benefit |
| *Sialogogues* | | | | |
| Salagen® | Stimulates saliva production from functioning salivary glands | Pilocarpine | Adult dosage: 5 mg 3 times daily | Investigational use for patients with radiation-induced xerostomia Contraindicated in patients with uncontrolled asthma or narrow-angle glaucoma; use caution with cardiovascular disease |

*(continued)*

**TABLE 29-15**   Prevention and Management of Perioral Complications of Cancer Treatment (continued)

### RELIEF OF PAIN AND INFLAMMATION

Pain from isolated areas of mucositis or ulceration is best managed with localized topical anesthetics and coating agents; topical rinses may be helpful for confluent, generalized ulcerations

Systemic analgesics may be necessary to alleviate moderate to severe oral pain and enhance oral intake

| Plan | Action | Active Ingredient | Schedule | Comments |
|---|---|---|---|---|
| *Coating Agents*<br>Orabase® | Topical anesthetic for localized areas of pain | Benzocaine 20% | Dry lesion(s) and apply as needed for pain | Quick onset of action—30 sec, but short duration of action—5–15 min<br>Does not change consistency after application |
| Hurricane® | Topical anesthetic | Benzocaine 20% | Apply as needed to lesion(s) for pain | Available as spray, liquid, or gel<br>Onset of action—30 sec, duration 15 min<br>No systemic absorption |
| Oratect-gel® | Topical anesthetic | Benzocaine 20% | Dry lesion(s) and apply as needed up to 4 times daily | Gel dries in about 30–60 sec to form a protective film<br>Maximum protection lasts about 2 hr<br>Film dissipates gradually over 6 hr<br>Do not try to mechanically remove<br>Mild, transient stinging when applied |
| Zilactin® | Provides a protective coating and leads to pain relief | Tannic acid 7% | Dry lesion(s) and apply 4 times daily | Forms protective film over oral ulcers that can last 5 hr<br>Gel forms an opaque white film inside the mouth and a transparent film extraorally when dried<br>Mild, transient burning sensation with application of gel |
| *Topical Anesthetic Rinses*<br>Xylocaine viscous 2% solution | Topical anesthetic for generalized areas of pain | Lidocaine HCl | 15 ml swish and spit every 3 hr as needed for pain (not to exceed 120 ml in 24 hr) | Onset of action is 5 min<br>Duration of action is approximately 20 min<br>Systemically absorbed<br>Watch for CNS and cardiac toxicity<br>Swish and swallow for brief pain relief (e.g., before meals) |
| Dyclonine Hydrochloride 0.5% or 1% solution | Topical anesthetic for generalized areas of pain | Dyclone | 15 ml swish and spit as needed for pain | Minimally absorbed<br>Decreasing potential for CNS and cardiac toxicity |
| Combination "mixtures" (e.g., viscous xylocaine 2%, Benadryl® elixir 12.5 mg/ml, Maalox®) | Topical anesthetics for general areas of pain | Lidocaine Diphenhydramine Magnesium hydroxide | 15 ml swish for 1 min, then spit or swallow 4 times daily | Benadryl may exacerbate xerostomia |

**TABLE 29-15** Prevention and Management of Perioral Complications of Cancer Treatment (continued)

| Plan | Action | Active Ingredient | Schedule | Comments |
|---|---|---|---|---|
| Ulcerease® | Anesthetic mouthrinse | Buffered solution of glycerin and liquified phenol (0.6%) | 15 ml swish for 15 sec, then spit every 2 hr as needed | Contains no alcohol Use full strength May apply directly to ulcers with cotton swab after rinsing |
| Sucralfate suspension | Binds to ulcerated tissue protecting it from further insult and may promote healing | Sucralfate (sulfated sucrose and aluminum hydroxide) | 1 g/15 ml swish (pc and hs) 15 ml 4 times daily—swish for 1–2 min, then spit | No anesthetic action Suspension may aggravate nausea |
| Vitamin E | Promotes healing of mouth ulcers and controls pain | Tocopherol | 1 ml (400 mg/ml) of vitamin E oil applied topically to oral lesions twice daily | Anecdotal and research-based studies conclude vitamin E may help speed healing of chemotherapy-induced stomatitis |
| *Systemic Analgesics*<br>Nonsteroidal anti-inflammatory agents (e.g., Trilisate®) | Mild to moderate pain | Choline magnesium trisalicylate | 1500–3000 mg | Longer duration of action than aspirin No effect on platelets Minimal GI side effects |
| Narcotic agents (e.g., morphine) | Moderate to severe pain | Morphine sulfate | | |

increase in mucositis, staining of teeth, and taste alterations.[63] As yet, the optimum mouthwash for stomatitis has not been determined.

Stomatitis can have a great impact on a patient's quality of life and compliance with therapy. A standard of nursing care to assess, plan, intervene, and evaluate is necessary to prevent or minimize this distressing side effect, to decrease the incidence of infection, and to prevent nutritional deficits.

Although the treatment of stomatitis remains palliative and symptom-oriented, studies are ongoing to evaluate prophylactic measures to alleviate this side effect. Several clinical trials have focused on appropriate measures to prevent this side effect. A pilot study by Clark and Slevin[68] found allopurinol rinses beneficial in decreasing the severity of stomatitis in six out of six patients receiving 5-FU alone. In a subsequent study, 77 patients treated with 5-FU with or without leucovorin were randomly assigned to use either a placebo or allopurinol mouthwash. Results were convincingly negative and demonstrated no protective effect of allopurinol; furthermore, a nonsignificant trend toward more mucositis was observed with those patients rinsing with allopurinol.[69] Further investigation is warranted before incorporating this procedure into routine clinical practice.

The use of oral cryotherapy has proved beneficial in minimizing oral stomatitis due to doxorubicin as well as 5-FU and leucovorin. In a study by Mahood et al,[70] 95 patients receiving 5-FU and leucovorin on five consecutive days were randomized to no treatment or ice chips

for 30 minutes beginning five minutes prior to chemotherapy. Those in the treatment group experienced less stomatitis. It would appear that ice effectively causes vasoconstriction, thereby minimizing blood flow to the oral cavity and preventing uptake of 5-FU by oral mucosal cells. Both doxorubicin and 5-FU have a short half-life, which makes cryotherapy a logical approach to prevention of stomatitis.

The efficacy of topical sucralfate suspension for prophylaxis of chemotherapy-induced mucositis has been alluded to previously. Sucralfate is thought to work by binding to the inflamed areas of the mucosa, thereby forming a protective barrier against further mucosal damage.[71] A placebo-controlled study evaluated treatment with sucralfate in patients receiving cisplatin and continuous 5-FU for five days. A significant reduction ($p = .04$) in objective measurements of mucositis was seen among 23 evaluable patients as well as a trend in patient preference for the sucralfate rinse.[72]

Of interest is the role that growth factors may play in stomatitis prevention. Research trials with colony-stimulating factors (e.g., G-CSF) administered to patients undergoing chemotherapy have incidentally reported a decrease in the occurrence and severity of stomatitis along with restoration of neutrophil counts and function.[73]

Other preventive measures reported in the literature include supplemental beta carotene and prostaglandin E compounds. Prophylactic use of antimicrobial rinses will be discussed in the next section.

## Infections of the Oral Cavity

Infection is the most clinically significant oral problem secondary to treatment with chemotherapy and/or localized radiation therapy. The mouth, inhabited by both normal and opportunistic pathogens, provides ideal conditions for microbial growth, particularly in the granulocytopenic patient. The risk of serious infection is directly related to the degree and duration of granulocytopenia.

Integral to the pathogenesis of infection in the cancer patient is impairment of normal host-defense mechanisms. Cytotoxic therapy weakens host defenses by changing the oral flora to become primarily gram-negative and reducing salivary and mucous gland function. An overgrowth of normal oral microorganisms results in invasion of both endogenous and exogenous pathological organisms capable of producing oral infections. Mucosal disruption becomes an important portal of entry and compromises the integrity of the oral mucosa as the first line of defense. Pathogenic organisms can further contaminate the lungs and the GI tract, disseminating infection systemically.

Pathogenicity of normal oral flora increases with poor oral hygiene and in the presence of oral disease. It has been shown that as oral hygiene measures are decreased, the presence of microbial populations increases. Periodontitis, a common oral disease in the general population, causes a tenfold increase in bacterial and fungal organisms in the mouth.[74] The discomfort and pain associated with stomatitis from either chemotherapy or radiotherapy often result in decreased intake of nutrients and fluids, which can lead to malnutrition and dehydration. Depletion of protein stores and malnutrition increase the risk of infection by altering the integrity of the epithelial barrier and depressing the immune system. Research suggests that adequate nutritional status as evidenced by normal serum albumin levels and optimal pretherapy weight may decrease the rate of oral infection.

Immunosuppression due to the treatment of cancer or the cancer itself further increases a patient's susceptibility to oral infection. Specifically, immunosuppression depresses phagocytic activity, interferes with the inflammatory response, abolishes antibody production, and inhibits the development of delayed hypersensitivity.

Bacterial, fungal, and viral infections are all common; *Streptococcus* species, *Candida* species, and herpes simplex virus are the major oral infectious pathogens.[75] Each infection has certain clinical features, such as the white or "cottage-cheese" appearance of *Candida albicans* or the painful vesicular lesions of herpes simplex, that assist in identification of the pathogen. However, the task is difficult at times, particularly when one is trying to differentiate between noninfectious therapy-induced lesions and those caused by pathogenic organisms. Ultimately, proper identification of the responsible pathogen requires culture. Management will vary depending on the pathogenic organism.

The most frequent cause of oral infection is fungal. *C albicans* is the predominating organism and pseudo-membranous candidiasis (oral thrush) the most common clinical manifestation. Due to discoloration by tobacco and food stains, oral thrush occasionally appears as a thick brown coating on the tongue surface.

Oral *Candida* infections are traditionally treated with topical antifungal agents such as nystatin oral rinses, or clotrimazole troches. The nystatin liquid must be swished in the mouth for five minutes and then spit or swallowed, four times daily. The troche, given five times a day, must be sucked in the mouth until dissolved (approximately 30 minutes). Long-term use of oral troches should be avoided as they contain large quantities of sugar that may result in dental caries. If xerostomia secondary to radiation is present, the troche will take a longer time to dissolve. Patients should be instructed to cleanse the mouth before administering the agent and not to eat or drink for at least 30 minutes after application. This will permit drug contact with the mucosal surfaces to exert an antifungal effect. The increased contact time is necessary to control the organism. Denture wearers should be instructed to soak their appliance overnight with 100 ml nystatin suspension. The plastic can act as a reservoir to reinfect the treated mucosa.

Alternatives for oropharyngeal candidiasis refractory to topical treatment are the systemic oral antifungal agents: ketoconazole 200 mg daily or fluconazole 100 mg daily.[76] Fluconazole is also available for intravenous use. Increased compliance due to once-a-day dosing is an advantage; however, fluconazole is potentially liver-toxic. Absorption of ketoconazole is dependent on gastric acidity; therefore, patients are instructed to avoid the use of antacids and other medications that alter gastric pH within two hours of taking ketoconazole. A course of low-dose intravenous amphotericin B is indicated for nonresponsive infection and in severe esophageal and disseminated candidal infections.

Herpes simplex virus (HSV) is the most common viral pathogen affecting the oral cavity. Since the appearance of HSV resembles other infectious lesions or therapy-induced stomatitis, culturing of suspicious lesions is mandatory. Optimally, vesicle fluid should be obtained for culture. When no vesicles are present, the base of the lesion should be swabbed using a viral culture swab. Swabs used for nasopharyngeal cultures (calcium alginate swabs) inactivate the virus and should not be used. Furthermore, gloves should always be worn when swabbing suspicious lesions as HSV is highly infective.

Reactivation of latent HSV is the cause of the majority of HSV infections. Immunocompromised patients who are seropositive are at risk. The more intense the immunosuppression, the greater the risk (e.g., BMT patients are at high risk). For patients with limited tissue involvement, acyclovir ointment can be applied topically every three to six hours while awake. Patients should be instructed to use gloves or cotton swabs when applying ointment, since autoinoculation with the virus can occur. Extensive tissue involvement or disseminated herpes requires systemic acyclovir therapy either orally or parenterally. Acyclovir prophylaxis may be used to prevent infection in selected high-risk patient populations (e.g., seropositive BMT or leukemic patients).[77] Optimum dose and schedule for prophylaxis have not been determined.

The vast majority of bacterial infections may affect three sites in the mouth: the gingiva, the mucosa, or the teeth. A bacterial culture isolate and positive blood culture confirm the diagnosis; however, clinical features (e.g., pain, fever, oral lesions) may be present without a positive blood culture. Parenteral antibiotic therapy based on causative organism is the treatment of choice. The effectiveness of chlorhexidine rinses in the prevention of local and systemic infections in immunocompromised patients has been reported differently in the literature. Results are inconclusive because of variances in the study design, including differences in the concentration of chlorhexidine used, duration of use, and concomitant use of broad-spectrum antibiotics. Table 29-16 outlines the clinical features, diagnosis, and management of oral infections.

## Esophagitis

Histologically, the mucosal lining of the esophagus is the same as the oral cavity and is lined with stratified squamous epithelial cells. Destruction and inadequate replacement of these epithelial cells by radiotherapy or chemotherapeutic agents result in an inflammatory response called *esophagitis*. Similar to stomatitis, esophagitis can progress to include ulceration, hemorrhage, and secondary infection and can cause sufficient pain to make eating very difficult. Treatment may be discontinued temporarily to allow recovery of these cells, which parallels recovery of the white blood cell count.

The most common early symptoms of esophagitis include dysphagia (difficulty in swallowing), odynophagia (painful swallowing), and epigastric pain. Esophageal pain that worsens and becomes continuous and substernal indicates progressing esophagitis.

### Radiation-induced esophagitis

Radiation used to treat esophageal cancer, Hodgkin's disease, head and neck, breast, and lung cancer often requires that the esophagus receive a radiation dose high enough to induce esophagitis. Esophagitis is a common and expected transient side effect. It occurs as a result of vascular changes and an inability for cell renewal to keep up with epithelial cell loss. This results in erythema and mucosal irritation.

Onset of esophagitis is dose-related and my be enhanced or hastened by concomitant chemotherapy or dietary indiscretions, especially alcohol. Symptoms often begin with a report of difficulty in swallowing liquids and a feeling as though there is a "lump in the throat." After two to three weeks of therapy, symptoms may progress to pain, often caused by swallowing; a burning sensation; and dysphagia. If the reaction becomes severe, the pain and burning sensation may be continuous and debilitating. A treatment break may be necessary to prevent or correct dehydration and malnutrition.

Treating esophageal cancer requires higher doses delivered directly to the esophagus. This places these patients at a higher risk for developing an esophageal ulceration, perforation, and/or fistula during or after treatment completion. Careful treatment planning, often utilizing an esophagram, is therefore employed in an attempt to predict and prevent this complication.

While resolution of the acute esophageal effects of radiation usually begins two to three weeks following treatment completion, late effects may be seen one to five years later. Late complications include epithelial thickening, microvascular changes, and fibrosis of muscle and connective tissue. Ulceration is seen less frequently,

**TABLE 29-16**   Infections of the Oral Cavity

| Infection | Clinical Features | Diagnosis | Management | Comment |
|---|---|---|---|---|
| **Bacterial** | | | | |
| Gingival | White, necrotic pseudo-membrane<br>Pain<br>Fever<br>Lymphadenopathy | + bacterial culture<br>± blood culture | Parenteral antibiotics (gram-negative coverage plus beta-lactam antibiotics)<br>Local debridement of bacterial plaques<br>Aggressive oral hygiene<br>Prophylactic chlorhexidine mouthrinse for high-risk patients | Resembles acute necrotizing ulcerative gingivitis (ANUG). More common in patients with preexisting periodontal disease<br>Calculus and plaque removal recommended prior to therapy |
| Odontogenic | Tooth pain<br>Fever | Dental examination including radiographs<br>± blood culture | Extraction of infected tooth<br>Fluoride treatment | Third molars are most often involved<br>Pretreatment dental examination and extraction are recommended |

*(continued)*

**TABLE 29-16** Infections of the Oral Cavity (continued)

| Infection | Clinical Features | Diagnosis | Management | Comment |
|---|---|---|---|---|
| Mucosal | Painful ulceration<br>Fever | + bacterial culture<br>+ blood culture | Broad-spectrum parenteral antibiotics<br>Aggressive oral hygiene<br>Prophylactic chlorhexidine mouthrinse for high-risk patients | Normal signs of inflammation and infection may be absent in neutropenic patients |
| Gram-negative bacilli (e.g., *pseudomonas* spp.) | Raised dry, yellowish lesion encircled by a reddened halo; center turns purple to black with necrosis | | | |
| Gram-positive cocci (e.g., *Streptococcus* spp.) | Yellowish-white exudate enclosed by an erythematous halo | | | |
| Fungal<br>*Candida albicans* | Pseudomembranous: white, raised cottage cheeselike plaques<br>Painless when undisturbed<br>Raw, bleeding, painful surface results when scraped off<br><br>Atrophic: localized to confluent erythema of oral mucosa<br>Patchy depapillation of dorsum of tongue<br>Painful<br><br>Fever rare with only oral involvement | + fungal culture for *Candida* spp.<br><br>+ smears:<br>Gram-stained<br>Potassium hydroxide<br>Wet preparation | Antifungal agents<br><br>Topical:<br>Nystatin oral rinse/troche<br>Clotrimazole troche<br><br>Systemic:<br>Oral ketoconazole<br>Oral fluconazole/intravenous<br><br>Nonresponsive:<br>Parenteral amphotericin B<br><br>Value of prophylactic antifungal agent is controversial<br>Chlorhexidine mouthrinse may be effective in modifying candidal infections | Patients with oral *Candida* are at significant risk for spread to esophagus and systemically<br><br>Radiation-induced xerostomia predisposes oral mucosa to fungal infection |
| Viral<br>Herpes simplex (HSV) | Prodromal symptoms of tingling, itching pain followed by eruption of small vesicles that ulcerate and become encrusted<br><br>Common areas of occurrence: lips and circumoral region<br><br>Fever, malaise, and lymphadenopathy may be present | + viral culture<br>↑ HSV serum titer | Antiviral agent:<br>Acyclovir<br><br>Topical:<br>Acyclovir ointment (e.g., lip lesions or herpes labialis)<br><br>Systemic:<br>Acyclovir<br><br>Prophylactic:<br>Acyclovir for high-risk seropositive patients | Reactivation of HSV is the most common cause of viral infection in the neutropenic cancer patient<br><br>Seropositive patients for HSV are at greater risk |
| Varicella zoster | Unilateral vesicular lesions along trigeminal nerve | | | |

with the incidence increasing when doses greater than 70 Gy have been delivered. If fibrosis and luminal stenosis become severe, repeated esophageal dilation may become necessary. If this procedure is unsuccessful, a gastrostomy may be necessary for nutritional intake and adequate hydration.

## Nursing considerations

Risk factors for developing esophagitis include alcohol consumption, tobacco use, ulcer disease, and esophageal exposure to radiation.

Ongoing assessments should be performed at least

weekly and should include weight, dietary and hydration status, and blood chemistry if indicated. This along with the patient's report of pain or difficulty in swallowing, should be carefully documented. Use of a grading scale such as that in Table 29-3 will help to ensure consistency in assessment and documentation.

Patients and their significant others must be educated regarding the possible acute and late side effects of therapy, probable time frame for their onset and duration, and self-care measures to help alleviate the side effects. Table 29-17 offers self-care guidelines to assist patients experiencing esophagitis and dysphagia. Compliance with recommended guidelines should be assessed and the importance frequently reinforced during a patient's treatment course.

Although management of esophagitis varies greatly, all management is directed at symptom relief and supportive care. Interventions are initiated to minimize irritation and promote comfort. This is best accomplished through dietary manipulation, topical anesthesia, and systemic analgesia when needed.

If nutritional status becomes compromised, patients may benefit from commercially prepared supplements. A nutritionist may be helpful in determining which products would best meet the individual needs of the patient. Some patients may require a feeding tube, usually gastrostomy, if esophagitis becomes severe. Occasionally, a tube will be placed prior to initiating treatment if nutritional problems are anticipated.

Local anesthetics are often used to help alleviate the pain associated with esophagitis. Temporary relief may occur after using over-the-counter preparations such as liquid antacids, Aspergum® (Plough, Inc.), and children's acetaminophen elixir. For moderate to severe esophagitis, numerous "cocktail" recipes exist. Most contain common ingredients including viscous lidocaine 2% to anesthetize and liquid antacids to coat and soothe. Many contain diphenhydramine elixir to reduce inflammation; however, this may burn and cause an increase in the dryness of already compromised mucous membranes. As an alternative, nonsteroidal anti-inflammatory agents may be used, if not contraindicated by existing gastric ulcers or thrombocytopenia. Patients using viscous lidocaine should be aware that their gag reflex may be diminished. Local anesthetics are usually prescribed every three to four hours as needed and/or 15–30 minutes before meals.

Sucralfate suspension is also used to treat radiation- and chemotherapy-induced esophagitis. It is suggested that it promotes comfort and possibly healing by binding to proteinaceous exudate in exposed mucosa. The ingredients of sucralfate suspension are sucralfate 12 g dissolved in 60 ml water, Benylin® syrup 60 ml, and Maalox suspension to a total of 180 ml. Patients are instructed to use 15 ml after meals and at bedtime—swish in clean mouth for two minutes and then swallow.[78]

If pain and discomfort are not relieved with topical anesthetic preparations, it may be necessary to add narcotic analgesics. Acetaminophen with codeine or morphine elixirs are often utilized as tablets and may be

## TABLE 29-17   Self-Care Guidelines for Esophagitis (Sore Throat) and Dysphagia (Difficulty Swallowing)

While receiving chemotherapy or radiation to the neck or chest, you may begin to develop a sore throat or a feeling like food is getting stuck when you swallow. This usually begins gradually after about 2 weeks of treatment and may become more severe as treatment continues. It is <u>temporary</u> and will begin to gradually get better about 2 weeks after treatment is finished.

The following guidelines were designed to help you to be more comfortable during treatment and to make sure that you are eating and drinking enough liquids.

1. Tell your nurse or doctor if you have a sore throat or are having trouble swallowing.
2. Change your diet to include foods that are soft and moist. Using sauces and gravies is helpful.
3. Avoid foods that are spicy, salty, dry, or rough in texture.
4. Drink at least eight glasses of liquid each day. Fruit nectar is often very soothing. Avoid alcoholic beverages, citrus juices, and carbonated beverages—they will irritate your throat.
5. Avoid very hot foods.
6. Eat or drink cold foods such as ice cream, frozen juice bars, and Jell-O. This may help to soothe the throat, especially before eating a meal.
7. Take small bites and chew foods well.
8. Use a straw to make swallowing easier.
9. Avoid using commercial mouthwashes because they often contain alcohol, which can irritate your throat.
10. Try not to smoke. It can be difficult to stop smoking during a stressful time, but your nurse or doctor can provide you with some helpful suggestions.
11. Placing a cool air humidifier with tap water in the room where you spend most of your time during the day and where you sleep at night may help to keep your mouth and throat from getting dry.
12. If your doctor prescribes medicine to help with the pain and discomfort, do not be afraid to take it. Taking this medicine will make you more comfortable and help you to eat and drink.
13. Notify your nurse or doctor if taking pills becomes difficult. Some, but not all, pills can be crushed and taken in ice cream or applesauce.
14. Keep your mouth fresh and clean. Baking soda (1 tsp mixed in 1 qt of water) works well to rinse your mouth and gargle. This can be done every 2 hr.
15. If it becomes more difficult to eat, change your foods to include very soft, blended, and/or liquid foods. Your nurse or doctor may suggest liquid food supplements.
16. Tell your nurse or doctor if you notice any of the following:
    - being unable to drink fluids
    - dizziness, extreme tiredness, or weakness
    - chills or fever of 100.8 °F or higher
    - urinating small amounts of dark urine

difficult to swallow. The alcohol content of elixirs may further irritate mucosa.

Superimposed *Candida* infections may also present significant problems for cancer patients. *Candida* esophagitis may or may not be symptomatic. Symptoms, when they exist, are often difficult to distinguish from treatment-induced esophagitis and may include dysphagia and pain. Prompt and appropriate medical treatment is necessary in order to prevent a systemic spread. Esophageal candidiasis is most commonly treated using ketoconazole, fluconazole, or nystatin oral suspension.[79]

### Chemotherapy-induced esophagitis

Any patient who develops oral mucositis following chemotherapy is at risk for spread to the esophageal mucosal tissue. Prior or concurrent radiation may augment the severity and extent of mucosal injury. Some drugs such as dactinomycin and doxorubicin potentiate radiation injury to the esophagus, while others including 5-FU, hydroxyurea, procarbazine, and vinblastine produce an additive toxic effect with irradiation. It is not uncommon for a stomatotoxic agent to be discontinued during treatment with radiation and restarted once radiation is completed.

Both infectious and noninfectious causes may result in clinically significant esophagitis. In immunocompromised patients who are granulocytopenic and receiving antibiotics, an infectious esophagitis is most common. Fungal, viral, and bacterial organisms can all be responsible. *Candida* is the most likely cause and can be fatal if disseminated systemically. Herpes simplex should also be considered in the differential diagnosis. Patients who have received extensive chest wall or mediastinal radiation can present with symptoms clinically identical to an infectious esophagitis.[80]

It is essential to determine the cause of esophagitis so that appropriate therapy can be given. Flexible endoscopy with brushings is more accurate than radiographic examination of the esophagus to identify the correct cause in immunocompromised patients. Biopsy, culture, and histologic examination are necessary for definitive diagnosis. If a biopsy is not possible, a trial course of empiric therapy can be given.

Nursing management is discussed in the preceding section on radiation-induced esophagitis.

## Enteritis

### Radiation-induced enteritis

Treatment of pelvic and abdominal malignancies usually necessitates inclusion of a portion of the bowel within the radiation treatment field. Although improvements in equipment, localization techniques, and treatment planning have significantly reduced the severity of acute and chronic radiation enteritis, its occurrence remains a common effect of treatment.

Cells of the epithelial lining of the intestinal mucosa have a short life cycle. Rapid mitosis is necessary in order to maintain a balance between cell renewal and cell death that occurs as a result of the frequent, normal trauma from passage of feces. This renders the intestinal mucosa quite radiosensitive and vulnerable to treatment-induced enteritis. Radiation doses necessary for tumor control

range from 47 to 75 Gy or more, which exceeds the normal tissue tolerance.[5]

Radiation enteritis can be classified as acute, occurring during treatment; and chronic or persistent, with symptoms at greater than six months. A lack of acute enteritis does not preclude the development of chronic radiation enteritis; however, there is a positive correlation between the occurrence of severe acute enteritis and the development of chronic radiation enteritis.

Several factors influence the degree, onset, and duration of radiation-induced acute and chronic enteritis.[4,81]

1. *Dose per fraction:* Higher doses given over shorter time periods result in greater toxicity.
2. *Volume of tissue (field size):* Treatment delivered to larger volumes will cause more side effects. Boost techniques or coning down reduces the volume of tissue included in the treatment field after a predetermined dose has been delivered.
3. *Treatment technique/plan:* The use of a four-field technique (anterior, posterior, right, and left laterals) helps to spare a portion of the bowel. Use of pretreatment contrast studies and computer-assisted planning to provide more individualized dosimetry decreases the incidence of chronic radiation enteritis.
4. *Bowel displacement techniques:* Attempts to move part of the small bowel out of the radiation field may include:
   a. treatment with a full bladder to elevate the small bowel
   b. patients lying in a prone position on a Styrofoam platform or "belly board" that has a cut-out area designed to allow abdominal contents to fall forward
   c. surgical placement of an omental sling or pedicle flap to support the small bowel in the upper abdomen (this technique is less commonly used due to the surgical procedure required)
5. *Previous abdominal surgery and/or radiation therapy:* These predispose patients to developing adhesions.
6. *Concomitant chemotherapy:* Significant enhancement of intestinal injury has been reported with actinomycin D, doxorubicin, 5-FU, and cisplatin.
7. *Patient-related considerations:* Factors including compromised nutritional status, preexisting bowel disorders, diabetes, and hypertension may enhance enteritis.

Consideration of these factors is important in anticipating toxicities and educating patients. Table 29-12 reviews GI toxicities.

Most patients receiving radiation therapy to the abdomen or pelvis will develop some degree of enteritis due to the highly radiosensitive nature of the epithelium. The severity ranges from a mild change in frequency and consistency to excessive diarrhea and cramping. Most patients report an increase in frequency to three to five bowel movements daily and a loose or watery consistency. Diarrhea accompanied by tenesmus may occur during or soon after abdominal or pelvic irradiation.

Radiation enteritis is the result of cellular and vascular

changes, alterations in absorption, and a decrease in enzyme activity. Morphological changes seen with increasing doses include an increased rate of cell loss from intestinal villi that exceeds the capability of reproduction by crypt cells and a shortening of the villi resulting in a reduction in the total epithelial surface.[82]

Although temporary, acute radiation enteritis can cause significant problems. A frequent need and sense of urgency can prevent patients from participating in work and social activities. If severe, a reduction in daily fraction size or an interruption in treatment may be necessary, and fluid and electrolyte imbalances may require intravenous support. Attempts should be made to prevent the potentially serious complications associated with acute radiation enteritis.

The role of the nurse in managing a patient at risk for developing acute radiation enteritis includes assessment, symptom management, and patient education. An initial assessment should include normal patterns of elimination as well as recent changes including frequency, amount, color and consistency, history of bowel disorders, use of laxatives and antidiarrheals, and food intolerances. Nutritional and hydration status must also be determined. Careful and complete documentation of the initial assessment will serve as a baseline for future comparison.

Ongoing assessment should occur at least weekly and includes any changes in elimination, abdominal tenderness, bowel sounds, weight, and hydration status. A complete blood count and chemistry panel may be indicated. In addition, assessment of the skin and mucous membranes of the perianal areas should be performed as diarrhea may further compromise these tissues. Documentation of toxicities can be accomplished by using a standard scale such as that found in Table 29-3.

Patients and their significant others should be educated as to the potential side effects of treatment including diarrhea, cramping, and mucosal irritation as well as the usual time of onset and resolution. Patients must understand the need to report changes and should also be reassured that appropriate interventions will be employed when the side effects occur. The importance of maintaining adequate food and fluid intake must be stressed.

Treatment of acute radiation enteritis begins when symptoms begin and is dependent upon the severity. Dietary changes, specifically a low-fat, low-fiber diet, are usually initiated at the first sign of radiation enteritis and are often the only treatment necessary. Table 29-18 includes dietary guidelines for managing enteritis.

Some patients develop a lactose intolerance during treatment. If this occurs, reducing or eliminating lactose in the diet is necessary. Products such as lactaid or lactose-free milk may be recommended to ensure adequate intake of calcium and riboflavin.

If dietary changes do not sufficiently control acute radiation enteritis, pharmacological management is implemented (see Table 29-19). Conservative treatment with mild antidiarrheals such as Pepto Bismol® or Kaopectate® may be helpful initially. Diphenoxylate (Lomotil®)

**TABLE 29-18** Dietary Guidelines for Enteritis

This diet is planned to help reduce the chance that you will develop diarrhea during radiation therapy or to lessen its effects should it develop. Please start this diet as soon as you are instructed.

This diet restricts the intake of foods that are (1) *high in roughage* (the indigestible parts of plants); (2) *fatty foods* such as fats, oils, fatty meats, fried foods, or rich desserts that may be poorly absorbed; and (3) foods that might cause increased intestinal activity, such as hot peppers, regular coffee, and alcohol.

Follow this diet for at least 2 weeks after your course of treatment is completed. Slowly and cautiously resume your normal eating pattern. By adding one new food at a time, you will know if a certain food causes diarrhea. Simply leave that food out of your diet for another month and then try it again.

### FOOD GROUPS

*Vegetables*
Include: Cooked young vegetables such as beets, carrots, green pepper; strained tomatoes; peeled squash; tomato paste, sauce, and puree; potato without skins

Avoid: Raw vegetables; cooked broccoli; cabbage; green beans; cauliflower; brussels sprouts; celery; peas and dried beans (of all kinds); spinach; onions; corn; any vegetables cooked in butter, margarine, or cream sauces

*Fruits and Juices*
Include: Cooked or canned fruit without seeds or skins and fresh ripe bananas; fruit nectars; apple, grape, or cranberry juices with added vitamin C

Avoid: Raw fruits (except bananas); dried fruits such as currants, raisins, and prunes; orange and grapefruit juice

*Bread, Muffins, Crackers, Cereals, Other Grains*
Include: Enriched bread without seeds; melba toast; muffins (plain, corn, and English); plain crackers; refined cereals (Cream of Wheat, rice, cornflakes, etc); converted white rice; pasta; plain pancakes or waffles

Avoid: Whole-grain breads such as whole wheat, sprouted wheat, or bran; breads with seeds, nuts, fruit skins; whole grains such as bran or whole wheat; crackers with seeds such as sesame, etc

*Fats*
All foods should be baked, broiled, or boiled without added fats. Meat should be well trimmed. Use butter, margarine, or mayonnaise *sparingly* on bread, vegetables, and starches.

*Meats, Fish, Poultry, Eggs, and Other Protein Foods*
Include: All chicken, turkey, fish, lean beef, lamb, and veal; liver; tofu (broil, bake, *do not fry*); eggs; cheese such as low-fat cottage cheese; processed skim milk cheeses; part-skim mozzarella and ricotta; Velveeta; American string cheese; Parmesan

Avoid: Fried foods; sour cream; cream cheese; poultry skin; fatty meats; nuts; gravies

*(continued)*

**TABLE 29-18** Dietary Guidelines for Enteritis (continued)

| | |
|---|---|
| *Desserts* | |
| Include: | Frozen juice bars; sherbet; pudding made with nonfat milk; Jell-O; angel food cake; arrowroot cookies; ginger snaps; vanilla wafers; frozen yogurt; hard candies; jelly beans |
| Avoid: | Frostings made with milk or fats; pies; puddings; custards made with whole milk; whipped toppings; chocolate cake |
| *Beverages* | |
| Include: | Water; weak or decaffeinated tea; ginger ale or 7-Up–type soft drinks; decaffeinated colas and Gatorade®. All should be iced and stirred to reduce the fizz. |
| Avoid: | Regular coffee; Dr. Pepper; Mountain Dew; alcohol |
| *Milk* | |
| Include: | Skim milk; low-fat milk; powdered skim milk; buttermilk; evaporated skim milk; low-fat yogurt; vanilla ice milk; frozen yogurt |
| Avoid: | Whole milk; evaporated milk; cream; ice cream; chocolate milk |

or loperamide (Imodium®) may also be prescribed. Anticholinergics, antispasmodics, and/or bile salt sequestrating agents may also be prescribed when appropriate.

Management of severe diarrhea may include the use of opiates such as opium tincture, paregoric elixir, and codeine to decrease peristalsis. Sandostatin® given subcutaneously may also be used to control diarrhea by suppressing the secretion of serotonin and gastroenteropancreatic peptides possibly contributing to diarrhea. Based on the presumption that radiation increases prostaglandin secretion and evidence that certain prostaglandins may be responsible for diarrhea in some patients, antiprostaglandin compounds such as salicylates and choline magnesium trisalicylate are now under study. Clinical trials are under way to determine if these agents may be useful in preventing or managing acute and chronic radiation enteritis.

Nursing care must also focus on skin care in the perianal area. Table 29-4 offers skin care guidelines for use during and after completion of radiation therapy. Should dry or moist desquamation occur, methods should be employed to promote healing and comfort (Table 29-5).

While the diagnosis of acute radiation enteritis is easily made based on clinical findings, the diagnosis of chronic enteritis is not. It can occur months to years following treatment, and its clinical features are often attributed to a recurrence of a malignancy. In any patient who received previous abdominal pelvic irradiation, chronic radiation enteritis should be suspected and attempts made to establish the diagnosis. Unfortunately, there are no specific noninvasive screening tests available to make this diagnosis, and those utilized are often inconclusive for various reasons. Diagnostic tests utilized include small bowel fol-

low-through, single-contrast barium infusion, and biochemical and hematologic testing. Correlation of test results with the clinical history and presentation is necessary to establish the diagnosis.

Chronic radiation enteritis most frequently occurs six months to five years following completion of treatment, although it may occur earlier or much later in some patients. It is estimated that 5%–15% of patients who received a dose greater than 55 Gy to the abdomen or pelvis may develop chronic enteritis.[82]

Progressive endarteritis is thought to be responsible for chronic changes in the alimentary tract. Mucosal ulceration and infarction necrosis may occur, and partial or complete obstruction may develop as a result of adhesions.

Conservative treatment of chronic radiation enteritis is preferred unless a patient presents with an acute problem requiring surgical intervention, such as complete obstruction or perforation. Diets low in fat and residue and free of gluten and lactose are frequently used to manage diarrhea and malabsorption problems. Antidiarrheal agents, antispasmodics, bile sequestrating agents, and broad-spectrum antibiotics may be used to treat obstructive and malabsorption symptoms.

Although resolution is usually temporary, a conservative approach is often used in treating patients with a partial bowel obstruction. Surgical intervention may become necessary as symptoms tend to recur without treatment of the underlying problem. Conservative treatment includes decompression with a nasogastric tube and support with parenteral fluids. This is followed by maintenance on a soft-liquid diet.

Repeated episodes of partial bowel obstruction often occur, necessitating surgical intervention. Intractable diarrhea and abdominal pain are also indications for surgery. It is important to note that there is often an increased risk of surgical complications including poor vascularity and impaired wound healing in irradiated tissue. When possible, patients should be free of infection and nutritionally stable at the time of surgery.

Controversy exists over the choice of surgical procedure to employ when attempting to repair chronic radiation enteritis. The choice of procedure is often dependent upon the presenting symptoms as well as clinical findings at the time of surgery. If extensive disease is found, a bypass procedure is usually recommended. However, if only a single discrete area of disease is found, resection and primary anastomosis is the preferred treatment.

Patient assessment should focus on abdomen and bowel status. Any changes or complaints indicative of progressing enteritis require prompt attention. This would include abdominal pain, hypo- or hyperactive bowel sounds, nausea and/or vomiting, a change in bowel movements, rectal bleeding, and impaired nutrition/hydration status.

Dietary changes should be reviewed with special attention placed on those items that can be included, as opposed to just those that must be avoided. If medications are prescribed, written instructions on use and potential side effects should be provided.

**TABLE 29-19**   Suggested Pharmacological Management of Diarrhea

| Drug | Active Ingredient | Adult Dosage | Comments |
|---|---|---|---|
| | | OVER-THE-COUNTER DRUGS | |
| *Nonspecific Therapy*<br>Kaopectate®<br>  Caplet—750 mg<br>  Liquid—600 mg/15 ml | Attapulgite | Initial: 2 caplets or 30 ml<br>Repeat as needed after each loose stool (maximum: 12 caplets in 24 hr) | Attapulgite is a clay-containing material<br>Acts as an adsorbent<br>Does not decrease gastric motility |
| Donnagel®<br>  Tablet—600 mg<br>  Liquid—600 mg/15 ml | Attapulgite plus three anticholinergics (atropine, scopolamine, hyoscyamine) | Initial: 2 tablets or 30 ml, then 1 tablet or 15 ml every 3 hr as needed | Adsorbent plus anticholinergic activity<br>Useful in diarrhea associated with abdominal cramping |
| Pepto-Bismol®<br>  Tablet<br>  Liquid<br>  (one tablet = 15 ml liquid) | Bismuth subsalicylate | Initial: 2 tablets or 30 ml<br>Repeat every ½–1 hr as needed (maximum: 8 doses in 24 hr) | Antisecretory and adsorbent<br>May temporarily turn stool black or darken tongue<br>Contains salicylates, caution advised when taken with oral anticoagulants<br>Also relieves associated abdominal cramping |
| Metamucil®<br>  Flavored powder<br>  Wafers | Psyllium<br>Hydrophilic mucilloid | One to three doses daily prepared per product label instructions | Absorbent<br>Bulk-forming natural fiber<br>Encourage additional fluids for optimal benefit |
| Imodium A-D®<br>  Caplet—2 mg<br>  Liquid—1 mg/5 ml | Loperamide HCl | Initial: 2 caplets or 20 ml, then 1 caplet or 10 ml after each loose stool (maximum: 4 caplets or 40 ml/24 hr, unless otherwise directed by physician) | Antiperistaltic activity<br>No central opioid activity found at normal therapeutic doses<br>Also available as prescription drug |
| Amphojel®<br>  Suspension 320 mg/5 ml | Aluminum hydroxide gel | 20–40 ml 4 times daily | Absorbent<br>Popular use as an antacid—alternate with magnesium-containing antacids to avoid swings from diarrhea to constipation |
| *Specific Therapy*<br>Bacid, Lactinex<br>  Capsule<br>  Chewable tablet<br>  Powder packets | *Lactobacillus* cultures | Bacid: 2 capsules 2–4 times/day, preferably with milk<br>Lactinex: 4 tablets or 1 packet 3–4 times/day | Help to restore normal intestinal flora after antibiotic use<br>Refrigeration necessary<br>Contraindications: allergy to milk or sensitivity to lactose |
| | | PRESCRIPTION DRUGS | |
| *Nonspecific Therapy*<br>Imodium®<br>  Capsule—2 mg | Loperamide HCl | Initial: 2 capsules, then 1 capsule after each unformed stool (maximum: 8 capsules in 24 hr) | Nonnarcotic<br>Antiperistaltic activity<br>Unlike Lomotil® and codeine, no central opioid activity found at normal therapeutic doses<br>Also available as over-the-counter drug (Imodium A-D) |
| Lomotil®<br>  Tablet<br>  Liquid<br>  One tablet = 5 ml | Diphenoxylate HCl (2.5 mg) plus atropine sulfate (0.025 mg) | 1–2 tablets (5–10 ml) 3–4 times daily (maximum: 8 tablets/40 ml in 24 hr) | Opiate<br>Schedule V controlled drug<br>Atropine added to discourage drug abuse<br>High doses (40–60 ml) may cause opioid activity including euphoria and respiratory depression |

*(continued)*

**TABLE 29-19** Suggested Pharmacological Management of Diarrhea (continued)

| Drug | Active Ingredient | Adult Dosage | Comments |
|---|---|---|---|
| Codeine<br>Tablet—15 mg, 30 mg, 60 mg | Codeine sulfate | PO: 30–60 mg every 4–6 hr as needed | Opiate<br>Schedule II controlled drug<br>More constipating than morphine<br>30 mg equivalent to 5 mg Lomotil or 2 mg Imodium |
| Tincture of opium<br>Liquid: 10% opium, 19% alcohol base | Opium | PO: 0.6 ml every 4–6 hr as needed | Opiate<br>Schedule II controlled drug<br>6 mg morphine equivalent per 0.6 ml dose (do not confuse with paregoric)<br>Anise flavor<br>Dilute with 30 ml water prior to taking |
| Paregoric<br>Liquid: camphorated tincture of opium 0.4%, 45% alcohol base | Opium | PO: 5–10 ml taken 1–4 times daily | Opiate<br>Schedule III controlled drug<br>2 mg morphine equivalent per 5 ml dose<br>Brown liquid appears milky when water is added |
| Sandostatin<br>1 ml ampuls in 3 strengths<br>.05 mg/ml<br>0.1 mg/ml<br>0.5 mg/ml | Octreotide acetate | SQ: 50–200 μg given 2–3 times daily<br>IV: 150 μg/hr by continuous infusion | Antisecretory<br>Side effects: pain at injection site, nausea, headache<br>Effective for 5-FU induced diarrhea |
| *Specific Therapy*<br>Antimicrobial agents | — | — | Specific to causative organism and susceptibility tests<br>May increase diarrhea if no bacteria present |
| Questran<br>Bulk powder | Cholestyramine | 16—32 g/day in 2–4 divided doses (before or during meals and at bedtime) | Binds unabsorbed bile salts in the gut<br>Give with at least 120 ml water or uncarbonated beverage<br>Take other drugs 1 hr before or 4 hrs after |
| VioKase, Pancrease, Cotazym<br>Tablet<br>Capsule<br>Powder packets | Pancreatin or pancrelipase | 1–3 tablets or capsules or 1–2 packets of powder with meals and snacks | Pancreatic enzyme used only for replacement<br>Do not change brands without physician approval<br>Capsules/tablets should not be chewed or crushed |

Absorbents—decrease fluidity of stool by absorbing water.

Adsorbents—hold noxious substances (toxins, bacteria) on drug surface preventing their absorption.

Opiates—decrease intestinal motility, thereby reducing stool frequency.

Antisecretory—inhibit GI endocrine secretion and/or inhibit secretion of fluids and electrolytes.

### Chemotherapy-induced enteritis

Destruction of rapidly proliferating cells of the intestinal mucosa by chemotherapeutic agents may also lead to enteritis and diarrhea. Epithelial cells in the small intestine (villi and microvilli) are more vulnerable to destruction than cells in the sigmoid colon, which have a longer cell cycle time. Epithelial damage occurs histologically in three stages:

1. initial injury (cellular atypia and maturation arrest)
2. progressive injury (cellular necrosis and epithelial denuding)
3. regeneration (resumption of mitotic activity and mucosal repair)

A rapid transit of intestinal contents is stimulated by these alterations and diarrhea results; adequate absorption of nutrients, fluids, and electrolytes is prevented. Without complications and supervening infections, normalization of the mucosa occurs seven to ten days after initial injury.

*Diarrhea,* an increase in the frequency, fluidity, or volume of bowel movements relative to one's usual pattern of bowel elimination, is often accompanied by abdominal cramping and rectal urgency. With excessive passing of stools, initiation and breakdown of anal tissue can occur and become a source of infection. Severity is documented through the use of a grading scale and can range from minimal symptoms (two to three stools over baseline) to bloody diarrhea. Diarrhea is also differentiated by the duration of the condition. Acute episodes are sudden in onset, lasting less than two weeks; chronic diarrhea lasts longer than two weeks.

In the cancer patient, diarrhea can be caused by the cancer itself (e.g., GI tumors) or can be tumor-related (e.g., partial intestinal obstruction). However, diarrhea most often results from the immediate previous therapies including chemotherapy, radiation therapy to fields that include the bowel, or GVHD following bone marrow transplantation. Other contributing factors include medications (antibiotics, antacids), dietary modifications (tube feedings, food intolerance), fecal impaction, anxiety, and increased stress. Since most diarrheas are not the result of a single mechanism, the key to management is knowing the multiple causes.

Chemotherapy-induced diarrhea most often results from the cytotoxic effects of the antimetabolites (5-FU and methotrexate) and the antitumor antibiotics (dactinomycin and doxorubicin). Of these, 5-FU associated diarrhea is the most toxic.[83]

The degree and duration of diarrhea depend on the drug, dose of drug, and intensity of drug administration. For example, weekly administration of 5-FU causes less toxicity than 5-FU given over five consecutive days or when given by continuous infusion. 5-FU's toxic effect is also potentiated when modulating compounds such as leucovorin are used to augment cytotoxicity. Asbury et al[84] report a 58% incidence of enteritis in metastatic colon cancer patients treated with 5-FU and high-dose leucovorin. Diarrhea was severe enough to cause hospitalization in seven patients (30%) and fatalities in two (9%). In an attempt to further improve therapeutic efficacy without worsening toxicity, the addition of thymostimulin to the 5-FU/leucovorin combination was tested.[85] A therapeutic advantage of the three-drug combination was demonstrated, with less toxicity than with leucovorin/5-FU alone.

Cancer patients treated with chemotherapy are frequently immunocompromised and susceptible to opportunistic infections. Invasion of mucosal walls by common microorganisms (e.g., *Escherichia coli*) can result in infectious diarrhea. If suspected, based on a careful patient history to rule out other causes, stools should be examined for pus, blood, fat, ova, or parasites; *Clostridium difficile* toxin; and culture and sensitivity. Antidiarrheal drugs that inhibit gut motility should be used cautiously or avoided until infectious causes are ruled out because they could slow elimination of pathogens from the GI system. Treatment of infectious diarrhea is based on the causative agent.

Since many cancer patients require antibiotic therapy at some point in their course of therapy, they are also at risk for antibiotic-associated colitis (pseudomembranous colitis). The cause is overgrowth of *C difficile* in the colon; almost all antibiotics can be responsible. Various classes of chemotherapeutic agents, most commonly methotrexate, have been reported to induce *C difficile* colitis, without recent exposure to antibiotics or GI surgery.[86] At high risk are leukemia and pediatric cancer patients.[87] Neutropenia may be responsible for the increased incidence of *C difficile* in leukemia patients. Neutropenic enterocolitis is a rare condition that can occur during treatment of hematologic malignancies, mainly lymphomas and leukemias; however, it may occur in any patient who is neutropenic and receiving chemotherapy. Clinical symptoms are nonspecific and include fever, diarrhea, bloody stools, and abdominal pain in the lower quadrant.

Intestinal candidiasis is rarely documented antemortem. A high index of suspicion is warranted in patients receiving any combination of chemotherapy, radiotherapy, corticosteroids, and antibiotics. Diagnosis requires elimination of other causes of diarrhea. A negative fungal culture of the oropharynx should not rule out involvement distally in the GI tract. The best diagnostic tool when possible is endoscopy with brushings and biopsy. Clinically stable, nonneutropenic patients may be treated initially with oral fluconazole (Diflucan); neutropenic or unstable patients require systemic amphotericin B.[88]

The treatment of chemotherapy-induced diarrhea is generally nonspecific, with the aim of restoring normal elimination patterns, maintaining adequate fluid intake and electrolyte balance, and reducing the discomfort and inconvenience of frequent bowel movements. The majority of chemotherapy-induced diarrhea episodes are mild and resolve within a week or less of stopping the causative agent unless other etiologies are identified.

Usually only simple supportive measures are required for mild and intermittent diarrhea. Measures include increasing fluid intake to 3 quarts daily; avoiding eating high-roughage, greasy, and spicy foods; avoiding using milk and caffeine products; and following prescribed medication schedules. The BRAT (banana, rice, applesauce, and toast) diet can be used temporarily. Patients who develop moderate to severe diarrhea should report these findings immediately. Considerably more attention and support are required. Interventions may include tube feedings, oral rehydration fluids, as well as intravenous hydration and nutritional support.

Patients often seek advice and/or prescriptions for relief of symptoms (nonspecific therapy) or relief of the underlying cause of the symptom (specific therapy) (Table 29-20). Until now the mainstay of nonspecific therapy has been the opiates and opiate derivatives. Of these, diphenoxylate and loperamide are the most widely pre-

**TABLE 29-20** Radiation-Induced Genitourinary Toxicities

| Tissue Response | Onset/Duration | Clinical Presentation | Physiological Rationale |
|---|---|---|---|
| Cystitis Acute | 30–40 Gy Resolution—2 wk after treatment completion | Bladder irritation, dysuria, frequency and urgency | Mucosal and submucosal inflammation. Capillary engorgement. |
| Chronic | 6 mo after high-dose radiation (65–70 Gy) | Frequency | Bladder volume diminished due to chronic replacement of detrusor muscle with fibrous deposits. |
| | | Hemorrhagic cystitis | Decreased capillary permeability results in increased pressure of blood flow. |
| Urethritis | 30–40 Gy Resolution—2 wk after treatment completion | Pain and burning with urination | Mucosal and submucosal inflammation. |
| | | | Epithelial cells are destroyed without sufficient replacement cells being produced. |
| Vaginitis | May begin during treatment and is chronic | Vaginal discharge, spontaneous and contact bleeding, dyspareunia, pruritus, dysuria, or pain | Epithelial cell loss results in thinning of the vaginal lining and loss of elasticity. |
| | | Fibrosis and stenosis | Diminished estrogen production is a direct result of radiation change. |
| | | | Adhesion formation. |

scribed. These drugs are effective in decreasing diarrhea by slowing peristaltic movements in the small and large intestines.

Psyllium preparations (e.g., Metamucil®) and adsorbent products (e.g., Kaopectate®) are other nonspecific agents sometimes used. Available over-the-counter, these agents may have no therapeutic effect in control of diarrhea. However, in milder cases they may help solidify the stool and decrease its frequency, thus allowing for more voluntary control of elimination.

Specific drug therapy (antibiotics) for treatment of acute infectious diarrhea is recommended in select cases based on the causative organism.[89] Octreotide acetate, a synthetic polypeptide analogue of somatostatin, has been used in the last decade to manage diarrhea associated with a number of secretory diarrheal disorders such as carcinoid and AIDS-related syndromes as well as acute GVHD following BMT. Recent preliminary data support the use of octreotide for treatment of chemotherapy–(5-FU and cisplatin)–related diarrhea.[87,90,91]

Complete resolution of diarrhea was reported by Petrelli et al[90] in 15 of 16 metastatic colorectal cancer patients given a continuous high-dose infusion of octreotide (150 μg/hr). All patients previously failed treatment with diphenoxylate plus atropine (Lomotil®). In a randomized trial Gebbia et al[91] supported subcutaneous (SQ) octreotide dosed at 0.5 mg three times per day to be more effective than oral loperamide (Imodium) 4 mg given three times per day in controlling 5-FU–induced diarrhea (grades 3 to 4). Resolution of diarrhea within four days

of treatment occurred in 83% of patients randomized to the octreotide arm versus 31% in the loperamide group. Octreotide is reported to be safely administered up to a maximum tolerated dose of 2000 mg SQ three times daily.[92] Although investigators suggest a dose-response effect, further clinical trials are warranted.

The efficacy of octreotide to prevent cisplatin-induced diarrhea has also been investigated.[93] Cisplatin-associated diarrhea generally occurs on the day of therapy and lasts no longer than 24 hours. Patients receiving cisplatin were randomized to receive placebo versus octreotide 0.1 mg, 15 minutes and 6 hours after cisplatin administration. Those given octreotide experienced less diarrhea (5% vs. 75%, $p = .01$). Although it appears from these studies that octreotide is effective in managing diarrhea associated with 5-FU and cisplatin, octreotide is costly. Ongoing randomized clinical trials are necessary to confirm its efficacy as well as justify its use as standard treatment for chemotherapy-induced diarrhea compared with the more common and less expensive antidiarrheal agents.

### Intestinal graft-versus-host disease

After allogeneic BMT, diarrhea is a prominent manifestation of intestinal involvement with GVHD. In its most severe form, acute GVHD causes profuse watery diarrhea (up to 15+ liters/day), protein and electrolyte loss, and marked debilitation. Available therapy with opiates is usually unsuccessful. Octreotide has been shown to be a useful agent in acute GVHD management. Ely et al[94] treated six BMT patients with SQ octreotide 50–250 µg three times a day. Three of six patients had significant responses within one to three days of starting octreotide therapy. Further studies are necessary to validate effectiveness.

Viral infections, herpes simplex, and varicella zoster are common after BMT, although acute GVHD is the most common cause of diarrhea. Treatment choice is acyclovir.

## ALTERATIONS OF THE GENITOURINARY MUCOUS MEMBRANES

### Radiation-Induced Cystitis and Urethritis

Radiation therapy employed to treat cancers of the genitourinary system, such as prostate, cervix, and bladder cancers, often results in a temporary irritation of the bladder and/or urethra. This irritation can be annoying and can cause considerable discomfort. Acute reactions tend to subside within two to three weeks after treatment completion (see Table 29-20). Due to the similarity of symptoms to a urinary tract infection, a clean-catch urine specimen is sent for culture and sensitivity, and antibiotics are prescribed as needed. A positive culture is unusual.

Treatment is directed at reducing irritation. Patients should be instructed to increase fluid intake as dilute urine will cause less irritation. Urinary anesthetics (Pyridium®) and antispasmodics (Urispas®, Ditropan®) are frequently used for symptom management.

Chronic cystitis is much less common, with an occurrence of about 15% in patients who have received high-dose irradiation (65–70 Gy). These patients will have considerable bladder contraction and submucosal hemorrhage. While no preventive treatment is available, the risk decreases when physical irritation is minimized. Trauma from infection and mechanical instrumentation and catheterization should be avoided.

### Radiation-Induced Vaginitis

Radiation therapy used in the treatment of gynecologic and colorectal malignancies frequently results in significant acute and chronic alterations in the vaginal mucosa. The rapidly proliferating cells of the mucosa as well as its secretory glands are quite radiosensitive, similar to those of the oral mucosa. This, coupled with the high doses needed to control these malignancies, places the vagina at high risk for radiation-induced complications.

The effects of radiation on the vaginal mucosa include erythema, inflammation, atrophy, fibrosis, hypopigmentation, telangiectasia, inelasticity, and ulceration. Clinical

manifestations are reviewed in Table 29-20. The physiological rationale for these changes is quite similar to that of the skin and GI mucous membranes. If preventive measures are not taken following pelvic irradiation, partial or complete vaginal occlusion can occur as a result of stenosis and adhesion formation. This combined with vaginal dryness can have serious implications in that sexual intercourse and pelvic examination become difficult, painful, and occasionally not feasible. Surgical intervention may become necessary to restore patency.

Fibrosis and vaginal stenosis may develop as a result of adhesions and can manifest as early as during the immediate postirradiation period when acute reactions are beginning to resolve. Women who are able to continue having intercourse during treatment have considerably less adhesion formation.[11,95] Adhesions develop most frequently at the areas receiving the highest doses of radiation. This includes the area between the ectocervix and vaginal mucosa, and the anterior and posterior surfaces of the upper third of the vagina. If adhesions are left unmanaged, they can result in occlusion, stenosis, and vaginal shortening. Stenosis is generally limited to the upper third of the vagina.

Patients at greatest risk for developing radiation vaginitis are those who have received treatment for cervical cancer. These patients often receive doses in excess of 100 Gy with a combination of external beam and brachytherapy. Direct effects of high-dose radiation on the vaginal mucosa and estrogen production combined with mechanical trauma induced by brachytherapy applicators and packing can result in severe trauma to the vaginal mucosa and underlying tissue.

Less commonly seen, but nonetheless the most serious complication of high-dose radiation, is tissue necrosis. A result of trauma and severe vascular damage, necrosis can result in vesicovaginal and/or rectovaginal fistula formation and hemorrhage. Conservative management is usually attempted for necrosis. This includes estrogen cream, antibiotic therapy, debridement, and antiseptic douches.[96] Tissue necrosis can cause severe pain that is often unresponsive to systemic therapy. Use of nonpharmacological pain interventions may be beneficial when combined with systemic therapy.

Fistula formation and hemorrhage often require surgical management; however, outcomes are often poor due to the severely damaged vasculature of irradiated tissue. Urinary or bowel diversion or total pelvic exenteration is occasionally necessary.

Postirradiation vaginitis can have significant consequences if not managed appropriately. Nursing interventions begin early, prior to treatment, to prevent or minimize its debilitating effects. The goals of intervention are to promote comfort and sexual expression and to ensure that complications do not impede medical follow-up.

Nurses also need to be cognizant of the increased risk of vaginal infections in patients who have received radiation to the pelvic area and should assess for signs and symptoms of an infection. Patients should be instructed to always report fever, changes in vaginal drainage, and pain. Early identification of an infection and prompt medical intervention will help to alleviate discomfort and prevent serious complications.

Discussing sexuality and the sexual organs can be very difficult for many people, and so it is often avoided. The implications of this can be fear and anxiety when patients complete treatment; anger because they were not aware of potential long-term consequences; and poor compliance with interventions. Patients and their significant others must be educated prior to radiation therapy as to the acute and late effects of radiation, as well as to the planned treatment for postirradiation vaginitis.

Treatment for radiation vaginitis usually begins two weeks after the completion of radiation when the acute reactions have begun to subside. Management is by vaginal dilatation and use of vaginal estrogen preparations. Dilatation can be accomplished through sexual intercourse and/or use of a vaginal dilator designed to minimize fibrosis and stenosis. Because dryness and some fibrosis may have already begun to occur, patients should be instructed to use a water-soluble lubricant during vaginal intercourse to reduce discomfort and to prevent irritation and trauma.

Vaginal estrogen preparations such as Premarin® and Estrace® may be used in the form of a cream or vaginal suppository. They are relatively easy to use and appear safe in the treatment of radiation vaginitis. However, vaginal estrogen preparations are absorbed systemically and result in high sustained levels of estrogen in the systemic circulation; therefore, their use should be avoided in patients with medical or oncological conditions in which systemic estrogen therapy is contraindicated. Patients need to know that the use of estrogen preparations will need to be permanent as high-dose pelvic radiation results in chronic estrogen deprivation. Patients treated prophylactically with estrogen preparations after radiation have been found to have less bleeding, dyspareunia, and narrowing of the vaginal caliber. Its use promotes epithelial regeneration and helps to prevent mucosal atrophy.[97]

Vaginal dilatation should take place at least three times per week, and its importance reinforced to the patient. Maintaining vaginal patency is essential for follow-up examinations as well as for sexual intercourse.

The use of a dilator may be quite distressing for some women. Fear of pain as well as a connotation of masturbation can reduce compliance. Nurses need to assess patients' feelings regarding its use and correct any misconceptions. Sensitivity and compassion are of utmost importance when reviewing the procedure with patients. Patients should be given verbal and written instructions on proper use of the dilator and should be encouraged to express any fears or concerns regarding its use. If possible, a dilator should be provided by the radiation oncology department. This will prevent the embarrassment often experienced when purchasing one. Table

29-21 includes patient instructions for using a vaginal dilator.

If patients are sexually active and have intercourse at least three times per week, use of a dilator is not necessary. If they are sexually active but have intercourse less than three times per week, use of a dilator is necessary.

Patients are encouraged to continue having intercourse; however, body image changes and fear of pain often interfere. Speaking with a patient's significant other, with the patient's permission, may be beneficial. Occasionally, the fragile vaginal mucosa is irritated by semen. Use of a nonlubricated condom and water-soluble lubricant may help prevent irritation. Water-soluble lubricants must always be used. Reinforcement of the need to continue vaginal dilatation should be provided at each follow-up visit. Review of proper technique is often necessary.

## Chemotherapy-Induced Vaginitis

Potentially any drug known to cause oral mucositis may also be associated with painful irritation and inflammation of the vagina. Because the vagina is near the vulva, women may experience both vulvar and vaginal irritation (vulvovaginitis). Other factors contributing to vaginitis besides cytotoxic therapy include exposure to pelvic irra-

**TABLE 29-21　Use of a Vaginal Dilator**

Vaginal dilatation is recommended for all women who have received radiation to the pelvis. This is to reduce the scar tissue that may form after treatment, which can cause the vagina to narrow. Dilatation can be accomplished through sexual intercourse and/or use of a vaginal dilator. Dilators are designed to keep the vagina open so that pelvic examination and/or sexual intercourse is not uncomfortable.

Vaginal dilators come in different sizes. Your nurse or doctor will decide which size you should use and if or when you need to change to a different size. Use the dilator three times each week.

1. Insert the dilator either lying in bed with knees bent or by standing with one foot up on a step or the toilet. Both positions will allow for relatively easy insertion.
2. Before you insert the dilator, apply a *water-soluble lubricant* on the dilator. Recommended lubricants include, but are not limited to: Astroglide®, K-Y Jelly®, Lubrin®, and Replens®.
3. Gently insert the rounded tip of the dilator into the vagina. Insert it as far as possible and hold the dilator in place.
4. Leave the dilator in place for 10–15 minutes. You should not feel pain or discomfort when the dilator is in.
5. Remove the dilator and rinse it with soap and water. Do not be alarmed if you notice a small amount of blood when you use the dilator the first few times.
6. Use the dilator three times a week unless you have sexual intercourse more than three times a week.

Please let your nurse or doctor know if you do not think you will be able to insert the dilator, if you have difficulty using the dilator, or if you have any increased bleeding or pain.

diation, antibiotic therapy, immunosuppressive therapy, and change in pH of the vagina.

Symptoms may occur three to five days after chemotherapy is given and resolve seven to ten days later. The nurse should inquire as to whether the patient is experiencing any discomfort because such information may not be easily volunteered. Signs and symptoms to report include vaginal discharge, itching, odor, pain, soreness, bleeding, or dyspareunia. The vulvar and vaginal membranes should be inspected for signs of impaired integrity such as erythema, swelling, or ulceration.

Nursing interventions are directed toward measures to decrease inflammation of mucous membranes, to increase comfort, and to minimize complications. Comfort can be provided with cold compresses or cool sitz baths for relief of pruritus and warm compresses for severe inflammation. Patients are instructed to wear cotton underpants and to avoid pantyhose and tight-fitting clothes. Analgesics may be needed for severe discomfort or pain. Exposure to physical and chemical irritants (e.g., tampons, genital deodorant sprays, deodorant-containing vaginal pads or liners) should be avoided to decrease inflammation of the mucous membranes.

The importance of recognizing specific treatable causes such as *Candida* vaginitis must be emphasized. Laboratory tests and cultures are valuable to determine causative organisms (e.g., potassium hydroxide–prepared slide identifies *Candida*). Medical treatment is based on etiology and includes topical and systemic medications.

The treatment of choice for *Candida* vaginitis is miconazole nitrate (Nystatin®) or clotrimazole (Gyne-Lotrimin®) cream or suppositories. When vaginal creams are prescribed, patients should be taught not to use tampons, which will absorb the medication. If a suppository is ordered, the patient should be instructed where it is to be placed (i.e., vaginally, not rectally). The importance of completing the course of therapy should be stressed since recurrence is common if therapy is stopped early. *Trichomonas* vaginitis is treated systemically with metronidazole (Flagyl); it is further recommended that the partner also receive therapy.

Prevention of chemotherapy-induced vaginitis includes educating the patient regarding good personal hygiene measures. The nurse's goal is to help the patient maintain a healthy vagina, thereby reducing the potential for secondary vaginal infections. The perineum should be cleansed following each urination and bowel movement with mild soap and water and then pat- or air-dried. Soap and water remove most odors from noninfectious causes; persistent genital odor should be investigated. An unresearched but popular hygiene practice recommends front-to-back wiping to prevent vaginal and urethral contamination with fecal organisms. Routine douching is not recommended.

Patient and family education should also include sexual activity guidelines. The patient is instructed to use a water-based lubricant during vaginal intercourse to avoid mucosal irritation. Condoms should be used to prevent transmission of organisms through nonintact mucosa. Vaginal intercourse should be avoided in the presence of mucosal ulcerations and while neutrophil and platelet counts are low. Alternative methods of sexual activity should be suggested.

# MALIGNANT WOUNDS

## Description

Malignant wounds can be one of the most debilitating and frustrating sequelae of cancerous infiltration of the epithelium. In addition to the detrimental effect on quality of life, if unmanaged these wounds can be the source of anemia, electrolyte imbalances, and a portal for infection.

Fortunately, these wounds are uncommon; however, when they do occur they are challenging and difficult to manage. Malignant wounds are most often seen in patients with cancers of the breast, stomach, lung, uterus, kidney, ovary, colon, and bladder; melanoma; sarcoma; and lymphoma. Mucosis fungoides is a T-cell lymphoma involving the skin that can develop into fungating lesions.

Malignant wounds are characterized by excessive purulent drainage, odor, and infection. They develop from local extension or tumor embolization into the epithelium and its supporting structures. Vascular permeability is altered in malignant wounds, persisting to provide a constant source of nutrients and oxygen to cells, thereby enhancing unregulated growth. Malignant cells continually secrete growth factors and have platelet-type functions that continually add new vasculature and collagen to support malignant growth. As the lesion increases in size, it "outgrows" and loses its vasculature, resulting in fragile capillaries. Poor vascular perfusion and altered collagen synthesis result in tissue ischemia and necrosis.[98,99]

Malignant wounds may develop at the primary cancer site or at a distant site due to metastasis. The latter, coupled with variability in appearance, often results in misdiagnosis until a lesion has become large and fungating.

A variety of treatments used alone or in combination have been reported. Choice of treatment is often based upon whether the disease is local or disseminated and whether the goal is to cure or simply palliate.

When definitive treatment is planned, local control is usually attempted with surgery, radiation, and/or hyperthermia. Surgical extirpation with or without radiotherapeutic sterilization is often successful in providing pain relief and eliminating infection, drainage, and odor. This procedure is contraindicated in patients with extensive disseminated disease.

Hyperthermia used alone or in conjunction with radiation therapy and cytotoxic drugs has shown impressive response. Hyperthermia has direct cytotoxic effects on heat-sensitive hypoxic cells, sensitizes cells to radiation, and enhances the cytotoxic effect of some radiosensitizing agents.

Microwaves or ultrasound are used to deliver local heat. The goal is to maintain a temperature of 42 °C–44 °C for 30–60 minutes. Hyperthermia should be delivered 30 minutes before or 30 minutes after radiation. The procedure is repeated two to three times per week. More frequent application has been shown to cause thermotolerance of some cells. Technical problems and an inability of some patients to tolerate heat often limit the use of hyperthermia.

## Nursing Considerations

The nurse's role in caring for a patient with a malignant wound is profound. Care requires flexibility, creativity, knowledge of normal wound healing and the pathophysiology of malignant wounds, and often unending patience. Unfortunately, little has been published regarding malignant wounds and their management. These wounds have a very poor prognosis for healing. Malignant wounds do not undergo normal healing due to the inability of epithelial cells to migrate over active tumors and their altered vascularity. Nonetheless, principles of normal wound healing and management should be the basis for planning care.

The goals of management should include minimizing the negative impact on quality of life, promoting comfort, maintaining an environment conducive to healing, maintaining and promoting the integrity of the skin surrounding the wound, and preventing fluid and electrolyte imbalance from excessive drainage.

Nursing responsibilities in managing this patient population include assessment, planning, evaluation, and patient education. Initial assessment and documentation should include wound characteristics—amount of drainage, presence of odor and infection, and measurement.

Based on assessment and principles of wound healing, a wound management program should be planned. Patients and their significant others should be encouraged to participate in the planning, implementation, and evaluation of care. They need to understand the difficulty in managing these wounds, have a realistic expectation for intervention, and realize that many changes in treatment strategy may be necessary. An acceptable and realistic plan of care will improve patient compliance and improve quality of life.

Considerations in developing a wound care regimen include goal of therapy (e.g., odor control, infection control, minimizing drainage), financial resources, product availability, ease of treatment, patient's ability to perform intervention, and availability of caregivers. Poor compliance will occur if patients cannot afford or obtain supplies; therefore, creative management is necessary. Table 29-6 includes many classifications of agents used in wound management, the rationale for their use, and product examples. The information is by no means exhaustive. A decision to use any product or combination of products is acceptable if based on principles of wound healing. Unless otherwise indicated, products should be used according to the package insert.

In order to maintain an optimal environment with control of infection, odor, and drainage, certain interventions are required. The following discussion will include debridement, infection control, hemostasis, wound care, and odor control.

### Debridement

Malignant wounds often contain large amounts of necrotic tissue and eschar that contribute to infection and odor and therefore should be removed. Debridement may be chemical or mechanical. Chemical debridement may be appropriate in the presence of a moderate amount of necrotic tissue or eschar. Great care must be used in ensuring that caustic agents do not disrupt normal tissue.

Gentle mechanical debridement is usually preferred and may be accomplished with vigorous wound irrigation using a large syringe. Wet to dry dressings are contraindicated as they are counterproductive and may induce trauma and bleeding when removed. If eschar is dense, it may act as a splint to prevent wound contraction. This may require surgical removal. Maintaining a debrided state will help to prevent infection, control odor, and reduce drainage.

### Infection control

Malignant wounds frequently become infected from bacterial infiltration. *E coli, Pseudomonas aeruginosa,* and strains of *Staphylococcus, Proteus,* and *Klebsiella* are common in these wounds, especially those with incomplete debridement. It is important to differentiate between normal wound inflammation with the presence of colonizing microorganisms and the presence of invading microorganisms. Organisms found in wound fluid are not necessarily invading. A positive wound culture of $>10^5$ bacteria is indicative of infection. In this case, antibiotics are appropriate and may be ordered based upon the specific organism. Topical antibiotics are often more successful due to the diminished vasculature and presence of necrotic tissue that may impede systemic therapy.[13] Proper wound care and cleaning will help to prevent infection.

### Hemostasis

Malignant wounds frequently bleed due to fragile vasculature and capillary oozing. If not managed, this can result in acute or chronic anemia. Bleeding is most often a result of trauma and can usually be prevented by proper wound care. Trauma can be greatly reduced by keeping wounds moist and using nonadherent dressings. If a wound and its dressing do become dry, soaking the dressing in normal saline before removal will help to prevent trauma.

Hemolytic agents may be necessary to arrest small-vessel bleeds. If unable to arrest bleeding with these agents or if bleeding is severe, radiation delivered in doses of 2–4 Gy per day may be given until bleeding stops.

### Cleansing

Wounds must be kept clean and free of debris if infection, drainage, and odor are to be controlled. Cleansing with a mild soap and water or nontoxic cleanser will help to remove necrotic tissue with minimal trauma.

Antiseptic agents commonly used in the past are not considered appropriate for most patients due to the caustic effect on cells and the rapid inactivation by many body fluids. If used, great care must be employed to protect healthy tissue. Agents should be rinsed thoroughly from the wound with water or normal saline.[98]

### Wound dressing

Maintaining a moist wound environment is necessary in order to prevent trauma from drying and fissuring, stimulate epithelial cell migration over any normal tissue, and facilitate resurfacing. Angiogenesis of tumors can be enhanced by fibrinolysis, which is stimulated by a moist environment. This tumor vascularization, in turn, can enhance the effectiveness of radiation and chemotherapy.

Moist wound environments can be attained using any number of wound care products. Wound fillers are very absorbent and can be used on noninfected wounds. Epithelial-stimulating wound gels such as aloe vera hydrogel, if applied liberally and not allowed to dry, also maintain a moist, pH-adjusted environment. Calcium alginate dressings can absorb large amounts of exudate and are easily removed without pain.[100] Occlusive hydrocolloid dressings have limited use in this type of wound due to their uneven texture, which makes application and occlusion difficult. Petroleum-impregnated dressings should be avoided as they inhibit aeration and increase anaerobic bacterial growth.

Dressings should be chosen that conceal and collect drainage and minimize odor and unnecessary expense. Nonadherent dressings should be used to prevent trauma to the wound bed during dressing changes. Cost-effective alternatives include sanitary pads and disposable diapers with nonadherent linings. These items are inexpensive, easy to obtain, and very absorbent. Care should be taken to avoid plastic placed next to the skin.

Maintaining the normal tissue surrounding the wound is important. Irritation by caustic agents, wound drainage, and tape used to secure dressings should be avoided.

Skin barriers and creative alternatives to tape can be used to prevent irritation. Montgomery straps, oversized sports bras, tube dressings, and flexible netting are alternatives. If it is necessary to use tape, hydrocolloid dressings can be applied to healthy skin and used as a base for securing tape.

### Odor management

Odor can be the most debilitating consequence of malignant wounds as it greatly impacts quality of life and normalcy. Patients often withdraw and avoid social situations because of the offensive odor.

The odor of these wounds is a result of bacterial invasion and the presence of debris and necrotic tissue. Attempts should be made to eliminate the cause of odor or, when this is not possible, to disguise the odor.

Frequent cleansing using a handheld shower (two to three times a day) will help to eliminate bacteria and excessive drainage. Cleansing with a dilute Dakin's solution 0.25% is useful to dissolve necrotic tissue. Chlorhexidine gluconate 4% (Hibiclens®, Stuart Pharmaceuticals, Wilmington, DE) is also effective. Chlorophyll-containing ointment and solution (Chloresium®) applied directly to the wound may significantly decrease or eliminate odor. If used, patients, caregivers, and health care team members should be aware of its green color. It has also been suggested that chlorophyll tablets taken orally may help control odor. No detrimental effects have been reported from the use of these agents. Nitronidazole (25 mg orally three times a day) has been used systemically as well as topically to control the odor caused by anaerobic infection. A 1% metronidazole solution can be used to irrigate the wound, followed by application of a 0.75% metronidazole gel (MetroGel®, Galderma Laboratories Inc., Fort Worth, TX) either once or twice daily.[101]

If the cause of odor cannot be eliminated, various deodorizing sprays and solutions and charcoal-containing dressings are available that may help to reduce offensive odors. Charcoal dressings tend to be quite expensive, which may limit their acceptability for long-term use. Suggesting that patients reserve use of these dressings for times when frequent dressing changes are not possible or when fear of odor is especially profound (as in social situations) may be financially feasible and help to promote socialization.

Although unconventional, odor control using yogurt or buttermilk, either applied topically or taken orally, has been found to be useful. Although the mechanism is not clear, it is postulated that the low pH of lactobacilli directly affects wound odor by inhibiting the growth of odor-producing organisms that require an alkaline medium for growth.

The psychosocial implications of malignant wounds cannot be overstated. Patients often are unable to separate wound from self and may feel as though their body is rotting. Isolation may result from embarrassment, shame, and guilt. Health care providers must treat patients with respect and compassion in order to improve self-concept.

In order to provide optimal care for patients with malignant wounds, nurses need to report successful interventions. Only through study and dissemination of information will health care providers be successful in managing malignant wounds and their subsequent consequences and in ensuring patients' optimal quality of life.

# REFERENCES

1. Stenn KS, Bhawan J: The normal histology of the skin, in Farmer ER, Hood AF (eds): *Pathology of the Skin.* Norwalk, CT, Appleton and Lange, 1990, pp 3–36

2. Jaworsky C: Dermatopathology of hair, in Murphy G (ed): *Dermatopathology: A Practical Guide to Common Disorders.* Philadelphia, Saunders, 1995, pp 371–393

3. Holbrook KA: Structure and development of the skin, in Soter NA, Baden HP (eds): *Pathophysiology of Dermatologic Diseases* (ed 2). New York, McGraw-Hill, 1991, pp 3–44

4. Perez CA, Brady LW: *Principles and Practice of Radiation Oncology.* (ed 2). Philadelphia, Lippincott, 1992

5. Hall EJ, Cox JD: Physical and biologic basis of radiation therapy, in Cox JD (ed): *Moss' Radiation Oncology: Rationale, Technique, Results,* (ed 7). St. Louis, Mosby, 1994, pp 3–66

6. Shimm DS, Cassady RJ: The skin, in Cox JD (ed): *Moss' Radiation Oncology: Rationale, Technique, Results,* (ed 7). St. Louis, Mosby, 1994, pp 99–118

7. Sitton E: Early and late radiation-induced skin alterations: Part I. Mechanisms of skin changes. *Oncol Nurs Forum* 19: 801–807, 1992

8. Sitton E: Early and late radiation-induced skin alterations: Part II. Nursing care of irradiated skin. *Oncol Nurs Forum* 19:907–912, 1992

9. Dow KH, Hilderley LJ: *Nursing Care in Radiation Oncology.* Philadelphia, Saunders, 1992

10. Margolin SG, Breneman JC, Denman DL, et al: Management of radiation-induced moist skin desquamation using hydrocolloid dressings. *Cancer Nurs* 13:71–80, 1990

11. McDonald A: Altered protective mechanisms, in Dow KH, Hilderley L (eds): *Nursing Care in Radiation Oncology.* Philadelphia, Saunders, 1992, pp 96–125

12. Winchester D, Cox JD: Standards for breast conservation. *CA Cancer J Clin* 42:134–162, 1992

13. Eaglstein W, Rudolph R, Shannon ML: New directions in wound healing. *Wound Care Manual* 1:1–99, 1990

14. Ratliff C: Impaired skin integrity related to radiation therapy. *J Entero Ther* 17:193–198, 1990

15. Hutchinson JJ, McGuckin M: Occlusive dressings: A microbiologic and clinical review. *Am J Infect Control* 18:257–268, 1990

16. Hardy MA: The biology of scar formation. *Phys Ther* 69: 1014–1024, 1989

17. Million R, Parsons J, Mendenhall W: Scar tissue, in Vaeth J, Meyer J (eds): *Radiation Tolerance of Normal Tissue.* New York, Karger, 1989, pp 83–100

18. DeSpain JD: Dermatologic toxicity, in Perry MC (ed): *The Chemotherapy Source Book.* Baltimore, Williams and Wilkins, 1992, pp 531–547

19. Siegel RD, Schiffman FJ: Systemic toxicity following intracavitary administration of bleomycin. *Chest* 98:509, 1990

20. Rest EB, Horn TD: Dermatology, in Armitage JO, Antman KH (eds): *High-Dose Cancer Therapy* (ed 2). Baltimore, Williams and Wilkins, 1995, pp 578–608

21. Clavell LA, Gelber RA, Cohen HJ, et al: Four-agent induction and intensive asparaginase therapy for treatment of childhood acute lymphocytic leukemia. *N Engl J Med* 315: 657–663, 1986

22. Weiss RB: Hypersensitivity reactions, in Perry MC (ed): *The Chemotherapy Source Book.* Baltimore, Williams and Wilkins, 1992, pp 553–569

23. Canal P, Bugot R, Chatelut E, et al: Phase I pharmacoki-

netic study of intraperitoneal teniposide (VM26). *Eur J Cancer Clin Oncol* 25:815–820, 1989

24. Lokich JJ, Moore C: Chemotherapy associated palmar plantar erythrodysesthesia syndrome. *Ann Intern Med* 101: 798–800, 1984

25. Burgdorf WHC, Gilmore WA, Garick RG: Peculiar acral erythema secondary to high dose chemotherapy for acute myelogenous leukemia. *Ann Intern Med* 97:61–62, 1982

26. Seiz AM, Yarbro CH: Pruritus, in Groenwald S, Frogge M, Goodman M, Yarbro CH (eds): *Cancer Symptom Management* (ed 3). Boston, Jones and Bartlett, 1996, pp 137–150

27. Bord MA, McCray ND, Shaffer S: Alteration in comfort: Pruritus, in McNally JC, Somerville ET (eds): *Guidelines for Oncology Nursing Practice* (ed 2). Philadelphia, Saunders, 1991, pp 143–147

28. Dangel R: Pruritus and cancer. *Oncol Nurs Forum* 13(1): 17–21, 1986

29. Serrano G, Aliaga A, Febrer I: Dacarbazine-induced photosensitivity. *Photoderm* 6:140–141, 1989

30. Ayres S: Hair transplantation, in Epstein ED (ed): *Skin Surgery* (ed 6). Philadelphia, Saunders, 1987, pp 198–279

31. Freedman TG: Social and cultural dimensions of hair loss in women treated for breast cancer. *Cancer Nurs* 17: 334–341, 1994

32. Baker BW, Wilson CL, Davis AL, et al: Busulfan/cyclophosphamide conditioning for bone marrow transplantation may lead to failure of hair regrowth. *Bone Marrow Transplant* 7:43–47, 1991

33. Hennessey JD: Alopecia and cytotoxic drugs. *BMJ* 2:1138, 1966 (letter)

34. Lovejoy NC: Preventing hair loss during adriamycin therapy. *Cancer Nurs* 2:117–121, 1979

35. Luce JK, Raffetto TJ, Crisp IM, et al: Prevention of alopecia by scalp cooling of patients receiving adriamycin. *Cancer Chemo Rep* 57:108–109, 1973 (abstr)

36. Dean JC, Griffith KS, Cetas TC, et al: Scalp hypothermia: A comparison of ice packs and the Kold Kap in the prevention of doxorubicin-induced alopecia. *J Clin Oncol* 1:33–37, 1983

37. Guy R, Parker H, Shah S, et al: Scalp cooling by thermocirculator. *Lancet* 1:937–938, 1982

38. Tollenaar RAEM, Liefers GJ, Repelaer Van Driel OJ, et al: Scalp cooling has no place in the prevention of alopecia in adjuvant chemotherapy for breast cancer. *Eur J Cancer* 30:1448–1453, 1994

39. Cline BW: Prevention of chemotherapy-induced alopecia: A review of the literature. *Cancer Nurs* 7:221–228, 1984

40. Wittman G, Cadman E, Chen M: Misuse of scalp hypothermia. *Cancer Treat Rep* 65:507–508, 1981

41. Middleton J, Franks D, Buchanan RB, et al: Failure of scalp hypothermia to prevent hair loss when cyclophosphamide is added to doxorubicin and vincristine. *Cancer Treat Rep* 69:373–375, 1985

42. Perlin E, Amin D: Protection from chemotherapy-induced alopecia. *Med Pediatr Oncol* 19:129–130, 1991

43. Sorrell DC: Scalp hypothermia devices: Current status. *ONS News* 6(8):1, 5, 1991

44. Hussein AM, Jimenez JJ, McCall CA, et al: Protection from chemotherapy-induced alopecia in a rat model. *Science* 249: 1564–1566, 1990

45. Hussein AM: Interleukin 1 protects against I-B-D arabino-furanosylcytosine-induced alopecia in the newborn rat animal model. *Cancer Res* 15:3331–3333, 1991

46. Granai CO, Frederickson H, Gajewski W, et al: The use of Minoxidil to attempt to prevent alopecia during chemo-

therapy for gynecologic malignancies. *Eur J Gynaecol Oncol* 12:129–132, 1991

47. Duvic M, Valero V, Hymes S, et al: Minoxidil for chemotherapy-induced alopecia. *J Invest Dermatol* 102:568, 1994
48. Ehmann JL, Sheehan A, Decker GM: Intervening with alopecia: Exploring an entrepreneurial role for oncology nurses. *Oncol Nurs Forum* 18:769–773, 1991
49. Eilers J: Alopecia article well received. *Oncol Nurs Forum* 16:155, 1989 (letter)
50. Brown BJ, Wilson-Shah SM: A scarf bank can boost cancer patients' self-confidence. *Cope* Sept/Oct: 35, 1995
51. Anderson MS, Johnson J: Restoration of body image and self-esteem for women after cancer treatment: A rehabilitative strategy. *Cancer Pract* 2:345–349, 1994
52. National Institute of Health Consensus Development Panel: Consensus statement: Oral complications of cancer therapies. *NCI Monogr* 9:3–8, 1990
53. Raybould TP, Ferretti GA: Oral care of the cancer patient, in Macdonald JS, Haller DG, Mayer RJ (eds): *Manual of Oncologic Therapeutics*. Philadelphia, Lippincott, 1995, pp 456–466
54. Lockhart PB, Sonis ST: Relationship of oral complications to peripheral blood leukocyte and platelet counts in patients receiving cancer chemotherapy. *Oral Surg* 48:21–28, 1979
55. Dreizen S, McCredie KB, Bodey GPN, et al: Quantitative analysis of the oral complications of antileukemic chemotherapy. *Oral Surg* 62:650–653, 1986
56. Beck SL: Prevention and management of oral complications in the cancer patient, in Hubbard SM, Greene PE, Knofb MT (eds): *Current Issues in Cancer Nursing Practice Updates*. Philadelphia, Lippincott, 1992, pp 1–11
57. Peterson DE, Schubert MM: Oral toxicity, in Perry MC (ed): *The Chemotherapy Source Book*. Baltimore, Williams and Wilkins, 1992, pp 508–528
58. Poon MA, O'Connell MJ, Moertel CG, et al: Biochemical modulation of fluorouracil: Evidence of significant improvement on survival and quality of life in patients with advanced colorectal carcinoma. *J Clin Oncol* 7:1407–1418, 1989
59. Schubert MM, Sullivan KM: Recognition, incidence, and management of oral graft-versus-host disease. *NCI Monogr* 9:135–141, 1990
60. Sonis ST, Woods PD, White BA: Pretreatment oral assessment. *NCI Monogr* 9:29–32, 1990
61. Cooper SJ: Carcinomas of the oral cavity and oropharynx, in Cox JD (ed): *Moss' Radiation Oncology: Rationale, Technique, Results* (ed 7). St. Louis, Mosby, 1994, pp 169–211
62. Ingall JF, Saper JR, Kish J, et al: Rehabilitation of head and neck cancer patients. *Head Neck* 1:1–13, 1992
63. Foote RL, Loprinz C, Frank A, et al: Randomized trial of a chlorhexidine mouthwash for alleviation of radiation-induced mucositis. *J Clin Oncol* 12:2630–2633, 1994
64. Makkonen TA, Bostrom O, Vilja P, et al: Sulcralfate mouthwashing in the prevention of radiation-induced mucositis: A placebo-controlled doubleblind randomized study. *Int J Radiat Oncol Biol Phys* 30:177–182, 1994
65. Johnson JT, Ferretti GA, Nethery JW: Oral pilocarpine for post-irradiation xerostomia in patients with head and neck cancer. *N Engl J Med* 329:390–395, 1993
66. Eilers J, Berger AM, Petersen MC: Development, testing, and application of the oral assessment guide. *Oncol Nurs Forum* 15:325–330, 1988
67. Kenny SA: Effect of two oral care protocols on the incidence of stomatitis in hematology patients. *Cancer Nurs* 13:345–353, 1990
68. Clark PI, Slevin ML: Allopurinol mouthwash and 5-fluorouracil induced oral toxicity. *Eur J Surg Oncol* 11:267–268, 1985
69. Loprinzi CL, Cianflore SG, Dose AM, et al: A controlled evaluation of an allopurinol mouthwash as prophylaxis against 5-FU–induced stomatitis. *Cancer* 65:1879–1882, 1990
70. Mahood D, Dose AM, Loprinzi C, et al: Inhibition of fluorouracil-induced stomatitis by oral cryotherapy. *J Clin Oncol* 9:449–452, 1991
71. Barker G, Loftus L, Cuddy P, et al: The effects of sucralfate suspension and diphenhydramine syrup plus kaolin-pectin on radiotherapy-induced mucositis. *Oral Surg Oral Med Oral Pathol* 71:288–293, 1991
72. Pfeiffer P, Madsen EL. Hansen O, et al: Effect of prophylactic sucralfate suspension on stomatitis induced by cancer chemotherapy. *Acta Oncol* 29:171–173, 1990
73. Chi KH, Chen SY, Chan VK, et al: Effect of granulocyte-macrophage colon stimulating factor (GM-CSF) on oral mucositis in head and neck cancer patients after cisplatin, 5-FU leucovorin chemotherapy. *Proc ASCO* 13:428, 1994 (abstr 1469)
74. McElroy TH: Infection in the patient receiving chemotherapy for cancer: Oral considerations. *JAMA* 109:454–456, 1984
75. Wingard JR: Infectious and noninfectious systemic consequences. *NCI Monogr* 9:21–26, 1990
76. Meunier F, Aoun M, Gerald M: Therapy for oropharyngeal candidiasis in the immunocompromised host: A randomized double-blind study of fluconazole vs. ketoconazole. *Rev Infect Dis* 12:364–367, 1990 (suppl 3)
77. Saral R: Management of acute viral infections. *NCI Monogr* 9:107–110, 1990
78. Wilkes GM: Sucralfate suspension for mucositis. *Oncol Nurs Forum* 13:71–72, 1986
79. Francis P, Walsh T: Current approaches to the management of fungal infections in cancer patients. *Oncology* 6:81–90, 1992
80. Pizzo PA, Meyers J: Infections in the cancer patient, in DeVita VT Jr, Hellman S, Rosenberg SA (eds): *Cancer: Principles and Practice of Oncology* (ed 3). Philadelphia, Lippincott, 1989, pp 2088–2133
81. Snijders-Keilholz A, Trimbos JB: A preliminary report on new efforts to decrease radiotherapy-related small bowel toxicity. *Radiol Oncol* 22:206–208, 1991
82. Crook J, Esche BA: The uterine cervix, in Cox JD (ed): *Moss' Radiation Oncology: Rationale, Technique, Results* (ed 7). St. Louis, Mosby, 1994, pp 617–682
83. Perry MC: Toxicity: Ten years later. *Semin Oncol* 19:453–457, 1992
84. Asbury RF, Boros L, Brower M, et al: 5-FU and high-dose folic acid treatment for metastatic colon cancer. *Am J Clin Oncol* 10:47–49, 1987
85. Mustacchi G, Pavesi L, Milani S, et al: High-dose folinic acid (FA) and fluorouracil (FU) plus or minus thymostimulin (TS) for treatment of metastatic colorectal cancer: Results of a randomized multicenter clinical trial. *Anticancer Res* 14:617–620, 1994
86. Anand A, Glatt AE: Clostridium difficile infection associated with antineoplastic chemotherapy: A review. *Clin Infect Dis* 17:109–113, 1993
87. Cascinu S: Drug therapy in diarrheal diseases in oncology/hematology patients. *Crit Rev Oncol Hematol* 18:37–50, 1995

88. Francis P, Walsh TJ: Current approaches to the management of fungal infections in cancer patients. *Oncology* 6: 81–92, 1992

89. Thielman NM, Guerrant RL: Acute infectious diarrhea, in Rakel RE (ed): *Conn's Current Therapy.* Philadelphia, Saunders, 1995, pp 9–16

90. Petrelli NJ, Rodriguez-Bigas M, Rustum Y, et al: Bowel rest, intravenous hydration, and continuous high-dose infusion of octreotide acetate for the treatment of chemotherapy-induced diarrhea in patients with colorectal carcinoma. *Cancer* 72:1543–1546, 1993

91. Gebbia V, Carreca I, Testa A, et al: Subcutaneous octreotide versus oral loperamide in the treatment of diarrhea following chemotherapy. *Anticancer Drugs* 4:443–445, 1993

92. Wadler S, Haynes H, Wiernik PH: Phase I trial of the somatostatin analog octreotide acetate in the treatment of fluoropyrimidine-induced diarrhea. *J Clin Onc* 13:222–226, 1995

93. Cascinu S, Fedeli A, Luzi Fedeli S, et al: Control of chemotherapy-induced diarrhea with octreotide: A randomized trial with placebo in patients receiving cisplatin. *Oncology* 5170–5174, 1994

94. Ely A, Dunitz J, Rogosheske J, et al: Use of a somatostatin analogue, octreotide acetate, in the management of acute gastrointestinal graft-versus-host disease. *Am J Med* 90: 707–710, 1991

95. Dow KH: Altered patterns of sexuality, in Dow KH, Hilderley LJ (eds): *Nursing Care in Radiation Oncology.* Philadelphia, Saunders, 1992, pp 149–159

96. Chamorro T: Cancer and sexuality, in Baird SB, Donehower MG, Stalsbroten VL: *A Cancer Source Book for Nurses* (ed 6). Atlanta, American Cancer Society, 1991, pp 141–149

97. Grigsby PW, Russell A, Bruner D, et al: Late injury of cancer therapy on the female reproductive tract. *Int J Radiat Oncol Biol Phys* 31:1281–1299, 1995

98. Ivetic O, Lyne PA: Fungating and ulcerating malignant lesions: A review of the literature. *J Adv Nurs* 15:83–88, 1990

99. Bunn PA, Fuks Z: Cutaneous lymphomas, in DeVita VT Jr, Hellman S, Rosenberg S (eds): *Cancer: Principles and Practice of Oncology* (ed 3). Philadelphia: Lippincott, 1989, pp 1799–1807

100. McDonald AE: Skin ulceration, in Groenwald S, Frogge M, Goodman M, Yarbro CH (eds): *Cancer Symptom Management.* Boston, Jones and Bartlett, 1996, pp 364–376

101. Rice T: Metronidazole use in malodorous skin lesions. *Rehabilitation Nursing* 17:224–245, 1990

# Chapter 30

# Late Effects of Cancer Treatment

Ida Marie (Ki) Moore, RN, DNSc

Kathleen S. Ruccione, RN, MPH

## SCOPE OF THE PROBLEM

More than 8 million Americans with a history of cancer are alive today; 5 million of these cases were diagnosed five or more years ago. At least half these individuals can be considered biologically cured.[1] For children, in particular, 63% survive five years or more from the time of diagnosis, an improvement of 40% since the early 1970s. In fact, the current estimate is that by the year 2010, 1 in every 250 young adults between the ages of 15 and 45 will be a survivor of childhood cancer.[2]

*Biological cure* refers to a patient who has no evidence of disease, has the same life expectancy as a person who never had cancer, and ultimately dies of unrelated causes.[3] Given the state of the art in cancer treatment, this cure is not without consequences. These consequences, or *late effects,* result from physiological changes related to particular treatments or to the interactions among the treatment, the individual, and the disease. In contrast to the acute side effects of chemotherapy and radiation that are due to the death of proliferative cells in tissues with relatively rapid renewal, late biological toxicity is believed to progress over time and by different mechanisms.

Late effects can appear months to years after treatment and can be mild to severe to life-threatening. They can be clinically obvious, clinically subtle, or subclinical. Their impact depends on the age and developmental state of the patient. Young people may rebound from the acute toxicities of treatment better than adults, but the growing child may be more vulnerable to the effects of delayed toxicities. A great unknown is what will happen to individuals who received intensive treatment in their youth as they age. Although we may not be able to detect any obvious side effects soon after the completion of treatment, the effect of even subtle tissue damage on the process of aging is unknown. For adults the cumulative effects of mild but permanent treatment toxicity in hearts, lungs, and kidneys when combined with hereditary predisposition to particular health problems and environmental exposure to pollutants are unknown. This chapter summarizes what is currently known about the long-term consequences of treatment on organ systems and on the development of second malignancies. The treatments associated with specific late effects and individual risk factors are discussed. Researchers are learning more about the specific pathophysiological mechanisms associated with late toxicities. This information is included whenever possible. Finally, early detection, treatment, and prevention strategies are discussed. This is included whenever possible.

## CENTRAL NERVOUS SYSTEM

Neuropsychological, neuroanatomic, and neurophysiological changes can occur as a result of central nervous system (CNS) treatment. These late effects have been observed in children with acute lymphoblastic leukemia (ALL) and brain tumors and in patients with small cell carcinoma of the lung (SCCL), all of whom received CNS treatment for the primary tumor or as prophylaxis against meningeal disease.

### Neuropsychological Effects

The most frequently described neuropsychological late effects of CNS treatment include significant decrements (10–20 points on the *WISC-R*) in general intellectual potential and academic achievement scores,[4–10] as well as specific deficits in visual-motor integration, attention, memory, and visual-motor skills.[6,11–20] Nonverbal, or performance, skills seem to be particularly vulnerable to the deleterious effects of CNS treatment,[15–17] and deficits in these areas may be among the first to appear. Children who receive antileukemia CNS therapy have also been found to have language deficits when compared with age- and sex-matched controls.[21,22]

An important hallmark of neuropsychological late effects is that they do not become apparent until 24–36 months following treatment.[4,7,8] For example, Obetz et al[23] found that 48% of children with ALL who had received treatment that involved the CNS more than two years prior to the time of evaluation had neuropsychological or neuroanatomic abnormalities. This latency between CNS treatment and the manifestation of neuropsychological late effects also has been observed in other patient populations.[10,18,19,20]

To overcome the problem of obtaining reliable pretreatment measures of intellectual functioning, several studies of children treated with cranial radiation have used healthy siblings' scores as a baseline estimate because the intelligence scores of siblings show high correlation. The findings from these studies demonstrated that children whose treatment involved the CNS were functioning at a significantly lower level than their healthy brothers and sisters[24–28] and that the differences became more marked over time.[24]

The type of CNS treatment that has been most closely associated with neuropsychological deficits is cranial radiation in combination with intrathecal (IT) chemotherapy. Numerous studies have compared children with ALL who received 2400 cGy of whole-brain radiation in combination with IT methotrexate with those who received only IT methotrexate for CNS prophylaxis. The findings provide strong evidence that radiation is closely linked to long-term functional problems.[3,7,11,18,23,26,28–30] Although less is known about the effects of chemotherapy, several reports suggest that the deficits are less severe.[29,31] Methotrexate, high-dose BCNU, cytosine, arabinoside, fludarabine, and spiromustine have been associated with acute and chronic neurotoxicities.[32]

There may be a synergistic effect between cranial radiation and chemotherapy that increases the magnitude of the toxicity. Robison et al[5] found that longer duration of chemotherapy was closely associated with lower intelligence quotient (IQ) scores in children with ALL who were treated with 2400 cGy, and Duffner et al[10] reported that adjuvant chemotherapy was a significant risk factor associated with declines in IQ in patients with brain tumors who received radiation. The schedule of administration of intrathecal methotrexate when used in combination with whole-brain radiation may influence intellectual function. Balsom and associates[33] found that full, performance, and verbal scale IQ scores were consistently higher in girls who received IT methotrexate prior to and during cranial radiation than in the corresponding control group who received IT methotrexate concurrent with whole-brain radiation.

It is difficult to systematically determine if a radiation-dose response relationship exists for neuropsychological sequelae. There is modest evidence that young children who received whole-brain radiation doses of less than 1000 cGy in preparation for bone marrow transplantation are neurologically and intellectually normal.[34–36] Tameroff et al[37] reported that children who received either 1800 or 2400 cGy of whole-brain radiation and IT methotrexate had significantly lower full and performance IQ and visual motor integration test scores than those who received only IT methotrexate; however, there were no significant differences between the scores of children in the two radiation groups. In contrast, higher doses of radiation (e.g., 2400–4800 cGy), which frequently are used in the treatment of brain tumors or micrometastasis in SCCL, tend to result in more severe impairments.[28,38–41]

Age at the time of CNS treatment is an important risk factor for neurological sequelae.[4,7,8,11,27] Children who receive at least 2400 cGy of cranial radiation before the age of three,[10,27] four,[41,42] or five[6,18] years are at greatest risk for neuropsychological late effects. This age-at-time-of-treatment effect has been attributed to the deleterious effects of radiation and chemotherapy on the processes of brain development that occur during early childhood.[43,44] There are no reported studies of the significance of age at the time of CNS treatment with lower doses of radiation. In addition to age, recent evidence suggests that girls are more severely affected than boys in terms of general cognitive performance such as IQ scores.[45] Balsom et al[33] found that the protective effect of preirradiation IT methotrexate was most significant in girls less than five years of age at the time of CNS treatment.

## Neuroanatomic Effects

Computed tomography (CT) and magnetic resonance imaging (MRI) have been used to evaluate structural changes after CNS treatment. Brouwers et al[46] found that the CT scans of 13 of 23 (57%) long-term survivors of ALL who received 2400 cGy of whole-brain radiation showed abnormalities. Similarly, there are reports that 73% of children with brain tumors[47] and from 70% to 100% of those with SCCL[12,19] treated with higher radiation doses have neuroanatomic changes that are unrelated to the tumor itself.

Atrophy and decreased subcortical white matter are the most frequently reported abnormalities. Atrophy usually is manifested as ventricular dilatation and widening of the subarachnoid spaces; it has been reported in 25%–51% of patients treated with cranial radiation.[47–50] Periventricular hypodensity, believed to represent decreased white matter, has been documented in 26% of patients with brain tumors[47] and 45% of those with SCCL;[19] however, it has occurred less frequently in patients with ALL who received 1800–2400 cGy of radiation.[44,48,51]

Other less common neuroanatomic abnormalities include calcification[28,37,48,50] and leukoencephalopathy.[12,38] As with neuropsychological effects, these neuroanatomic changes are associated most closely with cranial radiation, although mild indications of atrophy and white matter degeneration have been reported in up to 20% of children who received only IT methotrexate.[49,50]

These studies of neuroanatomic pathological conditions suggest that higher radiation doses result in a greater incidence and severity of abnormalities. Age at the time of CNS treatment also may be important. Davis et al[47] reported that children with brain tumors who receive irradiation before the age of three years are at greatest risk for abnormalities, and Tsurada et al[52] found that the highest incidence of white matter degeneration in adult patients with brain tumors occurred in those older than 60 years of age. This finding is of interest because it suggests that the aging, as well as the developing, brain may be more vulnerable to the deleterious effects of cancer treatment involving the CNS.

## Mechanisms of Pathogenesis

The pathogenesis of delayed injury to normal tissue after treatment of the CNS is not well understood. Sheline et al[53] suggest that demyelination may be important in the early stages of delayed injury, with ischemia becoming progressively significant over time. Oligodendroglia, the myelin-producing cells in the CNS, are proliferative during early childhood and therefore radiosensitive. Damage to or a reproductive loss of glial cells from radiation can disrupt the myelin membrane that insulates axons. Antigens released from the damaged glial cells initiate an autoimmune response that can also contribute to the pathogenesis of delayed tissue damage.[54]

A synergistic relationship between radiation and methotrexate may account for progressive demyelination.[55,56] The reduction of dihydrofolate to tetrahydrofolate, which is necessary for 1-carbon transfers in phospholipid synthesis, is inhibited by methotrexate. Procarbazine, which frequently is used in combination with methotrexate in the treatment of SCCL, can further this neurotoxicity by potentiating the methotrexate-induced depletion of the 1-carbon pool.[11] The result is disruption and loss of integrity in phospholipid membranes, such as the myelin sheath. An interference with phospholipid synthesis has been hypothesized as the underlying mechanism of demyelination[56] and a contributing factor to the pathogenesis of delayed tissue damage.[57] Degenerative changes of glial cells, disruption of myelin sheaths, thickened capillary walls, and necrotizing and sclerotic microangiopathy have been documented in children who died of leukoencephalopathy (progressive white matter destruction) and had been treated with a cumulative dose of 2000 cGy of cranial radiation and intravenous methotrexate.[57]

Myelin basic protein (MBP) has been used as a marker for the disruption in synthesis or increased breakdown of myelin following CNS treatment. Elevated MBP has been measured in the cerebral spinal fluid of patients with ALL who have clinical and neuroradiological evidence of leukoencephalopathy.[58,59] In one study the persistent release of MBP correlated with the progression of neurotoxicity.[59] Patients with elevations in MBP had received CNS treatment involving either 2400 cGy of whole-brain radiation in combination with IT methotrexate or triple IT therapy with methotrexate, hydrocortisone, and cytosine arabinoside. Children without evidence of leukoencephalopathy, however, did not have elevations in MBP in the cerebral spinal fluid with neuropsychological and/or neuroanatomic sequelae.

Damage to the endothelial cells of the microvasculature is believed to play an important role in the pathogenesis of delayed injury following CNS treatment.[55,56,60,61] These cells may be particularly vulnerable to the damaging effects of radiation because of their replicating capacity.[60] The consequences of endothelial cell damage include increased synthesis and density of collagenous tissue and loss of the tight intracellular junctions that form the blood-brain barrier. These pathological changes result in decreased perfusion, increased blood-brain barrier permeability, and disruption of active transport mechanisms. The net effect is inflammation, ischemia, and loss of parenchymal tissue function. Vascular changes have been documented in animals treated with low to moderate doses of radiation[62] and in human beings who received 1500–6000 cGy.[57,63]

## Vision and Hearing

In addition to the long-term effects of CNS treatment involving neuropsychological function and neuroanatomy, visual deficits and hearing loss also can occur. Enucleation, which may be necessary in the treatment of ocular tumors such as retinoblastoma, is the most disabling visual deficit. Cataracts have been associated with cranial irradiation and long-term corticosteroid therapy.[64] They may be detected on a visual examination or require a slit-lamp examination. Retinopathy can occur following radiation to the eye, orbit, nasal cavity, paranasal sinus, or nasopharyngeal area.[65,66] The mean time to onset of symptoms in one study was 2.8 years, and the earliest symptom was usually diminished vision.[65] The risk of radiation retinopathy increased with doses in the 45–55 Gy range. However, concurrent chronic illness, such as diabetes mellitus, may increase the risk.[65] In children who receive radiotherapy as conservative therapy for retinoblastoma, a dose-per-fraction effect may be important. In one study, hypofractionation was found to increase the risk of subsequent retinopathy.[66] The pathogenesis of radiation retinopathy involves obstruction of small vessels with resulting ischemia, edema, and neovascularization of the optic disk.[66]

Hearing loss in the high-tone range is most closely associated with cisplatin.[67] Recent evidence from a limited study of children with brain tumors suggests that treatment with high doses of cranial irradiation within ten months of cisplatin administration increases the sensitivity to the ototoxic effects of this drug in young children. Profound hearing loss occurred in all frequency ranges.[68] The investigators postulated that postirradiation hyperemia may have increased the sensitivity of the cochlea to cisplatin damage. Concurrent ifosfamide therapy can also exacerbate cisplatin-induced hearing loss. Patients who receive ifosfamide in combination with cisplatin are more likely to require amplification than those who receive cisplatin in combination with other drugs such as methotrexate and doxorubicin.[69] Recurrent otitis media, a common problem in children receiving chemotherapy, as well as the use of antibiotics that are ototoxic, also can contribute to hearing loss.

## ENDOCRINE SYSTEM

Cancer treatment can adversely affect a number of endocrine functions, including metabolism, growth, secondary sexual development, and reproduction. These late effects result from damage to the target organ (i.e., thyroid, ovary, and testis), and/or the hypothalamic pituitary axis. Table 30-1 summarizes the major endocrine sequelae, related risk factors, and recommendations for evaluation and treatment.[70]

## Thyroid

Direct damage to the thyroid gland causes primary hypothyroidism with a decreased production of thyroxine ($T_4$) and triiodothyronine ($T_3$). These hormones have biological effects on oxygen consumption, the central and peripheral nervous systems, skeletal and cardiac muscle, carbohydrate and cholesterol metabolism, and growth and development.[71] Primary hypothyroidism can be compensated when there is only partial organ damage and

**TABLE 30-1** Endocrine Late Effects and Associated Risk Factors

| Ovaries | Chemotherapy | Radiation | High Risk | Evaluation | Treatment |
|---|---|---|---|---|---|
| Ovaries | Procarbazine Cyclophosphamide Nitrogen mustard Busulfan (age-dependent) | 400–800 cGy Age-dependent | Older > younger age Abdominal and pelvic tumors Hodgkin's disease Spinal radiation (ALL, brain tumors) | LH FSH Estradiol | Oophoropexy before treatment Replacement hormones |
| Testes | Procarbazine Cyclophosphamide Nitrogen mustard Busulfan | ≤ 400 cGy: Azoospermia with recovery possible ≥ 600 cGy: Permanent azoospermia ≥ 2400 cGy: Leydig cell damage (↓ testosterone) | Pelvic tumors Testicular tumors Testicular leukemia Hodgkin's disease | LH FSH Testosterone | Sperm banking before treatment Transposition of testicles before treatment Replacement hormones |
| Thyroid | None currently identified | > 2000 cGy overt or compensatory hypothyroidism: Graves' disease ≥ 750 cGy TBI for BMT: hypothyroidism | Younger > older age Hodgkin's disease Head and neck tumors Brain tumors Leukemia (cranial rad) Bone marrow transplantation | Free triiodothyronine Thyroxine Antithyroid and antichromosomal autoantibodies (follow-up to 15 yr) | Replacement hormones |
| Hypothalamic: pituitary axis | None currently identified | ≥ 2400 cGy: Hypothalamic dysfunction ≥ 4000 cGy: Pituitary dysfunction | CNS tumors Head and neck tumors Leukemia with CNS irradiation | Growth chart Growth hormone   Pulsatile test   Stimulation test Somatomedin-C LH, FSH Prolactin | Replacement hormones Bromocriptine |

*ALL* = acute lymphocytic leukemia; *BMT* = bone marrow transplantation; *FSH* = follicle-stimulating hormone; *LH* = luteinizing hormone; *TBI* = total-body irradiation; *CNS* = central nervous system.

Hobbie WL, Schwartz CL: Endocrine late effects among survivors of cancer. *Semin Oncol Nurs* 5:15, 1989. Reprinted with permission.

some function is preserved. The compensated state is maintained by an increased production of thyrotropin releasing factor (TRF) and thyroid-stimulating hormone (TSH) from the hypothalamus and pituitary. This chronic overstimulation is of concern because it is believed to increase the risk of malignant transformation in previously damaged cells.

Overt or compensated primary hypothyroidism has been documented in 4%–80% of patients who received radiation to the neck for Hodgkin's disease, other lymphomas, and carcinomas.[72-78] Damage to the thyroid gland usually occurs after radiation doses of more than 2000 cGy in multiple fractions. In general, the incidence and severity of thyroid dysfunction appear to increase with higher radiation doses and may be due to damage to thyroid follicular cells, thyroid vasculature, or connective tissue. There are no chemotherapeutic agents that have been associated with long-term thyroid damage.

The importance of age at time of irradiation has been difficult to assess. Although hypothyroidism usually devel-

ops 3–4 years after treatment, it can occur as late as 7–14 years afterward.[78,79] Glatstein et al[72] reported a higher incidence of dysfunction in patients treated before the age of 20 years, which was attributed to an increased sensitivity of the thyroid in younger individuals or to an induced sensitivity from prolonged iodine release in the contrast used in lymphangiograms. Others have found that age at time of irradiation is not a significant risk factor.[80,81]

When the hypothalamic pituitary axis is in the field of radiation to the nasopharynx of the CNS, secondary hypothyroidism can occur. Decreased levels of TRF, TSH, $T_3$, and $T_4$ have been reported in patients who received at least 5500 cGy of external beam radiation for nasopharyngeal, paranasal sinus, or brain tumors that did not involve the hypothalamus or pituitary.[81,82] These studies found no difference in the development of secondary hypothyroidism between children and adults; however, the majority of subjects were adults. As with primary thyroid dysfunction, secondary hypothyroidism may not develop until years after the completion of therapy.

## Growth

Growth hormone deficiency with short stature is one of the most common long-term endocrine consequences of radiation to the CNS in children.[83] Growth impairment with deficient growth hormone release and decreased linear growth rate has been found in 50%–100% of children with brain tumors who received 2400 cGy or more of cranial or craniospinal radiation.[39,84-87] Children with ALL who received radiation for CNS prophylaxis have demonstrated a similar pattern of growth disturbances.[88,89] Pituitary dysfunction requires radiation doses of at least 4000 cGy, but damage to the hypothalamus occurs with lower doses.[90] Although the belief has been that growth disturbances as a result of hypothalamic damage require doses of at least 2400 cGy,[90,91] Starceski et al[92] observed a 25% decline in height percentile in children treated with 2400 cGy and 14% in children treated with 1800 cGy. In both groups, growth velocity decreased significantly over three years following treatment and did not recover. Sanders et al[93] observed partial growth hormone (GH) deficiency in 6 of 18 children who received total-body irradiation in preparation for bone marrow transplantation. A dose-response relationship has been demonstrated, with higher doses resulting in more significant growth abnormalities. Clayton and Shalet[94] found that dose of whole-brain radiation (from 27–47.5 Gy) and time from irradiation were significant predictors of GH deficiency. The overall incidence of GH deficiency (74%) five years after treatment was comparable across radiation doses; however, children who received 30 Gy or more of radiation developed GH deficiency earlier. The fewer the number of fractionations for a given radiation dose, the greater the risk of long-term sequelae. Children treated with cranial radiation before the age of five years are believed to be more susceptible to growth deficits, which may become most apparent during periods of rapid growth.[95] Growth retardation may be more pronounced in children who receive cranial and spinal irradiation because of spinal shortening.[86]

Chemotherapy in combination with cranial radiation may increase the risk for growth failure. In a study of 38 prepubertal children who survived medulloblastoma, those who received chemotherapy plus radiation had significantly poorer growth over a four-year period than those who received only radiation.[96]

## Secondary Sexual Development and Reproduction

Chemotherapy, specifically alkylating agents (e.g., cyclophosphamide, mechlorethamine, busulfan, and procarbazine), can cause permanent damage to the gonads. Primary ovarian failure, with amenorrhea, decreased estradiol, and elevated gonadotropins (luteinizing hormone and follicle-stimulating hormone [FSH]), has been reported in women who received these agents for Hodgkin's disease, breast cancer, and ovarian germ cell tumors.[97-99] In younger patients, ovarian damage is manifested as failure to develop secondary sexual characteristics or as arrested pubertal development.[70] Shalet[100] observed ovarian dysfunction in 4 of 12 girls with ALL who received cyclophosphamide. In three patients, normal pubertal development subsequently occurred, which suggests that both transient and permanent damage can occur.

Damage to the germinal epithelium of the testis with decreased or absent spermatogonia can occur in males treated with alkylating agents.[101] Leydig cell damage is unusual; thus, testosterone production and pubertal development are not affected. Testicular damage with azoospermia is most frequent in males with Hodgkin's disease who received MOPP (mechlorethamine, vincristine, procarbazine, and prednisone) but also has been observed in males with ALL or rhabdomyosarcoma treated with cyclophosphamide and cytosine arabinoside.[102,103] Impaired testicular function has also been documented in men who received higher-dose cisplatin and etoposide for germ cell cancer.[104]

Age at time of treatment, sex, total drug dose, and the use of combinations of alkylating agents are important risk factors for gonadal failure. The quiescence of the prepubertal gonad provides some protection, whereas the incidence of gonadal damage increases with age and stage in pubertal development. The testis appears to be more sensitive than the ovary to the damaging effects of therapy. Rivkees and Crawford[102] reported that the incidence of gonadal dysfunction increased from 0% in prepubertal girls and 14% in prepubertal boys to 71% in sexually mature women and 95% in mature men. Byrne et al[105] found that the fertility of men treated with alkylating agents was half that of the fertility of control subjects, whereas the fertility of women was unimpaired.

The risk of gonadal failure also increases with greater total doses of alkylating agents and the use of more than one drug, such as in MOPP therapy. Cumulative cyclophosphamide dose is an important risk factor for recovery of spermatogenesis. In a recent study of 11 men treated for non-Hodgkin's lymphoma, 53% of men who received doses greater than 9.5 g/m² had persistent azoospermia.[104]

Radiation is another cause of gonadal dysfunction. Pathological changes in women who receive radiation to the ovaries include reduced numbers of oocytes, inhibited follicle development, atrophic ovaries, and strong fibrohyalinization.[106,107] Older women are at greater risk for ovarian failure following radiation. The ovaries may be preserved in women who receive 800 cGy; however, ovarian failure has been reported in 100% of women older than 40 years of age treated with 400 cGy.[107]

The testis is extremely sensitive to the damaging effects of radiation. The threshold dose required to damage the germinal epithelium is as low as 300–900 cGy,[108] whereas the Leydig cells are more resistant, with permanent damage occurring following doses at 2000 cGy.[109]

Scatter to the ovaries and testes as a result of abdominal or craniospinal irradiation also can result in long-term damage.[104,108–110] In a large retrospective cohort study of 2283 survivors of childhood cancer, Byrne et al[105] found that radiation therapy directed below the diaphragm depressed fertility in men and women by approximately 25%, and combined therapy involving infradiaphragmatic radiation and alkylating agents reduced fertility to almost 50% of that in the control subjects. However, testicular damage and ovarian failure occur infrequently after treatment for leukemia with regimens that do not include alkylating agents or cytosine arabinoside, and there does not appear to be an increased frequency of adverse pregnancy outcome (i.e., spontaneous abortions and stillbirths) compared with the general population.[111] In addition to the damaging effects of chemotherapy and radiotherapy on stem cells, retroperitoneal lymph node dissection can contribute to ejaculatory dysfunction.[103]

Radiation to the cranium or nasopharynx can damage the hypothalamic pituitary axis, causing secondary gonadal failure. Subnormal levels of luteinizing hormone (LH), FSH, and prolactin inhibiting factor (PIF) have been found in both sexes treated for head and neck tumors with 400–7800 cGy of radiation.[81,112] In addition to the effects of low LH and FSH levels on ovarian and testicular function, the decrease in PIF and resultant increase in prolactin caused irregular menses, anovulatory periods, low testosterone, reduced libido, and impotence.[81,113] In children, cranial radiation is thought to disrupt CNS mechanisms influencing puberty. The result is early puberty, and the most profound disturbance occurs in children irradiated at a young age.[114]

## IMMUNE SYSTEM

Immunosuppression has long been recognized as one of the most serious acute toxic effects of chemotherapy and radiation. A more recent discovery is that certain aspects of immune function can be adversely affected for years after the completion of treatment. These immunologic late effects have been studied most thoroughly in patients treated for leukemia, Hodgkin's disease, and breast cancer, and following bone marrow transplantation.

Persistent immunologic impairments following radiation and chemotherapy can occur. The lymphopenia that occurs immediately after radiation usually involves both cellular (T cell) and humoral (B cell) immunity. The time required for recovery of these cell populations, however, varies.[115–118] The B-lymphocytes gradually repopulate within 12 months,[117,118] whereas T-lymphocyte depletion is much more prolonged. Of particular significance is the finding that suppressor T cells recover more rapidly than T-helper cells, which seem to be particularly radiosensitive. The result is an inversion of the helper-to-suppressor ratio that can persist for as long as ten years

following local radiation for breast cancer,[117] nodal radiation for Hodgkin's disease,[118] and total-body irradiation prior to bone marrow transplantation.[119] High-dose chemotherapy followed by bone marrow transplantation has been found to induce a profound and prolonged impairment of hematopoiesis. The impairment involves a quantitative defect with the hematopoietic system. Diminished stem cell self-renewal and low levels of erythroid and megakaryocyte progenitors have been reported.[120] Decreased lymphocyte proliferative capacity, natural killer cells, and immunoglobulin production associated with defective suppressor-cell immunoregulation and an abnormal helper-to-suppressor cell ratio also have been observed in patients treated with multiagent chemotherapy for Hodgkin's disease[121] and leukemia.[122,123] In addition, a pronounced long-term effect on plasma cell and immunoglobulin production, with a possible effect on T-cell function, also has been observed in children with ALL.[123]

The immunosuppressive effects of specific chemotherapeutic agents are not well known. The use of radiation in conjunction with multiagent chemotherapy can result in more frequent and more severe immune system impairment.[124] Larger volumes of irradiated bone marrow and greater total radiation doses result in more severe hematopoietic depression and more prolonged recovery. In a study of 32 patients with lymphoma who received either mantle or mantle with inverted Y radiation, bone marrow recovery was observed following doses of 2000 cGy,[125] but recovery was markedly limited after 4000 cGy. Compensation by hyperactivity of the nonradiated marrow persisted for up to ten years after radiation.

The clinical significance of these long-term alterations in immune function is not well understood. There is no evidence that patients with persistent immunologic abnormalities are at greater risk for infections. One group of patients who is at increased risk of infections are those who have undergone splenectomy. Overwhelming bacterial infections, primarily pneumococcal, are a major concern to these individuals because of the protective role of the spleen against encapsulated organisms. Persistent immune defects have not been linked to the occurrence of second malignancies. This may change, however, as survival time increases for larger numbers of patients.

## CARDIOVASCULAR SYSTEM

The use of anthracyclines, such as daunorubicin and doxorubicin, has improved survival in patients with acute leukemias, lymphomas, pediatric solid tumors, and other cancers. One of the most serious late effects of these drugs is cardiac toxicity, which typically presents as cardiomyopathy, with clinical signs of congestive heart failure.[126] Recent evidence, however, indicates that structural damage to the heart can occur in the absence of clinical signs.

Steinherz et al[127] detected abnormalities of contractility and rhythm, apparently related to myocardial fibrosis, on echocardiograms obtained 4 to 20 years after anthracycline therapy. These investigators also have documented cardiac failure, dysrhythmias, and sudden deaths many years following completion of therapy. Some of the patients with these late complications had no early symptoms. Myocardial fibrosis was present on autopsy in all cases of sudden death.[127]

The risk of cardiotoxicity is related to cumulative dose,[127,128] schedule of administration (continuous versus intermittent), and presence of other factors such as mediastinal irradiation. Cumulative doses of 550 mg/m² have been associated with cardiac toxicity;[128] similar abnormalities can occur after lower doses in adults and children. Lipshultz and colleagues[128] found that 57% of children with acute leukemia treated with doxorubicin developed abnormalities of left ventricular afterload or contractility. The cumulative dose of doxorubicin was the most significant predictor of abnormal cardiac function. Table 30-2 includes a summary of cardiotoxicity, methods of assessment, and suggestions for intervention.[129]

Individuals who received radiation therapy to a field that includes the heart, such as mediastinal radiation for Hodgkin's disease or other lymphomas, also are at risk for cardiotoxicity. Radiation-induced cardiotoxicity is manifested primarily as congestive heart failure.[130,131] An acceleration of coronary artery disease that results in angina and myocardial infarction may occur in some patients. Pericardial damage secondary to mediastinal irradiation is another cardiovascular complication. Patients may have overt symptoms and/or abnormalities that are visible on x-ray examination. Pericardial damage may be self-limiting, but life-threatening pericardial effusions also can occur.[132] In general, peripheral vascular disease is a rare cardiovascular late effect. However, approximately 50% of patients with germ cell tumors of the testes treated with cisplatin, vinblastine, and bleomycin report having Raynaud's phenomenon.[131] A case of episodic complete heart block after high-dose cyclophosphamide and thiotepa has been reported.[133]

## Prevention

The mechanisms of cardiac damage following anthracyclines include inhibited expression of genes encoding for cardiac muscle protein, binding to membranes rich in cardiolipin, and the formation of free radicals.[126] The heart is particularly sensitive to free radical–induced damage because of low levels of free radical scavengers. Recently, drugs that prevent the formation of superhydroxide radicals, and thereby prevent doxorubicin-induced cardiotoxicity, have been investigated and demonstrate encouraging results in animal and human studies.[134,135]

**TABLE 30-2** Biological Late Effects on Selected Organ Systems

| Body System | Health Problem | Associated Treatment Modality | Method of Assessment | Management and Nursing Considerations |
|---|---|---|---|---|
| Cardiovascular | Cardiomyopathy | Anthracycline chemotherapy Risk increased with lifetime cumulative dose >550 mg/m², mediastinal irradiation | Detection is difficult: ECG, echocardiogram, scans may be inadequate Monitor with clinical observation for shortness of breath, weight gain, edema | Careful monitoring of anthracycline dosage to limit lifetime dose If congestive heart failure develops, support care with digitalis, diuretics, sodium restriction, provision of adequate rest periods |
| | Pericardial damage | Mediastinal irradiation (e.g., 4000–6000 cGy) | Clinical observation for chest pain, dyspnea, fever, paradoxic pulse, venous distention, friction rub, Kussmaul's sign Abnormalities visible on chest film | May be self-limiting If pericardial effusion occurs, treatment may include anti-inflammatory agents, pericardiectomy |
| | Peripheral vascular disease | Vinblastine | History of digital cold sensitivity | Avoidance of cold |
| Respiratory | Pulmonary fibrosis | Lung irradiation Some chemotherapeutic agents Risk increased with larger lung volume in radiation field, dose: 4000 cGy, radiation-sensitizing chemotherapeutic agents | Clinical observation for dyspnea, rales, cough, decreased exercise tolerance, pulmonary insufficiency Monitor with physical examination, chest film, pulmonary function tests | Health education for smoking prevention/cessation Supportive care with provision of adequate rest periods Vigilance re: development of pulmonary infection |

**TABLE 30-2**   Biological Late Effects on Selected Organ Systems (continued)

| Body System | Health Problem | Associated Treatment Modality | Method of Assessment | Management and Nursing Considerations |
|---|---|---|---|---|
| Musculoskeletal | Scoliosis, kyphosis | Radiation therapy for intra-abdominal tumor in which vertebrae absorb radiation unevenly | Regular physical examination May not become apparent until adolescent growth spurt | Referral to orthopedist for rehabilitative measures, instruction regarding normal weight Maintenance to make problem less noticeable |
| | Spinal shortening (decrease in sitting height) | Spinal irradiation (e.g., for medulloblastoma); direct effect of radiation on growth centers of vertebral bodies | Serial measurements of sitting height (crown to rump) | Referral to orthopedist Anticipatory teaching regarding disproportion between shorter-than-usual trunk and normal leg length as full growth is attained; reassurance that disproportion probably will not be obvious to others but may be a problem in fitting clothing |
| | Increased susceptibility to fractures, poor healing, deformities, or shortening of extremities | Irradiation to lesions in long bones (e.g., Ewing's sarcoma) | Regular physical examination | Referral to orthopedist Teaching about protective measures such as avoiding rough contact sports |
| | Facial asymmetry | Surgery plus irradiation to head and neck area (e.g., for rhabdomyosarcoma) causing altered growth in facial bones | Physical examination Early evaluation by reconstructive surgeon | Anticipatory guidance regarding possible adjustment problems with visible deformity Referral to family counseling to manage or prevent adjustment and behavior problems |
| | Dental problems: gingival irritation and bleeding; tooth loosening, migration (can lead to peridontal disease); delayed/arrested tooth development | Radiation therapy to maxilla mandible areas; chemotherapy | Clinical observation with dental examination | Many dental problems can be minimized or prevented with good oral hygiene with flossing/brushing, gingival massage, use of plaque-disclosing tablets/solutions; preradiation therapy fluouride prophylaxis; dental evaluation 2 wk postradiation; orthodontic treatment for malocclusion; extraction of damaged, nonfunctional teeth |
| Gastrointestinal | Chronic enteritis | Radiation therapy Risk increased with doses > 5000 cGy, previous abdominal surgery, radiation-sensitizing chemotherapeutic agents | Clinical observation for pain, dysphagia, recurrent vomiting, obstipation/constipation, bloody or mucus-containing diarrhea, malabsorption syndrome | Nutritional consultation for diet plan to diminish symptoms while providing adequate nutrition for growth and development to fit family routine, ethnic or cultural customs; dietary modifications may include low-fat, low-residue, gluten-free, free of milk and milk products If enterostomy is performed, coordination with enterostomal therapist for patient/family teaching about stoma care |

*(continued)*

**TABLE 30-2** Biological Late Effects on Selected Organ Systems (continued)

| Body System | Health Problem | Associated Treatment Modality | Method of Assessment | Management and Nursing Considerations |
|---|---|---|---|---|
| | Hepatic fibrosis, cirrhosis | Radiation therapy Some chemotherapeutic agents | Clinical observation for pain, hepatomegaly, jaundice Monitoring with liver function tests and liver scans may be inconclusive, thus, periodic liver biopsy may be necessary | Supportive care with nutritional consultation |
| Kidney and urinary tract | Chronic nephritis (may lead to renal failure, cardiovascular damage) | Radiation to renal structures Risk increased with concomitant chemotherapy | Clinical observation and monitoring with blood pressure readings, urinalysis, CBC, BUN | If progressive renal failure develops, supportive care (possibly dialysis and/or transplantation) |
| | Chronic hemorrhagic cystitis | Chemotherapy (cyclophosphamide) Risk increased with pelvic radiation, inadequate hydration before, during, and after chemotherapy | Clinical observation for dysuria, urinary frequency, hematuria Monitoring with urinalysis | Ensure adequate hydration before, during, and after chemotherapy (3000 ml/m² /24 hr) Bladder hemorrhage may be treated with formalin instillation and/or fulguration of bleeding sites |
| | Unilateral kidney | Nephrectomy for Wilms' tumor | Clinical observation for dysuria, urinary frequency, flank pain, hematuria Monitoring with urinalysis | Health education to avoid injury to remaining kidney (e.g., contact sports) If urinary tract infection develops, identification of causative organism, antibiotic treatment, repeat urinalysis Medic-Alert identification bracelet/tag |

Adapted from Ruccione K, Weinberg K: Late effects in multiple body systems, *Semin Oncol Nurs* 5:6–8, 1989. Reprinted with permission.

# PULMONARY SYSTEM

Pneumonitis and pulmonary fibrosis are the major biological late effects of treatment to the pulmonary system (see Table 30-2). These problems can be caused by chemotherapy, radiation therapy, and recurrent respiratory infections in immunosuppressed patients.[136,137]

Alkylating agents, primarily busulfan, and the nitrosourea agents (e.g., lomustine and carmustine) also have been associated with the development of pulmonary fibrosis. The mechanisms of bleomycin injury include formation of free radicals and lipid peroxidation of phospholipid membranes. Subsequently interstitial edema and damage to type 1 pneumocytes occurs. Late lung injury is characterized by progressive fibrosis and collapse of alveoli.[136]

Pulmonary fibrosis is the most common type of chronic lung damage following radiation therapy. Obstructive lung disease also can occur. Pulmonary damage is more likely when higher radiation doses are used and when larger lung volumes are irradiated. Radiation therapy also can potentiate the long-term toxicity induced by other agents such as bleomycin and nitrosoureas. The late phase of fibrosis is characterized by a loss of capillaries and type I pneumocytes, and an increased deposition of collagen.[137] Recent evidence suggests that the activation of cells, such as the macrophage, that produce mediators such as cytokines and growth factors is an important mechanism of radiation-induced lung injury. For example, the synthesis of tumor necrosis factor-alpha and fibroblastic growth factors is increased in in vitro studies.[137]

# GASTROINTESTINAL SYSTEM

Radiation and radiation-enhancing chemotherapeutic agents can have long-term effects on the gastrointestinal tract and the liver. Late effects of radiation on the esophagus result primarily from damage to the esophageal wall, although mucosal ulcerations may also persist.[138] The major significant late effect of gastric irradiation is ulceration due to destruction of mucosal cells of the gastric mucosa. Although rare, vascular abnormalities and altered digestive system activity can result in malabsorption. Late effects in the liver are more common and include hepatic fibrosis, cirrhosis, and portal hypertension. Radiation therapy in combination with radiation-enhancing agents, such as actinomycin D and possibly vincristine, can result in hepatic fibrosis. Portal hypertension can occur if the fibrosis is severe. Methotrexate also has been linked to hepatic fibrosis and cirrhosis (although the use of citrovorum factor may minimize or prevent these effects), and methotrexate in combination with 6-mercaptopurine can result in cirrhosis with portal hypertension.[139] Hepatic arterial infusion chemotherapy for management of liver metastases can result in significant hepatotoxicity. In a recent study, 30 women with metastatic breast carcinoma to the liver underwent systemic chemotherapy alone (n = 6) or in combination with 3–5 cycles of hepatic arterial infusion chemotherapy. Morphological changes in the liver that were attributed to the toxic effects of treatment were identified in 27 women. These included fatty changes, severe cirrhotic changes, and localized atrophy.[140] Chemotherapy-induced hepatic injury is usually due to the breakdown of drugs into free radicals that impair cell function and result in cell death.[140]

Late radiation injury to the small and large intestine can result in fecal frequency, bleeding, pain, fistula formation, and obstruction, especially in the small intestine. The damage extends beyond the mucosa and can involve the entire intestinal wall.[138] Although chemotherapy can augment acute gastrointestinal radiation toxicity, the effect of chemotherapy on late toxicity is not well established. Finally, the administration of blood products as part of the supportive care of myelosuppressed patients can cause chronic hepatitis. Table 30-2 includes a summary of late biologic toxic effects in the gastrointestinal tract.

## RENAL SYSTEM

Nephritis and cystitis are the major long-term renal toxicities that result from cancer treatment (see Table 30-2). Damage to the nephrons and bladder has been documented in patients treated with cyclophosphamide, ifosfamide, and cisplatin. The hemorrhagic cystitis that can occur following cyclophosphamide therapy may persist, and the risk is increased by concurrent pelvic radiation. Acrolein, a metabolite of cyclophosphamide, is thought to be responsible for hemorrhagic cystitis. MENSA, a sulfhydryl compound, binds to acrolein within the urinary tract, and thereby decreases the incidence of renal toxicity with cyclophosphamide and ifosfamide.[141]

Children with unilateral nephrectomy who receive ifosfamide may develop Fanconi's syndrome. Renal phosphate and amino acid loss, renal tubular acidosis, and

dehydration can occur, and result in metabolic bone disease, growth failure, and decompensated renal tubular insufficiency.[142] Radiation also can damage the kidneys. Radiation doses of 2000 cGy or less may minimize the risk of renal toxicity, whereas concurrent administration of radiation-enhancing drugs increases the risk. Clinical manifestations of nephritis include proteinuria, hypertension, anemia, and progressive renal failure, although early detection and intervention may prevent irreversible damage. The compensatory hypertrophy of the remaining kidney following nephrectomy for renal tumors such as Wilms' tumor has not been associated with any biological consequences. However, urinary tract infections or trauma to the remaining kidney obviously can be a serious problem. Children with bilateral Wilms' tumor are at risk for renal failure, and in these patients kidney parenchymal sparing procedures offer the potential advantage of decreasing the risk of end-stage renal failure.[143]

## MUSCULOSKELETAL SYSTEM

The treatment most frequently associated with late effects in the musculoskeletal system is radiation. Stature already achieved at the time of radiotherapy, radiation dose, and volume of tissue irradiated are all risk factors.[143] Children treated at an early age (younger than 6 years) and those undergoing puberty are at high risk because of rapid growth and development. Uneven irradiation to the vertebrae, soft tissue, and muscles (e.g., radiation to one side of the body) for the treatment of intra-abdominal tumors frequently results in scoliosis or kyphosis, or both. Silber and colleagues[144] have developed a mathematical model for predicting adult stature in children successfully treated for cancer outside the CNS. The model is based on radiation dose adjusted for radiation site and attained height at the time of irradiation. Although more recent therapies have been modified to minimize these problems, skeletal abnormalities may occur in some children and tend to become more apparent during periods of rapid growth such as the adolescent growth spurt. In a recent study of 31 children successfully treated for Wilms' tumor with surgery, chemotherapy, and radiation (orthovoltage or megavoltage), ten children developed an orthopedic abnormality requiring intervention or a scoliotic curve greater than 20.[145] There were no orthopedic defects among children treated with megavoltage radiation. Other factors associated with the occurrence of significant late orthopedic problems were higher radiation dose (mean dose of 2890 cGy) and larger irradiated field (150 cm$^2$).

Spinal shortening, another radiation-related effect, is caused by damage to the growth centers in the vertebral bodies.[146] Children who receive spinal radiation frequently do not achieve their full height potential; those who receive craniospinal irradiation are at great risk for growth retardation because of central (hypothalamic-pituitary), as well as direct (skeletal), effects.

The late effects on long bones include functional limitations, shortening of the extremity, osteonecrosis, increased susceptibility to fractures, and poor healing. Radiation is the treatment most commonly associated with these problems; however, prolonged use of corticosteroids also can have degenerative effects. Finally, surgical procedures such as amputation or limb disarticulation have obvious immediate and lasting cosmetic, as well as physical, consequences.

Altered growth of facial bones following maxillofacial or orbital irradiation or surgery causes facial asymmetry. This is a difficult problem that frequently occurs in children treated for tumors such as rhabdomyosarcoma. Maxillofacial irradiation also can cause a number of dental problems such as foreshortening and blunting of the roots, incomplete calcification, delayed or arrested tooth development, caries, and loosening.[146] Recently, dental problems in patients who were treated with chemotherapy have been reported and include abnormal occlusion, hypoplasia, enamel opacities, and radiological abnormalities.[147]

Men who receive chemotherapeutic agents that impair gonadal function may lose bone mineral density. In a study of 29 men previously treated for Hodgkin's disease, a significant reduction in forearm cortical bone mineral content and in lumbar spine bone mineral density was identified. Length of time since completion of therapy (1.1–6.8 years), type of chemotherapy, and number of cycles were not related to bone mineral density.[148] The investigators hypothesize possible causes to include mild hypogonadism as a result of chemotherapy-induced Leydig cell function, a direct effect of chemotherapy on bone, or an effect of high-dose glucocorticoid on bone.[148]

Late radiation damage to muscle can occur, especially following treatment of soft tissue sarcomas of the extremities. Mechanisms of injury that have been identified primarily from animal studies include a direct effect on myocytes resulting in cell death; vascular damage with ischemia; atrophy and fibrosis; and inflammation with a preferential increase in type III collagen.[149] Muscle damage can progress over time; the risk increases with larger radiation doses and decreases with dose fractionation.

# SECOND MALIGNANT NEOPLASMS

It has been clearly established that adults and children who have received chemotherapy or radiation therapy, or both, for a primary malignancy are at increased risk for the development of a second malignant neoplasm. For example, in patients with Hodgkin's disease there is a 77-fold increased risk of the development of leukemia within four years of initial treatment.[150] For children the overall risk is estimated to be at least ten times greater than the cancer incidence among age-matched children.[151] Among a cohort of 981 children who were followed up 4.3–26.5 years after completion of ALL therapy, the estimated cumulative risk of second malignant neoplasms within 20 years was 2.9% and the corresponding risk for cases with radiation therapy was 8.1%, compared with 0.3% for those who received only chemotherapy.[152] Malignant transformation of normal cells is due to nonlethal damage to the DNA that is not repaired. Alkylating agents and ionizing radiation are the treatments most closely linked to a second malignant neoplasm. In addition to the type and dose of treatment received, the risk of the development of a second cancer depends on several predisposing factors. Some tumors have a common underlying etiologic factor. For example, patients with bladder cancer are at greater risk for the development of lung cancer because both tumors are associated with smoking.[152,153] Genetic susceptibility is a second factor.[151] Children with the genetic form of retinoblastoma (which is usually bilateral) have a much higher incidence of sarcomas (as a second malignant neoplasm) than those with the nongenetic form of the disease.[154]

## Second Malignancies Following Chemotherapy

Acute nonlymphocytic leukemia (ANL) following treatment with alkylating agents is the most common chemotherapy-related second malignant neoplasm. The disease usually is preceded by a period of prolonged pancytopenia and can occur as early as 1.3 years following the initiation of chemotherapy for the primary malignancy. The incidence of treatment-related ANL peaks at five years and plateaus at ten years following treatment.[155]

ANL following Hodgkin's disease has been studied intensively in large cohorts of patients.[155–160] The overall cumulative risk has been reported to be 3.3% at 15 years postdiagnosis but varies from 0.6% in patients who received only radiation therapy to 17% in those treated with combination chemotherapy.[155,161] The treatment regimen with the greatest leukemogenic potential is MOPP, presumably due to the mechlorethamine and procarbazine.[153,157–161] A dose-response relationship between alkylating agents and the occurrence of a second malignant neoplasm has been reported;[161] Aisenberg[157] has suggested that leukemia is most likely to develop in patients who received more than six cycles of MOPP or similar drug regimens that contain alkylating agents. The addition of radiation to the MOPP regimen does not appear to significantly increase the risk of ANL,[161] whereas the recent use of ABVD (doxorubicin, bleomycin, vinblastine, and dacarbazine) and a regimen involving procarbazine, melphalan, and vinblastine have not been found to carry an increased risk of acute leukemia, which is attributed to lower total dose of alkylating agents.[155,161] The risk of ANL in children previously treated for Hodgkin's disease has been associated with disease relapse, treatment with alkylating agents and radiation, and splenectomy.[162,163]

In patients with multiple myeloma the risk or the

development of ANL is unusually high, more than 200 times that of the incidence in the general population. The drug most closely associated with ANL was melphalan, although multiple myeloma may also be associated with an increased risk of ANL that is unrelated to treatment.[160]

Although the incidence is not as great as with Hodgkin's disease or multiple myeloma, treatment-related acute leukemia has occurred in patients with non-Hodgkin's lymphoma,[164,165] breast cancer,[166] gastrointestinal cancer,[167] lung cancer,[168,169] germ cell tumors in men,[170] and ovarian cancer[171] and in survivors of childhood cancer.[172-174] Alkylating agents, primarily cyclophosphamide and melphalan, have been linked to the occurrence of ANL. ANL was two to three times more likely to develop in women who received melphalan for the treatment of ovarian cancer than in those who received cyclophosphamide, which suggests that, of the two drugs, melphalan has the greater leukemogenic potential.[175] There is also concern among some cancer researchers that etoposide may increase the risk for ANL.[169] Intercalating topoisomerase II inhibitors (doxorubicin, dactinomycin), when combined with alkylating agents and radiation, may cause secondary AML. A review of 3696 patients treated for cancer at St. Jude Children's Research Hospital between 1980 and 1992 revealed 36 cases of secondary AML. Chromosomal abnormalities (11q23 and/or 21q22) were identified with alkylating agents and intercalating agents. Four cases with the chromosomal abnormalities had not received epipodophyllotoxin treatment.[174]

## Second Malignancies Following Radiation

Sarcomas of the bone and soft tissue are the most common second malignant neoplasm after radiation therapy. Although the latency period can be as short as five months, it ranges from 10 to 20 years following radiation.[176] The incidence has been found to peak at 15–20 years after the initial diagnosis.[152,176] Malignant transformation can occur in doses ranging from 1000 to 8000 cGy. The relative risk increases from 8 following doses of 1000–2000 cGy to 40 following doses of 6000 cGy.[176] It has been postulated that the decreased risk following doses of 8000 cGy is due to the phenomenon of cell killing rather than nonlethal cell damage.

In a large study of 9170 survivors of childhood cancer, 48 cases of bone cancer occurred as opposed to the 0.4 expected (relative risk 133).[176] The risk was highest among children treated for retinoblastoma (relative risk 999) and Ewing's sarcoma (relative risk 649) but also was increased significantly in patients treated for rhabdomyosarcoma, Wilms' tumor, and Hodgkin's disease. Of the patients with sarcoma, 84% had received radiation, and 83% of the subsequent tumors occurred within the field of radiation. Nygaard and colleagues[152] found the cumulative risk of second malignancies in children treated for ALL to be 2.9% by 20 years after diagnosis. The risk factor was higher for ALL patients who had received only chemotherapy (8.1% compared with 0.3%, $p = .05$).

Three brain tumors and two basal cell carcinomas of the scalp occurred in the 895 patients who received cranial radiation.

ANL following radiation therapy is uncommon but has been reported in childhood cancer[161] and non-Hodgkin's lymphoma.[158] Women with breast cancer treated with postoperative radiation also have a slightly increased risk of ANL.[166] In addition to sarcomas and leukemia, a variety of other solid tumors have been linked to treatment with radiation. Carcinomas of the breast can occur in girls treated with pulmonary irradiation,[161] and a slightly excessive number of tumors of the bladder, rectum, uterus, bone, and connective tissue has been reported in women who received radiation for gynecologic cancer.[177,178] Brain tumors can occur after cranial irradiation for CNS prophylaxis in childhood ALL.[152, 179,180] Finally, lung cancer following mantle radiation for Hodgkin's disease has been reported.[181] The average latency period was seven years, and smoking was a contributing factor in only 53% of patients. Table 30-3 summarizes the findings from selected studies on the risk of ANL in patients treated for various types of cancer.

Twenty-four second malignant neoplasms of the CNS were found in a cohort study of 9720 children treated for ALL.[180] This represented a 22-fold excess of CNS tumors. All CNS tumors developed in children treated with cranial radiation; the risk was greatest in children who were 5 years of age or younger at the time of diagnosis.[180]

## EARLY DETECTION AND PREVENTION

Early detection and prevention of late toxicities is a relatively recent area of investigation. If early indicators of late tissue damage are identified, interventions designed to diminish the severity and overall impact of the toxicity can be developed and tested. Knowledge of the mechanisms responsible for delayed tissue damage following radiation and chemotherapy is increasing, and provides the basis for interventions designed to inhibit specific pathways or scavenge toxic by-products. Recently, cooperative organizations that initiate and coordinate multicenter clinical trials have formed specific subcommittees to develop standard criteria for monitoring late injury to normal tissue. The SOMA scales (Subjective, Objective, Management, and Analytical evaluation of injury) are intended to address the need for sensitive and uniform criteria for monitoring late reactions.[182] The SOMA scales include the following evaluative criteria: Subjective: assessment of the injury as perceived by the patient; Objective: extent of morbidity; this may include signs of tissue injury that are below the threshold that will result in symptoms; Management: interventions that have been initiated in an attempt to ameliorate symptoms; and Analytic: methods by which tissue function can be assessed more objectively than by physical examination, including biological assessment techniques. For each of the catego-

**TABLE 30-3**   Selected Studies of Risk of Acute Nonlymphocytic Leukemia in Patients Treated for Several Types of Cancer

| Series | Total Number of Patients | Number of Leukemias Observed | Relative Risk | Cumulative Risk (no. yr follow-up) |
|---|---|---|---|---|
| Hodgkin's disease | | | | |
| Tucker et al[155] | 1507 | 28 | 66 | 3.3% ± 0.6% (15) |
| Valagussa et al[156] | 1329 | 27 | | 3.6% ± 0.9% (12) |
| Coleman et al[158] | 730 | 8 | 86 | |
| Blayney et al[159] | 193 | 12* | 96 | 10% ± 3% (15) |
| Ovarian cancer | | | | |
| Greene et al[175] | 3363 | 28 | 23.5 | 8.4% ± 1.6% (10)† |
| Non-Hodgkin's lymphoma | | | | |
| Greene et al[165] | 517 | 9 | 105 | 7.9% ± 3.2% (10) |
| Breast cancer | | | | |
| Fisher et al[166] | 8483 | 43* | NA | <2% (10) |
| Gastrointestinal cancer | | | | |
| Boice et al[167] | 3633 | 17* | | 3.2% (7) |
| Lung cancer | | | | |
| Chak et al[168] | 158 | 3 | 316 | 25% ± 13% (3.1) |
| Ratain et al[169] | 119 | 4 | NA | 44% ± 24% (2.5) |

*Includes myelodysplastic disorders.
†Cumulative risk among women treated with chemotherapy only.
‡Risk not statistically significant.
NA, data not available.
Adapted from Fraser MC, Tucker MA: Second malignancies following cancer therapy, *Semin Oncol Nurs* 5:43–55, 1989. Reprinted with permission.

ries, there are four degrees of injury ranging from grade 1, representing the most minor symptoms that require no intervention, to grade 4, representing irreversible functional damage, necessitating major therapeutic intervention.[182] SOMA scales have been developed for irradiated skin, breast, lung, muscle, peripheral nerves, and the gastrointestinal tract.[136,138,183,184] Similar grading scales are being developed for late cardiac damage.[130,131]

In vitro and in vivo methods for early detection of late toxicities are also being developed. For example, plasma transforming growth factor-beta (TGF-B) was measured in 52 women undergoing autologous bone marrow transplant for stage II breast cancer. Pretransplant TGF-B$_1$ was significantly higher in patients who later developed hepatic veno-occlusive disease and pulmonary drug toxicity.[185] The findings suggest that early detection can lead to early prevention of serious organ toxicities. Assays for predicting sensitivity of normal cells to radiation and chemotherapy are being investigated, and are based on the premise that radiosensitivity is genetically based, and a major factor in the development of delayed injury in other normal tissues. Cultured cells, such as fibroblasts, marrow cells, or lymphocytes, could be exposed to radiation and chemotherapy. The normal cells could be studied for survival, cytotoxicity, genetic damage, and loss of DNA repair proteins.[186–188]

Strategies for preventing late effects are also emerging. Drugs that bind intracellular iron and inhibit the formation of free radicals, such as Dexrazone, minimize anthracycline-induced cardiac toxicity.[126,134] An adrenocorticotropic hormone [ACTH (4-9)] analogue, Org 2766, has been found to minimize cisplatin neuropathy in men treated for testicular cancer. Preliminary evidence suggests that Org 2766, a neuropeptide, does not protect against the neurotoxic effects of cisplatin but ameliorates the neuropathy by enhancing endogenous nerve repair mechanisms.[189] Results from a preliminary study of six children with methotrexate-induced neurotoxicity unresponsive to standard treatment suggest that aminophylline may be beneficial. Four of the six children given 2.5 mg/kg of intravenous aminophylline had complete resolution of symptoms within 30 minutes of the infusion.[190] One of the effects of methotrexate on the CNS is intracellular accumulation of 5-aminoimidazole-4-caroxamide ribonucleotide (AICAR), which increases the release and accumulation of adenosine. Aminophylline is a competitive antagonist for adenosine receptors, and therefore may block adenosine-mediated neurotoxicity.

## CONCLUSION

This chapter has provided a comprehensive review of the biological late effects that can be caused by curative cancer therapy. Long-term surveillance for these toxic effects is a recent and challenging area for oncology nurses and physicians. A long-range perspective is essential because the latency period for some late toxicities is many years after completion of treatment and the consequences of permanent tissue damage across the life span are unknown.

General recommendations for long-term follow-up include an annual physical examination with a complete blood cell count and urinalysis. Evaluation of specific toxicity to organ systems and second malignancies depends on the initial diagnosis, type and amount of treatment received, and host risk factors. For some late toxicities, surveillance guidelines have been standardized. The Cardiology Committee of the Children's Cancer Study Group recently published guidelines for cardiac monitoring of children during and after anthracycline therapy.[191] Recommendations for late cardiac follow-up include (1) an electrocardiogram (ECG) and echocardiogram every two to three years and (2) a radionuclide angiocardiogram and 24-hour continuous taped ECG every six years posttherapy.[191] These recommendations may serve as a model for establishing long-term evaluation guidelines for all late toxicities. However, for all biological late effects a careful balance must be struck between monitoring and the creation of needless anxiety that could hinder the patient's overall rehabilitation and emotional adjustment.

# REFERENCES

1. *Cancer Facts and Figures: 1996.* Atlanta, American Cancer Society, 1996

2. Bleyer A: The impact of childhood cancer on the United States and the world. *CA Cancer J Clin* 40:355–376, 1990

3. van Eys J: Living beyond cure: Transcending survival. *Am J Pediatr Hematol Oncol* 9:114–118, 1987

4. Meadows AT, Massari DJ, Fergusson J, et al: Declines in IQ scores and cognitive dysfunctions in children with acute lymphoblastic leukemia treated with cranial irradiation. *Lancet* 2:1015–1018, 1981

5. Robison LL, Nesbit ME, Sather HN, et al: Factors associated with IQ scores in long-term survivors of childhood acute lymphoblastic leukemia. *Am J Pediatr Hematol Oncol* 6:115–121, 1984

6. Moore IM, Kramer JH, Ablin AR: Late effects of central nervous system prophylactic leukemia therapy on cognitive functioning. *Oncol Nurs Forum* 13:45–51, 1986

7. Lansky SB, Cairns NU, Lansky LL, et al: Central nervous system prophylaxis. *Am J Pediatr Hematol Oncol* 6:183–190, 1984

8. Stebhens JA, Kisker CT: Intelligence and achievement testing in childhood cancer: Three years postdiagnosis. *J Dev Behav Pediatr* 5:184–188, 1984

9. Moehle KA, Berg RA, Ch'ien LT, et al: Language-related skills in children with acute lymphocytic leukemia. *J Dev Behav Pediatr* 4:257–261, 1983

10. Duffner PK, Cohen ME, Parker MS: Prospective intellectual testing in children with brain tumors. *Ann Neurol* 23:575–579, 1988

11. Chak LK, Zatz IM, Wasserstein P, et al: Neurologic dysfunction in patients treated for small cell carcinoma of the lung: A clinical and radiological study. *Int J Radiat Oncol Biol Phys* 12:385–389, 1986

12. Frytak S, Earnest F, O'Neill B, et al: Magnetic resonance imaging for neurotoxicity on long-term survivors of carcinoma. *Mayo Clin Proc* 60:803–813, 1985

13. Pfefferbaum-Levine B, Copeland DR, Fletcher JM, et al: Neuropsychological assessment of long-term survivors of childhood leukemia. *Am J Pediatr Hematol Oncol* 6:123–128, 1984

14. Fletcher JM: Neurobehavioral effects of central nervous system prophylactic treatment of cancer in children. *J Clin Exp Neuropsychol* 10:495–538, 1988

15. Goff JR, Anderson HR, Cooper PF: Distractability and memory deficits in long-term survivors of acute lymphoblastic leukemia. *J Dev Behav Pediatr* 1:158–163, 1980

16. Kramer JH, Moore IM: Verbal learning deficits in long-term survivors of acute lymphoblastic leukemia. *Proc Am Psychol Assoc* 97:401, 1985 (abstr)

17. Kramer JH, Moore IM: Age at time of treatment effect on mnemestic functioning following CNS irradiation and intrathecal methotrexate. *J Clin Exp Neuropsychol* 7:627, 1985 (abstr)

18. Copeland DR, Fletcher JM, Pfefferbaum-Levine B, et al: Neuropsychological sequelae of childhood cancer in long-term survivors. *Pediatrics* 75:745–753, 1985

19. Ellison N, Bernath A, Kane R, et al: Disturbing problems of success: Clinical status of long-term survivors of small cell lung cancer. *Proc Am Soc Clin Oncol* 1:149, 1982 (abstr)

20. Rodgers J, Britton PG, Morris RG, et al: Memory after treatment for acute lymphoblastic leukemia. *Arch Dis Child* 67:266–268, 1992

21. Buttsworth DL, Murdoch BE, Ozanne AE: Acute lymphoblastic leukaemia: Language deficits in children post-treatment. *Disabil Rehabil* 15(2):67–75, 1993

22. Waber D, Tarbell N, Kahn C, et al: The relationship of sex and treatment modality to neuropsychologic outcome in childhood acute lymphoblastic leukemia. *J Clin Oncol* 10:810–817, 1992

23. Obetz SW, Smithson WA, Groover RV, et al: Neuropsychological follow-up of children with acute lymphoblastic leukemia. *Am J Pediatr Hematol Oncol* 1:207–213, 1979

24. Twaddle V, Britton PG, Craft AC, et al: Intellectual function after treatment for leukaemia or solid tumors. *Arch Dis Child* 58:949–952, 1985

25. Taylor HG: Postirradiation treatment outcomes for children with acute lymphoblastic leukemia: Clarification of risks. *J Pediatr Psychol* 12:395–411, 1987

26. Moss HA, Nannis ED, Poplack DG: The effects of prophylactic treatment of the central nervous system on the intellectual functioning of children with acute lymphocytic leukemia. *Am J Med* 71:47–52, 1981

27. Jannoun L: Are cognitive and educational development affected by age at which prophylactic therapy is given in acute lymphoblastic leukemia? *Arch Dis Child* 58:953–958, 1983

28. Silverman CL, Palkes H, Talent B, et al: Late effects of radiotherapy on patients with cerebellar medulloblastoma. *Cancer* 54:825–829, 1984

29. Rowland JH, Glidewell OJ, Sibley RF, et al: Effects of different forms of central nervous system prophylaxis on neuropsychological function in childhood leukemia. *J Clin Oncol* 2:1327–1335, 1984

30. Pavlovsky S, Castano J, Leiguda R, et al: Neuropsychologi-

cal study in patients with ALL. *Am J Pediatr Hematol Oncol* 5:79–128, 1983

31. Tamaroff M, Miller DR, Murphy ML: Immediate and long-term post-therapy neuropsychologic performance in children with acute lymphoblastic leukemia treated without central nervous system radiation. *J Pediatr* 101:524–529, 1982

32. Hussain M, Wozniak AJ, Edelstein MB: Neurotoxicity of antineoplastic agents. *Crit Rev Oncol Hematol* 14:61–75, 1993

33. Balsom WR, Bleyer WA, Robinson LL, et al: Intellectual function in long-term survivors of childhood acute lymphoblastic leukemia: Protective effect of pre-irradiation methotrexate. A Children's Cancer Study Group study. *Med Pediatr Oncol* 19:486–492, 1991

34. Kaleita T, Tesler A, Feig SA: Prospective neurodevelopmental studies: Two children treated with total body irradiation and bone marrow transplantation for acute leukemia in infancy. *Prog Bone Marrow Transplant* 1:157–164, 1987

35. Smedler AC, Bergman H, Bolme P, et al: Neuropsychological functioning in children treated with bone marrow transplantation. *J Clin Exp Neuropsychol* 10:325–326, 1988

36. Halberg F, Wara W, Kramer JH, et al: Total body irradiation in infancy: Effect on growth and development after bone marrow transplant for SIDS. *Int J Radiat Oncol Biol Phys* 15: 154, 1988 (abstr)

37. Tameroff M, Salwen R, Miller D, et al: Neuropsychological sequelae in irradiated (1800 rads [r] and 2400 r) and non-irradiated children with acute lymphoblastic leukemia (ALL). *Proc Am Soc Clin Oncol* 4:C-644, 1985 (abstr)

38. Duffner PK, Cohne ME, Thomas PR, et al: The long-term effects of cranial irradiation on the central nervous system. *Cancer* 56:1841–1846, 1985

39. Berry MP, Jenkins DT, Green GW, et al: Radiation treatment for medulloblastoma. *J Neurosurg* 55:43–51, 1981

40. Mulhern RK, Crisco JJ, Kim LE: Neuropsychological sequelae of childhood brain tumors: A review. *J Child Clin Psychol* 12:66–73, 1983

41. Packer RJ, Zimmerman RA, Bilaniuk LT: Magnetic resonance imaging in the evaluation of treatment-related central nervous system damage. *Cancer* 58:635–640, 1986

42. Chin HW, Maruyama Y: Age at treatment and long-term performance results in medulloblastoma. *Cancer* 53: 1952–1958, 1984

43. Dobbing J, Sands J: Quantitative growth and development of the human brain. *Arch Dis Child* 48:757–767, 1973

44. Davison AN, Dobbing J: Myelination as a vulnerable period in brain development. *BMJ* 22:40–44, 1966

45. Waber DP, Tarbell NJ, Kahn CM, et al: The relationship of sex and treatment modality to neuropsychologic outcome in childhood acute lymphoblastic leukemia. *J Clin Oncol* 10:810–817, 1992

46. Brouwers P, Riccardi R, Fedio P, et al: Long-term neuropsychological sequelae of childhood leukemia: Correlation with CT brain scan abnormalities. *J Pediatr* 106:723–728, 1985

47. Davis PC, Hoffman JC, Pearl GS, et al: CT evaluation of effects of cranial radiation therapy in children. *Am J Neuroradiol* 7:639–644, 1986

48. Peylan-Ramu N, Poplack DG, Pizzo PA, et al: Abnormal CT scans of the brain in asymptomatic children with acute lymphoblastic leukemia after prophylactic treatment of the central nervous system with radiation and intrathecal chemotherapy. *N Engl J Med* 298:815–818, 1978

49. Ochs JJ, Berger P, Brecher ML, et al: Computed tomography brain scans in children with acute lymphoblastic leuke-mia receiving methotrexate alone as central nervous system prophylaxis. *Cancer* 45:2274–2278, 1980

50. Ochs JJ, Parvey LS, Whitaker JN, et al: Serial cranial computed tomography scans in children with leukemia given two different forms of central nervous system therapy. *J Clin Oncol* 1:793–798, 1983

51. Kramer JH, Norman D, Brant-Zawadski M, et al: Absence of white matter changes on magnetic resonance imaging in children treated with CNS prophylaxis therapy for leukemia. *Cancer* 61:928–930, 1988

52. Tsurada JS, Kortman KE, Bradley WG, et al: Radiation effects on cerebral white matter: MR evaluation. *Am J Radiat* 149:165–171, 1987

53. Sheline GE, Wara WM, Smith V: Therapeutic irradiation and brain injury. *Int J Radiat Oncol Biol Phys* 6:1215–1228, 1980

54. Caveness WF: Experimental observations: Delayed necrosis in the monkey brain, in Gilbert MA, Kagan AR (eds): *Radiation Damage to the Nervous System.* New York, Raven Press, 1980, pp 1–38

55. Cassarett G: Basic mechanisms of permanent and delayed radiation pathology. *Cancer* 37:1002–1010, 1976

56. Committee for Radiation Oncology Studies: Normal tissue tolerance and damage. *Cancer* 37:2046–2055, 1976

57. Price RA, Jamieson PA: The central nervous system in childhood leukemia: II. Subacute leukoencephalopathy. *Cancer* 35:306–318, 1975

58. Mahoney DH, Fernbach DJ, Glaze DG, et al: Elevated myelin basic protein level in the cerebral spinal fluid of children with acute lymphoblastic leukemia. *J Clin Oncol* 2: 58–61, 1984

59. Gangji D, Reaman GH, Cohen SR, et al: Leukoencephalopathy and elevated levels of myelin basic protein in the cerebral spinal fluid of patients with acute lymphoblastic leukemia. *Medical Intelligence* 303:19–21, 1980

60. Packer R, Meadows AT, Rorke L, et al: Long-term sequela of cancer treatment on the central nervous system in childhood. *Med Pediatr Oncol* 15:241–253, 1987

61. Hopewell JW: Late radiation damage to the central nervous system: A radiobiological interpretation. *Neuropathol Appl Neurobiol* 5:329–343, 1979

62. Tiller-Borcich JK, Fike JR, Phillips TL, et al: Pathology of delayed radiation brain damage: An experimental canine model. *Radiat Res* 110:161–172, 1987

63. Deck MD: Imaging techniques in the diagnosis of radiation damage to the central nervous system, in Gilbert HA, Kag AR (eds): *Radiation Damage to the Nervous System.* New York, Raven Press, 1980, pp 107–127

64. Wharam MD: Radiation therapy, in Altman AJ, Schwartz AD (eds): *Malignant Diseases of Infancy, Childhood and Adolescence.* Philadelphia, Saunders, 1983, p 103

65. Parsons JT, Bova FJ, Fitzgerald CR, et al: Radiation retinopathy after external-beam irradiation: Analysis of time-dose factors. *Int J Radiat Oncol Biol Phys* 30:765–773, 1994

66. Coucke PA, Schmid C, Balmer A, et al: Hypofractionation in retinoblastoma: An increased risk of retinopathy. *Radiother Oncol* 28:157–161, 1993

67. Piehl IJ, Meyer D, Perlia CP, et al: Effects of cisdiammine dichloroplatinum (NSC-119875) on hearing function in man. *Cancer Chemother Rep* 58:871–875, 1974

68. Walkwe DA, Pillov J, Waters KD, et al: Enhanced cisplatin ototoxicity in children with brain tumors who have received simultaneous or prior cranial irradiation. *Med Pediatr Oncol* 17:48–52, 1989

69. Meyer WH, Ayers D, McHaney VA, et al: Ifosfamide and

exacerbation of cisplatin-induced hearing loss. *Lancet* 341: 754–755, 1993

70. Hobbie WL, Schwartz CL: Endocrine late effects among survivors of cancer. *Semin Oncol Nurs* 5:14–21, 1989

71. Ganong WF: The thyroid gland, in Ganong WF (ed): *Review of Medical Physiology.* Palo Alto, CA, Appleton and Lange, 1987, pp 262–275

72. Glatstein E, McHardy-Young S, Brast N, et al: Alterations in serum thyrotropin (TSH) and thyroid function following radiotherapy in patients with malignant lymphoma. *J Clin Endocrinol Metab* 32:838–841, 1971

73. Shalet SM, Rosenstock JD, Beardwell CT, et al: Thyroid dysfunction following external irradiation to the neck for Hodgkin's disease in childhood. *Radiology* 28:511–515, 1977

74. Smith RE, Adler RA, Clark P, et al: Thyroid function after mantle radiation in Hodgkin's disease. *JAMA* 245:46–49, 1981

75. Donaldson SS, Glatstein E, Rosenberg SA, et al: Pediatric Hodgkin's disease: II. Results of therapy. *Cancer* 37: 2436–2447, 1976

76. Ramsay N, Kim T, Coccia P, et al: Thyroid dysfunction in pediatric patients after mantle field radiation therapy for Hodgkin's disease. *Proc Am Soc Clin Oncol* 19:331, 1978 (abstr)

77. Mortilmer RH, Hill GE, Galligan JP, et al: Hypothyroidism and Graves' disease after mantle irradiation: A follow-up study. *Aust N Z J Med* 16:347–351, 1986

78. Josensuu H, Viikari J: Thyroid function after postoperative radiation therapy in patients with breast cancer. *Acta Radiol Oncol* 25:167–170, 1986

79. Constine LS, Rubin P, Woolf PD: Hyperprolactinemia and hypothyroidism following cytotoxic therapy for central nervous system malignancies. *J Clin Oncol* 5:1841–1851, 1987

80. Nelson DF, Reddy KV, O'Mara RE, et al: Thyroid abnormalities following neck irradiation for Hodgkin's disease. *Cancer* 42:2553–2562, 1978

81. Schimpff SC, Diggs CH, Wiswell JG, et al: Radiation-related thyroid dysfunction: Implications for the treatment of Hodgkin's disease. *Ann Intern Med* 92:91–98, 1980

82. Samaan NA, Vieto R, Scholtz PN, et al: Hypothalamic, pituitary and thyroid dysfunction after radiotherapy to the head and neck. *Int J Radiat Oncol Biol Phys* 8:1857–1867, 1982

83. Sklar CA, Constine LS: Chronic neuroendocrinological sequelae of radiation therapy. *Int J Radiat Oncol Biol Phys* 31:1113–1121, 1995

84. Davies HA, Didcock E, Didi M, et al: Disproportionate short stature after cranial irradiation and combination chemotherapy for leukaemia. *Arch Dis Child* 70:472–475, 1994

85. Kao GD, Willi SM, Goldwein J: The sequellae of chemoradiation therapy for head and neck cancer in children: Managing impaired growth, development, and other side effects. *Med Pediatr Oncol* 21:60–66, 1993

86. Braumer R, Rappaport R, Prevot C, et al: A prospective study of growth hormone deficiency in children given cranial irradiation, and its relation to statural growth. *J Clin Endocrinol Metab* 68:346–351, 1989

87. Oberfield SE, Allen JC, Pollack J, et al: Long-term endocrine sequelae after treatment of medulloblastoma: Perspective study of growth and thyroid function. *J Pediatr* 108: 219–223, 1986

88. Hakami N, Mohammad A, Meyer J: Growth and growth hormone of children with acute lymphoblastic leukemia following central nervous system prophylaxis with and with-

out cranial irradiation. *Am J Pediatr Hematol Oncol* 2: 311–316, 1985

89. Robison LL, Nesbit ME, Sather HN, et al: Height of children successfully treated for acute lymphoblastic leukemia: A report from the late effects study committee of Children's Cancer Study Group. *Med Pediatr Oncol* 13:13–21, 1985

90. Shalet SM, Bearwell CG, Pearson E, et al: The effect of varying doses of cerebral irradiation on growth hormone production in childhood. *Clin Endocrinol* 5:287–290, 1976

91. Cicognani A, Cacciari E, Veechi V, et al: Differential effects of 18- and 24-Gy cranial irradiation on growth rate and growth hormone release in children with prolonged survival after acute lymphoblastic leukemia. *Am J Dis Child* 141:550–552, 1986

92. Starceski PJ, Lee PA, Blatt J, et al: Comparable effects of 1800- and 2400-rad cranial irradiation on height and weight in children treated for acute lymphoblastic leukemia. *Am J Dis Child* 141:550–552, 1987

93. Sanders JE, Pritchard S, Mahoney P, et al: Growth and development following marrow transplantation for leukemia. *Blood* 68:1129–1135, 1986

94. Clayton PE, Shalet SM: Dose dependency of time of onset of radiation-induced growth hormone deficiency. *J Pediatr* 118:226–227, 1991

95. Brauner R, Czernichow P, Rappaport R: Greater susceptibility to hypothalamopituitary irradiation in younger children with acute lymphoblastic leukemia. *J Pediatr* 108:3332, 1986

96. Olshan JS, Gubernick J, Packer RJ, et al: The effects of adjuvant chemotherapy on growth in children with medulloblastoma. *Cancer* 70:2013–2017, 1992

97. Andrieu J, Ochoa-Molina ME: Menstrual cycle, pregnancies and offspring before and after MOPP therapy for Hodgkin's disease. *Cancer.* 52:435–438, 1983

98. Jordan VC, Fritz NF, Tormey DC: Endocrine effects of adjuvant chemotherapy and long-term tamoxifen administration on node-positive patients with breast cancer. *Cancer Res* 47:624–630, 1987

99. Gershenson DM: Menstrual and reproductive function after treatment with combination chemotherapy for malignant ovarian germ cell tumors. *J Clin Oncol* 6:270–275, 1988

100. Shalet SM: The effects of cancer treatment on growth and sexual development. *Clin Oncol* 4:223–238, 1985

101. Hensle T, Burbige K, Shepard B, et al: Chemotherapy and its effect on testicular morphology in children. *J Urol* 131: 1142–1144, 1982

102. Rivkees SA, Crawford JD: The relationship of gonadal activity and chemotherapy-induced gonadal damage. *JAMA* 259:2123–2125, 1988

103. Heyn R, Raney RB, Hays DM, et al: Late effects of therapy in patients with paratesticular rhabdomyosarcoma. *J Clin Oncol* 10:614–623, 1992

104. Petersen PM, Hansen SW, Giwercman A, et al: Dose-dependent impairment of testicular function in patients treated with cisplatin-based chemotherapy for germ cell cancer. *Ann Oncol* 5:355–358, 1994

105. Byrne J, Mulvihill JJ, Myers MH, et al: Effects of treatment on fertility in long-term survivors of childhood or adolescent cancer. *N Engl J Med* 317:1315–1321, 1987

106. Nicosia S, Matus-Ridley M, Meadows AT: Gonadal effects of cancer therapy in girls. *Cancer* 55:2364–2372, 1985

107. Fischer B, Bheung A: Delayed effect of radiation therapy with or without chemotherapy on ovarian function in

women with Hodgkin's disease. *Acta Radiol Oncol* 23:43–48, 1984

108. Shalet SM, Beardwell CG, Jacobs JG, et al: Testicular function following irradiation of the human prepubertal testis. *Clin Endocrinol* 9:483–490, 1978

109. Shalet SM, Horner A, Ahmed SR, et al: Leydig cell damage and testicular function combination chemotherapy in childhood for acute lymphoblastic leukemia. *Med Pediatr Oncol* 13:65–68, 1985

110. Hamre MR, Robison LL, Nesbit ME, et al: Effects of radiation on ovarian function in long-term survivors of childhood acute lymphoblastic leukemia: A report from the Children's Cancer Study Group. *J Clin Oncol* 5:1759–1765, 1987

111. Green DM, Hall B, Zevon M: Pregnancy outcome after treatment for acute lymphoblastic leukemia during childhood or adolescence. *Cancer* 64:2335–2339, 1989

112. Saman N, Vieto R, Schultz B, et al: Hypothalamic, pituitary and thyroid dysfunction after radiotherapy to the head and neck. *Int J Radiat Oncol Biol Phys* 8:1857–1867, 1982

113. Buvat J, LeMarie A, Burat-Herbaut M, et al: Hyperprolactinemia and sexual function in men. *Horm Res* 22:196–203, 1984

114. Ogilvy-Stuart AL, Clayton PE, Shalet SM: Cranial irradiation and early puberty. *J Clin Endocrinol Metab* 78:1282–1286, 1994

115. Job G, Pfreundschuh M, Baner M, et al: The influence of radiation therapy on T lymphocyte subpopulations defined by monoclonal antibodies. *Int J Radiat Oncol Biol Phys* 10:2077–2081, 1984

116. Rotstein S, Blomgren H, Petrini B, et al: Long-term effects on the immune system following local radiation therapy for breast cancer: I. Cellular composition of peripheral blood lymphocyte population. *Int J Radiat Oncol Biol Phys* 11:921–925, 1985

117. Rotstein S, Blomgren H, Petrini B, et al: Long-term effects on the immune system following local radiation therapy for breast cancer: IV. Proliferative responses and induction of suppressor activity of the blood lymphocyte population. *Radiother Oncol* 6:223–230, 1986

118. Haas GS, Halperin E, Poseret D, et al: Differential recovery of circulating T cell subsets after nodal irradiation for Hodgkin's disease. *J Immunol* 132:1026–1030, 1981

119. Ueda M, Harada N, Shiobara S, et al: T lymphocyte reconstitution in long-term survivors after allogeneic and autologous transplantation. *Transplantation* 3:552–556, 1981

120. Domenech J, Linassier C, Gihana E, et al: Prolonged impairment of hematopoiesis after high-dose therapy followed by autologous bone marrow transplantation. *Blood* 85:3320–3327, 1995

121. Van Rijswijk RF, Sybesma JPH, Kater L: A prospective study of the changes in the immune status before, during and after multiple agent chemotherapy for Hodgkin's disease. *Cancer* 51:637–644, 1983

122. Layward L, Ledvinsky RJ, Butler M: Long-term abnormalities in T and B lymphoblastic leukemia. *J Haematol* 49:251–258, 1981

123. Katz J, Walter BN, Bennetts GA, et al: Abnormal cellular and humoral immunity in childhood acute lymphoblastic leukemia in long-term remission. *West J Med* 146:179–187, 1988

124. Workman ML: Immunologic late effects in children and adults. *Semin Oncol Nurs* 5:36–42, 1989

125. Parmentier L, Morardet N, Tubina M: Late effects on human bone marrow after extended field radiotherapy. *Int J Radiat Oncol Biol Phys* 9:1303–1311, 1983

126. Hershko C, Link G, Tzahor M, et al: The role of iron and iron chelators in anthracycline cardiotoxicity. *Leuk Lymphoma* 11:207–214, 1993

127. Steinherz LJ, Steinherz P, Tan G, et al: Cardiac toxicity 4–20 years after completing anthracycline therapy. *Proc Am Soc Clin Oncol* 8:296, 1989 (abstr)

128. Lipshultz SE, Colan SD, Gelber RD, et al: Late cardiac effects of doxorubicin therapy for acute lymphoblastic leukemia in childhood. *N Engl J Med* 324:808–815, 1991

129. Ruccione K, Weinberg K: Late effects in multiple body systems. *Semin Oncol Nurs* 5:4–13, 1989

130. Stewart JR, Fajardo LF, Gillette SM, et al: Radiation injury to the heart. *Int J Radiat Oncol Biol Phys* 31:1205–1211, 1995

131. Benoff LJ, Schweitzer P: Radiation therapy–induced cardiac injury. *Am Heart J* 129:1193–1196, 1995

132. Roth BJ, Greist A, Kubilis PS, et al: Cisplatin-based combination chemotherapy for disseminated germ cell tumors: Long-term follow-up. *J Clin Oncol* 6:1239–1247, 1988

133. Ramireddy K, Kane KM, Adhar GC: Acquired episodic complete heart block after high-dose chemotherapy with cyclophosphamide and thiotepa. *Am Heart J* 127:701–704, 1994

134. Seifert CF, Nesser ME, Thompson DF: Dexrazoxane in the prevention of doxorubicin-induced cardiotoxicity. *Ann Pharmacother* 28:1063–1072, 1994

135. Basser RL, Green MD: Strategies for prevention of anthracycline cardiotoxicity. *Cancer Treat Rev* 19:57–77, 1993

136. McDonald S, Rubin P, Phillips TL, et al: Injury to the lung from cancer therapy: Clinical syndromes, measurable endpoints, and potential scoring systems. *Int J Radiat Oncol Biol Phys* 31:1187–1203, 1995

137. Morgan GW, Breit SN: Radiation and the lung: A reevaluation of the mechanisms mediating pulmonary injury. *Int J Radiat Oncol Biol Phys* 31:361–369, 1995

138. Coia LR, Myerson RJ, Tepper JE: Late effects of radiation therapy on the gastrointestinal tract. *Int J Radiat Oncol Biol Phys* 31:1213–1236, 1995

139. Jaffee N: Late sequelae of cancer therapy, in Sutow SS, Fernbach DJ, Vietti TJ (eds): *Clinical Pediatric Oncology*. St Louis, Mosby, 810–832, 1984

140. Shirkhoda A, Baird S: Morphologic changes of the liver following chemotherapy for metastatic breast carcinoma: CT findings. *Abdom Imaging* 19:39–42, 1994

141. Efros MD, Ahmed T, Coombe N, et al: Urologic complications of high-dose chemotherapy and bone marrow transplantation. *Urology* 43:355–360, 1994

142. Rossi R, Kleinebrand A, Gödde A, et al: Increased risk of ifosfamide-induced renal Fanconi's syndrome after unilateral nephrectomy. *Lancet* 341:755, 1993

143. Ritchey M, Green DM, Thomas P, et al: Renal failure in Wilms' tumor patients: A report from the national Wilms' tumor study group. *Med Pediatr Oncol* 26:75–80, 1996

144. Silber JH, Littman PS, Meadows AT: Stature loss following skeletal irradiation for childhood cancer. *J Clin Oncol* 8:304–312, 1990

145. Rate WR, Bulter MS, Robertson WW, et al: Late orthopedic effects in children with Wilms' tumor treated with abdominal irradiation. *Med Pediatr Oncol* 19:265–268, 1991

146. Shalet SM, Gibson B, Swindell R, et al: Effect of spinal irradiation on growth. *Arch Dis Child* 62:461–464, 1987

147. Maguire A, Craft AW, Evans RGB, et al: The long-term

effects of treatment on the dental conditions of children surviving malignant disease. *Cancer* 60:2570–2575, 1987

148. Holmes SJ, Whitehouse RW, Clark ST, et al: Reduced bone mineral density in men following chemotherapy for Hodgkin's disease. *Br J Cancer* 70:371–375, 1994

149. Gillette EL, Mahler PA, Powers BE, et al: Late radiation injury to muscle and peripheral nerves. *Int J Radiat Oncol Biol Phys* 31:1309–1318, 1995

150. Roller AC, Pembrook L, Plese L, et al: One-in-five Hodgkin's patients still at risk after 15 years. *Oncol Nurs Update* 2:13, 1987

151. Meadows AT: Second malignant neoplasms in childhood cancer survivors. *J Assoc Pediatr Oncol Nurs* 6:7–11, 1989

152. Nygaard R, Garwicz S, Haldorsen T, et al: Second malignant neoplasms in patients treated for childhood leukemia. *Acta Paediatr Scand* 80:1220–1228, 1991

153. Fraser MC, Tucker MA: Second malignancies following cancer therapy. *Semin Oncol Nurs* 5:43–55, 1989

154. Tucker MA, D'Angio GI, Boice JD, et al: Bone sarcomas linked to radiotherapy and chemotherapy in children. *N Engl J Med* 317:588–593, 1987

155. Tucker MH, Coleman CN, Cox RS, et al: Risk of second cancers after treatment for Hodgkin's disease. *N Engl J Med* 318:76–81, 1988

156. Valagussa P, Santoro A, Fossati-Bellani F, et al: Second acute leukemia and other malignancies following treatment for Hodgkin's disease. *J Clin Oncol* 4:830–837, 1986

157. Aisenberg AC: Acute nonlymphocytic leukemia after treatment for Hodgkin's disease. *Am J Med* 75:449–454, 1983

158. Coleman M, Easton DF, Horwich A, et al: Second malignancies and Hodgkin's disease: The Royal Marsden Hospital experience. *Radiother Oncol* 11:229–238, 1988

159. Blayney DW, Longo DL, Yound RC, et al: Decreasing risk of leukemia with prolonged follow-up after chemotherapy and radiation for Hodgkin's disease. *N Engl J Med* 316:710–714, 1987

160. Green MH: Epidemiologic studies of chemotherapy related acute leukemia, in Castellani A (ed): *Epidemiology and Quantitation of Environmental Risk in Humans from Radiation and Other Agents.* New York, Plenum, 1985, pp 499–514

161. Meadows AT: Second malignant neoplasms. *Clin Oncol* 4:217–261, 1985

162. Pui CH, Hancock ML, Raimondi SC, et al: Myeloid neoplasia in children treated for solid tumors. *Lancet* 336:417–421, 1990

163. Meadows AT, Obringer AC, Marrero O, et al: Second malignant neoplasms following childhood Hodgkin's disease: Treatment and splenectomy as risk factors. *Med Pediatr Oncol* 17:477–484, 1989

164. Pedersen-Bjergaard J, Ersboll J, Sorensen HM, et al: Risk of acute nonlymphocytic leukemia and preleukemia in patients treated with cyclophosphamide for non-Hodgkin's lymphomas. *Ann Intern Med* 103:195–200, 1985

165. Greene MH, Yound RC, Merrill JM, et al: Evidence of a treatment dose response in acute nonlymphocytic leukemias which occur after therapy of non-Hodgkin's lymphoma. *Cancer Res* 43:1891–1898, 1983

166. Fisher B, Rockete H, Fisher ER, et al: Leukemia in breast cancer patients following adjuvant chemotherapy or postoperative radiation: The NSABP experience. *J Clin Oncol* 3:1640–1658, 1985

167. Boice JD, Greene MH, Killen JY, et al: Leukemia and preleukemia after adjuvant chemotherapy of gastrointestinal cancer with semustine (methyl-CCNU). *N Engl J Med* 309:1079–1084, 1983

168. Chak LY, Sikie BL, Tucker MA, et al: Increased incidence of acute nonlymphocytic leukemia following therapy in patients with small cell carcinoma of the lung. *J Clin Oncol* 2:385–390, 1984

169. Ratain MJ, Kaminer LS, Bitran JD, et al: Acute nonlymphocytic leukemia following etoposide and cisplatin combination chemotherapy for advanced non-small cell carcinoma of the lung. *Blood* 70:1412–1417, 1987

170. Redman JR, Vugrin D, Arlin ZA, et al: Leukemia following treatment of germ cell tumors in men. *J Clin Oncol* 2:1080–1087, 1984

171. Kaldor JM, Day NE, Pettersson F, et al: Leukemia following chemotherapy for ovarian cancer. *N Engl J Med* 322:1–6, 1990

172. Tucker MA, Meadows AT, Boice JD Jr, et al: Leukemia after therapy with alkylating agents for childhood cancer. *J Natl Cancer Inst* 78:459–464, 1987

173. Moss TS, Stauss LC, Das L, et al: Secondary leukemia following successful treatment of Wilms tumor. *Am J Pediatr Hematol Oncol* 11:158–161, 1989

174. Sandoval C, Pui CH, Bowman LC, et al: Secondary acute myeloid leukemia in children previously treated with alkylating agents, intercalating topoisomerase II inhibitors, and irradiation. *J Clin Oncol* 11:1039–1045, 1993

175. Greene MH, Harris EL, Gershenson DM, et al: Mephalan may be a more potent leukemogen than cyclophosphamide. *Ann Intern Med* 105:360–367, 1986

176. Tucker MA, D'Angio GJ, Boice JD, et al: Bone sarcomas linked to radiotherapy and chemotherapy in children. *N Engl J Med* 317:588–593, 1987

177. Boice JD Jr, Blettner M, Kleinerman RA, et al: Radiation dose and second cancer risk in patients treated for cancer of the cervix. *Radiat Res* 116:3–55, 1988

178. Storm HH: Secondary primary cancer after treatment for cervical cancer: Late effects of radiotherapy. *Cancer* 61:679–688, 1988

179. Rimm IJ, Li FC, Tabell NJ: Brain tumors after cranial irradiation for childhood acute lymphoblastic leukemia: A 13 year experience from the Dana Farber Cancer Institute and The Children's Hospital. *Cancer* 59:1506–1508, 1987

180. Neglia JP, Meadows AT, Robison LL, et al: Second neoplasms after acute lymphoblastic leukemia in childhood. *N Engl J Med* 325:1330–1336, 1991

181. List AF, Doll DC, Greco A: Lung cancer in Hodgkin's disease: Association with previous radiotherapy. *J Clin Oncol* 3:215–221, 1985

182. Pavy JJ, Denekamp J, Letschert J, et al: Late effects toxicity scoring: the SOMA scale. *Int J Radiat Oncol Biol Phys* 31:1043–1047, 1995

183. Archambeau JO, Pezner R, Wasserman T: Pathophysiology of irradiated skin and breast. *Int J Radiat Oncol Biol Phys* 31:1171–1185, 1995

184. Gillette EL, Mahler PA, Powers BE, et al: Late radiation injury to muscle and peripheral nerves. *Int J Radiat Oncol Biol Phys* 31:1309–1318, 1995

185. Murase T, Anscher MS, Petros WP, et al: Changes in plasma transforming growth factor beta in response to high-dose chemotherapy for stage II breast cancer: Possible implications for the prevention of hepatic veno-occlusive disease and pulmonary drug toxicity. *Bone Marrow Transplant* 15:173–178, 1995

186. Bentzen SM, Overgaard M, Overgaard J: Clinical correla-

tions between late normal tissue endpoints after radiotherapy: Implications for predictive assays of radiosensitivity. *Eur J Cancer* 29A:1373–1376, 1993

187. Busch D: Genetic susceptibility to radiation and chemotherapy injury: Diagnosis and management. *Int J Radiat Oncol Biol Phys* 30:997–1002, 1994

188. Johansen J, Bentzen SM, Overgaard J, et al: Evidence for a positive correlation between in vitro radiosensitivity of normal human skin fibroblasts and the occurrence of subcutaneous fibrosis after radiotherapy. *Int J Radiat Oncol Biol Phys* 66:407–412, 1994

189. van Gerven JMA, Hovestadt A, Moll JW: The effects of an ACTH (4-9) analogue on development of cisplatin neuropathy in testicular cancer: A randomized trial. *J Neurol* 241:432–435, 1994

190. Bernini JC, Fort DW, Griener JC, et al: Aminophylline for methotrexate-induced neurotoxicity. *Lancet* 345:544–547, 1995

191. Steinherz LS, Graham T, Hurwitz R, et al: Guidelines for cardiac monitoring of children during and after anthracycline therapy: Reports of the Cardiology Committee of the Children's Cancer Study Group. *Pediatrics* 89:942–949, 1992

# PART V

# The Care of Individuals with Cancer

# Chapter 31

# AIDS-Related Malignancies

**Theresa A. Moran, RN, MS**

## INTRODUCTION

For decades, scientists and medical researchers have attempted to prove or disprove the hypothesis of immune surveillance and the evolution of cancer. As research in this area continues, it appears that human immunodeficiency virus (HIV) infection contributes yet another piece of evidence that supports the hypothesized link. The devastation wreaked by HIV on the immune system, particularly the cell-mediated arm, results in the diagnosis of a malignancy at some point during the illness in approximately 30%–70% of those with acquired immunodeficiency syndrome (AIDS).[1] Neoplasms of all organs and body systems also have been reported in patients whose serum is positive for HIV antibody. The four most common malignancies in AIDS are Kaposi's sarcoma (KS), non-Hodgkin's lymphoma (NHL), primary central nervous system (CNS) lymphoma, and invasive squamous cell cancer (SCC) of the cervix. These diseases have been referred to as *opportunistic* malignancies because they occur in patients with preexisting immunodeficiency, for example, in individuals with primary immunodeficiency, in those who undergo therapeutic immunosuppression, and now in those with HIV infection. Because these individuals are immunosuppressed, the aforementioned cancers proliferate rapidly.

## KAPOSI'S SARCOMA

In 1872 Dr. Moritz Kaposi first described the lesions of Kaposi's sarcoma in seven men of Mediterranean or Jewish ancestry. In 1947 the literature indicated that only 500 cases had been reported, and by 1960 only 1200 total cases had been documented in the 100 years since the disease was first described. The incidence in the general population was estimated to be two to six cases per 100 million people; thus, dermatologists and oncologists were not likely to diagnose this rare malignancy in the course of their professional careers. Beginning in the 1970s, however, the incidence of KS increased dramatically. As more sophisticated technologic advances brought on the era of organ transplantation, an increasing number of reports documented the occurrence of this malignancy in patients who were chemically immunosuppressed to prevent organ rejection.[1,2] With the development of new drugs, oncologists began seeing KS in patients treated with antineoplastic agents. Reports from Africa in the late 1970s revealed that KS was endemic in certain areas of the continent. In 1981 KS was reported in yet another population, that of previously healthy, young, homosexual men who were neither receiving chemotherapy nor undergoing organ transplantations.[3,4] This outbreak of what was once believed to be a rare skin cancer initially was considered an isolated anomaly, but as other cities

in the United States began noting the increasing numbers of young men with KS, it became obvious that a new phenomenon was occurring. Some controversy continues to exist over whether KS is a malignancy at all or simply a highly dysplastic phenomenon; however, it is generally accepted and treated as a malignancy.[5,6] In addition to KS, other opportunistic infections, primarily *Pneumocystis carinii* pneumonia, were diagnosed in this same population.[3,4]

In an effort to determine the cause of this KS outbreak, researchers began examining the immune systems of these young homosexual men. All were found to have some degree of immunosuppression.[4] In 1982 these findings led to the clinical definition of a new disease, acquired immunodeficiency syndrome (AIDS), in which the underlying immunodeficiency resulted in the appearance of indicator diseases.[7] One of the indicator diseases was the diagnosis of KS in a person younger than 60 years of age. In 1987 the diagnosis of AIDS was expanded to include the advent of KS in a person of any age who is seropositive for HIV antibody.[8]

### Epidemiology

Before the occurrence of HIV infection, KS was divided into the following categories: classic KS (nonAfrican), African KS (endemic), and KS that occurred in transplant recipients. Cases of classic KS are found in the United States and Europe. Predominantly a disease that occurs in men, it has a male/female ratio of 10–15:1 and primarily affects men of Mediterranean or Jewish ancestry in the fifth to eighth decades of life.[2] This malignancy is characterized as an indolent, slow-growing cutaneous nodule or plaquelike lesion. In 88% of those diagnosed, lesions will be confined to the lower extremities, distal to the knee, without invasive or disseminated disease. Treatment generally is not indicated because of its indolent nature. It is predictably a chronic, fairly benign malignancy that is rarely fatal.[2]

In contrast, African KS (endemic) is a malignant disease that affects persons of all ages, including children, and is found almost exclusively in black Africans. Cases of KS appear to cluster near the equator in the eastern half of the continent. African KS affects men twice as often as women, with a male/female ratio of 2.5:1.[9] Clinical presentations range from one similar to that observed in classic KS (nodular and indolent skin lesion) to a florid, infiltrative, and highly aggressive lymphadenopathic form that progresses rapidly and is frequently fatal.[9]

Transplant recipients experience an increased incidence of KS as high as 150 to 200 times the number of cases found in the general population.[10] Transplant KS also affects men at a higher incidence than women (2–3:1), and presentations can range from localized skin lesions to disseminated visceral and mucocutaneous disease. A correlation seems to exist between the degree of immunosuppression and the incidence of KS. The more depressed the immune system, the greater the incidence of KS. Spontaneous remissions have been documented in transplantation patients whose immunosuppression has been reversed.[10]

A fourth category, AIDS-associated KS, was first described in 1981 and is distinctly different from the other categories of KS (Table 31-1).[11] It is 20,000 times more likely to occur in an HIV-infected individual than in the general population and 300 times more likely than in other immunosuppressed groups.[12] Additionally, within the HIV-infected population it seems that those patients who acquire HIV through sexual transmission are more likely to develop KS than those whose source is injection drug use. Twenty-one percent of homosexual/bisexual men have an index diagnosis of KS, compared to only 1% of hemophiliacs affected with HIV. Interestingly, women are four times more likely to develop KS if their partners are bisexual. This suggests that, in addition to HIV infection, another sexually transmitted organism may play an important role in the development of KS.[12]

Clinical presentation ranges from localized skin lesions to disseminated disease that involves multiple body organs. KS that occurs with AIDS tends to be a highly aggressive disease. Interestingly, it appears that patients diagnosed with KS later than July 1984 may have a more severe form of the disease. Patients with KS diagnosed before then had a mean survival duration of 122.9 weeks, while those diagnosed after July 1984 have a mean survival duration of 71.9 weeks.[13] The reasons for this difference are unclear. Northfelt et al[13] did not elaborate on demographic data of the population or on any concomitant infection. The authors hypothesized that patients diagnosed earlier in the epidemic had a more intact immune system than those diagnosed later. Despite the aggressiveness of AIDS-related KS, patients rarely die as a direct result of KS. Overall, the mortality rate in this group is

approximately 41%, with more than 60% of all patients alive at one year and more than 50% alive at 22 months. This rate contrasts with the average survival rate of 18 months for all persons diagnosed with AIDS.[1] Patients with only KS and no opportunistic infections tend to live longer, and there are a number of anecdotal reports of persons with AIDS-related KS who have survived from three to seven years.[10] The cause of death in patients with AIDS-related KS is usually from concomitant opportunistic infections or the pathological effects of HIV itself.

## Etiology

Earlier in the epidemic, there appeared to be a strong link between immunosuppression and KS, even though the degree of immunosuppression provided no predictive ability. In 1990, Friedman-Kien et al reported on the appearance of KS in six HIV-negative gay men.[14] This report supported the hypothesis that a sexually transmitted agent may in fact be responsible for the development of KS and may be more readily expressed in the presence of HIV. There may also exist a large population infected with this KS-causing agent that remains symptom-free unless they become immunosuppressed.[14] Chang et al, in 1994, described an eloquent piece of research they conducted in which representation difference analysis was used to isolate a new viral genome.[15] The result of this research was the identification of a new human herpes virus that has some homology to Epstein-Barr virus and greatly resembles Saimiri herpes virus. This new virus is being called both Kaposi's sarcoma herpesvirus (KSHV) or human herpes virus type 8 (HHV8). Since the original paper, further research has demonstrated the presence of this virus in >90% of AIDS-related KS tissue samples.

**TABLE 31-1**   Clinical Features of Kaposi's Sarcoma

| Groups | Clinical Features | Response to Therapy |
|---|---|---|
| Classic: elderly men, especially of Jewish, Mediterranean ancestry | Indolent; cutaneous lesions of legs, feet; immunologic attrition of aging | Local radiation: good control; rarely fatal. |
| Endemic: black Africans | Variable; children: aggressive, lymphadenopathic; adults: usually indolent, affects extremities; no underlying immunodeficiency | Systemic chemotherapy; poor response in lymphadenopathic form; excellent response in indolent, adult form. |
| Renal transplant recipients | Aggressive, localized to visceral involvement; chemotherapy-induced immunosuppression | Controlled by stopping immunosuppressive medications |
| AIDS-related | Aggressive, disseminated disease with cutaneous, visceral, and lymphadenopathic involvement; virally induced immunodeficiency | Systemic chemotherapy: response rates of 25%–50%<br>Radiation therapy: good response but recurrence common: palliative not curative<br>Treatment selection is complex; need to control tumor without exacerbating immunodeficiency. |

Adapted from Volberding PA: Kaposi's sarcoma in AIDS, in Levy JA (ed): *AIDS, Pathogenesis and Treatment.* New York, Dekker, 1989, p 349.

To add credence to the role of this virus in the development of KS, tissue surrounding KS lesions has been examined for evidence of this virus, and none has been found. Of interest is the fact that this virus has also been found in tissue samples of classic KS lesions, non-HIV KS lesions, as well as in some AIDS lymphomas, specifically the body cavity lymphoma. Among the questions yet to be answered is what role this virus plays in the development of KS. Is it merely a passenger virus, does it directly transform cells, or trigger transformation through another mechanism?[16–18]

When KS was first reported, it was the initial indicator disease in 30%–35% of all diagnosed cases of AIDS. A steady decline has been noted, however, in the proportion of AIDS-KS cases among total AIDS cases.[19] It appears that in the gay population a decline of 20% per year has been noted; in other populations with AIDS-KS, a 10% decline per year has been reported. It has been suggested that this decline reflects behavior change, as correlated with a decreased risk of developing sexually transmitted diseases.[13] In light of the identification of a new virus, this indeed may be the explanation; however, it is important to keep in mind that a causal relationship has yet to be established between KSHV and the development of KS. Other possible explanations for this reduction in incidence of initial diagnosis include medical advancements that enable opportunistic infections to be diagnosed earlier than KS and the elimination of a cofactor that promotes the development of KS. Some researchers link the decreased incidence of KS to the decreased use of "poppers," or amyl nitrate, believed to be a cofactor in the development of AIDS-related KS.[20] This connection was suggested in several studies; however, large enough cohorts have not been collected and studied to document a causal relationship. Another group of researchers believes that hereditary or genetic predisposition plays an important role in the development of KS in both immunocompetent and immunodeficient populations. These researchers postulate that men infected with HIV who carry the human leukocyte antigen (HLA)-DR5 allele may be at an increased risk for KS development. Again, a causal relationship has not been established, and the postulate remains controversial.[21]

KS seems to be a disease found predominantly in homosexual and bisexual men with AIDS. Other groups diagnosed with AIDS (women, children, or men who are heterosexual or intravenous drug users, or both) do not have as high an incidence of KS as homosexual men with AIDS.[22,23] One study found the DNA of cytomegalovirus (CMV) in the nucleus of cells of KS lesions, which suggests a viral cause of KS.[24] Serological testing demonstrates that as many as 94% of all homosexual men may have been infected by CMV, as evidenced by antibodies to CMV.[25] CMV also has been isolated from the blood, semen, gastrointestinal tract, central nervous system (CNS), and lungs of patients with AIDS, which suggests the possible role of latent CMV infection in AIDS-related KS. In fact, a decline in CMV seroconversion also has been noted in recent years. Together with high CMV antibody seroprevalence, this viral link was once thought to be an explanation for the predominance of KS in homosexual men.

It is also important to remember that statistics for KS are kept only on initial diagnosis of AIDS. There are few reports that examine the development of KS at any point during the AIDS illness. Northfelt et al,[13] however, reported the San Francisco experience and indeed did note a decline in the report of KS at any time during the illness. This may reflect, however, the expanded definition of AIDS and the increased number of AIDS cases being reported under that expanded definition.

## Detection

Detection of KS is typically by self-observation of cutaneous or mucocutaneous lesions. This makes patient education in lesion identification an important method of detection. Additionally, all health care providers should routinely perform a careful visual examination of cutaneous surfaces of all persons who are seropositive for HIV or who are in a high-risk group for AIDS. Visual inspection includes the skin of the head (including the sclera), neck, torso, extremities, perirectal area, palms of the hands, soles of the feet, and the oral cavity. Biopsy specimens of suspicious lesions are examined. KS also may be a differential diagnosis in patients with enlarged lymph nodes, or with pulmonary symptoms, and/or a chest film with abnormal findings.

## Pathophysiology

After histological examination the pathologist has the responsibility of diagnosis. All types of KS (endemic, classic, transplantation-induced, and epidemic) are microscopically similar. Descriptions of lesions include interlacing bands of spindle cells with vascular structures in a network of reticular and collagen fibers. As the integrity of this network is lost, clefts usually occur among the vascular structures, which allows the extravasation of red blood cells. Lymphatic and blood vessels are present throughout the lesion and on its periphery. The nuclei of the spindle cells are frequently pleomorphic. Hemosiderin, extravasated red cells, and red cells that phagocytose the hemosiderin may be found between spindle cells. An inflammatory response involving histiocytes, lymphocytes, and plasma cells also may be seen.

Diagnosis can be difficult, especially in early or immature lesions. This stage has been referred to as the *macular stage*. Changes in this stage may be subtle, and the pathologist may observe only abnormally dilated vessels surrounding normal superficial vasculature. There may be little or no inflammatory response at this stage. Nuclear pleomorphism may be seen in mitosis, with nuclear atypia. As the lesion matures and becomes a plaque, it demonstrates more extensive neoplastic involvement, with proliferation through many layers, including the dermis and occasionally the adipose layers. A marked inflammatory response occurs at this stage, with a corresponding increase in numbers of spindle cells and extravasation of red cells. The prominence of hemosiderin deposits also is noted at this time. As the lesion advances toward nodular formation, these effects become more exaggerated. Spindle cells are dense, with considerable reticulum deposition.[21,26–28]

## Clinical Manifestations

The clinical presentation of AIDS-related KS resembles that of KS in transplant recipients. Multicentric skin lesions may be observed on any part of the body—the disseminated mucocutaneous and visceral disease frequently affects the lymphatic, pulmonary, gastrointestinal, cardiac, renal, biliary, and adrenal systems. There is no characteristic site of initial involvement as there is in the classic form of the disease. Lesions can be found on almost any skin surface, including the palms of the hands, soles of the feet, genitals, and head and neck. These lesions generally do not metastasize; instead, they are multicentric (i.e., each lesion is a primary lesion unto itself). The lesions range in pigmentation from brown, brown-red, purple, dark red, to violet; in rare cases they may appear to be deep blue-purple, resembling ecchymosis. They may be raised bullous nodules or flat plaquelike lesions. In either presentation they do not blanch when pressure is applied and are not painful unless they are responsible for structural damage or impinge on vital organs or nerves. Black patients commonly have nodular lesions, and white patients tend to have either nodular or plaquelike lesions. As with HIV infection, the average age range for AIDS-related KS is from 20–40 years. The patient may give a history of the KS lesions developing ("blossoming," "exploding") shortly after a bout with an opportunistic infection or treatment with steroids. The reason for this is unclear, but is an anecdotally observed phenomena. One possible explanation may be the associated deterioration of the immune system in the presence of an opportunistic infection and treatment with steriods. (Personal communication, Kaplan L, January 16, 1996)

This tumor can involve not only the skin but also the mucocutaneous surface of the buccal mucosa, the hard and soft palate, and the gums, as well as the sclera of the eyes. In fact, at the time of initial diagnosis of KS, approximately 72% of patients will already have involvement of one or more organ systems.[1] Internal organs most frequently affected include lymph nodes (81%), gastrointestinal tract (33%), and the lungs (11%).[29–32] KS in these organ systems can cause severe morbidity. Lesions also have been found in the liver, pancreas, adrenal glands, spleen, testes, and heart. Symptoms caused by these lesions usually are minimal.[1,24]

As HIV infection progresses, the immune system becomes increasingly suppressed; with it the occurrence and severity of KS also increase. Increasing numbers of skin lesions may be found all over the body surface. The multicentric skin lesions continue to enlarge, frequently coalescing with each other to form one large confluent lesion, often encompassing as large an area as the thigh, shin, or forearm. Malignant cells may involve the lymph nodes, thus compromising lymphatic drainage and blood circulation, resulting in severe edema distal to the affected area and stasis ulcers from edematous tissue. The lymph node involvement may be so severe as to cause major shifts in body fluids, limiting the flow of vital protein from lymph to plasma. The patient may succumb to anasarca, which is due to internal coalesced lesions and a decreased total serum protein/albumin resulting from the shift of fluid.

Additionally, when the gastrointestinal tract is involved, the patient may have a protein-losing enteropathy.[33] In this instance, protein is not absorbed from the gastrointestinal tract, which results in a decreased total serum protein/albumin level. Chronic anemia may also be observed in patients with KS in their gastrointestinal tract, as the lesions may ooze blood. In cases where progression of KS involves the lung, symptoms include dyspnea and shortness of breath, eventually culminating in fatal respiratory distress.[30,32]

## Staging

The ability to classify patients with similar stages of the disease would enable researchers to compare data and patient outcome, and to this end Laubenstein,[34] Krigel et al,[35] and later Mitsuyasu[19] proposed staging systems for AIDS-related KS (Table 31-2)[21,34] These researchers recognized that there are some patients with KS whose prognosis is better than others. The reasons are not clear, nor have all the variables been examined. Some studies have correlated the relationship between the absolute CD4 lymphocyte count and prognosis. For example, the lower the CD4 value in a patient with KS, the poorer the prognosis. A person with a helper/suppressor (H:S) ratio of greater than 0.5 (>1:2) and a CD4 lymphocyte count of greater than 300/mm³ has a relatively good prognosis. A helper/suppressor ratio of less than 0.2 (1:5) and a CD4 lymphocyte count of less than 100/mm³ indicates a very poor prognosis. The area in between these values is of unclear prognostic value.[35–39] Other data also indicate that patients with head and neck involvement,[39] patients with prior or concomitant opportunistic infections, and patients exhibiting "B" symptoms (weight loss, fevers, chills, night sweats, diarrhea) all have a shorter life expectancy than those without these factors. With the exception of the lung, organ involvement does not seem to influence prognosis, nor does tumor burden correlate with prognosis.[40]

In 1989 the Oncology Committee of the National Institute of Allergy and Infectious Diseases (NIAID) sponsored AIDS Clinical Trials Group (ACTG) developed a proposal for uniform evaluation, response, and staging criteria for KS. This system, similar to the tumor-node-metastasis (TNM) system, utilized the extent of tumor, the immune status, and other systemic illnesses (TIS)

**TABLE 31-2**   Staging of Epidemic Kaposi's Sarcoma

| Stage | NYU Staging System* | Mitsuyasu Staging System† |
|---|---|---|
| I | Cutaneous, locally indolent | Limited cutaneous (<10 lesions or one anatomical area) |
| II | Cutaneous, locally aggressive with or without regional lymph nodes | Disseminated cutaneous (>10 lesions or more than one anatomical area) |
| III | Generalized mucocutaneous and/or lymph node involvement‡ | Visceral only (GI, lymph node) |
| IV | Visceral | Cutaneous and viscera, or pulmonary KS |
| Subtype | | |
| A | No systemic signs or symptoms | No systemic signs or symptoms |
| B | Systemic signs; weight loss (10%) or fever (>100°F orally, unrelated to an identifiable source of infection lasting >2 wk) | Fevers >37.8°C unrelated to identifiable infection lasting >2 wk, or weight loss >10% of body weight |

* Kringel RL, et al: Kaposi's sarcoma: A new staging classification. *Cancer Treat Rep* 67:531, 1983

† Mitsuyasu RT, Groopman JE: Biology and therapy of Kaposi's sarcoma. *Semin Oncol* 11:53, 1984

‡ Generalized—more than upper or lower extremities alone; includes minimal GI disease defined as <5 lesions and <2 cm in combined diameters.

Groopman J, Broder S: Cancer in AIDS and other immunodeficiency states, in DeVita VT, Hellman S, Rosenberg SA (eds): *Cancer Principles and Practice of Oncology* (ed 3). Philadelphia, Lippincott, 1989, p 1962

**TABLE 31-3**   Recommended Staging Classification

| | Good Risk (0) (All of the Following) | Poor Risk (1) (Any of the Following) |
|---|---|---|
| Tumor (T) | Confined to skin and/or lymph nodes and/or minimal oral disease* | Tumor-associated edema or ulceration; extensive oral KS; gastrointestinal KS; KS in other nonnodal viscera. |
| Immune system (I) | CD4 cells ≥200/mm³ | CD4 cells ≤200/mm³ |
| Systemic illness (S) | No history of opportunistic infection or thrush; no "B" symptoms†; performance status ≥70 (Karnofsky) | History of opportunistic infection and/or thrush; "B" symptoms; performance status <70 (Karnofsky); other HIV-related illness (e.g., neurological disease; lymphoma) |

* Minimal oral disease is nonnodular KS confined to the palate.
† "B" symptoms: unexplained fever, night sweats, >10% involuntary weight loss, or diarrhea persisting more than 2 weeks.

Krown S, Metroka C, Wernz J: Kaposi's sarcoma in the acquired immune deficiency syndrome: A proposal for uniform evaluation, response, and staging criteria. *J Clin Oncol* 7:1206, 1989 (Reprinted with permission.)

that were AIDS-related to determine the stage of disease (Table 31-3).[41] Patients are assigned to either a good risk or poor risk category depending on the extent of the tumor, immune system status, and other systemic illnesses. In addition to the staging system developed by the NIAID-ACTG, this group also developed criteria for a standardized format of documenting the extent of KS on both initial and subsequent evaluation, as well as response definitions that include assessments of lesion nodularity and tumor-associated edema, supplementing the more traditional method for evaluating tumor response. This new system should allow for more accurate assessment of patients with KS and more meaningful outcomes from research studies.

## Assessment

A complete history and physical examination is indicated, including the patient's past history of drug use, sexual practice, and ethnic ancestry, along with close examina-

tion of the sclera, oral cavity, and integumentary system. Suspicious lesions must be biopsied before a diagnosis can be established. Visual inspection of lesions alone is insufficient to establish a diagnosis. Experienced physicians who care for patients with AIDS reflect anecdotally on lesions that appeared to be symptomatic of KS but were not histologically confirmed; conversely, examination of tissue from lesions that did not resemble those of KS proved to be diagnostic of KS. A lesion that visually suggested KS may be an immature lesion and thus does not show the distinctive pathological changes that are diagnostic of KS. Repeat biopsies of other suspicious lesions at a later date (e.g., in 2 weeks) may in fact yield a diagnosis of KS. It is worth noting that not every lesion that resembles KS is in fact KS. Lesions most often confused with KS are those associated with bacillary angiomatosis. Also, KS may not be the only pathology derived from the biopsy.[42] In one biopsy specimen, not only was KS identified, but so were bacillary angiomatosis, lymphoma, fungus, and herpes simplex virus. (Personal communication, Abrams D, June 12, 1993)

Examination of preparations from a 3-, 4-, or 6-mm punch biopsy of skin lesions is the most common method of diagnosis. Patients with KS involvement of the oral cavity should be referred to an oral surgeon for a diagnostic biopsy. Suspicious lymph nodes are best evaluated by means of an open (excisional) biopsy. Suspected KS involvement of other organs requires more invasive diagnostic procedures. For example, documentation of lung involvement requires a bronchoscopic examination. Similarly, documentation of gastrointestinal lesions requires endoscopic examination of the upper or lower tract. Lesions visualized by means of bronchoscopy or endoscopy may be examined by biopsy, but because of the submucosal and highly vascular nature of the tumor, removal of tissue from these sites may cause bleeding and increased morbidity. For this reason, visual inspection and identification may be adequate for diagnosing lung or gastrointestinal involvement.

Documenting organ involvement by other means can be difficult. KS that involves the lung cannot be diagnosed or distinguished from other causes of respiratory distress by means of chest films. An upper gastrointestinal series may demonstrate lesions in the gut, but the cause remains unknown without visual inspection by endoscopy or tissue biopsy. Because it appears that the presence or absence of organ involvement, with the exception of the lung, does not affect survival, documentation of extent of disease is not useful in treatment decisions. If treatment of a specific site is to be initiated (e.g., radiation therapy to treat enlarged lymph nodes), then tissue diagnosis must be determined.[38,39] There are several reports in the literature of patients having both KS and another malignancy in the same lymph node.

Patients with AIDS-related KS also may show laboratory abnormalities that probably are more related to HIV infection than to KS. These include elevated erythrocyte sedimentation rate (ESR), mild anemia, and leukopenia. Depressed test results with cosyntropin stimulation, elevated serum transaminase levels, and depressed platelet count may result from KS involvement of the adrenal glands, liver, or spleen respectively.

## Treatment

### Medical

Before the epidemic of AIDS and HIV infection, the KS seen in the United States was primarily classic KS (i.e., indolent, slow growing, and chronic), which required little or no treatment. In the transplant recipient the reversal of immunosuppression by withdrawing immunosuppressive drugs resolved the problem in 25%–50% of cases. In AIDS-related KS, treatment of the malignancy provides only temporary remission or stabilization of disease and does not improve survival rate. The main goal of treatment is to lessen morbidity.

As with other malignancies, three treatment options exist: surgery, radiation therapy, and chemotherapy, either local or systemic. Other than enabling the provider to establish a diagnosis, surgery has almost no role in the treatment of KS. Radiation therapy is highly effective and plays a role in local control of lesions and in cosmetic effect. This treatment, however, is not free of side effects and affects patients with KS in the same manner as it does others who receive radiation therapy. Irradiation of

tonsillar or oral lesions, for example, may cause severe stomatitis because of a preexisting *Candida* infection or poor dentition. Chemotherapeutic agents are useful in the treatment of AIDS-related KS when a systemic effect is necessary and the benefits of treatment outweigh the risks to the patient. Guidelines for treatment of AIDS-related KS are outlined in Table 31-4.[11,19,43]

Patients with aggressive or extensive disease who have an absolute neutrophil count greater than $1000/mm^3$ may receive weekly single-agent chemotherapy. Those single agents include doxorubicin, 10–15 $mg/m^2$; vinblastine, 0.1 $mg/kg$; vincristine, 2 mg; or etoposide 150 $mg/m^2$. A patient with rapidly progressing disease, with disease unresponsive to single-agent therapy, or with lung involvement may be offered combination chemotherapy consisting of doxorubicin, bleomycin, and vincristine, administered every other week on the basis of the patient's complete blood cell count (CBC) or single-agent etoposide either orally or intravenously.[44,45] Liposomal doxorubicin has been approved for treatment of those patients with refractory KS or who are intolerant of chemotherapy side effects. Use of liposomal doxorubicin has resulted in a 66% partial response rate. The usual dosage is 10–20 $mg/m^3$ every 2–3 weeks.[46–48] Overall, lung involvement is a poor prognostic sign. Patients who are unable to tolerate aggressive chemotherapy because of a low CBC receive a weekly course of either bleomycin or vincristine, alternating with vinblastine every other week.[11,20,43]

Interferon also has shown efficacy in the treatment of AIDS-related KS. Trials of recombinant alfa-interferon began in 1981, and since that time a select group of patients has been identified as favorable responders to alfa-interferon.[49] Their characteristics include CD4 counts greater than $200/mm^3$, no prior AIDS-defining diagnosis, and no "B" symptoms. Objective responses in this group of patients ranged from 42%–79%.[50,51] Recommended dosages range from 18–30 million units subcutaneously injected every day, 5 days a week. Due to both subjective (fevers, chills, myalgias) and objective side effects (neutropenia, thrombocytopenia, transient elevated transaminases), the usual dose tolerated is approximately one-quarter to one-half the recommended dose. To minimize systemic side effects, investigators also have explored the use of intralesional recombinant tumor necrosis factor and intralesional vinblastine for local control. Results from using intralesional recombinant tumor necrosis factor (rTNF) were disappointing. While 15 of the 16 patients treated with intralesional rTNF evidenced objective responses, the intense local inflammatory response was thought to be the cause of tumoricidal activity rather than the rTNF.[52]

Intralesional vinblastine can also be used to treat small localized lesions. The dosage is 0.4mg/cc administered directly into the lesion. The patient experiences mild pain on administration, and 3–5 days later the lesion begins to ulcerate. Overall effectiveness is good, lesions frequently need to be treated more than once, and a hyperpigmented area often remains after treatment.[53]

**TABLE 31-4** Guidelines for Therapy in AIDS-Related Kaposi's Sarcoma

| Group | Recommendations | Regimen |
|---|---|---|
| Minimal KS; <25 cutaneous lesions, stable disease, no history of opportunistic infections and/or "B" symptoms | No treatment with expectant observation for disease progression *or* | No treatment |
| | Experimental immunomodulators and/or antiviral drugs *or* | Alfa-interferon, 20–50 million units qd; SQ, IM or IV *or* Azidothymidine, 200 mg q 4hr, PO Vinblastine, 4–8 mg/wk, IV or |
| | Vinblastine or other single-agent therapy | Vincristine, 2 mg/wk or qowk, IV Doxorubicin, 15–20 mg/m²/wk, IV Vinblastine/vincristine, doses as above; each drug used individually on an alternating weekly basis |
| Minimal KS; <25 cutaneous lesions, stable disease, prior history of opportunistic infections and/or "B" symptoms | Vinblastine or other single-agent therapy *and* | Vinblastine; doses as above, or vincristine; doses as above, or doxorubicin; doses as above, or vinblastine; vincristine; doses as above |
| | Experimental immunomodulators and/or antiviral drugs if used in conjunction with cytotoxic agents | Alfa-interferon or azidothymidine; doses as above |
| Advanced KS; extensive disease, prior to history of opportunistic infection and/or "B" symptoms | Etoposide or doxorubicin as single-agent therapy *or* | Etoposide, 150 mg/m² qd × 3 days, then 28 days, IV doxorubicin; doses as above |
| | Multiple-agent chemotherapy with doxorubicin, bleomycin, and vinblastine | Doxorubicin, 40 mg/m² q wk–28 days, IV; bleomycin, 15 units/m² q 15 days, IV; vinblastine, 6 mg/m² q 21 days, IV |
| KS with severe neutropenia or thrombocytopenia | Vincristine with or without bleomycin | Vincristine; doses as above with or without bleomycin; doses as above |
| Pulmonary KS | Etoposide or doxorubicin with or without radiation therapy | Etoposide; doses as above |
| Localized, bulky KS lesion of oral cavity, face, legs, or lymph nodes | Radiation therapy | Local therapy, 800–3000 cGy; fractionation or slow dose administration to oral cavity or oropharynx |

Volberding PA: Kaposi's sarcoma in AIDS, in Levy JA (ed): *AIDS, Pathogenesis, and Treatment,* New York, Dekker, 1989, pp 352–354; Mitsuyasu RT: Kaposi's sarcoma in the acquired immunodeficiency syndrome, in Sande MA, Volberding PA (eds): *The Medical Management of AIDS.* Philadelphia, Saunders, 1988, pp 296–302

The response of KS lesions to chemotherapy can be dramatic. The lesions frequently will decrease in size, flatten, and lose their pigmentation; however, they do not completely go away. The area remains pigmented, even after treatment with chemotherapy, or radiation therapy, or both.

## Nursing

Nursing care includes assessment of the patient in terms of the health–illness continuum. Consideration is given to the psychosocial aspects of the disease, as well as to the physical status of the patient. A determination of the patient's risk group and whether KS is the patient's first diagnosis or one in a long line of indicator diseases will help the nurse establish a plan of care.

Although great strides have been made to reduce phobia concerning AIDS and homosexual men, it is important to remember that the patient may be explaining his sexual preference to his family for the first time and informing them that he has a fatal disease. Emotional support is crucial. If the patient is an intravenous drug user, philosophical dilemmas may arise concerning the patient entering drug rehabilitation programs. Realistic goals are necessary in this patient population because of both drug-seeking and manipulative behavior.

The complications associated with the use of chemotherapeutic agents in patients with KS are similar to the complications experienced by other patient populations receiving the same agents. Nausea, vomiting, anorexia, stomatitis, and alopecia all occur with the same frequency as in other populations. What appears to differ in the AIDS population is the severity of the complications. For this reason, nurses should be aggressive in the assessment of potential complications, alert the physician promptly, and implement appropriate nursing interventions. It also should be remembered that these patients have an underlying illness that predisposes them to other opportunistic infections and malignancies.

Patients with KS, on receiving the first dose of vinca alkaloids, may experience severe jaw pain. Although this reaction is a reported side effect of treatment with the vinca alkaloids, patients with AIDS and KS seem to have an increased incidence. Treatment with vinca alkaloids should be discontinued in patients with this reaction because they may cause irreversible nerve damage. (Personal communication, Lua J, August 3, 1989)

## NON-HODGKIN'S LYMPHOMA

### Epidemiology

Beginning in 1982, physicians in San Francisco, Los Angeles, and New York noted an increased incidence of NHL in homosexual patients. Because they believed that this incidence of NHL was somehow linked to the same immunodeficiency seen in AIDS, they began to prospectively collect blood for evaluation of the immune system. In fact, the immune deficiencies found in these patients with NHL were similar to those found in other patients with AIDS. Because cancer in and of itself is immunosuppressive, this finding alone did not establish a diagnosis of AIDS. It did, however, initiate further investigation. When the HIV antibody test became available, these patients with NHL were found to be seropositive. Thus, the link to HIV disease was demonstrated, and a new category of malignancy was added to the case definition of AIDS. NHL in a person who also is seropositive for HIV antibody or has positive culture results is considered to affirm a diagnosis of AIDS.[54–56]

It is difficult to determine the impact of HIV-related NHL on cancer statistics. Approximately 52,700 cases of NHL were diagnosed in 1996,[57] however, the percentage of those cases that are HIV-related cannot be determined because statistics concerning tumors do not account for HIV status. Because the reporting of AIDS cases to the Centers for Disease Control (CDC) now is required by law, the incidence of HIV-related NHL eventually may become known. It has been estimated that NHL has been diagnosed in 4%–10% of patients with AIDS. It is important to remember, however, that the CDC requires reporting of index diagnosis only and that HIV testing of all NHL has not become part of the standard workup. In one review by the French Registry of HIV-associated tumors, 33% of NHL occurred in patients already diagnosed with AIDS (56/168).[58] If U.S. statistics parallel the French data, one can assume that there has been a fair amount of underreporting. Of interest in the French review is the histology of the tumors. They reported three distinct categories of AIDS-related NHL: large cell lymphoma (LCL), immunoblastic lymphoma (IL), and Burkitt's lymphoma (BL). They also associated the first two lymphoma histologies with severe immune suppression, defined as a median CD4+ of 99 cells/μmL and compared with BL, with a median CD4+ of 270 cells/μml. This finding has significance in the pathogenesis of NHL. It is known that LCL and IL are associated with immune suppression, while BL is not, suggesting perhaps another reason for the development of BL in HIV-positive persons.[58]

A brief mention should be made of the controversy that exists around antiretroviral agents, specifically azidothymidine (AZT) and the development of NHL. The question continues to be asked whether the use of AZT increases the likelihood of developing NHL. While AZT has been shown to cause malignancies in laboratory animals, the dosages administered were 3 to 24 times higher than the recommended human dose. It is now generally recognized that the increased survival attributed to AZT increases the likelihood of developing NHL. Data exist showing that the incidence of developing NHL in long-term survivors of HIV is comparable whether the patient takes AZT or not.[59]

### Etiology

The connection between cancers and viruses has not been fully established; however, there are some malignancies in which a causative viral agent has been isolated. One such association exists between the malignancy known as African lymphoma, or Burkitt's lymphoma, which is a type of high-grade NHL, and Epstein-Barr virus (EBV). In 1962 Dr. Dennis Burkitt described a malignant lymphoma in African children that was typically extranodal in origin, with an affinity for facial bones. There appeared to be an increased incidence of this malignancy in regions of high temperature and rainfall. This suggested to Burkitt some type of insect vector as a method of infection (or transmission). Since then, serological studies and tissue cultures have established a constant association with the DNA-containing herpes virus known as EBV and the development of Burkitt's lymphoma.[46] Although the significance of the geographic distribution remains unclear, it has been hypothesized that malaria or some other insect-borne infection results in a reticuloendothelial hyperplasia that may be a necessary cofactor for the oncogenic virus in the development of the malignancy. EBV also has been implicated as the causative agent in nasopharyngeal carcinoma and in the development of NHL in transplant recipients; it also has been suggested as an important etiologic agent in AIDS-NHL.[46] Of interest is that similar research involving patients with AIDS could not causally link EBV to HIV-related NHL. Although the EBV genome has been isolated in 30%–50% of the DNA of HIV-positive patients with NHL, a direct relationship is not apparent.[60,61] The role of EBV in the development of NHL remains unclear; however, even though the viral link cannot be causally established, it is strongly suspected. Ziegler[62] hypothesized that once infection with HIV occurs, EBV may trigger lymphocyte proliferation that remains unchecked as a result of immune dysfunction caused by HIV. This proliferation, in turn, may allow the expression of two oncogenes, resulting in a polyclonal or monoclonal NHL.[63] Confusingly, Kaplan et al[64] report on EBV-positive serum in a small series of AIDS-NHL patients. In the 14 patients whose tissue was tested, four specimens were EBV-positive, and in a fifth patient EBV was recovered from one tumor site but not the second tumor site, leading Kaplan et al to hypothesize that EBV may be a "passenger" virus and not responsible for malignant transformation. There also seem to be distinct differences in EBV positivity between tumor histology and site of involvement. MacMahon et al[61] reported that large cell lymphomas were more frequently EBV-positive (65%), whereas the small, noncleaved cell (Burkitt's-like) lymphomas are less likely to be EBV-positive (20%) in the HIV-infected individuals. They also reported a consistent association of EBV to primary CNS lymphoma in the HIV-infected individual. Twenty-one specimens of brain tissue from HIV-positive CNS lymphoma patients were examined for EBV, and all 21 tested positive, suggesting a different pathogenesis from the systemic form of the disease.

New research by Chang et al identifying a new viral genome has led to the discovery of this new virus in certain lymphoma tissue specimens, specifically those of body cavity lymphomas.[15,17,18] The significance of this is unclear and further research is needed. It is now known that therapeutic immunosuppression increases the risk of lymphoma development. For example, the risk for transplant recipients has been estimated to be between 35 and 200 times greater than that for the general population.[65]

## Pathophysiology

AIDS-associated NHLs are predominantly B-cell malignancies, typically intermediate to high grade. However, there have been a few isolated reports of lymphomas that are T cell in origin in men who show HIV seropositivity. The significance of these few cases is unclear; the numbers are small and may simply represent the normal distribution of T-cell lymphoma in the general population. Only through an increase in the frequency of this type of lymphoma can significance be determined. In the meantime it remains an interesting phenomenon.[66,67]

Most cases of AIDS-NHL also have been associated with a previous history of persistent generalized lymphadenopathy. Benign follicular hyperplasia is a typical histological finding upon biopsy, which suggests that this lymphoma may arise from a polyclonal B-cell activation.

This polyclonal B-cell lymphoproliferation may be a complex result of EBV and HIV infection.[50,68–71] Current research is underway on the role of human T-lymphotropic virus type I as a coinfecting retrovirus in the development of lymphomas in AIDS.[72] Few patients have been identified as being coinfected, and it appears that their course of disease is determined more by their HIV infection. (Personal communication, McGrath M, August 3, 1989)

If the process of AIDS-associated NHL begins in a lymph node, the growing tumor causes structural damage, including effacement of the normal node architecture, replacement of normal cellularity by uniform and/ or grossly abnormal cells, and the random extension of cellular proliferations beyond the original structural confines of the node. Development of lymphoma, however, is not limited to lymph nodes or the spleen; all organs have lymphocytes within their boundaries that are capable of transforming and forming tumors.

## Clinical Manifestations

In the general population the earliest sign of NHL unrelated to AIDS is usually a painless, enlarged, discrete lymph node located in the neck. Although most patients have no symptoms, approximately 20% may experience "B" symptoms, including fever, night sweats, and weight loss.[60] Patients who do not have AIDS frequently have a history of intermittent lymphadenopathy that has been present for several months. Although axillary or inguinal lymph nodes may be the first to enlarge, this enlargement is not common. Frequently, there is involvement of Waldeyer's ring, epitrochlear nodes, the testes, and the gastrointestinal tract. The liver and bone marrow may be involved. There is a higher incidence of CNS involvement in patients with NHL unrelated to AIDS who have bone marrow involvement. The disease will be localized in fewer than 10% of patients who do not have AIDS.[73] Because of the diffuse presentation of lymphoma, non-AIDS NHL should be included in the differential diagnosis of patients with superior vena cava syndrome, acute spinal cord compression, solitary thyroid nodules, isolated tumor nodules of the skin, bone tumors, unexplained anemias, testicular masses, or solitary brain lesions.

In contrast to the presentation just described, patients with HIV-related NHL have very advanced disease, which frequently involves extranodal sites. In one of the first studies[73] of 90 cases of AIDS-NHL, 19% were classified as intermediate-grade diffuse large cell; 28% as high-grade, large-cell immunoblastic; and 36% as high-grade, small, noncleaved lymphomas. This presentation remains unchanged, with greater than 50% of patients presenting as high grade.[58,64] Extranodal sites most commonly involved include the CNS, bone marrow, bowel, and the anorectum; less commonly involved is the myocardium. In addition, these extranodal sites may be the only site of disease; that is, peripheral lymphadenopathy may be absent. If nodal sites are involved, there does not appear to be any predisposition to specific nodes.[70–73] In addition, these patients also may have underlying signs and symptoms of HIV infection, AIDS-related complex, or AIDS, including wasting, anorexia, nausea, vomiting, and fever, which confounds the workup and makes diagnosis difficult.

## Assessment

The diagnosis and classification of lymphoma can be made only by means of a biopsy specimen that is examined by a pathologist. Fine-needle aspirations may be helpful in differentiating a benign versus a malignant process, but, because of insufficient tissue yield, they are not useful in classifying the lymphoma. To fully assess HIV-related NHL, the patient's status must be staged and graded.

Staging—that is, determining the extent of disease involvement—is accomplished by means of the Ann Arbor staging classification system (see chapter 43). The staging workup includes a careful history, which notes the presence or absence of "B" symptoms, and a complete physical examination with special attention to Waldeyer's ring, the liver, and the spleen. Laboratory tests include CBC, differential cell and platelet count, sedimentation rate, serum chemistries, and liver function tests. The laboratory tests are not specific to lymphoma; they can indicate the overall wellness of the patient and are helpful in screening for hypercalcemia, hyperphosphatemia, and hyperuricemia. A chest film and computed tomography (CT) scans of the chest, abdomen, and pelvis also are indicated. These usually are not indicated for patients with NHL in the general population, but because of the extensive extranodal involvement characteristic of HIV-related NHL, they are extremely important. A bilateral bone marrow biopsy and aspiration, as well as a lumbar puncture, should be performed. Once all the tests are complete, the patient is assigned a staging number that can help predict responsiveness to treatment. It should be noted, however, that the Ann Arbor staging system was developed specifically for staging Hodgkin's disease and it's predictability of NHL is somewhat diminished.

Grading is a histological assessment of tumor type, recognizing that different cell types behave differently. Grading a tumor also gives the provider some sense of the tumor's aggressiveness.

If AIDS has not been previously diagnosed, an HIV antibody test is indicated. It is important to note that not all swollen lymph nodes are malignant; benign reactive lymphadenopathy is a common finding in this HIV-seropositive population and is postulated to be an adaptive physiological response to HIV insult. Abdominal masses or lymph nodes in a person who is HIV seropositive could be related to *Mycobacterium avium-intracellulare* infection; thus, it is essential to obtain a biopsy specimen and compare it with normal tissue before a diagnosis is made. It is unusual for patients with HIV-related NHL to present at a stage lower than stage III.[64,74,75]

## Treatment

### Medical

Once the disease is staged and graded, treatment for NHL may begin. Treatment options can be determined on the basis of method (surgery, radiation therapy, and chemotherapy), as well as by grade of tumor. Low-grade tumors are uncommon in the population infected with HIV; in the general population the tumors are indolent and slow growing, requiring no treatment until they impinge on a vital structure or cause symptoms. At that time, radiation therapy to the affected site usually is sufficient to treat the tumor, although chemotherapy may be used as well. Intermediate-grade tumors are more common in the population infected with HIV and may account for as much as 50% of HIV-related NHL. This grade of tumor in the general population can be treated with either chemotherapy or radiation therapy, depending on the stage at presentation.

The remaining HIV-related NHL occurs as high-grade, advanced stage disease. DiCarlo et al[74] found that 41% of patients with HIV-related NHL had high-grade disease. Ahmed et al[75] found that all patients with HIV-related NHL in their review had either intermediate or high-grade disease.

The treatment of choice for advanced intermediate/high-grade lymphoma is combination chemotherapy with CNS prophylaxis. The most active and effective single agent used in the treatment of NHL is cyclophosphamide. Other drugs that are effective include methotrexate, doxorubicin, vincristine, vinblastine, prednisone, and cytosine arabinoside. Generally, these agents are used in some combination. The most common regimens include M-BACOD (methotrexate, doxorubicin, cyclophosphamide, vincristine, dexamethasone), MACOP-B (methotrexate, doxorubicin, cyclophosphamide, vincristine, prednisone, bleomycin), and CHOP (cyclophosphamide, doxorubicin, vincristine, prednisone) (see chapter 43 for a description of these regimens). The patient also receives intrathecal methotrexate or cytosine arabinoside in an effort to prevent a CNS recurrence. Initial responses to chemotherapy usually are dramatic, with shrinkage of the tumor noted within 24 hours. But the response is not usually long-lived. Typically, patients remain disease-free while receiving chemotherapy; relapse occurs within 4–6 weeks after the discontinuation of chemotherapy. Once chemotherapy is reinstituted, response rates are somewhat diminished. The neutropenia that results from treatment may be severe (attributed to poor bone marrow reserve as a result of either HIV or to an intercurrent opportunistic infection such as *M. avium intracellulare*) and sometimes precipitates an opportunistic infection. Research trials being conducted by the ACTG are examining the use of growth factors to support the bone marrow in AIDS-related NHL patients being treated with chemotherapy. Kaplan et al recently reported the results of ACTG-142.[76] The study randomized patients with HIV-related NHL to either low dose m-BACOD or standard dose m-BACOD with growth factor support. Little difference was demonstrated between the two arms of the study, and the authors concluded that low dose therapy produced equivalent survival with the benefit of reduced toxicity when compared with standard dose therapy.[76] It is important to remember that these patients have an underlying immune disorder and that, whatever the outcome, they still have HIV infection and AIDS.

Radiation therapy may be useful for patients with limited bulky disease, for those who are unable to tolerate chemotherapy either because of poor health or low blood counts, for local control, or in some instances, for CNS prophylaxis. Surgery plays no role in the treatment of NHL other than to obtain a biopsy specimen.

### Results and prognosis

As with other types of cancer, a group of patients can be identified who will respond better to treatment and demonstrate a better prognosis. Kaplan et al identified a "good" prognosis category that included indicators such as prior AIDS diagnosis, Karnofsky performance status, site of disease, and CD4 count (Table 31-5). In addition, they identified a treatment-related indicator, the dose of cyclophosphamide received by the patient; however, they caution that these indicators were not the result of a randomized trial, and that many confounding variables exist.

### Nursing

Nursing care of patients with AIDS-related NHL is no different from the care of those patients in the general

population with non-AIDS-related NHL, with the exception of the emotional (psychosocial) aspect.

It should be noted that patients with large, bulky, high-grade disease are at high risk for tumor lysis syndrome. The exact numbers of patients with tumor lysis syndrome are unknown; some clinicians estimate that it may occur in as many as 10% of patients, whether or not their NHL is related to HIV. Anecdotally, it appears that patients with HIV-related NHL have a high incidence of this phenomenon, as they tend to present with larger, bulkier tumors. Tumor lysis syndrome generally occurs when the patient is initially treated. It is the result of the lysing of rapidly growing tumor cells that spill their contents into the general circulation, causing a metabolic imbalance. This results in hypocalcemia, hyperkalemia, hyperphosphatemia, and hyperuricemia. If left uncorrected, this condition may result in renal failure and death. The treatment of choice is prevention. Therefore, any patient suspected of being at high risk for tumor lysis, as determined by an elevated uric acid and lactate dehydrogenase level, should receive vigorous hydration (300–500 ml/hr) and may receive sodium bicarbonate to alkalinize the urine and prevent hyperuricemia nephropathy. However, sodium bicarbonate interferes with phosphate excretion and should be stopped prior to the administration of chemotherapy. In addition, allopurinol, a drug that blocks the conversion of metabolic wastes to uric acid, should be administered either intravenously or orally. The patient's urine output needs to be monitored every hour, and the physician should be alerted to any sign of urinary insufficiency. Serum chemistry levels are monitored every six hours in patients who are at high risk for tumor lysis, and in some cases the patient may need to be transferred to the intensive care unit. Dialysis may be necessary if the patient's electrolyte levels continue to rise and renal function deteriorates. Generally, there is less morbidity if the patient receives dialysis before renal failure occurs.

Although tumor lysis occurs in most patients 48–72 hours after the initiation of chemotherapy, some patients with HIV-related NHL may have this phenomenon sooner, usually within 24 hours. (Personal communication, Kaplan L, June 29, 1992) However, all patients with HIV-related NHL should be observed for a full 72-hour period for any sign of tumor lysis syndrome. These signs and symptoms include decreased urine output and increased lethargy. If the patient is being monitored by telemetry, arrhythmias may be noted. It also should be noted that some patients with HIV-related NHL have some form of tumor lysis before they receive treatment. This may be due to the tumor cells replicating and dying at an extraordinary rate, spilling their cellular contents into the general circulation.[77] These patients also may have tumors that produce lactic acid, causing metabolic acidosis before treatment.[77]

The complications of this group are the same as those experienced by all patients with NHL: neutropenia-related sepsis, thrombocytopenia, and untreated tumor lysis syndrome.

**TABLE 31-5** Prognosis and Survival Trends in Treated Patients with AIDS-Associated NHL

| Good Prognosis | Median Survival (months) | Poor Prognosis | Median Survival (months) |
|---|---|---|---|
| No prior AIDS diagnosis | 8.3 ± 1.5 | Prior AIDS diagnosis | 2.2 ± 7.7 |
| KPS <70% | 6.8 ± 1.7 | KPS >70% | 3.8 ± 1.1 |
| No extranodal sites | 12.2 ± 3.0 | Extranodal nodal | 3.4 ± 1.0 4.2 ± 1.3 |
| CD4 + >100 | 24 ± 3 | CD4 + <100 | 4.1 ± 1.0 |
| Treatment | | | |
| Cyclophosphamide (CTX) <1 g | 12.2 ± 1.7 | CTX >1 g | 4.6 ± 1.3 |

Adapted from Kaplan L, Abrams D, Feigal E, et al: AIDS-associated non-Hodgkin's lymphoma in San Francisco. *JAMA* 261:719–724, 1989

# PRIMARY CENTRAL NERVOUS SYSTEM LYMPHOMA

## Epidemiology

Primary CNS lymphoma is a rare malignancy, accounting for 0.3%–2% of all newly diagnosed lymphomas.[78] Although it can affect immunocompetent hosts, most of those diagnosed with primary CNS lymphoma are immunocompromised. Therefore, those with primary immunodeficiency, acquired immunodeficiency, and iatrogenic immunologic abnormalities (organ transplant recipients) are at increased risk for the development of primary CNS lymphoma.[79–81] In the case of organ transplant recipients, primary lymphoma involving the brain accounts for 50% of lymphomas in this population; it is common enough to predict its occurrence 28 months after transplantation.[81] It is not surprising then that primary CNS lymphoma develops in those infected with HIV who have subsequent severe immune dysfunction, defined as CD4 counts less than 75/mm³. Before the AIDS epidemic, primary CNS lymphomas were noted in the 50–70-year-old age range.[82] In the general population the average time from onset of symptoms to disease is 1–2 months. Unfortunately, patients with AIDS are also at risk for the development of infectious CNS disease. Cryptococcosis and toxoplasmosis are AIDS-related opportunistic infections of the CNS. The differential evaluation of these diseases can prolong and complicate the diagnostic process; yet, in the setting of HIV infection, a complete evaluation of all possible pathological causes is required.

The early medical literature reflects the confusion encountered in attempting to identify the cell of origin for primary CNS lymphoma. Perithelial sarcoma, reticulum cell sarcoma, and microglioma were a few of the names used to classify primary lymphoma involving the brain. It is now accepted that the cell of origin is the same as that causing NHL elsewhere in the body. The transformed cell, which multiplies in an area that does not allow expansion, is the cause of most presenting symptoms. In approximately 30% of all cases, this neoplasm will be multicentric, arising in several different areas of the brain at the same time.[80] This presentation is similar to that described in either spontaneously occurring tumors or in tumors arising in immunodeficient states.

## Clinical Manifestations

Two retrospective reviews[82,83] of a total of 26 patients revealed that the most frequently observed symptoms of HIV-associated CNS lymphomas included confusion, lethargy, and memory loss (12/26), and alterations in personality and behavior (5/26). Of the 26 patients, hemiparesis or aphasia was seen in seven, three patients had seizures, two had cranial nerve palsy, one had head-ache as the only symptom, one had headache associated with a lack of coordination, and one had no symptoms. Further review by So et al[82] revealed that although only three patients had seizures initially, seizures later developed in four additional patients. More than half the patients also reported more specific symptoms that consisted of focal seizures and progression of focal neurological symptoms over days or weeks. In a review by Gill et al,[83] all six patients studied had disease within the cranium; four had disease in the frontoparietal region, and two had involvement of the pons cerebellum.

These clinical manifestations are typical of spontaneous primary CNS lymphoma. They also are typical symptoms caused by other mass lesions in the CNS. This similarity in symptomatology often makes it difficult to distinguish between CNS lymphoma and vascular and infectious disorders. The most common explanation for a mass lesion in the CNS is toxoplasmosis, which occurs in 10% of patients with AIDS.[84] Because of the morbidity associated with brain biopsy, primary CNS lymphoma is usually a diagnosis of exclusion. That is, the patient with CNS symptoms and a demonstrated brain mass will generally be treated empirically for toxoplasmosis for approximately 2 weeks. If the lesion fails to respond to treatment, the diagnosis of primary CNS lymphoma will then be considered. At this point a brain biopsy could yield a definitive diagnosis; however, due to the invasiveness of the procedure, the degree of immune suppression usually present, and the dismal response of primary CNS lymphoma to treatment, a presumptive diagnosis may be established.

In most patients the radiographic findings from the CT and magnetic resonance imaging (MRI) examinations will reveal single or multiple discrete lesions. Prior to the use of a contrast medium on CT scanning, low-density lesions will appear, and a shift of midline structures also may be apparent. After the administration of contrast material, the lesion characteristically will appear enhanced. Reports differ on the type of enhancement; both uniform and patchy nodular enhancement with varying degrees of surrounding edema have been reported.[82,83] Primary CNS lymphoma usually appears as single or multiple discrete lesions and exhibits a characteristic pre- and postcontrast appearance. Some primary CNS lymphoma patients, however, have demonstrated ring-enhancing lesions on CT scan that are frequently indistinguishable from lesions seen in patients with cerebral toxoplasmosis. It is important to remember that a diagnosis of lymphoma cannot be determined by scans alone. In addition, MRI does not contribute to the differential diagnosis, although MRI may be useful in revealing lesions undetectable by the CT scan and may provide alternate biopsy sites.[82,83] Examination of cerebral spinal fluid (CSF) may reveal some abnormalities; however, the results are nonspecific and useful only in that they indicate some abnormality in the CNS. Tests ordered on CSF include toxoplasmosis titers, the Venereal Disease Research Laboratory (VDRL) test, and cytological examination. Cytological findings will be positive in approximately 50% of patients who have CNS lymphoma.[85] This result, however, tends to depend on the volume of CSF obtained. Toxoplasmosis titers and VDRL results can help rule out toxoplasmosis and syphilis as causes for behavioral changes and altered mental status.

## Treatment

### Medical

It appears that whether or not patients with AIDS-associated CNS lymphoma are treated, the outcome remains the same. In a review by So et al[82] they noted that in one study six patients experienced a highly aggressive course and died within two weeks. In another, 7 of 20 patients underwent treatment with radiation therapy.[83] Doses ranged from 3000–6000 cGy. Of the four patients who had CT scans after radiation therapy, three showed dramatic improvement. However, only 2 of 7 patients were alive at two months. Most patients die of the concomitant opportunistic infections frequently experienced in AIDS. In a review by Gill et al,[83] four patients were treated with subtotal resection of the tumor, followed by whole brain radiation and systemic chemotherapy. One patient remained alive at 28 months after diagnosis. It should be noted that the diagnosis of this particular patient was based on a pathological finding of low-grade lymphoma. The other patients survived less than two months. An average survival time of 1.7–2.7 months has been reported.[83] In a third retrospective review, 55 patients with primary CNS lymphoma who were treated with whole-brain radiation were evaluated. Complete radiological responses were reported in 17%, with 52%, of patients achieving a partial response. Clinical improvement was evidenced in 76%. Although responses were good, they were short-lived. In one group of 29 patients, the median survival was 119 days. Cause of death in the majority of patients was an opportunistic infection. There were no deaths attributable to unchecked primary CNS lymphoma.[86] Short survival was also reported by Formenti et al.[91] In this review, 6 of 10 patients with primary CNS lymphoma had a prior history of opportunistic infection and, treated with whole-brain irradiation, demonstrated complete responses. Again, the responses were not durable. Median survival in this group was 5.5 months.[87]

### Nursing

Nursing responsibility in the care of these patients includes a thorough assessment, paying particular attention to any focal findings, motor incoordination, and cognitive deficits. Safety in the environment must be considered in both the acute care setting and the home. Provisions for activities of daily living also must be anticipated and a long-term plan developed. For example, if the patient cannot be maintained at home, plans should be made for transfer to a skilled nursing care facility. Providing emotional support to the patient and family is essential, whether this be through referrals to counselors or by the nurse. Ethical issues may be encountered when treatment is discussed. A determination should be made as to whether the patient is mentally competent to make decisions; if not, it should be determined who is the next of kin or whether someone has been given power of attorney. If the patient is deemed incompetent, has no next of kin, or has not transferred power of attorney, then a legal guardian will need to be appointed by a court of law to make decisions for the patient.

## Complications

The most frequent complication in the treatment of AIDS-associated CNS lymphoma is the patient's mental deterioration to the point of becoming moribund and comatose. The reason for this downhill course associated with treatment is unclear. Unfortunately, there appears to be no preventive intervention. It may be a function of general debilitation caused by HIV, by HIV involvement of the brain, by the treatment itself, by a combination of these, or by another factor that has yet to be explored. Current research is not encouraging. Combining chemotherapy and radiation therapy in an attempt to control or eliminate the primary CNS lymphoma is currently being explored, but the research is confounded by the low numbers of enrollable patients and their rapid deterioration. As a result, the hope is for an effective antiviral agent that will control the HIV infection and for regeneration of the immune system through the use of immunomodulators.

## INVASIVE SQUAMOUS CELL CANCER OF THE CERVIX

Kaposi's sarcoma, non-Hodgkin's lymphoma, and primary CNS lymphoma account for approximately 95% of all cancers diagnosed in patients with AIDS, but they are not the only malignancies seen in persons who are seropositive for HIV antibody.[88,89] Nor are they the only malignancies that develop in the presence of immune dysfunction. It is reported in the transplant population that there is a 100-fold increase in the development of vulvar and anal cancers and a 14-fold increase in cervical cancer.[90] It was reasonable, therefore, to expect that patients immune suppressed as a result of HIV would be at risk of developing anogenital malignancies, in particular, invasive squamous cell cancer of the cervix. And indeed, beginning in 1989 reports began appearing in the literature documenting an unusually high prevalence of cervical intraepithelial neoplasi (CIN) and human papilloma virus (HPV) in women infected with HIV. What alarmed researchers was not only the incidence of HPV infection in women who were HIV positive, but also the degree of cervical intraepithelial neoplasia found. Early reports showed an increased HPV positivity in HIV-infected women (49%) compared with 25% of the general population. In addition, women who are both HIV/HPV infected are 42 times more likely to have cytological changes.[91] In one study, the cervical cytology of 35 HIV infected women and 23 uninfected women was evaluated by one cytologist who was blinded to the patient's HIV status. Squamous atypia was found in 4% of the seronegative women, while 31% of HIV infected had evidence of atypia.[92] In fact, numerous anecdotal reports published over the past five to six years repeatedly confirmed this phenomenon. Perhaps the most important study in this area was conducted by Maiman et al.[91] They reported on a group of seropositive women in New York with invasive and preinvasive cervical neoplasia. When compared to a group of women with similar characteristics who were seronegative, the researchers found the HIV infected women were more likely to have advanced disease at presentation, recur, have evidence of HPV infection, and to have perianal involvement. As the evidence for association of invasive squamous cell cancer (SCC) cervix and HIV mounted, the CDC in 1993 added this diagnosis to the surveillance definition of AIDS.[91,93]

## Epidemiology

Prior to HIV, several characteristics had been identified as risk factors for the development of SCC cervix. These included low socioeconomic status, young age at first sexual experience, multiple sexual partners, multiple pregnancies, prostitutes, DES daughters, and smoking. These risk factors, while well studied and correlated in the general population, appear not to correlate in the HIV population.[92]

## Etiology

HPV 16 and 18 have both been implicated in the development of SCC cervix in women who are not HIV positive, as has HSV type 2. Mounting evidence suggests that HPV plays a role in the development of invasive SCC cervix in women who are HIV positive.[91]

## Pathophysiology

Generally speaking, SCC cervix is a preventable disease; it is always preceded by dysplasia and squamous intraepithelial lesions (SIL). It arises from the squamoclumnar junction in the cervix, the area referred to as the transition zone (T-zone). The lesion is considered invasive when the malignant epithelial cells break through the basement membrane, enter the stroma, and spread by direct extension. In the non-HIV population this invasion occurs in 10–20 years, with 66% of SIL progressing if untreated within 10 years.[94] This process occurs more rapidly in the HIV population. In addition, it appears that HIV itself al-

ters cervical immunity, both humoral and cellular components. Evidence of cervical immunity is demonstrated by the fact that specific IgA antibodies directed against HIV can be isolated from vaginal secretions. In addition, both subepithelial T cells and langerhans cells have been identified within the cervix.[95] Infection of these cells with HIV may lead to decreased immune surveillance and to more rapid replication of HPV or reactivation of latent infection. The exact sequence of events is yet to be defined; it is unclear whether infection with HPV makes the cervix more susceptible to HIV or if the reverse is true.[99]

## Clinical Manifestations

Because so few cases of invasive SCC cervix have been reported, any differences between the clinical manifestations in a noninfected woman and the woman who is seropositive have not been defined. Please see chapter 39 for an in-depth discussion.

## Treatment

Several important pieces of information were obtained from Maiman et al's research.[91] First was the observation that there was a relationship between immune status and CIN. Women whose CD4 counts were less than 500 were at high risk of developing recurrent disease, while those with a relatively intact immune system still had twice the risk of recurrence when compared with women who were HIV negative. The second piece of information that the data suggested was that the mode of HIV acquisition correlated strongly with recurrent disease. That is women who acquired HIV through a sexual route were more likely to develop recurrent disease compared with women who acquired HIV through injection drug use. The final result reported was that traditional therapy used in the HIV infected population produced significantly shorter mean time intervals until disease recurrence and death. Currently, there is no standard recommendation for treatment.

### Nursing

Perhaps the most important role nurses can play in caring for women infected with HIV is that of strong advocate. Women are infected at a faster rate than men, and it is estimated that by the year 2004 the number of women infected will equal the number of infected men.[96] While the epidemic in women is thought to lag five years behind that in men, research in women is believed to trail closer to ten years behind. Women have been understudied and underdiagnosed. It is known that women will defer receiving care for themselves to care for a sick child or spouse; that women are more likely to be unemployed and on federal assistance programs causing problems of access to care; and that up to 15% of women are unaware of their risk factors for HIV, making screening difficult.

Women are also less likely to receive antiretroviral therapy or prophylactic treatment when compared to men, and in 1990, the CDC reported that 65% of women infected with HIV died without an AIDS defining diagnosis.[97]

Nursing can have an impact by recognizing two things. First, that it is not how one labels oneself that puts them at risk of developing HIV, but rather one's behavior, whether that be through sexual behavior or the use of injection drugs. Second, women with HIV will require more time and energy to acheive the same goals as men.

## OTHER MALIGNANCIES AND HIV

Hodgkin's disease, squamous cell cancers of the rectum, nasopharyngeal cancers, malignant melanomas, and multiple myelomas have all been reported in patients infected with HIV. The difference between the indicator malignancies (KS, NHL, and primary CNS lymphoma) and other malignancies in individuals with HIV is the frequency with which they occur. There is a significantly greater incidence of the indicator malignancies in those who are seropositive for HIV. The same is not true for the other malignancies described in AIDS patients. Although these cancers may be seen in AIDS patients, no epidemiologic link or direct causal relationship has been established. HIV positivity does not prevent the development of any other cancer at the same rate seen in those who are seronegative. It is useful to know, however, the HIV status of a patient with a malignancy because response to therapy is typically poor in the person with HIV infection. It is reasonable to expect an increasing incidence of virally linked malignancies (e.g., hepatomas and cervical cancer) as the incidence of AIDS and HIV infection continues to rise.[89] HPV has also been isolated from rectal pap smears of men. This is of concern because men who are HIV/HPV positive are also more likely to have cytological changes. Thirty-nine percent of men examined had abnormal anal cytologies, and in 54% of these patients, the DNA of HPV was identified in the cytology.[98]

## CONCLUSION

The care of patients with a malignant disease who also are infected with HIV presents a demanding challenge for nurses. In addition to the already difficult task of managing the care of a patient receiving chemotherapy, infection with an immunosuppressive virus must be taken into account. The patient also may be receiving antiviral agents or immunomodulators, or both. Sorting out the side effects, as well as providing a comprehensive plan of care for these patients, presents a major nursing challenge.

## REFERENCES

1. Longo DL, Seis RG, Lane HC, et al: Malignancies in the AIDS patient: Natural history, treatment strategies, and preliminary results. *Ann NY Acad Sci* 437:421–430, 1984
2. Steis R, Broder S: A general overview, in DeVita VT, Hellman S, Rosenberg SA (eds): *AIDS Etiology, Diagnosis, Treatment and Prevention.* Philadelphia, Lippincott, 1985, pp 299–338
3. Centers for Disease Control: Kaposi's sarcoma and *Pneumocystis* pneumonia among homosexual men—New York City and California. *MMWR* 30:305–308, 1981
4. Centers for Disease Control: Follow-up on Kaposi's sarcoma and *Pneumocystis* pneumonia. *MMWR* 30:409–410, 1981
5. Brooks JJ: Kaposi's sarcoma: A reversible hyperplasia. *Lancet* 2:1309–1311, 1986
6. Costa J, Rabson AS: Generalized Kaposi's sarcoma is not a neoplasm. *Lancet* 1:58, 1983
7. Centers for Disease Control: Update on acquired immune deficiency syndrome (AIDS)—United States. *MMWR* 31:507–514, 1982
8. Centers for Disease Control: Revision of the CDC surveillance case definition for acquired immunodeficiency syndrome. *MMWR* 35:3S–15S, 1987
9. Rosenberg SA, Suit H, Baker L, et al: Sarcomas of the soft tissue and bone, in DeVita VT, Hellman S, Rosenberg SA (eds): *Cancer Principles and Practice of Oncology.* Philadelphia, Lippincott, 1982, pp 1036–1093
10. Krigel R, Friedman-Kien A: Kaposi's sarcoma in AIDS, in DeVita VT, Hellman S, Rosenberg SA (eds): *AIDS Etiology, Diagnosis, Treatment, and Prevention.* Philadelphia, Lippincott, 1985, pp 185–212
11. Volberding P: Kaposi's sarcoma in AIDS, in Levy J (ed): *AIDS, Pathogenesis and Treatment.* New York, Dekker, 1989, pp 349–358
12. Beral V, Peterman T, Berkleman R, et al: Kaposi's sarcoma among persons with AIDS: A sexually transmitted infection. *Lancet* 335:123–127, 1990
13. Northfelt D, Kahn J, Volberding P: Treatment of AIDS-related Kaposi's sarcoma. *Hematol Oncol Clin North Am* 5:297–310, 1991
14. Friedman-Kien A, Saltzman B, Cao Y, et al: Kaposi's sarcoma in HIV-negative homosexual men. *Lancet* 335:168–169, 1990
15. Chang Y, Cesarman E, Pessin M, et al: Identification of herpesvirus-like DNA sequences in AIDS-associated Kaposi's sarcoma. *Science* 266:1865–1869, 1994
16. Schalling M, Ekman M, Kaaya E, et al: A role for a new herpesvirus (KSHV) in different forms of Kaposi's sarcoma. *Nat Med* 1:705–706, 1995
17. Cesarman E, Chang Y, Moore P, et al: Kaposi's sarcoma associated herpesvirus-like DNA sequences in AIDS-related body-cavity-based lymphomas. *New Engl J Med* 332:1186–1191, 1995
18. Cesarman E, Moore P, Rao P, et al: In vitro establishment and characterization of two acquired immunodeficiency syndrome-related lymphoma cell lines (BVC-1 and BC-2) containing Kaposi's sarcoma associated herpesvirus-like (KSHV) DNA sequences. *Blood* 86:2708–2714, 1995
19. Mitsuyasu RT: Kaposi's sarcoma in the acquired immunodeficiency syndrome. *Infect Dis Clin North Am* 2:511–523, 1988
20. Haverdos HW, Pinsky PF, Drotman DP, et al: Disease manifestation and homosexual men with acquired immunodeficiency syndrome: A possible role of nitrites in Kaposi's sarcoma. *Sex Transm Dis* 23:203–208, 1985

21. Groopman J, Broder S: Cancer in AIDS and other immuno-deficiency states, in DeVita VT, Hellman S, Rosenberg SA (eds): *Cancer Principles and Practice of Oncology* (ed 3). Philadelphia, Lippincott, 1989, pp 1953–1970

22. Garrett T, Lange M, Ashford A, et al: Kaposi's sarcoma in heterosexual intravenous drug users. *Cancer* 55:1146–1158, 1985

23. Nissenblatt M: Cancers and AIDS, in Gong V (ed): *Understanding AIDS.* New Brunswick, NJ: Rutgers University Press, 1985, pp 65–74

24. Urmacher C, Myskowski P, Ochoa M, et al: Outbreak of KS with CMV infection in young homosexual men. *Am J Med* 74:569–575, 1982

25. Drew L, Mintz L, Miner R: Prevalence of cytomegalovirus in homosexual men. *J Infect Dis* 143:188–192, 1981

26. McNutt N: Kaposi's sarcoma, in Theirs B, Dobson R (eds): *Pathogenesis of Skin Disease.* New York, Churchill Livingstone, 1986, pp 459–474

27. Caro W, Bronstein B: Tumors of the skin, in Moschella S, Hurley H (eds): *Dermatology* (vol 2) (ed 2). Philadelphia, Saunders, 1985, pp 1639–1671

28. MacKie R: Tumors of the skin, in Rook A, Ebling F, Wilkinson E, et al (eds): *Textbook of Dermatology* (vol 3). London, Blackwell Scientific Publications, 1986, pp 2375–2478

29. Meduri G, Stover D, Lee M, et al: Pulmonary Kaposi's sarcoma in the acquired immune deficiency syndrome: Clinical, radiographic and pathologic manifestations. *Am J Med* 81:11–18, 1986

30. Kaplan L, Hopewell P, Jaffe H, et al: Kaposi's sarcoma involving the lung in patients with acquired immunodeficiency syndrome. *J AIDS* 1:25–31, 1988

31. Ognibene F, Steis R, Macher A, et al: Kaposi's sarcoma causing pulmonary infiltrates and respiratory failure in acquired immunodeficiency syndrome. *Ann Intern Med* 102:471–475, 1985

32. Brown R, Huberman R, Vanley G: Pulmonary features of KS. *Am J Radiol* 139:659–660, 1986

33. Laine L, Plitoske E, Pardash G: Protein-losing enteropathy in acquired immunodeficiency syndrome due to intestinal Kaposi's sarcoma. *Arch Intern Med* 147:1174–1175, 1988

34. Laubestein L: Staging and treatment of Kaposi's sarcoma in patients with AIDS, in Friedman-Kien A, Laubestein L (eds): *AIDS: The Epidemic of Kaposi's Sarcoma and Opportunistic Infections.* New York, Masson, 1984, pp 51–56

35. Krigel R, Laubestein L, Muggia F: Kaposi's sarcoma: A new staging classification. *Cancer Treat Rep* 67:531–534, 1983

36. Krigel R: Prognosic factors in Kaposi's sarcoma, in Friedman-Kien A, Laubenstein L (eds): *AIDS: The Epidemic of Kaposi's Sarcoma and Opportunistic Infections.* New York, Masson, 1984, pp 69–72

37. Taylor J, Afrasia R, Fahey J, et al: Prognostically significant classification of immune changes in AIDS with Kaposi's sarcoma. *Blood* 76:666–671, 1986

38. Afrasiabi A, Mitsuyasu R, Nishanian R, et al: Characteristics of a distinct subgroup of high-risk persons with KS and good prognosis who present with normal T4 cell number and T4: T8 ratio and negative HTLV/LAV serologic test results. *Am J Med* 81:969–973, 1986

39. Gnepp D, Chandler W, Hyams V: Primary Kaposi's sarcoma of the head and neck. *Ann Intern Med* 100:107–114, 1984

40. Safai B, Sarngadharan M, Koziner B, et al: Spectrum of KS in the epidemic of AIDS. *Cancer Res* 45:6465–6485, 1985 (suppl 9)

41. Krown A, Metroka C, Wernz J: Kaposi's sarcoma in the acquired immunodeficiency syndrome: A proposal for uni-form evaluation, response, and staging criteria. *J Clin Oncol* 7:1201–1207, 1989

42. Cole M, Cohen P, Satra E, et al: The concurrent presence of systemic disease pathogens and cutaneous Kaposi's sarcoma in the same lesion. Histoplasma capsulatum and Kaposi's sarcoma coexisting in a single skin lesion in a patient with AIDS. *J Am Acad Dermatol* 26:285–287 1992

43. Mitsuyasu R: Kaposi's sarcoma in the acquired immunodeficiency syndrome, in Sande M, Volberding P (eds): *The Medical Management of AIDS.* Philadelphia, Saunders, 1988, pp 296–302

44. Laubenstein L, Krigel R, Odajnk C, et al: Treatment of epidemic Kaposi's sarcoma with etoposide or a combination of doxorubicin, bleomycin, and vinblastine. *J Clin Oncol* 2:1115–1120, 1984

45. Safai B: Kaposi's sarcoma and other neoplasms in acquired immunodeficiency syndrome, in Gallin J, Fauci A (eds): *Advances in Host Defense Mechanism* (vol 5), *Acquired Immunodeficiency Syndrome (AIDS).* New York, Raven Press, 1985, pp 59–73

46. Harrison M, Tomlinson D, Stewart S: Liposomal-entrapped doxorubicin: An active agent in AIDS-related Kaposi's sarcoma. *J Clin Oncol* 13:914–920, 1995

47. Sturzl M, Zietz C, Eisenburg B, et al: Liposomal doxorubicin in the treatment of AIDS-associated Kaposi's sarcoma: Clinical, histological and cell biological evaluation. *Res Virol* 145:261–269, 1994

48. Uziely B, Jeffers S, Isacson R, et al: Liposomal doxorubicin: Antitumor activity and unique toxicities during two complimentary phase I studies. *J Clin Oncol* 13:1777–1785, 1995

49. Krown A: The role of interferon in the therapy of epidemic Kaposi's sarcoma. *Semin Oncol* 14:24–33, 1987 (suppl 3)

50. Volberding P, Gotlieb M, Rothman J, et al: Therapy of Kaposi's sarcoma in acquired immunodeficiency syndrome (AIDS) with alpha-2 recombinant IFN. *Proc Am Soc Clin Oncol* 2:53, 1983(abstr)

51. Volberding P: Therapy of Kaposi's sarcoma in AIDS. *Semin Oncol* 11:60–67, 1984

52. Kahn J, Kaplan L, Volberding P, et al: Intralesional recombinant tumor necrosis factor-γ for AIDS-associated Kaposi's sarcoma: A randomized double blind trial. *J AIDS* 2:217–221, 1989

53. Newman S: Treatment of epidemic Kaposi's sarcoma (KS) with intralesional vinblastine injection (IL-VLB). *Proc Am Soci Clin Oncol* 7:5, 1988 (Abstr 19)

54. Kaplan L, Wofsy C, Volberding PA: Treatment of patients with acquired immunodeficiency syndrome and associated manifestations. *JAMA* 257:1367–1372, 1987

55. Diffuse, undifferentiated non-Hodgkin's lymphoma among homosexual males—United States. *MMWR* 31:277–279, 1982

56. Aisenberg A: Malignant lymphoma. *N Engl J Med* 288:883–890, 1973

57. *Cancer Facts and Figures: 1996* Atlanta, American Cancer Society, 1996

58. Roithmann S, Tourani J, Andrieu J: AIDS-associated non-Hodgkin's lymphoma. *Lancet* 338:884–885, 1991

59. Chapman M, Minor J: Lymphoma in AIDS patients receiving long-term antiretroviral therapy. *Am J Hosp Pharm* 49:174–175, 1992

60. DeVita VT, Jaffe E, Mauch P, et al: Lymphocytic lymphomas, in DeVita VT, Hellman S, Rosenberg SA (eds): *Cancer Principles and Practice of Oncology* (ed 3). Philadelphia, Lippincott, 1989, pp 1953–1970

61. MacMahon E, Glass J, Hayward S, et al: Epstein-Barr virus

in AIDS-related primary central nervous system lymphoma. *Lancet* 338:969–973, 1991

62. Ziegler J: AIDS and cancer. *Ann Inst Pasteur Immunol* 138: 253–260, 1987

63. Kaplan L, Abrams D, Feigal E, et al: AIDS-associated non-Hodgkin's lymphoma in San Francisco. *JAMA* 261:719–724, 1989

64. Kaplan L: AIDS-associated lymphomas, in Sande M, Volberding P (eds): *The Medical Management of AIDS*. Philadelphia, Saunders, 1988, pp 307–315

65. Frizzera G, Hanto D, Gaji-Peczalska K, et al: Polymorphic diffuse B-cell hyperplasia and lymphomas in renal transplant recipients. *Cancer Res* 41:4262–4279, 1981

66. Nasr S, Brynes R, Garrison C, et al: Peripheral T-cell lymphoma in a patient with acquired immune deficiency disease. *Cancer* 61:947–951, 1988

67. Presant C, Gala K, Wiseman C, et al: Human immunodeficiency virus associated with T-cell lymphoblastic lymphoma in AIDS. *Cancer* 60:1459–1461, 1987

68. Yarchoan R, Redfield R, Broder S: Mechanisms of B-cell activation in patients with acquired immunodeficiency syndrome. *J Clin Invest* 78:439–447, 1986

69. Ziegler J: Lymphomas and other neoplasms associated with AIDS, in Levy J (ed): *AIDS, Pathogenesis and Treatment*. New York, Dekker, 1989, pp 359–370

70. Knowles D, Chamulak G, Subar M, et al: Lymphoid neoplasia associated with the acquired immunodeficiency syndrome (AIDS): The New York University Medical Center experience with 105 patients (1981–1986). *Ann Intern Med* 108:744–753, 1988

71. Italian Cooperative Group for AIDS-Related Tumors, 1988: Malignant lymphomas in patients with or at risk for AIDS in Italy. *J Natl Cancer Inst* 80:855–860, 1988

72. Pieri KL, Murphy E: The clinical significance of HTLV-I and HTLV-II infection with the AIDS epidemic, in Volberding P, Jacobson M (eds): *AIDS Clinical Review 1991*. New York, Dekker, 1991, pp 39–57

73. Ziegler J, Beckstead J, Volberding P, et al: Non-Hodgkin's lymphoma in 90 homosexual men—relation to generalized lymphadenopathy and the acquired immunodeficiency syndrome. *N Engl J Med* 311:565–570, 1984

74. DiCarlo E, Amberson J, Metroka C, et al: Malignant lymphomas and the acquired immunodeficiency syndrome. *Arch Pathol Lab Med* 110:1012–1016, 1986

75. Ahmed S, Wormser G, Stahl R, et al: Malignant lymphomas in a population at risk for acquired immune deficiency syndrome. *Cancer* 60:719–723, 1987

76. Kaplan L, Staus D, Testa M, et al: Randomized trial of standard dose mBACOD with GM-CSF vs. reduced dose mBACOD for systemic HIV-associated lymphoma: ACTG-142. *Proc Amer Soc Clin Oncol*, 288, 1995 (abstr 818)

77. Warrell R Jr, Bockman R: Oncologic emergencies, in DeVita VT, Hellman S, Rosenberg SA (eds): *Cancer Principles and Practice of Oncology* (ed 3). Philadelphia, Lippincott, 1989, pp 1996–1997.

78. Henry J, Heffner R, Dillard S, et al: Primary malignant lymphomas of the central nervous system. *Cancer* 34: 1293–1302, 1987

79. Frizzera G, Rosai J, Dehner L, et al: Lymphoreticular disorders in primary immunodeficiency: New findings based on

an up to date histologic classification of 35 cases. *Cancer* 46: 692–699, 1980

80. Good A, Russo R, Schnitzer B, et al: Intercranial histiocytic lymphoma in rheumatoid arthritis. *J Rheumatol* 5:75–78, 1978

81. Levin V, Sheline G, Gutin P: Neoplasms of the central nervous system, in DeVita VT, Hellman S, Rosenberg SA (eds): *Cancer Practice and Principles of Oncology* (ed 3). Philadelphia, Lippincott, 1989, pp 1557–1611

82. So Y, Beckstead J, Davis R: Primary central nervous system lymphoma in acquired immunodeficiency syndrome. A clinical and pathological study. *Ann Neurol* 20:566–572, 1986

83. Gill P, Levine A, Meyer P, et al: Primary central nervous system lymphoma in homosexual men. *Am J Med* 78: 742–748, 1985

84. Mills J: *Pneumocystis carinii* and *Toxoplasmosis gondii* infections in patients with AIDS. *Rev Infect Dis* 8:1001–1011, 1986

85. Casciato D, Lowitz B: Neuromuscular complication, in Casciato D, Lowitz B (eds): *Manual of Clinical Oncology*. Boston, Little, Brown, 1988, pp 468–483

86. Baumgartner J, Rachlin J, Beckstead J, et al: Primary central nervous system lymphomas: Natural history and response to radiation therapy in 55 patients with acquired immunodeficiency syndrome. *J Neurosurg* 73:206–211, 1990

87. Formenti S, Gill P, Lean E, et al: Primary central nervous system lymphoma in AIDS: Results of radiation therapy. *Cancer* 63:1101–1107, 1989

88. Levine A: Non-Hodgkin's lymphomas and other malignancies in the acquired immune deficiency syndrome. *Semin Oncol* 14:34–39, 1987 (suppl 3)

89. Friedman S: Gastrointestinal and hepatobiliary neoplasms in AIDS. *Gastroenterol Clin North Am* 17:465–486, 1988

90. Penn I: Secondary neoplasms as a consequence of transplantation and cancer therapy. *Cancer Detect Prevent* 12: 39–57, 1988

91. Maiman M, Fruchter R, Serur E, et al: Human immunodeficiency virus infection and cervical neoplasia. *Gynecol Oncol* 38:377–382, 1990

92. Schrager L, Friedland G, Maude D, et al: Cervical and vaginal squamous abnormalities in women infected with human immunodeficiency virus. *J Acquir Immune Defic Syndrome* 2: 570–575, 1989

93. CDC: 1993 Revised classification system for HIV infection and expanded surveillance case definition for AIDS among adolescents and adults. *MMWR* 41:1–19, 1992

94. Kohn E, Liotta L: Tumor invasion and metastases, in Hoskins W, Perez C, Young R (eds): *Principles and Practice of GYN-Oncology*. Philadelphia, Lippincott, 1992 pp 69–86

95. Spinillo A, Tenti P, Zappatore R, et al: Langerhans cell counts and cervical intrepithelial neoplasian in women with human immunodeficiency virus infection. *Gynecol Oncol* 48: 210–213, 1993

96. CDC: AIDS in women: United States. *MMWR* 39:845–846, 1990

97. Chu S, Buehler J, Berkelman R: Impact of the human immunodeficiency virus epidemic on mortality in women of reproductive age—United States. *JAMA* 264:225–229, 1990

98. Palefsky J, Gonzales J, Greenblatt R, et al: Anal intraepithelial neoplasia and anal papilloma-virus infection among homosexual males with group IV HIV disease. *JAMA* 263: 2911–2916, 1990

# Chapter 32

# Bone and Soft-Tissue Sarcoma

Patricia A. Piasecki, RN, MS

## INTRODUCTION

Bone and soft tissue malignancies are so uncommon that they are not listed among the five leading cancer sites. They occur in all age-groups. Diagnosis and treatment of these lesions are complex. Key members of the health care team include the patient and family, the orthopedic surgeon, medical oncologist, radiologist, pathologist, radiation oncologist, thoracic surgeon, physical therapist, nurse, prosthetist, and social worker. Increased knowledge about bone and soft tissue sarcomas and a multidisciplinary approach to treatment have improved the results of bone and soft tissue tumor treatment in recent years.

## EPIDEMIOLOGY

The incidence of primary malignant bone and soft tissue tumors is remarkably low. These tumors constitute a small percentage of malignant tumors diagnosed in the United States.[1] The American Cancer Society estimated in 1995 that 2070 new cases of bone cancer were discovered. Incidence is slightly higher for men. The estimated number of deaths that occurred in 1995 from bone cancer is 1280. In 1995, 6000 new cases of soft tissue cancer were discovered. The estimated death toll from soft tissue tumors was 3600.[1]

## ETIOLOGY

At present, relatively little is known regarding the cause of primary bone and soft tissue tumors. Consequently, prevention and detection of bone and soft tissue sarcoma remain difficult because few risk factors have been identified. Prior cancer therapy in the form of high-dose irradiation has been linked to the development of bone and soft tissue sarcoma. Chemicals such as vinyl chloride gas, arsenic, and dioxin or Agent Orange have been associated with the formation of soft tissue sarcomas. Exposure to alkylating agents such as melphalan, procarbazine, nitrosoureas, and chlorambucil predisposes patients to sarcomas.[2] Immunosuppressed patients such as renal transplant recipients and persons with autoimmunodeficiency syndrome (AIDS) have a higher risk for soft tissue sarcomas. Neurofibromatosis patients have a 10% chance of one of their tumors transforming to a neurofibrosarcoma.[3] Prolonged lymphedema following a mastectomy can lead to a lymphangiosarcoma.[4]

Evidence of a familial tendency in bone cancer has been demonstrated by reports of siblings with osteosarcoma, Ewing's sarcoma, and chondrosarcoma. Bone and soft tissue sarcomas may be only part of a complex of different tumors that cluster in families.[5] These findings suggest that common susceptibility may be the critical factor in predisposition to diverse forms of cancer.

Malignant bone neoplasms have been associated with a number of preexisting bone conditions. Paget's disease predisposes individuals primarily to osteosarcoma but occasionally to fibrosarcoma, chondrosarcoma, and giant cell tumor. The incidence of sarcomas in patients with symptoms of Paget's disease is 0.8%.[6] It has been proposed that the mechanisms responsible for the relationship are prolonged growth, an overstimulated metabolism, or both. These mechanisms are also implicated in the occurrence of bone tumors associated with hyperparathyroidism, chronic osteomyelitis, old bone infarct, and fracture callus.

Other factors such as syndromes of skeletal maldevelopment and skeletal growth patterns have been implicated in the etiology of bone cancer. These factors are discussed here in conjunction with the specific bone tumor type to which they apply.

Molecular genetics are being studied in musculoskeletal tumors, and hopefully genetic therapy will be a trend in the next decade. Osteosarcomas are noted to occur if both alleles at the RB1 and P53 are altered; these are tumor-suppressor genes.[7,8] Similar studies in chondrosarcoma cell lines are being performed. Neurofibrosarcoma patients have a loss of tumor-suppressor gene on chromosome 17P.[9] There is also ongoing research in this area.

## PREVENTION, SCREENING, AND EARLY DETECTION

Due to the relative low incidence of malignant bone and soft tissue tumors, there are no screening tests available for these tumors. For individuals with a family history of sarcoma or predisposing conditions such as neurofibromatosis or exposure to dioxin, annual physical exams are a prudent routine to adopt. Routine radiographic screenings are not advised. If bone pain or a mass is discovered it should be evaluated even if there is no predisposing condition.

## PATHOPHYSIOLOGY

Primary malignant bone and soft tissue tumors are derived from the cells that have a common ancestry, namely, the mesoderm or ectoderm. One group of bone and soft tissue tumors is produced by cells characterized by their ability to produce collagen. This group includes the osteogenic tumors arising from osteoblasts, the chondrogenic tumors arising from chondroblasts, and the fibrogenic tumors arising from fibroblasts. Another group originates in the bone marrow reticulum and includes round cell tumors such as Ewing's sarcoma and reticulum cell sarcoma. The third group arises in blood vessels of the bone and includes the angiosarcomas. Soft tissue sarcomas such as alveolar soft part sarcomas and epithelioid sarcomas have no known cellular origins.

Little can be said regarding the pathophysiology of bone and soft tissue tumors in general because of the individualized behavior demonstrated by the different types of tumors. Nearly every bone and soft tissue in the skeleton may be affected; however, individual tumors have a predilection for certain locations. Most often soft tissue sarcomas arise in the extremities but can involve head and neck and retroperitoneal areas. In addition, there are differences in cellular characteristics and in the progression of disease. In general, bone and soft tissue tumors tend to involve contiguous tissue and muscle aggressively and metastasize early to the lungs via the hematogenous route. Occasionally, soft tissue sarcomas can spread to regional lymph nodes.

## CLINICAL MANIFESTATIONS

Bone and soft tissue sarcomas can manifest with one or more of the following presentations:

1. painful area on the musculoskeletal system
2. pain at rest
3. soft tissue or bony mass that may not be painful

## ASSESSMENT

### Patient and Family History

The evaluation of pain assumes a major focus in the interview. Obtaining information regarding the location, onset, duration, and quality of the pain assists in the differential diagnosis. It is important to rule out a traumatic injury to the area, which could result in a condition such as hematoma or myositis ossificans that can resemble tumors. More commonly, an injury merely brings a preexisting neoplasm to the attention of the individual. Bone tumor pain often has a gradual onset and may be present for a few months before the person seeks medical advice. An abrupt onset of pain does not necessarily rule out the presence of bone tumor because a pathological fracture may be the presenting symptom. Pain can be radicular. For example, a tumor of the hip can radiate pain via the obturator nerve and present with knee pain. Musculoskeletal tumor pain often is constant and worse at night. The severity of pain steadily increases as the tumor enlarges. Over-the-counter medications may not relieve the pain.

Soft tissue sarcomas present as painless masses unless they are impinging on nerves, blood vessels, or viscera. Other presenting symptoms such as a history of swelling

need to be assessed during the patient interview. Attention is given to symptoms suggestive of pulmonary disease such as hemoptysis, chest pain, or cough. Family history of any cancer diagnosis and subsequent treatment, toxic substance exposure, and prior orthopedic conditions such as Paget's disease or neurofibromatosis should be noted.

To determine potential problems and needs, a psychosocial assessment should be incorporated into the initial interview. The individual may have a life-threatening tumor. The nature of family, peer, and love relationships and other support systems is explored. It often is helpful to identify the person in whom the patient most frequently confides as well as the person's usual coping strategies when confronting stress. To further delineate possible resources, the significance of personal relationships, work, and leisure activities is assessed.

### Physical Examination

The physical examination of the individual with a suspected bone or soft tissue lesion involves inspection and palpation of the affected area. Inspection may reveal a visible mass or swelling. Dilated surface veins may be evident. A firm, nontender, warm enlargement may be palpated over the affected portions, although malignant bone tumors are not always visible or palpable. Dimensions of the soft tissue mass should be noted. Evaluation for adenopathy and hepatomegaly also is performed. Limitations in motion of proximal joints are noted. Muscle atrophy can occur in a chronic setting and can be documented by measuring the affected and nonaffected limb. Analysis will most likely reveal an antalgic gait for a lower extremity tumor, as the patient will shorten the time spent on the affected limb. An assessment of neurovascular function of the affected limb is done.

### Diagnostic Studies

Evaluation of the individual with symptoms suggestive of bone or soft tissue sarcoma necessitates the collaboration of the radiologist, orthopedic surgeon, and pathologist. Before any diagnostic conclusions are made, the person's clinical history is reviewed, as well as the radiological and histological features of the lesion.

Radiographs, although they frequently do not yield a specific diagnosis, provide the opportunity to view the location and the anatomy of the bony lesion, as well as the status of surrounding tissue (Figure 32-1). In general, radiographic changes can be appreciated only when the tumor is far advanced. Three basic patterns of tumor destruction that may be viewed radiographically are described as geographic, moth-eaten, or permeative. These patterns (Figure 32-2) may be correlated with the pathological aggressiveness or quiescence of the tumor and may occur alone or in combination with one or both of the other patterns.[10] The geographic pattern indicates

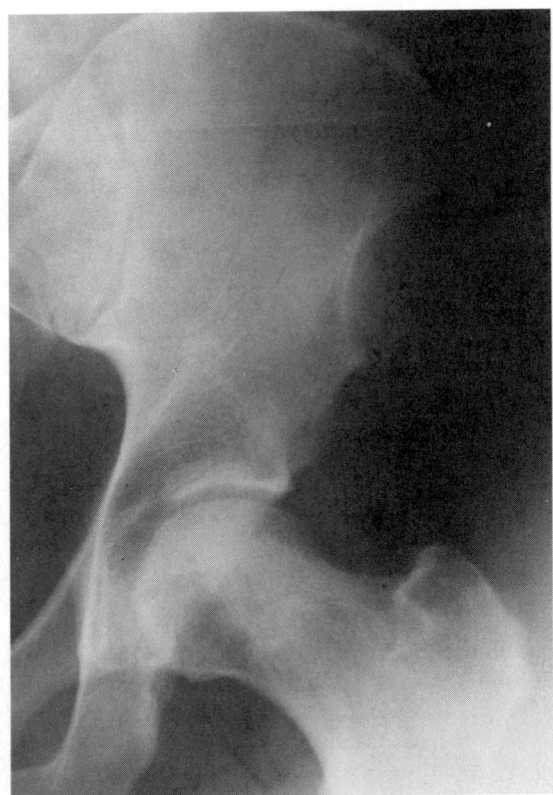

**FIGURE 32-1**    Radiograph of a 67-year-old man with primary osteosarcoma of the femur.

that the tumor has a slow rate of growth. It is characterized by a large, well-defined hole in which the edge of completely destroyed bone interfaces with the edge of bone that is completely intact. The moth-eaten pattern indicates a moderately aggressive tumor. It is characterized by multiple holes that tend to coalesce. This pattern implies severe cortical destruction. Finally, the permeative pattern indicates an aggressive tumor with a strong capacity for infiltration. It is characterized by multiple tiny holes in cortical bone. These holes diminish in size and number in the peripheral areas of the lesion. The moth-eaten pattern indicates that the tumor has breached the cortex and has extended longitudinally within the bone. Soft tissue sarcomas may have negative radiographs because radiographs best image bony tissue and poorly image the soft tissues.

Several other radiological methods may be used in the evaluation of primary malignant bone and soft tissue cancer. These include bone scans, arteriography, computed tomography (CT), fluoroscopy, and magnetic resonance imaging (MRI). A bone scan is not helpful in distinguishing one bone condition from another but is useful in verifying the presence of abnormal bone when plain radiographs show normal findings. A bone scan helps to detect or exclude the presence of additional lesions in the skeleton. Likewise, arteriography is not diagnostic but aids in the planning of surgical, radiation, and perfusion chemotherapy treatments by outlining tumor margins and mapping arterial blood supply to the tumor. CT provides an evaluation of the true bony extent of the disease. Fluoroscopy is used in the operating room to document the location in the bony lesion from which the biopsy specimen is taken.

MRI uses a magnetic field to produce an image. The MRI is superior to a CT scan in demonstrating the tumor extent in marrow and soft tissue and in detecting recurrence in the presence of surgical clips and metallic prostheses.[11] Ultrasonography is useful in determining size and density of the soft tissue mass. It measures the reflection of continuous high-frequency sound waves.

Biopsy is crucial for diagnosis. The biopsy should include the most representative section of the lesion as determined by the imaging. Biopsy tissue may be obtained by use of an open (incisional) or closed (needle) technique.

Open, or incisional, biopsy is the most common type of biopsy used for bone and soft tissue lesions. With the patient under general, regional, or local anesthesia, an incision is made over the tumor mass and through to the soft tissue. Bone biopsies are more painful, weaken the bone, and need to be processed in the pathology department for a few days before diagnosis is made. Incisional biopsy yields a larger volume of tissue for examination but may cause larger hematoma, potentially spilling malignant cells.

The location and size of the incision are equally important to the surgeon and radiation oncologist. If resection of the tumor is performed, the site of the biopsy incision is removed en bloc with the tumor. The radiation oncologist includes the incision site in the field of treatment. Therefore, it is advisable for the orthopedic oncologist rather than the referring surgeon to perform the biopsy.

Frozen sections are done during incisional biopsy to ensure that representative material has been obtained. In circumstances in which clinical and radiological findings are highly suggestive of a particular lesion, frozen sections are obtained with the intention of performing surgery while the patient is still anesthetized. For many bone tumors, however, it is advisable to await permanent paraffin sections.

Closed, or needle, biopsy is utilized on the basis that it is technically simple, involves minimal patient risk, is cost- and time-effective, may be repeated without any ill effects, and makes it possible to extract material from different depths of the tumor. This biopsy can be done by the surgeon under local anesthetic; in some centers radiologists perform CT-guided needle biopsies using sedation. In addition, it is always possible to do incisional biopsy if the diagnosis remains unclear. Although positive results of biopsy nearly always are accurate, biopsy yields a 20% false-negative rate. For this reason, needle biopsy generally is not the preferred method except in individuals with known metastatic disease.[12]

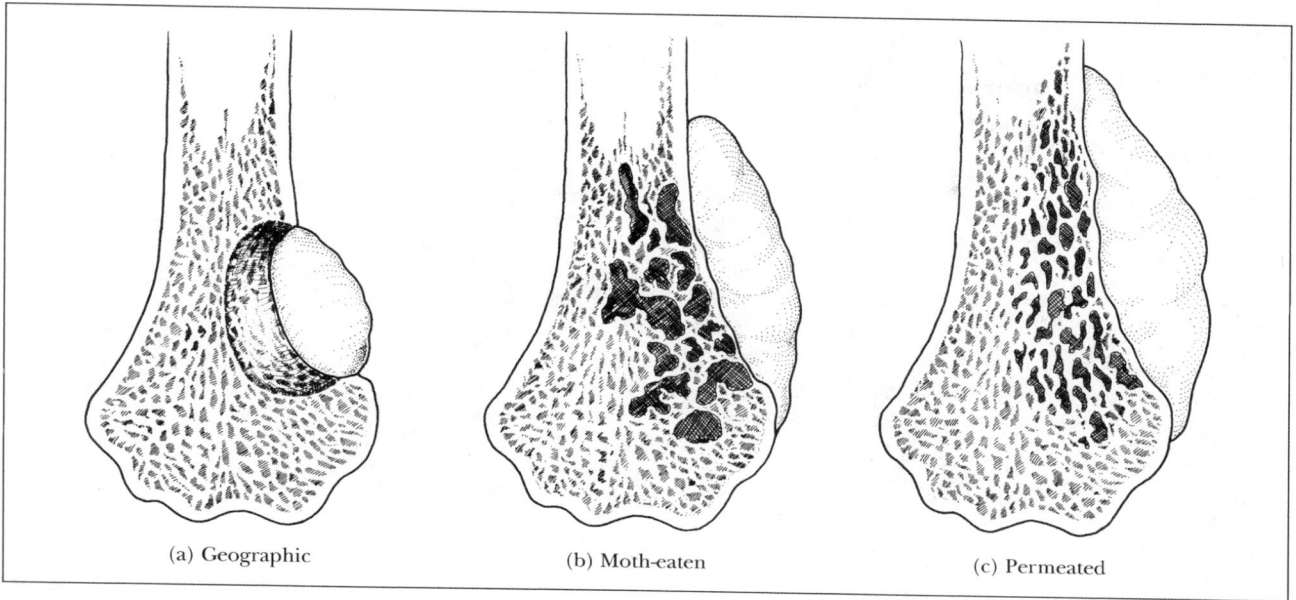

**FIGURE 32-2** Radiographic patterns of tumor destruction. (a) Geographic pattern, indicating a slow rate of tumor growth. (b) Moth-eaten pattern, indicating moderately aggressive tumor growth. (c) Permeative pattern, indicating aggressive tumor growth. (Lodwick GS: Solitary malignant tumors of the bone. *Semin Roentgenol*, 1:293–313, 1966).

In general, laboratory studies are not helpful in the diagnosis of musculoskeletal tumors. There are a few exceptions, which will be addressed in conjunction with the specific tumor type to which they apply.

Metastatic disease is screened for with a CT of the chest and regional lymph nodes. Node exam is done only if the node is palpable on physical examination.

## Prognostic Indicators

The prognosis for individuals with bone and soft tissue sarcoma is worse if the grade of the tumor is high, the location deep, and the tumor large. If there is distant metastasis to the lymph nodes, lungs, or other bones, the prognosis is also lowered. Nonresponsive tumors may be measured by use of serial thallium scintigraphy throughout treatment. This technique is still under investigation.[13]

## CLASSIFICATION AND STAGING

The classification of bone and soft tissue tumors currently is based on histological patterns, which in general correlate with the gross appearance, radiological features, and biological behavior of the tumor. Uncertainty with regard to the definition of terms used in pathological nomencla-ture and classification not only complicates the treatment of bone tumors but also impedes research efforts aimed at the development of staging classification for musculoskeletal tumors. Consequently, the American Joint Committee on Cancer has recommended that the *International Histological Classification of Tumors*, published by the World Health Organization, be used for specific definitions of histological typing.[14]

The World Health Organization scheme of classification (Table 32-1) is based on the type of differentiation shown by the tumor cells and the type of intracellular material they produce.[15] The main types of primary bone and soft tissue tumors are listed according to whether they are bone-forming, cartilage-forming, marrow-forming, vascular-forming, nerve-forming, or other connective tissue type.

The surgical staging system for musculoskeletal sarcomas includes surgical grade, surgical site, and presence of metastases (Table 32-2).[14] Stage I includes low-grade lesions with low incidence of metastases, such as periosteal osteosarcoma and giant cell tumors. Stage II includes high-grade lesions with high incidence of metastases, such as classic osteosarcoma and angiosarcoma. The site is noted to be "A," which indicates an intracompartmental lesion, or "B," which indicates an extracompartmental lesion. Anatomic compartments have barriers to tumor extension. In bone these barriers are cortical bone and articular cartilage; in joints, articular cartilage and joint capsule; and in soft tissue, the major fascial septa and the tendinous origins and insertions of muscle. Lesions that involve the neurovascular bundle are extracompart-

**TABLE 32-1** Histologic Typing of Primary Bone Tumors

| | |
|---|---|
| Bone-forming tumors<br>  Benign<br>    Osteoma<br>    Osteoid osteoma and osteoblastoma<br>  Malignant<br>    Osteosarcoma<br>    Surface osteosarcoma<br>      Periosteal<br>      Periosteal or juxtacortical<br><br>Cartilage-forming tumors<br>  Benign<br>    Chondroma<br>    Osteochondroma (osteocartilaginous exostosis)<br>    Chondroblastoma (benign chondroblastoma; epiphyseal chondroblastoma)<br>    Chondromyxoid fibroma<br>  Malignant<br>    Chondrosarcoma<br>    Juxtacortical or periosteal chondrosarcoma<br>    Mesenchymal chondrosarcoma<br>    Clear cell chondrosarcoma<br>    Dedifferentiated chondrosarcoma<br><br>Giant cell tumor<br><br>Marrow tumors<br>  Ewing's sarcoma<br>  Neuroectodermal tumor of bone<br>  Bone lymphoma<br>  Myeloma | Vascular tumors<br>  Benign<br>    Hemangioma<br>    Lymphangioma<br>    Glomus tumor (glomangioma)<br>  Intermediate or indeterminate<br>    Hemangioendothelioma<br>    Hemangiopericytoma<br>  Malignant<br>    Angiosarcoma<br>    Malignant hemangiopericytoma<br><br>Other connective tissue tumors<br>  Benign<br>    Benign fibrous histiocytoma<br>    Lipoma<br>  Intermediate<br>    Desmoplastic fibroma<br>  Malignant<br>    Fibrosarcoma<br>    Liposarcoma<br>    Malignant mesenchymoma<br>    Undifferentiated sarcoma<br>    Malignant fibrous histiocytoma<br>    Leiomyosarcoma<br><br>Other malignant tumors<br>  Chordoma<br>  Adamantinoma<br><br>Other benign tumors<br>  Neurilemmoma (schwannoma, neurinoma)<br>  Neurofibroma<br><br>Tumor-like lesions<br>  "Brown tumor" of hyperparathyroidism |

Schajowicz F: *Tumors and Tumor-like Lesions of Bone: Pathology, Radiology and Treatment* (ed 2). New York, Springer-Verlag, 1994.

**TABLE 32-2** Surgical Stages of Musculoskeletal Sarcomas

| Stage | Grade | Site |
|---|---|---|
| IA | Low (G₁) | Intracompartmental (T₁) |
| IB | Low (G₁) | Extracompartmental (T₂) |
| IIA | High (G₁) | Intracompartmental (T₁) |
| IIB | High (G₁) | Extracompartmental (T₂) |
| III | Any (G)<br>Regional or distant metastasis | Any (T) |

Enneking WF, Spanier S, Goodman M: A system for surgical staging of musculoskeletal sarcomas. *Clin Orthop* 153: 105–119, 1980.

mental. Stage III includes any site or grade lesion with metastases.[16] Another system developed by the American Joint Committee on Cancer includes surgical grade, site, presence of metastases, and nodal involvement (Table 32-3).[12]

## THERAPEUTIC APPROACHES AND NURSING CARE

The goals of treatment of primary malignant bone and soft tissue cancer include eradication of the tumor, avoidance of amputation when possible, and preservation of maximum function. The primary lesion is managed by surgery, radiotherapy, or chemotherapy, or a combination of these therapies. To a limited extent, immunotherapy is being evaluated for its usefulness as an adjuvant treatment. Treatment is highly individualized because an optimal treatment program has not been identified for each histological subtype.

### Surgery

Surgical management of primary neoplasia of the bone is strongly influenced by the histopathologic features, the anatomic site, and the physical size of the lesion. Clinical and radiographic data also are considered because they

**TABLE 32-3**   Anatomic Staging

| Rules for Classification |
| --- |

*Clinical staging.* Clinical staging includes physical examination, clinical laboratory tests, and biopsy of the sarcoma for microscopic diagnosis and grading.

*Pathological staging.* Pathological staging consists of the removal of the primary tumor, nodes, or suspected metastases.

**Primary tumors (T)**

| | |
| --- | --- |
| Tx | Primary tumor cannot be assessed |
| T0 | No evidence of primary tumor |
| T1 | Tumor 5 cm or less in greatest dimension |
| T2 | Tumor more than 5 cm in greatest dimension |

**Regional lymph nodes (N)**

| | |
| --- | --- |
| NX | Regional lymph nodes cannot be assessed |
| N0 | No regional lymph node metastasis |
| N1 | Regional lymph node metastasis |

**Distant metastasis (M)**

| | |
| --- | --- |
| MX | Presence of distant metastasis cannot be assessed |
| M0 | No distant metastasis |
| M1 | Distant metastasis |

**Tumor grade (G)**

| | |
| --- | --- |
| GX | Grade cannot be assessed |
| G1 | Well differentiated |
| G2 | Moderately well differentiated |
| G3–4 | Poorly differentiated; undifferentiated |

**Stage grouping**

| | | | | |
| --- | --- | --- | --- | --- |
| Stage IA | G1 | T1 | N0 | M0 |
| Stage IB | G1 | T2 | N0 | M0 |
| Stage IIA | G2 | T1 | N0 | M0 |
| Stage IIB | G2 | T2 | N0 | M0 |
| Stage IIIA | G3–4 | T1 | N0 | M0 |
| Stage IIIB | G3–4 | T2 | N0 | M0 |
| Stage IVA | Any G | Any T | N1 | M0 |
| Stage IVB | Any G | Any T | Any N | M1 |

American Joint Committee on Cancer: *Manual for Staging of Cancer,* (ed 5). Philadelphia, Lippincott, 1995.

provide further information about the biological behavior of a given lesion.

In the past 20 years, research has indicated that no procedure short of ablation would control or eradicate aggressive forms of osteosarcoma, fibrosarcoma, and chondrosarcoma.[17] Historically, the amputation included the joint above the tumor. Tumors in inaccessible areas such as the pelvis, spine, or skull pose unique and difficult problems, with treatment frequently aimed at palliation.

In 1984 the National Institutes of Health held a conference to evaluate the efficacy of limb-sparing surgery. Experts reported their experiences with 2000 individuals diagnosed with sarcoma. The same disease-free survival rate was reported for individuals who underwent limb-sparing surgery as for those who underwent amputation.[18]

The traditional contraindications for limb salvage are as follows: (1) inability to attain adequate surgical margin, (2) neurovascular bundle involved by tumor, and (3) age-group, that is, children younger than ten years, because of resultant limb length discrepancy.

An expandable prosthesis was developed in the early 1980s. The implantation of this prosthesis into the resected bone allows retention of the skeletally immature child's limb. Surgery is performed every 6 to 12 months to expand the prosthesis. The long-term outcome of these implants is unknown.[19]

Another option for skeletally immature patients with malignant neoplasm is the Van Nes rotationplasty. The procedure is utilized for distal femur lesions that otherwise would require an above-knee amputation. First, the bone and soft tissue of the thigh are resected while preserving the sciatic nerve. The proximal tibia is internally fixed to the proximal femur after rotating it 180°. The foot is backward. The foot is then used to fit a below-knee prosthesis.[20] The bone takes approximately three months to heal, and the prosthetic fitting ensues. Due to the unusual anatomy, prosthetic fitting and rehabilitation can be prolonged. The advantage of this surgery is that the limb is retained and, therefore, function is improved in terms of both energy and rigorous physical endeavors. The disadvantage of the surgery is the unusual limb appearance when the prosthesis is off. Complications include nonunion and infection.[21] It is another surgical option for young sarcoma patients.

Limb salvage is indicated for lesions that tend to metastasize late such as surface osteosarcoma and chondrosarcomas that have not invaded soft tissue. Wide resection is necessary in limb surgery to ensure adequate tumor excision.

If the tumor extends to the incision surface at any point or cannot be removed entirely, amputation at a more proximal level may be indicated. Amputation also is indicated if a nonfunctional limb would result from a salvage procedure.

### Radical resection with reconstruction

In the preoperative period, it is necessary to discuss with the patient and family the postoperative management and rehabilitation of patients with radical resection and reconstruction. The patient, especially a younger one, needs to be aware that implant failure may occur and further surgery, including amputation, may be necessary. In one study only 67% of the metallic implants were functioning at ten years.[22]

Postoperative management in terms of levels of activity, mobilization, joint motion, weight bearing, the use of bracing devices, or external immobilization will vary according to the amount of bone and soft tissue resected, the location, and the stability of the implant or graft. When more extensive surgery is done, the actual function cannot be predicted as readily as when an amputation is planned. It is important to clarify this postoperatively.

Prevention of postoperative complications begins with preoperative teaching in conjunction with follow-up after surgery. The extensive nature of most resections requires longer exposure to anesthesia, necessitating attention to pulmonary hygiene. In the preoperative period the individual is familiarized with the pulmonary regimen. The patient is also instructed in isometric exercises and ankle pumps to prevent venous stasis. Malignancies, along with immobilization, increase the risk of deep vein thrombosis and pulmonary embolism.

The nurse conducts a baseline assessment of neurovascular function distal to the surgical site. Because nerve injury may occur during the surgical procedure or postoperatively due to swelling, the assessment provides the opportunity to observe for changes in sensation and motor function that occur. A splint may be ordered until the nerve recovers.

Blood loss and anemia can result from extensive tumor resection and reconstruction. These patients may be somewhat anemic preoperatively due to adjuvant treatments. Patients with malignancies cannot donate autologous blood but may elect to have their families and friends donate the 4–6 units of blood that may be necessary. Banked blood from the hospital is also available. A drainage tube is placed in the wound for 24–48 hours to prevent hematomas or seromas. Iron supplementation may

be prescribed. The nurse monitors the patient's vital signs and laboratory values.[23]

Position restrictions are determined by the surgeon based on operative findings and personal management philosophies. Limb evaluation, length of bedrest, and other restrictions are noted in the chart. Patients who undergo hip arthroplasty return from surgery with an abductor pillow. For approximately six weeks postoperatively, patients are restricted from flexing the hip over 90°, leg crossing, or side lying without a pillow between the legs. If these positions are not followed, a dislocation of the hip may occur, which is very painful, and often the leg shortens. The patient will need to have his or her hip relocated under sedation or general anesthesia. Occasionally an open reduction is required. Following a dislocation, a hip spica cast or hip orthosis is applied for six weeks to allow the soft tissue to heal.

Postoperative pain occurs after these extensive procedures. Initially pain is managed with epidural catheter continuous infusions of narcotics or a patient-controlled analgesic pump. As pain decreases, milder narcotic tablets such as hydrocodone and nonsteroidal anti-inflammatory tablets are prescribed. Patients are frequently discharged on these oral medications.

Wound necrosis can occur if large flaps are used to close the wound, especially if the surgical site was previously irradiated. Conservative treatments such as debridement and frequent dressing changes may also be utilized. Plastic surgeons may be required to employ a muscle flap or split thickness skin grafts to close the wound that does not heal primarily.

Postoperative infection remains a significant concern because adjuvant therapies such as chemotherapy may adversely affect patient immunity. Patients are given broad-spectrum antibiotics for 48° or longer after surgery. Patients are advised in lifelong prevention of implant infection, which could result from a hematogenous source. For example, an abscessed tooth could spill bacteria into the bloodstream and infect the implant. Written instructions are given to the patient (Table 32-4). Considerable bone damage can occur before detection of infection. Once infection is identified, treatment involves removal of the graft or implant, insertion of drains, immobilization, intravenous antibiotic therapy for six weeks, and or/antibiotic therapy for 6–12 months. Amputation of the limb is a possibility if complications occur. The nurse must be vigilant in observing for signs of infection and in teaching patients about signs and symptoms to report.

Assessment for pneumonia, pulmonary embolism, and deep vein thrombosis is done during the postoperative period. Prophylactic anticoagulation with warfarin, low-molecular-weight heparin, sequential compressive embolic devices, and antiembolic stockings are often utilized.

Functional independence and a gradual adaptation to the changes in body image are the goals of rehabilitation. Resection often involves muscle tissue; therefore, physical therapy regimens often are used to improve and develop muscle tone. Assistive walking and brace devices may be

**TABLE 32-4**  Implant Infection Precautions

| Source of Infection | What to Do |
|---|---|
| 1. Invasive procedures:<br>Surgery<br>Proctoscopy<br>Cystoscopy<br>Endoscopy | Notify your doctor so antibiotics can be given to protect your implant. |
| 2. Dental procedures:<br>Cleaning<br>Extraction<br>Root canal<br>Drilling | Notify your doctor or dentist prior to your appointment so antibiotics can be started before your exam. |
| 3. Wound or abrasion that is red or pus-filled; fever, chills | Immediately see your doctor to determine if antibiotics are needed. |
| 4. Infection in urinary tract, ears, throat, etc. | Immediately see your doctor to determine if antibiotics are needed. |

needed if motor function is limited temporarily or permanently. For lower extremity resections, leg length discrepancies may necessitate gait retraining or may be managed simply through the use of shoe lifts. Finally, the importance of safety within the home environment cannot be overemphasized. The length of hospital stay ranges from five to ten days. Most patients who are discharged to their previous home environment are able to negotiate stairs. Lifelong activity restrictions, such as no jogging, heavy lifting, or racquet sports, may be imposed and thereafter alter the individual's career and recreation.

After wide resection, reconstruction to provide stability can be accomplished through the use of metal and synthetic materials; the use of bone *autografts,* which are those transplanted from one area to another in the same individual; or the use of bone *allografts,* which are those transferred between two genetically different members of the same species. The three most common methods of reconstruction after sarcoma resection are arthrodesis, arthroplasty with metallic or allograft implant, and intercalary allograft reconstruction. Careful consideration should be given to type of reconstruction, particularly in view of the patient's functional needs.

*Arthrodesis,* or fusion, results in a stiff joint, which is a handicap for the individual. This form of reconstruction, however, is sturdy and permits activities such as running and jumping. Revision surgery is less likely with this procedure. There are a variety of surgical techniques for arthrodesis that use metallic implants, allograft implants, or autograft bone (Figure 32-3). Complications include infection and nonunion. In 1985 Otis and colleagues[24] found that patients who underwent segmental replacement have lower energy cost during gait than those with above-the-knee amputation, which could be a consideration in elderly patients who frequently have compromised cardiac status.

Arthroplasty with metallic or bone allograft implant or a combination of metal and allograft allows mainte-

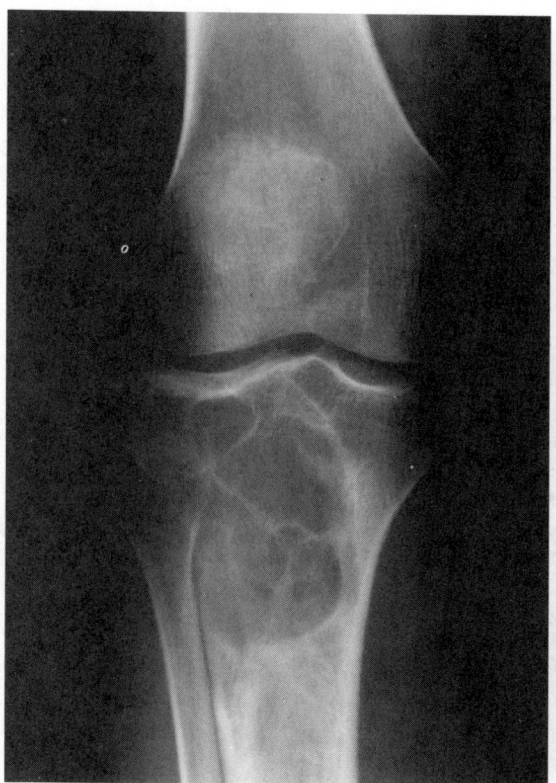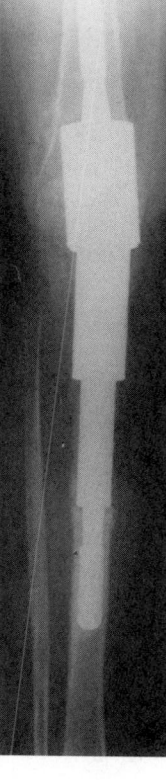

**FIGURE 32-3**  Radiograph of a 30-year-old woman with fibrosarcoma of the proximal tibia who underwent a wide excision of the tumor and received a segmental arthrodesis. She is disease-free after 6 years.

nance of joint function (Figure 32-4). The implant, however, is an artificial joint and will not tolerate percussive activities such as jogging and racquet sports or heavy lifting. Complications include infection, implant fracture, loosening of the implant, and nonunion. In any limb salvage surgery, muscle flaps and skin grafting may be necessary to assist in wound closure.

### Allografts

The use of allograft bone in tumor reconstruction has gained acceptance since the 1960s. In 1990, according to the American Association of Tissue Banks, an estimated 450,000 patients received transplants of bone, tendon, ligaments, and connective tissue. Allograft tissue can be custom sized in the surgical suite. There is no donor site morbidity or size limitation. Joint stability and function are improved by suturing allograft soft tissue attachments to host tissue. This is not possible with metallic implants. Allograft or cadaveric bone is procured in an operating room after consent is obtained from the next of kin. Often the donors have been involved in a motor vehicle accident or other fatal event. They may also donate heart, heart valves, lungs, liver, kidneys, corneas, and blood vessels. The donors are healthy and under 60 years of age. Thorough history and serological tests are performed to screen for viral or bacterial contamination. The chance of transplanting a human immune deficiency virus (HIV) allograft is calculated to be over one in a million.[25]

The bone is frozen, which diminishes its immune response. Bone allograft recipients do not require immuno-suppressive agents, which are often given to organ recipients.[26] Freezing does inhibit cartilage viability, even when cryopreservation agents such as glycerol are applied to the articular surfaces. In a recent study by Enneking and Mindell,[27] 16 retrieved cadaveric allografts were found to have no chondrocytes. When a bone is needed by a surgeon, the medical director of the tissue bank selects an appropriate-sized allograft utilizing recipient and allograft radiographs. Tissue typing is not performed. The tissue serves as a scaffold for the new host bone to grow into. The term *osteoconduction* describes this growth of capillaries and osteoprogenitor cells of the host into the allograft.

Osseous and osteochondral intercalary allografts provide a theoretically superior alternative to metallic implants because they provide joint mobility and are biological materials.

In an intercalary allograft the allograft is placed between two segments of the host bone (Figure 32-5). The allograft actually heals to the host bone after being secured by metallic plates and screws. Research indicates successful results in the replacement of long bone tumors with fresh-frozen allografts.[28–30] Degenerative arthritis can occur in osteoarticular allografts but can be managed by nonsteroidal anti-inflammatory medications, another osteoarticular allograft, or composite implant.[31,32,35]

Long-term activity restrictions for individuals undergoing allografts are the same as for those receiving metallic implants. However, the individual needs to limit weight bearing and often must wear a cast or brace, sometimes for up to 6 to 12 months, until the allograft is healed to

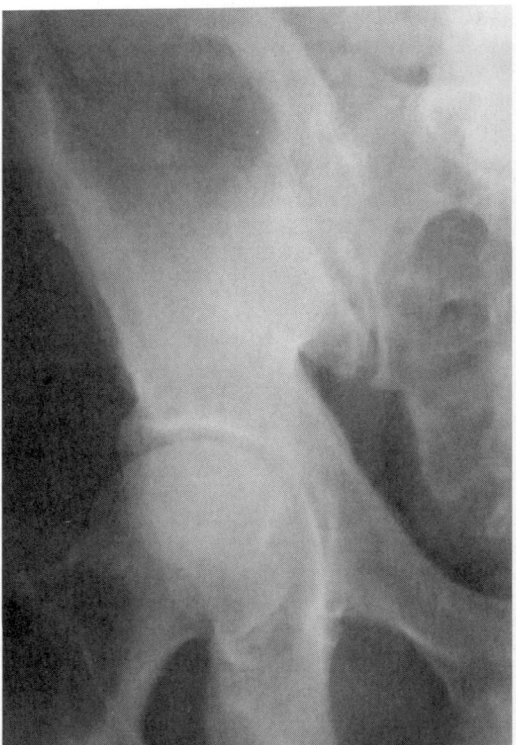
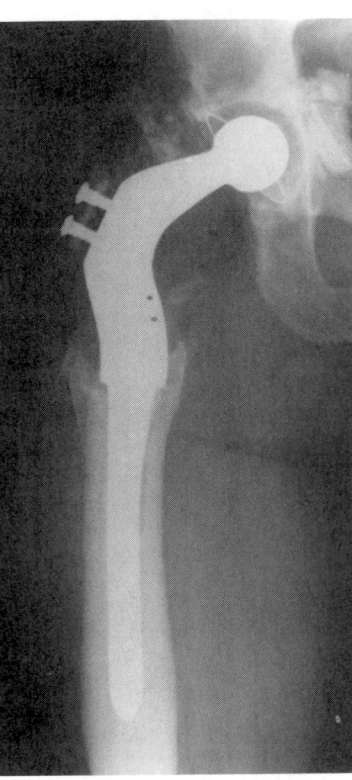

**FIGURE 32-4**  Radiograph of a 25-year-old man with osteosarcoma of the proximal femur, who underwent a wide excision of the tumor with proximal one-third femoral replacement with a metallic implant. He is disease-free after 10 years.

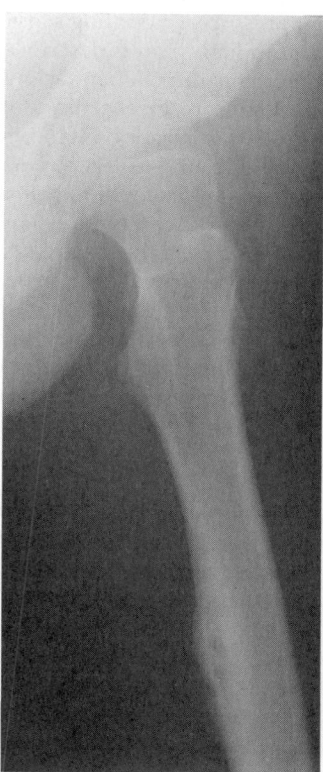
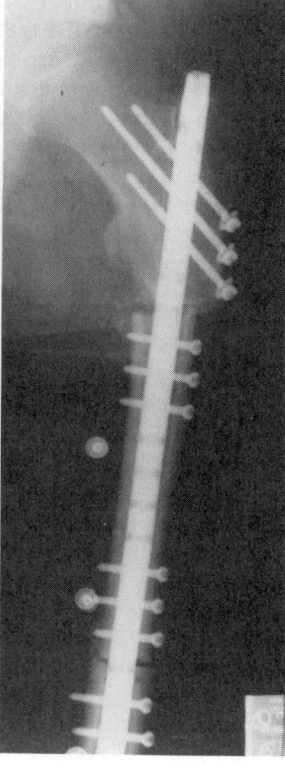

**FIGURE 32-5** Radiograph of an 18-year-old man with periosteal osteosarcoma of the diaphysis of the femur. He underwent a wide excision of the tumor with an intercalary allograft reconstruction. In the postoperative radiograph, it is difficult to detect the junction between the allograft and host bone. The individual is disease-free after 5 years.

the host bone. Complications of this procedure include infection, allograft fracture, and nonunion. The incidence of infection is reported to be 5%.[33] Nonunion may require an autogenous iliac bone graft for one year following surgery. Chemotherapy retards allograft healing; postoperative chemotherapy increased complications from 44% to 51% in three series of studies.[29,34,36] The future of allograft reconstruction appears promising for individuals whose bone is destroyed by malignant tumors.

### Metastatic sarcoma

The role of surgery in the management of disseminated disease has gained support in recent years. Sarcomas frequently metastasize to the lung before involving other sites. If untreated, most patients with pulmonary metastases will die within 18 months. Individuals in whom lung metastases develop are good candidates for resection, provided the primary tumor is controlled, there is no indication of other visceral metastatic disease, and the pulmonary nodules are resectable. CT of the chest and chest roentgenogram are performed at the time of diagnosis and every three months to assess for extent of dis-

ease. Wedge excision is the preferred procedure for lung lesions.[36] The nodule is adequately resected without compromising lung function. The only factor predictive of survival after relapse is if the patient can be rendered surgically disease-free. Patients generally recover rapidly after a thoracotomy. The five-year actuarial survival cure is 50%.[37]

### Radical resection without reconstruction

In soft tissue sarcomas and in bone sarcomas in expendable bones such as a fibula, clavicle, and sections of the pelvis, the resection is performed without any need for reconstruction. Nursing care is similar to that for patients with reconstruction. No lifelong infection concerns exist as no implants are placed.

### Amputation

The psychological needs of the individual who undergoes amputation should be considered during preoperative preparation. It is reasonable to assume that the person facing an amputation has fears regarding death, disability, and deformity. In addition, the person may be concerned about the potential loss of social and economic self-sufficiency. These fears and concerns may lead to changes in self-esteem, which can be manifested by anxiety and depression. All these factors will affect the individual's readiness to learn and ability to participate in rehabilitation. Consequently, the plan of care includes interventions aimed at minimizing fear, decreasing anxiety, and promoting realistic optimism. The individual and family may wish to express their fears and doubts. Efforts are made to integrate their expectations with reality by providing accurate information from nursing and medical staff regarding the postoperative recovery period and future rehabilitation.

The person may harbor fears concerning sexual adequacy. A woman needs to be reassured that pregnancy and normal delivery are possible after hemipelvectomy surgery. A decision concerning future pregnancies, however, may be influenced by the fact that the prosthesis cannot be worn during pregnancy. Impotence in a man often is related to age. Loss of erectile power is due primarily to a decrease in blood supply; however, pelvic nerve function may be compromised following hemipelvectomy. Most men recover potency over time. The younger the individual, the more rapid the recovery of potency.

To reduce anxiety it sometimes is helpful for the person undergoing surgery to meet preoperatively those individuals who will be involved in his or her postoperative care. Depending on the institution's program, this may include physical and occupational therapists, the prosthetist, the social worker, and the psychologist. Likewise, in some instances it may be helpful to arrange a preoperative visit from a person with an amputated limb who has mastered his or her prosthesis and achieved independence. Information regarding local organizations that train such volunteers can be obtained from the American Cancer Society. Care is taken in assessing which individuals could benefit by interaction with these resources. An overload of information may serve only to increase the person's anxiety and fear.

The nurse consults social service personnel to inform the patient and family about financial resources and rehabilitation programs available in the state. In general the available resources for individuals with cancer tend to be underutilized. Other support is available through groups such as the American Cancer Society and the American Handicapped Association.

It is important for the nurse to help establish realistic expectations regarding the patient's postamputation function. Many individuals who have lower extremity amputation can expect a return to full function and a relatively normal active life through the use of a lower limb prosthesis and occasional walking aids. Amputees resume activities such as downhill skiing, swimming, basketball, and cycling with or without recreational prosthesis. It is estimated that 20,000 amputees participate in sporting activities, with more than 5000 participating in organized competition.[38] The person who has a hemicorporectomy is wheelchair-bound. Hemipelvectomy prostheses will approximate only soft tissue, and the use of a walker or crutches will be necessary for additional stability. Because of the significantly increased energy expenditure required, it may be necessary for the person with a more proximal amputation to spend more time in a wheelchair. Elderly patients or those with cardiac conditions may find prosthetic use tiring and may need to use at least a cane.

Ideally, the goal for the individual is independent function with the use of prostheses. In evaluating rehabilitation potential, the nurse considers other factors such as age, effects of adjuvant therapy, the existence of unrelated disease, and the patient's attitude. Prosthetic rehabilitation requires cooperation, coordination, and tremendous physical energy, and a comfortable prosthesis.[39] Lane and colleagues[40] have found that amputees who have received doxorubicin and bleomycin have greater resting heart rates, decreased walking velocity, and increased oxygen requirements. The longer the stump, the lower the energy cost. With this information, they have found patients with lightweight prosthetic devices and three-times-a-week supervised cardiovascular training increased their gait velocity and reduced net energy cost.[40]

***Phantom limb phenomenon*** Preoperative teaching includes a discussion of phantom limb sensation and pain. It is a frightening experience for an individual with a recent amputation to feel sensation or pain, or both, in a limb that no longer exists. Consequently, the person who is not adequately prepared may neglect to report the occurrence of the phantom limb phenomenon and may harbor doubts about his or her sanity.

All individuals who have had an amputation can expect to feel some phantom limb sensation, whereas only 35% experience phantom limb pain.[41] Phantom limb sensation is described as an awareness of the position or existence of the limb. Itching, pressure, or tingling sensations may be described. Phantom limb pain is described as severe cramping, throbbing, or burning pain in various areas of the amputated limb. Phantom limb sensations usually are experienced shortly after surgery. Phantom limb pain usually occurs for one to four weeks after surgery and may be triggered by fatigue, excitement, sickness, weather change, stress, and other stimuli. The incidence and severity of phantom limb pain are greater when the amputation site is more proximal. For many individuals, phantom limb pain resolves gradually in a few months. However, the pain becomes worse over the years for 5%–10% of those who have amputations of limbs. It is suggested that increased severity of phantom limb pain after a few months may be a symptom of locally recurrent cancer in a stump, or it may be a sign of a neuroma.

Phantom limb pain is poorly understood but seems to depend on a combination of physical and emotional factors. The physical component relates to the surgical interruption of neural reflex pathways, with resultant transmission of abnormal patterns of nerve impulses. Melzack[41] noted a correlation between the length of time a person experiences limb pain before surgery and the incidence and duration of phantom limb pain. Other factors that contribute to phantom pain include the maladaptive use of pain for secondary gain, the availability of support systems, and the ability to cope with loss.[42]

A variety of measures are used to alleviate phantom limb pain. Relief may be obtained simply by applying heat to the stump or by pressure, such as with elastic bandages. Distraction and diversion techniques may decrease the person's awareness of the pain. Tranquilizers, local anesthesia, or muscle relaxants are occasionally effective in managing the pain. Psychotherapy and behavioral therapy also may be useful. Procedures that are available for intractable pain include hypnosis, nerve blocks, sympathectomy, cordotomy, acupuncture, biofeedback, and transcutaneous nerve stimulation. In rare cases revision of the stump with reamputation at a higher level may be done.

***Amputation of the lower extremity*** Preoperative preparation of the individual having a lower extremity amputation incorporates all considerations routinely given to any person undergoing surgery. The individual who is to have a hemipelvectomy will need to know that a urethral catheter will be inserted. A preoperative bowel cleansing will be given to decrease the content of the intestinal tract because of the slight chance that bowel would be penetrated intraoperatively.

General strengthening measures and mobility training should be initiated preoperatively by a physical therapist, if time and disease allow. Pull-ups provide preparation for walking with crutches. Active and active resistive exercises of the unaffected extremities maintain and increase muscle strength. The person also should be instructed in transfer maneuvers from bed to chair to commode. Finally, the person should be instructed to ambulate with the use of a walker or crutches. Control of weight bearing on the affected side should be emphasized.

The goals of postoperative care are to use modern prostheses, to achieve the highest level of function possible, and to minimize the negative psychosocial consequences of amputation. The actual postoperative care varies according to whether the individual has had an immediate prosthetic fitting or a conventional delayed prosthetic fitting.

Immediate postsurgical prosthetic fittings consist of a rigid dressing and cast applied to the stump at the time of surgery. A socket on the distal end of the cast is designed so that a pylon prosthetic unit may be attached to the cast (Figure 32-6). Restraining straps that go over the shoulder or attach to the waistband contribute to controlled pressure, improved stump shaping, and tissue support provided by the cast.

If a conventional delayed prosthesis fitting is planned, the patient will return from surgery with the stump covered with a dressing and an elastic bandage. To shrink and shape the stump, elastic bandages or elastic stump shrinkers are used until the first fitting (Figure 32-7). The individual is fitted with a temporary or intermediate prosthesis at approximately three to six weeks, when acute swelling has decreased. An intermediate prosthesis, however, lacks a cosmetic covering. Ambulation with weight bearing is encouraged as tolerated. Approximately three months after surgery, the individual is fitted with a permanent prosthesis, with or without immediate postsurgical fitting.

The relative advantages and disadvantages of immediate and delayed prosthesis fitting are summarized in Table 32-5. With the conventional delayed fitting, drains frequently are inserted during surgery to remove blood and serous drainage. The nurse observes for signs of hemorrhage such as excessive bleeding through the dressing or an increase in pain, tenderness, or swelling of the stump. The stump usually is elevated for 24 hours after surgery to prevent edema and promote venous return. To prevent hip contractures, the individual is assisted into the prone position three to four times a day for a minimum of 15 minutes and encouraged to assume that position for sleep. Exercises to maintain muscle tone and prevent edema, joint contractures, and muscle atrophy are initiated on the first postoperative day. Exercises include active range of motion, strengthening exercises for the upper extremities, and hyperextension of the stump.

Stump care involves frequent wrapping with elastic bandages or stump shrinkers to facilitate stump shrinking. Dangling transfer to a chair and crutch walking are encouraged on the first postoperative day. For the individual having a hemipelvectomy, mobilization also is possible on the second or third postoperative day. Length of stay varies from two to seven days, depending on level of amputation. Below-knee amputees may have a two-day stay, while hip disarticulation patients may need seven

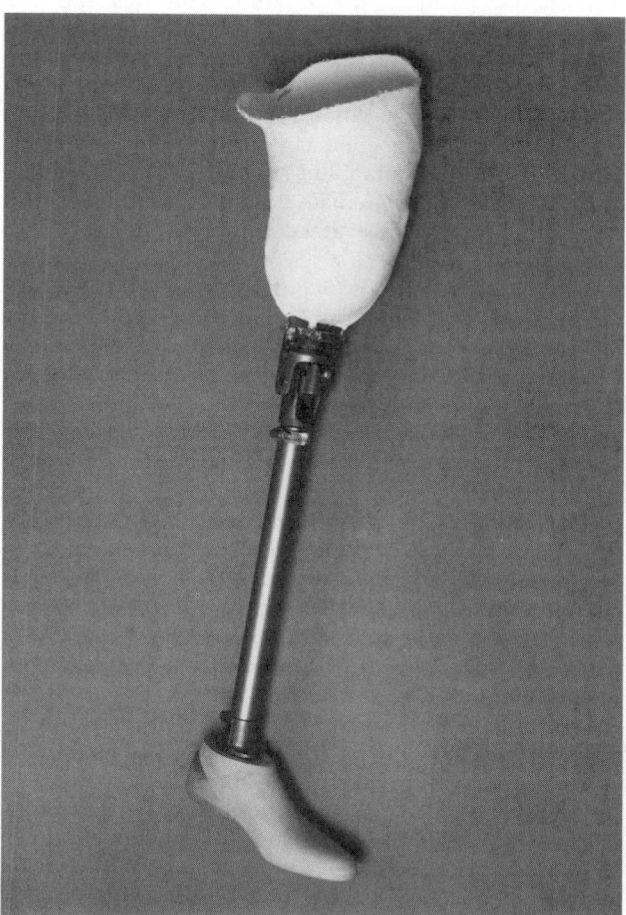

**FIGURE 32-6**   Immediate postsurgical prosthetic fitting with a pylon prosthetic unit attached to the cast.

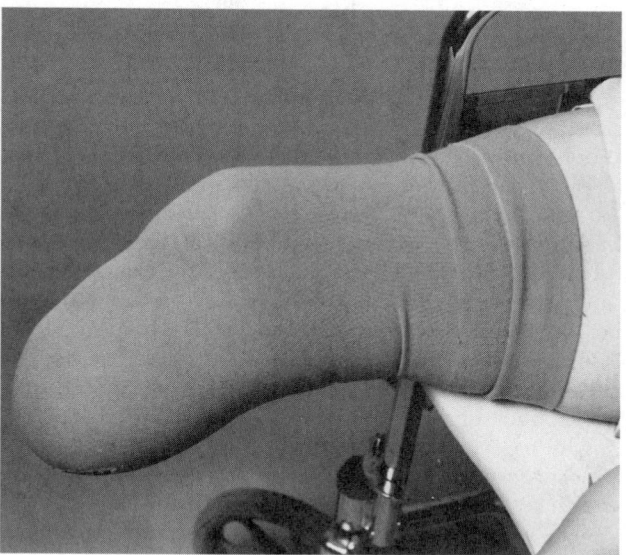

**FIGURE 32-7**   Elastic stump shrinker applied to shape stump.

**TABLE 32-5** Relative Advantages and Disadvantages of Delayed Versus Immediate Prosthetic Fitting

|  | Delayed Fitting | Immediate Fitting |
|---|---|---|
| Advantages | Wound can be inspected for healing. Skin can be conditioned by Ace wraps and stump shrinkers. | Better emotional adjustment with immediate substitute limb. Motivation increased with early ambulation with limb. Decreased stump edema, pain, phantom limb pain, and contractures (caused by pressure of device). |
| Disadvantages | Edema delays shrinking and shaping of stump. Continuous rewrapping with elastic bandages is required. Attention must be given to prevention of contractures and other complications of immobility. | Wound cannot be visualized. Temporary prosthesis is heavy. Poor gait pattern can develop because of heavy prosthesis and discomfort in early ambulation period. Prosthetist must go to operating room to apply. |

days. Sutures or staples are removed approximately two weeks after surgery. Temporary prosthetic fitting will occur at three to six weeks. The permanent prosthesis may be fitted within 12 weeks. A sitting or bucket prosthesis may be needed for an individual with a hemipelvectomy because of the absence of an ischium on which to sit. Until the bucket prosthesis is fabricated, a pillow is placed under the surgical site for balance.

With immediate prosthetic fitting, hemorrhage is less likely because of the compression effects of the cast. However, evidence of blood staining on the cast should be noted. The rigid cast also minimizes acute swelling; however, the stump is routinely elevated for 24 hours. Care must be taken to prevent the cast from slipping off the stump, which would rapidly lead to edema and wound disruption. Should this occur, the stump should be wrapped with an elastic bandage and the surgeon notified. Because the wound cannot be seen, it is important to monitor for signs of infection such as fever, increased white blood cell count, and significant stump pain. Such symptoms would necessitate immediate removal of the cast for wound inspection.

Nursing management includes cast care. The skin near the edges of the cast should be inspected for friction rubs, swelling, or discoloration. In addition, the cast should be inspected routinely for cracks. The rigid cast assists in the prevention of hip and joint contractures.

Ambulation with the pylon and crutches or walker is initiated on the first day. The length of time permitted for ambulation increases gradually. The individual advances to the use of parallel bars and to crutches while bearing touch-down weight on the pylon. Length of stay is similar to that for amputees without pylon. The sutures and cast are removed. A stump shrinker is applied two weeks after surgery. After the swelling is diminished, fitting for a permanent prosthesis is undertaken at 12 weeks after surgery. Chemotherapy may increase stump swelling and delay fitting of the permanent prosthesis.

The nurse makes the appropriate referrals to those professionals in the community who will become involved in the person's total rehabilitation. This may include a referral to a home nurse, home physical therapist, and local rehabilitation programs involved with vocational rehabilitation. Most individuals with amputated limbs are capable of eventually returning to work with restrictions.

Teaching the individual how to care for the stump is an essential element of the rehabilitation program. The patient needs to perform daily stump hygiene with the use of a mild soap and water. The patient also should be instructed to avoid the use of skin creams, oils, and rubbing alcohol. Daily inspection for redness, blisters, or abrasions should be incorporated into the patient's routine. The stump socks or elastic wraps should fit properly and be changed daily. When the wound has healed, the individual can prevent edema by putting on the prosthesis immediately after arising and keeping it on all day. The individual with an immediate postsurgical prosthetic fitting also should be instructed regarding cast care and inspection for fit.

The individual also is taught how to put on and care for the prosthesis. The prosthesis socket is wiped out daily with a damp, soapy cloth. Care is taken to thoroughly remove the soap and dry the socket to prevent a source of skin irritation and prosthesis rust. The individual is taught the importance of never attempting to make mechanical adjustments to the prosthesis. Discomfort or difficulties necessitate an immediate visit to the prosthetist.

The physical therapist reviews the exercises that contribute to achieving the highest level of functioning. Exercises that contribute to balance and movement patterns include standing, weight shifting, heel and toe balance, rocking, hip hiking, and stair climbing. The patient is advised to practice these home exercises after discharge from the hospital.

The physician and prosthetist collaborate in planning the construction of the prosthetic device. The prosthetist is responsible for the construction and fit of the prosthesis and should be certified by the American Board for Certification of Prosthetists. Lower limb prostheses generally consist of a socket, suspension such as a waistband or suction or latex sleeve, knee joint, ankle joint, and foot (Figure 32-8). Many varieties of these components are available; consequently, numerous combinations can be developed to meet the needs of each individual. For ex-

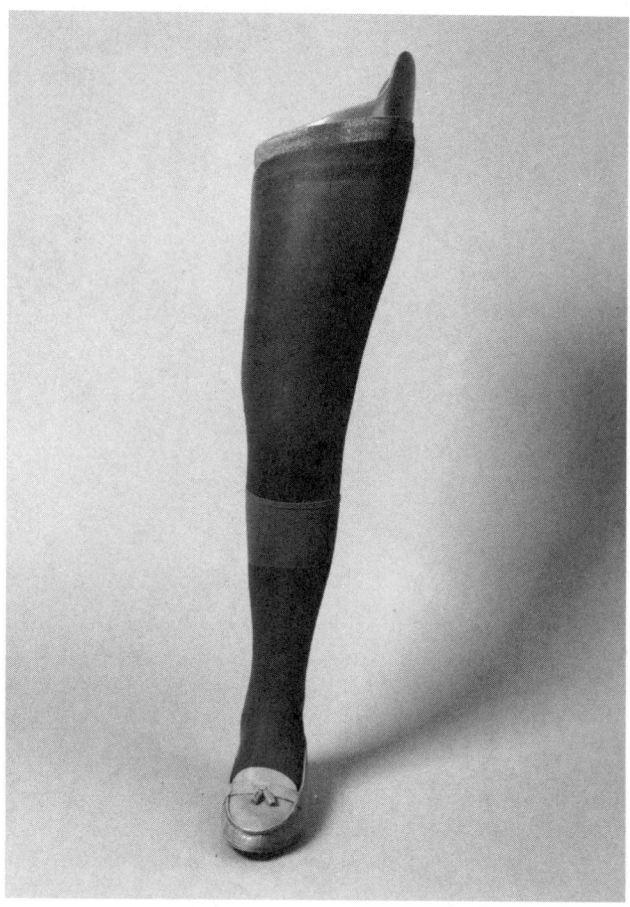

**FIGURE 32-8**  Lower limb prosthesis for an above-knee amputation showing the socket, suction suspension, joints, and foot.

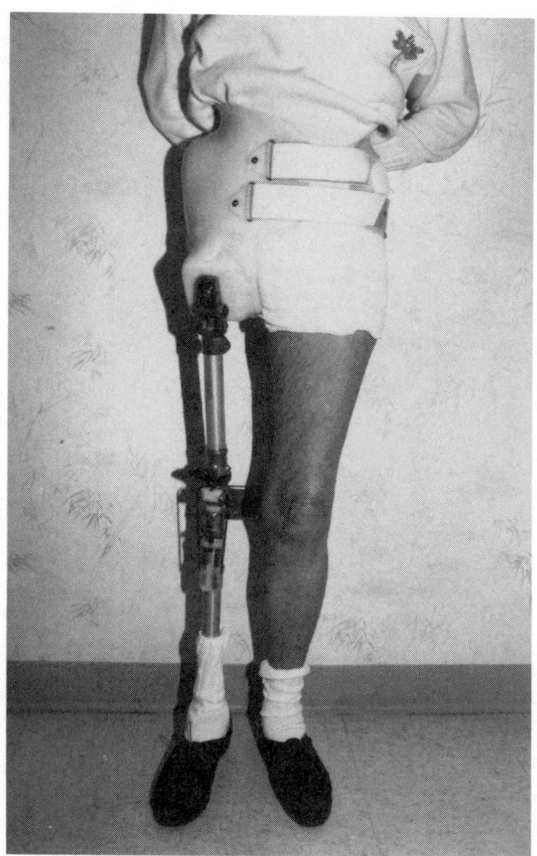

**FIGURE 32-9**  Hemipelvectomy endoprosthesis.

ample, knee joints are available that provide either mechanical or hydraulic assistance in controlling the swing phase of walking and provide increased stability during standing. Energy-storage prosthetic feet such as the Seattle foot are made with a flexible heel that releases the energy of foot fall at terminal stage to help initiate swing phase. These features, however, increase weight, cost, and maintenance. An above-knee prosthesis weighs approximately 3 kg and a below-knee prosthesis 1 kg. In designing the prosthesis, consideration is given to the person's age, ability, endurance, financial status, occupational goals, and motivation as well as comfort, fit, alignment, safety, ease of application, and appearance. The primary nurse can assess these factors and communicate them to the prosthetist. Figure 32-9 shows an endoprosthesis for the individual with a hemipelvectomy before application of the cosmetic urethane foam cover pictured in Figure 32-10.

After discharge, the individual with an amputation should be seen by the prosthetist every four to six weeks for the first year. The home health nurse and physical therapist observe for problems related to fit, comfort,

physical stress, or psychological maladjustment. These problems then should be explored with the individual and/or the prosthetist or physician. The rehabilitation process is complete when the individual has attained an optimal level of independence and has successfully incorporated the prosthesis into his or her body image.

***Amputation of the upper extremity***   Many of the considerations concerning preoperative, postoperative, and rehabilitative care that were discussed in the preceding section apply to individuals having an upper extremity amputation. There are, however, some significant differences.

Upper limb prostheses are far less satisfactory in both appearance and function than those created for lower extremities. The functional capabilities of the prosthesis for upper extremity amputation decrease as the level of amputation becomes more proximal. Power and motion are supplied in only a comparatively gross fashion. The most functional terminal(hand) device is a hook. The development of a substitute for the complex actions of the intricate muscles of the hand has thus far been impossible. Adequate cosmetic appearance can be obtained at the expense of function. Polyvinyl cosmetic gloves with realistic skin creases, veins, and hair are available. Skin tones are matched; shade changes that occur in the nor-

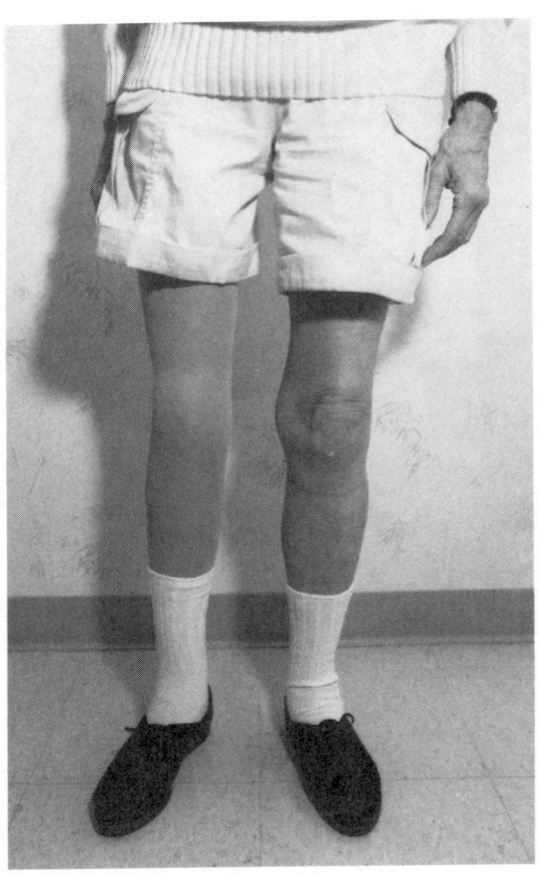

**FIGURE 32-10** Hemipelvectomy endoprosthesis with cosmetic urethane foam cover.

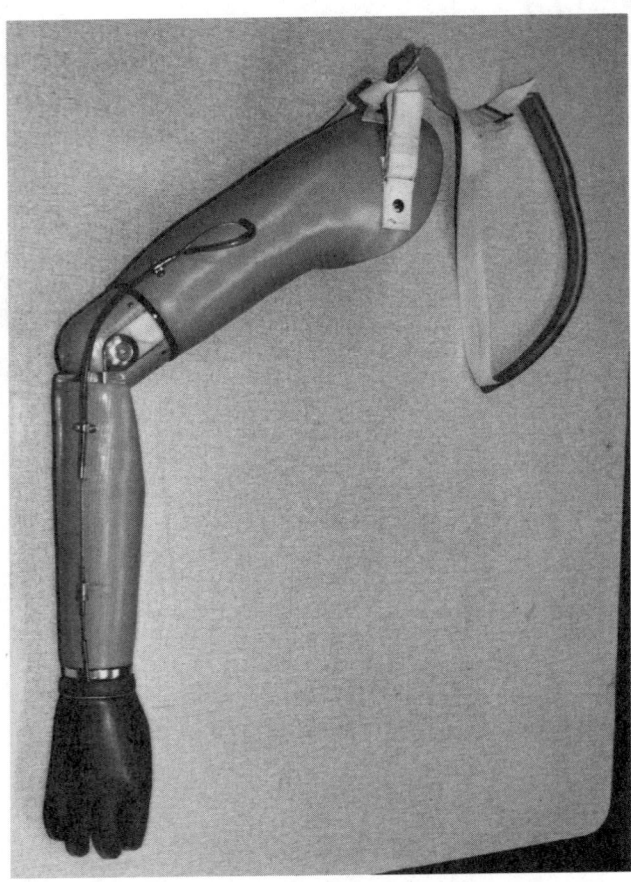

**FIGURE 32-11** Upper extremity prosthetic device showing a cable system, elbow joint, and hand terminal device.

mal hand as a result of position and season cannot be reproduced. In addition, the glove must be replaced frequently because ink, newsprint, and other stains are impossible to remove.

Conventional prostheses for the upper extremities consist of a hand terminal device, a harness to supply force from the proximal muscles, appropriate segments between them, including a socket for the stumps, and a cable system that provides motion at the terminal device and/or the elbow (Figure 32-11). Abduction of the scapula or flexion of the shoulder on the side of the prosthesis initiates movement. Flexion and extension of the wrist usually are omitted, although wrist units in flexed or extended positions are available. Pronation and supination are achieved by rotating the terminal device with the opposite hand. Likewise, opening and closing of the terminal device are accomplished through the use of the opposite hand.

Prostheses for interscapulothoracic amputations are fitted over the upper portion of the chest. Motion is severely limited because sources of power are unavailable. Some force can be initiated from the opposite shoulder and chest expansion. The primary function of the prosthesis, however, is cosmetic. Rejection of the upper extremity prosthetic devices occurs more often than with

prostheses of the lower extremity because of a combination of poor function, low cosmetic value, and lack of motivation.

Upper extremity prosthetic research has been directed at the development of myoelectric limb substitution. In this system, electrical impulses from the contraction of extensor and flexor muscle in the stump are picked up by electrodes in the socket and are in turn amplified, switching on and off electrical motors in the prosthesis. An external battery pack may be worn to provide an additional electrical supply. Opening and closing of the terminal device, pronation and supination, and elbow flexion can be provided. The individual must be assessed first for the ability to elicit and control myoelectric signals. The advantages include an increase in control with less energy expenditure and improved physical appearance. The disadvantages include the cost of the device, and electrical interference or inadvertent contraction of the muscles when the user coughs or stretches.

The inadequacy of available upper limb prostheses can be disappointing for the person with an upper limb amputation. The nurse, in conjunction with the physician, provides realistic information regarding the functional and cosmetic features of the upper extremity prostheses. It is important to discuss with the individual the negative social stigma attached to the hook, as well as its functional capabilities. Equal emphasis should be placed on the functional limitations and cosmetic value of the glove. Some individuals are willing to sacrifice function to obtain the best cosmetic replacement.

As with lower extremity amputations, immediate or delayed postsurgical prosthesis fitting is possible. When delayed fitting is planned, the individual will return from surgery with a soft dressing and elastic bandages covering the stump. Compression of the surgical area is to be avoided until healing takes place.

As with the lower extremity amputation, independence and an adapted body image can be facilitated through the provision of psychological support, patient and family education, and appropriate referral to community resources. Rehabilitation goals emphasize use of the remaining arm for activities of daily living. The patient should be evaluated preoperatively by an occupational therapist for information on one-handedness. Vocational rehabilitation assumes particular importance for the individual with an upper extremity amputation because the ensuing disability could prevent the resumption of previous employment.

## Radiotherapy

The use of radiotherapy in the management of primary or metastatic malignant bone or soft tissue sarcoma depends on the radiosensitivity of the particular tumor type. Most bone tumors are relatively unresponsive to radiation. Consequently, radiation is reserved for palliation and may be used in conjunction with chemotherapy for inoperable tumors or in conjunction with surgery to reduce the tumor load of partially resectable tumors. Conventional radiation doses for palliative treatment of primary bone tumors often result in fibrosis and contractures that lead to amputation even if the tumor is controlled. Neutron beam therapy, however, which is produced by heavy particle accelerators, can deliver higher doses with fewer complications. At the Fermilab Neutron Therapy Facility in Batavia, Illinois, 25 individuals were treated with neutron beam therapy for bone sarcoma in the axial skeleton or when surgery was refused for cosmetic or emotional reasons. The local control rate was 44%, and the crude survival rate was 39%.[43] Neutron beam irradiation may be an effective option for nonresectable sarcoma.

In contrast, radiotherapy plays an integral role in the management of Ewing's sarcoma and soft tissue sarcomas. Complications of treatment include tendon contractures, edema of the involved extremity distal to the site of irradiation, cessation of growth of the extremity, and nonhealing fractures. Brachytherapy or loading catheters in surgical wounds may be used for the soft tissue sarcoma.

Regional hyperthermia is a technique of raising the temperature in a tumor to 42 °C for approximately one hour. In a study of 40 patients with advanced sarcoma, regional hyperthermia along with ifosfamide plus etoposide was employed. There were 38 assessable patients, of whom only 6 had a complete response.[44] The treatment can be painful, with high systematic temperature and tachycardia occurring during the procedure. Complications include local infection, thrombosis, burns, and hematoma. Regional hyperthermia is not commonly utilized in the United States for sarcoma.

## Chemotherapy and Immunotherapy

Since the addition of postoperative chemotherapy to the treatment of bone sarcomas in the early 1970s, survival rates have increased from 20% to more than 50%.[45] Currently chemotherapy is given preoperatively as well as postoperatively. The rationale for preoperative chemotherapy is to treat the micrometastasis, to decrease the primary tumor size, thereby increasing the likelihood of limb salvage surgery, and to assess the effectiveness of the chemotherapeutic agents for two to three months.[46] The route of chemotherapy is either intravenous or intra-arterial. The duration of treatment ranges from 6 to 12 months. Adjuvant chemotherapy for soft tissue sarcomas is considered experimental; it will be discussed further in a later section.

Toxic effects are decreased by administering agents to counter the effects. Ifosfamide can cause hemorrhagic cystitis, but mesna, a sulphydryl scavenger, can inactivate metabolites in urine and prevent this complication.[47] High-dose methotrexate can cause renal toxicities, but calcium leucovorin or citrovorium factor can ameliorate this toxicity. The systemic effects of chemotherapy such as neutropenia and thrombocytopenia may create wound complications.[48] Neutropenia may increase incidence of infection but not necessarily impede wound healing. Administration of granulocyte stimulators diminishes the severity of neutropenia, allowing increasing the chemotherapeutic effect of a drug. Chemotherapy is tremendously important in the treatment of sarcoma, and ensuing complications are treated.

## CLASSIFICATION OF CERTAIN SARCOMAS

### Osteosarcoma

Osteosarcoma is the most common osseous malignant bone tumor. Its incidence is greatest in individuals between 10 and 25 years of age, and it affects males twice as often as females. The incidence of osteosarcoma peaks again in older adults with Paget's disease. The increased incidence of osteosarcoma during adolescence has been correlated with skeletal growth patterns, which in turn may account for the greater overall occurrence in males.[15]

There are two broad classifications: central and surface. Central osteosarcoma includes the classic high-grade tumor.

Osteosarcoma appears to arise from primitive bone-forming mesenchyma in the medullary cavity. Proliferating connective tissue generally gives rise to tumor osteoid and bone directly. The proliferating connective tissue also may form some tumor cartilage that undergoes rapid osseous transformation.

Surface osteosarcoma includes these two tumor types.[49] Periosteal osteosarcoma, a variant of osteosarcoma, was originally described by Unni et al.[50] It occurs as a hard mass on the bone surface, especially the tibia and knee. The tumor is confined to the periosteum and cortex without a medullary component. Tumors are low to intermediate grade and usually nonmetastatic. Parosteal or juxtacortical osteosarcomas occur also on bony surfaces, especially the posterior femur and humerus. They are often low grade.

The histological pattern of osteosarcoma is so variable that no two specimens are exactly alike. Specimens have varying mixtures of malignant bone, malignant cartilage, and malignant stroma. Consequently, the tumor may be described as osteoblastic, chondroblastic, or fibroblastic, depending on which component is dominant. Whatever the pattern, the essential criteria for the diagnosis of osteosarcoma are the presence of frankly sarcomatous stroma and the formation of tumor osteoid and bone by malignant connective tissue.

The most frequent sites of osteosarcoma include the distal end of the femur, the proximal end of the tibia, and the proximal end of the humerus. Osteosarcomas may be discovered in the iliac bone, vertebral column, mandible, and in rare cases the scapula, clavicle, or bones in the hands and feet. Humeral and tibial lesions have a better prognosis.[51]

Metastatic spread occurs primarily to the lungs by the hematogenous route. Radiological evidence of pulmonary or bony metastases usually appears within 24 months of the definitive surgery. Late metastasis in one or more of the other bones occurs occasionally, often in the presence of pulmonary metastases.

Half of the individuals with osteosarcoma have an elevated serum alkaline phosphatase level. This level, which represents osteoblastic activity, tends to decline after removal of the tumor and to return to the initially high level in the presence of pulmonary metastasis. In the normal growing child the levels are elevated. Other laboratory data do not appear to be significant in the diagnosis of osteosarcoma.

The classic radiological features of osteosarcoma include cortical bone destruction, extension of the tumor into soft tissue, and periosteal new bone formation that may appear in a perpendicular striated, or "sunburst," pattern. These findings can be diagnostic on plain radiographs.

The five-year survival rate for individuals treated with surgery alone or irradiation and surgery has been approximately 10%.[52] The high mortality rate is due principally to pulmonary metastasis, which is assumed to be present microscopically at the time of presentation. Reports evaluating adjuvant chemotherapy after surgery for osteosarcoma indicate a significant prolongation of the disease-free interval. Reports from the 1970s show that the five-year survival rate increased from 40% to 60% with the use of adjuvant chemotherapy using single agents.[53] Current chemotherapy protocols have used doxorubicin, high-dose cyclophosphamide, or high-dose methotrexate with leucovorin rescue. Most agents are given on an outpatient basis either intravenously or intra-arterially. Bacci and colleagues[52] and Glasser and Lane[51] demonstrated an 87% disease-free state at two years to 77% at five years. When preoperative or primary chemotherapy is used, effectiveness is assessed at the time of tumor resection. This regimen allows an in vivo study of the tumor cells. During the 8–20 weeks of preoperative chemotherapy, physical examination of the tumor site is performed to assess for effectiveness of treatment by indices such as decreased pain and swelling. If there is 90% tumor necrosis, the high-dose methotrexate regimen is continued postoperatively for six months. The greater the necrosis, the greater the survival. If tumor necrosis is less, the chemotherapy is changed to ifosfamide and etoposide. The course is extended to 8–12 months.

The improved results of chemotherapy have sparked interest in limb salvage resections. The chemotherapy can result in a decrease in the soft tissue component and ossification of the bony component. Surgery is planned after preoperative chemotherapy. The limb salvage criteria apply to these patients. Amputations are indicated for patients with large and invasive tumors. It is advisable to obtain a second opinion if an amputation is recommended. Local recurrence is as frequent in amputation surgery as in limb salvage surgeries (under 5%).[52] Resumption of chemotherapy after definitive surgery is delayed for one to two weeks.

Significant improvement of patient survival with metastatic disease was demonstrated in the 1980s. Of patients with osteosarcoma who had thoracotomies for metastases, 40% were free of disease more than two years after surgery.[45] No patients survived the development of pulmonary metastases unless they had surgical resection of gross disease. In these cases, chemotherapy is given after thoracotomy to eradicate microscopic disease.

Radiation is reserved for palliation or inoperable cases. Significant morbidity and mortality were reported when irradiation alone was used for treatment of the primary tumor.

## Chondrosarcoma

Chondrosarcoma accounts for approximately 14% of malignant bone tumors. The incidence is greatest in individuals between 30 and 60 years of age and among males.[15]

The occurrence of chondrosarcomas has been associated with syndromes of skeletal maldevelopment. Transformation of osteochondroma, multiple enchondromas,

Ollier's disease, or chondroplasia to chondrosarcoma has occurred. Chondrosarcoma arises from the cartilage and never has osteoid tissue.

There are both primary and secondary chondrosarcomas. The former include central chondrosarcomas that arise in the medullary cavity. The latter includes those chondrosarcomas that arise from benign tumors.

The diagnosis of chondrosarcoma is based on cytological changes of the cartilage cells. A cartilage tumor is considered malignant in the presence of many cells with plump nuclei, that is, more than a few cells with two such nuclei or clumps of chromatin.

The most frequent sites of chondrosarcoma include the pelvic bone, long bones, scapula, and ribs. Less frequent sites include bones of the hand and foot, the nose, the maxilla, and the base of the skull.

Most chondrosarcomas do not tend to metastasize early but rather remain slow-growing and locally invasive. When advanced chondrosarcoma does become aggressive, it tends to metastasize via venous channels to the lungs and heart. Regional lymph nodes or other bones occasionally may be involved.

Individuals with chondrosarcoma usually have a relatively long but unremarkable history. Medical advice often is sought for a slow-growing mass with intermittent dull, aching pain at the tumor site.

Radiographs of chondrosarcoma show a lobular pattern with or without calcification. If calcification is present, it usually is seen in a circular or semicircular pattern. Central chondrosarcomas in the long bones may show thickening of the cortex because of swelling of the shaft. The peripheral chondrosarcoma may demonstrate a vast, dense, blotchy appearance. Ragged, irregular, radiopaque streaks extending away from the central part of the lesion may be seen.

When the diagnosis of chondrosarcoma has been established, surgery is indicated. If the tumor is of central origin and has not extended through the cortex, wide resection and reconstruction are considered. Limb salvage surgery and amputation are options.

At present, chondrosarcoma remains nearly totally refractory to chemotherapeutic efforts inasmuch as chondrosarcomas usually have a poor blood supply. Consequently, drugs given intravenously do not reach the tumor in concentrations that are high enough to be effective. The benefit of chemotherapy as an adjunct to surgery has not been established.

Radiotherapy, usually neutrons, has limited effectiveness and is reserved for palliation of advanced or inoperable chondrosarcomas.

Individuals with a diagnosis of chondrosarcoma have a considerably better prognosis than those with osteosarcoma. The overall survival rate of individuals treated with wide resection or amputation has been reported to be 67% at five years and 50% at ten years.[54] In this series survival correlated well with the designated histological grade of the lesion. The estimated ten-year survival rate of individuals with grade 1 tumors is 87% and that of individuals with grade 2 tumors is 41%. For those with grade 3 lesions, the five-year survival rate is 44%, and the ten-year survival rate is 27%.

## Fibrosarcoma

Fibrosarcoma is rare, accounting for fewer than 7% of primary malignant bone tumors.[15] This type of neoplasm may occur at any age but is rare in children. There is no evident sex predominance.

Paget's disease may be a predisposing factor in the development of fibrosarcoma. In addition, the tumor may develop as a sequel to therapeutic irradiation or may develop at the site of an old bone infarct. Chronic osteomyelitis or fibrous dysplasia also may be a predisposing factor in the development of fibrosarcoma.

Fibrosarcoma is a malignant fibroblastic tumor that fails to develop tumor osteoid or bone in its local invasive growth site or in its metastatic foci. Periosteal new bone may be laid down as a direct extension of the tumor.

Like osteosarcoma, fibrosarcoma usually originates within the medullary cavity. It eventually penetrates the overlying cortex and extends into the periosteum and muscle. Occasionally a fibrosarcoma may arise periosteally and extend into the interior of contiguous bone.

Histological findings show that fibrosarcomas range from well differentiated to poorly differentiated. Rapidly growing tumors reflect cytological changes such as moderate anaplasia, cell irregularity, and many mitotic figures, and they tend to metastasize early. Less aggressive fibrosarcomas develop more slowly, taking longer to penetrate the cortex of the bone. Some fibrosarcomas are surprisingly indolent in their growth patterns and may show very little change over a period of years.

The femur and the tibia, the most common sites of occurrence, account for 50% of all fibrosarcomas. The neoplasm also may be observed in the humerus, radius, ulna, skull, and facial and pelvic bones. Metastasis occurs primarily to the lungs.

Individuals with fibrosarcoma, like those with other primary bone tumors, usually have pain and swelling of the affected area.

When the diagnosis of fibrosarcoma has been established, surgery is indicated. Limb and salvage amputations are options. Fibrosarcoma is considered to be radioresistant; consequently, the use of radiotherapy is reserved for inoperable tumors. Adjuvant chemotherapy programs after surgical treatment are being evaluated for reducing the incidence of microscopic residual metastatic disease.[15]

The prognosis for fibrosarcoma is guarded. The five- and ten-year survival rates after radical surgery have been reported at 28% and 21.8%, respectively.[15]

## Ewing's Sarcoma

Ewing's sarcoma accounts for 6% of all malignant bone tumors.[15] Eighty percent of such tumors are diagnosed in individuals between 5 and 15 years of age, with more males affected than females. These patients are younger than any other patient affected by primary malignant bone tumors. The development of Ewing's sarcoma has not been strongly linked to any specific etiologic factor.

Ewing's sarcoma is a primitive, multicentric tumor that appears to be derived from the mesenchymal connective tissue framework of bone marrow. The tumor usually arises in the marrow spaces in the shaft of long bones and rarely involves the epiphysis.

On microscopic examination, Ewing's sarcoma is characterized by the presence of uniform cells with indistinct borders. These cells are packed closely together and contain prominent round or ovoid nuclei and have finely divided chromatin.

No one site seems to predominate in the development of Ewing's sarcoma. The tumor commonly is situated in the pelvis and the diaphyseal or metadiaphyseal regions of long bones. Ewing's sarcomas metastasize early and most frequently involve the lungs. The lymph nodes and the skull are other frequent sites of metastasis. On autopsy, a considerable portion of skeleton is affected. It is unclear whether these bone lesions represent metastatic spread or independent development of disease in multiple sites. Metastasis may be present in nearly 20% of individuals at the time of diagnosis.

Many individuals have fever, anemia, high erythrocyte sedimentation rates, and sometimes leukocytosis at presentation. These symptoms can lead to an incorrect diagnosis of osteomyelitis. It has been observed that such findings result in a fulminating disease course that ends in death within a few months. Individuals who did not initially have such findings tended to survive longer. Bacci and colleagues[55] noted that normal lactic dehydrogenase, small distal primary lesion (<8 cm), and absence of metastasis were better prognostic factors for the patient with Ewing's sarcoma.

Radiographs of Ewing's sarcoma show bone destruction that involves the shaft. Varying amounts of periosteal thickening may be present, with "onion" layers of laminated subperiosteal new bone. A large soft tissue mass frequently will be visualized as well. Initially treatment consisted of radiation with chemotherapy. Local recurrence rates of 21%–30% were theorized to be caused by small foci of persistent tumor retained in each lesion.[55,56] Integrated therapy with radiation and/or surgery in combination with chemotherapy is the treatment of choice for Ewing's sarcoma.

Surgery or radiation alone will prevent neither the appearance of tumor foci elsewhere in the skeleton nor pulmonary metastasis. Consequently, primary chemotherapy, as prophylactic therapy for micrometastases and to decrease tumor bulk in order to lessen the need for local therapy, is used as part of the initial treatment for all patients. Using actinomycin, doxorubicin, vincristine, and cyclophosphamide, Bacci et al and Wilkins et al[55,56] reported an actuarial five-year disease-free survival rate of 40%–74%. Ifosfamide is an agent with a response rate approaching 50%.[57] Treatment usually takes place for 6–12 months and is often administered in an outpatient setting. Local treatment (surgery and/or radiation) begins approximately three months after the beginning of chemotherapy.

The tumor is extremely radiosensitive and capable of being cured locally with 50–60 Gy by means of shrinking fields. The National Cancer Institute reports a 3% incidence of radiation-induced sarcoma after combined chemotherapy and radiation in Ewing's patients.[58]

If margins are close, surgery followed by radiotherapy improves the local control rate.[59] Limb salvage and amputation are both options to be considered. The goal is to eradicate the tumor and maintain function.

Patients with metastases at the time of presentation are similarly treated, with a five-year survival rate of 30%. Ifosfamide is often utilized as a single agent for patients who have relapsed. There is ongoing research to evaluate its effectiveness as part of standard therapy for relapsed Ewing's sarcoma patients.

## Soft Tissue Sarcomas

The histological subtypes of soft tissue sarcomas include malignant fibrous histiocytoma, liposarcoma, fibrosarcoma, synovial sarcoma, rhabdomyosarcoma, and leiomyosarcoma. (Kaposi's sarcoma will be discussed in chapter 16.) They occur over 50% of the time in extremities; the remainder occur in the head and neck and retroperitoneum.

Soft tissue sarcomas invade surrounding tissue along the anatomic planes. They compress surrounding tissue and form a pseudocapsule, which contains tentacles of tumor. A marginal excision will never cure a soft tissue sarcoma. The local recurrence rate of this procedure is close to 100%.

Nodal metastases are common with a small amount of subtypes: synovial sarcomas (17%), epithelioid sarcoma (20%), and rhabdomyosarcoma (12%).[60] Lymph node involvement is a poor prognostic sign.

The more proximal lesions are usually larger since, in the retroperitoneum, buttock, or thigh, they can be disregarded until they are massive. A tumor that is superficial and smaller than 5 cm is felt to have a better prognosis.

Some histological subtypes such as rhabdomyosarcomas, synovial sarcomas, and malignant histiocytomas are considered poor prognosticators due to their high grade. However, any high-grade soft tissue sarcoma is ominous. Detectable pulmonary metastasis is more common in the high-grade soft tissue sarcomas. Typically, the first two years will reveal metastases and local recurrences. However, rhabdomyosarcomas in children are very sensitive to chemotherapy.

The five-year survival percentages of soft tissue sarcomas range from 30% to 95% based on subtype and grade.[9] The range for extremity sarcomas is 90%–95%, for trunk sarcomas 50%–75%, and for retroperitoneal lesions

30%–50%. In each of the three locations, higher-grade sarcomas have a poorer survival rate.

It is not uncommon for the surgeon to surgically remove a mass and, after routine pathological examination, learn it is a malignant sarcoma. In this situation microscopic tumor is usually found at the surgical site. It is recommended that a reexcision of the tumor bed be performed immediately following the definitive diagnosis of sarcomas. Occasionally, the second surgical excision will reveal no evidence of microscopic tumor cells. It is vital to ensure that no cells are left behind in order to avoid a local recurrence.[61]

In the optimal situation, imaging (Figures 32-12, 32-13) is performed prior to biopsy of the tumor. If the tumor is small and superficial, a primary myectomy (en bloc resection of tumor) may be recommended. The patient is informed that no biopsy will be done prior to the resection. The advantage behind this surgical decision is preventing cells leaking during biopsy and also avoiding a second surgery. The disadvantage is that occasionally the final histology will reveal a benign diagnosis, which could have been removed in a less radical manner. In most cases an incisional biopsy is performed.

The timing of surgery is based on the need for radiation. If radiation is deemed unnecessary, as in a subcutaneous or intramuscular tumor with no impingement on neurovascular structure, a salvage or amputation surgery is performed. Larger tumors may be excised after pretreatment with radiation.

A wide excision is defined as more than 3 cm of normal tissue. This procedure controls local disease in 90% of persons. If the pathologist notes a lesser margin, radiation is given.

The advantage of postoperative radiation is that it allows for thorough histological grading and diagnosis. There is no delay in surgery. Wound healing is uncomplicated. At the time of surgery, the tumor margin can be outlined with a radiopaque clip. Currently, this radiation timing is utilized for sarcomas that are widely resected with or without a close margin. The dose is 60–65 Gy to the tumor bed with 45–50 Gy to all tissues disrupted during the procedure.

Preoperative radiation has the advantage of a small treatment area with fewer complications. It does require more preplanning with the surgeon and the radiation oncologist. The patient may be rendered a candidate for limb salvage surgery with preoperative irradiation if the tumor has regressed. A series of radiation administered preoperatively has a 24% wound complication rate, which is higher than postoperative radiation programs.[62] This may reflect patient selection with larger tumors. Surgery is delayed for three to six weeks following the cessation of radiation. If margins are close, additional radiation may be ordered.

Another theoretical advantage of preoperative radiation is that the pseudocapsule surrounding the tumor becomes thicker in an experimental swarm rate.[63] A tumor with a thicker rind or encapsulation is easier and safer to remove.

Eilber and colleagues[64] developed a regime of preoperative doxorubicin and irradiation. The chemotherapy was given intra-arterially, followed by 35 Gy of radiation.

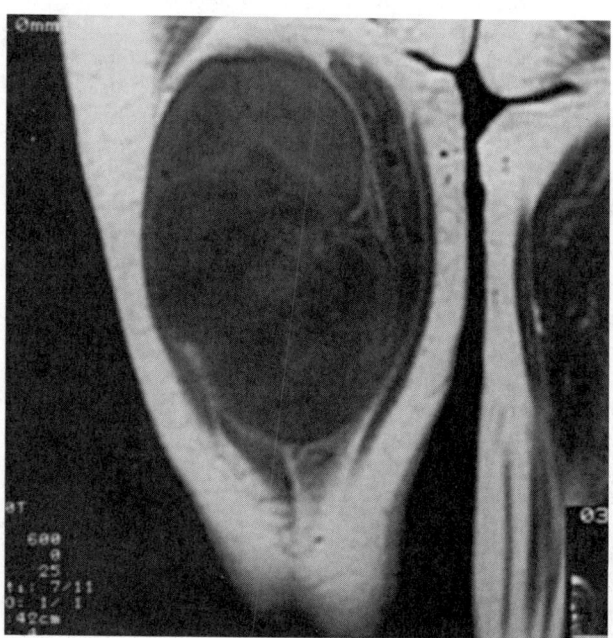

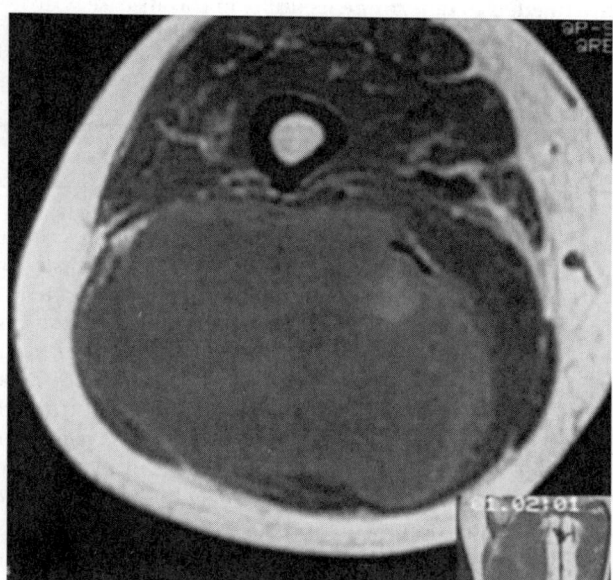

**FIGURES 32-12, 32-13** MRI imaging of a 62-year-old female with an enlarging posterior thigh mass. Biopsy revealed a liposarcoma. Both axial (32-12) and coronal (32-13) views reveal the large mass, which was treated with preoperative irradiation and limb salvage surgery.

Local tumor control approached 90%, but the complication rate was very high at 35% and consisted of wound sloughs and fractures. Lowering the radiation dose only reduced the complication to 25%. Nevertheless, some centers continue to use this method.

Brachytherapy is a technique in which catheters are placed in the tumor bed during surgery and one to two days later loaded with radioactive sources such as iridium 192. This method is utilized with large, deep tumor that is close to a neurovascular bundle. It is a technically tedious procedure. In a randomized prospective study, 117 patients who received brachytherapy were found to have decreased local recurrence as compared with patients who received external beam.[65] The wound complication rate is 22%, which is significantly higher than in the external beam group. This treatment may be given in lower doses to minimize complications.

Patients with soft tissue sarcomas often achieve improved local control but frequently develop distant metastases. Initially, studies using chemotherapy, specifically doxorubicin, were solely for patients with metastatic soft tissue sarcoma. These patients had prolonged survival. However, cardiac toxicity is a concern.

Based on these results, trials were designed to examine the role of adjuvant chemotherapy in the management of soft tissue sarcoma. Single-agent studies utilizing doxorubicin showed no improvement in disease-free survival or survival.[66] In the search to find better chemotherapy agents, multiagent trials for soft tissue sarcoma were initiated. One study showed improved disease-free survival but no improvement in overall survival utilizing doxorubicin and cyclophosphamide.[67] Recently, ifosfamide has been effective. The role of chemotherapy in the adjuvant setting for soft tissue sarcoma is still in its infancy. Further trials are needed to determine its utility in this disease. Cardioprotectant may improve our ability to raise doses safely.

# METASTATIC BONE TUMORS

Half of the million cancers diagnosed in the United States each year metastasize to bone. The three mechanisms by which a tumor spreads from the primary site to bone are direct extension to adjacent bones, arterial embolization, and direct venous spread through the pelvic and vertebral veins known as *Batson's plexus*. The common tumor locations include breast, lung, prostate, kidney, and thyroid. Other primary sites can metastasize but are less common. The mechanism for spread explains the affinity for bony metastasis to occur in the spine, pelvis, ribs, skull, and proximal long bones.

The patient commonly presents with skeletal pain that worsens with rest and a prior cancer history, and is greater than 40 years of age. An individual can experience a pathological fracture, in some reports up to 90%.[68] Individuals with spinal metastasis may have radicular pain, paresthesias, heaviness of limbs, leg buckling, and episodes of dropping items.[69] Compression of the spinal cord, which needs immediate treatment to prevent progressive neurological injury, includes symptoms of pain, hyperreflexia, weakness of lower limbs, sensory loss, and loss of bowel and bladder control. In addition, individuals can present with hypercalcemia due to extensive bone lysis (see chapter 25). Tumor invading bone marrow can result in abnormal production of leukocytes, thrombocytes, and erythrocytes. Transfusions and antibiotic treatments or prophylaxis may be needed (see chapter 22).

Diagnostic testing includes a biopsy if the individual has no known primary tumor. This biopsy is usually performed with a needle. A solitary lesion needs to be worked up as if it is a primary tumor, with local radiographic imaging such as a CT scan or MRI and a biopsy.[70] Other tests include laboratory tests such as serum acid phosphatase, which may lead to the primary site. A technetium bone scan is utilized to determine which bones are involved. Plain radiographs of areas positive on bone scan as well as any painful sites are done. Half of trabecular bone is destroyed before plain radiographs reveal lesions. MRI is useful for imaging spinal lesions as well as spinal cord compression.[71]

Chemotherapy for the primary site may result in pain reduction, decrease in the size of bony lesions, and stabilization of the number of lesions (see chapter on specific cancer). Other treatments must be timed appropriately if myelosuppression occurs. Surgical wounds need one to two weeks to develop collagen synthesis before chemotherapy is reinstituted.

Radiation is most commonly given by the external beam route to the involved sites. The goal of this treatment is to relieve pain, improve bone strength, and improve neurological deficits. In 1982, 49 U.S. institutions were studied to determine that the median dose was 30 Gy utilizing 10 fractions.[72] Pain relief occurred any time from 48 hours to eight weeks. Early pain relief can be attributed to release of chemical pain mediators and later pain cessation contributed to tumor lysis. Systemic radiation for diffuse bony metastasis can be given with radioisotopes such as strontium 89.[73] Repeat visits to the radiation department are avoided by administering the medication as a single dose. Pain relief is over 60% for those persons. Radiation may be utilized solely or combined with surgery.

Extremity lesions are managed by either arthroplasty or stabilization surgery. Pathological fractures preclude an individual's ability to walk, to maintain independence, and to experience pain relief. In addition, lesions greater than 2.5 cm in diameter and involving 50% of the cortex are at risk of fracture and need prophylactic stabilization.[74] Other authors propose predicting risk of pathological fracture by estimating load-bearing requirements.[75] It is recommended that impending fractures be fixed to decrease surgical morbidity and decrease the hospitalization time. The surgical procedures can range from an intramedullary stabilizing device, internal fixation, or a prosthetic arthroplasty with or without an allograft. Bone cement or methylmethacrylate can be used to fill the cavity created by the tumor to further stabilize the implant. Rarely, an amputation may be done to relieve pain or to treat a nonhealing fracture. The surgical goal is to permit patients full weight bearing.

Spinal lesions require surgery if conservative treatment such as steroids, radiation, and bracing have failed, progressive neurological symptoms develop, and/or spinal instability is present. Bracing is rarely comfortable if the person has rib, pelvis, or other spine lesions. The procedure consists of debulking the tumor followed by stabilization using instrumentation such as Cotrel-Dubousset, Isola, or Moss. Vertebral body replacement may range from a Moss cage filled with methylmethacrylate, bone from patients (autograft), bone from another human (allograft), or a vertebral fiber-metal prosthesis.[76] The goal of surgery is to improve function, optimally without use of a brace, and to improve ambulation.

The ongoing concern of those providing care to patients with metastatic bone tumors is prevention of fracture. In a study of 54 individuals with skeletal metastasis while undergoing rehabilitation, all were found to have a low risk of fracture during rehabilitation. Fractures did occur while persons were in bed.[77] Therefore, rehabilitation was recommended for this group. Nurses should be aware of bony involvement in order to plan nursing care, especially transfers. Carefully executed care is not a guarantee against pathological fractures.[78] Equally important is thoughtful ongoing pain management utilizing opioid and nonsteroidal anti-inflammatory medication.[79]

## SYMPTOM MANAGEMENT AND SUPPORTIVE CARE

### Pain

Pain is often the presenting symptom of a bone sarcoma and, at times, a soft tissue sarcoma. It may be severe enough to interfere with sleep. Pain management may begin with nonsteroidal anti-inflammatories, progress to mild narcotics such as codeine, and eventually need opiates such as morphine or methadone. Administering these medications on an outpatient basis and with concurrent treatment such as chemotherapy and radiation is a complex endeavor. Multiple phone calls are needed to assess the effectiveness of pain medication as well as medication side effects. Attention must be given to the patient's other responsibilities, i.e., career, home responsibilities such as child care, driving a vehicle. Use of walking aids may also be ordered to take weight off the involved limb for pain relief and to prevent a fracture.

### Limitations of Mobility

The tumor may limit motion of a joint and/or the ability to use the limb. Assistive devices such as a sling, crutches, or a cane may be necessary to support the involved area and prevent fracture. These devices may cause other disabilities such as inability to work, attend school, clean house, use public transportation, or go to the grocery store. The nurse or other health care provider may need to supply the individual with interventions such as handicapped license plates to park closer to stores, a letter to work requesting light duty, arrangements for a home aide to assist with housekeeping, and possibly encouragement to the patient to arrange transportation with family members. Hopefully, these limitations will decrease, but the treatments may lead to additional limitations of mobility. Continued assessment of the limitations of mobility need to be made, with appropriate interventions as needed.

## CONTINUITY OF CARE: NURSING CHALLENGES

One of the ongoing issues in the care of orthopedic oncology patients is negotiating for care out of system from the insurance plan. Multiple contacts and at times contracts with this insurance carrier are needed. Oncology nurses, especially in the outpatient setting, are frequently the insurance contact. Many states have one or two orthopedic oncology centers that have expert surgeons, oncologists, radiologists, pathologists, and nurses. The insurance carrier may not allow radiographic studies to be done at the center but will allow surgery. Physical therapy, either at home or on an outpatient basis, may be approved only by the insurance provider. It is important but nevertheless time-consuming to keep these communication lines open and convey information to the patient and his or her family.

Hospitalizations are becoming shorter. Discharge planning starts before admission and is a daily consideration. Modifying goals such as walking short distances instead of walking long distances and flexing the knee to 90° allows lengths of stay to be shorter. However, insurance carriers are less familiar with this population than with a breast cancer patient. Additional verbal and written communication may be needed to justify even shortened lengths of stay. Utilizing home services such as home nurses and home transfusion services are other methods to return the patient home.

Certain patients are too weak, immobile, or experiencing too much pain to be discharged to the home. Alternative plans such as having the patient go to a family member's home or transfer to a skilled nursing facility or rehabilitation facility may be necessary. Again, obtaining approval of the insurance carrier is crucial.

Many treatments are administered in ambulatory areas, including the vast majority of radiation treatment, biopsies, and much of chemotherapy. Coordination of appointments around friends' and family's schedules, work schedules, school schedules, and around other doctor and treatment appointments is time-consuming but crucial to keep multidisciplinary treatments on track.

Home care, as previously mentioned, is available for nearly all treatments such as initiating and discontinuing chemotherapy infusion pumps, setting up devices known as continuous passive movement devices to facilitate range of motion after limb salvage surgery, and assisting the patient in doing complex dressing or even monitoring wounds. Making the decision to use these services must entail obtaining insurance approval, patient approval, and an understanding of the cost and quality of the services. Having a home nurse going in for a wound assessment twice a week is not necessary if the patient is in the chemotherapy clinic twice a week and could have a wound check there. Frequent phone calls are another method to assess status of pain, wound drainage, and other problems if the patient and family are able to accurately describe these problems.

Care of self has been previously discussed under limitations of mobility. One of the most difficult aspects of self-care is that these previously independent individuals have short- and long-term periods in which they need family or professional assistance in the home. Some adjustment is to be expected.

## CONCLUSION

The treatment of bone and soft tissue sarcomas is complex. The overall survival rates have improved since the late 1970s. Progress can be attributed to factors such as improved staging, adjuvant chemotherapy, and pulmonary resections. With the advent of limb salvage surgery, fewer patients are having amputations, without altering their survival rates. It is hoped that ongoing studies of chemotherapy, surgery, radiation, and molecular genes will continue to show improved survival rates for bone and soft tissue sarcoma.

## REFERENCES

1. Parker SL, Tong T, Wingo P, Bolden B: Cancer statistics, 1996. *CA: Cancer J Clin* 46:5–29, 1996
2. Tucker M, D'Angio G, Boice J, et al: Bone sarcomas linked to radiotherapy and chemotherapy in children. *N Engl J Med* 317:588–593, 1987
3. Sorenson SA, Mulvihill J, Nielsen A: Long-term follow-up of Von Recklinghausen neurofibromatosis survival and malignant neoplasms. *N Engl J Med* 314:1010–1015, 1986
4. Hajdu SI, Rosen G: Sarcomas, in Calabresy P (ed.): *Medical Oncology: Basic Principles and Clinical Management.* New York, Macmillan, 1985, pp 1193–1225
5. Miller RW: Deaths from childhood leukemia and solid tumors among twins and other sibs in the United States, 1960–67. *NCI Monogr* 46:203–209, 1971
6. Uhthoff H: *Current Concept of Diagnosis and Treatment of Bone and Soft Tissue Tumor.* Berlin, Springer-Verlag, 1984, pp 195–236
7. Hansen M: Molecular genetic consideration in osteosarcoma. *Clin Orthop* 270:237–246, 1991
8. Araki N, Uchida A, Kimura T, et al: Involvement of the retinoblastoma gene in primary osteosarcomas and other bone and soft tissue tumors. *Clin Orthop* 270:271–277, 1991
9. Mazanet R, Antman K: Sarcomas of soft tissue and bone. *Cancer* 68:463–473, 1991
10. Lodwick G: Solitary malignant tumors of bone. *Semin Roentgenol* 1:293–313, 1966
11. Zimmer W, Berquist T, McLeod R, et al: Bone tumor magnetic resonance imaging versus computed tomography. *Radiology* 155:709–718, 1985
12. Shives T: Biopsy of soft tissue tumors. *Clin Orthop* 289:32–35, 1993
13. Ramanna L, Waxman A, Binney G, et al: Thallium-201 scintigraphy in bone sarcoma: Comparison with gallium-67 and technetium-MDP in evaluation of chemotherapeutic response. *J Nucl Med* 31:567, 1990
14. American Joint Committee on Cancer: *Manual for Staging of Cancer* (ed 4). Philadelphia, Lippincott, 1992, p 127–137
15. Schajowicz F: *Tumors and Tumor-like Lesions of Bone: Pathology, Radiology and Treatment* (ed 2). New York, Springer-Verlag, 1994
16. Enneking WF, Spanier S, Goodman M: A system for surgical staging of musculoskeletal sarcomas. *Clin Orthop* 153:105–119, 1980
17. Unni K: *Dahlin's Bone tumors* (ed 5). New York, NY, Lippincott-Raven, 1996, pp 143–217
18. Consensus Conference: Limb-sparing treatment of adult soft tissue sarcoma and osteosarcomas. *JAMA* 254:1791–1794, 1985
19. Lewis M: The use of an expandable and adjustable prosthesis in the treatment of childhood malignant bone tumors of the extremity. *Cancer* 57:499–502, 1986
20. Krajbich J: Modified Van Nes rotationplasty in the treatment of malignant neoplasms in the lower extremities of children. *Clin Orthop* 262:74–77, 1991
21. Cammisa F, Glasser D, Phil M, et al: The Van Nes tibial rotationplasty. *J Bone Joint Surg* 72A:1541–1547, 1990
22. Malawer M, Chou L: Prosthetic survival and clinical results with use of large segment replacements in treatment of high-grade sarcoma. *J Bone Joint Surg* 77A:1154–1165, 1995
23. Piasecki P: The nursing role in limb salvage surgery. *Nurs Clin North Am* 26:33–41, 1991
24. Otis J, Lane J, Kroll M, et al: Energy cost during gait in osteosarcoma patients after resection and knee replacement and after above-the-knee amputation. *J Bone Joint Surg Am,* 67:606–610, 1985
25. Buck B, Malinin T, Brown M: Bone transplantation and human immunodeficiency virus. *Clin Orthop* 249:129–136, 1989
26. Piasecki P, Rodts M: Bone banking: Its role in skeletal tumor reconstruction. *Orthop Nurs* 4(5):56–60, 1985
27. Enneking WF, Mindell ER: Observations on massive retrieved human allografts. *J Bone Joint Surg* 73A:1123–1142, 1991
28. Parrish FF: Allograft replacement of all or part of the end of a long bone following excision of a tumor: Report of twenty-one cases. *J Bone Joint Surg Am,* 55:1–22, 1973
29. Gebhardt M, Flugstad D, Springfield D, et al: The use of bone

allografts for limb salvage in high-grade extremity osteosarcoma. *Clin Orthop* 270:181–196, 1991

30. Gitelis S, Heligman D, Quill G, et al: The use of large allograft for tumor reconstruction and salvage of the failed total hip arthroplasty. *Clin Orthop* 231:62–70, 1988

31. Piasecki P: Update in orthopaedic oncology. *Orthop Nurs* 11(6):36, 38–43, 1992

32. Power R, Wood D, Tomford W, et al: Revision osteoarticular allograft transplantation in weight-bearing joints. *J Bone Joint Surg* 73B:595–599, 1991

33. Tomford W, Thongphasuk J, Mankin H, et al: Frozen musculoskeletal allografts. *J Bone Joint Surg* 72A:1137–1150, 1990

34. Eilber FR, Morton DL, Eckardt J, et al: Limb salvage for skeletal and soft tissue sarcomas. *Cancer* 54:2579–2589, 1984

35. Dick H, Malinin T, Mnaymneh W, et al: Massive allograft implantation following radical resection of high-grade tumor requiring adjuvant chemotherapy treatment. *Clin Orthop* 197:88–95, 1985

36. Goorin A, Shuster J, Baker A, et al: Changing pattern of pulmonary metastases with adjuvant chemotherapy in patients with osteosarcoma: Results from the multiinstitutional osteosarcoma study. *J Clin Oncol* 9:600–605, 1991

37. Snyder C, Saltzman D, Ferrell K, et al: A new approach to the resection of pulmonary osteosarcoma metastases. *Clin Orthop* 270:247–253, 1991

38. Michael J, Gailey R, Bowker J: New developments in recreational prostheses and adaptive devices for the amputee. *Clin Orthop* 256:64–75, 1990

39. Williamson V: Amputation of the lower extremity: An overview. *Orthop Nurs* 11(2):55–65, 1992

40. Lane J, Kroll M, Rossbach P: New advances and concepts in amputee management after treatment for bone and soft tissue sarcoma. *Clin Orthop* 256:22–28, 1990

41. Melzack R: *The Challenge of Pain.* New York, Basic Books, 1983, pp 265–355

42. Sherman R, Ernst J, Barja R, et al: Phantom pain: A lesson in the necessity for careful clinical research on chronic pain problems. *J Rehabil Res Dev* 25(2):7–10, 1988

43. Cohen L, Hendrickson J, Mansell J, et al: Response of sarcomas of bone and of soft tissue to neutron beam therapy. *Int J Radiat Oncol Biol Phys* 10:821–824, 1984

44. Issels R, Prenninger S, Nagele A, et al: Ifosfamide plus etoposide combined with regional hyperthermia in patients with locally advanced sarcomas. *J Clin Oncol* 8:1818–1829, 1990

45. Burk C, Belasco J, O'Neill J, et al: Pulmonary metastases and bone sarcomas. *Clin Orthop* 262:88–92, 1991

46. Malawer M: Impact of short course of neoadjuvant chemotherapy and the choice of surgical procedure for high grade sarcoma of extremities. *Proc Am Soc Clin Oncol* 8:320, 1989

47. Elias A, Ryan L, Aisner J, et al: Ifosfamide, mesna, doxorubicin, dacarbazine regime for adults with advanced sarcoma. *Semin Oncol* 17(2):41–49, 1990

48. Wornom I, Bochman S: *Bone and Cartilaginous Tissue.* In Cohen I, Piegelman R, Lindblad W (eds): *Wound Healing.* Philadelphia, Saunders, 1992, pp 356–383

49. Raymond K: Surface osteosarcoma. *Clin Orthop* 270:140–148, 1991

50. Unni KK, Dahlin DC, Baebout JW: Periosteal osteogenic sarcoma. *Cancer* 3:2476–2485, 1976

51. Glasser D, Lane J: Stage IIB osteogenic sarcoma. *Clin Orthop* 270:29–39, 1991

52. Bacci G, Picci P, Pignatti G, et al: Neoadjuvant chemotherapy for non-metastatic osteosarcoma of the extremities. *Clin Orthop* 270:87–98, 1991

53. Sutow WW, Gehan E, Dyment P, et al: Multidrug adjuvant chemotherapy of osteosarcoma: Interim report of Southwest Oncology Group studies. *Cancer Treat Res* 62:265–270, 1978

54. Gitelis S, Bertoni S, Picci P, et al: Chondrosarcoma of bone. *J Bone Joint Surg Am,* 63:1248–1257, 1981

55. Bacci G, Toni A, Maddelena A, et al: Long-term results in 144 localized Ewing's sarcoma patients treated with combined therapy. *Cancer* 63:1477–1486, 1989

56. Wilkin R, Pritchard P, Burgert E, et al: Ewing's sarcoma of bone: Experience with 140 patients. *Cancer* 58:2551–2555, 1991

57. Magrath I, Sandlund J, Raynor A, et al: A phase II study of ifosfamide in treatment of recurrent sarcomas in young people. *Cancer Chemother Pharmacol* 18(2):25–28, 1986 (suppl)

58. Donaldson S: The value of adjuvant chemotherapy in the management of sarcomas in children. *Cancer* 55:2184–2197, 1985

59. O'Connor M, Pritchard D: Ewing's sarcoma. *Clin Orthop* 262:78–87, 1991

60. Rosenthal H, Terek R, Lane J: Management of extremity soft tissue sarcoma. *Clin Orthop* 289:66–72, 1993

61. Rydholm A, Gustafson P, Rooser B, et al: Limb-sparing surgery without radiotherapy based on anatomic locale of soft tissue sarcoma. *J Clin Oncol* 9:1757–1765, 1991

62. O'Connor M, Pritchard D, Gunderson M: Integration of limb-sparing surgery, brachytherapy and external beam irradiation in treatment of soft tissue sarcoma. *Clin Orthop* 289:73–80, 1993

63. Gitelis S, Thomas R, Templeton A, et al: Characterization of the pseudocapsule of soft tissue sarcomas. *Clin Orthop* 246:285–292, 1989

64. Eilber F, Morton D, Eckardt J, et al: Limb salvage for skeletal and soft tissue sarcomas, multidisciplinary preoperative therapy. *Cancer* 53:2579–2590, 1984

65. Shiu M, Hilaris B, Harrison H, et al: Brachytherapy and functional saving resection of soft tissue sarcoma arising in limb. *Int J Radiat Oncol Biol Phys* 21:1485–1492, 1991

66. Eilber I, Giuliano A, Huth J, et al: A randomized prospective trial using postoperative adjuvant chemotherapy in high-grade extremity sarcoma. *Am J Clin Oncol* 11:39–45, 1988

67. Elias A: Chemotherapy for soft tissue sarcoma. *Clin Orthop* 289:94–105, 1993

68. Malawer M, Delaney T: Treatment of metastatic cancer to bone, in DeVita V, Helman S, Rosenberg S (eds.): *Cancer: Principles and Procedures of Oncology.* Philadelphia, Lippincott, 1989, pp 2225–2245

69. Weinstein J: Differential diagnosis and surgical treatment of pathological spine fractures, in Eilert R (ed.): *Instructional Course Lecture,* vol 41. Rosemont, IL: American Association of Orthopedic Surgeons, 1992, pp 301–315

70. Frassica F, Gitelis S, Sim F: Metastatic bone disease: General principles, pathophysiology, evaluation and biopsy, in Eilert R (ed.): *Instructional Course Lecture,* vol 41. Rosemont, IL American Association of Orthopedic Surgeons, 1992, pp 293–300

71. Trail Z, Richards M, Moore N: Magnetic resonance imaging of metastatic bone disease. *Clin Orthop* 312:76–88, 1995

72. Tong D, Gallick L, Hendrickson F: The palliation of symptomatic osseous metastases: Final results of the study by the Radiation Therapy Oncology Group. *Cancer* 50:893–899, 1982

73. Lehing A, Ackery D, Bayly R, et al: Strontium-89 therapy for pain palliation in prostatic skeletal malignancy. *Br J Radiol* 64:816–822, 1991

74. Sim F: Metastatic bone disease of the pelvis and femur, in

Eilert R (ed): *Instructional Course Lecture,* vol 41. Rosemont, IL: American Association of Orthopedic Surgeons, 1992, pp 317–327

75. Hipp J, Springfield D, Hayes W: Predicting pathological fracture risk in the management of metastatic bone defects. *Clin Orthop* 312:120–135, 1995

76. Hammerberg K: Surgical treatment of metastatic spine disease. *Spine* 17:1148–1153, 1992

77. Bunting R: Rehabilitation of cancer patients with skeletal metastases. *Clin Orthop* 312:76–88, 1995

78. Piasecki P: Nursing care of the patient with metastatic bone disease. *Orthop Nurs* 15(4):25–33, 1996

79. Twycross R: Management of pain in skeletal metastases. *Clin Orthop* 312:187–196, 1995

# Chapter 33

# Bladder and Kidney Cancer

**Julena Lind, RN, MN, MA, PhD(c)**

**Lynne Hagan, RN, BSN, CETN**

# BLADDER CANCER

## Epidemiology

Bladder cancer is the second most common genitourinary cancer after prostate cancer. It accounts for 4%–5% of cancers in the United States.[1]

The four major variables related to bladder cancer incidence are race, gender, age, and geographic location. In the United States the most outstanding epidemiological feature is the high incidence among white men. The age-adjusted bladder cancer rate in white men is twice the rate for black men.[2] In whites the bladder cancer ratio of men to women is 3:1. Average age at diagnosis is 65 years. There is a high incidence of squamous cell carcinoma of the bladder in certain areas of the world, notably Egypt. This is linked to the parasite *Schistosoma haemotobium.*

## Etiology

Bladder cancer is a multistep process of initiation and promotion. The exact genetic events leading to this transformation are unknown but probably involve activation of oncogenes and inactivation of cancer-suppressor genes. There is well-documented evidence of genetic changes in bladder cancer. High-grade bladder cancers have been noted to have an increased expression of the c-Ha-ras oncogene product *p21*, and the loss of genetic material on the long arm of chromosome 9 happens in all grades of bladder cancer.[3]

Human bladder cancer initiators and promoters have been identified which cause an alteration of the normal transfer of genetic information.

There are four etiologic hypotheses related to bladder cancer: cigarette smoking, occupational exposure to industrial chemicals, ingestion of other physical agents, and exposure to *S haemotobium.*

In the United States, only cigarette smoking and occupational exposure to aromatic amines are well-established risk factors.[2] Cigarette smoking was first associated with bladder cancer in 1956.[4] Since that time, most case-controlled studies report a twofold relative risk for cigarette smokers as compared with nonsmokers.[5] However, there are apparent inconsistencies between the case-controlled studies and supporting demographic evidence. For example, the incidence of smoking in women is increasing, while the incidence of bladder cancer in women is decreasing. Certain populations that have been studied for bladder cancer incidence, such as Polynesian men and American blacks, have a very high rate of cigarette smoking and a low incidence of bladder cancer.[2] Despite the inconsistencies, the overwhelming statistical evidence points to cigarette smoking as a prime epidemiological factor, accounting for as much as 50% of all bladder cancer in American

men and 31% in women.[3] The effect of cigarette smoking on bladder tissue seems to be different from that on lung cancer and is likely to be influenced by metabolic and genetic factors.

Among occupational exposure agents, arylamine(s), used in the synthetic textile dye industry, the rubber industry, hair dyes, and as paint pigment, is the class of chemical most strongly related to bladder cancer.[2] Beta-naphthylamine and benzidine are two examples of this chemical class. Occupations with relative risk estimates for bladder cancer of 2 or greater include janitors and cleaners, mechanics, miners, and printers.[5]

Ingestion of other physical agents, such as coffee, alcohol, saccharin, and phenacetin, have been weakly linked to bladder cancer. None of these agents has consistently been related to bladder cancer incidence in humans. The results of studies looking at coffee drinking as a possible etiologic factor in bladder cancer have generally been inconsistent, and the associated increases in risk are generally small.[2] A 1987 study of 823 men and 2469 age-matched controls showed no association between bladder cancer and alcohol.[5] Animal studies have shown that saccharin may cause bladder cancer in rodents.[2] However, several studies have failed to confirm any association.[3] Heavy regular use of phenacetin has also been suggested as an etiologic link; however, the results of various studies have been confusing.[2]

Schistosomiasis is rare in the United States but common in many African countries, especially Egypt. In areas where schistosomiasis is endemic, the incidence of squamous cell carcinoma of the bladder is much higher. In these areas a high percentage of the individuals with squamous cell bladder cancer are found to have *S haemotobium* ova in the bladder wall.[2]

## Pathophysiology

### Cellular characteristics

The urinary bladder is lined by transitional epithelium, often called the *urothelium.* About 90%–95% of bladder tumors in North America are transitional cell carcinomas that arise in the epithelial layer of the bladder. The epithelial layer rests on the basement membrane. Approximately 7% are squamous cell (associated with *S haemotobium*), and 2% are adenocarcinomas.[6]

Bladder cancer is a multifaceted problem. Major variables in the systems of classification are patterns of growth (in situ versus papillary versus solid), the presence or absence of invasion (the stage), and the degree of differentiation (the grade).[7]

Papillary tumors, although they may have a low cytological grade and be noninvasive, have a propensity for recurrence. Carcinoma in situ is usually multifocal and is associated with high recurrence rate and multicentricity, which necessitate aggressive follow-up after initial diagnosis and treatment.[7]

### Progression of disease

Many of these tumors arise on the floor of the bladder and may involve one or both of the ureteral orifices.[6] The growth rate varies depending on the histological type and grade of the tumor. The most important growth feature is the depth of penetration into the bladder wall.

Some tumors spread rapidly to the regional lymph nodes, which are the pelvic nodes just below the bifurcation of the common iliac arteries. Others grow more slowly and spread directly into pelvic tissues.

Growth occurs inward into the hollow aspect of bladder (in papillary tumors) and outward from the urothelial mucosa to the submucosa and to the detrusor muscle.

Metastasis takes place via direct extension out of the muscle of the bladder into the perivesicle fat (or serosa). Depending on the location of the tumor, it may obstruct the ureters or bladder neck and prostatic urethra. Figure 33-1, which shows the staging of bladder cancer, also depicts the anatomic spread within the bladder. Cancer can also spread by direct extension to involve other adjacent structures, particularly the sigmoid colon, the rectum, and/or the prostate, as well as the uterus and vagina. Hematogenous spread occasionally occurs to the bones, liver, and lungs.[6]

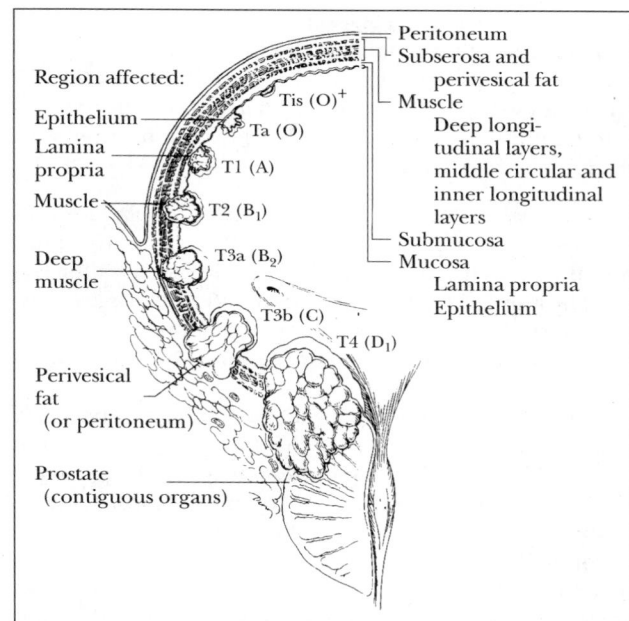

**FIGURE 33-1**   Staging of bladder cancer. (Caroll PR: Urothelial carcinoma: Cancers of the bladder, ureter, and renal pelvis, in Tanagho EA, McAninch JW (eds): *Smith's General Urology* [ed 14]. Norwalk, CT, Appleton and Lange, 1995, p 355.)

## Clinical Manifestations

Gross hematuria is the most common presenting symptom of bladder cancer. Painless hematuria is usually present through the entire stream of urine. This bleeding is rarely profuse, often microscopic, and usually intermittent.

Another symptom is irritability of the bladder. This manifests itself as dysuria, urinary frequency, and urgency and burning on urination if infection is present.

Symptoms associated with large tumor growth or metastasis also may be present. If the tumor is pushing on the internal urethral orifice, symptoms of bladder neck obstruction may be present, including urinary hesitancy and decrease in the force and caliber of the stream. Obstruction of the ureters can cause flank pain and results in hydronephrosis.

Pain in the suprapubic region, rectum, or back, as well as symptoms of lung, bone, or liver metastasis, occurs occasionally in individuals with advanced disease.

## Assessment

### Physical examination

There are no early signs of bladder cancer on physical examination. An invasive mass in the trigonal area occasionally may be revealed by rectal examination.

### Diagnostic studies

*Cytology*   Exfoliative urinary cytology is a relatively simple diagnostic tool in the assessment of bladder cancer. Many experts recommend the collection of a total voided specimen obtained in the late morning or early afternoon and sent immediately for cytology to reduce the chance of obscuring the results. Bladder washings obtained through saline irrigation of the bladder produce even more reliable results.[8]

*Flow cytometry*   For superficial transitional cell bladder cancer, identification of patients who are at risk of recurrent disease and/or progression to a higher stage is critical to assessment. Flow cytometry, which is a technique used to examine the DNA content of urine cells, has been useful in providing prognostic information beyond grading and staging. In this technique the interaction of fluorochromes or dyes with DNA causes the emission of light on exposure to high-intensity light (like a laser). Machines are able to analyze large numbers of urine samples, sort the urine cells by size, and indirectly measure the DNA content. This procedure can also be done on biopsy specimens and bladder washings.[9] Aneuploidy, or large numbers of DNA per cell, is an indication of high-grade, high-stage transitional cell tumors.[9]

*Excretory urogram (intravenous pyelogram)*   Excretory urogram (intravenous urogram) should be done prior to cystoscopy to help in evaluating the upper tracts at the same time.[4] Although it is not a conclusive diagnostic tool, excretory urography can help evaluate a suspected bladder tumor by possibly showing the tumor itself or by showing evidence of ureteral obstruction (hydronephrosis). Urethral obstruction also may be demonstrated with excretory urography.

***Cystoscopy*** Although initial diagnosis of bladder cancer is usually made using office cystoscopy and topical anesthesia, definitive evaluation requires general or spinal anesthesia.[8] Cystoscopic examination can serve several purposes: tumor visualization, an opportunity for biopsy, and an opportunity for bimanual examination of the bladder.

Once the tumor is visualized, a deep biopsy specimen is taken from the center of the tumor and its outside border. The goal of these biopsies is to assess the presence or absence of muscle invasion. Multiple biopsy specimens of the rest of the bladder wall, the bladder neck, and the trigone also may be taken to diagnose carcinoma in situ or atypia. Selected mucosal biopsy can also be an effective adjunct to the management of superficial bladder cancer.[7]

The development of the flexible fiberoptic cystoscope has made outpatient cystoscopy easier, reduced the morbidity, and made possible the use of local or regional anesthesia.[8]

Bimanual palpation performed under anesthesia may detect a palpable tumor or induration, which could indicate deep muscle invasion, inflammation of the tumor site, or extension of the tumor into the serosa.

***Tumor markers*** The expression of blood-group antigens on the surface of bladder cancer cells has proved to be a useful prognostic determinant. Tumors that elaborate A, B, or H antigens are often associated, stage for stage, with a better prognosis than tumors that do not express antigens.[3]

Recently it has been found that epidermal growth factor (EGF), a potent mitogen and tumor promoter, is overexpressed in late-stage bladder cancer. The presence of EGF and its receptor, epidermal growth factor receptor (EGFR), could prove to be useful molecular markers of tumor persistence, recurrence, and treatment response.[10] Overexpression of the *p53* nuclear oncoprotein has also been associated with a poorer prognosis.[11]

***Ultrasound, computerized tomography, magnetic resonance imaging*** Both abdominal and transurethral ultrasound have been used to define the local extension and the degree of involvement of the bladder wall.

Advocates of using computerized tomography (CT) scans in staging bladder cancer feel that they aid in defining the extent of the local tumor and in identifying pelvic lymph node metastasis.[6]

Magnetic resonance imaging (MRI) has been successful in distinguishing cancer from the normal bladder wall, as the tumor generates a higher signal intensity.[12] It has also been used to identify the presence of pelvic lymph node involvement.

The main advantage of CT and MRI is to distinguish organ-confined disease from extravesical extension.[3]

## Classification and Staging

Two staging systems for bladder cancer are currently in widespread use, the Jewett-Strong system (modified by Marshall) and the TNM system developed by the American Joint Committee for Cancer Staging and End Results Reporting (Table 33-1, Table 33-2, and Figure 33-1). A compilation of these systems is depicted in Figure 33-1.

Another factor sometimes considered in treatment but not included in the staging systems is the grade of the tumor, or its degree of cell differentiation.

Grading of bladder tumors is commonly done to predict the speed of recurrence and the progression to invasion and metastases. The more well-differentiated bladder tumors (low-grade) generally have a slower growth rate and therefore a better prognosis. The grades for cancer of the bladder are usually referred to as grade I, II, III, or IV, with IV designating the least well differentiated.

## Treatment

### Carcinoma in situ

Transurethral resection (TUR) and fulguration are the most common and conservative forms of management. Intravesicle treatment with thiotepa, mitomycin C, doxorubicin, or bacillus Calmette-Guerin (BCG) is used for patients with multiple tumors.[13] Radiotherapy has no proven value in the treatment of carcinoma in situ.[14]

### Superficial, low-grade tumors

More than 70% of the patients with bladder cancer present initially with superficial tumors (stages T0, Tis,

**TABLE 33-1    Jewett/Marshall Bladder Staging System**

| Stage 0 | Carcinoma in situ (CIS) or superficial papillary tumor confined to the mucosa with invasion |
|---|---|
| Stage A | Papillary tumor invading the lamina propria |
| Stage B1 | Tumor with superficial muscle invasion |
| Stage B2 | Tumor with deep muscle invasion |
| Stage C | Invasion of the perivesical fat |
| Stage D1 | Involvement of adjacent viscera and/or pelvic nodes |
| Stage D1 | Involvement of nodes above the aortic bifurcation or distant spread |

Adapted from Carroll PR: Urothelial carcinoma—cancers of the bladder, ureter, and renal pelvis, in Tanagho EA, McAninch JW (eds): *Smith's General Urology* (ed 14). Norwalk, CT: Appleton & Lange, 1995, pp 354–355

**TABLE 33-2** TNM Bladder Classification

| T = PRIMARY TUMOR | |
| --- | --- |
| TX | Primary tumor cannot be assessed |
| T0 | No evidence of primary tumor |
| Tis | Carcinoma in situ |
| Ta | Noninvasive papillary carcinoma |
| T1 | Tumor invades submucosa/lamina propria |
| T2 | Tumor invades superficial muscle |
| T3a | Tumor invades deep muscle |
| T3b | Tumor invades perivesical fat |
| T4 | Tumor invades adjacent organs |
| **N = REGIONAL LYMPH NODES (BELOW AORTIC BIFURCATION)** | |
| NX | Regional lymph nodes cannot be assessed |
| N0 | No regional lymph node metastasis |
| N1 | Metastasis in single node less than 2 cm |
| N2 | Metastasis in single node more than 2 cm but less than 5 cm, or multiple nodes less than 5 cm |
| N3 | Metastasis in nodes more than 5 cm |
| **M = DISTANT METASTASES** | |
| MX | Presence of distant metastasis cannot be assessed |
| M0 | No distant metastasis |
| M1 | Distant metastasis |

From: Beahrs OH, Henson DE, Hutter RVP, et al: *American Joint Committee on Cancer: Manual for Staging of Cancer.* Philadelphia: JB Lippincott Company, 4th ed., 1992, 197–201

Ta, and T1).[7] Superficial tumors of the bladder remain in the epithelium and lamina propria. In 80% of these patients, invasive tumors do not develop.[7] Standard treatment of these tumors is transurethral surgery with resection and fulguration (if there are multiple small lesions), laser therapy, or cystectomy. The overall five-year survival rate of patients with superficial bladder cancer treated with transurethral resection alone is approximately 80%.[7] Because the chance of recurrence is so great, intravesical chemotherapy is often given following surgery.

***Intravesical treatment*** Several agents have shown some effectiveness when instilled into the bladder, including thiotepa, mitomycin C, doxorubicin, and BCG. These agents are typically instilled into the bladder through a urethral catheter for two hours weekly for six weeks. To date there is no uniform consensus on the choice of drug, the timing for the start, the duration of treatment, or the schedule.[15] The most widely used drug for this purpose in the United States has been thiotepa. Dosages

vary from 30 to 60 mg diluted in equal amounts of sterile water. It is generally instilled and retained for one to two hours every week for six to eight weeks and in some instances at monthly intervals for two years thereafter. The drug's side effects include severe bladder irritability, myelosuppression, and renal failure if there is reflux.[15]

Mitomycin C also has been used in the treatment of superficial disease. Because it has limited intravesical absorption, myelosuppression is rare, and the major side effects are chemical cystitis and skin reactions from contact with the drug.[15] If, as some believe, the benefits of mitomycin C and thiotepa are comparable, the deciding factor might be the greater expense of using mitomycin C.

BCG is a live, attenuated culture preparation of the bacillus Calmette-Guerin strain of mycobacterium bovis. Unlike conventional intravesical chemotherapeutic agents that attack tumor cells directly, BCG is a biologic response modifier that is believed to exert its antitumor effect by stimulating various immune responses in the host. While the exact mechanism of action is unknown, it appears that direct contact between tumor cells and BCG is essential. Treatment with BCG has delayed progression and decreased the risk of death from bladder cancer.[16] This treatment is considered both safe and effective in treating superficial bladder cancer and in reducing transitional cell recurrences. It is considered the most successful adjuvant treatment for superficial recurrent bladder cancer.

A typical regimen begins one to two weeks after biopsy or transurethral resection of tumor and is repeated once a week for six treatments. For some patients a single six-week course of intravesical BCG is not sufficient and an additional six-week course is given.[3,7] Other protocols require BCG intravesically weekly for six weeks, then every other week times three, again at six months, and every six months for up to four years.[6,16] Most patients tolerate BCG instillation reasonably well, although side effects are expected as the patient becomes sensitized to the BCG. Side effects include dysuria, frequency of urination, and urgency, which occur three or four hours after the instillation. Mild hematuria associated with cystitis happens in about 50% of the patients and tends to occur after the third or fourth treatment.[3,16] Occasional influenza-like symptoms happen in about 25% of patients.[16]

***Laser therapy*** Small superficial bladder tumors have also been treated by laser beams. One of the most useful lasers is the neodymium yttrium-aluminum-garnet laser (Nd:YAG). This outpatient photodynamic therapy can be done through a small cystoscope, without causing bleeding or the stimulation of the obturator nerve, while the patient is under local anesthesia. The advantages are that it may be less likely than fulguration to promote tumor dissemination within the bladder, it can be performed under local anesthesia, it reduces the chance of bladder perforation, and an indwelling catheter is not necessary following the procedure.[3]

However, photodynamic therapy can be associated

with quite severe side effects, including inflammation of the bladder mucosa. Other disadvantages are that no tumor tissue is retrieved for histology, and it is not clear whether it offers substantial advantage over more conventional treatment.[7] Patients with recurrent superficial papillary tumors (Ta), who are at low risk for tumor progression, are good candidates for laser therapy.[15]

Partial (or segmental) cystectomy is advocated by some authorities but only for individuals with diffuse unresectable tumors or tumors that have not responded to intravesical therapy.[18] The success of partial cystectomy is much higher with stage A, grade I or II lesions. The greatest disadvantage of partial cystectomy is a high tumor recurrence rate.[18]

### Invasive tumors

Because of invasion of the bladder muscle, high-stage, high-grade tumors have dramatically altered prognoses. High-stage tumors are generally described as stages T2 to T4 or B1 to D1. Standard treatment options for invasive bladder cancer include radical cystectomy with or without pelvic lymph node dissection; external-beam irradiation (for nonsurgical candidates and other selected cases); interstitial implantation of radioisotopes alone and/or before/after external-beam irradiation; TUR with fulguration (in selected patients); segmental cystectomy (in selected patients); or combined external-beam irradiation with cisplatin.[3,6,19,20] Many protocols are under investigation, including chemotherapy (often methotrexate, vinblastine, doxorubicin, and cisplatin [MVAC] before or after cystectomy, or in conjunction with external-beam radiotherapy.[3,21-23]

***Radical cystectomy*** The term *radical cystectomy* in men is usually synonymous with prostatocystectomy. The procedure includes excision of the bladder with the pericystic fat, the attached peritoneum, and the entire prostate and seminal vesicles (Figure 33-2).

In women, radical cystectomy includes removal of the bladder and entire urethra, the uterus, ovaries, fallopian tubes, and the anterior wall of the vagina (Figure 33-3).

Including pelvic lymphadenectomy with this surgery is controversial. The evidence that it improves survival is sparse and inconclusive. Some surgeons have demonstrated that adding a meticulous lymph node dissection has resulted in a low incidence of pelvic recurrence compared with results for simple total cystectomy without dissection or preoperative radiation therapy.[6]

Complications of this surgical procedure include ureterocutaneous fistula, wound dehiscence, partial small bowel obstruction, wound infection, loss of sexual function, and small bowel fistula.[3]

***Cystectomy with urinary diversion*** Until the 1980s nearly all men who underwent radical cystectomy became impotent. To help patients overcome the problem of impotence after pelvic surgery, Walsh[24] described the neurovascular anatomy of the bladder and prostate more clearly and developed a surgical approach in which nerves

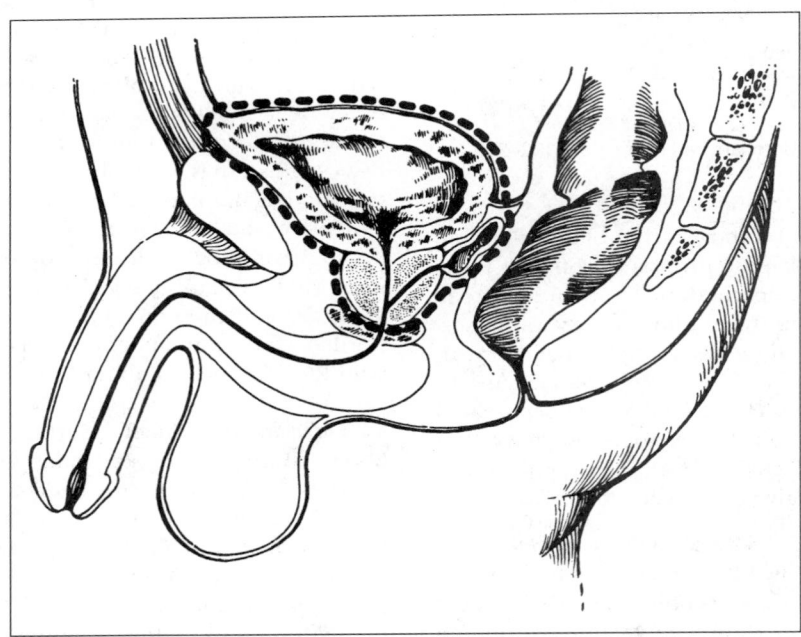

**FIGURE 33-2** Surgical boundaries of radical cystectomy in a man. The specimen includes the bladder, the prostate, and the seminal vesicles. (Swanson D: Cancer of the bladder and prostate: The impact of therapy on sexual function, in von Eschenbach AC, Rodriguez D (eds): *Sexual Rehabilitation of the Urologic Cancer Patient.* Boston, Hall, 1981, p 102.)

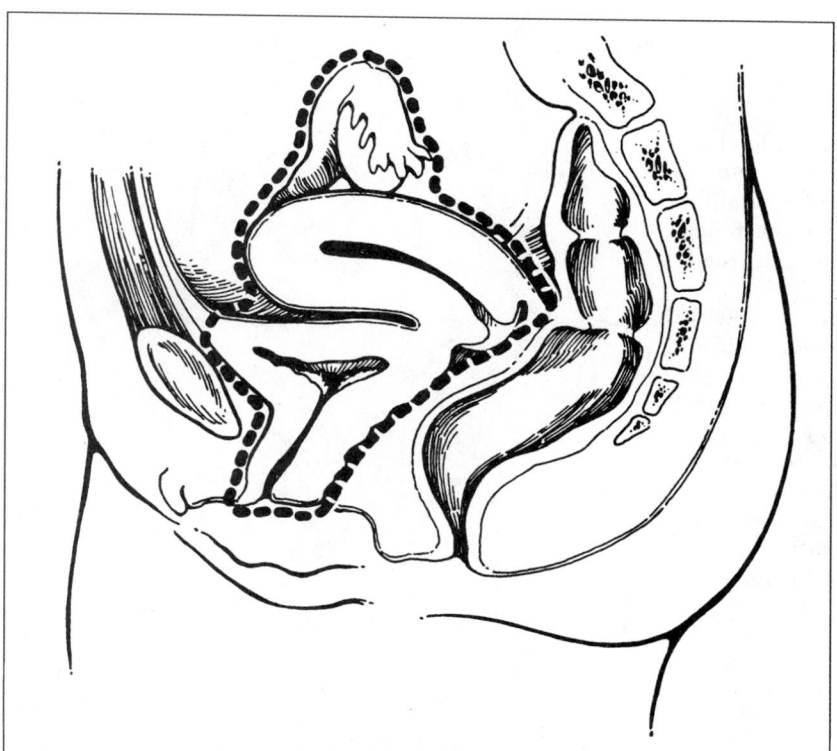

**FIGURE 33-3**   Surgical boundaries of radical cystectomy in a woman. The specimen includes the bladder and entire urethra, uterus, ovaries, fallopian tubes, and the anterior wall of the vagina. (Swanson D: Cancer of the bladder and prostate: The impact of therapy on sexual function, in von Eschenbach AC, Rodriguez D (eds): *Sexual Rehabilitation of the Urologic Cancer Patient.* Boston, Hall, 1981, p 103.)

crucial to the mechanisms of penile erection are spared. Although the majority of published experience relates to the management of prostate cancer, the removal of bladder cancer has also been performed in this way, and erectile potency has been preserved in 80% of young men.[7,24]

*Ileal conduit*   Since the early 1950s the Bricker ileal conduit has been a popular method of diverting urinary flow in the absence of bladder function. This procedure involves isolating a piece of terminal ileum, closing the proximal end, bringing the distal end out through a hole in the abdominal wall at a previously marked site, and suturing it to the skin, creating a stoma. It is important for proper functioning that the segment reach from the retroperitoneum to the skin comfortably and without tension on the distal (stoma) end.[25] The ureters are implanted into the ileal segment, urine flows into the conduit, and peristalsis propels it out through the stoma (Figure 33-4). Urinary stents may occasionally be threaded into the ureters to allow for free-flowing urine in the early postoperative period. Urinary stents are usually left in place for seven to ten days but may be left in longer at the physician's discretion.[25] Other portions of the bowel also have been used to divert the urine. Portions of the sigmoid colon are used infrequently as conduits in urinary diversions associated with bladder cancer. Construction of any of these conduits necessitates that the person wear an external collection appliance.

Complications are related to stoma construction and placement and to the possibility of long-term kidney damage. Stomas placed in skin creases, scars, or bony promi-

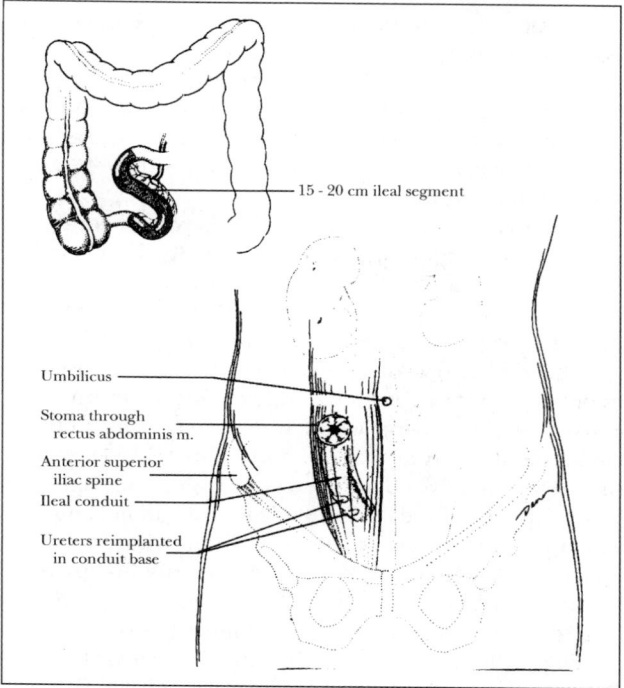

15 - 20 cm ileal segment

Umbilicus

Stoma through rectus abdominis m.

Anterior superior iliac spine

Ileal conduit

Ureters reimplanted in conduit base

**FIGURE 33-4**   Ileal conduit. (Caroll PR, Barbour S: Urinary diversion and bladder substitution, in Tanagho EA, McAninch JW (eds): *Smith's General Urology* [ed 14]. Norwalk, CT, Appleton and Lange, 1995, p 427.)

nences have difficulty with appliance adherence. Stomas that are flush with the skin and recessed have problems with appliance fit. Other complications include stomal stenosis, which has a host of sequelae, including pain, stones, and potential pyelonephritis. Recent studies have indicated a high incidence of ureteral reflux and ascending infection that results in late kidney deterioration. Despite the long-term complications, the Bricker ileal conduit is still the most widely used form of urinary diversion.[3,26]

*Ureterosigmoidostomy*   Ureterosigmoidostomy involves implanting the ureters into the sigmoid colon utilizing an antirefluxing anastomosis. The urine is then excreted through the rectum. Before Bricker described the ileal conduit in 1950, the ureterosigmoidostomy was the most popular form of urinary diversion. The early and late complications include metabolic acidosis because of the absorptive quality of the sigmoid colon, potassium depletion, anastomotic stenosis, and ascending infection, particularly in individuals with impaired renal function. This surgical procedure is rare today.

***Continent urinary diversion***   In recent years there has been a surge of enthusiasm for continent urinary diversions. Continent urinary diversions were created in an attempt to better substitute for the functions of the lower urinary tract. Ideally, voiding of urine should be under voluntary control at convenient intervals, and the upper renal tract should be protected from both obstruction and urine reflux. Continent diversions offer the patient opportunity for control of voiding and urinary reflux by the creation of low-pressure reservoirs and the use of one-way valves.[26]

There are several types of continent urinary diversions currently being performed. They differ, largely, in the portion of intestine used to create the pouch; the presence, absence, and/or number of valves; and the location of the urinary outlet.

*Kock pouch*   Figure 33-5 illustrates a type of continent reservoir technique originated by Nils Kock in Sweden and first reported in the United States in 1982 by Kock and associates.[27] Urinary diversion through a continent ileal reservoir provides an intra-abdominal pouch for storage of urine and two nipple valves that maintain continence and prevent ureteral reflux. One procedure for constructing the urinary pouch describes using a 60–70-cm segment of ileum, isolated approximately 50 cm from the ileocecal valve. The ureters are anastomosed to a short segment of the ileum that leads into an ileal nipple, which prevents reflux of the urine to the kidneys. Proximal to this segment, two 22-cm segments are used to create the reservoir pouch itself. The remaining segment is used for the continence nipple and the stoma.[28]

The outlet for the reservoir may be brought to the skin, urethra, and/or rectum. Since 1985 male patients have been candidates for the Kock pouch to the urethra. In 1991 the procedure was also modified for female patients.[29]

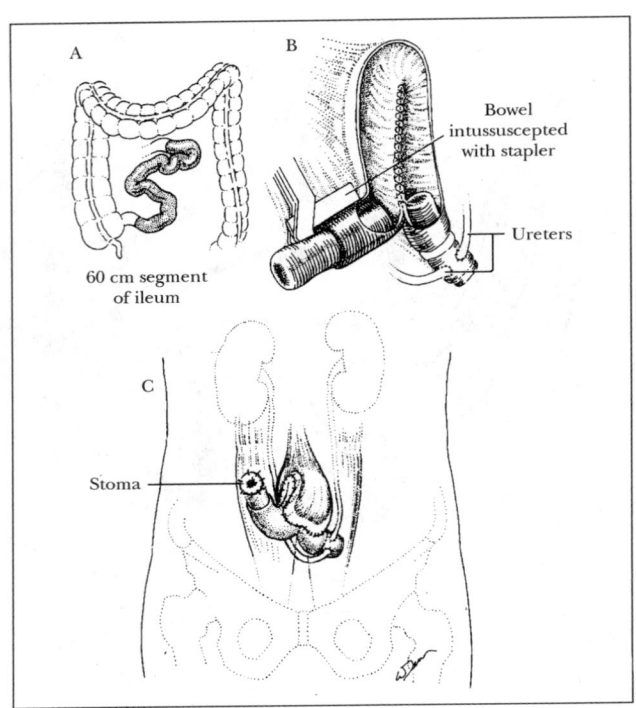

**FIGURE 33-5**   Kock pouch urinary reservoir. (A) 60 cm of small intestine selected. (B) Afferent (nonrefluxing) limb or ureteral reimplantation and efferent limb for stoma fashioned using stapling devices. (C) Completed reservoir. (Caroll PR, Barbour S: Urinary diversion and bladder substitution, in Tanagho EA, McAninch JW (eds): *Smith's General Urology* [ed 14]. Norwalk, CT, Appleton and Lange, 1995 p 454.)

When the lengthy surgical procedure is almost complete, a number 30 Medena tube (for a Kock pouch to the skin) or a 24 french Foley catheter (for a Kock pouch to the urethra) is passed into the pouch and positioned so that the drainage holes are several centimeters beyond the efferent nipple. This tube is sutured in place to secure it for three weeks. A flat latex drain called a *Penrose drain* is passed through a stab wound on the abdomen. Inside the abdomen, the drain is placed just beneath the newly created Kock pouch. It is secured to the skin with sutures and covered with a drainage bag to collect the fluid.

To prevent mucus obstruction postoperatively, the Medena tube should be irrigated every four hours or more with 30–60 ml of normal saline. Three weeks following surgery the reservoir is checked radiographically for any signs of extravasation. If the reservoir is patent the Medena tube is removed and the patient is taught self-catheterization technique, or the Foley catheter is removed and the patient is instructed on voiding techniques, beginning at two- to three-hour intervals.

Late complications usually involve problems with continence or catheterization, such as urinary leakage at the stoma or through the urethra, difficult catheterization, electrolyte abnormalities, pyelonephritis, hydronephrosis, and stone formation.

*Indiana reservoir*   The Indiana reservoir is another type of continent diversion. It is constructed from the cecum, the ascending colon, the ileocecal valve, and the terminal ileum. The colon is opened for its entire length in order to eliminate the normal peristaltic motion of the intestine and to create the pouch. The ureters are tunneled into the wall of the bowel. The ileocecal valve and the terminal ileum are fashioned into a structure that serves as a natural continence mechanism, preventing the outflow of urine.[30] The creation of an Indiana reservoir is technically less difficult than the Kock pouch because it does not require the creation of nipple valves from bowel.[30]

*Other continent urinary reservoirs*   There are many other reservoirs being constructed that are modifications of the Indiana reservoir. Some of these modifications include the Mainz pouch (right colon, cecum, and adjacent ileum) and the Florida pouch (right colon, distal ileum, ileocecal valve). These reservoirs differ from the Kock pouch in that they use different segments of the bowel to construct the pouch and to fashion the continent valves.[30] Table 33-3 illustrates the differences in construction of the pouches.

The Camey procedure is a technique of bladder substitution that uses a 40-cm segment of the ileum that is anastomosed directly to the urethra and to the ureters above the iliac vessels.[31]

***Postsurgical sexuality***   A radical cystectomy with urinary diversion, performed in the traditional manner, particularly if accompanied by a lymphadenectomy, can affect many aspects of sexual functioning. The etiology of physiological sexual dysfunction in men is similar to that associated with treatment for prostatic cancer. In addition, the psychological impact of a stoma and external appliance may contribute to changes in body image and libido.[32]

Erectile impotence that results after radical cystectomy (or radical prostatectomy) may be helped by the insertion of a penile prosthesis.[33] There are several types, all of which continue to be refined. The semirigid prostheses are malleable plastic rods that are inserted into the corpus cavernosa. The result is a permanent semierection that is not painful and does not interfere with daily activi-

ties. The Jonas prosthesis is an example of the semirigid type (Figure 33-6). There are also several types of inflatable prostheses that make it possible to control erectile function. The single-component inflatable prosthesis (FlexiFlate and Hydroflex) has inflating and deflating mechanisms contained in one cylinder, which is implanted in the scrotum. There are also two- and three-piece inflatable prostheses.[34]

In women, removal of the ovaries and uterus will result in sexuality changes similar to those following hysterectomy and oophorectomy for gynecologic malignancies. Psychological problems may occur as a result of the external urinary stoma and/or perceived losses related to hysterectomy and oophorectomy or may result from hormonal changes that occur as a result of surgery. A more direct physiological effect, however, involves removal of the anterior wall of the vagina. The vagina is

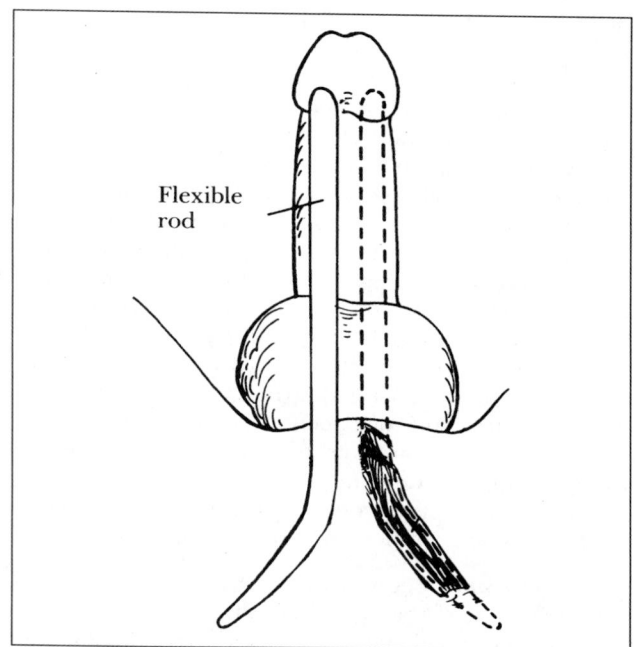

Flexible rod

**FIGURE 33-6**   Penile prosthesis. Semirigid prosthesis consisting of flexible rods. (Adapted from Luckmann J, Sorenson K: *Medical-Surgical Nursing—A Psychophysiologic Approach.* Philadelphia, Saunders, 1978, p 1843.)

**TABLE 33-3**   Continent Urinary Diversions

|  | Cutaneous Kock Reservoir | Kock Reservoir to Urethra | Indiana Reservoir |
|---|---|---|---|
| Structure | Ileum | Ileum | Ileum, ileocecal valve, cecum, ascending colon |
| Valves | Two | One | Ileocecal |
| Construction | Intussuscepted and stapled | Intussuscepted and stapled | Ileocecal |
| Advantages | Continence; prevents ureteral reflux | Continence and natural voiding through urethra | Continence; prevents uretheral reflux |

closed after surgery and therefore retains its original shape. However, if more than the anterior third of the vaginal wall is removed, the diameter of the introitus and the vaginal barrel can be severely compromised, and intercourse may be restricted. In addition, because of its close proximity to the urethral meatus, the clitoris may be injured or have compromised function because of scarring and fibrosis after surgery.[32] The physiological changes can result in an alteration in sensation and potential for orgasm and impairment of the ability to permit insertion of the penis into the vagina.

**Definitive radiotherapy** External beam radiotherapy of approximately 60 Gy delivered in fractions to the pelvis in five to eight weeks is an alternative to radical cystectomy. Although there has been controversy about the efficacy of definitive radiotherapy for invasive bladder cancer, many studies have shown its ability to eradicate tumors and permanently control tumors, while preserving bladder and sexual function.[6] The problem is that the disease often recurs after years of local control. Treatment with concurrent chemotherapy and radiotherapy has been associated with improved rates of local control compared with radiotherapy alone.[35]

The most common approach includes the entire bladder, the perivesical soft tissues, and pelvic lymphatics, while minimizing the dose to the rectum and anus. The exact tumoricidal dose is unknown, but many successful protocols recommend giving 65 Gy at a daily single dose of 180–200 cGy to the tumor region and a lesser dose of 47–55 Gy to the whole bladder and perivesical area.[6]

The acute (and self-limiting) side effects of fractionated treatment are dysuria, diarrhea, and/or urinary frequency in 50%–70% of patients. These can usually be treated symptomatically, and treatment usually does not have to be stopped. Long-term complications can happen as early as three years after treatment and include chronic urinary frequency or hematuria causing incontinence.[3,6]

**Chemotherapy** Because of the frequency of distant metastases, chemotherapy given preoperatively to decrease the presumed micrometastases is under evaluation in clinical trials. In trials chemotherapy is used as neoadjuvant (prior to surgery or radiotherapy) or adjuvant (following surgery or radiotherapy) treatment of invasive bladder cancer.[6] Results from clinical studies show that combined-modality treatment with neoadjuvant methotrexate, vincristine, doxorubicin (Adriamycin), and cisplatin (M-VAC), or with methotrexate, vinblastine, and cisplatin (MVC) can produce complete responses.[21,23,36,37]

### Advanced bladder cancer

Advanced bladder cancer (T4b, any T with N1–N3, or any T, any N with M1) may be present at diagnosis, or a result of recurrence. Treatment options include radical cystectomy with or without preoperative radiotherapy for select patients; external beam radiation; cystectomy or urinary diversion for palliation; or chemotherapy as an adjunct to local therapy.[20,21,23,37,38] A very small fraction of patients with advanced bladder cancer can be cured. Those with involvement of the pelvic organs by direct extension or small-volume metastases to the regional lymph nodes could be considered to be candidates for radical cystectomy with or without preoperative radiotherapy.

The focus of care for most patients with advanced bladder cancer is palliation of symptoms from a bladder tumor that often is very large. Urinary diversion may be indicated for palliation (for example, for severe irritative symptoms) or for preservation of renal function. Common chemotherapy regimens are M-VAC or CMV. Other drugs under clinical evaluation include paclitaxel (given with granulocyte colony-stimulating factor), ifosfamide, gallium nitrate, and gemcitabine.[39,40]

Radiotherapy can improve the problem of hemorrhage in the individual with advanced bladder cancer and certainly plays an important role in treating bony metastases. But local irritative symptoms can be made worse by radiotherapy.

## Results and Prognosis

Five-year survival rates (adjusted for normal life expectancy) as reported by the American Cancer Society can be seen in Table 33-4.

## Nursing Care of Individuals with Bladder Cancer

### Preoperative nursing care

When a diagnosis of bladder cancer has been confirmed and the treatment of choice includes urinary diversion, the type of diversion best suited for the individual must be chosen. The decision is based on each patient's needs, anatomy, history, and prognosis. Most urinary diversions have similar preoperative nursing considerations.

Bowel preparation begins with a low-residue diet two

**TABLE 33-4** Approximate Five-Year Survival Rates for Bladder Cancer

| Stage | |
|-------|---|
| Localized | 92% |
| Regional | 48% |
| Distant | 8% |
| All stages | 80% |

Reprinted from American Cancer Society: *Cancer facts and figures—1995.* Atlanta, GA, American Cancer Society, January 1995.

days before surgery. The day before surgery, antibiotics, cathartics, and a clear diet are administered.

Support to the patient and family should include thorough preoperative teaching that covers a description of the surgical procedure to be performed; the appearance of the abdomen after surgery, including drains, tubes, and midline incision; and pre- and postoperative care routines, including the progression of the return of bowel function after surgery, diet, pain control, and ambulation. Printed materials with explicit directions and illustrations are especially helpful preoperatively. It is important, if possible, to involve another family member or significant other. If indicated, the nurse can arrange for a preoperative visit by someone who has had similar surgery and has adjusted well.

The selection of a stoma site is an important preoperative consideration; the type of urinary diversion to be performed will dictate to some extent the stoma site selected. Any diversion that requires the wearing of an external appliance for the collection of urine must have an adequate surface for the adherence of the appliance. Ideally, the stoma site is selected and marked before surgery. It is of utmost importance that an appropriate site be chosen only after discussing with the patient his or her personal habits pertaining to work and recreational activities. The abdomen is examined and the individual observed while standing, sitting, and reclining. This is done to find an area at least 3 inches in diameter that is free of wrinkles and slightly convex. The site chosen should be visible to the individual and away from bony prominences, old scars or creases, and belt lines.

The Kock pouch, a continent ileal reservoir, needs no external collecting device, but the stoma must be placed for easy catheterization access by the patient.

There are several methods of marking the site selected. After the site is cleansed with alcohol, an insoluble dye such as gentian violet or methylene blue can be applied subdermally, or the dye can be tattooed into the midpoint of the selected site. Any method of marking the site that will remain visible after the surgical scrub is acceptable.

## General postoperative care

Postoperative care will vary depending on the method of urinary diversion or bladder substitution. As with all patients who have undergone major abdominal surgery, early ambulation, use of elastic stockings, and incentive spirometry may be used to prevent pulmonary emboli or respiratory complications. A nasogastric tube or gastrostomy tube is left in place until intestinal peristalsis resumes. Serum electrolytes and creatinine should be monitored postoperatively for the development of metabolic abnormalities that may occur after urinary diversion, such as hyponatremia, hypochloremia, or hyperkalemic metabolic acidosis.[31]

Continent urinary reservoirs and bladder substitutes produce much mucus. They should be irrigated regularly in the early postoperative period to prevent mucus accumulation. Mucus production will decrease over time and irrigation will become unnecessary.

Ultrasound or intravenous urography will be performed on a regular basis to check the upper urinary tract for hydronephrosis.[31]

Unlike a fecal diversion that is subject to an adynamic ileus, the urinary diversion should produce urine from the time of surgery. As mentioned in the treatment section, the continent ileal reservoir will be intubated with a Medena silastic catheter, which has been sutured to the skin line and connected to gravity drainage. An ileoconduit may have stents threaded through the ureteral ileo-anastomosis to provide for adequate urinary drainage while the anastomosis heals. If ureteral stents have been placed, they are usually removed sometime after postoperative day 5. The urinary flow should be rather continuous, and, in the case of an ileal conduit, a urinary appliance is needed to contain the drainage and to provide for accurate measurement. The appliance is then connected to the bedside gravity drainage.

## Nursing care following urinary diversion with an ileal conduit

***Stoma characteristics***   The intestinal stomal tissue can be compared with the mucosal lining of the mouth. The stoma may bleed when rubbed because of the capillaries in the area. A small amount of bleeding from the stoma is not serious, but it must be determined that the blood is from the stoma and not from the urine. Table 33-5 describes various stoma types and their specific problems and appliances.

Ideally, a urinary stoma should protrude 0.5–0.75 inch above the skin to allow the urine to drain into the aperture of an appliance. Flush stomas allow the urine to drain at skin level. This frequently is the cause of leakage and skin breakdown. The ileoconduit stoma is usually placed in the lower right quadrant. If a suitable area is not available to support an appliance there, it can be placed on the right side (within the confines of the rectus muscle to support the stoma).

Viability of the stoma is assessed by its color. This should be checked regularly, especially in the early postoperative period. Normal color of the stoma is deep pink to dark red. A dusky appearance ranging from purple to black may develop if circulation is seriously impaired. The appearance of a necrotic stoma may occur immediately after surgery or as late as five to seven days after surgery.[41] The dusky appearance of the stoma immediately after surgery may change in a few hours and appear viable. Sustained color change of the stoma should be reported to the surgeon.

A necrotic stoma may develop from abdominal distention causing tension on the mesentery, from twisting of the conduit at the time of surgery, or from arterial or venous insufficiency.[30] To determine the depth of the necrosis, a clear test tube can be inserted into the stoma

**TABLE 33-5** Stoma Types and Their Specific Problems and Appliances

| Stoma Type | Appliance Needed | Problems Seen |
|---|---|---|
| Nipple or bud | Any pouch | Minimal |
| Flush | May need convex skin barrier with belt | Skin irritation and insecurity<br>Inability to see stoma when applying the pouch<br>Occlusion of the stoma by the pouch<br>Decreased wearing time causing higher costs |
| Retracted | Rigid faceplate or convex skin barrier with belt | As above |
| Prolapsed | Flexible skin barrier so as to not constrict base of stoma | Ischemia or erosion of exposed bowel |

Carroll MD, Barbour S: Urinary diversion and bladder substitution, in Tanagho EA, McAninch JW (eds): *Smith's General Urology* (ed 14). Norwalk, CT, Appleton and Lange, 1992, p 436.

with the use of a small flashlight directed into the tube. The viable bowel will transilluminate the level of the necrosis. If the tissue at skin level is viable, surgical revision may be unnecessary. However, if necrotic, the tissue will slough, leaving a flush, retracted, or stenotic stoma. This leads to difficult management problems.

Stoma edema is normal in the early postoperative period as a result of surgical manipulation. This should not interfere with stoma functioning, but a larger opening will need to be cut in the appliance to prevent pressure or constriction of the stoma. Most stomas continue to shrink down over the next several months, and some will continue to decrease in size slightly for a year. Teaching the individual to continue to measure the stoma with a weekly change of appliance should alleviate the problem of the person wearing an appliance with an aperture too large for the stoma. The stoma needs only a space of 0.0625–0.125 inch to allow for expansion during peristalsis.

***Mucus production*** The intestine normally produces mucus, and mucus will be present in all diversions using segments of the bowel for a conduit or continent pouch. The amount of mucus produced varies with individuals and will cause the urine to appear cloudy. Excessive mucus also may be produced by an inflamed mucosa if infection is present. Some urinary appliances provide larger outlets to assist with the free flow of urine. Increasing fluid intake to 2 liters/day also will help by acting as a natural irrigant.

***Pouching a urinary stoma*** The fairly continuous flow of urine from a conduit requires the individual to wear an appliance at all times. In the early postoperative period, any one of the many clear, disposable urinary pouches may be used. The selection of a particular type of pouch may be governed by the availability in the facility or the surgeon's choice.[41]

The skin around the stoma should be clean and thoroughly dry before positioning the appliance over the stoma. The importance of dry skin cannot be emphasized enough. Very small amounts of moisture may cause adherence problems and leakage. The pouch should initially

be positioned to the patient's side so that it can be attached to bedside drainage without placing stress on the seal. The flange can then be "picture framed" with microporous tape to enhance the seal.

Many of the urinary pouches today are manufactured with an antireflux valve. This is double the thickness of the pouch, which prevents the urine from returning to the stoma. If stents are used to maintain patency, it may be necessary to thread them through the antireflux valve. The stoma should be clearly visible through the pouch.

Although not always possible, an effective urinary pouch should adhere at least three days. If no leakage occurs, the same pouch can remain adhered to the skin for ten days. It should then be changed for hygienic reasons and to observe the peristomal area. Table 33-6 describes common peristomal skin problems and their management.

Today there is a constant and ever-changing supply of new appliances. Materials and design are being updated rapidly to provide the consumer with the best protection and easiest care.

***Patient teaching for continuing care of a conduit*** The initial care rendered to the patient with a new conduit is extremely important both physiologically and psychologically. Before the individual is able to actively participate in self-care, the nurse or enterostomal therapist can teach by example. Procedures are "talked" through as they are being performed. Applied pouches should remain in place without leakage for three to five days. Peristomal skin should remain intact without irritation. This reinforces the attitude that a normal life is possible with a conduit. As the individual's condition improves, he or she should be encouraged to verbalize concerns and fears. A visit from a person who has been rehabilitated with a similar diversion may be arranged to give reassurance. The patient should be given the opportunity to handle the equipment and do as much of the needed care as possible. All the procedures necessary for continuing care of the stoma should be written down. Names and addresses where future supplies may be purchased should be included. Names and telephone numbers of

**TABLE 33-6**  Common Peristomal Skin Problems and Their Management*

| Problem | Cause | Management |
|---|---|---|
| Fungal infections—*Candida albicans* (Monilia) | • Urine accumulating under barrier (seen more frequently with diabetes mellitus and concurrent antibiotic use) | • Apply nystatin powder<br>• Dry skin thoroughly (use hair dryer)<br>• Prevent leakage under wafer |
| Allergic contact dermatitis | • Sensitivity to solvents, adhesives, detergents, wafers | • Identify irritant (skin patch test) and discontinue product<br>• Apply hydrocortisone cream (avoid prolonged use)<br>• Avoid solvents and soaps |
| Mechanical trauma | • Frequent or "excessive" pouch changing leading to skin stripping<br>• Pressure from belts<br>• Overuse of adhesive strips around the faceplate or barrier | • Minimize pouch changes<br>• Encourage gentle skin care<br>• Consider nonadhesive pouches (used with belt)<br>• Minimize use of sealants and adhesives |
| Pseudoverrucous skin lesions | • Urine contact with skin over extended time | • Ensure that the barrier and pouch are the correct size |

*The patient should see an enterostomal therapist nurse, if available.

Adapted from Carroll PR, Barbour S: Urinary diversion and bladder substitution, in Tanagho EA, McAninch JW (eds): *Smith's General Urology* (ed 14). Norwalk, CT: Appleton & Lange, 1995, p 458.

resource people to call if emergencies arise are a source of reassurance to the individual. The United Ostomy Association is an excellent resource for the patient in need of information and support.[41]

***Follow-up nursing care*** Many complications of a urinary diversion can be averted by a periodic reevaluation of both the stoma and the function of the conduit. The stoma may continue to decrease in size for several months or more. The size of the appliance opening should reflect this change. An opening too large for the stoma will permit peristomal skin to be exposed to urine, causing maceration and denudation of the skin. Openings that are too large also can permit the formation of hypertrophic lesions, which are referred to as *epitheliomatous hyperplasia*. Epitheliomatous hyperplasia can appear as smooth epithelium that extends onto the stoma mucosa or as a rough keratosis that is warty in appearance.[42] It can be painful to the individual and lead to poor adherence of the appliance because of the weeping or oozing, which in turn will cause continued leakage.

Alkaline encrustations around the stoma can lead to stoma stenosis as a result of skin contact with alkaline urine. Because bacteria thrive in an alkaline environment, infections can develop more readily when the pH of urine is allowed to become alkaline and is accompanied by serious weeping of the skin. Nurses have traditionally recommended that patients increase the intake of cranberry juice to help maintain a more acidic urine. However, research has not been able to support the efficacy of this intervention. Currently, patients in some settings are advised to take 500–2000 mg of vitamin C per day, along with at least a quart of acidic fruit juice such as orange, grapefruit, or cranberry juice, to lower bacteria counts in urinary diversions.

Stenosis, or narrowing, can occur in the stoma at the level of the skin, muscle, fascia, or any level of the ileal segment. Stenosis interferes with drainage and can lead to stasis, dilatation of the intestine, and infection.

The urinary component of a conduit is formed by the kidneys and their collecting systems, the renal pelvis and ureters. Ureteral angulation, stenosis, obstruction, or lithiasis leads to hydronephrosis, or irreparable renal damage. Periodic evaluation by means of excretory pyelography or loopography can detect this before irreparable damage occurs. Urine for analysis and culture should not be collected from the external appliance because the specimen collected will show bacteria and will not reflect the true conditions in the conduit.

## Nursing care of the individual with a continent ileal reservoir for urinary diversion

The patient remains in the hospital for seven to ten postoperative days. It is during this period that initial recovery and teaching begins. Discharge instructions for a Kock pouch with a Medena tube are found in Table 33-7.

Three weeks after surgery, the individual will be readmitted to the hospital. A radiographic picture of the pouch will be taken to confirm that there is no extravasation or reflux of urine from the pouch, and then the Medena tube and ureteral stents will be removed. The patient is taught to intubate/catheterize the pouch using a #20 French or #22 French coudé red-rubber catheter every two hours during the day and every three hours at night during the first week after the Medena tube is removed. This is increased gradually (by 1 hour each week) until the pouch is being intubated and drained approximately three or four times in 24 hours. In approximately six weeks the patient should be able to do catheter-

**TABLE 33-7**   Discharge Instructions for Patients with Kock Pouch with a Medena Tube

*PURPOSE:*
Irrigations are done to maintain patency of the catheter. Mucus and small blood clots can obstruct the catheter.

*SUPPLIES:*
Discharge pack for Kock pouch with Medena catheter:
1. 20 French coudé-tip red Robinson catheter
2. Small package of K-Y Jelly
3. One roll cloth adhesive tape
4. One roll paper adhesive tape
5. Large package of 4 × 4 gauze dressings
6. Urinary leg bag
7. Urinary drainage bag
8. Irrigation set
9. 2 quarts normal saline
10. Nonsterile specimen cup

*RECIPE FOR NORMAL SALINE:*
Mix 2 teaspoons of table salt to 1 quart of distilled water.

*INSTRUCTIONS:*
You will be discharged with a Penrose drain and Medena catheter sutured in place.

*PENROSE DRAIN CARE:*
You will be discharged with a plastic bag covering your Penrose drain. This bag collects the draining fluid. You may shower with the bag on.
1. Empty the bag when it becomes 1/3 to 1/2 full, or at least once daily.
2. Measure the output. Record the date, time, and amount.
3. If the draining fluid is a very small amount, or nothing at all, you may remove the bag. The bag is removed by peeling the adhesive, or waxy, surface off your skin.
4. You may then shower and allow the water to run over your Penrose drain. Clean your skin—you may use soap on your skin around the drain. Rinse thoroughly and pat dry. Apply a clean, dry gauze dressing pad over the drain. Tape in place.

*INSTRUCTIONS FOR IRRIGATION OF THE MEDENA CATHETER:*
You will be discharged with your Medena tube sutured in place.
1. The Medena catheter should be irrigated with 30 ml normal saline every 4 hours during the day only, following the method taught in the hospital. (Refer to Table 33-9, steps 2-9, for irrigation procedure.)
2. If you experience problems with the Medena catheter, drainage, or pain, you should irrigate to make sure the catheter is not plugged with mucus.
3. Sutures around the Medena tube might dry out and may result in the Medena tube slipping out of the pouch. If this should happen:
   A. Remove the sterile catheter from the package.
   B. Lubricate the catheter with K-Y Jelly.
   C. Slip the catheter through the stoma into the pouch. You may notice bleeding when you pass the catheter through the stoma—this is normal and will stop on its own. The catheter is into the pouch when you see some mucus and urine return.
   D. Tape the catheter in place to the skin securely. Reconnect it to the continuous gravity drainage.
   E. Call the physician for further orders, or earlier if you have any problems passing the catheter into the pouch.
   *HOSPITAL PHONE NUMBER (24 hours a day):*

USC/Kenneth Norris Jr. Cancer Hospital, Department of Nursing Services.

---

ization every six hours during the day and not at all at night. The method of draining the pouch is simple, there is no need to wear an external appliance, and the time intervals between emptying the pouch can duplicate normal bladder function. Table 33-8 describes patient instructions for home care of a Kock urinary reservoir.

Patient teaching accompanied by written instruction and periodic reevaluation of all components of the urinary diversion should facilitate the rehabilitation of the individual with minimal complications. The nurse's teaching efforts should focus on catheterization of the pouch, stoma care, and care of the catheter.

Basic principles of care for the continent diversions are similar. However, the nurse must have a thorough understanding of the method used to construct the continent valve. In the case of the Kock pouch, the valve is made of intussepted bowel. The structure of this valve allows the patient to digitally locate the tract should catheterization become difficult.[42] This is not the case with the Indiana reservoir or its modifications. The use of the ileocecal valve to form the continent valve mandates that a much smaller catheter be used to access the pouch and prohibits digitalization.[30] Table 33-3 describes the differences in the procedures. Patients are instructed to wear medical alert identification to inform health care personnel of care needed in case of emergency.[43]

### Nursing care for a Kock pouch to the urethra

The patient who has chosen the continent urinary Kock reservoir to be anastomosed to the urethra following a radical cystectomy is cared for in much the same way postoperatively as the patient who has had a continent reservoir procedure. The difference is that he has a #24 French Foley catheter inserted through the urethra into the reservoir for three weeks. Irrigations are done to keep the temporary Foley catheter open and functioning well. Table 33-9 describes discharge instructions for the patients. Three weeks postoperative the patient will be readmitted for Kock pouch training. After his radiographic study, if the reservoir is negative for extravasation, the Foley catheter and stents will be removed. Then the patient will be taught Kegel exercises and to stop and start the stream. He or she will void on a schedule night and day until the reservoir has expanded and continence is obtained. It takes a very motivated person three to six weeks to obtain total control during the day. It may take longer to obtain good control at night. Discharge instructions after removal of the Foley catheter are included in Tables 33-10 and 33-11.

### Nursing care of the individual receiving intravesical bacillus Calmette-Guerin

This treatment is usually given two to four weeks after transurethral resection of the bladder. The drug should be prepared using sterile technique while wearing gloves and a mask. The drug itself and all materials used in drug instillation containing the attenuated BCG mycobacterium should be treated as infectious waste.

**TABLE 33-8** Patient Home Care Instructions for Patients with Kock Urinary Diversion Without a Medena Catheter

---

### HOME CARE INSTRUCTIONS

*EQUIPMENT*
1. *Three resealable plastic bags*
2. *Four coudé-tip red-rubber catheters, 20 or 22 French*
3. *Clean paper towels*
4. *Stoma coverings (e.g., Nice & Natural Maxi Shields or Always panty liner cut into ½ or ⅓'s), or 2 × 2 gauze and paper tape)*
5. *Povidone-Iodine solution (Betadine)*
6. *Water-soluble lubricant (i.e., K-Y Jelly)*

*CATHETERIZATION TECHNIQUE:*
1. Wash hands prior to catheterizing.
2. Swab stoma with povidone-iodine solution on tissue or wipes to remove mucus.
3. Insert the catheter into the stoma of the Kock pouch and drain completely. If the catheter drains slowly or not at all, remove the catheter and run it under hot water to remove mucus plugs and reinsert it into the stoma to drain pouch of urine.
4. The mucosal lining of the stoma stays moist, so most patients do not need lubricating jelly. If lubrication is needed, use only water-soluble types such as K-Y Jelly or Lubafax. Never use Vaseline.
5. Tape your preferred stoma covering over stoma. Always have a waterproof covering to protect clothing.

*Catheterization Schedule:*
1. 1st Week: Catheterization should be done every 2 hours during the day and every 3 hours at night.

   2nd Week: Catheterize every 3 hours during the day and every 4 hours at night.

   3rd Week: Catheterize every 4 hours during the day and every 5 hours at night.

   4th Week: Catheterize every 5 hours during the day and every 6 hours at night.

   5th Week: Catheterize every 6 hours during the day and not at all during the night.
2. Irrigate the Kock pouch once a day, following your catheterization procedure, for 2 months after your discharge from the hospital. Use a 60-ml syringe full of normal saline or tap water and attach to the catheter to remove excess mucus. If a 60-ml syringe is not available, use a turkey or meat baster.
3. After two months, you can irrigate if you notice an increase in mucus or a change in the odor of your urine.
4. Pressure or discomfort can be felt when the pouch is overdistended. If this happens, catheterize your pouch. Never go longer than 7–8 hours without catheterization.
5. To make your own normal saline solution: Add 2 teaspoons of table salt to 1 quart of distilled water.

*Catheter Care:*
1. Cleanse used catheters in warm, soapy water. Be sure the water runs freely through the center of the catheter. Repeat this procedure, using clear water to rinse the catheter. Pour a small amount of Betadine solution through the inside of the catheter. Do not rinse the solution out.
2. Place catheter on a clean paper towel to air dry.
3. Place the clean, air-dried catheter in a clean, covered plastic container. A Tupperware celery container works well.
4. Make a kit up to use away from home. For example, female patients may use a cosmetic bag; male patients may use a pipe tobacco pouch.

**TABLE 33-8** (continued)

---

### HOME CARE INSTRUCTIONS

Place two dry, clean catheters into double-bagged resealable sandwich bags. In the outer bag keep extra stoma dressings and Betadine swabs. Place this equipment into the cosmetic or tobacco pouch. Strips of paper tape may be adhered to the outer plastic bag to eliminate carrying a roll of tape.
5. When catheterizing in a public restroom:
   a. Remove old dressing from stoma.
   b. Swab stoma off with Betadine swab.
   c. Insert catheter and drain reservoir completely.
   d. Dry catheter off with toilet tissue and place dirty catheter into the outside resealable sandwich bag to be cleaned when returning home.
   e. Cover the stoma with dressing of choice.

*NOTE:*
Patients with a urinary diversion need to wear a Med-Alert band with the following inscription:

"My stoma is a Continent Urinary Kock Pouch, catheterized every 4 to 6 hours with a 20Fr—*NON* Foley type catheter"

USC/Kenneth Norris Jr. Cancer Hospital, Department of Nursing Services.

The drug is given via catheter using strict aseptic technique to prevent infection. It is important that the catheterization procedure itself not cause urethral or bladder trauma. If there is evidence of traumatic catheterization, the drug should not be given.

Following instillation, the patient should be encouraged to retain the drug in his or her bladder for two hours (if possible). During the first hour the patient should lie first on his or her stomach for 15 minutes, then supine for 15 minutes, then on each side for 15 minutes each. A sitting position can be resumed during the second hour. Patients with a small bladder capacity may experience increased local irritation with the usual dose of BCG. If the instillation is given at home, the toilet should be disinfected with undiluted household bleach (1:1 for urine volume) for every voiding during the first six hours following drug instillation. The bleach should stand in the toilet for 15 minutes before flushing. This procedure deactivates the attenuated mycobacterium.[44]

The patient and family should be taught to watch for side effects of the treatment. These include a cough that develops following treatment, which could possibly indicate a BCG infection. Fever is common, and a fever over 101 °F should be treated with acetaminophen. A persistent fever above 101 °F for over two days or severe malaise could be further evidence of a systemic BCG infection. The patient and family should understand the importance of monitoring for signs of an inflammatory response in the bladder (urgency, dysuria, hematuria). These symptoms usually begin after two to three instillations and increase with the frequency and number of instillations. Bladder irritability can be treated with acetaminophen, propanthe-

**TABLE 33-9**   Discharge Instructions for Patients with a Kock Pouch to the Urethra

---

*PURPOSE:*
Irrigations are done to keep the temporary Foley catheter open and draining well (mucus and small blood clots can obstruct the catheter).

*EQUIPMENT:*
1 roll paper tape
2 quarts normal saline solution
4 ABD dressings
Urinary leg bag
Large package of 4 × 4 sterile dressing
Irrigation set
Nonsterile specimen cup
Urinary drainage bag
Recipe for normal saline solution: To every quart of distilled water, add 2 teaspoons of table salt. Mix thoroughly.

*INSTRUCTIONS:*
You will be discharged with the catheter and Penrose drain sutured in place. (Refer to Table 33-7 for care of Penrose drain.)
1. The Foley catheter should be irrigated at home every 4 hours during the day only. Follow the instructions taught to you in the hospital.
2. Wash your hands.
3. Fill a 60-ml catheter tip syringe with normal saline solution.
4. Disconnect the Foley catheter from the gravity drainage tubing.
5. Insert the catheter tip syringe into the catheter and slowly push in normal saline.
6. Aspirate with syringe and dispose of the returned solution.
7. Repeat these steps one more time or until fluid comes back clear.
8. This procedure may be repeated at any time if you feel discomfort, a decrease in drainage, or an increase in Penrose drain output.
9. Clean equipment with warm soapy water, pull syringe apart, and allow to air dry.

---

USC/Kenneth Norris Jr. Cancer Hospital, Department of Nursing Services.

---

**TABLE 33-10**   Discharge Instructions for Patients with a Kock Pouch to the Urethra Without a Foley Catheter

---

**DISCHARGE INSTRUCTIONS**
**Kock Pouch Training for Kock Pouch to the Urethra**

*PURPOSE:*
Instructing continent ileourethrostomy diversion patients to regain control of urinary elimination and return to a state of continency.

*DISCHARGE PACK INCLUDES:*
1. Incontinent pads: Attends, Chux
2. 18 French red Robinson catheter, K-Y Jelly, Betadine wipe prep.
3. Urinal

*INSTRUCTIONS:*
Your catheter has been removed. Now your new urinary reservoir (Kock pouch) has to be trained:
1. You will start to leak urine after removing the catheter. Try to empty the reservoir by sitting down on commode, bearing down, and/or using gentle pressure over the lower abdomen with your hands. Empty the reservoir as completely as possible.
2. Urinate on a schedule of every 2 hours during the day and every 3 hours at night. Try to increase the time between urination every week by ½–1 hour. If leaking starts before that scheduled time, try to empty the reservoir as instructed.
3. Kegel exercises are also of help with improving muscle tone.
   A. Kegel exercise:
      Isometric exercise involving a series of voluntary contractions of the pelvic muscles and perineum to improve the retention of urine.
   B. Directions:
      1. Relax abdominal muscles when doing the exercises.
      2. Contract and relax pelvic muscles 10 times in a row.
      3. Do the contractions while sitting, standing, and lying.
      4. 1st week hold contractions for 3 seconds.
         2nd week hold contractions for 5 seconds.
         3rd week hold contractions for 7–10 seconds.
      Do these exercises every other hour during the day or at least 4–6 times per day until continence has been obtained.
4. Your Kock pouch has to learn to expand and hold adequate amounts of urine. IT TAKES TIME AND PATIENCE TO RETURN TO A STATE OF CONTROL AND CONTINENCY.
5. Your Penrose drain has also been removed. Allow warm water to run over site in the shower. Pat dry. Apply dry 4 × 4 gauze dressing over site until there is no more drainage from site. Change dressing as needed.

---

USC/Kenneth Norris Jr. Cancer Hospital, Department of Nursing Services.

---

line, or phenazopyridine. Most patients develop varying degrees of nausea and vomiting after BCG instillation and occasionally systemic hypersensitivity reactions, which can be treated with diphenhydramine.[44]

### Follow-up care

Radiological studies are used to confirm the integrity of the pouch, to test the competence of the nipple valves, and to ensure complete emptying of the reservoir.[43] Intravenous pyelogram is performed to view the upper tracts. Renal function can be checked by the usual laboratory tests. The evaluations of the urea nitrogen, serum creatinine, urinary pH, and specific gravity or osmolality are the most useful tests of renal function. If urine is to be tested for culture, it is important to remember that continent diversions are not closed, sterile systems as is the bladder. The diversions are often colonized with bacteria, and the presence of bacteria does not necessarily indicate pathology.

# CANCER OF THE KIDNEY

## Epidemiology

There are two major types of kidney cancer. *Renal cell cancer* is the most common form. It occurs in the parenchyma of the kidney and also has been known as *renal cell carcinoma, renal adenocarcinoma, cancer of the kidney, renal parenchymal neoplasm,* and *hypernephroma.* The diversity of

**TABLE 33-11**   Discharge Instructions for Self-Catheterization

---

### DISCHARGE INSTRUCTIONS
#### "Self-Catheterization"

---

*PURPOSE:*

Three weeks after surgery the Foley catheter is removed and you begin voiding through your urethra. The urethra could become plugged with mucus and cause problems when you urinate. If this should occur, you would have to pass a catheter into the Kock pouch to drain it.

Self-catheterization is taught before surgery so that you will know how to pass a catheter into your urinary reservoir (Kock pouch).

*EQUIPMENT:*

- a moist towelette or soap and water
- a dry hand towel
- water-soluble lubricant
- 18 french coudé catheter

*INSTRUCTIONS: SELF-CATHETERIZATION:*

1. Wash your hands thoroughly with soap and water and dry.
2. Position yourself comfortably either in front of the toilet or sitting on the toilet.
3. Cleanse the urethral opening.
   *For women:* with one hand, separate the labia and wash from front to back with soap and water or a moist towelette.
   *For men:* hold the penis up with one hand and wash the tip of the penis to the base of the glans with soap and water or a moist towelette. You should wash in a circular motion starting at the urethra and working outward.
4. Lubricate the catheter end that will go into your urethra. Use a water-soluble lubricant such as K-Y Jelly. Do not use Vaseline or petroleum jelly.
5. Insert the catheter into the urethra until the urine begins to flow.
   *For women:* approximately 1–1.5 inches
   *For men:* approximately 6–8 inches
   Then insert the catheter about 1 inch farther and hold it there until urine stops flowing.
6. Take this opportunity to irrigate, or wash out, your Kock pouch. Leaving the catheter in place, instill normal saline or tap water with a 60-ml syringe or turkey baster. Draw the fluid out with the syringe, repositioning the catheter if necessary. Repeat until clear.
7. Slowly withdraw the catheter, stopping each time more urine drains out.
8. Pinch the catheter and remove.
9. Check the color, odor, and clarity of the urine to be aware of any changes that you may need to report to your doctor or nurse. For example, cloudy, foul-smelling, or bloody urine should be reported.

*CATHETER CARE:*

1. Wash the catheter with warm, soapy water.
2. Rinse thoroughly with clear water, including through the center of the catheter.
3. Dry the catheter. Allow it to sit out on a clean surface so that the center of the catheter can air dry.
4. Store the catheter in a clean, dry container of your choice.

USC/Kenneth Norris Jr. Cancer Hospital, Department of Nursing Services.

---

nomenclature reflects the early confusion regarding the histopathology of renal cell cancer.[45] The second major type is *cancer of the renal pelvis.*

Kidney cancer is not common in the United States, accounting for only about 3% of all cancers. Renal cell carcinoma accounts for about 85% of kidney cancers.[45]

There is a 2:1 male predominance in kidney cancer, especially in renal cell cancer. The incidence of renal cancer is equivalent between whites and blacks. However, Hispanic men and women have kidney cancer rates more than one-third higher than those of white Americans.[46]

There seem to be striking geographic differences, with the rate of kidney cancer being quite high in Scandinavian countries (about 11% of all cancers).[47] Japan has a low incidence, and the United States and most Western European countries appear to have an intermediate risk. Interestingly enough, Scandinavians who migrate to Los Angeles do not have higher than expected rates of either cancer of the kidney or cancer of the renal pelvis.[48]

One of the most important demographic risk factors for both renal cell cancer and cancer of the renal pelvis is age. Both are rare in people under 35 years of age, and thereafter the incidence increases with age. Renal cell cancer occurs most frequently in the fifth to sixth decade.[46]

## Etiology

### Cigarette smoking

The causes of kidney cancer remain obscure. The only risk factor that has been linked persistently to kidney cancer by both cohort studies[48–50] and epidemiological case-controlled studies[51–53] is cigarette smoking. For renal cell cancer, a consistent relationship between the number of cigarettes consumed and the risk of cancer has not been established. But for cancer of the renal pelvis there does appear to be a strong association between the number of cigarettes smoked and the risk for cancer.[46] It is not clear how cigarette smoking might induce kidney cancer, but studies have shown numerous mutagenic chemicals in the urine of cigarette smokers.[50]

### Occupation

Kidney cancer seems to be associated with certain occupational exposures. Exposures to asbestos[54] and lead (pigment in colored printing ink)[48] have each demonstrated a slightly increased risk for renal cell cancer than might otherwise be expected. But currently, occupational exposure is associated with only a very small proportion of all renal cancers.[46]

### Analgesic use

Heavy use of analgesics, specifically aspirin, phenacetin, or acetaminophen-containing products, has been shown to increase the risk of cancer of the renal pelvis.[46,48] A possible association between analgesics and renal cell cancer has been reported but not conclusively substantiated.[46,51]

### Other factors

A strong association between renal cell cancer and obesity in women was first identified in 1974.[52] Others have found similar associations,[51,55] but there remains the question of whether the increased incidence in women is related to obesity or to hormonal (estrogen) influences.[46]

An increased incidence of acquired cystic disease of the kidney and of renal cell carcinoma has been reported in patients undergoing dialysis. A 1990 study reported the risk of renal cell cancer in patients undergoing dialysis to be 57–134 times higher than in the general population.[56]

Epidermal and other growth factors have also been associated with renal cell carcinoma. Many patients have systemic effects, such as pyrexia, cachexia, abnormal liver function, hypercalcemia, and polycythemia, believed to be associated with abnormal growth factors.[57] Recent studies have shown that an overexpression of the epidermal growth factor receptor is associated with tumor initiation and progression of renal cell carcinoma[58–60] and cancer of the renal pelvis.[61] The overexpression has been associated with distant metastasis, venous invasion, or lymph node involvement. It is believed that the determination of epidermal growth factor receptor could become an important prognostic factor for the biological behavior of renal cell cancer.[58,59]

### Genetic factors

There is also a genetic link to renal cell cancer. Like many cancers, renal cell carcinoma occurs in both familial and nonfamilial (sporadic) forms. Rare family constellations have been described in which multiple family members develop renal cell cancer, and predisposition to the disease is inherited in an autosomal dominant fashion. Patients with familial renal cell cancer have a translocation of the short arm of chromosome 3 and the long arm of chromosome 8; unaffected members do not carry those translocations.[57,62]

A second form of hereditary renal cell cancer is seen as part of von Hipple–Landau (VHL) disease. This rare disease is a cancer syndrome in which affected patients are predisposed to develop multiple, bilateral renal cysts and carcinomas, bilateral pheochromocytomas, retinal angiomas, hemangioblastomas of the central nervous system, pancreatic cysts and tumors, and/or epididymal cysts. Recent studies have found that the same gene is involved in both the sporadic and the familial form of renal cell carcinoma.[62]

## Pathophysiology

### Cellular characteristics

Renal cell carcinoma is the most common form of kidney cancer, accounting for about 75%–85% of kidney cancers. Although the histology is diverse from tumor to tumor, renal cell carcinoma can be separated into two broad groups: clear cell tumors and granular cell tumors.

Renal cell carcinoma arises from tubular epithelial cells that are found in the parenchyma of the kidney. Tumors of the renal pelvis generally arise from epithelial tissue anywhere in the renal pelvis and are often papillary. These tumors often have independent, multifocal origins.[3]

Cancer of the renal pelvis accounts for about 5%–9% of all kidney cancers. The mucosal lining of the renal pelvis and ureter is similar to that of the urinary bladder, being composed of transitional epithelium.[3] Thus, the two major cell types in tumors of the renal pelvis are transitional cell cancer (most common) and squamous cell cancer. Grading is similar to that of bladder cancer. Papillomas account for 15%–20% of cases.[3]

### Progression of disease

Renal cell cancers tend to grow toward the medullary portion of the kidney, whereas tumors of the renal pelvis often grow at the ureteropelvic junction and invade the underlying submucosa and muscular coats.

Cancer of the renal pelvis and renal cell carcinoma spread through the venous and lymphatic routes. Hematogenous spread most often involves the lungs, bones, and liver. Lymphatic drainage of the kidneys is to the nodes in the ipsilateral renal hilus. These nodes then drain into the regional lymph nodes.

Renal cell carcinoma also spreads by direct extension to the renal vein and sometimes farther into the vena cava. It can also extend by growing up through the renal capsule into the perinephric fat or the adjacent visceral structures.[45]

Cancer of the renal pelvis grows by extension, as mentioned, down into the ureter and out through the muscular coats. Although the majority of upper urinary tract transitional cell cancers are localized at diagnosis, the most common metastatic sites are regional lymph nodes, bone, and lung.[3]

Exact numbers vary, but somewhere between 30% and 50% of individuals with kidney cancer have metastasis at diagnosis.[57]

## Paraneoplasia and Renal Cell Carcinoma

Renal cell carcinoma has a considerable association with certain paraneoplastic syndromes. The term *paraneoplastic syndrome* is used to describe systemic effects of a tumor on the host. The effects are not directly related to the tumor presence (such as compression or obstruction from a solid tumor) or to a particular metastatic lesion (for example, brain or bone metastasis). Rather, paraneoplastic syndromes are thought to be associated with compounds that the malignant cells synthesize that are not normally synthesized by cells of that type (see chapter 26). Although uncommon in general, renal cell carcinomas seem to have a higher association with paraneoplasia, particularly that which is related to the endocrine system.[63] Some of the ectopic (or inappropriately secreted) hormones that have been ascribed to tumors of renal origin are parathyroid hormone, erythropoietin, renin, gonadotropins, and adrenocorticotropic hormone.[57]

## Clinical Manifestations

### Renal cell carcinoma

In 40% of individuals diagnosed with renal cell carcinoma the initial symptom is gross hematuria. The hematuria appears uniform throughout the urinary stream, and lower tract discomfort is not present. Pain (which is usually dull and aching) is also a common presenting symptom, as is a palpable abdominal mass.[45] These three symptoms—hematuria, pain, and a palpable abdominal mass—represent the classic triad of symptoms of renal cell carcinoma. However, their simultaneous appearance on presentation is infrequent. Because of the well-protected anatomic position of the kidney, the presence of a tumor is unfortunately often concealed until advanced stages. Other more generalized symptoms also have been described with cancer of the kidney, including fever, weight loss, an elevated erythrocyte sedimentation rate (ESR), or anemia.

### Cancer of the renal pelvis

Only a few individuals with cancer of the renal pelvis present with the classic triad of symptoms. Most tumors of the renal pelvis originally present with hematuria (gross or microscopic). Some individuals may have both hematuria and flank pain, which is probably caused by the passage of blood clots or by obstruction of the ureteropelvic junction.[57] A palpable mass in a tumor of the renal pelvis almost always occurs either because the tumor has extended outside the kidney or because of massive hydronephrosis (resulting from a ureteropelvic junction obstruction).

Techniques for early detection have not been identified for either renal cell carcinoma or cancer of the renal pelvis.

## Assessment

### Renal cell carcinoma

The first step in diagnosis of renal cell cancer is to differentiate the more common benign renal cysts. Tests used in diagnosis and staging include kidney, ureter, and bladder (KUB) radiographs; nephrotomograms; excretory urogram; retrograde urogram; renal ultrasound (US); renal CT; and renal angiography. MRI examinations help to evaluate adjacent organ invasion and major vascular involvement, to identify renal cysts more readily,

and to distinguish solid renal masses from normal renal parenchyma.[57]

Excretory urograms have traditionally been known as *intravenous pyelograms*. The prefix *pyelo-* implies, however, that only the renal pelvis is shown. *Excretory urogram* is probably a more apt name because the test does show the entire urinary tract. Excretory urogram and renal tomography are considered by most to be the screening tests of choice for suspected renal mass lesions, although they are only 70%–75% accurate in differentiating benign cysts from malignant lesions.[64]

Renal US, which is generally the next step in the assessment of a renal mass, has the apparent advantage of being easy to do, noninvasive, and relatively inexpensive, and requiring a minimal physical expenditure on the patient's part. It can generally differentiate solid from cystic masses. Individuals who have solid or questionable masses should undergo further tests.

Renal US coupled with CT makes it possible to diagnose small tumors suggestive of malignancy. A CT scan can accurately evaluate a questionable lesion, determine the local extent of the cancer, identify the presence of enlarged regional lymph nodes, and describe the presence of tumor within the main renal vein and the inferior vena cava.[45,65] A CT scan of the abdomen, chest, and brain also can aid in detecting distant metastases.

Historically, renal angiography has been a standard part of the diagnosis of a suspicious renal mass. Recently, contrast-enhanced CT scans have, in some cases, replaced the use of renal angiography.

DNA flow cytometry has also added information in predicting the prognosis of renal cell cancer. Aneuploid tumors were found to be more likely to develop to invasive lesions than diploid tumors.[66]

### Cancer of the renal pelvis

Excretory urogram, retrograde urogram, and urinary cytology are the most useful techniques for establishing a diagnosis of cancer of the renal pelvis. Angiography is not useful in evaluating these tumors. US may help identify a mass density in the central region of the kidney, a CT scan might detect the presence of a soft-tissue mass in the renal hilum, and using MRI with CT can aid in the detection of regional lymph node involvement.[3]

From 20% to 30% of low-grade renal pelvic cancers and 60% of higher-grade lesions can be detected on urinary cytology.[3] Urinary cytology can be done on a freshly voided urine specimen or on washings from the renal pelvis obtained during a retrograde urogram.

## Classification and Staging

### Renal cell carcinoma

Staging for renal cell carcinoma, as with all cancers, is founded on those aspects that influence survival, including regional lymph node involvement, invasion through the renal capsule, extension to contiguous organs, and distant metastases.[67] The size of the primary tumor is not strongly correlated with survival and may not be a significant factor in staging.

The system used most often for classifying renal cell carcinoma is a modification of the system of Flocks and Kadesky,[68] a staging system based on gross physical characteristics of the tumor. Robson proposed modifications of the system that took into account the degree of vascular involvement, and it is that system that is most widely used (Figure 33-7). The TNM system (Table 33-12) more accurately classifies the magnitude of tumor involvement.

### Cancer of the renal pelvis

Staging of renal pelvic cancers is based on an accurate assessment of the degree of tumor infiltration and parallels the staging system developed for bladder cancer.[3] Table 33-13 outlines the TNM system for staging cancer of the renal pelvis.

## Treatment of Renal Cell Carcinoma

### Surgery

A radical nephrectomy is the standard, often curative, treatment for renal cell cancer. This routinely includes removal of the kidney, Gerota's fascia, the ipsilateral adrenal, the proximal one-half of the ureter, and lymph nodes in the renal hilar area. More recently it has been demonstrated that removal of the ipsilateral adrenal gland is not routinely necessary.[69,70]

Various surgical approaches have been used for radical nephrectomy. The abdominotransperitoneal approach can be performed with a midline or subcostal

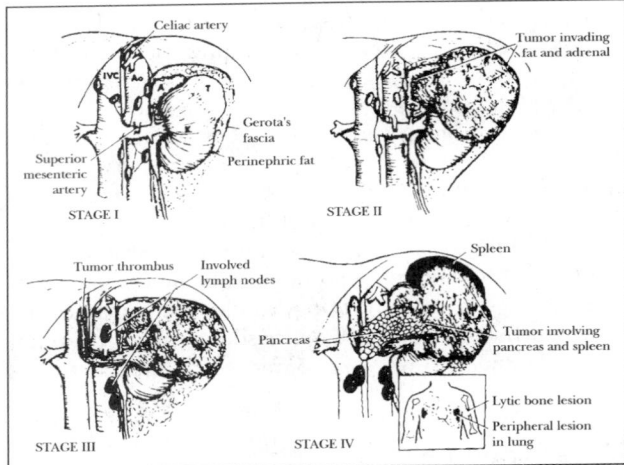

**FIGURE 33-7** Robson staging system for renal cell carcinoma. In stage A, IVC is inferior vena cava; Ao, aorta; A, left suprarenal gland; T, tumor; K, left kidney. (Dreicer R, Williams RO: Renal parenchymal neoplasms, in Tanagho, EA, McAninch JW (eds): *Smith's General Urology* [ed 14]. Norwalk, CT, Appleton and Lange, 1995, p 376.)

**TABLE 33-12    TNM Staging System for Cancer of the Kidney**

| PRIMARY TUMOR (T) | |
|---|---|
| TX | Primary tumor cannot be assessed |
| T0 | No evidence of primary tumor |
| T1 | Tumor 2.5 cm or less in greatest dimension limited to the kidney |
| T2 | Tumor more than 2.5 cm in greatest dimension limited to the kidney |
| T3 | Tumor extends into major veins or invades adrenal gland or perinephric tissues but not beyond Gerota's fascia |
| T3a | Tumor invades adrenal gland or perinephric tissues but not beyond Gerota's fascia |
| T3b | Tumor grossly extends into renal vein(s) or vena cava |
| T4 | Tumor invades beyond Gerota's fascia |

| LYMPH NODE (N) | |
|---|---|
| NX | Regional lymph nodes cannot be assessed |
| N0 | No regional lymph node metastasis |
| N1 | Metastasis in a single lymph node, 2 cm or less in greatest dimension |
| N2 | Metastasis in a single lymph node, more than 2 cm but not more than 5 cm in greatest dimension, or mulitple lymph nodes, none more than 5 cm in greatest dimension |
| N3 | Metastasis in a lymph node more than 5 cm in greatest dimension |

| DISTANT METASTASIS (M) | |
|---|---|
| MX | Presence of distant metastasis cannot be assessed |
| M0 | No distant metastasis |
| M1 | Distant metastasis |

| SITES OF DISTANT METASTASIS | |
|---|---|
| Pulmonary | PUL |
| Osseous | OSS |
| Hepatic | HEP |
| Brain | BRA |
| Lymph nodes | LYM |
| Bone marrow | MAR |
| Pleura | PLE |
| Peritoneum | PER |
| Skin | SKI |
| Other | OTH |

Beahrs OH, Henson DE, Hutter RV, Myers MH (eds): *American Joint Committee on Cancer: Manual for Staging of Cancer* (ed 4). Philadelphia, Lippincott, 1992.

**TABLE 33-13** TNM Staging System for Cancer of the Renal Pelvis and Ureter

| PRIMARY TUMOR (T) | |
|---|---|
| TX | Primary tumor cannot be assessed |
| T0 | No evidence of primary tumor |
| Tis | Carcinoma in situ |
| Ta | Papillary noninvasive carcinoma |
| T1 | Tumor invades subepithelial connective tissue |
| T2 | Tumor invades beyond muscularis into periureteric or peripelvic fat or renal parenchyma |
| T4 | Tumor invades adjacent organs or through the kidney into perinephric fat |

| LYMPH NODE (N) | |
|---|---|
| NX | Regional lymph nodes cannot be assessed |
| N0 | No regional lymph node metastasis |
| N1 | Metastasis in a single lymph node, 2 cm or less in greatest dimension |
| N3 | Metastasis in a lymph node more than 5 cm in greatest dimension |

| DISTANT METASTASIS (M) | |
|---|---|
| MX | Presence of distant metastasis cannot be assessed |
| M0 | No distant metastasis |
| M1 | Distant metastasis |

| STAGE GROUPING | | | |
|---|---|---|---|
| 0 | Tis | N0 | M0 |
| | Ta | N0 | M0 |
| I | T1 | N0 | M0 |
| II | T2 | N0 | M0 |
| III | T3 | N0 | M0 |
| IV | T4 | N0 | M0 |
| | Any T | N1 | M0 |
| | Any T | N2 | M0 |
| | Any T | N3 | M0 |
| | Any T | Any N | M1 |

Beahrs OH, Henson DE, Hutter RV, Myers MH (eds): *American Joint Committee on Cancer: Manual for Staging of Cancer* (ed 4). Philadelphia, Lippincott, 1992.

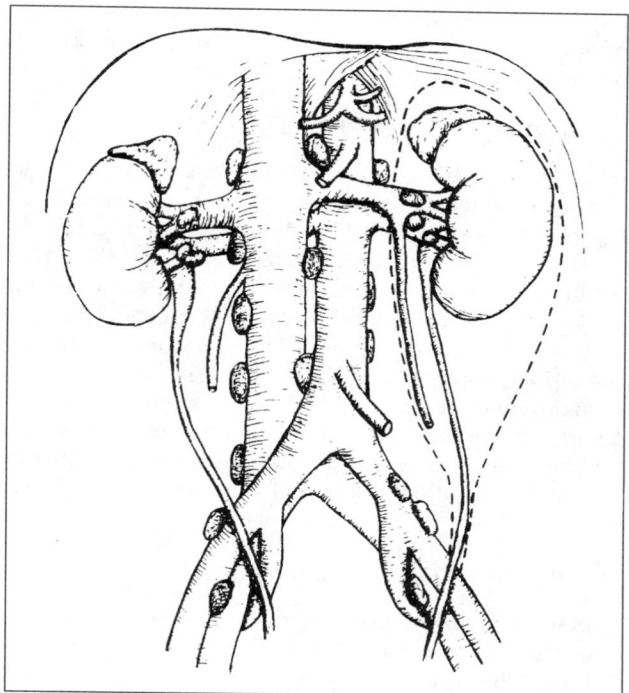

**FIGURE 33-8** Boundaries of a left radical nephrectomy. Dotted line represents both the surgical margin and Gerota's fascia. (Drecier R, Williams RO: Renal parenchymal neoplasms, in Tanagho EA, McAninch JW (eds): *Smith's General Urology* [ed 14]. Norwalk, CT, Appleton and Lange, 1995, p 381.)

abdominal incision. The thoracoabdominal approach may also be used. Figure 33-8 displays the boundaries of a left radical nephrectomy.

### Vena cava involvement

About 5%–9% of individuals with renal cell carcinoma have varying degrees of tumor extension into the vena cava.[57] Because of the shorter right renal vein, tumor thrombus occurs more often on the right side. To prevent tumor embolization, a tumor thrombus in the vena cava is removed in continuity with the renal tumor. Tumor invasion of the wall of the vena cava is no longer thought to be a completely incurable situation, and while the surgical treatment is complicated, published experience indicates a positive outcome for many of these patients if they are free of distant metastases.[71] Recently, management of extensive vena cava involvment has been treated with cardiopulmonary bypass with circulatory arrest and hypothermia.[72]

### Lymphadenectomy

Regional lymphadenectomy remains controversial.[73] Those who argue against lymphadenectomy feel that it does not improve survival; that its staging value in terms of predicting survival is limited because the cancer can spread via the venous system alone; and that because there is as yet no effective adjuvant therapy, identification of lymph node metastases is not important. There are no controlled clinical trials demonstrating that this procedure impacts the disease-free or overall survival of patients.[74]

Some settings routinely perform lymphadenectomy on all patients with stage I, II, or III disease. Those who favor lymphadenectomy feel that it offers the best chance of survival to those for whom radical nephrectomy is potentially curative.[57]

### Bilateral tumors or tumors in a solitary kidney

In the unusual case of bilateral tumors or cancer in a solitary kidney, two treatment options are available. In bilateral tumors where there is a larger tumor in one kidney than in the other, partial nephrectomy is performed on the kidney with the smaller tumor, and several weeks later radical nephrectomy is carried out on the kidney with the larger tumor. In cases where there is a tumor in a solitary kidney with no evidence of metastasis, partial nephrectomy or radical nephrectomy with subsequent chronic hemodialysis or renal transplantation are treatment alternatives. Nephron-sparing surgery is being accepted more often in situations where radical nephrectomy would leave a person anephric.[70]

### Radiotherapy and chemotherapy

Renal cell carcinomas and their metastases are usually radioresistant, and radiotherapy's treatment role is controversial, but pre- and postoperative radiotherapy have been combined with nephrectomy. Adjuvant chemotherapy has not demonstrated any improvement in survival rates over what may be accomplished without chemotherapy.[68] Vinblastine has been used as a single agent, with response rates reported in the 15% range.[45]

## Treatment of Advanced Renal Cell Carcinoma

About 30% of individuals with renal cell carcinoma present with metastases at the time of diagnosis. Another 50% will develop metastases after radical nephrectomy.[57] Since most patients with advanced renal cell cancer (T4, or any T with M1) are not candidates for curative treatment, the goal of therapy generally is palliation of symptoms. External-beam radiotherapy, angioinfarction, and nephrectomy can relieve many of the symptoms associated with the primary tumor or related ectopic hormone production. Spontaneous regressions occasionally occur with this tumor.[75]

Responses to systemic therapy using conventional chemotherapy have been disappointingly low, but recently more promising results have been achieved using biological therapies. For decades one approach to treating renal cell cancer was hormonal therapy using medroxyprogesterone acetate. The rationale for this treatment was based on preclinical studies of estrogen-induced renal cell cancer in hamsters.[57] Unfortunately, there has not been any clinical evidence to support a beneficial effect of adjuvant progesterone therapy and no evidence of a correlation between hormone receptor content and response.[57]

### Radiotherapy

Radiation therapy is an important modality in the palliation of patients with metastatic renal cell cancer. Despite the belief that this is a radioresistant tumor, effective palliation of metastatic disease to the bone, brain, and lungs is reported in up to two-thirds of patients. External-beam radiation therapy has occasionally been used to palliate patients with gross hematuria pain, but without significant efficacy.[45] Doses most commonly used are 40–50 Gy.[57]

### Surgery

Adjunctive or palliative nephrectomies have been described as approaches for individuals with metastatic renal cell carcinoma. Adjunctive nephrectomy is done to improve survival, whereas palliative nephrectomy is done to relieve symptoms of the primary renal tumor.

Individuals whose survival is improved by adjunctive nephrectomy are those who have the best performance status and the least amount of tumor before surgery.[70]

Palliative nephrectomy may be justifiable for individuals who have severe disabling symptoms such as local pain, bleeding, or endocrinopathy but who otherwise have a reasonable life expectancy of greater than six months.[70] Radiotherapy might relieve these symptoms equally well.

Angioinfarction of the kidney is used with and without nephrectomy to decrease vascularity before surgery or to lessen tumor bleeding, pain, or other systemic symptoms in patients with unresectable tumors.[57] Short-term embolization can be done with alcohol, autologous blood clot, or gelatin sponge pads (Gelfoam). Other inert substances such as stainless steel pellets or steel coils are used to embolize the renal artery. A postinfarction syndrome of pain, fever, and gastrointestinal complaints happens in most patients.[57]

### Chemotherapy

Chemotherapy has had no great impact on metastatic renal cell carcinoma.[63] Some clinicians, however, feel that chemotherapeutic trials might be appropriate for certain individuals because metastatic renal cell carcinoma presents so few options. Vinblastine is one chemotherapeutic agent that has demonstrated some success in achieving tumor responses.[45,70]

### Biologic response modifiers

Various biological therapies have been evaluated in the treatment of metastatic renal cell carcinoma since it was first reported in 1985 that antitumor responses could be achieved using high doses of interleukin-2 (IL-2) and large numbers of lymphokine-activated killer (LAK) cells.[76] Alfa-interferon has approximately a 15% objective response rate in appropriately selected individuals (nonbulky pulmonary and/or soft-tissue metastases, excellent performance status, no weight loss).[77,78] The alfa-interferon doses used in studies reporting good responses have been in an intermediate range (6–20 mu, SQ, tiw). These responses are rarely complete or durable. More promising are treatments using interleukin-2 (IL-2). Administration of IL-2, with or without LAK lymphocytes, appears to have a similar overall response rate to alfa-interferon, but with some durable complete remissions in approximately 5% of selected patients.[79]

These are toxic, complex biotherapies that act by stimulating host immunologic responses against cancer. Ongoing clinical trials are attempting to decrease toxicity and ease of administration of the agents by giving low doses of IL-2 subcutaneously.[80] There is interest today in using a combination of low-dose IL-2 with alfa-interferon. Trials have shown favorable response rates and much lower toxicity, allowing the treatment to be given on an outpatient basis.[81,82]

Common side effects of alfa-interferon and IL-2 include flulike symptoms, fatigue, cognitive dysfunction, myelosuppression, abnormal liver function, and anorexia.[83–86] IL-2 has the additional side effects of nausea and vomiting, diarrhea, edema and fluid retention, hypotension, tachycardia, decreased systolic blood pressure, skin rash, erythema, and inflammatory reactions at injection sites.[83] See chapter 17 for a more in-depth discussion of biological therapy.

## Treatment of Cancer of the Renal Pelvis

Treatment of renal pelvic cancers should be based on tumor grade, stage, and position. The standard treatment has been nephroureterectomy. To avoid recurrence in this segment, a radical nephrectomy, including the kidney, all perinephric tissue, regional lymph nodes, the ureter, and a small cuff of the bladder, is performed. Proponents of this radical procedure feel it is necessary to treat the secondary ureteral and vesical tumors that may be present.[3] Others who argue for more conservative kidney-sparing approaches to surgical treatment of this cancer stress the poor prognosis associated with advanced lesions and the mortality risks of radical procedures.[87]

Radiation therapy has not proved to be an effective adjunct for the control of residual tumor, local recurrence, or unresectable disease. Although controversial, postoperative radiotherapy has been used to decrease recurrence rates and improve survival in patients with deeply infiltrating cancer.[3,88] Chemotherapeutic agents that have been used with limited results include doxorubicin, cisplatin, methotrexate, and vinblastine.[89,90]

New treatment strategies for cancer of the renal pelvis include percutaneous or ureteroscopic resection of the tumors followed by laser irradiation or supplemental intracavitary BCG or epidoxorubicin.[57,91]

## Results and Prognosis

Survival rates for renal cell cancer depend on the stage of the disease. For patients with tumor confined to the kidney (T1 and T2) the five-year survival is approximately 92%–95%; for T3 tumors it is approximately 18%; for metastatic disease (T4, or any T with M1) the five-year survival is low, ranging from 0% to 20%. Overall five-year survival is 40%.[57]

The prognosis of cancer of the renal pelvis is relatively poor and is closely correlated with the degree of differentiation and extent of the tumor. Low-grade and low-stage cancers of the renal pelvis have 60%–90% five-year survival rates, compared with 0%–33% for tumors of a higher grade or those that have penetrated deep into or through the renal pelvic or ureteral wall.[3]

## Nursing Care of Individuals with Cancer of the Kidney

Individuals who are undergoing diagnostic procedures or treatments for kidney malignancy are extremely anxious. Some individuals equate the loss of a kidney with imminent death. Others worry that the remaining kidney will not be able to meet the body's total need for urine elimination. The alert nurse can help by providing correct information to the individual and family. The nurse should assess the individual's knowledge and feelings about the disease and its treatment to help the patient set realistic goals for dealing with the malignancy.

In general, the principal treatment of primary renal carcinoma is surgical excision. Radical nephrectomy is performed on all resectable lesions in stage I to III and is sometimes done palliatively for symptoms such as pain and bleeding for individuals with advanced disease. The pre- and postoperative nursing management of the person undergoing radical nephrectomy is similar to that of the individual undergoing laparotomy.

***Preoperative nursing care*** A renal infarction may be done two to three days prior to surgery in an attempt to decrease surgical hemorrhage by decreasing tumor vascularity. Following this procedure, the individual may experience considerable pain, fever, nausea, and vomiting. Those symptoms may persist for up to 36 hours. Analgesic and antiemetic medications should be administered for symptomatic control. Intravenous fluid supplementation may be necessary if the individual has severe fluid loss. Emotional support and reassurance during this time can be comforting to the patient and family.

***Postoperative nursing care***
*Pain relief* The primary objectives during the postoperative period are the management of pain and the prevention of postoperative complications. Pain can be quite severe after nephrectomy. For lower pole renal tumors, the flank incision (retroperitoneal) approach is generally used, and the individual is placed in a hyperextended side-lying position. The thoracoabdominal incision approach is generally used for larger and upper pole lesions. In this approach the person is placed in an oblique position with rolled towels situated to elevate the flank.

As a result of the position on the operating table, the individual undergoing nephrectomy experiences not only incision pain but also muscular aches and pains.

The nurse should administer adequate pain medication on a regular schedule for the first 48 hours after surgery and only gradually decrease the frequency and strength of analgesics according to the patient's needs per the physician's order. When establishing an effective pain management program after nephrectomy, it is important to remember that this is a painful surgery.

The use of moist heat, massage, and pillows to support the back while the patient is on his or her side also can provide relief. The individual should be turned from side to side at least every two hours or whenever desired.[41]

*Prevention of atelectasis and pneumonia* Because of the close proximity of the incision to the diaphragm, deep breathing and coughing can be extremely uncomfortable. The patient needs to be taught how to splint the incision while coughing. Use of analgesics at proper intervals will help the patient perform deep breathing and coughing more effectively. The nurse should instruct the individual to take at least ten deep breaths each hour while awake. The use of an incentive spirometer also may be beneficial. Intermittent positive pressure ventilation is not indicated for the average patient.[41]

*Monitoring renal function* If an indwelling catheter is in place, urine output should be monitored every hour immediately after surgery. The urine will be slightly blood-tinged for the first few hours after surgery. Urine output should be greater than 30 ml/hour. If the individual does not have a urinary catheter and has not voided within eight–ten hours after surgery, catheterization must be done to determine renal status. Accurate recording of fluid intake and output and weight should be done daily to determine the person's overall fluid balance status.

*Paralytic ileus* Paralytic ileus is fairly common following renal surgery. It is thought to be due to a reflex paralysis of intestinal peristalsis. The individual is usually allowed nothing to eat or drink by mouth for the first 24–48 hours after surgery. Oral food and fluids are avoided until bowel sounds are heard and gas is passed. The symptoms of paralytic ileus are abdominal distention, pain, and absence of bowel sounds. Nothing is given by mouth, and a nasogastric tube and/or rectal tube is used to relieve abdominal distention. Other measures such as ambulation, turning the patient, and use of a heating pad on the abdomen may also assist the individual in expelling flatus.

*Hemorrhage* Although not a frequent complication, postnephrectomy hemorrhage is a danger because the kidney is a highly vascular organ. Acute massive hemorrhage manifests itself by profuse drainage and distention at the suture line or internally. It can be reflected in an elevation of pulse rate and a drop in blood pressure. However, slow bleeding may not manifest itself in such obvious changes in vital signs. The nurse should observe the individual closely for symptoms of hemorrhage and shock. The patient should be turned and the underlying sheet examined for blood when the nephrectomy dressing is checked.

*Wound care* Wound care after nephrectomy is fairly routine. Frequently no drain is inserted. The frequency of dressing changes depends on the condition of the incision and the amount of drainage.

*Potential for pneumothorax* When the thoracoabdominal incision approach has been used for nephrectomy, the individual will have a chest tube placed during surgery to remove air and fluid from the thoracic cavity and to reexpand the lung. The nurse must maintain the chest tube under water drainage and keep it free of kinks.[41]

*Discharge planning* Discharge planning begins as soon as the individual is admitted to the hospital and is frequently updated. Arrangements should be made to have the patient visited by a home health nurse. Prior to discharge, the nurse should discuss with the individual the importance of continued liberal oral intake of fluids (at least 2500 ml/day) and the need to avoid any fad diets, which may result in excess protein catabolism. Individuals who are prone to hypertension should be encouraged to have frequent blood pressure checks because the nephrotic pressure gradient may change when only one kidney is present. Individuals who have had surgery to remove a renal tumor should be advised to have a complete physical examination and chest radiograph annually to rule out lung metastasis and to have an intravenous pyelogram yearly to check for contralateral tumors. The person also should be educated to report any symptoms of respiratory distress, hemoptysis, pain, or fracture of an extremity. These symptoms may signify metastasis. Last but not least, the person should be reassured that life with one kidney can be normal.

For nursing care of the individual undergoing chemotherapy refer to chapter 16. Refer to chapter 17 for nursing care associated with biotherapy.

## CONCLUSION

The two urinary tract cancers discussed in this chapter are relatively rare, together accounting for only about 6% of all cancers. Smoking is an etiologic factor for both types of cancers, as are certain genetic factors, although there are additional, differing risk factors for each cancer as well. Surgery is the usual choice of treatment for cure in the United States for most bladder and kidney cancers; however, radiation therapy is the mainstay of treatment for bladder cancer in many other countries.

Advances in treatment include the reemergence of intravesical BCG to prevent tumor progression and death from superficial bladder cancer; improved surgical procedures for continent urinary diversions following cystectomy for invasive bladder cancer; and neoadjuvant and adjuvant combined-modality treatment for invasive bladder cancer. Late-stage kidney cancer has recently shown improved response rates and lower toxicity to treatment with a combination of alfa-interferon and IL-2.

# REFERENCES

1. American Cancer Society: *Cancer Facts and Figures—1995.* Atlanta, American Cancer Society, 1995
2. Ross RK, Paganini-Hill A, Henderson BE: Epidemiology of bladder cancer, in Skinner DG, Lieskovsky G (eds): *Diagnosis and Management of Genitourinary Cancer.* Philadelphia, Saunders, 1988, pp 23–31
3. Carroll PR: Urothelial carcinoma: Cancers of the bladder, ureter, and renal pelvis, in Tanagho EA, McAninch JW (eds): *Smith's General Urology* (ed 14). Norwalk, CT, Appleton and Lange, 1995, pp 353–371
4. Lillienfeld AM, Levin ML, Moore GE: The association of smoking with cancer of the urinary bladder in humans. *Arch Intern Med* 98:129–135, 1956
5. Brownson RC, Chang JC, Davis JR: Occupation, smoking, and alcohol in the epidemiology of bladder cancer. *Am J Public Health* 77:1298–1300, 1987
6. Fair WR, Fuks ZY, Scher HI: Cancer of the bladder, in Devita VT, Hellman S, Rosenberg S (eds): *Cancer: Principles and Practice of Oncology* (ed 4). Philadelphia, Lippincott, 1993, pp 1052–1072
7. Raghavan D, Shipley WU, Garnick MG, et al: Biology and management of bladder cancer. *N Engl J Med* 322:1129–1138, 1990
8. Hossan E, Striegel A: Carcinoma of the bladder. *Semin Oncol Nurs* 9:252–266, 1993
9. Wheeless LL, Reeder JE, Han R: Consensus review of the clinical utility of DNA flow cytometry in bladder cancer. *Cytometry* 14:478, 1993
10. Mellon K, Wright C, Horne CH, et al: Long-term outcome related to epidermal growth factor receptor status in bladder cancer. *J Urol* 153:919–925, 1995
11. Lipponen PK: Over-expression of p53 nuclear oncoprotein in transitional-cell bladder cancer and its prognostic value. *Int J Cancer* 52:365–370, 1993
12. Javadpour N, Lalehzarian M: Magnetic resonance imaging (MRI) in bladder cancer. *Prog Clin Biol Res* 260:265–270, 1989
13. Holmang S, Hedelin H, Anderstrom A, et al: The relationship among multiple recurrences, progression and prognosis of patients with stages TA and T1 transitional cell cancer of the bladder followed for at least 20 years. *J Urol* 153:1823–1827, 1995
14. Hudson MA, Herr HW: Carcinoma in situ of the bladder. *J Urol* 153:564–572, 1995
15. Bono AV: Superficial bladder cancer: State of the art. *Cancer Chemother Pharmacol* 35:S101–S109, 1994 (suppl)
16. Herr HW, Schwalb DM, Zhang ZF, et al: Intravesical bacillus Calmette-Guerin therapy prevents tumor progression and death from superficial bladder cancer: Ten-year follow-up of a prospective randomized trial. *J Clin Oncol* 13:1404–1408, 1995
17. Coplen DE, Marcus MD, Myers JA, et al: Long-term follow-up of patients treated with 1 or 2, 6-week courses of intravesical bacillus Calmette-Guerin: Analysis of possible predictors of responses free of tumor. *J Urol* 144:652–657, 1990
18. Amling CL, Thrasher JB, Frazier HA, et al: Radical cystectomy for stages TA, TIS, and T1 transitional cell carcinoma of the bladder. *J Urol* 151:31–36, 1994
19. Richie JP: Surgery for invasive bladder cancer. *Hematol Oncol Clin North Am* 6:129–145, 1992

20. Jahnson S, Pederson J, Westman G: Bladder carcinoma: A 20-year review of radical irradiation therapy. *Radiother Oncol* 22:111–117, 1991
21. Tester W, Caplan R, Heaney J, et al: Neoadjuvant combined modality program with selective organ preservation for invasive bladder cancer: Results of Radiation Therapy Oncology Group phase II trial 8802. *J Clin Oncol* 14:119–126, 1996
22. Housset M, Maulard C, Chretien Y, et al: Combined radiation and chemotherapy for invasive transitional-cell carcinoma of the bladder: A prospective study. *J Clin Oncol* 11:2150–2157, 1993
23. Skinner DG, Daniels JR, Russell CA, et al: The role of adjuvant chemotherapy following cystectomy for invasive bladder cancer: A prospective comparative trial. *J Urol* 145:459–467, 1991
24. Walsh PC: Technique of radical retropubic prostatectomy with preservation of sexual function: An anatomic approach, in Skinner DG, Lieskovsky G (eds): *Diagnosis and Management of Genitourinary Cancer.* Philadelphia, Saunders, 1988, pp 753–778
25. Esrig D, Freeman J, Stein J, et al: Surgery in the management of bladder cancer. *Compr Ther* 21:20–24, 1995
26. Webster GD, Khoury JM: Continent urinary diversion, in Devita VT, Hellman S, Rosenberg SA (eds): *Important Advances in Oncology.* Philadelphia, Lippincott, 1992, pp 137–155
27. Kock NG, Nilson AE, Nilsson LO, et al: Urinary diversion via a continent ileal reservoir: Clinical results in 12 patients. *J Urol* 128:469–475, 1982
28. Skinner DG, Boyd SD, Lieskovsky G: Creation of the continent Kock ileal reservoir as an alternative to cutaneous urinary diversion, in Skinner DG, Lieskovsky G (eds): *Diagnosis and Management of Genitourinary Cancer.* Philadelphia, Saunders, 1988, pp 653–674
29. Stein J, Stenzl A, Esrig D: Lower urinary tract reconstruction following cystectomy in women using the Kock pouch ileal reservoir with bilateral urethrostomy: Initial clinical experience. *J Urol* 152:1404–1408, 1994
30. King LR, Stone AR, Webster GD (eds): *Bladder Reconstruction and Continent Urinary Diversion.* St Louis, Mosby Year Book, 1991, pp 306–318
31. Carroll PR, Barbour S: Urinary diversion and bladder substitution, in Tanagho EA, McAninch JW (eds): *Smith's General Urology* (ed 14). Norwalk, CT, Appleton and Lange, 1995, pp 448–461
32. Ofman US: Psychosocial and sexual implications of genitourinary cancers. *Semin Oncol Nurs* 9:286–292, 1993
33. Lue TF: Male sexual dysfunction, in Tanagho EA, McAninch JW (eds): *Smith's General Urology* (ed 13). Norwalk, CT, Appleton and Lange, 1992, pp 696–713
34. Boyd SD: Management of male impotency, including technique of penile prosthesis placement, in Skinner DG, Lieskovsky G (eds): *Diagnosis and Management of Genitourinary Cancer.* Philadelphia, Saunders, 1988, pp 675–683
35. Coppin C, Gospodarowicz M, Dixon P, et al: Improved local control of invasive bladder cancer by concurrent cisplatin and preoperative or radical radiation. *Proc Am Soc Clin Oncol* 11:Abstract 607, 198, 1992
36. Schultz PK, Herr HW, Zhang ZF, et al: Neoadjuvant chemotherapy for invasive bladder cancer: Prognostic factors for survival of patients treated with M-VAC with 5-year follow-up. *J Clin Oncol* 12:1394–1401, 1994
37. Kaufman DS, Shipley WU, Griffin PP, et al: Selective bladder

preservation by combination treatment of invasive bladder cancer. *N Engl J Med* 329:1377–1382, 1993

38. Thrasher JB, Crawford ED: Current management of invasive and metastatic transitional cell carcinoma of bladder cancer. *J Urol* 149:957–972, 1993

39. Raghavan D, Huben R: Management of bladder cancer. *Curr Probl Cancer* 19:1–64, 1995

40. Roth BJ: Preliminary experience with paclitaxel in advanced bladder cancer. *Semin Oncol* 22:1–5, 1995

41. Smeltzer SC, Bare BG: *Brunner and Suddarth's Textbook of Medical-Surgical Nursing* (ed 8). Philadelphia, Lippincott-Raven, 1996, pp 1168–1225

42. Razor BR: Continent urinary reservoirs. *Semin Oncol Nurs* 9:272–286, 1993

43. Greig BJ: Interventions of the ET nurse with the continent urinary Kock pouch patient. *J Enterostom Ther* 13:226–231, 1986

44. Kelly LP, Miaskowski C: An overview of bladder cancer: Treatment and nursing implications. *Oncol Nurs Forum* 23:459–476, 1996

45. Dreicer R, Williams RD: Renal parenchymal neoplasms, in Tanagho EA, McAninch JW (eds): *Smith's General Urology* (ed 14). Norwalk, CT, Appleton and Lange, 1995, pp 372–382

46. Paganini-Hill A, Ross RK, Henderson BE: Epidemiology of renal cancer, in Skinner DG, Lieskovsky G (eds): *Diagnosis and Management of Genitourinary Cancer*. Philadelphia, Saunders, 1988, pp 32–39

47. Mellemgaard A, Carstensen B, Nrgaard N, et al: Trends in the incidence of cancer of the kidney, pelvis, ureter and bladder in Denmark 1943–88. *Scand J Urol Nephrol* 27:327–332, 1993

48. Ross RK, Paganini-Hill A, Landolph J, et al: Analgesics, cigarette smoking and other risk factors for cancer of the renal pelvis and ureter. *Cancer Res* 49:1045–1048, 1989

49. Weir JM, Dunn JE: Smoking and mortality: A prospective study. *Cancer* 25:105–112, 1970

50. Doll R, Petro R: Mortality in relation to smoking: 20 years' observations on male British doctors. *BMJ* 2:1525–1536, 1976

51. McLaughlin JK, Mandel JS, Blot WJ, et al: A population-based case-control study of renal cell carcinoma. *J Natl Cancer Inst* 72:275–284, 1984

52. Wynder E, Mabuchi K, Whitmore W: Epidemiology of adenocarcinoma of the kidney. *J Natl Cancer Inst* 53:1619–1634, 1974

53. La Vecchia C, Negri E, D'Avanzo B, et al: Smoking and renal cell carcinoma. *Cancer Res* 50:5231–5233, 1990

54. Selikoff IJ, Hammond EC, Seidman HP: Mortality experience of insulation workers in the United States and Canada, 1943–1976. *Ann N Y Acad Sci* 330:91–116, 1979

55. Maclure M, Willett W: A case-control study of diet and risk of renal adenocarcinoma. *Epidemiology* 1:430–440, 1990

56. Ishikawa I, Saito Y, Shikura N, et al: Ten-year retrospective study on the development of renal cell carcinoma in dialysis patients. *Am J Kidney Dis* 16:452–458, 1990

57. Linehan WM, Shipley WU, Parkinson DR: Cancer of the kidney and bladder, in Devita VT, Hellman S, Rosenberg S (eds): *Cancer: Principles and Practice of Oncology* (ed 4). Philadelphia, Lippincott, 1993, pp 1023–1051

58. Stumm G, Eberwein S, Rostock-Wolf S, et al: Concomitant overexpression of the *EGFR* and *erbB-2* genes in renal cell carcinoma (RCC) is correlated with dedifferentiation and metastasis. *Int J Cancer* 69:17–22, 1996

59. Yoshida K, Tosaka A, Takeuchi S, et al: Epidermal growth factor receptor content in human renal cell carcinomas. *Cancer* 73:1913–1918, 1994

60. Kobayashi T, Honke K, Gasa S, et al: Epidermal growth factor elevates the activity levels of glycoprotein sulfotransferases in renal-cell-carcinoma cells. *Int J Cancer* 55:448–452, 1993

61. Imai T, Kimura M, Takeda M, et al: Significance of epidermal growth factor receptor and c-erbB-2 protein expression in transitional cell cancer of the upper urinary tract for tumor recurrence at the urinary bladder. *Br J Cancer* 71:69–72, 1995

62. Gnarra J, Lerman M, Zbar B, et al: Genetics of renal-cell carcinoma and evidence for a critical role for von Hippel–Lindau disease in renal tumorigenesis. *Semin Oncol* 22:3–8, 1995

63. Davis M: Renal cell carcinoma. *Semin Oncol Nurs* 9:267–271, 1993

64. Boswell WD: Diagnostic imaging in genitourinary cancer, in Skinner DG, Lieskovsky G (eds): *Diagnosis and Management of Genitourinary Cancer*. Philadelphia, Saunders, 1988, pp 237–263

65. McClennan BL: Oncologic imaging-staging and follow-up of renal and adrenal carcinoma. *Cancer* 67:1199–1208, 1991

66. Ljungberg B, Larsson P, Stenling R, et al: Flow cytometric deoxyribonucleic acid analysis in stage I renal cell carcinoma. *J Urol* 146:697–699, 1991

67. Pritchett TR, Lieskovsky G, Skinner DG: Clinical manifestations and treatment of renal parenchymal tumors, in Skinner DG, Lieskovsky G (eds): *Diagnosis and Management of Genitourinary Cancer*. Philadelphia, Saunders, 1988, pp 337–361

68. Flocks RH, Kadesky MC: Malignant neoplasms of the kidney: An analysis of 353 patients followed 5 years or more. *J Urol* 79:196–198, 1958

69. Thrasher JB, Robertson JE, Paulson DF: Expanding implications for conservative renal surgery in renal cell carcinoma. *Urology* 43:160–168, 1994

70. Novick AC: Current surgical approaches, nephron-sparing surgery, and the role of surgery in the integrated immunologic approach to renal-cell carcinoma. *Semin Oncol* 22:29–33, 1995

71. Hatcher PA, Anderson EE, Paulson DF, et al: Surgical management and prognosis of renal cell carcinoma invading the vena cava. *J Urol* 145:20–24, 1991

72. Janosko EO, Powell CS, Spence PA, et al: Surgical management of renal cell carcinoma with extensive intracaval involvement using a venous bypass system suitable for rapid conversion to total cardiopulmonary bypass. *J Urol* 154:555–557, 1991

73. Phillips E, Messing EM: Role of lymphadenectomy in the treatment of renal cell carcinoma. *Urology* 41:9–15, 1993

74. Peters PC, Brown GL: The role of lymphadenectomy in the management of renal cell carcinoma. *Urol Clin North Am* 18:705–709, 1991

75. Oliver RT, Nethersell AB, Bottomley JM: Unexplained spontaneous regression and alpha-interferon as treatment for metastatic renal carcinoma. *Br J Urol* 63:128–131, 1989

76. Rosenberg SA, Klotze MT, Muul LM, et al: Observations on the systemic administration of autologous lymphokine-activated killer cells and recombinant interleukin-2 with metastatic cancer. *N Engl J Med* 313:1485–1492, 1985

77. Krown SE: Interferon treatment of renal cell carcinoma: Current status and future prospects. *Cancer* 59:647–651, 1987 (suppl 3)

78. Muss HB: The role of biologic response modifiers in meta-

static renal cell carcinoma. *Semin Oncol* 15:30–34, 1988 (suppl 5)

79. Fyfe G, Fisher RI, Rosenberg SA, et al: Results of treatment of 255 patients with metastatic renal cell carcinoma who received high-dose recombinant interleukin-2 therapy. *J Clin Oncol* 13:688–696, 1995

80. Rosenberg SA, Yang JC, Topalin SL, et al: Treatment of 283 consecutive patients with metastatic melanoma or renal cell cancer using high-dose bolus interleukin 2. *JAMA* 271:907–913, 1994

81. Atkins MB, Spatano KA, Fisher RI, et al: Randomized phase II trial of high-dose interleukin-2 either alone or in combination with interferon alfa-2b in advanced renal cell carcinoma. *J Clin Oncol* 11:661–670, 1993

82. Ravaud A, Negrier S, Cany L, et al: Subcutaneous low-dose recombinant interleukin 2 and alpha-interferon in patients with metastatic renal cell carcinoma. *Br J Cancer* 69:1111–1114, 1994

83. Sandstrom SK: Nursing management of patients receiving biological therapy. *Semin Oncol Nurs* 12:152–162, 1996

84. Bender CM: Cognitive dysfunction associated with biological response modifier therapy. *Oncol Nurs Forum* 21:515–523, 1994

85. Skalla K: The interferons. *Semin Oncol Nurs* 12:97–105, 1996

86. Wheeler VS: Interleukins: The search for an anticancer therapy. *Semin Oncol Nurs* 12:106–114, 1996

87. Taneja SS, Pierce W, Figlin R, et al: Management of disseminated kidney cancer. *Urol Clin North Am* 21:625–637, 1994

88. Maulard-Durdux C, Dufour B, Hennequin C, et al: Postoperative radiation therapy in 26 patients with invasive transitional cell carcinoma of the upper urinary tract: No impact on survival? *J Urol* 155:115–117, 1996

89. Igawa M, Urakami S, Shiina H, et al: Long-term results with M-VAC for advanced urothelial cancer: High relapse rate and low survival in patients with a high complete response. *Br J Cancer* 76:321–324, 1995

90. Kobayashi H, Obata K: Results of adjuvant chemotherapy for invasive urothelial cancer with lymph-node metastasis. *Cancer Chemother Pharmacol* 35:s14–s17, 1994 (suppl)

91. Ponchietti R, Neri B, DiLoro F, et al: Endoluminal instillation of epidoxorubicin as adjuvant treatment for upper urinary tract urothelial tumors. *Anticancer Res* 16:537–539, 1996

# Chapter 34

# Breast Cancer

Dianne D. Chapman, RN, MS, OCN®

Michelle Goodman, RN, MS, OCN®

## INTRODUCTION

Breast cancer is the most common cancer in women and the leading cause of death for women 40–44 years of age. It is second to lung cancer as the leading cause of all cancer deaths in women. The incidence of breast cancer increases rapidly with age until menopause, after which time it increases more slowly with advancing years.[1,2] Over 70% of all breast cancer occurs in women who are 50 years of age or older. The National Institutes of Health consensus development conference statement emphasized that in the next decade, more than 1.8 million women (184,000 in 1996) in the United States will be newly diagnosed with invasive breast cancer and, of that number, 30% will die of their disease.[3] Screening methods, particularly mammography, have become more precise, permitting earlier diagnosis which in part accounts for the dramatic increase in incidence in breast cancer between 1982 and 1987, and likely is also responsible for the current slight decrease in mortality figures.[1,2] However, more research in the area of chemoprevention, systemic therapies, and access to preventive health care and early detection for the socioeconomically disadvantaged are needed to change the current mortality rates from this disease.[4]

In 1963, the lifetime risk of breast cancer was about 5.5%, or 1 in every 18 women with an estimated life span of 72 years.[5] Current statistics indicate that the average woman in her early 60s has a projected lifetime risk of almost 14% of developing breast cancer. In general, breast cancer incidence varies across the country, but is about 1 in every 8 women.[6] This increasing incidence is predominantly in women under 55 years of age and in black women. Possible reasons for this increased incidence are that there are more women who are living longer into the cancer-prone years, there is better statistical reporting, and there are better screening methods. In addition, changes in dietary and socioeconomic habits, and increasing exposure to carcinogens, may contribute to this increased incidence of breast cancer.[6,7]

While the incidence of breast cancer has increased over the past 30 years, the mortality rate has recently demonstrated a slight decrease, reflecting better cure rates for earlier staged lesions. This apparent progress may in part be related to a better understanding of the natural history of breast cancer, as well as reflect the benefit of early detection methods. The utilization of screening tools and community awareness of the signs and symptoms of breast cancer has probably been influential in reducing the average size of a breast tumor at diagnosis (2.74 cm in 1983 to 2.17 in 1991).[6] This decrease is more evident among white women than black women (Figure 34-1). It is imperative that nurses are acquainted with various cultural and economic barriers that may keep women from utilizing screening tools and benefitting from community education programs.

Historically, breast cancer has been considered a disease that remains localized until some time in which metastasis occurs via the lymph nodes and later spreads beyond regional nodes to distant sites. The possibility that hematogenous spread would occur early, prior to lymph node involvement, was proposed nearly two decades ago and supports the concept that breast cancer is a systemic disease at the time of clinical diagnosis.[8]

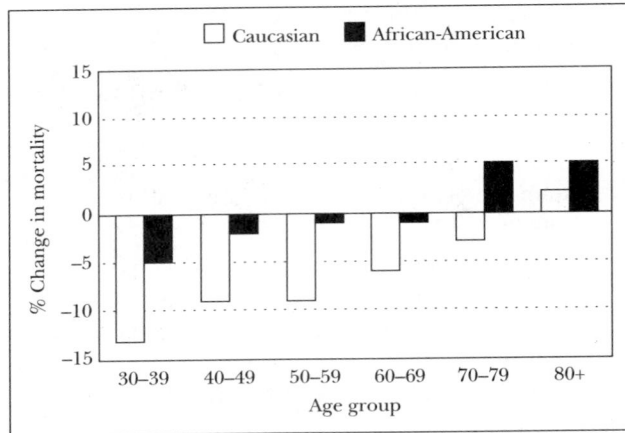

**FIGURE 34-1**    Breast cancer mortality 1989–1993. Data from *Cancer Letter* 22:4, 1996

It is now widely accepted that breast cancer is not one disease but rather protean, differing in histological, biological and immunologic characteristics. Phenotypic heterogeneity exists within individual breast neoplasms such that drug resistance, both intrinsic and acquired, occurs, rendering unresponsive cell lines unopposed and capable of establishing metastatic sites. Whether or not the individual with breast cancer survives the disease is determined by numerous factors, but the outcome primarily depends upon the intrinsic growth rate of the tumor, which varies dramatically; the age of the woman at diagnosis; and numerous biological parameters that ultimately define the natural history of the disease.

The interdisciplinary team utilizes various clinical, histological, and pathological findings to define, as precisely as possible, the particular characteristics of a breast cancer that will determine the most appropriate treatment plan for a given patient. This approach integrates the physical examination with the histopathological characteristics of the tumor, and incorporates the patient's personal bias based on her emotional needs and physical preferences. As a member of this team, the nurse must be aware of the factors affecting the selection of the treatment plan and appropriately educate the patient regarding the various treatment strategies in order to prevent and manage complications of the disease and its treatment.

## ETIOLOGY

### Risk Assessment

Experimental and clinical data indicate that the development of breast cancer is not a chance event. The genesis of breast cancer seems to be a multiphasic process involving many factors that are influential in the ongoing duel between tumor growth potential and host resistance.

Attempts are being made to reveal the etiology of breast cancer through an intense study of its epidemiology. As populations are identified in whom the incidence of the disease is increased, a genetic, hormonal, or biochemical factor may be identified that is considered significant in etiology. Epidemiological features, when statistically correlated with incidence of disease, designate a particular factor as a "risk factor." Each risk factor merely serves as one piece of the puzzle because there are so many different factors that either increase or decrease a woman's risk of developing breast cancer. Table 34-1 separates current risk factors for breast cancer according to their degree of importance in our understanding of the etiology of breast cancer.

## Hormonal Factors

The hormone environment has long been recognized as a major factor in the development of breast cancer. This is well demonstrated in that gender is the most significant

**TABLE 34-1**    Risk Factors

| PRIMARY | |
|---|---|
| Female | |
| Age >50 | |
| Country of origin: | North America Northern Europe |
| Family history: | Personal history of breast cancer |
| | Two or more first-degree relatives with breast cancer |
| | Bilateral/premenopausal breast cancer in first-degree relative |
| Biopsy histology: | Atypical hyperplasia |
| | Carcinoma in situ (DCIS and LCIS) |

| SECONDARY |
|---|
| Postmenopausal obesity |
| Early menarche (<12) coupled with late menopause (>55); onset of regular cycles within 1 year of menarche |
| First full-term pregnancy >30 years of age |
| Use of oral contraceptives prior to age 20 and persisting for 6 or more years |
| Ionizing radiation to chest with exposure occurring prior to age 35 |
| Benign breast disease |

| OTHER |
|---|
| Nulliparous |
| Estrogen replacement therapy |
| Alcohol |
| Diet |

risk factor for the development of the disease. Women are 100 times more likely to develop breast cancer than men. Additionally, after a diagnosis of breast cancer has been made, the relationship of the tumor estrogen receptor with the response to hormonal manipulation strongly suggests a hormonal connection. The significance of early menarche (before age 12), nulliparity or parity after age 30 and late menopause (after age 55) are well-known events that are considered risk factors for development of breast cancer. All of these events are linked to the type and duration of exposure to endogenous hormones that may have an impact on the development of breast cancer.

The relevance of breast cancer risk to early menarche and/or late menopause is correlated with the length of ovarian function. Additionally, women who experience early menarche with onset of regular cycles within a year are proposed to be at three times the normal risk. A woman with 40 or more years of ovarian function has twice the risk compared with those who have ovarian function for 30 or fewer years. Conversely, those with natural or surgical menopause before the age of 45 without replacement therapy are believed to have two times a reduction in risk.[9] Women who have their first full-term pregnancy after the age of 35 have a greater risk than nulliparous women.

Hormones play a significant role in the development of breast cancer, though the extent to which this role affects the genesis and outcome of the disease is relatively unknown at this time. While hormones themselves are not inherently mutagenic, it is surmised that they may act as initiators or promoters in that they alter cell proliferation, differentiation, and atrophy.[10,11]

The endocrine system circulates three estrogens in a woman's body; estriol, estrone, and estradiol. Estriol is not considered to be a factor in cancer genesis. In fact, it is thought to have an oppositional effect to the carcinogenic action of estrone and estradiol. Estrone may be used in the treatment of hormone deficiencies. It is considered to be less active than estradiol. Estradiol is a potent estrogen that is the primary ingredient in exogenous hormone therapy. Estradiol is the dominant hormone present during the premenopausal years, and estrone may play a significant role during the postmenopausal years.

Several studies have considered the relationship between the role of endogenous estrogens and breast cancer. A comprehensive review of hormone profiles in women with breast cancer has identified several commonalities. Premenopausal women tend to exhibit decreased adrenal androgen levels. Increased testosterone production and estradiol levels appear in both pre- and postmenopausal women.[11]

More recent speculation involves the effect of progesterone on the risk of breast cancer. Breast epithelial mitosis, which varies significantly within the menstrual cycle, peaks during the luteal phase.[12,13] This finding has suggested that progesterone and estrogen may contribute to the risk of breast cancer. However, studies that have measured progesterone in premenopausal women found that progesterone levels were decreased rather than increased in patients with breast cancer.[11]

Pregnancy (full term) has been reported to exert a deterrent effect on the development of breast cancer. This is generally thought to be based on the change in the hormonal milieu. The exact mechanism is unknown, but speculation includes the effects of the alteration of prolactin and/or estriol. Prolactin has been recognized as having a direct effect on the growth of human breast epithelial tissue and is associated with the generation of mammary tumors in the rat. The decrease in prolactin levels during pregnancy may account for this protective effect.[11] Furthermore, there is a significant increase in estriol compared with estrone and estradiol during pregnancy.

This preventive effect may be more pronounced with pregnancies at a young age (<20) and is enhanced by subsequent pregnancies.[14] Additionally, the benefit conferred on these women continues to be a positive factor during the extent of their lifetime. Lactation and breast feeding have historically been considered protective mechanisms for breast cancer development. Although the theory remains controversial and the benefit may only be related to parity, there have been several studies that correlate a progressive risk reduction in premenopausal women with the number of breast feeding years.[15–18]

The role that endogenous estrogens may play in the development of breast cancer suggests that exogenous therapy may be instrumental in the development of breast cancer. Animal studies have shown that exogenous estrogens, some progesterones, and some estrogen/progesterone combinations cause mammary tumors in rats and mice.[19] The information on the use of hormone therapy is limited in its consistency, owing to the disparity of dosages and duration as well as the current inability to assess cohort lifetime effects as well as multigenerational effects.

Oral contraceptives have been marketed since the 1960s. The question of a connection between oral contraceptives (OC) and breast cancer has resulted in inconsistent and controversial reports. Although studies investigating OC are often difficult to interpret, some basic risk information has been extrapolated. In general, nulliparous women who began using contraceptives before age 20 and continued uninterrupted use for more than six years, have a minimal increased risk of developing breast cancer. It has been suggested the risk may be more significant for black women but further studies must be done to determine if a racial difference exists.[20–25]

The literature also suggests the use of OC during the middle reproductive years seems to pose no additional risk. Another increase in risk has been associated with the use of OC during the perimenopausal years.[22] The risk possibly may be due to delaying menopause by creating and maintaining a hormonal environment that mimics that of a menstruating woman.[9]

The question of risk in relation to hormone replacement therapy (HRT) is equally murky, with little replicated evidence of increased risk. A review of the literature has demonstrated that HRT users either exhibit no increase or a minimal increase in risk attributable to dosage and duration of use. In summarizing the results, it appears that the risk is negligible for most users and increases slightly for those using HRT before 1958, long-term users (10 + years), and those who have also used OC.[26–33]

Current evidence suggests either no effect on breast cancer risk from HRT or an elevation in risk of less than twofold with very long-term use or relatively high doses. Any potential effect of HRT on breast cancer risk must be considered with the therapy's established protective effect against osteoporotic fractures and increased risk of endometrial cancer and probable decreased risk for coronary artery disease.[7]

The concern surrounding prescribing HRT for breast cancer survivors will undoubtedly become an increasingly problematic issue for clinicians. The number of survivors has steadily increased, including a growing population of women who are "forced" into a medical menopause through chemotherapeutic agents. The premenopausal women who experience an acute, early menopause seem to report more severe symptoms than premenopausal women who experience gradual, natural hormonal decreases over time. Although a majority of these women will enjoy disease-free survival, their quality of life may likely be compromised by somatic complaints (hot flashes, dyspareunia, labile mood swings, etc.)[34] and physical manifestations (heart disease and/or osteoporosis).[35,36] Hormone replacement therapy is known to remedy or reduce these problems, but physicians are reluctant to prescribe it. Giving breast cancer survivors estrogen therapy is a controversial issue, since the current standard of practice generally precludes prescribing these hormonal agents.[37–41]

Several articles have addressed the problem and the need for quantitative data, and prospective randomized studies are being launched to begin to answer this complicated issue. One such study has begun and another has been approved through ECOG (Eastern Cooperative Oncology Group). Vassilopoulou-Sellin and Theriault[39] have initiated a study designed to determine if HRT constitutes a cancer recurrence risk versus the benefit of reducing bone demineralization, thereby preventing or arresting the disabling effects of osteoporosis. Eligible patients for this study are selected from those with stage I or II disease who are disease-free for at least two years if their tumors are estrogen receptor-negative, or ten years if their tumors are estrogen receptor-positive or unknown. The differences in the interval reflects the historical hypothesis which suggests that exposure to estrogen stimulates cancer growth.

Another study initiated by Cobleigh et al[41] has been approved for a pilot study through the ECOG. The study will be initially restricted to breast cancer survivors who are currently taking tamoxifen for six or more months and are considered to be disease-free. The ultimate goal is to examine the quality of life issues surrounding the menopausal symptoms and the effect of HRT and tamoxifen on breast and endometrial tissue, mammographic images, bone density, and development of coronary heart disease. One of the questions asked by Cobleigh et al concerns the likelihood of breast cancer patients agreeing to participate in such a clinical trial. Anecdotally, the answer was overwhelmingly apparent soon after a report of this protocol was published in the *New York Times*. Within a few weeks, women from almost every state called, wishing to participate. Personal accounts of severe somatic complaints, consisting mainly of multiple hot flashes, vaginal atrophy causing dyspareunia, and emotional lability spanned every age group. Clearly, there is a definite if not desperate need for studies addressing the issues of HRT.

## Family History

Along with age and gender, family history of breast cancer is a contributing factor to the potential risk of developing the disease. Many people, including physicians, erroneously estimate risk factors. This is due to the wide range of risk associated with a family history of breast cancer dependent upon the age and known risk factors of the patient, the ages and number of first- and second-degree relatives with unilateral or bilateral breast cancer, and the presence of autosomal dominant gene mutations. Many studies have tried to extrapolate risk based on personal and family history.[37,42–45] Claus et al[46] using data from the Cancer and Steroid Hormone Study, developed a model which gives age-specific risk for a woman with a family history of one or more relatives. The Claus study provided confirmation that the risk of breast cancer not only is related to a positive family history but also is strongly correlated to the number and ages of affected relatives and can vary significantly. Examples of this variance are illustrated by a woman with a lifetime risk of 44% because she has two first-degree relatives diagnosed with cancer in their thirties versus a woman with a lifetime risk of 11% because two first-degree relatives were diagnosed in their seventies.[45]

The issue of lifetime risk is inferred in virtually all of these studies and is assumed to be true. The question of lifetime risk was addressed by examining data from 9000 women to determine if risk associated with family history remained stable or varied with age. Roseman et al[47] found that family history may not be a determinant for women over 60 and the Claus study[47] suggests that risk decreases with age for those with an autosomal dominant allele. Aside from those with genetic mutations, risk does seem to increase with age.[44]

Most women (approximately 70%) who develop breast cancer have no known risk factors. Familial and hereditary breast cancer account for a very small proportion of the diagnosed cases (20% and 9% respectively). The majority of breast cancers are considered to be *sporadic*, which is defined as no history of breast cancer through two generations. *Familial* or *polygenic* breast cancer is described as a family history of one or more first-degree relatives with breast cancer. *Hereditary* or *genetic* breast cancer is defined as a positive family history, often with related cancers (e.g., ovarian), consistent with an autosomal dominant factor that includes onset at an early age (less than 40), an excess of bilaterality, and other multiple cancers. Two autosomal dominant gene mutations have been isolated, one on the long arm of the 17th chromosome and another on the long arm of chromosome 13. The ultimate goal of gene mapping is to be able to identify a crucial gene, characterize it, and thereby gain an understanding of the molecular predisposition of breast cancer in families. This information should conceivably lead to new methods of breast cancer therapy.

Many of the genes responsible for inherited familial cancers seem to be tumor suppressor genes which are actively involved in supressing malignant growth during the cell cycle. When these genes undergo mutation(s), the normal function is altered, causing abnormal proliferation resulting in neoplastic and malignant cell growth.

Epidemiologists and physician researchers began to look for patterns within families having an abnormal incidence of breast cancers among the members. A major breakthrough was announced in the early 1990s when several papers were published identifying the presence and subsequent mapping and cloning of a breast cancer tumor suppressor gene on the long arm of chromosome 17 (17q12-21).[48–50] Mutations to genes occur through physical, environmental, or genetic influences resulting in abnormal cell proliferation and culminating with neoplastic development.

Inheritance of the *BRCA1* susceptibility gene is associated with a strong penetrance (likelihood that the effect of the mutation will result in the disease) for families with multiple breast and ovarian cancers (90%) as well as those with breast cancers diagnosed before the age of 45 (70%). There is also an associated risk with colon and prostate cancers. Of note, men who carry the mutated *BRCA1* do not seem to be at an increased risk for developing breast cancer (less than 1%).[51] Although this inherited gene mutation identifies only a very small proportion of the breast cancer population (5%–8%), the hope is that the information gleaned from this and other inherited genes will provide additional information to understand the complex puzzle known as sporadic breast cancer, affecting approximately 70% of those diagnosed.[52] Another breast cancer susceptibility gene, *BRCA2*, has been identified on the long arm of chromosome 13 (13q12-13).[52] This mutation seems to be associated with male breast cancer and early-onset female breast cancer.[53]

Another tumor suppressor gene, *p53*, also may become a promising marker for predicting breast cancers. This gene mutation has been identified in breast cancer and is often associated with a poor prognosis.[54,55] This gene has also been identified in various tissues ranging from normal to peritumoral.[56,57] These findings suggest that *p53* mutations may be present in varying degrees as the cells evolve from normal to malignant and, therefore,

*p53* could conceivably become an important risk assessment tool.

For the woman who has breast cancer, there is a 2%–14% risk of developing a second primary breast cancer.[29] Some variabilities that may alter the risk of developing a contralateral breast cancer are a personal early age of onset or having a first-degree relative with early-onset or bilateral disease. Treatment with chemotherapy and/or hormones for breast cancer may reduce the development of a second breast cancer.[42,58,59]

An increased risk of breast cancer also may be associated with primary ovarian or endometrial cancer, but this risk is low, estimated at less than two times the normal.

## Diet

The wide range of variance in breast cancer rates worldwide and dramatic increases in migrant populations may reflect one or several factors that influence the risk of breast cancer. The risk of breast cancer is greatest in developed countries, especially those of North America and northern Europe. The risk is lowest in developing third-world countries. Apart from a genetic influence, diet has been investigated as the most plausible variant.

Japan is known to have a low incidence of breast cancer. However, when Japanese women migrate from Japan to Hawaii where the incidence of breast cancer is high, they experience a significant increase in breast cancer incidence. By the second generation, the incidence rate parallels that of daughters of Japanese women born in Hawaii, suggesting a dietary influence. Diet, however, may not be the only factor in cancer genesis of migrants. The new culture may provide accessibility to risk factors that may not have been an issue in the country of origin. Changes in exercise habits, alcohol and drug use, hormone therapy, and smoking may be experienced, which could confound the diet correlation.

Diets high in fats have been implicated in countries that have shown a sudden increase in incidence rates, as well as high-risk countries. Reports of positive correlations with meat and dairy products have been issued, but additional case studies have largely failed to support the data.[59,60]

A potential answer to these questions may be provided by the Women's Health Initiative, sponsored by the National Institutes of Health. This study has begun accruing approximately 100,000 women representing multicultural and multisocioeconomic backgrounds. The study will examine the effects of reducing dietary fat, adding calcium supplements, and hormone replacement to determine if any intervention reduces the expected incidence of breast and colorectal cancer, osteoporosis, and heart disease. This will be accomplished through clinical trials, observational studies, and community educational programs.[61,62]

There is still controversy regarding at which time of life dietary habits may be most influential in the development of breast cancer. Looking at current diet regimens in relation to breast cancer would not be helpful if perimenarchal diet were the determining factor. The possible significance of diet at this time of a woman's life corresponds to a physical environment of accelerated growth and development of the breasts. These mammary tissues may potentially be altered by or sensitized to hormones produced by an excess of dietary fat.

The relationship of dietary fats and breast cancer is largely based on consistent findings in animal studies. Rats ingesting a high-fat diet demonstrated an increase in breast malignancies over those on a low-fat diet but other studies in animals suggest that the risk is associated with the amount of calories ingested rather than a specific food type.[63] It has been speculated that this connection may be linked to the amount and ratios of hormones produced by the endocrine system. The proliferation of breast tissue may be altered by changes in estrogen, pituitary, and thyroid function, which are sensitive to dietary changes.

## Obesity

Obesity confers a slight increased risk overall, but demonstrates more of a risk for those women who are postmenopausal than any other age group.[64,65] A history of weight gain in early adult life may be associated with an increased risk. Although further studies are needed for confirmation, this weight gain may impact risk most if it occurs during the third decade.[66,67] Obese women, in general, may be more at risk for recurrence, but this may be explained by detection bias owing to the large amount of body fat that could obscure clinical findings.

A possible explanation of the discrepancy between pre- and postmenopausal risk may be linked to hormonal influences. Obesity during childbearing years has been associated with a decrease in the level of progesterone, which reduces cell proliferation in the breast. Obese postmenopausal women have no ovarian function and have both higher rates of conversion of androstenedione to estrogen in adipose tissue and lower levels of sex hormone–binding globulin than do thinner women.[65] Additionally, the enzyme responsible for converting estrone to estradiol is present in adipose breast tissue, and the rate of conversion has been positively correlated to body weight.

## Alcohol

According to a meta-analysis,[68,69] the literature favors a positive association between alcohol and breast cancer risk. The biological mechanisms of the association are not known. Whether the increased risk involves exposure to circulating cytotoxic by-products of alcohol, its effect on hepatic function, a possible alteration in the cell membrane permeability in breast tissue, or other mechanisms is yet to be determined. The most compelling evidence

suggests that the relationship between alcohol and breast cancer risk is greatest for women who consume more than two drinks per day.[69–71] However, this connection is not strong enough at this point to conclude a causality exists between the use of alcohol and breast cancer. Women who consume alcohol should be counseled regarding the potential cancer risks versus benefits based on known and family risk factors.

## Radiation

The carcinogenic effect from both low- and high-dose ionizing radiation has been well documented. Survivors of the atomic bombs exhibited an increase in breast as well as other cancers. A risk of breast cancer has been associated with radiation therapy for a broad spectrum of health problems including chronic mastitis, tuberculosis, tinea capitis, thymus disorders, and adult and childhood cancers.[71,72] The risk increases with dosage, especially if a woman is exposed in the period of young adulthood. Mantle radiation for Hodgkin's disease is associated with an increased risk relative to age during treatment. Hancock et al reviewed 885 women and calculated a relative risk of 4.1 overall and a relative risk of 136 for women treated before age 15. This risk remains increased for those radiated before the age of 30 and negligible for those treated after 30.[73]

The concern about the effects of radiation has generated some apprehension regarding the potential harm of repeated mammograms and chest radiographs. The doses for these procedures are extremely small, and the potential benefit far outweighs the risk. A mammogram emits a dose of .15 cGy, and a chest film generates approximately .002 cGy to each breast.[73] The radiation exposure from a mammogram is similar to the radiation exposure incurred from flying 400 miles in an airplane.

## Nonproliferative Disease

Approximately 70% of biopsies reflect cellular changes that impart no risk or a very small risk to the patient and are often referred to as fibrocystic change. These include usual, moderate, or florid hyperplasia; sclerosing adenosis; and papilloma, which have been addressed previously. In addition, some nonproliferative changes are recognized to bestow a very slight or no increased risk to the patient. These are adenosis, apocrine change, duct ectasis, and usual mild epithelial hyperplasia.[74]

Apocrine change is often accompanied with the diagnosis of a cyst. These cells may form tufted or papillary clusters instead of the characteristic single cell layer. *Adenosis* and *duct ectasia* refer to an increase in the number of cells in a gland and a dilation of a duct. Epitheliosis or mild epithelial hyperplasia is associated with common configurations seen with slightly increased number of cells at the basement membrane.[75]

## Proliferative Disease

The presence of proliferation on a pathology slide indicates a presence of increased cell growth. According to Page and DuPont, the term *proliferative breast disease* "indicates that proliferative alterations are noted by histology and that they indicate a disease by their demonstrated link to an increased risk of subsequent carcinoma."[76,p.119] These risks have been categorized as *slight*, which is associated with one and one-half to two times the normal risk; *moderate*, which is associated with four to five times the normal risk; and *marked*, which is associated with eight to ten times the normal risk.

Proliferative disease without atypia falls into the slightly increased risk category. This classification includes examples of common types of epithelial hyperplasia, which may be subcategorized as mild, moderate, or florid. The degree refers to the number of cells present relative to the basement membrane of a lobular unit or duct. Since two cells are usually present above the basement membrane, the presence of three or more cells is described as mild hyperplasia. The presence of five or more cells constitutes moderate hyperplasia, and an increased progression of these changes characterizes florid hyperplasia. Twenty percent of breast biopsies contain moderate or florid hyperplasia. The presence of papilloma and sclerosing adenosis also falls in the slight risk category.[73–77]

The moderate risk category includes atypical ductal hyperplasia and atypical lobular hyperplasia. These risk statistics are not lifetime estimates, but are limited to approximately 18 years after biopsy, which is the limit of most benign breast disease follow-up. Atypical hyperplasia has some, but not all, of the characteristics of carcinoma in situ.[76]

## Carcinoma in Situ

Carcinoma in situ has been referred to as a "precancerous condition." This definition reflects the potential capabilities of the cells, rather than the histopathological characteristics. The nomenclature of *carcinoma in situ* refers to a localized process describing cells that are still within the site of origin. A carcinoma in situ that remains in the breast is capable of transforming to an invasive cancer but does not necessarily do so.

Ductal carcinoma in situ (DCIS) and lobular carcinoma in situ (LCIS) are characterized by an eight- to tenfold increased risk of developing invasive cancer.[78,79] DCIS lesions are often singular, and conservative treatment with local excision is an accepted treatment. Lobular carcinoma in situ may be associated with increased risk within both breasts. LCIS is usually not detected by palpation or mammography, and is most often an incidental microscopic finding when breast tissue is removed for another reason.[75] Current evidence suggests that LCIS functions as a marker of increased risk for developing an invasive ductal or lobular cancer. Mastectomy for LCIS should be considered a prophylactic procedure rather than therapeutic.[80] Mastectomy with close follow-up of the other breast has often been the treatment of choice, but clinicians increasingly feel LCIS may be treated with local excision and close follow-up that employs mammograms twice a year and clinical exam every three to four months. Improvements in mammography sensitivity have made this approach more feasible. Women who are unable or unwilling to comply with frequent monitoring may opt for a unilateral or bilateral mastectomy with or without reconstruction.

## PREVENTION OF BREAST CANCER

While it is conceivable to determine the possibility of developing breast cancer based on risk factors, it is virtually impossible to predict with certainty who will or will not develop breast cancer in a lifetime. The unknown etiology of breast cancer coupled with conflicting data regarding the identification of risk factors as well as how these risk factors influence the genesis of breast cancer makes preventive action difficult. To prevent an event from occurring, one must know the cause. Unfortunately, there is a paucity of information regarding the origin of breast cancer. As mentioned earlier in this chapter, some elements have been recognized to be primary risk factors in the development of breast cancer and others may be secondary or possible risk factors. Even this information is limited at best, because 70% of the women with breast cancer have no identifiable risk factors.

Research concerning prevention and early detection of breast cancer is critically important in the reduction of mortality from breast cancer. Of the more than 184,000 women diagnosed yearly, only 50% will be diagnosed with stage I disease, and approximately 30% of all women with breast cancer will subsequently die of their disease. Current evidence has indicated that the disease is often present in the breast six to eight years before it becomes mammographically or clinically evident. Newer, even more sophisticated methods of detecting breast cancer or preventing further proliferation of these undetectable pathological breast cancers are becoming the forefront of clinical research efforts. As nurses, our role in educating the public, promoting research, and recruiting women into these research studies cannot be overemphasized.

### Chemoprevention

Chemoprevention is the use of a chemical agent to prevent or alter the development of cancer. The development of a chemoprevention agent should be based on a disease model which identifies progressive development over several years and involves multiple factors which can be reversed. These interventions must be based on a biological rationale and have minimal toxic effects.[81–83]

Chemoprevention for breast cancer has been proposed to possibly alter the course of disease for those with known risk factors. Several dietary micronutrients have been touted for their presumed protective capabilities in animal studies, but they remain controversial for human use. Vitamin A and its retinoid derivatives offer some promise for chemoprevention. Vitamin A can affect the growth and differentiation of epithelial tissue. Breast cancer is considered a disease of the breast epithelial cells, and the retinoids may have the capacity to alter the oncogenic course.[84] Studies examining the effects of the synthetic retinoid 4-HPR in preventing breast cancer in high-risk women and preventing a second primary cancer in the contralateral breast are being conducted. Vitamins A, E, and C in foods act as antioxidants, which defend against free radicals and aid in stimulating the immune response. However, it is difficult to attribute these qualities to specific micronutrients because of the multiple components of vegetables and fruits.[84,85]

The most promising breast cancer prevention study to date is NSABP P-1, the randomized study using tamoxifen vs. a placebo to determine if breast cancer can be prevented in women with known high risk.

The influence of hormones in breast cancer is uniformly recognized. Because of this known association, physicians and scientists have long entertained the possibility of an antiestrogen that may prevent breast cancer. Tamoxifen was introduced in the 1970s and is the most widely used drug for breast cancer in the United States. It was first introduced as a treatment for advanced breast cancer in postmenopausal women.[86] Since then, tamoxifen has been found to be effective in the treatment of premenopausal women with advanced disease.[87] It has also been found to increase disease-free survival in node-negative, ER-positive disease,[88] as well as node-positive disease.[89] Women taking tamoxifen for primary breast cancer have experienced a reduction in the expected incidence of contralateral breast cancer. This strengthens the possibility of a chemoprotective effect, and has led to its use in a large prevention trial.

The enrollment into this study is based on the number of risk factors and the relative weight each factor is assigned.[90] Because of the increased risk with advancing age, any woman over 60 is eligible. No one below the age of 35 is eligible. Women over 35 with diagnoses of LCIS that have been treated with local excision are eligible. A woman between the ages of 35 and 59 must have a risk of developing breast cancer equal to a 60-year-old woman.

The study will last for a minimum of five years. The participants will be expected to comply with the schedule for daily medication, clinical examinations, and mammography.

Side effects are an important consideration when any drug is taken electively. The common toxicities reported are similar to menopausal symptoms; hot flashes, vaginal discharge, and irregular menses. Rare events include ocular changes, thromboembolic disease, and second primary cancers of the liver and endometrium.

Although tamoxifen is considered an antiestrogen and, therefore, an antagonist, it may also act as an agonist. As an antagonist, tamoxifen competes with estradiol for the receptor sites in the nucleus. This mechanism causes an estrogen blockade and impedes growth of malignant cells. Although the exact action of the drug is unknown, several explanations have been postulated. Tamoxifen may alter the growth factors that regulate breast cell proliferation,[91] bind to cytoplasmic antiestrogenic binding sites thereby increasing intracellular drug levels,[92] inhibit the amount of free estrogen available to the cell,[93] stimulate natural killer cells, or affect the endocrine regulation of breast cancer cells.[94]

Tamoxifen also exhibits agonist activity, which was recognized in the early trials. This agonist mechanism suggests beneficial action regarding osteoporosis and cardiovascular disease, both of which are significant factors of morbidity and mortality in postmenopausal women.[95]

Nurses across the country are instrumental in the identification of women who are eligible for the Breast Cancer Prevention Trial, the education of the public, recruitment of women to the study, and compliance with the treatment, as well as assessment of toxicity and data collection. Clinicians and families are enthusiastic about the potential outcome of this study, which may provide information on the possible feasibility of chemoprevention and innovative insights into the causal pathway of breast cancer.

## Exercise

The role of exercise in the prevention of breast cancer has not been widely studied. The endorsement of exercise is usually presented in the context of reducing or counteracting known risk factors. Women who exercise tend to have less body fat, which impacts their hormone milieu. Ovarian function is altered by strenuous exercising, which may delay menarche or create irregular menses or an amenorrheic state. Exercising may reduce the risk of breast cancer for postmenopausal obese women by reducing the amount of free estrogen stored in body fat.

The few studies which have looked at exercise as a protective agent have been generally inconclusive. This is possibly related to the presence of confounding risk factors, inaccurate activity measures, or alteration of activity over time.[96,97] Recently, two papers have suggested exercise confers a direct protective effect on the development of breast cancer. Bernstein et al[98] found that young women (menarche to early middle age) who vigorously exercised three to eight hours or more per week, experienced a 58% reduction in risk. Mittendorf et al[99] conducted a large case-controlled study which showed a modest effect for young women who reported any strenuous activity and a 50% reduction for those who vigorously exercised daily. While more studies are necessary, these similar findings support the hypothesis that physical activity may reduce the risk of breast cancer.

## Prophylactic Mastectomy

A *prophylactic mastectomy*,—the removal of the majority of breast tissue including total breast, tail of Spence, and nipple areola complex—may be warranted in certain high-risk women; however, controversy exists over how much risk is enough to justify performing this procedure. Women for whom a prophylactic mastectomy may be indicated have been identified as those with some or all of the following conditions.[94]

1. A family history of documented hereditary breast cancer consistent with an autosomal dominant factor. Women who are presumed to be gene carriers may have a breast cancer risk ranging from 50%–100% depending on family history.
2. A personal risk of at least 50% for developing breast cancer.
3. A proven history of breast cancer in one breast and extreme nodularity or cystic changes in the opposite breast. The incidence of a second breast cancer in the opposite breast is estimated to be 15%–20%.
4. Chronic cystic mastitis or a diagnosis of atypical hyperplasia with repeated surgical biopsies.
5. An overwhelming fear of breast cancer such that the possibility of developing breast cancer interferes with her daily life.

Since prophylactic mastectomies have been done for various reasons, not only for high risk, it is difficult to quantify the reduction in breast cancer risk.[100,101] Breast cancer has been known to occur in the chest wall or axillary region. It is therefore important for a woman to realize some risk of developing breast cancer exists after a prophylactic mastectomy.[100]

The patient must be presented with a clear, in-depth evaluation of her current and potential risk, stressing that a 50% risk also carries a 50% possibility of *not* developing the disease. It is important for the woman to take adequate time in weighing the risk versus benefit of this procedure. The complications are similar to those for a mastectomy. However, if reconstruction is added to this procedure, capsular contracture is another possibility.

Optimally, women at high risk for breast cancer should be followed by close surveillance utilizing mammograms and frequent clinical examinations, preferably through a comprehensive breast center. Provided such surveillance is feasible, this alternative is an important, even reassuring, alternative for the woman considering prophylactic mastectomy.

## SCREENING

Chemoprevention only applies to high-risk women at this time. Consideration needs to be directed to the 70% of women without significant risk factors who will develop breast cancer. In addition to research into more sophisticated methods to detect subclinical disease, efforts need to be directed toward educating the public to use the health promotions available to provide for early detection. The standard of breast care should include monthly breast self-examination (BSE), regular clinical exams by trained professionals, and periodic mammography.

Early detection reduces the mortality of breast cancer and provides a 90% survival rate for five years. The survival rate decreases significantly with regional and distant metastatic disease. The early detection efficacy of breast self-examination, clinical exam, and mammography has been well documented. Unfortunately, the literature reveals that BSE and mammography are generally grossly underutilized; strides need to be made in these areas before dramatic reductions in mortality will be seen.

## BSE

It is estimated that monthly BSE is performed by approximately one-third of adult women. Lack of proficiency is one of the most consistent barriers to BSE practice. This can be alleviated through an education process that provides verbal and written information as well as demonstration and return demonstration. Many women find the use of demonstration models helpful in increasing confidence and proficiency.

Women should be instructed by a trained professional to begin monthly BSE at age 20. Since 90% of breast lumps are found by the woman or her partner, BSE has the capability to be the primary screening tool for many women. Proficient self-examiners have the potential of finding cancers at an earlier stage, thereby improving prognosis and increasing survival.

Several studies have examined ways of encouraging women to continue performing monthly BSE after receiving instruction. Champion[102] reported belief and informational counseling increased frequency and proficiency. Lierman et al[103] found support strategies based on selected partnerships within a group increased frequency of BSE and predicted ongoing support dyads. Grady[104] suggests that frequency of BSE among elderly women may be increased with simplified instructions.

The nurse can play a major role in the educational process by promoting and initiating instruction of BSE in the community as well as the health care environment and reinforcing the skill by asking for a return demonstration immediately and each time the patient presents to the office or clinic. The American Cancer Society endorses three methods of self-examination; circular, vertical, and wedge. Regardless of style preference, it is important to note that BSE training should have three basic components: (1) a visual exam using a mirror; (2) a palpation exam in the shower and in the supine position on the bed; and (3) proper technique emphasized during the instructional and return demonstration session (i.e., area, motion, number and position of fingers, and pressure type) (Figure 34-2).

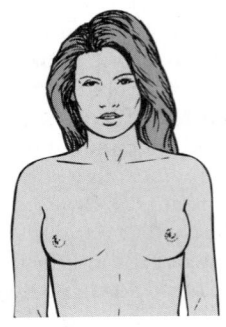

1. Stand before a mirror. Inspect both breasts for anything unusual such as any discharge from the nipples or puckering, dimpling, or scaling of the skin.

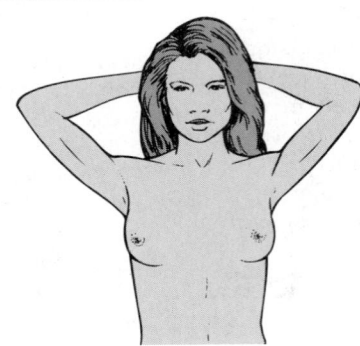

*The next two steps are designed to emphasize any change in the shape or contour of your breasts. As you do them, you should be able to feel your chest muscles tighten.*

2. Watching closely in the mirror, clasp you hands behind your head and press your hands forward.

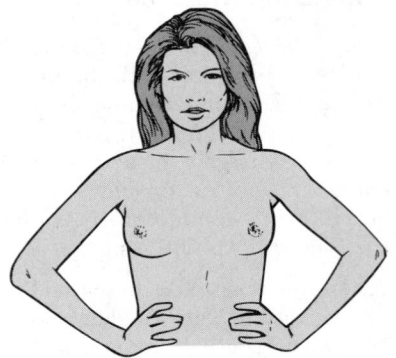

3. Next, press your hands firmly on your hips and bow slightly toward your mirror as you pull your shoulders and elbows forward.

*Some women do the next part of the exam in the shower because fingers glide over soapy skin, making it easy to concentrate on the texture underneath.*

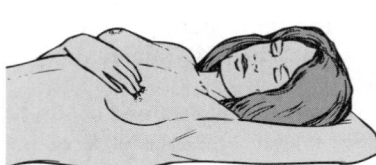

4. Lying on the bed, raise your left arm. Use three or four fingers of your right hand to explore your left breast firmly, carefully, and thoroughly. Beginning at the outer edge, press the flat part of your fingers in small circles, moving the circles slowly around the breast. Gradually work toward the nipple. Be sure to cover the entire breast. Pay special attention to the area between the breast and the underarm, including the underarm itself. Feel for any unusual lump or mass under the skin. Next, lower your arm and examine the armpit using the same technique and repeat on the opposite breast.

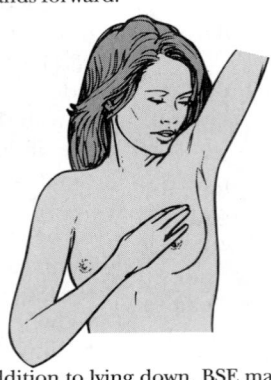

5. In addition to lying down, BSE may also be done in the shower for a thorough and complete exam.

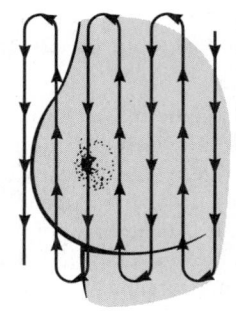

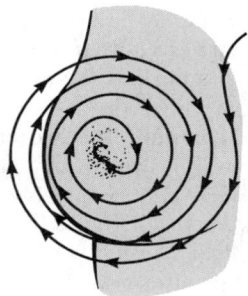

6. Examples of patterns.

**FIGURE 34-2**    Breast self-examination instructions.

The monthly exam should be done one to two days after menses stops in premenopausal women or on an appointed day of the month for postmenopausal women. It may be helpful to instruct these women to do BSE on the day that corresponds to their date of birth or the day retirement or Social Security checks arrive. This method is easier to remember than the first or last day of the month. Emphasizing one exam a month cannot be stressed enough. Women who examine themselves more than once (some may examine daily, thinking this offers them better protection) confuse the issue because breast tissue changes can vary from slight to dramatic during the month and they may be unable to determine the normal architecture of their breasts when a problem does arise.

The exam should begin with a visual inspection before

a mirror. The woman stands before a mirror with arms relaxed, looking for any changes in breast symmetry, size, and shape, including changes in the skin or nipple/areolar complex (e.g., puckering, dimpling, color of skin). The woman should turn to the side to inspect the lateral aspect of each breast as well. The visual inspection is repeated with arms overhead and with arms pressing on the hips. The reason for these position changes is that the pressure on the underlying muscle alters the appearance of the breast tissue, which may enhance the detection of an abnormality. The visual exam is concluded with the woman leaning forward to inspect the breasts while they are suspended.

BSE is best performed lying on the bed. Large breasted women may wish to place a towel beneath the shoulder to distribute the breast tissue more evenly. Raising the arm, use the flat pads of the first three fingers to examine the breast with small circular motions. The area below the collarbone and beside the breastbone should also be included. When one breast is completed, relax and lower the arm to the side and use the same motion to examine the armpit. The woman may choose the circular, vertical (up-and-down), or wedge method. Some studies have reported that the up-and-down pattern may result in a more thorough exam. Regardless of the technique, the important issue is to make sure all the breast and armpit tissue is examined.

Following the pattern chosen, begin at the outermost top edge of the breast and glide the fingers along without lifting the hand away, noticing any lumps or areas of thickness. Use light, moderate, and firm pressure with each overlapping motion to ensure examining all the tissue. It is generally not useful to squeeze the nipple, looking for discharge. Worrisome discharge is most often spontaneous, unilateral, and has a pink, red, or bloody hue. Examine the other breast in the same manner. Lubricating the hand and breast with lotion or powder beforehand helps the fingers to slide more easily over the skin.

In addition to doing BSE lying down, the woman may wish to examine herself in the shower to provide a complete and thorough monthly examination of the breasts. This complete self-exam is not a substitute for periodic examinations by a qualified physician or nurse.

## Mammography

Many groups, including the AMA, NCI, and ONS, have agreed to recommend guidelines for breast cancer screening. Their recommendations note that mammography and clinical breast exams provide the best protection for early detection and both must be incorporated for maximum benefit[105] (see Table 34-2). Asymptomatic women should begin screening mammography by the age of 40 and continue with screening mammography and clinical exams every one to two years as recommended by their physician. These organizations believe these guidelines will have a significant effect on the early detection rate for the 40–49 age group. Women 50 and

**TABLE 34-2** Breast Screening Guidelines

| Screening Method* | Age | Frequency† |
|---|---|---|
| BSE | >20 | Monthly |
| Professional clinical exam | 20–40 | Every 3 years |
| | >40 | Every 1–2 years |
| | >50 | Every year |
| Mammogram | >40 | Every 1–2 years |
| | >50 | Every year |

*All three components must be present to ensure early detection.

†The clinician may recommend mammography at an earlier age and/or more frequent clinical examinations for women with increased risk factors.

older are encouraged to have yearly screening mammography and clinical exams.

There has been recent controversy regarding the usefulness of regular screening for women aged 40–49. The NCI currently no longer recommends routine screening based on no significant decrease in mortality associated with mammography in this age group.[106] This policy change was based largely in part on the National Breast Screening Study of Canada. This study has been criticized by experts who questioned the selection of patients, the quality of the mammography, and expertise of personnel.[105] Recent information from SEER supports screening women in this age group. DCIS cases which are often found on mammogram have increased 216% and small stage I cancers (<1 cm) which generally are considered curable have increased 80%. Of particular note is the incidence of invasive metastatic cancers, which has decreased 38%.[107]

Mammograms are generally not recommended for women under age 35 because younger breasts tend to be dense, which causes the mammogram to appear white and contain very little contrast. After the age of 35, a woman's breast begins to be replaced by fat, which can be easily imaged.

Although it is accepted that young women's breasts are difficult to image, there has been an increase in the number of mammograms ordered for woman under 30. A retrospective study was conducted that evaluated the clinical influence of mammograms of 76 patients aged 18–29.[108] The patients were referred for evaluation of a palpable mass or a primary complaint other than a dominant mass (e.g., lumpy breasts, family history of breast cancer, discharge, enlarged lymph nodes). The study indicated that the radiographic findings did not influence clinical management and recommended alternative diagnostic tools be used including sonography and fine-needle aspiration.

Screening mammography has been proven to be beneficial in studies conducted in the United States and Europe.[105,109–112] These studies confirmed reductions in mortality as well as technical improvements in the detection of malignancies. Because mammography is considered to be such an integral part of the screening and detection process, the NCI has set a goal for an 80% utilization rate for screening mammography by the year 2000.[112] There are reasonable doubts whether this goal may be attained. While the use of mammography for women over 40 increased 200% in the 1980s, a significant number of women have never had a mammogram.[113]

Several possible explanations for this lack of mammography screening have been elicited from patients and physicians. There seems to be a general lack of awareness on the part of physicians and patients regarding the benefits and recommended guidelines for screening. Physicians expressed concern about radiation risk, noncompliance of patients, and overtreatment (i.e., unnecessary biopsies). Patients relate fear of discovering a malignancy, concern about discomfort during mammography, and cost of the examination.

Many of these issues may be addressed by educating patients and members of the health care field about the demonstrated value of mammography. Part of this educational process must address health behaviors which influence attitudes toward mammography, as well as stress the advantages of early detection that often increases survival and results in saving the breast through conservation surgery.[114]

Equipment and technical issues are easily addressed. The risk of harmful radiation from a mammogram is negligible, and the benefit far outweighs the perceived risk to the patient. Discomfort from breast compression has been generally considered to be a barrier to mammography. Several surveys have looked at discomfort as a possible deterrent to mammography. One study reported that patients who understood the procedure usually found the compression acceptable.[115] Another study indicated that the expected compression complaints were of a short duration, and, therefore, acceptable.[116] Nielsen et al[116] revealed that pain may be a deterrent for some women from certain ethnic and socioeconomic backgrounds. Education is an important component in addressing these issues and encouraging screening.[117] Women with tender breasts may wish to schedule the mammogram at the end of their menses to reduce discomfort.[116] Additionally, an analgesic may be taken a half hour before the mammogram to further minimize pain.

Cost is an issue that is difficult to address. The cost may vary from approximately $50.00 to $200.00. The high end reflects diagnostic mammograms, which are recommended when a clinical or prior mammographic abnormality is known to exist. Screening mammograms are less expensive and appropriate for the asymptomatic woman. Medicare now will cover screening mammograms for women every other year. Some city and county facilities offer free screening mammograms. Businesses interested in health promotion have begun providing on-site mobile mammography units free of charge or at a nominal fee. Facilities and centers may offer a reduced price to coincide with Breast Cancer Awareness Month in October.

Women who "shop" for their yearly mammogram may be doing themselves a disservice if the mammogram is taken at a different facility each time. Facilities may differ with respect to the expertise of the radiologist and the technique employed. Potentially, an abnormality could be overlooked or a stable abnormality will be recommended for biopsy because comparison films are not available. This problem can be avoided by always bringing old films for comparison or having yearly mammograms at the same institution.

## Ultrasound

Ultrasound is not considered an adequate screening tool because of its limited sensitivity compared to mammography. Ultrasound does have a role when mammography is not useful or advised. Extreme breast density due to various reasons will render a mammogram useless. Generally, mammograms for pregnant women are not recommended due to the radiation scatter. Additionally, pregnancy increases the vascularity and water content of the breast which, in turn, also increases the density of the breast. Lactating mothers or women who naturally have very dense breasts may need ultrasound as an additional or alternative screening tool.

## MULTIDISCIPLINARY BREAST CENTERS

The increasing public awareness of breast cancer treatment options and the recognized controversies in breast cancer detection and management, together with oncologists' and institutions' commitment to provide optimum care, have spearheaded the concept of the multidisciplinary breast center. The design of these centers is, in essence, a response to the fact that treatment of breast cancer has become a complicated process necessitating specialized, collaborative management that is often beyond the scope of an individual practitioner. The purpose and goals of a multidisciplinary breast center include, but are not limited to, the following:

1. To provide a comprehensive interdisciplinary evaluation and planning in the management of all aspects of breast disease.
2. To provide prompt and timely evaluation and diagnosis of potential breast disease implementing current methodology and state-of-the-art diagnostic tools.
3. To participate in and support national protocol studies that investigate new surgical and adjuvant treatment modalities as well as maintaining a patient database for retrospective and prospective in-house studies.
4. To provide risk assessment, genetic counseling, and careful surveillance of women at high risk for breast cancer, thereby minimizing the anxiety associated with the knowledge that one has an increased risk for developing the disease as well as reducing the risk of patients being lost to follow-up.

5. To provide educational materials and the opportunity to learn about early detection measures (e.g., BSE) and the possibility of participating in breast cancer prevention studies as well as research studies aimed at early detection and management of malignant breast cancer.

6. To provide educational opportunities for medical students, Fellows, general practitioners, nurses, and others involved in the care of the woman with breast disease as well as providing a mechanism for peer review of the oncologist in practice.

7. To provide highly specialized assessment and diagnostic procedures that enable prompt decision making in the evaluation of a breast mass, which conceivably minimizes unnecessary surgical biopsies.

8. To provide the woman and family with the necessary information to allow her to make an informed decision regarding her choices for treatment in a prompt and timely manner.

9. To offer educational programs to the community that include instruction in BSE and information on risk factors and the importance of utilizing the current methods available to promote early detection.

Ideally, the comprehensive breast center should have a full complement of disciplines available to provide an expert opinion regarding assessment of diagnostic and histopathological data; prognostic indicators; genetic assessment and evaluation; and surgical diagnostic and treatment options including systemic chemo/endocrine therapy, radiation treatment, and surgical reconstructive techniques when warranted. A psycho-oncologist and social worker provide counseling regarding body image issues, sexual concerns, and anticipated changes in lifestyle for those patients dealing with a potentially life-threatening disease.

As science and biotechnology continue to identify chromosomal abnormalities which confer a high probability for developing breast cancer, breast centers will be expected to provide risk assessment for families as well as genetic counseling and testing. The information emanating from the Human Genome Project will possibly overwhelm and definitely challenge a primary care physician in assessing and referring patients for genetic abnormalities. The primary physician will often be responsible for referring a patient for further evaluation and, therefore, must possess a basic working knowledge of the personal and familial histories which may suggest a genetic link. According to Peters and Stopfer,[118] genetic counseling should assist the patient/family in understanding the medical information pertinent to the disease(s), comprehending how heredity causes or predisposes one to the disease, and the personal risk of developing it, as well as creating a plan for follow-up which may include several treatment modalities.

Creating and implementing a breast genetic counseling program must include the following: a database and an assessment model based on known and accepted risk factors; genetic counselor(s) who carefully interview, screen, and educate the patient and family; a psychosocial support staff to address the emotional and physical consequences of the counseling and testing process; and clinicians, nurses and researchers who share clinical[119] responsibilities and actively participate in treatment protocols and prevention trials for breast cancer. Additionally, once risk has been established, the patient and family members should receive specific recommendations tailored to the needs of the individual (see Table 34-3).

Technological advances historically precede the ethical and moral issues which may arise from this data. Confidentiality, informed consent, and insurance issues should be carefully addressed by the staff. The institution's risk management team may play an active or consultant role, providing advice and counsel for current problems and future dilemmas. The Ethical, Legal, and Social Implications branch of the Human Genome Project has a principal role in addressing the basic rights of the individual seeking counseling and the role of the government, as well as moral and religious conflicts that will arise.

The American Society of Clinical Oncology (ASCO)[120] issued a position paper regarding genetic testing for cancer susceptibility. The ASCO paper recognizes that identifying those with the highest risk will certainly increase early detection and may ultimately lead to the prevention of many cancers. However, ASCO cites the importance of addressing the actual and potential risks of testing without extensive patient/family counseling and education and endorses testing within a research protocol format which includes a national registry, long-term outcomes, and psychological ramifications.

Very sensitive, often heretofore unknown, information may come to light that may challenge and alter relationships forever. DNA testing irrefutably identifies maternity and paternity. A man may discover one or more of his children have another father. As the demand for testing increases, it is imperative that people become skilled in the assessment and interpretation of the results.

An oncology nurse who receives additional education in the field of genetics will provide a wealth of information for the patient and family. All those who seek genetic counseling for breast cancer may or may not necessarily be at high risk. It is important for the staff to educate the patient and family as well as the referring physician regarding family and personal history assessments.

The oncology clinical nurse specialist is often viewed as the coordinator of the comprehensive breast center. It is imperative that this professional possesses specialized knowledge in all aspects of breast cancer and its treatment as well as a compassionate, yet controlled, approach to the evaluation of a suspected breast cancer. It is not uncommon for women to telephone the breast center, frantic with fear and apprehension, expressing a need to be seen as soon as possible. Regardless of the schedule, this is exactly what needs to occur if possible. Such understanding and prompt attention to the woman's needs and concerns will help to establish a trusting and caring relationship, which is vital considering the possible diag-

**TABLE 34-3**   Cancer Risk Evaluation Program: Breast and Ovarian Screening Guidelines

| LOW RISK ≤ 15% LIFETIME CUMULATIVE RISK | |
|---|---|
| Follow standard ACS recommendations | |
| Mammography | Baseline at age 35<br>Every other year ages 40–50<br>Every year age 50 and on |
| Clinical breast exam | Every year |
| Breast self-examination | Every month |

| MODERATE RISK 15%–30% LIFETIME CUMULATIVE RISK | |
|---|---|
| Start following the standard ACS guidelines at any age when breast cancer risk is ≥ to the risk of an average 50-year-old woman. (1 in 50 or 2%) | |

| HIGH RISK ≥ 30% LIFETIME CUMULATIVE RISK | |
|---|---|
| Mammography | Baseline at age 30<br>Next mammogram depending on informativeness |
| Clinical breast exam | Every 6 months |
| Breast self-examination | Every month |

| KNOWN BRCA1/BRAC2 MUTATION CARRIERS | |
|---|---|
| Mammography | Baseline at age 25<br>Every 6–12 months thereafter |
| Clinical breast exam | Every 6 months |
| Breast self-examination | Every month |
| Consider prophylactic mastectomy | |
| Consider prophylactic oophorectomy after childbearing | |

Cancer Risk Evaluation Program, University of Pennsylvania Cancer Center. Reprinted with permission. These are guidelines that may change as new data become available, and must be individualized.

nostic outcome. This approach to patient management is critical to the success of a comprehensive breast center.

The nurse coordinator ensures that all materials (slides, x-rays) necessary for a comprehensive evaluation are present at the time of the consultation. The nurse informs the patient and family of the sequence of events once the appointment is established. This includes which doctor(s) the patient will see and when, how materials will be reviewed, and the critical role the patient plays in the decision-making process. Emphasis is placed on the fact that often there is more than one approach to management of the problem and that once informed of her options, the patient is the ultimate decision maker. The nurse can be instrumental in ensuring that information is delivered in a manner that will enhance the patient's understanding and ability to make an informed decision.

In addition to facilitating the process of informed consent and decision making, the nurse is also instrumental in providing BSE instruction to all patients. The nurse also will be called on to answer questions regarding diagnostic tests, therapy regimens, clinical trials, postoperative events, and potential complications of treatment. The

nurse may see patients postoperatively in the hospital to provide continuity of care as well as instruction concerning general postoperative care including infection precautions. Ideally, the nurse coordinator will be able to provide exercise instruction prior to surgery and evaluate understanding and potential for compliance during the period following hospitalization. Additionally, the nurse utilizes every opportunity to lecture to professionals and the public concerning breast cancer as a health issue and methods available for early detection. In addition, time should be set aside specifically to accept or return phone calls concerning questions related to breast cancer risk specifically as well as other pertinent issues.

The design of a comprehensive breast center should reflect the goals of providing a complete, efficient, yet personal evaluation of the patient. The exam rooms should be large enough to accommodate the patient, family/significant other, as well as the team of physicians. The clinical area should have additional smaller consult rooms where the patient may be seen by individual consultants based on her individual concerns and needs.

A physician conference room should be available to

provide an area for viewing films, pathology slides, and reports. Diagnostic tests and outpatient surgery suites positioned on site facilitate a quick and efficient diagnostic process.

These centers are successful because they meet a growing need for a multidisciplinary and comprehensive approach to the care of the woman with breast disease and because they are philosophically based on the premise that women are entitled to all the information available to make an informed decision regarding their choice of treatment.[121]

## PATHOPHYSIOLOGY

### Cellular Characteristics

The majority of primary breast cancers are adenocarcinomas located in the upper outer quadrant of the breast (Figure 34-3). The most common types of breast tumors are summarized in Table 34-4. Infiltrating ductal carcinoma may take various histological forms; either well differentiated and slow growing, poorly differentiated and infiltrating, or highly malignant and undifferentiated with many mitoses. Adenocarcinoma can occur at any age, but highly malignant varieties with rapidly dividing cells affect more women in their early 50s. The overall 10-year survival rate is 50%–60%.

Invasive lobular carcinoma occurs in the same age range as ductal carcinoma, accounts for 5%–10% of all breast cancers, and is frequently bilateral. The prognosis is similar to ductal carcinoma.

Tubular carcinoma is fairly uncommon and represents a well-differentiated adenocarcinoma of the breast. These cancers typically occur in women aged 55 and

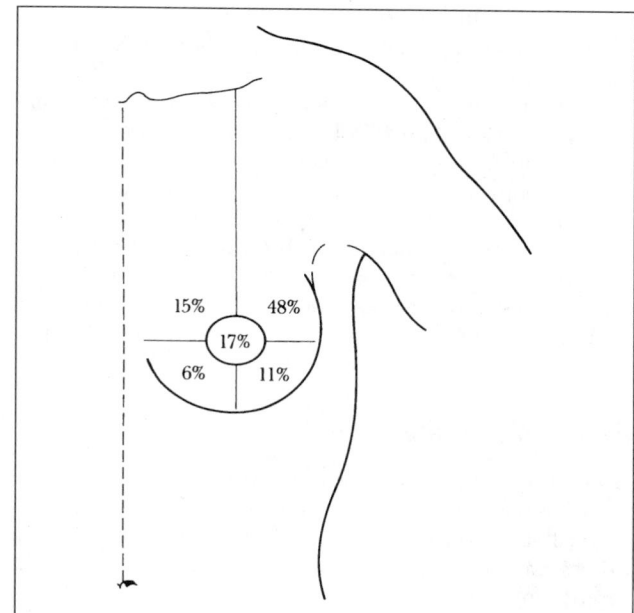

**FIGURE 34-3** Incidence of breast cancer according to location.

older. The presence of microcalcification is characteristic and facilitates early mammographic discovery. Axillary metastasis is uncommon.

Medullary carcinomas account for 5%–7% of malignant breast tumors, occurring most commonly in younger women (<50 years of age). These tumors may be quite large and circumscribed and may be bilateral.

Mucinous or colloid carcinoma is uncommon, occurring in women 60–70 years of age. This tumor type is characterized by the presence of large pools of mucin

**TABLE 34-4** Histological Types of Invasive Breast Cancers

| Histological Type | Percentage of Occurrence | Clinical Features | Metastatic Pattern | Prognosis |
|---|---|---|---|---|
| Infiltrating ductal carcinoma | 75% | Stony hardness to palpation<br>Prominent lump<br>Malignant cells have invaded through the walls of the duct<br>May have a spiculated appearance on mammogram | Axillary lymph nodes (common)<br>Bone<br>Lung<br>Liver<br>Brain | Poor |
| Infiltrating lobular carcinoma | 5%–10% | Diffuse, ill-defined thickness<br>Multicentric<br>Bilaterality (30%) | Axillary lymph nodes (common)<br>Occult lymph node micrometastasis may occur | Poor |
| Tubular | 2% | May be quite large | Axillary lymph nodes (uncommon)<br>Distant metastases uncommon | Favorable |
| Medullary | 5%–7% | Well circumscribed<br>Rapid growth rate<br>Bilaterality | Approximately 40% of cases demonstrate lymph node involvement at diagnosis | Favorable |
| Mucinous (Colloid) | 3% | Slow growing, bulky | Axillary lymph node involvement in less than ⅓ of cases at diagnosis | Favorable |

interspersed with small islands of tumor cells. Metastasis to axillary lymph nodes occurs in about one-third of patients and distant metastasis occurs late.

Inflammatory breast cancer occurs infrequently and accounts for less than 4% of breast cancers. Inflammatory breast cancer often presents with skin edema, redness, warmth, and induration of the underlying tissue and is often mistaken for cellulitis. Even though it appears to be localized it is associated with a poor prognosis.

Other malignant tumors of the breast include sarcomas, papillary carcinoma, apocrine, invasive cribriform, and Paget's disease.

## Patterns of Metastasis

Breast cancers behave differently from one woman to the next. Even among women with the same histological type, clinical stage, and treatment some will be cured, while others have emergence of metastatic disease within six months of therapy. There is no known reason for this disparity among individuals; however, there appears to be different cell clones, with diverse growth rates and metastatic potential which may in part account for the differences seen in clinical behavior. Research concerning the role of angiogenesis in tumor growth and its specific relevance in transformation, progression, and metastasis of breast cancer is ongoing. While the process of metastasis is a complex and poorly understood phenomenon, there is evidence to suggest that angiogenesis (neovascularization) of the tumor plays an important role in the biological aggressiveness of breast cancer.[122] The degree of intratumoral vascularization in primary breast cancer is a significant and possibly an independent prognostic factor.[123] Tumor-induced neovascularization appears to be a critical step in the oncogenic and metastatic cascades and may have important implications for the evaluation and therapy (anti-angiogenic) of patients with breast cancer. Anti-angiogenesis research is an exciting development in breast cancer and recent studies have suggested that specific anti-angiogeneic agents might be effective and safe, and preliminary clinical trials now are being planned to test these drugs.[122]

Breast cancer metastasizes widely and to almost all organs of the body, but primarily the bone, lungs, nodes, liver, and brain. The first site of metastasis is usually local or regional involving the chest wall or axillary supraclavicular lymph nodes or bone. Women with ER(−) disease are more likely to have recurrences in visceral organs whereas women with ER(+) disease have recurrences in skin and bone. Patients with metastatic disease generally present with symptoms specific to that organ. For instance, women with metastatic disease to bone often complain of bone pain or in the case of liver metastases, anorexia, weight loss, malaise, and occasionally right upper quadrant pain. CNS metastases may present with specific neurological damage or relate to specific neurological damage such as cranial nerve palsies (double vision), motor dysfunction, or spinal cord symptoms.

# CLINICAL MANIFESTATIONS

## Diagnostic Studies

Routine mammography may reveal a large spectrum of breast pathology ranging from equivocal benign conditions, to those that may mimic suspicious or malignant processes, to those that are considered malignant until proven otherwise. The appearance of these lesions is often a coincidental finding on a screening mammogram of an asymptomatic woman. However, if there is a palpable abnormality, additional diagnostic tools will be utilized to isolate the abnormality and provide more specific information for the clinician.

The diagnostic evaluation of breast lesions may be a simple one-step procedure or it may progress to a multilevel process. There are several noninvasive and low-invasive diagnostic tools that aid the clinician in identifying lesions within the breast. There are a series of steps that may be taken before determining which lesions actually need open (excisional) biopsy. Figures 34-4 and 34-5 describe the steps involved in the diagnostic evaluation of a nonpalpable and a palpable breast mass.

Clinical manifestations that are more suspicious of malignant disease are nipple retraction or elevation, which may be due to tumor fixation or infiltration into the underlying tissues. Skin dimpling or retraction also may be present and is possibly due to invasion of the suspensory ligaments and fixation to the chest wall. Heat and erythema of the breast skin may be related to inflammation, but they are also signs of inflammatory breast carcinoma. Skin edema, or *peau d'orange*, the French term for "skin of the orange" (Figure 34-6), is characteristic of malignant disease. The edema is thought to be due to the invasion and obstruction of dermal lymphatics by tumor. Ulceration of the skin with secondary infection may be present. The presence of isolated skin nodules indicates invasion of blood vessels and lymphatics. This often results in implantation of tumor emboli in adjacent tissues and indicates that distant metastases are likely. Clinical presentation may also include, or be limited to, signs of local or distant metastatic disease.

### Mammograms

***Screening mammograms*** Screening mammograms are used for routine breast surveillance for the asymptomatic patient. The goal of screening mammography is to detect a malignancy before it becomes clinically apparent. It is important to have an appreciation for what mammography can accomplish. A 10-mm tumor containing $10^9$ or 1 billion cells may be palpable by clinical examination. Mammography can improve this by about six or seven doublings, or approximately 20% of the life of the tumor. Detection at $10^7$ by mammography or $10^9$ by palpation (usually by a trained professional) occurs still earlier than

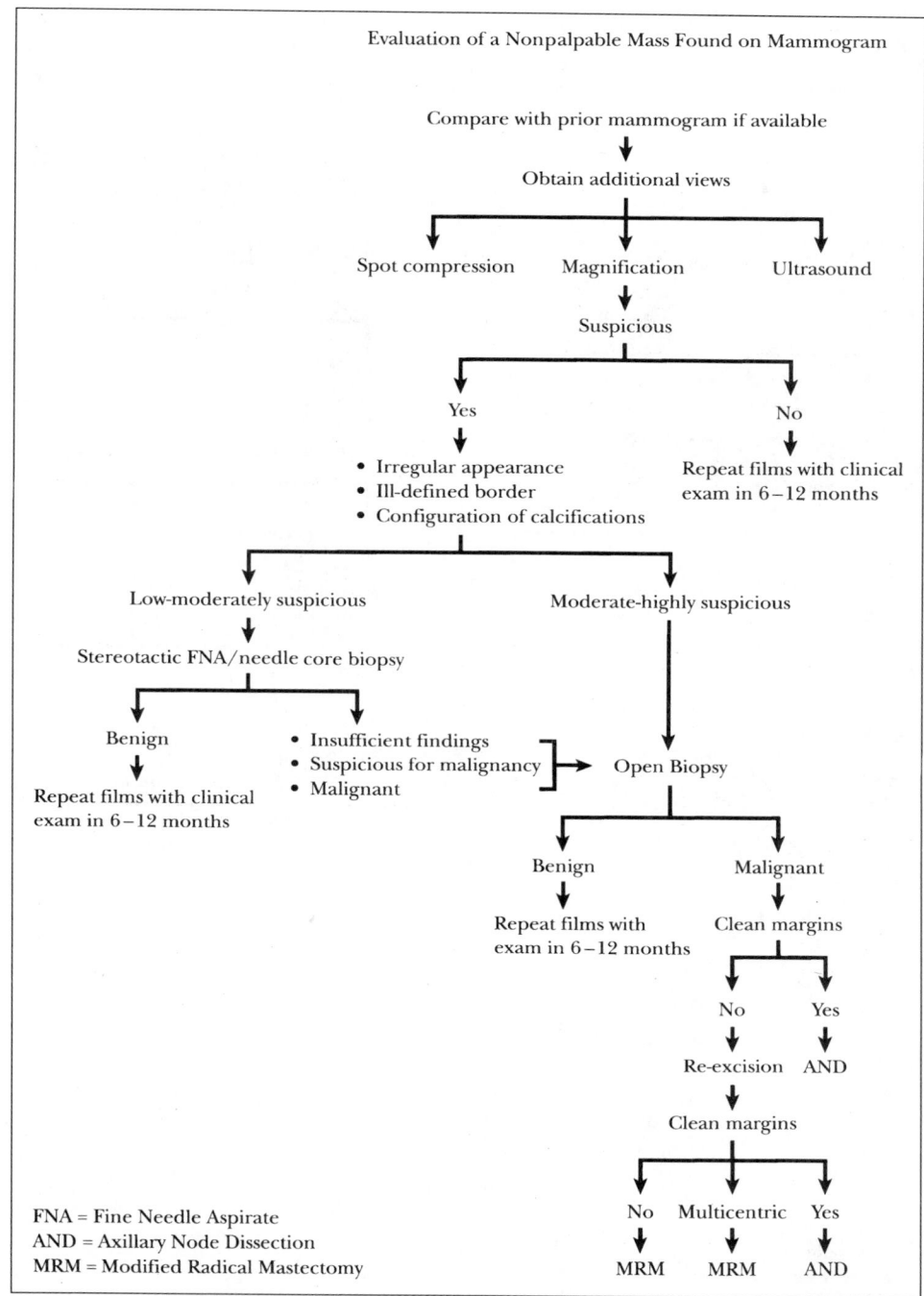

**FIGURE 34-4**   Evaluation of a nonpalpable mass found on mammogram.

the discovery of a tumor of the size ordinarily encountered in clinical practice (BSE).[124]

Clinical detection through the use of BSE generally occurs when a tumor is approximately the size of a walnut, and is by no means early in the biological history of the cancer. Therefore, mammography is an important consideration in the triad of early detection of breast cancer.

The routine screening mammogram provides a high-sensitivity study at the lowest possible cost. A highly sensi-

tive study enables the radiologist to detect any discrete abnormality, thereby reducing the false-negative reports. Film-screen mammography allows a high quality image with a minimum of radiation. Although xeromammography has been used in the past it is no longer utilized.

A woman should consider the institution where the mammogram is performed. Since 1994, all facilities except Veterans hospitals must comply with standards regarding equipment, personnel, record keeping, and must

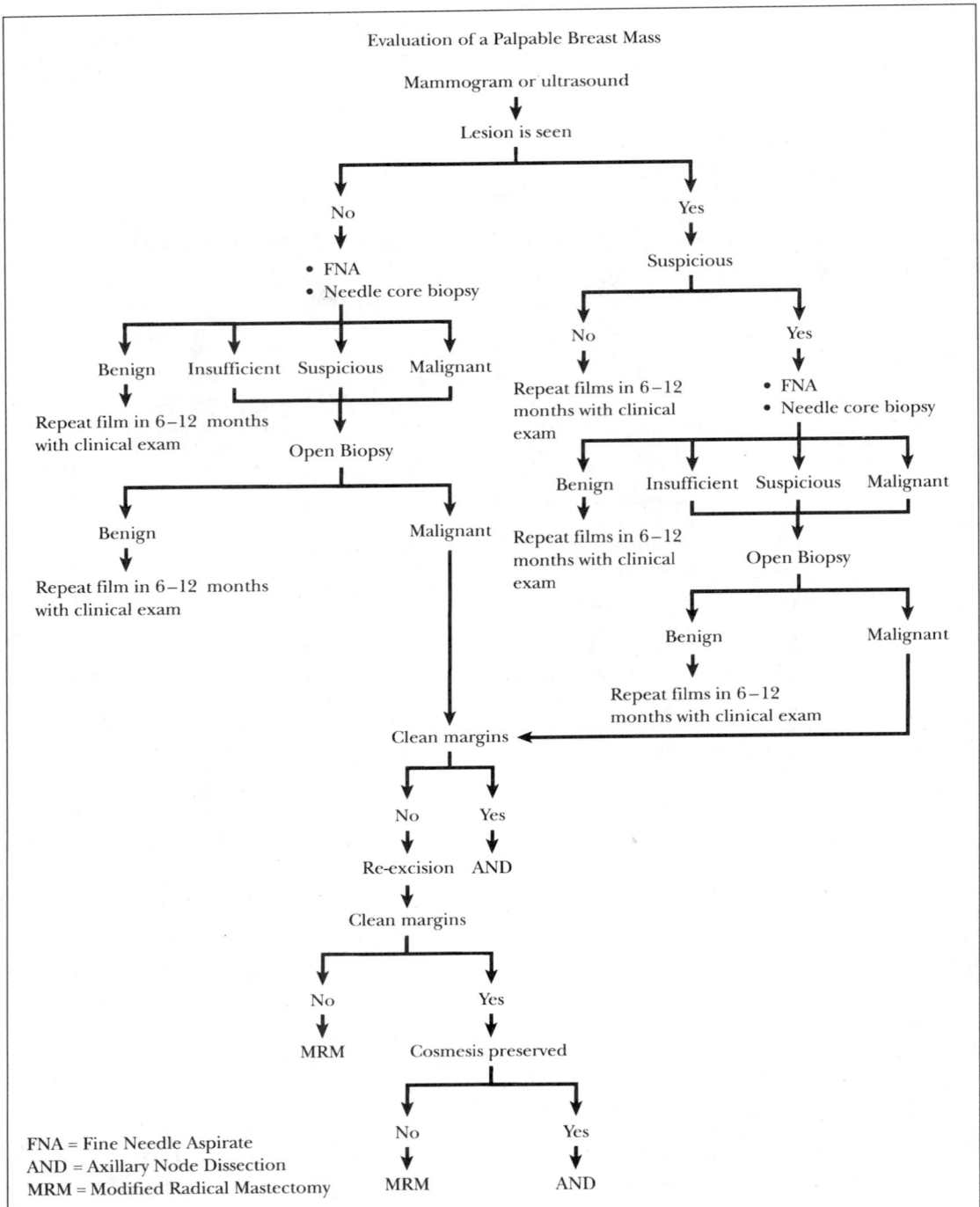

**FIGURE 34-5**    Evaluation of a palpable breast mass.

be certified by the FDA through an FDA-accredited body, such as the American College of Radiology.[125] One can call 1-800-ACR-LINE for current information on accredited hospital and clinics.

The screening mammogram usually consists of four views, two per breast (Figures 34-7 and 34-8). A mediolateral oblique and a craniocaudal view of each breast en-

ables the technologist to image as much breast as possible (i.e., the axillary tail and pectoralis muscle).

A screening mammogram allows the radiologist to detect characteristic benign and malignant masses. Benign masses include cysts, fibroadenomas, and inframammary lymph nodes, all of which have defined borders. Malignant lesions may present as spiculated or ill-defined

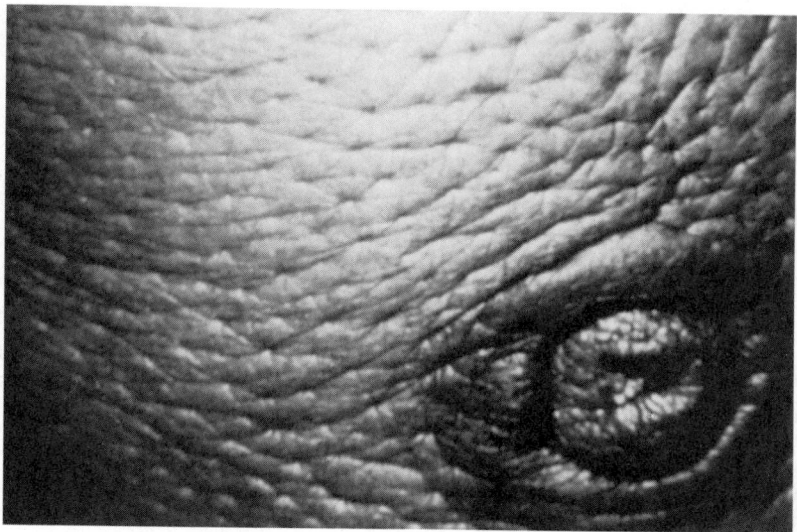

**FIGURE 34-6**   *Peau d'orange;* characteristic of lymphatic and dermal invasion by adenocarcinoma (inflammatory carcinoma).

masses, architectural distortion, asymmetric densities, and microcalcifications (Figures 34-9 and 34-10). Additionally, subtle abnormalities may be noted by the radiologist that require further studies to determine if pathology exists.[123]

***Diagnostic mammograms***   A diagnostic mammogram is performed when the patient reports specific symptoms, suspicious clinical findings exist, or an abnormality has been found on a screening mammogram. A diagnostic film uses additional views of the affected breast as well as the possibility of localized compression and magnifica-

tion views to increase the specificity of identifying the abnormality.[111] The area in question is locally compressed and/or magnified, which enables the radiologist to comment more accurately on the lesion (Figures 34-11 and 34-12).

Diagnostic mammography provides the radiologist with additional detail to render a more specific diagnosis, which may preclude the need for an open biopsy. However, if the diagnosis is nonspecific and the lesion has a low-suspicion threshold and is felt to be benign, the radiologist may recommend repeat films in six months to ensure the area in question has not changed. This

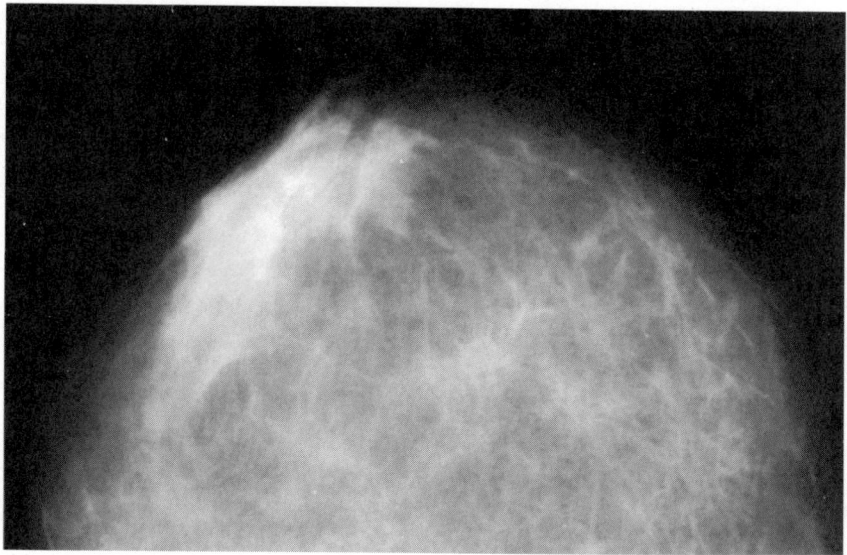

**FIGURE 34-7**   Screening mammography of an asymptomatic breast from above (craniocaudal view).

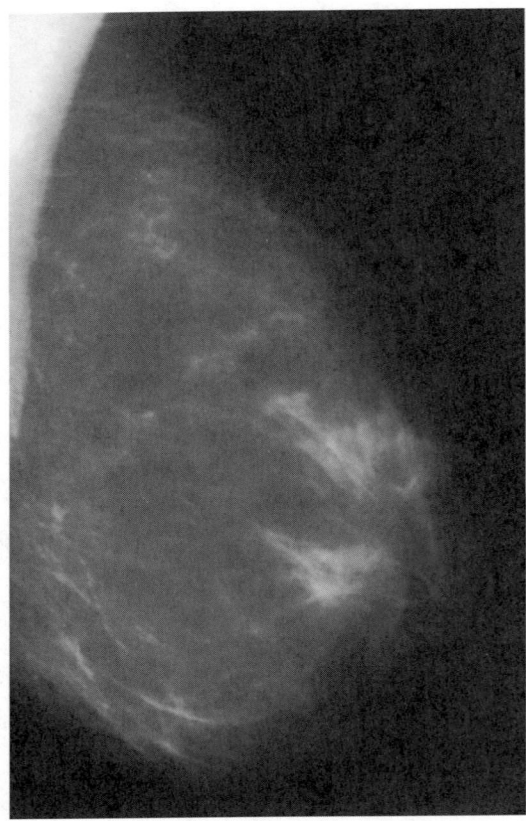

**FIGURE 34-8**  Screening mammography of an asymptomatic breast from the side (mediolateral view). Note the inclusion of the axilla and the pectoralis muscle, which ensures that the entire breast is imaged.

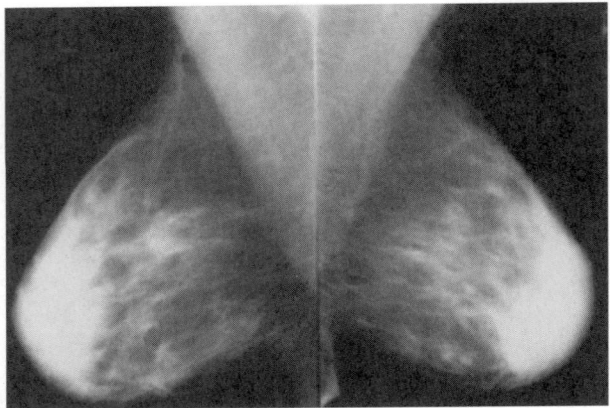

**FIGURE 34-9**  The mediolateral views show the appearance of an asymmetric density.

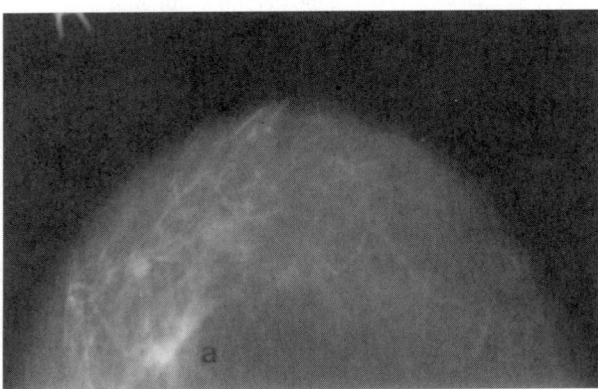

**FIGURE 34-10**  A craniocaudal view demonstrates the presence of spiculated nodules.

information must be discussed with the patient as some people are uncomfortable waiting to be reexamined mammographically and may prefer to have the abnormality sampled or excised.

***Digital mammography and computer assisted diagnosis (CAD)***  Digital mammography is currently an investigational tool that may hold promise as an adjunct to conventional mammography. The advantages of digital technology over film-screen mammography are listed by Adler and Wahl[126] and Schmidt and Nishikawa[127]; (1) digital technology allows for more variations in exposure, (2) radiologist's performance is increased by virtue of a second look, (3) differences in tissue contrast are more easily seen, (4) images can be transmitted and easily stored.

CAD utilizes a software program to target potentially suspicious lesions for the radiologist to review and interpret. The computer identification involves an algorithm from a preset database generated from probability tables. There are several promising outcomes which may result from this method of imaging. The specificity of the image is enhanced by real-time evaluation on a screen, allowing

for manipulation of contrast which enhances detection and permits more rapid interventional procedures. Additionally, this real-time evaluation will improve mobile systems in remote areas. Expert consultation may be immediately accessed via satellite, while the unit is still on site.[128]

### Sonogram

A sonogram or ultrasound is used to determine whether a lesion is solid or cystic. It can also be used to guide interventional procedures such as cyst aspiration, abscess drainage, FNA, needle core biopsies, or presurgical localization.[129,130] Ultrasounds are appropriate to investigate palpable lesions in young women whose breasts have the dense fibroglandular tissue that may obscure a lesion in the breast. Ultrasound are also useful in pregnant women, who need to be spared radiation when an

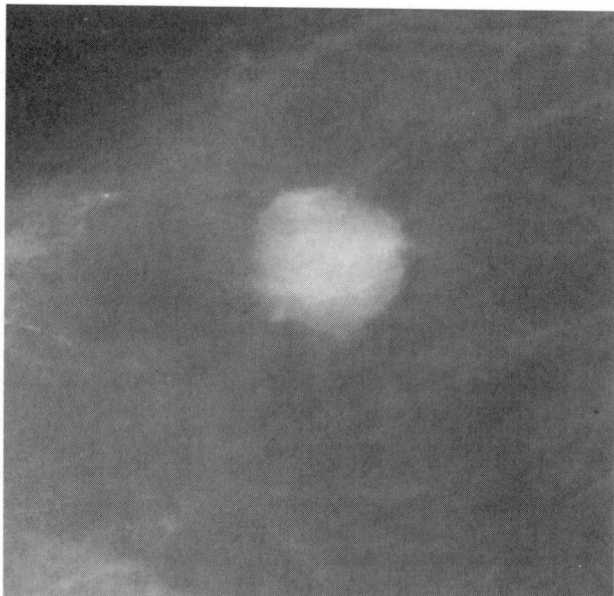

**FIGURE 34-11**  Magnification of the nodule provides a more accurate picture of the irregular border noted on screening mammogram. Note that the border is not clearly defined, but appears fuzzy or hazy, which is especially demonstrated on the left side. The irregular appearance makes this nodule suspicious for cancer.

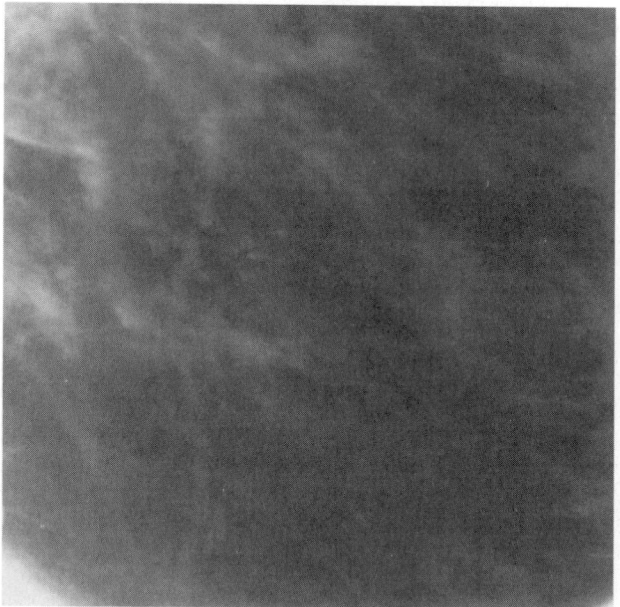

**FIGURE 34-12**  New microcalcifications were seen on a routine mammogram. The radiologist requested magnified views, which revealed a small area of clustered microcalcifications (top) as well as microcalcifications that tend to branch (below). Both are suspicious for cancer.

abscess or galactocele is suspected, or in recently lactating women whose breasts are extremely dense.

While sonograms are useful in determining if a lesion is solid or cystic, the sensitivity and specificity are not the same caliber as mammograms. They should generally not be used for screening purposes (Figure 34-13).

### MRI

MRI (or MRM, magnetic resonance mammography) of the breast is a relatively new procedure that may allow for earlier detection based on the ability of this test to determine smaller lesions and finer detail. MRI has become a highly accurate though costly tool, now that specificity is enhanced by contrast infusion. It is superior to ultrasound in imaging the parenchyma, axilla, or chest wall. MRI evaluates the rate at which the contrast initially enters the breast tissue. Malignant lesions tend to exhibit an increased enhancement within the first two minutes. It is limited in the detection of calcifications, which excludes its use for many nonpalpable lesions. MRI may be best viewed as a complement to mammography and clinical exam to distinguish between a benign or malignant lesion in the hope of preventing benign biopsies. MRI may also be utilized to identify recurrences, as well as to evaluate implant integrity.[126,131,132]

### PET

Positron emission tomography (PET) employs metabolic activity to image the breast tissue. The glucose radio-

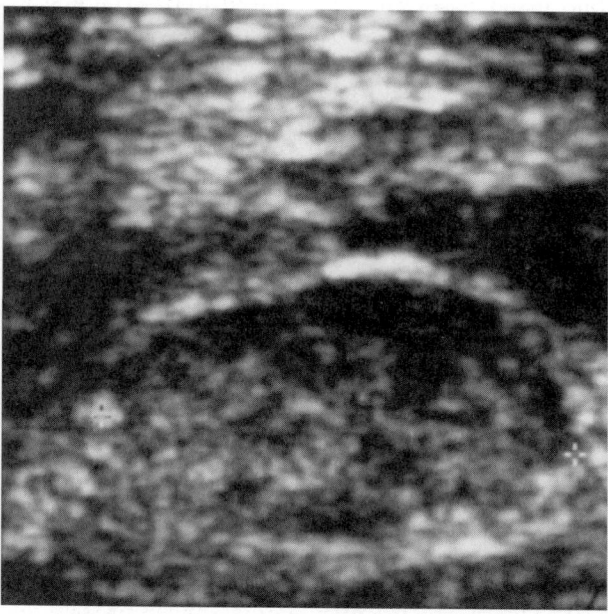

**FIGURE 34-13**  An ultrasound of a palpable mass reveals the characteristics of a fibroadenoma (between the crosses), which is a benign nodule.

pharmaceutical, 2-deoxy-2-[18F]-fluoro-D-glucose (FDG) has been reported most useful as a metabolic tracer which quantifies the over-consumption of glucose by a tumor cell.[126,133]

PET may be superior to MRI in identifying viable tumor versus scar tissue, benign and malignant axillary nodes, and tumors >1 cm. PET may also be utilized to locate primary, regional, and systemic metastases, and may play a future role in chemotherapy planning. The major limitations of PET are the high cost of the scanners and limited availability, as well as the short half-life of the radiopharmaceuticals.[131] Currently, PET is being used in research settings for various cancers and will not be available as a screening tool until more definitive data becomes available.

### Scintimammography

Scintimammography uses a variety of radioisotopes to image the breast. The most promising to date are thallium-201 (TI-201) and technetium-99M sestamibi (MIBI). This imaging tool is best known from the media reports which lauded it as the breakthrough needed to reduce unnecessary biopsies of the breast. While initial reports with small study numbers show sensitivity ranging from 89% to 95%, and specificity ranges from 72% to 87%, larger prospective trails need to be conducted to determine its diagnostic and prognostic role before widespread clinical use is advocated.[134-138]

### Fine-needle aspiration

Fine-needle aspiration (FNA) is employed when an abnormality is known to be solid or to determine if the lump is a cyst. FNA may also be used to confirm a clinically apparent positive diagnosis. FNA is a simple office procedure that can be performed with or without local anesthetic using a small 20- or 22-gauge needle.

If the lump in question is a cyst, the lump should disappear after the aspiration is completed. Cysts may return in the same area or in other areas of the breast and the patient may require repeated aspirations over time. If a lump is solid, it is possible to obtain a cytology sample by making several passes into the lesion using the same entry point. This method will retrieve small cell samples from several sites within the lesion and reduce the false-negative result.

It should be mentioned that a lesion that does not demonstrate a malignant histology may still remain clinically suspicious to the physician. In cases such as these, a biopsy will often be recommended.

### Stereotactic needle-guided biopsy

The increasing use of mammography in the past decade has resulted in a subset population of very small breast lesions needing tissue sampling. The stereotactic needle-guided biopsy (SNB) is mainly used to target and identify mammographically detected nonpalpable lesions in the breast. SNB is appropriate for sampling most nonpalpable lesions; however, it is less suitable for very small lesions or areas of calcification, superficial lesions, or those on the extreme medial or lateral area of the breast.[139,140]

While mammography offers the best detection of early breast cancer, mammography often cannot distinguish between benign or malignant tumors. Approximately 60%–80% of recommended biopsies are for benign abnormalities. The stereotactic biopsy permits diagnosis of benign disease without the trauma or scarring of an open biopsy. This procedure has been improved over time to yield sufficient tissue for diagnosis more than 97% of the time when performed by an experienced practitioner. It also results in a definite cost saving over excisional biopsy.[141-144] The basic principle of stereotactic biopsy is to immobilize the breast from fixed horizontal and vertical coordinates to calculate the exact position of the lesion within a three-dimensional field.[139]

The procedure takes place in a specially equipped operating room. The room contains breast-imaging equipment and an examination table that has an opening at the front end through which the breast is suspended as the patient lies in a prone position. This positioning is necessary to examine and target the precise area to be sampled. (See Figure 34-14.)

After proper placement is confirmed by stereoradiographs or digital mammograms, the breast is locally anesthetized and a small incision is made to penetrate the subcutaneous fibrous tissue. A needle (14g-20g) is placed in a spring-loaded biopsy gun which is mounted and stabilized. The gun emits a loud "pop" and it is helpful to fire the gun before placing the needle to reduce the risk of startling the patient.[144]

The needle is inserted several times, which allows two or three core biopsy samples to be taken. Histology samples are then sent to the pathology department, and results are usually reported in one to two days. Cytology specimens may also be taken at this time.

Stereoradiographs are taken again to identify the exact area from which the samples are taken to ensure entire removal.

After the procedure, pressure with or without an ice pack is applied for five minutes. The area is then cleaned and a sterile bandage is applied. The patient may shower the next day, but should avoid bathing for two days. The patient is then given instructions regarding notification of results.[144]

### Wire localization biopsy

The preparation for the wire-localized biopsy is somewhat similar to the stereotactic method. The difference lies in the goal of the procedure. The aim of this biopsy procedure is to assist the surgeon in locating the nonpalpable lesion for the purpose of excisional biopsy and to minimize the volume of tissue removed to avoid unnecessary deformity. The character of the abnormality is identified after biopsy. See Figure 34–15.

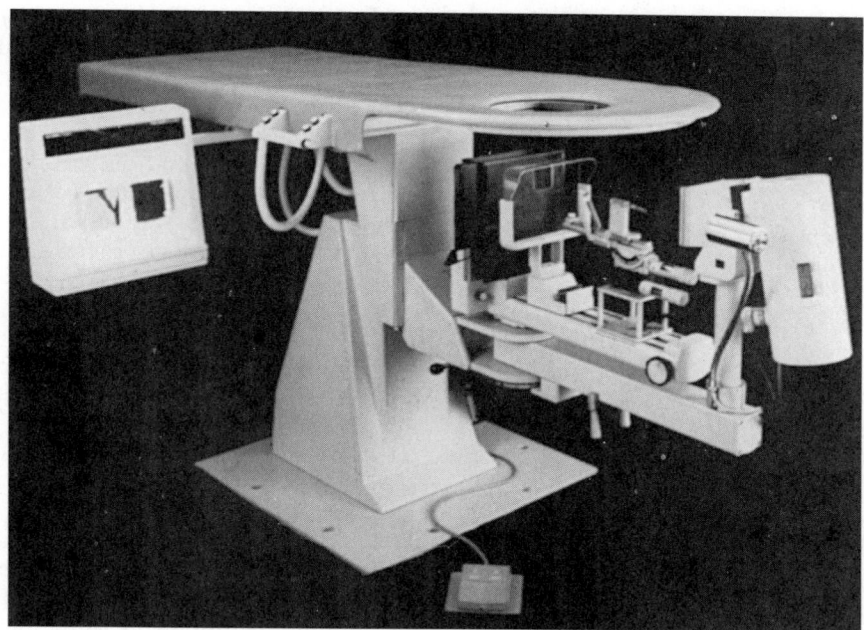

**FIGURE 34-14**  The stereotactic table allows for localization of the nonpalpable lesion between the Plexiglas plates below the opening from which the breast hangs down. Some machines allow for the procedure to be done in a sitting position, which is less favorable due to the possibility of syncope. (Photo courtesy of Fisher Imaging, Denver, CO.)

The needle-localized biopsy targets the area via mammography usually using a 90 degree view to determine the depth of the abnormality along with possible craniocaudal and/or mediolateral oblique views. Once the area is anesthetized, a double-lumen needle is inserted into the area that has been calculated by the planes of the mammograms. Multiple lesions may be localized at one time using several wires.[145] A set of repeat mammograms is then taken to ensure proper placement.

Once proper placement has been determined, the outer needle is removed, leaving a thin hook wire marking the area of concern (Figure 34–16). This wire is then taped to the skin of the breast to prevent dislodgement. The patient is sent to the operating room with the mammograms that note the area to be excised.[137] After the biopsy a specimen mammogram of the tissue is taken to ensure the abnormality has been removed.

### Open biopsy

The excisional biopsy is the most invasive diagnostic procedure. There are several reasons for recommending an excisional biopsy; (1) Sonogram findings show the lesion to be solid and indeterminant, (2) the cytology and/or histology results are insufficient, (3) the clinical or mammographic findings are suspicious, or (4) the patient with a probable low-risk lesion requests a biopsy to allay her anxiety.

The objective of this biopsy is to remove the lump or area identified, along with a small amount of surrounding normal tissue. This is done by using a curvilinear or circumareolar incision over the lesion after the area has been anesthetized. The use of circumareolar incisions for distant lesions is not recommended, and radial incisions should generally not be used because of poor cosmetic results. After the tumor is removed, the skin is closed without approximating breast tissue or fat. This method results in less deformity at the biopsy site. The excised tissue is identified and sent to pathology for histopathological diagnosis.

An incisional biopsy that removes only part of the lesion is rarely performed. If the tumor is very large and a diagnosis is needed, FNA or needle-core biopsy is usually sufficient and an incisional biopsy is not necessary.

## Prognostic Indicators

Pathologist and clinicians continue to attempt to identify morphological and phenotypic characteristics of tumors that will reflect the innate biological aggressiveness of the individual breast cancer. The identification of various prognostic indicators is valuable because such efforts help define the natural history of breast cancer, identify various subsets of women who might benefit most from adjuvant systemic therapies, as well as establish prognosis with increasing accuracy. Molecular technology is being used to study breast cancer and may one day provide valuable information about the mechanisms that give rise to breast cancer and help explain its clinical behavior.

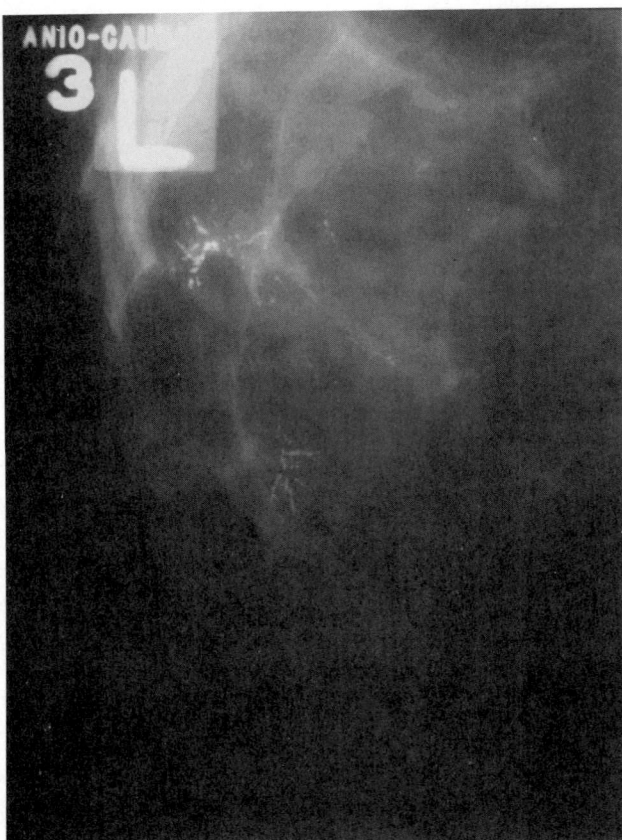

**FIGURE 34-15** Magnification view of two areas of suspicious microcalcifications.

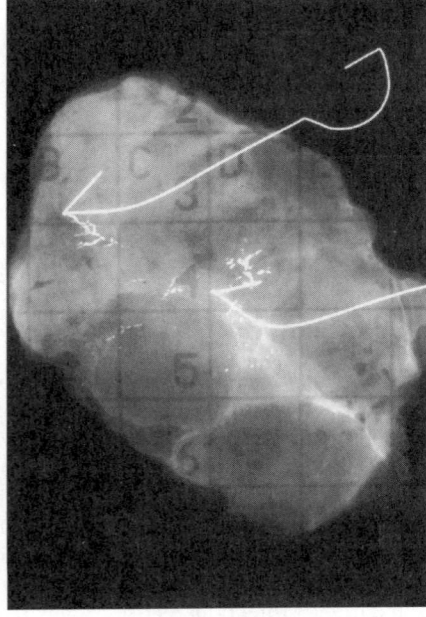

**FIGURE 34-16** Specimen mammogram: Hook-wires were placed in each area of calcification. They were removed with good margins of surrounding tissue.

Valuable parameters for determining the prognosis for patients with breast cancer include the status of the axillary lymph nodes, size of the tumor, the invasive nature of the neoplasm, multicentricity, nuclear grade, estrogen-progesterone receptor levels, and histological type.

Cell proliferative indices, DNA ploidy, Her-2/*neu* oncogene, and the amplification of specific genes (*C-myc*) are areas of investigation and are not currently considered to be independent prognostic indicators.

### Axillary lymph node status

The presence or absence of axillary node status has long been recognized as a key feature in determining prognosis in breast cancer (Figure 34-17). Clinical assessment of the axillary nodes carries a 30% false-positive and false-negative rate. Pathological staging of the lymph nodes is mandatory. However, in one study, 17% of stage I breast cancer patients initially diagnosed with no evidence of metastatic disease in lymph nodes had occult axillary metastatic disease when reexamined pathologically.[146] Once involvement is determined, important issues are whether the metastases are microscopic or macroscopic, the number of nodes involved, the levels of involvement, and whether the lymph node capsule has been invaded.[146] Extranodal extension is significant prognostically only when the metastases are confined to one to three nodes.[147] Staging of axillary nodes requires pathological view of at least four axillary nodes.[148]

Seventy percent of patients with negative nodes survive 10 years. Prognosis worsens as the number of positive lymph nodes increases. Recurrence of disease is seen in approximately 75% of women with many positive nodes. Metastases to the internal mammary nodes have the same significance as those to the axillary nodes. Internal mammary node metastasis occurs more readily in patients who have medial lesions. Internal mammary nodes are not commonly sampled but are invaded in 10% of patients when axillary nodes are negative. This may help to explain the recurrence patterns in some axillary node-negative women.[149]

The correlation between survival and number of involved nodes has been expanded from that originally used (i.e., 0, 1–3, 4 +) to include additional fractions of 4–6, 7–9, and 10 or more involved nodes (Table 34-5).[150]

### Tumor size

Prior to the more widespread use of mammography, less than 8% of women with node-negative breast cancer had tumors that were less than 1 cm in diameter with a relative overall five-year survival of nearly 99%. Patients with tumors measuring 1–3 cm have a relative five-year survival of approximately 91%, while those with tumors measuring more than 3 cm have a five-year survival of 85%.[151] Recurrence rates for patients with tumors greater than 3 cm is more than 50%, however.

Table 34-6 demonstrates a clear relationship between increase in systemic risk of recurrence and increasing

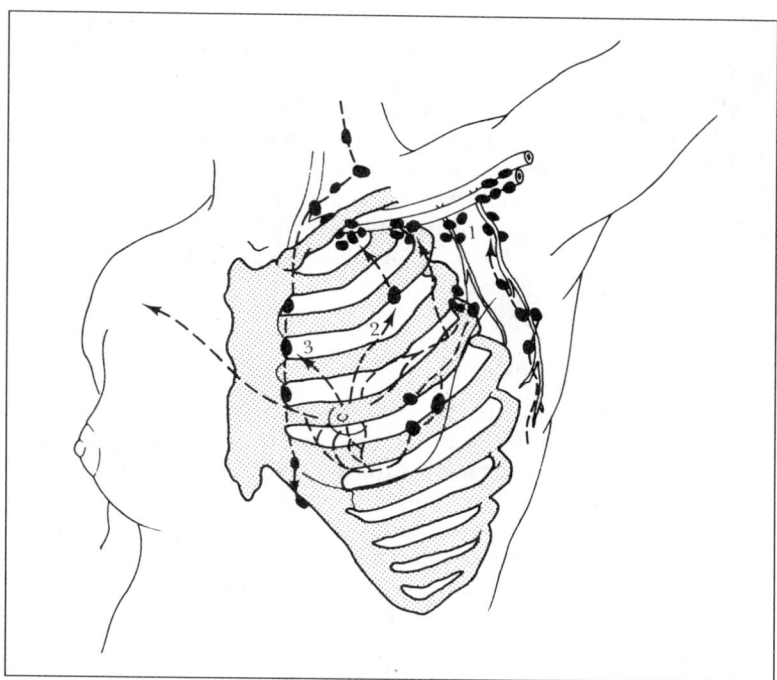

**FIGURE 34-17** Lymphatics of the breast leading to (1) axillary nodes, which are distributed over a large area from the lateral aspects of the breast proper to the axillary vessels; (2) interpectoral chain leading to interpectoral node (circle detail) and to high nodes in the axilla; and (3) chain of the internal mammary leading frequently to nodes in second interspace and to supraclavicular and cervical nodes. The lymphatics of the breast may empty into the opposite axillary nodes.

**TABLE 34-5** Recurrence Rates in 20,547 Women with Breast Cancer According to the Number of Histologically Involved Axillary Nodes

| Number of Positive Nodes | Recurrence at 5 Years |
|:---:|:---:|
| 0 | 25% |
| 1–3 | 40% |
| 4–6 | 49% |
| 7–9 | 58% |
| 10 + | 78% |

Adapted from Nemoto T, et al.[150]

**TABLE 34–6** Tumor Size and Recurrence-free Survival in Node-negative Breast Cancer Without Chemotherapy

| Tumor Size (cm) | Recurrence-free Survival (%) | |
|:---|:---:|:---:|
| | 10 years | 20 years |
| ≤ 1.0 | 91 | 88 |
| 1.1–2.0 | 77 | 72 |
| 2.1–3.0 | 75 | 71 |
| 3.1–5.0 | 62 | 59 |

Adapted from Rosen PP, et al.[152]

tumor size.[152] In addition, the presence of peritumoral vascular invasion is a marker of both local recurrence and future distant metastases. Consideration of other prognostic indicators is often necessary to determine the appropriate approach to systemic therapies.

### Hormone receptor status

The major benefit to hormone receptor status concerns its value in predicting which patients will respond to hormone manipulation. Its value in the prognostic assessment of breast cancer patients concerning risk for recurrence is less clear. It would appear that the lack of these receptors may be more predictive of early relapse.[153] According to information gained from the National Surgical Adjuvant Breast and Bowel Project (NSABP) there is a clear correlation between estrogen receptor positivity and an improved disease-free interval and overall survival.[154]

### Cell proliferative indices and DNA ploidy

Research indicates that assessment of cell proliferative potential may have important prognostic significance, especially in node-negative breast cancer. Using flow cytometry it is possible to measure DNA content and proliferative activity (S-phase fraction) of a tumor. Patients whose tumors have an abnormal amount of DNA are aneuploid. Those with normal DNA are diploid. Although different instruments have different norms, in general, about 6% is the break point. A high S-phase calculation (= 6%) consistently predicts a poorer outcome compared to those patients with an S-phase calculation <6%.[155]

Tumors with positive estrogen receptor protein tend to demonstrate a low proliferative activity (low S-phase fraction) and tend to be more diploid than aneuploid. Comparatively, tumors that are estrogen receptor negative tend to have a high S-phase fraction reflecting a more aggressive metastatic potential.

### Histological differentiation

The more differentiated the tumor cells, the better the prognosis. Tumors are generally classified as well differentiated, (grade I), moderately well differentiated, (grade II), or poorly differentiated (grade III) according to their degree of anaplasia. Such factors as nuclear size and shape, mitotic figures, and degree of tubule formation determine differentiation and likewise predict aggressiveness and metastatic potential of tumor cells. Approximately 10% of patients have grade 1 tumors and, of these patients, greater than 90% have estrogen receptor positive tumors; the majority are diploid and have a five-year disease-free survival rate of over 90%.[156] Therefore, in node-negative disease, grade may be a reliable tool for assessing the need for adjuvant therapy.

### Epidermal growth factor receptor

The idea that estrogen plays a significant role in the pathogenesis and initial proliferation of breast cancer is an accepted one. The fact that some cells develop estrogen independence during proliferation in part accounts for variance in clinical behavior and response to treatment in estrogen dependent (ER +) and estrogen independent (ER −) breast cancer. Mori et al[157] found that patients' breast cancer tissue that stained positive for epidermal growth factor tended to be estrogen receptor negative, suggesting that estrogen may exert inhibitory action on epidermal growth factor receptor (EGFR) production through binding to the estrogen receptor. In the absence of this inhibition, the EGFR may actually increase proliferation of breast cancer cells. Research in this area may lead to new approaches to controlling the growth and development of breast cancer cells.

### Her-2/*neu* oncogene

A frequently studied proto-oncogene in breast cancer is c-*erb* B-2. Overexpression or amplification of this oncogene occurs in about 20% of human breast cancers and correlates positively with a poor prognosis in node-positive disease. Studies concerning the relative prognostic importance of the Her-2/*neu* oncogene are conflicting. Gullick et al[158] demonstrate that the prognostic effect of this oncogene is equivalent in node-positive and node-negative patients, but they point out that, in order to reliably demonstrate prognostic effect of Her-2/*neu* expression, large numbers of patients are required. This is because node-negative patients have a better prognosis than node-positive patients. They relapse and die less frequently. In addition, the Her-2/*neu* oncogene is expressed relatively infrequently.[158]

Overexpression of Her-2/*neu* occurs more frequently in more advanced tumors that are more poorly differentiated.[159] Findings of Allred et al[160] indicate that overexpression of Her-2/*neu* oncogene is associated with poor clinical outcome (40% disease-free survival at five years compared to 80% in patients with Her-2/*neu* negative tumors) in a subset of node-negative patients with small, ER-positive, invasive tumors. The possibility that Her-2/*neu* could function as a growth factor receptor supports the idea that this oncogene also plays a role in drug resistance. Therefore the development of an antibody could restore sensitivity to resistant Her-2/*neu* overexpressing cells and enhance the cytotoxicity of certain drugs (i.e., cisplatin and doxorubicin) if given in combination.[161] Such an antibody has been developed and is in clinical trials.

### Cathepsin D

Cathepsin D is a lysosomal enzyme that is synthesized in normal tissues but that may be overexpressed and secreted in certain breast cancers and appears to have a direct role in invasion and metastasis.[162] High cathepsin D levels increase the probability of recurrence (60% at five years) and poor survival in aneuploid node-negative breast cancer.[162,163] Table 34-7 summarizes information concerning possible prognostic indicators in breast cancer.

## CLASSIFICATION AND STAGING

Once a breast cancer has been diagnosed, a complete evaluation of the disease is initiated to establish stage of disease and the most appropriate approach to treatment. Such planning and evaluation are optimally orchestrated through the auspices of a comprehensive breast center where all disciplines consult with the patient and family concerning her decisions regarding therapy.

In the initial evaluation, the diagnostic mammogram is utilized to look for evidence of tumor multicentricity or for evidence of bilaterality. The history and physical exam; routine blood work including complete blood counts, liver function tests, and serum calcium; and a chest film are complete prior to the initial planning session. A bone scan and/or bone films are only indicated if there is a suspicious area suggesting tumor involvement. Likewise, a liver scan would only be indicated if liver function tests were abnormal.

Following the pretreatment evaluation, the patient is clinically staged on the basis of the characteristics of the primary tumor, the physical examination of the axillary nodes, and the presence of distant metastases. As previously mentioned, the clinical evaluation is inaccurate and, because of the prognostic significance of axillary node involvement, a pathological stage is necessary to determine stage of disease.[170]

The pathological staging recommended by the American Joint Committee on Cancer (AJCC)[171] is described in Table 34-8 (page 946). This system is relatively complicated and can be simplified in terms of the most critical components, that is, whether or not nodes are involved and whether distant metastases are known to be present.

**TABLE 34-7** Prognostic Indicators in Breast Cancer

| Clinical/Pathological Parameter | Method of Analysis | Value | | Ref. # | Significance/Additional Comments |
|---|---|---|---|---|---|
| | | No. of involved nodes | Recurrence at 3 years (%) | | |
| Axillary lymph node status | Surgical pathological examination | 0<br>1–3<br>4–10<br>> 10 | 19<br>33<br>47<br>66 | 146–150 | Axillary lymph node status is the most important predictor of disease recurrence and survival. Approximately 30% of women with surgical/pathological negative nodes will experience recurrence of their breast cancer following local therapy. |
| Occult micrometastatic lymph node involvement | Immunohistochemical methods and serial sectioning | | | 164 | Detection of occult micrometastatic disease in axillary nodes of node-negative disease correlates with a poorer prognosis. |
| Tumor size | | ≤ 1 cm<br>1.1–2 cm<br>2.1–3 cm<br>3.1–5 cm | | 156<br><br><br><br>165,166 | In tumors less than 1 cm (node-negative), local therapy is usually adequate (5-year relapse-free survival 96%).<br>In node-negative disease, tumors 1–2 cm in diameter with a high S-phase fraction have a 5-year relapse-free survival of 52%.<br>In tumors greater than 3 cm, there is substantial relapse rate and aggressive therapy is generally indicated. |
| DNA analysis (content)<br>  Diploid<br>  Aneuploid | Flow cytometric analysis or Static cytophotometry | Diploid—DNA index of 1 (normal)<br>Aneuploid—DNA index of >1.2 (abnormal) | | 155 | S-phase fraction alone or in combination with ploidy may be more important prognostically than ploidy alone. |
| Proliferative indicators (measure growth fraction)<br>  S-phase fraction (SPF) | Titrated thymidine labeling<br>Flow cytometry<br>Immunohistochemistry | Low % of cells in S-phase (variable: generally <10%)<br>High % of cells in S-phase (variable: >10%) | | <br><br><br>168<br><br>167 | A high-S-phase fraction is associated with a rapidly proliferating tumor and a worse prognosis.<br>Diploid tumors have a lower risk for recurrence than aneuploid tumors.<br>SPF provides useful prognostic information for predicting disease-free survival for node-negative breast cancer patients with small ER positive tumors. |
| Histological grade (differentiation) | Histopathological examination | grade I—well differentiated | | 166 | The presence of glands is a strong indicator of good prognosis. |

(continued)

**TABLE 34-7** Prognostic Indicators in Breast Cancer (continued)

| Clinical/Pathological Parameter | Method of Analysis | Value | Ref. # | Significance/Additional Comments |
|---|---|---|---|---|
| A combined histological grading system takes into account mitotic activity, nuclear pleomorphism, and tubule formation | | grade II—moderately well differentiated grade III—poorly differentiated | 156 | The presence of mitoses is a strong indicator of poor prognosis. High histological grade is strongly associated with a high SPF. |
| Growth rate (tumor doubling time [dt]) | Serial mammography | Tumor doubling time (dt) <75 to >130 days | | The tumor growth rate correlates with the incidence of metastases 3 years following local treatment. Tumors with a dt of >130 days tend to be ER+, grade I, whereas tumors with a dt between 75–100 days tend to be ER−, grade III. |
| Epidermal growth factor receptor (EGFR) | Immunocytochemical assay | EGFR <20 fm/mg protein (favorable) >25 fm/mg protein (unfavorable) | 157 | May potentially facilitate proliferation of breast cancer cells in estrogen receptor-negative breast cancer. |
| c-erb B-2 protein (Her-2 *neu* oncogene) | Immunohistochemical staining of cell surface membranes of tumor cells Immunoblotting | <2000 fm/mg protein Overexpression is reported as present or absent | 158 | Overexpression of Her-2/*neu* protein may directly contribute to the malignant conversion of cells and have a direct impact on cellular growth control. |
| | | | 159 | Overexpression of c-erb B-2 is more common among tumors with poor nuclear grade and advanced stage. |
| | | | 160 | Overexpression of c-erb B-2 is associated with an increased mortality and may be an independent prognostic variable for survival in node-positive patients. Controversy exists whether this oncogene is a reliable predictor of prognosis in node-negative women. |
| Cathepsin-D autocrine growth factor | Western blot analysis Immunohistochemical assay | Negative: <30 fm/mg protein (favorable) Positive: >60 fm/mg protein (unfavorable) | | May be an important indicator of metastatic potential; may facilitate spread of cancer cells. |
| | | | 162 | High levels of cathepsin-D correlate with early relapse. |
| | | | 162,163 | Node-negative patients with high cathepsin-D aneuploid tumors have a higher rate of relapse compared to cathepsin-D-negative tumors. |

**TABLE 34-7**  Prognostic Indicators in Breast Cancer (continued)

| Clinical/Pathological Parameter | Method of Analysis | Value | Ref. # | Significance/Additional Comments |
|---|---|---|---|---|
| Cytoplasmic P24 protein P24 is an estrogen-regulated secretory protein that is generally not detectable in normal breast tissue | Immunocytochemical analysis using a monoclonal antibody to P24 protein | Positive: >10% of cells show cytoplasmic staining for P24 protein Negative: <10% of cells show cytoplasmic staining for P24 protein | 169 | Patients with P24-positive tumors have significantly higher response to treatment, more prolonged duration of response, and duration of survival from diagnosis of metastatic disease compared to P24-negative disease. ER-positive tumors commonly stain positive for P24 protein compared to ER-negative tumors. P24 positivity occurs more commonly in histological grade I and II tumors. |
| ER and PR receptors | Immunocytochemical staining (ER-ICA) Tumors that are positive for both ER and PR have a 75% response rate. ER+/PR− tumors have a response rate of only 30% | ER − <10 fm/mg protein ER + >10 fm/mg protein PR − <10 fm/mg protein PR + >10 fm/mg protein | 153  170 | About 60%–70% of primary breast cancers contain ER and 40%–50% have PR. Receptor content may change over time. Patients with receptor (+) tumors have a lower rate of recurrence and longer survival than those with receptor (−) tumors. |

Stage I—Tumor 0–2 cm in size; negative lymph nodes and no evidence of metastasis

Stage II—Describes a small tumor with positive lymph nodes or a larger tumor with negative lymph nodes.

Stage III—more advanced locoregional disease with suspected but undetectable metastases

Stage IV—distant metastases are present

# THERAPEUTIC APPROACHES AND NURSING CARE

## Local-Regional Disease

The current hypothesis governing the design of treatment alternatives for the woman with breast cancer contends that invasive breast cancer is potentially a systemic disease involving complex host–tumor interactions and that variations in local regional therapy are unlikely to affect survival outcomes.[172] This hypothesis has been tested, and studies confirm that the vast majority of women, including those with stage I and II breast cancer with positive or negative nodes, can be treated by mastectomy or breast conservation procedures (lumpectomy, partial mastectomy, segmental resection, or quadrantectomy) and breast irradiation.[173,174] Patients who die from breast cancer have distant occult metastases at the time of local therapy or metastases from inadequately treated local or regional disease.[174] To this end, the possibility of multicentric tumors and the presence of nodal involvement become critical.

In NSABP B-06 patients with stage I or stage II breast cancer (tumor size ≤4 cm) were randomized to total mastectomy, or to segmental mastectomy, or segmental mastectomy plus radiation, provided that margins of resection were free of tumor. All patients had axillary dissection. Results indicate that disease-free and overall survival were similar in all groups; however, those having breast radiation had significantly fewer breast recurrences compared to those having segmental mastectomy alone (10% vs. 39%).[173] These findings confirm the now standard approach to breast preservation, employing adjuvant radiation therapy. Most surgeons will advocate a wide local excision or partial mastectomy with a 1–2-cm margin of normal tissue as breast preservation surgery, but the NSABP trials have shown that any margin is adequate. The principal objective of this procedure is a cosmetic one, and if clean margins are not obtained, or the mammogram reveals extensive macrocalcifications, or the tumor is multicentric, or there is a sub-areolar mass, or cosmesis is unacceptable because of the tumor/breast mass ratio, then a total mastectomy or modified radical mastectomy is appropriate.

The extent of axillary dissection is generally determined by the size of the primary tumor and the presence of palpable nodes. A low-level dissection is appropriate

**TABLE 34-8** Pathological Staging System

| PRIMARY TUMOR (T) | |
|---|---|
| Tx | Primary tumor cannot be assessed |
| T0 | No evidence of primary tumor |
| Tis* | Carcinoma in situ: intraductal carcinoma, lobular carcinoma in situ, or Paget's disease of the nipple with no tumor |
| T1 | Tumor 2 cm or less in greatest dimension<br>T1a—0.5 cm or less in greatest dimension |
| T | T1b—more than 0.5 cm, but not more than 1 cm in greatest dimension |
| 1 | T1c—More than 1 cm, but not more than 2 cm in greatest dimension |
| T2 | Tumor more than 2 cm, but not more than 5 cm in greatest dimension |
| T3 | Tumor more than 5 cm in greatest dimension |
| T4† | Tumor of any size with direct extension to chest wall or skin<br>T4a—Extension to chest wall |

| PRIMARY TUMOR (T) | |
|---|---|
| T4† | T4b—Edema (including *peau d'orange*) or ulceration of the skin of the breast or satellite skin nodules confined to the same breast<br>T4c—Both (T4a and T4b)<br>T4d—Inflammatory carcinoma |

| REGIONAL LYMPH NODES (N) | |
|---|---|
| NX | Regional lymph nodes cannot be assessed (e.g., previously removed) |
| N0 | No regional lymph node metastasis |
| N1 | Metastasis to movable ipsilateral axillary lymph node(s) |
| N2 | Metastasis to ipsilateral axillary lymph node(s) fixed to one another or to other structures |
| N3 | Metastasis to ipsilateral internal mammary lymph node(s) |

| DISTANT METASTASIS (M) | |
|---|---|
| MX | Presence of distant metastasis cannot be assessed |
| M0 | No distant metastasis |
| M1 | Distant metastasis (includes metastasis to ipsilateral supraclavicular lymph node(s)) |

**TABLE 34-8** (continued)

| STAGE GROUPING | | | |
|---|---|---|---|
| Stage 0 | Tis | N0 | M0 |
| Stage I | T1 | N0 | M0 |
| Stage IIA | T0 | N1 | M0 |
| | T1 | N1 | M0 |
| | T2 | N0 | M0 |
| Stage IIB | T2 | N1 | M0 |
| | T3 | N0 | M0 |
| Stage IIIA | T0 | N2 | M0 |
| | T1 | N2 | M0 |
| | T2 | N2 | M0 |
| | T3 | N1,N2 | M0 |
| Stage IIIB | T4 | Any N | M0 |
| | Any T | N3 | M0 |
| Stage IV | Any T | Any N | M1 |

*Paget's disease associated with a tumor is classified according to the size of the tumor.
†Chest wall includes ribs, intercostal muscles, and serratus anterior muscle, but not the pectoral muscle.
From the American Joint Committee on Cancer: *Handbook for Staging of Cancer*. Philadelphia, Lippincott, 1993, p 161

for in situ carcinoma where microinvasion is noted on pathological examination of the primary lesion. Patients with invasive breast cancer usually require a level I or II dissection. More extensive dissections are associated with breast and arm edema, especially when radiation is also used. Efforts to improve clinical assessment of axillary node involvement include computerized tomography and positron emission tomography. These diagnostic tests may help to determine the need for more extensive axillary dissection.

A modified radical mastectomy involves the removal of all breast tissue and nipple areola complex, and level I and II axillary node dissection. The pectoralis muscle is preserved. A horizontal incision is made because it is cosmetically more acceptable. Modified radical mastectomy is indicated for larger, multicentric disease or where cosmesis is otherwise not achievable. Modified radical mastectomy may also be employed as definitive treatment following local recurrence in patients who fail conservative surgery and radiation. In general, patients with noninvasive or locally invasive tumors have excellent prognoses following salvage mastectomy. However, patients with predominantly invasive recurrent tumors are at significant risk for further relapse.[173]

Carcinoma in situ is becoming more of an issue in local control of breast cancer, owing to the success of mammography in detecting these small cancers. Lobular carcinoma in situ is distinctive in that it does not present in any discernible clinical or mammographic manner, but is usually discovered by the pathologist during the removal of a benign condition. In 20%–30% of cases, lobular carcinoma in situ may be bilateral.

Intraductal carcinoma or DCIS generally presents as clustered microcalcifications on mammography and rarely carries risk of axillary node involvement. Options for treatment include total mastectomy, wide excision followed by radiation, or wide excision alone. Because ductal carcinoma in situ frequently extends beyond the area of microcalcifications, a wide excision should include tumor-free margins around this area. Invasive carcinoma develops in about 20% of patients within ten years when excisional biopsy alone is selected as definitive treatment.[174,175]

The role of radiation in the treatment of localized breast cancer has evolved over the years and is now standard treatment, making breast preservation a realistic possibility. In selected patients, irradiation of the regional lymph node areas may reduce regional recurrence and distant dissemination. With an equivalent survival rate and preservation of the breast, conservative surgery plus radiation is now considered preferable to mastectomy for the majority of women. The major criteria for selecting patients for breast-conserving surgery and radiation therapy are, first, the feasibility of resecting the primary tumor without causing major cosmetic deformity and, second, the likelihood of tumor recurrence in the breast. Mammography will usually reveal the extent of microcalcifications and whether or not multiple tumors in the breast can be removed without sacrificing cosmesis.

Local recurrences following mastectomy usually occur within three years of surgery. Recurrences at or near the primary site are classified as a true recurrence whereas those remote from the primary site are usually thought to represent a second primary breast cancer. Both tumors will be examined by the pathologist to determine the nature of the second tumor.

Radiation doses to the breast are delivered using supervoltage equipment and tangential fields to minimize lung and heart exposure. The whole-breast dose ranges from 45–50 Gy delivered in about 6 weeks. Whether or not a boost is given depends upon the type of local excision and risk for local recurrence. The morbidity of a boost of moderate size and dose delivered either by electron beam or interstitial implantation is small.[176]

The cosmetic result following partial mastectomy and radiation therapy is generally considered to be good.[176] Some immediate side effects of radiation therapy are transient breast edema, erythema, and dry or wet desquamation. Later effects include telangiectasia, which is seen less often and arm edema which usually results from radiating the axilla for multiple positive nodes.

Radiation following modified radical mastectomy is reserved for patients with a high risk of local recurrence. Risk factors include tumors greater than 5 cm in diameter, positive axillary nodes, tumor involvement at the surgical resection, tumor invasion of muscle, or extranodal extension into the axillary fat. Patients who require chemotherapy will have radiation therapy either concurrently or after chemotherapy, depending on the regimen.[177]

## Adjuvant Systemic Therapy

### Early stage I and II breast cancer

Approximately 20 years of clinical research concerning the natural history of breast cancer supports the biological hypothesis concerning the presence of micrometastatic disease at diagnosis. Table 34-9 describes the factors influencing the design of adjuvant chemotherapy trials in curable breast cancer.[178] Scientific efforts have concentrated on finding optimal regimens of systemic therapy that can potentially destroy circulating tumor cells. The need for such research is paramount considering that nearly 90% of women newly diagnosed with breast cancer are potentially curable. Of that number, nearly 50%, or 85,000 women diagnosed each year will have node-negative disease.[179] The results of prospective clinical trials suggest that the rate of disease recurrence in patients with node-negative breast cancer can be reduced 20%–50% by adjuvant therapy.[174,180–182] This led to the conclusion at the NIH Consensus Development Conference on Early Stage Breast Cancer held in 1990 that, although "the majority of patients with node-negative breast cancer are cured by breast-conserving treatment or total mastectomy and axillary node dissection, the rate of local and distant relapse following local therapy for node-negative breast cancer is decreased by both combination cytotoxic chemotherapy and by tamoxifen."[183,p.4]

The Early Breast Cancer Trialists' Collaborative Group involved a worldwide meta-analysis of the results of ran-

**TABLE 34-9** Factors Influencing the Beginning of Modern Adjuvant Chemotherapy for High-Risk Operable Breast Cancer

By the time cancer becomes clinically detectable, it is advanced (near 30 doublings), and has had ample opportunity to establish distant micrometastasis.

Frequency of metastatic disease is directly related to tumor mass, and surgical cure rates drop as tumor volume at surgery increases.

Tumor growth fraction is inversely related to population size.

Effective drug kill follows first-order reaction kinetics.

Combination of drugs is superior to single agents and can eradicate 10–100 times as many cells.

In transplantable tumors, surgical adjuvant chemotherapy increases the long-term cure rates.

The optimal kinetic conditions to achieve cure exist when microscopic foci of disease are present after curative surgery and/or radiotherapy.

With permission from Bonadonna G: Evolving concepts in the systemic adjuvant treatment of breast cancer. *Cancer Res* 52:2127–2138, 1992.

domized trials involving 75,000 women with early (stage I and II) breast cancer and results were updated in 1992.[184] This large statistical analysis demonstrated that overall optimal use of adjuvant therapy can significantly improve long-term survival in women with stage I and II breast cancer and has the potential to save more lives from this disease than any other malignancy. In women <50 years of age, adjuvant chemotherapy alone reduces the annual odds of recurrence by 27%. Adjuvant chemotherapy is less effective in postmenopausal women >50. Treatment for this group reduces the annual odds of recurrence 22% and the annual odds of death 14%. In addition, tamoxifen as well as ovarian ablation was shown to significantly reduce the incidence of contralateral breast cancer. Table 34-10 summarizes pertinent findings of the meta-analysis.

The ability of adjuvant chemotherapy to increase disease-free intervals has been observed in clinical trials, but its effect on overall survival has not been demonstrated until recently. The meta-analysis demonstrates a clinically relevant reduction in tumor mortality due to adjuvant chemotherapy.

***Stage I (node-negative) breast cancer*** In certain subsets of women with node-negative breast cancer, the incidence of metastatic disease approaches 50%.[185] Combination chemotherapy can effectively reduce the annual odds of recurrence by at least 30% in this population. To accomplish this, 70% of patients will receive therapy unnecessarily because they have been cured by surgery alone.

Currently, there are important prognostic indicators that help to determine a woman's risk of recurrence, such as ploidy, proliferative indices, and tumor grade, but no one parameter is predictive of recurrence (Table

**TABLE 34-10** Early Breast Cancer Trialists' Collaborative Group (Meta-Analysis)

| |
|---|
| 14% overall reduction in the odds of death for those who received chemotherapy |
| CMF reduced the odds of death 23% (37% reduction in women younger than 50 years of age and a 9% reduction for older women) |
| 16% overall reduction in the odds of death for women who took tamoxifen (20% reduction among women 50 years of age or older) |
| A longer duration of chemotherapy (12 months) was no better than 6 months of chemotherapy |
| At the 10-year analysis, polychemotherapy increased survival over that seen at 5 years |
| In women <50, ovarian ablation was associated with significant improvement in overall survival (25%) |
| Adjuvant immunotherapy (BCG) had no influence on recurrence-free or overall survival |

Data from Early Breast Cancer Trialists' Collaborative Group.[113]

34-11). Most clinicians agree that many women with node-negative breast cancer should receive adjuvant chemotherapy, especially those with larger tumors,[172] although not all agree with this approach.[178] Women with the lowest risk of recurrence are those with tumors less than 2 cm, a grade I malignancy, positive estrogen/progesterone receptors, and a low proliferative rate. In contrast, those with tumors larger than 3 cm, grade III malignancy, negative estrogen/progesterone receptors, and a high rate of proliferation are most at risk for recurrence. Table 34-12 summarizes selected clinical trials involving therapy of women with node-negative breast cancer.

Node-negative and node-positive patients may benefit from preoperative chemotherapy. Because the chemotherapy is given prior to surgery, it is possible to evaluate the response of the tumor and to correlate this to disease-free survival and overall survival. It is also possible that the chemotherapy will permit more conservative surgery and decrease the incidence of ipsilateral tumor recurrence.

The NSABP protocol B-19 compared two different chemotherapy regimens known to be effective in node-negative breast cancer. One regimen involves methotrexate followed in 1 hour by 5-fluorouracil (M-F). Leukovorin calcium (L) is begun 24 hours after the methotrexate. This regimen was compared to standard cyclophosphamide, methotrexate, and 5-fluorouracil (CMF) therapy. Recent analysis of this study indicates that both regimens offer at least a 30% risk reduction for recurrence, but CMF was superior to M-F + L in risk reduction. The M-F + L appears to be less toxic in terms of myelosuppression and hair loss and does not have the leukemogenic potential of an alkylating agent–containing regimen. In premenopausal women, M-F + L does not affect gonadal function.

In a previous study, tamoxifen was found to be useful in premenopausal and postmenopausal, estrogen-positive, node-negative patients, representing a 30% reduction in risk of recurrence.[186] NSABP protocol B-20 asks whether chemotherapy (CMF or M-F + L) added to tamoxifen is superior to tamoxifen alone in women with node-negative, ER-positive tumors. Results of this study are not yet available.

NSABP protocol B-21 considers whether or not long-term treatment with tamoxifen (with or without breast irradiation) is effective in prolonging disease-free survival in patients with occult invasive cancer less than 1 cm. Previous studies have demonstrated that tamoxifen reduces the incidence of local recurrence after lumpectomy and radiation and significantly decreases the incidence of contralateral breast cancer.[186] The results of this study will help to determine whether radiation is necessary after lumpectomy as well as the impact of tamoxifen on recurrence.

Intergroup study 0102 asks whether a doxorubicin-based regimen (cyclophosphamide, doxorubicin, 5-fluorouracil—CAF) is superior to CMF in node-negative women deemed to be at high risk on the basis of tumor

**TABLE 34-11**   Cooperative Studies of Adjuvant Systemic Therapy in Node-Negative Disease

| Study and Patient Eligibility Criteria | Design | Primary Research Question |
|---|---|---|
| NSABP B-18: ER/PR status unknown, node-negative or node-positive patients with palpable operable breast cancer whose diagnosis is established by FNA or core biopsy (all patients who have lumpectomy receive radiation) | Total mastectomy or lumpectomy + axillary dissection + AC × 4<br>vs.<br>AC × 4 followed by total mastectomy or lumpectomy plus axillary dissection | Will preoperative chemotherapy effectively prolong disease-free survival and overall survival compared to the same regimen given postoperatively?<br><br>Will preoperative chemotherapy permit more conservative surgery and decrease the incidence of ipsilateral breast cancer recurrence?<br><br>Will response of the primary tumor to preoperative chemotherapy correlate in any way to disease-free survival and overall survival? |
| NSABP Protocol B19: ER-negative, lumpectomy or total mastectomy and axillary dissection | M–F + L<br>vs.<br>CMF | Is there a universally standard chemotherapy regimen for node-negative, ER-negative breast cancer? Recent findings indicate that CMF is superior to M–F + L. |
| NSABP Protocol B20: ER-positive, lumpectomy or total mastectomy and axillary dissection | TAM alone<br>vs.<br>TAM + M–F + L<br>vs.<br>TAM + CMF | Does the addition of tamoxifen to chemotherapy increase disease-free survival and overall survival significantly more than tamoxifen alone in ER-positive breast cancer? |
| NSABP Protocol B21: Occult invasive disease <1 cm, ER/PR status unknown, lumpectomy | TAM alone<br>vs.<br>TAM + RT<br>vs.<br>RT alone | What is appropriate therapy for clinically occult invasive breast cancer? |
| Intergroup Study 0102: ER-positive, high SPF, <2 cm tumor or ER-positive, ≥ 2 cm tumor or ER-negative tumors regardless of size | CAF ± TAM<br>vs.<br>CMF ± TAM | Is cyclophosphamide, doxorubicin, and 5-fluorouracil superior to standard CMF in high-risk, node-negative patients with breast cancer with or without tamoxifen? |

Abbreviations: *TAM* = tamoxifen; *RT* = radiation, *CMF* = cyclophosphamide, methotrexate, 5-fluorouracil; *AC* = adriamycin, cyclophosphamide; *CAF* = cyclophosphamide, adriamycin, 5-fluorouracil; *M–F + L* = methotrexate, 5-fluorouracil plus leucovorin.

size (2 cm or larger) and proliferative activity (S-phase fraction).

***Stage II (node-positive) breast cancer*** Women with tumor involving the lymph nodes are recognized as hav-ing a greater likelihood for distant recurrence and death. Adjuvant chemotherapy, especially for premenopausal women age 50 and younger, is widely accepted.

Early clinical trials using CMF confirmed the impor-tance of nodal extent.[187,188] These studies also demon-

**TABLE 34-12**   Cooperative Studies of Adjuvant Systemic Therapy in Node-Positive Breast Cancer

| Study and Patient Eligibility Criteria | Design | Primary Research Questions |
|---|---|---|
| ECOG 4188 (intergroup 0100): Postmenopausal, ER-positive, mastectomy ± radiation | TAM<br>vs.<br>CAF × 6 cycles + TAM for 5 years<br>vs.<br>CAF × 6 cycles followed by TAM for 5 years | How does TAM alone compare with chemoendocrine therapy in postmenopausal ER-positive patients? Is there a difference in response rate between patients who receive TAM concurrent with chemotherapy compared with those who receive TAM after the last course of chemotherapy? |
| ECOG 5188 (intergroup 0101): Premenopausal, ER-positive, lumpectomy + axillary dissection ± radiation, mastectomy ± radiation | CAF × 6 cycles<br>vs.<br>CAF followed by goserelin acetate × 5 years<br>vs.<br>CAF followed by goserelin acetate ± TAM for 5 years | Is the addition of goserelin acetate to CAF with or without TAM superior to CAF alone? |

*(continued)*

**TABLE 34-12** Cooperative Studies of Adjuvant Systemic Therapy in Node-Positive Breast Cancer (continued)

| Study and Patient Eligibility Criteria | Design | Primary Research Questions |
|---|---|---|
| NSABP protocol B-25:<br>All age groups, node positive (1 or more) ER positive or negative, lumpectomy + axillary dissection + RT or mastectomy ± RT | AC: comparison of three dose schedules every three weeks<br><br>I: A—60 mg/m² × 4<br>   C—1200 mg/m² × 4<br>vs.<br>II: A—60 mg/m² × 4<br>   C—2400 mg/m² × 2<br>vs.<br>III: A—60 mg/m² × 4<br>   C—2400 mg/m² × 4<br>plus<br>TAM × 5 years (all patients >50) | Will giving larger but fewer doses of cyclophosphamide (dose intensification) in combination with adriamycin and colony stimulating factors effectively prolong disease-free survival and overall survival more than the same cumulative dose of cyclophosphamide given over a prolonged period of time?<br><br>Will increasing dose intensity as well as cumulative dose of cyclophosphamide more effectively prolong disease-free survival and survival than the same dose intensity but for a shorter period of time? |
| NSABPB-27:<br>Palpable breast cancer confined to the breast and/or lymph nodes; node-negative patients are eligible. | AC × 4 cycles Q 21 days + TAM preoperative<br>vs.<br>AC × 4 cycles Q 21 days + TAM preoperative followed by preoperative docetaxel Q 21 days × 4<br>vs.<br>AC × 4 cycles Q 21 days + TAM preoperative followed by surgery followed by docetaxel Q 21 days × 4 cycles followed by RT if appropirate | To determine whether 4 cycles of preoperative or postoperative docetaxel given after 4 cycles of preoperative AC will more effectively prolong DFS and survival than do 4 cycles of AC alone. |
| ECOG (intergroup study):<br>Doxorubicin dose escalation with or without paclitaxel for node-positive operable disease.<br>Adjuvant postoperative chemotherapy | I: Adriamycin—60 mg/m²<br>  cyclophosphamide—600 mg/m²<br>  Q 21 days × 4 cycles<br>vs.<br>II: Adriamycin—37.5 mg/m² days 1 & 2<br>  cyclophosphamide—600 mg/m² day 1<br>  Q 21 days × 4 cycles<br>vs.<br>III. Adriamycin—45 mg/m² days 1 & 2<br>  cyclophosphamide—600 mg/m² day 1<br>  Q 21 days × 4 cycles + G–CSF and ciprofloxicin<br><br>Each group is then randomized to receive Taxol 175 mg/m² 3 hour infusion q 21 days × 4 cycles or no Taxol | To determine whether higher doses of adriamycin with standard dose cyclophosphamide in patients with early breast cancer will increase DFS and overall survival<br><br>To determine whether paclitaxel after AC will improve DFS and survival regardless of the dose of adriamycin |

strate the efficacy of 6 months versus 12 months of CMF. CMF for six months has been the standard approach to node-positive breast cancer against which other regimens have been and are being compared. One such clinical trial was NSABP B-15. In this study, patients who received adriamycin and cytoxan (AC) every three weeks for four courses did as well as those who received CMF for six months. While patients receiving AC experienced more immediate and profound hair loss, they experienced less nausea over time, visited health professionals one-third as often, and completed their therapy in much less time compared to those receiving CMF.

The efficacy of chemotherapy in postmenopausal women has been sufficiently demonstrated. Tamoxifen has proven efficacy and in a study involving almost 1200 patients, tamoxifen plus chemotherapy (AC) has shown greater benefit than tamoxifen alone.[189] In addition, this study failed to demonstrate an unfavorable interaction between chemotherapy and tamoxifen when administered simultaneously.

In a summary study, intergroup study 0100 compared CAF and concurrent or delayed tamoxifen with tamoxifen alone in postmenopausal, ER-positive, node-positive patients. This study will help to confirm or deny the worth of tamoxifen as standard therapy for this subset as well as to further delineate the role of tamoxifen in the prevention of contralateral breast cancer.

Intergroup study 0101 was designed for premenopausal women with ER-positive tumors. All women entered on the study received six months of chemotherapy. The luteinizing hormone-releasing hormone (LHRH) agonist, goserelin acetate (Zoladex: ICI Pharma, Wilmington, DE) with or without tamoxifen was given following chemotherapy. Because tamoxifen does not totally block the effects of circulating estrogen, the addition of Zoladex may help to create a total estrogen blockade in these ER-positive patients. The results of this and other studies will help to clarify the role of ovarian ablation as adjuvant therapy.

Efforts to improve outcome in node-positive patients have focused on the development and application of new drugs in combination with systemic therapy. Dose intensification may effectively increase intracellular drug concentration. With the addition of colony stimulating factors, it may be possible to ameliorate the dose-limiting toxicity of myelosuppression, possibly preventing the need for dose reductions or treatment delays. Giving optimal doses at regular frequent intervals is also an important strategy in preventing resistance and ultimate recurrence of disease.

The NSABP recently completed accrual into protocol B-18 which compares preoperative versus postoperative administration of four cycles of doxorubicin and cyclophosphamide (AC) in patients with operable breast cancer. Preliminary results indicate an overall response rate of 80%.[190] There was a highly statistically significant correlation between tumor response to preoperative chemotherapy and the type of surgery performed.

The NSABP has begun accrual for NSABP B-27, another preoperative trial, that uses standard doses of AC plus docetaxel, a drug known to be noncross-resistant to doxorubicin. It seeks to determine whether four cycles of preoperative or postoperative docetaxel given after four cycles of preoperative AC will prolong survival and disease-free survival compared to four cycles of preoperative AC alone.

A phase III intergroup study will examine the efficacy of dose-escalated doxorubicin and the addition of paclitaxel to the standard combination of AC in women with node-positive breast cancer. If there is dose response to adriamycin, this will be correlated with the presence or absence of overexpression of the Her-2/*neu* oncogene. There is some evidence that women whose tumors are positive for the Her-2/*neu* oncogene respond better to doxorubicin than those whose tumors are negative for the Her-2/*neu* oncogene.[191] This study will also determine whether the addition of paclitaxel has benefit.

In 1989, the NSABP began Protocol B-22, the goal of which was to evaluate the effect of dose intensification and increased cumulative dose of postoperative adriamycin and cytoxan (AC). The study involved node-positive women regardless of ER status.

The NSABP B-25 is a sequel to B-22 that looks at the value of not only dose intensification but also escalation of cytoxan.[192] All patients received standard dose adriamycin. All patients received colony stimulating factors. Tamoxifen is begun on day 1, continuing for five years (50 years and over age group). This is an important study because it will help to delineate the role of dose-intensive chemotherapy in high-risk women. In addition, because colony stimulating factors are given, it is hoped there will be fewer dose reductions and less myelosuppression. (Table 34-12 summarizes selected studies in node-positive breast cancer.)

### Locally advanced breast cancer (stage III)

Locally advanced breast cancer is associated with high risk of developing distant metastases. The larger the size of the primary tumor and the greater the number of histologically positive lymph nodes, the greater the risk of metastasis and death.[193,194] These tumors, by virtue of their size (>5 cm), are not amenable to treatment by breast-conserving surgery, and modified radical mastectomy is generally the treatment of choice if surgery is possible. Clinical characteristics of locally advanced disease include large or unresectable primary tumors, fixed axillary nodes, and the classic inflammatory carcinoma. While distant metastases are presumed to be present, they are not clinically apparent at staging.

If the tumor is fixed to the chest wall, inflammatory carcinoma is present, significant ulceration exists, or the axillary nodes are fixed to one another or other structures, the situation is generally considered to be inoperable due to the almost certain risk of recurrence.[194] The presence of supraclavicular lymph nodes is considered distant metastasis rather than locally advanced breast cancer; however, in the absence of more distinct distant metastasis, these patients are often grouped with locally advanced breast cancer.

The prognosis of patients with locally advanced disease is rarely improved by local therapy alone, and while many physicians approach these patients with a purely palliative intent, the role of systemic therapy is becoming more widely accepted. Results are superior when chemotherapy and radiation are included in the treatment plan.[195,196] The use of primary (neoadjuvant) chemotherapy has resulted in significant tumor regression in 60%–90% of women.[195] The advantage of this approach includes in vivo assessment of response. Significant tumor shrinkage may permit resection in previously unresectable disease, allowing for less extensive surgical procedures. Primary chemotherapy also provides immediate treatment to presumed metastasis that would otherwise be delayed by local therapy. Primary chemotherapy also prevents/avoids the postsurgery growth spurt of metastatic disease observed in animals. Combined modality therapy employing chemotherapy, surgery, and radiation may result in complete disappearance of disease in many patients including those with inflammatory cancer.[197]

High-dose chemotherapy with peripheral blood stem cell autologous bone marrow transplant and hematopoietic growth factor support is currently an option for treatment for women with high-risk advanced disease.

According to the North American Blood and Bone Marrow Transplant Registry breast cancer is now the most common diagnosis among patients who receive high-dose chemotherapy and autologous bone marrow transplant. It is estimated that ten times more women receive ABMT/PBSCT, usually with high-dose chemotherapy, off protocol than on protocol. Two randomized trials of high-dose chemotherapy with ABMT/PBSCT support have been initiated and are designed to address definitively the role of these therapies in early breast cancer. Both studies involve women with 10 or more positive nodes. In the CALGB study women are randomized to receive standard CAF followed by standard dose cyclophosphamide, cisplatin, and carmustine or CAF followed by high doses of the same drugs combined with bone marrow support. All patients receive tamoxifen and radiation. The ECOG/intergroup study randomizes patients to CAF followed by radiation and tamoxifen or to CAF followed by high-dose cyclophosphamide plus thiotepa with bone marrow support, tamoxifen, and radiation. The therapeutic benefit of ABMT or peripheral blood stem cell transplant have yet to be definitively established in breast cancer. The toxicities of this treatment are significant, with a mortality rate of up to 20%. The principal causes of death include infection, hemorrhage, and organ damage. Table 34-12 describes chemotherapy regimens commonly used to manage advanced local disease.[170]

***Adjuvant tamoxifen therapy*** Tamoxifen is a nonsteroidal antiestrogen that binds competitively to the estrogen receptor present in tumor cells. By blocking the binding of estrogen to the estrogen receptor it blocks cell cycle transit in G1 and inhibits tumor growth. According to the findings of the meta-analysis tamoxifen produced a 25% reduction in the odds of recurrence and a 16% reduction in the odds of death.[184] The benefit with adjuvant tamoxifen is similar for node-negative and node-positive patients, but is most evident in women over 50 years of age. Tamoxifen is especially attractive for treating women at a lower risk of disease recurrence as well as those who are elderly, experiencing concomitant illness, or those who refuse chemotherapy. The optimal duration of tamoxifen therapy is not known. Oncologists routinely prescribe tamoxifen 20 mg/day for five years and longer.

Undesirable consequences of the estrogen-like effects include stimulation of the endometrium. Tamoxifen therapy improves disease outcome and decreases the risk of contralateral cancer by 40%.[184] According to the findings of the NSABP B-14 trial, which randomized 2644 node-negative patients with ER + tumors to tamoxifen, 10 mg twice daily versus placebo, hot flashes occurred in 57% of women on tamoxifen compared with 40% of those on placebo.[186] About 20% of women on tamoxifen report severe hot flashes, compared with 3% of the placebo group. Vaginal discharge and irregular menses are also associated with tamoxifen therapy. Ocular toxicity (retinopathy or keratophy) has been reported in women taking conventional doses of tamoxifen, but in general ocular toxicity is not a clinically significant danger of tamoxifen therapy.[198] After tamoxifen withdrawal ocular abnormalities are usually found to be reversible. Currently the recommendation is to continue treatment unless visual symptoms are present. Patients might benefit from routine eye examination, especially those with other preexisting ophthalmologic conditions. There is also concern that tamoxifen may act as a promoter of endometrial cancer due to its estrogen agonist effects.[186] Fornander et al[199] in a study of 1846 women of whom 931 were randomized to therapy with 40 mg of tamoxifen daily observed a relative risk of 2.7 in those receiving tamoxifen as compared with controls. Further analysis using 20 mg per day of tamoxifen has not revealed a strong association between tamoxifen, endometrial cancer, and duration of therapy.[129] Moreover, the benefits of tamoxifen in lives saved exceeds the incidence of endometrial cancer.[200]

## Nursing Considerations in the Care of the Woman with Localized Breast Cancer

Women today are active health consumers who frequently seek information regarding their early options. It is not uncommon for the nurse to be called upon for advice concerning where a woman might go for a consultation concerning how a suspicious mass should be investigated. If a comprehensive breast center is available in the area, the woman should be referred to the center for an opinion. Women should not delay in seeking medical attention; indeed, most women view the need for a definitive diagnosis as a psychological emergency. Fortunately, nurses and physicians who specialize in breast cancer realize this and generally mobilize resources to provide a swift and accurate assessment of the breast problem. While a breast cancer diagnosis causes significant emotional, social, economic/vocational upheaval, such distress eases over time as therapy is planned and carried out. Most women actively participate in the decision-making process and are able to clearly articulate their need for information throughout treatment planning and months of therapy. To be a supportive advocate for the woman and her family, the nurse must be knowledgeable concerning the options for therapy, the goals of therapy, measures to minimize complications of treatment, and the various resources that may need to be mobilized throughout the treatment period and beyond.

For rehabilitation to be optimal, the nurse should pay careful attention to the woman's expressed need for information at each juncture of treatment. Seeking information is a valuable coping device and yet rarely useful unless the woman recognizes the need for it. The right amount of accurate information will help the woman formulate questions and will facilitate decision making, decrease anxiety, and enhance overall adjustment to the illness and treatment.[201]

How well a woman adjusts psychologically and socially to the diagnosis and treatment will depend upon her previous coping strategies and emotional stability. In addition, social support has consistently been found to influence a woman's adjustment through treatment.[202] The threat to emotional, social, sexual, and physical well-being is multifaceted, and the relative impact of these factors on adjustment varies from patient to patient and assumes varying degrees of importance at different stages of treatment.

A strong source of social support will be extremely valuable throughout all phases of treatment. While the most important sources of social support are the woman's spouse, her family, and friends, other sources of support may also be needed to maintain a strong social network.[203] The roles of the psycho-oncologist, the social worker, and various support groups are important resources in the care of these women and their families.

The patient's need for information will vary considerably throughout each phase of treatment. It is not uncommon for the treatment plan to include surgery, radiation, and chemotherapy. For many women the time of active treatment lasts at least six months and most do not feel rehabilitated for up to a year following their diagnosis. If reconstruction is planned, this rehabilitation phase will be extended.

### Surgical considerations

The current options for surgical management of stage I and II breast cancer include breast-preserving surgery and radiation or modified radical mastectomy.

The cosmetic result of breast-preserving surgery is generally considered to be acceptable, as body image is maintained. Prior to surgery, it is important to emphasize that the breast will appear different from the other breast depending on the size of the breasts and amount of tissue removed. Scar tissue may form causing some contracture over time, but most women find the cosmetic result acceptable, especially when wearing a bra.

Complications following breast-preserving surgery include arm edema, seroma formation and wound infection, shoulder dysfunction, upper extremity weakness, fatigue, and limitations in mobility.[204,205]

Postoperative complications following mastectomy include wound infection, flap necrosis, and seroma forma-

tion. A transverse incision is associated with less skin flap necrosis in the upper quadrants while vertical incisions are better in the lower quadrants. Seromas occur in about 10% of patients and generally resolve following aspiration. Antibiotics may be indicated to manage infection.

Lymphedema following mastectomy may be transient or permanent and may occur in the early postoperative period or much later. Lymphedema is more likely to occur in women who have postoperative radiation to the axilla, infection, seroma formation, flap necrosis, or who are obese.

Nursing care of the postmastectomy patient centers on wound care, with special attention to maintaining functioning wound drains. If drains become blocked, the wound is more likely to develop a seroma/hematoma leading to infection and possibly flap necrosis. To maintain suction and an adherent flap drains may be "milked" to remove small clots. Drains are usually removed within two to four days following surgery. Patients may be discharged with drains intact.

Postmastectomy exercises to maintain shoulder and arm mobility may begin as early as 24 hours after surgery. The woman is instructed to maintain the affected arm in the adducted position but to perform limited exercises involving the wrist and elbow. Flexing fingers and touching the hand to the shoulder are encouraged. Squeezing a ball is discouraged, as it increases blood flow and, if done too vigorously, leads to swelling in the early postoperative period (see Table 34-13—"Postmastectomy Exercises" and Table 34-14—"Hand and Arm Precautions").

Prior to discharge, the patient should have clear instructions regarding wound care. Initial care of the wound involves maintaining a clean incision with dressing changes daily if indicated. A return appointment is usually made to assess the wound and if necessary remove stitches. At that time the patient should receive specific instructions regarding postmastectomy exercises. A mild analgesic may be indicated to promote arm mobility during exercises and prevention of shoulder dysfunction.

Complaints of a stiff shoulder are common and are due primarily to postoperative immobility. It is not uncommon for a tightness to develop under the axilla extending to the elbow. This cord-like substance is thought to be sclerosed lymphatics which gradually dissipate two to three months after surgery. ROM exercises and massage therapy are beneficial.

Care of the axilla involves avoiding the use of depilatory creams, strong deodorants, and shaving under the arm for approximately two weeks following surgery.

Instructions regarding breast self-exam and follow-up are best given during the first outpatient visit after surgery. Introducing the patient to various prostheses and mastectomy bras can occur in the hospital, but women are generally more ready to receive this information once the surgery is behind them. Most are not advised to wear a prosthesis until the wound has healed completely (six to ten weeks). In this time period, the woman may want to meet with a Reach to Recovery or Y-ME volunteer who

**TABLE 34-13**    Postmastectomy Exercises

| When to Begin | Purpose | Exercises: Perform Exercises 5–10 Times Each, Three Times a Day |
|---|---|---|
| Postoperatively days 1–5 | Prevent and/or reduce swelling | • Position arm against your side in a relaxed position. Elbow should be level with your heart, and the wrist just above the elbow when resting.<br>• Rotate wrist in a circular fashion.<br>• Touch fingers to shoulder and extend arm fully. |
| After drains are removed | Promote muscle movement without stretching | • While standing, brace yourself with your other arm and bend over slightly, allowing your affected arm to hang freely. Swing the arm in small circles and gradually increase in size. Make 10 circles—rest—repeat in the opposite direction.<br>• Swing arm forward and back as far as you can without pulling on the incision.<br>• While standing, bend over slightly and swing arms across the chest in each direction.<br>• While sitting in a chair, rest both arms at your side. Shrug both shoulders, then relax.<br>• While sitting or standing, pull shoulders back, bring the shoulder blades together. |
| After sutures are removed | To stretch and regain full range of motion. To gain mobility of your shoulder, you must move it in *all* directions, several times a day | • While lying in bed with arm extended, raise arm over your head and extend backwards.<br>• While lying in bed, grasp a cane or short pole with both hands across your lap. Extend arms straight up and over your head and return.<br>• Repeat, rotating the cane clockwise and then counterclockwise while over your head.<br>• While standing, extend arm straight over your head and down.<br>• Extend your elbow out from your side at a 90° angle—hold it for 10 seconds—relax.<br>• Extend your arm straight out from your side even with your shoulder—extend arm straight up toward the ceiling.<br>• Stand at arms' length facing a wall. Extend arms so your fingertips touch the wall. Creep fingers up the side of the wall, stepping forward as necessary. Repeat the procedure going down the wall—keep arms extended.<br>• Stand sideways to the wall. Extend arm out so fingers touch the wall. Creep up the wall a little more each day.<br>• Use hand and arm normally (see Table 34-14). |
| After 6 weeks | To strengthen arm and shoulder and to regain total use of arm and shoulder | • Begin water aerobics.<br>• Begin overall fitness program.<br>• Begin aerobics, Jazzercise, or other resistive exercises.<br>• Avoid using weights as these may increase arm edema and subsequent swelling. |

will assist her in learning about resources in her area for purchasing a prosthesis. There are many different kinds of prosthesis; some are foam filled, liquid silicone filled, or are the more permanent self-adhering variety. It is important that the prosthesis fits properly and that the weight is similar to the remaining breast. Insurance pays for most prostheses provided a prescription or letter demonstrating medical necessity is submitted.

The woman alone or together with her husband or spousal designate should have the opportunity to discuss any physical or emotional concerns regarding sexual relations. Evidence is mounting to support the contention that, while the diagnosis of breast cancer and the loss of a breast are certainly emotionally distressing for all concerned, they do not result in an increased prevalence of psychiatric disorders or sexual dysfunction.[206,207] The

**TABLE 34-14**   Patient Information—
Hand and Arm Precautions

Do not permit injections (chemotherapy), blood samples, or vaccinations to be done on your affected arm unless approved by your physician.

When trimming cuticles, take extra care not to tear hangnails. Professional manicures *are* recommended.

Wear heavy gloves when gardening and digging or handling thorny plants.

Always use a thimble when sewing to avoid pinpricks, and wear rubber gloves while washing dishes.

Protect your arm from burns, especially from small appliances such as irons or frying pans, and from the sun.

Be sure your hand and arm are well protected with an elbow-length mitt when reaching into a hot oven.

Always have blood pressure measurements taken on the opposite arm.

Avoid arm constriction from tight elastic, sleeves, or jewelry.

Do not carry a heavy purse or other objects—especially grocery bags or luggage—with your affected arm.

Avoid strenuous upper body aerobics unless arm is supported by a properly fitted antilymphedema compression sleeve. Lifting weights of any kind is not recommended.

Apply a good lanolin cream several times daily if your skin appears dry.

Treat cuts and scratches by washing the area well and applying an antiseptic. Contact your physician if signs of infection, redness, warmth, or swelling occur.

woman's overall psychological health, relationship satisfaction, and prior sexual relations are far stronger predictors of sexual health than the extent of breast surgery. As a group, however, younger women have consistently been found to experience more episodes of depression, anger, resentment, sexual problems, and fears of recurrence compared to older women.[208,209]

### Chemotherapy

An important consideration is the occurrence of sexual dysfunction in the months following surgery. This may be in part due to the effects of chemotherapy and hormone therapy. Many premenopausal women who receive chemotherapy will experience ovarian failure and early menopause, especially if a larger cumulative dose of an alkylating agent is included in the treatment regimen. The probability of premature menopause occurring and being permanent increases for women over age 35. For most, menses cease during therapy or become erratic over two to three years, and amenorrhea occurs. Levels of follicle stimulating hormone (FSH) increase gradually and remain elevated for two to five years. FSH levels of >30 ng/L are usually considered diagnostic for ovarian failure. Estradiol levels decrease and testosterone levels

decrease by 60% which may account for the reports of lessened sexual desire and arousability.[210,211]

Premenopausal women who receive chemotherapy should be clearly informed of their risk for temporary or permanent ovarian failure. Women experiencing ovarian failure generally experience less subjective desire and arousability, vaginal dryness, vulvar/vaginal soreness, a burning pain, and light spotting after intercourse. Women should be encouraged to use a water-soluble lubricant (Astroglide or K-Y Jelly) during vaginal intercourse to minimize discomfort.

Other menopausal symptoms that commonly occur in women receiving chemo/hormonal therapy include hot flashes, night sweats, and irregular menses. Hot flashes and profuse perspiration may be most troublesome at night and may interfere with sleep. Some women may benefit from lowering the thermostat in the home, especially where they sleep. Avoiding highly seasoned foods, caffeine, and alcohol may minimize the frequency of hot flashes. Dressing in loose-fitting cotton clothing and in layers, so a sweater or jacket can be removed during a hot flash is advised. Women can try vitamin E, 800 IUs per day or, if this is ineffective, Bellargel-S®, one tablet twice daily[212] may be prescribed. A low-dose clonidine patch (Catapress Transderm®) may effectively control hot flashes. Side effects of clonidine include a dry mouth, headache, irritability, and dizziness.[213] Although no significant changes in blood pressure or pulse have been noted with low-dose clonidine, the patient's blood pressure should be checked once or twice a week during the first few weeks on clonidine therapy.

Weight gain is a troublesome side effect of therapy and is commonly felt by patients to occur because of water retention. In fact, it is due to increased caloric intake.[214] Significant correlations exist between weight gain and subjective feelings of unhappiness, worry, and increased distress regarding appearance when these women were compared to women who lost or maintained their weight. Factors contributing to weight gain include prednisone, oral cyclophosphamide, taste changes, increased appetite, depression, mild nausea that is relieved by eating, and psychological distress.[214–216]

Women need to receive nutritional counseling regarding the avoidance of weight gain at the outset of therapy. Some gain as much as 15 pounds and find it very difficult to lose once therapy is over. This adds to their increased distress and is avoidable with counseling.

Fatigue is a common subjective complaint associated with adjuvant therapy, and symptoms such as total body tiredness, forgetfulness, and wanting to rest increase over time throughout therapy.[216] Women should be encouraged to interject rest periods into their normal schedule and, if possible, to begin a regular exercise program such as walking or water aerobics. In addition to combating fatigue, exercise helps to minimize nausea associated with treatment. Nausea and vomiting with chemotherapy is predictable based on the type of chemotherapy or hormone therapy treatment. Patients on methotrexate and 5-FU experience less nausea and vomiting than women receiving CMF. Oral cyclophosphamide is associated with more prolonged nausea compared to intravenous cyclophosphamide. Women on higher doses of adriamycin and cyclophosphamide experience intense nausea and vomiting for 48–72 hours following therapy if appropriate antiemetics are not employed. Most women will usually not experience nausea and vomiting on the first day of their therapy especially when given a serotonin antagonist such as ondansetron or granisetron plus 20 mg of dexamethasone over 45 minutes as a single dose. However, the nausea and vomiting are worse on the second and third day posttreatment. Therefore, patients need a clear plan for managing these unpleasant symptoms for at least 72 hours posttreatment. Ondansetron, 8 mg orally every six to eight hours, prochlorperazine, 15-mg spansules, and lorazepam, 1 mg every 12 hours for 2 days following therapy, are effective in minimizing these symptoms.

Adriamycin and cytoxan (AC) are commonly used in curable breast cancer, which means many women experience total alopecia within 2 to 3 weeks of beginning therapy. This is highly distressing and contributes greatly to feelings of loss and body image changes. Women need to be aware of when and how hair loss will occur and have a plan to manage hair loss. Some women prefer shaving their heads or cutting the hair very short to minimize the constant and annoying shedding of their hair. The American Cancer Society's "Look Good, Feel Better" program is an excellent support and resource for women experiencing not only hair loss but body image changes in general.

Women on methotrexate-5-fluorouracil therapy do not lose significant amounts of hair and rarely require a wig. Women receiving CMF experience gradual thinning over the six to eight months of therapy and may require a wig only towards the end of treatment. Hair begins to grow back within a month of ending therapy at a rate of ¼ inch per month with some variation. Women, especially younger ones, often are able to go without a wig or head covering within four months of therapy. Large earrings, a little more makeup, and hair mousse enable a woman to feel attractive and stylish in the early recovery period (see chapter 33 for a more complete discussion of alopecia).

### Radiation

Radiation generally begins within three to four weeks following chemotherapy. Women commonly experience fatigue, some nausea, but primarily skin changes and arm and breast swelling. Breast edema is unique to patients undergoing breast-preserving surgery and radiation and usually appears during the treatment or within one to six months of treatment. Breast edema is more common in women who have had an axillary dissection where more than 11 nodes are removed and in those also receiving adjuvant chemotherapy. Skin reactions occur in all patients and generally present as itching, dryness, scaling, redness, and tenderness. The breast may feel sore and warm to touch. Patients are instructed not to use soap to wash the area and to pat dry. Dry desquamation can progress to a moist desquamation with infection. (For a complete discussion on skin care changes during radiation see chapter 33.)

Arm edema occurs more commonly in patients who have axillary dissection followed by RT to the axilla. Symptomatic pneumonitis characterized by a dry cough and low-grade fever is infrequent, but can appear within two to three months of therapy and is more common in women receiving methotrexate-5-FU concurrently. Brachial plexopathy manifesting as paresthesias, with or without arm and hand weakness, may be transient or permanent, but is an infrequent complication. Rib fractures and cardiac complications are also rare and relate to dose and whether concurrent chemotherapy is also given.

## BREAST RECONSTRUCTION

Initially, surgery was regarded as a primary curative modality with the emotional and psychological effects being virtually ignored or regarded as the "price a woman must pay." Consequently, many women experienced feelings of loss, depression, and alterations in body image. These responses may be lessened now that breast reconstruction has come to be regarded as a viable and acceptable component in the treatment of breast cancer. In the past decade, improved procedure techniques and advances in the manufacture of implants have enabled many women to retain their self-confidence and body image, thereby enhancing their quality of life. Prior to the advent of plastic surgery for the treatment of breast cancer, many women found the external prostheses cumbersome and consequently felt it necessary to alter their activity and/or selection of clothing due to fear of displacement or discomfort of the prosthesis.

Despite the recent findings equating the two surgical procedures (mastectomy vs. lumpectomy plus radiation), in terms of survival, many women either choose or are advised to have a mastectomy. This decision may be based on a variety of circumstances including histological findings, emotional or body image issues, financial considerations, or accessibility of medical resources.

A woman who presents with diffuse microcalcifications or multicentric disease throughout the breast is not considered a suitable candidate for breast preservation. Some patients are troubled by the fact that, although the cancer appears to have been removed, an occult lesion may remain, and consequently they will choose to remove the breast. Additionally, cosmesis may be compromised because too great a proportion of breast tissue needs to be removed to ensure clear margins. Patients who are responsible for a substantial portion of their medical bills may forego the cost of radiation treatments and choose mastectomy. Other women find that suitable medical facilities for radiation treatments may require extensive travel time or are geographically unavailable.

Implants are considered to be safe and effective treatment despite recent media comments to the contrary.[217] Citing the potential harmful effects of silicone implants revealed in an ongoing investigation, the FDA imposed a moratorium on the use of silicone implants for augmentation and issued guidelines to limit the use of silicone implants for reconstruction.

To qualify for placement of silicone implants, certain criteria must be met. The surgeon informs the patient of the possible side effects as well as documents that the patient fulfills an "urgent need" that has been predetermined by the FDA. Additionally, the patient is enrolled in a registry to aid in the long-term tracking of these patients.

Initially, the criteria were very stringent, but the revised guidelines issued in August 1992 expanded the eligibility regulations. The patient must be 18 years of age or older. Women who have experienced cancer, other disease, or trauma may have immediate or delayed reconstruction. Implants may be placed in any woman who currently has silicone implants and needs replacement or revision for medical or health reasons resulting from augmentation or mastectomy surgery. Women with congenital defects or severe asymmetry are considered candidates for silicone implants. Additionally, women who require augmentation of the unaffected breast for any of the preceding reasons may have an implanted silicone prosthesis. Additional information on current guidelines issued by the FDA is available from the American Society for Aesthetic and Plastic Surgery or the American Society of Plastic and Reconstructive Surgeons at 1-800-635-0635.

The patient exclusion criteria include pregnancy or lactation, tissue abnormalities, and increased risk due to other treatment or psychological issues. Women who demonstrate active infection, lupus, scleroderma, or uncontrolled diabetes are not candidates for the procedure. Patients experiencing radiation damage, problems with vascularization, or who have inadequate tissue available are considered to be ineligible. The surgeon may declare any patient unsuitable who possesses any other physical or psychological condition that will compromise compliance and/or success of the surgical procedure. Because of the adverse publicity of silicone gel implants, many women and physicians are choosing saline-filled implants which reduces the risk of silicone contamination if rupture should occur. These implants, however, do not have the same suppleness and natural feel of silicone gel implants. Alternative implants, that are filled with a radiolucent material that is compatible with surrounding tissue and absorbable by the body, should be available soon.[217,218]

Although implants are considered a viable and acceptable choice, other avenues continue to be explored. Autologous transplants have provided a suitable alternative to the inert prosthesis in certain circumstances. These procedures include latissimus dorsi flap, TRAM (transverse rectus abdominis muscle) flap, and free transfer of abdominal or gluteal tissue.[219]

The silicone implant was introduced in the 1960s, and the basic design remains relatively unchanged today. The saline tissue expander is used as a temporary device or may function as a more permanent implant to remain in place until more is known regarding the potential risk of the silicone implants.

The timing of the consultation is very important because of the myriad of considerations to be addressed prior to surgery. In the past the general rule of thumb was to delay reconstruction, sometimes waiting months to years. Currently, surgeons who recognize that the psychological trauma associated with the loss of a breast may be lessened by more timely reconstruction will, after careful assessment, offer the patient immediate reconstruction. However, the woman's general health and/or treatment plan may indicate that a delay in reconstruction be considered.

The ideal candidate is one who has early-stage disease. However, the absolute limiting factor of this surgery is a medical condition that may compromise the patient's safety during or post surgery.[140] Heavy smokers may be advised to quit smoking or significantly reduce daily use to ensure an adequate blood supply. The surgeon will also attempt to identify those who may be subject to additional problems such as hypotension or hypoxia, which may compromise circulation and impact on the success of the surgical procedure.[218] Patients who present with extensive local or metastatic disease may need further evaluation regarding chemotherapy and/or radiation therapy, which may necessitate a minor or significant delay in reconstruction due to immunosuppression and/or skin changes.

During the initial consultation the surgeon additionally evaluates and addresses the patient's and family's expectations of surgery. This may be done through the use of before and after pictures as well as the surgeon's frank explanation of the expected outcome. A patient with realistic expectations is well informed and more likely to accept the expected imperfections when these aspects are known prior to surgery. The goals of reconstructive surgery are to achieve "acceptable" symmetry and softness, correct any deformity caused by prior treatment, and construct an adequate nipple areolar complex.

## Silicone Implants

Silicone implants are used for reconstruction when the surgeon has ascertained that adequate skin is or will be available postmastectomy. The surgery is usually done in stages (i.e., the implant is placed during one procedure, the nipple areolar complex is constructed during another procedure, and some additional surgery may be needed subsequently to attain the desired cosmetic result).

An ideal candidate for a silicone implant is a woman who is small breasted with a minimum of ptosis on the contralateral breast. If the patient's opposite breast needs revision to achieve symmetry, an implant placement and/or mastopexy will be performed at the same time.

The procedure entails incising part of the mastectomy

scar or using the mastectomy incision to form a pocket beneath the chest wall muscles and inserting the silicone prothesis. Placing the implant beneath the chest wall muscles helps counteract the expected firmness due to capsular contraction and supports the implant.[140]

The complications that may arise are progressive contracture, hematoma, infection, and flap necrosis. Contracture is an expected sequela of silicone implants and is the result of scar tissue enveloping the prothesis. However, some patients will experience increasing contracture that alters and deforms the breast. New implants are being designed with an attempt to reduce the incidence of contracture, which has decreased from 35%–55% to 2%–11% today. However, approximately 5% of implants need to be removed due to severe contracture.[220] Hematomas occur infrequently and are most often surgically drained. Infections happen rarely and are most often successfully treated with antibiotics or removal of the implant in extreme cases. Flap necrosis can be serious and, if extensive, may necessitate the removal of the prosthesis. Usually, the necrosis involves a small amount of tissue that is excised.[218]

## Saline Tissue Expanders

Saline expanders are used when an inadequate supply of skin is available at the mastectomy site or when a large and/or ptotic breast is required. Tissue expansion is the most frequently used reconstructive procedure.[140] The expander is placed behind the chest wall muscles using the lines of the mastectomy incision.

The expanders have a filling port that is either located remotely or on the anterior of the implant. After allowing sufficient time for wound healing, a series of injections is performed as an office procedure. The saline expanders, which are partially filled at the time of insertion, usually require 60–200 cc injections on a weekly or biweekly basis. The expansion continues until the device is overinflated by approximately 50%, usually in six to eight weeks,[174] but may take as long as six months.[140,221] The overfilled expander is left in place for several months to allow for accommodation of the stretched tissue. This overfilling helps to promote a more natural, supple contour of the reconstructed breast (Figure 34-18). The expander is then removed and a permanent prosthesis of lesser fluid volume is placed.

Contracture is a complication that may hinder or prevent further expansion. Deflation can occur spontaneously or as a result of needle puncture. Expanders with remote ports are less likely to be accidentally deflated.

## Latissimus Dorsi Flap

The latissimus dorsi is a large fan-shaped muscle that is considered an expendable unit because alternative muscle groups are able to adduct the humerus and posteriorly rotate the shoulder.[140] The latissimus dorsi flap is used

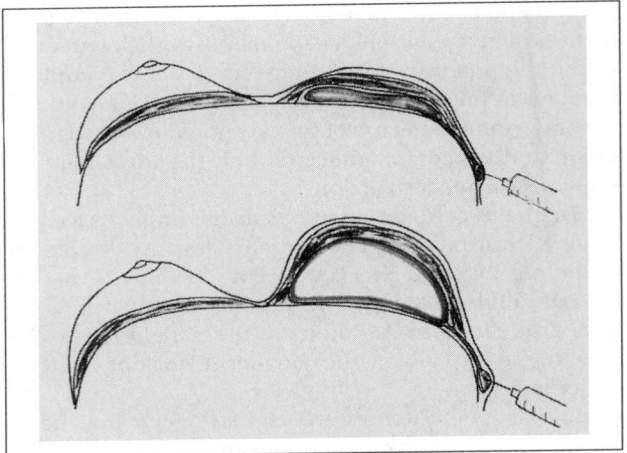

**FIGURE 34-18**   The horizontal view illustrates the overexpansion that is needed to allow for a more natural suppleness when the permanent prosthesis is implanted. (Courtesy of Dr. Craig Bradley, MD, Senior Attending, Plastic and Reconstructive Surgery, Rush Presbyterian St. Luke's Medical Center, Chicago.)

when inadequate skin is available at the mastectomy site and/or if additional tissue is needed to fill the supraclavicular hollow and create an anterior axillary fold following a radical mastectomy (Figure 34-19). An ellipse of skin along with the latissimus dorsi muscle is rotated onto the mastectomy site. The viability of the tissue is maintained through the thoracodorsal vessels (Figure 34-19).

Flap necrosis is rare due to the abundant vascularization of the area. The donor defect is often unnoticeable relative to the scar being beneath the bra-line.[140] This surgery takes three to four hours, approximately double the time needed for an implant procedure.

## TRAM Flap

The transverse rectus abdominis muscle flap has been commonly referred to as the "tummy tuck." During this procedure a low transverse ellipse incision is made and abdominal muscle and fat are tunneled under the abdominal skin to the mastectomy site. Tissue viability and perfusion are retained by the abdominal rectus muscle (Figures 34-20 and 34-21).

Possible complications are hernia at the donor site, which can be remedied by the placement of synthetic mesh, and flap necrosis, which may be largely avoided by careful selection of the candidates. Obese patients (> 20% overweight), those with circulatory problems, diabetes mellitus, prior history of liposuction, smokers, and those over age 65 generally are not considered eligible for this procedure.[218]

## Free Flap

The free flap represents the newest technique in reconstructive surgery. This procedure entails removing a por-

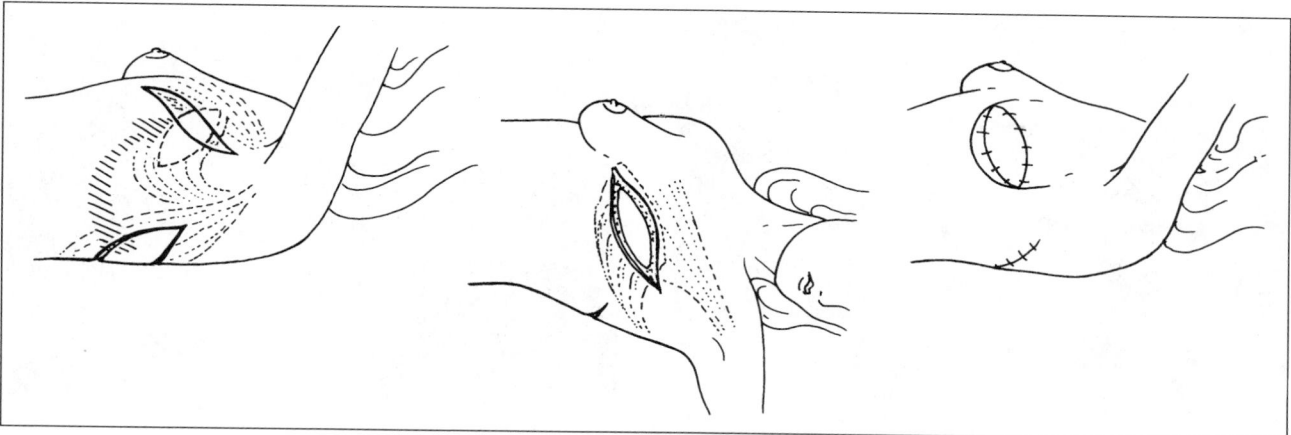

**FIGURE 34-19**  A diagram of the latissimus dorsi procedure. (Courtesy of Dr. Craig Bradley, MD, Senior Attending, Plastic and Reconstructive Surgery, Rush Presbyterian St. Luke's Medical Center, Chicago.)

tion of the skin and fat from the buttocks or lower abdomen and grafting it to the mastectomy site with microvascular anastomoses. This is a complicated procedure that demands microsurgical technique from two teams of surgeons; one to remove the flap and one to prepare the recipient vessels. The free TRAM flap has been reported to reduce complications, require shorter hospitalizations, and enhance the cosmetic outcome over pedicled tissue.[219] The success of this operation depends on the reliability of the anastomoses of the vessels to ensure adequate nourishment of the tissues. The main complication is failure to maintain sufficient perfusion in the postop period. Tissue death will ensue within six hours if flow is interrupted and cannot be sustained.[219]

### Gluteus Maximus Free Flap

If a TRAM flap is unavailable or inadequate in size, a portion of the buttock skin and muscle can be an alternative donor source. The skin and muscle are taken from the lower crease where the scar is less visible. Complications include posterior thigh numbness, possible flap necrosis, and a slight risk of infection. This surgery takes three to six hours to complete and requires a hospital stay of approximately one week with resumption of full activity in three to six months.[218]

### Nipple-Areolar Construction

The nipple-areolar complex is the final phase of the reconstruction process. The symmetry and cosmetic result of the breast mound should be satisfactory before this procedure is performed. The nipple should closely match the opposite side in size and pigment.

Tissue may be taken from the opposite breast if there is an adequate supply or if mastopexy has been performed. Previously, the nipple was often "banked" to the patient's thigh or groin to be used later. This method has fallen out of favor due to the risk of introducing potentially malignant tissue to the disease-free breast.

Tattooing is the primary method for creating the darker pigment of the areola.[219] Another option is a skin graft from the inner thigh. However, grafts are uncomfortable and can fade, requiring tattooing, so most women prefer to forgo this surgery and have the area tattooed.[218] (See Figures 34-22 and 34-23.)

Maintaining projection is a challenge that has been met by construction of pedicle flaps. These techniques employ folding the skin to achieve a slightly protuberant nipple. The most popular methods are the skate flap and c-v flap technique, in which the skin is raised and folded to achieve a natural nipple profile.

Complications are rare with this reconstruction, but those that may occur are failure to maintain suitable projection of the nipple, graft failure, and fading of the pigmented areas.

## METASTATIC BREAST CANCER

Despite improved screening techniques and increased awareness of breast cancer as a major health threat approximately 10% of women diagnosed with breast cancer have metastatic disease at clinical presentation. Approximately 30% of women diagnosed with an early stage node-negative disease and roughly 60% with node-positive disease will relapse despite adjuvant therapy.[222] The majority of patients who relapse (80%) do so within two years of the diagnosis. The median survival time for stage IV disease is two to three years; however, reports of five-year survival range from 12%–35% and ten-year survival from 5%–22%.[179]

Race may influence survival in breast cancer. African-American women tend to be diagnosed with more advanced disease than white women, and they have a 29%

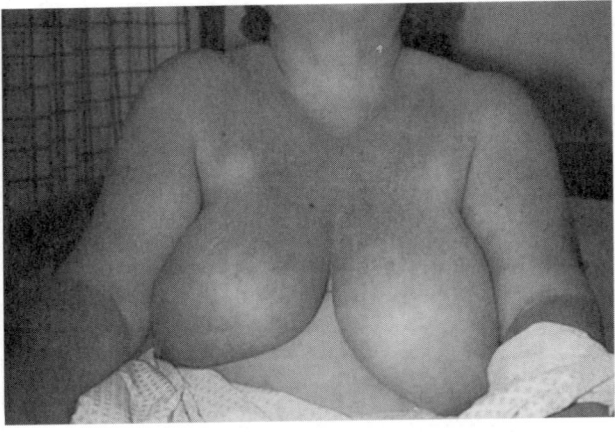

A

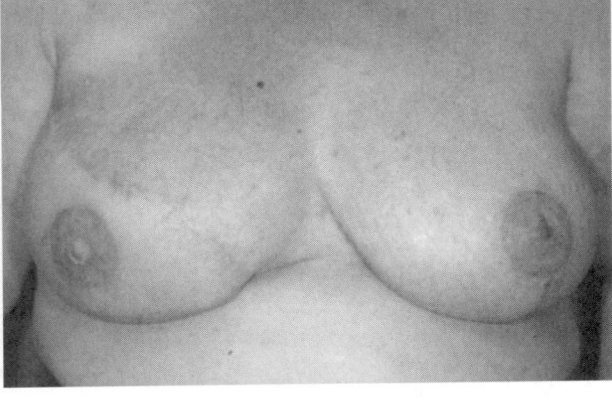

C

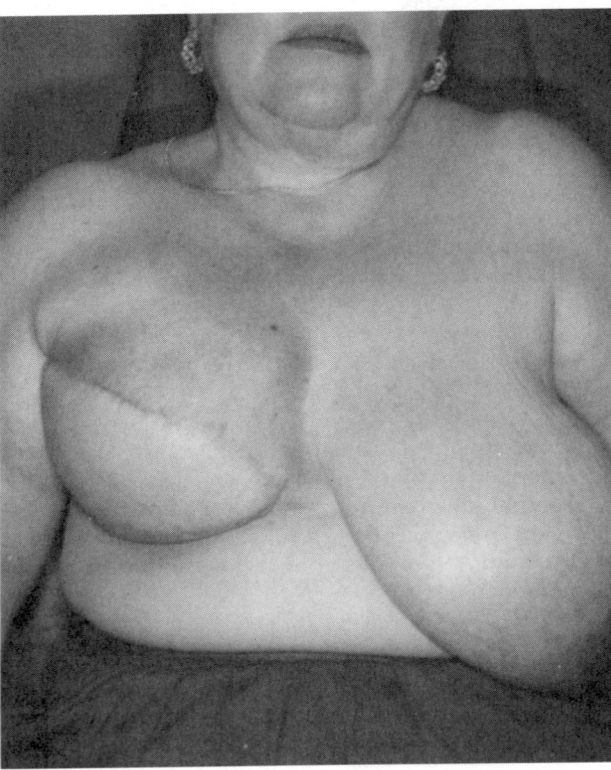

B

**FIGURE 34-20**   Three pictures illustrate a large woman (A) before the procedure, (B) after the mastectomy and latissimus dorsi flap, and (C) after mastopexy was performed to reduce the size of the other breast. Note the appearance of the tattooed nipple, which closely resembles the reduced breast. (Courtesy of Dr. Craig Bradley, MD, Senior Attending, Plastic and Reconstructive Surgery, Rush Presbyterian St. Luke's Medical Center, Chicago.)

higher death rate.[224] Differences in economic status, social factors, access to medical care, education levels, awareness of early detection measures, and willingness to comply with medical recommendations may contribute to this difference in survival. However, as yet unidentified biological factors may also account for these differences. Findings of Elledge and colleagues[225] revealed that African-American and Hispanic women were more likely to present with advanced disease and more likely to have ER-negative tumors and a high S-phase fraction compared to whites. These underserved minorities require intensive community screening programs aimed at education and assurance of access to care.

## Routes of Metastasis

The most common mode of metastasis is via the lymphatics, whereby the cells may be transported to local and more distant regional nodes. Conversely, breast cancer cells may enter the lymphatics by direct penetration. More virulent cancer cells can directly enter the blood vessels and spread to distant sites without evidence of lymph involvement. Once blood borne, malignant cells adhere to the vascular endothelium, stimulating endothelial retraction and exposing the underlying basement membrane, whereby a metastatic deposit and invasion of the structure occurs.

Breast cancer most commonly metastasizes to bone (> 50% of patients), specifically the spine, ribs, and proximal long bones. Patients will commonly complain of localized, deep-seated, unrelenting pain. Pathological fracture of the proximal femur may occur spontaneously despite efforts to protect the weakened bone. Likewise, persistent back pain may herald a compression fracture and possible neurological impairment. Hypercalcemia may reflect bone resorption due to tumor growth and resultant osteoclastic stimulation. Bone marrow metastasis occurs frequently in patients with extensive multifocal bone disease, generally presenting as bone marrow failure or as fleeting nocturnal pain.[226]

Loss of appetite and abnormal liver function tests are early symptoms of liver involvement. Late symptoms include pain, abdominal distention, nausea, emesis, periodic fever, jaundice, and generalized weakness. Pulmonary involvement may begin as a subtle, nonproductive cough or shortness of breath. Lymphangitic pulmonary

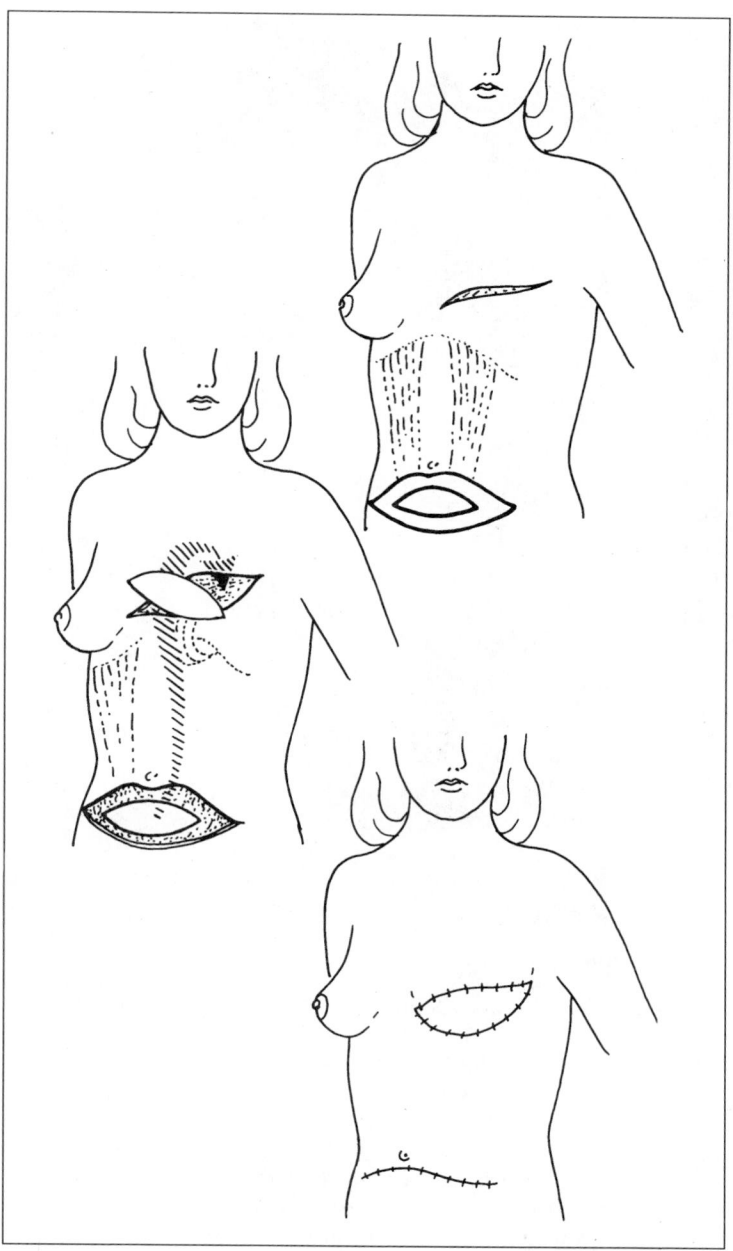

**FIGURE 34-21**  A diagram of the TRAM flap procedure. (Courtesy of Dr. Craig Bradley, MD, Senior Attending, Plastic and Reconstructive Surgery, Rush Presbyterian St. Luke's Medical Center, Chicago.)

spread is an ominous sign of rapidly progressive disease. Pleural effusions can progress slowly over time and respond temporarily to drainage and sclerosing. Renal involvement generally presents as oliguria and/or uremia in a woman with deteriorating mental status. Brain metastasis usually occurs in the supratentorial region, multiple sites, or as carcinomatous meningitis presenting as cranial nerve palsies, altered mentation, seizures, and/or focal paresis. Local cancer spread to the chest wall usually presents as a painless subcutaneous nodule along the mastectomy scar and adjacent chest wall areas. These lesions may respond well to local therapy, but distant disease is presumed to be present.

If the disease recurs locally after breast-conserving sur-

gery plus radiation, mastectomy is usually indicated. If recurrence is evident in the axilla, surgery and radiation are usually successful. However, evidence of disease in a supraclavicular node or recurrence in the scar or chest wall after mastectomy generally indicates metastatic spread beyond the breast and systemic therapy is warranted.

The management of patients with metastatic breast cancer is aimed at judicious use of local and systemic measures that control and/or palliate symptoms and improve quality of life.

The initial choice of therapy is generally the one that is the least toxic and carries with it the highest response rate. The basic strategy is to achieve optimal control of the disease and temporize for as long as possible. Local

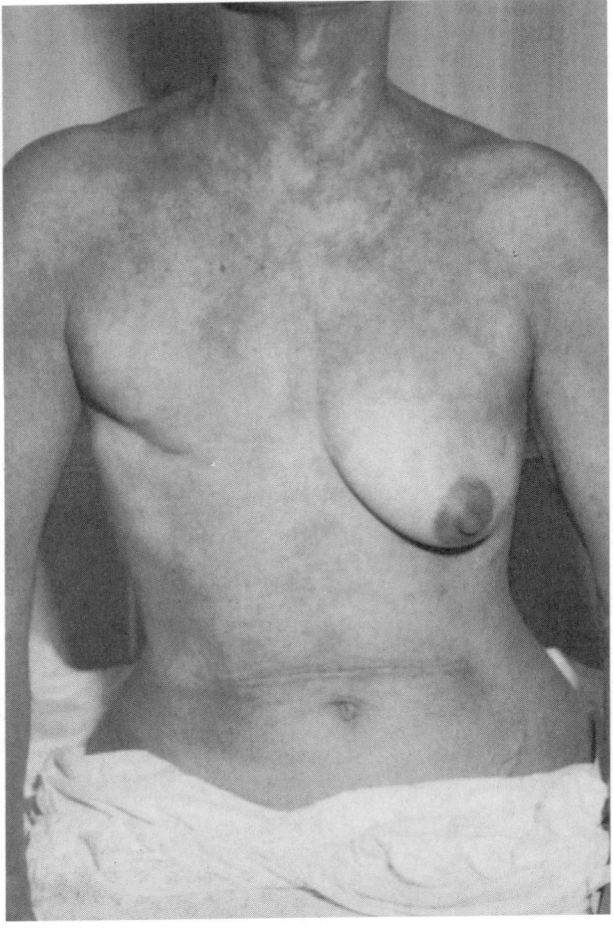
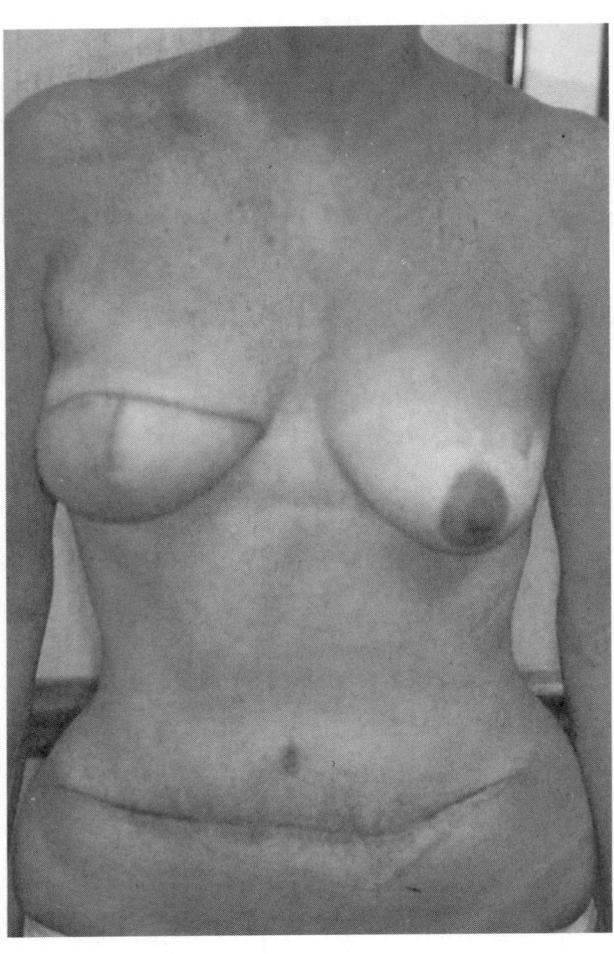

A                                              B

**FIGURE 34-22**    First picture shows a patient (A) after mastectomy and before the TRAM flap. The second and third pictures show the (B) anterior and (C) lateral view of the same patient shortly after the procedure. The scars will fade with time. (Courtesy of Dr. Craig Bradley, MD, Senior Attending, Plastic and Reconstructive Surgery, Rush Presbyterian St. Luke's Medical Center, Chicago.)                                                                                    *(continued)*

and systemic therapies are added periodically as needed until they have outworn their usefulness. For many women, especially those with hormone receptor positive disease, this can mean many years of quality of life. (See Table 34-15.)

It may be difficult for a woman with metastatic disease to understand why her doctor is not recommending more aggressive treatment. The idea that a new or different treatment is introduced only with evidence of disease or troublesome symptoms causes some women to ask why the treatment was not given to prevent the problem before it occurred. The answer is based on the desire not to make the woman more ill than her disease is making her and the knowledge that these therapies, including chemotherapy, have only a small effect on the median survival of women with metastatic disease. The goal is to get as much mileage out of each therapy as possible without compromising quality of life unless temporarily and absolutely necessary. However, an exception involves

the patient who is asymptomatic or minimally symptomatic, is desirous of therapy, and is not likely to require significant palliation for three to six months. In this situation it is entirely appropriate and optimal that the woman be introduced to innovative and experimental treatment protocols including high-dose chemotherapy and bone marrow transplant. Such therapies are available in cancer centers and cooperative cancer study groups. Their participation in studies involving dose-intensive, multidrug regimens may be appropriate and is critically important to women who desire more than what is currently available as well as to the overall research effort in breast cancer.

## Defining Extent of Disease

An assessment of the extent of disease is made to determine the most appropriate therapeutic approach and to

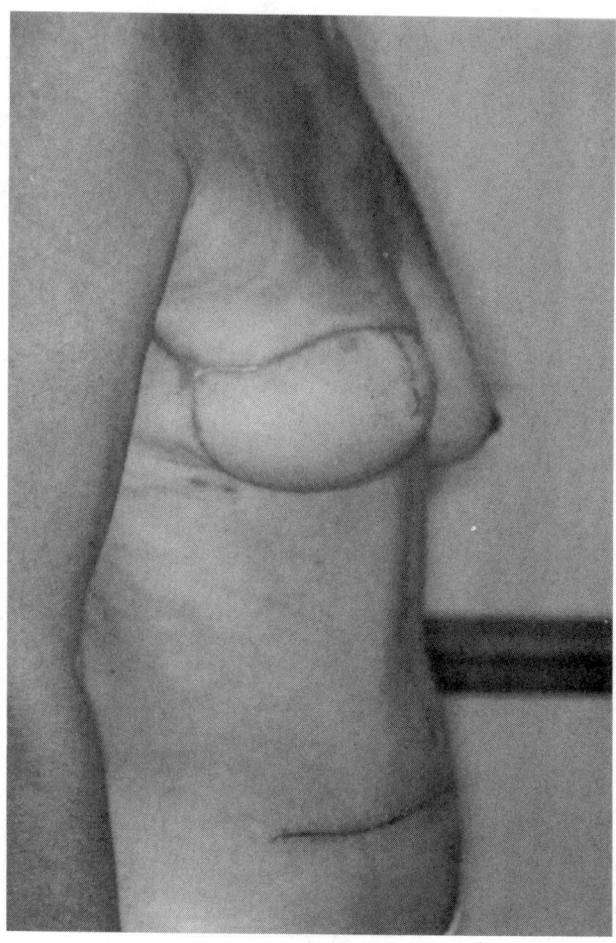

C

**FIGURE 34-22** *(continued)*

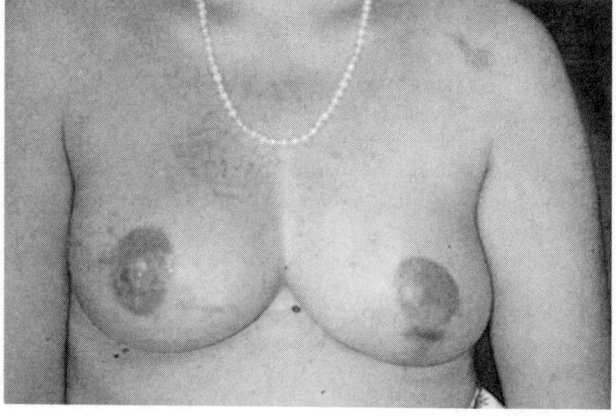

**FIGURE 34-23** Right breast reconstruction following a modified radical mastectomy. Unilateral nipple tattoo on the right is compared to the patient's own unaffected nipple on the left following mastoplexy. (Courtesy of Dr. Craig Bradley, MD, Senior Attending, Plastic and Reconstructive Surgery, Rush Presbyterian St. Luke's Medical Center, Chicago.)

determine response to therapy. Such clinical studies as chest film, liver scan, bone scan, MRI, CT or PET scan and cytological analysis of the cerebral spinal fluid may be indicated based on the woman's symptoms. Tumor measurements are taken periodically to determine response to therapy. Serum carcinoembryonic antigen (CEA) and CA 15-3 are important markers that indicate tumor activity often before clinical symptoms appear.

### Chemotherapy

Women who have a disease-free interval of less than two years, have hormone receptor negative disease, are refractory to hormone therapy, or have aggressive disease in the liver or pulmonary system are candidates for chemotherapy[170] (Table 34-15).

Combination chemotherapy results in higher response rates compared to single agents. Response rates vary from 50%–70% and can last for 9–12 months. The rate of complete response (percentage of individuals in whom all evidence of disease disappears) consistently has been only 10%–20% of cases.[227]

Currently, methotrexate-5-fluorouracil plus leucovorin, cytoxan-methotrexate-5-fluorouracil, mitoxantrone-thiotepa, or cytoxan-adriamycin-5-fluorouracil are among the more commonly used regimens. Doxorubicin-containing regimens have shown a 10%–20% better response rate, but currently offer no significant survival advantage over combinations not containing doxorubicin. For women who are elderly and prefer a regimen that does not cause hair loss or significant nausea, mitoxantrone and thiotepa or methotrexate-5-fluorouracil plus leucovorin are available. For women who fail on first line therapy, 5-FU may be given as a continuous infusion with or without leucovorin with good results, even in those who previously failed on 5-FU.[228,229]

Individuals with slow-growing disease and those with rapidly progressing disease will benefit from chemotherapy. The response of women to cytotoxic agents is not significantly related to the predominant site of disease. Women with visceral metastases as well as those with bony involvement will respond. Although radiological evidence of bone healing may take as long as six months, subjective improvement occurs within a shorter time.

## Endocrine Therapy

Women who have estrogen receptor positive breast cancer demonstrate a consistently superior survival after recurrence compared to women who are estrogen receptor negative. Endocrine therapy is one of the major forms of treatment of the woman with metastatic breast disease. It is well known that the growth of normal mammary tissue is influenced by a variety of steroid hormones. Normal mammary cells contain cytoplasmic receptor sites for each of the hormones known to influence the growth and function of the mammary gland, specifically, estrogen, progesterone, and prolactin.

**TABLE 34-15** Cytotoxic Therapy for Advanced Breast Cancer

| Acronym/Brand | Drugs | Dose (mg/m²) | Response Rate (%) | Median Duration of Response (months) |
|---|---|---|---|---|
| CMF ± P | Cyclophosphamide<br>Methotrexate<br>5-fluorouracil<br>Prednisone | 100, PO days 1 to 14<br>40, IV days 1 and 8<br>600, IV days 1 and 8<br>40, PO days 1 to 14; repeat every 28 days | 49%–59% | 5–8 |
| FAC | 5-fluorouracil<br>Doxorubicin<br>Cyclophosphamide | 500, IV days 1 and 8<br>50, IV day 1<br>500, IV day 1; repeat every 21 days | 50%–75% | 6–10 |
| AC | Doxorubicin<br>Cyclophosphamide | 40, IV day 1<br>200, PO days 3 to 6; repeat every 21 days | 40%–80% | 6–12 |
| CAF | Cyclophosphamide<br>Doxorubicin<br>5-fluorouracil | 100, PO days 1 to 14<br>30, IV days 1 and 8<br>500, IV days 1 and 8 | 60%–80% | 10–12 |
| Novantrone | Mitoxantrone | 12–14 every 21 days | 17%–35% | 4–5 |
| Taxol | Paclitaxel | 175 IV every 21 days | 30% | 6 |
| Taxotere | Docetaxel | 100 | 41% | 6 |

Adapted from Ravdin PM, Osborne CK: Breast cancer, in Wittes RE (ed): *Manual of Oncologic Therapeutics*, Philadelphia, Lippincott, 1995.

Steroid hormones can promote the growth of a breast cancer if the cells are hormonally dependent. In a woman who has a hormonally dependent tumor, estrogen enters the cell and binds to a specific cytoplasmic receptor protein called *estrophillin* or estrogen-receptor protein. The estrogen-receptor hormone complex is then believed to undergo transformation and enter the cell nucleus to promote tumor growth. It is thought that if the source of estrogens is removed by surgical ablation or medication manipulation, or if the hormone's access to the estrogen-receptor protein is blocked by antiestrogens, the chain of action is broken and the tumor regresses. Tumor cells that lack the cytoplasmic estrogen-receptor protein should not be expected to regress with hormonal or antiestrogen therapy.

The amount of estrogen-receptor protein present in a tumor remains relatively constant throughout the course of a woman's disease, and its measurement provides information about the degree of hormone dependency of a tumor.

Premenopausal women have a lower incidence of receptor-positive tumors (30%) than postmenopausal women (60%), and perimenopausal women have the lowest rate (10%).

Receptor-negative disease is usually associated with a short disease-free interval and more aggressive disease. Receptor-positive tumors are generally associated with a long disease-free interval between initial treatment and recurrence. These women often have slow growing disease, usually in soft tissue or bone.

In summary, treatment with hormonal therapy, either additive or ablative, is indicated when there are metastases, the metastases are not amenable to treatment by surgery or radiotherapy, the disease is not life-threatening, and the tumor is estrogen-receptor positive. Because endocrine therapies generally have the same efficacy, the least toxic is used first (Figure 34-24).

### Antiestrogen therapy

Tamoxifen is a synthetic antiestrogen and is the most widely used hormonal therapy. Tamoxifen acts by binding to the estrogen receptor thereby blocking the effects of endogenous estrogens. Tamoxifen has a long half-life (seven days) and takes four weeks to reach a steady state drug concentration. Once this steady state is reached, patients may take it once a day rather than twice a day which promotes compliance. Women on tamoxifen may experience a transient "tumor flare" which may cause increased bone pain, hypercalcemia, swelling, or erythema of superficial lesions within the first two weeks of treatment. These symptoms are managed with anti-inflammatory agents and will abate with subsequent tumor response.

In premenopausal women tamoxifen is equivalent to ovarian ablation. Women who respond initially to tamoxifen and subsequently become resistant are likely to respond to ovarian ablation. The most common side effects of tamoxifen include hot flashes, mild nausea, fluid retention, vaginal cornification, and postmenopausal bleeding.

### Estrogens

In women who are five or more years past menopause, the administration of pharmacological doses of estrogens (diethylstilbestrol [DES], 5 mg orally two or three times

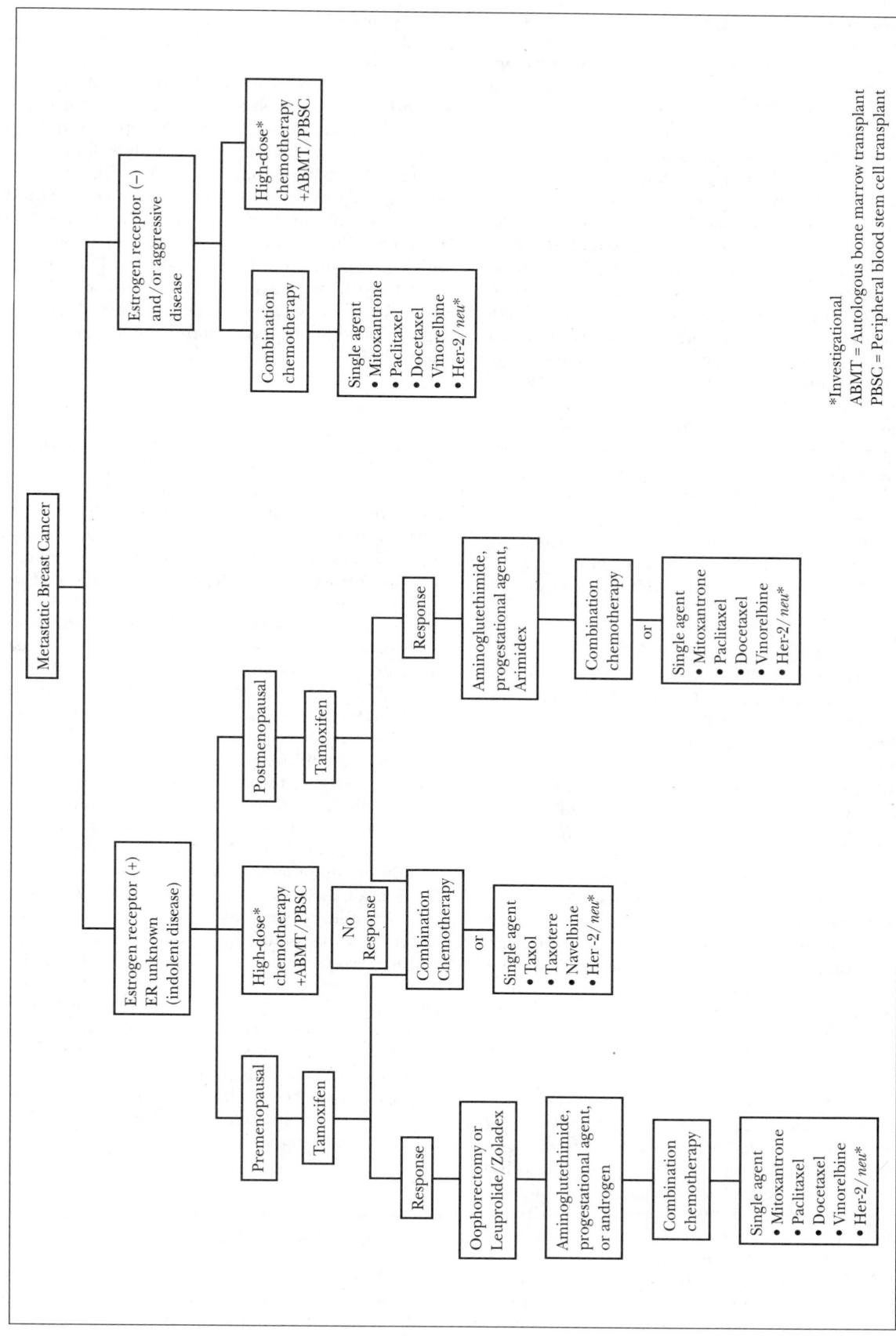

**FIGURE 34-24** Metastatic breast cancer: systemic approaches to management.

*Investigational
ABMT = Autologous bone marrow transplant
PBSC = Peripheral blood stem cell transplant

per day) can result in an objective remission in about 35% of the cases, lasting several months to many years. Administration of high doses of exogenous estrogens suppresses pituitary follicle-stimulating hormone (FSH) and luteinizing hormone (LH) and therefore the production of endogenous estrogens.

At the initiation of therapy, nausea and occasional vomiting may occur for a few days. Nausea and vomiting accompanied by progressive lethargy or polyuria are symptoms of hypercalcemia, which may occur with the initiation of therapy but is not necessarily an indication for discontinuing therapy. The woman taking estrogens should be instructed to limit sodium intake and be aware that she is likely to retain fluid and have decreased bladder tone as a result of estrogen administration. Diuretics are frequently needed to control fluid retention. Increased pigmentation of the nipples and areolas and enlargement of the breasts are other side effects.

Objective evidence of tumor regression is seen most often in women with soft tissue disease. When the disease is reactivated, estrogen therapy is terminated. Estrogen withdrawal occasionally will result in a reinduction of a brief partial remission. Individuals may experience uterine bleeding with estrogen withdrawal. Women who respond to estrogen therapy and then experience a relapse may benefit from other forms of endocrine therapy.

### Androgens

Androgens are most effective in women who are five or more years postmenopause. The overall response rate is 20%. Androgens block pituitary gonadotropin secretion thereby opposing endogenous estrogens. Androgen therapy may be added to oophorectomy in women under 35 years of age, but response rates are low. In the postmenopausal woman, androgens are indicated for the treatment of soft tissue or bone metastases and may result in "tumor flare" with initiation of treatment. Danazol is a synthetic steroid and is more commonly used because it has less virilizing effects (hirsutism, hair loss, acne, deepening of the voice, and increased libido) compared to testosterone or fluoxymesterone (Halotestin). Generally, because of the toxicity profile, androgens are reserved for use after most other forms of hormonal manipulation are exhausted.

### Progestins

The precise mechanism of action of progestins is unclear but they appear to inhibit the stimulator effect of estradiol on tumor growth. Megestrol acetate is a progestational agent with a response rate of 26%–30%, with a median duration of up to 22 months.[222] The standard dose of megestrol acetate is 160 mg a day. This drug is generally tolerated as well as tamoxifen and is comparable in efficacy but it is usually used only after women have failed on tamoxifen. The mechanism of action of megestrol acetate is thought to include interference in binding of estrogen to the estrogen receptor, and interference of the aromatization of androgens to estrogens. Megestrol acetate effectively decreases FSH and LH as well as estradiol levels.

Antiprogestins including RU486 (mifepristone) and Onapristone are investigational agents. Each is thought to bind to both the progesterone receptor and the glucocorticoid receptor. RU486 is generally well tolerated and associated with some nausea, hot flashes, and dizziness. Studies using these agents in breast cancer are hindered by the societal implications of its use as an abortifacient in Europe. The most important side effect is weight gain, which occurs in up to 50% of patients. This weight gain is related primarily to increased food intake and increases with higher doses. Other side effects include hot flashes, vaginal bleeding, hypercalcemia, tumor flare, and thrombophlebitis.

### Aromatase inhibitors

An important option for treatment of women with advanced, estrogen-receptor positive breast cancer is through the reduction of circulating estradiol levels by inhibiting aromatization of adrenal androgens to estrogens. In premenopausal women, the primary source of estradiol is the ovary. In postmenopausal women, estrogens are formed from androgens (primarily androstenedione) in extra glandular tissues, (i.e. fat, liver, and muscle). Androstenedione, and to a more limited extent testosterone, are converted to estrone in a reaction catalyzed by the aromatase enzyme complex. After aromatization of androstenedione to estrone, the enzyme 17-hydroxysteroid dehydrogenase converts estrone to estradiol in peripheral tissues, including the liver.

Aminoglutethimide is an aromatase inhibitor that was developed as an alternative to adrenalectomy. It acts by blocking the conversion of androstenedione to estrone. In the adrenal gland it blocks the conversion of cholesterol to pregnenolene which is the precursor of androstenedione thereby blocking adrenal steroid synthesis. The overall response to aminoglutethimide (Cytadren) is comparable to surgical ablation without the risks of surgery. Because of its effects on adrenal steroidogenesis, hydrocortisone replacement is needed. The side effects of aminoglutethimide include lethargy, orthostatic hypotension, dizziness, depression, hypothyroidism, and rash.

Arimidex is an aromatase inhibitor that has been well tolerated without evidence of effect on mineralocorticoids or glucocorticoids. It has been found to effectively suppress estradiol levels similar to other aromatase inhibitors. Side effects include slight headache, hot flashes, tiredness, and fatigue.

## MALE BREAST CANCER

It was estimated that 1000 new cases of breast cancer would be diagnosed in men in 1996 and 300 men would die of their disease.[230] Male breast cancer accounts for less than 1% of all breast cancers.[230] The anatomic structures of the male breast are the same as those of the female breast. It is the hormonal stimulation present in the female breast and absent in the male breast that accounts for the development and physiological differences between the male and female breast. This lack of hormonal stimulation also may explain the comparatively low incidence of male breast cancer. However, the disease in both sexes is similar in terms of epidemiology, natural history, and response to therapy. Family history of breast cancer is present in about 30% of males with breast cancer.[231,232] Various factors contributing to the development of male breast cancer include undescended testes, orchiectomy, orchitis, late puberty, infertility, obesity, hypercholesteremia, and estrogen use.[233]

The incidence of breast cancer is increased in men who have undergone sex-change procedures. The administration of estrogens results in lobular development and enlargement of the male breast. Hormonal imbalance (androgen deficiency) and gynecomastia are characteristic of Klinefelter's syndrome, and the incidence of breast cancer is increased in men 20 to 66 times that of an average male, with a risk of breast cancer of 3%.[234]

The administration of DES to men with carcinoma of the prostate has been associated with male breast cancer but is a rare occurrence. While it is true that large numbers of men receiving DES for prostatic carcinoma do not exhibit an increased incidence of breast cancer, it is important to note that the life expectancy of these men is relatively short, and breast cancers may indeed be present but not yet manifested.

Breast cancer occurs most frequently in men aged 50–70 years with the peak incidence occurring at 60 years of age. It appears that after 40 years of age, the Sertoli cells (elongated cells in the seminiferous tubules) secrete increasing amounts of estrogens. The majority of male breast cancers (75%) are known to be estrogen-receptor positive and approximately 30% will respond to hormonal manipulation. They typically arise from ductal elements and present as infiltrating ductal carcinoma, which is commonly fixed to underlying fascia and skin. Nipple retraction and a bloody discharge may be present.

A painless, centrally located subareolar mass is usually the first symptom that brings the man to seek medical attention. Pectoral fixation, involvement of skin, nipple changes, and discharge are commonly present because of limited breast disease and delay in seeking medical attention. These factors may account for the increased frequency of widespread disease and early invasion of local and regional lymphatics. Ulceration may occur early in the course of the disease and carries a relatively poor prognosis. A bloody discharge from the nipple and nipple inversion may be present. Because of its relatively central location, male breast cancer can be expected to metastasize to the internal mammary nodes. The lungs and bony skeleton are the most common metastatic sites.

Because of the low incidence and relatively small number of patients, it is difficult to conduct controlled clinical trials to aid in establishing appropriate therapy. The treatment of male breast cancer is based in principle on the treatment of female breast cancer. The modified radical mastectomy has been the mainstay of therapy. The skin and underlying fascia are frequently involved, requiring skin grafting. Adjuvant radiotherapy, hormonal manipulation, and chemotherapy are the main methods of treatment.

With evidence of extensive disease, hormonal manipulation (orchiectomy, aminoglutethimide, or tamoxifen) is indicated unless the disease is life-threatening or aggressive, in which case chemotherapy would be indicated. The response rate to chemotherapy is about 44%.[235]

Orchiectomy appears to remove the source of estrogen and androgen in recurrent male breast cancer and can result in a prompt remission. With recurrent disease, further hormonal manipulation, including tamoxifen, aminoglutethimide, progestin, and DES, may be beneficial. Aminoglutethimide, tamoxifen, and other forms of hormone manipulation are relatively ineffective without orchiectomy. However, Buserelin, or goserelin acetate, effectively reduces testosterone to castration levels and may be an important alternative to men who refuse orchiectomy.

## SYMPTOM MANAGEMENT AND SUPPORTIVE CARE

### Bone Metastasis

Many individuals with breast cancer will, throughout the course of their illness, experience pain due to bony destruction by tumor. The individual may complain of pain over the rib cage, which is aggravated by a cough, or pain in the leg when rising from a sitting position. The person may also report feeling as if his or her back was strained while bending to pick something off the floor. In general, the pain is constant and grows progressively more severe. Pain at night and pain not relieved by rest are especially suspicious. A radiograph of the area may demonstrate lytic bony destruction with sclerotic foci and may be the first sign of metastasis or progression of disease. Bone pain may precede the development of skeletal radiographic changes by several weeks. Destructive bone lesions must be 1.0–1.5 cm in diameter and associated with a 30%–50% loss of bone mineral content before they can be detected with conventional radiography. A bone scan is therefore indicated to determine the extent of disease. A more sensitive method than radiography for detecting metastatic disease, a bone scan should be obtained in all individuals with symptoms suggesting skeletal involvement. However, routine screening in the asymptomatic woman is not indicated since while earlier detection of metastatic disease may occur, the overall five year survival rate will go unchanged.

In addition to radiography, examination of peripheral blood or serum chemistries may indicate metastatic disease. Anemia, thrombocytopenia, leukocytosis, and immature forms of circulating nucleated red blood cells may indicate metastasis to the bone marrow. Elevation of the serum, acid and alkaline phosphatase level may be observed with bone involvement. CA 15-3, a human breast tumor-associated antigen is a sensitive marker in breast cancer metastases and may be used as a screening test for bone metastases.

Increased osteoclastic activity results in dissolution of bone matrix. Dissolution of bone matrix releases the breakdown products of bone into the circulation. The serum calcium level also may be increased and indicates significant bone destruction. Individuals who complain of back pain should have a thorough neurological examination as well as radiographic evaluation of the spine. An MRI may be necessary to determine whether spinal cord compression is present or imminent.

For the individual who has had a long disease-free interval, a bone biopsy may be needed to document metastatic disease in bone. This is particularly true for the person who has no evidence of other metastatic deposits.

In addition to being painful, destructive lesions involving the femur or the humerus are highly susceptible to fracture. If fracture of the diseased bone should occur, severe vascular or neurological damage may ensue, as well as immobility and severe pain. Treatment is aimed at relieving pain, preventing development of pathological fractures, enhancing mobility and function, and thereby improving survival. Irradiation in doses of 30–40 Gy to symptomatic areas often results in effective pain relief and recalcification of bone. If a fracture is pending or has occurred, surgery to stabilize the bone by internal fixation or replacement of the femoral head may be necessary. This is followed by 25–30 Gy of irradiation. This palliative surgery should allow the individual to remain ambulatory, thus decreasing the hazards of immobility such as hypercalcemia, deep vein thrombosis, and pneumonia. Physical therapy is instituted in the postoperative period and after discharge to ensure optimal rehabilitation.

In individuals with widespread bone involvement, radiation is given to areas that are painful and disabling. In cases where one or more fractures are pending, surgery is indicated and offers the least morbidity. The nurse should be particularly aware of the vulnerability of a person with metastatic bone lesions. Simply turning the person in bed can result in fracture of the affected area. The customary ways of repositioning patients in bed are contraindicated for the individual with disease in the clavicle. Lifting beneath the person's arms puts pressure on the clavicle and may cause a fracture. A pull sheet should be used to reposition the person with known disease in the hip, ribs, or vertebrae. At least two people are needed to reposition the patient properly so that correct body alignment is ensured. The nurse also should be aware of the intense pain often associated with a frac-

ture and institute an aggressive pain management protocol.

In the presence of significant osteoclastic activity and bone resorption due to dissolution of bone matrix, destruction of the microarchitecture of the bone leads to increased risk of fracture and hypercalcemia. Bisphosphonates are analogues of pyrophosphate which is a natural inhibitor of bone demineralization. Bisphosphonates (etidronate, clodronate, pamidronate) result in stabilization of bone mineral which inhibits bone mineral dissolution. In an open randomized trial of oral pamidronate reductions in episodes of hypercalcemia, bone pain, fractures, and the need for palliative radiation therapy were demonstrated in patients with metastatic disease.[236] (See chapter 25, Hypercalcemia.)

## Epidural Spinal Cord Compression

Epidural metastases most commonly arise from metastases to the vertebral column. Spinal cord compression constitutes an emergency because of the potential for developing paraplegia. Compression may be secondary to epidural tumor or altered bone alignment due to pathological fracture. The initial signs and symptoms may be extremely subtle. Pain may be referred, radicular, or local and is usually present for several weeks before the development of additional neurological symptoms. Pain is usually worsened by lying supine. The vertebral column is the most frequent site of metastases to bone because cancers of the breast are in communication with the Batson vertebral plexus, a low-pressure valveless venous system that fills when thoracoabdominal pressure is raised (e.g., by maneuvers such as coughing, straining, lifting).[237] Most epidural metastases are situated anterior or anterolateral to the spinal cord, and occur most commonly in the thoracic spine partly due to the pattern of drainage from the Batson plexus and the proximity of the primary tumor to the thoracic vertebrae. Imminent compression should be suspected in individuals who have known bone metastases, progressive back pain associated with weakness, paresthesias, bowel or bladder dysfunction, or gait disturbances. An MRI is performed as soon as the diagnosis is suspected to determine the exact level of the compression and identify other occult extradural lesions.

If the individual is found to have compression with an isolated extradural mass, radiotherapy combined with corticosteroids may produce optimal results and return of ambulation. The person is usually fitted with a brace or maintained on bed rest throughout the course of radiotherapy. Decompression laminectomy may be indicated for individuals who develop spinal cord compression and in whom the diagnosis of epidural metastasis is in doubt, or whose neurological deficits continue to worsen while they receive radiotherapy. However since most lesions appear on the anterior or anterolateral location, the posterior approach of a laminectomy often does not relieve the compression. Surgery is associated with a higher rate of complication compared to radiation and steroid therapy. The degree of recovery of function correlates directly with the length of time the patient experiences symptoms prior to therapeutic interventions. Individuals who are ambulatory before treatment usually remain so; however, only 18%–69% of nonambulatory patients regain the ability to walk.[238,239] The mean survival of patients with breast cancer who develop epidural spinal cord compression is 4–13 months posttreatment. Ambulatory status is the most important factor influencing survival in patients with breast cancer.[238,240]

## Brain Metastasis and Leptomeningeal Carcinomatosis

Brain metastasis occurs in about 30% of individuals diagnosed with breast cancer and is often associated with devastating physical and emotional problems. The most frequent signs and symptoms of intracranial metastasis are headaches, seizures, visual defects, motor weakness, and mental changes. Symptoms generally subside with total brain irradiation and chronic steroids. Leptomeningeal metastases (covering of the brain and spinal cord) occur in approximately 2%–5% of women with metastatic breast cancer.

Most chemotherapeutic agents do not achieve a therapeutic concentration in the brain or cerebral spinal fluid (CSF). This is why the central nervous system may be considered a potential sanctuary for tumor cells. Leptomeningeal metastases occur most likely by hematogenous spread through the capillary structure of the choroid plexus or by rupture of cerebral metastases that subsequently involve the subarachnoid space. Leptomeningeal metastases occur most commonly on the spine with complaints of lower limb weakness and paresthesias. The diagnosis of leptomeningeal metastases is made by lumbar puncture and analysis of the CSF. Headache and changes in mental status are the most common symptoms of cerebral meningeal carcinomatosis. Cranial nerve dysfunction also may be present. Ocular muscle paresis and diplopia are common cerebral symptoms as are facial weakness, hearing loss, and vision loss. The definitive method of diagnosing leptomeningeal metastases is by detection of malignant cells in the CSF and use of MRI to determine the presence of bulky disease.

Treatment generally involves total brain irradiation (24–30 Gy in eight to ten fractions), and radiation to areas of bulky disease in the spine. This is commonly followed by intraventricular-intrathecal chemotherapy given through an Ommaya reservoir. Methotrexate, cytosine arabinoside, steroids, and thiotepa may safely be given intrathecally. Treatment usually includes methotrexate and thiotepa given twice weekly initially, then once a week until there is no evidence of metastatic cells in the CSF. Radiation may enhance neurotoxicity of chemotherapy and is reserved for patients with evidence of brain or cranial nerve compression.

## Chronic Lymphedema

The overall prevalence of lymphedema in breast cancer is 20%. The magnitude of the surgical excision and axillary irradiation are important factors in the development of lymphedema. Scatter radiation from the breast field can be absorbed at the level of the dissected axillary lymphatic tissue and contribute to lymphedema. Lymphedema is most common in women who have had axillary dissection followed by radiation in excess of 46 Gy.[241] With the recent trend toward more conservative surgical resection with minimal axillary dissection for the individual undergoing mastectomy, the problem of massive lymphedema is less common. When axillary dissection is done, there may be transient edema initially; however, 24% of patients may report edema more than three months after surgery.[242]

Beyond the extent of the surgical procedure, the most common causes of chronic or late lymphedema are infection and tumor recurrence, or tumor enlargement in the axilla. Lymphedema occurs because of an increased resistance to venous flow and a disturbance in oncotic pressure that develops in the affected arm. Protein accumulation in the tissues results in increased interstitial colloid oncotic pressure, leading to more fluid accumulation and tissue fibrosis. Anything that increases blood flow to the affected arm contributes to the incidence and degree of lymphedema. Heat, strenuous exercise, lifting objects weighing more than five to ten pounds will contribute to lymphedema. Lymphedema is especially noted in women who have mastectomy and axillary dissection on their dominant side because they use that arm more. The longer the edema persists, the more difficult it is to manage. Lymph is an excellent culture medium, and infections such as cellulitis and lymphangitis can flourish. The individual is instructed to elevate the hand above the elbow and the forearm higher than or level with the heart whenever possible. If edema persists or worsens, the individual is instructed in the use of an elastic stockinette to aid in venous flow. The stockinette is measured precisely to ensure that it fits properly and does not constrict venous flow. The individual wears the stockinette when out of bed. While the individual is sleeping, the arm is positioned to aid venous flow. Therapeutic retrograde massage is also a useful form of conservative treatment. The individual is instructed to care for the skin and fingernails very carefully to avoid infection. Infection enhances lymphedema and slow regeneration of lymphatics. Individuals with chronic lymphedema are also instructed to control their weight and, in some situations, to lose weight.

For the individual who has massive edema without evidence of infection, a program of intermittent compression with an extremity pump may be necessary. The arm usually is treated daily as tolerated for three to four hours in the morning and three to four hours in the afternoon. When the arm reaches 1 + pitting edema, the treatment is discontinued and the arm is measured for a compression support to help maintain the displaced fluid. A compression pump is strictly contraindicated when there is evidence of acute phlebitis, perivascular lymphangitis, or cellulitis.

The lymphedematous arm is cosmetically unattractive and can be functionally useless. The arm can cause tremendous strain on the neck and shoulder muscles, which can result in pain. The woman may have difficulty adjusting her wardrobe to provide for the increasing size of her arm. Furthermore, the edematous arm can rarely be concealed adequately and can renew feelings of disfigurement and depression associated with the mastectomy that the woman may have resolved before the lymphedema occurred. When function of the arm is affected, the woman may not be able to work or perform activities of daily living. These limitations may not have been imposed on the woman following her mastectomy. Efforts should be made to discuss the goals and rationale of management with the woman, thereby enlisting her cooperation and participation in the planned treatment regimen.[243]

# PREGNANCY AND BREAST CANCER

## Pregnancy and the Woman with Curable Breast Cancer

The fact that women are delaying parenting into their mid-30s, the increasing incidence of cancer in premenopausal women, early detection measures, and successful treatment outcome make the issue of pregnancy and breast cancer a particularly important topic. Having a diagnosis of breast cancer is frightening and makes one poignantly aware of mortality and the experiences one truly wants in life before dying. Parenting is something some women have an intense desire to experience. Approximately 25% of all breast cancer patients will develop their disease during their childbearing years.[244] Approximately 7% of premenopausal women have one or more pregnancies after treatment for breast cancer, with 70% of these occurring within the first five years after treatment.[244]

The most important considerations in the potential effect of pregnancy in a woman with a history of breast cancer are whether or not the hormonal changes from pregnancy might stimulate growth of occult disease, the risk for genetic alterations in offspring, the woman's overall risk for recurrent breast cancer, and the risk of a second primary breast cancer.

While it is true that hormone changes of pregnancy may potentially influence the behavior of a breast cancer, there are no data to suggest that pregnancy subsequent to successful breast cancer treatment worsens a woman's prognosis.[245,246] In fact, there is some evidence that women who become pregnant subsequent to breast cancer have a better survival than women who do not become preg-

nant.[247] In women who have node-negative disease, it is unreasonable and scientifically unfounded to encourage a delay of two years before attempting pregnancy. These women may gain nothing but lost time by waiting. Even early-stage patients who experience a local recurrence following breast conservation therapy remain curable by mastectomy. On the other hand, for patients at high risk for recurrence, there is no time span beyond which their risk lessens, although most women who recur do so within two years of treatment.

Counseling the woman who wishes to become pregnant following successful breast therapy involves, above all else, attention to what is known concerning prognosis as it relates to pregnancy and the individual woman's prognosis. The decision must be reinforced as hers alone. The best service the professional can offer is to help the patient and her family understand the uncertainties and risks involved.

## Pregnancy and Breast Cancer as a Simultaneous Event

The literature reports the incidence of concurrent pregnancy or lactation and breast cancer to be 0.2%–3.8%.[247] The diagnosis of breast cancer during pregnancy occurs in about 10% of eligible patients. This number is likely to rise as many women delay pregnancy into their late 30s and early 40s, ages when breast cancer is more common.

The prognosis of women diagnosed with breast cancer during pregnancy has generally been poor, not necessarily because of excessive estrogen stimulation but because pregnancy-associated breast cancer is more often diagnosed at a more advanced stage. When pregnancy-associated breast cancer patients are evaluated with nonpregnant controls, the pregnancy-associated group has an equivalent survival rate.

Although the techniques of early detection and diagnosis in a pregnant patient can be difficult to perform because of the physiological changes in the breast, they are no less essential. Breast examinations should be performed as a regular part of prenatal care, and all women should be encouraged to practice BSE throughout the duration of the pregnancy. Any suspicious lump should receive a prompt workup as previously outlined. The effectiveness of mammography may be compromised by the increased density of the breast and, if it is performed, the fetus should be shielded. The risk to the fetus in the event a breast biopsy is needed is minimal.

The treatment of breast cancer in this population of women is determined by the extent of the disease present and the term of pregnancy or lactation. In general, the same treatment principles apply. However the metastatic workup is usually curtailed somewhat to avoid radiation exposure to the fetus. A bone scan would therefore be delayed until after delivery. Magnetic resonance imaging (MRI) has been used and appears to be safe for the fetus.[248] Chest x-ray with shielding of the fetus is safe especially during the third trimester. Early-stage disease should be surgically treated with little risk to the fetus. Radiation therapy is not recommended due to potential hazards to the fetus. Chemotherapy, if indicated, should not be administered during the first trimester, but can be more safely used in the second and third. Antimetabolites, specifically folic acid antagonists, when given during the first trimester, have consistently been shown to be teratogenic. As exposure to a drug increases over time, the frequency and severity of the teratogenic effects also increase.[247] There is also a threshold effect, meaning that below a certain dose the incidence of death, malformation, growth retardation, or functional deficit is not greater than controls. Research concerning the use of antiemetics in pregnancy are understandably limited. Metaclopramide has been compared with prochlorperazine or a placebo to treat hyperemesis of pregnancy. Metaclopramide was somewhat superior to prochlorperazine and placebo. Ondansetron is associated with minimal toxicities, and while there are no human data, reproductive studies have been done in rats with no evidence of harm to the fetus. Overall, it appears that antiemetics cause minimal toxicity.[249]

A therapeutic abortion during the first trimester is not necessary, nor has it been found to be therapeutically beneficial. A more advanced disease stage needs effective, urgent palliation and may indicate the need for termination of an early pregnancy to promptly begin treatment for the breast cancer. If the diagnosis is made in the third trimester, local therapy is carried out and adjuvant therapy is instituted once the child is born. When chemotherapy is deemed crucial because of more aggressive disease, cesarean section at the earliest opportunity may be recommended. There is no evidence that chemotherapy given in the latter months of pregnancy will harm the fetus. However, while infants may be described as phenotypically normal, subtle impairments in growth and development may go unnoticed, increasing the need for these children to be followed over time.[250,251]

## CONTINUITY OF CARE

### Support Systems

Women with breast cancer may find a need for different support systems as they maneuver through the different phases of their diagnosis, treatment, and survival. Initially, the prediagnosis worry is often shared with friends and family who then continue to provide ongoing support through the diagnosis, treatment, and survivorship. Many people find support through their faith and the people with whom they worship. Health professionals, often called upon to demonstrate support and encouragement during emotionally difficult times, may or may not be always up to the task. Many people have found comfort, validation, and information by joining a support group. Support groups are recognized as valuable sources of hope, encouragement, and education for the individual with breast cancer as well as other chronic diseases.[202]

Although the prognosis for breast cancer is constantly improving, the psychological impact of the disease may result in feelings of anxiety, depression, suicidal ideation, insomnia, and fear of recurrence and death which directly impacts sexuality and ability to function.[252–254] Seeking out and participating in a support group often helps to reduce and alleviate some of these feelings of loss of control and vulnerability.

Most cancer support groups rely on mutual aid or interdependence to attain a common goal, and individual participation is usually grounded in the needs of the individual and what goals she hopes to accomplish. Cella and Yellen[253] listed basic needs most people are seeking. These are hope, honesty, emotional freedom, and the ability to discuss death and dying. Cella and Yellen also recognize retaining each person's social identity, the importance of providing education, emotional, and environmental support, and a social connection as commonly shared goals of most support groups.

Many successful groups such as Alcoholics Anonymous are archetypical of people with specific needs who come together to help one another. The common bond associated with these groups is providing a forum where essential needs can be addressed which include assistance, personal insights, support, and belonging. Additionally, these groups may have needs and goals that vary according to the organizational components. Some organizations, such as Y-ME, try to offer groups specific to the organizational make up and/or type of surgery or current disease status. Spouses find comfort and freedom to ask questions and hear the experiences of other men. Spanish-speaking women are able to be more expressive and forthcoming speaking in their native language. Women who have been treated with mastectomy have concerns and questions that differ from a woman who has had breast preservation. Women with metastatic disease have needs and issues beyond those who are disease-free.

Another recent advance in information and support exists through on-line web pages. Many computers are equipped with a modem and software allowing access to the Internet and World Wide Web. This accessibility allows women who are isolated by geographic or physical constraints to communicate with sources on an international basis. Information is provided by a wide spectrum of health care workers as well as patients and families. The sharing of stories and experiences creates a helpful and inspiring chronicle and many have found posing a question will often initiate a multitude of responses.

Examples of these on-line services are Avon's Breast Cancer Awareness Crusade at http://www.pmedia.com/avon.html, National Cancer Information Service at http://wwicicc.nci.nih.gov/, and GO CANCER on CompuServe. For more information on different web sites, call CompuServe at (800) 848-8199 or America On Line at (800) 827-6364. There is an Internet discussion line for children and young adults who have a friend or relative with cancer. The address is CaringKids-Request@-sjuvm.stjohns.edu. In addition, one can access journal searches through medical libraries that contain Medline and Cancerlit or by purchasing the software. A call to a local medical library will provide the information needed to locate the software.

## Nursing Challenges

Possibly the greatest challenge in the care of the woman with breast cancer is to recognize rehabilitation goals throughout the trajectory or natural history of the disease as the individual woman experiences it. When the woman is first diagnosed with breast cancer her initial fear of the disease is eased with the task of formulating a plan of care by consulting with a team of experts including a surgeon, plastic surgeon, medical oncologist, radiation oncologist, and clinical nurse specialist. When managed through the auspices of a comprehensive breast center she and her family come to value the combined efforts of the team assembled to help manage her disease. With a thorough explanation of the disease and treatment plan, she may choose to proceed or to seek other opinions before making her decision. The task of seeking other opinions for treatment is worthwhile because she learns more about her disease and can feel most confident in her decision once she has had time to evaluate all options. This time may be particularly stressful since often she will have a number of treatment options and feel she is not prepared to choose. The nurse can be particularly helpful at this time to clarify the differences between the various approaches to management, why such differences exist, and essentially give the woman and her family the opportunity to explore all options including appropriate research studies. Throughout this time the nurse concentrates on helping the woman find information and make contact with individuals who will help her make her own decision regarding treatment.

Once the plan of care is decided, the nurse formulates rehabilitation goals which are accomplished through further education regarding what the woman can expect and by teaching the woman self-care measures. Initially these goals will include postoperative care of the wound and appropriate exercises to regain optimal function of the arm and shoulder. Such instructions are written with personalized directions regarding how to perform the exercises and minimize pain through adequate use of analgesics. Some women will benefit from the assistance of a physical therapist trained specifically in the rehabilitation of the woman who has had a mastectomy. Often women have no difficulty performing their exercises, however some are reluctant to exercise to the point of discomfort and need additional support and encouragement. Others will exercise more than is recommended and experience pain and arm swelling in the postoperative period. Women need frequent follow-up in the post-

operative period to be certain they are progressing to the best of their abilities.

In the initial six weeks following mastectomy the woman will be instructed not to wear a prosthesis. Instead she usually wears a soft cotton form in her bra which will not irritate the incision. During this time she can be fitted for a prosthesis and explore the type she prefers. Women need referrals to stores that specialize in these garments and breast forms. Nurses need to keep up-to-date records on the specialty stores since surgeons rarely will address this issue with their patients. The American Cancer Society's Look Good Feel Better program is especially helpful to these women to help them look and feel their best. The Y-ME organization is another invaluable resource for women experiencing breast cancer and looking for advice concerning prostheses and the manner in which others have sought out and utilized resources.

When chemotherapy is incorporated into the treatment plan the nurse instructs the patient and family regarding the side effects of chemotherapy and management strategies. Depending on the treatment plan this would include prevention and management of nausea and vomiting, ways to minimize fatigue, managing hair loss, oral hygiene, and prevention of infection. Eventually other problems may arise including difficulty sleeping, complaints of fatigue and lack of energy, as well as menopausal symptoms. The nurse maintains close contact with the woman usually through phone contact since most if not all patients are treated on an outpatient basis. The primary nursing model is critically important to the care of the woman with breast cancer since problems arise months later and with consistent nursing care and a close and trusting relationship the woman is less reluctant to seek assistance for whatever problem she is experiencing.

The primary goal for the woman with localized breast cancer is to finish therapy and resume her life goals and re-establish the routines she enjoyed prior to her illness. For most women this process takes about a year at which time she feels more energetic with fewer sleepless nights. Often the hair has grown back and she feels more like herself. She may begin to inquire about breast reconstruction if she has not already done so. Most women should realize this is major surgery and will again require an extended time period for recovery. It is often associated with a six-month period of fatigue and complaints of exhaustion. However, this is normal and should not in any way discourage a woman from having the reconstructive procedures done.

While most women fear recurrence of their disease, seeing the physician (surgeon and/or medical oncologist) every three months for the first year and every six months for two years and yearly after that usually is frequent enough to be reassuring. Some will prefer to be seen at more frequent intervals. If the cancer does recur it is devastating. The disappointment and fears are often more intense than with her initial diagnosis. She feels betrayed by everyone, especially her own body. Most women have worked very hard to be well and comply with all their doctors and nurses recommend, so when the disease comes back the woman feels she has little control and begins initially to lose hope in her ability to once again be courageous. At this time many will need the counsel of a psycho-oncologist trained specifically in the care of the cancer patient. The recurrence is as devastating to the family as it is to the woman and they too will need to talk about their fears as therapy is once again discussed. Other supports include the woman's religious organization and an appropriate patient support group.

Goals for the woman who has recurring cancer center on helping her and her family understand the treatment goals and recognize how the treatment is helping. Remaining hopeful and supportive throughout with emphasis on the success of therapy and numerous options available is reassuring. Few women will need home care at this time since most recurrences are not debilitating unless the individual is elderly and the disease recurs in the brain or liver. When the disease begins to effect a woman's ability to perform activities of daily living, the need for home care should be introduced to determine the woman's options for insurance coverage. The family needs to be encouraged to identify their needs and whether or not they need assistance in her care on a daily basis or two or three times per week. Establishing a relationship with a nursing service that also has a hospice component is worthwhile because there is a smooth transition when hospice is deemed appropriate. Hospice should be introduced as an option for care once treatment is felt to be strictly palliative and the woman is thought to have less than six months to live.

Bereavement counselling is a component of hospice care and usually continues for at least a year. The nurse also is seen as a pivotal person capable of helping the family through the grieving process and the months to follow.

## REFERENCES

1. Miller BA, Feuer EJ, Hankey BF: Recent incidence trends for breast cancer in women and relevance of early detection: An update. *CA: Cancer J Clin* 43:27–41, 1993
2. Parker SL, Tong T, Bolden, et al: Cancer statistics. *CA: Cancer J Clin* 46:5–28, 1996
3. Conference Statement: Treatment of Early Stage Breast Cancer. Bethesda, MD, National Institutes of Health, 1990
4. Kirkman-Liff B, Kronenfeld J: Access to cancer screening devices for women. *Am J Public Health* 82:733–735, 1992
5. Shimkin MB: Cancer of the breast. *JAMA* 183:358, 1963
6. American Cancer Society: *Cancer Facts and Figures—1996.* Atlanta, American Cancer Society, 1996
7. Kelsey JL, Gammon MD: The epidemiology of breast cancer. *CA: Cancer J Clin* 41:146–165, 1991
8. Fisher B: Biology and clinical considerations regarding the use of surgery and chemotherapy in treatment of primary breast cancer. *Cancer* 40:574–587, 1977
9. Henderson BE, Bernstein L: Endogenous and exogenous hormonal factors, in Harris JR, Lippman ME, Morrow M. and Hellman S: (eds): *Diseases of the Breast.* Philadelphia, Lippincot-Raven, 1996, pp 185–200
10. Hulka BS, Liu ET, Lininger RA: Steroid hormones and the risk of breast cancer. *Cancer* 74:1111–1124, 1994 (suppl 3)
11. Zumoff B: Hormone profiles in women with breast cancer. *Obstet Gynecol Clin North Am* 21:751–772, 1994
12. Potten CS, Watson RJ, Williams GT: The effect of age and menstrual cycle upon proliferative activity of the normal human breast. *Br J Cancer* 58:163–170, 1988
13. Bernstein L, Ross RK: Endogenous hormones and breast cancer risk. *Epidemiol Rev* 15:48–65, 1993
14. Bruzzi P, Negri E, LaVecchia C, et al: Short term increase in risk of breast cancer after full term pregnancy. *Br J Med* 297:1096–1098, 1988
15. Yang CP, Weiss NS, Band PR, et al: History of lactation and breast cancer risk. *AM J Epidemiol* 138:1050–1056, 1993
16. Yoo KY, Tajima K, Karoishi T, et al: Independent effect of lactation against breast cancer: A case-control study in Japan. *AM J Epidemiol* 135:726–733, 1992
17. Land CE, Hayakawa N, Machado SG: A case-control interview study of breast cancer among Japanese A-bomb survivors. II. Interactions with radiation dose. *Cancer Causes Control* 5:167–176, 1994
18. Newcomb PA, Stover BE, Longnecker MP, et al: Lactation and a reduced risk of premenopausal breast cancer. *N Engl J Med* 330:81–87, 1994
19. Petitti DB: Animal models of sex steroid hormones and mammary cancer: Lessons for understanding studies in humans, in Institute of Medicine, Division of Health Promotion and Disease Prevention: *Oral Contraceptives and Breast Cancer.* Washington, DC, National Academy Press, 1991, pp 152–164
20. Holmberg L, Lund E, Bergstrom R, et al: Oral contraceptives and prognosis in breast cancer: Effects of duration, latency, frequency, age at first use and relation to parity and body mass index in young women with breast cancer. *Eur J Cancer* 30A:351–354, 1994
21. Rookus MA, vanLeeuwen FE: Oral contraceptives and risk of breast cancer in women aged 20–54 years. *Lancet* 344:844–851, 1994
22. Lipnick RJ, Buring JE, Hennekens CH, et al: Oral contraceptives and breast cancer. *JAMA* 255:58–61, 1986
23. LaVecchia C, Negri E, Francaschi S, et al: Oral contraceptives and breast cancer, a cooperative Italian Study. *Int J Cancer* 60:163–167, 1995
24. Palmer JR, Rosenberg L, Rao RS, et al: Oral contraceptive use and breast cancer risk among African-American women. *Cancer Causes and Control* 6:221–231, 1995
25. Mayberry RM: Age specific patterns of association between breast cancer and risk factors in black women, ages 20 to 39 and 40 to 54. *Ann Epidemiol* 4:205–213, 1994
26. Schlesselman JJ: Net effect of oral contraceptive use on the risk of cancer in women in the U.S. *Obstet Gynecol* 85:793–801, 1995
27. Bergkvist L, Adami HO, Persson I, et al: The risk of breast cancer after estrogen and estrogen-progestin replacement. *N Engl J Med* 321:293–297, 1989
28. Dupont WD, Page DL, Rogers LW: Influence of exogenous estrogens, proliferative breast disease and other variables on breast cancer risk. *Cancer* 63:948–957, 1989
29. Mills PK, Beeson L, Phillips RL, et al: Prospective study of exogenous hormone use and breast cancer in Seventh Day Adventists. *Cancer* 64:591–597, 1989
30. Colditz GA, Egan KM, Stampfer MJ: Hormone replace-

ment therapy and risk of breast cancer: Results from epidemiologic studies. *Am J Obstet Gynecol* 168:1473–1480, 1993

31. Maguire PJ: Estrogen replacement therapy and breast cancer. *J Reprod Med* 38:183–185, 1993

32. Zumoff B: Biological and endocrinological insights into the possible breast cancer risk from menopausal estrogen replacement therapy. *Steroids* 58:196–204, 1993

33. Wilklund I, Holst J, Kurlberg, et al: A new methodological approach to the evaluation of quality of life in postmenopausal women. *Maturitas* 14:211–224, 1992

34. Schover LR: Sexuality and body image in younger women with breast cancer. *Monogr Natl Cancer Inst* 16:177–182, 1994

35. Theriault RL, Sellin RV: A clinical dilemma: Estrogen replacement therapy in postmenopausal women with a background of primary breast cancer. *Ann Oncol* 2:209–217, 1991

36. Davidson J: The need for a randomized trial of hormone replacement therapy in women with breast cancer. *Med J Aust* 157:429, 1991

37. Henderson IC: Risk factors for development of breast cancer. *Cancer* 71:2127–2140, 1993 (suppl)

38. Marchant DJ: Estrogen replacement therapy after breast cancer. *Cancer* 71:2169–2176, 1993

39. Vasselopoulou-Sellin R, Theriault RL: Randomized prospective trial of estrogen-replacement therapy in women with a history of breast cancer. *Monogr Natl Cancer Inst* 16:153–159, 1994

40. Sattin RW, Rubin GL, Webster L, et al: Family history and the risk of breast cancer. *JAMA* 253:1908–1913, 1985

41. Cobleigh MA, Berris RF, Bush T, et al: Estrogen replacement therapy in breast cancer survivors. *JAMA* 272:540–545, 1994

42. Bernstein JL, Thompson WD, Risch N, et al: The genetic epidemiology of secondary breast cancer. *Am J Epidemiol* 136:937–948, 1992

43. Gail MH, Brinton LA, Byar DP, et al: Projecting individualized probabilities of developing breast cancer for white females who are being examined annually. *J Natl Cancer Inst* 81:1879–1886, 1989

44. Kelsey JL, Horn-Ross PL: Breast cancer: Magnitude of the problem and descriptive epidemiology. *Epidemiol Rev* 15:7–16, 1993

45. Kelsey JL, Whittemore AS: Epidemiology and primary prevention of cancers of the breast, endometrium and ovary: a brief overview. *Ann Epidemiol* 4:89–95, 1994

46. Claus EB, Risch N, Thompson WD: Autosomal dominant inheritance of early-onset breast cancer: Implications for risk prediction. *Cancer* 73:643–651, 1994

47. Roseman DL, Straus AK, Shorey W: A positive family history of breast cancer: Does its effect diminish with age? *Arch Intern Med* 150:191–194, 1990

48. King MC, Rowell S, Love SM: Inherited breast and ovarian cancer. What are the risks? What are the choices? *JAMA* 269:1975–1980, 1993

49. Mikki V, Swensen J, Slattuck-Eidens D, et al: A strong candidate for the breast and ovarian cancer susceptibility gene *BRCA1. Science* 266:66–71, 1994

50. Futreal PA, Quingyron L, Shattuck-Eidens D, et al: *BRCA1* mutations in primary breast and ovarian carcinomas. *Science* 266:120–122, 1994

51. Weber B: Genetic testing for breast cancer. *Sci Am* 3:12–21, 1996

52. Wooster R, Neuhauser SL, Mangion J, et al: Localization of breast cancer susceptibility gene (*BRCA2*) to chromosome 13q 12–13. *Science* 265:2088–2090, 1994

53. Thorlacius S, Tryggvadottir L, Olafdottir G, et al: Linkage to *BRCA2* in hereditary male breast cancer. *Lancet* 346:544–545, 1995

54. Harris C, Holstein M: Clinical implications of the *p53* tumor supression gene. *N Engl J Med* 329:1318–1327, 1993

55. Saitoh S, Gunningham J, Devries EMG, et al: *p53* gene mutations in breast cancer in midwestern U.S. women: Null as well a missense-type mutations are associated with poor prognosis. *Oncogene* 9:2869–2875, 1994

56. Aguilar F, Harris C, Sun T, et al. Geographic variation of *p53* mutational profile in non-malignant human liver. *Science* 264:1317–1319, 1994

57. Nees M, Homann N, Sicher H, et al: Expression of mutated *p53* occurs in tumor-distant epithelia of head and neck cancer patients. A possible molecular basis for development of multiple tumors. *Cancer Res* 53:4189–4196, 1993

58. Berstein JL, Thompson WD, Risch N, et al: Risk factors predicting the incidence of second primary breast cancer among women diagnosed with a first primary breast cancer. *Am J Epidemiol* 136:925–936, 1992

59. Berstein JL: Risk factors predicting the incidence of a second primary breast cancer. *Dis Abstract Int* 54:195, 1993

60. Wilett WC, Hunter DJ: Prospective studies of diet and breast cancer. *Cancer* 74:1085–1089, 1994 (suppl)

61. Rose D: Introduction to the proceedings of a workshop on new developments on dietary fat and fiber in carcinogenesis. *Prev Med* 16:449–450, 1987

62. Pinn VW: The role of the NIH's Office of Research on women's health. *Acad Med* 69:698–702, 1994

63. Howe GR: Dietary fat and breast cancer risk: An epidemiologic perspective. *Cancer* 74:1078–1084, 1994 (suppl 3)

64. Cummings NB: Women's health and nutritional research: U.S. governmental concerns. *J Am Coll Nutr* 12:329–336, 1993

65. Deslypere JP: Obesity and cancer: *Metabolism*: 44:24–27, 1995 (suppl 3)

66. Stoll BA: Timing of weight gain in relation to breast cancer risk. *Ann Oncol* 6:245–248, 1995

67. Kumar NB, Aziz NM, Schapira DV, et al: Weight at age 30 and breast cancer risk. *Proc Am Soc Clin Oncol* 13:A469, 1994

68. Morabia A, Wynder EL: Epidemiology and natural history of breast cancer. *Surg Clin North Am* 70:739–752, 1990

69. Longnecker MP: Alcoholic beverage consumption in relation to risk of breast cancer: Meta-analysis and review. *Cancer Causes Control* 5:73–82, 1994

70. Giovannucci E, Stampfer MJ, Colditz GA, et al: Recall and selection bias in reporting past alcohol consumption among breast cancer cases. *Cancer Causes Control* 4:441–448, 1993

71. Plant ML: Alcohol and breast cancer: A review. *Int J Addict* 27:107–128, 1992

72. John EM, Kelsey J: Radiation and other environmental exposures and breast cancer. *Epidemiol Rev* 15:157–162, 1993

73. Hancock SL, Tucker MA, Hoppe RT: Breast cancer after treatment of Hodgkin's disease. *J Natl Cancer Inst* 85:25–31, 1993

74. Page DL, Dupont WD: Anatomic markers of human malignancy and risk of breast cancer. *Cancer* 66:1326–1335, 1990

75. Page DL, Dupont WD: Premalignant conditions and mark-

ers of elevated risk in the breast and their management. *Surg Clin North Am* 70:831–850, 1990

76. Page DL, Dupont WD: Anatomic indicators (histologic and cytologic) of increased breast cancer risk. *Breast Cancer Res Treat* 28:157–166, 1993

77. Dupont WD, Parl FF, Hartman WH, et al: Breast cancer risk associated with proliferative breast disease and atypical hyperplasia. *Cancer* 71:1258–1265, 1993

78. Page DL, Dupont WD: Indicators of increased breast cancer risk in humans. *J Cell Biochem* 16G:175–182, 1992

79. Morrow M, Schmitt JS: Lobular carcinoma in situ, in Harris J, Lippman ME, Morrow M, Hellman S (eds): *Diseases of the Breast*. Philadelphia, Lippincott-Raven, 1996, pp 369–373

80. Bilimoria MM, Murrow M: The woman at increased risk for breast cancer: Evaluation and management strategies. *CA: Cancer J Clin* 45:263–278, 1995

81. Kelloff GJ, Johnson JR, Crowell JA, et al: Approaches to development and marketing approval of drugs that prevent cancer. *Cancer Epidemiol Biomarkers Prev* 4:1–10, 1995

82. Love RR: Prevention of breast cancer in premenopausal women. *Monog Natl Cancer Inst* 16:L61–65, 1994

83. Kelloff GJ, Boone CW, Steele VE, et al: Mechanistic considerations in chemopreventive drug development. *J Cell Biochem* 20:1–24, 1994 (suppl)

84. Lippman SM, Benner SE, Hong WK: Chemopreventive strategies for the control of cancer. *Cancer* 72:984–990, 1993 (suppl 3)

85. Lippman SM, Benner SE, Hong WK: Cancer chemoprevention. *J Clin Oncol* 12:851–873, 1994

86. Cole MP, Jones CT, Todd ID: The new anti-estrogenic agent in late breast cancer: An early clinical approach of ICI 46474. *Br J Cancer* 25:27–275, 1971

87. Sawka CA, Pritchard KI, Paterson HG, et al: Role and mechanism of action of tamoxifen in premenopausal women with metastatic breast carcinoma. *Cancer Res* 46:3152–3156, 1986

88. Fisher B, Constantino J, Redmond C, et al: A randomized clinical trial evaluating tamoxifen in the treatment of patients with node-negative breast cancer who have estrogen-receptor positive tumors. *N Engl J Med* 320:479–484, 1989

89. Cummings JF, Gray R, Tormey DC, et al: Adjuvant tamoxifen versus placebo in elderly women with node-positive breast cancer: Long term follow-up and causes of death. *J Clin Oncol* 11:29–35, 1993

90. NSABP Protocol P-1: *A Clinical Trial to Determine the Worth of Tamoxifen for Preventing Breast Cancer*. Pittsburgh, National Surgical Adjuvant Breast and Bowel Project, 1992

91. Jaiyesimi IA, Buzdar AU, Decker DA, et al: Use of tamoxifen for breast cancer: Twenty-eight years later. *J Clin Oncol* 13:513–529, 1995

92. Knabbe C, Lippman ME, Wakefield LM: Evidence that transforming growth factor-β is a hormonally regulated negative growth factor in human breast cancer cells. *Cell* 48:417–428, 1987

93. Jordan VC, Fritz NF, Tormey DC: Long-term adjuvant therapy with tamoxifen: Effects on sex hormone binding globulin and antithrombin III. *Cancer Res* 47:4517–4519, 1987

94. Vogel VG: Prevention of breast cancer: Clinical considerations in breast cancer prevention, in Harris JR, Lippman MC, Morrow M, Hellman S (eds): *Diseases of the Breast*. Philadelphia, Lippincott-Raven, 1996, pp 341–354

95. Vogel VG: High-risk populations as targets for breast cancer prevention trials. *Prev Med* 20:88–100, 1991

96. Paffenbarger RS Jr, Lee I-M, Wing AL: The influence of physical activity on the incidence of site specific cancers in college alumni, in Jacobs MM (ed): *Exercise, calories, fat and cancer*. New York, Plenum, 1992

97. Dogan JF, Brown C, Barrett M, et al: Physical activity and the risk of breast disease in the Framingham Heart Study. *Am J Epidemiol* 139:662–669, 1994

98. Bernstein L, Henderson BE, Hanisch R, et al: Physical exercise and reduced risk of breast cancer in young women. *J Natl Cancer Inst* 86:1403–1408, 1994

99. Mittendorf R, Longnecker MP, Newcomb PA, et al: Strenuous exercises in young adulthood and risk of breast cancer. *Cancer Causes Control* 6:347–353, 1995

100. Ziegler LD, Kroll SS: Primary breast cancer after prophylactic mastectomy. *Am J Clin Oncol* 14:151, 1991

101. Berger K, Bostnick JB: Preventive mastectomy for the woman at risk, in Berger K, Bostwick JL (eds): *A Woman's Decision: Breast Care Treatment and Reconstruction* (ed 4). St Louis, Quality Medical Publishing, 1994, pp 288–298

102. Champion VL: Results of a nurse-delivered intervention on proficiency and nodule detection with breast self-examination. *Oncol Nurs Forum* 22:819–824, 1995

103. Lierman LM, Young HM, Powell-Cope G, et al: Using social support to promote breast self-examination performance. *Oncol Nurs Forum* 21:1051–1056, 1994

104. Grady KE: Efficacy of breast self-examination. *J Gerontol* 47:69–74, 1992

105. Mettlin C, Smart CR: Breast cancer detection guidelines for women 40–49 years. Rationale for the American Cancer Society reaffirmation of recommendations. *CA: Cancer J Clin* 44:248–255, 1994

106. Volkers N: NCI replaces guidelines with statement of evidence. *J Natl Cancer Inst* 86:14–15, 1994

107. Mettlin C: Encouraging trends in breast cancer incidence. *Cancer* 72:637–638, 1993

108. Williams SM, Kaplan PA, Petersen JC, et al: Mammography in women under age 30: Is there clinical benefit? *Radiology* 161:49–51, 1986

109. Smart CR, Hartmann WH, Beahrs OH, et al: Insights into breast screening of younger women: Evidence of the 14 year follow-up of breast cancer detection demonstration project. *Cancer* 72:1449–1456, 1993

110. Tabar L, Duffy SW, Barhenne LW: New Swedish breast cancer detection results for women 40–49. *Cancer* 72:1437–1448, 1993

111. Bassett LW, Manjikian V, Gold RH: Mammography and breast cancer screening. *Surg Clin North Am* 70:775–800, 1990

112. Kopans DB: Breast cancer screening: Women 40–49 years of age. *PPO Updates* 8:1–11, 1994

113. Newcomb PA, Lantz PM: Recent trials in breast cancer incidence, mortality and mammography. *Breast Cancer Res Treat* 28:97–106, 1993

114. Champion VL: Strategies to increase mammography utilization. *Med Care* 32:118–129, 1994

115. Rutter DR, Calnan M, Vaile MSB, et al: Discomfort and pain during mammography: Description, predictor and prevention. *Br Med J* 305:443–445, 1992

116. Nielsen B, Miaskowski C, Dibble SL: Pain with mammography: Fact or fiction? *Oncol Nurs Forum* 20:639–642, 1992

117. Peart O: Helping women overcome the fear of mammography. *Radiol Technol* 66:34–38, 1994

118. Peters JA, Stopfer JE: Role of the genetic counselor in familial cancer. *Oncology* 10:159–166, 175, 1996

119. Lynch HT: Genetic counseling in cancer: a status report—part 2. *Oncology,* 10:131–134, 1996

120. Statement of the American Society of Clinical Oncology: *Genetic Listing for Cancer Susceptibility.* Philadelphia, American Society of Clinical Oncology, 1996

121. Durant JR: How to organize a multidisciplinary clinic for the management of breast cancer. *Surg Clin North Am* 70: 977–983, 1990

122. Gasparini G, Harris AL: Clinical importance of the determination of tumor angiogenesis in breast carcinoma much more than new prognostic tool. *J Clin Oncol* 12:765–782, 1995

123. Hayes DF: Angiogenesis and breast cancer. *Hematol Oncol* 8:51–69, 1994

124. Dodd GD: American Cancer Society Guidelines from Past to Present. *Cancer* 72:1429–1432, 1993

125. Garms R: Mammography quality standards act of 1992. *J Oncol Management* 3:64–65, 1994

126. Adler DD, Wahl RL: New methods for imaging the breast: techniques, findings, potential. *Am J Radiol* 164: 19–30, 1995

127. Schmidt RA, Nishikawa RM: Clinical use of digital mammography: The present and the prospects. *J Digit Imaging* 81:74–79, 1995 (suppl)

128. Adler DD, Wahl RL: New methods for breast cancer imaging, in Harris JR, Lippman ME, Murrow M, Hellman S (eds): *Diseases of the Breast.* Philadelphia, Lippincott-Raven, 1996, pp 84–98

129. Venta LA, Dudiak CM, Salomon CG, et al: Sonographic evaluation of the breast. *Radiographics* 12:29–50, 1994

130. Mendelson EB: Interventional breast ultrasonography, in Dershaw DD (ed): *Interventional Breast Procedures.* New York, Churchill-Livingston, 1996, pp 129–153

131. Orel SG, Schnall MD, Powell CM, et al: Staging of suspected breast cancer: Effect of MRI imaging and MR-guided biopsy. *Radiology* 196:16–28, 1995

132. Harms SE, Flamig DP, Evans WP, et al: MR imaging of the breast current status and future potential. *Am J Radiol* 163: 1039–1047, 1994

133. Crowe, Adler LP, Shenk RR, et al: Positron emission tomography and breast masses: Comparison with clinical mammographic and pathologic findings. *Am J Radiol:* 132–140, 1994

134. Kotz D: Scintimammography: Magic bullet or false promise? *J Nucl Med* (Newsline) 36:15–20, 1995.

135. Stuntz ME, Khalkhali I, Moss JF, et al: Breast imaging techniques and their application in breast disease. *Breast J* 1:285–294, 1996

136. Waxman A, Nagaraj N, Ashok G, et al: Sensitivity and specificity of TC-99m meltoxy isobutal isonitrile (MIBI) in the evaluation of primary carcinoma of the breast: Comparison of palpable and non-palpable lesions with mammography. *J Nucl Med* 35:22, 1994 (abstr)

137. Khalkhali I, Cutrone J, Mena I, et al: Scintimammography (SSM) versus mammography: The complementary role of TC-99 sestamibi prone breast imaging for the diagnosis of breast carcinoma. *Radiology* 196:421–426, 1995

138. Picolo S, Lastoria S, Mainolfi C, et al: Role of TC-99M. MDP scintigraphy in the diagnosis of primary breast cancer. *J Nucl Med* 35:22, 1994 (abstr)

139. Dowlatshahi K, Danaher M, Snider H, et al: Diagnosis of non-palpable lesions by stereotaxic needle biopsy and interval mammography. *Proc Am Soc Clin Oncol* 12:A118, 1993

140. Silen W, Matory E, Love S (eds): *Atlas of Techniques in Breast Surgery.* Philadelphia, Lippincott-Raven, 1996

141. Lieberman L: Stereotaxic biopsy techniques, in Dershaw DD (ed): *Interventional Breast Procedures.* New York, Churchill-Livingstone, 1996, pp 129–153

142. Gisvold JJ, Goellner JR, Grant CS, et al: Breast biopsy: A comparative study of stereotaxically-guided core and excisional technique. *Am J Radiol* 162:815–820, 1994

143. Mikhael RA, Nathan RC, Weiss M, et al: Stereotactic core needle biopsy of mammographic breast lesions as a viable alternative to surgical biopsy. *Ann Surg Oncol* 1:363–367, 1994

144. Lieberman L, Fahs MC, Dershaw DD, et al: Impact of stereotactic core breast biopsy on cost of diagnosis. *Radiology* 195:633–637, 1995

145. Dershaw DD: Needle localization for breast biopsy, in Dershaw DD (ed): *Interventional Breast Procedures.* New York, Churchill-Livingstone, 1996, pp 129–153

146. Leis HP: Prognostic parameters for breast carcinoma, in Bland KI, Copeland EM (eds): *The Breast: Comprehensive Management of Benign and Malignant Disease.* Philadelphia, Saunders, 1991, pp 331–346

147. Mambo NC, Gallagher HS: Carcinoma of the breast: The prognostic significance of extranodal extension of axillary disease. *Cancer* 39:2280–2285, 1977

148. Kinne DW: Staging and follow-up of breast cancer patients. *Cancer* 67:1196–1197, 1991

149. Donegan WL: Prognostic factors: Stage and receptor status in breast cancer. *Cancer* 70:1755–1764, 1992

150. Nemoto T, Vana J, Bedwani RN, et al: Management and survival of female breast cancer: Results of a national survey by the American College of Surgeons. *Cancer* 45:2917–2924, 1980

151. Carter CL, Allen C, Henson DE: Relation of tumor size, lymph node status, and survival in 24,740 breast cancer cases. *Cancer* 63:181–187, 1989

152. Rosen PP, Groshen S, Kinne DW, et al: Factors influencing prognosis in node-negative breast carcinoma analysis of 767 $T_1N_0M_0/T_2N_0M_0$ patients with long-term follow-up. *J Clin Oncol* 11:2090–2100, 1993

153. Ravdin PM: A practical view of prognostic factors for staging, adjuvant treatment planning and as baseline studies for possible future therapy. *Hematol Oncol Clin North Am* 8: 197–212, 1994

154. Fisher B, Redmond C, Fisher E, et al: Relative worth of estrogen or progesterone receptor and pathologic characteristics of differentiation as indicator of prognosis in node-negative breast cancer patients: Findings from the NSABP B-06. *J Clin Oncol* 6:1076–1087, 1988

155. Dressler L: Are DNA flow cytometry measurements providing useful information in the management of node-negative breast cancer patients? *Cancer Invest* 5:477–486, 1992

156. McGuire WL, Clark GM: Prognostic factors and treatment decisions in axillary node-negative breast cancer. *N Engl J Med* 326:1756–1760, 1992

157. Mori T, Morimoto T, Komaki K, et al: Comparison of estrogen receptor and epidermal growth factor receptor content on primary and involved nodes in human breast cancer. *Cancer* 68:532–537, 1991

158. Gullick WJ, Love SB, Wright C, et al: c-erb B-2 protein overexpression in breast cancer is a risk factor in patients with involved and uninvolved lymph nodes. *Br J Cancer* 63: 434–437, 1991

159. Lovekin C, Ellis IO, Locker A, et al: c-erb B-2 oncoprotein

expression in primary and advanced breast cancer. *Br J Cancer* 63:439, 1991

160. Allred DC, Clark GM, Tandon AK: Her-2/*neu* in node-negative breast cancer: Prognostic significance of overexpressing influenced by the presence of in situ carcinoma. *J Clin Oncol* 10:559–605, 1992

161. Tripathy D, Benz C: Growth factors and their receptors. *Hematol Oncol Clin North Am* 8:29–47, 1994

162. Rochefort H, Capony F, Garcia M: Cathespin D in breast cancer: From molecular and cellular biology to clinical application. *Cancer Cells* 2:383–388, 1990

163. Isola J, Weitz S, Visakorpi T, et al: Cathepsin D expression detected by immunohistochemistry has independent prognostic value in axillary node-negative breast cancer. *J Clin Oncol* 11:36–43, 1993

164. International Breast Cancer Study Group: Prognostic importance of occult axillary lymph node micrometastases from breast cancer. *Lancet* 335:1565–1568, 1990

165. O'Reilly SM, Camplejohn RS, Barns DM, et al: Node-negative breast cancer: Prognostic subgroups defined by tumor size and flow cytometry. *J Clin Oncol* 8:2040–2046, 1990

166. Page DL: Prognosis and breast cancer: Recognition of lethal and favorable prognostic type. *Am J Surg Pathol* 15:334–349, 1991

167. Clark GM, Matheiu MC, Owens MA: Prognostic significance of S-phase fraction in good risk node-negative breast cancer patients. *J Clin Oncol* 10:428–432, 1992

168. Frierson HF: Ploidy analysis and S-phase fraction determination by flow cytometry of invasive adenocarcinomas of the breast. *Am J Surg Pathol* 15:358–367, 1991

169. Seymour L, Bezwoda WR, Meyer K: Tumor factors predicting for prognosis in metastatic breast cancer. *Cancer* 66:2390–2394, 1990

170. Ravdin PM, Osborne CK: Breast Cancer, in MacDonald JS, Haller DG, Mayer RJ (eds): *Manual of Oncologic Therapeutics* (ed 3). Philadelphia; Lippincott-Raven, 1995, pp 153–161

171. Fisher B: Laboratory and clinical research in breast cancer: A personal adventure: The David A Karnofsky Memorial Lecture. *Cancer Res* 40:3863–3874, 1980

172. Fisher B: A biological perspective of breast cancer: Contributions of the National Surgical Adjuvant Breast and Bowel Project Clinical Trials. *CA: Cancer J Clin* 41:97–111, 1991

173. Fisher B, Redmond C, Poisson R, et al: Eight year results of a randomized clinical trial comparing total mastectomy and lumpectomy with or without irradiation in the treatment of breast cancer. *N Engl J Med* 320:822–828, 1989

174. Moore MP, Kinne DW: The surgical management of primary invasive breast cancer. *CA: Cancer J Clin* 45:279–289, 1995

175. Marcial VA: Primary therapy for limited breast cancer. *Cancer* 65:2159–2164, 1990

176. Recht A, Come SE, Gelman RS, et al: Integration of conservative surgery, radiotherapy, and chemotherapy for the treatment of early-stage, node-positive breast cancer: Sequencing, timing, and outcome. *J Clin Oncol* 9:2662–2667, 1991

177. Harris JR, Morrow M: Treatment of early stage breast cancer, in Harris JR, Lippman ME, Morrow M, Hellman S (eds): *Diseases of Breast*. Philadelphia: Lippincott, 1996, pp 487–547

178. Bonadonna G: Evolving concepts in the systemic adjuvant treatment of breast cancer. *Cancer Res* 52:2127–2137, 1992

179. Andersson I, Aspegren K, Jamzon L, et al: Mammographic screening and mortality from breast cancer: Malmo-mammographic screening trial. *Br Med J* 297:943–948, 1998

180. Fisher B, Constantino J, Redmond C, et al: Randomized clinical trial evaluating tamoxifen in the treatment of patients with node-negative breast cancer who have estrogen-receptor-positive tumors. *N Engl J Med* 320:479–484, 1989

181. Fisher B, Redmond C, Nikolay V, et al: A randomized clinical trial evaluating sequential methotrexate and fluorouracil in the treatment of patients with node-negative breast cancer who have estrogen-receptor-negative tumors. *N Engl J Med* 320:473–478, 1989

182. Mansour EG, Gray R, Shatila AH, et al: Efficacy of adjuvant chemotherapy in high-risk node-negative breast cancer. *N Engl J Med* 320:485–490, 1989

183. Door FA (ed): Proceedings of the NIH Consensus Development Conference on Early Stage Breast Cancer. *Monogr Natl Cancer Inst* 1–9, 1990

184. Early Breast Cancer Trialists' Collaborative Group: Systemic Treatment of Early Breast Cancer by Hormonal Cytoxic or Immune Therapy: Part I and II. *N Engl J Med* 339:1–15, 71–85, 1992

185. Winchester DP: Adjuvant therapy for node-negative breast cancer. *Cancer* 67:1741–1743, 1991

186. Fisher B, Constantino J, Redmond C, et al: A randomized clinical trial evaluating tamoxifen in the treatment of patients with node-negative breast cancer who have estrogen receptor positive tumors. *N Engl J Med* 320:479–484, 1989

187. Bonadonna G: Conceptual and practice advances in the management of breast cancer: Karnofsky Memorial Lecture. *J Clin Oncol* 7:1380–1937, 1989

188. Bonadonna G, Valagussa P, Rossi A, et al: Ten year results with CMF-based adjuvant chemotherapy in resectable breast cancer. *Cancer Res Treat* 5:95–115, 1985

189. Fisher B, Redmond C, Legault-Poisson S, et al: Postoperative chemotherapy and tamoxifen compared with tamoxifen alone in the treatment of positive-node breast cancer patients aged 50 years and older with tumors responsive to tamoxifen: Results from the National Surgical Adjuvant Breast and Bowel Project B-16. *J Clin Oncol* 8:1005–1018, 1990

190. Fisher B, Rockette H, Robidoux A, et al: Effect of preoperative therapy for breast cancer (BC) on local-regional disease: First report of NSABP B-18. *Proc Am Soc Clin Oncol*, 13:64, 1994 (abstr 57)

191. Muss H, Thor A, Jute T, et al: *erb* B-2 (c-*erb* B-2; Her-2/*neu*) and S-phase fraction (SPF) predict response to adjuvant chemotherapy in patients with node-positive breast cancer. CAIGB Trial 8869. *Proc Amer Soc Clin Oncol* 12:72, 1993

192. Swain SM: Chemotherapy: Toxicities of adjuvant therapy and high dose therapy with autologous bone marrow transplant. *12th Annual International Breast Conference* March 1995 (abstr)

193. Duggan D: Local therapy of locally advanced breast cancer. *Oncology* 5:67–72, 1991

194. Carter CL, Allen C, Henson DE: Relation of tumor size, lymph node status and survival in 24,470 breast cancer cases. *Cancer* 63:181–187, 1989

195. Swain S, Lippman M: Systemic therapy of locally advanced breast cancer: Review and guidelines. *Oncology* 3:21–28, 1989

196. Osborne CK, Clark GM, Ravdin P: Adjuvant systemic therapy of breast cancer, in Harris J, Lippman M, and Morrow M (eds): *Diseases of the Breast*. Philadelphia: Lippincott-Raven, 1996, pp 548–578

197. Hortobagi GN, Buzdar AN: Locally advanced breast cancer: A review including the M.D. Anderson experience, in Ragaz T, Ariel T (eds): *High Risk Breast Cancer.* Berlin-Heidelberg: Springer Verlag, 1991, pp 382–413

198. Longstaff S, Siguardsson H, O'Keeffe M, et al: A controlled study of the ocular effects of tamoxifen in conventional dosage in the treatment of breast carcinoma. *Eur J Cancer* 25:1805, 1989

199. Fornander T, Rutquist LE, Wilking N: Effects of tamoxifen on the female genital tract. *Ann NY Acad Sci* 622:469–476, 1991

200. Jordan VC, Assikis VJ: Endometrial carcinoma and tamoxifen: Clearing up a controversy. *Clin Cancer Res* 1:467–472, 1996

201. Knobf MK: Symptoms and rehabilitation needs of patients with early-stage breast cancer during primary therapy. *Cancer* 66:1392–1401, 1990

202. Wolter J: Support programs, in Harris JR, Lippman M, Morrow M, Hellman (eds): *Diseases of the Breast.* Philadelphia: Lippencott-Raven, 1996, pp 948–951

203. Gellert GA, Maxwell RM, Siegel BS: Survival of breast cancer patients receiving adjunctive psychosocial support therapy. *J Clin Oncol* 11:66–69, 1993

204. Fowble B: Local-regional treatment options for early invasive breast cancer, in Fowble B, Goodman RL, Glick JH, Rosato EF (eds): *Breast Cancer Treatment: A Comprehensive Guide to Management.* St Louis: Mosby Year Book, 1991, pp 25–88

205. Cooley ME, Erikson B: Rehabilitation, in Fowble B, Goodman RL, Glick JH, Rosato EF (eds): *Breast Cancer Treatment: A Comprehensive Guide to Management.* St. Louis: Mosby Year Book, 1991, pp 511–583

206. Schover LR: The impact of breast cancer on sexuality, body image and intimate relationships. *CA: Cancer J Clin* 4:112–119, 1991

207. Psychological Aspects of Breast Cancer Study Group: Psychological response to mastectomy: A prospective comparison study. *Cancer* 69:189–196, 1987

208. Vinokur AD, Threatt BA, Vinokur-Kaplann D, et al: The process of recovery from breast cancer for younger and older patients: Changing during the first year. *Cancer* 65:1242–1254, 1990

209. Schover LR: Sexuality and body image in younger women with breast cancer. *Monogr Natl Cancer Inst* 16:177–182, 1994

210. U.S. Congress Office of Technology Assessment: The menopause, hormone therapy and women's health. Washington, DC, U.S. Government Printing Office, May 1992

211. Goodman M: Menopausal symptoms, in Groenwald SL, Frogge MH, Goodman M, Yarbro CH (eds): *Cancer Symptom Management.* Boston: Jones and Bartlett, 1996, pp 77–93

212. Bergmans M, Merkos J, Corbey R, et al: Effect of bellargel regard on climacteric complaints: A double blind placebo controlled study. *Maturitas* 9:227–234, 1987

213. Magamani M, Kelver M, Smith E: Treatment of menopausal hot flashes with transdermal administration of Clonidine. *Am J Obstet Gynecol* 156:561–565, 1987

214. Grindel CG, Cahill CA, Walker A: Food intake of women with breast cancer during the first 6 months of chemotherapy. *Oncol Nurs Forum* 16:401–407, 1989

215. Knobf MT: Physical and psychological distress associated with adjuvant chemotherapy in women with breast cancer. *J Clin Oncol* 4:678–684, 1986

216. Knobf M, Mullen J, Xistris D, et al: Weight gain in women with breast cancer receiving adjuvant chemotherapy. *Oncol Nurs Forum* 10:28–33, 1983

217. Duffy MJ, Woods JE: Health risks of failed implants: A 30-year clinical experience. *Plast Reconstr Surg* 95:1129–1131, 1995

218. Berger K, Bostwick J, III: *A Woman's Decision—Breast Care Treatment and Reconstruction* (ed 2). St. Louis: Quality Medical Printing, 1995

219. Mackay GJ, Bostwick J, III: Breast reconstruction-reconstructive breast surgery, in Harris JR, Lippman ME, Morrow M, et al: *Diseases of the Breast.* Philadelphia: Lippincott-Raven, 1996, pp 601–619

220. Baker RR, Niederhubert J: Breast reconstruction, in Baker RR, Niederhuber J (eds): *The Operative Management of Breast Disease.* Philadelphia: Saunders, 1992, pp 117–129

221. Handel N: Current status of breast reconstruction after mastectomy. *Oncology* 5:73–83, 1991

222. Honig SF: Hormonal therapy and chemotherapy, in Harris JR, Lippman ME, Morrow M, Hellman S (eds): *Diseases of the Breast.* Philadelphia: Lippincott-Raven, 1996, pp 669–718

223. Smith IA: Recurrent disease, in Harris JR, Hellman S, Henderson IC (eds): *Breast Diseases.* Philadelphia, Lippincott, 1987, pp 369–384

224. Boring CC, Squires TS, Heath CW: Cancer statistics for African-Americans. *CA: Cancer J Clin* 42:7–14, 1992

225. Elledge RM, Clark GM, Chamnes GC, et al: Tumor biologic factors and breast cancer prognosis among white, Hispanic, and black women in the United States. *Int J Cancer* 86:705–709, 1994

226. Nicolson GL, Hug V: Breast cancer growth and metastases. *MD Anderson Oncol Case Rep Rev* 5:1–11, 1990

227. Canellos GB: Systemic therapy of breast cancer. *Med J Aust* 148:88–91, 1988

228. Jabboury K, Holmes FA, Hortobagyi G: 5-fluorouracil rechallenge by protracted infusion in refractory breast cancer. *Cancer* 64:793–797, 1989

229. Loprinzi CL: 5-fluorouracil with leukovorin in breast cancer. *Cancer* 63:1045–1047, 1989

230. Boring C, Squires T, Tong T, et al: Cancer statistics 1994. *CA Cancer J Clin* 44:18, 1994

231. Rosenblatt K, Thomas D, McTiernan A, et al: Breast cancer in men: Aspects of familial aggregation. *J Natl Cancer Inst* 83:849–853, 1991

232. Donegan WL: Cancer of the breast in men. *CA: Cancer J Clin* 41:339–352, 1991

233. Thomas DB, Jiminez LM, McTiernan A, et al: Breast cancer in men: risk factors with hormonal implications. *Am J Epidemiol* 135:734–739, 1992

234. Evans DB, Crichlow RW: Carcinoma of the male breast and Klinefelter's syndrome: Is there an association? *CA: Cancer J Clin* 37:246–251, 1987

235. Patel HZ, Buzdar AU, Hortobagi GN: Role of adjuvant chemotherapy in male breast cancer. *Cancer* 64:1583–1585, 1989

236. Van Holten-Verzantroort ATM, Kroon HM, Bijvoet OLM, et al: Palliative pamidronate treatment in patients with bone metastases from breast cancer. *J Clin Oncol* 11:491–497, 1993

237. Batson OV: The vertebral venous system: Caldwell lecture, 1956, in Weiss L, Gilbert AA (eds): *Bone Metastasis.* Boston, GK Hall, 1981, p 21

238. Hill ME, Richards MA, Gregory WM, et al: Spinal cord compression in breast cancer: A review of 70 cases. *Br J Cancer* 68:969–972, 1993

239. Kim RY, Spencer SA, Meridith RF, et al: Extradural spinal cord compression analysis of factors determining functional prognosis: prospective study. *Radiology* 176:279–283, 1990

240. Maranzano E, Latini P, Checcaglini F, et al: Radiation therapy of spinal cord compression caused by breast cancer: A report. *Int J Radiat Oncology Biol Phys* 240:201–206, 1992

241. Larsen D, Weinstein M, Goldberg I, et al: Edema of the arm as a function of the extent of axillary surgery in patients treated with stage I–II carcinoma of the breast treated with primary radiotherapy. *Int J Radiat Oncol Biol Phys* 16:1575–1582, 1986

242. Maunsell E, Brisson J, and Deschenes L: Arm problems and psychological distress after surgery for breast cancer. *Can J Surg* 36:315–320, 1992

243. Humble CA: Lymphedema: Incidence, pathophysiology, management and nursing care. *Oncol Nurs Forum* 22:1503–1509, 1995

244. Danforth DN: How subsequent pregnancy affects outcome in women with prior breast cancer. *Oncology* 5:23–29, 1992

245. VonSchoultz E, Johansson H, Wilking N, et al: Influence of prior and subsequent pregnancy on breast cancer prognosis. *J Clin Oncol* 13:430–434, 1995

246. Petrek JA: Breast cancer and pregnancy, in Harris J, Lippman ME, Morrow M, Hellman S (eds): *Diseases of the Breast.* Philadelphia: Lippincott-Raven, 1996, pp 883–892

247. Doll DC, Ringenberg QS, Yarbro JW: Antineoplastic agents and pregnancy. *Semin Oncol* 16:337–346, 1989

248. Mattison DR, Argtuaco T: Magnetic resonance imaging in prenatal diagnosis. *Clin Obstet Gynecol* 31:353–355, 1988

249. Leathem AM: Safety and efficacy of antiemetics used to treat nausea and vomiting in pregnancy. *Clin Pharmacol* 5:660–668, 1986

250. Garber JE: Long-term follow-up of children exposed in vitro to antineoplastic agents. *Semin Oncol* 16:337–344, 1989

251. Zemlickis D, Lishner M, Degendorfer P, et al: Fetal outcome after in utero exposure to cancer chemotherapy. *Arch Inter Med* 152:573–576, 1992

252. Katz AH, Maida CA: Health and disability self-help organizations, in Powell TJ (ed): *Working with Self-help.* Silver Springs, MD: National Association of Social Workers, 1990, pp 141–155

253. Cella DF, Yellen SB: Cancer support groups: the state of the art. *Cancer Prac* 1:56–61, 1993

254. Riessman F, Carroll D: Self-help and the new health agenda, in Reismann F, Caroll D (eds): *Redefining Self-help.* San Francisco: Josey Bass, 1995, pp 83–108

# Chapter 35

# Central Nervous System Cancers

Karen Belford, RN, MS, OCN®, CCRN

# INTRODUCTION

Cancer of the central nervous system (CNS) includes primary and metastatic tumors of the brain and spinal cord. The incidence of these tumors is thought to be increasing, particularly the metastatic tumors. CNS cancers are not uncommon and are associated with significant morbidity and mortality. Whether benign or malignant, primary or secondary, CNS tumors can drastically affect an individual's life and impede the ability to function. Knowledge of the various tumor types and their differences, associated neuroanatomy and neurophysiology, and the many issues related to treatment is essential to provide accurate assessment, ongoing intervention, and supportive management for these individuals.

# EPIDEMIOLOGY

Primary CNS cancers represent 2% of all reported malignancies, and an estimated 17,900 new cases were diagnosed in the United States in 1996.[1] Neurological cancers are found in people of all ages, with a peak incidence occurring in the first, fifth, sixth, and seventh decades. The incidence is slightly higher in men than in women with the exception of meningiomas, which occur more often in women. CNS cancers are the second most common cancer diagnosed in children, second only to leukemia.

Malignant CNS tumors are responsible for approximately 2.5% of all cancer-related deaths. In women between the ages of 15 and 34, CNS neoplasms are the fourth-leading cause of cancer mortality. In men between the ages of 15 and 34 they are the third, and in men between 35 and 54 years, CNS cancers are the fourth-leading cause of cancer-related mortality.[1] Most intracranial tumors, however, occur in individuals older than 45 years.[2] Over the past three decades, the incidence of primary malignant brain tumors appears to have increased in the elderly.[3] This apparent increase may be attributed to possible environmental carcinogens found in industrialized nations, improved diagnostic capabilities, changing attitudes toward the care of the elderly, and medical support programs.[4] The increase is established only for primary central nervous system lymphoma (PCNSL).

The most prevalent CNS malignancy is the metastatic brain tumor, which is increasing in frequency and occurs at least four to five times more often than primary brain tumors. The most common primary brain tumor is the malignant glioma, accounting for more than half of all primary CNS cancers. The incidence of spinal cord tumors is about 15% of that of brain tumors, with metastatic spinal tumors representing more than half of this group of neoplasms.

# ETIOLOGY

## Genetic Factors

Specific causes and risk factors for the majority of CNS tumors have not been identified. Fewer than 5% of CNS tumors are associated with specific genetic disorders. Neurofibromatosis type 1 (NF-1) is an autosomal dominant disorder occurring in 1 out of 3000 individuals.[5] The most common CNS tumors associated with NF-1 are optic nerve gliomas, astrocytomas, ependymomas, meningiomas, and neurofibromas, reported in 4%–45% of individuals with NF-1.[6] Neurofibromatosis type 2 (NF-2), also an autosomal dominant disorder, occurs less frequently and is characterized by an increased incidence of cranial and spinal nerve root tumors, most commonly schwannomas.[6,7] Tuberous sclerosis, or Bourneville's disease, also an autosomal dominant disorder in skin, CNS, and kidney abnormalities, has been associated with a variety of gliomas.[2,6] The Li-Fraumeni syndrome is a rare autosomal dominant disorder associated with an increased incidence of many different types of cancer including gliomas.[5,6] Gliomas, medulloblastomas, and pituitary adenomas have been observed in individuals with Turcot syndrome, an autosomal dominant syndrome of CNS tumors in individuals with adenomatous polyposis coli (APC). Approximately 5% of families with APC have this syndrome.[2,5] Finally, those with the autosomal dominant von Hippel–Lindau disease are at risk for developing cerebellar or spinal hemangioblastomas.[7,8] In addition to the genetic disorders listed here, various tumor types have been linked to chromosomal abnormalities specifically on chromosomes 22, 17, and 10.[9,10] Recent advances in molecular biology have identified both the expression of activated oncogenes and the inactivation of tumor-suppressor genes in a variety of brain tumors.[11]

## Chemical and Environmental Factors

Although many chemicals are carcinogenic in animals and produce CNS tumors, the possible association of chemical exposure and CNS tumors has not been truly established and is limited to a few occupations. Various studies of each of these occupations and chemicals conflict and require confirmation. Agricultural workers exposed to multiple chemicals in pesticides, herbicides, and fertilizers have had a higher than expected incidence of gliomas.[11,12] Several studies suggest a relationship between CNS tumors and such industries as synthetic rubber, petrochemical, aeronautics, and nuclear energy.[13,14] Excess risk of gliomas and meningiomas has been associated with precision metal work.[11,15] Workers exposed to polyvinylchloride may be at increased risk for gliomas. Other substances that may be implicated in the development of brain tumors are organic solvents, phenols, formalin, polycyclic aromatic hydrocarbons, and nitrosoureas.[11,13]

## Viral Factors

Viruses have been directly implicated in the development of CNS tumors in animals only. However, individuals with autoimmunodeficiency syndrome (AIDS)-related PCNSL have been found to have a high rate of infection with the Epstein-Barr virus (EBV), and evidence of EBV has been isolated from the tumor tissue. It is not understood why PCNSL is often associated with acquired immunosuppression. Individuals with AIDS have an increased risk for developing PCNSL and possibly gliomas.

## Radiation

Therapeutic irradiation of the head has been linked to the subsequent appearance of CNS tumors. This has been seen in individuals who have received radiation therapy (RT) during childhood for treatment of acute lymphoblastic leukemia[16] and tinea capitis[17] and in adults who have received cranial irradiation for treatment of pituitary adenomas.[18] An increased incidence of both primary and metastatic tumors, including PCNSL, has been found following immunosuppressive therapy.[19,20]

Although disputed, epidemiological studies suggest a possible association between exposure to extremely-low-frequency electromagnetic fields (ELF-EMFs) and increased incidence of cancer.[21–23] Exposure to ELF-EMFs is almost universal today in industrialized nations. While empirical evidence is inconsistent, several occupational studies have suggested a higher than expected incidence of CNS tumors, specifically gliomas, among electricians, electronics and communications workers,[11,24] railway workers, and welders.[23] Occupational exposure may be just a fraction of the total ELF-EMF exposure. Other ELF-EMF sources outside the workplace include residential heating, and proximity to power lines and electrical appliances in the home.[23] Residential studies have focused primarily on ELF-EMF and the two most common cancers in children, leukemia and CNS cancers; while positive associations between the two have been reported,[25–27] the evidence is inconsistent.

## PREVENTION, SCREENING, EARLY DETECTION PROGRAMS

No prevention, screening, or early detection programs exist for CNS cancers. However, individuals with specific hereditary syndromes that may predispose them to CNS tumors may be informed of their genetic risks.

## PATHOPHYSIOLOGY

### Anatomy and Physiology

#### Brain

The embryonic development of the nervous system begins at approximately three weeks and originates from the ectodermal layer of the embryo. As the ectoderm rapidly develops, it folds inward, thickens, and begins to fuse, forming the neural tube,[28] which will later develop into the various structures of the brain. The neural tube cells form two cell types: the *neuroblasts*, which give rise to the neurons, and the *spongioblasts*, which give rise to the neuroglia (glia) cells. The neurons are the basic anatomic and functional unit of the nervous system. The glial cells provide structural support, nourishment, and protection for the neurons. Approximately 40% of the brain and spinal cord is composed of glial cells.[29] Six types of glial cells are in the nervous system: astrocytes, oligodendrocytes, ependymal cells, Schwann cells, microglia, and satellite cells. These cells can undergo anaplasia and are the major source of primary tumors of the CNS. The specific tumor type is derived from the glial cell of origin. For example, ependymal cells develop into the brain tumor ependymoma.

The brain is divided into three main areas: the cerebrum, the brain stem, and the cerebellum. The cerebrum contains the two cerebral hemispheres and the diencephalon. The cerebral hemispheres are connected by a large area of white matter, the corpus callosum, which allows each portion of one hemisphere to connect with its corresponding portion of the other hemisphere. It essentially allows communication between the two hemispheres.[30] Each cerebral hemisphere is divided into four lobes: frontal, parietal, temporal, and occipital (Figure 35-1).[31] The diencephalon is composed of the thalamus, hypothalamus, and basal ganglia. The pituitary gland is connected to the hypothalamus. The brain stem is made up of the midbrain, pons, and medulla. The cerebellum

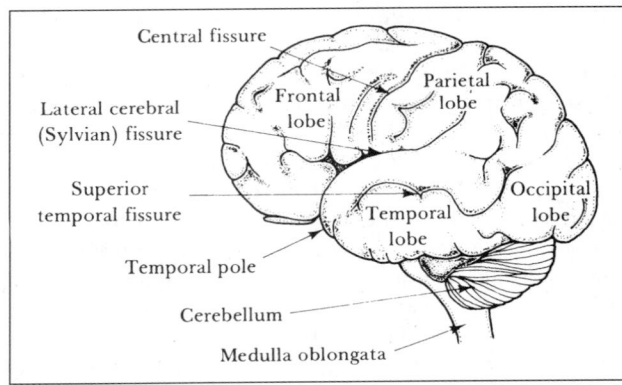

**FIGURE 35-1**    The four lobes of the cerebral hemispheres.[31]

has two hemispheres and is connected to the brain stem by three pairs of cerebellar peduncles. The functions of these areas are listed in Table 35-1 during the discussion of clinical manifestations.

Twelve pairs of cranial nerves (CNs) have fiber pathways entering and exiting the brain. Each pair of CNs has a specific function and is identified by Roman numerals (Figure 35-2). The functions of these nerves are listed in table 35-4. Symptoms of cranial nerve dysfunction (cranial nerve palsy) can provide valuable information for localizing an intracranial tumor.

The brain is encased within the rigid bony structure of the skull. The skull, with the meninges and cerebrospinal fluid (CSF), helps to support and protect the brain. The meninges are the membranes covering the brain and spinal cord. The cranial meninges are shown in Figure 35-3.[32]

There are three layers of meninges: the *dura mater,* *arachnoid,* and *pia mater.* The outermost layer, the dura mater, is a double-layered, whitish, thick fibrous membrane that lines the interior of the skull.[29] The outer layer of the dura is the periosteum of the cranial bones. The inner dural layer contains arteries and veins and folds in on itself to create anatomic compartments. The falx cerebri, the tentorium cerebelli, and the falx cerebelli

are three such folds. The falx cerebri, a double fold of dura, descends vertically and separates the two cerebral hemispheres. The tentorium cerebelli, a tentlike fold of dura running between the occipital lobes of the cerebrum and the cerebellum, divides the skull into the supratentorial space and the infratentorial space. Structures and tumors that lie above the tentorium (cerebral hemispheres, diencephalon, and basal ganglia) are located in the supratentorial compartment, and those lying below the tentorium (cerebellum and brain stem) are in the infratentorial compartment (Figure 35-4). A third fold of dura, the falx cerebelli, separates the two lobes of the cerebellum.

The middle meningeal layer, the arachnoid, is a thin, delicate avascular transparent membrane that loosely surrounds the brain. The subarachnoid space lies beneath the arachnoid and separates it from the pia mater, the innermost layer of the meninges. CSF circulates throughout the subarachnoid space. The pia mater is a meshlike vascular membrane that adheres directly to the surface of the brain. The pia dips down between the convolutions of the brain surface.

The ventricular system consists of a series of interconnected chambers and pathways responsible for the production and circulation of CSF around the brain and

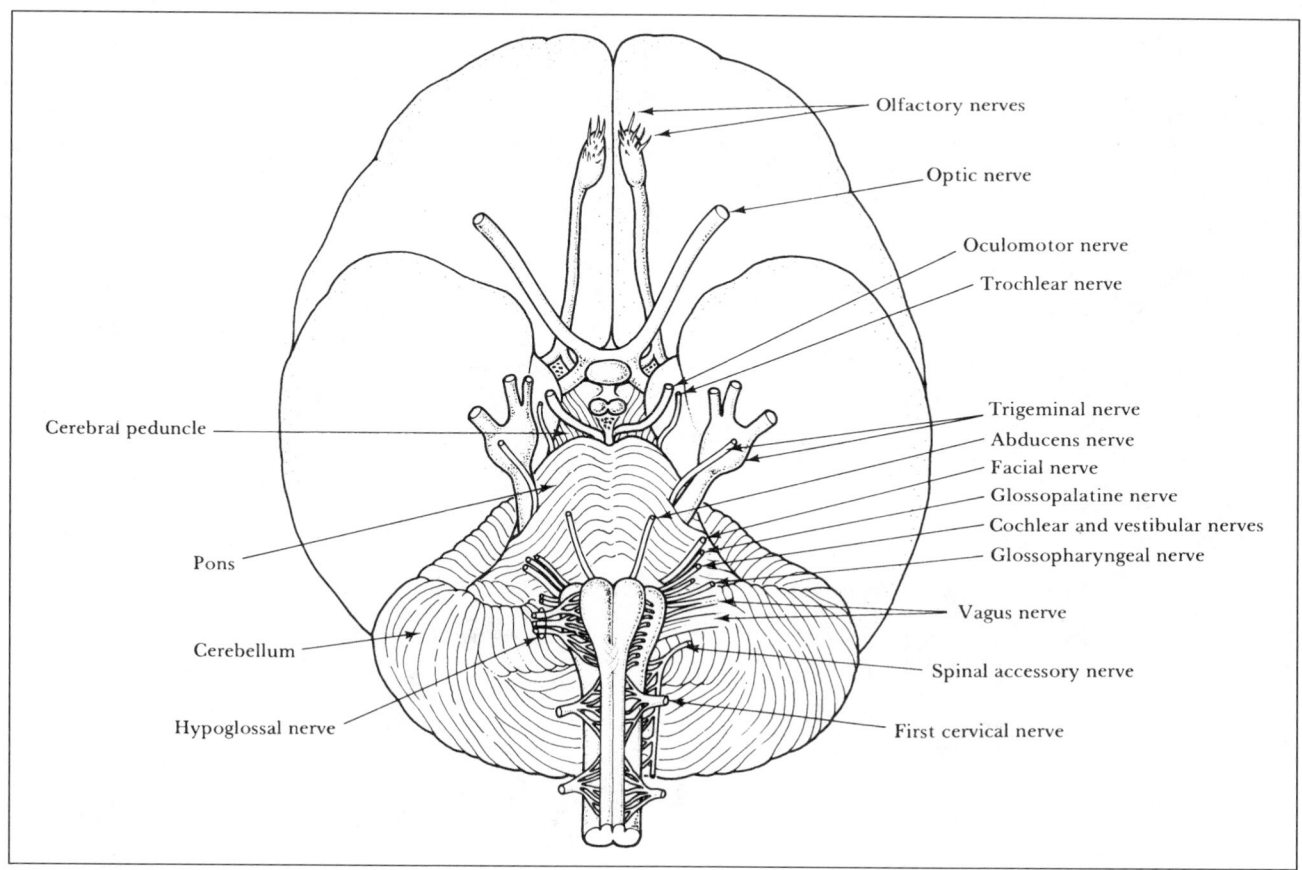

**FIGURE 35-2**   Cranial nerves from the base of the brain.[31]

**TABLE 35-1**   Clinical Manifestations of Intracranial Tumors

| Location | Function | Abnormality |
|---|---|---|
| Frontal lobes | Intellect | Intellectual deterioration |
| | Personality | Personality changes |
| | Judgment | Impaired judgment |
| | Abstract thinking | |
| | Mood and affect | Emotional liability, flat affect |
| | Long-term memory | Memory loss |
| | Voluntary motor activity (contralateral) | Muscle weakness or paralysis |
| | |   Babinski's sign |
| | |   Increased deep tone reflexes |
| | | Bowel and bladder incontinence |
| | Language expression (dominant side) | Expressive aphasia |
| | |   (Broca's aphasia) |
| | | Seizures |
| Parietal lobes | Sensory integration (contralateral) | Decrease or loss of sensation (pain, temperature, pinprick, |
| | Sensory interpretation (contralateral) |   light touch, proprioception, vibration, two-point |
| | |   discrimination, stereognosis, graphesthesia) |
| | | Seizures |
| | | Inability to write |
| Temporal lobes | Hearing | Hearing changes, hallucinations |
| | Short-term memory | Memory loss |
| | Language comprehension (dominant side) | Receptive aphasia |
| | |   (Wernicke's aphasia) |
| | Interpretation of memory | Intellectual impairment |
| | Emotion | Emotional lability |
| | | Seizures |
| Occipital lobes | Vision | Visual field defects, blindness |
| | Visual interpretation | Hallucinations |
| | | Inability to identify objects or symbols or meaning of written |
| | |   words |
| | | Seizures |
| Thalamus | Sensory relay station | Sensory abnormality |
| | Conscious awareness of pain | Neuropathic pain |
| | Sleep-wake cycle | Hydrocephalus |
| | Focusing of attention | Increased ICP |
| | Emotion | Inattentiveness |
| | | Emotional lability |
| Hypothalamus | Coordination of autonomic nervous system | |
| |   function | |
| | Temperature regulation | Hypo or hyperthermia |
| | Regulation of water metabolism | |
| | Regulation of hormone secretions | Endocrine dysfunction |
| | Regulation of appetite | |
| | Control of thirst center | |
| | Regulation of part of sleep-wake cycle | |
| | Mediation of affective behavior | Flat affect |
| | | Emotional lability |
| Basal ganglia | Fine motor control | Weakness or paralysis |
| | | Intention tremors |
| Brain stem | Point of origin for cranial nerves III through XII | Cranial nerve dysfunction |
|   midbrain | Vital reflex centers | Hydrocephalus |
|   pons | Maintenance of consciousness | Cerebellar dysfunction |
|   medulla | Provision of nerve pathway | Vomiting |
| | | Headache |
| Cerebellum | Coordination | Ataxia |
| | Fine motor control | Action tremor |
| | | Nystagmus |
| | | Dysarthria |
| | Balance (ipsilateral) | Loss of balance, wide-base gait |
| | | Hydrocephalus |

Modified from Wegmann JA[31]

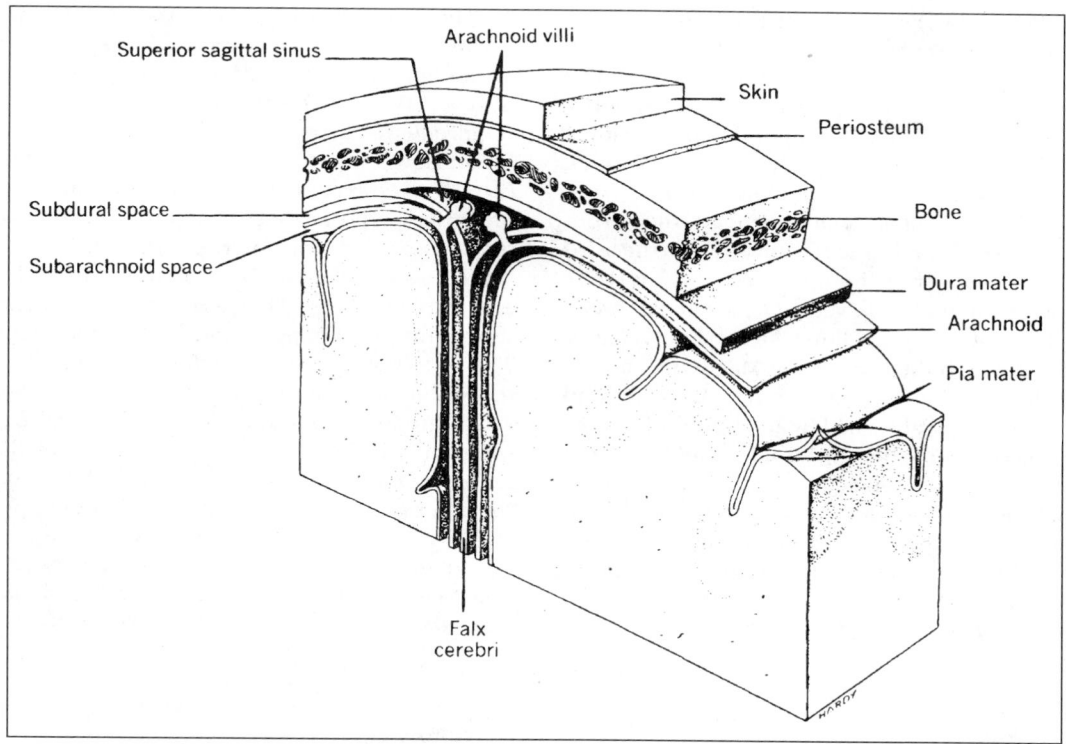

**FIGURE 35-3**   The cranial meninges. (Reprinted with permission from Hickey JV: The Clinical Practice of Neurological and Neurosurgical Nursing. Philadelphia, Lippincott, 1992. Originally published in Chaffee EE, Lytle IM: *Basic Physiology and Anatomy*. Philadelphia, Lippincott Company, 1980.[32])

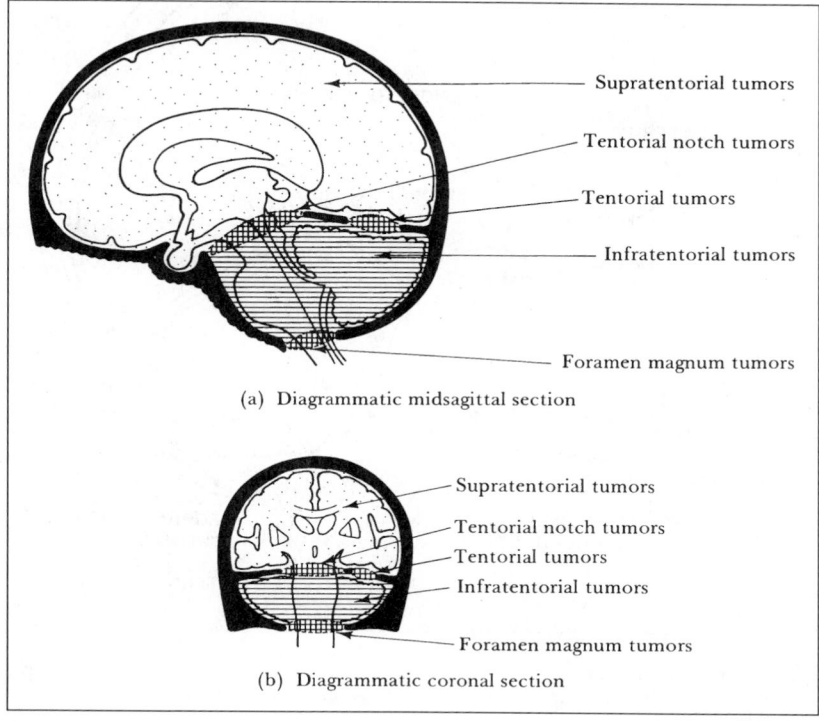

(a)  Diagrammatic midsagittal section

(b)  Diagrammatic coronal section

**FIGURE 35-4**   Localization of intracranial tumors.[31]

spinal cord (Figure 35-5).[33] The majority of CSF is formed in the choroid plexuses, the cauliflower-like structures located in the third, fourth, and lateral ventricles. The lateral ventricles, located in the cerebral hemispheres, are divided into the frontal, temporal, and occipital horns. CSF flows from the two lateral ventricles through the intraventricular foramina (foramina of Monro) into the third ventricle, which is situated beneath the corpus callosum and surrounded by the thalamus. From the third ventricle, CSF flows through the aqueduct of Sylvius (cerebral aqueduct) into the fourth ventricle, located between the hemispheres of the cerebellum. The CSF then leaves the ventricles through the foramen of Magendie and the foramina of Luschka to circulate around the brain and spinal cord. CSF is then absorbed by arachnoid villi, small fingerlike projections of the arachnoid membrane, into the dural venous sinuses. The superior sagittal sinus is a major site of CSF reabsorption. There are expanded areas of the subarachnoid space called *cisterns* where CSF may be aspirated. The major cisterns are the *cisterna magnum,* located between the medulla and the cerebellar region, and the *lumbar cistern,* between vertebrae L-2 and S-2.[29]

The cerebral circulation is the body's most complex vascular network. The brain receives approximately 20% of the body's resting cardiac output. This large amount of blood flow reflects the brain's tremendous metabolic requirements, particularly for oxygen and glucose.[34] Blood flow to the brain is supplied by the two internal carotid arteries (anterior circulation) and the two vertebral arteries (posterior circulation). The internal carotids bifurcate to form the anterior and middle cerebral arteries. These arteries supply blood to the frontal, temporal, and parietal lobes. They also have subdivisions, which supply the basal ganglia and part of the diencephalon. The vertebral arteries enter the base of the skull through the foramen magnum and unite to form the basilar artery, which subdivides into the posterior cerebral arteries. The vertebral arteries and their branches supply the cerebellum, the brain stem, the spinal cord, the occipital lobes, the inferior and medial aspects of the temporal lobes, and a portion of the diencephalon.[29]

Collateral circulation to the brain is provided by an intact circle of Willis (Figure 35-6). The circle of Willis, located at the base of the brain, connects the anterior

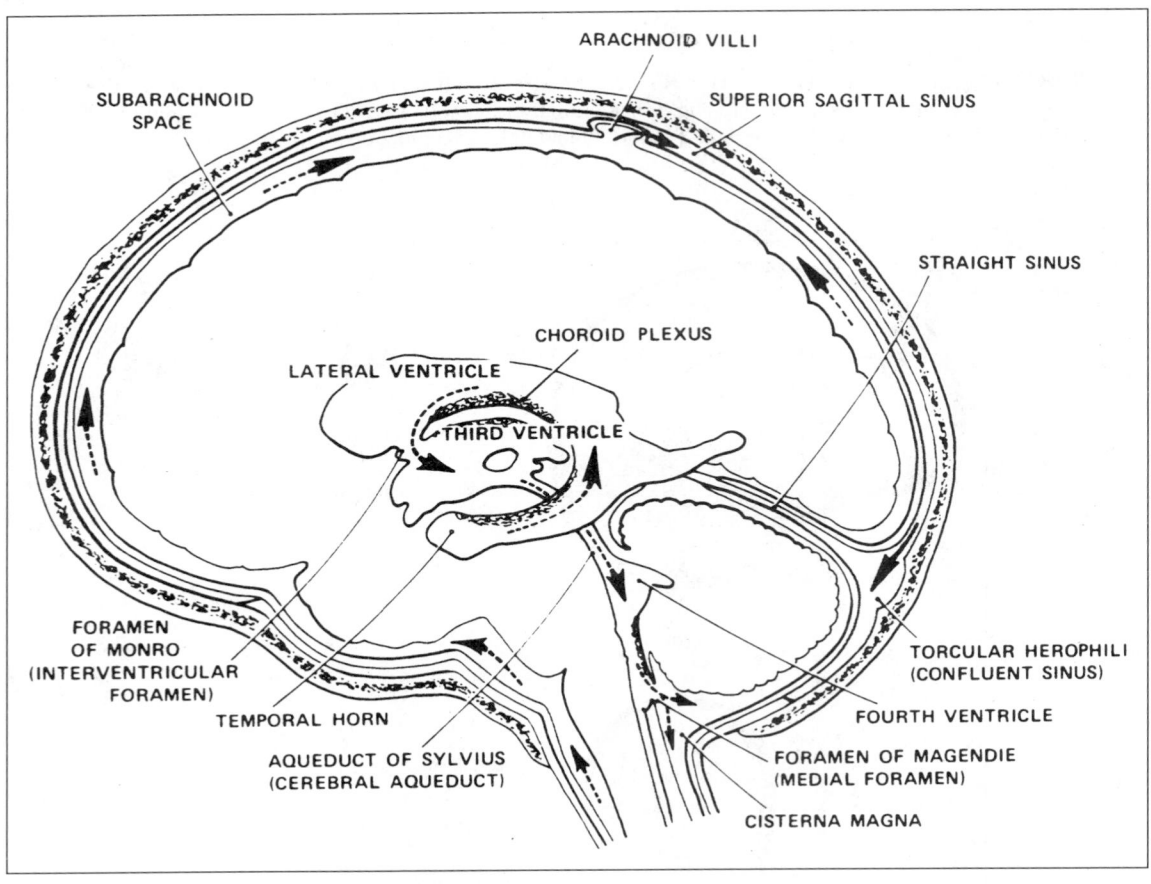

**FIGURE 35-5**   Circulation of cerebrospinal fluid. The foramina of Luschka are not shown. (Reprinted with permission from Gilman S, Newman SW: *Manter and Gatz's Essentials of Clinical Neuroanatomy and Neurophysiology* [ed 8]. Philadelphia: F.A. Davis Company, 1992.[33])

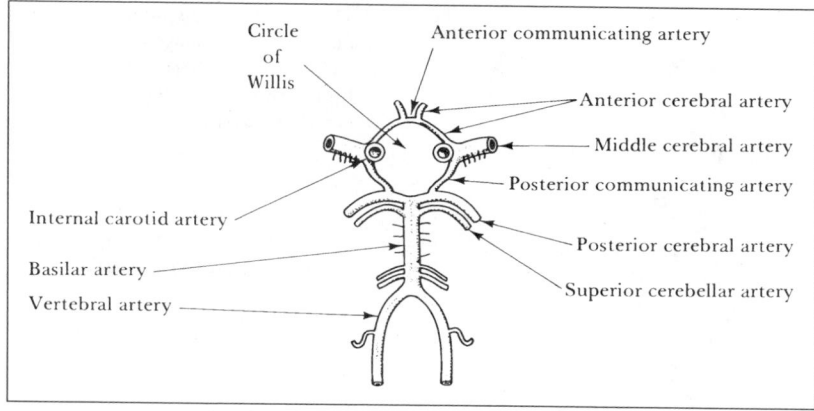

**FIGURE 35-6**  Circle of Willis.[31]

and posterior circulations. The circle is completed by the two posterior communicating arteries, which connect the internal carotid and posterior cerebral arteries, and the anterior communicating artery, which connects the two anterior cerebral arteries. Blood can be shunted from one area to another, allowing an adequate blood supply to reach all parts of the brain. However, collateral circulation depends on the presence and patency of all the components of the circle. Anatomic variations are common, especially with the communicating arteries. Blood vessels in the meninges also help to ensure collateral circulation in the brain.

### Spinal cord

The spine is a flexible column formed by a series of vertebrae, each stacked one upon another to support the head and trunk. The vertebral column shown in Figure 35-7 consists of 33 vertebrae: 7 cervical, 12 thoracic, 5 lumbar, 5 sacral, and 5 coccygeal. The five sacral vertebrae fuse to form the sacrum, and the four coccygeal vertebrae fuse to form the coccyx. A thoracic vertebra is shown in Figure 35-8. Each vertebra has an anterior solid segment or body and a posterior segment or arch.[29] Two pedicles and two laminae supporting seven processus (four articular, two transverse, and one spinous) make up the arch. The two pedicles are short, thick pieces of bone. The concavity above and below the pedicles creates the intervertebral foramen through which the spinal nerves exit the vertebral column. The intervertebral foramina are narrow, and the nerves may easily be compressed at this site by a protruding disk or arthritic spurring.[34] The two laminae are broad plates of bone. They complete the neural arch by fusing in the midline and enclosing the vertebral foramen through which the spinal cord passes, thus providing protection for the spinal cord. The spinous process projects backward from the laminae and serves as the attachment for muscles and ligaments.[29] The spinous process is palpable beneath the skin in most individuals.

The four articular processus and two transverse processus provide stability for the spine.

The spinal cord, housed within the vertebral canal, is an elongated mass of nerve tissue less than an inch in diameter and approximately 17–18 inches in length. The spinal cord, arising from the medulla oblongata, begins at the foramen magnum and extends down to the lower border of the first lumbar vertebra, where it ends in a tapered, conelike structure called the *conus medullaris*. The spinal cord is about 10 inches shorter than the vertebral column, and the lower segments of the spinal cord, therefore, are not aligned opposite corresponding vertebrae. Thus, the lumbar and sacral spinal nerves have very long roots. These roots descend in a bundle from the conus, and because of its resemblance to the tail of a horse, this formation is called the *cauda equina*.[33]

There are 31 pairs of spinal nerves exiting from the spinal cord through the intervertebral foramina: 8 cervical, 12 thoracic, 5 lumbar, 5 sacral, and 1 coccygeal. Each spinal nerve has a dorsal root by which afferent (sensory) impulses enter the cord and a ventral root by which efferent (motor) impulses leave the spinal cord. The dorsal roots convey sensory input from skin segments that represent specific areas of the body known as *dermatomes* (Figure 35-9).[35] Interruption of one sensory nerve root may result in paresthesia or pain in that dermatomal area. The ventral roots convey motor impulses from the spinal cord to the body, innervating specific areas of muscle groups called *myotomes* (Table 35-2).

The meningeal system in the cranial cavity is contiguous within the spinal canal to support and protect the spinal cord. The spinal dura is a continuation of the inner layer of the cerebral dura. The outer dural layer ends at the foramen magnum, being replaced by the periosteal lining of the vertebral canal. The spinal dura encloses the spinal roots and the spinal nerves and terminates at the level of the sacrum. The arachnoid layer of the spinal meninges is a continuation of the cerebral arachnoid. The pia mater in the spinal cord is thicker, firmer, and

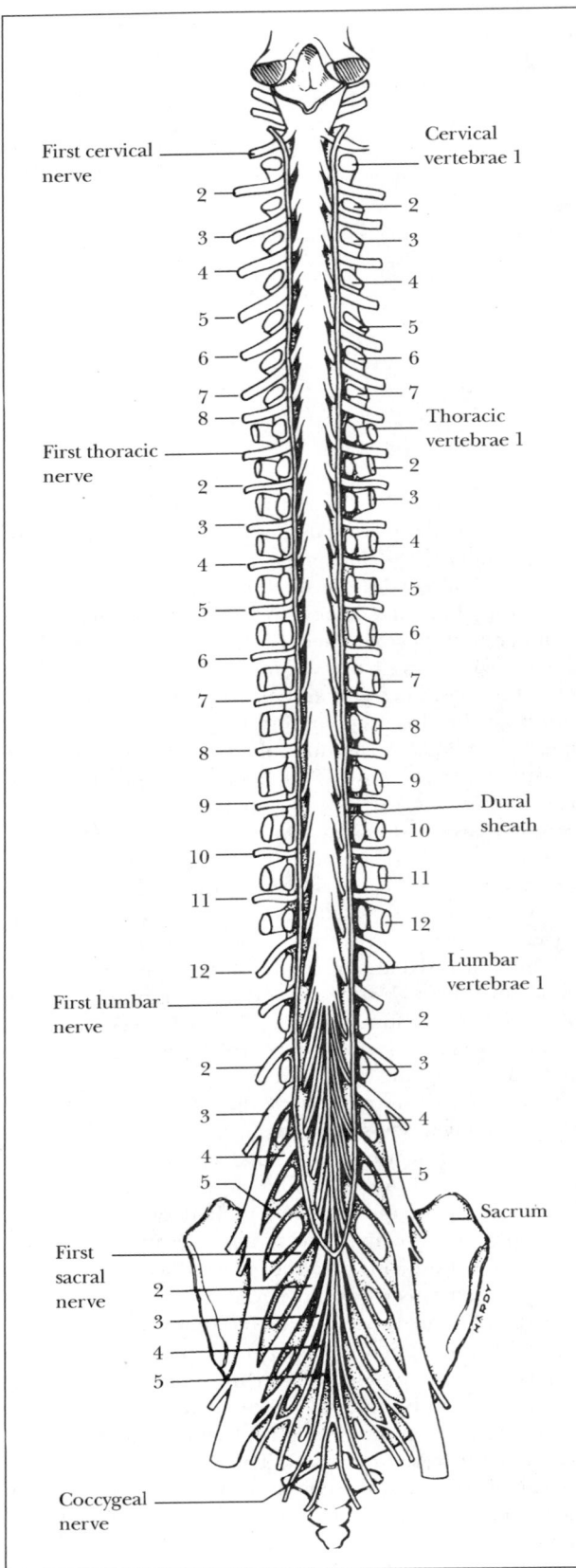

First cervical nerve

Cervical vertebrae 1

First thoracic nerve

Thoracic vertebrae 1

Dural sheath

Lumbar vertebrae 1

First lumbar nerve

First sacral nerve

Sacrum

Coccygeal nerve

**FIGURE 35-7** The spinal cord lying within the vertebral canal. Spinal nerves are numbered on the left side, and the vertebrae are numbered on the right side. (Reprinted with permission from Chaffee EE, Lytle IM: *Basic Physiology and Anatomy.* Philadelphia, Lippincott, 1980.[32])

less vascular than that of the brain.[29] The spinal meninges are shown in Figure 35-10.

### Physiology of intracranial pressure

An understanding of the normal physiology of intracranial pressure is essential in understanding the pathophysiology of brain tumors. Intracranial pressure (ICP) is the pressure exerted within the skull and meninges by brain tissue, CSF, and cerebral blood volume. The skull and meninges form a rigid compartment holding the three major components: brain tissue (comprising 80% of the total volume), CSF (constituting 10%), and the blood volume (accounting for the remaining 10%). The modified *Monro-Kellie hypothesis* is helpful in understanding the pathophysiology of ICP. It states that the rigid vault formed by the skull and meninges is filled to capacity with essentially noncompressible contents, which remain relatively constant, and therefore is unyielding to any increases in volume. If any one component increases in volume, a concomitant decrease in the volume of one or both of the remaining components must occur to maintain normal ICP. If the reciprocal compensation does not occur, ICP rises. The normal ICP is 4–15 mm Hg or 80–180 cm $H_2O$.

The mechanism by which this secondary decrease in volume occurs is called *compensation*. The compensatory mechanisms to decrease volume are as follows

- displacement of CSF from the cranial subarachnoid space to the spinal subarachnoid space

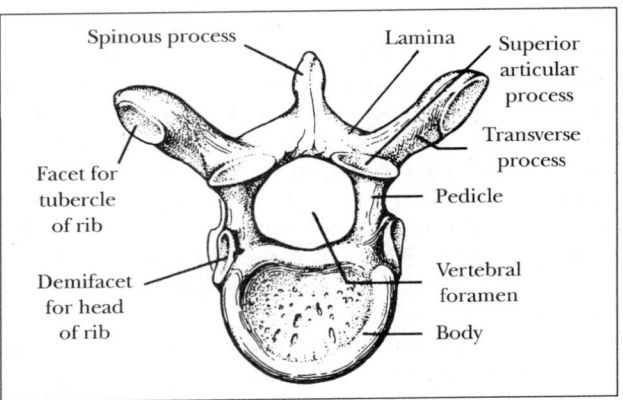

Spinous process

Lamina

Superior articular process

Transverse process

Facet for tubercle of rib

Pedicle

Demifacet for head of rib

Vertebral foramen

Body

**FIGURE 35-8** Thoracic vertebra. (Reprinted with permission from Hickey JV: *The Clinical Practice of Neurological and Neurosurgical Nursing* [ed 3]. Philadelphia, Lippincott, 1992.[29])

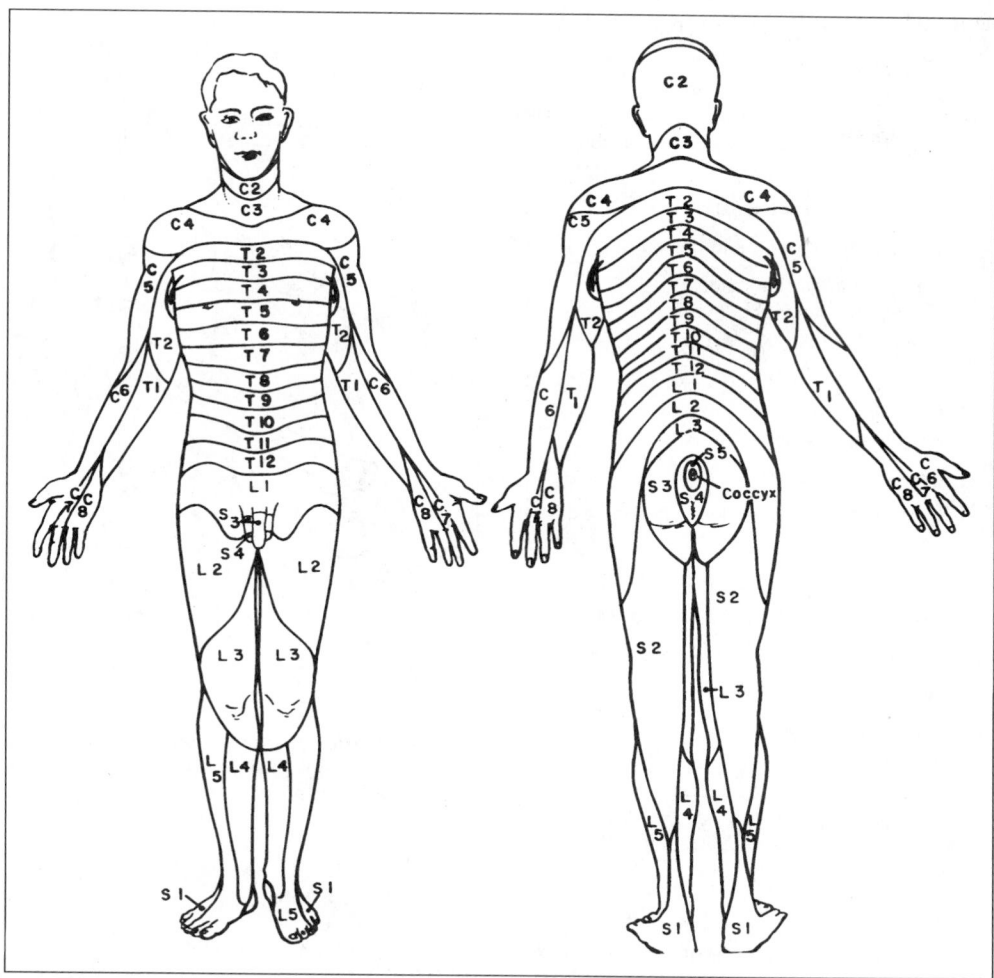

**FIGURE 35-9**   Cutaneous distribution of the spinal nerves (dermatomes). (Reprinted with permission from Barr ML and Kiernan JA: *The Human Nervous System* [ed 5]. Philadelphia, Lippincott, 1988.[35])

- a decrease in the CSF production by the choroid plexus
- an increase in the CSF absorption by the arachnoid villi
- shunting of venous blood from the affected area into the venous sinuses

These compensatory mechanisms are finite and eventually become exhausted. Once all the compensatory mechanisms are depleted, relatively small increases in volume result in large increases in ICP.

Small volume increments can be compensated far more readily than large volume increments. Increases in volume made over long periods can be accommodated more easily than a comparable quantity introduced within a much shorter interval. An individual with an acute subdural hematoma, a rapidly enlarging lesion, will develop signs and symptoms of increased ICP much more rapidly than a person with a large, slow-growing brain tumor.[29] The individual with the slow-growing tumor may not exhibit clinical signs and symptoms until the compensatory mechanisms have been exhausted.

Another important concept relating to ICP is *autoregulation*. Autoregulation maintains a normal ICP despite fluctuations in arterial pressure and venous drainage. It assures a constant cerebral blood flow when the mean systemic arterial pressure is between 60 and 160 mm Hg. Cerebral blood flow and cerebral blood volume are controlled through adjustments in the size of blood vessels.[31] In the presence of an increased systemic arterial pressure, autoregulatory vasoconstriction occurs, leading to an increased cerebral vascular resistance and a decreased cerebral blood flow. Likewise, a decreased systemic arterial pressure produces vasodilation and results in a decreased cerebral vascular resistance and an increased cerebral blood flow.[36]

Another consideration is that the cerebral venous system does not have valves as do other venous vessels in

**TABLE 35-2** Motor Nerve Roots (Myotomes) and Areas They Innervate

| Spinal Nerves | Muscles |
| --- | --- |
| C-1 to C-4 | Neck (flexion, lateral flexion, extension, rotation) |
| C-3 to C-5 | Diaphragm (respirations) |
| C-5 and C-6 | Shoulder movement and flexion of elbow |
| C-5 to C-7 | Forward thrust of shoulder Thumb and index finger (C-6) |
| C-5 to C-8 | Adduction of arm from front to back Middle finger (C-7) |
| C-6 to C-8 | Extension of forearm and wrist Ring and pinky fingers (C-8) |
| C-7, C-8, T-1 | Flexion of wrist |
| T-1 to T-12 | Control of thoracic, abdominal, and back muscles |
| L-1 to L-3 | Flexion of hip |
| L-2 to L-4 | Extension of leg and adduction of thigh |
| L-4, L-5, S-1, S-2 | Abduction of thigh and flexion of lower leg |
| L-4 to L-5 | Dorsal flexion of foot |
| L-5, S-1, S-2 | Plantar flexion of foot |
| S-2, S-3, S-4 | Perineal area and sphincters |

Data reprinted with permission from Hickey JV: *The Clinical Practice of Neurological and Neurosurgical Nursing* (ed 3). Philadelphia, Lippincott, 1992.[29]

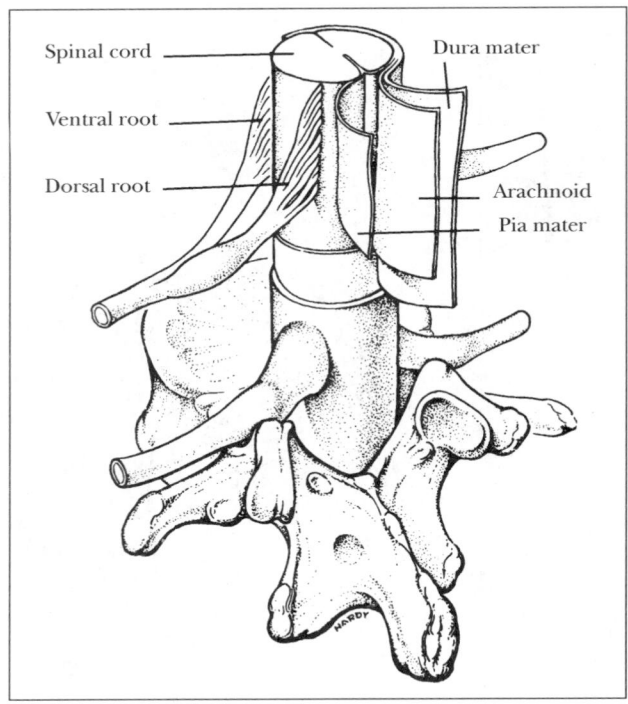

**FIGURE 35-10**   The spinal meninges. (Reprinted with permission from Hickey JV: *The Clinical Practice of Neurological and Neurosurgical Nursing* [ed 3]. Philadelphia, Lippincott, 1992.[29])

the body. Any condition that obstructs or compromises the venous outflow may also increase cerebral blood volume because more blood is backed up in the intracranial cavity.[29] Activities such as coughing, sneezing, or performing the Valsalva maneuver increase intrathoracic and intra-abdominal pressures that increase ICP by decreasing cerebral venous outflow via the jugular veins.[36] Rotation and extreme flexion or extension of the neck may also obstruct venous outflow and arterial inflow. Positive end-expiratory pressure (PEEP) treatments, hip flexion, and lying on the abdomen also increase thoracic and abdominal cavity pressures.[31] Elevating the head of the bed facilitates venous drainage.

The autoregulatory mechanism also responds to certain metabolic factors. The cerebral blood vessels vasodilate in response to increased $PaCO_2$ and decreased pH, leading to an increased cerebral blood flow and cerebral blood volume. A decreased $PaCO_2$ and increased pH lead to a decreased cerebral blow flow and cerebral blood volume.

## Gliomas

Gliomas are the most common primary brain tumor in adults and include the astrocytomas, oligodendrogliomas, ependymomas, and mixed gliomas.

### Astrocytomas

The majority of gliomas are astrocytomas, accounting for approximately 60% of all primary brain tumors. Astrocytomas arise from the star-shaped supportive tissue of the CNS, the astrocytes. These tumors are graded to describe their degree of malignancy. Grade is based on the tumor's microscopic appearance and indicates its similarity to normal cells, its tendency to spread, and its growth rate. Numerous grading systems exist for astrocytomas, with most of them using three or four grades of malignancy. The four-grade system describes these tumors as grade I through grade IV. In this system grade I tumors tend to be benign and grade IV tumors are the most malignant. The three-grade system divides this group of tumors into astrocytoma, anaplastic astrocytoma, and glioblastoma multiforme (GBM). The three-tiered grading system has been shown to be more closely related to prognosis and is widely used in grading astrocytomas today.[37]

Although it is generally recognized that higher grades of malignancy are associated with a poorer prognosis, the grading criteria for astrocytomas and for all gliomas appear to be somewhat inexact because patients differ. The prognosis for individuals with a specific tumor grade may be difficult to predict on the basis of grade alone. Clinically, astrocytomas with similar histological features may behave in a dissimilar fashion. The cellular composition of some tumors may be considered heterogeneous. There is a remarkable diversity of cells between different areas of the same tumor and between similar tumors of different individuals,[38] especially in those with the tumor GBM. Location of the astrocytic tumors may also have important implications for treatment and prognosis. Tumors located in vital or inaccessible areas may be difficult to treat despite their histologically benign character.

Increasing grades of malignancy within the astrocytoma group are often associated with patient age. Low-grade astrocytomas are most common in individuals between 20 and 40 years of age, anaplastic astrocytomas in individuals who are between 30 and 50, and GBM, the most malignant glioma, in those who are 50 or older.[37,39] Low-grade astrocytomas rarely occur in those over 50, whereas glioblastomas can occur in younger individuals and children. There is a slightly higher incidence of astrocytomas in males than in females.

Astrocytomas generally arise in the cerebral hemispheres. The lobar distribution of these tumors is similar to the amount of white matter present in each lobe, with the highest frequency occurring in the frontal lobes. Low-grade astrocytomas show an increased cellularity and have mild nuclear pleomorphism compared with normal brain tissue. Other features of anaplasia such as mitotic activity, vascular proliferative changes, and necrosis are absent. Some astrocytomas may be cystic, and microcalcifications can be present. These tumors are slightly discolored yellow or gray and have indistinct margins with the surrounding brain.[37] They are diffusely infiltrative tumors, although their invasion is largely limited to white matter.

The treatment of low-grade astrocytomas is controversial. Large symptomatic and progressive tumors are usually surgically resected. Some low-grade astrocytomas present with well-controlled seizures and are relatively small, asymptomatic, and indolent lesions. Many individuals with these tumors can be safely observed and closely monitored without surgery or other treatment. Intervention would be indicated if the tumor progressed, if the radiographic appearance changed (such as the development of new contrast enhancement), or if the individual developed new or uncontrolled symptoms.[40] In a retrospective study Recht et al[41] reported on a group of individuals with low-grade astrocytomas who were monitored without intervention other than anticonvulsants. When compared with another group of similar individuals who received immediate treatment with surgery and RT, there was little difference noted in either survival or quality of life. Delayed treatment postpones the risks of surgery and the side effects of RT. These astrocytomas are rarely cured because they cannot be completely excised. In addition, a large percentage of these tumors undergo malignant transformation to a higher tumor grade over time.

The high-grade gliomas are anaplastic astrocytoma and GBM. The histological features of the anaplastic astrocytoma are similar to the low-grade astrocytomas but are more abundant and exaggerated. Cellularity is increased, as are nuclear and cellular pleomorphism. Mitotic activity and proliferative vascular changes are found within the tumor. These changes may occur in the endothelial cells or in the cells of the vessel wall itself.[37] Necrosis

is not present. The GBM has these characteristics plus necrosis. Necrosis is the distinguishing factor between anaplastic astrocytoma and GBM. Glioblastomas infiltrate the brain extensively but rarely spread to distant locations. Anaplastic astrocytomas account for less than one-third of the gliomas, whereas the GBM is the most common adult primary brain tumor and represents more than 50% of the gliomas. Individuals with anaplastic astrocytoma have a significantly better prognosis than those with glioblastomas. Median survival for anaplastic astrocytoma is approximately 36 months, compared with 10–12 months for GBM.[42,43] Standard treatment for these high-grade gliomas includes surgery, RT, and chemotherapy.

### Oligodendrogliomas

Oligodendrogliomas represent between 3% and 7% of all primary brain tumors and 10%–15% of the gliomas. Oligodendrogliomas arise from the oligodendrocyte cell responsible for the development and maintenance of the myelin sheath.[44] About 50% of these tumors contain oligodendrocytes, astrocytes, and ependymal cells and are referred to as *mixed gliomas*. These tumors most frequently occur in middle-aged individuals, with a peak incidence between 25 and 49 years.[45]

These tumors typically present as well-defined, spongy, vascular masses, usually located in the frontal or temporal lobes of the cerebral hemispheres. Approximately 50% of oligodendrogliomas have calcifications within the tumor and adjacent brain tissue,[31,45] and up to 20% are cystic. Like astrocytomas, oligodendrogliomas vary in malignancy. Pure oligodendrogliomas are relatively low-grade and well-differentiated, with cells that appear only slightly abnormal. They tend to be slow-growing and are often present for many years before diagnosis. Malignant forms, or anaplastic oligodendrogliomas, have highly abnormal-looking cells and usually grow faster. Anaplastic features include areas of necrosis and proliferation of blood vessels.[31,44] Other grading systems such as A–D or I–IV may also be used to describe these tumors. They are graded by the most malignant type of cell found in the tumor tissue.

Clinically these tumors present in the same fashion as other similarly located tumors. However, two features separate the oligodendrogliomas: the antecedent (prodromal) history, averaging seven to eight years, tends to be longer, and seizures are more common, occurring in 70%–90% of patients by the time of diagnosis.[45] The standard treatments for oligodendrogliomas have been surgery, when a good neurological outcome is possible, and RT. Large symptomatic, unresectable, or incompletely resected tumors should be treated with RT.[46] The role of postoperative RT is controversial for well-differentiated tumors. Oligodendrogliomas are chemosensitive tumors. The PCV (procarbazine, CCNU, vincristine) regimen developed by Levin et al[45] is particularly effective, although responses have also been seen with carmustine (BCNU), melphalan, and thiotepa. Responses to PCV have also been reported in low-grade oligodendrogliomas.[47] The unique response this tumor shows to chemotherapy has led to additional clinical trials to determine the most effective treatment.

### Ependymomas

Ependymomas represent less than 5% of all adult primary brain tumors and 9% of the gliomas.[48] They occur in all age-groups but are most often seen in young adults and children. Ependymomas arise from these ependymal cells, which form the lining of the ventricles and the central canal of the spinal cord.

The majority of intracranial ependymomas are infratentorial and usually arise from the fourth ventricle. Supratentorial tumors develop from the ependymal lining of the third and lateral ventricles or may be located deep in the cerebral hemispheres without visible connection to the ventricles.[44,45] Ependymomas may be differentiated and low-grade or anaplastic and high-grade. The characteristic histological pattern of low-grade ependymomas consists of epithelial-like arrangements of cells around an irregular open space or a radiating, tapering process of tumor cells surrounding a blood vessel.[48] In addition to the typical pattern of low-grade tumors, malignant or anaplastic ependymomas also have cellular pleomorphism, necrosis, mitoses, and multinucleation.[49]

High-grade and infratentorial tumors are more likely to spread through the CSF pathways. Signs and symptoms vary depending on the location of the tumor. Ependymomas are often associated with obstructive hydrocephalus, and a ventriculoperitoneal shunt may be required to relieve the increased ICP.

Standard treatment of ependymomas is surgery and RT. Maximal surgical resection should be performed when possible. Low-grade tumors are treated with local RT unless there is evidence of disseminated disease, which requires full craniospinal radiation. Malignant ependymomas are generally treated with craniospinal radiation, but there is an increasing tendency to treat these tumors locally because the majority recur at the primary site. Chemotherapy is used primarily for recurrent ependymomas. A variety of agents used alone or in combination have been investigated, including CCNU, BCNU, carboplatin, cisplatin, procarbazine, vincristine, and cytoxan.

### Meningiomas

Meningiomas, the most common benign brain tumors, account for up to 20% of all adult intracranial tumors. They arise from the cap cells of the arachnoid layer of the meninges and are often located near major venous sinuses, large cerebral blood vessels, and the skull base.[50,51] Meningiomas occur twice as often in women as in men and tend to occur late in life, with a peak incidence in the sixth decade for men and the seventh decade for women. The incidence of meningiomas is also higher in individuals with breast cancer.[52,53]

Most meningiomas are differentiated with low proliferative capacity and limited invasiveness and have well-defined borders. The traditional classification divides meningiomas into various subtypes, but this distinction has little prognostic significance with the possible exception of the malignant meningioma. The malignant meningioma contains abundant mitoses, nuclear pleomorphism, necrosis, high nuclear to cytoplasmic ratio, loss of normal architecture, and invasion of surrounding brain tissue.[54] Malignant meningiomas account for 12% of all meningiomas, occur more often in men, are frequently multifocal, cause systemic metastases in up to 24% of patients,[52,55] and generally have a high recurrence rate.

Meningiomas produce symptoms by compression of surrounding brain tissue rather than by infiltration. Individuals may present with seizures, headache, increased ICP, focal neurological deficits such as altered mentation and hemiparesis, and cranial neuropathies. The precise clinical features vary depending on the exact location of the tumor.

The primary treatment modality for meningiomas is surgery, with the extent of surgical resection the primary factor influencing the recurrence rate. Factors that impede the possibility of complete resection are tumor location, size, consistency, vascular and cranial nerve involvement, and, in the case of recurrence, prior surgery, radiotherapy, or both. Better understanding of neuroanatomy and improved neurosurgical techniques allow many previously unresectable meningiomas to be surgically excised today. RT is indicated for individuals with inoperable, partially resected, and recurrent meningiomas. Chemotherapy for malignant meningiomas using varied regimens has been generally unsuccessful. There have been occasional responses to alpha-interferon.[50]

The growth of meningiomas may be influenced by hormones and growth factors. Approximately 30% of meningiomas have estrogen receptors, and 70%–80% have progesterone receptors.[52,56] Treatment with antiestrogens such as tamoxifen has been ineffective,[52,57] but antiprogesterone agents have shown promise.[52,58] Current studies are under way to investigate the possibility of medical therapy as treatment for meningioma.

### Vestibular Schwannomas (Acoustic Neuromas)

Vestibular schwannomas, traditionally called *acoustic neuromas*, are benign tumors arising from the Schwann cells at the vestibular portion of the eighth cranial nerve (vestibulocochlear or acoustic nerve). They account for approximately 10% of all intracranial tumors and commonly occur in individuals between the ages of 30 and 60 years. These are very slow-growing tumors whose symptoms are related to compression and stretching of cranial nerves, causing interference with their function.[59] As the tumor expands from its origin on the vestibular nerve, it extends into the area between the cerebellum, pons, and medulla known as the ***cerebellopontine angle.*** The cochlear, trigeminal, and facial nerves are compressed. As the tumor continues to grow, it ultimately compresses the cerebellar peduncles, cerebellum, brain stem, and cranial nerves IX, X, and XI (glossopharyngeal, vagus, and spinal accessory nerves).[52] The most common presenting symptom is a unilateral sensorineural hearing loss. Other initial symptoms are tinnitus, vertigo, and disequilibrium. Late clinical features are facial palsy, facial numbness, headache, ataxia, diplopia, dysphagia, and hydrocephalus.[52,54]

Diagnostic tests include audiometry and brain stem auditory evoked potentials followed by magnetic resonance imaging (MRI) with gadolinium. Surgery and radiosurgery are the primary treatment modalities for most individuals with vestibular schwannomas. The goal of surgery is to completely remove the tumor while preserving facial nerve function and hearing. Because most of these tumors lie around the vestibular portion of the eighth cranial nerve, the nerve will most likely be severed during surgery in order to remove the entire tumor.[60] Vertigo occurs as a result. When Wiegand and Fickel[61] surveyed postoperative acoustic neuroma patients, 90% reported some degree of vertigo, while 8% rated vertigo as a severe handicap. For those tumors not completely resected or in individuals who do not undergo surgery, radiosurgery may be used.

## Primary Central Nervous System Lymphomas

PCNSL is an aggressive non-Hodgkin's lymphoma that arises within and is confined to the CNS.[62] Until recently, PCNSL has been a rare tumor, accounting for only 2% of all intracranial cancers.[63,64] However, it is increasing in both immunocompetent and immunosuppressed individuals. The number of cases of PCNSL in otherwise healthy individuals has more than tripled in recent years and cannot be attributed to new and improved diagnostic techniques, the adoption of a uniform classification system, or a similar rise in the number of systemic lymphomas diagnosed.[63,65] PCNSL is often associated with acquired or congenital immunosuppression. The highest incidence occurs in patients with AIDS where PCNSL develops in up to 6% of cases.[62,66] This number may actually be higher because up to 50% of AIDS-related PCNSLs are diagnosed only at autopsy.[67] PCNSL is the second most common brain lesion and the fourth most common cause of death in AIDS patients.[64] Other populations at risk include organ transplant recipients, individuals with collagen vascular diseases, and those with congenital immunodeficiencies.

PCNSL is almost always disseminated within the CNS. The sites involved are the brain, leptomeninges, eyes, and (rarely) the spinal cord. Ninety-five percent of patients diagnosed with PCNSL have a brain lesion, and 50% of these lesions are multifocal. The lesions are often periventricular and involve the leptomeninges. As a result, seeding within the CSF often occurs. Positive cytology is found in approximately one-third of patients at diagnosis, and an additional one-third have a suspicious cytology.[68] The eyes are a direct extension of the nervous system and are involved in up to 20% of patients at diagnosis. Lymphoma may begin in the eye only. Eventually more than one-half of these patients will go on to develop brain lymphoma.[69]

These non-Hodgkin's lymphomas are primarily of B-cell origin and are of the intermediate- to high-grade type. PCNSL is a stage $I_E$ lymphoma, i.e., confined to a single extranodal site. These patients show no evidence of a systemic lymphoma. The EBV ·has been found in pathology specimens of AIDS patients with PCNSL, but it is not yet known what role this plays in the development of PCNSL.

Most PCNSLs involve the frontal lobes. Common symptoms include the following:

- changes in level of consciousness (lethargy, confusion)

- changes in personality (apathy, flat affect)

- signs of increased ICP (headache, nausea, vomiting)

- motor symptoms (hemiparesis or hemiplegia)

- visual disturbances

- seizures (rarely)

Diagnostic workup includes MRI, CSF analysis, ophthalmologic exam, and a systemic workup to rule out systemic lymphoma. In immunocompetent individuals, PCNSL has a typical appearance on MRI that can help distinguish it from other processes. The lesions are usually multifocal, uniformly enhance with contrast, and are located near the ventricles, basal ganglia, and corpus callosum. If a diagnosis is made from positive CSF cytology or a positive biopsy of the vitreous of the eye, a brain biopsy is unnecessary. The most successful treatments to date in immunocompetent individuals have been with intra-Ommaya and high-dose intravenous (IV) methotrexate followed by focal RT,[68] blood-brain barrier disruption with mannitol followed by intra-arterial and systemic chemotherapy without RT,[70] and the combination of procarbazine, lomustine, and vincristine (PCV),[71] yielding a mean survival of 41–44.5 months. The behavior of PCNSL in the immunosuppressed population differs from that in immunocompetent individuals, thereby creating specific diagnostic and therapeutic challenges.

## Metastatic Brain Tumors

Approximately 80,000–100,000 metastatic brain tumors are diagnosed each year.[72] Twenty-four percent of patients with systemic cancer develop brain metastases.[73,74] The incidence of brain metastases is increasing as patients are living longer, there is better control of systemic cancer, and cancers that commonly metastasize to the brain, e.g., lung and breast, are also on the rise. Other contributing factors to this phenomenon are advances in neuroimaging, use of routine staging tests that assess the CNS, and perhaps the sanctuary effect provided by the blood-brain barrier, which may isolate the nervous system tissue from the antitumor effects of systemic chemotherapy.[75]

Brain metastases occur at three sites: the brain parenchyma itself, the skull and dura, and the leptomeninges. Parenchymal brain metastases occur in more than 60% of these cases, with dural and leptomeningeal metastases accounting for the remainder.[74,76] The majority of brain metastases are a result of hematogenous spread from the primary tumor. The lung is the most common site of origin. If the primary tumor is not pulmonary, it may have metastasized to the lungs before reaching the brain. In addition, the majority of metastatic brain tumors of unknown primary cancer are of the lung. From the lungs, cancer cells may enter the pulmonary veins and reach the left atrium and ventricle. Tumor cells transported in this manner are widely dispersed and are ultimately deposited in the arterial circulation, where the tumor cells can readily travel to the brain.[31] Other cancers that commonly metastasize to the brain include breast cancer, melanoma, colon cancer, and renal cancer. Breast and lung cancers are prevalent in the population, whereas melanoma accounts for only 1% of all cancers diagnosed. Yet melanoma has the highest propensity of all systemic cancers to metastasize to the brain. Almost 40% of patients with melanoma develop brain metastases,[74,77] making it, despite the rarity of melanoma as a primary tumor, the third-most-frequent cause of brain metastases.

When neurological symptoms of brain metastases develop, the individual often has widespread systemic disease. Brain metastases are characterized by severe peritumoral edema, which contributes to the neurological symptoms. The presenting signs and symptoms of metastatic brain disease are dependent upon the lesion's location in the brain and can be identical to those of other space-occupying lesions. Most brain metastases occur in the cerebral hemispheres. Symptoms include signs of increased ICP (headache, nausea, vomiting), change in level of consciousness, diminished cognitive function, personality changes, hemiparesis, language problems, and seizures. Seizures occur as the initial presenting symptom in 15%–20% of patients. Because these lesions are often hemorrhagic, seizures are particularly common in metastatic melanoma, occurring 50% of the time.[74,78]

Approximately half of the patients with brain metastases have a single metastatic lesion, and an additional 20% have only two lesions.[74,76,77] With early diagnosis and management, brain metastases often respond to therapy. Most patients benefit from palliative treatment; an increasing number of patients experience a prolonged remission or, rarely, are cured of their cerebral disease. Neurological function may be preserved and quality of life maintained. Thus, systemic cancer rather than neurological disease usually limits life expectancy.[75,79]

For many years WBRT has been the standard treatment for both single and multiple brain metastases. Patchell et al[80] compared surgery plus WBRT versus WBRT alone in a randomized prospective study and found a significantly prolonged survival in the individuals who received surgery and WBRT. In addition, those undergoing surgery maintained a higher performance status and improved quality of life for a longer period of time compared with those receiving WBRT alone.[81,82] While surgery may be considered the first therapeutic intervention for many individuals with a single cerebral metastatic lesion,[74] some physicians advocate radiosurgery in its place. Current treatment options include WBRT, surgery and WBRT, radiosurgery and WBRT, and occasionally adjuvant chemotherapy. Current clinical trials are evaluating WBRT alone compared with WBRT and radiosurgery.

Tumors that metastasize to the bone, particularly metastatic tumors of the breast, prostate, and lung, may infiltrate the skull or dura by direct extension and may compress the venous sinuses or underlying brain tissue. Signs and symptoms include headache, a palpable mass, seizures, and other common symptoms of a parenchymal brain mass. Treatment may be RT or surgical resection.

Leptomeningeal metastasis, once thought to be a rare complication of cancer, is increasing in frequency. Leptomeningeal metastasis, or meningeal carcinomatosis, is a diffuse or multifocal seeding of cancer cells throughout the meninges and CSF. The seeding pattern of growth covers the surface of the brain and spinal cord.[83]

Although the exact incidence of leptomeningeal metastasis is difficult to determine, studies have found an overall incidence of up to 8%.[76] While any systemic cancer can seed the meninges, the most common cancers leading to meningeal carcinomatosis are leukemia, lymphoma, melanoma, and breast, lung, and gastrointestinal (GI) cancers. The incidence of meningeal leukemia has decreased, while leptomeningeal metastases from breast and lung cancer are increasing. Clinical manifestations are headache, mental status changes, gait disturbances, hydrocephalus, cranial nerve palsies, back pain, radiculopathies, weakness, and paresthesias. Diagnosis is established by close examination of the CSF and MRI of the brain and spinal cord. Repeated lumbar punctures are often required to identify malignant cells in the CSF. Other CSF findings are elevated CSF pressure, increased white blood cell (WBC) count, elevated protein, and decreased glucose. Treatment includes RT to symptomatic areas only because radiation to the entire neuroaxis leads to bone marrow depression. This is followed by chemotherapy administered directly into the CSF. Chemotherapy can be injected directly into the lateral ventricle of the brain by using an Ommaya reservoir, thus ensuring optimal consistent CSF levels. Common chemotherapeutic agents include methotrexate, cytarabine, and thiotepa. Reports of median survival range from 7 to 24 weeks.[76]

## Spinal Cord Tumors

Primary spinal cord tumors occur less frequently than primary brain tumors, accounting for only 15% of all primary CNS tumors. They occur most often in individuals between 20 and 60 years of age, and with the exception of meningiomas, which occur more often in women, spinal cord tumors are found with equal frequency in men and women. Spinal tumors are classified by their cell of origin and their anatomic location. The major anatomic consideration of spinal cord tumors relates to the tumor's location in relation to the spinal dura mater (Figure 35-11).[84] The classification and frequency of spinal cord tumors are found in Table 35-3. Extradural tumors lie outside the dura. Most of these tumors are caused by metastatic cancer to the vertebral column, a common site of bone metastasis. Metastatic spinal cord tumors most often originate from cancers of the breast, lung, prostate, and kidney and from multiple myeloma. Less common are cancers of the GI tract, thyroid, and melanoma. However, other tumor types can lead to vertebral body metastases as well. The neurological symptoms seen with extradural tumors result from compression rather than invasion of the spinal cord. The spinal cord is usually compressed anteriorly because the tumors develop between the dura and periosteum. This compression leads to edema and ischemia of the spinal cord and mechanically distorts and damages the neural tissue. Spinal cord compression (SCC) occurs either by direct extension of the tumor into the epidural space, by vertebral collapse

**TABLE 35-3**   Classification and Frequency of Spinal Cord Tumors

| EXTRADURAL (45%) |
| --- |
| Metastatic (from solid tumors) |
| Sarcoma |
| Lymphoma |
| Myeloma |
| Chrodoma |

| INTRADURAL (55%) |
| --- |
| Extramedullary (35%) |
|   Schwannoma |
|   Meningioma |
| Intramedullary (20%) |
|   Ependymoma |
|   Astrocytoma |
|   Oligodendroglioma |
|   Hemangioblastoma |
|   Mixed glioma |

and displacement of bone into the epidural space, or by direct extension through the intervertebral foramina.

The thoracic spine is the most frequent location of epidural SCC, followed by the lumbosacral and cervical

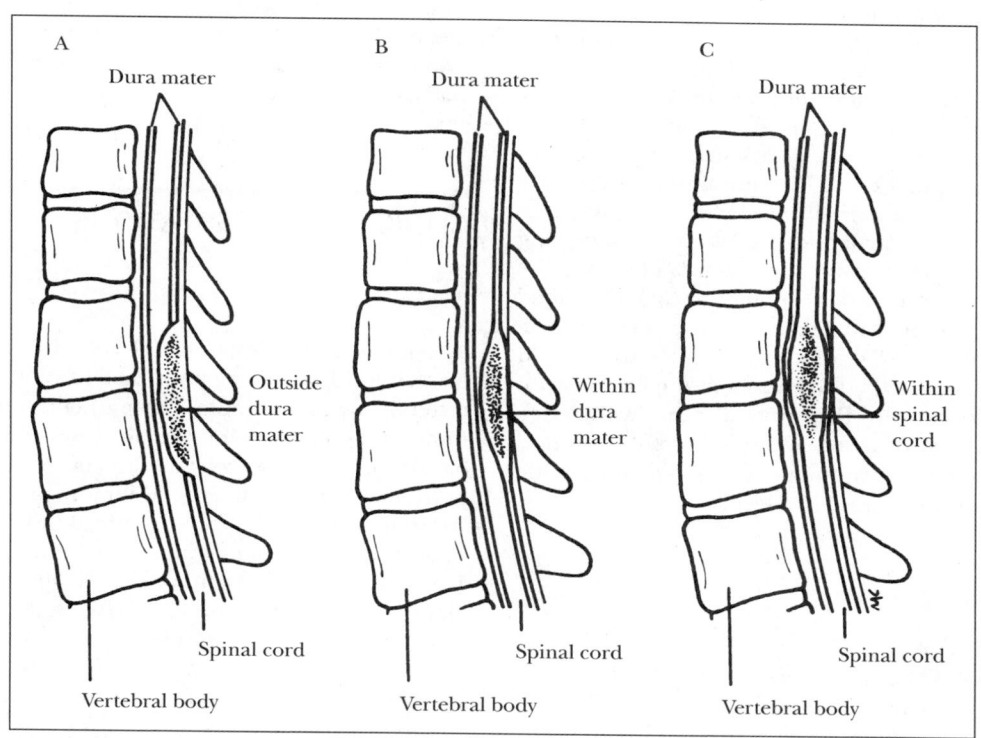

**FIGURE 35-11**   Possible locations of spinal tumors in a lateral longitudinal section of the vertebrae and spinal cord. The shaded area indicates tumor sites. (Schott GD: Spinal tumors I: Classification. *Nurs Times* 71:2055–2057, 1975.[84] A: Extradural lesion. B: Intradural or extramedullary lesion. C: Intramedullary lesion. Reproduced by kind permission of *Nursing Times* where this figure first appeared with the article "Spinal Tumours I: Classification" on December 25, 1975.)

spine. Lung and breast cancer most often cause thoracic compression, whereas prostate, renal, and GI tumors are more likely to affect the lower thoracic or lumbosacral vertebrae.

Epidural SCC is a relatively common neurological complication of cancer. It occurs in 5%–10% of cancer patients and is considered an oncological emergency. The incidence of SCC may actually be increasing because patients are living longer and the incidence of cancers that commonly spread to the bone is rising. Epidural SCC usually occurs late during the course of metastatic cancer, often during its terminal stages.[76]

Lymphomas may be a cause of SCC because they can extend directly through the intervertebral foramina. Other tumors such as sarcoma and chordoma may arise as primary extradural tumors. The chordoma is a slow-growing but highly invasive tumor. It often occurs in the sacrum but can also be found in the cervical spine and intracranially at the base of the skull. This tumor erodes bone and soft tissue extensively, and even though it is histologically benign, it is difficult to remove in its entirety.[85]

Intradural tumors arise from the nerve roots or coverings of the spinal cord (intradural, extramedullary) or develop in the spinal cord itself (intradural, intramedullary). Schwannomas are the most common extramedullary tumor, followed by meningiomas. They account for 90% of these tumors, and both types occur most commonly in the thoracic spine. The majority of intramedullary tumors are ependymomas, followed next by astrocytomas and then oligodendrogliomas. Ependymomas are frequently located in the lumbosacral area, whereas astrocytomas are distributed more evenly throughout the spinal cord. The intradural tumors are histologically identical to their intracranial counterparts; however, the grade of malignancy is often lower, making the majority of primary spinal cord tumors benign.

Spinal cord tumors are also anatomically described based on their location in relation to the vertebral column. Approximately 50% of spinal tumors are located in the thoracic spine, 30% are located in the lumbosacral region, and 20% involve the cervical spine. Knowledge of the specific level of involvement is helpful in understanding the signs and symptoms in relation to the specific dermatomes and myotomes involved.

## Pattern of Spread

The pattern of spread of CNS cancers differs from that of other tumors. While these tumors may spread to other parts of the CNS, metastases outside the brain and spinal cord are rare. Metastases outside the CNS may occur when tumor cells are transferred to the scalp, cerebral blood vessels, or dural sinus during an operative procedure. Once they invade the cerebral blood vessels, tumor cells enter the circulation. Once the tumor cells have traveled outside the CNS, they can also spread through the lymphatic system.[28] The spread of glial tumor cells through ventriculopleural and ventriculoperitoneal shunts has also been reported.

It is more common for CNS cancers to spread to other areas in the CNS. Brain tumors grow by expansion, infiltration, or both. While gliomas rarely metastasize to distant sites outside the CNS, they do invade locally. Glioma cells are sometimes found at intracranial sites distant from the main tumor, making many of these lesions seem multifocal. Cancers of the CNS may seed the CSF and spread through the subarachnoid space. Seeding occurs along the surface of the brain and spinal cord, and "drop metastases" can occur. Some tumors, including PCNSLs, ependymomas, and medulloblastomas, seed the CSF more often than others.

Most metastatic brain tumors develop from hematogenous spread of tumor cells, usually through the arterial circulation. In some cases tumor cells may reach the brain via the Batson's plexus. Batson's plexus is a valveless system of veins that runs the length of the vertebral column from the pelvic veins to the large venous sinuses of the skull.[31]

The most common mechanism of spread for extradural spinal metastases is thought to be by hematogenous arterial spread to bone marrow, which results in vertebral body collapse and formation of an anterior epidural mass. A second mechanism of spread is by direct invasion through the intervertebral foramina. Another probable mechanism of metastatic epidural spinal cord compression is by retrograde venous spread from the primary site via Batson's plexus.[86]

## CLINICAL MANIFESTATIONS

### Brain Tumors

The clinical manifestations of a brain tumor can vary tremendously from one individual to another and among different types of tumors. The particular signs and symptoms with which an individual presents are dependent on the location, size, type, method of expansion, and rate of tumor growth. Intracranial tumors produce signs and symptoms by creating a mass effect and increasing ICP, by infiltrating and damaging normal brain tissue, or both. The clinical manifestations can be divided into three major categories: generalized effects of increased ICP, focal effects, and effects caused by displacement of brain structures. Often a combination of these effects produces signs and symptoms simultaneously (Figure 35-12).

#### Generalized effects of increased ICP

Brain tumors increase ICP by their size, cerebral edema, or obstruction of CSF pathways. The presence of increased ICP and the speed at which it develops can be

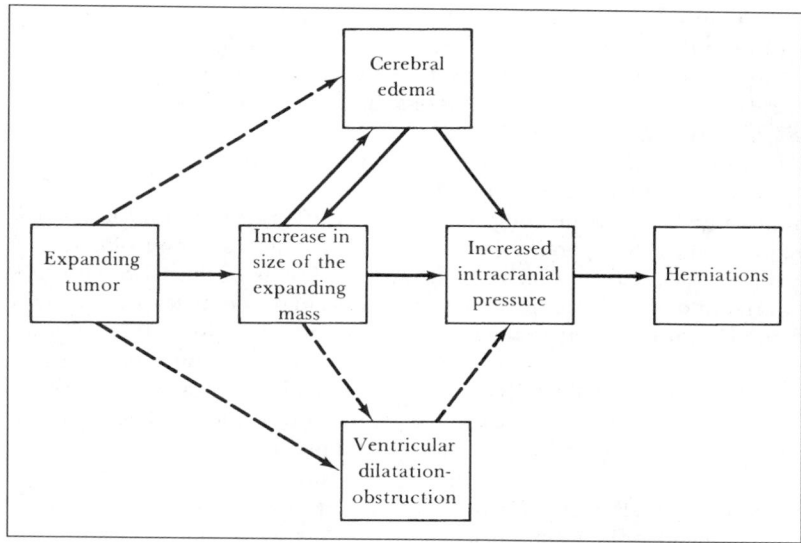

**FIGURE 35-12**  Mechanisms responsible for the clinical manifestations of intracranial tumors.[31]

variable. In some locations of the brain, a very small tumor can lead to marked elevations of ICP. For example, a relatively small tumor near the third or fourth ventricle can obstruct the CSF flow. In other areas of the brain, however, large, extensive tumors may not initially cause ICP to rise, as in some tumors of the frontal or temporal lobes. A rapidly developing tumor with extensive edema will raise ICP sooner than a slower-growing lesion with little edema.

Signs and symptoms result from the effects of increasing pressure on nerve cells, blood vessels, and the dura. Sustained increases in ICP ultimately cause nerve cell damage and cell death. An expanding tumor (or other space-occupying lesion) can create a vicious cycle of intracranial hypertension (Figure 35-13). After the brain's normal compensatory mechanisms have been exhausted, the increased ICP results in a decreased cerebral blood flow. The cerebral blood flow drops because the autoregulatory system fails. Failure of the autoregulatory system means that cerebral blood flow will now fluctuate passively with the systemic arterial pressure, unlike the healthy brain, where cerebral blood flow is relatively constant. Increases in systemic blood pressure will now directly affect ICP. A reduction in the brain's blood supply leads to tissue hypoxia because the brain does not receive sufficient oxygen. The diminished blood supply also interferes with the removal of carbon dioxide and lactic acid. These metabolic by-products act as potent vasodilators. Vasodilation of the cerebral blood vessels leads to further edema. As a result, the total volume within the cranium increases, ICP rises further, and the cycle repeats itself.[31]

The signs and symptoms of increased ICP include change in the level of consciousness or cognition, headache, pupillary changes and papilledema, motor and sensory deficits, vomiting, and changes in vital signs.

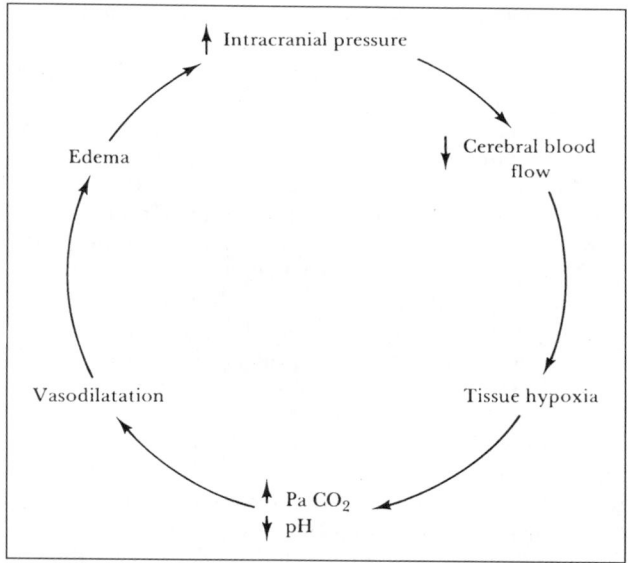

**FIGURE 35-13**  Cycle of intracranial hypertension.[31]

Increased ICP may cause additional effects by displacing brain tissue.

Level of consciousness can be an extremely sensitive index of neurological status[30] and ranges from alert and oriented, restless, confused, unable to follow simple commands, lethargic, to comatose. An individual may have short-term memory loss, impaired judgment, or difficulty concentrating, or may be forgetful. He or she may be drowsy or may exhibit personality changes or diminished cognitive ability. Sleeping more is the most commonly reported early sign of the tumor. Many of the initial changes have a gradual onset and can be so subtle that they are evident only to the family or a skilled observer.[31] Families may report that the individual just isn't himself or herself. If the increased ICP is not treated, the level of consciousness deteriorates further.

Headache is a common presenting symptom in individuals with intracranial tumors. The location and characteristics of the headache must be evaluated to distinguish them from other common types of headache (migraine, tension, muscle contraction). The brain parenchyma itself does not contain pain sensors. The headache pain is attributed to pressure or traction on pain-sensitive structures such as the dura, venous sinuses, blood vessels, and cranial nerves.

The headache is usually bilateral in the frontal, temporal, or retro-orbital areas. Typically, the pain occurs in the early morning, subsides after arising, and recurs the following morning. The pain can be described as dull, sharp, or throbbing. Some individuals complain of an uncomfortable feeling in the head rather than a headache. Bending over, coughing, or performing a Valsalva maneuver often aggravates or initiates the pain. The headaches gradually increase in frequency, duration, and severity until, in their later stages, they are almost constant and may be associated with other signs and symptoms of increased ICP.[76]

Papilledema is considered a cardinal sign of increased ICP, but it may be a late finding. The edema of the optic disk results from compression around the optic nerve impeding the outflow of venous blood. The presence of papilledema should be assessed by a trained individual using an ophthalmoscope. Other visual signs and symptoms can occur, including blurry vision, visual field deficits, and changes in pupillary size and reaction to light.

Motor signs of increased ICP include hemiparesis or hemiplegia on the contralateral side of the tumor, diminished reflexes, or the development of pathological reflexes. Decorticate and decerebrate posturing can occur in the late stages of increased ICP when the diencephalon and brain stem become compressed. Decorticate posturing is an abnormal flexion of the arms with extension of the legs. Decerebrate posturing is an abnormal extension of the arms and legs. Sensory symptoms consist of impaired sensation, inability to interpret sensory information, or both.

Vomiting as a sign of increased ICP occurs more commonly in children and in individuals with infratentorial tumors.[2] Vomiting may be preceded by nausea, or it may be sudden, unexpected, and projectile. It is not related to food ingestion. Increased pressure on the vomiting center of the medulla is believed to precipitate this symptom.[31]

Changes in vital signs occur late in the course of increased ICP. They result from increased pressure on the vasoactive centers of the medulla in the brain stem. Systolic blood pressure rises and diastolic blood pressure drops, thus widening the pulse pressure. Bradycardia and an abnormal respiratory pattern (usually slowed and irregular respirations) develop. This combination of hypertension, bradycardia, and abnormal respirations, referred to as *Cushing's triad*, is a very late sign of increased ICP. By the time Cushing's triad is identified, the patient is usually already comatose.

### Focal effects

Intracranial tumors also cause localized or focal signs and symptoms of neurological dysfunction. Specific anatomic areas in the CNS have unique functions, and the neurological deficits produced are directly related to the particular area involved. Performing a careful neurological examination and possessing knowledge of neuroanatomy and neurophysiology can assist in identifying the location of a lesion based on the neurological findings (Table 35-1).

Tumors of the frontal lobe can cause a variety of symptoms, including inability to concentrate, inattentiveness, difficulty with abstraction, impaired memory, personality changes, quiet flat affect, inappropriate behavior, lack of social control, indifference, emotional lability, and loss of initiative. Tumors of the motor strip cause hemiparesis or hemiplegia on the contralateral (opposite) side of the tumor. Deep tendon reflexes increase on the paretic side, and a positive Babinski sign is present. Broca's area is located in the frontal lobe. Damage to this area in the dominant hemisphere results in the inability to express oneself in words even though the individual may comprehend speech and language. Broca's aphasia has been referred to as *expressive aphasia* and can be extremely frustrating for individuals.

Most people have one cerebral hemisphere that is more developed or dominant than the other with respect to language. In right-handed individuals and most left-handed people, the dominant hemisphere is the left. This is important to distinguish because the left side of the brain controls language and the right hemisphere (nondominant side in the majority of people) is the nonverbal or perceptual hemisphere, which processes temporospatial information.

Parietal lobe tumors affect sensory and perceptual functions more than motor function, although mild hemiparesis is sometimes seen with these tumors.[2] Tumors in either lobe can cause mild to severe disturbances. Common symptoms include impaired sensation, paresthesias, loss of two-point discrimination, inability to recognize an object by feeling its size and shape (astereognosis), inability to locate or recognize parts of the body (autotopagnosia), loss of awareness or denial of a motor or sensory defect in the affected body part (anosognosia), inability to write (agraphia) or to calculate numbers (acalculia), and inability to execute learned movements in the absence of weakness or paralysis (apraxia).

Tumors of the temporal lobe can cause impairment of recent memory, aggressive behavior, and psychomotor seizures. Psychomotor seizures are described as visual, auditory, or olfactory hallucinations and may begin with an aura. These seizures may be characterized by automatism and behavioral changes. Involvement of the dominant side can lead to an inability to recall names (dysnomia), impaired perception of verbal commands, and Wernicke's or receptive aphasia. In this type of aphasia (more appropriately called dysphasia), the patient speaks easily, appears to be making an effort to communicate, and is easily engaged in conversation. However, little meaning is conveyed. The patient may speak in phrases or complete sentences, but the listener is usually unable to make sense of the content.

Occipital lobe tumors produce visual symptoms, including homonymous hemianopia (visual loss in half of each visual field on the contralateral side of the lesion) and visual hallucinations. Tumors located in this area can also interfere with the ability to interpret what is seen.

Tumors located in or near the thalamus can lead to hydrocephalus, mild sensory disturbances or paresthesias and neuropathic pain, emotional lability, and sleep pattern disturbances. Hypothalamic tumors typically lead to endocrine dysfunction. These tumors can also affect water metabolism, appetite, sexual behavior, regulation of temperature, and sleep-wake patterns.

Brain stem tumors can produce dire consequences, since the centers that control respiration and heart rate are located here. The points of origin of cranial nerves III through XII are also located here, and dysfunction is common.

Tumors located in the cerebellum have a classic presentation. Individuals may have a wide-based ataxic gait, a dysarthric speech pattern, and nystagmus. They may exhibit clumsiness, balance difficulty, or tremors. Symptoms of increased ICP such as early morning headache and vomiting are often present.

Seizures, another common clinical manifestation in both primary and metastatic brain tumors, are seen primarily with supratentorial tumors. Seizures may occur in 70%–90% of individuals with low-grade gliomas and oligodendrogliomas, and in 20%–30% of individuals with other tumor types. They may be the initial presenting symptom in a number of patients, sometimes occurring months to years before the clinical diagnosis is made.

Seizures can also occur as a treatment-related complication.

The focal effects of a tumor, causing cerebral edema and alterations in the electrical potential of normal nerve cells, result in hyperactive cells. This hyperactivity, in turn, produces abnormal, paroxysmal discharges or seizure activity that can be focal or generalized.[29] Focal or partial seizures involve a particular area of the brain, whereas generalized seizures involve both cerebral hemispheres. Focal seizures are more common and can aid in localizing the tumor, depending on the pattern of seizure activity.

### Displacement of brain structure

The cranial cavity is divided into several compartments by an infolding of the rigid dura mater. The falx cerebri divides the brain into the right and left hemispheres, and the tentorium cerebelli separates the occipital lobes from the cerebellum, thus creating the supratentorial and infratentorial spaces. Normally pressure is distributed equally between the compartments (Figure 35-14a). A growing tumor mass and the associated edema cause pressure to increase within the cranial compartment. Initially the brain's compensatory mechanisms attempt to accommodate the pressure by decreasing the amount of CSF, blood volume, or both within the brain. Once these mechanisms are exhausted, the increased pressure can cause the brain tissue in one compartment to protrude into another compartment. The brain tissue shifts or herniates from the high-pressure compartment into the lower-pressure compartment. This process, called *herniation*, is a life-threatening neurological emergency.[31]

The shifting brain tissue compresses other neural tissue and structures, further increases the edema, causes ischemia from damage to blood vessels, and can obstruct CSF pathways, leading to hydrocephalus. These compressive, ischemic, vascular, and obstructive changes all add to and aggravate the original problem of increased ICP. The potentially reversible complications of an expanding tumor become irreversible.[31]

There are two major classifications of herniation: *su-*

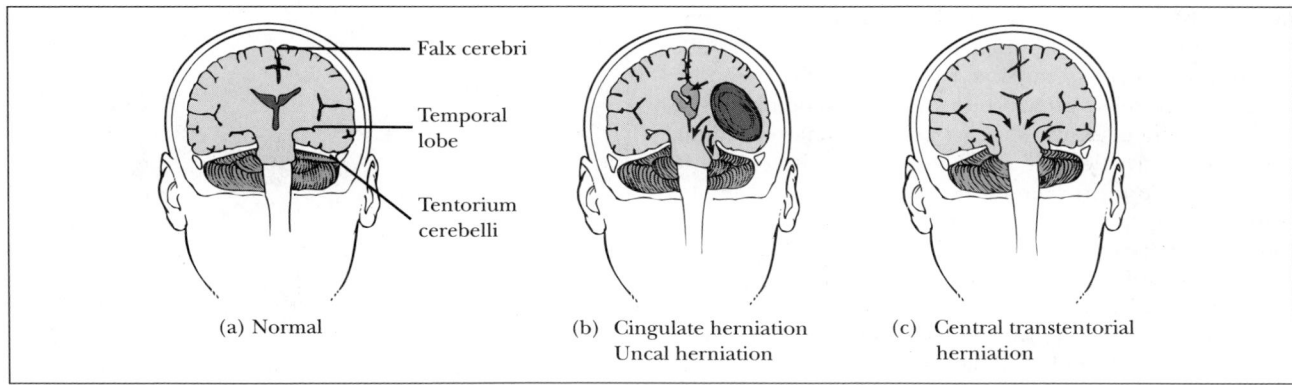

(a) Normal

(b) Cingulate herniation
    Uncal herniation

(c) Central transtentorial
    herniation

Falx cerebri

Temporal lobe

Tentorium cerebelli

**FIGURE 35-14**   Displacement of brain structures. (Modified from Wegmann JA[31])

*pratentorial* and *infratentorial*. The clinical manifestations of the two types differ. Supratentorial herniation generally causes a change in the level of consciousness and ocular, motor, and respiratory signs, whereas infratentorial herniation leads to a loss of consciousness and respiratory and cardiac changes. The expanding tumor mass is capable of displacing tissue distant from the tumor site. The resulting neurological signs and symptoms may not have true localizing value.[31]

There is usually an orderly progression of abnormal clinical signs. Careful neurological assessment in patients at risk for herniation may facilitate early identification of this potentially life-threatening complication. However, herniation can occur with little warning. A sudden change in the ICP or contents (as in an acute hemorrhage or the performance of a lumbar puncture) will rapidly lead to brain stem compression.

Supratentorial tumors, located above the tentorium cerebelli, can lead to cingulate, uncal, or central transtentorial herniation. Herniation of the cingulate gyrus under the falx cerebri compresses the contralateral frontal lobe and the anterior cerebral arteries (Figure 35-14b). Such herniation can cause bilateral frontal ischemia, urinary incontinence, leg weakness, and mental status changes. The diencephalon is shifted to the contralateral side, compresses itself and the third ventricle, and leads to diminished consciousness.[76]

Uncal herniation, usually occurring with expanding temporal lobe tumors, forces the medial portion of the temporal lobe (the uncus) into the tentorial notch (Figure 35-14b). The midbrain is compressed laterally. The herniated uncus compresses the third cranial nerve, the posterior cerebral artery, and the diencephalon. Compression of the third cranial nerve, the oculomotor nerve, initially causes the pupil to sluggishly react to light. With further compression the pupil dilates and becomes unreactive. With midbrain compression, the motor pathways of the cerebral peduncle produce a contralateral hemiparesis. Sometimes uncal herniation compresses the opposite cerebral peduncle against the opposite tentorial notch (opposite the side of herniation). This is called *Kernohan's notch* and causes a hemiparesis that is ipsilateral to the side of the lesion (and to the third cranial nerve palsy). This is a false localizing sign that may lead to confusion in determining the location of the lesion. The tumor is on the same side as the third nerve palsy.[31] A positive Babinski's sign may be seen with the hemiparesis. The enlarging mass also shifts the diencephalon, leading to a progressive loss of consciousness beginning with drowsiness and proceeding to stupor and finally to coma.[76] Compression of the posterior cerebral artery can cause ischemia or infarction of the ipsilateral occipital lobe. Later findings in uncal herniation include decorticate followed by decerebrate posturing, and impaired oculocephalic and oculovestibular reflexes. Oculocephalic reflexes are tested by holding the patient's eyelids open and briskly rotating the head from side to side or by briskly flexing and extending the neck (doll's eyes

phenomenon). Oculovestibular reflexes are tested by injecting ice water into the external ear canal. In the comatose patient, testing these reflexes assesses for the presence of brain stem function.

Central or transtentorial herniation results from the downward displacement of the cerebral hemispheres and basal ganglia onto the diencephalon and midbrain, which are then forced through the tentorial notch (Figure 35-14c). Initially, there will be a change in the level of consciousness or behavior. The person becomes drowsy, inattentive, or agitated. Pupil size is reduced. There may be deep sighing or yawning with respirations.[30] As the tumor continues to displace tissue downward, the individual becomes stuporous and eventually progresses to coma. Pupils become nonreactive, eye movements disconjugate, and as the brain stem becomes compressed, decorticate posturing deteriorates to decerebrate in response to noxious stimuli. Oculocephalic and oculovestibular reflexes may be absent.

Both central and uncal herniations cause changes in the respiratory pattern. Irregular depth and rhythm often are more significant than changes in respiratory rate alone. Initially, respirations may be irregular with occasional pauses, sighs, or gasps. Later respiratory pattern changes include Cheyne-Stokes breathing, sustained hyperventilation, ataxic breathing, apnea, and finally, respiratory arrest.[31] The classic vital sign changes of Cushing's triad are seen during the terminal phase of herniation.

Tumors of the posterior fossa can lead to an infratentorial herniation causing displacement of the cerebellum either upward through the opening in the tentorium cerebelli or downward through the foramen magnum (Figure 35-15). In upward transtentorial herniation, the cerebellum compresses the midbrain. Obstruction and

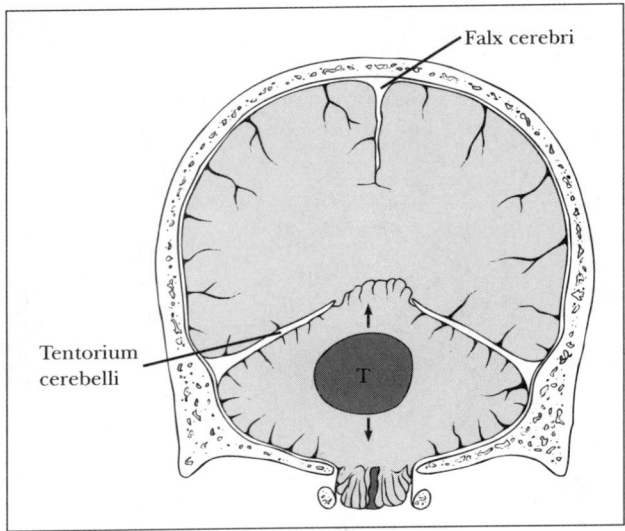

**FIGURE 35-15** An infratentorial tumor causing upward and downward shifts of the cerebellum. (Modified from Wegmann JA[31])

blockage of CSF pathways may occur. The individual may lose consciousness immediately. This may be accompanied by hyperventilation; pinpoint, fixed, and unequal pupils; upward gaze paralysis; vomiting; and decerebration.[30]

Downward cerebellar tonsillar herniation is more common and results in the downward protrusion of the cerebellar tonsils through the foramen magnum. The lower brain stem is compressed; when the compression is acute, it can cause sudden loss of consciousness followed by respiratory arrest. This may be precipitated by events causing a sudden rise in ICP such as sneezing, coughing, or performing a Valsalva maneuver. The outflow of CSF from the fourth ventricle becomes blocked, leading to obstructive hydrocephalus. Other signs include lower cranial nerve dysfunction, suboccipital headache, vomiting, and neck pain. Altered consciousness with resulting coma may be an early sign. Later signs of medullary compression include abnormal respiratory patterns, fluctuating blood pressure and heart rate, and cardiac dysrhythmias. In both types of infratentorial herniation, respiratory arrest, cardiac arrest, or both will occur if untreated.

## Spinal Cord Tumors

The clinical manifestations associated with spinal cord tumors result from compression and, much less frequently, invasion of the spinal cord. Extramedullary tumors affect the cord by compression, causing traction on or irritation of the spinal nerve roots, displacement of the spinal cord itself, interference with the spinal blood supply, or obstruction of CSF circulation. Intramedullary tumors invade and destroy the spinal cord itself. When spinal cord compression occurs, the normal physiology involved in providing an adequate blood supply, maintaining stable cellular membranes, and facilitating afferent and efferent impulses for specific sensory, motor, and reflex functions of the spinal cord and related spinal nerves is altered.[29] Edema results, causing additional deficits.

The clinical manifestations seen with spinal cord tumors are dependent on the tumor's rate of growth and the level of the spinal cord affected. A slow-growing tumor better allows the cord to accommodate the mass. Tumors can be present for years, compressing the cord into a thin ribbonlike structure without causing significant neurological deficits. On the other hand, the spinal cord cannot accommodate a sudden mass or rapidly growing lesion such as a hematoma or a malignant or metastatic tumor. The spinal cord has little ability to compensate such lesions that increase pressure and create extensive edema causing sudden neurological dysfunction. The signs and symptoms of spinal cord tumors are pain, motor weakness, sensory impairment, and autonomic dysfunction involving bowel and bladder function.

Pain is the most common presenting symptom of a spinal cord tumor. In epidural metastases, back or neck pain may be present for weeks or months, and intradural tumors can cause pain for years before the correct diagnosis is established. Often the pain is initially dismissed as arthritis, back strain, or disk disease, and until other more obvious neurological manifestations appear, the diagnosis of a spinal cord tumor is usually not considered. Back or neck pain in cancer patients, especially those with tumor types that commonly metastasize to bone, should be evaluated for spinal metastases (Figure 35-16).[87]

The pain may be localized or radicular. Localized pain and tenderness are common over the involved area, particularly with epidural metastases. Radicular pain may be described as bandlike and follows the distribution of the spinal nerve roots (dermatomes). The pain can vary from mild to severe and from dull to sharp or burning. The pain almost always becomes more severe with time. Pain may be worse at night; a recumbent position often aggravates it. Pain that is aggravated by movement and relieved with immobility may indicate spinal instability. Activities that produce a Valsalva maneuver such as sneezing, coughing, and straining increase the spinal pressure and cause intensification of pain.

Weakness is the most readily identified objective finding and may follow the appearance of sensory symptoms. The level of impairment determines the muscle groups involved (myotomes). The weakness is often associated with hyperreflexia, spasticity, and a positive Babinski sign. The weakness will eventually progress to complete paraplegia unless treatment is initiated.

Specific sensory deficits will depend on where the tumor is on a cross section of the spinal cord. A lateral tumor will affect pain and temperature, causing symptoms of coldness, numbness, and tingling. Awareness of vibration and proprioception of body parts are affected if the posterior aspect is involved. Anterior tumors lead to weakness and an uncoordinated ataxic gait. The compression affects function below the lesion; therefore, it is important to determine the highest functional level. A sensory assessment begins at the toes and moves upward to determine the level at which function remains, which is generally the level of the tumor. However, there may be a discrepancy between the level of remaining function and apparent tumor location. The lesion may actually be one or two vertebrae above the level of compression. The tumor level is often accompanied by a narrow band of hyperesthesia directly above it.[29]

The effects may be symmetrical and bilateral, asymmetrical, and even unilateral. A combination of sensory and motor deficits may also be seen. A loss of touch, vibration, position sense, and motor ability on the same side as the lesion with contralateral loss of pain and temperature is called the Brown-Séquard syndrome. This occurs in approximately 20% of patients.[2]

Later symptoms are bowel dysfunction, bladder dysfunction, or both, and include constipation, fecal incontinence, urgency, difficulty in initiating urination, urinary retention, and urinary incontinence. These symptoms may be present earlier with an intramedullary tumor.

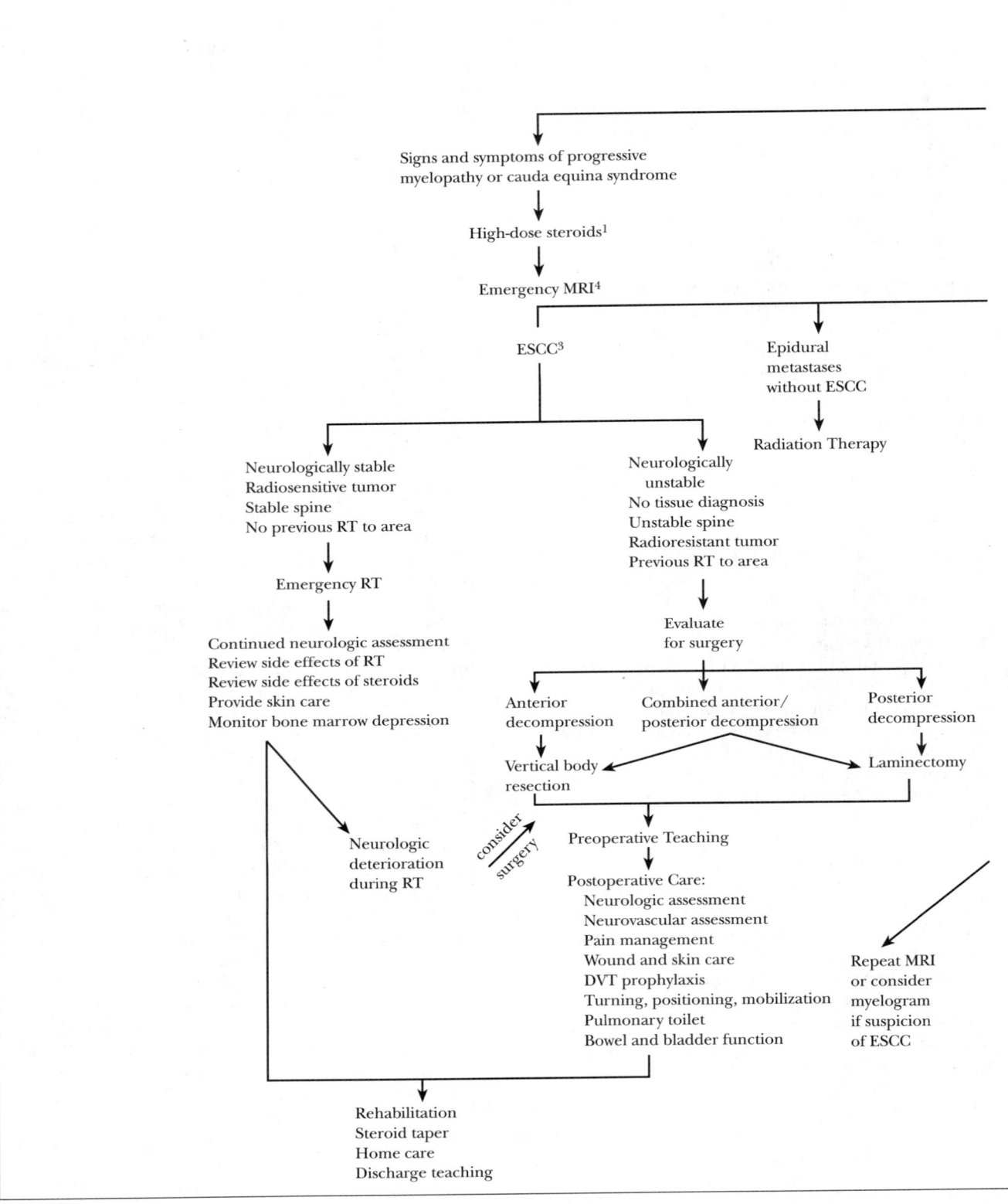

**FIGURE 35-16** Algorithm for the assessment and treatment of back pain in the cancer patient. Adapted from Foley KM: Pain syndromes in patients with cancer. In Portenoy RK, Kanner RM: *Pain Management: Theory and Practice.* © 1996, F. A. Davis Company, Philadelphia, PA.[87]

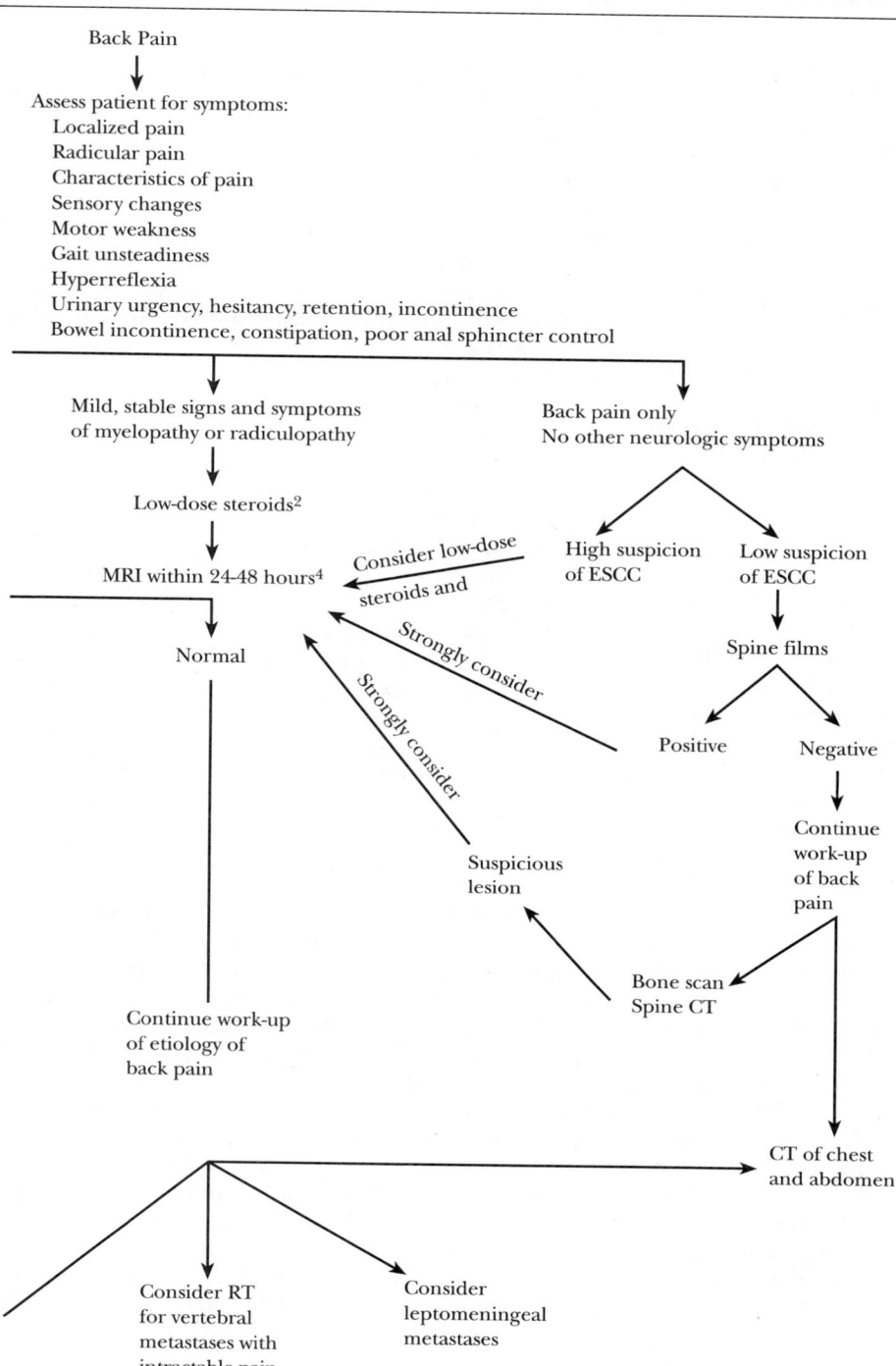

Back Pain

Assess patient for symptoms:
  Localized pain
  Radicular pain
  Characteristics of pain
  Sensory changes
  Motor weakness
  Gait unsteadiness
  Hyperreflexia
  Urinary urgency, hesitancy, retention, incontinence
  Bowel incontinence, constipation, poor anal sphincter control

Mild, stable signs and symptoms
of myelopathy or radiculopathy

Low-dose steroids[2]

MRI within 24-48 hours[4]

Normal

Continue work-up
of etiology of
back pain

Back pain only
No other neurologic symptoms

Consider low-dose steroids and

High suspicion
of ESCC

Low suspicion
of ESCC

Spine films

Strongly consider

Strongly consider

Positive        Negative

Suspicious
lesion

Continue
work-up
of back
pain

Bone scan
Spine CT

CT of chest
and abdomen

Consider RT
for vertebral
metastases with
intractable pain

Consider
leptomeningeal
metastases

Key:
[1]Example of high-dose steroid regimen = dexamethasone 100 mg IV stat followed by dexamethasone 24 mg q6h, with slow taper over weeks.
[2]Example of low-dose steroid regimen = dexamethasone 16 mg followed by dexamethasone 4 mg q6h, with slow taper over weeks.
[3]ESCC = epidural spinal cord compression.
[4]In patients with known metastatic disease, a complete spinal MRI is recommended because additional lesions may be discovered.

**FIGURE 35-16**   (continued)

## ASSESSMENT

Assessment of the individual with a known or suspected CNS tumor begins by obtaining the individual's medical history. The description and duration of symptoms, when they occur, the presence of exacerbating or relieving factors, and the order of their appearance are important pieces of information. This is followed by a complete neurological examination. An initial neurological assessment is essential because it provides a baseline knowledge of the individual's neurological function. Future assessments will be evaluated in comparison with the initial examination, allowing the detection of any changes or abnormalities.

The neurological exam begins with an assessment of the patient's level of consciousness and mental status. In most instances the first, earliest, and most sensitive indicator of dysfunction will be a change in the level of consciousness. Level of consciousness is the ability of the person to interact appropriately within the context of the immediate environment.[30] The individual whose level of consciousness is impaired must be sufficiently stimulated to be able to appropriately describe the degree of alteration. Various levels of alteration may occur, ranging from full consciousness to deep coma. Common descriptions include alert and oriented, confused, lethargic, stuporous, obtunded, semicomatose, and comatose. Many institutions have included components of the Glascow Coma Scale, a tool that assesses neurological function in comatose patients as part of their vital sign sheets or neurological assessment sheets. An example of such a tool, shown in Figure 35-17, allows graphic representation of an individual's neurological status at any point in time.

Mental status and cognitive ability are assessed by conversing with and observing the individual. One should note the person's behavior, appearance, mood, affect, and speech patterns. Observation of actions, posture, facial expressions, and responses to conversation provide information regarding general cerebral function. Orientation, general knowledge, recent and remote memory, attention span, immediate recall, abstract reasoning, and judgment are also part of the assessment of cognitive function. The presence of aphasia (the inability to understand or express one's own language), agnosia (the inability to recognize common objects through the senses of sight, touch, and sound), and apraxia (the inability to perform a skilled motor act in the absence of weakness or paralysis) is noted.

Motor and sensory function are also evaluated. A motor exam assesses whether the individual moves normally or abnormally, what the level of response is, and the strength of both the upper and lower extremities against gravity and resistance. A motor exam also tests gait, posture, and reflexes. Deep tendon reflexes (DTRs) and superficial reflexes are examined. Sensation is assessed by introducing various stimuli to different parts of the body with the eyes closed. Light touch, pain, temperature, and position sense are evaluated bilaterally. The motor and sensory examinations are particularly important for the person with a spinal cord tumor, as is the presence of bowel and bladder dysfunction.

Assessment of cerebellar function focuses on the ability to coordinate movement and to maintain normal muscle tone and equilibrium. The person is asked to perform the finger-to-finger, finger-to-nose, hand patting, Romberg, and tandem walking tests.

Testing of cranial nerve function can be the most intimidating portion of the neurological assessment. The 12 pairs of cranial nerves, their function, method of testing, and desired response are listed in Table 35-4.

The performance of the initial assessment is as important for the individual newly diagnosed with a CNS tumor as it is for the person with recurrent or progressive disease. The presence and severity of generalized and focal signs and symptoms are documented. The history of the symptoms is important to ascertain from the patient and family. Any change in symptom characteristics should be identified, along with possible exacerbating or relieving factors. Seizures are another area that warrants investigation. The nurse determines whether the individual has had seizures, the frequency and pattern of occurrence, and whether the person experiences an aura before the seizure. Changes in the neurological assessment, the development of new symptoms, or both can indicate increased ICP, spinal cord compression, recurrent disease, or side effects of treatment.

Realistically, it is not always possible to perform a full neurological assessment on every individual with a CNS tumor each time he or she is evaluated. After the initial assessment is done to provide a baseline, it is possible to complete a modified assessment with specific emphasis on the abnormal components or those indicating particular functions.[30] For example, the individual with a spinal cord tumor should have a complete motor and sensory exam rather than an examination of the cranial nerves. The person with a cerebellar tumor who is completely oriented might have follow-up testing of cerebellar function. Again, an understanding of relative neuroanatomy and neurophysiology is essential when caring for individuals with CNS tumors.

## Diagnostic Studies

Developments in neuroimaging have dramatically improved the ability to diagnose, localize, and treat individuals with CNS cancers. Computed tomography (CT) and MRI have become standard imaging techniques. Positron emission tomography (PET) and single-photon emission computed tomography (SPECT) are being used to distinguish tumor from radiation necrosis and to increase the understanding of the metabolism of malignant tumors.[88] These and the remaining procedures used to detect the presence of CNS tumors require nursing intervention to educate the individual in the procedure and, when necessary, the postprocedural routine.

**Memorial Hospital for Cancer and Allied Diseases**

**Neurological Assessment**

Patient Identification

| | | | | | | | | | | | | | | |
|---|---|---|---|---|---|---|---|---|---|---|---|---|---|---|
| Date | | | | | | | | | | | | | | |
| Time | | | | | | | | | | | | | | |
| Initial | | | | | | | | | | | | | | |

**COMA SCALE**

1. Eyes Open
   eyes closed
   by swelling = c
   - Spontaneously
   - To Speech
   - To Touch
   - To Pain
   - None

2. Best verbal response
   - Oriented
   - Confused
   - Inappropriate
   - Incomprehensible
   - None

3. Best Motor Response
   - Obeys commands
   - Localizes Pain
   - Withdraws
   - Decorticate (Flexion)
   - Decerebrate (Extension)
   - None

4=Normal Strength
3=Lifts and Holds
2=Lifts and Falls Back
1=Moves on Bed
0=No Movement

| | |
|---|---|
| Arm | Rt. |
| Leg | Rt. |
| Arm | Lt. |
| Leg | Lt. |

PUPILS    2mm  3mm  4mm  5mm
N=Normal
S=Sluggish   6mm   7mm   8mm
F=Fixed

| | |
|---|---|
| Size | Rt. |
| Size | Lt. |
| React. | Rt. |
| React. | Lt. |

CONSCIOUSNESS

RESPIRATIONS

**CODES**

**ORIENTATION**
3 ORIENTED X 3 SPHERES
2 ORIENTED X 2 SPHERES
1 ORIENTED X 1 SPHERE

**CONSCIOUSNESS**
4 ALERT
3 LETHARGIC
2 RESTLESS, AGITATED
1 STUPOROUS
0 COMATOSE

ˇ **BLOOD PRESSURE**
ˆ
• **PULSE**

200
190
180
170
160
150
140
130
120
110
100
90
80
70
60
50
40
30
20

/11.050

**FIGURE 35-17**  Neurological assessment form. (Memorial Sloan-Kettering Cancer Center, Division of Nursing.)

**TABLE 35-4**  Examination of Cranial Nerves

| Cranial Nerve | Major Function | Method of Testing | Desired Response |
|---|---|---|---|
| I. Olfactory | Smell | Inhalation of commonly recognized aromatic substance such as cloves; avoid use of ammonia or alcohol because these stimulate the trigeminal nerve and evoke a pain response | Identification of the substance with each nostril |
| II. Optic | Vision | Direct ophthalmoscopy; use finger movement and eye charts to test visual acuity and fields | Note the appearance of the optic disk, vessels, and retina; correct eye movement and chart identification with each eye separately |
| III. Oculomotor | Movement of eyes in 4 of the 6 cardinal directions of gaze (inward, upward, downward, upward and outward); pupillary constriction and accommodation; elevation of upper eyelid | Individual follows the examiner's finger with the eyes to test eye movement; check pupil response to light; observe for ptosis of the eyelid | Movement of eyes should be equal in the cardinal directions of gaze; pupils react to direct and consensual response to light; eyes are symmetric at rest and move conjugatively |
| IV. Trochlear | Movements of eyes (downward and inward) | Individual follows the examiner's finger with the eyes to test eye movement | Movement of eyes should be equal |
| V. Trigeminal | Muscles of mastication and eardrum tension; general sensations from anterior half of head including face, nose, mouth | Individual clamps the jaw, opens the mouth against resistance and masticates to check motor division of the nerve; touch both sides of the person's face, checking for pain, touch, and temperature response; gently touch the person's cornea with a cotton wisp to check the corneal reflex | Correct identification of sensations; rapid blinking |
| VI. Abducens | Movement of eyes (outward) | Individual follows the examiner's finger to test eye movement (oculomotor, trochlear, and abducens are tested together) | Movement of eyes should be equal |
| VII. Facial | Muscles of facial expression and tension on ear bones; lacrimation and salivation; taste to anterior two-thirds of tongue | Observe for facial symmetry and the person's ability to contract muscles to check motor division; individual tastes sweet, sour, salty, and acidic flavors | Person smiles, frowns, wrinkles nose and brow, closes eyes tightly with symmetry, correct identification of tastes |
| VIII. Acoustic (cochlear and vestibular) | Hearing; balance and equilibrium | Test hearing ability with the use of whispered voice and tuning fork at various distances from the ear to check the cochlear nerve; check the vestibular nerve by having the person stand on one foot with eyes closed | Recognition of sound; maintenance of balance |
| IX. Glossopharyngeal | Gag and swallowing, salivation, taste to posterior third of tongue | Check the gag reflex by touching the pharynx with a tongue depressor | Gag response |
| X. Vagus | Gag and swallowing, laryngeal control, parasympathetic to thoracic and abdominal viscera | Check the individual's swallowing ability; ask person to cough and speak; Glossopharyngeal and vagus nerves are examined together because of overlapping innervation of the pharynx | Speak without hoarseness or weakness |
| XI. Spinal Accessory | Movement of head and shoulders | Ask the individual to elevate the shoulders, turn the head, and resist the examiner's attempts to pull the chin back to midline; check the symmetry of the trapezius and sternocleidomastoid muscles | Equal bilateral strength; atrophy may indicate nerve dysfunction |
| XII. Hypoglossal | Movement of tongue | Ask the individual to protrude the tongue | Absence of deviations, atrophy, or tremors |

Modified from Wegmann JA[31]

Another area that warrants investigation is seizures. The nurse determines whether the individual has a history of seizures; if so, the frequency and pattern of occurrence are then determined, along with whether the individual had experienced an aura before the seizure.

CT scan is a computer-calculated image that results from absorption of an x-ray beam as it passes through cross sections of bone and tissue in a single plane. The degree to which the beam is absorbed is determined by the density of the bone and cranial contents, which allows differentiation between bone, brain tissue, blood, and CSF.[30] Hyperdense structures such as blood appear as white areas on the two-dimensional display. Other hyperdense areas may indicate vascularity, tumor, or calcification. CSF is hypodense and appears as black areas on the display. Other hypodense regions may reflect infarction, edema, air, or necrosis. The normal brain is isodense and appears as various shades of gray.[29,30]

CT is highly sensitive to blood within the brain and is the technique of choice for evaluating the presence of acute hemorrhage. Bony structures are extremely well visualized on a CT scan and can be used to evaluate skull metastases and other bony pathology.[89] CT is widely available in most facilities and is generally less expensive than MRI. It can be conducted more rapidly than MRI, an important consideration in emergency situations or when sedation may be contraindicated.[31,90]

CT is the usual preliminary study in an individual with signs and symptoms suggesting a brain tumor. The scan is first done without the injection of an iodinated radiopaque contrast material. Noncontrast CT is necessary to determine the presence of calcium or hemorrhage. Contrast is then administered to delineate the margins and extent of blood-brain barrier disruption.[89] Contrast enhancement is due to extravasation of dye into the extracellular space, which is normally prevented by the blood-brain barrier.[88] If the tumor enhances the contrast material, breakdown of the blood-brain barrier and a more active tumor are likely. Once a lesion is identified, MRI is usually performed for anatomic detail and tissue characterization.

MRI is the more definitive and preferred imaging study for the individual with a CNS tumor. MRI is a precise scanning technique that uses powerful magnetic fields and radio frequency pulses to produce computer-calculated three-dimensional images of organs and tissues from different planes.[30] MRI has much better resolution than CT scans and is much more anatomically detailed. In addition, it is possible to differentiate between solid tumor, edema, and fluid collection. MRI imaging provides superior definition of the borders of a CNS tumor, and the extent of the tumor and its invasiveness can be better demonstrated by MRI than by CT[31,90] (Figure 35-18). The use of the contrast-enhancing material gadolinium-DTPA results in remarkable improvement in the image resolution and illustrates not only blood-brain barrier breakdown but changes in tissue metabolism as well.[29,91]

MRI also demonstrates an increased sensitivity for small (<1 cm) lesions[31] and can detect CT-occult tumors.[75]

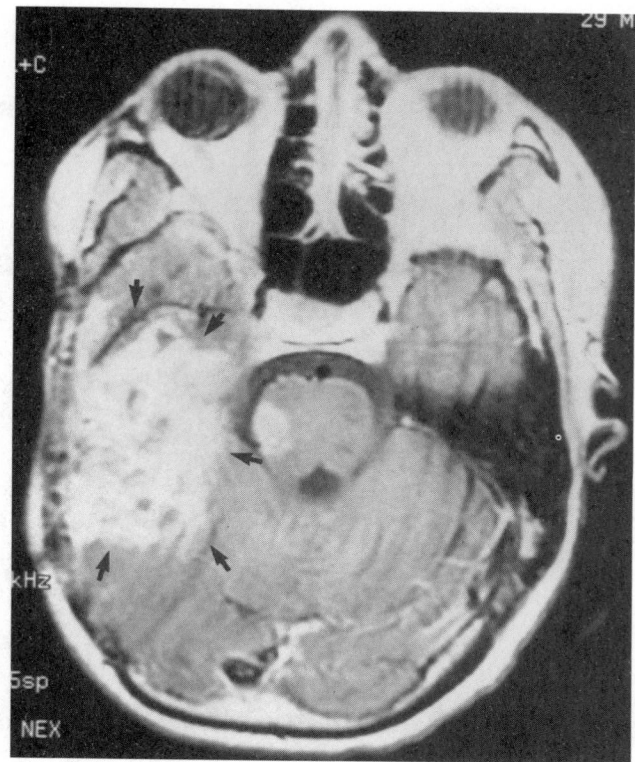

**FIGURE 35-18**   MRI of the brain with gadolinium. The axial view T1-weighted image depicts a malignant glioma. This contrast-enhancing lesion is located in the right temporal lobe. A second enhancing lesion is found in the brain stem. (Reprinted with permission from Memorial Sloan-Kettering Cancer Center, Department of Neurology.)

An MRI may be positive when the CT is negative; this may sometimes be seen with low-grade tumors and PCNSL lesions. It is also superior to CT scan in imaging the posterior fossa because bone artifact is not present in MRI. MRI can also more readily identify leptomeningeal metastases (Figure 35-19).

Because MRI involves powerful magnetic fields, some metal objects must be excluded from the magnet. This procedure may be contraindicated for individuals with certain metallic implants such as pacemakers, specific types of aneurysm clips, intravascular coils, filters, otologic implants, and orthopedic devices. To assure firm implantation into the vessel wall, some intravascular coils, filters, and stents require a minimum two-week wait postplacement before an MRI is performed. Thereafter, it would be highly unlikely that they would be moved or dislodged by magnetic forces.

Cerebral angiography may be used to confirm that the lesion in question is a vascular malformation or an aneurysm rather than a neoplasm. In other situations, for example, with large meningiomas, angiography may be useful before surgery to determine the blood supply so that it can be embolized during the arteriography procedure or obliterated during the surgical procedure,

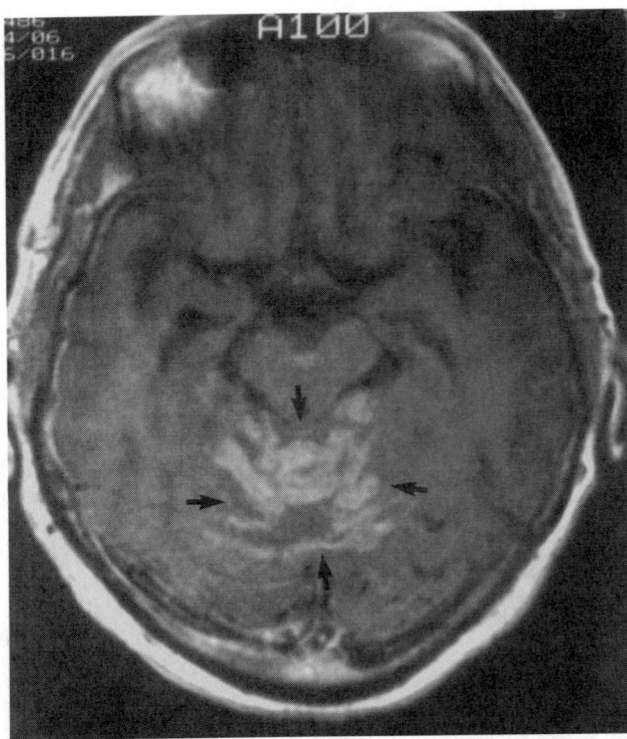
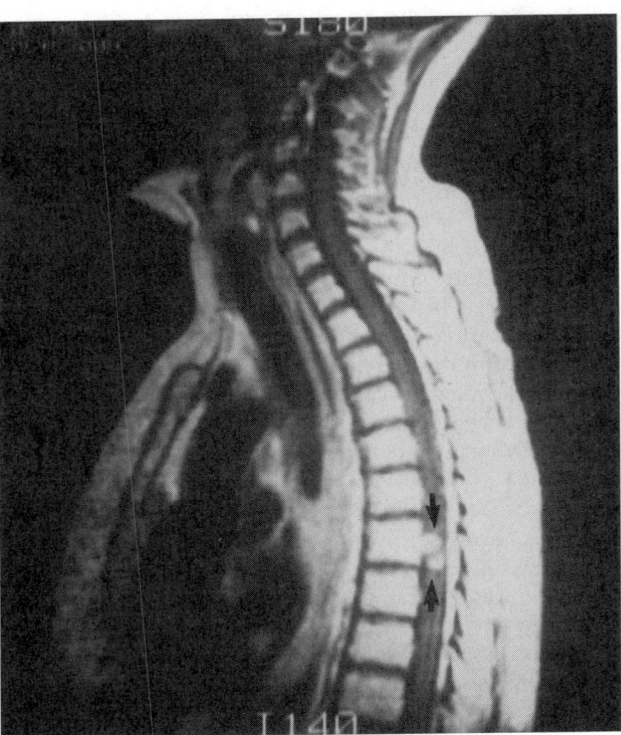

**FIGURE 35-19**    Leptomeningeal metastases. (Left) MRI of the brain with gadolinium. This axial view T1-weighted image illustrates diffuse meningeal enhancement, depicting meningeal carcinomatosis. (Right) MRI of the cervico-thoracic spine with gadolinium. This sagittal view illustrates nodular leptomeningeal tumors or drop metastases. (Reprinted with permission from Memorial Sloan-Kettering Cancer Center, Department of Neurology.)

or both.[2] Cerebral angiography involves percutaneous puncture of the femoral artery with injection of radiopaque medium to visualize the cerebral vasculature. It allows the circle of Willis and the large blood vessels that enter the cerebrum to be visualized by serial imaging of the transit of the contrast medium through the vasculature.[30,31] Neurological and neurovascular assessments are performed frequently after the procedure to identify signs and symptoms of weakness, stroke, seizures, or interrupted vascular integrity. Invasive cerebral angiography is being used much less frequently because of the increasing availability of less invasive MR angiography.

Another diagnostic study that may be performed in individuals with CNS tumors is a lumbar puncture. CSF is often examined for malignant cells in individuals with tumors such as medulloblastomas, ependymomas, and PCNSL that have the propensity to seed the subarachnoid space and spread throughout the CSF pathways. CSF studies are also evaluated in individuals with known or suspected leptomeningeal metastases. A lumbar puncture should be performed after neuroimaging studies such as MRI and CT scan, especially in an individual with a suspected tumor, because of the risk of herniation.[2]

PET is a functional imaging technique that may also be used in individuals with brain tumors, specifically malignant gliomas. This technique provides dynamic information on cerebral blood flow and metabolism rather than the precise anatomic localization seen in CT scanning and MRI. PET combines the properties of nuclear scanning with physical characteristics of positron-emitting isotopes of naturally occurring atoms.[31,89] Radioactive isotopes produced in a cyclotron are incorporated into a chosen brain metabolite and injected intravenously. These isotopes disintegrate and form a positively charged electron (a positron). The positron travels until it comes together with an electron and then converts into a pair of photons traveling in opposite directions. A ring of collimators surrounding the patient's head records these events, computers calculate measurements, and a reconstruction algorithm produces an axial view of brain uptake. In addition, by monitoring the arterial concentration of radioactivity via an arterial line, the absolute metabolic rate of areas in the brain can be calculated.[89]

Most PET studies have used [18]F-fluorodeoxyglucose (FDG), a fluorinated glucose analogue to measure glucose metabolism, which is increased in tumor cells.[88,92] The amount of FDG uptake correlates with the degree of malignancy, i.e., low-grade gliomas tend to have lower uptake (hypometabolic) and malignant gliomas have higher uptake (hypermetabolic). Figure 35-20 compares an MRI and a PET scan of a malignant glioma. In addition to determining tumor grade, this technique has become the standard imaging modality to distinguish between tumor recurrence and radiation necrosis. PET has also

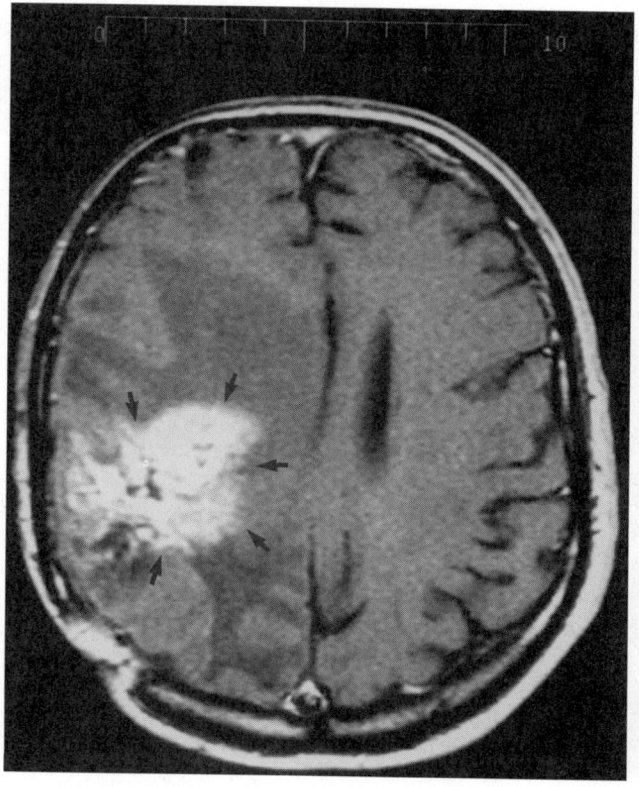
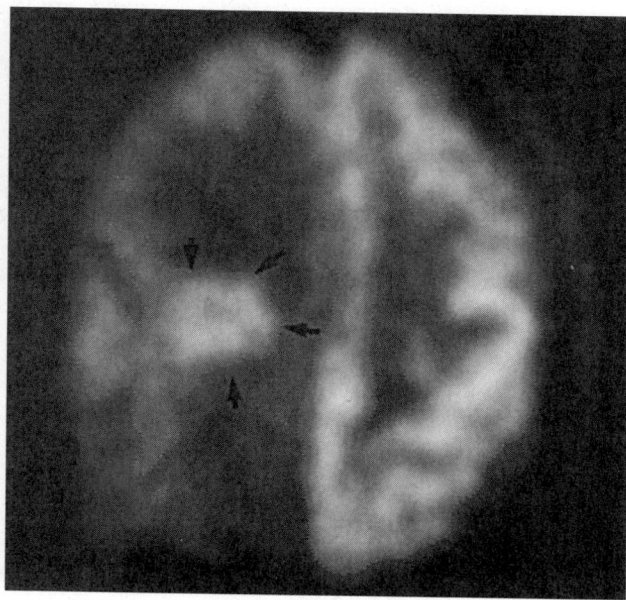

**FIGURE 35-20**   Comparison of MRI of the brain with gadolinium (left) and PET scan (right) of a malignant glioma. (Left) This axial view T1-weighted image illustrates a large contrast-enhancing lesion in the parietal lobe representing a glioblastoma multiforme. (Right) A region of hypermetabolism (higher uptake of the FDG analogue) corresponds with the enhancing region on MRI which is suggestive of a malignant tumor. (Reprinted with permission from Memorial Sloan-Kettering Cancer Center, Departments of Neurosurgery and Nuclear Medicine.)

been used to localize areas of probable tumor for biopsy, differentiate residual tumor after surgery from postoperative changes, and study the metabolic effects of chemotherapy, radiation therapy, and steroids on tumor metabolism.[88,92]

PET is not used routinely to diagnose brain tumors but can complement information obtained by CT and MRI. Its use is limited by its high cost and restricted availability. Individuals having PET scans using the glucose analogue FDG should not receive dextrose intravenous solutions and should not eat for several hours prior to the test because glucose metabolism is being measured.

SPECT is used for the imaging of functional neuroanatomy. This technique involves the intravenous administration of isotopes taken up by the brain and tumor cells. These isotopes emit photons that are detected by a rotating gamma camera. Standard tomography reconstruction algorithms are then used to generate cross-sectional images of the brain.[92] Thallium 201 is a potassium analogue that does not normally enter the brain parenchyma. In regions with a disrupted blood-brain barrier, however, the thallium that is taken up through an adenosine triphosphate cell membrane pump distinguishes the tumor from the surrounding brain.[88,89] Regions of intense thallium uptake usually represent solid

active tumor recurrence, whereas low thallium uptake generally represents radiation necrosis. This technique has also been shown to be effective in distinguishing the presence of infiltrating tumor from solid tumor.[89] SPECT has also proved effective in differentiating lymphoma from toxoplasmosis in AIDS patients, which may lead to earlier diagnosis and treatment. While SPECT is more widely available than PET, it presently provides only an indirect measure of brain metabolism. Also, SPECT is used only to complement the information obtained by CT scanning or MRI, as is PET, and is not used in the initial diagnosis of brain tumors. Recent developments have allowed SPECT to overlap on MRI data using computer processing techniques, so that it is possible to directly correlate anatomic and functional information.[89]

CT myelography has been the standard method for identifying the location and level of spinal cord and nerve root compromise resulting from spinal tumors. Extradural, intradural extramedullary, and intramedullary spinal tumors are distinguished by characteristic myelographic patterns. Contrast medium is injected into the subarachnoid space, usually by means of a lumbar puncture, and CT images of the spinal cord and vertebral column are taken to determine if a partial or complete obstruction is present. When the level of a complete block identified by lumbar myelography is uncertain, a cisternal myelogram should be performed to determine the extent of the lesion or to identify multiple levels of involvement.

After a CT myelogram has been performed, the individual must be assessed for any neurological changes and positioned appropriately (usually supine, with the head of the bed elevated at a prescribed level). Possible complications include allergic reaction to the contrast agent, meningeal irritation, headache, nausea, vomiting, infection, and seizure.

MRI is replacing myelography as the diagnostic procedure of choice for the evaluation of both intramedullary and extramedullary spinal cord tumors (Figure 35-21). MRI provides superb anatomic detail of the spinal cord, is noninvasive, and has fewer risks than myelography. It is helpful for planning radiation therapy and surgery as well.

## Prognostic Indicators

The prognosis for an individual with a CNS tumor varies considerably depending on the specific type and location of the tumor. Generally, the prognosis for a malignant brain glioma, the most common adult CNS tumor, is dismal. However, several important prognostic factors have been identified that may affect the eventual outcome. Young age, lower histological grade, and high performance status are favorable prognostic indicators for astrocytomas. In adults, younger patients do better and live longer than older patients even when adjusted for the other prognostic factors. Individuals younger than 40 with a GBM have a 50% 18-month survival rate, compared with 20% for those between 40 and 60 years of age and 10% for those older than 60.[92] Age appears to be a more important prognostic indicator than even histology.[42]

The more aggressive tumors, or those with a higher histological grade, have a poorer prognosis. As mentioned previously, individuals with anaplastic astrocytoma have a significantly better prognosis than those with GBM. The median survival for anaplastic astrocytoma is approximately 36 months, compared with 10–12 months for glioblastoma. The survival rate for individuals with low-grade gliomas is 50%–60% at five years and 30%–40% at ten years with standard treatment.[46] A lower histological grade is also a favorable factor for tumors other than astrocytomas, for example, the oligodendroglioma. Approximately 75% of patients with nonanaplastic oligodendroglioma will survive five years from the time of diagnosis, with a median survival reported to be in the range of six to ten years. The median survival for those with the higher-grade oligodendroglioma, the anaplastic oligodendroglioma, decreases to three to four years.[93]

The prognosis of individuals with high-grade gliomas, as with most of the CNS tumors, decreases as their functional status decreases. Those who have severe neurological deficits or are debilitated generally do not tolerate treatment as well as those with a higher performance status. They are generally more susceptible to complications as well. Individuals with high-grade astrocytomas whose Karnofsky Performance Status (KPS) is greater than 70 have been reported to have a 34% 18-month survival, compared with 13% for those with a KPS less than 60.[42]

The extent of surgical resection is another important prognostic factor. Most of the retrospective studies have demonstrated a delay in tumor recurrence and an increased survival for those individuals undergoing a complete surgical resection compared with those having a partial resection or biopsy alone. Although this may not be universally accepted, the recent trend in the literature has been to support the strategy of removing as much tumor as possible in malignant gliomas.[94] The extent of tumor resection is also an important prognostic indicator for other types of tumors. For example, completely excised meningiomas and pituitary tumors have lower recurrence rates.

Other favorable prognostic factors have been suggested for many brain tumors but may not be universally accepted. They include a long duration of symptoms before diagnosis, the presence of seizures, a normal neurological examination, a cystic component to the tumor, location of the tumor (frontal lobe), and small preoperative tumor size.

Brain metastases are generally associated with a poor prognosis. However, more favorable outcomes are associated with a high KPS, absent or controlled primary tumor, age under 60 years, metastatic spread limited to the brain, and a single surgically accessible lesion.

The prognosis is far better for intradural spinal cord tumors than for extradural. The majority of extradural spinal tumors result from metastatic disease. Metastatic cancer generally carries a poorer prognosis because of the more advanced stage of disease. Many survive less than a year, and death is often a result of the widespread systemic cancer rather than the epidural tumor. However, subgroups of patients—for instance, those with breast cancer, limited systemic disease, and radiosensitive tumors—survive for longer periods.

Rapid onset and quick progression are worse prognostic factors for recovery. Tumors causing neurological dysfunction that develop over hours to days carry a worse prognosis than those that evolve more slowly. The faster the spinal cord compression develops, the less likely neurological recovery is after treatment. The outcome of spinal cord compression relates to the neurological status at the time of treatment. The severity of weakness is the most significant prognostic factor for neurological recovery. Eighty percent of those who are ambulatory at the time of diagnosis remain so after treatment. As the neurological dysfunction increases, the likelihood of recovery diminishes. Only 30%–45% of patients who are initially paraparetic and nonambulatory become ambulatory, and those who are paraplegic at diagnosis are likely to remain so, with only 5% regaining the ability to walk.[86] In addition, those who do not regain or retain ambulation have

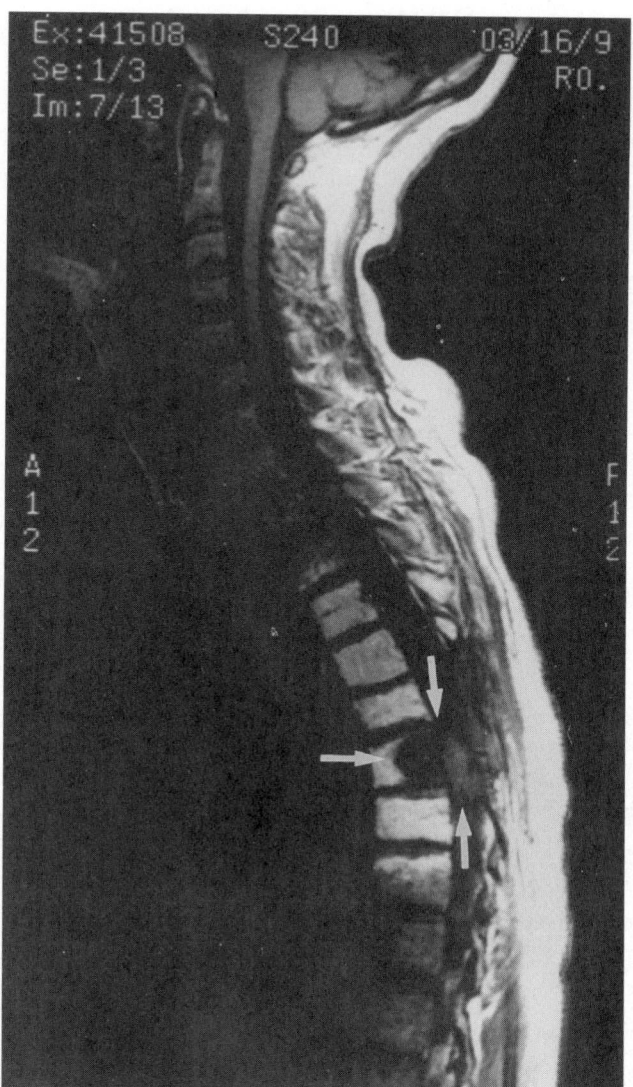

**FIGURE 35-21**   Tumors involving the spinal cord. (Left) This sagittal view of a cervico-thoracic MRI of the spine with gadolinium demonstrates an extradural metastatic lesion involving the T7 vertebral body causing spinal cord compression. (Right) Axial view of the involved area shows the spinal cord compression. (Printed with permission from Memorial Sloan-Kettering Cancer Center, Department of Neurosurgery.)

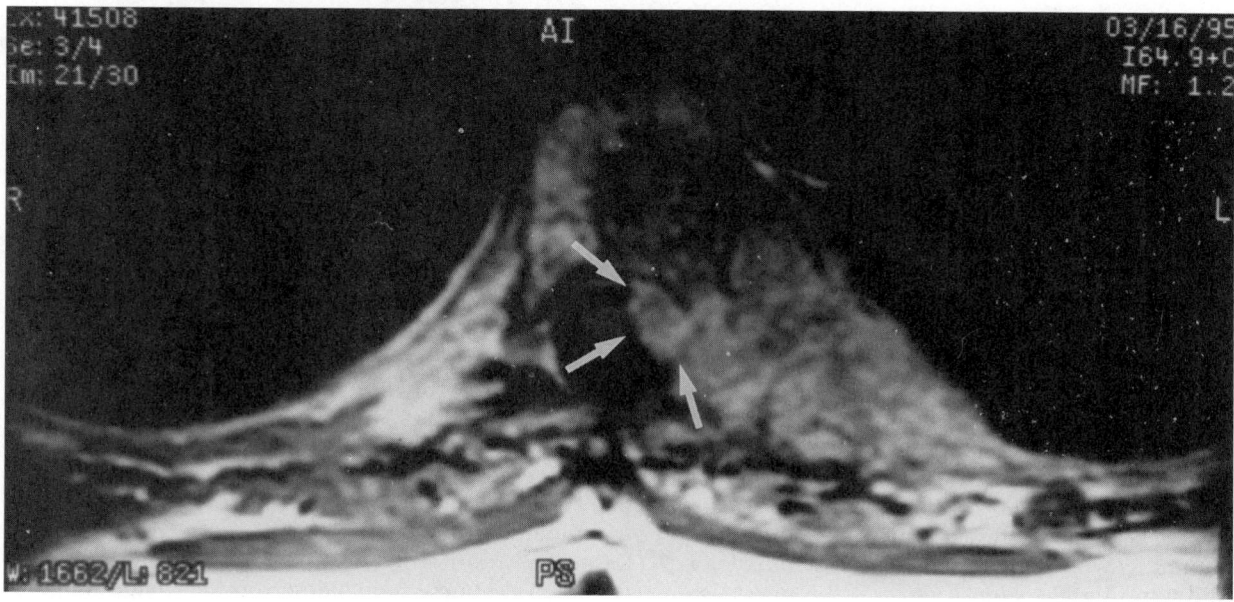

a substantially shorter survival than those who do. The shorter survival results in part from complications of paraplegia.[76]

Favorable prognostic factors for the intradural tumors include extent of surgical resection, histological grade, and, as in extradural tumors, slow onset of neurological dysfunction. Schwannomas, meningiomas, and ependymomas have a low recurrence rate if completely resected. The same cannot be said for astrocytomas. The available literature has failed to demonstrate a significant correlation between prognosis and degree of surgical resection.[95,96] A higher-grade spinal astrocytoma carries a poorer prognosis as in brain tumors. Those with malignant astrocytomas of the spinal cord generally do not survive longer than eight months.[2]

lower grade. Low-grade tumors can also transform and become more anaplastic over time.

The distinction between benign and malignant tumors can be misleading when discussing classification of CNS tumors. The term *benign* suggests that a cure is possible, whereas *malignant* implies a poor prognosis. Histological features alone do not determine malignancy in the CNS. Some tumors that are histologically benign may produce malignant responses. They may not be surgically resected because of their location in an inaccessible or vitally important area or their adherence to a critical structure. These tumors may then continue to grow, producing neurological deficits, compressing other tissues or structures, leading to increased ICP, spinal cord compression, and even causing death.

## CLASSIFICATION AND STAGING

CNS neoplasms represent a diverse heterogeneous group of primary and metastatic tumors of the brain and spinal cord. The classification of CNS tumors is based on the premise that each type of tumor results from the abnormal growth of a specific cell type. The consistent naming and grouping of similar tumor types are extremely important when gathering information and statistics on the incidence, etiology, effectiveness of treatment, and prognosis of CNS tumors. Several classification systems are presently in use for CNS tumors, particularly the astrocytomas, which contributes to the complexity in grading and understanding these tumors.

The most critical feature in the classification of CNS tumors is histopathology.[31,97] Recently, the World Health Organization (WHO) revised its classification of CNS tumors. This system first characterizes a tumor histologically by its cell of origin and then designates a grade based on its similarity to normal cells. Grading assesses the degree of malignancy or aggressiveness of the tumor cells by comparing the cellular anaplasia, differentiation, and mitotic activity with normal counterparts.[98] Tumor classification has clinical implications, dictates the choice of therapy, and predicts prognosis. The WHO system provides a comprehensive, uniform, internationally recognized method to categorize CNS tumors. The WHO classification of CNS tumors is found in Table 35-5.[99]

The TNM staging system classifies solid tumors by the anatomic extent of disease and evaluates the extent of the primary *tumor,* regional *lymph nodes,* and *metastases.* While the CNS does not contain lymphatic structures, metastases may occur, although rarely. The TNM classification of brain tumors is found in Table 35-6.[97]

Tumors of the CNS can often contain several types and grades of cells. The highest or most malignant grade of cell found during microscopic examination determines the tumor grade, even if most of the tumor is a

## THERAPEUTIC APPROACHES AND NURSING CARE

Many factors influence the treatment of CNS cancers, including type, grade, and location of the tumor; age, general condition of the patient; and the patient's wishes. Conventional treatment of the high-grade gliomas is usually a combination of surgery, RT, and chemotherapy. Low-grade gliomas and most benign tumors are generally treated with surgery and, in some cases, RT. Spinal cord tumors are treated with surgery, radiation, or both. The therapy for recurrent tumors is based on the previous types of therapy the individual has already received.

### Brain Tumors

#### Surgery

Surgery remains the initial treatment for the majority of individuals with brain tumors. Recent technical advances in neuroimaging and instrumentation have made the surgical treatment of brain tumors safer and more effective. The goal of surgery is often multipurpose. It establishes a diagnosis by providing tissue for histological examination. It provides relief of symptoms by quickly reducing the tumor bulk. This helps to alleviate ICP and the mass effect caused by compression or infiltration of brain tissue. Decreasing the tumor burden may also increase the effectiveness of adjuvant therapies by decreasing the number of tumor cells that must be treated, altering cell kinetics, removing radioresistant hypoxic cells, and removing areas of the tumor inaccessible to chemotherapy.[100] Low-grade tumors can transform to higher-grade tumors. Reducing the tumor bulk decreases the number of tumor cells remaining that may be at risk for genetic transformation. Surgery also provides access for other treatment modalities. In some tumors surgery

**TABLE 35-5**   World Health Organization Classification of CNS Tumors

| NEUROEPITHELIAL TUMORS OF THE CNS | |
|---|---|
| **Astrocytic tumors**<br>  Astrocytoma (WHO grade II)<br>  Anaplastic astrocytoma (WHO grade III)<br>  Glioblastoma multiforme (WHO grade IV)<br>  Pilocytic astrocytoma (WHO grade I)<br>  Subependymal giant cell astrocytoma (WHO grade I)<br>  Pleomorphic xanthoastrocytoma (WHO grade I)<br><br>**Oligodendroglial tumors**<br>  Oligodendroglioma (WHO grade II)<br>  Anaplastic oligodendroglioma (WHO grade III)<br><br>**Ependymal cell tumors**<br>  Ependymoma (WHO grade II)<br>  Anaplastic ependymoma (WHO grade III)<br>  Myxopapillary ependymoma<br>  Subependymoma (WHO grade I)<br><br>**Mixed gliomas**<br>  Mixed oligoastrocytoma (WHO grade II)<br>  Anaplastic oligoastrocytoma (WHO grade III)<br>  Others (e.g., ependymo-astrocytoma)<br><br>**Neuroepithelial tumors of uncertain origin**<br>  Polar spongioblastoma (WHO grade IV)<br>  Astroblastoma (WHO grade IV)<br>  Gliomatosis cerebri (WHO grade IV)<br><br>**Tumors of the choroid plexus**<br>  Choroid plexus papilloma<br>  Choroid plexus carcinoma<br><br>**Neuronal and mixed neuronal-glial tumors**<br>  Gangliocytoma<br>  Dysplastic gangliocytoma of cerebellum<br>  Ganglioglioma<br>  Anaplastic ganglioglioma<br>  Desmoplastic infantile ganglioglioma<br>  Central neurocytoma<br>  Dysembryoplastic neuroepithelial tumor<br>  Olfactory neuroblastoma (esthesioneuroblastoma)<br><br>**Pineal parenchymal tumors**<br>  Pineocytoma<br>  Pineoblastoma<br>  Mixed pineocytoma/pineoblastoma | **Tumors with neuroblastic or glioblastic elements (embryonal tumors)**<br>  Medulloepithelioma<br>  Primitive neuroectodermal tumors<br>    Medulloblastoma<br>    Cerebral primitive neuroectodermal tumor<br>  Neuroblastoma<br>  Retinoblastoma<br>  Ependymoblastoma<br><br>**Other CNS Neoplasms**<br>  Tumors of the sellar region<br>    Pituitary adenoma<br>    Pituitary carcinoma<br>    Craniopharyngioma<br>  Hematopoietic tumors<br>    Primary malignant lymphomas<br>    Plasmacytoma<br>    Granulocytic sarcoma<br>**Germ cell tumors**<br>  Germinoma<br>  Embryonal carcinoma<br>  Yolk sac tumor<br>  Choriocarcinoma<br>  Teratoma<br>  Mixed germ cell tumors<br>**Tumors of the meninges**<br>  Meningioma<br>  Atypical meningioma<br>  Anaplastic meningioma<br>**Nonmeningothelial tumors of the meninges**<br>  Benign mesenchymal<br>  Malignant mesenchymal<br>  Primary melanocytic lesions<br>  Hemopoietic neoplasms<br>  Tumors of uncertain histogenesis (hemangioblastoma)<br>**Tumors of cranial and spinal nerves**<br>  Schwannoma (neurinoma, neurilemoma)<br>  Neurofibroma<br>  Malignant peripheral nerve sheath tumor<br>**Local extensions from regional tumors**<br>  Metastatic tumors<br>  Unclassified tumors<br>  Cysts and tumorlike lesions |

Reprinted with permission from Kleiheus P, Burger PC, Sheithauer BW: Histological typing of tumours of the central nervous system. *World Health Organization, International Histological Classification of Tumours.* Berlin, Heidelberg, Springer-Verlag, 1993.[99]

provides a cure. Surgical intervention is often indicated in cases of metastatic brain tumors as well.

When evaluating an individual for surgery, many factors must be considered: size and location of the tumor, relationship of the tumor to functional brain regions, presence of widespread or multiple sites of disease, and the individual's age and neurological status. For example, a tumor with well-defined margins or one that is encapsulated in the nondominant hemisphere lends itself to an extensive resection. A rapidly growing infiltrative tumor that extends across the midline and is located in a deep vital structure or within the motor or sensory cortex may not be completely excised. In these cases a biopsy or

partial resection may be a safer option than a radical procedure. An individual with a single accessible brain metastasis may be a better surgical candidate than one with multiple metastatic lesions. PCNSL, a tumor often widely disseminated throughout the CNS, is not usually surgically resected. This tumor is often best managed by biopsy alone, followed by adjuvant therapy.

A biopsy removes sufficient tissue to establish a histological diagnosis. Different biopsy procedures may be performed. A needle biopsy is usually CT- or MRI-guided and is obtained through a burr hole drilled in the skull. An open biopsy, by way of a craniotomy, increases the accuracy of tissue samples, since the tumor can be visualized. Repeated tissue samples are obtained through a small cortical incision.[38] A stereotactic biopsy is the most precise means of obtaining a tissue sample and is the most widely used method today. Stereotaxis precisely locates areas in the brain with the use of three-dimensional coordinates.[91] It provides precise information about tumor location without direct visual access. Using a stereotactic frame such as the Brown-Roberts-Wells (BRW) device (Figure 35-22),[101] the patient's head is secured to the head ring with four skull pins to provide rigid skull fixation. A localizing cage composed of vertical and diagonal graphite rods is secured in the head ring and an imaging study is performed. The lesion is referenced to the nine x- and y-coordinates of the localizing cage, and these points are transformed to three-dimensional space. The localizing cage is removed, and a sterile arc guidance system is fixed to the head ring. The center of the arc depicts the target lesion, which can be approached from any angle or point on the arc quadrant. The biopsy probe or needle is accurately directed to within 1–2 mm of the target.[91,94] Regardless of the biopsy procedure used, the possibility of sampling error exists. The potential complications after a brain biopsy include hemorrhage at the biopsy site and exacerbation of cerebral edema occurring in few patients.[93]

There are indications for a brain biopsy alone in some individuals: when the diagnosis is uncertain despite good-quality MRI studies, the individual is unable to undergo craniotomy because of medical and anesthetic risks, the lesion involves deep brain structures, multiple lesions are present, there is a question of radiation necrosis versus tumor recurrence, or suspected tumor progression must be histologically verified.[94]

Stereotactic procedures can also be used to remove tumors. Kelly et al[102] originally described computer-assisted stereotactic resection. This method combines the concepts of radical surgery and stereotaxis to perform image-guided surgery. A stereotactic frame is used, and the tumor is resected through a speculum inserted and repositioned under computerized guidance. A laser is used to vaporize the tumor. Stereotactic craniotomies may be beneficial for small, deep tumors or in the case of multiple brain metastases because several resections can be performed in one sitting.[100,103]

External stereotactic frame systems have limitations and benefits. Frames are awkward and can obstruct access to patients' craniums. Adjusting the frames can be time-consuming and difficult. Because they report discomfort with the head frame, especially during placement, patients usually require premedication. In adults, stereotactic biopsy is generally performed under local anesthesia. This may decrease complications associated with general anesthesia but requires patient cooperation to perform the procedure. The need for patient cooperation with these systems discourages their use in pediatric patients and patients with dementia.[104] These individuals typically require general anesthesia. Associated mortality and morbidity may be decreased with stereotactic procedures, and

**TABLE 35-6** TNM Classification of Brain Tumors

| PRIMARY TUMOR (T) | |
|---|---|
| TX | Primary tumor cannot be assessed |
| TO | No evidence of primary tumor |

| SUPRATENTORIAL TUMOR | |
|---|---|
| T1 | Tumor 5 cm or less in greatest dimension; limited to one side |
| T2 | Tumor more than 5 cm in greatest dimension; limited to one side |
| T3 | Tumor invades or encroaches upon the ventricular system |
| T4 | Tumor crosses the midline, invades the opposite hemisphere, or invades infratentorially |

| INFRATENTORIAL TUMOR | |
|---|---|
| T1 | Tumor 3 cm or less in greatest dimension; limited to one side |
| T2 | Tumor more than 3 cm in greatest dimension; limited to one side |
| T3 | Tumor invades or encroaches upon the ventricular system |
| T4 | Tumor crosses the midline, invades the opposite hemisphere, or invades supratentorially |

| REGIONAL LYMPH NODES (N) | |
|---|---|
| This category does not apply to this site. | |

| DISTANT METASTASIS (M) | |
|---|---|
| MX | Presence of distant metastasis cannot be assessed |
| MO | No distant metastasis |
| M1 | Distant metastasis |

| HISTOPATHOLOGIC GRADE (G) | |
|---|---|
| GX | Grade cannot be assessed |
| G1 | Well-differentiated |
| G2 | Moderately well-differentiated |
| G3 | Poorly differentiated |
| G4 | Undifferentiated |

| STAGE GROUPING | | | |
|---|---|---|---|
| Stage IA | G1 | T1 | MO |
| Stage IB | G1 | T2 | MO |
| | G1 | T3 | MO |
| Stage IIA | G2 | T1 | MO |
| Stage IIB | G2 | T2 | MO |
| | G2 | T3 | MO |
| Stage IIIA | G3 | T1 | MO |
| Stage IIIB | G3 | T2 | MO |
| | G3 | T3 | MO |
| Stage IV | G1,2,3 | T4 | MO |
| | G4 | Any T | MO |
| | Any G | Any T | M1 |

Data from Behars OH, Henson DE, Hutter R, et al: *Manual for Staging of Cancer* (ed 4), Philadelphia, Lippincott, 1992, pp 247–252.[97]

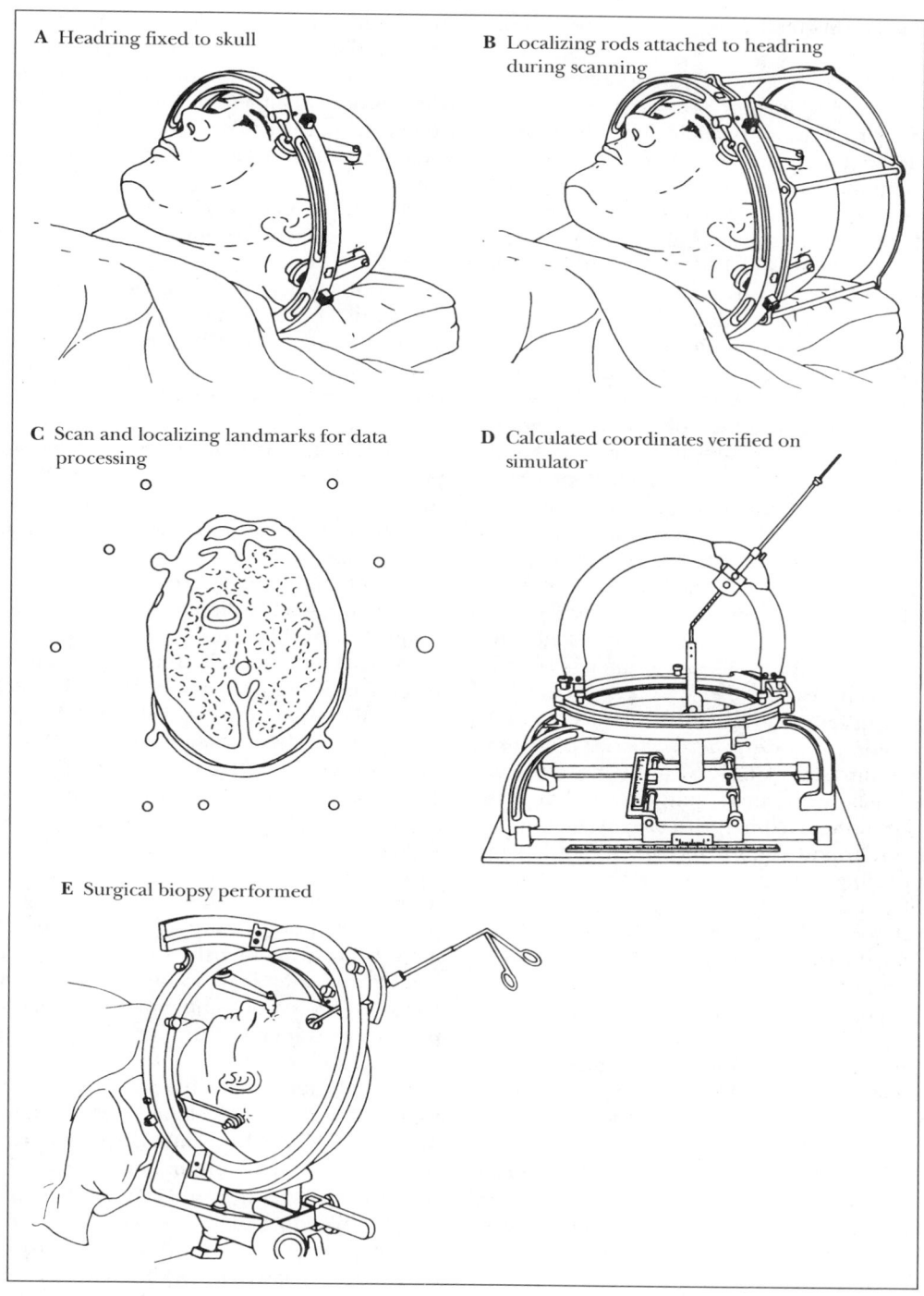

A Headring fixed to skull

B Localizing rods attached to headring during scanning

C Scan and localizing landmarks for data processing

D Calculated coordinates verified on simulator

E Surgical biopsy performed

**FIGURE 35-22**  Stereotaxic surgery. Diagrams show the sequence of steps using the BRW stereotaxic guidance system. A: The head ring is fixed to the skull. B: The localizing rod system is attached to the head ring for scanning. C: A sample localizing scan from which x-y coordinates of nine localizing rod and intracranial target images are determined for computation by the calculator. D: Computed arc settings are verified for correct trajectory and depth to target on the simulator. E: Arc guidance system is attached to the head ring, and intracranial procedure is performed. (Reprinted with permission from Heilbrun MP, Roberts TS, Apuzzo MLJ, et al: Preliminary experience with Brown-Roberts-Wells (BRW) computerized tomography stereotaxic guidance system. *J Neurosurg* 59:217–222, 1983.[101])

hospital stays may be shorter, leading to decreased hospitalization costs.

The aim of brain tumor surgery is to remove the tumor completely and ultimately provide a cure. However, surgical cure is often not possible, as in the case of most gliomas. Reduction of tumor bulk or partial resection during a craniotomy decompresses the brain and becomes the next goal. Partial tumor resection will generally improve the person's neurological condition by decreasing local compression and ICP. This should be the first therapeutic modality for most tumors. Surgical resection is complicated and may not always be possible when tumors are located deep within the brain or in areas that control vital functions. Another factor adding to the complexity of tumor removal is the difficulty in determining where the tumor ends and the normal brain begins. Preoperative imaging studies readily identify tumors and some of their characteristics. They are unable to precisely define the margins of a solid tumor, the surrounding areas of infiltrating tumor cells and peritumoral edema, and the normal adjacent brain.[100,105] Recent advances in neurosurgery have helped to address these issues so that most individuals with brain tumors today can safely undergo successful resections.[100,106] These advances include intraoperative monitoring devices and frameless stereotactic surgical procedures.

Typically, the surgeon has relied on consistency and color of the tumor to guide the resection.[94] The use of intraoperative ultrasound (IOUS) gives the surgeon immediate feedback during the craniotomy and depicts images that assist in the maximal resection of the tumor. Intraoperative ultrasound helps to define the borders of tumors by delineating both the tumor and its transition toward normal tissue and differentiating edema from solid tumor and normal brain.[100,107] In addition, IOUS is useful in planning the route or approach through normal tissue to reach the tumor.[100]

Functional mapping of the brain is another type of intraoperative monitoring. Brain mapping can facilitate a more complete tumor resection, with decreased morbidity in some patients. Once the dura is opened, electrodes are placed on the surface of the brain. By stimulating the electrodes, the motor cortex and, in awake patients, the speech centers can be located. Once these functional areas are located, the resection continues and the tumor is removed, keeping the mapped areas intact and reducing the neurological deficits. This type of procedure can also be used to detect the origin of seizure foci in persons with refractory seizures. Brain mapping is useful in surgery in the dominant hemisphere, the motor and sensory regions, and the speech centers.

Frameless stereotactic surgical procedures have recently been used with success in brain tumor surgery. Frameless stereotactic neurosurgery provides neurosurgeons with precise preoperative and intraoperative patient information. A pointing device, such as the viewing wand, is used to quickly communicate surgical locations to a computer system.[104] At any time during the surgery, the surgeon can place the probe on a structure and, by viewing the screen, determine its location in relation to surrounding structures and the angle of the approach to the tumor.[100] Such a navigational tool allows the surgeon to perform a safe, more effective, and less invasive tumor excision, which translates into improved patient outcomes.

The introduction of intraoperative monitoring devices, stereotactic surgical procedures (framed and frameless), complex imaging techniques, and new and improved surgical instruments for tumor removal have helped make tremendous advances in the surgical management of brain tumors. Many tumors traditionally considered unapproachable are being biopsied, partially resected, and sometimes completely removed with success.

Surgery also provides access for other adjuvant therapies. A stereotactic surgical procedure may be used to place radioactive sources within the tumor. Chemotherapy wafers may be implanted surgically within a tumor to slowly and continuously release chemotherapy directly into the brain. Ommaya reservoirs may be placed to deliver chemotherapy directly into the CSF, as discussed in chapter 15 of this text.

Nursing interventions for patients undergoing neurosurgical procedures begin preoperatively. A baseline neurological examination is essential and includes assessment of general cerebral function, including level of consciousness and cognitive function, motor and sensory function, coordination, gait, and cranial nerves. Neurological assessment is conducted on an ongoing basis to identify any variations that may signify potential complications such as increased ICP. Patient and family preoperative teaching consists of education in the planned surgical procedure, postoperative routines, the probable need for monitoring in an intensive care unit, measures to prevent complications, and medications that will be administered. Figure 35-23 is an example of a documentation tool for pre- and postoperative teaching for patients undergoing neurosurgery.

Complications after neurosurgery include intracranial bleeding, cerebral edema, further neurological impairment, electrolyte imbalance, infection, seizures, venous thromboembolism, and hydrocephalus. Hemorrhage at the operative site can occur within hours after surgery. Bleeding may also occur from traction on the bridging veins between the brain and the dura, leading to a subdural hematoma.[31] Additional areas where bleeding may occur are the epidural space, the subarachnoid space, or within the ventricles.

Postoperative cerebral edema is especially severe when there is residual tumor, but it occurs even after complete tumor removal. It results from the surgical manipulation of the surrounding brain tissue, changes in regional blood flow, or brain injury caused by excessive retraction.[100] The amount of edema varies in each individual but generally reaches its maximum peak at 48–72 hours postoperatively. Cerebral edema is treated with corticosteroids, usually dexamethasone, careful fluid man-

**MEMORIAL SLOAN-KETTERING CANCER CENTER**
**PATIENT EDUCATION DOCUMENTATION FORM**

**PATIENT IDENTIFICATION**

| DATE | **LEARNING NEEDS ASSESSMENT** |
|---|---|
| **INITIALS** | Check any of the following that impact teaching/learning:<br>— Physical disability    — Religion<br>— Cognitive changes    — Culture<br>— Emotional issues    — Language<br>— Lack of agreement with learning objectives |

Date and initial all entries.
Document all comments on the reverse side; indicate by circling your initials in the appropriate column.

Taught to: _____ patient _____ other _____

| | | Teaching Sessions | | | | | | Outcome Achieved | |
|---|---|---|---|---|---|---|---|---|---|
| | **EXPECTED OUTCOMES** | **1** | | **2** | | **3** | | | |
| | THE PATIENT / FAMILY IS ABLE TO: | Date | Initials | Date | Initials | Date | Initials | Date | Initials |
| 1. | Describe the operative procedure to be performed. | | | | | | | | |
| 2. | Describe any significant physical changes likely to result from surgery (i.e., incision, skull defect, motor/sensory loss, speech loss). | | | | | | | | |
| 3. | State that aspirin or products containing aspirin must be discontinued 10 days before surgery. | | | | | | | | |
| 4. | State that the physician should be notified if any new illness develops before surgery (i.e., cold, flu, fever, sore throat). | | | | | | | | |
| 5. | State that he/she will be NPO after midnight. | | | | | | | | |
| 6. | State that valuables (dentures, etc.) will be removed before he/she leaves the unit to go to the O.R. | | | | | | | | |
| 7. | Demonstrate proper technique for coughing and deep breathing. | | | | | | | | |
| 8. | Demonstrate proper use of the incentive spirometer. | | | | | | | | |
| 9. | Demonstrate proper technique for leg exercises. | | | | | | | | |
| 10. | State the reason for log rolling while on bedrest (laminectomy only). | | | | | | | | |
| 11. | State the reason for the use of Venodyne® boots. | | | | | | | | |
| 12. | State that he/she might remain in PACU overnight. | | | | | | | | |
| 13. | State the reason for NICU stay and probable length of stay in NICU. | | | | | | | | |
| 14. | Describe catheters/tubes that he/she may have upon return from surgery (i.e., Foley®, IV/arterial lines, Jackson Pratt®, chest tube, nasogastric tubes). | | | | | | | | |
| 15. | Describe how and where family can obtain information on patient's status during surgery. | | | | | | | | |
| 16. | State the importance of taking pain medication. | | | | | | | | |
| 17. | State that pain medication will not be given automatically and describe how to obtain it. | | | | | | | | |
| 18. | State the reason for not giving sleeping medication immediately after surgery. | | | | | | | | |
| 19. | State that P.O. fluids will be restricted. | | | | | | | | |
| 20. | State the reason that he/she will be awakened every hour for 12 hours and then every two hours through the first night after surgery. | | | | | | | | |

**TEACHING BEFORE NEUROSURGERY**

Revised January 1995
MRC approved 1/26/95

**SEE BACK FOR COMMENTS/NOTES/SIGNATURE/RESOURCES**
56-11330

**B**59

**FIGURE 35-23**  Patient education documentation form. (Reprinted with permission from Memorial Sloan-Kettering Cancer Center, Division of Nursing.)

agement, and osmotherapy when necessary. The effects of osmotic diuretic therapy on ICP are best evaluated by the use of an intracranial pressure monitor.[31] Other techniques for controlling ICP are hyperventilation, CSF drainage, hypothermia, and the use of anesthetic agents. Activities that can exacerbate ICP should be avoided. The head of the bed is generally elevated 30°–45° for supratentorial surgeries and 10° for infratentorial surgeries. Patients are assessed frequently to identify increased ICP. The signs and symptoms of cerebral edema may be similar to those of intracranial bleeding: decreased level of consciousness, progressive focal neurological deficit, increased ICP, seizures, and possible herniation.

A transient increase in neurological deficit can occur immediately after surgery as a result of swelling, retraction, or resection. Rambo and Sawaya[100,108] reported this complication in approximately 10% of patients.

Electrolyte imbalance, namely hyponatremia, can occur and is treated with fluid restriction. Some authors recommend limiting total fluid administration to 1500 ml/day after craniotomy.[102] Infection is often prevented by the prophylactic use of antibiotics for 24–48 hours postoperatively.

Seizures are managed with prophylactic anticonvulsants and maintenance of therapeutic serum levels. It is generally accepted that all patients undergoing supratentorial craniotomy receive seizure prophylaxis. Phenytoin is the most commonly used agent. A CT scan is indicated after a postoperative seizure to rule out hematoma, increased cerebral edema, or pneumocephalus.[102]

Venous thromboembolism is a particular concern in neurosurgery patients because of the length of surgery, immobility of some postoperative patients, and tumor-related hypercoagulable states.[100] The incidence of this complication is reduced by the use of pneumatic compression stockings.

Postoperative hydrocephalus may be caused by tumor, periventricular swelling, or intraventricular blood. When severe, it is usually treated with ventriculostomy or ventriculoperitoneal shunting.

## Radiation therapy

Radiation therapy plays a central role in the treatment of adult brain tumors.[109] Early randomized studies by the Brain Tumor Cooperative Group (BTCG) firmly established the role of postoperative RT in patients with malignant gliomas, the most common adult primary brain tumor. Individuals who received postoperative RT had a significantly prolonged survival as compared with those who received only postoperative supportive care. These studies were so convincing that almost all subsequent clinical trials evaluating adjuvant therapy for malignant brain tumors have included RT in all treatment arms.[110] Radiotherapy also has an important role in the treatment of patients with low-grade gliomas, inoperable, partially resected, or recurrent benign brain tumors, and metastatic brain tumors.

The amount of brain tissue to include within the treatment field has been the subject of considerable debate. Radiotherapy for malignant gliomas historically was delivered to the whole brain (WBRT). This was due in part to the belief in the diffuse nature of these tumors and that treatment failure was due to inadequate tumor coverage. Neuroimaging studies have shown that the majority of tumors recur within 1–2 cm of their original location. In addition, many individuals who survive for extended periods after WBRT develop significant treatment-related morbidity.[43,111,112] Therefore, partial brain irradiation or local field radiotherapy (LFRT) is now accepted as the standard treatment approach.[43,113] Conventional external beam RT is given in divided doses (fractions) over a long period of time. This allows normal tissue a chance to repair any radiation damage. Tumor tissue, however, is less capable of repair. It is believed that cells deep within the tumor are hypoxic. Since radiation is more damaging to cells with oxygen, dividing the RT into multiple doses may allow hypoxic tumor cells the opportunity to obtain oxygen, making them more susceptible to the next dose of radiation. The radiation is generally administered once daily over six weeks to deliver 60 Gy to the tumor and a 3-cm margin of tissue surrounding the perimeter.[43,109,114] Higher doses have not improved the outcome and have led to increased toxicity. WBRT is usually reserved for multifocal disease.

Other primary brain tumors may be treated with RT. Benign brain tumors such as meningiomas and pituitary adenomas are often surgically cured. In tumors that cannot be completely excised or that recur despite aggressive resection, RT is an important adjuvant therapy. Completely resected benign meningiomas and pituitary adenomas have a low risk of recurrence, and postoperative RT is not generally recommended. In contrast, the risk of recurrence in partially resected tumors is much higher, and studies have demonstrated that postoperative RT may delay recurrence, ultimately improving survival, or, in some patients, provide a cure. A dose of 55 Gy is recommended for benign tumors. Individuals with malignant meningiomas generally receive postoperative RT, regardless of the extent of resection, and the dose is increased to 60 Gy.[2]

The role of RT in low-grade gliomas is not as clearly defined.[115] Shaw et al concluded that postoperative RT should be routinely given to all patients with low-grade gliomas. The rationale for early intervention is based on the poor long-term survival in these individuals, the likelihood that low-grade tumors will transform into high-grade tumors, and the decreased morbidity of modern RT.[115,116] Others, though, prefer observation alone and defer RT until progression or recurrence of disease occurs. Recht et al[41] compared two groups with low-grade gliomas, one group who received RT after surgery and the other group who received observation alone, and found no difference in survival. Those in favor of observation alone base their opinion on the lack of proven benefit and the potential long-term effects of RT in these patients.[115,117] A dose of 55 Gy is generally administered,[2] although 45–65 Gy may be considered reasonable.[115] Several clinical trials evaluating delayed versus immediate treatment in low-grade gliomas are in progress and will hopefully help define the optimal therapy for these individuals.

Radiation therapy is the standard treatment for metastatic brain tumors. Although up to 50% of individuals with metastatic brain tumors have single lesions, many will not be surgical candidates. The lesion may be surgically inaccessible, or widespread systemic disease may be present. These individuals and those with multiple metastases typically undergo RT. WBRT is preferred because multiple metastases may be present even if some are too small to be detected on imaging studies. There is no consensus on the optimal radiation dose and schedule for the treatment of brain metastases. Currently, typical radiation treatment schedules for metastatic brain tumors consist of a total dose of 30–50 Gy delivered over a short period of time (7–15 days).[118] This type of schedule minimizes the duration of treatment while still delivering an adequate radiation dose to the tumor. Lower daily fractions and a more protracted course may be indicated in persons with a better prognosis.[76,117] As with primary tumors, response rates vary with the histological characteristics of the primary tumor. For example, metastases from breast and lung cancers respond better to RT than metastases from melanoma or renal or colon cancers.[31,76]

A number of new approaches in RT have been and continue to be evaluated in an attempt to improve the results obtained with conventional RT in individuals with brain tumors. These are the use of radiosensitizers, alternative methods of fractionation, focal dose escalation, hyperthermia, particle therapy, and boron neutron capture therapy (BNCT).

Malignant gliomas are radioresistant. It is believed that the radioresistance of gliomas may be due in part to the presence of hypoxic tumor cells. Hypoxia protects the tumor cells from the effects of RT. The radiation dose would have to be increased by about three times to obtain the same effect in hypoxic cells that is achieved in fully oxygenated cells. This large amount of radiation, however, would cause unacceptable side effects and damage to normal brain tissue. Radiosensitizers are chemicals that increase the lethal effects of radiation. Hypoxic cell sensitizers sensitize the hypoxic tumor cells without increasing the radiation effect on the well-oxygenated normal tissue. The compounds metronidazole and misonidazole, along with RT, have shown no improvement in survival over RT without the sensitizers. Other hypoxic cell sensitizers being investigated are etanidazole and pimonidazole.[109,111]

Another class of radiosensitizers, the halogenated pyrimidines, are also being evaluated. Two of these compounds, 5-bromodeoxyuridine (BUdR) and 5-iododeoxyuridine (IUdR), appear to work as sensitizers by substituting for one of the essential ingredients needed by cells to repair radiation damage. Only actively dividing tumor cells incorporate these drugs. The substitution of these drugs may potentiate the effectiveness of RT at these sites of incorporation only. Initial studies of BUdR with RT indicated a significant improvement in survival for patients with anaplastic astrocytoma. Randomized studies are currently in progress comparing BUdR-sensitized RT with nonsensitized RT in individuals with anaplastic astrocytoma.[109]

Alternative forms of fractionation are hyperfractionation and accelerated fractionation. In hyperfractionation two or more treatments are administered daily using fraction sizes that are smaller than conventional dose fractions to increase the total dose given over the same period of time. It is known that damage to normal brain tissue is related not only to a higher total radiation dose but also to the size of the fraction administered and to the amount of brain irradiated. If the amount of each fraction is lowered or the volume of tissue radiated is decreased, an increase in the total dose may not cause excessive damage. This approach allows a higher dose to be given to the tumor while maintaining the normal brain tissue at or below tolerance levels.[109] In accelerated fractionation, conventional dose fractions are administered two to three times daily and reduce the overall treatment time. This fractionation scheme may be appropriate for individuals with a shorter life expectancy such as the elderly. In addition, the more frequent fractions administered in these techniques may increase the possibility of catching the tumor cells in a vulnerable stage of the cell cycle.

Conventional doses of radiation fail to locally control the majority of malignant gliomas. These tumors generally recur within two centimeters of the original site in 80%–90% of cases.[119] New techniques have been developed that allow focal dose escalation to the tumor while decreasing the radiation exposure to normal brain tissue. These include interstitial brachytherapy, stereotactic radiosurgery, and three-dimensional conformal RT.

Brachytherapy involves the temporary implantation of radioactive sources directly into the brain tumor. Catheters are placed into the tumor using CT- and MRI-guided stereotactic surgical techniques, and the radiation seeds or pellets are then placed in the catheters. The radiation sources generally used are iodine 125 ($^{125}$I) or iridium 192 ($^{192}$Ir) and are removed after several days or weeks. The area of tumor receives the highest dose, since the sources are directly within the area to be irradiated. Surrounding normal brain tissue is spared because there is a rapid falloff in dose as the distance from the radiation source increases.[109] The advantage to interstitial brachytherapy is that the effect on normal tissue is greatly reduced, thus decreasing some of the resulting side effects.

Only about 30% of individuals with malignant gliomas are usually eligible for brachytherapy. Individuals with tumors that are large or multifocal, that cross the midline, that are inaccessible or located in functionally vital areas, or whose performance status is low are not candidates for this form of therapy. The initial studies using brachytherapy demonstrated an increased survival in individuals with recurrent GBM. These results led to trials with [125]I implants as a component of primary therapy along with conventional external beam RT. Gutin et al[120] reported a median survival from diagnosis of 88 weeks in a group of newly diagnosed individuals with GBM who received conventional RT followed by brachytherapy boost as part of initial treatment. In a similar trial Wen et al[92] reported a median survival of 18 months. Another significant finding was the increased two-year survival of 39% and 34%, respectively.

Another method of focal dose escalation is stereotactic radiosurgery, which uses an imaging-compatible stereotactic device to precisely localize an intracranial target and delivers a high radiation dose in a single session without delivering significant radiation to the surrounding normal brain tissue.[43] This technique is performed using a modified linear accelerator, gamma knife unit, or cyclotron. Radiosurgery has become increasingly available, with over 200 facilities in the United States currently treating patients.

Radiosurgery was initially used for small arteriovenous malformations (AVMs), benign brain tumors, and brain metastases. Initially, malignant tumors were not considered appropriate for radiosurgery because of their invasiveness and large size. Recently, however, there has been a growing interest in the use of radiosurgery in the treatment of primary and recurrent malignant brain tumors, and some of the initial results are encouraging. Shrieve and associates[114] reported on a group of individuals with recurrent GBM treated with radiosurgery. The median survival was 10.2 months, with a 19% two-year survival. In another study, 69 newly diagnosed individuals with GBM received radiosurgery as a boost following surgery and external beam RT. Median survival was 19.7 months, and two- and three-year survival rates were 31% and 20%.[109,121] Unfortunately, the majority of individuals with malignant gliomas also would not be eligible for this type of therapy because of their functional status, tumor size, or tumor shape. A prospective randomized trial by the RTOG is in progress to evaluate the role of radiosurgery in the initial management of those with malignant gliomas. Patients are randomized to receive either conventional RT and BCNU alone (standard therapy) or preceded by a radiotherapy boost.[43]

The major complication of both brachytherapy and radiosurgery is the development of symptomatic radiation necrosis requiring prolonged administration of steroids and reoperation. The rate of reoperation is 30%–40%, usually within six months. There has not been a randomized trial comparing radiosurgery and brachytherapy in the treatment of either primary or recurrent GBM. Although the outcomes for brachytherapy and radiosurgery are similar, radiosurgery offers several advantages. Radiosurgery is a noninvasive single-day procedure usually performed in an outpatient setting. Thus the risk of hemorrhage and infection and a prolonged hospitalization can be avoided. Radiosurgery can be used for

lesions that may be unsuitable for brachytherapy because of their location. Radiosurgery may also be used to retreat patients with small, previously irradiated lesions.[43]

Stereotactic radiotherapy (SRT) uses the planning technology of stereotactic radiosurgery but delivers the treatment using standard fractionation doses. Stereotactic radiosurgery hardware and software and head frames that can be relocalized daily in a nontraumatic and reproducible fashion are used.[43] Standard fractionation avoids the toxicities associated with large single doses, and tumors located near critical structures may be more successfully treated with the precision of the stereotactic technique. This approach is being used for some benign tumors and gliomas.

Three-dimensional conformal radiation therapy (3D-CRT) is a new method of high-precision RT. It utilizes CT information and powerful computer technology to plan and deliver external beam radiation treatments that shape the prescription dose distribution to conform to the anatomic boundaries of the tumor in its entire three-dimensional configuration.[43] Until recently, 3D-CRT was not practical because the highly complex software required for treatment planning and for computer-controlled dose delivery was unavailable. This method provides complete anatomic and dose information for the entire tumor volume and its surrounding normal tissue. The selection of beam shapes and the direction they travel confine the radiation dose to the tumor target, while minimizing the dose to the surrounding normal tissue. Comparative two-dimensional and three-dimensional treatment planning studies in brain tumor patients have demonstrated a 30% reduction in the amount of normal brain irradiated when the 3D-CRT method is used.[43,122] This method not only decreases the risk of normal tissue injury but may also allow higher than traditional doses to be safely administered to patients with malignant gliomas. Dose escalation studies are in progress.

Hyperthermia is heat therapy. While heat is cytotoxic to both normal and malignant cells, several characteristics of brain tumor cells may make them more susceptible to heat damage. Hypoxic cells and cells in the S phase are sensitive to heat; heat inhibits the repair of sublethal radiation damage and, therefore, has an additive effect when combined with RT;[111] heat may also augment the effect of some chemotherapeutic agents.

Various methods can be used to produce the heat, including radio frequency, microwave antennae, ultrasound, and electromagnetic techniques. Hyperthermia is usually performed during a surgical procedure. However, the inability to homogeneously heat the tumor mass and the ineffective monitoring of intratumoral and normal brain temperatures have been limitations of this method.[111] Several studies have evaluated the use of hyperthermia in CNS tumors as single therapy, in combination with RT, and in combination with chemotherapy in small series of patients. Sneed et al[123] reported a median survival of 47 weeks in a group of patients with recurrent

GBM treated with brachytherapy and hyperthermia, and a 65% 18-month survival in patients with recurrent anaplastic astrocytoma treated with brachytherapy and hyperthermia. The therapeutic effect of this type of therapy remains to be seen.

Particle therapy refers to the use of subatomic particles rather than photons as a form of radiation. These particles, which include neutrons, protons, helium ions and heavier nuclei, and pions, are produced by cyclotrons. Charged particles allow for better dose localization of their beams to the tumor volume. This decreases damage to normal tissue. Charged particles also have a greater biological effect than photons; that is, they are more effective in killing tumor cells.[111] Research in this newer form of therapy continues.

In BNCT a boron compound is administered systemically and is theoretically incorporated only into dividing cells such as tumor cells. A type of nonionizing radiation, focused thermal neutron irradiation, is administered. The neutrons react with the boron and release high-energy alpha particles, cytotoxic to the cells in which the reaction occurs, namely, the boron-containing cells. The normal brain cells are not affected because the radiation causes a reaction only in the boron-containing cells.

The widespread use of this technique has been limited by the high cost, limited availability of nuclear reactors, and the lack of suitable boron compounds that do not have harmful side effects. In addition, the biodistribution of boron limits significant concentrations of this compound in infiltrating cells. Therefore, this is only a focal therapy at present. Tumor cells in areas away from the tumor mass will not incorporate the boron and will then not be sensitive to the neutrons. Early studies in astrocytoma patients did not improve survival and were associated with significant toxicity. However, interest in this therapy is growing again.

Side effects of RT can be classified as acute reactions, early delayed reactions, and late delayed reactions. The acute reactions occur during the course of treatment and are temporary. They result from an increase in cerebral edema; the administration of corticosteroids usually decreases or alleviates symptoms. Other acute adverse effects are nausea, vomiting, anorexia, fatigue, alopecia, and skin irritation.

The early delayed reactions generally develop one to three months after completion of therapy. These, too, are of a temporary nature. Symptoms include anorexia, sleepiness, lethargy, and an increase in neurological deficits. These effects are thought to result from the temporary disruption of myelin formation, which helps speed the relay of nerve signals. It takes approximately six weeks for myelin to repair.

Late effects of RT usually occur 6–24 months after completion of treatment. These effects are irreversible and often progressive. They result from direct injury to brain tissue and blood vessels. Leukoencephalopathy, degeneration of the white matter, occurs at the tumor site and surrounding irradiated brain. The risk of developing leukoencephalopathy increases with the concomitant use of neurotoxic chemotherapeutic agents, particularly methotrexate. The clinical manifestations range from mild cognitive neurological impairment to dementia to death. The onset and progression can be quite variable. Radiation necrosis occurs more commonly after brachytherapy and radiosurgery but can occur after conventional RT as well. Those at increased risk for long-term radiation effects are children under 2 years of age and adults over 50. Long-term effects can be initially managed to some degree with corticosteroids and surgery to remove necrotic tissue. Other long-term effects include loss of vision, development of secondary malignancies, and endocrine disturbances.

### Chemotherapy

Although it does not produce a cure or substantial numbers of long-term survivors, chemotherapy plays an important adjuvant role in the treatment of adult primary brain tumors. The most widely studied group of tumors has been the malignant glioma because it is the most common adult primary brain tumor and accounts for the majority of deaths in individuals with brain tumors. Many studies have evaluated a variety of single chemotherapeutic agents and multiple drug regimens. However, some studies have reported conflicting results and some results are difficult to interpret; as a result, ambiguities exist as to current treatment recommendations.[124]

It has been historically difficult to accrue large numbers of individuals with primary brain tumors into clinical trials. Early trials often contained heterogeneous patient populations and failed to separate participants according to prognostically significant variables such as age, tumor histology, and performance status. A younger person with a malignant glioma will generally respond better than an older individual with the same tumor. A person with an anaplastic astrocytoma has a better prognosis than a person with a GBM, and those with a higher performance status generally do better than those with a low performance status. Another problem is the lack of uniform response criteria to facilitate the interpretation and comparison of data from the many clinical trials. Different pathological grading criteria have been used in different studies, also making it difficult to compare results.

Despite these methodological problems, Fine et al[110] performed a meta-analysis to find out if adjuvant chemotherapy improved survival in individuals with malignant gliomas. They compared the results from 16 randomized clinical trials and found a statistically significant survival advantage for those who received adjuvant chemotherapy. The BTCG also concluded that standard treatment of individuals with malignant gliomas should include chemotherapy with a nitrosourea.[125]

Many factors affect the responsiveness of brain tumors to chemotherapy. These include tumor histology, tumor blood flow, the presence of inherent and acquired mechanisms of drug resistance, and the concentrations of the chemotherapeutic agent delivered to the tumor.[126]

The delivery of adequate concentrations of chemotherapy to tumors within the CNS is limited by the presence of the blood-brain barrier (BBB). The BBB is made of a continuous lining of endothelial cells that are connected by tight junctions (Figure 35-24).[31] The passage of substances across the lipid membranes of endothelial cells depends on molecular weight, lipid solubility, and ionization state.[126] Large, water-soluble, charged particles and compounds bound to plasma proteins are unable to penetrate the BBB. This vascular barrier normally protects the brain by limiting the entry of potentially toxic substances into brain tissue. Unfortunately, the BBB also effectively prevents the majority of chemotherapeutic agents from entering brain tissue. If the BBB did not exist, it is possible that CNS toxicity rather than myelosuppression or gastrointestinal toxicity would be the dose-limiting factor for most chemotherapeutic agents[2] because more drug would reach brain tissue.

Although the BBB can be a potential obstacle to the delivery of chemotherapy to these tumors, the most malignant brain tumors are often associated with marked disruption of this barrier. The cause of this BBB dysfunction is not well understood. Tumor angiogenesis may produce vessels that are not capable of forming a functional barrier.[127] Ultrastructural studies have shown ab-

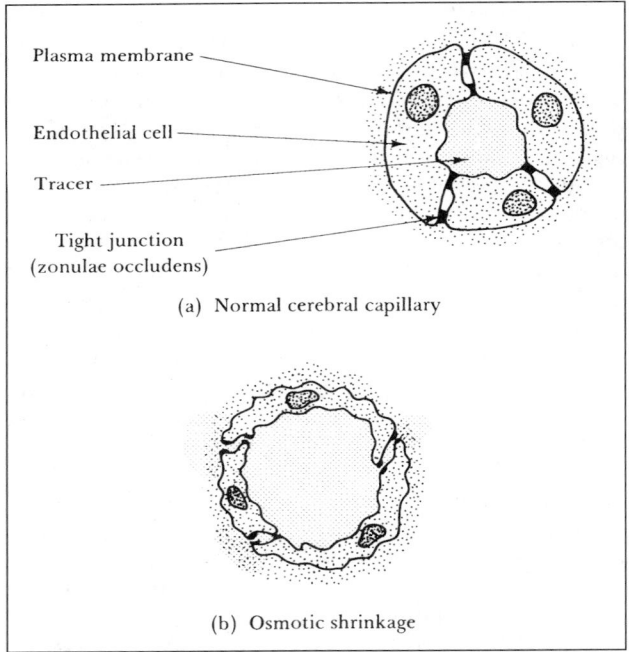

Plasma membrane

Endothelial cell

Tracer

Tight junction
(zonulae occludens)

(a)  Normal cerebral capillary

(b)  Osmotic shrinkage

**FIGURE 35-24** Schematic representation of the blood-brain barrier.[31] (a) Normal cerebral capillary showing tight junctions. (b) Blood-brain barrier opening by widening of the interendothelial tight junctions. When the endothelial cells shrink in a hypertonic environment, the permeability of the junctions is increased.

normally tight junctions and a disrupted endothelial surface in brain tumor vasculature.[128] Also, astrocytomas appear to produce a substance capable of altering the permeability of the cerebral blood vessels.[129] Regardless of the mechanism involved, water-soluble contrast agents administered with CT or MRI are able to cross the normally impermeable BBB and enter the brain in the region of the tumor. The surrounding normal brain, however, continues to exclude the contrast material because its BBB remains intact. Thus, the enhancing masses seen on CTs and MRIs represent regions of tumor with a substantially disrupted BBB. Malignant cells, however, often infiltrate adjacent tissue and spread to distant sites. Contrast enhancement usually does not occur in the surrounding normal brain that typically contains micrometastatic disease.[128] The BBB is therefore at least partially intact in many brain tumors, particularly in the periphery of the tumor and around infiltrating tumor cells.

Small, water-soluble chemotherapeutic agents, normally excluded from the brain by an intact BBB, may reach enhancing areas of a tumor. Systemically administered water-soluble agents have been shown to produce a response in some tumors, but treatment with only water-soluble agents is of limited value since these tumors extend beyond the regions of contrast enhancement.[127] For this reason, initial chemotherapeutic agents studied in individuals with malignant gliomas were lipid-soluble agents that readily cross the BBB such as the nitrosoureas, mainly carmustine (BCNU). After years of study and many trials, no other chemotherapeutic agent or combination of agents has been shown to be more effective than carmustine for those with GBM. Other agents that have shown some activity against gliomas include procarbazine, cisplatin, carboplatin, etoposide, cyclophosphamide, vincristine, iproplatin, nimustine, lomustine, and hydroxyurea.[126,127] In some studies the combination of procarbazine, lomustine, and vincristine (PCV) has been found to be more effective than carmustine alone for those with anaplastic astrocytoma. Levin et al[45] demonstrated an increased median survival of 151 weeks in individuals with anaplastic astrocytoma treated with PCV as opposed to 82 weeks for those who received BCNU. This regimen (PCV), as opposed to BCNU, is being increasingly used as adjuvant chemotherapy for persons with anaplastic astrocytoma.

Recently the oligodendrogliomas have been found to be chemosensitive. The PCV combination has been the most widely studied regimen for these tumors, and positive results have been obtained for both newly diagnosed and recurrent tumors. This regimen is now the treatment of choice for these tumors.[124] Mixed gliomas also appear to respond to these agents.

Individuals with many of the less common brain tumors many also be treated with chemotherapy. PCNSL and germ cell tumors are highly sensitive to chemotherapy. The germ cell tumors respond to a number of regimens containing cisplatin. Some of the successful agents include cyclophosphamide, doxorubicin, vincristine, vinblastine, bleomycin, etoposide, and carboplatin. The optimal chemotherapy for PCNSL has yet to be established, but promising results have been reported with a number of combination regimens. Medulloblastomas, occurring more often in children, have been treated with a variety of single-agent and combination chemotherapies. Anecdotal reports suggest that chemotherapy may be useful in a small percentage of patients with pineal tumors or ependymomas.[126] Finally, chemotherapy may be used in select groups of individuals with metastatic disease whose primary tumors are chemosensitive.

Unfortunately, the addition of adjuvant chemotherapy has added little improvement to the survival of individuals with malignant brain tumors, particularly those with GBM. New approaches have been explored in an attempt to increase the efficacy of the currently available chemotherapeutic agents by circumventing the BBB and delivering more drug to the tumor. These include IV continuous-infusion chemotherapy, intrathecal or intraventricular chemotherapy, intra-arterial chemotherapy, high-dose chemotherapy with autologous bone marrow transplantation, and interstitial chemotherapy. These strategies can selectively deliver higher concentrations of chemotherapy to the tumors. Unfortunately, the neurotoxicity of these approaches may correlate with the drug levels in the normal brain surrounding the tumor.[128]

As mentioned previously, water-soluble contrast agents used to image tumors on CT or MR scans are able to pass through the disrupted BBB near the area of tumor, producing contrast enhancement at the outer ring of the tumor. The inner portion of the tumor does not initially enhance. Bolus infusions of water-soluble agents with short plasma half-lives might treat the contrast-enhancing tumor ring but may never reach therapeutic concentrations within the center of the tumor. The observation that contrast enhancement, after hours of sustained blood levels, can reach the center of the tumor suggests that continuous infusions of water-soluble chemotherapeutic agents might result in a more uniform drug distribution within brain tumors.[128] Several studies combining lipid and water-soluble agents administered as a 72-hour continuous infulsion (BCNU and cisplatin) demonstrated partial responses in 50%–70% of participants and survival rates of 64% and 12% at one and three years, respectively.[128,130,131] A randomized study comparing this type of regimen with standard therapy of RT and BCNU is being evaluated.

The instillation of chemotherapy directly into the CSF is an important method of administering chemotherapy for individuals with leptomeningeal metastases, leukemic or lymphomatous meningitis, PCNSL, and primary CNS tumors such as medulloblastomas where the subarachnoid space is involved. A lumbar puncture for intrathecal chemotherapy administration has been performed safely in select persons. However, chemotherapy instilled directly into the ventricular CSF by way of the Ommaya reservoir has been found to produce better drug distribution throughout the CSF and more consistent drug levels.

Thus, the Ommaya reservoir is the preferred method of delivering chemotherapy into the CSF. It allows for greater ease of administration and less discomfort for the patient. Complications occurring with the use of this device include infection, catheter blockage, catheter leakage, and, after the administration of chemotherapy, a chemical meningitis.

Intra-arterial chemotherapy involves the catheterization of the carotid or vertebral arteries, which provide the arterial supply to brain tumors for the administration of chemotherapeutic agents. Agents that have been evaluated in this approach include BCNU, cisplatin, carboplatin, ACNU, and methotrexate. This method increases the amount of chemotherapy delivered to the tumor while decreasing the systemic toxicity. Although a number of small studies, using a variety of agents, have recorded encouraging results, it is not clear whether intra-arterial chemotherapy is more effective than conventional chemotherapy.[124] It is clear, however, that this method of drug delivery has significant toxicities. Shapiro et al[125] reported on the large BTCG study evaluating intra-arterial BCNU as one treatment arm that was discontinued early because of unacceptable toxicity. Fifteen percent of patients developed ipsilateral vision loss, and 10% had severe neurotoxicity. Moreover, survival rates were worse for those treated with intra-arterial BCNU than for those who received conventional IV BCNU.

Another approach to intra-arterial chemotherapy is to transiently disrupt the BBB with an osmotic agent such as mannitol just before the administration of the intra-arterial chemotherapy. Hypertonic mannitol causes a loss of fluid from the capillary endothelial cells, causing the endothelial cells to shrink and the tight junctions (zonulae occludens) to break, resulting in osmotic shrinkage (Figure 35-24).[31] Large molecular-sized materials or water-soluble agents may then diffuse through the opened junctions into the surrounding brain. Neuwelt and colleagues[132] treated 38 glioblastoma patients with IV cyclophosphamide followed by intra-arterial mannitol, methotrexate, and oral procarbazine, and the median survival achieved was 17.5 months. Gumerlock and associates,[133] in a more recent study, treated 37 glioblastoma patients with the same regimen and described a 22-month median survival rate. These prolonged survival rates compare favorably with the 10- to 12-month survival rate for those glioblastoma patients treated with conventional therapy. However, BBB disruption can be associated with significant toxicity. This procedure is performed monthly for 12 cycles under general anesthesia. In addition to the risks of general anesthesia, intra-arterial chemotherapy with BBB disruption produced worsening of neurological deficits in up to 56% and seizures in up to 44% of patients.[132] One reason for this toxicity is that mannitol also increases the permeability of normal capillaries, which significantly increases the vulnerability of the normal brain tissue to the toxic effects of chemotherapy.

High-dose chemotherapy followed by autologous bone marrow transplantation has also been evaluated in individuals with malignant gliomas in the hope of delivering more chemotherapy to the tumor. Most of the studies have used BCNU alone or in combination with other agents, including thiotepa and etoposide, as the preparative regimen. BCNU is the most effective agent to date for GBM, and its delayed and cumulative bone marrow depression is the dose-limiting toxicity. BCNU also has a steep dose-response curve, and these factors make it a good agent to consider for dose intensification followed by bone marrow rescue.[126] Although some long-term survivors were noted, median survival for newly diagnosed patients undergoing autologous bone marrow transplantation was 12–17 months. This approach was associated with significant morbidity, including fatal pulmonary toxicity, hepatotoxicity, and progressive neurological deterioration.[124] Studies evaluating the effectiveness of autologous bone marrow transplantation in individuals with a variety of brain tumors are in progress to determine whether this form of treatment will improve survival.

Interstitial chemotherapy involves the use of biodegradable polymers impregnated with chemotherapeutic agents and is a promising approach in chemotherapy delivery for brain tumors. These polymers are placed intraoperatively in the walls of the tumor cavities after resection and continuously release high local concentrations of chemotherapeutic agents. Chemotherapy delivered directly to the tumor bypasses the variably disrupted BBB, results in high local drug concentrations, and minimizes systemic toxicity. Chemotherapeutic agents, including 5-Fluorouracil, methotrexate, bleomycin, cisplatin, and ACNU, have been administered directly into the tumor in patients with high-grade gliomas without benefit.[126] Implantation of BCNU wafers, however, was found to prolong median survival to 46 weeks in a group of patients with recurrent high-grade gliomas.[134] A follow-up randomized, double-blind, placebo-controlled clinical trial was conducted at 27 medical centers in 222 patients with malignant glioma.[135,136] In this study the polymers containing BCNU modestly improved survival and did not cause significant adverse effects as compared with the many toxic effects commonly experienced by patients treated with systemic or intra-arterial BCNU. The safety and efficacy with which the polymers permit intracranial BCNU administration suggest that this drug delivery method could be used for a wide array of therapeutic agents that have not been successfully used in the past for treatment of brain tumors.[135] Future studies are planned to evaluate the effectiveness of higher doses of carmustine and the use of polymer implants as initial therapy for malignant brain tumors. This new route of administration may allow the use of new and established chemotherapeutic agents that previously could not be efficiently, safely, or effectively delivered to the brain.

Progress in the development of new chemotherapeutic agents for malignant brain tumors has been slow. Recently, however, several promising new agents for malignant gliomas have entered clinical trials. Partial responses were found in 40%–50% of individuals with newly diagnosed and recurrent high-grade gliomas treated with an oral agent, temozolomide. Other agents being studied include topotecan, a topoisomerase I inhibitor with excellent CNS penetration, and paclitaxel, which acts as a radiosensitizer and has direct antiglioma activity.[124,128]

Nursing management of the individual receiving chemotherapy includes assessment and evaluation of side effects, patient and family education regarding treatment schedules and routines, possible side effects, and interventions to enhance tolerance and maintain functional ability. Side effects of chemotherapeutic agents used for CNS cancers are listed in Table 35-7.

### Biotherapy

To date, biotherapy has had little success in the treatment of malignant brain tumors. However, there has been a renewed interest in this form of therapy. Recent studies have included the use of cytokines, adoptive immunotherapy with lymphokine-activated killer (LAK) cells and interleukin-2 (IL-2), monoclonal antibodies, and gene therapy.

The interferons have been evaluated in the treatment of gliomas more than any other cytokine. Response rates of up to 20% for alpha-interferon and 50% for beta-interferon have been reported.[42,137] However, these responses were short-lived and associated with significant neurotoxicity. Additional cytokines are being evaluated.

One method of adoptive immunotherapy that has been studied in gliomas is the infusion of LAK cells and IL-2 into the brain tissue surrounding the tumor during craniotomy, or into the tumor bed via a modified Ommaya reservoir. Although various responses have been reported, the results of this form of therapy have been disappointing in part because of the associated toxicity and the inability of the LAK cells to reach and kill the infiltrating tumor cells.[42,137] However, Hayes and associates[138] reported a 53-week median survival in patients with recurrent GBM who were treated with this approach. This compares favorably with the four to six-month average median survival for patients with recurrent GBM.

Research continues in the area of monoclonal antibodies for the treatment of CNS tumors. To date they have not been very effective because of the heterogeneity of CNS tumor cells, lack of tumor-specific antigens, poor ability of the antibodies to cross the BBB, and the development of neutralizing antibodies.[42,139]

A novel immunologic approach to the treatment of malignant brain tumors is gene therapy, which can be defined as the targeted transfer of genetic information for the purpose of effecting a change in a pathophysiological process.[137] Brain tumors appear to be a good choice for this type of therapy because they are relatively localized and rarely metastasize outside the CNS, and because well-established methods of drug delivery directly into the tumor (stereotactic injection, Ommaya reservoir, and intra-arterial injection) already exist.

The initial gene therapy trials for high-grade gliomas began in 1991 and used a retrovirus to carry one of the

**TABLE 35-7**  Chemotherapeutic Agents for CNS Cancers and Related Side Effects

| Chemotherapeutic Agents | Side Effects |
|---|---|
| Carboplatin | Myelosuppression<br>Nausea and vomiting<br>Peripheral neuropathy (less than cisplatin)<br>Ototoxicity<br>Alopecia |
| Carmustine (BCNU) | Delayed myelosuppression<br>Cumulative bone marrow toxicity<br>Pain and burning at intravenous site<br>Facial flushing<br>Brown discoloration of skin<br>Pulmonary fibrosis<br>Nausea and vomiting |
| Cisplatin | Nephrotoxicity<br>Ototoxicity<br>Nausea and vomiting<br>Myelosuppression<br>Peripheral neuropathies<br>Hypomagnesemia |
| Cyclophosphamide | Myelosuppression<br>Nausea and vomiting<br>Hemorrhagic cystitis<br>Cardiomyopathy<br>Pulmonary fibrosis<br>Syndrome of inappropriate secretion of anti-diuretic hormone (SIADH)<br>Alopecia |
| Cytarabine (ARA-C) | Myelosuppression<br>Cerebellar dysfunction<br>Chemical conjunctivitis<br>Nausea and vomiting |
| Etoposide (VP16) | Myelosuppression<br>Hypotension<br>Nausea and vomiting<br>Bronchospasm<br>Alopecia |
| Lomustine (CCNU) | Myelosuppression<br>Nausea and vomiting<br>Nephrotoxicity<br>Pain and burning at intravenous site<br>Hepatotoxicity |
| Methotrexate | Myelosuppression<br>Stomatitis<br>Diarrhea<br>Nephrotoxicity<br>Hepatotoxicity<br>Photosensitivity<br>Alopecia<br>Neurotoxicity |
| Methotrexate intraommaya intrathecal | Headache<br>Nuccal rigidity<br>Fever<br>Confusion |

**TABLE 35-7**  (continued)

| Chemotherapeutic Agents | Side Effects |
|---|---|
| Procarbazine | Nausea, vomiting, and diarrhea<br>Myelosuppression<br>Hypertensive crisis with tyramine-containing foods<br>Hepatotoxicity<br>Neurotoxicity |
| Thiotepa | Myelosuppression<br>Headache<br>Fever<br>Dizziness |
| Vincristine | Peripheral neuropathies<br>Constipation<br>Myelosuppression (mild)<br>Alopecia<br>Nausea and vomiting |

herpes simplex virus genes, the *thymidine kinase (TK)* gene, into tumor cells. The tumor cell becomes genetically like the herpes virus, divides, and produces more such cells. When an antiviral agent, gancyclovir, is administered, the tumor cells are killed. While the initial gene therapy trials are encouraging, many questions remain, including how to improve the gene transfer and how to reach more tumor cells.

A final area of investigation is in the inhibition of angiogenesis, which is the growth of new blood vessels. Tumor growth is dependent on the development of a new vascular supply. Endothelial proliferation is a characteristic feature of astrocytomas. The inhibition of tumor-associated new vessel growth could retard tumor growth and become a potentially useful treatment modality. Until recently, there have not been any selective nontoxic, powerful inhibitors of angiogenesis available. However, several new agents are now being investigated.[137]

## Spinal Cord Tumors

### Surgery

Surgery is the primary treatment modality for most intradural tumors. Intradural, extramedullary tumors such as schwannomas and meningiomas can often be completely resected today with microsurgical techniques and modern neurosurgical instruments. As in brain tumor surgery, intraoperative monitoring assists the surgeon in maximizing the resection while protecting the spinal cord. In most cases these tumors can be removed through a posterior (laminectomy) approach. The uncommon tumor directly anterior to the spinal cord must sometimes be approached anteriorly.[2] The risk of recurrence is estimated to be approximately 10% for complete resections, while recurrence rates increase to approximately 20% for incompletely resected tumors.[95] Recurrences are generally treated with repeat surgical resection unless the tumor extends beyond what is surgically accessible.

Surgery is the initial treatment for intramedullary tumors (ependymomas and astrocytomas) with the exception of the malignant astrocytomas. The determining factor in the successful surgical treatment of these tumors is the degree of infiltration of the surrounding spinal cord by the tumor. As with intracranial glial tumors, indistinct tumor margins can prevent complete tumor removal. Ependymomas of the spinal cord have a longer natural history than astrocytomas. Recurrence of ependymomas may be delayed up to 12 years, whereas astrocytomas that recur generally do so within three years.[2]

In extradural tumors, surgery is generally indicated only in cases where the cause of spinal cord compression is unknown, there is spinal instability or bone collapse into the spinal canal, a recurrence cannot be retreated with additional RT, the tumor is known to be radioresistant, or the individual is rapidly deteriorating neurologically, perhaps during the course of RT. Two common surgical procedures are posterior decompressive laminectomy and anterior vertebral body resection.

Laminectomy generally only decompresses the spinal cord. The surgeon is often unable to remove the bulk of the tumor during this approach because the tumor is usually located anterior to the spinal cord. If the tumor has invaded the epidural space posteriorly, a modified approach can sometimes allow considerable tumor removal. In a vertebral body resection, most or all of the tumor can be removed, and the resected vertebra is replaced with either bone or a synthetic substance such as methylmethacrylate. The spinal column is often further stabilized anteriorly, for example, with Steinmann pins or plates screwed into intact bone, or posteriorly with instruments such as Harrington rods or hooks.[76] Stabilization procedures require intact bone above and below the site of compression to accept, support, and maintain the fixation devices.[95] Patients with spinal instability typically must remain in bed until they can undergo a stabilization procedure or be fitted for a brace.

Complications related to surgical intervention include standard surgical risks (stroke, hemorrhage, development of a hematoma, deep vein thrombosis, pulmonary embolism, and infection) as well as neurological deficits, CSF leak, and wound dehiscence. The most significant complication to treat is a new neurological deficit in which the neurological function often may not return. This complication is typically related to vascular insult of or manipulation to the spinal cord during surgery.[95] A CSF leak may develop because the dura is not completely sealed or a tear was not repaired. A CSF leak is usually treated with lumbar drainage for several days. If the leakage continues, surgery may be required to repair the leak. A CSF leak increases the risk of infection and may lead to meningitis. Many individuals who develop spinal cord compression late in the course of their cancer may be debilitated and have often been on steroids. As a result, wound healing is poor, and they are at risk for wound dehiscence.[76]

### Radiation therapy

RT is generally not recommended for completely resected intradural (intramedullary and extramedullary) spinal cord tumors. Extramedullary tumors may be treated with RT on recurrence if surgical resection is not feasible. Intramedullary tumors that initially cannot be completely excised are generally irradiated with 50–55 Gy with good results. In patients with ependymomas who received adjuvant RT, five- and ten-year survival rates range from 60%–100% and 86%–93%, respectively. The ten-year relapse-free survival rates are 60%–90% and 40%–90%, respectively.[2,139] For those individuals with a high-grade astrocytoma, RT is often the only therapy available, and even so, the prognosis is poor.

RT and steroids are the most widely used therapy for extradural tumors. The treatment technique depends on the region of spinal involvement. The sensitivity of the spinal cord to radiation limits the prescribed dose. Spinal cord tolerance has been considered to be approximately 45–50 Gy delivered in 180-cGy fractions, between 35 and 37.5 Gy in 250-cGy fractions and between 30 and 33 Gy in 300-cGy fractions.[140] The usual dose administered is 30 Gy in 300-cGy fractions.[76] Often, higher doses are administered for the initial treatments, especially if there is evidence of neurological dysfunction.

Spinal RT does not cause acute clinical symptoms.[76] The major complication of spinal cord radiation—radiation myelopathy—results from demyelination and white matter necrosis or intramedullary microvascular injury. Radiation myelopathy may present as an early-delayed or a more severe late-delayed reaction. The transient early-delayed myelopathy is clinically manifested by momentary electrical shock–like paresthesias or numbness radiating from the neck down to the extremities, and it is precipitated by flexing the neck (Lhermitte's sign). This syndrome develops after an average of 3–4 months following treatment and resolves within 6–12 months without the need for intervention.[2]

The more severe late-delayed radiation myelopathy generally occurs 12–28 months following RT. The clinical manifestations are irreversible; they begin with weakness and can progress to a complete functional loss from the level of the radiation portal down. The number of individuals who develop this late myelopathy would be higher were it not for the fact that many succumb to their primary disease before the myelopathy becomes clinically evident.

### Chemotherapy

Chemotherapy does not play a large role in the treatment of spinal cord tumors. It may be considered for metastatic extradural tumors in individuals with chemosensitive tumors. There have been no trials of chemotherapy for intramedullary tumors. Drugs active against intracranial gliomas would logically be assumed to be effective against these same histologies in the spinal cord. There have been anecdotal reports of chemotherapy for primary spinal cord tumors.[2]

# SYMPTOM MANAGEMENT AND SUPPORTIVE CARE

Individuals with CNS tumors frequently suffer from disabling symptoms that dramatically affect their ability to function. Many of these symptoms are directly related to the tumor. Neural structures are destroyed or compressed, leading to increased ICP or spinal cord compression. Other symptoms, however, are only indirectly related to the cancer. These include side effects of medications used for symptom relief, such as corticosteroids and anticonvulsants, and the psychological symptoms resulting from the devastating effects of the nervous system tumor itself (e.g., aphasia, paralysis, incontinence, cognitive dysfunction).[141] The care of these individuals continues to shift to the home and community, regardless of prognosis. Supportive nursing measures assume importance in all areas of patient care.[31] Table 35-8 describes common nursing diagnoses, suggests causes of the problems, and offers some of the associated nursing interventions for the care of these individuals.

Brain tumors increase ICP by their size, cerebral edema, or obstruction of CSF pathways. Cerebral edema can often be managed with corticosteroids such as dexamethasone. Dramatic improvements in neurological function are often seen along with reduction in ICP within hours to days following the initiation of steroids, particularly in those individuals with tumors producing substantial edema.[34] Malignant intracranial tumors typically cause disruption of the BBB. The leaky blood vessels allow extravasation of plasma proteins into the surrounding area, which then pulls water into the area as well. Although the mechanism is unclear, the steroids act to reestablish the BBB,[78] thus decreasing edema.

In situations where ICP is acutely elevated, corticosteroids alone are insufficient and osmotic diuretics, also referred to as hyperosmolar agents, are required. The high concentration of the drug causes water to be drawn from the normal tissue. The principle of water diffusion depends on the presence of a semipermeable membrane. The direction of flow is from the hypoconcentrated to the hyperconcentrated solution. When a hyperosmolar drug, usually mannitol, is given, the flow of fluid is from the brain to the blood. The extracellular fluid of the edematous brain is hypotonic in relation to the hyperconcentration created by the drug in the blood. The fluid crosses the semipermeable cell membrane, moving into the blood and decreasing the edema in the brain.[29] Diure-

sis occurs within one to three hours and lasts up to approximately eight hours. An indwelling urinary catheter, strict recording of intake and output, and monitoring of electrolytes are necessary. Corticosteroids are administered concurrently. Other methods to help control increased ICP include fluid restriction, hyperventilation, sedation, and control of temperature. Valsalva maneuvers, isometric muscle contractions, coughing, sneezing, straining, and the use of PEEP should be avoided as they can further aggravate increased ICP. A decrease in venous outflow will increase the total blood volume within the intracranial space, leading to elevated ICP. Head and neck positions that impair venous outflow include jugular compression, head rotation, neck flexion, and neck extension. The head of the bed should be elevated to promote venous drainage. Lying prone and flexing the hips should also be avoided because these positions increase intra-abdominal and intrathoracic pressures, also leading to elevations in ICP. When turning or positioning in bed, the head and neck should be maintained in a neutral position. Alert individuals should be instructed not to turn themselves. Many patients unintentionally perform a Valsalva maneuver or grab the side rails tightly (isometric muscle contraction) when turning.[31]

Unfortunately, many nursing interventions, although necessary, can further aggravate increased ICP. These include turning and positioning, range-of-motion exercises, suctioning, and pulmonary hygiene. Although many of these activities cannot be avoided, they can be better spaced over time. It is a common practice to group these activities together. For example, when a patient is bathed, he or she is turned several times, receives range-of-motion exercises and pulmonary toileting, and is repositioned. The patient is probably suctioned, medicated, and may have a dressing or two changed before the nurse leaves the room to attend to other patients or responsibilities. While this is often considered necessary to manage time and remain efficient and organized, it is not always in the best interest of the patient with increased ICP. Spacing the activities and care can decrease sustained elevations of increased ICP.

Blocked CSF pathways lead to hydrocephalus and increases in ICP. Often the tumor bulk and accompanying peritumoral edema are responsible for the elevated ICP. A ventriculoperitoneal shunt or temporary ventriculostomy may be required. A tumor compressing the ventricle that may be completely removed will probably not require shunting. An unresectable tumor causing hydrocephalus will often require placement of a ventriculoperitoneal shunt. A ventriculostomy is indicated when the etiology of the hydrocephalus is believed to be of a temporary nature. Patients with a ventriculostomy require correct head positioning in relation to the level of the drainage system. The drainage system drip chamber level is ordered by the physician and is usually positioned level with the external auditory meatus. The level is changed based on the patient's clinical condition and the amount of CSF drainage. The procedure of leveling the drip chamber at,

**TABLE 35-8**  Nursing Management of an Individual with a CNS Tumor

| Nursing Diagnosis | Possible Cause | Nursing Interventions |
|---|---|---|
| Altered cerebral tissue perfusion | Tumor size<br>Cerebral edema | Neurological assessment<br>Corticosteroid administration<br>ICP monitoring<br>Avoid cumulative activities |
|  | Obstruction of CSF pathways<br>Decreased cranial venous outflow | Ventriculostomy<br>Elevate head of bed<br>Avoid head rotation, neck flexion and extension |
|  | Increased intraabdominal and intrathoracic pressure<br>Increased systemic arterial blood pressure | Avoid hip flexion and prone position<br>Avoid Valsalva maneuvers, isometric muscle contractions, coughing, emotional arousal |
| High risk for seizures | Disturbance of intracranial contents | Prophylactic anticonvulsants<br>Institute seizure precautions<br>Maintain safe environment<br>Be aware of concurrent medications that interfere with anticonvulsant action, absorption, or both |
|  | Electrolyte abnormality | Correct electrolyte abnormalities |
| Impaired cognition:<br>  Memory<br>  Judgment<br>  Thought process | Frontal tumor<br>Cerebral edema<br>Hydrocephalus<br>Radiation therapy<br>Medication effects | Maintain safe environment<br>Reorient individual<br>Utilize calendars, clocks, labels, photographs, etc. as visual cues or reminders<br>Maintain as close to normal function as possible<br>Encourage use of remaining functional ability<br>Encourage social activities<br>Instruct family members<br>Provide written instructions |
| Impaired physical mobility:<br>  Hemiparesis<br>  Hemiplegia<br>  Paraparesis<br>  Paraplegia<br>  Ataxic gait<br>  Level of consciousness | Frontal tumor<br>Parietal tumor<br>Spinal tumor<br>Spinal RT<br>Steroids | Maintain maximal activity level<br>Provide assistance as necessary for ambulation, transfer, ADL's.<br>Encourage proper footwear (nonskid soles, enclose the foot)<br>Maintain safe environment<br>Keep needed objects close at hand<br>Physical and occupational therapy<br>Range of motion exercises<br>Teach proper use of assistive devices (brace, cane, walker)<br>Institute measures to prevent complications such as DVT, pressure ulcer, foot drop, pneumonia<br>Develop specific interventions to compensate for deficits<br>Instruct patient and family in safety measures and above techniques<br>When preparing for discharge, obtain necessary equipment for home (wheelchair, bed, commode, walker, guardrail for bathroom, stool for shower)<br>Assess home for physical setup and safety (stairs, rugs) |
| Alteration in sensory/perceptual ability | Occipital tumor<br>Parietal tumor<br>Frontal tumor<br>Spinal cord tumor<br>Peripheral neuropathy | Monitor sensory function<br>Identify highest level of intact sensory function<br>Instruct patient and family on methods of compensation (checking position of involved areas visually, turning head completely to scan area)<br>Occupational therapy for assistive devices<br>Instruct patient and family in safety measures, proper clothing, and footwear |
| Knowledge deficit:<br>  Disease<br>  Treatment<br>  Medications<br>  Discharge | New diagnosis<br>Anxiety | Provide education to patient and family appropriately<br>Encourage questions<br>Clarify misconceptions<br>Refer to resources as needed<br>Provide written materials and written instructions |

**TABLE 35-8**  Nursing Management of an Individual with a CNS Tumor (continued)

| Nursing Diagnosis | Possible Cause | Nursing Interventions |
|---|---|---|
| Alteration in comfort:<br>Headache<br>Back pain | Intracranial tumor<br>Increased ICP<br>Spinal cord compression<br>Steroid withdrawal | Assess for verbal and nonverbal indicators of pain<br>Have patient rate pain using 0-10 scale, if possible<br>Administer analgesics, steroids, or other non-narcotic agents and evaluate effectiveness<br>Encourage relaxation techniques or meditation<br>Encourage diversional activities |
| High risk for impaired skin integrity | Immobility<br>Sensory changes<br>Poor nutrition | Assess skin condition frequently<br>Position changes<br>Frequent, thorough skin care<br>Use of pressure relieving devices<br>Maximize nutrition<br>Instruct patient and family on measures to prevent skin breakdown (proper positioning techniques, lotion, massage, bathing, nutritious snacks & meals) |
| Alteration in urinary elimination:<br>Retention | Immobility<br>Spinal cord tumor | Monitor intake and output<br>Assist into effective position to void<br>Assess for bladder distension<br>Encourage increased fluids<br>Intermittent catheterization<br>If necessary, instruct patient or family member in catheterization technique |
| Incontinence | Overflow due to retention<br>Frontal tumor<br>Spinal cord tumor<br>Diminished LOC | Assess for urinary retention<br>Skin care<br>Attempt toileting schedule<br>Bladder training |
| Alteration in bowel elimination:<br>constipation | Decreased mobility<br>Spinal cord tumor<br>Narcotics<br>Steroids<br>Inadequate diet | Assess bowel sounds and normal pattern of elimination<br>Institute bowel regimen<br>Encourage increased fluids and foods high in fiber<br>Allow sufficient time and privacy<br>Assist to proper position |
| Anxiety<br>Individual<br>Family | New diagnosis<br>Treatment protocols<br>Functional loss<br>Anticipatory grieving<br>Poor prognosis | Assess for verbal and nonverbal signs of anxiety<br>Allow individual, family, or both, to verbalize feelings and source of anxiety<br>Provide emotional support<br>Keep individual and family updated on treatment plans, condition, etc.<br>Refer to appropriate resources as necessary |

Other possible nursing diagnoses:
  Self-care deficit
  High risk for falls
  Alteration in nutrition
  Ineffective individual coping
  Ineffective family coping
  Alteration in comfort:
    nausea and vomiting
  Alteration in oral mucosa
  Fatigue
  Altered protective mechanisms:
    myelosuppression
  Anticipatory grieving

above, or below the external auditory meatus minimizes the risk of both excessive CSF drainage leading to collapse of the ventricles and insufficient CSF drainage leading to hydrocephalus. The level of the drip chamber is continuously monitored, the amount and consistency of CSF are assessed hourly, and the patient is evaluated for any neurological changes and signs of infection.

Individuals with spinal cord tumors also receive corticosteroids, especially when SCC has developed. Once the condition is determined or even clinically suspected, corticosteroids are initiated immediately, often in high doses. Steroids decrease the edema of the spinal cord and rapidly relieve back pain in many patients. Dexamethasone is the most commonly used steroid. For patients without neurological symptoms except for pain, low doses of steroids can be administered, usually 4 mg four times daily. The dose can be increased if pain persists, new symptoms develop, or a definitive diagnosis is made. For patients with severe pain or with neurological symptoms, high doses are given, usually 100 mg as an IV bolus followed by 24 mg every six hours for several days.[76] The dose should be tapered as the patient is treated with other treatment modalities, usually beginning within several days.

More than 95% of individuals with SCC report pain. While the addition of steroids provides pain relief for many individuals, others require additional analgesics. Effective analgesia needs to be established early on and dosages adjusted as the steroids and treatment further reduce the pain. The variety of available analgesics and the different methods of administration assist the nurse in providing adequate pain relief for spinal cord–compressed individuals.

Neurological symptoms of SCC other than pain usually evolve quickly. If prompt treatment is not initiated, weakness leading to paralysis will occur. If diagnosis and treatment are delayed until the patient becomes paraplegic, functional recovery is rare. However, patients who are ambulatory at the onset of treatment will most likely retain that ability. Individuals are taught to report signs and symptoms to assure prompt treatment. The goal of treatment is to preserve and maintain existing neurological function. Patient assessment is therefore crucial throughout this period to evaluate neurological status. This assessment includes monitoring motor, sensory, bowel, and bladder function. Changes in the neurological exam or the development of new deficits must be followed up immediately.

Glucocorticoid hormones are the most widely used drug in neuro-oncology.[140] Unfortunately, they have many unwanted side effects. Some of the common side effects, while distressing to the individual, are considered mild. These include insomnia, fatigue, increased appetite, hiccups, blurry vision, behavioral changes, acne, edema, abdominal bloating, and the characteristic moon face (caused by the redistribution of fat). Other effects can be more serious: GI bleeding, bowel perforation, hyperglycemia, hallucinations, psychosis, myopathy, op-

portunistic infections, osteoporosis, and acute adrenal insufficiency resulting from steroid withdrawal. Individuals receiving steroids should be observed for the previously mentioned side effects. Immunosuppression caused by prolonged steroid administration can lead to opportunistic infections, particularly *Pneumocystis carinii* pneumonia (PCP). For this reason many individuals on prolonged steroids also receive PCP prophylaxis with either trimethoprim and sulfamethoxazole or pentamadine. PCP prophylaxis generally continues for one month after the steroids have been discontinued. Ongoing assessment is necessary because neuro-oncology patients often receive steroids for prolonged and repeated periods of time. Patients and families need to be instructed on the side effects to observe for and possible measures to take, indications to call their physicians, and the absolute necessity of taking the prescribed dose. Sudden withdrawal of steroids can lead to adrenal insufficiency. Symptoms of this condition include fatigue, muscular weakness, joint pain, fever, anorexia, nausea, and orthostatic hypotension.[31] Steroid dosages are tapered slowly to prevent these symptoms of withdrawal. Patients should be given instructions about the schedule of the steroid taper. They should be monitored for increased neurological symptoms as the dose is decreased. Some individuals may become steroid-dependent and do not tolerate even a slow taper. It is also important to be familiar with the drug interactions of steroids and other medications the individual may be taking. Drugs such as phenytoin, phenobarbitol, and perhaps carbamazepine increase the metabolic clearance of steroids and may decrease their therapeutic effect. Therefore, some individuals on stable doses of steroids may develop increased symptoms when they are coincidently started on these medications[141] and may need to have their steroid dose increased.

Common anticonvulsants used to prevent seizures in individuals with primary and metastatic brain tumors include phenytoin, phenobarbitol, carbamazepine, and valproate. These agents all cause drowsiness and cognitive dysfunction. Worsening neurological symptoms occur at toxic therapeutic levels. These effects can add to already existing neurological dysfunction. Patients receiving these agents should have periodic blood levels assessed for therapeutic range. However, seizures may be controlled at levels below the therapeutic range; conversely, seizures may occur despite therapeutic levels. Also, some individuals may not exhibit signs of toxicity at high therapeutic levels.

Many individuals with CNS cancers suffer anxiety and depression. This is often thought to be a natural response to the illness and disabling neurological deficits and is sometimes overlooked. The presence of excessive anxiety or depression should be evaluated. Often, antidepressants and antianxiolytics help improve the psychological symptoms an individual with a CNS cancer can experience. Many individuals and families benefit from counseling as well.

## CONTINUITY OF CARE: NURSING CHALLENGES

Planning for discharge from the hospital for the individual with a CNS tumor should begin early. An accurate assessment of neurological deficits and functional limitations is made. The patient and family are assisted in setting realistic goals. For example, the paraplegic patient will not be able to walk up stairs. Rehabilitation potential is always viewed with hope and optimism, and the attitude of realistic hope must be conveyed to the individual and family.[31] Rehabilitation for the CNS-impaired individual has undergone tremendous change. A modified program of home physical therapy is often available for those with brain tumors even though they may be considered to have a shortened survival. Rehabilitation is important for the individual with a primary spinal cord tumor because many of these individuals have extended periods of time between recurrences.

The home should be assessed for its physical setup and safety. Maintaining a safe environment must be constantly reinforced. At some point during the course of the disease, the individual with a brain tumor often has cognitive impairment. Continuous supervision may become necessary to prevent harm. Stairs, rugs, and the shower are often a potential source of injury. Obstacles should be cleared from common pathways to avoid falls. The individual may need to remain on the ground floor, making room changes necessary. Reality-orientation devices (clocks, calendars, written instructions, photographs) need to be readily visible. Daily roles and routines may need to be altered to accommodate the individual who now has neurological deficits.

Once the individual with a CNS tumor is discharged, coordination of care assumes an even greater role. Just as the primary nurse in the inpatient setting coordinated the patient's care among the many disciplines involved, the nurse in the outpatient setting must do the same. Follow-up appointments, diagnostic tests, travel arrangements, treatment schedules, special instructions, side effects of medications, treatments, or both, home care issues, insurance company issues, and communication between the various disciplines involved are some of the many issues the outpatient nurse manages daily. It is important that the patient and family know there is one person who is familiar with their history and is managing their disease in its entirety. This provides a sense of continuity and can often allay anxiety. Many of these individuals develop progressive disease, and as their neurological deficits increase they will require additional support. Many may travel a great distance for their cancer therapy. These patients then must have a local physician who can provide emergency care and manage the day-to-day issues and problems that arise. For example, many patients on steroids develop diabetes and require frequent insulin dosage adjustments as the steroids are being tapered.

Many persons with CNS tumors can rapidly deteriorate as their disease advances. Their neurological function, physical status, and support systems will need to be reevaluated frequently and adjustments made. There may be issues related to young children at home, employment, and finances. New goals and plans should be formulated. Family members may need to take on added responsibilities such as physical care of the individual, medication administration, and assessment of their condition. Additional resources may need to be accessed, such as other family members, friends, community agencies (e.g., Visiting Nurse Service, American Cancer Society, or Cancer Care), local community programs, and support groups. Table 35-9 provides a list of additional resources available for those with CNS cancers. Life expectancy at home may not be of long duration. The person with progressive CNS involvement generally is at a terminal stage, and hospice care is an appropriate resource for families for both physical and emotional concerns.[142]

## CONCLUSION

Malignancies of the CNS present tremendous challenges for individuals, families, and caregivers. Because the clinical manifestations, course of treatment, and complications vary with the type and site of tumors, individuals with CNS cancers require a highly individualized plan of care. Supportive care takes on a role of utmost importance and encompasses the entire course of illness from diagnosis through the terminal phase of disease. Even with advances in overall therapeutic modalities, successful treatment of CNS cancers remains elusive.[142] Outcomes can range from cure to permanent disability to life prolonged by a few days, weeks, or months. The ongoing physical and emotional support necessary for both the individual and the family create a challenging role for oncology nurses. The neurological symptoms and complications produced by CNS cancers are, unfortunately, pro-

**TABLE 35-9**   Resources for Individuals with CNS Cancers

American Brain Tumor Association
Acoustic Neuroma Association
The Brain Tumor Society
National Cancer Institute - Cancer Information Service
Central Brain Tumor Registry of the United States
Epilepsy Foundation of America
National Brain Tumor Foundation
National Familial Brain Tumor Registry
National Institute of Neurological Disorders and Stroke
National Neurofibromatosis Foundation
National Tuberous Sclerosis Association
Pituitary Tumor Network Association
von Hippel–Lindau Family Alliance

foundly disabling and impact severely on quality of life. Assisting the individual to manage problems of daily living, maintain normal function to the best of his or her ability, and attain quality of life are our ultimate goals.

# REFERENCES

1. Parker SL, Tong T, Bolden S, et al: Cancer statistics 1996. *CA: Cancer J Clin* 46:5–27, 1996

2. Levin VA, Gutin PH, Leibel S: Neoplasms of the central nervous system, in DeVita VT, Hellman S, Rosenberg SA (eds): *Cancer: Principles and Practice of Oncology* (ed 4). Philadelphia, Lippincott, 1993, pp 1679–1737

3. Riggs JE: Rising primary malignant brain tumor mortality in the elderly. *Arch Neurol* 52:571–575, 1995

4. Modan B, Wagener DK, Feldman JJ, et al: Increased mortality from brain tumors: A combined outcome of diagnostic technology and change of attitude toward the elderly. *Am J Epidemiol* 135:1349–1357, 1992

5. Watkins D, Rouleau GA: Genetics, prognosis and therapy of central nervous system tumors. *Cancer Detect Prev* 18:139–144, 1994

6. Bondy M, Wiencke J, Wrensch M, et al: Genetics of brain tumors: A review. *J Neurooncol* 18:69–81, 1994

7. Salcman M: Surgical decision-making for malignant brain tumors. *Clin Neurosurg* 35:285–313, 1989

8. Martz CH: von Hippel–Lindau Disease: A genetically transmitted multisystem neoplastic disorder. *Semin Oncol Nurs* 8:281–287, 1992

9. Wilson CB: Meningiomas: Genetics, malignancy, and the role of radiation in induction and treatment. *J Neurosurg* 81:666–675, 1994

10. Mikkelson T: Recent advances in brain tumor molecular biology. *Curr Opin Oncol* 6:229–234, 1994

11. Berleur MP, Cordier S: The role of chemical, physical, or viral exposures and health factors in neurocarcinogenesis: Implications for epidemiologic studies of brain tumors. *Cancer Causes Control* 6:240–256, 1995

12. Musicco M, Filippini G, Bordo BM, et al: Gliomas and occupational exposure to carcinogens: Case-control study. *Am J Epidemiol* 116:782–787, 1982

13. Thomas LT, Waxweiler JR: Brain tumors and occupational risk factors: A review. *Scand J Work Environ Health* 12:1–15, 1986

14. Keyser A: Epidemiology of neuro-oncological disease, in Twijnstra A, Keyser A, Ongerboer de Visser BW (eds): *Neuro-Oncology.* Amsterdam, Elsevier, 1993, pp 1–12

15. Preston-Martin S, Mack W, Henderson BE: Risk factors for gliomas and meningiomas in males in Los Angeles County. *Cancer Res* 49:6137–6143, 1989

16. Neglia JP, Meadows AT, Robinson LL, et al: Second neoplasms after acute lymphoblastic leukemia in childhood. *N Engl J Med* 325:1330–1336, 1991

17. Ron E, Modan B, Boice JD, et al: Tumors of the brain and nervous system after radiotherapy in childhood. *N Engl J Med* 319:1033–1039, 1988

18. Tsang RW, Laperriere NJ, Simpson WJ, et al: Glioma arising after radiation therapy for pituitary adenoma. *Cancer* 72:2227–2233, 1993

19. Penn I: Cancer as a complication of severe immunosuppression. *Surg Gynecol Obstet* 162:603–609, 1986

20. DeAngelis LM: Primary central nervous system lymphoma as a secondary malignancy. *Cancer* 67:1431–1435, 1991

21. Washburn EP, Orza MJ, Berlin JA, et al: Residential proximity to electricity transmission and distribution equipment and risk of childhood leukemia, childhood lymphoma, and childhood central nervous system tumors: Systematic review, evaluation, and meta-analysis. *Cancer Causes Control* 5:299–309, 1994

22. Poole C, Trichopoulos D: Extremely low-frequency electric and magnetic fields and cancer. *Cancer Causes Control* 2:267–276, 1991

23. Floderus B, Persson T, Stenkind C, et al: Occupational exposure to electromagnetic fields in relation to leukemia and brain tumors: A case-control study in Sweden. *Cancer Causes Control* 4:465–476, 1993

24. Sahl JD, Kelsh MA, Greenland S: Cohort and nested case-control studies of hematopoietic cancers and brain cancers among electric utility workers. *Epidemiology* 4:104–114, 1993

25. Tomenius L: 50-Hz electromagnetic environment and the incidence of childhood tumors in Stockholm County. *Bioelectromagnetics* 7:191–207, 1986

26. Savitz DA, Wachtel H, Barnes FA, et al: Case-control study of childhood cancer and exposure to 60-Hz magnetic fields. *Am J Epidemiol* 128:21–38, 1988

27. Wertheimer N, Leeper E: Electrical wiring configurations and childhood cancer. *Am J Epidemiol* 109:273–284, 1979

28. Willis D: Intracranial astrocytoma: Pathology, diagnosis and clinical presentation. *J Neurosci Nurs* 23:7–14, 1991

29. Hickey JV: *The Clinical Practice of Neurological and Neurosurgical Nursing* (ed 3). Philadelphia, Lippincott, 1992

30. Leahy NM: *Quick Reference to Neurological Critical Care Nursing.* Rockville, MD, Aspen Publishers, 1990

31. Wegmann JA: Central nervous system cancers, in Groenwald SL, Frogge MH, Goodman M, Yarbro CH (eds): *Cancer Nursing: Principles and Practice* (ed 3). Boston, Jones and Bartlett, 1993, pp 959–983

32. Chaffee EE, Lytle IM: *Basic Physiology and Anatomy.* Philadelphia, Lippincott, 1980

33. Gilman S, Newman SW: *Manter and Gatz's Essentials of Clinical Neuroanatomy and Neurophysiology* (ed 8). Philadelphia, Davis, 1992

34. Marshall SB, Marshall LF, Vos HR, et al: *Neuroscience Critical Care.* Philadelphia, Saunders, 1990

35. Barr ML, Kiernan JA: *The Human Nervous System* (ed 5). Philadelphia, Lippincott, 1988

36. Andrus C: Intracranial pressure: Dynamics and nursing management. *J Neurosci Nurs* 23:85–92, 1991

37. Bruner JM: Neuropathology of malignant gliomas. *Semin Oncol* 21:126–138, 1994

38. Adams BA, Clancey JK, Eddy M: Malignant glioma: Current treatment perspectives. *J Neurosci Nurs* 23:15–19, 1991

39. Burger PC, Scheithauer BW, Vogel FS: Brain: Tumors, in *Surgical Pathology of the Nervous System and Its Coverings* (ed 3). New York, Churchill Livingstone, 1991, pp 194–376

40. Macdonald DR: Low-grade gliomas, mixed gliomas, and oligodendrogliomas. *Semin Oncol* 21:236–248, 1994

41. Recht LD, Lew R, Smith TW: Suspected low-grade glioma: Is deferring treatment safe? *Ann Neurol* 31:431–436, 1992

42. Wen PY, Fine HA, Black PM, et al: High-grade astrocytomas, in Wen PY, Black PM (eds): *Neurologic Clinics: Brain Tumors in Adults.* Philadelphia, Saunders, 1995, pp 875–900

43. Leibel SA, Scott CB, Loeffler JS: Contemporary approaches to the treatment of malignant gliomas with radiation therapy. *Semin Oncol* 21:198–219, 1994

44. Slooff JL: Primary tumors of the brain: Neuropathology,

in Twijnstra A, Keyser A, Ongerboer de Visser BW (eds): *Neuro-Oncology.* Amsterdam, Elsevier, 1993, pp 101–116

45. Levin VA, Silver P, Hannigan J, et al: Superiority of post-radiotherapy adjuvant chemotherapy with CCNU, procarbazine, and vincristine (PCV) over BCNU for anaplastic gliomas: NCOG 6G61 final report. *Int J Radiat Oncol Biol Phys* 18:321–324, 1990

46. Macdonald DR: New therapies of primary CNS lymphomas and oligodendrogliomas. *J Neurooncol* 24:97–101, 1995

47. Mason WP, DeAngelis LM: Procarbazine, CCNU, vincristine (PCV) chemotherapy for benign oligodendrogliomas. *Neurology* 44:A262, 1994 (abstr) (suppl 2)

48. Schiff D, Wen PY: Uncommon brain tumors, in Wen PY, Black PM (eds): *Neurologic Clinics: Brain Tumors in Adults.* Philadelphia, Saunders, 1995, pp 953–974

49. Cohen ME, Duffer PK: Ependymomas, in Cohen ME, Duffer PK (eds): *Brain Tumors in Children* (ed 2). New York, Raven Press, 1994, pp 219–239

50. DeMonte F: Current management of meningiomas. *Oncology* 9:83–96, 1995

51. Schrell UMH, Fahlbusch R, Adams EF: Meningiomas and neurofibromatosis for the oncologist. *Curr Opin Oncol* 6:247–253, 1994

52. Black PM: Benign brain tumors, in Wen PY, Black PM (eds): *Neurologic Clinics: Brain Tumors in Adults.* Philadelphia, Saunders, 1995, pp 927–954

53. Rubenstein AB, Schein M, Reichenthal E: The association of carcinoma of the breast with meningioma. *Surg Gynecol Obstet* 169:334–336, 1989

54. Black PM: Brain tumors. *N Engl J Med* 324:1555–1564, 1991

55. Younis GA, Sawaya R, DeMonte F, et al: Aggressive meningeal tumors: Review of a series. *J Neurosurg* 82:17–27, 1995

56. Carroll R, Glowacka D, Dashner K, et al: Progesterone receptor in meningiomas. *Cancer Res* 53:1312–1316, 1993

57. Goodwin JW, Crowley J, Stafford B, et al: A phase II evaluation of tamoxifen in unresected or refractory meningiomas: A Southwest Oncology Group study. *J Neurooncol* 15:75–77, 1993

58. Lamberts SWJ, Tanghe HLJ, Avezaat CJJ, et al: Mifepristone (RU 486) treatment of meningiomas. *J Neurol Neurosurg Psychiatry* 55:486–490, 1992

59. Campbell C: Acoustic neuroma: Nursing implications related to surgical management. *J Neurosci Nurs* 23:50–60, 1991

60. Young JS: Acoustic neuroma: Postoperative vertigo and the mechanisms of compensation. *J Neurosci Nurs* 24:194–198, 1992

61. Wiegand D, Fickel V: Acoustic neuroma: The patient's perspective: Subjective assessment of symptoms, diagnosis, therapy, and outcomes in 541 patients. *Laryngoscope* 99:179–186, 1989

62. DeAngelis LM: Primary central nervous system lymphoma. *Recent Results Cancer Res* 135:155–169, 1994

63. Eby NL, Grufferman S, Flannelly CM, et al: Increasing incidence of primary brain lymphoma in the US. *Cancer* 62:2461–2465, 1988

64. O'Neill BP, Illig JJ: Primary central nervous system lymphoma. *Mayo Clin Proc* 64:1005–1020, 1989

65. Selch MT, Shimizu KT, DeSalles AF, et al: Primary central nervous system lymphoma. *Am J Clin Oncol* 17:286–293, 1994

66. Rosenblum ML, Levy RM, Bredesen DE, et at: Primary central nervous system lymphoma in patients with AIDS. *Ann Neurol* 23:513–516, 1988

67. Forsyth PA, Yahalom J, DeAngelis LM: Combined-modality therapy in the treatment of primary central nervous system lymphoma in AIDS. *Neurology* 44:1473–1479, 1994

68. DeAngelis LM: Current management of primary central nervous system lymphoma. *Oncology* 9:63–71, 1995

69. DeAngelis LM, Yahalom J, Heinemann MH, et al: Primary CNS lymphoma: Combined treatment with chemotherapy and radiotherapy. *Neurology* 40:80–86, 1990

70. Neuwelt EA, Goldman DL, Dahlborg SA, et al: Primary CNS lymphoma treated with osmotic blood-brain barrier disruption: Prolonged survival and preservation of cognitive function. *J Clin Oncol* 9:1580–1590, 1991

71. Chamberlain MC, Levin VA: Primary central nervous system lymphoma: A role for adjuvant chemotherapy. *J Neurooncol* 14:271–275, 1992

72. Laws ER, Thapar K: Brain tumors. *CA Cancer J Clin* 43:263–271, 1993

73. Posner JB, Chernik NL: Intracranial metastases from systemic cancer. *Adv Neurol* 19:579–592, 1978

74. DeAngelis LM: Management of brain metastases. *Cancer Invest* 12:156–165, 1994

75. O'Neill BP, Buckner JC, Coffey RJ, et al: Brain metastatic lesions. *Mayo Clin Proc* 69:1062–1068, 1994

76. Posner JB: *Neurologic Complications of Cancer.* Philadelphia, Davis, 1995

77. Delattre JY, Krol G, Thaler HT, et al: Distribution of brain metastases. *Arch Neurol* 19:579–592, 1978

78. Byrne TN, Cascino TL, Posner JB: Brain metastasis from melanoma. *J Neurooncol* 1:313–317, 1983

79. Posner JB: Surgery for metastases to the brain. *N Engl J Med* 322:544–545, 1990

80. Patchell RA, Tibbs PA, Walsh JW, et al: A randomized trial of surgery in the treatment of single metastases to the brain. *N Engl J Med* 322:544–545, 1990

81. Flickinger JC, Loeffler JS, Larson DA: Stereotactic radiosurgery for intracranial malignancies. *Oncology* 8:81–98, 1994

82. Patchell RA: Brain metastases. *Neurol Clin* 9:817–824, 1991

83. Wujcik D: Meningeal carcinomatosis: Diagnosis, treatment, and nursing care. *Oncol Nurs Forum* 10:35–40, 1983

84. Schott GD: Spinal tumours I: Classification. *Nurs Times* 71:2055–2057, 1975

85. Kornblith PJ, Walker MD, Cassady JR: *Neurologic Oncology.* Philadelphia, Lippincott, 1987

86. Grant R, Papadoppoulos SM, Sandler HM, et al: Metastatic epidural spinal cord compression: Current concepts and treatment. *J Neurooncol* 19:79–92, 1994

87. Portenoy RK, Kanner RM: *Pain Management: Theory and Practice.* Philadelphia, Davis, 1996

88. Byrne TN: Imaging of gliomas. *Semin Oncol* 21:162–171, 1994

89. Schwartz RB: Neuroradiology of brain tumors, in Wen PY, Black PM (eds): *Neurologic Clinics: Brain Tumors in Adults.* Philadelphia, Saunders, 1995, pp 723–756

90. Jaeckle KA: Neuroimaging for central nervous system tumors. *Semin Oncol* 18:150–157, 1991

91. Arbour RA: Stereotactic localization and resection of intracranial tumors. *J Neurosci Nurs* 25:14–21, 1993

92. Wen PY, Alexander E III, Black PM, et al: Long term results of stereotactic brachytherapy used in the initial treatment of patients with glioblastomas. *Cancer* 73:3029–3036, 1994

93. Peterson K, Cairncross JG: Oligodendrogliomas, in Wen PY, Black PM (eds): *Neurologic Clinics: Brain Tumors in Adults.* Philadelphia, Saunders, 1995, pp 861–873

94. Berger MS: Malignant astrocytomas: Surgical aspects. *Semin Oncol* 21:172–185, 1994

95. Abernathey CD: Spinal intradural extramedullary tumors,

in Rengachary SS, Wilkins RH (eds): *Principles of Neurosurgery*. London, Wolfe Publishing, 1994, pp 38-1–38-8

96. Minehan KJ, Shaw EG, Scheithauer BW, et al: Spinal cord astrocytoma: Pathological and treatment considerations. *J Neurosurg* 83:590–595, 1995

97. Beahrs OH, Henson DE, Hutter R, et al: *Manual for Staging of Cancer* (ed 4). Philadelphia, Lippincott, 1992, pp 247–252

98. O'Mary SS: Diagnostic evaluation, classification, and staging, in Groenwald SL, Frogge MH, Goodman M, Yarbro CH (eds): *Cancer Nursing: Principles and Practice* (ed 3). Boston, Jones and Bartlett, 1993, pp 161–174

99. Kleihues P, Burger PC, Scheithauer BW: Histological typing of tumours of the central nervous system, in *World Health Organization, International Histological Classification of Tumours*. Berlin, Heidelberg, Springer-Verlag, 1993, pp 5–10

100. Sawaya R, Rambo WM, Hammond MA, et al: Advances in surgery for brain tumors, in Wen PY, Black PM (eds): *Neurologic Clinics: Brain Tumors in Adults*. Philadelphia, Saunders, 1995, pp 757–771

101. Heilbrun MP, Roberts TS, Apuzzo MLJ, et al: Preliminary experience with Brown-Roberts-Wells (BRW) computerized tomography stereotaxic guidance system. *J Neurosurg* 59:217–222, 1983

102. Kelly PJ, Alker GJ, Goerss S: Computer-assisted stereotactic laser microsurgery for the treatment of intracranial neoplasms. *Neurosurgery* 10:324–331, 1982

103. Moore MR, Black PM, Ellenbogen R, et al: Stereotactic craniotomy: Methods and results using the Brown-Roberts-Wells stereotactic frame. *Neurosurgery* 25:572–577, 1989

104. League D: Interactive, image-guided, stereotactic neurosurgery systems. *AORN J* 61:360–370, 1995

105. Kelly PJ, Daumas-Duport C, Kispert DB, et al: Imaging-based stereotaxic serial biopsies in untreated glial neoplasms. *J Neurosurg* 66:865–874, 1987

106. Nazzaro JM, Neuwelt EA: The role of surgery in the management of supratentorial intermediate and high-grade astrocytomas in adults. *J Neurosurg* 73:331–344, 1990

107. Gooding GA, Edwards MS, Rabskin AE, et al: Intraoperative real-time ultrasound in the localization of intracranial neoplasms. *Radiology* 146:459–461, 1983

108. Rambo WM, Sawaya RE: Neurosurgical treatment of brain tumors. *Cancer Bull* 45:320–325, 1993

109. Shrieve DC, Loeffler JS: Advances in radiation therapy for brain tumors, in Wen PY, Black PM (eds): *Neurologic Clinics: Brain Tumors in Adults*. Philadelphia, Saunders, 1995, pp 773–793

110. Fine HA, Dear KB, Loeffler JS, et al: Meta-analysis of radiation therapy with and without adjuvant chemotherapy for malignant gliomas in adults. *Cancer* 71:2585–2597, 1993

111. Laperriere NJ, Bernstein M: Radiotherapy for brain tumors. *CA Cancer J Clin* 44:96–108, 1994

112. Shapiro WR: Therapy of adult malignant brain tumors: What have the clinical trials taught us? *Semin Oncol* 13:38–45, 1986

113. Vick NA, Paleologos NA: External beam radiotherapy: Hard facts and painful realities. *J Neurooncol* 24:93–95, 1995

114. Shrieve DC, Alexander E III, Wen PY, et al: Comparison of stereotactic radiosurgery and brachytherapy in the treatment of recurrent glioblastoma multiforme. *Neurosurgery* 36:275–284, 1995

115. Shaw EG, Scheithauer BW, O'Fallon JR: Management of supratentorial low-grade gliomas. *Oncology* 7:97–111, 1993

116. Shaw EG: Low grade gliomas—to treat or not to treat? The

117. Cairncross JG, Laperriere NJ: Low-grade glioma—to treat or not to treat? *Arch Neurol* 46:1238, 1990

118. Patchell RA: Metastatic brain tumors, in Wen PY, Black PM (eds): *Neurologic Clinics: Brain Tumors in Adults*. Philadelphia, Saunders, 1995, pp 915–925

119. Malkin MG: Interstitial irradiation of malignant gliomas. *Rev Neurol* 148:448–453, 1992

120. Gutin PH, Prados MD, Philips TL, et al: External irradiation followed by an interstitial high activity iodine-125 implant "boost" in the initial treatment of malignant gliomas: NCOG study 6G-82-2. *Int J Radiat Oncol Biol Phys* 21:601–606, 1991

121. Addesa AE, Shrieve DC, Alexander A III, et al: Stereotactic radiosurgery as primary adjuvant treatment for glioblastoma: The JCRT update (abstract). In *Proc Am Soc Clin Oncol*, 31st Annual Meeting, Los Angeles, May 20–23, 1995, p 144

122. Thorton AF, Hegarty TJ, Ten Haken RK, et al: Three-dimensional treatment planning of astrocytomas, a dosimetric study of cerebral irradiation. *Int J Radiat Oncol Biol Phys* 20:1309–1315, 1991

123. Sneed PK, Larson DA, Gutin PH: Brachytherapy and hyperthermia for malignant astrocytomas. *Semin Oncol* 21:186–197, 1994

124. Conrad CA, Milosavljevic VP, Yung WK: Advances in chemotherapy for brain tumors, in Wen PY, Black PM (eds): *Neurologic Clinics: Brain Tumors in Adults*. Philadelphia, Saunders, 1995, pp 795–812

125. Shapiro WR, Green SB, Burger PC, et al: Randomized trial of three chemotherapy regimens and two radiotherapy regimens in postoperative treatment of malignant glioma. *J Neurosurg* 71:1–9, 1989

126. Lesser GJ, Grossman SA: Tumor review: The chemotherapy of adult primary brain tumors. *Cancer Treat Rev* 19:261–281, 1993

127. Moynihan TJ, Grossman SA: The role of chemotherapy in the treatment of primary tumors of the central nervous system. *Cancer Invest* 12:88–97, 1994

128. Lesser GJ, Grossman S: The chemotherapy of high-grade astrocytomas. *Semin Oncol* 21:220–235, 1994

129. Oshini T, Sher PB, Posner JB, et al: Capillary permeability factor secreted by malignant brain tumors: Role in peritumoral brain edema and possible mechanism for anti-edema effect of glucocorticoids. *J Neurosurg* 72:245–251, 1990

130. Grossman SA, Sheidler V, Weissman D, et al: Continuous infusion therapy for primary brain tumors: A new approach with a high response rate. *Proc Am Soc Clin Oncol* 6:72, 1987

131. Grossman SA, Wharam M, Sheidler V, et al: BCNU/Cisplatin (B/C) followed by radiation in poor-prognosis patients with high-grade astrocytomas (HGA). *Proc Am Soc Clin Oncol* 11:149, 1992

132. Neuwelt EA, Howieson J, Frenkel EP, et al: Therapeutic efficacy of multiagent chemotherapy with drug delivery enhancement of blood-brain barrier modification in glioblastoma. *Neurosurgery* 19:573–582, 1986

133. Gumerlock MK, Belshe BD, Madsen R, et al: Osmotic blood-brain barrier disruption and chemotherapy in the treatment of high grade malignant glioma: Patient series and literature review. *J Neurooncol* 12:33–46, 1992

134. Olivi A, Brem H: Interstitial chemotherapy with sustained

release polymer systems for the treatment of malignant gliomas. *Recent Results Cancer Res* 135:149–154, 1994

135. Sipos EP, Brem H: New delivery systems for brain tumor therapy, in Wen PY, Black PM (eds): *Neurologic Clinics: Brain Tumors in Adults.* Philadelphia, Saunders, 1995, pp 813–826

136. Brem H, Piantadosi S, Burger PC, et al: Intraoperative controlled delivery of chemotherapy by biodegradable polymers: Safety and effectiveness for recurrent gliomas evaluated by a prospective multi-institutional placebo-controlled clinical trial. *Lancet* 345:1008–1012, 1995

137. Fine HA: Novel biologic therapies for malignant gliomas, in Wen PY, Black PM (eds): *Neurologic Clinics: Brain Tumors in Adults.* Philadelphia, Saunders, 1995, pp 827–846

138. Hayes RL, Koslow M, Hiesiger EM, et al: Improved long term survival after intracavitary interleukin-2 and lymphokine-activated killer cells for adults with recurrent malignant gliomas. *Cancer* 76:840–851, 1995

139. Linstadt DE, Wara WM, Leibel SA: Postoperative radiotherapy of primary spinal cord tumors. *Int J Radiat Oncol Biol Phys* 16:1397–1402, 1989

140. Grant R, Papadopoulos SM, Sandler HM, et al: Metastatic epidural spinal cord compression: Current concepts and treatment. *J Neurooncol* 19:79–92, 1994

141. Posner JB: Supportive care of the neuro-oncology patient, in Hildebrand J (ed): *Management in Neuro-Oncology.* Berlin, Springer-Verlag, 1992, pp 89–99

142. Wegmann JA: CNS tumors: Supportive management of the patient and family. *Oncology* 5:109–113, 1991

## Chapter 36

# Colon and Rectal Cancer

**Linda Hoebler, RN, MSN**

# INTRODUCTION

Colorectal carcinoma is a prevalent malignancy throughout the world, particularly in the Western Hemisphere. The United States ranks 23rd among 48 selected countries in the world for death rates from colorectal cancer.[1] Within the past few decades improvements have been made in survival that may be attributable to earlier diagnosis and a decrease in treatment-related mortality.[2] One of the most significant factors influencing improved outcomes is early diagnosis. The percentage of neoplasms of the colon and rectum diagnosed at a localized or regional stage is 37%.[1]

Risk factors for colorectal cancer reflect a cadre of biological, environmental, and lifestyle factors. Genetic factors are in the forefront of research today with specific gene defects identified as promoters for colorectal cancer. First-degree relatives of persons with colorectal cancer are at high risk. The World Health Organization has recently revised screening recommendations for high-risk individuals.

Surgery continues to be the first line intervention for colorectal carcinoma. Laparoscopic surgery and cryosurgery for metastatic disease have evolved into two of the newer techniques being implemented. Radiation therapy, chemotherapy, and immunotherapy are used in various combinations to improve long-term survival and quality of life. Adjuvant therapy is now being used to treat earlier stages of the disease.

As advances in diagnostic and therapeutic techniques continue to be developed and refined, clinical outcomes will subsequently improve. Epidemiological studies, genetic mapping, new imaging techniques, surgical innovations, and adjuvant clinical trials afford health care professionals the capabilities to provide state of the art treatment and care.

# EPIDEMIOLOGY

Cancer of the colon and rectum is the third most commonly diagnosed malignancy in the United States. Colon and rectal cancer is also the third leading cause of death from a malignancy for both men and women.[1] In 1996 it was estimated that there would be a total of 134,500 newly diagnosed cases and 54,900 deaths from colorectal carcinoma.

The probability of developing colon or rectal cancer increases with age. Although one of the youngest documented cases of colon cancer was a nine-month-old infant,[3] the disease predominantly affects the older population. For men between the ages of 60 to 79 years, there is a 4.35% chance of being diagnosed with colorectal cancer.[1] For women between the ages of 60 to 79 years, there is a 3.28% chance of being diagnosed.[1]

The incidence and mortality rates for colorectal cancer have remained constant among males for the past 40 years. The incidence and mortality rates for colorectal cancer among females have declined slightly.[4] Reproductive factors are suspected to reduce the incidence of colorectal cancer in women. Oral contraceptives and hormone replacement therapy are being investigated for potential protective effects relative to specific subsites in the colon.[5]

Overall, incidence and mortality rates have reflected a downward trend over the past decade.[6] The five-year survival rate for all stages of colorectal disease between 1986 and 1991 was 62%. There have been some reports of racial differences in mortality from colorectal cancer. The mortality rates from 1973 to 1987 reflected a decline among the white population, but an increase among black men. During the same period, the mortality rate for black women remained unchanged. It has been postulated that the differences in these mortality rates may be attributable to differences in health care access.[7] However, similar mortality rates were demonstrated by the Surveillance, Epidemiology and End Results Program with an analysis of the population of middle-class blacks who reportedly did not have the health care accessibility issue.[8] More recent statistics reported from 1992 indicate that blacks have a lower mortality rate than whites from cancer of the colon and rectum.[1] The reasons for this change are not yet known.

# ETIOLOGY

Many etiological factors impact upon the pathogenesis of colorectal carcinoma. Age, genetics, diet, environment, inflammatory bowel conditions, radiation proctocolitis, and surgery may each play a role in the development of colorectal cancer.

## Age

The number of individuals diagnosed with colorectal carcinoma begins to increase steadily after the age of 40. The risk of colorectal cancer then rises sharply at the age of 50 to 55 and doubles each decade thereafter up to the age of 75. The greatest number of cancer deaths in males from cancer of the colon and rectum occurs between the ages of 55 and 74.[1] The greatest number of cancer deaths in females from cancer of the colon and rectum occurs at age 75 and older.[1] Years of exposure to carcinogens in the large intestines and rectum may promote the development of this malignancy.

## Genetics

Genetic studies suggest that the development of colorectal cancer may be secondary to an inheritable susceptibility to the disease.[9] Individuals who have a first-degree relative with colorectal cancer have double the risk for developing adenomatous polyps.[10,11] Adenomatous polyps are considered to be precursors of colorectal carcinoma. In addition, an inheritable autosomal dominant trait is found in families with a high incidence of colon cancer.

Cancers of the colon with a genetic component generally fall into two categories: *adenomatosis polyposis coli* syndrome, and *hereditary nonpolyposis colorectal cancer* (HNPCC) syndrome. In the polyposis syndrome category, there is an absence of chromosome 5. It has been suggested that as a result of this missing genetic material, there is a lack of tumor suppressor genes that retard neoplastic growth.[4] Polyposis syndromes include diseases such as Gardner's syndrome, Turcot's syndrome, Puetz-Jagher's syndrome, and juvenile polyposis. In the nonpolyposis syndrome category there is an abnormality of chromosome 2. The aberration in chromosome 2 is a DNA instability in which nucleotides are lost or gained during the course of tumor development.[12] The average age for the diagnosis of nonpolyposis syndrome is 45 years. Individuals who have nonpolyposis syndrome are considered to be at a 50% risk for developing cancer of the colon. Nonpolyposis syndrome can be further subdivided into Lynch I syndrome and Lynch II syndrome. Lynch I syndrome is site-specific nonpolyposis syndrome. Lynch II syndrome is a cancer family type of nonpolyposis syndrome.

Another inherited autosomal dominant trait found in families with a higher incidence of colon cancer is familial adenocarcinomatosis. In familial adenocarcinomatosis there is a higher incidence found within families of a variety of different primary adenocarcinomas, such as colon, breast, gastric, and endometrial.

## Diet

A diet high in fat content is considered to be a risk factor and promoter of colon carcinogenesis.[13] Populations within the Western Hemisphere typically consume diets with 40%–45% of food calories from fat. Diets high in fat increase the production of, and change the composition of, bile salts. These altered bile salts are converted into potential carcinogens by intestinal flora. While the exact mechanism by which bile salts act as a promotor for colorectal cancer is unknown, researchers suggest that the process is mediated by diacylglycerol.[14] Phospholipids are converted to diacylglycerol by intestinal bacteria. Diacylglycerol then enters the epithelial cell of the colon and activates protein kinase C, which has a role in cell growth and tumor promotion.

Dietary fiber has been found to decrease the effects of fatty acids.[15] The protective mechanism of dietary fiber is exerted in a number of ways, such as increasing fecal bulk, which changes the bacterial composition of the feces and accelerates the transit time in the intestinal tract. Not all dietary fiber is equally beneficial. Wheat bran and cellulose are the most protective fibers, while oat and corn bran seem to have little protective capabilities.[16]

## Alcohol

Alcohol has been considered a risk factor in the development of colorectal cancer. Beer consumption places males at statistically significant higher risk for developing rectal carcinoma.[17] Other studies also suggest a positive correlation between alcohol consumption and bowel cancer.[17,18] Alcohol may stimulate gastrointestinal cell proliferation and promote carcinogenesis secondary to an excess of unabsorbed carcinogens, such as nitrosamines found in beer and whiskey.[19]

## Environment

Occupational risk factors are not regarded as significant for cancer of the colon and rectum. Some studies, however, have shown a correlation between colorectal cancer and the occupation of the individual. Solvents, abrasives, and fuel oils are substances that may increase the risk for developing this malignancy.[20] Automotive pattern and model workers were found to have twice the mortality from colon and rectal cancers as compared to the general population.[21] There also may be an increased risk from occupational exposure to formaldehyde and particulate compounds.[22]

## Inflammatory Bowel Conditions

Ulcerative colitis places an individual at risk for cancer of the colon. The risk is influenced by a number of different factors, including duration of the colitis, extent of the colitis, age of onset, presence of chronic symptoms, and severity of the initial attack.[23] In individuals with ulcerative colitis, irrespective of age, the predisposition to develop colon cancer is five to ten times higher than that of the general population.[11] Colon cancer in individuals with ulcerative colitis usually develops earlier in life, is anaplastic, and is aggressive in nature.

Crohn's disease is also considered to be a risk factor for carcinoma of the colon. This inflammatory disease usually involves all layers of the intestinal mucosa. While the incidence of colon cancer in the population with Crohn's disease is not comparable to that of ulcerative colitis, those with Crohn's disease can present with adenocarcinoma of the colon at a younger age.[24]

## Radiation

Radiation therapy to the pelvis for treatment of other primary malignancies correlates with an increased risk for developing carcinoma of the colon and rectum. Individuals previously treated with external beam radiation to the pelvis may develop this second malignancy years after the initial treatment.[25] It is hypothesized that radiation may induce carcinogenic activity. There is no consensus as to whether or not the risk is associated with specific radiation doses. Some studies indicate a higher risk if the individual has received low dose radiation.[26]

## Ureterosigmoidostomy

Ureterosigmoidostomy is performed for a number of benign and malignant conditions. There have been reports in the literature of a 5% to 10% increased incidence of colon carcinoma occuring 15 to 30 years after the initial surgery.[4] The most common site of the colon cancer is distal to the surgical site where there has been chronic exposure of the intestinal mucosa to both urine and feces.

# PREVENTION, SCREENING, EARLY DETECTION

The premise for chemoprevention is to minimize the effects of potential carcinogens with the ultimate intent of preventing the occurrence of a malignancy. Many food substances, medications, vitamins, and elements have received attention recently as chemopreventive agents.

Antioxidants are included in the category of chemoprevention because they block oxidative damage to cellular DNA. Vitamins E and C inhibit the formation of nitrosamine, a known carcinogen. Another antioxidant, N acetyl-L-cysteine, reduces the formation of DNA carcinogens.[27]

Nonsteroidal anti-inflammatory drugs (NSAIDs) are being studied as potential chemopreventative agents. Sulindac (Clinoril) produced regression of colon polyps[28] and piroxicam (Feldene) administration inhibited colon tumor development in experimental trials.[29] The mechanism of chemopreventive action for NSAIDs is related to a reduction in endogenous prostaglandin. For NSAIDs to be beneficial, research indicates they should be taken for at least three consecutive months and for at least 16 days each month. If such a regimen is followed, then it is hypothesized that the risk of developing colon and rectal cancer could be reduced by one-half.[30]

Epidemiological studies indicate that the incidence of colon cancer can be decreased with regular use of aspirin. A study conducted by the American Cancer Society demonstrated a 40% reduction in the mortality rate of colorectal cancer for those who used aspirin on a regular basis.[31,32] Regular aspirin use is defined in some trials as two times per week as a chemopreventive agent.

Calcium, taken orally, has been shown to decrease the risk of developing colon cancer. Calcium binds bile and fatty acids so that there is less exposure of gastrointestinal cells to these potentially harmful compounds.[33] Calcium supplementation may be most beneficial when initiated prior to the development of any neoplastic alteration.[34]

Postmenopausal hormone replacement is currently receiving attention as a potentially chemopreventative regimen. The use of exogenous estrogen appears to exert a protective mechanism and decreases the risk of colon cancer in women.[35] Several studies have indicated a significant statistical decrease in the risk of colon cancer in women who are postmenopausal and taking hormonal replacement therapy.[35,36] While it is believed that endocrine factors play a role in colorectal carcinogenesis, the exact mechanism of action has yet to be identified.

Updated guidelines for the prevention of colorectal cancer were recently published by the World Health Organization (WHO) in collaboration with Memorial Sloan Kettering Cancer Center.[37] These guidelines for primary prevention included recommendations for:

1. The primary prevention of colorectal cancer
2. The screening for average-risk individuals
3. The screening for relatives of individuals with colorectal cancer
4. The surveillance of individuals with colorectal polyps
5. The surveillance of individuals with chronic ulcerative colitis

Adenomas are considered to be premalignant precursors of colorectal carcinoma. Colonoscopy and removal of these adenomatous polyps reduces the risk of developing colon cancer.[38] Complete colonoscopy is recommended for those with adenomas of any size. The updated WHO guidelines recommend that individuals who have adenomatous polyps removed should then have a follow-up colonoscopy three years later. The rationale for this guideline is to detect missed adenomas or subsequent adenomas. Colonoscopy after this initial follow-up may then be performed approximately every five years.

Genes play a major role in individuals and families who are prone to developing colorectal carcinoma. The Kirsten rat sarcoma viral oncogene homologue (K-*ras*) is a proto-oncogene that is absent in normal colon tissue. However, adenomas larger than one centimeter in diameter have K-*ras* mutations in 60% of cases, and the K-*ras* mutation occurs in 30%–50% of colorectal carcinomas.[39] The *adenomatous polyposis coli* (APC) gene, the *deleted in colorectal carcinoma* (DCC) anti-oncogene, and the *hereditary nonpolyposis colorectal cancer* (HNPCC) gene can be used as indicators to identify a colorectal malignancy.[40] Laboratory tests for gene mutations may soon be commercially available, thus making it easier to screen individuals at increased risk for developing colorectal cancer.[41] Genetic counseling for populations at risk could then include gene testing for increased accuracy and earlier identification of the colorectal malignancy.

Three tests are recommended by the American Cancer Society and the National Cancer Institute in the screening for colorectal cancer.[42] The first screening test is the digital rectal examination. It is suggested that every man and woman have a digital rectal examination annually after the age of 40. The second screening method recommended is the Hemoccult® test. A recent clinical trial conducted by the Minnesota Colon Cancer Control Study group revealed that an annual fecal occult blood test using rehydrated Hemoccult® slides could reduce mortality from colorectal cancer by 33%.[43] Stool samples need to be obtained and checked for occult blood from three consecutive bowel movements. Specific dietary guidelines restricting peroxidase-containing foods may be recommended. Peroxidase-containing foods include red meat, fresh fruit, and raw vegetables. Consensus does not exist as to whether these dietary restrictions need to be followed. Stool samples should be checked for occult blood on an annual basis for men and women over the age of 50. The third recommended screening tool is flexible sigmoidoscopy. Guidelines indicate that this examination should be performed every three to five years for men and women beginning at the age of 50. If numerous risk factors are present in an individual, then the sigmoidoscopy should be done more frequently.

## PATHOPHYSIOLOGY

### Cellular Characteristics

The most common histological type of colorectal neoplasm is adenocarcinoma.[44] Other tumors such as lymphoma, sarcoma, melanoma, and carcinoid are relatively rare in the large bowel. Some reports indicate that the most common anatomical sites affected are the descending and sigmoid colon.[45] However, the National Cancer Data Base has reported that there is increasing incidence of adenocarcinoma occurring in the proximal portion of the bowel.[46] Thirty-six percent of the malignancies were found in the ascending colon and 33% of the malignancies were discovered in the distal portion of the colon.[46] Studies hypothesize that the increasing incidence in proximal colon carcinoma may be attributable to the aging population, especially women.[47,48]

Colorectal lesions exhibit different characteristics depending upon their location in the bowel. Right-sided tumors present as cauliflower-like fungating masses that progress to become ulcerative and necrotic. Right-sided tumors are usually well differentiated and have a better prognosis. Left-sided or descending sigmoid colon lesions present as ulcerative tumors with everted edges. These tumors tend to infiltrate the bowel wall and have a poorer prognosis than right-sided tumors. Rectosigmoid tumors present as villous, frondlike lesions. Early rectal cancer symptoms include a change in the caliber of the stool and rectal bleeding. Advanced cancer symptoms include tenesmus and rectal pain.

### Progression of Disease

Adenocarcinoma of the colon and rectum develops in the bowel mucosa. After the initial mucosal growth, the tumor will invade locally usually by direct extension protruding into the lumen of the bowel wall. Once the tumor has traversed the muscularis mucosa and infiltrates the submucosa, it is termed invasive. Submucosal involvement with a tumor commonly leads to further infiltration via the extensive lymph and vascular network. Direct extension may also occur into the peritoneal surfaces. The lymphatic flow within the colon is via the pericolic, intermediate, and principle lymph node chains.[4] Metastasis into the lymph nodes is more commonly seen in colorectal tumors of a higher histological grade.

The major site for visceral spread is the liver. The liver is the initial site for metastasis in approximately one-third of recurring colorectal cancers. Although colorectal carcinoma can spread to the lungs, bone, and brain, this is rare without first evidencing liver involvement. The median survival for individuals with distant metastasis ranges from six to nine months.[4]

Implantation of tumor cells at other sites can occur as a result of surgical manipulation of the tumor, intraluminal spread, or the shedding of tumor cells into the peritoneum. Intraperitoneal seeding and carcinomatosis may occur even without lymphatic or visceral spread.

## CLINICAL MANIFESTATIONS

The clinical manifestations of colorectal cancer relate to the anatomic location of the tumor. There are no signs and symptoms of early colorectal carcinoma. Symptoms are usually vague and nonspecific. The duration of the symptoms does not necessarily correlate with the severity of the disease.

Lesions in the ascending colon may have clinical manifestations of fatigue, palpitations, and iron deficiency anemia. Because stool in the ascending colon is liquid, obstruction rarely occurs secondary to the tumor. Alterations in bowel habits usually are not seen. A mass may be palpable in the affected quadrant.

Tumors in the transverse colon can present the clinical picture of constipation alternating with diarrhea. Because the stool has a more solid consistency and the bowel lumen narrows at the splenic and hepatic flexures, bowel obstruction may occur. Melena may also be detected if the mass is in the transverse colon.

Masses in the sigmoid colon are more obstructive in nature. The individual may complain of nausea and vomiting.[49] The most common symptoms found in individuals with cancer of the sigmoid colon are abdominal pain (72%) and melena (53%).[44] Perforation becomes more of a concern with tumors in this anatomic location. Radiographical studies of the abdomen typically depict annular constricting lesions.

Cancer of the rectum clinically results in bright red rectal bleeding and a change in bowel habits. There may be the feeling of inability to completely empty the bowel.

Unexplained constipation or a report of a change in the caliber of stools are also common clinical complaints.

Unfortunately, the first symptoms arising from colorectal carcinoma may be from metastatic disease. Jaundice, pruritis, and ascites could indicate metastatic liver involvement.[50] Hepatomegaly may be detected upon physical examination. As the liver enlarges and distends due to tumor growth, pain may become problematic.

As cancer of the colon and rectum progress, obstruction and perforation of the bowel become more likely. Approximately 15% of individuals with colon cancer present with large bowel obstruction.[44] The primary symptom of intestinal obstruction is abdominal pain. Patients who present with obstruction or perforation have a poorer prognosis than those who do not. Fistula formation, general peritonitis, and abscess are the sequelae of perforation.

Lung metastases may be revealed upon chest x-ray showing scattered densities in the lung fields. Spread into the pelvis may cause renal impairment or sacral or sciatic pain.

Individuals will often complain of weight loss at the time of initial presentation. Anorexia and weight loss can be significant with advanced colorectal carcinoma. Anorexia may be intensified by lesions that partially obstruct the bowel. Obstructive lesions can cause crampy abdominal pain exacerbated by the intake of food.

**TABLE 36-1   Areas to Include When Taking a Family History for Colorectal Cancer Evaluation**

| Risk Factor Evaluation | Symptom Evaluation |
|---|---|
| A. Inflammatory Bowel Disease<br>  1. Ulcerative colitis<br>  2. Crohn's disease<br>B. Familial Polyposis Syndrome<br>  1. Gardner's syndrome<br>  2. Turcot's syndrome<br>  3. Juvenile polyposis<br>  4. Puetz-Jagher's syndrome<br>C. Familial Nonpolyposis Syndrome<br>  1. Lynch I syndrome<br>  2. Lynch II syndrome<br>D. Familial Adenocarcinomatosis<br>  1. Colorectal cancer<br>  2. Breast cancer<br>  3. Endometrial cancer<br>  4. Gastric cancer<br>E. Occupational History<br>F. Dietary History<br>G. History of Radiation Treatments to Pelvis<br>H. Surgical History | A. Recent Weight Loss/Gain<br>B. Change in Appetite<br>C. Change in Color, Shape, Consistency of Stools<br>  1. Constipation<br>  2. Diarrhea<br>D. Nausea/vomiting<br>E. Blood Noted in the Stools<br>  1. Bright red blood<br>  2. Dark colored stools<br>F. Abdominal Pain<br>G. Abdominal Bloating<br>H. Excessive Fatigue<br>I. Heart Palpitations<br>J. Unusual Coloration of the Skin or Sclera<br>K. Unusual Itching of the Skin |

# ASSESSMENT

## Patient and Family History

The nurse needs to elicit a complete history and perform a thorough physical examination. Careful review of initial clinical symptoms and astute evaluation of any physiological changes can provide invaluable information. A thorough history would include individual and family risk factors that could contribute to colorectal cancer (Table 36-1).

## Physical Assessment

A thorough abdominal assessment should progress through inspection, auscultation, percussion, and palpation.[51]

Inspection of the abdominal wall should include the skin to note any distention or dilated veins. The contour of the abdomen should be noted for the presence of any bulging, displacement, or irregularities caused by a mass.

Auscultation should occur in all four quadrants. The frequency and character of the bowel sounds should be recorded. Bowel sounds may be increased with diarrhea or absent with a bowel obstruction.

Percussion should produce a tympanic sound over the abdomen. Suprapubic dullness should be heard over the bladder. Percussion of the liver should also produce the sound of dullness. Normally liver dullness is 4 to 8 centimeters midsternally and 6 to 12 centimeters in the midclavicular area. The dullness increases if hepatomegaly is present.

Palpation should be done in all four quadrants of the abdomen. Masses or tender areas need particular scrutiny and extensive description. While the liver is usually palpable, the spleen is normally not. Inguinal palpation should be included, to check for lymph node enlargement.

The digital rectal examination is part of the physical assessment. The perianal area should be inspected for the presence of fissures or hemorrhoids. The anal canal should be palpated for any masses or nodular areas. The rectal wall should be examined after the finger has been advanced further up into the rectum. Once the exam is complete, it is advisable to check the stool for occult blood.

## Diagnostic Studies

If there is suspected colorectal pathology, then a diagnostic workup including laboratory and radiological studies should be pursued. A stool sample for fecal occult blood testing needs to be obtained. This test is relatively inexpensive and easy to accomplish. Many different fecal occult blood screening tests are available on the market. Most cancer screening programs utilize the Hemoccult II, a guaiac-based test; however, for asymptomatic colorectal malignancies the sensitivity is unsatisfactory.[52] Comparisons of the sensitivity of four fecal occult blood tests have been conducted. The four fecal occult blood tests included Hemoccult II and HemoccultSensa (both guaiac tests), Hemiselect (immunochemical test), and HemoQuant (heme-porphyrin test). Results indicated that the Hemeselect and HemoccultSensa had a higher sensitivity for detecting colorectal neoplasms.[53]

The proctosigmoidoscopy, with the fiberoptic sigmoidoscope, provides an optimal diagnostic visualization of up to 60 centimeters of colon, far enough into the colon to detect 55% of colorectal tumors.[54] Examination with the flexible fiberoptic sigmoidoscope results in a 60%–80% decrease in the risk of adenocarcinoma of the colon and rectum, in comparison to individuals who have never received such screening.[55,56]

The barium enema is commonly used in the diagnostic workup for colorectal cancer. Double contrast barium enemas are considered to be diagnostically superior to the single contrast exam. Double contrast tests have a rate of 98% accuracy for detecting colorectal cancers larger than 15 millimeters. In many cases, this examination has replaced the colonoscopy and is considered to have an equivalent diagnostic capability to detect colorectal carcinoma and polyps.[57]

A chest x-ray is part of the clinical evaluation for the detection of metastatic lesions in the lung. The computed tomography (CT) scan of the abdomen and pelvis is helpful in defining the extent of the tumor and in identifying metastatic areas.

Hematologic studies include a CBC to determine the presence of an anemia secondary to blood loss or hepatic involvement. Liver function studies also aid in the evaluation of liver involvement. The plasma tumor marker carcinoembryonic antigen (CEA) is measured preoperatively and postoperatively for therapeutic effectiveness.[58] The CEA level does not specifically correlate with tumor burden and may be elevated in the presence of tumors of the breast, lung, pancreas, ovary, and other adenocarcinomas. Individuals who smoke may also have an elevated CEA. Medical conditions such as bronchitis and colitis will also cause the CEA to rise. The monoclonal antibody CA 19-9 has also been used to indicate tumor activity in colorectal carcinoma. Though CA 19-9 has specificity for pancreatic cancer, it has been used cautiously in monitoring colorectal cancer.

The malignant potential of cells can be studied by evaluating their DNA content. An endoscopic biopsy of colorectal tissue can be obtained and the chromosomal patterns and division phases of the cells evaluated by flow cytometry. Flow cytometry allows for the measurement of ploidy and growth rate of cells in the S-phase. Chromosomal patterns are evaluated based upon diploidy (the normal number of chromosomes) and aneuploidy (an abnormal number of chromosomes). Aneuploidy is observed when a colorectal malignancy is present.[59–61] The analysis of cellular DNA content for diploidy or aneuploidy can further enhance clinical diagnosis of the presence of a colorectal carcinoma.

## Prognostic Indicators

The prognosis for an individual with colorectal carcinoma is directly related to the stage of the disease at the time of diagnosis.[62] At the time of diagnosis, 37% of colorectal carcinomas are localized, 37% are regional, and 19% are distant.[1] Recent data from the National Cancer Institute (NCI) reflects a five-year survival rate of 92% for localized colorectal cancer, 63% for regional colorectal cancer, and 7% for distant colorectal cancer.[1] The overall survival rate for all stages is 62%.[1] There has been an increased five-year survival rate for this malignancy seen over the past twenty-five years. This increased survival rate has been attributed to the advances in diagnostic techniques, the increased understanding of gastrointestinal epithelial transformation, the decrease in surgical mortality, the innovation of surgical techniques, and the initiation of adjuvant therapy for high-risk patients after the primary surgical intervention. The use of hormonal replacement therapy by postmenopausal women also contributes to the increased survival rate.

## CLASSIFICATION AND STAGING

The Dukes' staging system has been the traditional format for staging colorectal cancer since 1932.[63] The Dukes' system is based upon classifying the depth of penetration from the tumor as well as lymph node involvement. Dukes' stages of classification are A, B, C, and D. This system has been modified numerous times over the years with additional prognostic variables included (Table 36-2).

The American Joint Commission on Cancer (AJCC)

**TABLE 36-2** Dukes' Classification and Corresponding Five-Year Survival Rate

| Dukes' Stage | Pathological Description | Five-Year Survival Rate |
|---|---|---|
| A | Cancer confined to mucosa and submucosa | > 90% |
| B₁ | Cancer extends into the muscularis | 85% |
| B₂ | Cancer extends into or through the serosa | 70%–85% |
| C | Cancer involves the regional lymph nodes | 30%–60% |
| D | Cancer has metastasized to distant organs or structures | 5% |

Mayer RJ: Tumors of the large and small intestine, in Isselbacher KJ, Braunwald E, Wilson JD, et al: *Harrison's Principles of Internal Medicine* (ed 13). New York, McGraw-Hill, 1994, p 1428

has developed another commonly used staging system for colorectal cancer. Many health care professionals feel that one system, the AJCC system, should be adopted as the standard for the staging of colorectal carcinoma.[64] The AJCC classification indicates the degree of penetration of the gastrointestinal mucosa by primary tumor (T), the number and site of lymph nodes involved by regional lymph nodes (N), and the presence or absence of metastases by distant metastasis (M)[65] (Table 36-3).

## THERAPEUTIC APPROACHES AND NURSING CARE

The management of colorectal cancer involves a multifaceted therapeutic approach. Surgical intervention remains the first line treatment for this malignancy. Surgical techniques have evolved to include laparoscopic techniques for colon resection or cryosurgery for metastatic liver disease. Following postoperative recovery, additional treatment regimens are implemented including radiation therapy, chemotherapy, and immunotherapy. Adjuvant treatment is being recommended to enhance long-term survival.

**TABLE 36-3**   TNM Classification of Colon and Rectal Cancer

| | |
|---|---|
| **T: Primary tumor** | |
| TX | Primary tumor cannot be assessed |
| TO | No evidence of primary tumor |
| Tis | Carcinoma in situ |
| T1 | Tumor invades submucosa |
| T2 | Tumor invades muscularis propria |
| T3 | Tumor invades through the muscularis propria into the subserosa, or into nonperitonealized pericolic or perirectal tissues |
| T4 | Tumor perforates the visceral peritoneum, or directly invades other organs or structures[a] |
| **N: Regional lymph node involvement** | |
| NX | Regional lymph node cannot be assessed |
| NO | No regional lymph node metastasis |
| N1 | Metastasis in 1 to 3 pericolic or perirectal lymph nodes |
| N2 | Metastasis in 4 or more pericolic or perirectal lymph nodes |
| N3 | Metastasis in any lymph node along the course of a named vascular trunk |
| **D: Distant metastasis** | |
| MX | Presence of distant metastasis cannot be assessed |
| MO | No distant metastasis |
| MI | Distant metastasis |

[a]Direct invasion of other organs or structures includes invasion of other segments of colorectum by way of serosa (e.g., invasion of the sigmoid colon by a carcinoma of the cecum).

From Beahrs OH, Henson DE, Hutter RVP, et al (eds): *American Joint Committee on Cancer: Manual for Staging of Cancer.* (ed 4). Philadelphia, Lippincott, 1992.

## Surgery

The mainstay of therapy for colorectal cancer is surgery. While surgical techniques continue to evolve and be refined, adequate margins and complete excision of the tumor provide the individual with the best long-term survival.[66,67] The location and extent of the malignancy will determine the type of surgical resection (see Figure 36-1).

The ideal surgical margin surrounding the neoplasm is five centimeters. Wider margins may be indicated if the carcinoma is poorly differentiated or anaplastic. Excision of the regional lymphatics or lymphadenectomy relates to the anatomic site of the colectomy. Regional lymphadenectomy assists in adequately staging the disease and determining who will benefit from adjuvant therapy. Evidence indicates improved survival in individuals with node-positive disease that receive postoperative systemic chemotherapy.[68]

Preoperative preparation includes the cleansing of the colon and rectum. The most common infective organisms in the bowel are aerobic *E. coli* and anaerobic *Bacteroides fragiles.*[69] The colon never can be completely cleansed of bacteria, but the goal is to reduce the population of organisms as much as possible. The commonly used mechanical bowel preparation is an isotonic lavage solution, such as Golytely®. Usually the surgical candidate is asked to drink four liters of this bowel preparation the evening before surgery. Clear liquids are recommended for the evening meal and nothing by mouth after midnight. In addition to using a mechanical bowel preparation, antibiotics are also prescribed to minimize colorectal bacteria. Broad-spectrum antibiotics are taken orally at specific times the day before the surgery and intravenous antibiotics are ordered on call to the operating room the day of the surgery.

The usual surgical intervention for tumors in the cecum and ascending colon is the right hemicolectomy. This procedure includes removal of a segment of the terminal ileum, the cecum, and the right half of the transverse colon. The accompanying mesocolon and lymphatic channels are also excised. The ileum and left transverse colon are then anastomosed. An attempt is made not to excise more than 50 centimeters of the terminal ileum so that Vitamin $B_{12}$ and bile salt absorption are affected as little as possible.[70] Lack of $B_{12}$ may result in a pernicious anemia and lack of adequate bile salt absorption may result in malabsorption of nutrients and chronic diarrhea.

A transverse colectomy is the procedure of choice when the lesion involves the middle and left transverse colon. The middle colic artery is resected to the base of the mesentery to interrupt lymphatic drainage to the area. An anastomosis of the ileum and proximal descending colon is then performed.

Carcinomas of the descending and sigmoid colon are surgically resected by left hemicolectomy. This operation removes the distal, transverse, descending, and sigmoid

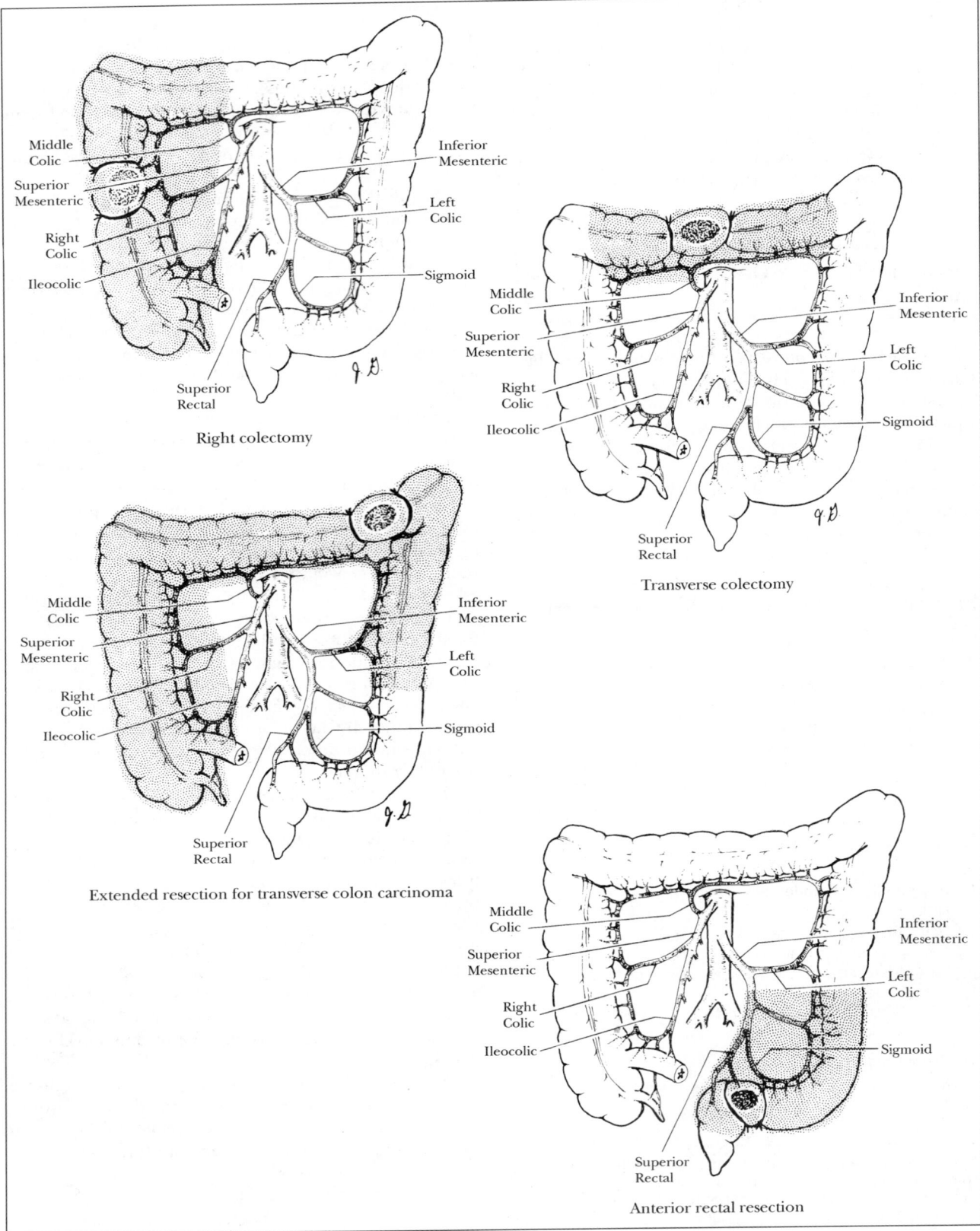

**FIGURE 36-1**   The choice of surgical procedure relates to the location and extent of the tumor. (Ahlgren JD, Macdonald JS (eds): *Gastrointestinal Oncology.* Philadelphia, Lippincott, 1992.)

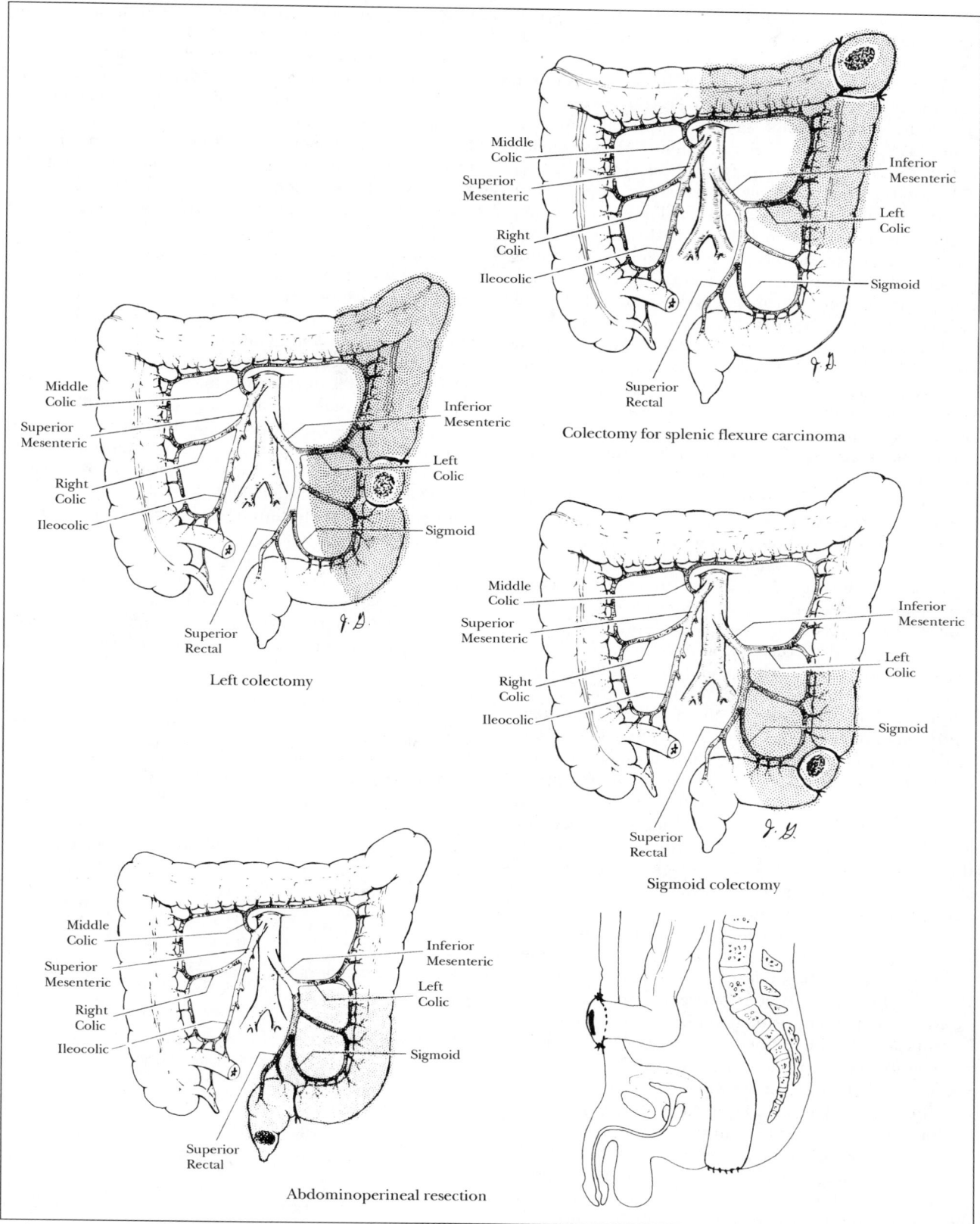

Left colectomy

Colectomy for splenic flexure carcinoma

Sigmoid colectomy

Abdominoperineal resection

**FIGURE 36-1** (continued)

colon as well as the associated mesocolon. In this procedure, the right transverse colon is anastomosed to the distal sigmoid.

A method now being used for bowel resections is laparoscopic colorectal surgery. In a recent survey of the American Society of Colon and Rectal Surgeons, approximately 47% of the respondents stated they used laparoscopic procedures for certain types of colorectal surgery.[71] The criteria used to select laparoscopic surgery were based upon the diagnosis of early colorectal carcinoma or for the purpose of palliation of this disease. Most laparoscopic interventions are undertaken for ascending or sigmoid carcinomas secondary to ease of accessability.[72] Long-term management and survival will need to be evaluated for this new laparoscopic intervention.

The surgical intervention for rectal carcinoma has changed during the last decade. For proximal and mid-rectal adenocarcinomas, a low anterior resection has become the technique of choice. This surgical approach still provides adequate proximal, distal, and radial margins without sacrificing sphincter control. Concern about the low anterior resection involves the possibility of submucosal lymphatic or suture line recurrence of the rectal malignancy. However, researchers have shown that an adequate margin is considered 2–2½ centimeters distal to the tumor.[73]

By using this surgical technique, there is no need for a permanent colostomy because external anal sphincter control is preserved. Yet, internal anal sphincter control may be impaired by the low anterior resection due to surgical damage of the nerve supply. Even if the external anal sphincter remains intact, complete continence may be altered. Stool frequency, urgency, and continency could potentially be compromised with nerve damage to the internal anal sphincter, although bowel function continues to improve for 12 to 18 months after surgery.[69]

Abdominoperineal resection is usually used for poorly differentiated adenocarcinoma and more advanced disease. If anal sphincter function cannot be preserved and the anus must be included in the surgical resection, then an abdominoperineal resection is indicated. If the rectum and sphincter muscles must be removed, a permanent colostomy is needed. The selection for the colostomy site is done best prior to surgery. This permits the stoma placement to be accessible for individual care and not within a fold of adipose tissue or over a bony prominence.

Radiolabeled monoclonal antibodies are being given intraoperatively to identify occult disease and metastatic areas in individuals with colorectal carcinoma. Radioactive isotopes are used in the operating room to detect occult disease.[74] This technique allows for improved detection and more complete surgical eradication of colorectal adenocarcinoma. Though limited at this time, the technique of using radiolabeled antibodies is promising.

For smaller tumors of the colon and rectum, laser therapy is being delivered to the tumor bed through a colonoscope or flexible sigmoidoscope. The YAG laser vaporizes tissue to a depth of 5 mm.[69] The laser procedures are generating great interest among surgeons because they are easier, quicker, and less complicated.

Prophylactic oophorectomy is recommended for some women diagnosed with adenocarcinoma of the colon and rectum. There is a 6% reported incidence of ovarian metastasis in females with colorectal carcinoma.[75] If the disease is disseminated at the time of diagnosis, then prophylactic bilateral oophorectomy may be suggested as a means of decreasing morbidity and preventing ovarian metastasis. This treatment becomes a particular area for consideration if the woman is young and premenopausal.

Acute complications of colorectal surgery are listed in Table 36-4. The nurse plays a critical role in detecting these complications early and providing appropriate intervention for the resolution of postoperative problems. Anastomotic leak and genitourinary tract injury require immediate surgical intervention. Intra-abdominal abscess and large bowel obstruction may be managed initially with more conservative measures such as antibiotics or continuous nasogastric drainage; however, these complications may also require surgical intervention. Staphylococcal enteritis can rapidly progress to include hypovolemia, dehydration, and electrolyte abnormalities. Immediate administration of broad spectrum antibiotics is the appropriate treatment.

Long-term effects following an abdominoperineal resection include sexual dysfunction and impotence. Because the surgical intervention is extensive, injury to sympathetic and parasympathetic nerve fibers may occur. Sexual dysfunction may vary from partial to complete

**TABLE 36-4** Complications of Colorectal Surgery

| Complications | Signs and Symptoms |
| --- | --- |
| Anastamotic leak | Intra-abdominal pain<br>Pelvic abscess<br>Peritonitis |
| Intra-abdominal abscess | Recurring or persistent fever more than 72 hours postoperatively<br>Leukocytosis with elevated bands<br>No abdominal pain |
| Staphylococcal enteritis | Diarrhea<br>Prostration<br>Sepsis |
| Large bowel obstruction | Constipation<br>Abdominal pain<br>Nausea/vomiting<br>Abdominal distention |
| Injury to the genitourinary tract | Leakage of urine through the incision<br>Oliguria<br>Anuria |

Hoebler L, Irwin MM: Gastrointestinal tract cancer: Current knowledge, medical treatment, and nursing management. *Oncol Nurs Forum* 19:1403–1415, 1992

impotence. The incidence of sexual dysfunction ranges from 15%–100%.[2] The degree of dysfunction is related to surgical technique, the age of the individual, and any preexisting medical or surgical conditions that impact on sexual function. Sexual function may return gradually during the postoperative recovery period (about one year). If there is no return or incomplete return of sexual functioning, the individual may consider improving sexual function through use of a penile prosthetic device. See chapter 28 for additional information.

The individual who undergoes surgery for colorectal carcinoma may also require a colostomy. The type of colostomy and character of the stoma is related to the anatomic site surgically removed. The single barrel colostomy is formed when the proximal portion of the colon is exteriorized. The double barrel colostomy has two separate stomas. The proximal stoma excretes the stool; the distal stoma secretes mucus. The loop colostomy is formed by bridging the fascia under the bowel loop or looping the large bowel over a supporting bridge device. The character of the stool is dependent upon the placement of the stoma within the intestinal tract. Ascending colostomies excrete loose, liquid stool. Transverse stomas excrete semisolid or pasty stool. Descending or sigmoid colostomies excrete soft, formed stools. Individuals may still experience mucous secretions from the rectum despite the presence of the colostomy.

The most common site for metastatic involvement from colorectal carcinoma is the liver. The liver has an integral and extensive network of vascular and lymphatic channels that likely enable the dissemination of colon cancer. Five-year survival rates following hepatic resection for metastatic colorectal disease are estimated at 20%–25%.[76] Individuals older than 60 years with less than 24 months between the initial colorectal surgery and hepatic resection have the poorest outcome.[77] Cryosurgery is also being used to treat liver metastasis from colorectal carcinoma. Cryosurgery employs a repeated freezing and thawing process via probes placed in the metastatic hepatic lesions. A 32% five-year survival rate was documented in a study of cryosurgery used to treat hepatic colorectal metastases.[77]

## Chemotherapy

The cornerstone of chemotherapy for cancer of the colon and rectum is 5-fluorouracil (5-FU). It is the most commonly used cytotoxic agent for this malignancy.[11,49,78] This drug is administered by a variety of different routes: oral, intravenous, intraperitoneal, and intra-arterial. Various doses and lengths of infusion are used. The major side effects associated with the administration of 5-FU are hematological and gastrointestinal: anorexia, nausea, vomiting, stomatitis, and diarrhea. Leukopenia, thrombocytopenia, and anemia can occur with this chemotherapeutic agent. The nadir period is seven days postadministration.

Though 5-fluorouracil is the cytotoxic agent of choice for colorectal cancer, it is most commonly administered in combination with other drugs, particularly with leucovorin (folinic acid). Leucovorin enhances the cytotoxic effect of 5-FU. Individuals with Dukes' B and C stage disease given 5-FU and leucovorin experienced a 37% three-year disease-free survival rate.[79] Individuals with advanced colon carcinoma with liver metastases had a response rate of 36%, which was better than when 5-FU was used as a single agent drug.[80] Other researchers have reported a response rate of 23% for 5-FU and leucovorin.[81] Side effects from combination therapy with 5-FU and leucovorin include: nausea, vomiting, diarrhea, mucositis, fever, leukopenia, thrombocytopenia, and hypotension.[80]

A campthotecin derivative CPT-11 (Irinotecan) is currently being evaluated for efficacy against colorectal carcinoma, particularly refractory metastatic disease previously treated with 5-FU. This drug is still in clinical trials but has demonstrated an overall survival for metastatic condition of 11.9 months in some studies.[82] The major side effects from Irinotecan are diarrhea, neutropenia, nausea, and vomiting.[83,84] Another campthotecin derivative being evaluated for activity against colorectal cancer is topotecan. Initial trials have yielded partial responses in patients. The dose-limiting toxicity is myelosuppression.

Advanced colorectal cancer is treated with 5-FU. Intravenous administration is preferred to oral administration. Leucovorin and 5-FU in combination are also used to treat metastatic disease. Improved tumor response has been noted in individuals with this malignancy receiving 5-FU and leucovorin where 5-FU alone had previously failed to produce a tumor response.[85]

Intraportal chemotherapy administered through the portal vein or hepatic artery into the liver has also shown evidence for improved survival. One of the more traditional drugs given by intraportal infusion is floxuridine (FUDR). The response rate for individuals with metastasis to the liver receiving intraportal chemotherapy is approximately 40%.[86] The major toxicity associated with hepatic infusion is chemical hepatitis. Elevated transaminase levels and jaundice indicate the onset of chemical hepatitis and the need for therapy to be halted.[86] These symptoms are reversible and chemotherapy may be reinstituted once the symptoms subside.

Research has indicated that for individuals with metastatic colorectal cancer, chemotherapy provides prolonged survival and enhanced quality of life in comparison to individuals who received supportive care only.[87]

## Immunotherapy

Levamisole is an immunomodulator originally used as a veterinary antithelminthic. In humans, a 30% improved survival rate for colon cancer has been demonstrated with the use of a combination of 5-FU and levamisole for one year postoperatively.[88] Levamisole enhances the efficacy of 5-FU for the treatment of colorectal carcinoma.[11] Data support the use of these two drugs for adjuvant treatment of Stage III (Dukes' C) colon cancer.[89,90]

Alfa- and gamma-interferon are also being used as immunotherapy for advanced cancer of the colon and rectum. Alfa-interferon combined with 5-FU yielded better response rates than when 5-FU was used alone.[91] Response rates ranged from 23%–38%.[92] While this combination has demonstrated cytotoxicity, significant toxic effects have also been encountered. Central nervous system side effects including aphasia and seizures have necessitated dosage reductions with these two drugs.[93] Gamma-interferon has been used as an adjuvant therapy in individuals with stage II, III, and IV colon cancer. However, gamma-interferon used as a single agent modality was felt to produce no significantly enhanced survival.[94]

Interleukin-2 (IL-2) is being evaluated in clinical trials for efficacy against advanced colon cancer. While these studies have provided needed information on toxicities and optimal dose range, efficacy against this malignancy is still being established.

Bacillus Calmette-Guerin (BCG) and autologous tumor cell vaccines are also being employed in the treatment of colorectal cancer. BCG is now being incorporated into a specific active vaccine because the initial vaccine failed to demonstrate any benefit. Efficacy is still under investigation.

## Radiation Therapy

Radiation therapy has been used in preoperative, intraoperative, and postoperative treatment of colorectal cancer. Radiation therapy is used primarily, however, to treat rectal adenocarcinoma. The rationale for using radiation therapy is to decrease the incidence of local recurrence after surgical resection. Such local recurrences are believed to occur as a result of inadequate surgical margins. Local recurrence is more common with rectal adenocarcinoma because of the retroperitoneal anatomic location. Radiation doses delivered to the pelvis range from 4400–5000 cGy.

Preoperative radiation is given with the intent of decreasing the existing tumor burden. Research supports decreased local recurrence when preoperative radiotherapy is used in individuals with rectal cancer.[89,95] Preoperative radiation therapy can also reduce tumor cell dissemination during surgery. Radiation enteritis is rarely a complication because preoperative radiation doses are small. The duration of these preoperative regimens varies from five days (2500 cGy) to five weeks (4500 cGy).[11]

Intraoperative radiation therapy can be used to treat advanced, recurrent, or inoperable rectal cancer. Intraoperative radiation therapy is typically used to treat rectal adenocarcinoma if there is surgical difficulty in attaining adequate disease-free margins. Some studies have demonstrated a lower local failure rate as well as a prolonged survival rate of three years for individuals with cancer of the rectum when intraoperative radiation is used.[95]

Postoperative irradiation is used most frequently in the treatment of rectal carcinomas. Local recurrence rates are decreased if postoperative radiation therapy is used.[2] The combined modality of external beam radiation and 5-FU has also demonstrated a decrease in local recurrence and improvement in survival.[96,97]

Adenocarcinomas of the colon and rectum are radiosensitive and respond well to radiation therapy. Tumors that are not surgically resectable may be treated with palliative radiation. Symptom management can also be aided by external beam radiation. Control of bleeding and/or pain can be attained in 90% of cases.[98]

The most common injury to the large bowel that occurs following radiotherapy is proctosigmoiditis.[99] Bleeding, tenesmus, and pain are manifestations of proctosigmoiditis. If symptoms do not subside with time, surgical intervention for bowel diversion may be necessary. Other commonly encountered side effects secondary to radiation to the large bowel include increased bowel motility, which creates abdominal cramping and loose, watery stools. Occasionally, nausea and vomiting become problematic. Acute side effects generally resolve after the cessation of therapy.[100] Chronic radiation enteritis can produce bowel mucosal thinning and inflammation, eventually resulting in ulceration. In the colon, fibrosis and stricture can occur that could eventually lead to obstruction. These problems may arise up to five years after radiation therapy.

# SYMPTOM MANAGEMENT AND SUPPORTIVE CARE

## Hepatic Metastases

Approximately one in four individuals with colorectal carcinoma have liver metastases at the time of initial presentation and approximately 70% have metastatic disease to the liver by the time they die.[101] Predominant symptoms from liver metastases are right upper quadrant abdominal pain, weight loss, anorexia, changes in bowel habits, and hepatomegaly. Between 25% and 30% of these individuals may experience ascites and jaundice.[102]

Liver metastases may be suspected if serial serum CEA levels begin to rise. Serum liver function studies may also be elevated and indicate metastases. Ultrasound and CT scan of the abdomen are important imaging techniques. For detection by CT scan, the hepatic lesion needs to be 1–2 cm in size and by ultrasound less than 1 cm in size.

Treatment for hepatic metastases can involve a myriad of treatment regimens. Surgical resection is still believed to be the major modality. Cryotherapy may also be used with the intent of eradicating the metastatic colorectal lesion with subzero temperatures. In one study, cryosurgery resulted in a 29% disease-free survival rate two years after the intervention.[103] Chemotherapy, radiotherapy, and immunotherapy are also used to treat liver metastases from colorectal carcinoma.

Palliation of symptoms is important in the management of hepatic metastases. One of the measures is to treat the underlying etiology with one of the above mentioned strategies. Ascites can be palliatively treated with intermittent paracentesis or the insertion of an intraperitoneal Tenchoff® catheter for intermittent drainage. Intraperitoneal sclerosing with agents such as Bleomycin has been tried with the goal of preventing further fluid accumulation in the abdominal cavity. Diuretics are not effective in the treatment of malignant ascites. For further discussion about ascites, see chapter 27.

Pain secondary to hepatic metastases occurs from tumor pressure on the liver capsule. Treatment of the underlying disease to shrink the neoplasm is optimal for pain relief. Pharmacological approaches to pain management need to be consistently implemented to provide optimal comfort. Specific analgesic interventions are discussed at length in chapter 20.

Pruritis may also be problematic secondary to liver metastases. Pruritis results from chemical irritation caused by excessive accumulation of bile salts in the system. Interventions to manage pruritis include increasing fluid intake, promoting capillary constriction, and applying topical anesthetic preparations. The use of antihistamines such as Benadryl has also proven beneficial in the control of pruritis.

## Bowel Obstruction

Bowel obstruction secondary to advanced colorectal carcinoma may be extrinsic or intrinsic. Extrinsic compression of the bowel may occur as a result of abdominal carcinomatosis or tumor studding along the bowel. Intrinsic compression of the bowel can result from growth and progression of the tumor within the lumen of the bowel itself.

Signs and symptoms of bowel obstructions are nausea and vomiting, abdominal distention, abdominal pain, progressive constipation, and absence of bowel sounds over the affected area. Vomitus is usually bilious in nature. The individual may also complain of early satiety and anorexia.

Diagnosis of a bowel obstruction is confirmed by an abdominal obstruction series film. The film proximal to the obstruction will reveal a colon dilated and gas-filled while distal to the obstruction no gas will be visualized in the colon. Sonography is also helpful in determining the level and cause of the obstruction.[104]

Initial management of a bowel obstruction associated with advanced colorectal disease is medically conservative. The placement of a nasogastric tube to decompress the gastrointestinal tract is standard. There are situations whereby bowel obstructions can resolve spontaneously without further intervention.

If the individual has had little nutritional intake prior to the insertion of the nasogastric tube or it is anticipated that nutritional intake will be impaired for a period of time, total parenteral nutrition may be a consideration. In an individual who is already in a negative metabolic state, hyperalimentation provides needed nutritional support.

If there is no spontaneous resolution of the bowel obstruction, then the insertion of a gastrostomy tube may be needed for palliation. The gastrostomy tube permits not only a vehicle for intermittent decompression but also for nutritional support if total parenteral nutrition is not an option.

## Ureteral Obstruction

Individuals with adenocarcinoma of the colon and rectum have ureteral obstruction in 38% of cases.[105] Genitourinary manifestations occur more frequently in individuals with metastatic colorectal carcinoma than upon primary presentation.[105] The five-year survival rate for individuals with genitourinary involvement from colorectal cancer approximates 30%.[104]

Bilateral ureteral obstruction can occur with advanced colorectal malignancies secondary to direct tumor compression of the ureters. Individuals present with oliguria and an elevated serum creatinine. A cystoscopy and bilateral retrograde pyelogram are the most reliable diagnostic tools for determining ureteral obstruction.[106] These exams determine whether the obstruction is intrinsic to the ureter or extrinsic, as would be seen with an advancing colorectal lesion.

Treatment of ureteral obstruction may be accomplished at the time of the retrograde pyelogram. Urinary stents can be inserted into the ureters to establish patency and prevent further compression by the tumor. Stents circumvent the need for a surgical procedure. If the ureteral stents become occluded, the stent can usually be changed via cystoscopy. There are situations when urinary stents cannot be utilized because of ureteral strictures or inability to visualize the ureters. In such cases, percutaneous nephrostomy tubes can be used to treat the obstruction. Nephrostomy tubes are placed directly into the kidney via a percutaneous approach to allow for adequate urinary drainage directly from the renal pelvis.

## Pulmonary Metastases

While endobronchial metastases are rare, colorectal carcinoma is one of the most common primary tumors with pulmonary metastases.[107] Tumors that metastasize to the lungs may present as solitary masses or multiple nodules. Individuals who experience pulmonary metastases from a colorectal primary may present with symptoms of dyspnea. It has been estimated that 85% of pulmonary metastases are asymptomatic.[108]

Most colorectal metastases to the lungs are detected by routine chest x-ray. More definitive evaluation can be accomplished by CT scan of the chest, which further defines the number and location of the lesions.

Pulmonary resection of the metastic area provides the best long-term survival for individuals. Pulmonary wedge resection is best undertaken if the lesion is isolated. Individuals with four or fewer metastatic pulmonary lesions have a better prognosis than individuals with four or more.[109] Individuals with metastatic lung involvement from colon cancer have been found to have a 31% five-year survival rate after surgical resection of the metastatic lesion.[110]

## CONTINUITY OF CARE: NURSING CHALLENGES

In today's health care environment, the delivery of care takes place in an accelerated fashion. The time span between presentation, physiological workup, diagnosis, acute intervention, and follow-up treatment can be encapsulated into a month. Often there are a multitude of health care professionals involved in the individual's care, and communication and coordination of the treatment plan become paramount. It has been estimated that 62% of whites and 53% of blacks diagnosed with colon cancer will attain the five-year survival rate.[1] Similarly 60% of whites and 52% of blacks diagnosed with rectal cancer will be alive at the five-year mark.[1] The course of colorectal carcinoma, including follow-up, can span many years and there needs to be a provision for the continuity of care.

At the time of initial presentation the individual's entry into the health care system is usually through the primary care physician either for a routine physical exam or because of troublesome symptoms. A physical exam and diagnostic testing ensues and once the appropriate results are evaluated, referral is made to a gastrointestinal surgeon. Additional testing takes place, and should a colorectal biopsy be done, tissue pathology may already be available before the individual goes to the operating room. If a final tissue diagnosis is not available, the surgeon shares his or her suspicions with the individual prior to any surgical intervention. Close collaboration between the individual, family, primary care physician, and surgeon facilitates the flow of consistent information and treatment planning. This is especially crucial when the individual is obtaining needed information on an outpatient basis. Once the decision has been reached regarding operative intervention, the individual and family need to gain an understanding from the surgeon as to what to expect. The anticipated surgical preparation, day of surgery, length of surgery, potential complications, anticipated outcome, and length of hospital stay need to be reviewed. The individual/family needs to have a general understanding about the incision line, surgical drains, Foley catheter, nasogastric tube, potential for colostomy, and provisions for pain management. It is optimal to provide the patient and caretakers with the name and phone number of a specific health care professional for reassurance and reference should any questions or issues arise prior to the surgical date.

The average length of stay for someone who has had a surgical resection secondary to colorectal carcinoma is less than five days. At the time of admission, the appropriate referrals need to be made. Should the individual have a colostomy, the enterostomal therapist needs to be involved. A registered dietician lends support for caloric calculations, hyperalimentation guidelines, and dietary specifics at the time of discharge. Social service may need to be consulted as dictated by the individual's home and support situation. Home care is also a consideration to meet specific health care needs once the individual is discharged.

Upon discharge the individual needs to be clear about when to call the physician for problems such as fever, chills, shortness of breath, or hemoptysis. Should any change occur with the incision such as erythema, drainage, or wound separation, the surgeon also needs to be notified. Information about discharge medications and resuming previous medications needs to be reviewed and clarified. Optimally, the specific name and number of the same health care professional needs to be given to the individual and family for questions or difficulties that may arise before the return appointment to the surgeon.

Upon return for the postoperative check, an overall physical assessment takes place and the final pathology is shared with the individual and family if the tissue diagnosis was not available at the time of discharge. The general plan for follow-up treatment can be discussed as well. While additional adjunctive therapy may not begin for another few weeks, the appropriate referrals to the radiation oncologist or oncologist need to be made in a timely fashion. Appointments with the appropriate physicians providing additional treatment could be made prior to departure from the surgeon's office.

Coordination of all of these services and the provision for continuity of care is imperative. The individual is confronted with an oncological diagnosis, recovery from surgery, and treatment follow-up. A health care professional is an integral player in assisting with organizing, scheduling, interpreting, and managing the treatment plan.

If the disease is advanced, palliation of symptoms is also part of the spectrum of care. The individual and family need to be educated regarding the gradual progression of the disease, what to expect from a physiological standpoint, and options available for the treatment of these symptoms. The individual and family can be offered the services and support of hospice. Options for interventions need to be explored so that an informed decision can be made. Symptom management techniques secondary to the metastatic site from colorectal carcinoma have been previously discussed in this chapter. Most symptoms can be handled within the comfort of the individual's home if so desired. Should a hospital admission become necessary, however, decisions regarding life support measures need to be explored with the individual and family.

## CONCLUSION

Over the past 30 years there has been a downward trend in the incidence, morbidity, and mortality associated with colorectal carcinoma. Current screening mechanisms, diagnostic techniques, surgical interventions, and adjuvant therapy regimens have enabled individuals diagnosed with this malignancy to experience improved long-term survival and enhanced quality of life.

Factors that contribute to the pathogenesis of this disease are multifactorial. Age, genetics, diet, alcohol, environment, inflammatory bowel conditions, prior radiation therapy, and surgery are risk factors for colorectal cancer. Genes are the focus of attention at present. The presence or absence of certain genetic factors increases the risk for the development of this malignancy.

Surgery continues to be the mainstay of therapy for colorectal adenocarcinoma. Some literature supports the premise that more extensive surgery lends itself to improved cure and long-term survival.[111] Combination modality therapy continues to be implemented in the treatment of this neoplasm. Chemotherapy, radiation therapy, and immunotherapy continue to be utilized preoperatively, intraoperatively, and postoperatively to achieve better long-term survival.

In today's health care environment things continue to change rapidly. More is accomplished on an outpatient basis and hospital lengths of stay dwindle. A multitude of physician specialities are employed to care for the individual with colorectal carcinoma. The coordination and quality of this care needs to be paramount as we move toward earlier diagnosis and better long-term survival for this disease.

## ACKNOWLEDGMENT

The author wishes to acknowledge the professional contribution of William Beaumont and Chris Workman in the development of this manuscript.

## REFERENCES

1. Parker SL, Tong T, Bolden S, et al: Cancer statistics 1996. *CA Cancer J Clin* 65:5–27, 1996

2. Beart, RW: Colon and rectum, in Abeloff MD, Armitage JO, Lichter AS, Niederhuber JE: *Clin Oncol.* New York, Churchill Livingston, 1995, pp 1267–1286

3. Kern WH, White WC: Adenocarcinoma of the colon in a 9-month old infant. *Cancer* 11:855–857, 1958

4. Mayer RJ: Tumors of the large and small intestine, in Isselbacher KJ, Braunwald E, Wilson JD, Martin JB, Fauci AS, Kasper DL: *Harrison's Principles of Internal Medicine* (ed 13). New York, McGraw-Hill, 1994, pp 1424–1429

5. Devesa SS, Chow WH: Variation in colorectal cancer incidence in the United States by subsite of origin. *Cancer* 71:3819–3826, 1993

6. DeCosse JJ, Tsioulias GJ, Jacobson JJ: Colorectal cancer. *Cancer* 44:27–42, 1994

7. Greenwald P: Colon cancer overview. *Cancer* 70:1206–1215, 1992 (suppl 5)

8. Cordice JW Jr, Johnson H Jr: Anatomic distribution of colonic cancers in middle-class black Americans. *J Natl Med Assoc* 83:730–731, 1991

9. Fearon ER, Vogelstein B: A genetic model for colorectal tumorigenesis. *Cell* 61:759–767, 1990

10. Bazzoli F, Fossi S, Sottilis M, et al: The risk of adenomatous polyps in asymptomatic first-degree relatives in persons with colon cancer. *Gastroenterology* 109:783–788, 1995

11. Haskell CM, Lavey RS, Ramming KP: Colon and rectum, in Haskell CM: *Cancer Treatment* (ed 4). Philadelphia, Saunders, 1995, pp 469–497

12. D'Emilia JC, Rodriguez-Bigas MA, Petrelli NJ: The clinical and genetic manifestations of hereditary nonpolyposis colorectal carcinoma. *Am J Surg* 169:368–372, 1995

13. Vargas PA, Alberts DS: Colon cancer: The quest for prevention. *Oncology* 7:33–40, 1993

14. Morotomi M, Guillem JG, LoGerfo P, et al: Production of diacylglycerol, an activator of protein kinase C, by intestinal microflora. *Cancer Res* 50:3595–3599, 1990

15. Steinmetz KA, Kushi LH, Bostick RM, et al: Vegetables, fruit and colon cancer in the Iowa Woman's Health Study. *Am J Epidemiol* 139:1–15, 1994

16. Reddy BS, Engle A, Katsifis S, et al: Biochemical epidemiology of colon cancer. *Cancer Res* 49:4629–4635, 1980

17. Kune GA, Vitetta L: Alcohol consumption and the etiology of colorectal cancer: A review of the scientific evidence from 1957 to 1991. *Nutr Cancer* 18:97–111, 1992

18. Newcomb PA, Storer BE, Marcus PM: Cancer of the large bowel in women in relation to alcohol consumption: A case-control study in Wisconson. *Cancer Causes Control* 4:405–411, 1993

19. Meyer F, White E: Alcohol and nutrients in relation to colon cancer in middle-aged adults. *Am J Epidemiol* 138:225–236, 1993

20. Spiegelman MS, Wegman DH: Occupational-related risk factors for colorectal cancer. *J Natl Cancer Inst* 75:813–820, 1985

21. Tilley BC, Johnson CC, Schultz LR, et al: Risk of colorectal cancer among automotive pattern and model makers. *J Occup Med* 32:541, 1990

22. Stewart PA, Schairer C, Blair A: Comparison of jobs, exposures and mortality for short- and long-term workers. *J Occup Med* 32:703, 1990

23. Takahashi T, Mori T, Moossa AR: Tumors of the Colon and rectum: clinical features and management, in Moossa AR, Schimpff SC, Robson MC: *Comprehensive Textbook of Oncology* (ed 2). Baltimore, Williams and Wilkins, 1991, pp 904–933

24. Greenstein AJ, Sachar DB, Smith H, et al: Patterns of neoplasia in Crohn's disease and ulcerative colitis. *Cancer* 46: 403–407, 1980

25. Jao SW, Beart RW, Reiman HM, et al: Colon and anorectal cancer after pelvic irradiation. *Dis Colon Rectum* 30:953–958, 1987

26. Levitt MD, Millar DM, Stewart JO: Rectal cancer after pelvic irradiation. *J R Soc Med* 83:152–154, 1990

27. DeFlora S, Izzoti A, D'Agostini F, et al: Antioxident activity and other mechanisms of thiois involved in chemoprevention of mutation and cancer. *Am J Med* 91:122S, 1991 (suppl 3c)

28. Rigau J, Pique JM, Rubin E, et al: Effects of long-term sulindac therapy on colonic polyposis. *Ann Int Med* 115: 952, 1991

29. Reddy BS, Nayini J, Tokumo K, et al: Chemoprevention of colon carcinogenesis by dietary piroxicam, a nonsteroidal anti-inflammatory drug with D, L-a-difluoromethylornithine, an ornithine decarboxylase inhibitor in diet. *Cancer Res* 50:2562, 1990

30. Rosenberg L, Palmer JR, Zauber AG, et al: A hypothesis: Nonsteroidal anti-inflammatory drugs reduce the incidence of large bowel cancer. *J Natl Cancer Inst* 83:355, 1991

31. Thun MJ, Namboodiri MM, Calle EE, et al: Aspirin use and reduced risk of fatal colon cancer. *N Engl J Med* 325: 1593–1596, 1991

32. Gridley G, McLaughlin JK, Ekbom A, et al: Incidence of cancer among patients with rheumatoid arthritis. *J Natl Cancer Inst* 85:307–311, 1993

33. Welberg JW, Monkelbaan JF, de-Vries EG, et al: Effects of supplemental dietary calcium on quantitative and qualitative fecal fat excretion in man. *Ann Nutr Metab* 38:185–191, 1994

34. Buras RR, Shabahang M, Davoodi F, et al: The effect of extracellular calcium on colonocytes: Evidence for differential responsiveness based upon degree of cell differentiation. *Cell Prolif* 28:245–262, 1994

35. Calle EE, Miracle-McMahill HL, Thun MJ, et al: Estrogen replacement therapy and risk of fatal colon cancer in a prospective cohort of postmenopausal women. *J Natl Cancer Inst* 87:517–523, 1995

36. Newcomb PA, Storer BE: Postmenopausal hormone use and risk of large bowel cancer. *J Natl Cancer Inst* 87: 1067–1071, 1995

37. Winawer DJ, St John JH, Bond P, et al: Prevention of colorectal cancer: Guidelines based on new data. *Bull World Health Organ* 73:7–10, 1995

38. Winawer SJ, Zauber AG, Ho MN, et al: Prevention of colorectal cancer by colonscopic polypectomy: The National Polyp Study Work Group. *N Engl J Med* 329:1977–1981, 1993

39. Vogelstein B, Fearon ER, Hamilton SR, et al: Genetic alterations during colorectal tumor development. *N Engl J Med* 319:525–532, 1988

40. Loescher, L: Genetics in cancer prediction, screening and counseling: Part 1, genetics in cancer prediction and screening. *Oncol Nurs Forum* 22:10–15, 1995

41. Brown ML, Kessler LG: The use of gene tests to detect hereditary predisposition to cancer: Economic considerations. *J Natl Cancer Inst* 87:1131–1136, 1995

42. Mahon SM: Using brochures to educate the public about the early detection of prostate and colorectal cancer. *Oncol Nurs Forum* 22:1413–1420, 1995

43. Lang CA, Ranschoff DF: Fecal occult blood screening for colorectal cancer. *JAMA* 271:1011–1013, 1994

44. Steele G, Tepper J, Motwani B, et al: Adenocarcinoma of the colon and rectum, in Holland JF, Frei E, Bast R, Kufe SN, Morton DL, Weichselbaum RR: *Cancer Medicine* (ed 3). Philadelphia, Lea & Febiger, 1993, pp 1493–1522

45. Ahlquist DA, Wieand HS, Moertal CG, et al: Accuracy of fecal occult blood screening for colorectal neoplasia. *JAMA* 269:1262–1267, 1993

46. Steele GD, Jessup LM, Winchester DP, et al: Clinical highlights from the National Cancer Data Base: 1995. *CA Cancer J Clin* 45:102–113, 1995

47. Cordice JW Jr, Johnson H Jr: Anatomic distribution of colonic cancers in middle-class black Americans. *J Natl Med Assoc* 83:730–731, 1991

48. Fleshner P, Slater G, Aufes A Jr: Age and sex distribution of patients with colorectal cancer. *Dis Colon Rectum* 32: 107–111, 1989

49. Hoebler L, Irwin MM: Gastrointestinal tract cancer: Current knowledge, medical treatment and nursing management. *Oncol Nurs Forum* 19:1403–1415, 1992

50. Fry RD, Fleshman JW, Kodner IJ: Cancer of colon and rectum. *Clin Symp* 41:2–32, 1989

51. Bates B: The abdomen anatomy and physiology, in Bates B: *A Guide to Physical Examination* (ed 5). Philadelphia, Lippincott, 1991, pp 339–362

52. Allison JE, Feldman R, Tekawa IS: Hemoccult screening in detecting colorectal neoplasms: Sensitivity, specificity, and predictive value. Long-term follow-up in a large group practice setting. *Ann Intern Med* 112:328–333, 1990

53. St John DJ, Young GP, Alexeyeff MA, et al: Evaluation of new occult blood tests for detection of colorectal neoplasia. *Gastroenterology* 104:1661–1668, 1993

54. Yeatman T, Bland K: Malignant lesions of the colon, rectum and anus, in Moody FG: *Surgical Treatment of Digestive Diseases* (ed 1). Chicago, Yearbook Medical Publishers, 1990, pp 799–816

55. Selby JV, Friedman GD, Quesenberry CP, et al: A case-controled study of screening sigmoidoscopy and mortality from colorectal cancer. *N Engl J Med* 326:653–657, 1992

56. Newcomb PA, Norfleet RG, Storer BE, et al: Screening sigmoidoscopy and colorectal cancer mortality. *J Natl Cancer Inst* 84:1572–1575, 1992

57. Dodd GD: The role of the barium enema in the detection of colonic neoplasms. *Cancer* 70:1272–1275, 1992

58. Ehlke G: Gastrointestinal tumors, in Baird S, McCorkle R, Grant M (eds): *Cancer Nursing: A Comprehensive Textbook* (ed 1). Philadelphia, Saunders, 1991, pp 1485–1497

59. Saccani JG, Fontanesi M, Orsi N, et al: DNA content in human colon cancer and non-neoplastic adjacent mucosa. *Int J Biol Markers* 10:11–16, 1995

60. Nori D, Merimsky O, Samala E: Tumor ploidy as a risk factor for disease recurrence and short survival in surgically treated Dukes' B2 colon cancer patients. *J Surg Oncol* 59: 239–242, 1995

61. Nishida K, Takano H, Yoneda M, et al: Flow cytometric analysis of nuclear DNA content in tissues of colon cancer using endoscopic biopsy specimens. *J Surg Oncol* 59:181–185, 1995

62. Fleshner P, Slater G, Autes A: Age and sex distribution of patients with colorectal cancer. *Dis Colon Rectum* 32: 107–111, 1989

63. Dukes CE: The classification of cancer of the rectum. *J Pathol* 35:323–332, 1932

64. Steele GD: The National Cancer Data Base report on colorectal cancer. *Cancer* 74:1979–1989, 1994

65. Williams ST, Beart RW: Staging of colorectal cancer. *Semin Surg Oncol* 8:89–93, 1992

66. Imbembo AL, Lefor AT: Carcinoma of the colon, rectum, and anus, in Sabiston DC: *Textbook of Surgery, The Biological Basis of Modern Surgical Practice.* Philadelphia, Saunders, 1991, pp 948–958

67. Steele G: Colorectal cancer, in McKenna RJ, Murphy GP: *Cancer Surgery* (ed 1). Philadelphia, Lippincott, 1994, pp 125–184

68. Steele G: Adjuvant therapy for patients with colon and rectal cancer: clinical indications for multimodality therapy in high risk groups and specific surgical questions for future multimodality trials. *Surgery* 112:847–849, 1992

69. Kodner IJ, Fry ID, Fleshman JW, et al: Colon, rectum, and anus, in Schwartz SI: *Principles of Surgery* (ed 6). New York, McGraw-Hill, 1994, pp 1272–1307

70. Kettlewell MG: Colorectal cancer and benign tumours of the colon, in Morris PJ, Malt RA: *Oxford Textbook of Surgery* (ed 1). New York, Oxford University Press, 1994, pp 1060–1087

71. Wexner SD, Cohen SM, Ulrich A, et al: Laparoscopic colorectal surgery: Are we being honest with our patients? *Dis Colon Rectum* 38:723–727, 1995

72. Ortega AE, Beart RW, Steele GD, et al: Laparoscopic bowel surgery. *Dis Colon Rectum* 38:681–685, 1995

73. Jessup JM, Steele G: Rectal and Anal Cancer, in Steele G: *General Surgical Oncology* (ed 1). Philadelphia, Saunders, 1992, p 171

74. Brumley CL, Kuhn JA: Radiolabeled monoclonal antibodies. *AORN J* 62:343–347, 1995

75. Birnkrant A, Sampson J, Sugarbaker PH: Ovarian metastasis from colorectal cancer. *Dis Colon Rectum* 29:767, 1986

76. Cole DJ, Ferguson CM: Complications of hepatic resection for colorectal carcinoma metastasis. *Am Surg* 58:88–91, 1992

77. Gayowski TJ, Iwatsuki S, Madariaga JR: Experience in hepatic resection for metastatic colorectal cancer: Analysis of clinical and pathologic risk factors. *Surgery* 116:703–711, 1994

78. Reynolds T: Issues remain for treating colorectal cancer. *J Natl Cancer Inst* 87:480, 1995

79. Wolmark N, Rockette H, Fisher B: The benefit of leucovorin modulated fluorouracil as postoperative adjuvant therapy for primary colon cancer. *J Clin Oncol* 11:1879–1887, 1993

80. Pensel R, Giangiacomo G, Breier S: 5-fluorouracil (5-FU) associated to folinic acid (FA) for the treatment of advanced colon cancer (ACC). *Proc Annu Meet Am Soc Clin Oncol* 10:A 446, 1991

81. Ilson DH, Kelsen DP: Adjuvant postoperative therapy of gastrointestinal malignancies. *Oncology* 8:75–83, 1994

82. Bugat R, Rougier P, Douillard JY, et al: Efficacy of Irinotecan HCL (CPT 11) in patients with metastatic colorectal cancer after progression while receiving a 5-FU based chemotherapy. *Proc Am Soc Clin Oncol* 14:A 567, 1995

83. Rougier P, Culine S, Bugat R, et al: Multicentric phase II study of first line CPT-11 (irinotecan) in advanced colorectal cancer: Preliminary results. *Proc Am Soc Clin Oncol* 13:A 585, 1994

84. Armand JP: Irinotecan (CPT 11): recent clinical development and future direction. *Ann Oncol* 5:A 360, 1994 (suppl 5)

85. Bruckner HW, Motwani BT: Chemotherapy of advanced cancer of the colon and rectum. *Semin Oncol* 18:443, 1991

86. Macdonald DS: Gastrointestinal Cancers, in Wittes RE: *Manual of Oncologic Therapeutics 1991/1992* (ed 1). Philadelphia: Lippincott, 1991, pp 161–174

87. Scheithauer W, Rosen H, Kornek GV, et al: Randomized comparison of combination chemotherapy plus supportive care with supportive care alone in patients with metastatic colorectal cancer. *Br Med J* 306:752–755, 1993

88. Moertel C, Fleming T, Macdonald J: Levamisole and fluorouracil for adjuvant therapy of resected colon carcinoma. *N Engl J Med* 322:352–358, 1990

89. Dahl O, Horn A, Morild I, et al: Low dose preoperative radiation postpones recurrences in operable rectal cancer. *Cancer* 66:2286–2294, 1990

90. Dobelbower RR, Loeffler RK, Merrick HW, et al: Radiation therapy in cancer management: New frontiers, in Moosa AR, Schimpff SC, Rosen MC: *Comprehensive Textbook of Oncology* (ed 2). Baltimore, Williams & Wilkins, 1991, pp 502–522

91. Sparano JA, Wadler S, Schwartz EL, et al: Clinical and pharmacologic studies of interferon and chemotherapy in gastrointestinal and breast cancer. *Int J Clin Pharmacol Res* 13:1–9, 1993

92. Pazdur R, Abbruzzese J, Faintuch J, et al: Phase II study of recombinant interferon alpha and 5-fluorouracil in patients with advanced colorectal carcinoma. *Proc Am Soc Clin Oncol* 9:117, 1990

93. Wadler S, Schwartz EL, Goldman M, et al: Fluorouracil and recombinant alfa-2a-interferon; an active regimen against advanced colorectal carcinoma. *J Clin Oncol* 7:1769, 1989

94. Wiesenfeld M, O'Connell MJ, Wieand HS, et al: Controlled clinical trial of interferon-gamma as postoperative surgical adjuvant therapy for colon cancer. *J Clin Oncol* 13:2324–2329, 1995

95. Minsky DB: Preoperative combined modality treatment for rectal cancer. *Oncology* 8:53–58, 1994

96. Pahlman L, Glimelius B: Preoperative and postoperative radiotherapy and rectal cancer. *World J Surg* 16:858–865, 1992

97. Lopez M: Adjuvant therapy of colorectal cancer. *Dis Colon Rectum* 34:86–91, 1994 (suppl)

98. Beart RW: Colorectal Cancer, in Holleb AH, Fink DJ, Murphy GP: *American Cancer Society Textbook of Clinical Oncology* (ed 1). Atlanta, American Cancer Society, 1991, pp 213–218

99. Shank B: Radiotherapy: Implications for general patient care, in Wittes RE: *Manual of Oncologic Therapeutics 1991/1992* (ed 1). Philadelphia, Lippincott, 1991, pp 60–65

100. Rostock RA, Zajac AJ, Gallagher MJ: Radiation therapy in the treatment of colorectal cancer, in Ahlgren J, Macdonald J: *Gastrointestinal Oncology* (ed 1). Philadelphia, Lippincott, 1992, pp 359–381

101. Fong Y, Blumgart LH, Cohen AM: Surgical treatment of colorectal metastases to the liver. *CA Cancer J Clin* 45:50–62, 1995

102. Ravikumar TS, Steele G: Liver metastases, in Moosa AR, Schimpff SC, Robson MC: *Comprehensive Textbook of Oncology* (ed 1). Baltimore, Williams & Wilkins, 1991, pp 1625–1637

103. Ravikumar TS, Steele G, Kane R, et al: Experimental and clinical observations on hepatic cryosurgery for colorectal metastases. *Cancer Res* 51:6323–6327, 1991

104. Lim LH, Ko YT, Lee DH, et al: Determining the site and causes of colonic obstruction with sonography. *Am J Roentgenol* 163:1113–1117, 1994

105. Lee PH, Khauli RB, Baker S, et al: Prognostic and therapeu-

tic observations of manifestations in the genitourinary tract of adenocarcinoma of the colon and rectum. *Surg Gynecol Obstet* 169:511–518, 1989

106. Lieber MM: Urologic emergencies, in Wittes RE: *Manual of Oncologic Therapeutics* (ed 1). Philadelphia, Lippincott, 1991, pp 336–338

107. McCormick PM, Martini N: A current view of surgical management of pulmonary metastases, in Economou SG, Witt TR, Deziel DJ, et al: *Adjuncts To Cancer Surgery* (ed 1). Philadelphia, Lea & Febiger, 1991, pp 246–251

108. DePadt G, Delacrois R, Meuretta J, et al: Surgical treatment of pulmonary metastases: problems and prospects, in Hell-man K, Eccles SA: *Proceedings.* Philadelphia, Taylor and Francis, 1985, pp 5–8

109. Avis F: Surgical treatment of isolated metastases to the liver, lungs, and brain, in Wittes RE: *Manual of Oncologic Therapeutics* (ed 1). Philadelphia, Lippincott, 1991, pp 308–309

110. Mountain CF, McMurtrey MJ, Hermes KF: Surgery for pulmonary metastasis: A 20 year experience. *Ann Thorac Sur* 38:323–330, 1984

111. Peloquin AB: Cancer of the colon and rectum: Comparison of the results of three groups of surgeons using different techniques. *Can J Surg* 16:28–34, 1988

# Chapter 37

# Endocrine Malignancies

Rita Wickham, RN, PhD(c) AOCN

Kimberly Rohan, MS, RN, OCN®

# INTRODUCTION

Approximately 17,000 individuals in the United States were diagnosed with an endocrine malignancy in 1996, and 1900 deaths resulted from these cancers.[1] Thyroid malignancies are the most common, constituting approximately 90% of these cancers. Endocrine malignancies arise from glands that secrete endocrine hormones, that is, chemical signals released into the bloodstream to exert their effects at sites distant from their origin. Although it is now recognized that virtually very organ possesses some endocrine function,[2] the classic endocrine glands include the pituitary, the thyroid, the parathyroids, the adrenal glands, the gonads, and the islets of Langerhans. This chapter will focus on malignancies arising in the thyroid, parathyroid, pituitary, and adrenal cortex and medulla (pheochromocytoma), as well as multiple endocrine neoplasia (MEN) syndromes. Individuals who inherit an autosomal dominant gene or genes that code for a MEN syndrome may experience a particular constellation of endocrine tumors, which tend to occur earlier in life than in individuals who develop sporadic endocrine tumors.

# THYROID TUMORS

The thyroid is a small organ that lies below the cricoid cartilage at the base of the neck and around either side of the trachea. The thyroid normally weighs between 15 and 20 g but is capable of massive enlargement in disease states.[3] Follicles, the functional units of the thyroid, are epithelial cells arranged in a tubelike fashion and are interspersed with parafollicular cells (also known as C cells). Groups of follicles are bound tightly together to form lobules. The follicular cells produce the thyroid hormones thyroxine ($T_4$) and triiodothyronine ($T_3$), and

C cells produce calcitonin, all of which hold large amounts of iodine. The thyroid synthesizes its hormones in response to thyroid-stimulating hormone (TSH) released by the anterior pituitary gland.

Virtually all of the body's cells require thyroid hormones for optimal functioning, and thyroid hormones affect growth, metabolism, and the regulation of body temperature. Thyroid hormone acts as a growth factor to promote bone formation and skeletal maturation, and is required for the production of growth hormone (GH). In addition, thyroid hormones play a critical role in the maturation of the central nervous system (CNS) of infants, and modulate the actions of the autonomic nervous system throughout life.[3] The role of thyroid hormones in oxidative metabolism is reflected in the basal metabolic rate (BMR); the thyroid helps to maintain a steady body temperature through heat production or conservation when appropriate via this process. Carbohydrate metabolism, in particular, is positively affected by $T_3$, and lipid metabolism is affected by thyroid hormones in concert with insulin. The excess or absence of thyroid hormones increases or decreases the synthesis and degradation of body proteins.

## Epidemiology

Fewer than 14,000 cases of thyroid cancer were diagnosed in the United States in 1995, and about 1120 deaths occurred as a result of these tumors.[4] Thyroid malignancies are most commonly diagnosed in individuals aged 40–49, and women are three times as likely as men to develop a thyroid tumor. Age is an important determinant of prognosis, as five-year survival with thyroid cancer is 95% in patients younger than 59 years but only 64% in those older than 70 years.

## Etiology

Ionizing radiation to the head and neck is the only clearly identified causative agent for papillary thyroid cancer,[5]

but other factors may play a role. These include benign thyroid disease, hormonal and reproductive factors in women,[6] and a diet deficient in iodine.[7-9] The carcinogenic risk of radiation is dose-dependent: minimal risk exists with exposure to very small doses (6.5–80 cGy), and risk increases linearly to a dose of 2000 cGy. At doses > 2000 cGy, the risk for thyroid cancer falls off as the thyroid cells die and the gland becomes "sterile."[5,8]

A great deal of knowledge about the carcinogenic effect of radiation has been gained by following children treated with radiation (prior to the mid-1960s) for enlarged thymus glands, tonsillitis, adenoid hypertrophy, pharyngitis, and skin diseases of the face and neck.[10] Risk is inversely related to age; that is, infants and young children are more susceptible to the carcinogenic effect of radiation to the neck region than are older children.[11,12] Furthermore, the carcinogenic effect of radiation may persist for as long as four decades after exposure, and this effect is also more pronounced in younger children.[8,13]

Two examples highlight the risks for children receiving high doses of therapeutic or accidental radiation to the thyroid. Children who receive total-body irradiation for allogeneic bone marrow transplantation are at increased risk for papillary thyroid malignancy, and thus should be followed on a regular basis for thyroid tumors.[6,14] Likewise, thyroid cancer has increased dramatically in children exposed to high levels of radioactive fallout from the Chernobyl nuclear plant disaster. Before the accident at Chernobyl in 1986, the rate of thyroid cancer was 1 child per million, but nine years later was 36 per million in the surrounding three countries. In the region just north of the reactor, the incidence has reached 100 cases per million.[15]

High rates of follicular and papillary tumors are noted in areas of endemic goiter.[16] This supports the hypothesis that iodine insufficiency, especially in women, adolescents, and young adults, is a causative factor for thyroid malignancy.[17]

## Pathophysiology

There are four types of endocrine thyroid neoplasms: papillary, follicular, medullary, and anaplastic. Papillary and follicular tumors arise from the follicle, medullary tumors arise from parafollicular cells, and anaplastic tumors arise from differentiated papillary or follicular cells.

### Papillary and follicular tumors

Tumors consisting only of papillary cells, as well as those consisting of mixed papillary and follicular cells, are classified as papillary carcinomas because they behave similarly. Papillary carcinomas occur in three times as many females as males and constitute 60%–70% of the thyroid malignancies in adults and children.[10] Papillary carcinomas are characteristically well differentiated and

indolent, and they have a good prognosis. Tumors are often more aggressive in males and in older patients.[13,16]

Papillary tumors are typically multifocal and infiltrate local tissues. Forty percent of patients have regional lymph node metastases at the time of diagnosis, a finding not related to tumor size.[16] Vascular invasion and metastasis to a distant site, such as bone and lung, are more common in papillary tumors than in follicular tumors.[13,18] Patients may survive for decades even when they have metastatic disease.[13]

Follicular thyroid cancer, diagnosed in about 20% of all cases, is more aggressive than papillary cancer. Age, tumor size, and blood vessel invasion are significant prognostic indicators.[18] Follicular cancer is most often diagnosed in persons in their 50s, but those younger than 40 have the best prognosis.[5,13] Indicators of poor prognosis include large tumor size (> 6 cm) and blood vessel invasion. Hürthle cell carcinoma, a subtype of follicular carcinoma occurring in older persons, may retain the necessary enzymes for thyroid hormone synthesis and thus may cause hyperthyroidism.[11,13]

### Medullary tumors

Medullary thyroid tumors, which constitute 5%–10% of thyroid tumors, occur equally in men and women over the age of 50.[5,19] Eighty percent of medullary tumors are sporadic, while the remainder occur because of germline mutations that lead to MEN syndrome.[8] Fifty percent of patients have tumor spread to their cervical lymph nodes at the time of diagnosis.[5,13] Regional lymph node spread is an ominous prognostic sign; ten-year survival is only 42% in patients with involved lymph nodes but is 90% in patients with negative regional lymph nodes. Medullary tumors metastasize via the bloodstream and lymphatics to lung, liver, and bone.

### Anaplastic tumors

Between 5% and 10% of thyroid malignancies are anaplastic.[5,8,13,16] These tumors usually grow "explosively." Patients typically present with a rapidly growing firm or hard neck mass invading the structures of the neck to cause dysphagia and dysphonia. Most individuals are in their 60s when this tumor is diagnosed, and males and females have about the same risk for tumor development.[20,21] Anaplastic tumors have the best prognosis when the tumor is completely resectable.[21] Unfortunately, this is often not the case, and most patients live for only 4–12 months following diagnosis. Metastasis is an early event, and sites may include lymph nodes, bone, and lung.[22] Treatment of these tumors with radiation and/or chemotherapy has not significantly altered survival rates, which are 1.0%–7.1% at five years.[20,21]

## Clinical Manifestations

Thyroid malignancies often do not cause symptoms until the disease is advanced. Patients may seek medical attention when they notice that their necks look larger, or because their neck mass is painful and noticeably enlarging. In other instances they may be experiencing local symptoms such as recent-onset dysphagia, dysphonia, or hoarseness.[9] Approximately 20%–30% of patients who have medullary thyroid carcinoma experience persistent diarrhea secondary to hypersecretion of calcitonin by their tumor.[5]

## Assessment

Diagnostic procedures for thyroid malignancies include history and physical examination, and in some instances laboratory and imaging procedures. The history may provide clues to the diagnosis, especially information about radiation exposure to the neck in early childhood. A thorough family history is important, especially if familial medullary carcinoma related to MEN is suspected.

Young patients with a thyroid mass tend to present with painless anterior cervical adenopathy. In older patients the first manifestation is usually regional lymph node metastasis or, rarely, distant metastasis.[23] Thyroid masses are commonly found either by the patient or by a health care provider during routine physical examination. Upon gentle palpation of the neck, normal thyroid lobes are small, smooth, and free of nodules, and the thyroid rises freely with swallowing. Any deviations from normal require further investigation.

Thyroid function tests are not included as part of the workup for thyroid cancer because most tumors do not alter the thyroid's functional capacity. One exception is elevated serum calcitonin levels, which are strongly suggestive of medullary hyperplasia or carcinoma.[24] Medullary tumor cells, which arise from parafollicular C cells, continue to secrete calcitonin that may be a useful tumor marker to monitor the effectiveness of treatment and disease recurrence.[13] Carcinoembryonic antigen (CEA) levels are occasionally elevated in medullary tumors, but not other cell types.

Ultrasonography and radionuclide scanning cannot accurately distinguish between benign and malignant nodules but can provide useful information about tumors. Ultrasound distinguishes cystic, solid, and mixed lesions, and because it does not employ ionizing radiation, is safe for children and pregnant women. Radionuclide scans after injection of iodine ($^{123}$I) or technetium are used to visualize the thyroid. Of the two,$^{123}$I is preferable because it will confirm a suspicious nodule's ability not only to trap iodine but to incorporate it. Technetium, on the other hand, only demonstrates a nodule's ability to trap iodine.[25] Most malignant nodules scan "cold," that is, they are nonfunctional. However, a small percentage of functional ("hot") nodules prove to be malignant on biopsy.[26]

If a thyroid nodule is discovered, the patient may be treated with a trial of TSH-suppressive drugs that may cause a benign nodule to shrink while a malignant nodule will not.[8] Unfortunately, there are side effects to the drugs, and successful suppression of growth does not guarantee the nodule is benign. Thus biopsy and histopathological examination of tumor tissue are ultimately needed to confirm the diagnosis.

Fine-needle aspirate (FNA) biopsy is the procedure of choice to confirm thyroid malignancy.[27–30] When done by an experienced and proficient surgeon, FNA biopsy is highly sensitive. It accurately diagnoses thyroid malignancy 95% of the time and has only a 5%–10% false-negative rate.[26,28] FNA helps eliminate unnecessary surgery for benign lesions and allows appropriate treatment in the event a malignant tumor is found. If the FNA is negative it may be repeated with ultrasound guidance to confirm that the lesion is indeed benign.[27,31] This procedure is relatively inexpensive, can be performed in outpatient settings, and causes minimal complications. Another advantage is that sufficient tissue is obtained for DNA analysis, which may provide further information about how aggressive the tumor is.

## Classification and Staging

Histological diagnosis and age are important determinants of prognosis. The American Joint Committee on Cancer (AJCC) has thus developed a staging system for thyroid cancer that incorporates these two factors (Table 37-1).[32]

## Therapeutic Approaches and Nursing Care

### Surgery

Treatment decisions are complicated by the fact that most thyroid tumors are indolent. Because of the protracted clinical course, many clinicians do not recommend treatment until the patient is symptomatic.[8] While surgery is the treatment of choice for thyroid tumors, there is no consensus about how extensive surgical resection should be for well-differentiated tumors. Studies comparing total, subtotal, and partial thyroidectomy have found that subtotal resection of small tumors (<1 cm) in patients under the age of 45 results in similar recurrence and survival rates as more extensive surgery.[8,23] When cure is possible, more aggressive surgery (near-total thyroidectomy, tumor resection, and neck dissection) is advocated for medullary and anaplastic tumors.[9] Table 37-2 summarizes recommended therapeutic approaches in the management of thyroid tumors.

Postoperative complications of thyroidectomy include vocal cord paralysis with subsequent respiratory embarrassment, thyroid storm, hemorrhage, and hypothyroidism.[33] Thyroid storm, or thyrotoxic crisis, is an acute episode of thyroid overactivity that is characterized by high fever, tachycardia, delirium, dehydration, and extreme excitability. Vocal cord paralysis related to damage to the laryngeal nerve during surgery is a rare occur-

**TABLE 37-1** Staging Classification of Thyroid Carcinomas

PRIMARY TUMOR (T)

All categories may be subdivided: (a) solitary; (b) multifocal—measure the largest classification

| | |
|---|---|
| TX | Primary tumor cannot be assessed |
| T0 | No evidence of primary tumor |
| T1 | Tumor 1 cm or less in greatest dimension limited to the thyroid |
| T2 | Tumor more than 1 cm but not more than 4 cm |
| T3 | Tumor more than 4 cm in greatest dimension limited to the thyroid |
| T4 | Tumor of any size extending beyond the thyroid capsule |

LYMPH NODES (N)

Regional nodes are the cervical and upper mediastinal lymph nodes

| | |
|---|---|
| NX | Regional lymph nodes cannot be assessed |
| N0 | No regional lymph node metastasis |
| N1 | Regional lymph node metastasis |
| N1a | Metastasis in ipsilateral cervical lymph nodes |
| N1b | Metastasis in bilateral, midline, or contralateral cervical or mediastinal lymph nodes |

DISTANT METASTASIS (M)

| | |
|---|---|
| MX | Presence of distant metastasis cannot be assessed |
| M0 | No distant metastasis |
| M1 | Distant metastasis |

STAGE GROUPING

Separate stage groupings are recommended for papillary and follicular, medullary and undifferentiated

Papillary or Follicular

| *Under 45 Years* | | *45 Years and Over* | |
|---|---|---|---|
| Stage I | Any T, any N, M0 | Stage I | T1, N0, M0 |
| Stage II | Any T, Any N, M1 | Stage II | T2, N0, M0 |
| | | | T3, N0, M0 |
| | | Stage III | T4, N0, M0 |
| | | | Any T, N1, M0 |
| | | Stage IV | Any T, any N, M1 |

Medullary

| | |
|---|---|
| Stage I | T1, N0, M0 |
| Stage II | T2, N0, M0 |
| | T3, N0, M0 |
| | T4, N0, M0 |
| Stage III | Any T, N1, M0 |
| Stage IV | Any T, any N, M1 |

Undifferentiated

All cases are stage IV

| | |
|---|---|
| Stage IV | Any T, any N, any M |

Reprinted from the *AJCC Manual for Staging of Cancer* with permission from the American Joint Committee on Cancer (AJCC).

**TABLE 37-2** Recommended Treatment Approaches for Thyroid Tumors

| Tumor Type | Age | Size of Lesion | Recommended Therapy | Comments |
|---|---|---|---|---|
| Papillary and follicular: Differentiated | < 45 | < 2 cm | Thyroid lobectomy or near-total thyroidectomy, followed by suppressive therapy | Suppression with thyroxine is used to decrease serum levels of TSH |
| Differentiated | < 45 | > 2 cm | Near-total or total thyroidectomy plus [131]I ablation | Therapeutic dose of [131]I is dependent upon uptake during diagnostic whole-body scan |
| Differentiated | ≥ 45 | < 4 cm | Near-total or total thyroidectomy with suppression and [131]I ablation | |
| Differentiated | Any | > 4 cm | Near-total or total thyroidectomy plus suppression and [131]I ablation, plus or minus local radiation therapy | Local radiation therapy is used to control symptoms |
| Medullary | Any | Any | Near-total or total thyroidectomy with modified neck dissection if extrathyroidal disease present | Chemotherapy may be effective to control disease |
| Anaplastic | Any | Any | Near-total thyroidectomy or tumor dissection, if possible, followed by chemotherapy plus or minus radiation therapy | Use of chemotherapy or radiation therapy is controversial because of limited effectiveness |

Data from Norton et al 1993;[8] DeGroot and Sridama 1989.[9]

rence. Because of the possibility of hemorrhage, the nurse monitors output from drains and assesses the patient for symptoms of impending shock.

Temporary or permanent hypoparathyroidism is a major complication, occurring in 1% of patients undergoing near-total thyroidectomies and up to 6%–8% having total thyroidectomies.[8,23] Hypothyroidism results in hypocalcemia that requires the administration of exogenous thyroid hormone to prevent the clinical effects of hypothyroidism. Postoperative nursing management requires keen assessment for the signs and symptoms of tetany, for hypocalcemia, and for other complications (Table 37-3).[33,34]

### Radiation therapy

Brachytherapy with oral [131]I is used to treat some cases of papillary and follicular tumors but not medullary and anaplastic tumors, which do not concentrate and retain iodine. Four to six weeks after surgery, oral [131]I is administered to ablate any remaining functioning thyroid tissue and residual tumor (primary and metastatic). Destruction of functional thyroid accomplishes the initial therapeutic goal, which is to increase circulating TSH levels. This in turn causes [131]I to be taken up into well-differentiated tumors. A whole-body scan is done two to three months after treatment to determine whether any tumor and functioning thyroid tissue remain, and is repeated at four- to six-months intervals as necessary.[5] If any tumor remains, [131]I is repeated until the whole-body scan is negative.

Side effects of [131]I include nausea and vomiting, fatigue, headache, bone marrow suppression, salivary gland inflammation, and infrequently leukemia and radiation-induced pulmonary fibrosis.[35] The reader can refer to chapter 13 for specific information regarding the care of the patient receiving brachytherapy with [131]I. Nursing care includes minimizing the sense of isolation for the patient and providing radiation safety for staff and visitors. Patient and family education, included in Figure 37-1, is extremely important to clarify misconceptions regarding [131]I treatment.

External-beam radiation is occasionally used to attempt local control of anaplastic tumors, but these tumors are usually radioresistant so success rates are low.[13] Successful treatment with combined radiotherapy and chemotherapy has been reported.[36] One clear indication for external-beam radiation is to palliate painful bone metastasis.

### Chemotherapy

There are very few reports of chemotherapy for refractory, metastatic, and anaplastic thyroid cancers, and the results are generally discouraging. Doxorubicin has shown the greatest activity against thyroid malignancies.[37–39] Response rates vary, ranging from 14% to about 31% for anaplastic tumors and well-differentiated medullary tumors, respectively. Combination therapy with 5-fluorouracil (5-FU) plus streptozocin or dacarbazine for patients with metastatic medullary thyroid cancer resulted in partial responses or long-term stabilization of disease in 17 of 20 patients.[40] These agents may thus warrant further investigation.

**TABLE 37-3** Care Plan for the Patient Undergoing Thyroid Surgery

| Problem/Diagnosis | Nursing Observations/Actions | Comments |
|---|---|---|
| Potential for ineffective airway clearance related to:<br>• Hematoma<br><br>• Vocal cord paralysis | Assess respiratory status every 1 hr × 12 hr, then every 4 hr × 48 hr<br>Assess vital signs every 4 hr × 48 hr<br>Observe for:<br>• Hoarseness<br><br>• Inability to speak<br><br>• Retraction of neck muscles<br><br>• Crowing respirations<br><br>• Dyspnea<br><br>• Cyanosis<br><br>• Hematoma formation<br>Keep trach basket at bedside<br>Keep head of bed >45° at all times.<br>Maintain neck support by placing hands behind neck with elbows raised when sitting or moving<br>Assist with turn, cough, and deep breathing every 2 hr | Notify physician immediately for:<br>• Signs and symptoms of vocal cord paralysis<br><br>• Respiratory distress<br><br>• Patient complaints of neck tightness, fullness or pressure (indicates possible internal bleeding) |
| Potential for decreased serum calcium level related to impaired parathyroid function, secondary to removal or reimplantation | Observe for signs and symptoms of tetany every 4 hr × 7 days<br>Monitor serum calcium levels every day<br><br><br><br><br><br><br><br><br><br>Administer calcium gluconate as ordered<br><br><br><br><br><br>Teach patient to avoid foods that suppress calcium absorption (e.g., spinach, Swiss cheese, beets, bran, and whole grain cereals) | • Numbness, tingling, cramps in extremities or around mouth<br><br>• Stiffness, twitching, or spasms in hands or feet<br><br>• Positive Chvostek's sign (twitching of nose, mouth, and eye induced by sharp tapping over facial nerve anterior to ear)<br><br>• Trousseau's sign: carpopedal spasm induced by inflation of BP cuff to 200 mm Hg after 1 min<br><br>• Odorless and tasteless<br><br>• Administer parenterally or orally.<br><br>• Warm IV solutions to body temperature and administer slowly (0.5–2 ml/min) to prevent cardiac arrythmias |
| Potential for thyrotoxic crisis (thyroid storm), related to partial thyroidectomy | Observe patient every 4 hrs for signs and symptoms of thyroid storm:<br>• Sudden temperature increase<br><br>• Extreme restlessness or irritability<br><br>• Delirium<br><br>• Tachycardia<br><br>• Widening pulse pressure followed by hypotension<br><br>• Nausea and vomiting, diarrhea, and warm flushed skin<br><br>In case of thyroid storm:<br>• Administer prescribed IV fluid, vitamins, and glucocorticoids | Notify physician immediately if oral temperature rises to >99 °F orally, or 100 °F rectally, because this may be the first sign of thyroid storm |

*(continued)*

**TABLE 37-3**    Care Plan for the Patient Undergoing Thyroid Surgery (continued)

| Problem/Diagnosis | Nursing Observations/Actions | Comments |
|---|---|---|
| | • Administer prescribed antithyroid medication (propylthiouracil)<br><br>• Administer prescribed iodine medication<br><br>• Employ measures to reduce body temperature, such as cooling blanket, tepid sponge bath | |

Data from Servé P 1986;[33] Lehne RA 1994.[34]

# PARATHYROID TUMORS

The parathyroid glands are located on the posterior thyroid, either on the surface or imbedded in the thyroid. Most people have four glands, but the normal range is two to eight. The major functional cells are chief cells, which are exquisitely sensitive to extracellular calcium levels. The chief cells produce parathyroid hormone (PTH), which is critical to maintain normal serum calcium balance. PTH increases calcium resorption from bone when serum calcium is low and simultaneously increases urinary excretion of phosphate. When serum calcium levels are high, the opposite effect occurs.[41]

## Epidemiology

Greater than 95% of parathyroid tumors are benign,[42] and malignant tumors account for less than 1% of primary hyperparathyroidism.[43,44] Parathyroid adenomas occur equally in males and females, who are usually diagnosed in their 40s and 50s.[8,42,43] Parathyroid tumors are most commonly linked to familial MEN 1 and less frequently to MEN 2A.[10]

## Etiology

No definitive risk factors have been identified for the development of parathyroid carcinoma.[42] For instance, only rare individuals diagnosed with parathyroid carcinoma have received radiation to the neck area. One suggestion proposes a relationship between chronic renal failure, which may cause secondary hyperparathyroidism, and parathyroid carcinoma.

## Pathophysiology

It may be difficult to establish whether a parathyroid mass is a benign tumor, a malignant tumor, or even hyperplasia because all of these may appear histopathologically simi-lar. At diagnosis, carcinomas may be hard, lobulated, and larger than benign tumors, and 50% will have invaded adjacent structures.[45] Both benign and malignant parathyroid tumors are usually biochemically functional, that is, they hypersecrete PTH and cause hypercalcemia.[43] Flow cytometry DNA analysis may help differentiate benign from malignant tumors, as malignant tumors often produce human chorionic gonadotropin (HCG) subunits alpha and beta, while benign tumors do not.[42]

Carcinomas tend to be indolent and to recur locally after surgical resection. Metastasis of parathyroid carcinoma is most often a late event, but 20% of patients have cervical lymph node disease, and 16% have distant metastases to the lungs, bone, liver, and other organs at diagnosis.[45]

## Clinical Manifestations

Hypercalcemia is the hallmark of parathyroid tumors. The patient's serum calcium is usually greater than 14 mg/dl and is accompanied by signs and symptoms of hypercalcemia (see chapter 25).[42,43] Symptoms of parathyroid carcinoma may reflect renal and bone involvement, as well as organ effects of hypercalcemia (neuromuscular, rheumatologic, gastrointestinal, and cardiovascular symptoms, and calcification of the cornea and other soft tissues).[8] Fewer than 10% of patients experience hoarseness, and 42% have a palpable neck mass.[42]

## Assessment

The diagnosis of parathyroid tumor is essentially confirmed by the signs and symptoms of parathyroid hyperplasia or tumor. A search for parathyroid carcinoma begins with the identification of unexplained hypercalcemia. Immunoassay typically reveals markedly increased levels of PTH.[46] Most patients do not have a palpable mass, so visualization procedures (nuclear and computerized tomography [CT] scans) are used most often to localize and evaluate tumor masses after surgery.[47] Radiographs or bone scans are useful to confirm bone metasta-

---

### ¹³¹I Treatment

**What is ¹³¹I?**

¹³¹I is radioactive iodine that goes to the thyroid gland and thyroid cancer cells. It is toxic to these cells, and the aim of treatment is to kill cancer cells. It will also kill normal thyroid cells.

**Where will I go to get the ¹³¹I treatment?**

You will have to go to the hospital to get this treatment. While in the hospital, you will wear only hospital gowns, robe, and slippers. Do not bring things from home.

**How will I take the ¹³¹I?**

You will be given a special container of ¹³¹I, and you will drink it through a straw.

**Will I be able to have visitors while I am in the hospital?**

You may have adult visitors while you are in the hospital, but because you will be radioactive there are some rules:

1. No pregnant women can visit
2. Visitors will only be able to stay for 30 minutes or less for the first 48 hours

**Will I have any side effects from the ¹³¹I?**

Possible side effects may include nausea and vomiting, tiredness, headache, a sore mouth, and a lowered white blood count after you get the treatment. Your nurse will give you medicine for the nausea or the headache if you have them, and your doctor may want you to get a blood test after you go home. You will also have a metallic taste in your mouth for several days after taking ¹³¹I.

**Will I still be radioactive when I go home?**

Yes, you will be radioactive for a few days. For three days after you go home, you should:

1. Sleep alone
2. Not hold children close

**How can I help my body get rid of the ¹³¹I?**

You need to drink as much fluid as you can (at least 2 quarts per day) for several days after getting the ¹³¹I. This can include water, juices, and sodas. The ¹³¹I will pass out of your body in your urine, so when you go to the bathroom:

1. Both men and women should sit on the toilet to urinate so urine does not splash anywhere
2. You should flush the toilet three times after you pass urine

**How will my doctor know if the thyroid cancer is gone?**

You doctor will schedule you for a body scan in about three to six months. If the scan shows that there aren't any more thyroid cancer cells, you will not need any more ¹³¹I. If there are any thyroid cancer cells that show up on the scan, you will get another ¹³¹I treatment.

**If you have any other questions, please write them down on the back so you remember to ask your doctor or your nurse.**

---

**FIGURE 37-1** Teaching sheet for the patient receiving ¹³¹I.

ses, which occur in about 50% of patients.[46] Soft-tissue radiography of the finger bones may be done because subperiosteal bone resorption occurs in hyperparathyroid carcinoma. FNA to confirm the diagnosis before surgery is not recommended because of the risk of tumor spillage and local spread.

## Therapeutic Approaches and Nursing Care

### Surgery

Surgery is the treatment of choice for parathyroid tumors, but radical surgery may not change the course of the disease.[43,44] This is because the tumor's intrinsic biological behavior is the most important prognostic determinant.[47] Radiotherapy and chemotherapy are ineffective in treating primary and metastatic disease.

Surgery for localized parathyroid adenomas and carcinomas includes unilateral neck dissection.[47] The primary tumor is resected in toto with the ipsilateral thyroid lobe and isthmus. The surgeon is careful to avoid rupture of the parathyroid capsule, which may result in local seeding of tumor.[43] Extensive surgery may be necessary to remove all tumor from the trachea, involved central lymph nodes, and any contiguous tissues to which the tumor adheres.[8,43] If the recurrent laryngeal nerve is involved, this too must be resected. Patients who have indolent disease may benefit from further resection of metastatic disease. Because parathyroid tumors grow slowly, they may recur two to three years after the original surgery.

The focus of postoperative nursing care is monitoring calcium levels and teaching the patient and family self-care management. After surgery, "hungry bone syndrome" signifies successful extirpation of tumor. In this syndrome calcium and phosphorus are rapidly deposited into bone, which results in symptomatic hypocalcemia (see Table 37-3).[43] The patient requires supplemental intravenous calcium and calcitrol until the remaining parathyroid glands recover. After that, serum calcium and PTH levels are monitored every three months for elevation, which signifies recurrent local and/or metastatic disease.

### Chemotherapy

Because parathyroid malignancy is so rare, no studies involving chemotherapy have been done, and anecdotal reports of limited success are few. Bukowski and others[48] reported that one patient with metastatic disease had a five-month remission after receiving 5-FU, cyclophosphamide, and dacarbazine. Similarly, Chahinian and colleagues[49] reported that a patient who had mediastinal metastases and pleural effusion responded to a combination of methotrexate, doxorubicin, cyclophosphamide, and lomustine for 18 months. Overall, however, chemotherapy has been judged ineffective for parathyroid carcinomas.

Control of hypercalcemia in patients with parathyroid

tumors is often difficult because the condition is caused by tumor recurrence. When surgery is not feasible, recurrent hypercalcemia is treated with the same drugs used to treat other instances of hypercalcemia. Calcium levels may remain persistently elevated despite attempts to inhibit the effects of tumor PTH with calcitonin, gallium nitrate, mithramycin, or bisphosphonates, which may be partially effective for a limited time.[8,42,43,50] Chronic, uncontrolled hypercalcemia remains the cause of death in most patients.

# PITUITARY TUMORS

The pituitary is a 1-cm organ that lies in the sella turcica, a bony cavity in sphenoid bone, at the base of the brain. It consists of two anatomically and physiologically distinct portions: the anterior and the posterior pituitary. The anterior pituitary, from which tumors arise, secretes six physiologically important hormones that control functions of the thyroid, adrenal glands, gonads, and mammary glands, as well as growth by secreting trophic hormones. These include TSH, which controls the rate by which the thyroid secretes thyroxine; adrenocorticotropin, which controls some of the adrenocortical hormones (ACTH); prolactin, which promotes the development of breast tissue and milk production; and growth hormone (GH), which promotes growth and affects many metabolic processes throughout the body. Other hormones that are secreted include melanocyte-stimulating hormone, follicle-stimulating hormone, and luteinizing hormone. Each hormone is secreted by a different type of cell.

Secretion of trophic hormones is regulated by negative feedback influenced by the CNS, predominantly the pituitary and the hypothalamus, and the target organs. The pituitary is connected to the hypothalamus by the pituitary stalk. The hypothalamus plays a critical role in regulating trophic hormones by releasing hypothalamic-releasing and inhibitory hormones. These are conducted directly from the hypothalamus to the pituitary via the hypothalamic-hypophysial portal vessels.[51]

## Epidemiology

Pituitary tumors constitute 5%–16% of all diagnosed brain tumors.[52,53] These tumors remain small and hormonally silent in many persons; therefore, many are discovered as incidental findings upon autopsy. The female-to-male incidence varies with tumor type. For instance, the rate of prolactinomas is 1:1050 in women but only 1:2800 in men.[54] Pituitary adenomas occur at all ages, but 70% occur in individuals between 30 and 50 years of age.[55]

## Etiology

Pituitary tumors arise from epithelial cells in the anterior pituitary, but their exact pathogenesis is unknown. There are two hypotheses of tumorigenesis: the pituitary hypothesis and the hypothalamic hypothesis. The pituitary hypothesis holds that tumors arise from the spontaneous development of a transformed clone of particular cells within the pituitary. Studies have shown that most pituitary tumors are monoclonal in origin, which strongly supports somatic mutation as a key event in transformation.[54] Moreover, mutations in genes that code for growth factors for pituitary cells have been identified in persons with some pituitary tumors.[55]

The hypothalamic hypothesis proposes that some change in hormonal equilibrium, such as hypersecretion of releasing factors or a lack of inhibitory factors from the hypothalamus, causes the development of a pituitary tumor.[52] There is evidence that both events occur, which is congruent with the multistage theory of tumorigenesis.[53] In this view the initial congenital or acquired mutation is the initiator, which remains physiologically silent unless intervening stimulatory (or lack of inhibitory) endocrine factors promote tumor growth.

## Pathophysiology

Most pituitary tumors are localized, benign adenomas that are incapable of metastasizing.[52] Adenomas consist of transformed cells that grow by expansion and cause mass effects. In addition, both benign and malignant tumors usually express altered gene products for neurotransmitters and hypothalamic hormones that cause physiological effects. True pituitary carcinomas, that is, malignant tumors that have the ability to metastasize, are rare.[56] Carcinomas may invade the subarachnoid space and metastasize to the brain and spinal cord through lymphatic or vascular channels, and to the liver and bone through the cervical lymphatics.[57,58]

## Clinical Manifestations

Signs and symptoms of pituitary adenomas result from secretion or depression of particular hormones in most cases, and to mass effects in some cases. Considering the variety of tumors that arise, a corresponding number of syndromes may occur. These relate to the hypersecretion of prolactin, GH, ACTH, or, less commonly, to other hormones.

### Hormone effects

***Prolactinomas***   In women, prolactinomas cause galactorrhea, menstrual irregularities including amenorrhea or oligomenorrhea, or infertility. In men the same tumor produces decreased libido or impotence, and in some cases, galactorrhea.[52,54] Women tend to notice these symptoms earlier, while men may attribute them to advancing age; thus women with prolactinomas tend to be diagnosed when their tumors are smaller.

*Growth hormone–secreting tumors*   Almost all cases of GH-secreting tumors arise in the pituitary. These tumors induce acromegaly in adults and gigantism in prepubescent children. GH-secreting tumors progress slowly, and the average time from onset of symptoms to diagnosis is 6.5 years.[59] Early symptoms are nonspecific and include fatigue or lethargy, paresthesia, and headache. As tumors enlarge, excessive GH leads to enlargement of bone, organs, and soft tissues. The result is the characteristic disfigurement of the face (Figure 37-2),[59] arthropathies, and neuropathies (from soft-tissue swelling) that interfere with normal activities. Other symptoms include weight gain, excessive perspiration, insulin resistance, and decreased glucose tolerance leading to diabetes.[52,60] Death often results from cardiac complications, cerebrovascular accidents, or infection.[59]

*Cushing's syndrome*   From 70% to 80% of all cases of Cushing's syndrome result from the sustained hypersecretion of ACTH by a pituitary adenoma.[54,61] Cushing's syndrome is characterized by several signs. Greater than 90% of affected individuals have the characteristic moon face, and 80%–90% have truncal obesity, hypertension, impaired glucose tolerance, and hypogonadism (menstrual irregularities, loss of libido).[62] Other common symptoms include hirsutism (in women), congestive heart failure, purple striae, muscular weakness, pedal edema, skeletal pain, and psychological changes.[52,54] Figure 37-3 demonstrates the physical appearance in severe Cushing's syndrome. Less commonly patients experience easy bruising, infection, poor wound healing, osteoporosis and fractures, polyuria with polydipsia, and renal calculi. The onset of symptoms is often subtle, and there is usually a long lag time between onset of symptoms and the diagnosis of Cushing's syndrome. It is not unusual for patients to be treated for individual symptoms, such as obesity, menstrual irregularities, or depression, before the constellation of symptoms is noted.[62] Even if caused by a benign adenoma, Cushing's syndrome is a severe disease. As many as 50% of patients will die within five years from cardiovascular disease, infection, or suicide secondary to severe depression if treatment is not instituted.

### Mass effects

Many critical structures surround the sella turcica, and if the tumor enlarges beyond the sella, mass effects occur.[54] Extension into the optic chiasm is most common. This leads to compression of the optic nerve and bilateral visual field loss, most often beginning with the superior temporal quadrants. If cranial nerves III, IV, and VI are compressed by lateral tumor extension, abnormalities in extraocular muscle function occur. Tumor extension superiorly through the diaphragma sellae may cause compression of the hypothalamus or pituitary stalk. Secretion of posterior pituitary hormones may be altered, resulting in increased appetite, diabetes insipidus, or other changes in anterior pituitary hormone secretion.

Compression of the pituitary stalk leads to altered anterior pituitary control and sequential loss of hormone secretion, which begins with growth hormone or the gonadotropins, luteinizing hormone, and follicle-stimulating hormone, followed by depressions of TSH and corticotropin.[52,54] The end result is hormone insufficiency.

Enlargement beyond the sella may also cause generalized signs of increased intracranial pressure, headache, seizures, or cerebrospinal fluid (CSF) rhinorrhea. A rare cause of hypofunction is pituitary apoplexy, in which hemorrhage into a large tumor causes infarction. Signs and symptoms may include sudden decline of pituitary function, headache, vomiting, changes in visual fields and in visual acuity, and altered level of consciousness.[63] Prompt surgical decompression may reverse neurological problems and restore partial pituitary function.

## Assessment

Diagnosis of pituitary tumors includes the history and physical examination, endocrinologic testing, radiological findings, and histopathologic examination. The history focuses on questions regarding subtle changes that have occurred over a long period of time, as most pituitary tumors are slowly progressive.[56] Many drugs and physical conditions, which are included in Table 37-4, can elevate serum prolactin, although elevations from drugs or physiological factors are not as great as those induced by tumors.[64–66] Physical examination includes testing of peripheral visual fields and cranial nerve function.

Diagnostic procedures for all patients with suspected pituitary tumor focus on the most frequent tumors and may include evaluation of gonadal, thyroid, and adrenal functioning. Gonadal tests for women include evaluating luteinizing hormone, follicle-stimulating hormone, and plasma estradiol. Plasma testosterone is evaluated in men. Thyroid function tests include $T_3$, $T_4$, and TSH. Basal plasma or urinary steroids are sampled to evaluate adrenal functioning. More specific tests for stimulation and suppression of pituitary hormones are done in some cases to detect tumors and to evaluate response to therapy.[52,54,59,67,68] These are outlined in Table 37-5.

Radiological tests may confirm abnormalities in and about the pituitary. Plain radiographs of the head can show only gross enlargement of the sella turcica. Magnetic resonance imaging (MRI) and/or CT more clearly demonstrate in three dimensions the tumor size and extension preoperatively and after surgery.[69] Some tumors, such as those that cause Cushing's disease, may be so small as to elude detection.[70] In the future, positron emission tomography (PET) may also be used to evaluate pituitary tumors.

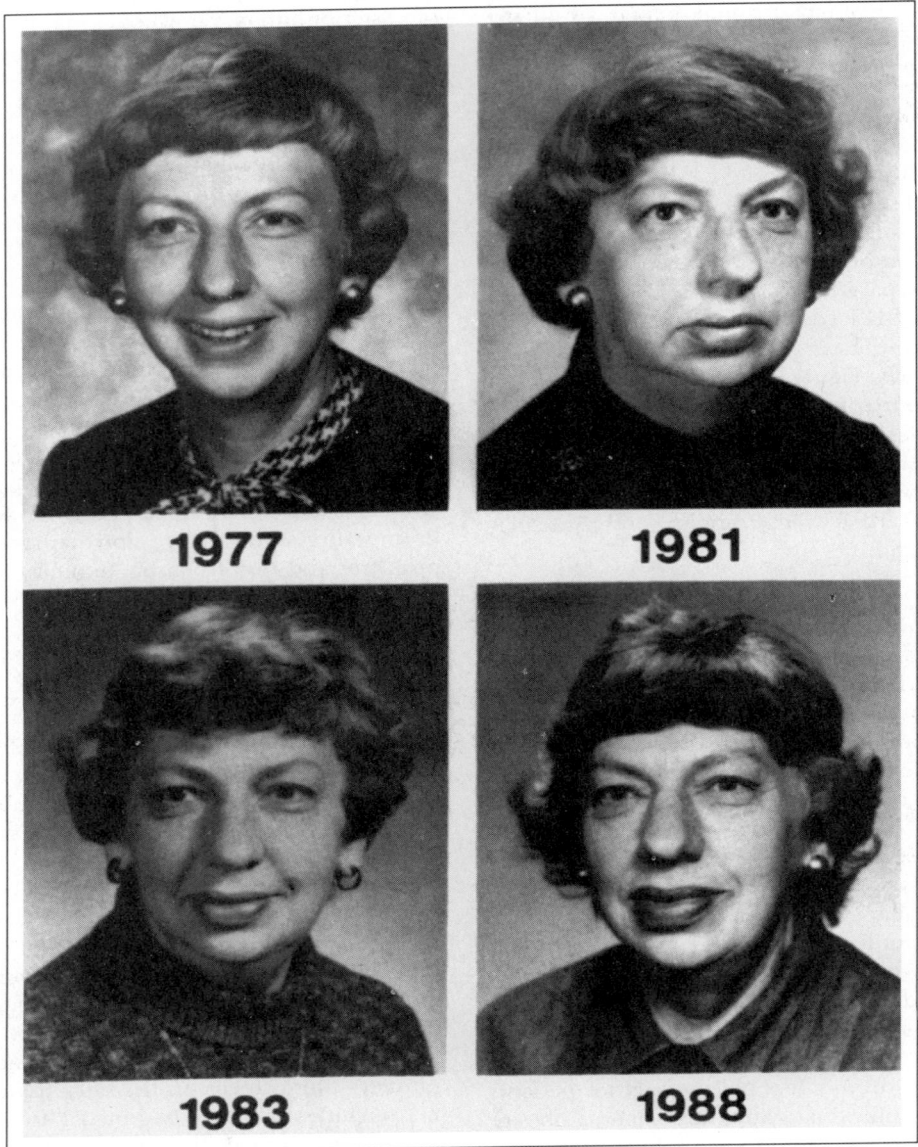

**FIGURE 37-2**   A 64-year-old woman with acromegaly. Photographs reveal gradual changes over 11 years. At the time she presented to a physician, she also had hypertension, arthropathy, and enlargement of her hands. (Reprinted with permission from Molitch ME: Clinical manifestations of acromegaly. *Endocrinol Metab Clin North Am* 21:597–614, 1992.)

## Classification and Staging

In addition to classification by the hormone that is secreted, pituitary adenomas are classified according to their secretory ability, size, and invasiveness. Most tumors are functioning, that is, they secrete a given hormone and cause the corresponding clinical syndrome. Other tumors do not secrete an excessive amount of hormone, or else secrete biological inactive molecules or hormone precursors, and are thus considered to be nonfunctioning.[54] The most common tumors are prolactinomas, which are diagnosed in 40% of cases. Nonfunctioning

tumors constitute 30% of pituitary tumors, while GH-secreting tumors (acromegaly) occur in 20% and ACTH-secreting (Cushing's syndrome) in 10% of patients; 10% of tumors secrete more than one hormone.[65]

Microadenomas are tumors that are less than 10 mm in diameter, while macroadenomas are greater than 10 mm. The signs and symptoms induced often predict whether a tumor will be diagnosed when it is smaller or larger. For instance, women of childbearing age are more likely to report symptoms of prolactinoma, while men may attribute decreased libido to normal aging. Thus women are more likely to have a microadenoma, while macroadeno-

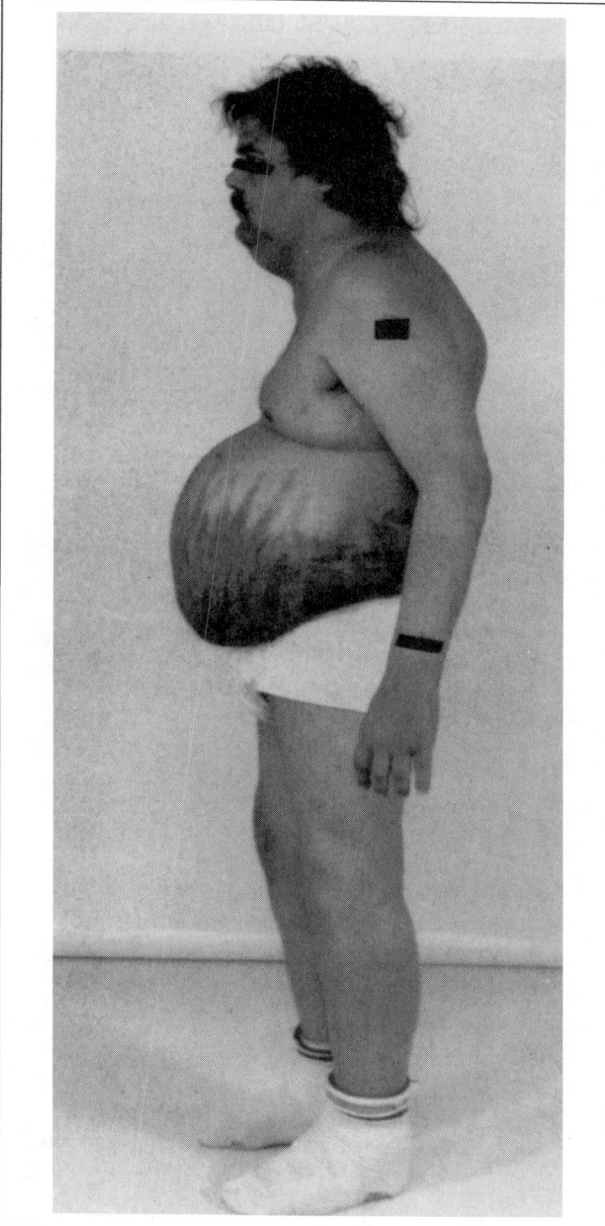

**FIGURE 37-3**  Side view of a patient with Cushing's syndrome. Note protuberant abdomen, marked abdominal striae, and buffalo hump. (Reprinted with permission from Gumowski J, Proch M, Kessler CA: Endocrinopathies of hyperfunction: Cushing's syndrome and aldosteronism. *AACN Clin Issues Crit Care Nurs* 3:331–347, 1992.)

mas are diagnosed more often in men. ACTH-secreting tumors tend to be diagnosed while they are microadenomas, while 70% of GH-secreting tumors are macroadenomas. Tumors are also characterized as intrasellar and extrasellar, depending on their ability to expand outside the sella turcica, and as noninvasive or invasive, depending on whether they can infiltrate into the dural and osseous walls.[53]

**TABLE 37-4**  Other Causes of Elevated Serum Prolactin

| DRUGS |
| --- |
| Dopamine antagonists: metoclopramide, phenothiazines (i.e., prochlorperazine, thiethylperazine, chlorpromazine), butyrophenones (i.e., haloperidol) |
| Reserpine |
| α-methyldopa, carbidopa, benserazide |
| Estrogens |
| Opioids (i.e., codeine, morphine) |
| Cimetidine |
| Tricyclic antidepressants |
| Verapamil |
| Amphetamines |

| PHYSICAL AND OTHER CAUSES |
| --- |
| Chronic renal failure |
| Cirrhosis |
| Hypothyroidism |
| Trauma or surgery involving the pituitary stalk |
| Nursing or stress to the chest wall |
| Exercise |

Data from Delitala 1992;[64] Chong and Newton 1993;[65] Sarapura 1995.[66]

## Therapeutic Approaches and Nursing Care

Surgery, radiation therapy, and drug therapy may be used singly or in combination to treat symptomatic pituitary tumors. Treatment decisions are based on the necessity for immediate relief of mass effect or endocrinologic abnormalities, the potential that the therapy will lead to long-term control, and the adverse effects induced by the therapy. If the tumor is small and is not producing excess hormone, the physician may choose to monitor the patient with MRI or CT scans at yearly intervals.[56] The optimal treatment goal is total tumor removal and rapid normalization of hormone levels, without secondary pituitary insufficiency.[54]

### Surgery

Surgery is the treatment of choice for almost all tumors except prolactinomas.[53] Surgery is done to remove or debulk large tumors that are compressing vital structures about the sella (optic chiasm or cranial nerves),[56] as well as to confirm the histological diagnosis. In other instances surgery will be done to evacuate a cyst about the tumor, decompress a hemorrhagic tumor, or reduce obstructive hydrocephalus.[54] The transsphenoidal route is most often used because it is most likely to allow for tumor removal and preservation of pituitary function. In this procedure the surgical incision is made behind the upper lip, and the maxillary sinus and nasal septum are displaced. The neurosurgeon then opens the sella and microsurgically resects the tumor (Figure 37-4).[71] The surgeon then packs the sella with adipose tissue harvested from the abdomen or other body site in order to decrease

**TABLE 37-5**   Laboratory Tests for Pituitary Tumors

| Diagnostic Test/Tumor | Normal Values | Test Procedure | Comments |
|---|---|---|---|
| Glucose tolerance test/ GH-secreting (acromegaly) | • Growth hormone = 2–6 ng/ml (in A.M. after 8 hr of sleep)<br>• GH suppressed to < 2 ng/ml after glucose tolerance test | • Fasting test (do in A.M.)<br>• Administer 75–100 g of oral glucose (lemon juice may increase palatability)<br>• Blood samples collected 1, 2, and 3 hr later | • In normal individuals GH causes increased blood glucose, which increases resistance to insulin; hypoglycemia leads to GH release and hyperglycemia to GH suppression<br>• Acromegaly: GH not suppressed to <0.5 $\mu$g within 20–120 min<br>• 60% of individuals with acromegaly have a paradoxical increase of GH |
| Urinary excretion of GH/ GH-secreting (acromegaly) | | • 24-hr urine collection<br>• Store collection bottle in refrigerator to decrease bacterial growth | • Increased in some patients with acromegaly |
| Plasma insulin-like growth factor 1/GH-secreting (acromegaly) | • Normal values vary in males and females; children, adolescents, and adults | • Blood sample | • Normal values, males: preadolescent 60.8–724 ng/ml, adolescent 112.5–450 ng/ml, adult 141.8–389.3 ng/ml females: preadolescent 65.5–841 ng/ml, adolescent 83.3–378.5 ng/ml, adult 54.0–328.5 ng/ml |
| Dexamethasone suppression test/ACTH-secreting (Cushing's syndrome) | • Serum cortisol suppressed to <5 $\mu$/dl<br>• Fasting, 8 A.M.–noon, 5–25 $\mu$/dl | • Administer 1 mg po dexamethasone at 11 P.M.<br>• Draw plasma cortisol at 9 A.M. the following day | • In normal individuals increased corticosteroid suppresses ACTH release and subsequently cortisol production<br>• To confirm results, test may be repeated for 3 days while administering larger doses of dexamethasone<br>• Sensitive test, but not specific for tumors only |
| Urinary free cortisol/ ACTH-secreting tumor | • 20–70 $\mu$/24 hr<br>• 25–95 ng/mg of creatinine | • Give dexamethasone 0.5 mg Q 6 hr for 2 days<br>• Then collect 24-hr urine sample (refrigerate) | • More specific than dexamethasone suppression test<br>• Single best screening test for ACTH-secreting tumor<br>• Spironolactone and quinacrine may affect accuracy |
| Plasma prolactin/ prolactinoma | • Women (nonlactating): 0.48–0.9 IU/liter or 0–15 ng/ml<br>• Pregnancy 1st trimester: <80 ng/ml 2nd trimester: <160 ng/ml 3rd trimester: <400 ng/ml<br>• Values increase during lactation<br>• Men: 0–15 ng/ml | | • Values <1 U/liter are rarely clinically significant<br>• Values <2.5 U/liter usually indicate nonfunctioning tumor<br>• Values >6 U/liter usually indicate a macroprolactinoma<br>• Tests repeated because of normal variations in serum prolactin levels |

Data from Croughs 1992;[54] Lamberts 1992;[60] Samuels 1995;[67] Corbett 1996.[68]

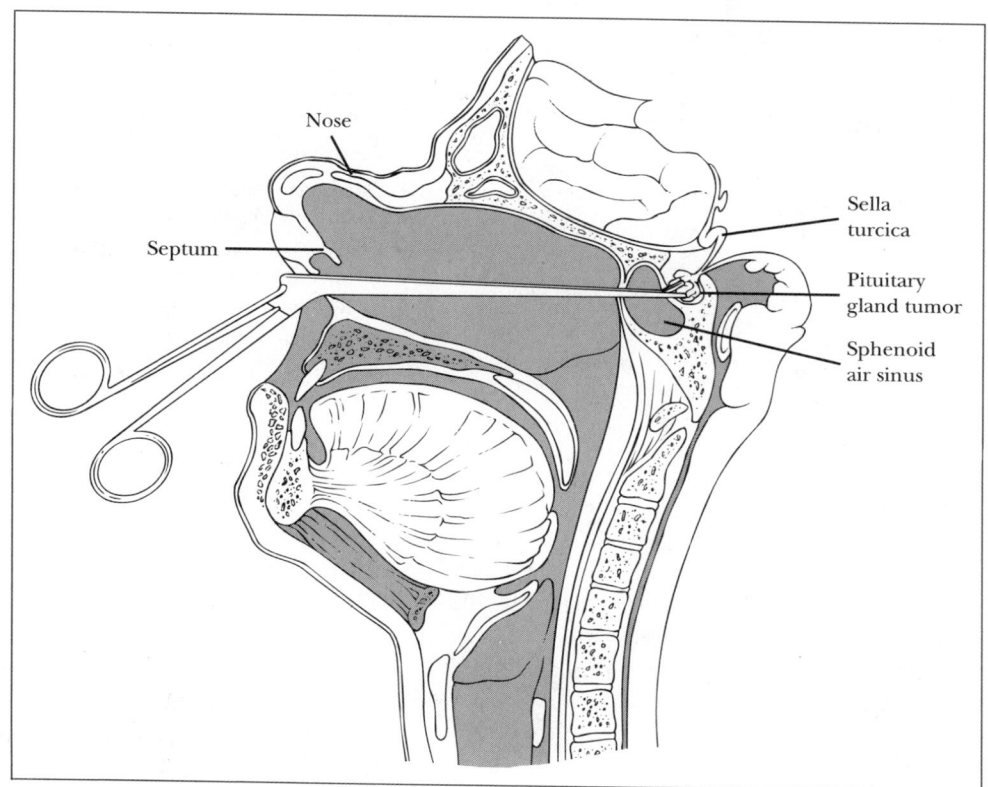

**FIGURE 37-4**   Transsphenoidal surgical resection of a pituitary tumor. The upper lip is retracted and an incision is made in the gingival mucosa. After displacing the septal cartilage, the surgeon removes the anterior wall of the sphenoid sinus and the floor of the sella turcica. The pituitary tumor is removed using the microsurgery technique in an attempt to preserve normal pituitary structure and function.

the risk of CSF leak. The septum and maxillary sinus are then reapproximated and the nares packed.

### Radiation therapy

External-beam radiation is used for patients who refuse surgery or those who cannot tolerate surgery, and also in some cases of subtotal resection.[54,69] Treatment fields are designed to treat the tumor while minimizing the dose to adjacent structures. Usual total doses are 5000 cGy. Lower doses may not control the tumor, and higher total doses or fractions greater than 200 cGy per day cause more complications (e.g., injury to the optic nerves/chiasm and hypopituitarism). Disadvantages of radiation include the possibility that the therapeutic effect may be too slow for patients whose tumors secrete excessive hormone and the tendency, in rare instances, for radiation to induce second CNS malignancies.[54] Furthermore, 38% of patients develop long-term complications such as pituitary dysfunction or, less often, visual deterioration.[69]

### Drug therapy

Antineoplastic chemotherapy is not used for pituitary tumors. Other drugs are indicated as first-line therapy

for microadenomas or macroadenomas before surgery or radiation in some instances, and following therapy in others. Dopamine agonists and octreotide are used to treat hormone oversecretion (Table 37-6). Dopamine agonists, such as bromocriptine, are the usual primary treatment for prolactinomas because they rapidly reduce elevated serum prolactin levels in most patients.[54,72,73] Estrogen replacement or oral contraceptives may be used to restore ovulation and menses in women with microprolactinomas.[74] Estrogen has the advantages of being less expensive than bromocriptine and preventing bone loss, which bromocriptine does not.

Octreotide is a parenteral agent that effectively reduces GH secretion in patients with acromegaly.[59,72,73] It may be used before surgery to reduce the size of the tumor and make complete resection more likely, as well as to strengthen diminished cardiac functioning.[75] Either dopamine agonists or octreotide may be helpful for gonadotropin-secreting pituitary tumors.[54]

### Nursing care

Nursing care for patients with pituitary tumors centers on the diagnostic, postsurgical, and follow-up phases. During the diagnostic phase, the nurse explains the pur-

**TABLE 37-6**   Drug Therapy of Pituitary Adenomas

| Drug | Indication | Adverse Effects | Comments |
|---|---|---|---|
| Bromocriptine | Prolactinoma GH-secreting tumor (acromegaly) May be helpful for gonadotropin-secreting tumor | • Dizziness<br>• Headache<br>• Nausea and vomiting<br>• Orthostatic hypotension<br>• Nasal congestion<br>• Constipation<br>• Peripheral vasoconstriction<br>• Psychiatric reactions | • First-line treatment for prolactinoma<br>• Normalizes plasma prolactin levels in 90% of patients<br>• Headache, nausea, and orthostatic hypotension are most frequent and limit use in 10%–20% of patients<br>• Menses resume within 2 months; use barrier birth control until then; birth control pills may be used after periods resume<br>• Resistance occurs in about 10%<br>• Side effects are less if doses are escalated gradually and taken with food<br>• 5% continue to have side effects<br>• May decrease GH secretion and acromegaly, improve glucose tolerance in acromegalic patients<br>• Long-acting depot |
| Pergolide mesylate | Prolactinoma GH-secreting tumor | • Suppression of GI motility and secretion<br>• Flatulence<br>• Abdominal discomfort | • Parolel LAR (long acting repeatable) injection available; administered once a month |
| Octreotide | GH-secreting tumor (acromegaly) May be helpful for gonadotropin-secreting | | • Used similarly to bromocriptine<br>• Parenteral drug administered 3 times per day<br>• 100 µg is usual dose, but optimal dose is variable and doses may be as high as 500 µg<br>• Injections may be painful<br>• Used before surgery to shrink macroadenomas, then after surgery if elevated serum GH persists<br>• 40%–50% of patients develop gallstones with long-term treatment, managed with drug-free interval or ureodeoxycholic acid (allows normal contraction of gallbladder) |

Data from Croughs 1992;[54] Lamberts 1992.[60]

poses and procedures of the tests and reinforces the explanation with written materials. Immediately after surgery, the patient will be cared for on a neurosurgical or surgical intensive care unit. Postoperative complications, which are usually transient but may be long-lasting, include diabetes insipidus (DI), CSF leak, meningitis, damage to cranial nerves III, IV, V, and VI, optic nerve or optic chiasm damage, and sinusitis.[71,76,77] Damage to cranial nerves, optic nerves, or the optic chiasm may lead to complete or partial visual loss or visual field defects. Sinusitis can occur from the intranasal trauma or if the nasal packing is left in too long, so the nasal packing is removed within 24–48 hours unless the patient has epistaxis.

Surgical trauma may cause transient swelling of the pituitary and pressure on the pituitary stalk or posterior pituitary. This causes temporary DI followed by water intoxication, dehydration, and hypernatremia. The nurse must thus closely monitor the patient's fluid and electrolyte status. Mild DI is usually managed with isotonic intravenous fluids, and vasopressin is administered in more severe cases.[58] The usual dose of vasopressin is 5 units subcutaneously every four to six hours until urine volume becomes normal. If the patient develops hyponatremia, fluid restriction is instituted until DI resolves, usually within ten days. Desmopression (DDAVP), 0.1 ml intranasally, is administered once or twice a week in patients in whom DI persists. Teaching includes the symptoms of DI, how to administer DDAVP, and the symptoms of DDAVP overdosage. CSF leak presents as persistent postnasal drip, so the nurse teaches the patient to report a dripping sensation in the back of the throat. If CSF leak is confirmed, the patient is treated by elevating the head of the bed and maintaining bedrest to decrease pressure.

Patients having transsphenoidal surgery may be discharged from the hospital within three to four days. Clearly written discharge instructions must include information about diet, activities, analgesics, antibiotics, hydrocortisone, and any other medications. The patient is instructed to notify the surgeon for any fever over 101 °F, any symptoms of meningitis (e.g., headache, stiff neck), CSF leak (clear drainage from the nose), infection at the surgical site, and hormone insufficiency (e.g., hypothyroidism, cortisone deficiency, and GH deficiency).[77,78] The nurse also reinforces the importance of physician follow-up after the postsurgical period. Patients must be carefully monitored at regular intervals because complications of therapy, especially hypopituitarism and tumor recurrence, can occur as late as 30 years after treatment.

There is little scientifically based knowledge of patients' responses to the diagnosis and treatment of a pituitary tumor. Gotch[79] surveyed patients with Cushing's disease and found they experienced great distress from unexplained fatigue, depression, changes in appearance, and decreased ability to work. Similar findings would probably be found in patients with acromegaly, and other changes in persons with different pituitary tumors. Specific suggestions for nurses to help patients cope included helping them find support, offering specific suggestions for energy conservation, and offering suggestions that would increase bone density and prevent fractures.

# ADRENAL TUMORS

The adrenal glands, paired organs that lie atop each kidney, consist of a cortex and a medulla. Both the cortex and the medulla are critical in maintaining homeostasis in the face of multiple internal and external stressors. The medulla acts rapidly and secretes catecholamines within seconds of a stressful incident. When the stressor is eliminated, the catecholamine effects disappear rapidly and catecholamines return via a re-uptake mechanism to sympathetic nerve endings. The cortex, on the other hand, releases its hormones more slowly, and the actions of the hormones are long-lived. In essence, the medulla and the cortex act in concert, as the medulla rapidly responds to changes in the environment and the cortex amplifies and sustains the response.

The functional cells of the adrenal medulla are chromaffin cells, which are modified postganglionic neurons. The medulla is part of the sympathetic nervous system (SNS), which is responsible for the "fight or flight" reaction to stress. The adrenal medulla synthesizes catecholamines, particularly epinephrine and norepinephrine (ratio about 5:1) from dopamine. Catecholamines have both positive and inhibitory effects on almost all body tissues.[80]

Adrenocortical tumors arise from the cortex, and pheochromocytomas arise from the medulla. Both types of tumors are most often benign, but both benign and malignant tumors can alter quality of life and may be life-threatening. Because they occur in essentially different organs, the tumors will be discussed separately.

# ADRENOCORTICAL TUMORS

A functioning adrenal cortex, which makes up about 90% of the adrenal gland, is essential to life. The cortex synthesizes several corticosteroids in response to signals from the pituitary gland or other systems. The most important of these are the glucocorticoid cortisol (also known as hydrocortisone) and the mineralocorticoid aldosterone, as well as small amounts of androgens (including testosterone) and estradiol.

Corticosteroids play critical roles in many body processes, including glucose, protein and lipid metabolism, wound healing, myocardial contractility, and arteriolar tone. Corticosteroids oppose the inflammatory response by reducing the formation of inflammatory mediators (prostaglandins, leukotrienes, histamine, etc.). They cause an overall general immunosuppression and specifically inhibit interleukins 1 and 2 (IL-1 and IL-2), and may inhibit the synthesis of antibodies and B lymphocytes.[80,81]

Mineralocorticoids are critical to maintaining normal serum sodium balance and, to a lesser degree, potassium balance. The primary stimulus for the synthesis of aldosterone is fluid loss, but the pituitary plays a small role as well. Aldosterone induces the kidney to reabsorb sodium and, in turn, water.[80]

## Epidemiology

Adrenocortical tumors are extremely rare. The risk of cortical carcinomas is 0.5–2 per million,[82] and these tumors constitute only 0.05% of all neoplasms.[83] Overall, adrenocortical tumors occur most frequently in children under 10 years of age, and in adults in their 50s. Women are more likely to have a hypersecreting tumor, whereas men more often have nonfunctioning tumors.[82] Cushing's disease usually occurs between the ages of 20 and 60.[62]

## Etiology

There are no known risk factors for adrenal tumors. Pathogenesis is thought to be a multistep process in which initiation of a single cell occurs as a random mutation, or from chronic stimulation of the adrenal cortex by pituitary hormones. The evidence that supports this thesis is that DNA from adrenal neoplasms demonstrates single-cell transformation, that is, tumors are monoclonal.[84] Furthermore, mutations in tumor-suppressor and growth factor genes on chromosome 11 have been documented. Deletions of alleles at the 15 locus, a dominant suppressor gene, are associated with overexpression of an insulin-like growth factor and are often seen in malignant tumors but rarely in adenomas.[83,85] Similarly, mutations of the *p53* suppressor gene have been documented in adults and children with adrenocortical carcinomas.[86,87]

## Pathophysiology

Tumors of the cortex are characterized as functional or nonfunctional. Functional tumors are further characterized by the hormone(s) they produce in excess. Fifty percent of tumors hypersecrete cortisol (Cushing's syndrome), 25% secrete estradiol or testosterone and cause feminizing or masculinizing effects, respectively, and only rare tumors secrete aldosterone (Conn's syndrome).[88] Approximately 20%–25% of Cushing's syndrome results from benign or malignant adrenocortical tumors. Nonfunctional tumors do not produce cortical hormones and are called *incidentalomas*. These are usually discovered on radiological scans done for other reasons or at autopsy.

Adrenal tumors do not produce hormones as efficiently as normal adrenal glands, so tumors usually become large before they cause clinical symptoms and are detected.[88] The pathologist often has difficulty in differentiating whether a tumor is benign or malignant. As a rule, very large tumors are malignant, and malignant tumors have a greater number of mitotic figures than do benign tumors. The number of mitoses observed also correlates with prognosis, so a greater number is associated with a shorter life span.

## Clinical Manifestations

The signs and symptoms of adrenocortical tumors vary depending upon the hormone or hormones secreted. Cushing's syndrome induced by adrenal tumors causes similar symptoms to those induced by pituitary tumors (see previous discussion of pituitary tumors). Patients with aldosterone hypersecreting tumors will present with hypertension, hypokalemia, hypernatremia, and suppressed renin activity.[61] Hypokalemia may cause the most serious effects, such as cardiac arrythmias, abnormal changes on electrocardiogram (ECG), digitalis toxicity, weakness, polydipsia, and visual disturbances.

Women are likely to have virilizing tumors and have symptoms reflecting hypersecretion of androgen. Progressive hirsutism (increased hair on the face, trunk, and limbs) is the most frequent symptom. Acne, clitoral hypertrophy, menstrual abnormalities, deepening of the voice, frontal baldness, and increased libido may also occur.[89,90] Tumors that hypersecrete estradiol are the rarest adrenal tumors and generally occur in young to middle-aged men, who experience diminished libido, testicular atrophy, and gynecomastia.[91] Sex hormone–secreting tumors in children are manifested by precocious puberty.

## Assessment

Diagnosis of adrenal tumors is often protracted and delayed because symptoms are usually nonspecific and slowly progressive. In addition, adrenal tumors are so rare that they are not likely to be high on an initial list of differential diagnoses. Diagnosis is confirmed by correlating physical findings with laboratory values and localization procedures. Laboratory tests focus on abnormally high adrenocortical hormones in the blood and high amounts of their metabolites in the urine. Urinary excretion tests are frequently done because hormone metabolites are excreted in the urine; these noninvasive tests are highly sensitive. No test is 100% sensitive, so two or more tests are necessary. Tests are summarized in Table 37-7.[88,90,92] Localization or imaging examination of the adrenal cortex may include CT or MRI.

## Classification and Staging

It is often difficult to determine whether an adrenal tumor is benign or malignant at initial diagnosis. While small tumors are more likely to be benign and large masses malignant, there is considerable overlap, and size alone is not a reliable indicator of pathology.[83] Malignant tumors are more likely to have a high mitotic rate, atypical and hyperchromatic nuclei, and greater tumor necrosis than benign tumors. In addition, malignant tumors may grow more rapidly and may cause abdominal pain, fever, and weight loss.[88] The most reliable indicator of malignant disease is the presence of local recurrences or metastases to lung, liver, or peritoneum, and rarely brain and lung.

Cortical tumors have been staged using the TNM system. Stage I and stage II tumors are localized, with the tumor being up to 5 cm and greater than 5 cm, respectively. Stage III and IV are considered advanced disease and include positive regional lymph nodes and metastatic disease, respectively. Overall prognosis of adrenocortical carcinomas is poor. Median survival is 4–30 months, and fewer than 25% of patients survive for five years.[93]

## Therapeutic Approaches and Nursing Care

### Surgery

Whenever possible, surgical removal of local and metastatic disease is recommended because surgery offers the only chance for cure of malignant adrenal tumors. Cure is likely only with stage I or II tumors. Unfortunately, at diagnosis only 2% of tumors are stage I, while approximately 80% are stage III or IV.[88] Radiation is reserved for palliative treatment of metastatic disease, such as bone metastases.

### Chemotherapy

Chemotherapy is given in some instances of cortical tumors. Mitotane, an analogue of the insecticide DDD that can cause adrenal necrosis, is the usual first-line agent.[37] Response rates to mitotane are generally about 35%, but responses are rarely prolonged or complete, and survival does not increase.[82,94] Some investigators have suggested that higher doses of mitotane would be more effective, but most patients do not tolerate such doses. Gastrointestinal and neuromuscular toxicities are considerable and unacceptable. Significant nausea and vomiting, diarrhea, an-

**TABLE 37-7**  Laboratory Values of Adrenal Tumors

| Tumor/Syndrome | Test | Implications/Comments |
|---|---|---|
| Cushing's disease | • Dexamethasone suppression test (see Table 37-4) | • Tumor-induced cortisol or metabolites will not be suppressed by feedback mechanisms |
| | • 24-hr urine for free cortisol | • Plasma cortisol will be elevated the morning after administration to >80–100 μg |
| | • 2-day, high-dose dexamethasone suppression test | • Metabolites of adrenocortical steroids, 17 ketosteroids, are not suppressed |
| | | • Normal values vary with gender and age |
| | • Plasma ACTH immunoassay | • Suppressed to less than normal because of negative feedback loop (increased adrenocortisol leads to decreased ACTH release by pituitary) |
| | | • Normal 6–76 ng/ml |
| Virilizing | • Basal serum testosterone | • Elevated; nonsuppressible with dexamethasone administration (usually suppresses adrenocortical hormone production) |
| | | • Normal: women = 20–90 ng/dl, men = 250–1000 ng/dl |
| Conn's syndrome (aldosterone-secreting) | • Plasma aldosterone | • Elevated with tumor or hyperplasia, which increase production |
| | | • Normal: 7 A.M. supine <16 ng/ml, 9 A.M. upright 4–316 ng/ml |
| | • Urinary aldosterone | • Elevated: >20 μg in 24 hr |
| | • Plasma renin activity | • Suppressed because increased plasma aldosterone has not been induced by low extracellular fluid volume induction of renin/angiotensin system |
| | | • Normal: supine 0.5–1.6 ng/ml, upright 1.9–3.6 ng/ml |
| Pheochromocytoma | • Plasma catecholamines (dopamine, epinephrine, norepinephrine) | • Elevated by tumor production |
| | | • Antihypertensives and antidepressants may invalidate test; confirm drug history |
| | • 24-hr urine for metanephrines | • Metabolites of catecholamines, elevated to 1.5–2 times greater than normal |
| | | • Normal: 0.0–0.9 μ/24 hr |
| | • 24-hr urine for normetanephrines | • Elevated to 1.5–2 times greater than normal |
| | | • HCl is added to urine specimen bottle to maintain pH ≤3 |
| | | • BP, height, and weight are recorded on laboratory requisition |
| | | • Patient must be instructed to collect entire 24-hr collection, or results may be false-negative |

Data from Corbett 1996;[68] Findling 1992;[70] Müller 1990;[90] Brennan and Pommier 1991;[88] Derksen et al 1994;[92] Werbel and Öber 1995;[97] Gerlo and Sevens 1994;[101] Lenders et al 1995.[102]

orexia, lethargy, somnolence, and depression progressing to suicidal ideation have been reported.[88,94] Patients may also experience prolonged bleeding times.[93]

There are a few anecdotal reports of combination chemotherapy of mitotane plus other agents including cisplatin, doxorubicin, cyclophosphamide, etoposide, and 5-FU,[93,95] and one prospective trial of mitotane plus cisplatin.[96] Results are similar to those of single-agent mitotane, that is, about 30% of patients respond and median survival is less than 12 months. Side effects are more numerous and severe with combination chemotherapy.

## Symptom management and supportive care

Because of delays in diagnosis, many patients with adrenal tumors have progressive disease that does not respond to treatment. Palliative treatment for these persons includes medications to reduce symptoms produced by hormone excess. Thus drugs for Cushing's syndrome may be ketoconazole, aminoglutethimide, or metyrapone, which block the synthesis of corticosteroids.

# PHEOCHROMOCYTOMA

## Epidemiology

Pheochromocytomas are tumors that arise from chromaffin cells. From 85% to 95% arise from the adrenal medulla, but these tumors may also arise from other sympathetic nervous system cells.[97] Approximately 90% of tumors occur sporadically, and the others occur as part of the MEN syndrome. About 90% of pheochromocytomas in adults are benign, whereas children often have malignant tumors.[98] The incidence of pheochromocytomas is unknown. Males and females are at equal risk to develop pheochromocytomas, which are diagnosed at any age.[97]

## Etiology

Almost nothing is known about the etiology of pheochromocytomas. It is known that hyperplasia precedes tumor development. It is hypothesized that some genetic defect in neural crest cells occurs, and this ultimately results in a pheochromocytoma.[88]

## Pathophysiology

Both benign and malignant pheochromocytomas hypersecrete catecholamines, predominantly norepinephrine, or less often epinephrine. This is the inverse of normal adrenal secretion.[99] The diagnosis of a tumor as benign or malignant cannot be made by histological appearance or size but depends on the absence or presence of metastases. Poor prognosis is predicted by tetraploid or aneuploid DNA, large tumor size, or local tumor extension. Malignant tumors may metastasize to lymph nodes, bone, lung, liver, brain, and omentum.[97]

## Clinical Manifestations

Hypertension is the hallmark of pheochromocytoma, and may occur in the classic triad including pounding headache and profuse perspiring.[97,98] Hypertension occurs in one of three patterns: indistinguishable from essential hypertension, normal blood pressure with superimposed paroxysmal hypertension, or sustained hypertension with extreme paroxysms.[88] Up to two-thirds of patients experience significant postural hypertension.[97] Patients describe the paroxysms as "attacks."[100] They may be brought on by many factors, including exercise, passing urine or stool, intercourse, pain, and pressure on or palpation of the abdomen. Surgery and chemotherapy can also cause extreme hypertension. Anticholinergic drugs may cause perilous tachycardias, and several drugs, including dopamine antagonists (metoclopramide and phenothiazines), tricyclic antidepressants, and naloxone, may precipitate extreme hypertension.[88,98]

Catecholamine effects occur in all organ systems, and tumors that produce large amounts of epinephrine cause many symptoms. These may include headache, tachycardia, palpitations, sweating, tremulousness, anxiety, nausea and vomiting, and pain. Patients may experience several mental status changes, such as acute anxiety and altered thought processes (personality changes, emotional lability, and frank psychosis).[98] Excessive smooth muscle effects are manifested as constipation. Cardiovascular complications are common and include myocarditis, congestive heart failure, symptoms similar to myocardial infarction, and cardiovascular accidents.[88] The most severe complication is pheochromocytoma crisis, which leads to encephalopathy that may progress to coma, shock, and multiple organ system failure, including renal and hepatic failure, disseminated intravascular clotting, seizures, and possibly death.[97,98]

## Assessment

The diagnosis of pheochromocytoma is often delayed because hypertension is much more likely to have other causes. For instance, only 0.1%–0.2% of all cases of hypertension are due to pheochromocytoma.[87] Diagnosis is confirmed by correlating physical findings with laboratory values and localization procedures. Urinary excretion tests for the catecholamine metabolites metanephrine and normetanephrine are the most sensitive in detecting pheochromocytomas (Table 37-7).[70,88,101,102]

CT, MRI, and nuclear scans may be useful to localize cortical tumors. Nuclear scan after injection of iodine[131] meta-iodobenzylguanidine (MIBG) is used for localized or metastatic pheochromocytomas. MIBG is taken up by catecholamine storage vessels in normal and tumor cells, and can localize highly active tumor cells.[97] Patients are pretreated with a saturated solution of potassium iodide (SSKI) to prevent uptake of the $^{131}I$ by the thyroid.

## Classification and Staging

As mentioned earlier, most pheochromocytomas are benign in adults. However, they also cause the same problems as malignant pheochromocytoma. As with cortical tumors, metastasis is the most reliable indicator of malignancy. The five-year survival for medullary tumors is 44%.[88] Most patients with benign or malignant tumors die from complications related to excessive catecholamine effects on normal systems, such as cardiovascular disease, hypertension, cerebrovascular accident, renal disease, or diabetes mellitus.

## Therapeutic Approaches and Nursing Care

### Surgery

The treatment of choice for pheochromocytoma is surgery, as cure is most likely with resectable disease.[88] Radiation therapy is indicated only for palliation of metastatic disease. Surgery or other invasive procedures can precipitate severe and uncontrolled hypertension, and patients require alpha-adrenergic blockade beforehand. Some patients may require beta-adrenergic blockade as well.

### Chemotherapy

Few reports of chemotherapy for pheochromocytoma are found in the literature. Patients may respond to drugs that are effective for other neuroendocrine neoplasms.[97] There are case reports of chemotherapy causing severe hypertension that occurred three to six hours after the administration of cyclophosphamide, vincristine, and dacarbazine.[103] One patient's blood pressure rose to 195/124, and she experienced headache and vomiting. A second patient's blood pressure rose to 280/140, and he also had substernal chest pain and pulmonary edema. The authors suggested that chemotherapy may induce tumor lysis, which rapidly releases catecholamines stored in tumor cells into the bloodstream. Thus they recommend that these patients have adequate alpha-adrenergic blockade before chemotherapy starts, and that patients' hemodynamic status be closely and continuously monitored during the first cycle of therapy.

Treatment to induce alpha-adrenergic blockade is started at least one to two weeks before surgery or chemotherapy. Phenoxybenzamine is usually the drug of choice, and the dose is escalated until the patient's blood pressure is normal and he or she has moderate, asymptomatic postural hypotension without paroxysms.[88] If the patient has persistent tachycardia (pulse > 140 per minute), extrasystoles, or a history of arrhythmias, propranolol may be added only after the alpha-blockade is complete to induce beta-adrenergic blockade. Nursing actions for these patients include teaching them how to take their drugs and monitoring blood pressure. Close monitoring during chemotherapy, as mentioned, is critical. Nifedipine 10-mg tablets are kept at the bedside; these may be administered sublingually or orally to temporarily abort hypertensive crisis.[103]

### Symptom management and supportive care

Metyrosine is useful to decrease catecholmaine synthesis in pheochromocytoma, and is given in combination with phenoxybenzamine and propranolol. Side effects are sedation, fatigue, depression, hallucinations, Parkinson's symptoms, and sleep disturbances.[98]

# MULTIPLE ENDOCRINE NEOPLASIA

Multiple endocrine neoplasia (MEN) includes syndromes in which several endocrine malignancies occur. These are broadly classified as MEN type 1 and type 2. While MEN syndromes may occur sporadically, they most often are familial and are inherited as an autosomal dominant gene. MEN tumors produce the same symptoms as sporadic tumors. However, tumors tend to occur earlier, are multicentric, and are more likely to be bilateral than sporadic endocrine tumors. Characteristics of MEN syndromes are included in Table 37-8.[104]

## Multiple Endocrine Neoplasia Type 1 (MEN 1)

The endocrine tumors that occur with MEN 1 are parathyroid, pituitary, and pancreatic islet cell. It is not possible to predict how these will present, but patients may have one, two, or all three tumors. Parathyroid neoplasms are the most frequent, occurring in 90% of patients at the average age of 19 (mean 12–28 years).[105] Pituitary adenomas are not as clinically important. These tumors, which may be diagnosed when the patient is in his or her 40s, may or may not secrete hormones. Pituitary tumors are often not discovered until autopsy.

On the other hand, 30%–75% of patients who develop pancreatic tumors experience symptoms because their tumors secrete one of several pancreatic peptides. Gastrin, the most frequently secreted peptide, causes hypersecretion of gastric acid (Zollinger-Ellison syndrome).[106] In patients who manifest MEN 1, the mean age at diagnosis of pancreatic tumors is 25. If MEN 1 is not diagnosed early, the majority of patients die in their 60s from gastrointestinal bleeding or metastatic pancreatic cancer.[105,107]

## Multiple Endocrine Neoplasia Type 2 (MEN 2)

Men and women with MEN 2 develop hyperplasia or tumors of the thyroid, parathyroid, and adrenal glands. Three separate forms, or subtypes, may arise: MEN 2A, MEN 2B, and familial medullary thyroid cancer (MTC).

### MEN 2A

The hallmark tumor of MEN 2A is hyperplasia of thyroid C cells that progresses to MTC. Tumors have been detected in patients as young as 10 and as old as 80.[5] About 60% of patients develop clinically evident MTC by the time they are 70 years old.[108] When an individual

**TABLE 37-8** Characteristics of Multiple Endocrine Neoplasia Types 1, 2A, and 2B

| Organ | Tumor | Hormone | Common Presenting Symptom |
|---|---|---|---|
| | | **MEN 1** | |
| Pituitary | Prolactinoma, somatotropinoma | Prolactin, growth hormone | Galactorrhea, acromegaly |
| Pancreas (islet) | Gastrinoma, insulinoma, VIPoma | Gastrin, insulin, VIP | Peptic ulcer, hypoglycemia, diarrhea |
| Parathyroid | Adenoma | Parathyroid hormone | Hypercalcemia, urolithiasis |
| | | **MEN 2A** | |
| Thyroid | Medullary thyroid carcinoma (MTC) | Calcitonin | Diarrhea |
| Adrenal medulla | Pheochromocytoma | Catecholamines | Hypertension, palpitations |
| Parathyroid | Adenoma | Parathormone | Hypercalcemia, urolithiasis |
| | | **MEN 2B** | |
| Thyroid | Medullary thyroid carcinoma | Calcitonin | Diarrhea |
| Adrenal medulla | Pheochromocytoma | Catecholamines | Hypertension, palpitations |
| Parathyroid (rare) | Adenoma | Parathormone | Hypercalcemia, urolithiasis |
| Oral mucosa, conjunctiva, intestinal mucosa | Ganglioneuromas | — | Constipation, diarrhea, vomiting, difficulties in swallowing |

Reprinted with permission from Ponz de Leon M: Multiple endocrine neoplasia (MEN) types 1, 2A, and 2B: Organ involvement, type of tumor, main hormones, and symptoms, in *Familial and Hereditary Tumors*. New York, Springer-Verlag, 1994, pp 68–83.[104]

is identified as a MEN gene carrier, the rate of C-cell hyperplasia and/or MTC rises to 100%.[109] Long-term prognosis depends upon the treatment of MTC.[110] The cure rate is near 100% if elevated calcitonin levels are not accompanied by palpable tumor but decreases to 17% if the tumor is palpable.[8]

Pheochromocytomas occur in 20%–50% of patients with MEN 2A.[108–110] Between 50% and 80% of patients present with bilateral disease, and another 10% require adrenalectomy of the remaining gland within five years.[110,111] Hypertension is the most frequent symptom, as with sporadic pheochromocytoma, and is a major cause of death.

Parathyroid adenomas occur in 10%–20% of persons with MEN 2A. These tumors occur much later in patients with MEN 2A than in those with MEN 1, and are not usually significant. Patients appear to be physically normal.

### MEN 2B

Patients who have MEN 2B may be identified because of their physical appearance (Figure 37-5). From 85% to 95% have a marfanoid appearance and several musculoskeletal abnormalities, including pes cavus, or an abnormally high arch of the foot (persons who have Marfan syndrome have pes planus, or flat feet). Other abnormalities include kyphosis, scoliosis, lordosis, increased joint looseness, proximal muscle weakness, and delayed puberty.[108,112,113] Facial features are characteristic and include enlarged and bumpy lips from ganglioneuromatomas, which exist throughout the entire gastrointestinal tract, from mouth to colon. Patients may have neuromas on other mucosal surfaces, such as the eyelids. MTC occurs much earlier in MEN 2B, on average at age 20.[109]

### Assessment

Ongoing screening is the major focus of management for families known to express MEN. Current recommendations include annual screening for laboratory evidence of hypersecreting tumor. Negative tests do not guarantee that an individual does not have the syndrome. Because tumors occur at varying ages, a negative test indicates only that they do not yet have detectable disease.[112]

Screening for MEN 2 begins in early childhood and focuses on identifying elevated serum calcitonin, which may be a marker for early MTC. Provocative tests for calcitonin, which include the injection of pentagastrin or calcium, are done. Serum calcitonin is measured at baseline and at two to three minutes, and then five to ten minutes, after injection. Reproducible serum calcium elevations above a normal range are an indication to

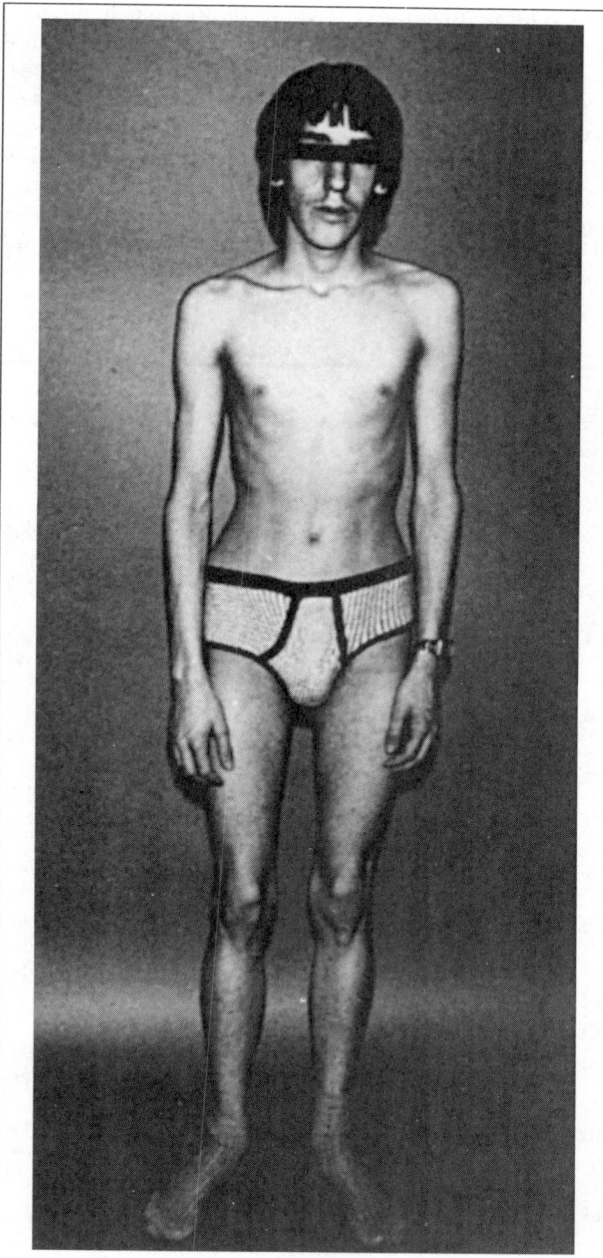

**FIGURE 37-5**  Typical appearance of a patient with MEN 2B, demonstrating marfanoid habitus, thickening of the lips (ganglioneuromatomas), and elongated face. (Reprinted with permission from Frank K, Raue F, Gottswinter J, et al: The importance of early diagnosis and followup in sporadic MEN II. *Eur J Pediatr* 143:112, 1984.)

proceed to total thyroidectomy. Those patients whose calcitonin levels are borderline are retested within three to six months.[109] Problems exist with the calcitonin provocation tests in that both false-negatives and false-positives can occur. A false-negative result may erroneously lull the patient into a sense of security, while a false-positive may result in an unnecessary total thyroidectomy.[114]

## Genetic Basis of MEN 1 and MEN 2

Patients with familial MEN 1 or 2 develop their tumors because they have inherited a mutated gene that codes for a tumor-suppressor gene or proto-oncogene from one of their parents. This autosomal dominant gene is present in the germ line, and thus in all body cells. Afflicted individuals are predisposed to develop adenomas and malignant tumors much earlier and much more frequently because the gene expresses a high, but variable, rate of penetrance and requires only mutation in the allele inherited from the nonaffected parent for transformation. Mutations of several other genes that code for suppressor genes, oncogenes, and growth factors are undoubtably involved in progression to malignancy. For instance, it is estimated that 35% of the children who have the MEN 2 gene will develop clinically significant disease.[112]

### MEN 1

Gene linkage and marker studies indicate that the gene responsible for MEN 1 is located on the long arm of chromosome 11 q13. There are genes in this area that may be tumor-suppressor genes (anti-oncogenes), but the actual gene causing MEN 1 has not been identified.[116,117]

If individuals affected with MEN are identified, it is now possible to use DNA analysis to determine whether their blood relatives (siblings, children) are at risk. Even though the actual gene responsible for MEN 1 has not yet been identified, DNA analysis using flanking markers about the region containing the gene assumed to cause MEN 1 can identify whether a family member has the mutation specific to that family.

### MEN 2

The *RET* proto-oncogene, located on chromosome 10, has been clearly identified to be responsible for MEN 2.[109,118,119] It is active during fetal life and is expressed during the development of neural crest structures; it is expressed postnatally in parathyroid, thyroid (C cells), adrenal medulla, enteric ganglia, and the urogenital system.[112]

Genetic testing for *RET* in families with a known risk for MEN 2 (A and B) is now recommended as the diagnostic method of choice.[114,118] Specific mutations in the *RET* proto-oncogene are identified in family members confirmed to have MEN 2. Then a single blood sample is drawn from blood relatives and their DNA is compared with that of the known carriers. If no mutations are identified in family members at risk, they will not develop MEN. DNA analysis of the *RET* gene for mutations has been demonstrated to be highly reliable. Thus far, there have been no false-positive or false-negative results.[120,121] Individuals in whom the mutation exists will require annual screening, as outlined previously, starting in early childhood.[112,117] Unaffected individuals, however, are spared unnecessary expensive screening.

## Therapeutic Approaches and Nursing Care

Preventive adrenalectomy or thyroidectomy for MEN 1 and total thyroidectomy for MEN 2 are standard therapy.[122,123] In MEN 2, prophylactic thyroidectomy may be done as early as age 5.[121] Patients whose adrenal gland or thyroid is resected will require lifelong hormone replacement.

A major difference in the treatment of parathyroid tumors in MEN 1, as opposed to sporadic tumors, is that all of the parathyroid tissue must be located and removed. Thus the procedure is always bilateral and includes extensive exploration of the tissues surrounding the thyroid. A small, normal-appearing parathyroid gland must be preserved to maintain calcium homeostasis. It is transplanted away from the thyroid into a muscle in the neck or forearm. Tissue in these sites is easier to monitor, and the patient will not need a subsequent reexploration of the previous surgery site if the tumor recurs.[124] Periodic screening of serum calcium will always be required in these patients.

Many issues have arisen with the ability to identify persons who are likely to develop a disease because of confirmed genetic risk. These include family members' emotional responses and concerns, and the lack of health care providers who are educated to provide genetic counseling. One study has reported the results from 87 persons in 19 large MEN 2 families.[125] Many family members expected they would not be identified as carriers of the gene because of past normal clinical tests, because they were older, because of mistaken ideas of disease transmission, or because they resembled family members without the disease. Patients were dissatisfied with their physicians' inadequate knowledge about MEN 2 and about genetic testing, and the information and medical support they received. Patients had to wait about four months to find out the results of their tests and were generally shocked to find out that they were carriers. Upon disclosure of their actual status, both those who received news that they were MEN carriers and those who did not had increased complaints of anxiety (54% and 38%), depression (42% and 31%), somatic problems (46% and 33%), and sleep disturbances (58% and 46%). By one year after disclosure anxiety had decreased to 14% and 24%, respectively, depression to 14% in both groups, somatic complaints to 21% and 14%, and sleep complaints to 7% and 10%.

## CONCLUSION

Endocrine tumors are rare and varied. They are most often benign, but both benign and malignant tumors may cause significant morbidity and negatively affect quality of life. As with other malignancies, early detection of small tumors that are surgically resectable affords the best prognosis. The relative rarity of these tumors has hampered the ability to scientifically test the effectiveness of chemotherapy in most instances. Many endocrine tumors are detected late in their course and cause the affected person's death because of mass effects or because of physiological effects induced by hypersecretion of an endocrine hormone. Nursing care for patients with endocrine tumors requires knowledge of the hormones secreted and their effects on body systems, and often focuses on symptom assessment and management.

## REFERENCES

1. Parker SL, Tong T, Bolden S, et al: Cancer statistics: 1996. *CA: Cancer J Clin* 65:5–27, 1996
2. Goodman HM: Introduction, in *Basic Medical Endocrinology* (ed 2). New York, Raven Press, 1994, pp 1–27
3. Goodman HM: Thyroid gland, in *Basic Medical Endocrinology* (ed 2). New York, Raven Press, 1994, pp 46–70
4. Steele G, Jessup LM, Winchester DP, et al: Clinical highlights from the National Cancer Data Base. *CA Cancer J Clin* 45:102–111, 1995
5. Greenfield LD, Luk KH: Thyroid, in Perez CA, Brady LW (eds): *Principles and Practice of Radiation Oncology* (ed 2). Philadelphia, Lippincott, 1992, pp 1356–1381
6. Hallquist A, Hardell L, Degerman A, et al: Medical diagnostic and therapeutic radiation and the risk of thyroid cancer: A case-control study. *Eur J Cancer Prev* 3:259–267, 1994
7. Franceschi S, La Vecchia C: Thyroid cancer. *Cancer Surv* 19/20:293–322, 1994
8. Norton JA, Levin B, Jensen RT: Cancer of the endocrine system, in DeVita VT, Hellman S, Rosenberg SA (eds): *Cancer: Principles and Practice of Oncology* (ed 4). Philadelphia, Lippincott, 1993, pp 1333–1435
9. DeGroot LJ, Sridama V: Thyroid neoplasia, in DeGroot LJ, Besser GM, Cahill GF Jr, Marshall JC, Nelson DH, Odell WD (eds): *Endocrinology* (ed 2). Philadelphia, Saunders, 1989, pp 758–776
10. Chrousos GP: Endocrine tumors, in Pizzo PA, Poplack DG (eds): *Principles and Practice of Pediatric Oncology* (ed 2). Philadelphia, Lippincott, 1993, pp 889–912
11. Fraker DL: Radiation exposure and other factors that predispose to human thyroid neoplasia. *Surg Clin North Am* 75:365–375, 1995
12. Ron E, Lubin JH, Shore RE, et al: Thyroid cancer after exposure to external radiation: A pooled analysis of seven studies. *Radiat Res* 141:259–277, 1995
13. Wittes RE: Endocrine system, in Wittes RE (ed): *Manual of Oncologic Therapeutics*. Philadelphia, Lippincott, 1991, pp 221–229
14. Uderzo C, van Lint MT, Rovelli A, et al: Papillary thyroid carcinoma after total body irradiation. *Arch Dis Child* 71: 256–258, 1994
15. Thyroid cancer soars in kids near Chernobyl reactor. *Chicago Tribune*, Nov. 21, 1995, sect 1, p 8
16. Mendelsohn G: Pathology of thyroid disease, in Mendelsohn G (ed): *Diagnosis and Pathology of Endocrine Diseases*. Philadelphia, Lippincott, 1988, pp 37–117
17. Galanti MR, Sparen P, Karlsson A, et al: Is residence in

areas of endemic goiter a risk factor for thyroid cancer? *Int J Cancer* 61:615–621, 1995

18. Segal K, Arad A, Lubin E, et al: Follicular carcinoma of the thyroid. *Head Neck* 16:533–538, 1994

19. Doniach I: Carcinoma of the thyroid, in Besser GM, Cudworth AG (eds): *Clinical Endocrinology: An Illustrated Text.* Philadelphia, Lippincott, 1987, pp 14.1–14.10

20. Demeter JG, DeJong SA, Laurence AM, et al: Anaplastic thyroid carcinoma: Risk factors and outcome. *Surgery* 110:956–963, 1991

21. Tan RK, Finley RK, Driscoll D, et al: Anaplastic carcinoma of the thyroid: A 24-year experience. *Head Neck* 17:41–48, 1995

22. Farndon JR: Endocrine tumours, in McArdle CS (ed): *Surgical Oncology: Current Concepts and Practice.* London, Butterworths, 1990, pp 97–114

23. Cady B: Neoplasms of the thyroid, in Holland JF, Frei E, Bast RC, Kufe DW, Morton DL (eds): *Cancer Medicine* (ed 3). Philadelphia, Lea and Febiger, 1993, pp 1138–1147

24. Lennquist S: The thyroid nodule: Diagnosis and surgical treatment. *Surg Clin North Am* 67:213–232, 1987

25. Mazzaferri EL: Management of a solitary thyroid nodule. *N Engl J Med* 328:553–559, 1993

26. Boigon M, Moyer D: Solitary thyroid nodules: Separating benign from malignant conditions. *Postgrad Med* 98:73–80, 1995

27. Rosen IB, Azadian A, Walfish PG, et al: Ultrasound-guided fine-needle aspiration biopsy in the management of thyroid disease. *Am J Surg* 166:346–349, 1993

28. McHenry CR, Rosen IB, Walfish PG, et al: Influence of FNA biopsy and frozen section examination on the management of thyroid cancer. *Am J Surg* 166:353–356, 1993

29. Hamburger JI: Extensive personal experience. Diagnosis of thyroid nodules by fine needle biopsy: Use and abuse. *J Clin Endocrinol Metab* 79:335–339, 1994

30. Piromalli D, Martelli G, Del Prato I, et al: The role of fine needle aspiration in the diagnosis of thyroid nodules: Analysis of 795 consecutive cases. *J Surg Oncol* 50:247–250, 1992

31. Dwarakanathan AA, Staren ED, D'Amore MJ, et al: Importance of repeat fine-needle biopsy in the management of thyroid nodules. *Am J Surg* 166:350–352, 1993

32. Beahrs OH: *Manual for Staging of Cancer* (ed 4). Philadelphia, Lippincott, 1992, pp 53–56

33. Servé P: Thyroidectomy, in Brown MH, Kiss ME, Outlaw EM, Viamontes CM (eds): *Standards of Oncology Nursing Practice.* New York, Wiley, 1986, pp 197–201

34. Lehne RA: *Pharmacology for Nursing Care* (ed 2). Philadelphia, Saunders, 1994, pp 673–685

35. Baker KH, Feldman JE: Thyroid cancer: A review. *Oncol Nurs Forum* 20:95–104, 1993

36. Tennvall J, Lundell G, Hallquist A, et al: Combined doxorubicin, hyperfractionated radiotherapy, and surgery in anaplastic thyroid carcinoma. *Cancer* 74:1348–1354, 1994

37. Stephens RL: Chemotherapy of endocrine tumors, in Perry MC (ed): *The Chemotherapy Source Book.* Baltimore, Williams and Wilkins, 1992, pp 998–1007

38. Shimaoka K, Schoenfeld DA, DeWys WD, et al: A randomized trial of doxorubicin versus doxorubicin plus cisplatin in patients with advanced thyroid cancer. *Cancer* 56:2155–2158, 1985

39. Droz JP, Schlumberger M, Rougier P, et al: Chemotherapy in nonmetastatic thyroid cancer: Experience at the Institut Gustave-Roussy. *Tumori* 76:480–483, 1990

40. Schlumberger M, Abdelmoumene N, Delisle MJ, et al: Treatment of advanced medullary thyroid cancer with an alternating combination of 5FU-streptozocin and 5FU-dacarbazine. *Br J Cancer* 71:363–365, 1995

41. Goodman HM: Hormonal regulation of calcium metabolism, in *Basic Medical Endocrinology* (ed 2). New York, Raven Press, 1994, pp 175–202

42. Averbuch SD, Baylin SB, Chahinian AP, et al: Neoplasms of the neuroendocrine system, in Holland JF, Frei E, Bast RC, Kute DW, Morton DL, et al (eds): *Cancer Medicine.* Philadelphia, Lea and Febiger, 1993, pp 1153–1180

43. Shane E: Parathyroid carcinoma, in Bilezikian JP, Marcus R, Levine MA (eds): *The Parathyroids: Basic and Clinical Concepts.* New York, Raven Press, 1994, pp 575–581

44. Hakaim AG, Esselsytn CB: Parathyroid carcinoma: 50-year experience at the Cleveland Clinic Foundation. *Cleve Clin J Med* 60:331–335, 1993

45. Wang CA, Gaz RD: Natural history of parathyroid carcinoma: Diagnosis, treatment and results. *Am J Surg* 149:522–527, 1985

46. Fujimoto Y, Obara T: How to recognize and treat parathyroid carcinoma. *Surg Clin North Am* 67:343–357, 1987

47. Sloan DA, Schwartz RW, McGrath PC, et al: Diagnosis and management of thyroid and parathyroid hyperplasia and neoplasia. *Curr Opin Oncol* 7:47–55, 1995

48. Bukowski RM, Sheeler L, Cunningham J, et al: Successful combination chemotherapy for metastatic parathyroid carcinoma. *Arch Intern Med* 144:399–400, 1994

49. Chahinian AP: Chemotherapy for metastatic parathyroid carcinoma. *Arch Intern Med* 144:1889, 1984 (letter)

50. Warrell RP, Isaacs M, Alcock NW, et al: Gallium nitrate for treatment of refractory hypercalcemia from parathyroid carcinoma. *Ann Intern Med* 107:683–686, 1987

51. Goodman HM: Pituitary gland, in *Basic Medical Endocrinology* (ed 2). New York, Raven Press, 1994, pp 28–45

52. Ureles AL, Chang Y-C, Constine LS, et al: Cancer of the endocrine glands: Thyroid, adrenal, and pituitary, in Rubin P, McDonald S, Qazi R (eds): *Clinical Oncology: A Multidisciplinary Approach for Physicians and Students* (ed 7). Philadelphia, Saunders, 1993, pp 531–555

53. Faglia G, Ambrosi B: Hypothalamic and pituitary tumours: General principles, in Grossman A (ed): *Clinical Endocrinology.* Boston, Blackwell Scientific Publications, 1992, pp 113–122

54. Croughs RJM: Pituitary tumors: Diagnosis and treatment. *Anticancer Drugs* 3:555–565, 1992

55. Faglia G: Epidemiology and pathogenesis of pituitary adenomas. *Acta Endocrinol* 129:1–5, 1993 (suppl 1)

56. Molitch ME: Evaluation and treatment of the patient with a pituitary incidentaloma. *J Clin Endocrinol Metab* 80:8–11, 1995

57. Frost AR, Tenner S, Tenner M, et al: ACTH-producing pituitary carcinoma presenting as the cauda equina syndrome. *Arch Pathol Lab Med* 119:93–96, 1995

58. McDermott MT: Nonfunctioning pituitary tumors, in McDermott MT (ed): *Endocrinology Secrets.* Philadelphia, Handley and Belfus, 1995, pp 99–101

59. Molitch ME: Clinical manifestations of acromegaly. *Endocrinol Metab Clin North Am* 21:597–614, 1992

60. Lamberts SWJ: Acromegaly, in Grossman A (ed): *Clinical Endocrinology.* Boston, Blackwell Scientific Publications, 1992, pp 154–168

61. Gumowski J, Proch M, Kessler CA: Endocrinopathies of hyperfunction: Cushing's syndrome and aldosteronism. *AACN Clin Issues Crit Care Nurs* 3:331–347, 1992

62. von Werder K, Müller OA: Cushing's syndrome, in Grossman A (ed): *Clinical Endocrinology*. Boston, Blackwell Scientific Publications, 1992, pp 442–456

63. Reversible hypopituitarism. *Lancet* 337:276, 1991 (brief communication)

64. Delitala G: Hyperprolactinaemia: Causes, biochemical diagnosis and tests of prolactin secretion, in Grossman A (ed): *Clinical Endocrinology*. Boston, Blackwell Scientific Publications, 1992, pp 123–131

65. Chong BW, Newton TH: Hypothalamic and pituitary pathology. *Radiol Clin North Am* 31:1147–1181, 1993

66. Sarapura V: Prolactin-secreting pituitary tumors, in McDermott MT (ed): *Endocrinology Secrets*. Philadelphia, Hanley and Belfus, 1995, pp 102–105

67. Samuels MH: Cushing's syndrome, in McDermott MT (ed): *Endocrinology Secrets*. Philadelphia, Hanley and Belfus, 1995, 116–121

68. Corbett JV: *Laboratory Tests and Diagnostic Procedures with Nursing Diagnoses*. Stamford, CT, Appleton and Lange, 1996

69. Andrews DW: Pituitary adenomas. *Curr Opin Oncol* 6:53–59, 1994

70. Findling JW: Cushing syndrome: An etiologic workup. *Hosp Pract* 27 (10):107–112, 114–118, 1992

71. Chipps E: Transsphenoidal surgery for pituitary tumors. *Crit Care Nurse* 12:30–39, 1992

72. McCutcheon IE: Management of individual tumor syndromes: Pituitary neoplasia. *Endocrinol Metab Clin North Am* 23:37–51, 1994

73. Levy A, Lightman SL: Diagnosis and management of pituitary tumours. *BMJ* 308:1087–1091, 1994

74. Loriaux DL, Wild RA: Contraceptive choices for women with endocrine complications. *Am J Obstet Gynecol* 168: 2021–2026, 1993

75. Stevenaert A, Beckers A: Presurgical octreotide treatment in acromegaly. *Acta Endocrinol* 129:18–20, 1993 (suppl 1)

76. McEwen DR: Transsphenoidal adenomectomy. *AORN J* 61: 321–337, 1995

77. Smith-Rooker JL, Garrett A, Hodges LC: Case management of the patient with pituitary tumor. *MedSurg Nurs* 2: 265–274, 1993

78. Shiminski-Maher T: Patient/family preparation and education for complications and late sequelae of craniopharyngiomas. *Pediatr Neurosurg* 21:114–119, 1994 (suppl 1)

79. Gotch PM: Cushing's syndrome from the patient's perspective. *Endocrinol Metab Clin North Am* 23:607–617, 1994

80. Goodman HM: Adrenal glands, in *Basic Medical Endocrinology*. New York, Raven Press, 1994, pp 71–112

81. Vinson GP, Whitehouse BJ, Hinson JP: The structure and function of the adrenal cortex, in Grossman A (ed): *Clinical Endocrinology*. Boston, Blackwell Scientific Publications, 1992, pp 373–392

82. Wooten MD, King DK: Adrenal cortical carcinoma: Epidemiology and treatment with mitotane and a review of the literature. *Cancer* 72:3145–3155, 1993

83. Medeiros LJ, Weiss LM: New developments in the pathologic diagnosis of adrenocortical neoplasms: A review. *Am J Clin Pathol* 97:73–83, 1992

84. Beuschlein F, Reincke M, Karl M, et al: Clonal compositions of human adrenocortical neoplasms. *Cancer Res* 54: 4927–4932, 1994

85. Gicquel C, Bertagna X, Schneid H, et al: Rearrangements at the 11p15 locus and overexpression of insulin-like growth factor–11 gene in sporadic adrenocortical tumors. *J Clin Endocrinol Metab* 78:1444–1453, 1994

86. Reincke M, Karl M, Travis WH, et al: *p53* Mutations in human adrenocortical neoplasms: Immunohistochemical and molecular studies. *J Clin Endocrinol Metab* 78:790–794, 1994

87. Wagner J, Postwine C, Rabin K, et al: High frequency of germline *p53* mutations in childhood adrenocortical cancer. *J Natl Cancer Inst* 86:1707–1710, 1994

88. Brennan MF, Pommier RF: Management of adrenal neoplasms. *Curr Probl Surg* 28:663–739, 1991

89. Coonrod DV, Rizkallah TH: Virilizing adrenal carcinoma in a woman of reproductive age: A case presentation and literature review. *Am J Obstet Gynecol* 172:1912–1915, 1994

90. Müller J: Adrenocortical tumors: Clinical and diagnostic findings. *Recent Results Cancer Res* 118:106–112, 1990

91. Paja M, Díez S, Lucas T, et al: Dexamethasone-suppressible feminizing adrenal adenoma. *Postgrad Med J* 70:584–588, 1994

92. Derksen J, Nagesser SK, Meinders AE, et al: Identification of virilizing adrenal tumors in hirsute women. *N Engl J Med* 331:968–973, 1994

93. Haak HR, Hermans J, van de Velde CJH, et al: Optimal treatment of adrenocortical carcinoma with mitotane: Results in a consecutive series of 96 patients. *Br J Cancer* 69: 947–951, 1994

94. Vassilopoulou-Sellin R, Guinee VF, Klein MJ, et al: Impact of adjuvant mitotane on the clinical course of patients with adrenocortical cancer. *Cancer* 71:3119–3123, 1993

95. Schlumberger M, Brugieres L, Gicquel C, et al: 5-fluorouracil, doxorubicin, and cisplatin as treatment for adrenal cortical carcinoma. *Cancer* 67:2997–3000, 1991

96. Bukowski RM, Wolfe M, Levine HS, et al: Phase II trial of mitotane and cisplatin in patients with adrenal carcinoma: A Southwestern Oncology Group study. *J Clin Oncol* 11: 161–165, 1993

97. Werbel SS, Ober PO: Pheochromocytoma: Update on diagnosis, localization, and management. *Med Clin North Am* 79:131–153, 1995

98. Agana-Defensor R, Proch M: Pheochromocytoma: A clinical review. *AACN Clin Issues Crit Care Nurs* 3:309–318, 1992

99. Saeger W: Tumours of the adrenal gland. *Recent Results Cancer Res* 118:79–96, 1990

100. Bravo EL, Gifford RW: Pheochromocytoma. *Endocrinol Metab Clin North Am* 22:329–341, 1993

101. Gerlo EAM, Sevens C: Urinary and plasma catecholamines and urinary catecholamine metabolites in pheochromocytoma: Diagnostic value of 19 cases. *Clin Chem* 40:250–256, 1994

102. Lenders JWM, Keiser HR, Goldstein DS, et al: Plasma metanephrines in the diagnosis of pheochromocytoma. *Ann Intern Med* 123:101–109, 1995

103. Wu L-T, Dicpinigaitis P, Bruckner H, et al: Hypertensive crises induced by treatment of malignant pheochromocytoma with a combination of cyclophosphamide, vincristine, and dacarbazine. *Med Pediatr Oncol* 22:389–392, 1994

104. Ponz de Leon M: Multiple endocrine neoplasia, in Ponz de Leon M (ed): *Familial and Hereditary Tumors*. New York, Springer-Verlag, 1994, pp 68–83

105. Skogseid B, Rastad J, Öberg K: Multiple endocrine neoplasia type I. *Endocrinol Metab Clin North Am* 23:1–17, 1994

106. DeLellis RA: Multiple endocrine neoplasia syndromes revisited: Clinical, morphologic, and molecular features. *Lab Invest* 72:494–505, 1995

107. Skogseid B, Larsson C, Lindgren P-G, et al: Clinical and genetic features of adrenocortical lesions in multiple endocrine neoplasia type I. *J Clin Endocrinol Metab* 75:76–81, 1992

108. Raue F, Frank-Raue K, Grauer A: Multiple endocrine neoplasia type 2. *Endocrinol Metab Clin North Am* 23:137–156, 1994

109. Vasen HFA, Vermey A: Hereditary medullary thyroid carcinoma. *Cancer Detect Prev* 19:143–150, 1995

110. van der Vaart CH, Heringa MP, Dullaart RPF, et al: Multiple endocrine neoplasia presenting as phaeochromocytoma during pregnancy. *Br J Obstet Gynaecol* 100:1144–1145, 1993

111. Casanova S, Rosenberg-Bourgin M, Farkas D, et al: Phaeochromocytoma in multiple endocrine neoplasia type 2 A: Survey of 100 cases. *Clin Endocrinol* 132:532–537, 1993

112. Mulligan LM, Ponder BAJ: Genetic basis of endocrine disease: Multiple endocrine neoplasia type 2. *J Clin Endocrinol Metab* 80:1989–1995, 1995

113. Frank K, Raue F, Gottswinter J, et al: The importance of early diagnosis and followup in sporadic MEN II. *Eur J Pediatr* 143:112–116, 1984

114. Lynch HT: The Grosfeld et al article reviewed. *Oncology* 10:146, 152, 1996

115. Goodfellow PJ: Mapping the inherited defects associated with multiple endocrine neoplasia type 2A, multiple endocrine neoplasia type 2B, and familial medullary thyroid carcinoma to chromosome 10 by linkage analysis. *Endocrinol Metab Clin North Am* 23:177–185, 1994

116. Larsson C, Friedman E: Localization and identification of the multiple endocrine neoplasia type 1 disease gene. *Endocrinol Metab Clin North Am* 23:67–79, 1994

117. Thakker RV: The role of molecular genetics in screening for multiple endocrine neoplasia type I. *Endocrinol Metab Clin North Am* 23:117–135, 1994

118. Statement of the American Society of Clinical Oncology: Genetic testing for cancer susceptibility. *J Clin Oncol* 14:1730–1736, 1996

119. Grosfeld FJM, Lips CJM, Beemer FA: Psychosocial consequences of DNA analysis for MEN type 2. *Oncology* 10:141–146, 1996

120. Lips CJM, Landsvater RM, Höppener JWM, et al: Clinical screening as compared with DNA analysis in families with multiple endocrine neoplasia type 2a. *N Engl J Med* 331:828–835, 1994

121. Wells SA, Chi DD, Toshima K, et al: Predictive DNA testing and prophylactic thyroidectomy in patients at risk for multiple endocrine neoplasia type 2a. *Ann Surg* 220:237–250, 1994

122. Kousseff BG: Multiple endocrine neoplasia 2 (MEN 2)/MEN 2a (Sipple syndrome). *Dermatol Clin* 13:91–97, 1995

123. Holloway KB, Flowers FP: Multiple endocrine neoplasia 2b (MEN 2b)/MEN 3. *Dermatol Clin* 13:99–103, 1995

124. Mallette LE: Management of hyperparathyroidism in the multiple endocrine neoplasia syndromes and other familial endocrinopathies. *Endocrinol Metab Clin North Am* 23:19–35, 1994

125. Grosfeld FJM, Lips CJM, ten Kroode HFJ, et al: Psychosocial consequences of DNA analysis for MEN type 2. *Oncology* 10:141–146, 1996

# Chapter 38

# Esophageal, Stomach, Liver, Gallbladder, and Pancreatic Cancers

**JoAnn Coleman, RN, MS, CRNP, OCN®**

Of all the organ systems in the body, the gastrointestinal tract accounts for the highest incidence of malignant tumors. More than 25% of cancer deaths are attributed to cancer of the gastrointestinal tract every year in the United States; there are approximately 222,500 new cases of gastrointestinal cancer and 125,400 deaths.[1] The incidence of cancer at different sites along the gastrointestinal tract presents an interesting pattern when incidence among men is compared with that among women (Table 38-1). Incidence in men decreases from the esophagus to the large intestine, whereas the opposite is true for women. No clear explanations exist for this pattern, but researchers are studying this finding.

The problems common to all gastrointestinal cancers stem from delay in clinical presentation. Gastrointestinal tumors proliferate insidiously and extend locally, presenting signs and symptoms that can be misdiagnosed or self-treated for a long time. As the tumor grows, it can exceed the distensible capacity of the gastrointestinal lumen and result in obstruction. The metastasis of gastrointestinal tumors typically occurs by local spread, blood vessel invasion, and dissemination through the lymphatic system. Prognosis depends on the tumor size, degree of cellular differentiation, extent of metastases, treatment efficacy, and the individual's general health status. Most tumors of the gastrointestinal tract are adenocarcinomas, with the exception of the esophagus and anus, where squamous cell carcinomas predominate. The prognosis for individuals with gastrointestinal tumors varies according to site.

**TABLE 38-1** Gastrointestinal Tumors: Percentage Distribution by Sex

| Site | Total Cases | Percentage of Males | Percentage of Females |
|---|---|---|---|
| Esophagus | 12,300 | 76 | 24 |
| Stomach | 22,800 | 61 | 39 |
| Pancreas | 26,300 | 47 | 53 |
| Liver | 19,900 | 54 | 46 |
| Small intestine | 4,600 | 52 | 48 |
| Colon-rectum | 13,500 | 51 | 49 |

Parker SL, Tong T, Bolden S, et al: Cancer statistics 1996. *CA Cancer J Clin* 46:5–27, 1996.

# ESOPHAGEAL TUMORS

## Introduction

Many people with esophageal cancer mistakenly attribute its signs and symptoms to more common disorders that affect older adults, for example, indigestion, heartburn, and decreased appetite. If the individual has delayed seeking medical attention, the tumor may be advanced and obstruct the lumen. He or she can be dehydrated, malnourished, and debilitated as a result of inadequate nutrition and inappropriate self-treatment. Esophageal tumors that obstruct the lumen can cause a spillover of food, fluid, and saliva into the tracheobronchial tree, resulting in aspiration pneumonia. The physician and nurse are faced with the challenge of a candidate at poor risk for aggressive therapy. Because cancer of the esophagus grows rapidly, metastasizes early, and is diagnosed late, survival rates are poor.

## Epidemiology

Esophageal cancer is uncommon in the United States compared with other parts of the world. It constitutes only 1% of all forms of cancer and is responsible for only 2% of total deaths from cancer. There are approximately 12,300 new cases and 11,200 deaths from cancer of the esophagus in the United States annually.[1] The most alarming fact about esophageal cancer is that only 7% of those affected will be alive five years after diagnosis. This is one of the poorest survival rates among malignant diseases. The incidence of esophageal cancer is much higher in African-Americans than in whites. In the United States the age-adjusted mortality rate for carcinoma of the esophagus per 100,000 persons is higher among white men (5.0) than among white women (1.2) and is significantly increased among African-American men (14.4)

and African-American women (3.8).[2] Carcinoma of the esophagus develops at a younger age in African-Americans than in whites.[3] Most individuals with this disease are 50–70 years of age.

A puzzling feature of esophageal cancer is the remarkable difference in incidence according to geographic location, sometimes varying more than 100-fold.[4] No other tumor demonstrates such variation, and there is no unifying concept that explains the intriguing differences. There are countries in which the incidence of esophageal cancer is 400 to 500 times that of the United States.[5]

## Etiology

Although a variety of relationships yield clues to the etiology of esophageal cancer, the factors are complex and not well understood. Variations in incidence by geographic location point to nutritional and environmental factors. Individuals with esophageal cancer typically have a history of heavy alcohol intake, heavy tobacco use, and poor nutrition.[6-9] Cirrhosis, micronutrient deficiency, anemia, and poor oral hygiene may be contributing etiologic factors. Nitrosamines in food and vitamin deficiencies are among the factors associated with the high incidence of esophageal cancer in different regions of the world.[10,11]

Medical conditions of chronic irritation have been cited as possible etiologic factors: hiatal hernia, reflux esophagitis, and diverticula. In some cases esophageal cancer has developed in individuals with long-standing injuries such as lye-induced strictures, in whom the cancer usually appeared 40 or more years after the agent was ingested.[12] Chronic consumption of hot or heavily seasoned foods and liquids has been associated with this disease.

Individuals with long-standing achalasia have an increased incidence of esophageal cancer, but controversy exists as to whether there is a connection; the issue is still being debated.[13] Barrett's esophagus, which develops from chronic esophageal reflux, is recognized as an important risk factor for the development of adenocarcinoma of the esophagus.[14] Because dysphagia is the only reliable indicator of early malignant changes, antireflux therapy and periodic endoscopic surveillance of Barrett's esophagus are recommended for early detection.[14-17] An associated risk of adenocarcinoma exists in approximately 10% of these individuals despite therapy.[18] Tylosis palmaris et plantaris, a rare inherited syndrome characterized by hyperkeratosis of the palms or soles and papillomas of the esophagus, has a strong association with esophageal cancer.[19,20] Approximately 95% of persons with tylosis develop esophageal cancer by the age of 65.[21] Reports of cancer of the upper esophagus have been associated with esophageal webs, which are usually associated with iron deficiency anemia, glossitis, and esophagitis and are referred to as the *Plummer-Vinson* or *Paterson-Kelly syndrome.*[22]

Dietary deficiencies of certain mineral elements are

considered risk factors for esophageal cancer. In areas with a high incidence of esophageal cancer, dietary deficiencies of selenium are correlated with esophageal cytological changes. Because selenium potentially increases resistance to cancer, a deficiency may signal a high-risk individual.[23]

Esophageal cancers may also develop as a second primary tumor in individuals with other primary tumors, particularly of the upper aerodigestive tract. When a second primary tumor appears, survival from the first tumor is adversely affected.[24]

## Prevention, Screening, Early Detection Programs

Early detection of esophageal cancer can be enhanced by appropriate health education. The nurse's role in the prevention and detection of esophageal cancer can influence early identification of this aggressive tumor. Any individual with risk factors for esophageal cancer should be instructed both on the importance of health care follow-up and on ways to reduce or eliminate risk factors. Counseling on nutrition, alcohol, and tobacco is an important measure for prevention. Chronic users of over-the-counter medications for gastrointestinal upsets should be encouraged to seek medical attention to evaluate potential problems.

There are no cost-effective screening methods to permit early diagnosis in the United States. Certain endemic areas of the world have been successful in screening for esophageal cancer. Use of screening techniques seems prudent for individuals known to be at risk for the development of esophageal carcinoma, such as those with Barrett's esophagus.

## Pathophysiology

Malignant lesions occur at all levels of the esophagus. The site of esophageal tumors is an important factor in detection and prognosis. The distribution of occurrence generally follows this pattern:

- cervical esophagus 15%

- upper and middle thoracic esophagus 50%

- lower thoracic esophagus 35%[2]

### Cellular characteristics

Squamous cell carcinoma and adenocarcinoma are the two major histological types of esophageal cancer. Squamous cell carcinoma represents greater than 85% and adenocarcinoma represents about 10% of esophageal tumors. The esophagus is almost entirely lined with squamous epithelium; thus it follows that squamous cell carcinoma would dominate the area from the pharynx to within a few centimeters of the esophagogastric junc-

tion. In the distal few centimeters of the esophagus, adenocarcinomas and squamous cell carcinomas appear equally. However, tumors in the area of the esophagogastric junction usually are primary gastric adenocarcinomas that have extended from the stomach into the lower esophagus. The occurrence of adenocarcinoma of the esophagus is rapidly increasing in the United States, with some reports indicating a shift upward to 20% of esophageal cancers.[18,25]

Carcinoma of the esophagus may be grossly classified as polypoid, ulcerative, or infiltrative.[26] An infiltrative pattern of tumor growth enriches and thickens the wall, thus leading to marked luminal narrowing. Most often the tumor has a polypoid mass projecting into the esophageal lumen. When tumor proportions exceed the distensible capacity of the esophageal wall, complete obstruction occurs. The ulcerative lesion is elevated and has irregular, nodular edges. Because the ulcerative lesion expands in the submucosa, the lesion can be elevated to such an extent that it obstructs the lumen. Some lesions will remain localized, whereas others will extend over a wide area of the esophagus.

Squamous cell carcinomas and adenocarcinomas exhibit a range of cellular differentiation. Some lesions are so poorly differentiated that it is difficult to ascertain cellular origin. At present, studies are being conducted to determine if there is a correlation between the degree of differentiation and factors such as rapidity of growth, invasiveness, metastases, response to therapy, and prognosis. Histopathologic characteristics,[27] flow cytometric analysis of DNA content,[28] epidermal growth factor receptors,[29] and karyometric measurements of cell contents[30] are some of the parameters being studied as possible predictors of extent of disease and response to therapy.

### Progression of disease

Because there is no serosal covering to the esophagus, tumors can spread into the adjacent mediastinal tissues early in the disease. Squamous cell carcinomas extend beyond the lumen wall to invade adjoining structures in about 60% of cases.[31] Tumors of the cervical esophagus may directly involve the carotid arteries, pleurae, recurrent laryngeal nerves, trachea, or larynx. Tumors of the upper thoracic esophagus may involve the left main stem bronchus, thoracic duct, aortic arch, or pleurae. In the lower portion of the thoracic esophagus, tumors may invade pericardium, pleurae, descending aorta, and diaphragm. If the phrenic nerve is involved, paralysis of the diaphragm can result. Tumor invasion of adjacent structures may be extensive enough to prevent surgical resection, thereby necessitating alternative therapies.

### Patterns of spread

Tumors of the esophagus metastasize principally by way of the lymphatic system. This occurs early and is common on presentation. The rich lymphatic drainage of the esophagus is complex, and the lack of a serosal barrier permits early regional extension and dissemination of esophageal carcinoma before clinical signs appear. Lesions of the cervical and upper thoracic esophagus usually metastasize upward to the supraclavicular and anterior jugular lymph nodes. In the middle thoracic esophagus, tumor cells may metastasize to the mediastinum and subdiaphragmatic lymph nodes. Tumors in the lower part of the esophagus will disseminate to the abdominal lymph nodes, especially those around the celiac axis.

Hematogenous spread of tumor cells or tumor emboli is another mode of metastasis. Tumor emboli may dislodge into the caval system and become embedded in the lung or liver. Distant metastases to the lung, liver, adrenal glands, bone, brain, and kidney are common with advanced disease.

## Clinical Manifestations

Early symptoms of esophageal carcinoma may be nonspecific and cause little concern. Symptoms may be present for only weeks or a few months, yet the esophageal carcinoma can be advanced. Initial symptoms include a vague sense of pressure, fullness, indigestion, and occasional substernal distress.

Dysphagia and weight loss extending over three to six months are classic symptoms in almost 90% of cases.[2,32,33] A significant characteristic of esophageal cancer is the progressive nature of the dysphagia. Because the esophagus initially will distend to allow liquid or food to pass the tumor, the individual will unconsciously masticate solid food more thoroughly and will substitute soft and liquid food to relieve the dysphagia. Most individuals complain of food sticking in their throat and point to the level of the sternal notch. When tumor size exceeds a critical luminal circumference, saliva, food, and liquids may spill over into the lungs, causing aspiration pneumonia. Pain on swallowing occurs in about 50% of individuals with esophageal cancer.[2]

Weight loss inevitably follows and is a dramatic symptom, equaled in frequency only by pancreatic cancer. A loss of 10%–20% of initial body weight is common. Anorexia, anemia, and dehydration may add to an individual's already debilitated state.

The tumor is locally aggressive and produces symptoms that suggest invasion. A characteristic cough-swallow sequence may indicate aspiration of food or a tracheoesophageal fistula. Substernal and epigastric pain often mimics heartburn. Fever can signal pulmonary involvement by tumor or aspiration pneumonia. Supraclavicular or cervical adenopathy may be palpated. Superior vena cava obstruction, pleural effusion, and hepatomegaly may also occur. Tumor involvement of the recurrent laryngeal nerve can result in laryngeal paralysis and hoarseness.[34]

## Assessment

### Patient and family history

The diagnosis of esophageal cancer depends on a thorough patient history, with particular attention to the sequelae of symptoms and nutritional alterations.

### Physical examination

Physical examination reveals few findings for the definitive diagnosis, except in cases of advanced disease. Individuals with advanced disease usually exhibit profound dysphagia and weight loss, palpable enlarged lymph nodes, and enlarged or displaced organs. Systemic manifestations such as aspiration pneumonia are also present. For an individual with an early presentation, a high level of suspicion should be maintained, and the individual should proceed immediately with diagnostic studies.

### Diagnostic studies

***Radiological examination***    In addition to routine chest x-ray, the double-contrast barium study can provide the initial assessment of the extent of the disease in the esophagus as well as any involvement of other thoracic structures. The typical changes noted with a barium esophagram or swallow are mucosal irregularity, displacement, narrowing, and stricture. Advanced lesions produce a characteristic annular apple-core pattern. Ulceration is difficult to visualize but is indicated by irregularity, angulation, and distortion of the linear mucosal folds. In cases of near-complete obstruction, antispasmodics are used to enhance visualization. Barium will leave the stomach within two to six hours. In consideration of the individual's poor nutritional state, the nurse should be certain that laxatives or an enema is given after the test to prevent a barium impaction.

Computed tomography (CT) scan is an excellent modality for staging but is not appropriate to screen for esophageal cancer. CT scan can evaluate the presence of nodal involvement and invasion of adjacent structures, as well as metastatic spread to lung, liver, or celiac nodes.[35,36] Magnetic resonance imaging (MRI) is less valuable to assess esophageal cancers due to cardiac and aortic motion. MRI does not offer a diagnostic advantage over CT scan for detection of this disease.

***Endoscopy and biopsy***    Endoscopic visualization plays an important role in the differential diagnosis of esophageal tumors. It is performed to confirm the diagnosis of esophageal cancer in those individuals who have an abnormal barium swallow. Direct biopsy of the tumor can be performed during esophagoscopy. Following instrumentation, the individual will receive nothing to eat or drink and will remain with the head elevated until the anesthetic dissipates and the gag reflex has returned. Nursing observations should be directed toward signs of esophageal perforation, fluid aspiration, and laryngospasm. Visualization of lesions by endoscopy has limitations and is therefore complemented by cytological examination. A diagnosis can be made by cytological brushing with an accuracy rate of 90%.[37] During endoscopy, samples for cytology are obtained by washings or by brushing the tumor directly. In China, endoscopy and cytology brushings are being used for mass screening to detect early lesions and to monitor high-risk individuals.[38]

Endoscopic ultrasound (EUS) also has an important role in determining the stage of the tumor.[39] Endoscopic ultrasound enables direct visualization of the tumor and determines the depth of penetration through the wall and into surrounding structures as well as any presence of adenopathy.[40,41] For the diagnosis of recurrent tumor following surgical resection, the EUS can produce detailed images.[42]

Biopsy of lymph nodes is a definitive diagnostic tool; however, nodes are not always accessible. If a laparotomy is performed as part of the therapeutic approach, extensive biopsy of the entire area is done, since the rich network of lymph nodes often is a metastatic site.

Bronchoscopy may be done to rule out invasion of the left main stem bronchus found mostly with tumors in the middle third of the esophagus. Assessment of vocal cord function is also performed with this procedure.[35] If metastatic disease is suspected, CT scan of the liver and/or a bone scan is recommended, depending on the individual's signs and symptoms.[43]

### Prognostic indicators

The proximity of the esophagus to the aorta and trachea influences prognosis. Any invasion into these contiguous viscera is an indication of advanced disease. Diagnostic studies, pathological staging, and histological examination assist with staging the disease as well as defining the prognosis. The depth of invasion, involvement of lymph nodes, and metastatic spread to other viscera are the most important variables affecting survival. There are no tumor markers to assess in diagnosing or monitoring esophageal cancer.

## Classification and Staging

Unlike more accessible cancers, clinical staging of esophageal cancer is difficult to accomplish without invasive measures. The extent of tumor growth (T) cannot be fully assessed by radiographic or endoscopic examination. The lymph node status (N) can be evaluated noninvasively only in cervical esophageal lesions. By the time a diagnosis is established, disease frequently has metastasized (M) to the liver, lungs, or bone. The aggressiveness of the therapeutic approach is based on an evaluation of the individual and the extent to which the disease has progressed. Esophageal tumors are staged clinically by anatomic extent of the primary tumor as determined by pretreatment studies. Pathological staging is based on

surgical exploration and histological examination of the resected specimen and its lymph nodes.[43]

For purposes of classification and end results, the American Joint Committee for Cancer Staging and End-Results Reporting has developed a standardized classification system listed in Table 38-2.[44]

## Therapeutic Approaches and Nursing Care

### Treatment planning

***Selection of the treatment plan***   In view of the biological nature and poor prognosis of esophageal carcinoma, the goal of interdisciplinary planning is to select the therapies most appropriate for the extent of the tumor and for the individual. Despite advances in surgery, radiotherapy, and chemotherapy, esophageal carcinoma has a poor outcome, with approximately 7%–11% of individuals surviving five years.[1] Careful multidisciplinary planning is needed to define the extent of the disease, to assess the

**TABLE 38-2**   TNM Classification System for Cancer of the Esophagus

| PRIMARY TUMOR (T) | |
|---|---|
| TX | Primary tumor cannot be assessed |
| T0 | No evidence of primary tumor |
| Tis | Carcinoma in situ |
| T1 | Tumor invades lamina propria or submucosa |
| T2 | Tumor invades muscularis propria |
| T3 | Tumor invades adventitia |
| T4 | Tumor invades adjacent structures |

| REGIONAL LYMPH NODES (N) | |
|---|---|
| NX | Regional lymph nodes cannot be assessed |
| N0 | No regional lymph node metastasis |
| N1 | Regional lymph node metastasis |

| DISTANT METASTASIS (M) | |
|---|---|
| MX | Presence of distant metastasis cannot be assessed |
| M0 | No distant metastasis |
| M1 | Distant metastasis |

| STAGE GROUPING | | | |
|---|---|---|---|
| Stage 0 | Tis | N0 | M0 |
| Stage I | T1 | N0 | M0 |
| Stage IIA | T2 | N0 | M0 |
| | T3 | N0 | M0 |
| Stage IIB | T1 | N1 | M0 |
| | T2 | N1 | M0 |
| Stage III | T3 | N1 | M0 |
| | T4 | Any N | M0 |
| Stage IV | Any T | Any N | M1 |

From Beahrs OH, Henson DE, Hutter RVP, et al (eds): *American Joint Committee on Cancer: Manual for Staging of Cancer* (ed 4). Philadelphia, Lippincott, 1992.

individual's physiological status, and to discuss alternatives completely with the individual before the course of treatment is selected. The nurse is in a valuable position to assess the patient's understanding and reaction to the anticipated therapy.

Surgical resection, radiotherapy, and chemotherapy are used to treat esophageal cancer. A combination of these treatment methods appears to offer the greatest hope of cure or control. The most effective combination or sequence of therapies has yet to be established. Preoperative radiation therapy and chemotherapy have been shown to improve resectability rates but not long-term survival rates. It is hoped that cooperative group trials in progress will help to resolve the issue of the best multimodality therapy. Progress in surgical approaches and care has markedly reduced operative mortality rates to 5%–10%.[45,46] In light of the nature of this disease, aggressive efforts aimed at either cure or palliation are justifiable and constitute the only hope in many cases.

The optimal candidate for curative treatment should be free of any renal, cardiac, and pulmonary diseases, be relatively well nourished, and have a tumor that is localized, responsive, and accessible to treatment (i.e., stage I or II). The interdisciplinary team will develop a plan that can include single or combined modalities of surgery, radiation, or chemotherapy.

The historical trend has been to treat lesions of the cervical esophagus initially with radiotherapy. Surgery is performed three to four weeks later.[2] Surgical resection is limited by the location of the tumor and problems with reconstruction. Improvements in restoring the continuity of the cervical esophagus have been reported.[45]

Although controversial, certain findings will preclude an individual from consideration for curative treatment:

- fixed lymph nodes (N3)
- a fixed tumor mass (T3)
- extension of the tumor outside the esophagus (T3, M1)
- recurrent laryngeal nerve involvement (T3, M1)

In cases of advanced disease, the quality of life can be improved by restoration or maintenance of a patent gastrointestinal tract. Treatment can be radiotherapy, surgical resection or bypass, dilation, prosthetic device implants, or systemic chemotherapy. Although long-term survival is rarely affected, aggressive therapy can be tolerated by many individuals and results in an improvement in the individual's quality of life.

***Preparation for treatment***    If an aggressive treatment plan has been selected, ideally the individual will undergo pretreatment preparation to improve general health and nutrition. If the disease is advanced and the symptoms and manifestations are severely debilitating, palliative therapy may need to be initiated immediately and supportive measures introduced whenever possible.

Progressive dysphagia affects about 90% of individuals with esophageal tumors. The degree of weight a person loses can be correlated with prognosis.[2] Because of difficulty with swallowing, protein-calorie malnutrition, cachexia, muscle wasting, and negative nitrogen balance may be present. Intensive nutritional therapy, which can include total parenteral nutrition, enteral tube feedings, or high-calorie protein liquid supplements, may be given to improve therapeutic outcome.

The high incidence of aspiration that occurs in individuals with esophageal cancer dictates that pulmonary hygiene be a priority in pretreatment care. Since many individuals with this disease are heavy smokers, this will further necessitate intensive chest physiotherapy. The individual is taught to breathe deeply and cough, with careful attention to expectorating secretions. As an aid to achieving pulmonary toilet, the individual is instructed to bend forward when coughing and to expectorate into a tissue, cloth, or basin. Expectorants, antibiotics, or bronchial dilators can be used to facilitate pulmonary hygiene. Esophageal lavage via a nasogastric tube placed above the obstruction may be necessary to prevent aspiration of accumulated food or secretions.

The individual with a large esophageal tumor usually cannot swallow saliva and thus will drool and expectorate frequently. The nurse must be acutely aware of the physiological impact of this embarrassing problem and change in body image. Assist the person to establish an acceptable method for controlling secretions (e.g., a nearby basin, use of oral suction equipment, abundant tissues, room air filter).

The period of treatment preparation is an excellent time to begin teaching the individual and family about the proposed therapy and anticipated course of the disease and to establish supportive relationships.

### Radiation

Squamous cell carcinoma of the esophagus is more responsive than adenocarcinoma to radiotherapy. Radiation can result in rapid relief of an obstruction. Radiotherapy can be used alone, as preoperative, intraoperative, or postoperative therapy, or as palliative therapy. Radiotherapy alone is not being used now because few individuals are being diagnosed in the early stages when radiation can be effective for cure. Methods of therapy combining chemotherapy, radiation, and surgery are providing better results than radiation alone.[47] Radiation is an excellent therapeutic alternative for a patient with advanced disease or for an elderly or severely debilitated patient who could not withstand the rigor of aggressive therapy.

The most important factor in determining the appropriateness of radiation is whether the individual is potentially curable or whether palliation is the only option. Small localized lesions (<5 cm) with no evidence of metastases can be treated for cure with radiotherapy alone or in combination.[48] Doses of 5000–7000 cGy are administered over six to eight weeks to destroy the tumor.

Unfortunately, about 60% of esophageal cancers are beyond potential cure at diagnosis because of distant spread.[49] Radiotherapy is the treatment favored by many clinicians for stage I and II cervical esophageal lesions since surgical mortality rates are high and the larynx can be preserved with radiation. Tumors located in the cervical esophagus are complex to treat because of their proximity to the spinal cord. Tumors located in the upper thoracic esophagus respond well to radiotherapy. Lesions of the lower thoracic esophagus usually are treated with multimodality therapy.

Complications and side effects of radiotherapy relate to tissue tolerance, site and amount of radiation, and adjuvant therapy. Esophageal fistula, stricture, hemorrhage, radiation pneumonitis, and pericarditis are possible problems. Side effects expected during therapy are swallowing difficulties, such as burning, pain, and dryness, and skin reactions. Nursing management should be aimed at anticipating and preventing complications of the radiation therapy and concomitant therapies, maintaining adequate nutritional intake, and minimizing the discomfort of esophageal and skin irritation. Nursing care of individuals who receive radiotherapy is discussed in detail in chapter 13. The nurse or dietitian must plan an intensive dietary program based on the constraints of an obstructive tumor, the degree of nutritional deficit, and the patient's preferences.

***Preoperative radiation therapy***   Preoperative radiation therapy in doses of 3000–6000 cGy can reduce tumor bulk and improve surgical resectability. It can also enable individuals with esophageal tumors to swallow and significantly improve nutritional status and reduce operative risk. Preoperative radiation therapy can potentially eradicate local microscopic disease and reduce the risk of dissemination of tumor cells during surgery.

Clinical studies lend credibility to the effectiveness of the combination of preoperative radiation and surgery.[50-54] Increased resectability rates and decreased operative mortality rates occur when combination therapy is used. The limitation to the aggressiveness of preoperative radiation or preoperative chemoradiation is toxicity.

***Postoperative radiation therapy***   Postoperative radiation therapy is administered to eradicate residual tumor cells in the area of the surgical site. These cells may have been implanted during surgery or could be residual cells in the unresected tumor or adjacent tissue. If the tumor is an unresectable advanced esophageal cancer, postoperative radiotherapy can be effective for local control. The surgeon can mark the involved area with radiopaque clips to enable more precise delivery of the radiation. If the tumor is resected and the stomach or colon is used to restore intestinal continuity, there will need to be a more limited radiation dose (4000–5000 cGy) in order to avoid tissue injury.[2]

Postoperative radiotherapy does not affect surgical mortality, but it may not be as effective as chemoradiation prior to surgical resection. Further investigation is needed to determine the most effective sequence of radiation therapy in the treatment pattern.

***Intracavity radiation***   Through the use of intraluminal brachytherapy, it is possible to provide a therapeutic boost to the local area involved. Implants are placed by an endoscope or through high-dose afterloading techniques. Intracavity radiation can be useful for retreatment after external-beam therapy.[55]

### Surgery

Surgical intervention is employed selectively for lesions at all three levels of the esophagus. The goal of surgery may be cure or palliation, depending on the stage of the tumor and the overall condition of the individual. Curative surgery attempts to eradicate the tumor and reestablish esophageal continuity, whereas palliative surgery may aim to maintain esophageal patency. Surgery can be used alone or in combination with chemotherapy or radiation.

Preoperative indications for curative surgery include a satisfactory nutritional state, a resectable tumor without evidence of invasion of adjacent structures (stages I and II), no distant metastases, and no serious concomitant diseases. Age is not an issue, unless the person's general health is unsatisfactory. Curative surgery can be attempted if it is expected that the tumor will be removed completely and esophageal patency reestablished. If possible, blood, fluid, electrolyte, and nutritional balance should be established before aggressive surgical resection is performed. Impaired wound healing and increased incidence of infection are associated with hypoalbuminemia.[56] Before surgery, chest physiotherapy includes respiratory exercises and incentive spirometry. The individual is requested to refrain from smoking for two to three weeks before surgery.

***Surgical approaches***   The surgical technique and approach to esophageal resection depend on the location of the tumor. Surgical options include curative and palliative resections as well as bypass procedures to restore normal swallowing. Surgery is the best treatment for control of a local tumor and is the best treatment to provide relief of dysphagia. Surgical risks and length of hospitalization have decreased to acceptable levels.[57-61] The lack of a serosal covering of the esophagus makes it impossible to suture esophagus to esophagus, necessitating a complete excision of the tumor as well as the remaining distal esophagus. Usually a portion of the proximal stomach is removed along with the esophagus, which gives rise to the term *total* or *partial esophagogastrectomy*.

Currently, four surgical approaches are being used: left thoracoabdominal approach, combined abdominal and right thoracotomy approach (Ivor-Lewis), transhiatal approach, and radical esophagectomy (en bloc resection). For cancers near the gastroesophageal junction or lower third of the esophagus, the left thoracoabdominal approach facilitates esophageal dissection, especially when the extent of gastric invasion is unclear, and the approach yields superb exposure and maximizes reconstruction options. For cancer of the upper and middle third of the esophagus, the abdominal and right thoracotomy is used to optimize exposure of the esophagus in the thorax. Once the esophagus is mobilized, a partial esophagogastrectomy is performed, and the esophagus is replaced by stomach, colon, or—less frequently—jejunum. The advantage of this technique is the excellent exposure of the esophagus, and the disadvantage is related to the thoracotomy, which increases the potential for an anastomotic leak in the chest. Transhiatal partial esophagogastrectomy has become a popular surgical approach that does not require a thoracotomy and places the esophageal anastomosis in the neck, where the consequences of anastomotic leak are minimized. Radical esophagectomy involves removal of a tissue block that is completely surrounded by normal tissue and incorporates removal of abdominal and mediastinal lymph nodes.[33]

Partial esophagogastrectomy is the most widely used surgical procedure for resection aimed at potential cure. Because lymph node involvement can occur at a distance from the primary esophageal cancer, complete removal of the esophagus and adjacent lymph nodes is considered the procedure of choice.[46] Whenever there is evidence that cure is a strong possibility, a more extensive radical esophagectomy is performed.

Reconstruction following esophagectomy can be achieved by various procedures. Elevating the stomach to create an esophagogastrostomy is the most widely used reconstructive procedure (Figure 38-1 and 38-2). If a gastrectomy has previously been performed or the stomach is not suitable as a reconstructive organ, a colon

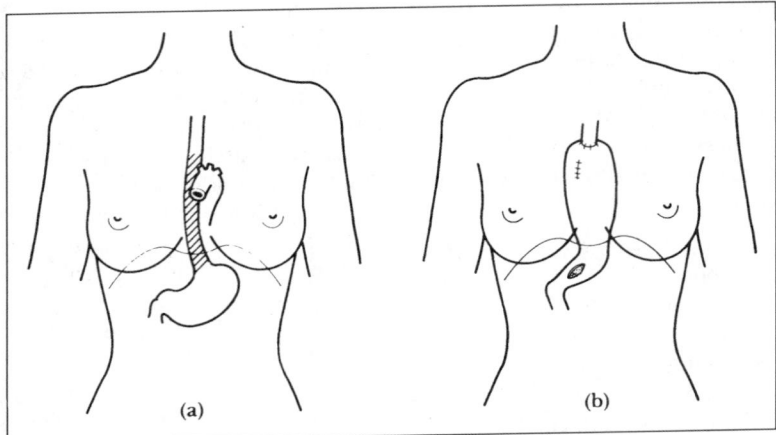

**FIGURE 38-1**   The technique of esophagectomy for cancers involving the mid-esophagus. (a) The extent of esophagus removed is shown by the darkened area. (b) The esophagogastrostomy above the aortic arch and pyloroplasty is illustrated.

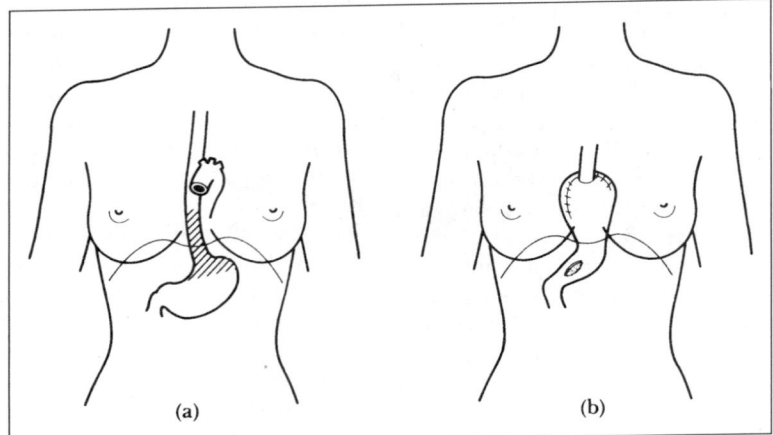

**FIGURE 38-2**   Esophagectomy for lesions of the lower esophagus. In most cases the procedure can be performed through the left thoracic incision. The midline abdominal incision is used when the duodenum must be mobilized to permit the esophagogastrostomy to be performed. (a) The extent of esophagus and stomach removed is shown by the darkened area. The lymph nodes at the celiac axis are removed with the specimen. (b) The esophagogastrostomy is illustrated. A pyloroplasty is also done.

interposition may be done (Figure 38-3). A gastric tube sometimes is created from the greater curvature of the stomach, reversed, and elevated to reconstruct the esophagus (Figure 38-4).

*Special considerations: cervical esophagus* Tumors of the cervical esophagus are the least common. Resection of lesions and reconstruction of the cervical esophagus require careful planning because of the difficulties imposed by its location. Surgery is extensive and is recommended only if cure is the goal. Tumors of the cervical esophagus that do not have laryngeal involvement can sometimes be resected completely without removing the larynx. The surgical procedure consists of a radical neck dissection and partial cervical esophagectomy. However, most tumors of the cervical esophagus are first detected at a more advanced stage and require more extensive surgery. Usually, resection of cervical esophagus lesions involves removing all or part of the pharynx, larynx, thyroid, and proximal esophagus.[2]

Reconstruction of intestinal patency is a major consid-eration, especially with irradiated tissue. The reconstructive procedure may be done at the time of the initial resection or later as a second-stage procedure. At present, cervical esophageal continuity usually is reestablished by anastomosing the stomach to the pharynx, called a *gastric pull-up*. In some instances the colon is interposed and anastomosed to the pharyngeal stump.[2]

A satisfactory, functional result can be achieved with these procedures, but the postoperative period can be plagued with complications of fistula, anastomotic leak, strictures, respiratory insufficiency, pulmonary embolism, obstruction, and infection.[2] Postoperative mortality ranges from 3% to 26%,[46,47] depending on the skill and experience of the surgeon.

*Postoperative care* Respiratory complications, fistulae, and anastomotic leaks constitute the bulk of complications following surgical resection for esophageal cancer.[62] Severe atelectasis, pneumonia, pulmonary edema, and adult respiratory distress syndrome contribute to postoperative morbidity and mortality.[45] Lengthy

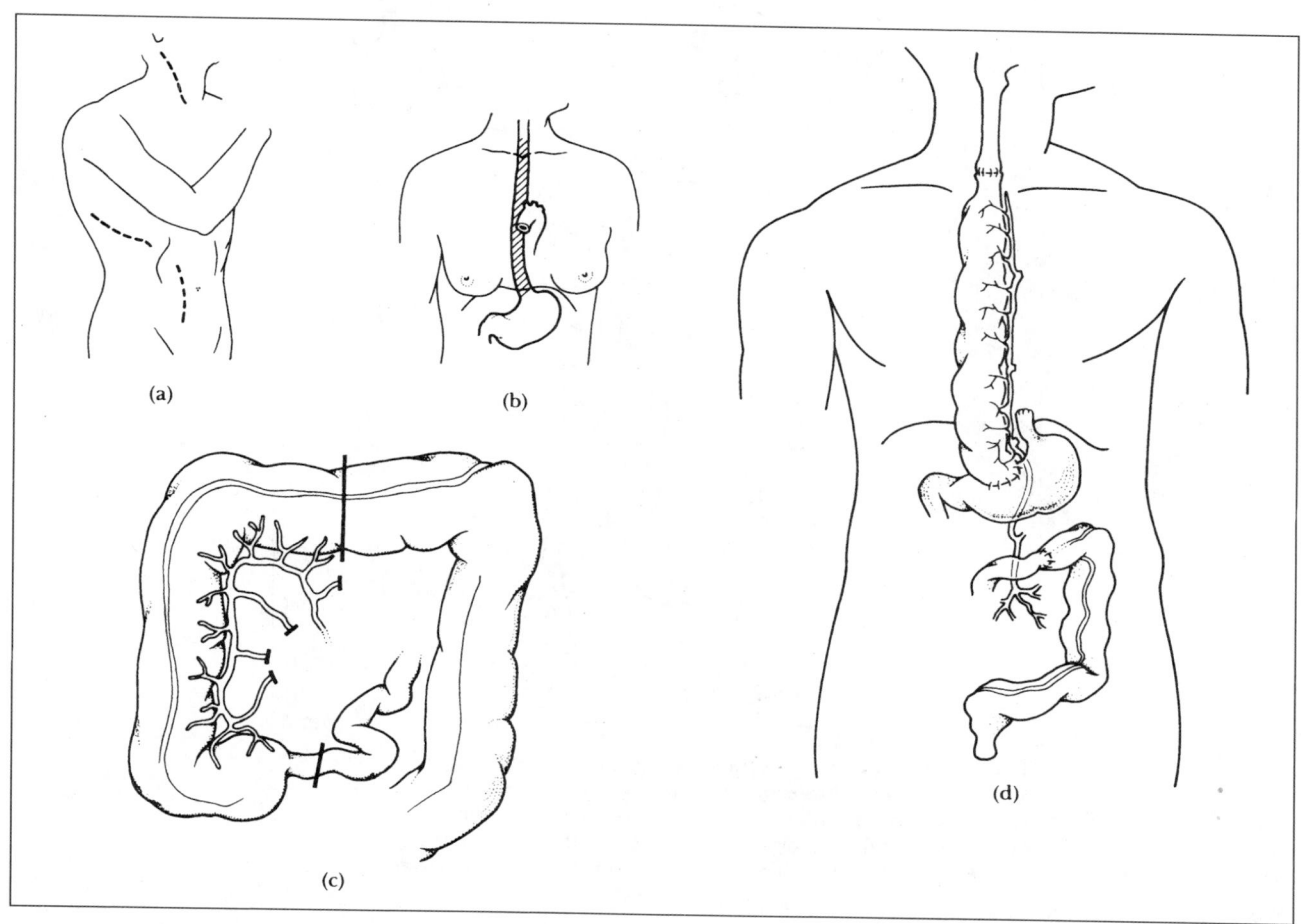

(a)

(b)

(c)

(d)

**FIGURE 38-3** A right colon substernal transplant and total esophagectomy. (a) The cervical and abdominal incisions are made at the first stage of the operation. The right thoracic incision is used at the second stage to remove the esophagus. (b) The extent of esophageal resection is shown. (c) The right colon on a pedicle consisting of the midcolic artery and vein is illustrated. (d) The completed operation is shown.

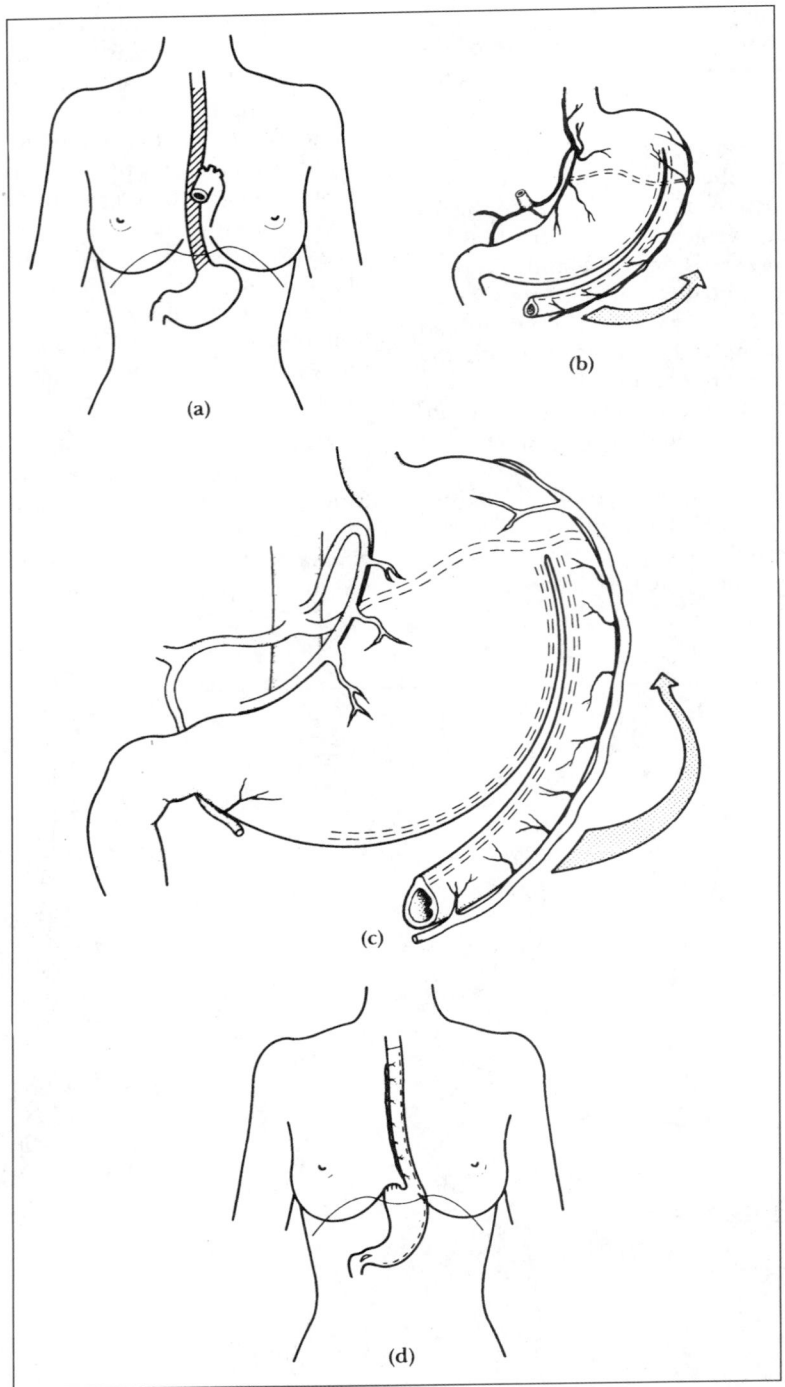

**FIGURE 38-4**   Reversed gastric tube and total esophagectomy. (a) The extent of esophageal resection is shown. (b) The reversed gastric tube created from two parallel rows of staples is shown. (c) The gastroepiploic vessels are carefully preserved and vascularize the gastric tube. (d) The completed operation, with gastrostomy and pyloroplasty, is shown.

surgical procedures (five to eight hours) and a compromised preoperative pulmonary condition can precipitate problems, such as hypothermia and hypovolemia. Because most individuals who undergo surgery for an esoph-ageal tumor are in a poor nutritional state, protein depletion and generalized muscle weakness are common. Ability to breathe deeply and cough is compromised by weakness and incisional pain. Aggressive respiratory care can include tracheal intubation, chest physiotherapy, tracheobronchial aspiration, prevention of fluid overload, and antibiotic therapy. Early ambulation and mild exercise can improve respiratory status.

The esophagus is a thin-walled organ drawn upward with each swallow, so an anastomosis involving the esophagus has more of a risk of developing dehiscence and anastomotic leak than any other area of the gastrointestinal tract.[59,63] Decompression tubes, nasogastric or gastrostomy, must be patent at all times to prevent pressure or tension on the anastomotic site. Chest tubes must be placed to facilitate full reexpansion of the lungs and extraesophageal drainage. Bloody, purulent, or brown, malodorous drainage from the chest tubes indicates leakage. Fever or pain is usually the earliest sign of wound dehiscence or anastomotic leak.[64] The nurse should routinely auscultate the individual's chest to identify any changes in lung expansion or accumulation of fluid. Contrast studies can be done four to six days after surgery to evaluate anastomotic healing. Small leaks usually close spontaneously if decompression is adequate, whereas large leaks may require surgical intervention before mediastinitis or empyema occurs. Intrathoracic anastomotic leaks usually are managed with chest tube drainage, aggressive antibiotic therapy, cessation of oral intake, and open thoracotomy if the disruption is large.[65]

Infections are a serious threat to recovery. Virulent mouth organisms and overgrowth of pathogenic bacteria on ulcerating lesions may be a source of wound and intracavitary infections. If the individual has had preoperative radiation therapy, the risks of tissue breakdown, poor wound healing, and fistula are greatly increased. Nursing assessments for signs of infection and fistula include inspection of suture lines, monitoring vital signs with particular attention to temperature, pulmonary auscultation, and close attention to drainage, urinary output, and hematologic parameters.

Meticulous attention to suture lines and constant monitoring for signs of inflammation, drainage, and edema are necessary. Esophagocutaneous fistulae usually appear in raised, reddened, or necrotic areas along the suture line. The individual should be observed carefully during swallowing as a leak may occur at the suture line. Chylous fistulae produce a milky white secretion that gradually increases in amount. Systemic signs of fistula are fever, malaise, and increased respirations and pulse rate. The individual is maintained in proper body alignment to reduce tension on anastomoses. Suction catheters are not introduced into the oropharyngeal cavity without knowledge of the location of the suture line as disruption may occur. The nasogastric tube should be advanced or manipulated only with the aid of fluoroscopy.

If the individual had a cervical esophagectomy in conjunction with a laryngectomy, the nursing care needs are complex. The nursing care of the individual with a laryngectomy is discussed in detail in chapter 40.

The postoperative nursing care of the individual with an esophagogastrectomy includes anticipation and prevention of reflux aspiration and esophagitis. The head of the bed should be elevated at all times. After the individual is discharged, a foam rubber wedge or correctly aligned multiple pillows will work well at home. Snacks or liquids after the evening meal should be avoided so the stomach will be relatively empty at bedtime. The individual should ingest all food and fluids in small amounts in an upright position and should remain upright for 20–30 minutes after eating.[65,66] The individual should be instructed to avoid bending over from the waist and especially to avoid any exercise or lifting that would increase intra-abdominal and thoracic pressure and cause reflux.[67] Squatting to lift objects will displace the stress to the legs rather than to the abdomen.

Feeding jejunostomy tubes may have been placed preoperatively or at the time of surgery. Individuals must be taught routine care of the tube along with signs and symptoms of complications from the tube. Whenever the feeding tube is placed, the individual must be given proper instruction to maintain the security and patency of the tube. Administration of enteral nutrition supplements is taught to the individual. Tube feedings may be started after surgery to maintain nutrition and prevent bacterial translocation as a source of sepsis. The nurse must monitor for any clog or obstructed flow of fluids through the tube. Measures should be taken immediately to unclog the tube upon noting the cease of flow. The use of carbonated beverages and enzymes has proved effective in declogging feeding tubes. Feeding tubes should be flushed with an adequate amount of water at least every four hours to prevent clogging.

When a segment of colon is used to reconstruct or bypass part of the esophagus, the individual will have complex nursing care needs in addition to those discussed previously for esophagectomy. Pulmonary hygiene, prevention of infection, control of odor, and nutrition are nursing priorities.

Prior to surgery for colon interposition, a regimen of oral antibiotics is begun to suppress bacterial flora in the intestine. Despite efforts to sterilize and prepare the bowel for transposition, contamination of the peritoneal cavity and infection leading to fistula formation can occur and present serious complications. Gram-negative bacteria can produce endotoxic shock, evidenced by rapid pulse, decreased blood pressure, increased respirations and temperature, warm, dry skin, and confusion. The suture lines should be observed for signs of infection, vital signs monitored regularly, and careful lung assessments performed to detect an anastomotic leak or extraesophageal accumulation of fluid.

Foul-smelling breath is a distressing consequence of having used a segment of bowel to reconstruct the esophagus. The extensive program of preoperative bowel preparation will reduce but not eliminate fecal odor. Frequent, meticulous oral care is necessary in the postoperative period and after discharge. The individual should be instructed to avoid foods that cause belching, because the eructated air will have fecal odor that could embarrass the person. The individual can prepare a small, discreet travel kit that includes such items as a toothbrush, toothpaste, mouthwash, mint candies, and charcoal carbonate tablets. Some individuals find that commercially available breath sprays are useful. Charcoal carbonate tablets taken regularly will help to control odor.

### Chemotherapy

Chemotherapy in the treatment of esophageal tumors has assumed an increasingly important role. It is no longer used only to palliate metastatic disease but has become an integral part of the management of the individual with locally confined disease.[33] Cisplatin, 5-fluorouracil (5-FU), mitomycin C, mitoguazone, doxorubicin, bleomycin, and vindesine have demonstrated cytotoxic activity with esophageal tumors.[68,69] Combination regimens are more effective than single-agent therapy.[33,70–72] Cisplatin plus infusional 5-FU is the most commonly used regimen for the treatment of either adenocarcinoma or squamous cell carcinoma of the esophagus. The identification of vinorelbine and paclitaxel as active agents offers the potential for developing more effective therapies.[33]

Sequenced chemotherapy and its use in multimodality treatment approaches offer the most promising areas to explore at this time. Theoretically, neoadjuvant chemotherapy exposes micrometastatic cells at a time of maximum sensitivity and minimal resistance. Preoperative chemotherapy could enable a surgical resection with less chance of metastatic disease recurrence. Current clinical trials of preoperative chemotherapy include various combinations of active agents. Neoadjuvant therapy has produced significant response rates, but impact on survival has been modest.[43]

Preoperative chemoradiation therapy delivers local and systemic therapy simultaneously. The radiation therapy component will improve resectability, and the chemotherapy is expected to reduce systemic micrometastases. Together, a higher rate of tumor sterilization is induced. Protocols include combination chemotherapy, usually cisplatin and 5-FU, and fractionated radiation doses that total 3000–5000 cGy before surgery.[47,73,74] Tumor regression is effected in most cases. Cisplatin and 5-FU may act as radiosensitizers to improve therapeutic effect. The toxicities associated with the extensive combination of chemotherapy, radiation therapy, and surgery are compounded and may be intolerable for some individuals, but most appear to tolerate the therapy.[73] Severe mucositis and myelosuppression are the major toxicities noted. Operative morbidity and mortality have not been increased.[73] Some chemotherapeutic agents, such as doxorubicin, actinomycin D, and daunorubicin, can produce radiation-recall esophagitis and skin reactions in individuals who have received previous irradiation. To reduce the severity of this effect, chemotherapy should not be initiated for several weeks after radiotherapy. It is not yet known whether this approach to esophageal cancer will improve long-term disease-free intervals.

Chemoradiation alone, without surgery, has received attention.[75,76] Results with early-stage cancers indicate that a better response is achieved with chemoradiation alone than with surgery or radiation alone. Optimal management of esophageal cancer is an area that requires further study.

## Symptom Management and Supportive Care

The objective of palliative therapy is to relieve the distressing symptoms of esophageal cancer, thereby improving the quality of the individual's life. Progressive dysphagia is probably the most debilitating of the symptoms, occurring in about 90% of individuals with advanced disease. Selection of a particular form of palliative therapy will depend on the individual's preference, nutritional status, hematologic status, and ability to tolerate palliative therapy.

Palliative radiotherapy provides rapid symptomatic and objective relief. Usually, 3000–5000 cGy will be given to decrease the size of the tumor or reduce bleeding or both.[77] Intracavity brachytherapy has also been used. Because of its noninvasive nature, many oncologists will select palliative radiotherapy over other forms of supportive treatment.

Laser therapy is being used more frequently to alleviate esophageal obstruction or severe dysphagia. The laser photocoagulation process is delivered via endoscope. It is generally well tolerated and rapidly relieves tumor blockage.[78–80] Generally, repeated treatments are needed to achieve the desired result and maintain a patent esophageal lumen.[78,81,82] Survival in individuals who have laser therapy is thought to be due to tumor debulking, improved nutritional status, decrease in aspiration pneumonia, enhanced sense of well-being, and a person's motivation.[78]

In selected individuals with advanced disease, palliative resection with reconstruction or surgical bypass of the esophagus will be done to relieve severe symptoms of the disease or reduce the size of the tumor. Limited resection or bypass of the tumor can be achieved by elevation of the stomach, substernal or subcutaneous colon interposition, or a tube formed from the greater curvature of the stomach.[2] In some instances esophagectomy may be performed as a palliative procedure for esophageal disruption. This type of surgery is usually done as an emergency for perforation caused by palliative therapy or by the tumor itself. The nurse must recognize the signs and symptoms of acute perforation: chest pain, respiratory distress, tachycardia, hypotension, and elevated temperature. A CT scan can verify the findings. The individual will need to be quickly prepared for emergency surgery. Now an individual who was not originally a candidate for surgery will have a major operation and be a nursing challenge postoperatively, with all the inherent problems of a poor surgical candidate.

A number of synthetic esophageal funnel prosthetic tubes have been designed to create an open passage for swallowing when the esophagus is obstructed by an inoperable tumor. The two most common techniques for placing the tube are the push-through method and the pull-through method. With the push-through method, the tube is placed blindly or with the aid of an endoscope.[83] The pull-through method involves pulling the tube into place by means of a guide wire or gastrostomy. Radiological dilation before tube placement can reduce complications. Comparison of these two intubation techniques in individuals with esophageal cancer has shown the endoscopic push-through technique to be safer. Esophageal perforation is a complication that occurs in about 5%–10% of individuals.[83] Dislodgement and/or obstruction with food occurs frequently. Satisfactory palliative results achieved with either type of tube are limited; however, increased food intake after tube placement occurs in about 80% of individuals.[83] Overgrowth of the tube with cancer can occur but can be relieved with laser ablation.[84]

Nursing care of the individual with an endoprosthesis is aimed at preventing complications and maintaining tube patency. Individuals need to understand the purpose, function, and care of the esophageal prosthesis. With the prosthesis in place, reflux of gastric contents can lead to pneumonia. Nursing care measures to prevent reflux include elevating the head of the bed at all times, ensuring patency of decompression tubes, and pursuing aggressive pulmonary hygiene.[85] Strategies to prevent reflux should be developed when the individual is able to begin eating, usually the day after placement. The individual is instructed to take all meals and liquids in an upright position. The first attempts at swallowing may be uncomfortable, but encouragement by the nurse can greatly increase the individual's confidence. It may be necessary to ingest smaller amounts of liquid or food with each swallow. If food becomes lodged in the tube because it is too large or inadequately chewed, it usually can be dislodged carefully with a nasogastric tube. Discharge teaching should include instructions to drink at least a half glass of water or carbonated beverage at the end of the meal to clear the tube completely.

Other palliative treatments include hyperthermochemoradiotherapy,[86] high-dose photoirradiation,[87] and laser therapy to reduce the obstructive mass. Laser therapy is also used to reduce esophageal stricture that may be caused by a tumor.[88]

Gastrostomy and jejunostomy tubes are alternative palliative procedures for individuals with esophageal cancer. Although they permit nutritional maintenance, they do not relieve the debilitating problem of inability to swallow solids, liquids, or saliva. Nursing measures to increase tolerance of tube feedings are discussed in chapter 24. Nursing management of the individual with advanced esophageal cancer includes control of pain, nutritional support, and psychological support. Because esophageal cancer grows rapidly and disseminates early, the nurse can be most helpful by anticipating problems and providing support to the individual and family.

## Continuity of Care: Nursing Challenges

The nurse assumes the role of educator, advocate, and caregiver for the individual with esophageal cancer as the disease progresses. Therapies are chosen to best meet the needs of the individual, always with the hope that the treatment will improve quality and quantity of life. It is important for the individual to understand toxicities and complications of therapy to meet the challenges that can occur. Hope should always be rendered to any person with such a devastating cancer.

In light of the dreary outlook on esophageal cancer, it is important for the nurse to consider what the future may hold for individuals with this disease. Nutrition becomes a central focus of the patient and family. The nurse needs to anticipate problems and provide support to the patient and family as the patient succumbs to the vicious spiral of inability to eat, weight loss, malnutrition, and muscle wasting. Progression of the tumor may also lead to other sequelae if erosion into other major organs or vessels occurs.

# STOMACH TUMORS

## Introduction

At the beginning of this century, gastric cancer was the leading cause of cancer death in the United States, but the incidence has declined progressively since 1930.[1,89] No major advances in diagnosis or treatment have been made during this period. Although there has been a decrease in gastric cancers, the number of patients with proximal gastric and gastroesophageal adenocarcimonas has increased during the past 15 years.[18] Other countries have not seen a decreased rate of gastric cancer. It is epidemic in Japan, Eastern Europe, and portions of Central and South America. Japan has the highest incidence of gastric cancer, which is the number one cause of death nationally.[90]

The prognosis for individuals diagnosed with stomach cancer in the United States is extremely poor, with the five-year survival rate ranging from 5% to 15%. In Japan, despite the epidemic incidence of gastric cancer, there has been a decline in mortality rates over the past 25 years. This is due to aggressive screening programs and national efforts toward early detection of this serious problem for the Japanese.[89] Gastric cancer is insidious in its onset and development, usually infiltrates rapidly, and can be disseminated throughout the body before overt signs are manifested. Gastric cancer mimics several other gastrointestinal maladies and diseases, such as polyps, ulcers, dyspepsia, and gastritis. The most challenging aspects of prevention and early detection are informing and motivating people at risk for developing gastric cancer to seek medical attention for chronic "stomach problems."

Inappropriate use of home remedies, self-medication, and misdiagnosis are major challenges.

## Epidemiology

Japan has the highest incidence in the world of gastric cancer for both men and women, and the disease is the country's major cause of death.[91,92] In the United States the incidence of gastric cancer is low.[1] The dramatic differences in geographic patterns of incidence throughout the world remain an enigma to epidemiologists.[93]

The United States has approximately 23,000 new cases and 14,000 deaths from gastric cancer each year.[1] This reflects a 65% decrease in incidence within the past 35–40 years, with the greatest decline occurring among whites. In the United States, African-Americans, Japanese, Chinese, and native Hawaiian individuals have a higher incidence and mortality rate than do whites.[96] There is also great variation of incidence among the Native Americans of New Mexico, Hispanic Americans, and non-Hispanic whites.[94] Gastric cancer is found more commonly in individuals between 50 and 70 years of age. It is predominantly a disease of men worldwide, occurring about twice as often in men as in women. A small increased incidence has been noted in the direct relatives of individuals who had gastric cancer. A study of Japanese immigrants to the United States and their offspring suggests that exposures early in life, rather than a genetic influence, are the major causative factors in gastric cancer.[95]

## Etiology

Factors believed to contribute to or be associated with gastric cancer are largely environmental and genetic. The fact that immigrants exhibit incidence rates similar to those of their country of origin has led researchers to accept exogenous influences such as environment and diet. A high intake of smoked or salted meats and fish and nitrates, along with low consumption of fresh vegetables and fruits, have all correlated with increased gastric cancer risk in populations. High intakes of grains and low intakes of animal fats and proteins appear to be associated with a decreased risk. Diets rich in vitamins A and C are associated with a low risk for gastric cancer.[96] Controversy exists over the role of nitrates found in soil-grown foods, drinking water, and prepared foods. Because refrigeration and a high intake of ascorbic acid inhibit the formation of nitrates, it is postulated that the presence of these factors may account for the decrease in gastric cancer in the United States. Decreases in incidence may also be due to the ingestion of greater amounts of fresh fruits, vegetables, and grains. Neither smoking tobacco nor drinking alcohol has been demonstrated to increase the risk of gastric carcinoma.[97,98]

Those at greatest risk for the development of gastric cancer are older than 40 years of age and exhibit one or several of the following factors:[99]

- low socioeconomic status[100]
- poor nutritional habits[101]
- vitamin A deficiency
- family history[102,103]
- previous gastric resection for benign disease[104,105]
- pernicious anemia[106]
- *Helicobacter pylori* infection[107–109]
- gastric atrophy and chronic gastritis
- occupation (rubber and coal workers)

Individuals whose occupations appear to place them at risk for gastric cancer are coal miners, nickel refiners, rubber and timber processors, and asbestos workers.[97]

## Prevention, Screening, Early Detection Programs

In high-incidence areas such as Japan, mass screening programs for gastric cancer have proved successful. Screening tests usually include barium x-ray or upper endoscopy, which has 90% sensitivity and specificity. The detection of early gastric cancer in the screened populations has been substantial and has resulted in a high cure rate.[110,111]

Because the initial symptoms of gastric cancer are vague, it is not unusual for misdiagnosis or treatment delay to occur. Although the incidence of gastric cancer is decreasing, aggressive preventive health care in high-risk individuals is necessary to ensure that this decline continues.

## Pathophysiology

### Cellular characteristics

Approximately 95% of gastric cancers are adenocarcinomas.[97,112,113] Other less common neoplasms of the stomach are leiomyosarcoma and lymphoma. It is essential that differentiation between adenocarcinoma and lymphoma of the stomach be made because staging, treatment strategies, and prognosis will differ according to cell type.[114] Most gastric cancers arise in the antrum, the distal third of the stomach. The predominant site of gastric cancer occurrence has changed over the last 30 years.[89,115] A larger number of tumors involving the proximal stomach and the gastroesophageal junction have been found. Usually, adenocarcinomas of the gastroesophageal junction are primary cancers of the stomach that have extended to the distal esophagus. The lesser curvature of the stomach is more frequently involved than the greater curvature. There are different male-to-female and ethnic distribution patterns.[97,116] Gastric tumors may be grossly classified as polypoid, scirrhous, ulcerative, or superficial.

### Progression of disease

Because initial symptoms are vague, gastric cancer is usually locally advanced or metastatic when an individual is first symptomatic. Gastric tumors can cause ulceration, obstruction, hemorrhage, or manifestations of metastatic involvement.

### Patterns of spread

There are four characteristic routes by which gastric carcinoma spreads and metastasizes: (1) by direct extension into adjacent structures such as the pancreas, liver, or esophagus; (2) local or distant nodal metastases mostly on the left side of the neck (Virchow's node); (3) bloodstream metastases; and (4) intraperitoneal dissemination, particularly to the ovary (Krukenberg tumor), perirectal area (Blumer's rectal shelf), and periumbilical nodules (Sister Mary Joseph nodule). The pattern of metastatic spread of gastric cancer correlates with the size and location of the tumor. Lesions of the distal portion of the stomach usually will metastasize to infrapyloric, inferior gastric, and celiac lymph nodes. Tumors in the proximal portion often metastasize to pancreatic, pericardial, and gastric lymph nodes. Distant metastatic sites are the lung, adrenals, bone, liver, rectum, and peritoneal cavity.[97]

## Clinical Manifestations

The initial symptoms of gastric cancer are vague and nonspecific, with variable duration.[18] Individuals usually will delay several months between the onset of symptoms and initial medical consultation. Pain in the epigastrium, back, or retrosternal area is often cited as an early symptom that was ignored or that responded temporarily to self-treatment. The individual may complain of a vague, uneasy sense of fullness, a feeling of heaviness, and moderate distention after meals. Antacids and home remedies are employed successfully for a while until more definitive signs and symptoms appear. As the disease advances, progressive weight loss can result from disturbances in appetite, nausea, and vomiting. Individuals who have weight loss appear to have a significantly shorter survival than those without weight loss.[117] Weakness, fatigue, and anemia are common findings. Dysphagia may occur with tumors of the proximal portion of the stomach. Persistent vomiting can occur with a distal stomach cancer obstructing the pylorus. Hematemesis, melena, or a change in bowel pattern is sometimes reported. Unfortunately, many individuals are diagnosed with gastric cancer after the development of ascites, jaundice, or a palpable mass, indicating the disease is already locally advanced or metastatic.[89]

## Assessment

A complete history and physical examination can provide valuable findings to direct the sequence of diagnostic studies. Endoscopy, radiography, and laparotomy may be necessary to establish a diagnosis of gastric carcinoma. Health care providers must be keenly aware of the vague initial signs and symptoms of this disease.

### Patient and family history

To establish a clinical picture, a complete assessment of the individual's nutritional status, physical examination, and social and family history should be obtained. An in-depth nutritional assessment and history aids in identifying subtle changes in dietary habits or contributory signs such as pain or bowel changes. Areas to include in a nutritional history and assessment are as follows:

1. food and fluid intake patterns (types, amount, number, calories)
2. symptoms associated with eating (pain, eructation, dysphagia, nausea, fullness, reflux)
3. change in dietary habits or appetite (food intolerance, aversions, volume, types of food)
4. weight (actual, usual, ideal)
5. bowel patterns and habits (frequency, consistency, color, flatulence)
6. medications (over-the-counter, home remedies, prescriptions)
7. previous and/or concurrent illness (childhood, adult, transient maladies)

### Physical examination

The physical examination includes palpation of the abdomen and lymph nodes, particularly the supraclavicular and axillary lymph nodes. Palpation for any nodules around the umbilicus should also be performed. An abdominal mass and/or hepatomegaly may be palpated. Enlarged lymph nodes and hepatomegaly indicate the need for biopsy. A large ovarian mass or a large shelf of metastatic deposits may be felt on pelvic or rectal examination. If an obstruction exists in the pyloric area, peristaltic activity moving in a left-to-right direction may be detected. Advanced gastric cancer can result in anemia and jaundice.

### Diagnostic studies

Any signs and symptoms suggestive of gastric cancer should be investigated by diagnostic procedures. Upper endoscopic gastroduodenoscopy (EGD) is now considered the study of choice to establish a diagnosis of gastric cancer. Biopsy and brushings for cytology can be performed at the same time with an accuracy rate of greater than 90%.[89,118] Direct visualization of the esophagus, stomach, and duodenum during EGD can provide important information about the extent of disease. The tumor size, location, morphology, extent of spread, and any other mucosal abnormalities can be evaluated. Usually, six to ten biopsy samples need to be obtained to yield an accurate diagnosis.[119] Linitus plastica is a gastric tumor that is difficult to diagnose endoscopically because mucosal abnormalities are not obvious. The diagnosis of linitus plastica may be suspected if the stomach fails to distend normally when insufflated with air during endoscopy.[120]

Flexible endoscopic gastroscopy is more comfortable for the individual and less traumatic to the gastrointestinal tissues. Topical anesthetics, analgesics, or sedatives (conscious sedation) are administered to facilitate endoscopic instrumentation and to make the individual more comfortable. Nursing measures should be employed to prevent aspiration or trauma for two to four hours following the procedure. The individual receives nothing to eat or drink until the gag reflex returns. Hoarseness from throat irritation can be relieved by lozenges or warm saline gargles after the effects of anesthesia dissipate. The individual should be observed closely in the first few hours for signs of perforation: abdominal pain or distention, fever, dyspnea, cyanosis, or subcutaneous crepitus.

A double-contrast upper gastrointestinal series will reveal the mucosal pattern, character of mobility, distensibility, and flexibility of the stomach wall. Filling defects and rigidity of walls suggest malignant involvement. Following radiographic examinations involving barium, care must be taken to administer laxatives to prevent barium impaction. CT scanning is useful in defining tumor extension and systemic metastases.[121]

EUS has been used to accurately stage gastric cancers. The depth of invasion of the tumor and the presence of lymph nodes can be estimated using this technique. The instruments for EUS still need to be refined to allow passage through small diameters such as those found in gastroesophageal strictures.[89] CT scan and EUS are presently used as complementary tests to enhance staging of gastric cancers. Laparotomy for staging may also be considered. Tissue diagnosis can also be established from easily accessible nodular metastases such as those found around the umbilicus or in peripheral lymph nodes.

Laboratory analyses include hematologic profiles, which may reveal anemia resulting from gradual blood loss in both gastric cancer and chronic gastric ulcer. Malignancy is highly probable when there is a chronic unresponsive gastric ulcer, a gastric ulcer on the greater curvature of the stomach, obstruction in the presence of an ulcer, or achlorhydria and positive cytological findings.

## Prognostic indicators

Karyometric studies of DNA content have correlated high-ploidy gastric tumors with a higher incidence of lymphatic and vascular invasion.[122] Several tumor markers have been investigated (CA 50, CEA, tissue polypeptide antigen [TPA]), but none has proved to be significant for clinical practice.[123]

The Japanese have led in the early diagnosis and radical surgical treatment for gastric cancer. Their survival statistics are consistently better for individuals with nodal metastases compared with like individuals in the United States. Strong predictors of outcome in gastric cancer have been shown to be lymph node metastases and the number of positive lymph nodes at the time of surgery.[124]

## Classification and Staging

Treatment planning ensues once a diagnosis is confirmed and the extent of involvement is known. The prognosis and treatment plan depend on the stage of the disease and the general well-being of the individual. The American Joint Committee for Cancer Staging and End-Results Reporting has established and adopted the TNM classification system listed in Table 38-3.

**TABLE 38-3** TNM Classification for Gastric Carcinoma

| PRIMARY TUMOR (T) | |
|---|---|
| TX | Primary tumor cannot be assessed |
| T0 | No evidence of primary tumor |
| Tis | Carcinoma in situ: intraepithelial tumor without invasion of the lamina propria |
| T1 | Tumor invades lamina propria or submucosa |
| T2 | Tumor invades the muscularis propria or the subserosa |
| T3 | Tumor penetrates the serosa (visceral peritoneum) without invasion of adjacent structures |
| T4 | Tumor invades adjacent structures |

| REGIONAL LYMPH NODES (N) | |
|---|---|
| NX | Regional lymph node(s) cannot be assessed |
| N0 | No regional lymph node metastasis |
| N1 | Metastasis in perigastric lymph node(s) within 3 cm of the edge of the primary tumor |
| N2 | Metastasis in perigastric lymph node(s) more than 3 cm from the edge of the primary tumor, or in lymph nodes along the left gastric, common hepatic, splenic, or celiac arteries |

| DISTANT METASTASIS (M) | |
|---|---|
| MX | Presence of distant metastasis cannot be assessed |
| M0 | No distant metastasis |
| M1 | Distant metastasis |

| STAGE GROUPING | | | |
|---|---|---|---|
| Stage 0 | Tis | N0 | M0 |
| Stage IA | T1 | N0 | M0 |
| Stage IB | T1 | N1 | M0 |
| | T2 | N0 | M0 |
| Stage II | T1 | N2 | M0 |
| | T2 | N1 | M0 |
| | T3 | N0 | M0 |
| Stage IIIA | T2 | N2 | M0 |
| | T3 | N1 | M0 |
| | T4 | N0 | M0 |
| Stage IIIB | T3 | N2 | M0 |
| | T4 | N1 | M0 |
| Stage IV | T4 | N2 | M0 |
| | Any T | Any N | M1 |

From Beahrs OH, Henson DE, Hutter RVP, et al (eds): *American Joint Committee on Cancer: Manual for Staging of Cancer* (ed 4). Philadelphia, Lippincott, 1992.

## Therapeutic Approaches and Nursing Care

Prior to initiation of a treatment plan, the individual and family should receive a thorough explanation of the anticipated course and expected outcomes. The overall plan of therapy for gastric cancer depends on the stage of the disease and current advances in surgery, radiotherapy, and chemotherapy.

Localized gastric carcinomas are treated with aggressive surgery alone or in combination with chemotherapy or radiotherapy for curative intent. Approximately 50% of individuals are candidates for curative resection.

Advanced tumors that are partially resectable, unresectable, or disseminated are treated with combination therapy including surgery and chemotherapy, with or without radiotherapy, and palliative surgery. Palliative procedures such as esophagojejunostomy or partial gastric resection alleviate obstructive tumors and restore intestinal continuity. If the individual cannot medically withstand or elects not to have such a procedure, less traumatic palliative procedures may be done such as a bypass gastrojejunostomy or insertion of a percutaneous jejunal feeding tube. Combinations of chemotherapeutic agents have produced transient improvements with advanced tumors.[89] Despite advances in both operative and postoperative management, overall survival rates are still low.

### Surgery

Surgery is the only treatment modality that can potentially cure localized gastric cancer. It is also the most effective approach for palliation.[125] Definitive or palliative gastrectomy should always be considered, even in individuals with known metastatic disease. Consideration for surgery is given to any individual with a good performance status and no major medical contraindications. Issues that should be weighed by health care providers and the individual considering surgery include morbidity, postoperative rehabilitation, and potential nutritional problems.[97]

Measures to prepare an individual for surgery include correction of fluid and electrolyte imbalances, correction of anemia from chronic blood loss, and attention to nutritional status. Weight loss, emaciation, and malnutrition can adversely affect therapy and require aggressive intervention. Improvement of the nutritional status of the individual with gastric cancer by enteral nutrition is preferred.

Controversy exists among proponents of radical surgical approaches to cure gastric cancer and those who support a more conservative resection. The cure rates with both surgical approaches are comparable, but there are differences in operative mortality and surgical morbidity that need ongoing investigation.[126,127] The choice of surgical procedure is based on location and extent of disease.

Gastric cancers should not be considered unresectable or incurable based on the size of the tumor. Some researchers have achieved cure with resection of extensive lesions.[128] The types of surgical approaches for gastric cancer are total gastrectomy, radical subtotal gastrectomy, and proximal subtotal gastrectomy. The benefits from extended lymph node resection, total gastrectomy for tumors of the body or antrum of the stomach, and prophylactic splenectomy are being investigated.[89]

***Total gastrectomy*** A total gastrectomy may be performed for a resectable lesion located in the midportion or body of the stomach. Linitus plastica is usually treated with a total gastrectomy because of the extensive involvement of the gastric wall. The entire stomach is removed en bloc, along with supporting mesentery and lymph nodes. The esophagus is anastomosed to the jejunum. A thoracic approach is sometimes necessary to perform the esophagojejunostomy. Pneumonia, infection, anastomotic leak, hemorrhage, and reflux aspiration are possible complications. Overall mortality rates are 10%–15% for individuals who have a total gastrectomy.[128] The Japanese have been proponents of a more radical resection that includes an extended lymph node dissection and extended regional resection.[91,129]

***Radical subtotal gastrectomy*** Lesions located in the middle and distal portions of the stomach are treated by radical subtotal gastrectomy. A Billroth I or Billroth II operation will be performed. A Billroth I, or gastroduodenostomy, involves resection of the distal stomach, pylorus, first portion of the duodenum, and supporting circulatory and lymph vessels. The remaining stomach is anastomosed to the duodenum (Figure 38-5). The Billroth I involves a limited amount of resection, and as a result generally produces lower cure rates than a Billroth II. A Billroth I is usually selected if the individual is debilitated and needs restricted intraoperative time.

A Billroth II is a wider resection that includes about 75% of the stomach, thereby decreasing the possibility of nodal or metastatic recurrence. A Billroth II involves removal of the antrum, pylorus, first portion of the duodenum, supporting circulatory structures, and all visible

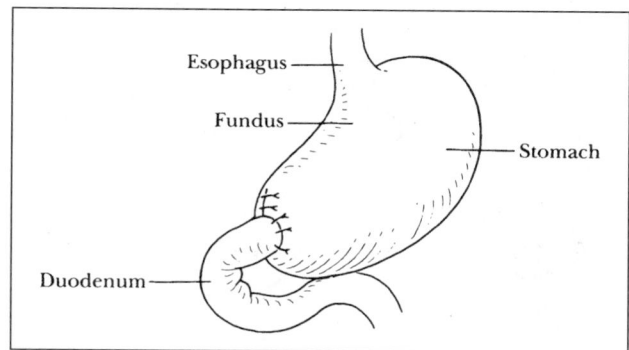

**FIGURE 38-5**  A Billroth I, or gastroduodenostomy, involves resection of the proximal duodenum, distal stomach, pylorus, and supporting structures.

and palpable lymph nodes. The remaining stomach is anastomosed end-to-side to the jejunum. The duodenal stump is oversewn with sutures (Figure 38-6).

Gastric emptying is altered by the Billroth I and II procedures. Potential complications and resultant sequelae are the same as with all postgastrectomy syndromes: dumping syndrome, nausea, vomiting, diarrhea, steatorrhea, weight loss, vitamin deficiency, and anastomotic leak. There is also a chance of duodenal stump leak following a Billroth II procedure.

***Proximal subtotal gastrectomy***  A proximal subtotal gastrectomy may be performed for a resectable tumor located in the proximal portion of the stomach or cardia. In some cases a total gastrectomy and distal esophagectomy will be selected for a more extensive resection. Following resection of the stomach and a portion of the esophagus, the esophagus is anastomosed to the duodenum or jejunum. Potential complications include pneumonia, anastomotic leak, infection, reflux aspiration, and esophagitis.[130]

***Surgical palliation***  Unfortunately, many individuals with gastric cancer are not candidates for curative resection. Most individuals with advanced gastric cancer have symptoms that significantly affect their quality of life and require palliative intervention. Obstruction, bleeding, and pain are common problems. Gastric perforation can also result in the need for emergency surgical intervention.[130]

Resection is the most effective palliative treatment for advanced gastric cancer if the individual is a suitable candidate for the procedure.[125] Although the survival time with palliative surgery is disappointing, it appears to be longer than without resection.[130] Relief of gastrointestinal symptoms, such as vomiting, can be achieved with a palliative resection.[131] Palliative surgery may increase the effectiveness of adjuvant therapy.[132] Placement of an esophageal stent can restore the individual's ability to swallow, particularly liquids, and also help prevent aspiration of saliva. Palliative procedures such as gastric or esophageal bypass, gastrostomy, or jejunostomy temporarily alleviate symptoms but do not prolong life expectancy.[133,134] Laser therapy has been used for palliation of unresectable obstructing lesions of the esophagus and the gastroesophageal junction with satisfactory results.[135]

***Postoperative care***  Nursing measures for the person with gastric cancer who undergoes surgical resection do not differ from those for other individuals who undergo gastric surgery. The nurse must be acutely aware of the preoperative status of the individual and must employ nursing measures necessary to maintain or improve the person's preoperative condition. Pneumonia, infection, anastomotic leak, hemorrhage, and reflux aspiration are frequent complications following radical gastric surgery. Occasionally, an individual will experience bezoar formation (ingested fibrous food clumping), causing gastric outlet obstruction. A bezoar can be dissolved with enzymes, such as papain, or broken up by endoscopic intervention.

Dumping syndrome is a potential sequela of subtotal gastrectomy and total gastrectomy that affects many but not all individuals. Small, frequent feedings of low-carbohydrate, high-fat, high-protein foods are recommended. It is important to restrict liquids for 30 minutes before and after a meal to avoid the effects of dumping syndrome.[136] Antispasmodics and antiperistaltics can reduce diarrhea. Vitamin $B_{12}$ deficiency will occur in an individual with a total gastrectomy. Monthly parenteral replacement therapy is necessary to prevent pernicious anemia.

### Radiation

Gastric adenocarcinomas are generally radiosensitive. Radiation therapy is somewhat prohibitive because the stomach lies deep in the abdomen and tumor is often widely disseminated. Dose-limited organs, such as stomach, liver, kidney, and spinal cord, restrict the use of radiotherapy. Radiation therapy can be administered as adjuvant therapy along with chemotherapy and surgery. It is useful for treating individuals with inoperable cancer or with locally advanced or recurrent local disease. Great care must be taken in treating individuals after gastrectomy because they often suffer from nutritional deficiency that may be aggravated by the anorexia, nausea, vomiting, abdominal cramps, and diarrhea produced by radiotherapy. Excessive weight loss is the main dose-limiting toxicity that can delay or halt treatment.[137]

Radiotherapy is used to augment locoregional control of residual or unresectable gastric cancer. Multimodality approaches using radiation and chemotherapy for individuals with unresectable disease have been documented to improve survival compared with treatment with either radiotherapy or chemotherapy alone.[89,137] The sequence of administering radiotherapy and chemotherapy could

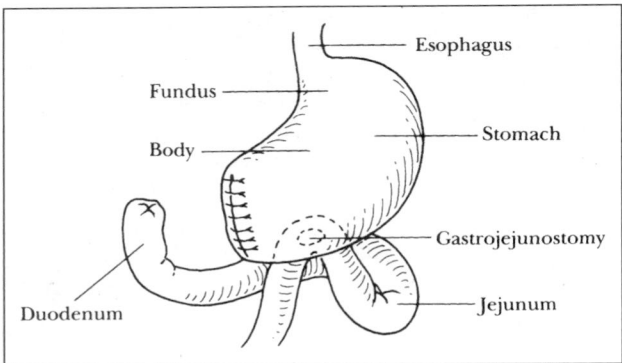

**FIGURE 38-6**  A Billroth II, or gastrojejunostomy, is a wider resection than the Billroth I. Up to 75% of the stomach can be resected. The remaining stomach is then anastomosed end-to-side to the jejunum.

take advantage of any radiosensitization effect, diminished repopulation between treatments, or synergistic effect.[138] Radiotherapy may contribute to the palliation of symptoms and prolongation of survival in individuals with gastric cancer.

Intraoperative radiotherapy (IORT) has been used extensively in Japan.[137,139] The advantages of delivering radiotherapy intraoperatively are the direct visualization of the site to be irradiated and the opportunity to move the radiosensitive tissues away from the field during the radiation.[139] The disadvantages of this treatment approach are the need for special equipment and a specially prepared operating room. Extensive professional collaboration is required. IORT is provided by only a few institutions in the United States. Its role in the management of gastric cancer has not been studied well enough to know the full impact of this approach.

### Chemotherapy

Interest in chemotherapy has increased in the last two decades, since a number of therapy regimens appear to have significant activity in gastric cancer. No specific chemotherapeutic regimen alone has been able to establish a clear impact on survival from gastric cancer. Single agents (5-FU, doxorubicin, cisplatin, etoposide, and mitomycin C) have been studied, but combination drug therapy appears to be superior. Single agents typically produce response rates in 20% of cases, whereas combination chemotherapy can result in 30%–50% response rates.[140,141]

The combination regimens used most commonly are FAM (5-FU, doxorubicin mitomycin C); FAP (5-FU, doxorubicin, platinol); FAMTX (5-FU, doxorubicin, leucovorin); and EAP (etoposide, doxorubicin, cisplatin).[141–143] Other drugs used in combination regimens include cisplatin, its analogues, and nitrosoureas.[144,145] Toxicities depend on the drug and dose. Regimens involving combination chemotherapy are presently a major focus of investigation. Alternative methods of delivery are being investigated, such as intrahepatic and intraperitoneal administration of chemotherapeutic agents.[146,147]

Neoadjuvant chemotherapy has been considered in the treatment of gastric cancer to control the primary tumor and distant metastases as well as to identify those individuals who could benefit from postoperative chemotherapy. Potential problems with this modality include the emergence of resistant tumor cells, a delay in local control, and uncertainty as to extent of surgical resection. Individuals who respond to neoadjuvant chemotherapy may then refuse surgery or irradiation.[89,137]

Combining chemotherapy and biotherapy has little therapeutic benefit.[148] Survival time has been increased when chemotherapy is used in combination with surgery or radiotherapy.[149] At present, chemotherapy is not standard clinical treatment for gastric cancer as the response rates are low. Therapy regimens that are active in individuals with advanced disease are needed.

## Symptom Management and Supportive Care

Advanced gastric cancer can result in an individual's rapid deterioration. Medical and nursing management is aimed at controlling symptoms and maintaining optimal function. As gastric cancer advances, nutrition becomes a serious problem, because of disruption of stomach continuity or stomach dysfunction. Lack of gastric secretions leads to enzyme and nutrient deficiencies. The resulting malnutrition decreases the individual's ability to withstand therapy, fight infection, and perform self-care activities. Nutritional surveillance and aggressive approaches to maintaining a high level of nutrition are nursing priorities. The reader is referred to chapter 24 for suggestions on management of nutritional problems. From the time of diagnosis until death due to gastric cancer, nutrition will be the most challenging management problem.

When gastric cancer spreads to the most common metastatic sites (regional lymph nodes, intraperitoneal cavity, liver, pancreas, lung, and bone), the manifestations of disease in those areas will require the anticipatory and symptomatic nursing measures discussed in the chapters on specific manifestations of cancer. Individuals with gastric cancer commonly die of bronchopneumonia or lung abscess secondary to malnutrition or immobility. Other causes of death seen with gastric cancer are deep vein thrombosis, pulmonary emboli, anastomotic rupture, or a second primary tumor.[126]

Many individuals and their families feel a strong sense of guilt and negligence if the individual has delayed seeking medical attention or has self-medicated for any length of time. The nurse can support the individual and family by dispelling misconceptions and promoting a realistic sense of hope.

## Continuity of Care: Nursing Challenges

The nurse provides care and support to the individual with gastric cancer. Providing information and clarifying and explaining the multiple treatment modalities can help the individual and the family understand options and make informed decisions. The nurse can help the individual and the family deal with physical problems and obtain help for psychosocial and economic issues. Good nurse-to-nurse communication across settings can ensure a smooth transition for care because individuals with gastric cancer usually receive combined therapies. A thorough understanding of the entire continuum of care for an individual with gastric cancer is necessary for all members of the health care team. No matter what treatments are chosen, the nurse needs to advocate for the individual. The nurse constantly assesses the individual with gastric cancer for signs and symptoms of problems to help prevent or treat complications that may hinder treatment. Finally, compassionate care for the individual with terminal gastric cancer can help ease the pain, physically and emotionally, of such a devastating cancer.

# LIVER TUMORS

## Introduction

Hepatocellular cancer is one of the ten most common cancers in the world. Liver cancer is the main cause of cancer death in Africa and Asia.[150] In the United States, primary liver cancer is relatively uncommon in children and adults. Liver cancers have unusual clinical and pathological features; they are commonly diagnosed at an advanced stage, negating curative surgery. Furthermore, any surgery may be impeded by the association of the cancer with cirrhosis and reduced hepatic reserve. Many critical questions about this disease remain unanswered. At present, no specific treatment effectively controls this aggressive malignancy, and the outlook remains poor. Early detection is critical, along with advances in diagnosis and combined treatment modalities.

## Epidemiology

An unusual epidemiological aspect of liver cancer is its geographic distribution. While the incidence of liver cancer is low in North America and Europe, there is a high incidence of the disease in China, Korea, and Africa below the Sahara.[151] Liver cancer is the most common cause of death in males worldwide. In all populations, the incidence rate increases with age.[152,153] In regions where there is a high incidence of the disease, there is a marked shift toward the younger age-group, with the average age being 40–50 years.[154] In Taiwan it is reported as the fifth most common malignancy of children.[155] In contrast, the average age of onset is 60–70 years in the United States. Approximately 19,900 new cases and 15,200 deaths from primary liver cancer are seen in the United States each year.[1]

## Etiology

Hepatocellular carcinomas are associated with environmental and hereditary factors. A close relationship has been identified between liver cancer and infection with hepatitis B and hepatitis C viruses. Viral hepatitis infection causes liver damage and cirrhosis and appears to increase the risk of developing liver cancer.[156–159] There is a suggested carcinogenic interaction between hepatitis B virus and transforming growth factor-alpha, which is expressed at high levels in individuals with liver cancer.[160]

Aflatoxins, produced by the molds *Aspergillus flavus* and *Aspergillus parasiticus,* are among the naturally occurring substances that have become suspect as etiologic agents.[161,162] Aflatoxin B occurs in foods and grains stored under humid conditions. It has the highest potential among the aflatoxins to be a toxin and a carcinogen.[163]

There is a close correlation with hepatocellular carcinoma and cirrhosis. The macronodular cirrhosis associated with chronic hepatitis B virus is a major risk factor for liver cancer.[164] It is also thought that cirrhosis is an independent risk factor, not requiring hepatitis B infection to be present. Studies show that cirrhosis clearly increases the risk of liver cancer in the individual infected with hepatitis B virus. The risk of hepatocellular carcinoma is much lower with the micronodular cirrhosis of alcoholic liver disease. Alcoholic cirrhosis is a common risk factor for cancer in the United States.[165,166] It is suggested that the chronic liver injury and subsequent continuous regeneration associated with cirrhosis precipitate a loss of normal cellular controls, eventually leading to liver neoplasia.

Ingestion of estrogens, androgens, and oral contraceptives has been reported to be associated with liver tumors. Short-term use of these hormones appears to have no association.[167–170] Thorotrast, a radiographic contrast agent no longer in use, may have produced progressive liver damage, which after a latent period of approximately 20 years may develop into liver cancer.[171] Metabolic conditions such as hemochromatosis, alpha$_1$-antitrypsin deficiency, porphyria cutanea tarda, tyrosinemia, glycogen storage diseases, and Wilson's disease may also increase the risk.[172–174] However, the association between these factors and primary liver cancer is unclear and the evidence is not convincing. The association between etiologic factors and the development of liver cancer is still being investigated but is hindered by the limited number of cases. Environmental, clinical, and genetic factors have all been suggested. It is hoped that further studies will provide definitive explanations.

## Prevention, Screening, Early Detection Programs

Convincing evidence linking liver cancer with chronic hepatitis B and hepatitis C viruses, aflatoxin exposure, and alcoholic cirrhosis indicates that preventive measures to avoid these factors could reduce the incidence of hepatocellular cancer. Efforts are under way in parts of China to reduce or eliminate hepatocellular carcinoma by aggressive programs to vaccinate newborns against hepatitis B virus.[175] It will take many years to observe a decrease in the incidence and measure the effect of these programs.[176] The present recommendation in the United States to vaccinate all newborns against hepatitis B virus may prevent future cases of hepatocellular carcinoma.

Prevention of hepatitis B and hepatitis C infection is the ideal measure. But when an individual is infected with the virus, the administration of an antiviral therapy to prevent or reverse the chronic situation is the only option. Interferon therapy has been useful in the treatment of these individuals,[176–178] but it is far more effective to prevent the infection through vaccination programs or through public health measures.

Health education is important in high-risk populations. Improvement in food and grain storage can reduce exposure to aflatoxins. Hepatitis transmission can be reduced with the use of sterile needles for mass immunization programs. This precaution is not practiced in many countries. Routine sensitive screens of blood products are needed to reduce the incidence of posttransfusion hepatitis. Educating children and adults about the many risks related to chronic alcohol consumption is also needed.[163]

The National Cancer Institute (NCI) held a workshop on screening for hepatocellular carcinoma to determine which populations might benefit. Those areas with a high prevalence for hepatitis B virus infection represented the group most in need of screening. In the United States those with the greatest risk are hepatitis B–positive males with a family history of the disease, individuals older than 45 years, or individuals who have cirrhosis.[179]

Ultrasound (US) and serum alfa-fetoprotein (AFP) tests are inexpensive and relatively effective tools to screen for hepatocellular carcinoma in high-risk populations. Elevated serum AFP levels in high-risk populations have detected small liver tumors, increasing the number of surgically resectable lesions and improving survival rates. In North America and Europe this approach is not useful due to the low incidence of hepatocellular carcinoma. It is recommended that regions of the world with moderate to high risk use tests of serum AFP level combined with US to screen for primary cancer of the liver.[180] Studies have shown that US is more accurate than AFP levels in detecting small tumors (<3 cm).[181]

Even if high-risk individuals are screened as recommended by the NCI, any changes that will affect outcomes of hepatocellular cancer will more likely come from prevention strategies, including universal hepatitis B virus vaccination.[182]

## Pathophysiology

Tumors of the liver may be a primary cancer of the liver or secondary tumors that have metastasized from other sites. One of the most important issues in the diagnosis and treatment of liver cancer is to differentiate whether the cancer is a primary tumor or a metastatic lesion.

### Cellular characteristics

***Primary liver cancer*** Most primary tumors of the liver are adenocarcinomas of two cell types: about 90% are hepatocellular carcinomas arising from the liver cells; about 7% are cholangiocarcinomas arising from the bile ducts; and a very small proportion are hepatoblastomas, angiosarcomas, or sarcomas.[156,183] Another important variant is fibrolamellar carcinoma, which usually presents as a large, solitary mass arising in a noncirrhotic liver, and tends to occur in younger individuals, with a slight female predominance. Fibrolamellar cancer has a more indolent course, is more frequently resectable, and has a better prognosis than most primary liver cancer.[184]

The macroscopic appearance of primary hepatocellular carcinoma is either nodular, massive, or diffuse. The *nodular* type consists of multiple, similarly sized, widely dispersed clusters of cells. The *massive* type often has a single dominant large mass with associated satellite nodules. The *diffuse* form is characterized by an extensive pattern of infiltration that may involve the entire liver. All three forms of hepatocellular carcinoma originate mainly in the right lobe of the liver. The tumor may be multicentric in origin, as commonly seen in cirrhotic livers, or it may start with a single focus that subsequently develops satellite lesions. Hepatocellular carcinomas generally are soft and highly vascular, which can lead to rupture and hemorrhage. Parts of the liver may be dull gray or green as a result of the presence of bile. There may also be areas of necrosis and hemorrhage. Cholangiocarcinomas also exhibit nodular or diffuse forms but usually appear as a solitary grayish white mass. The firm, fibrous tumor may secrete mucin but does not form bile. Cholangiocarcinomas tend to invade surrounding parenchyma in a disorderly, irregular manner and tend to metastasize late.

Liver tumors are often well-differentiated lesions with clearly defined margins and cells that are larger than normal parenchymal cells. About 50% of individuals with primary liver cancer will not develop extrahepatic spread of tumor.[34] When metastases occur, they usually affect the diaphragm and neighboring tissues or the portal and/or hepatic veins. Regional lymph node metastasis is uncommon—a definite characteristic of liver cancer. Tumor encapsulation and longer doubling time may be used as indicators of survival.[185,186]

***Secondary liver cancer*** The liver is a repository for metastatic deposits from nearly all sites and is 20 times more likely to harbor a metastatic deposit than a primary liver cancer.[187] Metastases to the liver usually are from the following high-incidence sites: lung, breast, kidney, and the intestinal tract (gallbladder, extrahepatic bile ducts, pancreas, stomach, colon, rectum).[188] Metastases may occur as a single mass, but metastatic deposits more often are multiple masses in the liver. Spread within the rest of the liver is through the extensive venous system. Metastatic tumors in the liver usually indicate that the primary cancer is incurable. However, if a localized metastasis in the liver can be resected or controlled with chemotherapy, then the primary tumor can be aggressively pursued. It is uncommon for a cancer to metastasize to a cirrhotic liver, possibly because the tissue damage precludes a favorable environment for metastases.[189]

### Progression of disease

As liver cancer advances, serious complications arise and multiple body systems are affected. Liver failure and hemorrhage have been cited as the cause of death in about 50% of individuals with liver cancer.[190] It is postulated that if the portal vein becomes obstructed rapidly, as occurs with tumor emboli, there is insufficient time for the collateral branches of the hepatic circulatory system to compensate. As a result, the tamponade effect can lead to necrosis, rupture, and hemorrhage. Esophageal varices and unrelenting ascites are common sequelae of either primary or secondary liver cancer.

Because of the late onset of definitive signs, liver cancer can be far advanced by the time of diagnosis. The prognosis is poor, with an overall five-year survival rate of about 5%. If the disease is untreated, death usually occurs within six to eight weeks following diagnosis. The cause of death from liver cancer most often is pneumonia, malnutrition, thromboemboli, hepatic failure, or hemorrhage.[171,190]

### Patterns of spread

Liver cancer tends to advance by direct extension within and around the liver. The tumor will enlarge within the lobules that have been weakened by pressure and derangement of the blood supply. Venous invasion commonly accounts for the multinodular appearance of hepatocellular carcinoma. The tumor grows along the veins as a solid mass to distal parts of the liver. About 50% of individuals with liver cancer will have distant metastases to regional lymph nodes, lungs, bone, adrenal glands, and brain.[156,171]

Normal liver tissue receives its blood supply from both the hepatic artery and the portal vein and drains by way of the hepatic vein. Liver tumors typically alter the pattern of blood flow within the liver. Tumors receive their blood supply almost exclusively from the hepatic artery and drain from the hepatic vein.[191] Within the liver the tumor may spread by emboli or direct permeation of the hepatic and portal vein, resulting in rapid spread of the tumor throughout the liver. Portal vein occlusion is common.[156]

## Clinical Manifestations

The natural history of carcinoma of the liver is insidious. The tumor can grow to huge proportions before symptoms appear. In adults the most common presenting complaint is right upper quadrant abdominal pain that is not severe, but rather dull and aching. The pain may radiate to the right scapula. The continuous pain may become more troublesome, prevent sleep, and be aggravated if the individual lies on the right side or experiences jolting movements. Profound, progressive weakness and fatigue are characteristic of liver cancer. Fullness in the epigastrium, especially after meals, and constipation or diarrhea are common manifestations. Anorexia and weight loss are indicators of advanced disease.[192]

Mild jaundice may be present, caused either by obstruction from massive liver involvement by tumor compressing major intrahepatic bile ducts or by hepatocellular dysfunction.[192] Cirrhosis is found in 30%–70% of

persons with hepatocellular carcinoma.[171] On palpation, the liver is an enlarged, hard, nodular mass; a raised, protruding tumor occasionally can be felt. Enlargement of the liver may be diffuse or limited to one lobe, usually the right. Liver cancer should be suspected in all persons with cirrhosis who experience a sudden or unexpected deterioration in health.

Ascites and signs of portal hypertension that result from portal vein compression frequently accompany advanced disease. Hematemesis secondary to esophageal varices or tumor invasion of the stomach can occur. A variety of paraneoplastic manifestations may occur, such as hypoglycemia, erythrocytosis, hypercalcemia, leukocytosis, carcinoid-like syndrome, porphyria, and coagulation abnormalities.[183]

## Assessment

Primary liver cancer is silent for a long period before it produces signs and symptoms that prompt the individual to seek medical attention. He or she may be treated initially for a disorder that mimics liver cancer, such as gastritis. Primary liver cancer must be distinguished from secondary liver cancer due to metastases. The only definitive diagnostic tool is tissue diagnosis. Unfortunately, the risk of hemorrhage following needle biopsy is significant; therefore, noninvasive measures are relied on heavily. The choice of therapy will be based on the location and extent of tumor involvement, whether extrahepatic spread has occurred, and the individual's general condition.

### Patient and family history

The most significant information gathered from the individual relates to any exposure to the etiologic factors that would predispose to liver cancer. A history of cirrhosis, hepatitis B or hepatitis C virus infection, or exposure to mycotoxins or other agents that cause chronic liver failure will aid in confirming the diagnosis. A hereditary disorder that causes liver damage may also contribute to making a definitive diagnosis.

### Physical examination

A complete physical examination usually reveals a painful, enlarged liver and such manifestations as ascites, edema, an audible arterial bruit, jaundice, and splenomegaly.[171] Muscle wasting related to anorexia and weight loss can be found on examination. A persistent temperature elevation may be related to tumor necrosis and release of pyrogenic compounds.[192] Endocrine changes, such as menstrual disorders, testicular atrophy, and gynecomastia, may be observed.

### Diagnostic studies

A simple radiograph of the abdomen may establish hepatomegaly and displacement or deformity of adjoining structures. An upper gastrointestinal series may show stomach displacement by an enlarged liver. Plain films are useful in advanced disease but are not useful for early diagnosis.

US of the abdomen, CT scan of the abdomen and lungs, and MRI are noninvasive techniques used in the diagnostic evaluation of liver cancer. These three studies are complementary in the diagnosis and staging of primary liver cancer and metastatic disease because no one study is 100% accurate. US is safe, portable, and relatively inexpensive. It can detect masses and help determine the extent of invasion of the vasculature of the liver as primary liver cancer has a propensity for vascular invasion. With advances in Doppler imaging and intravenous US contrast agents, the ability to detect and precisely diagnose hepatic lesions may be improved.[193] CT scan, especially with contrast, is able to demonstrate small lesions and vascular derangements as well as detecting metastatic disease. CT scan is useful for diagnosing underlying cirrhosis associated with a liver tumor. This study is also helpful in assessing response to therapy by tumor volumetrics.[194] MRI is more accurate than CT scan in detecting and delineating liver tumors, but CT scan is more readily available, less expensive, and better for staging disease outside the liver.[195]

Radionuclide scanning is an effective noninvasive technique for outlining primary and metastatic tumors of the liver. It is unlike most other imaging modalities, as it uses specific physiological and biochemical properties of each pathological entity that affects the liver. Hepatic scintigraphy is widely available, noninvasive, and relatively low in cost; it is proving to be a powerful adjunct to other imaging techniques in the evaluation of liver masses. Small lesions (<2.5 cm in diameter) may be missed by the photoscanning device. The single-photon emission computed tomography (SPECT) imaging equipment has increased the rate of detection. SPECT and US are frequently complementary techniques, each identifying lesions not detected by the other. Positron emission tomography (PET) scan is a newer, more specialized technique that may prove to be the most useful.[196] Immunoscintigraphy is another new and promising diagnostic technique. Monoclonal and polyclonal antibodies labeled with [131]I have been successful in detecting primary and metastatic deposits of primary liver cancer.[197]

Selective hepatic arteriography is the best way to delineate hepatic artery anatomy and the presence of vascular invasion or encasement to plan surgical resection, arterial catheter placement for regional infusion, or chemoembolization. Combining CT scan with an arteriogram (CTA), which requires bolus infusion of contrast medium into the hepatic artery during a dynamic CT scan of the liver, can help detect lesions less than 1 cm in diameter. CT arterial portography (CTAP) requires injection of contrast medium into the superior mesenteric artery followed by a dynamic CT scan of the liver to detect small primary or metastatic tumors, which are occult on conventional CT scan or MRI.[198,199] Any arteriography is associated with increased risks due to the placement of an arterial catheter. These procedures are also time-consuming and expensive.

The individual undergoing arteriography must have any coagulopathy corrected before the invasive procedure. The individual must be monitored carefully after the procedure for signs of hemorrhage from a weakened or perforated vessel. Arteriograms may be done as outpatient procedures; therefore, discharge teaching and written instructions for any signs and symptoms of complications must be reviewed with the individual and the person who has come to assist the individual home after conscious sedation.

*Laboratory studies* The hematologic profiles and liver function tests of individuals with localized primary cancer who do not have cirrhosis will show normal findings. In the absence of cirrhosis, tumor growth can extensively involve parenchyma before liver function is impaired. Liver enzyme levels and liver function tests are not definitive diagnostic aids but can alert the clinician to a possible tumor. In advanced cases of liver cancer, decreases in platelet and white blood cell counts may signal portal hypertension and associated hypersplenism. Prothrombin time, partial thromboplastin time, and albumin levels reflect hepatic synthetic function and should be measured.

AFP is a tumor marker that is elevated in the serum of 70%–90% of individuals with primary hepatocellular carcinoma.[156,171,183] AFP disappears one to two weeks after successful resection of hepatocellular cancer. A reappearance of AFP can indicate recurrence. Serial monitoring of AFP levels and carcinoembryonic antigen (CEA) is used to follow response to treatment or to screen for recurrent disease following hepatic resection. Other serum tumor markers are being investigated with liver cancer, such as alpha-L-fucosidase.[200] Not all liver cancers secrete AFP, so other early indicators are needed. Elevated levels of CEA are not indicative of primary liver cancer but may signify metastatic involvement. Colon cancer often metastasizes to the liver and will produce elevated CEA levels.

*Biopsy* Biopsy is required to establish a histological diagnosis. Many clinicians feel strongly that needle biopsy should be avoided at all cost if there is a chance for curative resection. They believe that the needle violates the tumor capsule, thereby potentially seeding and spreading the cancer. If a tumor appears to be resectable, tissue can be obtained during surgery, thus avoiding potential problems with bleeding.[201] If the tumor appears to be unresectable, a percutaneous needle biopsy can be performed, usually as a fine-needle aspiration (FNAB) with US or CT scan guidance. Needle biopsy should be performed only on a cooperative individual with normal hemostatic function. The individual must be monitored closely for intra-abdominal hemorrhage following needle biopsy. Potential complications following liver biopsy are hemorrhage, shock, peritonitis, and pneumothorax. This biopsy can also be performed as an outpatient procedure.

The nursing care is directed at careful postprocedure assessment and education regarding potential complications that must be reported to the physician immediately if encountered after discharge.

## Classification and Staging

A staging system has been developed for liver cancer that incorporates tumor size, location within the liver, extent of disease within and external to the liver, and metastatic sites (Table 38-4). The staging system has not been universally accepted but is available for use.

## Therapeutic Approaches and Nursing Care

### Treatment planning

Treatment of liver cancer provides a twofold challenge. First, the limited number of cases of primary liver cancer makes prospective systematic investigation of therapy difficult. Second, the dismal outlook for individuals with liver cancer has led to misconceptions about the effectiveness of various treatments, which have taken years to dispel. Surgery, radiotherapy, and chemotherapy play a significant role in the treatment of both primary and secondary liver cancer. At present, biological and hormonal therapies are being investigated.

The five-year survival rate for individuals with primary liver cancer is less than 2%. However, for individuals with solitary, localized liver cancer, advances in surgery, radiotherapy, and chemotherapy offer hope of cure or palliation. The choice of treatment depends on a number of factors: type and extent of tumor, concomitant diseases, liver function and reserve, individual/family preference, hematologic status, nutritional status, age, and skill of the principal clinicians. Assessment of the individual's learning ability, coping mechanisms, and compliance potential are important, especially if long-term therapy is anticipated.

***Pretreatment therapy*** Prior to the initiation of any therapeutic modality, physiological parameters are examined carefully. Most individuals with primary liver cancer have some degree of anemia, which must be corrected. Efforts are made by the nurse and other health care workers to conserve the individual's energy and to begin instruction on appropriate measures to help minimize the anemia.

Depending on the extent of liver dysfunction produced by tumor involvement, deficits in clotting mechanisms can exist. Vitamin K is administered, fluid and electrolyte imbalances are corrected, and measures to prevent trauma or bleeding are taken.

Vitamins A, C, D, and B complex can be given to reduce the effect of jaundice. Pruritus, which frequently accompanies jaundice, is precipitated by irritation of the

**TABLE 38-4** TNM Classification System for Liver Cancer

| PRIMARY TUMOR (T) | |
|---|---|
| TX | Primary tumor cannot be assessed |
| T0 | No evidence of primary tumor |
| T1 | Solitary tumor 2 cm or less in greatest dimension without vascular invasion |
| T2 | Solitary tumor 2 cm or less in greatest dimension with vascular invasion, *or* Multiple tumors limited to one lobe, none more than 2 cm in greatest dimension without vascular invasion, *or* A solitary tumor more than 2 cm in greatest dimension without vascular invasion |
| T3 | Solitary tumor more than 2 cm in greatest dimension with vascular invasion, *or* Multiple tumors limited to one lobe, none more than 2 cm in greatest dimension, with vascular invasion, *or* Multiple tumors limited to one lobe, any more than 2 cm in greatest dimension, with or without vascular invasion |
| T4 | Multiple tumors in more than one lobe *or* Tumor(s) involve(s) a major branch of portal or hepatic vein(s) |

| REGIONAL LYMPH NODES (N) | |
|---|---|
| NX | Regional lymph nodes cannot be assessed |
| N0 | No regional lymph node metastasis |
| N1 | Regional lymph node metastasis |

| DISTANT METASTASIS (M) | |
|---|---|
| MX | Presence of distant metastasis cannot be assessed |
| M0 | No distant metastasis |
| M1 | Distant metastasis |

| STAGE GROUPING | | | |
|---|---|---|---|
| Stage I | T1 | N0 | M0 |
| Stage II | T2 | N0 | M0 |
| Stage III | T1 | N1 | M0 |
| | T2 | N1 | M0 |
| | T3 | N0, N1 | M0 |
| Stage IVA | T4 | Any N | M0 |
| Stage IVB | Any T | Any N | M1 |

From Beahrs OH, Henson DE, Hutter RVP, et al (eds): *American Joint Committee on Cancer: Manual for Staging of Cancer* (ed 4). Philadelphia, Lippincott, 1992.

cutaneous sensory nerve fibers by accumulated bile salts. Meticulous skin hygiene and efforts to reduce itching are instituted. The use of deodorant soaps should be avoided since they tend to dry skin and intensify pruritus. Relief is sometimes obtained with oil-based lotions, antihistamines, or cholestyramine. The only effective measure for relief of pruritus is resolution of the jaundice.

Most individuals with liver cancer are in a poor nutritional state and benefit from a diet high in proteins and carbohydrates and moderate in fats. If there has been significant weight loss, enteral feedings or total parenteral nutrition may be used to correct the nutritional imbalance. If treatment is expected to adversely affect nutritional status, aggressive nutritional regimens are begun early.

### Objectives of treatment

*Primary liver cancer* Cure is the objective of the therapy if the primary liver tumor is a localized, solitary mass without evidence of regional lymph node involvement or distant metastases. Surgical excision of the primary liver cancer is the only definitive treatment for cure. Only about 25% of individuals with primary liver cancer are candidates for radical resection.[156] Aggressive efforts toward eradicating residual cancer cells and possible micrometastases with adjuvant chemotherapy and radiotherapy usually are initiated.[202]

If the tumor is multicentric, involves a large portion of the liver, or involves extrahepatic areas, control of tumor growth is the objective of therapy. Control can be achieved by surgical resection to remove or debulk the tumor, by radiotherapy, or by specific vascular ligation or cannulation followed by aggressive use of chemotherapeutic agents.[203]

Palliation of the disabling effects of liver cancer may be the objective of treatment for advanced disease. Surgery, chemotherapy, and radiotherapy are used selectively to increase the individual's comfort and quality of life.

*Secondary liver tumors* When metastatic deposits occur in the liver, cure of the primary cancer is difficult. Aggressive therapy is employed if the metastatic deposit is a solitary or well-defined mass in a single lobe of the liver. Treatment of metastatic tumors of the liver may be surgical excision, arterial infusion of chemotherapeutic agents, ligation or embolization of the hepatic artery, radiotherapy, or cryotherapy.[204–208] The aim of aggressive treatment of metastatic tumors in the liver is to control the tumor, increase survival time, and palliate debilitating symptoms such as jaundice, anemia, and pain. An individual with colorectal cancer that has metastasized to the liver is the typical candidate for resection, since the liver usually is the first metastatic site for colorectal tumors.[204,205]

### Surgery

Surgical excision is the most definitive treatment for primary liver tumors and depends mainly on tumor size, location, and the condition of the uninvolved liver.[204] If cirrhosis is present, the surgical risk is directly proportional to the degree of cirrhosis. Current series of liver resections for primary liver cancer show the operative mortality rate is less than 10% as a result of better preoperative evaluation of functioning liver tissue, increased experience of the surgeons, and improved operative techniques.[209]

A hepatic lobectomy can be safely performed if the opposite lobe of the liver appears free of tumor. If cirrhosis is moderately advanced, left lobectomy can be considered; however, right hepatic lobectomy would be difficult and potentially life-threatening. Local resection, US-guided cryosurgery, or laser surgery may be possible.[210–212] Individuals with severe cirrhosis are not candidates for surgery.

Extensive assessment must be done prior to hepatic resection to identify any possible contraindications. In addition to severe cirrhosis, contraindications to major hepatic resection include the following:[171,183]

1. Distant metastases in the lung, bone, or lymph nodes indicate that an attempt at cure or control would likely be futile. Multiple discrete tumor nodules throughout both anatomic lobes would rule out definitive surgery as the treatment of choice.
2. Although not always the case, jaundice could indicate tumor extension or obstruction of the common bile duct. Palliative resection of the tumor can be done to relieve progressive jaundice.
3. Ascites usually indicates liver failure and inability to tolerate a surgical procedure. The ascites may result from tumor cell seeding in the peritoneal cavity and/or cirrhosis. In either case it is preferable to control the ascites medically; surgery could be considered but it is associated with risks.
4. Poor visualization on angiographic studies jeopardizes the certainty with which the surgeon resects the tumor. Because the liver is a highly vascular organ, intraoperative hemorrhage is a great risk in all hepatic surgical procedures.
5. Biochemical changes that indicate poor liver function lower the probability of survival.
6. Involvement of the inferior vena cava and the portal vein bifurcation by tumor makes surgical excision hazardous.

Therefore, if the tumor is localized, solitary, and can be defined anatomically, a wide en bloc surgical excision is the initial treatment of choice for both primary and secondary liver tumors. Greater than three-quarters (80%–85%) of the noncirrhotic liver can be removed safely unless the tumor is in the posterior segment of the right lobe, where the hepatic veins are embedded. Because the hepatic veins can be difficult to isolate, resection is considered a dangerous procedure.[183] Right or left hepatic lobectomy, trisegmentectomy (also called an *extended right lobectomy*), and lateral segmentectomy are the classic liver resections, as seen in Figure 38-7. Partial resections (segmentectomy or nonanatomic wedge resection) may be performed on individuals with isolated, discrete metastases. Individuals with mild cirrhosis may tolerate a partial liver resection. The reader is referred to specific references for detailed information about the techniques of hepatic surgical procedures.[213,214]

Cryosurgery with liquid nitrogen has been employed for local destruction of tumors in individuals with multiple primary or metastatic tumors in both lobes of the liver.[211,212,215] The tumors are destroyed by rapid freezing,

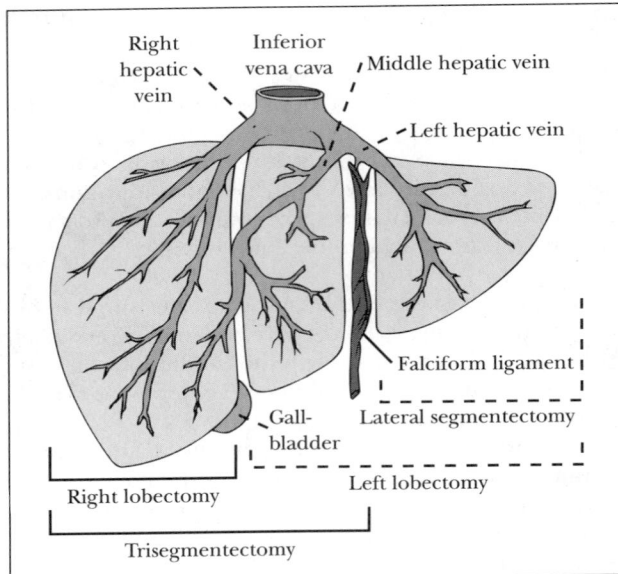

Right hepatic vein

Inferior vena cava

Middle hepatic vein

Left hepatic vein

Falciform ligament

Gall-bladder

Lateral segmentectomy

Right lobectomy

Left lobectomy

Trisegmentectomy

**FIGURE 38-7**  Major hepatic resections for primary liver tumors (with demonstration of hepatic venous drainage). Adapted by permission of *Surgery, Gynecology and Obstetrics*, now known as the *Journal of the American College of Surgeons*.

causing cell death by a combination of mechanisms. Intraoperative US is used to determine the number and location of tumors as well as to follow the freeze-and-thaw cycle, which takes approximately 20 minutes.[216]

Individuals undergoing cryoablation need to understand the risks and benefits of the procedure as well as that of any major abdominal surgery. The individual needs routine preoperative assessment and teaching. Postoperatively, most individuals develop a symptomatic pleural effusion. A mild elevation in white blood cell count and elevated liver function tests (alkaline phosphatase, lactic dehydrogenase, alanine aminotransferase, and aspartate aminotransferase) are common but transient, and usually return to normal by five days after treatment. Temperature elevations to as high as 39 °C are common during the first three to five days following the procedure because of acute tubular necrosis. The most serious complications of hepatic tumor cryoablation include major hemorrhage from the cryoprobe tract, bile duct fistula, hepatic abscess, subphrenic abscess, and renal insufficiency related to myoglobinuria. Nursing interventions are focused on educating the individual and providing emotional and psychosocial support. In addition to routine postoperative nursing care, astute assessment, close hemodynamic monitoring, early detection of potential surgical complications, and promotion of healing are required. Prevention, early recognition, and intervention for complications are important.[217]

Liver transplantation is controversial and fraught with a high incidence of recurrent cancer in the transplanted liver.[218,219] The necessary use of immunosuppressant drugs after liver transplantation has been suspected of increasing the rate of growth of micrometastases by suppression of immunity of the primary tumor.[220] Neoadjuvant and postoperative chemotherapy have been used in attempts to decrease the rate of cancer recurrence following liver transplant.[221] Multimodality treatment protocols are being tried to improve the overall prognosis of individuals with primary liver cancer. For rare types of liver tumors, such as fibrolamellar tumors, and very selected cases, liver transplant may be a worthwhile treatment option.[222,223]

Improvements in intraoperative decision making, surgical techniques, and instrumentation have combined to improve the selection of individuals likely to benefit from resection for liver cancer, and to reduce intraoperative blood loss and postoperative mortality. Control of blood loss and the use of special instruments, such as the ultrasonic dissector, that cauterize the cut surface of the liver, help reduce the incidence of postoperative bleeding and bile leaks. These technological advances have permitted difficult resections or nonanatomic resections that preserve normal liver tissue.[224]

Primary cancers of the liver develop a new vascular network arising exclusively from the hepatic artery. Hepatic artery occlusion or embolization is used to deprive the tumor of its blood supply, causing tumor necrosis.[225] Embolization can be induced with injection of nondegradable particles such as polyvinyl alcohol and cellulose. Degradable products such as starch microspheres and Gelfoam® cubes are used for temporary occlusion. Chemotherapeutic agents absorbed onto Gelfoam® cubes or microspheres have also been tried.[226–229] Hepatic artery occlusion has been used alone or in combination with intra-arterial chemotherapy.

Percutaneous injections of liver tumors with ethanol under US guidance have been used as both palliative and curative treatments. Injection of absolute alcohol into the tumor produces tumor cell cytotoxicity and necrosis of the tumor mass. This therapy is particularly useful for individuals with small tumors and coexisting cirrhosis.[230–232] Other approaches include suspension of chemotherapy in an oily contrast medium to enhance retention of the drug in the microvasculature of the liver for prolonged tumor-drug exposure.[233]

***Postoperative care***    Overall surgical mortality (individuals who do not survive the hospitalization period) is less then 10% with hepatic resection.[209] Individuals who have had hepatic resection require intensive medical and nursing support. The principal concerns in the care of an individual after hepatic surgery are control of hemorrhage, replacement of blood loss, prevention of infection and pneumonia, and appropriate supportive care. The individual with cirrhosis will have greater difficulty in the postoperative period than the individual who is not cirrhotic. Knowledge of the potential complications, expected reactions, and anticipatory nursing care will aid immeasurably in the postoperative period. The major complications following liver resection include the following:

- hemorrhage

- biliary fistula

- subphrenic abscess

- infection

- pneumonia

- atelectasis

- transient metabolic consequences

- portal hypertension

- clotting defects

### Postoperative complications

*Hemorrhage* The abundant vascularity of the liver cannot be overemphasized. Despite preventive measures to control bleeding, intra-abdominal hemorrhage must be recognized early, i.e., before the condition is irreversible. Hemorrhage usually will appear within the first 24 hours following surgery. Nursing observations and assessments should include frequent monitoring of vital signs; central venous pressure monitoring; examination of the skin and extremities for perfusion; accurate measurement of abdominal girth; frequent checks for bleeding from incision sites, urine, and stool; and close attention to fluid and electrolyte levels and blood profiles. In addition, cirrhotic individuals should be watched closely for overt and subclinical signs of bleeding disorders, due to their predisposition to hematologic complications.

*Biliary fistula* The placement of a T-tube in the common bile duct may be performed at the time of a hepatic resection. A properly placed T-tube normally will drain about 700 ml of bile per day. The T-tube can become dislodged from the common bile duct and may continue to drain small amounts of bile, thus masking its malposition. Bile leaking into the abdomen can cause peritonitis, abscess, and sepsis. Wound drains are also placed near the edge of the surgical resection. A subhepatic drain is usually placed, and a small amount of bile is expected to drain from necrosis on the edge of the liver. Excessive drainage of bile through the subhepatic drain could indicate a biliary fistula pouring large amounts of bile into the subhepatic space. Fever, pain, distended abdomen, and altered vital signs may accompany a biliary fistula.

*Subphrenic abscess* Incomplete or insufficient drainage of the surgical defect can precipitate a subphrenic abscess. Close attention to vital signs and to the function and output of the drainage tubes should continue for an extended period because an abscess can appear later in the postoperative course. Auscultation of the base of the lungs could detect the presence of an abscess and/or fluid. Development of sharp, piercing right upper quadrant pain later in the postoperative course and a low-grade fever are other warning signs.

*Infection* Individuals with cirrhosis are more prone to infection following hepatic resection than individuals without cirrhosis. The mortality associated with serious infection is high. Frequent monitoring of vital signs and assessment of the wound and drainage tubes will provide early clues of impending infection. Constant, intermittent, or remittent hyperthermia or hypothermia secondary to infection requires aggressive intervention.

*Pneumonia and atelectasis* Nursing care directed toward prevention of respiratory complications is similar to that for any other individual following abdominal or thoracic surgery. Aggressive pulmonary toilet is especially important. These individuals will be reluctant to comply because respiratory exercises cause significant incisional pain. Early ambulation, administration of analgesics prior to pulmonary exercise, incisional support, and avoidance of contact with persons with respiratory infections are important nursing care measures.

*Transient metabolic consequences* Jaundice is common during the first postoperative week. It may result from the temporary inability of the remaining liver to handle bile, but the condition usually subsides by the third week, when the liver regenerates. More often, jaundice results from multiple blood transfusions and anoxia of the hepatocytes caused by vascular occlusion during surgery. If jaundice in an individual without cirrhosis does not subside after ten days, mechanical obstruction should be suspected. Nursing measures to relieve the discomforts of jaundice are discussed earlier in the section on pretreatment planning.

*Portal hypertension* Another transient postoperative consequence of hepatic resection that the nurse should anticipate is portal hypertension. Portal hypertension is the result of the surgical rerouting of portal venous flow through a small remnant of liver, which leads to sequestration in the splanchnic circulation. Fortunately, the liver has a great potential for increasing blood flow if it is given adequate time to compensate. Central venous pressure monitoring is a good indicator of blood volume. Bleeding episodes from any cavity, wound, or puncture site require immediate attention.

*Clotting defects* The prothrombin time may be delayed during the first postoperative week. Severe coagulopathies may develop during the operative period and usually are not a concern postoperatively. The nurse should take measures to prevent and/or detect complications from deficiencies in the clotting mechanisms, such as applying pressure to injection sites, monitoring abdominal girth, and testing urine and stool for blood.

## Chemotherapy

The majority of individuals with primary liver cancer are not candidates for curative or palliative surgery; therefore, chemotherapy may be the treatment of choice. Metastatic tumors to the liver also can be treated with chemotherapeutic agents, but surgical excision is the preferred therapy. Systemic administration of single-agent therapy has produced poor results; however, current trials of combination therapy are more promising. Chemotherapeutic agents can be administered by two approaches: systemic administration of single or combination drug regimens, and regional infusion into a hepatic artery or portal vein.[171] Chemotherapeutic agents used with primary and secondary liver cancer include doxorubicin, floxuradine (FUDR), 5-FU, cisplatin, streptozocin, etoposide, mitomycin C, folinic acid, mitoxantrone, epirubicin, methyl CCNU, and teniposide.[234]

Because a significant number of individuals with liver cancer have bulky, unresectable disease that does not extend beyond the liver, regional therapy is a treatment alternative. Regional therapy provides a high concentration of drug directly and continuously to the tumor, with minimal systemic exposure.[234–236] Dose limitations are related to hepatic toxicity and upper gastrointestinal toxicity (ulcer, gastritis).[235,237,238] Continuous infusion pumps and implantable pumps have renewed clinicians' interest in regional therapy.[239] Development of selective angiography has greatly aided the clinician in determining the pattern of blood flow to the tumor and to normal liver tissue. In addition, advances in surgical techniques for catheter placement have improved outcomes, including the laparoscopic approach. Catheters are placed into the specifically defined vessels identified as the major source of blood supply to the tumor.[237] Drugs that have been used for regional chemotherapy administration include 5-FU, cisplatin, doxorubicin, mitomycin C, nitrogen mustard, and methotrexate.[234]

In general, regional infusion is considered superior to systemic chemotherapy.[237] Administration of drug into the hepatic artery could increase local drug delivery to the tumor as well as lower systemic toxicity. The combination of regional infusion and systemic therapy has been studied, with promising results for prolonging survival.[163,240] Regional infusions have been combined with radiotherapy. However, if more than 50% of the liver is involved with tumor or if the major vessels to the liver are narrowed or nonfunctional, systemic chemotherapy usually is the selected route of administration.

Intraperitoneal administration of 5-FU has been well tolerated by individuals and produces results comparable to those with regional therapy.[241] Further investigation is needed to explore the role of intraperitoneal chemotherapy in liver cancer.

### Radiation therapy

To date, because of the poor tolerance of normal liver tissue, the role of radiotherapy in liver cancer therapy is limited to palliation. Many questions still are unanswered regarding how high a dose of radiation can be tolerated by normal liver. Relief of pain, improvements in strength, increased appetite, and increased liver function have been reported with doses ranging from 1900 cGy to 3100 cGy over a period of 2–20 days.[171] Radiation therapy has been enhanced without damage to normal liver tissue by the use of [131]I-Lipidiol, a radiolabeled iodinated contrast medium. When injected intra-arterially, the agent is trapped selectively in the microvasculature and has been reported to produce up to 40% objective response.[242]

Radiosensitizing agents have also been tried in the treatment of liver cancer, but clinical trials are needed to determine their role.[243]

Radiotherapy is used in conjunction with surgery or chemotherapy to palliate symptoms or to eradicate micrometastases. Researchers are investigating the effectiveness of concurrent chemotherapy and radiotherapy and are finding that such regimens have been well tolerated in individuals with secondary liver cancer.[244] The major side effects of radiotherapy to the liver are nausea, vomiting, anorexia, and fatigue. The effects usually are compounded when two or more treatment modalities are combined.

### Biological and hormonal therapy

Interferons have been used in combination with chemotherapeutic agents in randomized trials showing tumor regression and longer survival than in those individuals who received no antitumor therapy. Toxicity was also tolerable. The interferon was administered intramuscularly several times per week. It remains to be seen whether this expensive regimen given by a painful route of administration will be used in other clinical trials.[245,246] Hormonal therapy has been used alone and in combination with chemotherapeutic agents in both controlled and uncontrolled studies with variable results. Antiandrogens have been used in several trials, but antitumor effects do not appear significant.[247,248]

## Symptom Management and Supportive Care

The prognosis for the individual with liver cancer is dismal. Most individuals die within six months of diagnosis. The tumor proliferates rapidly and is difficult to detect and treat. Individuals in advanced stages of the disease may experience pain, severe ascites, hepatic failure, infection, bleeding diathesis, weight loss, weakness, and pneumonia. The individual and family should be kept informed of the treatment plans and assured that efforts will be made to provide relief of symptoms.[249]

Pain is one of the most difficult problems to manage. In later stages the pain is severe, worsens at night, and often radiates to the right scapular or subscapular area. Position, activity, coughing, and deep breathing make the pain worse. Pulmonary hygiene can be attempted only when pain relief measures are most effective.

Ascites can become severe in advanced disease. Palliative measures to control ascites include fluid and sodium restriction, diuretic therapy, paracentesis, and albumin administration.

Anorexia and vomiting may be late-stage manifestations in liver cancer. Antiemetics, vitamin supplements, antidepressants, and tranquilizers have helped some individuals. Relief sometimes is afforded by manipulating the environment or food presentation, or with distraction techniques. Significant weakness, muscle atrophy, and immobility can eventually lead to pulmonary congestion, atelectasis, pneumonia, and death.

Jaundice with pruritus may present an ongoing problem, and routine nursing measures may be of little benefit as the individual progresses to end-stage liver failure. Hepatic coma occurs with profound liver dysfunction as the liver fails to work and toxins accumulate in the body. This may be compounded by any bleeding disorders that have resulted from liver dysfunction. Pain medications may also contribute to hepatic coma because the liver cannot metabolize the drugs, which leads to a buildup in the body. Dehydration from poor fluid intake and infection can accelerate liver failure. Anticipatory management of the rapidly developing symptoms and individual and family support are the major goals of nursing care in advanced disease.

## Continuity of Care: Nursing Challenges

As more multimodality therapies are being investigated to treat individuals with liver tumors, coordination of care across disciplines will be challenged. The nurse will be in a pivotal position to manage the care of the individual through more complicated regimens. Communication and education between the nurse and the individual as well as among all other clinicians and the individual will be most important. The nurse can assess the impact of the therapies on the individual and his or her family and help support them through both positive and negative outcomes. Anticipatory management will be necessary when an individual fails or no longer desires aggressive therapy. The nurse can ease the transition to the terminal phase of the disease through caring and support.

The nurse may encounter an individual who has a rapidly progressing disease, in which case the need for care will be brief. Other individuals may have a protracted course through various treatments and surgeries. Regardless of the length of the encounter, there will always be the need for nursing across the continuum of care for the individual with liver cancer.

# GALLBLADDER CANCER

## Introduction

The two most common malignancies of the biliary tree are adenocarcinoma of the gallbladder and bile ducts (cholangiocarcinoma). There is some overlap in the diagnosis and treatment of these two cancers. Carcinoma of the gallbladder is a rare form of cancer and as such has a distinct etiology, pathophysiology, clinical presentation, and treatment.

## Epidemiology

Although gallbladder cancer is a rare form of cancer, it is the most common cancer of the liver and biliary passages. Approximately 6000 cases are diagnosed in the United States each year. The incidence of gallbladder cancer in the United States is 2.5 per 100,000 residents.[1] Wide variations in incidence exist in different regions of the United States, as well as across the world. In the United States, gallbladder cancer incidence is highest in New Mexico,[250,251] where the occurrence is most frequent among southwestern American Indian women. Other countries with high rates of gallbladder cancer include Israel, Mexico, Bolivia, Chile, and northern Japan. In contrast, gallbladder cancer rates are low in India, Nigeria, and Singapore.[252]

Women develop gallbladder cancer three times more often than men, which is similar to the incidence of gallstones.[253] Gallbladder cancer is rare in individuals under 50 years of age, with the average age at diagnosis being 60 years.[254]

## Etiology

Several factors are associated with an increased risk for gallbladder cancer. Gallstones are the most common factor, probably due to the high prevalence in the general population. More than 90% of individuals with gallbladder cancer have coexistent chronic cholecystitis (inflamed gallbladder) and cholelithiasis (gallstones).[163] Gallbladder cancer is more likely to occur in individuals with a single large gallstone than with multiple smaller stones.[252] It is presumed that the large gallstones have been present for a long period of time, causing chronic irritation of the gallbladder wall, thus predisposing to the development of carcinoma. Of all the individuals who have a cholecystectomy for gallstones, approximately 1% will be found to have an unsuspected gallbladder cancer.[255]

Individuals with a choledochal cyst may develop carcinoma throughout the biliary tree, but most tumors arise in the gallbladder. The chance of developing an associated gallbladder or bile duct cancer increases with age.[256] Recent studies have suggested that an anomalous pancreatobiliary duct junction (APBDJ) is associated with an increased incidence of gallbladder cancer in individuals with a choledochal cyst.[256,257] This common channel abnormality between the common bile duct and pancreatic duct allows reflux of pancreatic juice into the biliary tree. The question still remains as to whether it is the regurgitation of pancreatic juice or the relationship of the abnormal junction to bile stasis and the subsequent retention of carcinogens within the biliary tree that cause gallbladder cancer.[252]

Various chemical carcinogens have been suspected to cause biliary cancers because excretion in the bile is a common way of clearing toxic metabolites. An increased incidence of gallbladder cancer has been reported in rubber plant workers.[258] Animal studies have suggested that azotoluene and nitrosamines can cause gallbladder cancer.[259,260] An association between gallbladder cancer and obesity and estrogens has been suggested in epidemiologic studies.[260]

Typhoid carriers have an increased risk of gallbladder and bile duct cancers. The higher incidence of gallbladder cancer in chronic typhoid carriers is also thought to result from chronic irritation.[261] Calcification of the gallbladder wall, the so-called porcelain gallbladder, is associated with a 25%–60% incidence of gallbladder cancer.[262] Gallbladder polyps are also a risk factor for cancer. Polyps greater than 1 cm are most likely to become malignant and are an indication for cholecystectomy.[263,264] Adenomatous polyps of the gallbladder in individuals with Peutz-Jeghers syndrome are also associated with gallbladder cancer.[265]

## Prevention, Screening, Early Detection Programs

At present there is no effective method of screening for gallbladder cancer as it is such a rare tumor and is often confused with other biliary cancers. The presenting symptoms of the disease usually occur with advanced disease, making early detection almost impossible. Effective ways to eliminate the formation of gallstones in the general population and especially in high-risk individuals would be beneficial for many reasons, one of which is decreased gallbladder cancer. Heightened awareness of the incidence of gallbladder cancer through education of high-risk individuals may lead to routine surveillance and early detection.

## Pathophysiology

### Cellular characteristics

The vast majority of gallbladder cancers are adenocarcinomas, which occur in 85% of individuals.[266] Cancers of the gallbladder can be one of several histological types with varying degrees of invasion including papillary, nodular, tubular, poorly differentiated, and combinations. Histological grades of gallbladder carcinoma include well-differentiated, moderately differentiated, poorly differentiated, and undifferentiated.[252]

### Progression of disease

Since most individuals with cancer of the gallbladder present with disease at an advanced stage, it is difficult to know the exact progression of the disease. Gallbladder cancer is a locally invasive tumor that may extend directly into the gallbladder bed in the liver, extrahepatic bile ducts, duodenum or transverse colon, portal vein, hepatic artery, or pancreas.[267]

### Pattern of spread

The pattern of spread predictably follows lymphatic and venous drainage of the gallbladder. Venous drainage of the gallbladder is directly into the adjacent liver. The most common pattern of spread of gallbladder cancer is through direct extension into the liver. The lymphatic drainage of the gallbladder is to the cystic duct lymph node, periportal lymph nodes, and then to celiac and superior mesenteric lymph nodes. These tumors can spread into and around the cystic duct and can extend into the common bile duct, causing biliary obstruction (Figure 38-8). Thus, jaundice may be the first clinical manifestation of a problem. Distant metastasis is possible but is less common.[268]

## Clinical Manifestations

The signs and symptoms of gallbladder cancer are similar to those of gallstones. Right upper quadrant pain, discomfort, and dyspepsia can result from both. Individuals with gallbladder cancer commonly have advanced disease and present with nonspecific signs of malaise, weight loss, nausea, vomiting, and anorexia. Almost half of individuals with gallbladder cancer will present with jaundice in addition to the clinical symptoms suggestive of biliary tract disease. In advanced stages of the disease, individuals may present with a palpable mass in the right upper quadrant resulting from obstruction and distention of the gallbladder. Tumor invasion of the cystic duct can cause cystic duct obstruction, resulting in the development of acute cholecystitis. Jaundice occurs when the tumor extends into the common bile duct. Diagnosis often is made not preoperatively but at the time of surgery for jaundice or acute cholecystitis.[252,268]

## Assessment

### Patient and family history

The individual may have had no previous symptoms or vague, chronic complaints of right upper quadrant pain. A change in character of the symptoms may bring the individual to seek medical attention. Any individual who is at high risk for gallbladder cancer or who has a family history of the disease should receive a thorough examination.

### Physical examination

Jaundice with pruritus may be evident in individuals with an obstructing gallbladder cancer. In advanced carcinoma of the gallbladder, an individual may have a visibly palpable gallbladder when supine. Severe weight loss as well as a palpable liver from metastatic disease may be evident.

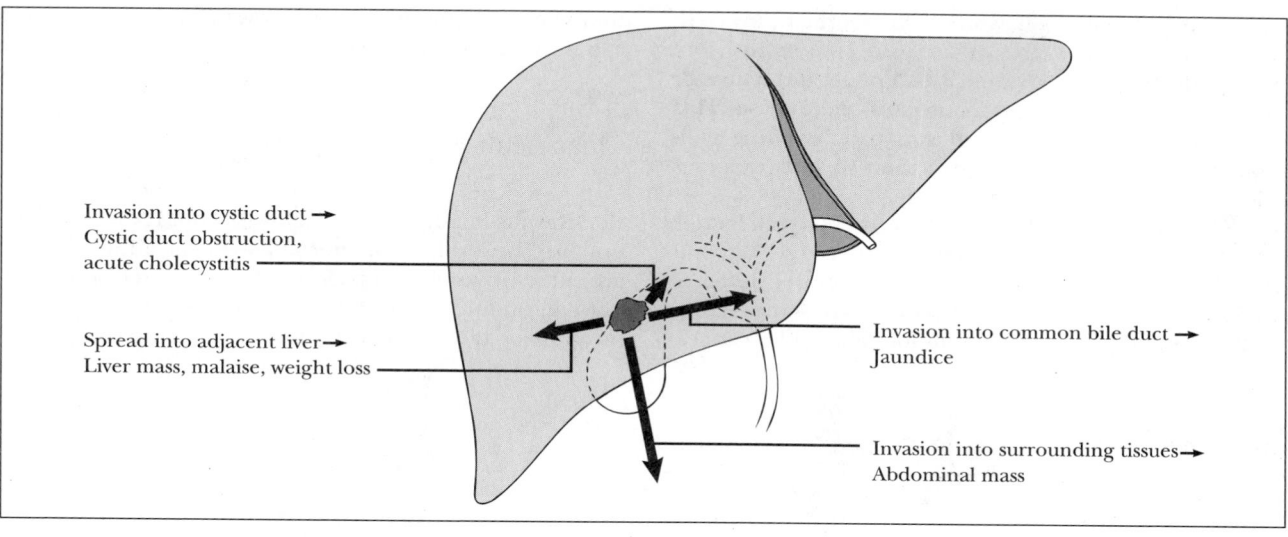

Invasion into cystic duct →
Cystic duct obstruction,
acute cholecystitis

Spread into adjacent liver→
Liver mass, malaise, weight loss

Invasion into common bile duct →
Jaundice

Invasion into surrounding tissues→
Abdominal mass

**FIGURE 38-8**   Tumor spread and presenting signs in gallbladder cancer. Gallbladder cancer commonly spreads by direct extension into surrounding tissues. This tumor extension results in the clinical presentations of jaundice, acute cholecystitis, abdominal mass, and weight loss. Adapted from Norwold DL, Dawes LG: Biliary neoplasms. In Greenfield LJ et al (eds): *Surgery: Scientific Principles and Practice* (ed 2). Philadelphia, Lippincott, 1997, pp 1056–1067.

### Diagnostic studies

With the exception of jaundice, no specific laboratory abnormalities are present. Between 10% and 20% of gallbladder cancers are discovered only after pathological examination of a gallbladder for symptomatic gallstones.[252,253,272]

Ultrasonography, CT scan, MRI, cholangiography, and angiography may all be helpful in evaluating individuals with suspected gallbladder cancer. In approximately 50% of individuals, US is used to identify a mass protruding into the gallbladder either filling or replacing the gallbladder.[273,274] CT scan can demonstrate a gallbladder cancer as an intraluminal mass, a mass replacing the gallbladder, or a mass extending from the gallbladder. CT scan is also accurate in demonstrating early invasion of the liver or liver metastases.[275,276] Limited experience exists with the use of MRI in the evaluation of gallbladder cancer. New magnetic resonance cholangiography and vascular enhancement techniques make it possible to visualize biliary obstruction, obstruction and/or encasement of the portal vein, and hepatic involvement.[277]

Cholangiography can be useful for diagnosing gallbladder cancer in an individual with jaundice.[278] Percutaneous transhepatic cholangiography (PTC) or endoscopic retrograde cholangiopancreatography (ERCP) may both be beneficial. The typical finding on either study is a long stricture of the common hepatic duct. Angiography may be the most useful radiological study for staging gallbladder cancer as it can define the presence of tumor vessels in the wall of the gallbladder and encasement of the portal vein or hepatic artery. Angiography is used to determine resectability through assessment of vascular encasement. However, new spiral CT scan and MRI techniques may provide this same information.

If radiological studies suggest that the gallbladder cancer may be resectable or if palliative surgery is considered, tissue diagnosis is not required before surgery. Likewise, if resection is not deemed possible due to extensive liver invasion, liver or peritoneal metastases, or encasement of the main portal vein, a biopsy of the tumor is necessary to help establish a diagnosis and confirm the stage of tumor. A liver biopsy by US or CT scan guidance can be obtained to assist in establishing the diagnosis. Brushings of obstructed bile ducts or bile cytology via PTC or ERCP has a low yield of sample for diagnosis.[255] Laparoscopy may also be used to obtain a biopsy of the liver, peritoneum, or tissue around the gallbladder.

### Prognostic indicators

The histological grade has significant prognostic implications. The presence or absence of metaplasia is an important prognostic factor in gallbladder cancer. Individuals with metaplasia have a better prognosis.[269] Metaplasia is more common in women. Poorly differentiated infiltrating tumors have a strong association with gallstones, lymph node metastasis, and direct extension into the liver.[266] Papillary tumors are less likely to directly invade the liver and have a lower incidence of lymph node metastasis. They are also less likely to have associated gallstones. Nodular forms of tumor are more likely to infiltrate early, to invade the liver, and to have lymph node metastasis along with a higher incidence of gallstones. Tubular tumors are in the midrange with respect to their aggressive metastatic behavior.[252] The degree of invasion by the tumor is predictive of survival. Tumors with the best prognosis are those found incidentally at the time of cholecystectomy for symptomatic gallstone disease. This emphasizes the importance of surgically opening gallbladders at the time of cholecystectomy so any suspicious lesions can be examined immediately.

CEA and AFP have been associated with gallbladder cancer.[270,271] The markers are not considered to be good screening tests since the incidence of elevated levels is low and their specificity is poor. When these tumor markers are elevated prior to resection for gallbladder cancer,

they may be important in the follow-up and early identification of recurrent disease.[252]

## Classification and Staging

The American Joint Committee for Cancer Staging and End-Results Reporting has established the TNM classification listed in Table 38-5. Alternative classification schemes are currently used in Europe and Japan. Both histological grading on the basis of differentiation and the degree of invasion of the tumor are important factors in staging

**TABLE 38-5**  TNM Classification System for Gallbladder Cancer

| PRIMARY TUMOR (T) | |
|---|---|
| TX | Primary tumor cannot be assessed |
| T0 | No evidence of primary tumor |
| Tis | Carcinoma in situ |
| T1 | Tumor invades mucosa or muscle layer<br>T1a  Tumor invades the mucosa<br>T1b  Tumor invades the muscle layer |
| T2 | Tumor invades the perimuscular connective tissue; no extension beyond the serosa or into the liver |
| T3 | Tumor perforates the serosa (visceral peritoneum) or directly invades into one adjacent organ, or both (extension 2 cm or less into the liver) |
| T4 | Tumor extends more than 2 cm into the liver and/or into two or more adjacent organs (stomach, duodenum, colon, pancreas, omentum, extrahepatic bile ducts, any involvement of the liver) |

| REGIONAL LYMPH NODES (N) | |
|---|---|
| NX | Regional lymph nodes cannot be assessed |
| N0 | No regional lymph node metastasis |
| N1 | Metastasis in cystic duct, pericholedochal, and/or hilar lymph nodes (i.e., in the hepatoduodenal ligament) |
| N2 | Metastasis in peripancreatic (head only), periduodenal, periportal, celiac, and/or superior mesenteric lymph nodes |

| DISTANT METASTASIS (M) | |
|---|---|
| MX | Presence of distant metastasis cannot be assessed |
| M0 | No distant metastasis |
| M1 | Distant metastasis |

| STAGE GROUPING | | | |
|---|---|---|---|
| Stage I | T1 | N0 | M0 |
| Stage II | T2 | N0 | M0 |
| Stage III | T1 | N1 | M0 |
|  | T2 | N1 | M0 |
|  | T3 | N0, N1 | M0 |
| Stage IVA | T4 | Any N | M0 |
| Stage IVB | Any T | Any N | M1 |

From Beahrs OH, Henson DE, Hutter RVP, et al (eds): *American Joint Committee on Cancer: Manual for Staging of Cancer* (ed 4). Philadelphia, Lippincott, 1992.

gallbladder cancers and determining survival. Almost all known survivors of gallbladder cancer have had well-differentiated tumors. The higher the histological grade, the greater the association with advanced stage and rapid disease progression. No ideal staging system exists that adequately correlates all aspects of gross and histological pathology conditions of cancer of the gallbladder.

## Therapeutic Approaches and Nursing Care

The individual and the stage of the tumor must be considered when deciding on the appropriate treatment of cancer of the gallbladder. An individual's general medical condition is more important than chronological age. Several factors must be considered before surgery. Special attention must be given to any liver problems, as cirrhosis and portal hypertension will increase the risk from surgery. Obstructive jaundice may alter organ and immune function and should be addressed preoperatively if liver resection is being considered.[279] Altered renal function, poor nutritional status, and sepsis are other parameters that increase the risk for a poor surgical outcome in individuals who are jaundiced.[280]

Local invasion of the adjacent liver is a common finding that can sometimes be managed with a wedge resection of the liver. More extensive liver involvement may require a larger liver resection. Extension of the tumor into the colon may require a colon resection. Extension into the duodenum or pancreatic head can be resected with a pancreaticoduodenectomy. Multiple metastases in both lobes of the liver, or peritoneal or distant metastases are considered contraindications to resection of the primary gallbladder tumor.

### Surgery

Less than 25% of cancers of the gallbladder are resectable, but the most effective treatment for cancer of the gallbladder is resection of the primary tumor and areas where it has locally invaded. The tumor may spread locally by venous, lymphatic, or direct extension. In this way the tumor may spread into the adjacent liver, into lymph nodes along the common bile duct toward the pancreas or the celiac axis, or into the duodenum, pancreas, or transverse colon. In addition, liver and/or peritoneal metastases may be present when the individual presents with the disease.

Cholecystectomy is the primary treatment of stage I gallbladder carcinoma.[254,263,281] Many gallbladder cancers are found incidentally at the time of elective cholecystectomy. Prognosis depends on the depth of invasion of the gallbladder wall. If the tumor is limited to the mucosa, simple cholecystectomy is sufficient therapy and has a very good prognosis. Position of the tumor within the gallbladder wall may also dictate further therapy. If the tumor is next to the liver bed with minimal invasion, the recurrence rate may be high. Likewise, if the tumor is superficial and away from the liver, cholecystectomy may be an adequate operation.[281–283] If the tumor penetrates the serosa, a simple cholecystectomy is not adequate.

Laparoscopic removal of the gallbladder is not recommended. Tumor implantation at the trocar sites has been found when gallbladder cancer was removed laparoscopically. Laparoscopic manipulation of the tumor could also lead to tumor dissemination in the abdomen.[284]

When the cancer involves deeper layers of the gallbladder wall, the prognosis is grim. A radical or extended cholecystectomy has been recommended in the hopes of improving survival rates for those individuals who have gallbladder cancer. The procedure consists of a cholecystectomy with a wide resection of the liver around the gallbladder bed and a major lymph node dissection,[252] (Figure 38-9). If the gallbladder cancer is near the cystic duct or if the bile duct is involved with tumor, a bile duct resection may be performed at the time of extended cholecystectomy. Studies have shown a five-year survival of 70%–85% with this approach for gallbladder cancer.[285–287] Even when the serosa is involved, extended cholecystectomy provides a better survival advantage over simple cholecystectomy. This extensive resection should be considered the therapy of choice for preoperatively recognized and potentially resectable gallbladder cancer. More extensive resections that include both the liver and the duodenum or pancreas have been advocated by some Japanese groups, but there is considerable morbidity and mortality with these operations.[285,286,288]

Survival after surgical resection depends on tumor stage and the operation performed. For stage I tumors, the five-year survival after routine cholecystectomy is greater than 85%. For stage II, III, and IV tumors, five-year survivals are approximately 25%, 10%, and 2%, respectively. Individuals with stage II tumors treated with an extended cholecystectomy may be expected to have a five-year survival of better than 65%.[252] The best survival for individuals with advanced tumors has been attained in Japan with more radical surgery.

***Postoperative care***   Routine postoperative care is necessary for an individual having simple cholecystectomy. The surgery may be done on an outpatient basis or with a hospitalization of only a few days. For an extensive surgery involving the removal of any part of the liver or surrounding tissues, more intensive monitoring and assessment are needed. The nursing care required for these individuals is the same as for anyone having a major liver resection. The main concerns in the care of an individual following hepatic surgery are control of hemorrhage, replacement of blood loss, prevention of infection and pneumonia, and appropriate supportive care. Postoperative complications include hemorrhage, biliary fistula, infection, transient metabolic consequences, subphrenic abscess, pneumonia, atelectasis, portal hypertension, and clotting defects. These complications are discussed in the section on liver cancer. Knowledge of the potential complications, expected reactions, and anticipatory nursing care will aid greatly in the postoperative period.

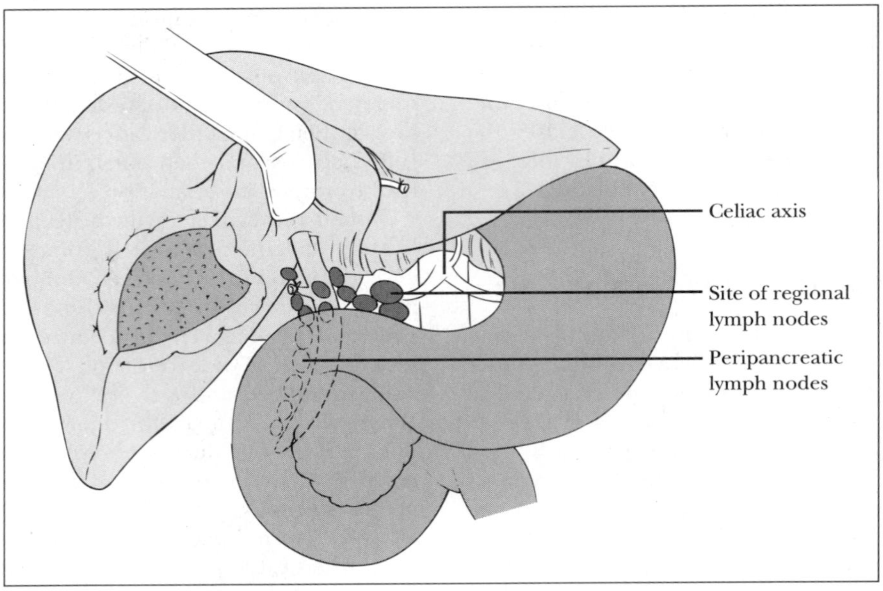

**FIGURE 38-9** Treatment for invasive gallbladder cancer is cholecystectomy and a wedge resection of the liver along with a regional lymphadenectomy. The wedge resection of the liver is illustrated along with the lymph node regions that drain the gallbladder and that should be removed during operation for gallbladder cancer. Adapted from Norwold DL, Dawes LG: Biliary neoplasms. In Greenfield LJ et al (eds): *Surgery: Scientific Principles and Practice* (ed 2). Philadelphia, Lippincott, 1997, pp 1056–1067.

Hospitalization is minimal after surgery today. The nurse can review and explain postoperative treatment options. Treatment modalities are limited, and it can be disconcerting to the individual to know there is little to offer with any proven benefit for advanced cancer of the gallbladder.

### Palliative therapy

Most therapies for gallbladder cancer are palliative.[253,263,281] Most individuals are unable to be resected with negative margins. If a tissue diagnosis can be obtained through percutaneous liver biopsy or by laparoscopy, nonoperative palliation should be considered. Many individuals with gallbladder cancer will have obstructive jaundice, which can be relieved and managed with an endoscopic or percutaneous transhepatic biliary catheter. One complication with percutaneous stenting is the development of acute cholecystitis, which subsequently may require percutaneous drainage of the gallbladder and intravenous antibiotics.[289] Recurrent jaundice and cholangitis are problems that may recur during the course of the disease due to tumor obstruction of the biliary tree or biliary tubes.

Pain should be treated aggressively to improve the individual's quality of life. Opiates are given as indicated. Radiation therapy may be helpful to palliate the pain. Percutaneous celiac nerve block may also be helpful in reducing pain and reducing the need for pain medication. Nerve blocks can be repeated. Unfortunately, individuals who require nonoperative palliation usually do not survive more than three months.

Operative palliation may be helpful to establish a diagnosis, remove the gallbladder to prevent acute cholecystitis, relieve or prevent pain, and treat or prevent gastric outlet obstruction. A gastrojejunostomy bypass may be performed to relieve or prevent a gastric outlet obstruction. The individual is then placed on acid antisecretory agents for the rest of his or her life. The management of jaundice depends on the extent of the disease. If metastatic disease is found, the jaundice may be relieved by preoperatively placed percutaneous transhepatic biliary catheters, which may be left in place or changed to an internal stent. If the tumor is locally unresectable without extension to adjacent organs (duodenum or pancreas), a Roux-en-Y choledochojejunostomy (anastomosis of a loop of jejunum to the common bile duct proximal to the obstruction) may be performed, which can be stented with transhepatic silastic catheters to relieve biliary obstruction.[252] Nursing care is the same as for any abdominal surgery.

The addition of any internal-external percutaneous transhepatic biliary stents depends on the extent of disease and the choice of the physician in treating jaundice. The individual and the family will need to be taught the care and flushing of these stents as they will be maintained for the rest of the person's life. The stents are usually flushed twice a day with sterile normal saline solution. Daily cleansing of the stent site is required. Signs and symptoms of complications of the stents must be reviewed to alert the individual and family to notify the clinician promptly to avoid problems and unnecessary hospitalization. Percutaneous transhepatic biliary catheters are discussed in the section on pancreatic cancer.

The majority of individuals with gallbladder cancer have unresectable disease at the time of diagnosis. Less than 5% of all individuals with gallbladder cancer are alive after five years. Individuals with unresectable stage III tumors have a median survival of six months. The median survival for an individual with stage IV gallbladder cancer with liver or peritoneal metastases at the time of presentation is only one to three months.[252]

### Radiation therapy

Radiation therapy has been used to treat individuals with resected gallbladder cancer as well as unresectable tumors. There has been no proven survival advantage with external-beam radiation alone after surgery. In unresectable cancer, external-beam radiation has been used to help relieve pain or to relieve biliary obstruction. Intraoperative radiation has also been used at some centers, but the advantage of this technique combined with resection and/or external-beam radiotherapy has not been proved.[290,291] Likewise, the role of radiation sensitizers, such as 5-FU, and the addition of leucovorin to intraoperative or external-beam radiation therapy has yet to be studied in individuals with gallbladder cancer.[252]

### Chemotherapy

Chemotherapy agents for the treatment of gallbladder cancer have been limited due to poor tumor response to the agents. Mitomycin C and 5-FU have been most commonly used. In individuals suspected of having microscopic disease after resection, chemotherapy may be considered as adjuvant therapy, but its effectiveness has been difficult to document.[252] Intra-arterial and intraperitoneal delivery of chemotherapeutic agents has been tried in limited studies with varying results.

## Symptom Management and Supportive Care

Individuals with advanced cancer of the gallbladder usually have disease involving the liver and biliary tree. Obstructive jaundice, liver abscess, and liver failure are potential complications. Management of any drains or percutaneous transhepatic biliary catheters is taught to the individual and his or her family. Teaching the individual and family the signs and symptoms of potential problems resulting from the tumor or any tubes and drains may allow for earlier interventions and less hospitalization. Persistent pain, fever, chills, and recurrent jaundice may be symptoms of a liver abscess caused by obstructed bile ducts. Malfunctioning endoscopic or percutaneous biliary catheters can also present as fever, chills, and recurrent jaundice.

With progressive liver failure, ascites and increased abdominal girth may cause problems with pain, discomfort, and dyspnea. Supportive measures include aggressive pain management and proper body positioning. Ascites can be controlled by fluid and sodium restriction along with diuretic therapy. Intra-abdominal spread of tumor can cause pain and palpable or visible tumor.

Nutritional intake is poor in the individual with gallbladder cancer and jaundice. Elevated bilirubin levels cause changes in taste, leading to a decrease in appetite and weight loss. Food prepared with spices that enhance taste can be tried. Plastic silverware can be used if the individual complains of a metallic taste in the mouth. Small, frequent snacks and a change in the environment may be helpful. Nausea, vomiting, and anorexia can also hinder nutrition. Antiemetics and vitamin supplements may help.

Liver failure usually develops as the disease progresses. Liver failure follows a progression of lethargy and weakness to encephalopathy and hepatic coma. Renal failure is also common at this time. The nurse can assist the family by explaining what to expect as the symptoms develop. Individual and family support are the major goals of nursing care.

## Continuity of Care: Nursing Challenges

Most individuals present at an advanced stage and rapidly decline from gallbladder carcinoma. The nurse who provides care during therapy must be aware of the individual's physical and psychosocial status. Communication from the radiation therapy or chemotherapy nurse to home care and hospice nurses can be invaluable to assist with delivering quality care to an individual with a rapidly changing condition. Transition to hospice care with attention to individual and family needs can be easy when information is shared by the nurses who know the most about the individual. The burden to the family and their experience with cancer can be greatly eased by anticipatory management and supportive care by the nurse.

# PANCREATIC CANCER

## Introduction

Cancer of the pancreas is the fifth-leading cause of death from cancer in the United States. It is ninth among all cancers in incidence in the United States. During the past two decades, the incidence has peaked and plateaued, with a current estimate of 26,000 new cases of pancreatic cancer each year and an equal number of deaths from pancreatic cancer in the United States. It is a disease with a poor prognosis, considered by many to be one of the deadliest malignancies. Less than 20% of affected individuals survive one year after diagnosis, and the overall five-year survival is only 3%.[1]

Pancreatic cancer is one of the most difficult tumors to detect or diagnose because of its anatomic location and the biological nature of the tumor. Its onset is insidious, with signs and symptoms that occur late, are vague and misleading, and mimic other diseases. The individual with pancreatic cancer typically will ignore the initial signs and symptoms or rely on self-treatment for months until jaundice or other prominent and intolerable signs appear.

Recent progress in both surgical management of individuals with pancreatic cancer and improved responses to combined therapy have begun to improve overall results.[292,293] A growing understanding of the biology and molecular genetic origins of pancreatic cancer will hopefully provide opportunities for advances in prevention, earlier tumor detection, and more effective therapy.

## Epidemiology

Pancreatic cancer accounts for 2% of new cancer cases in the United States as well as worldwide. The incidence of pancreatic cancer increases with age, with peak incidence between ages 60 and 70. Although cancer of the pancreas can occur in individuals younger than 40 years of age, it is quite unusual. In the past, pancreatic carcinoma was more common in males than females,[294] but for unknown reasons the incidence currently is nearly the same in both sexes. The incidence of pancreatic cancer is slightly higher in African-Americans.[1]

## Etiology

Multiple studies have identified various environmental factors that may be associated with increased risk of pancreatic cancer. Cigarette smoking has been the strongest risk factor associated with the development of pancreatic cancer.[295–297] The risk increases as the number of cigarettes smoked increases, but risk decreases after cessation of smoking.[298] Alcohol and coffee consumption have been implicated in some studies, but there is insufficient evidence to confirm these observations.[299–301]

Previously, the results of studies on work environments suggested that increased chemical exposures were associated with increased rates of pancreatic cancer. Recent studies have failed to confirm these earlier observations and found no association between occupation or workplace and an increased risk of pancreatic cancer.[302–305] A diet high in animal fat has been associated with an increased risk of pancreatic cancer.[303,306] Likewise diets high in fresh fruits and vegetables appear to provide a protective effect.[306,307]

Diabetes mellitus and chronic pancreatitis have been identified in some studies as additional risk factors for pancreatic cancer.[296,297,308,309] However, the findings from these studies are inconclusive, as both diabetes and pancreatitis may be early manifestations of the cancer, rather than a risk factor for the malignancy.[310,311]

## Prevention, Screening, Early Detection Programs

Prevention of pancreatic cancer will require better identification of factors demonstrated to cause or place individuals at a high risk of developing pancreatic cancer. Reduction or elimination of exposure to these risk factors will be necessary to prevent cancer of the pancreas. Cancer of the pancreas is an insidious disease, with little known about the best treatment, much less the cause. Not until recently have researchers embarked on any studies to learn more about pancreatic cancer.

A growing understanding of the biology and molecular genetic origins of pancreatic cancer will hopefully provide opportunities for earlier tumor detection and perhaps prevention. Gene mutations and other acquired chromosomal abnormalities are being delineated. Abnormalities in the expression of the tumor-suppressor gene *p53* and the oncogene *K-ras* seem to be the most common mutations recognized, with each occurring in over 70%–80% of individuals. How mutations or abnormalities in gene expression relate to the pathogenesis of pancreatic cancer is unknown. However, the general hypothesis being tested is that pancreatic cancer represents a disease of progressive, acquired somatic mutations. Strategies for screening, early detection, and specific therapies are fast approaching as the knowledge of cell biology and nuclear control of cellular proliferation increases.[312,313]

Total DNA content has been investigated as a prognostic factor for long-term survival in many neoplasms, including pancreatic cancer. Studies have suggested that individuals with diploid tumors have a more favorable survival advantage over those with nondiploid tumors.[314–316]

Familial cases of pancreatic cancer are being studied to identify genetic alterations that are inherited through the germ line. Genetic analyses could be used to establish the prognosis for an individual with pancreatic cancer and, it is hoped, eventually could be used to detect and treat pancreatic cancer.[317,318]

## Pathophysiology

The most common pathological form of pancreatic cancer is an adenocarcinoma that originates from the cells lining the pancreatic duct.[319] Tumors of the pancreas develop in both the endocrine and the exocrine parenchyma. Approximately 90% of tumors arise from the exocrine pancreas, which contains two major types of epithelium: acinar and ductal. The acinar cells of the pancreas produce digestive enzymes, whereas the cells lining the pancreatic duct are responsible for the secretion of fluid and electrolytes and the conveyance of pancreatic juice to the duodenum.

Cystic neoplasms of the pancreas also arise from the exocrine pancreas. These tumors are classified as either benign serous cystadenomas, potentially malignant mucinous cystadenomas, or malignant cystadenocarcinomas.

Cystic tumors are less common than ductal adenocarcinomas, are found throughout the entire gland, and tend to occur in women.[320]

Endocrine or islet cell tumors constitute the remainder of pancreatic malignant tumors. Many islet cell tumors secrete excessive hormones, resulting in significant clinical manifestations. Nonfunctional islet cell tumors do not produce obvious clinical manifestations and are usually detected because of their space-occupying characteristics or as an incidental finding.[321] Pancreatic lymphomas are rare, but early recognition is important because of their dramatic response to chemotherapy.[322]

### Cellular characteristics

Adenocarcinomas of the pancreas usually are tannish, hard, nodular, firm masses with a large amount of fibrosis. These tumors may vary from well differentiated to undifferentiated and exhibit variable gland formation, irregular cell size, and variable nuclear changes. Often, pancreatic lesions are associated with an extensive desmoplastic reaction that can make diagnosis on the basis of needle biopsy difficult.[323–325]

Although uncommon (<5%), islet cell tumors arise from the endocrine parenchyma. The tumors usually occur as small, well-circumscribed, reddish-orange tissue that rarely extends beyond the pancreas. On microscopy, islet cell tumors are well vascularized and encapsulated, usually compressing adjacent parenchyma. Fibrosis and calcification may be seen. Malignant islet cell tumors are difficult to distinguish because they closely resemble normal islet cells and retain secretory or synthetic functions. The presence of metastases is the most reliable criterion for establishing malignancy.[321] Chapter 37 presents a more detailed discussion of endocrine tumors.

### Progression of disease

Pancreatic cancer arises in the head of the pancreas in 60%–70% of cases. About 15% of tumors develop in the body of the gland, another 10% develop in the tail, and the remaining 5%–15% are diffuse. Extension beyond the confines of the pancreas is the rule rather than the exception with ductal carcinoma of the pancreas.

There is no apparent explanation for the tendency of pancreatic cancer to develop in the head of the gland. Tumors in the head of the gland are often detected at a small size (2–3 cm). The bile duct is invaded early in the course of the disease, causing obliteration of the tissue and obstruction of the flow of bile. This accounts for easily recognized symptoms, such as jaundice, which enables detection of smaller tumors. Tumors tend to invade local structures, such as the duodenum and retroperitoneum, either directly or via the course of autonomic nerves of the celiac plexus. Some degree of perineural invasion is present in 90% of cases. The portal or superior vein may also be invaded. Venous invasion or encasement by tumor growth may result in obstruction, thrombosis, ascites, and portal hypertension. Vascular encasement and neural in-

filtration can contribute to severe back pain. Involvement of the mesenteric vessels may preclude resection of these tumors.

In the body and tail of the pancreas, tumors are often larger than 5 cm before they produce symptoms and are detected. Cancer of the body and tail of the pancreas can invade the splenic vein with resultant thrombosis and development of gastric varices.

### Patterns of spread

At the time of detection, large tumor masses may be fixed to tissues behind the pancreas or to the vertebral column. The tumor may directly invade surrounding organs, such as kidney, spleen, or diaphragm. Invasion of the celiac nerve plexus may account for unrelenting pain. Other sites of local invasion, which tends to occur later, include the superior mesenteric and splenic arteries, transverse colon, stomach, kidneys, and left adrenal gland.[323] Obstruction of the portal vein and tributaries can lead to portal hypertension and esophageal varices.

Characteristically, tumors of the pancreas grow slowly, with late signs and symptoms of pathology. At the time of diagnosis, 90% of cases have perineural invasion, 70%–80% have lymphatic spread, 50% have venous involvement, and 20%–25% have duodenal invasion. The liver, peritoneum, and regional lymph nodes are the most commonly involved structures.[326] Supraclavicular nodes may be involved more frequently with carcinoma of the body and tail of the pancreas. Metastatic deposits reach the liver through the portal bloodstream or lymphatics. Peritoneal seeding by metastatic deposits also occurs. The frequency of lymph node metastasis correlates with the size of the primary tumor.[327]

## Clinical Manifestations

The early signs and symptoms of pancreatic cancer are vague, nonspecific, and gradual, which often contributes to a delay in diagnosis by both the individual and the physician. Early diagnosis of pancreatic cancer requires a low index of suspicion and appropriate aggressiveness in pursuing the diagnosis. Specific symptoms usually develop only after invasion or obstruction of a nearby structure. Careful assessment and extensive inquiry into the character, onset, duration, and modulators of presenting signs and symptoms will greatly aid definitive diagnosis. Manifestations of disease differ according to the location of the tumor.

Weight loss and abdominal pain are the most prominent symptoms. These symptoms are usually nonspecific, and a clinical suspicion of pancreatic cancer must be high to identify the presence of a tumor. Individuals found to have resectable pancreatic cancer tend to present with few symptoms. The delay in diagnosis from the onset of symptoms may contribute to the overall poor prognosis in individuals with pancreatic cancer.

Weight loss and clinical wasting are classic symptoms

of cancer of the pancreas, particularly when it is located in the head of the gland. The weight loss initially may not cause concern and may be attributed to gastric maladies. As the disease advances, significant weight loss is common and often accelerated by pain, anorexia, flatulence, nausea, and vomiting. Duodenal obstruction, with nausea and vomiting, is a late manifestation of pancreatic cancer. Tumor involvement of the pancreas prevents secretions of the digestive pancreatic enzymes and may diminish insulin production. Malabsorption can lead to diarrhea, constipation, steatorrhea, and muscle weakness.[328] New onset of diabetes is found in 15%–20% of individuals.[329] The onset of glucose intolerance in an elderly person with vague gastrointestinal symptoms should alert the clinician to the possibility of pancreatic cancer.[328] Metabolic disturbances such as hyperglycemia, glycosuria, and hypoalbuminemia may occur.

A combination of factors probably causes the weight loss associated with pancreatic cancer. An increase in resting energy expenditure,[330] a decrease in consumption of calories, and fat malabsorption exist in individuals with pancreatic cancer.[331]

Pain is often vague and nonspecific. A dull, intermittent pain in the epigastric region is initially experienced by most individuals, which may be attributed to indigestion or gaseous distention. The pain may become more distinctive. It may be continuous and frequently radiates to the back or right upper quadrant of the abdomen.

It may be colicky, dull, or vague. The intensity of the pain is affected by activity, eating, and posture. The pain is often ameliorated when the individual sits forward or lies in the fetal position.[332] Pain is a more prevalent symptom in individuals with tumors in the body and tail of the pancreas. These tumors are larger at presentation and are located in the retroperitoneum, which contributes to earlier nerve involvement, resulting in pain. Although intractable pain frequently is associated with pancreatic cancer, it seldom is an early manifestation. Recent studies suggest that fewer than one-third of individuals with cancer of the pancreas report moderate to severe pain. Severe pain usually indicates local invasion of splanchnic nerves, suggestive of advanced disease.[333]

### Head of pancreas

When carcinoma involves the head of the pancreas, the signs and symptoms often appear earlier than a tumor in the body or tail of the pancreas (Figure 38-10). A classic triad of symptoms is seen in individuals with cancer of the head of the pancreas: jaundice, pain, and weight loss.

Jaundice, caused by obstruction of the distal common bile duct as it passes through the head of the pancreas, is the presenting symptom in 80% of cases of cancer of the pancreas. Regardless of whether jaundice is the initial

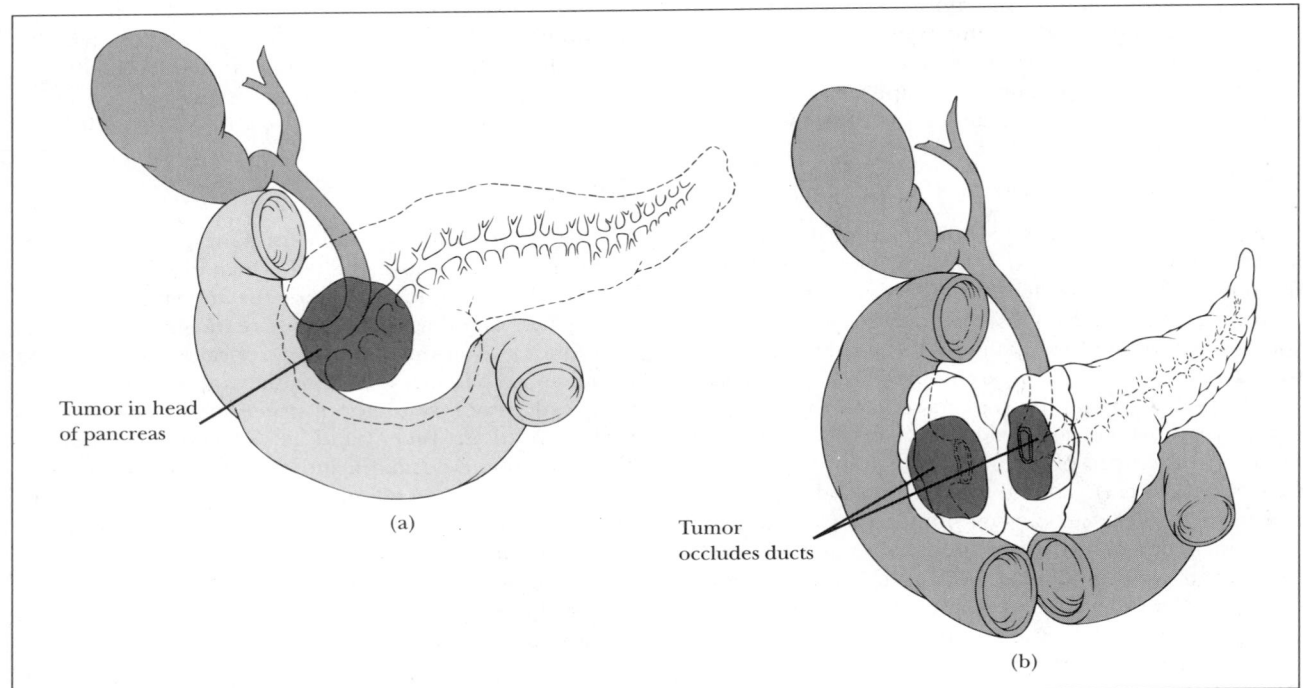

(a)

Tumor in head of pancreas

Tumor occludes ducts

(b)

**FIGURE 38-10**   Pancreatic cancers originate in the duct when they are located in the head of the pancreas (a) they will occlude the distal common bile duct (b). Note the proximity of the pancreatic duct and common bile duct, explaining the characteristic cutoff at the "knee" of the distal bile duct on cholangiography. Adapted from Bastidas JA, Niederhuber JE: Pancreas, in Aberhoff MD et al (eds): *Clinical Oncology*. New York, Churchill Livingstone, 1995, p 1380.

symptom or follows the onset of pain, it is the symptom that invariably causes individuals to seek medical attention. Jaundice along with pain is far more common than painless jaundice.[334] Obstructive jaundice leads to severe pruritus, dark urine, and clay-colored stools. Jaundice does not necessarily indicate extensive disease and unresectability.

Other symptoms are less common and nonspecific. These include weakness, food intolerance, and anorexia. Two unusual symptoms include depression and superficial thrombophlebitis. Depression and anxiety may be part of the initial presentation of pancreatic cancer, independent of pain and other somatic symptoms. These symptoms predate the diagnosis of a pancreatic tumor in approximately 50% of individuals. A triad of depression, anxiety, and feelings of impending doom has been described.[335] This increased incidence of depression is significantly higher than that seen in individuals with other intra-abdominal malignancies.[336] The significance of findings of this triad of symptoms may indicate the presence of neuroendocrine agents in pancreatic cancer that circulate and target the central nervous system. Thrombophlebitis (Trousseau's sign) occurs in fewer than 5% of individuals with pancreatic cancer.

### Body of pancreas

Tumors in the body of the pancreas produce signs and symptoms late in the disease process, making early detection virtually impossible. By the time it is brought to the attention of a physician, the tumor may be large enough to palpate. Severe epigastric pain usually is the first and predominant symptom. The individual may experience intense epigastric pain three to four hours after a meal. This is caused by the space-occupying tumor displacing the stomach or by encroachment at the ligament of Treitz. The pain often is excruciating and accompanied by vomiting. Relief is brought about by sitting up, leaning forward, or lying on the right side with both knees drawn up to the chest. These episodes of pain are short in duration and are most severe at night.[332] Cancer located in the body and tail produce more pain and weight loss than lesions in the head of the pancreas.[337] There is no jaundice with tumors of the body and tail of the pancreas. An enlarged spleen may be found on palpation, caused by tumor pressing on the splenic vein and resulting in splenic vein thrombosis and splenomegaly.

### Tail of pancreas

Cancer in the tail of the pancreas has the most silent and insidious progression of disease. Individuals with carcinoma of the tail of the pancreas may complain of left upper quadrant abdominal pain, generalized weakness, vague indigestion, anorexia, and unexplained weight loss. Metastatic disease is usually present when cancer in the tail of the pancreas is diagnosed. Upper gastrointestinal bleeding, splenomegaly, and signs of portal hypertension and ascites may result from thrombosis of the portal system or extensive liver damage. In rare cases a bruit may be ascultated in the left upper quadrant of the abdomen from splenic artery compression or involvement by tumor.[338]

## Assessment

### Patient and family history

Careful attention to an individual's presenting symptoms and risk factors, and a heightened awareness of the possibility of pancreatic cancer by the clinician are important. Eliciting a family history of pancreatic cancer could help to detect genetic abnormalities and perhaps aid in better treatments for family members in the future.

### Physical examination

Physical examination of the pancreas is virtually impossible because it is an inaccessible organ, lying behind the stomach and in front of the vertebral column. It has been called the "hermit organ" because of its hidden location in the abdomen. There are few signs on presentation except in those individuals presenting with obstructive jaundice. A palpable liver is the most common finding on physical exam in 30%–50% of individuals. A hard, well-defined, mass palpable in the left upper quadrant of the abdomen is found in individuals presenting with lesions in the body and tail of the pancreas and is uncommon in lesions in the head of the pancreas. Fewer than one-third of individuals with cancer of the head of the pancreas present with an enlarged, palpable gallbladder (Courvoisier sign).[339]

### Diagnostic studies

A number of diagnostic studies are available to assist in the identification of pancreatic cancer and to assess for resectability by preoperative staging. If definitive diagnosis cannot be made with these studies, exploratory laparotomy and biopsy may be necessary.

***Radiological examination.*** US of the abdomen can be used as an initial diagnostic test when pancreatic cancer is suspected, especially for lesions in the head of the pancreas. It is a marginal study for visualization of the body, tail, and uncinate process of the pancreas. US can detect intrahepatic and extrahepatic bile duct obstruction, a pancreatic mass, liver metastases greater than 1 cm in diameter, and ascites. It is not sensitive in defining local nodal spread or involvement of the major blood vessels in the area.

CT scan is the diagnostic procedure of choice for the jaundiced individual with a suspected malignancy, especially in older individuals. CT scan is as sensitive as US in defining biliary structures and is superior in defining the level of obstruction, demonstrating the presence of a pancreatic mass, and detecting liver metastases or local vascular invasion.[340] Currently the use of dynamic intravenous and oral contrast-enhanced spiral CT scan offers the best form of imaging of the pancreas.[341] Likewise, CT scanning is more accurate in the diagnosis of unresectability. CT scan findings that indicate the tumor is unlikely to be resected for cure include vascular invasion, enlarged lymph nodes outside the boundaries of the resection, ascites, distant metastases (e.g., liver), and organ invasion.[342] MRI has no apparent advantage over CT scan.[343]

Cholangiography is indicated in the evaluation of the jaundiced individual to define the site of biliary obstruction, by either the endoscopic or the percutaneous approach. Using ERCP, both biliary and pancreatic ductal systems can be visualized. In addition to delineating the site of obstruction, biopsy specimens for cytological analysis can be obtained. A pancreatogram may be important if the differential diagnosis includes chronic pancreatitis. In most cases of pancreatic carcinoma, the pancreatic ductal system will be obstructed, a finding not usually seen in pancreatitis. ERCP may be most useful in the nonjaundiced individual with vague gastrointestinal symptoms in whom an early nonobstructing cancer is suspected. The percutaneous transhepatic approach to the biliary tree is technically easier if there is a dilated biliary tree and is most helpful in defining the proximal biliary system in cases of bile duct cancer (cholangiocarcinoma). PTC with percutaneous transhepatic biliary drainage (PTBD) is usually reserved for those individuals who fail ERCP.

A biliary stent to alleviate jaundice can be placed through the obstructing lesion by either the endoscopic or the percutaneous approach. The use of biliary stents preoperatively has not been shown to improve overall operative risk.[344,345] In selected individuals with severe malnutrition, sepsis, or correctable medical conditions, preoperative biliary drainage is useful. Theoretically, the internal drainage of biliary secretions may provide an immunologic advantage, leading to decreased perioperative complications of sepsis. Finally, percutaneously placed biliary catheters can be used in the operative management of individuals with pancreatic cancer either for resection or for palliation.[346]

Individuals with an endoscopically placed stent need to be informed of the procedure. This procedure, an ERCP with stent placement, is performed under conscious sedation and the person can be discharged the same day. Antibiotics are usually administered intravenously as prophylaxis against cholangitis due to manipulation within the biliary tract. The benefit of a stent drainage catheter is that there is no external tube to manage. The individual needs to be taught the signs and symptoms of possible complications of the stent, such as recurrent jaundice and cholangitis (shaking chills and fever). Any manifestation of these signs or symptoms needs to be reported to the physician immediately, since the individual is prone to bacteremia and sepsis.

The individual having a PTC with placement of a PTBD catheter needs to be taught about the procedure as well as the care and management of the external biliary

catheter. This interventional radiological procedure is performed under conscious sedation. An internal-external catheter is placed. Prophylactic antibiotics are given to prevent biliary sepsis. Individuals are monitored for 24 hours to assess patency of the catheter and assure bile drainage. Initially, the biliary catheter is attached to a bile bag, for external drainage, to allow the obstructed biliary tree to decompress. The bile bag is removed and the biliary catheter is capped off to allow internal drainage and the free flow of bile into the bowel. The care of a percutaneously placed biliary catheter to maintain a properly functioning catheter is an important aspect of patient teaching. Signs and symptoms of any complications, such as fever, chills, recurrent jaundice, bleeding at the exit site or through the biliary catheter, dislodgment of the catheter from its original site, or inability to flush the catheter, must be reported immediately to the physician to prevent problems. Teaching protocols are important for consistent and correct information. Written instructions given to the individual as a handout or video to take home are also very helpful.

Preoperative angiography is performed selectively to determine vascular invasion and to delineate the important vascular anomalies that might alter the operative approach.[347] The study may also be done when the CT scan suggests vascular abnormalities. Modern CT scanning has replaced angiography in the identification of pancreatic tumors.

EUS is a relatively new technique in which a high-frequency US transducer is placed in close contact with the pancreas through the gastrointestinal lumen to provide images of the pancreas and adjacent organs. This procedure can establish the size of the tumor, its extension into adjacent structures, local and regional nodal involvement, and any vascular involvement.[348] This technique may be helpful in staging periampullary cancers and for identifying individuals who may not be optimal surgical candidates.[349]

Laparoscopy and direct visualization are best used for staging cancer of the pancreas. Biopsy of metastatic lesions can be performed at the same time. This minimally invasive procedure can help prevent an unnecessary laparotomy for diagnosis and staging of pancreatic cancer, particularly in individuals with advanced disease and limited survival. Laparoscopy can be performed as an outpatient procedure, or it may be done as an initial procedure at the time of proposed resection to evaluate for resectability.[350,351]

Percutaneous FNAB of pancreatic tumors is useful in selected individuals, especially when guided by CT scan or US. This technique is safe and reliable, but it is not indicated in individuals who are candidates for resection or surgical palliation.[352,353] FNAB may not be useful in potentially resectable tumors because it has a false-negative rate of 20%, because smaller and more curable tumors are most likely to be missed by the needle, and because the tumor can be seeded either along the needle tract[354] or via intraperitoneal spread.[355] The pancreas is a vascular organ with a rich lymphatic network. Unnecessary manipulation can disseminate a cancer that already has a high propensity for local invasion and vascular permeation.[334] FNAB is primarily used in an individual with an unresectable mass in the body or tail of the pancreas, based on CT scan evidence. This technique is also useful in individuals with cancer in the head of the pancreas who are not surgical candidates and whose disease can be palliated nonoperatively.[328] FNAB would be useful for diagnosis and staging in neoadjuvant protocols and can be performed as an outpatient procedure. Education with written follow-up instructions for signs and symptoms of complications is necessary.

*Laboratory tests*   Routine laboratory tests are generally within the normal range, except for those individuals presenting with obstructive jaundice. Increased serum bilirubin, alkaline phosphatase, and often elevated levels of aminotransaminases are found. Mild coagulopathy, as evidenced by prolonged prothrombin time and anemia, may also be evident. Serum and urine amylase concentrations will be elevated when a pancreatic tumor is obstructing the pancreatic duct causing a secondary pancreatitis.[356] New-onset diabetes mellitus may be found in an individual with elevated glucose levels, which may or may not be controlled with oral hyperglycemic agents. An individual with previously diagnosed and orally treated diabetes may find that insulin administration is required to control his or her glucose level, or an individual may need increasing amounts of insulin to control erratic glucose levels. A pancreatic problem should be investigated in an individual with previously controlled diabetes who exhibits any unexplained changes in glucose control.

*Tumor markers*   At present, no serum tumor marker has been found as sufficiently sensitive or specific to be considered cost-effective and 100% reliable for screening purposes. A wide variety of serum tumor markers have been proposed for use in the diagnosis and follow-up of pancreatic carcinoma. The carbohydrate antigen 19-9 (CA 19-9) is tumor-associated, not tumor-specific, and has been the most useful and important tumor marker. This serological test is widely available but is nonspecific for pancreatic carcinoma because it also is elevated in individuals with jaundice and other gastrointestinal carcinomas.[357,358] Also, CA 19-9 is not produced by individuals without the Lewis antigen (5%–10% of the Western population).[359] The levels of CA 19-9 are usually normal in the early stages of pancreatic cancer; thus CA 19-9 is not suitable as a screening test.[360] Elevated CA 19-9 levels may be useful in differentiating benign diseases from pancreatic cancer.[361] After resection of pancreatic cancer, CA 19-9 levels fall and the antigen may be useful for prognosis and follow-up surveillance.[362] Combining CA 19-9 with other tumor-associated antigens, particularly CA 242, has improved specificity for pancreatic cancer, with approximately 80% of pancreatic cancers being correctly diagnosed.[363]

CEA levels are not elevated in early pancreatic cancer

and are not specific to pancreatic cancer.[364] CA 494, a glycogen antigen, has shown promise as a marker for pancreatic cancer. It is more specific for differentiation between chronic pancreatitis and pancreatic cancer. It is not elevated in individuals with type I or type II diabetes without malignant pancreatic neoplasms.[365] Other tumor markers (CA 50, DU-PAN-2, CA 12-5, CA 72-4, and SPAN-1) are being evaluated but thus far have not been as reliable as CA 19-9 in the diagnosis and monitoring of pancreatic cancer. Oncoproteins are a new category of tumor markers being investigated for clinical relevance.[334]

## Classification and Staging

The goal of staging of cancer of the pancreas is to determine the optimal treatment for each individual, with minimal risks and in a cost-effective manner. The aim is to determine which tumors are potentially resectable, which cannot be resected but are still localized, and which have already metastasized to distant sites.[361]

The staging of pancreatic carcinoma is based on the tumor-node-metastases (TNM) system, which classifies tumors according to the extent of the primary tumor, the status of the regional lymph nodes, and the presence or absence of metastases. The primary tumor status (T) is defined by the presence and degree of extension through the pancreatic capsule; the nodal status (N) is defined by the presence or absence of regional pancreatic lymph node involvement; metastases (M) are defined by the presence or absence of distal peritoneal or visceral metastatic disease. Utilizing these definitions, four stages have been described for use in the diagnosis of pancreatic cancer by the Cancer of the Pancreas Task Force of the American Joint Commission on Cancer Staging and End-Results Reporting; they are listed in Table 38-6. These parameters represent the most important factors influencing resectability and prognosis.

## Treatment

Every individual diagnosed with cancer of the pancreas should be carefully evaluated prior to initiation of any therapy. With advances in diagnosing and staging the disease, progress has been made in the efficacy of the surgical and nonsurgical approaches to treatment and palliation. An individual must be adequately prepared physiologically and psychologically before undergoing any therapy. The poor prognosis of individuals with pancreatic cancer has caused many clinicians to have a dismal outlook, and thus they are reluctant to treat the disease aggressively.[366] Recent reports on surgical outcomes are encouraging,[367,368] and it is hoped that renewed investigation into the pathogenesis of cancer of the pancreas will lead to better screening, prevention, diagnosis, and treatment. The overall current perspective on the disease is changing.

Surgery, radiotherapy, and chemotherapy are the

**TABLE 38-6**   TNM Classification System for Cancer of the Pancreas

| PRIMARY TUMOR (T) | |
|---|---|
| TX | Primary tumor cannot be assessed |
| T0 | No evidence of primary tumor |
| T1 | Tumor limited to the pancreas |
| | T1a   Tumor 2 cm or less in greatest dimension |
| | T1b   Tumor more than 2 cm in greatest dimension |
| T2 | Tumor extends directly to any of the following: duodenum, bile duct, or peripancreatic tissues |
| T3 | Tumor extends directly to any of the following: duodenum, stomach, spleen, colon, or adjacent large vessels |

| LYMPH NODE (N) | |
|---|---|
| NX | Regional lymph nodes cannot be assessed |
| N0 | No regional lymph node metastasis |
| N1 | Regional lymph node metastasis |

| DISTANT METASTASIS (M) | |
|---|---|
| MX | Presence of distant metastasis cannot be assessed |
| M0 | No distant metastasis |
| M1 | Distant metastasis |

| STAGE GROUPING | | | |
|---|---|---|---|
| I | T1 | N0 | M0 |
| | T2 | N0 | M0 |
| II | T3 | N0 | M0 |
| III | Any T | N1 | M0 |
| IV | Any T | Any N | M1 |

From Beahrs OH, Henson DE, Hutter RVP, et al (eds): *American Joint Committee on Cancer: Manual for Staging of Cancer* (ed 4). Philadelphia, Lippincott, 1992.

major treatment modalities used for pancreatic cancer. Surgical resection still remains the best therapeutic option even though few individuals are cured. Most surgical procedures are palliative as nonresectable pancreatic cancer predominates. Only about 10% of malignancies of the head of the pancreas are resectable and potentially curable at surgery.[337] The three-year and five-year survival after resection of the head of the pancreas are only 35% and 21%, respectively. The resection and survival rates for tumors in the body and tail are much lower.

Multimodality therapy that combines surgery, radiation therapy, and chemotherapy is being studied to determine if survival time can be lengthened. Available therapeutic interventions include surgery, usually in combination with radiation therapy and chemotherapy with single agents or in combination for either cure or palliation. Various regimens of chemotherapeutic agents alone or in combination with radiation therapy are also used for nonoperative cancer of the pancreas. A longer palliation is usually achieved with combined modalities.

Once a diagnosis has been made, the extent of the tumor involvement established, and complete assessment of the individual's physical status made, a treatment plan

will be presented to the individual. If surgery is an option, the individual's physical ability to undergo general anesthesia and a major abdominal operation must be considered; advanced age is not necessarily a negative factor. Nutritional status, hematologic status, liver function, concomitant disease, and skill of the principal clinicians all contribute to the choice of therapy.

Cure is the objective if the tumor is localized and not fixed to other structures, and if there is no evidence of regional or distant metastases. Complete resection of the tumor will be performed and supplemented with adjuvant radiation and/or chemotherapy.

Control or palliation is the goal of therapy if the tumor is unresectable or has metastasized to regional or distant nodes or to other organs. Unfortunately, 90% of all cases of pancreatic carcinoma are diagnosed after the tumor is unresectable. In a considerable number of individuals, operative palliation for bypassing bile and/or gastric outlet obstruction may be indicated for optimal long-term management.[328] Other treatments aimed at palliating devastating symptoms may be selected, including radiotherapy, chemotherapy, percutaneous pain block, percutaneous or endoscopic biliary decompression to relieve obstruction and pressure, and gastric decompression for gastric outlet obstruction. Nutritional supplementation to achieve adequate total protein levels helps to decrease surgical risk, puts the individual in a better metabolic state for having any treatment modality, and increases the overall general state of well-being.

No matter what treatment is selected, it is important to understand an individual's goal of therapy, method of family coping, and pattern of communication. When all members of the health care team, along with the individual, agree upon a course of treatment, communications are enhanced and issues or problems can be identified and addressed. Identifying the support network and understanding the coping mechanisms of an individual can promote the uniqueness of the individual as disease and illness has a special meaning to each person. Living with cancer of the pancreas and dealing with the knowledge that the disease has a poor prognosis, regardless of what treatment is undertaken, can create many unforeseen problems. Patience and understanding are paramount.

### Surgery

Surgical resection of pancreatic carcinoma still remains the best therapeutic option. Pancreatic resection provides the only opportunity for cure. Most surgical procedures for cancer of the pancreas are palliative. Only about 10% of carcinomas of the head of the pancreas are resectable and potentially curable at surgery. The survival rate for tumors in the body and tail is much lower. There is limited prospective research evaluating surgical procedures for cancer of the pancreas.

Recent reports from institutions with large series of patients have reported increasing survival periods following resection.[361,367,368] Operative mortality rates have decreased to less than 5% in most experienced centers. A decrease in complications is attributed to refinements in surgical technique, anesthesia, critical care, and preoperative and postoperative care. Other reasons for improvement with surgical management include the operation being performed by surgeons who are experienced in the surgical management of pancreatic carcinoma, concentration of patients in centers of excellence, and improved methods to diagnose and treat complications.[369] Most surgical results report collective overall outcomes; however, individuals with small (< 2 cm) tumors experience 30% five-year survival rates, and the survival rates increase for those with no residual disease or without lymphatic involvement.[361] The crux of the problem is late detection of pancreatic tumors. Until improvements in early detection and diagnosis are made, curative surgery will be limited to very few candidates, and palliative procedures will continue as the mainstay of therapy.

The surgical approach most used when cure is the objective is a pancreaticoduodenectomy (Whipple procedure). Total pancreatectomy may be performed for tumor involvement of the entire gland. An extended or radical pancreaticoduodenectomy has also been performed as a modification of the original regional pancreatectomy. The regional pancreatectomy has been evaluated and found to have higher morbidity and mortality rates, with no improvement in survival over the standard pancreaticoduodenectomy.[370] Controversy exists over the advantages, disadvantages, and long-term results of each operation (Table 38-7). In order to determine the best operation for resectable pancreatic cancer, data from prospective randomized studies comparing standard versus radical pancreaticoduodenectomy in individuals are needed.

Despite sophisticated preoperative staging methods, many individuals with adenocarcinoma of the head of the pancreas that appears to be resectable preoperatively are found to have metastatic or locally invasive disease at laparotomy, thus precluding resection. Resectability is determined by the absence of distant metastases (e.g., to the liver, peritoneal surfaces, distant lymph nodes) as well as whether the tumor has grown to involve adjacent major vascular structures (superior mesenteric and portal veins, superior mesenteric and hepatic arteries). Although preoperative studies may help with assessment for resectability, only surgical exploration is definitive.

***Pancreaticoduodenectomy (Whipple procedure)*** The Whipple procedure is the most commonly performed operation for carcinoma of the pancreas. The classic Whipple procedure includes resection of the distal stomach, gallbladder, distal common bile duct, head of the pancreas, and duodenum. Gastrointestinal continuity is restored by anastomosing the common bile duct and the remaining pancreas to the jejunum proximal to the gastrojejunostomy. Some surgeons anastomose the remaining pancreas to the back of the stomach because they believe it is safer and decreases the potential for pancreatic fistula formation.[371–373] The gastrojejunostomy is performed to allow alkaline bile and pancreatic juices to enter the jejunum before acidic gastric secretions (Figure 38-11). This decreases the potential of ulceration at the gastrojejunostomy. The distal gastrojejunostomy also reduces reflux of intestinal contents into the bile duct and pancreas. Many surgeons no longer perform a truncal vagotomy to reduce the risk of marginal ulceration as part of the Whipple procedure as the incidence has been found to be low. Individuals are managed prophylactically with acid antisecretory agents instead.[374]

A modification of the original Whipple procedure, called a *pylorus preserving pancreaticoduodenectomy*, is preferred by some surgeons. This procedure preserves the entire stomach, including the pylorus, and a small cuff of proximal duodenum (Figure 38-12). It has the advantage of maintaining a normal gastric reservoir and potentially avoiding nutritional problems associated with the classic Whipple procedure such as weight loss, dumping syndrome, diarrhea, and anastomotic ulcer. This procedure is less time-consuming and technically easier to perform.[375] The complication of delayed gastric emptying that may occur from this operation generally resolves over time with conservative treatment (gastric decompression, parenteral or enteral nutrition, and prokinetic agents). Erythromycin, a motilin agonist, also has been used to improve gastric emptying after surgery.[376] Concern continues that the pylorus preserving pancreaticoduodenectomy is not an adequate cancer operation because of limited surgical margins and inadequate removal of lymph nodes in the area draining cancer, which may compromise cure. Studies are being conducted to compare the two procedures with respect to morbidity and survival.

Pancreatic fistula and delayed gastric emptying are the most common serious complications after a pancreaticoduodenectomy. The pancreas, attached to the jejunum, is technically the most difficult of the anastomoses. If the pancreas does not heal properly, a pancreatic fistula may develop. Although fistulae and leaks were previously associated with significant mortality because pancreatic juices eroded into major blood vessels, the situation has changed. The incidence and severity of pancreatic anastomotic leaks appear to have decreased with improved surgical technique, intravenous nutritional support, modern antibiotics, and appropriate wound drainage systems.[367,375] The use of the somatostatin analogue octreotide, which decreases pancreatic secretion, may also be useful in the management of postoperative pancreatic fistulae.[377,378] Intra-abdominal infection, bile leak, gastrointestinal bleeding, and intra-abdominal hemorrhage occur less frequently.[379]

It is important for the nurse to know exactly what surgical procedure was performed in order to know what to assess from various drains and tubes placed at the time of surgery. Bile duct-to-jejunum anastomosis may be stented with either a preoperatively placed percutaneous transhepatic biliary catheter or with an operatively placed T-tube for decompression of the jejunum and to allow the free flow of bile. This stent also provides direct access into the biliary tree to assess for an anastomotic leak,

**TABLE 38-7**  Comparison of Types of Pancreatic Resections for Malignancy

| | Classic Pancreatico-duodenectomy (Whipple) | Pylorus Preserving (PP) Pancreatico-duodenectomy (Whipple) | Extended or Radical Pancreatico-duodenectomy | Total Pancreatico-duodenectomy (May Be Classic or PP) | Distal Pancreatectomy |
|---|---|---|---|---|---|
| Indications | Periampullary or lo-calized carcinoma of head, neck or un-cinate process of pancreas | Periampullary or lo-calized carcinoma of head, neck or un-cicate process of pancreas | Periampullary or lo-calized carcinoma of head, neck or un-cinate process of pancreas | Diffuse carcinoma of entire gland or a multicentric tumor | Carcinoma localized to body or tail of gland |
| Tissues removed | Head, neck and un-cinate process Duodenum Gastric antrum and pylorus Common bile duct Gallbladder Lymph nodes in pancreaticoduode-nal groove | Head, neck and un-cinate process Duodenum (except most proximal por-tion) Common bile duct Gallbladder Lymph nodes in pancreaticoduode-nal groove | Head, neck and un-cinate process Duodenum Gastric antrum and pylorus Common bile duct Gallbladder Extensive lymph node and tissue dis-section Vascular resection may be included | Entire pancreas Duodenum (Gastric antrum and pylorus) Common bile duct Gallbladder Spleen Peripancreatic nodes Lymph nodes in pancreaticoduode-nal groove | Distal pancreas Spleen Peripancreatic lymph nodes |
| Anastomoses | Hepaticojejunos-tomy or choledo-chojejunostomy Gastrojejunostomy Pancreaticojejunos-tomy or pancreatic-ogastrostomy | Hepaticojejunos-tomy or choledo-chojejunostomy Duodenojejunos-tomy Pancreaticojejunos-tomy or pancreatic-ogastrostomy | Hepaticojejunos-tomy or choledo-chojejunostomy Gastrojejunostomy Pancreaticojejunos-tomy or pancreatic-ogastrostomy | Choledochojejunos-tomy or hepaticojej-unostomy Gastrojejunostomy or duodenojejunos-tomy | None |
| Potential advan-tages | Pancreatic remnant may prevent diabe-tes and malabsorp-tion Better cancer oper-ation? | Pancreatic remnant may prevent diabe-tes and malabsorp-tion Normal gastric res-ervoir Less disruption of digestion Reduced marginal ulceration at duode-nojejunostomy | Extensive regional nodal dissection Pancreatic remnant may prevent diabe-tes and malabsorp-tion Better cancer oper-ation? | Excision of entire pancreas may re-move multifocal tumor More complete peripancreatic nodal dissection No pancreatic en-teric anastomsis | Pancreatic remnant may prevent diabe-tes and malabsorp-tion No pancreatic or bili-ary enteric anasto-mosis |
| Potential disad-vantages | Partial pancreatic resection may leave residual tumor in body or tail of gland. Issue of multicen-tricity Dumping syndrome secondary to loss of pylorus Nutritional prob-lems Leak at pancreatic anastomosis | Partial pancreatic resection may leave residual tumor in body or tail of gland Leak at pancreatic anastomosis Delayed gastric emptying | Partial pancreatic resection may leave residual tumor in body or tail of gland Leak at pancreatic anastomosis Dumping syndrome secondary to loss of pylorus Nutritional prob-lems Chylous leak Longer operation | Insulin-dependent diabetes and com-plete exocrine ab-sence Need for insulin and enzyme replace-ment Postsplenectomy state | Limited resection may leave residual tumor (Postsple-nectomy state) |

Modified from Sindelar WF, Kinsella TJ, Mayer RJ: Cancer of the pancreas, in DeVita VT, Hellman S, Rosenberg SA (eds): *Cancer: Principles and Practice of Oncology* (ed 2). Philadelphia, Lippincott, 1985, pp 691–739.

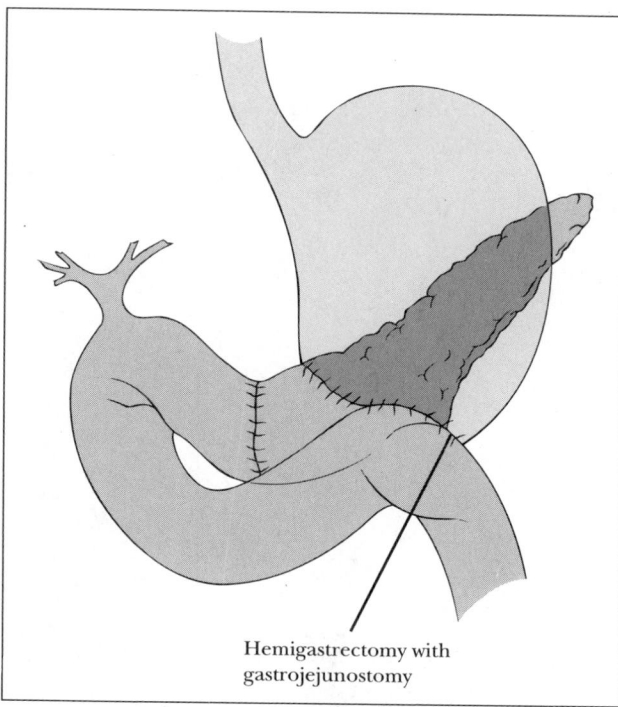

Hemigastrectomy with
gastrojejunostomy

**FIGURE 38-11**   Reconstructive alternatives. Classic
Whipple procedure with end-to-end pancreaticojejunostomy
and hemigastrectomy, with gastrojejunostomy.

obstruction, or stricture. Likewise, wound drains are
placed adjacent to the pancreatic anastomosis to enable
rapid assessment of bile or pancreatic juice leakage or
bleeding. The use of various feeding tubes placed at the
time of surgery depends on the preference of the surgeon.

Nutritional assessment is important to establish that
the person has adequate protein and calories for wound
healing. Most individuals will receive postoperative adjuvant therapy; therefore, good nutritional status along with
physical and psychological readiness are essential. Immediate postoperative pain management can be successfully
provided by intravenous or epidural patient-controlled
analgesia (PCA).

*Extended pancreaticoduodenectomy*   This operation
consists of a pancreaticoduodenectomy or sometimes a
total pancreatectomy, along with an extensive retroperitoneal lymph node and soft-tissue resection. Resection of
the superior mesenteric vein, portal vein, or superior
mesenteric artery may also be included. The extended
pancreaticoduodenectomy has been supported since data
suggest that lymph node involvement is an important
prognostic factor in individuals with carcinoma of the
head of the pancreas. Evidence suggests that wide lymphatic resections, wider than those commonly performed
with the standard Whipple procedure, may prolong survival.[380–382] The available data are retrospective, and no
prospective, randomized studies between the standard

and the extended pancreaticoduodenectomy have been
reported. An appropriately designed study needs to be
done before modification of the standard pancreaticoduodenectomy is adopted.

*Total pancreatectomy*   A total pancreatectomy includes
an en bloc resection of the distal stomach, duodenum,
gallbladder, and distal common bile duct, along with the
entire pancreas, spleen, and a wide margin of peripancreatic tissue including lymph nodes. Total pancreatectomy eliminates the problem of residual tumor at the
margins of the pancreas, tumor spillage when the pancreas is divided, and pancreatic fistula. This operation
has shown no reduction in mortality or morbidity[358,374] nor
evidence of any increase in survival when it is performed
routinely.[383] Individuals who have total pancreatectomy
develop pancreatic endocrine and exocrine insufficiency
and as a result are brittle diabetics with difficult-to-control
glucose levels. Pancreatic enzyme supplementation is necessary for a lifetime. This operation is usually reserved
for selected cases, particularly when there is evidence of
tumor throughout the entire pancreas.

*Distal pancreatectomy*   In rare cases, tumors of the
body and tail of the pancreas are detected early enough
to be considered curable. In these cases a distal pancreatectomy with a splenectomy is performed. The prognosis
is poor, with few persons surviving for more than two
years. Lesions of the body and tail rarely cause gastrointestinal obstructive symptoms and as a result are not recognized until the tumor has become unresectable.[384] Most
individuals with adenocarcinomas of the body or tail of
the pancreas are unresectable and survive for only a short
period. The only change in the management of these
individuals has been a diminished need for exploratory
laparotomy to establish tissue diagnosis.[339] The use of
laparoscopy and FNAB to determine metastatic or unresectable disease spares these individuals an unnecessary
laparotomy.

*Palliative procedures*   Currently, only approximately
15% of individuals with pancreatic cancer are resectable
for cure at the time of presentation. Therefore, palliation
of symptoms to maximize the quality of life is the primary
goal for these individuals.[385] These individuals present
challenging management problems because optimal palliation of symptoms is difficult. Obstructive jaundice, duodenal obstruction, and pain are the most frequent
symptoms requiring intervention.[328] Operative and nonoperative techniques are available to provide relief of
symptoms. The management of most individuals with
unresectable pancreatic cancer can be tailored to the
individual's clinical presentation, prognosis, and overall
medical condition.[385] A choice must be made between
operative and nonoperative palliation. Individuals should
have operative palliation who are deemed appropriate
surgical candidates, have a good performance status, and
are expected to survive for longer than six months. Individuals in poor health or those not expected to live for

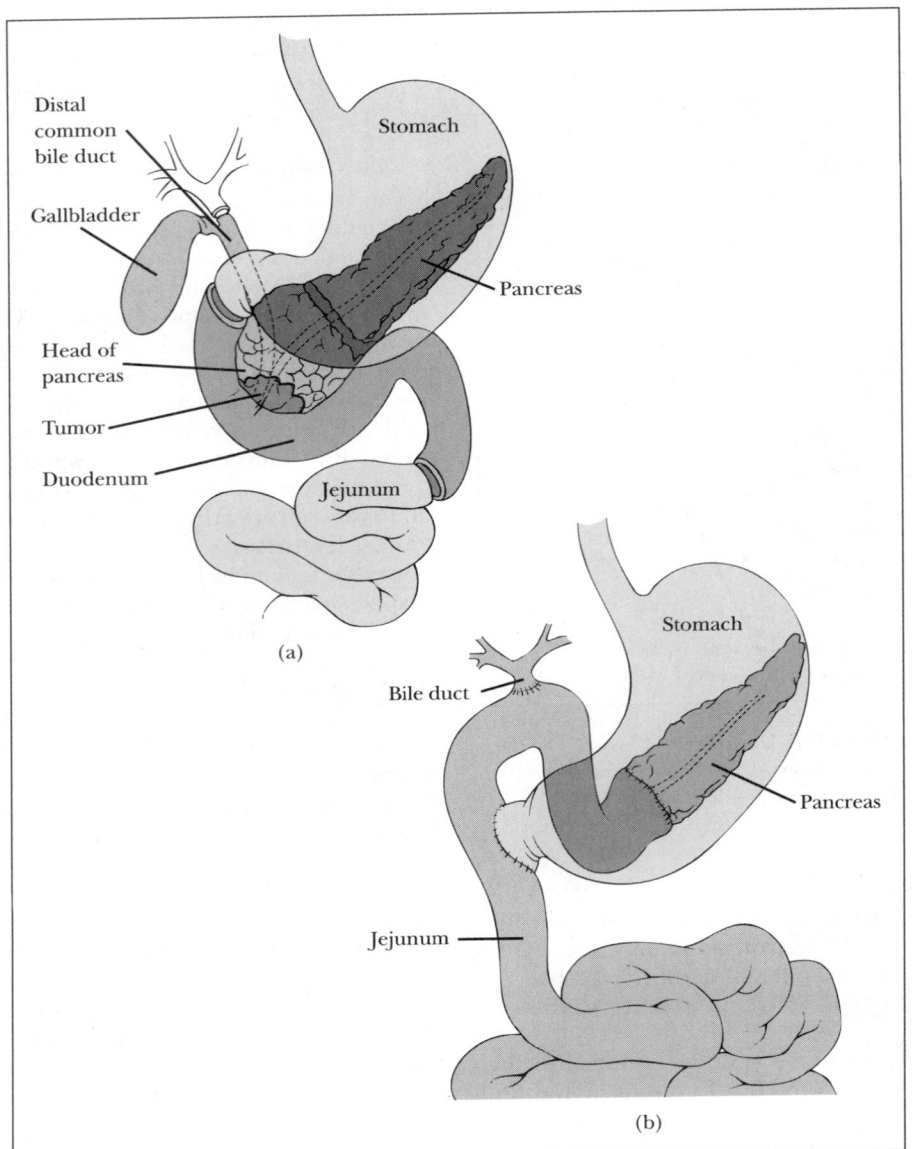

**FIGURE 38-12** Pylorus-preserving pancreaticoduodenectomy. Anatomy of the resected area (a) and reconnected digestive tract with end-to-end pancreaticojejunostomy (b). Adapted from Pitt HA: Curative treatment for pancreatic neoplasms. *Surg Clin N Am* 75:891–904, 1995.

a prolonged time should be considered for nonoperative palliation.[328]

Conventional surgical palliation for an individual with a tumor in the head of the pancreas is directed toward relief of obstructive jaundice, gastric outlet obstruction, and pain. Operative procedures designed for palliation include biliary-enteric drainage, gastrojejunostomy, and chemical splanchnicectomy. Individuals with body and tail lesions of the pancreas are less likely to have jaundice or duodenal obstruction, and pain is the major symptom.

Obstructive jaundice is the most common presenting symptom in the majority of cancers of the head of the pancreas. If untreated, obstructive jaundice results in progressive liver dysfunction, culminating in liver failure and early death. In addition, the pruritus associated with obstructive jaundice can be unbearable and is seldom responsive to medications. The jaundiced individual usually experiences anorexia, nausea, and progressive malnutrition.[385] Relief of jaundice can provide improvement in an individual's overall well-being.

The surgical options for palliation of obstructive jaundice include an internal biliary bypass by means of a choledochojejunostomy (common bile duct to jejunum) or a cholecystojejunostomy (gallbladder to jejunum). In most individuals, bypass of the obstructed biliary tree to the jejunum is preferred and is necessary if the gallbladder is surgically absent.

Nonoperative palliation of obstructed jaundice by either percutaneous or endoscopic drainage methods is also effective. Placement of a biliary tube through the area of biliary obstruction stents the bile duct and allows the free flow of bile internally into the duodenum. Compared with operative decompression, biliary stents reduce the length of initial hospitalization, appear to be associated with lower complication rates and lower procedure-related mortality, and are significantly less expensive.[386-388]

Endoscopically placed biliary stents offer an advantage over the percutaneous technique, with fewer procedure-related complications and better individual acceptance. The major problem is stent occlusion associated with recurrent jaundice and sepsis. This can require stent replacement every three to four months.[388] Prolonging stent patency is now being addressed with the development and use of large-diameter expandable metallic stents, which require fewer endoscopic interventions, a safer and cost-effective alternative.[389] These metallic stents appear to stay patent for a time that closely approximates the length of survival of the individual.[390] Endoscopic stents are also preferred for individuals with ascites.

Percutaneous biliary drainage is indicated in individuals in whom endoscopic biliary drainage is unsuccessful and in individuals with recurrent jaundice following surgical bypass.[390] An internal-external drainage catheter is placed by an interventional radiologist. The biliary catheter requires daily maintenance by the individual or caregiver. Daily catheter flushing and dressing of the catheter entry site are needed. The presence of an external limb of the catheter is a constant reminder to the individual of the disease. Bile leakage around the catheter, skin irritation, catheter dislodgment, and catheter occlusion may also occur. In individuals with ascites, leakage of ascitic fluid around the catheter almost always occurs and is difficult to control. Because all catheters placed within the biliary tree eventually will occlude, percutaneous biliary catheters are exchanged approximately every three months to prevent development of catheter obstruction, recurrent jaundice, or cholangitis. This exchange can be easily performed as an outpatient procedure. Complications related to percutaneous biliary drainage are transient bacteremia or sepsis, hemobilia, and bile peritonitis.

Duodenal obstruction occurs in a significant number of individuals when unresectable disease progresses. Obstruction from cancer in the head of the pancreas typically occurs at the duodenal C loop. A large tumor in the body or tail of the pancreas will usually obstruct the junction of the duodenum and jejunum at the ligament of Treitz.[385] A gastrojejunostomy can be performed to treat or prevent gastric outlet obstruction. Controversy exists as to the value of the procedure as a prophylactic measure in individuals with unresectable pancreatic cancer. Evidence suggests that the individual's morbidity or mortality is not increased when gastrojejunostomy is performed as either a therapeutic or a prophylactic measure.[391,392] If an individual is not a surgical candidate because of recurrent tumor or is in the terminal stage of disease, duodenal obstruction can be alleviated by placement of a percutaneous endoscopic gastrostomy (PEG) decompression tube. This tube is not used for feeding, but it is effective in relieving gastric distention and may improve the comfort of the individual in the terminal stages of the disease.

Pain is the most significant symptom for individuals with pancreatic cancer. The severity and persistence of pain correlate well with the stage of the disease. For most individuals with pancreatic cancer who are not surgical candidates, the appropriate use of oral agents can successfully manage pain.[393,394] Chemical splanchnicectomy (alcohol block) is an alternative therapy available to those individuals who do not benefit from oral analgesia or cannot tolerate oral intake due to gastric outlet obstruction. It is performed using a spinal needle to inject alcohol on each side of the aorta at the level of the celiac axis (Figure 38-13). Percutaneous celiac nerve block, with either fluoroscopic or CT scan guidance, can be per-

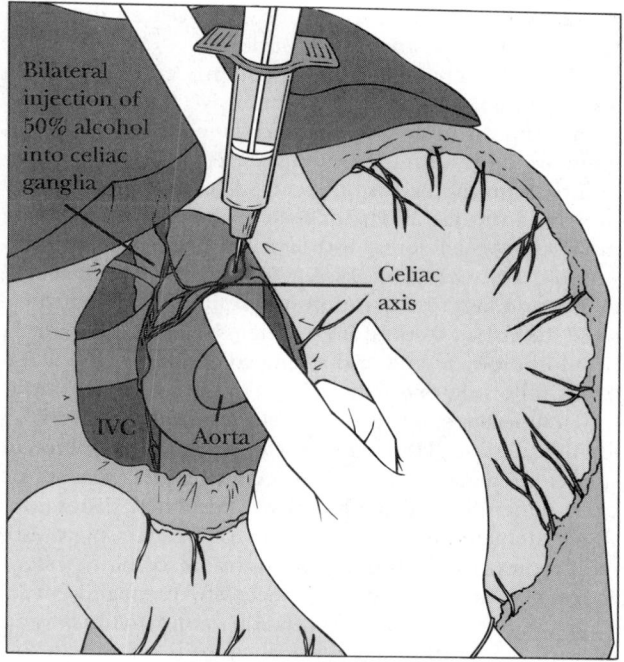

**FIGURE 38-13** Chemical splanchnicectomy was performed using a syringe and a 20- or 22-gauge spinal needle. Solution (20 cc) was injected on each side of the aorta at the level of the celiac axis. Adapted from Lillemoe KD, Cameron JL, Kaufman HS, et al: Chemical splanchnicectomy in patients with unresectable pancreatic cancer: A prospective randomized trial. *Ann Surg* 217:447–457, 1993.

formed to reduce pain and to reduce the need for oral narcotics. Nerve blocks can be done as an outpatient procedure or at the time of surgery for those individuals undergoing a palliative operation. Percutaneous nerve blocks can be repeated in individuals with previous blocks that have subsequently worn off.[395,396] Orthostatic hypotension is the most common complication after the block. Intraoperative celiac injection of alcohol has been shown to both relieve pain and prevent the development of pain. A recent prospective study has clearly documented efficacy and safety of intraoperative nerve block. The improvement in pain control was associated with prolonged survival. This observation shows the importance of effective pain control and its contribution to quality of life.[395]

Another modality used for control of pain due to unresectable pancreatic cancer is external-beam radiation.[366] Finally, transthoracic splanchnicectomy can be performed by thoracotomy or thoracoscopy to relieve pain due to unresectable pancreatic cancer in selected individuals.[397]

***Postoperative care***    Postoperative medical and nursing management of individuals who undergo pancreatic resection is critical for reducing surgical morbidity and mortality. Careful assessment, anticipatory management, and complete patient and family teaching will greatly enhance recovery and rehabilitation.[398] Hemorrhage, hypovolemia, and hypotension pose the greatest threats in the immediate postoperative period.

Following a pancreatic resection procedure, individuals are initially admitted to an intensive care unit, where hemodynamic monitoring is performed. Stabilizing and maintaining fluid requirements are essential. Careful attention is given to signs of bleeding, security and patency of wound drains, and pain management. Pain management can be achieved with opiates delivered by intravenous or epidural PCA. Following endotracheal extubation, aggressive pulmonary toilet is needed to reduce the risk of respiratory problems. Ideally, individuals should be out of bed and sitting in a chair within a few hours following extubation.

Hemorrhage in the early postoperative period can be life-threatening. Hemorrhage can occur from failure of surgical hemostasis, from leakage at the anastomosis, or from generalized coagulopathy. Abdominal distention, shock, hematemesis, bloody drainage from gastrointestinal decompression tubes, wound drains, or bloody stool warrant immediate attention. Successful management requires correction of coagulation abnormalities and prompt reoperation if a surgical cause is suspected.[394]

Hypovolemia can develop from fluids lost during extensive surgery, through decompression tubes and wound drains, or from the shift of fluid from the vascular space to the interstitial space (third spacing). Low levels of circulating plasma proteins secondary to malnutrition and hypoalbuminemia usually account for the third spacing syndrome. The first phase of fluid compartment shifting begins immediately after surgery and can last 48–72 hours. Signs of fluid shift are as follows:

- decreased blood pressure
- increased pulse rate
- low central venous pressure
- decreased urine output
- increased specific gravity
- low levels of serum albumin
- hemoconcentration

When the plasma protein is replaced and levels return to normal, fluid reabsorption follows. Urine output will dramatically increase and will greatly exceed intake. The individual is closely monitored for signs of circulatory overload. The reabsorption phase will reach equilibrium within 24–48 hours.

Hypotension is a potential postoperative complication that is believed to result from severance of the sympathetic nerve fibers of the mesenteric complex. Vital signs and urine output should be monitored frequently to detect alterations. Vasopressor drugs and liberal intravenous fluids may be administered.

Pulmonary complications following surgery usually result from immobility and inadequate lung expansion secondary to pain and splinting. In addition, those individuals who are malnourished and protein-deficient are susceptible to pneumonia. The importance of vigorous pulmonary hygiene and early ambulation cannot be overemphasized. Parenteral nutrition may also be needed to correct nutritional deficiencies.

Careful attention is given to wound drains for any sudden change in amount, color, or consistency of drainage. Abdominal wound drains are observed for evidence of bile or clear pancreatic juice that would suggest anastomotic leakage. Pancreatic juice that changes color to milky or brown with a foul odor suggests a pancreatic fistula. The somatostatin analogue octreotide may be given to reduce pancreatic secretion.[377,378]

Prolonged ileus and delayed gastric emptying are also potential complications. These generally resolve by taking a conservative approach with nasogastric suction, maintenance of parenteral or enteral nutrition, and the use of prokinetic agents, such as metoclopramide, or a motilin agonist, such as erythromycin.[376] The surgical incision must be examined routinely for any signs of infection as this complication can be synergistic with a pancreatic fistula or delayed gastric emptying.

Following resection of the pancreas, exocrine and endocrine functions will be temporarily or permanently altered, depending on the amount of viable pancreatic tissue remaining. In the immediate postoperative period, laboratory tests are useful for monitoring protein, fat, and glucose levels. Prior to discharge, the individual and family must become familiar with and able to recognize the signs and symptoms of exocrine and endocrine abnormalities such as hyperglycemia, hypoglycemia, steatorrhea, stupor, and lethargy.

Endocrine function, the secretion of insulin, and the production of glucagon may be altered after a pancreatic resection. Usually, a nondiabetic individual will not develop diabetes after a pancreaticoduodenectomy (occurring in < 10% of cases).[399] Individuals who have a total pancreatectomy will develop significant hyperglycemia and are usually managed in the immediate postoperative period with an insulin drip infusion. Endocrine consultants should be contacted soon after surgery to assist with glucose management and insulin adjustment, particularly when the individual is taking oral foods and fluids. Serum glucose levels are monitored at least every six hours, and a sliding-scale insulin dose is administered as needed if the individual can take nothing by mouth. These individuals generally require only moderate amounts of insulin and are not prone to ketoacidosis. However, they are particularly brittle and easily develop life-threatening hypoglycemia.[391] Discharge teaching and home therapy programs, including self-administration of insulin, knowledge of signs and symptoms of hyper- or hypoglycemia, diabetic diet, meticulous hygiene, and the importance of routine follow-up with an endocrinologist or a medical physician for diabetes management are the same as for individuals with diabetes. Inability to control glucose levels could indicate recurrence of disease.

Alteration of exocrine function by removal of pancreatic tissue can result in a malabsorption syndrome characterized by an inability to use ingested forms of fat and protein. The caloric requirements of the individual following surgery exceed 3000 calories per day; therefore, adequate nutritional intake is essential to recovery. Oral ingestion of food is the best means of maintaining essential nutrients, but ileus or delayed gastric emptying may prohibit this mode. Parenteral or enteral alimentation may be necessary to replace calories lost as a result of the surgically induced malabsorption of fats and proteins until the individual can be advanced to an oral diet. Pancreatic enzymes are replaced with oral enzyme supplements. Pancreatic enzyme supplements contain lipase, amylase, and trypsin. The most frequently used forms are pancreatin and pancrelipase. Pancreatin and pancrelipase supplements are made from extracts of hog or beef pancreas enriched with bile salts and plant and fungal enzymes. The usual therapeutic dose is three to six tablets with each meal and one to two tablets with a fatty snack. The enzymes are taken with or during the meal.[400] It may require several adjustments before the most appropriate dosage for each person is determined, because eating patterns and individual responses vary.[401] The individual should be informed that steatorrhea will decrease but may not be eliminated.

After pancreatic surgery when the individual is able to tolerate food, several small feedings consisting of foods that are low in fat and high in carbohydrates and protein are tolerated better than large meals. Restrictions include overindulgence (which places a great demand on the pancreas), caffeine, and alcohol. It is advantageous for the clinical dietitian to consult with the individual to select the most agreeable diet plan based on individual needs and lifestyle. The individual and family should be instructed on how to monitor the individual's tolerance to the diet and pancreatic enzyme replacement therapy. The stool should be examined daily for the characteristic signs of steatorrhea; frothy, floating, foul-smelling stool with fat particles floating in the water. If these are observed, it should be reported to the physician or nurse for dietary and/or pancreatic enzyme adjustment.[400]

### Chemotherapy

Because most individuals present with unresectable cancer of the pancreas, the use of chemotherapeutic agents has been tried. The overall survival results have been dismal as these individuals have metastatic disease and are already in a debilitated state, making benefit from antineoplastic therapy unlikely. Individuals with pancreatic cancer exhibit precarious physiological conditions, which makes it difficult to differentiate the side effects of therapy from the natural progression of the disease. Response to therapy is also difficult to evaluate.

Some chemotherapeutic agents have been used as single agents in the treatment of pancreatic cancer: 5-FU, mitomycin C, streptozocin, ifosfamide, and doxorubicin. The results have been minimally effective with single agents. It was hoped that combinations of chemotherapeutic agents with regimens such as SMF (streptozocin, mitomycin C, 5-FU) and FAM would produce higher response rates. Unfortunately, combination chemotherapy has shown no survival advantage over treatment with single agents. Chemotherapy as adjuvant treatment for pancreatic cancer is still being investigated. The high rate of mortality associated with metastatic disease indicates that systemic therapy is needed as part of multimodality treatment. Current applications of chemotherapy have failed to produce significant results.

A more realistic objective of treatment may be the improvement in the quality of life, with prolonged survival being a secondary benefit. Drug efficacy in pancreatic cancer may be better judged by the alleviation of tumor-related symptoms than by measuring tumor shrinkage. A new cytotoxic agent, gemcitabine, has been evaluated in the treatment of individuals with unresectable pancreatic cancer. Clinical benefit response is a novel approach to assess the clinical effectiveness of gemcitabine based on marked improvement in pain control, analgesic consumption, and performance status. Prolonged survival was a secondary end point. The drug has been found to be well tolerated, with a relatively mild toxicity profile. This new therapeutic paradigm for measuring response may serve as a model for the development of other effective therapies for individuals with advanced pancreatic cancer.[402] It is hoped that new chemotherapeutic agents, new sequencing of therapies, or new drug combinations will improve outcomes.

### Radiation therapy

Radiation therapy has been used for both palliation and curative therapy of pancreatic cancer. Directed radiation to the pancreas is difficult because of the limited radiation tolerance of adjacent organs in the upper abdomen, including the kidney, liver, stomach, small bowel, and spinal cord.[403] The technique usually used to treat pancreatic cancer is external-beam radiotherapy. More specialized methods of radiotherapy have been used, such as intraoperative radiotherapy[404] and brachytherapy,[405] but no benefit over external-beam irradiation has been found.[406]

Radiation therapy in combination with surgery has been used to improve local disease control and survival. Radiation therapy is given postoperatively as tumor may still remain in adjacent tissue and lymph nodes. It may also be given preoperatively to reduce tumor size to permit subsequent resection.[364,392] For those individuals with unresectable pancreatic cancer, radiation therapy can palliate signs and symptoms of local disease, especially pain.[407,408]

The benefit of using adjuvant combined chemotherapy and radiation therapy after surgical resection for pancreatic cancer was demonstrated by the Gastrointestinal Tumor Study Group (GITSG).[293] Radiation therapy is directed at the region from which the tumor was resected or where the greatest tumor burden lies, and chemotherapy is used to address the smaller or microscopic tumor burden that may remain. The use of external-beam radiation combined with 5-FU significantly increased survival when compared with controls who had curative resection without adjuvant therapy. Likewise, for individuals with locally unresectable disease, the use of chemoradiation provides modest benefit, as suggested by the GITSG trials.[409] Adjuvant therapy is now recommended for all individuals with pancreatic cancer as part of multimodality therapy.

A number of clinical trials are under way, including preoperative chemoradiation protocols. Current results suggest that preoperative chemoradiation therapy does not increase the morbidity or mortality of the subsequent surgical resection.[410,411] Although improvement in local control of the disease is obtained, long-term survival rates as compared with controls are not improved at this time.[412]

Newer combinations and means of administering radiation therapy and chemotherapy may provide better local control and survival for individuals with resectable and locally unresectable disease.[413] The development of more promising adjuvant therapies, such as combining chemoradiation with immunotherapy, may further enhance survival of individuals with pancreatic cancer.

## Symptom Management

The individual who has had surgery for pancreatic cancer usually dies of locally recurrent disease. The most common harbingers of imminent demise are recurrence of pain, jaundice from obstruction or intrahepatic metastases, and the development of ascites. These symptoms require symptomatic or palliative treatment.[364] Likewise, the individual who is diagnosed with advanced cancer of the pancreas, either locally or due to metastases, may present with the following:

- pain
- obstructive jaundice, which can lead to intrahepatic abscess
- infection
- ascites
- liver failure
- hemorrhage
- malnutrition from bowel obstruction
- anorexia
- early satiety
- cachexia
- nausea and vomiting
- change in bowel habits (constipation or diarrhea)
- dyspnea

The goal of palliative therapy is to reduce the debilitating symptoms of the disease and to improve the quality of remaining life. This is best accomplished by treating the individual with respect to his or her wishes and not just treating the tumor.[414]

Relief of pain is a primary objective, particularly in advanced disease. The pain syndrome associated with cancer of the pancreas is usually related to the anatomic location of the tumor in the organ and subsequent impingement on other structures: tissues, blood vessels, bile or pancreatic ducts, or body organs. The complex nerve fibers and ganglions that affect the pancreas and related organs and structures contribute to the pain associated with pancreatic cancer.[415] Pain associated with tumors in the head of the pancreas may be due to pancreatitis. Tumors located in the body and tail of the pancreas often present later, are larger, and tend to cause pain by invading the stomach, retroperitoneum, and nerves.

The nature of pain will evolve and change throughout the progression of the disease. Treatment approaches must address the current, specific complaints of pain using all available modalities.[415] Eliminating the source of the pain is the first objective, as in bile duct decompression or relief of duodenal obstruction. The most effective approach to pain therapy in individuals with advanced disease is to prevent the pain from peaking by routinely administering the selected relief measures. Oral, parenteral, or transdermal opiates, sedatives, nerve blocks, relaxation therapy, and proper positioning may provide pain relief. Radiotherapy in combination with chemotherapy has also been used to reduce pain.[409] Concomitant use of analgesics, celiac nerve blocks, and radiotherapy should be considered as palliative treatments. An aggressive pain treatment plan should be devised and started immediately. The goal of pain management should be to permit an acceptable level of functioning and to allow the individual to die as free of pain as possible.[416] Continuous pain assessment facilitated by good communication and trust between the individual and the clinician is necessary for effective pain management.

Nutritional status affects an individual's quality of life in regard to self-image, ability to perform activities of daily living, and overall life satisfaction. An individual's ability to socialize and interact with friends and family is affected by his or her ability or desire to eat.[417] Malnutrition, cachexia, muscle weakness, and fatigue all contribute to depression, causing a cycle of difficulties. Reduced activity and bedrest lead to constipation and more muscle wasting.[400]

Nutritional support may pose a difficult problem as a result of the obstructive nature of advanced pancreatic cancer. Supportive nutritional efforts for individuals undergoing active treatment can decrease complications, shorten hospital stays, reduce costs, and improve the individual's sense of well-being. Oral feedings should be maintained as long as the individual can meet caloric requirements. Frequent, small feedings and supplemental mixtures may be tolerated better than larger meals. Antiemetics prior to eating may assist in controlling nausea and vomiting. Metoclopramide, megestrol acetate, and cannabinoids are some of the pharmacological agents used to manage anorexia.[418,419] Individuals with pancreatic cancer complain of sensory changes that interfere with food intake. The sense of smell may be profoundly affected. Sensitivity to food odors as well as aversions to perfumes and soaps can also occur. Serving food cold instead of hot may be helpful in decreasing the aroma. Cooking odors can be minimized by using covered pots, boiling bags, or a kitchen fan. Taste changes are common, particularly complaints that food has a metallic taste. The use of plastic eating utensils and nonmetal cooking containers can help alleviate this problem. The use of parenteral nutrition in end-stage disease is controversial due to the high cost, high risk of complications, and lack of proven benefit.[419]

If the individual is diagnosed with a bowel obstruction, the cause must be elicited. Bowel obstruction can be from a mechanical or a functional problem. Immediate management consists of nasogastric suction for control of nausea and large-volume emesis along with hydration by intravenous fluids. Bowel obstruction caused by tumor may necessitate the placement of a gastric tube for decompression. The tube can be placed surgically or endoscopically. Removal of the nasogastric tube and allowing small amounts of liquids by mouth are the most humane course. Somatostatin has also been used in treating individuals with bowel obstruction, as it reduces intestinal secretions and the dose can be titrated to control the volume of secretions. Prokinetic agents should not be used in individuals with known bowel obstruction.

Opiate-induced bowel obstruction must also be considered. This can be avoided by the aggressive use of laxatives and an established bowel regimen along with appropriate education of the individual and family for symptoms suggestive of bowel obstruction: pain, nausea, vomiting, abdominal distention, and change in bowel elimination.

The administration of continuous subcutaneous opiate infusions by means of a PCA pump has the advantage of delivering analgesics to individuals with impaired gastrointestinal function and for whom oral analgesics are not appropriate. The pump can also provide optimal analgesia in those individuals who develop a bowel obstruction and are not able to take food or liquids by mouth.[414]

The cause of constipation can usually be delineated by a careful bowel history and abdominal examination. Prevention of opioid-induced constipation can best be accomplished by the use of an established bowel program.[420] Diarrhea is associated with tumors in the head of the pancreas; its management depends on identifying the cause. Malabsorption may result from steatorrhea and pancreatic exocrine insufficiency. Lactose intolerance may also be seen. Treatment consists of a diet high in protein and carbohydrate and replacement of pancreatic enzymes.

Individuals with cancer of the pancreas frequently have liver involvement, resulting in abdominal distention from malignant ascites. The treatment is difficult, but symptom control can be accomplished with the careful use of diuretics. Spironolactone and furosemide can reduce ascites, improve the person's comfort, and hopefully decrease the need for paracentesis.[414] Dyspnea may result not directly from the tumor itself but from disease complications, as seen in an individual with ascites and a diminished lung capacity. Individuals with dyspnea from pancreatic cancer will have a shortened survival.[421]

Jaundice due to ductal obstruction or liver damage is a debilitating symptom that occurs in the majority of individuals with pancreatic cancer. It causes severe pruritus and dry skin. The individual should be instructed to use soap sparingly, preferably using mild soaps and oil-based lotions, calamine lotion, or cocoa butter, or to bathe in sodium bicarbonate to relieve pruritus.

Palliation of obstructive jaundice can be provided with endoscopic or percutaneous procedures. Insertion of internal biliary stents by endoscopy can relieve jaundice and its concomitant symptoms. Percutaneously placed internal-external biliary drainage catheters also can provide relief of jaundice. The catheter and insertion site must receive daily care and routine flushing. Unrelieved biliary obstruction can cause recurrent infection in the biliary tree as well as lead to liver abscess that can cause pain and sepsis. Liver abscesses are treated by percutaneous insertion of a drain and intravenous antibiotics.

Jaundice not relieved by biliary decompression is usually a sign of liver failure. Liver failure results in progressive weakness, lethargy, encephalopathy, and eventual coma with imminent demise of the individual. Renal failure usually occurs as the liver fails (hepatorenal failure).

The individual is more prone to coagulation problems and bleeding as the liver continues to fail. Hemorrhage may also occur from metastatic tumor eroding into blood vessels in the liver or local tumor eroding into nearby vessels. These individuals die of massive internal hemorrhage.

Almost 90% of individuals with pancreatic cancer die within a year of diagnosis. The course of the disease can be rapid. It is important that the individual and family understand that some form of treatment or another medication will always be available to make the person as comfortable as possible.

## Continuity of Care: Nursing Challenges

Whatever the course of treatment chosen by the individual, both physiological and psychological preparation are necessary. By discerning patterns of family support, coping, and communication, the nurse can adopt a teaching style that suits the individual. Listening is vital to good communication in order to understand and be sensitive to the individual's needs. Education by the nurse can increase compliance as well as prepare the individual and family for side effects of both the disease and its treatment. The nurse is the constant figure of hope, understanding, and support through all the diagnostic tests, from the time an individual is told of the diagnosis of cancer of the pancreas, continuing through whatever treatment modalities are performed as the disease progresses, assisting with symptom management, and helping the individual and his or her family in the terminal stages of the disease.

The individual with terminal pancreatic cancer can be cared for at home by family or a caregiver with hospice support. The hospice nurse assists the individual and the caregiver in the terminal stages of the disease by educating them as to what to expect and helps to manage symptoms. Individuals in the terminal stage of pancreatic cancer may not wish to eat, may become extremely cachectic, and may have decreased or no urine output as hepatorenal failure ensues. Helping the family and especially the caregiver to deal with the eventuality of the disease is a primary nursing concern.

## CONCLUSION

Much research is now being done on all aspects of gastrointestinal cancer. Discoveries in the field of molecular genetics hold promise for earlier detection, possibly using gene-based diagnostic modalities. The ability to predict tumor biology in order to customize the treatment of individuals with gastrointestinal cancer brings hope for improved survival. New vaccines aimed at activating an individual's immune system to fight his or her cancer are currently being developed and tested.

There has been a reduction in morbidity and mortality associated with surgical resection for gastrointestinal cancer. This has led to more aggressive surgical therapy. These changes, along with improved responses to multimodality therapy and the potential for earlier diagnosis, lead to cautious optimism in the treatment of gastrointestinal cancer.

## REFERENCES

1. Parker SL, Tong T, Bolden S, et al: Cancer statistics 1996. *CA: Cancer J Clin* 46:5–27, 1996
2. Roth JA, Lichter AS, Putnam JB, et al: Cancer of the esophagus, in De Vita VT, Hellman S, Rosenberg SA (eds): *Cancer: Principles and Practice of Oncology* (ed 4). Philadelphia, Lippincott, 1993, pp 776–817
3. Blot WJ, Fraumeni JF: Trends in esophageal mortality among US blacks and whites. *Am J Public Health* 77:296–298, 1987
4. Klump TR, Macdonald JS: Esophageal cancer: Epidemiology and pathology, in Ahlgren JD, Macdonald JS (eds): *Gastrointestinal Oncology*. Philadelphia, Lippincott, 1992, pp 77–80
5. Qui S, Yang G: Precursor lesions of esophageal cancer in high-risk populations in Honan Province, China. *Cancer* 62:551–557, 1988
6. Zeigler RG: Alcohol-nutrient interaction in cancer etiology. *Cancer* 58:1942–1948, 1986
7. Gray JR, Coldman AJ, MacDonald WC: Cigarette and alcohol use in patients with adenocarcinoma of the gastric cardia or lower esophagus. *Cancer* 69:2227–2231, 1992
8. Choi SY, Kahyo H: Effect of cigarette smoking and alcohol consumption on the etiology of cancers of the digestive tract. *Int J Cancer* 49:381–386, 1991
9. Kato I, Nomura AM, Stemmermenn GN, et al: Prospective study of the association of alcohol with cancer of the upper aerodigestive tract and other sites. *Cancer Causes Control* 3:145–151, 1992
10. Ghardirian P, Ekoe JM, Thouez JP: Food habits and esophageal cancer: An overview. *Cancer Detect Prev* 16:163–168, 1992
11. Mock G, Patterson B, Suber A: Fruit, vegetables, and cancer prevention: A review of the epidemiologic evidence. *Nutr Cancer* 18:1–29, 1992
12. Applequist P, Salmo M: Lye corrosion carcinoma of the esophagus. *Cancer* 45:2655–2658, 1980
13. Aggestrup S, Holm JC, Sorensen HP: Does achalasia predispose to cancer of the esophagus? *Chest* 102:1012–1016, 1992
14. Kuster GG, Foroozan P: Early diagnosis of adenocarcinoma developing in Barrett's esophagus. *Arch Surg* 124:925–927, 1989
15. Nishimake T, Holscher AH, Schuler M, et al: Histopathologic characteristics of early adenocarcinoma in Barrett's esophagus. *Cancer* 68:1731–1736, 1991
16. Sarr MG, Hamilton SR, Marrone GC, et al: Barrett's esophagus: Its prevalence and association with adenocarcinoma in patients with symptoms of gastroesophageal reflux. *Am J Surg* 149:1878–1892, 1985
17. Hamilton SR, Smith RL: The relationship between colum-

nar epithelial dysplasia and invasive adenocarcinoma arising in Barrett's esophagus. *Am J Clin Pathol* 87:301–312, 1987

18. Blot WJ, Devesa SS, Kneller RW, et al: Rising incidence of adenocarcinoma of the esophagus and gastric cardia. *JAMA* 265:1287–1289, 1991
19. Harper PS, Harper RMJ, Howel-Evans AW: Carcinoma of the esophagus with tylosis. *Q J Med* 34:317, 1970
20. Helm F: *Cancer Dermatology*. Philadelphia, Lea and Febiger, 1979, pp 48–49
21. Howel-Evans AW, McConnell RB, Clarke CA, et al: Carcinoma of the esophagus with keratosis palmaris et plantaris (tylosis): A study of two families. *Q J Med* 27:413–429, 1958
22. Mizroch S: Epidemiology of esophageal cancer. *JAMA* 239:2340, 1978
23. Jaskiewicz K, Marass WF, Rossouw JE, et al: Selenium and other mineral elements in populations at risk for esophageal cancer. *Cancer* 62:2635–2639, 1988
24. Cooper JS, Pajak TF, Rubin P, et al: Second malignancies in patients who have had head and neck cancer: Incidence, effect on survival and implications based on the ROTG experience. *Int J Radiat Oncol Biol Phys* 17:449–456, 1989
25. Hesketh PJ, Clapp RW, Doos WG, et al: The increasing frequency of adenocarcinoma of the esophagus. *Cancer* 64:526–530, 1989
26. Livstone EM, Skinner DB: Tumors of the esophagus, in Berk JE (ed): *Gastroenterology*. Philadelphia, Saunders, 1985, pp 818–840
27. Goseki N, Koike M, Yoshida M: Histopathologic characteristics of early stage esophageal carcinoma. *Cancer* 69:1088–1092, 1992
28. Jin-Ming Y, Li-Hua Y, Guo-Qian, et al: Flow cytometric analysis of DNA content in esophageal carcinoma. *Cancer* 64:80–82, 1989
29. Ozawa S, Ueda M, Ando N, et al: Prognostic significance of epidermal growth factor receptor in esophageal squamous cell carcinoma. *Cancer* 64:2169–2173, 1989
30. Stephens JK, Bibbo M, Dytch H, et al: Correlation between automated karyometric measurements of squamous cell carcinoma of the esophagus and histopathologic and clinical features. *Cancer* 64:83–87, 1989
31. Anderson LL, Lad TE: Autopsy findings in squamous cell carcinoma of the esophagus. *Cancer* 50:1587–1590, 1982
32. Moses FM: Squamous cell carcinoma of the esophagus. *Gastroenterol Clin North Am* 20:703–716, 1991
33. Heitmiller RF, Forastiere AA: Esophagus, in Abeloff MD, Armitage JO, Lichter AS, Neiderhuber JE (eds): *Clinical Oncology*. New York, Churchill Livingstone, 1995, pp 1189–1208
34. Ojala K, Sorri M, Jokinin K, et al: Symptoms and diagnostic delay in patients with carcinoma of oesophagus and gastric carcinoma: A retrospective study of 225 patients. *Postgrad Med J* 58:264–267, 1982
35. Inculet TI, Keller SM, Dwyer A, et al: Evaluation of noninvasive tests for preoperative staging of carcinoma of the esophagus: A preoperative study. *Ann Thorac Surg* 40:561–651, 1985
36. Becker CD, Barbier P, Porcellini B: CT evaluations of patients undergoing transhiatal esophagectomy for cancer. *J Comput Assist Tomogr* 10:607, 1986
37. Winaiwer SJ, Sherlock P, Belladonna JA, et al: Endoscopic brush cytology in esophageal cancer. *JAMA* 232:1358, 1975
38. Huang CJ: Esophageal cancer. *Jpn J Surg* 11:399, 1981
39. Ziegler K, Sanft C, Friedrich M, et al: Evaluation of endosonography in TN staging of oesophageal cancer. *Gut* 32:16–20, 1991

40. Aibe T, Ito T, Yoshia T, et al: Endoscopic ultrasound of lymph nodes surrounding the upper GI tract. *Scand J Gastroenterol* 21:164–169, 1986
41. Takemoto T, Aibe T, Fuji T, et al: Endoscopic ultrasound. *Clin Gastroenterol* 15:305–329, 1986
42. Lightdale CJ, Botet JF, Kelsen DP, et al: Diagnosis of recurrent upper gastrointestinal cancer at the surgical anastomosis by endoscopic ultrasound. *Gastrointest Endosc* 35:407–412, 1989
43. Peacock JL, Asbury RF, Keller JW: Alimentary cancer, in Rubin P, McDonald S, Qazi R (eds): *Clinical Oncology: A Multidisciplinary Approach for Physicians and Students* (ed 7). Philadelphia, Saunders, 1993, pp 557–596
44. Beahrs OH, Henson DE, Hutter RV, et al (eds): *American Joint Committee on Cancer: Manual for Staging of Cancer* (ed 4). Philadelphia, Lippincott, 1992
45. Gomes MN: Esophageal cancer: Surgical approach, in Ahlgren JD, Macdonald JS (eds): *Gastrointestinal Oncology*. Philadelphia, Lippincott, 1992, pp 89–121
46. Davydov MI, Akhvlediani GG, Stilidi IS, et al: Surgical aspects in the treatment of esophageal cancer. *Semin Surg Oncol* 8:4–8, 1992
47. Orringer MB, Forastiere AA, Perez-Tamayo C, et al: Chemotherapy and radiation therapy before transhiatal esophagectomy for esophageal carcinoma. *Ann Thorac Surg* 49:348–355, 1990
48. Ellis FH: Esophageal carcinoma, in Steele G, Bady B (eds): *General Surgical Oncology*. Philadelphia, Saunders, 1992, pp 87–106
49. Harter KW: Esophageal cancer: Management with radiation, in Ahlgren JD, Macdonald JS (eds): *Gastrointestinal Oncology*. Philadelphia, Lippincott, 1992, pp 123–134
50. Kelsen DP, Minsky B, Smith M, et al: Preoperative therapy for esophageal cancer: A randomized comparison of chemotherapy versus radiation therapy. *J Clin Oncol* 8:1352, 1990
51. Petrovich Z, Lam K, Langholz B, et al: Surgical therapy and radiotherapy for carcinoma of the esophagus. *J Thorac Cardiovasc Surg* 98:614–617, 1989
52. Mamontov AS, Kiseleva ES, Kucharenko VM, et al: Combined therapy of thoracic esophageal cancer. *Semin Surg Oncol* 8:21–26, 1992
53. Pirogov AI, Krasnitsky YN: Successive radiation and surgical treatment of esophageal cancer. *Semin Surg Oncol* 8:37–40, 1992
54. Gill PG, Denham JW, Jamieson GG, et al: Patterns of treatment failure associated with the treatment of esophageal carcinoma with chemotherapy and radiotherapy either as sole treatment or followed by surgery. *J Clin Oncol* 10:1037–1043, 1992
55. Sur RK, Singh DP, Sharma SC, et al: Radiation therapy of esophageal cancer: Role of high dose rate brachytherapy. *Int J Radiat Oncol Biol Phys* 22:1043–1046, 1992
56. Naini AB, Dickerson JW, Brown MM: Preoperative and postoperative levels of plasma protein and amino acid in esophageal and lung cancer patients. *Cancer* 62:355–360, 1988
57. Ellis PH, Gibb SP, Watkins E: Limited esophagogastrectomy for carcinoma of the cardia. *Ann Surg* 208:354–361, 1988
58. Mitchell RL: Abdominal and right thoracotomy approach as a standard procedure for esophagogastrectomy with low morbidity. *J Thorac Cardiovasc Surg* 93:205–211, 1987
59. Mathisen DJ, Grillo HC, Wilkins EW, et al: Thoracic esophagectomy: A safe approach to carcinoma of the esophagus. *Ann Thorac Surg* 45:137–143, 1988

60. Orringer MB, Stirling MC: Esophagectomy for esophageal disruption. *Ann Thorac Surg* 49:35–43, 1990

61. Bremmer RM, DeMeester TR: Surgical treatment of esophageal carcinoma. *Gastroenterol Clin North Am* 20:743–763, 1991

62. Tsutsui S, Moriguchi S, Morita M, et al: Multivariate analysis of postoperative complications after esophageal resection. *Ann Thorac Surg* 53:1052–1056, 1992

63. Patil PK, Patel SG, Mistry RC, et al: Cancer of the esophagus: Esophagogastric anastomotic leak—A restrospective study of predisposing factors. *J Surg Oncol* 49:163–167, 1992

64. Hoebler L, Irwin MM: Gastrointestinal tract cancer: Current knowledge, medical treatment, and nursing management. *Oncol Nurs Forum* 19:1403–1415, 1992

65. Medvec BR: Esophageal cancer: Treatment and nursing interventions. *Semin Oncol Nurs* 4(4):246–256, 1988

66. Morton KA, Karwande SV, Davis RK, et al: Gastric emptying after gastric interposition for cancer of the esophagus or hypopharynx. *Ann Thorac Surg* 51:759–763, 1991

67. Cameron M: What patients need most before and after thoracotomy. *Nursing* 8(5):28–36, 1978

68. Leichman L, Berry BT: Experience with cisplatin in treatment regimens for esophageal cancer. *Semin Oncol Nurs* 18:64–72, 1991

69. Ahlgren JD: Esophageal cancer: Chemotherapy and combined modalities, in Ahlgren JD, Macdonald JS (eds): *Gastrointestinal Oncology*. Philadelphia, Lippincott, 1992, pp 135–147

70. Vikram B, Malamud S, Gold J, et al: Chemotherapy rapidly alternating with accelerated radiotherapy for advanced carcinomas of the hypopharynx and upper esophagus: A feasibility study. *Head Neck* 13:415–419, 1991

71. Ajani JA, Roth JA, Ryan B, et al: Evaluation of pre- and postoperative chemotherapy for resectable adenocarcinoma of the esophagus or gastroesophageal junction. *J Clin Oncol* 8:1231–1238, 1990

72. Kelsen D, Lovett D, Wong J, et al: Interferon alfa-2 and fluorouracil in the treatment of patients with advanced esophageal cancer. *J Clin Oncol* 10:269–274, 1992

73. Stewart FM, Harkins BJ, Hahn SS, et al: Cisplatin, 5-fluorouracil, mitomycin C, and concurrent radiation therapy with and without esophagectomy for esophageal carcinoma. *Cancer* 64:622–628, 1989

74. Urba SG, Orringer MB, Perez-Tamayo C, et al: Concurrent preoperative chemotherapy and radiotherapy in localized esophageal carcinoma. *Cancer* 69:285–291, 1992

75. Herskovic A, Martz K, Al-Sarraf M, et al: Combined chemotherapy and radiotherapy compared with radiotherapy alone in patients with cancer of the esophagus. *N Engl J Med* 326:1593–1598, 1992

76. Rotman MZ: Chemoirradiation: A new initiative in cancer treatment. *Radiology* 184:319–327, 1992

77. Reed CE, Marsh WH, Carlson LS, et al: Prospective, randomized trial of palliative treatment for unresectable cancer of the esophagus. *Ann Thorac Surg* 51:552–556, 1991

78. Siegel HI, Laskin KJ, Dabezies MA, et al: The effect of endoscopic laser therapy on survival in patients with squamous-cell carcinoma of the esophagus. *J Clin Gastroenterol* 13:142–146, 1991

79. McCaughan L: Lasers in photodynamic therapy. *Nurs Clin North Am* 25:725–738, 1990

80. Isaac JR, Sim EK, Ngoi SS, et al: Safe and rapid palliation of dysphagia for carcinoma of the esophagus. *Am Surg* 57:245–249, 1991

81. Buset M, des Marez B, Baize M, et al: Palliative endoscopic management of obstructive esophagogastric cancer: Laser or prothesis. *Gastrointest Endosc* 124:225–228, 1987

82. Suzuki H, Miho O, Watanabe Y, et al: Endoscopic laser therapy in the curative and palliative treatment of upper gastrointestinal cancer. *World J Surg* 13:158–163, 1989

83. Cusumano A, Ruol A, Segalin A, et al: Push-through intubation: Effective palliation in 409 patients with cancer of the esophagus. *Ann Thorac Surg* 53:1010–1014, 1992

84. Sargeant IR, Loizou LA, Tulloch M, et al: Recanalization of tube overgrowth: A useful new indication for laser in palliation of malignant dysphagia. *Gastrointest Endosc* 38:165–169, 1992

85. Mackety CJ: Caring for a cancer patient who has an esophageal endoprothesis. *RN* 40:51–53, 1977

86. Maehara Y, Kuwano H, Kitamura K, et al: Hyperthermochemoradiotherapy for esophageal cancer. *Anticancer Res* 12:805–810, 1992

87. Karanov S, Shopova M, Getov H: Photodynamic therapy in gastrointestinal cancer. *Lasers Surg Med* 11:395–398, 1991

88. Loizou LA, Rampton D, Atkinson M, et al: A prospective assessment of the quality of life after endoscopic intubation and laser therapy for malignant dysphagia. *Cancer* 7:386–391, 1992

89. Alexander HR, Kelsen DP, Tepper JE: Cancer of the stomach, in DeVita VT, Hellman S, Rosenberg SA (eds): *Cancer: Principles and Practice of Oncology* (ed 4). Philadelphia, Lippincott, 1993, pp 818–848

90. Mishima Y, Hirayama R: The role of lymph node surgery in gastric cancer. *World J Surg* 11:406–411, 1987

91. Maruyama K, Okabayashi K, Kinoshita T: Progress in gastric cancer surgery in Japan and its limits of radicality. *World J Surg* 11:418–425, 1987

92. Nakamura K, Ueyama T, Yao T, et al: Pathology and prognosis of gastric carcinoma. *Cancer* 70:1030–1037, 1992

93. Horm JW, Asire AJ, Young JL, Pollack ES (eds): *SEER Program: Cancer Incidence and Mortality in the United States 1973–1981*. NIH publication No. 85-1837. Bethesda, MD, National Cancer Institute, 1984

94. Wiggins CL, Becker TM, Key CR, et al: Stomach cancer among New Mexico's American Indians, Hispanic whites, and non-Hispanic whites. *Cancer Res* 49:1595–1599, 1989

95. Lawrence W: Gastric neoplasms, in Holleb AI, Fink DJ, Murphy GP (eds): *American Cancer Society Textbook of Clinical Oncology*. Atlanta, American Cancer Society, 1991, pp 245–253

96. Hotz J, Goebel H: Epidemiology and pathogenesis of gastric carcinoma, in Meyer HJ, Schmoll HJ, Hotz J (eds): *Gastric Carcinoma*. New York, Springer-Verlag, 1989, pp 3–15

97. Macdonald JS, Hill MC, Roberts IM: Gastric cancer: Epidemiology, pathology, detection, and staging, in Ahlgren JD, Macdonald JS (eds): *Gastrointestinal Oncology*. Philadelphia, Lippincott, 1992, pp 151–158

98. Nomura A, Grove JS, Stemmermann GN, et al: A prospective study of stomach cancer and its relation to diet, cigarettes, and alcohol consumption. *Cancer Res* 50:627–631, 1990

99. Moller H, Toftgaard C: Cancer occurrence in a cohort of patients surgically treated for peptic ulcer. *Gut* 32:740–744, 1991

100. Boeing H: Epidemiological research in stomach cancer: Progress over the last ten years. *J Cancer Res Clin Oncol* 117:133–143, 1991

101. Risch HA, Jain M, Choi NW, et al: Dietary factors and incidence of cancer of the stomach. *Am J Epidemiol* 122: 947–959, 1985

102. LaVecchia CL, Negir E, Frannceschi S, et al: Family history and the risk of stomach and colorectal cancer. *Cancer* 70: 50–55, 1992

103. Correa P: Clinical implications of recent developments in gastric cancer pathology and epidemiology *Semin Oncol* 12: 2–10, 1985

104. Giarelli L, Melato M, Stanta G, et al: Gastric resection: A cause of high frequency of gastric carcinoma. *Cancer* 52: 1113–1116, 1983

105. Stalnikowicz R, Benbassat J: Risk of gastric cancer after gastric surgery for benign disorders. *Arch Intern Med* 150: 2022–2026, 1990

106. Hoffman NR: The relationship between pernicious anemia and cancer of the stomach. *Geriatrics* 25:90–95, 1970

107. Rugge M, Cassaro M, Leandro G, et al: *Helicobacter pylori* in promotion of gastric carcinogenesis. *Dig Dis Sci* 41:950–955, 1996

108. Burstein M, Monge E, Leon-Barua R, et al: Low peptic ulcer and high gastric cancer prevalence in a developing country with a high prevalence of infection of *Helicobacter pylori. J Clin Gastroenterol* 13:154–156, 1991

109. Parsonnet J, Friedman GD, Vandersteen DP, Chang Y, et al: *Helicobacter pylori* infection and the risk of gastric carcinoma. *N Engl J Med* 325:1127–1131, 1991

110. Kaneko E, Nakamura T, Umeda N, et al: Outcome of gastric carcinoma detected by gastric mass survey in Japan. *Gut* 18:626–630, 1977

111. Murakami R, Tsukuma H, Ubukata T, et al: Estimation of validity of mass screening program for gastric cancer in Osaka, Japan. *Cancer* 65:1255–1260, 1990

112. Blomjous JG, Hop WC, Langenhorst BL, et al: Adenocarcinoma of the gastric cardia. *Cancer* 70:569–574, 1992

113. MacDonald WC, MacDonald JB: Adenocarcinoma of the esophagus and/or gastric cardia. *Cancer* 60:1094–1098, 1987

114. Haber DA, Mayer RJ: Primary gastrointestinal lymphoma. *Semin Oncol* 15:154–169, 1988

115. Powell J, McConkey CC: Increasing incidence of adenocarcinoma of the gastric cardia and adjacent sites. *Br J Cancer* 62:440–443, 1990

116. Roubein LO, Levin B: Trends in gastric cancer diagnosis including diagnosis of early cancer, in Doughlass HO (ed): *Gastric Cancer.* New York, Churchill Livingstone, 1988, pp 87–107

117. Dewys WD, Begg D, Lavin PT: Prognostic effect of weight loss prior to chemotherapy in cancer patients. *Am J Med* 69:491–499, 1980

118. Muruyama M: Comparison of radiology and endoscopy in the diagnosis of gastric cancer, in Preece PE, Cuschierie A, Wellwood JM (eds): *Cancer of the Stomach.* San Diego, Grune and Stratton, 1986, pp 123–144

119. Graham DY, Schwartz JT, Cain GD, et al: Prospective evaluation of biopsy number in the diagnosis of esophageal carcinoma. *Gastroenterology* 82:228–231, 1982

120. Levine MS, Rubesin SE, Karstaedt RE, et al: Double contrast upper gastrointestinal examination: Technique and interpretation. *Radiology* 168:593–602, 1988

121. Halvorson R, Thompson W: Primary neoplasms of the hollow organs of the gastrointestinal tract: Staging and follow-up. *Cancer* 67:1181–1188, 1991

122. Ohyama S, Yonemura Y, Miyazaki I: Proliferative activity and malignancy in human gastric cancers. *Cancer* 69:314–321, 1992

123. Wobbes T, Thomas CM, Segers MF, et al: Evaluation of seven tumor markers (CA 50, CA 19-9, CA 19-9 TruQuant, CA 72-4, CA 195, carcinoembryonic antigen, and tissue polypeptide antigen) in the pretreatment sera of patients with gastric carcinoma. *Cancer* 69:2036–2041, 1992

124. Okusa T, Makane Y, Boku T, et al: Quantitative analysis of nodal involvement with respect to survival rate after curative gastrectomy for carcinoma. *Surg Gynecol Obstet* 170: 488–494, 1990

125. Douglass HO, Nava HR: Gastric adenocarcinoma: Management of the primary disease. *Semin Oncol* 12:32–45, 1985

126. Cady B: Gastric cancer, in Steele G, Cady B (eds): *General Surgical Oncology.* Philadelphia, Saunders, 1991, pp 139–147

127. Monson JR, Donohue JH, McIlrath DC, et al: Total gastrectomy for advanced cancer. *Cancer* 68:1863–1868, 1991

128. Hoerr SO. Long-term results in patients who survived five or more years after gastric resection for primary carcinoma. *Surg Gynecol Obstet* 153:820–822, 1981

129. Kodama Y, Sugimachi K, Soejima K, et al: Evaluation of extensive lymph node dissection for carcinoma of the stomach. *World J Surg* 5:241–248, 1981

130. Vezeridis MP, Wanebo HJ: Gastric cancer: Surgical approach, in Ahlgren JD, Macdonald JS (eds): *Gastrointestinal Oncology.* Philadelphia, Lippincott, 1992, pp 159–170

131. Stern JL, Denman S, Elias EG, et al: Evaluation of palliative resection in advanced carcinoma of the stomach. *Surgery* 77:291–298, 1975

132. Moertel CG, Mittelman JA, Bakermeier RF, et al: Sequential and combination chemotherapy of advanced gastric cancer. *Cancer* 38:678–682, 1976

133. ReMine WH: Palliative operations for incurable gastric cancer. *World J Surg* 3:721–729, 1979

134. Ellis HF, Gibb SP, Watkins E: Esophagogastrectomy: A safe and widely applicable and expeditious form of palliation for patients with carcinoma of the esophagus and cardia. *Ann Surg* 198:531–540, 1983

135. Hunter JG: Endoscopic laser applications in the gastrointestinal tract. *Surg Clin North Am* 69:1146–1166, 1989

136. Wang JF: Stomach Cancer. *Semin Oncol Nurs* 4(4):257–264, 1988

137. Caudry M: Gastric cancer and approaches to locally unresectable or recurrent disease, in Ahlgren JD, Macdonald JS (eds): *Gastrointestinal Oncology.* Philadelphia, Lippincott, 1992, pp 181–193

138. O'Connell MJ, Gunderson LL, Moertel CG, et al: A pilot study to determine clinical tolerability of intensive combined therapy for locally unresectable gastric cancer. *Int J Radiat Oncol Biol Phys* 11:1827–1831, 1985

139. Abe M, Shibamoto Y, Takahashi M, et al: Intraoperative radiotherapy in carcinoma of the stomach and pancreas. *World J Surg* 11:459–464, 1987

140. Macdonald JS, Gohmann JJ: Chemotherapy of advanced gastric cancer: Present status, future prospects. *Semin Oncol* 15(3):42–49, 1988 (suppl)

141. Havlin KA, Macdonald JS: Gastric cancer: Chemotherapy of advanced disease, in Ahlgren JD, Macdonald JS (eds): *Gastrointestinal Oncology.* Philadelphia, Lippincott, 1992, pp 171–179

142. Kelsen D, Atiq OT, Saltz L, et al: FAMTX versus etoposide,

doxorubicin, and cisplatin: A random assignment trial in gastric cancer. *J Clin Oncol* 10:541–548, 1992

143. Lerner A, Gonin R, Steele GD, et al: Etoposide, doxorubicin, and cisplatin chemotherapy for advanced gastric adenocarcinoma: Results of a phase II trial. *J Clin Oncol* 10: 436–540, 1992

144. Epelbaum R, Haim N, Stein M, et al: Treatment of advanced gastric cancer with DDP (cisplatin), Adriamycin, and 5-fluorouracil (DAF). *Oncology* 44:201–206, 1987

145. Allum WH, Hallissey MT, Kelly JA: Adjuvant chemotherapy in operable gastric cancer. *Lancet* 1:517–574, 1989

146. Schlag P: Adjuvant chemotherapy in gastric cancer. *World J Surg* 11:473–477, 1987

147. Raab K: Intraperitoneal techniques offer daring alternative for abdominal cancer. *Oncol Biotech News,* August 1989, p 19

148. Pazdur R, Ajani JA, Winn R, et al: A phase II trial of 5-fluorouracil and recombinant alpha-2a-interferon in previously untreated metastatic gastric carcinoma. *Cancer* 69: 878–882, 1992

149. Maehara Y, Emi Y, Moriguchi S, et al: Postoperative chemotherapy for patients with advanced gastric cancer. *Am J Surg* 163:577–580, 1992

150. Beasley R: Hepatitis B virus: The major etiology of hepatocellular carcinoma. *Cancer* 61:1942, 1988

151. Rustgi VK: Epidemiology of hepatocellular carcinoma. *Gastroenterol Clin North Am* 16:545–551, 1987

152. Lai C, Gregory P, Wu P, et al: Hepatocellular carcinoma in Chinese males and females. *Cancer* 60:1107–1110, 1987

153. Yeh F, Yu M, Mo D, et al: Hepatitis B virus, aflatoxins, and hepatocellular carcinoma in southern Guangxi, China. *Cancer Res* 49:2506–2509, 1989

154. Beazley RM, Cohn I: Tumors of the liver, in Holleb AI, Fink DJ, Murphy GP (eds): *American Cancer Society Textbook of Clinical Oncology.* Atlanta, American Cancer Society, 1991, pp 237–244

155. Ni YH, Chang MH, Hsu HY, et al: Hepatocellular carcinoma in childhood. *Cancer* 68:1737–1741, 1991

156. Lotze MT, Flickinger JC, Carr BI: Hepatobiliary neoplasms, in DeVita VT, Hellman S, Rosenberg SA (eds): *Cancer: Principles and Practice of Oncology* (ed 4). Philadelphia, Lippincott, 1993, pp 883–914

157. Gumaste VV: Hepatocellular carcinoma and hepatitis B. *Gastroenterology* 109:1400–1402, 1995

158. Weimann A, Oldhafer KJ, Pichlmayr R: Primary liver cancers. *Curr Opin Oncol* 7:387–396, 1995

159. Riegler JL: Preneoplastic conditions of the liver. *Semin Gastrointest Dis* 7:74–87, 1996

160. Hsia CC, Axiotis CA, Bisceglie AM, et al: Transforming growth factor-alpha in human hepatocellular carcinoma and coexpression with hepatitis B surface antigen in adjacent liver. *Cancer* 70:1049–1056, 1992

161. McLean M, Dutton MF: Cellular interactions and metabolism of aflatoxin: An update. *Pharmacol Ther* 62:163–192, 1995

162. Chen CJ, Wang LY, Lu SN, et al: Elevated aflatoxin exposure and increased risk of hepatocellular carcinoma. *Hepatology* 24:38–42, 1996

163. Curley SA, Levin B, Rich TA: Liver and bile ducts, in Abeloff MD, Armitage JO, Lichter AS, Neiderhuber JE (eds): *Clinical Oncology.* New York, Churchill Livingstone, 1995, pp 1305–1372

164. Sherman M, Peltekian KM, Lee C: Screening for hepatocellular carcinoma in chronic carriers of hepatitis B virus.

Incidence and prevalence of hepatocellular carcinoma in a North American urban population. *Hepatology* 22:432–438, 1995

165. Ohnishi K, Shinji I, Shosuke I, et al: The effect of chronic habitual alcohol intake on the development of liver cirrhosis and hepatocellular carcinoma: Relation to hepatitis B surface antigen carriage. *Cancer* 49:672–677, 1982

166. Yu MC, Tong MJ, Govindarajan S, et al: Nonviral risk factors for hepatocellular carcinoma in a low-risk population, the non-Asians of Los Angeles County, California. *J Natl Cancer Inst* 83:1820–1826, 1991

167. Sherman M: Hepatocellular carcinoma. *Gastroenterologist* 3: 55–66, 1995

168. Palmer JR, Rosenberg L, Kaufman DW, et al: Oral contraceptive use and liver cancer. *Am J Epidemiol* 130:878–882, 1989

169. World Health Organization Collaborative Study of Neoplasia and Steroid Contraceptives. *Int J Cancer* 43:254–259, 1989

170. Coe JE: Hormonal influence on hepatocarcinogenesis. *Prog Clin Biol Res* 394:399–421, 1996

171. Oberfield RA, Steele G, Gollan JL: Liver cancer. *CA Cancer J Clin* 39:206–218, 1989

172. Colombo M: Hepatocellular carcinoma. *J Hepatol* 15:225–236, 1992

173. Kew MC, Popper H: Relationship between hepatocellular carcinoma and cirrhosis. *Semin Liver Dis* 4:136–146, 1984

174. Okuda K: Hepatocellular carcinoma: Recent progress. *Hepatology* 15:948–963, 1992

175. Eddleston A: Modern vaccines: Hepatitis. *Lancet* 335: 1142–1145, 1990

176. Perrillo R, Schiff E, Davis G, et al: A randomized, controlled trial of interferon alfa-2b alone and after prednisone withdrawal for the treatment of chronic hepatitis. *N Engl J Med* 323:295–301, 1990

177. Saracco G, Rosini F, Abate ML, et al: Long-term follow-up of patients with chronic hepatitis C treated with different doses of interferon-alpha 2b. *Hepatology* 18:1300–1305, 1993

178. Kobayashi Y, Watanabe S, Konishi M, et al: Quantitation and typing of serum hepatitis C virus RNA in patients with chronic hepatitis C treated with interferon-β. *Hepatology* 18:1319–1325, 1993

179. McMahon BJ, London T: National Cancer Institute workshop on screening for hepatocellular carcinoma. *J Natl Cancer Inst* 83:916–919, 1991

180. Ramsey WH, Wu GY: Hepatocellular carcinoma: Update on diagnosis and treatment. *Dig Dis* 13:81–91, 1995

181. Cattone M, Turri M, Caltagirone M, et al: Early detection of hepatocellular carcinoma associated with cirrhosis by ultrasound and alfa-fetoprotein: A prospective study. *Hepatogastroenterology* 35:101–103, 1988

182. Hoofnagle JH. Toward universal vaccination against hepatitis B virus. *N Engl J Med* 9:1333–1334, 1989

183. Ahlgren JD, Wanebo HJ, Hill MC: Hepatocellular carcinoma, in Ahlgren JD, Macdonald JS (eds): *Gastrointestinal Oncology.* Philadelphia, Lippincott, 1992, pp 417–436

184. Renard V, Merlet C, Hagege H: Fibrolamellor liver cell carcinoma. *Ann Gastroenterol Hepatol* 27:314–321, 1991

185. Ng IO, Lai EC, Ng MM, et al: Tumor encapsulation in hepatocellular carcinoma. *Cancer* 70:45–49, 1992

186. Okazaki N, Yosshino M, Yoshida T, et al: Evaluation of the prognosis for small hepatocellular carcinoma based on tumor volume doubling time. *Cancer* 63:2207–2210, 1989

187. Saddler D: Focus on the patient with metastatic disease. Hepatic metastasis: A nursing perspective. *Dimens Oncol Nurs* 1:4–6, 1985

188. Ong GB: Techniques and therapies for primary and metastatic liver cancer. *Curr Probl Cancer* 2:1–48, 1977

189. Melato M, Laurino L, Mucli E, et al: Relationship between cirrhosis, liver cancer, and hepatic metastases. *Cancer* 64:455–459, 1989

190. Lee YTN: Primary carcinoma of the liver: Diagnosis, prognosis, and management. *J Surg Oncol* 22:17–25, 1983

191. Bierman HR, Byron RL, Kelley KH, et al: Studies on blood supply of tumors in man: Vascular patterns of liver by hepatic arteriography in vivo. *J Natl Cancer Inst* 12:107–131, 1951

192. Kassiandes C, Kew MC: The clinical manifestations and natural history of hepatocellular carcinoma. *Gastroenterol Clin North Am* 16:553–562, 1987

193. Nisenbaum HL, Rowling SE: Ultrasound of focal hepatic lesions. *Semin Roentgenol* 30:324–346, 1995

194. Jacobs JE, Birnbaum BA: Computed tomography imaging of focal hepatic lesions. *Semin Roentgenol* 30:308–323, 1995

195. Schnall M: Magnetic resonance imaging of focal liver lesions. *Semin Roentgenol* 30:347–361, 1995

196. Kinnard MF, Alavi A, Rubin RA, et al: Nuclear imaging of solid hepatic masses. *Semin Roentgenol* 30:375–395, 1995

197. Goldenberg DM, Goldenberg H, Higginbotham-Ford E, et al: Imaging of primary and metastatic liver cancer with [131]I monoclonal and polyclonal antibodies against alphafetoprotein. *J Clin Oncol* 5:1827–1835, 1987

198. Soulen MC: Angiographic evaluation of focal liver masses. *Semin Roentgenol* 30:362–374, 1995

199. Sitzmann JV, Coleman J, Pitt HA, et al: Preoperative assessment of malignant hepatic tumors. *Am J Surg* 159:137–143, 1990

200. Giardina MG, Matarazzo M, Varriale A, et al: Serum alpha-L-fucosidase. *Cancer* 70:1044–1048, 1989

201. McGill DB, Zinsmeister AR, Ott BJ: Liver biopsy: Increased risks in patients with cancer. *Gastroenterology* 89:1396–1400, 1990

202. Sitzmann JV, Abrams R: Improved survival for hepatocellular cancer with combination surgery and multimodality treatment. *Ann Surg* 217:149–154, 1993

203. Tang ZY, Yu YQ, Zhou XD, et al: Treatment of unresectable primary liver cancer: With reference to cytoreduction and sequential resection. *World J Surg* 19:47–52, 1995

204. McDermott WV, Jenkins RL, Cady B, et al: Primary and metastatic cancer of the liver, in Steele G, Cady B (eds): *General Surgical Oncology*. Philadelphia, Saunders, 1992, pp 185–194

205. Scheele J, Stang R, Altendorf-Hofmann A et al: Resection of colorectal metastases. *World J Surg* 19:59–71, 1995

206. Mayer RJ: Chemotherapy for metastatic colorectal carcinoma. *Cancer* 70:1414–1424, 1992

207. Kemeny N, Cohen A, Seiterk, et al: Randomized trial of hepatic arterial floxuridine, mitomycin and carmustine versus floxuridine alone in previously treated patients with liver metastases from colorectal cancer. *J Clin Oncol* 11:330–335, 1993

208. Weaver ML, Atkinson D, Zemel R: Hepatic cryosurgery in treating colorectal metastases. *Cancer* 76:210–214, 1995

209. Nagorney DM, van Heerden JA, Ilstrup DM, et al: Primary hepatic malignancy: Surgical management and determinants of survival. *Surgery* 106:740–749, 1989

210. Pichlmayr R, Ringe B, Bechstein WO, et al: Approach to primary liver cancer. *Recent Results Cancer Res* 110:65–73, 1988

211. Ravikumar TS, Steele GD: Hepatic cryosurgery. *Surg Clin North Am* 69:433–440, 1989

212. Cance W: Cryosurgery in the treatment of hepatic tumors. *Curr Surg* 126:183–187, 1992

213. Cameron JL: *Atlas of Surgery*, vol 1. Toronto, Decker, 1990

214. Zollinger RM Jr, Zollinger RM: *Atlas of Surgical Operations* (ed 7). New York, McGraw-Hill, 1993

215. Shafir M, Shapiro R, Sung M, et al: Cryoablation of unresectable malignant liver tumors. *Am J Surg* 171:27–31, 1996

216. Kruskal JB, Kane RA: Intraoperative ultrasonography of the liver. *Crit Rev Diagn Imaging* 36:175–226, 1995

217. Brandt BT, DeAntonio P, Dezort MA, et al: Hepatic cryosurgery for metastatic colorectal carcinoma. *Oncol Nurs Forum* 23:29–36, 1996

218. Yokoyama I, Carr B, Saitsu H, et al: Accelerated growth rates of recurrent hepatocellular carcinoma after liver transplantation. *Cancer* 68:2095–2100, 1991

219. Yokoyama I, Sheahan DG, Carr B, et al: Clinicopathologic factors affecting patient survival and tumor recurrence after orthotopic liver transplantation for hepatocellular carcinoma. *Transplant Proc* 23:2194–2196, 1991

220. Lohmann R, Bechstein WO, Langrehr JM, et al: Analysis of risk factors for recurrence of hepatocellular carcinoma after orthotopic liver transplantation. *Transplant Proc* 27:1245–1246, 1995

221. Stone MJ, Klintmalm GBG, Polter D, et al: Neoadjuvant chemotherapy and liver transplantation for hepatocellular carcinoma: A pilot study in 20 patients. *Gastroenterology* 104:196–202, 1993

222. Senninger N, Langer R, Klar E, et al: Liver transplantation for hepatocellular carcinoma. *Transplant Proc* 28:1706–1707, 1996

223. Ringe B, Canelo R, Lorf T: Liver transplantation for primary liver cancer. *Transplant Proc* 28:1174–1175, 1996

224. Hodgson WJB, Morgan J, Byrne D, et al: Hepatic resections for primary and metastatic tumors using the ultrasonic dissector. *Am J Surg* 163:246–251, 1992

225. Ikeda K, Kumada H, Saitoh S, et al: Effect of repeated transcatheter arterial embolization on the survival of patients with hepatocellular carcinoma. *Cancer* 68:2150–2154, 1992

226. Bismuth H, Morino M, Sherlock D, et al: Primary treatment of hepatocellular carcinoma by arterial chemoembolization. *Am J Surg* 163:387–394, 1992

227. Bronowicki JP, Boudjema K, Chone L, et al: Comparison of resection, liver transplantation and transcatheter oily chemoembolization in the treatment of hepatocellular carcinoma. *J Hepatol* 24:293–300, 1996

228. Beppu T, Ohara C, Yamaguchi Y, et al: A new approach to chemoembolization for unresectable hepatocellular carcinoma using aclarubicin in combination with cisplatin suspended in iodized oil. *Cancer* 68:2555–2560, 1991

229. Civalleri D, Pellicci R, Decaro G, et al: Palliative chemoembolization of hepatocellular carcinoma with mitoxantrone, Lipiodol, and Gelfoam: A phase II study. *Anticancer Res* 16:937–941, 1996

230. Livraghi T, Bolondi L, Lazzaroni S, et al: Percutaneous ethanol injection in the treatment of hepatocellular carcinoma in cirrhosis. *Cancer* 69:925–929, 1992

231. Ohto M, Yoshikawa M, Saisho H, et al: Nonsurgical treatment of hepatocellular carcinoma in cirrhotic patients. *World J Surg* 19:42–46, 1995

232. Livraghi T, Giorgio A, Marin G, et al: Hepatocellular carcinoma and cirrhosis in 746 patients: Long-term results of percutaneous ethanol injection. *Radiology* 197:101–108, 1995

233. Takayasu K: Interventional angiography for primary and secondary hepatic malignancies. *Jpn J Clin Oncol* 20: 225–231, 1990

234. Farmer DG, Rosove MH, Shaked A, et al: Current treatment modalities for hepatocellular carcinoma. *Ann Surg* 219:236–247, 1994

235. Neiderhuber JE, Grochow LB: Status of infusion chemotherapy for the treatment of liver metastases. *PPO Updates* 3:1–9, 1989

236. Patt YZ, Mavligit GM: Arterial chemotherapy in the management of colorectal cancer: An overview. *Semin Oncol* 18: 478–490, 1991

237. Sterchi JM, Richards F, White DR, et al: Chemoinfusion of the hepatic artery for metastases to the liver. *Surg Gynecol Obstet* 168:291–295, 1989

238. Wong E, Khardori N, Carrasco CH, et al: Infectious complications of hepatic artery catheterization procedures in patients with cancer. *Rev Infect Dis* 113:583–586, 1991

239. Atiq OT, Kemeny N, Niedzwiecki D, et al: Treatment of unresectable primary liver cancer with intrahepatic fluorodeoxyuridine and mitomycin C through an implantable pump. *Cancer* 69:920–924, 1992

240. Safi F, Bittner R, Roscher R, et al: Regional chemotherapy for hepatic metastases of colorectal carcinoma (continuous intraarterial versus continuous intraarterial/intravenous therapy). *Cancer* 64:378–387, 1989

241. Andersson R, Holmberg A: Intraperitoneal 5-fluorouracil in the management of colorectal liver cancer. *Eur J Surg Oncol* 18:152–155, 1992

242. Raoul JI, Bretagne JF, Caucanas JP, et al: Internal radiation therapy for hepatocellular carcinoma. *Cancer* 69:346–352, 1992

243. Hellman K, Goold M, Higgins N, et al: Responses of liver metastases to radiotherapy and razoxane. *J R Soc Med* 85: 136–138, 1992

244. Miller RL, Bukowski RM, Andersen S, et al: Phase II evaluation of sequential hepatic artery infusion of 5-fluorouracil and hepatic irradiation in metastatic colorectal carcinoma. *J Surg Oncol* 37:1–4, 1988

245. Gastrointestinal Tumor Study Group: A prospective trial of recombinant human interferon alpha 2β in previously untreated patients with hepatocellular carcinoma. *Cancer* 66:135–139, 1990

246. Lai CL, Lau JY, Wu PC, et al: Recombinant interferon-α in inoperable hepatocellular carcinoma: A randomized controlled trial. *Hepatology* 17:389–394, 1993

247. Farinati F, Salvaginini M, de Maria N, et al: Unresectable hepatocellular carcinoma: A prospective controlled trial with tamoxifen. *J Hepatol* 11:297–301, 1990

248. Gupta S, Korula J: Failure of ketoconazole as anti-androgen therapy in nonresectable primary hepatocellular carcinoma. *J Clin Gastroenterol* 10:651–654, 1988

249. O'Mary SS: Liver cancer: Primary and metastatic disease. *Semin Oncol Nurs* 4:265–273, 1988

250. Black WC, Key CR, Carmany TB, et al: Carcinoma of the gallbladder in a population of southwestern American Indians. *Cancer* 39:1267–1279, 1983

251. Lowenfels AB, Lindström CG, Conway MJ, et al: Gallbladder and risk of gallbladder cancer. *J Natl Cancer Inst* 75: 77–83, 1985

252. Pitt HA, Dooley WC, Yeo CJ, et al: Malignancies of the biliary tree. *Curr Probl Surg* 32:11–36, 1995

253. Nagorney DM, Mcpherson GAD: Carcinoma of the gallbladder and extrahepatic bile ducts. *Semin Oncol* 15: 106–116, 1988

254. Jones RS: Carcinoma of the gallbladder. *Surg Clin North Am* 70:1419–1428, 1990

255. Anderson JH, Cooper WJ, Williamson CN: Adenocarcinoma of the extrahepatic biliary tree. *J R Coll Surg England* 67:139–143, 1985

256. Aoki H, Sugaya H, Shimazu M: A clinical study on cancer of the bile duct associated with anomalous arrangements of the pancreaticobiliary ductal system: Analysis of 569 cases collected in Japan. *J Bile Tract Pancreas* 8:1539–1551, 1987

257. Tanaka K, Nishimura A, Yamada K, et al: Cancer of the gallbladder associated with anomalous junction of the pancreatobiliary duct system without bile duct dilatation. *Br J Surg* 80:622–624, 1993

258. Mancuso TF, Brennan MJ: Epidemiological consideration of cancer of the gallbladder, bile ducts and salivary glands in the rubber industry. *J Occup Med* 12:333–338, 1970

259. Kowalewski K, Todd EF: Carcinoma of the gallbladder induced in hamsters by insertion of cholesterol pellets and feeding dimethylnitrosamine. *Proc Soc Exp Biol Med* 136: 482–486, 1971

260. Hasegawa R, Ogawa K, Takaba K, et al: 3,2'-Dimethyl-4-aminobiphenyl–induced gallbladder carcinogenesis and effects of ethinyl estradiol in hamsters. *Jpn J Cancer Res* 83: 1286–1292, 1992

261. Welston JC, Marr JS, Friedman SM: Association between hepatobiliary cancer and typhoid carrier. *Lancet* 1:791–794, 1979

262. Sons HU, Borchard F, Joel BS: Carcinoma of the gallbladder: Autopsy findings in 287 cases and review of the literature. *J Surg Oncol* 28:199–206, 1985

263. Piehler JM, Crichlow RK: Primary carcinoma of the gallbladder. *Surg Gynecol Obstet* 147:929–935, 1978

264. Yamagiwa H: Mucosal dysplasia of gallbladder: Isolated and adjacent lesions to carcinoma. *Jpn J Cancer Res* 80: 238–245, 1989

265. Koichi W, Masao T, Koji T, et al: Carcinoma and polyps of the gallbladder. *World J Surg* 15:315–321, 1991

266. Sumiyoshi K, Nagai E, Chijiiwa K, et al: Pathology of carcinoma of the gallbladder. *World J Surg* 15:315–321, 1991

267. Keller JW, Peacock JL, Smith JL: Cancer of the major digestive glands: Pancreas, liver, bile ducts, gallbladder, in Rubin P (ed): *Clinical Oncology: A Multidisciplinary Approach for Physicians and Students* (ed 7). Philadelphia, Saunders, 1993, pp 597–615

268. Nahrwold DL, Dawes LG: Biliary neoplasms, in Greenfield LJ, Mulholland M, Oldham KT, Zelenock GB, Lillemoe KD (eds): *Surgery: Scientific Principles and Practice* (ed 2). Philadelphia, Lippincott-Raven, 1997, pp 1056–1066

269. Yamamoto M, Nakajo S, Tahara E: Carcinoma of the gallbladder: The correlation between histogenesis and prognosis. *Arch Pathol Anat* 414:83–90, 1989

270. Maxwell P, David RI, Sloan JM: Carcinoembryonic antigen (CEA) in benign and malignant epithelium of the gallbladder, extrahepatic bile ducts, and ampulla of Vater. *J Pathol* 170:73–76, 1993

271. Brown JA, Roberts CS: Elevated serum alpha-fetoprotein levels in primary gallbladder carcinoma without hepatic involvement. *Cancer* 70:1838–1840, 1992

272. Lokich JJ, Kane RA, Harrison DA, et al: Biliary tract obstruction secondary to cancer: Management guidelines and selected literature review. *J Clin Oncol* 5:969–981, 1987

273. Tsuchiya Y: Early carcinoma of the gallbladder: Macroscopic features and US findings. *Radiology* 179:171–175, 1991

274. Hederstroma E, Forsberg L: Ultrasonography in carcinoma of the gallbladder, diagnostic difficulties and pitfalls. *Acta Radiol* 28:715–718, 1987

275. Smathers RL, Lee JKT, Heiken JP: Differentiation of complicated cholecystitis from gallbladder carcinoma by computed tomography. *Am J Roentgenol* 143:255–259, 1984

276. Arake T, Hihara T, Karikomi M, et al: Intraluminal papillary carcinoma of the gallbladder: Prognostic value of computed tomography and sonography. *Gastrointest Radiol* 13: 261–265, 1988

277. Wilbur AC, Gyi B, Renigers SA: High-field MRI of primary gallbladder carcinoma: Imaging findings in 50 patients with pathologic correlation. *Gastrointest Radiol* 16:142–144, 1988

278. McNulty JG: Preoperative diagnosis of carcinoma of the gallbladder by percutaneous transhepatic cholangiography. *Am J Roentgenol* 101:605–610, 1967

279. Pitt HA: The changing role of preoperative biliary decompression. *Perspect Gen Surg* 1:113–126, 1990

280. Little JM: A prospective evaluation of computerized estimates of risk in the management of obstructive jaundice. *Surgery* 102:473–476, 1987

281. Eckhauser FE, Raper SE, Mulholland MW, et al: Carcinoma of the gallbladder, in Neiderhuber JE (ed): *Current Therapy in Oncology.* St. Louis, Mosby–Year Book, 1993, pp 402–409

282. Donohue JM, Nagorney DM, Grant CS, et al: Carcinoma of the gallbladder. *Arch Surg* 125:237–241, 1990

283. Cubertafond P, Gainant A, Cucchiaro G: Surgical treatment of 724 carcinomas of the gallbladder: Results of the French Surgical Association survey. *Ann Surg* 219:275–280, 1994

284. Clair DG, Lautz DB, Brooks DC: Rapid development of umbilical metastases after laparoscopic cholecystectomy for unusual gallbladder carcinoma. *Surgery* 113:355–358, 1993

285. Ogura Y, Mizumoto R, Isaji S, et al: Radical operations for carcinoma of the gallbladder: Present status in Japan. *World J Surg* 6:337–342, 1991

286. Yamaguchi K, Enjoji M: Carcinoma of the gallbladder. *Cancer* 62:1425–1432, 1988

287. Nakamura GH, Sakaguchi S, Suzuki S, et al: Aggressive surgery for carcinoma of the gallbladder. *Surgery* 106: 467–472, 1989

288. Nimura Y, Hayakawa N, Kamiya J, et al: Hepatopancreaticoduodenectomy for advanced carcinoma of the biliary tract. *Hepatogastroenterology* 38:170–175, 1991

289. Lillemoe KD, Pitt HA, Kaufman HS, et al: Acute cholecystitis occurring as a complication of percutaneous transhepatic drainage. *Surg Gynecol Obstet* 168:348–352, 1989

290. Busse PM, Cady B, Bothe A, et al: Intraoperative radiation therapy for gallbladder cancer. *World J Surg* 15:352–356, 1991

291. Todoroki T, Iwasaki Y, Orii K, et al: Resection combined with intraoperative radiation therapy (IORT) for stage IV gallbladder carcinoma. *World J Surg* 15:357–366, 1991

292. Crist DW, Cameron JL: The current status of the Whipple operation for periampullary carcinoma. *Adv Surg* 25:21–49, 1992

293. Gastrointestinal Tumor Study Group: Further evidence of effective adjuvant combined radiation and chemotherapy following curative resection of pancreatic cancer. *Cancer* 59:2006–2010, 1987

294. Aoki K, Ogawa H: Cancer of the pancreas: International mortality trends. *World Health Stat Rep* 31:2–13, 1978

295. Zheng W, McLaughlin JK, Gridley G, et al: A cohort study of smoking, alcohol consumption, and dietary factors for pancreatic cancer. *Cancer Causes Control* 4:447–482, 1993

296. Kalapothaki V, Tzonou A, Hseih CC, et al: Tobacco, ethanol, coffee, pancreatitis, diabetes mellitus, and cholelithiasis as risk factors for pancreatic carcinoma. *Cancer Causes Control* 4:375–382, 1993

297. Friedman GD, van den Eeden SK: Risk factors for pancreatic cancer: An exploratory study. *Int J Epidemiol* 22:30–37, 1993

298. Chyou PH, Nomura AM, Stemmermann GN: A prospective study on the attributable risk of cancer due to cigarette smoking. *Am J Public Health* 82:37–40, 1992

299. Lyon JL, Mahoney AW, French TK, et al: Coffee consumption and the risk of cancer of the exocrine pancreas: A case control study in a low-risk population. *Epidemiology* 3: 164–170, 1992

300. Adami HO, McLaughlin JK, Hsing AW, et al: Alcoholism and cancer risk: A population-based cohort study. *Cancer Causes Control* 3:419–425, 1992

301. Bueno de Mesquita HB, Maisonneuve P, Moerman CJ, et al: Lifetime consumption of alcoholic beverages, tea and coffee and exocrine carcinoma of the pancreas: A population-based case control study in the Netherlands. *Int J Cancer.* 50:514–522, 1992

302. Mack TM, Peters JM, Yu MC, et al: Pancreas cancer is unrelated to the workplace in Los Angeles. *Am J Ind Med* 7:253–266, 1985

303. Gold EB, Gordis L, Diener MD, et al: Diet and other risk factors for cancer of the pancreas. *Cancer* 55:460–467, 1985

304. Falk RT, Pickle LW, Fontham ET, et al: Occupation and pancreatic cancer risk in Louisiana. *Am J Ind Med* 18: 565–576, 1990

305. Hearne FT, Pifer JW, Grose F: Absence of adverse mortality effects in workers exposed to methylene chloride: An update. *J Occup Med* 32:234–240, 1990

306. Kalapothaki V, Tzonou A, Hseil CC, et al: Nutrient intake and cancer of the pancreas: A case-control study in Athens, Greece. *Cancer Causes Control* 4:383–389, 1993

307. Olsen GW, Mandel JS, Gibson RW, et al: Nutrients and pancreatic cancer: A population-based case-control study. *Cancer Causes Control* 2:291–297, 1991

308. Gullo L, Peziylli R, Morsell-Labate AM, et al: Diabetes and the risk of pancreatic cancer. *N Engl J Med* 331:81–84, 1994

309. Lowenfels AB, Maisonneuve P, Cavallini G, et al: Pancreatitis and the risk of pancreatic cancer. *N Engl J Med* 328: 1433–1437, 1993

310. O'Mara BA, Byers T, Schoenfeld E: Diabetes mellitus and cancer risk: A multisite case-control study. *J Chron Dis* 38: 435–441, 1985

311. Gold EB, Cameron JL: Chronic pancreatitis and pancreatic cancer. *N Engl J Med* 328:1485–1486, 1993

312. Hahn SA, Kern SE: Molecular genetics of exocrine pancreatic neoplasms. *Surg Clin North Am* 75:857–869, 1995

313. Kern SE, Pietenpol JA, Thiagalingam S, et al: Oncogene forms of *p53* inhibit *p53*-regulated gene expression. *Science* 256:827–830, 1992

314. Bui HX, Ballouk F, del Rosario A, et al: Nuclear DNA content and clinical follow-up in resected pancreatic adenocarcinoma. *Anal Quant Cytol Histol* 15:389–395, 1993

315. Allison DC, Bose KK, Hruban RH, et al: Pancreatic cancer cell DNA content correlates with long-term survival after pancreaticoduodenectomy. *Ann Surg* 214:648–656, 1991

316. Sciallero S, Giaretti W, Geido E, et al: DNA aneuploidy is an independent factor of poor prognosis in pancreatic and peripancreatic cancer. *Int J Pancreatol* 14:21–28, 1993

317. Lynch HT, Fusaro L, Lynch JF: Familial pancreatic cancer: A family study. *Pancreas* 7:511–515, 1992

318. Lumadue JA, Griffin CA, Osman M, et al: Familial pancreatic cancer and the genetics of pancreatic cancer. *Surg Clin North Am* 75:845–855, 1995

319. Poston GJ, Gillespie J, Guillou PJ: Biology of pancreatic cancer. *Gut* 32:800–812, 1991

320. Fernandez-del Castillo C, Warshaw AL: Cystic tumors of the pancreas. *Surg Clin North Am* 75:1001–1016, 1995

321. Bieligk S, Jaffe BM: Islet cell tumors of the pancreas. *Surg Clin North Am* 75:1025–1040, 1995

322. Webb TH, Lillemoe KD, Pitt HA, et al: Pancreatic lymphoma: Is surgery mandatory for diagnosis or treatment? *Ann Surg* 209:25–30, 1989

323. Bastidas JA, Niederhuber JE: Pancreas, in Abeloff MD, Armitage JO, Lichter AS, Neiderhuber JE (eds): *Clinical Oncology*. New York, Churchill Livingstone, 1995, pp 1373–1400

324. Kern HF, Elsasser HP: Fine structure of human pancreatic adenocarcinoma, in Go VLW, Dimagno EP, Gardner JD, Lebenthal E, Reber HA, Scheele GA (eds): *The Pancreas: Biology, Pathobiology, and Disease* (ed 2). New York, Raven Press, 1993, pp 857–869

325. Kloppel G: Pathology of nonendocrine pancreatic tumors, in Go VLW, Dimagno EP, Gardner JD, Lebenthal E, Reber HA, Scheele GA (eds): *The Pancreas: Biology, Pathobiology, and Disease* (ed 2). New York, Raven Press, 1993, pp 871–897

326. Cubilla AL, Fitzgerald PJ: Cancer of the exocrine pancreas: The pathological aspects. *CA Cancer J Clin* 35:2–18, 1985

327. Nagakawa T, Kobayashi H, Veno K, et al: The pattern of lymph node involvement in carcinoma of the head of the pancreas: A histologic study of the surgical findings in patients undergoing extensive nodal dissections. *Int J Pancreatol* 13:15–22, 1993

328. Lillemoe KD: Current management of pancreatic carcinoma. *Ann Surg* 221:133–148, 1995

329. Rosa JA, Van Linda BM, Abourizk NN: New-onset diabetes mellitus as harbinger of pancreatic carcinoma. *J Clin Gastroenterol* 11:211–215, 1989

330. Falconer JS, Fearon KC, Plester CE, et al: Cytokines, the acute phase response, and resting energy expenditures in cachectic patients with pancreatic cancer. *Ann Surg* 219:325–331, 1994

331. Perez MM, Newcomer AD, Moertel CH, et al: Assessment of weight loss, food intake, fat metabolism, malabsorption, and treatment of pancreatic insufficiency in pancreatic cancer. *Cancer* 52:346–352, 1983

332. Ventafridda GV, Caraceni AT, Sbanotto AM, et al: Pain treatment in cancer of the pancreas. *Eur J Surg Oncol* 16:1–6, 1990

333. Hudis C, Kelsen D, Niedzwieck D, et al: Pain is not a prominent symptom in most patients with early pancreas cancer. *Proc Annum Meeting Am Soc Clin Oncol* 10:326, 1991

334. Moossa AR, Gamagami RA: Diagnosis and staging of pancreatic neoplasms. *Surg Clin North Am* 75:871–890, 1995

335. Green AL, Austin CP: Psychopathology of pancreatic cancer: A psychobiologic probe. *Psychosomatics* 34:208–221, 1993

336. Frias I, Litin EM, Pearson JS: Comparison of psychiatric symptoms of carcinoma of the pancreas with those in some other intra-abdominal neoplasms. *Am J Psychiatry* 123:1553–1562, 1967

337. Raijman I, Levin B: Exocrine tumors of the pancreas, in Go VLW, Dimagno EP, Gardner JD, Lebenthal E, Reber HA, Scheele GA (eds): *The Pancreas: Biology, Pathobiology, and Disease* (ed 2). New York, Raven Press, 1993, pp 889–913

338. Nordback IH, Cameron JL: Periampullary cancer, in Cameron JL (ed): *Current Surgical Therapy*. St Louis, Mosby–Year Book, 1992, pp 441–448

339. Nordback IH, Hruban RH, Boitnott JK, et al: Carcinoma of the body and tail of the pancreas. *Am J Surg* 164:26–31, 1992

340. Balthazar EJ, Chako AC: Computed tomography of pancreatic masses. *Am J Gastroenterol* 85:343–349, 1990

341. Wyatt SH, Fishman EK: Spiral CT of the pancreas. *Semin Ultrasound CT MR* 15:122–132, 1994

342. Moossa AR: Tumors of the pancreas, in Moossa AR, Schimpff SC, Robson MC (eds): *Comprehensive Textbook of Oncology* (ed 2). Baltimore, Williams and Wilkins, 1991, pp 958–988

343. Sterner E, Stark DD, Hahn PF, et al: Imaging of pancreatic neoplasms: Comparison of MRI and CT. *Am J Roentgenol* 152:487–491, 1989

344. Pitt HA, Gomes AS, Lois AF, et al: Does preoperative percutaneous biliary drainage reduce operative risk or increase hospital cost? *Ann Surg* 201:545–553, 1985

345. Lygidakis NJ, Van Der Heyde MN, Lubler MJ: An evaluation of preoperative biliary drainage in the surgical management of pancreatic head carcinoma. *Acta Chir Scand* 153:665–668, 1987

346. Crist DW, Kadir S, Cameron JL: The value of preoperatively placed percutaneous biliary catheters in reconstruction of the proximal part of the biliary tract. *Surg Gynecol Obstet* 165:421–424, 1987

347. Biehl TR, Traverso LW, Hauptmann E, et al: Preoperative visceral angiography alters intraoperative strategy during the Whipple procedure. *Am J Surg* 165:607–612, 1993

348. Palazzo L, Roseau G, Gayet B, et al: Endoscopic ultrasonography and endoscopic pancreatography in pancreatic diagnosis. *Endoscopy* 25:143–150, 1993

349. Tao TL, Tytgat GN, Cikot RJ, et al: Ampullopancreatic carcinoma: Preoperative TNM classification with endosonography. *Radiology* 175:455–461, 1990

350. Lightdale CJ: Diagnostic laparoscopy in the era of minimally invasive surgery. *Gastrointest Endosc* 38:392–393, 1992

351. Warshaw AL, Gu ZY, Wittenberg J, et al: Preoperative staging and assessment of resectability of pancreatic cancer. *Arch Surg* 125:230–233, 1990

352. Parsous L, Palmer LH: How accurate is fine-needle biopsy in malignant neoplasia of the pancreas? *Arch Surg* 124:681–683, 1989

353. Al-Kaisi N, Siegler EE: Fine needle aspiration cytology of the pancreas. *Acta Cytol* 33:145–182, 1989

354. Rashleigh-Bilcher HJC, Russell RCG, Lees WR: Cutaneous seeding of pancreatic carcinoma by fine-needle aspiration biopsy. *Br J Radiol* 59:182–183, 1986

355. Weiss SM, Skibber JM, Mohiuddinn, et al: Rapid intra-abdominal spread of pancreatic cancer. *Arch Surg* 120:415–416, 1985

356. Fabris C: Urinary enzyme excretion in pancreatic diseases. *J Clin Gastroenterol* 14:281–284, 1992

357. Steinberg W: The clinical utility of the CA 19-9 tumor-associated antigen. *Am J Gastroenterol* 85:350–355, 1990

358. Robles-Diaz G, Diaz-Sanchez V, Fernandez-del Castillo C, et al: Serum testosterone: Dihydrotestosterone ratio and CA 19-9 in the diagnosis of pancreatic cancer. *Am J Gastroenterol* 86:591–594, 1991

359. Bell RH: Neoplasms of the exocrine pancreas, in Greenfield LJ, Mulholland M, Oldham KT, Zelenock GB, Lillemoe KD (eds): *Surgery: Scientific Principles and Practice* (ed 2). Philadelphia, Lippincott, 1997, pp 901–915

360. Frebourg T, Bercoff E, Mouchon N, et al: The evaluation of CA 19-9 antigen level in the early detection of pancreatic cancer. *Cancer* 62:2287–2290, 1988

361. Warshaw AL, Fernandez-del Castillo C: Pancreatic carcinoma. *N Engl J Med* 326:455–465, 1993

362. Glenn J, Steinberg WM, Kurtzman SH, et al: Evaluation of the utility of a radioimmunoassay for serum CA 19-9 levels in patients before and after treatment of carcinoma of the pancreas. *J Clin Oncol* 6:462–468, 1988

363. Rothlin MA, Joller H, Largiader F: CA 242 is a new tumor marker for pancreatic cancer. *Cancer* 71:701–707, 1993

364. Brennan MF, Kinsella TJ, Casper ES: Cancer of the pancreas, in DeVita VT, Hellman S, Rosenberg SA (eds): *Cancer: Principles and Practice of Oncology* (ed 4). Philadelphia, Lippincott, 1993, pp 849–882

365. Friess H, Buchler M, Auerbach B, et al: CA 494: A new tumor marker for the diagnosis of pancreatic cancer. *Int J Cancer* 53:759–763, 1993

366. Ahlgren JD, Hill MC, Roberts IM: Pancreatic cancer: Patterns, diagnosis, and approaches to treatment, in Ahlgren JD, Macdonald JS (eds): *Gastrointestinal Oncology*. Philadelphia, Lippincott, 1992, pp 197–214

367. Cameron JL, Pitt HA, Yeo CJ, et al: One hundred and forty-five consecutive pancreaticoduodenectomies without mortality. *Ann Surg* 217:430–438, 1993

368. Yeo CJ, Cameron JL, Lillemoe KD, et al: Pancreaticoduodenectomy for cancer of the head of the pancreas: 201 patients. *Ann Surg* 221:721–733, 1995

369. Gordon TA, Burleyson GP, Tielsch JM, et al: The effects of regionalization on cost and outcome for one high-risk surgical procedure. *Ann Surg* 221:43–49, 1995

370. Sindelar WF: Clinical experience with regional pancreatectomy for adenocarcinoma of the pancreas. *Arch Surg* 124:127–132, 1989

371. Morris DM, Ford RS: Pancreaticogastrostomy: Preferred reconstruction for Whipple resection. *J Surg Res* 54:122–125, 1993

372. Takao S, Shimazu H, Maenohara S, et al: Modified pancreaticogastrostomy following pancreaticoduodenectomy: Current management. *Am J Surg* 165:317–321, 1993

373. Yeo CJ, Cameron JL, Maher MM, et al: A prospective randomized trial of pancreaticogastrostomy versus pancreaticojejunostomy after pancreaticoduodenectomy. *Ann Surg* 222:580–592, 1995

374. Grace PA, Pitt HA, Tompkins RK: Decreased morbidity and mortality after pancreaticoduodenectomy. *Am J Surg* 151:141–149, 1986

375. Braasch JW, Deziel DJ, Rossi RL, et al: Pyloric and gastric preserving pancreatic resection: Experience with 87 patients. *Ann Surg* 204:411–418, 1986

376. Yeo CJ, Barry MK, Sauter PK, et al: Erythromycin accelerates gastric emptying after pancreaticoduodenectomy: A prospective, randomized, placebo-controlled trial. *Ann Surg* 218:229–238, 1993

377. Kwan D, Aufses AH: Short-term administration of SMS

378. Buchler M, Friess H, Klempa I, et al: Role of octreotide in the prevention of postoperative complications following pancreatic resection. *Am J Surg* 163:125–131, 1992

379. Yeo CJ: Management of complications following pancreaticoduodenectomy. *Surg Clin North Am* 75:913–924, 1995

380. Ishikawa O, Ohhigashi H, Sasaki Y, et al: Practical usefulness of lymphatic and connective tissue clearance for carcinoma of the pancreas head. *Ann Surg* 208:215–220, 1988

381. Manabe T, Ohshio G, Baba N, et al: Radical pancreatectomy for ductal cell carcinoma of the head of the pancreas. *Cancer* 64:1132–1137, 1989

382. Tashiro S, Uchino R, Hiraoke T, et al: Surgical indication and significance of portal vein resection in biliary and pancreatic cancer. *Surgery* 190:481–487, 1991

383. van Heerden JA, McIlrath DC, Ilstrup DM, et al: Total pancreatectomy for ductal adenocarcinoma of the pancreas: An update. *World J Surg* 12:658–662, 1988

384. Dalton RR, Sarr MG, van Heerden JA, et al: Carcinoma of the body and tail of the pancreas: Is curative resection justified? *Surgery* 111:489–494, 1992

385. Lillemoe KD, Barnes SA: Surgical palliation of unresectable pancreatic carcinoma. *Surg Clin North Am* 75:953–968, 1995

386. Cotton PB: Nonsurgical palliation of jaundice in pancreatic cancer. *Surg Clin North Am* 69:613–627, 1989

387. Speer AG, Cotton PB, Russell RCG: Randomized trial of endoscopic versus percutaneous stent insertion in malignant obstructive jaundice. *Lancet* 2:57–62, 1987

388. Proctor H, Mauro M: Biliary diversion for pancreatic carcinoma: Matching of the methods and the patient. *Am J Surg* 159:67–71, 1990

389. Lichtenstein DR, Carr-Locke DL: Endoscopic palliation for unresectable pancreatic carcinoma. *Surg Clin North Am* 75:969–988, 1995

390. Kaufman SL: Percutaneous palliation of unresectable pancreatic carcinoma. *Surg Clin North Am* 75:989–999, 1995

391. Ashley SW, Reber HA: Surgical management of exocrine pancreatic cancer, in Go VLW, Dimagno EP, Gardner JD, Lebenthal E, Reber HA, Scheele GA (eds): *The Pancreas: Biology, Pathobiology, and Disease* (ed 2). New York, Raven Press, 1993, pp 913–930

392. Lillemoe KD, Sauter PK, Pitt HA, et al: Current management of surgical palliation of periampullary carcinoma. *Surg Gynecol Obstet* 176:1–10, 1993

393. Saltzburg D, Foley KM: Management of pain in pancreatic cancer. *Surg Clin North Am* 69:629–649, 1989

394. Levy MH: Pharmacologic treatment of cancer pain. *N Engl J Med* 335:1124–1132, 1996

395. Lillemoe KD, Cameron JL, Kaufman HS, et al: Chemical splanchnicectomy in patients with unresectable pancreatic cancer: A prospective randomized trial. *Ann Surg* 217:447–455, 1993

396. Lee MJ, Mueller PR, vanSonnenberg E, et al: CT-guided celiac ganglion block with alcohol. *Am J Roentgenol* 161:633–636, 1993

397. Worsey J, Ferson PF, Keenan RJ, et al: Thorascopic pancreatic denervation for pain control in irresectable pancreatic cancer. *Br J Surg* 80:1051–1052, 1993

398. Coleman J: Supportive management of the patient with pancreatic cancer: Role of the oncology nurse. *Oncology* 10:23–25, 1996 (suppl)

399. Doty JE, Fink AS, Meyer JH: Alterations in digestive func-

tion caused by pancreatic disease. *Surg Clin North Am* 69: 447–465, 1989

400. Ottery F: Supportive nutritional management of the patient with pancreatic cancer. *Oncology* 10:26–32, 1996 (suppl)

401. Spross JA, Manalatos A, Thorpe M: Pancreatic cancer: Nursing challenges. *Semin Oncol Nurs* 4(4):274–284, 1988

402. Rothenberg ML: New developments in chemotherapy for patients with advanced pancreatic cancer. *Oncology* 10: 18–22, 1996 (suppl)

403. Abrams RA, Grochow LB: Adjuvant therapy with chemotherapy and radiation therapy in the management of carcinoma of the pancreatic head. *Surg Clin North Am* 75: 925–938, 1995

404. Zerbi A, Fossati V, Parolini D, et al: Intraoperative radiation therapy adjuvant of resection in the treatment of pancreatic cancer. *Cancer* 73:2930, 1994

405. Mohiuddin M, Rosato F, Barbot D, et al: Long-term results of combined modality treatment with I-125 implantation for carcinoma of the pancreas. *Int J Radiat Oncol Biol Phys* 23:305–311, 1992

406. Dobelbower RR, Konski AA, Merrick HW, et al: Intraoperative electron beam radiation therapy (IOEBRT) for carcinoma of the exocrine pancreas. *Int J Radiat Oncol Biol Phys* 20:113–119, 1991

407. Matsuno S, Sato T: Surgical treatment for carcinoma of the pancreas. *Am J Surg* 152:499–504, 1986

408. Whittington R, Dobelbower RR, Mohiuddin M, et al: Radiotherapy of unresectable pancreatic carcinoma: A six year experience with 104 patients. *Int J Radiat Oncol Biol Phys* 7:1639–1644, 1981

409. Gastrointestinal Tumor Study Group: Therapy of locally unresectable pancreatic carcinoma: A randomized comparison of high dose (6000 rads) radiation alone, moderate dose radiation (4000 rads + 5-fluorouracil) and high dose radiation + 5-fluorouracil. *Cancer* 48:1705–1710, 1981

410. Evans DB, Rich TA, Byrd DR, et al: Preoperative chemoradiation and pancreaticoduodenectomy for adenocarcinoma of the pancreas. *Arch Surg* 127:1335–1339, 1992

411. Staley CA, Lee JE, Cleary KR, et al: Preoperative chemoradiation, pancreaticoduodenectomy, and intraoperative radiation therapy for adenocarcinoma of the pancreatic head. *Am J Surg* 171:118–125, 1996

412. Yeung RS, Weese JL, Hoffman JP, et al: Neoadjuvant chemoradiation in pancreatic and duodenal carcinoma: A phase II study. *Cancer* 72:2124–2133, 1993

413. Coia L, Hoffman J, Scher R, et al: Preoperative chemoradiation for adenocarcinoma of the pancreas and duodenum. *Int J Radiat Oncol Biol Phys* 30:161–167, 1994

414. Walsh D: Palliative management of the patient with advanced pancreatic cancer. *Oncology* 10:40–44, 1996 (suppl)

415. Alter CL: Palliative and supportive care of patients with pancreatic cancer. *Semin Oncol* 23:229–240, 1996

416. Foley KM: Supportive care and the quality of life of the cancer patient, in DeVita VT, Hellman S, Rosenberg SA (eds): *Cancer: Principles and Practice of Oncology* (ed 4). Philadelphia, Lippincott, 1993, pp 2417–2448

417. Padilla GV: Psychological aspects of nutrition and cancer. *Surg Clin North Am* 66:1121–1135, 1986

418. Walsh D: Palliative care: Management of the patient with advanced cancer. *Semin Oncol* 21:100–106, 1994 (suppl)

419. Watanabe S, Bruera E: Anorexia and cachexia, asthenia, and lethargy. *Hematol Oncol Clin North Am* 10:189–206, 1996

420. Portenoy RK: Constipation in the cancer patient: Causes and management. *Med Clin North Am* 71:303–311, 1987

421. Krech RL, Walsh D: Symptoms of pancreatic cancer. *J Pain Symptom Manage* 6:360–367, 1991

# Chapter 39

# Gynecologic Cancers

Janet Ruth Walczak, RN, MSN

Paula R. Klemm, RN, DNSc, OCN®

Carol Guarnieri, RN, MSN, AOCN

## INTRODUCTION

Gynecologic cancers account for about 14% of all cancers in women. In 1996 it was estimated that there would be approximately 82,100 new cases of invasive female genital cancer and 65,000 new cases of carcinoma in situ or intraepithelial neoplasia in the United States (Table 39-1). Approximately 26,000 women were estimated to die of gynecologic malignancies in 1996.[1] This constitutes about 10% of cancer deaths in women. Although gynecologic cancers can occur at any age, the majority occur in the middle years (cervical), perimenopausal years (ovarian), and postmenopausal years (endometrial, vulvar, and vaginal). Like many other malignancies, cancers of the female genital tract can be cured if diagnosed in early stages. Unfortunately, only cervical cancer has a specific and sensitive screening tool that can be applied to large numbers of women safely and inexpensively. As a result, many women, particularly those with ovarian cancer, are diagnosed in later stages when the ability to achieve cure is limited by the lack of effective therapy.

The major gynecologic cancers are reviewed in this chapter. Cancer of the uterine corpus, or endometrial cancer, is the predominant cancer of the female genital tract and usually occurs in the postmenopausal years. Regular gynecologic visits that include a screening endometrial biopsy in high-risk women could increase early detection of curable adenocarcinoma of the endometrium. Ovarian cancer is usually disseminated at diagnosis. Localized disease is asymptomatic in the vast majority of cases and routine pelvic examinations frequently fail to detect ovarian tumors in this group. Efforts to define methods of detection are still in progress. Because ovarian cancer is usually diagnosed in late stages, it is the fifth leading cause of cancer death.

Cervical cancer predominantly occurs during the reproductive years when women are more likely to receive regular gynecologic care, including Pap smear testing. Therefore, the majority of cervical lesions are diagnosed in the preinvasive stages of intraepithelial neoplasia when the disease is curable. Vulvar and vaginal cancers usually occur in the postmenopausal years when many women feel that they no longer need to be seen by a gynecologist. These cancers are frequently preceded by preinvasive intraepithelial neoplasia and are readily curable if diagnosed in early stages.

**TABLE 39-1**  Gynecologic Cancer in the United States—1996

| Cancer Site | Estimated New Cases | Estimated Deaths |
|---|---|---|
| Cancer of the cervix | 15,700 | 4900 |
| Cancer of the endometrium | 34,000 | 6000 |
| Cancer of the ovary | 26,700 | 14,800 |
| Other gynecologic cancers | 5700 | 1200 |

Parker SL, Tong T, Bolden S, et al: Cancer Statistics, 1996. *CA Cancer J Clin* 46:5–27, 1996

## ENDOMETRIAL CANCER

### Epidemiology

Cancer of the endometrium is the predominant cancer of the female genital tract. While there were an estimated

34,000 new cases of endometrial cancer diagnosed in the United States in 1996, only approximately 6000 women died of the disease in 1996. This low mortality rate reflects the fact that 79% are diagnosed with localized disease.[1] Survival rates for endometrial cancer by stage are 76% for stage I, 50% for stage II, 30% for stage III, and 9% for stage IV.[2]

Endometrial cancer is primarily a disease of post-menopausal women. The median age at diagnosis is 61 years, with the majority of women diagnosed between 50 and 59 years of age. Only about 5% of women will be diagnosed before 40 years of age, and 20%–25% will be premenopausal.[3]

## Etiology

Multiple risk factors have been associated with the development of endometrial cancer. These include obesity (> 20 pounds overweight), nulliparity, late menopause (after age 52), diabetes, hypertension, infertility, irregular menses, failure of ovulation, a history of breast or ovarian cancer, adenomatous hyperplasia, and prolonged use of exogenous estrogen therapy. An obese, nulliparous woman who experiences menopause after 59 years of age appears to have a five-fold greater risk of developing endometrial cancer.[3,4] Additionally, Feldman et al identified that the nulliparous, diabetic woman over 70 years of age who presents with abnormal vaginal bleeding has an 87% risk of developing endometrial cancer or hyperplasia, while the woman who presents with abnormal bleeding and has none of the other factors has only a 3% risk.[5]

Excessive endogenous estrogen metabolism or production has been implicated in the development of endometrial cancer. Several hormonal aberrations can be linked to obesity. Increased body size plays a role in androgen conversion to estrogen.[4,6,7] Additionally, obese women with an upper body fat pattern have a 5.8-fold increase in risk over women who are nonobese or have a lower body fat pattern.[8] Fat cells are an excellent storage depot for estrogen, and the chronic slow release of estrogen from these cells may account for the increased risk. In obese postmenopausal women, secretion of serum sex hormone-binding globulin (SHBG) is depressed, leaving higher concentrations of free estradiol in the blood. Obese women have endocrine malfunctions that cause anovulatory cycles with irregular menses. This results in failure of progesterone to oppose chronic estrogen effects on the endometrium. Another source of endogenous estrogen can be feminizing ovarian tumors (e.g., granulosa cell tumors).[4,6,7]

Use of unopposed exogenous estrogen has been linked to an increased incidence of endometrial cancer since the mid-1970s.[9] This problem virtually can be eliminated by cycling estrogen and progesterone and by histologically sampling the endometrium for early detection.[3,10] Tamoxifen, which acts as an antiestrogen on breast tissue, has a weak estrogenic effect on endometrial tissue and has been associated with thickening of the endometrium and changes from polyps to hyperplasia and cancer.[11–16] More data are needed to define endometrial screening criteria and management of women with breast cancer who are being treated with tamoxifen and women participating in the breast cancer chemoprevention with tamoxifen trials.

Either exogenous or endogenous estrogen may lead to endometrial hyperplasia. While adenomatous hyperplasia is considered a risk factor of endometrial cancer, it is unclear if it is a precursor, unless atypia accompanies the hyperplasia.[3]

## Prevention, Screening, Early Detection

Two factors appear to have a protective effect against the development of endometrial cancer: oral contraceptives and cigarette smoking. Oral contraceptive usage for at least 12 months decreases the woman's risk of developing endometrial cancer, and this protection seems to persist for up to 15 years in nulliparous women. Similarly, smoking has been correlated with a reduction in risk, especially in women over 50 years old. However, the risks of developing lung cancer and other health problems well outweigh any protection gained against endometrial cancer.[3,17–20]

Unfortunately, there is no sensitive and specific screening test for endometrial cancer. The Pap smear will only occasionally detect an endometrial cancer. Though endometrial biopsy is 90% effective in detecting a cancer and can be accomplished in the outpatient setting, it is not without morbidity and cost and should not be applied as a screen at this time to the general population. The American Cancer Society and the American College of Obstetricians and Gynecologists currently recommend that women should have an annual pelvic examination and Pap smear; that an endometrial biopsy should be obtained at menopause and before beginning hormone replacement therapy or tamoxifen; and that an endometrial biopsy be obtained in women at high risk for the development of endometrial cancer.[21,22]

## Pathophysiology and Cellular Characteristics

The uterine corpus is a muscular, hollow, pear-shaped organ with an endometrial lining composed of ciliated epithelial cells. Throughout the epithelium are small, tubular glands that extend to the myometrium, or muscle wall of the corpus. Endometrial cancer develops in the epithelial layer. Tumors that arise in the lower uterine segment involve the cervix sooner and have a higher incidence of pelvic and para-aortic lymph node involvement than do tumors that arise higher in the fundus. Similarly, tumors that have deep myometrial invasion tend to be more aggressive and have a poorer survival rate.[3]

Over 90% of endometrial cancers are adenocarcinomas. Three types of adenocarcinomas account for 88% of histological patterns: pure adenocarcinomas, adenoacanthoma (adenocarcinoma with a benign squamous component), and adenosquamous (where both components are malignant). The less frequent patterns include clear cell (mesonephroid) carcinoma, undifferentiated carcinoma, and the papillary carcinomas, which include the endometrioid and serous types. The clear cell and serous patterns are more aggressive than the other carcinomas.[3,19]

## Clinical Manifestations

Multiple factors affect the natural history and prognosis of endometrial cancer. These include histological type and differentiation, uterine size, stage of disease, myometrial invasion, peritoneal cytology, lymph node metastasis, and adnexal metastasis.[3,23]

Cancer usually starts in the fundus and may spread to involve the entire endometrium. Through direct extension and infiltration, the cancer spreads to the myometrium, endocervix, cervix, fallopian tubes, and ovaries. Adnexal spread is infrequent but is found at surgery in about 10% of women with clinical stage I disease. Recurrence appears in 38% of women with adnexal spread versus 11% of those without such involvement.[3]

Metastatic spread is usually to pelvic and para-aortic lymph nodes and has been positively correlated with tumor differentiation, stage of disease, and amount of myometrial invasion. Pelvic and para-aortic lymph node metastases can be present, even in women with stage I disease (Figure 39-1) when about 10% will have positive pelvic nodes, and stage II disease when 36% will have positive nodes.[3,24] Less common sites of metastases include the vagina, peritoneal cavity, omentum, and inguinal lymph nodes. Hematogenous spread often involves the lung, liver, bone, and brain. The size of the uterus, measured by uterine sound, has been an indicator of survival. However, since large uterine size can be secondary to intercurrent disease, such as fibroids, this factor is no longer included in the staging and prognosis of endometrial cancer. Even so, the five-year survival rate for women with a normal-sized uterus is 84%, whereas for women with an enlarged uterus it is 67%.[25]

Histological differentiation is one of the most sensitive indicators of metastases and prognosis. The less differentiated the tumor, the poorer the prognosis. Grade 1 tumors are highly differentiated, grade 2 tumors are moderately differentiated, and grade 3 tumors are mostly solid or undifferentiated carcinomas.[26] Overall five-year survival rates are 96% for patients with grade I tumors, 79% for those with grade II tumors, and 70% for those with grade III tumors.[2,3]

Another prognostic indicator, the degree of myometrial invasion, is generally classified as: none (localized to the endometrium), superficial (invasion <50%), or deep (>50%).[2] The greater the invasion, the poorer the

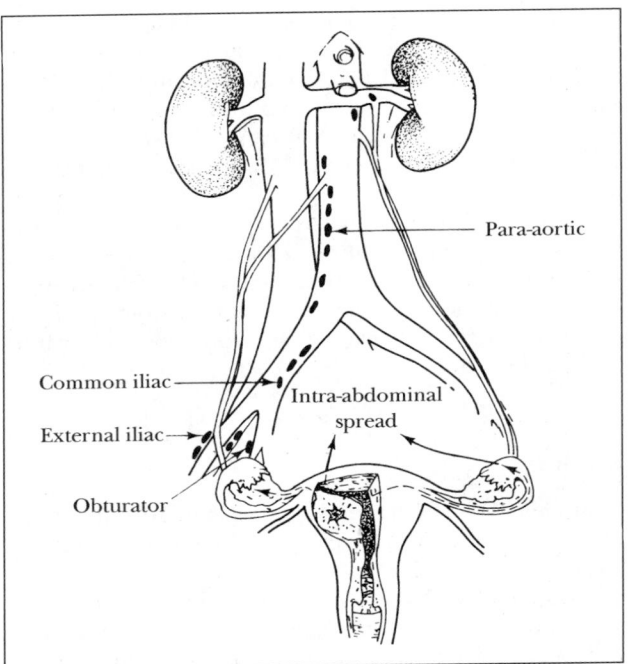

**FIGURE 39-1**   Spread pattern of endometrial cancer, with particular emphasis on potential lymph node spread. Pelvic and para-aortic nodes are at risk, even in stage I disease. (DiSaia PJ, Creasman WT: *Clinical Gynecologic Oncology.* St Louis, Mosby, 1989.)

prognosis. Additionally, the less differentiated the tumor, the greater the chance of myometrial invasion. Thus, the grade of the tumor is combined with the degree of myometrial invasion to estimate survival.

During laparotomy, samples of peritoneal fluid or washings of the peritoneal cavity are obtained for staging purposes, but the results also have prognostic significance. Women with positive washings are at a higher risk for pelvic recurrence. DiSaia and Creasman[3] reported a 15% rate of positive washings in women with stage I disease. Recurrence developed in 34% of these individuals, compared with 10% among patients showing negative cytological change.

## Assessment

Fortunately, the abnormal vaginal bleeding associated with endometrial cancer causes women to seek medical attention promptly. Postmenopausal bleeding should always be evaluated, even though only 20% of women with this symptom will have cancer. Any serosanguinous vaginal discharge or new heavy bleeding also needs evaluation. Premenopausal onset of irregular or heavy menstrual flow may be significant, especially if the patient is infertile with anovulatory cycles. Other more infrequent symptoms are pyometria and hematometria, particularly in the older woman, and lumbosacral, hypogastric, or pelvic pain in women with more advanced disease.[26]

In women suspected of having endometrial cancer, a thorough pelvic examination is performed. A Pap smear will only occasionally detect an endometrial cancer.[16] A more reliable technique is endometrial biopsy, which allows histological rather than cytological examination. This procedure is 90% effective in detecting endometrial cancer and can be performed in the outpatient setting.[3] If the endometrial biopsy is negative and symptoms persist, a fractional dilatation and curettage (D & C) is performed.[3]

Other diagnostic tests include chest radiograph, intravenous pyelogram (IVP), complete blood count (CBC), and blood chemistry profiles. Cystoscopy, barium enema, and proctoscopy are performed if bladder or rectal involvement is suspected. Other studies that may be used to evaluate pelvic, abdominal, and nodal disease status include hysterography, hysteroscopy, lymphangiography, and computerized axial tomogram scan.[27] Although magnetic resonance imaging (MRI) cannot distinguish benign from malignant neoplasms, it is effective in detecting the degree of myometrial invasion.[28–30]

## Classification and Staging

Endometrial cancer is staged surgically (Table 39-2) in patients who are surgical candidates, that is, if medical condition and intra-abdominal disease permit. Staging helps to define primary tumor size and location as well as extent of spread beyond the uterus. Approximately 75% of tumors are diagnosed in stage I, 13% in stage II, 9% in stage III, and 3% in stage IV.[2]

Surgical staging and treatment can involve an extensive evaluation of the abdomino-pelvic cavity and use of the following procedures: bimanual examination under anesthesia, peritoneal cytology, inspection and palpation of all peritoneal surfaces, biopsy of suspicious areas, selective pelvic and para-aortic lymphadenectomy, total abdominal hysterectomy (TAH), bilateral salpingo-oophorectomy (BSO), and possible omentectomy and

**TABLE 39-2** Corpus Cancer Staging

### CARCINOMA OF THE UTERINE CORPUS

The Committee decided that corpus cancer should be surgically staged and as a result additional factors of prognostic importance are included in the staging. The Committee also decided to change the current definitions of tumor grading to coincide with the new recommendations of the International Society of Gynecological Pathologists. The recommended staging is as follows:

#### STAGE

| | | |
|---|---|---|
| IA | G123 | Tumor limited to endometrium |
| IB | G123 | Invasion to <1/2 myometrium |
| IC | G123 | Invasion to >1/2 myometrium |
| IIA | G123 | Endocervical glandular involvement only |
| IIB | G123 | Cervical stromal invasion |
| IIIA | G123 | Tumor invades serosa and/or adnexa and/or positive peritoneal cytology |
| IIIB | G123 | Metastases to pelvic and/or para-aortic lymph nodes |
| IVA | G123 | Tumor invasion of bladder and/or bowel mucosa |
| IVB | | Distant metastases including intra-abdominal and/or inguinal lymph nodes |

### HISTOPATHOLOGY: DEGREE OF DIFFERENTIATION

Cases of carcinoma of the corpus should be grouped with regard to the degree of differentiation of the adenocarcinoma as follows:

G1 5% or less of a nonsquamous or nonmorular solid growth pattern
G2 6%–50% of a nonsquamous or nonmorular solid growth pattern
G3 More than 50% of a nonsquamous or nonmorular solid growth pattern

### NOTES ON PATHOLOGICAL GRADING

(1) Notable nuclear atypia, inappropriate for the architectural grade, raises the grade of a grade I or grade II tumor by one.
(2) In serous adenocarcinomas, clear-cell adenocarcinomas, and squamous-cell carcinomas, nuclear grading takes precedence.
(3) Adenocarcinomas with squamous differentiation are graded according to the nuclear grade of the glandular component.

### RULES RELATED TO STAGING

(1) Since corpus cancer is now surgically staged, procedures used previously for the differentiation of stages are no longer applicable (e.g., using dilatation and curettage findings to differentiate between stage I and stage II). (It is appreciated that there may be a small number of patients with corpus cancer who will be treated primarily with radiation therapy. If that is the case, the clinical staging adopted by FIGO* in 1971 would still apply but designation of that staging system would be noted.)
(2) Ideally, the thickness of the myometrium should be measured along with the depth of tumor invasion.

*FIGO, International Federation of Gynecology and Obstetrics.
FIGO News, *Int J Gynecol Obstet* 28:189–193, 1989

resection of tumor implants.[31,32] Tissue from the primary tumor is obtained for analysis of estrogen and progesterone receptors, although the results are not used in the staging process.

## Therapeutic Approaches and Nursing Care

### Primary

Primary surgical staging prior to any radiation therapy is advantageous since many women with early-stage disease will not need additional postoperative therapy and thus can avoid the time, effort, and morbidity associated with pelvic radiation therapy. Also, the pathologist is better able to evaluate untreated tissue for the histological indicators of prognosis (histological type, grade, and myometrial invasion).

Selection of adjuvant radiation therapy for early endometrial cancer is determined by stage, histology, and cytopathology. In patients with positive peritoneal cytology, intraperitoneal radioactive colloidal phosphorous ($^{32}$P) may be helpful in preventing or delaying recurrence if no other therapy is indicated. However, prospective data are not available to support or refute this approach.

Patients with stage I, grade 1 disease and no myometrial invasion require no further treatment after TAH, BSO. Patients with stage I, grade 2 disease and less than 50% myometrial invasion require intravaginal radiation to reduce the risk of central recurrence. Indications for pelvic external beam radiation therapy include disease localized to the pelvis, a high-grade tumor, or greater than 50% myometrial invasion. Whole-pelvis radiation, in contrast to intravaginal radiation, allows treatment of all pelvic tissue including nodes and lymphatics. The role of whole-abdominal radiation in the treatment of serous and clear cell carcinomas and advanced adenocarcinomas is still under investigation.[3,19,23,32,33]

Adjuvant hormonal therapy in endometrial cancer is considered unproven and remains controversial.[26] Kauppila et al[34] reported on over 1100 patients who received adjuvant progestin therapy for two years after primary treatment for endometrial cancer; recurrence occurred even in women with stage I disease.

### Advanced or recurrent disease

Endometrial cancer is one of the most difficult cancers to treat if metastasis or recurrence has occurred.[35] Women with vaginal recurrences can be treated successfully with surgery or radiotherapy. These individuals do well and usually are long-term survivors.[3] However, women with recurrences outside the upper vagina (pelvis or distant) are not easily treated. Radiotherapy has a limited role in recurrent disease, although palliative radiation can be employed to control heavy vaginal bleeding in patients who present with advanced, incurable disease. Hormonal therapy or chemotherapy is essential to treat recurrent and advanced disease.[3]

*Hormonal therapy*    The most commonly used systemic therapy for recurrent endometrial cancer has been synthetic progestational agents. Response rates range from 30%–37%, and response seems to be related to histological grade of the tumor, length of the disease-free interval, the woman's age, and presence of areas of squamous metaplasia within the primary tumor.[26] Receptor status can also predict which tumors will respond to progestins. Positive estrogen and progesterone receptor status correlates with a better response to progestin therapy regardless of the grade of the tumor. If both receptors are positive, there is a 77% response rate associated with progestin therapy, compared with only a 9% response rate if both receptors are negative.[36]

Side effects of progestational agents include fluid retention, phlebitis, and thrombosis. Side effects are usually minimal unless high doses are employed. Patients have reported feelings of well-being as well as weight gain while taking progestins.[26]

Oral preparations of megestrol acetate or intramuscular medroxyprogesterone acetate are effective agents against endometrial cancer.[26] The progestins are continued until the disease progresses. At that time, chemotherapy is considered.

The antiestrogen tamoxifen, which can cause hot flashes, vaginal dryness, and infrequently emotional lability, has been used to treat advanced endometrial cancer in an attempt to induce progesterone receptor positivity. No improvement in length of response was seen, although the drug was shown to increase the number of receptors per tumor.[37] The use of tamoxifen is still experimental.[2] Quinn and Campbell[38] suggested using a combination of tamoxifen and progestogen as the first choice of hormonal therapy.

*Chemotherapy*    Cytotoxic agents have a limited role in advanced endometrial cancer since only a few agents have demonstrated activity equal to or greater than progestin therapy. In single-agent trials, the most promising results were obtained by Thigpen et al[39] using 60 mg/m$^2$ of doxorubicin every three weeks. These researchers reported a 37% response rate, with 26% complete responses. Prognostic factors did not correlate with the probability of response.

Administration of high doses (100 mg/m$^2$) of cisplatin has achieved response rates of 46% in women with no prior chemotherapy.[40] However, when cisplatin was used as a second-line treatment, the results were not impressive (4% response rate).[41] Thigpen et al[42] studied 49 women with advanced or recurrent endometrial carcinoma who had not received prior chemotherapy and who were no longer controllable with other treatment modalities. Patients were treated with cisplatin, 50 mg/m$^2$ intravenously, every three weeks. Forty-five percent exhibited stable disease for at least two months, while 35% had disease progression in less than two months after beginning chemotherapy.

Combination therapy has been studied to a limited

degree; in one study cisplatin, doxorubicin, and cyclophosphamide resulted in an overall response rate of 45% in 209 patients.[43] Other studies have shown little improvement over response rates seen with single agents. In addition, the profile of side effects experienced with single agents is more limited.[44,45] There is little evidence at present to support the use of combination chemotherapy in the management of endometrial carcinoma.[42] Newer approaches such as circadian-timed chemotherapy administration and the use of biologics, need to be further studied.[46,47] Additional well-controlled clinical trials examining the role of combination chemotherapy in patients with advanced or recurrent endometrial carcinoma are needed.[2]

Though the majority of women are diagnosed with early-stage disease, women still die from recurrent or advanced disease. Ongoing efforts strive to define adjuvant therapy to further improve survival and reduce recurrence. The role of [32]P in early-stage disease with positive pelvic cytology needs to be defined in a prospective clinical trial. However, as better methods for control of central disease are achieved, patients who then fail to respond to primary therapy will recur outside of the pelvis. The role of whole-abdominal radiation therapy in preventing or treating recurrences is not yet defined; however, the Gynecologic Oncology Group continues to conduct prospective clinical trials.[32,48] Also, prospective clinical trials to identify cytotoxic drugs and drug regimens with improved response and survival rates continue.

The role of estrogen and progesterone receptor status in the choice of therapy and as a predictor of response needs to be defined. With the availability of assays for receptors, more information can be collected. Early studies showed a positive correlation between the presence of progesterone receptors and clinical response to progestin therapy.[49] This information also could be correlated with other prognostic factors to pinpoint more specifically those women who will respond. Theoretically, women with positive estrogen receptors should respond to antiestrogen therapy. If both estrogen receptors and progesterone receptors are positive, future trials could employ combination hormonal therapy. However, actual treatment models for hormonal therapy are yet to be defined.[50] Utaaker et al[51] reported that steroid receptors were found in more than 85% of primary endometrial carcinomas. Highly differentiated tumors were more often estrogen receptor and progesterone receptor rich than were poorly differentiated ones, but receptor status was not significantly associated with surgical stage.

Estrogen replacement therapy (ERT), while historically contraindicated in women with endometrial cancer, also needs further investigation in order to identify the appropriate candidate for ERT. For women with stage I disease, low-grade tumors, and no myometrial invasion, the benefits of ERT in decreasing the risk of cardiovascular disease and osteoporosis may outweigh the associated risk of breast cancer and recurrent endometrial cancer. Finally, as younger women develop endometrial cancer,

conservative therapy for early-stage, low-grade disease needs to be prospectively evaluated for long-term outcomes. The nursing care of the patient with endometrial cancer includes those issues discussed in the chapters devoted to the specific treatment modalities such as surgery, radiation therapy, and chemotherapy. The other major area for assessment and intervention is knowledge related to health maintenance behaviors, therapeutic interventions, and psychosocial concerns. These issues are summarized in Table 39-3.

## Symptom Management and Continuity of Care

For the vast majority of women with endometrial cancer, the major nursing challenges are those that relate to regular follow-up. Since most patients will be cured with their primary surgery, regular follow-up will be the basis of their care. Education about the importance of follow-up as well as a healthy lifestyle must be stressed. Follow-up usually involves regular pelvic examinations, at least quarterly in the initial years after diagnosis, and CT scans at least annually. A healthy lifestyle includes weight reduction if appropriate, regular exercise, and regular screening for other cancers, including mammography.

For those women who present with advanced disease or who have a recurrence, the challenges of care will vary according to the type of therapy they are receiving, and the specifics can be found in the appropriate chapters. Certainly, educational issues are still crucial to their care and should focus on information about the side effects of therapy and how to manage them; self care issues such as care of a venous access device, nutritional intake, and pain control; and community resources for assistance including home care resources, support groups, and counseling available. The issue of quality of life is also important to discuss with the woman and her family, focusing on physical changes and functional status, psychosocial concerns such as changes in roles within the family, economic concerns, and spiritual and religious concerns. The reader is referred to the chapters on quality of life, home care, and hospice care for more detailed information.

## OVARIAN CANCER

### Epidemiology

In 1996 there were approximately 26,700 new cases of ovarian cancer diagnosed in the United States and over 14,800 deaths from the disease. Ovarian cancer accounts for approximately 33% of all gynecologic cancers and 55% of deaths from cancer of the female genital tract. It is the most common cause of death from gynecologic

**TABLE 39-3** Information Needs Related to Endometrial Cancer

| Topic | Information |
|---|---|
| **Health maintenance issues that affect risk** | |
| Estrogen replacement therapy (ERT) | Indications: |
| |     Vaginal atrophy with infection or sexual dysfunction |
| |     Loss of pelvic support with incontinence |
| |     Postmenopausal osteoporosis |
| |     Perimenopausal emotional lability |
| |     Early surgical or radiation castration |
| |     Vasomotor instability |
| |     Lowered morbidity and mortality for cardiovascular disease |
| | Estrogen cycled with progesterone |
| | Annual pelvic exam |
| | Regular histological sampling of endometrium |
| | Annual mammogram |
| | Seek medical attention if any abnormal vaginal bleeding occurs including postmenopausal bleeding (PMB) |
| Breast self-examination (BSE) | Importance of BSE in conjunction with ERT |
| | Determine schedule to aid in compliance |
| | Technique for performing BSE and demonstration of skill |
| Diet and weight control | Low-fat, calcium-rich diet |
| | Maintain weight within normal range |
| | Large amounts of caffeine and fiber may decrease calcium absorption |
| | Weight-bearing exercises to decrease bone loss, (e.g., walking) |
| Abnormal vaginal bleeding | Seek medical attention for new onset of abnormal bleeding, including intramenstrual and PMB |
| | PMB and abnormal bleeding in the infertile patient with anovulatory cycles must be evaluated, even though only 20% of PMB is associated with malignancy |
| | Evaluation of abnormal bleeding includes pelvic exam and endometrial biopsy |
| **Therapeutic interventions** | |
| Surgery | Types of surgery planned, what will be removed, change in anatomy and function anticipated |
| | Clarify, reinforce informed consent |
| | Role in postoperative care to facilitate recovery, e.g., progressive ambulation, respiratory care |
| | Discharge planning related to self-care issues, need for assistance, and appointment for postoperative follow-up |
| Radiation | Type of therapy planned |
| | Inpatient versus outpatient therapy |
| | Associated morbidity, e.g., GI, GU |
| | Appointments for follow-up |
| Hormonal | Schedule for medications |
| | Expected side effects |
| Chemotherapy | Types of drugs and regimen planned |
| | Side effects and toxicities of drugs |
| | Inpatient versus outpatient versus home chemotherapy |
| | Duration of therapy |
| | Need for venous access device |
| | Regular appointments to monitor response |
| **Psychosexual concerns** | |
| Role functioning | Dispel myths related to perceived loss of femininity due to removal of uterus, tubes, and ovaries, e.g., weight gain, loss of sexual interest/enjoyment, aging, mental deterioration |
| | Help redefine self in terms other than reproduction |
| Sexual functioning | Review anatomy, physiology, and sexual functioning preoperatively |
| | Complete sexual assessment |
| | Alteration in sexual response secondary to hysterectomy: |
| |     Cervix contributes to but is not essential for orgasm |
| |     Uterus elevates during excitement phase and contracts rhythmically during orgasm |
| | Alteration in sexual functioning secondary to radiation: |
| |     Vaginal dryness and stenosis may result in patient who is not sexually active, unless vaginal dilators and lubricants are employed |
| |     Use of water-soluble lubricants during intercourse, such as Astroglide® or nonhormonal moisturizers used three times a week, such as Replens® |

cancers and the fifth leading cause of cancer death in women in the United States.[1] Ovarian cancer is a leading cause of death in industrialized countries (except Japan) but is rare in developing nations.[27]

It is estimated that 1 of every 71 women will develop ovarian cancer, with most cases seen in women between 55 and 59 years of age.[52,53] Only 7%–8% of ovarian carcinomas occur in women under 35 years of age.[54]

The overall five-year survival rate for women with ovarian cancer is between 30% and 35% and has not changed over the past 30 years. The poor survival rate is due in part to several factors: (1) it is difficult to diagnose ovarian cancer early (60%–70% of tumors are stage III or IV at diagnosis); (2) treatment, although intensive, has not been curative; (3) a high-risk population has not been clearly defined; and (4) the etiology is essentially unknown.

## Etiology

Little is known regarding the etiology of ovarian cancer, but multiple risk factors have been identified including environmental, hormonal, menstrual, reproductive, dietary, and hereditary indicators. Environmental factors seem to play an important role since the industrialized nations, except Japan, have the highest incidence of ovarian cancer. The relationship between educational level, socioeconomic level, childbearing practices, and environment cannot be ignored. Women with higher educational and socioeconomic levels tend to delay childbearing, have fewer children, and have a higher incidence of ovarian cancer.[55] Additionally, the incidence of ovarian cancer in Japanese immigrants to the United States approaches that of white women in the United States by the second generation.[3]

Reproductive issues associated with ovarian cancer include age at first pregnancy, number of pregnancies, and use of oral contraceptives. Increased risk has been identified in nulliparous women and to a lesser degree in women who first became pregnant after age 35. Risk seems to be inversely related to the cumulative time that ovulation is suppressed during the childbearing years due to pregnancy, lactation, or oral contraceptives. The use of oral contraceptives not only has a protective effect against ovarian cancer, but this effect seems to persist for at least 15 years after use has stopped.[56] These factors support the theory that "incessant ovulation" produces chronic irritation to the ovarian epithelium. Gonadotropin levels, which are low during pregnancy and with the use of oral contraceptives, become elevated in the postmenopausal years and may be a factor in the increased incidence in women over 45 years of age.[57,58]

Recently other hormonal or endocrine abnormalities have been reported. Whittemore et al[59] found that it was not the time over which ovulation occurred but the inability to conceive in ovulating women that increased risk. Early menarche, late menopause, and hormonal therapy have also been identified as impacting the risk

for ovarian cancer. However, conflicting data exist so that the actual risk, if any, still needs to be defined. Talc has been examined as a potential etiologic agent. It has been suggested that talc may act as a tumor promotor by direct contact with the ovaries and peritoneal cavity after retrograde flow through the reproductive tract from the vagina.[53,60]

The relationship of ovarian cancer to diet is controversial. Some authors state that there is no relationship between ovarian cancer and dietary practices,[61] while others state that ovarian cancer is associated with a diet high in fats.[52,53]

Women with a family history of ovarian cancer are at an increased risk of developing the disease, though only 5%–10% of women with ovarian cancer have a genetic predisposition. Hereditary ovarian cancer is associated with ovarian cancer families, breast and ovarian cancer families, and the Lynch II syndrome of breast, ovarian, and colon cancer. The predisposition can be passed through both maternal and paternal lineages. A family history of breast cancer doubles the risk of ovarian cancer,[60] as does a history of cancer of the colon, particularly in conjunction with breast cancer.[61] Hereditary cancer is considered to be an autosomal dominant trait that imposes a 50% risk of developing the disease in affected families compared with a 1.4% risk in the general population.[62] Women with two or more first-degree relatives with ovarian cancer have a threefold increase in risk.[52,53] However, familial cancer may be more common than was previously indicated, and further data are needed to quantify the risk in daughters of women with ovarian cancer.[63]

## Prevention, Screening, Early Detection

Prevention of ovarian cancer may be achieved, at least temporarily, with the use of oral contraceptives;[56] however, even the prophylactic removal of the ovaries does not provide absolute protection. In addition, avoiding the use of talc and maintaining a diet low in fat may be preventative.

There are no sensitive and specific tests for screening for ovarian cancer. Routine pelvic examination will detect one ovarian carcinoma in 10,000 examinations of asymptomatic women. Despite this, pelvic examinations remain the most usual method for detecting early disease. Also any ovary that can be palpated in a woman more than 3–5 years after menopause should raise suspicions of an ovarian neoplasm,[3] referred to as the "postmenopausal palpable ovary syndrome."[52] The use of transvaginal ultrasound in conjunction with CA-125, a tumor-associated antigen, is gaining popularity but needs further investigation as a screening method.[64–66] The use of transvaginal color flow imaging to identify malignant ovarian neoplasms is also being investigated and shows promise as a specific and sensitive technique for detecting ovarian cancer.[67,68] Sonographic morphology indexing of ovarian tumors may also increase the differentiation of malignant from benign ovarian tumors and is being further studied.[69] Currently, sonographic indexing techniques are being applied in investigational settings or are being used with high risk women, particularly those with a strong family history of ovarian cancer. These techniques will need to demonstrate high sensitivity, specificity, and predictive value before they will be more widely implemented. Current screening tools for ovarian cancer have not detected disease at a stage when treatment could alter the outcome. While relatively inexpensive as diagnostic tests, these techniques are relatively expensive as screening tools; thus specific criteria for screening will need to be defined. Currently, the American Cancer Association and the American College of Obstetricians and Gynecologists do not have specific recommendations for screening for ovarian cancer but an annual pelvic examination including a rectal-vaginal examination is a general recommendation.[21,22]

## Pathophysiology and Cellular Characteristics

Epithelial ovarian cancers arise from a malignant transformation of the ovarian surface epithelium. How this transformation occurs is not known, but there have been hypotheses suggested by the analysis of phenotypically malignant cells. Alterations in DNA quantities and structure have been demonstrated with the study of ovarian cancer cells by cytogenetics. These changes may correlate with alterations in cellular oncogene activities (including c-myc, H-ras, K-ras, and neu oncogenes) and growth factor signal transformations. Study of cytogenetics, oncogenes, and growth factor regulation has occurred in cultured tissue from patients with advanced ovarian cancer, but information about the early phases of the malignant transformation of the ovarian surface epithelium is not defined. Current knowledge of abnormal chromosomes and oncogenes associated with ovarian cancer indicates that carcinogenesis in ovarian cancer is a complex, multistage process that requires further investigation to define.[70,71] Ovarian cancer includes several histological types that may occur in different age groups, exhibit different methods of spread, and respond to different therapeutic regimens. Epithelial, stromal, and germinal cells give rise to the major subsets of ovarian cancer: epithelial, germ cell, and stromal tumors.

Epithelial tumors constitute 80%–90% of all malignant ovarian neoplasms.[52,60,72] The histological categories of these tumors include serous, mucinous, endometroid, clear cell (mesonephroid), Brenner, and undifferentiated carcinomas. Epithelial histological cell types have similar presentation and dissemination patterns. Histological type itself has little prognostic value except for the clear cell type, which is more aggressive.[60]

Epithelial ovarian tumors of low malignant potential (LMP) constitute a separate clinical and pathological entity between benign and invasive disease and represent about 15% of epithelial tumors. These tumors are described as neoplasms with no invasion of the ovarian stroma, yet they have greater cellular proliferation than the benign cystadenomas.[52,53] Tumors of LMP usually occur in women less than 40 years of age and have a favorable prognosis regardless of stage.[57] Malignant germ cell tumors account for 4% of ovarian malignancies and are most often encountered in children and premenopausal women. The remaining 6% of ovarian malignancies are sex cord or stromal tumors. This chapter focuses only on the epithelial ovarian cancers.

Histological grade is an important predictor of treatment response and survival.[39] Although important in all stages of disease, grade seems to be of greater prognostic significance in stage I and II disease, where the more differentiated tumors respond better to treatment.[72]

## Clinical Manifestations

Knowledge of the natural history of ovarian cancer is essential to appreciate the difficulties in staging and treatment. Most ovarian malignancies originate from the epithelial surface of the ovary. As the tumor grows, it invades the stromal tissue and penetrates the capsule of the ovary. The most common mechanisms of spread are by direct extension and peritoneal seeding. Direct extension occurs when tumor cells on the surface of the ovary invade the adjacent structures, including fallopian tubes, uterus, bladder, and rectosigmoid and pelvic peritoneum. Peritoneal seeding occurs when cells exfoliate into the peritoneal cavity, where they are carried in fluid via the posterior paracolic spaces to the subdiaphragmatic surfaces. Tumor nodules or seeds may be found on the peritoneal surfaces of the liver, diaphragm, bladder, and large and small bowel. The diaphragmatic and substernal lymphatics that drain the peritoneal cavity may become obstructed, and peritoneal fluid subsequently accumulates in the abdominal cavity.[72] Although intraperitoneal spread is the most common method of dissemination, ovarian lymphatics may also have a role. The ovary contains an extensive lymphatic network that flows cephalad toward the aortic nodes. Piver et al[73] found a 10% incidence of aortic and pelvic lymph node metastasis in stage I and II ovarian cancer. These nodes must be sampled during surgery to ensure proper staging. Hematogenous spread of disease is the least common method of dissemination. The most frequently encountered distant sites are the liver, lung, and pleura.[72]

Death is usually secondary to intra-abdominal tumor dissemination. Bowel and mesentery are most commonly involved, producing multiple areas of malfunction, malabsorption, varying degrees of alteration in peristalsis, and eventually obstruction. Women with intra-abdominal tumor dissemination gradually deteriorate and eventually die of electrolyte imbalance, sepsis, or cardiovascular collapse. Other contributory causes of death include toxicities of treatment, intercurrent medical problems, and pulmonary embolus.[61]

## Assessment

Unfortunately, there are typically no early manifestations of ovarian cancer. Localized disease limited to the ovary is asymptomatic in the majority of women. As the mass enlarges, the woman may experience abdominal discomfort, dyspepsia, indigestion, flatulence, eructations, loss of appetite, pelvic pressure, or urinary frequency. These vague complaints are often attributed to personal stresses and midlife changes and may precede other symptoms by months.[53] A physician examining a 40–70-year-old woman with these persistent symptoms should include ovarian cancer in the differential diagnostic work-up. Unfortunately, because these nonspecific complaints are not disabling, physicians may not initially pursue the search for ovarian cancer. Often evaluation does not occur until the woman has a palpable mass or ascites. As a result, the cancer has spread beyond the ovary in 75% of patients at the time of diagnosis.[3,72] Once the diagnosis is suspected, routine diagnostic tests may help rule out another primary tumor as the source of the pelvic mass. A complete physical examination is carried out, with careful attention to the pelvis, abdomen, and breasts. A barium enema may be done to rule out primary rectosigmoid cancer, which can metastasize to ovaries. A proctosigmoidoscopy and gastrointestinal series can also be useful if the woman has intestinal symptoms.

Chest radiography helps to determine the presence of pleural effusion or parenchymal metastases. An IVP aids in determining the location of the pelvic mass relative to the ureters. Ultrasound (US) and computed tomography (CT) scans are used to evaluate the size and location of the mass. Also, MRI may be helpful to detect lesions smaller than either US or CT can identify. MRI will probably be most helpful for monitoring response to therapy.[53] Paracentesis is avoided because of the risk of rupturing an encapsulated ovarian mass and causing malignant cells to spill into the peritoneal cavity. Tumor cells can also seed along the needle tract. Whether or not the ascitic fluid is malignant, a laparotomy is necessary to confirm the diagnosis and to adequately determine the stage or extent of disease.

## Classification and Staging

The staging of ovarian cancer is based on surgical evaluation and forms the basis for planning subsequent therapy.[74]

Approximately 15%–20% of patients present as stage I, 10%–15% as stage II, 60%–70% as stage III, and 10%–15% as stage IV.[2] Table 39-4 summarizes the surgical staging for ovarian cancer.

The initial surgical exploration enables the surgeon to determine the precise diagnosis and accurate stage and to perform optimal debulking. Careful evaluation of all peritoneal surfaces is required to ensure accurate staging. The subdiaphragmatic surfaces need to be evaluated and scraped for cytopathology if no tumor is palpable. Similarly, all intra-abdominal organs, surfaces, and retroperitoneal nodes are palpated to determine extent of disease. The surgeon then attempts cytoreduction of the tumor volume. Size of residual disease is an important prognostic factor. Maximally reducing the tumor size to <1 cm in diameter offers the patient a better chance of response with additional therapy.[52,60,75,76]

Unfortunately, accurate surgical staging is not obtained in all patients presenting with early ovarian cancer.[59] Only about 25% of women in the United States with stage I and II disease have a surgical incision adequate to allow evaluation of the entire pelvis and abdominal cavity. Often a lower abdominal transverse incision is used, particularly if ovarian cancer is not the preoperative diagnosis. Understaging is common. Thirty-three percent of patients thought to be free of disease following initial surgery actually have persistent, residual disease, and about 75% have disease that has spread intra-abdominally.[77]

## Therapeutic Approaches and Nursing Care

Initial ovarian cancer therapy includes thorough evaluation, staging, and cytoreduction. A TAH-BSO, omentectomy, selected pelvic and para-aortic lymph node sampling, and maximal cytoreduction are performed when surgically feasible[3] (Figure 39-2).[78] Other surgical approaches such as laparoscopic staging of early ovarian cancer, and aortic and pelvic lymphadenectomy for advanced disease are being investigated.[79,80] Because the majority of women with epithelial ovarian cancer are diagnosed in the late stages, additional therapy is indicated. Selection of the appropriate therapy is based on stage, grade, size and location of residual tumor, and presence of ascites or peritoneal washings that contain malignant cells.[81]

### Stage I

Patients with stage I, grade 1 tumors have a greater than 90% survival with surgery alone.[82] If fertility is a concern, conservative surgical treatment may be acceptable in this select population.[3] There is no standard adjuvant therapy defined for other stage I ovarian cancers; therapies vary and are still under investigation. The therapies used include: no therapy, chemotherapy, intraperitoneal radioisotopes, and external radiotherapy. A platinum-based chemotherapy regimen is considered beneficial for patients with stage IC, grade 3 tumors who are at high risk for recurrence.[82–84]

Early studies of localized ovarian cancer did not always include careful surgical staging and thus were not conclusive in determining optimum treatment.[60] Generally, after the initial surgery, patients received no additional therapy, although pelvic irradiation or intermittent chemotherapy was occasionally given. Relapse after pelvic

**TABLE 39-4**  Staging Classification of Malignant Ovarian Tumors

| PRIMARY TUMOR (T) | | |
|---|---|---|
| TNM | FIGO | Definition |
| T1a | IA | Tumor limited to one ovary; capsule intact, no tumor on ovarian surface, no malignant cells in ascites or peritoneal washings |
| T1b | IB | Tumor limited to both ovaries; capsules intact, no tumor on ovarian surface, no malignant cells in ascites or peritoneal washings |
| T1c | IC | Tumor limited to one or both ovaries with any of the following: capsule ruptured, tumor on ovarian surface, malignant cells in ascites or peritoneal washings |
| T2 | II | Tumor involves one or both ovaries with pelvic extension |
| T2a | IIA | Extension and/or implants on the uterus and/or tube(s); no malignant cells in ascites or peritoneal washings |
| T2b | IIB | Extension to other pelvic tissues; no malignant cells in ascites or peritoneal washings |
| T2c | IIC | Pelvic extension (2a or 2b) with malignant cells in ascites or peritoneal washings |
| T3 and/or N1 | III | Tumor involves one or both ovaries with microscopically confirmed peritoneal metastasis outside the pelvis and/or regional lymph node metastasis |
| T3a | IIIA | Microscopic peritoneal metastasis beyond the pelvis |
| T3b | IIIB | Macroscopic peritoneal metastasis beyond the pelvis 2 cm or less in the greatest dimension |
| T3c and/or N1 | IIIC | Peritoneal metastasis beyond the pelvis more than 2 cm in the greatest dimension and/or regional lymph node metastasis |
| M1 | IV | Distant metastasis (excludes peritoneal metastasis) |

**REGIONAL LYMPH NODES (N)**

| | |
|---|---|
| NX | Regional lymph nodes cannot be assessed |
| N0 | No regional lymph node metastasis |
| N1 | Regional lymph node metastasis |

**DISTANT METASTASIS (M)**

| TNM | FIGO | Definition |
|---|---|---|
| MX | — | Presence of distant metastasis cannot be assessed |
| M0 | — | No distant metastasis |
| M1 | IV | Distant metastasis (excludes peritoneal metastasis) |

**STAGE GROUPING**

| AJCC/UICC | | | | FIGO |
|---|---|---|---|---|
| Stage IA | T1a | N0 | M0 | Stage IA |
| Stage IB | T1b | N0 | M0 | Stage IB |
| Stage IC | T1c | N0 | M0 | Stage IC |
| Stage IIA | T2a | N0 | M0 | Stage IIA |
| Stage IIB | T2b | N0 | M0 | Stage IIB |
| Stage IIC | T2c | N0 | M0 | Stage IIC |
| Stage IIIA | T3a | N0 | M0 | Stage IIIA |
| Stage IIIB | T3b | N0 | M0 | Stage IIIB |
| Stage IIIC | T3c | N0 | M0 | Stage IIIC |
| | Any T | N1 | M0 | |
| Stage IV | Any T | Any N | M1 | Stage IV |

Reprinted from *American Joint Committee on Cancer: Manual for Staging of Cancer* (ed 4). Philadelphia, Lippincott, 1992.

irradiation was 30%, while relapse with observation alone was 17%, and with intermittent oral melphalan was 6%.[60] Carefully controlled studies are now being performed to determine the best approach for treating stage I ovarian cancer patients, since approximately 20% of patients with early-stage disease still relapse and die.[2,85]

### Stage II

Following the surgical staging and cytoreduction, intraperitoneal $^{32}P$, whole-abdominal radiation, single-agent chemotherapy, or platinum-based combination chemotherapy may be employed.[3,53] Data on the therapy of stage II ovarian cancer are sparse because few women are diagnosed at this stage.

### Stage III, IV

When the patient is a surgical candidate, aggressive staging and cytoreductive surgery are advocated to reduce the tumor burden and amount of residual disease. This debulking may involve dissection of multiple masses and the creation of a colostomy to prevent intestinal obstruction. If the tumor is cytoreduced and the patient

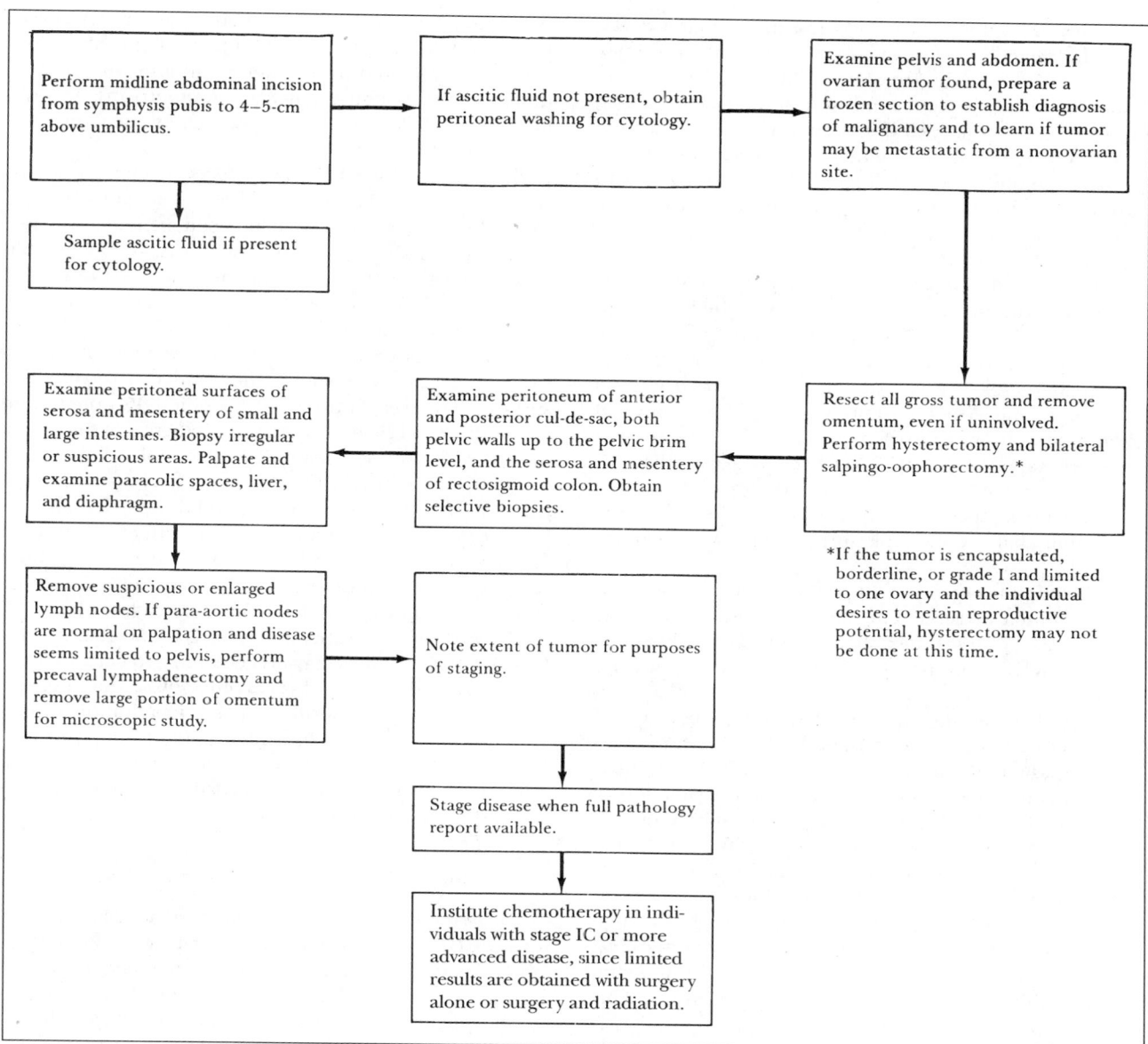

**FIGURE 39-2** Surgery for ovarian carcinoma. (Bristol Laboratories, Division of Bristol-Myers Co: Platinol: Effective palliation therapy in metastatic ovarian cancer. Syracuse, NY, Bristol Laboratories, 1982.)

has no area of residual disease greater than 1 cm in diameter, she may be treated with a platinum-based paclitaxel regimen of chemotherapy or whole-abdominal and pelvic radiation. While survival rates are comparable for chemotherapy and radiation, morbidity is significantly greater with radiation therapy.[3,86]

Platinum-based combination chemotherapy including paclitaxel is administered for stage III with residual disease greater than 1 cm and for stage IV disease.[86] The use of neoadjuvant chemotherapy and subsequent cytoreductive surgery remains controversial. At the current time, survival is unchanged regardless of the timing of the surgical intervention relative to the institution of chemotherapy.[60,87]

### Recurrent or persistent disease

Once a woman has persistent or recurrent disease following initial therapy, the benefits of salvage therapy are limited. Many chemotherapeutic agents have been used, with varying responses and limited duration of response. High-dose chemotherapy with autologous bone marrow rescue has been used in this population but remains investigational.[88–90] Other treatment modalities employed include immunotherapy, intraperitoneal chemotherapy, and biologic therapy.

***Second-look surgery*** A second-look operation is performed on patients who have a complete clinical response following the full course of chemotherapy (usually 6 to

12 cycles) as evidenced by a negative tumor marker (CA-125) and negative CT scan or US. This surgery is advocated for the following reasons: (1) to determine if the patient had a complete remission and therapy can be stopped, (2) to assess the response and determine whether a change in the therapy is indicated, and (3) to perform secondary cytoreductive surgery to attempt to prolong survival. Controversy exists over the actual therapeutic value in doing a second-look laparotomy and when it should be done.[52,60,91,92] Sonnendecker[93] challenged whether second-look laparotomy was justified, especially in patients with initial stage I disease, since he found that 71.8% of patients had no gross or microscopic evidence of disease at the time of second-look surgery. He proposed that second-look surgery should be limited to clinical trials to define either optimum or minimum doses of chemotherapy or to assess new single or combination chemotherapeutic agents.[43] Barber[53] suggests that patients live longer and more comfortably, even though there are no prospective randomized clinical studies demonstrating that second-look surgery adds to long-term survival.

A second-look operation is performed through a vertical abdominal incision. The surgeon evaluates whether there is more or less tumor than was present at the initial laparotomy. If gross tumor is found, it is resected. If no gross disease is present, a thorough staging evaluation is performed, including peritoneal washings, biopsies of any irregularities or adhesions, multiple biopsies of areas where residual tumor was located at the initial operation, precaval lymphadenectomy, and thorough evaluation of the intestine. TAH-BSO and omentectomy should be performed if not done previously. Usually, 26 to 30 biopsy specimens are obtained.[83] Use of the Nd:YAG laser or the ultrasonic surgical aspirator is helpful for resecting tumors that are retroperitoneal, or fixed to the diaphragm, sacrum, pelvic side wall, or pubic symphysis.[94–96] If the second-look operation yields negative results, the woman is followed regularly for signs of recurrence. Further therapy is indicated if the second-look operation is positive for tumor. If the disease is microscopic, whole-abdominal and pelvic irradiation may be considered. If gross disease remains, second-line chemotherapy or investigational treatment is initiated. Additional controlled clinical trials will further delineate the role of second-look surgery. Peritoneoscopy may also be used in certain situations rather than laparotomy.[72]

***Tumor-associated antigens*** If tumor-associated antigens specific for epithelial ovarian cancer could be detected in the bloodstream, they would provide a means for diagnosis at an early stage when patients could be cured. Tumor-associated antigens would also provide a means of monitoring tumor response during therapy and potentially allow discrimination between benign and malignant pelvic masses.[97] One monoclonal antibody that reacts with epithelial ovarian cancer cells has been developed and studied extensively.[98] It can detect an antigen (CA-125) in the blood of women with ovarian cancer. However, CA-125 is not specific for ovarian cancer alone and can be elevated from other conditions that produce inflammatory responses, such as endometriosis. Approximately 83%–96% of ovarian cancer patients have elevated serum CA-125 levels.[99]

Elevations of CA-125 have preceded clinical disease recurrence by 1–11 months.[97,100,101] A negative CA-125 value does not indicate that the patient is disease-free, since almost half will have persistent disease.[60] CA-125 is being used to supplement standard methods of disease monitoring. Jager et al[102] propose that second-look surgery be done when serum CA-125 levels have fallen or returned to normal and also that patients with rising serum CA-125 levels should not undergo second-look surgery. However, Potter et al[103] studied 45 women and found that CA-125 levels were not predictive of the potential for resection of disease at second-look.

CA-19-9 is another tumor marker used in combination with CA-125. It is a monosialoganglioside originally isolated from a colonic tumor cell.[104] Fioretti et al[105] studied CA-125 and CA-19-9 levels in 21 patients receiving both surgical and chemotherapeutic treatment of ovarian carcinoma. They found an 89.7% correlation of CA-125 levels with disease status and a 72.2% correlation with CA-19-9. Rising values may precede the clinical and ultrasonographic detection of recurrence by several months. They think that measuring CA-19-9 in addition to CA-125 could offer some benefit in monitoring patients. Neunteufel and Breitenbecker[99] also advocated using more than one tumor marker, but this remains controversial and requires further study.

### Chemotherapy

***Single-agent therapy*** The mainstay of adjuvant therapy for stage III and IV epithelial ovarian cancer is chemotherapy. Historically, standard therapy consisted of single-alkylating agents: melphalan, chlorambucil, thiotepa, cyclophosphamide, and the nitrosoureas. In the United States the agent of choice was usually melphalan because it could be given orally and rarely caused alopecia or nausea.[106] Response rates seen with alkylating agents varied from 33%–65%.[71] A small number of women (5%–10%) were cured with single-alkylating agent therapy.[72] Because of the risk of leukemia from alkylating agents, other drugs were evaluated. No improvement in response was realized with other single agents such as hexamethylmelamine and doxorubicin, with response rates of 20%–35%. Cisplatin is now considered the single most active agent for treatment of ovarian cancer, with response rates reported as high as 55% depending on dose.[55,72]

A new drug, paclitaxel, has demonstrated a 30% response in previously treated patients. The diterpene plant product is a unique antimicrotubule agent that acts by shifting the equilibrium between tubulin dimers and microtubules toward polymerization, which has the effect of creating overly stable and nonfunctional microtubules. Paclitaxel has quickly gained popularity and is considered to be an important drug in the initial treatment of advanced ovarian cancer.[86,107–109]

Topotecan, or hycamptamine, inhibits the enzyme topoisomerase I and leads to DNA cleavage. Drugs that are active with topoisomerase seem to be so in levels proportional to the target enzyme available. This is the opposite effect of other drugs, such as the antimetabolites that effect target enzyme systems. Activity of topotecan in phase I and II trials has led to further investigation of topotecan alone and in combination with other active agents and is now known to be an active agent in the treatment of refractory ovarian cancer.[110] Docetaxel, a semisynthetic taxoid, has also demonstrated significant activity in ovarian cancer with responses in phase II trials ranging from 25% to 41%. Further investigation in phase III trials is ongoing.[111]

Other single agents that may have some activity in advanced ovarian cancer include ifosfamide, AZQ, VP-16 (etoposide), Peptichemio, and low-dose mitomycin C (Table 39-5).[112]

***Combination chemotherapy***  Combination chemotherapy for advanced ovarian cancer has been studied extensively. It is difficult to compare the studies because of great variation in patient selection, prognostic factors, and response criteria. However, the studies generally compared single agents to combination chemotherapy and to salvage chemotherapy regimens for those women who did not respond to previous therapy.[72]

The overall response rates for combination chemotherapy vary, with clinical complete remission seen in up to 40%–50% of women. Selected regimens for combination chemotherapy are summarized in Table 39-6. Half of the women who have a complete clinical remission demonstrate residual disease at second-look laparotomy.[39] The optimal combination regimen and duration of therapy remains elusive.[113]

The first study that demonstrated significantly improved survival using combination chemotherapy compared HexaCAF (hexamethylmelamine, cyclophosphamide, methotrexate, and 5-fluorouracil [5-FU]) with melphalan alone. The four-drug combination yielded better results, with an overall response rate of 75% versus 54%, a complete response rate of 33% versus 16%, and median survival of 29 months versus 17 months.[72,114] Several studies followed, showing that combination therapy is more beneficial than single-agent therapy in advanced ovarian cancer. The addition of cisplatin into combination chemotherapy regimens markedly improved response rates.[115,116] It appears that the platinum-based combination regimen given without dose modification offers the best chance for response (up to 80%) and for achieving a complete remission (20%–50%) in women with advanced ovarian carcinoma.[72,117]

In a meta-analysis of data from 1194 patients in four clinical trials comparing cisplatin-doxorubicin-cyclophosphamide (CAP) with cisplatin-cyclophosphamide (CP), a survival advantage was demonstrated with the CAP regimen ($P = 0.02$), as well as significant improvement in the number of negative second-look laparotomies with the CAP (CAP = 30%, CP = 23%; $P = 0.01$). It was unclear to the investigators whether the improvement in survival and response at second-look was due to the addition of doxorubicin or to the dose intensity in three of the four trials.[118]

A number of studies with cisplatin have demonstrated the important relationship of response rate being proportional to the dose administered. Patients who were refractory to initial therapy or had recurrent disease, and those patients not previously treated, have received various schedules and ranges of high-dose cisplatin. The major dose-limiting toxicity of high-dose cisplatin is neurotoxicity. Results of these studies are not clear in terms of survival, but it does appear that the high-dose chemotherapy regimen is markedly effective in rapidly debulking tumors in patients who present with advanced-stage disease and large abdominal tumors.[60] However, one randomized trial comparing dose intensity with standard doses failed to demonstrate survival advantage in the dose intensity arm, and showed that toxicities were significantly more frequent and severe than in the standard arms.[119] Further investigation of dose intensity is warranted.

Carboplatin, a platinum analogue, is an alternative to cisplatin. Pharmacological techniques to decrease some of the toxicities associated with the platinum compounds are being investigated. A randomized trial comparing a CHAP-5 regimen (cisplatin 20 mg/m² daily × 5; doxorubicin 35 mg/m² on day 1, hexamethylmelamine 150 mg/m²; cyclophosphamide 100 mg/m² orally on days 14 to 28) with CHAC-1 (carboplatin 350 mg/m² on day 1; all

**TABLE 39-5**  Single Agents Active in Advanced Ovarian Adenocarcinoma

| | |
|---|---|
| **Alkylating agents** | **Plant alkaloids** |
| Melphalan | Vinblastine |
| Chlorambucil | VP-16 |
| Thiotepa | Paclitaxel |
| Cyclophosphamide | Docetaxel |
| Mechlorethamine | Topotecan |
| Ifosfamide | |
| AZQ | **Miscellaneous** |
| | Hexamethylmelamine |
| **Antimetabolites** | Cisplatin |
| 5-fluorouracil | Carboplatin |
| Methotrexate | Dianhydrogalacticol |
| | Peptichemio |
| **Antitumor antibiotics** | |
| Doxorubicin (adriamycin) | |
| Mitomycin C | |

AZQ = Aziridinyl benzoquinone; *VP-16* = etoposide.
Adapted from Young R, Perez CA, Hoskins WJ: Cancer of the ovary, in DeVita VT, Hellman S, Rosenberg SA (eds): *Cancer: Principles and Practice of Oncology* (ed 4). Philadelphia, Lippincott, 1993, p 1246.

**TABLE 39-6**　Selected Regimens for Combination Chemotherapy in Advanced Ovarian Cancer

| Regimen | Schedule | Response |
|---|---|---|
| HexaCAF | | CR and PR = 75% |
|   Hexamethylmelamine | 150 mg/m² orally days 1–14 | |
|   Cyclophosphamide | 150 mg/m² orally days 1–14 | |
|   Methotrexate | 40 mg/m² IV day 1, 8 | |
|   5-fluourouracil | 600 mg/m² IV day 1, 8 | |
| CAP | | pCR = 33% |
|   Cisplatin | 50–70 mg/m² IV | |
|   Doxorubicin | 30–60 mg/m² IV | |
|   Cyclophosphamide | 500–600 mg/m² IV | |
| CP | | pCR = 23% |
|   Cyclophosphamide | 500–1000 mg/m² IV | |
|   Cisplatin | 50–70 mg/m² IV | |
| CHAP-5 | | pCR = 30% |
|   Cyclophosphamide | 100 mg/m² orally days 15–28 | cCR = 23.5% |
|   Hexamethylmelamine | 150 mg/m² orally days 15–28 | |
|   Doxorubicin | 35 mg/m² IV day 1 | |
|   Cisplatin | 20 mg/m² IV days 1–5 | |
| CHAC-1 | | CR = 24.4% |
|   Cyclophosphamide | 100 mg/m² orally days 15–28 | |
|   Hexamethylmelamine | 150 mg/m² orally days 15–28 | |
|   Doxorubicin | 35 mg/m² IV day 1 | |
|   Carboplatin | 350 mg/m² IV day 1 | |
| TC | | CR = 51% |
|   Taxol | 135 mg/m² IV over 24 hours day 1 | pCR = 26% |
|   Cisplatin | 75 mg/m² IV day 2 | |

CR = complete response; PR = partial response; pCR = pathological complete response; cCR = clinical complete response.
Adapted from Young R, Fuks Z, Hoskins HJ: Cancer of the ovary, in DeVita VT, Hellman S, Rosenberg SA (eds): *Cancer: Principles and Practice of Oncology* (ed 3). Philadelphia, Lippincott, 1989, p 1181.

other drugs the same as CHAP-5) showed that antitumor activity did not appear to have any statistical differences between the two regimens but that the toxicity pattern observed in patients treated with CHAC-1 was much milder and more tolerable.[120] Like cisplatin, carboplatin has a significant dose-response relationship and can be given to patients who are not platinum refractory yet can no longer tolerate the neurotoxicity or nephrotoxicity associated with cisplatin. As a result, carboplatin has become an important drug in the treatment of ovarian cancer.[121] Diethyldithiocarbamate (DDTC) may protect against the myelosuppression of carboplatin and the dose-limiting neurotoxicity of cisplatin without changing the antitumor effect. If this is so, dose escalation could be achieved without increased toxicity.[61] Rothenberg et al[122] studied 21 patients with relapsed or refractory ovarian cancer who were treated with high-dose carboplatin followed three hours later with DDTC (4g/m²). The overall response rate was 19%; however, the regimen was associated with clinically significant hematologic and autonomic toxic effects. Colony stimulating factors (CSF) may allow higher doses of myelosuppressive drugs and are currently being incorporated into treatment regimens.[123] Another approach to enable the administration of high

doses of myelosuppressive drugs is the use of autologous bone marrow rescue. Drugs used with the bone marrow or peripheral blood stem cell rescue include cyclophosphamide, melphalan, and carboplatin. This approach remains investigational but has been used in patients with persistent disease.[88,90,124–126]

Since the majority of patients suffer disease recurrence despite response to initial chemotherapy, efforts continue to identify active new second-line agents. Current single-agent response rates range from 0%–6% in women who have received prior cisplatin therapy. Generally the responses are partial and of short duration.[126]

Alberts et al[127] treated 25 relapsed ovarian cancer patients with mitomycin-C 10 mg/m² intravenously on day 1 every six weeks and 5-FU 500 mg/m² intravenously daily on days 1–3 every three weeks. The overall objective response rate was 40%, and the most prevalent toxicity was bone marrow suppression. They suggest further trials of this combination. They also recommend the addition of cisplatin for first-line therapy in patients with clinically measurable diseases.[127]

***Drug resistance***　The development of multidrug resistance severely limits the effectiveness of chemotherapy.

Patients with ovarian cancer die from chemotherapy-refractory disease. Drug resistance is likely due to multiple factors, including: (1) alterations in drug transport across cell membranes, (2) presence of the MDR-1 gene with its protein product, (3) the P-170 glycoprotein, (4) the elevation of sulfhydryl molecules such as intracellular glutathione (GSH), and (5) increased DNA repair.[72] It may be possible to pharmacologically reverse drug resistance,[72,128] and clinical trials using verapamil and buthionine sulfoximine (BSO) are underway to determine this.[72]

Debulking surgery to reduce tumor burden to aggregates of 1 cm or less improves the response to postoperative chemotherapy by reducing the potentially refractory disease. Moreover, complete responses are associated with significant increases in survival. Combination chemotherapy is associated with higher overall response rates and, more importantly, with an increase in complete responses. New combinations, alternate dosing schedules, and sequential and continuous infusion administration techniques to reduce drug resistance continue to be investigated.[129,130]

***Intraperitoneal chemotherapy***   Because ovarian cancer usually remains confined to the abdominal cavity, one approach to chemotherapy administration is the intraperitoneal (IP) method. Intraperitoneal chemotherapy has been used for many years to control malignant ascites;[72] however, the current aim of the IP approach is to increase cytotoxic drug levels to the tumor sites. Patients who will benefit most from IP therapy are those with: (1) minimal residual disease (microscopic or ≤0.5 cm in diameter) following systemic therapy with or without secondary surgical cytoreduction, (2) high-grade tumors with a surgically defined complete response, (3) high-grade stage I/II with the risk of covert disease in the upper abdomen, (4) advanced disease with all or some drugs administered IP, and (5) advanced disease with IP therapy following a limited course of intravenous therapy with or without secondary surgical debulking.[131–133]

Researchers have used methotrexate,[134] doxorubicin,[135] 5-FU,[136] cisplatin with systemic thiosulfate protection,[137] mitomycin-c,[138] mitoxantrone,[139] cytarabine,[140] and recombinant alpha-interferon.[141] Aclacinomycin (an analogue of adriamycin) and carboplatin are also being evaluated to determine their efficacy as IP drugs.[132] Paclitaxel via the intraperitoneal route has also been evaluated, but further investigation is necessary to define its role and the appropriate regimen for treatment of ovarian cancer.[142,143] Intraperitoneal combination chemotherapy approaches are also being studied in clinical trials.[144,145] While further study is needed, a recent randomized trial demonstrated improved response and survival with intraperitoneal cisplatin and intravenous cyclophosphamide in optimally debulked stage III patients.[145]

Investigations of IP use of biologic agents including gamma-interferon, tumor necrosis factor, interleukin-2, and monoclonal antibodies have been conducted.[146–148] Intraperitoneal delivery of antineoplastic agents in 10% dimethyl sulfaoxide (DMSO) may also be useful with certain ovarian cancers.[149]

The technique for IP administration includes placement of a semipermanent Tenckhoff dialysis catheter or implanted port system into the abdominal cavity so that a large volume of fluid can be instilled. A volume of up to 2 liters of fluid is instilled intraperitoneally to ensure optimal distribution throughout the abdomen. The chemotherapeutic agent and fluids in the abdominal cavity are slowly absorbed into the general circulation. When daily treatments are required, alteration in the volume of fluid infused may be necessary in order to minimize the discomfort experienced by the patient from the volume of residual fluid left from the previous treatment.[133]

The Tenckhoff dialysis catheter and the infusion port both have problems associated with their use. In approximately 20% of cases a fibrin sheath forms that will not allow outflow and occasionally inhibits delivery of the drug.[60,131,132,144] A new catheter, designed specifically for IP chemotherapy, would allow improvement in drug administration and distribution and removal of any ascites prior to the IP chemotherapy infusion.[148,150] Concerns persist about IP therapy related to the delivery of the drug to the tumor sites, toxicities specific to the IP route (such as infection secondary to bowel perforation), and the risk of chronic and long-term consequences (such as adhesions and bowel obstruction).[132] Ozols and Young[60] point out some unresolved clinical issues related to IP chemotherapy: (1) Can IP chemotherapy produce a significant objective response rate? (2) In what clinical situations should it be used? (3) What is the optimum drug to use? (4) What role do drug combinations have? and (5) What is the optimum technique to deliver IP drugs? While the use of IP cisplatin or carboplatin in selected patients who responded to an initial intravenous platinum-based regimen is appropriate, other applications of this method of administration do not have adequate data to support its use. Randomized trials are needed to demonstrate that the theoretical and pharmacological advantages also correlate with survival advantages for this patient population.[133]

## Hormone therapy

Hormone therapy for ovarian cancer has resulted in uneven responses.[151] Tamoxifen has been investigated as a second-line drug in individuals who have failed combination chemotherapy.[27,152] Belinson et al[153] randomly treated 33 patients with either megestrol acetate alone or megestrol acetate and tamoxifen. Doses were 160 mg/day of megestrol and 20 mg/day of tamoxifen. There was no demonstrated tumor regression, but 39% of patients showed stabilization of disease from 4 to more than 16 months. Kavanagh et al[151] used leuprolide acetate (1 mg subcutaneously daily for a minimum of 8 weeks) for patients with refractory epithelial ovarian cancer and found better responses in patients with grade 1 disease. Further clinical trials are needed to define the role of hormonal therapy in ovarian cancer.

### Radiotherapy

Radioactive chromic phosphate ($^{32}$P) and radioactive gold ($^{198}$Au) have been used as adjuvant therapy in women with stage I ovarian cancer (Figure 39-3).[3] Colloidal gold is not presently available for therapy. Complications of $^{32}$P can include small bowel obstruction and stenosis and are higher in women who have uneven distribution of the radioactive material in the peritoneal cavity.[57,72,154] Prior to instilling $^{32}$P, even distribution is verified by infusing radiopaque technitium sulfur colloid.[3]

Potter et al[155] treated 59 patients with intraperitoneal chromic phosphate and concluded that it is an alternative to chemotherapy or external radiation in the primary treatment of early-stage ovarian lesions. It may also be useful for second-line therapy of early-stage or low-grade ovarian lesions after a positive second-look surgery, but only if microscopic disease remains. In general, reported cure rates with chromic phosphate in stage I tumors have been in the range of 90%, but there is no evidence that these results are better than those that might be achieved in the same patients without radiotherapy.[57]

The role of external beam radiotherapy in advanced disease has also been explored, and its effectiveness is directly related to the volume of disease at the time radiation is administered.[2,60] Patients who have less than 2 cm of disease have an approximately equivalent result with either combination chemotherapy or total abdominal radiation. Whole-abdominal radiation (WAR) appears to be most effective in those selected individuals with little or no gross residual disease.[91,156]

The use of WAR as salvage therapy for patients with persistent or progressive disease after combination chemotherapy who have been explored and have residual cancer (<2 cm) has also been studied.[91,156–159] Associated morbidity has been significant.[158] Schray et al[157] found that patients with well- to moderately differentiated tumors or those with small-volume residual disease after the initial operation had a significantly better outcome from salvage radiation therapy. They suggest further randomized study to determine the best option for patients with poor prognostic factors.

### Biologic therapy

The role of chemoimmunotherapy has been investigated by two cooperative groups. The Gynecologic Oncology Group[160] compared melphalan with melphalan plus *Corynebacterium parvum*. The response rate with melphalan alone was 55%, whereas the response rate with melphalan plus *C. parvum* was 65%. The Southwest Oncology Group[161] compared doxorubicin-cyclophosphamide alone and in combination with bacillus Calmette-Guerin (BCG). The response rates were 43% and 51%, respectively. In contrast, Alberts et al[162] reported that the use of BCG did not add to the efficacy of a doxorubicin, cyclophosphamide, and cisplatin (DCP) regimen in patients with measurable stage III or IV disease.

Immunotherapy, including monoclonal antibodies, adoptive cellular immunotherapy, and interferon, may soon become the fourth modality of therapy for ovarian cancer (in addition to surgery, radiation, and chemotherapy).[146] These promising agents have cytotoxic mechanisms that are probably unrelated to the other treatment modalities and are most likely different enough from each other to enable sequential use. They can remain in the peritoneal cavity for prolonged periods when administered intraperitoneally, are most likely not mutagenic, and have manageable toxicities.[146] Immunotherapy using IP lymphokine-activated killer cells (LAK), interferons, and interleukin-2 (IL-2) is being examined in the treatment of women with minimal residual disease ovarian cancer.[2,60,146] Since immunotherapy is nonspecific, results have been unpredictable. It is hoped that nonspecific immunotherapy will soon be replaced by specific vaccines.[53]

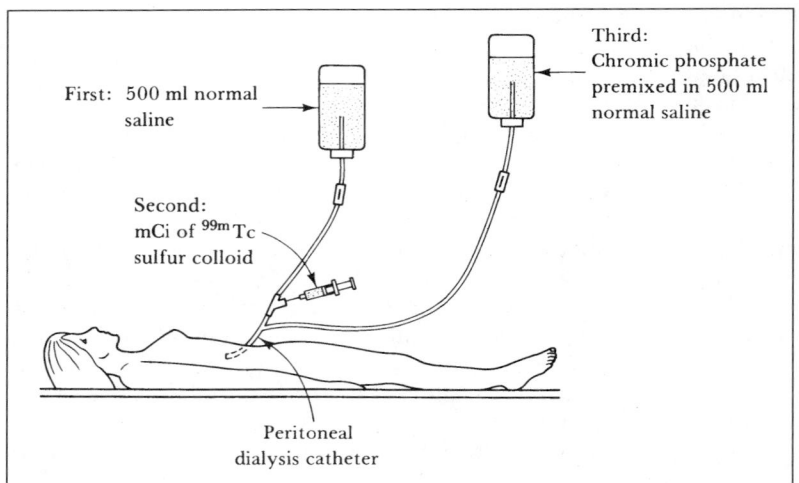

First: 500 ml normal saline

Second: mCi of $^{99m}$Tc sulfur colloid

Third: Chromic phosphate premixed in 500 ml normal saline

Peritoneal dialysis catheter

**FIGURE 39-3** Method of administration of radioactive colloidal chromic phosphate into the peritoneal cavity. (DiSaia PJ, Creasman WT: *Clinical Gynecologic Oncology.* St Louis, Mosby, 1989.)

A phase II study with human leukocyte interferon suggested possible antitumor activity in epithelial ovarian cancer.[163] Recombinant alfa-interferon has shown some promise in patients with small-volume residual disease who were given the drug intraperitoneally.[145] Combination therapy of alfa-interferon and doxorubicin produced complete and partial responses with acceptable toxicity in 7 of 24 ovarian cancer patients with recurrent disease.[164] Lichtenstein et al[165] conducted a phase I study using IP recombinant alfa-interferon for 11 patients with persistent epithelial ovarian cancer at second-look surgery and found that 45% experienced a surgically documented antitumor response. Further study is needed to more clearly define the role of biologics in the treatment of ovarian cancer.

Despite aggressive multimodality therapy, the overall survival rate of ovarian cancer remains poor. Efforts to define new and more effective means of treating this disease continue. New drug development and testing needs to be continued. Tetraplatin is an organoplatinum (IV) compound that is not cross-resistant with cisplatin. Preclinical results suggest that tetraplatin has greater antitumor activity than either cisplatin or carboplatin. A phase II study is anticipated.[166] Biologic therapies are also being pursued. Mullerian inhibitory substance (MIS) is a growth factor that has inhibited in vitro clonogenic growth of some ovarian cancer cells. Further study is needed to determine if MIS has potential as an anticancer agent.[69] Radiolabeled antibodies may be able to demonstrate the presence of tumor, thus avoiding second-look laparotomy. Immunotoxins, antitumor antibodies conjugated to potent plant or bacterial toxins, are also under clinical trial. Antibodies conjugated to cytotoxic chemotherapeutic agents may improve the therapeutic index.[146,167]

Another investigational approach is to define methods of overcoming intrinsic or acquired drug resistance. Buthionine sulfoximine and ethacrynic acid are currently being studied.[168,169] However, other means of overcoming drug resistance, such as gene therapy, must be pursued. Biologics and gene therapy are exciting treatment modalities that are developing and will be further investigated in ovarian cancer.[167]

The patient with ovarian cancer has many diverse needs. Some are no different than those that other cancer patients experience while undergoing extensive surgery and toxic chemotherapy or radiation therapy. The nursing management of patients receiving surgery, radiation, or chemotherapy for cancer is reviewed in previous chapters. Table 39-7 summarizes some common nursing management issues specific to the woman with ovarian cancer.

## Symptom Management and Continuity of Care

The overwhelming issue in caring for women with ovarian cancer is that the majority are diagnosed in late stages when the hope for cure is grim. Although some women will have long-term responses to their initial therapy, most will not. Many women will have to deal with abdominal ascites either as a presenting sign or as a sign of recurrent, progressive disease. In addition to the care issues discussed in Table 39-8, these women will need to learn self-care measures such as the care of a peritoneovenous shunt, monitoring weight gain, and measuring for increase in abdominal girth. Diversional activities and guided imagery are often useful in assisting the woman to cope with the increasing ascites. Nausea and vomiting can also develop either due to the increasing fluid compressing the gastrointestinal organs or due to tumor encasing the organs and causing obstruction or dysfunction. Often surgical correction is not warranted with advanced disease and the woman is faced with these debilitating symptoms for the remainder of her life. The use of gastric tubes for the purpose of drainage to prevent vomiting is often necessary as a comfort measure.

Because of the generally poor survival rates and the ongoing need for treatment and support, the patient and her family will become well known to the health care team. Their emotional needs as well as the woman's physical problems will need to be addressed. A caring, comprehensive approach that focuses on continuity of care will enable the patient and her family to achieve optimal quality of life. Home care and eventually hospice referral may be helpful to promote optimal self care, symptom relief, and respite care for the caregivers.

In considering future areas for research, prevention and early detection cannot be ignored. Efforts need to continue to define sensitive and specific screening methods that can be widely applied. Research to further define risk factors, etiology, and carcinogenesis will be the only comprehensive means of reducing the morbidity and mortality from ovarian cancer.

# CERVICAL CANCER

## Epidemiology

Throughout the world, cervical cancer is a significant cause of morbidity and mortality for women. It is the primary cause of death among women in Kenya and ranks second as a cause of cancer death among Chinese women.[170,171] Overall, the highest incidence of invasive cervical cancer is reported in the Latin American countries (see Table 39-9).

According to the American Cancer Society, 15,700 new cases of invasive cervical cancer were diagnosed in the United States in 1996, and approximately 4900 women died of the disease.[1] The incidence of invasive cervical cancer has steadily decreased as a result of the Pap smear, which can diagnose the disease in a preinvasive state. The number of deaths from cervical cancer has decreased in women over age 45, while mortality in women under 35 years has increased.[3,172] However, cervi-

**TABLE 39-7**  Nursing Issues in the Care of the Woman with Ovarian Cancer

| Treatment/Disease | Physical, Psychosocial Issues | Interventions |
|---|---|---|
| Diagnosis/staging laparotomy | Preoperative testing | Give information regarding preoperative testing |
| | Operative procedure planned | Reinforce information regarding operative procedure |
| | Facing extensive exploratory and cytoreductive surgery | Role in postoperative care, including promoting respiratory function, progressive ambulation, careful monitoring of vital signs, intake and output, electrolytes, GI function, renal function |
| | Facing potentially terminal disease | Encourage verbalization of fears, concerns from patient, family; clarify misconceptions; discuss additional therapy planned |
| Chemotherapy | Combination platinum-based regimen is therapy most ovarian cancer patients receive. Side effects include nausea, vomiting, diarrhea, bone marrow depression, alopecia, neurotoxicity, liver/renal toxicity | Instruct patient about types of therapy (standard or investigational), method of administration, drugs, side effects, frequency, and duration |
| | Most side effects can be managed | Monitor side effects and develop plan to minimize effects, including antiemetic regimen, colony stimulating factors, hematological monitoring |
| | | Nutritional needs may require small frequent meals, dietary supplements, and continued antiemetics to overcome nausea, vomiting, anorexia |
| | Routine for blood testing, scans, and physical examinations | Develop schedule for appointments and follow-up |
| | Roles and relationships within the family may change due to therapy | Assist in coping with disease and treatment; assess need for referrals for additional support, e.g., to other cancer patients, support groups, psychotherapy |
| Radiation therapy | $^{32}$P: acute side effects, IP route of administration, follow-up | Instruct patient about planned regimen, method of administration, side effects, duration of therapy, follow-up |
| | Whole-abdominal radiation: schedule, treatment ports, side effects (acute and chronic), and follow-up | Monitor side effects and develop plan to minimize effects; medication can help reduce side effects; nutritional support with antiemetics, antidiarrheals, antispasmodics, small frequent low-fiber meals, dietary supplements |
| | Roles and relationships within the family may change due to therapy | Assist in coping with disease and treatment Assess need for referrals for additional support, e.g., to other radiation patients, support groups, psychotherapy |
| Progressive disease | Salvage therapy offers little response in chemotherapy-refractory disease | Instruct patient about salvage therapy: regimen, side effects, hope for response |
| | Parenteral hyperalimentation may address nutritional needs of patient but may not improve quality of life due to progressive disease; inability to eat is a great source of fright and frustration for patient and family | Nutritional support with dietary supplements or enteral feedings |
| | Disease progression leads to lymphatic obstruction, edema, anasarca, massive peritoneal effusions, and pleural effusions | Focus on symptom control, comfort measures |
| | Ascites/pleural effusions are source of discomfort, respiratory compromise, and GI dysfunction (Table 39-8); effusions may be drained and pleural space sclerosed | Encourage verbalization by patient and family of fears/concerns regarding progressive/terminal disease |
| | Women often remain mentally alert despite deteriorating physical status | Encourage diversional therapy to enable patient to focus on other means of comfort that may reduce tension/anxiety experienced by patient and family |

**TABLE 39-8** Nursing Care of the Patient with Malignant Ascites

| Symptom/Distress | Assessment | Intervention |
|---|---|---|
| Abdominal distension | Bulging abdomen and flanks; everted umbilicus; shiny skin | Daily abdominal girths, weights; palpate for fluid wave; percuss for sounds of shifting dullness. |
| Respiratory compromise | Dyspnea; shortness of breath; tachypnea; use of accessory muscles | Elevate head of bed; provide rest periods; restrict activities as tolerated; oxygen as needed; analgesics as ordered. |
| Fluid and electrolyte imbalance | Signs and symptoms of dehydration; lymphedema of lower extremities; signs of hypokalemia, hyponatremia, hypomagnesemia | Monitor serum protein, albumin, electrolytes, fluid replacements as ordered; daily weight, abdominal girth; monitor intake and output, vital signs; high-protein diet; minimize sodium and fluid intake; diuretics as ordered; compression stockings, boots; assist patient in maintaining mobility. |
| Peritoneovenous shunting | Pain; infection; bleeding; skin integrity at operative site; DIC, tumor embolus | Teach patient and family about surgical procedure, operating room routine, methods of maintaining patency of shunt; provide shunt care; monitor fluid, electrolytes, and coagulation profile. |

Reprinted with permission from Eriksson JH, Walczak JR: Ovarian cancer. *Semin Oncol Nurs* 6:225, 1990.

cal cancer remains a significant health problem in women aged 65 years and older.[173]

Though the incidence of invasive cancer has decreased by nearly 50%, the incidence of carcinoma in situ (CIS) has climbed dramatically since 1945. More than 65,000 new cases of CIS were diagnosed in 1996.[1] Women in their 20s are most often diagnosed with cervical dysplasia; those aged 30 to 39 with in situ cancer; and those over age 40 with invasive cancer.[174]

## Etiology

Many personal risk factors have been associated with precancerous lesions of the cervix (Table 39-10).[170,175] A

**TABLE 39-9** Age-Adjusted Cervical Cancer Death Rates per 100,000 Population: 15 Countries with Highest Death Rates

| Country | Death Rate |
|---|---|
| Mexico | 15.9 |
| Chile | 12.5 |
| Costa Rica | 10.4 |
| Romania | 10.3 |
| Venezuela | 9.7 |
| Poland | 7.9 |
| Hungary | 6.8 |
| Cuba | 6.5 |
| Ecuador | 5.8 |
| Czechoslovakia | 5.6 |
| Denmark | 5.3 |
| USSR | 5.2 |
| Uruguay | 4.7 |
| Scotland | 4.6 |
| Argentina | 4.6 |

Adapted from *CA: Cancer J Clin* 45:28–9, 1996.

higher incidence of the disease occurs in lower socioeconomic groups; smokers; blacks; Hispanics; women who become sexually active prior to age 17, have many sexual partners, and are multiparous.

Cervical dysplasia, carcinoma in situ, and cervical cancer have been designated as AIDS-defining illnesses by the Center for Disease Control. Women with HIV infection are at higher risk for developing squamous intraepithelial lesions (SIL) of the cervix.[175–177] In HIV infected females, cervical cancer may manifest itself in unusual ways, be more aggressive, and run a more fulminant course.[176,178–180] Conversely, cervical carcinoma is infrequent in women who are nulliparous, and those who are lifetime celibates or lifetime monogamous.[26,175,181–183] Females exposed to diethylstilbestrol (DES) in utero have a higher incidence of clear cell adenocarcinoma of the cervix and vagina.[184,185]

Human papillomaviruses (HPV) are members of the family of DNA tumor viruses that can cause cellular hyperproliferation and a variety of warty infections. In women, the genital variety of HPV is called *papilloma acuminata* and is sexually transmitted. More than 70 distinct types of HPV have been identified but only some types of HPV are associated with genital warts, precancerous lesions, or invasive cervical carcinoma.[170,186–192] About 20 types of HPV have been associated with high-grade cervical intraepithelial lesions or invasive cancer. Nine types (16,18,31,33,35,45,51,52,56) are linked to cervical cancer while only five types (6,11,42–44) are linked to condyloma acuminatum.[193] Both HPV 16 and 18 are associated with high-grade cervical (squamous) intraepithelial lesions or invasive cancer.[192,194,195] There is evidence linking HPV 6 and 11 to intraepithelial neoplasia of the cervix.[195,196] HPV 18 is associated with 15% to 50% of invasive cervical cancer lesions. The prevalence of HPV 16 appears to increase with the severity of the lesion.[197] Several researchers, utilizing a DNA hybridization technique, indicated

**TABLE 39-10**　Malignancies of the Lower Genital Tract: Risk Factors and Preventive Measures

| Risk Factors | Preventive Measures |
| --- | --- |
| **CERVICAL CANCER** | |
| HIV | Pap smears per ACS guidelines |
| HSV2 | Pelvic examinations |
| HPV | Barrier contraception |
| Abnormal transformation zone | Limit number of sexual partners |
| Sex prior to age 17 | Sex after age 17 |
| Multiple sexual partners | Stop smoking |
| History of smoking | Hygienic environment for sexual activity |
| Chemicals in cigarette smoke | Assess occupational risk |
| Spouse whose previous wife had cervical cancer | |
| Maternal use of DES | |
| Immunosuppression | |
| Multiparous | |
| Socioeconomic status | |
| Race/ethnic background | |
| Spouse with cancer of penis | |
| Partner's occupation | |
| Number of sex partners of husband | |
| Sperm, semen | |
| **VULVAR CANCER** | |
| HSV2 | Routine vulvar examination |
| HPV | Pap smear |
| Condylomato | Barrier contraception |
| Immunosuppression | |
| Chronic vulvar disease | |
| Exposure to coal tar derivatives | |
| History of breast, cervical, endometrial malignancies | |
| **VAGINAL CANCER** | |
| Cervical CIN | Pap smear |
| HPV | Barrier contraceptives |
| Vaginal trauma | Limit number of sexual partners |
| Previous abdominal hysterectomy for benign disease | |
| Radiotherapy for cervical cancer | |
| Increased age | |
| Race | |
| Lower socioeconomic status | |
| Education | |

HIV, human immunodeficiency virus
HSV2, herpes simplex virus type 2
HPV, human papillomavirus

that HPV 18 is the most common papillomavirus found in women with adenocarcinoma of the cervix, while HPV 16 was more commonly associated with squamous carcinomas.[198–200]

Herpes simplex virus type 2 (HSV2) has been shown to be carcinogenic in animals. Women with cervical cancer usually have higher HSV2 specific antibody titers than controls, but several prospective studies have failed to show an association between development of HSV2 antibodies and development of cervical cancer.[26,201,202] Still, HSV2 may be a contributing factor in the development of cervical neoplasia.[203]

The male plays a role in the etiology of cervical cancer. Women married to men whose previous spouses had cervical cancer seem to be at a higher risk of developing cervical cancer, but the cause for this apparent relationship has not yet been determined.[170,204] The male partner's age at first coitus, smoking habits, visitation of prostitutes, and number of sexual partners also may affect relative risk.[175,196,204] In addition wives of men with cancer of the penis are at increased risk for the development of cervical cancer.[189] Women married to men who are sailors, laborers, textile workers, chemical workers or gardeners/ sports workers have higher mortality rates from cervical cancer.[175] Women who work as maids, cleaners, and cooks may have a slightly elevated risk of developing invasive disease.[205] These findings are most likely related to women being directly exposed to occupational carcinogens or indirectly exposed via sexual contact with men in the cited occupations. Several factors may lower a woman's risk of developing preinvasive lesions as precursors to invasive cervical cancer. These include barrier-type contraception, vasectomy, recommended daily allowances of vitamin A, beta carotene, vitamin C, limiting the number of sexual partners, and initiating sexual activity at a later age.[175, 189]

Several researchers have cited the use of vitamins as chemopreventive agents.[206–208] Creek et al[206] noted that diets deficient in vitamin A and/or beta-carotene have been associated with an increased risk of cervical cancer. Childers et al[207] designed a phase III study to determine if folic acid given p.o. played a role in preventing cervical cancer. The researchers found after six months of treatment that there was no significant difference between the groups with regard to improvement in Pap smear or colposcopic findings.

Meyskens et al[209] applied all-trans-retinoid acid (RA) topically to treat women with CIN. Results indicated that locally applied RA can effectively reverse CIN II, but is not effective for CIN III. Other researchers have studied the ability of retinoids and cytokines to prohibit cellular proliferation.[210–212] Further study is needed to define the role of these approaches in cervical neoplasia. Recently, researchers found that melatonin had an inhibitory effect on human cervical cancer cell growth in vitro.[213]

## Pathophysiology

### Cellular characteristics

Histologically, 80%–90% of cervical tumors are squamous, 10%–20% are adenocarcinomas, and a very small number are of other types including adenosquamous, glassy cell, sarcomas, and melanomas.[3,26] Adenocarcinomas, generally in younger women, impose a greater risk because the tumor arises within the endocervical mucus-producing gland cells. The tumor can become quite bulky before it becomes clinically evident. The bulkiness makes the tumor harder to treat, and thus has a high rate of local recurrence.[186,214] Adenocarcinomas appear to be increasing in prevalence.[186,214] Less is known about the epidemiology of adenocarcinoma of the cervix than squamous cell cancer of the cervix. In addition, adenocarcinomas are more difficult to detect than squamous carcinoma; there is no consistent definition of this histological type; no uniform reporting method; and no clear cut histological pattern for correlation of cytological features.[186] Oral contraceptives may be associated with higher rates of adenocarcinoma in younger women. This may be especially true if oral contraceptives are used during adolescence when the cervix has not fully ma-

tured. This connection, however, needs to be studied further. Prognosis seems to be related to tumor volume and nodal metastasis.[186]

### Progression of disease

The cervix, the lower part of the uterus, extends from the isthmus into the vagina and is divided into two major parts: the endocervix and the exocervix. The endocervix is contiguous to the exocervix, which includes the external os and extends to the vaginal fornix. The *squamo-columnar junction* refers to the area where the columnar epithelium of the endocervix joins the squamous epithelium of the exocervix at the os.[3,215]

Cancer of the cervix is a culmination of a progressive disease that begins as a neoplastic alteration of the squamocolumnar junction. Over time, these abnormal cells can progress to involve the full thickness of the epithelium and invade into the stromal tissue of the cervix. The initial preinvasive or premalignant changes are called cervical intraepithelial neoplasia (CIN).

The term *cervical intraepithelial neoplasia* (CIN) was introduced in the mid-1960s to better define epithelial cervical abnormalities. CIN classification demonstrates the progression of the disease process rather than delineating distinctly different abnormalities. As such, each step in the cervical disease spectrum merges imperceptibly into the next.[172,185] CIN is divided into three categories: CIN I, CIN II, and CIN III.

The term *CIN I* is used to describe dysplasia or atypical changes in the cervical epithelium involving less than one-third the thickness of the epithelium. *CIN II* describes neoplastic changes involving up to two-thirds the thickness, and *CIN III* or *carcinoma in situ* describes a lesion that has neoplastic changes involving up to full thickness of the epithelium with no areas of stromal invasion or metastases (Figure 39-4).[3,183,216,217] Once the disease progresses beyond the basement membrane and invades the cervical stroma, the disease is considered invasive or malignant.

In 1988, a workshop sponsored by the National Cancer Institute was held in Bethesda, Maryland to address problems inherent in the Papanicolaou system. Clinical experts felt that the Pap system, introduced in the 1930s,

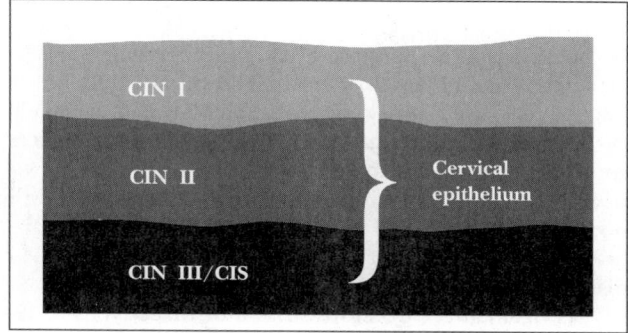

**FIGURE 39-4** Atyical changes in the cervical epithelium.

did not: (1) reliably communicate information relevant to the clinician, (2) include diagnostic histopathologic terminology, (3) provide diagnoses for noncancerous lesions, or (4) afford uniformity in reporting diagnostic interpretations.[218,219] The goal was to review existing terminology and to make recommendations for a more effective method of reporting. The outcome of this conference was the Bethesda System which is used to report cervical/vaginal cytological diagnoses.[218–222]

The Bethesda System (Table 39-11) addresses the following elements: (1) a statement of the adequacy of the cytological specimen (satisfactory, less than optimal, unsatisfactory); (2) a general categorization of the diagnosis (within normal limits, other); and (3) a descriptive diagnosis which includes two new terms: low-grade and high-grade squamous intraepithelial lesions (SIL). The descriptive diagnosis allows cytopathologists to list reactive and reparative changes (e.g., changes secondary to inflammatory processes, treatment [chemotherapy, radiotherapy], or contraceptive devices). By 1992, 85% of cytology laboratories were utilizing the Bethesda System terminology. As a result of the strict format used in reporting cytological abnormalities, the number of women identified with abnormal Pap smears has increased.[223,224]

Low-grade SIL includes cellular changes associated with HPV or mild dysplasia (CIN I). High-grade SIL includes lesions formerly designated as moderate dysplasia (CIN II) and severe dysplasia or CIS (CIN III). The use of the word *grade* as it is utilized with the SIL terminology does not imply invasive carcinoma.[218,221]

Although use of the Bethesda System is becoming more widespread, there is still opposition to it. Some clinicians argue against using only one diagnostic category (SIL) with two subcategories (low-grade and high-grade SIL) for all intraepithelial lesions, even though qualifying terms may be added to the cytological reports.[225,226] Several researchers have questioned the inclusion of CIN II and CIN III in the high-grade SIL category.[225] They felt that lumping CIN II and III together implied similar management, which may not be the case. Others have expressed the fear that women may be over diagnosed and given unnecessary treatment.[225,227]

Due to a lack of consensus on a system for reporting cervical/vaginal cytological diagnoses, the terms CIN and SIL are both seen in the literature.

### Patterns of spread

Each type of SIL (CIN) lesion can regress, persist, or become invasive. High-grade SIL (CIN III) is more likely to progress than the milder forms, which may regress spontaneously to normal. Because there is no way to predict which lesions will become invasive and which will not, all patients should be treated as soon as lesions are discovered. Most authorities believe that SIL is a venereal disease which has a prolonged incubation period.[185,228]

Cervical cancer develops in one of three types of lesions: exophytic, excavating (or ulcerative), or endo-

phytic. Exophytic lesions[3,229] are the most common and appear as cauliflowerlike, fungating cancers which are very friable and bleed easily. The lesions may involve a small area of the cervix, or be quite extensive, involving the entire cervix and upper vagina.

The excavating or ulcerative lesion[3,229] is a necrotic lesion that replaces the cervix and upper vagina with an ulcer or crater that bleeds easily. These are often associated with local infection and purulent discharge.

The endophytic lesion[229] is located within the endocervical canal and is without visible tumor or ulceration. The cervix appears normal or enlarged and barrel-shaped and is hard to the touch. If there is parametrial involvement, the parametrium also may be hard and nodular.

Once invasive, cervical cancer spreads by three routes: direct extension, via lymphatics, and by hematogenous spread. Direct extension is the most common route and the lesion may spread in any direction.[186] The lesion begins on the endocervix and spreads throughout the entire cervix, into the parametrium, and through the vesicovaginal and rectovaginal septae into the bladder and rectum. The upper vagina and corpus of the uterus may also become involved.

Involvement of the lymph nodes is fairly predictable. The primary nodes involved in the spread of cervical cancer include the obturator, external iliac, and hypogastric. The secondary group of lymph nodes involved are the parametrial, inferior gluteal, and presacral nodes.[186] (See Figure 39-5.) Lymph node involvement can be correlated with stage of disease. The prevalence of positive nodes is 15% to 20% in stage I, 25% to 40% in stage II, and at least 50% in stage III.[3]

Hematogenous spread through the venous plexus and the paracervical veins occurs less frequently than lymphatic spread but is relatively common in the more advanced stages. The most common sites of metastasis are the lungs, mediastinal and supraclavicular nodes, liver, and bone.

## Clinical Manifestations

Cervical cancer is usually asymptomatic in the preinvasive and early stages, although women may notice a watery vaginal discharge. In the majority of cases the disease is discovered by PAP smears during routine examinations. The later symptoms which often prompt the woman to seek medical attention in cervical cancer are postcoital bleeding, intermenstrual bleeding, or heavy menstrual flow. If this bleeding is chronic, the woman may complain of symptoms related to anemia. A common complaint in advanced cervical malignancy is that of a serous foul smelling vaginal discharge.[3,186,216]

Other late symptoms, which are indicative of advanced disease, include pain in the pelvis, hypogastrium, flank, or leg. This is secondary to involvement of the pelvic wall, ureters, lymph nodes, or sciatic nerve roots. Urinary

**TABLE 39-11** The 1988 Bethesda System for Reporting Cervical/Vaginal Cytological Diagnoses

**Statement on Specimen Adequacy**

Satisfactory for interpretation
Less than optimal
Unsatisfactory

Explanation for less than optimal/unsatisfactory specimen:

- Scant cellularity
- Poor fixation or preservation
- Presence of foreign material (e.g., lubricant)
- Partially or completely obscuring inflammation
- Partially or completely obscuring blood
- Excessive cytolysis or autolysis
- No endocervical component in a premenopausal woman who has a cervix
- Not representative of the anatomic site
- Other

**General Categorization**

Within normal limits
Other:
*See "Descriptive Diagnoses"*
Further action recommended

**Descriptive Diagnoses**

*INFECTION*
Fungal
Fungal organisms morphologically consistent with *Candida* species
Other
Bacterial
Microorganisms morphologically consistent with *Gardnerella* species
Microorganisms morphologically consistent with *Actinomyces* species
Cellular changes suggestive of *Chlamydia* species infection, subject to confirmatory studies
Other
Protozoan
*Trichomonas vaginalis*
Other
Viral
Cellular changes associated with cytomegalovirus
Cellular changes associated with herpesvirus simplex
Other
(Note: for human papillomavirus (HPV), refer to "Epithelial Cell Abnormalities, Squamous Cell")
Other

*REACTIVE AND REPARATIVE CHANGES*

Inflammation
Associated cellular changes
Follicular cervicitis
Miscellaneous (as related to patient history)
Effects of therapy

Ionizing radiation
Chemotherapy
Effects of mechanical devices (e.g., intrauterine contraceptive device)
Effects of nonsteroidal estrogen exposure (e.g., diethylstilbestrol)
Other

*EPITHELIAL CELL ABNORMALITIES*

Squamous Cell

- Atypical squamous cells of undetermined significance (recommended follow-up and/or type of further investigation: specify)
- Squamous intraepithelial lesion (SIL) (comment on presence of cellular changes associated with HPV if applicable)
  Low-grade squamous intraepithelial lesion, encompassing:
    Cellular changes associated with HPV
    Mild (slight) dysplasia/cervical intraepithelial neoplasia grade 1 (CIN I)
  High-grade squamous intraepithelial lesion, encompassing:
    Moderate dysplasia/CIN II
    Severe dysplasia/CIN III
    Carcinoma in situ/CIN III
- Squamous cell carcinoma

Glandular Cell

- Presence of endometrial cells in one of the following circumstances:
  Out of phase in a menstruating woman
  In a postmenopausal woman
  No menstrual history available
- Atypical glandular cells of undetermined significance (recommended follow-up and/or type of further investigation: specify)
  Endometrial
  Endocervical
  Not otherwise specified
- Adenocarcinoma
  Specify probable site of origin: endocervical, endometrial, extrauterine
  Not otherwise specified
- Other epithelial malignant neoplasm: specify

*NONEPITHELIAL MALIGNANT NEOPLASM: SPECIFY*

*HORMONAL EVALUATION (APPLIES TO VAGINAL SMEARS ONLY)*

- Hormonal pattern compatible with age and history
- Hormonal pattern incompatible with age and history: specify
- Hormonal evaluation not possible
  Cervical specimen
  Inflammation
  Insufficient patient history

*OTHER*

Adapted from *J Natl Cancer Inst* 82:989, 1990.

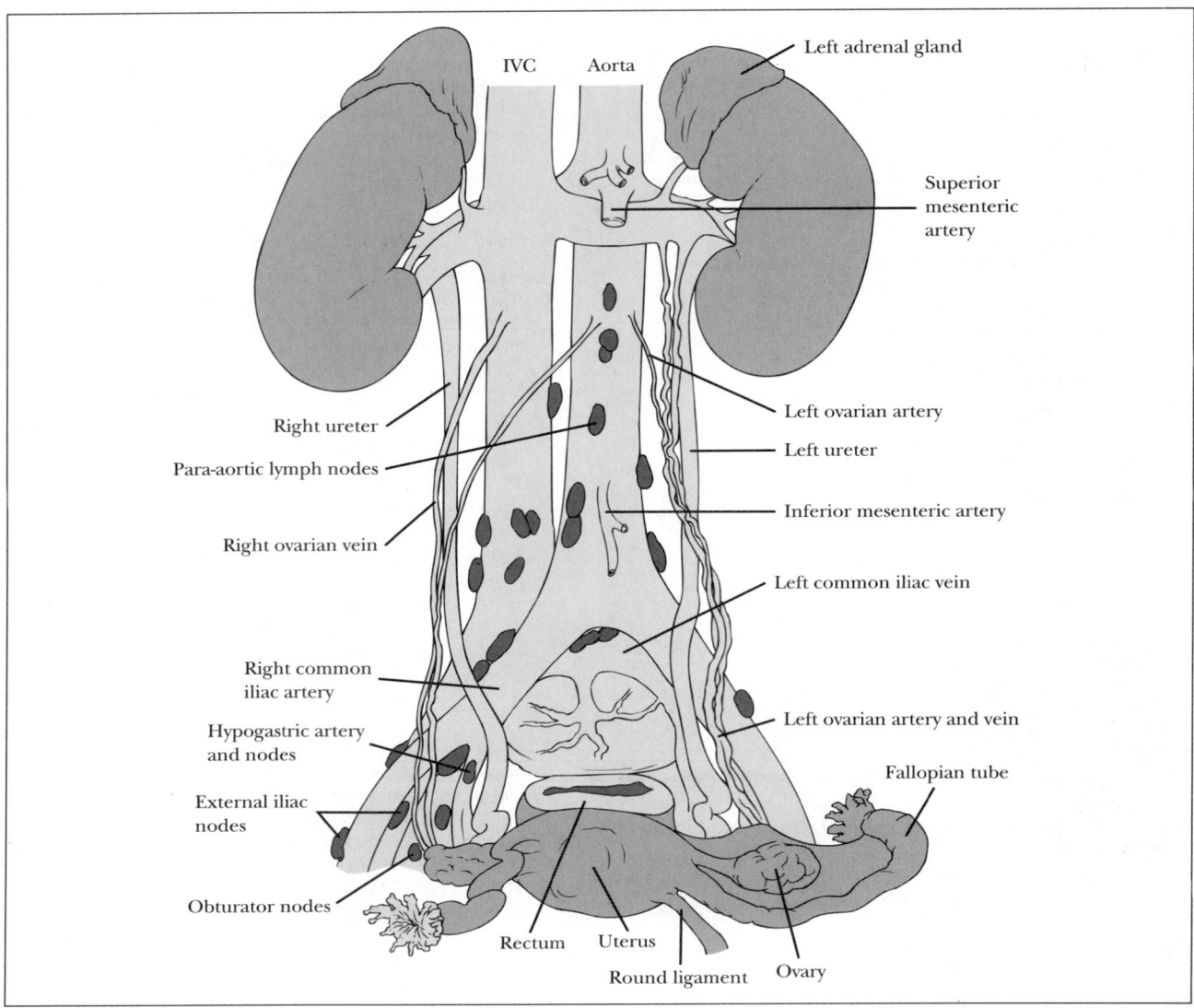

**FIGURE 39-5**    The pelvic and para-aortic lymph nodes and their relationship to the major retroperitoneal vessels. (Reproduced, with permission, from Hacker NF, Moore JG (eds): *Essentials of Obstetrics and Gynecology.* Philadelphia, Saunders, 1986, p 8.)

and rectal symptoms may indicate invasion of these structures by tumor. End-stage disease may be characterized by edema of the lower extremities due to lymphatic and venous obstruction. Massive vaginal hemorrhage and development of renal failure may result from local invasion of blood vessels and bilateral ureteral obstruction by tumor.[3,186,216]

## Assessment—SIL

The Pap smear is an effective, accurate, and economical screening technique to detect cervical neoplasia. Accuracy of the examination depends on the sampling method, staining, and microscopic examination.[186,230,231] Automated interpreters can be useful in detection of

cervical abnormalities and can lower false-negative rates. High-resolution video scanners distinguish between normal and abnormal cytological specimens and can decrease mistakes due to human error.[193]

The American Cancer Society recommends that all women who are or have been sexually active or who are 18 years or older should have an annual Pap test and pelvic examination. After a woman has had three or more consecutive normal annual examinations, the Pap test may be performed less frequently at the discretion of her physician.[232] The American College of Obstetricians and Gynecologists, The National Cancer Institute, The American Academy of Family Physicians, and the American Medical Association recommend annual examinations that begin with the onset of sexual activity or at 18 years of age.

Sexually active women should have annual Pap smears. Those who have any pelvic symptoms such as pain, vaginal discharge, or abnormal bleeding should be evaluated by their physician promptly. False-negative Pap smears occur and are thought to be due to sampling inefficiency.[186,233] A negative Pap smear offers no guarantee that the woman is free of cervical cancer.[186,233]

The correlation between cytological diagnosis and subsequent histological examination is over 90%.[234] Although SIL is becoming the standard terminology for cervical (squamous) intraepithelial lesions, many cytology laboratories still use CIN terminology and a few may even use the old I-V class system when reporting. The relationship between the three is depicted in Table 39-12.

When the Pap smear report shows SIL, referral for biopsy, colposcopy, and/or treatment is indicated.[235] Colposcopy is a diagnostic test to evaluate the cervix after an abnormal PAP smear, and is done on an outpatient basis. A colposcope is a stereoscopic, binocular microscope that illuminates and magnifies the view of the cervix.[185,236] During this procedure the cervix is swabbed with 3% acetic acid solution, which accentuates the abnormalities and differentiates between normal or metaplastic areas.[230] The epithelium of the cervix is visualized and the abnormal areas biopsied.

## Therapeutic Approaches and Nursing Care—SIL

It is critical that the extent of the disease is determined as accurately as possible before treatment begins. The Pap smear, colposcopy, and biopsy determine the extent and severity of the cervical lesion, differentiating between SIL and invasive carcinoma of the cervix. Treatment for SIL may include a direct cervical biopsy, electrocautery/cryosurgery, laser surgery, electrosurgery, cone biopsy, or hysterectomy.[230,236]

Cryosurgery, the most commonly used method for outpatient treatment of SIL in the United States, makes use of a portable probe to induce freezing of cervical tissue. It is a cost-effective and painless treatment with low morbidity that can be performed in the office. Patients most often complain of a watery discharge for 2 to 4 weeks after treatment.

Research studies[186,237-239] show that approximately 80% to 90% of SIL can be eradicated by laser. The laser is mounted on the colposcope, and the laser beam is directed under colposcopic control. The advantage of using the laser is that significantly less disease-free tissue is removed with the entire lesion. Patients may experience a little more discomfort than with cryosurgery, but there is usually less vaginal discharge, and complete healing occurs in about two weeks.[3,236,240] One disadvantage of the laser is that it may cause thermal damage to tissue, making it difficult to rule out invasive cancer.[186]

Treatment of SIL using the loop electrosurgical excision procedure (loop diathermy excision) is an increasingly popular alternative. In selected patients this approach may allow for diagnosis and treatment of SIL during one out-patient visit. The loop electrosurgical excision procedure (LEEP) utilizes a thin wire loop electrode which allows excision of affected tissue with minimal ablation.[186,241] The advantage of LEEP is that there is less likelihood of tissue ablation than with the use of other procedures such as the laser. The laser

**TABLE 39-12** Cytological Report Correlations

| Class | CIN Terminology | Description | Bethesda Terminology |
|---|---|---|---|
| I | | Smear normal, no abnormal cells | Normal |
| II | | Atypical cells present below the level of cervical neoplasia | Other infection reparative |
| III | CIN I, CIN II | Smear contains abnormal cells consistent with dysplasia—mild: CIN I; severe: CIN II | SIL low-grade high-grade |
| | CIN III | Smear contains abnormal cells consistent with severe dysplasia: CIN III | SIL high-grade |
| IV | CIS | Carcinoma in situ | SIL high-grade |
| V | ICC | Invasive squamous carcinoma | Squamous cell carcinoma |

CIN = cervical intraepithelial neoplasia.
SIL = squamous intraepithelial neoplasia
CIS = carcinoma in situ
ICC = invasive squamous carcinoma

Adapted from Nelson JH and Richard RM: Cervical intraepithelial neoplasia and carcinomas in situ and early invasive cervical carcinoma. *CA Cancer J Clin* 39:157–178, 1989.

may cause thermal damage to tissue, making it difficult to rule out invasive cancer. Complications of LEEP are similar to those seen with laser treatment.[241,242]

Conization involves removal of a cone-shaped piece of tissue from the exocervix and endocervix (Figure 39-6).[3,236] This procedure, performed under general anesthesia as an outpatient, can be used as a diagnostic or therapeutic technique. The exact size of the cone depends on the colposcopic findings. Conization is performed in specific situations: (1) for diagnosis, if no lesion of the cervix is noted and an endocervical tumor is suspected; (2) to determine extent of the lesion if microinvasion is diagnosed on biopsy, or if the entire lesion cannot be seen with the colposcope, (3) if there are discrepancies between the cytological report (Pap smear) and the histological appearance of the lesions on biopsy, and (4) when the patient cannot be relied upon for long term follow-up.[243] Major immediate complications of conization include hemorrhage, uterine perforation, and complications of anesthesia. Delayed complications include bleeding, cervical stenosis, infertility, cervical incompetence, and increased chances of preterm (low birth weight) delivery. In general, complications of conization are related to the amount of endocervix that is removed.[236,240]

Total vaginal hysterectomy (TVH) may be employed for treatment of individuals with high-grade SIL (CIS). Total abdominal hysterectomy is appropriate for individuals with high-grade SIL (CIS) who have completed childbearing. These individuals must be followed as closely for recurrence as those treated with more conservative measures.[3]

Ultimately, the therapy selected is based on the extent of the disease, the patient's wishes to preserve ovarian and reproductive function, and the physician's experience. Women with low-grade or high-grade SIL (CIN I or II) who wish to maintain optimum fertility can be considered for electrocautery, laser therapy, or cryosurgery. High-grade SIL (CIN III) also can be treated in this manner as long as the woman is aware that there is a slightly higher incidence of recurrence with this treatment method.[3]

Interferon (IFN) has been used sparingly in the treatment of low-grade SIL, but more research needs to be done on this methodology.[244,245] The use of IFN for the treatment of SIL is inferior to surgical methods when cure rate is considered. The advantage to using IFN is that it does not deform the cervix or interfere with a normal pregnancy. Therefore it may be appropriate for use in selected females during the childbearing years.

Figure 39-7 summarizes the appropriate management of a patient with an abnormal Pap smear.[3] Regardless of the type of treatment selected for SIL, frequent follow-up is essential.

### Continuity of care: Nursing challenges

The primary nursing responsibilities for women with SIL focus on education. This educational process includes defining the disease, explaining treatment, and stressing the importance of close follow-up.

If the biopsy indicates SIL, the woman may erroneously think that she has invasive cancer. The nurse assures the patient that she does not have cancer and that SIL is an easily treated premalignant condition. In women treated for SIL, self-esteem was lowest and anxiety highest during the initial and postsurgical visits. In addition, women expressed fear of losing sexual functioning.[246] The nurse helps the woman to understand the type of treatment recommended. The nurse explains the nature and purpose of treatment, and side effects of the therapy.

Following treatment, the nurse instructs the woman on how to care for herself at home. Douching, tampons, and sexual intercourse are prohibited for at least two to four weeks, depending on the treatment. A return visit must be scheduled for two to four weeks, then every three months for a year, and every six months thereafter. The importance of this follow-up must be stressed because there is a possibility of treatment failure or recurrence of the SIL. Minimal bleeding and vaginal discharge may be present for a week or longer after biopsy, cryosurgery, or laser and for several weeks following conization.

Information concerning sexual functioning and fertility should be discussed with women undergoing treatment for SIL, although electrocautery, cryosurgery, laser therapy, and conization rarely cause physiological sexual dysfunction.[241,247] Most women report no change in libido, orgasm, coital frequency, or overall satisfaction with their sex life. Fertility is usually maintained, but difficulty with conception may occur. Table 39-13 summarizes issues specifically related to nursing management.

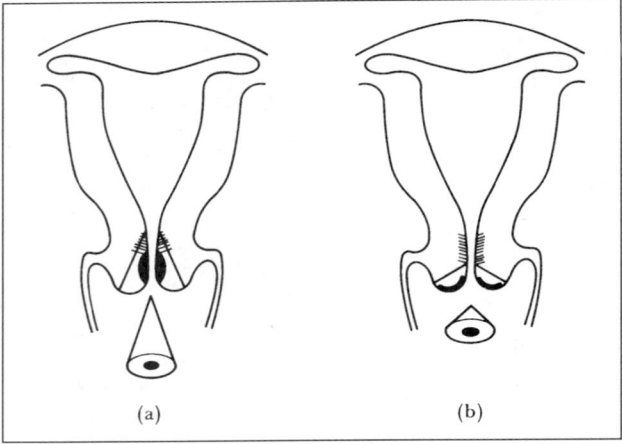

**FIGURE 39-6**  (a) Cone biopsy for endocervical disease. (b) Cone biopsy for CIN of the exocervix. CIN = cervical epithelial neoplasia. (DiSaia PJ, Creasman WT: *Clinical Gynecologic Oncology.* St Louis, Mosby, 1989.)

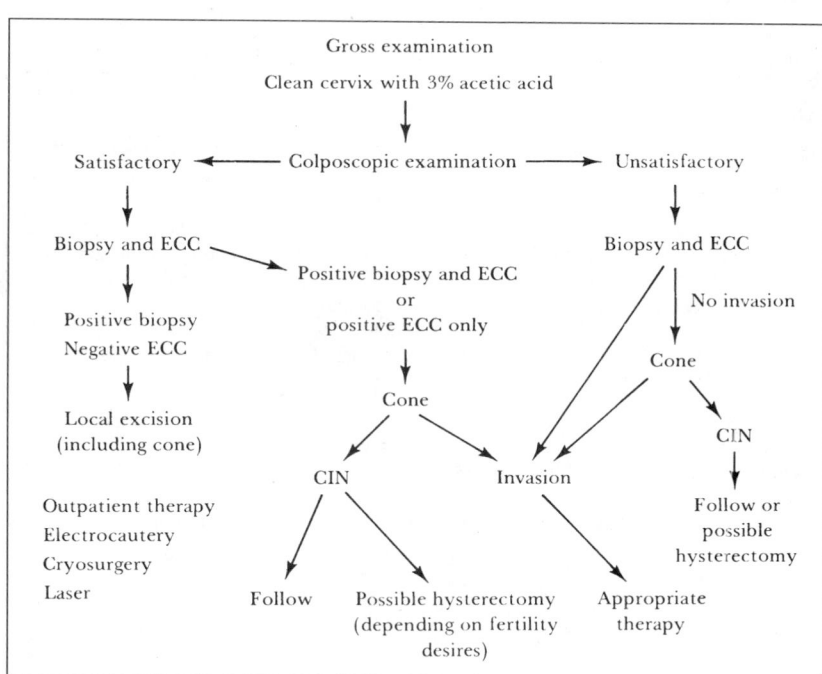

**FIGURE 39-7** Evaluation and management schema for individual with abnormal Pap smear. (DiSaia PJ, Creasman WT: *Clinical Gynecologic Oncology.* St. Louis, Mosby, 1989.)

## Assessment—Invasive Disease

### Diagnostic studies

A thorough clinical examination under anesthesia includes cervical biopsies, endocervical curettage, cystoscopy, and proctosigmoidoscopy. Additional diagnostic tests may include chest radiograph, IVP, barium enema, CBC, and blood chemistries. If liver enzymes are elevated, a liver scan (or CT scan) is indicated.[186,236,248]

Lymphangiogram may be indicated in selected individuals. The use of lymphangiography has been controversial due to a high false-negative rate. Twenty-one percent of patients with lymphangiograms interpreted as normal are found to have histologically positive nodes at laparotomy. If enlarged nodes are seen on lymphangiogram, fine-needle aspiration may be done. Lymphangiogram may also be valuable in outlining abnormal lymph nodes to be included in radiotherapy ports.[186,216,249]

Additional studies that are helpful in defining the extent of disease but do not alter clinical staging include CT and MRI. Computerized axial tomograms may be used to determine the extent of pelvic disease, define radiotherapy portals, and to evaluate lymph node status. The main use of CT is to help identify enlarged lymph nodes in the pelvis and paraaortic areas.[186] Magnetic resonance imaging offers no advantage over CT in evaluating lymph node metastasis or assessment of parametrial disease.[186] However, researchers found that MRI offered improved evaluation of tumor size, stromal invasion, and extent of disease as compared to CT.[250] Both CT and MRI were able to evaluate lymph node metastasis (86% each) MRI has been used to assess the response of cervical cancer to neoadjuvant chemotherapy, but was not as precise as surgical staging in these cases.[251] Verification of tumor volume (the most important prognostic factor for survival of the patient with cervical cancer) by MRI may help the physician to determine the best treatment modality.[252] Positron emission tomography (PET) may be able to detect disease not seen on CT or MRI. In addition PET, if used in conjunction with CT and MRI, may be better able to determine extent of local disease and nodal involvement.[186]

Clinical staging is not changed on the basis of surgical findings, but treatment may be altered. In selected cases where lymphangiogram or CT are equivocal, a selected pelvic and periaortic lymphadenectomy may be performed. Surgical staging has been included in some investigational chemotherapy/radiation protocols to better define extent of disease and select appropriate radiation therapy.[253,254]

Supraclavicular node biopsy is done if one of these nodes is palpable or if paraaortic nodes are positive. The left node is most often positive because this is where the thoracic duct enters into the subclavian vein. Positive supraclavicular nodes are often associated with a positive aortic node. In such cases a blind scalene node biopsy is recommended. If this is positive, systemic therapy is necessary. Following a thorough evaluation, the clinical stage is determined (Table 39-14).[186,255]

Tumor markers are not used extensively by oncologists, though several researchers have advocated their use. Borras et al[256] found elevated CEA levels in 33%, CA-19.9 in 32%, and CA-125 in 21.5% of women studied with invasive cervical carcinoma. The researchers concluded that CEA, CA-125, and CA-19.9 were useful in detecting cervical cancer and monitoring the course of cervical

**TABLE 39-13** Nursing Management of the Woman with Cervical, Vulvar, or Vaginal Cancer

| Disease/Therapeutic Modality | Treatment Issues | Psychosocial Concerns |
|---|---|---|
| **Preinvasive disease (CIN, VIN, VAIN) treated by:** | | |
| Local therapies (e.g., laser, cryosurgery, electrocautery, electrosurgery, conization, interferon cream) | Prepare patient by explaining the disease<br>Explain treatment to patient<br><br>Instruct patient in self-care after treatment (no douching, tampons, sexual intercourse for 2–4 weeks)<br>Stress importance of follow-up | Assure patient that CIN, VIN, VAIN are *not* cancer<br>Educate patient on possible complications of the treatment<br>Address patient concerns related to sexual functioning, changes in libido, orgasm, coital frequency, fertility<br>Discuss possibility of treatment failure or recurrence<br>Assess for anxiety, depression, changes in self- or body image |
| **Invasive disease treated by:** | | |
| Surgery | Preoperative testing<br>Operative procedure planned<br>Review bowel preparation procedure<br>Instruct patient in use of incentive spirometer; importance of turning, coughing, deep breathing, abdominal splinting, and use of antiembolic stockings<br>Review need for IV, urinary catheter, colostomy, ileal conduit as indicated<br><br>Stress availability of pain medication<br><br>Stress importance of early ambulation<br><br>Provide wound care postoperatively<br><br>Assess religious and cultural beliefs as related to treatment (e.g., no blood transfusions, avoidance of drugs, dietary restrictions, etc.)<br>Monitor:<br>  Vital signs<br>  Respiratory function<br>  Cardiac function<br>  Circulatory function<br>  Neurological function<br>  Renal function<br>  Fluid and electrolytes<br>Assess:<br>  Nutritional status, lymphedema, skin integrity, hazards of immobility, alteration in sleep and rest patterns<br>Assess for deep vein thrombosis<br>Assess for alteration in sexual functioning | Assess level of understanding<br><br><br>Have patient give a return demonstration as indicated<br><br><br>Begin ostomy teaching preoperatively as indicated and involve family or significant others in teaching sessions<br>Review use of patient-controlled analgesia pump as indicated<br>Explore with patient nonpharmacological pain relief measures<br>Encourage patient to participate in wound care<br>Assess for changes in self- or body image<br>Assess spiritual needs/concerns<br><br><br>Preoperatively assess woman's knowledge of anatomy, physiology, and sexual function<br>Preoperatively assess information on support systems, coping strategies, attitudes about self<br>Assess for anxiety, depression<br>Assess usual coping mechanisms; mutually devise ways to deal with current stress<br><br><br><br><br>Assess preoperative expectations of sexual outcome<br>Assist patient to realize her intrinsic worth and dignity<br>Assess effects of treatment on quality of life<br>Assess psychological effects of loss of reproductive function<br>Assess psychological response to loss of sexually responsive tissue<br>Assist patient to redefine self-concept in ways other than reproduction<br>Initiate a comprehensive counseling approach involving the patient and her sexual partner and make referrals as needed |

**TABLE 39-13** Nursing Management of the Woman with Cervical, Vulvar, or Vaginal Cancer (continued)

| Disease/Therapeutic Modality | Treatment Issues | Psychosocial Concerns |
|---|---|---|
| Radiotherapy | Review treatment procedure (external beam, intracavitary, interstitial, etc.)<br>Review side effects of therapy<br>Assess skin integrity<br>Assess G.I. function<br>Monitor hematologic values<br>Assess for deep vein thrombosis<br>Explain mobility restrictions with intracavitary, interstitial radiotherapy<br>Assess pain related to radiation applicators<br>Assess for placement of radiotherapy applicators<br><br>Assess religious and cultural beliefs as related to treatment (e.g., no blood transfusions, avoidance of drugs, dietary restrictions) | Assess level of understanding<br>Assess information on support systems<br>Encourage patient to express fears, concerns<br>Begin teaching about prevention of vaginal stenosis as indicated<br><br>Encourage diversional activities to relieve boredom<br>Emphasize availability of traditional pain relief measures<br>Explore with patient nonpharmacological pain relief measures (music, T.V., massage, etc.)<br>Assess spiritual needs/concerns<br>Assess for anxiety, depression<br>Assist woman to realize her intrinsic worth and dignity<br>Encourage patient to express concerns related to fertility, sexuality, body/self-image<br>Assess effects of treatment on quality of life<br>Initiate a comprehensive counseling approach involving the patient and her sexual partner and refer as needed |
| Chemotherapy | Explain the treatment to the patient: rationale, name of drug(s), mechanism of action, dose, frequency of administration, nadir, method of administration, side effects<br><br><br><br><br><br><br><br>Assess religious and cultural beliefs as related to treatment (e.g., no blood transfusions, avoidance of drugs, dietary restrictions, etc.) | Assess evidence of learning<br>Address patient concerns about side effects and treatment of side effects<br>Assess emotional status of patient and family<br>Encourage patient to express fears, concerns<br>Assess information on support systems<br>Assess for anxiety, depression, changes in self- or body image<br>Assess usual coping mechanisms; mutually devise ways to deal with current stress<br>Assess effects of treatment on quality of life<br>Assess spiritual needs/concerns |

neoplasia. CA-125 and CA-19.9 were most useful in women with adenocarcinoma. Research has indicated that squamous cell carcinoma (SCC) antigen and CA-125 are useful markers for progression of disease because the markers increased about three months before clinical evidence of disease recurrence.[257] CA-125 is more likely to be elevated in women with adenocarcinoma.

DNA subtyping has been conducted to evaluate HPV-associated lesions and holds promise of enhancing screening for cervical malignancies.[186,258] Antibodies against HPV 16 have been found in the sera of women with cervical cancer. In one study, forty-four percent of SIL lesions (CIN II/III) were found by HPV testing, although cytology was negative. However, 25% of SIL (CIN II/III) lesions were not detected by the HPV tests. The researchers concluded that HPV testing could augment, but not replace current cytologic testing.[259]

Specimens from over 1000 women with cervical cancer from 22 countries were collected in order to determine if the association between genital HPV infection and cervical cancer is consistent worldwide. HPV DNA was detected in 93% of the malignancies. HPV 16 was found most frequently in all countries with the exception of Indonesia where HPV 18 was most common. Less common types of HPV differed by geographic location. The development of vaccines targeted at genital HPVs could help reduce the incidence of cervical cancer worldwide.[198]

## Classification and Staging—Invasive Disease

Cervical cancer is staged clinically, with confirmation obtained from examinations completed with the patient under anesthesia. This allows for a more accurate staging including visualization of the upper vagina and palpation of parametrial and lateral side wall tissues.[186] Evaluation under anesthesia usually occurs at the same time as the planned surgical intervention or when radiation implants are inserted. The clinical stage is not changed if disease recurs. The initial staging is one of the best prognostic indicators. Approximate 5-year survival rates are: stage I,

**TABLE 39-14** FIGO* Staging for Carcinoma of the Cervix Uteri

| Stage | Description |
|---|---|
| 0 | Carcinoma in situ, intraepithelial carcinoma |
| I | The carcinoma is strictly confined to the cervix. |
| IA | Invasive cancer identified only microscopically. All gross lesions even with superficial invasion are Stage IB cancers. Invasion is limited to measured stromal invasion with maximum depth of 5 mm and no wider than 7 mm. |
| IA1 | Measured invasion of stroma no greater than 3 mm in depth and no wider than 7 mm |
| IA2 | Measured invasion of stroma greater than 3 mm and no greater than 5 mm in depth, and no wider than 7mm |
| IB | Clinical lesions confined to the cervix or preclinical lesions greater than Stage IA |
| IB1 | Clinical lesions no greater than 4 cm in size |
| IB2 | Clinical lesions greater than 4 cm in size |
| II | The carcinoma extends beyond the cervix but has not extended to the pelvic wall. The carcinoma involves the vagina but not as far as the lower third. |
| IIA | No obvious parametrial involvement |
| IIB | Obvious parametrial involvement |
| III | The carcinoma has extended to the pelvic wall. On rectal examination, there is no cancer-free space between the tumor and the pelvic wall. The tumor involves the lower third of the vagina. All cases with a hydronephrosis or nonfunctioning kidney are included unless they are known to be due to other causes. |
| IIIA | No extension to the pelvic wall |
| IIIB | Extension to the pelvic wall and/or hydronephrosis or nonfunctioning kidney |
| IV | The carcinoma has extended beyond the true pelvis or has clinically involved the mucosa of the bladder or rectum. A bullous edema as such does not permit a case to be allotted to stage IV |
| IVA | Spread of the growth to adjacent organs |
| IVB | Spread to distant organs |

*FIGO, International Federation of Gynecology and Obstetrics, 1995.

80.5%; stage II, 59%; stage III, 33%; and stage IV, 7%.[2,260] Unfortunately when clinical and surgical stage are compared, 30%–40% of cases are understaged.[2]

## Therapeutic Approaches and Nursing Care—Invasive Disease

Once invasive cervical cancer is diagnosed and the stage is established, treatment is based on the woman's age, general medical condition, extent of the cancer, and the presence of any complicating abnormalities. Either surgery or radiation therapy can be used equally effectively for patients with early-stage disease. With either radiotherapy or surgery, the 5-year survival rate for stage I is 85%.[261] Radiotherapy can be used for all individuals, whereas surgery is indicated only for women who are considered good surgical candidates.[186,262] Key components include being treated in an institution with the appropriate personnel and equipment for either type of treatment and multidisciplinary planning.[216] In general, patients with stage IIb to IV are treated with radiotherapy.

### Stage Ia

Stage Ia disease (microinvasive carcinoma) has been divided into Ia1 and Ia2. Stage Ia1 should be treated by TAH or TVH if the patient is healthy and does not desire further childbearing. Conization can be done for those who are poor surgical risks or who wish to preserve fertility, as long as the biopsy margins are free of disease and the patient is followed closely.[216,236,263,264] Intracavitary radiation may also be utilized to treat cervical cancer in this stage.[236,263,264]

Stage Ia2 disease is treated by TAH or TVH if invasion is less than 3 mm and there is no lymphovascular involvement. If the invasion is greater than 3 mm or there is lymphovascular invasion, the disease is managed the same as a Stage Ib. Five-year survival in patients with properly staged Ia cervical cancer is close to 100%.[216,236,261,264] Conservative measures are recommended to treat stage Ia1, but more aggressive measures are indicated for stage Ia2 because of the higher risk of lymphovascular involvement.[265,266]

### Stage Ib and IIa

In 1995 FIGO divided stage Ib into stage Ib1 (lesions no greater than 4 cm in size) and Ib2 (lesions greater than 4 cm in size). The choice of therapy for patients with Stage Ib and IIa disease remains controversial, and the choice of surgery or radiation depends on the gynecologist and radiation oncologist involved as well as the woman's condition and the characteristics of the lesion.

Stage Ib and Stage IIa disease can be treated with radical abdominal hysterectomy and pelvic lymphadenectomy or with definitive radiation, which may include external beam and/or intracavitary insertions.[171,264,267] Cure rates for stage Ib using radiation or surgery are almost identical.[3,186]

Surgery is preferred to radiotherapy by some gynecologic oncologists since ovarian function can be preserved. The vagina usually remains more pliable after surgery than with radiation, the overall treatment time is shorter, and long-term radiation complications to pelvic tissue can be avoided. Using radiation therapy has the advantages of avoiding major intraoperative and postoperative complications, and the patient can receive the therapy as an outpatient.[216]

Patients with bulky disease (barrel-shaped cervix) have a higher incidence of central recurrence, pelvic and paraaortic lymph node metastases, and distant dissemination. An increased dose of radiation to the central pelvis or radical hysterectomy, or both, have been advocated in patients with bulky disease.[216,264] The use of combined radical surgery followed by radiation remains controversial.

### Stage IIb, III, and IVa

Women with stage IIb, III, and IV cervical cancer are usually treated with high doses of external pelvic radiation, with parametrial boosts, intracavitary radiation, or a pelvic exenteration. Radiation doses of 5500 cGy to 6000 cGy to the whole pelvis over 5 to 7 weeks are recommended.[186,261] Interstitial parametrial implants may also be used to supplement standard radiation techniques.[216,264] The 5-year survival rates of patients with stage IIb cancer are 60%–79%, while those with stage III have survival rates of 25%–50%, and those with stage IV have less than 10%.[186,216,268] The advantages of radiation over surgery for advanced disease is that radiation can be given as an outpatient, avoids surgery, and is suitable for women who are poor surgical candidates.[186,216] However, Shingleton and Orr[186] assert that radical surgery for stage IIb disease may offer better cure rates than radiation.

The number of total pelvic exenterations has decreased dramatically in the past twenty years because the incidence of isolated pelvic recurrence has decreased. This procedure is utilized only in a selected group of patients. Candidates for pelvic exenteration include women previously treated with radiation who have recurrent centralized disease not adherent to pelvic sidewalls and not involving lymph nodes. In addition, candidates for exenteration should be psychologically able to adjust to the changes in body function and body image.[186,216,261]

Surgical staging of advanced disease before initiating treatment is advocated in an attempt to gain a more precise evaluation of the extent of the disease.[253,254,269] Arguments for pretreatment laparotomy include the following: (1) the extent of the disease can be ascertained, (2) patients who have disease not curable by radiation may be offered palliative therapy, and (3) those patients most likely to benefit from extended field radiation are identified. Arguments against pretreatment laparotomy are that: (1) surgical staging can cause morbidity and mortality, (2) many patients with para-aortic nodal metastases also have systemic disease not detected by surgery, (3) there is only minimal improvement in net survival, and (4) surviving patients have high morbidity. Some surgeons are using alternative extraperitoneal staging methods to determine extent of disease. One approach involves making a small incision near the umbilicus and outside of the proposed radiation field. This allows sampling of the aortic and/or common ileac nodes, collection of peritoneal fluids for cytology, and palpation of pelvic structures.[186]

At present, chemotherapy alone has not proved useful as initial therapy for women who are at high risk for recurrence, but continues to be investigated. Chemotherapy is usually reserved for patients with recurrent disease or metastasis. Recently, interest in the use of neoadjuvant chemotherapy for advanced squamous cell carcinoma of the cervix has increased. Neoadjuvant chemotherapy is the use of chemotherapeutic agents to shrink tumors prior to surgery or radiotherapy.[270–272] Even though neoadjuvant chemotherapy may make more cervical tumors resectable, cure rates are not improved over definitive radiotherapy used alone.[273]

### Recurrent or persistent disease

Approximately 35% of women with invasive cervical cancer will have recurrent or persistent disease.[3] Therefore, thorough, regular follow-ups after treatment are mandatory and critical to early detection of recurrence.[3] Recurrent cervical cancer is difficult to diagnose. Clinical and cytological evaluation of an irradiated cervix is problematic because the cells and configuration of the cervix are distorted from the radiation. Therefore, histological confirmation of recurrence is essential.

Almost 80% of recurrences manifest within two years after therapy;[186,261] however, the signs and symptoms may be subtle and varied. They may include unexplained weight loss, leg edema (excessive and often unilateral), pelvic or thigh and buttock pain, serosanguinous vaginal discharge, progressive ureteral obstruction, supraclavicular lymph node enlargement (usually of the left side), or cough, hemoptysis, and chest pain. If the woman presents with the triad of weight loss, leg edema, and pelvic pain, the outlook is grim. Evaluation after histological confirmation will usually include chest radiograph, IVP, CBC, and blood chemistries. Some physicians will include a CT scan, lymphangiography or fluoroscopically-directed needle biopsies to evaluate the status of the regional lymph nodes, liver, and kidneys. These procedures have replaced more elaborate operative procedures to provide histological confirmation of recurrence.[3] Tumor recurrence and radiation fibrosis may also be differentiated with fine-needle CT-guided aspiration.[274] This may save the woman unnecessary surgery.

Following surgery or radiotherapy as primary treatment for patients with cervical cancer, about 75% of all recurrences are local (cervix, uterus, vagina, parametrium, and regional lymph nodes). The remaining 25% involve distant metastases to the lung, liver, bone, mediastinal, or supraclavicular lymph nodes.[275]

The prognosis for patients with persistent or recurrent carcinoma of the cervix is dismal. One-year survival rates are 10% to 15%.[3] Survival averages 6 to 10 months once recurrent cervical cancer is diagnosed.[214] The aim of treatment in recurrent disease is palliation because control or cure is rare.

***Surgery*** When cervical cancer recurs centrally following radiotherapy, pelvic exenteration may be considered. Total pelvic exenteration includes radical hysterectomy, pelvic lymph node dissection, and removal of the bladder and rectosigmoid colon. Occasionally, a posterior exenteration (which preserves the bladder) or anterior exenteration (which preserves the rectum) can be performed.[3,186,276] Partial pelvic exenterations are usually not done because the bladder and rectum may have residual radiation effects and are prone to complications.

Because the goal of the surgery is curative, only a small percentage of women with recurrence are candidates for pelvic exenteration. Women with disease outside the pelvis or with the triad of unilateral leg edema, sciatic pain, and ureteral obstruction are not candidates for pelvic exenteration. Obesity, severe medical problems, and advanced age also may be reasons that this surgery is contraindicated.[3,186,261]

Extensive preoperative evaluation must be done to ensure that there is not disease outside the pelvis and that renal function is adequate. Studies usually performed include chest radiography, IVP, blood chemistries, creatinine clearance, CT scan, bone scan, and liver-spleen scan. Some clinicians also order lymphangiography as well as abdominal CT scan to evaluate the regional lymph nodes. If lymphadenopathy is present, a needle aspiration of the nodes may be done. If the aspirate is positive for malignancy, the woman may be spared an unnecessary laparotomy. A blind scalene node biopsy may be recommended to complete the evaluation. Preoperative evaluation of nutritional status is important in this population. Up to 50% of hospitalized patients may exhibit laboratory or clinical evidence of malnutrition. This percentage is generally increased in cancer patients.[186,277,278]

At laparotomy, the entire abdomen and pelvis is explored for metastases. A selective para-aortic lymphadenectomy, bilateral pelvic lymphadenectomy, and biopsies of the pelvic sidewalls are done and sent for frozen section. If any of these is positive, the exenteration is usually aborted because the disease is considered incurable.[3] However, some surgeons support the use of pelvic exenterations in patients with recurrent disease complicated by pelvic lymph node metastases.[269,279]

The use of the end-to-end anastomotic (EEA) stapling device has resulted in patients' not needing a permanent colostomy after pelvic exenteration.[276] The EEA also reduces the risk of anastomotic leaks, fistula formation, and late strictures, and decreases operative time. Permanent colostomy can also be avoided by using a segment of sigmoid colon as a rectal substitute.[280,281]

Immediate postoperative problems include pulmonary embolism, pulmonary edema, cardiovascular accident, hemorrhage, myocardial infarction, sepsis, and small bowel obstruction. Long-term problems include fistula formation, urinary obstruction, infection, and sepsis. The use of pelvic exenteration had been limited to a highly select group of candidates, since reports indicate a 5-year survival of 23%–50% and an operative mortality of approximately 9.8%.[186,216] In studying 104 women undergoing pelvic exenteration, Torres-Lobaton et al[279] found that women under 35 years of age had a better prognosis when compared to those over 35 years. Psy-

chosexual and social rehabilitation of surviving patients is a major challenge.[186,269,282,283] Vaginal reconstruction at the time of exenteration and psychological support in the postoperative period can help patients adjust.

*Radiotherapy* In previously irradiated individuals, metastatic disease outside the initial radiation field may be treated cautiously with radiation to provide local control and relieve symptoms. In selected cases, radiation within previously treated areas may be used.[3,216] For women treated initially with surgery, full-dose radiotherapy using a combination of external and intracavitary implants may afford excellent palliation or even cure.[216]

Intraoperative radiation therapy given concomitantly with extensive surgical dissection was performed on 22 women with recurrent cervical cancer. The 5-year survival and local control rates were 43% and 48%. The researchers suggested that intraoperative radiation therapy could be beneficial in selected cases of recurrent cervical cancer involving the pelvic wall.[284] Other approaches that are being studied in conjunction with radiotherapy are hyperthermia,[185,285] hyperbaric oxygen,[286] and photodynamic therapy.[287]

*Chemotherapy* In general, surgery or radiation will not be curative in women who have recurrent cervical cancer. Thus, chemotherapy may be the only hope for cure in these cases.[186,216,288] Chemotherapy for patients with cervical carcinoma is complicated because these patients frequently have decreased pelvic vascular perfusion, a limited bone marrow reserve, and poor renal function related to previous radiation or surgery, and ureteral obstruction from tumor or scarring.[2,3,36]

Response rates for patients with recurrent cervical cancer treated with single-agent and investigational chemotherapy[216,289] range from 0% to 48%, with most less than 20% (Table 39-15). In general, there is no long-term benefit, with responses lasting four to eight months with variable lengths of survival.[3,186,288] Response rates are higher in patients who have received no prior radiotherapy or chemotherapy. Documented activity has been shown for doxorubicin dibromoducitol, ifosfamide, CHIP (iproplatin), doxorubicin, vincristine, and carboplatin.[186,262,288,290,291] Of the single agents, cisplatin remains the drug with the greatest antineoplastic activity although carboplatin may be used as first-line treatment as well.[186,262,290,291] Even so, objective response rates with cisplatin only range between 17%–30% and provide no increase in survival time for patients.

Combination chemotherapy has not been proven more effective than single agents. Higher response rates may be achieved with combination therapy, but survival is not affected.[292,293] The drugs most commonly used are bleomycin, 5-FU, mitomycin C, methotrexate, cyclophosphamide, doxorubicin, and cisplatinum. Complete response rates of up to 36% suggest some enhancement of effect using a combination of drugs. However, median survival rates range between 4–10.5 months.[186] Many clinical trials using combination chemotherapy have had rela-

**TABLE 39-15** Single-Drug Therapy for Squamous Cell Carcinoma of the Cervix

| Drug | Prior Therapy | Response (%) | Drug | Prior Therapy | Response (%) |
|---|---|---|---|---|---|
| **ALKYLATING AGENTS** | | | **ANTIMETABOLITES** | | |
| Cyclophosphamide | Mixed | 38/251 (15) | 5-fluorouracil | Mixed | 29/142 (20) |
| Chlorambucil | Mixed | 11/44 (25) | 5-fludarabine phosphate | Mixed | 7/34 (21) |
| Melphalan | Mixed | 4/20 (20) | 5-fludarabine phosphate | Mixed | 0/20 (0) |
| Ifosfamide | No | 7/46 (15) | Methotrexate | Mixed | 17/96 (18) |
| Ifosfamide | Yes | 3/27 (11) | 6-mercaptopurine | Mixed | 1/18 (5) |
| Ifosfamide | Mixed | 25/84 (29) | Dichloromethotrexate | No | 3/37 (8) |
| Dibromodulcitol | No | 16/55 (29) | Baker's antifol | Mixed | 5/32 (16) |
| Dibromodulcitol | No | 7/47 (15) | Trimetrexate | Yes | 0/27 (0) |
| Galactitol | Mixed | 7/36 (19) | | | |
| Semustine | Mixed | 7/94 (7) | **PLANT AKLALOIDS** | | |
| Lomustine | Mixed | 3/63 (5) | | | |
| Yoshi 864 | Yes | 0/18 (0) | Etoposide | Mixed | 0/31 (0) |
| | | | Teniposide | Yes | 3/22 (14) |
| **HEAVY METAL COMPLEXES** | | | Vincristine | Mixed | 10/55 (18) |
| | | | Vinblastine | Yes | 0/33 (0) |
| Cisplatin | No | 182/785 (23) | Vinblastine | Mixed | 5/21 (24) |
| Cisplatin | Yes | 8/30 (27) | Vinblastine | Yes | 0/33 (0) |
| Carboplatin | No | 27/175 (15) | Vindesine | Mixed | 5/21 (24) |
| Iproplatin | No | 19/177 (11) | Maytansine | Yes | 1/29 (3) |
| | | | | | |
| | | | **OTHER AGENTS** | | |
| **ANTIBIOTICS** | | | | | |
| | | | Hydroxyurea | Mixed | 0/14 (0) |
| Doxorubicin | No | 12/61 (20) | ICRF-159 | Mixed | 5/28 (18) |
| Doxorubicin | Mixed | 33/205 (16) | Aminothiadiazole | Yes | 1/21 (5) |
| Mitoxantrone | Yes | 2/26 (8) | AMSA | Yes | 1/25 (4) |
| Epirubicin | Mixed | 5/27 (18) | PALA | Yes | 0/36 (0) |
| Epirubicin | Mixed | 18/38 (48) | Diaziquone | Yes | 1/26 (4) |
| Esorubicin | Yes | 0/28 (0) | N-methylformamide | Yes | 0/20 (0) |
| Menogaril | Yes | 0/14 (0) | Spriogermanium | Yes | 0/18 (0) |
| Piperazinedion | No | 5/38 (13) | Hexamethylmelamine | No | 12/64 (19) |
| Echinomycin | Yes | 2/28 (7) | Didemnin B | Mixed | 0/24 (0) |
| Porfiromycin | No | 17/78 (22) | Didemnin | Mixed | 0/16 (0) |
| | | | Amonafide | Yes | 0/15 (0) |
| | | | CPT-11 | Mixed | 13/55 (25) |

Shingleton HM and Orr JW: Cancer of the Cervix. Philadelphia, Lippincott, 1995, p 301.

tively small sample sizes, making it difficult to determine their usefulness in treating advanced cervical cancer.[3,186,293–296] Pelvic intra-arterial chemotherapy using a variety of drugs (e.g., cisplatin FUDR and cisplatin; and adriamycin, cisplatin, and bleomycin) in conjunction with radiation therapy or radical surgery has been studied in advanced cervical cancer. While some results have been promising, further investigation is warranted to define its role in treating cervical cancer.[297–300]

In treating 54 patients with stage Ib and II bulky disease, Kim et al[301,302] used a regimen of vinblastine, bleomycin, and cisplatin followed by radical hysterectomy and found that it was effective in reducing tumor volume, the stage of disease, and lymph node involvement and in improving the 2-year survival rate. In a phase II study of 14 women diagnosed with advanced or recurrent cervical cancer, Kredentser et al[303] utilized etoposide (VP-16), ifosfamide/MESNA, and cisplatin. They found an overall response rate in eight of the 14 patients (57%) and three were disease free up to 24 months posttreatment.

Chemotherapy can be used as a radiation sensitizer, particularly hydroxyurea.[186,264,304,305] This approach may be most useful in women who have large hypoxic tumors confined to the pelvis.[186] Several studies have shown improved survival rates from the concurrent administration of radiation and hydroxyurea.[304,306] Results have also indicated that patients experienced an increased incidence of hematologic toxicity with hydroxyurea. Weekly low-dose cisplatin with radiation has been associated with a modest improvement is disease-free survival without any significant increases in toxicity.[216] Kuske et al[307] utilized cisplatin and 5-FU as radiosensitizers and reported that 52% of patients in the study were disease free one to three years after treatment, while 39% experienced pelvic recurrence. Thigpen et al[291] advocated the use of radiation plus a combination of cisplatin and 5-FU over radiation alone in advanced or recurrent disease to increase progression-free interval and survival. A recent study found that paclitaxel (Taxol) acted as a modest radiosensitizer in human cervical cancer in vitro.[308] Additional studies need to be conducted to explore this. Other agents used as radiosensitizers are SR2508, RO 03-8700 (pimonidazole), misonidazole, and biologic modifiers such as LC9018 sizofiran and interferon.[186]

A recent Phase I study[309] utilized methoxymorpholinyldoxorubicin, an analogue of doxorubicin, in 53 patients with refractory solid tumors. One patient with cervical cancer had a complete response. No cardiotoxicity was noted in this sample. Current research involves the use of second-generation topoisomerase I inhibitors, irinotecan (CPT-11) and topotecan, and the taxanes, Taxol and Taxotere.

The use of chemoradiotherapy in the treatment of cervical cancer has been reported recently in the literature. Lin et al[310] completed a study of 22 women with IIb and IIIb cervical cancer who were treated with etoposide, cisplatin, and bleomycin in conjunction with external radiotherapy and intracavitary brachytherapy. Twenty-one women had a complete response which lasted during the median 12 month follow-up. A second study to confirm the benefits of this approach is underway. Thirty-five women with stage Ib, IIb, and II-IVa were treated with chemoradiation followed by colpohysterectomy with lymphadenectomy or pelvic exenteration. Two-year survival rates were reported to be 61% and 66% for stage Ib-IIb and 77% and 65% for stage III-IVa. Additional research is recommended to confirm these results.[311] In treating 17 women with advanced cervical cancer, Morris et al[312] administered simultaneous chemoradiotherapy with carboplatin. Seventy-six percent of the sample achieved a complete remission.

Initial treatment of cervical cancer with chemotherapy is generating increased interest. Vogl[313] proposed its use in tumor debulking, spatial restoration, as a radiation sensitizer, and as adjuvant therapy. Because radiotherapy works better on a smaller tumor volume, induction chemotherapy may debulk the tumor before other therapies are started. This might reduce the incidence of pelvic recurrence. Studies continue to support the use of chemotherapy in the initial treatment of cervical cancer.[294,295,314,315] Other recent studies have evaluated the efficacy of new protocols utilizing combination chemotherapy,[271,316] chemoradiation and surgery,[311] chemotherapy and radiation,[317–319] and surgery and radiation.[320–322]

Chemotherapy has not been shown to be useful as adjuvant therapy after definitive treatment in high-risk women (e.g., women with positive nodes, bulky lesions, or adenocarcinomas). A recent research study described the use of epirubicin and cisplatin followed by pelvic radiation in 260 women with stage IIb and IVb cervical cancer. For women with bulky disease, treatment results with radiation have been disappointing. It was hoped that the administration of chemotherapy prior to radiation might increase local control and survival as compared to the use of radiation alone. Results indicated a significant tumor response, but local control of disease and overall survival were not improved.[323]

*Biologic response modifiers*   One group of researchers reported a case study of a woman with recurrent cervical cancer treated with tumor infiltrating lymphocytes, tumor necrosis factor, and radiation. The tumor decreased markedly in size and the condition of the woman improved. They believe that antitumor biological therapies have the potential to be effective agents in the treatment of cervical malignancies.[324]

***Complications of surgery***   Radical hysterectomy involves removal of the uterus, upper third of the vagina, entire uterosacral and uterovesical ligaments, all of the parametria and pelvic node lymphadenectomy. This is a complex procedure because the organs removed are proximal to many vital body structures: the bladder, ureters, rectum, and great vessels of the pelvis.[171,186,233,261] The major complications of radical hysterectomy include ureteral fistulas, bladder dysfunction, pulmonary embolus, lymphocysts, pelvic infection, bowel obstruction, rectovaginal fistulas, and hemorrhage.[233,268]

***Complications of radiotherapy***   Morbidity resulting from properly administered radiotherapy in cervical cancer is usually manageable. There are reported adverse reactions when poor technique is used, but these reactions occur infrequently in properly treated women. The higher the dose of radiation, the greater the rate of complications. Some morbidity attributed to radiation is secondary to uncontrolled tumor or compounded effects of multiple therapies and not a direct result of radiation alone. Major complication rates for stage I and IIa disease range from 3% to 5%, respectively, and are 10% to 15%, respectively, for patients with stage IIb and III disease.[264,325,326]

The major complications related to radiotherapy include vaginal stenosis, fistula formation, sigmoid perforation or stricture, uterine perforation, rectal ulcer or proctitis, intestinal obstruction, fistulas, ureteral stricture, severe cystitis, pelvic hemorrhage, and pelvic abscess. Other problems related to radiation therapy include nausea, vomiting, diarrhea, and rarely, radiation myelitis.

Sexual dysfunction secondary to vaginal atrophy, stenosis, and lack of lubrication is a known effect of the radiation therapy. Radiation causes thinning of the vaginal epithelium and the vagina may become shortened, less flexible, and partially obliterated. Vaginal intercourse may cause dyspareunia and bleeding.[186,327] Women who are not sexually active experience greater incidence of atrophy and stenosis than do sexually active women. The use of vaginal dilators and water soluble lubricants can minimize the radiation effects.

***Complications of chemotherapy***   The complications of chemotherapy may manifest themselves in any organ system and depend on the agent, dose, and route utilized. In addition, chemotherapy may adversely affect psychological, emotional, and psychosocial aspects of the cancer patient's life. The reader is referred to the chapters on chemotherapy in this text for in-depth information related to these issues.

## Continuity of Care: Nursing Challenges

Although mortality rates for cervical cancer have decreased over the past 40 years, the rates among nonwhites and Hispanics are higher than those among whites due to decreased utilization of screening methods by women in these populations.[328–334] Access to cervical cancer screening for blacks, Hispanics, older women of all races, and those who are economically disadvantaged should be a priority for health care professionals. Several researchers have undertaken creative approaches to increase cervical cancer screening for underserved groups including a church-based model,[335] use of nurse practitioners,[336] a nurse-delivered program to reduce barriers,[337] and in-home educational interventions.[337] In summary, nurses are in a unique position to educate women about the risks and benefits of cancer screening. It is through repeated, creative interventions with patients and their families that nurses can have an impact on the morbidity and mortality of cervical cancer.

Given the complexity of treatment modalities provided in the hospital environment, outpatient setting, and in the home, continuity of care across health care settings should be a priority for all women with gynecologic malignancies. In addition, prevention and/or control of side effects secondary to treatment are vital to maintaining patient quality of life during treatment. Table 39-13 summarizes issues related to the nursing management of women with malignancies of the lower genital tract.

# VULVAR CANCER

## Epidemiology

Vulvar carcinoma accounts for 3%–4% of all gynecologic cancers. It is a disease of elderly women, with peak incidence occurring in the seventh decade of life. Vulvar cancer rarely occurs in women under 40 years of age.[26,339,340] Vulvar cancer is categorized as either VIN or invasive. Vulvar intraepithelial neoplasia (VIN) is a term that describes epithelial abnormalities of the vulva. VIN is divided into categories I, II, or III that differentiate the degree of epithelial involvement by neoplastic cells.[341] Although the incidence of VIN has dramatically increased during the most recent decades, the incidence of invasive vulvar carcinoma has remained stable. Most commonly, VIN is seen in postmenopausal women in their fifties and sixties, but it can develop at any age. The frequency of VIN appears to be increasing among younger women.[3,342]

## Etiology

The etiology of VIN and invasive vulvar cancer is largely unknown. Even the relationship of VIN to invasive disease remains unclear. The human papillomavirus (HPV), particularly HPV type 16, is associated with VIN and invasive vulvar cancer. HPV has been found in 50%–80% of VIN III lesions. However, HPV is present in only 15% of vulvar carcinomas that are not associated with VIN III. For this reason, the relationship between HPV, VIN, and vulvar cancer remains unclear.[343–345] Recently, studies have identified risk factors for vulvar cancer: multiple sexual partners, venereal warts, and cigarette smoking.[345,346] Herpes simplex type 2 has been identified as a risk factor for vulvar cancer.[347] A history of chronic vulvar disease and previous malignancies of the lower genital tract are also seen in women with vulvar cancer. In addition, a history of breast, cervical, or endometrial malignancy is associated with invasive vulvar carcinoma[348] (Table 39-16).

## Pathophysiology

### Cellular characteristics

VIN commonly presents in a multifocal pattern. Discoloration of the vulva with white, gray, red, or brown lesions is usual. The lesions may be macular or papular and often present with a roughened surface.[240] Histologically, squamous cell cancer accounts for about 90% of vulvar malignancies. The remaining 10% include malignant melanoma, basal cell, Pagets, Bartholins gland, adenocarcinoma, and sarcoma.[240,341]

### Progression of disease

VIN is divided into three categories: VIN I, VIN II, and VIN III. The term VIN I is used to describe mild dysplasia. VIN II describes moderate dysplasia. VIN III, or carcinoma in situ (CIS), describes severe dysplasia and suggests full thickness changes of the epithelium. VIN III of the vulva does not appear to have the same malignant

**TABLE 39-16** Clinical Features of the Patient with Vulvar Cancer

| |
|---|
| Advanced age (>60 years) |
| Chronic vulvar disease |
| Previous malignancy of lower genital tract |
| History of breast cancer |
| HPV |
| HSV2 |
| Chronic irritation |
| Exposure to coal tar derivatives |

HPV = human papillomavirus; HSV2 = herpes simplex virus type 2.

potential as CIN III of the cervix. VIN III/CIS of the vulva is most likely to progress to invasive disease if the patient is elderly or immunosuppressed.[240]

### Patterns of spread

Although primary disease can develop anywhere on the vulva, the labia are the most common sites, followed by the clitoris. The lesions occur three times more frequently on the labia majora than on the labia minora.[349] Vulvar cancer usually remains a localized disease with well-defined margins.

The most common routes of metastatic spread are through direct extension and lymphatic dissemination to regional lymph nodes. Metastatic lesions spread predictably to the inguinal lymph nodes, followed by spread to the pelvic nodes. The overall incidence of positive lymph nodes is 46% in patients with vulvar cancer. Inguinal node metastases can occur in 35%–40% of patients, and the incidence of pelvic node metastases is 5%–10%. With the possible exception of vulvar melanoma, vulvar cancer does not usually spread by the blood stream to distant sites.[349]

## Clinical Manifestations

The symptoms of VIN and invasive vulvar carcinoma are variable and insidious. In VIN, 50% of women are asymp-tomatic whereas others may complain of vulvar pruritus or burning (vulvodynia).[350] Up to 20% percent of women with vulvar cancer are asymptomatic, with lesions detected only during routine pelvic examination. The most common complaint is the presence of a mass or growth in the vulvar area. Other symptoms include vulvar bleeding and pain.[351]

Delay in diagnosing the woman with vulvar cancer may occur because she may be too embarrassed to seek medical assistance due to the intimate area of the body that is involved. As result a woman may have symptoms for 2 to 16 months before seeking medical attention.[352] Another reason for a delay in definitive treatment may be that symptomatic topical treatment for vulvar lesions may continue for up to 12 months or longer before being biopsied for definitive diagnosis.[3,353] Most recent studies report smaller lesions being diagnosed and treated, which may suggest that patients with vulvar cancer are being biopsied earlier.

## Assessment—VIN

Careful inspection of the vulva during routine gynecologic examination is imperative. This remains the most productive diagnostic measure. The entire vulva, perineum, and perianal area should be evaluated. A 1% toluidine blue solution can be used to stain suspicious areas but this technique has a high false-positive rate. The diag-

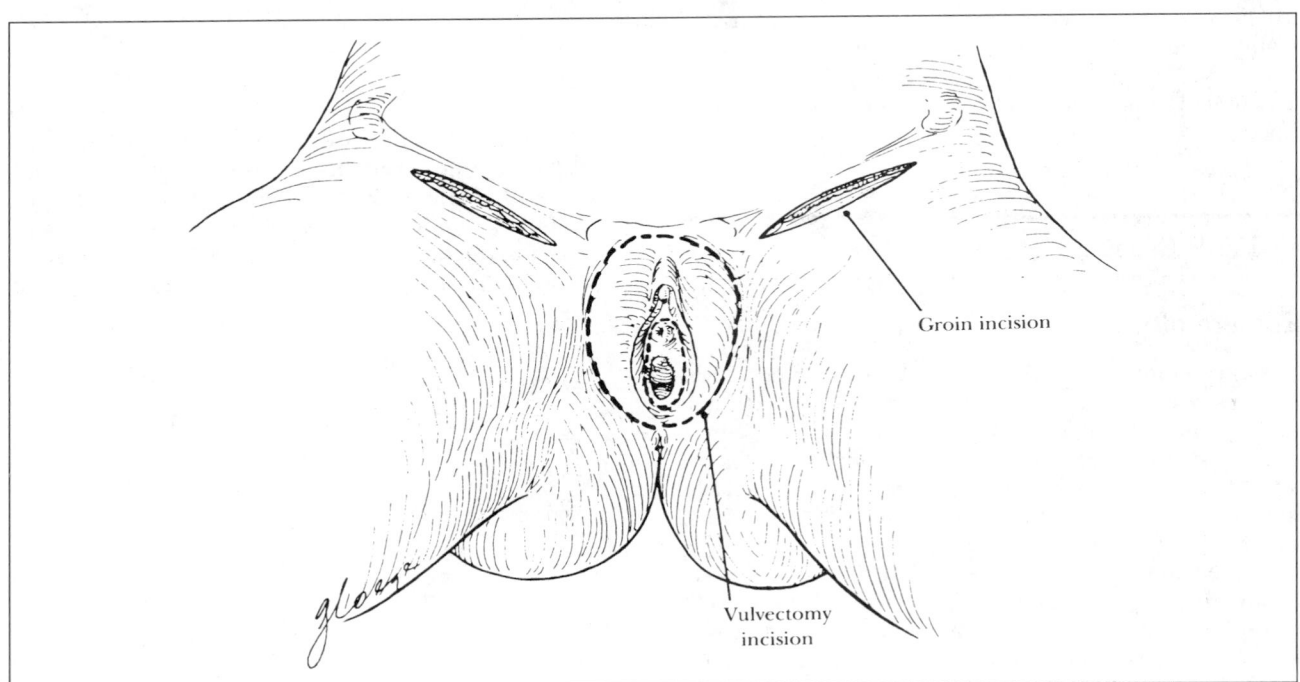

**FIGURE 39-8**  Skin incision for groin dissection through a separate incision. A line is drawn 1 cm below and parallel to the groin crease and a narrow ellipse of skin is removed. (Hacker NF: Vulvar cancer, in Berek JS, Hacker NF (eds): *Practical Gynecologic Oncology.* Baltimore, Williams & Wilkins, 1989, p 404. © 1989, the Williams & Wilkins Co., Baltimore, MD.)

nosis of VIN can be subtle. To avoid delay, multiple vulvar biopsies should be done if lesions are noted.[3]

## Therapeutic Approaches and Nursing Care—VIN

Some controversy exists about the treatment of choice for patients with VIN. Current treatment is a wide local excision followed by primary-closure skin flaps or skin graft to restore normal anatomy. This surgical procedure successfully controls the disease with recurrence rates of only 9%–12%.[354,355] For multicentric disease, a skinning vulvectomy (Figure 39-8)[3] is performed in which the vulvar skin is excised while conserving the fat, muscle, and glands below the skin. A split thickness skin graft reconstruction from the thigh or buttock is performed. The wide local excision and skinning vulvectomy provides excellent cosmetic and functional results.[3,26] A skinning vulvectomy may not be an option for elderly women since the healing of the skin graft after a skinning vulvectomy requires prolonged bed rest.

An alternative to excision of the vulvar lesion is to treat it locally with cautery, laser surgery, or cryosurgery. The advantages of these surgical techniques are outpatient management, sparing effect on surrounding tissue, and minimal scarring. However, the procedures can result in painful ulcers and require several sequenced treatments.[356,357] Topical 5% 5-FU may be used for VIN. However, this requires daily applications and can produce painful, slow healing ulcers.

### Continuity of care: Nursing challenges

For women with VIN, education is an essential responsibility of nursing. Explaining the difference between VIN and invasive cancer is key. The nurse can help women understand the type of treatment recommended. Follow-up care by the nurse includes teaching the woman how to care for herself at home. When sexual intercourse is resumed, in approximately four to six weeks, a water soluble lubricant can be used. Sexual satisfaction is possible and nurses can mutually explore with the woman methods to maintain sexual activity. Close follow-up should be stressed. Table 39-13 summarizes issues specifically related to the nursing management of women diagnosed with cervical, vulvar, or vaginal cancer.

## Assessment—Invasive Disease

Vulvar cancer is diagnosed by local excisional biopsy of the lesions. Colposcopy is useful for defining areas to biopsy. Pap smear of the cervix is essential since 10% of women with vulvar neoplasia also have cervical SIL or invasive cancer. Examination under anesthesia may be needed to fully evaluate the cervix, vagina, and pelvis. Careful physical examination with attention to the inguinal lymph nodes is mandatory. Metastatic evaluation includes chest radiograph, proctosigmoidoscopy, cystoscopy, barium enema, IVP, and biochemical profile. Computerized axial tomography or MRI of the pelvis may help to evaluate retroperitoneal nodal areas.[3,26]

## Classification and Staging

An International Federation of Gynecology and Obstetrics (FIGO) staging system for vulvar cancer was adopted in 1988 (Table 39-17). The 5-year survival rate for vulvar cancer can be correlated with stage and nodal involvement. Overall 5-year survival rate is between 70%–75% for all stages. For patients with stage I and II disease, the survival rate is 85%–90%; and for those with stage III disease 51%–74%. Stage IV disease carries a poor prognosis of only 18%–30%.[358] Groin lymph node status is the best indicator of survival in patients with vulvar carcinomas. Regardless of stage, if negative lymph nodes are

**TABLE 39-17** FIGO* Staging of Vulvar Cancer

| TNM | Stage | Description |
|---|---|---|
| T1 N0 M0 | I | Tumor confined to vulva or perineum, 2 cm or less in diameter |
| T2 N0 M0 | II | Tumor confined to vulva or perineum, more than 2 cm in greatest dimension |
| T3 N0 M0<br>T3 N1 M0<br>T1 N1 M0<br>T2 N1 M0 | III | Tumor of any size that spread to (1) any of the following: lower urethra, vagina, anus, and/or (2) unilateral regional lymph metastasis |
| T1 N2 M0<br>T2 N2 M0<br>T3 N2 M0<br>T4 any N M0 | IVa | Tumor invades any of the following: upper urethra, bladder or rectal mucosa, pelvic bone and/or bilateral regional lymph node metastasis |
| Any T any N M1 | IVb | Tumor of any size, location with distant metastasis |

*FIGO = International Federation of Gynecology and Obstetrics.
FIGO News: *Int J Gynecol Obstet* 28:189–193, 1989.

present, there is about a 95% survival rate, which decreases to 65% if positive nodes are present.[359,360]

## Therapeutic Approaches and Nursing Care—Invasive Disease

### Surgery

The traditional treatment for women with cancer of the vulva has been surgical: *en bloc* dissection of the tumor and contiguous skin, subcutaneous fat, regional inguinal and femoral nodes, and vulva (labia minora, labia majora, clitoris, and perineal body). Some physicians recommend routine pelvic node dissection also be done. Many surgeons have abandoned the *en bloc* approach and are now performing the nodal dissections through separate groin incisions (see Figure 39-8). In addition, pelvic node dissection is reserved for women with positive groin nodes or large lesions.[361,362] The trend has been away from radical surgery that has been associated with disturbances in sexual function and body image. Recently, there is more emphasis on individualized treatment of the patient, taking into account age, location of disease, extent of disease, and psychosocial consequences.[363,364]

Stage I carcinomas of the vulva are treated with modified radical vulvectomy or hemivulvectomy with ipsilateral inguinofemoral lymphadenectomy. For patients with midline lesions, bilateral node dissections are performed.[2,26,27]

Stage II lesions may require more extensive surgery. This usually involves a radical vulvectomy and bilateral inguinal femoral lymphadenectomy.[361] With stage III disease, the tumor has spread to the urethra, vagina, anus, or to the lymph nodes in the inguinal area. For stage III patients, radical vulvectomy often involves removal of a portion of the distal urethra or vagina and may require excision of a portion of the anus. If the inguinal nodes contain cancer, patients usually undergo postoperative pelvic irradiation.[26,356,365] Patients with stage IV disease may require pelvic exenteration in addition to radical vulvectomy if the bladder or rectum is involved. If the tumor is fixed to the bone or distant metastases have occurred, treatment is usually palliative and mainly consists of radiotherapy.[366]

The major immediate complication after radical surgery is groin wound infection, necrosis, and breakdown. With the use of separate incision approach for nodal resection, the incidence of wound breakdown decreased to about 44%. Major wound breakdown occurs in about 14% of patients. With the *en bloc* operation, wound breakdown was reported to be as high as 85%. Other postoperative complications include urinary tract infection, deep venous thrombosis, and pulmonary embolism[358] (see Table 39-18).

The major late complication of radical surgery is chronic leg edema which has been reported to occur in up to 30% of patients. The use of elastic stockings is recommended for 12 months after surgery to allow development of collateral pathways for lymph drainage. Recur-

**TABLE 39-18**  Reported Complications After Radical Surgery for Vulvar Cancer

| Complication | Percentage of All Cases |
|---|---|
| Wound breakdown or infection | 54% |
| Chronic leg edema | 30% |
| Lymphocyst | 10% |
| Genital prolapse | 7% |
| Stress incontinence | 5% |
| Thrombophlebitis | 3.5% |
| Grafting of skin flaps | 1.7% |
| Hernia (femoral, inguinal) | 1.5% |
| Pulmonary embolus | 1.2% |
| Ruptured femoral artery | 1.9% |
| Hospital deaths | 3.3% |

Adapted from Morrow CP, Townsend DE (eds): *Synopsis of Gynecologic Oncology* (ed 3). New York, Wiley, 1987, pp 57–89.

rent cellulitis of the leg, urinary stress incontinence, and genital prolapse may also occur.

### Radiation

The role of radiation therapy in the management of carcinoma of the vulva is still evolving. Radiation therapy is being used more often in combination with surgery. Patients who have undergone a resection of the primary lesion and are considered at high risk for recurrence due to inadequate resection margins or positive nodes may be good candidates for postoperative irradiation. Postoperative irradiation should consist of at least 4500–5000 cGy. Higher doses of irradiation (6000–7000 cGy) can be given to known areas of gross residual tumor. Other treatment approaches include preoperative radiation for patients with advanced disease and radiation as primary therapy for patients with small primary tumor or unresectable primary tumor.[3,26,367]

Patients who receive external radiation to the vulva can develop severe erythema and swelling. Maintaining skin integrity and management of pain and discomfort is the aim of nursing care. Radiation cystitis may also occur with radiation treatment in the pelvis. The patient should be encouraged to increase fluid intake and be referred for medical evaluation.[368]

### Chemotherapy

To date, chemotherapy has not been effective in the treatment of vulvar cancer. The use of concurrent radiation and chemotherapy for initial therapy is being studied. Hopefully, this will allow a more conservative approach to surgery. Chemoradiation also appears to enhance locoregional control in recurrent or advanced disease.[369,370] Further research needs to be done in order to fully define and develop the use of chemotherapy in the treatment of vulvar cancer.

About 80% of recurrences will develop within the first two years after initial treatment, which demands initial close follow-up. Patients with less than three positive nodes generally have a low incidence of recurrence, while high recurrence rates are correlated with patients who have more than three positive nodes.[359,366] Over half of the recurrences are local and in close proximity to the original lesion. In many instances, local recurrences can be successfully treated using wide local excision with adequate tumor-free margins. Radiation therapy also may be used in conjunction with surgery.[3] Distant recurrences are difficult to treat, with an 8% survival rate at five years. A combination of radiation and chemotherapy may be used as a palliative measure in metastatic disease.[370]

## Continuity of Care: Nursing Challenges

Because cancer of the vulva primarily affects elderly women and as a result of the radical surgery involved, coordination of care from hospital to home is essential. The patient may face problems such as chronic leg edema, urinary difficulties, and wound infection. Nurses in all settings can assist patients in dealing with the physical, psychological, and social implications of a radical vulvectomy. Sexual satisfaction is low among postvulvectomy patients. Nurses can help with open discussions about sexual concerns with the patient and her partner. Approaches for helping the woman with issues of sexuality are covered in chapter 28.

# VAGINAL CANCER

## Epidemiology

Carcinoma of the vagina, a rare malignancy, accounts for 1%–2% of gynecologic malignancies.[26,371,372] Usually, the vagina is a secondary site of malignant dissemination from primary cancers of the cervix or other sites.[368,372] The peak incidence of squamous carcinoma of the vagina, the most common cell type, occurs in women between 50 and 70 years of age. In contrast, the peak incidence for clear cell adenocarcinoma of the vagina occurs in women aged 18–19.

Vaginal intraepithelial neoplasia (VAIN) is much less common than cervical (CIN) (SIL) or vaginal (VIN). However, the incidence of VAIN is climbing and the mean age at diagnosis is decreasing.[240,373] VAIN is usually seen in women who have been treated for CIN (SIL) or after radiotherapy for invasive cervical cancer. Up to 30% of patients with primary vaginal carcinoma have a history of in situ or invasive cervical cancer treated at least five years earlier.[372,374] VAIN is divided into three categories (I, II, III) with each higher number indicative of increasing epithelial involvement. Unlike CIN (SIL), VAIN is generally multifocal in nature.[3]

## Etiology

Incidence of squamous cell cancer of the vagina increases with age. Rates are higher in the black population and persons of low socioeconomic level. Other related risk factors include a history of HPV, vaginal trauma (douching with preparations other than water or vinegar), previous abdominal hysterectomies for benign disease, and absence of regular PAP smears. Prior radiation therapy may also be a predisposing factor in primary vaginal carcinoma.[375] This may be particularly important in young patients who live long enough to develop a second neoplasm in the irradiated vagina.

Like squamous cell carcinoma of the vagina, adenocarcinoma is usually a disease of older women. However, since 1971 the study of adenocarcinoma of the vagina has focused on young women who were exposed to diethylstilbestrol (DES) in utero and who seemed to have an unusual incidence of vaginal cancer. DES was used in the management of diabetic pregnancies, threatened abortion, habitual abortion, and other high-risk obstetric problems. From the late 1940s to 1970, an estimated 2 million pregnant women received DES.[376] The risk of developing vaginal cancer in women exposed to DES in utero is about 1 in 1000. Of greater risk is the development of cervicovaginal dysplasia, which has been estimated to be as high as 18% in this population.[377]

## Pathophysiology

### Cellular characteristics

Squamous cell carcinoma makes up 75%–95% of the cases.[378,379] Other histological types include adenocarcinoma, melanoma, sarcoma, and verrucous carcinoma.[341,373,375]

### Patterns of spread

Vaginal cancers occur most commonly on the posterior wall of the upper third of the vagina. The second most common site is the anterior wall in the lower one-third of the vagina.[368,372] The tumor may spread along the vaginal wall to involve the cervix or vulva. However, if the cervix is involved, the tumor is considered a primary cervical lesion. Anterior vaginal lesions penetrate into the vesicovaginal septum during early stages. Posterior lesions can invade the rectum, but this is usually in the late stages. The tumor spreads by direct extension into the obturator fossa, cardinal ligaments, lateral pelvic walls, and uterosacral ligament.[26]

The lymphatic drainage of the vagina consists of a vast, interconnecting network that facilitates drainage into any of the local nodal groups regardless of the location of the vaginal lesion. The incidence of lymph node metastasis is directly proportional to the stage of the vaginal cancer. The overall incidence of positive nodes is about 21%. Metastasis to the lungs or supraclavicular nodes in squamous cell carcinoma tends to occur in more advanced stages.[380] However, in clear cell carcinoma, metastasis to the lungs and supraclavicular nodes occurs more frequently.[26]

Extension or metastasis of other malignancies to the vagina occurs more frequently than primary cancer of the vagina. Spread of cervical cancer to the vagina is the most common, but cancers of the endometrium, ovary, urethra, bladder, rectum, and malignant trophoblastic disease may also spread or metastasize to the vaginal area.[3]

## Clinical Manifestations

An abnormal Pap smear is usually the event that initiates the search for a definitive diagnosis because many lesions are asymptomatic. Colposcopic examination is done and biopsies taken. If left untreated, VAIN lesions may spontaneously regress, persist, or progress to vaginal cancer.[381]

The most frequent initial symptoms of invasive vaginal cancer are abnormal vaginal bleeding, foul-smelling discharge, and dysuria. Even in early-stage disease, urinary symptoms are more common when vaginal tumors are in close proximity to the bladder neck and compress the urethra.[3,368]

## Assessment

Clinical diagnosis of a vaginal neoplasm is made by careful visual examination and palpation of the vagina. Pap smear is helpful for squamous carcinoma, but not for adenocarcinoma because it is often subepithelial. Colposcopy is particularly helpful for directed biopsies of abnormal vaginal areas.[26]

Women with invasive vaginal cancer should be investigated in the same manner as those with cervical cancer. All patients should have a history and physical examination, chest radiograph, biochemical profile, IVP, barium enema, cystoscopy, and proctosigmoidoscopy. Optional, but often helpful, are CT, MRI, and lymphangiogram.[26,381]

Colposcopic exam, which allows visualization and determination of location, number, and size of lesions, is essential for planning appropriate therapeutic management.[374] The disease may be then evaluated and staged under anesthesia by the gynecologic oncologist and radiation therapist, and additional vaginal and cervical biopsies taken. Negative biopsies of the cervix are necessary to rule out cervical cancer and confirm the diagnosis of primary vaginal carcinoma.

## Classification and Staging

Vaginal cancer is staged clinically using the staging classification system shown in Table 39-19.[382] The overall 5-year

**TABLE 39-19** Staging Classification for Carcinoma of the Vagina

| PRIMARY TUMOR (T) | | |
|---|---|---|
| TNM | FIGO | Definition |
| TX | | Primary tumor cannot be assessed |
| T0 | | No evidence of primary tumor |
| Tis | 0 | Carcinoma in situ |
| T1 | I | Tumor confined to vagina |
| T2 | II | Tumor invades paravaginal tissues but not to pelvic wall |
| T3 | III | Tumor extends to pelvic wall |
| T4 | IVa | Tumor invades mucosa of bladder or rectum and/or extends beyond the true pelvis |
| M1 | IVb | Distant metastasis |

| LYMPH NODES (N) | |
|---|---|
| NX | Regional lymph nodes cannot be assessed |
| N0 | No regional lymph node metastasis |
| *Upper two-thirds of vagina:* | |
| N1 | Pelvic lymph node metastasis |
| *Lower one-third of vagina:* | |
| N1 | Unilateral inguinal lymph node metastasis |
| N2 | Bilateral inguinal lymph node metastasis |

| DISTANT METASTASIS (M) | | |
|---|---|---|
| TNM | FIGO | Definition |
| MX | | Presence of distant metastasis cannot be assessed |
| M0 | | No distant metastasis |
| M1 | IVb | Distant metastasis |

| STAGE GROUPING | | | |
|---|---|---|---|
| Stage 0 | Tis | N0 | M0 |
| Stage I | T1 | N0 | M0 |
| Stage II | T2 | N0 | M0 |
| Stage III | T1 | N1 | M0 |
| | T2 | N1 | M0 |
| | T3 | N0, N1 | M0 |
| Stage IVA | T1 | N2 | M0 |
| | T2 | N2 | M0 |
| | T3 | N2 | M0 |
| | T4 | Any N | M0 |
| Stage IVB | Any T | Any N | M1 |

Reprinted from *American Joint Committee on Cancer: Manual for Staging of Cancer* (ed 4). Philadelphia, Lippincott, 1992.

survival rate for all stages of squamous vaginal carcinoma is between 40%–50%. The survival rate is 80% for patients with stage I, 48% for those with stage II, 30% for those with stage III, and 6% for those with stage IV.[372,378,381] The 5-year survival rate in patients with adenocarcinoma is 75%. This may be related to the fact that females exposed to DES in utero have been followed closely due to their risk for developing adenocarcinoma, and are often diagnosed early in the disease.[3]

Clinical stage is the most important prognostic indicator in vaginal cancer. A better prognosis is associated with early diagnosis, small tumor burden, and negative nodal involvement. Other prognostic factors include age of the patient, location of the lesion, and differentiation of tumor. Well-differentiated tumors respond better to treatment and overall survival is improved.[381] Eighty percent of women who recur have pelvic recurrences within two years of primary treatment.[26]

## Therapeutic Approaches and Nursing Care—VAIN

Location of the lesion, the size of the lesion, and whether it is a single focus or multiple foci are considered in determining the treatment option.[26] Local excision is appropriate for single lesions or for several lesions clustered in a single portion of the vagina.[26] Surgery for diffuse multiple lesions may result in a shortened or absent vagina.[383]

Local application of 5-FU cream can completely eradicate preinvasive lesions.[373,383,384] Care must be taken to insure direct contact with the entire lesion and to avoid contact with the vulva. Laser therapy can cure between 69% and 80% of patients with vaginal intraepithelial lesions.[373] The use of radiation therapy is rarely indicated. However, for some patients who are poor surgical candidates, irradiation of the vagina using intracavitary and interstitial sources alone produced excellent response rates.[385]

## Therapeutic Approaches and Nursing Care—Invasive Disease

The anatomic position of the vagina, located between the urethra and bladder anteriorly and the rectum posteriorly, is the predominant factor in treatment planning. Radiotherapy is the treatment of choice for most invasive vaginal cancers, especially for patients with stage I and II disease.[3,381] Small lesions may be treated with local irradiation while larger lesions can require both local and regional treatment. In general, radiation treatment provides good control of tumor with limited morbidity.[381,386] In stages III and IVA results with radiation therapy decrease to only 25%–30% survival rates.[26]

If the tumor is adenocarcinoma, surgery may be used in stage I. A radical hysterectomy and vaginectomy with radical lymph node dissection is performed.[387] All other stages of adenocarcinoma can be treated with radiation therapy.

Lesions of any cell type that fail to respond to radiation can be treated effectively with surgery. Depending on the extent of disease, surgery for recurrence may range from wide local excision to total pelvic exenteration.[388] With advanced disease in older women, surgery is often impossible if adjacent structures have been invaded and disease is too extensive.[366] In these cases, radiation may be the best treatment option.

For women receiving radiation therapy to the vagina, vaginal fibrosis and scarring with a loss of blood supply and elasticity is a major adverse effect. Frequent intercourse can minimize these effects. For patients who are not sexually active, the use of a vaginal dilator with water soluble lubricants or prescribed estrogen cream starting two weeks after treatment are effective prophylactic measures to minimize functional loss.[368]

For women who had a reconstructed vagina, sexual intercourse or the use of vaginal dilators is also encouraged because the neovagina can be narrow. Open communication between the nurse and the patient about sexual concerns is essential. Sexual satisfaction can be achieved for women posttreatment for cancer of the vagina. See chapter 28 for additional information.

## Continuity of Care: Nursing Challenges

Women with cancer of the vagina face physical and emotional challenges. Nurses in all settings should address with each woman changes in body image, alteration in sexuality, and coping mechanisms. Coordination of care from the hospital, to outpatient, to home care is key in helping women with vaginal cancer meet these challenges.

## CONCLUSION

Gynecologic cancer represents about 13% of all cancers in women and results in 10% of all female cancer deaths.[1] The potential for cure is enhanced when the disease is diagnosed in early stages. Only cervical cancer has an effective screening method for early detection. Continued research is essential in order to identify sensitive and specific screening methods for early detection and to decrease the incidence of endometrial and ovarian cancers. Treatment modalities for women with gynecologic malignancies are often very aggressive regardless of whether the approach is surgery, radiotherapy, chemotherapy, or biological therapy. This may result in profound physical, sexual, and psychosocial demands on the woman and her family. Additionally, when recurrences appear, expectations for cure are unrealistic and effective palliation remains a challenge. Until improved methods of screening for early detection are developed to reduce the incidence of gynecologic cancers, the search for more effective treatment to reduce mortality remains a priority.

Finally, there are nursing management issues related to the care of the woman with gynecologic cancer that need to be investigated. A study conducted by the Oncology Nursing Society[389] indicated that quality of life and symptom management were the top research priorities identified by oncology nurses. These were followed by outcome measures for interventions, pain control and management, cancer survivorship, prevention and early detection, research utilization, cancer rehabilitation, cost containment, and economic influences. Certainly, all of these issues are relevant to the care of the woman with gynecologic cancer. In addition, a survey of research priorities was conducted by the Gynecologic Oncology Group Nursing Research Subcommittee. The top ranked categories for nursing research included identifying means of enhancing the patient's control of the illness and treatment, and quality of life issues.[390,391] The issue of defining toxicities for new treatments and interventions to reduce morbidity need to be continued. Quality of life related to the aggressive nature of the disease and the physically and emotionally demanding therapies need to be pursued. Finally, women with gynecologic malignancies may need to address changes in body image, alterations in sexuality, and coping and stress management. All of these issues are important for the nurse researcher to pursue and are relevant in preventing cancer or assisting women and their families to live with the disease and its treatment.

# REFERENCES

1. Parker SL, Tong T, Bolden S, et al: Cancer statistics, 1996. *CA Cancer J Clin* 46:5–27, 1996
2. Young RC: Gynecologic cancers, in Wittes RE (ed): *Manual of Oncologic Therapeutics: 1989/1990*. Philadelphia, Lippincott, 1989, pp 270–291
3. DiSaia PJ, Creasman WT: *Clinical Gynecologic Oncology*. St. Louis, Mosby, 1993
4. MacMahan B: Risk factors for endometrial cancer. *Gynecol Oncol* 2:122–129, 1974
5. Feldman S, Cook EF, Harlow BL, et al: Predicting endometrial cancer among older women who present with abnormal vaginal bleeding. *Gynecol Oncol* 56:L367–381, 1995
6. Smith DB: Gynecological cancers: Etiology and pathophysiology. *Semin Oncol Nurs* 2:270–274, 1986
7. Ewertz M, Schou G, Blice JD Jr: The joint effect of risk factors on endometrial cancer. *Eur J Cancer* 24:189–194, 1988
8. Elliott EA, Matonoski GM, Rosenshein NB, et al: Body fat patterning in women with endometrial cancer. *Gynecol Oncol* 39:253–258, 1990
9. Persson I, Adami HO, Bergkvist L, et al: Risk of endometrial cancer after treatment with oestrogens alone or in conjunction with progestogens: Results of a prospective study. *Br Med J* 298:147–151, 1989
10. Hulka BS: Replacement estrogens and risk of gynecologic cancers and breast cancer. *Cancer* 60:1960–1964, 1987
11. Fisher B, Costantino JP, Redmond CK, et al: Endometrial cancer in tamoxifen-treated breast cancer patients: Findings from the National Surgical Adjuvant Breast and Bowel Project (NSABP) B-14. *J Natl Cancer Inst* 86:527–537, 1994
12. Fornander T, Rutquist LE, Cedarmark B, et al: Adjuvant tamoxifen in early breast cancer: Occurrence of new primary cancers. *Lancet* 1:117–129, 1989
13. Cohen I, Beyth Y, Tepper R, et al: Adenomyosis in postmenopausal breast cancer patients treated with tamoxifen: A new entity? *Gynecol Oncol* 58:86–91, 1995
14. Cohen I, Rosen DJT, Shapira J, et al: Endometrial changes with tamoxifen: Comparison between tamoxifen-treated and nontreated asymptomatic postmenopausal breast cancer patients. *Gynecol Oncol* 52:185–190, 1994
15. Barakat RR, Wong G, Curtin JP, et al: Tamoxifen use in breast cancer patients who subsequently develop corpus cancer is not associated with a higher incidence of adverse histologic features. *Gynecol Oncol* 55:164–168, 1994
16. Robinson DC, Bloss JD, Schiano MA: A retrospective study of tamoxifen and endometrial cancer in breast cancer patients. *Gynecol Oncol* 59:186–190, 1995
17. Franks AL, Kendrick JS, Tyler CW Jr: Postmenopausal smoking, estrogen therapy, and the risk of endometrial cancer. *Am J Obstet Gynecol* 156:20–23, 1987
18. The Cancer and Steroid Hormone Study of the Centers for Disease Control and the National Institute of Child Health and Human Development. *JAMA* 257:796–800, 1987
19. Hubbard JL, Holcombe JK: Cancer of endometrium. *Semin Oncol Nurs* 6:206–213, 1990
20. Parazzini F, LaVecchia C, Negri E, et al: Smoking and risk of endometrial cancer: Results from an Italian case-control study. *Gynecol Oncol* 56:195–199, 1995
21. American Cancer Society: *Cancer Fact and Figures–1993*. publication No. 93–15M. Philadelphia, American Cancer Society, 1993
22. American College of Obstetricians and Gynecologists: *Routine Cancer Screening*. Technical Bulletin No. 128. Washington, D.C., 1993
23. Hacker NF: Uterine Cancer, in Berek JS, Hacker NJ (eds): *Practical Gynecologic Oncology*. Baltimore, Williams & Wilkens, 1989, pp 285–326
24. Morrow CP, DiSaia PJ, Townsend DE: Current management of endometrial carcinoma. *Obstet Gynecol* 42:399–406, 1973
25. Jones HW: Treatment of adenocarcinoma of the endometrium. *Obstet Gynecol* 30:147–169, 1975
26. Hoskins WJ, Perez C, Young RC: Gynecologic tumors, in DeVita VT Jr, Hellman S, Rosenberg SA (eds): *Cancer: Principles and Practice of Oncology* (ed 4). Philadelphia, Lippincott, 1993, pp 1152–1225
27. Beecham JB, Helmkamp BF, Rubin P: Tumors of the female reproductive organs, in Rubin P (ed): *Clinical Oncology: A Multidisciplinary Approach*. New York, American Cancer Society, 1983, pp 428–480
28. Yazigi R, Cohen J, Munoz AK, et al: Magnetic resonance imaging determination of myometrial invasion in endometrial carcinoma. *Gynecol Oncol* 34:94–97, 1989
29. Belloni C, Vigano R, delMaschio A, et al: Magnetic resonance imaging in endometrial carcinoma staging. *Gynecol Oncol* 37:172–177, 1990
30. Atsukawa H, Saski H, Tada S: A multivariate analysis of assessment of myometrial invasion of endometrial carci-

noma by magnetic resonance imaging. *Gynecol Oncol* 54: 298–306, 1994

31. Shepherd JH: Revised FIGO staging for gynaecological cancer. *Br J Obstet Gynaecol* 96:889–892, 1989
32. Axelrod JH, Bundy B, Roy T, et al: Advanced endometrial carcinoma treated with whole abdominal irradiation: A Gynecologic Oncology Group (GOG) Study. *Gynecol Oncol* 56:135–136, 1995
33. Piver MS, Hempling RE: A retrospective trial of postoperative vaginal radium/cesium for grade 1–2 less than 50% myometrial invasion and pelvic radiation therapy for grade 3 or deep myometrial invasion in surgical stage I endometrial adenocarcinoma. *Cancer* 66:94–97, 1989
34. Kauppila A, Gornroos N, Nieminen U: Clinical outcome in endometrial cancer. *Obstet Gynecol* 60:473–480, 1982
35. Edmonson JH, Krook JE, Hilton JF, et al: Randomized phase II studies of cisplatin and a combination of cyclophosphamide-doxorubicin-cisplatin (CAP) in patients with progestin-refractory advanced endometrial carcinoma. *Gynecol Oncol* 28:20–24, 1987
36. Thigpen T, Vance R, Lambuth B, et al: Chemotherapy for advanced or recurrent gynecologic cancer. *Cancer* 60: 2104–2116, 1987
37. Weintraub NT, Freedman ML: Gynecologic malignancies of the elderly. *Clin Geriatr Med* 3:669–696, 1987
38. Quinn MA, Campbell JJ: Tamoxifen therapy in advanced/recurrent endometrial carcinoma. *Gynecol Oncol* 32:1–3, 1989
39. Thigpen T, Buchsbaum HJ, Mangan C, et al: Phase II trial of adriamycin in treatment of advanced or recurrent endometrial carcinoma. *Cancer Treat Rep* 63:21–27, 1979
40. Seski JC, Edwards CL, Herson J, et al: Cisplatin chemotherapy for disseminated endometrial cancer. *Obstet Gynecol* 59: 225–228, 1982
41. Thigpen T, Shingleton H, Homesley H, et al: Phase II trial of cisplatinum in the management of advanced or recurrent endometrial carcinoma. *Proc Am Soc Clin Oncol* 22:469, 1981
42. Thigpen JT, Blessing JA, Homesley H, et al: Phase II trial of cisplatin as first-line chemotherapy in patients with advanced or recurrent endometrial carcinoma: A Gynecologic Oncology Group Study. *Gynecol Oncol* 33:68–70, 1989
43. Turbow MM, Thornton J, Ballon S, et al: Chemotherapy of advanced endometrial cancer with platinum, adriamycin, and cyclophosphamide. *Proc Am Soc Clin Oncol* 1:108, 1982
44. Long HJ, Langdon RM Jr, Cha SS, et al: Phase II trial of methotrexate, vinblastine, doxorubicin, and cisplatin in advanced/recurrent endometrial carcinoma. *Gynecol Oncol* 58:240–243, 1995
45. Burke TW, Gershenson DM, Morris M: Postoperative adjuvant cisplatin, doxorubicin, cyclophosphamide (PAC) chemotherapy in women with high risk endometrial carcinoma. *Gynecol Oncol* 55:47–50, 1994
46. Rossiello F, Nardone FDeC, Dell'Acqua: Interferon B increases the sensitivity of endometrial cancer cells to cell-mediated cytoxicity. *Gynecol Oncol* 55:130–136, 1994
47. Gallion HH, Hrushesky WJ, Cibull M: A randomized study of doxorubicin plus cisplatin versus circadian timed doxorubicin plus cisplatin in patients with primary stage III and IV, recurrent endometrial carcinoma: A Gynecologic Oncology Group study No 139, Philadelphia, 1993
48. Randall ME, Spertos N, Dvoretsky P, et al: Whole abdominal radiotherapy versus combination doxorubicin-cisplatin chemotherapy in advanced endometrial carcinoma. A Gynecologic Oncology Group Study No. 122. Philadelphia, 1992
49. Creasman WT, McCarty KS Sr, McCarty KS Jr: Clinical correlation of estrogen, progesterone binding proteins in human endometrial adenocarcinoma. *Obstet Gynecol* 55: 363–370, 1980
50. Satyaswaroop PG: Development of a preclinical model for hormonal therapy of human endometrial carcinomas. *Ann Med* 25:105–111, 1993
51. Utaaker E, Iversen OE, Skaarland E: The distribution and prognostic implications of steroid receptors in endometrial carcinomas. *Gynecol Oncol* 28:89–100, 1987
52. Runowicz CD: Ovarian cancer. *Mediguide Oncol* 7:1–5, 1987
53. Barber HRK: Ovarian cancer. *CA Cancer J Clin* 36:149–184, 1986
54. Hubbard SM: Ovarian carcinoma: An overview of current concepts in diagnosis and management. *Cancer Nurs* 1: 115–128, 1978
55. Barber HRK: *Ovarian Carcinoma: Etiology, Diagnosis, and Treatment* (ed 2). New York, Masson, 1982
56. Parazzini F, Franceschi S, LaVecchia C, et al: Review: The epidemiology of ovarian cancer. *Gynecol Oncol* 43:9–23, 1991
57. Richardson GS, Scully RE, Nikrui N, et al: Common epithelial cancer of the ovary. *N Engl J Med* 312:474–483, 1985
58. Heintz APM, Hacker NF, Lugasse LD: Epidemiology and etiology of ovarian cancer: A review. *Obstet Gynecol* 66: 127–135, 1985
59. Whittemore AS, Wu ML, Paffenbarger RS, et al: Epithelial ovarian cancer and the ability to conceive. *Cancer Res* 49: 4047–4052, 1989
60. Ozols RF, Young RC: Ovarian cancer. *Curr Probl Cancer* 11: 57–122, 1987
61. McGowan L: Ovarian cancer, in McGowan L (ed): *Gynecologic Oncology*. New York, Appleton-Century-Crofts, 1978
62. de Leon MP: Hereditary and familial ovarian cancer. *Recent Results Cancer Res* 136:133–145, 1994
63. Piver MS, Baker TR, Piedmonte M, et al: Epidemiology and etiology of ovarian cancer. *Semin Oncol* 18:177–185, 1991
64. Higgins RV, VanNagell JR, Woods CH, et al: Interobserver variation in ovarian measurements using transvaginal sonography. *Gynecol Oncol* 34:402–406, 1989
65. Campbell S, Bhan V, Royston J, et al: Screening for early ovarian cancer. *Lancet* 1:710–711, 1988
66. Bourne TH, Campbell J, Reynolds K, et al: The potential role of serum Ca-125 in an ultrasound-based screening program for familial ovarian cancer. *Gynecol Oncol* 52: 379–389, 1994
67. Weiner Z, Thaler I, Beck D, et al: Differentiating malignant from benign ovarian tumors with transvaginal color flow imaging. *Obstet Gynecol* 79:159–162, 1992
68. Kawai M, Kano T, Kikkawa F, et al: Transvaginal doppler ultrasound with color flow imaging in the diagnosis of ovarian cancer. *Obstet Gynecol* 79:163–167, 1992
69. DePriest PD, Varner E, Powell J, et al: The efficacy of a sonographic morphology index in identifying ovarian cancer: A multi-institutional investigation. *Gynecol Oncol* 55: 174–178, 1994
70. Perez RP, Godwin AK, Hamilton TC, et al: Ovarian cancer biology. *Semin Oncol* 18:270–291, 1991
71. Kim JW, Cho YH, Kwon DJ, et al: Aberrations of *p53* tumor suppressor gene in human epithelial ovarian carcinoma. *Gynecol Oncol* 57:199–204, 1995

72. Young R, Perez CA, Hoskins WJ: Cancer of the ovary, in DeVita VT, Hellman S, Rosenberg SA (eds): *Cancer: Principles and Practice of Oncology* (ed 4). Philadelphia, Lippincott, 1993, pp 1226–1263

73. Piver MS, Barlow JJ, Lele SB: Incidence of subclinical metastasis in stage I and II ovarian carcinoma. *Obstet Gynecol* 52: 100–104, 1978

74. Beahrs OH, Henson DE, Hutter RVP, et al: Philadelphia, Lippincott, 1992; pp155-180 American Joint Committee on Cancer: *Manual for Staging of Cancer* (ed 4).

75. Eriksson JH and Walczak JR: Ovarian cancer. *Semin Oncol Nurs* 6:214–227, 1990

76. Smith JP and Day TG: Review of ovarian cancer at the University of Texas Systems Cancer Center, M.D. Anderson Hospital and Tumor Institute. *Am J Obstet Gynecol* 135: 984–993, 1979

77. Young RC: Initial therapy for early ovarian carcinoma. *Cancer* 60:2042–2049, 1987

78. Bristol Laboratories, Division of Bristol-Myers Co: *Platinol: Effective palliation therapy in metastatic ovarian cancer.* Syracuse, NY, Bristol Laboratories, 1982

79. Pomel C, Provencher D, Dauplat J, et al: Laparoscopic staging of early ovarian cancer. *Gynecol Oncol* 58:301–306, 1995

80. Spiritos NM, Gross GM, Freddo JL, et al: Cytoreductive surgery in advanced epithelial cancer of the ovary: The impact of aortic and pelvic lymphadenectomy. *Gynecol Oncol* 56:345–352, 1995

81. Stanhope CR and Smith JP: *Ovarian cancer: The current approach to diagnosis and treatment.* Syracuse, NY, Bristol Laboratories, 1981

82. Young RC, Walton LA, Ellenberg SS, et al: Adjuvant therapy in stage I and stage II epithelial ovarian cancer. *N Engl J Med* 322:1021–1027, 1990

83. Dottino PR, Plaxe SC, Cohen CJ: A phase II trial of adjuvant cisplatin and doxorubicin in stage I epithelial ovarian cancer. *Gynecol Oncol* 43:203–205, 1991

84. Monga M, Carmichael JA, Shelley WE, et al: Surgery without adjuvant chemotherapy for early epithelial ovarian carcinoma after comprehensive surgical staging. *Gynecol Oncol* 43:195–197, 1991

85. Gallion HH, van Nagell JR, Donaldson ES, et al: Adjuvant oral alkylating chemotherapy in patients with stage I epithelial ovarian cancer. *Cancer* 63:1070–1073, 1989

86. McGuire WP, Hoskins WJ, Brady MF, et al: Cyclophosphamide and cisplatin compared with paclitaxel and cisplatin in patients with stage III and stage IV ovarian cancer. *N Engl J Med* 334:1–6, 1996

87. Jacob JH, Gepshenson DM, Morris M, et al: Neoadjuvant chemotherapy and interval debulking for advanced epithelial ovarian cancer. *Gynecol Oncol* 42:146–150, 1991

88. Dauplat J, Legros M, Condat P, et al: High-dose melphalan and autologous bone marrow support for treatment of ovarian carcinoma with positive second look operation. *Gynecol Oncol* 34:294–298, 1989

89. Shpall EJ, Clarke-Rearson D, Soper JT, et al: High-dose alkylating agent chemotherapy with autologous bone marrow support in patients with stage III/IV epithelial ovarian cancer. *Gynecol Oncol* 38:386–391, 1990

90. Stiff PJ, McKenzie RS, Alberts DS, et al: Phase I clinical and pharmacokinetic study of high-dose mitoxantrone combined with carboplatin, cyclophosphamide, and autologous bone marrow rescue. *J Clin Oncol* 12:176–183, 1994

91. Solomon JH, Atkinson KH, Coppleson JVM, et al: Ovarian carcinoma: Abdominopelvic irradiation following reexploration. *Gynecol Oncol* 31:396–401, 1988

92. Lawton FG, Redman CW, Luesley DM, et al: Neoadjuvant (cytoreductive) chemotherapy combined with intervention debulking surgery in advanced, unresected epithelial ovarian cancer. *Obstet Gynecol* 73:61–65, 1989

93. Sonnendecker EWW: Is routine second-look laparotomy for ovarian cancer justified? *Gynecol Oncol* 31:249–255, 1988

94. Brand E, Wade ME, Lagasse LD: Resection of fixed pelvic tumors using the Nd: YAG laser. *J Surg Oncol* 37:246–251, 1988

95. Deppe G, Malviya VK, Doike G, et al: Use of cavitron surgical aspirator for debulking of diaphragmatic metastases in patients with advanced carcinoma of the ovaries. *Gynecol Obstet* 168:455–456, 1989

96. Deppe G, Malviya VK, Malone JM, et al: Debulking of pelvic and para-aortic lymph node metastases in ovarian cancer with the cavitron surgical aspirator. *Obstet Gynecol* 76: 1140–1142, 1990

97. Bast RC Jr, Hunter V, Knapp RC: Pros and cons of gynecologic tumor markers. *Cancer* 60:1984–1992, 1987

98. Bast RC, Klug TL, St. John E, et al: A radioimmunoassay using a monoclonal antibody to monitor the course of epithelial ovarian cancer. *N Engl J Med* 309:883–887, 1983

99. Neunteufel W, Breitenbecker G: Tissue expression of CA 125 in benign and malignant lesions of ovary and fallopian tube: A comparison with CA 19-9 and CEA. *Gynecol Oncol* 33:297–302, 1989

100. Niloff JM, Bast RC Jr, Schaetzl EM, et al: Predictive value of CA 125 antigen levels at second-look procedures in ovarian cancer. *Am J Obstet Gynecol* 151:981–986, 1985

101. Berek JS, Knapp PC, Malkasian GD, et al: CA 125 serum levels correlate with second-look operations among ovarian cancer patients: A prospective multi-institutional study. *Obstet Gynecol* 67:685–689, 1986

102. Jager W, Adam R, Wildt L, et al: Serum CA-125 as a guideline for the timing of a second-look operation and second-line treatment in, ovarian cancer. *Arch Gynecol Obstet* 243: 91–99, 1988

103. Potter ME, Moradi M, To ACW, et al: Value of serum CA 125 levels: Does the result preclude a second look? *Gynecol Oncol* 33:201–203, 1989

104. MacDonald F, Bird R, Stokes H, et al: Expression of CEA, CA 125, CA 19-9 and human milk fat globule membrane antigen in ovarian tumours. *J Clin Pathol* 41:260–264, 1988

105. Fioretti P, Gadducci A, Ferdeghini M, et al: Correlation of CA 125 and CA 19-9 serum levels with clinical course and second-look findings in patient with ovarian carcinoma. *Gynecol Oncol* 28:278–283, 1987

106. Tobias JS, Griffiths CT: Management of ovarian carcinoma. *N Engl J Med* 294:818–823, 1976

107. McGuire WP, Rowinsky EK, Rosenshein NB, et al: Taxol: A unique antineoplastic agent with significant activity in advanced ovarian epithelial neoplasms. *Ann Intern Med* 111:273–279, 1989

108. McGuire WP, Rowinsky EK: Old drugs revisited, new drugs and experimental approaches in ovarian cancer therapy. *Semin Oncol* 18:255–269, 1991

109. Thigpen JT, Blessing JA, Ball H, et al: Phase II trial of paclitaxel in patients with progressive ovarian carcinoma after platinum-based chemotherapy: A Gynecologic Oncology Group study. *J Clin Oncol* 12:1748–1753, 1994

110. Rowinsky E, Grochow L, Hendricks C, et al: Phase I and

pharmacologic study of topotecan: A novel topoisomerase I inhibitor. *Proc Am Soc Clin Oncol* 10:240, 1991

111. Cortes JE, Pazdur R: Docetaxel. *J Clin Oncol* 13:2643–2655, 1995

112. Francis P, Schneider J, Hann L, et al: Phase II trial of docetaxel in patients with platinum refractory advanced ovarian cancer. *J Clin Oncol* 12:2301–2308, 1994

113. Gershenson DM, Taylor Wharton J, Copeland LJ, et al: Treatment of advanced epithelial ovarian cancer with cisplatin and cyclophosphamide. *Gynecol Oncol* 32:336–341, 1989

114. Young RC, Chabner BA, Hubbard SM: Prospective trials of melphalan (L-PAM) versus combination chemotherapy (Hexa-CAF) in ovarian adenocarcinoma. *N Engl J Med* 299: 1261–1266, 1978

115. Bruckner HW, Cohen CJ, Feuer E, et al: Prognostic factors: Cisplatin regimens for patients with ovarian cancer after failure of chemotherapy. *Obstet Gynecol* 69:114–120, 1987

116. Vogl SE, Pagano M, Kaplan BH, et al: Cisplatin-based combination chemotherapy for advanced ovarian cancer. *Cancer* 51:2024–2030, 1983

117. Thigpen JT, Blessing JA, Vance RB, et al: Chemotherapy in ovarian carcinoma: Present role and future prospects. *Semin Oncol* 16:58–65, 1989

118. Ovarian Cancer Meta-Analysis Project: Cyclophosphamide plus cisplatin versus cyclophosphamide, doxorubicin, and cisplatin chemotherapy of ovarian carcinoma: A meta-analysis. *J Clin Oncol* 9:1668–1674, 1991

119. McGuire WP, Hoskins WJ, Brady MF, et al: Assessment of dose intensity in suboptimally debulked ovarian cancer: A Gynecologic Oncology Group study. *J Clin Oncol* 13: 1589–1599, 1995

120. ten Bokkel Huinink WW, van der Berg MEL, van Oosterom AT, et al: Carboplatin in combination therapy for ovarian cancer. *Cancer Treat Rev* 15:9–15, 1988 (suppl B)

121. Yarbro CH: Carboplatin: A clinical review. *Semin Oncol Nurs* 15:63–69, 1989 (suppl)

122. Rothenberg ML, Ostchega Y, Steinberg SM, et al: High-dose carboplatin with diethyldithiocarbamate chemoprotection in treatment of women with relapsed ovarian cancer. *J Natl Cancer Inst* 80:1488–1492, 1988

123. Reed E, Janik J, Bookman M, et al: High-dose chemotherapy and rGM-CSF in refractory ovarian cancer. *Proc Am Soc Clin Oncol* 9:157, 1990

124. Mulder PO, Willemse H, Aalders JG, et al: High-dose chemotherapy with autologous bone marrow transplantation in patients with refractory ovarian cancer. *Eur J Cancer* 25: 645–649, 1989

125. Shea T, Graham M, Bernard S, et al: A clinical and pharmacokinetic study of high-dose carboplatin, paclitaxel, granulocyte stimulating factor, and peripheral blood stem cells in patients with unresectable or metastatic cancer. *Semin Oncol* 22:80–85, 1995 (suppl 2)

126. Stiff PJ, McKenzie RS, Alberts DS, et al: Phase I clinical and pharmacokinetic study of high-dose mitoxantrone combined with carboplatin, cyclophosphamide, and autologous bone marrow rescue: High response rate for refractory ovarian carcinoma. *J Clin Oncol* 12:176–183, 1994

127. Alberts DS, Garcia-Kendall D, Surwit EA: Phase II trial of mitomycin C plus 5-FU in the treatment of drug-refractory ovarian cancer. *Semin Oncol* 15:22–26, 1988 (suppl 4)

128. Fojo A, Hamilton TC, Young RC, et al: Multidrug resistance in ovarian cancer. *Cancer* 60:2075–2080, 1987

129. Donehower RC, Rosenshein NB, Rotmensch J, et al: Se-

quential methotrexate and 5-fluorouracil in advanced ovarian carcinoma. *Gynecol Oncol* 27:90–96, 1987

130. Goodman HM, Dottino PR, Kredenster D, et al: Continuous infusion fluoropyrimidines as salvage therapy for patients with advanced ovarian carcinoma. *Gynecol Oncol* 29: 348–355, 1988

131. Markman M: Intraperitoneal chemotherapy as treatment of ovarian carcinoma: Why, how and when? *Obstet Gynecol Surv* 42:533–539, 1987

132. Ozols RF: Intraperitoneal chemotherapy. *Mediguide Oncol* 5:1–5, 1986

133. Markman M: Intraperitoneal chemotherapy. *Semin Oncol* 18:248–254, 1991

134. Jones RB, Collins JM, Myers CE, et al: High volume intraperitoneal chemotherapy with methotrexate in patients with cancer. *Cancer Res* 41:55–59, 1981

135. Ozols RF, Young RC, Speyer JL, et al: Phase I and pharmacological studies of adriamycin administered intraperitoneally to patients with ovarian cancer. *Cancer Res* 42:4265–4269, 1982

136. Speyer J, Collins JM, Dedrick RL, et al: Phase I and pharmacological studies of 5-FU administered intraperitoneally. *Cancer* 40:567–572, 1980

137. Howell SB, Pfeifle CL, Wung WE, et al: Intraperitoneal cisplatin with systemic thiosulfate protection. *Ann Intern Med* 97:845–851, 1982

138. Monk BJ, Surwit EA, Alberts DS, et al: Intraperitoneal mitomycin C in the treatment of peritoneal carcinomatosis following second-look surgery. *Semin Oncol* 15:27–31, 1988

139. Loeffler T, Freund W: Pharmacokinetics of mitoxantrone intraperitoneal. *Proc Am Assoc Cancer Res* 27:175, 1986

140. King ME, Pfeifle CE, Howell SB: Intraperitoneal cytosine arabinoside in ovarian carcinoma. *J Clin Oncol* 2:662, 1984

141. Berek JS, Hacker NF, Lichtenstein A, et al: Intraperitoneal recombinant alpha-interferon for "salvage" immunotherapy in stage III epithelial ovarian cancer: A Gynecologic Oncology Group study. *Cancer Res* 45:4447–4453, 1985

142. Markman M. Intraperitoneal paclitaxel in the management of ovarian cancer. *Semin Oncol* 22:86–87, 1994 (suppl 2)

143. Francis P, Rowinsky E, Schneider J, et al: Phase I feasibility and pharmacologic study of weekly intraperitoneal paclitaxel: A Gynecologic Oncology Group pilot study. *J Clin Oncol* 13:2961–2967, 1995

144. Piccart MJ, Abrams J, Dodion PF, et al: Intraperitoneal chemotherapy with cisplatin and melphalan. *J Natl Cancer Inst* 80:1118–1124, 1988

145. Alberts DS, Liu PY, Hannigan EV, et al: Phase III study of intraperitoneal (IP) cisplatin (CDDP)/intravenous (IV) cyclophosphamide (CPA) vs in CDDP/IV CPA in patients (pts) with optimal disease stage III ovarian cancer: A SWOG-GOG-ECOG intergroup study (int0051). *Proc Am Soc Clin Oncol* 14:273, 1995 (abstr 760)

146. Hamilton TC, Ozols RF, Longo DL: Biologic therapy for the treatment of malignant common epithelial tumors in the ovary. *Cancer* 60:2054–2063, 1987

147. Chapman PB, Hakes T, Gabrilove JL, et al: A phase I pilot study of intraperitoneal rIL-2 in ovarian cancer. *Proc Am Soc Clin Oncol* 5:23, 1986

148. Smith LH, Tend NNH: Clinical applications of monoclonal antibodies in gynecologic oncology. *Cancer* 60:2068–2074, 1987

149. Pommier RF, Woltering EA, Milo G, et al: Synergistic cytotoxicity between dimethyl sulfoxide and antineoplastic

agents against ovarian cancer in vitro. *Am J Obstet Gynecol* 159:848–852, 1988

150. Rubin SC, Hoskins WJ, Markman M, et al: Long-term access to the peritoneal cavity in ovarian cancer patients. *Gynecol Oncol* 33:46–48, 1989

151. Kavanagh JJ, Roberts W, Townsend P, et al: Leuprolide acetate in the treatment of refractory or persistent epithelial ovarian cancer. *J Clin Oncol* 7:115–118, 1989

152. Weiner SA, Alberts DS, Surwit EA, et al: Tamoxifen therapy in recurrent epithelial ovarian carcinoma. *Gynecol Oncol* 27:208–213, 1987

153. Belinson JL, McClure M, Badger G: Randomized trial of megestrol acetate vs. megestrol acetate/tamoxifen for the management of progressive or recurrent epithelial ovarian carcinoma. *Gynecol Oncol* 28:151–155, 1987

154. Pezner RD, Stevens KR Jr, Tong D, et al: Limited epithelial carcinoma of the ovary treated with curative intent by intraperitoneal instillation of radiocolloids. *Cancer* 42:2563–2571, 1978

155. Potter ME, Partridge EE, Shingleton HM, et al: Intraperitoneal chromic phosphate in ovarian cancer: Risks and benefits. *Gynecol Oncol* 32:314–318, 1989

156. Weiser EB, Burke TW, Heller PB, et al: Determinants of survival of patients with epithelial ovarian carcinoma following whole abdomen irradiation (WAR). *Gynecol Oncol* 30:201–208, 1988

157. Schray MF, Martinez A, Howes AE, et al: Advanced epithelial ovarian cancer: Salvage whole abdominal irradiation for patients with recurrent or persistent disease after combination chemotherapy. *J Clin Oncol* 6:1433–1439, 1988

158. Bolis G, Zanaboni F, Vanoli P, et al: The impact of whole abdominal radiotherapy on survival in advanced ovarian cancer patients with minimal residual disease after chemotherapy. *Gynecol Oncol* 39:150–154, 1990

159. Linstach DE, Stern JL, Quirey JM, et al: Salvage whole abdominal irradiation following chemotherapy failure in epithelial ovarian carcinoma. *Gynecol Oncol* 36:327–330, 1990

160. Creasman WT, Yale SA, Blessing JA, et al: Chemoimmunotherapy in the management of primary stage III ovarian cancer: A Gynecologic Oncology Group study. *Cancer Treat Rep* 63:319–323, 1979

161. Alberts DS, Moon TE, Stephens RA, et al: Randomized trials of chemoimmunotherapy for advanced ovarian carcinoma: A preliminary report of a Southwest Oncology Group Study. *Cancer Treat Rep* 63:325–331, 1979

162. Alberts DS, Mason-Liddil N, O'Toole RV, et al: Randomized phase III trial of chemoimmunotherapy in patients with previously untreated stages III and IV suboptimal disease ovarian cancer: A Southwest Oncology Group study. *Gynecol Oncol* 32:8–15, 1989

163. Einhorn N, Cantell K, Einhorn S, et al: Human leukocyte interferon therapy for advanced ovarian cancer. *Am J Clin Oncol* 5:167–172, 1987

164. Welander CE: Use of interferon in the treatment of ovarian cancer as a single agent and in combination with cytotoxic drugs. *Cancer* 59:617–619, 1987

165. Lichtenstein A, Spina C, Berek JS, et al: Intraperitoneal administration of human recombinant interferon-alpha in patients with ovarian cancer: Effects on lymphocyte phenotype and cytotoxicity. *Cancer Res* 48:5853–5859, 1988

166. Alberts DS, Garcia D, Roe D, et al: Lack of tetraplatin cross resistance with cisplatin against epithelial ovarian cancers

obtained from more than 70 patients with advanced disease. *Proc Am Assoc Cancer Res* 32:2434, 1991

167. Bookman MA, Bast RC: The immunobiology and immunotherapy of ovarian cancer. *Semin Oncol* 18:270–291, 1991

168. Hamilton T, O'Dwyer P, Young R, et al: Phase I trial of buthionine sulfoximine (BSO) plus melphalan (L-PAM) in patients with advanced ovarian cancer. *Proc Am Soc Clin Oncol* 9:73, 1990

169. Shilder RJ, Nash S, Tew KD, et al: Phase I trial of thiotepa (TT) in combination with the glutathione transferase inhibitor ethacrynic acid (EA). *Proc Am Assoc Cancer Res* 31:177, 1990

170. Lovejoy NC, Anastasi JK: Squamous cell cervical lesions in women with and without AIDS: Biochemical risk factors, prevention, and policy. *Cancer Nurs* 17:294–307, 1994

171. Guo WD, Hsing AW, Li JY, Chen JS, Chow WH, Blot WJ: Correlation of cervical cancer mortality with reproductive and dietary factors, and serum markers in China. *Int J Epidemiol* 23:1127–1132, 1994

172. Anderson M: The pathology of tumors of the cervix, in Blackledge GRP, Jordan JA, Shingleton HM (eds): *Textbook of Gynecologic Oncology*. Philadelphia, WB Saunders, 1991, pp 265–283

173. Celentano DD, Shapiro S, Weisman CS: Cancer: Preventive screening behavior among elderly women. *Prev Med* 11:454–463, 1982

174. Spano WJ, King A, Keeney E, et al: Age as a prognostic factor in carcinoma of the cervix. *Gynecol Oncol* 35:66–68, 1989

175. Lovejoy NC: Precancerous and cancerous cervical lesions: The multicultural "male" risk factor. *Oncol Nurse Forum* 21:497–504, 1994

176. Stratton P, Ciacco KH: Cervical neoplasia in the patient with HIV infection. *Curr Opin Obstet Gynecol* 6:86–91, 1994

177. Braun L: Role of human immunodeficiency virus infection in the pathogenesis of human papillomavirus-associated cervical neoplasia. *Am J Pathol* 144:209–214, 1994

178. Korn AP, Landers DV: Gynecologic disease in women infected with human immunodeficiency virus type I. *J Acquir Immune Defic Syndr* 9:361–370, 1995

179. Singh GS, Aikins JK, Deger R, et al: Metastatic cervical cancer and pelvic inflammatory disease in an AIDS patient. *Gynecol Oncol* 54:372–376, 1994

180. Northfelt DW: Cervical and anal neoplasia and HPV infection in persons with HIV infection. *Oncology (Huntingt)* 8:38–41, 1994

181. Hildesheim A, Reeves WC, Brenton LA, et al: Association of oral contraceptive use and human papillomaviruses in invasive cervical cancers. *Int J Cancer* 45:860–864, 1990

182. Parazzini P, La Vecchia C, Negri E, et al: Oral contraceptive use and invasive cervical cancer. *Int J Epidemiol* 19:259–263, 1990

183. Herrero R, Brinton LA, Reeves WC, et al: Risk factors for invasive carcinoma of the uterine cervix in Latin America. *Bull Pan Am Health Organ* 24:263–283, 1990

184. Cuzick J, Boyle P: Trends in cervix cancer mortality. *Cancer Surv* 7:417–439, 1988

185. Burke L, Antonioli DA, Ducatman BS: *Colposcopy: Text and Atlas*. Norwalk, CT, Appleton & Lange, 1991

186. Shingleton HM, Orr JW: *Cancer of the Cervix*. Philadelphia, Lippincott, 1995

187. Koss LG: Cytologic and histologic manifestations of human papillomavirus infection of the female genital tract and their clinical significance. *Cancer* 60:1942–1950, 1987

188. Syrjanen K, Vayrynen M, Saarikoski S, et al: Natural history of cervical human papillomavirus (HPV) infections based on prospective follow-up. *Br J Obstet Gynaecol* 92:1086–1092, 1985

189. Meanwell CA, Blackledge G, Cox MF, et al: HPV 16 DNA in normal and malignant cervical epithelium: Implications for the etiology and behavior of cervical neoplasia. *Lancet* 1:703–707, 1987

190. Howley PM, Schlegel R: The human papillomaviruses. *Am J Med* 85:155–158, 1988 (suppl 2A)

191. Richart RM: Causes and management of cervical intraepithelial neoplasia. *Cancer* 60:1951–1959, 1987

192. Lorincz AT, Reid R, Jenson AB, et al: Human papillomavirus infection of the cervix: relative risk associations of 15 common anogenital types. *Obstet Gynecol* 79:328–337, 1992

193. Schiffman MH, Kiviat NB, Burk RD, et al: Accuracy and interlaboratory reliability of human papillomavirus DNS testing by hybrid capture. *J Clin Microbiol* 33:545–550, 1995

194. Pao CC, Lin CY, Chang YL, et al: Human papillomaviruses and small cell carcinoma of the uterine cervix. *Gynecol Oncol* 37:151–164, 1990

195. Berumen J, Unger ER, Casas L, Figueroa P: Amplification of human papillomavirus types 16 and 18 in invasive cervical cancer. *Hum Pathol* 26:676–681, 1995

196. Wright TC, Richart RM: Role of human papillomavirus in the pathogenesis of genital tract warts and cancer. *Gynecol Oncol* 37:151–164, 1990

197. McCance DJ, Campion MJ, Clarkson PK, et al: Prevalence of human papillomavirus type 16 DNA sequences in cervical intraepithelial neoplasia and invasive carcinoma of the cervix. *Br J Obstet Gynaecol* 92:1101–1105, 1985

198. Bosch FX, Manos MM, Munoz N, et al: Prevalence of human papillomavirus in cervical cancer: a worldwide perspective. International biological study on cervical cancer (IBSCC) study group. *J Natl Cancer Inst* 87:796–802, 1995

199. Hadjimichael O, Janerich D, Lowell DM, et al: Histologic and clinical characteristics associated with rapidly progressive invasive cervical cancer: A preliminary report from the Yale Cancer Control Research Unit. *Yale J Biol Med* 62: 345–350, 1989

200. Tase T, Okagaki T, Manias DA, et al: Human papilloma virus types and localization in adenocarcinomas and adenosquamous carcinoma of the uterine cervix: A study by in situ DNA hybridization. *Cancer Res* 48:993–998, 1988

201. Meanwell CA: The Epidemiology and Etiology of Cervical Cancer, in Blackwell GRP, Jordan JA, Shingleton HM (eds): *Textbook of Gynecologic Oncology*. Philadelphia, Saunders, 1991, pp 250–264

202. Vonka V, Kanka J, Jelinek J, et al: Prospective study on the relationship between cervical neoplasia and herpes simplex type-2 virus. I. Epidemiology characteristics. *Int J Cancer* 33:49–60, 1984

203. Munoz N, Kato I, Bosch FX, et al: Cervical cancer and herpes simplex virus type 2. *Int J Cancer* 60:438–442, 1995

204. Eddy DM: Screening for cervical cancer. *Ann Intern Med* 113:214–226, 1990

205. Savitz DA, Andrews KW, Brinton LA: Occupation and cervical cancer. *J Occup Environ Med* 37:357–361, 1995

206. Creek KE, Geslani G, Batova A, et al: Progressive loss of sensitivity to growth control by retinoic acid and transforming growth factor-beta at late stages of human papillomavirus type 16-initiated transformation of human keratinocytes. *Adv Exp Med Biol* 375:117–135, 1995

207. Childers JM, Chu J, Voigt LF, et al: Chemoprevention of cervical cancer with folic acid: a phase III Southwest Oncology Group Intergroup study. *Cancer Epidemiol Biomarkers Prev* 4:155–159, 1995

208. Kelloff GJ, Boone CW, Steele VE, et al: Progress in cancer chemoprevention: perspectives on agent selection and short-term clinical intervention trials. *Cancer Res* 54: 2015s–2024s, 1994 (suppl 7)

209. Meyskens FL, Survit E, Moon TE, et al: Enhancement of regression of cervical intraepithelial neoplasia II (moderate dysplasia) with topically applied all-trans-retinoic acid: a randomized trial. *J Natl Cancer Inst* 86:539–543, 1994

210. Bollag W: Experimental basis of cancer combination chemotherapy with retinoids, cytokines, 1,25-dihydroxyvitamin D3, and analogs. *J Cell Biochem* 56:427–435, 1994

211. Widschwendter M, Daxenbichler G, Marth C, et al: Interaction of interferon with retinoic acid. *Gynakol Geburtshilfliche Rundsch* 34:168–170, 1994

212. Eckert RL, Agarwal C, Hembree JR, et al: Human cervical cancer. Retinoids, interferon, and human papillomavirus. *Adv Exp Med Biol* 375:31–44, 1995

213. Chen LD, Leal BZ, Reiter RJ: Melatonin's inhibitory effect on growth or ME-180 human cervical cancer cells is not related to intracellular glutathione concentrations. *Cancer Lett* 91:153–159, 1995

214. Brand E, Berek JS, Hacker NF: Controversies in the management of cervical adenocarcinoma. *Obstet Gynecol* 71: 261–269, 1988

215. Anthony CP: *Textbook of Anatomy and Physiology*. St. Louis, Mosby, 1983

216. Hopkins MP: Diseases of the vulva, in Wilson JR, Carrington LR (eds): *Obstetrics and Gynecology*. Baltimore, Mosby, 1991, pp 550–563

217. Jones HW, Jones GS: *Novak's Textbook of Gynecology*. Baltimore, Williams & Wilkins, 1981

218. Lundberg GD: The 1988 Bethesda System for reporting cervical/vaginal cytological diagnoses. *JAMA* 262:931–934, 1989

219. Koss LG: The New Bethesda System for reporting results of smears of the uterine cervix. *J Natl Cancer Inst* 82: 988–991, 1990

220. Soloman D: The 1988 Bethesda System for reporting cervical/vaginal cytologic diagnoses. *J Reprod Med* 34:779–783, 1989

221. Kurman RJ, Malkasian GD, Sedlis A, et al: From Papanicolaou to Bethesda: The rationale for a new cervical cytologic classification. *Obstet Gynecol* 77:779–782, 1991

222. Shepherd JC, Fried RA: Preventing cervical cancer: the role of the Bethesda system. *Am Fam Physician* 51:434–440, 1995

223. Jones HW: Impact of the Bethesda System. *Cancer* 76: 1914–1918, 1995 (suppl)

224. Mahon SM: The Bethesda system for classification of Pap smears: The clinical experience of one cancer screening center. *Cancer Nurs* 18:458–466, 1995

225. Herbst AL: The Bethesda System for cervical/vaginal cytologic diagnoses: A note of caution. *Obstet Gynecol* 76: 449–450, 1990 (editorial)

226. Bottles K, Reiter RC, Steiner AL, et al: Problems encountered with the Bethesda System: The University of Iowa experience. *Obstet Gynecol* 78:410–413, 1991

227. Vooijs GP: Does the Bethesda System promote or endanger the quality of cervical cytology? *Acta Cytol* 34:455–456, 1990

228. Cox JT: Epidemiology of cervical intraepithelial neoplasia:

The role of human papillomavirus. *Clin Obstet Gynaecol* 9: 1–37, 1995

229. Caputo TA: *Uterine cervical cancer: The current approach to diagnosis and treatment.* Syracuse, NY, Bristol Laboratories, 1979

230. Cashavelly BJ: Cervical dysplasia: An overview of current concepts in epidemiology, diagnosis, and treatments. *Cancer Nurs* 10:199–206, 1987

231. Shy K: Concepts in the application of cervical cytology, in Greer BE, Berek JS (eds): *Gynecologic Oncology: Treatment Rationale and Techniques.* New York, Elsevier, 1991, pp 13–32

232. Fink DJ: Change in American Cancer Society checkup guidelines for detection of cervical cancer. *CA Cancer J Clin* 38:127–128, 1988

233. Schwartz PE, Merino MJ, McCrea Curnen MG: Clinical management of patients with invasive cervical cancer following a negative Pap smear. *Yale J Biol Med* 61:327–338, 1988

234. Kern WH, Zivolich MR: The accuracy and consistency of the cytologic classification of squamous lesions of the uterine cervix. *Acta Cytol* 21:519–523, 1977

235. Learmonth GM, Durcan CM, Beck JD: The changing incidence of cervical intra-epithelial neoplasia. *S Afr Med J* 77: 637–639, 1989

236. Hatch K, Helm CW: Cancer of the cervix—surgical treatment, in Blackledge GRP, Jordan JA, Shingleton HM (eds): *Textbook of Gynecologic Oncology.* Philadelphia, Saunders, 1991, pp 313–327

237. Masterson BJ, Krantz KE, Calkins JW, et al: The carbon dioxide laser in cervical epithelial neoplasia: A five-year experience in treating 230 patients. *Am J Obstet Gynecol* 139: 565–567, 1981

238. Burke L: The use of carbon dioxide laser in the therapy of cervical intraepithelial neoplasia. *Am J Obstet Gynecol* 144: 337–340, 1982

239. Anderson MC: Treatment of cervical intraepithelial neoplasia with the carbon dioxide laser: Report of 543 patients. *Obstet Gynecol* 59:720–725, 1982

240. Reid R: Preinvasive disease, in Berek JS, Hacker NF (eds): *Practical Gynecologic Oncology.* Baltimore: Williams & Wilkins, 1989, pp 195–239

241. Chen RJ, Chang DY, Yen ML, et al: Loop electrosurgical excision procedure for conization of the uterine cervix. *J Formos Med Assoc* 93:196–199, 1994

242. Tabbara S, Saleh ADM, Andersen WA, et al: The Bethesda Classification for Squamous Intraepithelial Lesions: Histologic, Cytologic, and Viral Correlates. *Obstet Gynecol* 79: 338–346, 1992

243. Nelson JH, Averette HE, Richart RM: Cervical intraepithelial neoplasia (dysplasia and carcinoma in situ) and early invasive cervical carcinoma. *CA Cancer J Clin* 39:157–178, 1989

244. Yliskoski M, Cantell K, Syrjanen K, et al: Topical treatment with human leukocyte interferon of HPV 16 infections associated with cervical and vaginal intraepithelial neoplasias. *Gynecol Oncol* 36:353–357, 1990

245. Iwasaka R, Hayashi Y, Yokoyama M, et al: Interferon y treatment for cervical intraepithelial neoplasia. *Gynecol Oncol* 37:96–102, 1990

246. McDonald TW, Neutens JJ, Fischer LM, et al: Impact of cervical intraepithelial neoplasia diagnosis and treatment on self-esteem and body image. *Gynecol Oncol* 34:345–349, 1989

247. Lamb MA: Sexual dysfunction in the gynecologic oncology patient. *Semin Oncol Nurs* 1:9–17, 1985

248. Chan KK: The presentation of carcinoma of the cervix, in Blackledge GRP, Jordan JA, Shingleton HM (eds): *Textbook of Gynecology Oncology.* Philadelphia, Saunders, 1991, pp 306–312

249. Greer BE, Berek JS: *Gynecologic Oncology: Treatment Rationale and Techniques.* New York, Elsevier, 1991

250. Subak LL, Hricak H, Powell CB, Azizi L, Stern JL: Cervical carcinoma: computed tomography and magnetic resonance imaging for preoperative staging. *Obstet Gynecol* 86: 43–50, 1995

251. Vives A, Castelo-Branco C, Iglesias X, et al: Is MRI helpful in evaluating the response of cervical cancer to neoadjuvant chemotherapy? *Acta Obstet Gynecol Scand* 74:467–471, 1995

252. Burghardt E, Hofmann HMH, Ebner F, et al: Magnetic resonance imaging in cervical cancer: A basis for objective classification. *Gynecol Oncol* 33:61–67, 1989

253. Rose PG, Watkins E, Amyot K, et al: A randomized comparison of hydroxyurea *versus* hydroxyurea, 5-FU infusion, and bolus cisplatin *versus* weekly cisplatin as adjunct to radiation therapy in patients with stage IIb, III, IVa carcinoma of the cervix and negative paraaortic nodes. Philadelphia, Gynecology Oncology Group Study, 1992

254. Varia MA, Remmenga S, Evers C, et al: Extended field radiation therapy with concomitant 5-FU infusion and cisplatin chemotherapy in patients with cervical carcinoma metastatic to paraaortic lymph nodes. Philadelphia, Gynecology Oncology Group Study, 1992

255. Hatch KD: Cervical Cancer, in Berek JS, Hacker NF (eds): *Practical Gynecology Oncology.* Baltimore, Williams & Wilkins, 1989, pp 241–284

256. Borras G, Molina R, Xercavins J, et al: Tumor antigens CA 19-9, CA 125, and CEA in carcinoma of the uterine cervix. *Gynecol Oncol* 57:205–211, 1995

257. Gocze PM, Vahrson HW, Freeman DA: Serum levels of squamous cell carcinoma antigen and ovarian carcinoma antigen (CA 125) in patients with benign and malignant diseases of the uterine cervix. *Oncology* 51:430–434, 1994

258. Stoian M, Repanovici R: Identification of antibodies against human papillomavirus type 16 E4 and E7 proteins in sera of patients with cervical neoplasias. *Rev Roum Virol* 45: 185–192, 1994

259. Cuzick J, Szarewski A, Terry G, et al: Human papillomavirus testing in primary cervical screening. *Lancet* 345: 1533–1536, 1995

260. Hernandez E, Rosenshein NB: *Manual of Gynecologic Oncology.* New York, Churchill Livingstone, 1989

261. Fowler J, Montz FJ: Malignancies of the uterine cervix, in Cameron RB (ed): *Practical Oncology.* Norwalk, CT, Appleton & Lange, 1994, pp 364–376

262. Omura GA: Chemotherapy of cervix cancer, in Blackledge GRP, Jordon JA, Shingleton HM (eds): *Textbook of Gynecologic Oncology.* Philadelphia, Saunders, 1991, pp 361–368

263. Kolstad P: Follow-up study of 232 patients with stage 1a1 and 411 patients with stage 1a2 squamous cell carcinoma of the cervix (microinvasive carcinoma). *Gynecol Oncol* 33: 265–272, 1989

264. Perez CA: Radiation treatment of carcinoma of the uterine cervix, in Blackledge GRP, Jordan JA, Shingleton HM (eds): *Textbook of Gynecologic Oncology.* Philadelphia, Saunders, 1991, pp 328–360

265. Orlandi C, Costa S, Terzano P, et al: Presurgical assessment and therapy of microinvasive carcinoma of the cervix. *Gynecol Oncol* 59:255–260, 1995

266. Morris M: Conization for microinvasive carcinoma of the cervix. *Contemp OB/GYN* 40:79–99, 1995

267. Kinney WK, Alvarez RD, Reid GC, et al: Value of adjuvant

whole-pelvis irradiation after Wertheim Hysterectomy for early-stage squamous carcinoma of the cervix with pelvic nodal metastasis: A matched-control study. *Gynecol Oncol* 34:258–262, 1989

268. Clarke-Pearson DL, Soisson AP, Wall LL: Surgical treatment of early-stage cervical cancer, in Greer BE, Berek JS (eds): *Gynecologic Oncology: Treatment Rationale and Techniques.* New York, Elsevier, 1991, pp 187–206

269. Jones WB: Surgical approaches for advanced or recurrent cancer of the cervix. *Cancer* 60:2094–2103, 1987

270. Berek JS, Hacker NF: *Practical Gynecologic Oncology.* Baltimore, Williams and Wilkins, 1994

271. Eddy GL, Manetta A, Alvarez RD, et al: Neoadjuvant chemotherapy with vincristine and cisplatin followed by radical hysterectomy and pelvic lymphadenectomy for FIGO stage Ib bulky cervical cancer: a Gynecologic Oncology Group pilot study. *Gynecol Oncol* 57:412–416, 1995

272. Nevin J, Bloch B, Van-Wijk L, et al: Primary chemotherapy with bleomycin, ifosfamide and cisplatinum (BIP) followed by radiotherapy in the treatment of advanced cervical cancer. A pilot study. *Eur J Gynaecol Oncol* 16:30–35, 1995

273. Corn BW, Lanciano RM: Combined modality treatment for carcinomas of the uterine cervix and vulva. *Curr Opin Oncol* 6:524–530, 1994

274. Lewis E: The use and abuse of imaging in gynecologic cancer. *Cancer* 60:1993–2009, 1987

275. Henriksen E: The lymphatic spread of carcinoma of the cervix and the body of the uterus. *Am J Obstet Gynecol* 58:924–942, 1949

276. Osborne RJ, Murphy KJ, DePetrillo AD: Pelvic exenteration, in Greer BE, Berek JS (eds): *Gynecologic Oncology: Treatment Rationale and Techniques.* New York, Elsevier, 1991, pp 207–226

277. Schulmeister L: Nutrition, in Otto SE (ed): *Oncology Nursing.* Baltimore, Mosby, 1994, pp 641–657

278. Hardin TC, Page CP: Nutritional care, in Weiss GR (ed): *Clinical Oncology.* Norwalk, CT, Appleton & Lange, 1993, pp 50–58

279. Torres-Lobaton A, Bastida-Blanco A, Marquez-Acosta G, et al: Pelvic exenteration for cancer of the uterine cervix (prognostic factors). *Ginecol Obstet Mex* 62:189–193, 1994

280. Lagasse LD, Johnson GH, Smith ML, et al: Use of sigmoid colon for rectal substitution following pelvic exenteration. *Am J Obstet Gynecol* 116:106–110, 1973

281. Hatch KD, Shingleton HM, Potter ME, et al: Low rectal resection and anastomosis at the time of pelvic exenteration. *Gynecol Oncol* 31:262–267, 1988

282. Shell JA: Impact of cancer of sexuality, in Otto SE (ed): *Oncology Nursing.* Baltimore, Mosby, 1994, pp 737–760

283. Andersen BL, Lamb MA: Sexuality and cancer, in Murphy GP, Lawrence W, Lenhard RE (eds): *American Cancer Society Textbook of Clinical Oncology.* Atlanta, The American Cancer Society, 1995, pp 699–713

284. Stelzer KJ, Koh WJ, Greer BE, et al: The use of intraoperative radiation therapy in radical salvage for recurrent cervical cancer: outcome and toxicity. *Am J Obstet Gynecol* 172:1881–1886, 1995

285. Feldmann HJ, Seegenschmiedt MH, Molls M: Hyperthermia—its actual role in radiation oncology. Part III: Clinical rationale and results in deep seated tumors. *Strahlenther Onkol* 171:251–264, 1995

286. Fleming ID, Brady LW, Mieszkalski GB, et al: Basis for major current therapies for cancer, in Holleb GP, Lawrence W, Lenhard RE (eds): *American Cancer Society Textbook of Clinical Oncology.* Atlanta, 1995, pp 96–134

287. Untch M, Korell M, Kirschstein M, et al: The synergistic effect of delta-aminolevulinic acid and photodynamic laser therapy based on an in vitro model of the ATP tumor chemosensitivity test. *Gynakol-Geburtshilfliche-Rundsch* 35:85–89, 1995

288. Alberts DS, Garcia DJ: Salvage chemotherapy in recurrent or refractory squamous cell cancer of the uterine cervix. *Semin Oncol* 21:37–46, 1994 (suppl 7)

289. Thigpen JT: Chemotherapy, in Marrow CP, Townsend DE (eds): *Synopsis of Gynecologic Oncology.* New York, Wiley & Sons, 1987, pp 409–458

290. Hannigan EV, Dinh TV, & Doherty MG: Ifosfamide with Mesna in squamous carcinoma of the cervix: Phase II results in patients with advanced or recurrent disease. *Gynecol Oncol* 43:123–129, 1991

291. Thigpen R, Vance RB, Khansur T: Carcinoma of the uterine cervix: current status and future directions. *Semin Oncol* 21:43–54, 1994 (suppl 2)

292. Paredes-Espinoza M, Lippman SM, Kavanaph JJ, et al: Treatment of 32 cervico-uterine cancer patients with 13-cis-retinoic acid and interferon alpha. *Rev Invest Clin* 46:105–111, 1994

293. Stornes I, Mejlholm I, Jakopsen A: Phase II trial of ifosfamide, 5-fluorouracil, and leucovorin in recurrent uterine cervical cancer. *Gynecol Oncol* 55:123–125, 1994

294. Cervellino JC, Araugo CE, Sanchez O, et al: Cisplatin and ifosfamide in patients with advanced squamous cell carcinoma of the uterine cervix. A phase II trial. *Acta Oncol* 34:257–259, 1995

295. Fanning J, Ladd C, Hilgers RD: Cisplatin, 5-fluorouracil, and ifosfamide in the treatment of recurrent or advanced cervical cancer. *Gynecol Oncol* 56:235–238, 1995

296. Ng HT, Yuan CC, Kan YY, et al: An evaluation of chemotherapy in patients with cancer of the cervix and lymph node metastases. *Arch Gynecol Obstet* 256:1–4, 1995

297. Sueyama H, Nakano M, Sakumoto K, et al: Intraarterial (I-A) chemotherapy with cisplatin via uterine artery prior to definitive radiotherapy. *Gynecol Oncol* 59:327–332, 1995

298. Morris M, Eifel PJ, Burke TW, et al: Treatment of locally advanced cervical cancer with concurrent radiation and intraarterial chemotherapy. *Gynecol Oncol* 57:72–78, 1995

299. Scarabelli C, Zarrelli A, Gallo A, et al: Multimodal treatment with neoadjuvant intraarterial chemotherapy and radical surgery in patients with stage IIIb and IVa cervical cancer: A preliminary study. *Cancer* 76:1019–1026, 1995

300. Tsuji K, Yamada R, Kawabata M, et al: Effect of balloon occluded arterial infusion of anticancer drugs on the prognosis of cervical cancer treated with radiation therapy. *Int J Radiat Oncol Biol Phys* 32:1337–1345, 1995

301. Kim DS, Moon H, Kim KT, et al: Two-year survival: Preoperative adjuvant chemotherapy in the treatment of cervical cancer stage Ib and II with bulky tumor. *Gynecol Oncol* 33:225–230, 1989

302. Kim DS, Moon H, Hwang YY, et al: Preoperative adjuvant chemotherapy in the treatment of cervical cancer stage Ib, IIa, and IIb with bulky tumor. *Gynecol Oncol* 29:321–332, 1988

303. Kredentser DC: Etoposide (VP-16); Ifosfamide/Mesna, and Cisplatin chemotherapy for advanced and recurrent carcinoma of the cervix. *Gynecol Oncol* 43:145–148, 1991

304. Piver MS, Barlow JJ, Vongtama V, et al: Hydroxyurea and radiation therapy in advanced cervical cancer. *Am J Obstet Gynecol* 120:969–972, 1974

305. Stehman FB, Bundy BN, Thomas G, et al: Hydroxyurea versus misoidazole with radiation in cervical carcinoma:

long term follow-up of a gynecologic oncology group trial. *J Clin Oncol* 11:1523–1526, 1993

306. Hreshchyshyn MM, Aron BS, Boronow RC, et al: Hydroxyurea or placebo combined with radiation to treat stage IIIB and IV cervical cancer confined to the pelvis. *Int J Radiat Oncol Biol Phys* 5:317–322, 1979

307. Kuske RR, Perez CA, Grigsby PW, et al: Phase I/II study of definitive radiotherapy and chemotherapy (cisplatin and 5-fluorouracil) for advanced or recurrent gynecologic malignancies. *Am J Clin Oncol* 12:467–473, 1989

308. Rodriguez M, Sevin BU, Perras J, et al: Paclitaxel: a radiation sensitizer of human cervical cancer cells. *Gynecol Oncol* 57:165–169, 1995

309. Vasey PA, Bissett D, Strolin-Benedetti M, et al: Phase I clinical and pharmacokinetic study of 3′-deamino-3′-(2-methoxy-4-morpholinyl) doxorubicin (FCE 23762). *Cancer Res* 55:2090–2096, 1995

310. Lin JC, Ho ES, Jan JS, et al: Concomitant chemoradiotherapy for advanced epidermoid carcinoma of the uterine cervix: a preliminary report. *Chung-Hua-I-Hsueh-Tsa-Chih-Taipei* 54:26–32, 1994

311. Resbeut M, Cowen D, Viens P, et al: Concomitant chemoradiation prior to surgery in the treatment of advanced cervical carcinoma. *Gynecol Oncol* 54:68–75, 1994

312. Morris M, Gershenson DM, Burke TW, et al: A phase II study of carboplatin and cisplatin in advanced or recurrent squamous carcinoma of the uterine cervix. *Gynecol Oncol* 53:234–238, 1994

313. Vogl SE: Chemotherapy of squamous cell carcinoma of the uterine cervix: Progress and potential. *Curr Concepts Oncol* 5:10–11, 15–17, 1983

314. Chambers SK, Lamb L, Kohorn EI: Chemotherapy of recurrent/advanced cervical cancer: results of the Yale University PBM-PFU protocol. *Gynecol Oncol* 53:161–169, 1994

315. Murad AM, Triginelli SA, Ribalta JC: Phase II trial of bleomycin, ifosfamide, and carboplatin in metastatic cervical cancer. *J Clin Oncol* 12:55–59, 1994

316. Alberts DS, Garcia DJ: Salvage chemotherapy in recurrent or refractory squamous cell cancer of the uterine cervix. *Semin Oncol* 21:37–46, 1994 (suppl 7)

317. Kumar L, Kaushal R, Nandy M: Chemotherapy followed by radiotherapy versus radiotherapy alone in locally advanced cervical cancer: a randomized study. *Gynecol Oncol* 54:307–315, 1994

318. Marayama Y, Bowen MG, Van-Nagell JR, et al: A feasibility study of 252Cf neutron brachytherapy, cisplatin + 5-FU chemoadjuvant and accelerated hyperfractionated radiotherapy for advanced cervical cancer. *Int J Radiat Oncol Biol Phys* 29:529–534, 1994

319. Brock A, Prager W, Bohme R, Pohlmann S: The methods and results of simultaneous radiochemotherapy with carboplatin in advanced cervical carcinomas. *Strahlenther Onkol* 170:264–268, 1994

320. Frigerio L, Busci L, Rabaiotti E, Mariani A: Adjunctive radiotherapy after radical hysterectomy in high risk early stage cervical carcinoma. Assessment of morbidity and recurrences. *Eur J Gynaecol Oncol* 15:132–137, 1994

321. Husseinzadeh N, Shrake P, DeEulis R, et al: Chemotherapy and extended-field radiation therapy to paraaortic area in patients with histologically proven metastatic cervical cancer to paraaortic nodes: a phase II pilot study. *Gynecol Oncol* 52:326–331, 1994

322. Fang FM, Yeh CY, Lai YL, et al: Radiotherapy following simple hysterectomy in patients with invasive carcinoma of the uterine cervix. *J Formos Med Assoc* 92:420–425, 1993

323. Tattersall MH, Lorvidhaya V, Vootiprux V, et al: Randomized trial of epirubicin and cisplatin chemotherapy followed by pelvic radiation in locally advanced cervical cancer. *J Clin Oncol* 13:444–451, 1995

324. Goto S, Sakai S, Kera J, et al: A case report of recurrent cervical cancer which responded to a combination of biological therapies. *Eur J Gynaecol Oncol* 15:235–240, 1994

325. Perez CA, Breaux S, Bedwinek JM, et al: Radiation therapy alone in treatment of the uterine cervix. II. Analysis of complications. *Cancer* 54:235–246, 1984

326. Eifel PJ, Levenback C, Wharton JT, et al: Time course and incidence of late complications in patients treated with radiation therapy for FIGO stage IB carcinoma of the uterine cervix. *Int J Radiat Oncol Biol Phys* 32:1289–1300, 1995

327. Cartwright-Alcarese F: Addressing sexual dysfunction following radiation therapy for a gynecologic malignancy. *Oncol Nurs Forum* 22:1227–1232, 1995

328. Freeman HP: Cancer in the socioeconomically disadvantaged. *CA Cancer J Clin* 39:266–288, 1989

329. Wilkes G, Freeman H, Prout M: Cancer and poverty: breaking the cycle. *Semin Oncol Nurs* 10:79–88, 1994

330. Devesa S: Cancer patterns among women in the United States. *Semin Oncol Nurs* 11:78–87, 1995

331. Boring CC, Squires TS, Heath CW: Cancer statistics for African Americans. *CA Cancer J Clin* 42:7–18, 1992

332. Calle EE, Flanders WD, Thun MJ, et al: Demographic predictors of mammography and Pap smear screening in US women. *Am J Public Health* 83:53–60, 1993

333. Whitman S, Ansell D, Lacey L, et al: Patterns of breast and cervical cancer screening at three public health centers in an inner-city urban area. *Am J Public Health* 81:1651–1653, 1991

334. Berman BA, Bastani R, Nisenbaum R, et al: Cervical cancer screening among a low-income multiethnic population of women. *J Women's Health* 3:33–43, 1994

335. Davis DT, Bustamante A, Brown CP, et al: The urban church and cancer control: a source of social influence in minority communities. *Public Health Rep* 109:500–506, 1994

336. Mitchell H: Pap smears collected by nurse practitioners: a comparison with smears collected by medical practitioners. *Oncol Nurs Forum* 20:807–810, 1993

337. Ansell D, Lacey L, Whitman S, et al: A nurse-delivered intervention to reduce barriers to breast and cervical cancer screening in Chicago inner city clinics. *Public Health Rep* 109:104–111, 1994

338. Sung JF, Coates RJ, Williams JE: Cancer screening intervention among black women in inner-city Atlanta—design of a study. *Public Health Rep* 107:381–388, 1992

339. Crum CP: Carcinoma of the vulva: epidemiology and pathogenesis. *Obstet Gynecol* 79:448–454, 1992

340. Cavanagh D, Fiorica JV, Hoffman MS, et al: Invasive carcinoma of the vulva. *Am J Obstet Gynecol* 163:1007–1014, 1990

341. Rollason TP: Vulva and vagina: Pathology of malignant tumors, in Blackledge CRP, Jordan JA, Shingleton HM (eds): *Textbook of Gynecologic Oncology.* Philadelphia, Saunders, 1991, pp 390–411

342. Hording U, Junge J, Poulsen H, et al: Vulvar intraepithelial neoplasia III: A viral disease of undetermined progressive potential. *Gynecol Oncol* 56:276–279, 1995

343. Nuovo GJ, Delvenne P, MacConnell P, et al: Correlation of histology and detection of human papillomavirus DNA in vulvar cancers. *Gynecol Oncol* 43:275–280, 1991

344. Anderson WA, Franquemont DW, Williams J, et al: Vulvar squamous cell carcinoma and papillomaviruses: Two separate entities? *Am J Obstet Gynecol* 165:329–336, 1991

345. Hording U, Junge J, Daugaard S, et al: Vulvar squamous cell carcinoma and papillomaviruses: Indications for two different etiologies. *Gynecol Oncol* 52:241–246, 1994

346. Britton LA, Nasca PL, Mallin K, et al: Case control study of cancer of the vulva. *Obstet Gynecol* 75:859, 1990

347. Friedrich EJ, Wilkinson EJ, Fu YS: Carcinoma in situ of the vulva: A continuing challenge. *Am J Obstet Gynecol* 136: 830–843, 1980

348. Morrow CP, Townsend DE (eds): *Synopsis of Gynecologic Oncology* (ed 3). New York, Wiley, 1987

349. Plentl AA, Friedman EA: *Lymphatic system of the female genitalia: The morphologic basis of oncologic diagnosis and therapy.* Philadelphia, Saunders, 1971

350. DiPaola GR, Belardi MG: Squamous vulvar intraepithelial neoplasia, in Knapstein PG, DiRe F, DiSaia P (eds): *Malignancies of the vulva.* New York, Thieme Medical Publishers, 1991, pp 57–72

351. Buscema J, Woodruff JD, Parmley TH, et al: Carcinoma in situ of the vulva. *Obstet Gynecol* 55:225–230, 1980

352. Rubin D: Gynecologic cancer: cervical, vulvar, and vaginal malignancies. *RN* May:56–63, 1987

353. Monaghan JM: Presentation of carcinoma of the vulva, in Blackledge GRP, Jordan JA, Shingleton HM (eds): *Textbook of Gynecologic Oncology.* Philadelphia, Saunders, 1991, pp 412–418

354. Forney JP, Morrow CP, Townsend DE, et al: Management of carcinoma in situ of the vulva. *Am J Obstet Gynecol* 127: 801–806, 1977

355. Dean RE, Taylor ES, Weisbrod DM, et al: The treatment of premalignant and malignant lesions of the vulva. *Am J Obstet Gynecol* 119:59–68, 1974

356. Higgins RV, Van Nagell JR Jr., Donaldson ES, et al: The efficacy of laser therapy in the treatment of cervical intraepithelial neoplasia. *Gynecol Oncol* 36:79, 1990

357. Baggish MS, Dorsey JH: $CO_2$ laser for the treatment of vulvar carcinoma in situ. *Obstet Gynecol* 57:371–375, 1981

358. Hacker NF: Vulvar cancer, in Berek JS, Hacker NF (eds): *Practical Gynecologic Oncology* (ed 2). Baltimore, Williams and Wilkins, 1994, pp 403–439

359. Bjerregaard B, Andreasson B, VisFeldt J, et al: The significance of histology and morphometry in predicting lymph node metastases in patients with squamous cell carcinoma of the vulva. *Gynecol Oncol* 50:323–329, 1993

360. Burger MP, Hollema H, Emanuels AG: The importance of the groin node status for survival of $T_1$ and $T_2$ vulval carcinoma patients. *Gynecol Oncol* 57:327–334, 1995

361. Siller BS, Alvarez RD, Conner WD, et al: $T_{2-3}$ vulvar cancer: A case-control study of triple incision versus en bloc radical vulvectomy and inguinal lymphadenectomy. *Gynecol Oncol* 57:335–339, 1995

362. Farias-Eisner R, Cirisano FD, Grouse D, et al: Conservative and individualized surgery for early squamous carcinoma of the vulva: The treatment of choice for stage I and II ($T_{1-2}N_{0-1}M_0$) disease. *Gynecol Oncol* 53:55–58, 1994

363. Hacker NF: Management of stage I vulvar cancer, in Snapstein PG, Dire F, DiSaia P, et al (eds): *Malignancies of the Vulva* (ed 1). New York, Thieme Medical Publishers, 1991, pp 80–98

364. Cavanagh D, Fiorica JV, Hoffman MS, et al: Invasive carcinoma of the vulva. *Am J Obstet Gynecol* 163:1007–1014, 1990

365. Homesley HD, Bundy BN, Sedlis A, et al: Radiation therapy versus pelvic node resection for carcinoma of the vulva with positive groin nodes. *Obstet Gynecol* 69:733–740, 1986

366. Durrant KR: Tumors of the vulva and vagina: Treatment of advanced disease, in Blackledge GRP, Jordan JA, Shingleton HM (eds): *Textbook of Gynecologic Oncology.* Philadelphia, Saunders, 1991, pp 426–431

367. Greer BE, Berek JS: Evolution of the primary treatment of invasive squamous cell carcinoma of the vulva, in Greer BE, Berek JS (eds): *Gynecology Oncology: Treatment, Rationale and Techniques.* New York, Elsevier, 1991, pp 227–238

368. Chamorro T: Cancer of the vulva and vagina. *Semin Oncol Nurs* 6:198–205, 1990

369. Thomas G, Dembo A, DePetrillo A, et al: Concurrent radiation and chemotherapy in vulvar carcinoma. *Gynecol Oncol* 59:51–56, 1995

370. Eifel PJ, Morris M, Burke TW, et al: Prolonged continuous infusion cisplatin and 5-flurouracil with radiation for locally advanced carcinoma of the vulva. *Gynecol Oncol* 59: 51–56, 1995

371. Podczaski E, Herbst AL: Cancer of the vagina and fallopian tube, in Knapp RS, Berkowitz RS (eds): *Gynecologic Oncology,* New York, MacMillan, 1986, pp 339–424

372. Davis KP, Stanhope CR, Garton GR, et al: Invasive vaginal carcinoma: Analysis of early stage disease. *Gynecol Oncol* 42: 131–136, 1991

373. Audet-Lapointe P, Body G, Vauclair R, et al: Vaginal intraepithelial neoplasia. *Gynecol Oncol* 36:232–239, 1990

374. Rubin SC, Young J, Mikuta JJ: Squamous carcinoma of the vagina: Treatment complications and long-term follow-up. *Gynecol Oncol* 20:346, 1985

375. Binton LA, Nasca PC, Mallin K, et al: Case-control study of in situ and invasive carcinoma of the vagina. *Gynecol Oncol* 38:49–54, 1990

376. Auclair CA: Consequences of prenatal exposure to diethylstilbestrol. *J Gynecol Nurs* 8:35–39, 1979

377. Robboy SJ, Noller KL, O'Brien P, et al: Increased incidence of cervical and vaginal dysplasia in 3980 diethylstilbestrol-exposed young women. Experience of the National Collaborative Diethylstilbestrol Adenosia Project. *JAMA* 252: 2979–2983, 1984

378. Sulak P, Barhill D, Heller P, et al: Nonsquamous cancer of the vagina. *Gynecol Oncol* 29:309–320, 1988

379. Plentl AA, Friedman EA: *Lymphatic System in the Female Genitalia.* Philadelphia, Saunders, 1971

380. Aho M, Vesterinen E, Meyer B, et al: Natural history of vaginal intraepithelial neoplasia. *Cancer* 68:195–197, 1991

381. Kucera H, Vavra N: Radiation management of primary carcinoma of the vagina: Clinical and histopathological variables associated with survival. *Gynecol Oncol* 40:12–16, 1991

382. American Joint Committee on Cancer: *Manual of Staging of Cancer,* (ed 4). Chicago, AJCC, 1992

383. Nolke S, Hanjani P: Intraepithelial neoplasia of the lower genital tract. *Semin Oncol Nurs* 6:181–189, 1990

384. Woodruff JD, Parmley TH, Julian CG: Topical 5-fluorouracil in the treatment of vaginal carcinoma-in-situ. *Gynecol Oncol* 3:124–132, 1975

385. Perez CA, Camel HM: Long-term follow-up in radiation therapy of carcinoma of the vagina. *Cancer* 49:1308–1315, 1982

386. Nanavanti PJ, Fanning J, Hilgers RD, et al: High-dose-rate brachytherapy in primary stage I and II vaginal cancer. *Gynecol Oncol* 51:67–71, 1993

387. Herbst AL, Robboy SJ, Sculley RE, et al: Clear-cell adenocarcinoma of the vagina and cervix in girls: Analysis of 170 registry cases. *Am J Obstet Gynecol* 119:713–724, 1974

388. Geisler JP, Look KY, Moore DA, et al: Pelvic exenteration for malignant melanomas of the vagina or urethra with over 3mm of invasion. *Gynecol Oncol* 59:338–341, 1995

389. Mooney KH, Feukell BR, Nail LM, et al: 1991 Oncology Nursing Society Research Priorities Survey. *Oncol Nurs Forum* 18:1381–1388, 1991

390. Walczak JR, Nolte S, Eriksson JH: A survey of research priorities in gynecologic (GYN) nursing. Poster of NAACOG Ninth National Meeting, Minneapolis, 1992

391. Nolte S, Walczak JR, Eriksson JH: A model for developing a nursing research program in a national cooperative group. *Proc Oncol Nurs Soc 17th Congress, 1992* (in press)

# Chapter 40

# Head and Neck Malignancies

Connie Yuska Bildstein, RN, MS, CORLN

Carol Blendowski, RN, BS, OCN®

## INTRODUCTION

The challenges for the patient presented by a diagnosis of head and neck cancer are significant. No other tumor site is exposed so completely to society's view. The patient not only must cope with extreme physiological changes in structure and function but also must incorporate changes in body perception as well. In addition, nurses need to understand the magnitude of the rehabilitation needs based on the structural and functional changes that result. It is important to understand the normal anatomic and functional relationships that exist in the head and neck area so that the extent of subsequent deficits created by surgery or tumor can be predicted and rehabilitation planned.

The challenge for the nurse caring for the patient with head and neck cancer is to understand the disease process and available treatment options. In addition, the ability to clearly predict and support rehabilitation needs is paramount. The purpose of this chapter is to provide a comprehensive review of the disease process as it presents in various anatomic sites in the head and neck area and to discuss treatment options and care.

## EPIDEMIOLOGY

It is estimated that approximately 70,800 new cases of head and neck cancer were diagnosed in the United States in 1996, an annual incidence rate of approximately 17 per 100,000. This figure represents about 4% of all malignant tumors in the United States. However, the disease is much more prevalent in other parts of the world. The frequency of distribution of primary tumors in the anatomic sites are as follows: 40% oral cavity, 25% larynx, 15% oro/hypopharynx, 7% major salivary glands, and

13% in remaining sites. The ratio of male to female incidence remains 3:1. However, the incidence of squamous carcinomas of all sites of the upper aerodigestive tract has risen in females. This rise can be attributed to an increased incidence of consumption of alcohol and tobacco in this group.[1] The incidence increases markedly after age 50, averaging about 45 in 100,000 during the sixth decade and 65 in 100,000 during the seventh and eighth decades. For males the incidence increases to 70 in 100,000 in the seventh decade and 100 in 100,000 during the eighth decade.[1]

In some tumors of the head and neck, pain occurs very late, causing a delay in medical treatment. On initial presentation, 80%–90% of oral cancers are 2 cm or more in diameter. More than 60% of the 70,800 individuals in whom head and neck cancer is diagnosed each year in the United States will have advanced disease. Complicating this picture is the fact that the development of head and neck tumors is associated with the personal habits of smoking and drinking alcohol. Although the intake of these substances is under the control of the individual, the presentation of a patient who has a history of addiction to cigarettes and alcohol is consistent with the denial of symptoms and a subsequent delay in seeking medical treatment.

## ETIOLOGY

Tobacco use remains the primary risk factor in the development of head and neck cancer. This includes not only cigarette use but the use of smokeless tobacco as well. The sites at greatest risk for developing cancer from tobacco use are the areas in which direct contact with tobacco and tobacco smoke occur. Those sites are the oral cavity, pharynx, larynx, and esophagus. The relative risk and development of disease will vary according to the daily consumption, type, and manner of tobacco use.[2]

The use of smokeless tobacco increased significantly during the 1970s because it was promoted as a "safe" alternative to smoking. The group of tobacco users changed from men over 50 years of age and older women living primarily in the South to white, male adolescents and young adults in the age range of 14–29 years.[3]

Over 95% of the cases of head and neck cancer can be attributed to the use of tobacco and alcohol together.[4] The combination of alcohol and tobacco potentiates carcinogenesis and creates a significantly higher risk than does either one alone.[5] Some studies have also shown an association with exposure to wood, metal, leather, or textile dust. In addition, poor oral hygiene and possibly chronic mechanical irritation from ill-fitting dentures and plates or sharp, jagged teeth have been predisposing factors in the development of carcinoma of the tongue as well as the gingiva and other sites in the oral cavity. As many as 15% of patients with head and neck cancer may have a viral etiology associated with the development of their tumors.[6] The Epstein-Barr virus (EBV) has long been associated with the development of nasopharyngeal cancers as suggested by the high incidence of elevated EBV titers in patients with nasopharyngeal cancer.[7]

Nutritional deficiencies are also seen in patients with head and neck cancer. Plummer-Vinson syndrome, in which iron deficiency anemia occurs, has been associated with cancers of the tongue, hypopharynx, and esophagus. This syndrome is characterized by generalized nutritional deficiencies, anemia, achlorhydria, chronic dysphagia, and splenic enlargement. Atrophy of the mucous membranes in the mouth and pharynx may also be presenting symptoms. Vitamin A deficiencies and retinoids may play a role in the development of disease as well. Other associated risk factors are listed in Table 40-1.

**TABLE 40-1**   Risk Factors in the Development of Head and Neck Cancer

| Risk Factor | Associated Site |
| --- | --- |
| Tobacco use (cigarettes, snuff) | Oral, pharyngeal, laryngeal |
| Heavy alcohol intake | Oral, pharyngeal, laryngeal |
| Poor oral hygiene | Oral |
| Jagged teeth | Oral |
| Improperly fitting dentures | Oral |
| Exposure to wood dust | Nasopharyngeal |
| Leather manufacturing | Oral, pharyngeal, laryngeal |
| Mustard gas | Oral, pharyngeal, laryngeal |
| Betel nut chewing | Oral |
| Exposure to metals (nickel, chromium) | Oral, pharyngeal, laryngeal |
| Exposure to the sun | Lip |

## PREVENTION, SCREENING, EARLY DETECTION PROGRAMS

### Primary Prevention

Avoiding use of tobacco and alcohol is key to prevention of head and neck cancer. As public awareness of the dangers of tobacco use grows and a negative image of smoking is portrayed in the media, it is anticipated that the incidence of head and neck cancer will decrease. Nurses can play an active role in community education by participating in health fairs and corporate health-related events and by contacting the media to emphasize the dangers of tobacco use. In 1989 a coordinated, nationwide campaign was launched by the American Academy of Otolaryngology, Head and Neck Surgery, Inc., and the National Cancer Institute to dissuade our nation's youth from using smokeless tobacco. The campaign is titled "Through with Chew" and is primarily directed toward young boys aged 11–17. Nurses and other health professionals can participate in this and other community awareness programs by presenting lectures at local area schools.

Nurses, primary care physicians, and other health care providers are frequently in positions where they see children and parents together. This presents an opportunity to provide education regarding the serious health effects presented by smoking and by inhaling secondhand smoke. A strong message can be sent to smokers who have children or other nonsmoking members in the household. In addition, the health care professional can discuss ways a parent can discourage smoking by their children. For example, the parent can quit smoking, deny the child access to tobacco, express disapproval of smoking, and explain the serious health effects that result from smoking. In discussing this subject with teenagers, one effective approach is to discuss the undesirable cosmetic effects that result from long-term use of tobacco. Moreover, if the teen is an athlete, discussing the adverse effects on athletic performance can be a motivating factor in either stopping smoking or never taking up the habit. Nurses can use every encounter with a child or young adult to make the point that smoking is a dangerous, addictive, and unhealthy habit.[8]

### Retinoids

Isotretinoin has shown some activity in suppressing oral premalignancies and in preventing second primary tumors in patients with squamous cell cancer of the head and neck. One hundred and three patients who received prior treatment for oral cavity carcinoma were either randomized to placebo or to 50–100 mg/m³/d of isotretinoin orally for one year. Although there was no significant difference in recurrence rate of primary cancers, 4% of patients in the isotretinoin group had second primaries at 32 months, compared with 24% of those in the placebo group. Despite these promising results, further clinical trials are needed to identify the ideal chemopreventive approach to treating oral cancers.[9]

## Screening and Early Detection

The role of the nurse in early detection clinics is becoming even more important as health care institutions and payors emphasize "wellness care." This includes periodic screening of high-risk individuals. Nurses in early detection clinics can perform thorough head and neck exams and collect comprehensive patient histories. Referrals can be made to smoking-cessation programs to decrease the chance of individuals developing head and neck malignancy.

Early detection remains the key to successful control of disease. Five-year disease-free cure rates remain about 30%–40%, regardless of tumor site. These poor results are related to size of tumor at diagnosis as well as the presence of regional lymph node disease and distant metastases. More than 60% of individuals diagnosed each year with head and neck cancer have advanced disease upon presentation. Diagnosis may be delayed because pain may not be present and denial of symptoms and a fear of treatment are common.

Often, metastasis to regional lymph nodes has already occurred when the patient first seeks medical care. Head and neck cancers typically are very aggressive locally and spread initially to anatomic sites within the head and neck area. This pattern of spread makes treatment more complex and the subsequent course of rehabilitation more challenging.

## PATHOPHYSIOLOGY

Approximately 95% of all head and neck carcinomas are squamous cell in origin. Arising from the epithelium that lines the upper aerodigestive tract, the typical mucosal lesion can appear as an ulceration, roughened or thickened area, cauliflowerlike lesion, or a combination of all of these. Submucosal lesions can begin in epithelial invaginations such as the tonsils or tongue base, or from the ducts of minor salivary glands. Early lesions generally have either a reddish (erythroplasia) or whitish (leukoplakia) color. As the tumor grows, infection, necrosis, or bleeding may occur.

The majority of head and neck tumors invade locally, deep into underlying structures as well as along tissue planes (including perichondrium or periosteum) or nerves. Direct invasion into bone occurs late in the course of the disease, through preexistent anatomic openings. Perineural and lymphatic spread contribute to the metastasis of malignant cells beyond the primary site.

Lymphatic spread occurs both locally at the primary site and regionally through lymphatic channels when tumor implantation into the lymph nodes occurs. Enlarged cervical lymph nodes combined with a diagnosis of a head and neck malignancy reflects this implantation and may be the presenting symptom. Poorly differentiated tumors tend to metastasize early to regional lymph nodes and beyond. Lymphatic drainage of the head and neck area is depicted in Figure 40-1.

The presence or absence of histologically proven lymph node metastasis is an important factor in determining prognosis. As the number of nodes involved with tumor increases, the degree of lymph node involvement and the presence of soft tissue spread after penetration of the lymph node capsule are other factors that affect prognosis. As tumor spreads to lower nodes in the neck, there appears to be a related reduction in the five-year survival rate. The prognosis and survival rates are the lowest for individuals with involvement in the lower third of the neck and with three or more positive nodes.

The greatest risk of a second primary tumor occurs within the initial three-year period following treatment for primary cancer. Approximately 30% of individuals with head and neck cancer will have a second primary cancer; in many cases the lung will be the site of a second

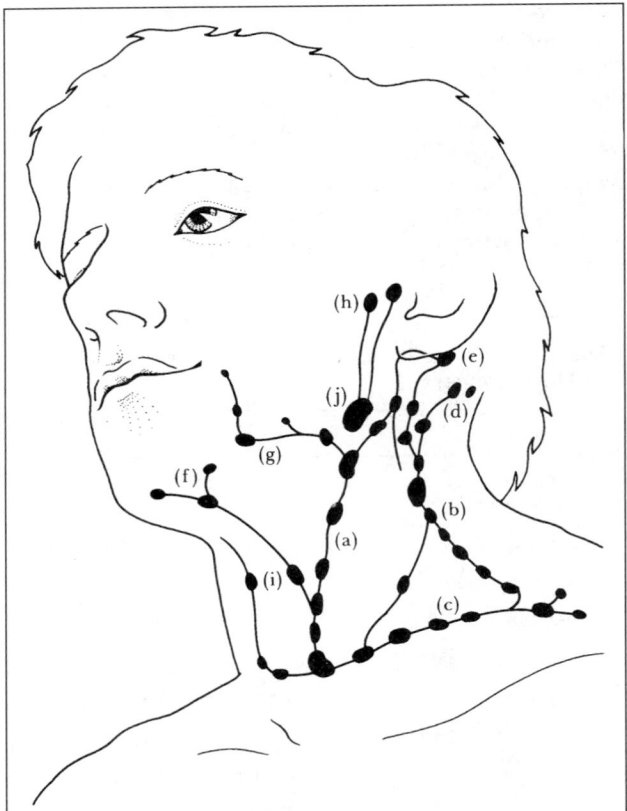

**FIGURE 40-1** Lymphatic drainage of the head and neck. (a) Lateral cervical midjugular. (b) Midposterior cervical. (c) Supraclavicular. (d) Occipital. (e) Posterior auricular. (f) Submental. (g) Submandibular. (h) Preauricular. (i) Anterior cervical. (j) Subdigastric.

primary. For this reason it is recommended that the patient be examined at regular intervals for the first three to five years following treatment.

---

## CLINICAL MANIFESTATIONS

### Carcinoma of the Nasal Cavity and Paranasal Sinuses

Eighty percent of cancers in the nasal cavity and paranasal sinus area are squamous cell in origin. The remainder are adenocarcinomas. The maxillary sinus is the most common tumor site in this area and most tumors are squamous cell in origin. Adenocarcinoma is more commonly diagnosed in the ethmoid sinus, which accounts for the remainder of tumors in the area. Primary carcinomas are rarely seen in the frontal or sphenoid sinuses. Most patients are over the age of 40 at diagnosis, and there is a 2:1 male predominance over females.[10]

The incidence of nasal cavity carcinoma is increased in persons with occupations in nickel plating, furniture manufacturing, and leather working. In addition, exposure to chromate compounds, hydrocarbons, nitrosamines, and dioxane has proven to be a risk. Other occupational exposures include mustard gas, isopropyl alcohol, and petroleum.

Symptoms may be similar to those of chronic sinusitis, although in the early stages of disease the patient may be asymptomatic. Other symptoms include a stuffy nose, history of sinus headache, dull facial pain, rhinorrhea, epistaxis, cheek hypoesthesia, trismus, and loose teeth. Physical findings may include diplopia, proptosis, a submucosal palatal mass, maxillary fullness, or a cranial nerve deficit. General prognosis is more favorable if tumors are located anterior and inferior to a plane connecting the medial canthus to the angle of the mandible. Tumors that are posterior and superior to this plane, such as those that are closer to the orbit and cranium, carry a less favorable prognosis. Cervical adenopathy is also an unfavorable finding that occurs in 10% of patients at diagnosis.[10]

### Carcinoma of the Nasopharynx

Symptoms of nasopharyngeal carcinoma may include nasal obstruction (with or without epistaxis), hearing impairment and tinnitus secondary to obstruction of the eustachian tube, and otitis media. An enlarged node in the neck may be the first indication of nasopharyngeal carcinoma in many patients. Poorly localized headache and facial pain are symptoms that occur late in the course of disease and can signify bony erosion and pressure on the fifth cranial nerve. Invasion of tumor through the base of the skull results in cranial nerve involvement; therefore, cranial nerve abnormalities provide important diagnostic information (Table 40-2). Double vision will occur when the third, fourth, and sixth cranial nerves are involved. The presence of Horner's syndrome represents

**TABLE 40-2**  Symptoms of Cranial Nerve Compression from Nasopharyngeal Carcinoma

| Nerve | Symptoms |
|---|---|
| Olfactory (I) | Seldom occurs; difficult to assess unilateral deficiency to olfaction |
| Optic (II) | Complete unilateral blindness |
| Oculomotor (III) | Paralysis of the upper, lower, and inner rectus muscle of the eye; complete fixation of the eye except for its lateral movement |
| Trochlear (IV) | Paralysis of the superior oblique muscles of the eye |
| Trigeminal (V) | Neurological pain of supraorbital and superior maxillary regions; painful anesthesia of half of the tongue, floor of the mouth, and buccal mucosa; compression of the mandibular branch results in paralysis of the temporal, internal pterygoid, and masseter muscles; lack of corneal reflex |
| Abducens (VI) | Paralysis of the external rectus muscle of the eye and diplopia |
| Facial (VII) | Peripheral facial paralysis; seldom occurs |
| Acoustic (VIII) | Loss of hearing and vertigo; seldom occurs |
| Glossopharyngeal (IX) | Difficulty swallowing, partial loss of taste, hoarseness, hemi-anesthesia of the soft palate |
| Vagus (X) | Anesthesia of the soft palate, pharynx, and larynx; tachycardia and tachypnea |
| Spinal accessory (XI) | Paralysis and atrophy of the trapezius and sternocleidomastoid muscles; hemiparesis of the soft palate and larynx |
| Hypoglossal (XII) | Rapid atrophy of the affected side of the tongue, which, when protracted, deviates toward the affected side |
| Cervical sympathetic nerve | Constriction of the pupil, retraction of the eye into the orbit, and narrowing of the palpebral fissure (Horner's syndrome) |

tumor invasion of the sympathetic nerve fibers accompanying the carotid artery as it passes intracranially. The syndrome is characterized by ptosis, miosis, and anhidrosis.[11] Epistaxis may occur with necrosis of the tumor and vessel walls. Malignant tumors of the nasopharynx are one of the few tumors in the head and neck that metastasize widely. Frequent sites of metastasis include the lung, liver, and bone.

## Carcinoma of the Oral Cavity

If diagnosed early when tumor size is small, cure rates for cancer of the oral cavity improve dramatically. In 1996 an estimated 29,490 people in the United States developed cancer of the oral cavity, and approximately 8,260 of those succumbed to the disease.[12] Cancer of the oral cavity and oropharynx account for 4% of all cancers in men and 2% of all cancers in women.[13]

The assessment and finding of oral cavity lesions are frequently first made in the dentist's office and are then referred to the otolaryngologist/head and neck cancer surgeon. The following positive findings in the history should alert the clinician to the possibility of an oral malignancy: history of smoking (cigarettes, cigars, and pipes), alcohol abuse, use of smoking tobacco (chewing tobacco and snuff), and systemic syphilis. Other potential factors include a history of poor oral hygiene; poorly fitting dentures and dental appliances; and, particularly in India (or among individuals of Indian descent), a habit of chewing betel nuts. Also, a custom in India that is associated with a higher incidence of hard palate carcinomas, is the habit of reverse smoking of cigarettes, or "chuttas," in which the lighted end is placed in the mouth.[14]

Alcohol also acts as an irritant to the oral mucosa. Alcohol is thought to act synergistically with tobacco in causing oral cavity cancers. In addition, it may act indirectly by promoting malnutrition and cirrhosis. These two side effects may indirectly stimulate activity of oral carcinogens.

*Field cancerization* is the development of multiple primary cancers that occur either concurrently or subsequently in the same patient. The mechanism of action is unclear; however, it is suggested that groups of cells are stimulated to form lesions in an appropriate tissue environment. The continuance of the habits of smoking and alcohol consumption contribute to the provision of a suitable environment for the development of cancer. As many as 37% of patients with oral cavity cancers have been reported to develop multiple tumors. Tumors can involve separate organ systems; however, most seem to involve the same organ area. The initial three-year period following therapy for the primary lesion is the period of greatest risk for the development of a second primary.[15]

More than 90% of oral cavity tumors are squamous cell carcinomas. Adenocarcinomas rank second in frequency. Squamous cell cancers are more often seen in men and older age groups, while adenocarcinomas predominate in younger-aged women.[16] However, it is important to remember that oral cavity carcinomas are neither age- nor sex-specific.

## Carcinoma of the Hypopharynx

Patients with cancer of the hypopharynx typically present with: odynophagia (painful swallowing), referred otalgia (usually unilateral), and dysphagia (difficulty swallowing). Advanced tumors of the pyriform sinus and pharyngeal wall with extension into the larynx may have the associated symptoms of hoarseness or aspiration. The patient often reports a history of difficulty swallowing even liquids and has a sensation of a foreign body in the throat as evidenced by repeated attempts to clear the throat. If these symptoms have persisted for some time, there is often an accompanying weight loss and an alteration in the nutritional status.

## Carcinoma of the Larynx

Cancer of the larynx cannot be considered one disease, but, rather, as cancer involving different areas within the larynx such as the glottis (space between the true cords), supraglottis (area and structures above the glottis), and subglottis (area and structures below the glottis). Tumors in each region involve distinct signs and symptoms, treatment regimens, and, most important, rehabilitation measures.

### Subglottic carcinoma

The subglottic area is the area from the lower border of the vocal cords to the cervical trachea. Subglottic tumors, like as supraglottic tumors, are more likely to be poorly differentiated when compared to glottic carcinomas. Poorly differentiated tumors also metastasize more often and are cured less often.

### Glottic carcinoma

The glottic area includes the upper surface of the vocal fold (horizontal plane at the floor of the ventricle) and extending 1 cm below this plane. This area includes the true vocal folds and the anterior and posterior glottic commissures. Tumors in this area tend to be well-differentiated, grow slowly, and metastasize late. Because there are limited lymphatics in the cord, metastasis usually occurs only when the disease infiltrates muscle or has spread beyond the limits of the true cord. The lesion may extend across the midline to the opposite cord or may invade the thyroid cartilage. In addition, spread may occur superiorly into the ventricles, ventricular bands, and aryepiglottic fold. Inferior extension may occur into the subglottic space. If vocal cord motion is impaired, it may indicate extension of posteriorly situated cord lesions into the cricoarytenoid articulation and arytenoid region.

Important diagnostic information includes the mobility of the cords, evidence of fixation of the cord, involvement of the anterior commissure, and involvement of cervical lymphatic vessels.

### Supraglottic carcinoma

Lesions that lie superior to a horizontal plane passing through the floor of the ventricles and including the epiglottis, aryepiglottic folds, arytenoids, and ventricular bands (false cords) are classified as supraglottic tumors. Supraglottic tumors account for 35% of laryngeal cancers and are characterized by aggressive growth patterns, both by direct extension and lymph node metastases. Approximately one-half of these patients will present with lymph node involvement, which occurs because lymphatic channels drain into the jugulodigastric, mid, and inferior levels of the internal jugular chain.[10]

Supraglottic cancer is often advanced when first detected because there are few early symptoms. The patient may complain of pain and poorly defined throat and neck discomfort that occurs during swallowing. Many patients complain of referred otalgia in combination with throat pain. Glottic hoarseness may occur in advanced disease and usually means that vocal cord fixation has occurred from tumor extension. The presence or absence of vocal cord fixation is an important factor in deciding on therapy.

## ASSESSMENT

A thorough review of the patient's medical history should be done, with particular emphasis on exposure to carcinogens as well as a positive family history of cancer. A review of lifestyle habits and occupation should also be included. In addition, a thorough review of current symptomatology should be included. The following symptoms are all significant: unilateral nasal obstruction or discharge, persistent ulceration, persistent hoarseness, odynophagia, dysphagia, sore throat, and cervical adenopathy. Persistent symptoms lasting longer than three weeks should be promptly reported to a physician.[3]

A thorough assessment should be performed using inspection and palpation techniques. The following equipment will be necessary: a good light source, gloves, tongue blade, nasal speculum, laryngeal mirror, and otoscope.

### Physical Exam

Bimanual examination is essential in assessing the oral cavity and neck. Careful attention must be directed toward the exam of the oral cavity. The buccal mucosa should be retracted and the U-shaped floor of the mouth should be closely inspected. The areas of the oral cavity

and oropharynx are generally considered high-risk areas and should be assessed carefully. Regional metastasis in the neck is the *only* presenting symptom in more than one-third of patients with head and neck cancers. The examination of the neck should assess the presence or absence of palpable adenopathy, number, location, and size of palpable lymph nodes. In addition, the presence of extracapsular extension of disease such as fixation of the overlying skin or soft tissue or paralysis of the cranial nerves should be noted.[4] The most common lymph node groups involved will be the jugular and posterior cervical chains and the submandibular lymphatics. In particular, the subdigastric nodes including the upper jugular and tonsillar nodes most frequently will be involved.[4]

In addition to a thorough history and physical exam, an indirect mirror examination of the pharynx and larynx will be performed. Advances in optics technology have allowed greater visualization of the hypopharyngeal and laryngeal areas with flexible fiberoptic endoscopes. This exam is easily performed in the physician's office using local anesthetics.

## Diagnostic Studies

An even more thorough exam of the entire head and neck area is next performed under either local or general anesthesia in the operating room. Biopsies of suspicious areas are obtained to confirm a histological diagnosis. In addition, conventional radiography, computerized tomography (CT), magnetic resonance imaging (MRI), and positron emission tomography (PET) are valuable tools in performing a comprehensive evaluation and assessment of response to therapy. The use of PET has been helpful in differentiating malignancy from normal tissue. The technique is not yet widely used and is expensive; however, the technology shows promise in the field of diagnostics for head and neck cancer. Open biopsy of a neck mass should be considered only as a last resort when a primary site cannot be identified. Normal anatomical relationships and structural function of specific sites in the head and neck area will be discussed individually.

Unless the patient is symptomatic, an extensive metastatic workup for distant disease is seldom indicated. The incidence of distant metastasis at initial presentation is so low that a comprehensive metastatic workup usually is not cost-effective.[1]

## CLASSIFICATION AND STAGING

It is essential to stage all tumors prior to initiating therapy because accurate staging provides the framework for selection of the appropriate therapy. Head and neck tumors are classified and staged according to the TNM classification system proposed by the American Joint Committee on Cancer and the International Union Against Cancer.[17]

The $T$ (tumor) indicates the extent of the primary tumor; $N$ (node) indicates regional lymph node involvement, $M$ (metastasis) indicates spread outside the head and neck region. Generally, tumors of the oral cavity and oropharynx are staged by their surface dimensions. Tumors of the larynx, nasopharynx, and hypopharynx are staged by their local extent to adjacent anatomic sites and regions. However, the lymph node staging is uniform for all sites in the head and neck region.[4] Because of anatomic considerations, the specific details for each site differ; however, the general interpretations remain the same. An overview of the distinctions in the TNM method is outlined in Table 40-3.

## THERAPEUTIC APPROACHES AND NURSING CARE

### Surgery

A multidisciplinary approach to the treatment of head and neck cancer has advanced the treatment of these malignancies. Surgery and radiation given alone and in combination therapy remain the standard treatment options for this disease. Over the past decade, advances in the combination therapies of chemotherapy and radiation have changed how large tumors are treated.[18] Surgery and radiotherapy are equally effective in the treatment of early-stage disease. The choice of treatment depends on the location, size, and histology of the primary tumor and the involvement of cervical lymph nodes. Other factors that should influence the choice of treatment include cost, potential complications, and competence and compliance of the patient with posttreatment care.[4]

Advances in reconstructive surgical techniques have changed the attitude of the surgeon performing the tumor resection. With advanced techniques, the surgeon now has the ability to restore both hard and soft tissue as well as motor and sensory functions with the use of various flaps at the time of resection. These advances have enabled surgeons to perform major ablative procedures with resultant minimal dysfunctional and cosmetic defects.[4]

In addition, conservation and partial surgical procedures have been developed for both primary tumors and disease in the local/regional area. These procedures meet criteria for sound oncological procedures, but with minimal resultant defect when compared with procedures done in the past. Examples of these procedures include partial laryngopharyngectomy, vertical and horizontal laryngeal surgery, and marginal mandibulectomy. Salvage surgery remains the most effective treatment after prior therapy. Prior irradiation and combination therapy no longer serve as a contraindication to salvage surgery.[4]

**TABLE 40-3**   TNM Classification System for Head and Neck Tumors: Nodal and Distant Sites

| NODAL INVOLVEMENT (N) CLASSIFICATION FOR ALL HEAD AND NECK MALIGNANT NEOPLASMS | |
| --- | --- |
| NX | Nodes cannot be assessed |
| N0 | No clinically positive nodes |
| N1 | Single clinically positive homolateral node 3 cm or less in diameter |
| N2 | Single clinically positive homolateral node 3–6 cm in diameter |
| N2a | Single clinically positive homolateral node 3–6 cm in diameter |
| N2b | Multiple clinically positive homolateral nodes, none more than 6 cm in diameter |
| N3 | Massive homolateral node(s), bilateral nodes, or contralateral node(s) |
| N3a | Clinically positive homolateral node(s), none more than 6 cm in diameter |
| N3b | Bilateral clinically positive nodes (each side of the neck is clinically staged separately) |
| N3c | Contralateral clinically positive node(s) only |

| DISTANT METASTASIS (M) CLASSIFICATION FOR ALL HEAD AND NECK MALIGNANT NEOPLASMS | |
| --- | --- |
| MX | Not assessed |
| M0 | No known distant metastasis |
| M1 | Distant metastasis present; specify site and degee of organ impairment |

| STAGE GROUPING | |
| --- | --- |
| Stage I | T1, N0, M0 |
| Stage II | T2, N0, M0 |
| Stage III | T3, N0, M0<br>T1 or T2 or T3, N1, M0 |
| Stage IV | T4, N0 or N1, M0<br>any T, N2 or N3, M0<br>any T, any N, M1 |

From Beahrs OH, Henson DE, Hutter RVP, et al (eds): *American Joint Committee on Cancer: Manual for Staging of Cancer* (ed 4). Philadelphia, Lippincott, 1992

### Carcinoma of the nasal cavity and paranasal sinuses

***Anatomy***   The nasal cavity is separated into two chambers by the nasal septum. This area communicates with four pairs of sinus cavities: sphenoid, ethmoid, frontal, and maxillary. The lateral margin is formed by the frontal sinus, cribiform plate, and sphenoid sinus. The cavity is

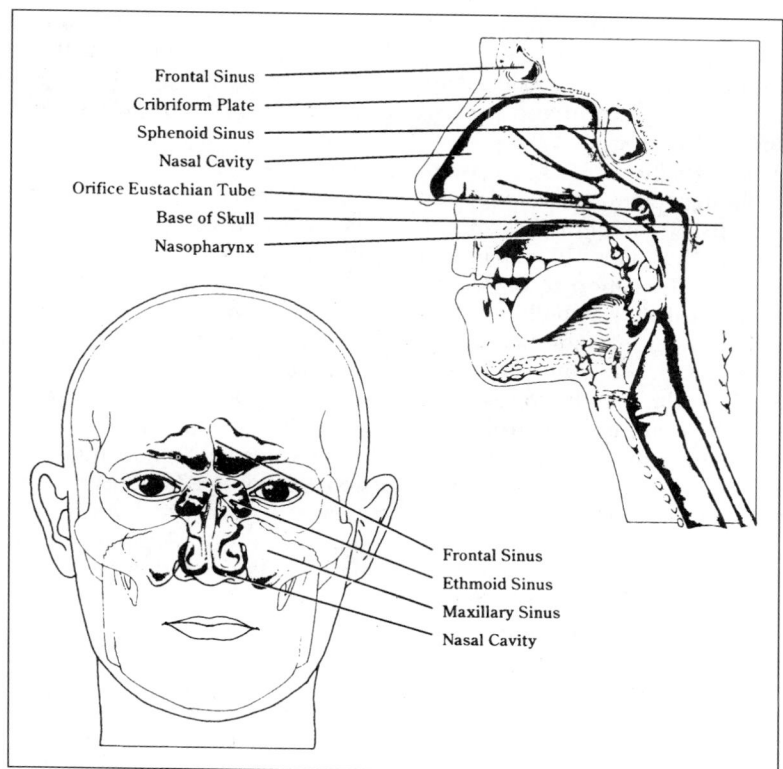

Frontal Sinus
Cribriform Plate
Sphenoid Sinus
Nasal Cavity
Orifice Eustachian Tube
Base of Skull
Nasopharynx

Frontal Sinus
Ethmoid Sinus
Maxillary Sinus
Nasal Cavity

**FIGURE 40-2**   The nasal cavity and the paranasal sinuses.

divided internally into the vestibule, septum, floor, roof, cribiform, and lateral wall or turbinates (Figure 40-2).

The triangular-shaped maxillary sinus forms the floor of the orbit superiorly and the palate inferiorly. Together, the right and left maxilla form the upper jaw. The ethmoid sinus forms a portion of the medial wall of the maxillary sinus and the entire medial wall of the orbit. The medial wall of the sinus is the middle turbinate and the roof is the fovea ethmoidalis. Symptoms of ethmoid sinus involvement can include decreased vision, epiphora (excessive tearing), medial orbital swelling, and olfactory changes. Distant metastasis from the paranasal and nasal cavity area can occur, but death is usually caused by tumor extension to the brain. The frontal sinus is an extension of the ethmoid sinus into the frontal bone. The anterior portion is the medial forehead, while the posterior portion separates the sinus from the anterior cranial fossa. The floor of the frontal sinus forms the medial roof of the orbit to the midline.

The sphenoid sinus is in the sphenoid bone and consists of a cubicle body in the center of the skull. Three processes extend from the body of the sphenoid—the lesser wing, greater wing, and pterygoid process. The optic canal passes through the root of the lesser wing.[19] Tumor extension in the area of the sphenoid sinus can cause compression of the third, fourth, and sixth cranial nerves, resulting in diplopia. In addition, pressure on the optic nerve can result in gradual loss of vision.

***Treatment***   Early carcinomas of the nasal cavity and paranasal sinuses can be effectively treated with either surgery or radiation therapy. However, most tumors are not discovered until they are advanced. In those situations, loco-regional control may be best achieved by a combination approach of surgery and radiation therapy.

Maxillectomy remains the treatment of choice for tumors in the maxillary sinus. More extensive disease with invasion into the floor of the orbit may necessitate combining radical maxillectomy with orbital exenteration.

Before surgical excision the maxillofacial prosthodontist will take an impression of the hard and soft palate to create an obturator, which is placed following resection and before the patient leaves the operating room suite. The obturator restores oronasal continuity and allows the patient to speak and eat immediately following surgery. Moreover, the obturator enhances the patient's comfort by protecting the wound from irritation and debris. Approximately five days after surgery, the packing that was placed in the defect is removed and the obturator is replaced.

The patient is instructed about meticulous wound care before discharge from the hospital. Mucosal drying and atrophic changes will occur in the maxillectomy cavity following surgery. The skin grafts that line the defect are subject to crusting and drying. The problems of drying, crusting, and superficial infection are increased if the patient has had prior irradiation. It is imperative that the defect be kept clean. An oral irrigating device with controlled pressure of the jet stream will effectively cleanse the cavity. A solution that has an alkaline base is recommended to increase ciliary action and prevent drying. A solution of saline and baking soda can provide adequate cleansing and will not burn. After irrigation, the patient can instill a solution containing the following: 5 ml of mineral oil, 2 drops of camphor, 2 drops of eucalyptol, and 2 drops of menthol. This will help loosen crusts and decrease oral odors. Irrigation of the defect should be done after each meal and at bedtime. The patient who is receiving chemotherapy, radiotherapy, or both should be particularly alert for mucositis and report this to both the oncologist and the prosthodontist. The patient should not remove the obturator for prolonged periods because atrophic changes may occur. A permanent obturator is usually made six months after the initial surgery to allow time for complete healing and consolidation of scar tissue.

There is minimal facial deformity following maxillectomy because the incision along the nose generally blends in with facial lines and fades over time. However, if an orbital exenteration is performed, the patient loses the eyeball and orbital contents. A skin flap is generally used to provide coverage and reconstruct the area. If the orbit has been removed and the cheek is intact, the patient may choose to wear a patch or be fitted with an external orbit prosthesis, which is cosmetically acceptable, especially when worn with glasses.

***Cranial base surgery***   Tumors located in the skull base were once believed inaccessible to surgical intervention and were treated only with radiation therapy. Today, advances in surgical techniques combined with technological advances offer new hope to what once was considered a very dismal situation.

The craniofacial approach, one of the most challenging areas of head and neck surgery, is used to resect tumors involving the skull base. Benign intracranial tumors and low-grade malignant tumors of the skull base with extension to the nasal cavity, paranasal sinuses, orbit, or infratemporal fossa may be reached by the intracranial approach. In addition, benign and malignant diseases of the nose and paranasal sinuses, nasopharynx, or infratemporal fossa may be resected via the craniofacial approach. Other potential candidates include patients whose disease, such as esthesioneuroblastoma and ethmoid and nasopharyngeal carcinoma,[20] has failed to respond to radiation therapy or to limited surgical resection.

Cranial base surgery often combines the talents of the otolaryngologist, microvascular surgeon, and neurosurgeon to offer a comprehensive approach to the treatment of skull base tumors. The cranial or skull base is divided into three regions: the anterior, middle, and posterior regions. The ethmoid sinuses, frontal sinuses, and superior hemisphere of the orbits are included in the anterior region. The greater and lesser wings of the sphenoid bone, the infratemporal fossa, the optic apex, and chiasm are contained in the middle region. Finally, the clivis, posterior fossa, jugular foramen, and internal auditory canal are included in the posterior cranial base.

The surgical approach depends upon the location of the tumor. The transpalatal and transoral approaches are often employed, as well as the subtemporal-infratemporal approach.[21]

The patient and family must understand the potential dangers and complications of cranial base surgery. In addition, any expected functional sequelae should be explained. Expected outcomes will depend upon the surgical approach, anatomic location of the tumor, and the biological behavior of the tumor being treated. For example, orbital exenteration may be necessary and will result in loss of vision. Temporary facial paralysis resulting from dissection in the infratemporal fossa can commonly occur. Anesthesia of the middle or lower face can occur as well. Loss of smell will result from transection of olfactory nerves. If midface or maxillary defects are created by the resection, preoperative plans need to be made for postoperative rehabilitation. Although the potential for central nervous system complications is great, the incidence should approach zero when surgical techniques are carefully executed. When surgical intervention, anesthesia, and postoperative care have been carefully planned, craniofacial resection may be no more stressful than a standard maxillectomy.[20]

***Nursing considerations***   Following cranial base surgery the patient is on bed rest with the head of the bed elevated 20–30 degrees. A lumbar subarachnoid drain is left in place 24–48 hours postoperatively with the drainage bag suspended at the level of the orbit to maintain a low-normal cerebrospinal fluid pressure.[20] Typically, these patients are monitored very closely in the neurosurgical intensive care unit. Intravenous antibiotics are given as long as the cavity packing is in place. The cavity packing is removed on postop day 5–8 if split thickness skin grafts were done. The packing may be removed in four to five days if no skin graft has been applied.

Careful monitoring of fluid balance must be done because of the effects of extreme fluctuations in blood pressure on cerebral blood flow, such as inadequate cerebral perfusion and vasoconstriction.[22]

A thorough neurological assessment is performed preoperatively to establish a baseline for the frequent monitoring that occurs postoperatively. In addition to careful monitoring of the neurological status, another nursing concern is the monitoring and maintenance of the lumbar spinal drain. The purpose of a lumbar drain is to relieve pressure at the operative site through cerebral spinal fluid decompression. Typically, 50 cc of spinal fluid are ordered to be drained from the patient every eight hours. The cerebrospinal fluid must be monitored closely, and any changes in appearance of the fluid, lack of drainage, or disruption in drainage system sterility should be promptly reported. Management of headache pain that can accompany the presence of a lumbar drain is generally controlled with a mild narcotic that does not interfere with monitoring the patient's level of consciousness.[21]

## Carcinoma of the nasopharynx

***Anatomy***   The nasopharynx is cuboidal shaped and continuous with the nasal cavities, lying just posterior to the nasal passages. This area is called the posterior choanae. The superior portion is attached to the base of the skull and slopes downward to become the posterior pharyngeal wall. The orifice of the eustachian tube is the most prominent landmark on the lateral wall. Between the cartilaginous medial end of this tube and the posterior wall is the fossa of Rosenmueller. This is a cleftlike space whose apex reaches the anterior margins of the carotid canal. A rich, capillary lymphatic system drains into ipsilateral and contralateral nodes. Metastasis occurs most often to the cervical triangle, the entire jugular chain, and the supraclavicular nodes.

The diagnosis of nasopharyngeal carcinoma is made by careful examination of the area using a head-mirror, tongue depressor, and laryngeal mirror to visualize the area. CT scans and other radiological evaluations can determine extensiveness of spread. Angiography can assist in determining potential collaterizations in the cerebrovascular tree.

***Treatment***   Radiotherapy remains the primary treatment for nasopharyngeal carcinoma; however, surgical treatment following radiation is gaining credibility.[11] The course of radiation usually involves laterally opposed fields through which a dose of 60–75 Gy is delivered to the primary site over a six- to nine-week period. Special care must be taken to provide a minimal dose to the brain and spinal cord. Radioactive implants may also be used to boost the dosage.

Information about the efficacy of chemotherapy for patients with recurrent or metastatic carcinoma of the nasopharynx is scarce. However, recent retrospective reviews of patients treated with cisplatin-based combinations suggest the following: (1) carcinoma of the nasopharynx should be considered a malignant neoplasm that is distinct from squamous cell cancer of the head and neck, and (2) selected patients with recurrent or metastatic carcinoma of the nasopharynx should receive aggressive combination chemotherapy.[23]

The patient with advanced disease often has severe pain and headaches resulting from bony invasion and erosion. In addition, the patient may experience multiple cranial nerve palsies, visual problems, sensory losses, anorexia, severe weight loss, respiratory difficulty secondary to vagal nerve paralysis, and laryngopharyngeal edema.

## Carcinoma of the oral cavity

***Anatomy***   The anatomic boundaries of the oral cavity are outlined in Table 40-4 and Figure 40-3. The following discussion is limited to the behavior of squamous cell tumors in the oral cavity. Squamous cell carcinomas generally grow along mucosal surfaces. They can first appear as a white, patchy lesion or an oral ulcer that fails to heal. In advanced lesions, infiltration into deeper structures is seen. Due to their surface friability, some lesions ulcerate

**TABLE 40-4**   The Oral Cavity

| Site | Anatomic Borders |
|---|---|
| Lip | Begins at the junction of vermillion border. Well defined into upper and lower lip, which are joined laterally at the commissure of the mouth. |
| Buccal mucosa | Membranous lining of the inner surface of the cheeks and lips from the line of contact of the opposing lips to the line of attachment of mucosa of the alveolar ridge. |
| Lower alveolar ridge | Includes alveolar process of the mandible and its covering mucosa. Extends from the line of attachment of mucosa in the buccal gutter to the line of free mucosa of the floor of the mouth. Posteriorly ascends to the ascending ramus of the mandible. |
| Upper alveolar ridge | Upper ridge is the alveolar process of the maxilla and covering mucosa. Extends from upper gingival-buccal gutter to junction of hard palate. Posterior margin is upper end of pterygopalatine arch. |
| Retromolar trigone | Attached mucosa overlying the ascending ramus of the mandible from the level of the posterior surface of the last molar tooth to the apex superiorly. Adjacent to the tuberosity of the maxilla. |
| Floor of the mouth | Semilunar space of the mylohyoid and hypoglossus muscles. Extends from inner surface of lower alveolar ridge to undersurface of the tongue. Posterior boundary forms base of anterior pillar of the tonsil. Anterior portion divided into two sides by frenulum of the tongue. Contains the ostia of the submandibular and sublingual salivary glands. |
| Hard palate | Semilunar area between the upper alveolar ridge and the mucous membrane covering the palatine process of the maxillary palatine bones. Extends from inner surface of superior alveolar ridge to posterior edge of palatine bone. |
| Oral tongue | Anterior two-thirds is freely mobile and extends anteriorly from line of circumvallate papilla to the undersurface of the tongue at the junction of the floor of the mouth. Composed of four areas: tip, lateral borders, dorsum, and undersurface. |

Rice D, Spiro R: *Current Concepts in Head and Neck Cancer.* New York, American Cancer Society, 1989

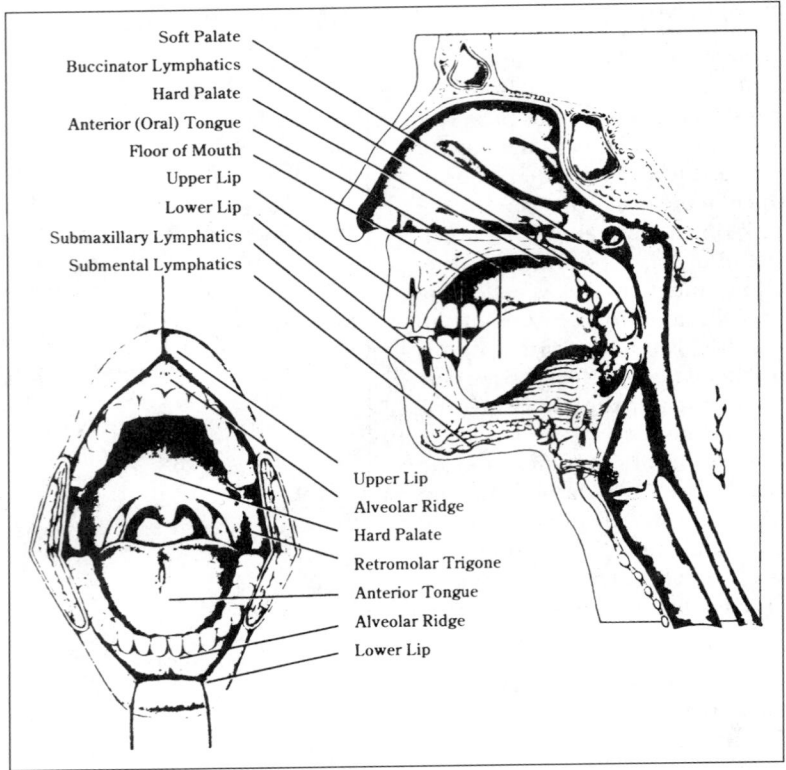

Soft Palate
Buccinator Lymphatics
Hard Palate
Anterior (Oral) Tongue
Floor of Mouth
Upper Lip
Lower Lip
Submaxillary Lymphatics
Submental Lymphatics

Upper Lip
Alveolar Ridge
Hard Palate
Retromolar Trigone
Anterior Tongue
Alveolar Ridge
Lower Lip

**FIGURE 40-3**   The oral cavity.

easily and suffer trauma from mechanical actions such as chewing. Figure 40-4 illustrates a tumor in the posterior oral cavity.

A steady, persistent growth pattern is demonstrated by most squamous cell tumors. As deep invasion occurs, spread may be evident along preformed pathways of muscle fascia or nerves. In addition, as the tumor grows, regional lymph node metastasis frequently occurs. Generally, the upper cervical nodes are affected, with the submandibular and upper jugular nodes most commonly involved. Contralateral cervical metastases can frequently result from lesions in the floor of the mouth and tongue.

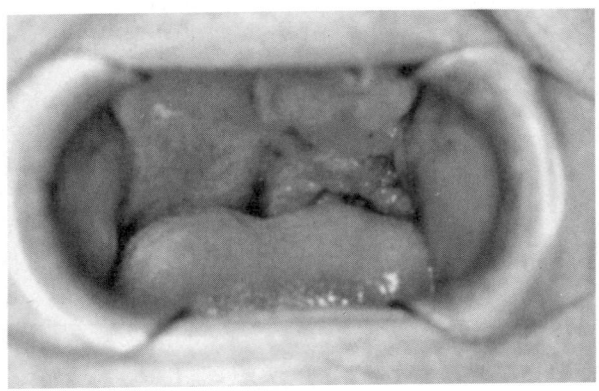

**FIGURE 40-4**   Posterior oral cavity tumor.

The mechanism of action is that tumor cells from oral lesions pass through lymphatics that cross the midline from the primary tumor. A second route of spread can occur from ipsilateral regional nodes via collateral lymph flow resulting in contralateral node involvement.

In general, tumor metastases occur when a primary lesion has been present for some time. However, when primary tumors are poorly differentiated and clinically aggressive, metastases occur in relatively short periods of time.[14] Distant metastases occur from cancer cells spreading through the lymphatic system or by blood vessel embolization.[24] When underlying bone is affected, the destruction is secondary to tumor invasion.

***Treatment***   One may postulate that diagnosis of oral tumors would occur expeditiously since the area is immediately accessible to the examiner. However, delays in treatment may occur if the lesion is treated initially as benign. In the past, such treatment has included topical medications, antibiotics, dental extractions, and dental adjustment. Fortunately, over the past two decades the dental community has become keenly aware of the hazards of delaying a diagnosis of oral cancer and now includes a screening exam in routine visits.

Unfortunately, many patients will delay seeking treatment due to denial of symptoms. The most common historical complaint may be a painless lesion that has existed for some time. Pain may or may not be present at the primary site. It is commonly reported as referred pain to the ear or jaw. Referred pain is an important sign that can indicate induration, ulceration, or pressure affecting adjacent nerves. As the lesion increases in size, the individual may experience difficulty chewing foods and swallowing.

Treatment options will be determined by the size of the tumor. Surgery and radiation alone have comparable cure rates in early-stage lesions. The choice of treatment in early-stage lesions depends on functional and cosmetic results, the patient's general health, and patient preference. While chemotherapy alone cannot cure oropharyngeal cancer, complete and partial response rates as high as 90% have been demonstrated for platinum-based combinations. However, these responses are rarely of long duration, and studies continue to investigate the effect of combination therapy on survival.[25]

*Surgery*   Surgical resection in this area involves a neck dissection in continuity with the tumor and regional tissues. An ipsilateral neck dissection is often done because there is a high frequency of metastasis to ipsilateral nodes.[26-28] If the mandible is involved, the appropriate portion is included in the resection.[29] The guiding principle of surgical resection is removal of the primary tumor with adequate margins that are free from tumor involvement. Resection of 2 cm of surrounding normal tissue is usually considered adequate to ensure clear margins. Surgical treatment of stage III and IV lesions often results in a greater degree of tissue resection and thus greater dysfunction and disfigurement.[26] Depending on the location of the tumor, speaking and swallowing can be greatly affected.

A typical resection may include removal of the base of the tongue, a portion of the posterior pharyngeal wall, and a segment of the mandible. In this case, reconstruction would be completed with the use of a large tissue flap such as a pectoralis major myocutaneous flap. Reconstructive techniques will be discussed later in this chapter.

The individual's rehabilitation needs after surgery are dependent upon the extent of the resection. Patients who have had large surgical resections will have a temporary tracheostomy for approximately seven to ten days. In addition, an enteral feeding tube will be placed and the patient will be NPO for 10 days to two weeks or until all intraoral suture lines are healed. The patient and family will need assistance coping with any alterations in facial contour that may have occurred with the surgical resection.

*Laser therapy*   One of the single most important advances in the treatment of head and neck lesions over the past decade has been the increasing use of the laser in surgical excision of early-stage oral cavity, pharyngeal, and laryngeal cancers. The $CO_2$ laser has the advantage of being very precise, and it contributes to decreased possibility of tumor spread by sealing lymphatics as tissue is removed. The use of the laser has resulted in reduced patient morbidity, decreased hospital stay, and an improved recovery.[30]

Another advancement in surgical technology that has contributed to decreased morbidity is the use of preoperative internal carotid occlusion with placement of intraluminal balloons. The use of this technology results in relatively safe ligation and excision of the common and internal carotid artery, decreasing the rate of stroke to less than 5%.[30]

### Cancer of the hypopharynx

*Etiology*   Common etiologic factors that contribute to the development of hypopharyngeal cancer include excessive smoking and alcohol consumption. In northern Europe, a high incidence of Plummer-Vinson syndrome has been associated with a higher incidence of postcricoid carcinoma, particularly noteworthy because this occurs in nonsmoking women.

Most lesions in the hypopharynx are squamous cell in origin. There is a tendency for submucosal spread, often resulting in what appears to be multiple separate primary tumors. Carcinoma of the hypopharynx tends to metastasize superiorly to the base of the skull via the parapharyngeal lymphatics. Inferiorly the spread is seen toward the tracheo-esophageal lymph nodes and then to the mediastinum.

*Anatomy*   There are three distinct regions in the hypopharynx—the hypopharynx, the posterior surface of the larynx (the postcricoid area), and the lower posterior pharyngeal wall.

The two recesses on both sides of the larynx are called the *pyriform sinuses*. The superior border of each sinus is the pharyngo-epiglottic fold, and the inferior border is the upper border of the cricoid cartilage. On either side of the pyriform sinuses lie the aryepiglottic fold and the arytenoid cartilages. The postcricoid area extends from the posterior aspect of the arytenoid cartilages and their connecting folds to the inferior limit of the cricoid cartilage. The area is bounded laterally by the pyriform sinuses.[10] The remaining portion of the hypopharynx consists of the posterior and lateral walls (Figure 40-5).

The physical examination includes visualization of the pharyngeal wall and pyriform sinus area using a laryngeal mirror and a tongue depressor. The pyriform sinuses are best visualized during phonation. When the mirror is angled against the soft palate, adequate visualization of the posterior and lateral pharyngeal is possible. It is seldom possible to visualize the inferior tip of the pyriform sinus and the area below the superior aspect of the postcricoid area. This area is best examined with a flexible laryngoscope. A flexible laryngoscope is also helpful to examine a patient with a hyperactive gag reflex.

Diagnostic studies include CT, which can help to define the extent of the primary tumor and may demonstrate nonpalpable metastases in the lateral or retropharyngeal cervical lymph nodes. Direct laryngoscopy and biopsy are performed to confirm a tissue diagnosis. Because pyriform sinus tumors tend to be necrotic, multiple deep biopsies may be necessary to ensure an adequate tissue sample. Esophagoscopy with biopsy may be neces-

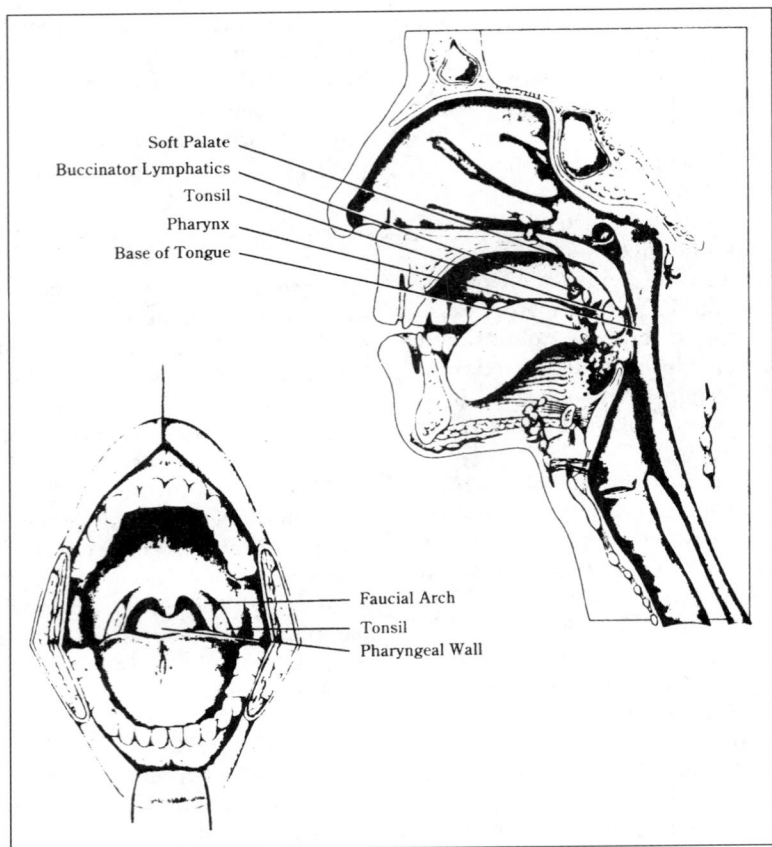

Soft Palate
Buccinator Lymphatics
Tonsil
Pharynx
Base of Tongue

Faucial Arch
Tonsil
Pharyngeal Wall

**FIGURE 40-5**    The hypopharynx.

sary if posterior invasion of the esophagus appears evident on pharyngoscopy.

Pertinent findings that may indicate cervical esophageal extension and thereby influence treatment planning include the following:

**1.** *Presence or absence of laryngeal involvement by tumor.* If both cords are mobile, invasion by tumor has not occurred, and the lesion is exterior to the larynx. If one cord is fixed, the individual may be a candidate for a partial laryngectomy in continuity with the primary site.

**2.** *Tumor invasion and mucosal involvement of the posterior wall of the pharynx.* The posterior pharynx is often used to reconstruct the site after resection, but involvement by tumor would obviate its use for reconstruction, and alternate tissues would need to be used.

**3.** *Pooling of saliva in or around the pyriform sinus and pharynx.*

These findings could indicate cervical esophageal extension or obstruction of the opening of the cervical esophagus, which would require aggressive treatment.

Treatment planning is based on the stage of disease, as outlined in Table 40-5.

***Treatment***    The majority of patients with carcinoma of the hypopharynx will present with advanced primary tumors. The management of these tumors is particularly difficult due to the anatomic location of the tumor and the impact on physiological function. In addition, accurate assessment of these tumors is difficult because of

**TABLE 40-5**    TNM Classification System for Carcinoma of the Hypopharynx

| T1 | Tumor confined to the site of origin |
|----|--------------------------------------|
| T2 | Extension of tumor to adjacent region or site, without fixation of the hemilarynx |
| T3 | Extension of tumor to adjacent region or site, with fixation of the hemilarynx |
| T4 | Massive tumor invading bone or soft tissue of the neck |

From Beahrs OH, Henson DE, Hutter RVP, et al (eds): *American Joint Committee on Cancer: Manual for Staging of Cancer* (ed 4). Philadelphia, Lippincott, 1992.

submucosal spread. Typically, these tumors will involve adjacent structures such as the larynx and base of the tongue.[18]

A combination approach using surgery, radiation therapy, and chemotherapy is often necessary to control the disease. Surgery is generally done first, followed by radiation therapy. Currently, postoperative radiation therapy is preferred in most centers because it allows the surgeon to deal with tumor margins that have not been altered by treatment. In addition, it reduces the chance of delayed healing and other problems that typically occur when irradiated tissues are resected.

Because most hypopharyngeal tumors are locally advanced, either partial or total pharyngectomy is required. It may be necessary to combine this procedure with a partial or total laryngectomy and neck dissection. Approximately 75% of patients with hypopharyngeal cancer present with cervical metastases and require a radical or bilateral neck dissection to be done along with resection of the primary tumor.

The method of reconstruction following laryngopharyngectomy depends on the amount of tissue removed from the pharynx and esophageal areas. If sufficient pharyngeal tissue remains, direct closure is the easiest method. If primary closure is performed, great care must be taken to avoid tension on the suture line in order to avoid a postoperative fistula. If a greater amount of tissue is needed to facilitate closure, a myocutaneous flap from either the pectoralis major or latissimus dorsi areas can be utilized to close the pharyngeal defect. If the full circumference of the pharyngeal wall must be resected to achieve adequate margins, alternative reconstructive procedures may include the following: posterior tongue flap with dermal graft; tubed pectoralis major or latissimus dorsi myocutaneous flap; or gastric pull-up, colon interposition, free jejunal interposition, or other free flaps.[31]

Because of the poor prognosis associated with hypopharyngeal lesions, organ-preserving surgical procedures have been introduced. One technique introduced by Steiner is that of $CO_2$ laser microsurgery.[32] Effective tumor ablation with satisfactory functional results can be achieved with the technique. Most importantly, this minimally invasive surgery often allows the integrity of the alimentary tract to be maintained, most commonly without the need for a tracheotomy.

***Rehabilitation needs***  Swallowing is often a problem following surgical resection for hypopharyngeal carcinoma. The surgical resection may involve the pharyngeal constrictors, which assist with control of a food bolus with resultant delivery into the esophagus during swallowing. If more than half of the middle and lower constrictors are resected and reconstructed, scar contracture can interfere with swallowing, necessitating swallowing rehabilitation. If aspiration becomes a chronic problem, a total laryngectomy may be necessary.

Patients who have undergone surgical resection will

be at increased risk for fistula formation. The risk is increased if the patient has had previous radiation therapy. Because surgery in this area involves opening of the upper digestive tract, this becomes a contaminated procedure. For this reason, the individual will receive antibiotic therapy postoperatively. In addition, postoperative assessments will include observing for signs of fistula formation such as an elevated temperature and saliva draining through the suture line. If infection or fistula should develop, the integrity of the carotid artery is severely compromised.

Postoperatively these patients will have a temporary tracheostomy, enteral feedings, and wound care consisting of suture line care. If an orocutaneous fistula develops, the area may be packed with betadine-soaked or iodoform gauze and be allowed to close spontaneously. Large fistulas are generally repaired with flap reconstruction.

Speech rehabilitation will depend on the clinical status of the patient. Patients who have had a pharyngolaryngectomy will rarely be able to learn esophageal speech. This may be due in part to the method of reconstruction, which can interfere with the muscular vibratory activity necessary to produce sound. The options for these patients may be the electrolarynx or a tracheoesophageal puncture procedure.

### Cancer of the larynx

The staging of glottic laryngeal cancer is based on the assessment of the depth of tumor invasion and the extent of mucosal disease (Table 40-6). Computed tomography (CT) is a reliable indicator of cartilagenous involvement. Magnetic resonance imaging (MRI) can be equally effective in assessing tumor infiltration in the cartilage. Moreover, MRI can be more accurate in assessing soft-tissue involvement.[33]

**TABLE 40-6**  TNM Classification System for Glottic Carcinoma

| TIS | Carcinoma in situ |
|---|---|
| T1 | Tumor confined to the vocal cord(s) with normal mobility (includes involvement of anterior or posterior commissures) |
| T1a | Tumor limited to one vocal cord |
| T1b | Tumor involves both vocal cords |
| T2 | Supraglottic and/or subglottic extension with normal or impaired cord mobility |
| T3 | Tumor confined to the larynx with cord fixation |
| T4 | Massive tumor with thyroid cartilage destruction and/or extension to other tissues beyond the larynx (e.g., oropharynx, soft tissues of the neck) |

From Beahrs OH, Henson DE, Hutter RVP, et al (eds): *American Joint Committee on Cancer: Manual for Staging of Cancer* (ed 4). Philadelphia, Lippincott, 1992.

T1 lesions of the membranous cord are treated with equal success by both radiotherapy and conservation surgery. The advantage of radiation therapy in the treatment of early glottic lesions is preservation of excellent vocal quality. Early lesions have also been successfully treated with microlaryngoscopy and vocal cord stripping as well as laser excision. When there is no evidence of cord fixation, a conservative laryngeal resection is usually the treatment of choice. Conservative surgery for glottic cancer includes laryngofissure, partial laryngectomy, or hemilaryngectomy.

### Surgery

*Early disease (T1 or T2)* When tumor extends forward to the anterior commissure or posteriorly to or beyond the vocal process, the surgery that is most effective is hemilaryngectomy. The anatomical limits of the surgery are outlined in Table 40-7.

Following hemilaryngectomy, the individual will have a temporary tracheostomy and receive enteral feedings. Decannulation will occur between the 10th and 14th postoperative days. The nasogastric tube is removed and the patient is started on feedings by mouth following healing of all incisions, usually 10 to 14 days after surgery. Postoperatively the patient will have a hoarse but serviceable voice. Vocalization is accomplished by the adduction of the remaining cord against the scar tissue that eventually takes the place of the resected cord. Damage to the superior and recurrent laryngeal nerves can lead to persistent aspiration. In this case a total laryngectomy may be indicated to prevent recurrent aspiration pneumonia.

Radiotherapy is utilized as an option for cure in early lesions. The usual dosage is 55–70 Gy over six to seven weeks. If there is no response after 40 Gy, the therapy may be discontinued and surgery may be indicated.

*Advanced disease (T3 to T4)* A total laryngectomy is reserved for patients who have persistent or recurrent disease after radiotherapy or who present with advanced disease. In either case, vocal cord mobility is impaired and/or the tumor may extend outside of the glottis and destroy the thyroid cartilage. The procedure of total laryngectomy involves removal of all laryngeal structures between and including the thyroid bone, thyroid cartilage, cricoid cartilage, and two to three tracheal rings. Radical neck dissection is indicated for any patient who

**TABLE 40-7** Hemilaryngectomy (Vertical Partial Laryngectomy)

| Structure Removed | Structures Remaining | Postoperative Outcome |
|---|---|---|
| One vocal cord and underlying cartilage, false vocal cord | Epiglottis and set of vocal cords on unaffected side | Hoarse but serviceable voice |
| Arytenoid on affected side | | Minimal swallowing problems |

presents with obvious metastasis to the lateral neck nodes. This is most frequently seen in patients with larger, high-grade tumors or vocal cord fixation. The major effects of removal of the larynx are permanent loss of voice and alteration in the airway. Because these losses are considerable, the patient and family should be provided every opportunity to express their fears and anxieties. In addition, coping strategies that have been successful in the past should be identified and a multidisciplinary plan established to assist the patient and family in the coping process.

Preoperative counseling with a speech therapist is essential to review potential methods of speech rehabilitation. Approaches that may be used to facilitate communication in the immediate postop period range from writing and use of communication boards to the use of artificial larynges. The patient should be an active participant in selecting the method that seems most comfortable.

Use of an electrolarynx, esophageal speech, and esophageal prosthetic voice restoration are three options for speech on a long-term basis.[34] Each method produces a vibration that is introduced as sound into the vocal tract. The sound is then shaped by tongue and lip movements into intelligible speech.[34]

In the early postoperative period the speech-language pathologist may give the patient an electrolarynx to use while in the hospital. Following a period of healing, the patient may choose to learn esophageal speech. This requires that the patient learn to produce sound by injecting air into the esophagus by movements of the tongue and lips. The air is trapped in the esophagus, causing tissue at the top of the esophagus to vibrate. Through practice of specific exercises, the patient learns to prolong the esophageal voice, refine it, and ultimately produce esophageal speech. This process can take as long as a year or more. If the patient has scarring in the area of the pharynx or tumor recurrence, it may be impossible to ever learn intelligible esophageal speech.

In some centers, tracheoesophageal (TE) puncture is done in combination with total laryngectomy. As a result of this procedure the patient can divert exhaled pulmonary air through a surgically constructed fistula tract directly into the esophagus. The exhaled air causes the cricopharyngeus muscle at the top of the esophagus to vibrate, producing sound. There is not as much effort exerted as there is to learn the often complicated method of air injection required by esophageal speech; however, the patient must learn to insert, clean, and replace the small prosthesis that fits into the fistula tract, preventing food and fluid from back-flowing into the trachea.

It is ideal if patients are given an opportunity to see and learn about all three types of speech that can be used. It is important for the patient to have choices concerning different methods of speech rehabilitation at a time when he or she may feel the situation is uncontrollable. Many patients may ultimately use all three methods at different times in the rehabilitation period: artificial larynx immediately after surgery; esophageal voice therapy a month or so after surgery; and, after a few months, surgical voice restoration or TE puncture.[35]

*Postoperative care*   In the immediate postoperative period, most patients will have a laryngectomy tube placed. The decision to place a tube will depend on the surgical technique used to create the stoma and the amount of contracture that occurs as healing progresses. The tube will help prevent trauma to the tracheal mucosa due to suctioning and, most importantly, will maintain an adequate stoma size. Since the laryngectomy stoma is permanent, the tube may be removed and cleaned without fear of stomal closure. The stoma area underneath the tube should be kept clean and free of crusting. The presence of crusts from drainage of the stomal incision can lead to infection and increased scar formation. If the patient continues to experience stomal stricture over a period of time, the laryngectomy tube will need to be placed at night to help prevent further stricture.

The provision of adequate humidity will remain a lifelong concern for the laryngectomized patient. Because the airway is diverted and the patient no longer has the ability to warm, moisten, and filter the air through the nose, supplemental humidity will need to be provided, especially in dry climates. Generally a large room humidifier is recommended for use in the home. A small bedside humidifier may also be necessary. The humidity level in the home should be kept above 50%.

The patient should be aware of changes in secretions that could signal insufficient humidity, including blood-tinged sputum, an increase in thickness or tenacity of secretions, or increased difficulty mobilizing secretions. The patient should be taught how to instill 1–3 cc of normal saline into the stoma to keep secretions thin, moist, and easy to cough out. The frequency of instillation will depend on environmental humidity. For example, in the winter months the frequency of instillation may be hourly, while in the summer months when the humidity level is higher it may only be necessary three times a day. The goal of instruction should be an understanding of the concept of lack of humidity and the subsequent effect on the tracheal secretions. Another method to ensure rapid mobilization of secretions is to fill a room with steam from a shower and stand in the room for approximately 15 minutes. The patient should also be instructed to wear a stoma covering, especially in the winter. The covering will assist to warm, moisten, and filter dry, cold air. In addition, adequate fluid intake will assist in hydration, prevent changes in secretions, and prevent tracheitis. The oral ingestion of potassium iodine is also helpful in increasing the volume and viscosity of secretions. Cough effectiveness is significantly reduced because the laryngeal sphincter is absent and thus intrabronchial pressure cannot be elevated, making adequate mobilization of secretions even more of a challenge.

Hyposmia occurs to some degree in every laryngectomized patient. This is a permanent loss recognized early on by the patient. Some limited odor detection and recognition will develop in the accessory olfactory areas over time. The ability to taste, closely related to stimulation of olfactory cells, is also reduced. This combination of factors may affect the patient's appetite, indicating a need for early intervention and nutritional counseling to prevent long-term weight loss.

An enteral feeding tube is placed during surgery to allow for nutritional support until the suture lines have healed. Because the feeding tube rests on the incision line, it should not be manipulated in any way. If it should become dislodged or pulled out, the possibility of its being replaced without perforation of the suture line is limited. The tube remains in place for approximately seven days in the nonirradiated patient and for ten days in the previously irradiated patient.

If the patient has had previous irradiation, the potential for fistula formation is increased. This usually extends the hospital stay. Increased scarring in the suture line will contribute to later problems with esophageal stricture and dysphagia. Strictures can be treated effectively with periodic dilation, although occasionally a secondary surgical procedure is necessary. Other conditions that may interfere with swallowing may be pseudodiverticuli that develop at the base of the tongue. Submucosal masses on the posterior pharyngeal wall caused by contraction of the detached constrictor muscles can interfere with swallowing. Finally, dysphagia can also occur in the absence of stricture as a result of the uncoordinated contractions of the detached inferior constrictor muscles.

Most patients with a laryngectomy resume their preoperative lifestyle, with only a few limitations. Due to the absence of thoracic fixation after laryngectomy, the patient's ability to lift heavy objects is compromised. The patient is instructed not to lift more than ten pounds for four months after surgery. Heavy lifting and strenuous exercise may be performed gradually. A second precaution involves the avoidance of water sports. The laryngectomy patient cannot protect the airway during activities such as swimming and boating, and these activities should be avoided. Special precautions must be taken to avoid getting dust or dirt in the airway when performing activities such as gardening or housework. If the patient's occupation depends on speech communication, the pressure to communicate effectively using an alternate method increases. However, even executives who deliver speeches have returned to their positions and through perseverance in learning either esophageal speech or another method have been successful communicators.

### Supraglottic cancer

*Assessment*   The diagnosis of supraglottic cancer is usually made through indirect laryngoscopy, with direct laryngoscopy used for obtaining a biopsy specimen. Radiographs, CT, and MRI scans are helpful in determining the inferior extent of disease necessary for optimal staging of the disease (Table 40-8).

*Treatment*   All supraglottic tumors, with the exception of T1 epiglottic cancer, may metastasize to the neck. In addition, because many lesions are located in the midline, the chance for bilateral neck disease is high.[18]

**TABLE 40-8** TNM Classification System for Supraglottic Carcinoma

| TIS | Carcinoma in situ |
|-----|-------------------|
| T2 | Tumor confined to one subsite of supraglottis or glottis with normal cord mobility |
| T3 | Tumor limited to the larynx with vocal cord fixation and/or invades the postcricoid area, medial wall of the pyriform sinus, or preepiglottic space |
| T4 | Tumor invades through thyroid cartilage and/or extends to other tissues beyond the larynx (e.g., to cropharynx, soft tissues of the neck) |

From Beahrs OH, Henson DE, Hutter RVP, et al (eds): *American Joint Committee on Cancer: Manual for Staging of Cancer* (ed 4). Philadelphia, Lippincott, 1992.

Early supraglottic cancers can be treated effectively by irradiation or by surgery with the possible addition of irradiation to control the neck disease. Transoral $CO_2$ laser epiglottectomy has recently been recognized as effective treatment for selected T1 and T2 epiglottic lesions.[36] This technique involves resection of the epiglottis, one aryepiglottic fold, and in some cases, the ventricular band. One significant advantage of this technique over the traditional supraglottic laryngectomy is the patient will have no difficulty with aspiration. Hospital stays are shortened and morbidity is minimized.[18]

The standard supraglottic laryngectomy consists of resection of the following structures: the hyoid bone, epiglottis, pre-epiglottic space, thyrohyoid membrane, superior half of the thyroid cartilage, and the false vocal cords. The success of supraglottic laryngectomy is limited by the following: fixation of the arytenoid, thyroid cartilage invasion, pyriform fossa apex involvement, postcricoid involvement, impaired vocal cord mobility, glottic extension, bilateral arytenoid involvement, cricoid cartilage involvement, and extensive involvement of the base of the tongue.[37]

Postoperative airway obstruction is common following supraglottic laryngectomy due to edema in the surgical area. For this reason, patients will have a temporary tracheostomy tube placed at the time of surgery. The tube will be removed following successful swallowing without aspiration within 10 to 14 days after surgery. Some patients may be sent home with the tube in place until they are able to learn how to protect the airway during swallowing.

Aspiration during swallowing is one of the major complications following supraglottic laryngectomy. Because the epiglottis, which is a protective mechanism during swallowing, has been removed, the chances for chronic aspiration are increased. The patient must relearn to swallow without aspirating. A thorough evaluation and treatment plan is identified by the speech and swallowing therapist and is reinforced by the nursing staff. The mechanisms of action in the supraglottic swallow are outlined in Table 40-9. It is important to remember that the ap-

**TABLE 40-9** Standard Supraglottic Laryngectomy and Supraglottic Swallow

| Structure Removed | Structures Remaining | Post-operative Problem | Rehabili-tation Outcome |
|-------------------|---------------------|------------------------|-------------------------|
| Epiglottis Hyoid bone False vocal cords Superior half of thyroid cartilage | True vocal cords Arytenoids | Aspiration | Minimal aspiration |

**SUPRAGLOTTIC SWALLOW SEQUENCE***

| Action | Effect |
|--------|--------|
| Cough or clear throat | Clears airway of secretions |
| Inhale | Closes vocal cords |
| Valsalva maneuver | Forces food into esophagus |
| Place food in the mouth Swallow | |
| Cough or clear throat again | Vibration causes excess food to clear from vocal cords |
| Swallow again | Remaining food enters esophagus |

*Note: This sequence is modified by the speech therapist following a thorough swallowing assessment.
Thawley SE, Panje WR, Batsakis JG, Lindberg RD (eds): *Comprehensive Management of Head and Neck Tumors.* Philadelphia, Saunders, 1987

proach to the supraglottic swallow is individualized for each patient according to the extent of the resection. Further complicating the ability to swallow without aspirating is the fact that sensation in the area is destroyed when the supraglottic larynx and the internal laryngeal nerve are resected. In addition, if the arytenoid or a portion of the vocal cord is included in the resection, the aspiration rate increases significantly.

During normal swallowing, aspiration is prevented by three major sequential events: the epiglottis closes over the laryngeal inlet, the true vocal cords close, and the larynx elevates to oppose the base of the tongue. The procedure of supraglottic laryngectomy interferes with one or all of these variables. In some institutions, cricopharyngeal myotomy is performed in order to prevent failure of relaxation of the cricopharyngeal sphincter during swallowing. This allows food to pass more easily through this sphincter. Laryngeal suspension is another surgical technique that may be performed to decrease aspiration. This is accomplished by suturing the thyroid cartilage remnant to the mentum of the mandible. This results in lifting the larynx superiorly and tilting it posteriorly. There are conflicting reports regarding the ultimate success of this technique in improving the swallow. If the arytenoid or a part of it is included in the surgical resection, the remaining vocal cord should be fixed in the midline. If this is not done, the posterior glottic area will be incompetent during adduction of the vocal cords and aspiration will consistently result. Because of the difficulties associated with aspiration, elderly individuals or those with chronic bronchitis or decreased lung compliance may not be candidates for supraglottic laryngectomy. If aspiration becomes severe, meal times can become a period of frustration and anxiety for the patient and family. If pneumonia develops and aspiration persists, the patient may need to undergo total laryngectomy as a life-saving procedure.

A cine-esophogram and videofluoroscopy are usually obtained before the tracheostomy tube is removed to evaluate the patient's ability to swallow without aspirating. Commonly referred to as a "cookie swallow," this exam is often repeated at specified intervals to determine the progress of the swallowing therapy.

Liquids are the most difficult thing for the patient to swallow without aspirating. For this reason the patient should be started on foods that have a soft consistency such as mashed potatoes, applesauce, or baby food. The patient should be in a sitting position with minimal distractions during meal times. Small bites should be taken initially. The cuff of the tracheostomy tube should be deflated because it will inhibit elevation of the laryngeal remnant against the base of the tongue. If aspiration during meals is severe, the cuff will need to be inflated to protect the airway. Generally, in this situation the cuff will be inflated for meals and for approximately one-half hour following the meal. The swallowing therapist should initiate the swallowing plan and be present with the patient for the first meal and for following meals as indicated.

The nurse's role in swallowing therapy is one of support and collaboration. The nursing staff should be familiar with the specifics of the swallowing therapy so they can reinforce the steps of the swallow when the therapist is unable to be present. It is helpful to have the sequential steps written clearly on a large card that can be kept at the bedside and referred to by the patient during meal times. In addition, clinicians should remember that many patients are "silent aspirators" and will not cough during swallowing if aspiration occurs.

Relearning a basic function like swallowing is frustrating and often humiliating. The patient must be treated with patience and dignity during this process. Specific strategies may need to be outlined for the family to be supportive in this process as well. Often, in their quest to be helpful, they unknowingly exert undue pressure on the patient to be successful. As swallowing therapy progresses, the patient gradually learns to swallow solid foods, semisolids, and finally liquids.

Tracheal suctioning is especially important after supraglottic laryngectomy. There are an abundance of secretions caused by increased edema in the laryngeal area. Generally, the tracheal secretions are extremely thin and liquid. For this reason, more frequent tracheal suctioning may be necessary to prevent aspiration and pneumonia. The patient should also be encouraged to cough and breathe deeply every few hours and should be encouraged to ambulate outside the room at least four times a day.

## Methods of Reconstruction

The goal of reconstructive procedures in the head and neck is to restore function while simultaneously retaining socially acceptable cosmesis. There are a variety of reconstructive options available today for the head and neck cancer patient. The decision regarding which option to employ will depend on the location and extent of tissue resected. The decision regarding the method of reconstruction should be discussed with the patient and family prior to surgery; however, the precise outcome may not be known because the extent of tumor may not be able to be precisely identified preoperatively.

### Myocutaneous flap

The advent of the pectoralis major myocutaneous flap was a major breakthrough in reconstruction of the head and neck. Major surgical resections are now possible in which vital organs such as brain dura and the carotid artery are exposed without risking a high rate of meningitis, brain abscess, and carotid hemorrhage.

The myocutaneous flap is especially useful when large amounts of tissue have been resected and bulk is needed to reconstruct the defect. These flaps consist of muscle, skin, and blood supply and, in some cases, even contain bone or cartilage. The muscles most often used to reconstruct defects in the head and neck area include the pectoralis major, sternocleidomastoid, trapezius, and latissimus dorsi.

Another major breakthrough occurred with the use of the trapezius osseomyocutaneous flap for one-stage reconstructive procedures requiring reconstruction of a mandibular bony defect associated with a large soft tissue defect.[38] These flaps rely on well-vascularized muscles that receive their blood supply from a major arterial vessel. The pectoralis myocutaneous flap can be simply elevated from the anterior chest wall. The blood supply is provided by the pectoral branch of the thoracoacromial artery. In some cases an island of pectoral skin can be transported upon the pectoralis muscle to reach the oral cavity, and the vascularized muscle pedicle is placed beneath the neck skin. This flap is best utilized for reconstruction of larger defects of the oral cavity.

### Free flap

First used in the early and mid-1970s, the microvascular free flap was the first successful attempt at one-stage reconstruction in the head and neck.[39] The free flap is completely removed from its donor site and placed into the recipient site using microvascular anastomosis. Donor sites that have been used successfully include the groin and the radial forearm. Some of the major advantages of the free flap are that immediate functional reconstructive replacement of removed tissue is possible, the donor site is not exposed, and bulky exposed pedicles are avoided. Disadvantages of using this technique include prolonged operating time and the need for microsurgical expertise and two teams of operating surgeons.

### Deltopectoral flap

Popularized during the 1960s, the deltopectoral flap had the advantage of bringing well-vascularized tissue to a previously irradiated surgical bed from an area that had not been treated with radiation. There is no muscle included in the deltopectoral flap. It maintains its blood supply from its base and consists of skin and the blood supply only. The disadvantages of this flap include strictures, fistulae, and the fact that several stages are necessary. Due to its thinness, the deltopectoral flap has a limited role in head and neck reconstruction. However, it remains a useful tool for selected reconstructive needs such as resurfacing cutaneous defects of the neck.

### Nursing care of flaps and grafts

The goal of nursing care of any type of flap is to ensure flap viability. This is accomplished through frequent and thorough observation and assessment of the flap area. In addition, if a skin graft has been placed, both the donor and recipient site are observed closely for signs of adequate healing.

***Skin grafts*** Split-thickness skin grafts are used frequently to reconstruct a primary defect or to protect a major structure such as the carotid artery. Skin grafts are composed of a thin layer of epidermis and a small amount of dermis. The skin graft is resected completely from the donor site and sutured into the recipient site. A commonly used donor site is the anterior thigh on the operative side. Nursing assessment and care will include both the donor and recipient sites. The patient usually returns from the operating room with a protective covering placed over the donor site. This covering may differ from institution to institution depending upon the preference of the surgeon. If a transparent covering is used, observation of the area for complications such as bleeding can be easily done. If bleeding does occur, the physician may order small slits to be placed in the covering to release the pressure and allow the blood to escape. If a nontransparent covering is used, the area will be wrapped with a circular gauze dressing. This dressing generally stays in place for one to two days after surgery. Re-epithelialization occurs in the donor site area as the healing process takes place. The area must be kept free from infection during this process. This is accomplished by using sterile technique when caring for the wound and remaining alert for any signs of infection.

The patient will complain of pain in the donor site. This is due to exposure of nerve endings and bruising of the underlying muscle during resection of the graft.

It is helpful to avoid mechanical contact with the donor site area from pajama bottoms or other articles of clothing. In addition, the patient may require a mild analgesic every three to four hours to alleviate discomfort.

The donor site is often exposed to air while healing occurs. A heat lamp may be used to dry the area if excess drainage is present. The heat lamp generally is applied once every eight hours for one-half hour, with care taken to avoid overexposure. The heat lamp is positioned approximately two to three feet from the area. Once the donor site heals and the protective dressing dries, the dressing will come off on its own. If it is not easy to remove the dressing, saline-soaked gauze may be applied to the area to help loosen the dressing. Frequent application of saline soaks should assist in loosening the dressing until it can be easily pulled off. It is important, however, not to use force in removing the dressing because this can interfere with the healing process. If the dressing continues to adhere to the donor site, the patient is instructed to soak in the bathtub several times a day until the dressing is easily removed.

The recipient site should also be observed for signs of infection. The skin graft is sutured in place and a bolus of gauze impregnated with bismuth tribromophenate (XeroForm®) is placed over the graft. The bolus packing generally remains in place for five days. During this time, if the graft has been placed in the oral cavity, oral hygiene is avoided. The area is observed for odor and drainage. Once the packing is removed, oral hygiene can be performed four times a day using a solution of one-quarter part hydrogen peroxide in three-quarters parts water.

***Skin flaps*** The following principles should guide nursing assessment and interventions in performing flap care.

Circulation is very important. The viability of any flap depends on adequate vascularization. The blood supply coming into the flap area must be adequate, and, concurrently, the blood flowing out of the flap must not be obstructed. More flap deaths occur from venous blood that is unable to flow out of the flap than from not enough blood flowing into the flap. The following indicators should be assessed every two hours through postop day 2 and then every four hours until postop day 5:

1. *Color:* Color is usually the best indicator of adequate blood supply. The flap color is usually a pale pink in Caucasians. The color may not match surrounding skin exactly but should be close to the color of the skin at the donor site. A white color indicates a dearterialized flap that has lost its blood supply, and a blue color indicates venous congestion has occurred or the input of blood exceeds output. It may be more difficult to detect subtle changes in color in African-Americans.

2. *Temperature:* The flap should feel warm to the touch. Because the pads of the fingers can be less sensitive to temperature, the back of the fingers should be used to touch the flap area to assess the temperature. A flap

that is cool to the touch indicates that arterial inflow is decreased.

**3.** *Capillary refill:* The tissue of the flap should blanche with gentle pressure applied to the flap and return to normal color quickly.

The criteria of temperature and capillary refill are not applicable to the assessment of intraoral flaps. The color of the flap is one assessment that may be used as an indicator of viability. In addition, a doppler can be used to detect aberrations in blood flow that may signal danger to the viability of the flap.

Significant changes in any of the above indicators should be reported promptly to the physician. Flaps can tolerate only four hours of ischemia before irreversible tissue necrosis occurs. Figures 40-6 through 40-10 (Plates 15 through 19) illustrate the sequence of flap failure and repair.

External factors can also compromise flap viability. Care must be taken to avoid any circumferential pressure on the flap from either dressings or tracheostomy ties. It is for this reason that the physician may suture a tracheostomy tube and avoid neck tapes to secure the tube until flap viability is ensured. Proper positioning of the patient is essential to prevent tension or kinking of the pedicle of the flap. The proper position is dependent on flap location. This should be discussed with the surgeon and communicated clearly to all health care workers caring for the patient. It is also helpful to include the patient and family in these discussions, so the proper position can be maintained at all times.

Surgical drains are placed in the flap area for approximately four to six days after surgery. The drains will remove any accumulation of blood or fluid from underneath the flap area that could interfere with healing. When the drainage decreases to 50 cc or less in a 24-hour period, the drains are usually removed. After removal of the drains, the area should be inspected closely for any accumulation of blood or serum. If a hematoma occurs, the area may be drained at the bedside, or, depending on the size, the patient may need to return to the operating room for evacuation of the hematoma.

Incision lines in the flap area and in other areas should be cleansed with a solution of half-strength hydrogen peroxide and normal saline at least once a shift. An accumulation of dried blood and serum on the suture line can interfere with healing and provide an environment for infection.

The patient should be placed in a semi-Fowler's to high-Fowler's position. This position will help to decrease edema by gravitational drainage and will prevent hyperextension of the neck that could place excessive tension on neck flaps and compromise wound healing.[40]

## Chemotherapy

In the past, single-agent chemotherapy was reserved for palliating the symptoms of head and neck cancer. Currently, the role of chemotherapy in the treatment of localized, potentially curable head and neck cancer is controversial. The discussion centers around an apparent lack of evidence that the addition of chemotherapy increases overall survival compared to the standard therapies of surgery and radiation alone. However, it must be stressed that a prolonged disease-free survival means less morbidity and a longer life without the devastating effects of cancer. This obviously enhanced quality of life and lower health care cost seems worthwhile despite the lack of increased overall survival and remains an important goal of therapy. In the presence of metastatic or recurrent head and neck cancer the addition of chemotherapy is an appropriate standard approach to treatment.[41] The goals of chemotherapy in this situation are palliation of symptoms, in particular pain control, and an improved quality of life.

### Primary/neoadjuvant chemotherapy

The head and neck area was among the first cancer sites identified for the application of primary or induction chemotherapy.[42] Primary chemotherapy involves giving a specified number of chemotherapy cycles before standard, local, or regional therapy is instituted. The tumor response is evaluated after the chemotherapy is given and permits an objective measure of the effectiveness of chemotherapy for any given patient. Interestingly, response or resistance to chemotherapy appears to predict response or resistance to subsequent radiotherapy.[43] Patients with resectable tumors will have surgery and radiation therapy. Unresectable tumors are usually treated with radiation therapy.

Besides organ preservation, the goal of neoadjuvant chemotherapy is to decrease the size of the tumor, thereby enhancing disease control, and to increase the chance of cure (survival) with subsequent surgery and radiation. In addition, studies have shown a reduction in distant metastases when utilizing this approach.[44] However, no difference in survival or patterns of failure have been demonstrated with neoadjuvant chemotherapy.

### Adjuvant/concurrent chemotherapy

The fact that 60%–90% of patients with regionally advanced head and neck cancer will have local recurrences, usually within the first two years after initial therapy, makes this a logical population in which to explore adjuvant/concurrent chemotherapy.[43] This is especially true where organ/tissue preservation is a goal. The preservation of the functional ability to chew, swallow, and speak is a critically important goal of treatment. Surgical techniques continue to be refined, resulting in decreased morbidity. Chemotherapy added to the treatment regimen may allow a further decrease in the need for radical surgical intervention. There is strong evidence that chemotherapy allows increased larynx preservation without alteration of overall survival. While current trials of organ preservation have focused on the larynx, the outcomes of these studies will benefit others who are faced with a potential functional impairment due to radical surgery in the head and neck area.

According to a meta-analysis of prospective and randomized adjuvant and adjunctive chemotherapy trials in head and neck cancer it is apparent that concurrent chemotherapy with local definitive treatment is the approach most likely to produce a statistically significant improvement in survival and is therefore worth investigating where cure is possible.[45] However, the results of recent adjuvant chemotherapy studies in head and neck cancer have traditionally demonstrated a significant increase in morbidity without significant improvement in survival.[46] One explanation for this apparent lack of improvement in survival with enhanced toxicity might be the fact that head and neck cancer is typically a diffuse multifocal disease. The entire aerodigestive tract is exposed to the carcinogenic effects of environmental carcinogens causing a "field cancer" where various stages of epithelial neoplastic transformation occur over time progressing eventually to recurrent local disease. Additionally, the efficacy of chemotherapy is dependent upon adequate blood supply to the site of possible micrometastases. A significant drawback to the efficacy of adjuvant chemotherapy in the prevention of local recurrence is the fact that the vascular and lymphatic drainage pattern to and from the primary sites are altered following surgical resection and radiotherapy. As a result, drug delivery to the potential sanctuaries of residual disease may be compromised. Also, chemotherapy is considerably more toxic in head and neck cancers because of the sensitivities of the tissues and the anatomic proximity of structures in this area. Patients often experience anorexia, mucositis, xerostomia, dehydration, nausea, and vomiting with weight loss due to treatment and are therefore nutritionally and emotionally depleted. These factors greatly compromise the ability of the treatment team to deliver the optimal doses of chemotherapy that could have a direct effect on treatment outcome.

The goal of concomitant chemoradiotherapy is to enhance the efficacy of each modality without undue toxicity. Combining chemotherapy and radiation in patients with locally advanced solid tumor aims at overcoming radioresistance as a cause of local treatment failure. Further, since each mode of therapy has a different site of action early eradication of distant micrometastasis may prevent systemic treatment failure.[46] The combination can also shorten the overall treatment time and limit tumor repopulation and the debilitating effects of treatment. Each has a different toxicity profile, so while the combination may cause additional toxicities, the toxicity of each is not potentiated. In addition it appears that radiation sensitization decreases the ability of cells to repair themselves either through the direct interaction of chemotherapy and radiation or the direct cytotoxic activity of chemotherapy against radioresistant or hypoxic cells.[47]

The radiosensitizing effects of certain chemotherapy drugs (e.g., 5-fluorouracil, cisplatin, carboplatin, and paclitaxel) are known to enhance radiation effects. Phase II and III trials have shown that concomitant treatment results in improved local control and disease free status.[48] Two basic schedules of concomitant radiotherapy are used: continuous (synchronous) and interrupted or split-course (alternating radiation and chemotherapy). An example of interrupted chemoradiotherapy is a combination of hyperfractionated split-course radiotherapy and cisplatin, 5-FU, and hydroxyurea. Hydroxyurea is known to be active in head and neck cancer, but it is also known to have radiation-enhancing properties and the ability to modulate the activity of 5-FU.[49] Interrupted schedules permit the use of multiple agents, but may also result in delay in treatment (radiation) due to toxicity.

Alternating/sequential chemoradiotherapy for potentially curable disease is considered a standard approach to treatment in many settings. For example, alternating cisplatin at 20mg/m², daily for five consecutive days or infusional 5-FU (1-2 g/m²/d) for 72 hours with radiation over a total of ten weeks of treatment has resulted in a favorable treatment outcome.[50,51] Carboplatin may also be used in place of cisplatin. When used to treat patients with locally advanced disease three-year survival is only 50%.[43]

### Palliative chemotherapy

Chemotherapy may be used to effectively palliate the symptoms of advanced, nonresectable, or recurrent disease. Palliative therapy may consist of using drugs including methotrexate, carboplatin, cisplatin, bleomycin, or infusional fluorouracil as a single agent or in combination with cisplatin. Such approaches produce similar response rates in the range of 15%–30% with a median response duration of two to five months.[43] Newer agents such as paclitaxel, docetaxel, topotecan, and gemcitabine produce similar response rates but are encouraging because they present new possibilities in terms of combination chemotherapy. High-dose therapy utilizing agents such as methotrexate or cisplatin has not proven more effective than standard low-dose therapy and toxicity is markedly less with standard therapy. Given the cost of high-dose therapies and the lack of improvement in disease-free or overall survival, the cost of such therapies cannot be justified.

Intra-arterial or regional chemotherapy is a local way of delivering high drug levels to the tumor with less systemic toxicity. For example cisplatin given weekly for four weeks with systemic sodium thiosulfate protection has been shown to be relatively well tolerated and highly active.[52] Newer microcatheters and technology have reduced the morbidity of this procedure and therefore enhanced interest in intra-arterial therapy as a treatment option for locally advanced, nonresectable disease. Radiation may also be given either concurrently or sequentially to improve local control.

### Biologic response modifiers

Initial studies of the efficacy of IFN and IL-2 in the treatment of squamous cell cancer of the head and neck have indicated that this form of immunotherapy may result in tumor regression in some patients with advanced malignancies. Immunotherapy is of interest for head and neck cancer patients because they consistently demonstrate impaired cellular immunity.[53] Interleukin-2 (IL-2) has been used with chemotherapy but the ideal dosage and route of administration have yet to be determined. Interferon-alfa has been used to potentiate the activity of cisplatin and 5-FU, but the benefits of the addition of interferon to the overall treatment outcome is questionable. *Cis* retinoic acid and interferon are being studied for their effects as regrowth inhibiting agents. There is evidence that the proliferative rate of head and neck cancer plays an important role in determining the prognosis of the disease. Clinical observations have demonstrated that tumor regrowth during therapy is a major cause of treatment failure in head and neck cancers. Research into the role of these two agents and their ability to possibly affect tumor regrowth is an exciting area of research.[5,53]

Because the expected survival benefit is small regardless of the therapy, patients with head and neck squamous cell carcinoma should be encouraged to participate in clinical trials. This population is an ideal group for phase I or phase II drug development trials. Oncology nurses have the opportunity to seek information on the availability, potential benefits, and adverse toxicities of therapies, as patients and families will be looking to the nurse for information and guidance.

## Radiation Therapy

Radiation therapy has an important role as a treatment modality in head and neck cancer. Used as primary treatment in early lesions, radiation therapy is potentially an effective cure. When radiation is combined with surgery for advanced lesions, control of disease and decrease of subsequent recurrence are often achieved.

The mode of delivery can vary and will depend on the treatment plan. The following methods of treatment are most frequently seen: external beam, interstitial implantation, and intraoperative therapy. The ultimate goal of any radiation treatment is to eradicate tumor while preserving function and cosmesis.

Dosage decisions for planning external beam therapy are dependent upon the size and location of the tumor as well as neck node involvement. Standard radiation therapy consists of five daily treatments per week for five to seven consecutive weeks. The dose usually prescribed for treatment of microscopic disease is a total of 45–50 Gy delivered over a period of four to five weeks. To adequately treat disease that is visible, a dose of at least 65 Gy and up to 75 Gy, depending on the size of the tumor,

may be needed. The spinal cord is usually protected at doses of approximately 45 Gy.[54]

Recent research in tumor cell kinetics suggests that there may be a good reason to reconsider the fractionation usually planned for head and neck cancer radiation therapy. It may be necessary to destroy not only all of the tumor cells present at the beginning of the course of therapy, but also those that may result in cell divisions during the course. Therefore, the shorter the course of treatment, the less opportunity there is for cellular proliferation.[55] To achieve this goal, many different fractionation schedules of treatment have been tried. More than one fraction must be administered on each treatment day to give an increased number of treatments and to reduce the overall duration of treatment. This is referred to as combining hyperfractionation with treatment acceleration.[55]

The success of radiation therapy depends on cell death during division. The damage occurs in the DNA during cell division. Head and neck tumors are in the middle range of sensitivity to radiation. They can be controlled with radiation but will require a higher dose than other tumors such as lymphomas that are more radiosensitive.[56]

### Implant therapy (brachytherapy)

Implant therapy is the use of radioactive sources placed directly into the tumor. These low-energy sources deliver the radiation dose to the tumor bed while causing minimal morbidity to the surrounding tissues. The sources are placed using a procedure called *after-loading*. Under general anesthesia, hollow catheters are inserted in the tumor bed. These hollow catheters will hold the radioactive source, which is placed following the patient's return to his or her room. The radioactive material usually used is iridium 192, iodine 125, gold 198, or cesium 137. The implant is usually left in place for three to five days. This will deliver a total dose of 30–70 Gy.[56,57]

Implants may be used as a curative therapy for early-stage lesions in the floor of the mouth and anterior tongue or may be used to boost a tumor that has received prior external beam therapy. Lesions that can effectively be treated with interstitial implants include those on the lip, floor of the mouth, buccal mucosa, nasal vestibule, and skin.

Another common approach is to combine external beam therapy with intracavitary or interstitial implantation of radioactive sources. The external beam therapy is usually administered first to approximately 60%–70% of a conventional curative dose. Following a two to three week rest period during which treatment reactions are allowed to settle, the therapy can be completed with radioactive sources.

Radioactive seeds may also be implanted permanently at the time of surgery. Generally, seeds will be used at positive margins, neck nodes, or extension of the tumor into the base of the skull. The seeds have a low-level activity, with radiation being absorbed within the tumor with little or no exposure at the skin surface.[57]

### Hyperthermia with radiation

Hyperthermia is rarely used in head and neck cancer but may be combined with radiation to enhance tumor response. Heating the tumor superficially with ultrasound or microwave increases blood flow in the area and subsequently increases oxygen in the tumor bed, enhancing the radiation response. The area is generally heated to $41°$–$45°C$ for 45–60 minutes. The treatment is given once or twice weekly and is delivered through temperature sensors that are held in catheters that have been placed directly into the site. Patients may complain of a burning sensation, and blisters may appear in the treated area. The efficacy of this technique to enhance radiation response in head and neck cancers continues to be evaluated.

### Concomitant radiation therapy and chemotherapy

Head and neck cancer is a locally aggressive disease, with few patients presenting with clinically overt distant metastases at the time of diagnosis. Therefore, standard therapies have been aimed at control of local disease. However, there is a high regional recurrence rate even when surgery and radiotherapy are used together. The goal of therapy is to control regional disease, thereby decreasing the high incidence of persistent disease. The rationale for using radiotherapy with concomitant chemotherapy is to meet this goal. Chemotherapy can be successful at eliminating systemic micrometastases while concurrently enhancing the activity of radiotherapy in the irradiated field.[50]

The use of concomitant chemoradiotherapy has been studied in patients with head and neck cancer since the 1960s. Recently, studies have used combination chemotherapy schedules with split-course radiotherapy.

Cisplatin, 5-FU, and bleomycin have all been used as single agents in combination with radiotherapy. Results from trials using intermittent single-agent chemotherapy with concomitant radiotherapy have been promising; however, the numbers of patients that have received benefit from this approach do not at this time warrant making any of these approaches standard therapy.[50]

The use of chemotherapy with irradiation has shown promise as an alternative to total laryngectomy in patients with advanced laryngeal cancer. In a study published recently by the Veterans' Affairs Laryngeal Cancer Study Group, patients with advanced disease were randomized between the following treatments: induction chemotherapy (CDDP and 5-FU) and irradiation or total laryngectomy and postoperative radiation. Similar survival rates were shown between the two groups. Most importantly, the larynx was preserved in 64% of patients who received induction chemotherapy and radiotherapy.[58]

### Nursing management of patients undergoing radiation therapy

Nursing interventions in caring for the patient undergoing radiation therapy are aimed at helping the patient understand the goal of therapy, as well as dealing with both acute and long-term side effects. The patient is making daily trips during the week to receive treatments at the radiation facility. This often results in a five to seven week daily disruption in normal activities combined with increased fatigue as the course progresses.

The following side effects are usually experienced by any patient who receives radiation therapy to the head and neck area: mucositis, xerostomia, loss of taste, anorexia, fatigue, and local skin reaction. Nursing assessment and interventions can be extremely successful in abating and controlling symptoms during and after the treatment course.

***Mucositis***  Mucositis is an inflammatory response of the oral mucosa to radiation therapy. The soft palate, tonsillar pillars, buccal mucosa, pharyngeal walls, and lateral tongue are most susceptible. Mucositis can appear as early as the first week of treatment and generally will resolve within three weeks after the treatment is completed. The oral cavity will appear reddened and inflamed, and white patchy areas may be noted on oral exam. In addition, the patient will complain of a sore mouth and throat.

Oral care is essential during this time to alleviate discomfort and prevent infection. Commercial mouthwashes should be avoided because of their high alcohol content, which acts as a mucosal irritant. A mouthwash consisting of 1 teaspoon of salt and 1 teaspoon of baking soda in a glass of warm water will effectively rinse debris and soothe oral membranes. Viscous lidocaine may be prescribed to decrease discomfort. In addition, the patient should be instructed to avoid spicy foods, citrus juices, and fruits and vegetables such as grapefruit and tomatoes. (See chapter 29.)

***Xerostomia***  Xerostomia is a drying of the oral mucosa that results from loss of saliva due to damage that occurs to the salivary glands subsequent to radiation therapy to the head and neck. In the first week of treatment, salivary flow may decrease by 50%. Maximum dysfunction is usually reported after six weeks of therapy. In addition, salivary changes include a thicker saliva by the third week of treatment. These salivary changes are reported to persist for three months after treatment is completed in 43% of patients.[59]

To prevent dental caries, which can occur as a result of loss of the protective mechanisms of saliva, meticulous oral hygiene and prophylactic dental care should be initiated. A dental consult is indicated prior to the initiation of radiation therapy. Daily fluoride treatments that the patient performs at home can help to prevent dental caries. Artificial saliva products exist and can be recommended to the patient; however, the effect is only temporary and patients report equally satisfying relief from drinking frequent small sips of water. Although some salivary function can return following the cessation of treatment, the patient should understand that salivary function will never reach the preradiated level. Recently, oral pilocarpine has been approved for use as a stimulant to the exocrine glands. This results in diaphoresis, salivation, lacrimation, and gastric and pancreatic secretion. Administered in a dose of 5 mg orally three times a day, symptomatic improvements of xerostomia are found in 87% of users.[60,61]

***Loss of taste*** A side effect that frequently occurs with radiation to the head and neck is loss of or alteration in taste. This symptom occurs when the taste buds are included in the radiated field and is compounded by mucositis and xerostomia. Generally, alterations in taste are reported during the second week of treatment. Doses in the 50–65 Gy range cause maximum taste loss. The most severely affected taste qualities are salt and bitter. Sweet taste is generally least affected.[61] Patients will find eating very difficult at a time when maintenance of good nutritional status is paramount. Frequent meals that include high-protein, high-calorie foods should be encouraged. Because the patient may experience taste changes associated with favorite foods, bland foods may be better tolerated. High-calorie, high-protein malts and shakes generally are soothing to the oral mucosa and are not associated with any taste changes. Anorexia is an accompanying symptom that can interfere with an optimal nutritional status. Nutritional interventions will be discussed later in this chapter.

***Trismus*** If the posterior mandible is included in the irradiated field, the patient may experience jaw hypomobility or trismus. These patients should be taught exercises that increase the inter-arch distance by inserting several stacked tongue blades between the teeth and successively wedging in more blades until slight pain occurs.[61]

***Fatigue*** Fatigue is a frequently reported side effect of radiation therapy. Patients should be aware that this is a normal side effect that can occur at any time during the treatment course. Daily activities should be planned to include frequent rest periods for conservation of energy. In addition, depression and poor nutritional intake can also contribute to fatigue.

***Skin reactions*** Wet and or dry desquamation can occur in the tissues of the radiated site. This is frequently observed in areas of the neck that are subjected to frequent irritation, like the collar line. A variety of protocols exist for treatment of skin reactions. The radiation therapy department should determine the specific treatment approach. Generally, the patient should be instructed to avoid using harsh creams, lotions, or soaps in the radiated area. The area should be protected from the sun both during and after treatment. If the patient has a metal tracheostomy tube, it should be changed to a plastic one during treatment to prevent an enhanced reaction at the tracheostomy site.

The patient and family should understand the importance of radiation therapy in the treatment plan. Often, the symptoms experienced will be very difficult to endure and may affect the patient's ability to persevere to complete the treatment course. However, with support from family and health care workers and with information and suggestions for symptom control, the radiation course can be successfully completed.

# SYMPTOM MANAGEMENT AND SUPPORTIVE CARE

## Management of the Altered Airway

If the treatment plans include compromise of the upper airway or if the tumor affects the patient's ability to breathe, a temporary tracheostomy will be placed. The accompanying nursing care is a large portion of both caring for and teaching the head and neck cancer patient. Tracheostomy is effectively used in situations where airway obstruction or compromised pulmonary function is anticipated or already exists. In the postoperative patient with head and neck cancer, the massive edema that develops after oropharyngeal procedures necessitates tracheostomy at the time of surgery.

The procedure is usually performed under general anesthesia in the operating room. The patient is positioned with the neck hyperextended. A horizontal skin incision is made about 1½ mm below the level of the cricoid cartilage. A vertical incision (one of several types of incisions) is made through the second and third tracheal rings. A cuffed tracheostomy tube is then placed into the trachea and sutured into place. If the incision is made below the level of the third ring, the end of the tracheostomy tube can erode the innominate or right common carotid arteries, resulting in massive hemorrhage.[62]

### The tracheostomy tube

The type of tracheostomy tube utilized will depend on the surgical procedure performed and the clinical objectives to be achieved. A cuffed tracheostomy tube is the tube of choice for postoperative management of the patient. The standard parts of any tracheostomy tube and their functions are outlined in Table 40-10.

### Tracheal suction

The tracheal suctioning procedure is an important part of postoperative nursing care of the head and neck cancer patient. The procedure itself is often one of the most frightening procedures for the patient; however, with adequate preoperative teaching and discussion, fears and anxiety can be minimized. If the procedure is performed correctly, the patient should not experience pain.

**TABLE 40-10**  The Standard Tracheostomy Tube

| Part | Function |
| --- | --- |
| Obturator | Provides smooth tapered end during insertion to avoid tearing tracheal mucosa. Only used during insertion of outer cannula. |
| Outer cannula | Rigid structure inserted into tracheostoma. Curved between 70 and 95 degrees. |
| Inner cannula | Removed and cleaned (nondisposable type) or changed (disposable) to prevent accumulation of mucus plugs in outer cannula. Locks into outer cannula. |
| Cuff | Bonded to outer cannula. When inflated, provides seal between the tracheostomy tube and sides of tracheal wall. |

The suction catheter is passed gently into the trachea and a small "pill-rolling" motion performed on removal of the catheter. There is controversy as to whether suctioning a patient should be a sterile or a clean procedure. This author believes that sterile techniques should be employed until self-care teaching begins. Clean technique is always used in the home environment, and the patient is taught good hand washing and a procedure for cleaning and reusing suction catheters.

Each institution will have an approved procedure for suctioning the trachea, but all procedures should follow the same basic sequence:

1. Wash hands thoroughly.
2. Open sterile suction kit and/or tracheostomy tray.
3. Apply sterile gloves.
4. Attach catheter to source of negative pressure.
5. Fill basin with sterile water or saline solution.
6. Quickly insert catheter without pressure.
7. Apply suction and slowly withdraw catheter using a rotating motion.
8. Rinse saline or water through lumen of catheter.
9. Repeat procedure if secretions are profuse.

Some points to remember regarding suctioning a tracheostomy include the following:

- Only suction after a thorough respiratory assessment reveals that the patient cannot clear the airway effectively. Routine suctioning can produce tracheal trauma and irritation.

- Limit suctioning to 10 seconds or less at 120 mm Hg or less.

- Hyperoxygenation and hyperinflation of the lungs are advised both before and after the procedure to prevent suction-induced hypoxemia and subsequent arrhythmias.

## Inner cannula care

The inner cannula allows for removal and cleaning to maintain patency of the tracheostomy tube. The inner cannula should be removed and cleaned as needed but should be checked at least every four hours in the immediate postoperative period. Tubes that are constructed of a polyvinyl chloride or other plastic material can be cleaned with hydrogen peroxide and saline. Inner cannulas from metal tracheostomy tubes should be cleaned with saline or sterile water only. If metal tubes are cleaned with hydrogen peroxide, the oxidizing properties will tarnish the metal quickly.

## Tracheostomy site care

The tracheostomy site should be treated like any other surgical wound. The nurse must be alert to signs and symptoms that can signal infection such as erythema and purulent drainage from the site. The site should be cleansed with a cotton swab that has been dipped in half-strength hydrogen peroxide and then should be rinsed with a swab dipped in sterile water. Generally, site care is performed once every eight hours in the immediate postoperative period. The tracheostomy ties should be threaded through the slots in the flange of the tube and tied in a double knot on the uninvolved side of the neck. The ties should be secured at a tension that allows one finger to slip easily between the ties and the neck. The ties should be changed whenever they become soiled. The new ties should be in place before the soiled ties are cut and removed to prevent accidental dislodgement of the tube. The tracheostomy dressing should be placed under the flange of the tube and should also be changed whenever it becomes soiled. The dressing is always a gauze dressing that will absorb secretions and help to keep the tracheostomy area dry. If wound breakdown occurs at the tracheostomy site, care is directed toward promoting healing and preventing infection. It may be helpful to apply an occlusive material such as Stomahesive® to the skin adjacent to the tracheostomy site to promote healing. If there are flaps or grafts or a large amount of edema in the area, breakdown can occur at pressure points of the neck flange of the tube. Meticulous site care, relieving pressure by not tying the ties too tightly, and changing the tracheostomy dressing whenever it becomes soiled will help promote wound healing.

## Humidity

The concept of providing adequate humidity to the patient with an altered airway is one of the most important points for the patient and family to understand. It is important to remember that the patient with a tracheotomy has lost the functions of the nose in warming, moistening, and filtering the air when breathing. If supplemental humidity is not provided, the tracheal secretions become thick, tenacious, and difficult to clear from the airway. In the immediate postoperative period, high humidity (100%) with oxygen if indicated, or room air if oxygen is not indicated will prevent drying of the tracheal mucosa. In addition, the mucociliary transport process is not interrupted, and crusting of mucus along the airway passages is prevented. The most commonly used device to provide supplemental humidity in the immediate postoperative period is the tracheostomy high-humidity collar. In the home setting the patient should have a large, nine- to ten-gallon room humidifier in the living area of the home and a small bedside humidifier during the nighttime.

### Instillation of normal saline

Up to 5 ml of sterile normal saline may be instilled directly into the tracheostomy tube if secretions are tenacious and difficult to remove. The action of the saline is to lavage and irritate the trachea and bronchi: coughing is precipitated and secretions are mobilized. In addition, a nasal atomizer may be filled with saline and four or five "puffs" of saline sprayed into the tracheostoma on a regular basis to keep secretions thin and moist.

### Cuffed tracheostomy tubes

The purpose of a cuff on a tracheostomy tube is to protect the airway from aspiration of blood or secretions. A cuff should be used only if indicated and should not be overfilled. Cuffs on tracheostomy tubes are high volume and low pressure, exerting less than 25 mm Hg on the tracheal wall. Inflating a cuff beyond its maximal resting volume can cause tracheal necrosis and damage. The recommended procedure for cuff inflation, the "minimal leak technique," is as follows:

1. Using a hand-held resuscitation bag, simultaneously auscultate the neck.
2. Slowly inflate the cuff until a seal is obtained.
3. Withdraw 0.1 ml of air to create a small leak.

This procedure will ensure safe use of the tracheostomy cuff. Indications for use of a cuff may be the following:

- chronic aspiration
- bleeding in the head and neck area
- cardiopulmonary resuscitation
- positive pressure respiratory treatments
- emesis

A sample teaching plan that summarizes the specifics of preparing a patient to go home with a tracheostomy can be found in Table 40-11.

### Laryngectomy care

Care of the altered airway of the laryngectomy patient includes all of the respiratory care mentioned previously. If the patient has a laryngectomy tube, it will have an inner cannula that can be cleaned as previously described. If there is no tube in place, the edges of the laryngectomy

**TABLE 40-11**   Teaching Plan for Tracheostomy Care

| OBJECTIVE: To prepare the patient and family for performing tracheostomy care in the home. | | |
| --- | --- | --- |
| | Activity | Expected Outcome |
| DAY 1<br><br>*Equipment:*<br>Clean basin with $H_2O_2$ and water<br>Soft, lint free cloth to dry inner cannula<br>Trach brush | 1. Teach removal and cleaning of inner cannula:<br><br>If patient is going home with a *reusable* inner cannula, it will need to be removed and cleaned at least three times a day or as indicated by accumulation of secretions.<br><br>  Clean cannula in hydrogen peroxide using trach brush to remove secretions.<br><br>  Rinse with tap water.<br><br>  Replace. | Patient/significant other (S.O.) is able to unlock and remove cannula, stabilize neck plate during removal, and successfully clean cannula. |
| | If patient has a *disposable* inner cannula, it will need to be checked for secretions at *least* three times a day. If secretions have accumulated, discard soiled cannula and replace with clean cannula.<br><br>If patient has metal tube, use water instead of hydrogen peroxide, which will tarnish the metal. | Patient/S.O. uses snap-lock mechanism; removes and changes inner cannula. |

*(continued)*

**TABLE 40-11**   Teaching Plan for Tracheostomy Care (continued)

| | Activity | Expected Outcome |
|---|---|---|
| **DAY 2**<br><br>*Equipment:*<br>Suction machine<br>Suction catheters<br>Mirror<br>Small cup of saline<br>Small basin with soap and water<br>Lint-free towel to dry catheter | SUCTIONING THE TRACHEOSTOMY<br><br>1. Clean technique may be used.<br>2. Wash hands prior to performing procedure.<br>3. Attach appropriate-sized suction catheter to portable suction machine.<br>4. Turn machine on.<br>5. Occlude suction port; test suction in small cup of saline.<br>6. Introduce catheter into tracheostoma, keeping suction port *open.*<br>7. Occlude suction port to apply suction.<br>8. Slowly withdraw catheter using "pill-rolling" motion to facilitate suction of all secretions.<br>9. Suction saline through catheter to clear.<br>10. Catheter may be washed in mild liquid soap and stored in a clean, covered container for reuse.<br><br>INDICATIONS FOR SUCTIONING<br><br>1. Suction technique should be used whenever secretions become thick, tenacious, and difficult to mobilize by coughing. | Patient/S.O. will perform suction technique correctly and will understand indications for performing suction technique. |
| *Equipment:*<br>H₂O₂<br>Cotton-tipped applicator<br>Saline in small cup<br>Clean gauze dressing | TRACHEOSTOMY SITE CARE<br><br>1. Tracheostomy site should be cleaned at least daily and more frequently as indicated by accumulation of secretions.<br>2. Use hydrogen peroxide-soaked applicator to clean skin under neck plate close to stomal edges.<br>3. Follow by cleansing skin with saline-soaked applicator.<br>4. Report any signs of infection: erythema, purulent drainage, fever.<br>5. Change tracheostomy dressing whenever it becomes soiled. Tracheostomy dressing consists of a gauze dressing (noncotton back). | Patient/S.O. will carefully perform trach site care. He or she will understand rationale for frequency of cleaning as indicated by drainage. He or she will know signs and symptoms of infection to be reported. |
| **DAY 3** | IMPORTANCE OF SUPPLEMENTAL HUMIDITY<br><br>1. Supplemental humidity is required for any patient with a tracheostomy or laryngectomy.<br>2. Methods of administration of supplemental humidity include: instilling 1½–2 cc of normal saline into tracheostomy tube *or* using saline-filled nasal atomizer (four or five puffs to tracheostomy tube).<br>3. The humidity level in the home should be kept around 40%. A large 9–10 gallon room humidifier and a bedside humidifier will usually provide adequate humidity. | Patient/S.O. will understand the need to provide supplemental humidity. He or she will be able to manually perform instillation procedures and will be able to verbally relate signs and symptoms of inadequate humidity as well as actions to correct situation in which additional humidity is required. |

**TABLE 40-11**   Teaching Plan for Tracheostomy Care (continued)

| | Activity | Expected Outcome |
|---|---|---|
| | **CARE OF EQUIPMENT IN THE HOME** | |
| | 1. Suction catheters may be rinsed in mild soap and water and stored in a clean, covered container. They may be reused until discoloration in the catheter appears.<br>2. Follow manufacturer's recommendations for care of suction machine and humidifer. Generally, weekly cleaning is recommended.<br>3. One-quarter-inch seam binding, purchased from a fabric store, may be substituted for tracheostomy ties.<br>4. A second tracheostomy tube of the same size should be sent home with the patient. All parts to the tube should be kept together and not interchanged with second tube. | The patient/S.O. will understand that equipment may be reused in the home if cared for properly. Not only does this decrease cost, but it is safe in the home environment. |
| | **CHANGING THE TRACHEOSTOMY TUBE** | |
| *Equipment:*<br>New trach tube with ties<br>Water-soluble lubricant<br>Cotton-tipped swabs<br>Hydrogen peroxide one-quarter strength<br>Scissors<br>Mirror | 1. Change tracheostomy tube once a week or as directed by physician.<br>2. Tracheostomy tubes are only changed once the trach is firmly established. (Usually 2–3 weeks postoperatively)<br>3. Assemble equipment. Place clean trach tube with tie on clean cloth surface. Place obturator inside trach tube. Lubricate tip with water-soluble lubricant. Snip trach tie. Remove trach with downward curved motion. Cough—Wipe stoma with gauze. Inspect stoma. Cleanse with hydrogen peroxide and saline-soaked gauze. Insert clean trach tube into stoma. Lead with obturator tip in an upward curved motion into stoma. Immediately remove obturator. Secure with trach ties. Take a moment to catch your breath. Suction if necessary. | Patient/S.O. will demonstrate trach change on a model or patient as directed by physician. |
| | **PRECAUTIONS** | |
| | 1. The patient should avoid swimming and water sports and should exercise care in the shower to prevent water from entering the tracheostomy tube.<br>2. If difficulty breathing is experienced, the first action should be to remove the inner cannula—a mucus plug in the cannula could be obstructing the airway. If not relieved, suctioning should be performed. Finally, emergency assistance should be summoned and transportation to a local emergency room should be arranged. | The patient/S.O. will verbalize an understanding of precautions and potential emergency situations. |

stoma are kept clean and free from crusting with the same procedure indicated for tracheostomy site care. Suctioning occurs directly through the stoma in this instance as well.

The provision of adequate humidity is a lifelong concern for the laryngectomy patient. Seasonal variances and geographic location will affect the amount of humidity needed to keep secretions moist and easy to mobilize. In addition, the laryngectomy patient should take care to protect the stoma from dirt, dust, and other particulate matter. A variety of stoma covers that are attractive and effective in protecting the airway are available. The local branch of the American Cancer Society can be helpful in recommending vendors who supply laryngectomy appliances.

## Nutritional Management

Cancers of the head and neck by virtue of their location often impair the patient's ability to take nourishment by mouth. Often this results in a 15- to 20-pound weight loss that prompts the patient to seek medical treatment, presenting initially in a nutritionally compromised state. The discussion here will focus specifically on the interventions commonly utilized to improve the nutritional status in the patient with head and neck cancer.

### Enteral therapy

The primary goal of nutritional support in the patient with head and neck cancer is to correct nutritional imbalances and to maintain an adequate weight. Patients who undergo surgical resections will have compromised oral intake necessitating placement, at least temporarily, of a feeding tube.

Most patients with head and neck cancer have a gastrointestinal tract that is intact and functioning. Any obstruction in the GI tract is usually seen in the upper area of the tract, therefore requiring enteral support to be delivered below the level of the obstruction. There are several options available for enteral access. They include transnasal intubation, percutaneous endoscopic gastrostomy or jejunostomy, and surgical gastrostomy or jejunostomy. The chosen route will be dependent on the individual situation and need.[63] The type of feeding tubes that are most comfortable for the patient are small-bore, weighted tubes that are sized from 7 to 12 French. These tubes are flexible and have a low incidence of nasopharyngeal and nasogastric irritation. In addition, there is a decreased risk of reflux aspiration compared to large-bore tubes.[64] Small-bore tubes may be inserted with or without a stylet. Because there are inherent risks of esophageal perforation and pulmonary intubation with lung puncture, it is recommended that only experienced personnel place the tubes with a stylet. In addition, proper placement of the tube should be verified radiographically prior to the first feeding.

The feeding tube is placed during surgery for the surgical patient. Following return of bowel sounds, the patient is started on a continuous slow feeding of an isotonic commercial formula. Usually, feedings are started slowly at 25 cc/hour and gradually increased to 100 cc/hour or as tolerated. When the patient is more active and mobile, the feeding may be changed to intermittent feedings every four hours. The dietitian monitors the patient's nutritional status closely and makes appropriate changes in either the method of delivery or the formula.

If enteral support is anticipated to be necessary for a prolonged period of time, a feeding gastrostomy tube may be recommended. Gastrostomy tubes are frequently seen in the patient with head and neck cancer in the palliative setting. They are easily cared for in the home and can deliver nutrients that will increase the patient's comfort.

### Oral feeding

Prior to initiating oral feedings for the postoperative patient with head and neck cancer, an assessment of the patient's oral competence is necessary. Assessing a patient's ability to swallow is discussed in the swallowing rehabilitation section later in this chapter. In addition, nutritional counseling should include an evaluation of dietary intake and an explanation of the patient's requirement for calories and proteins. The teaching should include suggestions for dietary changes that will be necessary as the patient begins to experience difficulty in ingestion such as during radiation therapy. The movement from a regular to soft to blenderized diet may be gradual as the patient begins to experience dysphagia.

The psychosocial aspects of long-term enteral nutrition or even an altered method of eating should not be overlooked. The isolation that occurs from an inability to participate in meals and the body image changes associated with an alteration in eating pattern affect the quality of life for many patients.

## Oral Care

The provision of regular and thorough oral care is imperative in the patient with head and neck cancer. Not only can halitosis be a significant problem, but, more importantly, the surgical site of the oral cavity should be kept clean to prevent infection.

The method of oral care will depend upon the extent of surgical resection and the method of reconstruction. Oral care via lavage or power spray is most effective. A solution of hydrogen peroxide and water will adequately cleanse debris from the area and will not interfere with healing. Oral care should be delivered every four hours in the early postop period. As wound healing occurs, it can be performed once every eight hours to prevent odors and promote healing. A foul-smelling odor from the oral cavity could signal an infection in the area and should be investigated further. To avoid disruption of the suture line when using an oral power spray, the lowest setting on the machine should be used to deliver the treatment.

## Swallowing Rehabilitation

The act of swallowing involves transporting a bolus of food or liquid from the mouth to the stomach. During swallowing, food that has been placed in the mouth is broken down in preparation for the swallow. The act of swallowing is one that is taken for granted until impairment from surgery or neurological disease occurs.

The four phases of the normal swallow include: the oral preparation phase, the oral phase, the pharyngeal phase, and the esophageal phase.[35] The sequence of events in a normal swallow is outlined in Table 40-12.

There are two primary components of the swallowing evaluation: the bedside evaluation and the radiographic evaluation. Completed by the swallowing therapist, the bedside evaluation can alert the practitioner to alterations in the oral preparatory and oral stages of swallowing. This portion of the assessment process evaluates the labial, lingual, and palatal range of movement during both speech and swallowing exercises. The bedside exam will not provide accurate information on the pharyngeal stage of swallow. In addition, it will not indicate why a patient aspirates if there is clinical evidence of material entering the airway. During the bedside evaluation it is important to remember that the patient can aspirate material and show no evidence of it by coughing. Many patients who have problems with aspiration never cough.

The assessment of the oral and pharyngeal stages of swallow are completed by a modified barium swallow, or "cookie swallow," in which the patient ingests small amounts of liquid, paste, and semisolid materials that have been coated with barium. The modified barium swallow will detect aspiration. From this study the etiology of the problem can be defined and swallowing therapy can be initiated.

## Wound Care

The nursing responsibility in wound management lies initially in observation of dressings or the surgical site for any signs of infection or dehiscence. External suture lines are cleansed with cotton swabs soaked in a solution of half-strength hydrogen peroxide followed by sterile water or saline. This will help to loosen and remove crusting that accumulates following surgery. The use of an antibiotic or other ointment has been controversial and the physician should be consulted for preference.

A wound that requires debridement will be treated with wet to dry dressings. Gauze packing that has been soaked in saline is applied slightly wet, followed by application of a dry dressing as the outer dressing. Within three to four hours the packing will dry and it is gently removed, pulling necrotic tissue from the wound during the removal process. This procedure is repeated until all necrotic tissue is removed and evidence of tissue growth in the wound is seen. If an increased length of time for wound healing is projected, this procedure can be taught to the family and performed in the home.

### Wound breakdown

Wound breakdown with subsequent exposure of the carotid artery is one of the most serious and life-threatening sequelae of either the disease process itself or of surgical therapy. Rupture of the carotid artery or any other major artery in the head and neck is a medical emergency. All health care workers who interact with patients with head and neck cancer should be familiar with the procedures that are necessary to save a patient's life after carotid hemorrhage. The patient who is at risk for carotid hemorrhage should be identified to all as soon as there is evidence of wound breakdown in the area. In addition, emergency equipment should be placed at the bedside to manage the patient effectively until transport to the operating room for ligation can be arranged. An example of equipment needed is included in Table 40-13.

The nursing actions during a carotid hemorrhage focus on maintenance of the airway and control of bleeding. If the patient has a tracheostomy, the cuff should be inflated to prevent aspiration. The pressure from the cuff can also provide additional pressure internally to slow bleeding. The head of the bed is elevated to facilitate drainage of secretions, and the airway is suctioned to maintain patency. Firm pressure should be applied to the neck using a towel or dressing material. If an internal carotid bleed is suspected, a vaginal pack or fluff dressing should be used to tightly pack the oral cavity and oropharynx. The pressure should not be released during prepara-

**TABLE 40-12**   The Normal Swallow

| Phase | Action |
|---|---|
| Oral preparation phase | Food prepared for processing. Chewing occurs. Lip closure occurs to prevent drooling. |
| Oral phase | Bolus of food is propelled into pharynx. |
| Pharyngeal phase | Velopharyngeal valve closes to prevent nasal reflux. Soft palate retracts and elevates. Food enters pharynx. Tongue base retracts into pharynx. |
| Esophageal phase | Bolus approaches pyriform sinuses and enters esophagus. Cricopharyngeal muscle opens to allow entry. Larynx moves upward and forward. Peristalsis assists transport into the stomach. |

Logemann J: Swallowing and communication rehabilitation. *Semin Oncol Nurs* 5:205–207, 1989

**TABLE 40-13**  Carotid Precautions: Equipment

| |
|---|
| Sterile cotton dressings (6 packages 4 × 4s) |
| 2 cotton bath towels |
| Sterile bowl and normal saline solution |
| Ringer's lactate |
| Albumin |
| Type and crossmatch equipment (Vacutainer, holder, needle) |
| Completed requisitions for 2 units of blood |
| Two 20-ml syringes |
| Alcohol swabs |
| 1 cuffed tracheostomy tube if indicated |
| Suction equipment |

Adapted from Schwartz SS, Yuska CM: Common patient care issues following surgery for head and neck cancer. *Semin Oncol Nurs* 15:191–194, 1989.

tion and transport of the patient to the operating room. Hemorrhagic shock is avoided by rapid infusion of intravenous fluids. Preparations are made for administration of blood if needed. The patient is then transported to the operating room for ligation of the carotid artery. Unfortunately, patients generally remain conscious throughout this ordeal and are extremely frightened, not only by the sight of a large amount of blood but also by the intense level of activity that occurs rapidly around them. Measures to decrease the level of anxiety include speaking to the patient in a calm voice while explaining the activities that are occurring and emphasizing that the goal is to stop the bleeding.

The patient should be observed closely for subsequent hemorrhage or neurological deficits following a carotid artery ligation. Numbness or tingling of the extremities on the ipsilateral side, diplopia, blindness, progressive motor loss, and changes in the level of consciousness will alert the nurse to possible cerebral ischemia secondary to carotid artery ligation.[62]

### Carotid hemorrhage in the terminal patient

The goal following carotid hemorrhage in the patient who is terminal will not be ligation but providing an atmosphere that minimizes anxiety and ensures death with dignity. All of the previously mentioned precautions should be observed, with the exception of transportation of the patient to the operating room for ligation. Narcotics should be administered to relieve discomfort and distress. If the plan includes discharging the patient to home, the nurse should discuss precautions to prepare the patient and family for the event of carotid hemorrhage at home. The realization of the imminence of death will make the patient and family apprehensive, but an open and frank discussion regarding the goal of treatment and an empathetic and knowledgeable approach

by the nurse can facilitate a calm atmosphere at the time of death.

## Pain Management

The management of pain following surgery for head and neck cancer or in the palliative setting requires an understanding of the physiology involved as well as utilization of keen assessment skills. Nicolson and colleagues[65] reported that patients with head and neck cancer report less pain than do other cancer patients. In the immediate postoperative period this can be attributed to the severing of superficial nerves in the neck area, which results in a feeling of numbness in the surgical area rather than overt pain.

The type of pain usually experienced by the patient with head and neck cancer is described as "throbbing, pounding, or pressurelike." The rise in spinal fluid pressure that occurs with occlusion or ligation of the jugular vein contributes to this description.

As with any pain management regimen, the goal is to provide adequate relief while simultaneously allowing the patient to function at an optimum level or to die with minimal discomfort. There are a variety of products available that can achieve this goal. It is preferable to use an oral or enteral route for pain management on a long-term basis. In addition, concentrated doses can be administered to patients with dysphagia so there is a smaller volume of liquid to swallow.

## Psychosocial Issues

In addition to coping with a diagnosis of cancer and its subsequent treatment, the patient with head and neck cancer must also cope with an alteration in facial appearance and possible loss of speech, sight, taste, smell, and ability to swallow. This combination of adjustments is an enormous threat to the self-image. In addition, the patient's very identity and confidence are often threatened. Survival and adequate coping require great emotional strength. It is imperative that the practitioner working with the patient with head and neck cancer understand the process of reintegrating the alterations that have resulted from surgery and identify a plan to assist the patient in the process.

Anxiety and depression are commonly reported both prior to surgery and during the rehabilitative period. The psychological investment in the head and neck area is greater than that in any other part of the body. This is because social interaction and emotional expression depend greatly on the integrity of the face, especially the eyes.[65] This is of even greater concern for the head and neck cancer patient who cannot hide the structural changes that result from treatment and must therefore deal with constant exposure to others. It is expected that the patient will have fears regarding the reaction of family, friends, and strangers to the alteration in appearance.

Two parameters must be considered in the adjustment process: disfigurement and dysfunction. Although both may vary from minor to major, the health care worker must be sensitive to both issues. The degree of body image change required of the patient in adapting to the loss correlates with the extent of dysfunction and disfigurement. This can predict the severity of emotional response and can be helpful in constructing a plan of care.[66]

Dropkin has extensively studied the process of coping with disfigurement and dysfunction following head and neck cancer surgery. Regulations that limit the time a cancer patient may stay in the hospital have made it imperative to recognize maladaptive coping immediately and initiate appropriate interventions quickly. The Dysfunction/Disfigurement Scale developed by Dropkin and others at Memorial Sloan-Kettering Cancer Center can assist the nurse in developing a treatment plan to address these issues.[67] The results of Dropkin's study revealed important information about the way patients cope with disfigurement and dysfunction after head and neck cancer surgery. It was found that, generally, postoperative days four through six are pivotal in the recovery process in terms of acceptance of the defect. The measurements included assessment of self-care and amount of social affiliation that occurred between the patient and others. Acceptance of the defect, as demonstrated by the performance of self-care tasks, usually preceded social affiliative behaviors. Patients who do not cope effectively should receive more intensive interventions prior to discharge to prevent noncompliance with care at home. Moreover, failure to adequately cope with disfigurement and dysfunction can lead to pathological obsession with or denial of the defect, depression, or social isolation.[68]

## CONTINUITY OF CARE: NURSING CHALLENGES

The challenges of managing care for the patient with head and neck cancer in the 1990s are significant. Prospective payment systems are mandating shorter lengths of stay in hospitals and limiting the amount of home care that can be provided to the patient. Because patients are staying in the hospital for shorter periods of time, they often are sent home with only introductory contact with members of the rehabilitation team. In addition, because patients often are not physically strong when they are discharged, they may not be able to return to the hospital immediately for outpatient rehabilitation.[69] This creates a need for good communication between the hospital nurse and the home care or ambulatory care nurse. Ideally, a clinical pathway is developed that is specific to the care of the head and neck patient with identification of needs along the continuum of care. This pathway acts as a guide and a communication tool for health care professionals as the patient moves between the acute care facility and alternate site care.

## Home Care

Changes in reimbursement, technological advances, and consumerism have fostered the growth of home care over the past decade. Home infusion therapy is one area of home care that has seen significant growth. Chemotherapy protocols once delivered only in the hospital now are being safely administered in the home. The patient with head and neck cancer routinely receives either a portion of or the entire course of chemotherapy in the home.

As the patient with head and neck cancer moves through the various phases of treatment, the home care nurse is often the only health care professional with whom the patient routinely interacts.[70] The home care nurse can help to ensure coordination and communication with other members of the health care team, including the physician, the pharmacist, the office-based nurse, and the nurse in the radiation oncology clinic.

Discharge planning should begin either prior to or certainly upon admission. An assessment of the patient's home care needs should be noted in the plan of care. Typically, patients who go home with an altered airway, dressing changes, and enteral feedings will require a referral to a home care agency for follow-up care. Prior to discharge, the nurse should assess the patient's ability to perform self-care procedures. Any self-care tasks with which the patient continues to experience difficulty should be clearly communicated to the home care nurse for follow-up assessment in the home. If possible, an opportunity for the home care nurse to observe the patient's self-care procedures during hospitalization should be provided. In addition, the patient's insurance coverage for home care services must be verified to determine the patient's responsibility for payment.

The referral to the home care agency should be arranged as soon as possible. The home care agency can make plans for the needed supplies to be placed in the home prior to the patient's discharge and the home care nurse's first visit. The home care nurse can explore the available options in the community for reordering and stocking supplies. Referrals to other community services and agencies may also be beneficial to the patient upon discharge. Examples of these agencies include the following: the American Cancer Society (ACS) for assistance with medications, equipment, and supplies; the ACS support groups for psychosocial support in the home; and the Bureau of Vocational Rehabilitation.[40]

Emergency procedures for airway maintenance should also be reviewed with the patient and family prior to discharge. If the patient has a laryngectomy or tracheostomy and should require resuscitation, mouth-to-stoma rather than mouth-to-mouth resuscitation will be needed. Information on Medic-Alert identification should be provided and should indicate the patient is a "stoma breather."

Although most patients are anxious to leave the hospital and return home, there often is significant concern expressed by both the patient and family regarding their ability to perform self-care tasks in the home. Clearly communicating the expectations of the patient and family in the performance of self-care tasks as well as the knowledge of ongoing support provided by members of the health care team will greatly ease the transition home.

## Quality of Life in Head and Neck Cancer

Quality of life and performance status are two important outcomes to be considered in the development of a treatment plan for the head and neck cancer patient. The disease as well as the treatment options often have a negative impact on the patient's quality of life. As organ-preserving concomitant chemoradiotherapy is used more frequently and toxicities of treatment continue to vary, quality of life outcomes must continue to be well documented.[71] In a longitudinal assessment of quality of life in laryngeal cancer patients, rate and recovery of function were evaluated over a six-month period in 21 patients with laryngeal cancer. Patients were divided into three groups: total laryngectomy, hemilaryngectomy, and radiotherapy only. Although the three groups varied in patterns of performance recovery, there was little difference between the groups' overall quality of life over time. In addition, the results demonstrated no relationship between performance and emotional outcomes. This study needs to be replicated with a larger sample so that results can be used to establish benchmarks against which to evaluate performance of individual patients as they recover. Results of a larger study may also assist clinicians in preparing patients prior to and during the course of treatment.[71]

A diagnosis of head and neck cancer makes a significant impact on the patient's emotional as well as physical health. Multimodality therapy consisting of chemotherapy, radiotherapy, and surgery results in a number of health professionals participating at different intervals in the provision of care. A multidisciplinary approach is essential to provide quality care throughout the course of treatment as well as during the rehabilitation period. Optimally, the following members of the health care team should approach the diagnostic phase jointly: surgeon, radiation oncologist, and medical oncologist. The clinical case can be reviewed and a treatment plan outlined in a comprehensive manner. It may be helpful to structure a system that allows for all three physicians to evaluate the patient in a clinic setting prior to treatment planning as well as at predetermined intervals following each phase of treatment. This approach ensures comprehensive diagnosis and treatment planning throughout the patient's course of treatment. Ideally, appropriate members of the health care team should meet the patient and family prior to admission to the hospital. This often can be incorporated into the multidisciplinary clinic appointment. Additional members of the multidisciplinary team include: the nurse, social worker, chaplain, pharmacist, speech and swallowing therapist, discharge planner, dietitian, and prosthodontist.

Successful multidisciplinary teams find that regular meetings facilitate implementation of the plan of care as well as assist in preparing the patient and family for discharge. If major surgery that results in loss of speech or changes in facial contour is planned, the individual and family will have to adjust to these changes. In addition, the basic functions of eating and talking must often be relearned. It is not uncommon for the patient to experience feelings of anger and frustration during the immediate postoperative period. The members of the multidisciplinary team can assist the patient and family during this readjustment period.

## CONCLUSION

At no other time in our history has the health care industry experienced such dramatic change. Not only is the economic landscape of health care financing changing at breakneck speed, but advancements in technology are improving the options that may be offered to oncology patients. What does all this change mean for the individual with head and neck cancer?

Hospital stays for patients with head and neck cancer will continue to decline as managed care increases across the country. This change will continue to force more treatment to be delivered in the outpatient and home setting. Reinforcement of patient teaching will be done in the alternate site settings of the physician's office, radiation oncology clinic, or the home. Forums that enhance multidisciplinary communication across the continuum of sites of care will be required. The knowledge base of the nurse working with the head and neck cancer patient will become even more critical as the role of the nurse advances to one of case manager across the continuum. It will be imperative that nurses in all settings understand the disease process and treatment options for head and neck cancer.

The role of preventive education and assessment in the area of head and neck cancers will continue to increase. Public education on the hazards of smoking, drinking alcoholic beverages, and using smokeless tobacco will increase as health care continues to shift toward a focus on wellness. Broader implementation of smoke-free environments and improved methodologies in behavioral modification for individuals who do smoke or chew should result in fewer people at risk.[72]

Over the past decade, there have been significant advancements in treatment options for the patient with head and neck cancer. Unfortunately, there has been little impact on survival. The disease process as well as the treatment regimen continue to challenge the patient as well as the health care provider. Providing quality care to the patient with head and neck cancer in the next century will require an approach that crosses the many sites within the health care continuum. The role that nursing plays in providing assessment, education, and care to the patient with head and neck cancer will become even more critical in the years to come.

# REFERENCES

1. Parker SL, Tong T, Bolden S, et al: Cancer Statistics, 1996. *CA: Cancer J Clin* 46:5–29, 1996
2. Rothman KJ, Cann CI, Flanders D, et al: Epidemiology of laryngeal cancer. *Epidemiol Rev* 2:195–209, 1980
3. Schleper JR: Prevention, detection, and diagnosis of head and neck cancers. *Semin Oncol Nurs* 5:139–149, 1989
4. Shah J, Lydiatt W: Treatment of cancer of the head and neck. *CA Cancer J Clin* 45:352–368, 1995
5. Myers JN: Molecular pathogenesis of squamous cell carcinoma of the head and neck, in Myers EN, Suen JY (eds): *Cancer of the Head and Neck* (ed 3). Philadelphia, Saunders, 1996, pp 5–16
6. Steinburg BM: The role of HPV in benign and malignant lesions, *Cancer Treat Res* 74:1–16, 1995
7. Wei WI, Sham J: Cancer of the nasopharynx, in Myers EN, Suen JY (eds): *Cancer of the Head and Neck* (ed 3). Philadelphia, Saunders, 1996, pp 277–293
8. Bol D, Lloyd J, Manley M: The role of the primary care physician in tobacco use, prevention and cessation. *CA: Cancer J Clin* 45:369–373, 1995
9. Ryan D, Starr B: Vitamins in prevention and treatment of cancer. *Contem Oncol* 2:45–65, 1992
10. Spiro R, Rice D: *Current Concepts in Head and Neck Cancer.* New York, American Cancer Society, 1989
11. Nuss DW, Janecka IP: Cranial base tumors, in Myers EN, Suen JY (eds): *Cancer of the Head and Neck* (ed 3). Philadelphia, Saunders, 1996, pp 234–275
12. American Cancer Society: *Cancer Facts and Figures, 1996.* Atlanta, American Cancer Society, 1996
13. Hannon L: Cancer of the oral cavity. *Semin Oncol Nurs* 5:150–159, 1989
14. Alvi A, Myers EN, Johnson JT: Cancer of the oral cavity, in Myers EN, Suen JY (eds): *Cancer of the Head and Neck* (ed 3). Philadelphia, Saunders, 1996, pp 321–360
15. Lippman SM, Clayman GL, Huber MH: Biology and reversal of aerodigestive tract carcinogenesis, in Hong WK, Weber RS (eds): *Head and Neck Cancer.* Boston, Kluwer Academic Publishers, 1995, pp 89–115
16. Adams G, Haselow R: Oral and pharyngeal cancer—Early diagnosis for optimal treatment. Part I. *Hosp Med* 19:173, 1983
17. American Joint Committee on Cancer: *Manual for Staging of Cancer* (ed 4). Philadelphia, Lippincott, 1992
18. Wenig B: The role of surgery in head and neck cancer: Standard care and new horizons. *Semin Oncol* 21:289–295, 1994
19. Parsons JT, Stringer SP, Mancuso AA: Nasal vestibule, nasal cavity and paranasal sinuses, in Million RR, Cassisi NJ (eds): *Management of Head and Neck Cancer* (ed 2). Philadelphia, Lippincott, 1994, p 596
20. Schramm V: Craniofacial surgery for sinus tumors, in Thawley SE, Panje WR, Batsakis JG, Lindberg RD (eds): *Comprehensive Management of Head and Neck Tumors.* Philadelphia, Saunders, 1987, pp 390–407
21. Nestler A: Integral nursing interventions for cranial base surgical patients. *ORL-Head Neck Nurs* 10:7–10, 1992
22. Guyton AC: *Physiology of the Human Body.* Philadelphia, Saunders, 1979, pp 145–146
23. Chao R, Tannock I: Chemotherapy for recurrent or metastatic carcinoma of the nasopharynx. A review of the Princess Margaret Hospital experience. *Cancer* 68:2120–2124, 1991
24. Robbins SL, Angell M, Kumar V: *Basic Pathology* (ed 3). Philadelphia, Saunders, 1981
25. Oken MM: Chemotherapy in the treatment of head and neck cancer, in McQuarrie DG, Adams GL, Shons AR, Browne G (eds): *Head and Neck Cancer: Clinical Decisions and Management Principles.* Chicago, Year Book Medical, 1986, pp 133–143
26. Sessions DG: Composite resection and reconstruction with skin grafts for oral cavity and oropharynx cancer, in Chretien PB, John ME, Shedd DP, Strong E, Ward P (eds): *Head and Neck Cancer: Proceedings of the International Conference, July 22–24, 1984.* Philadelphia, Dekker, 1985, pp 187–193
27. Shah J, Sheman L, Strong E, et al: Buccal mucosa, alveolus, retromolar trigone, floor of mouth, hard palate, and tongue tumors, in Thawley SE, Panje WR, Batsakis JG, Lindberg RD (eds): *Comprehensive Management of Head and Neck Tumors.* Philadelphia, Saunders, 1987, pp 551–563
28. Jesse RH, Ballantyne AJ, Larson RL: Radical or modified neck dissection: Therapeutic dilemma. *Am J Surg* 136:516, 1978
29. Lingeman R, Shellhamer R: Surgical management of tumors of the neck, in Thawley SE, Panje WR, Batsakis JG, Lindberg RD (eds): *Comprehensive Management of Head and Neck Tumors.* Philadelphia, Saunders, 1987, pp 1325–1350
30. Sher N, Panje WR: New concepts in head and neck surgery. *Hematol Oncol Clin North Am* 5:627–634, 1991
31. Thawley S, Sessions D: Surgical therapy of hypo-pharyngeal tumors, in Thawley S, Panje WR, Batsakis JG, Lindberg RD (eds): *Comprehensive Management of Head and Neck Tumors.* Philadelphia, Saunders, 1987, pp 774–812
32. Steiner W: Results of curative laser microsurgery of laryngeal carcinomas. *Am J Otolaryngol* 14:116–121, 1993
33. Wenig BL, Ziffra K, Mafee MF: Magnetic imaging of squamous cell carcinoma of the larynx and hypopharynx. *Otolaryngol Clin North Am* (in press)
34. Edels Y (ed): *Laryngectomy: Diagnosis to Rehabilitation.* Rockville, MD, Aspen, 1983
35. Logemann J: Swallowing and communication rehabilitation. *Semin Oncol Nurs* 5:205–212, 1989
36. Zeitels SM, Vaughn CW, Domanowski GF: Endoscopic management of early supraglottic cancer. *Ann Otol Rhinol Laryngol* 99:951–956, 1990
37. Thawley S, Sessions D: Surgical therapy of supraglottic tumors, in Thawley S, Panje WR, Batsakis JG, Lindberg RD (eds): *Comprehensive Management of Head and Neck Tumors.* Philadelphia, Saunders, 1987, pp 959–991
38. Panje WR: Myocutaneous trapezius flap. *Head Neck Surg* 2:206–212, 1980
39. Ackland RD, Flynn MB: Immediate reconstruction of oral cavity and oropharyngeal defects using micro-vascular free flaps. *Am J Surg* 136:419, 1978
40. Sigler BA, Edwards A, Wilkerson J: Nursing care, in Myers EN, Suen JY (eds): *Cancer of the Head and Neck* (ed 3). Philadelphia, Saunders, 1996 pp 818–838
41. Vokes EE: Head and neck cancer, in Perry MC (ed): *Chemo-*

*therapy Source Book.* Baltimore, Williams & Wilkins, 1992, pp 918–931

42. Hong WK, Bromer R: Chemotherapy in head and neck cancer. *N Engl J Med* 308:75–79, 1983

43. Lippman SM, Hong WK: Chemotherapy and chemoprevention, in Myers EN, Suen JY (eds): *Cancer of the Head and Neck* (ed 3). Philadelphia, Saunders, 1996, pp 782–801

44. Vokes EE. Challenges in head and neck cancer. *Semin Oncol* 21:279–280, 1994

45. Stell PM, Rawson NSB: Adjuvant chemotherapy in head and neck cancer. *Br J Cancer* 61:779–787, 1990

46. Pinto HA, Jacobs C: Distant metastases from head and neck squamous cancer: The role of adjuvant chemotherapy, *Cancer Treat Res* 74:243–262, 1995

47. Merlano M, Vitale V, Rosso R, et al: Treatment of advanced squamous cell carcinoma of the head and neck with alternating chemotherapy and radiotherapy. *N Engl J Med* 327: 1115–1121, 1992

48. Vokes EE, Weichselbaum RR: Concomitant chemoradiotherapy: Rationale and clinical experience in patients with solid tumors. *J Clin Oncol* 8:911–934, 1990

49. Atanasiadis I, Vokes EE: Expanding the role of chemotherapy for head and neck squamous cell carcinoma. *Adv Oncol* 2:742–756, 1995

50. Haraf DJ, Weichselbaum RR, Vokes EE: Timing and sequencing of chemoradiotherapy, *Cancer Treat Res* 74:173–198, 1995

51. Taylor SG, Murthy AK, et al: Randomized comparison of neoadjuvant cisplatin and fluorouracil infusion followed by radiation versus concomitant treatment in advanced head and neck cancer. *J Clin Oncol* 12:385–395, 1994

52. Robbins KT, Vicario D, Seagren S, et al: A targeted supradose cisplatin chemoradiation protocol for advanced head and neck cancer. *Am J Surg* 168:419–422, 1994

53. Forastiere AA, Urba SG: Experimental therapeutic approaches for recurrent head and neck cancer, in Hong WK, Weber RS (eds): *Head and Neck Cancer.* Boston. Kluwer Academic Publishers, 1995, pp 263–281

54. Awan A, Vokes E, Weichselbaum R: Recent advances in radiation therapy for head and neck cancer. *Hematol Oncol Clin North Am* 5:635–655, 1991

55. Dische S: Radiotherapy-New fractionation schemes. *Semin Oncol* 21:304–310, 1994

56. Ang KK, Kaanders J, Peters LJ: in *Radiotherapy for Head and Neck Cancers Indications and Techniques.* Philadelphia, Lea and Febiger, 1994, pp 3–40

57. Bova FJ: Treatment Planning for Irradiation of Head and Neck Cancer, in Million RR, Cassisi NJ (eds): *Management of Head and Neck Cancer* (ed 2). Philadelphia, Lippincott, 1994, pp 291–310

58. The Department of Veterans Affairs Laryngeal Cancer Study Group: Induction chemotherapy plus radiation compared with surgery plus radiation in patients with advanced laryngeal cancer. *N Engl J Med* 324:1685–1690, 1991

59. King KB, Nail LM, Kreamer KK, et al: Patients' descriptions of the experience of receiving radiation therapy. *Oncol Nurs Forum* 12:55–61, 1985

60. LeVeque F, Montgomery M, et al: A multicenter, randomized, double-blind, placebo-controlled, dose titration study of oral pilocarpine for treatment of radiation-induced xerostomia in head and neck cancer patients. *J Clin Oncol* 11: 1124–1131, 1993

61. Strohl R: The etiology and management of acute and late sequelae of radiation therapy in persons with head and neck cancers. *ORL-Head Neck Nurs* 13:23–27, 1995

62. Johnson JT, Myers EN: Management of complications of head and neck surgery, in Myers EN, Suen JY (eds): *Cancer of the Head and Neck* (ed 3). Philadelphia, Saunders, 1996, p 708

63. Barbour L: Dysphagia, in Groenwald SL, Hansen-Frogge MH, Goodman M, Yarbro C (eds): *Cancer Symptom Management.* Boston, Jones and Bartlett, 1996, pp 197–217

64. Martyn-Nemeth P, Fitzgerald K: Tube feeding in the elderly. *J Gerontol Nurs* 18:30–36, 1992

65. Nicholsen BA, McGuire DB, Maurer VE: Assessment of pain in head and neck cancer patients using the McGill questionnaire. *J Soc Otorhino Head/Neck Nurs* 6:8–12, 1988

66. Breitbart W, Holland J: Psychosocial aspects of head and neck cancer. *Semin Oncol* 15:61–63, 1988

67. Dropkin M: Coping with disfigurement and dysfunction after head and neck cancer surgery: A conceptual framework. *Semin Oncol Nurs* 5:213–219, 1989

68. Nordlicht S: Facial disfigurement and psychiatric sequelae. *NY State J Med* 9:1282, 1384, 1979

69. Logemann J: Rehabilitation of the head and neck cancer patient. *Semin Oncol* 21:359–365, 1994

70. Salvaggio R: Meeting the challenge of home therapy for the patient with cancer. *Clin Pers Oncol Nurs* 1:1–12, 1995

71. List MA, et al: Longitudinal assessment of quality of life in laryngeal cancer patients. *Head and Neck.* 18:1–10, 1996

72. Hong W, Weber R (eds): *Head and Neck Cancer.* Boston, Kluwer Academic Publishers, 1995, pp 283–292

# Chapter 41

# Leukemia

**Debra Wujcik, RN, MSN, AOCN**

# INTRODUCTION

Leukemia is the name given to a group of hematologic malignancies affecting the bone marrow and lymph tissue. First described by the German pathologist Virchow in 1847 as simply "white blood," the term *leukemia* now includes abnormalities of proliferation and maturation in lymphocyte and myeloid (nonlymphocyte) cell lines. The acute leukemias are marked by an abnormal proliferation of immature blood cells with a short natural history (one to five months), while the chronic leukemias have an excessive accumulation of more mature-appearing but still ineffective cells and a slower, progressive course (two to five years). The excessive proliferation of the leukemia cells results in an overcrowding of the bone marrow, causing a decreased production and function of normal hemopoietic cells.

# EPIDEMIOLOGY

Leukemia represents 3% of the cancer incidence, with an estimated 27,600 new cases and 21,000 deaths expected in 1996.[1,2] Approximately one-half of the cases are acute and the remaining cases are chronic, but the number of new cases per year is greater in adults (24,800) than in children (2800). The most common types of leukemia in adults are acute myelogenous leukemia (AML) and chronic lymphocytic leukemia (CLL), while acute lymphocytic leukemia (ALL) accounts for 80% of all childhood leukemias.[3,4] The incidence of leukemia rose steeply from 1900 to the 1940s. Since then the incidence of AML has continued to increase steadily, both in the United States and developing countries, suggesting the influence of occupational and environmental exposure.[5]

# ETIOLOGY

The cause of leukemia is not known. The etiologic factors most commonly considered are genetic predisposition, radiation, chemicals, drugs, and viruses.

## Genetic Factors

The relationship of genetic factors to the incidence of leukemia has been suggested in certain high-risk families and specific hereditary syndromes. There is evidence of familial clustering with a four- to sevenfold increased risk in individuals with a family member diagnosed with leukemia.[6,7] Additionally, 10%–20% of monozygous twins of individuals with leukemia develop the disease.[6-8]

Certain genetic disorders are associated with increased incidence of leukemia. Children with Down's syndrome (trisomy 21) have an 18-fold to 20-fold increased incidence of acute leukemia.[9,10] Other disorders with chromosome abnormalities or fragilities also associated with acute leukemia are Bloom's syndrome, Fanconi's anemia, Kleinfelter's syndrome, and Ellis-Van Creveld syndrome.[3,11,12]

Diseases such as ataxia telangiectasia and congenital agammaglobulinemia are also prone to terminate in acute leukemia.[6,8] Although chromosomal abnormalities in these diseases are not detectable, deficiencies exist in humoral and cellular immunity. Whether congenital chromosomal defects cause or coexist with leukemia remains unclear; evidence of chromosomal abnormality and/or fragility appears to favor progression to a malignant state. In addition to certain genetic factors being associated with the development of leukemia, new techniques in chromosome analysis allow investigators to correlate chromosomal aberrations with survival rates.[12] This should allow the modification of therapy to include intensive or investigational therapy to improve outcome for those with low response rates.

## Radiation

Populations exposed to ionizing radiation have an increased incidence of leukemia, especially AML. Japanese survivors of the atomic bomb experienced a 20-fold increased incidence of AML and chronic myelogenous leukemia (CML). There appeared to be a direct relationship with the distance the individual was from the center of the explosion. The peak incidence was at five to seven years following exposure, and increased risks continued for 20 years.[13,14] In addition, early radiologists exposed to excessive irradiation experienced a higher incidence of leukemia.[15] Also, patients who were diagnosed with ankylosing spondylitis and treated with 2000 cGy had a 14-fold increase of AML when compared with similar patients who were not irradiated.[16] Radiation remains the most conclusively identified leukemogenic factor in human beings.

## Chemicals

Chronic exposure to certain chemicals has been associated with an increased incidence of pancytopenia and subsequent AML. Benzene, an aromatic hydrocarbon, is produced by natural processes and by industry (unleaded gasoline, rubber cement, cleaning solvents).[17] It was first implicated in the development of acute leukemia in Turkish cobblers in the early 1900s. Since then other populations have been identified as being at risk, including workers with explosives, distillers, dye users, painters, and shoemakers.[18,19]

## Drugs

Drugs that have demonstrated a relationship to the etiology of acute leukemia include certain alkylating agents, the antibiotic chloramphenicol, and phenylbutazone. AML is the most frequently reported second cancer following aggressive chemotherapy and is associated with treatment for Hodgkin's disease, multiple myeloma, ovarian cancer, non-Hodgkin's lymphoma, and breast cancer. Recently the epipodophyllotoxin etoposide has also been implicated as a leukemogen.[20-22]

Characteristics that distinguish therapy-related and *de novo* (with no known causative factors) leukemia are summarized in Table 41-1.[23] Secondary leukemias induced by alkylators are characterized by chromosome translocations such as t(9;22) or t(4;11), while leukemias arising after epipodophyllotoxin therapy are identified by 11q abnormalities. Therapy-related leukemia now represents 10%–15% of all AML patients,[24] and overall median survival is four to eight months.[25,26] The time of greatest risk appears to be the first ten years after treatment. Chloramphenicol and phenylbutazone are known to cause aplastic anemia and chromosomal breaks that eventually terminate in AML.[27,28]

## Viruses

The role of viruses in the etiology of human leukemia is unclear. The enzyme reverse transcriptase is present primarily in C-type viruses, a group of RNA viruses that can cause leukemia in animals. This enzyme reverses the usual transcription of genetic information from DNA to RNA, allowing the RNA tumor virus to produce oncogenic DNA within the host cells.[29] There is evidence of horizontal transmission of this leukemogenic virus from cat to cat.[30] Reverse transcriptase has been detected in human leukemic blood cells, but not in normal blood cells.

Adult T-cell leukemia in Japan and the Caribbean is associated with the human T-cell leukemia virus (HTLV-I). There is evidence for a role of HTLV-I in the etiology of adult T-cell leukemia in the United States.[31] HTLV-II has been identified in a rare form of hairy cell leukemia and is also prevalent in intravenous drug addicts.[32,33]

## CLASSIFICATION

Leukemias are classified as either chronic or acute and as either myeloid or lymphoid. In chronic leukemia the predominant cell is mature-appearing although it does not function normally. The disease has a gradual onset, prolonged clinical course, and a relatively longer survival time. The predominant cell in acute leukemia is undifferentiated or immature, usually a "blast" cell. The abrupt onset and rapid disease progression result in a short survival time. However, as progress is made in the treatment of children with acute lymphocytic leukemia and longer survival occurs, it may no longer be appropriate to describe acute leukemia as having a short survival.

Figure 41-1 presents the major classification of leuke-

**TABLE 41-1**   Characteristics of Treatment-Induced Acute Nonlymphocytic Leukemia (ANL) Compared to "Spontaneous" ANL

| Treatment-Related ANL | "Spontaneous" ANL |
| --- | --- |
| Related to prior exposure to alkylating agents and/or radiotherapy | Etiology largely unknown; small % related to chemical exposure (e.g., benzene) |
| Prolonged pancytopenia/preleukemia prior to onset | Approximately 30% present with preleukemia; rest have sudden onset |
| Latency period 2–5 years postexposure, with peak in incidence approximately 5 years | Latency period unknown |
| Dysplasia of one or more cell lines on marrow biopsy | May show dysplasia of cell lines |
| Specific cytogenetic abnormalities of chromosomes 3, 5, 7, 17 Approximately 90% have abnormalities of 5 and/or 7. Abnormalities of 11q are associated with epipodophyllotoxin exposure | Specific cytogenetic abnormalities of chromosomes 5, 7, 8, 11, 15, 16, 17, 21, (rarely 3, 4). Less than 5% have abnormalities of 5 and/or 7. |
| Refractory to treatment | Responsive to combination chemotherapy |
| Poor survival; almost uniformly fatal within a few months | Approximately 50% 1-year survival with some long-term survivors following BMT |
| Peak age varies depending on primary tumor, age of onset, about 5 years after treatment for first cancer | Peak age onset in 50s |

Reprinted from the *Oncology Nursing Forum* with permission from the Oncology Nursing Press. Fraser MC, Tucker MA: Late effects of cancer therapy: Chemotherapy-related malignancies. *Oncol Nurs Forum* 15:70, 1988.

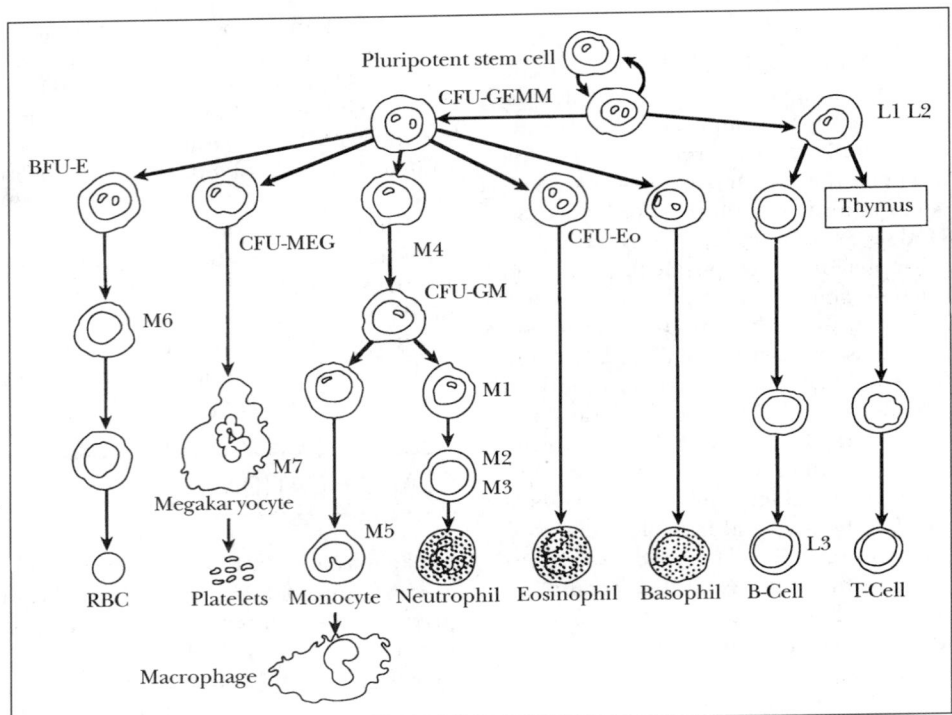

**FIGURE 41-1** Hematopoietic cascade with FAB classifications of acute nonlymphocytic leukemia and acute lymphocytic leukemia at proposed levels of arrested cell maturation. BFU = burst-forming unit; CFU = colony-forming unit; GM = granulocyte, macrophage; GEMM = granulocyte, erythrocyte, macrophage, megakaryocyte; Epo = erythropoietin; MEG = megakaryocyte; Eo = eosinophil; E = erythrocyte; M1 = undifferentiated myelocytic; M2 = myelocytic; M3 = promyelocytic; M4 = myelomonocytic; M5 = monocytic; M6 = erythroleukemia; M7 = megakaryocytic; L1 = childhood; L2 = adult; L3 = Burkitt's type.

mia according to the type of cell that predominates and the location of arrested cellular maturation. All cell lines arise from the same totipotent stem cell. From this cell, which has the potential to differentiate into a variety of cells, the myeloid and lymphocyte series are derived. The myeloid stem cell is pluripotent and gives rise to erythrocyte, thrombocyte, granulocyte, and monocyte progenitors, or committed cells. These are immature forms that mature into fully functional red blood cells, platelets, and white blood cells. The lymphoid stem cell matures in the thymus to form T-cell progenitors, or in the bone marrow to form B-cell progenitors.

The type of leukemia is named according to the point at which cell maturation is arrested. Although the terms *lymphocytic* and *myelogenous* (nonlymphocytic) leukemia are most commonly used, further specification within each class (for example, *promyelocytic, myelocytic*) describes the exact point at which arrest of maturation seems to occur.

In 1976 the French-American-British (FAB) Cooperative Group developed criteria for the classification of the acute leukemias[34] (Table 41-2). The purpose was to provide a systematic, objective system that would be feasible in most hematologic laboratories. The system, based on morphology and number of cells, has been revised and

**TABLE 41-2** French-American-British (FAB) Classification of Acute Leukemia

| Myeloid | | Lymphocytic |
|---|---|---|
| M1 | Undifferentiated myelocytic | L1, childhood (Pre B- and T-cell) |
| M2 | Myelocytic | |
| M3 | Promyelocytic | L2, adult (Pre B- and T-cell) |
| M4 | Myelomonocytic | L3, Burkitt's type (B-cell) |
| M5 | Monocytic | |
| M6 | Erythroleukemia | |
| M7 | Megakaryocytic | |

Data from Bennett JM et al.[34–36]

updated.[35,36] The additional information obtained through cytogenetics, identification of surface markers, and histochemical staining provides important therapeutic and prognostic information.

## PATHOPHYSIOLOGY

In the normal bone marrow, efficient regulatory mechanisms ensure that cell proliferation and maturation are adequate for the needs of the individual. In leukemia, control is missing or abnormal. The results are (1) arrest of the cell in an early phase of its maturation process, causing the accumulation of immature cells; (2) an abnormal proliferation of these immature cells; and (3) crowding of other marrow elements, resulting in inhibited growth and function of these elements and eventual replacement of the marrow by leukemic cells.

Manifestations of leukemia are related to three factors: (1) excessive proliferation of immature leukocytes within blood-forming organs such as the bone marrow, spleen, and lymph nodes, resulting in destruction of tissue; (2) infiltration of proliferating leukocytes into various organs of the body; and (3) decrease in the number of normal leukocytes, erythrocytes, and thrombocytes as a result of crowding of the bone marrow by proliferating leukemic cells. Table 41-3 summarizes possible leukemic manifestations, although these vary considerably with each type of leukemia.[37] The presenting manifestations, complications, course of disease, and treatment for each major type are discussed separately (Table 41-4).

## ASSESSMENT OF ACUTE LEUKEMIA

Factors that influence the symptoms and physical findings are: (1) the type of leukemic cell, (2) the degree of leukemic cell burden (early-stage or advanced disease), (3) the involvement of organs or systems outside of the bone marrow or peripheral circulation, and (4) the depression of normal marrow elements by the leukemic process. Since the presenting symptoms of AML and ALL are similar, the assessment parameters of acute leukemia will be discussed first. The classification and treatment of AML and ALL will be discussed individually. The chronic leukemias, CML and CLL, will be discussed separately.

### Patient History

Acute leukemia presents with a large and rapidly growing population of leukemic cells. Usually, signs and symptoms have been present for less than three months, and per-

haps for only a few days. Although the diagnosis cannot be made by history taking alone, many of the findings are typical and essential in guiding the diagnostic workup.

The most common complaints of the patient are nonspecific—that is, fatigue, malaise, weight loss, and fever. The presenting symptoms are the manifestations of the effects of leukemic cells on the normal marrow elements. Infections are recurrent in the common sites such as the skin, gingiva, perianal tissue, lung, and urinary tract. The patient may complain of sore throat and describe fever with or without signs of localized infection. Unexplained bleeding may occur with nose-bleeds, gingival bleeding, mid-cycle menstrual flow, or heavy bleeding with menses. Symptoms of progressive anemia include fatigue, palpitations, shortness of breath, and anorexia. Pain may arise from several sources: bones such as the sternum, enlarged lymph nodes, and hepatosplenomegaly.

Neurological complaints are frequent and may signal either leukemia infiltration (especially in ALL) or intracerebral hemorrhage. These include a history of headache, vomiting, visual disturbances, or seizures.

Review of the individual's past medical history may be noncontributory. However, it is of etiologic importance to note a history of recurrent infections or bleeding tendencies as well as the type and time of any drug exposure to try to document the approximate onset of leukemia. Similarly, the occupational (especially chemical and radiation) exposure and family history of genetic abnormalities or cancer contribute to the total epidemiological picture.

An essential part of the initial history that serves as a baseline for understanding the individual and planning care is the psychosocial profile. Questions that elicit details concerning past and present coping strategies with illness or other crises should be asked. Determination of significant others can be made by asking such questions as: "Who can you talk to most easily about your illness?" Finally, the nurse must ascertain how the patient and family perceive the illness and what their previous experience with hospitalization has been.

### Physical Examination

The physical findings of acute leukemia usually relate directly to the effects of pancytopenia. Vital signs may demonstrate fever, tachycardia, and tachypnea. The skin and mucous membranes generally appear pale, with readily apparent ecchymoses or petechiae. Generalized or localized adenopathy may be present due to leukemic infiltration or infection.

A comprehensive physical examination serves to validate findings elicited in a complete history and review of symptoms. Ophthalmoscopic examination may reveal retinal capillary hemorrhage or papilledema due to leukostatic or thrombocytopenic-induced bleeding and/or increased intracranial pressure. An oral infection with *Candida albicans* may be present. Examination of the lungs and heart may reveal the effects of anemia (cardiac mur-

**TABLE 41-3** Manifestations of Leukemia

|  | Organ | Manifestations |
|---|---|---|
| **PRIMARY MANIFESTATIONS** | | |
| Result from the proliferation of leukocytes within blood-forming organs | Bone marrow | Hyperplasia of abnormal cells<br>Hypoplasia of all normal cellular components<br>  Thrombocytopenia leads to bleeding<br>  Erythrocytopenia leads to anemia<br>  Granulocytopenia leads to infection |
|  | Spleen and liver | Hepatosplenomegaly<br>Changed consistency:<br>  Acute leukemia—soft<br>  Chronic leukemia—hard<br>Infarction causes pain<br>Hypersplenism leads to pancytopenia |
|  | Lymph nodes | Lymphadenopathy<br>May be painful<br>Obstruction of adjacent organs or structures |
| **SECONDARY MANIFESTATIONS** | | |
| Result from the infiltration of leukemic cells into body tissues *or* consequences of bone marrow suppression | Liver | Hepatomegaly<br>May be painful or tender |
|  | Bones, joints, and muscle | Enlargement of the cortex of the long bones in children with acute lymphoblastic leukemia<br>Osteolytic lesions<br>Goutlike symptoms<br>Pain<br>Swelling |
|  | Central nervous system | Thrombosis } paralysis<br>Hemorrhage }<br>Increased intracranial pressure<br>Headache<br>Vomiting |
|  | Skin | Purpura<br>Petechiae<br>Ecchymoses<br>Infection |
|  | Gastrointestinal system | Ulceration<br>Hemorrhage<br>Infection |
|  | Mouth, throat, and nose | Bleeding gums<br>Epistaxis<br>Ulceration<br>Necrosis<br>Infection |
|  | Lungs | Infarction<br>Infection<br>Pleural effusion |
|  | Eyes | Retinal hemorrhage<br>Subconjunctival hemorrhage<br>Papilledema<br>Visual disturbances |
|  | Kidneys | Bilateral asymmetric enlargement<br>Hyperuricemia<br>Rare pyelonephritis leads to renal failure |

**TABLE 41-4** Comparative Features of the Leukemias at Presentation

| Description | Median Age | Initial Remission Rate | Median Survival with Treatment | Splenomegaly | Infection | Adenopathy | Hemoglobin | White Blood Cell Count | Platelets |
|---|---|---|---|---|---|---|---|---|---|
| Acute myelogenous leukemia | 50–60 | 60%–70% | 10–15 mos | No | Yes | No | Low | Variable | Low |
| Acute lymphoblastic leukemia | 4 | Adult 70%; children 90% | Adult 2 years; children 5 years | Yes | Yes | Yes | Low | Variable | Low |
| Chronic myelogenous leukemia | 49 | 90% | 3 years | Yes | No | No | Low | 100,000–300,000 granulocytes | Normal or low |
| Chronic lymphocytic leukemia | 60 | 90% | 4–6 years | Yes | Yes | Yes | Low | 20,000 lymphocytes | Low |

murs) or infection (abnormal lung sounds). Abdominal palpation may demonstrate hepatosplenomegaly or enlarged kidneys due to leukemic infiltration, especially in children with ALL. Perirectal tissue may be tender and swollen and the only evidence of an abscess or a fistula. Finally, gentle palpation of bones and joints may reveal swelling and elicit pain.

## Diagnostic Studies

Laboratory and radiographic studies are essential for proper diagnosis. It is important to separate AML and ALL, since the treatment and prognosis differ markedly. An ongoing explanation to the patient and family of the plan and purpose of the exhaustive diagnostic workup will facilitate cooperation, decrease anxiety, and create an atmosphere of confidence and trust.

The diagnosis is suggested by the peripheral smear but requires a full examination of the bone marrow. The white blood cell count may be low, normal, or high, and 90% of patients have blast cells present in the peripheral blood. Neutropenia (absolute granulocyte count less than 1000 cells/mm³) is frequent, and thrombocytopenia is present in 40% of patients. Blood chemistry studies may reveal hyperuricemia and increased lactic dehydrogenase as well as altered serum and urine muramidase (greatly increased with monocyte and myelomonocytic leukemia, but normal to low in lymphoblastic leukemia). If acute promyelocytic leukemia ($M_3$) is suspected, laboratory evaluation should include plasma fibrinogen, fibrin split products, and prothrombin time.

Bone marrow contents are usually hypercellular, with 60%–90% blasts in the differential blood count. Auer rods are diagnostic of AML, and so are special stains (Sudan Black and peroxidase).

Improved techniques of cytogenetics (chromosome analysis) can provide information confirming the diagno-

sis and specific classification of the leukemia. Approximately half of patients with de novo acute leukemia exhibit nonrandom chromosome abnormalities,[12] and 40% of adults with leukemia have some cytogenetic translocations. Translocations are an adverse feature in ALL, while some translocations in AML indicate a better prognosis. These abnormalities in the leukemic cells serve as tumor markers that disappear during remission and reappear with recurrence of the leukemia.[38]

Cytogenetic analysis is performed at the time of diagnosis. Cells from the bone marrow or peripheral blood are collected and placed in culture for 24–72 hours. Cells are stimulated chemically to divide, then stopped in metaphase by the addition of drugs such as vinblastine or colchicine. After special stains are applied, the cells are examined for abnormalities in number and shape. These abnormalities are described as translocations, inversions, or loss or gain in chromosome number. Specific aberrations are related to a favorable or unfavorable outcome (see Table 41-5). The results of chromosome analysis are usually available within four weeks. Since this is also the time the patient is recovering from induction therapy, this information is useful in planning further treatment.

Further information is obtained from immunologic studies. Monoclonal antibodies reactive to immature cells can identify the predominant cell type and stage of arrested development in the leukemic cell line.[39] The use of surface marker antigens in patients with ALL has revealed the presence of markers for both lymphoid and myeloid cells. Mixed lymphoid and myeloid surface markers are found in 21% of patients with de novo ALL.[40] These hybrid leukemias may be biphenotypic where one cell line expresses characteristics of two lineages, or bilineal where two distinct populations may express either myeloid or lymphoid characteristics separately.[41] In general, patients with mixed lineage leukemia have a poor response to treatment and should be considered for other investigational therapies.

**TABLE 41-5** Prognostic Factors in Acute Leukemia

| | Poor Prognosis | Favorable Prognosis |
|---|---|---|
| Acute myelogenous leukemia | Age > 60 yr<br>FAB: M5, M6<br>Chromosome abnormalities:<br>−5/5q−;<br>−7/7q− t(6;9);<br>t(4;11); t(9;22)<br>Prior radiation/ chemotherapy<br>Prior MDS<br>Infection at diagnosis | Age < 60 yr<br>FAB: M3<br>Chromosome abnormalities:<br>t(15;17); t(8;21); inversion 16 |
| Acute lymphocytic leukemia | Age > 10 yr<br>FAB: L3<br>WBC > 25,000/mm³<br>Male<br>Immunophenotype: T-cell with tumor bulk<br>Pre-B, B-cell<br>cALLa −<br>Cytogenetics: hypodiploidy chromosome abnormalities:<br>t(9;22); t(4;11); t(8;14)<br>CNS involvement<br>Late achievement of CR | Age < 10 yr<br>FAB: L1, L2<br>WBC < 10,000/mm³<br>Female<br>Immunophenotype: Pre pre B-cell<br>cALLa +<br>Cytogenetics: hyperdiploidy |

Data from Champlin R;[45] Keating MJ, et al;[61] Priesler HD, et al;[62] Foon KA, Todd RF;[68] Hoelzer D, Gale RP.[76]

# ACUTE MYELOGENOUS LEUKEMIA

## Classification

Acute myelogenous leukemia (AML), also referred to as acute nonlymphocytic leukemia (ANLL), is a disease of the pluripotent myeloid stem cell. The malignant clone arises in the myeloid, monocyte, erythroid, or megakaryocyte lines. The exact event that triggers the malignant transformation is not known.

The leukemic cells have more abundant cytoplasm and granulation in the cytoplasm is usually but not always present. Auer rods, which are abnormal lysosomal granules, are present and pathognomonic for AML. Multiple nucleoli are present and tend to vary in size.

As previously stated, the type of leukemia is named for the predominant cell. The most common myeloid leukemia is acute myelocytic leukemia ($M_1$). Acute promyelocytic leukemia (APL) ($M_3$) is associated with an increased risk of disseminated intravascular coagulation. This is due to the release of procoagulants from granules

within the leukemic promyelocyte, especially during remission induction therapy.[25] Patients with acute monocytic ($M_5$) or myelomonocytic ($M_4$) leukemia often exhibit extramedullary leukemic infiltration with gingival hypertrophy, cutaneous leukemia, and liver, spleen, and lymph enlargement.[10]

Erythroleukemia ($M_6$), which was first described by DiGugliolmo, has both a chronic and acute form.[3] As the erythroleukemia progresses, the morphological picture resembles that of myelocytic or myelomonocytic leukemia. Megakaryocytic leukemia ($M_7$) is quite rare and less responsive to chemotherapy.[42]

By the time an individual is diagnosed with AML, the bone marrow and peripheral blood contain up to $10^{12}$ leukemic cells.[43] The accumulation within the bone marrow space results in inhibition and crowding out of normal marrow stem cells and infiltration of other organs by myeloblasts. Anemia, thrombocytopenia, and neutropenia result. If the disease is left untreated, death occurs within a few months due to infection or uncontrolled bleeding.

## Treatment

The goal of antileukemic treatment for AML is the eradication of the leukemic stem cell. Complete remission is defined as the restoration of normal peripheral counts and <5% blasts in the bone marrow.[41] Treatment regimens capable of inducing a complete remission are composed of several drugs, each of which is known to be effective against leukemic myeloblasts. The course of therapy is divided into two stages: (1) induction and (2) postremission therapy.

### Induction therapy

The goal of induction therapy is to cause severe bone marrow hypoplasia. At diagnosis the leukemic cells are proliferating more slowly than normal myeloid precursors. Therefore, the myeloid stem cells repopulate the depleted marrow faster than leukemic cells. The cornerstone for remission induction is the cell cycle-specific antimetabolite cytosine arabinoside plus an anthracycline (daunorubicin, doxorubicin, mitoxantrone, amsacrine, or idarubicin).[44-46] It is theorized that a drug that is noncycle-specific will have a synergistic effect when given sequentially with a cell cycle-specific drug by causing proliferating cells to enter the cell cycle concurrently. Cytosine arabinoside is administered continuously for seven days and the anthracycline is given for three days. The continuous infusion of cytosine arabinoside ensures that slowly cycling leukemia cells are adequately exposed to the drug during the synthesis phase of the cell cycle.[47] This protocol is called "7 + 3,"[48] but variations include 5-day or 10-day infusions of cytosine arabinoside. Gale and Foon,[49] in a review of the results of eight clinical studies, reported a complete response rate of 50%–75%, with the best results in the protocols with seven days of cytosine arabinoside.

The impact of the chemotherapy is assessed at one week after the completion of therapy with a bone marrow biopsy and aspiration on the 14th day. If residual leukemia is present, a second course is begun. Bone marrow recovery usually takes 14–21 days after the end of the chemotherapy with median time to complete recovery at 28–32 days. Complete response rates are now observed in 65%–80% of patients.[41,50,51] Unfortunately, in spite of improving remission rates, only 20% of patients remain in complete remission. Relapse occurs in the remaining cases within 1–2 years.[52,53] Thus, postremission therapy is essential.

### Postremission therapy

By the addition of postremission therapy, the median duration of remission can be increased from 4–8 months to 10–15 months.[50] Wolff et al[54] have used high-dose cytosine arabinoside to increase the continuing complete remission rate to 51%. The goal of further therapy is to prevent leukemic recurrence related to undetectable, resistant disease, also called *minimal residual disease*. Postremission therapies include consolidation, intensification, maintenance, and allogeneic or autologous bone marrow transplant.[55,56] None has emerged as the clear-cut, optimal therapy. (See Figure 41-2.)

Consolidation therapy consists of one or two courses of very high doses of the same drugs used for induction. Up to 30 times induction doses of cytosine arabinoside are used to consolidate the remission.[53] Although the patient is in a healthier state for this part of the treatment, the toxicities are substantial, with extended myelosuppression, cerebellar dysfunction, dermatitis, hepatic dysfunction, and conjunctivitis. The longest remissions appear to occur after two or more courses of consolidation therapy, with a median remission of one to two years.[45]

Intensification may be initiated right after remission induction (early intensification) or several months later (late intensification). Different drugs are used with the hope that they will be non–cross-resistant with the induction drugs. Mitoxantrone is less cardiotoxic and has less extramedullary toxicity than daunorubicin. With a steep dose-response curve, mitoxantrone is good for dose intensification.[56] Another combination being used for postinduction therapy is ICE (idarubicin, cytosine arabinoside, and etoposide).[57]

Maintenance therapy is treatment with lower doses of the same or other drugs given monthly for a prolonged period of time. Maintenance therapy is not currently recommended in the treatment of AML.[50,55]

Because microscopic disease is being treated in postremission therapy, it is difficult to know how much treatment is enough. Investigation continues to determine the optimal curative treatment.

Patients who relapse after induction and postinduction chemotherapy have a 30%–60% likelihood of achieving a second remission.[49,58] Leukemic cells acquire increasing resistance to chemotherapy. The cellular kinetics change due to an increased growth fraction and shortened generation time, resulting in a decreased doubling time.[38] The second and subsequent remissions are influenced by prior treatment, length of remission, and initial response to therapy. Patients who relapse quickly or who have resistant leukemia should be considered for clinical trials or bone marrow transplant.[58]

The role of bone marrow transplant (BMT) in the treatment of AML remains controversial.[59,60] The first issue is the availability of an HLA-matched donor. In the general population, a potential donor exists in less than 40% of cases.[59] Other options may include a matched unrelated donor BMT obtained through the National Marrow Donor Program. There are increased risks of graft-versus-host disease (GVHD) and lack of engraftment from these histocompatible but unrelated cells. A purged autologous BMT may be performed in a young patient with no HLA match. In patients less than 30 years of age, BMT may offer a higher cure rate than standard

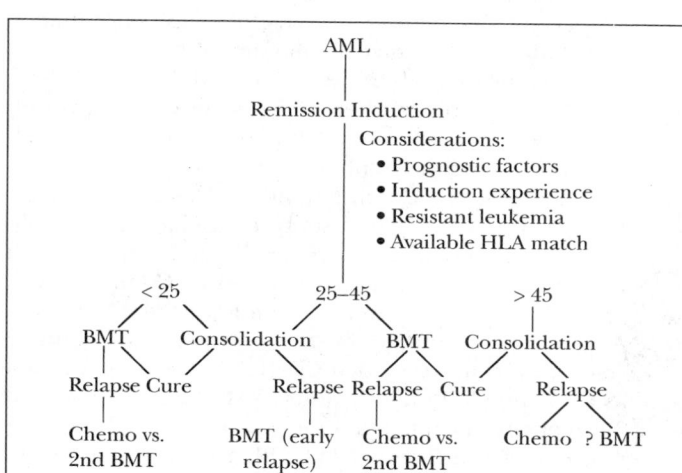

**FIGURE 41-2** Treatment considerations and options for patients with acute myelogenous leukemia.

treatment. In patients in the fourth decade, the results of chemotherapy versus BMT vary. Transplant centers usually do not admit patients over the age of 50. Because allogeneic BMT carries the risk of GVHD, interstitial pneumonia, and infection with cytomegalovirus, the decision for BMT is not easy. The question of the optimal timing for transplant remains unanswered. In addition, patients who relapse after allogeneic BMT can be treated with a second BMT or an infusion of donor buffy coat to stimulate the graft-versus-leukemia effect.[60] (See chapter 18 for an in-depth discussion of bone marrow transplantation.)

Another consideration in the treatment of AML is the significance of prognostic indicators, which may be useful in determining the best course of therapy (Table 41-5).[4,45,61,62] For example, patients with unfavorable factors such as older age or multiple chromosomal abnormalities may be treated with high-dose or investigational drugs. A patient who had a poor response to initial therapy and other medical problems is unlikely to benefit from reinduction therapy. Such patients may benefit from a less aggressive approach, with transfusion support and oral hydroxyurea to control the WBC count. In a younger patient with an unfavorable morphological subtype, BMT may be preferred to consolidation therapy.

A newer strategy being applied to patients with risk factors, early relapse, or resistant leukemia is drug therapy to overcome multidrug resistance (MDR). MDR is the phenomenon by which a cancer becomes resistant to multiple drugs that have little similarity in their chemical structure and mechanism of action.[63] MDR can be kinetic in origin, meaning the malignant cells are resistant at the onset of the disease. MDR is also acquired when drugs that were initially effective are no longer effective. Acquired MDR is associated with P-glycoprotein, which acts as a pump to transport drugs in and out of malignant cells. P-glycoprotein is associated with the MDR phenotype. The MDR1 message or its P-glycoprotein product is expressed in 10%–20% of cases of newly diagnosed AML. In addition, more than 50% of cases with relapsed AML express P-glycoprotein.[64,65]

The anthracyclines, specifically daunomycin and doxorubicin, are associated with acquired MDR. One strategy to overcome P-glycoprotein resistance is to use cyclosporine, a lipophilic endoecapeptide with immunosuppressive properties. Cyclosporine restores daunorubicin sensitivity in drug-resistant tumor cell lines.[65]

Strategies altering cellular kinetics to overcome de novo MDR are being explored. High-dose therapy with etoposide by continuous infusion for 29–69 hours along with cyclophosphamide on 3–4 days produced a complete remission (CR) in 42% of 40 patients with AML, including six patients with resistance to high-dose cytosine arabinoside.[66] Hematopoietic colony stimulating factors (CSF) such as granulocyte (G-CSF), granulocyte-macrophage (GM-CSF), and interleukin 3 (IL3) can enhance recruitment of cells into synthesis phase and optimize the cytotoxicity of cytosine arabinoside.[38,47,67,68]

A new therapeutic option is available for patients with APL. During the past several years, all-trans retinoic acid (RA), a derivative of vitamin A, has been used to induce remissions in some patients.[69,70] The break point for the chromosome region abnormality characteristic in APL (15;17) is clustered near the location of the retinoid acid receptor-alpha. The administration of RA seems to induce terminal differentiation and subsequent death of the previously arrested leukemic cells. Recently, RA was approved for remission induction in patients with APL who are refractory to chemotherapy or who have relapsed after prior chemotherapy. Once remission is obtained, treatment switches to chemotherapy because patients quickly develop resistance to RA.[71] Patients unable to tolerate conventional chemotherapy (older or with concomitant illness) also benefit from RA therapy. The most commonly used dosage is 45 mg/m²/day administered orally BID for remission induction. About one-half of patients experience the complications of disseminated intravascular coagulopathy, but few hemorrhagic deaths occur. Common side effects include headache, dry skin, xerostomia, cheilitis (cracking at the corners of the lips), and bone pain.

## ACUTE LYMPHOCYTIC LEUKEMIA

Acute lymphocytic leukemia (ALL) is a malignant disease of the lymphoid progenitors. The abnormal clone originates in the marrow, thymus, and lymph nodes, but the exact etiologic event is unknown. The leukemic lymphoblast is nongranular, with little cytoplasm. The round nucleus resembles a normal lymphoblast. Although the defect does not involve the myeloid cell lines, the secondary effect of the high leukemic cell burden on the bone marrow interferes with normal hematopoietic activity.

### Classification

The FAB classification for ALL is based upon several cell properties: size ratio of nucleus to cytoplasm; number, size, and shape of nucleoli; and amount and basophilia of the cytoplasm (Table 41-2).[34–36] In childhood ALL, 85% have L1 morphology, whereas the majority of adults with ALL have L2 morphology. Patients with L3 ALL, which resembles Burkitt's lymphoma, are rare.

Another classification system for ALL is based upon immune features.[68,72] Four subtypes are identified by the presence of certain markers on the cell surface. T-cell leukemias make up 20% of all ALL. Common ALL (cALL) is the most frequent and least differentiated ALL.[73] It is identified by the common ALL antigen (cALLa) recently renamed CD 10.[41] T-cell antigens such as CD5 and CD7 identify other T-ALL. Both cALLa and T-cell antigens contain another marker, terminal deoxynucleotidyl transferase (TdT). Other surface and cell immunoglobulins denote the rare B-cell ALL which accounts for 80% of ALL. Finally, about one-fourth are pre pre B (formally null) leukemias that do not have any identifiable surface markers.

Lymphoblasts have a propensity for organ infiltration and may remain sequestered in sanctuary sites even after remission has been achieved. Leukemic cells infiltrate into the central nervous system (CNS) early in the disease.[74] Because drugs used for treatment penetrate poorly into the cerebrospinal fluid, the leukemic cells are sheltered from the cytotoxic effects of the drugs. Over time, the leukemic cells proliferate and cause relapse. Cells can also be harbored in the testes.[4] In addition, 80% of patients have lymphadenopathy and/or splenomegaly at the time of diagnosis due to the infiltration of these organs by leukemic cells.[10]

The prognosis for long-term survival is more favorable for individuals with ALL than AML since drugs are available that are uniquely effective against lymphocytes—for example, prednisone. CNS prophylaxis is used in ALL and has proven successful.

As with AML, long-term survival and cure for individuals with ALL is possible only if a complete remission is achieved. This is documented by a bone marrow aspirate containing <5% lymphoblasts and the disappearance of all peripheral manifestations of the disease.

## Treatment

In contrast to AML, current chemotherapeutic regimens proven effective against ALL contain drugs that are selectively toxic to lymphoblasts and relatively sparing of normal hematopoietic stem cells. Therefore, the patient experiences hypoplasia that is less severe and of shorter duration with greater leukemic cell kill. In addition, relapses may be more effectively treated because the marrow is better able to recover.

The focus of therapy for ALL is to eradicate all leukemic cells from the marrow and lymph tissue and eliminate any residual foci of disease within the CNS. Treatment is divided into three stages: (1) induction, (2) CNS prophylaxis, and (3) postremission therapy. (See Figure 41-3.)

### Induction therapy

Although it is possible to achieve complete remission in 93% of children with ALL by using a combination of vincristine, prednisone, and L-asparaginase,[75] the same drugs even with the addition of an anthracycline produce remission rates of only 70%–75% in adults with ALL.[75,76] Between 35%–40% achieve long-term disease-free survival.[74] Therapy usually begins in the hospital, but hypoplasia is shorter than with AML treatment. Once remission is documented, the therapy is completed on an outpatient basis.

### CNS prophylaxis

Meningeal leukemia is present at diagnosis in about 2% of patients and is known to occur in up to 50% of patients with ALL in the absence of CNS prophylaxis.[73,77] By comparison, in patients with AML the incidence is less than 5%. Leukemic lymphoblasts enter the leptomeninges either by direct extension from the blood of the meningeal vessels or by seeding from thrombocytopenic bleeding. The cells extend deeply into the cerebral sulci and nerve sheaths, causing a mechanical obstruction of the cerebral spinal fluid (CSF). If unchecked, hydrocephaly and death occur. Several factors may explain the increased incidence of CSF infiltration with ALL.[78] There is a selective tendency for lymphoblasts rather than myeloblasts to enter the CNS. Drugs used in ALL enter the CSF slowly or in concentrations too low to be cytotoxic. The slower proliferation of lymphoblasts in the CSF may require longer drug exposure. Signs and symptoms of CNS leukemia include headache, blurred vision, nausea/vomiting, and cranial nerve palsies.[73]

CNS prophylaxis should start within a few weeks of

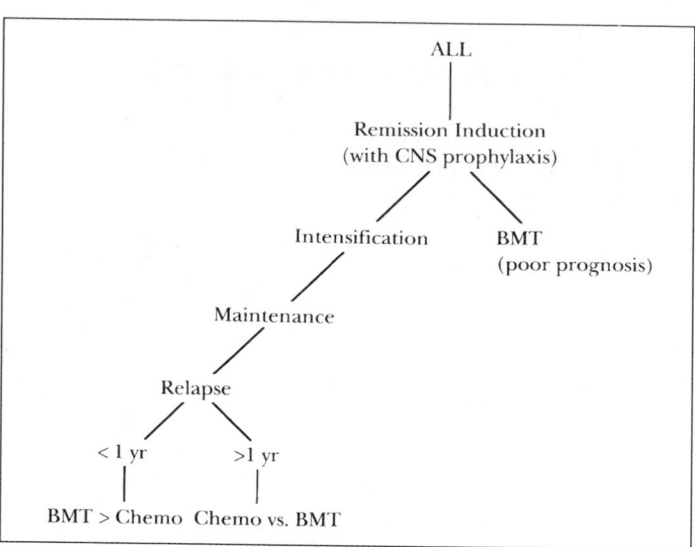

**FIGURE 41-3** Treatment considerations and options for patients with acute lymphocytic leukemia.

the initiation of therapy. Treatment usually includes intracranial radiation and intrathecal methotrexate.[45,74,79] Cranial radiation delivered in fractionated doses of 200 cGy up to a total dose of 2400 cGy produces predictable penetration of leukemic cells regardless of CSF dynamics. This therapy can also kill or sterilize cells not undergoing cell division. However, this therapy has recognized side effects, including somnolence, chemical meningitis, paraparesis, and leukoencephalopathy.[73]

### Postremission therapy

As in AML, even after complete remission, patients with ALL harbor remaining leukemic cells. Relapse occurs in two to three months if there is no continuing therapy. Prolonged chemotherapy may lead to a 40% overall cure rate, but the type and duration are not completely defined.[74] Currently many patients receive some type of intensification with high-dose chemotherapy or the use of multiple new drugs.[4,80] Methotrexate and 6-mercaptopurine may be added to the drugs used during induction. Maintenance therapy often continues for two to three years.

The outlook for patients in whom relapse occurs during therapy is quite poor, and younger patients with an HLA-matched donor should be immediately referred for BMT.[79] If relapse occurs after the completion of therapy, treatment is continued with high-dose methotrexate, tenoposide, and cytarabine, or high-dose cytosine arabinoside with an anthracycline or amsacrine. Second remission can be achieved in up to 50% of cases.[76] An analysis of eight studies using high-dose cytosine arabinoside in relapsed patients with ALL revealed a mean CR of 38%.[81] This same researcher reviewed 19 other studies that combined high-dose cytosine arabinoside (HDCA) with anthracyclines, vincristine, and/or prednisone and determined the CR rates to be 36%–63%[81] Idarubicin and HDCA induced second remissions in 65% of adults with ALL.[56]

Prognostic factors (summarized in Table 41-5) are also important in planning treatment for ALL.[74,76] Because patients treated with allogeneic BMT show a trend toward longer survival if the transplant is performed during the first remission,[59] it is important to identify patients with an unfavorable prognosis in the early stages of disease.

## MYELODYSPLASTIC SYNDROMES

Myelodysplastic syndromes (MDS) are a group of hematologic disorders with an increased risk of transformation to AML. They are characterized by a change in the quantity and quality of bone marrow products. Hematologic disorders that preceded acute leukemia were first reported in the late 1940s and referred to as *preleukemia anemia*.[82] Other terms used are *preleukemia, hematopoietic dysplasia, refractory anemia with excessive myeloblasts, subacute myeloid leukemia, oligoblastic leukemia,* and *dysmyelopoietic syndromes.*[83]

Currently MDS are divided into five subtypes according to the FAB group classification: refractory anemia (RA), refractory anemia with ringed sideroblasts (RARS), refractory anemia with excessive blasts (RAEB), refractory anemia with excessive blasts in transformation (RAEB-t), and chronic myelomonocytic leukemia (CMML).[84] Table 41-6 lists each type, along with diagnostic criteria, risk of evolution into acute leukemia, and average survival time.[83,84]

MDS are believed to occur as the result of an altered stem cell. The cause is unknown. Chromosome abnormalities are present at the level of the totipotent hematopoietic stem cell. Since MDS can progress to AML, ALL, or a mixed cell leukemia, it is thought that both myeloid and lymphoid progenitors are involved.[85]

Approximately 30% of patients diagnosed with AML initially present with preleukemic syndrome.[10] MDS may be considered to be different stages of the same disease. Cases have been noted of transition from one type of

**TABLE 41-6**  Classification of Myelodysplastic Syndrome with Percentage of Blast Cells, Leukemia Risk, and Average Survival

| Category | BLASTS (%) | | Risk of Evolution to Acute Leukemia (%) | Survival (months) |
|---|---|---|---|---|
| | Blood | Bone Marrow | | |
| RA | <1 | <5 | 0–25 | 18–71 |
| RARS | <1 | <5 | 8 | 14–76+ |
| RAEB | <5 | ≥5 | 20–44 | 7–16 |
| RAEB-t | >5 | 20–30 | 27–60 | 2.5–20 |
| CMML | <5 | 1–20 | 14 | 9–60 |
| | >10⁹ Monocytes | | | |

RA = refractory anemia; RARS = refractory anemia with ringed sideroblasts; RAEB = refractory anemia excess blasts; RAEB-t = refractory anemia with excess blasts in transformation; CMML = chronic myelomonocytic leukemia

Data from Buzaid AC, et al;[83] Bennett JM, et al.[84]

MDS to another before transition to AML.[95] Even if the evolution to acute leukemia never occurs, life-threatening anemia, thrombocytopenia, and/or neutropenia invariably occur. The defect is usually noted in the erythrocyte line first, then in the granulocytes and megakaryocyte.

Twenty percent of patients diagnosed with MDS are older than 50 years of age, with a median age of 60. The incidence is slightly higher in males than females.[86] A bone marrow biopsy and aspirate usually reveal dyshematopoiesis in all cell lineages. Ringed sideroblasts, abnormal nuclear shapes, cytoplasmic abnormalities, and maturation defects of RBCs indicate dyserythropoiesis. Evidence of dysmegakaryocytopoiesis includes atypical shapes; multiple, small nuclei; and increased or decreased numbers of platelets. Dysgranulocytopoiesis is seen with hypogranular cells, nuclear abnormalities, and maturation defects of granulocytes. A hypocellular bone marrow with one or more of these lineage defects provides a diagnosis of MDS.

About half of patients with MDS develop AML. Historically patients with MDS do not respond as well from antileukemic therapy as do those with de novo AML. However, a subset of patients with MDS (RAEB and RAEB-t) do respond to AML-type chemotherapy.[87] Survival for MDS ranges from several months to years, with median survival of 28 months. Poor prognostic indicators include excessive blast cells in the bone marrow, small clusters of immature myeloid precursors, pancytopenia, and complex chromosome abnormalities.[85] Death usually occurs within two years from complications related to bone marrow depression or transformation to acute leukemia.

Treatment for MDS is as aggressive as the course of the disease.[83] Serial bone marrow and peripheral blood examinations allow the physician to monitor the pace of the disease.[83] Supportive therapy includes replacement of RBCs or platelets and antibiotics for infection. Continuous infusion of low-dose cytosine arabinoside (20 mg/m²/day) is thought to induce differentiation of immature myeloid cells in 25%–35% of patients with MDS.[85] Other differentiation inducers include retinoic acid, dimethyl sulfoxide (DMSO), and vitamin D derivatives.[88] A synthetic androgen, danazol, is sometimes used to elevate platelet levels.[89] For the rare group of patients less than 40 years of age with an HLA-matched donor, BMT is the treatment of choice.[85]

# CHRONIC MYELOGENOUS LEUKEMIA

Chronic myelogenous leukemia (CML), also called chronic granulocytic leukemia, is a disorder of the myeloid stem cell characterized by marked splenomegaly and an increased production of granulocytes, especially neutrophils.[90] Approximately 90% of patients with CML have a diagnostic marker, the Philadelphia chromosome (Ph¹). The G group chromosome, number 22, is missing a portion of the long arm (q), which has been translocated to the long arm of number 9.[91,92] The significance of the marker is that a proto-oncogene is activated. When the proto-oncogene *c-abl* is translocated from chromosome 9 to 22, a new oncogene, *bcr-abl*, is formed. This gene produces a protein that is associated with triggering growth factor receptors.[93,94] It is speculated that this gene may induce uncontrolled growth of leukemic cells. Patients with Ph¹-negative CML have been found to have activation of this same gene even though no visible chromosome change is present.[95] In addition, as long as the marker is present, the patient is not cured of the disease.

There is no known specific cause for CML, except exposure to ionizing radiation.[92] The peak incidence is in the third and fourth decades, and both sexes are affected equally.[90]

The natural course of CML is divided into a chronic and terminal phase. The initial chronic phase is characterized by excessive proliferation and accumulation of mature granulocytes and precursors. There is an absence of lymphadenopathy, but 90% of patients have palpable splenomegaly.[90] Within 30–40 months the disorder transforms into a terminal phase consisting of accelerated and blastic phases. The accelerated phase includes progressive leukocytosis with increasing myeloid precursors (including blasts), increasing basophils, splenomegaly, weight loss, and weakness. There is increasing resistance to therapy, and serial cytogenetic studies indicate progressive chromosomal abnormalities.[92]

The blastic phase resembles AML, with 30%–40% of the bone marrow cells being blasts or promyelocytes. A crisis occurs as blast cell counts rise rapidly, often exceeding 100,000/dl. Leukostatic lesions caused by the high cell count result in occlusion of the microvasculature of the CNS or lungs.[90] The majority of patients have myeloblastic transformation, but some have lymphoblastic transformation, evidenced by the presence of TdT or cALLa. Median survival after the onset of the terminal phase is 3 months.[91]

## Assessment

CML in up to 20% of affected individuals is diagnosed in the absence of any symptomatology.[92] Most patients, however, present with a history that reflects the gradual accumulation of a white blood cell mass that is 10–150 times normal.

### Patient history

The initial symptoms or illness typically include symptoms related to massive splenomegaly due to infiltration of the spleen by leukemic cells: left upper quadrant pain, early satiety, and vague abdominal fullness may be the presenting complaints. Leukemic infiltration of joints may also cause bone and joint pain. A history of malaise, fatigue, weight loss, and fever caused by a gradually worsening hypercatabolic state may precede more acute symptoms of anemia.[96]

To a lesser extent than with acute leukemia, epidemiological clues may be provided by a complete past medical and family history, such as a history of exposure to ionizing radiation or a positive family history for leukemia.

### Physical examination

The vast majority of people are diagnosed during the chronic phase of their disease. The anemic individual appears pale. Examination of the eyes, ears, nose, and throat may reveal leukemic infiltration. Splenomegaly and hepatomegaly are common.

The physical examination of the patient in blast crisis is similar to that for the patient with acute leukemia. In blast crisis, blastic transformation of the leukemic granulocytes has replaced the bone marrow, causing an acute illness with pancytopenia, infection, and hypercatabolism. Rapid diagnosis and treatment to reduce the number of proliferating blasts are essential.

### Diagnostic studies

A complete blood count in the chronic phase reveals anemia and severe leukocytosis (WBC >100,000 mm$^2$). The differential count of the leukocytes demonstrates WBCs in every stage of maturation, with a predominance of more mature cells. The presence of functional but leukemic granulocytes in these individuals accounts for the low incidence of infection during the chronic phase. There is usually moderate anemia and thrombocytosis. The anemia is normocytic and normochromic with a median hemoglobin of 9–10 gm/dl.[92]

Other laboratory studies reveal high serum B$_{12}$ levels and a low leukocyte alkaline phosphatase level (LAP).[91,97] Both may return to normal with successful therapy.[90] Bone marrow biopsy demonstrates hyperplasia, with a myeloid to erythroid ratio of 15:1 and normal to increased megakaryocytes (platelet precursors). If the abnormal Ph$^1$ chromosome is found in the granulocytic, erythrocytic, and megakaryocytic series of the marrow, the diagnosis of CML is confirmed.[91]

Another tool has become useful in confirming the diagnosis of CML. Polymerase chain reaction (PCR) probes are used to separate RNA from viable cells for analysis.[98] This process of reverse transcripterase-PCR (RT-PCR) is used to detect the fusion genes that result from chromosome translocations. In the case of patients with CML, RT-PCR detects the BCR-ABL fusion gene. In some cases, the PCR data showed the presence of the BCR-ABL fusion gene after successful response was indicated by the Ph chromosome negativity. It is hoped that PCR will be a better diagnostic indicator than relying on the presence of the Ph chromosome alone.[91]

## Treatment

The only chance for cure of CML is with ablation of the Ph$^1$ chromosome and absence of the BCR-ABL fusion gene. Currently this occurs after high-dose therapy followed by allogeneic BMT. CML is a chronic disease and usually is suppressed by chemotherapy with hydroxyurea or busulfan. Late in the disease or at blastic crisis, investigational drugs are used. Recently, interferon has been approved for patients in chronic phase CML.[99,100]

### Chronic phase

The standard therapy during the chronic phase is single-agent oral chemotherapy.[91,97] Busulfan, an alkylating agent, is active against primitive hematopoietic stem cells. The WBC count begins to drop 10–14 days after starting therapy. To prevent prolonged or severe myelosuppression, treatment is stopped if the WBC is less than 20,000/mm$^3$. Long-term side effects include skin hyperpigmentation and pulmonary or retroperitoneal fibrosis. Hydroxyurea is cytostatic to cycling cells and inhibits ribonucleotide reductase. It acts on late progenitor stem cells causing rapid disease control, but it requires frequent monitoring of blood levels. Since hydroxyurea does not have the long-term toxicities on pulmonary and bone marrow tissue, it may be a better choice if a future BMT is a possibility.[91] Although both of these drugs decrease the leukemic cell mass and improve the quality of life, the progression to a terminal, refractory stage is not altered.

Interferon-alfa (IFN) is approved for previously untreated or pretreated patients with chronic phase, Ph positive CML. It is recommended that therapy begin within one year of diagnosis. The dose is 9 million international units daily, administered subcutaneously or intramuscularly. Patients who achieve a hematologic response (defined as a normalization of blood counts) and a cytogenetic response (absence of the ABL-BCR gene) should continue with treatment until disease progression. Those who achieve only hematologic response should continue for up to two years to maximize the possibility of achieving a cytogenetic response.[100]

Side effects associated with IFN therapy in this population are similar to others previously reported. The most common are flu-like symptoms such as fever, chill, malaise, fatigue, headache, and myalgias.[101] Lowered blood counts occur with neutropenia (22%), thrombocytopenia (27%), and anemia (15%) that quickly reverses when therapy is held.[100] A large study compared IFN with standard chemotherapy.[102] The overall response rate for patients treated with IFN was 30% compared to standard chemotherapy at 5%. Median survival with IFN versus chemotherapy was 72 months versus 52 months and time to progression of disease was >72 months with IFN versus 45 months with chemotherapy.

### Terminal phase

CML is a chronic neoplasm with a 100% incidence of blastic transformation.[91] This transformation, also described as a metamorphosis, is a gradual failure of response to treatment and failure of production of erythrocytes and platelets. Serial cytogenetic analyses can reveal signs of blastic transformation three to four months before clinical signs are evident. However, bone marrow aspirations are required, which are costly and uncomfortable for the patient.[91] The current trend is to treat the accelerated phase by continuing chronic phase therapy until evidence of the blastic phase appears. Because the transformation from benign to malignant appears to be random in length, it is difficult to predict survival, although life expectancy is less than 1 year.[96]

Blast crisis requires intensive chemotherapy, similar to that used in the treatment of AML. If the transformation is myeloblastic, therapy includes cytosine arabinoside, an anthracycline, and thioguanine. If lymphoblastic transformation has occurred, vincristine and prednisone are added. Patients who develop lymphoblastic transformation are more responsive to treatment and live longer.[103]

Although BMT remains the only chance for cure, it is an option for only 25% of patients.[97] The best results have been obtained in patients receiving allogeneic BMT during the chronic phase, with 55%–70% being disease-free at three to five years.[105]

The proposed sequence of treatment for patients with CML is outlined in Figure 41-4.[104] Patients less than 50 years old in chronic phase are immediately evaluated for an allogeneic BMT. Older patients with a high WBC receive hydroxyurea until the WBC <20,000/mm³. Therapy is then changed to IFN which continues until complete cytogenetic response or if no response until six months. Then the patient without an allogeneic donor,

those who do not respond to initial therapy, and those who relapse after therapy are considered for a matched unrelated donor transplant, autologous BMT, or other investigational therapy. Interferon is not usually helpful in patients with advanced disease. However effectiveness is noted in patients with advanced disease when interferon is given after cytotoxic therapy has decreased the tumor load.[105]

## CHRONIC LYMPHOCYTIC LEUKEMIA

A progressive accumulation of morphologically normal but functionally inert lymphocytes is found in chronic lymphocytic leukemia (CLL).[106] As the disease progresses, the abnormal lymphocytes accumulate in the bone marrow, spleen, liver, and lymph nodes. In 95% of the cases, there is clonal (from a single cell) expansion of neoplastic B-lymphocytes.[107] The median age at diagnosis is 60 years; the majority of cases are male.[92,108]

The pathological cells are usually small lymphocytes with markers of B-lymphocytes and surface IgM or IgD.[43] Approximately one-half of individuals with CLL experience frequent viral and fungal infections due to hypogammaglobulinemia.[107,108] For more than 95% of patients the diagnosis is an incidental finding during routine examination. Anemia, lymphadenopathy, or infection may be present. Coomb's positive autoimmune hemolytic anemia occurs in 25% of patients.[43]

The clinical course is variable, and, as with other hematologic malignancies, many attempts have been made to correlate a staging system with prognosis.[109–112] The two most commonly used systems are Rai and Binet. The Rai staging system has five levels based on the extent of tissue involvement and compromise of bone marrow function.[106] The Binet system identifies three groups, each with a subsequently worsening prognosis.[106] The International Workshop on CLL (IWCLL) attempted to combine the two systems (Table 41-7).[113] Binet et al[110] reviewed numerous systems and concluded that all staging systems defined a high-risk group of patients with anemia and/or thrombocytopenia.[110] In general, treatment is withheld until the patient shows evidence of

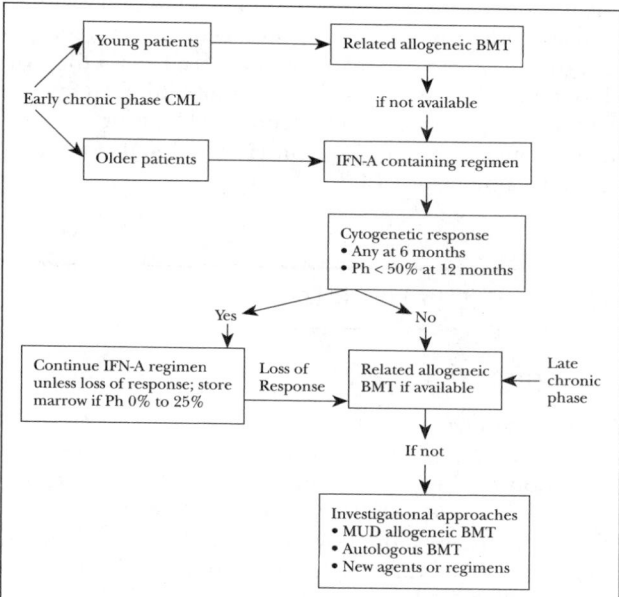

**FIGURE 41-4** Proposed treatment approach for patients with chronic myelogenous leukemia. BMT = bone marrow transplant; IFN-A = interferon-alfa; Ph = Philadelphia chromosome; MUD = matched unrelated donor. Reprinted from *Blood* with permission. Kantarjian HM, Deisseroth A, Kurzrock R, et al: Chronic myelogenous leukemia: A concise update. *Blood* 82:691–703, 1993.

**TABLE 41-7** Three Systems for the Classification of Chronic Lymphocytic Leukemia

| Rai | Binet | IWCLL* | Prognosis |
|-----|-------|--------|-----------|
| 0 | A | A(0), A(I), A(II) | Good: >10 yr |
| I | B | B(I), B(II) | Intermediate: <7 yr |
| II | C | C(III), C(IV) | Poor: <2 yr |
| III | | | |
| IV | | | |

*IWCLL: International Workshop on Chronic Lymphocytic Leukemia

Data from Binet JL, et al.[113]

hemolytic anemia, cytopenia, disfiguring or painful lymphadenopathy, symptomatic organomegaly, or marked systemic symptoms.[42]

## Assessment

One-fourth of individuals with CLL are diagnosed during a routine physical examination. Clues that alert the clinician early on, however, may be provided by a complete health history.

### Patient history

Early CLL may be asymptomatic. However, because CLL is a disease of immunoglobulin-secreting cells, a history of recurrent infections, especially of the skin and respiratory tract, may be elicited. The onset, location, duration, and response to treatment for infection should be documented.

Progressive infiltration and accumulation in nodal structures and the bone marrow gradually produce the symptoms that are typical of more advanced disease. Vague complaints of malaise, anorexia, and fatigue are common, as is noticeable and bothersome lymphadenopathy. Splenomegaly may cause early satiety and abdominal discomfort. The past medical history should focus on the documentation of any underlying autoimmune or immune-deficiency diseases, bleeding tendencies, and infectious episodes.

### Physical examination

The individual with early CLL appears well. Splenomegaly may be the only clinical finding. In advanced disease there may be evidence of infection, fever, and rashes. Lymphadenopathy occurs in 60% of patients, especially in the cervical, axillary, inguinal, and femoral nodes. The nodes are described as mobile, discrete, and nontender.[107]

### Diagnostic studies

Peripheral blood examination reveals lymphocytosis with normal or immature lymphocytes. The lymphocyte count is greater than 20,000/mm³ in early disease and may be over 100,000/mm³ in advanced disease. Protein electrophoresis documents the hypogammaglobulinemia that occurs in approximately 50% of patients. Bone marrow aspirate reflects the lymphocytosis seen peripherally, with varying degrees of infiltration. The severity of infiltration depends on the severity of the disease. Although early CLL causes patchy or focal infiltrates of the mature-appearing lymphocytes, progressive disease leads to a "packed marrow" with few normal hematopoietic cells. Lymph node biopsy may be interpreted as well-differentiated lymphocytic lymphoma if the blood count and bone marrow findings are unknown to the pathologist.

## Treatment

In general, treatment consists only of observation until the patient is symptomatic with cytopenias or organomegaly.[107,108] The rate of progressive lymphocytosis directs the frequency of observation and start of therapy. Patients may show a fluctuating moderate lymphocytosis for many years with no treatment at all.

Chlorambucil and cyclophosphamide are two alkylating agents used to treat CLL.[108,114] Chlorambucil is most effective in suppressing growth of well-differentiated, small lymphocytes. Cyclophosphamide suppresses growth of less mature lymphocytes with relative sparing of neutrophils and platelets. These drugs provide a response rate of 60%, with complete remission in 10%–20% of patients. There is a concern, however, that prolonged use of alkylating agents may induce secondary development of AML.[114,115]

Corticosteroids are used to control leukocytosis and immune-mediated cytopenias. When the patient no longer responds to steroid therapy, splenectomy may provide relief of symptoms.[114]

Radiation therapy may be used to treat lymphadenopathy or painful splenomegaly. Total body irradiation (TBI) and extracorporeal irradiation of blood to reduce lymphocyte counts are treatment options that may induce a temporary remission. TBI causes severe bone marrow depression, which limits usefulness.[107,108]

For patients with advanced disease (stage III or IV) and anemia or thrombocytopenia, combination therapy is recommended.[110] This includes cyclophosphamide, vincristine, doxorubicin, and prednisone. Fludarabine is the newest agent approved for use in B-cell CLL and is especially promising in patients refractory to alkylator therapy. Fludarabine is given as a daily 30-minute infusion for five days and is generally well tolerated.[91,116] Future studies include the use of interferon and monoclonal antibodies in the treatment of CLL.[114,117]

# HAIRY CELL LEUKEMIA

## Etiology

An unusual variant of the chronic leukemias is *hairy cell leukemia (HCL)*, so named for the prominent cytoplasmic projections on circulating mononuclear cells. Golomb[118] suggested that these cells share a common stem cell origin with histiocytes or monocytes and that the malignant cell is an immunoglobulin-bearing B-lymphocyte. HCL is also called *leukemic reticuloendotheliosis*.

Clinically, HCL may be difficult to distinguish from CLL or malignant lymphoma. The distinguishing characteristics are massive splenomegaly and little or no adenopathy. The characteristic hairy cells stain positively for tartrate-resistant acid phosphatase.[43] Two-thirds of individuals with HCL have pancytopenia, with symptomatic anemia, bleeding, and infection.

## Treatment

The goal of therapy in HCL has progressed from palliation to cure with the use of nucleoside analogues and interferon. Historically, patients without cytopenias required no immediate treatment. However, since infection is the primary cause of death, patients with HCL are monitored closely. Splenectomy is the treatment of choice for patients with marked pancytopenia, recurrent infections, massive splenomegaly, or rapid disease progression and may allow prolonged survival of up to 15 years.[118,119] Recently, complete remissions have been obtained in HCL with 2'-deoxycoformycin and 2-chlorodeoxyadenosine. Normalization of pheripheral blood counts occurs with absence of hairy cells in the bone marrow.[120,121] Recombinant alfa-interferon is considered the treatment of choice for those in whom disease progresses either before or after splenectomy.[91,118,122] Administered daily by intramuscular or subcutaneous injection, alfa-interferon decreases the need for transfusions, reduces risk of infection, and improves overall quality of life.

## SUPPORTIVE THERAPY

The increase in the length and quality of survival experienced by most individuals with leukemia is due not only to advances in antileukemic therapy but also to improved blood product and antimicrobial support and specialized nursing care. The complex means of providing effective supportive care include medical management to maintain physiological homeostasis as well as an interdisciplinary approach to the health care plan.

Effective nursing participation in the supportive care of any patient with leukemia depends on an understanding of the staging and natural history of each of the leukemias. From this base of knowledge the nurse contributes to the care of the patient with leukemia in each of the areas of education, physical care, symptom management, and psychosocial adaptation.

## Education

Providing information related to the disease process and treatment is clearly a standard in oncology nursing.[123] The nurse caring for the patient with AML has the unique opportunity of providing information to the patient and family because the patient is usually hospitalized throughout the course of therapy. The teaching plan for all patients includes pertinent information about the diagnosis, strategies for self-care in the prevention and treatment of side effects both in the hospital setting and at home, and methods to facilitate coping and adaptation to the illness.

For all patients with leukemia it is helpful to include the basic physiology of the bone marrow in the teaching plan. A hematologic malignancy is not as easy to understand as the concept of a solid tumor. Describing the bone marrow as the center of the bone where all blood products are made is a simple start. Further explanation includes the type, function and abnormalities of the blood cells (see Figure 41-5). From this base, individualized instruction related to the specific leukemia is given. Educational materials can be obtained from the Leukemia Society, American Cancer Society, and the National Cancer Institute. Information for contacting the organizations is found in chapter 66.

## Physical Care

The physical care needs of patients with leukemia require nurses who are skilled in physical assessment. Patients with AML receive intensive therapy aimed at producing bone marrow aplasia for several weeks. Those with ALL have defective lymphocytes producing altered immunocompetence. The drugs received are cytotoxic. The hypogammaglobulinemia associated with CLL increases the patient's susceptibility to viral and fungal infections. In any type of leukemia the incidence of infection is high, but the usual signs and symptoms of infection are diminished or absent. Therefore, the nurse must regularly conduct a thorough physical examination in order to detect any evidence of infection. Subtle changes in vital signs and mentation may indicate early sepsis. Oozing of blood from gums and intravenous sites may be the first sign of disseminated intravascular coagulation. Cerebellar toxicity related to chemotherapy may be manifested as slightly altered responses in the neurological examination. Each of these situations may be life-threatening, and the astute skills of the experienced nurse may be the crucial factor in initiating appropriate treatment.

In addition to having good assessment skills, the nurse caring for the patient with acute leukemia must be experienced in the use of right atrial catheters (RACs) and vascular access devices (VADs).[124] Patients undergoing aggressive induction therapy in the hospital often have a double or triple lumen RAC placed prior to the start of therapy. The RAC is used for blood sampling as well as for the infusion of fluids, chemotherapy, antibiotics, total parenteral nutrition, and blood products.[125] Patients who require ongoing treatment but less frequent blood sampling and no simultaneous infusion of multiple fluids may have a VAD placed subcutaneously.[126] The advantages, disadvantages, and nursing procedures associated with RAC and VAD are beyond the scope of this chapter. However, since most patients with acute leukemia have one of these devices, it is important for the nurse to become familiar with them.

## Symptom Management

Certain side effects associated with antileukemic therapy and disease-related complications can best be amelio-

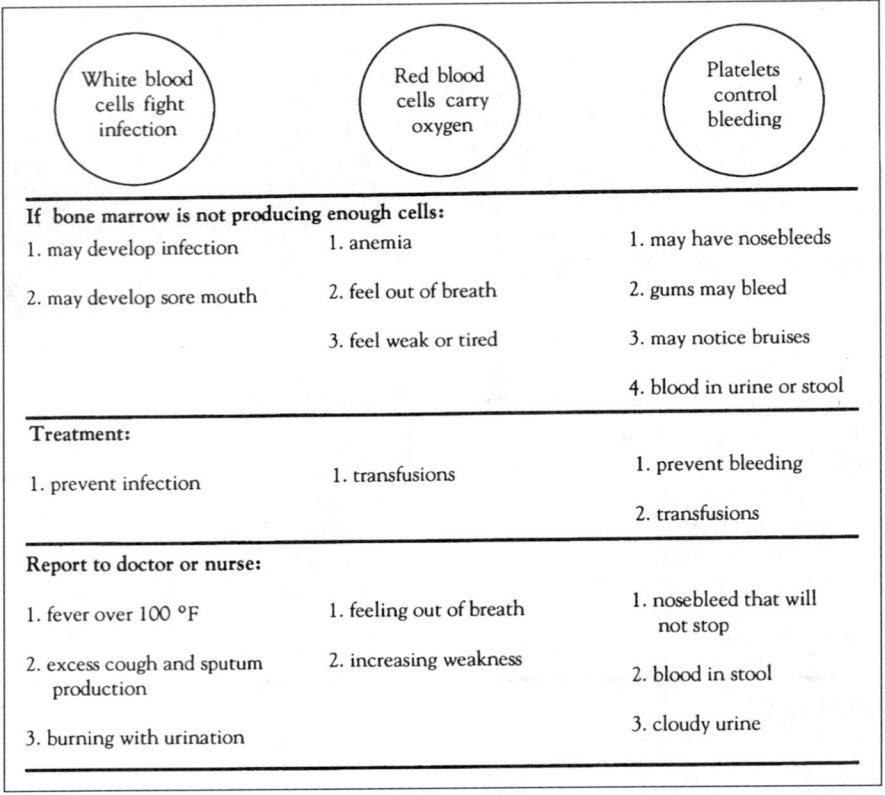

**FIGURE 41-5**   Patient teaching sheet for blood cell function.

rated if detected early and treated promptly. Knowing which side effects are expected and when they may occur allows the nurse to focus care appropriately.

### Bone marrow depression

The desired effect of cytotoxic therapy is bone marrow hypoplasia. The duration of pancytopenia is variable, depending on the type of therapy and the person's ability to recover. However, individuals with acute leukemia in the induction phase or individuals with CML in blast crisis may remain severely hypoplastic for months.

*Neutropenia*   It takes 9–10 days for immature cells formed in the bone marrow to become mature granulocytes. Because granulocytes circulate for only six to ten hours, any interruption in their production quickly places the patient at risk for developing an infection. Infection is the major complication for leukemia patients, with up to 20%–30% mortality.[52,127,128] Neutropenia is commonly defined as an absolute neutrophil count less than 1000/mm³. Since the neutrophils are responsible for phagocytosis, neutropenia eliminates one of the body's first lines of defense against infection. The patient with leukemia is particularly at risk due to a rapid drop in WBC with the initiation of therapy, a continuing decrease until the nadir (lowest point) is reached, and a prolonged time for recovery.[128]

Approximately 60% of neutropenic individuals develop infection. One-third have documented bacteremia, another third have documented infection without bacteremia, and the final third have apparent infection with no microbiologically documented pathogen. The risk of infection rises as the neutrophil count decreases, with 100% incidence of infection if the neutrophil count remains <100/mm³ for three weeks.[129,130] Other factors that add to the risk of infection are corticosteroids, hospital environment, antibiotic usage leading to increased colonization, and mucosal alteration.[129,131]

Adrenal corticosteroids are frequently used as part of the chemotherapeutic regimen or as supportive therapy. Steroids cause lysis of lymphocytes, suppression of antibody production, protein malnutrition, and suppression of inflammatory responses. As a result, the use of corticosteroids predisposes the patient to infection.

Most infections are due to organisms endogenous to the host or present in the environment.[129] The most common sites of infection are the alimentary tract (pharynx, esophagus, anorectum), sinuses, lungs, and skin.[129,132,133] The alimentary mucosa is directly damaged by the chemotherapy and the neutropenia allows colonization with yeasts and/or gram-negative bacilli. Perianal infection occurs in 25% of patients with AML. The only signs may be induration, erythema, and pain on defecation. Pneumonia can be caused by gram-negative organisms such as

*Pseudomonas aeruginosa, Klebsiella pneumonia,* or *Escherichia coli.* The most common gram-positive organism causing infection is *Staphylococcus epidermidis.*[129,133]

More serious infections associated with prolonged neutropenia are fungal infections such as *Candida* tropicalis, *Aspergillus* spp, *Fusarium* spp, and *Trichosporon* spp[127] or protozoa such as *Pneumocystis carinii.* When these infections occur during severe aplasia and immune depression, recovery of the blood counts is the best hope for survival.

Empiric antibiotic therapy is used to treat high-risk (neutropenic and febrile) patients until an infecting organism is identified. Early empiric antibiotic therapy includes drugs to cover both gram-negative and gram-positive organisms. The usual combinations include an aminoglycoside plus an extended-spectrum cephalosporin or a broad-spectrum antipseudomonal penicillin.[129,131,133] There is currently a trend toward initial broad-spectrum monotherapy.[134]

Amphotericin B is used to treat life-threatening fungal infections in myelosuppressed, immunosuppressed individuals. It is indicated if fever continues for five to seven days after the start of antibiotic therapy, if there is no identified source of infection, and continued neutropenia is expected.[130,135] Side effects of this toxic therapy include fever, chills, and rigors (80%–90%); nephrotoxicity (90%); headache (45%); anorexia (50%); vomiting (20%); and anemia.[135,136] Because anaphylaxis is a risk, a test dose of 1 mg is administered over 30 minutes. If the patient does not experience cardiopulmonary or mental changes, the starting dose is given. Fever is not a contraindication when the patient has recurrent fevers prior to the therapy. The dose is escalated daily until the desired dose is reached, and therapy continues for weeks to months, depending on the organism being treated and the patient's response.

Symptom management includes the following interventions to prevent or treat fever, chills or rigors: premedication with corticosteroids, acetaminophen, or diphenhydramine, and adding 10–15 mg hydrocortisone sodium succinate to the infusion. Intravenous meperidine 25–50 mg is given at the onset of chills or as a premedication.[136,137] Increasing room temperature, adding extra covers, using relaxation and hypnosis, and isometric leg and arm movements are other suggested comfort measures.[137] Potential nephrotoxicity due to a decreased glomerular filtration rate requires close monitoring of blood urea nitrogen, creatinine, sodium, and magnesium as well as evaluation of fluid balance. Peripheral phlebitis can be avoided by adding heparin to the solution. The anemia associated with amphotericin B is reversible and problematic only in that it compounds the existing myelosuppression.

There are currently a number of clinical trials evaluating the administration of amphotericin B in lipid vehicles.[127] The lipid vehicles do not enhance efficacy of the drug but seem to reduce the toxicities, thus allowing higher doses to be administered.

Some centers now place patients on prophylactic fluconazole and itraconazole[127] to prevent disseminated infections in patients expected to have prolonged neutropenia.[138]

Because the neutropenic patient does not produce an adequate inflammatory response to infection, the usual signs and symptoms are absent. Fever is usually the first sign of infection that leads to closer inspection of high-risk areas (perirectal area, oral mucosa, IV sites). Patients are often unable to produce sputum; thus, the early indications of pneumonia are shortness of breath or cough. Vital signs are assessed every four hours. At the onset of fever over 100°F in the neutropenic patient, blood, urine, and sputum cultures are obtained and empiric antibiotic therapy is initiated. The importance of prompt reporting of fever and initiation of therapy cannot be overemphasized since delay of only a few hours can allow the patient to go into septic shock.

Prevention of infection focuses on restoring host defenses, decreasing invasive procedures, and decreasing colonization of organisms. Treatment and remission induction will restore normal defenses against infection. Decreasing invasive procedures includes avoiding the use of Foley catheters. If catheterization is necessary, the smallest lumen possible should be used, and the catheter should be anchored. Other measures are meticulous care of IV or RAC exit sites and aseptic technique for any invasive procedures.

To decrease the number of gram-negative organisms, uncooked fruits and vegetables are avoided, especially salads. *P. aeruginosa* can be decreased by removing aerators from faucets, using ice machines in which the ice falls directly into the cup, and by frequently changing stagnant water sources such as oxygen humidifiers. Proper hand-washing techniques by everyone in contact with the patient can eliminate the main source of gram-positive organisms. Fungi that are found in food or the air can also be decreased by cooking foods and eliminating live plants or flowers from the patient's room. A private room is necessary, and visitors are restricted. All of these measures are to be practiced by the health care team and taught to the patient and family.[129,139,140] Further information is provided in chapter 21.

In certain circumstances such as BMT, total reverse isolation may be used. The patient is kept in a sterile laminar air-flow room. Nonabsorbable antibiotics are used to sterilize the alimentary canal. Normal skin flora is decreased by frequent cleansing with hexachlorophene or an iodine-base soap.[8,52]

Granulocyte transfusions may be indicated for patients with profound neutropenia and documented infections not responding to antibiotics.[133,141] However, the hazards of this therapy (increased alloimmunization and refractoriness to platelet transfusions) and its high cost make it a controversial therapy.

Colony stimulating factors have been used in the treatment of patients with leukemia. Both granulocyte (G-CSF) and granulocyte-macrophage (GM-CSF) have been administered to patients after completion of standard induction therapy to shorten the period of neutropenia.[142,143] Because myeloid leukemia cells have receptors for CSFs and have demonstrated increased growth in response to CSFs in vitro,[143] there is concern about administering myeloid CSFs to patients with AML. There is, however, some evidence of decreased myelosuppression and infection.

*Erythrocytopenia*    Individuals undergoing intensive chemotherapy develop a tolerance for chronic low-grade anemia. However, in severe cases of hypoplasia, sudden blood loss due to bleeding, or symptomatic anemia, support with transfusions of RBCs is provided. Premedication with acetaminophen and diphenhydramine can decrease the febrile response to antibodies to white cells that occurs after multiple transfusions. Leukocyte-poor RBCs may be used to decrease the antibody production against antigens on the leukocytes.[144,145]

*Thrombocytopenia*    Thrombocytopenia is the abnormal decrease in the number of circulating platelets. The potential for bleeding occurs when levels reach $\leq$50,000 platelets/mm$^3$, and spontaneous bleeding occurs at levels of $\leq$20,000 platelets/mm.[3,146] The first evidence of bleeding may be petechiae or ecchymoses on the skin of dependent limbs or on mucous membranes or oozing from gums, nose, or IV site.

Random donor platelets are given to keep the platelet count above 20,000/mm$^3$. Once antibodies to the platelets develop, refractoriness to random donor platelets occurs. When blood counts one hour posttransfusion reveal poor increments, the patient may require HLA-matched single-donor platelets.[132] Because chills and fever can destroy circulating platelets, the patient is premedicated with acetaminophen and diphenhydramine.[146] Additional measures used to prevent bleeding include maintaining skin integrity, preventing trauma, and avoiding medications that have the potential to induce or prolong bleeding.[116] Stool softeners will prevent the Valsalva maneuver and rectal tears. Further detail is given in chapter 22.

### Complications

Certain complications of the specific leukemic process or therapy may be singled out as untoward but not unexpected side effects. Knowledge of these occurrences assists the nurse in anticipating problems in high-risk individuals. These complications include leukostasis, disseminated intravascular coagulation, retinoic acid-APL (RA-APL) syndrome, oral complications, and cerebellar toxicity.

*Leukostasis*    Individuals with extremely high numbers of circulating blasts are at risk of leukostatic-induced hemorrhage. This occurs most often in patients with ALL. Leukostasis occurs as leukemic blasts accumulate and invade vessel walls, causing rupture and bleeding. Because of the extensive capillary network and the limited vascula-

ture space of the brain, intracerebral hemorrhage is the most common and most lethal manifestation of this complication. Therefore, early detection of patients at risk (WBC >50,000 cells/mm$^3$) and immediate efforts to reduce the number of circulating cells are imperative. Treatment consists of high doses of cytotoxic drugs to reduce the burden of circulating cells. Leukapheresis and cranial irradiation may be used to provide immediate treatment.[3]

*Disseminated intravascular coagulation*    Disseminated intravascular coagulation (DIC) is most frequently associated with acute promyelocytic leukemia, although it may occur with any acute leukemia.[52] During induction therapy there is excessive release of procoagulants from granules within the leukemic promyelocyte. (See chapter 22 for a discussion of the pathophysiology of DIC.)

Correction of the coagulopathy in DIC depends on the successful treatment of the leukemia. Therapy usually includes heparin and replacement of plasma factors and platelets. Nursing care focuses on the prevention of injury, administration of prescribed therapy, and monitoring of the appropriate laboratory results.[146,147]

*Retinoic acid-APL syndrome*    Another toxicity associated with treatment of APL is RA-APL syndrome. This syndrome appears clinically similar to the capillary leak syndrome associated with interleukin-2 therapy and is characterized by fever, respiratory distress, pulmonary infiltrates on chest x-ray, and weight gain. The incidence of RA-APL is 25% and the etiology is unknown. Early identification and treatment with high dose intravenous steroids has decreased the mortality associated with this syndrome.[148] Nursing care is focused on early detection of fluid retention (with measurement of weight, abdominal girth, orthostatic blood pressure, intake and output), fever (vital signs), and pulmonary distress.[149]

*Oral complications*    Oral complications of leukemia may be the result of the disease or the therapy. Gingival hypertrophy due to massive infiltration by leukemic cells is associated with acute myelomonocytic and monocytic leukemia.[10] The gingiva may be swollen, necrotic, and/or superinfected. The most effective treatment is therapy for the leukemia. Stomatitis due to the direct toxicity of chemotherapeutic agents such as the anthracyclines or methotrexate, combined with prolonged neutropenia and antibiotic therapy, renders the patient at high risk for oral infection.

Oral care consists of regular cleansing with a solution of one quart of water with one teaspoon each of salt and sodium bicarbonate, treatment of infection with nystatin mouth rinses, and appropriate analgesia as needed.[150]

*Cerebellar toxicity*    Cerebellar toxicity is a CNS toxicity associated with the administration of high-dose cytosine arabinoside (HDCA). Conventional dosages are 100–200 mg/m$^2$, whereas HDCA is $\geq$3 g/m$^2$. The incidence of neurotoxicity is 11%–28% at dosages of 3 g/m$^2$ and as high as 67% in dosages up to 4.5 g/m$^2$.[151,152] This toxicity is also age-related, with an increased risk in patients over

50 years of age.[153] The syndrome may begin with signs of ataxia and nystagmus and progress to dysarthria (difficulty in articulating words) and adiadochokinesis (inability to perform rapid alternating movements). This toxicity may be irreversible if not detected early. Therefore, it is essential that prior to each dose of HDCA the nurse completes a full neurological assessment.[154] Any changes are reported and the dosage is held until the physician evaluates the patient.

## PSYCHOSOCIAL SUPPORT

Individuals and their significant others are at risk for ineffective coping during the diagnostic workup for malignancy and during subsequent treatments.[155] A primary objective of supportive care must be to facilitate the most effective coping mechanisms for the individual and family as well as to enable the patient to live as full and normal a life as possible. Several factors should be taken into consideration as the nurse coordinates the care plan for psychological and physical rehabilitation.

The age of the individual at the time of diagnosis may vary from infancy to old age. Issues may range from concern about fertility or the risk of a second malignancy in the young adult to fear of job stigma in the middle-aged individual. The elderly patient may be dealing with increasing physical decline in addition to the debilitating effects of cancer. Assessment of the individual's needs and degree of stress will facilitate the planning of suitable intervention.[156]

The stage and "curability" of the disease are other factors to be considered. It is imperative that the nurse understand the implications of the planned therapy and assist the patient in making appropriate decisions. For example, a young mother undergoing intensive chemotherapy for AML may need to make the necessary arrangement for child care and housekeeping for six to eight weeks. A patient undergoing BMT may need to discuss with his or her employer the need to be on extended sick leave. The emotional ups and downs related to multiple remission inductions and relapses are exhausting to the patient and family.[157] As survival with leukemia increases, patients must deal with many issues such as fear of relapse, return to an independent state, and an uncertain future.[158,159] Ongoing support from the health care team is essential to overcome these fears. Education and reassurance by consistent nursing staff can help the individual regain a sense of control and hopefulness.

## CONCLUSION

The care of the individual with a diagnosis of leukemia requires a multidisciplinary approach that considers many factors. The classification of acute or chronic and myeloid or lymphoid determines diverse treatment plans and prognoses that are quite variable. The age of the patient and the stage of the disease determine the aggressiveness of therapy. Newer diagnostic studies allow the identification of both favorable and high-risk subsets of patients. As research continues, more durable cure rates may be achieved.

The role of the nurse providing direct care for patients with leukemia includes education, physical care, symptom management, and psychosocial support. In addition, contributions to research studies are essential. Although the nurse has an indirect impact on the prognosis through correct administration of therapy and management of side effects, the direct result of continuous support and education is an improved quality of life.

## REFERENCES

1. *Cancer Facts and Figures 1996.* New York, American Cancer Society, 1996, p 16
2. Parker SL, Tong T, Bolden S, et al: Cancer Statistics, 1996. *CA Cancer J Clin* 46:5–27, 1996
3. Henderson ES: Acute leukemia: General considerations, in Williams WJ, Beutler E, Erslev AJ, Lichtman MA (eds): *Hematology.* New York, McGraw-Hill, 1983, pp 221–253
4. Maguire-Eisen ME, Edmonds KS: Leukemias, in Clark JC, McGee RF (eds): *Core Curriculum for Oncology Nursing.* Philadelphia, Saunders, 1992, pp 480–487
5. Sandler OP: Epidemiology and etiology of acute leukemias: An update. *Leukemia* 6:3–5, 1992 (suppl)
6. Miller RW: Relation between cancer and congenital defects: An epidemiological evaluation. *J Natl Cancer Inst* 40:1079, 1968
7. Keating MJ, Freireich EJ, McCredie KB, et al: Acute leukemia in adults, 1977. *CA Cancer J Clin* 27:2–25, 1977
8. Gunz FW: Genetic factors in human leukemia, in Gunz FW (ed) *Leukemia* (ed 4). New York, Grune & Stratton, 1983, pp 313–328
9. Rosner F, Lee SL: Down's syndrome and acute leukemia: Myeloblastic or lymphoblastic? *Am J Med* 53:203–218, 1972
10. Keating HJ, Estey E, Kantarjian H: Acute leukemia, in DeVita VT, Hellman S, Rosenberg SA (eds): *Cancer: Principles and Practice of Oncology* (ed 4). Philadelphia, Lippincott, 1993, pp 1938–1964
11. Zuelzer WW, Cox DE: Genetic aspects of leukemia. *Semin Hematol* 6:228, 1969
12. Bloomfield CD, de la Chapelle A: Chromosome abnormalities in acute nonlymphocytic leukemia: Clinical and biological significance. *Semin Oncol* 14:372–383, 1987
13. Brill AB, Tomonaga M, Heyssell RM: Leukemia in man following exposure to ionizing radiation: Summary of findings in Hiroshima and Nagasaki and a comparison with other human experience. *Ann Intern Med* 56:590–609, 1962
14. Kamada N, Tanaka K, Oguma N, et al: Cytogenetic and molecular changes in leukemia among atomic bomb survivors. *J Radiat Res* 32:257–265, 1991
15. Matanowski GM, Seltser R, Sartwell PE: The current mortality rates of radiologists and other physician specialists: Specific causes of death. *Am J Epidemiol* 101:199-210, 1975

16. Court-Brown WM, Doll R: Mortality from cancer and other causes after radiotherapy for ankylosing spondylitis. *Br Med J* 2:1327–1332, 1986

17. Rinsky RA, Smith AB, Horning R, et al: Benzene and leukemia. *N Engl J Med* 316:1044–1050, 1987

18. Thorpe JJ: Epidemiologic survey of leukemia in persons potentially exposed to benzene. *J Occup Med* 16:375–382, 1974

19. Snyder P, Kalf GF: A perspective on benzene leukemogenesis. *Crit Rev Toxicol* 24:177–209, 1994

20. Whitlock JA, Greer JP, Lukens JN: Epipodophyllotoxin-related leukemia. *Cancer* 68:600–604, 1991

21. Pedersen-Bjergaard J, Daugaard G, Hansen SW, et al: Increased risk of myelodysplasia and leukemia after etoposide, cisplatin, and bleomycin for germ-cell tumours. *Lancet* 338:359–363, 1991

22. Domer PH, Head DR, Renganathan N, et al: Molecular analysis of 13 cases of MLL/11q23 secondary acute leukemia and identification of topoisomerase II consensus–binding sequences near the chromosomal breakpoint of a secondary leukemia with the t(4;11). *Leukemia* 9:1305–1312, 1995

23. Fraser MC, Tucker MA: Late effects of cancer therapy, chemotherapy related malignancies. *Oncol Nurs Forum* 15:67–77, 1988

24. Keating M, Cork AL, Broach Y, et al: Towards a clinically relevant cytogenetic classification of acute myelogenous leukemia. *Leuk Res* 11:119–133, 1987

25. Foon KA, Gale RP: Controversies in the therapy of acute myelogenous leukemia. *Am J Med* 72:963–978, 1982

26. Kantarjian HM, Keating M: Therapy related leukemia and myelodysplastic syndrome. *Semin Oncol* 14:435–443, 1987

27. Dougan L, Woodleff AJ: Acute leukemia associated with phenylbutazone treatment. *Med J Aust* 1:217–219, 1965

28. Brauer MJ, Dameshek W: Hypoplastic anemia and myeloblastic leukemia following chloramphenicol therapy. *N Engl J Med* 277:1003–1005, 1967

29. Gallagher RE, Gallo RC: Type of C RNA tumor virus isolated from cultured human acute myelogenous leukemia cells. *Science* 187:350–353, 1975

30. Jarrett W, Essex M, Mackey L, et al: Horizontal transmission of leukemia virus and leukemia in the cat. *J Natl Cancer Inst* 51:833–84l, 1973

31. Heath CW: Epidemiology and hereditary aspects of acute leukemia, in Wiernick PH (ed): *Neoplastic Diseases of the Blood* (vol 1). New York, Churchill-Livingstone, 1985, pp 183–200

32. Kalyanaraman VS, Sarngadharan MG, Robert-Guroff M, et al: A new subtype of human T-cell leukemia virus (HTLV-II) associated with a T-cell variant of hairy cell leukemia. *Science* 218:571–573, 1982

33. Rosenblatt JD, Plaeger-Marshall S, Giorgi JV, et al: A clinical, hematologic, and immunologic analysis of 21 HTLV-II-infected intravenous drug users. *Blood* 76:409–417, 1990

34. Bennett JM, Catovsky D, Daniel MT, et al: Proposals for the classification of the acute leukemias. *Br J Haemat* 33:451–458, 1976

35. Bennett JM, Catovsky D, Daniel MT, et al: Criteria for the diagnosis of acute leukemia of megakaryocyte lineage (M7). *Ann Intern Med* 103:460–462, 1985

36. Bennett JM, Catovsky D, Daniel MT, et al: Proposed revised criteria for the classification of acute myeloid leukemia. *Ann Intern Med* 103:626–629, 1985

37. Johnson BL: Leukemias, in Groenwald S (ed), *Cancer Nursing, Principles and Practice.* Boston, Jones and Bartlett, 1987, pp 654–670

38. Arlin ZA, Heddeman W, Feldman E, et al: Further thoughts on "cell kill" in acute leukemia. *Acta Haematol* 85:1–5, 1991

39. Griffin JD, Davis R, Nelson DA: Use of surface marker analysis to predict outcome of adult myeloblastic leukemia. *Blood* 68: 1232–1241, 1986

40. Sobel RE, Mick R, Royston I: Clinical importance of myeloid antigen expression in adult acute lymphoblastic leukemia. *N Engl J Med* 316:1111–1117, 1987

41. Devine S, Larsen RA: Acute leukemia in adults: Recent developments in diagnosis and treatment. *CA: Cancer J Clin* 44:326–352, 1994

42. Peterson BA, Ellis EG: Uncommon subtypes of acute nonlymphocytic leukemia: Clinical features and management of FAB $M^5$ $M^6$ $M^7$. *Semin Oncol* 14:425–434, 1987

43. Champlin R, Golde DW: The leukemias, in Braunwald E, Isselbacher KJ, Petersdorf RG, Wilson JD (eds): *Harrison's Principles of Internal Medicine* (ed 11). New York, McGraw-Hill, 1987, pp 1541–1550

44. Larson RA, Daly KM, Choi RE, et al: A clinical and pharmacokinetic study of mitoxantrone in acute non-lymphocytic leukemia. *J Clin Oncol* 5:391–397, 1987

45. Champlin R: Acute myelogenous leukemia: Biology and treatment. *Mediguide Oncol* 8:1–9, 1988

46. Berman E, Heller G, Santorsa J, et al: Results of a randomized trial comparing idarubicin and cytosine arabinoside with daunorubicin and cytosine arabinoside in adult patients with newly diagnosed acute myelogenous leukemia. *Blood* 77:1666–1674, 1991

47. Brach MA, Henschler R, Martelsman R, et al: To overcome pharmacologic and cytokinetic resistance to cytarabine in the treatment of acute myelogenous leukemia by using recombinant interleukin-3. *Semin Hematol* 28:39–43, 1991

48. Preisler H, Davis RB, Kirshner J, et al: Comparison of three remission induction regimens and two postinduction strategies for the treatment of acute nonlymphocytic leukemia: A cancer and leukemia Group B study. *Blood* 69:1441–1449, 1987

49. Gale RP, Foon KA: Therapy of acute myelogenous leukemia. *Semin Hematol* 24:40–54, 1987

50. Mayer RJ: Current chemotherapeutic treatment approaches to the management of previously untreated adults with de novo acute myelogenous leukemia. *Semin Oncol* 14:384–396, 1987

51. Arlin ZA, Hagenbeek A, Feldman E, et al: Implications of leukemia "cell kill" for the treatment of acute myelogenous leukemia (AML): Can the cure rate be increased? *Acta Haematol* 82:175–178, 1989

52. Foon KA, Gale RP: Controversies in the therapy of acute myelogenous leukemia. *Am J Med* 72:963–978, 1982

53. Wolff SN, Marion J, Stern RS, et al: High dose cytosine arabinoside and daunorubicin as consolidation therapy for acute nonlymphocytic leukemia in first remission: A pilot study. *Blood* 65:1407–1411, 1985

54. Wolff SN, Herzig RH, Phillips CL, et al: High dose cytosine arabinoside and daunorubicin as consolidation therapy for acute nonlymphocytic leukemia in first remission: An update. *Semin Oncol* 14:12–17, 1987 (suppl)

55. Bloomfield CD: Post remission therapy in acute myeloid leukemia. *J Clin Oncol* 3:1570–1572, 1985 (editorial)

56. Arlin ZA, Feldman ET, Finger LR, et al: Short course high dose mitoxantrone with high dose cytarabine is effective

therapy for adult lymphoblastic leukemia. *Leukemia* 5: 712–714, 1991

57. Bassan R, Barbui T: Remission induction therapy for adults with acute myelogenous leukemia: Towards the ICE age. *Haematologica* 80:82–90, 1995

58. Grever MR: Treatment of patients with acute nonlymphocytic leukemia not in remission. *Semin Hematol* 14:416–424, 1987

59. Zittoun RA, Mandelli F, Willemze R, et al: Autologous or allogeneic bone marrow transplantation compared with intensive chemotherapy in acute myelogenous leukemia. *N Engl J Med* 332:217–223, 1995

60. Barrett AJ, Locatelli F, Treleave JG, et al: Second transplants for leukemia relapse after bone marrow transplantation: High early mortality but favorable effect of chronic GVHD on continued remission, a report by the EBMT Leukaemia Working Party. *Br J Haematol* 79:567–574, 1991

61. Keating MJ, Gehan EA, Smith TL, et al: A strategy for evaluation of new treatments in untreated patients: Application to a clinical trial of AMSA for acute leukemia. *J Clin Oncol* 5:710–721, 1987

62. Priesler HD, Raza A, Barcos M, et al: High dose cytosine arabinoside as the initial treatment of poor-risk patients with acute nonlymphocytic leukemia: A leukemia intergroup study. *J Clin Oncol* 5:75–82, 1987

63. Dalton WS, Miller TP: Multidrug resistance. *PPO Updates* 5:1–13, 1991

64. Herweijer H, Sonneveld P, Baas F, et al: Expression of *mdr1* and *mdr3* multidrug-resistence genes in human acute and chronic leukemias and association with stimulation of drug accumulation by cyclosporine. *J Natl Cancer Inst* 82:1133–1140, 1990

65. Nooter K, Sonneveld P, Oostrum R, et al: Overexpression of the *mdr1* gene in blast cells from patients with acute myelocytic leukemia is associated with decreased anthracycline accumulation that can be restored by cyclosporine. *Int J Cancer* 45:262–268, 1990

66. Brown RA, Herzig RH, Wolff SN, et al: High dose etoposide and cyclophosphamide without bone marrow transplantation for resistant hematologic malignancy. *Blood* 76:473–479, 1990

67. Cannistra SA, Groshek P, Griffin JD: Granulocyte-macrophage-colony-stimulating factor enhances the cytotoxic effects of cytosine arabinoside in acute myeloblastic leukemia and in the myeloid blast crisis phase of chronic myeloid leukemia. *Leukemia* 3:328–334, 1989

68. Foon KA, Todd RF: Immunologic classification of leukemia and lymphoma. *Blood* 68:1–31, 1986

69. Castaigne S, Chomienne C, Daniel MT, et al: All-trans retinoic acid as a differentiation therapy for acute promyelocytic leukemia. I. Clinical results. *Blood* 76:1704–1709, 1990

70. Warrell RP, Frankel S, Miller WH, et al: Differentiation therapy of acute promyelocytic leukemia treated with tretinoin (all-trans retinoid acid). *N Engl J Med* 324:1385–1393, 1991

71. Roche Laboratories: Vesanoid® (tretinoin) capsules (package insert). Nutley, NJ, 1995

72. Foon KA, Gale RP, Todd RF: Recent advances in the immunologic classification of leukemia and lymphoma. *Semin Hematol* 23:257–283, 1986

73. Henderson ES: Acute leukemia: General considerations, in Williams WJ, Beutler E, Erslev AJ, Lichtman MA (eds): *Hematology.* New York, McGraw-Hill, 1990, pp 236–251

74. Kantarjian HM: Adult acute lymphocytic leukemia: Critical review of current knowledge. *Am J Med* 97:176–184, 1994

75. Ortega JA, Nesbit ME, Donaldson MH, et al: L-asparaginase, vincristine and prednisone for induction of first remission in acute lymphocytic leukemia. *Cancer Res* 37:535–540, 1977

76. Hoelzer D, Gale RP: Acute lymphoblastic leukemia in adults: Recent progress, future directions. *Semin Hematol* 24:27–39, 1987

77. Law IP, Blum J: Adult acute leukemia—Frequency of CNS involvement in long-term survivors. *Cancer* 40:1304–1306, 1977

78. Kuo AH, Yataganas X, Galicich YY, et al: Proliferative kinetics of central nervous system leukemia. *Cancer* 36:232–239, 1975

79. Preti A, Kantarjian HM: Management of adult acute lymphocytic leukemia: Present issues and key challenges. *J Clin Oncol* 12:1312–1322, 1994

80. Hoelzer D: Acute lymphoblastic leukemia in adults, in Hoffman R, Benz EJ, Shattel SI, Furie B, Cohen HJ (eds): *Hematology: Basic Principles and Practice.* New York, Churchill Livingstone, 1991, pp 793–804

81. Hoelzer D: High-dose chemotherapy in adult acute lymphoblastic leukemia. *Semin Hematol* 28:84–89, 1991

82. Hamilton-Paterson JL: Preleukemia anemia. *Acta Haematol* 2:309–316, 1949

83. Buzaid AC, Garewal HS, Greenberg BR: Management of myelodysplastic syndromes. *Am J Med* 80:1149–1157, 1986

84. Bennett JM, Catovsky D, Daniel MT, et al: The French-American-British (FAB) Cooperative Group: Proposals for the classification of the myelodysplastic syndromes. *Br J Haematol* 51:189–199, 1982

85. Tricot GJ, Lauer RC, Appelbaum FR, et al: Management of the myelodysplastic syndromes. *Semin Oncol* 14:444–453, 1987

86. Greenberg PL: The smoldering myeloid leukemic states: Clinical and biologic features. *Blood* 61:1035–1044, 1983

87. Estey E, Pierce H, Kantarjian H, et al: Treatment of myeloblastic syndromes with AML-type chemotherapy. *Leuk Lymphoma* 11:59–63, 1993

88. Yoemans AC, Harle MT: Myelodysplastic syndromes. *Semin Oncol Nurs* 6:9–16, 1990

89. Cines DB, Cassileth PA, Kiss JE: Danazol therapy in myelodysplasia. *Ann Intern Med* 103:58–60, 1985

90. Adamson JW: The myeloproliferative disease, in Braunwald E, Isselbacher KJ, Petersdorf RG, Wilson JD (eds): *Harrison's Principles of Internal Medicine* (ed 11). New York, McGraw-Hill, 1987, pp 1527–1533

91. Morrison VA: Chronic leukemias. *CA Cancer J Clin* 44:353–377, 1994

92. Hughes TD, Goldman JM: Chronic myeloid leukemia, in Hoffman R, Benz EJ, Shattil SJ, Furie B, Cohen HJ (eds): *Hematology: Basic Principles and Practice.* New York, Churchill-Livingstone, 1991, pp 854–869

93. Eisbruch A, Blick M, Evinger-Hodges MJ, et al: Effect of differentiation-inducing agents on oncogene expression in a chronic myelogenous leukemic cell line. *Cancer* 62:1171–1178, 1988

94. Fitzgerald PH, Morris CM: Ph-negative chronic myeloid leukemia: The nature of the breakpoint junction and mechanism of ABL transposition. *Leuk Lymphoma* 6:277–287, 1992

95. Deisseroth AB, Andreef M, Champlin R, et al: Chronic

leukemias, in Devita VT, Hellman S, Rosenberg SA (eds): *Cancer: Principles and Practice of Oncology*. Philadelphia, Lippincott, 1993, pp 1965–1983

96. Spiers AS: Chronic granulocytic leukemia. *Med Clin North Am* 68:713–727, 1984

97. Griffin JD: Management of chronic myelogenous leukemia. *Semin Hematol* 23:20–26, 1986 (suppl 1)

98. Lee MS, Kantarjian H, Talpaz M, et al: Detection of minimal residual disease by polymerase chain reaction in Philadelphia chromosome-positive chronic myelogenous leukemia following interferon therapy. *Blood* 79:1920–1923, 1992

99. Morra E, Lazzarino M, Aliména G, et al: The role of interferon in the treatment of chronic myelogenous leukemia: Results and prospects. *Leuk Lymphoma* 6:305–315, 1992

100. Roche Laboratories: Roferon®-A (interferon alfa-2a, recombinant) (package insert). Nutley, NJ, 1995

101. Moldawar NP, Figlin R: The interferons, in Rieger PT (ed): *Biotherapy: A comprehensive overview*. Boston, Jones and Bartlett, 1995, pp 69–92

102. Italian cooperative study group on chronic myeloid leukemia: Interferon alfa-2a as compared with conventional chemotherapy for treatment of chronic myeloid leukemia. *N Engl J Med* 330:820–825, 1994

103. Champlin RE, Goldman JM, Gale RP: Bone marrow transplantation in chronic myelogenous leukemia. *Semin Hematol* 25:74–80, 1988

104. Kantarjian HM, Deisseroth A, Kurzrock R, et al: Chronic myelogenous leukemia: A concise update. *Blood* 82:691–703, 1993

105. Shalrid M, Lugussy G, Berrebi A: High response rate to recombinant interferon alpha in chronic myeloid leukemia after intensive cytoreductive chemotherapy. *Blood* 74:370A, 1989

106. Rai KR, Montserat E: Prognostic factors in chronic lymphocytic leukemia. *Semin Hematol* 24:252–256, 1987

107. Rai KR, Sawitsky A, Jagathambal K, et al: Chronic lymphocytic leukemia. *Med Clin North Am* 68:697–711, 1984

108. Silbar R, Stahl R: Chronic lymphocytic leukemia and related diseases, in Williams WJ, Beutler E, Erslev AJ, Lichtman MA (eds): *Hematology*. New York, McGraw-Hill, 1990, pp 1005–1025

109. Lipshutz MD, Mu R, Rai KR, et al: Bone marrow biopsy and clinical staging in chronic lymphocytic leukemia. *Cancer* 46:1422–1427, 1980

110. Binet JL, Chastang C, Dighiero G, et al: Prognostic and therapeutic advances in CLL management: The experience of the French Cooperative Group. *Semin Hematol* 24:275–290, 1987

111. Lee JS, Dixon DO, Kantarjian HM, et al: Prognosis of chronic lymphocytic leukemia: A multivariate regression analysis of 325 untreated patients. *Blood* 69:929–936, 1987

112. Mandelli F, DeRossi G, Mancini P, et al: Prognosis in chronic lymphocytic leukemia: A retrospective multicenter study from the GIMEMA Group. *J Clin Oncol* 5:398–406, 1987

113. Binet JL, Cavotsky D, Chandra P, et al: Chronic lymphocytic leukemia: Proposals for a revised prognostic staging system. *Br J Haemal* 48:365–367, 1981

114. Foon KA, Gale RT: Staging and therapy of chronic lymphocytic leukemia. *Semin Hematol* 24:264–274, 1987

115. Pape LH: Therapy related acute leukemia: An overview. *Cancer Nurs* 11:295–302, 1988

116. Cheson BD: New modalities of therapy in chronic lymphocytic leukemia. *Crit Rev Oncol Hematol* 11:167–177, 1991

117. Foon KA, Bunn PA: Interferon treatment of cutaneous T-cell lymphoma and chronic lymphocytic leukemia. *Semin Oncol* 13:35–39, 1986 (suppl 5)

118. Golomb HM: Hairy cell leukemia: An unusual lymphoproliferative disease. *Cancer* 42:946–956, 1978

119. Steis RG, Longs DL: Update on the treatment of hairy cell leukemia. *PPO Updates* 2:1–12, 1982

120. Piro LD, Carrera CJ, Carson DA, et al: Lasting remissions in hairy-cell leukemia induced by a single infusion of 2-chlorodeoxyadenosine. *N Engl J Med* 322:1117–1121, 1990

121. Spiers AS, Moore D, Cassileth PA, et al: Remissions in hairy-cell leukemia with pentostatin (2'-deoxycoformycin). *N Engl J Med* 316:825–830, 1987

122. Quesada JR, Reuben J, Manning JT, et al: Alpha interferon for induction of remission in hairy-cell leukemia. *N Engl J Med* 310:15–18, 1984

123. Somerville ET: Knowledge deficit related to chemotherapy, in McNally JC, Stair JC, Somerville ET (eds): *Guidelines for Cancer Nursing Practice*. Philadelphia, Saunders, 1985, pp 57–61

124. Hadaway LC: Comparison of vascular access devices. *Semin Oncol Nurs* 11:154–166, 1995

125. Winslow MN, Trammell L, Camp-Sorrell D: Selection of vascular access device and nursing care. *Semin Oncol Nurs* 11:167–173, 1995

126. Goodman MS, Wickham R: Venous access devices: An overview. *Oncol Nurs Forum* 11:16–23, 1984

127. Bodey GP: What's new in fungal infections in leukemic patients. *Leuk Lymphoma* 11:127–135, 1993

128. Oniboni AC: Infection in the neutropenic patient. *Semin Oncol Nurs* 6:50–60, 1990

129. Bodey GP: Infection in cancer patients. *Cancer Treat Rev* 2:89–129, 1975

130. Carlson AC: Infection prophylaxis in the patient with cancer. *Oncol Nurs Forum* 12:56–64, 1985

131. Reheis CE: Neutropenia: Causes, complications, treatment, and resulting nursing care. *Nurs Clin North Am* 20:219–225, 1985

132. Scheffer CA, Wade JC: Supportive care: Issues in the use of blood products and treatment of infection. *Semin Oncol* 14:454–467, 1987

133. Young LS: Management of infections in leukemia and lymphoma, in Ruben RH, Young LS (eds): *Clinical Approach to Infection in the Compromised Host*. New York, Plenum Medicare Book, 1981, pp 461–497

134. Hathorn JW, Ruben M, Pizzo PA: Empirical antibiotic therapy in the febrile neutropenic cancer patient: Clinical efficacy and impact of monotherapy. *Antimicrob Agents Chemother* 31:971–977, 1987

135. Bodey CP: Topical and systemic antifungal agents. *Med Clin North Am* 72:637–659, 1988

136. Mahon SM: Taking the terror out of amphotericin B. *Am J Nurs* 88:961–966, 1988

137. Rutledge DN, Holtzclaw RJ: Amphotericin B-induced shivering in patients with cancer: A nursing approach. *Heart Lung* 17:432–440, 1988

138. Freifeld A, Pizzo P: New developments in the antimicrobial supportive care of the immunocompromised patient. *PPO Updates* 5:1–14, 1990

139. Bruce JL, Grove SK: Fever: Pathology and treatment. *Crit Care Nurs* 12:40–49, 1992

140. Wujcik D: Infection, in Groenwald SL, Frogge MH, Goodman M, Yarbro CH (eds): *Cancer Symptom Management*. Boston, Jones and Bartlett, 1996, pp 289–307

141. Frelreich EJ: White cell transfusions born again. *Leuk Lymphoma* 11:161–165, 1993

142. Ohno R, Tomonoage M, Kobayaski T, et al: Effect of granulocyte colony stimulating factor after intensive induction therapy in relapsed or refractory acute leukemia. *N Engl J Med* 323:871–877, 1990

143. Karp JE, Gruke DH, Donehower RC: Effects of the rhGM-CSF on intracellular ara-c pharmacology in acute myelocytic leukemia: Comparability with drug induced humorol stimulatory activity. *Leukemia* 4:553–556, 1990

144. Pruett J: Bleeding, in Groenwald SL, Frogge MH, Goodman M, Yarbro CH (eds): *Cancer Symptom Management.* Boston, Jones and Bartlett, 1996, pp 269–288

145. Erickson JM: Blood support for the immunocompromised patient. *Semin Oncol Nurs* 6:61–66, 1990

146. Fuller AK: Platelet transfusion therapy for thrombocytopenia. *Semin Oncol Nurs* 6:123–128, 1990

147. Rooney A, Hawley C: Nursing management of disseminated intravascular coagulation. *Oncol Nurs Forum* 12:15–22, 1985

148. Frankel SR, Eardley A, Lauwers G, et al: The "retinoic acid syndrome" in acute promyelocytic leukemia. *Ann Intern Med* 117:292–296, 1992

149. Wujcik D: Update on the diagnosis of and therapy for acute promyelocytic leukemia and chronic myelogenous leukemia. *Oncol Nurs Forum* 23:478–487, 1996

150. Beck SL: Mucositis, in Groenwald SL, Frogge MH, Goodman M, Yarbro CH (eds): *Cancer Symptom Management.* Boston, Jones and Bartlett, 1996, pp 308–323

151. Sylvester RK, Fisher AJ, Lobell M: Cytarabine-induced cerebellar syndrome, case report and literature review. *Drug Intel Clin Pharm* 21:177–179, 1987

152. Herzig RH, Lazarus GP, Herzig PF, et al: Central nervous system toxicity with high dose cytosine arabinoside. *Semin Oncol* 12:233–236, 1985 (suppl)

153. Herzig RH, Hines JD, Herzig GP, et al: Cerebellar toxicity with high dose cytosine arabinoside. *J Clin Oncol* 5:927–932, 1987

154. Conrad KJ: Cerebellar toxicities associated with cytosine arabinoside: A nursing perspective. *Oncol Nurs Forum* 13:157–59, 1986

155. Doublisky J: Ineffective individual coping, in McNally JC, Stair JC, Somerville ET (eds): *Guidelines for Cancer Nursing Practice.* Philadelphia, Saunders, 1985, pp 66–72

156. Smith K, Lesko LM: Psychosocial problems in cnacer survivors. *Oncol* 2:33–40, 1988

157. Scott DW, Goode WL, Arlin ZA: The psychodynamics of multiple remissions in a patient with nonlymphoblastic leukemia. *Cancer Nurs* 6:201–206, 1983

158. Levinson JA, Lesko LM: Psychiatric aspects of adult leukemia. *Semin Oncol Nurs* 6:76–83, 1990

159. Yeager KA, Miaskowski C: Advances in understanding the mechanisms and management of acute myelogenous leukemia. *Oncol Nus Forum* 21:541–548, 1994

# Chapter 42

# Lung Cancers

Rebecca J. Ingle, RN, MSN, FNP, AOCN

## INTRODUCTION

Lung cancer is the most frequent cause of cancer death in men and women in North America. At the beginning of the twentieth century, lung cancer was a rare disease; over the next 40 years it reached epidemic proportions for men, and is now considered to be an epidemic among women.[1-4] Although many factors have been associated with this major national and worldwide health problem, cigarette smoking has been estimated to cause 80%–90% of all lung cancer deaths.[1,3,5]

Despite the use of multimodality treatments for lung cancer, overall cure rates remain a discouraging 14%.[6] There is reason for cautious optimism, however, with the clinical investigation of several new promising chemotherapeutic agents, new diagnostic techniques, and improving feasibility of primary and secondary prevention measures that must receive preferential emphasis if progress is to be made in the control of this deadly disease.

## EPIDEMIOLOGY

In 1996, 177,000 new cases of lung cancer and 158,700 deaths from lung cancer were estimated to occur.[6] These alarming numbers are in stark contrast to the 956 cases reported in 1920.[7] Today, lung cancer kills more women than any other cancer in the United States (Figure 42-1), and worldwide, U.S. women are second only to those in Denmark in age-adjusted death rates for lung cancer per 100,000 population.[6] Although the mortality rate for men with lung cancer began to decline in the mid-1980s, lung cancer continues to cause over 2.5 times more deaths in men than prostate cancer, the second leading cancer killer among men in the United States (Figure 42-2).[6] Peak exposure to tobacco among women occurred in the 1960s, more than a decade later than for men. Because lung cancer incidence and mortality rates are highest about 35 years after peak exposure, the mortality rates

in women will not decline until after the year 2010, when incidence rates plateau.[1,8]

Lung cancer is rare among Native Americans. Mortality rates among African-American men are slightly higher than for white men, but are comparable among African-American and white women.[2] The highest incidence of lung cancer is in the elderly, peaking at 75 years of age, probably due to longer lifetime carcinogen exposure.[1]

## ETIOLOGY

### Cigarette Smoke

The causal relationship between lung cancer and cigarette smoking has been well established.[1,4,7,9] The risk of lung cancer development in heavy smokers is estimated to be 10–25 times the risk of nonsmokers.[1,7] Risk from smoking is determined by multiple factors: number of cigarettes smoked per day, duration of smoking, age at which smoking began, inhalation patterns, and tar content of cigarettes.[1,2,7,10-12] Several studies have shown that reducing tar exposure can reduce the risk of lung cancer.[11] However, others have documented that when smokers choose a lower-tar content cigarette they often compensate by inhaling more deeply, thereby negating the benefit of less tar.[13,14] Age at beginning to smoke appears to be related more to duration of smoking than to an increased susceptibility at a younger age.[2]

Chyou and colleagues were able to compute attributable risk due to cigarette smoking in a large cohort of men. Attributable risk estimates how much risk might be reduced if cigarette smoking was discontinued or never initiated. Their findings showed an attributable risk of 85% among current smokers, and they estimated that if current smokers had quit smoking, 60% of their risk for lung cancer could have been eliminated.[9] Others concur that benefit from smoking cessation begins five years after quitting and increases steadily over time, although the risk for lung cancer among former smokers will remain higher than the risk for lifetime nonsmokers.[2,8,10,12]

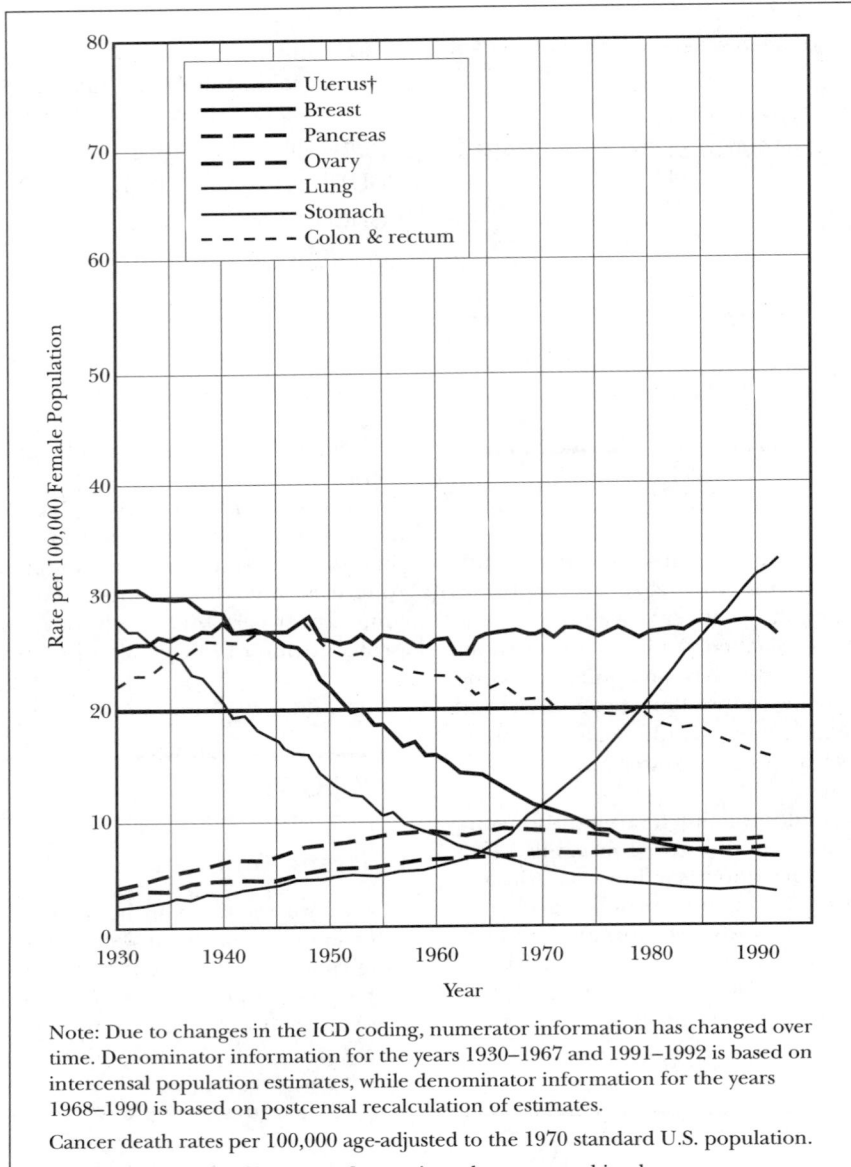

**FIGURE 42-1** Age-adjusted cancer death rates: Females by site, United States, 1930–1991. (From Parker SL, Tong T, Bolden S, et al: Cancer statistics, 1996. *CA: Cancer J Clin* 46:5–27, 1996.)

Cigarette smoke is known to contain over 4000 chemical compounds, which insult the bronchial epithelium when smoke is inhaled. Tar, the most carcinogenic compound, causes basal cell hyperplasia, then dysplasia with displacement of the normal, healthy ciliated and mucus-secreting cells. With repeated exposure to smoke a lung cell may undergo neoplastic transformation.[8]

Tobacco smoke is a complete carcinogen, containing both initiator and promoter substances. Initiators can cause irreversible gene mutations. Repeated exposure to promoters may cause a cell to exhibit malignant behaviors, although cellular repair may occur if promoters are withdrawn. Eventually tumor progression ensues and the cellular damage is irreversible.

## Passive Smoke

Considerable attention has been given in the past two decades to the effects of environmental tobacco smoke (ETS), also called sidestream smoke, involuntary smoke, or passive cigarette smoke.[11] Sidestream smoke contains

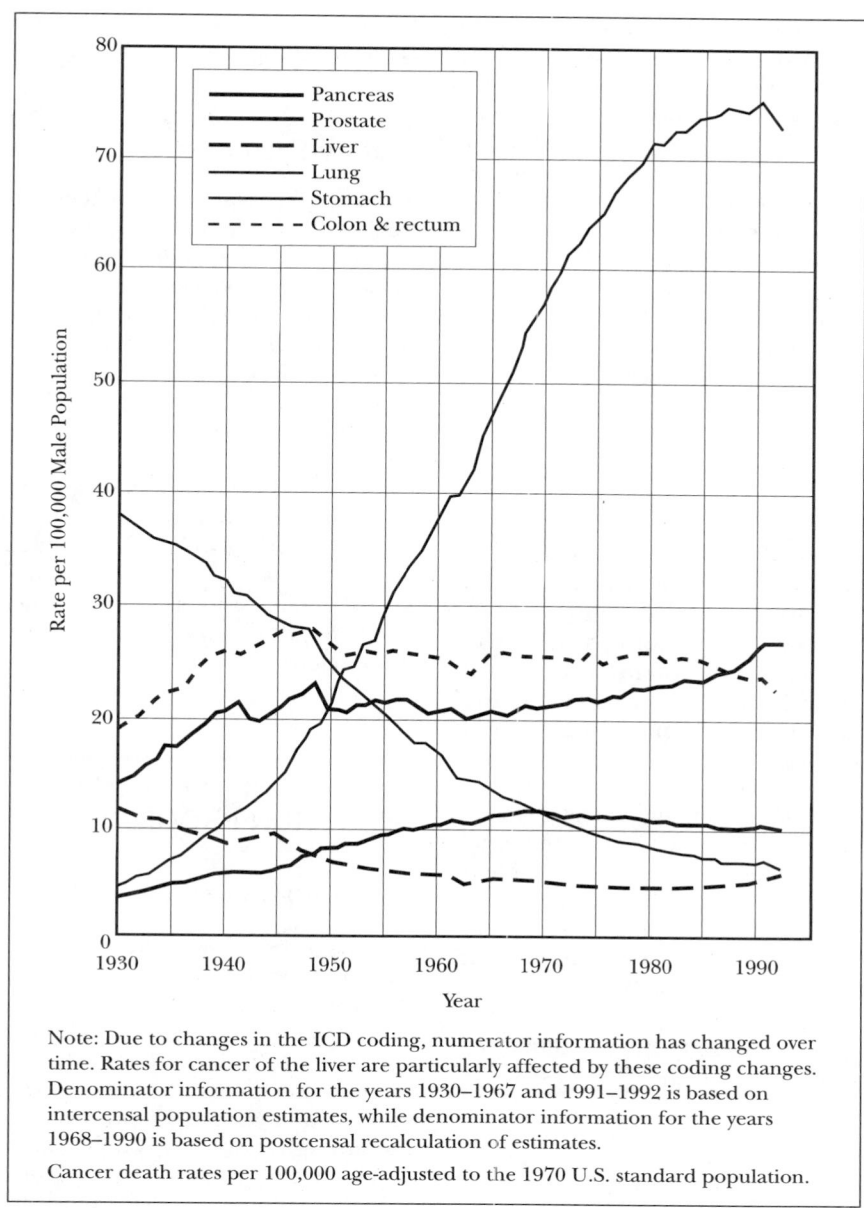

Note: Due to changes in the ICD coding, numerator information has changed over time. Rates for cancer of the liver are particularly affected by these coding changes. Denominator information for the years 1930–1967 and 1991–1992 is based on intercensal population estimates, while denominator information for the years 1968–1990 is based on postcensal recalculation of estimates.

Cancer death rates per 100,000 age-adjusted to the 1970 U.S. standard population.

**FIGURE 42-2** Age-adjusted cancer death rates: Males by site, United States, 1930–1991. (From Parker SL, Tong T, Bolden S, et al: Cancer statistics, 1996. *CA: Cancer J Clin* 46:5–27, 1996)

nearly all of the carcinogens contained in mainstream smoke inhaled by smokers, but because it is not filtered, greater numbers of carcinogens are inhaled passively.[15] Even though ETS increases the risk for lung cancer less than active smoking, a causal relationship has been firmly established and the Environmental Protection Agency (EPA) considers ETS to be a human carcinogen.[16,17] In a study of exposure to passive smoke in the household, Janerich and colleagues found that the risk of lung cancer doubled for persons exposed to 25 or more years of passive smoke during childhood and adolescence. Exposure to ETS accounts for 17% of lung cancers among nonsmokers.[18] In contrast, the risk for lung cancer did not increase in adult nonsmokers exposed to ETS at home or in the workplace. Other epidemiological studies have shown statistically significant increased risks for persons living with smoking spouses.[15] These data suggest that 30% of all lung cancers are caused by exposure to ETS.[11]

## Asbestos

Asbestos exposure is the most common occupational etiology of lung cancer,[1] causing 3%–4% of all cases.[19] *Asbes-*

*tos,* a general term describing fibrous silicates with different properties, is divided into two groups of fibers: chrysotile and amphibole. Although the sharp, needle-like amphibole asbestos bodies are more likely to cause disease due to deeper penetration into the lung,[11] both groups have been implicated in lung cancer development. In a study of 158 Japanese subjects exposed to asbestos, squamous cell carcinoma was seen most frequently and small-cell lung cancer was rare.[20]

Asbestos and smoking have a synergistic effect on lung cancer promotion. Compared with nonexposed nonsmokers, the incidence of lung cancer is increased 5-fold in nonsmokers exposed to asbestos and a startling 80–90-fold in exposed smokers.[1]

## Radon

Radon gas is an inert, natural product of uranium decay. Its effects were studied initially in underground uranium mine workers. During the radioactive decay process, radon products emit heavily ionizing alpha particles that, when inhaled, deliver intense radiation to the bronchial epithelium.[12,19] Radon particles act as both initiators and promoters, causing nonlethal events in cell nuclei. Synergy with cigarette smoke has been reported.[11]

Because radon is present in rock and soil and is known to seep into homes and office buildings through basements and crawl spaces, it has become an environmental concern. The amount of radon in a home is dependent upon ventilation and distance from the source. Although the residents of over 1 million U.S. homes have radon exposure similar to that of uranium miners, insufficient data exist at this time to predict their risk of developing lung cancer.[1,19] Nevertheless, the U.S. EPA estimates that over 14,000 lung cancer deaths per year are caused by radon, mostly in smokers.[2]

## Occupational Agents

An increased incidence of lung cancer has been documented in individuals working with arsenic, copper, silica, lead, zinc, gold, chloromethyl ether, diesel exhaust, chromium, coal, hydrocarbons, nickel, ionizing radiation, cadmium, and beryllium.[2,10,12] Fur handlers and vineyard workers are also known to have increased risk.[12] Evidence linking these occupational agents to cigarette smoking is limited, and no conclusions can be drawn.

## Indoor Air Pollution

In developing countries, exposure to carcinogenic cooking oil aerosols has been associated with lung cancer.[3,4] Indoor environments may be contaminated with other harmful pollutants including radon, cigarette smoke, building materials, household aerosol products, combus-tion devices, and the entry of outdoor air contaminants.[2] Data regarding risk are inconclusive.

## Dietary Factors

Although the relationship of diet to lung cancer requires further investigation, early evidence suggested an inverse relationship between lung cancer risk and consumption of vitamin A or beta-carotene, vitamin C, vitamin E, and selenium.[2,3,19] It was proposed that these nutrients may prevent carcinogenesis by acting as scavengers of free oxygen radicals produced by tobacco smoke, solvents, and pollutants.[2,19] However, clinical trials of oral beta-carotene administered in populations at high risk for lung cancer were ceased in early 1996 due to the finding of increased lung cancer in the population receiving beta-carotene.[21] Hennekens and colleagues found neither harm nor benefit relative to incidence of malignancies in a 12-year study of beta-carotene supplementation in healthy men.[22] Other nutrients such as watercress are also being investigated as inhibitors of a tobacco-specific carcinogen.[1]

## PREVENTION, SCREENING, EARLY DETECTION PROGRAMS

### Primary Prevention

Primary prevention of lung cancer depends on identifying successful strategies for smoking prevention and cessation. If smoking were totally eliminated, 85% of lung cancers would disappear. Multiple economic, political, and social factors continue to impede progress toward this goal. Smoking dates back to the ancient Mayan civilization. Its medicinal qualities, addictive properties, and use through the years in ritual and ceremony have made acceptance of its harmful properties more difficult.

After automobiles, cigarettes are the second most heavily advertised product in the United States.[23] Women, children, and persons in developing countries have become primary targets of cigarette company marketing.[11] Cigarette smoking was considered to be socially unacceptable for women prior to the 1920s. As marketing strategies associated smoking with beauty, thinness, and independence, large numbers of women began to smoke. Today's death rate from lung cancer in women is 500% higher than that of 1935.[24] Over 22 million women in the U.S. smoke, including 25% of those who are pregnant.[25]

Perhaps the most vulnerable groups targeted by cigarette advertisers are children and adolescents. Cartoon characters such as Old Joe Camel appeal to children, and have been found to be as familiar to small children as Mickey Mouse.[26] Of the 1 million Americans who become smokers each year, most are children or adolescents. Ninety percent of smokers begin smoking before they are 20 years old,[11,25] and most are girls.[3] Tobacco companies take advantage of adolescent vulnerability to the tune of over $4 billion a year spent in advertisement and promotional fees related to cigarettes and smoking.[11]

As antismoking efforts have gained acceptance in developed countries, tobacco companies have sought to develop new markets in underdeveloped countries. Tobacco is a prized export of the United States, and American cigarettes are a status symbol in some countries.[8] In these countries, little emphasis is placed on the harmful effects of smoking, and warning labels on cigarette packages may not be required.

In the United States, higher smoking rates are seen in individuals of a lower socioeconomic status, particularly women, although male blue-collar workers continue to be the heaviest smokers. Smoking is more common in African-Americans than in whites. Though fewer cigarettes are smoked by African-Americans, smoking cessation rates are also lower.[27] Education appears to be inversely related to smoking rates.[8,25]

Efforts to prevent smoking must focus on antismoking education, legislation, and taxation of cigarettes. Given the propensity for young people to smoke, education must begin early. Many nonprofit organizations, including the American Cancer Society, the American Lung Association, and the American Heart Association, promote smoking prevention programs through the distribution of a variety of educational materials about smoking. Nurses should incorporate education about smoking across the continuum of care, working within communities to promote healthy lifestyle behaviors. School-based programs to promote a tobacco-free environment should be encouraged. Educational efforts that target high-risk populations should emphasize the association between smoking and lung cancer. Repetition of the message may help individuals to internalize its meaning.

Antismoking legislation appeared in the 1960s following the 1964 surgeon general's report on the dangers of smoking. Laws were passed requiring health warnings on cigarettes, and cigarette advertisements in the broadcast media were banned. During the 1970s, 1980s and 1990s, significant progress was made to limit and/or ban smoking in the workplace, on airplanes, in U.S. government buildings, and in other public places. In 1995 President Clinton approved a Food and Drug Administration regulatory plan to restrict seductive advertising directed at minors and to reduce easy access to cigarettes by banning vending machines except in areas of adult entertainment, banning free sample distribution, eliminating the sale of "singles" and "kiddie packs," and requiring proof of age to purchase cigarettes. The tobacco industry opposed the regulations and immediately filed lawsuits attempting to block the actions, accusing the president of government meddling in private choice decisions.[28] Resolution is pending, but regulations are expected to go into effect in early 1997. Almost all states have passed legislation prohibiting the sale of tobacco to minors, and campaigns are under way to impose a high excise tax on each pack of cigarettes sold.[11] Increasing the cost of cigarettes and enforcing age restrictions are thought to be the most effective strategies in reducing the number of minors who smoke.[29]

## Secondary Prevention

### Smoking cessation

While primary prevention is the most effective means of controlling lung cancer, the elimination of all tobacco products is not a realistic goal. Smoking cessation, as secondary prevention, can reduce the risk for lung cancer in a smoker, depending on how much and how long the person smoked. Up to 90% of smokers say they would like to quit, and as many as 60% have made serious attempts to stop smoking.[30-32] Those who are successful usually have a strong desire to quit, use behavioral techniques to quit, and are supported in their efforts by family, friends, and/or health care providers.[31-33]

In 1996 the Agency for Health Care Policy and Research (AHCPR), an agency of the United States Department of Health and Human Services, published clinical practice guidelines for smoking cessation.[34] A multidisciplinary panel of tobacco addiction and smoking cessation experts compiled and reviewed data from over 3000 research articles and abstracts. Specific step-by-step strategies for primary care clinicians, including those discussed in the following sections, are provided in the guidelines.

Because it has been shown that smokers respond to direct, unequivocal messages from nurses and physicians to quit smoking, such messages should be given at every opportunity.[32,35,36] Failure to ask about smoking may give the false impression that smoking cessation is not a priority. Fiore has proposed that smoking status be the "new vital sign," measured each time vital signs are taken in the outpatient follow-up setting.[37] Two simple questions asked by the care provider—"Do you smoke now?" and "Have you ever smoked in the past?"—offer many opportunities to promote smoking cessation and to reinforce attention to the issue. Such brief intervention has been associated with 5% quit rates lasting more than one year.[30,31,35]

Smokers must believe that they are personally vulnerable before they are ready to quit. The nurse can point out that symptoms such as cough, bronchitis, or decreased energy are associated with smoking.[31] If cancer has already been diagnosed, benefits of cessation should be discussed. These include decreased rate of cancer recurrence, less risk of second primary tumors, improved tolerance of therapy, and lower risk of pulmonary infections.[30]

Smoking cessation behaviors have been described as occurring in stages,[38] each with opportunities for nursing intervention. The first stage is precontemplation, during which there is no plan to quit smoking. The smoker does not recognize the risks of smoking to self or others. The nurse can assess the smoker's knowledge, beliefs, and attitudes about smoking and can raise risk awareness through education.

In contemplation, the second stage, the smoker expresses a desire to quit within the next six months and may ask for educational materials. Fears associated with quitting such as nicotine withdrawal, weight gain, and fear of failure may be verbalized. The nurse can express support and respect for the addiction while personalizing the benefits of quitting. It may be helpful to identify specific barriers to quitting and to suggest strategies for overcoming those barriers. Help the smoker set a quit date and reinforce the idea that smoking as a learned behavior can be unlearned.

Preparation is the third stage, during which the smoker plans to stop smoking within the next month. Behavioral therapy during this stage may help the smoker to identify reasons for smoking and for wanting to quit, to substitute alternative behaviors as a distraction from smoking behaviors, to learn to cope with urges and withdrawal symptoms, and to develop and implement a plan of action. Referral to a structured, behavioral smoking cessation program is appropriate in this stage, although as many as 95% of smokers prefer to quit without a structured program.[30,31] The smoker should consider nicotine replacement therapy, and pertinent educational materials should be provided. The nurse should arrange for follow-up by mail, telephone, or visits.

Action, the fourth phase, involves efforts to quit and prevent relapse. Relapse is common, and usually occurs during the first week after cessation when nicotine withdrawal symptoms are most pronounced.[31] Smokers often quit several times before they achieve long-term success. The nurse provides nonjudgmental support, framing the relapse as a "rehearsal" for the next cessation attempt.

The last phase, maintenance, begins when the smoker has been smoke-free for six months or longer. The risk for relapse lessens, although stressful life events may trigger a relapse.[30] Follow-up with physician and nurse counseling in frequent face-to-face contacts contributes to maintenance of smoking cessation.[35] Lerman and colleagues propose the use of biological markers as a motivation for success.[38] Other investigators have demonstrated that measuring carbon monoxide (CO) levels and correlating them with physical symptoms such as nausea, headaches, and reduced exercise tolerance has tripled quit rates as compared with a standard nursing educational intervention.[39] Measurement of cotinine, a more sensitive indicator of tobacco exposure, is another potential motivational intervention for smoking cessation.[40] In addition, markers of abnormal cytological changes such as the CVP2D6 enzyme have been related to lung cancer susceptibility and show promise as a component of smoking cessation programs.[38]

Smoking cessation rates after behavioral interventions alone have been discouraging, as low as 13% at six months and lower than 5% at one year.[36,38] Success rates of 20% or more for a particular program are considered a good outcome.[31] Nicotine withdrawal symptoms often contribute to relapse. Symptoms, including irritability, restlessness, craving to smoke, impatience, hunger, wakefulness, anxiety, lowered heart rate, headache, and altered bowel habits, peak several days after cessation and last up to four weeks.[8,11,31] Nicotine replacement using chewing gum or the transdermal patch has been shown to relieve withdrawal symptoms and has improved success rates to as high as 27.5% at one year when combined with smoking cessation counseling.[32,41]

The best candidates for nicotine replacement are smokers who are physically addicted to nicotine. The Fagerstrom Test for Nicotine Dependence, a brief, eight-item scale, can be used to measure degree of addiction.[42] When nicotine gum or patch replacement therapy is used, careful instructions are given regarding usage to avoid adverse effects. Nicotine replacement can be very expensive; cost information should be provided to the individual smoker.

New research findings reported by Fowler and colleagues give clues about the addictive properties of smoking.[43] They found that the brains of living smokers had significantly lower levels of the enzyme monoamine oxidase B (MAO B) than the brains of nonsmokers and former smokers. MAO B helps break down dopamine, a neurotransmitter involved in feelings of pleasure associated with many substances of abuse, including nicotine. Because nicotine stimulates the release of dopamine, it is thought that this action is synergistic with that of low levels of MAO B in boosting dopamine levels, thereby enhancing the addictive effects of the nicotine. The causative substance of lower levels of MAO B in smokers has not been identified, although it is known that it is not nicotine.[43] These findings have exciting implications for potential smoking cessation strategies.

### Chemoprevention

Chemoprevention as a secondary prevention measure appears to show promise for current or former smokers. Chemoprevention, also called *chemoprophylaxis*, is treatment with agents that may prevent or reverse the promotion phase of carcinogenesis.[44–46] It is based on the concept of field cancerization, which holds that the entire area of epithelium exposed to carcinogens such as cigarette smoke is susceptible to cancer development, and that individuals who develop one malignancy are at high risk for developing a second primary tumor (SPT) later in the same epithelial field.[44] Survivors of small-cell lung cancer may have a cumulative risk of 50% at ten years for SPT development.[44–47] The risk for SPTs in non–small-cell lung cancer patients may exceed 10%, and in one study 26% of persons with laryngeal cancer developed a secondary lung cancer.[48] The leading cause of death in early-stage lung cancer is SPTs.[45]

Chemoprevention agents are being investigated as a means of preventing primary or secondary cancer development after carcinogen exposure. The most commonly studied groups of chemoprevention agents are the retinoids and carotenoids, which, as synthetic analogues of vitamin A, regulate normal and malignant cell growth and differentiation. In a landmark 1990 chemoprevention trial at MD Anderson, Hong and colleagues studied the effects of 13-*cis* retinoic acid (13-cRA) versus placebo in patients with head and neck cancers.[49] Although the agent had no effect on recurrence, patients receiving 13-cRA had significantly fewer SPTs. Low-dose 13-cRA has been well tolerated with significantly less toxicity compared with high-dose 13-cRA.[45]

Dietary intake of beta-carotene and vitamin A has been associated with a decreased risk of lung cancer. Studies have shown a stronger correlation of decreased risk of lung cancer with vegetable consumption as compared with equivalent carotenoid intake, suggesting that other dietary factors play a role in risk reduction.[44] However, a large-scale randomized trial of beta-carotene plus retinol versus placebo in smokers and asbestos-exposed smokers was stopped when it was discovered that the individuals receiving beta-carotene were experiencing a higher rate of lung cancer development.[21]

The most common end point for chemoprevention trials has been the appearance of a malignancy, which often takes many years to develop. In order to more quickly evaluate promising new chemopreventive agents, investigators are searching for cell markers that might verify the effects of these agents before a malignancy actually develops. These markers could also be used to identify high-risk individuals, who might benefit from chemoprevention by the detection of early changes associated with carcinogenesis.[44,46,47,50] Markers under investigation include suppressor oncogenes such as *p53* and the retinoblastoma gene *Rb*, dominant oncogenes such as *ras* and *myc*, and several growth factors.[47]

## Screening and Early Detection

In the early 1970s the National Cancer Institute (NCI) Early Lung Cancer Group screened 30,000 male smokers with chest radiograph and sputum cytology. The results of these large trials showed that even though lung cancers identified by the screening methods were more frequently early-stage, long-term survival rates did not improve.[29,33,50,51] European trials have confirmed that screening can detect lung cancer at an earlier stage but does not improve survival. Therefore, mass screening for lung cancer using currently available techniques is not recommended. However, scientific trials are under way to identify mutated genes in lung cancer cells that may represent early events in carcinogenesis and offer opportunities for interventions to cure or reverse the disease.[50,52] Tockman and colleagues developed a monoclonal antibody that successfully identified sputum abnormalities in 20 of 25 subjects who later developed lung cancer.[53] Ongoing trials are further evaluating these findings.

Two groups of oncogenes are involved in lung cancer development and are included in the early detection research. Dominant oncogenes, whose expression promotes neoplastic growth, include the *ras* and *myc* families. The *ras* oncogenes appear to function early in the process of carcinogenesis and may be a good target for early detection. However, their screening usefulness will be limited since only about 15% of lung cancers exhibit a *ras* mutation. Expression of the *myc* oncogene is a late event and thus might not be effective as a target for early detection.[50]

The recessive oncogenes, or tumor-suppressor genes, inhibit cellular growth. When they are absent or reduced, neoplastic growth can occur. Mutations of the *Rb* suppressor gene are present in over 90% of small-cell lung cancers. Difficulties in defining this gene have limited its usefulness as an early detection marker.[50]

## PATHOPHYSIOLOGY

### Cellular Characteristics

During normal embryogenesis a branched tracheobronchial tree forms by the 10th week. It is lined with a single layer of cells from which the respiratory mucosa develops. All lung cancers are thought to arise from a pluripotent stem cell originating from this primitive endodermal structure, eventually differentiating into multiple different histological subtypes.[19,51]

Normally the bronchial epithelium is composed of pseudostratified columnar cells, some of which are ciliated. Others are mucus-secreting goblet cells. Basal cells and neuroendocrine cells containing secretory granules complete the epithelial stratification, which has a protective function. Repeated carcinogenic irritation to the bronchial epithelium may cause increased rates of cellular replication. Healthy ciliated cells are replaced with a proliferation of basal cells, eventually resulting in hyperplasia, dysplasia, or carcinoma in situ[54] (Figure 42-3).[55,56]

Bronchogenic cancers have been grouped into two broad categories: small-cell lung cancer (SCLC) and the non–small-cell lung cancers (NSCLC), which include squamous cell carcinoma, adenocarcinoma, and large-cell carcinoma. Each of these subtypes has distinct cellular characteristics upon which diagnosis and management are based. Because all types of lung cancer arise from a pluripotent stem cell, many tumors are heterogeneous, containing cells from more than one histological type, which makes accurate classification more difficult.[19,54] A discussion of cellular characteristics of each subtype follows.

#### Small-cell lung cancer

SCLC was recognized as an epithelial tumor in 1926. Prior to that time it was believed to be a sarcoma.[57] SCLC invades the submucosa and is thought to arise from Kulchitsky cells, neuroendocrine cells that secrete peptide hormones. Most SCLC tumors are centrally located, developing around a main bronchus as a whitish gray growth that invades surrounding structures, eventually compressing the bronchi externally.[1,10,12,57,58] Necrosis and areas of

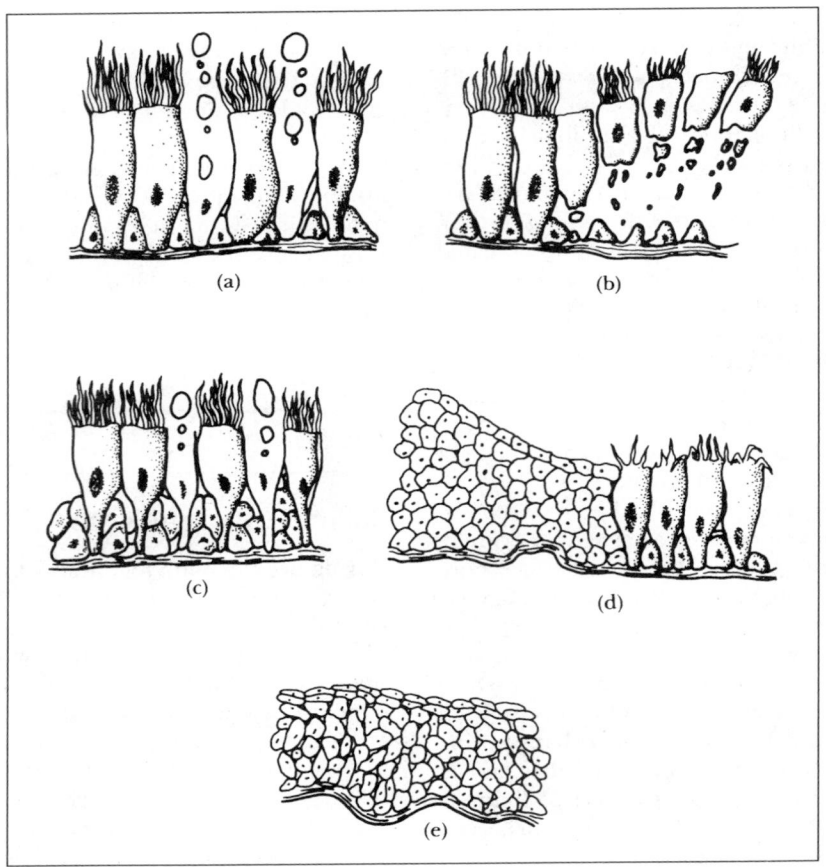

**FIGURE 42-3**  Response of bronchial epithelium to chronic irritation.
(a) Normal bronchial epithelium. (b) Ciliated airway cells are continuously shed and replaced in response to irritant exposure. (c) Ciliated cells regenerate from basal cells. (d) Chronic irritation results in an increased turnover proliferation. (e) Continuation of irritation may produce bronchial epithelial dysplasia and carcinoma in situ. (From Elpern EH: Lung cancer, in Groenwald SL, Frogge MH, Goodman M, Yarbro CM (eds): *Cancer Nursing: Principles and Practice* (ed 3). Boston, Jones and Bartlett, 1993, pp 1174–1199. Illustration adapted from Kotin P: Carcinogenesis of the lung, in Liebow AA, Smith DE (eds): *The Lung.* Baltimore, MD, Williams and Wilkins, 1968.)

hemorrhage are frequently seen, although SCLC usually does not cavitate. Responsible for 25% of all lung cancers, SCLC is an aggressive tumor and often is metastatic at the time of diagnosis. Its doubling time, shorter than that of any other lung cancer type, is slightly less than two months.[1,12]

The World Health Organization has classified SCLC into three subtypes:[57,58] (1) oat cell, which accounts for 90% of cases; (2) intermediate; and (3) combined (oat cell with adenocarcinoma or squamous cell carcinoma component). This classification was intended to show a link between small-cell and large-cell carcinomas, although the clinical significance of the subtypes is controversial. In many instances no difference in subtypes is seen relative to response to treatment or survival.[57] Other classifications have been proposed, each striving for diagnostic and clinical significance.[58]

Although morphologically the cells of each subtype differ from each other, all SCLC cells are several times larger than a mature lymphocyte, have scant cytoplasm, and show multiple atypical mitoses.[57,58] Many genetic abnormalities have been identified, including absence of two suppressor genes, the retinoblastoma (*RB*) gene and the *p53* gene. There is evidence that suppression of the *RB* gene may play a role in the initiation or progression of SCLC. Mutations of the *p53* gene appear to occur in response to cigarette smoke and radon exposure.[59]

Amplification of the *myc* family of proto (dominant) oncogenes, including *c-myc, n-myc,* and *l-myc,* has also been observed in SCLC.[10,12,57,59] Amplification is the process in which the DNA is duplicated many times, thereby activating the proto-oncogene and releasing it from normal growth-controlling mechanisms.[59] While *myc* amplification is not thought to be a primary contributor to the pathogenesis of lung cancer, *c-myc* amplification has been correlated with a shorter duration of survival in SCLC patients. *Myc* amplification, which occurs in up to 24% of SCLC tumors, occurs less frequently in NSCLC cells.[57,59]

It has long been recognized that about 70% of SCLCs produce neuroendocrine markers, including neuron-specific enolase, L-dopa decarboxylase, chromogranin A, synaptophysin, and bombesin.[10,12,59] While these markers are not specific to SCLC, they help explain many of the paraneoplastic syndromes that occur in SCLC patients. Early identification of neuroendocrine markers may aid in the diagnosis and management of SCLC, and may have prognostic significance.[10]

Lung cancer cells can produce autocrine growth factors, which are peptide hormones that stimulate their own growth by binding to their own receptors. The most common autocrine growth factor is gastrin-releasing peptide (GRP). Studies have shown that the growth factor receptor sites can be blocked by a monoclonal antibody developed in the laboratory against bombesin, a GRP analogue from frog skin.[57,60] Figure 42-4 illustrates autocrine growth in lung cancer cells and the mechanism of monoclonal antibody blockage, which inhibits growth of the SCLC cells.[60]

### Non–small-cell lung cancer

***Squamous cell carcinoma*** Squamous cell carcinomas constitute 30% of all lung cancers and are more common in males than in females.[55] These tumors arise from the basal cells of the bronchial epithelium and usually present as masses in large bronchi. Growth into adjacent structures, cavitation, and extension centrally are common, causing atelectasis and pneumonitis.[12] When detected early, squamous cell cancers are often resectable.

Squamous tumors may be well differentiated or poorly differentiated. Well-differentiated tumors may show pearly formation, while poorly differentiated tumors are characterized by keratinization. Other cellular characteristics of squamous cell carcinomas include intercellular bridges and inflammation.[1] Because cells of these tumors are easily shed, sputum cytologies may be positive at an early stage, long before a lesion can be detected on a chest radiograph.[19]

Squamous cell carcinoma has a doubling time of 90–100 days.[1] Because it is a relatively slow-growing tumor, several years may elapse between the development of a carcinoma in situ and clinical detection. In about 8% of cases, mutations in the *ras* family of oncogenes are seen.[59] Squamous cell cancers have been associated with ectopic production of a parathyroid hormone–type substance, causing hypercalcemia.

***Adenocarcinoma*** Adenocarcinoma is the most common lung cancer in males, in females, and in nonsmokers, accounting for 40% of all tumors.[1,19] Its increasing incidence in recent years has been attributed to more accurate histological distinction between adenocarcinoma and undifferentiated large-cell carcinoma. Adenocarci-

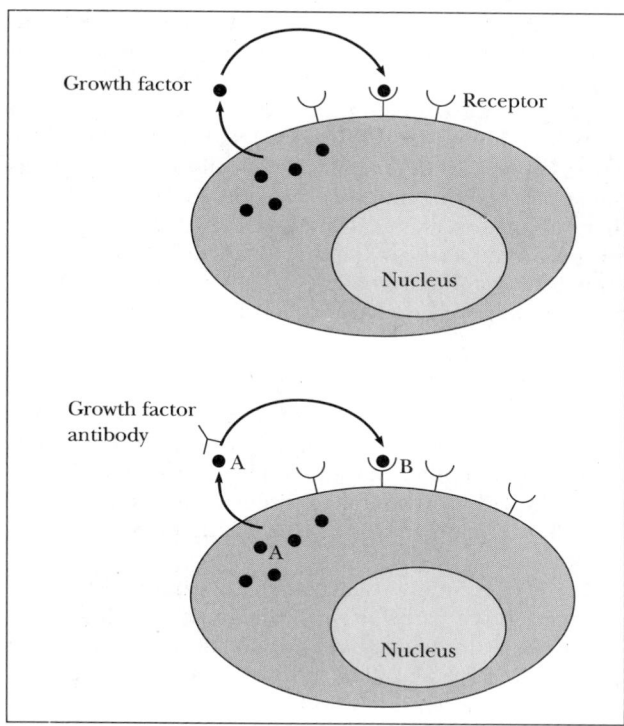

**FIGURE 42-4**  A. Autocrine growth in lung cancer. The cell produces peptide hormones or growth factors (represented as dark circles), that are secreted from the cell, bind to receptors on its surface, and stimulate their own growth. B. Blocking autocrine growth with antibodies in lung cancer. The figure diagrammatically shows the mechanism that has been used successfully to interrupt the autocrine growth loop. The monoclonal antibody directed against growth factors (A) prevents the growth factor from binding to its receptor and (B) thereby blocks the autocrine growth of the cell. (Reprinted from *Lung Cancer*, Vol. 12, Johnson BE, Kelley MJ, Biology of small cell lung cancer, S5–S16, 1995 (suppl), with kind permission from Elsevier Science Ireland Ltd., Bay 15K, Shannon Industrial Estate, Co. Clare, Ireland.)

noma arises from the bronchial epithelium and may form in lung scars or fibrous tissue. Adenocarcinoma usually presents as a single peripheral nodule, although rapidly progressive multifocal disease may be present at diagnosis. This malignancy may be quite silent initially, producing few symptoms,[12] and is often detected radiographically before sputum cytologies are positive.[1]

Most adenocarcinomas form glands and produce mucin. They tend to metastasize early through hematogenous spread, and nearly half of the tumors are considered to be unresectable at the time of diagnosis.[1] Areas of metastasis commonly include the brain, liver, bone, and adrenal glands. Adenocarcinomas have the longest doubling time of all lung cancers, approximately six months.[1]

Mutations of the *K-ras* oncogene are seen in approximately one-third of adenocarcinoma cases and represent about 90% of all mutations seen in these tumors.[51,59] In several studies, identification of the *K-ras* oncogene in all non–small-cell lung cancers has been associated with shortened survival and therefore may prove to be an important prognostic marker for adenocarcinoma.[51,59]

The World Health Organization (WHO) has classified adenocarcinomas of the lung by four histological subtypes: (1) acinar, (2) papillary, (3) solid carcinoma with mucus formation, and (4) bronchoalveolar, although there is controversy regarding whether the latter should be considered a separate entity. Bronchoalveolar tumors show little glandular change, usually present as solitary or multiple peripheral lesions, and are slow-growing tumors.[1,19]

***Large-cell carcinoma***    Large-cell carcinoma is the least common type of lung cancer, representing approximately 10%–15% of cases.[19] Although large-cell carcinoma is larger than adenocarcinoma, other features common to the two types have sometimes precluded accurate diagnosis. Often diagnosis is made by eliminating other cell types.

Large-cell tumors usually arise as peripheral nodules and metastasize early, often to the gastrointestinal tract. The average doubling time is about three months. The tumor cells have abundant cytoplasm and enlarged nuclei.[1] *Ras* mutations are found in about 23% of large-cell cancer cases.[59]

Large-cell carcinomas are classified by the WHO into two types: (1) clear cell and (2) giant cell. The rare giant cell tumors have the poorest prognosis. In general, large-cell tumors have the same prognosis as adenocarcinomas of the lung.[19]

## Progression of Disease

Repeated carcinogenic exposure results in epithelial cell transformations that progress from a benign to a malignant phenotype. Manifested initially as atypical metaplasia, then carcinoma in situ, and finally invasive carcinoma of the lung, invasion of deeper tissues follows until the malignancy is clinically detectable. A lung tumor has undergone about 30 doublings, or three-quarters of its natural history, by the time it is large enough to be detected on chest radiograph or sputum cytologies.[1] Many tumors metastasize in the preclinical phase, as evidenced by the dismal 14% overall cure rates for lung cancer.[6]

## Patterns of Spread

Lung cancers spread by direct extension, lymphatic invasion, and hematogenous routes. In SCLC, metastasis to distant sites has already occurred in up to 63% of cases at the time of diagnosis.[57] The most common metastatic sites for SCLC are the bone, liver, central nervous system, lymph nodes, pleurae, and subcutaneous tissue, although metastases to nearly every organ system have been found.[10]

Non–small-cell lung cancers are more likely to spread initially by direct extension or lymphatic invasion. Tumors may grow into and around the bronchial lumen, extending in plaquelike fashion or completely occluding the lumen. Other pulmonary structures may be compressed, including vasculature, lymphatic channels, nerves, and alveolar tissue. Extension to the pleurae, chest wall, and diaphragm may occur. Rich mediastinal lymphatic drainage offers routes for tumor invasion into the bronchopulmonary, mediastinal, and supraclavicular lymph nodes. Once vascular invasion occurs, metastasis is seen most frequently to bone, liver, adrenal glands, pericardium, and the brain.[19]

# CLINICAL MANIFESTATIONS

Clinical manifestations of lung cancer are dependent upon the location of the tumor and the extent of spread. Only 6% of patients are asymptomatic at the time of diagnosis.[12] Symptoms may be divided into three categories: local-regional symptoms, symptoms due to extrathoracic involvement, and systemic symptoms with or without paraneoplastic syndromes. A summary of symptoms associated with lung cancer is presented in Table 42-1.

## Local-Regional Symptoms

Lung tumors may be present for as long as five years before symptoms are experienced. The most common symptoms of local-regional disease include cough, dyspnea, hemoptysis, wheezing, chest pain, and postobstructive pneumonia. Cough occurs in 75% of patients and often is attributed to a cold, especially if fever is present. It is not uncommon for a patient to be treated empirically with several courses of antibiotics before further diagnostic investigation is done. Hemoptysis is seen in 50%–70% of patients and should always raise the suspicion of a malignancy.[12,51]

Although peripheral tumors cause chest pain in as many as 50% of patients, central tumors are more likely to cause symptoms associated with airway obstruction, such as wheezing, stridor, dyspnea, atelectasis, and pneumonia.[61] As the tumor grows, intrathoracic involvement of adjacent structures produces other symptoms, particularly those related to nerve involvement. Involvement of the left recurrent laryngeal nerve may produce hoarseness, a poor prognostic sign, and phrenic nerve involvement may cause hiccups.[62] Apical tumors may involve the cervical and first thoracic nerves, producing shoulder and arm pain; first and second rib destruction; and Horner's syndrome, characterized by ptosis, pupil contraction, miosis, enophthalmos, and ipsilateral decreased sweating.[61] Pleural effusions are seen commonly with pleural involvement.[19] Bloody pleural fluid is likely due to metastasis and is a poor prognostic sign.[61] Pericar-

**TABLE 42-1**   Clinical Manifestations Associated with Lung Cancer

| | |
|---|---|
| Local-Regional Manifestations | Cough |
| | Dyspnea |
| | Hemoptysis |
| | Wheezing |
| | Chest pain |
| | Stridor |
| | Hoarseness |
| | Hiccups |
| | Atelectasis |
| | Pneumonia |
| | Pancoast's syndrome |
| | Horner's syndrome |
| | Pleural effusion |
| | Pericardial effusions |
| | Superior vena cava syndrome |
| Manifestations of Extrathoracic Involvement | Bone pain |
| | Headache |
| | Central nervous system disturbances |
| | Gastrointestinal disturbances |
| | Jaundice |
| | Hepatomegaly |
| | Abdominal pain |
| Systemic Symptoms | Weakness |
| | Fatigue |
| | Anorexia |
| | Cachexia |
| | Weight loss |
| | Anemia |
| | Symptoms associated with paraneoplastic syndromes |

dial effusions due to pericardial invasion may also be seen.

As a lung tumor with mediastinal involvement grows, it may eventually compress the superior vena cava, causing superior vena cava syndrome (SVCS). Occlusion of the superior vena cava causes reduced venous return to the right atrium, resulting in increased venous pressure, venous hypertension, and venous stasis in the head, arms, and upper chest. Initial symptoms include cough, dyspnea, stridor, hoarseness, edema in the face, neck, and arms, and neck and chest vein distention. The conjunctiva may also be engorged. If the compression is untreated, neurological symptoms related to increased intracranial pressure may ensue, including headache, dizziness, visual disturbances, and occasionally alterations in mental status. Symptoms are most pronounced when the patient is prone and may disappear after the patient is upright for several hours.

SVCS is rarely an emergency, but if untreated the syndrome progresses from venous congestion to thrombosis, cerebral edema, pulmonary complications, and possibly death. If the SVCS develops gradually, the collat-

eral circulation shunts enough blood to minimize complications.[63]

In addition to clinical evidence, a radiograph of the chest usually reveals a mediastinal mass or adenopathy. In the rare case that SVCS is diagnostic and tissue diagnosis has not been made, fractionated irradiation of the mediastinum is the treatment of choice. Radiation doses of 300–400 cGy/day are administered initially, followed by 200-cGy doses to achieve a cumulative dose of 3000–3500 cGy to the obstructing tumor site. In most cases, tissues diagnosis has been made, and the SVCS is treated by standard therapy to the underlying tumor.

Catheter-induced SVCS, most often the result of thrombosis, is treated with fibrinolytic therapy such as streptokinase or urokinase and possibly catheter removal. Streptokinase has more frequent complications such as hemorrhage, pyrexia, and allergic reaction. One approach to the treatment of SVCS due to thrombosis is the use of tissue type plasminogen activator (rTPA) rather than traditional fibrinolytic agents.[64]

Surgical intervention is rarely used for the treatment of malignant SVCS. One of two approaches, superior vena cava bypass graft or stent placement, may be performed for the patient with a good prognosis who has chronic or recurrent SVCS for whom other treatment options have been exhausted. The graft creates a new vessel that circumvents the obstruction; the stent is inserted into the superior vena cava to dilate and expand the narrowed lumen of the vessel.

Nursing care of patients experiencing SVCS is directed toward maintaining adequate cardiopulmonary status, monitoring the progression of SVCS, assisting with medical intervention, and reducing the patient's anxiety. Figure 42-5 describes the clinical pathway for SVCS and highlights critical decisions and interventions for this syndrome.[65]

## Symptoms Due to Extrathoracic Involvement

Signs and symptoms of extrathoracic metastases depend upon the site of involvement. Bone pain due to metastases occurs in approximately 37% of patients. Pathological fractures are rare.[57] Central nervous system metastases produce symptoms 90% of the time, including headache, seizures, confusion, gait disturbances, and personality changes.[57,62] Liver involvement may manifest in jaundice, hepatomegaly, abdominal pain, and gastrointestinal disturbances. Although adrenal metastases are fairly common, signs of adrenal insufficiency are rarely seen.

## Systemic Symptoms with or without Paraneoplastic Syndromes

Systemic symptoms of lung cancer include generalized weakness and fatigue, anorexia, cachexia, weight loss, and anemia. The mechanisms for these symptoms are poorly

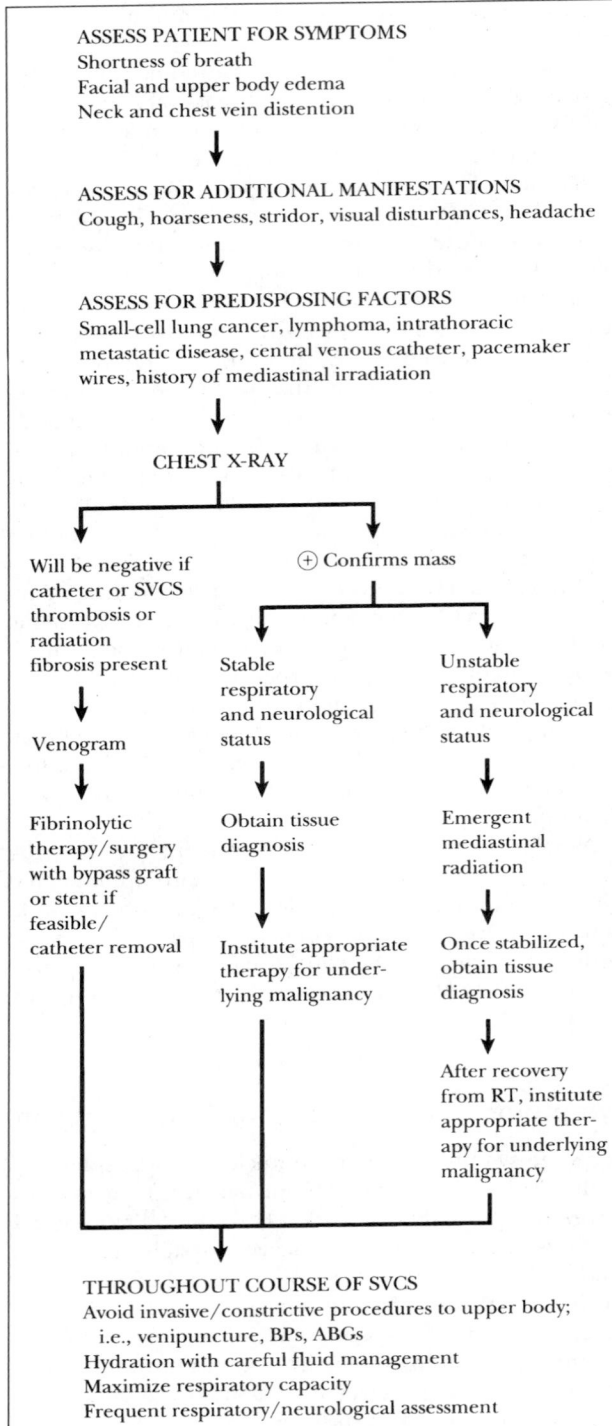

ASSESS PATIENT FOR SYMPTOMS
Shortness of breath
Facial and upper body edema
Neck and chest vein distention

ASSESS FOR ADDITIONAL MANIFESTATIONS
Cough, hoarseness, stridor, visual disturbances, headache

ASSESS FOR PREDISPOSING FACTORS
Small-cell lung cancer, lymphoma, intrathoracic
metastatic disease, central venous catheter, pacemaker
wires, history of mediastinal irradiation

CHEST X-RAY

Will be negative if
catheter or SVCS
thrombosis or
radiation
fibrosis present

⊕ Confirms mass

Venogram

Stable
respiratory
and neurological
status

Unstable
respiratory
and neurological
status

Fibrinolytic
therapy/surgery
with bypass graft
or stent if
feasible/
catheter removal

Obtain tissue
diagnosis

Emergent
mediastinal
radiation

Institute appropriate
therapy for under-
lying malignancy

Once stabilized,
obtain tissue
diagnosis

After recovery
from RT, institute
appropriate ther-
apy for underlying
malignancy

THROUGHOUT COURSE OF SVCS
Avoid invasive/constrictive procedures to upper body;
    i.e., venipuncture, BPs, ABGs
Hydration with careful fluid management
Maximize respiratory capacity
Frequent respiratory/neurological assessment

**FIGURE 42-5**  Clinical pathway for superior vena cava syndrome. Reprinted from Dietz et al.[65]

**TABLE 42-2**  Paraneoplastic Syndromes Associated with Lung Cancer

| Type of Cancer | Associated Paraneoplastic Syndrome |
|---|---|
| Small-Cell Lung Cancer | Ectopic ACTH (Cushing's syndrome) Syndrome of inappropriate antidiuretic hormone (SIADH) secretion Lambert-Eaton myasthenic syndrome (LEMS) |
| Non–small-Cell Lung Cancer | Humoral hypercalcemia of malignancy Hypertrophic pulmonary osteoarthropathy Nephrotic syndrome |
| All Lung Cancers | Hypercoagulable state Erythrocytosis, granulocytosis Neurological syndromes Dermatologic syndromes (acanthosis nigricans) |

unrelated to the spread of cancer. Some syndromes are related to ectopic hormone production; others involve autoimmune mechanisms. Some syndromes are specific to a particular type of lung cancer, while other syndromes may be associated with all lung cancers.

Small-cell lung cancer is associated with paraneoplastic syndromes more frequently than the non–small-cell tumors. Cushing's syndrome, resulting from ectopic secretion of adrenocorticotropic hormone (ACTH), is seen in 5% of SCLC patients and manifests in edema, proximal myopathy, elevated cortisol levels, hypokalemia, and hyperglycemia.[10] The syndrome of secretion of inappropriate antidiuretic hormone (SIADH) results from ADH secretion by the tumor. The incidence of SIADH in SCLC is 5%–10%. Symptoms include hyponatremia and low serum osmolality, characterized by mental status changes, lethargy, seizures, and confusion.

The Lambert-Eaton myasthenic syndrome (LEMS) can be documented in 6% of patients with SCLC.[66] LEMS is thought to be an autoimmune disorder in which the release of acetylcholine by the motor nerve terminals is impaired. Symptoms include proximal muscle weakness, especially in the pelvis, thighs, arms, and shoulders; dry mouth; and double vision.[67,68] LEMS may be the presenting symptom of SCLC.

Humoral hypercalcemia of malignancy, the most frequent paraneoplastic syndrome in NSCLC, commonly is associated with squamous cell carcinomas. It is caused by ectopic production of a parathyroid hormone–like substance.[62] Hypertrophic pulmonary osteoarthropathy, a paraneoplastic condition associated with periostitis of the long bones and clubbing of the fingers and toes, can cause pain, tenderness, and swelling in the joints.[61]

understood. They occur with equal frequency among the various types of lung cancer.

Lung cancer has been associated with many paraneoplastic syndromes (Table 42-2), with manifestations

## ASSESSMENT

### Patient and Family History

An accurate health history is an important means of gathering information needed to establish a diagnosis. This part of the health assessment will help guide decisions regarding diagnostic testing, and can give early clues to the diagnosis.

The patient is asked first to describe the problem(s) that prompted the health care visit. Questions eliciting a full description of each complaint or symptom should be asked, helping the person to describe the onset, duration, location, character, severity, frequency, and measures that aggravate or alleviate each symptom. The nurse should ascertain how the symptoms have had an impact on the quality of the patient's life.

An assessment of past history and family history should also be included, related particularly to smoking, prior respiratory problems, lung cancer history, and exposure to other carcinogens known to increase the risk of lung cancer. Smoking history for all family members should include age of starting to smoke, number of years as a smoker, average amount smoked per day, and type of tobacco smoked. Although a genetic link to lung cancer is not firmly established, a family history of lung cancer may increase a person's risk for developing the disease.

After a determination of coping abilities, strengths, and available supportive resources is gleaned from a thorough psychosocial history, a review of systems completes this part of the health assessment.

### Physical Exam

The physical exam, the second component of the assessment process, focuses on a thorough examination of the pulmonary and lymphatic systems. The systematic assessment should include inspection, palpation, percussion, and auscultation.

#### Inspection

Inspection can provide information about the pattern of respirations, symmetry and integrity of the thorax, and thoracic configuration. Dyspnea, although a subjective observation, is a general indication of inadequate respiration. Pleuritic chest pain may be manifested by rapid, shallow breathing. Intercostal retractions on inspiration indicate obstruction to air inflow, while bulging interspaces on expiration are associated with outflow obstruction; either may be an indication of tumor.[69] Stridor is a manifestation of extrathoracic airway obstruction. The use of accessory muscles for breathing, labored, prolonged expiration, and wheezing may indicate obstruction of intrathoracic airways.

Clubbing of the fingers; skin changes consistent with weight loss; visible signs of Horner's, Pancoast's, and SVC syndromes; and joint swelling consistent with hypertrophic pulmonary osteoarthropathy are also noted.

#### Palpation

Palpation is used to assess areas of tenderness, thoracic expansion, tactile fremitus, position of the trachea, and abnormal areas identified by inspection. Asymmetrical thoracic excursion may be indicative of pulmonary pathology. Decreased tactile fremitus may be associated with pleural effusion and tumors of the pleural cavity, while increased tactile fremitus may indicate a lung mass.[70] Tracheal deviation from midline may be a result of tumor growth, lymphadenopathy, or pleural effusion.[61,69]

#### Percussion

Percussion is used in the thoracic exam to determine the presence or distribution of air, fluid, or areas of consolidation in the lungs, and to delineate the boundaries of other organs. In a normal lung, percussion produces resonant sounds that are loud, low in pitch, and long in duration. Short dull sounds heard on percussion indicate the presence of consolidation, masses, and pleural effusions.[70]

#### Auscultation

Auscultation of the lungs through a stethoscope gives the examiner information about the flow of air throughout the tracheobronchial tree. The lungs are systematically assessed by auscultating the apices and the posterior, lateral, and anterior chest. Absent or decreased breath sounds can be heard when normal lung tissue is replaced by tumor, or when the patient has a pleural effusion. Wheezing and rhonchi may be heard in the presence of bronchial obstruction. A pleural friction rub may be indicative of an inflammatory response to invading tumor. Any abnormal or adventitious breath sounds are described relative to pitch, intensity, quality, and duration of inspiratory and expiratory phases.

### Diagnostic Studies

When a lung malignancy is suspected, diagnostic studies are crucial in making an accurate determination of tumor type, location, and extent of disease. Selection of appropriate tests will provide the necessary information for making treatment decisions. The nurse should become familiar with each test so that education and guidance can be provided to the patient and family.

#### Imaging studies

*Chest radiograph*   The chest radiograph is probably the most helpful diagnostic study for lung cancer. Peripheral nodules usually can be detected when 1 cm or larger in size.[1,61] Central lesions may manifest as a variety of radiographic changes, such as atelectasis or hilar changes.[1] Mediastinal changes on radiograph may suggest lymphadenopathy or pleural effusions, and an elevated diaphragm may be seen with phrenic nerve involvement.[51,61]

***Computed tomography and magnetic resonance imaging*** Computed tomography (CT), introduced in the late 1970s, has greatly improved the precision of lung cancer staging.[51] Lesions not seen on chest radiograph can be detected on CT, and previously identified lesions can be more clearly defined. The chest CT can be particularly helpful in evaluating mediastinal lymph nodes that, if enlarged, should be evaluated further in the staging process before treatment decisions are made.[19,51] Upper abdominal scanning is done along with the chest CT scan to evaluate the liver and adrenals for signs of metastasis.

Magnetic resonance imaging (MRI) of the chest does not offer an advantage over CT scanning and is not used routinely as part of the diagnostic workup. However, MRI may be superior in evaluating the perihilar and paravertebral regions and may be employed when CT scan results are not definitive.[1,19,51]

### Tissue diagnostic studies

***Sputum cytology*** When lung cancer is suspected, the sputum cytology test can be a simple, cost-effective means of obtaining a pathological diagnosis. Early-morning sputum samples are collected for three to five days; deep coughing is recommended since coughing dislodges cancer cells into the sputum. The diagnostic yield for sputum cytologies is up to 80% for central tumors but drops to below 20% for small peripheral tumors.[51] Squamous cell carcinomas are the most frequent type diagnosed by sputum cytology; adenocarcinomas are least often diagnosed by this test. Although the false-positive rate is extremely low at less than 1%, the false-negative rate can be as high as 43%. Therefore, a negative sputum cytology does not rule out malignancy.[1]

***Bronchoscopy*** Fiberoptic bronchoscopy is a procedure in which a flexible bronchoscope is passed through the trachea into the bronchi to collect samples for cytological or histological examination. When central lesions can be visualized, the diagnosis can be made more than 90% of the time from biopsies, brushings, and washings.[19] Even peripheral lesions and suspicious areas where no lesion is seen can be evaluated through the use of needles, cytology brushes, or biopsy forceps introduced via a bronchoscope. Sputum cytology yields are often higher after bronchoscopy.

Recent advances have included the measurement of tumor markers in the bronchoalveolar fluid obtained by bronchoscopy[1] and use of the bronchoscope to sample mediastinal lymph nodes.[29] Complications from bronchoscopy, including hypoxemia, arrhythmias, and mild hemorrhage, are usually minor and occur in less than 10% of cases.[71]

***Fine-needle aspiration*** Percutaneous fine-needle aspiration is used when lung lesions cannot be visualized by bronchoscopy but are accessible percutaneously. A needle guided by CT or fluoroscopy is inserted into the lesion for aspiration of cells. A positive diagnosis can be made up to 95% of the time.[51] Pneumothorax is the most common complication, with an increased risk in persons with chronic obstructive pulmonary disease.[1]

***Mediastinoscopy*** Mediastinoscopy is an invasive procedure used primarily for staging, although it can also be used diagnostically. Mediastinoscopy allows for direct visualization and palpation of mediastinal lymph nodes. A small incision is made in the suprasternal fossa through which the surgeon inserts a finger to evaluate the size and consistency of the lymph nodes; a mediastinoscope is then passed to view and biopsy the nodes.[72]

Mediastinoscopy is indicated in patients who have enlarged mediastinal lymph nodes on CT scan because up to 45% of the time those nodes will be benign.[73] Accurate nodal assessment is vital in determining which patients are candidates for surgery or multimodality protocols. Even when the CT scan is negative for enlarged lymph nodes, mediastinoscopy may be performed if risk factors for occult mediastinal involvement are present.

***Video-assisted thoracoscopic surgery*** Video-assisted thoracoscopic surgery (VATS) has been used in recent years for the staging and diagnosis of lung cancer. Small thoracotomy incisions are made through which thoracoscopic instruments are inserted (Figure 42-6).[72] Visualization of the chest and mediastinum and assessment of pleural effusions are superior to that achieved using older scopes, which may help improve diagnostic accuracy. Although VATS will probably not replace mediastinoscopy, it may prove to be highly effective in evaluating suspicious peripheral nodules. In some centers VATS is being used successfully to perform resections such as lobectomies.[72]

***Thoracotomy*** On rare occasion thoracotomy is necessary to make a diagnosis of lung cancer. Adequate tissue samples are almost always obtained by thoracotomy, although morbidity and mortality are higher than with mediastinoscopy.[61]

## Prognostic Indicators

### Small-cell lung cancer

The most favorable prognostic factor in SCLC is limited-stage disease. In addition, there appears to be some benefit in extensive-stage disease when metastases are limited to a single organ and when there is no liver or brain involvement.[57] Ambulatory performance status, female gender, and a normal serum lactic dehydrogenase (LDH) are also favorable prognostic factors for SCLC.[1]

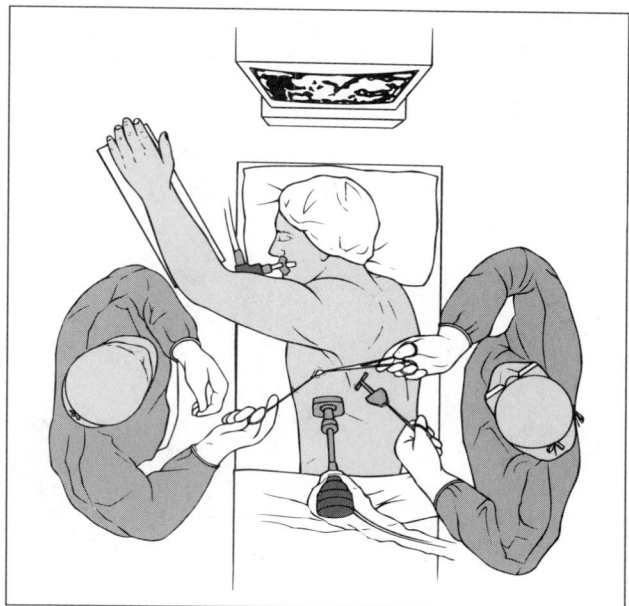

**FIGURE 42-6**  A video-assisted, left-sided thoracoscopic procedure. Two surgeons working with thoracoscopic instruments through a small thoracotomy incision using a video monitor (VATS). (From Sugarbaker DJ, Strauss GM: Advances in surgical staging and therapy of non–small-cell lung cancer. *Semin Oncol* 20:163–172, 1993.)

In some studies, weight loss and impaired immunocompetence as measured by delayed hypersensitivity skin testing have been unfavorable prognostic factors.[57] Cushing's syndrome has been associated with a poorer clinical outcome. Data regarding the effects of SIADH and other paraneoplastic syndromes are inconclusive.[74]

Studies have shown that the tumor marker neuron-specific enolase (NSE) is a promising prognostic indicator. Other markers under investigation include thymidine kinase and tissue polypeptide antigen (TPA).[74] Although amplification of the *c-myc* oncogene has been associated with more aggressive tumor growth, the clinical significance of this finding is yet to be defined.[51]

SCLC has the poorest survival rates of all lung cancer types. Untreated, survival averages 6–12 weeks.[75] With treatment for limited- and extensive-stage disease, two-year survivals of 12%–21% and 1%–4%, respectively, can be expected.[1]

#### Non–small-cell lung cancer

Stage of disease is the most significant prognostic factor for NSCLC, with early-stage cancers responding better to treatment and demonstrating longer survival.[76] The presence of mediastinal lymph node metastases usually indicates a very poor prognosis, although patients with ipsilateral node involvement may be curable with multimodality treatment.[77] Factors associated with shortened survival include weight loss, poor performance status, male gender, elevated serum LDH, and bone or liver metastases. Although diploid tumors have been associated with longer survival, aneuploidy may have a negative survival impact on squamous cell carcinomas.[19]

Several neuroendocrine markers have been studied relative to their prognostic value for NSCLC, including NSE, chromogranin, and *Leu-7*. A positive NSE is associated with improved response to treatment in patients with adenocarcinoma but has had no effect on survival.[19] Point mutations of the *K-ras* oncogene also appear to be an important prognostic factor for NSCLC, especially adenocarcinoma. Their presence has been associated with resistance to radiation and chemotherapy treatment, high risk for relapse, and shortened survival.[19,51]

Survival rates for NSCLC depend upon the extent of disease at diagnosis and the treatment modalities used. Five-year survival for resectable tumors may exceed 70%, whereas rates for locally advanced and metastatic NSCLC are, at best, 0%–30% at five years.[57]

## CLASSIFICATION AND STAGING

### Non–Small-Cell Lung Cancer

In 1986 the American Joint Committee on Cancer (AJCC) revised the staging system for lung cancer to more accurately reflect extent of disease and treatment subsets.[77] The system uses the TNM letters. T designates primary tumor and is divided into categories relative to size, location, and invasion. N, with three categories, represents regional lymph node status. M designates the absence or presence of distant metastases (Table 42-3).[78] Lung cancer is divided into six stages (Table 42-4),[78] each of which is distinct relative to treatment and five-year survival statistics. Accurate staging is crucial in determining appropriate curative or palliative treatment for the patient with lung cancer.

### Small-Cell Lung Cancer

Although the AJCC has always recommended that SCLC be staged using the TNM classification system, most clinicians use the simple two-stage system. Since most SCLC patients have metastatic disease at the time of diagnosis, this system describes the extent of disease as either "limited" or "extensive." *Limited-stage disease* is defined as tumor confined to one hemithorax and regional lymph nodes with or without pleural effusion. It is meant to include all tumor that can be encompassed within a single radiotherapy portal. *Extensive-stage disease* refers to tumor that has spread beyond the boundaries of limited disease. This system has been meaningful in identifying groups of SCLC patients that differ from each other relative to

**TABLE 42-3** TNM Definitions for Lung Cancers

| Primary Tumor (T) | |
|---|---|
| TX | Primary tumor cannot be assessed, or tumor proved by the presence of malignant cells in sputum or bronchial washings but not visualized by imaging or bronchoscopy |
| T0 | No evidence of primary tumor |
| Tis | Carcinoma in situ |
| T1 | Tumor 3 cm or less in greatest dimension, surrounded by lung or visceral pleura, without bronchoscopic evidence of invasion more proximal than the lobar bronchus (i.e., not in the main bronchus)* |
| T2 | Tumor with any of the following features of size or extent: More than 3 cm in greatest dimension Involving main bronchus, 2 cm or more distal to the carina Invading the visceral pleura Associated with atelectasis or obstructive pneumonitis that extends to the hilar region but does not involve the entire lung |
| T3 | Tumor of any size that directly invades any of the following: chest wall (including superior sulcus tumors), diaphragm, mediastinal pleura, or parietal pericardium; or tumor in the main bronchus less than 2 cm distal to the carina but without involvement of the carina; or associated atelectasis or obstructive pneumonitis of the entire lung |
| T4 | Tumor of any size that invades any of the following: mediastinum, heart, great vessels, trachea, esophagus, vertebral body, carina; or tumor with a malignant pleural effusion** |

| Regional Lymph Nodes (N) | |
|---|---|
| NX | Regional lymph nodes cannot be assessed |
| N0 | No regional lymph node metastasis |
| N1 | Metastasis in ipsilateral peribronchial and/or ipsilateral hilar lymph nodes, including direct extension |
| N2 | Metastasis in ipsilateral mediastinal and/or subcarinal lymph node(s) |
| N3 | Metastasis in contralateral mediastinal, contralateral hilar, ipsilateral or contralateral scalene or supraclavicular lymph node(s) |

| Distant Metastasis (M) | |
|---|---|
| MX | Presence of distant metastasis cannot be assessed |
| M0 | No distant metastasis |
| M1 | Distant metastasis |

*Note: The uncommon superficial tumor of any size with its invasive component limited to the bronchial wall, which may extend proximal to the main bronchus, is also classified as T1.

**Note: Most pleural effusions associated with lung cancer are due to tumor. However, there are a few patients in whom multiple cytopathological examinations of pleural fluid are negative for tumor. In these cases, fluid is nonbloody and is not an exudate. When these elements and clinical judgment dictate that the effusion is not related to the tumor, the effusion should be excluded as a staging element and the patient should be staged as T1, T2, or T3.

Reprinted with permission from Beahrs OH, Henson DE, Hutter RVP, Kennedy BJ (eds): *Handbook for Staging of Cancer* (ed 4). Philadelphia, Lippincott, 1993.

**TABLE 42-4** Stage Grouping

| Occult | TX | N0 | M0 |
|---|---|---|---|
| Stage 0 | Tis | N0 | M0 |
| Stage I | T1 | N0 | M0 |
| | T2 | N0 | M0 |
| Stage II | T1 | N1 | M0 |
| | T2 | N1 | M0 |
| Stage IIIA | T1 | N2 | M0 |
| | T2 | N2 | M0 |
| | T3 | N0 | M0 |
| | T3 | N1 | M0 |
| | T3 | N2 | M0 |
| Stage IIIB | Any T | N3 | M0 |
| | T4 | Any N | M0 |
| Stage IV | Any T | Any N | M1 |

Reprinted with permission from Beahrs OH, Henson DE, Hutter RVP, Kennedy BJ (eds): *Handbook for Staging of Cancer* (ed 4). Philedelphia, Lippincott, 1993.

survival length. The TNM system is sometimes helpful in identifying the rare SCLC surgical candidate.

# THERAPEUTIC APPROACHES AND NURSING CARE

## Surgery

Surgical resection is considered standard treatment for stage I and stage II NSCLC and is performed with the intent to cure the patient. Over 50,000 operations for lung cancer are performed each year in the United States.[79] Despite advances in early diagnosis, 50% of all lung cancer cases are inoperable at diagnosis, and another 25% of patients have tumors that cannot be completely resected.[80] The five-year survival rates following surgical resection exceed 50% for stage I and 35% for stage II tumors.[19] Decreased survival has been shown for stage I patients who had any symptom at the time of diagnosis.[81]

Controversy exists regarding the appropriate treatment for stage IIIa patients, particularly those who have ipsilateral mediastinal lymph node involvement ($N_2$ disease). Mediastinal lymph node involvement is a poor prognostic sign, especially when diagnosed preoperatively.[19] However, carefully selected patients with $N_2$ disease have achieved cure rates of up to 29% after complete surgical resection.[82] Most surgeons consider individuals with stage IIIb and stage IV lung cancer to be inoperable, which includes tumors that invade the mediastinum, heart, great vessels, trachea, esophagus, or carina, and any tumors that present with distant metastases.[80] In selected cases, solitary metastatic lesions can be resected, particularly lung and brain lesions.[82] Resection of solitary brain lesions is associated with prolonged survival and improved quality of life, and five-year survival is 5%–10%.[51]

Surgical resection may be an option for the limited number of SCLC patients who present with a small, solitary mass, no lymph node involvement, and no distant metastases. Since many SCLC cancers recur in the chest, surgery is thought to offer increased cure benefit when combined with radiation and chemotherapy in those patients with $T_1N_0M_0$ disease.[80,82]

Because of the high risk of complications following thoracic surgery, candidates should be carefully selected. Cardiopulmonary status is evaluated to determine whether the patient can tolerate pulmonary resection. Pulmonary function tests are done. Increasing emphasis is being given to cardiac studies to more accurately identify patients at risk for postoperative cardiopulmonary complications. In general, if the ratio of the forced expiratory volume in 1 second ($FEV_1$) to forced vital capacity (FVC) is below 75% of the predicted value, postoperative complications increase dramatically. Unacceptable morbidity and mortality are associated with $FEV_1$/FVC ratios of less than 50% of the predicted value.[19] The patient's ability to perform pulmonary toilet measures and upper extremity range-of-motion exercises postoperatively should be evaluated in a preoperative education session.

### Surgical procedures

***Pneumonectomy*** Although it was the standard surgical lung cancer procedure for many years, pneumonectomy is now performed only if a tumor cannot be completely excised by lobectomy.[19] Pneumonectomy is chosen when the tumor involves the proximal bronchus, is widespread throughout the lung, or is fixed to the hilum.[51,80]

Pneumonectomy can be a simple or radical procedure. A simple pneumonectomy involves removal of the affected lung with suturing or stapling of the bronchus. The radical procedure includes removal of the mediastinal lymph nodes. After either procedure, mediastinal shift is prevented by allowing the empty thoracic space to consolidate gradually with fluid (Figure 42-7a). The average mortality rate for pneumonectomy is 6%.[19]

***Lobectomy*** Lobectomy is the most common surgical procedure performed for primary lung cancer confined to a single lobe of the lung. It includes dissection and excision of the affected lobe from the remaining lung tissue, with closure of the bronchial stump (Figure 42-7b). Two chest tubes are placed in the pleural cavity on the operative side to drain fluid, blood, and air. The remaining lung tissue expands to fill the space left by the resected lobe. Because noncancerous lung tissue is conserved, morbidity with lobectomy is lessened and the mortality rate, at 3%, is half that of pneumonectomy.[19,51]

***Sleeve resection with bronchoplastic reconstruction*** When the tumor is confined to the bronchus or pulmonary artery and there is no evidence of metastasis, the affected area can be removed and the bronchus reattached with cure rates comparable to those for pneumo-

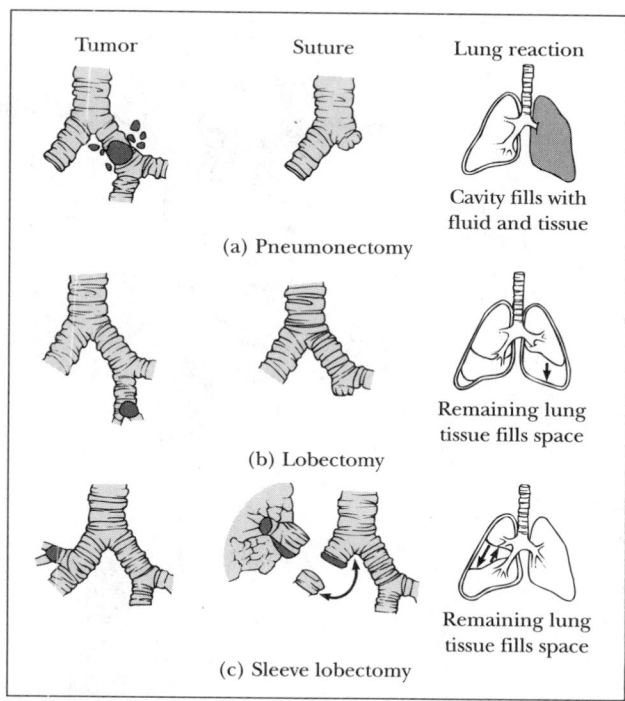

**FIGURE 42-7** Approaches to lung resection. (a) Pneumonectomy: The lung alone is removed (simple pneumonectomy) or the lung and involved adjacent nodes are removed (radical pneumonectomy). (b) Lobectomy: A single pulmonary lobe is resected. (c) Sleeve lobectomy: The tumor-bearing lobe is resected together with a segment of the main bronchus, followed by an end-to-end anastomosis. Classic indication is a carcinoma of the right upper lobe bronchus. (From Elpern EH: Lung cancer, in Groenwald SL, Frogge MH, Goodman M, Yarbro CH (eds): *Cancer Nursing: Principles and Practice* (ed 3). Boston, Jones and Bartlett, 1993, pp 1174–1199.)

nectomy for similar patients.[19] Sleeve resection can also be successfully combined with lobectomy (Figure 42-7c). This lung-conserving operation improves the quality of life and reduces morbidity and mortality.

***Segmental resection (Segmentectomy)*** Segmental resection is the partial removal of a lobe of the lung, including the bronchovascular segment supplying the resected area (Figure 42-8a). The role of this procedure has yet to be clearly defined. A well-designed trial by the Lung Cancer Study Group of limited resection versus lobectomy in stage I NSCLC showed a threefold increase in local recurrence in the limited resection group, although mortality and morbidity were equal in both groups.[83] At the present time, limited resections are reserved for those patients with cardiopulmonary compromise who are not suitable candidates for more extensive surgery.[81,82] The mortality rate for segmental resection averages 1%.[51]

***Wedge resection*** Wedge resection, the most conservative surgical approach, is done to remove small peripheral nodules or as the procedure of choice in individuals

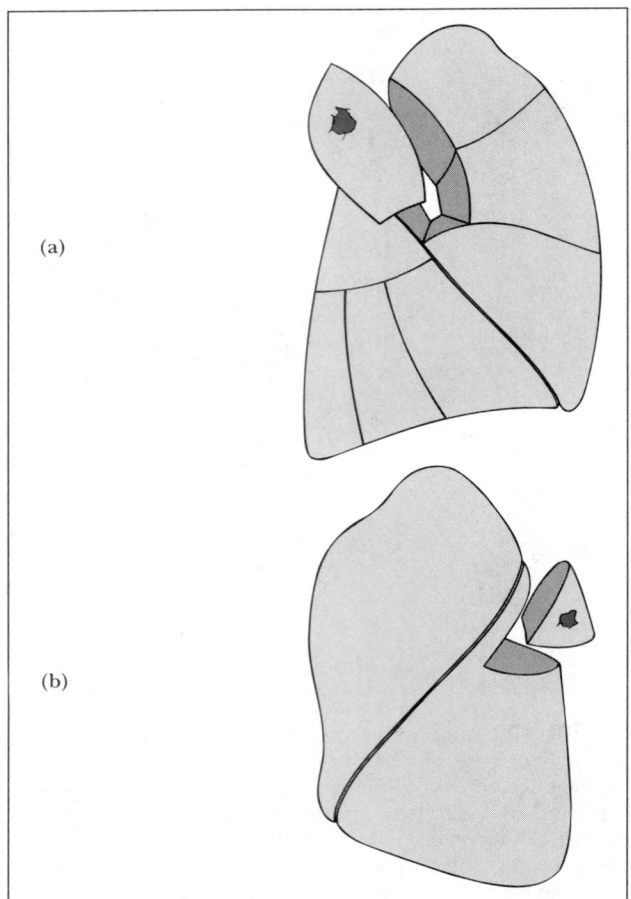

**FIGURE 42-8** (a) Segmentectomy: Partial removal of a lobe of the lung. (b) Wedge resection: Removal of a small area of disease.

whose physical condition will not permit more extensive surgery. The procedure involves removing the small area of disease without removing the bronchovascular segment of the lobe (Figure 42-8b). As with the other limited resection procedures, mortality is low at 1% but local recurrence rates average 15%, three times higher than with lobectomy.[19,82]

***Types of incisions*** Pulmonary resection can be accomplished through a variety of operative approaches, depending on the size and location of the tumor and the type of procedure to be performed. The most common approach is the posterolateral thoracotomy, in which a curved incision is made from the submammary fold to slightly below the scapula along the underlying rib. This incision gives the surgeon access to both the lung and the mediastinum.[80]

The anterolateral thoracotomy incision extends from the sternal border between the fourth and fifth intercostal spaces to the midaxillary line. Limited exposure of the lung lessens its usefulness.

The median sternotomy, which is used to gain access to both lungs and/or to tumor in the mediastinum, has

been associated with less postoperative pain than with other procedures.[80,84] An incision is made from the sternal notch to the xiphoid or umbilicus. The sternum is then split with an oscillating saw and spread with retractors to provide maximum exposure. After the resection, the sternum is closed with heavy steel wires.

The axillary incision, from the anterior to the posterior axillary line, is used in patients with lateral peripheral lesions easily accessible by this approach.

### Complications

Complications associated with surgical resection of the lung are largely dependent upon the physical status of the patient, the extent of disease, and the surgical procedure performed. Perioperative complications may include air leak, bleeding, atelectasis, and the myriad of other well-known intraoperative complications.

The most common postoperative complications are pain and atelectasis. Postthoracotomy incisional pain can be severe and is aggravated by the presence of chest tubes. Inadequate pain control prevents effective coughing and mobilization, and atelectasis may result. Complications that cause impaired gas exchange include pneumothorax, bronchospasm, pulmonary embolus, bronchopleural fistula, and adult respiratory distress syndrome.

Infection and sepsis may also complicate the postoperative course. Wound infections may develop at the incision or chest tube insertion sites; empyema and pneumonia are not uncommon, especially with prolonged intubation. Invasive monitoring devices, urinary catheters, and a generally compromised physical state also increase the risk of infection. Some surgeons recommend preoperative bronchoscopy cultures to assess the bacterial flora of the patient so that appropriate treatment can be initiated before infection manifests.[84]

Cardiac arrhythmias and myocardial infarction may occur postoperatively, and preoperative digitalization is sometimes employed as a preventive measure.[81,84] Sequential compression devices on the lower extremities both during and after surgery help to prevent pulmonary emboli.

### Nursing care

Surgery for lung cancer is a major procedure with the potential for significant morbidity and discomfort for the patient. Meticulous nursing care is essential in preventing postoperative complications and in promoting comfort. A plan of care or critical pathway should be developed based on nursing diagnoses and appropriate nursing interventions.

***Knowledge deficit*** The patient must be fully engaged in the treatment process to increase the chance for successful recovery. Preoperative education about the surgical procedure and what the patient will experience before, during, and after surgery are provided, with particular emphasis on the patient's participation in pulmonary toilet activities. Demonstration and return demonstration of cough, deep breathing, and splinting techniques are included. Anticipatory guidance about the intensive care unit, monitoring devices, and ventilatory support is provided to minimize fear and anxiety related to the initial postsurgical period. Ongoing education about self-care measures to be used after discharge is provided throughout the hospitalization.

***Alteration in comfort*** Pain is assessed frequently to evaluate the effectiveness of analgesics. Intravenous or epidural infusion of narcotic analgesics is necessary for control of incisional pain, which is severe initially and has been shown to last as long as four years in up to 50% of cases.[79] Teaching the patient position changes and exercises to do in bed can also promote comfort and help to prevent "frozen shoulder," which occurs when pain impairs mobility in the arm and shoulder on the operative side. Range-of-motion exercises should be encouraged.

Nausea due to anesthesia or analgesic medications can occur. Antiemetics should be offered and their effectiveness evaluated.

***Potential for impaired gas exchange*** Postsurgical complications can be life-threatening, and early recognition of these by the nurse can assure appropriate intervention. Vital signs and arterial blood gases are monitored. Sputum production is assessed for amount, color, and consistency. Patency of chest tubes is assessed, and drainage amount measured and recorded. The patient is encouraged to cough and deep breathe frequently, using incentive spirometry or respiratory treatments to help mobilize secretions.

***Potential for infection*** The incision and chest tube insertion sites are inspected regularly for signs of infection, including erythema, induration, and drainage. Preventive nursing measures regarding wound management are instituted. Attention to signs and symptoms of other types of infections are a regular part of the nursing assessment.

***Alterations in bowel elimination*** Both diarrhea and constipation can occur in the postoperative period. Diarrhea is most often related to enteral feedings or stress and may be treated with antidiarrheal agents and by addressing the causative factors. Consulting a dietitian can be helpful in developing a nutritional plan that is less likely to cause diarrhea. Constipation may result from narcotic analgesics, immobility, and decreased dietary intake. Dietary fiber should be increased, and a bowel protocol established early in the postoperative course.

***Potential for ineffective coping/anxiety*** Fear and anxiety are normal manifestations of the stress associated with lung cancer and surgery. The patient and family members are encouraged to express their feelings and concerns. Realistic information and reassurance are given, and referrals to other members of the health care team, including the social worker, clinical nurse specialist, case manager, or chaplain, are made as appropriate. Discharge planning should begin on admission, utilizing available resources in the institution and the community to facilitate a smooth transition to the use of self-care measures in the home.

## Radiation Therapy

### Non–small-cell lung cancer

Radiation therapy (RT) is an important treatment in the management of individuals with NSCLC. The usual dosage of external beam chest irradiation is 50–60 Gy delivered in fractions of 1.8–2.0 Gy five days a week over five to six weeks.[85] Although surgery offers the best chance for cure for stage I and stage II disease, RT offers a potentially curative alternative in patients who refuse surgery or are not surgical candidates. Postoperative RT is not commonly used for early-stage NSCLC because even though it decreases the incidence of local recurrence, it has not improved overall survival.[19,51]

Postoperative RT is the standard of care for selected stage IIIa patients undergoing surgical resection, and is thought to prolong disease-free survival, although not long-term survival.[19] RT is also the standard treatment for patients with unresectable stage III disease. However, when used alone, the effectiveness of RT is limited, with median survival of eight to ten months and five-year survival of 5%–7%.[86,87] In an effort to improve survival rates in patients with regionally advanced NSCLC, new methods of fractionation of RT dosages are being tested. With continuous hyperfractionated accelerated RT (CHART), three fractions per day of less than 1.8 Gy each are given over 12 consecutive days with an interval of at least six hours between fractions. The total CHART dosage is greater than standard dosages, and the short interval between fractions prevents cancer cell repopulation. The lower dosage per fraction enhances normal repair of sublethal tissue damage.[85,87] Several studies have shown impressive one- and two-year survival rates with CHART compared with conventional RT.[86,87] Esophagitis is the most common toxicity, occurring at around day 18 when treatment is completed.

Multimodality treatment of stage III patients combining chemotherapy and radiation therapy is a current area of considerable interest. A landmark study by Sause and colleagues showed a statistically significant survival advantage for unresectable stage III patients treated with chemotherapy followed by RT versus standard RT alone or hyperfractionated radiation therapy.[88] Chemotherapy treatment for NSCLC is discussed in greater detail later in this chapter.

### Small-cell lung cancer

SCLC is quite sensitive to both radiation and chemotherapy. Most oncologists consider thoracic RT in combination with chemotherapy for limited-stage disease to be the standard of care.[57,87] Combined-modality treatment results in lower recurrence rates and appears to confer a modest survival advantage over chemotherapy alone.[87] The usual dosage of chest RT for SCLC is 45–50 Gy over three to four weeks. Conventional and hyperfractionation schedules have been used. Concurrent or alternating treatment appears to improve response rates over sequential chemotherapy and RT, although toxicity is more intense with concurrent therapy.[89]

Prophylactic cranial irradiation (PCI) in limited-stage SCLC is an area of considerable debate. Because of the potentially serious long-term side effects of PCI, including dementia, gait disturbances, and intellectual impairment, benefit must be weighed against risk.[90] Some argue that because there is a 50% chance of central nervous system recurrence with SCLC, PCI is worth the risk of toxicity, particularly if (1) it is given only to individuals who have a complete response to initial therapy; (2) it is not given concurrently with any drugs; and (3) standard or lower dosages are used.[87]

Others argue that because PCI reduces brain recurrence but does not improve overall survival, the associated morbidity does not justify brain irradiation unless a metastatic brain lesion develops.[91] Figure 42-9 illustrates this point. Group A patients who received PCI were compared with group B patients who received cranial RT only when a brain metastasis developed. The ultimate outcomes were the same. Twenty percent of patients were left with unresolved symptomatic brain metastases, although most patients in group B were spared the toxicity of PCI. PCI is not recommended for patients who do not have a complete response to therapy because it does not reduce the risk of brain recurrence in those patients. Chest irradiation in extensive-stage SCLC offers no survival advantage and is not recommended.[57]

### Palliative radiation therapy for all lung cancer types

RT can be used as an effective palliative treatment for many of the distressing symptoms caused by metastatic lung cancer. Duration and toxicity of the treatment relative to expected survival of the patient should always be considered and treatment decisions individualized.

Bone metastases can be irradiated to alleviate pain, prevent pathological fractures, and prevent spinal cord compression. Individuals with SVCS often experience relief within one to two days after RT is initiated. Radiation to metastatic brain lesions can also promote improved function and symptomatic relief.

One of the most common indications for palliative RT is major airway obstruction by endobronchial lesions. External beam irradiation and brachytherapy have been used. Most recently, high-dose-rate (HDR) brachytherapy has been used to palliate symptoms of obstruction such as cough, hemoptysis, and dyspnea.[92] During the HDR brachytherapy procedure a catheter is placed bronchoscopically beyond the distal margin of the tumor (Figure 42-10). A radioactive source is delivered into the tumor via the catheter providing a high dose of therapy in a short period of time, usually minutes.[93] The onetime treat-

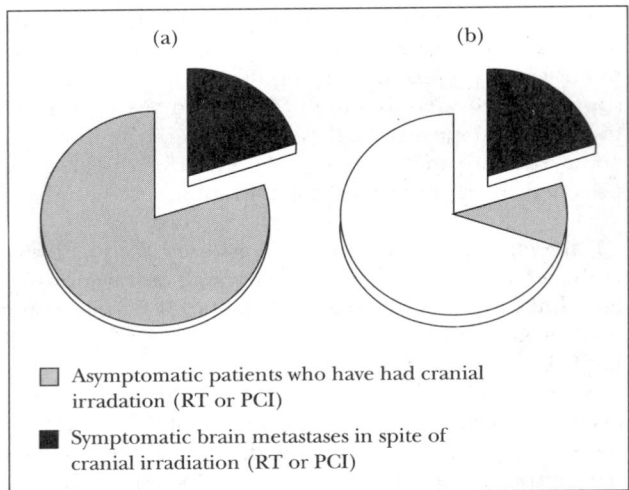

Asymptomatic patients who have had cranial irradiation (RT or PCI)

Symptomatic brain metastases in spite of cranial irradiation (RT or PCI)

**FIGURE 42-9**   Schematic presentation of two different scenarios in the management of SCLC. Each cycle represents the groups of complete responders (CR) with small-cell lung cancer. (A) All CR patients receive prophylactic cranial irradiation (PCI) and approximately 20% relapse in the brain, with very limited chances of further palliation (black area). (B) Cranial irradiation is withheld until a manifest brain relapse occurs. This happens in 30% of CR patients, of whom 40% achieve a complete symptomatic alleviation of some duration. Approximately 20% are left with symptomatic brain metastases (black area). (Reprinted from *Lung Cancer,* Vol. 12, Kristjansen PEG, Hansen HH, Prophylactic cranial irradiation in small cell lung cancer—an update, S23–S40, 1995, with kind permission from Elsevier Science Ireland Ltd., Bay 15K, Shannon Industrial Estate, Co. Clare, Ireland.)

ment can be given safely in the outpatient setting. Although side effects of HDR brachytherapy are usually minimal, pneumothorax and bronchoesophageal fistulae have been reported, and in one study, massive fatal hemoptysis was reported in 6 of 12 patients.[94]

### Side effects of radiation therapy for lung cancer and nursing care

Side effects of RT are generally related to the area being irradiated. Most patients experience uncomfortable side effects. The most common side effects of chest RT include skin irritation; esophagitis, manifested by dysphagia; radiation pneumonitis, manifested by dry cough, dyspnea on exertion, and fever; pericarditis, with chest pain, electrocardiogram abnormalities, and a pericardial friction rub; and fatigue. Acute side effects usually begin during the second to third week of therapy;[57] long-term effects such as pericarditis may not develop for more than a year after therapy completion.[85] Larson and colleagues reported that outcomes related to weight, body mass index, and multidimensional functional status were no different for persons over 65 than for those younger than 65 after RT for lung cancer.[95] This study suggests that age should not be the only determinant of ability to manage

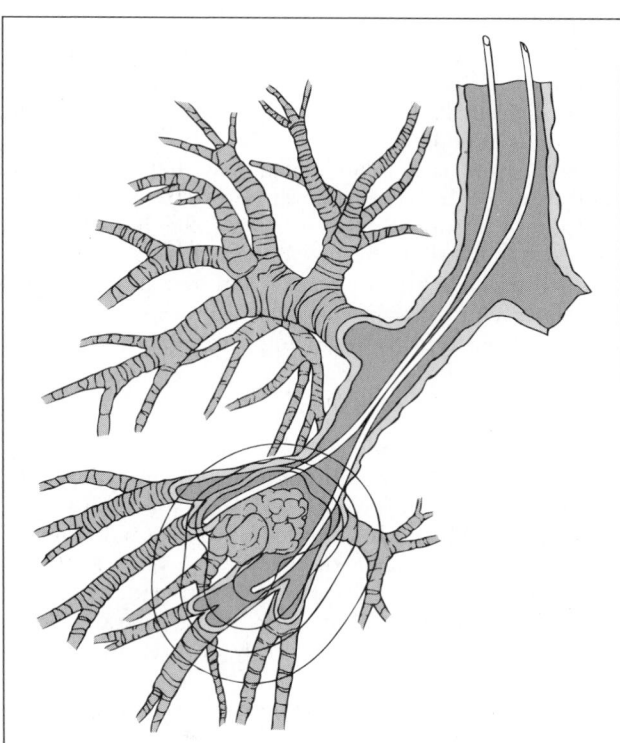

**FIGURE 42-10**  Lung implant for delivery of radiation. Two brachytherapy catheters surround the tumor and deliver a high dose of radiation directly to the tumor. (From the Nucletron-Oldelft Corporation, Columbia, MD.)

demanding treatment. Weight loss after RT for lung cancer is common, and was found to be greater in men, current smokers, and the elderly.[96] These findings can be used to identify individuals at high risk for weight loss and to guide early nutritional intervention. Nursing care of the person receiving RT is discussed in detail in chapter 13.

## Chemotherapy

### Non–small-cell lung cancer

Fifty to seventy-five percent of all patients with NSCLC will present with regionally advanced or metastatic disease and are not candidates for surgery.[97,98] Eighty percent of those who present with resectable disease relapse with distant metastases.[47] If progress is to be made in survival rates of individuals with NSCLC, improvements in systemic treatment must be realized. Although adjuvant chemotherapy for stage I and stage II disease has not shown a survival benefit and is not the standard, continued clinical trials with new drugs are currently under way.[47,99]

Chemotherapy is used to treat stage III and stage IV patients. Response rates of 50%–70% are seen in stage III patients when chemotherapy is added to surgery or RT, and some chemotherapeutic agents act as radiation sensitizers.[98,99] A survival advantage has been demon-

strated in stage III individuals treated with chemotherapy followed by RT versus RT alone.[88] Cisplatin-based chemotherapy protocols are the standard of treatment.[98]

Neoadjuvant therapy—chemotherapy with or without RT prior to surgery—has been an area of interest in recent years for patients with stage III disease. Neoadjuvant therapy is based on the premise that eradicating micrometastatic disease and debulking the tumor prior to surgery may improve the chance of a complete resection and cure. Survival rates after neoadjuvant therapy have been higher than with other treatments.[100] Although neoadjuvant treatment shows promise, it can be quite difficult for the patient, with increased operative complications and higher morbidity and mortality.

Although multimodality treatment is the emerging standard of care for stage III NSCLC, patients with distant metastases (stage IV) have traditionally been treated with either chemotherapy alone or supportive care.[101] Agents used in the past ten years have included ifosfamide, vinblastine, vindesine, cisplatin, etoposide, and mitomycin. Given the intrinsic resistance to chemotherapy manifested by NSCLC cells, use of these drugs has been repeatedly questioned. Response rates with chemotherapy average 15%, and median survival time is only 25–30 weeks.[102,103]

Palliation of symptoms, quality of life, and length of survival, in addition to response rates, must be evaluated when chemotherapy is given for metastatic NSCLS. Chemotherapy has been compared with best supportive care (BSC) in many clinical trials. In these trials BSC has included measures for pain control, symptom management, palliative RT, and antibiotics, but no chemotherapy.[47] Chemotherapy extended survival and also improved symptoms such as cough, hemoptysis, bone pain, malaise, and weight loss.[96,104] A cost analysis performed by the National Cancer Institute of Canada revealed that chemotherapy saved health care dollars when compared with BSC because symptoms improved and patients spent less time in the hospital.[96] With the widespread use of improved antiemetic drugs, chemotherapy has become a more acceptable option for patients with advanced NSCLC.

Despite skepticism over the past few decades about the relative efficacy of chemotherapy in NSCLC, a number of promising new chemotherapeutic agents are available (Table 42-5). Many of these agents have mechanisms of

**TABLE 42-5**  Promising New Chemotherapeutic Agents Used in the Treatment of NSCLS

| | |
|---|---|
| Camptothecin analogues: | Topotecan<br>Irinotecan (CPT-11) |
| Taxanes: | Paclitaxel (Taxol)<br>Docetaxel (Taxotere) |
| Vinca alkaloid: | Vinorelbine |
| Antimetabolites: | Gemcitabine<br>Edatrexate (10-EDAM) |

action different from those of standard drugs. Some have shown more activity as a single agent than standard combination chemotherapy. A discussion of each new agent follows.

***Camptothecin analogues*** The camptothecins, including topotecan and irinotecan (CPT-11), are plant alkaloids extracted from a large-leafed tree common in southeastern China. They exert their cytotoxic action by inhibiting topoisomerase I, an enzyme necessary for DNA replication.[99]

Results of topotecan clinical trials with NSCLC have not been encouraging.[105] CPT-11, studied extensively in Japan, has shown promising activity in NSCLC. Response rates of up to 41% as a single agent and 54% when combined with cisplatin have been reported.[98] Dose-limiting toxicities include diarrhea and myelosuppression. Nausea, vomiting, alopecia, anorexia, stomatitis, and anemia have also been reported.[105] Because the diarrhea can be life-threatening, the importance of patient education about the recommendations for diarrhea management cannot be overemphasized.

***Taxanes*** Paclitaxel and docetaxel exert their effects by stabilizing microtubules so that the cell cannot progress beyond the $G_2$ or M phase of the cell cycle into cell division.[98,99] Using paclitaxel as a single agent, response rates of over 20% have been seen.[47] In a landmark study by Langer and colleagues, paclitaxel and carboplatin together in advanced NSCLC yielded an astonishing 62% response rate, with 9% complete responses.[106] The one-year survival rate was 54%. The regimen was fairly well tolerated: severe myelosuppression was less than 22% with the use of filgrastim. Other reported side effects included anemia, thrombocytopenia, neuropathy, myalgias, and arthralgias. Paclitaxel alone may also cause nausea and vomiting, stomatitis, diarrhea, and a rare hypersensitivity reaction.[98]

Docetaxol has also shown promise, with response rates of up to 33% in early trials.[101,105] Side effects are similar to those of paclitaxel, including neutropenia, skin reactions, hypersensitivity, neuropathy, edema, stomatitis, alopecia, and weakness.

***Vinorelbine*** Vinorelbine, the newest drug in the vinca alkaloid class, inhibits cellular replication by interfering with the assembly of microtubules. In patients with advanced NSCLC, vinorelbine in combination with cisplatin has shown a survival advantage over vindesine and cisplatin and vinorelbine alone.[104,107] Many oncologists believe that vinorelbine plus cisplatin should be considered as the initial therapy for stage IV NSCLC, although a "best" regimen has yet to be defined.[104] Neutropenia is the dose-limiting toxicity. Other side effects include nausea, vomiting, and diarrhea, although neurotoxicity has been less severe than with the other vinca alkaloids.[98]

***Investigational antimetabolites*** Gemcitabine and edatrexate (10-EDAM) are two new antimetabolites. Gemci-

tabine has consistently shown response rates of about 20%. A relatively mild side effect panel, including minimal myelosuppression and a flulike syndrome, make it an attractive drug to combine with other more myelosuppressive regimens.[47,99,101]

Edatrexate is a folate antagonist that is similar to methotrexate. In patients never before treated with chemotherapy, response rates of up to 32% have been reported.[99] Mucositis is the dose-limiting toxicity. Other side effects include fatigue, nausea, vomiting, and myelosuppression. Edatrexate in combination with other chemotherapy drugs is currently being investigated.

### Small-cell lung cancer

SCLC is initially much more sensitive to chemotherapy than NSCLC. Chemotherapy, with or without RT, has been the mainstay of treatment for many years. Despite complete response rates of up to 90% in limited-stage disease, long-term survival at five years is 10% at best, and almost 0% for patients with extensive-stage SCLC.[103] Eventual resistance to chemotherapy is acquired over time and is currently an area of vigorous investigation.

Several chemotherapy regimens have emerged as effective options for treatment (Table 42-6), although a single best regimen is yet to be defined. In the 1970s and 1980s the CAV regimen (cyclophosphamide, doxorubicin, and vincristine) was most commonly used, with high response rates and occasional cures.[108] Later, etoposide emerged as an extremely active agent in SCLC and became the cornerstone of new regimens. Currently, etoposide and cisplatin (EP regimen) are standard induction therapy for SCLC. They appear to be synergistic, have comparable efficacy to CAV, and combined side effects are less severe than with CAV.[108,109]

**TABLE 42-6** Chemotherapy Regimens Commonly Used for Small-Cell Lung Cancer

| Regimen | Drug Names |
|---|---|
| CAV | Cyclophosphamide, doxorubicin, vincristine |
| EP CAV alternating with EP | Etoposide, cisplatin |
| Oral EP | Oral etoposide, cisplatin |
| EC | Etoposide, carboplatin |
| CAE | Cyclophosphamide, doxorubicin, etoposide |
| CAVE | Cyclophosphamide, doxorubicin, vincristine, etoposide |
| CODE | Cisplatin, vincristine, doxorubicin, etoposide |
| ICE (VIP) | Ifosfamide, cisplatin, etoposide |

More recently, carboplatin and etoposide have been reported to exhibit activity equal to that of EP, with significantly less nausea, vomiting, nephrotoxicity, mucositis, neurotoxicity, neutropenia, and sepsis events.[110] The CODE regimen (cisplatin, vincristine, doxorubicin, etoposide), currently under investigation, has shown promise when combined with RT in patients with extensive SCLC, with response rates of 94% and two-year survival of 30%.[108] Because myelosuppression is the dose-limiting toxicity for many of the drugs active in SCLC, the use of hematopoietic growth factors has shortened the duration of neutropenia and enabled safer administration of higher-dose regimens. Whether or not these regimens extend survival is a question still to be answered.

Many of the drugs used in the treatment of SCLC are poorly tolerated by elderly individuals. Potential nephrotoxicity with the EP regimen is a concern, and tolerance for myelosuppression may be decreased. The elderly often are excluded from clinical trials because of the fear that they will experience undue toxicity. In this group of patients, oral etoposide has been shown to be an excellent alternative to more aggressive therapy, with overall response rates of up to 85%.[111] Neutropenia is still a concern, although less so than with other therapies.

Chemotherapy for SCLC is usually given for four to six months. Maintenance chemotherapy beyond this time is not recommended because it does not improve survival.[57] Although autologous bone marrow transplantation in patients with SCLC has been studied for over a decade, results are inconclusive.[109]

### Complications of chemotherapy and nursing care

Complications associated with chemotherapy for lung cancer are many and are dependent upon the drugs given. Side effects may be acute or chronic. Acute side effects include myelosuppression, nausea, vomiting, diarrhea, mucositis, constipation, anorexia, alopecia, skin changes, hemorrhagic cystitis, hypersensitivity reactions, myalgias, and arthralgias. Potential long-term effects include organ toxicities such as cardiomyopathy, hepatotoxicity, nephropathy, peripheral neuropathy, pulmonary toxicity, ototoxicity, and infertility.[112] Specific aspects of nursing care related to side effects are described in chapter 16.

Many patients with lung cancer are symptomatic at diagnosis and present in a debilitated state. Chemotherapy usually adds to debilitation, at least temporarily, and some of the side effects can be life-threatening.

Education for the patient and family about chemotherapy begins early. Emphasis is placed on teaching self-management of side effects since most side effects will be experienced in the home setting. Early referrals to supportive resources are made, encouraging the patient to attend to the emotional as well as the physical aspects of the illness. Because accessibility of the health care providers is extremely important and reassuring to the patient during treatment, phone numbers for the nurse and physician should be provided.

## Biotherapy

In general, results of clinical trials with biological therapies have not been encouraging. Response rates with alfa-interferon alone in both SCLC and NSCLC have been less than 15%.[47] Beta-interferon is thought to be synergistic with RT, and in one study produced an overall response rate of 81% in 25 patients with stage III NSCLC.[98] Continued clinical trials to evaluate efficacy and toxicity of this combination are under way. Alfa-interferon with cisplatin or carboplatin does not appear to be superior to chemotherapy alone,[99] although data from current trials are pending. Interleukin-2, studied as a treatment for NSCLC, has resulted in poor response rates with significant toxicity.[99,113]

Because lung cancer is known to impair both cellular and humoral immunity, restoration of immune function has been targeted in recent studies. Intrapleural bacillus Calmette-Guerin (BCG) was studied with no observed improvement in treated patients. Likewise, treatment with levamisole, an immunomodulator, did not produce results more favorable than in the control arm of the study.[113]

The hematopoietic growth factors have been the most useful biologic response modifiers in treatment of lung cancer. Both granulocyte (G) and granulocyte-macrophage (GM) colony-stimulating factors (CSFs) decrease myelosuppression, febrile episodes, and number of hospital days when given in conjunction with chemotherapy. Although the CSFs do not affect survival, their impact on cost and quality of life has been profound.[51]

## Photodynamic Therapy

Photodynamic therapy (PDT) has been used in an investigational setting to treat lung cancer.[114] PDT is performed under general anesthesia. After the patient is given a photosensitizer such as porfimer sodium, light generated from a laser is transmitted through a bronchoscope to tumor on the bronchial surface. A "cleanup" bronchoscopy is done several days later to remove cellular debris and mucus that is too thick for the patient to expectorate. If residual tumor is seen at that time, the PDT procedure may be repeated.

PDT is most useful in early-stage lung cancer. Several studies in Japan showed that 90% of small superficial tumors can be completely eradicated with PDT.[114] Complete response rates have been as high as 89%. PDT is not used to treat regional lymph nodes, and is not effective for bronchial stump recurrences.

PDT has been compared with yttrium aluminum garnet (YAG) laser therapy in treating bronchial obstruction from intraluminal tumors. While both treatments are equally effective, relief of obstruction is quicker with YAG laser therapy. YAG should be used in acute cases of bronchial obstruction. The porfimer sodium used with PDT can cause skin photosensitivity for up to several months. However, time to treatment failure has been slightly longer after PDT than after YAG laser therapy.[114]

Brachytherapy continues to be the treatment of choice for patients with advanced obstructive bronchial tumors invading the submucosa. Studies combining PDT with external beam radiation have shown promise in achieving better local control than RT alone.

Complications for PDT and YAG laser therapy are similar. Fatal hemorrhage, respiratory failure, or cardiac arrest occurs in 1.5% of patients. Less severe complications occur in less than 0.5% of cases.[115]

# SYMPTOM MANAGEMENT AND SUPPORTIVE CARE

Suffering has been defined as a negative state that results from events or situations perceived to be physically or psychologically painful, uncomfortable, or distressing.[116] Lung cancer is synonymous with suffering for many people. Up to 90% of patients report some degree of suffering relative to physical, emotional, or psychosocial dysfunction. While the nursing care challenges are significant, so too are the opportunities for meaningful intervention. Symptom management and supportive care for this population of patients, discussed in the following, require our most finely honed nursing skills.

## Cough

A chronic cough may result from stimulation of irritant receptors in the bronchial mucosa through tumor infiltration. Hypersecretion of mucus also may cause coughing. Persistent coughing may increase pain, prevent adequate rest, and promote fatigue, and it can cause rib fractures when bone metastases are present.[55] The dry, irritating cough must be distinguished from the productive cough. Although it may be appropriate to suppress a dry, persistent, and debilitating cough, this should not be attempted at the expense of removal of secretions.

The goal of nursing interventions is to promote comfort. Narcotic medications, specifically codeine preparations, are generally used for cough suppression. Inspired air is warmed and humidified and cigarette smoking discouraged. Deep breathing and effective coughing techniques are taught and reinforced as necessary. Tracheal suctioning is to be used only if the individual's cough is ineffective in removing secretions. A chronic, nonproductive cough in a patient with underlying chronic obstructive lung disease may respond to inhaled bronchodilators.[55]

## Hemoptysis

Mild hemoptysis is common and is caused by erosion of the pulmonary vasculature by tumor. If the volume of bleeding is less than 50 ml in 24 hours, the patient usually is treated conservatively on an outpatient basis.[55] If hemoptysis is exacerbated by coughing, cough suppressants may be prescribed. Although death from exsanguination is rare, the fear of bleeding to death is often expressed by patients. Accurate information and reassurance should be provided.

Hospitalization and careful monitoring are required for patients with profound hemoptysis. Bleeding of over 200 ml in 24 hours requires immediate attention. The patient should be positioned with the suspected bleeding lung in a dependent position to prevent blood spillage into the unaffected lung.[55] Emergency surgery may be required.

## Dyspnea

Dyspnea and the sensation of smothering can be a terrifying experience for the patient, and is much more common in advanced lung cancer than was previously recognized.[118] Dyspnea may be associated with destruction of lung tissue by tumor, pleural effusions, airway obstruction by endobronchial lesions, and increased mucus production. Palliation of dyspnea can be achieved in many cases with appropriate treatment.

Helping the patient cope with and manage dyspnea is a primary goal of nursing care. Teach the patient to assess patterns of occurrence including precipitating factors, duration, and relief measures. Help plan coping strategies including interventions such as relaxation techniques, controlled coughing techniques, oxygen administration, or position changes. Help the patient identify ways to conserve energy and minimize fatigue.[117]

Dyspnea in the individual with lung cancer is often associated with pleural effusion. Not all pleural effusions are malignant, and etiology should be established before palliative treatment is initiated. Large volumes of fluid can be removed by thoracentesis, which results in lung reexpansion unless the lung has become trapped by tumor.

When pleural effusions reaccumulate, as is often the case, pleurodesis is the recommended therapy.[119,120] A chest tube is inserted to completely drain the pleural space; then a sclerosing agent is instilled into the pleural space to obliterate the space and prevent reaccumulation of fluid. Agents used for pleurodesis include bleomycin, talc, doxycycline, and minocycline.[119] Tetracycline, formerly the most frequently used sclerosing agent, is no longer available in the injectable form. Because pleurodesis is a painful procedure, appropriate analgesics should be administered by the nurse. In cases of recurrent effusion, a pleuroperitoneal shunt can be inserted to divert fluid from the chest cavity to the abdomen[119] (see chapter 27).

## Pain

Pain is experienced by most individuals with lung cancer, and the prevalence increases as the disease advances.[121] Chest pain occurs in half of all patients with lung cancer and may be caused by mediastinal extension of tumor, pleural effusions, bronchial obstruction, or infection.[117] Bone pain is common, as is pain related to metastases to other distant sites. Many patients with lung cancer experience pain for more than a year prior to death. While not all patients experience pain as suffering, adequate pain control is clearly a key goal in promoting quality of life. Guidelines for cancer pain management have been published by the Agency for Health Care Policy and Research[122] and promote a well-researched approach to pain management with pharmacological and nonpharmacological interventions. Narcotic analgesics commonly used include morphine, hydromorphone, and fentanyl. Nonsteroidal anti-inflammatory drugs have been effective for metastatic bone pain.[123]

The key to pain management is its accurate assessment. Visual analogue scales, multidimensional instruments such as the McGill Pain Questionnaire, and pain flow sheets are helpful in assessing pain and evaluating the effectiveness of interventions. Wilkie and colleagues investigated if coaching patients to communicate pain in ways that clinicians recognize would reduce the discrepancy between patients' self-report of sensory pain and nurses' assessment of pain.[121] A trend toward improvement in percent agreement between patients and nurses was reported. A continued larger study now under way may have implications for patient education relative to communication of pain (see chapter 20).

## Fatigue

Disability related to fatigue and weakness has been reported to be the source of greatest suffering among persons with lung cancer.[116] Serious disruptions in physical functioning occur as the disease progresses. Difficulty with household chores, interference with work, reduced energy, and problems with ambulation and recreation are reported commonly.[124,125] These disruptions are often stressful and are a burden borne by the whole family. Anticipating difficulties can help the nurse prepare the patient and family for the course ahead of them.

The individual's feeling of fatigue is influenced by many factors—physiological, pathological, psychological, and behavioral. Significant correlations have been reported between pain and fatigue in individuals with lung cancer, and between fatigue and mood states as measured by the Profile of Mood States.[126] Regular assessments for fatigue should be performed regardless of age, stage of disease, or treatment. Interventions to control factors contributing to fatigue, such as pain, should be planned and implemented so that energy is restored rather than depleted. Patients' satisfaction with their level of functioning is the ultimate goal for quality of life (see chapter 23).

## Gastrointestinal Disturbances: Nausea/Vomiting, Anorexia/Cachexia, and Elimination

Nausea and vomiting related to the disease process in the person with lung cancer have several etiologies, including gastrointestinal obstruction, liver metastases, increased intracranial pressure from brain metastases, and narcotic analgesics. Metabolic disturbances related to paraneoplastic syndromes also may cause nausea. Often, treatment of the underlying causes can alleviate the symptoms. The array of effective antiemetic drugs in use today may also relieve nausea and promote comfort.

Anorexia and cancer cachexia are common manifestations of lung cancer.[127] The disease process itself, treatment complications, and psychological factors may all contribute to anorexia. Pain, fatigue, and dyspnea also interfere with the desire to eat. The cancer cachexia syndrome, manifested by weight loss, anorexia, taste changes, emaciation, and muscle wasting, is poorly understood. The patient may experience an increase in the basal metabolic rate and alterations in protein, fat, and carbohydrate metabolism.

As many as 50% of all individuals with lung cancer lose weight prior to their diagnosis, which is generally considered to be a poor prognostic factor.[128] Weight loss from cachexia is thought to first occur in the skeletal muscle and then adipose tissue, which helps explain the rapid impairment of functional status. In a study by Sarna and colleagues, weight loss in persons with lung cancer was greater in adults under 65, in patients with SCLC, and in those receiving chemotherapy.[127] Those who had experienced greater weight loss at the initiation of the study reported greater functional impairment and symptom distress. These findings can help the nurse identify individuals at high risk for weight loss and initiate early support strategies. Because eating and enjoyment of food are equated with health and wellness in our society, anorexia and weight loss can be particularly distressing to the patient and family. A thorough nutritional assessment and appropriate nutritional counseling and education can help to promote an improved quality of life. In addition to nursing strategies known to promote appetite, the drug megestrol acetate has been found to improve appetite and contribute to weight gain when administered orally to individuals with cancer.[123]

Constipation may occur as a result of any combination of factors such as medication side effects, inactivity, poor fluid intake, and lack of dietary fiber.[117] The patient taking narcotic analgesics is at high risk for constipation. Information obtained in the nursing assessment includes normal bowel patterns and any deviation from that pattern, medications, dietary factors that might affect elimination, and measures that relieved constipation in the past. The abdomen is examined for the presence of bowel sounds and any sign of distention.

Natural laxatives and dietary measures such as increased fiber and fluids can be recommended for mild constipation. For moderate to severe constipation, stronger laxatives, enemas, or digital disimpaction may be needed. The key to managing constipation is prevention. Many health care settings have implemented prophylactic bowel protocols developed by the multidisciplinary team.

## Psychosocial Issues

Given the current lack of success with curative treatment for lung cancer, many patients and their families will be confronted with the myriad of stressors and traumas that accompany a rapidly progressive fatal disease. Therefore, attention to psychosocial issues and care takes on great importance.[118]

The goal of nursing care relative to psychosocial issues is to foster appropriate coping responses of the patient and family members.[129] Identifying factors that have an impact on psychosocial adjustment can help guide nursing interventions. Klemm reported that patients who experienced greater demands of illness, including physical symptoms, issues of family functioning, and treatment issues, had lower psychosocial adjustment scores.[130] In a study of patients with SCLC, Cella and colleagues found that psychological distress was higher as performance status and extent of disease worsened.[131] Findings from a study of causal attribution, perceived control, and adjustment in patients with lung cancer suggest that when coping with a difficult disease like lung cancer it is the discovery of meaning in the disease that gives one a sense of mastery, regardless of whether the meaning or attributed cause of the cancer is external or internal. Helping the patient to talk and make sense of his or her experience may be the primary nursing intervention in promoting that sense of mastery.[132]

Fear and anxiety are common among individuals with lung cancer and have been associated with high degrees of suffering.[116] They may occur at various times throughout the illness, and one may precipitate the other. Specific fears may include fear of pain, fear of abandonment, fear of recurrence, fear of dependency, and fear of death.[129] Reassurance about the effectiveness of pain control measures can be of help to the patient and family. Fear of abandonment and separation from family, friends, and health care workers is pervasive. The patient should be encouraged to verbalize feelings of loss and grief related to unfulfilled desires and dreams, and leaving loved ones.

The recurrence of lung cancer can be a greater crisis than the initial diagnosis. Hope, often synonymous with life and living, is not as strong, and the patient and family may be at high risk for depression during this time.[129] Social withdrawal is common due to the disability associated with lung cancer,[133] and fears of inability to care for oneself and becoming dependent on loved ones may be particularly anxiety-provoking. Anxiety may be alleviated somewhat by emphasizing benefits of palliative treatment and by recognizing and affirming healthy, intact parts of the patient.[129]

Often the fear of dying is not as profound as the fear of suffering in the process of dying. An assessment of resources available to the patient and family and referral to supportive resources such as hospice or home health care may be appropriate. The patient should be allowed to explore fears, concerns, and wishes regarding death. Attentive listening and guidance can provide comfort and emotional healing. Sometimes just the quiet, accepting presence of the nurse can help ease the pain associated with fear and anxiety.

Major depression has been reported with greater frequency in persons with lung cancer than in healthy people.[133] Correlates of depression have included psychiatric history and the presence of metastatic disease. It is sometimes difficult for the clinician to distinguish between biological and psychological etiologies for depression in individuals with lung cancer. Side effects from the disease or treatment such as extreme fatigue, anorexia, and sleep disorders may be confused with symptoms of depression, and vice versa. Brain metastases cause symptoms that are mistaken for psychological distress. In SCLC, ectopic corticotropin production can produce manic episodes.[133] All possibilities should be considered when the patient presents with altered mood or behavior.

Although the database relating to psychological distress in persons with lung cancer is small, experience with this population indicates that the needs are great. Unfortunately, current lung cancer educational materials do not adequately address psychosocial issues and require tenth-grade or higher-level reading skills.[134] Early intervention using a multidisciplinary team approach can assure that the patient and family receive thorough education on all aspects of the disease and treatment, referrals for counseling and support groups, and information about other resources that promote psychological, social, and spiritual well-being.

## CONTINUITY OF CARE: NURSING CHALLENGES

With the current chaos in health care delivery systems, challenges to continuity of care have never been greater. Central to the challenge is seamless access to high-quality care for the patient and family and a systematic flow of information to all care providers from diagnosis until resolution of the illness. Access to care can be impeded by competition for patients and territoriality among agencies. In addition, individuals without insurance or with restricted coverage may have to go without much-needed services or pay out of pocket.[135] The nurse caring for the patient with lung cancer is often at the organizational hub of the care continuum and can play a major role in ensuring that appropriate communication and coordination of care take place and that, through collaboration, effective negotiation around barriers to care can occur.

Most individuals with lung cancer will have episodic

care in the hospital. A plan for continuity of care should be initiated on admission. While there are many care delivery models, continuous communication among all members of the health care team should be a priority. Communication is promoted through the use of multidisciplinary discharge planning team conferences, case management critical pathways, multidisciplinary documentation tools, and written communication to referral agencies upon discharge. Many acute care agencies use a discharge planning nurse or a case manager to assume primary responsibility for coordination of care. Gaps in care may occur when appropriate referrals are not made or when important information is not communicated in a timely manner to subsequent care providers.

Today, most treatment for lung cancer is administered in the outpatient setting. The complexity of treatment requires that the nurse not only be skilled technically but also be able to perform a comprehensive patient and family assessment to develop a plan of care for the patient to follow at home.[136] Education about self-care must be provided, and other care resources coordinated. Many larger cancer centers utilize a comprehensive approach to the treatment of lung cancer by having practitioners from multiple disciplines collaborate on a treatment and follow-up plan.[137] State-of-the-art services, including rehabilitation and support services, can be tailored to the individual needs of the patient.

It is the nurse in the ambulatory care setting who is positioned to facilitate continuity of care over a period of months or years. Since transitions into new care settings can be particularly stressful for the patient as the illness progresses, the outpatient or office nurse can be a familiar and comforting touchstone, providing reassurance and preventing feelings of abandonment and despair. Often a referral to home health care or hospice is appropriate for the person with lung cancer. Arranging opportunities for contact with the new agency before the transition actually takes place creates a linkage between the care settings and promotes a feeling of control and orientation for the patient and family. Most home care nurses are trained to administer chemotherapy in the home setting, and all are required to manage the complex symptoms and side effects that are associated with lung cancer and its treatment. Communication back to the referring physician is vital in maximizing opportunities for successful management of care in the home.

When medical care for the person with lung cancer shifts from curative to palliative, the patient and family must choose a care setting. Home or hospice care can provide familiar surroundings, feelings of normalcy, involvement of family, and less cost,[117] although not all individuals have family members or friends who are willing or able to provide care. Although hospice has proved to be an extremely effective model for terminal care, referrals to a hospice often are not made until the final days or hours of life. The difficulty lies in predicting when death will occur, since Medicare reimbursement requires that a hospice patient have a life expectancy of six months

or less. A case manager or other nurse responsible for coordination of care can help to make more timely referrals to hospice because of familiarity with the patient and improved communication among all care providers.

Regardless of the setting, self-care should be promoted along the continuum of care. Most effects of lung cancer and its treatment will be experienced in the home, and the patient and family must be taught how to manage them. A learning needs assessment should be conducted, with particular attention to willingness, desire, and ability to learn. Barriers to learning, such as illiteracy and environmental and social factors, should be assessed. Supportive resources for self-care should be provided as required by the individual situation. Patients will be able to manage less self-care as the disease progresses, and family members will require education with demonstration of care techniques, return demonstration, and opportunities for questions and verbalization of feelings about caring for the one who is ill.

## CONCLUSION

Despite discouraging survival statistics for lung cancer, there is reason for optimism as one considers the disease trajectory. Emphasis on primary and secondary prevention will decrease the incidence and prevalence. Discoveries in chemoprevention and early identification of premalignant lung cells increase our hope for effective early intervention. Promising new chemotherapeutic agents and multimodality treatments are improving cure and control rates. Increasingly effective strategies for palliative care, including pain control, symptom management, and emotional support, are serving to promote comfort and well-being during the final days of life. The nurse has opportunities at every juncture of the patient's care for clinical practice, education, and research. Each role will have increasing importance as the fight against this epidemic disease escalates.

## REFERENCES

1. Lee-Chiong TL, Matthay RA: Lung cancer in the elderly patient. *Clin Chest Med* 14:453–472, 1993
2. Samet JM: The epidemiology of lung cancer. *Chest* 103: 20S–29S, 1993 (suppl)
3. Dumas L: Lung cancer in women. *Nurs Clin North Am* 27: 859–869, 1992
4. Gilliland FD, Samet JM: Lung Cancer. *Cancer Surv* 19: 175–195, 1994
5. American Cancer Society: *Cancer Facts and Figures—1996.* Atlanta, American Cancer Society, 1996
6. Parker SL, Tong T, Bolden S, et al: Cancer statistics, 1996. *CA Cancer J Clin* 46:5–27, 1996

7. Nathan FE: Introduction. *Semin Oncol* 20:103–104, 1993

8. Franklin RA: Smoking. *Nurs Clin North Am* 27:631–642, 1992

9. Chyou P, Nomura AM, Stemmermann GN: A prospective study of the attributable risk of cancer due to cigarette smoking. *Am J Public Health* 82:37–40, 1992

10. Glover J, Miaskowski C: Small cell lung cancer: Pathophysiologic mechanisms and nursing implications. *Oncol Nurs Forum* 21:87–95, 1994

11. Potanovich LM: Lung cancer: Prevention and detection update. *Semin Oncol* 9:174–179, 1993

12. Seale DD, Beaver BM: Pathophysiology of lung cancer. *Nurs Clin North Am* 27:603–613, 1992

13. Wynder E, Kabat GC: The effect of low yield cigarette smoking on lung cancer risk. *Cancer* 62:1223–1230, 1988

14. Davis R: Current trends in cigarette advertising marketing. *N Engl J Med* 316:725–732, 1987

15. Tredaniel J, Boffetta P, Saracci R, et al: Exposure to environmental tobacco smoke and risk of lung cancer: The epidemiological evidence. *Eur Respir J* 7:1877–1888, 1994

16. U.S. Environmental Protection Agency: *Respiratory Health Effects of Passive Smoking: Lung Cancer and Other Disorders.* EPA/600/6–90/006 F. Washington, DC, Office of Research and Development, 1992

17. Burns DM: Environmental tobacco smoke: The price of scientific certainty. *J Natl Cancer Inst* 84:1387–1388, 1992

18. Janerich DT, Thompson WD, Varela LR, et al: Lung cancer and exposure to tobacco smoke in the household. *N Engl J Med* 323:632–636, 1990

19. Ginsberg RJ, Kris MG, Armstrong JG: Non–small cell lung cancer, in DeVita VT, Hellman S, Rosenberg SA (eds): *Cancer: Principles and Practice of Oncology* (ed 4). Philadelphia, Lippincott, 1993, pp 673–722

20. Kishimoto T, Okada K: The relationship between lung cancer and asbestos exposure. *Chest* 94:486–490, 1988

21. Omenn GS, Goodman GE, Thornquist MD, et al: Effects of a combination of beta carotene and vitamin A on lung cancer and cardiovascular disease. *N Engl J Med* 334:1150–1155, 1996

22. Hennekens CH, Buring JE, Manson JE, et al: Lack of effect of long-term supplementation with beta carotene on the incidence of malignant neoplasms and cardiovascular disease. *N Engl J Med* 334:1145–1149, 1996

23. MacKenzie TD, Bartecchi CE, Schrier RW: The human costs of tobacco use: Part II. *N Engl J Med* 330:975–980, 1994

24. Itri L: Women and lung cancer. *Public Health Rep Suppl* 102:92–96, 1987

25. Ernster VL: Women and smoking. *Am J Public Health* 83:1202–1203, 1993 (editorial)

26. Fischer PM, Schwartz MP, Richards JW, et al: Brand logo recognition by children, aged 3 to 6 years: Mickey Mouse and Old Joe the camel. *JAMA* 266:3145–3153, 1991

27. Fiore MC, Novotny TE, Pierre JP, et al: Trends in cigarette smoking in the United States: The changing influence of gender and race. *JAMA* 261:49–55, 1989

28. Carroll-Johnson RM: Smoke screen. *Oncol Nurs Forum* 22:1331, 1995 (editorial)

29. Aisner J, Belani CP: Lung cancer: Recent changes and expectations of improvements. *Semin Oncol* 20:383–393, 1993

30. Rose MA: Intervention strategies for smoking cessation: The role of oncology nursing. *Cancer Nurs* 14:225–231, 1991

31. Risser NL: The key to prevention of lung cancer: Stop smoking. *Semin Oncol Nurs* 3:228–236, 1987

32. Miller NH: Tips for smoking cessation. *Heart Dis and Stroke* 2:5–7, 1993

33. Stanislaw A, Wewers ME: A smoking cessation intervention with hospitalized surgical cancer patients: A pilot study. *Cancer Nurs* 17:81–86, 1994

34. The Agency for Health Care Policy and Research Smoking Cessation Clinical Practice Guideline. *JAMA* 275:1270–1280, 1996

35. Manley M, Epps RP, Husten C, et al: Clinical interventions in tobacco control: A National Cancer Institute training program for physicians. *JAMA* 266:3172–3173, 1991

36. Hollis JF, Lichtenstein E, Vogt TM, et al: Nurse-assisted counseling for smokers in primary care. *Ann Intern Med* 118:521–525, 1993

37. Fiore MC: The new vital sign: Assessing and documenting smoking status. *JAMA* 266:3183–3184, 1991

38. Lerman C, Orleans CT, Engstrom PF: Biological markers in smoking cessation treatment. *Semin Oncol* 20:359–367, 1993

39. Risser NL, Belcher DW: Adding spirometry, carbon monoxide, and pulmonary symptom results to smoking cessation counseling: A randomized trial. *J Gen Intern Med* 5:16–22, 1990

40. Velicer WF, Prochaska JO, Rossi JS, et al: Assessing outcome in smoking cessation studies. *Psychol Bull* 111:35–41, 1992

41. Hurt RD, Lowell CD, Fredrickson PA, et al: Nicotine patch therapy for smoking cessation combined with physician advice and nurse follow-up. *JAMA* 271:595–600, 1994

42. Heatherton TF, Kozlowski LT, Frecker RC, et al: The Fagerstrom test for nicotine dependence: A revision of the Fagerstrom tolerance questionnaire. *B J Addict* 86:1119–1127, 1991

43. Fowler JS, Volkow ND, Wang GJ, et al: Inhibition of monoamine oxidase B in the brains of smokers. *Nature* 379:733–736, 1996

44. Huber MH, Lee JS, Hong WK: Chemoprevention of lung cancer. *Semin Oncol* 20:128–141, 1993

45. Lippman SM, Benner SE, Hong WK: Chemoprevention strategies in lung carcinogenesis. *Chest* 103:15S–19S, 1993 (suppl)

46. Goodman GE: Chemoprophylaxis strategies in high-risk groups with an emphasis on lung cancer. *Chest* 103:60S–62S, 1993 (suppl)

47. Bunn PA: Future directions in clinical research for lung cancer. *Chest* 106:399S–407S, 1994 (suppl)

48. Christenson P, Joergensen K, Munk J, et al: Hyperfrequency of pulmonary cancer in a population of 415 patients treated for laryngeal cancer. *Laryngoscope* 97:612–614, 1987

49. Hong WK, Lippman SM, Itri LM, et al: Prevention of second primary tumors with isotretinoin in squamous-cell carcinoma of the head and neck. *N Engl J Med* 323:795–801, 1990

50. Szabo E, Birrer MJ, Mulshine JL: Early detection of lung cancer. *Semin Oncol* 20:374–382, 1993

51. Feld R, Ginsberg RJ, Payne DG, et al: Lung, in Abeloff MD, Armitage JO, Lichter AS, Niederhuber JE (eds): *Clinical Oncology.* New York: Churchill Livingstone, 1995, pp 1083–1152

52. Mulshine JL, Treston AM, Brown PH, et al: Initiators and promoters of lung cancer. *Chest* 103:4S–9S, 1993 (suppl)

53. Tockman MS, Gupta PK, Myers JD, et al: Sensitive and specific monoclonal antibody recognition of human lung cancer antigen on preserved sputum cells: A new approach to early lung cancer detection. *J Clin Oncol* 6:1685–1693, 1988

54. Chia MM, Gazdar AF, Carbone DP, et al: Biology of lung cancer, in Murray JF, Nadel JA (eds): *Textbook of Respiratory Medicine* (ed 2). Philadelphia, Saunders, 1994, pp 1485–1503

55. Elpern EH: Lung cancer, in Groenwald SL, Frogge MH, Goodman M, Yarbro CH (eds): *Cancer Nursing: Principles and Practice* (ed 3). Boston, Jones and Bartlett, 1993, pp 1174–1199

56. Kotin P: Carcinogenesis of the lung, in Liebow AA, Smith DE (eds): *The Lung*. Baltimore, Williams and Wilkins, 1968 pp 203–225

57. Ihde DC, Pass HI, Glatstein EJ: Small cell lung cancer, in DeVita VT, Hellman S, Rosenberg SA (eds): *Cancer: Principles and Practice of Oncology* (ed 4). Philadelphia: Lippincott, 1993, pp 723–758

58. McCue PA, Finkel GC: Small-cell lung carcinoma: An evolving histopathological spectrum. *Semin Oncol* 20:153–162, 1993

59. Richardson GE, Johnson BE: The biology of lung cancer. *Semin Oncol* 20:105–127, 1993

60. Johnson BE, Kelley MJ: Biology of small cell lung cancer. *Lung Cancer* 12:S5–S16, 1995 (suppl)

61. Epps ME: Diagnostic testing for patients with lung cancer. *Nurs Clin North Am* 27:615–629, 1992

62. Holmes CE, Livingston R, Turrisi A: Neoplasms of the thorax, in Holland JF, Frei E, Bast RC, Kufe DW, Morton DL, Weichselbaum RR (eds): *Cancer Medicine* (ed 3). Malvern, PA, Lea and Febiger, 1993, pp 1285–1336

63. Murray MJ, Stewart JR, Johnson DH: Superior vena cava syndrome, in Abeloff MD, Armitage JO, Lichter AS, Niederhuber JE (eds): *Clinical Oncology*. New York, Churchill Livingstone, 1995, pp 609–618

64. Greenberg S, Kosinski R, Daniels J: Treatment of SVC thrombosis with rTPA. *Chest* 99:1298–1301, 1991

65. Dietz KA, Flaherty AM: Oncologic emergencies, in Groenwald SL, Frogge MH, Goodman M, Yarbro CH (eds): *Cancer Nursing: Principles and Practice* (ed, 3). Boston, Jones and Bartlett, 1993, pp 800–839

66. Pancrazio JJ, Viglione MP, Tabbara IA, et al: Voltage-dependent ion channels in small-cell lung cancer cells. *Cancer Res* 49:5901–5906, 1989

67. Sanders DB: Lambert-Eaton myasthenic syndrome: Pathogenesis and treatment. *Semin Neurol* 14:111–117, 1994

68. Struthers CS: Lambert-Eaton myasthenic syndrome in small cell lung cancer: Nursing implications. *Oncol Nurs Forum* 21:677–683, 1994

69. Assessment of the respiratory system, in Malasanos L, Barkauskas V, Stoltenberg-Allen K (eds): *Health Assessment* (ed 4). St. Louis, Mosby, 1990, 297–324

70. Patient assessment, in DesJardins T, Burton GG (eds): *Clinical Manifestations and Assessment of Respiratory Disease* (ed 3). St. Louis, Mosby-Year Book, 1995, pp 3–118

71. Shure D: Fiberoptic bronchoscopy: Diagnostic applications. *Clin Chest Med* 8:1–13, 1987

72. Sugarbaker DJ, Strauss GM: Advances in surgical staging and therapy of non–small-cell lung cancer. *Semin Oncol* 20: 163–172, 1993

73. Rea HH, Sherland JE, House AJS: Accuracy of computed tomographic scanning in assessment of the mediastinum in bronchial carcinoma. *J Thorac Cardiovasc Surg* 81:825–829, 1981

74. Buccheri G, Ferrigno GB: Prognostic factors in lung cancer: Tables and comments. *Eur Respir J* 7:1350–1364, 1994

75. Souhami RL, Law K: A report to the lung cancer subcommittee of the United Kingdom coordinating committee for cancer research. *Br J Cancer* 61:584–589, 1990

76. Shepherd FA: Treatment of advanced non–small cell lung cancer. *Semin Oncol* 21:7–18, 1994 (suppl 7)

77. Stitik FP: The new staging of lung cancer. *Radiol Clin North Am* 32:635–647, 1994

78. Lung, in Beahrs OH, Henson DE, Hutter RVP, Kennedy BJ (eds): *Handbook for Staging of Cancer* (ed 4). Philadelphia, Lippincott, 1993, pp 132–133

79. Lederle FA, Niewoehner DE: Lung cancer surgery: A critical review of the evidence. *Arch Intern Med* 154:2397–2400, 1994

80. Langston WG: Surgical resection of lung cancer. *Nurs Clin North Am* 27:665–679, 1992

81. Harpole DH, Herndon JE, Young WG, et al: Stage I non-small cell lung cancer: A multivariate analysis of treatment methods and patterns of recurrence. *Cancer* 76:787–796, 1995

82. Pearson FG: Current status of surgical resection for lung cancer. *Chest* 106:337S–339S, 1994 (suppl)

83. Ginsberg RJ, Rubinstein L: The comparison of limited resection to lobectomy for T1N0 non–small cell lung cancer: LCSG 821. *Chest* 106:318S–319S, 1994

84. Beattie EJ, Harvey JC, Pisch J: Lung, in Beattie EJ, Bloom N, Harvey J (eds): *Thoracic Surgical Oncology*. New York, Churchill Livingstone, 1992, pp 27–185

85. Stewart GS: Trends in radiation therapy for the treatment of lung cancer. *Nurs Clin North Am* 27:643–651, 1992

86. Belani CP: Multimodality management of regionally advanced non–small-cell lung cancer. *Semin Oncol* 20: 302–314, 1993

87. Hazuka MB, Turrisi AT: The evolving role of radiation therapy in the treatment of locally advanced lung cancer. *Semin Oncol* 20:173–184, 1993

88. Sause WT, Scott C, Taylor S, et al: Radiation Therapy Oncology Group (RTOG) 88-08 and Eastern Cooperative Oncology Group (ECOG) 4588: Preliminary results of a phase III trial in regionally advanced, unresectable non–small cell lung cancer. *J Natl Cancer Inst* 87:198–205, 1995

89. Turrisi AT: Innovations in multimodality therapy for lung cancer: Combined modality management of limited small-cell lung cancer. *Chest* 103:56S–59S, 1993 (suppl)

90. Harris DT: Prophylactic cranial irradiation in small-cell lung cancer. *Semin Oncol* 20:338–350, 1993

91. Kristjansen PEG, Hansen HH: Prophylactic cranial irradiation in small cell lung cancer: An update. *Lung Cancer* 12: S23–S40, 1995 (suppl)

92. Gustafson G, Vicini F, Freedman L, et al: High dose rate endobronchial brachytherapy in the management of primary and recurrent bronchogenic malignancies. *Cancer* 75:2345–2350, 1995

93. Jordan LN, Mantravadi R: Nursing care of the patient receiving high dose rate brachytherapy. *Oncol Nurs Forum* 18:1167–1171, 1991

94. Khanavkar B, Stern P, Alberti W, et al: Complications associated with brachytherapy alone or with laser in lung cancer. *Chest* 99:1062–1065, 1991

95. Larson PJ, Lindsey AM, Dodd MJ, et al: Influence of age on problems experienced by patients with lung cancer

undergoing radiation therapy. *Oncol Nurs Forum* 20: 473–480, 1993

96. Brown JK: Gender, age, usual weight, and tobacco use as predictors of weight loss in patients with lung cancer. *Oncol Nurs Forum* 20:466–472, 1993

97. Evans WK: Management of metastatic non–small-cell lung cancer and a consideration of cost. *Chest* 103:68S–71S, 1993

98. Feigal EG, Christian M, Cheson B, et al: New chemotherapeutic agents in non–small-cell lung cancer. *Semin Oncol* 20:185–201, 1993

99. Shepherd FA: Future directions in the treatment of non–small cell lung cancer. *Semin Oncol* 21:48–62, 1994 (suppl 4)

100. Faber LP: Current status of neoadjuvant therapy for non–small cell lung cancer. *Chest* 106:355S–358S, 1994 (suppl)

101. Livingston RB: Current management of unresectable non–small cell lung cancer. *Semin Oncol* 21:4–13, 1994

102. Johnson DH, Einhorn LH: Paclitaxel plus carboplatin: An effective combination chemotherapy for advanced non–small-cell lung cancer or just another Elvis sighting? *J Clin Oncol* 13:1840–1842, 1995 (editorial)

103. Doyle LA: Mechanisms of drug resistance in human lung cancer cells. *Semin Oncol* 20:326–337, 1993

104. Vokes EE: Integration of vinorelbine into chemotherapy strategies for non–small-cell lung cancer. *Oncology* 9: 565–582, 1995

105. Eckardt J, Eckhardt G, Villalona-Calero M, et al: New anticancer agents in clinical development. *Oncology* 9: 1191–1199, 1995

106. Langer CJ, Leighton JC, Comis RL, et al: Paclitaxel and carboplatin in combination in the treatment of advanced non–small-cell lung cancer: A phase II toxicity, response, and survival analysis. *J Clin Oncol* 13:1860–1870, 1995

107. Viallet J, Ayoub J, Rousseau P, et al: Vinorelbine (Navelbine) in the adjuvant and neoadjuvant treatment of non–small cell lung cancer. *Semin Oncol* 21:64–72, 1994 (suppl 10)

108. Johnson DH: Recent developments in chemotherapy treatment of small-cell lung cancer. *Semin Oncol* 20:315–325, 1993

109. Blackstein ME: Advances in chemotherapy for small cell lung cancer. *Semin Oncol* 21:38–42, 1994

110. Kosmidis PA, Samantas E, Fountzilas G, et al: Cisplatin/etoposide versus carboplatin/etoposide chemotherapy and irradiation in small cell lung cancer: A randomized phase III study. *Semin Oncol* 21:23–30, 1994

111. Johnson DH: Treatment of the elderly patient with small-cell lung cancer. *Chest* 103:72S–74S, 1993 (suppl)

112. Pate RW: The role of chemotherapy in the treatment of lung cancer. *Nurs Clin North Am* 27:653–663, 1992

113. Fishbein GE: Immunotherapy of lung cancer. *Semin Oncol* 20:351–358, 1993

114. Lam S: Photodynamic therapy of lung cancer. *Semin Oncol* 21:15–19, 1994

115. Gelb AF, Epstein JD: Laser in treatment of lung cancer. *Chest* 86:662–666, 1984

116. Benedict S: The suffering associated with lung cancer. *Cancer Nurs* 12:34–40, 1989

117. Turner JT: Nursing care of the terminal lung cancer patient. *Nurs Clin North Am* 27:691–702, 1992

118. Bernhard J, Ganz PA: Psychosocial issues in lung cancer patients (part 1). *Chest* 99:216–223, 1991

119. Keller SM: Current and future therapy for malignant pleural effusion. *Chest* 103:63S–67S, 1993 (suppl)

120. Sahn SA: Malignant effusions. *Emerg Med* 23(5): 119–126, 1991

121. Wilkie DJ, Williams AR, Grevstad P, et al: Coaching persons with lung cancer to report sensory pain. *Cancer Nurs* 18: 7–15, 1995

122. Management of Cancer Pain Panel: *Management of Cancer Pain.* U.S. Department of Health and Human Services, Agency for Health Care Policy and Research publication No. 94-0593. Rockville, MD, 1994

123. Schmitt R: Quality of life issues in lung cancer: New symptom management strategies. *Chest* 103:51S–55S, 1993 (suppl)

124. Sarna L: Functional status in women with lung cancer. *Cancer Nurs* 17:87–93, 1994

125. Sarna L: Fluctuations in physical function: Adults with non–small cell lung cancer. *J Adv Nurs* 18:714–724, 1993

126. Blesch KS, Paice JA, Wickham R, et al: Correlates of fatigue in people with breast or lung cancer. *Oncol Nurs Forum* 18: 81–87, 1991

127. Sarna L, Lindsey AM, Dean H, et al: Nutritional intake, weight change, symptom distress, and functional status over time in adults with lung cancer. *Oncol Nurs Forum* 20: 481–489, 1993

128. Dewys WD, Begg C, Lavin PT, et al: Prognostic effect of weight loss prior to chemotherapy in cancer patients. *Am J Med* 69:491–497, 1980

129. Houston SJ, Kendall JA: Psychosocial implications of lung cancer. *Nurs Clin North Am* 27:681–690, 1992

130. Klemm PR: Variables influencing psychosocial adjustment in lung cancer: A preliminary study. *Oncol Nurs Forum* 21: 1059–1062, 1994

131. Cella DF, Orofiamma B, Holland JC, et al: The relationship of psychologic distress, extent of disease, and performance status in patients with lung cancer. *Cancer* 60:1661–1667, 1987

132. Berckman KL, Austin JK: Causal attribution, perceived control and adjustment in patients with lung cancer. *Oncol Nurs Forum* 20:23–30, 1993

133. Bernhard J, Ganz PA: Psychosocial issues in lung cancer patients (part 2). *Chest* 99:480–485, 1991

134. Sarna L, Ganley BJ: A survey of lung cancer patient-education materials. *Oncol Nurs Forum* 22:1545–1550, 1995

135. Beddar SM, Aikin JL: Continuity of care: A challenge for ambulatory oncology nursing. *Semin Oncol Nurs* 10: 254–263, 1994

136. Rostad M: Advances in nursing management of patients with lung cancer. *Nurs Clin North Am* 25:393–403, 1990

137. An update on the new USC/Norris Lung Cancer Management Center. *Cope,* July/August, 1995, 16–17

# Chapter 43

# Malignant Lymphomas

Connie Henke Yarbro, RN, MS, FAAN

Mary Ellen McFadden, RN, MLA, OCN®

## INTRODUCTION

The malignant lymphomas constitute a diverse group of neoplasms that arise from the uncontrolled proliferation of the cellular components of the lymphoreticular system. This complex network of specialized cells and organs defends the body against infection. Malignancies of the immune system may present locally; however, the majority are widespread at the time of diagnosis, presumably because of the natural ability of the immune cells to circulate. Based on histologic characteristics, the lymphomas are divided into two major subgroups—Hodgkin's disease (HD) and non-Hodgkin's lymphoma (NHL). Some suggest that the term *lymphocytic lymphoma* be ascribed to the latter because it emphasizes the essential role that lymphocyte transformation has in its ontogeny. However, both terms are equally acceptable, and since *NHL* is used most frequently in practice and in the literature, it is selected for this chapter.

Lymphomas are among the most studied human tumors, and determination of their immunophenotypes, gene rearrangements, cytogenetic abnormalities, and oncogene activation are providing valuable clues about the inherent mechanisms of the neoplastic process itself. Also, some are considered to be among the most curable of all malignancies. Impetus for this clinical success is provided by therapeutic advances using combination chemotherapy, chemotherapy plus radiation therapy, and ablative chemotherapy followed by bone marrow transplantation in patients with refractory disease.

Despite a number of shared superficial similarities, the distinctions between HD and NHL are important because their clinical courses, prognoses, and treatments are substantially different. Indeed, controversy truly begins at the cellular level with an unresolved debate about their respective cells of origin. Although several distinct T-cell lymphomas have been identified, B-cell neoplasms account for the majority of non-Hodgkin's lymphomas. A variety of candidates have been proposed for the originating cell in HD, including lymphocytes (T and B), monocytes-macrophages, and interdigitating reticulum cells.[1] At least some HD have a B-lymphocyte as the cell of origin based on immunoglobulin gene rearrangements.[2] The Epstein-Barr virus (EBV) seems to be related to transformation in some but not all cases of HD.[3]

The clinical behavior of the malignant lymphomas is highly variable. Some patients follow a rapid downhill course, with progressive generalized adenopathy, fever, night sweats, splenomegaly, and infiltration of the bone marrow, lungs, liver, and other organs with proliferative neoplastic cells. Death occurs within one to two years of diagnosis and usually results from infection, hemorrhage due to tumor-induced destruction of the bone marrow, or systemic failure of vital organ function. Other individuals follow a more indolent course in which the disease is apparently limited to the lymph nodes for many years. Eventually the malignant process becomes more aggressive, and invasion of extranodal organs requires a revision in management strategies.

Recent statistical analysis indicates that the incidence of lymphomas, particularly NHL, is escalating, and it has now become the fifth most common cancer in the United States. Incidence in 1996 is estimated at nearly 53,000 newly diagnosed cases and the annual mortality rate is expected to reach 23,310.[4] A major factor contributing to this increase is the established association between NHL and the acquired immunodeficiency syndrome (AIDS) caused by the retrovirus known as human immunodeficiency virus (HIV). Advances in antiviral therapy and treatment or prophylaxis against opportunistic infections have resulted in the prolonged survival of AIDS patients, and a substantial increase in secondary NHL has been noted in the AIDS population. Gail et al[5] estimated that between 8% and 27% of all 1992 cases of NHL would be attributable to this syndrome. There is, in addition to the NHL in the AIDS population, an independent and dramatic increase in NHL that began before the AIDS epidemic, the cause of which is unknown.[6] Thus, this malignancy truly has the potential to become an increasing burden and challenge to health care systems well into the twenty-first century.

In an effort to help oncology nurses effect optimal patient care and education, this chapter will provide comprehensive information about the etiology, classifications, clinical manifestations, staging, diagnosis, and therapeutic management of HD and NHL. Treatment and disease-related complications as well as important issues related to survivorship will also be addressed.

## THE IMMUNE SYSTEM AND NEOPLASIA

The immune system is a highly integrated, complex mechanism that has evolved to help the body protect itself against foreign tissues and invading microbes such as viruses, bacteria, fungi, and parasites. It distinguishes such threats from normal tissue by recognizing invasive antigens or foreign molecules as "nonself" and seeks to eliminate or destroy them by mounting an appropriate response via the formation of antigen-specific protein antibodies.[7] The organs of the immune system are scattered throughout the body and are generally referred to as *lymphatic* or *lymphoid* organs because they are concerned with the growth, development, and deployment of T- and B-lymphocytes. These white blood cells are the key operatives of immune function and the primary cellular component of malignant lymphomas. The lymphoid organs as illustrated in Figure 43-1 include the spleen, bone marrow, thymus, lymph nodes, tonsils, adenoids, appendix, and clumps of lymphoid tissue in the small intestine known as Peyer's patches. The blood and lymphatic vessels that transport lymphocytes also can be considered part of this system.

Lymph is derived from interstitial fluid and flows

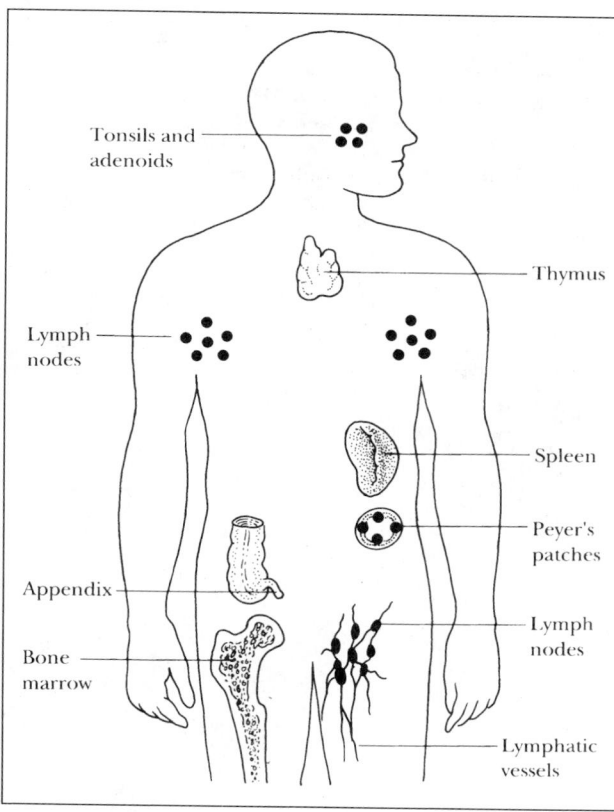

**FIGURE 43-1** Organs of the immune system. (Illustrated by J. Thommen.)

through lymphatic vessels transporting immune cells and foreign antigens to the circulatory system via the thoracic duct. Along its course, detritus is filtered out of lymph by the lymph nodes. These small, encapsulated clusters in the neck, axilla, abdomen, and groin (Figure 43-2) have a very specific structure and contain specialized compartments that facilitate lymphocyte maturation and differentiation. T-lymphocytes are selectively concentrated in the paracortical regions of the lymph node and within the periarterial lymphoid sheaths of the spleen. Small numbers of T-cells are also found within the follicles, where they facilitate B-cell differentiation. On the other hand, B-lymphocytes are concentrated in the follicles and medullary cords of the lymph nodes and in the follicles of the spleen. The lymphoid follicles represent the proliferative site of the B-cell system, and the medullary cord region represents its secretory component. Monocytes circulate in the peripheral blood, while histiocytes are preferentially found in the subcapsular and medullary sinuses of the lymph nodes and the red pulp of the spleen. Figure 43-3 depicts normal lymph node architecture and the areas associated with lymphoid localization and malignant transformation.

Lymphomas are preeminently a malignancy of the lymphocyte, and the process by which a lymphoid neoplasm is generated may be thought of as a series of cellular changes whereby a once normal lymphoid cell (or cell clone) becomes refractory to the regulation of its differentiation and proliferation. These changes are, of necessity, genetic, whether induced by mutation, chromosomal translocation/deletion, or insertion of foreign genes (e.g., viral genes) into the cell. Translocations generally result in altered expression of an adjacent gene. Deletions may cause loss of genes necessary for appropriate cellular regulation and differentiation. Mutations could stimulate either of these effects, while viruses are likely to enhance modification of adjacent genes by viral promotion/enhancement or of distant genes via viral transactivation.[7]

Once transformed, the new clone of malignant cells follows the behavior pattern of the stage at which lymphocyte alteration took place. For example, if the function of the maturing lymphocyte is secretion of an antibody protein, the tumor cells will continue to secrete the normal protein, albeit in abnormal quantities. In this case a faulty regulatory mechanism and not abnormal cell proliferation is responsible for the neoplastic change. However, if the function at the time of transformation is for the lymphocytes to form maturing nodules in the lymph nodes, their excessive production will result in nodular lymphoma.

The association of certain malignancies with congenital or acquired immunodeficiency diseases and the bimodal distribution of cancer in the very young and the very old suggests that an immature or debilitated immune system predisposes to neoplasia.[8] Malignant lymphomas are linked strongly with congenital immunodeficiency disorders such as Wiskott-Aldrich syndrome, Klinefelter syndrome, and ataxia telangiectasia. The chronic inflammatory process activated by many autoimmune diseases (e.g., rheumatoid arthritis, systemic lupus erythematosus, and Sjögren syndrome) predisposes an individual to lymphomas of extranodal origin. Renal, cardiac, and other organ transplants also have been found to increase risk.[9] Such tumors usually occur in the first year following transplant; they are rapidly progressive and frequently involve the central nervous system. Definitive cause of these lymphomas is unknown, but viral infection, drug-induced immunosuppression, and chronic antigenic stimulation from the graft may be contributing factors.

## MATURATION OF THE LYMPHOCYTE

The origin of the lymphocyte can be traced to a pluripotent stem cell in the bone marrow that has the potential to develop into any of the cells that normally circulate in the blood. At each step along the path of differentiation, a cell loses its capacity to proceed along an alternate route. In the first step, the stem cell matures so that it is either the precursor of the lymphocyte series or of all the other cellular series of the blood (erythrocyte, megakaryocyte, polymorphonuclear neutrophil, or monocyte). The lymphocyte precursor then develops into one of a number

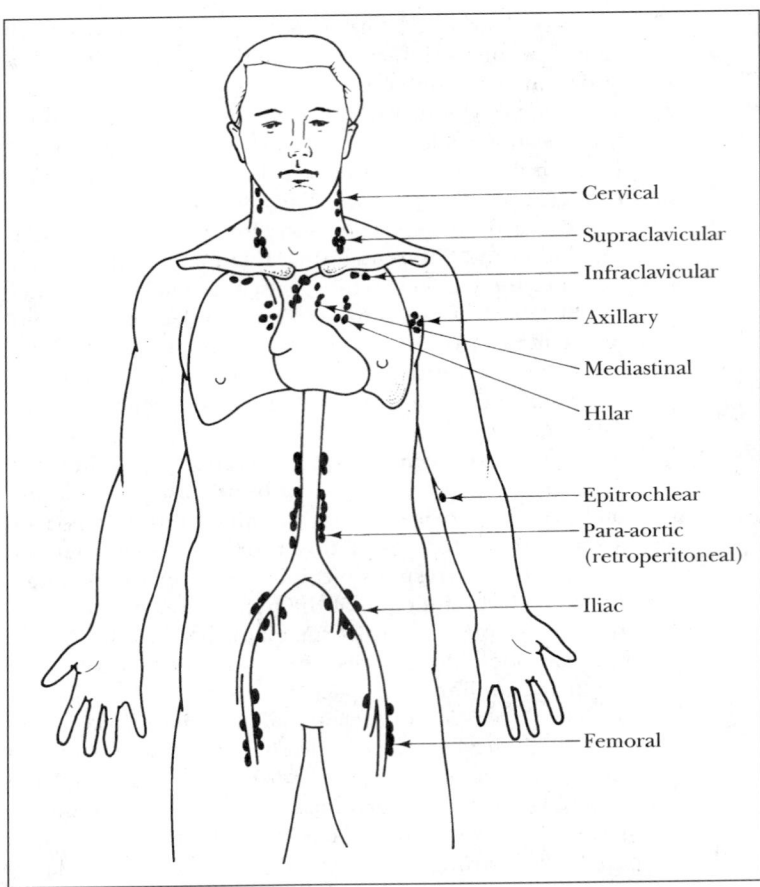

**FIGURE 43-2** Major lymph node groups. (Yarbro CH: Lymphomas, in Groenwald SL, Frogge MH, Goodman M, Yarbro CH [eds]: *Cancer Nursing: Principles and Practice* [ed 2]. Boston, Jones and Bartlett, 1990. Reprinted with permission.)

Cervical
Supraclavicular
Infraclavicular
Axillary
Mediastinal
Hilar
Epitrochlear
Para-aortic (retroperitoneal)
Iliac
Femoral

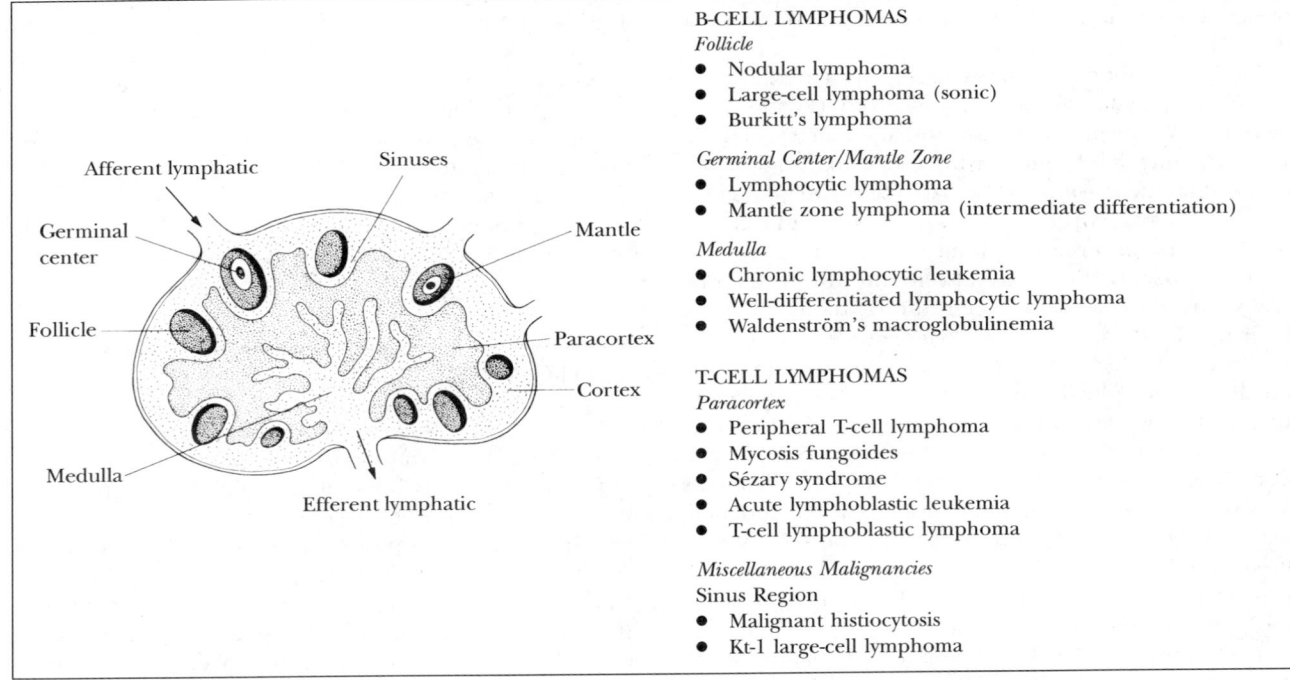

Afferent lymphatic
Sinuses
Germinal center
Mantle
Follicle
Paracortex
Cortex
Medulla
Efferent lymphatic

**B-CELL LYMPHOMAS**

*Follicle*
- Nodular lymphoma
- Large-cell lymphoma (sonic)
- Burkitt's lymphoma

*Germinal Center/Mantle Zone*
- Lymphocytic lymphoma
- Mantle zone lymphoma (intermediate differentiation)

*Medulla*
- Chronic lymphocytic leukemia
- Well-differentiated lymphocytic lymphoma
- Waldenström's macroglobulinemia

**T-CELL LYMPHOMAS**

*Paracortex*
- Peripheral T-cell lymphoma
- Mycosis fungoides
- Sézary syndrome
- Acute lymphoblastic leukemia
- T-cell lymphoblastic lymphoma

*Miscellaneous Malignancies*
Sinus Region
- Malignant histiocytosis
- Kt-1 large-cell lymphoma

**FIGURE 43-3** Sites of lymphocyte transformation in the lymph node. (Illustrated by J. Thommen.)

of types of mature lymphocytes. Figure 43-4 demonstrates the maturation sequence of the immunocompetent lymphocyte.

Lymphocytes are responsible for the two arms of the immunologic defense system: the humoral arm, which consists of plasma cells that produce circulating antibodies against foreign antigens, and the cellular arm, which consists of circulating lymphocytes that have developed specificity against foreign antigens. These two arms of the immune process are distinct, but they function jointly in defending the host against foreign proteins. An early step in the differentiation of the maturing lymphocyte occurs when the cell is programmed either by the bone marrow (bursa equivalent) or by the thymus to become a B-lymphocyte or a T-lymphocyte respectively. Humoral immunity is provided by the B-lymphocytes, which, when exposed to an appropriate foreign antigen, mature into plasma cells and produce antibodies against that antigen. T-lymphocytes, when similarly exposed to a foreign antigen, develop into killer lymphocytes that will attack and destroy the foreign antigen without benefit of an antibody intermediary, thus providing cellular immunity. In addition, some T-lymphocytes develop specific regulator roles in which they either suppress or stimulate immune functions (suppressor cells and helper cells).

Eighty percent of lymphomas manifest B-cell origin, and most patients initially present with disease involving bone marrow or lymph nodes. Nonlymphoid tissue exten-

sion is also common, particularly in the thyroid, gastrointestinal tract, salivary glands, and conjunctiva. Diagnosis is usually straightforward because of characteristic monoclonal immunoglobulin elevations and/or distinct morphological features. In general, B-cell neoplasms tend to follow a more indolent course than those induced by T-cell transformation.[10]

Lymphomas derived from T-lymphocytes are a complex group of diseases with marked biological and clinical heterogeneity. These neoplasms usually arise in bone marrow, thymus, lymph nodes, and skin. They may produce abnormal amounts of lymphokines or may markedly activate histiocytes (macrophages) throughout the body. These activated cells often destroy normal blood cells causing anemia, thrombocytopenia, and/or leukopenia.[11] T-cell lymphomas are generally more aggressive and grow more rapidly than their B-cell counterparts.

## HODGKIN'S DISEASE

### Historical Perspective

In 1832, Dr. Thomas Hodgkin, an English physician, described clinical data and postmortem findings of seven patients with a relentlessly progressive, ultimately fatal

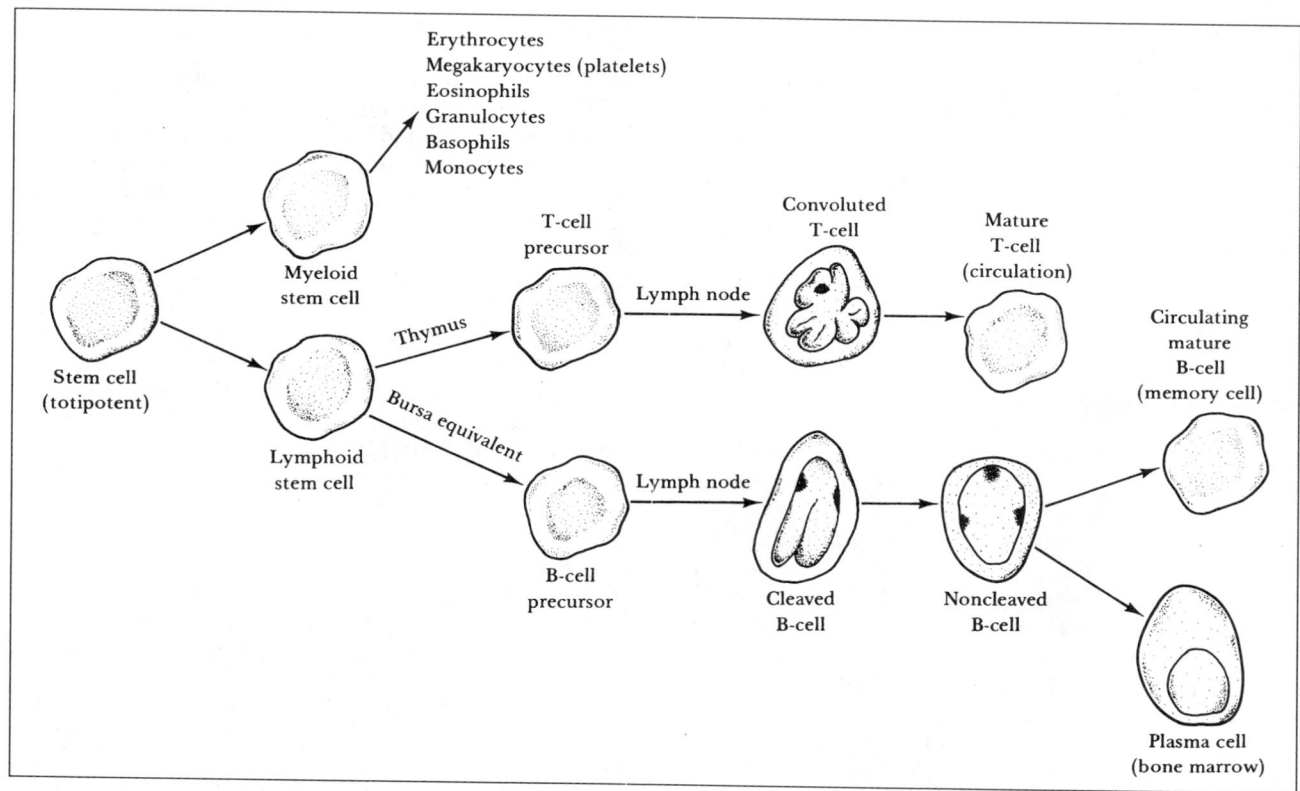

**FIGURE 43-4**  Maturation sequence of the lymphocyte. (Illustrated by J. Thommen.)

tumorous enlargement of the lymph nodes, liver, and spleen.[12] His recognition that these pathological changes represented a primary proliferation inherent in the nodal tissues themselves rather than a reactive, inflammatory process was extremely important and insightful. Prior to that time, lymphomas often had been mistaken for a common infectious disease, tuberculosis of the lymph nodes.

More than three decades after Hodgkin's paper was presented, Samuel Wilks rediscovered the original manuscript and, after further clinical clarification and elaboration, he attached the eponym "Hodgkin's disease" in 1865.[13] A review of the original tissues nearly 100 years later[13] demonstrated that Hodgkin's cases actually represented examples of what we now call Hodgkin's disease as well as non-Hodgkin's lymphoma. All lymphomas were called HD until around the turn of the century when the giant, multinucleated cells in the nodal material of HD patients were characterized by Reed[14] and Sternberg,[15] and their names have been associated with the pathognomonic cell of HD ever since. Subsequently, those lymphomas demonstrating the Reed-Sternberg cell were classified as HD and those in which the cell was absent were called lymphosarcoma or reticulum cell sarcoma and later NHL. Although the nature and origin of the Reed-Sternberg cell remain uncertain, it is clear that this cell is useful in prognosis since lymphocytic malignancies that are similar in pathological appearance behave differently according to the presence or absence of this cell. Today, diagnosis of HD requires two components. First, the presence of Reed-Sternberg cells must be verified. Second, the diagnostic cells must be identified within an appropriate cellular background that is composed of a polymorphous mixture of apparently normal inflammatory cells in various proportions.

## Epidemiology

Hodgkin's disease currently accounts for approximately 15% of the malignant lymphomas and less than 1% of all cancers. However, because a disproportionate number of HD victims are young adults, it is viewed as a particularly serious problem. The American Cancer Society estimates that in 1996, 7500 new cases (4000 male and 3500 female) and over 1500 deaths will occur.[4] The disease has a world wide distribution, and its most prominent epidemiological feature pertains to the distinct age-related incidence patterns that have been observed. In developed countries the incidence of HD is clearly bimodal. In these areas the disease is infrequent in children under 10 years old. Incidence rises rapidly in adolescence and has its first peak among young adults aged 20–30. Subsequently, it falls until after age 45; then the incidence of new cases begins to climb steadily. This second upslope continues throughout the seventh and eighth decades.[16] Similar bimodality appears to exist in less developed countries except that the young adult age peak is shifted closer to childhood. Of interest is the fact that as underdeveloped geographic areas become increasingly progressive, their incidence patterns of HD change as well. Histological category and anatomic distribution also vary with age. The nodular sclerosis form of the disease predominates in young adults, while mixed cellularity is more common in middle age and lymphocyte-depleted HD is the predominant histology in the elderly.

It has been suggested that HD is really two separate entities and that the first incidence peak may represent a disease of viral etiology, more common in middle-class than in lower-class families and more common in developed than in undeveloped countries.[17] These characteristics are consistent with a virus that is widely disseminated under conditions of poor hygiene and which, if contracted, rarely leads to severe illness. Such a pattern favors the evolution of a subclinical or asymptomatic process in low socioeconomic groups and undeveloped countries because children in such circumstances are antigenically exposed at a very early age, when they are resistant and able to develop immunity. In middle-class families and developed nations, however, improved hygiene delays such exposure until adolescence or young adulthood. Indeed, the general level of home hygiene has been found to correlate inversely with incidence—the better the general sanitation, the higher the risk of HD among children in the household. The second incidence peak of HD in those over 45 years of age appears to be relatively similar across all societal groups.[16]

## Etiology

Although many theories have been proposed, the etiology of HD remains unclear. Because of clinical manifestations such as fever, chills, and leukocytosis and because of histological similarity to a granulomatous process, an infectious source has long been a topic of speculation. The Epstein-Barr virus (EBV) is now recognized as being associated with several forms of lymphoma. It was initially described in Burkitt's lymphoma in Africa. Subsequently it was described in association with AIDS-related NHL and more recently EBV antigens have been found in the Reed-Sternberg cells of HD.

The exact manner in which EBV interacts to transform lymphocytes to malignant growth has not yet been elucidated. EBV is the etiological agent of infectious mononucleosis, in which it infects B-lymphocytes and causes them to proliferate. This polyclonal proliferation is subsequently brought under control by T-lymphocytes in subjects with a normal immune system. Presumably, with immune suppression, EBV-induced proliferation is not controlled and subsequently the polyclonal proliferation is transformed by unknown mechanisms into a malignant monoclonal proliferation.

EBV is identified in Reed-Sternberg cells more commonly in children than in adults, more commonly in under-developed countries than in the United States, and more commonly in some histological types of HD than in others.[18-20] This is consistent with the hypothesis that there may be different etiologies of HD in adults and children and with different histological types. EBV is detected more frequently in HIV associated than in non-HIV associated HD.[21]

Genetic and occupational predispositions for HD may also exist. Familial patterns have been documented, and HD clearly occurs with increased frequency in first-degree relatives of HD patients.[22,23] Although such findings might also be expected to lend support to the notion of an infectious vector, increased incidence has not been documented in marital partners or health care professionals caring for HD patients.[24] In contrast to other forms of cancer, evidence is sparse that chemical exposures are a significant factor in the development of HD. Persons employed in woodworking and using benzene compounds may be at increased risk, but current data are not convincing.[22]

## Cellular Abnormalities

Although humoral immunity appears to remain relatively intact, patients in all stages of HD exhibit a molecular defect characterized by markedly reduced cellular immunity. This deficit is manifested by impaired delayed hypersensitivity skin reactions and reduced T-cell proliferation following antigenic stimulation. They also display increased susceptibility to infectious complications from opportunistic pathogens such as herpes zoster, cytomegalovirus, and *Pneumocystis carinii*.[25]

Elucidation of the biochemical mechanisms of HD has been difficult and data are sometimes conflicting. The *bcl-2* oncogene is able to prevent apoptosis and this promotes malignant growth because cells with genetic damage continue to proliferate rather than die as is normally the case. In nodular NHL there is a translocation t(14;18) which activates *bcl-2*. Activation of *bcl-2* is seen in some cases of HD but the t(14;18) translocation is seen only rarely. However, EBV infection may activate *bcl-2* and it has been suggested that in at least some cases of HD the pathogenesis involves EBV infection, subsequent activation of *bcl-2*, followed by suppression of apoptosis.[26,27] This mechanism seems common in most forms of HD, but is probably not the case in the nodular lymphocyte predominant form.[28,29] Thus there are probably at least two mechanisms involved in the development of HD and this is consistent with the data showing that EBV may be involved in virtually all pediatric cases and most adult cases in under-developed countries but is far less frequent in developed countries.[30]

## Clinical Manifestations

A typical HD patient presents with a slow, insidious, superficial lymphadenopathy. Characteristic nodes of variable size (from 1 cm to several centimeters) are firm, rubbery, and freely movable. Occasionally their size varies spontaneously over a period of several days. The enlarged nodes may be unilateral or bilateral, and most are located in the cervical and supraclavicular areas. Axillary and inguinal involvement is reported in less than 10% of the patients. A second common presentation, mediastinal adenopathy, is often recognized during routine chest roentgenogram. Overall, the adenopathy is usually painless unless lymph node growth is rapid. However, pain does occur in about 20% of the cases following ingestion of alcohol.

Constitutional symptoms of fever, malaise, night sweats, weight loss (>10% of normal body weight), and pruritus appear in about 40% of affected individuals. These manifestations, called *B symptoms*, are more common in patients with advanced disease.

The spread of HD is via contiguous nodal groups, and the pattern is quite predictable. In general, symptomatology and prognosis are related to the location and number of disease sites. Local pressure symptoms may arise from enlarged mediastinal nodes causing cough, dyspnea, dysphagia, pleural effusions, and, in extreme situations, superior vena cava syndrome. An enlarged spleen may result in left upper quadrant pain. Jaundice may evolve due to hepatic extension or extra-hepatic bile duct obstruction. Retroperitoneal adenopathy often induces gastrointestinal and genitourinary dysfunction, abdominal pain, and ascites. Bone pain and fractures may be caused by secondary skeletal involvement of the vertebrae, ribs, and sternum. Herpes zoster infections are a relatively frequent finding and usually indicate impending epidural involvement. Exfoliative dermatitis and intense pruritus develop when the lymphatics of the skin are involved; indeed, they are often the first subjective symptoms to be reported.[31]

## Assessment

The diagnosis of HD can be established only by biopsy of involved tissue, usually a lymph node. Cervical nodes are preferable to axillary and inguinal nodes because the latter often reveal evidence of chronic inflammatory changes. Occasionally, multiple biopsies are necessary for proper evaluation since reactive hyperplasia of nodes adjacent to those involved with tumor may provide equivocal results. It is important to remember that there are many causes of lymphadenopathy, especially in younger individuals. These include upper respiratory infections (bacterial or viral), infectious mononucleosis, allergic reactions, and other nonspecific causes. Older persons with cancers of the head and neck also may present initially with enlarged cervical nodes.

When an abnormal node is palpated during routine physical examination or when the patient reports such a complaint, a careful history and physical examination should be performed. If there is evidence of a recent infection or other nonmalignant process, the physician may choose to delay biopsy and observe the clinical course. In most cases, lymphadenopathy of infectious origin will usually resolve in a few days or weeks. When the adenopathy persists or the etiology is not apparent, a biopsy is generally indicated. Because a family history of HD increases the risk to other siblings, this, too, may be a factor in the decision process. In the absence of fever or overt systemic complaints, the detection of an enlarged lymph node in the neck of an older person is an indication that a careful search of the mouth, pharynx, and larynx for the presence of a malignant process should be made. Once a diagnosis is confirmed, it is necessary to obtain accurate histological typing and staging of the disease in order to determine the precise prognosis and selection of therapy.

## Histopathology

Hodgkin's disease is distinguished from other lymphomas by the presence of the Reed-Sternberg cell. This is a large, bizarre cell with two or more mirror-image nuclei, each containing a single prominent nucleolus. Unlike most cancers, this characteristic cell represents only a small fraction of the cells in a malignant lymph node. Normal lymphocytes, plasma cells, and fibrous stroma comprise the bulk of palpable tissue. Although Reed-Sternberg cells are essential for the diagnosis of HD, they also have been reported in other conditions such as lymphoid hyperplasia, infectious mononucleosis, nonlymphoid malignancies (carcinomas and sarcomas), and phenytoin (Dilantin) therapy.[32]

The current histopathologic classification of HD was established in 1966 by an international conference in Rye, New York.[33] Four distinct subtypes of HD were enumerated: nodular sclerosis, lymphocyte-predominant, mixed cellularity, and lymphocyte-depleted. Each category has well-defined characteristics and manifests certain features of natural history (Table 43-1). Prior to the availability of highly curative chemotherapy and radiation therapy, these subtypes also implied notable differences in expected survival. However, recent therapeutic advances have rendered each of them potentially curable.

*Nodular sclerosis (NS)*, with its unique age incidence (between ages 15 and 34) and its different sex incidence (females more commonly than males), has a singular histological makeup that does not fit into the spectrum presented by the other three types. In NS-HD, the lymph node is divided into nodules by sclerosing bands of collagen. Lymphocytes within these collagen-bound nodules may be of various types, from predominantly small lymphocytes to large histiocytic forms. A variation of the Reed-Sternberg cell, the lacunar cell, is an identifiable feature of this subtype. Most patients are asymptomatic at presentation and exhibit stage I or II disease. They also tend to be clustered in the urban areas of developed countries. Anterior mediastinal involvement is exceedingly common and ultimately may involve cervical, supraclavicular, and upper abdominal lymph nodes as well as the spleen. Bulky mediastinal disease often contributes to metastatic infiltration of the lung parenchyma.

The other three histological types of HD exhibit a range of prognoses from good to poor. The *lymphocyte-predominant (LP)* is characterized by sheets of mature-appearing small lymphocytes and few Reed-Sternberg cells. Patients usually present with localized stage I or II disease, primarily in the cervical lymph nodes. Peak incidence occurs in the fourth or fifth decades, and B symptoms are uncommon. Its natural history is usually indolent. Outcome is quite favorable.

*Mixed cellularity (MC)* HD is intermediate between lymphocyte-predominant and lymphocyte-depleted in terms of histology and prognosis. Disorderly fibrosis may be seen, but the broad fibrous bands indicative of the NS subtype are absent. There is a wide age range that peaks in the 30–40-year-old age group, and male cases predominate. More than 50% of the patients have stage III or IV disease and the majority manifest B symptoms. Extranodal abdominal extension is common.

*Lymphocyte-depleted (LD)* HD is the most aggressive of the four Rye classifications. It is marked by a paucity of small lymphocytes and an increased number of Reed-Sternberg cells. Two slightly different variants have been identified—reticular and diffuse fibrosis. Reticular LD-HD patients often present with bone marrow infiltration and peripheral lymphadenopathy. Those with diffuse fibrosis are more likely to exhibit lymph node and visceral involvement. Patients in this group are usually elderly males with advanced-stage disease and B symptoms. Prior to the advent of combination therapy, it carried a very poor prognosis. It is interesting to note that in some retrospective histological studies, up to one-third of LD-HD tumors have been reclassified as NHL.

## Staging

After the diagnosis of HD has been established on the basis of lymph node biopsy and the histological type has been determined in accordance with the outlined criteria, the next step in patient management is the careful determination of the extent of the disease. This process is referred to as *staging* and it indicates the degree of systemic progression and the intensity of treatment that

**TABLE 43-1**    Rye Classification of Hodgkin's Disease

| Histology | Frequency (%) | Features |
|---|---|---|
| Nodular sclerosis | 30–70 | Stage I and II disease<br>Young females predominate |
| Lymphocyte-predominant | 10–15 | Middle-age peak<br>Males predominate<br>Localized stage I and II disease |
| Mixed cellularity | 20–40 | Males predominate<br>Intermediate prognosis<br>B symptoms common |
| Lymphocyte-depleted | 5–15 | Older males predominate<br>Widespread dissemination<br>Poor prognosis |

will be required; it also allows the clinician to draw an inference with regard to the disease process.

Beginning in 1970, most HD patients were staged according to the Ann Arbor Classification System.[34] Over time, however, adherence to its guidelines became less strict due to: (1) new features of recognized prognostic importance, (2) questions concerning the need for staging laparotomy, and (3) advances in diagnostic imaging techniques that facilitated recognition of occult disease sites. In an effort to address these issues, a meeting was convened in Cotswolds, England, in 1989. Specialists in attendance approved criteria for a new system that retained the original Ann Arbor framework but included modifications incorporating designations for number of sites and bulk of disease.[35] Figure 43-5 provides a schematic representation of the new Ann Arbor–Cotswolds classification system created for both HD and NHL.

Lymph node involvement in just one area is designated as stage I disease. Involvement of two or more areas confined to one side of the diaphragm constitutes stage II. In stage III, lymph node groups above and below the diaphragm are affected. The spleen may be involved (stage IIIs), and this often precedes widespread hematogenous dissemination. In HD, stage III is subdivided further into stage III$_1$ for disease limited to the upper abdomen (spleen and splenic, hilar, celiac, and/or porta hepatic nodes), and stage III$_2$ for disease involving the lower abdomen (periaortic, pelvic, or inguinal nodes). Stage IV is marked by diffuse extralymphatic progression that may affect, for example, the liver, bone marrow, lung, and skin. A subscript $E$ in stages I, II, and III indicates localized extranodal extension from a nodal mass, and designation of a stage as either $A$ or $B$ indicates the absence *(A)* or presence *(B)* of unexplained weight loss greater than 10% of body weight in the preceding six months and/or fever of greater than 38°C and/or night sweats. Subscript $X$ is indicative of bulky disease.

The adoption of this classification schema implies a dual system of stage designation according to both clinical and pathological criteria. Clinical staging (CS) rests on

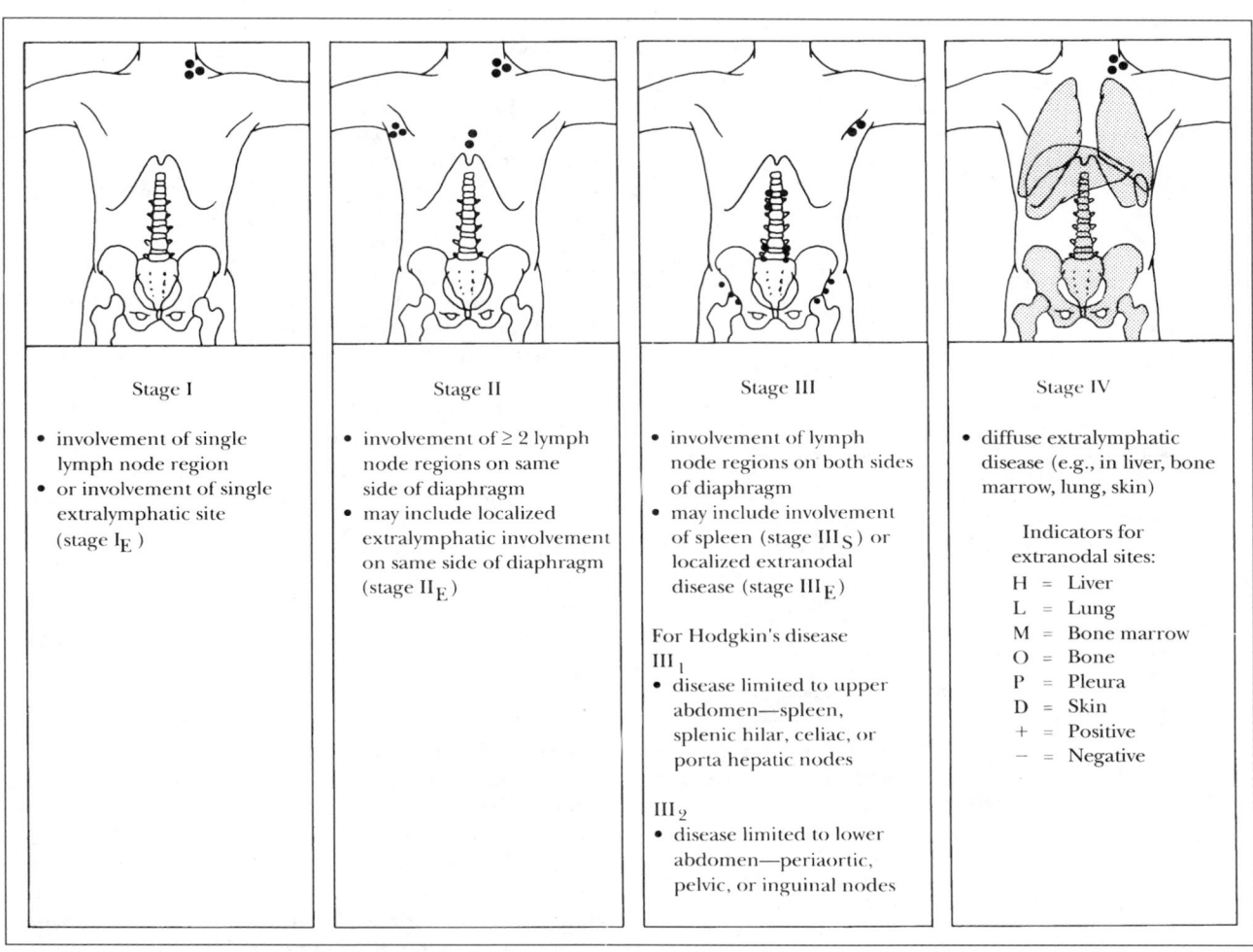

**Stage I**
- involvement of single lymph node region
- or involvement of single extralymphatic site (stage I$_E$)

**Stage II**
- involvement of ≥ 2 lymph node regions on same side of diaphragm
- may include localized extralymphatic involvement on same side of diaphragm (stage II$_E$)

**Stage III**
- involvement of lymph node regions on both sides of diaphragm
- may include involvement of spleen (stage III$_S$) or localized extranodal disease (stage III$_E$)

For Hodgkin's disease
III$_1$
- disease limited to upper abdomen—spleen, splenic hilar, celiac, or porta hepatic nodes

III$_2$
- disease limited to lower abdomen—periaortic, pelvic, or inguinal nodes

**Stage IV**
- diffuse extralymphatic disease (e.g., in liver, bone marrow, lung, skin)

Indicators for extranodal sites:

| | | |
|---|---|---|
| H | = | Liver |
| L | = | Lung |
| M | = | Bone marrow |
| O | = | Bone |
| P | = | Pleura |
| D | = | Skin |
| + | = | Positive |
| − | = | Negative |

**FIGURE 43-5**   Ann-Arbor staging system for Hodgkin's disease. (*Atlas of Diagnostic Oncology*, Second Edition by A.T. Skarin, 1996. Mosby-Wolfe Limited, London, U.K.) Philadelphia, Lippincott, 1991. Reprinted with permission.)

history, physical examination, initial diagnostic biopsy, laboratory tests, and radiographic evidence. Pathological staging (PS) adds definitive histopathologic information obtained through biopsy of strategic sites.[36] It is customary to specify whether a stage is determined on the basis of clinical signs alone (e.g., an abdominal lymphangiogram) or on the basis of pathological examination of a biopsy section. Thus, a patient may be referred to as having "clinical" stage III (CS III) or "pathological" stage III (PS III), depending on the strength of the evidence. The nurse should be familiar with the essential procedures and terms used in diagnostic staging (Table 43-2) in order to help a patient follow the sequence and understand the significance of the evaluative workup.

A controversial component of the staging process is the exploratory laparotomy, an extensive surgical procedure that includes splenectomy, wedge and needle liver biopsies, anterior iliac crest bone marrow biopsy, and extensive biopsy and dissection of abdominal lymph nodes. Although surgical mortality is quite uncommon, morbidity may include wound infection, subphrenic abscess, pulmonary embolus, stress ulcer, gastrointestinal bleeding, and wound dehiscence. In addition, splenec-

**TABLE 43-2   Staging Evaluation for Hodgkin's Disease**

| |
|---|
| Adequate surgical biopsy reviewed by an experienced hemopathologist. In primary extranodal lymphomas, biopsy should also include a lymph node when palpable. |
| Detailed history with special attention to the presence or absence of systemic symptoms |
| Careful physical examination, emphasizing node chains, size of liver and spleen, Waldeyer's ring inspection, and bony tenderness |
| Routine laboratory tests: complete blood count, erythrosedimentation rate, liver function tests, serum uric acid, serum copper |
| Chest roentgenogram (posteroanterior and lateral) with measurement of mass/thoracic ratio |
| Bilateral lower extremity lymphogram |
| Chest MRI |
| Abdominal and pelvic CT scan |
| Radioisotopic evaluation with gallium 67 when the results of other conventional diagnostic procedures are inconclusive |
| Core needle biopsy of bone marrow from posterior iliac crest. Biopsy should be bilateral, especially in the presence of CS III and in patients with systemic symptoms. |
| Needle or surgical biopsy of any suspicious extranodal (e.g., hepatic, splenic, osseous, pulmonary, cutaneous) lesion(s) |
| Cytologic examination of any effusion |
| Staging laparotomy with splenectomy, needle and wedge biopsy of liver, and biopsies of para-aortic, mesenteric, portal, and splenic hilar lymph node in CS I to II patients only if change in stage will change treatment plan. |

Data from DeVita et al,[24] Bonadonna et al.[36]

tomy patients face the lifelong risk of a septic event from encapsulated organisms. Current recommendations advocate that staging laparotomy be utilized only when the surgical findings will either (a) alter the extent of radiation therapy to be administered or (b) make chemotherapy rather than radiation therapy the primary treatment modality. With more recent movement toward a combined modality approach, especially in patients with bulky stage II disease or confirmed stage III$_2$ A disease, the need for laparotomy to define possible sites of occult intraabdominal disease has become limited.[16]

## Treatment

The initial treatment plan for HD is crucial in determining eventual outcome because the overwhelming majority of patients, even those in the most advanced disease stages, are potentially curable if optimal therapy is employed. A comprehensive approach is essential and requires input from a variety of disciplines (radiology, surgery, pathology, medical oncology) working together collaboratively as an interdisciplinary team.

Association with multiple physicians and the complexity of the staging procedures often cause a patient to feel confused and overwhelmed. In many cases the nurse may be the only constant contact this individual has with the diagnostic and treatment teams. Therefore, it is essential that psychological support be provided as the individual adjusts to the full ramifications of a malignant diagnosis. The diverse procedures to which the patient will be subjected may require clarification and repeated explanations. These should be given with understanding, empathy, compassion, and tact.[37]

Current treatment recommendations are relatively noncontroversial and guidelines for stage-specific therapies are outlined on Table 43-3. In all instances, the primary objective is to cure the most patients with the least therapy in order to avoid complications to the greatest extent possible. Since nearly one-third of all HD patients die without evidence of lymphoma at autopsy, the prevention of iatrogenic complications must be of paramount importance.[36]

Radiation therapy is curative in most patients with limited disease. Several important factors impact upon its effectiveness—skilled use of linear accelerators, careful field simulation, administration of tumoricidal doses, and comprehensive follow-up. The radiation fields commonly employed in HD may be divided into three volumes: the mantle, the para-aortic, and the pelvis (Figure 43-6). In order to achieve high cure rates, each of these fields generally must be extended to include adjacent, clinically negative nodal sites. Carefully constructed field shapes and blocks are used to protect the lungs, heart, spinal cord, larynx, kidneys, iliac crests, and gonads. All standard radiation treatments employ an opposed field, usually anterior-posterior, technique to provide homogenous dose distribution and to minimize potential radiation damage.

**TABLE 43-3**   Guidelines for Treatment of Hodgkin's Disease

| Stage | Recommended Therapy | Alternative Therapy |
|---|---|---|
| I, II (A or B, negative laparotomy) | Subtotal lymphoid irradiation | Irradiation to involved field with combination chemotherapy |
| I, II (A or B, with mediastinal mass >⅓ diameter of the chest) | Combination chemotherapy followed by irradiation to involved field | Subtotal lymphoid irradiation followed by chemotherapy |
| III A₁, (minimal abdominal disease) | Total lymphoid irradiation | Combination chemotherapy with irradiation to involved sites |
| III A₂, (extensive abdominal disease) | Combination chemotherapy with irradiation to involved sites | Total lymphoid irradiation or combination chemotherapy alone |
| III B | Combination chemotherapy | Combination chemotherapy with irradiation to involved sites |
| IV (A or B) | Combination chemotherapy | Combination chemotherapy with irradiation to involved sites |

Reprinted with permission from Eyre HJ, Farver ML: Hodgkin's disease and non-Hodgkin's lymphoma, in Holleb AI, Fink DJ, Murphy GP (eds): *Textbook of Clinical Oncology.* Atlanta, The American Cancer Society, 1991.

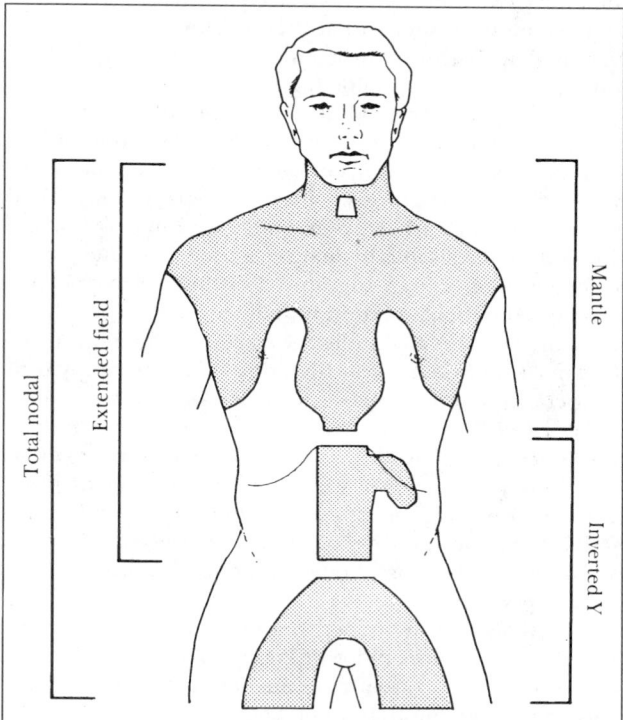

**FIGURE 43-6**   Standard radiation fields for Hodgkin's disease. Mantle—from mandible to diaphragm. Lungs, heart, spinal cord, and humeral heads are shielded. Inverted Y—from diaphragm to ischial tuberosities, including the spleen if not removed; spinal cord, kidneys, bladder, rectum, and gonads are shielded. Extended Field—involves mantle zone and uppermost inverted Y zone; does not include the pelvic, inguinal, or femoral nodes. Total Nodal—mantle zone and complete inverted Y zone.

For stage I A and II A disease above the diaphragm, without bulky mediastinal extension, mantle irradiation to a total dose of 3500–4400 cGy over a period of four to six weeks is advocated. Paraaortic lymph nodes are usually included except in those with mediastinal involvement or those with lymphocyte predominant histology. Stage III₁ A patients having only splenic involvement may be treated with total or subtotal nodal irradiation. Generally, total nodal irradiation is considered inappropriate for stage III₂ A individuals.[38] If careful laparotomy staging has been conducted, patients with stage II B disease may receive total or subtotal nodal radiotherapy; otherwise, chemotherapy is indicated. When bulky mediastinal disease is known to be present, combination radiation and chemotherapy are unequivocally required. In addition, the combined approach is usually indicated for patients with adverse prognostic factors such as B symptoms, bulky masses, or disease involving nodes in the lower abdomen.

Whereas radiotherapy is curative in local and regional HD, chemotherapy may be curative in both early and advanced disease. The use of both modalities together is sometimes required for cure, but because multimodality therapy is associated with a much higher complication rate, especially second malignancies, there is controversy as to when to combine these modalities.[39,40]

Because of their high response and durable remission rates, the MOPP regimen (Table 43-4) and the ABVD regimen (Table 43-5) have become the benchmarks for combination chemotherapy in HD. Both regimens are routinely administered in 28-day cycles for a minimum of six cycles. As a rule, chemotherapy is continued for two cycles after complete remission is documented. Each combination can be expected to produce remissions in more than 80% of previously untreated patients, and 60%–70% of those who achieve complete remission will be alive with no evidence of disease after 10 years, presumably cured.

**TABLE 43-4**    The MOPP Regimen for Hodgkin's Disease

| Drug | Dosage | Schedule |
|------|--------|----------|
| Nitrogen mustard | 6 mg/m² IV | Days 1 and 8 |
| Vincristine (Oncovin) | 1.4 mg/m² IV | Days 1 and 8 |
| Procarbazine | 100 mg/m² PO | Days 1 through 14 |
| Prednisone (cycles 1 and 4 only) | 40 mg/m² PO | Days 1 through 14 |

Repeat cycle every 28 days for a minimum of six cycles. Complete remission must be documented before discontinuing therapy.

Overall, either MOPP or ABVD can be expected to produce a complete remission in more than half of the patients who have recurrent disease after treatment with the other combination. At present, there is no evidence that maintenance therapy adds to cure for patients in remission. It is important to note that recent studies indicate ABVD may actually be superior to MOPP because it minimizes the leukemogenesis and permanent male sterility associated with regimens containing alkylating agents.[41]

The combination of MOPP and ABVD in various ways shows evidence of being superior to either regimen alone. The underlying principle of increasing the number of drugs in a combination is the Goldie-Coldman hypothesis, which postulates that multiple drugs reduce the chance of failure due to development of drug resistance by tumor cells.[42] MOPP/ABVD has been shown to improve failure free survival in randomized trials, but there is no improvement of overall survival compared to ABVD alone.[43,44] At present the standard of therapy is either ABVD or a MOPP/ABVD hybrid regimen.

The success of aggressive chemotherapeutic regimens is quite dependent on the dosage and timing of drug administration because even minor alterations can have a substantial impact on efficacy. The reduction of doses and omission of drugs to avoid nausea and vomiting, with its attendant loss of curative potential, is truly a poor bargain for any patient. Nursing can play a pivotal role in promoting patient compliance by providing emotional

**TABLE 43-5**    The ABVD Regimen for Hodgkin's Disease

| Drug | Dosage | Schedule |
|------|--------|----------|
| Doxorubicin | 25 mg/m² IV | Days 1 and 15 |
| Bleomycin | 10 units/m² IV | Days 1 and 15 |
| Vinblastine | 6 mg/m² IV | Days 1 and 15 |
| Dacarbazine (DTIC) | 375 mg/m² IV | Days 1 and 15 |

Repeat cycle every 28 days for a minimum of six cycles. Complete remission must be documented before discontinuing therapy.

support, effective symptom management, and reassurance about the finite nature of the treatment program.

Refinements in treatment protocols have led to the identification of specific subsets of patients who appear to benefit from combined chemotherapy and radiation therapy.[45] These patients present with what has been called "bulky" disease, usually defined as adenopathy greater than one-third the width of the chest on x-ray examination. This pattern of disease has a high recurrence rate after radiotherapy alone and poses some risk in exploratory laparotomy because the mediastinal mass may complicate anesthesia.[46,47] It is probably best for chemotherapy to be used as an adjunct after radiotherapy in these patients.[48]

Residual or recurrent disease poses a unique challenge. For patients with a favorable prognosis (e.g., limited disease at recurrence, good performance status, absence of B symptoms, age <60 years, slow-growing residual tumor), salvage therapy is a potential option.[36,49] Those who relapse following irradiation can be treated with chemotherapy, and, under certain circumstances, additional radiation may be possible. When relapse occurs after chemotherapy, the extent of the disease-free interval is very important. If relapse takes place more than 12 months after initial therapy, the patient can be retreated with the same agents and the probability of long-term survival remains high.[50]

When relapse occurs less than 12 months after initial remission or patients are refractory to initial therapy, the prognosis is grave. Conventional salvage regimens are rarely effective. High dose chemotherapy with stem cell rescue, utilizing either autologous bone marrow or peripheral stem cells, has been investigated as an alternative to conventional salvage therapy.[51] Results tend to be better in relapsed patients than in initially refractory patients,[52] probably because of the degree of tumor chemosensitivity. There is evidence that high-dose chemotherapy with stem cell rescue is effective with disease-free survival at two years of 75%, although treatment related complications account for a 13% mortality.[53] There were three independent prognostic variables: the number of prior chemotherapy regimens, prior radiotherapy, and extranodal disease at the time of high-dose therapy. Of these the number of prior chemotherapy regimens was the most important.

It is likely that high-dose therapy will be used increasingly in the future and will be applied earlier in the disease in order to treat patients before tumors acquire resistance to chemotherapeutic agents.

## NON-HODGKIN'S LYMPHOMAS

### Historical Perspective

The non-Hodgkin's lymphomas are a diverse group of neoplasms derived from the different developmental and functional subdivisions of the lymphoreticular system. Although these malignancies have many features in common, they also reflect the diversity of their normal counterpart cells and exhibit a wide range of immunologic and biological characteristics. There is no precise definition of NHL that is universally accepted, and although many meet the criteria that have been proposed for neoplasia, others lurk in a nebulous arena between benign lymphoproliferation and true malignancy.[54]

Throughout the nineteenth century, scientists used a variety of terms (e.g., *giant follicle lymphoma, lymphosarcoma,* and *reticulum cell sarcoma*) to categorize these tumors, and "pseudoleukemia" became a catchall for a host of conditions that exhibited lymphadenopathy and splenomegaly. Use of these designations persisted into the twentieth century and did much to obscure the delineation and subclassification of NHL.[55]

Recent technological refinements have enabled pathologists and clinicians to classify NHL according to a number of individual determinants including their ability to reproduce the same cytoarchitecture (follicular versus diffuse), cell size (small or large), nuclear characteristics (cleaved or noncleaved, convoluted or cerebriform), and immunological ontogeny (T-cell or B-cell lymphocytes). Today the most accurate definition of lymphoma type is one that includes each of these elements. Further differentiation appears to be on the horizon, and future designations will likely include genetic markers as well.

## Epidemiology

In the United States, NHL is diagnosed nearly six times as often as HD, and its death rate is 13 times greater. American Cancer Society statistics for 1996 indicate that 52,700 new cases and 23,300 deaths will occur.[4] Age-adjusted incidence is somewhat higher in males than in females (29,900 to 22,800), and the white population is affected more than the black population. Age-specific analyses reveal a preadolescent peak, a late teenage drop, and then a logarithmic rise with increasing age that persists into the eighth decade. The current mean is in the fifth decade. Like HD, higher mortalities are associated with higher socioeconomic status and urban residence.[56]

Because of the many available classification schemes for NHL, it is difficult to compare the incidence or frequency of the histological subtypes of lymphoma in different parts of the world. However, a rising incidence appears to be noted internationally; there has been a one- to twofold increase in most Western countries since 1960.

## Etiology

The heterogeneity of NHL suggests that a variety of factors including viral infections, genetic abnormalities, and immune disturbances interact in the pathogenesis. The most convincing evidence of a viral etiology of malignant lymphoma has come from the studies of adult T-cell leukemia/lymphoma (ATL). A unique RNA retrovirus, human T-cell leukemia/lymphoma virus type I (HTLV-I), has been isolated from lymphocytes of patients with ATL in endemic areas of southwestern Japan, the Caribbean, and southeastern United States. ATL is primarily a disease of adults over 40 years old. Its manifestations include a high frequency of cutaneous infiltration, hepatosplenomegaly, lymphadenopathy, and hypercalcemia.[57]

Epstein-Barr virus (EBV), a DNA herpes virus, is the most likely etiologic agent for another form of NHL, Burkitt's lymphoma (BL). This neoplasm is confined almost exclusively to endemic areas of Africa and New Guinea, and, indeed, evidence of EBV infection is found in 96% of African cases of BL. In Africa, BL is a malignancy of childhood. The mean age at presentation is 7 years, and males are affected twice as often as females. The children usually present with large extranodal tumors involving the bones of the jaw (72%) and abdominal organs (56%), particularly the ovaries, kidneys, and retroperitoneum. Although the etiology of BL is unknown, a current hypothesis focuses on an acute malarial infection as the environmental factor that interacts with a susceptible host immune system to predispose an individual to EBV-induced lymphoma.[58,59] Recently, EBV has been linked to neoplastic proliferation in a variety of congenital, iatrogenic, and acquired immunodeficient conditions.[60,61]

Environmental factors and exposure to chemicals in the workplace also are implicated in the pathogenesis of NHL. Pesticides and fertilizers have been suspected because of increased lymphoma incidence among midwestern farmers born after 1900 and dying before age 65 years. Vinyl chloride workers in the U.S. tire manufacturing industry exhibit increases, as do anesthetists, chemists, and workers in petroleum refining, asbestos, and herbicide industries. Japanese survivors of the atomic bomb and patients receiving ionizing radiation for congenital disorders and HD also face increased neoplastic potential.[62]

One form of lymphoma, gastric lymphoma of mucosa-associated lymphoid tissue (MALT), has recently been reported to be due to the same bacteria that induces gastric ulcers, *Helicobacter pylori*. In its early stages it may be cured by eradication of the bacteria with antibiotics.[63] The fuel implications of this exciting observation are not yet understood.

## Cellular Abnormalities

A consideration of the molecular pathogenesis of both B- and T-cell origin in NHL reveals several consistent features. In most cases, chromosomal translocations facilitate the identification of the genetic lesion responsible for oncogenesis. Nearly all individuals with Burkitt's lymphoma (BL) have one of three translocations involving the *c-myc* proto-oncogene. These include chromosomes 8 and 14 (t 8;14), chromosomes 2 and 8 (t 2;8), and chromosomes 8 and 22 (t 8;22). Eighty-five percent of follicular lymphomas and 20% of diffuse lymphomas have the characteristic t(14;18) translocation that activates the *bcl-2* gene which suppresses apoptosis.[64] Mantle cell lymphomas, also called centrocytic or intermediate lymphomas, have a characteristic t(11;14) translocation that activates the *bcl-1* gene causing cyclin D1 protein overexpression leading to very rapid proliferation and resistance to cure by conventional chemotherapy.[65]

Cytogenetic analysis of lymphoma cells has identified other abnormalities as well. Deletions on chromosome 6 are found in a significant portion of patients with large-cell lymphoma. Such a loss of chromosomal material may lead to deleterious effects via the elimination of functional suppressor or growth inhibitory genes. Gains of one or more whole chromosomes are common, and trisomy of chromosomes 2,3,7,18, and 21 have been described.[66] At present the sequence of events that explains the transformation of a normal lymphocyte into a lymphomatous cell is unknown. Optimally, a better understanding of the genetic mechanisms of malignancy will translate eventually into new strategies of treatment based on the biology of the disease.[67]

## Clinical Manifestations

The non-Hodgkin's lymphomas encompass a spectrum of neoplasms ranging from indolent tumors, which can occasionally undergo spontaneous regression, to rapidly progressive tumors, which may be fatal within weeks if untreated. They are usually generalized diseases and can involve almost any organ or tissue, thus resulting in a wide array of systemic manifestations (Table 43-6). Some of the clinical features may be caused by chemical mediators produced by the lymphoma cells, by metabolic changes resulting from a high rate of cell death in the tumor, or by secondary events such as opportunistic infections, immunosuppression; and paraneoplastic electrolyte abnormalities.[68] In contrast to HD, 80% of patients with NHL present to their physicians with advanced disease (stage III or IV). This is usually reflected by painless, generalized lymphadenopathy. Systemic B symptoms (fever, night sweats, and/or weight loss) are the initial complaint in as many as 20% of the cases.[69] Although their presence signifies advanced disease, it is not as predictive of prognosis as in HD.

Extranodal lymphoma is seen in nearly 20% of individuals during initial evaluation and it generally is confirmed in more than 50% of cases at autopsy.[56] Gastrointestinal involvement is fairly common at presentation; the most frequent sites of infiltration are the stomach and small intestine. Malignancies originating in Waldeyer's ring of the nasopharynx have a particular propensity for gastric extension. Common clinical signs are pain, abdominal mass, and anorexia and, less commonly, nausea, vomiting, bleeding, diarrhea, or obstruction.

Pulmonary parenchymal disease is related most often to lymphatic tumor spread from hilar and mediastinal nodes, and cough, dyspnea, and chest pain are quite indicative of lung infiltration. Central lymphatic obstruction or pleural seeding with tumor may result in superior vena cava syndrome or pleural effusion. Lytic bone lesions are seen in the femurs, pelvis, vertebrae, ribs, and skull. Lymphomas occasionally infiltrate the skin as red or purplish nodules, primarily in the head and neck region, while tumorous replacement of the bone marrow can result in a leukemia-like picture in the peripheral blood. Liver involvement often occurs without signs or symptoms, and, unlike the situation in HD, splenic extension need not occur concomitantly. Solitary brain lymphomas

**TABLE 43-6** Systemic Alterations in Non-Hodgkin's Lymphoma

| System | Manifestations |
| --- | --- |
| Lymphoid system | Lymphadenopathy—peripheral or central<br>Hepatosplenomegaly<br>Thymic (anterior superior mediastinal) mass<br>Waldeyer's ring involvement<br>Bone marrow involvement |
| Gastrointestinal system | Abdominal or pelvic mass<br>Upper or lower gastrointestinal bleeding<br>Malabsorption<br>Intussusception<br>Perforation<br>Fistula<br>Biliary obstruction<br>Pancreatic mass<br>Ascites<br>Salivary gland swelling |
| Genitourinary system | Renal mass, ureteric obstruction<br>Testicular mass<br>Ovarian mass<br>Vaginal bleeding |
| Nervous system | Meningeal involvement<br>Cranial nerve palsies<br>Intracranial mass (extradural or intracerebral)<br>Paraspinal mass<br>Intraorbital, periorbital, or ocular mass<br>Peripheral neuropathy<br>Progressive multifocal leucoencephalopathy |
| Endocrine system | Thyroid mass<br>Adrenal mass |
| Other | Bone involvement<br>Paranasal sinus involvement<br>Jaw involvement<br>Skin infiltration<br>Venous or (rarely) arterial obstruction<br>Pericardial effusion<br>Pulmonary infiltration |
| General | Pyrexia/night sweats<br>Weight loss<br>Lethargy |

Reprinted with permission from Magrath IT, Wilson W, Horvath K, et al: Clinical features and staging, in Magrath IT (ed): *The Non-Hodgkin's Lymphomas*. Baltimore, Williams & Wilkins, 1990.

are being reported with increasing frequency. They are often associated with AIDS or iatrogenic immunosuppression. These mass lesions may induce headaches, seizures, and changes in mental status. Another common central nervous system manifestation is leptomeningeal spread, which results in cranial nerve palsies, meningeal irritation, and increased intracranial pressure.[69]

## Assessment

Because every enlarged lymph node does not necessarily represent NHL, careful histological evaluation is the most important first step toward initiating proper care of the patient. When a lymphoma is suspected, the pathologist should be notified so that special processing procedures including cytogenetics, surface markers, immunohistochemistry stains, and molecular biological studies can be used in addition to routine histology of biopsied specimens. Since NHL occurs more commonly in extranodal sites than HD, needle biopsies may be more diagnostically helpful; widespread visceral extension or occult retroperitoneal disease may require open biopsy or laparotomy for confirmation.

A careful history and physical examination should be precise in evaluating abnormal clinical manifestations and the length of time they have been present. This is particularly important in patients who present with vague constitutional complaints or with derangements referable to more than one organ system. In general, the principles governing assessment of NHL are the same as those previously identified for HD.

## Histopathology

Few areas of pathology have evoked as much controversy and confusion as the classification of NHL, and the lack of consistent standardization makes international analysis and comparison extremely difficult.[69] The first widely accepted classification was proposed by Rappaport et al[70] in 1956. This scheme separates lymphomas on the basis of two morphological features: (1) pattern of growth (nodular or diffuse depending on the macrostructure of the lymph node); and (2) the degree of cytological differentiation of the predominant malignant cell. Tumors composed of cells similar in size and morphology to normal lymphocytes are considered *well-differentiated,* whereas those composed of irregularly shaped lymphocytes are referred to as *poorly differentiated.* If tumor cells are two to three times larger than small lymphocytes and have abundant cytoplasm, they are called *histiocytes* because of their resemblance to macrophages. *Undifferentiated* lymphomas are composed of intermediate-sized cells that fail to demonstrate evidence of either lymphoid or histiocytic origin. *Mixed lymphomas* are tumors formed by poorly differentiated lymphocytes and histiocytes.[71] Over the years, the Rappaport classification has been popular with clinicians because it is reproduced easily

and correlates well with clinical observations. However, it gives little insight into the underlying pathophysiology.

As knowledge accumulated, additional categories were added. Lukes and Collins[72] proposed an immunologic classification system that provides important correlations with the pathophysiology of the lymphoreticular system. Their approach relates lymphoma cell morphology to the sequential stages in the histogenesis of normal B- and T-lymphocytes (Figure 43-3), and the observations are reinforced by the identification of specific T- or B-cell markers on the cell surfaces.

By the late 1970s, in addition to the schemes of Rappaport and Lukes and Collins, four other classifications were in use throughout the world. The alternatives included those of the British National Lymphoma Group, Dorfman, the World Health Organization, and Kiel. A study funded by the National Cancer Institute developed what was hoped would become an international standard of classification for NHL. The Working Formulation[73] was proposed as a means of translation among the various systems to facilitate clinical comparisons and therapeutic trials. The major classifications in the Working Formulation and their pathological counterparts in the Rappaport and Lukes-Collins systems are compared in Table 43-7. The low-grade lymphomas are predominantly B-cell tumors; intermediate-grade lymphomas include B-cell and some T-cell neoplasms; immunoblastic malignancies are predominantly B-cell in origin, while the lymphoblastic group usually is composed of T-cell tumors. Burkitt's and non-Burkitt's lymphomas manifest B-cell origin, and the rare, true histiocytic lymphomas most likely are derived from the monocyte/macrophage line. Mycosis fungoides is a T-cell neoplasm.

Although the diagnosis of NHL in the Working Formulation is based solely on morphological features, it has predictive value for survival. Tumors with a good prognosis include all the low-grade NHLs and some of the intermediate-grade tumors with long natural histories. Tumors with a poor prognosis include the rapidly progressive high-grade tumors as well as the diffuse large-cell malignancies from the intermediate-grade group. However, because of their biological behavior and clinical course, most treatment protocols recognize only two major groups—low-grade and high-grade.

Recently, yet another classification of NHL has been proposed, the Revised European-American Lymphoma (REAL) classification.[74] This system is not yet accepted although it offers some advantages in that it includes several types of lymphoma (e.g., Mantle cell lymphoma) not included by the Working Formulation.

### Low-grade lymphomas

The low-grade category includes three tumors: small lymphocytic lymphoma; follicular, predominantly small cleaved cell lymphoma; and follicular mixed (small cleaved and large-cell) lymphoma. These malignancies occur predominantly in older individuals (median age is 55 years), and they affect males and females equally. The

**TABLE 43-7** Non-Hodgkin's Lymphoma Nomenclature: Comparative Classifications

| Working Formulation | Rappaport System | Lukes-Collins System |
|---|---|---|
| **LOW-GRADE** | | |
| A  Small lymphocytic | Diffuse, well-differentiated lymphocytic | Small lymphocytic B-cell or T-cell |
| B  Follicular, small cleaved | Nodular, poorly differentiated lymphocytic | Follicular, small cleaved FCC |
| C  Follicular, mixed small cleaved, and large-cell | Nodular, mixed lymphocytic and histiocytic | Follicular, mixed small cleaved and large FCC |
| **INTERMEDIATE-GRADE** | | |
| D  Follicular, large-cell | Nodular histiocytic | Follicular, large cleaved and/or non-cleaved FCC |
| E  Diffuse, small cleaved | Diffuse, poorly differentiated lymphocytic | Diffuse, small cleaved FCC |
| F  Diffuse, mixed small and large | Diffuse, mixed lymphocytic and histiocytic | Diffuse, mixed small and large cleaved or noncleaved FCC |
| G  Diffuse, large-cell | Diffuse histiocytic | Diffuse, large cleaved or noncleaved FCC |
| **HIGH-GRADE** | | |
| H  Immunoblastic, large-cell | Diffuse histiocytic | Immunoblastic sarcoma, B-cell or T-cell |
| I  Lymphoblastic | Lymphoblastic | Convoluted T-cell |
| J  Small, noncleaved Burkitt's | Undifferentiated, Burkitt's and non-Burkitt's | Small, noncleaved FCC |
| **MISCELLANEOUS** | | |
| | Composite<br>Mycosis fungoides<br>Histiocytic<br>Extramedullary plasmacytoma<br>Unclassifiable<br>Other | |

FCC = follicular center cell

majority of patients are asymptomatic. The usual presenting problems are connected with a painless, progressive, often symmetrical generalized lymphadenopathy. Except for liver and bone marrow involvement, extranodal extension is uncommon.

Like normal lymphocytes, low-grade B-cell lymphomas often circulate; thus, patients generally present with widespread stage III or IV disease. Some patients describe a history of lymph nodes that wax and wane in size for many years prior to diagnosis. Host immunity has been invoked to explain this phenomenon, and, in some cases, clinical regression has been preceded by a viral or bacterial infection.[69]

Most low-grade lymphomas have a long natural history (median survival is seven to nine years) that appears to be largely unaffected by treatment. As the disease progresses, patients may complain of increasing fatigue, malaise, low-grade fever, night sweats, and weight loss. Eventually the general pace of the disease accelerates and the majority of indolent lymphomas transform from low-grade to in-

termediate- or high-grade malignancies. Treatment strategies must then be modified to be appropriate for aggressive lymphomas. Death usually results from progressive growth and eventual tumorous replacement of hematopoietic and lymphoid tissues, thereby producing multiple systemic dysfunctions. Although the overall picture for these lymphomas seems optimistic, the disease is usually fatal; median survival generally is less than one year after such transformation.

### Intermediate-grade lymphomas

There are four neoplasms under the intermediate-grade category in the Working Formulation—an uncommon tumor with a follicular architecture and three others with a diffuse pattern. The follicular, predominantly large-cell NHL has a more aggressive clinical course than that of the other more indolent subtypes of follicular lymphomas. Most patients have advanced disease at the time of diagnosis. Peripheral blood involvement is unusual. Immunologically, these are neoplasms of B-lymphocytes, and almost all cases exhibit translocations of chromosomes 14 and 18.

Because they share similar clinical, histological and immunologic features, the three diffuse subgroups in the Working Formulation can be grouped together. These lymphomas occur mainly in adults, and, unlike follicular NHL, patients with diffuse neoplasms often present with disease limited to one side of the diaphragm. Although nodal presentation is common, these subtypes frequently involve extranodal progression to the gastrointestinal tract, skin, and bone. Privileged sites such as the testes and central nervous system also may be involved. If left untreated, diffuse NHLs are invariably fatal and survival is less than two years. However, these malignancies are responsive to chemotherapy and a significant chance for cure exists, particularly in patients with localized disease.

### High-grade lymphomas

High-grade lymphomas consist of three quite distinct diseases that are grouped together in the Working Formulation because of their aggressive clinical behavior and poor prognosis. The first of this group are immunoblastic lymphomas. The term *immunoblast* refers to an activated lymphocyte. Under the influence of mitogens and/or antigens to which the individual has been previously exposed, T and B cells transform from small or dormant lymphocytes to large, metabolically active, dividing forms.[71] The majority of immunoblastic tumors are of B-cell origin, although a small percentage with T-cell ontogeny are related to peripheral T-cell lymphomas. These neoplasms usually occur in adults over 50 years old. Anemia, B symptoms, and advanced stage are common at presentation, and a high incidence of cutaneous disease has been reported. It is of interest to note that approximately 50% of B-immunoblastic lymphomas are associated with a previous history of immunologic impairment such as that seen in Sjögren's syndrome or with states of immunosuppression as in transplant recipients or patients with AIDS. Poor responses to chemotherapy and poor survival are characteristic of this group.

Lymphoblastic lymphoma is a high-grade, usually T-cell malignancy that is closely related to T-cell acute lymphocytic leukemia. Adolescents and young adults account for the majority of cases; 40% of childhood lymphomas fall into this category. Males outnumber females by a 2:1 ratio. Approximately two-thirds of the patients present with a prominent anterior mediastinal mass suggestive of a thymic origin. There is usually widespread involvement of lymph nodes, and lytic bone lesions are not uncommon. Unless effectively treated, patients have a rapidly progressive, downhill course with dissemination of tumor to the bone marrow, blood, cerebrospinal fluid, and central nervous system. Recent attempts to treat this malignancy with aggressive leukemic protocols and bone marrow transplantation offer new encouragement.[75]

Within the category of small, noncleaved cell lympho-mas are two distinct subtypes. Burkitt's lymphoma (BL) occurs endemically in tropical Africa and New Guinea, where it is associated with the Epstein-Barr virus. This lymphoma is more common in males than females, and the average age at onset is seven years. Massive involvement of the jaw, ovaries, kidneys, liver, mesentery, and central nervous system is a prominent feature. U.S. cases of BL are not associated with EBV and arise in slightly older children (11 years). Involvement of the ileocecal region of the bowel is common and often results in obstruction and intussception. Children older than 13 years of age at onset have a poorer prognosis. In general, Burkitt's tumors are highly sensitive to chemotherapeutic agents, and their response is often dramatic and enduring.

Non-Burkitt's lymphoma is a relatively uncommon malignancy. The median age is 34 years, and incidence is equal for males and females. Peripheral lymphadenopathy is a common clinical manifestation, and bone marrow, liver, central nervous system, and gastrointestinal tract are major sites for extranodal progression. In patients who have undergone treatment for HD and in those with AIDS, this type of lymphoma often occurs, as a complicating factor.[76] Because the disease disseminates rapidly, even multiagent chemotherapy is generally ineffective, and the median survival is approximately one year.

Typically, aggressive lymphomas exhibit rapid tumor growth and a high mitotic index. Without treatment, survival is usually less than 18 months. However, because these neoplasms respond better to chemotherapy than the indolent, low-grade lymphomas, they have a greater potential for cure, especially if complete remissions are sustained for at least two years. From a prognostic perspective, clinical evaluation of NHLs at the National Institutes of Health has revealed that the following features independently have an adverse effect on survival: male sex, poor performance status, B symptoms, anemia (hemoglobin <12 g/dl), high serum lactate dehydrogenase (>500 U), bone marrow involvement, liver involvement, large (>10 cm) abdominal mass, and age greater than 65 years.[71]

### Mycosis fungoides (cutaneous T-cell lymphoma)

Among the miscellaneous group of lymphomas, the best characterized is a rare disorder referred to in older literature as *mycosis fungoides* and in current reviews as *cutaneous T-cell lymphoma (CTCL)*. Involvement of the skin is a hallmark of this malignancy that results from the clonal proliferation of T-lymphocytes. CTCL tends to be initially indolent, but it may evolve into a widely disseminated malignancy. The disease occurs in middle age, and males are affected more often than females. Histologically, there is infiltration of the epidermis and upper dermis with neoplastic T-cells, which have an extremely unusual cerebriform nucleus. Clinically, the lesions exhibit three distinct cutaneous stages. The initial premycotic stage is characterized by superficial inflammatory skin eruptions and generalized pruritus. In this stage,

CTCL may be confused with other dermatologic disorders such as psoriasis and eczema. Eventually the disease progresses through an aggravated plaque stage to one with nodular tumors. In most patients with extensive disease, extracutaneous manifestations and visceral dissemination develop and ultimately lead to a fatal outcome. A variety of CTCL, the Sézary syndrome, presents with generalized exfoliative erythroderma and circulating leukemia-like cerebriform lymphocytes. The full implication of detecting circulating neoplastic cells has not been fully determined. In general, however, CTCL patients with a high percentage of circulating Sézary cells have a shorter survival compared to those with a lower percentage.[77]

### Mantle cell lymphoma

Mantle cell lymphoma, also called centrocytic or intermediate lymphoma, is a distinct clinical and pathological entity comprising about 5%–15% of NHL. These cases were formerly classified in the Working Formulation as group E (diffuse small cleaved). There is a very aggressive clinical course due to the high proliferative rate of the lymphoma cells. None of the usual chemotherapeutic regimens seems curative and these lymphomas have the worst prognosis of the common lymphomas.[65] High-dose chemotherapy regimens with or without stem cell rescue may be the treatment of choice.

## Staging

Once a histological diagnosis of NHL has been confirmed by biopsy, a careful, comprehensive staging workup is essential to determine the extent of the disease, the bulk of the tumor mass, and the imminence of potential complications. The workup enables the physician to provide an accurate prognosis and to plan effective treatment. Both the condition of the patient and the histopathologic classification of the tumor direct the type and speed of staging procedures to be performed. For example, an individual with a rapidly progressive, high-grade lymphoma whose natural history can be measured in weeks requires immediate initiation of therapy with only essential procedures performed beforehand. On the other hand, an indolent, low-grade lymphoma can be staged at the convenience of the patient and physician.[78]

Baseline studies for all patients should include complete history and physical examination with particular emphasis on all lymphoid tissue including liver, spleen, Waldeyer's ring, and lymph nodes. Also required are complete blood counts, blood chemistries including liver and kidney function tests, erythrocyte sedimentation rate, uric acid, serum immunoglobulins, and bone marrow biopsy. The latter is an important evaluative component because there is a high incidence of marrow involvement in stage III and IV disease in the low-grade lymphomas and an equal distribution of stage I and II versus stage III and IV with less marrow involvement in the intermediate- and high-grade groups.

Unlike HD, where the disease sites are more predictable and orderly, the multiplicity of potential NHL locations and the variety of their clinical presentations forestall the adoption of a single radiological scheme. All patients require a chest x-ray to facilitate detection of hilar adenopathy, mediastinal mass, parenchymal lung infiltration, or pleural/pericardial effusions. Computed tomography (CT) of the chest is advised when the x-ray is suspicious. Abdominal and pelvic CT should be performed on all individuals because nodal and extranodal masses in these regions occur frequently in some subgroups.[68] The CT scan is replacing lymphangiography (LAG) in many patients because of its usefulness in detecting upper retroperitoneal and mesenteric nodes, as well as hepatic and splenic extension. These are important areas of assessment in most cases of NHL. LAG does have one distinct advantage: The dye often remains in nodal tissues for 6 months or more, so abnormal nodes can be closely monitored during treatment and follow-up.

Additional studies that may be appropriate in certain circumstances include multiple biopsies of the liver, removal of the spleen for pathological study, and exploratory laparotomy for biopsy of multiple lymph node groups. As a rule, surgical evaluation of the abdomen should be undertaken only if it clearly makes a major difference in the treatment selection. However, in patients with extensive gastrointestinal disease, a staging laparotomy can be helpful in reducing the risk of perforation and/or bleeding complications. A recent study indicates that refinements in endoscopic technology may eliminate the need for gastrectomy and its associated sequelae during the initial treatment phase of gastric lymphomas.[79] Table 43-8 outlines the current suggestions for staging procedures in NHL.

After clinical evaluation is complete, patients are classified according to the criteria previously outlined for HD in the Ann Arbor–Cottswolds staging system (Figure 43-5). It is important to note that this system is not as useful in directing the management of NHLs because these malignancies are characterized by early hematogenous dissemination and their natural history is poorly described by staging criteria based primarily on anatomic distribution. However, the clinical stage within each histological subtype does appear to carry reliable prognostic significance.[78]

## Treatment

The treatment of NHL usually requires a multidisciplinary approach to effect an optimal cure rate. This approach is determined by several key factors: histology of the tumor, stage of the disease, and physiological performance status of the patient. The histological grades of the Working Formulation represent a spectrum of survival in untreated patients that ranges from just weeks in the highly aggressive lymphomas to years in the indolent

**TABLE 43-8** Staging Procedures for Non-Hodgkin's Lymphoma

---

### REQUIRED

1. Adequate surgical biopsy, reviewed by an experienced hematologist
2. A detailed history recording duration and the presence or absence of fever, unexplained sweating and its severity, unexplained pruritus, and unexplained weight loss
3. A careful and detailed physical examination; special attention to all node-bearing areas, including Waldeyer's ring (indirect laryngoscopy is the procedure of choice) and determination of size of liver and spleen
4. Necessary laboratory procedures
   a. Complete blood count, including an erythrocytic sedimentation rate
   b. Serum alkaline phosphatase
   c. Evaluation of renal function
   d. Evaluation of liver function
5. Radiologic studies include
   a. Chest roentgenogram (posteroanterior and lateral)
   b. Bilateral lower extremity lymphogram
   c. Abdominal-pelvic computed axial tomographic scan
6. Bilateral bone marrow needle biopsies (not just aspirates; biopsy should be performed before aspirate, if both are done together)

---

### VARIABLE

1. Whole-chest tomography if any abnormality is noted or suspected on the routine chest roentgenogram
2. Abdominal ultrasonogram, inferior cavography, intravenous pyelogram or upper or lower GI contrast studies to supplement lymphographic findings or investigate sites of unexplained symptoms
3. Plain bone radiographs of symptomatic or tender areas
4. Head or spinal CT for neurologic signs or symptoms
5. Exploratory laparotomy and splenectomy, if management decision will depend on the identification of abdominal involvement. Note: Decision to proceed with laparotomy requires knowledge of treatment plan used at institution of record
6. Magnetic resonance imaging
7. Gallium whole-body scans
8. Skeletal scintigrams
9. Hepatic and splenic scintigrams
10. Serum chemistries to include serum calcium and uric acid for overall management of patient
11. Estimates of the patient's delayed hypersensitivity of the tuberculin type

---

Adapted with permission from Longo DL, DeVita VT, Jaffe ES, et al: Lymphocytic lymphomas, in DeVita VT, Hellman S, Rosenberg SA (eds): *Cancer: Principles and Practice of Oncology*, (vol 2) (ed 4). Philadelphia, Lippincott, 1993.

grades. Thus, the primary determinant in any treatment program is the natural history of the histological subtype.

The second major consideration is the extent of disease. Unlike HD, with its organized progression via contiguous nodal groups, most NHLs are widely disseminated at diagnosis. Therefore, in order to be of any practical use, their staging must always be modified according to histology.

Evaluation of individual performance status is the final component in treatment planning. Because the primary goal for many lymphomas is cure, the majority of therapeutic regimens are quite toxic. However, the observed toxicities are nearly always dose-related and predictable. Although the patient's physical status, age, and underlying medical problems should be taken into consideration when planning aggressive therapy, it is important to remember that advanced age per se is not a contraindication to using an effective program. "Patients with aggressive lymphomas will have a short and unpleasant life because of the lymphoma. Those with potentially curable disease should therefore not be treated gently out of fear of causing toxicities."[69]

### Indolent lymphomas

There is no area of lymphoma treatment that is more controversial than what, if any, approach can alter the natural history of indolent or low-grade NHLs and induce their long-term, disease-free survival. This concern is quite understandable because the natural history of these malignancies has been such that, despite any therapeutic intervention, most patients live with their disease and eventually die from it. Some physicians advocate a policy of "watchful waiting" until systemic symptoms require intervention. When symptoms develop, patients are managed with sufficient chemotherapy or radiotherapy to control the disease, at which point the program of "watchful waiting" is resumed.

An alternate approach is the use of intensive combination chemotherapy regimens to induce a complete remission. The patient is then observed until the time of recurrence. These regimens almost never produce a cure as in the treatment of aggressive lyhmphoma. Total body irradiation will produce a complete remission, but the average duration is only two to three years and it is doubtful if this is superior to combination chemotherapy.

High-dose chemotherapy with stem cell rescue has been tried in low-grade lymphoma and some feel it is beneficial, but at the present time there are no data to show that any particular therapeutic strategy is superior to "watchful waiting."[80] Given the long, benign course of this disease, even though it is ultimately fatal, a conservative approach may be best.

New agents such as fludarabine may offer promise. Fludarabine is highly active in indolent lymphoma and its use in combination with other agents has not been thoroughly explored.[81]

### Aggressive lymphomas

Patients with unfavorable histology (intermediate- and high-grade lymphomas) have a much more aggressive disease process, which usually results in a rapid, downhill progression. Thus, there is no place for administration of single agents in the primary treatment plan. Historically, RT has been used with moderate success in those with stage I and II disease.

The recognized treatment of choice for advanced-stage aggressive NHL is combination chemotherapy.[82] Over the past 20 years, therapeutic regimens of increasing intensity have evolved (Table 43-9). The initial combination of an alkylating agent, a vinca alkaloid, and a corticosteroid (CVP or COP) has been enhanced by the addition of doxorubicin and other agents, resulting in such protocols as CHOP, BACOP, and C-MOPP. These are usually given as monthly cycles for six to nine months and produce long-term remissions in 35%–45% of cases.[69] The major problems associated with these combinations involve tumor regrowth between cycles and central nervous system relapse.[83]

Because of their ability to cross the blood-brain barrier, second-generation regimens such as M-BACOD, m-BACOD, PROMACE/MOPP, and COP-BLAM have been designed. These combinations use methotrexate with leucovorin rescue or cytosine arabinoside to prevent lymphomatous extension to the central nervous system. In an attempt to defeat the intrinsic drug resistance of tumor cell populations, they also utilize a staggered dose schedule for myelotoxic and nonmyelotoxic agents.

Attempts to refine programs with even more intense protocols have led to third-generation combinations such as MACOP-B, PROMACE/CYTABOM, and COP-BLAM III. The two major principles that have influenced their design are the Goldie-Coldman[42] hypothesis and the Hryniuk[84] dose-intensity hypothesis. The former theory estimates that a larger fraction of patients will be cured if they are exposed to the largest number of agents at full doses as early as possible in the treatment course. The latter predicts that the best results will occur when a maximum rate of drug delivery is maintained.

The second- and third-generation regimens for aggressive NHL were developed and tested in non-randomized trials. Before they could be accepted as standard therapy it was necessary to compare them to CHOP, which was the accepted standard. This was done in a series of randomized studies with rather surprising results. CHOP was either superior to or equivalent to the more intensive

**TABLE 43-9** Chemotherapeutic Regimens for Aggressive Lymphomas

| Regimen | Dose and Route | Day | Frequency |
|---|---|---|---|
| CVP | | | |
| C—cyclophosphamide | 400 mg/m² PO | 1–5 | Repeat every 21 days |
| V—vincristine (Oncovin) | 1.4 mg/m² IV | 1 | |
| P—prednisone | 100 mg/m² PO | 1–5 | |
| C-MOPP | | | |
| C—cyclophosphamide | 650 mg/m² IV | 1, 8 | Repeat every 28 days |
| O—vincristine (Oncovin) | 1.4 mg/m² IV | 1, 8 | |
| P—procarbazine | 100 mg/m² PO | 1–14 | |
| P—prednisone | 40 mg/m² PO | 1–14 | |
| BACOP | | | |
| B—bleomycin | 5 u/m² IV | 15, 22 | Repeat every 28 days |
| A—doxorubicin (Adriamycin) | 25 mg/m² IV | 1, 8 | |
| C—cyclophosphamide | 650 mg/m² IV | 1, 8 | |
| O—vincristine (Oncovin) | 1.4 mg/m² IV | 1, 8 | |
| P—prednisone | 60 mg/m² PO | 15–28 | |
| CHOP | | | |
| C—cyclophosphamide | 750 mg/m² IV | 1 | Repeat every 21 days |
| H—doxorubicin (Adriamycin) | 50 mg/m² IV | 1 | |
| O—vincristine (Oncovin) | 1.4 mg/m² IV (max 2.0 mg) | 1 | |
| P—prednisone | 100 mg PO | 1–5 | |
| COMLA | | | |
| C—cyclophosphamide | 1500 mg/m² IV | 1 | Repeat every 91 days |
| O—vincristine (Oncovin) | 1.4 mg/m² IV (max 2.0 mg) | 1, 8, 15 | |
| M—methotrexate | 120 mg/m² IV (bolus) | 22, 29, 36, 43, 50, 57, 64, 71 | |
| L—leucovorin | 25 mg/m² PO × 4 | 24 hours after methotrexate | |
| A—cytarabine | 300 mg/m² IV | Same as methotrexate | |
| COP/BLAM | | | |
| C—cyclophosphamide | 400 mg/m² IV | 1 | Repeat every 21 days |
| O—vincristine (Oncovin) | 1 mg/m² IV | 1 | |
| P—prednisone | 40 mg/m² PO | 1–10 | |
| BL—bleomycin | 15 u/m² IV | 15 | |
| A—doxorubicin (Adriamycin) | 40 mg/m² IV | 1 | |
| M—procarbazine | 100 mg/m² PO | 1–10 | |

**TABLE 43-9**    Chemotherapeutic Regimens for Aggressive Lymphomas (continued)

| Regimen | Dose and Route | Day | Frequency |
|---|---|---|---|
| **M-BACOD** | | | |
| M—methotrexate* | 3000 mg/m² IV (over 40–60 minutes) | 14 | Repeat every 21 days |
| B—bleomycin | 4 u/m² IV | 1 | |
| A—doxorubicin (Adriamycin) | 45 mg/m² IV | 1 | |
| C—cyclophosphamide | 600 mg/m² IV | 1 | |
| O—vincristine (Oncovin) | 1 mg/m² IV | 1 | |
| D—dexamethasone (Decadron) | 6 mg/m² PO | 1–5 | |
| **m-BACOD** | | | |
| m—methotrexate* | 200 mg/m² IV (over 15 minutes) | 8, 15 | Repeat every 21 days |
| B—bleomycin | 4 u/m² IV | 1 | |
| A—doxorubicin (Adriamycin) | 45 mg/m² IV | 1 | |
| C—cyclophosphamide | 600 mg/m² IV | 1 | |
| O—vincristine (Oncovin) | 1.4 mg/m² IV | 1 | |
| D—dexamethasone (Decadron) | 6 mg/m² PO | 1–5 | |
| **ProMACE-MOPP** | | | |
| Pro—prednisone | 60 mg/m² PO | 1–14 | Repeat every 28 days |
| M—methotrexate* | 1500 mg/m² IV (over 12 hours) | 15 | |
| A—doxorubicin (Adriamycin) | 25 mg/m² IV | 1, 8 | |
| C—cyclophosphamide | 650 mg/m² IV | 1, 8 | |
| E—etoposide | 120 mg/m² IV | 1, 8 | |
| *Followed by MOPP after maximal response* | | | |
| M—mechlorethamine | 6 mg/m² IV | 1, 8 | Repeat every 28 days |
| O—vincristine (Oncovin) | 1.4 mg/m² IV | 1, 8 | |
| P—procarbazine | 100 mg/m² PO | 1–14 | |
| P—prednisone | 40 mg/m² PO | 1–14 | |
| **ProMACE-CytaBOM** | | | |
| Pro—prednisone | 60 mg/m² PO | 1–14 | Repeat every 21 days |
| A—doxorubicin (Adriamycin) | 25 mg/m² IV | 1 | |
| C—cyclophosphamide | 650 mg/m² IV | 1 | |
| E—etoposide | 120 mg/m² IV | 1 | |
| Cyta—cytarabine | 300 mg/m² IV | 8 | |
| B—bleomycin | 5 u/m² IV | 8 | |
| O—vincristine (Oncovin) | 1.4 mg/m² IV | 8 | |
| M—methotrexate* | 120 mg/m² IV bolus | 8 | |
| **ProMACEd1/MOPPd8** | | | |
| Pro—prednisone | 60 mg/m² PO | 1–14 | Repeat every 28 days |
| M—methotrexate* | 500 mg/m² IV (over 1 hour) | 15 | |
| A—doxorubicin (Adriamycin) | 25 mg/m² IV | 1 | |
| C—cyclophosphamide | 650 mg/m² IV | 1 | |
| E—etoposide | 120 mg/m² IV | 1 | |
| M—mechlorethamine | 6 mg/m² IV | 8 | |
| O—vincristine (Oncovin) | 1.4 mg/m² IV | 8 | |
| P—procarbazine | 100 mg/m² PO | 8–14 | |
| **MACOP-B** | | | |
| M—methotrexate* | 400 mg/m² IV (100 mg/m² IV bolus, then 300 mg/m² IV over 4 hours) | 8, 36 64 | Repeat every 84 days |
| A—doxorubicin (Adriamycin) | 50 mg/m² IV | 1, 15, 29, 43, 57, 71 | |
| C—cyclophosphamide | 350 mg/m² IV | 1, 15, 29, 43, 57, 71 | |
| O—vincristine (Oncovin) | 1.4 mg/m² IV (max. 2.0 mg) | 8, 22, 36, 50, 64, 78 | |
| P—prednisone | 75 mg/m² PO | 1–84 | |
| B—bleomycin | 10 u/m² IV | 22, 50, 78 | |

*Leucovorin rescue is given for 24 hours after each methotrexate dose.

IV = intravenously; PO = by mouth.

Reprinted with permission from Gaynor ER, Fisher RI: Diffuse aggressive lymphomas in adults, in Magrath IT (ed): *The Non-Hodgkin's Lymphomas.* Baltimore, Williams & Wilkins, 1990.

regimens.[85-87] It was concluded that CHOP was the best treatment for intermediate-grade and high-grade NHL.

High-dose chemotherapy with stem cell rescue was suggested as appropriate for patients who had slow responses to initial therapy and thus were at high risk of early relapse. When this approach was compared in a randomized fashion to conventional CHOP in patients who achieved only a partial remission after three cycles of CHOP, no difference in disease-free survival was noted.[88] It was concluded that high-dose marrow ablative chemoradiotherapy with autologous bone marrow transplantation did not improve the outcome in patients with aggressive NHL that responds slowly to first-line CHOP chemotherapy.

## Salvage Therapy

Relapsed indolent lymphomas are rarely resistant to treatment unless they undergo histological progression. Thus, retreatment with the same induction program often produces additional responses. In contrast, however, the outlook for nonresponsive or relapsed aggressive lymphomas is dismal. Despite the fact that most of the tumors originally are sensitive to chemotherapeutic combinations at the time of relapse, refractoriness to treatment is the rule rather than the exception; thus, cure is rarely possible with recurrent aggressive NHL. Patients who relapse generally have a reduced bone marrow reserve as a result of primary therapy (whether radiotherapy or chemotherapy) and tolerate secondary treatment poorly. These individuals require platelet transfusions as the chemotherapy drives their platelet counts into the danger zone below 20,000/mm³. Overall, sepsis is a major cause of morbidity and mortality.

With the advent of high-dose therapy followed by autologous bone marrow transplantation (ABMT), a substantial number of relapsed patients with aggressive lymphoma are achieving durable second complete remissions.[89,90] The induction regimen usually consists of high-dose cyclophosphamide followed by total body irradiation, and it appears that other agents such as cytosine arabinoside and etoposide can be added without significant increase in toxicity.[91] Clinical trials seem to indicate that allogeneic bone marrow transplantation may provide an alternative to conventional chemotherapy for those with poor-prognosis Burkitt's lymphoma.[92] In patients with positive marrow disease, a new technique for collecting stem cells from peripheral blood provides a viable transplant option.[93,94]

Biological response modifiers have shown initial promise in the treatment of select malignancies and presumably work by boosting an endogenous antitumor immune response. In an attempt to provide better treatment outcomes for patients with lymphoma, a number of these agents (e.g., interferons, monoclonal antibodies, interleukin-2, and colony stimulating factors) have been used.[95-97] Current results from clinical trials, although promising in some instances, remain generally inconclusive.

## COMPLICATIONS OF TREATMENT

Radiotherapy often causes complications during treatment (acute) or following the completion of treatment (subacute or late). The most common reactions associated with mantle irradiation are loss of taste, dry mouth, redness of skin, dysphagia, loss of hair at the nape of the neck, nausea, and vomiting. Because the amount of saliva is decreased, these individuals are at increased risk of dental caries. Therefore, instructions in proper dental hygiene, which includes routine examination and cleaning every four to six months, should always be given.

Inverted-Y port irradiation usually results in nausea, vomiting, anorexia, diarrhea, and malaise. Bone marrow depression may occur and must be monitored by frequent complete blood counts. Total nodal irradiation leads to all the side effects noted previously and particularly to severe bone marrow depression.

The various combinations of chemotherapy used in the treatment of HD and NHL will invariably result in acute and chronic side effects. The nature of these responses depends on the drugs used, but many are common to most anticancer agents. The most frequent side effect is nausea and vomiting. Although the severity of this reaction varies from one individual to another, it is generally transient and can often be effectively controlled by antiemetics. Depending on the particular drug regimen administered, other reactions can include alopecia, myalgia, chills, fever, euphoria, fluid retention, stomatitis, gastrointestinal disturbances, hemorrhagic cystitis, and mental depression. The most serious side effect produced by all combination regimens is bone marrow suppression, which renders the individual susceptible to infection and hemorrhage. Specific aspects of nursing care related to these side effects are covered elsewhere in this text.

## CONSEQUENCES OF SURVIVAL

Oncological advances in diagnostic technology, therapeutic regimens, and supportive interventions have shown great progress in the past two decades, and many lymphoma patients face a future in which long-term survival is a reasonable expectation. However, the cost of such progress is yet to be determined. While acute toxicities of established treatment modalities are well documented, clinical evaluation studies are just beginning to investigate the delayed effects and iatrogenic risks associated with surgery (splenectomy/laparotomy), radiation therapy, and chemotherapy. The delayed toxicities tend to produce lifelong problems and may vary in severity from relatively minor to potentially fatal.[98] Table 43-10 highlights a number of long-term complications that may develop in those cured of malignant lymphomas.

It is important to stress that no organ system is immune to alteration. An extension of injury to the lungs is common in mantle irradiation, and it may develop as early as one to three months after RT is completed. Resulting complications can include pneumothorax, radiation pneumonitis, pulmonary fibrosis, and superimposed pulmonary and parenchymal infections. In addition, nitrosoureas, high-dose busulfan, and bleomycin are known to induce fibrotic lung damage.[99]

Tumors on the right side of the superior mediastinum have the potential to obstruct the return of blood to the heart from the superior vena cava. This produces a characteristic syndrome of edema in the upper half of the body that is associated with prominent collateral cir-

**TABLE 43-10**   Long-Term Complications in Patients Cured of Malignant Lymphoma

| Complication | Etiology and Risk Factors | Management and Prevention |
|---|---|---|
| Immunologic dysfunction | Underlying disease, therapy | Appropriate vaccinations |
| Herpes zoster-varicella | Underlying disease, therapy | Systemic antiviral therapy, zoster immune globulin |
| Pneumococcal sepsis | Splenectomy | Pretherapy pneumonococcal vaccine, selected |
|  | Functional asplenia postradiation therapy (RT) | antibiotic prophylaxis, avoid unnecessary staging splenectomy |
| Nonlymphocytic leukemia | Therapy, age above 40 | Avoid combined modality therapy for HD; supportive care; low-dose chemotherapy; aggressive therapy +/− bone marrow transplant |
| Myelodysplastic syndromes | Therapy, age above 40 | Same as above |
| Non-Hodgkin's lymphoma | Therapy | Aggressive combination CT (e.g., MACOP-B) |
| Solid tumors | Direct or indirect RT exposure | Conventional management |
| Thymic hyperplasia | Underlying disease, therapy | Resection |
| Hypothyroidism | Direct or indirect RT exposure | Hormone replacement, thyroid suppression during therapy (?) |
| Thyroid cancer | Direct or indirect RT exposure, chronic thyroid stimulation | Thyroid suppression |
| Male infertility | Therapy, underlying disease | Attempt sperm storage, testicular shielding during RT, suppression of spermatogenesis during CT (?), alternative chemotherapy regimens |
| Male impotence | Therapy, underlying disease | Counseling, trial of testosterone |
| Female infertility | Therapy | Oophoropexy, ovarian suppression during therapy (?), cyclic estrogen replacement |
| Female impotence | Therapy, underlying disease | Counseling, cyclic estrogen replacement |
| Pericarditis, acute | Mediastinal RT, recall with chemotherapy (CT) post-RT | Appropriate RT shielding and technique; avoid doxorubicin post-RT; anti-inflammatory medication; pericardiocentesis |
| Pericarditis, chronic | Mediastinal RT | Appropriate RT shielding and technique, pericardiectomy |
| Cardiomyopathy | Mediastinal RT, doxorubicin, recall with CT post-RT | Appropriate RT shielding and technique; avoid doxorubicin post-RT; monitor for early signs of toxicity; limit cumulative doxorubicin dose; supportive medical management |
| Pneumonitis, acute | Direct or indirect RT, bleomycin, nitrosoureas, recall with CT post-RT | Appropriate RT shielding and technique, monitor for early signs of toxicity, avoid known toxic drugs, avoid excessive pO$_2$ |
| Pneumonitis, chronic | Same as above | Supportive management |
| Avascular necrosis | Steroid therapy, underlying disease (?) | Anti-inflammatory medications, joint surgery |
| Growth retardation | Pediatric RT | Minimize RT, use symmetric RT fields |
| Dental caries | Salivary change post-RT | Maintain good oral hygiene, daily fluoride treatment |

Reprinted with permission from DeVita VT, Mauch PM, Harris NL: Hodgkin's disease, in DeVita VT, Hellman S, Rosenberg SA (eds): *Cancer: Principles and Practice of Oncology* (ed 2). Philadelphia, Lippincott, 1997.

culation. Lung cancer, especially the oat cell variety, is the most common cause of this complication, but the lymphomas represent the second most common precipitating factor. This is an oncological emergency that necessitates prompt therapy aimed at relieving pressure on the superior vena cava. External beam radiation therapy has been the traditional approach, especially in the management of an acute-onset syndrome.[100]

Both RT and chemotherapy promote toxic effects on the heart and peripheral blood vessels. Acute and chronic pericarditis are not uncommon, and a patient often presents with a spectrum of symptoms ranging from cough and chest pain to edema, paradoxical pulse, cardiac tamponade, and hemodynamic compromise. Coronary artery disease and cardiomyopathy are also seen following extensive mediastinal radiation. Similar risks have been noted with doxorubicin, whose cumulative dose effect often is potentiated when drug administration follows RT.[101]

The multiagent regimens used most in HD (MOPP and ABVD) appear to induce little nephrotoxicity. However, glomerulonephritis is considered a paraneoplastic syndrome of this malignancy. Despite improvements in shielding techniques, radiation damage to the kidneys is possible in retroperitoneal NHL. Limiting the radiation dose to 2000 cGy or less may minimize the risk of a functional deficit. Cyclophosphamide induces topical damage to the bladder, and hemorrhagic cystitis is a potentially serious complication of all chemotherapeutic regimens using this drug.[102]

Because both chemotherapy and radiotherapy are immunosuppressive, bacterial as well as other unusual infections may occur. The most common gram-negative organisms in individuals with lymphoma are *Escherichia coli, Pseudomonas aeruginosa,* and *Klebsiella.* Various species of *Staphylococcus* are also becoming increasingly prevalent infectious agents in these patients. Although fever as a presenting complaint may be attributable to the lymphoma itself, fever in a patient who has been treated (especially one who is neutropenic) must always be considered a sign of potentially life-threatening sepsis until proven otherwise. Thus, appropriate cultures should be obtained and empiric antibiotic therapy must be started immediately.

The two fungal infections diagnosed most often are candidiasis and aspergillosis. *Pneumocystis carinii* is a rare protozoal infection in immunologically normal individuals, but it is frequently pathogenic in lymphoma patients. Currently it is recognized as one of the leading causes of death in the AIDS population.

Herpes zoster is a troublesome complication that is often seen in individuals with HD and NHL. It results from the reactivation of latent foci of chickenpox virus, presumably secondary to the immunosuppression caused by the lymphoma and/or its treatment. The virus is usually localized, but on occasion a life-threatening fulminant process may occur. This infection may be seen at any time during the course of illness, from initial treatment to relapse. In addition, patients who have undergone

splenectomy face a lifelong risk of activation by encapsulated organisms.

Chronic progressive radiation myelopathy is a disabling neurological problem associated with mantle radiation. Symptoms include paresthesias, weakness, and bowel/bladder dysfunction. Peripheral neuropathies are associated with vincristine and vinblastine, and the incidence of central nervous system lymphoma is increasing dramatically in the AIDS population.

Rare as a presenting symptom but commonly seen in progressive lymphoma, compression of the spinal cord represents a complication that is dreaded because of its potential to cripple with paraplegia a person who might otherwise have many productive years remaining. This oncological emergency develops swiftly, with weakness of the lower extremities, increased tendon reflexes, positive Babinski signs, and the development of a sensory "level" below which sensation is lost. Precise localization of the compression by myelogram is essential. Recently, MRI has offered the promise of a non-invasive diagnostic technique, but myelography remains the current diagnostic standard. Early diagnosis is critical to prevention of neurological impairment. Patients who have already developed compromised neurological status usually do not have a return of function after treatment.[103] Consequently the nurse must be sensitive to complaints of leg weakness or bowel and bladder dysfunction, especially in patients with back pain.

Two of the most devastating complications associated with lymphoma treatment are sterility and carcinogenesis. Because many of the patients are less than 40 years old when initially diagnosed, these tragic consequences not only confer physical alterations; they also create severe psychological distress as the individual is forced to face a lack of procreative potential and another malignant threat to life.

During RT, men will experience transient aspermia, but recovery of spermatogenesis has been documented when careful testicular shielding is employed. Women who have not had an oophoropexy or shielding of the ovaries may undergo artificial menopause. At the time of exploratory laparotomy, surgical fixation of the ovaries to the uterus is often performed in young female patients to preserve their ovarian function.

Transient and sometimes permanent male sterility is a recognized complication of induction chemotherapy for lymphoma As a group, the alkylating agents are the most toxic to the testicular germ cells. In general, reversible changes occur up to a given threshold level; irreversible germinal aplasia develops once that threshold has been exceeded. Individuals with HD who are treated with MOPP have a greater than 80% likelihood of developing germinal aplasia, azoospermia, and testicular atrophy with elevated serum follicle-stimulating hormone levels.[104] Chapman and colleagues[105] reported 100% infertility during the first 12 months after therapy in 74 men who received this regimen. Return of active spermatogenesis was seen in only 4 of 64 men 15–51 months after therapy stopped. ABVD, an alternative chemotherapy program for HD, may be as effective as MOPP, but it is less toxic to germinal epithelial cells. The use of combination chemotherapy in women also produces ovarian dysfunction, with those older than 35–40 years of age being the most susceptible. In the case of MOPP therapy, only 40%–50% of the women experienced ovarian failure.[104] Clearly, the complications of gonadal dysfunction may result in considerable psychosocial problems in both men and women being treated for cure.[6] Thus, reproductive counseling and procreative alternatives are essential components of nursing care to consider for this patient population.[106]

Second malignancies may develop after curative treatment for lymphoma.[107] Acute nonlymphocytic leukemia is the most common and well-recognized long-range complication of exposure to radiation or alkylating anticancer drugs. Cumulative risk varies according to the intensity and nature of the treatment and the period of observation. It may range from less than 1% to well over 10%.[108] If both radiation and chemotherapy are used, the risk of subsequent leukemia is greatest. It is generally believed that the alkylating agents are more leukemogenic than other anticancer drugs; thus, a regimen such as ABVD might be associated with a lower rate of leukemia than MOPP.

## SUPPORTIVE CARE

Supportive care of the lymphoma patient begins at diagnosis with an explanation of the disease, a description of the steps that will be taken for staging and treatment, and a generation in the patient of a feeling of confidence in the multidisciplinary team responsible for care. Regardless of whether the primary treatment is radiotherapy or chemotherapy, it is certain that the clinical course will be lengthy and highly toxic. The individual must be prepared to cope with this reality. The person who presents with constitutional symptoms and receives several cycles of chemotherapy often becomes completely asymptomatic. Because symptoms are relieved, the patient might question why he or she should proceed with a treatment program that causes adverse side effects. This follow-up period is crucial if a positive outcome is to be achieved. The nurse can play a major role by providing the understanding and emotional support the patient needs and by making sure the patient understands that although small foci of disease cause no symptoms, they will, if untreated, lead to recurrence.

After the primary treatment there will be a prolonged period (months to years) during which the patient must be observed for a recurrence of disease. This is a particularly trying period because the individual has already, in his or her own mind, been very close to death by virtue of having dealt with the diagnosis of cancer. The treatment has (as a rule) produced complete remission, but each visit to the clinic now carries with it the threat that the disease may have relapsed and the nightmare must begin all over again. The nurse must be aware that whereas the treatment team views this as a "routine" visit for a patient who has responded very well to therapy, the individual perceives every word or facial expression as a potential clue that the cancer has recurred. The reader is referred to chapters 48, 49, and 50 for a review of cancer survivorship issues.

## CONCLUSION

The lymphomas comprise more than a dozen separate neoplasms that exhibit a wide gamut of clinical presentations ranging from slow, indolent growth to rapidly fatal progression. Some lymphomas are highly curable with appropriate therapy, while others show no increase in survival following treatment. These malignancies are separated from each other on the basis of subtle differences and require expert interpretation and evaluation. Megavoltage radiotherapy and combination chemotherapy have provided improved management techniques, leading to the expectation of cure in well over 50% of all individuals with lymphoma. However, the skillful application of the complex and toxic treatments requires a precise delineation of histological type and extent of disease in accordance with rigorously established principles of staging.

Although the etiology of the lymphomas remains elusive, tantalizing hints are provided by the strong suggestion of Epstein-Barr virus–induced Burkitt's lymphoma and other lymphomas, the viruslike epidemiological pattern of nodular sclerosing Hodgkin's disease, and the clear association between malfunction of the immune defense system and the development of non-Hodgkin's lymphoma.

Effective diagnosis, staging, and multimodal management of the lymphomas require the collaborative efforts of multiple health care disciplines. The contributions of the nurse are vital to the achievement of a positive outcome. It is the nurse who, to a greater extent than others on the team, must respond to the patient's deepest need for support and understanding; it is the nurse who must meet the patient's need for careful explanation of the complex diagnostic and therapeutic methods designed to deal with a life-threatening malignancy; and it is the nurse who constantly must be alert to the possible complications of both the disease and its treatment.

The ultimate goal of any therapeutic regimen should be to return the individual to as healthy a lifestyle as possible. Because the cohort of cancer survivors continues to increase, the scope of nursing practice must expand as well. Now that cure is no longer beyond our grasp, emphasis must shift to the rehabilitation arena, where attention that complements the goals of the acute care setting can be directed toward the individual's functional, psychological, vocational, and economic limitations. Although many iatrogenic effects cannot always be anticipated or reversed, early identification of rehabilitation issues and timely intervention by an expert caregiver can help minimize potential disability and enhance overall quality of life. Patients who have struggled to overcome their cancer experience and those who supported them make such efforts meaningful and worthwhile.

# REFERENCES

1. Urba WJ, Longo DL: Hodgkin's Disease. *N Engl J Med* 326: 678–687, 1992

2. Kuppers R, Rajewsky K, Zhao M, et al: Hodgkin's disease: Hodgkin and Reed-Sternberg cells picked from histological sections show clonal immunoglobulin gene rearrangements and appear to be derived from B-cells at various stages of development *Proc Natl Acad Sci USA* 91: 10962–10966, 1994

3. Kadin ME: Pathology of Hodgkin's disease. *Curr Opin Oncol* 6:456–463, 1994

4. Parker SL, Tong T, Bolden S, and Wingo PA: Cancer Statistics, 1996. *CA Cancer J Clin* 65:5–27, 1996

5. Gail MH, Pluda JM, Rabkin CS, et al: Projections of the incidence of non-Hodgkin's lymphoma related to acquired immunodeficiency syndrome. *J Natl Cancer Inst* 83:695–701, 1991

6. Carli PM, Boutron MC, Maynadie M, et al: Increase in the incidence of non-Hodgkin's lymphomas: evidence for a recent sharp increase in France independent of AIDS. *Br J Cancer* 70:713–715, 1994

7. Magrath IT: Lymphocyte ontogeny: A conceptual basis for understanding neoplasia of the immune system, in Magrath IT (ed): *The Non-Hodgkin's Lymphomas.* Baltimore, Williams and Wilkins, 1990, pp 29–48

8. Appelbaum JW: The role of the immune system in the pathogenesis of cancer. *Semin Oncol Nurs* 8:51–62, 1992

9. Opelz G, Henderson R: Incidence of non-Hodgkin's lymphoma in kidney and heart transplant recipients. *Lancet* 342:1514–1516, 1993

10. Parker JW, Lukes RJ: Neoplasms of the immune system, in Stites DP, Terr AI (eds): *Basic and Clinical Immunology.* Norwalk, CT, Appleton and Lange, 1991, pp 599–631

11. Rahr VA, Tucker R: Non-Hodgkin's lymphoma: Understanding the disease. *Cancer Nurs* 13:56–91, 1990

12. Hodgkin T: On some morbid appearances of the absorbent glands and spleen. *Med Chir Tran* 17:68–114, 1832

13. Wilks S: Cases of enlargement of the lymphatic glands and spleen, or Hodgkin's disease. *Guy's Hosp Rep* 11:56–67, 1865

14. Reed DM: On the pathological changes in Hodgkin's disease, with especial reference to tuberculosis. *Johns Hopkins Rep* 10:133–196, 1902

15. Sternberg C: Über eine eigenartige unter dem Bilde der Pseukoleukamie verlaufende: Tuberculose des lymphatischen apparates. *Z Heilkd* 19:21–90, 1898

16. Parker BA, Green MR: Hodgkin's disease, in Moosa AR, Schimpff SC, Robson MC (eds): *Comprehensive Textbook of Oncology* (vol 2) (ed 2). Baltimore, Williams and Wilkins, 1991, pp 1257–1267

17. Cole P, MacMahon B, Aisenberg A: Mortality from Hodg-kin's disease in the United States: Evidence for the multiple etiology hypothesis. *Lancet* 2:1371–1376, 1968

18. Ambinder RF, Browning PJ, Lorenzana I, et al: Epstein-Barr virus and childhood Hodgkin's disease in Honduras and in the United States. *Blood* 81:462–467, 1993

19. Preciado MW, De Matteo E, Diez B, et al: Presence of Epstein-Barr virus and strain type assignment in Argentine childhood Hodgkin's disease. *Blood* 86:3922–3929, 1995

20. Armstrong AA, Alexander FE, Paes RP, et al: Association of Epstein-Barr virus with pediatric Hodgkin's disease. *Am J Pathol* 142:1683–1688, 1993

21. Siebert JD, Ambinder RF, Napoli VM, et al: Human immunodeficiency virus-associated Hodgkin's disease contains latent, not replicative, Epstein-Barr virus. *Hum Pathol* 26: 1191–1195, 1995

22. Grufferman S, Delzell E: Epidemiology of Hodgkin's disease. *Epidemiol Rev* 6:76–106, 1984

23. Robertson SJ, Lowman JT, Grufferman S, et al: Familial Hodgkin's disease. *Cancer* 59:1314–1319, 1987

24. DeVita VT, Mauch PM, Harris NL: Hodgkin's disease, in DeVita VT, Hellman S, Rosenberg SA (eds): *Cancer: Principles and Practice of Oncology* (ed 5). Philadelphia, Lippincott, 1997, pp 2242–2283

25. Slivnick DJ, Nawrocki JF, Fisher RI: Immunology and cellular biology of Hodgkin's disease. *Hematol Oncol Clin North Am* 3:205–220, 1989

26. Hell K, Lorenzen J, Fischer R et al: Hodgkin cells accumulate mRNA for *bcl-2*. *Lab Invest* 73:492–496, 1995

27. Bhagat SK, Medeiros LJ, Weiss LM, et al: *bcl-2* expression in Hodgkin's disease: Correlation with the t(14;18) translocation and Epstein-Barr virus. *Am J Clin Pathol* 99:604–608, 1993

28. Alkan S, Ross CW, Hanson CA, et al: Epstein-Barr virus and *bcl-2* protein overexpression and not detected in the neoplastic cells of nodular lymphocyte predominance Hodgkin's disease. *Mod Pathol* 8:544–547, 1995

29. Schlaifer D, March M, Krajewski S, et al: High expression of the *bcl-x* gene in Reed-Sternberg cells of Hodgkin's disease. *Blood* 85:2671–2674, 1995

30. Weinreb M, Day PJR, Niggli F, et al: The consistent association between Epstein-Barr virus and Hodgkin's disease in children in Kenya. *Blood* 87:3828–3836, 1996

31. Seiz AM, Yarbro CH: Pruritus. In Groenwald SL, Frogge MH, Goodman M, Yarbro CH (eds). *Cancer Symptom Management.* Boston, Jones and Bartlett, 1996, pp. 137–150

32. Strum SB, Dark JK, Rappaport H: Observations of cells resembling Sternberg-Reed cells in conditions other than Hodgkin's disease. *Cancer* 26:176–190, 1970

33. Craver LF, Hall TC, Rappaport H, et al: Report of the nomenclature committee. *Cancer Res* 26:1311, 1966

34. Carbone PP, Kaplan HS, Musshoff K, et al: Report of the committee on Hodgkin's disease staging. *Cancer Res* 31: 1860–1861, 1971

35. Lister TA, Crowther D, Sutcliffe SB, et al: Report of a committee convened to discuss the evaluation and staging of patients with Hodgkin's disease: Cotswolds meeting. *J Clin Oncol* 7:1630–1636, 1989

36. Bonadonna G, Wiernik PH, Santoro A: Clinical treatment of Hodgkin's disease, in Wiernik PH, Canellos GP, Kyle RA, Schiffer CA (eds): *Neoplastic Diseases of the Blood* (ed 2). New York, Churchill-Livingstone, 1991, pp 701–727

37. McFadden ME: Lymphomas, in Groenwald SL, Frogge MH, Goodman M, Yarbro CH (eds): *Cancer Nursing: Princi-*

*ples and Practice* (ed 3). Boston, Jones and Bartlett, 1993, pp 1200–1228

38. Lister TA, Dorreen MS, Faux M, et al: The treatment of Stage III A Hodgkin's disease. *J Clin Oncol* 1:745–759, 1983

39. Longo DL: The case against the routine use of radiation therapy in advanced-stage Hodgkin's disease. *Cancer Invest* 14:353–360, 1996

40. Prosnitz LR, Wu JJ, Yahalom J: The case for adjuvant radiation therapy in advanced Hodgkin's disease. *Cancer Invest* 14:361–370, 1996

41. Santoro A, Bonadonna G, Valagussa P, et al: Long-term results of combined chemotherapy-radiotherapy approach in Hodgkin's disease: Superiority of ABVD plus radiotherapy versus MOPP plus radiotherapy. *J Clin Oncol* 5:27–37, 1987

42. Goldie JH, Coldman AJ, Guaduskus GA: Rationale for the use of alternating non-cross-resistant chemotherapy. *Cancer Treat Rep* 66:439–449, 1982

43. Somers R, Carde P, Henry-Amar M, et al: A randomized study in stage IIIB and IV Hodgkin's disease comparing eight courses of MOPP versus an alternation of MOPP with ABVD. *J Clin Oncol* 12:279–287, 1994

44. Cannellos GP, Anderson JR, Propert KJ, et al: Chemotherapy of advanced Hodgkin's disease with MOPP, ABVD, or MOPP alternating with ABVD. *N Engl J Med* 327:1478–1484, 1992

45. Henkelmann GC, Hagemester FB, Fuller LM: Two cycles of MOPP and radiotherapy for Stage III, A and III, B Hodgkin's disease. *J Clin Oncol* 6:1293–1302, 1988

46. Schomberg PJ, Evans RG, O'Connell MJ, et al: Prognostic significance of mediastinal mass in adult Hodgkin's disease. *Cancer* 53:324–328, 1984

47. Prakash U, Abel MD: Mediastinal mass and tracheal obstruction during general anesthesia. *Mayo Clin Proc* 63:1004–1011, 1988

48. Leopold KA, Canellos GP, Rosenthal D, et al: Stage IA-IIB Hodgkin's disease. Staging and treatment of patients with large mediastinal adenopathy. *J Clin Oncol* 7:1059–1065, 1989

49. Fisher R, DeVita VT, Hubbard S, et al: Prolonged disease-free survival in Hodgkin's disease with MOPP reinduction after first relapse. *Ann Intern Med* 90:761, 1979

50. Jotti GS, Bonadonna G: Prognostic factors in Hodgkin's disease: Implications for modern treatment. *Anticancer Res* 8:749–759, 1988 (review)

51. Jones RJ, Piantadosi S, Mann RB, et al: High-dose cytotoxic therapy and bone marrow transplantation for relapsed Hodgkin's disease. *J Clin Oncol* 8:527–537, 1990

52. Ager S, Wimperis JZ, Tolliday B, et al: Autologous bone marrow transplantation for Hodgkin's disease—a five-year single centre experience. *Leuk Lymphoma* 13:263–272, 1994

53. Nademanee A, O'Donnell MR, Snyder DS, et al: High-dose chemotherapy with or without total body irradiation followed by autologous bone marrow and/or peripheral blood stem cell transplantation for patients with relapsed and refractory Hodgkin's disease: Results in 85 patients with analysis of prognostic factors. *Blood* 85:1381–1390, 1995

54. Magrath IT: The non-Hodgkin's lymphomas: An introduction, in Magrath IT (ed): *The Non-Hodgkin's Lymphomas* Baltimore, Williams and Wilkins, 1990, pp 1–14

55. Aisenberg AC: A historical overview of malignant lymphoma, in Wiernik PH, Canellos GP, Kyle RA, Schiffer CA (eds): *Neoplastic Diseases of the Blood* (ed 2). New York, Churchill-Livingstone, 1991, pp 597–607

56. Lester EP, Ultmann JE: Lymphoma, in Williams WJ, Beutler E, Erslev AJ, Lichtman MA (eds): *Hematology* (ed 1). New York, McGraw-Hill, 1990, pp 1067–1087

57. Purtilo DT, Stevenson M: Lymphotropic viruses as etiologic agents of lymphoma. *Hematol Oncol Clin North Am* 5:901–923, 1991

58. Urba WJ, Longo DL: Burkitt's lymphoma, in Moosa AR, Schimpff SC, Robson MC (eds): *Comprehensive Textbook of Oncology* (vol 2) (ed 2). Baltimore, Williams and Wilkins, 1991, pp 1296–1301

59. Wright DH: Pathogenesis of non-Hodgkin's lymphoma: Clues from geography, in Magrath IT (ed): *The Non-Hodgkin's Lymphomas*. Baltimore, Williams and Wilkins, 1990, pp 122–134

60. Shapiro RS: Epstein-Barr virus-associated B-cell lymphoproliferative disorders in immunodeficiency: Meeting the challenge. *J Clin Oncol* 8:371–373, 1990 (editorial)

61. Joncas JH, Russo P, Brochu P, et al: Epstein-Barr virus polymorphic B-cell lymphoma associated with leukemia and with congenital immunodeficiencies. *J Clin Oncol* 8:378–384, 1990

62. Urba WJ, Longo DL: Lymphocytic lymphomas: Epidemiology, etiology, pathology, and staging, in Moosa AR, Schimpff SC, Robson MC (eds): *Comprehensive Textbook of Oncology* (vol 2) (ed 2). Baltimore, Williams and Wilkins, 1991, pp 1268–1276

63. Roggero E, Zucca E, Pinotti G, et al: Eradication of *Helicobacter pylori* infection in low-grade gastric lymphoma of mucosa-associated lymphoid tissue. *Ann Intern Med* 122:767–769, 1995

64. Yang E, Korsmeyer SJ: Molecular thanatopsis: A discourse on the *BCL2* family and cell death. *Blood* 88:386–401, 1966

65. Segal GH, Masih AS, Fox AC, et al: CD5 expressing B-cell non-Hodgkin's lymphomas with *bcl-1* gene rearrangement have a relatively homogeneous immunophenotype and are associated with an overall poor prognosis. *Blood* 85:1570–1579, 1995

66. Levine EG, Bloomfield CD: Cytogenetics of malignant lymphomas, in Wiernik PH, Canellos GP, Kyle RA, Schiffer CA (eds): *Neoplastic Diseases of the Blood* (ed 2). New York, Churchill-Livingstone, 1991, pp 689–700

67. Peng JW, Lee EC: Cytogenetics, in Magrath IT (ed): *The Non-Hodgkin's Lymphomas*. Baltimore, Williams and Wilkins, 1990, pp 77–95

68. Magrath IT, Wilson W, Horvath K, et al: Clinical features and staging, in Magrath IT (ed): *The Non-Hodgkin's Lymphomas*. Baltimore, Williams and Wilkins, 1990, pp 180–199

69. Longo DL, DeVita VT, Jaffe ES, et al: Lymphocytic lymphomas, in DeVita VT, Hellman S, Rosenberg SA (eds): *Cancer: Principles and Practice of Oncology* (vol 2) (ed 4). Philadelphia, Lippincott, 1993, pp 1859–1937

70. Rappaport H, Winter WJ, Hicks EB: Follicular lymphoma: A reevaluation of its position in the scheme of malignant lymphomas, based on a survey of 253 cases. *Cancer* 9:792, 1956

71. Medeiros LJ, Jaffe ES: Pathology of malignant lymphomas, in Wiernik PH, Canellos GP, Kyle RA, Schiffer CA (eds): *Neoplastic Diseases of the Blood* (ed 2). New York, Churchill-Livingstone, 1991, pp 631–661

72. Lukes RJ, Collins RD: Immunologic characterization of human malignant lymphomas. *Cancer* 34:1488–1503, 1974

73. The Non-Hodgkin's Lymphoma Pathologic Classification Project: National Cancer Institute Sponsored Study of Classifications of Non-Hodgkin's Lymphomas. Summary and

description of a Working Formulation for clinical usage. *Cancer* 49:2112–2135, 1982

74. Harris NL, Jaffe ES, Stein H, et al: A revised European-American classification of lymphoid neoplasms: a proposal from the International Lymphoma Study Group. *Blood* 84:1361–1392, 1994

75. Sandlund J, Magrath IT: Lymphoblastic lymphomas, in Magrath IT (ed): *The Non-Hodgkin's Lymphomas.* Baltimore, Williams and Wilkins, 1990, pp 240–255

76. Skarin AT (ed): *Atlas of Diagnostic Oncology* (ed 2). London, U.K., Mosby-Wolfe Limited, 1996

77. McFadden ME: Cutaneous T-cell lymphoma. *Semin Oncol Nurs* 7:36–44, 1991

78. Vose JM, Bierman PJ, Armitage JO: Non-Hodgkin's lymphoma, in Wiernik PH, Canellos GP, Kyle RA, Schiffer CA (eds): *Neoplastic Diseases of the Blood* (ed 2). New York, Churchill-Livingstone, 1991, pp 739–751

79. Maor MH, Velasquez WS, Fuller LM, et al: Stomach conservation in Stages IE and IIE gastric non-Hodgkin's lymphoma. *J Clin Oncol* 8:266–271, 1990

80. Vose JM, Armitage JO: Role of autologous bone marrow transplantation in non-Hodgkin's lymphoma. *Hematol Oncol Clin North Am* 7:577–590, 1993

81. Zinzani PL, Bendandi M, Tura S: FMP regimen (fludarabine, mitxantrone, prednisone) as therapy in recurrent low-grade non-Hodgkin's lymphoma. *Eur J Haematol* 55:262–266, 1995

82. Gaynor ER, Fisher RI: Diffuse aggressive lymphomas in adults, in Magrath IT (ed): *The Non-Hodgkin's Lymphomas.* Baltimore, Williams & Wilkins, 1990, pp 317–329

83. Urba WJ, Longo DL: Lymphocytic lymphomas: Clinical course and management, in Moosa AR, Schimpff SC, Robson MC (eds): *Comprehensive Textbook of Oncology* (vol 2) (ed 2). Baltimore, Williams and Wilkins, 1991, pp 1277–1295

84. Hryniuk W, Bush H: The importance of dose intensity in chemotherapy of metastatic breast cancer. *J Clin Oncol* 2:1281–1287, 1984

85. Fisher RI, Gaynor ER, Dahlberg S, et al: Comparison of a standard regimen (CHOP) with three intensive chemotherapy regimens for advanced non-Hodgkin's lymphoma. *N Engl J Med* 328:1002–1006, 1993

86. Gordon LI, Harrington D, Andersen J, et al: Comparison of a second-generation combination chemotherapeutic regimen (m-BACOD) with a standard regimen (CHOP) for advanced diffuse non-Hodgkin's lymphoma. *N Engl J Med* 327:1342–1349, 1992

87. Cooper IA, Wolf MM, Robertson TI, et al: Randomized comparison of MACOP-B with CHOP in patients with intermediate grade non-Hodgkin's lymphoma. The Australian and New Zealand Lymphoma Group. *J Clin Oncol* 12:769–778, 1994

88. Verdonck LF, van Putten WL, Hagenbeek A, et al: Comparison of CHOP chemotherapy with autologous bone marrow transplantation for slowly responding patients with aggressive non-Hodgkin's lymphoma. *N Engl J Med* 332:1045–1051, 1995

89. Phillip T, Armitage JO, Spitzer G, et al: High dose therapy and ABMT after failure of conventional chemotherapy in one hundred adults with intermediate or high grade non-Hodgkin's lymphoma. *N Engl J Med* 316:1493–1498, 1987

90. Freedman AA, Takvorian T, Anderson KC: Autologous bone marrow transplantation in B-cell non-Hodgkin's lymphoma: Very low treatment-related mortality in 100 patients in sensitive relapse. *J Clin Oncol* 8:784–791, 1990

91. Gribben JG, Goldstone AH, Linch DC, et al: Effectiveness of high-dose combination chemotherapy and autologous bone marrow transplantation for patients with non-Hodgkin's lymphomas who are still responsive to conventional-dose therapy. *J Clin Oncol* 7:1621–1629, 1989

92. Troussard X, Leblond V, Kuentz M, et al: Allogeneic bone marrow transplantation in adults with Burkitt's lymphoma or acute lymphoblastic leukemia in first complete remission. *J Clin Oncol* 8:809–812, 1990

93. Takaue Y, Watanabe T, Kawano Y, et al: Isolation and storage of peripheral blood hematopoietic stem cells for auto-transplantation into children with cancer. *Blood* 74:1245–1251, 1989

94. Bitran JD, Williams SF, Moormeier J, et al: High-dose combination chemotherapy with thiotepa and autologous hematopoietic stem cell reinfusion in the treatment of patients with relapsed refractory lymphomas. *Semin Oncol* 17:39–42, 1990

95. Weber JS, Yang JC, Topalian SL, et al: The use of interleukin-2 and lymphokine-activated killer cells for the treatment of patients with non-Hodgkin's lymphoma. *J Clin Oncol* 10:33–40, 1992

96. Gisselbrecht C, Maranichi D, Pico JL, et al: Interleukin-2 treatment in lymphoma: A phase II multicenter study. *Blood* 83:2081–2085, 1994

97. Vuist WM, Levy R, Maloney DG: Lymphoma regression induced by monoclonal anti-idiotypic antibodies correlates with their ability to induce Ig signal transduction and is not prevented by tumor expression of high levels of *bcl-2* protein. *Blood* 83:899–906, 1994

98. Ruccione K, Weinberg K: Late effects in multiple body systems. *Semin Oncol Nurs* 5:4–13, 1989

99. Wickham R: Pulmonary toxicity secondary to cancer treatment. *Oncol Nurs Forum* 13:69–76, 1986

100. Baker GL, Barnes HJ: Superior vena cava syndrome: Etiology, diagnosis, and treatment. *Am J Crit Care* 1:54–64, 1992

101. Kaszyk LK: Cardiac toxicity associated with cancer therapy. *Oncol Nurs Forum* 13:81–88, 1986

102. Lydon J: Nephrotoxicity of cancer treatment. *Oncol Nurs Forum* 13:68–77, 1986

103. Wilson JK, Masaryk TJ: Neurologic emergencies in the cancer patient. *Semin Oncol* 16:490–503, 1989

104. Yarbro CH, Perry MC: The effect of cancer therapy on gonadal function. *Semin Oncol Nurs* 1:3–8, 1985

105. Chapman R, Rees L, Sutcliffe SB, et al: Cyclical combination chemotherapy and gonadal function: Retrospective study in males. *Lancet* 1:285–289, 1979

106. Kaempfer SH, Wiley FM, Hoffman DJ: Fertility considerations and procreative alternatives in cancer care. *Semin Oncol Nurs* 1:25–34, 1985

107. Jacquillat C, Khayat D, Desprez-Curely JP, et al: Occurrence of non-Hodgkin's lymphoma after therapy for Hodgkin's disease. *Cancer* 53:459–462, 1984

108. Fraser MG, Tucker MA: Second malignancies following cancer therapy. *Semin Oncol Nurs* 5:43–55, 1989

# Chapter 44

# Multiple Myeloma

Carol A. Sheridan, RN, MSN, AOCN

## INTRODUCTION

Waldenstrom's macroglobulinemia, monoclonal gammopathy of undetermined significance (MGUS), and multiple myeloma constitute the group of diseases classified as plasma cell disorders. These disorders are characterized by the overproduction of immunoglobulins.[1] In these diseases the malignant cell is the plasma cell, the functional mature cell that differentiates and develops from the B lymphocyte.[2,3] Multiple myeloma, the most common malignant plasma cell disorder, can affect the hematologic, skeletal, renal, and nervous systems.[4] Despite advances in our understanding and treatment of many hematologic malignancies, multiple myeloma remains a chronic and universally fatal disease.[5]

## EPIDEMIOLOGY

Within the United States, multiple myeloma represents 1% of all hematologic malignancies.[1] Although the incidence of multiple myeloma appears to be increasing in the United States, there is some evidence that the increased incidence may be due to earlier and improved diagnosis in older, high-risk populations.[6] The onset of multiple myeloma is late, with peak occurrence between the fifth and seventh decades of life.[7] Sixty-nine is the median age at diagnosis, but 2% of all cases occur before the age of 40.[1] Differences in disease incidence can be noted based on sex and race. Within the United States, multiple myeloma is more common among blacks than among whites by 2 to 1.[1] For all groups there is a male predominance, although black females have a higher incidence than white males. This racial difference persists with mortality rates, with both black and white females having a higher mortality rate than either whites or any other ethnic group (Native American, Chinese, Japanese, and Hispanic) within the United States.[8] Two explanations have been put forward for these racial differences. First, blacks have a higher circulating level of immunoglobulin G (IgG), representing a greater opportunity for B-cell malignant transformation.[1] The second explanation is more generic and involves exposure to pollutants (air, water, food) over time, promoting chronic antigenic stimulation of the immune system.[9] The African-American community within the United States is clearly at higher risk for morbidity and mortality associated with multiple myeloma. Worldwide, some Asian populations have the lowest incidence rates.[6]

## ETIOLOGY

The exact etiology of multiple myeloma is unknown, although a variety of factors have been associated with the development of the disease. In an attempt to better understand the etiologic factors, Potter[10] used an animal model and demonstrated that only specific strains of mice developed plasmacytomas following mineral oil injections. An analogous case for genetic linkage was made by Maldonado and Kyle,[11] who documented an increased frequency of plasma cell disorders among close relatives of individuals with multiple myeloma. First-degree relatives of patients with multiple myeloma appear to have a higher incidence of the disease.[3] Chromosomal abnormalities have also been documented in mice that underwent experimentally induced plasma cell disease. Although a specific chromosomal abnormality involving the immunoglobulin loci has not been detected in humans with multiple myeloma, frequent chromosomal abnormalities have been observed.[1] Chronic low level exposure to radiation has been associated with a two- to sixfold increase in the incidence of multiple myeloma, which may develop as late as 20 years after the radiation exposure.[7,12] Chronic antigenic stimulation, such as recurrent infections and drug allergies, may be part of the medical history in individuals who develop multiple myeloma. Occupational exposure to low-dose ionizing radiation, wood, textile, rubber, metal, petroleum products, and chemicals used as herbicides has been associated with the development of multiple myeloma.[7,12,13] No clear evidence demonstrating a common environmental or chemical etiologic factor has been established. In all such instances, further study is warranted to demonstrate a definitive risk relationship.

## NORMAL PHYSIOLOGY

The pluripotent stem cell resides within the bone marrow and has the ability to either self-replicate or differentiate into either the myeloid or lymphoid stem cell. The lymphoid stem cell is the earliest lymphoid cell. It resides within the bone marrow and retains the ability to self-replicate or differentiate into either T lymphocytes or B lymphocytes. T lymphocytes regulate the immune response and participate in cell-mediated immunity. B lymphocytes mature into plasma cells that manufacture and secrete large quantities of immunoglobulins. B lymphocytes are responsible for humoral immunity. Five classes of immunoglobulins are secreted: IgG, IgA, IgM, IgD, and IgE. IgM is the first immunoglobulin produced during a primary immune response and the first immunoglobulin produced in infants.[1] IgA is the primary immunoglobulin in saliva, tears, and the secretions of the gastrointestinal and respiratory tract. IgA plays a primary role in protecting these mucous membranes and vital organ systems by maintaining the first line of defense.[14] IgD and IgE are trace immunoglobulins found in the plasma. IgD acts as a cell-surface receptor that binds with antigen and triggers further B-lymphocyte differentiation and production. IgE can be elevated in response to parasitic infections and allergic response such as hay fever and asthma.

It is thought that IgE binds to receptors on basophils and mast cells and may stimulate these cells to release vasoactive substances as part of the allergic response.[1,14] IgG is the primary immunoglobulin in the serum. It has four subclasses (IgG 1–4) with slightly different physiological properties. IgG1 and IgG3 bind complement and mononuclear cells better than IgG2 and IgG4. When IgG1 and IgG3 are overproduced in multiple myeloma, the hyperviscosity syndrome may result. IgG is the only immunoglobulin that can cross the placenta and therefore confers passive immunity to newborns. In adults, IgG constitutes the largest proportion of immunoglobulin, followed by IgA and IgM.

The immunoglobulins are composed of four polypeptide chains, two heavy and two light. The heavy chains take their names from the class of immunoglobulin: IgG (gamma) IgA (alpha), and IgM (mu). The light chains are either lambda ($\lambda$) or kappa ($\kappa$).[7,12,14] Each immunoglobulin has a dual function: one end specific to a specific antibody that binds to complement or antigen; the other function is the constant region or Fc fragment that binds to membrane receptors.[14]

## PATHOPHYSIOLOGY

The plasma cell is derived from the B lymphocyte and is the functionally mature cell producing immunoglobulins; it has been thought to be the identifiable malignant cell in multiple myeloma.[15] Pilarski and colleagues demonstrated the expression of myeloid and megakaryocytic antigens on the plasma cell clone, causing the investigators to hypothesize that myeloma development may be programmed into cells prior to B-cell differentiation.[16] A final proposed model for myeloma development involves genetic and molecular defects in the early development of myeloma. A large number of chromosomal changes have been identified, and as many as one-third of all myeloma patients had chromosomal changes in one report.[7] These hypotheses require further investigation and may prove useful in developing future successful therapies.

Regardless of the exact location of the malignant change in multiple myeloma, there is abnormal overproduction of one immunoglobulin called the *M protein;* the *M* refers to monoclonal antibody, myeloma protein, or malignant protein. Although an excessive amount of immunoglobulin is being produced, the M protein is unable to effectively produce antibody necessary for maintaining humoral immunity. Approximately 80%–90% of all multiple myeloma patients will show evidence of the aberrant M protein in the serum.[3]

## The Role of Cytokines in the Pathogenesis of Multiple Myeloma

The exact site of the malignant transformation that causes multiple myeloma remains unknown. Within the past five years there have been advances in our understanding of the role many cytokines play in the development and growth of multiple myeloma (Table 44-1).[7,14,15]

Interleukin-6 (IL-6) has been identified by both in vitro and in vivo studies as one of the major growth factors involved in the development of multiple myeloma.[17] The paracrine growth function of IL-6 has been demonstrated. IL-6 is produced by the bone marrow stromal cells as well as by monocytes.[7,18] Reibnegger and associates demonstrated that serum IL-6 levels controlled C-reactive protein production and were prognostic in multiple myeloma patients.[19,20] An elevated IL-6 level was associated with increased C-reactive protein levels and associated with increased severity of multiple myeloma (i.e., hypercalcemia and poor survival). Other cytokines such as tumor necrosis factor (TNF) and interleukin-IB (IL-1B) have been shown to increase the bone marrow stromal cell production of IL-6.[7] Both IL1-B and TNF have been identified as the so-called osteoclast-activating factors responsible for the bone resorption and destruction associated with multiple myeloma.[1,7]

Investigational in vitro studies have demonstrated that IL-3, IL-5, and granulocyte-macrophage colony-stimulating factor (GM-GSF) have a synergistic effect with IL-6, promoting myeloma cell production. Future research directed at these early progenitor growth factors may increase our knowledge regarding the exact pathogenesis of multiple myeloma.

IL-10 has been identified as a differentiating factor promoting B cells into cells responsible for immunoglobulin production.[17] In vitro results demonstrate an increase in myeloma cell proliferation in short-term cultures of bone marrow cells from individuals with multiple myeloma. The exact role of IL-10 in vivo requires further investigation.

Alpha-interferon in vitro has been demonstrated to promote the growth of IL-6–dependent myeloma cells in culture.[17] The exact role and use of alpha-interferon in the treatment of multiple myeloma remains controversial. Future laboratory and clinical studies will clarify the exact role that cytokines play in the pathogenesis and progression of multiple myeloma.

**TABLE 44-1**   Cytokines Currently under Investigation in the Pathogenesis of Multiple Myeloma

| |
| --- |
| Interleukin-1B (IL-1B) |
| Interleukin-3 (IL-3) |
| Interleukin-5 (IL-5) |
| Interleukin-6 (IL-6) |
| Interleukin-10 (IL-10) |
| Tumor necrosis factor (TNF) |
| Granulocyte-macrophage colony-stimulating factor (GM-CSF) |
| Alpha-interferon |

## DIAGNOSIS AND STAGING

Once symptoms are present, untreated individuals with multiple myeloma have a median survival of seven months.[3] This can be extended with standard therapy to a median survival of two to three years.[2,3,21] Individuals with multiple myeloma may have a long prodromal, indolent, or asymptomatic period. However, once symptoms occur, systemic therapy becomes necessary. Patients may eventually enter a period in which their disease becomes refractory or unresponsive to conventional therapy, at which time investigational therapies are warranted.[22,23]

The most frequent symptom at presentation is bone pain. The clinical course of the disease is complicated by pathological fractures, pain, hypercalcemia, spinal cord compression, anemia, fatigue, thrombocytopenia, recurrent bacterial infections, and renal failure. The diagnosis of multiple myeloma can be confirmed by bone marrow biopsy with histological confirmation of increased (>10%) numbers of plasma cells and the presence of the monoclonal (M) protein in either the serum or the urine. Osteolytic "punched-out" lesions may or may not be present at initial diagnosis. The diagnostic workup for multiple myeloma is designed to determine the extent of involvement of other organs (Table 44-2). Serum $B_2$ microglobulin, platelet count, and the presence of either renal failure and/or infection have been identified as having a role in predicting prognosis when diagnosing, staging, and treating myeloma patients.[23-26]

Since 1975 the Durie/Salmon system has been proposed for use in staging multiple myeloma (Table 44-3).[27] This staging system integrates clinical and laboratory findings associated with multiple myeloma. In 1980 Durie and associates identified a process to quantitate the total-body myeloma cell mass.[28] The total-body myeloma cell number can be calculated by dividing the total-body M-component synthetic rate per myeloma cell. In examining a large series of individuals with multiple myeloma, the authors identified three stages of the disease.

**TABLE 44-2** Diagnostic Workup for Multiple Myeloma

| Diagnostic Exams | Purpose |
|---|---|
| Bone marrow aspirate/biopsy | Check % of plasma cells |
| Serum protein electrophoresis (SPEP) Immunoelectrophoresis (IEP) | Check for the presence of M protein |
| Serum chemistry | Check for evidence of hypercalcemia, renal dysfunction |
| Complete blood count (CBC) | Check for evidence of anemia, thrombocytopenia |
| Skeletal survey | Check for evidence of osteolytic bone lesions |

**TABLE 44-3** Myeloma Staging System

| Criteria | Measured Myeloma Cell Mass (Cells × 10$^{12}$/m²) |
|---|---|
| **Stage I** All of the following: Hemoglobin value > 10 g/dl Serum calcium value normal (< 12 mg/dl) On roentgenogram, normal bone structure (scale 0) or solitary bone plasmacytoma only Low M-component production rates IgG value <5 g/dl IgA value <3 g/dl Urine light chain M component on electrophoresis < 4 g/24 hr | <0.6 (low) |
| **Stage II** Overall data not as minimally abnormal as shown for stage I and no single value as abnormal as defined stage III | 0.6–1.20 (intermediate) |
| **Stage III** One or more of the following: Hemoglobin value <8.5 g/dl Serum calcium value >12 mg/dl Advanced lytic bone lesions (scale 3) High M-component production rates IgG value >7 g/dl IgA value >5 g/dl Urine light chain M component on electrophoresis >12 g/24 hr | >1.20 (high) |
| Subclassification A = relatively normal renal function (serum creatinine value <2.0 mg/dl) B = abnormal renal function (serum creatinine value ≥2.0 mg/dl) Examples Stage IA = low cell mass with normal renal function Stage IIIB = high cell mass with abnormal renal function | |

*IgA,* Immunoglobulin A; *IgG,* immunoglobulin G.

Reprinted with permission from Salmon SE and Cassady JR: Plasma cell neoplasms, in DeVita VT, Hellman S, Rosenberg SA (eds): *Cancer: Principles and Practice* (ed 3). Philadelphia, Lippincott, 1989.

First, stage I, or low cell mass, consists of less than 0.6 × 10$^{12}$ cells/m². Stage II, or intermediate cell mass, reflects more than 0.6–1.2 × 10$^{12}$ cells/m². Finally, stage III, or high cell mass, consists of greater than 1.2 × 10$^{12}$ cells/m².[1,4] Further staging is done based on renal status at the time of diagnosis. Group A consists of individuals with a normal renal function (creatinine level <2.0 mg/ml), and group B consists of individuals with evidence of renal dysfunction (creatinine level >2.0 mg/ml). In addition to renal function, infection, C-reactive protein,

B$_2$ microglobulin, and abnormal karyotype have been identified as prognostic in predicting response and overall survival.[24,29-31] The identification of the kinetic features of the predominant clone in the individual with myeloma is useful for both prognosis and treatment. The labeling index (LI) is the percentage of myeloma cells incorporating thymidine during a one-hour flash label.[3] To calculate the total number of myeloma cells in the compartment, one multiplies the LI by the total myeloma cell mass.

Individuals with a high cell mass and an LI >3% have a poor prognosis, with a median survival of less than six months.[3,5,17,26] In the future, these prognostic factors may be considered by clinicians when offering standard, intensive, or investigational therapy given the toxicity, morbidity, and overall survival.

## CLINICAL MANIFESTATIONS

### Skeletal Involvement

From 68% to 80% of individuals with multiple myeloma present with destructive, painful osteolytic lesions at the time of diagnosis.[9,32] Symptoms associated with these lesions include hypercalcemia (20%–40% of patients), pathological fractures with acute and chronic pain, decreased mobility, and an inability to fully participate in activities of daily living.[29-33] The bone lesions can be of three distinct types: (1) a solitary osteolytic lesion, (2) diffuse osteoporosis, and (3) multiple discrete osteolytic "punched-out" or "cannonball" lesions. The pathophysiology of the bone destruction is thought to be myeloma cell production of osteoclast activating factor (OAF). Once thought to be a single substance, OAFs have now been identified as a class of bone-resorbing factors (cytokines) produced by lymphocytes and monocytes.[34] Several OAFs have been purified and molecularly cloned, including lymphotoxin, TNF, the interferons, and IL-1.[1] Although the precise relationships and interactions between these cytokines have not been described, IL-1A, IL-1B, TNF, and IL-6 have been associated with an increase in both myeloma proliferation and osteoclast activity.[17,35,36]

Myeloma-associated bone lesions occur as a result of increased osteoclast activity and are most readily diagnosed by roentgenograms or bone surveys. Magnetic resonance imaging (MRI) is the test of choice for evaluating and diagnosing spinal cord compression.[4] If untreated, myeloma-induced osteolytic lesions can lead to compression fractures of the spine with irreversible neurological sequelae, refractory hypercalcemia compromising renal function, and possibly death.

### Infection

As with most cancer, 50%–70% of all multiple myeloma patients will die as a result of bacterial infection.[3,37] The two most common sites of infection are the respiratory and urinary tracts.[9,38] Common infectious organisms include *Staphylococcus aureus, Streptoccus pneumoniae, Escherichia* coli, *Pseudomonas,* and *Klebsiella.* In the 1980s, Savage and associates[39] demonstrated a biphasic pattern of infection in the person with multiple myeloma. *Streptococcus pneumoniae* and *Haemophilus influenzae* occurred early in the disease (within eight months of diagnosis) or in patients who responded early to chemotherapy, whereas infections caused by nonencapsulated gram-negative bacilli and *S. aureus* typically occurred in neutropenic patients or those individuals with unresponsive or refractory disease.[3,40]

A number of mechanisms have been identified as responsible for the immunosuppression and infection associated with multiple myeloma. These include a deficiency in the normal amount and function of immunoglobulins, neutropenia associated with plasma cell replacement in the bone marrow, qualitative defects in neutrophil and complement system functioning, and decreased physical activity as a result of symptoms and syndromes caused by the disease.

### Bone Marrow Involvement

A normocytic, normochromic anemia clinically manifested by fatigue and weakness occurs in over 60% of patients at initial diagnosis.[7,41] The anemia is initially caused by the excessive replacement of erythrocyte precursors with plasma cells in the bone marrow. Anemia can also be caused by increased red blood cell destruction. The M protein can coat normal erythrocytes, causing the red cells to line up similar to a roll of coins (rouleaux formation). This formation results in capillary sludging with associated hemolysis.[1,2,41] A multifactorial model for multiple myeloma–associated anemia has been postulated (Table 44-4).[3,5] It includes the replacement of erythrocyte precursors in the bone marrow with plasma cells; an increase in erythrocyte destruction; elevated levels of circulating immunoglobulins (IgG, IgA) with an increase in plasma volume, resulting in a falsely lowered hematocrit by approximately 5%–6%; chronic renal failure; low erythropoietin levels (<100 mU/ml); low iron stores (<50 μg/dl); and the in vivo activity in animals of IL-6 as a growth factor for multiple myeloma inducing

**TABLE 44-4** Multifactorial Basis for Multiple Myeloma–Associated Anemia

Replacement of erythrocyte precursors with plasma cells

Increased erythrocyte destruction (rouleaux formation)

Elevated levels of immunoglobulins increase plasma volume, and result in falsely lowered hematocrit

Chronic renal failure

Low erythropoietin levels (<100 mU/ml)

Low iron stores (<50 μg/dl)

Interleukin-6 (IL-6)

anemia and thrombocytosis.[17,42,43] As the myeloma cell burden increases or if the patient is treated with systemic chemotherapy, qualitative as well as quantitative defects in neutrophil and platelet function can occur. Bleeding can be caused by a decrease in the number of circulating platelets, by the M protein's effect on clotting factors, or by nonspecific coating of platelets with immunoglobulins.[1] The final result is platelet dysfunction and bleeding.

## Renal Insufficiency

At initial diagnosis, renal insufficiency is present in 29% of patients with multiple myeloma. During the course of the disease and its treatment, 50% of these individuals will experience renal failure, and 15% will die as a result of renal insufficiency.[5] The presence of renal insufficiency as a negative prognostic indicator in multiple myeloma has been well established.[2,25] Multiple myeloma can cause intrinsic renal lesions as well as renal failure precipitated by the sequelae of the disease (infection, hypercalcemia, and dehydration).[33] "Myeloma kidney" is the principal type of lesion associated with renal failure. In myeloma kidney, the renal tubules are filled with damaging, dense casts surrounded by multinucleated giant cells. These large, dense, tubular casts lead to the formation of precipitates in the tubules that can obstruct and rupture the tubular epithelium. In addition, interstitial inflammation, fibrosis, and tubular degeneration may occur, resulting finally in renal failure.[1,7] The tubular casts have been shown to contain characteristic light-chain immunoglobulins (Bence Jones proteins), which may be directly toxic to the renal tubular epithelium regardless of the presence of tubular casts.[9] The excretion of large amounts of Bence Jones proteins in the face of clinical dehydration with a low urine pH contributes to the risk of precipitation of light-chain proteins in the renal tubule and possible co-precipitating with calcium, further exacerbating acute renal failure.

Another renal lesion that occurs in approximately 10%–30% of myeloma patients is caused by amyloid deposits,[1,4] which can be found in the tubular basement membranes, renal blood vessels, interstitium, or glomerulus. Evidence of albuminuria and nephrotic syndrome strongly suggests amyloidosis, an adverse prognostic factor that can occur in up to 10% of myeloma patients.[2,9]

## Sequelae

Hypercalcemia as a clinical sequela of multiple myeloma has been described earlier. Untreated hypercalcemia in multiple myeloma patients can precipitate renal insufficiency by reducing the glomerular filtration rate, altering renal blood flow, changing the kidney's ability to concentrate urine, and precipitating calcium in the tubules or renal interstitium.

Hyperuricemia occurs in multiple myeloma patients as a result of a large tumor burden with an increased rate of cell death. Uric acid–induced nephropathy is caused by precipitation and crystallization of uric acid in the distal tubules, where the urine pH is low and the concentration of uric acid is high.[44] This syndrome can be exacerbated in patients who are dehydrated. If untreated, elevated uric acid levels will lead to further kidney damage.

Infection is the leading cause of death in multiple myeloma patients. Any episode of sepsis associated with hypotension or the use of nephrotoxic antibiotics (aminoglycosides with or without concurrent cephalosporins) should alert the clinician to closely monitor the individual for signs and symptoms of renal insufficiency.[44]

The treatment of renal insufficiency associated with multiple myeloma should be directed toward preventing or correcting the predisposing factors (dehydration, hypercalcemia, infection, hyperuricemia) and reducing the concentration and/or risk for precipitation of light-chain proteins in the renal tubules. A recent study demonstrated that aggressive approaches to treatment resulted in 51% of the patients achieving normal renal function.[29] The prognosis for multiple myeloma patients with renal insufficiency has clearly improved.

## Hyperviscosity Syndrome

Although rare (<5% of multiple myeloma patients), hyperviscosity syndrome can occur in individuals with IgM myeloma and occasionally in those with IgA, IgG1 and IgG3 myeloma.[1,45] It is caused by a high concentration of proteins that increase serum viscosity and result in vascular sludging. Initial clinical signs (blurred vision, irritability, headache, drowsiness, confusion) may indicate neurological impairment. Vascular sludging may also occur within the kidney, further compromising renal perfusion and increasing the risk of renal insufficiency. Plasmapheresis can be life-saving and is the treatment of choice for hyperviscosity syndrome.[38]

## Peripheral Neuropathy

Peripheral neuropathies have been recognized as part of the clinical sequelae associated with multiple myeloma.[46] In some cases the hyperviscosity syndrome has been identified as the causative factor.[45] Bosch and Smith recently postulated an autoimmune mechanism, with the IgM monoclonal antibody directed at peripheral nerve antigens.[47] Although evidence of this mechanism is developing, a definitive causal relationship between monoclonal proteins and peripheral neuropathies has not been established.

## ASSESSMENT

Since the exact pathogenesis of multiple myeloma remains elusive, no specific prevention, screening, or early detection programs for this rare hematologic malignancy have been developed. Clinicians providing primary care who recognize the risk factors associated with multiple myeloma (family history; agricultural or occupational exposure to wood, metal, rubber, or textiles; low-dose ionizing radiation; older African-American men and women) can utilize this knowledge to maintain a "high index of suspicion" when evaluating individuals who present with signs and symptoms that may be indicative of multiple myeloma.[1,6,12]

Physical examination findings may include bone pain, with or without a decrease in range of motion, an inability to bear weight, or signs and symptoms of spinal cord compression. This may be indicative of skeletal involvement, which can be diagnosed by radiological exams, MRI, or bone surveys.[1,7,9] Individuals with multiple myeloma may present with changes in mental status that could be related to hypercalcemia, hyperviscosity syndrome, or renal insufficiency. Routine chemistry laboratory values may be significant for elevations in blood urea nitrogen (BUN), creatinine, uric acid, and calcium. Serum protein immunoelectrophoresis (SPEP) can confirm the monoclonal spikes, and immunoelectrophoresis (IPEP) can also confirm the presence of M protein in the urine.[1,4] Individuals with multiple myeloma may appear pale and fatigued, and may show evidence of anemia on peripheral blood counts and evidence of plasmacytosis on bone marrow biopsy.[2,3]

A number of negative prognostic factors have been identified in the literature (Table 44-5).[1,14,24,25,26] Clinicians should consider these prognostic factors along with performance status and comorbid conditions when presenting treatment options to patients and their families.

## TREATMENT

### Chemotherapy

Patients with indolent, asymptomatic multiple myeloma are typically not treated with systemic therapy until clinical symptoms occur. There is no clinical evidence that initiating antineoplastic therapy in asymptomatic patients increases response rates or improves overall survival. There is widespread agreement that with the onset of symptoms (anemia, bone pain, and hypercalcemia), systemic antineoplastic therapy consisting of melphalan and

**TABLE 44-5** Negative Prognostic Findings in Multiple Myeloma

| |
|---|
| Infection |
| High labeling index |
| Elevated B$_2$ microglobulin |
| Renal insufficiency (hypercalcemia, hyperuricemia) |
| Plasmacytosis (>30%) in the bone marrow |

prednisone is the first line of therapy.[1,3,4,48,49] The response rate is 50%–60%, with a median survival of 24–36 months.[3,5,24,29] Melphalan is usually administered on an intermittent schedule (8 mg/m$^2$/day for 4 days) along with prednisone (75 mg/day for 7 days).[7] The treatment cycle is repeated every four weeks. This intermittent schedule allows patients to recover from the immunosuppressive effects of the drugs, is associated with fewer acute toxicities, and requires fewer blood counts. This chemotherapy protocol can be safely administered on an outpatient basis and allows the myeloma patient to remain in the community. Both agents are administered orally. Due to the uncertain absorption of melphalan from the gastrointestinal tract, patients should be encouraged to take this antineoplastic agent on an empty stomach,[5] unlike prednisone, where the patient should be instructed to take the medication with meals.[50] Alternately, patients may take a H$_2$-histamine receptor antagonist like famotidine designed to control gastric secretions and prevent the gastric distress associated with steroids.[4] Patients are monitored closely for signs of renal impairment (increased BUN and creatinine, proteinuria), and the dose of melphalan may need to be reduced based on the severity of renal toxicity. It is also important to closely monitor serial blood counts because the bone marrow–suppressive effects of melphalan may be cumulative in older patients. Although the addition of prednisone increases the response rate, it does not confer any benefit toward long-term survival; it is useful, however, in preventing bone resorption that could contribute to hypercalcemia and pathological fractures.[1] If the individual's myeloma is unresponsive, the melphalan dose may be escalated by 20% every five weeks provided there is no evidence of hematopoietic toxicity.[5] More recently, Samson and associates[51] demonstrated that VAD—vincristine (0.4 mg/24-hour continuous infusion × 4 days), doxorubicin (Adriamycin 9 mg/m$^2$/continuous infusion × 4 days), and dexamethasone (odd-number cycles 40 mg PO days 1–4, 9–12, 17–20; even-number cycles 40 mg PO days 1–4 only)—could be safely administered as first-line therapy, with an improved response rate (84%) and improved median survival (44 months). VAD is administered every 28 days. This regime has the added benefit of efficacy as both initial therapy and therapy for resistant disease.[4] Using it as initial therapy, Alexanian and Dimopoulos reported a higher response rate (55%) in newly diagnosed patients.[5] Unfortunately, this did not result in improved overall survival when compared with melphalan/prednisone. Clinically, this regime is beneficial to patients as first-line therapy because it can be used in patients with myeloma-associated renal dysfunction and has been shown to rapidly induce remission, which may translate into a decrease in hypercalcemia, renal failure, or bone disease.[5] Although initial response rates are slightly improved, clinicians need to administer this regime with caution in elderly patients (> 60 years old) because there is some evidence that the elderly experience more toxicity associated with high-dose steroid administration.[7,23] The VAD regime has gained widespread acceptance as treatment for resistant or refractory myeloma, with reported response rates between 65% and 75%.[3,7] Clinicians must monitor the total dose of doxorubicin and treat patients to a maximum tolerated dose of 450 mg/m². Patients will most likely require an implantable intravascular device to enable safe administration of these vesicants and close monitoring of blood counts. Depending on the patient's performance status and the available community services, this regime may require a four-day hospital stay or a referral to a skilled home care agency for safe administration of VAD in the home. Patients are closely monitored for signs and symptoms of steroid toxicity: severe dyspepsia, fluid and sodium retention, corticosteroid myopathy, acute pancreatitis, insulin-dependent hyperglycemia, and steroid psychosis. Patient and family education will include signs and symptoms of steroid-induced gastritis; if these persist or worsen (including nausea and vomiting with or without hematemesis), the treatment team should be contacted. Steroid gastritis that is not prevented, identified early, and appropriately treated can proceed to gastric ulceration and bleeding. Steroid-associated sodium and fluid retention is of particular concern, especially in elderly individuals with multiple myeloma who may have concurrent diseases like congestive heart failure. Monitoring the patient for weight gain and peripheral edema is imperative because these may precede rales and pulmonary compromise. Individuals with underlying insulin-dependent and non–insulin-dependent diabetes should be closely evaluated for signs and symptoms of steroid-induced hypoglycemia. Any one of these toxicities mandates at least a 50% reduction, if not complete discontinuation, of dexamethasone. Severe neurological toxicities (paresthesias or constipation) require at least a 50% reduction in the vincristine dose. In the face of progressive toxicity (paralytic ileus), vincristine must be discontinued. Prolonged thrombocytopenia and granulocytopenia require a 50%–100% reduction in the dose of doxorubicin. If the doxorubicin cannot be administered due to prolonged bone marrow suppression, the entire cycle may be delayed for one week and therapy resumed once the platelet count is above 50,000/mm³ and the absolute neutrophil count (ANC) is over 750. Hepatic toxicity characterized by a bilirubin greater than 2.0 requires reduction or discontinuation of both doxorubicin and vincristine, depending on the severity. If the bilirubin is greater than 5.0, both doxorubicin and vincristine are discontinued. If drug resistance emerges, cyclophosphamide is another, structurally different, alkylating agent that is cross-resistant with melphalan. Cyclophosphamide is also administered orally on an intermittent schedule. Patients are encouraged to increase their oral intake to avoid possible exacerbation of underlying renal dysfunction. Patients who may be concurrently receiving allopurinol should be carefully monitored, as this agent may enhance bone marrow suppression in patients receiving cyclophosphamide.

Thirty percent to 40% of myeloma patients will not respond to first-line therapy, while those who initially respond will eventually relapse.[1,9] Consequently, second-line combination chemotherapy regimens have been developed. The most consistently effective second-line therapy, resulting in a 70% response rate with projected survival greater than one year, is the combination of vincristine, doxorubicin and dexamethasone (previously described).[5,52] In an effort to minimize toxicity, increase response rates, and improve overall survival, investigators continue to combine agents such as doxorubicin and carmustine (BCNU); vincristine, carmustine, doxorubicin, and prednisone (VBAP); and vincristine, cyclophosphamide, doxorubicin, and prednisone (VCAP). To date, these clinical trials have been equivocal; further studies are warranted.[23,48,49,53]

## Interferon

In view of the equivocal results with combination chemotherapy for refractory multiple myeloma, it is not unreasonable for investigators to examine alternatives, such as alfa-interferon.[54] The specific mechanism of action of interferon in multiple myeloma is unknown but is thought to be multifactorial. Interferon exerts its biological effects by stimulating the host cells to indirectly affect tumor cells, specifically by inhibiting plasma cell growth and the ability of myeloma stem cells to self-replicate.[5,55] Despite this indirect effect on tumor cells, clinical investigators have demonstrated minimal to no effect in previously treated myeloma patients.[22] However, alfa-interferon has been proposed as a strategy to prolong remission duration and survival in multiple myeloma patients who initially respond to cytotoxic therapy.[56,57] Recently, investigators have begun to use interferon for maintenance therapy in patients who have responded to 12 courses of induction chemotherapy. The investigators concluded that they were able to prolong response and survival with minimal toxicity.[58] In contrast, in 1994 the Southwest Oncology Group reported a randomized prospective trial involving 522 previously untreated individuals with multiple myeloma who were randomized to three chemotherapy regimes with differing glucocorticoid doses.[59] A total of 193 patients achieved remission and were randomized to receive 3 million units of alfa-interferon three times per week or observation. The investigators drew two conclusions: that higher-dose glucocorticoids increase the frequency of response to chemotherapy and prolong survival in myeloma; and that there was no significant difference in overall survival between the interferon group and observation. In contrast, Browman and associates reported on a smaller perspective randomized trial that involved 402 newly diagnosed individuals with multiple myeloma who received melphalan and prednisone (M-P) as induction therapy.[55] In this trial, 176 responders were randomized to either 2 million units of alfa-interferon subcutaneously three times per week (n = 85) or no maintenance (n = 91). The conclusions include a statistically significant improvement in response duration and overall survival for interferon compared with no maintenance therapy. The second observation was that interferon toxicity caused 58% of the patients to reduce their dose, and 14% of the patients had to discontinue interferon treatment. The toxicity associated with alfa-interferon can be substantial (flulike syndrome, anorexia, fatigue, hepatotoxicity, thrombocytopenia, and neurological toxicity).[54,55] The patient is closely monitored by the treatment team for evidence of interferon toxicity. The dose-reduction schedule (50%–100%) and plan to discontinue interferon are dependent on the individual's response to the severity of the toxicity. Nurses play a key role in assessing and grading treatment-related toxicities and in assisting patients and their families in managing side effects. Oken and associates report similar findings from an Eastern Cooperative Oncology Group (ECOG) study in which 608 previously untreated individuals with multiple myeloma were randomized to three treatment arms.[60] First vincristine, BCNU, melphalan, cyclophosphamide, and prednisone (VBMCP); second, VBMPC and interferon (interferon 5 MU/m$^2$; 3×/week); third, in patients < 70 years old, cyclophosphamide 600 mg/m$^2$ was substituted for prednisone 100 mg/m$^2$ PO day 1–4 for cycles 3 and 5 of VBMCP (VBMCP and high-dose cyclophosphamide (HiCy)). The VBMCP/interferon arm had a higher complete response rate with a trend toward failure-free survival, but without an increase in survival. Clinically these improved response rates associated with maintenance therapy in individuals with multiple myeloma can translate into clinical improvement in symptoms associated with the disease (bone lesions, pain, renal dysfunction) and an overall improvement in the individual's functional ability and quality of life. To date, the results of randomized trials using interferon in the treatment of multiple myeloma remain equivocal. Some investigators have raised concerns regarding the controversial role of alfa-interferon in multiple myeloma. Laboratory data suggest that alfa-interferon is a potent myeloma cell growth factor. It induces the autocrine production of IL-6, thus promoting further myeloma cell growths.[3,17] The burden of proof rests with the scientists and clinicians to define the specific safe role for alfa-interferon in managing multiple myeloma.

## Radiation

Multiple myeloma is considered a disseminated disease with evidence of distant organ involvement at the time of diagnosis. However, in rare instances (<5%) the disease may be localized and present as a solitary bone plasmacytoma.[9] On biopsy the individual's bony lesion will show evidence of plasma cells. Bone marrow aspiration and biopsy, peripheral counts including complete blood counts (CBCs), and serum chemistry will be unremarkable and show no evidence of other organ involvement (i.e., renal). Although this clinical presentation is rare, Dimopoulos and colleagues present 45 cases followed over ten years where megavoltage irradiation (at least

3000 cGy) to the solitary lesion was curative.[61] Persistent myeloma protein was an adverse prognostic factor, and the reemergence of the myeloma protein heralded recurrence requiring systemic therapy. Multiple myeloma remains an extremely radiosensitive malignancy, and historically the goal of radiation therapy has been palliative. Radiation therapy has been effective in arresting local bone disease prior to the point of fracture, but it does not lead to bone repair and healing. This nonoperative approach to managing painful bony lesions is aimed at symptom relief for the individual, maintaining functional ability and promoting the individual's overall satisfaction with quality of life.[62]

Hemibody irradiation has been used in individuals with refractory or advanced multiple myeloma.[9] It involves a technique in which a single dose of radiation (500–800 Gy) is administered to a large body area at one time. The benefit of this approach is that it allows for the potential treatment of both halves of the body sequentially in doses that are higher than could be delivered with total-body irradiation.[63] This approach provides pain relief within 24–48 hours, and this time frame should be considered by clinicians when ordering and administering narcotic analgesics to manage pain. Treatment toxicity may be significant and dependent on the treatment field (upper hemibody field: head to the fourth lumbar vertebrae; midbody field: the abdomen and pelvis from the top of the diaphragm to the obturator foramina; and the lower hemibody: the torso below the iliac crest and extending to the ankles).[63] Providing patient education and managing symptoms such as nausea, vomiting, diarrhea, and bone marrow toxicity may include coordinating or administering premedications (corticosteroids, antiemetics, and narcotic analgesics) so that the individual will be able to comfortably complete his or her therapy in the radiotherapy department.[64]

## Bone Marrow Transplantation

Bone marrow transplantation (syngeneic, allogeneic, autologous) and peripheral stem cell support have been attempted in the treatment of multiple myeloma.[65-73] Age restrictions for both donor and recipient previously limited the appropriate use of this technology in elderly individuals (>60 years of age).

Jagannath and colleagues treated 55 previously treated myeloma patients with myeloablative chemoradiation and unpurged autologous bone marrow transplant.[66] They identified two pretransplant variables that were associated with negative patient outcomes:[65] a pretransplant elevated B$_2$ microglobulin level (>3 mg/liter) and the presence of non-IgG isotype myeloma. Response rates improved when investigators purged autologous marrow.[66,71]

Gahrton and colleagues reported a series of 90 myeloma patients who received allogeneic bone marrow transplant in 26 European centers.[67] The complete remission after bone marrow transplant was 43%, with a median duration of relapse-free survival of 48 months for complete responders. One clinically significant finding was that bone lesions were largely unaffected by the cytotoxic therapy used in the bone marrow transplant setting. Two posttransplant factors were useful in predicting individuals with better long-term survival; complete remission after transplant and grade 1 graft-versus-host disease. Gahrton and colleagues were the first to hypothesize a possible graft-versus-myeloma effect similar to the graft-versus-leukemia effect.[67] Five years later, Tricot and associates reported a case demonstrating direct evidence of graft-versus-myeloma effect in a 40-year-old individual with multiple myeloma who received a matched unrelated T-cell–depleted transplant after conditioning with total-body irradiation, thiotepa, and cyclophosphamide. The patient also received allogeneic peripheral blood mononuclear cells (stem cells) without further chemotherapy. The patient experienced severe acute and chronic graft-versus-host disease with a complete response duration greater than 14 months.[72]

Through the early 1990s investigators continued to design clinical trials aimed at improving response rates and duration of responses. Tura and Cavo reviewed allogeneic bone marrow transplant data and reported remission rates of 50%–60%.[68] Despite high mortality rates (40%–50%), Tura and Cavo suggested that allogeneic transplant be used earlier in the disease treatment as consolidation therapy, postulating that this might improve the number of long-term disease-free survivors.

In the early 1990s some investigators and treatment centers began to incorporate hematopoietic growth factors (granulocyte colony-stimulating factor [G-CSF], granulocyte macrophage colony stimulating factor [GM-CSF]) into clinical trials with transplant and stem cell support regimes to shorten the duration and depth of neutropenia after cytotoxic therapy. Within a very short time these technological and supportive care advances were incorporated into practice. Investigators are now reporting dramatic decreases in mortality rates (<5%) in autologous bone marrow transplant.[71]

Attal and colleagues reported the results of a European prospective randomized trial of autologous bone marrow transplant or conventional chemotherapy in multiple myeloma.[73] Two hundred previously untreated myeloma patients less than 65 years of age were randomly assigned to two treatment groups. The conventional dose treatment consisted of alternating cycles of VMCP/BVAP or high-dose therapy with autologous bone marrow transplant (Table 44-6). The investigators report a 81% response rate in the high-dose group and a 57% response rate in the conventional chemotherapy group (*p*<.001). Complete response rates were disappointing in both groups: high-dose (22%) and conventional (5%). Treatment-related mortality (<10%) was similar in the two groups. This study did not include the use of hematopoietic growth factors after transplant, and the investigators are considering the use of these agents in future treatment regimes.

**TABLE 44-6**  Treatment Schema for European Bone Marrow Transplant in Multiple Myeloma

| CONVENTIONAL TREATMENT—VMCP/BVAP* | |
|---|---|
| VMCP: | |
| Vincristine | 1 mg IV; day 1 |
| Melphalan | 5 mg/m² PO; days 1-4 |
| Cyclophosphamide | 110 mg/m² PO; days 1-4 |
| Prednisone | 60 mg/m² PO; days 1-4 |
| BVAP: | |
| Vincristine | 1 mg IV; day 1 |
| Carmustine | 30 mg/m² IV; day 1 |
| Doxorubicin | 30 mg/m² IV; day 1 |
| Prednisone | 60 mg/m² PO, days 1-4 |

Recombinant alfa-interferon (3 million U/m² SQ 3 times/week from cycle 9 until relapse.)

| HIGH-DOSE AS ABOVE |
|---|

Autologous bone marrow was collected after cycle 4 (200 million nucleated cells/kg body weight).

All patients received between 4 and 6 cycles of VMCP/BVAP; if their WHO (World Health Organization) performance status was <3 and a transplant facility was available the individual was transplanted.

Preparative regimen:   Melphalan 140 mg/m²
Total-body irradiation (8 Gy 4 fractions over 4 days with no lung shields)

Unpurged autologous bone marrow was readministered.

Alfa-interferon was administered from cycle 9 until relapse; after bone marrow transplantation hematologic recovery occurred (granulocyte count > 1500 cc/mm; platelet count > 75,000 cc/mm).

*Alternating cycles (every 3 weeks for 12 months; total 18 cycles).

Attal M, Harousseau JL, Stopp AM, et al: A prospective, randomized trial of autologous bone marrow transplantation and chemotherapy in multiple myeloma. *N Engl J Med* 335:91–97, 1996.

A number of questions remain unanswered regarding the appropriate use of transplantation in the treatment of multiple myeloma. Future clinical trials will attempt to determine the best time to do transplant (first remission versus at the time of disease progression). What type of transplant should be done (autologous bone marrow or peripheral stem cells versus allogeneic bone marrow or peripheral stem cells)? Have we identified all the prognostic factors that will identify the "best" patients or the patients most likely to benefit? As we learn more about the body's natural immune response and the specific pathogenesis of myeloma, we may be able to take advantage of new classes of cytotoxic agents: topoisomerase inhibitors, suramin, paclitaxel, retinoids, B-cell–directed immunotoxins, and vaccinations with idiotypes.[71,73]

## Long-Term Sequelae

The risk of developing a secondary malignancy or treatment-related malignancy after primary treatment for cancer has been recognized by the oncology community since the 1970s.[1] Reported risks for treatment-related malignancies range between 1.3-fold and 20-fold in comparison to the general public.[74] Recognizing this risk, oncology clinicians must monitor multiple myeloma patients for evidence of acute leukemia.[9] The precise pathogenesis of this leukemia remains obscure, but two hypotheses have been proposed. First, the chronic long term administration of alkylating agents (melphalan and cyclophosphamide) causes significant damage within the pluripotent stem cell compartment. The second hypothesis is that there is an inherent defect in the early bone marrow progenitor cells that causes the development of both malignancies (multiple myeloma and acute leukemia). Ongoing studies continue to show a low but significant risk for post–bone marrow transplant malignancies.[75] As myeloma patients continue intensive regimes requiring transplant support, clinicians will need to incorporate the risk for the development of acute leukemia into the informed consent process, the management, and the long-term follow-up of these patients. Secondary acute leukemia can be refractory to treatment. Treated patients have a dismal median survival of four to eight months.[76]

## NURSING MANAGEMENT

Multiple myeloma is a chronic disease with no known cure. The patient may experience indolent periods as well as acute episodes. In planning the nursing care it is imperative that the entire treatment team be knowledgeable of the patient's realistic prognosis. Initially and throughout the treatment trajectory, it is critical to incorporate the patient and his or her family when discussing therapeutic goals and treatment options. Goals can range from intensive treatment, preventing or delaying life-threatening complications, prolonging disease-free survival, palliation, or terminal care. Regardless of the goal, a symptom management approach to nursing care with a review of systems is useful in organizing assessments and interventions (Table 44-7).[77]

### Neurological

The most frequent symptom that myeloma patients present with is pain. Bone destruction from the myeloma results in osteoporosis and pathological fractures of long bones or vertebrae that may result in spinal cord compression that requires aggressive assessment and management of both acute and chronic pain.[62,78] Acute pain is characterized by a specific trauma (fracture) and is of short duration (less than six months), whereas chronic pain has no specific obvious initiation point and may occur over a protracted period. Interventions for pain include assessment and documentation of the individual's severity of pain (0–10 scale), proper positioning of affected limbs, use of supports and braces (cervical collar, back brace, sling) to prevent additional stress on bones, and consultation with physical and occupational therapists. The effective and appropriate utilization of narcotics and nonnarcotic analgesics, massage, heat, and/or cold where appropriate should be included.[79,80] Mental status changes can be an initial sign of hypercalcemia, hyperviscosity syndrome, or drug toxicity. Any change in mental status requires closer assessment to determine etiologic factors so that appropriate treatment can be promptly initiated. The nurse also plans for prevention of injury and maintaining the patient in a safe environment.[81] Depression, anxiety, and insomnia are but a few of the psychological responses that patients may exhibit in response to their disease and treatment.[82] Cognitive strategies (cognitive restructuring, assisting with problem solving, giving information in small amounts, listening, and expressing care and concern) have been recommended in selected individuals to assist in the adaptation to a cancer diagnosis.[83]

### Protective Mechanisms

Infection is the leading cause of death in patients with multiple myeloma. The supportive care of cancer patients with anemia, thrombocytopenia, and neutropenia is well documented in the nursing literature, and guidelines for the care of patients with anemia, infection, and bleeding are provided in chapters 21 and 22.[84–86] Guidelines for the care of neutropenic patients are principally aimed at the early recognition and/or prevention of infection; care of the thrombocytopenic patient is directed toward preventing bleeding; and care of the anemic patient is directed toward early recognition and treatment to prevent contributing to the fatigue-weakness state that may be a component of the disease and/or its treatment.[87] Blood product support will consist mainly of packed red blood cell and platelet transfusions. The clinical use of hematopoietic growth factors in the prevention of febrile neutropenia after myelosuppressive chemotherapy, in the treatment of anemia in cancer patients receiving chemotherapy, in patients undergoing peripheral blood progenitor cell (PBPC) collection, and in patients receiving bone marrow transplant is now established as supportive therapy in managing individuals with multiple myeloma. The American Society of Clinical Oncology's 1996 guidelines for the use of hematopoietic colony-stimulating factors adds two important risk factors (poor performance status and more advanced cancer) for consideration in the older population (>60 years) of individuals with multiple myeloma.[88] Clinicians may use these and other risk factors

**TABLE 44-7** Nursing Care of the Patient with Multiple Myeloma

| System | Signs and Symptoms | Patient Education |
|---|---|---|
| Neuromuscular | Pain (acute/chronic)<br>Hypercalcemia<br>Hyperviscosity syndrome<br>Spinal cord compression<br>Pathological fractures<br>Depression | Pain control measures<br>Signs and symptoms of hypercalcemia<br>Prevention of pathological fractures<br>Cognitive strategies<br>Counseling |
| Protective mechanisms | Anemia<br>Neutropenia<br>Thrombocytopenia | Exercise<br>Energy conservation activities<br>Prevention of infection<br>Prevention of bleeding<br>Self-administration of prescribed hematopoietic growth factors |
| Respiratory | Pneumonia | Prevention of pooling of pulmonary secretions<br>Increase gas exchange<br>Use of incentive spirometer |
| Gastrointestinal | Constipation | Preventive measures<br>Change in fluid and dietary intake |
| Genitourinary | Renal insufficiency | Increase fluid intake<br>Allopurinol administration<br>Recognition of signs of urinary tract infection |

when assessing patients prior to ordering hematopoietic growth factors for primary prophylaxis of febrile neutropenia after myelosuppressive chemotherapy.

## Respiratory

The respiratory system is the most frequent site of infection in myeloma patients. As a result, nursing care is directed toward teaching patients and their families activities to decrease pooling of pulmonary secretions and increase gas exchange (e.g., coughing and deep breathing exercises, use of incentive spirometers, avoiding family members with signs and symptoms of upper respiratory infection (URI)). Patients and families are instructed about the symptoms that are important to report to the clinician immediately, such as fever, cough, sore throat, and sputum production. Due to the underlying defect in humoral immunity induced by multiple myeloma, patients should be instructed not to receive vaccines with live organisms or be in close contact with others who may have received live organism vaccines that may be shedding organisms (i.e., children immunized with oral polio and MMR).[89]

## Gastrointestinal

Multiple myeloma patients are at risk for constipation as a result of decreased physical activity due to bone pain/pathological fractures, treatment of pain with narcotic analgesics, dehydration, and the use of vincristine. Although not considered a life-threatening clinical problem, this condition can influence nutritional intake,

comfort, and quality of life.[90] Nursing management includes the assessment of past and present bowel habits, changes in fluid and dietary intake, medication administration, activity changes, and patient and family education.

## Genitourinary

Renal insufficiency or failure can be exacerbated as a result of the primary disease, fluid and electrolyte abnormalities (hyperuricemia, hypercalcemia), dehydration, and/or infection.[91] Nursing care is directed at preventing or quickly reversing renal insufficiency. Maintaining adequate hydration, along with the administration of allopurinol, will protect the kidneys from uric acid nephropathy.[92] The nurse closely monitors the patient for early signs and symptoms of urinary tract infection (UTI) (fever, dysuria, frequency, urgency) and educates patients and families to recognize these symptoms and report them promptly to the physician.

## CONCLUSION

The last decade has witnessed dramatic improvements in the overall response rates for patients with multiple myeloma. The utilization of combination chemotherapy, earlier recognition of complications, and appropriate utilization of support therapies have all contributed to increasing patient survival. In the next decade we will witness increasing utilization of new technologies to better determine etiologic factors contributing to the development of multiple myeloma. The nursing care of multiple myeloma patients and their families offers the nurse an opportunity to care for patients experiencing both acute and chronic sequelae of disease. Nursing care can have a direct effect in early recognition of complications and managing toxicity. Patient and family education can lead to the early recognition and identification of complications, contributing to overall improvement in quality of life. Future areas for nursing research include studying specific nursing interventions aimed at symptom distress.

# REFERENCES

1. Bubley GJ, Schnipper LE: Multiple myeloma, in Murphy GP, Lawrence W, Lenhard RE. (eds): *American Cancer Society Textbook of Clinical Oncology.* Atlanta, American Cancer Society, 1995, pp 470–485

2. Jacobs P: Myeloma. *Dis Mon* 36:317–371, 1990

3. Hussein M: Multiple myeloma: An overview of diagnosis and management. *Cleve Clin J Med* 61:285–298, 1994

4. Sheridan CA: Multiple myeloma. *Semin Oncol Nurs* 12:1–12, 1996

5. Alexanian R, Dimopoulos MA: Management of multiple myeloma. *Semin Hematol* 32:20–30, 1995

6. Riedel DA: Epidemiology of multiple myeloma, in Wiernik PH (ed): *Neoplastic Diseases of the Blood.* New York, Churchill Livingstone, 1991, pp 347–372

7. Gautier M, Cohen MJ: Multiple myeloma in the elderly. *J Am Geriatr Soc* 42:653–664, 1994

8. American Cancer Society: Cancer Facts and Figures—1995. Atlanta, American Cancer Society, 1995

9. Shulman LN: Plasma cell diseases and related disorders, in Hadin RI, Lux SE, Stossel TP (eds): *Blood Principles and Practice of Hematology.* Philadelphia, Lippincott, 1995, pp 885–913

10. Potter M: Plasmacytomas in mice. *Semin Oncol* 13:275–281, 1986

11. Maldonado JE, Kyle RA: Familial myeloma: Report of eight families and a study of serum proteins in their relatives. *Am J Med* 57:875–884, 1974

12. Riedel DA, Pottern LM: The epidemiology of multiple myeloma. *Hematol Oncol Clin North Am* 6:225–247, 1992

13. Eriksson M, Karlsson M: Occupational and other environmental factors and multiple myeloma: A population-based case-control study. *Br J Ind Med* 49:95–103, 1992

14. Gallucci BB, McCarthy D: The immune system, in Reiger PT (ed): *Biotherapy: A Comprehensive Overview.* Boston, Jones and Bartlett, 1995, pp 15–42

15. Varterasian ML: Biologic and clinical advances in multiple myeloma. *Oncology* 9:417–424, 1995

16. Pilarski LM, Mant MJ, Ruether, BA: Pre-B cells in peripheral blood of multiple myeloma patients. *Blood* 66:416–422, 1985

17. Klein B: Cytokine receptors, transduction signals, and oncogenes in human multiple myeloma. *Semin Hematol* 32(1): 4–19, 1995

18. Klein B, Zhang XG, Luz Y, et al: Interleukin-6 in human multiple myeloma. *Blood* 85:863–872, 1995

19. Reibnegger G, Krainer M, Herold M, et al: Predictive value of interleukin-6 and neopterin in patients with multiple myeloma. *Cancer Res* 51:6250–6253, 1991

20. Pelliniemi TT, Irjala K, Mattila K, et al: Immunoreactive interleukin-6 and acute phase proteins as prognostic factors in multiple myeloma. *Blood* 85:765–771, 1995

21. MacLennan IC, Drayson M, Dunn J: Multiple myeloma. *BMJ* 308:1033–1036, 1994

22. Alexanian R, Barlogie B, Gutterman J: Alpha interferon combination therapy of resistant myeloma. *Am J Clin Oncol* 14(3):188–192, 1991

23. Friedenberg WR, Kyel RA, Knospe WH, et al: High-dose dexamethasone for refractory or relapsing multiple myeloma. *Am J Hematol* 36(3):171–175, 1991

24. Durie BG, Stock-Novak D, Salmon SE, et al: Prognostic value of pretreatment serum beta₂ microglobulin in myeloma: A Southwest Oncology Group Study. *Blood* 75:823–830, 1990

25. Cherng NC, Asal NR, Keubler JP, et al: Prognostic factors in multiple myeloma. *Cancer* 67:3150–3156, 1991

26. Kyle, RA: Newer approaches to the management of multiple myeloma. *Cancer* 72:3489–3494, 1993 (suppl 11)

27. Durie BGM, Salmon SE: A clinical staging system for multiple myeloma. *Cancer* 36:842–854, 1975

28. Durie BG, Salmon SE, Moon TE: Pretreatment tumor mass cell kinetics and prognosis in multiple myeloma. *Blood* 55: 364–372, 1980

29. Alexanian RJ, Barlogie B, Dixon D: Renal failure in multiple myeloma pathogenesis and prognostic implications. *Arch Intern Med* 150:1693–1695, 1990

30. Bataille R, Boccadoro M, Klein B, et al: C-reactive protein and B₂ microglobulin produce a simple and powerful myeloma staging system. *Blood* 80:733–737, 1992

31. Weh HJ, Gutensohn K, Selbach J, et al: Karyotype in multiple myeloma and plasma cell leukemia. *Eur J Cancer* 29: 1269–1273, 1993

32. Brage ME, Simon MA: Evaluation, prognosis, and medical treatment considerations. *Orthopedics* 15:589–596, 1992

33. Kaplan M: Hypercalcemia of malignancy: A review of advances in pathophysiology. *Oncol Nurs Forum* 21:1039–1048, 1994

34. Moscinski LC, Ballester DF: Recent progress in multiple myeloma. *Hematol Oncol* 12:111–123, 1994

35. Carter A, Merchau S, Silvian-Draxler I, et al: The role of interleukin-1 and tumor necrosis factor in human multiple myeloma. *Br J Haematol* 74:424–431, 1990

36. Bataille R, Chappard D, Klein B: Mechanisms of bone lesions in multiple myeloma. *Hematol Oncol Clin North Am* 6: 285–295, 1992

37. Jacobson DR, Zolla-Pazner S: Immunosuppression and infection in multiple myeloma, in Wiernik PH (ed): *Neoplastic Diseases of the Blood.* New York, Churchill Livingstone, 1991, pp 415–426.

38. Lawrence J: Critical care issues in the patient with hematologic malignancy. *Semin Oncol Nurs* 10:198–207, 1994

39. Savage DG, Lindenbaum J, Garrett TJ: Biphasic pattern of bacterial infection in multiple myeloma. *Ann Intern Med* 96: 47–50, 1982

40. Berthaud V, Milder J, el-Sadr W: Multiple myeloma presenting with *Hemophilus influenzae* septic arthritis: Case report and review of the literature. *J Natl Med Assoc* 85:626–628, 1993

41. Duff TP: The many pitfalls on the diagnosis of myeloma. *N Engl J Med* 326:394–396, 1992

42. Barlogie B, Beck T: Recombinant human erythropoietin

and the anemia of multiple myeloma. *Stem Cells* 11:88–94, 1993

43. Asano S, Okano A, Ozawa K, et al: In vivo effects of recombinant human interleukin-6 in primates: Stimulated production of platelets. *Blood* 75:1602–1609, 1990

44. Brasfield K: Renal disorders, in Thelan LA, Davie JK, Urden LD, Lough ME (eds): *Critical Care Nursing.* St. Louis, Mosby, 1994, pp 603–620

45. Paterson WP, Caldwell CW, Doll DC: Hyperviscosity syndromes and coagulopathies. *Semin Oncol* 17:210–216, 1990

46. Sidoti SP, Cherpack FJ: Neurologic involvement of multiple myeloma: Literature review and case report. *J Am Podiatr Med Assoc* 81:220–223, 1991

47. Bosch EP, Smith BE: Peripheral neuropathies associated with monoclonal proteins. *Med Clin North Am* 77(1): 125–139, 1993

48. Boccadoro M, Marmont F, Tibalto M, et al: Multiple myeloma: VMCP/VBAP alternating combination chemotherapy is not superior to melphalan and prednisone even in high-risk patients. *J Clin Oncol* 9:444–448, 1991

49. Gregory WM, Richards MA, Malas JS: Combination chemotherapy versus melphalan and prednisone in the treatment of multiple myeloma: An overview of published trials. *J Clin Oncol* 10:334–342, 1992

50. Skidmore-Roth L: *1996 Nursing Reference.* St. Louis, Mosby, 1996, pp 880–881

51. Samson D, Gaminara E, Newland A, et al: Infusion of vincristine and doxorubicin with oral dexamethasone as first-line therapy for multiple myeloma. *Lancet* 2:882–885, 1989

52. Kyle RA, Greipp PR, Gertz MA: Treatment of refractory multiple myeloma and considerations for future therapy. *Semin Oncol* 13:326–333, 1986

53. Oken MM: Standard treatment for multiple myeloma. *Mayo Clin Proc* 69:781–786, 1994

54. Rödjer S, Vikrot O, Wahlin A, et al: Effect of interferon alpha-2b in advanced multiple myeloma. *J Intern Med* 227: 45–48, 1990

55. Browman GP, Bergsagel D, Sicheri D, et al: Randomized trial of interferon maintenance in multiple myeloma: A study of the National Cancer Institute of Canada Clinical Trials Group. *J Clin Oncol* 13:2354–2360, 1995

56. Camba L, Durie BG: Multiple myeloma: New treatment options. *Drugs* 44:170–181, 1992

57. Borden EC: Innovative treatment strategies for non-Hodgkin's lymphoma and multiple myeloma. *Semin Oncol* 21: 14–22, 1994, (6 suppl 14)

58. Mandellia F, Avvisati G, Amador S, et al: Maintenance treatment with recombinant interferon alpha-2b in patients with multiple myeloma responding to conventional chemotherapy. *N Engl J Med* 322:1430–1434, 1990

59. Salmon SE, Crowley JJ, Grogan TM, et al: Combination chemotherapy, glucocorticoids and interferon alfa in the treatment of multiple myeloma: A Southwest Oncology Group Study. *J Clin Oncol* 12:2405–2414, 1994

60. Oken MM, Leong T, Kay NE, et al: The effect of adding interferon or high-dose cyclophosphamide to VBMCP to treat multiple myeloma: Results from an ECOG phase III trial. *Blood* 86:441a, 1995, (10 suppl 1)

61. Dimopoulos MA, Goldstein J, Fuller L, et al: Curability of solitary bone plasmacytoma. *J Clin Oncol* 10:587–590, 1992

62. Anderson MG: The lymphomas and multiple myeloma, in Baird SB, McCorkle R, Grant M (eds): *A Cancer Source Book for Nurses.* Atlanta, American Cancer Society, 1991, pp 286–295

63. Dudjak LA: Alternatives in dose fractionation and treatment volume, in Dow KG, Hilderley LJ (eds): *Nursing Care in Radiation Oncology.* Philadelphia, Saunders, 1992, pp 285–294

64. Hilderley LJ: Radiotherapy, in Groenwald SL, Frogge MH, Goodman M, Yarbro CH (eds): *Cancer Nursing: Principles and Practice,* (ed 3). Boston, Jones and Barlett, 1993, pp 235–269

65. Jagannath S, Barlogie B, Dicke K, et al: Autologous bone marrow transplantation in multiple myeloma: Identification of prognostic factors. *Blood* 76:1860–1866, 1990

66. Anderson KC, Barut BA, Ritz J, et al: Monoclonal antibody-purged autologous bone marrow transplantation therapy for multiple myeloma. *Blood* 77:712–720, 1991

67. Gahrton G, Tura S, Ljungman P, et al: Allogeneic bone marrow transplantation in multiple myeloma. *N Engl J Med* 325:1267–1273, 1991

68. Tura S, Cavo M: Allogeneic bone marrow transplantation in multiple myeloma. *Hematol Oncol Clin North Am* 6: 425–435, 1992

69. Copelan EA, Biggs JC, Szer J, et al: Allogeneic bone marrow transplantation for acute myelogenous leukemia, acute lymphocytic leukemia, and cyclophosphamide (BuCy2). *Semin Oncol* 20:33–38, 1993, (suppl 4)

70. Ballester OF: Allogeneic bone marrow transplantation for multiple myeloma. *Semin Oncol* 20:67–71, 1993, (suppl 6)

71. Barlogie B, Jagannath S, Vesole D, et al: Autologous and allogeneic transplants for multiple myeloma. *Semin Hematol* 32:31–44, 1995

72. Tricto G, Vesole DH, Jagannath S, et al: Graft-versus-myeloma effect: Proof of principle. *Blood* 87:1196–1198, 1996

73. Attal M, Harousseau JL, Stoppa AM, et al: A prospective, randomized trial of autologous bone marrow transplantation and chemotherapy in multiple myeloma. *N Engl J Med* 335:91–97, 1996

74. Bhatia S, Ramsay NKC, Steinbuch M, et al: Malignant neoplasms following bone marrow transplantation. *Blood* 87: 3633–3639, 1996

75. Deeg HJ, Witherspoon RP: Risk factors for the development of secondary malignancies after marrow transplantation. *Hematol Oncol Clin North Am* 7:417–423, 1993

76. Wujcik D: Leukemia, in Groenwald SL, Frogge MH, Goodman M, Yarbro CH (eds): *Cancer Nursing: Principles and Practice* (ed 3). Boston, Jones and Barlett, 1993, pp 1149–1173

77. McDaniel RW, Rhodes VA: Symptom experience. *Semin Oncol Nurs* 11:232–234, 1995

78. Held JL, Peahota A: Nursing care of the patient with spinal cord compression. *Oncol Nurs Forum* 20:1507–1514, 1993

79. Coyle N, Cherny N, Portenoy RK, Pharmacologic management of cancer pain, in McGuire DB, Yarbro CH, Ferrell BR (eds): *Cancer Pain Management.* Boston, Jones and Barlett, 1995, pp 89–130

80. Spross JA, Burke MW, Non-pharmacologic management of cancer pain, in McGuire DB, Yarbro CH, Ferrell BR (eds): *Cancer Pain Management.* Boston, Jones and Barlett, 1995, pp 159–205

81. Kanak MF: Interventions related to patient safety. *Nurs Clin North Am* 27:371–395, 1992

82. Valente SM, Saunders JM, Cohen MZ: Evaluating depression among patients with cancer. *Cancer Pract* 2:65–71, 1993

83. Hagopian GA: Cognitive strategies used in adapting to a cancer diagnosis. *Oncol Nurs Forum* 20:759–763, 1993

84. McNally JC, Stair J: Potential for infection, in McNally JC, Somerville ET, Miaskowski C, Rostad M (eds): *Guidelines for Oncology Nursing Practice.* Philadelphia, Saunders, 1991, pp 191–202

85. Alexander EJ: Potential for injury related to thrombocyto-penia, in McNally JC, Somerville ET, Miaskowski C, Rostad M (eds): *Guidelines for Oncology Nursing Practice.* Philadelphia, Saunders, 1991, pp 203–207

86. Rostad M: Potential for injury related to anemia, in McNally JC, Somerville ET, Miaskowski C, Rostad M (eds): *Guidelines for Oncology Nursing Practice.* Philadelphia, Saunders, 1991, pp 208–215

87. Nail LM, Winningham ML: Fatigue and weakness in cancer patients: The symptom experience. *Semin Oncol Nurs* 11: 272–278, 1995

88. The American Society of Clinical Oncology Health Services Committee: Update of recommendations for the use of hematopoietic colony-stimulating factors: Evidence-based clinical practice guidelines. *J Clin Oncol* 14:1957–1960, 1996

89. Wong DL: Health promotion of the infant and family, in Wong DL, Wilson D (eds): *Nursing Care of Infants and Children.* St Louis, Mosby, 1995, pp 514–573

90. Canty SL: Constipation as a side effect of opioids. *Oncol Nurs Forum* 21:739–745, 1994

91. Moore JM: Tumor lysis syndrome, in Gross J, Johnson BL (eds): *Handbook of Oncology Nursing.* Boston, Jones and Bartlett, 1994, pp 691–700

92. Hubbard SM, Galassi A: Chemotherapy, in Gross J, Johnson BL (eds): *Handbook of Oncology Nursing.* Boston, Jones and Bartlett, 1994, pp 55–94

# Chapter 45

# Prostate Cancer

**Jeanne Held-Warmkessel, RN, MSN, CS, AOCN**

## INTRODUCTION

Each year, the number of men diagnosed with prostate cancer increases. More and more, nurses in all practice settings will care for men with a potential or actual prostate cancer diagnosis. Up-to-date information is required by nurses to educate and care for these patients. This chapter will present current information regarding the diagnosis and management of prostate cancer. Screening and early detection are also discussed.

## EPIDEMIOLOGY

Prostate cancer is the most commonly diagnosed cancer in American males and the second-leading cause of cancer-related deaths. In 1996, an estimated 317,100 new cases of prostate cancer were diagnosed and 41,400 men died from the disease.[1] With aging, the risk of prostate cancer increases. The average age of the American male is increasing, which predisposes these men to a higher risk of prostatic cancer. Consequently, the incidence of prostate cancer will continue to rise.[2]

The incidence of prostate cancer is 37% higher for black men than white men.[1] Controlling for social class does not eliminate the difference in rates between black and white American males of the same age.[3] Japanese males have the lowest incidence and mortality rates from prostate cancer.[4,5] Globally, the incidence of prostate cancer found on autopsy is similar throughout same-aged but different racial groups. When males emigrate from Japan to the western United States, in approximately one to two generations the incidence of prostate cancer in Japanese-American males is similar to that in American males.[6,7] This observation indicates that multiple events are probably needed for the progression of an initiated tumor with histological characteristics diagnostic of a cancer into an invasive, potentially metastatic cancer.[5]

Two of the events that may be important are diet and serum testosterone levels. Japanese living in Japan consume a mostly vegetarian diet. When Japanese males emigrate, their diet becomes increasingly Americanized. The vegetarian diet reduces serum testosterone levels.[8] The loss of the vegetarian diet and increased fat consumption may help to explain the change in prostate cancer rates for Japanese-American males.[9]

Serum testosterone levels are on average 15% higher in black males than in white males.[10] This elevated level may explain the higher incidence of prostate cancer found in black men.

## ETIOLOGY

The cause of prostate cancer is unknown. Risk factors have been identified and relate primarily to lifestyle, age, and heredity.

Lifestyle factors include nutrition and exposure to carcinogens. Animal fat consumption appears to be related to the risk of death from prostate cancer.[4] Diets higher in animal fat may alter the hormonal environment and predispose a man to an increased cancer risk.[11] A hypothesized model explains that the risk of prostate cancer development begins in utero secondary to dietary fat consumption by the mother. It is known that black females have higher levels of testosterone during the first trimester.[12] This is hypothesized to have an impact on the incidence of prostate cancer in black males.

Reducing the consumption of animal fats may offer some protection from developing prostate cancer.[4,5,13] Increasing fiber consumption may also be beneficial.[14] Vitamin A is an essential fat-soluble vitamin that promotes normal cellular growth. Vitamin A derived from plant sources may reduce one's risk of prostate cancer, whereas that derived from animal sources may increase the risk of prostate cancer.[15]

Body fat composition may predispose one to prostate cancer development. Being 130%–241% of optimal weight increases the risk of fatal prostate cancer by 2.5 compared to those weighing 90%–109% of optimal weight.[16] Body fat distribution may also play a role. Men with prostate cancer had more upper body fat than normal controls.[17]

Exposure to carcinogens such as cigarette smoking, cadmium, or zinc may play a role in prostate cancer development.[18] Further research is needed into the roles diet, animal fat, fiber, vitamins, and trace elements play in prostate carcinogenesis.

The use of vasectomy for birth control may increase the risk of prostate cancer.[18] The risk appears to be greater for men who had a vasectomy more than 20 years ago.[19,20] The age-related relative risk of prostate cancer after vasectomy is 1.66.[19] If the vasectomy was done 22 years ago or more, the relative risk is 1.85. The etiology by which vasectomy may promote prostate cancer development is poorly understood but may relate to prostatic gland fluid stasis, which occurs postvasectomy as it does with aging. Other studies have failed to demonstrate an increased risk of prostate cancer.[21,22] Nurses should educate their patients who wish to undergo vasectomy for birth control that the procedure may increase the risk of prostate cancer; however, more research is needed to determine the etiologic relationship between vasectomy and carcinogenesis.[23] Men who do select this procedure should discuss and consider participating in annual prostate cancer screenings provided by their family doctor beginning at age 40.

Prostate cancer is clearly a disease of the older male. Before age 50, clinically evident prostate cancer is rare. The incidence after age 50 increases on a yearly basis to reach approximately 1000 cases per 100,000 males aged 65–69.[5] By ages 80–84, the incidence per 100,000 males is greater than 3000.

Hereditary prostate cancer is characterized by an early onset and the presence of an autosomal dominant pattern of inheritance.[24] The risk of cancer for a particular individual is greater if the family member with cancer is a first-degree relative (father, brother) and greatest if both first-degree and second-degree relatives (grandfather, uncle) had prostate cancer.[25]

Several oncogenes have been identified in prostate cancers, including the c-erbB-2 oncogene.[26] Chromosomal and gene rearrangements have also been found. The exact role these alterations play in prostate carcinogenesis requires additional research.

## PREVENTION, SCREENING, AND EARLY DETECTION

As the etiology of prostate cancer is unknown, specific recommendations regarding prevention cannot be made. Rather, based upon the known risk factors, several suggestions can be made. Consuming a low-fat, high-fiber diet may reduce one's risk of developing prostate cancer. Maintaining normal weight for height would also seem reasonable. Obtaining one's vitamins and trace minerals from vegetable sources, avoiding known carcinogens such as cigarette smoke, and considering alternative methods of contraception may also reduce one's risk of prostate cancer.

Screening for prostate cancer involves the use of digital rectal exam (DRE), analysis of prostate-specific antigen (PSA) level, and, if appropriate, evaluation of the gland using transrectal ultrasound (TRUS).

DRE involves palpation of the prostate gland and is the most commonly performed screening exam for prostate diseases.[27] The posterior and lateral glandular tissue is evaluated by the examiner's finger.[28] The exam assists in evaluating for lesions, texture, and symmetry of the gland. Limitations to DRE include failure to locate tumors in the anterior and midline of the prostate, where approximately 40% of cancers may be found.[29] Small lesions may be missed, especially those less than 1.5 cm.[30] DRE is recommended as part of an annual physical exam for men beginning at age 40.[31] Those with higher risk factors, such as black men, should begin screening at a younger age. Also recommended by the American Cancer Society are annual PSA determinations beginning at age 50, done in conjunction with DRE by one's family physician (see Table 45-1).

PSA is a glycoprotein found in normal prostatic tissue. The protein is found in higher concentrations within the gland than in the blood. A barrier layer of three tissues lies between the blood and the PSA found in prostate ducts.[32] Anything that destroys this natural tissue barrier allows PSA to enter the bloodstream, where it can be collected and evaluated in a laboratory. Procedures that can falsely elevate PSA levels, such as biopsy, urethral instrumentation, catheterization, and possibly rectal examination, should be avoided prior to obtaining PSA blood specimens.[33]

Tandem-R PSA assay (Hybritech Inc., San Diego, CA) uses a range of 0–4.0 ng/ml[3] as the normal value. The human prostate gland continues to grow in the adult male after the completion of puberty. As the prostate increases in size, the PSA also increases. Hyperplastic benign prostatic tissue can therefore be expected to produce a higher serum concentration of PSA both in the absence and presence of prostate cancer. One gram of benign prostate hyperplasia (BPH) may increase serum PSA levels by "about 0.3 ng/ml/gram of hyperplastic tissue."[34,p. 915] Also, conditions other than prostate cancer can give rise to elevated PSA levels. Oesterling and colleagues assessed 2119 healthy men in a prospective trial to determine the effect of BPH on PSA levels.[35] They determined that PSA levels are related to patient age and prostate volume and that prostate volume is related to

**TABLE 45-1** Summary of ACS Recommendations Regarding Prostate Cancer Screening[31,35]

| Test | Frequency | Beginning at Age | How Test is Performed |
|------|-----------|------------------|------------------------|
| Digital rectal exam (DRE)} | Annual | 40 | The examiner's gloved and lubricated finger is inserted into |
| Prostate exam (PE)} | Annual | 50 | the rectum while the patient bends over the examining table. |
| Prostate-specific antigen (PSA) | Annual | 50 | Blood work |

| Normal Results | Significance | | |
|----------------|--------------|---|---|
| DRE} No palpable abnormality PE } Prostate gland symmetry, texture, and no masses felt | Able to detect gland asymmetry, abnormal texture, and presence of lesions | | |
| PSA 0–4.0 ng/ml 0–2.5 ng/ml 0–3.5 ng/ml 0–4.5 ng/ml 0–6.5 ng/ml | Results may be age-related[35] Ages 40–49 Ages 50–59 Ages 60–69 Ages 70–79 | | |

All abnormal results require additional diagnostic studies.

patient age. The PSA concentration increases by 0.04 ng/ml/year. Based upon their study, the authors recommended a new range for PSA values based on patient age. For men aged 40–49, the new range is 0–2.5 ng/ml; ages 50–59, 0–3.5 ng/ml; ages 60–69, 0–4.5 ng/ml; ages 70–79, 0–6.5 ng/ml. These new ranges will improve the usefulness of PSA in identifying important cancers in younger and older patients (see Table 45-1).

TRUS is used to follow up abnormal DRE or elevated PSA levels. Its role in screening programs is not yet defined. The test can evaluate prostate volume and identify suspicious areas for biopsy.[36] An ultrasound probe is inserted into the rectum and can reveal hypoechoic areas and other abnormalities in the prostate. Needle biopsies of suspicious areas are then taken under ultrasonic guidance. Three additional directed biopsies from each lobe of the prostate are also routinely obtained.

No area of cancer research is as hotly debated as the issue of whether or not there should be mass public screenings to detect prostate cancer. A recent study reviewed the pathological features of 583 localized prostate cancers for the number that were clinically unimportant, clinically important, curable, or clinically important advanced.[37] The patients had either clinically-detected or cystoprostatectomy-detected cancers. Tumors detected by cystoprostatectomy were smaller, more likely to be confined to the prostate, and less likely to contain poorly differentiated cells. Most of these lesions were felt to be clinically unimportant. Tumors that had been clinically detected and then removed by radical prostatectomy were more likely to be clinically important. Fifty-five of the 583 patients had nonpalpable tumors but elevated PSA. The cancers in the latter group were of higher grade, and 40% of them extended outside the prostatic capsule. Patients with tumors palpable by DRE were more likely to be advanced than nonpalpable tumors (34% versus 11%). Another study determined that 84% of cancers detected by PSA were clinically significant.[38,39]

Additional support for the ability of PSA to detect clinically important cancer comes from the Physician's Health Study.[40] During ten-year follow-up, only 8.7% of the men with an elevated PSA did not develop clinical prostate cancer. In fact, it was determined that one PSA assessment would have found 80% of the important prostate cancers that became apparent in five years and would also have found approximately 50% of those that were identified in ten years. The authors therefore concluded that PSA is a valid tool for screening cancer.

Contradicting this evidence are new data from the American Cancer Society National Prostate Cancer Early Prostate Detection Program.[41] The study involves 2999 healthy men aged 55–70, who were followed annually for five years or until a cancer was diagnosed in the prostate. The annual exam included DRE, TRUS, and PSA. Biopsies were obtained via TRUS when a suspicious area was detected during DRE. Biopsies from 265 men were evaluated and were diagnostic for prostate cancer in 177 men. Seven men were diagnosed as having prostatic intraepi-thelial neoplasia (PIN), and the remainder as having atypical glands, atypical hyperplasia, or benign hyperplasia. The men with cancers were found to have low-grade tumors.

Currently, both nationally and internationally prospective randomized trials are evaluating the issues related to screening.[42] These results may answer questions about who should be screened for prostate cancer in the general population. Until then, the ACS guidelines should be utilized. Black males, because of their higher risk of prostate cancer, should be encouraged by nurses to participate in annual prostate cancer screening provided by their family physicians. Men who have first-degree relatives with prostate cancer should be educated regarding the need to participate in earlier screening.

## PATHOPHYSIOLOGY

The prostate gland, approximately the size of an inverted, triangularly shaped walnut sits beneath the bladder and anterior to the rectum. The section of the urethra that passes through the prostate is known as the prostatic urethra. Draining into the prostatic urethra are the prostatic ducts. Prostatic fluid drains into the prostatic ducts from the glandular elements of the prostate. This fluid aids in the fertilization process.[43] (See Figure 45-1.)

The prostate gland is composed of three major sections: the central zone, the peripheral zone, and the transitional zone. The larger peripheral zone that surrounds the central zone is the most common site for cancer.[44]

The prostate is well vascularized. Its major blood supply originates from the inferior vesical artery.[44] Venous drainage is through the inferior hypogastric venous system and the presacral prevertebral venous plexus; lymphatic drainage is via the external and internal iliac groups and obturator lymph nodes. These nodes and lymphatics then drain into the common iliac and preaortic lymph nodes.

### Cellular Characteristics

The vast majority of prostate cancers are adenocarcinomas. Of the 5% of prostate cancers that are not adenocarcinomas, greater than 90% are transitional cell carcinomas. A rare squamous cell carcinoma may also occur and is the third most common type. All prostate cancers arise from one cell of origin, the embryonic urogenital sinus epithelium.[45]

Two types of prostatic proliferative lesions have been identified.[45] One is described as "atypical adenomatous hyperplasia" or "adenosis."[45,46] The lesions are characterized by the development of new structural elements. The second is "prostatic intra-epithelial neoplasia" (PIN).[45,47]

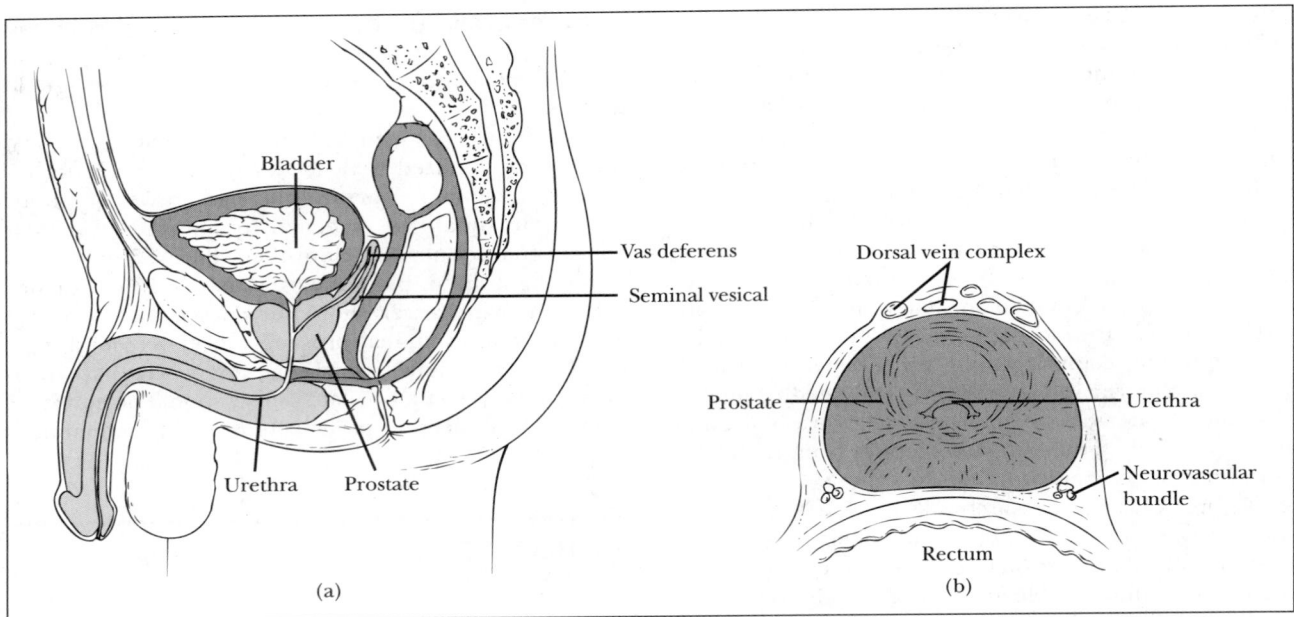

**FIGURE 45-1** (A) Regional anatomy of the pelvis. The prostate is located at the outlet of the urinary bladder and is accessible to palpation through the rectum. (B) A transverse section through the midportion of the prostate gland shows the proximity to the rectum and the relation of the neurovascular bundles to the prostate. The cavernous nerves, responsible for penile erections, accompany small vessels in the groove between the rectum and the posterolateral peripheral zone of the prostate, where most prostate cancers arise. Adapted from Figure 35-2, in DeVita V, Hellman S, Rosenberg S (eds): *Cancer: Principles and Practice of Oncology* (ed 4). Philadelphia, Lippincott, 1993.

These severely dysplastic lesions are likely precursors to prostate adenocarcinoma; the greater the amount of dysplasia present in PIN, the greater the risk of microinvasive carcinoma development.

Prostate tissue specimens are subjected to a type of pathological scoring based on cellular architecture known as Gleason's grade.[48] The majority of the tumor may be occupied by cells with one type of histological feature that is given a number of 1 to 5 based upon the severity of the cellular changes. The lower numbers are assigned to cellular patterns that are similar to prostatic tissue. The higher numbers are cellular patterns with more bizarre architectural features that look less like normal prostatic tissue. This primary number is added to a secondary number, which reflects the second most common type of cellular structure using the same scoring format. The sum of the two numbers gives the final total Gleason grade. Not all studies utilize the summed format. Tumors graded 1–3 are considered well differentiated and those 4 or greater are considered poorly differentiated carcinomas[45] (see Table 45-2). When the entire prostate is available for pathological review, the volume of tissue and the Gleason grade can predict the presence of lymph node metastases.[49] When the Gleason score is 4–5 (poorly differentiated), the risk of nodal metastases increases when the volume of cancer is more than 3.2 cc. The risk of nodal metastases is less than 1% when the cancer volume is less than 3.2 cc. Nodal metastases help predict survival.[50] Therefore, the Gleason system may be

**TABLE 45-2   Gleason Scoring System**

| Pattern 1 | Closely packed, single, separate, round, uniform glands; well-defined tumor margin |
|---|---|
| Pattern 2 | Single, separate, round, less uniform glands separated by stroma up to one gland diameter; tumor margin less well-defined |
| Pattern 3 | Single, separate, irregular glands of variable size; enlarged masses with cribriform or papillary pattern; poorly defined tumor margin |
| Pattern 4 | Fused glands in mass with infiltrating cords, small glands with papillary, cribriform, or solid patterns; cells small, dark, or hypernephroid (clear cells) |
| Pattern 5 | Few or no glands in background of masses with comedo pattern; cords or sheets of tumor cells infiltrating stroma |

*Gleason tumor grade = dominant pattern + secondary pattern.

Data from Hanks G, Myers G, Scardino P: Cancer of the prostate, in DeVita V, Hellman S, Rosenberg S (eds): *Cancer: Principles and Practice of Oncology* (ed 4). Philadelphia, Lippincott, 1993.

useful in predicting nodal metastases and subsequently survival.[49]

Prostate cancers can also be divided into those that are clinically important and those that are clinically unimportant.[51] Clinically important cancers include features such as large tumor volume, Gleason grade 3–5 (moderate to poor differentiation), an invasive, proliferative pattern of growth, elevated PSA, and origination in the peripheral zone. These cancers threaten the patient's life because they progress to fatal metastatic cancers. Cancers that do not threaten the patient's life are termed indolent or clinically unimportant. These indolent cancers comprise the vast majority of prostate cancers. These cancers are small with a Gleason's score of 1–2 (well differentiated), are noninvasive in their pattern of growth, do not elevate the PSA, originate in the transitional zone, and tend to fail to progress into invasive metastatic cancers. Clinically unimportant cancers should be monitored for rising PSA levels, which may indicate a change in the cancer's behavior to a more aggressive pattern of growth, requiring treatment.

## Progression of Disease

Prostate cancer is characterized by a slow pattern of growth. The tumor grows locally along tissue planes such as the boundary between the peripheral zone and the transitional zone.[52] The prostatic capsule is then penetrated via the perineural spaces.[53] Lymphatic metastases occur and involve the obturator-hypogastric and external iliac nodes.[54] After lymph node metastases, the next most commonly involved metastatic sites include the bones, lungs, bladder, and liver.[55] The cells spread to these distant sites via the bloodstream.

## CLINICAL MANIFESTATIONS

Prostate cancer may be asymptomatic in its early stages. An annual DRE is the most effective method of early detection.[56] Patients may present with urinary tract obstructive symptoms similar to benign prostatic hypertrophy (BPH), such as frequency, hesitancy, nocturia, and urgency.[57] Symptoms may be abrupt in their onset but otherwise are similar to BPH. Other symptoms may include a change in erectile capability. Advanced prostate cancer is evidenced by the appearance of ureteral obstruction caused by ureterovesical junction compression by tumor or nodal metastases.[58] Hydronephrosis can then ensue, threatening function of the associated kidney. Back pain may reveal the presence of vertebral body metastases with the potential for spinal cord compression.[59] There may also be local pain due to the presence of the cancer in the prostate gland and invasion into surrounding structures, and referred pain to the legs and abdomen. Bone pain can be problematic and is related to the presence of additional skeletal metastases. The hip, legs, neck, shoulders, and ribs are the next most common areas.[58] Additional symptoms related to advanced prostate growth include rectal obstruction from local growth, coagulation deficits related to the release of procoagulant into the bloodstream from the prostate

cancer cells, hypercalcemia, leg edema from nodal metastases, and pancytopenia from marrow metastases.[59,60]

## ASSESSMENT

### Patient and Family History

Nursing assessment of patients at risk for or with a diagnosis of prostate cancer should begin with questioning the patient about past medical problems or diagnoses of prostate diseases. The presence of a prostate cancer diagnosis in first- and second-degree relatives should be ascertained, and exposure to potential prostate carcinogens or risk factors need to be determined.

The nurse should evaluate the patient's voiding pattern and ask if the patient has problems with dysuria, frequency, nocturia, hematuria, and other signs of bladder outlet obstruction (see Table 45-3). The pelvic area should be percussed and palpated for bladder distention. A postvoiding residual measurement may be ordered by

**TABLE 45-3**   Questions Useful in Assessing Urinary Symptoms Associated with Prostate Cancer[79]

| Symptom | Assessment |
| --- | --- |
| Dysuria | Does the patient have difficulty initiating urination? If so, how often? Does the patient have difficulty maintaining or ending the urine stream? Does the patient need to apply pressure to the bladder to initiate urination? Does dribbling occur at the end of urination? Is there pain on urination? If so, how does the pain feel? Does it persist or is it intermittent? Are there bladder spasms? |
| Frequency | How often does the patient need to urinate? What is the volume of each voiding? Does the patient void and then need to void again a few minutes later? Is there a reduction in the urine volume produced? |
| Nocturia | How many times does the patient get out of bed each night to urinate? Is there incontinence at night? |
| Hematuria | Is there blood in the urine? Clots? What is the color of the urine? |
| Other | Does the urine have an odor? Is particulate matter present in the urine? When did the patient void most recently? Can the patient feel his bladder through the abdominal wall? Is there flank pain? How many urinary tract infections has the patient had in the last 12 months? Has there been a change in the strength of penile erections? |

the physician to evaluate the volume of residual urine in the bladder.

## Physical Exam

The patient is examined for evidence of local and distant metastases. Inguinal nodes are palpated, and the patient is asked about bone pain, specifically back pain. If back pain is present, the patient is questioned about signs of spinal cord compression, such as numbness, tingling and other indications of sensory loss, motor weakness, or bowel or bladder incontinence.[61] Other potential areas of pain include the rectum and local pelvic area. The patient is asked about the pain medications he has been using and their effectiveness and side effects. The patient's legs should be examined for edema and its severity and for indications of deep vein thromboses, such as unilateral leg edema, pain, local heat, and redness. The skin should be checked for petechiae and ecchymoses. The patient is weighed and asked about how much weight he has lost since the illness began.

## Diagnostic Studies

Once a presumptive diagnosis of prostate cancer is made, the patient will have a PSA level drawn and a DRE performed if these tests have not previously been performed. As PSA levels reflect the severity of the patient's disease,[57] PSA level may be drawn before and after therapeutic interventions and then periodically to monitor the status of the cancer. Additional blood tests include serum chemistries, including calcium, liver function tests, blood urea nitrogen (BUN), creatinine, and complete blood count (CBC). A urinanalysis is performed and a chest x-ray and an electrocardiogram (ECG) are completed. Computerized tomographic (CT) scans of the abdomen and pelvis are done to evaluate local and nodal metastasis and to determine the eligibility of the patient for treatment. A bone scan is frequently performed as part of the staging workup[62] to evaluate bone pain. TRUS may be used to assist in evaluating the extent of localized prostate cancer.[63] In patients being considered for curative surgery, a laparoscopic pelvic lymph node dissection may be done to evaluate the presence of nodal metastasis.[57]

## Prognostic Indicators

As mentioned previously, PSA levels reflect the extent of disease and the amount of cancer found in the prostate gland.[57] For example, PSA levels in stage A disease average 3.1 ng/ml; $A_2$—12.1 ng/ml; $B_1$—12.3 ng/ml; $B_2$—25 ng/ml; $B_3$—40 ng/ml; C—102 ng/ml; and $D_2$—563 ng/ml.[64] PSA levels are used to monitor the effectiveness of treatment and to monitor the patient for disease recurrence. Unfortunately, not all prostate cancers produce PSA, and other diagnostic studies, such as CT scan, may be needed

to monitor disease status. Baseline blood levels are obtained before and after treatment and usually are monitored every three months after treatment for one year and then every 6 to 12 months. Levels greater than 80 ng/ml reflect a large disease burden and often metastatic cancer. After undergoing primary therapy for any stage of prostate cancer, an increasing PSA level reflects disease progression.[65] After undergoing curative resection for prostate gland-confined cancer, PSA levels should be undetectable.[66] Doses of 5040–5400 cGy external beam radiation therapy are used to treat prostate cancer. PSA levels should be normal 3 to 18 months after completion of therapy. Failure of PSA to normalize often reflects localized disease recurrence.[67] Therefore, PSA is a highly useful tool for the monitoring of disease response to therapy and monitoring the patient for cancer relapse.

## CLASSIFICATION AND STAGING

The most commonly used staging system for prostate cancer is the American Urologic Association (AUA) System.[68] This system was originally developed by Whitmore and then updated by Jewitt. Recently, a tumor-node-metastasis (TNM) system was developed by the American Joint Committee on Cancer (AJCC). Although the AUA system is frequently used, many facilities use the TNM classification system. See Table 45-4 for a comparison of the two staging systems.

Small cancers found on transurethral resection of the

**TABLE 45-4** Comparison of the American Urologic Association (AUA) and TNM Classification Systems for Prostate Cancer

|  | TNM | AUA |
|---|---|---|
| Tumor is incidental histological finding | T1 | A |
| Three or fewer microscopic foci | T1A | A1 |
| More than three microscopic foci | T1B | A2 |
| Tumor is present clinically or grossly and limited to the prostate | T2 | B |
| Tumor <1.5 cm, with normal tissue on at least three sides | TA2 | B1 |
| Tumor >1.5 cm or in more than one lobe | T2B | B2 |
| Tumor invades the prostatic apex or into or beyond the prostatic capsule, bladder neck, or seminal vesicle, but is not fixed | T3 | C |
| No invasion of seminal vesicles | T3 | C1 |
| Invasion of seminal vesicles | T3 | C2 |
| Pelvic wall fixation | T4 | C2 |
| Lymph node metastasis | N | D |
| Distant metastasis | M | D |

Data from Hanks G, Myers G, Scardino P: Cancer of the prostate, in DeVita VT, Hellman S, Rosenberg SA (eds): *Cancer: Principles and Practice of Oncology* (ed 4). Philadelphia, Lippincott, 1993.

prostate for BPH are often asymptomatic and are staged as A. When the cancer is 1.5 cm or less and involves only one lobe of the gland, it is considered $B_1$ disease. $B_2$ cancer is larger than 1.5 cm and involves more than one lobe of the prostate. After the cancer has invaded into or beyond the prostate capsule, stage C disease is present. With metastasis to distant sites, the patient has stage D cancer.[69] Survival is stage dependent. Patients with stage A disease have survival at 10 years of 95%, stage B at 10 years—80%, stage C at 10 years—60%, stage D (nodal metastases)—40% and stage D (distant metastases)—10%.[51]

# THERAPEUTIC APPROACHES AND NURSING CARE

Treatment options available for a particular patient are based upon age, general medical condition, tumor grade, and tumor volume (stage).[70–72] A patient may be offered watchful waiting (periodic observation), surgery, radiation therapy, hormonal manipulation, chemotherapy, or investigational drugs.

## Watchful Waiting or Periodic Observation for Early Stage Prostate Cancer (Stages A and B)

Prostate cancer is a heterogenous disease. As indicated previously, prostate cancer is often slow growing. Men with small volume, well-differentiated cancers may die with, rather than from, prostate cancer. If one considers the male population in the United States, there exists a group of 8 million men over 50 years of age with a potentially diagnosable prostate cancer. Of these 8 million men, 7.9 million will have an autopsy-discoverable cancer. The remaining 100,000 men have a clinically diagnosable cancer.[51] Clinically diagnosable prostate cancer, untreated, will continue to grow and threaten the life of the patient. Latent or clinically unimportant cancers do not threaten the patient's life. Of men aged 50 or older, approximately one-third will have malignant cells in their prostate.[73] As men age beyond 50, the incidence of cancer cells in the prostate increases. However, only 3% of men who develop malignant cells in their prostate will die of the disease. For men with early stage A and $B_1$ prostate cancer, this observation has led some physicians to offer periodic observation as a method of cancer management. Periodic observation involves PSA level monitoring and physical examination every three to six months to determine if there has been clinical disease progression.

For patients over 70, watchful waiting may be an appropriate option.[70] Research has yet to demonstrate that for the approximately 60% of men who present with stage A or B cancer, treatment is more beneficial than watchful waiting.[74] For men under 70, a physician may often be reluctant to offer watchful waiting, and there is evidence

that for younger men with moderately or poorly differentiated localized prostate cancer, treatment may offer a survival advantage.[70] For patients over 70, treatment that produces side effects such as incontinence may be less beneficial.[70]

Treatment for localized prostate cancer may be offered in hopes of preventing metastatic disease from developing.[73] However, there is no evidence that this is true. Currently for younger men in their 40s and 50s, even with well-differentiated cancers, treatment is almost always offered. Prostate cancer may behave in a more aggressive manner because of higher grade tumors in younger men, and for this reason alone, treatment is offered. Also, younger men have the potential to live longer and thus develop metastases that may be life-threatening.

The option of watchful waiting may not gain widespread support without evidence from prospective randomized trials. Until the results are known, which will take years, standard therapy with surgery or radiation therapy will be offered to patients with localized prostate cancer. Three studies have been conducted that address the concept of watchful waiting, one in Sweden and two in the United States. However, all three of the studies contain methodological flaws.[73] Even though flawed, these studies are often cited as evidence that watchful waiting is an appropriate option in selected patients.[73] The Swedish study followed 223 patients with stage A or B prostate cancer.[75] Urinary symptoms were managed with transurethral prostatic resection (TURP), and if disease progression occurred, hormonal manipulation was initiated. At the ten-year mark, 124 of the original 223 patients were dead, but for only 8.5% of the patients the cause of death was related to the prostate cancer.[75]

Fleming and colleagues[76] examined the literature to identify risks and benefits of currently available therapy for men over 60. The following groups of men were identified as benefiting from watchful waiting: men with well-differentiated tumors and men over 75. The research also concluded that patients with moderately to poorly differentiated tumors should undergo treatment, as longer survival (3.5 years) may be achieved.

The last study evaluated data from 828 patients who participated in six nonrandomized trials. The men received observation and delayed hormone therapy for localized stage A and B cancer.[77] The cancers were graded 1 (well differentiated, Gleason score 2–4), 2 (moderately differentiated, Gleason score 5–7), or 3 (poorly differentiated, Gleason score 8–10). Grade 3 patients had a poorer survival ratio and at 10 years, 34% of these men were alive and 26% were free of metastatic disease. The authors concluded that for grade 1–2 clinically localized cancer in men with a life expectancy of less than 10 years, observation and delayed hormonal manipulation is an option for selected patients.

Patients may not be able to cope with the concept that "there is a cancer in my body and it can be removed; why should I continue to let it grow?" When watchful waiting is the option offered by the patient's physician, the nurse should support the patient by reinforcing current information, clarifying misconceptions, answering questions, providing support by encouraging verbalization, and, if appropriate, supporting the patient's decision to seek a differing medical opinion.

## Surgery

### Transurethral resection of the prostate (TURP)

Prostate cancer is not cured by TURP.[72] Rather, it is used to treat symptoms of bladder outlet obstruction and in some patients, provides pathological evidence that a cancer, previously unsuspected, is present. Using a transurethral resectoscope and electrocautery, the hypertrophic prostate is removed in pieces called "chips." The procedure is done under spinal anesthesia or general anesthesia with the patient in the lithotomy position. Potential immediate postoperative complications include clot retention, bleeding, and infection. The bladder is kept as free of blood and clots as possible using continuous saline irrigation through a three-way indwelling catheter. Bladder spasms can be problematic and patients may require analgesics and antispasmodics. After the bleeding decreases, bladder irrigation is discontinued. As the urine becomes more normal in appearance, the catheter is removed. Patients may have difficulty initiating urination after catheter removal and may require recatheterization.

Crucial aspects of managing patients include preoperative education as to routine aspects of anesthesia, such as coughing, deep breathing, and early ambulation. The patient needs to know he will have a catheter for several days after surgery and bladder irrigation for approximately 24 hours or less. Pain management approaches using oral and rectal medications are taught. The patient must drink large volumes of fluid, such as water, to promote urine formation. Accurate recording of intake and output is required until discharge. The patient needs to be aware that late complications, such as incontinence, impotence, and bladder neck contraction requiring urethral dilation, may occur[78] and will require physician notification for appropriate management. Patients may have problems with bladder outlet obstruction recurrence and may need to undergo repeat TURP. This will occur in approximately 5% of men (see Table 45-5 for management of the TURP patient).

### Radical prostatectomy

The use of radical prostatectomy has increased since 1985.[81,82] In 1984, 8.9% of patients with a newly diagnosed prostate cancer underwent radical prostatectomy. By 1990, the incidence of radical prostatectomy had increased to 21.4%.[83] The majority of procedures are done in younger men (aged 59 or younger) with localized

**TABLE 45-5**   Nursing Management of the Patient Undergoing a TURP[79,80]

| Nursing Diagnosis | Etiology | Outcome | Nursing Management |
|---|---|---|---|
| Knowledge deficit Surgery | Lack of prior experience with surgery | Patient will verbalize an understanding of preoperative and postoperative course. | 1. Assess patient's understanding of cancer diagnosis, planned surgery to remove obstructing section of prostate gland around prostatic urethra compressing urethra and impeding release of urine from the bladder, expected outcome that patient will be able to void with reduced difficulty, potential complications of surgery including incontinence.<br>2. Educate patient regarding:<br>• care of indwelling catheter<br>• continuous bladder irrigation (CBI)<br>• drinking fluids<br>• ambulating first day postop<br>• coughing and deep breathing<br>• pain management with belladonna and opium suppositories for bladder spasms, oral narcotics for pain<br>• signs/symptoms of urinary tract infection (UTI) to report to physician after surgery—pain, burning, frequency, hematuria<br>• need to notify physician after discharge of inability to void, continued incontinence |
| Incontinence | The urinary sphincter may be injured during surgery—may persist up to three months in elderly. | The patient will be able to manage incontinence. | • methods for managing incontinence (see Table 45-6) |

**TABLE 45-5** Nursing Management of the Patient Undergoing a TURP[79,80] (continued)

| Nursing Diagnosis | Etiology | Outcome | Nursing Management |
|---|---|---|---|
| Indwelling catheter care | The patient is unable to void after indwelling catheter is removed postop and requires recatheterization and discharge home with indwelling catheter. | The patient will demonstrate the skills necessary to maintain an indwelling catheter at home. | 3. Educate patient to:<br>• wash around urinary meatus with soap and water, to rinse and dry the area 2 times daily.<br>• utilize leg bag during day, how to attach, disconnect, empty and cleanse bag to maintain a clean environment inside the equipment.<br>• utilize straight drainage at night, how to cleanse bag to maintain a clean environment inside the equipment.<br>• maintain a clean bag environment by rinsing the equipment, washing it with soapy water, rinsing well, and allowing it to air dry. |
| Altered urinary elimination related to TURP and indwelling catheter | The patient has undergone TURP and requires catheter to maintain prostate urethra patency and elimination of urine and blood.<br><br>Clots have formed in the bladder, occluding the catheter/tubing lumen. As the bladder fills, clots slide down the outside of the catheter and out the meatus. | The catheter will remain patent. Urine output will be ≥ 30 ml/hr. | 1. Maintain accurate I & O.<br>2. Empty urinary drainage bag when ⅔ full.<br>3. Maintain CBI at prescribed rate using NSS 3-liter irrigation bags. Do not allow bags to empty. Keep NSS running at all times to maintain pink-colored drainage. CBI is usually discontinued 24 hours postop, but may by required for a longer period if some bleeding or clot formation persists beyond the first 24 hours.<br>4. Monitor for clots in the tubing, monitor for clot retention with subsequent bleeding around the catheter. Assess for bladder distention. Notify physician of clot retention. Irrigate Foley manually with saline until free of clots.<br>5. Maintain IV fluids at prescribed rate of infusion.<br>6. Encourage fluid intake, usually 2000 ml/24 hrs.<br>7. Maintain catheter tubing patency by unkinking tubing.<br>8. Two to three days postop, the catheter is removed. Accurately measure the first and each subsequent voiding until discharge. Notify physician if patient does not void in 8 hours. |
| Bleeding related to TURP | The prostate is highly vascularized. Cauterization during the surgery does not seal all the bleeding capillaries, therefore bleeding occurs in the postoperative period. | The patient will have prompt recognition of and immediate intervention for increased bleeding. Bleeding will decrease daily. | 1. Monitor H/H values. Notify physician of ≥ 1 gm reduction in hemoglobin.<br>2. Maintain traction with tape on catheter applied during surgery to assist in control of venous bleeding in prostatic bed.<br>3. Monitor color of urine. There should be a noted reduction in the amount of blood in the urine daily. If increased blood is present, notify physican.<br>4. Do not remove water from over-filled indwelling catheter balloon, as this helps to control bleeding.<br>5. Do not remove indwelling catheter until physician orders its removal. Premature removal may result in bleeding.<br>6. Monitor for bladder distention, which increases bleeding by pulling on capillaries. |
| Potential for infection related to surgery and indwelling catheter | The presence of an indwelling catheter may promote bladder infection. The patient has undergone surgery under general anesthesia and may develop postop atelectasis, which may develop into pneumonia. | The patient will not develop a fever or other sign of infection. | 1. Encourage Q1H coughing and deep breathing.<br>2. Use aseptic technique when emptying drainage bag and attaching new bladder irrigation bags.<br>3. Perform meatal care twice daily with soap and water.<br>4. Maintain catheter patency. Observe for clots, chips of tissue, mucus that can obstruct catheter lumen. Keep catheter and tubing straight and free of kinks. Keep drainage bag off floor. Hang with hook from bed.'<br>5. Notify physician of temp ≥ 38.5 °C, tachycardia, tachypnea, decreased BP, other signs of infection.<br>6. Obtain urine, blood, or other cultures as prescribed. |

*(continued)*

**TABLE 45-5** Nursing Management of the Patient Undergoing a TURP[79,80] (continued)

| Nursing Diagnosis | Etiology | Outcome | Nursing Management |
|---|---|---|---|
| Altered comfort related to pain, bladder spasms, or both | Pain or bladder spasms may be due to surgery, bladder distention, infection, clots, or the catheter balloon. | The patient will verbalize an acceptable level of analgesia. | 1. Assess quantity, quality, and duration of pain.<br>2. Check for bladder distention, kinked tubing, freely flowing drainage. Palpate bladder after turning off CBI. Restart CBI if patient not distended. Otherwise, notify physician.<br>3. Administer prescribed narcotic for pain.<br>4. Administer belladonna and opium suppository, oxybutynin or propantheline for bladder spasms.<br>5. Gently irrigate indwelling catheter if prescribed. Never force irrigation fluid—notify physician.<br>6. Remind patient not to tug or pull at the catheter. If the patient should pull out the catheter, notify physician immediately. |
| Potential for urethral stricture formation related to surgery | The urethra may heal with stricture formation if catheter is removed prematurely. | The patient will have a patent urethra. | 1. The catheter is never to be removed without a physician's order.<br>2. Monitor for signs of stricture, such as small urine stream, straining to void, and difficulty voiding. |
| Potential for urinary retention after catheter removal | The patient is not able to void after catheter is removed. | The patient will not develop urinary retention. | 1. The patient should void when he feels the urge and not wait, as this may produce urinary distention, which may cause retention. |
| Constipation related to antispasmodics used to manage bladder spasms | Anticholinergic drugs cause constipation. Straining can cause bleeding. | The patient will have an easy bowel movement. | 1. Administer stool softeners/laxatives to reduce constipation and promote easy colon evacuation.<br>2. Educate patient not to strain on bowel movement. |

disease as opposed to regional disease. More procedures are done in the Pacific region and the fewest in the mid-Atlantic and New England regions.[84] The increasing use of radical prostatectomy is related to the use of PSA to screen asymptomatic men.[85]

The procedure involves removal of the prostate gland, capsule, ejaculatory ducts, seminal vesicles, and possibly the lymph nodes if a laparoscopic nodal sampling has not been done as part of the staging workup to determine the patient's eligibility for the radical procedure. Radical prostatectomy is usually done on patients staged with A or B disease.[78] With stage C disease, it may be more difficult to obtain tumor-free margins. The patient is informed preoperatively by the physician about the potential for postoperative incontinence and impotence. Incontinence may occur after indwelling catheter removal. Up to 15% of men remain incontinent six months postoperatively.[79] Fifty incontinent men were evaluated for the impact of incontinence after radical prostatectomy on their quality of life.[86] Twenty-six percent of the 50 men reported that moderate to severe incontinence had a serious impact on their quality of life. Not only were physical activities reduced, but so were activities of daily living. In spite of the inconvenience of incontinence, 68% of the 50 men would still select the surgical intervention.

The autonomic nerves that control erectile function lie beneath the prostate. Surgery may damage or sever these nerves; however, the right or left neurovascular bundles now may be preserved[87] (see Figure 45-1). Walsh developed the method of sparing one of the neurovascular bundles responsible for an erection.[88] With this procedure, it is possible to spare potency; however, there will not be prostatic fluid and therefore no emission and ejaculation. The nerve-sparing procedure is recommended for patients with stage A or B disease who are eligible to undergo radical prostatectomy. The nerve-sparing procedure was performed in 503 men who were able to maintain an erection before surgery.[89] Sixty-eight percent of the patients were potent after surgery. Factors identified that promote sexual function after surgery are age less than 50, stage of disease, and the preservation of neurovascular bundles. In younger men (aged 50 and younger), lower stage and surgical procedure were the factors associated with potency. When one bundle is intact in patients younger than 50, potency is preserved. In patients over 70, only 22% will regain potency postoperatively, even if both neurovascular bundles are spared. If disease is more advanced and there is involvement of the prostatic capsule or seminal vesicles at the time of surgery, resection may involve removal of or damage to the nerves. In the patients with $B_2$ or C disease, 51% had one bundle left intact. Age again becomes important with men under 50 regaining potency and older patients having a reduced likelihood of potency.

Incontinence and impotence can place a heavy burden on male patients and their families. Increasingly research is addressing concerns related to quality of life (QOL). Compared with normal age-matched men living in the same location, men who have undergone treatment for localized prostate cancer are more likely to have problems related to sexual, urinary, or bowel function.[90] QOL issues may be amenable to nursing interventions, such as patient education, and nurses need to accept responsibility for the assessment, management, and evaluation of these issues.

Preoperative nursing care is similar to that provided to patients undergoing other surgical procedures of the abdomen and pelvis.[91] Many patients undergoing radical prostatectomy will be over age 50, and special attention should be paid to the patient's comorbid factors such as cardiopulmonary status. Additional routine preoperative care includes administering a bowel preparation to evacuate the colon, starting prescribed intravenous therapy, and ensuring that the patient eats or drinks nothing after midnight. Elderly patients may have longer postoperative recovery times and should be aware that their recovery will be slower than that of younger men.

Intraoperatively, the prostate and its surrounding structures are removed via a perineal, retropubic, or suprapubic incision.[92] One or more drains may be placed during surgery, and frequent dressing changes may be required to control drainage, reduce bacterial growth, and reduce the risk of skin maceration and resultant infection. The nurse must monitor incision and drainage sites for infection.

Depending upon the surgical approach and degree of intraoperative findings, such as disease greater than expected, the patient may be immobilized on the operating room table for several hours. He is thus at risk for the usual postoperative complications. The nurse needs to encourage coughing, deep breathing, use of analgesics, and moving around in bed to promote lower extremity venous return to the heart. Compression stockings are usual in the postoperative period to reduce the risk of thrombophlebitis and potentially fatal pulmonary embolus. In the presence of thrombophlebitis or suspected/proven pulmonary emboli, anticoagulant therapy is initiated with heparinization and a heparin drip.

An indwelling Foley catheter is placed in the operating room and will remain in place postoperatively. Attention is needed to reduce the risk of infection with good hand washing, use of aseptic technique when emptying the drainage bag, and monitoring the catheter for patency.

In addition to maintaining the indwelling catheter, the nurse needs to monitor the amount of hematuria. In the initial postoperative period, a nasogastric tube may be in place to control gastric distention and remove gastric secretions. Management includes monitoring the type and amount of drainage, providing mouth care to promote oral comfort, and maintaining tube patency.

Postoperatively, it is crucial that the patient maintain a urine output of greater than 30 ml/hr.[80] In addition to monitoring for hematuria and clots, maintaining a patent catheter and an accurate intake and output, the nurse should assess the bladder for urinary retention and ad-

minister parenteral fluids. Traction on the catheter is maintained by securely taping the catheter to the patient's upper leg.

Bladder spasms can be annoying and painful. The most frequent method of managing spasms is to administer antispasmodics such as oxybutynin, and if not contraindicated, belladonna and opium (B & O) suppositories. Be sure the catheter is not kinked and that urine is flowing freely as spasms can be due to bladder distention or from the catheter itself.[93]

Hematuria and clots are common for the first three to four postoperative days.[93] Frank bleeding is abnormal and requires physician notification. Frequent vital sign monitoring is needed to assess the patient for signs of excess blood loss and temperature elevation, which may indicate a wound or urinary tract infection.

The patient may be discharged with an indwelling catheter and needs to be educated in meatal care, attachment of a leg drainage bag, change to straight drainage bag at bedtime, clean technique, and signs of urinary tract infection that would require physician notification. After the catheter is removed, incontinence may be a problem for days, weeks, or months. A variety of management options are available. Simple devices, such as penile clamps or incontinence pads, may be suggested. Reducing the volume of fluid consumed after dinner may control problems with nighttime incontinence. Frequent emptying of the bladder (e.g., every hour) may provide a patient with enough control over his incontinence that he finds occasional incontinence more acceptable. Educating the patient to use Kegel exercises to strengthen the muscles also may be beneficial. Incontinence is a problem for not only patients undergoing prostate surgery but also for many other adults. The problem is so severe that the Agency for Health Care Policy and Research released urinary incontinence guidelines in 1992.[94] These guidelines provide an in-depth discussion of incontinence and its management (see Table 45-6).

An additional burden placed on postprostatectomy men is the development of altered sexuality. See chapter 28 for an in-depth discussion of the issue and suggestions for nursing management. See Table 45-7 for "Helpful Hints for Starting Sexual Activity After Prostate Surgery."

## Radiation Therapy

External beam radiation therapy (XRT) may be administered in curative doses to treat men with early prostate cancer ($A_2$, $B_1$, $B_2$) confined to the gland itself. Young men with $A_1$ disease usually are also offered treatment rather than periodic observation.[104] Radiation therapy is an option available if a patient wishes to avoid surgery or is not a surgical candidate due to preexisting medical problems. There is no evidence that either radiation therapy or surgery is superior to the other.[105] Node-negative patients have approximately 90% disease-free 5-year survival.[106] Radiation therapy may also be appropriate for stage C or $D_1$ disease.[107] The dose of radiation adminis-

**TABLE 45-6** Assisting Patients to Manage Urinary Incontinence After Prostate Surgery[79,94–100]

After prostate surgery, continence is maintained by the external urinary sphincter. It is this striated urethral sphincter that prevents urinary leakage after prostate surgery.[95] Damage to the muscle controlling the sphincter or damage to its nerve supply can result in postoperative incontinence. The retropubic approach to prostatectomy may result in a lower rate of incontinence by avoiding injury to the cavernous nerves of the pelvic plexus.[96,97] After radical prostatectomy, 92% of patients achieve urinary control, 8% experience stress incontinence, and 6% wear one or fewer incontinence pads per day. Approximately 1% of men are incontinent after a TURP.[98]

### Evaluation

Diagnostic studies are performed to evaluate incontinence after a history and physical exam are performed. Cystourethroscopy is used to evaluate the integrity of the external urinary sphincter under direct visualization. A voiding cystourethrogram looks for anatomic abnormalities while urodynamic studies evaluate physiology.[99]

### Management

Diapers, liners—These devices absorb urine. There are a variety available on the market. Liners are useful for light to moderate incontinence. Adult diapers are needed for heavy urine loss. All devices should be changed frequently to avoid odor and skin maceration. Fungal infections can occur, and in summer, diapers can be hot and uncomfortable.[100] Cost can become a factor when absorbent products need to be changed frequently; for people with a limited income, this can be a financial burden. Bulky items may be noticed under clothing.

Drip collectors—The penis is placed inside the collector which is worn underneath clothing in a garment holder designed to hold the disposable collecting device.[100]

Condom catheters—Latex self-adhesive condom-shaped external urine collecting device. Problems include adhesive loss, skin breakdown and urinary tract infections. The skin needs to be cleansed daily and monitored daily for irritation and infection.[94]

Indwelling catheters—Closed sterile system that includes a catheter with a retaining water-filled balloon inserted into the urethra attached to a collection bag. Often left in place after surgery, these devices require daily cleansing and skin care to reduce the risk of infection and skin necrosis. These are not useful for long-term management of incontinence unless no other approach is successful.

Penile clamps—External urethral compressive device that occludes the urethra to reduce incontinence. The position of the clamp must be changed every 3 hours to prevent skin necrosis. Other complications include pain, edema, penile and urethral erosion, and urethral obstruction.[94]

Ostomy pouch—Useful for a small or retracted penis. Clip the hair around where the adhesive is applied and attach pouch to a collection bag.

Fluid restriction—The patient who experiences incontinence mostly at night should restrict fluids after dinner to reduce the bladder urine volume and thus the risk of incontinence. Otherwise, 2 quarts of fluids per day are encouraged.

Timed voiding—At predetermined intervals, the patient empties the bladder. To develop a schedule, the patient needs to keep a diary for three or four days to identify times of incontinence. A schedule is then developed for the patient to void prior to the times identified as being at risk for incontinence.[94]

Kegel exercises—The pelvic floor muscles are crucial to maintaining continence. These muscles can be strengthened with exercise. The exercise consists of contracting the pelvic floor muscles by squeezing the pubococcygeus muscle.[94] Squeezing this muscle closes the urethra. The abdominal, pelvic, and thigh muscles must not be contracted during the exercises. Contracting the muscles involved in a bowel movement by pulling them in and holding for 10 seconds, followed by a 10 second rest, and repeated 30 to 80 times a day for a minimum of 6 weeks, can result in better bladder control.

Biofeedback—Used in conjunction with Kegel exercises and timed voiding, biofeedback helps the patient become attuned to his physiology. Instruments help the person learn about bladder control.

Bladder dysfunction (detrusor instability)—Treatment includes fluid restriction and medications:

**Anticholinergics**

Propantheline—blocks bladder contractions, dose 7.5 mg to 30 mg 3 to 5 times a day;[94] cost—inexpensive; effect—may reduce incontinence in up to 53% of patients; side effects—urinary retention, dry mouth, blurred vision, nausea, constipation, confusion, drowsiness. Hyoscyamine is a newer drug.

Oxybutynin—also relaxes smooth muscle, dose 2.5 to 5 mg 3 to 4 times a day; effect—may reduce incontinence in up to 56% of patients; side effects—dry skin, blurred vision, nausea, constipation.[94]

**Antidepressants**

Imipramine—anticholinergic properties, dose 10 to 25 mg 1 to 3 times a day; side effects—rare; effect—up to 77% of patients may have reduced incontinence.[94]

Sphincter incompetence—Treatment includes alpha-adrenergic agonist drugs and surgery. The drugs increase sphincter resistance:

Phenylpropanolamine—dose 50 mg twice a day; effect—up to 45% of patients are drier; side effects—nausea, dry mouth, rash, itching, restlessness, insomnia.[94]

Surgery—goal is urethral compression.[99] Artificial urinary sphincter—useful in patients with normal detrusor function and an incompetent sphincter[98] and after failure of previously discussed methods.[94] Approximately 80% of patients treated will be dry or almost dry requiring no incontinence pads.[98] Complications include infection, device malfunction, bleeding, erosion of cuff site, and urethral injury.[94] Injections of collagen or polytetrafluoroethyline may be useful in patients who are not surgical candidates.

---

tered is based on disease stage. For stage A disease, the dose delivered is 60 Gy; for stage B, 60–65 Gy; and for stage C, 66–70 Gy.[108] However, these doses are not universally accepted and variability in dosing can be expected.

The radiation portal includes the prostate, periprostatic tissue, and pelvic lymph nodes. Treatment is usually given to a wide pelvic field to 50 Gy and then the treatment area is reduced to the prostate and surrounding

**TABLE 45-7**  Helpful Hints for Men Starting Sexual Activity After Prostate Surgery[79,101–103]

With removal of the prostate, men may notice changes in their sexual functioning. Some men and their partners benefit from understanding these changes and learn how to adapt to them. Beginning with some definitions of the changes, methods of ways to adapt to these changes will be described.

Erection—stiff penis due to increased blood flow

Potency—ability to cause vaginal penetration

Orgasm—sexual climax or pleasure with ejaculation of semen

Semen—mixture of sperm, prostate secretions, and seminal vesicle fluid

Sperm—reproductive cells produced by testes

Radical prostatectomy—removal of prostate, seminal vesicles, and surrounding tissues to remove cancer. With removal of the prostate and seminal vesicles, the ejaculate will be reduced and may be retrograde into the bladder resulting in a dry ejaculation. The urine will become cloudy from the sperm. Orgasms may still occur without ejaculation but with the contractions that occur as part of ejaculation. Impotency can result from surgery or radiation therapy. This can be partial or complete inability to obtain an erection. Some men will regain potency postoperatively, especially those under 50 years old.

Nerve-sparing radical prostatectomy—Depending on the size and location of the tumor, the surgeon spares one or both nerve bundles responsible for an erection. In the majority of men under 50 potency returns after wound healing occurs and all edema from the surgery subsides. This can take up to two years. Older men, over age 70, will probably not regain an erection.

Orgasms after prostate surgery may be weaker but are rarely completely absent. Alternative methods of obtaining pleasure need to be pursued if there is impotency.

In order to begin sexual activity after prostate surgery, wound healing must be complete; therefore, the urologist's permission is needed. This may occur six weeks to three months after surgery. Open, honest discussion of sexual issues with one's physician, nurse, and partner will help explore avenues of sexuality not previously considered. Open communication with the partner is the cornerstone of sexual recovery. Explore alternative methods of pleasure such as kissing, stroking, cuddling, massage, gentle rubbing, and fondling. Consider sexual counseling with a therapist if open discussion with the partner and other methods of pleasure are not successful. Couples need to understand that there is more to sexuality and pleasure than penis-vagina intercourse. The intimacy that develops between two partners who love each other will permit exploration. Beginning exploration produces trust and more intimacy that promotes the desire to find ways to pleasure the partner that may not have been previously considered. Failure to communicate desires and needs to one's partner is the greatest barrier to regaining sexual relations. It must also be understood that cancer of the prostate cannot be transmitted during sex or in the sperm. Cancer of the prostate is not a sexually transmitted disease.

Alternate methods of obtaining an erection include external and internal devices. Men in stable relationships with a previously good sex life are the best candidates. However, many of these couples have been able to substitute other sexual activity if erections are not able to penetrate the vagina.[102]

External Devices

Suction apparatus—vacuum erection device fits over the penis and air is removed by pumping it out with the device. Blood flows into the penis, making it rigid. A band is placed at the base of the penis to prevent blood from leaving the penis after the device is removed. After intercourse, the band is removed.[101]

Injections of drugs into the spongy penile tissue increase blood flow to the area and produce an erection. Side effects include penile fibrosis and priapism. Drugs include prostaglandin E and papavernine.[79]

Internal Devices (implanted penile prostheses)

Semirigid—a variety of devices are available. The rod is placed in the spongy tissue of the penis but away from the urinary sphincter so that voiding is not affected. Heavy athletic undergarments will conceal the crotch bulge. Many of the devices available have a metal core that allows the device to be bent upward for sexual activity and downward for everyday activities.[101]

Self-containing prosthesis, semirigid—a self-contained device with a pump behind the head of the penis that is pumped to fill the rod with fluid from a reservoir. As the rod fills, an erection is produced. After sexual activity, a release valve drains the fluid back into the reservoir. Many of these devices can be placed under local anesthesia. Semirigid rods are the most commonly implanted penile prostheses. Success rates run about 95% for semirigid devices.[79]

Inflatable penile prosthesis—consists of inflatable rods, reservoir, tubing, and pump. The reservoir for the fluid which fills the inflatable rods is placed in the abdomen with the pump in the scrotum. When the pump is activated manually, the fluid exits the reservoir and enters the rods, producing an erection. To release the fluid and deflate the rods at the end of intercourse, the release valve is activated. Mechanical problems occur in 10% to 20% of devices placed.[79,101]

---

area to complete the prescribed dosage.[109] Radiation therapy also can be administered in the postoperative setting. Indications include positive surgical margins, "close" surgical margins, and seminal vesicle involvement.[110] Patients who relapse after prostatectomy may also benefit from radiation therapy.[111] Doses administered range from 60–65 Gy. This allows 74% of patients to achieve tumor control with 45% having five-year relapse-free survival. Radiation is also useful in managing complications of advanced prostate cancer including hematuria, urinary obstruction, ureteral obstruction, and pelvic pain. Some patients with recurrence after radiation therapy may be eligible to receive additional treatment with brachytherapy.

Radiation therapy side effects include impotence, urinary incontinence, bone marrow depression, lower extremity edema, cystitis, urethral strictures, diarrhea, proctitis, and rectal bleeding.[57,92] Diarrhea can be problematic, as a part of the colon and rectum lie within the pelvic field. The patient needs dietary counseling at the initiation of therapy. Teaching includes a low-residue diet and management of diarrhea through regulation of the quantity of fiber consumed. Antidiarrheals, such as loperamide HCl, may be used to control diarrhea. Severe diarrhea may require opioid therapy.

The skin in the perineal area is thin and easily damaged by radiation therapy. Skin integrity is maintained through frequent perineal care, including gentle washing of the rectal area with soap and water after each bowel movement and applying a radiation-approved gel such as Natural Care Gel (Bard Patient Care Division) or cream after treatment. All gels and creams should be washed off before treatment each day. The patient needs to avoid ointments and products that are difficult to remove until radiation therapy is completed. Silver sulfadiazine cream may be useful in promoting wound healing after radiation is completed.

Radiation cystitis can be managed through the use of urinary antispasmodics such as oxybutynin, urinary analgesics such as phenazopyridine, frequent voiding, and management of urinary tract infections with antibiotic therapy. Fluids should be consumed in large volumes and caffeine should be avoided.

Altered sexual functioning probably is related to damage to the blood supplying the corpora cavernosa.[112] Potency is maintained in approximately 30%–50% of patients receiving radiation[56,113] and may be related to age, with older men being at greater risk of impotency. Impotence begins months to years after completion of therapy. Cigarette smoking may have a negative impact on potency.[112] Diabetes and hypertension are also negative risk factors.[113]

Proctitis and rectal bleeding require medical management, including sigmoidoscopy, fulguration of bleeding vessels, and hydrocortisone enemas. Blood transfusions may be required if bleeding causes the hemoglobin to drop to 8 gm/dl.

Urethral strictures from inflammation are managed with periodic dilation or transurethral resection of the stenosis.[69] Repeated dilation may be needed. The incidence of urinary complications from radiation therapy is low and is related to the dose of radiation delivered and the volume of the radiation portal; the higher the dose and the larger the volume of tissue treated, the greater the risk of complication development.[114] In a study of 1000 patients undergoing radiation therapy for prostate cancer, 7.7% developed urinary complications and only 0.5% needed surgery.

Leg edema may occur following radiation therapy. Management includes leg elevation when sitting out of bed, leg exercises to promote venous and lymph return, compression stockings, and elevating the scrotum with a folded towel.[80]

### Brachytherapy

Recent improvements in the methods of using brachytherapy to treat prostate cancer are related to new technology and better knowledge of brachytherapy radiobiology.[115] Prostatic brachytherapy involves the placement of radioactive seeds directly into the prostate. A high dose of radiation is delivered to a smaller volume of tissue with reduced doses delivered to surrounding normal structures such as the bladder and rectum. Iodine-125 seeds are the most frequently used source of radiation.[116] With the patient under general anesthesia, in the lithotomy position, a template is placed on the perineal area and needles are placed into the target tissue. A radioactive seed is left in place. Early-stage patients may be offered brachytherapy as a single modality therapy, or it can be used in locally advanced disease as a boost to the primary therapy.[115]

After insertion of the source, the principles of time, distance, and shielding should be utilized as Iodine-125 emits gamma radiation. Hospitalization lasts until decay of the source is reduced to 30 millicuries or less.[116] Side effects include discomfort from the needle and seed insertion, dysuria, hematuria for 24 hours, and in rare cases, infection.[80,116] Urine should be strained to locate any dislodged radioactive seeds.[117] Routine predischarge instructions include teaching the patient to avoid close contact with children and pregnant women. A condom should be worn during sexual intercourse for two months after the implantation in case a radioactive seed is lost during intercourse.[117] The patient poses no danger as a radioactive source and the patient and his family must understand this concept before discharge to avoid issues related to self-imposed isolation for fear of exposing others to radiation.

### Hormonal Therapy

Advanced prostate cancer is frequently managed by altering the patient's hormonal status. Three different cell populations comprise both normal and malignant prostate tissues: hormone dependent, hormone sensitive, and hormone independent.[118,119] When the hormonal source is eliminated from hormone-dependent cells, they die, and the hormone-sensitive ones no longer divide.[120] Hormone-independent cells do not respond to the loss of hormones and continue to grow. The adrenal gland also produces hormones, which will continuously support hormone-independent cells.[69]

Androgen is the hormone on which hormone-dependent and hormone-sensitive cells are dependent. The vast majority of androgen is produced by the testes. Androgen secretion is dependent on luteinizing hormone-releasing hormone (LHRH) released from the hypothalamus. LHRH stimulates the pituitary gland to produce luteinizing hormone (LH), which in turn stimulates the testes to produce testosterone (androgen).[121,122] The goal of hormone therapy for prostate cancer is to reduce the level of circulating androgens, causing the death of hormone-dependent cells and inhibiting the growth of hormone-sensitive cells, thereby reducing tumor size. Hormonal manipulation is not curative therapy, but can provide many patients with symptom palliation.

There are surgical and medical approaches to reducing serum testosterone levels. The oldest method is bilateral orchiectomy. Testosterone levels are reduced quickly as 90%–95% of testosterone production is eliminated with removal of the testicles.[123]

Estrogen administration blocks LHRH and LH, resulting in reduced testosterone secretion. Diethylstilbestrol is a commonly used estrogen. The potential for cardiovascular side effects makes estrogen therapy less favorable in light of newer therapies available, which include LHRH agonists and antiandrogens.

LHRH agonists initially increase testosterone levels, but after several days of therapy, testosterone levels fall to castration level. The surge of testosterone production after initiation of an LHRH agonist is called a "flare." During a flare, patients need to be aware that symptoms can worsen and require prompt medical intervention. Pain may increase as well as symptoms of bladder outlet obstruction. Serious complications include spinal cord compression. Flutamide, an antiandrogen, may be administered prior to the initiation of an LHRH agonist to reduce the flare. Antiandrogens prevent the binding of testosterone to receptors on prostate cells.[124] Combining antiandrogenic therapy with an LHRH agonist, such as leuprolide or goserelin, is called total androgen ablation (TAA). TAA may improve survival and increase the amount of time before tumor progression.[121] When a patient is appropriate for hormonal manipulation, combination therapy is an often-used treatment option.[125]

All hormonal manipulations have the potential to produce side effects. The most common ones are hot flashes, impotence, and decreased libido.[126] Flutamide causes diarrhea if taken three times a day. It should be taken orally every eight hours to reduce the diarrhea. Patients on hormonal therapy may have problems with altered self-esteem, such as feelings of emasculation.[113] The loss of sexual potency may be a crisis for the patient and his sexual partner. Sensitive discussions allowing verbalization of feelings are required before and during treatment.

Leuprolide and goserelin are injections administered on a monthly basis. Leuprolide is given as an intramuscular injection. After mixing with provided diluent (1 ml), thoroughly shake the solution until the particles dissolve into a white liquid. Goserelin is given as a subcutaneous injection into abdominal fat as follows.[126] (1) Ascertain that the drug pellet is visible in its see-through chamber. (2) Cleanse the skin with alcohol and stretch the skin tautly. (3) Firmly grasp the syringe and insert the needle into the fat. (4) After the bevel enters the skin, move the syringe so the needle is parallel to the skin and insert the needle up to the hub and then back up 1 cm. (5) Press the plunger. (6) Withdraw the needle, apply pressure to the needle site, and examine the see-through chamber to confirm that the pellet has been administered. (7) Discard the syringe according to hospital policy. (8) Apply ice to the injection site to reduce some of the discomfort associated with the large needle gauge. (Bleeding is minimal.)

Patients will respond well to hormonal therapy 70%–89% of the time and responses can be several years in duration.[113] Progression of disease may be managed with palliative radiation therapy or second-line hormonal manipulation. Hormone-refractory prostate cancer may respond to the withdrawal of flutamide.[127] Discontinuing flutamide in 36 patients receiving flutamide plus an LHRH agonist resulted in 10 patients having reduced PSA levels and improved clinical symptoms. Aminoglutethimide and hydrocortisone combination therapy may be tried, or hydrocortisone may be used as a single agent.[128,129] Aminoglutethimide is administered orally (250 mg, twice a day). Testosterone levels are reduced. Adrenal suppression occurs with aminoglutethimide; therefore, hormonal replacement with hydrocortisone is required (20 mg, twice a day). Hydrocortisone alone, however, lowers testosterone levels, and as a single agent may be appropriate treatment for hormone-refractory men.

## Chemotherapy

For a patient with hormone-refractory prostate cancer, antineoplastic therapy may be an option. However, a review of 26 drug trials conducted from 1987 to 1991 failed to demonstrate the effectiveness of chemotherapy.[130] Remissions in the trials averaged 8.7% indicating that, for the most part, hormone-refractory prostate cancer is also chemotherapy resistant. Multidrug resistance is a possible explanation for the failure of patients to respond to chemotherapy.

The most effective single agents available for treating prostate cancer are vinblastine, trimetrexate, mitoquazone, and estramustine. Vinblastine, a mitotic inhibitor, has been studied in multiple protocols and produces responses in 15%–30% of treated patients.[69,131,132] Mitoquazone, an enzyme inhibitor, has undergone phase I and phase II trials and exhibited responses in up to 24% of patients.[133] Trimetrexate, an antifolate, has a partial response rate of 17%.[134]

The most effective drug combination consists of vinblastine and estramustine.[130,135,136] Response rates for the combination range from 3%–47%. The major side effect is granulocytopenia. PSA values decreased by 50% or more in almost half the patients studied. Only limited numbers of patients have been managed in these trials. Prospective randomized research studies are needed by cooperative groups to fully explore the impact of vinblastine and estramustine therapy in hormone-refractory prostate cancer.

Suramin may be a useful chemotherapeutic drug in the treatment of prostate cancer. A complex polysulfated polysaccharide with the ability to inhibit multiple unrelated enzymes,[137] Suramin's ability to block growth factor receptors may play a role in its antineoplastic activity. Highly protein bound, the drug is released slowly producing a half-life of 40–50 days.[138,139] Dose-limiting toxicities have been coagulopathies and neurotoxicities when the serum concentration exceeds 300 mcg/ml.[140,141] If serum concentration falls below 100 mcg/ml, the drug has minimal antitumor effect. Different drug administration schedules have been investigated with the goal of reducing the dose-limiting toxicities. By giving the drug as a two-hour infusion at 1000 mg/m² on day 1 and adjusting the dosage day 2–5 based on a model of "adaptive-control-with-feedback," toxicity can be reduced and the therapeutic blood level maintained.[142] This method involves measuring suramin blood levels before each subsequent infusion to determine dose to avoid toxicity but maintaining blood levels in the therapeutic range. Subsequently, it was determined that a fixed schedule can be used with a 200 mg test dose given on day 1. If no toxicity develops, it is followed by a 1000 mg/m² therapeutic dose given intravenously over two hours. Plasma levels are checked daily before treatment and 30 minutes after the infusion.[143] Additional side effects include anaphylaxis, pancytopenia, infection, hyperglycemia, rash, elevated BUN and serum creatinine, adrenal insufficiency, and myopathy.[137,144,145] Adrenal insufficiency which is due to adrenal cortex atrophy from suramin is managed with hydrocortisone (30–40 mg daily) replacement while the patient is on suramin treatment and may be required after treatment is terminated.[143] Anaphylaxis is rare and occurred at a rate of 0% in 100 patients treated.[145] Anaphylaxis has been reported in patients with suramin treated for its antiparasitic effect. Symptoms include nausea, vomiting, sweating, motor excitement, and loss of consciousness in 0.27% of patients.[146] Bone pain is reduced, PSA values decrease, and patients respond for about 26 weeks. Ongoing research with hydrocortisone in combination with vinblastine and suramin is needed.[147]

## SYMPTOM MANAGEMENT AND SUPPORTIVE CARE

Advanced prostate cancer patients require management of bone pain with narcotic analgesics, nonsteroidal anti-inflammatory drugs (NSAIDs), and laxatives and stool softeners to control narcotic-induced constipation. Bladder outlet obstructive symptoms may require catheterization and subsequent TURP to remove the obstructing tissue. Leg and scrotal edema may respond to leg and scrotal elevation but often proves difficult to control. Diuretics are effective infrequently and compression stockings may be needed to reduce the edema. All patients with bone metastasis are at risk for spinal cord compression. These men and their families need to be aware that worsening back pain, weakness of the lower extremities, or sensory deficits require immediate medical attention. Radiation therapy will be administered in most cases to control tumor impingement on the spinal cord. Unilateral leg edema may demonstrate the presence of a deep vein thrombosis requiring anticoagulant therapy. Monitoring for pulmonary embolism is needed. An inferior vena cava filter may be placed if anticoagulant

therapy is not indicated. Another complication requiring heparin therapy in prostate cancer is disseminated intravascular coagulation (DIC). Low-grade DIC detected by laboratory tests may not require treatment.

## Continuity of Care

The vast majority of prostate cancer patients will spend their time at home throughout the disease course. It is crucial that the patient be knowledgeable in all aspects of his care. Follow-up PSA values will be monitored to assess disease status throughout the patient's lifetime. Postprostatectomy patients may need nursing care at home for wound management, catheter maintenance, and assessment and monitoring for postoperative complications. Radiation therapy patients will need to manage diarrhea and prevent skin breakdown during the treatment period. Ambulatory care visits will include treatment with hormonal drugs and chemotherapy. Lastly, during the terminal phase, patients and their families can benefit from hospice interventions at home.

## CONCLUSION

As the incidence and prevalence of prostate cancer increases, it is imperative that nurses, especially those in advance practice roles, become active in early detection programs that target high-risk individuals, especially black males. Participation in public education programs in the workplace will further demonstrate the nurse's role as educator and patient advocate. Helping families to understand the controversies involved in the management of prostate cancer continues to be a nursing priority.

## REFERENCES

1. American Cancer Society: *Cancer Facts and Figures—1996.* Atlanta, American Cancer Society, 1996
2. Carter H, Coffey D: The prostate: an increasing medical problem. *Prostate* 16:39–48, 1990
3. Meikle A, Smith J: Epidemiology of prostate cancer. *Urol Clin North Am* 17:709–718, 1990
4. Rose D, Boyar A, Wynder E: International comparisons of mortality rates for cancer of the breast, ovary, prostate and colon and per capita food consumption. *Cancer* 58:2363–2371, 1986
5. Carter H, Piantadosi S, Isaacs J: Clinical evidence for and implications of the multistep development of prostate cancer. *J Urol* 143:742–746, 1990
6. Dunn J: Cancer epidemiology in populations of the United States—with emphasis on Hawaii and California—and Japan. *Cancer Res* 35:3240, 1975

7. Haenszel W, Kurihara M: Studies on Japanese migrants: I. Mortality from cancer and other diseases among Japanese in the United States. *J Natl Cancer Inst* 40:43, 1968

8. Hill P, Wynder E: Effect of a vegetarian diet and dexamethasone on plasma prolactin, testosterone and dehydroepiandrosterone in men and women. *Cancer Lett* 7:273–282, 1979

9. Hirayama T: Epidemiology of prostate cancer with special reference to the role of diet. *Monogr Natl Cancer Inst* 53: 149–155, 1979

10. Ross R, Bernstein L, Judd H, et al: Serum testosterone levels in healthy young black and white men. *J Natl Cancer Inst* 76:45–48, 1986

11. Ross R, Henderson B: Do diet and androgens alter prostate cancer risk via a common etiologic pathway? *J Natl Cancer Inst* 86:252–254, 1994

12. Henderson B, Bernstein L, Ross R, et al: The early in utero oestrogen and testosterone environment of blacks and whites: Potential effects on male offspring. *Br J Cancer* 57: 216–218, 1988

13. Giovannucci E, Rimm E, Colditz G, et al: A prospective study of dietary fat and risk of prostate cancer. *J Natl Cancer Inst* 85:1571–1579, 1993

14. Ross J, Pusateri D, Shultz T: Dietary and hormonal evaluation of men at different risks for prostate cancer: Fiber intake, excretion, and composition, with in vitro evidence for an association between steroid hormones and specific fiber components. *Am J Clin Nutr* 51:365–370, 1990

15. Mettlin C, Selenskas S, Natarajan N, et al: Beta-carotene and animal fats and their relationship to prostate cancer risk. A case-control study. *Cancer* 64:605–612, 1989

16. Snowdon D, Phillips R, Choi W: Diet, obesity and risk of fatal prostate cancer. *Am J Epidemiol* 120:244–250, 1984

17. Demark-Wahnefried W, Paulson D, Robertson C, et al: Body dimension differences in men with or without prostate cancer. *J Natl Cancer Inst* 84:1363–1364, 1992

18. Pienta K, Esper P: Risk factors for prostate cancer. *Ann Intern Med* 118:793–803, 1993

19. Giovannucci E, Ascherio A, Rimm E, et al: A prospective cohort study of vasectomy and prostate cancer in U.S. men. *JAMA* 269:873–877, 1993

20. Giovannucci E, Tostesone T, Speizer F, et al: A retrospective cohort study of vasectomy and prostate cancer in U.S. men. *JAMA* 269:878–887, 1993

21. Nienhuis H, Goldaere M, Seagroatt V, et al: Incidence of disease after vasectomy: a record linkage retrospective cohort study. *Br Med J* 304:743–746, 1992

22. Moller H, Knudsen L, Lynge E: Risk of testicular cancer after vasectomy: Cohort study of over 73,000 men. *Br Med J* 309:295–299, 1994

23. Mahon S, Casperson D: Focus on oncology: Vasectomy and the risk of prostate cancer. *J Urol Nurs* 12:599–602, 1993

24. Carter B, Beaty T, Steinberg G, et al: Mendelian inheritance of familial prostate cancer. *Proc Natl Acad Sci USA* 89:3367, 1992

25. Carter B, Bova S, Beaty T, et al: Hereditary prostate cancer: Epidemiologic and clinical features. *J Urol* 150:797–802, 1993

26. Kuhn E, Sesterhenn I, Chang E, et al: Expression of the c-*erb* B-2 (HER-2/*neu*) oncoprotein in human prostatic carcinoma. *J Urol* 150:1427–1433, 1993

27. Waldman A, Osborne D: Screening for prostate cancer. *Oncol Nurs Forum* 21:1512–1517, 1994

28. Thomas R, Clejan S: Digital rectal examination—associated alteration in serum prostate-specific antigen. *Am J Clin Pathol* 97:528–534, 1992

29. Littrup P, Lee F, Mettlin C: Prostate cancer screening: Current trends and future implications. *CA Cancer J Clin* 42:198–211, 1992

30. Lee F, Littrup P, Torp-Pedersen S, et al: Prostate cancer: comparison of transrectal US and digital rectal examination for screening. *Radiology* 168:389–394, 1988

31. Mettlin C, Jones G, Averette H: Defining and updating the American Cancer Society Guidelines for the cancer-related checkup: Prostate and endometrial cancers. *CA Cancer J Clin* 43:42–46, 1993

32. Ploch N, Brawer M: How to use prostate-specific antigen. *Urology* 43:27–35, 1994 (suppl)

33. Brawer M, Catalone W, McConnell J: Prostate cancer: Is screening the answer? *Patient Care* 26:55–68, 1992

34. Stamey T, Yang N, Hay A, et al: Prostate-specific antigen as a serum marker for adenocarcinoma of the prostate. *N Engl J Med* 317:909–916, 1987

35. Oesterling J, Jacobsen S, Chute C, et al: Serum prostate-specific antigen in a community-based population of healthy men. *JAMA* 270:860–864, 1993

36. Narayan P: Neoplasms of the prostate gland, in Tanagho E, McAninch J (eds): *Smith's General Urology* (ed 13). Norwalk, CT, Appleton & Lange, 1992, pp 378–412

37. Ohori M, Wheeler T, Dunn J, et al: The pathologic features and prognosis of prostate cancer detectable with current diagnostic tests. *J Urol* 152:1714–1720, 1994

38. Epstein J, Walsh P, Carmichael M, et al: Pathologic and clinical findings to predict tumor extent of nonpalpable (stage T1c) prostate cancer. *JAMA* 271:368–374, 1994

39. Epstein J, Walsh P, Brendler C: Radical prostatectomy for impalpable prostate cancer. The Johns Hopkins experience with tumors found on transurethral resection (stages T1A and T1B) and on needle biopsy (stage T1C). *J Urol* 152:1721–1729, 1994

40. Gann P, Hennekens C, Stampfer M: A prospective evaluation of plasma prostate-specific antigen for detection of prostate cancer. *JAMA* 273:289–294, 1995

41. Mostofi F, Murphy G, Mettlin C, et al: Pathology review in an Early Prostate Cancer Detection Program: Results from the American Cancer Society—National Prostate Cancer Detection Project. *Prostate* 27:7–12, 1995

42. Slawin K, Ohori M, Dillioglugil O, et al: Screening for prostate cancer: An analysis of the early experience. *CA: Cancer J Clin* 45:134–147, 1995

43. Guyton A: *Textbook of Medical Physiology* (ed 8). Philadelphia, Saunders, 1991

44. Tanagho E: Anatomy of the lower urinary tract, in Walsh P, Retik A, Stamey T, Vaugh E (eds): *Campbell's Urology* (ed 5). Philadelphia, Saunders, 1986, pp 62–64

45. Stamey T, McNeal J: Adenocarcinoma of the prostate, in Walsh P, Retik A, Stamey T, Vaugh E (eds). *Campbell's Urology* (ed 6). Philadelphia, Saunders, 1992, pp 1159–1221

46. Brawn P: Adenosis of the prostate: A dysplastic lesion that can be confused with prostate adenocarcinoma. *Cancer* 49: 826–833, 1982

47. Quinn B, Cho K, Epstein J: Relationship of severe dysplasia to stage B adenocarcinoma of the prostate. *Cancer* 65: 2328–2337, 1990

48. Gleason D: Histologic grading and staging of prostate carcinoma, in Tannenbaum M (ed): *Urologic Pathology: The Prostate*. Philadelphia, Lea & Febiger, 1971, pp 171–197

49. McNeal J, Villers A, Redwine E, et al: Histologic differentiation, cancer volume, and pelvic lymph node metastasis in adenocarcinoma of the prostate. *Cancer* 66:1225–1233, 1990

50. Kramer S, Spahr J, Brendler C, et al: Experience with Gleason's histopathologic grading in prostatic cancer. *J Urol* 124:223–225, 1980

51. Scardino P, Weaver R, Hudson M: Early detection of prostate cancer. *Hum Pathol* 23:211–223, 1992

52. McNeal J, Redwine E, Freiha F, et al: Zonal distribution of prostatic adenocarcinoma. *Am J Surg Pathol* 12:897–906, 1988

53. Viller A, McNeal J, Redwine E, et al: The role of perineural space invasion in the local spread of prostatic adenocarcinoma. *J Urol* 142:763–768, 1989

54. Fowler J, Whitmore W: The incidence and extent of pelvic lymph nodes metastases in apparently localized prostatic cancer. *Cancer* 47:2941–2945, 1981

55. Saitoh H, Hida M, Shimbo T, et al: Metastatic patterns of prostatic cancer: Correlation between sites and number of organs involved. *Cancer* 54:3078–3084, 1984

56. Gittes R: Carcinoma of the prostate. *New Engl J Med* 324:236–245, 1991

57. Garnick M: Prostate cancer: screening, diagnosis and management. *Ann Intern Med* 118:804–818, 1993

58. Surya B, Provent J: Manifestations of advanced prostate cancer: prognosis and treatment. *J Urol* 142:921–928, 1989

59. Payne R: Pain management in the patient with prostate cancer. *Cancer* 71:1131–1137, 1993 (suppl)

60. deKernion J, Lowitz B, Casciato D: Urinary tract cancers, in Casciato D, Lowitz B (eds): *Manual of Clinical Oncology* (ed 2). Boston, Little, Brown, 1988, pp 198–219

61. Held J, Peahota A: Nursing care of the patient with spinal cord compression. *Oncol Nurs Forum* 20:1507–1516, 1993

62. Smith P, Bono A, Calais de Silva F, et al: Some limitations of the radioisotope bone scan in patients with metastatic prostatic cancer. A subanalysis of EORTC Trial 30853. *Cancer* 66:1009–1016, 1991

63. Scardino P, Shinohara K, Wheeler T, et al: Staging of prostate cancer: Value of ultrasonography. *Urol Clin North Am* 16:713–734, 1989

64. Stamey T, Kabalin J: Prostate-specific antigen in the diagnosis and treatment of adenocarcinoma of the prostate. I. Untreated patients. *J Urol* 141:1070–1075, 1989

65. Andriole G: Serum prostate-specific antigen: Expanding its role as a measure of treatment response in patients with prostate cancer. *J Clin Oncol* 11:596–597, 1993

66. Morton R, Steiner M, Walsh P: Cancer control following anatomical radical prostatectomy: An interim report. *J Urol* 145:1197–1200, 1991

67. Ritter M, Messing E, Shanahan T, et al: Prostate-specific antigen as a predictor of radiotherapy response and patterns of failure in localized prostate cancer. *J Clin Oncol* 10:1208–1217, 1992

68. Whitmore W: National history and staging of prostate cancer. *Urol Clin North Am* 11:205–220, 1994

69. Hanks G, Myers G, Scardino P: Cancer of the prostate, in DeVita VT, Hellman S, Rosenberg S (eds): *Cancer: Principles and Practice of Oncology* (ed 4). Philadelphia, Lippincott, 1993, pp 1073–1113

70. Fleming C, Wasson J, Albertsen P, et al: A decision analysis of alternative treatment strategies for clinically localized prostate cancer. *JAMA* 269:2650–2658, 1993

71. Whitmore, W: Management of clinically localized prostatic cancer: An unresolved problem. *JAMA* 269:2676–2677, 1993

72. El-Mahdi A, Kuban D: Treatment of carcinoma of the prostate in the 1990s. *Compr Ther* 18:10–15, 1992

73. Garnick M: The dilemmas of prostate cancer. *Sci Am:* 72–81, 1994

74. Wasson J, Cushman C, Bruskewitz R, et al: A structured literature review of treatment for localized prostate cancer. *Arch Fam Med* 2:487–493, 1993

75. Johansson J, Adami H, Andersson S, et al: High 10-year survival rate in patients with early, untreated prostate cancer. *JAMA* 267:2191–2196, 1992

76. Fleming J, Wasson P, Albertsen M, et al: A decision analysis of alternative treatment strategies for clinically localized prostate cancer. *JAMA* 269:2650–2658, 1993

77. Chodak G, Thisted R, Gerber G, et al: Results of conservative management of clinically localized prostate cancer. *New Engl J Med* 330:242–248, 1994

78. Tanagho E, McAninch J: *Smith's General Urology* (ed 12). Norwalk, CT, Appleton-Lange, 1992

79. Black J, Matassarin-Jacobs E (eds): *Luckmann & Sorensen's Medical-Surgical Nursing: A Psychophysiologic Approach* (ed 4). Philadelphia, Saunders, 1993

80. Held J, Osborne D, Volpe H, et al: Cancer of the prostate: Treatment and nursing implications. *Oncol Nurs Forum* 21:1517–1529, 1994

81. Mettlin C, Murphy G, Menck H: Trends in treatment of localized prostate cancer by radical prostatectomy: Observations from the Commission on Cancer National Cancer Database 1985–1990. *Urology* 43:488–492, 1994

82. Lu-Yao G, Greenbud E: Changes in prostate cancer incidence and treatment in USA. *Lancet* 343:251–254, 1994

83. Mettlin C, Jones G, Murphy G: Trends in prostate cancer care in the United States, 1974–1990: Observations from the patient care evaluation studies of the American College of Surgeons Commission on Cancer. *CA Cancer J Clin* 43: 83–91, 1993

84. Lu-Yao G, McLerran D, Wasson J, et al: An assessment of radical prostatectomy: Time trends, geographic variation, and outcomes. *JAMA* 269:2633–2636, 1993

85. Kantoff P, Talcott J: The radical prostatectomy series: Apples are not oranges. *J Clin Oncol* 11:2243–2245, 1994

86. Herr H: Quality of life of incontinent men after radical prostatectomy. *J Urol* 151:652–654, 1994

87. Waxman E: Sexual dysfunction following treatment for prostate cancer: Nursing assessment and intervention. *Oncol Nurs Forum* 20:1567–1571, 1993

88. Walsh P: Nerve sparing radical prostatectomy for early stage prostate cancer. *Semin Oncol* 15:351–358, 1988

89. Quinlan D, Epstein J, Carter B, et al: Sexual function following radical prostatectomy: Influence of preservation of neurovascular bundles. *J Urol* 145:998–1002, 1991

90. Litwin M, Hays R, Fink A, et al: Quality of life in men treated for localized prostate cancer. *JAMA* 273:129–135, 1995

91. Maxwell M: Cancer of the prostate. *Semin Oncol Nurs* 9: 237–251, 1993

92. Heinrich-Rynning T: Prostatic cancer treatments and their effect on sexual functioning. *Oncol Nurs Forum* 14:37–41, 1987

93. Lind J, Kravitz K, Greig B: Urologic and male genital malignancies, in Groenwald SL, Frogge MH, Goodman M, Yarbro CH (eds): *Cancer Nursing: Principles and Practice* (ed 3). Boston, Jones and Bartlett, 1993, pp 1258–1313

94. Urinary Incontinence Guideline Panel: *Urinary Incontinence in Adults: Clinical Practice Guidelines.* AHCPR publication No. 92–0038. Rockville, MD, Agency for Health Care Policy and Research, 1992

95. Walsh P: Radical retropubic prostatectomy, in Walsh P, Retik A, Stamey T, Vaughan E (eds): *Campbell's Urology* (ed 6). Philadelphia, Saunders, 1992, pp 2865–2886

96. Steiner M, Morton R, Walsh P: Impact of anatomic radical prostatectomy on urinary continence. *J Urol* 145:512–515, 1991

97. Walsh P, Quinlan D, Morton, et al: Radical retropubic prostatectomy: Improved anastomosis and urinary continence. *Urol Clin North Am* 17:679–684, 1990

98. Marks J, Light J: Management of urinary incontinence after prostatectomy with the artificial urinary sphincter. *J Urol* 142:302–304, 1989

99. Foote J, Yun S, Leach G: Postprostatectomy incontinence: Pathophysiology, evaluation and management. *Urol Clin North Am* 18:229–241, 1991

100. Thayer D: How to assess and control urinary incontinence. *Am J Nurs* 94:42–47, 1994

101. Schrover L: *Sexuality and Cancer: For the Man Who Has Cancer, and His Partner.* American Cancer Society, 1988

102. Schrover L: Sexual rehabilitation after treatment for prostate cancer. *Cancer* 71:1024–1030, 1993

103. Bachers E: Sexual dysfunction after treatment for genitourinary cancers. *Semin Oncol Nurs* 1:18–24, 1985

104. Smith J, Cho Y-H: Management of stage A prostate cancer. *Urol Clin North Am* 17:769–777, 1990

105. Lange P: Controversies in management of apparently localized cancer of the prostate. *Urology* 34:13–18, 1989 (suppl 4)

106. Bagshaw M, Cox R, Ray G: *Status of Radiation Treatment of Prostate Cancer at Stanford University,* in NCI monograph No. 7. NIH publication No. 88–3005. Washington, DC, Government Printing Office, 1988

107. Lai P, Perez C, Shapiro S, et al: Carcinoma of the prostate stage B and C: Lack of influence of duration of radiotherapy on tumor control and treatment morbidity. *Int J Radiat Oncol Biol Phys* 19:561–568, 1990

108. Hanks G, Martz K, Diamond J: The effect of dose on local control of prostate cancer. *Int J Radiat Oncol Biol Phys* 15: 1299–1305, 1988

109. Hanks G: *External Beam Radiation Therapy for Clinically Localized Prostate Cancer: Patterns of Care Studies in the United States,* in NCI monograph No. 7. NIH publication No. 88–3005. Washington, DC, Government Printing Office, 1988

110. Pilepich M, Walz B, Baglan R: Postoperative irradiation in carcinoma of the prostate. *Int J Radiat Oncol Biol Phys* 10: 1869–1873, 1984

111. Perez C, Cosmatos D, Garcia D, et al: Irradiation in relapsing carcinoma of the prostate. *Cancer* 71:1110–1122, 1993

112. Goldstein I, Feldman M, Deckers P, et al: Radiation-associated impotence: A clinical study of its mechanism. *JAMA* 251:903–910, 1984

113. Keller J, Sahasrabudhe D, McCune C: Urologic and male genital cancers, in Rubin P, McDonald S, Qazi R (eds): *Clinical Oncology: A Multidisciplinary Approach for Physicians and Students* (ed 7). Philadelphia, Saunders, 1993, pp 419–452

114. Lawton G, Won M, Pilepich M, et al: Long-term treatment sequelae following external beam irradiation for adenocarcinoma of the prostate: Analysis of RTOG studies 7506 and 7706. *Int J Radiat Oncol Biol Phys* 21:935–940, 1991

115. Porter A, Blasko J, Grimm P: Brachytherapy for prostate cancer. *CA Cancer J Clin* 45:165–178, 1995

116. Dow K: Principles of brachytherapy, in Dow K, Hilderley L (eds): *Nursing Care in Radiation Oncology.* Philadelphia, Saunders, 1992, pp 16–29

117. Greenberg S, Peterson J, Hansen-Peters I, et al: Interstitially implanted I-125 for prostate cancer using transrectal ultrasound. *Oncol Nurs Forum* 17:849–854, 1990

118. Isaacs J, Schulze H, Coffey D: Development of androgen resistance in prostate cancer. *Prog Clin Biol Res* 243:21–31, 1987

119. Schulze H, Isaacs J, Coffey D: A critical review of the concept of total androgen ablation in the treatment of prostate cancer. *Prog Clin Biol Res* 243:1–19, 1987

120. Martikainen P, Kyprianou N, Tucker R, et al: Programmed death of nonproliferating androgen-independent prostatic cancer cells. *Cancer Res* 51:4693–4700, 1991

121. Crawford E, Nabors W: Total androgen ablation: American experience. *Urol Clin North Am* 18:55–63, 1991

122. Goodman M: Concepts of hormonal manipulation in treatment of cancer. *Oncol Nurs Forum* 15:639–647, 1988

123. Sogani P, Fair W: Treatment of advanced prostate cancer. *Urol Clin North Am* 14:353–371, 1987

124. McLeod D: Antiandrogenic drugs. *Cancer* 71:1046–1049, 1993

125. LaBrie F, Belanger A, Simard J, et al: Combination therapy for prostate cancer. *Cancer* 71:1059–1067, 1993 (suppl 3)

126. Taylor T: Endocrine therapy for advanced stage D prostate cancer. *Urol Nurs* 11:22–26, 1991

127. Scher H, Kelly W: Flutamide withdrawal syndrome: Its impact on clinical trials in hormone-refractory prostate cancer. *J Clin Oncol* 11:1566–1572, 1993

128. Dowsett M, Shearer R, Ponder B, et al: The effects of aminoglutethimide and hydrocortisone, alone and combined, on androgen levels in post-orchiectomy prostatic cancer patients. *Br J Cancer* 57:190–192, 1988

129. Plowman P, Perry L, Chard T: Androgen suppression by hydrocortisone without aminoglutethimide in orchiectomized men with prostatic cancer. *Br J Urol* 59:255–257, 1987

130. Yagoda A, Petrylak O: Cytotoxic chemotherapy for advanced hormone-resistant prostate cancer. *Cancer* 71: 1098–1109, 1993

131. Eisenburger M, Abrams J: Chemotherapy for prostatic carcinoma. *Semin Urol* 6:303–310, 1988

132. Dexeus F, Logothetis C, Samuels M, et al: Continuous infusion of vinblastine for advanced hormone-refractory prostate cancer. *Cancer Treat Rep* 69:885–886, 1985

133. Scher H, Yagoda A, Ahmed T, et al: Methyl glyoxal-bis guanylhydrazone (MGBG): an active drug in prostate cancer. *J Clin Oncol* 3:224–228, 1985

134. Scher H, Curley T, Geller N, et al: Trimetrexate in prostatic cancer: Preliminary observations of the use of the prostate-specific antigen and acid phosphatase as a marker in measurable hormone-refractory disease. *J Clin Oncol* 8: 1830–1838, 1990

135. Amato R, Logothetis C, Dexeus F, et al: Preliminary results of a phase II trial of estramustine and vinblastine for patients with progressive hormone-refractory prostate cancer. *Proc Am Assoc Cancer Res* 32:186, 1991

136. Seidman A, Scher H, Petrylak D, et al: Estramustine and vinblastine: Effects on serum prostate-specific antigen in hormone-refractory prostate cancer. *Proc Am Assoc Cancer Res* 32:187, 1991

137. Stein C, LaRocca R, Myers C: Suramin: an old compound with new biology. *PPO Updates* 4:1–12, 1990

138. Collins J, Klecker R, Yarchoan R, et al: Chemical pharmacokinetics of suramin in patients with HTLV-III/LAV infection. *J Clin Pharmacol* 26:22–26, 1986

139. Coleman M, Adjepon-Yamoah K: The disposition of suramin in the isolated perfused rate liver. *Biochem Pharmacol* 35:3389–3392, 1986

140. Horne M, Stein C, LaRocca R, et al: Circulating glycosaminoglycan anticoagulants associated with suramin treatment. *Blood* 71:273–279, 1988

141. LaRocca R, Meer J, Gilliatt R, et al: Suramin-induced polyneuropathy. *Neurology* 40:954–960, 1990

142. Jodrell D, Reyno L, Sridhara R, et al: Suramin: development of a population pharmacokinetic model and its use with intermittent short infusions to control plasma drug concentrations in patients with prostate cancer. *J Clin Oncol* 12:166–175, 1994

143. Eisenberger M, Sinibaldi V, Reyno L: Suramin. *Cancer Pract* 3:187–189, 1995

144. Myers C, Cooper M, Stein C, et al: Suramin: A novel growth factor antagonist with activity in hormone-refractory metastatic prostate cancer. *J Clin Oncol* 10:881–889, 1992

145. Scher H, Kelly W: Suramin: Defining the role in the clinic. *PPO Updates* 7:1–16, 1993

146. Kopp R, Pfeiffer A: Suramin alters phosphoinositide synthesis and inhibits growth factor receptor binding in HT-29 cells. *Cancer Res* 50:6490, 1990

147. Figg W, McCall N, Sartor O, et al: The in vitro activity of estramustine, vinblastine and suramin on PC-3, PC-3M, DU-145 and LNCa P cells and their potentiation when combined. *Proc Am Soc Clin Oncol* 14:253, 1995

# Chapter 46

# Skin Cancers

Lois J. Loescher, RN, MS

Marsha A. Ketcham, RN, OCN®

## INTRODUCTION

Cancers of the skin consist of basal cell carcinoma (BCC), squamous cell carcinoma (SCC), and malignant melanoma. BCC and SCC are often grouped together and referred to as *nonmelanoma skin cancer* (NMSC). Most melanomas are cutaneous (CM); others, which are rare, originate in the eye or viscera. Although cutaneous cancers share common etiologic factors, they vary in other regards. NMSCs have a higher incidence but have a low metastatic potential and mortality rate. The associated morbidity is of concern, as NMSC often requires costly, extensive, and repeated treatments that may result in cosmetic and functional damage. Conversely, melanoma has a much lower incidence rate but a mortality rate triple that of the NMSC. The increased mortality from melanoma is directly related to its high potential for metastasis. An understanding of skin cancer epidemiology, etiology, and pathogenesis will help oncology nurses recognize the subtle and major differences among different skin cancers. Knowledge of assessment, treatment, and prevention of nonmelanoma and melanoma skin cancers enables nurses to provide quality care for people with the disease and those at high risk.

## EPIDEMIOLOGY

Over 800,000 new skin cancers are reported annually, with most of those being BCC or SCC.[1] These statistics may underestimate the actual incidence of NMSC because most of these cancers are diagnosed and treated in physicians' offices or in outpatient clinics.[2] BCC is the most common form of skin cancer in whites and outnumbers SCC by a ratio of 3:1.[2] BCC more commonly occurs in men, but the gender difference has become less pronounced in recent years.[3] Although the incidence rate increases with each decade of age, NMSC generally occurs in adults over age 55.[4] It is, however, not surprising to see 30- and 40-year-olds with BCC.[2] NMSC has an overall five-year survival rate of 95% but still accounts for an estimated 2100 deaths per year.[1] One study estimated an age-adjusted NMSC mortality rate of 0.44/100,000 per year.[5]

Approximately 34,000 melanoma cases were reported in 1995.[1] Since 1973 the incidence of CM in whites has increased more than that of any other major cancer, except lung cancer in women.[6] Based on the age-adjusted cancer incidence rates reported by the Surveillance, Epidemiology, and End Results (SEER) program in 1994, CM is largely confined to whites, who have an incidence of about 11.5/100,000. From 1973 to 1991, white males and females of all ages experienced a 94% increased incidence of CM, and a yearly increased incidence of about 4%. Age-adjusted CM incidence rates among white males at all ages are higher than those for white females,

being approximately 14.5 and 10.9 per 100,000, respectively. Figure 46-1 shows the incidence of CM by age and gender in whites. Blacks have a much lower incidence of CM than whites. From 1973 to 1991, black males and females of all ages experienced a 42% increased incidence and a yearly increased incidence of 0.4%.[7]

Although CM represents only about 4% of skin cancers, its malignant potential must not be underestimated, as it accounts for an estimated 7200 cancer deaths annually.[1] The percent increase in mortality reported by SEER for both genders and all races from 1973 to 1991 was 35.2%, with an estimated annual change of 1.7%. Early detection and treatment, however, have steadily increased the overall five-year relative survival rates for whites of both genders from 60% to 68% during 1960–1973 to about 85% during 1983–1990. The five-year relative survival rate for blacks approximated 66% during 1974–1976, dropped to about 54% during 1977–1982, and increased to about 70% during 1983–1990.[7]

Skin cancers of any type are rare in children. The rate of CM in children is under 1 in 1 million per year; however, the incidence rate increases 100-fold by the midteen years, to 10 in 100,000 per year.[8] Similarly, BCC is no longer rare in young adults.[3]

## ETIOLOGY AND RISK FACTORS

Fraser et al[9] and Williams and Sagebiel[10] reviewed multiple etiologic factors associated with skin cancers (Table 46-1). Ultraviolet radiation (UVR) is the probable cause of most skin cancers, although other etiologic factors also are involved. UVR is a major cause of NMSCs, which are commonly found on sun-exposed areas of the body such as the head and neck, arms, upper back, and legs. The direct association of UVR with CM is controversial, as CM can also develop in non–sun-exposed areas. Marks and Whiteman[11] reviewed studies of sunburn and melanoma and suggested that there is an association between the two, but the increase in melanoma risk is modest. The authors also questioned whether melanoma risk related to sunburn is constant throughout life or whether there is a critical period during which UVR exposure is more harmful. Scotto and Fears[12] reported that the effect of UVR exposure on incidence of CM is significant.

Types of UVR harmful to the skin are UVB and UVA. UVB rays have short wavelengths and are absorbed by the top skin layer, causing sunburn. UVA rays have long wavelengths and can penetrate deeply into the lower levels of the skin, causing damage.[13] One research report suggested that 90%–95% of melanoma induction may be attributed to UVA rays.[14] The biological effects of UVR on the skin are most likely photochemical alterations of DNA, which trigger a cascade of events culminating in a state of antigen-specific, T-lymphocyte–mediated immunosuppression.[15]

Geographic, environmental, and lifestyle factors all

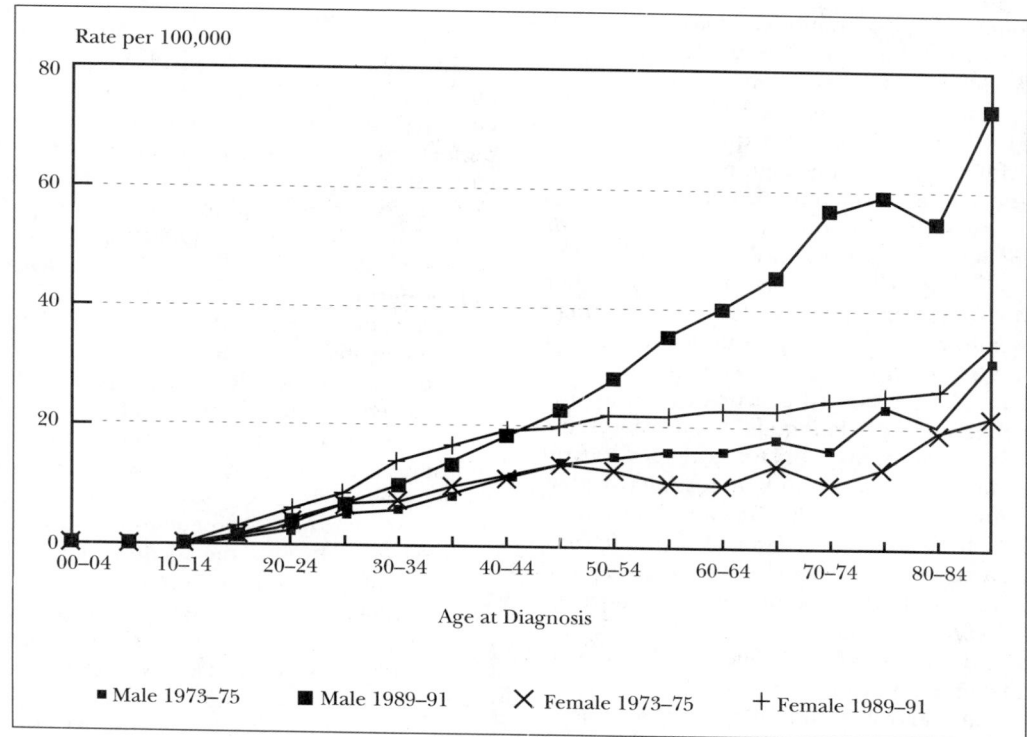

**FIGURE 46-1** Incidence of cutaneous melanoma by age and sex for whites (1973–1975 vs. 1989–1991). (Ries LAG, Miller BA, Hankey BF, Kosary CL, Harras A, Edwards BK [eds.]: *SEER Cancer Statistics Review 1973–1991: Tables and Graphs*. NIH publication No. 94-2789. Bethesda, MD, National Cancer Institute, 1994, p 299.)

affect human exposure to UVR. The incidence of both CM and NMSC is higher in latitudes closer to the equator that receive more UVR and lower in latitudes farther from the equator. UVR exposure increases at higher altitudes.

Chlorofluorocarbons (CFCs) are man-made pollutants that deplete stratospheric ozone, the atmospheric layer that shields the earth from UVR. The U.S. Environmental Protection Agency (EPA) reports that for every 1% de-

**TABLE 46-1** Examples of Etiologic Factors for Basal Cell Carcinoma, Squamous Cell Carcinoma, and Cutaneous Melanoma

| Factor | Examples |
|---|---|
| **Host factors** | |
| Pigmentation/phenotype | Light skin, hair, and eyes; easily sunburned; abnormal mole phenotype(‡) |
| Precursor lesions | Actinic keratosis,* arsenical keratosis,* Bowen's disease,* chronic radiation keratosis,* large congenital nevi‡ lentigo maligna‡ |
| Hereditary conditions | Nevoid basal cell syndrome,† Gorlin syndrome,† xeroderma pigmentosum, familial atypical mole or melanoma syndrome (FAMM)‡ |
| Genetic alterations | Mutations of *p16* gene or *p53* gene‡ |
| Immunosuppression | Organ transplant recipients* |
| **Environmental factors** | |
| Ultraviolet (UV) radiation | Solar UVA and UVB rays; artificial tanning devices |
| Pollutants | Chlorofluorocarbons (CFCs) |
| Chemicals | Polycyclic hydrocarbons,*† inorganic arsenic,*† psoralens† |
| Ionizing radiation | X-ray therapy for tinea capitis,*† enlarged thymus; radon,*† radium*† |
| Viruses | Human papillomavirus,* human immunodeficiency virus*† |
| Physical trauma | Cutaneous damage following burns |

*Only squamous cell carcinoma.

†Only basal cell carcinoma.

‡Only cutaneous melanoma.

crease in ozone, a 2% compounded increase in UVB reaching the earth will result. This translates into an additional 1%–3% increased skin cancer incidence per year.[13] The type of clothing worn as well as the time of day also affect the amount of UVR exposure.

Most individuals have many pigmented lesions on their bodies (nevi, freckles, birthmarks), and the average white adult averages 10–40 lesions. A few of these lesions may be present at birth, while others develop throughout life. Generally, the higher the number of nevi, the higher the risk of CM.[10] Almost all pigmented lesions are normal; however, a change in any one can be indicative of skin cancer.[9,10,16] A persistently changed or changing mole or presence of irregular pigmented precursor lesions (dysplastic nevi, congenital nevi, lentigo maligna) represents a major high-risk situation for CM. Dysplastic nevi (atypical nevi) are cutaneous markers of increased risk that may be transmitted in CM-prone families as an autosomal dominant gene. Individuals with familial dyplastic nevi (also called *familial atypical multiple mole or melanoma syndrome*) are several hundred times more likely to develop melanoma than controls in the general population.[17] Dysplastic nevi are discussed in more detail in the section "Cutaneous Melanoma" in this chapter.

Skin pigmentation is clearly important in the etiology of skin cancers in that American blacks and persons of African, Asian, or Mediterranean descent are known to have a lower incidence.[5] When these individuals do develop CM, it usually originates on the less densely pigmented areas of the body such as the palms, soles, and fingernails.[16] Whites with red hair and fair complexions who tend to sunburn or freckle easily have higher relative risks for all skin cancers, ranging from 2 to 4.[4]

Other possible risk factors for CM include age, hormonal factors, immunosuppression, and a previous history of melanoma.[6,10,16] Family history of CM increases its relative risk 2–12 times.[10] No conclusive evidence exists regarding the use of oral contraceptives and the increased risk of CM;[18–20] however, some physicians recommend that women with a history of melanoma use a nonhormonal contraceptive.

# NONMELANOMA SKIN CANCERS

## Basal Cell Carcinoma

### Pathogenesis

BCC, also called *basal cell epithelioma,* is the least aggressive type of skin cancer. BCC is an epithelial tumor with a disputed site of origin, believed to arise either from cells in the basal layer of the epidermis that have an impaired ability to mature and keratinize or from cells in the surrounding dermal structures.[3] BCC usually grows slowly by direct extension and has the capacity to involve and destroy local tissue, including nerves, lymphatics, blood vessels, cartilage, and bone.[3]

### Assessment

Differences in BCC classifications are determined clinically and histologically. Common classifications include nodular (also called nodulo-ulcerative), superficial, pigmented, morpheaform, and keratotic[3,4] (Table 46-2). Nodular BCC is the most common type. Histologically, nodular BCC consists of masses of tumor cells that have large oval nuclei, are uniform in appearance, and resemble basal cells of the epidermis. These cells descend from the epidermis and fill the dermis, with the peripheral cells resembling a picket fence pattern.[2,3] Clinically, nodular BCC begins as a small, firm, well-demarcated, dome-shaped papule. The color can be pearly white, pink, or skin-colored, with telangiectases often evident on the surface. As the lesion enlarges, it ulcerates peripherally or centrally and develops raised, pearly, well-circumscribed borders. Nodular BCC most commonly occurs on the face, head, and neck[2,4] (see Figure 46-2—Plate 20).

Superficial BCC is the second most common type, histologically exhibiting islands of irregular proliferating tumor tissue attached to the undersurface of the epidermis. Clinically, it is flat and has erythematous or pink scaling plaques or papules with well-defined margins and occasional shallow erosions or crusts.[3,4] Superficial BCC usually develops on the trunk and extremities and can be invasive.[3,4]

Pigmented BCC is less common and may be nodular or superficial. It has a melanin pigment concentrated in the center of a nest of BCC cells, causing a brown, black, or blue color that can be clinically mistaken for melanoma. Also present is a shiny, pearly, papulary border with well-defined margins, and telangiectases.[21,22] Biologically, the behavior of pigmented BCC is similar to that of nodular BCC.[22] Pigmented BCC most commonly occurs on the head, neck, and face.

Morpheaform BCC is the rarest type. Histologically, this tumor has many roots with branching strands embedded in dense fibrous stroma of collagen and elastic fibers.[3] Clinically, it is flat and ivory-colored or colorless, resembles a scar, lacks translucency, and has ill-defined margins. This lesion is more aggressive than nodular BCC, having increased invasiveness and destructiveness of surrounding tissues, particularly muscle, nerve, and bone. Morpheaform BCC develops primarily on the head and neck.[3,4]

Keratotic (or basosquamous) BCC contains basal cells and squamoid-appearing cells that keratinize. Unlike the other BCCs, this tumor grows aggressively, recurs locally, and is more likely to metastasize. Keratotic BCC develops in the pre- and postauricular sulcus.[3]

## Squamous Cell Carcinoma

### Pathogenesis

SCC is a tumor that may arise in any epithelium. Its behavior in the skin is similar to that of neoplasms arising from stratified squamous epithelium in other organ sites.

**TABLE 46-2**  Comparisons of the Classifications of Nonmelanoma Skin Cancers

| Type | Site | Clinical Description | Histological Factors |
|---|---|---|---|
| Nodular BCC (most common) | Face, head, neck | Small, firm, well-demarcated dome-shaped papule; pearly, white, pink, or flesh-colored with telangiectases; may ulcerate | Uniform masses of cells with large oval nuclei; resemble epidermal basal cells |
| Superficial BCC (2nd most common) | Trunk, extremities | Flat, erythematous or pink scaling plaques or papules; well-defined margins; occasional shallow erosions or crusts | A bud of irregular proliferating tumor attached under the epidermis |
| Pigmented BCC (less common) | Head, neck, face | Melanin-pigmented center; shiny, pearly, papulary border with well-defined margins and telangiectases; resembles melanoma | Similar to nodular |
| Morpheaform BCC (rare) | Head, neck | Flat, ivory-colored or colorless; scarlike, ill-defined margins | Many roots with branching strands embedded in collagen and elastic fibers |
| Keratotic BCC (basosquamous) | Pre- and postauricular sulcus | Similar to nodular BCC | Contains basal cells and squamous-appearing cells that keratinize |
| Squamous cell carcinoma | Areas exposed to UV radiation; common sites: nose, forehead, ear, back of hands, lower lip | Flesh-colored or erythematous; raised, firm papule; may ulcerate, indurate crust, and bleed | Well differentiated (similar to normal squamous epithelium, keratin pearls common); anaplastic (distorted nuclei, numerous mitoses, bizarre cells) |

BCC, basal cell carcinoma.

The cells of SCC vary from well differentiated to completely anaplastic. The well-differentiated tumor cell has a histological appearance similar to that seen in normal squamous epithelium in that it is a large polygonal cell with intercellular bridges and round nuclei. Some individual cell keratinization exists, and formation of keratin pearls is common. Keratinization and keratin pearl formation diminish as the tumor becomes less well differentiated and disappears with high-grade tumors. As the tumor cells become more anaplastic, the nuclei become distorted in shape, mitoses become more numerous, cell shapes become more bizarre, and cell numbers increase.[23] SCC is more aggressive than BCC as it has a faster growth rate, less-well-demarcated margins, and a greater metastatic potential.[4,23] The depth of SCC plays an important role in determining metastatic potential. In addition, the metastatic potential of SCC is increased in patients receiving immunosuppressive agents.[2,4] Metastatic disease is usually first noted in the regional lymph nodes.

### Assessment

SCC appears as a flesh-colored or erythematous raised, firm papule. It may be crusted with keratin products and in its early or late stages may ulcerate and bleed, becoming tender and painful. Infiltration of the tumor into normal surrounding skin produces induration around the nodule (Figure 46-3—Plate 21). SCC is usually confined to areas exposed to UVR. The most highly exposed areas of skin, such as the top of the nose, the forehead, the ear helices, the back of hands, and the lower lip, tend to be more affected. With the exception of the lower lip site, SCC on these areas is less likely to metastasize than lesions located on areas not exposed to UVR.[24,25] SCC can also arise in old radiation, thermal, or chemical burn scars; in areas of chronic inflammation or increased cell proliferation; and in mucous membranes. Tumors originating in these areas are more aggressive and have a high frequency of metastasis.

Several preexisting conditions may lead to invasive SCC. Intraepidermal SCC, also called *carcinoma in situ,* may develop in existing cutaneous lesions such as scar tissue, actinic keratoses, radiation keratoses, and Bowen's disease. Intraepidermal SCC remains in the epidermis for an extended time but unpredictably passes through the basement membrane and extends into the dermis. These lesions appear as slightly raised erythematous plaques with varying amounts of scaling and well-defined margins. Other conditions include keratoacanthomas, which are hyperkeratotic lesions morphologically similar to SCC, and epidermodysplasia verruciformis, characterized by multiple flat, wartlike lesions containing oncogenic type 5 and 8 human papillomavirus.[2,26]

## Treatment of Nonmelanoma Skin Cancers

Standard treatment for NMSC includes surgical excision, Mohs' micrographic surgery, curettage and electrodesiccation, radiation, cryotherapy, and topical chemotherapy. Factors to consider when choosing a treatment are tumor type, location, size, and growth pattern, and whether the tumor is primary or secondary. The patient's age and general health also should be considered. No single therapy is applicable to all tumors; however, the primary goals of treatment are cure, preservation of tissue and function, minimal operative risk, and optimal cosmetic results.

The four types of biopsy techniques used for NMSCs are the shave biopsy (a superficial part of the tumor is sliced with a scalpel), the punch biopsy (a deeper specimen is punched out by an instrument placed into the reticular dermis or subcutaneous tissue), the incisional biopsy (a portion of the tumor is removed with a scalpel), and the excisional biopsy (the entire lesion is removed for histological analysis). The biopsy technique should be individually selected to yield the optimum specimen for determining correct diagnosis.[2]

### Surgical excision

Surgical excision can be performed for any NMSC and may be simple or complex, depending on tumor size and location. An elliptical excision with suture closure of a small to moderate lesion using local anesthesia usually can be done on an outpatient basis. Surgical excision facilitates healing of large carcinoma sites where thin layers of subcutaneous tissue overlie bony areas such as the forehead, scalp, and distal extremities. Surgical excision also is beneficial in treating residual tumor and large carcinomas presenting in conjunction with late radiation dermatitis and those arising in scars and ulcers, as these areas cannot tolerate radiation therapy. In addition, excision of large carcinomas of the eyelid and lip preserves function and allows reconstruction by graft or flap.[2,4,21,27]

A skin graft or flap may be performed as an adjunct to surgical excision. A graft or flap is indicated when a lesion is large or located in an area where insufficient tissue for primary closure would result in deformity. A skin flap consists of skin and subcutaneous tissue transferred from one area of the body to another. A flap contains its own blood supply, whereas a graft is avascular and depends on the blood supply of the recipient site for its survival. Skin grafting or flapping requires hospitalization, and possible complications include graft failure, hematoma, scarring, and infection.

The advantages of surgical excision as a treatment are rapid healing, the fact that an entire specimen for histological examination can be obtained, and favorable cosmetic results. Disadvantages are that the procedure is time-consuming and requires a skilled physician to judge the exact extent of the tumor and risk of infection.[4,21,27]

### Mohs' micrographic surgery

Another type of surgical treatment available for select tumors is Mohs' micrographic surgery (also called *chemosurgery*). This procedure involves horizontal shaving and staining of tissue in thin layers with careful histological mapping of all specimen margins. This is the most accurate technique of assessing the actual extent of NMSC. Mohs' microsurgery is most often used as a first line of treatment for cancers in high-risk areas such as the nose and nasolabial folds, the medial canthus, and pre- and postauricular locations.[28] It is also used for lesions with unclear margins, recurrent lesions, aggressive tumors, and extensive lesions (usually larger than 2 cm). Skin grafting may need to accompany this treatment. The advantages of Mohs' microsurgery include preservation of the maximum amount of tissue for easier reconstruction, the ability to histologically map tumor margins, and performance of the procedure on an outpatient basis using a local anesthetic.[28,29] The disadvantages are the requirement of specialized training and equipment, the time-consuming nature of the procedure (4–6 hours), the need for daily wound care postoperatively, and the possibility of graft rejection and wound dehiscence.[28,29] Because most cutaneous carcinomas can be removed by routine surgery, chemosurgery should be used only for the specific indications mentioned earlier.[29]

### Curettage and electrodesiccation

Curettage and electrodesiccation (also called *electrosurgery*) treatment is used only for BCC skin cancers that are small (< 2 cm), superficial, or recurrent because of poor margin control. The tumor is destroyed by scraping out the tumor mass through curettage and treating the tumor base with electrodesiccation, or a low-voltage electrode. The physician uses the curettage to determine the tumor edges. As tumor tissue is softer and more friable than normal tissue, electrodesiccation maintains hemostasis and softens normal tissue so a safe margin can be curettaged.[22,23] Advantages of this treatment are its rapidity, good cosmetic results, preservation of normal tissue, and the opportunity to obtain a tissue specimen for histopathology. Disadvantages include no margin control, prolonged healing, the need for physician skill to seek out the tumor tissue by "feel," and persistent tumor in some anatomic areas.[22] In place of the low-voltage electrode physicians may use a carbon dioxide laser to vaporize tumor. When used with curettage, this treatment is beneficial for superficial BCC and nonaggressive BCC. Advantages of this alternative treatment are minimal thermal injury to adjacent cells, faster healing, and minimal pain.[21]

### Radiotherapy

Radiotherapy generally is recommended only for lesions that are inoperable; lesions located in sites such as the corner of the nose, eyelid, lip, and canthus; and those greater than 1 cm but less than 8 cm.[21,22] Patients who are poor surgical candidates may benefit from radiotherapy, but the treatment is not recommended for younger patients (less than age 45) since the irradiated area becomes more atrophic, erythematous, and irregular over the years.[4,22,27] Radiation is administered in fractional doses because increased skin tolerance may enhance its effectiveness.[4] Advantages of radiotherapy are painless treatment, preservation of normal anatomic contours, and the ability to extend treatment into areas surrounding the tumor if desired. Disadvantages include lack of histological tissue for margin control, long treatment periods (three to four weeks), the danger that the treatment itself may lead to BCC or SCC, and the need for clinical facilities with persons trained in radiotherapy.[21]

### Cryotherapy

Cryotherapy involves tumor destruction by using liquid nitrogen to freeze and thaw tumor tissue. The tumor is locally anesthetized; then liquid nitrogen is applied to the lesion by open spray, causing a quick, intense freezing of the tissue, which is then allowed to thaw slowly. This cycle is repeated, and tumor necrosis and erosion follow.

Cryotherapy can be used for small to large primary tumors, for certain recurrent lesions such as those in areas of prior radiation, for multiple superficial BCC, and for lesions needing palliative treatment. Only lesions with well-defined margins (both lateral and depth) benefit from this treatment.[30,31] A minimum of 3-mm margins should be used.[32] Cryotherapy is not recommended for the medial canthal area and the rim of the ears as frozen cartilage buckles during healing and recurrence rates are high.[25,30] Advantages to this treatment include the fact that it produces minimal discomfort (a burning or hot sensation is usually experienced), can be done on an outpatient basis, and can be performed quickly with good cosmetic results. Disadvantages include the need for wound care, prolonged healing time, possible temporary nerve damage, bleeding, and the lack of a specimen for pathology.[21,31,32,33] Careful follow-up is suggested for two years postoperatively to detect secondary tumors, which usually occur within 18 months.[32]

### Chemotherapy

Topical 5-fluorouracil (5-FU) applied to BCC for several weeks produces an inflammatory response that prevents DNA synthesis and cellular reproduction. Topical 5-FU is available as a lotion or a cream in strengths of 1%, 2%, or 5%. 5-FU is applied twice daily for four to six weeks.[3,4] Achieving the desired amount of inflammation does not necessitate causing discomfort in the patient—a mild to moderate erythematous response is sufficient. 5-FU has been shown to be quite effective in superficial BCC but ineffective in other types of BCC.[4]

### Other treatments

Investigational studies for NMSCs are currently ongoing. Those showing encouraging results for the preexcisional treatment of superficial or nodular BCC and SCC are intralesional alfa-2 interferon[4,34] and photodynamic therapy.[3,35] Topical application of photosensitizers such as meso-tetraphenylporphenesulphonate (TPPS) to superficial BCC, followed by exposing the tumors to the dye laser, has produced a complete response rate as high as 94%.[36,37]

## MELANOMA

### Cutaneous Melanoma

#### Pathogenesis

CM arises from melanocytes, which are cells specializing in the biosynthesis and transport of melanin. These pigment-producing cells migrate from the neural crest to the skin, uveal tract, meninges, and ectodermal mucosa by the third month of gestation.[6,38] Melanocytes are most commonly found in the basal layers of the epidermis and in the eye but are also found in the meninges, in the alimentary and respiratory tracts, and in the lymph nodes.[6] Melanocytes contain a melanosome, the specific organelle that synthesizes the melanin pigment. Melanin is synthesized using the tyrosinase enzyme in the melanin synthetic pathway.[6,38] The melanosome-melanin package migrates upward from the basal layer through the epidermis and may be visible in the skin as pigmented melanin granules.[38] (Figure 46-4—Plate 22). In melanomas, the melanosomes may be abnormal or even absent in amelanotic clones.[38] Melanocytes produce receptors for growth factors (e.g., nerve growth factor, epidural growth factor) that may have a critical role in the pathogenesis of melanoma.[6]

Three specific precursor lesions of CM that have been well studied are dysplastic nevi, congenital nevi, and lentigo maligna.

*Dysplastic nevi (DN)* DN are possibly the most controversial lesions in the practice of dermatology and pathology. Critics question their actual existence in terms of lesion size, number, and architecture, whereas proponents suggest they may represent a paradigm for the evolutionary sequence of all cancer.[10,39,40] Also known as *atypical moles*, DN may be familial (i.e., B-K mole syndrome; familial atypical multiple mole or melanoma syndrome) or nonfamilial (sporadic dysplastic nevi). The histological and clinical findings are similar for both.[41,42] Although familial DN is uncommon, members of affected families have a risk of developing CM that approaches 100%. The risk of nonfamilial DN in the general population is estimated at 5%–10%; however, the upper range of some risk estimates has been 50% or more. The magnitude of this risk is still under discussion.[43–46] One study of people with sporadic DN indicated they have a 6.8-fold risk of developing CM.[47]

DN are absent at birth. An early clinical indication may be the presence of an increased number of histologically normal nevi between the ages of 5 and 8 years, with dysplastic changes occurring after puberty.[17] When compared with typical nevi, DN tend to express melanocyte-associated antigens (e.g., epidermal growth factor receptor, nerve growth factor receptor), have a higher frequency of random chromosomal abnormalities (but not nonrandom chromosomal abnormalities observed in

CM), have a greater area of intraepidermal melanocytes, and have some abnormal DNA content of melanocytic nuclei. These changes support the role of DN as an intermediate stage of tumor progression between common typical nevi and CM.[40]

DN generally have one or more of the clinical features of CM (i.e., asymmetry, border irregularity, color variegation, and a diameter greater than 6 mm). A patient with "classic" DN has a triad of more than 100 moles, at least 1 mole 8 mm or larger in diameter, and at least 1 mole with CM features.[10,41] DN appear on the face, trunk, and arms but also may be seen on the buttocks, groin, scalp, and female breast. Pigmentation is irregular, with mixtures of tan, brown, and black, or red and pink. A distinctive feature is a "fried egg" appearance with a deep pigmented papular area surrounded by an area of lighter pigmentation. The lesion may have a macular and/or papular component and an indistinct, irregular border.[10] (Figure 46-5—Plate 23).

People with DN or suspected DN should be thoroughly questioned about family or personal history of melanoma, presence of immunosuppression, sun exposure, atypical pigmented lesions, and prior lesion excisions of any kind. Results of any prior skin biopsies should be obtained, if possible. The entire skin surface should be examined, including the scalp, axilla, genitalia, and between the toes and fingers. Williams and Sagebiel[10] suggested viewing the patient from a distance and clinically defining an abnormal mole phenotype as the presence of more than 100 nevi, with or without typical nevi, or the existence of more than 50 nevi with 1 or several clinically atypical nevi. Excision and biopsy of the most atypical lesions document the presence of histological dysplasia or CM.[10,40] Once a diagnosis of a DN has been established, the patient needs to have periodic skin examinations by a dermatologist, with accompanying total-body photographs every three to six months. Changing or new lesions suspicious for melanoma should be removed and biopsied. Individuals with DN and their first-degree relatives should be taught to examine their entire body every three to six months and should be educated about melanoma risk factors and preventive behaviors.[10]

***Congenital nevi***   Congenital nevi are present at birth or shortly thereafter. They are classified as large or small and range in size from 1.5–3.0 cm to large lesions covering extensive body surfaces such as the trunk, arm, or a hand. Large congenital nevi are uncommon, occurring in 1 in 500,000 newborns, but they carry a substantial lifetime risk for CM (relative risk, 5–15).[10,48] Congenital nevi of all sizes carry a lifetime risk of malignant transformation of 6%–7%.[43]

The color of a congenital nevus ranges from brown to black, and lesions may be slightly raised, with an irregular surface and a fairly regular border. Larger lesions may contain areas of nodularity.

A careful history and examination of congenital nevi are essential to management and should include dates of first appearance and subsequent changes. A biopsy should be obtained from any abnormal-appearing lesion to confirm its exact histology. Treatment consists primarily of surgical excision. Some debate exists as to whether small and large congenital nevi should be surgically removed early in life as a preventive measure.[48] Larger lesions may require several surgeries, which can be disfiguring depending upon their location and size. After treatment, regular follow-up examinations are essential.

***Lentigo maligna***   Lentigo maligna is detailed in a following section describing its very similar counterpart, lentigo maligna melanoma. Treatment of this precursor lesion is discussed in the melanoma treatment section.

## Assessment

A thorough patient history and physical examination are essential to identify individuals at high risk and for early detection of CM and suspicious lesions. Comments and complaints about a preexisting nevus or a new lesion should be investigated. Important questions to ask patients include the following:

1. When was the lesion first noted?
2. Is the lesion new or preexisting? How long has it been there?
3. What caused you to notice the lesion: change in color, size, or texture; bleeding; a different sensation such as burning, itching, tingling, etc.?
4. How long has the lesion been changing and over what time period?
5. Do you have a history of frequent or intense sun exposure, chemical or thermal injury, or skin trauma?
6. Do you have a family history of dysplastic nevus syndrome or melanoma?

Physical recognition of CM by practitioners and those at risk can be initiated by using the "ABCDE" rule.[49] In this rule, $A$ = asymmetry, $B$ = border irregularity, $C$ = color variation or dark black color, $D$ = diameter greater than 0.6 cm (pencil eraser size), and $E$ = elevation. Another assessment measure, the revised seven-point checklist, consists of three major features (change in size, shape, color) and four minor features (inflammation, crusting or bleeding, sensory change, and diameter $\geq$ 7 mm). Healsmith et al[49] compared sensitivity and specificity of the ABCDE system with the revised seven-point checklist and found that the seven-point checklist had greater sensitivity for detecting CM lesions.

The initial step of the physical examination includes a complete visual examination of the cutaneous surface, the questionable lesion(s), and the area surrounding the lesion to determine the presence of satellite lesions or in-transit metastases. All accessible lymph nodes, particularly those in the regional drainage sites, are palpated. A review of systems is obtained. The skin assessment is described in detail in the "Nursing Management" section of this chapter.

Melanoma can metastasize to virtually every organ in the body, and individuals with the diagnosis should undergo the recommended examinations for metastatic disease. Initially, a chest x-ray, a complete blood count, and serum chemistries with liver function tests are performed following diagnosis. Liver function tests have proved to be most useful in determining liver metastasis.[6,50] The combination of an elevated lactate dehydrogenase (LDH), serum glutamic-oxaloacetic transaminase (SGOT), and alkaline phosphatase suggests the possibility of liver involvement and indicate that a computerized tomography (CT) scan of the liver is necessary.[51] If clinical findings indicate possible involvement of other common metastatic sites such as skin, subcutaneous tissue, lymph nodes, lung, brain, and bone, a more extensive metastatic workup is performed. This may include skin or lymph node biopsy for new lesions; a chest x-ray for increased shortness of breath, new cough, or hemoptysis; a CT scan of the brain for neurological abnormality, headaches, mental deficits, or seizures; and a bone scan for undetermined bone pain.[6] Magnetic resonance imaging (MRI) scans offer clearer images and detect different characteristics of lesions than does a CT scan. Since the cost of MRI is high, it may be reserved for special situations.

Patients diagnosed with CM exhibit numerous chromosomal structural abnormalities, including deletions and translocations commonly involving chromosomes 1, 6, 7, 10, and 11.[52] Mutations in the protein *p16* (also called the *CDKN2* or *MTS1* [multiple tumor suppressor] gene), located on segment p21 of chromosome 9, have been identified consistently in patients with CM from some melanoma-prone families. *p16* is known to bind and inhibit normal activity of cyclin-dependent kinase (CDK) 4, which promotes normal passage through the cell cycle. Additional research needs to be done to further pinpoint the mutations of *p16* or to explore the possibility of another CM-associated tumor-suppressor gene on

9p21.[53,54] The tumor-suppressor gene *p53* has been infrequently implicated in CM.[6]

## Classification

Melanoma has been classified into several types: lentigo maligna (LMM), superficial-spreading (SSM), nodular, acral lentiginous (mucocutaneous), those in which the radial growth phase is not characteristic of SSN or LMM, those arising from congenital nevi, those arising from blue nevi, visceral, and ocular (oncology nurses likely would encounter patients with ocular melanoma that has metastasized). The four major types of CM described here include lentigo maligna, superficial-spreading, nodular, and acral lentiginous (Table 46-3). Each of these is characterized by a radial and/or vertical growth phase. In the radial growth phase, tumor growth is parallel to the surface of the skin. This phase may last several years. The propensity for the tumor to metastasize is very small, and surgical excision may be curative. In the vertical growth phase, however, there is focal, deep penetration of atypical melanocytes into the dermis and subcutaneous tissue. This penetration occurs rapidly, increasing the risk of metastasis.[6,55]

LMM, often called *Hutchison's melanotic freckle*, constitutes 4%–10% of all CM and is the least serious type.[43,54] It occurs on body areas heavily exposed to UVR, such as the face, neck, and occasionally the dorsal hands and lower legs. Early premalignant, in situ lesions often precede LMM and are termed *lentigo maligna*. Both lentigo maligna and LMM are large and are primarily tan with different shades of brown throughout (Figure 46-6—Plate 24). The predominant histological feature of lentigo maligna is proliferation of atypical melanocytes along the basal layer of the epidermis. This early radial growth

**TABLE 46-3** Comparisons of the Four Major Types of Cutaneous Melanoma

| Type | Site | Radial Growth Phase | Vertical Growth Phase | Characteristics |
|------|------|---------------------|------------------------|-----------------|
| Lentigo maligna melanoma | Face, neck, dorsal hands, lower legs; areas chronically exposed to sun | Yes (10–25 yr) | Yes (less aggressive) | Size: Large (10 cm)<br>Color: Tan/brown<br>Radial phase: Irregular mottling with regression<br>Vertical phase: Raised nodules on surface |
| Superficial-spreading | Men: trunk, back<br>Women: legs | Yes (1–5 yr) | Yes (aggressive) | Radial phase: Flat with fine crust/scaly surface; tan/brown color<br>Vertical phase: Shiny surface; tan/brown/black to red/white/blue color; borders irregular; raised nodules; ulceration |
| Nodular | Head, neck, trunk (may or may not be exposed to sun) | No | Yes (aggressive, 2–18 mo) | Vertical phase: Raised, dome-shaped blue-black/red color; ulcerations/bleeding may be present |
| Acral lentiginous | Palms, soles, nail beds, mucous membranes | Yes (2–5 yr) | Yes (aggressive) | Radial phase: Flat, tan/brown/black color similar to lentigo maligna<br>Nail bed: Tan/brown stain/streaking<br>Vertical phase: Elevated areas of nodularity |

phase usually lasts between 10 and 25 years, with the lesion growing as large as 10 cm. As soon as these melanocytes invade the dermis, the lesion becomes malignant. With increased growth of the LMM, irregular mottling or freckling may occur, along with regression in some areas. A portion of the lesion may begin a vertical growth phase, with accompanying raised nodules over the surface.[6,55]

SSM accounts for approximately 70% of CM.[43] In men this lesion is most commonly seen on the trunk, and in women, on the legs. SSM usually arises in a preexisting nevus. Early lesions are generally flat with a fine crust or scaly surface. The radial growth phase lasts between one and five or more years. As the lesion enters the vertical phase, a rapid increase of growth occurs, with a change in color ranging from a mixture of tan, brown, and black to a characteristic red, white, and blue appearance. As the lesion continues to grow, the borders become irregular and notched, and the surface becomes shiny and irregular, with raised nodules and ulceration[6,55] (Figure 46-7—Plate 25).

Nodular melanoma constitutes 15%–30% of CM.[43] This lesion appears as a raised, dome-shaped blue-black or red nodule on areas of the head, neck, and trunk that may or may not be exposed to the sun. Ulcerations and bleeding may be present (Figure 46-8—Plate 26). Nodular melanoma has only a vertically invasive component, making early diagnosis difficult. It is more aggressive than the other melanoma types and has a shorter clinical onset. Commonly, these lesions begin de novo in uninvolved skin rather than from a preexisting lesion. Because this lesion lacks a radial phase and is difficult to detect in early stages, there is an increased chance of metastasis being present at diagnosis.[6,55]

Acral lentiginous or mucocutaneous melanoma is the most frequent type of CM in people of color but accounts for less than 5% of CM in whites.[55] This lesion occurs on the palms, soles, nail beds, and mucous membranes. Acral lentiginous melanoma exhibits both a radial and a vertical growth phase. The radial growth phase may last for years and resembles an early lentigo maligna. In this phase the lesion is flat, with nonpalpable margins, and is haphazardly pigmented with tan, brown, and black. In subungual areas the radial growth phase appears as an irregular tan-brown stain of streaking in the nail bed (Figure 46-9—Plate 27). Acral lentiginous melanomas in the vertical phase become elevated, with areas of nodularity. A small percentage are flesh-colored. In the vertical phase, acral lentiginous melanomas are more aggressive and can metastasize.[6]

Juvenile melanomas occur before puberty. They are similar in appearance to CM of adults; however, they can be distinguished histologically by the presence of giant cells. Juvenile melanomas rarely metastasize; therefore, conservative surgery is appropriate treatment. There is, however, a rise in the ability of juvenile melanomas to metastasize after puberty, an event possibly related to hormonal activity.[48,56]

### Staging and prognostic factors

*Microstaging* is a term used to describe the level of invasion of the CM and maximum tumor thickness. Two systems are used in assessing the depth of invasion of melanoma (Figure 46-10). The first is the anatomic level of invasion, or the Clark level, and the second is the thickness of tumor tissue, or the Breslow level. The Clark system categorizes CM into five histological levels based on vertical depth of tumor invasion, with the deeper lesions having the worst prognosis for metastases and survival. When using the Clark system, subjective difficulties in classifying certain melanomas may occur, such as those located in thin-skinned areas (e.g., elbow, under the eye) and lead to poor reproducibility of classification among pathologists. To eliminate these problems, the Breslow system modified the Clark system by using an ocular micrometer to measure, in millimeters, the maximum vertical tumor thickness. This measurement is made from the top of the granular cell layer of the tumor to the deepest level of invasion of the melanoma.

The traditional three-stage system (Table 46-4) is still used, even though it does not include important disease criteria such as tumor thickness. The American Joint Committee on Cancer (AJCC) four-stage system for CM is preferable because it divides patients more evenly and allows for more consistent exchange of information (Table 46-5).[43,57] This staging system includes level of invasion and nodal involvement using the tumor-node-metastasis (TNM) nomenclature.

It is well documented that as CM thickness increases, survival rates decrease. Thus, the Breslow level has consistently proved to be a significant prognostic variable in stage I CM.[6,58,59] Other factors that predict survival are age, sex, and clinical and histological factors. Younger patients and women have a somewhat better prognosis. Clinically, survival related to the anatomic site of the CM is still controversial. With equivalent thicknesses, lesions on the hands, feet, and scalp may have a poorer prognosis.[43] One difficulty in determining prognosis related to feet and scalp lesions is that these lesions are not easily visible and are usually detected later. Histological factors that predict an unfavorable prognosis are the presence of microscopic satellites of tumor, high miotic activity, ulceration, vertical growth phase, and large tumor volume.[43]

Koh[43] reported that stage I LMM and SSM have better five-year survival rates (85%–90%) than do nodular (about 60%) and acral lentiginous melanomas. In stage II disease the five-year survival rates are 36%, but these rates vary according to the clinical status of nodes, the number of nodes involved, and the presence or absence of ulceration in the primary tumor. Stage III (AJCC stage IV) disease is generally incurable secondary to metastases. Median survival is approximately six months.[43]

### Treatment

***Surgery***    The initial surgical procedure for suspected CM is a biopsy. An excisional biopsy that removes a few

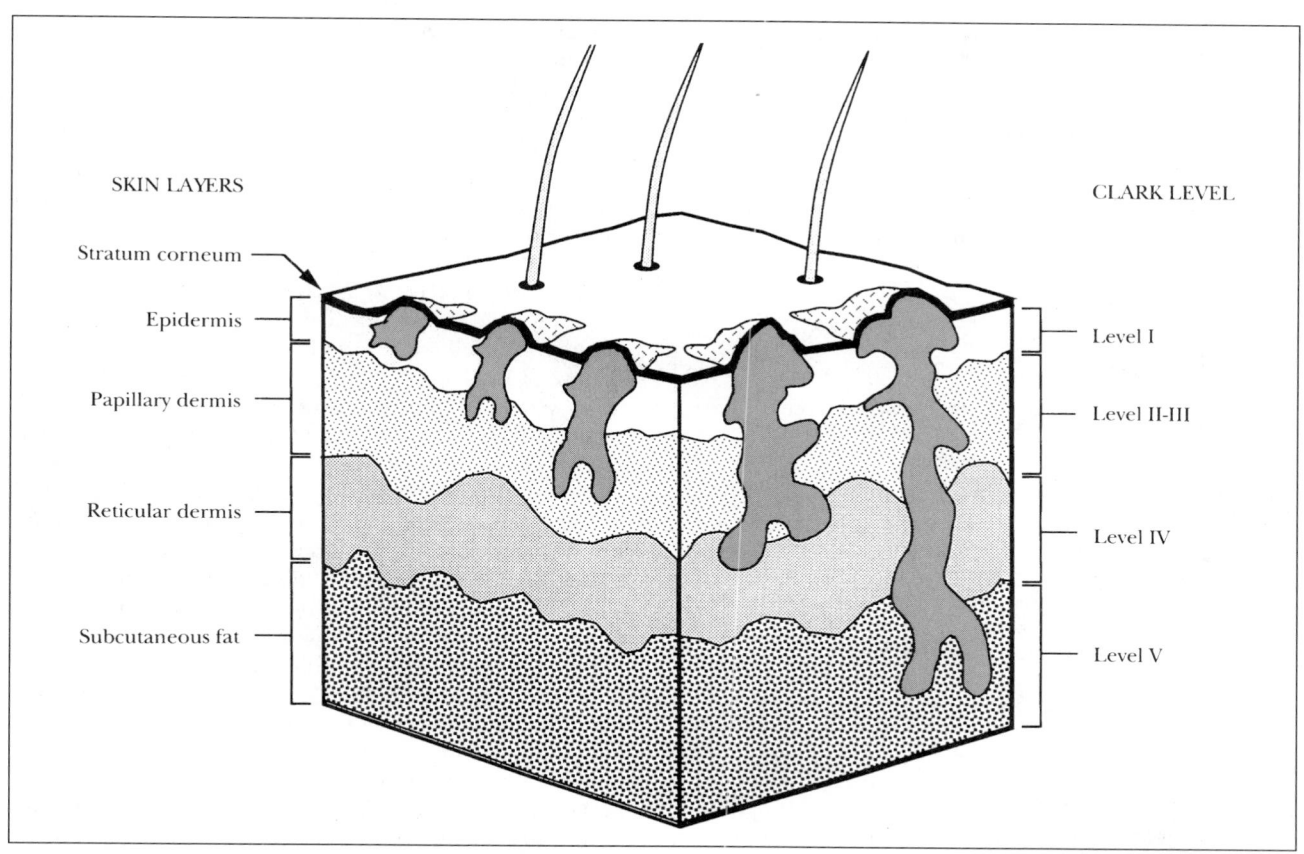

**FIGURE 46-10**  Microstaging (corresponding thicknesses of Clark and Breslow levels).

**TABLE 46-4**  The Traditional Three-Stage System for Cutaneous Melanoma

| Stage | Extent of Disease |
|-------|-------------------|
| I | Localized primary melanoma |
| IA | Local recurrence (satellite lesions) |
| II | Regional lymph node involvement or in-transit metastases |
| III | Distant metastases |

millimeters of normal tissue surrounding the lesion is preferable since it provides a definitive diagnosis along with microstaging information. An incisional biopsy can be used for lesions located in cosmetically sensitive areas or for large lesions. The incisional site should include any areas of change, particularly suspicious raised or nodular-appearing areas. Both techniques should remove a full thickness of the skin and some underlying subcutaneous fat.[60,61] Electrocoagulation, curettage, shaving, and burning should never be used to remove a suspicious mole.

For stage I CM the standard treatment is a wide excision. Debate exists as to the extent of the excision needed to achieve optimal control.[6,61–63] The common margin standard has been 3–5 cm of normal skin, but increasing evidence has shown that the risk of local recurrence correlates with the thickness of the lesion and that margin size does not influence survival.[6,58,60,61,63] Since a minimal risk of local recurrence exists for thin melanomas ($<0.76$ mm), only a 1-cm margin of clinically normal skin around the lesion, along with removal of underlying subcutaneous tissue down to the fascia, is recommended.[60,62–64] A 1-cm-wide excision margin is also suitable for LMM, which has a low metastatic potential. Thicker lesions require a 3–5-cm margin of normal skin with a split thickness graft.[60] For lesions in areas of sensitivity or where cosmesis is an issue, the surgeon determines the safest wide excision margin. Subungual lesions are treated by amputation.

Controversy exists over the use of elective lymph node dissection (ELND) in the treatment of stage I disease. ELND has a high degree of morbidity, and use of this procedure is debatable when no clinical evidence of nodal involvement exists. There is agreement that neither a primary CM lesion less than 0.76 mm nor a LMM requires an ELND. In addition, patients with large lesions ($>4$ mm) do not benefit from ELND because they most likely have microscopic metastases.[6,65–67] Proponents of

**TABLE 46-5** The AJCC's* Four-Stage System for Cutaneous Melanoma

| PRIMARY TUMOR (pT) | |
| --- | --- |
| pTX | Primary tumor cannot be assessed |
| pT0 | No evidence of primary tumor |
| pTis | Melanoma in situ (Clark's level I) |
| pT1 | Tumor ≤ 0.75 mm thick, invading papillary dermis (Clark's level II) |
| pT2 | Tumor 0.76–1.50 mm thick, invading papillary-reticular dermal interface (Clark's level III), or both |
| pT3 | Tumor 1.5–4.00 mm thick, invading reticular dermis (Clark's level IV), or both |
| pT3a | Tumor 1.51–3.00 mm thick |
| pT3b | Tumor 3.01–4.00 mm thick |
| pT4 | Tumor >4.00 mm thick, invading subcutaneous tissue (Clark's level V), or both, and/or satellite(s) within 2 cm of primary tumor |
| pT4a | Tumor >4.00 mm thick, invading subcutaneous tissue, or both |
| pT4b | Satellite(s) within 2 cm of primary tumor |

| REGIONAL LYMPH NODES (N) | |
| --- | --- |
| NX | Regional lymph nodes cannot be assessed |
| N0 | No regional lymph node metastasis |
| N1 | Metastasis ≤ 3cm in greatest dimension in any regional lymph node(s) |
| N2 | Metastasis >3 cm in greatest dimension in any regional lymph node(s) and/or in-transit metastasis |
| N2a | Metastasis >3 cm in greatest dimension in any regional lymph node(s) |
| N2b | In-transit metastasis |
| N2c | Both (N2a and N2b) |

| DISTANT METASTASIS (M) | |
| --- | --- |
| MX | Presence of distant metastasis cannot be assessed |
| M0 | No distant metastasis |
| M1 | Distant metastasis |
| M1a | Metastasis in skin, subcutaneous tissue, or lymph node beyond the regional lymph nodes |
| M1b | Visceral metastasis |

| STAGES | |
| --- | --- |
| I | pT1 or pT2, N0, M0 |
| II | pT3, N0, M0 |
| III | pT4, N0, M0 |
| | Any pT, N1 or N2, M0 |
| IV | Any pT, any N, M1 |

*AJCC, American Joint Committee on Cancer.

Beahrs OH, Henson DE, Hutter RVP, et al (eds): *American Joint Committee on Cancer: Manual for Staging of Cancer* (ed 4). Philadelphia, Lippincott, 1992.

ELND argue that 20%–30% of the clinically normal nodes contain malignant cells and that managing these nodes while the tumor burden is low will decrease the incidence of distant metastases. Opponents maintain that since nodal metastases are rare in patients with thinner melanomas, 70%–80% of these individuals will undergo unnecessary surgery.[64–66] Reviews of some nonrandomized, prospective studies have demonstrated improved survival in patients with intermediate-thickness extremity lesions treated with ELND.[6,62,66] Prospective randomized studies, however, have shown no survival benefit.[6,64] No prospective randomized trials have been performed addressing the use of ELND for CM of the trunk, head, and neck.[6,66] Retrospective studies are also inconclusive; however, some suggest that some patients with stage I CM of intermediate thickness (1–3.99 mm) may benefit from ELND.[6,61,62,68]

Standard surgical therapy of clinical stage II (clinical, but not histological, evidence of draining lymph node involvement) disease includes excision of the primary lesion, along with surgical dissection of the involved nodes.[6] In cases where the index of suspicion is low for metastatic disease, a palpable node may be biopsied by either the open or fine-needle approach.[6]

Surgery is also useful for palliation of disease and symptomatic involvement. Surgical removal of a solitary metastatic lesion is recommended if the lesion is easily accessible and if removal will enhance quality and duration of survival. For example, craniotomy is indicated for removal of a solitary brain metastasis, and thoracotomy is indicated for removal of an isolated lung lesion.[69]

***Chemotherapy*** Metastatic malignant melanoma is highly resistant to currently available systemic chemotherapeutic agents, indicating the need for further research in this area. Dacarbazine (DTIC) is the most active agent for disseminated melanoma, with overall response rates ranging from 15% to 28%.[6,62,70] Metastases to skin, subcutaneous tissues, and lymph nodes respond most favorably to DTIC. However, only 5% of patients achieve a complete response with a median duration of less than six months.[6,62,70] Other single agents with activity include the nitrosoureas (BCNU, CCNU, methyl-CCNU, and chlorozotocin), cisplatin, and paclitaxel, all having response rates no greater than that of DTIC and more toxicities.[43,70,71]

Drug combinations that show some promise for treatment of metastatic disease are DTIC, BCNU, cisplatin, and tamoxifen (DBPT or the Dartmouth regimen); bleomycin, vindesine, CCNU, and DTIC (BELD); DTIC, CCNU, bleomycin, and vincristine (BOLD); and combinations of cisplatin and DTIC with or without vinblastine. Responses of 40%–50% are primarily seen in patients with lung or soft-tissue metastases; survival benefit has not been shown.[70,71] These regimens are still investigational, and more information is needed to support their efficacy.[71] The toxicities of the most frequently used chemotherapeutic agents are discussed in chapter 16.

Isolated limb perfusion is a controversial adjuvant therapy for advanced melanoma confined to a limb or for disease involving melanoma satellites, in-transit metastasis, and poor-prognosis extremity lesions. The treatment consists of hyperthermia plus vascular perfusion of chemotherapy through an isolated region, enabling high concentrations of chemotherapeutic agents to be administered with minimal systemic toxicities. The agent most commonly used for this procedure is melphalan. Others used alone and in combination include thiotepa, dacarbazine, carmustine, cisplatin, and doxorubicin.[6,62,72,73] Complications of treatment include tissue necrosis, transient or persistent edema of the treated extremity, neurological disorders, wound infection, pain, and deep vein thrombosis.[72,74] Isolated limb perfusion remains expensive, investigational, and extremely controversial, since a limited number of control groups have been utilized in reported studies.[6,72,74,75]

Another technique that has been used is intra-arterial infusion chemotherapy without hyperthermia. This involves applying a tourniquet proximally and infusing the chosen chemotherapy agent intra-arterially. This method is simpler than the perfusion technique, but drug levels may not be as high or as evenly distributed.[71,76]

A newer approach is the use of high-dose chemotherapy followed by autologous bone marrow transplantation. This can obtain up to 48% response rates but is complicated by several treatment-related toxicities and significant morbidity, and the responses are usually short-lived. Its role in the treatment of CM requires further study.[70,71,77]

**Radiotherapy** Radiotherapy is most effective when tumor volume is low and when a high dose per fewer fractions radiation level is used (>4 Gy per fraction). Response rates range from a low of 0%–25% to a high of 45%–71%.[6,71] Radiotherapy is often used for palliation in disease with subcutaneous, cutaneous, and nodal metastases that are inaccessible for surgical removal.[6,78,79] Palliative radiation to the brain in conjunction with steroids offers considerable relief of neurological symptoms. Pending bone fractures and bone pain can also be reduced by radiation. Radiotherapy cannot be used to treat liver or lung metastases because of resultant loss of function.[6]

Hyperthermia may enhance the effect of radiation. Studies have shown that when heat (42 °C–43 °C) is applied to lesions for 30–45 minutes before or during radiotherapy, the complete response rate may increase by a factor of 1.5–2. These results have created new interest in this treatment.[70]

**Hormonal therapy** A hormonal influence on melanocyte and melanoma cell proliferation has been suggested by the usual occurrence of CM following puberty, increased incidence during menopause, and increased or decreased CM growth during pregnancy or after parturition.[19,79,81] Hormonal effects are also evidenced by the presence of estrogen and progesterone receptor sites on some CM cells, suggesting that endocrine therapy may be beneficial. Clinically, steroid hormones may directly affect CM growth or may indirectly be mediated by gonadotropins or other pituitary or hypothalamic factors modulated by steroids.[80] A high incidence of steroid binding in melanoma tissue has led to clinical trials demonstrating some tumor response with tamoxifen, diethylstilbestrol, estramustine phosphate, progesterone, and antiandrogens.[80] Another strategy in hormonal therapy is to use melanocyte-stimulating hormone (MSH) to target chemotherapeutic agents toward melanocytes.[80] A large prospective trial of megestrol acetate is under way.[82] Trials using endocrine therapy remain inconclusive.[6,71]

**Immunotherapy** Immunotherapy is a recent form of melanoma treatment with the rationale for use paralleling the natural history of CM, indicating that immunologic intervention by the host may alter the growth pattern of CM. This immunologic interaction is demonstrated by the occurrence of more spontaneous remission in CM than in other adult tumors. Additionally, specific tumor antigen antibodies have been found in patients with melanoma. Patients who have lymphocytic infiltrates at the tumor site have a more favorable prognosis.[6,82,83]

Immunotherapy is currently being investigated as adjuvant therapy and as treatment for metastatic disease. Phase II studies of melanoma vaccines have reported response rates of 13%–23% in patients with advanced disease.[82] Agents such as interferons, interleukins, levamisole, tumor necrosis factors, monoclonal antibodies, and bacillus Calmette-Guerin (BCG) are being studied either singly, in combination with each other, or in combination with chemotherapy (chemoimmunotherapy). The frequently used DTIC and BCG combination has better responses than when either drug is used alone.[71,82]

Adoptive immunotherapy involves obtaining lymphocytes from patients via leukapheresis, incubating the cells with interleukin-2 (IL-2) to generate and expand lymphokine-activated killer (LAK) cells and then reinfusing the LAK cells along with IL-2 into the patient. Response rates range between 15% and 25%. Unfortunately, the toxicities of this treatment, mainly capillary leak syndrome, hypotension, respiratory distress, anemia, and liver and renal dysfunction, have limited its use. Current research is striving to improve the remission rate and limit its toxicity.[43,83] Interferon use in CM remains a palliative measure with a chance of stabilization. Interferons can be used alone or in combination with chemotherapy after tumor removal in cases of high-risk melanoma or CM with early metastatic spread.[6,84–86]

**Gene transfer therapy** Now becoming known as the fifth modality for cancer treatment, gene therapy is being studied for its effect on CM. The patient's own immune system is stimulated to respond to a changing genetic structure within the malignant cell. Nabel et al[87] directly injected the gene for the human transplantation antigen, *HLA-B7*, into a patient who was negative for this antigen. They incorporated the *HLA-B7* gene into a liposomal vector and injected it directly into tumor nodules. The *HLA-B7* gene was accepted by some of the melanoma cells that subsequently were destroyed by cytotoxic T cells that reacted to the HLA-B7 antigen produced by the gene.[83] This modality is still under investigation, but in another phase I study based on Nabel et als trial, a 40% response rate in melanoma patients is being further evaluated.[88] The transfer of the tumor necrosis factor gene into tumor-infiltrating lymphocytes and the insertion of genes for other cytokines such as IL-2, IL-4, and gamma-interferon can cause destruction of melanoma tumor cells.[83]

**Other treatments**　Topical 5-FU has shown desirable results for extensive facial LMMs. In lentigo maligna CM with poor prognosis, preoperative treatment with topical 5-FU has been improving surgical results.[89] One small study indicated that topical tretinoin solution applied to dysplastic nevi may have a biological effect.[90]

Melanoma vaccines have been reported to slow the progression of metastatic lesions in some patients and delay recurrence after surgical excision in stage II disease.[41,91] They appear to be toxicity-free, with the exception of localized swelling. Ongoing trials with melanoma vaccines are being done to test efficacy; however, preliminary results are encouraging.[83]

# PREVENTION

## Primary Prevention

Many skin cancers can be prevented by reducing exposure to avoidable risk factors, particularly exposure to excessive UVR. The harmful effects of UVR exposure begin in childhood, and as UV-induced damage is cumulative, severe effects may be seen by young adulthood.[92] For example, Weinstock et al[93] found a significant association between blistering sunburns in young women aged 15–20 and increased melanoma risk after age 30. Holman et al[94] suggested that the type of swimsuit worn by young women aged 15–25 affects their later risk of developing CM. They estimated a 13-fold increased CM risk in women who wore bikinis or were nude bathers, compared with women who wore conservative, one-piece suits. Stern et al[95] estimated that using a sunscreen with a sun protection factor (SPF) of 15 during the first 18 years of life would reduce the lifetime incidence of NMSC by 78%. Thus, prevention behaviors for reducing exposure must start early in life. Loescher et al[96] conducted a study to determine whether a preschool curriculum about sun safety could facilitate very young children's ability to assimilate information about sun protection. They found that 4-year-olds had long-term retention of knowledge and understanding of basic sun safety concepts (i.e., cover up, find shade, ask for sunscreen), but they could not apply the information independently. Buller et al[97] studied parents with children under age 13 and found that the parents were more likely to practice skin cancer prevention for their children than for themselves and that parents'

own protection was positively related to protection for their children.

Specific sun protection behaviors recommended by the Skin Cancer Foundation[98] and the Arizona Sun Awareness Project[99] include the following:

1.　*Minimize sun exposure* during the hours of 10 A.M. to 3 P.M., when UVR is the strongest.

2.　*Cover up* with a wide-brimmed hat, long-sleeved shirt and long pants (made out of tightly woven material), and protective (UV-filtering) sunglasses.

3.　*Use a waterproof or water-resistant sunscreen with an SPF of 15 or more* before every exposure to the sun. Reapply after the protection time is up. Sunscreen should be applied even on overcast days because 70%–80% of UVR can penetrate cloud cover. Individuals with any risk factors for skin cancer should get into the habit of applying sunscreen on a daily basis. If an allergic reaction to a particular product develops, another brand with different active ingredients can be tried (e.g., PABA-free products). Sunscreens specially formulated for children can be used on children as early as 6 months of age, but perform a "patch test" to determine whether the child's skin is sensitive to the product.

4.　*Be aware of photosensitivity* caused by certain medications (e.g., tetracyclines, oral contraceptives) and cosmetics.

5.　*Be protected when on or near surfaces such as sand, snow, concrete, or water*, which can reflect more than half the UVR onto the skin. Sitting under a shade tree or beach umbrella near these surfaces does not guarantee any added protection from UVR.

6.　*Avoid artificial tanning* as UVA emitted by tanning lights and booths damages the deep skin layers, causing early skin aging and wrinkling.

7.　*Keep infants well protected* when outdoors.

People who work with substances known to cause skin cancer should wear protective clothing and use protective equipment to reduce their exposure.

## Chemoprevention

Randomized, controlled clinical trials that involve treatment of humans with precursor lesions for cutaneous cancers are ongoing. Retinoids (vitamin A and its derivatives) used as biological treatment agents have shown some effect as chemopreventive agents in persons with BCC, actinic keratosis, keratoacanthoma, epidermodysplasia verruciformis, and dysplastic nevi.[100,101] NCI-sponsored chemoprevention trials are currently being conducted using retinol in people with previous BCC or actinic keratosis and 4-hydroxyphenylretinamide (4-HPR) in patients with actinic keratosis. Retinoids used as dietary agents also exhibit potential anticancer effects.[102] A large trial of low-dose 13-*cis* retinoic acid (isotretinoin) in persons with NMSC did not demonstrate any risk reduction.[103] Carotenoids (beta-carotene) are also being studied as chemopreventive agents; however, in persons with recurrent NMSC, treatment with beta-carotene did not reduce the occurrence of new skin cancers over a five-year follow-up period.[104] Beta-carotene is currently under study in people with prior BCC and SCC. The mineral selenium may have some protective benefit against skin cancers.[105] The role of α-difluoromethylornithine (DFMO) in skin cancer prevention is currently being investigated.[105] Definitive results from these and other skin cancer chemoprevention studies will take several years.

## Screening

Early detection and diagnosis of skin cancers are of utmost importance. Most changes on the skin are easily visible and can be detected early, thereby improving chances for cure. One study showed that skin examination by a dermatologist has high sensitivity for CM detection that parallels the Pap smear, fecal occult blood test, and mammography for cervical, colorectal, and breast cancers, respectively.[106] Both the general public and health care professionals need to understand the importance of early evaluation of an unusual skin lesion. Figure 46-11 is an example of a patient education poster that describes these early changes.

## NURSING MANAGEMENT

Because skin cancers are reaching epidemic proportions, the involvement of the nurse in prevention, early detection education, screening, and management of these cancers continues to escalate. Important components of nursing management include interview, skin assessment, education, and posttreatment management.

## Interview

All individuals with skin cancer or those at risk should be questioned about their knowledge of skin cancers, past medical history, and exposure to risk factors. The diagnosis of skin cancer can be frightening for the patient and family members, and the interview elicits information about their knowledge and attitudes, potential fears, and coping mechanisms. Attitudes toward the disease can influence health practices; thus, the interview provides the patient and family with the opportunity to discuss any concerns or issues and to receive appropriate information and reassurance.[107,108] The interview should elicit information about environmental factors such as exposure to UVR, ionizing radiation, and chemicals. A review of systems may reveal information about changes in moles

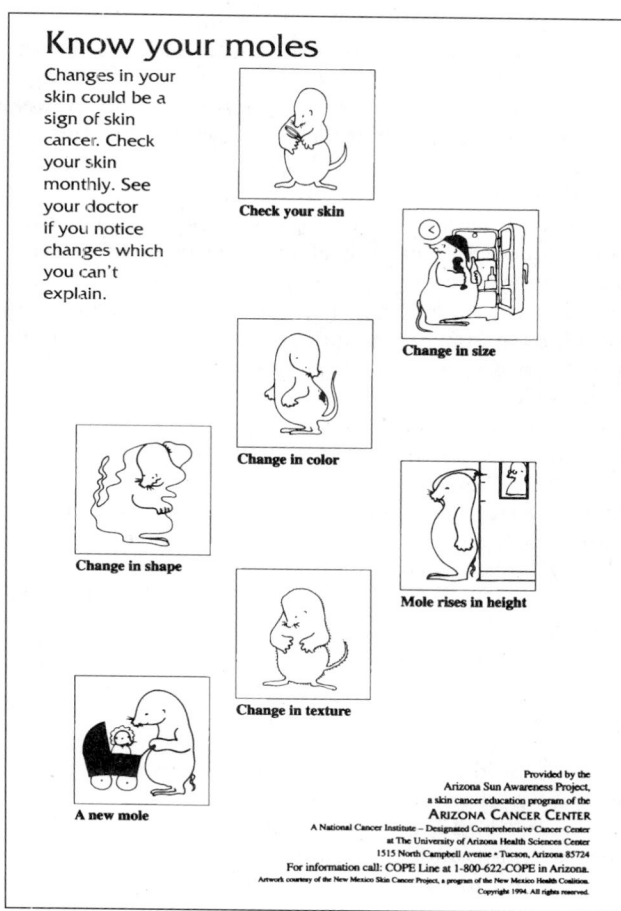

**FIGURE 46-11** Patient education poster describing mole changes that should be reported to a physician. (Printed by permission from the Arizona Cancer Center.)

or an overlooked cancer-related symptom.[109,110] Finally, nurses who are trained in pedigree assessment can complete a family pedigree to ascertain family history of skin cancers. The history and exposure to risk factors will determine how detailed a skin assessment should be.[111]

## Skin Assessment

Nurses working in hospitals, nursing homes, clinics, schools, and home care settings all have an opportunity to examine a person's skin.[110] A thorough nursing skin assessment can initially identify suspicious lesions. Good lighting (preferably bright, natural light) and magnification are essential for the examination. The patient is usually seated during formal skin assessment, although any opportunity such as bathing, dressing changes, or back rubs can be used to check a hospitalized patient's skin. Skin assessment consists of inspection and palpation to identify obvious lesions; visible swellings; adenopathy; alterations in normal borders and contour of nevi; discoloration in skin or mucosa; and areas of ulceration, scaling, crusting, and erosion. Tightly stretching the skin during the examination helps identify nodular and scaly lesions, as well as those within the dermis.[21]

Before the examination the person should undress totally or to his or her underpants, which can easily be pulled away from the body for inspection of the skin underneath.[112] The examination begins with the head and neck, including the entire scalp; eyelids; external ear and auditory canal; external and interior surfaces of the nose; the oral cavity; and the parotid, submaxillary, and sublingual glands. Next, the thyroid is palpated along with the regional lymph nodes of the neck. The examination then progresses to the chest, abdomen, back, and extremities, with special attention to intertrigous areas such as under pendulous breasts, between the buttocks, the chin, an obese abdomen, hairy areas, axillae, nail beds, webs between fingers and toes, and soles of the feet. External genitalia are also examined. The location and descriptive characteristics of suspicious lesions should be recorded on an anatomic chart.[109,111] Warts, moles, scars, vascularities, and birthmarks should also be documented.

## Education

Nurses have the opportunity to educate about skin cancer in many professional and social settings. Berwick et al[112] summarized educational models that could be used by nurses. In one model the nurse is an educator and support person for the dermatologist. Another model uses the nurse as an educator and "prescreener" who conducts the first assessment of the patient, then alerts the physician to the clinical findings and the potential need for referral to a dermatologist. Education for those at high risk for or diagnosed with skin cancers begins with an initial assessment of their knowledge deficit related to skin cancers. The nurse can assess educational background, readiness to learn, and patient and family response to education. Clear and accurate information related to the diagnosis is then given to the patient and repeated several times, if necessary. Photographs of normal moles and birthmarks compared with photographs of skin cancers can be used as teaching aids. Nurses can teach patients systematic skin self-assessment and encourage patients to examine their skin monthly.[107] Family members may assist in checking hard-to-see areas such as the scalp, back, ears, and soles. Examinations should be scheduled at least twice yearly with a dermatologist or oncologist specializing in skin cancers. The nurse needs to emphasize that with attentive self-care and medical management, most patients can lead relatively normal lives.[107] At the conclusion of any educational session, the nurse documents patient and family response to instruction, including comprehension and ability to perform skin self-examination.

Numerous public and professional education brochures describing various aspects of skin cancers and prevention are available from the American Cancer Society, American Academy of Dermatology, National Cancer Institute, Skin Cancer Foundation, pharmaceutical companies that manufacture sunscreens, and other agencies.[113] These teaching aids are usually free of charge.

## Posttreatment Management

Surgical excision is still the most common treatment for skin cancers, and postoperative nursing management is determined by the extent of the procedure. Patients who have had surgical excision only should be instructed to limit environment insults to the surgical site and to protect the site against exposure to irritants and mechanical trauma. Patients who have undergone skin grafting or flapping require careful and frequent observation for signs of infection and hemorrhage in both donor and recipient sites. The recipient site should be immobilized to prevent separation, and involved limbs should be elevated to minimize edema. Some sloughing of a graft site may occur but can be controlled by use of mineral oil or lanolin.[114]

Nursing management of patients receiving chemotherapy, radiotherapy, or immunotherapy is determined by the specific treatment regimen administered. General nursing care for patients receiving these therapies is described in parts III and V of this text.

Some clinicians believe that all patients diagnosed with melanoma should be evaluated at regular intervals for recurrence or metastatic disease (i.e., every three to four months for the first two years, every six months up to five years, and yearly thereafter), with follow-up intervals adjusted according to the risk of metastatic disease in any individual patient.[50,115] In a recent retrospective study of 145 patients who developed recurrent CM, Weiss et al[116] found that most of the recurrences were detected by history and/or physical examination. Their data indicated that routine blood analyses and chest x-rays have limited value in follow-up of patients with resected intermediate- and high-risk CM. Patients need to understand the importance of follow-up visits and testing and of informing the physician or nurse of any physical or mental changes that occur.

## CONCLUSION

This chapter has described three primary forms of skin cancer: basal cell carcinoma, squamous cell carcinoma, and cutaneous malignant melanoma. The best-known treatment to date for most skin cancers is prevention, and oncology nurses are in an ideal position to educate the public and other professionals about preventive behaviors. By practicing early detection, screening, and preventive behaviors themselves, oncology nurses can serve as role models for the general population and for those at high risk.

# REFERENCES

1. Wingo PA, Tong T, Bolden S: Cancer statistics, 1995. *CA Cancer J Clin* 45:8–30, 1995

2. Safai B: Cancers of the skin, in Devita VT, Hellman S, Rosenberg SA: *Cancer: Principles and Practice of Oncology.* Philadelphia, Lippincott, 1993, pp 1567–1611

3. Lang PG, Maize JC: Basal cell carcinoma, in Freedman RJ, Rigel DS, Kopf AW, Harris MN, Baker D (eds): *Cancer of the Skin.* Philadelphia, Saunders, 1991, pp 35–73

4. Preston DS, Stern RS: Nonmelanoma cancers of the skin. *N Engl J Med* 327:1649–1662, 1992

5. Weinstock MA, Bogaars HA, Ashley M, et al: Nonmelanoma skin cancer mortality: A population-based study. *Arch Dermatol* 127:1194–1197, 1991

6. Balch CM, Houghton AN, Peters LJ: Cutaneous melanoma, in Devita VT, Hellman S, Rosenberg SA (eds): *Cancer: Principles and Practice of Oncology.* Philadelphia, Lippincott, 1993, pp 1612–1661

7. Ries LAG, Miller BA, Hankey BF, Kosary CL, Harras A, Edwards BK (eds): *SEER Cancer Statistics Review, 1973–1991: Tables and Graphs.* NIH publication No. 94-2789. Bethesda, MD, National Cancer Institute, 1994

8. Sober AJ: Cutaneous melanoma: Opportunity for cure. *CA Cancer J Clin* 41:197–199, 1991

9. Fraser MC, Hartge P, Tucker MA: Melanoma and nonmelanoma skin cancer: Epidemiology and risk factors. *Semin Oncol Nurs* 7:2–12, 1991

10. Williams ML, Sagebiel RW: Melanoma risk factors and atypical moles. *West J Med* 160:343–350, 1994

11. Marks R, Whiteman D: Sunburn and melanoma: How strong is the evidence? *BMJ* 308:75, 76, 1994

12. Scotto J, Fears TR: The association of solar ultraviolet and skin melanoma incidence among Caucasians in the United States. *Cancer Invest* 5:275–283, 1987

13. National Institutes of Health Consensus Development Conference: *Sunlight, Ultraviolet Radiation, and the Skin.* Bethesda, MD, National Institutes of Health, 1991

14. Setlow RB, Grist E, Thompson K, et al: Wavelengths effective in induction of malignant melanoma. *Genetics* 90:6666–6670, 1993

15. Kripke ML: Ultraviolet radiation and immunology: Something new under the sun. Presidential address. *Cancer Res* 54:6102–6105, 1994

16. Rhodes AR, Weinstock MA, Fitzpatrick TB, et al: Risk factors for cutaneous melanoma. *JAMA* 258:3146–3154, 1987

17. Greene MH, Clark WH, Tucker MA, et al: Acquired precursors of cutaneous malignant melanoma: The familial dysplastic nevus syndrome. *N Engl J Med* 312:91–97, 1986

18. Rampen FHJ: Sex differences in survival from cutaneous melanoma. *Int J Dermatol* 23:444–452, 1984

19. Holly EA: Melanoma in pregnancy, in Gallagher RP (ed): *Recent Results in Cancer Research: Epidemiology of Malignant Melanoma.* New York, Springer-Verlag, 1986, pp 118–125

20. Schwartz BK, Zashin SJ, Spencer SK, et al: Pregnancy and hormonal influences on malignant melanoma. *J Dermatol Surg Oncol* 13:276–281, 1987

21. Vargo N: Basal and squamous cell carcinomas: An overview. *Semin Oncol Nurs* 7:13–25, 1991

22. McKinney P, Robinson JK: Basic principles in management of basal cell epithelioma. *Ill Med J* 173:105–111, 1988

23. Dzubow L, Grossman D: Squamous cell carcinoma and verrucous carcinoma, in Freedman RJ, Rigel DS, Kopf AW, Harris MN, Baker D (eds): *Cancer of the Skin.* Philadelphia, Saunders, 1991, pp 74–84

24. Edwards L, Levine N: Skin cancer: The best route to early diagnosis. *Mod Med* 54:42–54, 1986

25. Stegman SJ: Basal cell carcinoma and squamous cell carcinoma: Recognition and treatment. *Med Clin North Am* 70:95–107, 1986

26. Lynch P: Viral oncogenesis in cutaneous malignancy, in Freedman RJ, Rigel DS, Kopf AW, Harris MN, Baker D (eds): *Cancer of the Skin.* Philadelphia, Saunders, 1991, pp 85–94

27. Loeffler M, Hornblass A: Characteristics and behavior of eyelid carcinoma (basal cell, squamous cell, sebaceous gland, and malignant melanoma). *Ophthalmic Surg* 21:513–518, 1990

28. Roenigk RK: Mohs' micrographic surgery. *Mayo Clin Proc* 63:175–183, 1988

29. Darmstadt GL, Steinman HK: Mohs' micrographic surgery of the head and neck. *West J Med* 152:153–158, 1990

30. Tobinick EL: Basal cell carcinoma. *Am Fam Physician* 36:219–224, 1987

31. Torre D: Cryosurgery of basal cell carcinoma. *J Am Acad Dermatol* 15:917–929, 1986

32. Holt PJA: Cryotherapy for skin cancer: Results over a 5-year period using liquid nitrogen spray cryosurgery. *Br J Dermatol* 119:231–240, 1988

33. Wheeland RG, Bailin PL, Ratz JL, et al: Carbon-dioxide laser vaporization and curettage in the treatment of multiple superficial basal cell carcinomas. *J Dermatol Surg Oncol* 13:119–125, 1987

34. Greenway H, Cornell R, Tanner D, et al: Treatment of basal cell carcinoma with intralesional interferon. *J Am Acad Dermatol* 15:437–443, 1986

35. McCaughan J, Guy J, Hicks W, et al: Photodynamic therapy for cutaneous and subcutaneous malignant neoplasms. *Arch Surg* 124:211–216, 1989

36. Sacchini V, Melloni E, Marchesini R, et al: Preliminary clinical studies with PDT and TPPS administration in neoplastic skin lesions. *Lasers Surg Med* 7:6–11, 1987

37. Santoro O, Bandieramonte G, Melloni E, et al: Photodynamic therapy by topical mesotetraphenylporphinesulfonate tetrasodium salt administration in superficial basal cell carcinomas. *Cancer Res* 50:4501–4503, 1990

38. Worth AJ: Growth patterns in melanoma and its precursor lesions, in Gallagher RP (ed): *Epidemiology of Malignant Melanoma.* Berlin, Springer-Verlag, 1986, pp 1–7

39. Murphy GE, Halpern A: Dysplastic melanocytic nevi: Normal variants or melanoma precursors? *Arch Dermatol* 126:519–522, 1990 (editorial)

40. Barnhill RL: Moles and melanoma: New method in the madness. *West J Med* 160:381–383, 1994

41. Friedman R, Rigel D, Silverman M, et al: Malignant melanomas in the 1990's: Continued importance of early detection and role of physician examination and self-examination of the skin. *CA Cancer J Clin* 41:201–226, 1991

42. Roush GC, Barnhill RL: Correlation of clinical pigmentary characteristics with histopathologically-confirmed dysplastic nevi in nonfamilial melanoma patients: Studies of melanocytic nevi IX. *Br J Cancer* 64:943–947, 1991

43. Koh H: Cutaneous melanoma. *N Engl J Med* 325:171–182, 1991

44. Rigel DS, Rivers JK, Kopf AW, et al: Dysplastic nevi: Markers for increased risk for melanoma. *Cancer* 63:386–389, 1989

45. Piepkorn M, Meyer LJ, Goldgar D, et al: The dysplastic melanocytic nevus: A prevalent lesion that correlates

poorly with clinical phenotype. *J Am Acad Dermatol* 20: 407–415, 1989

46. Ackerman AB: Pathobabble: Confusing terminology in the language of melanocytic neoplasia, in Cascinelli N, Santinami M, Veronesi U (eds): *Cutaneous Melanoma Biology and Management.* Milan, Italy, Masson, 1990, pp 127–132

47. Halpern AC, DuPont G IV, Elder DE, et al: Dysplastic nevi as risk markers of sporadic (nonfamilial) melanoma. *Arch Dermatol* 127:995–999, 1991

48. Ceballos PI, Ruiz-Maldonado R, Mihm MC Jr: Melanoma in children. *New Engl J Med* 332:656–662, 1995

49. Healsmith MF, Bourke JF, Osborne JE, et al: An evaluation of the revised seven-point checklist for the early diagnosis of cutaneous malignant melanoma. *Br J Dermatol* 130: 48–50, 1994

50. Berdeaux DH, Moon TE, Meyskens FL: Management of stage I cutaneous melanoma. *Arizona Med* 40:768–772, 1983

51. Finck SJ, Giuliano AE, Morton DL: LDH and melanoma. *Cancer* 51:840–843, 1983

52. Trent JM, Meyskens FL, Salmon SE, et al: Relation of cytogenetic abnormalities and clinical outcome in metastatic melanoma. *N Engl J Med* 322:1508–1511, 1990

53. Kamb A, Gruis NA, Weaver-Feldhaus J, et al: A cell cycle regulator potentially involved in genesis of many tumor types. *Science* 264:436–440, 1994

54. Marx J: Link to hereditary melanoma brightens mood for *p16* gene. *Science* 265:1364–1365, 1994

55. Crotty K, Mihm MC: Cutaneous malignant melanoma: A photo atlas and review of types and stages. *Adv Oncol* 10(4): 10–16, 1994

56. Spitz S: Classics in oncology: Melanoma of childhood. *CA Cancer J Clin* 41:40–51, 1991

57. Beahrs OH, Hensen DE, Hutter RV, Kennedy BJ. (eds) Malignant melanoma, in *Handbook for Staging of Cancer.* Philadelphia, Lippincott, 1993, pp 158, 159

58. Rigel DS, Sober AJ, Friedman RJ: Prognostic factors influencing survival in persons with cutaneous malignant melanoma, in Freedman RJ, Rigel DS, Kopf AW, Harris MN, Baker D (eds): *Cancer of the Skin.* Philadelphia, Saunders, 1991, pp 198–206

59. Kopf AW, Welkovich B, Frankel RE, et al: Thickness of malignant melanoma: Global analysis of related factors. *J Dermatol Surg Oncol* 13:345–420, 1987

60. Urist MM, Balch CM, Milton GW: Surgical management of the primary melanoma, in Balch CM, Milton GW, Shaw HM, Soong SJ (eds): *Cutaneous Melanoma.* Philadelphia, Lippincott, 1985, pp 71–90

61. Meyer KL, Kenady DE, Childers SJ: The surgical approach to primary malignant melanoma. *Surg Gynecol Obstet* 160: 379–386, 1985

62. Harris MN, Roses DF: Malignant melanoma: Treatment, in Freedman RJ, Rigel DS, Kopf AW, Harris MN, Baker D (eds): *Cancer of the Skin.* Philadelphia, Saunders, 1991, pp 177–197

63. NIH Consensus Development Panel on Early Melanoma: Diagnosis and treatment of early melanoma. *JAMA* 268: 1314–1319, 1992

64. Dhawan M, Kirkwood JM: Melanoma therapy: A status report. *Contemp Oncol* 4:40–50, 1994

65. Sim FH, Taylor WF, Pritchard DJ, et al: Lymphadenectomy in the management of stage I malignant melanoma: A prospective randomized study. *Mayo Clin Proc* 61:697–705, 1986

66. Veronesi U: Delayed node dissection in stage I malignant melanoma: Justification and advantages. *Cancer Invest* 5: 47–53, 1987

67. Balch CM: The role of elective lymph node dissection in melanoma: Rationale, results, and controversies. *J Clin Oncol* 6:163–172, 1988

68. Day CL, Lew RA: Malignant melanoma prognostic factors 7: Elective lymph node dissection. *J Dermatol Surg Oncol* 11: 233–239, 1985

69. Wornon IL, Smith JW, Soong SJ, et al: Surgery as palliative treatment for distant metastases of melanoma. *Ann Surg* 204:181–185, 1986

70. Oratz R, Blum RH: Chemotherapy for malignant melanoma. *Adv Oncol* 10(4):26–29, 1994

71. Ho V, Sober A: Therapy for cutaneous melanoma: An update. *J Am Acad Dermatol* 22:159–176, 1990

72. Klein ES, Ben-Ari GY: Isolation perfusion with cisplatin for malignant melanoma on the limbs. *Cancer* 59:1068–1071, 1987

73. Muchmore JH, Carter RD, Krementz ET: Regional perfusion for malignant melanoma and soft tissue sarcoma: A review. *Cancer Invest* 3:129–143, 1985

74. Ghussen F, Kruger I, Groth W, et al: The role of regional hyperthermia cytostatic perfusion in the treatment of extremity melanoma. *Cancer* 61:654–659, 1988

75. Franklin HR, Koops HS, Oldhoff J, et al: To perfuse or not to perfuse? A retrospective comparative study to evaluate the effect of adjuvant isolated regional perfusion in patients with stage I extremity melanoma with a thickness of 1.5mm or greater. *J Clin Oncol* 16:701–708, 1988

76. Clark WH Jr, Elder DE, Guerry D IV, et al: Model predicting survival in stage I melanoma based on tumor progression. *Natl Cancer Inst* 81:1893–1904, 1989

77. Rogers GS, Kopf AW, Rigel D, et al: Hazard-rate analysis in stage I malignant melanoma. *Arch Dermatol* 122:999–1102, 1986

78. Rofstad EK: Radiation biology of malignant melanoma. *Acta Radiol* 25:1–10, 1986

79. Overgaard J: The role of radiotherapy in recurrent and metastatic malignant melanoma: A clinical radiobiological study. *Int J Radiat Oncol* 12:867–872, 1986

80. Meyskens FL: The endocrinology of malignant melanoma. *Rev Endocrine-Related Cancer* 9:5–13, 1981

81. Reintgen DS, McCarty KS, Vollmer R, et al: Malignant melanoma and pregnancy. *Cancer* 55:1340–1344, 1985

82. Barth A, Morton DL: The role of adjuvant therapy in melanoma management. *Cancer* 75:726–734, 1995

83. Ho RCS: Medical management of stage IV malignant melanoma. *Cancer* 75:735–741, 1995

84. Stadler R, Mayer-da-Silva A, Bratzke B, et al: Interferons in dermatology. *J Am Acad Dermatol* 20:650–656, 1989

85. Creagan ET, Ahmann DL, Frytak S, et al: Recombinant leukocyte A interferon in the treatment of disseminated malignant melanoma. *Cancer* 58:2576–2578, 1986

86. Bratzke B, Stadler R, Garbe C, et al: Interferon (rIFNa2nb-IFN) for postsurgical adjuvant treatment in stage II malignant melanoma. Seventh World Congress in Dermatology. Berlin. Abstracts vol. II:164, 1987

87. Nabel GJ, Nabel EG, Yang ZY, et al: Direct gene transfer with DNA-liposome complexes in melanoma: Expression, biologic activity, and lack of toxicity in humans. *Proc Natl Acad Sci USA* 90:11307–11311, 1993

88. Hersh E, Stopeck A, Harris E, et al: Long-term follow-up and retreatment studies on patients with metastatic malignant melanoma (MM) treated in a phase I/II study

of direct intratumoral injection of the HLA-B7/β2M gene (Allovectin-7) in a cationic lipid vector. *Proc Am Soc Clin Oncol* 15:235, 1996 (Abstr. 576)

89. Ryan R, Krementz E, Litwin M: A role for topical 5-fluorouracil therapy in melanoma. *J Surg Oncol* 38:250–256, 1988

90. Edwards L, Jaffe P: The effect of topical tretinoin on dysplastic nevi. *Arch Dermatol* 126:494–499, 1990

91. Dugan M, Oratz R, Bystryn JC: Immunotherapy in the treatment of malignant melanoma, in Friedman RJ, Rigel DS, Kopf AW, Harris MN, Baker D (eds): *Cancer of the Skin*. Philadelphia, Saunders, 1991, pp 569–579

92. National Cancer Institute: *Nonmelanoma Skin Cancers: Research Report*. NIH publication No. 88-2977. Bethesda, MD, National Cancer Institute, May 1988

93. Weinstock MA, Colditz GA, Willet WC, et al: Nonfamilial cutaneous melanoma incidence in women associated with sun exposure before 20 years of age. *Pediatrics* 84:199–204, 1989

94. Holman CDJ, Armstrong BK, Heenan PJ: Relationship of cutaneous malignant melanoma to individual sunlight exposure habits. *J Natl Cancer Inst* 76:403–414, 1986

95. Stern RS, Weinstein MC, Baker SG: Risk reduction for nonmelanoma skin cancer with childhood sunscreen use. *Arch Dermatol* 122:537–545, 1986

96. Loescher LJ, Emerson J, Taylor A, et al: Educating preschoolers about sun safety. *Am J Public Health* 85:939–943, 1995

97. Buller DBB, Callister MA, Reichert T: Skin cancer prevention by parents of young children: Health information sources, skin cancer knowledge, and sun-protection practices. *Oncol Nurs Forum* 22:1559–1566, 1995

98. *Simple Guidelines to Help Protect You from the Damaging Rays of the Sun*. New York, Skin Cancer Foundation, 1988

99. *Living Well in Arizona*. Tucson: Arizona Cancer Center, 1992

100. Lippman SM, Kessler JF, Meyskens FL: Retinoids as preventive and therapeutic anticancer agents (parts 1 and 2). *Cancer Treat Rep* 71:391–405, 493–515, 1987

101. Bertram JS, Kolonel LN, Meyskens FL: Rationale and strategies for chemoprevention of cancer in humans. *Cancer Res* 47:3012–3031, 1987

102. Ritenbaugh CK, Meyskens FL: Analysis of dietary associations of vitamin A with cancer, in Bland J (ed): *The Year in Nutritional Medicine*. New Canaan, CT, Keats, 1986, pp 263–291

103. Tangrea JA, Edwards BK, Taylor PR, et al: Long-term therapy with low-dose isotretinoin for prevention of basal cell carcinoma: A multicenter clinical trial. *J Natl Cancer Inst* 84:323–332, 1992

104. Greenberg ER, Baron JA, Stukel TA, et al: A clinical trial of beta carotene to prevent basal-cell and squamous-cell cancers of the skin. *N Engl J Med* 323:789–795, 1990

105. Loescher LJ, Meyskens FL: Chemoprevention of human skin cancers. *Semin Oncol Nurs* 7:45–52, 1991

106. Koh HK, Caruso A, Gage I, et al: Evaluation of melanoma/skin cancer screening in Massachusetts: Preliminary results. *Cancer* 65:375–379, 1990

107. Fraser MC: The nurse's role and malignant melanoma. *Cancer Nurs* 5:351–360, 1982

108. Fraser MC, McGuire DB: Skin cancer's early warning system. *Am J Nurs* 84:1232–1236, 1984

109. White LN, Spitz MR: Cancer risk and early detection assessment. *Semin Oncol Nurs* 9:188–197, 1993

110. Lawler PE, Schreiber S: Cutaneous malignant melanoma: Nursing's role in prevention and early detection. *Oncol Nurs Forum* 16:345–352, 1989

111. Schulmeister L: Screening for skin cancer: A necessary part of your assessment routine. *Nursing* 11:42–45, 1981

112. Berwick M, Bolognia JL, Heer C, et al: The role of the nurse in skin cancer prevention, screening, and early detection. *Semin Oncol Nurs* 7:64–71, 1991

113. Grossman DJ: Public and professional educational materials on skin cancer. *Am Acad Dermatol* 21:1012–1018, 1989

114. Stern C: Melanoma: The most lethal skin cancer. *RN* 50:53–57, 1987

115. Kibbi AG, Mihm MC, Sober AJ, et al: Diagnosis and management of malignant melanoma. *Compr Ther* 12:23–31, 1986

116. Weiss M, Loprinzi C, Creagan ET, et al: Utility of follow-up tests for detecting recurrent disease in patients with malignant melanomas. *JAMA* 274:1703–1705, 1995

# Chapter 47

# Testicular Germ Cell Cancer

Debra L. Brock, RNC, MSN, ANP, AOCN

Susan M. Fox, RN, MS, OCN®

## INTRODUCTION

Testicular cancer is a relatively rare cancer yet it is the most common cancer in men aged 15 to 35. The American Cancer Society estimates that there were 7100 newly diagnosed cases of testis cancer and 370 deaths due to testis cancer in 1996.[1] The incidence of testis cancer has shown a slight increase although reasons are unknown. According to Chilvers et al the incidence in frequency of cryptorchidism has also increased.[2] Even though testis cancer is highly curable, particularly when found in early stages, it has a profound impact on the economic, social, and emotional status of the young population it affects due to potential losses during the productive years of life.

## EPIDEMIOLOGY

Although the overall incidence of testicular cancer accounts for about 1% of all male cancers, the incidence is increasing in Caucasian males. Worldwide incidence of testis cancer is the greatest in Scandinavian countries with Denmark having one of the highest rates in the world. Testis cancer rarely occurs in African-American men. Africa and Asia have the lowest incidence of testicular cancers.[3]

Testis cancer most commonly affects those in the 20- to 30-year-old age group. It occurs less frequently in adolescents and in men over 40 years of age.

As a group, testicular germ cell cancers are comprised of seminomas and nonseminomatous cell types. Nonseminomatous germ cell tumors include teratoma, yolk sac, embryonal (endodermal sinus tumor), choriocarcinoma, or mixed combinations. Seminomas comprise a group within themselves. Males with pure seminoma tend to be older than those diagnosed with nonseminomatous cell types. The most common tumor is embryonal.

Men with testis cancer have a higher overall family incidence of testis cancer and of genitourinary anomalies.[4] Males diagnosed with testicular cancer also have about a 1%–2% chance of developing testicular cancer in the contralateral testicle.

Extragonadal germ cell tumors, which are neoplasms arising outside of the gonads, not only are rare but also can occur within the same age group. There are three primary sites for extragonadal germ cell tumors: mediastinal, retroperitoneal, and the pineal gland. Extragonadal germ cell tumors have a poorer prognosis than a primary testicular cancer. An association between mediastinal germ cell tumors and Klinefelter's syndrome has been identified.[5] Klinefelter's syndrome is characterized by small firm testes, azoospermia, gynecomastia, and elevated levels of plasma gonadotropins.

## ETIOLOGY

A definite etiology for germ cell tumors is unknown. Many factors such as hormonal drugs, diseases, age, genetic anomalies, trauma, occupation, and socioeconomics have been studied. Testis cancer is more likely to occur in men with a history of an undescended testicle. There is an overall 10–40-fold increased risk of developing testis cancer in the undescended testicle. However, only approximately 10% of all testicular cancers present with a history of a unilateral undescended testicle. In men with cryptorchidism, about 25% will develop testicular cancer in the contralateral testicle. Early orchipexy before the age of six may lessen the risk for testicular cancer.[6] One to two percent of all germ cell tumors are bilateral, which may occur simultaneously or at a later date. Therefore, it is most critical to stress the importance of testicular self exam (TSE) when educating men who have a history of testicular cancer.[7]

First-degree male relatives of men with testicular cancer have an overall greater incidence of cyptorchidism, inguinal hernias, hydroceles, and testicular cancer.[6,8] These data suggest that some genetic predisposition and/or in-utero environmental event(s) may result in several urothelial developmental abnormalities.

It has been recognized that a specific cytogenetic abnormality located on chromosome 12 is associated with testicular cancer and extragonadal tumors. This finding is thought to be helpful in classifying poorly differentiated neoplasms of obscure origin. Eighty percent of germ cell tumors will have the abnormality.[9] Hopefully, research into this area will provide further information regarding the etiology of testicular and extragonadal tumors.

The use of exogenous estrogens during pregnancy in the mothers of men with testicular cancer has been analyzed by several investigators. Interest in this as a possible etiology factor is based on the observation that murine testicular tumors can be produced experimentally by the administration of estrogen.[10] Male offspring of mothers treated with diethylstilbesterol (DES), a synthetic nonsteroidal estrogen, exhibit a number of urogenital developmental abnormalities, including testicular hypoplasia and maldescent.[11–13]

## PREVENTION, SCREENING, EARLY DETECTION

Due to the aggressive nature of testicular cancer and the high rate of cure, early detection is of utmost importance for a favorable outcome. A cancerous testis is commonly nonfunctioning and is most likely azoospermic or oligospermic. Although the exact cause is unknown, up to 80% of males with testicular cancer will be oligospermic at the time of diagnosis.[14] These findings suggest that men experiencing fertility problems should be evaluated for testicular cancer.

Nurses have a key role in the education of all males in the prevention and screening of testicular cancer. Because testicular cancer is a rare cancer, mass screening for the disease is not cost-effective or practical. To assist in the fight against testicular cancer and increase early detection, males are encouraged to perform monthly testicular self-examinations (TSE). Males should be instructed on how to perform monthly TSE by age 15. TSE should be performed immediately after a warm shower or bath when the scrotum is relaxed and abnormalities are more easily identified. While in a standing position, each testicle should be rolled between the thumb and fingers checking for lumps, swelling, or other changes. The normal testicle should feel egg shaped, smooth, and firm. A male should be instructed to report any mass to his health care provider.

Many states have adopted policies that require TSE be taught to high school males. The American Cancer Society provides literature, models, and video tapes regarding testicular self-exam that nurses can utilize in teaching.

## PATHOPHYSIOLOGY

The testicles are the male gonads. Early in the development of the male fetus the testes are located in the abdominal cavity. Before or soon after birth, the testes normally will descend into the scrotum. The testes produce sperm and are also the primary source of male hormones. The male hormones or androgens are responsible for secondary sex characteristics, development of the reproductive system, and the male sex drive.

As with other cancers, testicular cancer is a result of multiplying abnormal cells. Testicular cancer has a remarkably high tumor cell doubling-time, which unlike other cancers, is a factor in the favorable response to treatment.

The spread of testicular cancer occurs in an orderly progression. Testicular cancer cells metastasize through the lymphatics and the blood. Testicular cancer can spread to the abdominal retroperitoneal lymph nodes, lungs, bone, liver, and brain. Typical spread is from the testis to the retroperitoneal lymphatics, and to the lung. Testicular cancer is fairly aggressive and spreads quickly. An early diagnosis is important in order to realize a favorable outcome. Even those men with a high tumor volume and metastatic spread will have a 50%–60% chance of cure. Approximately 90% of men diagnosed with testicular cancer will be cured. Advanced disease at diagnosis involving the brain, liver, and bone is rare.

Testicular lymphatic drainage was first noted by Jamieson and Dodson, who documented that metastatic spread occurred from the testicular tumor to the ipsilateral retroperineal lymph nodes.[15] Metastatic lymph node spread occurs on the same side of the body as the primary testicular tumor.[15] Right-sided tumors drain to the paracaval, interaortocaval, and preaortic nodes while left-sided lesions drain to the para-aortic and preaortic nodes within the retroperitoneal cavity. Later dissemination is to the mediastinal and supraclavicular lymph nodes. Hematogenous spread is not uncommon. Sanctuary sites following treatment may include the central nervous system and the contralateral testicle. Late sites of dissemination may include lungs, liver, bone, and brain.

Testicular cancer is classified by two main histological cell types, seminomas and nonseminomas. Seminomas include classic and spermatocytic. Nonseminomas include embryonal, yolk sac, choriocarcinoma, and teratoma. (Table 47-1). Many of these subtypes will secrete alpha-fetoprotein (AFP) and/or beta human chorionic gonadotropin (BHCG). AFP and BHCG are considered meaningful tumor markers for testicular cancer. Seminomas are frequently associated with normal tumor markers; only 10%–20% of men will have an abnormal BHCG. Any elevation of AFP seen in a man diagnosed with "pure seminoma" would mean marker evidence of nonseminoma and therefore the tumor should be approached as a nonseminomatous tumor.

## CLINICAL MANIFESTATIONS

A mass in the scrotum accidentally discovered is often the presenting symptom of testicular cancer. Athletic males will often present with a recent history of an injury to the testicle. Although trauma does not cause testicular cancer, it does draw attention to the scrotal area resulting in discovery of the mass. The most common sign of testicular cancer is a small hard mass in the scrotum. However, a dragging sensation, swelling, dull aching or pain in the scrotal area also may be presenting symptoms. Germ cell tumors are often mistaken for epididymitis as well as other benign causes of testicular symptoms. (Table 47-2).[16] Frequently a complaint of low back pain is a presenting symptom indicating that the cancer has spread into the retroperitoneal lymph nodes. Gynecomastia also can be present due to an elevation of the serum beta subunit of human chorionic gonadotropin (BHCG). Advanced pulmonary metastasis can present with a history of cough, hemoptysis, dyspnea, and chest pain. Symptoms related to metastasis to the liver, bone, or brain are seldom presenting symptoms.

## ASSESSMENT

### Patient and Family History

A thorough history must be obtained that should include the past medical history and family history. Ascertaining

**TABLE 47-1**   Testicular Cancer Cell Types/Characteristics/Tumor Markers

| Neoplasm | Age | Percentage | Markers |
|---|---|---|---|
| **Seminomatous Tumors:** | | | |
| Classic | 40–50 | 93% | BHCG +/− AFP − |
| Seminoma | Median 65 | 7% | BHCG +/− AFP − |
| **Nonseminomatous Tumors:** | | | |
| Embryonal | 20–30 | 20%–25% | BHCG + AFP + |
| Yolk Sac | 0–5 | 1%–10% | BHCG − AFP + |
| | Relatively unaggressive | | |
| | In adults a virulent neoplasm | | |
| Choriocarcinoma | 13–25 | 1%–2% | BHCG + AFP − |
| | Pure chorio of adult testes is rare and the | | |
| | most aggressive of germ cell tumors. | | |
| Teratoma | Preschool | 5%–10% | BHCG − AFP − |

**TABLE 47-2**   Benign Causes of Testicular Cancer Symptoms

| | |
|---|---|
| Orchitis | Infections or inflammation of the testes due to epididymitis/mumps<br>*Symptoms:* Pain and swelling of the testicles; fever; scrotum often reddened and edematous |
| Epididymitis | Infection<br>*Symptoms:* Pain in the groin and scrotum; edema; redness, tenderness of the scrotum; chills, fever |
| Torsion of the appendix of testes | Swelling of the testes<br>*Symptom:* Painful and enlarged testes usually seen in the youths |
| Hydrocele | Abnormal accumulation of fluid in the scrotum and around the testes<br>*Symptoms:* None; swelling is usually painless |
| Varicocele | Engorgement of veins within the scrotum<br>*Symptoms:* Dragging sensation within the scrotum |
| Tuberculosis | Testicular involvement rarely seen until late stages of the disease<br>*Symptoms:* None; usually a nontender mass involving the epididymis |
| Syphilitic orchitis | Seen in tertiary stage of syphilis<br>*Symptoms:* Firm, hard testes, painless; serology positive for syphilis |

Reprinted with permission from Hubbard SM, Jenkins J: An overview of current concepts in the management of patients with testicular tumors of germ cell origin - Part I: Pathophysiology, diagnosis and staging. *Cancer Nurs* 6:43, Philadelphia, Lippincott, 1983

if there has been a previous history of testicular cancer either in the person currently being evaluated or in any family member is important information to obtain. Inquiring about cryptorchidism, previous congenital abnor-malities, and hormonal drug usage should also be documented as part of the medical history.

## Physical Exam

A physical exam should include an examination of the neck for supraclavicular adenopathy, lungs, breast for gynecomastia, the abdomen for retroperitoneal masses, and the testicles. Any testicular mass found on clinical exam should be transilluminated. (See chapter 8 for the technique of transillumination of the testicles.) If a testicular mass does not transilluminate, it should be considered suspicious for testicular cancer.

## Diagnostic Studies

Ultrasound is obtained to identify scrotal masses and to discriminate between hydroceles and solid mass. Inguinal orchiectomy remains the standard approach for definitive pathological diagnosis. A biopsy or a transcrotal approach orchiectomy can cause possible spread of tumor into the inguinal lymph nodes and therefore is not recommended.[17] Both a fine needle biopsy and a transcrotal approach are contraindicated because surgical violation can result in a high incidence of local recurrence and metastasis to the inguinal lymph nodes, thereby changing normal predictable metastatic patterns of spread and making subsequent follow-up and management more complex. Chest x-rays and chest scans are utilized to evaluate the possibility of lung metastasis and abdominal scans are diagnostic for retroperitoneal and pelvic metastasis. These tests together with serum tumor markers consisting of the beta subunit of human chorionic gonadotropin (BHCG) and alpha-fetoprotein (AFP) can be useful in the staging of testicular cancer, but also in documenting disease recurrence, as well as in monitoring response to treatment.[18] (See Table 47-1.) Overall, HCG, AFP, or both will be elevated in 85% of males with disseminated testicular and primary retroperitoneal nonseminomatous germ cell tumors.[19]

## Prognostic Indicators

Most men with seminoma have tumor limited to the testis at the time of diagnosis. These men generally receive radiotherapy and almost all will remain free of cancer. At least 95% of men with seminoma will survive their disease. Of individuals with limited stage II seminoma 80%–90% will remain free of cancer. In men with large volume stage II seminoma, about 60% will remain tumor free after initial chemotherapy, plus radiation.

Overall 95% or more of men diagnosed with stage I and II nonseminomatous germ cell tumors will survive their disease. Men with limited advanced disease—either nonseminoma or seminoma—have a favorable prognosis with greater than a 90% cure rate. Men with high tumor volume have a 50%–60% cure rate. In general, those with serum marker elevation only or small volume disease without visceral involvement are highly curable and have a very good prognosis. Approximately 70% of the males with testicular cancer will fall into this category.

## CLASSIFICATION AND STAGING

There are several available staging systems utilized for testicular cancer.[20] The most common clinical staging systems used for seminoma and nonseminomatous germ cell tumors are from Royal Marsden Hospital (Table 47-3). Indiana University Hospital has developed an exclusive staging system utilized for only disseminated disease (Table 47-4).

## THERAPEUTIC APPROACHES AND NURSING CARE

### Nonseminomatous Germ Cell Tumors

Nonseminomatous germ cell tumors have served as an extraordinary example of integrating both surgical resection and/or combination chemotherapy in successful management of testicular cancer. Early-stage disease primarily is approached surgically. Subsequent stages are treated with cisplatin-based chemotherapy with possible postsurgical resection of remaining tumor.

#### Stage I

The choice of management for stage I nonseminomatous germ cell testis cancer is one of the most controversial topics in urologic oncology. A retroperitoneal lymph

**TABLE 47-3**   Royal Marsden Hospital Staging Classifications of Seminoma and Nonseminomatous Testicular Germ Cell Tumors

| SEMINOMA | |
|---|---|
| Stage I: | Tumor confined to the testes |
| Stage II: | Abdominal disease<br>IIA disease < 2 cm<br>IIB disease 2-5 cm<br>IIC disease < 5 cm. |
| Stage III: | Supradiaphragmatic, but nodally-confined disease |
| Stage IV: | Extragonadal involvement of lung, bone, or other viscera |

| NONSEMINOMAS | |
|---|---|
| Stage I: | Tumor that is confined to the testes |
| Stage II: | Tumor that has spread beyond the testes<br>"A" less than six lymph nodes, with none larger than 2 cm<br>"B" greater than six lymph nodes, any lymph nodes greater than 2 cm<br>"C" massive retroperitoneal disease |
| Stage III: | Tumors that are disseminated |

**TABLE 47-4**   Indiana University Staging System for Disseminated Disease

**Minimal Disease***
1. Elevated markers after RPLND
2. Cervical nodes (+/− retroperitoneal disease <10 cm)
3. Unresectable, but <10 cm, retroperitoneal disease
4. Minimal pulmonary disease (< 5 pulmonary metastases per lung and largest <2 cm in size with +/− retroperitoneal disease <10 cm)

**Moderate Disease***
5. Retroperitoneal disease >10 cm as only anatomic site of disease
6. Moderate pulmonary metastasis (5 to 10 pulmonary metastases per lung and largest < 3 cm, or mediastinal mass <50% intrathoracic diameter, or solitary pulmonary metastasis and size >2 cm with +/− retroperitoneal disease <10 cm)

**Advanced Disease^**
7. Advanced pulmonary metastasis (mediastinal mass >50% intrathoracic diameter or >10 pulmonary metastasis per lung field or pulmonary metastasis >3 cm with +/− retroperitoneal disease <10 cm. Also any NSGCT or seminoma mediastinal primary of >50% intrathoracic diameter)
8. Retroperitoneal disease >10 cm, plus pulmonary metastasis +/− supraclavicular disease
9. Hepatic, bone, or CNS metastasis

*Both minimal and moderate disease are considered "good risk."

^Advanced disease is considered "poor risk."

node dissection (RPLND) has been the time-honored approach to the treatment of testicular cancer confined to the testis. Recently, however, this approach for patients with early-stage nonseminomatous germ cell tumors has been challenged.[21] Treatment options following orchiectomy include surgery with a RPLND or a nonoperative approach.

The rationale for surgery is well grounded. RPLND in low volume testis cancer is useful for staging because approximately 30% of patients with clinical stage I testis cancer are, in fact, pathological stage II. Surgery alone provides cure to approximately 90% of patients with pathological stage I testis cancer with less than 1% chance of local recurrence. Individuals who undergo a staging RPLND and are found to have pathologically negative lymph nodes are classified as pathological stage I. Ten percent of pathological stage I males will develop recurrent disease.[14] Most relapses will occur in the lungs since the lymph nodes within the retroperitoneum have been surgically removed. With close monthly follow-up the first year and every two months the second year, virtually all individuals who develop recurrent disease will have minimal disease, for which the cure rate with cisplatin-based chemotherapy is 99% or greater.[17] Therefore, RPLND is advantageous for two reasons, for staging and as a therapeutic modality.

The RPLND involves selection of a surgical approach to best visualize the nodal involvement. Normal abdominal surgical preparations are made preoperatively. A nasogastric tube and indwelling catheter are anchored. Central and arterial lines may be utilized to maximize feedback during and after surgery. Routine postoperative care is essential to a full recovery. Discharge is usually on the fifth postoperative day.[20] Postoperative evaluation occurs in approximately four to six weeks. Recommendations for follow-up include serum markers and chest x-rays monthly the first year, every other month the second year, every six months in years three through five, and yearly thereafter.

The major objection to RPLND has been the fertility consequences. Males who undergo full bilateral lymphadenectomy universally lose emission and the ability to ejaculate with resultant loss of fertility.[22] In an attempt to minimize ejaculatory dysfunction, "nerve-sparing" RPLND has been successfully refined. Donahue and colleagues demonstrated that the unilateral dissection is an acceptable alternative in individuals with grossly negative nodes.[23] Unilateral RPLND generally involves surgical dissection of lymph nodes on the same side as the primary lesion with limited intervention on the contralateral side. This innovation preserves the contralateral sympathetic efferent nerves and normal ejaculatory function in 75%–100% of males with testicular cancer.[24]

Selection for surveillance must be considered carefully for individuals with clinical stage I testicular cancer. Individuals must have normal serum BHCG and AFP following orchiectomy, plus normal x-rays and scans. Since it is known that approximately 30% of these individuals will relapse, primarily within the retroperitoneum,

individuals selected for this approach must be highly motivated and able, logistically and psychologically, to comply with consistent lifelong follow-up.[25]

### Pathological stage II A/B

Individuals who are thought to have clinical stage I testis cancer, but are found at RPLND to have metastasis to the retroperitoneum are considered to have pathological stage II disease with either microscopic (II A) or gross (II B) involvement. If no additional therapy is provided to pathological stage II patients postsurgery, approximately 30% of stage II A and 50% of stage II B will relapse.[25] Significant improvement in relapse rates have been seen with adjuvant cisplatin-based chemotherapy. Two immediate postoperative courses of adjuvant cisplatin-based chemotherapy—usually BEP (bleomycin, etoposide, cisplatin)—after complete resection of stage II disease prevent relapse in nearly 100% of men diagnosed with testicular cancer (Table 47-5).

### Clinical stage II B

Those individuals who have a nonpalpable (<2–3 cm) abdominal mass or fewer than five lymph nodes visualized on CT scan traditionally have undergone RPLND with complete resection followed by either observation or adjuvant chemotherapy, with outstanding results. However, based on the results of chemotherapy as primary treatment in disseminated disease, oncologists currently promote the use of initial combination cisplatin-based chemotherapy to achieve radiographic complete remission while hopefully avoiding the morbidity and expense of an RPLND. Chemotherapy alone will provide 98% of individuals with a complete remission, with less than one-fourth requiring RPLND postchemotherapy for residual disease or because of persistent serum marker elevation.[26]

### Disseminated disease

A palpable abdominal mass with lymph nodes >5 cm or involvement of more than five lymph nodes is desig-

**TABLE 47-5**  Testicular Germ Cell Cancer Chemotherapy Regimens

---

**Adjunct Chemotherapy (BEP)**
Bleomycin 30 units, weekly for 12 weeks
Cisplatin 20 mg/m$^2$, daily for 5 days
Etoposide 100 mg/m$^2$, daily for 5 days—every 28 days for 2 cycles

**Disseminated Disease Chemotherapy (BEP)**
Bleomycin 30 units, weekly for 9–12 weeks
Cisplatin 20 mg/m$^2$, daily for 5 days
Etoposide 100 mg/m$^2$, daily for 5 days—every 21 days for 3–4 cycles

**Salvage Chemotherapy (VeIP)**
Vinblastine 0.11 mg/kg on days 1 and 2
Ifosfamide 1.2 Gm/m$^2$, daily for 5 days plus Mesna
Cisplatin 20 mg/m$^2$, daily for 5 days—every 21 days for 4 cycles

nated as stage II C disease. Abdominal disease of this magnitude will prohibit initial surgical resection. Metastasis above the diaphragm, involvement of visceral organs, brain, or bone is classified as stage III. Approximately 70% of men with stage III disease will achieve a complete remission. An additional 10%–20% will normalize serum markers, but have persistent radiographic abnormalities and require subsequent surgery to achieve disease-free status.[27]

In men who present with advanced or bulky disease, chemotherapy is the mainstay of treatment. Following orchiectomy, initial cisplatin-based chemotherapy is recommended for cytoreduction and potential cure. The most widely used front-line regimen is BEP (see Table 47-5), consisting of bleomycin, etoposide, and cisplatin for three to four cycles, depending on whether an individual is deemed good- or poor-risk.[28] Chemotherapy should always be given on time regardless of myelosuppression, due to the rapidity of tumor cellular division and growth. Likewise, dose reductions should be avoided, and cytokines used when indicated. Since cisplatin is not myelosuppressive the dose is rarely, if ever, reduced.

Evaluation of men with disseminated germ cell tumors treated with BEP has led to various staging systems that estimate prognosis. The Indiana University Staging System (Table 47-3) separated those patients with minimal and moderate disease who were considered a "good-risk" with a greater than 90%–99% cure rate from those individuals with advanced disease considered at "poor-risk" with a 50%–60% cure rate.[14] Treatment strategies in advanced disease have focused on minimizing toxicity for men who are a good risk, and investigating innovative and intensive therapy for men who are a poor risk (Figure 47-1).

Research has shown that in men presenting with minimal to moderate disease, three cycles of BEP is the chemotherapy regimen of choice (Table 47-5). Multiple studies have demonstrated that three cycles of BEP are equivalent to four cycles of EP; BEP is better than EP alone (if bleomycin cannot be given for medical reasons, the individual should receive four cycles of EP); and finally carboplatin plus etoposide is less effective than EP.[14,29–31]

The present emphasis in the initial treatment of advanced disseminated poor-risk disease is the exploration of cisplatin-intense regimen and the incorporation of new innovative agents. Intensification of therapy has included both high-dose cisplatin as well as administering all five active agents within the same regimen (i.e., VIP/VeB—etoposide, ifosfamide, cisplatin, vinblastine, bleomycin).[32] Other intensification has included high-dose carboplatin and etoposide with either bone marrow transplantation or peripheral stem cell rescue.[33–35]

Cisplatin-based chemotherapy is not without morbidity. Selective 5HT-3 antagonists and other supportive care aspects have made the cisplatin-based chemotherapy utilized in testicular cancer relatively well-tolerated. While alopecia is universal, with good assessment, cisplatin-induced renal damage and bleomycin-induced lung damage are rare. Aggressive pre- and posthydration amelio-

rates nephrotoxicity, and careful pulmonary evaluation will pinpoint toxicity early. Febrile neutropenic episodes, rarely of major consequence due to empirical antibiotic therapy, occur in approximately 25% of patients. Thrombocytopenia is not common. Other manageable side effects may include diarrhea, mucositis, constipation/paralytic ileus, peripheral neuropathy, and hypomagnesemia.

Thirty percent of men who present with disseminated disease will require surgery postchemotherapy.[20] A postchemotherapy RPLND (PC RPLND) is indicated if a residual mass remains. Most commonly a full bilateral nodal dissection is performed with the subsequent loss of emission and antegrade ejaculation. A small percentage of men will qualify for a nerve-sparing procedure that may spare ejaculatory function. Postchemotherapy surgery patients have a higher incidence of side effects than primary RPLND patients and are usually admitted postoperatively to an intensive care unit.[20] Side effects of PC RPLND include pulmonary toxicity from the combination of bleomycin and anesthesia; temporary rise in serum creatinine and tachycardia from necessary fluid restrictions; noncardiogenic pulmonary edema; and ileus.[20,36] Hospitalization usually lasts about six days. For individuals with residual disease above the diaphragm, thoracic surgery may be necessary to remove residual disease. The scope of the thoracic surgery and potential for cure will depend on the amount and placement of residual disease present postchemotherapy.

### Late relapse testis cancer

Until recently, it has been generally accepted that if an individual was to relapse following surgical resection or chemotherapy-induced complete remission, it would occur within two years following completion of therapy. Late relapse in testicular cancer is thought to be a recurrence after greater than a 24-month disease-free interval. As an increased number of case reports of late relapse appeared, retrospective analysis of several large series were undertaken in an attempt to determine the true rate of relapse.[37–41] These series consistently describe a relapse rate following a complete remission of 2%–4% with recurrences as late as 18 years. In general after surgery, individuals recurring with mature teratoma have done well. Men with marker positive neoplasms have tended to recur with bulky disease and have had a less favorable response even when surgery has been combined with chemotherapy.

Indiana University retrospectively analyzed 81 men who had recurrence after two or more years.[42,43] Sixty percent of these men relapsed beyond five years, with the latest relapse being 16 years. Marker elevations were seen with 56% of individuals having an elevated AFP and 27% an elevated BHCG. Fifteen men (19%) had a recurrence of teratoma and eight remain free of disease. Four additional men are currently disease free. Overall, 65 individuals received cisplatin-based chemotherapy and 26% achieved disease-free status with chemotherapy with

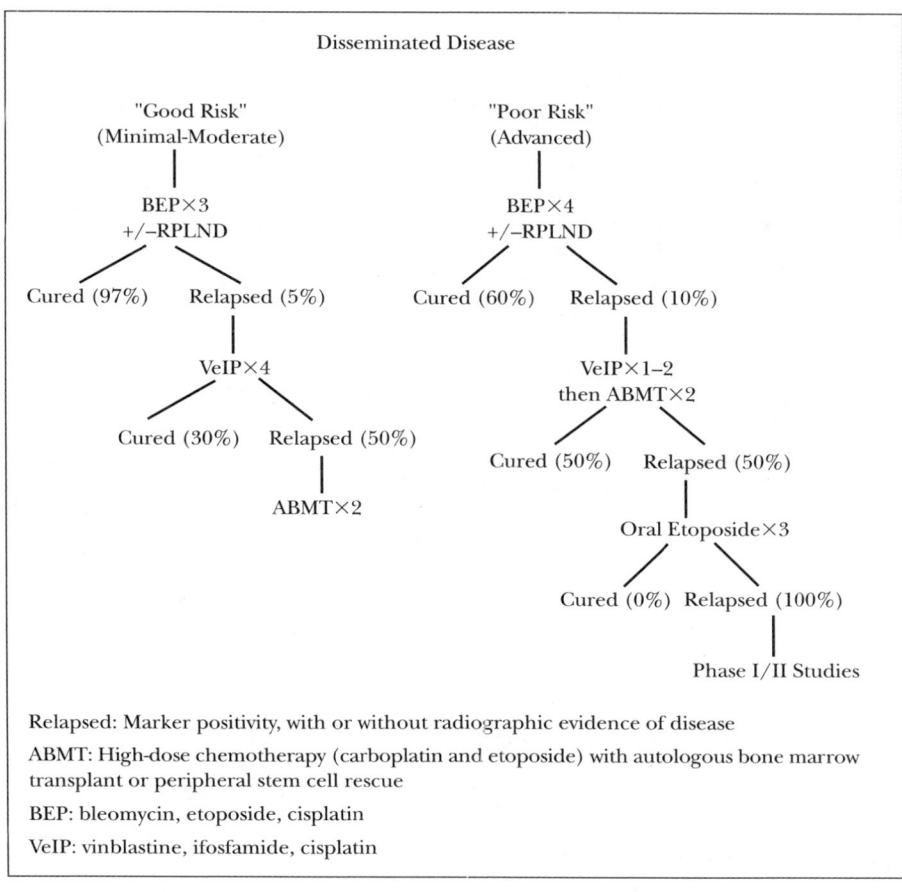

**Disseminated Disease**

"Good Risk"
(Minimal-Moderate)

BEP×3
+/−RPLND

Cured (97%)   Relapsed (5%)

VeIP×4

Cured (30%)   Relapsed (50%)

ABMT×2

"Poor Risk"
(Advanced)

BEP×4
+/−RPLND

Cured (60%)   Relapsed (10%)

VeIP×1–2
then ABMT×2

Cured (50%)   Relapsed (50%)

Oral Etoposide×3

Cured (0%)   Relapsed (100%)

Phase I/II Studies

Relapsed: Marker positivity, with or without radiographic evidence of disease

ABMT: High-dose chemotherapy (carboplatin and etoposide) with autologous bone marrow transplant or peripheral stem cell rescue

BEP: bleomycin, etoposide, cisplatin

VeIP: vinblastine, ifosfamide, cisplatin

**FIGURE 47-1**  Treatment for disseminated testicular cancer.

or without the addition of aggressive surgery. Twelve of these 17 men have relapsed. Only two individuals treated with chemotherapy alone are presently disease free; both were chemotherapy naive. Another series demonstrated similar results.[44]

The appearance of rapidly progressive, marker-positive cancer after more than two years has been puzzling. One possibility may be that residual, mature teratoma may have the ability to de-differentiate into malignant germ cell tumors after a length of time. The presence of teratoma in the original pathology may be a statistically significant predictor of late relapse. The tendency toward large-volume disease at the time of relapse may be a result of insufficient follow-up. Nurses need to educate patients that at least yearly medical evaluations should continue indefinitely for all men with a prior history of testicular cancer.

## Seminomas Germ Cell Tumors

Pure seminomas account for approximately 47% of all germ cell tumors of the testicles.[45] With the use of effective chemotherapy and radiotherapy, the overall cure rate for all stages is above 90%.[46] Fortunately, unlike nonsemi-

nomatous testicular tumors, 80% of seminomas present as clinical stage I disease (i.e., confined to the testis alone).[25]

Seminomas are known to be exquisitely sensitive to radiotherapy. Both stage I and stage II A/B are treated with external-beam irradiation. Chemotherapy is the primary treatment of bulky stage II C and disseminated disease. The management following chemotherapy remains controversial.

### Stage I and II A/B

A total dose of 25 Gy of radiotherapy is administered in 1.25 to 1.5 Gy daily fractions for individuals with stage I disease.[46] For stage II A/B, a boost dose of an additional 5–10 Gy to the involved nodes with a 5 cm margin is recommended. Both anterior and posterior fields are treated. The area of treatment includes the paracaval and para-aortic nodes extending superiorly to the level of T-10/11 and extending inferiorly to include the bilateral common iliac and the ipsilateral external iliac nodes. Elective radiation to the mediastinum is no longer indicated.[47] If the scrotum has been violated at the time of orchiectomy, if tumor spill has occurred, or if positive margins are present, the radiation field may be extended to include the ipsilateral hemiscrotum. If an inguinal approach to orchiectomy is utilized, the scrotum and contralateral testis are shielded to limit scatter irradiation to the remaining testicle. The bladder is also shielded. Although surveillance may be an option following orchiectomy for stage I seminoma, excellent results with minimal side effects and morbidity make radiation the treatment of choice.

Oligospermia or azoospermia may occur as a result of radiation even when appropriate radiation shields are employed. Spermatogenesis recovery is dose dependent. Recovery of pretreatment sperm counts may occur between nine months to five years with most men recovering within one year.[48] Other treatment-related side effects include mild nausea, myelosuppression, diarrhea, mild anorexia, and fatigue.

Long-term survival of more than 95% of men diagnosed with stage I disease is expected.[49–51] Eighty to ninety percent of men with evidence of retroperitoneal metastasis <5 cm (stage II A/B) will be cured.[52]

## Stage II C

Treatment of bulky, localized retroperitoneal disease is controversial. Both chemotherapy and radiotherapy are effective. It is known that radiotherapy alone provides cure to 30%–60% of patients with stage II C disease.[25] However, a direct correlation exists between the volume of disease and the anticipated cure rate with radiotherapy. Individuals who present with large abdominal masses (> 10 cm) have a high relapse rate with radiation alone. Initial combination cisplatin-based chemotherapy for men with bulky retroperitoneal disease allows for a greater than 90% cure rate.[45,46] In individuals with abdominal masses between 5–10 cm, equivalent results can be obtained with either radiotherapy or chemotherapy. A viable option may be to use chemotherapy for individuals with retroperitoneal disease >5 cm and radiation as a front-line, single modality treatment for those individuals with <5 cm retroperitoneal disease, retaining chemotherapy for the 30%–40% that will eventually relapse.[25]

## Stage III and IV

Initial radiotherapy for metastasis to distant sites and bulky abdominal masses produces survival rates of 20%–30% while cisplatin-based regimens will yield response rates of 60%–100%.[45,53–55] Stage IV, extranodal disease of the bone, lung, liver, or central nervous system has a cure rate of 60%–80% with chemotherapy. Bleomycin, etoposide, and cisplatin for three to four cycles, in identical doses to those used in nonseminomatous germ cell tumors, are standard treatment (Table 47-5).

Management of residual disease following chemotherapy remains debatable. Motzer et al support biopsy following chemotherapy if the residual mass is greater than 3 cm with possible resection.[56] Indiana University and other centers endorse close monthly observation versus surgery for two reasons. First, a retrospective review of patients at Indiana University revealed only a 10% incidence of significant pathological finding on biopsy with residual radiographic evidence of disease.[57] Secondly, following therapy, a dense desmoplastic reaction may occur at the tumor site making surgery difficult, therefore increasing morbidity.[25]

## Salvage Therapy in Recurrent Disease

Twenty to thirty percent of individuals will not achieve a complete remission with initial therapy, and ten percent will relapse following a complete remission.[29,58,59] Men in this cohort are candidates for second-line or "salvage" therapy (Figure 47-1). Testicular cancer is one of the few cancers where second-line chemotherapy offers a chance of cure. Men who fail to achieve a complete response with salvage therapy have a dismal probability for long-term survival. Greater than 50% of individuals will relapse following a complete remission from salvage therapy.[60] Present therapeutic strategies for salvage treatment include chemotherapy, surgical salvage, phase II agents, and high-dose chemotherapy with bone marrow rescue.

### Salvage chemotherapy

Evaluation for disease recurrence is a thought-provoking process. Occasionally individuals will be misdirected for salvage chemotherapy based on misleading radiographic evidence or rising serum markers (AFP, BHCG) that appear to demonstrate progressive disease. Benign, growing teratoma; false elevations of BHCG due to marijuana use; cross-reactivity with luteinizing hormone; hepatitis; and pseudonodules from bleomycin may all mimic presentation of metastatic disease. Likewise, persistent marker elevation may represent a cancer within the brain or remaining testis that can serve as sanctuary sites.

The combination of cisplatin, vinblastine (or etoposide, if not included in initial chemotherapy), and ifosfamide (VeIP) is the recommended front-line salvage regimen for recurrent disease when initial induction therapy was composed of cisplatin, etoposide (or vinblastine), and bleomycin (Table 47-5).[61–63] Einhorn and associates at Indiana University reported 45% achieved disease-free status and 23% remained disease-free with four cycles of VeIP.[64]

Phase I and II trials are in progress investigating agents for use in third-line chemotherapy. Oral etoposide is a schedule-dependent agent known to have activity in germ cell tumors.[65] Research has demonstrated a response in individuals who have failed to achieve a complete remission following salvage chemotherapy. Oral etoposide has also been shown to significantly prolong remission duration in men who have achieved a complete remission with salvage chemotherapy.[60,66] Recent evaluation of paclitaxel demonstrated a 26% response as second-line therapy in men who did not obtain disease-free status with primary chemotherapy. VIP/VeB (etoposide, ifosfamide, cisplatin, vinblastine, and bleomycin) in combination is being investigated. Other agents presently being explored include gemcitabine, vinorelbine, all-*trans* retinoic acid and the topoisomerase I inhibitors.

### Surgical salvage

Individuals with persistently elevated serum markers, indicative of persistent viable disease following salvage chemotherapy, have not usually been considered surgical candidates because of the presumed systemic nature of the disease. However, some of these men do have locoregional tumors amenable to resection.[67] Approximately 20% of carefully selected individuals achieve long-term survival with salvage surgery.[61]

## High-Dose Chemotherapy with Rescue

Individuals who recur following salvage chemotherapy or do not respond to first-line cisplatin therapy are considered cisplatin-refractory. These individuals are incurable by standard chemotherapy. Autologous bone marrow and/or peripheral blood stem cell rescue in conjunction with high-dose chemotherapy have been and continue to be investigated in this population. High-dose chemotherapy has been found to offer a better response than conventional chemotherapy.

Initially researchers explored the use of etoposide in high doses without cisplatin.[68,69] Etoposide was investigated in high dosages for the treatment of testicular cancer primarily because of efficacy, but also for its manageable side effects. Although complete responses occurred with etoposide alone, remissions were brief and no impact was made with regard to survival.

Subsequent research underscored the importance of combining etoposide with cisplatin due to synergy between the two drugs. Pico and colleagues demonstrated a continuous complete response in 31% of men with recurrent germ cell tumor with high-dose etoposide, cisplatin, and cyclophosphamide.[70] Unfortunately cisplatin, the most active agent in testicular cancer, is poorly suited to dose intensity due to the known side effects of nephrotoxicity and ototoxicity. Therefore, carboplatin, a second-generation platinum analogue, is better suited for dose intensification because its toxicity is largely confined to myelosuppression. A number of preclinical and clinical studies suggested similar anti-tumor activity in regard to carboplatin and cisplatin.[71] In 1989 Nichols and associates reported responses to high-dose etoposide and carboplatin in 14 of 33 men, including eight complete remissions and three men obtaining continuous disease-free survival for greater than one year.[63] All eligible individuals had extensive prior therapy and two-thirds were cisplatin-refractory. Other investigators at Indiana University have subsequently provided long-term follow-up for 40 individuals.[72,73] Overall, 60% of those men achieved an objective response with 30% in complete remission. Fifteen percent of the complete responders achieved and remained in

remission beyond two years. A large national study confirmed these responses.[74]

A logical next step has been to incorporate high-dose chemotherapy with rescue earlier in the treatment of poor-risk individuals. Seigert et al treated 55 men with conventional cisplatin, etoposide, and ifosfamide before initiating high-dose carboplatin.[75] Thirty-eight percent of individuals responded with disease-free survivals of between 3–26 months. Motzer and associates reported the use of two to three cycles of VAB-6 (bleomycin, cyclophosphamide, actinomycin D, vinblastine, cisplatin) followed by high-dose carboplatin and etoposide with bone marrow support, with 56% obtaining a complete response.[76]

It is established that a small but definite cure rate exists for heavily pretreated, refractory individuals. However, it remains unclear whether high-dose chemotherapy will become a part of standard initial therapy in poor-risk individuals with testicular cancer.[77]

## Sanctuary Sites

In advanced testis cancer the central nervous system (CNS) and contralateral testicle are the most common sanctuary sites.[25] CNS metastasis, whether it is present at diagnosis or as a manifestation of relapse, is approached with curative intent. Chemotherapy poorly penetrates the blood-brain barrier. Whole-brain radiation therapy of 50 Gy over five weeks in combination with chemotherapy for systemic disease is recommended for individuals with CNS metastasis and disseminated disease. Those individuals relapsing with a single CNS focus without evidence of systemic relapse undergo resection followed by radiotherapy and two postoperative cisplatin-based chemotherapy regimens. Occult CNS metastases should be suspected if in the presence of chest/abdominal radiological remission following therapy, new elevations or persistent tumor markers are present. In this situation, CAT scan or MRI of the brain should be obtained even in the absence of clinical symptoms.

It is questionable if chemotherapy penetrates the testicle which is why the testicle has long been considered a sanctuary site for tumor cells. Normally the testis primary tumor is surgically resected prior to treatment. However, in the presence of advanced disseminated disease and positive tumor markers, chemotherapy may be initiated prior to a tissue diagnosis. At the completion of chemotherapy the involved testis is removed. Whenever markers remain elevated following removal of the involved testicle (in the absence of radiographic evidence of disease) a second testis primary should be investigated.

## SYMPTOM MANAGEMENT AND SUPPORTIVE CARE

The time of diagnosis and initiation of treatment are stressful. Education must begin early. Careful explanation of the nature of the disease, its treatment, goal of therapy, and side effects is essential.[77] Information needs to be provided and repeated at various intervals along the treatment continuum. Comprehensive education is not an easy task as the patient's and family's anxiety level may be elevated from perceived and real threats of mortality and alterations in life roles and sexual identity. The individual with cancer should be included in all treatment-related options. All questions need to be answered fully with openness and honesty.

## Surgery

An inguinal orchiectomy performed to establish a histological diagnosis is an outpatient procedure. Nursing interventions should focus on postoperative teaching regarding pain management, activity level, and incisional wound care. Individuals and family need to learn how to change the dry, sterile dressing and to be alert to signs of infection and unusual bleeding. Men need to understand that neither sexual function nor fertility will be impaired or changed. However, an altered body image may result. Supportive interventions may be indicated to improve coping.

Care of the individual undergoing a RPLND, outside of the issues of fertility, is similar to other abdominal surgeries. However, for the person who has had chemotherapy, RPLND is associated with specific side effects, namely adult respiratory syndrome with pulmonary fluid overload, ileus, and fertility issues.

### Pulmonary complications

Men who have received bleomycin at a cumulative dose of greater than 200 mg/m² are at greater risk of pulmonary edema with subsequent respiratory failure or death during the postoperative recovery period.[78] Individuals with even mild bleomycin toxicity demonstrate to some degree arterial oxygen desaturation with high concentrations of inspired oxygen and an abnormal carbon monoxide diffusion capacity.[79] Special precautions are taken prior to surgery to safeguard patients, including baseline pulmonary function test, careful physical exam, radiographic imaging of the lungs, and alerting the anesthesiologist.

Rigid fluid restrictions imposed during surgery and a reduction in inspired oxygen to an $FiO_2$ of 0.24 has been shown to prevent mortality.[78] The day before surgery, individuals begin a clear liquid diet with nothing by mouth permitted after midnight. Intravenous fluid consisting of 50 cc/hr of synthetic volume expander and 25 cc/hr of $D_5$ 1/2 NS begin before surgery. Fluid restrictions continue postoperatively. However, following surgery 150–200 cc/hr of ice chips are usually allowed. A clear liquid diet is introduced when bowel sounds have been auscultated. Intravenous fluids are gradually decreased.

As a result of fluid restrictions, transient elevations of the serum creatinine and sinus tachycardia may occur. Kidney function is assessed through close monitoring of laboratory values, intake and output, and daily weight. Auscultation is routinely performed to assess cardiac function. Over time pulmonary function tests have been shown to return to baseline normal a median of four years after treatment.[80]

### Gastrointestinal complications

Ileus, a common side effect of abdominal surgery in general, may be prolonged for two to four days after an RPLND depending on the extent of the abdominal resection performed and length of time under anesthesia. Men are started on a clear liquid diet the day before surgery and undergo bowel preparation usually consisting of ingesting magnesium citrate or a full mechanical bowel preparation. A nasogastric tube is placed during surgery and will remain in place until normal bowel sounds are present. After auscultation of normal bowel sounds, a clear liquid diet will be initiated, advancing to a regular diet as tolerated.

### Fertility

The traditional bilateral RPLND results in the loss of antegrade ejaculation with resultant infertility from retrograde ejaculation. The ability to experience a normal orgasm is not impaired. The nerve-sparing modification of the classic RPLND has steadily increased postoperative ejaculatory rates. Ninety-eight percent of men undergoing nerve-sparing RPLND will have normal preoperative fertility. Awareness and sensitivity to the individual's and family's educational needs and initiating appropriate interventions to provide for psychosocial adjustment to the real or possible fertility changes will promote coping and acceptance. Sperm banking prior to initiation of treatment may be an option depending on the stage of disease and sperm count at diagnosis. Sperm banking can take weeks to obtain sufficient viable sperm. Men need to be aware of the possibility of treatment delay and cost-related issues involving collection and storage. Therefore, sperm banking may not be a viable option due to the aggressiveness of the disease.

## Radiation

The resultant toxicities of abdominal radiotherapy for testicular cancer are less severe than in the past due to improved equipment and computerized axial tomographic planning.[81] Sequelae that may be problematic include diarrhea, fatigue, nausea, fertility issues, myelosuppression, and occasionally bladder irritation and ulcers.

### Gastrointestinal complications

Loose stools may result from radiation. Individuals should be instructed to manage associated diarrhea with diet and over-the-counter drugs but to seek medical attention if diarrhea continues despite appropriate interventions. A prescriptive antidiarrheal may be indicated. Dietary modifications with a low residue diet may be helpful.[82] A low-residue diet is designed to reduce the amount of fiber in the intestinal tract by restricting indigestible carbohydrates such as milk products, high fat-content foods, fruit and vegetables with seeds or skins, and high-fiber breads.

Unlike radiation to other parts of the body, nausea and vomiting are not unusual with the first radiotherapy treatment. Oral antiemetics administered one hour prior to the radiotherapy treatment and as needed usually controls the associated mild nausea and vomiting.[82] Serotonin 5HT-3 antagonists used in combination with a steroid may be useful. Light meals prior to treatment should be encouraged.

### Fertility

Radiotherapy does not effect libido or potency but can lead to impairment of spermatogenesis.[83] During radiotherapy gonad shields are in place; however, scatter radiation can occur to the remaining testis, decreasing sperm production or resulting in azoospermia.[18] Individuals and families need to know that recovery to pretreatment sperm levels may take from 9 to 18 months or as long as five years.[84] The opportunity for sperm banking may be appropriate prior to radiation therapy.

### Myelosuppression

Radiation to the para-aortic lymph nodes and the pelvis often produces myelosuppression. Weekly complete blood counts with differential and platelets are monitored. Acute complications are uncommon. Information should be provided on the importance of seeking medical assistance for fever when neutropenia is present. Instruction should be provided to avoid medication that could potentially mask a fever. Individuals should be made aware that fatigue may interfere with normal activities. Pacing activities and frequent rest periods will help the patient cope with fatigue. Also, instructions should be given to call the physician's office if bruising or unusual bleeding occurs since these could be a sign of thrombocytopenia. However, the need for blood product support is unusual.

Between 4%–10% of individuals will experience dyspepsia with radiotherapy.[85] Small low-fat frequent meals, avoiding meals and snacks within one hour of bedtime, and the use of antacids may provide relief from dyspepsia. However, the use of over-the-counter antacids needs to be monitored since medical intervention for an active gastric ulcer may be indicated.

## Chemotherapy

The side effects of chemotherapy are specific to the drug combinations and the dosages administered, the volume of disease present, and history of prior therapy. Nursing management can best be approached with awareness and anticipation of potential side effects (Table 47-6).

## CONTINUITY OF CARE: NURSING CHALLENGES

The recent changes in health care delivery have modified certain aspects in the approach of care for testicular cancer. The shift from inpatient to primarily outpatient chemotherapy, the role of managed health care, continued shortening of inpatient hospitalization following surgery, and the increasingly important role of home care has impacted how care is provided to the individual with testicular cancer.

Nursing is challenged in a compressed time frame to provide the patient and family with the necessary explanations of testicular cancer, treatment, self-care, and long-term issues. The importance of a ready-made plan of care that can be individualized to identify specific patient issues, organize care, shorten planning time, and better utilize nursing time is essential. Critical or care pathways developed for testicular cancer are currently perceived as a method to manage individual needs within a multidisciplinary framework, identify outcomes and necessary resources, and direct interventions within the expected time frame. Pathways can be utilized by nursing, medicine, and support staff for specific aspects of treatment or across the health care continuum to provide individualized care and hopefully to balance quality care with cost-saving efficiency.[97]

Within the pathways health professionals can incorporate added support and referrals within the community, not only to assist coping, but also for transportation, child care, and financial assistance for identified individuals.

Home care can be of assistance with management of hydration including assessment of fluid intake and output; with phlebotomy to monitor lab results; with monitoring nausea and vomiting; with wound care; and with discharge postsurgery that may include administration of antibiotics. With the continued need for cost containment and the advent of managed-care, home care nurses may experience a more primary role in treatment and education. Hospice in the home environment is a preferable option for those with terminal disease.

## CONCLUSION

Although testicular cancer is a rare and devastating disease to the young population it affects, it also is one of the most highly curable cancers. Testicular self-exam

**TABLE 47-6** Nursing Care and Educational Needs of Patients Receiving Chemotherapy for Testicular Cancer

| Problem | Drug(s) | Nursing Interventions |
|---------|---------|----------------------|
| Nausea/vomiting | cisplatin ifosfamide | • Administer prophylactic antiemetics with 5 HT-3 antagonist and high-dose dexamethasone[86]<br>• Instruct how to take antiemetics<br>• Encourage and maintain adequate fluid intake<br>• Consider the use of music and relaxation therapy[87,88] |
| Constipation | vinblastine etoposide | • Assess bowel status prior to giving drug<br>• Encourage fluids and high-fiber diet<br>• Monitor bowel sounds<br>• Instruct patient to report significant bowel changes |
| Myelosuppression | ifosfamide vinblastine etoposide | • Monitor complete blood count<br>• Instruct patient to report signs of infection, fever, bleeding, shortness of breath, severe weakness, tachycardia<br>• Discuss avoiding crowds and individuals with active infections, bleeding precautions<br>• Inform patients with advanced disease that blood/platelet transfusions may be necessary |
| Nephrotoxicity | cisplatin ifosfamide | • Monitor renal function tests (creatinine and BUN), daily intake and output[89]<br>• Provide aggressive pre- and posthydration and increased oral intake<br>• Avoidance of aminoglycosides for the treatment of granulocytopenic fever when receiving cisplatin[90] |
| Hemorrhagic cystitis | ifosfamide | • Obtain urinalysis daily, if >10 RBCs per high-powered field, alert physician and hold drug<br>• Provide aggressive pre- and posthydration and instruct patient to increase oral intake<br>• Administer Mesna, a uroprotectant, as directed |
| Integumentary changes | ifosfamide bleomycin etoposide | • Prepare patient for hair loss, reinforcing its temporary nature[91]<br>• Alert patient regarding skin hyperpigmentation and nail changes |
| Reproduction | cisplatin etoposide bleomycin ifosfamide vinblastine | • Arrange for sperm banking if possible prior to chemotherapy<br>• Reinforce that ejaculation/impotence will not change<br>• Inform patients of azoospermia for at least 12 months with normal spermatogenesis returning in 50% of men within two years and those treated with 3–4 cycles of BEP are at higher risk for persistent semen abnormalities[14,17,92–94] |
| Neurological changes | cisplatin vinblastine bleomycin | • Instruct reporting of numbness and tingling of hands and feet (i.e., Raynaud's phenomenon)[95]<br>• Inform patients to wear gloves and dress warmly in cold weather<br>• Instruct patients to report hearing changes[90,96]<br>• Obtain baseline and serial audiometry for high-risk patients (i.e., >50 years, total dose of >400 mg cisplatin, abnormal renal function[77,96] |
| Pulmonary complications | bleomycin | • Assess for bibasilar rales, inspirational lag, and cough[14,20]<br>• Evaluate men at high risk for fibrosis (i.e., smokers, decreased renal function, previous chest irradiation, and >450 units)[14,92,94] |

remains the best available tool for early diagnosis and treatment. Most males today can be successfully treated with few adverse side affects unlike the situation 20 years ago. Today's high cure rate of testicular cancer can be attributed to dedicated clinical researchers who utilize combination modalities such as surgery, chemotherapy, radiation therapy, and bone marrow transplantation in the treatment of testicular cancer. Researchers continue to look for ways to improve current treatment modalities.

# REFERENCES

1. American Cancer Society: *Cancer Facts and Figures.* Atlanta, American Cancer Society, 1996

2. Chilvers C, Forman D, Pike M, et al: Apparent doubling of frequency on undescended testis in England and Wales in 1962–1981. *Lancet* 2:330–332, 1984

3. Van den Eden SK, Weiss NS: Is testicular cancer incidence in blacks increasing? *Am Public Health* 79:1553–1554, 1989

4. Tollured DJ, Blattner WA, Frasier MC: Familial testicular cancer and urogenital development anomalies. *Cancer* 55: 1849–1854, 1989

5. Nichols C, Heerema N, Palmer C, et al: Klinefelter's syndrome associated with mediastinal germ cell neoplasm. *J Clin Oncol* 5:1290–1294, 1987

6. Batata MA, Whitemore WFJ, Chu FCH: Cryptorchidism and testicular cancer. *J Urol* 124:382–387, 1980

7. Aristizabal S, Davis JR, Miller RC: Bilateral primary germ cell tumors. Report of four cases and review of the literature. *Cancer* 42:591–597, 1978

8. Martin DC: Germinal cell tumors of the testis. *J Urol* 121: 422–424, 1979

9. Atkin N, Baker M: Specific chromosomal marker in seminoma and malignant teratoma of the testes. *Cancer Genet Cytogenet* 10:199–204, 1983

10. Andervont H, Shimkin M, Canter H: Susceptibility of seven inbred strains of the F1 hybrids to estrogen-induced testicular tumors and occurrence of spontaneous testicular tumors in strain BALB/c mice. *J Natl Cancer Inst* 25:1069–1081, 1960

11. Cosgrove M, Benton B, Henderson B: Male genitourinary abnormalities and maternal diethystilbesterol. *Urology* 117: 220–222, 1977

12. Depue R, Pike M, Henderson B: Estrogen exposure during gestation and the risk of testicular cancer. *J Natl Cancer Inst* 71:1151–1155, 1983

13. Gill W, Schumaker G, Bibbo M: Structural and functional abnormalities in the sex organs of male offspring of mothers treated with DES. *Reprod Med* 16:147–153, 1976

14. Loehrer P: Testicular cancer, in Carbone P, Brain M (eds): *Current Therapy in Hematology-Oncology* (ed 4). Ontario, BC Dekker, 1992, pp 300–305

15. Jamieson J, Dobson J: The lymphatics of the testicle. *Lancet* 1:493, 1910

16. Hubbard SM, Jenkins J: An overview of current concepts in the management of patients with testicular tumors of germ cell origin—Part I: Pathophysiology, diagnosis, and staging. *Cancer News* 6:43–49, 1983

17. Roth B, Griest A, Kubilis P, et al: Cisplatin-based chemotherapy for disseminated germ cell tumors: Long term follow-up. *J Clin Oncol* 6:1239–1247, 1988

18. Einhorn L, Richie J, Shipley W: Cancer of the testis, in DeVita V, Hellman S, Rosenberg S (eds): *Cancer: Principles and Practices of Oncology* (ed 4). Philadelphia, Lippincott, 1993, pp 1126–1151

19. Nichols CR, Roth BJ, Einhorn LH: Managing testicular cancer. *Contemp Oncol* 1:13–30, 1991

20. Brock D, Fox S, Gosling G, et al: Testicular cancer. *Semin Oncol Nurs* 9:224–236, 1993

21. Donahue J, Thornhill R, Foster R, et al: Retroperitoneal lymphadenectomy for clinical stage A testis cancer (1965 to 1989): Modifications of technique and impact on ejaculation. *J Urol* 149:237–243, 1993

22. Donahue J, Rowland R: Complications of retroperitoneal lymphadenectomy. *J Urol* 125:338, 1981

23. Donahue J, Zachary J, Maynard B: Distribution of nodal metastasis in nonseminomatous testis cancer. *J Urol* 128:315, 1982

24. Donahue J, Foster R, Rowland R, et al: Nerve sparing retroperitoneal lymphadenectomy with preservation of ejaculation. *J Urol* 144:287, 1990

25. Roth B, Nichols C, Einhorn L: Neoplasms of the testis, in Holland J, Frei E, Bast R, Kufe D, Morton D, Weichselbaum R (eds): *Cancer Medicine,* vol 2 (ed 3). Philadelphia, Lea & Febiger, 1993, pp 1592–1619

26. Logeothetis C, Swanson D, Dexeus F, et al: Primary chemotherapy for clinical stage II nonseminomatous germ cell tumors of the testis: A follow-up of 50 patients. *J Clin Oncol* 5:906, 1987

27. Keller J, Sahasrabudhe D, McCune C: Urologic and male genital cancers, in Rubin P (ed): *Clinical Oncology* (ed 7). Philadelphia, Saunders, 1993, pp 442–453

28. Sturgeon J, Herman J, Jewlett M, et al: A policy for surveillance alone after orchiectomy for stage I nonseminomatous testis tumors. *Proc Am Soc Clin Oncol* 4:1199, 1986

29. Einhorn L, Williams S, Loehrer P, et al: Evaluation of optimal duration of chemotherapy in favorable prognosis disseminated germ cell tumors: A Southeastern Cancer Study Group protocol. *J Clin Oncol* 7:387–391, 1989

30. Levi J, Raghavan D, Harvey V, et al: Deletion of bleomycin from therapy for good prognosis advanced testicular cancer. *Proc Am Soc Clin Oncol* 5:97, 1986

31. Schmoll H, Schubert I, Arnold H, et al: Disseminated bulky disease: Results of a phase II study with cisplatin/ultra high dose/VP-16/Bleomycin. *Int J Androl* 10:311, 1987

32. Loehrer P, Lohnson D, Elson P, et al: Importance of bleomycin in favorable prognosis disseminated germ cell tumors: an Eastern Oncology Group study. *J Clin Oncol* 13:470–476, 1995

33. Droz J, Pico J, Ghosen M, et al: High complete remission and survival rates in poor prognosis nonseminomatous germ cell tumors with high-dose chemotherapy and autologous bone marrow transplant. *Proc Am Soc Clin Oncol* 8:130, 1989

34. Horwich A, Brada M, Nicholls J, et al: Intensive induction chemotherapy for poor risk nonseminomatous germ cell tumors. *Eur J Clin Oncol* 25:177, 1989

35. Wettlaufer J, Feiner A, Robinson W: Vincristine, cisplatin, and bleomycin with surgery in the management of advanced metastatic nonseminomatous testis tumors. *Cancer* 53:203, 1984

36. Bihrle R, Donahue J, Foster, R: Complications of retroperitoneal lymph node dissection. *Urol Clin North Am* 15:237–242, 1988

37. Terebelo H, Taylor G, Brown A, et al: Late relapse of testicular cancer. *J Clin Oncol* 1:566–571, 1983

38. Lianes P, Paz-Ares L, Rivera F, et al: Late recurrence in malignant germ cell tumors. *Ann Oncol* 3:165, 1992 (suppl 5) (abstr)

39. Deleo M, Greco F, Hainsworth J, et al: Late recurrence in long-term survivors of germ cell neoplasms. *Cancer* 62: 985–988, 1988

40. Charbner B, Cannellos G, Olweny C, et al: Late recurrence of testicular tumors. *N Engl J Med* 287:413, 1972

41. Blom J: Late recurrence of testicular tumor. *J Urol* 112:211, 1974

42. Nichols C, Baniel J, Foster R: Late relapse of germ cell tumors. *Proc Am Soc Clin Oncol* 13:1994 (abstr 497)

43. Baniel J, Foster R, Gonin R, et al: Late relapse of testicular cancer. *J Clin Oncol* 13:1170–1176, 1995

44. Gerl A, Clemm C, Hartenstein R, et al: Late relapse of nonseminomatous germ cell tumors (NSGCT) after cisplatin-based chemotherapy. *Proc Am Soc Clin Oncol* 13:229, 1994 (abstr 153)

45. Richie J: Detection and treatment of testicular cancer. *CA Cancer J Clin* 43:151–175, 1993

46. Hanks G, Peters T, Owen P: Seminoma of the testis: Long-term beneficial and deleterious effects. *Int J Radiat Oncol Bio Phys* 24:913–919, 1992

47. Thomas G, Rider W, Dembo A, et al: Seminomas of the testis: Results of treatment patterns and failures after radiation therapy. *Int J Radiat Oncol Bio Phys* 8:165–174, 1982

48. Bracken R: Cancer of the testis, penis and urethra: The impact of therapy on sexual function, in von Eschenbach A, Rodriguez D (eds): *Sexual Rehabilitation of the Urological Cancer Patient*. Boston, Hall, pp 108–127, 1981

49. Calman F, Peckman M, Hendy W: The pattern of spread and the treatment of metastases in testicular seminomas. *Br J Urol* 51:154, 1979

50. Cavelli F, Klepp O, Renard J, et al: A phase II study on oral VP-16-213 in nonseminomatous testis cancer. *Eur J Cancer* 17:245, 1981

51. Cavelli F, Sonntag R, Brunner K: Epipodophyllotoxin derivative (VP-16-213) in the treatment of solid tumors. *Lancet* 2:362, 1977

52. Gregory C, Peckman M: Results of radiotherapy for stage II testicular seminoma. *Radiother Oncol* 6:285, 1988

53. Einhorn L, Williams S: Chemotherapy of disseminated seminoma. *Cancer Clin Trials* 3:307–313, 1980

54. Vugrin D, Whitmore W, Batata M: Chemotherapy of disseminated seminoma with combination platinum and cyclophosphamide. *Cancer Clin Trials* 4:423–427, 1981

55. Wajsman Z, Beckley S, Pontes J: Changing concepts in the treatment of advanced seminomatous tumors *J Urol* 129:303–306, 1983

56. Motzer R, Bosl G, Heelan R, et al: An indication for further therapy in patients with advanced seminoma following chemotherapy. *J Clin Oncol* 5:1064, 1987

57. Schulz S, Einhorn L, Conces D, et al: Management of postchemotherapy residual mass in patients with advanced seminoma. *J Clin Oncol* 7:1497, 1989

58. Einhorn LH: Treatment of testicular cancer: A new and improved model. *J Clin Oncol* 8:1777–1781, 1990

59. Nichols C, Williams S, Loehrer P, et al: Randomized study of cisplatin dose intensity in poor risk germ cell tumors: A Southeastern Cancer Study Group and Southwest Oncology Group protocol. *J Clin Oncol* 9:1163–1172, 1991

60. Cooper M, Einhorn L: Maintenance chemotherapy with daily oral etoposide following salvage therapy in patients with germ cell tumors *J Clin Oncol* 13:1167–1169, 1995

61. Einhorn LH: Salvage theapy for germ cell tumors. *Semin Oncol* 21:47–51, 1994

62. Motzer R, Cooper K, Geller N, et al: The role of ifosfamide plus cisplatin-based chemotherapy as salvage therapy for patients with refractory germ cell tumors. *Cancer* 66:2476–2481, 1990

63. Nichols C, Tricot G, Williams S, et al: Dose intensive chemotherapy in refractory germ cell cancer—A phase I–II trial of high dose carboplatin and etoposide with autologous bone marrow transplantation. *J Clin Oncol* 7:932–939, 1989

64. Einhorn L, Weathers T, Loehrer P, et al: Second-line chemotherapy with vinblastine, ifosfamide, and cisplatin after initial chemotherapy with cisplatin, VP-16, and bleomycin in disseminated germ cell tumors: Long-term follow-up. *Proc Am Soc Clin Oncol* 11:169, 1992 (abstr)

65. Williams S, Einhorn L, Greco F, et al: Salvage chemotherapy for refractory germinal neoplasms. *Cancer* 46:2154–2158, 1980

66. Miller J, Einhorn L: Phase II study of daily oral etoposide in refractory germ cell tumors. *Semin Oncol* 17:36–39, 1990

67. Murphy B, Breeden E, Donohue J, et al: Suurgical salvage of chemo-refractory germ cell tumors. *J Clin Oncol* 11:324–329, 1993

68. Mulder P, DeVries E, Koops H, et al: Chemotherapy with maximal tolerated doses of VP-16-213 and cyclophosphamide followed by autologous bone marrow transplantation for the treatment of relapsed or refractory germ cell tumors. *Eur J Cancer Clin Oncol* 24:675–679, 1988

69. Wolff S, Hohnson D, Hainsworth J, et al: High dose VP-16-213 monotherapy for refractory germinal malignancies: A phase II study. *J Clin Oncol* 2:271–274, 1984

70. Pico J, Droz J, Gouyette A, et al: 25 high dose chemotherapy regimens (HDCR) followed by autologous bone marrow transplantation (ABMT) in refractory or relaplsed nonsem-innomatous germ cell tumors. *Proc Am Soc Clin Oncol* 5:111, 1986 (abstr)

71. Saxman S: Salvage chemotherapy in recurrent testicular cancer. *Semin Oncol* 19:143–147, 1992

72. Broun E, Tricot G, Fox E, et al: Long-term follow-up of salvage chemotherapy in relapse and refractory germ cell tumors using high dose carboplatin and etoposide with aotologous bone marrow transplant. *Proc Am Soc Clin Oncol* 10:167, 1991 (abstr)

73. Broun R, Nichols C, Kneebone P, et al: Long term outcome of patients with relapsed and refractory germ cell tumors treated with high dose chemotherapy and bone marrow rescue. *Ann Intern Med* 117:124–128, 1992

74. Nichols C, Anderson J, Lazarus H, et al: High dose carboplatin and etoposide with autologous bone marrow transplantation in refractory germ cell cancer: An Eastern Cooperative Oncology Group protocol. *J Clin Oncol* 10:558–563, 1992

75. Siegert W, Beyer J, Wersback V, et al: High dose carboplatin, etoposide, ifosfamide with autologous stem cell rescue for relapsed and refractory nonseminomatous germ cell tumors. *Proc Am Soc Clin Oncol* 10:163, 1991

76. Motzer R, Gulati S, Crown J, et al: High dose chemotherapy and autologous bone marrow rescue for patients with refractory germ cell tumors: Early intervention is better tolerated. *Cancer* 69:550–559, 1992

77. Higgs DJ: The patient with testicular cancer: Nursing management of chemotherapy. *Oncol Nurs Forum* 17:243–246, 1990

78. Goldiner P, Carlon G, Critkovic E, et al: Factors influencing postoperative morbidity and mortality in patients treated with bleomycin. *Br Med J* 1:1664, 1978

79. Lazo J, Chabner B: Bleomycin, in Chabner B, Longo D (eds): *Cancer Chemotherapy and Biotherapy: Principles and Practice* (ed 2). Philadelphia, Lippincott-Raven, 1996, pp 379–393

80. Osanto S, Bukman A, Van Hoek F, et al: Long-term effect of chemotherapy in patients with testicular cancer. *J Clin Oncol* 10:574, 1992

81. Boyer M, Raghavan D: Toxicity of germ cell tumors. *Semin Oncol* 19:128–142, 1992

82. Strohl R: Symptom management of acute and chronic reactions. *Oncol Nurs Forum* 15:429–434, 1988

83. Lind J, Irwin R: Genitourinary cancer, in Baird S, McCorkle R, Grant M (eds): *Cancer Nursing: A Comprehensive Textbook.* Philadelphia, Saunders, 1991, pp 477–480

84. Fossa S, Ous S, Abyholm T, et al: Post treatment fertility in patients with testicular cancer. *Br J Urol* 57:210–214, 1985

85. Marks L, Ansher M, Shipley W: Radiation therapy for testicular seminoma: Controversies in the management of early stage disease. *Oncology* 6:43–52, 1991

86. Fox S, Einhorn L, Cox E, et al: Ondansetron versus ondansetron, dexamethasone, and chlorpromazine in the prevention of nausea and vomiting associated with multiple-day cisplatin chemotherapy. *J Clin Oncol* 11:2391–2395, 1993

87. Cotanch P, Strum S: Progressive muscle relaxation as antiemetic therapy for cancer patients. *Oncol Nurs Forum* 14: 33–37, 1987

88. Frank J: The effects of music therapy and guided imagery on chemotherapy-induced nausea and vomiting. *Oncol Nurs Forum* 12:47–52, 1985

89. Nichols C, Roth B, Einhorn L: Managing testicular cancer. *Contemp Oncol* 1:13–30, 1991

90. Schweitzer V, Hawkins J, Lilly D, et al: Ototoxic and nephrotoxic effects of combined treatment with cisdiaminedichloroplatinum and karamycin in guinea pig. *Otolaryngol Head Neck Surg* 92:38–49, 1984

91. Wagner L, Bye M: Body image and patient experiencing alopecia as a result of chemotherapy. *Cancer Nurs* 2:365–369, 1979

92. Senturia Y, Peckham C, Peckham M: Children fathered by men treated for testicular cancer. *Lancet* 2:766–769, 1985

93. Roth B, Einhorn L, Griest A: Long-term complications of cisplatin based chemotherapy for testicular cancer. *Semin Oncol* 15:345–350, 1988

94. Stephenson W, Poirier S, Rubin L, et al: Evaluation of reproductive capacity in germ cell tumor patients following treatment with cisplatin, etoposide, and bleomycin. *J Clin Oncol* 13:2278–2280, 1995

95. Fox E, Loehrer PJ: Chemotherapy for advanced testicular cancer. *Hematol Oncol Clin North Am* 5:1173–1187, 1992

96. Schaefer S, Post J, Close L, et al: Ototoxicity of low and moderate dose cisplatin. *Cancer* 56:1934–1939, 1985

97. Lyons J: Models of nursing care delivery and case management: Clarification of terms. *Nurs Econ* 11:163–169, 1993

# PART VI

# Issues in Cancer Survivorship

# Chapter 48

# Psychosocial Responses to Cancer

**Andrea M. Barsevick, RN, DNSc**

**Judie Much, MSN, CRNP, AOCN**

**Carole Sweeney, RN, MSN, OCN®**

## INTRODUCTION

### The Need for Psychosocial Care

The prevailing western view is that cancer is a chronic treatable disease. Societal expectations for the individual with cancer include his or her accepting the diagnosis, seeking care, complying with treatment, and having "fighting" spirit. To the individual living through the experience, however, cancer is a greatly feared entity. It usually occurs without warning, may have an uncontrollable spread, may be incurable beyond a certain point, is assumed to be accompanied by pain and discomfort, and is a threat to quality of life. Persons with cancer are not confronted with a single stressor, but with a series of stressors. The stress is not limited to diagnosis and treatment but continues throughout survival with long-term physiological alterations, fears of relapse and death, dependence on caregivers, survivor guilt, and negative effects on families. It is paramount for the individual and those he or she shares life with to develop skills for managing the stresses associated with the cancer experience.

Cancer affects the functioning of the entire family unit. Its impact has been likened to dropping a stone into a pond.[1] The ripple effect changes the family and forces them to adjust their routines and basic functions including eating, sleeping, working, and communicating with each other. No family emerges unchanged.[2] Because of the transition of health care from the hospital to home, individuals with cancer rely on their families to assist them with complex medical regimens. Both family members and patients may have difficulty adjusting to role changes and lifestyle adaptations. If the cancer progresses, the family's role becomes more central. Families who are able to share their feelings and the work of caregiving may have less difficulty coping with the changes than families who function in isolation from each other.

In this chapter, we will address the stressful challenges faced by the individual and family dealing with cancer using a simple model of the stress-coping process. We will use a research base to describe factors influencing the stress-coping process, interventions to enhance coping efforts, and common problems of individuals and families. We will also address professional responses to cancer.

### A Model of the Stress and Coping Process

The stress and coping model of Lazarus and Folkman[3] provides the framework for this discussion of psychosocial issues related to cancer (Figure 48-1). This model provides the clinician with a useful framework for understanding the complex psychosocial problems of individuals and families when an individual has cancer. The model provides a basis for gathering information to conduct a psychosocial assessment and for selecting and designing interventions to assist and support the individual's coping efforts.

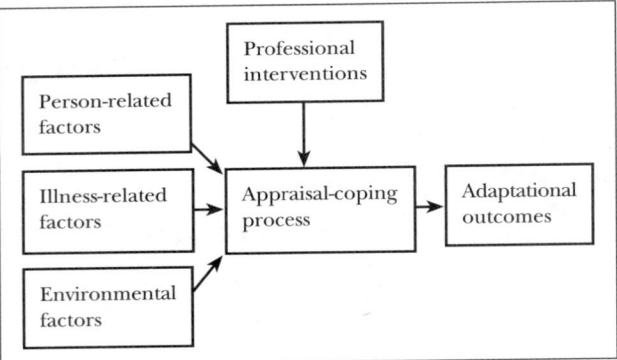

**FIGURE 48-1** The stress-coping process.

### The appraisal-coping process

Central to the model is the appraisal-coping process. Appraisal and coping are cognitive and behavioral processes people use to deal with a problem. Appraisal is a person's evaluation of the problem, including the definition of the problem; one's perception of it as a threat, loss, or challenge; and the resources available for dealing with it. Coping refers to the cognitive and behavioral strategies used to manage the stressful situation, including strategies directed toward management of the problem itself as well as those used to deal with the negative emotions that are aroused by the situation.

To describe appraisal and coping as a process means that we are describing what a person actually thinks and does within a specific context or situation. Process also suggests that thoughts and actions change as the situation unfolds, as information is obtained, and as the demands on the individual change. The dynamics and changes that occur are not random. They are a function of the individual's continuously changing appraisals of the situation and the resulting modification of coping efforts due to those changing appraisals. A process can be likened to a sailboat on the sea. The captain watches the horizon, the weather, and the water conditions. On the basis of these, he decides on a course, and constantly readjusts the rudder and fine-tunes the sails to stay on course. So it is with the coping process. The individual appraises a specific situation and puts in motion a set of coping strategies, constantly readjusting and fine-tuning the appraisal and coping strategies used as new information becomes available and as aspects of the situation change. Shifts in the information available to the individual lead to a reappraisal of what is happening, its significance, and what can be done. The reappraisal, in turn, determines subsequent coping efforts.

Coping serves two basic functions. Problem-focused coping efforts are directed at managing or altering the problem causing the stress, while emotion-focused coping strategies are directed at regulating emotional responses to the stressful situation. Problem-focused coping involves problem-solving efforts such as defining the problem, generating alternative solutions, weighing the alternatives with regard to their costs and benefits, choosing among them, and acting. Problem-focused coping also includes strategies for reducing environmental pressures or barriers, information-seeking, and learning new skills or behaviors. Emotion-focused coping includes strategies with the direct intent of reducing the emotional distress caused by the stressful problem. These include typical defense mechanisms such as denial, avoidance, distancing, or selective attention. Emotion-focused coping also may include expressions of emotion including humor, hope, grieving, and anxiety, since expressing feelings is often necessary to reduce distress.

Problem- or emotion-focused coping strategies can be used successfully or unsuccessfully (Table 48-1). The success of a coping strategy is determined by its outcome or intended outcome. The behavior of denial is "value neutral," meaning that it is not inherently adaptive or maladaptive. Its adaptiveness is determined by what it can or does achieve. An example of successful use of denial as a coping strategy involves a woman who, after hearing the diagnosis of breast cancer, refuses to discuss her diagnosis in the first weeks of treatment. This protective behavior allows her to assimilate information at her own pace, preventing despair. Later, this same woman becomes active in advocating breast health and serves as a visitor to other women having surgery for breast cancer. Conversely, if this woman's denial resulted in refusal or discontinuation of treatment, the potential negative outcome would have defined the coping behavior as maladaptive.

### Adaptational outcomes

The prime importance of the appraisal-coping process is that it affects adaptational outcomes. An outcome is commonly defined as a relevant end result.[4,5] The principal psy-chosocial outcomes of the appraisal and coping process in the health care context are the maximization of (1) physical health, (2) functioning in work and social living, and (3) psychological well-being. To the extent that the appraisal-coping process fosters one or more of these outcomes, it is adaptive; when it does not, it is maladaptive.

### Factors influencing the process

The appraisal-coping process does not occur in a vacuum. It is influenced by a variety of person-related, illness-related, and environmental factors. Knowing which factors influence the stress and coping process can help the clinician identify persons who may be at risk for developing psychological or behavioral problems. Identifying these individuals is critical so that resources can be directed to persons with the greatest need for them. Being aware of these factors can also provide cues to the clinician about how to approach the individual or family.

### Professional interventions

Professional interventions to support or enhance the appraisal-coping process are necessary if the individual's appraisal of the problem is inaccurate or distorted, if the individual has inadequate resources for dealing with it, or if the individual's coping efforts are inadequate or unlikely to achieve the desired outcome. Professional interventions may include preparatory information, teaching cognitive or behavioral skills, or providing supportive care.

## ASSESSMENT OF THE APPRAISAL-COPING PROCESS

Individuals and families, faced with a potential or actual cancer diagnosis, generally use the appraisal-coping process very effectively to deal with the problems they encounter. They gather information from health care providers, make decisions about diagnostic and treatment options, manage their emotional distress, and effectively make use of support systems. Professional nursing assessment is indicated at two junctures: (1) the initial contact between nurse and patient/family when a baseline assessment is performed, and (2) when the nurse observes difficulties indicating a breakdown in the effectiveness of the appraisal-coping process. In keeping with the tenets of the stress and coping model, an assessment of the appraisal-coping process must be viewed as a "snapshot" of one point in time since the process is constantly changing.

At the initial contact between nurse and patient, the nurse can use the concepts of the appraisal-coping process as a basis for an initial assessment (Figure 48-2). The individual's perception of a problem is a major component of his or her appraisal.[6] A probable diagnosis of cancer will be appraised differently depending on the specific circumstances of the individual facing the diagnosis. To a young

**TABLE 48-1** Successful and Unsuccessful Coping

| Strategy | Successful | Unsuccessful |
|---|---|---|
| Anger | Able to identify source<br><br>Able to resolve<br>Maintain sense of self | Depression, passivity, or aggression |
| Humor | Tension reducer<br>Decreases social distance | Masks feelings<br>Avoidance |
| Depression | Normal response | Persistent, pervasive feelings of loss<br>Suicide |
| Anxiety | Gradual understanding<br><br>Initially protective | Ignoring, refusing reality |
| Hopefulness | Comforting, sustaining<br>Belief that future good exists | Limited choices<br>Inability to mobilize energy |

- What are the major problems you face related to your cancer?
- For each problem identified:
  How difficult is the problem for you to handle?
  How do you feel about this problem?
  What resources do you have to help you deal with it?
  How are you coping with it?
  How are you coping with your feelings about it?
  What is the desired outcome of your efforts to deal with this problem?

**FIGURE 48-2** Assessment of the appraisal-coping process.

woman with small children, a diagnosis of breast cancer can be a devastating crisis not only because of the disease itself but also because of the threat it poses to her family. From her vantage point, the most stressful problem she faces may not be the diagnostic and treatment procedures but the uncertainty about her ability to care for her family in the immediate and long-term future. For an elderly woman who is the sole caretaker of her elderly mate, the stressful problem may be the diagnostic and treatment procedures that take her away from her caretaker responsibilities. It is important for the nurse to understand the individual's unique perception of the problems he or she faces in order to provide targeted and individualized interventions.

An important aspect of the individual's perception of the problem is his or her feelings about it. Lazarus and Folkman[3] indicate that a problem may be appraised as a threat, a loss, or a challenge, each suggesting different patterns of response based on perception. Individuals who perceive a problem as a threat are likely to experience anxiety or fear; those perceiving loss may experience grief or depression; and individuals who view a problem as a challenge could experience positive feelings such as eager anticipation or hopefulness.

Another important aspect of appraisal is the individual's perception of the resources he or she has for dealing with the problem. To say a person is resourceful means that she or he has tangible items or competencies to draw upon and is able to use them to manage difficult or complex situations. Tangible resources include people, information, equipment, and money. Internal resources include energy, positive beliefs, problem-solving skills, or social skills.

# FACTORS THAT INFLUENCE THE APPRAISAL-COPING PROCESS

## Person-related Factors

### Cultural background

A person's culture is the lens through which he or she perceives the world. Values, beliefs, and norms are culture-bound ideals that guide thinking, decision making, and actions[7] and explain many differences in behavior. When faced with the problem of cancer, persons from different cultures are likely to appraise and cope with it in diverse ways related to their cultural background.

The use of a stress and coping model requires that care be based on the individual's perception of the problem(s) he or she faces. Within a cultural context, the nurse must recognize that the individual's perceptions are culture-bound and culturally determined, as are the nurse's own. In a pluralistic society, nurses need to be prepared to work with individuals of varied cultural backgrounds to ensure that nursing care is culturally appropriate. Where there is a cultural difference between the nurse and the individual under his or her care, differences in key areas may need to be acknowledged and addressed.[7] Communication may be a problem if there are discrepancies between the nurse and patient with regard to language or their conceptions of health and illness. Space may also be a problem or source of discomfort since different cultures have different spatial needs. Time may be an issue since different cultures vary in their sense of urgency about time and in the degree to which they focus on the present or future. Social organizations must also be considered. Every culture determines acceptable ways for families to interact with and assist one another. The use of family resources called for by the stress and coping model must be evaluated within the cultural context. Religious affiliation must also be considered since cultural and religious values are often linked. Lastly, culturally determined health-seeking and sick role behaviors must be considered since cultures often differ in the behavioral expectations of individuals who are seeking health or illness care.

### Socioeconomic status

Differences in culture may be compounded by differences in socioeconomic status since minorities in the United States often have fewer financial and educational resources.[8–10] It has long been recognized that socioeconomic status has an important influence on morbidity and mortality due to cancer. Individuals with low annual incomes are three to seven times more likely to die of cancer than those with high annual incomes.[8] Not graduating from high school has been associated with death rates that are two to three times greater than college graduates. These factors are likely to have a profound effect on the appraisal and coping strategies used by persons of lower socioeconomic means. When examining psychological responses of persons with lower socioeconomic status, the clinician must recognize the influence of lack of education, unemployment, poor nutrition, lifestyle factors that increase risk, and difficulties with access to health care.

Illustrations of the influence of culture and socioeconomic status on people's appraisal of the problem of cancer are found in a study of a white working-class neighborhood in Philadelphia targeted for a cancer prevention program[11] and in a study of a group of black women from eastern North Carolina who had advanced breast cancer.[12] In both cultures, cancer was viewed as a powerful and unstoppable disease that was fatal and incurable. The people being studied could identify no particular cause for cancer, so they had no explanation for why one person fell victim to it and not another. Another important concept in both cultures was the desire not to tempt fate by engaging in cancer screening. For working-class Philadelphians, "to think about cancer, to try to prevent it, is to tempt fate."[11, p.16] One of the North Carolinians expressed it this way, "If you have a lump and it's not bothering you, leave it alone. You don't want to get it started."[12, p.795] For the North Carolina women, fatalism, lack of knowledge of risk factors for breast cancer, lower educational levels, and a strong belief in the effectiveness of folk medicine contributed to late-stage presentation of disease.[12]

When culture and/or socioeconomic status constitutes a barrier to care, the nurse could also consult with the ill individual and family members to gain a better understanding of the health values and behaviors of the unfamiliar culture and incorporate these values whenever possible into the plan of care. It may be useful to identify resources to help the nurse understand the values and behaviors of the individual in his or her care. Several textbooks are now available describing the health beliefs, values, and behaviors of a number of cultural groups in the United States.[7,13] (See also chapter 62 in this text.) It may also be helpful to involve a person who is culturally, linguistically, and socially similar to the person targeted for care. This individual could serve as an interpreter if there is a language barrier.

### Age

Age is a sociodemographic factor that is predictive of psychological adjustment to cancer. Yet health care professionals have misunderstood its influence, believing that older people have greater adjustment difficulties.[14] In fact, research has demonstrated that younger people report greater difficulties in comparison to their older counterparts.[14] At 12-month and 4-year follow-ups, women under 65 who were treated for breast cancer experienced greater emotional distress, poorer mental health, and greater deterioration of psychological well-being than older women.[15,16] Younger individuals with a variety of cancer also reported more problems with physical health, finances, communication with providers, and home care than older people.[14] This research underscores the need for clinicians to pay careful attention to the problems identified by each individual under his or her care, particularly younger people, who often undergo more aggressive therapy with greater threats to their quality of life.

### Psychological coping styles

Another important person-related factor is the enduring beliefs or traits that constitute an individual's person-

ality. Beliefs are personally formed or culturally shared cognitive ideas about reality that determine what is fact and shape the individual's understanding of reality.[3] Traits are relatively stable and enduring ways in which one individual differs from others and that exert generalized effects on behavior.[17] For example, the idea has been introduced that people differ in their beliefs about locus of control in health situations.[18] Such beliefs can buffer or exaggerate the individual's appraisal and subsequent coping efforts in a stressful situation. When a situation is highly ambiguous, the individual with an internal locus of control is more likely to appraise it as controllable than the person whose locus of control is external.

There is evidence that individual differences in stable coping styles serve as buffers in stressful situations. Traits such as personal control or optimism may give rise to an appraisal of challenge rather than threat or loss when a diagnosis of cancer is made. This could lower the individual's perceived stress during the diagnostic and treatment period in comparison to the stress experienced by those whose world view is pessimistic. Thus, traits can moderate an individual's appraisal of a problem. Another way that personality traits can influence the stress-coping process is by influencing the individual's choice of coping strategies. Although they may be distressed by the diagnosis of cancer, optimists have been found to make greater use of positive, adaptive coping strategies such as acceptance, positive reframing, and gaining comfort from one's religious beliefs and less use of denial or behavioral disengagement.[19] Likewise, information preference coping styles determine the extent to which individuals engage in and benefit from information-seeking behavior.[20,21] Individual differences or traits often are not immediately evident to the observer. However, measurement instruments are available that can aid the clinician.[22,23]

## Illness-related Factors

A history of comorbidity (whether psychiatric or medical) and the presence of more advanced disease increases the individual's risk for poor psychosocial outcomes after a cancer diagnosis. These factors do not constitute a guarantee of problems. However, they do alert the professional to observe and question the individual so that coping difficulties do not result in poorer outcomes.

A history of previous psychiatric diagnosis, particularly depressive disorders, increases the risk of developing depression after a cancer diagnosis.[24] Among women with breast cancer, two-thirds of those with a history of depression reported significant distress 18 months after diagnosis while only 14% of those without a psychiatric history reported distress.[25] Likewise, the presence of other comorbid conditions when cancer is diagnosed also seems to heighten the individual's risk for psychological problems. Results from the Medical Outcomes Study indicate that individuals with comorbid chronic illnesses have poorer social and role functioning, poorer mental health, and perceptions of poorer health than individuals without comorbid conditions.[26] Severity of disease has also been associated with poorer psychological adjustment. Women with more extensive surgery for breast cancer[15] and those with regional as opposed to local disease[25] reported higher levels of psychological distress and poorer long-term adjustment than women with less severe disease.

## Environmental Factors

Social networks have been found to have a protective effect with regard to psychosocial outcomes. Married people live longer and have lower mortality rates for all major causes of death than persons who have never been married or who are separated, widowed, or divorced.[27] Individuals with cancer who have support from a spouse or a social network are diagnosed at an earlier stage and receive more complete treatment than individuals without a social network.[28–31]

## PSYCHOSOCIAL INTERVENTIONS

A critical question with regard to the psychosocial management of the individual with cancer is, "What specific intervention is most effective for the individual with a specific problem, and under which set of circumstances is it effective?" Answering this question is difficult because "cancer" encompasses different diseases with disparate etiologies and outcomes. Examining psychological interventions in the context of the magnitude of the disease and treatment process, Andersen[32] concluded that those with advanced disease made more significant gains with the help of psychosocial interventions. Furthermore, they were more likely than individuals with localized disease to worsen without intervention.

Descriptive and intervention studies point to the effectiveness of crisis intervention and brief therapy models of intervention.[32] Both use similar approaches with regard to early assessment, present-day focus, limited goals, counseling direction, and prompt interventions. The components of this type of therapy include information about the disease and its treatment, an emotionally supportive context in which to address emotional concerns including fears and anxieties, instruction in cognitive and behavioral coping strategies including relaxation techniques, and focused interventions for specific problems such as sexual functioning in individuals with diseases affecting the sexual organs. Procedural variations such as whether the intervention is administered individually or in groups do not have an impact on the effectiveness of the intervention.

Andersen[32] also addresses the probable mechanism for intervention effectiveness. Interventions assist individuals to learn more about the stressor and to confront it in a positive coping state with active behavioral strategies. Using skills learned through the intervention process, the individual is able to reduce emotional distress, make a realistic appraisal of current and impending stresses, and enhance his or her self-efficacy and feelings of control early in the adjustment process. Gains have been found to continue and often increase during the first posttreatment year even when the therapy has been brief.

A variety of interventions are available to the oncology nurse, including education, counseling, storytelling, and relaxation. Each of these will be addressed.

## Education

In addition to the obvious benefits of increased knowledge, education assists the individual with cancer to reduce his or her sense of helplessness and inadequacy related to uncertainty.[33] A meta-analysis of 116 psychoeducational intervention studies for cancer patients examined the effect of educational interventions on anxiety, depression, mood, nausea, vomiting, pain, and knowledge.[34] Educational topics included specific information on type and stage of disease, treatment types, and how to live with cancer. Beneficial effects were found across all seven outcomes. The most effective intervention for knowledge acquisition was printed material, although other educational methods were also effective. Education can be effective when targeted to an individual or to a group. It may consist of written or oral content, including videotape, audiotape, or didactic methods.

## Counseling

The individual who is depressed or has difficulty coping with the disease is best managed with consistent emotional support and counseling within the context of a trusting relationship. The oncology nurse can help with problem solving, acknowledge the person's fears, and allow for control and decision making based on the person's unique needs. The goals of this intervention are to improve the individual's self-worth, correct misconceptions about the past and present, and integrate the present illness into the individual's self-concept. Active listening is used by the nurse to build trust and acceptance.[35] Good communication sets a stable tone and is supportive of hope.[36] Counseling involves the provision of support by the nurse and the identification of other social supports for the individual, such as family, friends, other patients, support groups, and community resources. It optimizes past strengths, supports past coping efforts, and mobilizes resources. Experienced oncology nurses weave this approach into their everyday activities, including self-care activities, examinations, phone calls, and treatment visits. There is evidence that just providing the opportunity to air their feelings helps individuals cope with the cancer experience.[37–40]

## Storytelling

Intervening in the individual's experience of cancer may cause the nurse to reach deep into the self for creativity. Storytelling can be an effective method of communicating with individuals for whom more direct methods of communication are ineffective.[41] Stories can be used to transmit knowledge, improve learning, and assist with problem solving.[42–44] Procedures and situations can be explained by way of stories containing metaphor and symbolism. Stories are perceived by individuals hearing or reading them as being "outside" themselves; therefore, the content or metaphor is easily taken in and is less likely to trigger a defensive response.[45] Techniques that can be used include prescribing a story to be read, telling a story, or using a metaphor. In order for storytelling to be successful, the story must "fit" the situation and the information must be given in a natural manner and only after rapport has developed. When the intervention is successful, it can provide the patient and family with a new perspective with which to view their situation. Patients and families can also derive satisfaction from telling or writing their stories. Using this technique, an individual may be able to verbalize endings that are either desired or greatly feared. Stories also may be written in a journal or letters that are kept.

## Relaxation

Progressive muscle relaxation is helpful in dealing with conditioned nausea associated with chemotherapy administration. It can also be used to manage anxiety related to stressful situations and physiological arousal. Relaxation techniques provide a means of distracting oneself from difficult situations and increase one's sense of control.

# PSYCHOSOCIAL OUTCOMES

## The Importance of Outcomes

The stress and coping model used to guide the discussion of psychosocial problems defines outcomes as the final variable in the process. Coping strategies used by individuals and their families are value-neutral—that is, they are not adaptive or maladaptive by virtue of any inherent properties. Their effectiveness is determined by the intended or actual outcome. Therefore, the type of nursing care required in a given set of circumstances is determined by the intended outcome(s) of that care and the effectiveness of the nursing care provided is evaluated by actual outcomes achieved. Without being aware of nursing outcomes, the nurse cannot be sure of the direction or the effectiveness of the care provided.

More importantly from a clinical standpoint, articulation of intended outcomes provides a means for the oncology nurse to communicate with the patient and family and make mutual decisions about the type and direction of care. It helps them to set the direction and course for their work together. For example, if the patient's goal is to minimize symptom burden (desired outcome) so he or she can continue working during treatment, then the nurse identifies the information and skills training that will be necessary to achieve this outcome. If the patient is elderly and is likely to need additional physical care during treatment to maintain comfort and satisfaction, the nurse begins the process of identifying the resources available to supply the instrumental and emotional support needed.

Another reason that outcomes are a critical focus of oncology nursing practice is that they define our practice. Medicine has defined survival and tumor response as critical outcomes of interest to their practice. As a result, the effectiveness of any medical intervention is evaluated with regard to its effect on these outcomes, and "cure" and survival rates are defined as the domain of medical practice. In the same way, nursing can use outcomes to define its domain of practice. Of course, this also means that oncology nurses need to take these outcomes off the pages of the text and begin measuring, tracking, and reporting them.

An even more critical reason for the emphasis on outcomes has to do with the atmosphere of cost containment and cost effectiveness in which oncology nurses practice. As a group, nurses need to be able to identify and quantify nursing's effect on patient outcomes in order to define their worth and position in patient care. If nurses do not document their stake in influencing outcomes, then the temptation will be great to reduce the number of nurses involved in patient care and turn it over to lesser-skilled providers.

## What Outcomes Are Important

The psychosocial care that oncology nurses provide to individuals with cancer is likely to influence a broad range of outcomes, including physical health, functional well-being, psychological well-being, and social well-being. Within each of these domains of outcomes are perhaps hundreds of individual factors that are measurable. But which of these individual outcomes or domains are of greatest importance to oncology nursing? How can we communicate about these outcomes in language that is understandable to the lay public and that includes, in a meaningful way, a variety of outcomes?

Quality of life (QOL) is a health care construct that incorporates these diverse outcomes.[22,23] Cella[46] defines QOL as the appraisal of and level of satisfaction with one's current state of well-being. QOL is complex in that it cannot be evaluated adequately by means of a single indicator or dimension, requiring indicators from several domains to adequately represent it. It is also subjective—that is, it can only be understood from the perspective of the individual experiencing it. This is because the individual's own cognitive processes determine his or her evaluation of QOL, including illness and treatment perceptions, expectations of self and outcomes, and appraisal of risk or harm.

The dimensions or domains of QOL have not been firmly established.[46] However, four dimensions that are typically represented include physical, functional, psychological, and social well-being. Each of these domains is relevant to nursing and, in some cases, nursing interventions have been associated with improvements in quality of life.

### Physical well-being

The physical dimension of QOL refers to perceived bodily dysfunction or disruption. Common examples in oncology are physical symptoms including pain, nausea, and fatigue. Our own discussion in this chapter of symptom management related to treatment suggests that preparatory information reduces the number and severity of symptoms experienced.[47–49] The provision of home nursing care for lung cancer patients has been found to delay the progression of symptoms in this population.[50]

### Functional well-being

Distinct from the physical dimension is the functional dimension of QOL. Functional status refers to the ability to perform activities related to one's personal care and role responsibilities.[46] It can refer to activities of daily living or the ability to carry out responsibilities related to family, home, or work. The use of preparatory information for individuals undergoing radiation treatment for prostate cancer has resulted in better functioning, particularly in recreational and leisure activities.[48,49]

### Psychological well-being

This domain refers to emotional state, including both positive and negative moods. For individuals with cancer, emotional distress is not a major problem.[51,52] However, blunting of positive emotions may occur.[46] The literature on psychosocial interventions indicates that a brief counseling or crisis intervention approach is beneficial to psychological well-being, especially in individuals with more advanced disease.[32] Whereas studies have shown that individuals with less advanced disease may improve emotionally without intervention, those with more advanced disease who received no counseling worsened.[39,50]

### Social well-being

Another dimension of QOL is social well-being, which includes social support, family functioning, and intimacy.

Abundant research has demonstrated that the diagnosis of cancer (particularly advanced cancer) has a negative impact on the family.[53] Social support groups benefit people by reducing isolation and loneliness.[54,55] A number of counseling interventions have demonstrated beneficial effects on sexual functioning.[56]

Overall, psychosocial care of cancer patients—including education, counseling, crisis intervention, social support, and behavioral skills training—has had favorable effects on many aspects of their QOL. Research has also shown that certain populations of individuals are more vulnerable to poor outcomes: these include individuals of low socioeconomic status, younger age, and more advanced disease. Nurses can begin to target their intervention efforts to individuals with these characteristics in order to make the most effective and efficient use of their services.

## COMMON PROBLEMS OF THE INDIVIDUAL/FAMILY WITH CANCER

### Making Decisions About Treatment

There are two issues the oncology nurse must consider: role preference in treatment decision making and desire for information. With regard to treatment decisions, individuals with cancer typically have played a passive role.[57,58] Yet increasingly, they are expressing a desire for greater participation in decision making about treatment, most notably women with breast cancer and persons with AIDS.

Three different role preferences have been identified among individuals with cancer.[59] Between 12% and 20% of cancer patients expressed a desire to take an active role in making the final selection of treatment. A second group of 32% to 59% preferred passivity, allowing the physician to make the final decision about treatment. A third group of 28% to 40% preferred to collaborate with the physician in making decisions.

It would seem to follow logically that individuals who wish to participate in decision making need sufficient illness- and treatment-related information to make informed decisions. But what of those who prefer a passive role in decision making? Do they need little or no information? When the desire for information of each of the role preference groups was examined, virtually all of the individuals who wanted to play an active or collaborative role also wanted detailed information about treatment alternatives, treatment procedures, and side effects.[57] There was also a group of persons desiring a passive role who wanted minimal information. However, a second group of passive patients wanted detailed medical information. Even though they were content to play a passive role in decision making, they still wanted to know what would be happening to them. These conclusions provide clear guidance to the oncology nurse in determining patient preference for involvement in decision making.

Newfeld and colleagues[60] determined preferences by asking individuals to sort five cards consisting of written statements and an illustrative drawing according to their preferred role in treatment decision making[57] (Figure 48-3). This approach is adapted easily for clinical use by simply asking individuals how involved they wish to be in making decisions about their treatment. For individuals who wish to participate, providing written information about specific aspects of their illness and treatment has been shown to enhance retention and recall of information and to reduce anxiety.[61,62] Individuals have also benefited from "coaching" on how to ask questions and negotiate decisions.[63] To summarize, active individuals should be encouraged to assert themselves and be furnished with detailed information about their care.

Research is less clear about how to deal with individuals who prefer a more passive role in decision making and who prefer minimal information. One might be tempted to say that passive individuals should have their information preferences respected. However, there is ample research demonstrating clear benefits of providing information to patients and families about what to expect.[47,49] For individuals who desire minimal information, there is some evidence that this preference is rooted in the individual's concern about the negative emotions that are likely to be aroused by an influx of information on a threatening topic such as cancer. It has been proposed that the professional must tease out the fears, anxieties, and concerns of these individuals and first teach them ways of coping with their negative emotions through relaxation techniques and cognitive restructuring procedures.[64] Once they have mastered the skills to deal with the negative emotions that are likely to be aroused, the nurse can begin the educational process.

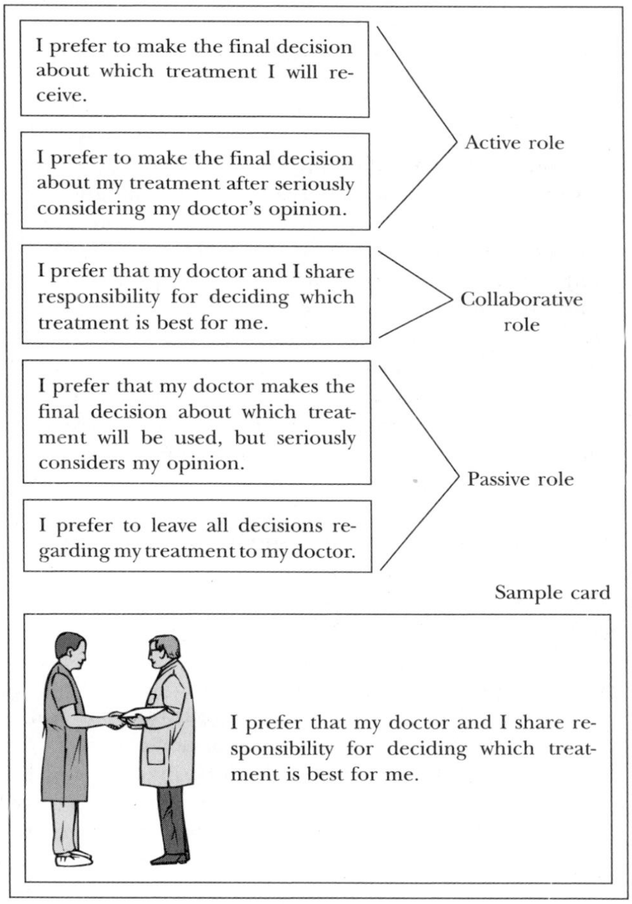

## Dealing with Uncertainty

Uncertainty is a common problem experienced by individuals and families dealing with cancer. The probabilistic nature of cancer diagnosis and treatment, the complexity of treatment and system of care, the lack of information about diagnosis and treatment, and the unpredictability of the disease course contribute to the uncertainty associated with cancer.[65] Uncertainty interferes with the formation of a realistic appraisal of a stressful problem because the individual is hampered in his or her efforts to recognize and classify information.

Appraisal in a situation of uncertainty involves the processes of inference and illusion. When using inference, the individual bases his or her appraisal on general knowledge and past experience by identifying examples from similar situations. The greater the similarity between the recalled event and the current situation, the greater the effect of recall on the formation of an appraisal.[66] Illusions—beliefs constructed in the absence of knowledge—may also be used to form an appraisal. The use of illusion can be valuable in protecting the individual when information is unavailable or when information is available but difficult to accept. The danger in using inference and illusion as a basis for making an appraisal of a threatening problem is that it may be flawed, distorted, or inaccurate. As shown in the example of the poor black women in North Carolina, the idea that a painless lump in the breast is best left alone has had enormous consequences in unnecessary disability and premature death for women of color.[12]

Under conditions of uncertainty, appraising a situation as threatening is likely to result in pessimism, elevated anxiety, or depression.[66] Coping efforts are directed to reducing the uncertainty and managing the emotion generated by an appraisal of threat. Direct action may be used to reduce uncertainty, although there is evidence that in catastrophic illnesses such as cancer, direct action is the least-used coping strategy. Vigilance in monitoring symptoms or health problems also may be used. However, the primary means for reducing uncertainty is information seeking. It is used to formulate probabilities and to create a framework for ordering illness-related experi-

**FIGURE 48-3**  Preferred roles in treatment decision making.
Newfeld KR, Degner LF, Dick JAM: A nursing intervention strategy to foster patient involvement in treatment decisions. *Oncol Nurs Forum* 20: 631–635, 1993

ences. Health care providers serve as information sources, and they also help to structure information. Significant others can also provide or reinforce expert information or they can interpret events. If these strategies are not effective in reducing uncertainty, then emotion-focused coping strategies are used to achieve this goal.

The goal of nursing is to reduce uncertainty whenever possible while recognizing that some aspects of uncertainty related to cancer may never be removed. Mishel[66], who has studied this phenomenon extensively, suggests that one way that health care professionals reduce uncertainty is by providing credible authority. Credible authority refers to the strength of the relationship and trust between an individual and a health care provider. Individuals may rely on professionals to provide a logical structure for interpreting their experiences as they proceed through them and to provide judgments and recommendations regarding the physical aspects of care, the efficacy of treatment, expectations about outcomes, and the performance of the health care system. The greater the nurse's credible authority, the greater his or her ability to reduce uncertainty related to cancer and its treatment.

The most common means of reducing uncertainty is by providing preparatory information about the specific aspects of the cancer experience faced by the individual. The content of the preparatory information is discussed elsewhere in this book. This section discusses the process of preparing people in a manner that enables them to cope more effectively with the experience. Research has demonstrated that the most effective information is that which helps people to form a realistic mental image of the experience they are about to undergo.[67–69] Both the subjective and objective characteristics of the experience should be described. Subjective features include physical sensations and experiences that can be verified only by the person experiencing them. This information must be obtained from people who have experienced a particular type of treatment and its effects.[70] Objective features include the temporal and spatial characteristics of an experience, such as how long a procedure lasts and what the environment looks like.

Several guidelines may be followed in the provision of this type of information. Physical sensations should be described without evaluation. For example, people may be told that after surgery, the incision will feel tender and sore and that they may feel pressure, aching, and pulling. They should be informed of the reasons for the sensations so they will be less likely to misinterpret them as evidence that something has gone wrong. This is especially true for individuals with cancer, because treatment-related symptoms can be confused with symptoms of the disease. Research has also shown that the use of emotionally charged words such as "pain" and descriptions of the magnitude of sensations such as the severity of pain are not helpful.[71]

Individuals who are properly informed are freed from the task of sorting through a large number of details about an experience to figure out the best way to handle it. Individuals are also less likely to misinterpret their experiences and choose inappropriate or inefficient methods of coping with them. This information has been found to have positive long-term effects on an individual's functional recovery from treatment procedures.[67,68,72]

## Managing the Side Effects of Treatment

Cancer treatment, whether curative, palliative, or prophylactic, does not come without a cost.[73] Treatment results in a variety of adverse side effects that can be debilitating and long-lasting, causing considerable distress for individuals and families dealing with cancer. Not surprisingly, many of the interventions that have been found effective in managing these side effects are psychosocial in nature, given that many of the side effects are stress-related.

King and associates[70] have pointed out that to be effective in managing the side effects of treatment, nurses need to be aware of the frequency, onset, duration, and severity of the symptoms presented by their patients in order to provide efficient and effective nursing assessment and interventions. For example, individuals receiving radiation therapy to the chest, head and neck, male genitourinary tract, or female reproductive system were queried about their experience of treatment-related symptoms.[70] Many of the symptoms reported by each of the groups occurred during the second and third weeks of treatment, and many of them could affect the individual's nutritional status (e.g., anorexia, nausea, fatigue, sore throat, changes in saliva, and diarrhea). The findings of this study suggest that a critical time for nursing assessment for this population is the second and third week of treatment. This information enables the nurse to allocate scarce nursing resources during the most critical time period without compromising patient care. Because many of these symptoms can affect nutritional status, it is critical that the nurse determine whether the experience of symptoms compromises the person's ability to maintain adequate intake of food or fluids. At-risk individuals, such as insulin-dependent diabetics or individuals taking potassium-depleting diuretics, should be scheduled for a symptom assessment at this time.

A variety of psychosocial interventions that prevent or alleviate treatment-related symptoms have been identified. Primary among these is preparatory information. Nursing interventions can be used to prepare individuals for treatment by informing them about what symptoms to expect, whether they will increase or decrease in severity, and how long they will last.[49] This information provides individuals with a standard for comparison with their own experience. The ability to anticipate side effects assists the individual in planning daily activities. Since fatigue was reported by a majority of individuals receiving radiation treatment, and a substantial number of people reported this symptom through the third month after treatment was completed, this information can be used to prepare people for the likelihood that they may need to continue to modify their usual activities for up to three months after treatment.[70]

The effectiveness of preparatory information for individuals with treatment-related symptoms is underscored by an investigation by Burish and associates.[47] They compared a general coping preparation procedure for individuals undergoing chemotherapy with a progressive muscle-relaxation training to determine the most effective means for reducing the conditioned side effects of chemotherapy and other types of treatment-related distress. The preparatory intervention consisted of one 90-minute class for patients and their families prior to the first chemotherapy treatment. A videotape presented the chemotherapy procedure, provided information dealing with typical questions, and showed a patient successfully dealing with the experience. A question and answer period followed, and a written summary of the session was provided.

The progressive muscle-relaxation training consisted of a 30-minute session in which the individual was trained to tense and relax ten major muscle groups followed by several minutes of relaxing imagery involving the use of a sequence of thoughts and mental pictures that facilitate or deepen relaxation. The specific imagery differed for each individual and was determined by a pretreatment interview. This training session was audiotaped so the individual could practice the relaxation techniques at home. Individuals were encouraged to practice the techniques frequently, especially during the days immediately following chemotherapy when the symptoms were most severe.

The results indicated that the preparatory information intervention was the most effective, reducing conditioned side effects, increasing individuals' knowledge of the disease and its treatment, reducing negative emotions, and improving general coping ability. The relaxation intervention decreased negative moods and vomiting but did not have the other beneficial effects of the preparatory information. A combination intervention did not have any advantage over the preparation intervention. Overall, the results indicate that preparatory information that oncology nurses can provide is more effective than a behavioral relaxation procedure requiring special training.[74]

Other interventions have also been identified that prevent or alleviate symptoms related to cancer treatment.[75] Stress reduction and distraction including relaxation, music, self-hypnosis, and massage have been effective for nausea and vomiting or pain.[76–82] Physical remedies have also been used: exercise[83] or oral ginger[84] for nausea and vomiting; extremity wraps for shivering[85]; and oral care for mucositis.[86]

## Responses of Families and Caregivers

Individuals with cancer are living longer with increasingly complex medical regimens. During periods of active treatment, patients frequently depend on their families for assistance with care, transportation, medical procedures, medication, and symptom management.[53] While the individual with cancer is under the family's care, a caregiver usually emerges. Most caregivers are older women caring for spouses or their parents. Caregivers often feel ultimately responsible for coordinating the care of the family member with cancer; they often feel they must be available 24 hours a day. When the caregiver requires assistance, most often it is obtained from another family member, rarely from a health care professional. A variety of caregiver needs and issues have been identified. These needs are most acute during the three-month period following hospitalization.[50,87,88] A major concern of caregivers is their own health and how they are going to manage all the demands on them. The caregiver who is employed often expresses concern about being able to maintain or return to his or her usual work pattern. Caregivers also report that providing emotional support to the individual with cancer is one of their most difficult tasks.[89] They also report a lack of time to develop supportive social relationships for themselves. Caregivers are unwilling to discuss their concerns with the cancer patient because of fears that it might be distressing to the patient and because of a need to "protect" him or her from becoming upset. The overwhelming demands and complexity of care for the individual with cancer can result in caregiver burden.[88–92]

In order to provide support to a husband or wife with cancer, a spouse must be able to see the situation from the other's perspective and to understand what he or she is experiencing. In an examination of the attitudes and experiences of Israeli spouses and patients about head and neck cancer, Chaitchik et al[93] found that, overall, spouses had little knowledge about the way in which their husband or wife experienced the stress of cancer. When relationships were examined between spouse and patient perceptions of health problems, social relationships, family functioning, work adjustment, or negative moods after diagnosis, few correlations were found between spouse and patient responses. However, when patients with low and high levels of information about their disease were compared, there was a significant correspondence between patient and spouse perceptions for patients with high information; whereas, for patients with low information, there was no correspondence between perceptions. The investigators concluded that the likely cause of low correspondence between patient and spouse responses is lack of information. When the individual with cancer knows little about his or her disease, the couple function under highly restrictive conditions of denial, fear, isolation, and conjecture.

Other research points to differences in the types of issues or concerns of cancer patients and their spouses. Patients receiving palliative care for advanced cancer reported that closeness with their partner was most important to their quality of life,[94] whereas spouses indicated that coping with marital situations was the major contributor to their QOL. The difference probably reflects a distinction of roles of the ill or healthy partner: the ill person is coming to terms with eventual death, while the healthy partner is coping with the concrete necessities of providing for the patient.

The research suggests that the nurse could play an important role in opening up channels of communication between the spouse and patient. The oncology nurse plays a critical role in informing the patient and spouse of the diagnosis and in deepening the spouse's understanding of the situation from the patient's perspective. This can be accomplished in several ways.[93] The nurse can converse with the patient and spouse alone and together. He or she can encourage the first discussion of disease-relevant issues in the presence of the nurse. The nurse who knows the patient and spouse well can describe for each partner how the other views the situation, thereby disclosing to the spouse the experience of the patient and suggesting to the patient the spouse's ignorance of his or her world. In doing this, the nurse would hope to evoke in each party enough curiosity about the world of the other to overcome the fear and despair that are likely to block effective communication. He or she can help them adopt a terminology for describing disease phenomena and referring to aspects of the situation. This process of patient and spouse education may help the parties to initiate a dialogue between them and then expand it.

In addition to his or her role in imparting information and supporting the communication efforts of patient and family, research has identified other important supportive roles for the oncology nurse. Twenty-four hour accessibility and availability of the hospice nurse was identified by family caregivers as critical in reducing their anxieties about caregiving.[95] Accessibility meant that there was always a respected, knowledgeable professional who could make helpful suggestions for changes in care or who would come in person if needed. As more complex regimens are being implemented at home, the need for such resources is likely to expand to more individuals and families.

## Changes in Sexual Functioning

Because of the seriousness of a cancer diagnosis, it is not surprising that professionals often do not address the likelihood of developing sexual dysfunction as a result of treatment. In addition, the ambivalence of Americans about discussing sexuality contributes to the silence that is often maintained by both professionals and patients. The oncology nurse has a pivotal role to play in preparing individuals for the consequences of treatment on sexual functioning, educating individuals about ways of coping with changes in sexual functioning, identifying individuals who are having difficulty coping with these changes, and making appropriate referrals. The need for timely professional nursing assessment is reinforced by research suggesting that the number of individuals reporting sexual dysfunction increases over time after cancer treat-

ment. In a group of women with breast cancer, 18% reported sexual dysfunction 3 months after surgery, 27% experienced it after 1 year, and 32% reported it at 24 months.[96] These findings suggest that earlier assessment could reduce coping difficulties associated with this problem.

Sexual dysfunction in cancer patients may be related to a variety of biological, psychological, or social factors. Diseases that affect the sexual organs, pelvis, or breasts are more likely to have consequences for sexual functioning than other cancers.[97] More invasive or disfiguring surgery and greater anatomical changes are more likely to result in sexual dysfunction. Hormonal changes including ovarian failure can result in loss of desire as well as problems with arousal. Not to be underestimated are the effects of chemotherapy on sexuality. Nausea and vomiting as well as hair loss affect body image and feelings of attractiveness. Low sexual desire, dyspareunia, and difficulty reaching orgasm are reported more frequently by women undergoing chemotherapy for breast cancer than by women who do not receive this treatment.[98] Also, concurrent medical conditions and/or treatments such as diabetes or the use of antihypertensive drugs can affect sexual functioning.

Psychological factors can also place an individual at risk for sexual difficulties. Negative moods, loss of personal control, cancer worries, relationship difficulties (such as poor communication or fear of rejection), and past psychiatric problems (including alcohol abuse) can contribute to sexual dysfunction.[99] Younger people, those without partners, and persons in relationships of shorter duration are at higher risk than older, longer-married patients.[100] People with traditional views of sexuality and gender role and those who are pessimistic about their future are more prone to sexual dysfunction after cancer treatment.[101]

Andersen[56] suggests that the overall extent of disease and treatment plays a major role in determining who is at risk for sexual morbidity after a diagnosis of cancer. More extensive disease is characterized by higher stage, more invasive or mutilating treatment, lack of applicability of reconstructive procedures (such as breast or vaginal reconstruction), and continuing stressors from disease or treatment. A review of several studies of women treated for cancer of the cervix, endometrium, or ovary revealed that persons with extensive disease had a 90%–100% risk of sexual morbidity, whereas those with limited disease had a risk of 20%–30%.[56] However, although individuals with limited disease had little disruption of overall quality of life, sexual functioning was the one life area at greatest risk of disruption. Furthermore, 30% of low-risk women reported that their partners had difficulty reaching orgasm, suggesting that partners of cancer patients need to be included in the plan of care for sexuality changes.

Assessment of sexual functioning must begin with information gathering and sexual history. Because health care professionals often feel uneasy about dealing with the topic of sexuality, a few general guidelines may be helpful. Privacy is important for discussions of sexuality.

It is useful for the nurse to assume a nonjudgmental attitude and not react emotionally to the discussion of sensitive issues. Moving from less-sensitive to more-sensitive issues can also help both the nurse and patient manage anxiety. The nurse must be aware of timing to ensure that this discussion is appropriate to the functional level and needs of the patient and/or partner.

Nurses are often wary of initiating discussions of sexuality with their patients because they feel they lack the necessary expertise to give advice. However, most discussions do not require a "sexuality expert."[102,103] What the individual needs is someone who is willing to discuss sexuality issues, who can offer advice about how to manage immediate problems (such as vaginal dryness), and who can identify resources for managing more difficult problems (such as a sex therapist or a physician who treats erectile dysfunction).

Three questions that can be incorporated into the general patient assessment at the beginning of treatment are recommended:[102,104]

- Has your cancer treatment interfered with being a spouse or parent?
  (Invites the individual to discuss his or her functional role in the family and how it has been altered by illness or treatment.)

- Has your cancer treatment changed the way you view yourself as a man or a woman?
  (Addresses the individual's sexual self-image.)

- Do you expect your sexual functioning/sex life to be changed by your cancer treatment?
  (Directly addresses sexual functioning.)

The nurse who conducts a nonthreatening and non-judgmental sexual history at the beginning of cancer treatment can do a lot to prevent and reduce the anxiety and guilt that can surround sexual concerns and problems. By initiating an early discussion of sexual issues, the nurse establishes both the legitimacy of these concerns and his or her willingness to discuss them. For example, a man anticipating an abdominoperitoneal resection who is encouraged to talk about sexual concerns in the preoperative period will probably be more comfortable initiating questions after treatment.

Annon[105] has described an approach to sexual rehabilitation known as the PLISSIT model that describes four levels of intervention for sexuality issues. At the first level, the nurse gives permission (P) to express sexual concerns. In some cases, the simple acknowledgment and discussion of a perceived change in sexual health may be sufficient to help the patient or partner resolve the problem. Providing limited information (LI) is the second level of the model. This may include information about sexual anatomy, the sexual response cycle, or specific sexual changes to be expected after treatment. The third level of intervention involves specific suggestions (SS) for communication of sexual concerns, alternative positions and techniques, the use of devices, and medical interventions to restore function or appearance. The fourth level, inten-

sive therapy (IT), is the only one that is more appropriately referred to a trained professional.

Health professionals often concentrate on issues for the individual with cancer, overlooking those of the partner. Cancer and its treatment may have consequences for the sexual partner of the individual with cancer although the needs of the partner have not been well researched.[99,101,106] Experts agree that more attention should be paid to the partner's responses and that both partners should be involved in treatment planning for sexual dysfunction to enhance recovery.[99]

Interventions for changes in sexual health generally combine education and counseling. A few empirical studies have addressed the effectiveness of such interventions.[107–110] The studies demonstrate that a brief therapy model is most effective in improving sexual outcomes, particularly for individuals with less extensive disease.[56] These interventions are characterized by early assessment of problems, present-day focus, limited goals, direction by the counselor, and prompt intervention. The interventions provide a supportive context for the discussion of varied concerns, information about specific problems related to disease and treatment, and focus on the development of cognitive and behavioral coping skills. The therapeutic components of the interventions have a greater impact on outcomes than their specific format. For example, both group and individual approaches were equally effective.[107] Likewise, involvement of sexual partners was not critical to the effectiveness of the interventions.[109,111] The research also indicates the need for interventions specifically focused on sexual functioning for individuals treated for cancer involving the genitals.[56] This includes information about sexuality, an explanation of the anticipated changes in sexual functioning resulting from treatment, a discussion of medical interventions that could restore functioning or appearance, and specific suggestions and strategies to improve sexual functioning.

## Problems of Cancer Survivors

Cancer survival rates have steadily improved over the past four decades[112] and have plateaued since the 1980s at about 50%. Increased survival means that more individuals complete treatment with the anticipation of being disease-free for an extended period of time. Yet survivors report a host of QOL problems, including difficulties with physical functioning, role adaptation, work productivity, social adaptation, and psychological distress.[113,114]

The experience of surviving cancer has been characterized as producing long-standing mental scars despite a lack of major or severe psychopathology.[115–117] Cancer survivors easily recall emotions related to illness and recovery, continuing concerns about mortality, and an enduring sense of vulnerability.[118] Even after definitive cure, cancer survivors are less certain about living a long life and have greater anxiety and mood changes.[119] The anniversary of a cancer diagnosis can trigger reactions that include reexperiencing the diagnosis and nightmares or flashbacks about the experience.[116,119] One year after diagnosis, breast cancer survivors express concern about whether the cancer will recur or progress, not being able to care for themselves in the future, and how their families will manage without them if they die. They also report difficulty communicating with their providers and families about these fears and worries.[63,120]

Survivors often experience stress during reentry into the "well role."[114] The intense outpouring of emotional support experienced during treatment may not be sustained when the individual no longer looks and acts sick. Friends and relatives engage in a sorting-out process, ultimately determining who remains close and who distances themselves from the survivor.[117] Likewise, marital stress that accumulates during treatment can produce marital disruption after the completion of therapy.[121] The issue of infertility caused by treatment can be a source of distress for childless couples.[122]

Employment-related problems have been identified by almost 40% of cancer survivors,[123] including denial of insurance or other benefits, not getting job offers, conflict with supervisors or coworkers, and termination of employment.[121] Despite difficulties, approximately 80% return to work after diagnosis.[124] Some survivors indicate that the experience of having had cancer has "locked" them into their jobs because of fears of lost medical coverage, pension rights, or other benefits. The Americans with Disabilities Act of 1994 has greatly increased the rights of workers with disabilities due to cancer.

Although it has not been well researched, survivors themselves have pointed to the need for education to restore and maintain their well-being. Survivors want to be informed of potential disruptions before they experience them. A number of specific learning needs have been identified for survivors.[121,125] One is the fact that fatigue or energy loss may be a problem for a year or more after therapy is completed, especially if the individual is elderly. Survivors also need information about the likelihood of marital stress after treatment is over. Likewise, employers may need information and input to understand the survivor's work-related limitations due to the cancer or its treatment. Fear of cancer recurrence is common, and education about the problem as well as strategies for overcoming it are necessary. In addition, survivors need information about how to cope with physical disabilities.

## PROFESSIONAL RESPONSES TO CANCER

Like individuals and families dealing with cancer, the oncology nurse must engage coping skills to adapt to the charged emotional environment in which they work. The professional needs to see the challenge of the cancer experience in a way that resonates with his or her own beliefs about life, death, and illness, so that caring for

this group of people does not become emotionally overwhelming. Generally, this adaptation occurs on both conscious and unconscious levels.[126]

Consciously, nurses engage their intellects to grasp the situation in which they find themselves, rejecting superstitions and myths about cancer. Examples of superstitions include beliefs about contagion and horrible deaths. Oncology nurses work with patients and families to solve problems, offer constructive feedback, and function under pressure with patients. Their emotional controls generally work effectively.

The unconscious, however, is less rational. Nurses may find themselves avoiding certain situations or responding to them irrationally. They believe that verbalizing their anxiety and acknowledging their fear of cancer renders them both vulnerable and nonprofessional. In turn, feelings of embarrassment, shame, guilt, and anger focused at themselves for their weaknesses are kept hidden.

These feelings are part of the normal adaptation to oncology nurses' professional lives, just as it is normal for patients and families to experience a wide range of emotions. Unless they have dealt with cancer extensively or experienced many losses, the professional education they have received leaves them less than optimally equipped to deal with the stresses they experience.

In a process parallel to that experienced by patients and families, there is a time component to experimenting with various coping strategies before resolving feelings in a comfortable manner. Anxiety related to working with cancer patients is greatest at the beginning of work life and is usually stabilized after about six months. During this time, nurses may experience transient cancerphobia—for example, having feelings of panic about swollen lymph nodes and fearing it is lymphoma.[126] Vachon[127] found that stress levels of nurses on a new palliative care unit were equal to those of recently widowed women. Stress levels returned to that of a control group not experiencing either of these challenges by the end of one year.

By accepting the lack of control over this disease and modifying their expectations of outcomes, nurses can begin to acknowledge the extent of their emotional reactions while caring for this population, and they may doubt their own sense of purpose. Questions such as "Why am I putting myself through this?" and "Why am I bothering if I can't cure this person?" are normal. At this time, nurses should mourn the losses and discover their inner strength. It is at this time that all experiences, both personal and professional, will be mixed together to shape character and influence what choices nurses make in their lives.[123] A minority of professional caregivers will be stuck in reactive anxiety and depression that, with proper support, can resolve spontaneously in weeks or months. Conversely, the nurse may decide it is better to transfer to another type of nursing.

In the same manner that patients and families choose coping behaviors that are successful or unsuccessful, the oncology nurse chooses from various strategies. Two concepts, distancing and caring, can be examined from the standpoint of being "value neutral" forms of coping. Either strategy employed to excess can have negative consequences for both the caregiver and the patient.

Distancing is a response used by professionals, either consciously or unconsciously, to those in their care. Typically, this has been a response to one who is dying.[128] It may manifest as less time spent with a particular individual, ignoring a call light, failure to communicate, and an unswaying "professionalism" in emotionally charged situations. Maguire et al[110] found that this was a strategy often used when a patient had not been fully informed of the diagnosis. Today, this strategy often is used with patients and families who are viewed as difficult, by caregivers uncomfortable with closeness, and among members of the health care team when conflicts arise. Distancing can be helpful in allowing the patient and family to try out their own problem-solving skills in a controlled situation before having to handle the problems alone, or by setting appropriate limits about the amount of nursing time or resources that realistically can be provided. Distancing becomes "unsuccessful" when it occurs over a long period of time and results in increased loneliness and isolation in those for whom one is caring.

Professionals also use caring as a response to cancer. Caring has been defined in a number of ways. In 1979, Watson[129] referred to caring as a process that helped a person attain or maintain health or a peaceful death. Benner and Wrubel[130] defined caring as an enabling condition of connection and concern. Caring is communicated by accepting the patient and respecting thoughts, feelings, and needs. It implies access. Generally speaking, caring describes the quality of the nurse-patient interaction. Caring, like distancing, can be given in excess, withheld, or used successfully as a technique to help the nurse and patient achieve goals.

Another way of thinking about caring and distancing is to describe "boundaries." Caring is the essence of the therapeutic use of self, such as empowering the patient and family through care, education, and guidance to gain control over the situation in which they find themselves.[131] In order for caring to be successful, professional boundaries need to be maintained; otherwise, potentially negative outcomes (such as overinvolvement and burnout) can develop for both the patient and professional. A boundary is a psychological term referring to one's sphere of influence. Boundaries can be rigid, diffuse, or clear (Figure 48-4). Interactions start at the point where nurses' boundaries touch those of others. If the boundaries are rigid, they will not touch or influence the boundaries of the other person with whom they are trying to relate. There will be a psychological gap between the patient and caregiver. Most nurses have encountered the "cool" or "hard" caregiver who never gets involved with the patient or family and seems untouched by the emotions around them.

If boundaries are diffuse, they overlap with the boundaries of others. Nurses may become enmeshed with their

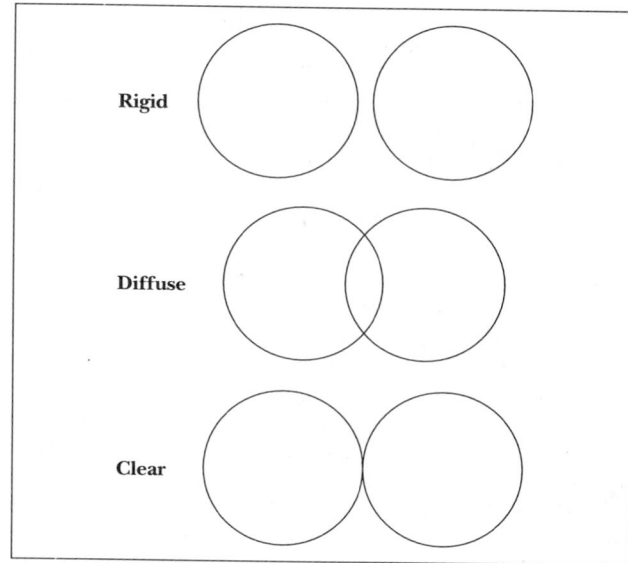

**FIGURE 48-4**  Professional boundaries.

patients and may become overinvolved in their care. The nurse in this scenario stays late often, believes he or she is the only one who can care adequately for this individual, and provides opinions about medical care and treatment decisions. As an example, the nurse may promote chemotherapy for a similarly aged woman with children because that is what the nurse would want if she had cancer. The nurse has become overinvested emotionally.

When psychological boundaries are clear, they touch another's but do not get mixed up with the other person's priorities or goals. Nurses relate and are empathetic but they do not impose their choices on others; rather, they help others decide what is in their own best interests. These are the kind of boundaries that professionals strive for. This is when caring is therapeutic.

Oncology nursing is full of situations that "hook" nurses into violating the boundaries of others. Examples include patients of the same age, those who remind nurses of family or loved ones, patients with circumstances similar to theirs, those similar to others they have cared for, and colleagues who are patients.

It is normal for the oncology nurse to "cross" boundaries periodically, either by being too close or too aloof in a particular situation. When the majority of interactions fall either one way or the other, the nurse should consider the ramifications of actions. Underinvestment leaves the nurse unfulfilled and the patient feeling alone and lost in the experience. Underinvestment may be the result of repeated overinvestment in the past. Conversely, overinvestment can leave the patient relying on the nurse for decision making, and the nurse feeling overextended and burned out. It is important to remember that when nurses become like "family" to a patient, they lose their value as a professional resource.

The nurse needs to ask the following questions: Is

my job satisfaction related to how much a patient or family needs me? Do I feel no one can care for the patient as well as I can? Is it difficult for me to leave my patients at the end of the day? If the answer to any of the questions is "yes," boundary difficulties may be present. Other questions can be asked either individually or of the institution as a whole: Are there "favorite" patients? What happens to those patients who are no one's favorite? Are nurses simultaneously maintaining professional and social relationships with patients and families? Are nurses assuming responsibility for some facets of care that might be better handled by families, social services, or community resources (e.g., buying items and bringing them in for patients, buying gifts or taking care of children while parents are hospitalized, or providing meals for patients and families during recovery after hospital discharge)?

Nurses with boundary problems usually come by it naturally, that is, they usually come from a family with similar conflicts about boundaries.[131] Therefore, nurses must recognize the type of family system they were brought up in. If everyone in a nurse's family is highly involved in his or her life to the point that individuality is compromised, the nurse is likely to become heavily invested in the lives of patients he or she cares for. If, however, the nurse grew up without closeness, she or he is likely to have a distant professional demeanor; conversely, he or she can overcompensate for the isolation experienced by becoming overinvolved with patients.

Issues related to boundaries are best handled through open, honest communication and discussions. This can be done by informal discussion, staff development programs, standards for professional nursing practice, and departmental guidelines. The approach taken should consider the institutional norms, the individual setting, the desire to change, the resources available, and the degree of administrative support.

Barnsteiner and Gillis-Donovan[131] reported on the method used by one urban pediatric center to develop standards for therapeutic relationships and culture modifications. Staff representation and nursing leadership collected sufficient data to define and conceptualize the problem, and then went on to write policy, train staff regarding concepts, and educate other departments. Mental health clinical nurse specialists were employed to help resolve issues as they were identified (issues of loss and grief for staff, close identification with patients/families, etc.). Systems were put into place to help provide for unique needs of patients or families so that an individual nurse would not need to provide for the patients.

Individually, nurses need to understand themselves and the dynamics of their family of origin; seek balance between their personal and professional lives; seek the counsel of their managers, peers, families, friends, or a mental health professional; take the time to recognize limitations and vulnerabilities; and let go of the illusion of controlling the whole situation.

## CONCLUSION

Cancer threatens both quantity and quality of life for the person who is faced with complex treatment plans, uncertainty of recurrence, and the prospect of alterations in self-concept, roles, and relationships with others. The oncology nurse can play a significant role in helping individuals and their families cope with the many stresses they face by assessing their needs and concerns and by being flexible in providing both educational and emotional support. The ultimate goal is to help individuals adjust to and achieve control over the stresses of the cancer experience.

## REFERENCES

1. Sabo D: Men, death anxiety, and denial: Critical feminist interpretations of adjustment to mastectomy, in Clark C, Fritz J, Reid P (eds): *Clinical Sociological Perspectives on Illness and Loss.* Philadelphia, Charles Press, 1990, pp 71–84
2. Northouse L: The impact of cancer on the family: An overview. *Int J Psychiatry Med* 14:215–242, 1984
3. Lazarus RS, Folkman S: *Stress, Appraisal, and Coping.* New York, Springer, 1984
4. Crane SC: A research agenda for outcomes research. *Proceedings of the State of the Science Conference sponsored by the National Center for Nursing Research.* In *Patient Outcome Research: Examining the Effectiveness of Nursing Practice.* NIH publication No. 93–3411. Bethesda, MD, Public Health Service, National Institutes of Health, 1992
5. Lang NM, Marek KD: Outcomes that reflect clinical practice. *Proceedings of the State of the Science Conference sponsored by the National Center for Nursing Research.* In *Patient Outcome Research: Examining the Effectiveness of Nursing Practice.* NIH publication No. 93–3411. Bethesda, MD, Public Health Service, National Institutes of Health, 1992
6. Aguilera DC: *Crisis Intervention Theory and Methodology* (ed 6). Philadelphia, Mosby, 1990
7. Giger JN, Davidhizar RE: *Transcultural Nursing: Assessment and Intervention.* Philadelphia, Mosby Year Book, 1991
8. Chen MS: Behavioral and psychosocial cancer research in the underserved. *Cancer* 74:1503–1508, 1994
9. Evans LA: Black and white differences: Narrowing the gap in cancer medicine. *In vivo* 6:429–434, 1992
10. Kerner JF, Dusenbury L, Mandelblatt JS: Poverty and cultural diversity: Challenges for health promotion among the medically underserved. *Ann Rev Public Health* 14:355–377, 1993
11. Balshem M: Cancer, control, and causality; a working-class community. *Am Ethnol* 18:152–172, 1991
12. Mathews HF, Lannin DR, Mitchell JP: Coming to terms with advanced breast cancer: Black women's narratives from Eastern North Carolina. *Soc Sci Med* 38:789–800, 1994
13. Frank-Stromborg M: *Carrier Prevention in Minority Populations.* St. Louis, Mosby, 1993
14. Kahn SB, Houts PS, Harding SP: Quality of life and patients with cancer: A comparative study of patient versus physi-

cian perceptions and its implications for cancer education. *J Cancer Educ* 7:241–249, 1992

15. Vinokur AD, Threatt BA, Caplan RD, et al: Physical and psychosocial functioning and adjustment to breast cancer: Long-term follow-up of a screening population. *Cancer* 63:394–405, 1989

16. Vinokur AD, Threatt BA, Vinokur-Kaplan D, et al: The process of recovery from breast cancer for younger and older patients: Changes during the first year. *Cancer* 65:1242–1254, 1990

17. Mischel W: *Personality and Assessment*. New York, Wiley, 1968

18. Smith RA, Wallston BS, Wallston KA, et al: Measuring desire for control of health care processes. *J Pers Soc Psychol* 47:485–492, 1984

19. Carver CS, Pozo C, Harris SD, et al: How coping mediates the effect of optimism on distress: A study of women with early stage breast cancer. *J Pers Soc Psychol* 65:375–390, 1993

20. Krantz DS, Baum A, Wideman M: Assessment of preferences for self-treatment and information in health care. *J Pers Soc Psychol* 39:977–990, 1980

21. Miller SM, Mangan CE: Interacting effects of information and coping style in adapting to gynecologic stress: Should the doctor tell all. *J Pers Soc Psychol* 45:223–236, 1983

22. Waltz CF, Strickland OL: *Measurement of Nursing Outcomes* (vol 1). New York, Springer, 1988

23. Strickland OL: Measures and instruments. *Proceedings of the State of the Science Conference sponsored by the National Center for Nursing Research*. In *Patient Outcome Research: Examining the Effectiveness of Nursing Practice*. NIH publication No. 93-3411. Bethesda, MD, Public Health Service, National Institutes of Health, 1992

24. Plumb M, Holland J: Comparative studies of psychological function in patients with advanced cancer: II. Interviewer-rated current and past psychological symptoms. *Psychosom Med* 43:243–254, 1981

25. Maunsell E, Brisson J, Deschenes L: Psychological distress after initial treatment of breast cancer. *Cancer* 70:120–125, 1992

26. Stewart AL, Greenfield S, Hays RD, et al: Functional status and well-being of patients with chronic conditions: Results from the medical outcomes study. *J Am Med Assoc* 262:907–913, 1989

27. Ortmeyer CF: Variation in mortality, morbidity, and health care by marital status, in Erhardt LL, Berlin JE (eds): *Mortality and morbidity in the United States*. Cambridge, MA, Harvard University Press, 1974, pp 159–184

28. Goodwin JS, Hunt WC, Key CR, et al: The effect of marital status on stage, treatment, and survival of cancer patients. *JAMA* 258:3125–3130, 1987

29. Berkman LF, Syme SL: Social networks, host resistance, and mortality: A nine year follow-up study of Alameda County residents. *Am J Epidemiol* 109:186–204, 1987

30. House JS, Hunt WC, Samet JM: The association of social relationships and activities with mortality: Prospective evidence from the Tecumseh community health study. *Am J Epidemiol* 116:123–140, 1982

31. Goodwin JS, Hunt WC, Samet JM: A population-based study of functional status and social support networks of elderly patients newly diagnosed with cancer. *Arch Intern Med* 151:366–370, 1991

32. Anderson BL: Psychological interventions for cancer patients to enhance the quality of life. *J Consult Clin Psychol* 60:552–568, 1992

33. Fawzy FI, Fawzy NW, Arndt LA, et al: Critical review of psychosocial interventions in cancer care. *Arch Gen Psychiatry* 52:100–113, 1995

34. Devine EC, Westlake SK: The effects of psychoeducational care provided to adults with cancer: Meta-analysis of 116 studies. *Oncol Nurs Forum* 22:1369–1381, 1995

35. McCabe MS: Psychological support for the patient on chemotherapy. *Oncology* 5:91–99, 1991

36. Herth KA: The relationship between level of hope and level of coping response and other variables in patients with cancer. *Oncol Nurs Forum* 16:67–72, 1989

37. Greer S: Psychological response to cancer and survivors. *Psychol Med* 21:43–49, 1991

38. Pettingale KW: Coping and cancer prognosis. *J Psychosom Res* 28:363–364, 1984

39. Spiegel D: *Living Beyond Limits: New Help and Hope for Facing Life-threatening Illness*. New York, Times Books/Random House, 1993

40. Temoshok L, Heller BW, Sagebiel RW, et al: The relationship of psychosocial factors to prognostic indicators in cutaneous malignant melanoma. *J Psychosom Res* 29:139–153, 1983

41. Heiney SP: The healing power of story. *Oncol Nurs Forum* 22:899–904, 1995

42. Cunningham M: The moral of the story, in Weaver M (ed): *Tales as Tools: The Power of Story in the Classroom*. Jonesborough, TN, National Storytelling Association Press, 1994, pp 11–14

43. MacDonald M: Making time for stories, in Weaver M (ed): *Tales as Tools: The Power of Story in the Classroom*. Jonesborough, TN, National Storytelling Association Press, 1994, pp 9–10

44. Schram P: Collections for the people of the story, in Weaver M (ed): *Tales as Tools: The Power of Story in the Classroom*. Jonesborough, TN, National Storytelling Association Press, 1994, pp 176–178

45. Bornstein EM: Therapeutic storytelling, in Zahourek RP (ed.): *Relaxation and Imagery: Tools for Therapeutic Communication and Intervention*. Philadelphia, Saunders, 1988, pp 101–120

46. Cella DF: Quality of life: Concepts and definition. *J Pain Sympt Management* 9:186–192, 1994

47. Burish TG, Snyder SL, Jenkins RA: Preparing patients for cancer chemotherapy: Effect of coping preparation and relaxation interventions. *J Consult Clin Psychol* 59:518–525, 1991

48. Johnson JE, Nail LM, Lauver D, et al: Reducing the negative impact of radiation therapy on functional status. *Cancer* 61:46–51, 1988

49. Johnson JE, Lauver DR, Nail LM: Process of coping with radiation therapy. *J Consult Clin Psychol* 57:358–364, 1989

50. McCorkle R, Benoliel JQ, Donaldson G, et al: Randomized clinical trial of home nursing care for lung cancer patients. *Cancer* 64:1375–1382, 1989

51. Barsevick AM, Pasacreta J, Orsi A: Psychological distress and functional dependency in colorectal cancer patients. *Cancer Pract* 3:105–110, 1995

52. Guadagnoli E, Mor V: Measuring cancer patients' affect: Revision and psychometric properties of the profile of mood states (POMS). *J Consult Clin Psychol* 1:150–154, 1989

53. Laizner AM, Yost LM, Barg FK, et al: Needs of family caregivers of persons with cancer: A review. *Semin Oncol Nurs* 9:114–120, 1993

54. Cella DF, Yellen SB: Cancer support groups: The state of the art. *Cancer Pract* 1:56–61, 1993

55. Spiegel D, Bloom JR: Group therapy and hypnosis reduce metastatic breast carcinoma pain. *Psychosom Med* 45:333–339, 1983

56. Anderson BL: Predicting sexual and psychologic morbidity and improving the quality of life for women with gynecologic cancer. *Cancer* 71:1678–1690, 1993

57. Hack TF, Degner LF, Dyck DG: Relationship between preferences for decisional control and illness information among women with breast cancer: A quantitative and qualitative analysis. *Soc Sci Med* 39:279–289, 1994

58. Oken D: What to tell cancer patients: A study of medical attitude. *J Am Med Assoc* 175:1120, 1961

59. Degner LF, Sloan JA: Decision-making during serious illness: What role do patients really want to play? *J Clin Epidemiol* 45:941, 1992

60. Newfeld KR, Degner LF, Dick JAM: A nursing intervention strategy to foster patient involvement in treatment decisions. *Oncol Nurs Forum* 20:631–635, 1993

61. North N, Cornbleet MA, Knowles G, et al: Information giving in oncology: A preliminary study of tape-recorder use. *Br J Clin Psychol* 31:357, 1992

62. Reynolds PM, Sanson-Fisher RW, Poole AD, et al: Cancer and communication: Information-giving in an oncology clinic. *Br Med J* 282:1449, 1981

63. Greenfield S, Kaplan S, Ware JE: Expanding patient involvement in care: Effect and patient outcomes. *Ann Intern Med* 102:520–528, 1985

64. Miller SM, Shoda Y, Hurley K: Applying cognitive social theory to health protective behavior: Breast self-examination in cancer screening. *Psychol Bull* (in press)

65. Mishel MH, Braden CO: Finding meaning: Antecedents of uncertainty in illness. *Nurs Res* 37:98–103, 1988

66. Mishel MH: Uncertainty in illness. *Image* 20:225–232, 1988

67. Johnson JE, Fuller SS, Endress MP, et al: Altering patients' responses to surgery: An extension and replication. *Res Nurs Health* 1:111–121, 1978

68. Johnson JE, Rice VH, Fuller SS, et al: Sensory information, instruction in a coping strategy, and recovery from surgery. *Res Nurs Health* 1:4–17, 1978

69. McHugh NG, Christman NJ, Johnson JE: Preparatory information: What helps and why. *Am J Nurs* 82:780–782, 1982

70. King KB, Nail LM, Kreamer K, et al: Patients' descriptions of the experience of receiving radiation treatment. *Oncol Nurs Forum* 12:55–61, 1985

71. Leventhal H, Brown D, Shacham S and Engquist G: Effects of preparatory information about sensations, threat of pain, and attention on cold pressor distress. *J Pers Soc Psychol* 37:688–714, 1979

72. Johnson JE: Psychological interventions and coping with surgery, in Baum A, Taylor SE, Singer JE (eds): *Handbook of psychology and health: Vol. 4. Social psychological aspects of health.* Hillsdale, NJ, Erlbaum, 1984, pp 167–187

73. Burish TG, Redd WH: Symptom control in psychosocial oncology. *Cancer* 74:1438–1444, 1994

74. Burish TG, Tope DM: Psychological techniques for controlling the adverse side effects of cancer chemotherapy: Findings from a decade of research. *J Pain Sympt Management* 7:287–301, 1992

75. Smith MC, Holcombe JK, Stullenbarger E: A meta-analysis of intervention effectiveness for symptom management in oncology nursing research. *Oncol Nurs Forum* 21:1201–1210, 1994

76. Cotanch PH, Strum S: Progressive muscle relaxation as antiemetic therapy for cancer patients. *Oncol Nurs Forum* 14:33–37, 1987

77. Lerman C, Rimer B, Blumberg B, et al: Effects of coping style and relaxation on cancer chemotherapy side effects and emotional responses. *Cancer Nurs* 13:308–315, 1990

78. Carty JL: Relaxation with imagery: An adjunctive treatment for anticipatory nausea and/or vomiting. Unpublished doctoral dissertation, Catholic University of America, Washington, DC, 1990

79. Weinrich SP, Weinrich MC: The effect of massage on pain in cancer patients. *Appl Nurs Res* 3:140–145, 1990

80. Beck SCL: The effect of the therapeutic use of music on cancer related pain. Unpublished doctoral dissertation, University of Utah, Salt Lake City, 1988

81. Zimmerman L, Pozehl B, Duncan K, et al: Effects of music in patients who had chronic cancer pain. *West J Nurs Res* 11:298–309, 1989

82. Dalton JA, Toomey T, Workman MR: Pain relief for cancer patients. *Cancer Nurs* 11:322–328, 1988

83. Winningham ML, MacVicar MG: The effect of aerobic exercise on patient reports of nausea. *Oncol Nurs Forum* 15:447–450, 1988

84. Pace JC: Oral ingestion of encapsulated ginger and reported self-care actions for relief of chemotherapy associated nausea and vomiting. Unpublished doctoral dissertation, University of Alabama at Birmingham, 1986

85. Holtzclaw BJ: Control of febrile shivering during amphotericin B therapy. *Oncol Nurs Forum* 17:521–524, 1990

86. Kenny SA: Effect of two oral care protocols on the incidence of stomatitis in hematology patients. *Cancer Nurs* 13:345–353, 1990

87. Oberst MT, James RH: Going home: Patient and spouse adjustment following cancer surgery. *Top Clin Nurs* 7:46–57, 1985

88. McCorkle R, Wilkerson K: Home care needs of cancer patients and their families. *Final Report (NR01914)*. Philadelphia, National Center for Nursing Research, 1991

89. Carey PJ, Oberst MT, McCubbin MA, et al: Appraisal and caregiving burden in family members caring for patients receiving chemotherapy. *Oncol Nurs Forum* 18:1341–1348, 1991

90. Siegel K, Raveis VH, Houts P, et al: Caregiver burden and unmet patient needs. *Cancer* 68:1131–1140, 1991

91. Jensen S, Given BA: Fatigue affecting family caregivers of cancer patients. *Cancer Nurs* 14:181–187, 1991

92. Given CW, Stommel M, Given B, et al: The influence of cancer patients' symptoms and functional states on patients' depression and family caregivers' reaction and depression. *Health Psychol* 12:277–285, 1993

93. Chaitchik S, Kreitler S, Rappoport Y, et al: What do cancer patients' spouses know about the patients? *Cancer Nurs* 15:353–362, 1992

94. Fuller S, Swensen CH: Marital quality and quality of life among cancer patients and their spouses. *J Psychosoc Oncol* 10:41–56, 1992

95. Hull MM: Hospice nurses: Caring support for caregiving families. *Cancer Nurs* 14:63–70, 1991

96. Morris J, Ingham R: Choice of surgery for early breast cancer: Psychosocial considerations. *Soc Sci Med* 27:1257, 1988

97. Schover LR: The impact of breast cancer on sexuality, body image, and intimate relationships. *Cancer* 41:112–120, 1991

98. Schover LR, Yetman RJ, Tuason LJ, et al: Partial mastectomy and breast reconstruction. *Cancer* 75:54–64, 1995

99. Dobkin PL, Bradley I: Assessment of sexual dysfunction in oncology patients: Review, critique, and suggestions. *J Psychosoc Oncol* 9:43–75, 1991

100. Andersen BL: Sexual functioning morbidity among cancer survivors: Present status and future research directions. *Cancer* 55:1835–1842, 1985

101. Schover LR, Evans RB, von Eschenbach AC: Sexual rehabilitation in a cancer center: Diagnosis and outcome in 384 consultations. *Arch Sex Behav* 16:445–461, 1987

102. Shell JA, Smith CK: Sexuality and the older person with cancer. *Oncol Nurs Forum* 21:553–558, 1994

103. Smith DB, Babaian R: The effects of treatment for cancer on male fertility and sexuality. *Cancer Nurs* 15:271–275, 1992

104. Lamb MA, Woods NF: Sexuality and the cancer patient. *Cancer Nurs* 4:137–144, 1981

105. Annon JS: *Behavioral Treatment of Sexual Problems: Brief Therapy*. New York, Harper & Row, 1976

106. Steinberg MS, Juliano MA, Wise L: Psychological outcome of lumpectomy versus mastectomy in the treatment of breast cancer. *Am J Psychiatry* 142:34–39, 1985

107. Cain EN, Kohorn EI, Quinlan DM, et al: Psychosocial benefits of a cancer support group. *Cancer* 57:183–189, 1986

108. Capone MA, Good RS, Westie KS, et al: Psychosocial rehabilitation of gynecologic oncology patients. *Arch Phys Med Rehabil* 61:128–132, 1980

109. Christensen DN: Postmastectomy couple counseling: An outcome study of a structured treatment protocol. *J Sex Marital Ther* 9:266–274, 1983

110. Maguire P, Hopwood P, Tarrier N, et al: Treatment of depression in cancer patients. *Acta Psychiatr Scand* 72: 81–84, 1985 (suppl 320)

111. Heinrich RL, Coscarelli-Schag C: Stress and activity management: Group treatment for cancer patients and their spouses. *J Consult Clin Psychol* 53:439–446, 1985

112. Horm JW: An overview of female breast cancer, in Engstrom PF, Rimber B, Mortensen LE (eds): *Advances in Cancer Control: Screening and Prevention Research: Proceedings of the Association of Community Cancer Centers 15th National Meeting*. Bethesda, MD, March 29-April 1, 1989. New York City, Wiley-Liss, 1990, pp 217–226

113. Schag CAC, Ganz PA, Polinsky ML, et al: Characteristics of women at risk for psychosocial distress in the year after breast cancer. *J Clin Oncol* 11:783–793, 1993

114. Welch-McCaffrey D, Hoffman B, Leigh SA, et al: Surviving adult cancers. Part 2: Psychosocial implications. *Ann Intern Med* 111:517–524, 1989

115. Mullan F: Seasons of survival: Reflections of a physician with cancer. *N Engl J Med* 313:270–273, 1985

116. Smith K, Lesko LM: Psychosocial problems in cancer survivors. *Oncology* 2:33–44, 1988

117. Cella DF: Cancer survival: Psychosocial and public issues. *Cancer Invest* 5:59–67, 1987

118. Shanfield SB: On surviving cancer: Psychological considerations. *Compr Psychiatry* 21:128–134, 1980

119. Cella DF, Tross S: Psychological adjustment to survival from Hodgkin's disease. *J Consult Clin Psychol* 54:616–622, 1986

120. Schag CAC, Heinrich RL, Aadland RL, et al: Assessing problems of cancer patients: Psychometric properties of the Cancer Inventory of Problem Situations. *Health Psychol* 9:83–102, 1990

121. Fobair R, Hoppe RT, Bloom J, et al: Psychosocial problems among survivors of Hodgkin's disease. *J Clin Oncol* 4: 805–814, 1986

122. Schover LR, Fife M: Sexual counseling of patients undergoing medical surgery for pelvic or genital cancer. *J Psychosoc Oncol* 3:21–41, 1985

123. Houts PS, Kahn SB, Yasko JM, et al: The incidence and causes of job-related problems among employed persons with cancer in Pennsylvania. *J Psychosoc Oncol* 1989 (in press)

124. Crothers HM: Employment problems of cancer survivors: local problems and local solutions, in *Proceedings of the Workshop of Employment Insurance and the Patient with Cancer*. New Orleans, American Cancer Society, 1986

125. Mullan F: Re-entry: The educational needs of the cancer survivor. *Health Educ Q* 10:88–94, 1984 (suppl)

126. Lederberg MS: Psychological problems of staff and their management, in Holland JC, Rowland JH (eds): *Handbook of Psycho-oncology: Psychological Care of the Patient with Cancer*. New York, Oxford University Press, 1990, pp 631–646

127. Vachon MLS: Motivation and stress experienced by staff working with terminally ill. *Death Educ* 2:113–122, 1978

128. Youll JW: The bridge beyond: Strengthening nursing practice in attitudes towards death, dying, and the terminally ill, and helping the spouses of critically ill patients. *Intensive Care Nurs* 5:88–94, 1989

129. Watson J: *Nursing: The Philosophy and Science of Caring*. Boston, Little, Brown, 1979

130. Benner P, Wrubel J: *The Primacy of Caring: Stress and Coping in Health and Illness*. Menlo Park, California, Addison-Wesley, 1989

131. Barnsteiner JH, Gillis-Donovan J: Being related and separate: A standard for therapeutic relationships. *Am J Matern Child Nurs* 15:223–228, 1990

# Chapter 49

# Physical, Economic, and Social Adaptation of the Cancer Survivor

**Karen Smith Blesch, RN, PhD**

## INTRODUCTION

The early literature dealing with the physical, emotional, and psychosocial issues facing cancer survivors focused on rehabilitation and functional adaptation to specific physical deficits (such as ostomies, amputations, or lymphedema) due to the disease and its treatment. It stressed realistic and measurable goal setting with the patient, social and emotional well-being, and use of interdisciplinary teams, as well as the notion that cancer rehabilitation begins at diagnosis and continues throughout the disease trajectory. Although the early literature raised issues such as returning to work, economic security, family relationships, job discrimination, sexuality, telling the patient his or her diagnosis, health care reimbursement, alterations in body image, and pain and symptom management, it did not consider them in depth because there was little knowledge about these issues at the time.[1-7]

The early literature was written largely by rehabilitation physicians, physical therapists, and counselors who saw specific applications of their work in cancer patients. Oncology nurses began contributing to the cancer rehabilitation literature in the late 1980s and early 1990s, when the growing cancer survivorship movement renewed interest in cancer rehabilitation concepts[8-10] and began to emphasize psychosocial as well as physical functioning aspects of cancer rehabilitation.[11-13]

In 1989 the Oncology Nursing Society defined cancer rehabilitation as "a process by which individuals, within their environments, are assisted to achieve optimal functioning within the limits imposed by cancer."[14] This definition allowed consideration of both the psychosocial and the physical functioning aspects of cancer rehabilitation, thus expanding the scope of needs and interventions that could be considered rehabilitative.[15-20] It allowed cancer rehabilitation to be considered as a conceptual approach to cancer care as well as a specific program of services that addresses survivorship issues.[21]

Many cancer patients do not fit the classic picture of a "rehabilitation patient," an individual whose functional status is limited by specific, easily identified neuromuscular or physical deficits that require specific training, adaptive devices, or prosthetics. The functional status of individuals with cancer is more often limited by pain, fatigue, nausea, disfigurement, and psychosocial problems rather than specific physical disabilities.[22] These types of problems are often more difficult to identify and manage effectively than concrete physical deficits.

Today cancer rehabilitation concerns any aspect of the individual's quality of life that is affected by the disease or its treatment. This includes psychological and social factors,[11-13,23,24] sexual functioning,[25,26] nutrition,[27] fitness and exercise,[28,29] pain and symptom management,[30-33] elimination and skin care,[34] as well as adaptation to physical and functional deficits.[35]

Integrating the work of multiple members of an interdisciplinary team is a classic aspect of rehabilitation. Like classic rehabilitation patients, cancer survivors may experience a wide array of both simple and complex barriers to optimal functioning. A diverse interdisciplinary cancer rehabilitation team such as that described by Frymark[36] is essential. The interdisciplinary team is composed of professionals and laypersons and includes physicians (possibly from several specialties); nurses (office-based, home care, acute care); clergy; community volunteers; family members; friends; physical, occupational, and/or speech therapists; nutritionist; teachers or tutors; social worker; vocational counselor; recreation, art, and/or music therapists; respiratory therapists; enterostomal therapists; psychologists and counselors; homemakers; and home health aides.

Very few specifically identified "cancer rehabilitation teams" actually exist. It is often the nurse's responsibility to be aware of the services that cancer survivors require as well as their availability, and to assemble the appropriate providers and coordinate their efforts according to the individual's needs. This is a complex task that requires thoroughly assessing, predicting, and documenting the patient's needs, as well as progress toward goals.

In the past, coordinating the efforts of an interdisciplinary team was one of many interventions that a nurse provided to a patient. It was often done rather informally and haphazardly, depending on the motivation and knowledge of the individual nurse. The recent development of "managed care" approaches to health care delivery in the United States stresses the importance of identifying and achieving predictable and measurable goals and outcomes for patients, and returning patients to optimal levels of functioning as efficiently as possible. This has led to the development of formalized "case manager" roles, which are often filled by nurses working for either a health care provider or a payer. While these roles are still evolving as part of the total evolution of managed care in the United States, the formalization of the "case management" role is an important step toward creating seamless systems of interdisciplinary care that optimize rehabilitation efforts.

This chapter discusses four main considerations affecting the adult cancer survivor's ability to achieve optimal physical, social, and psychological function: developmental considerations, disease trajectory considerations, physical function and cosmesis, and socioeconomic considerations.

## DEVELOPMENTAL CONSIDERATIONS FOR ADULT CANCER SURVIVORS

### Young Adulthood

Young adults (early 20s through age 45) have completed most of the developmental tasks of childhood, including achievement of independence from their parents and at least a basic education. Some primary concerns of young adults are employment, parenting, fertility, and sexuality. Being either a young adult survivor of a childhood cancer or a survivor of a cancer that occurred early in adulthood has a great impact on the individual's ability to be successful in these areas.

Much of the literature concerning cancer survivorship issues of adults in this age-group deals with employability, economic security, insurability, and discrimination in one form or another. In the past, adult cancer survivors may have been reluctant to admit their cancer history to employers, insurers, and even primary care providers.[37,38] Those who did faced multiple barriers. However, adult cancer survivors are more numerous and visible than ever before. It has been estimated that over 10 million people alive today, most of them adults, have a history of cancer, with 7 million of them diagnosed five or more years ago.[39] This represents about 4% of the U.S. population, or about 1 in every 25 individuals. Cancer and cancer survivorship are common topics in health news reports in the mass media. The increasing visibility of cancer survivors and cancer survivorship issues is bringing cancer patients and their needs into the full view of lawmakers, employers, insurers, and health professionals.

### Employment

The shift of cancer treatment from inpatient to ambulatory and home care settings has enabled many patients undergoing active treatment for some tumors to continue working successfully,[38] occasionally with a modified work schedule. It is important to help the patient and family balance the need to maintain a "normal" lifestyle during and after cancer treatment with any increased needs for rest, stress reduction, or other limitations imposed by cancer and its treatment.

Even when functional deficits are resolved, symptoms are well managed, and the patient is able to return to work, there may be barriers. Although the numbers, visibility, and activities of cancer survivors are increasing, individual workplaces and coworkers vary in their acceptance of individuals with chronic diseases such as cancer.[40–42] Several authors have emphasized the legal protection of employment and vocational rehabilitation that is available to individuals with cancer, although cancer patients may find it difficult to take advantage of these programs and resources.[42–46] For example, the Americans with Disabilities Act (ADA), which prohibits discrimination against individuals with serious illnesses, went into effect in 1992. However, filing a claim against an employer under the ADA can be a long, laborious, stressful process that a person with cancer may not be willing to undertake. In such a case, lawyers, vocational counselors, and other community supporters may make considerable contributions to the rehabilitation process.

### Insurance coverage

In the United States, health insurance coverage is closely tied to employment. While there may be legal protection of a patient's current job and opportunities for job retraining, job mobility may be limited by the patient's insurability. Thus, a young adult with a history of cancer may be forced to forgo professional growth and new work opportunities in order to keep his or her insurance coverage.[42,46] This situation also occurs when the cancer patient is the dependent child of an adult. Although there is currently much discussion in the United States regarding health care reform, some kind of "universal" or government-mandated health insurance does not appear to be imminent at this writing. However, federal legislation passed in 1996 has mandated that, as of July 1997, insurance companies can no longer deny coverage for or impose restrictive waiting periods on individuals with preexisting illnesses such as cancer.

### Parenting

Young adulthood is when parenthood begins and the raising of young children is a primary task. Cancer in a parent of young children may be more disruptive to the family than cancer in a young child. Cancer patients who are parents of young children may need assistance in talking with their children about their disease; balancing the demands of home, work, and cancer treatment; enlisting childrens' help with tasks and chores; and dealing with feelings of guilt and inadequacy regarding their ability as parents. Parenting issues are an area where the nurse may make a referral to some other members of the cancer rehabilitation team, such as a child's teacher, social worker, or psychologist for an identified problem or further assessment.

### Fertility

For young adults with cancer who have not had children or have future intentions of doing so, fertility is an important consideration. Reproductive organs are the fourth most common cancer site, and treatment of nonreproductive cancers can result in infertility and premature menopause.[47] Male infertility can occur directly with loss of spermatogenesis through surgery, radiation, or chemotherapy, or indirectly, through loss of erectile or ejaculatory ability. This latter complication may result from nerve damage during surgery involving the lower abdomen or pelvis.[48] While sperm can be retrieved and stored indefinitely for assisted reproduction attempts, there are no known methods of preserving eggs.

### Sexuality

Sexuality is an important issue for cancer rehabilitation at any age. Adult survivors of childhood cancer face many of the same issues surrounding sexuality and body image as those faced by individuals diagnosed in early adulthood. Issues concerning sexuality and cancer have been reviewed in detail.[47] The following factors may affect a cancer patient's sexual rehabilitation: presence of a partner during diagnosis and treatment; disclosure of history to new partners; uncertainty about cancer survival or recurrence; prior sexual activity; religious and cultural beliefs and values; obvious physical changes in anatomy, functioning, or appearance; presence of appliances or prostheses; changes or limitations in sexual and nonsexual (e.g., speech) functions; loss of reproductive organs; meaning of cancer diagnosis to patient and partner; and meaning of sexual activity to patient and partner.

The nurse should never assume that someone else has discussed these issues with the patient. Patients may be reluctant to raise issues of sexuality and fertility, particularly at the beginning of treatment, when the urgency of the cancer diagnosis and concerns about survival are foremost. Yet sperm should be banked and stored before treatment or early in treatment. Sexual health is an important and widely recognized aspect of optimal functioning, and should be a key aspect of any cancer rehabilitation plan. Bruner and Iwamoto provide excellent recommendations for managing the problems of altered sexual health in cancer patients.[49]

## Middle Adulthood

Middle age (45–64 years) is when cancer incidence rates begin to rise, and the more common cancers such as lung, breast, ovarian, and colorectal cancers begin to occur in larger numbers. By this age, the individual with cancer may already have lost friends or acquaintances to cancer or may know several people who have or have had it. Middle-aged adult cancer survivors are generally near the end of their reproductive years, although they may still be working very hard at the parenting of young and adolescent children. Important considerations for middle-aged adults are career advancement; job security; financial security; sexuality/body image; interpersonal relationships; sick role behaviors; being a member of the "sandwich generation" with caregiving responsibilities for aging parents as well as children; and well-being of children.

Middle age is a time of life when career advancement and stability are extremely important. Career advancement must occur by middle age if it is going to occur at all. As this was written, the United States was going through an unprecedented period of business downsizing and restructuring. Many of the individuals who lost jobs were middle-aged, midlevel managers, with little hope of returning to the type of job they had lost. Job retraining and "starting over" in middle adulthood are extremely difficult even without the added burdens of cancer. Although no data exist on the effects of corporate downsizing on middle-aged cancer survivors, job security is clearly an important issue.

Concerns about job security may negatively affect a middle-aged adult's ability to optimize treatment. He or she may be afraid to divulge the cancer diagnosis to an employer for fear of being laid off in an upcoming down-sizing. Reluctance to take time off from work for diagnosis, treatment, and necessary "sick time" may interfere with healing and treatment efforts.

While advances in cancer treatment have shifted much of cancer care from the hospital to home and ambulatory settings, allowing cancer patients more freedom of choice in how they live their lives during cancer treatment, including continuing to work, it is important to remember that these people are still sick. In our culture it is difficult to be sick and "out of commission" while at home and receiving outpatient treatment. Advances in telecommunications and use of home-based business machines and services may allow some individuals to continue working productively while they receive treatment at home. While there are distinct advantages to this arrangement, some "sick role" behaviors may be essential for optimal functioning and outcomes. It may be increasingly difficult for a middle-aged cancer patient to take essential time and energy away from work in order to devote it to cancer treatment. Helping patients achieve a balance between being sick and being well is an important nursing intervention.

There are many individuals whose jobs are not secure, not adaptable to telecommuting, and not adaptable to change. Some jobs carry sick time, disability benefits, and other forms of income and job protection, but many others do not. While there are some legal provisions in place to protect individuals with disabilities (including cancer) against discrimination and job loss, these do not apply in many situations and may be difficult for the individual to take advantage of in other situations.[42–46]

Financial security is an important issue in middle age. It can disappear quickly with loss of a job or when one is faced with necessary extraordinary expenses due to illness or some other problem. College or retirement "nest eggs" and equity in a home may need to be tapped to help meet expenses. Families who have never known financial security and with few resources to draw upon may be even further stressed.[50]

Sexuality, body image, and physical appearance continue to be important in middle age. Marital and family relationships may be stressed. The young children of adults with cancer have special needs. They may be asked to assume more "adult" family roles. They may feel guilty about their parent's illness, and family stresses may lead to social or school difficulties. Middle-aged adults are likely to be members of the sandwich generation. There is little knowledge about the effects of cancer and chronic disease on these life issues of middle age.

It is important to pay special attention to these areas when caring for middle-aged adults and to understand that they may all contribute to less than optimal functioning. Many of these potential rehabilitation needs are outside the range of the nurse's assessment and intervention skills. Therefore, identifying and making referrals to appropriate providers is a primary intervention for this age-group.

## Older Adulthood

The elderly (65 years and over) have lived the majority of their lives free of the direct influences of cancer and have fewer life tasks to complete as cancer survivors. While issues surrounding employment and the raising of young children are not as common in this age-group, hard-won financial security may be threatened by cancer. Health insurance is less of a problem once Medicare coverage begins at age 65. However, substantial costs may be incurred that are not covered by Medicare or supplemental insurance. While cancer incidence rates are at their highest in old age, cancer survival rates are lowest. Cancer rehabilitation considerations for the elderly have been reviewed,[51,52] and include the following: comorbid conditions; age-related declines in physiological reserves; social isolation; fragmented care; caregiving roles; functional status; and sexuality/body image.

The impact of cancer on an elderly patient's ability to achieve optimal functioning is much less clear than it is in younger individuals. Cancer rehabilitation efforts may be hampered by the presence of other chronic conditions such as heart disease, arthritis, or dementia. Studies of older women with breast cancer have found that the presence of comorbid conditions affects multiple aspects of their disease, including the stage at which cancer is diagnosed, treatment received, ability to resume activities of daily living, and survival.[53–55] Cross-sectional population-based studies show that common chronic conditions such as heart disease, osteoporosis, cerebrovascular disease, arthritis, diabetes, and atherosclerosis have a larger impact on disability than cancer.[56]

Age-related changes in bone marrow reserves, vital systems (heart, lungs, kidneys, liver), lean mass, body water, and fat distribution may play a significant part in an elderly patient's ability to tolerate, respond to, and recover from cancer treatment.[57] Cancer treatment decisions in many elderly individuals are not as clear-cut as they are for younger patients. A number of other physiological and psychosocial variables must be considered.[58,59]

Social networks provide three types of support: emotional, instrumental (assistance with tasks, transportation, etc.), and informational (assistance in obtaining or interpreting information).[60] They are essential to maintaining optimal functioning. The social networks of elderly persons are frequently compromised due to death, disease, or disability, and may not be able to provide the amount or type of support an elderly cancer patient needs in order to achieve optimal function.

In the elderly, fragmentation of care is common. Older individuals frequently see several different health providers for different problems. Cancer increases the physician and provider mix, and the question of who should be taking care of what problem often arises. A critical role of the nurse in this aspect of patient care is to help organize providers around the patient's needs.

Nearly one-third of all individuals over the age of 65 live alone.[61] An elderly person with cancer who has successfully lived alone may need to move in with a relative or other caregiver on at least a temporary basis. In other cases, some kind of long-term care facility may be needed. While individuals who live alone present special caregiving demands, those living with a spouse or others may also have caregiving needs. When the caregiver is also elderly or chronically ill, the caregiver's supportive capacity may be suddenly or quickly exhausted, necessitating other sources of care for both.

Caregiver role strain is another consideration. Caregiving often demands changes in established roles and interpersonal relationships within a family. These changes may result in severe emotional strain for all involved. Finally, if the elderly cancer patient has been serving as the caregiver for a spouse or relative, new caregiving arrangements may need to be made for both parties.

Important but often neglected aspects of caring for the elderly concern sexuality and body image. While the elderly are clearly beyond their reproductive years, they are not beyond sexual activity. Surgical disfigurement, hair loss, or weight gain or loss are as important to optimal functioning and normalcy in old age as they are at younger ages.[26,47]

## DISEASE TRAJECTORY CONSIDERATIONS

In addition to age, the individual's prognosis and the limitations imposed by cancer must be considered in determining goals and interventions to achieve optimal functional status. A young adult with a good prognosis and little residual disfigurement or disability has different rehabilitation needs than a young adult with significant disabilities and a good prognosis, or a poor prognosis. Wells[62] conceptualized cancer rehabilitation as having three levels, depending on the presence or absence of disfigurement or disability and life expectancy. Table 49-1 summarizes the three levels and rehabilitation goals and considerations for each level.

The patient with little or no disability or disfigurement and a good prognosis (level 1) will probably spend little time in the hospital and will receive most cancer care in an outpatient setting. The needs of patients at this level may be less apparent than at the other two levels, and there may not be a great deal of opportunity to assess the patient's and family's needs because of the intermittent nature of the patient's care. It is easy to overlook the rehabilitation needs of cancer patients at this level, yet they may face long lives as cancer survivors with significant social, workplace, and emotional issues that could benefit from nursing assessment and intervention.

The patient at level 2 may experience considerable changes in body image and functioning, or may have complex problems such as underlying physical or mental comorbidities that have been aggravated by cancer or that hamper cancer treatment. Although life expectancy at this level is still good, adaptation to the disease and

**TABLE 49-1**   Levels of Cancer Rehabilitation According to Disability/Disfigurement and Prognosis

| Type of Patient | Rehabilitation Goals |
|---|---|
| **LEVEL 1:   NO DISFIGUREMENT OR DISABILITY; LIFE EXPECTANCY GOOD** | |
| Local or in situ disease; generally healthy; no or minor residual defects from surgery; expect to return to full and active life | Promote recovery from acute episode; prevent treatment complications; return to level of functioning prior to illness in all areas of life including work, recreation, nutrition, sexuality, significant relationships |
| **LEVEL 2:   PHYSICAL OR PSYCHOLOGICAL DISABILITY/DISFIGUREMENT; LIFE EXPECTANCY GOOD** | |
| Localized or in situ disease; surgical treatment may leave noticeable changes in appearance or body function (mastectomy, colostomy, excision of melanoma, amputation); may require adjuvant chemotherapy or radiation therapy; may require speech, occupational, and/or physical therapy; may have underlying comorbid physical or mental conditions that have been brought on or aggravated by cancer diagnosis and treatment that require restabilization | As for Level 1, except that return to prior levels of functioning may not be possible in all life areas; adaptation to disabilities/disfigurements to promote optimal functioning within limitations; control of comorbid conditions |
| **LEVEL 3:   SHORTENED LIFE EXPECTANCY, WITH OR WITHOUT DISABILITY/DISFIGUREMENT** | |
| Advanced stage of disease; patient may experience remission of disease after initial treatment, but relapse and premature death are likely; aggressive cancer treatment at first, followed by second- and third-line treatment with relapses; ultimately followed by palliative/supportive care | Short-term return to normal functioning within limits imposed by disease if remission occurs; maintain adaptive functioning with relapse and terminal disease; focus on pain and symptom management, nutrition, elimination, skin care, and psychosocial needs |

its consequences may require more effort, and a complete return to normalcy may not be feasible. These patients' needs are more obvious than those of level 1 patients, and patients at level 2 will probably receive a higher level of care from a variety of professionals and therapists than will level 1 patients, depending on the specific disability or disfigurement.

Advanced stage at diagnosis is the most powerful predictor of cancer survival. A level 3 patient may have started out as a level 1 or level 2 patient whose disease progressed despite treatment, or the patient may be diagnosed at an advanced stage of disease. If the patient is young, it is likely that aggressive treatment will be given, in the hopes of inducing a remission.

Hospice care falls into this level of rehabilitation, once aggressive treatment is stopped.[63,64] Rehabilitation goals focus on physical and emotional comfort, control of symptoms, and overall quality of life.[65]

## PHYSICAL FUNCTIONING AND COSMESIS

Physical functioning and cosmesis are critical areas for individuals whose disease leaves them with functional deficits and cosmetic problems.[66] A computerized search of the medical literature using the terms *neoplasms* and *rehabilitation* found 267 scholarly articles published between 1993 and 1995. Most of these papers dealt with functional outcomes of surgical and medical interventions for cancer, and the negative and positive effects of the outcomes on quality of life. The most frequently mentioned tumor sites were head and neck (prostheses, speech, dentition, swallowing, breathing, appearance), breast (pain, lymphedema), musculoskeletal (appearance, limb salvage, prostheses), digestive (gastric resection, urinary and fecal diversions), and central nervous system (maintenance of intelligence, mobility, sensory function). Detailed discussion of measures to improve the physical functioning and cosmesis of cancer survivors can be found in parts IV and V of this text.

## SOCIOECONOMIC CONSIDERATIONS

The socioeconomic impact of cancer on the individual has been discussed throughout this chapter. Socioeconomic considerations are an important factor in all aspects of cancer care, from prevention and early detection through treatment and rehabilitation. The total costs of cancer in the United States are estimated to be $104 billion annually, or approximately 10% of the national health care bill.[39] The figure includes $35 billion for direct medical costs, $12 billion for lost productivity, and $57 billion for mortality. The figure does not include costs for cancer screening (approximately $3–$4 billion) or out-of-pocket costs not covered by insurance such as transportation, housing, child care, homemaker services, personal care, nonprescription medications, off-label drugs, lost time from work for caregivers, and other supplies and services that must be purchased by the individual or family in order to cope with the disease and its treatment.

Cancer imposes inordinate financial demands, regardless of socioeconomic status. For the very poor, government assistance programs such as Supplemental Security Disability Insurance or Medicaid are available but difficult to access. For the elderly, Medicare and Medicare supplemental insurances are not designed to deal with long-term care or chronic disease needs. There is little help available for the "working poor," who often have no insurance benefits or job security and face the double jeopardy of being financially responsible for the illness burden, plus job loss. For middle- and upper-class families with adequate health insurance and relatively secure jobs, out-of-pocket expenditures for deductibles, copayments, gaps in insurance coverage (for example, prostheses or restorative surgery), and support services not covered by insurance may be extraordinary, and can drive a family into poverty.[50,67,68] Inability to pay for services and supplies may mean that they are denied.

The setting of cancer care may also affect the socioeconomic impact of cancer on the family. Although the shift of cancer care from the inpatient, acute setting to outpatient and home care may be less expensive on a large scale, the financial benefits to patients and families are less clear. There may be significant out-of-pocket costs for caregiving, and some treatments that are fully covered by insurance when given in the hospital setting are not as well covered in a physician's office or outpatient center or when self-administered.[50,68]

As financial losses incurred by cancer increase, the personal resources of the family may be drained. Unmet financial needs or the necessity to liquidate long-term assets in order to pay short-term bills can have a significant impact on the patient's treatment and the family's overall functioning and quality of life.[50]

may have important roles. Economic, school, and workplace issues may arise. The seamless and efficient integration of the efforts of multiple individuals and organizations for the benefit of the patient is a major challenge that may be taken on by the nurse, either officially in a "case manager" position or unofficially as a patient care provider.

Interventions for many of the cancer rehabilitation needs discussed here may be complex and varied, and many fall outside the realm of nursing practice. A key nursing intervention, however, is the thorough assessment of the rehabilitation needs and potential of the patient and family. The assessment is an important first step in making referrals and determining goals and interventions. Instruments exist for this purpose,[66,69–71] although none are in widespread use.

Many oncology nurses are involved in various community-based cancer support and rehabilitation programs.[72–76] These programs offer a variety of social and motivational supports to patients and families. It is useful for nurses to be familiar with and involved in cancer support and rehabilitation programs in the communities they serve. When referrals are made, it is wise to follow up with the patient and the program to see if and how the patient's needs were met by the program.

More individuals than ever before are surviving for significant amounts of time after a cancer diagnosis. They are living with physical, emotional, and social problems of unprecedented complexity. The reality of living with a cancer diagnosis is extremely stressful and can have profound life-altering effects for patients and families.[77]

Rehabilitation implies a return to normalcy. For cancer survivors and their families, "normal" financial and work status, "normal" physical functioning, "normal" school abilities, "normal" sexual and reproductive functioning, and "normal" living may not be realistic goals. For some cancer survivors illness may be "normal" and wellness may be an "abnormal" state. Patients' and families' definitions of "normal" may have to change to accommodate the demands imposed by cancer. Adaptation to these changes in what is "normal" is a key goal for cancer survivors and their families.

## CONCLUSION

This chapter has stressed the importance of interdisciplinary teamwork in helping individuals with cancer achieve optimal functional status within the limits imposed by their disease. The role of the professional nurse in assessing and coordinating these efforts is evolving into a more formalized function with the advent of managed care approaches to health care delivery.

A cancer patient may be treated by a surgeon, radiation oncologist, medical oncologist, radiation oncology nurse, acute care nurse, home care nurse, outpatient oncology nurse, medical social worker, physical therapist, and chaplain. The patient's family and significant others

## REFERENCES

1. Lehman J, DeLisa J, Warren D, et al: Cancer rehabilitation: Assessment of need, development, and evaluation of a model of care. *Arch Phys Med Rehabil* 59:410–419, 1978
2. Northern California Cancer Program: *Western States Conference on Cancer Rehabilitation: Conference Proceedings.* San Francisco, 1982
3. Downie PA: *Cancer Rehabilitation: An Introduction for Physiotherapists and the Allied Professionals.* London, Faber and Faber, 1978
4. Hardy RE, Cull JG: *Counseling and Rehabilitating the Cancer Patient.* Springfield, IL, Charles C. Thomas, 1975

5. Dietz JH: *Rehabilitation Oncology.* New York, Wiley, 1981

6. Rusk H: *Rehabilitation Medicine* (ed 5). New York, Mosby, 1984

7. Gunn AE: *Cancer Rehabilitation.* New York, Raven Press, 1984

8. Leigh SA: Cancer rehabilitation: A consumer perspective. *Semin Oncol Nurs* 8:164–166, 1992

9. Loescher LJ, Clark L, Atwood JR et al: The impact of the cancer experience on long-term survivors. *Oncol Nurs Forum* 17:223–229, 1990

10. Leigh S, Logan C: The cancer survivorship movement. *Cancer Invest* 9:571–579, 1991

11. Brietbart W: Psycho-oncology: Depression, anxiety, delirium. *Semin Oncol* 21:754–769, 1994

12. Razavi D: Psychosocial rehabilitation: A new challenge for oncology. *Acta Clin Belg Suppl* 15:24–31, 1993

13. Hill DR, Kelleher K, Shumaker SA: Psychosocial interventions in adult patients with coronary heart disease and cancer: A literature review. *Gen Hosp Psychiatry* 14:28S–42S, 1992 (suppl 6)

14. Mayer D, O'Connor L: Rehabilitation of persons with cancer: An ONS position statement. *Oncol Nurs Forum* 16:433, 1989

15. Ganz PA: Current issues in cancer rehabilitation. *Cancer* 65: 742–751, 1990 (Suppl 3)

16. Mellett SJ: Cancer rehabilitation. *J Natl Cancer Inst* 85: 781–784, 1993

17. Friedman LC, Lehane D, Weinberg AD, et al: Physical and psychosocial needs of cancer patients. *Tex Med* 89:61–64, 1993

18. Mellett SJ, Blunk KL: Cancer rehabilitation. *Semin Oncol* 21: 779–782, 1994

19. Gamble GL, Brown PS, Kinney CL, et al: Cardiovascular, pulmonary, and cancer rehabilitation. 4. Cancer rehabilitation: Principles and psychosocial aspects. *Arch Phys Med Rehabil* 71:S244–247, 1990 (Suppl 4)

20. Watson PG: The optimal functioning plan: A key element in cancer rehabilitation. *Cancer Nurs* 15:254–263, 1992

21. Mayer DK: Introduction. *Semin Oncol Nurs* 8:163, 1992

22. Watson PG: Cancer rehabilitation: An overview. *Semin Oncol Nurs* 8:167–173, 1992

23. Barofsky J: The status of psychosocial research in the rehabilitation of the cancer patient. *Semin Oncol Nurs* 8:190–201, 1992

24. Hermann JF, Carter J: The dimensions of oncology social work: Intrapsychic, interpersonal, and environmental interactions. *Semin Oncol* 21:712–717, 1994

25. Cull AM: The assessment of sexual function in cancer patients. *Eur J Cancer* 28A:1680–1686, 1992

26. Shell JA, Smith CK: Sexuality and the older person with cancer. *Oncol Nurs Forum* 21:553–558, 1994

27. Ottery FD: Rethinking nutritional support of the cancer patient: The new field of nutritional oncology. *Semin Oncol* 21:770–778, 1994

28. Winningham ML: Walking program for people with cancer: Getting started. *Cancer Nurs* 14:270–276, 1991

29. Shephard RJ: Exercise in the prevention or treatment of cancer. *Sports Med* 15:258–280, 1993

30. Levy MH: Pharmacologic management of cancer pain. *Semin Oncol* 21:718–739, 1994

31. Rosen SM: Procedural control of cancer pain. *Semin Oncol* 21:740–747, 1994

32. Stroey P: Symptom control in advanced cancer. *Semin Oncol* 21:748–753, 1994

33. Gamble GL, Kinney CL, Brown PS, et al: Cardiovascular,

34. Frymark S: Cancer rehabilitation in the outpatient setting. *Oncol Issues* 5:12–17, 1990

pulmonary, and cancer rehabilitation. 5. Cancer rehabilitation: Management of pain, neurologic and other clinical problems. *Arch Phys Med Rehabil* 71:S248–S251, 1990, Suppl 4

35. Blesch KS: Rehabilitation of the cancer patient at home. *Semin Oncol Nurs* 12:219–225, 1996

36. Frymark SL: Rehabilitation resources within the team and community. *Semin Oncol Nurs* 8:212–218, 1992

37. Beyer DA: Cancer is a chronic disease. *Nurse Pract Forum* 6: 201–206, 1995

38. Herold AH, Roetzheim RG: Cancer survivors. *Prim Care* 19: 779–791, 1992

39. American Cancer Society: *Cancer Facts and Figures 1996.* Atlanta, American Cancer Society, 1996

40. van der Wouden JC, Greaves-Otte JG, Greaves J: Occupational reintegration of long-term cancer survivors. *J Occup Med* 34:1084–1089, 1992

41. Berry DL, Cantanzaro M: Persons with cancer and their return to the workplace. *Cancer Nurs* 15:40–46, 1992

42. Browne HG, Tai-Seale M: Vocational rehabilitation of cancer patients. *Semin Oncol Nurs* 8:202–211, 1992

43. National Institutes of Health: *Facing Forward: A Guide for Cancer Survivors.* NIH publication No. 90-2424. Washington, DC, U.S. Department of Health and Human Services, 1990

44. Conti J: Cancer rehabilitation: Why can't we get out of first gear? *Journal of Rehabilitation* 56:19–22, 1990

45. Taylor CM: The rehabilitation of persons with cancer: Is this the best we can do? *J Rehabil* 50:60–71, 1984

46. Leake AR: The economic impact of cancer. *Nurs Pract Forum* 6:207–214, 1996

47. Nishimoto PW: Sex and sexuality in the cancer patient. *Nurse Pract Forum* 6:221–227, 1995

48. Roth BJ, Einhorn LH, Greist A: Long-term complications of cisplatin-based chemotherapy for testis cancer. *Semin Oncol* 5:315–350, 1988

49. Bruner DW, Iwamoto RR: Altered sexual health, in Groenwald SL, Frogge MH, Goodman M, Yarbro CH (eds): *Cancer Symptom Management.* Boston, Jones and Bartlett, 1996, pp 523–551

50. Berkman BJ, Sampson SE: Psychosocial effects of cancer economics on patients and their families. *Cancer* 72: 2846–2849, 1993

51. O'Connor LM, Blesch KS: Life cycle issues affecting cancer rehabilitation. *Semin Oncol Nurs* 8:174–184, 1992

52. Blesch KS: Cancer survivorship: The older person, in *Surviving Cancer: Proceedings of the Sixth National Conference on Cancer Nursing.* Atlanta, American Cancer Society, 1992, pp 39–42

53. Satariano WA, Ragheb NE, Branch LG, et al: Difficulties in physical functioning reported by middle-aged and elderly women with breast cancer: A case-control comparison. *J Gerontol* 45:M3–M11, 1990

54. Satariano WA: Comorbidity and functional status in older women with breast cancer: Implications for screening, treatment, and prognosis. *J Gerontol* 47:24–31, 1992 (special issue)

55. Satariano WA, Ragland DR: The effect of comorbidity on 3-year survival of women with primary breast cancer. *Ann Intern Med* 120:104–110, 1994

56. Verbrugge L, Lepkowski JM, Imanaka Y: Comorbidity and its impact on disability. *Milbank Q* 67:450–484, 1990

57. Blesch KS: The normal physiological changes of aging and the impact on the response to cancer treatment. *Semin Oncol Nurs* 4:178–188, 1988

58. Cohen HJ: Oncology and aging: General principles of cancer in the elderly, in Hazzard WR, Bierman EL, Blass JP, Ettinger WH, Halter JB (eds): *Principles of Geriatric Medicine and Gerontology* (ed 3). New York, McGraw-Hill, 1994, pp 77–89

59. Wetle T: Age as a risk factor for inadequate treatment. *JAMA* 258:516, 1987

60. Berkman LF, Oxman TE, Seeman TE: Social networks and social support among the elderly: Assessment issues, in Wallace RB, Woolson RF (eds): *The Epidemiologic Study of the Elderly.* New York, Oxford University Press, 1992, pp 196–212

61. Kaspar JD: *Aging Alone, Profiles and Projections: A Report of the Commonwealth Fund Commission on Elderly People Living Alone.* New York; Commonwealth Fund, 1988

62. Wells RJ: Rehabilitation: Making the most of time. *Oncol Nurs Forum* 17:503–510, 1990

63. Miller RJ: Supporting a cancer patient's decision to limit therapy. *Semin Oncol* 21:787–791, 1994

64. Kinzbrunner BM: Hospice: What to do when anti-cancer therapy is no longer appropriate, effective, or desired. *Semin Oncol* 21:792–798, 1994

65. Yoshioka H: Rehabilitation for the terminal cancer patient. *Am J Phys Med Rehabil* 73:199–206, 1994

66. Fucile J: Functional rehabilitation in cancer care. *Semin Oncol Nurs* 8:186–189, 1992

67. Houts P, Lipton A, Harvey H, et al: Nonmedical costs to patients and their families associated with outpatient chemotherapy. *Cancer* 53:2388–2392, 1984

68. American Cancer Society: *Cancer and the Poor: A Report to the Nation.* Atlanta, American Cancer Society, 1991

69. O'Toole DM, Golden AM: Evaluating cancer patients for rehabilitation potential. *West J Med* 155:384–387, 1991

70. Schag CA, Ganz PA, Heinrich RL: Cancer rehabilitation evaluation system–short form (CARES-SF): A cancer specific rehabilitation and quality of life instrument. *Cancer* 68:1406–1413, 1991

71. Ganz PA, Schag CA, Lee JJ, et al: The CARES: A generic measure of health-related quality of life for patients with cancer. *Quality of Life Research* 1:19–29, 1992

72. MacMillan SC, Tittle MB, Hill D: A systematic evaluation of the "I Can Cope" program using a national sample. *Oncol Nurs Forum* 20:455–461, 1993

73. Pierce MS: American Cancer Society services for cancer patients. *Today's Operating Room Nurse* 14:35–38, 1992

74. Johnson JB, Kelly AW: A multifaceted rehabilitation program for women with cancer. *Oncol Nurs Forum* 17:691–695, 1990

75. Berglund G, Bolund C, Gustavsson UL, et al: Starting again: A comparison study of a group rehabilitation program for cancer patients. *Acta Oncol* 32:15–21, 1993

76. Yancey DG, Greger HA, Coburn P: Effects of an adult cancer camp on hope, perceived social support, coping, and mood states. *Oncol Nurs Forum* 21:727–733, 1994

77. Davidson KW: Social work with cancer patients: Stresses and coping patterns. *Soc Work Health Care* 10:73–82, 1985

# Chapter 50

# Spiritual and Ethical End-of-Life Concerns

Elizabeth Johnston Taylor, RN, PhD

# INTRODUCTION

"I had to do a crash course in spirituality, I mean you may be facing the end of your life . . . I started going back to church and trying to investigate my feelings about God, and about what would happen after I die. . . . At one point you're facing death, and then the next point you're like facing 'What am I going to eat for breakfast tomorrow morning?' . . . That's what I think I came to terms with after crying for six months, that you know, either this is it, and you might as well die right now, or you can have a life. It's your choice. So I said, 'OK, I'm going to have a life.' "

This 40-year-old woman's statement about living with breast cancer poignantly describes a pervasive experience among cancer survivors: when diagnosed with cancer, individuals inevitably become more aware of their personal mortality. And when confronted with death, individuals typically confront spiritual and ethical questions. Such spiritual and ethical concerns can be summed up in the following two questions: How shall I die? and How shall I live before I die? It is these two fundamental "end-of-life" decisions confronting cancer survivors (albeit with varying degrees of awareness) that this chapter will address.

To prepare the reader for a discussion of these questions, a review of literature discussing the relationship between imminent death and spirituality among persons with cancer will be presented. This discussion of the topic identifies factors within the cancer experience that help explain why imminent death can bring spiritual concerns into greater awareness. The chapter concludes by addressing ethical issues faced by cancer patients at the end of their lives, and identifying strategies for promoting spiritual well-being.

## Definitions

Before a discussion using easily misunderstood terms such as spirituality, religiosity, and ethics proceeds, such terms must be defined. *Spirituality* refers to that dimension of being human that motivates meaning-making and self-transcendence—or intra-, inter-, and transpersonal connectedness.[1,2] In nursing literature that defines related terms such as spiritual distress, need, or well-being, one will find spirituality described as an integrating energy, a life principle, an innate human quality.[3–5] Spirituality prompts individuals to make sense of their universe and to relate harmoniously with self, nature, and others—including any god/s (as conceptualized by each person).

In contrast to spirituality, *religiosity* often is viewed as a narrower concept.[5–7] Religion is the representation and expression of spirituality. A religion offers an individual a specific world view and an explanation that seeks to provide answers to the questions of ultimate meaning; it

also may recommend how one is to live harmoniously with self, others, nature, and god(s). Such explanations and recommendations are presented in a religion's belief system (e.g., myths/stories, doctrines, dogmas) and are remembered and appreciated with rituals and other religious practices or observances.[6,7] One's religion may or may not be of an institutional nature.[8]

*Ethics* involves reflecting systematically about "oughts," theorizing about right conduct and how to live as a good person.[9] Thus, an ethical dilemma or conflict arises when a choice must be made between the lesser of evils or the best of goods. In addressing such ethical conflicts, certain frameworks (e.g., utilitarianism, deontology) and principles (e.g., respect for autonomy, beneficence, nonmaleficence, justice, veracity) are considered during the decision-making process.[9,10]

Spirituality and ethics are closely related. This relationship is brought to awareness by such questions as the following: What is it that determines our oughts? Where do the values and meanings behind our ethical principles originate? What is this instinctual motivation to do right, not wrong? Where does it come from? As one considers the supreme values and ultimate meanings accompanying ethical issues, one is essentially exploring spiritual elements. Thus, ethical questions inevitably lead to spiritual questions.

## Spirituality and the Cancer Experience

Research and clinical observations suggest that there is heightened spiritual awareness among individuals surviving cancer.[8,11–14] This heightened awareness of personal spirituality may manifest itself as spiritual or existential distress[15–17] or increased spiritual well-being.[14,18–21] Numerous articles have been written by health care professionals regarding the spiritual and religious needs of individuals with cancer.[22–25] These articles imply that individuals surviving cancer have unique spiritual needs.

However, few empirical studies exist that directly support these clinical observations about the pervasiveness of spiritual distress. One study found that 32 of 50 consecutive cancer patients referred for a psychiatric consult were concerned with religious issues; these included recent loss of religious support, pressure to adopt a different religious position, conflict between religious views and view of illness, and preoccupation with the meaning of life and illness.[16] Other studies document that aspects of spirituality, such as meaningfulness and hopefulness, are threatened by the cancer experience—thereby creating the possibility of spiritual distress.[26–30]

In contrast, other research lends evidence to the possibility that the cancer experience may contribute to spiritual well-being. For example, Reed[19] observed that terminally ill cancer patients had greater spiritual perspective than did nonterminally ill hospitalized patients and healthy adults (N = 300). Furthermore, spiritual perspective has been found to be positively related to various indicators of psychosocial well-being among cancer survivors,[19,31–33] including anxiety about death.[34]

The research reporting that individuals with cancer frequently use spiritual and/or religious strategies to cope with their cancer-related experiences also indicates the heightened spiritual awareness among individuals with cancer. Studies of individuals surviving cancer document religious faith or prayer as a top-ranked coping strategy.[11,14,23,35–39] Sodestrom and Martinson[13] found that of 25 cancer patients, 88% used a variety of spiritual coping strategies; they also reported that these patients indicated an increase in the awareness and practice of their spiritual beliefs since diagnosis.

In summary, the literature indicates that individuals surviving cancer characteristically become more aware of their spirituality. This increased awareness may be experienced as painful and negative, and/or positive and pleasant. Indeed, within one individual, spiritual responses to cancer can be mixed and ambivalent.

## The Relationship between Spirituality and Imminence of Death

Why do individuals surviving cancer have a heightened sense of spiritual awareness? The fundamental answer appears to lie in the realization of personal mortality and vulnerability that a cancer diagnosis creates. Even if a survivor believes that "Cancer is a word, not a sentence," the reality of eventual death becomes vivid for those diagnosed with cancer. Moberg[40] expanded on this relationship between imminence of death and spirituality when he argued that they were integrally linked in three primary ways: "The avoidance of death is a spiritual phenomenon; the social meanings of death relate to spiritual issues; and the preparation for death is a spiritual task."[40,p140]

Whereas the literature reviewed earlier indicated that the experience of surviving cancer can bring an increased awareness of personal spirituality, there is also evidence of a direct relationship between spirituality and imminence of death; that is, the closer to death an individual with cancer gets, the more she or he will become aware and concerned with personal spirituality. This relationship between spirituality and imminence of death is empirically supported in a variety of ways. For example, Gotay[36] found that praying, having faith, and hoping were used as coping strategies more by women with advanced cancer than their counterparts with early-stage cancer. Reed[18] observed significantly greater religiousness among 57 terminally-ill cancer patients than among the 57 healthy matched counterparts. Filipp[41] observed from a post-hoc analysis of data collected from individuals with cancer that those who were soon to die used the "search for meaning in religion" as a coping strategy more often than did survivors. Also, health care professionals in oncology settings have written anecdotally of an increased spiritual awareness or sensitivity accompanying the end of life.[22,42,43]

What is it about the imminence of death that contributes to this increased spiritual awareness for persons with cancer? What are the "end-of-life" experiences that heighten one's sense of spirituality? Table 50-1 offers an incomplete list of possible answers. Such experiences of cancer can contribute to greater spiritual awareness—spiritual pain and/or pleasure.

Cancer survivors, especially those at the end of life, experience numerous and various losses and changes. These could include loss of mobility and independence, changes in social roles, loss of the future, and so forth. Social psychologists theorize that significant losses and changes cause individuals to search for meaning, as a way of trying to make sense of such a negative experience.[44–46] This process of searching for meaning often makes individuals reexamine their beliefs about their world, including religious beliefs.

A human response to the reality of death is to seek immortality.[47,48] Rather than accepting that their lives are finite or insignificant, humans are comforted by beliefs in an after-death life and by leaving legacies that benefit others. Leaving a legacy, whether it is a monetary endowment, an oral history, a work of art, or a baby blanket

**TABLE 50-1**  Possible Contributors to Increased Spiritual Awareness for Cancer Patients Facing Imminent Death

| Experiences Inherent in Facing Imminent Death | | Manifestations of Spirituality |
|---|---|---|
| Losses and changes | --------- > | Search for meaning |
| Realization of mortality | --------- > | Search for immortality (e.g., afterlife beliefs, leaving legacies) |
| Existential questions | --------- > | Search for answers, meaning, and purpose |
| Powerlessness and vulnerability | --------- > | Search for security and comfort; transcend self to seek a greater power |
| Isolation or loneliness | --------- > | Search for relatedness and love |
| Social disengagement | --------- > | Engagement with greater Other; self-transcendence |
| Guilt or shame | --------- > | Search for forgiveness and acceptance |
| Life review | --------- > | Joy and meaning, or anger and questions |

for a future grandchild, brings a sense of value and significance to a dying individual's life and work.

Anxiety and existential questions inherently arise for individuals confronting imminent death.[40,49–51] Indeed, it has been argued that death is the fundamental source of all anxiety.[52] The questions can be framed in a variety of ways, and reflect varying degrees of intellectual honesty. For some survivors, such questions may be too painful to acknowledge. Blatant existential questions a nurse may hear from an intellectually bold cancer survivor might include: "What is the purpose of my death? What was the purpose for my life? Why was I born if I was meant to die?" These questions often directly challenge an individual's spiritual or religious assumptions.

At the end of life, a person with cancer may be especially overwhelmed by pain, fatigue, anger, depression, and other difficult aspects of suffering and dying. Such aspects of suffering and dying characteristically leave an individual feeling powerless and vulnerable. Indeed, many individuals with cancer are heard to say that their illness experience teaches them that they are "not in control"—of their bodies, their world, or their future. While some respond to this lack of control with a sense of helplessness and perhaps hopelessness, others regain "control" by cognitively reframing the experience as positive (e.g., "Having cancer has taught me how to receive help from others" or "I've learned to take responsibility for the things I can change, and to not worry about the rest").[28,44,53] Powerlessness and vulnerability, and the subsequent emotional and cognitive responses to these states, reflect and draw from one's core, one's spirituality.

The experiences of suffering and dying also frequently contribute to isolation and loneliness. Whether one is institutionalized for death or surrounded at home by loved ones, dying can be a lonely experience. After all, no one can share the personal experience of irreversible death with a dying individual. Furthermore, the fear and denial of death prevalent in our society causes people to distance or remove themselves from those who are dying,[47,50,52] contributing to the isolation and loneliness. The self-transcendent nature of spirituality that prompts individuals to love and relate to others is thus stressed. Another related aspect of dying is disengagement; a social death often precedes biological death.[50] Because the human spirit provokes or requires love and relationship, a dying person may seek such love and relationship with a spiritual being or God, instead of, or in addition to, human relationships.

Some individuals with cancer may become increasingly aware of their spirituality at the end of life because of a sense of guilt or shame.[22] Whereas some may believe that their cancer is punishment for past "sins,"[54] others may feel guilty or shamed because of illness-related factors. For example, a person may feel guilty for being angry and doubtful about God, or for being a burden to family caregivers. Regardless of whether or not the guilt is appropriate or logical, one's desire to resolve this spiritual distress with acceptance and forgiveness demands attention.

## Summary

This discussion of Table 50-1 provides a beginning look at empirical evidence suggesting that spiritual awareness is sharpened as death becomes imminent. The spiritual issues cancer patients may face at the end of life can be summarized in two fundamental questions: How shall I die? and How shall I live before I die?

## FUNDAMENTAL "END-OF-LIFE" QUESTIONS

### How Shall I Die?

While this question is too disturbing for some to ask and answer openly, others consider it with directness and honesty. Regardless of whether an active or passive answer is given, a decision inevitably is made. For those who confront seriously the conditions of their death, several questions may be explicitly asked: Where do I want to die? (At home, in a hospice, or somewhere else?). When do I want to die? (When "nature takes its course," or before certain other conditions like pain or dementia reach an unbearable threshold? When should death be delayed, if at all? If delayed, to what extent should "heroic" and resuscitation measures be used?) How do I want to die? (Alone or with loved ones present? Naturally or with assistance? What would constitute a good or dignified death for me?)

Because life is valued as sacred by most humans, questions related to how one will die consequentially introduce ethical and spiritual issues. Is it right to hasten a death when suffering is unbearable? or even when it is bearable? Is it right to cause a death, or assist with a death, when life is present? These questions of suicide and euthanasia create debate not only for cancer nurses and other health care professionals, but for societies at large. End-of-life issues, debated for centuries, have received increased attention in contemporary American society, exemplified by organizations such as the Hemlock Society and Choice in Dying; self-help books such as *Final Exit*, which offer laypersons techniques for nonviolent death; and state initiatives proposing legalization of physician-assisted death.

*Suicide* is the intentional taking of one's own life. *Euthanasia,* translated from Greek as an easy or good death, refers to the act of assisting or enabling a sufferer's death, preferably without pain. Because suffering is thereby relieved by death, euthanasia is often called "mercy killing"; euthanasia is sometimes referred to as assisted suicide or assisted death. However, some may differentiate between assisted suicide or death and euthanasia, reserving the term euthanasia to describe a self-inflicted death. (For example, the physician who gives the lethal dose in contrast to the physician who provides the patient with a lethal dose to self-administer.) Active euthanasia refers to direct intervention causing death, whereas passive euthanasia refers to letting a sufferer die by withholding or withdrawing life-sustaining care. Passive or active euthanasia is voluntary if the sufferer requests it.

### Nurses' perspectives on end-of-life issues

The American Nurses' Association's (ANA) code for nurses begins by stipulating that "the nurse provides services with respect for human dignity and the uniqueness of the client."[55] The Oncology Nursing Society (ONS) is one of several nursing specialty organizations that have endorsed the ANA Code. Both nursing organizations support the role of the nurse as a patient advocate who is obligated to protect the moral and legal rights of care recipients. In 1991, the ONS passed a resolution in recognition of the need for cancer nurses to examine, understand, and respond to current ethical issues related to oncology practice, and to promote decision making based on patient-centered values.[56] In 1996, a resolution recognizing factors that interfere with provision of humane end-of-life care and affirming oncology nurses' commitment to quality end-of-life care was proposed to the ONS membership.[57] Assisted suicide and end-of-life decisions were identified as the two most important ethical issues by the Oncology Nursing Society Ethics Advisory Council and by 900 nurses surveyed by the ANA.[58] Clearly, cancer nurses recognize the importance of addressing end-of-life issues; they are dedicated to understanding how nursing values and ethics can be implemented in clinical practice.

Although often intimately involved in caring for cancer survivors making end-of-life decisions, oncology nurses hold diverse perspectives about such controversial decisions. Several researchers have explored cancer nurses' attitudes about end-of-life issues.[59–62] Young and colleagues[60] found that ONS members who responded to a questionnaire about physician-assisted dying (N = 1,210) held widely varying attitudes; that is, while some respondents stated that they believed it wrong and would refuse involvement, others indicated that it was a legitimate choice that they would support. Furthermore, the researchers found that many nurses were willing to lay aside their personal beliefs about the wrongness of physician-assisted death to support a patient who requested it. Richardson[62] also noted ambivalence among oncology nurses when she questioned them about voluntary active euthanasia; although some of the 200 nurses wrote about situations where they wished for a terminally ill person's rapid death, 40% indicated that they disagreed with voluntary active euthanasia for themselves or their loved ones. When Davis' research team[69] interviewed 80 nurses (many of whom were cancer nurses) about active euthanasia, only 17% justified it. While the rationale for nurses who opposed active euthanasia included personal and professional integrity, sanctity of life, and religious beliefs, the nurses who supported active euthanasia typically cited patient autonomy, families' wishes, severe suffering, and terminal illness as reasons for supporting active euthanasia. Interestingly, the same arguments and ethical principles were cited by nurses both for and against active euthanasia.

It is important to note that private religiosity does significantly influence oncology nurses' attitudes about end-of-life options.[60,62] Richardson[62] observed that nurses with "strong religious belief" disagreed with legalization of voluntary active euthanasia. Young and colleagues[60] reported that Roman Catholic nurses accepted physician-assisted death significantly less than did Protestant, Jewish, atheist, or agnostic nurses. Valente and colleagues[61] noted that "suicide was against their religion" for some cancer nurses. These findings underscore the subtle, yet strong, influence nurses' religious views can have on clinical practice. In contrast, a large survey of British individuals grieving the recent loss of a loved one to terminal illness observed that religiosity did not contribute to beliefs about euthanasia and whether their loved one should have died earlier.[63] Perhaps religious mores are overridden when one is forced to confront end-of-life issues in personal reality. (In such cases, religiosity may be overruled by instinctual or more fundamental ethical-spiritual principles.)

### Illness-related factors influencing end-of-life decisions

Compared with the general population, cancer survivors have been found to have a higher suicide rate.[64] Numerous factors appear to contribute to a cancer survivor's desire to end life with suicide or euthanasia;[61,65–67] these factors include medical, social, psychological, and spiritual concerns as follows:

- Advanced illness, poor prognosis
- Inadequately managed severe physical symptoms (pain, fatigue, exhaustion)
- Delirium, disinhibition
- Hospitalization
- Preexisting psychopathology
- Family history of suicide or personal suicide history
- Hopelessness, helplessness
- Depression
- Loss of self-esteem, loss of control
- Fear of abandonment
- Anxiety
- Existential distress
- Caregiver (family or health care professional) fatigue

Pain and other symptom distress are the most frequently addressed factors contributing to cancer-related suicide or euthanasia. Indeed, cancer pain is a prevalent and typically controllable problem. Pain plays a large role in determining quality of life because of its impact on sleep, mood, fatigue, hopelessness, and so forth. Several cancer clinicians suggest that if pain and other distressing cancer symptoms are adequately managed, requests for ending life will be unnecessary and will abate.[65–68]

Few researchers have explored the relationship between symptom distress and the desire to die among individuals with cancer.[69] A study of 185 cancer survivors with pain found that 17% had suicidal ideation.[70] From surveying over 4000 British individuals, Seale and Addington-Hall[63] determined that dying individuals' requests for euthanasia increased as symptom distress and dependency increased. For people dying of cancer, they found that the more pain experienced, the more their relatives were likely to say that it would have been better if the patient had died earlier.

### Ethical considerations

The spiritual urge to be and do right is reflected in the debate about what is the ethical response to end-of-life decisions.[59,69,71,72] On one side, there are those who posit euthanasia and suicide as immoral killing. They argue that euthanasia devalues life, and may lead to devaluation of other aspects of human life. Clinicians who oppose euthanasia argue that palliative care is a preferred alternative to euthanasia. They suggest that terminally ill individuals do not equate wanting to die with wanting to be killed.[67] Instead, the desire for euthanasia may actually be a response to fear—fear of loss of control, fear of pain, and so forth. Opponents further argue that euthanasia robs patients and their loved ones of the opportunity to allow closure of a life to be celebrated.

Those in favor of euthanasia contend that it can allow closure for a life. By having control over one's death, euthanasia allows one to have control over one's life. It allows death to occur with dignity, without the devaluing context of misery. The ethical principles of respecting the autonomy of the person, of self-determination and beneficence, and of promoting individual well-being are used by supporters of euthanasia.

Ogden[69] synthesizes this debate by suggesting that palliation and euthanasia may both be ethical end-of-life options: "Are palliative care and euthanasia really opposites, or are they on a continuum of health care? Is there only one morally right way to die?"[69,p. 82]

Regardless of how one decides to die, perhaps the proverb that says "One dies as one has lived" best summarizes how the person with cancer will respond to this debate.

## How Shall I Live Before I Die?

Living at the end of life, of course, poses many challenges. Two primary end-of-life challenges that cancer patients often deal with are spiritual and ethical in nature: (1) how to ascribe meaning to their life, illness, and death; and (2) how to relate to themselves and others (which might include a deity or other spiritual beings).

### Meaning making

Unless a person expects cancer and perceives it to be a nonthreatening, positive experience, he or she will search for meaning.[27,45,46,73] It is exceptional if a person with cancer does not search for meaning to some degree. That is, all individuals will attempt to make sense of their cancer experience by trying to find answers to questions about what caused the cancer, what is responsible for bad things happening to people, why the cancer happened to them in particular, and what the significance or meaningfulness of the cancer is.[74]

Perhaps the most frequent approach to meaning making is by attempting to attribute a cause to the cancer. Causes for cancer that individuals frequently consider include personal lifestyle factors (e.g., smoking or diet), environmental causes (e.g., polluted water or air), heredity, randomness, and stressors (e.g., work or poor family relations).[27,28,75–77] While some individuals immediately accept an explanation of cause with complete confidence, others are never certain as to what really caused their cancer.

Related to attributing a cause to cancer are the sensitive notions of responsibility and blame.[74,77,78] Individuals with cancer may find comfort in blaming themselves for their condition; this allows them to view their illness as controllable, thereby decreasing their sense of vulnerability.[79] Yet blaming the self may create a sense of shame, guilt, and spiritual distress. Indeed, some people with cancer question, and sometimes accept, the cancer as punishment for previous wrongdoing or sin.[27,54] Studies have also found that cancer patients occasionally identify "God" or "God's will" as a cause of cancer.[77,80–83]

The need to make sense of cancer is often expressed in the question "Why me?" This question of selective incidence[78] asks not only why something bad has happened, but why it has happened to "me" in particular. Some people appear to find comfort in answering this question with "I was chosen [by a deity]" whereas others deny this could be possible and seek other answers for comfort. Some respond to the question with another question: "Why not me?" Regardless of the answer conjectured, the person has a spiritual need to maintain a sense of self-respect. A sense of self-respect is illustrated in the following contrasting statements made to the author by women with breast cancer: "I was chosen because I was strong; God knew He could use me as a witness through this cancer." "I don't know why it happened to me; things just happen—but I do know it's not because I deserved it."

Another aspect of meaning making is construing benefit or ascribing a positive significance to the negative experience of cancer.[28,44,84] This cognitive reframing explains why some survivors comment that they are better for having had cancer. Several types of construed benefits may be described by a survivor: For example, because of cancer, (a) personal values and purpose were reconsidered, (b) profound appreciation and joy for life and nature resulted, (c) spiritual sensitivity increased, and/or, (d) self-knowledge and self-respect increased.

For survivors with a belief in an omnipotent god who

maintains whatever is in humankind's best interest, the suffering associated with cancer and death raises theodical questions (i.e., questions about the justification of God's ways when considering the problem of suffering). Foley[85] identified 12 attitudes toward personal suffering by which individuals explain such theodical issues (see Table 50-2). Regardless of a survivor's conjectures, answers to such theodical questions are ultimately unverifiable. This unknowing and mystery contributes to end-of-life spiritual and ethical struggles.

### Relating

When cancer patients face the end of life and reevaluate the meaning and values in their lives, they characteristically realize anew their intense appreciation for family and friends. This appreciation frequently is potentiated by the experience of receiving physical or emotional care from loved ones. As a result, people with cancer often attempt to restructure their lives so that more time can be spent with loved ones.

While receiving care and love from others has its joy, it also can create spiritual pain and ethical dilemmas. It is difficult to receive care and love when one cannot reciprocate. Hence, dependent cancer patients often perceive that they are "being a burden"—to their loved ones, if not to society. Being a burden challenges one's sense

**TABLE 50-2** Interpretations of Suffering

| Theodical Theory | Example |
| --- | --- |
| Punishment | "My pain is the result of my sins." |
| Testing | "God is testing my loyalty to Him." |
| Bad luck | "The odds are against me." |
| Submission to the laws of nature | "It's nature taking her course, and I've got to grin and bear it." |
| Resignation to the will of God | "God willed it—even though I don't know why, so there is no way that I can avoid it." |
| Acceptance of the human condition | "Pain is a part of life." |
| Personal growth | "This suffering is making me a better person." |
| Defensiveness and denial | "I just don't think about it." |
| Minimization | "It could be worse." |
| Divine perspective | "If I could see things from God's perspective, I know I'd see a reason for this pain." |
| Redemption | "There is joy in my suffering because it has increased my appreciation for Christ's suffering." |

Adapted from Foley[85]

of worth and purpose. It is this sense of being a burden that may bring an individual to conclude that suicide or euthanasia is appropriate.

Activities that can allow a person to return the gifts of love to others include: praying for others, listening to others, sharing personal wisdom gained from the cancer experience with others, creating legacy gifts such as poems, prose, taped oral histories, or crafts as functional ability permits. If such activities are valued and encouraged by those near to the care recipient, he or she will likely value the activity and find meaning and self-worth in doing it.

Because the cancer experience increases one's sense of the preciousness of each moment, it often teaches individuals to be more selective about the people with whom they spend time. Many individuals with cancer learn from their illness "who their friends really are." As a result, the friends and family members cancer patients continue to value are those who are not only compassionate, but emotionally and spiritually honest.

While individuals' relationships with others may change as a result of the cancer experience, so also may their relationship with their deity or spiritual beings. Indeed, many cancer survivors report intensified and satisfying relationships with God resulting from illness.[11,20,27] However, it is likely that cancer survivors' experiences with their deity and/or spiritual being are diverse. Relational experience with a deity may range from intensity and closeness to apathy and distance. For example, anger at one's deity/spiritual beings can facilitate closeness or distance. Assumedly, a survivor's experience with a deity/spiritual being is influenced by multiple factors such as place in the cancer trajectory, previous spiritual responses to critical life experiences, and degree of spiritual development.[86-88]

### Summary

The decisions relative to how to die and how to live before dying are multifaceted, spiritually and ethically challenging, and emotionally exhausting. Oncology nurses who assist people with such end-of-life issues not only demonstrate caring (the hallmark of nursing), but fulfill nursing mandates that require nurses to care for the whole person with attention to ethical and spiritual aspects of living and dying.[56,89-92] Presented next are various approaches and strategies available to oncology nurses to address these spiritual and ethical issues.

## APPROACHES TO MAKING SPIRITUAL AND ETHICAL END-OF-LIFE DECISIONS

When caring for a person confronted with any of these end-of-life decisions, the goal of nursing care is to facili-

**TABLE 50-3** Religious Perspectives on Death and Afterlife

### BAHA'I FAITH

Persons who recognize the Divine Manifestations (including Baha'u'llah) and obey their law and guidance will achieve salvation, which is a process of recognizing the reality of God and following God's guidance. Spiritual development continues after death; resurrection is spiritual, not physical. Heaven and hell are not literal places, but spiritual conditions reflecting closeness to God. Cremation is not allowed because the body has been a temple for the spirit and must be respected. Suicide is forbidden but those who do it are not beyond redemption.

### BUDDHISM

At death a person's consciousness leaves the body and takes rebirth soon thereafter, until Enlightenment is achieved. Place of rebirth depends on degree of virtuousness (especially just preceding death); there are numerous heavens and hells. Thus, someone who dies in an anguished or depressed state is apt to be subsequently propelled to a similarly unhappy situation.

### CHURCH OF JESUS CHRIST OF LATTER-DAY SAINTS (MORMON)

When a person's life ends, his or her spirit leaves the body and goes to a spirit world where he or she continues to grow spiritually and awaits resurrection and judgment. After resurrection (when the spirit is reunited with a perfected physical body), an individual progresses to one of the three degrees of glory (heavens). Individuals may obtain a lower degree of glory, or if they deny the Holy Ghost, be deprived of glory. Cremation is allowed. Christ is the judge of those who commit suicide.

### HINDUISM

Human beings are souls on an evolving spiritual journey; no soul is lost. At death, the soul enters one of seven heavens or seven nether worlds (relative planes of existence), to reap the results of their virtuous actions or to expiate through suffering the results of unrighteous actions. The soul then becomes reborn or reincarnated as a human. Cremation is common. Suicide is a heinous sin.

### ISLAM

Those who live ethically and believe in the oneness of Allah will be worthy of heaven. There are five clear requirements of believers, which if not met mean hell after death: verbal testimony of belief in Allah (God) and Mohammed, His prophet; prayer five times per day; fasting during the month of Ramadan; paying alms-tax; and at least one pilgrimage to the holy cities. After death there is a place where souls await fearfully the judgment. Cremation is not practiced, and suicide is considered a grave sin.

### JUDAISM

A life in which God's commandments, the mitzvoth, are obeyed is more important than seeking heaven. There is variation among Jews regarding beliefs about heaven, but generally the concept of hell is not addressed. Traditionally,

**TABLE 50-3** (continued)

suicide has been considered a major offense. Cremation is not permitted (except by Reformed Jews).

### ROMAN CATHOLICISM

Heaven is a condition of eternal fullness of life and intimacy with God, and is a gift that comes with salvation through Jesus Christ. Hell is a self-chosen alienation from God. At death, God accepts or rejects; a full resurrection and final judgment follow at the end of time. Purgatory is a condition of transition and adaptation for those entering heaven. Cremation and organ donation are permitted. Suicide is generally attributed to unbearable stress; thus victims are accordingly not refused Christian burial.

### PROTESTANT

After a judgment, those who believed in Jesus Christ, repented, and were baptized, will be saved and dwell with God in heaven. In contrast, the unrighteous will be cast in the (sometimes eternal) fires of hell. Heaven and hell are seen by some Protestants as literal, whereas others view them as metaphorical. A resurrection of spiritual and/or physical bodies will occur at the return of Jesus Christ to earth, which for many occurs after a millennium. Cremation is generally permitted. Suicide is often considered to be a violation of God's desires, but God may show mercy to those who commit suicide.

Data from Johnson and McGee[93]

tate and promote informed decision making. The nurse ultimately cannot make decisions for care recipients. A nurse can: (1) encourage activities that increase the individual's sense of meaningfulness, self-awareness, and spiritual sensitivity; (2) offer a caring relationship and openness to dialogue; and (3) provide information about decision making and the issues confronted. In these ways the nurse facilitates the building of an environment for making informed decisions.

The following approaches can assist individuals in addressing spiritual and ethical end-of-life decisions. Each approach must include respect for the unique personal spiritual perspective and religious background of the cancer patient. Various religious beliefs regarding death are summarized in Table 50-3.[93] Although an individual may state acceptance of a specific institutional religion, beliefs can vary widely even within a religion. Even though an individual may acknowledge affiliation with one religion, he or she may be strongly influenced by another (e.g., the religion of parents or spouse). The following approaches that can assist one in resolving spiritual and ethical issues are presented because they are appropriate regardless of the individual's beliefs about religion.

## Dedication to a Mission or Cause

The question of "How shall I make sense of my death, life, or illness?" can be answered by creating the answer, rather than by finding the answer.[94] One way to create a sense of meaningfulness and purpose is to dedicate oneself to a cause or mission.[95] This mission may be sociopolitical, artistic, or scientific in nature. For example, cancer survivors may become involved in advocating for cancer research funding, may become active in cancer support activities, may apply themselves to writing about the cancer experience, may begin to write the poetry they always had dreamed of writing but never did, may become more involved in campaigning against smoking, and so forth. Dedication to a cause not only provides survivors with a sense of purpose and "something to live for," but exposes them to "the larger picture"—it offers them perspective. A side benefit may be that it also offers distraction from personal suffering.

## Leaving a Legacy

Those who question how to confront mortality may find comfort and meaning in activities that leave a legacy. A poignant example of how one can leave a legacy was told to this author by a mother with breast cancer: "I'm cutting up my wedding dress. I'm going to make a christening dress with it. I figure, my son will marry someday, and someday have a child. When that grandchild that I'll never get to see is christened, he or she will be wearing my gown. In that way I can still be there for my offspring." Other ways people can leave legacies include writing or taping personal histories or messages for their descendants. A legacy can also be left for the world by the individual's dedication to a cause. Many people state that they "just want to leave the world a better place."

## Storytelling

Individuals' questions about the meaning of their lives can be answered in part by telling life stories and reminiscing. Churchill and Churchill defined storytelling as "the forward movement of description of actions and events which makes possible the backward action of self-understanding."[96, p 73] Stories of the past influence human thought and serve as a vehicle for transmitting beliefs and values, world views and frameworks for making meaning. Stories of the present enable a person to integrate the past with the present in order to find meaning for the future. Thus, stories assist people to make the past, present, and future meaningful.[97–99]

Storytelling promotes well-being in several ways. Encouraging people to tell their stories allows them to organize their thoughts and experiences, to reflect on their past, and to make sense of their life. Storytelling also allows them to share and connect with the listener, promoting intimacy. Finally, storytelling allows the individual to transmit values and leave a legacy.

Although storytelling has typically been used as an intervention for the aged, it is therapeutic for others as well.[97,100] Pickrell[100] outlined several activities for storytell-

ing used in counseling the terminally ill, including: diagramming one's life timeline with or without its peaks and valleys; family activities (e.g., members gather to discuss family memorabilia) creating a "This is your life" production; discussing life anecdotes; mind traveling (e.g., completing statements such as "I always wanted to. . . ."); or creating a collage or artwork to depict one's life.

## Prayer, Meditation, and Journal Writing

Prayer can develop inward awareness and spiritual sensitivity. "To pray is to listen to and hear the self who is speaking. This speech is primary because it is basic and fundamental, our ground. In prayer we say who in fact we are—not who we should be, nor who we wish we were, but who we are."[101, p 1] The inner awareness that prayer facilitates provides a basis for (self-) informed decision making about end-of-life issues.

Regardless of one's beliefs about religion, prayer (liberally defined) can be a resource to all. Of course, the philosophy and expression of prayer varies among religious traditions. Furthermore, the function and content of prayer will vary for an individual depending on the circumstances. One study of predominantly Christian North Americans identified four types of prayer expression; conversational and meditative types were more directly correlated with spiritual well-being than petitionary and ritualistic approaches.[102]

Considering that roughly 90% of North Americans pray,[102] it is no surprise that a number of studies have documented that cancer patients use prayer as a coping strategy for managing illness, distressing symptoms, and anxiety-provoking medical procedures.[11,35,38,39,103] Prayer is also used for maintaining hope among the critically and chronically ill.[104–106] Indeed, some cancer patients desire that nurses allow them time for prayer when they are hospitalized.[38,103]

During the terminal phase of life, individuals' prayers may reflect unique end-of-life issues.[103,107] Terminally ill patients often pray about salvation, that their deity will deem them worthy (e.g., for Heaven or for a better life when reincarnated). Some terminally ill individuals will pray about the circumstances of their death (e.g., that it will come soon, that it will be without pain). Likewise, the terminally ill often pray for the loved ones who will grieve their death.

In addition to the content of prayers reflecting end-of-life issues, individuals' prayers may change form. When the end of life brings severe emotional or physical distress, individuals may find comfort in very short repetitive prayers (e.g., "God, have mercy").[108] For survivors who are able, prayer may also be expressed while meditating, keeping a journal, or creating art. By keeping a journal or writing, the individual becomes reflective and aware.[99] Strength and insight can be gained by reading past entries. Similarly, when people express themselves in art (be it music, painting, poetry, quilting, or another art form), they can reflect on this creativity as an expression of the spiritual. They may seriously analyze it to learn from it, or simply bathe themselves in its beauty.[109]

## Spiritual Mentoring

Cancer survivors who have become increasingly aware of their inner spirituality may benefit from interactions with a spiritual director, mentor, or soul friend.[109,110] Similar to a psychological counselor who addresses psychological issues with a patient, a spiritual mentor can assist with spiritual issues. A spiritual mentor provides comfort, encouragement, and companionship, as well as guidance and prodding.

A spiritual mentor preferably has training in spiritual direction or pastoral counseling, and has personally received spiritual direction.[110] Regardless of training, a spiritual mentor must have a high level of self-awareness and spiritual maturity, as well as listening skills, honesty, and openness. Although religious centers and retreat houses often offer the services of spiritual directors, a person may have to (or want to) find such a resource elsewhere.

The individual with cancer and his or her spiritual director need to mutually agree on the nature, purpose, and frequency of their meetings together. Those experienced in spiritual direction recommend meetings at least once every six weeks, and suggest visits be limited to topics that are most related to spiritual issues. Although directly uninvolved in this process of spiritual mentoring, the nurse can initiate the process by providing the person with information.

## Cognitive Strategies

Janoff-Bulman[45] asserts that individuals each have a set of assumptions about themselves and their world. Specifically, individuals assume that the world is benevolent, meaningful, and that they have worth. Traumatic events such as a cancer diagnosis or recognition of an imminent death can shatter such assumptions. When individuals' assumptions about the world are shattered, they will work to reconstruct their world view so that it includes assumptions that are maturer and wiser, encompassing the trauma.

This work of reconstructing a world view involves a process of balancing thinking about the painful subject with avoiding painful thoughts (approach versus avoidance).[45] Cognitive strategies that individuals use for reconstructing the assumptions include making comparisons (e.g., "it could be worse"), self-blame (e.g., "because I caused it, I can prevent it from happening again"), and construing benefit and positive meaning from the suffering (e.g., "this cancer has made me a better person").

The individual must construe his or her own meanings for life's traumas and death. The nurse cannot do this cognitive work. However, a nurse can encourage a person to verbalize thoughts and feelings about the meaning of

cancer.[111] Using therapeutic techniques such as clarification and summarization, the nurse can assist a person in identifying and appreciating cognitive strategies that provide comfort and meaning (e.g., "I hear how emotionally distressing cancer has been for you; however, I also hear how you have learned to find good things that have come from your cancer experience").

The nurse can also instruct the patient regarding the process of searching for meaning. By understanding that searching for meaning is normal and a process, the distress of not finding satisfactory meaning immediately may be allayed.[46] Some people with cancer interviewed by this author suggest that it is beneficial to put boundaries on the rumination that can viciously circle about the "why?" questions. Some survivors also recognized the helpfulness of releasing unanswerable "why?" questions, and focusing on "how do I choose to respond?" These practical suggestions from cancer survivors complement Janoff-Bulman's[45] suggestion that individuals need to use both cognitive approach and avoidance when adapting to trauma.

## Confronting the Reality of Death

The influence of a death-denying society continues to have an impact on how individuals with cancer and their family and professional caregivers confront the realities of death.[47,50–52,112] While some individuals may initiate discussions about their death, others cannot. Some may wish to talk about their death, but are prevented from doing so by those around them (e.g., family or health care professionals). The oncology nurse must remain gentle, honest, and sensitive when discussing death-related topics with care recipients.

Recognizing the function and multifaceted nature of denial will also assist the nurse in addressing death at an appropriate level.[50] Breznitz[113] contends that denial, as a defense mechanism against a threat, protects an individual from additional threatening information. Although denial serves a useful function, extreme denial prevents hopefulness and the ability to recognize positive outcomes of stress. Table 50-4 offers Bresnitz's typology of denial with examples from the context of cancer-related death.

## Advance Directives

A recent intervention that presumably has increased patient-practitioner dialogues about death is the Patient Self-Determination Act (PSDA) passed by the United States Congress in 1990.[114,115] This legislation requires that all health care institutions receiving Medicare or Medicaid reimbursement ask the patients they admit if they have an advance directive. If patients do not, the institution is obligated to provide written information about such directives.[114]

Most state statutes support two types of advance direc-

**TABLE 50-4** Seven Kinds of Denial

| Kind of Denial | Example |
|---|---|
| Denial of information | "I don't really have cancer." |
| Denial of threatening information | "I have cancer, but it isn't a life-threatening kind." |
| Denial of personal relevance | "I have a life-threatening type of cancer, but I'm hardy; it isn't going to get me." |
| Denial of urgency | "I have a life-threatening type of cancer, but it's not going to affect me really until I get old anyway." |
| Denial of vulnerability or responsibility | "I have a life-threatening cancer, but I can cope with it and conquer it." |
| Denial of affect | "I have a life-threatening cancer, but it doesn't really scare me." |
| Denial of affect relevance | "I have a life-threatening cancer and I do get scared, but it's not because I think I'm going to die." |

Adapted from Bresnitz[113]

tives (ADs). An AD "is a statement made by a competent person that directs their medical care in the event that they become incompetent."[115,p. 891] A Directive to Physician, or Living Will (a less accurate label), allows individuals to state their wishes regarding medical treatment in the event they become unable to do so. A Durable Power of Attorney for Health Care allows an individual to designate an agent who will make health care decisions on his or her behalf in the event he or she becomes incompetent. Dimond[115] outlines the advantages of ADs for oncology nurses. ADs provide: clarification of individual's wishes and values, guidance for family members concerning patients' choices, direction for the health care team, and protection of patients' assets from depletion caused by futile, high-cost care.

In addition to informing patients about ADs, oncology nurses can also facilitate discussions about ADs and end-of-life issues between patients and their families. If a challenging end-of-life decision arises for a patient or family, the nurse may "step" them through a decision-making or problem-solving process such as the "nursing process." For instance, the nurse can assist those involved with making the decision to: identify the contributing factors (e.g., values, beliefs), specifically define the problem and/or the desired outcome, list the possible approaches to solving the problem, choose and implement the appropriate approach, and evaluate.

Hoffman[114] discusses several problems related to ADs that clinicians can encounter in practice:

1. Patients can confuse what a Living Will means; they do not specify disbursement of assets.
2. ADs do not address all possible medical situations; they generally address only terminal conditions due to illness or injury.

3. The words "artificial" and "extraordinary" are often used in an AD; however, these words can be interpreted differently.
4. A directive may not always be honored and implemented; technicalities can arise such as questions about the patient's competency when the AD was signed or the inability of medicine to determine the terminality of the patient's condition.
5. An AD is a one-person statement, not a legally binding contract.

## CONCLUSION

As death becomes imminent for a person with cancer, ethical and spiritual issues and questions arise. The oncology nurse can assist the person and his or her family to face and respond knowingly to such decisions. Addressing such concerns may not decrease morbidity or mortality, save health care dollars, or be evidenced by other outcome indicators; however, providing such care can certainly make a marked difference in the quality and worth of the lives of individuals with cancer, their family caregivers, and their nurses. Indeed, it is awareness of our death that contributes to the life that is present; as Koestenbaum stated, "it is a better understanding of death that makes us into individuals."[112,p. 31]

## REFERENCES

1. Hunglemann J, Kenkel-Rossi W, Klassen L, et al: Spiritual well-being in older adults: Harmonious interconnectedness. *J Relig Health* 24:147–153, 1985
2. Reed PG: An emerging paradigm for the investigation of spirituality in nursing. *Res Nurs Health* 15:349–357, 1992
3. Haase J, Britt T, Coward D, et al: Simultaneous concept analysis of spiritual perspective, hope, acceptance and self-transcendence. *Image* 24:141–147, 1992
4. Emblen JD: Religion and spirituality defined according to current use in nursing literature. *J Prof Nurs* 8:41–47, 1992
5. Mansen TJ: The spiritual dimension of individuals: Conceptual development. *Nurs Diag* 4:140–147, 1993
6. DeCraemer W, Vansina J, Fox RC: Religious movements in Central Africa. *Compar Stud Soc History* 18:458–475, 1976
7. Geertz C: *The Interpretation of Cultures.* New York, Basic Books, 1973
8. Munley A: Toward an understanding of spiritual support, in Munley A (ed): *The Hospice Alternative.* New York, Basic Books, 1983, pp 226–268
9. Fowler MDM: Introduction to ethics and ethical theory: A road map to the discipline, in Fowler MDM, Levine-Ariff J (eds): *Ethics at the Bedside.* Philadelphia, Lippincott, 1987, pp 24–38
10. Beauchamp TL, Childress JF: *Principles of Biomedical Ethics* (ed 3). New York, Oxford University Press, 1989
11. Sodestrom KE, Martinson IM: Patients' spiritual coping

strategies: A study of nurse and patient perspectives. *Oncol Nurs Forum* 14:41–46, 1987

12. Mermann AC: Spiritual aspects of death and dying. *Yale J Biol Med* 65:137–142, 1992

13. Burns S: The spirituality of dying. *Health Progress* 72:48–54, 1991

14. Highfield MF: Spiritual health of oncology patients: Nurse and patient perspectives. *Cancer Nurs* 15:1–8, 1992

15. Weisman AD, Worden JW: The existential plight in cancer: Significance of the first 100 days. *Int J Psychiatry Med* 7:1–15, 1976

16. Peteet JR: Religious issues presented by cancer patients seen in psychiatric consultation. *J Psychosoc Oncol* 3:53–66, 1985

17. Dobratz MC, Burns KM, Oden RV: Pain in home hospice patients: An exploratory descriptive study. *Hospice J* 5:117–132, 1989

18. Reed PG: Religiousness among terminally ill and healthy adults. *Res Nurs Health* 9:35–41, 1986

19. Reed PG: Spirituality and well-being in terminally ill hospitalized adults. *Res Nurs Health* 10:335–344, 1987

20. Coward DD: The lived experience of self-transcendence in women with advanced breast cancer. *Nurs Sci Q* 3:162–169, 1990

21. Fryback PB: Health for people with a terminal diagnosis. *Nurs Sci Q* 6:147–159, 1993

22. Vastyan EA: Spiritual aspects of the care of cancer patients. *CA: Cancer J Clin* 36:110–114, 1986

23. Johnson SC, Spilka B: Coping with breast cancer: The roles of clergy and faith. *J Relig Health* 30:21–33, 1991

24. Highfield MF, Cason C: Spiritual needs of patients: Are they recognized? *Cancer Nurs* 6:187–192, 1983

25. Epperly J: The cell and the celestial: Spiritual needs of cancer patients. *J Med Assoc Ga* 72:374–376, 1983

26. O'Conner AP, Wicker CA, Germino BB: Understanding the cancer patient's search for meaning. *Cancer Nurs* 13:167–175, 1990

27. Taylor EJ: The search for meaning among persons living with recurrent cancer. *Dissertation Abstr Int* 53:4036B, 1993

28. Taylor SE: Adjustment to threatening events: A theory of cognitive adaptation. *Am Psychol* 38:1161–1173, 1983

29. Ersek M: The process of maintaining hope in adults undergoing bone marrow transplantation for leukemia. *Oncol Nurs Forum* 19:883–889, 1992

30. Steeves RH: Patients who have undergone bone marrow transplantation: Their quest for meaning. *Oncol Nurs Forum* 19:899–905, 1992

31. Smith ED, Stefanek ME, Joseph MV, et al: Spiritual awareness, personal perspective on death, and psychosocial distress among cancer patients: An initial investigation. *J Psychosoc Oncol* 11:89–103, 1993

32. Acklin MW, Brown EC, Mauger PA: The role of religious values in coping with cancer. *J Relig Health* 22:322–333, 1983

33. Kaczorowski JM: Spiritual well-being and anxiety in adults diagnosed with cancer. *Hospice J* 5:105–116, 1989

34. Smith DK, Nehemkis AM, Charter RA: Fear of death, death attitudes, and religious conviction in the terminally ill. *Int J Psychiatry Med* 13:221–232, 1983

35. Peteet JR, Stomper PC, Ross DM, et al: Emotional support for patients with cancer who are undergoing CT: Semistructured interviews of patients at a cancer institute. *Radiology* 182:99–102, 1992

36. Gotay CC: The experience of cancer during early and advanced stages: The views of patients and their mates. *Soc Sci Med* 18:605–613, 1984

37. Yates JW, Chalmer BJ, St. James P, et al: Religion in patients with advanced cancer. *Med Pediatr Oncol* 9:121–129, 1981

38. Reed PG: Preferences for spiritually related nursing interventions among terminally ill and nonterminally ill hospitalized adults and well adults. *Appl Nurs Res* 4:122–128, 1991

39. Ferrell B, Taylor EJ, Grant M, et al: Pain management at home: Struggle, comfort, and mission. *Cancer Nurs* 16:169–178, 1993

40. Moberg DO: Spiritual well-being of the dying, in Lesnoff-Caravaglia G (ed): *Aging and the Human Condition.* New York, Human Sciences Press, 1982, pp 139–155

41. Filipp SH: Could it be worse? The diagnosis of cancer as a prototype of traumatic life events, in Montada S, Filipp SH, Lerner MJ (eds): *Life Crises and Experiences of Loss in Adulthood.* Hillsdale, NJ, Lawrence Erlbaum Associates, 1992, pp 23–56

42. Brown-Saltzman KA: Tending the spirit. *Oncol Nurs Forum* 21:1001–1006, 1994

43. Granstrom S: Spiritual care for oncology patients. *Top Clin Nurs* 7:39–45, 1985

44. Taylor SE, Wood JV, Lichtman RR: It could be worse: Selective evaluation as a response to victimization. *J Soc Issues* 39:19–40, 1983

45. Janoff-Bulman R: *Shattered assumptions: Towards a New Psychology of Trauma.* New York, The Free Press, 1992

46. Marris P: *Loss and Change.* London, Routledge & Kegan Paul, 1986

47. Aries P: *The Hour of Our Death.* New York, Knopf, 1981

48. VandeCreek L, Nye C: Trying to live forever: Correlates to the belief in life after death. *J Pastoral Care* 48:273–280, 1994

49. Bryant C: Said another way: Death from a spiritual perspective. *Nurs Forum* 26:31–34, 1991

50. Weisman AD: *On Dying and Denying.* New York, Behavioral Publications, 1972

51. Weisman AD: *Coping with Cancer.* New York, McGraw-Hill, 1979

52. Becker E: *The Denial of Death.* New York, Free Press, 1973

53. Rothbaum F, Weisz JR, Snyder SS: Changing the world and changing the self: A two-process model of perceived control. *J Pers Soc Psychol* 42:5–37, 1982

54. Mahon SM, Cella DF, Donovan MI: Psychosocial adjustment to recurrent cancer. *Oncol Nurs Forum* 17:47–52, 1990 (suppl)

55. American Nurses' Association: *Code for Nurses with Interpretive Statements.* Kansas City, MO, American Nurses' Association, 1985

56. Oncology Nursing Society: Oncology Nursing Society's support of the oncology nurse's role in dealing with ethical decision-making relative to client-centered care, and related legal issues. *Oncol Nurs Forum* 20:47, 1993 (suppl)

57. Oncology Nursing Society: Resolution for end-of-life care proposed. *ONS News* 10:8, 1995

58. Ersek M, Scanlon C, Glass E, et al: Priority ethical issues in oncology nursing: Current approaches and future directions. *Oncol Nurs Forum* 22:803–807, 1995

59. Davis AJ, Phillips L, Drought TS, et al: Nurses' attitudes toward active euthanasia. *Nurs Outlook* 43:174–179, 1995

60. Young A, Volker D, Rieger PT, et al: Oncology nurses' attitudes regarding voluntary, physician-assisted dying for

competent, terminally-ill patients. *Oncol Nurs Forum* 20: 445–451, 1993

61. Valente SM, Saunders JM, Grant M: Oncology nurses' knowledge and misconceptions about suicide. *Cancer Pract* 2:209–216, 1994

62. Richardson DS: Oncology nurses' attitudes toward the legalization of voluntary active euthanasia. *Cancer Nurs* 17: 348–354, 1994

63. Seale C, Addington-Hall J: Euthanasia: Why people want to die earlier. *Soc Sci Med* 39:647–654, 1994

64. Fox BH, Stanek EJ, Boyd SC, et al: Suicide rates among cancer patients in Connecticut. *J Chron Dis* 35:89–100, 1982

65. Foley KM: The relationship of pain and symptom management to patient requests for physician-assisted suicide. *J Pain Sympt Management* 6:289–297, 1991

66. Cherny NI, Coyle N, Foley KM: The treatment of suffering when patients request elective death. *J Palliat Care* 10:71–79, 1994

67. Coyle N: The euthanasia and physician-assisted suicide debate: Issues for nursing. *Oncol Nurs Forum* 19:41–46, 1992 (suppl)

68. Baile WF, DiMaggio JR, Schapira DV, et al: The request for assistance in dying: The need for psychiatric consultation. *Cancer* 72:2786–2791, 1993

69. Ogden R: Palliative care and euthanasia: A continuum of care. *J Palliat Care* 10:82–85, 1994

70. Breitbart WS: Assessing suicide risk in cancer patients, in Holland JC, Lesko LM, Massie MJ (eds): *Current Concepts in Psycho-oncology.* New York, Memorial Sloan-Kettering Institute, 1991, pp 115–119

71. Brock DW: Euthanasia. *Yale J Biol Med* 65:121–129, 1992

72. Fischer DS: Observations on ethical problems and terminal care. *Yale J Biol Med* 65:105–120, 1992

73. Thompson SC, Janigian AS: Life schemes: A framework for understanding the search for meaning. *J Soc Clin Psychol* 7:260–280, 1988

74. Taylor EJ: Whys and wherefores: Adult patient perspectives of the meaning of cancer. *Semin Oncol Nurs* 11:32–40, 1995

75. Berckman KL, Austin JK: Causal attribution, perceived control, and adjustment in patients with lung cancer. *Oncol Nurs Forum* 20:23–30, 1993

76. Mumma C, McCorkle R: Causal attribution and life-threatening disease. *Int J Psychiatry Med* 12:311–319, 1983

77. Bard M, Dyk RB: The psychodynamic significance of beliefs regarding the cause of serious illness. *Psychoanal Rev* 43: 146–162, 1956

78. Janoff-Bulman R, Lang-Gunn L: Coping with disease, crime, and accidents: The role of self-blame attributions, in Abramson LY (ed): *Social Cognition and Clinical Psychology.* New York, Guilford Press, 1988, pp 116–147

79. Meyerowitz B: Correlates of breast cancer. *Psychol Bull* 87: 108–131, 1980

80. Lowery B, Jacobsen B: Attributions, control, and adjustment to breast cancer. *Second National Conference on Cancer Nursing Research.* Baltimore, January 1992, p 65-C (abstr)

81. Linn MW, Linn BS, Stein SR: Beliefs about causes of cancer in cancer patients. *Soc Sci Med* 16:835–839, 1982

82. Gotay CC: Why me? Attributions and adjustment by cancer patients and their mates at two stages in the disease process. *Soc Sci Med* 20:825–831, 1985

83. Baider L, Sarell M: Perceptions and causal attributions of Israeli women with breast cancer concerning their illness: The effects of ethnicity and religiosity. *Psychother Psychosom* 39:136–143, 1983

84. Thompson SC, Pitts J: Factors relating to a person's ability to find meaning after a diagnosis of cancer. *J Psychosoc Oncol* 11:1–21, 1993

85. Foley DP: Eleven interpretations of personal suffering. *J Relig Health* 27:321–328, 1988

86. Stepnick A, Perry T: Preventing spiritual distress in the dying client. *J Psychosoc Nurs* 30:17–24, 1992

87. Reker GT, Peacock EJ, Wong PTP: Meaning and purpose in life and well-being: A life-span perspective. *J Gerontol* 42: 44–49, 1987

88. Fowler JW: *Stages of Faith: The Psychology of Human Development and the Quest for Meaning.* San Francisco, Harper & Row, 1981

89. Amenta MO: Nurses as primary spiritual care workers. *Hospice J* 4:47–57, 1988

90. Travelbee J: *Interpersonal Aspects of Nursing* (ed 2). Philadelphia, FA Davis, 1977

91. Ley DCH, Corless IB: Spirituality and hospice care. *Death Studies* 12:101–110, 1988

92. International Council of Nurses: *Code for nurses: Ethical Concepts Applied to Nursing.* Geneva, Imprimeries Populaires, 1973

93. Johnson CJ, McGee MG (eds): *Encounters with Eternity: Religious Views of Death and Life after Death.* New York, Philosophical Library, 1986

94. Baird RM: Meaning in life: Discovered or created? *J Relig Health* 24:117–124, 1985

95. Yalom ID: *Existential Psychotherapy.* New York, Basic Books, 1980

96. Churchill LR, Churchill SW: Storytelling in medical arenas: The art of self-determination. *Literature Med* 1:73–79, 1982

97. Tarmen VI: Autobiography: The negotiation of a lifetime. *Int J Aging Hum Dev* 27:171–191, 1988

98. Brody H: *Stories of Sickness.* New Haven, CT, Yale University Press, 1987

99. Cunningham AJ: Does cancer have "meaning"? *Advances* 9:63–69, 1993

100. Pickrel J: "Tell me your story": Using life review in counseling the terminally ill. *Death Studies* 13:127–135, 1989

101. Ulanov A, Ulanov B: *Primary speech: A Psychology of Prayer.* Atlanta, John Knox Press, 1982

102. Poloma MM, Gallup GH Jr.: *Varieties of Prayer: A Survey Report.* Philadelphia, Trinity Press International, 1991

103. Taylor EJ, Outlaw FH: The use of prayer among persons with cancer. Oncology Nursing Society, Anaheim, CA, 1995 (poster presentation)

104. Clark CC, Cross JR, Deane DM, et al: Spirituality: Integral to quality care. *Holistic Nurs Pract* 5:67–76, 1991

105. Raleigh EDH: Sources of hope in chronic illness. *Oncol Nurs Forum* 19:443–448, 1992

106. Miller JF: Hope-inspiring strategies of the critically ill. *Appl Nurs Res* 2:23–29, 1989

107. Lucas MA: Praying with the terminally ill. *Hosp Progress* 59: 66–70, 1978

108. Taylor EJ, Ersek M: Ethical and spiritual dimensions of cancer pain management, in McGuire D, Yarbro CH, Ferrell B (eds): *Cancer Pain Management* (ed 2). Boston, Jones and Bartlett, 1994, pp 41–60

109. Taylor EJ: Spiritual self-care after a cancer diagnosis. *Coping* 4:30–31, 1995

110. Jones A: *Exploring Spiritual Direction: An Essay on Christian Friendship.* San Francisco, Harper & Row, 1982

111. Wortman CB, Silver RC: Reconsidering assumptions about coping with loss: An overview of current research, in Mon-

tada L, Filipp S, Lerner MJ (eds): *Life Crises and Experiences of Loss in Adulthood*. Hillsdale, NJ, Lawrence Erlbaum Associates, 1992, pp 341–365

112. Koestenbaum P: *Is There an Answer to Death?* Englewood Cliffs, NJ, Prentice-Hall, 1976

113. Breznitz S: The seven kinds of denial, in Goldberger L, Breznitz S (eds): *Handbook of Stress: Theoretical and Clinical Aspects*. New York, Free Press, 1982, pp 257–286

114. Hoffman MK: Use of advance directives: A social work perspective on the myth versus the reality. *Death Studies* 18: 229–241, 1994

115. Dimond EP: The oncology nurse's role in patient advance directives. *Oncol Nurs Forum* 19:891–896, 1992

# PART VII

# Delivery Systems for Cancer Care

# Chapter 51

# Cancer Programs and Services

Luana Lamkin, RN, MPH, OCN®

## INTRODUCTION

The explosion of technology in cancer treatment, the economic constraints imposed by payers, and the growing sophistication of consumers have coalesced to form an unprecedented impetus for improving the integration of cancer care services. Consumers are frustrated by fragmented care that causes them to traverse the country or even their communities to access the complex services they require. They are seeking centers recognized for excellence in cancer care in their communities.

For the past 25 years, since the National Cancer Act in 1971, cancer programs have been aggressively developed in community hospitals in a more or less concerted fashion spurred on by oncologists educated and trained at university cancer treatment facilities. Community hospitals replicated many of the operational components (e.g., tumor boards and institutional review boards) that support and encourage multidisciplinary cancer patient management. Moreover, based on the cost-plus reimbursement system for hospitals, financial success was assured.[1]

Although the acute care hospital became the focal point for developing more comprehensive cancer programs, the introduction of diagnosis-related groups (DRGs) in the 1980s led to a shift from inpatient to outpatient care.[1] Subsequently, competition from entrepreneurial physician providers posed a major threat to the viability of community cancer care centers as hospitals began to slash budgets to deal with reduced revenues and inpatient volumes.

More recent political and economic trends have driven hospitals and physicians to develop new relationships, networks, and health care systems. A number of these health care systems are expanding to become fully integrated, full-service cancer care programs that span the continuum of cancer care (prevention, detection, genetic counseling, diagnosis, multidisciplinary treatment, supportive care, lifetime follow-up, research, rehabilitation, and hospice services). These integrated programs also are uniting the various caregivers and settings (e.g., physicians' offices, ambulatory chemotherapy clinics, radiation therapy centers, and cancer inpatient visits) to offer combined pricing and services to health care consumers and payers. Finally, integration efforts are affecting previously informal relationships among physicians and hospitals. Today, physicians are forming independent practice organizations or associations (IPO/As), hospitals are merging with one another to form health care systems, and hospitals and physician groups are developing physician/hospital organizations (PHOs), with varying degrees of commitment.

Which of these new entities will survive and thrive, and whether these care delivery networks will succeed in taking integrated cancer programs to their next logical iteration remains to be seen. What is clear is that merging large and small disparate systems while the entire health care industry is in a state of flux presents major challenges to nurses and other cancer care managers. These coalitions are challenged to provide cancer care with maximum efficiency, effectiveness, quality, and ease of accessibility.

Often, nurses are responsible for developing oncology programs. In a 1980 survey of cancer program administrators, 53% of the respondents were nurses.[2] The nursing process prepares nurses to be planners, implementors, and evaluators. The nurse chosen for program development generally has well-established relationships with pivotal physicians who can form vital coalitions of health care providers. Clinical nurses employed for such roles need to carefully define the new responsibilities to ensure enough time for administrative functions. Often, an outstanding clinical nurse is asked to accept a role in program-planning while maintaining patient responsibilities, which can result in an overwhelming workload and frustration for the nurse, the patients, and other program staff.

## FORCES AFFECTING CANCER CARE DELIVERY

### Forces in Health Care

The shifts in health care are a direct result of economic pressures from payers. Table 51-1 lists some of these changes. As the percentage of a business' expenses for health care benefits rises, employers have demanded cost controls. The overall cost of cancer care in the nation reached $104 billion in 1990.[3] Cancer potentially could represent 15%–20% of the country's health care expenditures in the future.[3] Managed care companies have responded to employer needs for reducing costs by developing health plans that require preauthorization and close utilization management. In 1993, Health Maintenance Organizations' (HMOs) penetration was 17% across the country.[4] Indemnity or fee-for-service enrollment within the private health insurance market has de-

**TABLE 51-1** Shifts in Health Care Delivery

| | | |
|---|---|---|
| Fee for service | → | Managed care |
| Inpatient care | → | Ambulatory care |
| Focus on illness | → | Focus on health |
| Oncology physician | → | Primary care physician |
| Independent physicians | → | Physician groups |
| Private, nonprofit hospitals | → | Investor-owned hospital systems |
| Primary care nursing | → | Multiskilled workers |

creased from 72% in 1988 to 33% in 1993, according to the most current national data available.[5]

These shifts away from indemnity care are evident at varying rates across the country. For example, HMO enrollment is only 17% nationally, but greater than 50% in isolated communities such as Minneapolis, MN; Madison, WI; and San Diego, CA.[4] Factors influencing accelerated growth are: the presence of a national employer, state initiatives to capitate Medicaid recipients, provider overcapacity, presence of PHO structures, a strong presence by Blue Cross-Blue Shield, emerging HMO companies, and the areas' demographics.[4]

With care being more tightly managed by payers, many have questioned the future of the specialized cancer center. National Cancer Institute (NCI)-designated comprehensive cancer centers are exempt from federal prospective payment systems, specifically Medicare. Instead, they are reimbursed at a flat rate for all discharges based upon their historical costs. Commercial payers could look unfavorably at contracting with these centers whose costs are generally higher due to sophisticated equipment, teaching programs, and heavy emphasis and expenditures on clinical research trials. Some individual centers, such as Fox Chase Cancer Center in Philadelphia, are establishing referral networks to maintain their volume of patients as well as their national presence.[6] A number of NCI-designated cancer centers are also forming a national preferred provider organization (PPO) for contracting purposes.

## Demographic Factors

Hospitals and physicians cite varying reasons for developing an integrated oncology program (as noted in Table 51-2). Cancer is a disease of older people and the demographic data show that the United States is becoming a country of older generations.[7] Three unprecedented demographic variables will affect U.S. health care services:[8]

- The senior boom—by 2040, life expectancy is projected to be 86 years for men and 91.5 years for women.

- The birth dearth—fertility in the United States plummeted to its lowest point ever in 1980 and has been hovering there ever since.

- The aging baby boomers—baby boomers are entering their 50s; this will cause the country to become focused on aging, as it was focused on the children in the 1950s. Baby boomers will have unprecedented political and social clout.

## Mission, Market, and Margin

Demographics aside, there are clear mission, margin, and marketing reasons for developing and expanding cancer care services to include inpatient, outpatient, and home

**TABLE 51-2**   Motivating Factors for Developing a Cancer Program

**Meet a community need**
- Population growth
- Population aging
- Quality of competitors
- Distance to other centers

**Create a service niche**
- Distinguish hospital's services from competitors
- Develop significant expertise

**Positively impact financial success**
- Maintain current market share
- Gain new market share

**Ensure continuity of care**
- Enhance communication
- Multidisciplinary team planning

**Integrate quality, cost containment, and databases**
- Shared services and supports

care. Nathanson and Lerman[9] cite three motivators for developing outpatient cancer centers: (1) economic incentives toward more profitable outpatient care, (2) establishment of a market niche, and (3) meeting patient demand for cancer care that is convenient and accessible.

Mission-driven hospitals look to provide continuity of care for patients with cancer, who face a confusing set of questions, emotions, and decisions following a cancer diagnosis. These patients confront a highly complex health care system, with numerous and changing caregivers, treatment settings, and treatment modalities. The program's ability to prevent additional dysfunction and inconvenience for the patient (and significant family members) is highly dependent upon a coordinated multidisciplinary program.[10] The ability to select treatments, plan multimodality treatment sequencing, and identify and meet a patient's supportive care needs is greatly enhanced when all team members belong to a program with structural and operational bonds. Physicians are often motivated to participate in developing and maintaining cancer programs by both their desire to make a wide range of treatments and services easily accessible to their patients, and their dependence (as subspecialists) on a strong base of referring physicians.

Currently, cancer accounts for the largest population of patients and the highest rate of reimbursement on a per-case basis from Medicare.[11] Despite the fact that oncology is not considered one of the most profitable service lines in health care, most facilities report at least breaking even in oncology.[1] The hospitals that are the most profitable offer radiation therapy.[1] If outpatient diagnostic records were coded to reflect the patient's primary diagnosis, most facilities would find their overall oncology programs financially successful.[12] As inpatient oncology volume shrinks and revenue declines, many hospitals, health systems, and networks are expanding into outpatient services to maintain market share.

Many organizations, especially those that have already invested the capital dollars for facility construction and renovation and for program expansion, will look for a return on these expenditures in coming years. These hospitals clearly will want a part of the $100 billion-plus expenditures anticipated in cancer care.

The clear economic incentive to be in the cancer care marketplace is seen in the emergence of outside investor groups eager to participate in what they seem to view as profitable ventures. In the new order, where payers are often afforded a superior position, large insurers want easy access for their members and a complete package of cancer care services through one contract (thus decreasing the number of providers they must contract with individually). This situation also leads to widespread integration of cancer program activities and services.

Marketing motivations abound in this era of the competitive health care model. While marketing issues are handled in detail in a later section, there are a number of marketing motivations driving providers to develop and maintain cancer care services. Cancer care services like cardiac services often exhibit a "halo effect," reflecting on the institution as a whole. The public seems to understand that excellent cancer care requires both sophisticated technology and highly skilled professionals. The halo effect manifests the public's assumption that an institution with an outstanding reputation for cancer care must deliver excellent care for other (perhaps less-feared) diseases and conditions. Thus, as F. Pritchard stated in a conversation (December 1995), a distinctive competency in cancer care, if recognized by target markets (including the general public), can be a measurable advantage as part of a marketing strategy designed to distinguish one institution from its competitors.

Finally, the development of an integrated cancer program can help an organization meet its goal of providing quality care in an environment of cost containment. The ability to measure quality within a system-integrated program often is easier because it is not hampered by individual department loyalties, turf battles, and variances in data keeping. Regulatory agencies and health care insurers are seeking measures that combine quality of care and cost competitiveness. By integrating the complex service delivery components of an oncology program, systemwide data and outcomes can be combined. Insurers are also now searching for "centers of excellence" for their clients. An integrated program can respond to the multiple needs for cost management, revenue management, and quality management.[10]

## Networks, Mergers, Affiliations

Health care is going through a period of amalgamating into larger and larger systems.[13] Consolidation of providers is taking place in three major forms: (1) hospitals are forming networks and other collaborations; (2) hospitals and physicians are integrating; and (3) small medical practices are consolidating into larger groups.[14]

Since the early 1980s, increased financial and competitive pressures have induced more hospitals to join systems (defined as two or more hospitals with a common form of ownership or alliance). In 1992, 45% of the nation's community hospitals belonged to systems.[15] Another 30% of hospitals belonged to looser networks, affiliations, or consortia.[16] Some experts have estimated that as many as 80% of community hospitals will be part of a network.[17] Hospitals are forming and joining larger alliances to gain economic and political advantages. This move toward larger integrated delivery systems is in response to insurers' (public or private) desire to write one check to cover the health care needs of a defined population. The assumption driving the integration is that it will be easier to manage the population's health and manage the distribution of income if the providers are all owned or employed by one single organization.[18] How successful these interorganizational networks will be in achieving their objectives and in meeting payer and patient needs remains to be seen.

Beckham has identified the cornerstones of the emergence of an integrated delivery system.[17] A regional approach to organizing and delivering health care means subordinating local focus while still identifying and meeting the needs of local communities and constituencies. A true economic partnership occurs as a result of a trust relationship between physicians and hospitals that includes financial risk-sharing. Attempts to link delivery of care and financing of that care are evident in hospital partnerships' efforts to develop and sell health insurance products.[17]

Fragmentation of care is something the oncology community has been concerned with for decades. It will be impossible to manage cost and quality as long as care delivery remains fragmented by physician specialty, care delivery sites, and organizational structure. Achieving smooth functioning along a continuum of care will require heavy financial and intellectual investment in information systems and standardized practice.[17]

Even though providers are clamoring to join networks, there is little solid evidence that they are more successful economically or in patient outcomes. Some would argue that the new superstructures for networks result in greater numbers of management levels, highly paid executives, and consultant contracts, and slowed decision making.[18] Networks, alliances, and systems require leaders to give up some autonomy, and to develop planning, marketing, financing, and information systems that cut across multiple delivery sites.[15]

For the individual charged with operating a merged or merging cancer program, the challenges of managing within a network will require communication, negotiation, and persuasion skills, as well as creativity to develop alternative organizational structures within untested alliances. A leader must be cognizant of how the oncology program fits into the broader strategy of the system. The needs, demand, and welfare of individual program components must be viewed within the context of an integrated health care system.

Today, however, the primary issues for leaders within integrating systems are the inevitable challenges of blending multiple cultures and organizational styles. This can mean reductions in staff, shifting of program components, outsourcing of services, and confusion generated by rapid, continual change.

Much of the integration of hospitals and physicians has been initiated by hospitals.[14] These collaborations are driven by managed care entities which dictate close collaborations between these two providers. These alliances are usually physician-hospital organizations (PHOs), management service organizations (MSOs), foundation models, or integrated health organizations (IHOs). There is some indication that physician-hospital organizations develop along a continuum, from one model to the next, with each subsequent model fostering much tighter integration between the parties.[19] Hurley identifies six reasons hospitals and physicians choose to form alliances.[20] The alliance will be more successful in securing economies of scale, acquiring assets, gaining political and organizational influence, gaining access to technical services, enhancing the revenue base, and strengthening market position.

Table 51-3 shows ten characteristics critical to successful integration.[21] Five of the ten key characteristics address the importance of integrating physicians. An examination of California mergers and alliances (e.g., Sharp in San Diego, Sutter in Sacramento, and UniHealth in metropol-

itan Los Angeles) clearly demonstrates that the hospital is not the center of the emerging health care delivery system. The center is somewhere inside the physician community.[18]

Goldsmith argues that there are two critical elements that will hold together physician-hospital alliances and make them profitable: (1) the operating system to which the parties agree, and (2) the financial incentives.[18] Hospital-physician alliance models currently are perceived as serving several purposes, including unified contracting with managed care organizations, improved access to capital and patients, and a strengthened competitive position.[19]

The physician's motivation to merge is driven by several factors they are now experiencing, such as lowered levels of payments for specialists, limitations on cost shifting, increased utilization review, and increased expense of operating their practice.[19] Currently, these factors have resulted in a flattening of net income for the physician. Moreover, patterns of referral are increasingly dictated by managed care contracts, causing many primary care physicians to switch from referring to specialists with whom they have historically had such relationships.

These forces and stresses are particularly difficult for solo practitioners and small groups. Often these small business entities do not have the financial resources to purchase, maintain, and operate the complex, multisite information systems needed to function today. Nor can small practices afford the sophisticated personnel with managed care contracting, marketing, and management expertise.[19] Consequently, physicians are forming and joining large practice groups.

It is estimated that at least 75% of medical oncologists practice in groups of three or fewer physicians.[22] This situation will change as physicians seek to reduce their uncertainty about the environment by banding together.[23] The current models for oncology practice alignment include the multispecialty network (including primary care physicians and specialists), larger-group, single-specialty practice (either medical or radiation oncologists), and oncology specialty practice groups (including all relevant oncological specialties). Distinctions between these models is sometimes blurry, since many physicians are independently developing models while others choose to sell or joint-venture their practices with investor-owned national or regional corporations. How physicians organize is becoming a critical determinant of how health care dollars will flow.

**TABLE 51-3**   Ten Keys to Successful Integration

1. Physicians play a critical role in the leadership of the organization.
2. Organizational structure facilitates common management and coordination of all elements of the system.
3. Primary-care doctors are economically integrated into the system.
4. Primary-care locations provide geographic coverage of the system's service area.
5. The system is appropriately sized; the number and mix of specialists as well as hospital capacity (primarily inpatient) matches the needs of the market.
6. Physicians are themselves integrated, often forming new or joining existing medical group practices.
7. The system owns its own health plan and/or has the ability to enter into "single-signature contracts" with other health plans or large employers.
8. Financial incentives of physicians, hospitals, and health plans are aligned.
9. Communications systems are in place to provide ready access to information.
10. The system has access to capital and the ability to shift financial resources.

Coddington DC, Moore KD, Fischer EA: Integrating? Hang in there—the odds are in your favor. *Healthcare Forum J* 38:72–76, 1995

## CANCER PROGRAM DEVELOPMENT

### Defining Cancer Programs

Several organizations track and support cancer programs in the United States. These include the National Cancer Institute (NCI), which has designated 26 cancer programs as Comprehensive Cancer Centers,[24] the American College of Surgeons' (ACoS) Commission on Cancer, which surveys and approves cancer programs (and at the end of 1995 had given approval status to 1405 programs); and the Association of Community Cancer Centers (ACCC), a paid-membership association with 489 institutional members and 275 individuals as of the end of 1995.[25]

A confusing list of descriptive titles for cancer programs exists. The NCI classifies cancer centers as comprehensive, clinical, basic science, or consortium programs.[26] As of September 1995 there were 55 cancer centers: 10 basic science centers, 18 clinical centers, 1 consortium, and 26 comprehensive centers.[26] The NCI restricts the use of the term *NCI-designated* to those centers that have been awarded funding through a core grant award and meet eight major criteria.

In 1976, the NCI began a program to enlist patients in community hospitals for clinical trials, the Cooperative Group Outreach Program (CGOP). The success of that program led to the initiation of the Community Clinical Oncology Program (CCOP) in 1983 to provide support for physicians to enter community-based patients into clinical research protocols. Today, there are 52 Community Clinical Oncology Programs throughout 30 states. Moreover, a number of CCOPs are consortiums of multiple hospitals which expand the geographic reach of each CCOP and of clinical trial participation. Each CCOP is required to enter a certain number of patients annually into clinical treatment and cancer control trials. Many community cancer programs choose to make their CCOP-NCI affiliation part of their marketing strategy.

Many facilities without NCI designation have chosen titles to distinguish themselves in their geographic areas, such as comprehensive cancer center, cancer center, oncology center, cancer institute, regional cancer center, and freestanding cancer center. For the purpose of this chapter, the terms *cancer center* and *cancer programs* are used interchangeably and are defined as hospital-based integrated cancer programs that offer the major treatment modalities, diagnostic and screening services, inpatient and outpatient treatment units, and clinical research trial opportunities.

## Strategic Planning

Strategic planning is the process used to determine and evaluate alternatives for an organization to achieve its mission and objectives.[27] Generally, a strategic plan spans three to five years and sets out the major initiatives that will require the bulk of human and financial resources over the specified time frame. The plan identifies the priorities for future decision making and also defines what initiatives will not be pursued. There are a variety of methods for developing a strategic plan.[27–34] Perhaps the single most important element in the strategic planning process is knowing the process and adhering to it.

Some authors argue that strategic planning is dead because external forces change so quickly and because classic strategic planning was done by professional planners, not the operational and clinical staff.[35] Perhaps the solution to keeping up with the pace of change today is to develop plans that have shorter time frames (one to three years), to ensure frequent updates, and to hold oncology leaders accountable for the plans with the aid of planners.

Johnson[30] simplifies the planning process into three phases: (1) clarify values and aspirations, (2) analyze information, and (3) develop a strategy to create the image. The central focus of a strategic plan relies upon shared values.[36] Generally, an organization undertaking a strategic planning process begins by evaluating and, perhaps, revising its mission. This is usually done by a heterogeneous group of staff, physicians, and board members. The mission spells out the organization's intent (e.g., "Provide the highest-quality, most cost-effective health care"), whom it serves (e.g., "to the people of Hawaii regardless of their ability to pay"), and through what means (e.g., "through inpatient and outpatient care, education, and research"). The mission statement clearly spells out the basis upon which care policies will be established, defines the market as a specific geographic area, and prioritizes patient care, education, or research. The strategic plan is then built upon these few critical phrases.

The next stage of strategic planning is to identify the service lines that will be the cornerstones of future development. Most organizations have many services vying for both human and financial resources. Service line data by payer and external growth potential will determine which services (oncology, cardiology, psychiatry) the organization will pursue. Strategic goals of the organization may be to develop centers of excellence in oncology and cardiology and to increase referrals from outlying geographic locations. It is not imperative that the entire organization embark upon a major planning effort for one service line to pursue its own strategic planning.

Identifying who will be involved in the planning process and who will serve as interim and final decision makers is imperative. The involvement of maximum numbers of staff and physicians is ideal for future commitment but impractical for working meetings. An alternative is to include a broad representation of professionals, administrators, patients, and community agencies in focus groups to gather information and ideas and then designate a small working group of six to eight people who actually evaluate data and develop a plan.[34]

One well-utilized framework for data gathering is the SWOT analysis to identify Strengths, Weaknesses, Opportunities, and Threats.[33] In general, an internal assessment results in a list of strengths and weaknesses, while the external assessment results in a list of opportunities and threats.

Internal assessment data for an oncology program include an evaluation of present services and sites such as nursing care areas, surgery, laboratory, pharmacy, diagnostics, radiation therapy, and patient education. Human resources are evaluated including availability, general reputation, and skill level. Assessment of current physician strengths and weaknesses using these same criteria is of great importance. An assessment is also made of the physical facilities including the condition, technological ability, location, accessibility, visibility, parking, and potential for renovation or expansion. Waterman[36] suggests further evaluation of the infrastructures and systems through which work is accomplished, such as the admitting or registration process. He also suggests evaluating the style or culture of the service area and the organizational structure under which it is managed.

A careful evaluation must be conducted with the financial department regarding present workload, payer mix, cost, charges, and revenue for all areas and sites where oncology care is delivered.[28] A growing number of organizations and systems are capable of providing these details for analysis for both inpatient and outpatient services. If estimates or extrapolations are made, they should be developed with the financial and planning personnel who can attest to their validity.

An assessment is made of the present cancer market in the service area, demographics, the number of patients, where they are treated, and by whom. Patient satisfaction with the present care and services and other major providers' current programs and plans for expansion should be taken into consideration. The assessment includes competitor analysis of services and geographic outreach.

Projections for future workload and revenue are as difficult to develop as they are imperative. Anticipated changes in practice patterns, potential mergers or networking, reimbursement policies of third-party payers, technology, personnel policies, shifts to managed care and capitation, and changes in physicians practicing at the facility all should be detailed as footnotes to market projections. Figure 51-1 depicts the progression of analysis for strategic planning.

The compiled list of strengths, weaknesses, opportunities, and threats will probably be long and require significant pondering. Can a strong reputation for inpatient nursing care be translated to an outpatient clinic to meet the growing shift to ambulatory care? Can the recruitment of a surgical oncologist meet the needs for specialized care of an aging population without alienating the general surgeons? The list of potential plans requires careful prioritization. One method of organizing these issues is to develop a position statement on each major issue and match the ideas to the full range of considerations.

The development of a strategic plan requires considerable time and the cooperation of a variety of people, many of whom care more about the organization as a whole than they do about any specific service. Garnering cooperation from associated departments and ultimately making the plan advantageous to the entire medical staff and board challenges the leadership of the oncology team.

The strategic plan defines the long-range target and the sequence of development. To realize the strategic goals—for example, to increase outpatient oncology revenue by 12% in two years—specific programs such as a breast health center may be developed. These specific plans are referred to as *business plans*.

The strategic planning process is an opportunity for individuals from divergent oncology groups to become a multidisciplinary team and develop a shared vision. The process itself can enable the oncology service to see itself as a united group that will work together to implement its plans. The process serves as the basis for integrating oncology services. The team must now begin planning for individual business units while not losing track of the overall mission and goals. The group should continue to meet regularly to evaluate progress and reevaluate internal and external projections.

## The Business Plan

After a list of potential business plans has been developed from the strategic plan's goals, it is wise to establish a small working group to design very specific business plans. Include the staff and physicians who will ultimately manage or utilize the service. Business plans generally have a time frame of one year or less and are specific in terms of financial projections, milestones for development, and evaluation criteria. A sample business plan outline is shown in Table 51-4. Most organizations have criteria for the development and approval of new plans. For instance, a new program requiring greater than $25,000 initial outlay and/or greater than one full-time equivalent (FTE) may require more rigorous financial assessment. Criteria for approval might include positive cash flow in 12 to 24 months.

A similar but more focused assessment of the internal and external environment is required to identify market share. Data for the assessment can be difficult to assemble. Some states have requirements for reporting data to health departments or health care associations. If the specific data required for the analysis do not exist and estimates must be made by extrapolating the information, document the assumptions initially made so trends can be followed over time using the same assumptions. For most oncology services, market share can only grow by capturing a competitor's market or by identifying an unserved or underserved market component. Part of a business plan's report should be quality related and part should be financially based.

## Improving Quality, Outcomes, and Cost Effectiveness

A major concern among health care practitioners is voiced by Kassirer[37] in the *New England Journal of Medicine*:

"Market-driven health care creates conflicts that threaten our professionalism. On one hand, doctors are expected to provide a wide range of services, recommend the best treatments, and improve patients' quality of life. On the other, to keep expenses to a minimum they must limit their

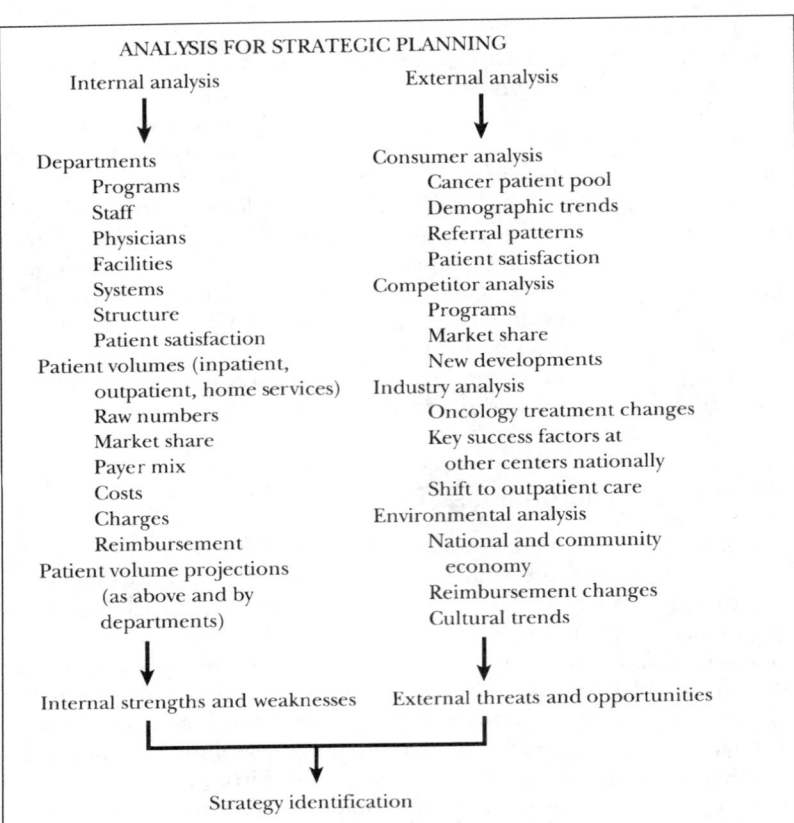

**FIGURE 51-1** Analysis for strategic planning.

services, increase efficiency, shorten the time spent with each patient, and use specialists sparingly."[37]

Many see in this a cost-versus-quality struggle. The public, particularly those with cancer, are seeking value. Value may not be equal to, but is at least proportional to, quality divided by cost. (Value = Quality/Cost). As we increase the quality while maintaining costs, we increase the value; as we reduce costs to provide services we increase the value as long as the quality remains unchanged. Goldsmith purports that the emerging business of health care systems is to conserve clinical resources and engineer value into the provision of care.[18]

Integrated cancer programs have an excellent opportunity to take the lead in establishing quality outcomes and cost effectiveness for cancer care. The multidisciplinary cancer team's day-to-day functional style provides the groundwork for the systems-oriented approach necessary for quality improvement. The cancer team is prepared to test quality indicators throughout the system. The active involvement of physicians is integral to successful quality improvement, and the cancer team's medical director can play a major role.[38] Finally, most cancer teams are familiar with the research process and appreciate that significant fact-finding must take place before system improvement solutions are identified and quality indicators are developed.

It is ideal to have one quality manager responsible for assisting the oncology team and its components to develop and monitor their quality improvement strategies. Problem areas such as pain control, patient education, and continuity of care involve more than one area, and the solutions frequently are available from within the team membership. Care pathways, critical paths, or standard treatment protocols span many areas and are more easily put into place via previously organized teams. Fiengold et al[38] report expected new profits of $600,000 for their 375-bed hospital after implementing oncology standard treatment protocols. Such protocols must span inpatient, outpatient, and home services to be effective along a continuum of care. Perhaps the most important tenet for the cancer program team to ensure is that the provision of care be monitored not only by financial parameters but also by patient satisfaction and quality parameters.

### Quality and outcome measurements

In chapter 55, Dorsett describes cancer program studies completed or underway in the areas of comfort, nutrition, coping, information, prevention, and detection. Many of these studies could be replicated in inpatient, outpatient clinic, radiation therapy, and support group settings of a cancer program. Dorsett also lists oncology-related indicators, predictors, and guidelines for care

**TABLE 51-4**   Sample Business Plan Outline

1. Description
   A. Title
   B. Description of proposal
   C. Service objectives
2. Relationship to strategic plan
3. Assessment of competition in service area
4. Degree of risk
   A. Financial
   B. Liability
5. Implementation
   A. Time line of major planning and implementation milestones
   B. Responsibility and authority
   C. Resources required:
      • human resources
      • capital expense (one-time expense over $500 for items with a life greater than 2 years, such as computers and furniture)
      • operational expense (ongoing annual expenses such as personnel, office supplies, and medical supplies)
      • space
6. Evaluation
   A. Measures of success
   B. Reporting requirements
7. Financial Analysis
   A. Projected workload
   B. Projected market share
   C. Projected payer mix
   D. FTE requirements
   E. Supplies and expenses
   F. Capital expense—equipment
   G. Renovations
   H. Overhead cost (e.g., housekeeping)
   I. Impact on other services (e.g., admissions)
   J. Rate setting, reimbursement forecast
8. Pro forma income statement (3–5 yrs)
9. Net present value analysis (3–5 yrs)
10. Recommendation

Reprinted with permission from Lamkin L: Assessment development and evaluation of cancer programs. *Semin Oncol Nurs* 9:22, 1993.

from the literature. The quality of programs is judged differently by different audiences. The organized oncology program also has the opportunity to conduct patient satisfaction surveys that evaluate the entire system and coordination of care, not just one department or service. Such a questionnaire can inquire about continuity of care in a complex organization from the patients' perspective. Wiggers et al[39] tested a 60-item satisfaction scale to assess the perception of 232 ambulatory cancer patients about the importance of and their satisfaction with nine dimensions of patient care that cut across delivery areas. Their data can be used to select questions that best meet the needs of the individual organization or system.

Outcomes and quality have become important to patients, payers, and providers. Accrediting agencies for oncology care have recently provided standards for cancer care practice. The Joint Commission on the Accreditation of Healthcare Organizations has identified important elements of care that mesh well with the American College of Surgeons' Commission on Cancer approvals program.[40] Oncology providers have also been in the forefront of providing quality of life outcome measures.[41]

Employers now provide their employees with outcome and process data supplied by competing insurance plans. It is hoped that these "report cards" provide information that employees use when choosing a payer, and therefore a provider.[42] Many communities now have formal reporting by all or most health care systems that are published in local newspapers.[43]

Specific items that a cancer program may consider reporting to interested parties are included as Table 51-5. For data to have meaning to any of the audiences (public, patients, payers, providers) it must be accompa-

**TABLE 51-5**   Potential Performance Indicators and Measures, Specific and Comparative Data

Data sets:
Number of beds dedicated to oncology
Number of oncology admissions
Number of oncology surgeries, inpatient and outpatient
Number of unexpected returns to surgery
Average oncology length of stay, overall and by DRG
Number of unexpected emergency department visits
Percent of oncologists on staff who are board-certified
Percent of oncology nurses who are certified
Number and percent of oncology discharges to rehabilitation facilities and average length of stay
Number and percent of oncology discharges to skilled nursing facilities and average length of stay
Average number of home care visits per oncology patient referral
Accreditations and scores
   JCAHO
   ACoS
   ACR
Oncology surgical mortality
Bone marrow transplant mortality
Number of people screened for cancer

Oncology/patient satisfaction related to:
Overall perceived outcome of stay or service
Pain management success
Access to care
Provision of information
Quality of staff
Response time of staff

Financial data:
Average cost/charge per oncology admission by DRG
Average cost/charge for specific radiation therapy course (e.g., prostate cancer)
Average cost/charge per home care visit and home care referral
Average cost/charge for autologous bone marrow transplant
Average cost/charge for first year of care by specific disease

nied by national or local comparative figures. National data banks with specific oncology data are extremely limited. The need for an integrated oncology database that includes quality, financial, and tumor registry data is paramount for the future of oncology programs and providers.

The care of a person with cancer offers special challenges to practitioners to ensure that care over the illness trajectory is not just a series of discrete events. Patients expect and should receive highly coordinated continuity of services and convenient access to services. Beddar and Aiken[44] offer no less than ten definitions of continuity of care for cancer patients. One simple, direct definition comes from O'Hare and Terry: "A standard of care in which there is planned coordination that results in improved outcomes for the patient."[45] Cancer programs usually provide a spectrum of services, from second opinion clinics to bereavement counseling services, but if there is minimal coordination between providers, there can be diminished benefit to the patient and family.

### Clinical care paths

The key to ensuring continuity of care is coordinated communication. The question is: How do we best coordinate and communicate with the myriad of caregivers the cancer patient sees? One excellent tool to consider is the clinical care path, critical path, or care Multidisciplinary Action Plan (MAP). These multidisciplinary tools lead to quality patient outcomes and appropriate utilization of resources. The benefits to developing paths are many: clearly stated goals to which both patient and provider agree, coordinated sequencing of treatment and services, outcome or variance analysis, and a scientifically-based practice.[46] Clinical paths are most common in the inpatient setting, but lend themselves to ambulatory care as well.

A great deal is written about how to implement paths; however, little is evident in the oncology literature in terms of examples and outcomes. To date, the most successful paths are those developed for discrete, planned surgical admissions. For example, the course of care is fairly predictable for a woman having a simple mastectomy that is preceded by teaching and followed by home care management of surgical drains.

Hawkins and Goldberg[47] describe a process by which they evaluated and resolved the system's problems associated with the efficient delivery of chemotherapy for an inpatient based on a care path. They demonstrated a reduction in length of stay from 6.7 to 2.1 days and a reduction in ancillary service utilization of 64%. To achieve these results they took the following actions: (1) ensured patients arrived with physician orders; (2) inserted vascular access devices prior to admission; (3) provided inpatient nurses with computer access to outpatient laboratory results; (4) instituted a decentralized pharmacy system; (5) installed an "express" admission process for repeated patient admissions; and (6) implemented an improved system for scheduling and holding beds on the oncology unit. This kind of process reengineering requires a multidisciplinary team dedicated to improving patient satisfaction and quality.

Katterhagen and Patton[48,49] have published the results of three clinical care paths developed for oncology. Physicians are crucial in the leadership role in developing and implementing paths. For the medical respiratory neoplasm DRG they demonstrated: (1) reduction in length of stay by 24%, (2) reduction in respiratory therapy charges by 58%, and (3) outcome goals met in 98% of patients.[48]

One major success factor embedded in the surgical pathway is attendance at preoperative preparation sessions or clinics. Surgical paths lend themselves to incorporation of preoperative teaching and postoperative follow-up by a manager of care other than the physician, specifically the nurse case manager.

### Case management

Case management has varied meanings requiring accurate definition. Traditionally case management has involved discharge planning and utilization review. When used as an approach to continuity of care, case management can take on much greater depth and breadth.[50] Oncology case management is usually provided by a registered nurse who is system-based or community-based, not hospital-based. The nurse works closely with the patient, family, and physicians to coordinate communication among the many care settings and care delivery personnel. The case manager spans the continuum of care by coordinating services and information between hospital, outpatient diagnostic and treatment settings, home care, hospice, and social support groups and organizations.

Progressive cancer programs anticipate their patients as they move through their system and provide case management services prior to or in collaboration with payer case managers. Case management systems include: patient self-care teaching, a documented plan shared by patients and caregivers, and a backup communication system when the patient is in physical or psychosocial stress.[51]

## Organization and Structure

### Standards for programs

Several resources are available to provide a framework or template for developing, monitoring, and measuring cancer care programs. Professional organizations and some national and state regulatory agencies have standards available to monitor and measure specific aspects or components of a multifaceted cancer care program.

The Joint Commission on Accreditation of Healthcare Organizations (JCAHO) provides general delivery of care standards and scoring guidelines that are not specific to cancer, but can apply to oncology care. The standards are framed as performance guidelines. As part of the JCAHO standard "Improving Organizational Performance," health care organizations are required to measure, assess, and improve their performance. The intent statement for this section exhorts hospitals to review and consider using relevant Joint Commission indicators.[52] Several clinical indicators relate directly to oncology patients. These indicators track information for patients with cancer of the lung, colon/rectum, and female breast. For example, one indicator is a measure of whether tumor staging was assigned by the managing physician for the purpose of establishing baseline information about the patient's disease upon which all cancer treatment should be designed.

The additional cancer-related indicators measure the use of multimodality therapy for female patients with stage II pathological lymph node-positive breast cancer, and track specific clinical events to assess surgical care for lung cancer.[52] JCAHO has also developed six indicators for home infusion patients.

The Association of Community Cancer Centers (ACCC) has developed a set of standards detailing a cancer program in a format that allows for self-assessment.[53] Though the specificity of the assessment criteria varies, the guidelines are helpful as a comprehensive blueprint for developing goals, building program elements, and evaluating program components. The ACCC standards are especially helpful to systems providing a spectrum of cancer services in that they deal with inpatient, outpatient, hospice, and home care. They also relate to a wide variety of services in those settings, such as nutrition, pastoral care, and research.[53]

The American College of Surgeons' (ACoS) Commission on Cancer is currently the only agency in the United States that accredits or approves cancer programs. In 1996 ACoS redesigned their program standards and survey techniques. The approvals program now encompasses the spectrum of cancer care from prevention to terminal care.[54] The expanded format includes ten areas of evaluation (see Table 51-6). Although these new standards broaden the scope of review for Commission-approved programs, they measure capacity to perform rather than actual performance. One notable exception is the section on quality management and improvement that has an outcome focus. The College also recognizes an array of

cancer programs within nine separate categories ranging from Affiliate Hospital Cancer Program to Comprehensive Cancer Program.

Another organization currently involved in external review and accreditation is the National Committee for Quality Assurance (NCQA). This accreditation body reviews organizations that deliver managed health care services, including traditional staff and group model HMOs, network and independent practice association (IPA) model HMOs, mixed models and open-ended HMOs, or point of service products.[55] Oncology group practices that contract with managed care organizations must be able to demonstrate to the managed care organization, as well as other external reviewers, compliance with the NCQA standards.

NCQA's goals are to improve quality of care and to provide quality information to purchasers of managed care systems.[55] NCQA uses specific measurement tools to provide purchasers with data on clinical performance, quality of service, and member (patient) satisfaction.

A number of other organizations review, accredit, or otherwise issue standards that relate to cancer care. For example, as noted in personal communication with T. Tappert (January 1996), the JCAHO Ambulatory Healthcare Accreditation Program reviews and accredits a wide range of freestanding facilities and services, including ambulatory surgery centers and radiation therapy centers. The standards for ambulatory care are similar in format to the JCAHO Accreditation guidelines for hospitals and also are used to accredit individual physicians' office-based practices. The American College of Radiology has standards and accredits diagnostic radiology services (e.g., mammography) as well as radiation therapy facilities. The Accreditation Association for Ambulatory Health Care also accredits freestanding, ambulatory health care entities (e.g., surgery centers and radiation therapy centers).

Finally, the Oncology Nursing Society (ONS) publishes many useful resources to assist managers in planning and monitoring individual programs. The *Resource Manual for Oncology Nurse Managers and Administrators*[56] provides an update on 57 oncology-specific topics and an extensive bibliography.

## Structure for oncology program development

Oncology leaders are inventing new models of structure and are caught in what Stuart Davidson calls "the theory-to-practice time warp."[57] Payer changes are whittling down inpatient revenues and threatening the structure and organizations that were built primarily to support inpatient services. In the integrated health system, hospitals are cost centers; inpatient units are small; and the majority of cancer patients are not only ambulatory but are served in a variety of outpatient settings as part of an organized network.

Spallina proposes several characteristics and components that may point to the future.[58] He asserts that organizing the cancer program as a business with an

**TABLE 51-6**   American College of Surgeons Commission on Cancer—Cancer Program Standards

1. Institutional and programmatic resources
2. Program management and administration
3. Clinical management
4. Inpatient and outpatient care
5. Supportive care services
6. Research
7. Quality management and improvement
8. Cancer data management
9. Public education prevention and detection
10. Professional education and staff support

From Commission on Cancer: *Cancer Program Standards, Vol. II.* Chicago, American College of Surgeons, 1996

adequate infrastructure will be vital.[58] This infrastructure includes:

- a program director

- a medical director (and medical staff)

- a program board charged with implementing strategy

- a case management system

- uniformity in quality and outcomes management across treatment settings

- uniformity in medical records and financial systems

- minimal intranetwork competition and duplication of resources

- uniform strategic and financial objectives for all providers across all treatment settings

- coordinated planning and strategy development across the cancer program continuum

The program board is a multidisciplinary group of oncologists, referring physicians, surgeons, and system executives who focus planning, technology, credentialing, and managed care.[59] The program board also monitors the clinical and program activities of the cancer committee, as well as the continuous quality improvement process.

An unanswered question in this model is who will pay for the organizational structure (including the program board, medical director, and program director) the costs of which historically have been absorbed by the acute care hospital. It is clear that maintaining a valuable marketplace position in cancer care, even within an integrated system, will require medical and clinical champions, administrative leadership, and budgetary disbursements.[59] Most health care providers have a long way to go before their current organizations have integrated sufficiently to manage effectively several providers across geographically dispersed delivery sites. Beckham[60] warns that duplicating outmoded functional hospital organizations across a broader geography is a significant step in the wrong direction.

***Product line management model***   One option for structuring cancer programs used by a number of organizations is product line or service line management. Product line management (PLM) became popular in the early 1980s. A single administrator is responsible for strategy formulation, coordination of resources, monitoring of production, and marketing, budgeting, and measuring results for the product line.[40] A broader definition is the bundling together of systems and services related to cancer management to enhance market success.[61] Nackel et al[62] define product line management as the organizational structure, management control system, and delivery strategies for health care services structured around case types or major clinical services.

Figures 51-2, 51-3, and 51-4 illustrate three different PLM structures for oncology programs. Zelman and Parham[63] developed a typology of PLM alternatives, labeling them transitionalist, market driven, product driven, and the czar approach. With the czar approach, every oncology-related department and function reports to the PLM manager. The other three alternatives are variations of matrix structures. Within a matrix structure, the PLM manager has responsibility for many program-related outcomes, but specific departments (e.g., nursing, pharmacy, laboratory) maintain a functional relationship only with the cancer program. In these matrix structures, PLM has not eliminated functional management structure but has been superimposed on it. Some form of matrix reporting relationship was the most frequent organizational structure found in oncology programs surveyed in 1990.[64] Product line managers do not usually have total budget authority over all cancer-related services.[65]

Some cancer programs rely on the tumor registrar to coordinate a limited number of cancer care activities. The tumor registrar will typically coordinate the four traditional components of an American College of Surgeons' approved Cancer program: tumor registry/data collection, the cancer committee, tumor board, and patient care evaluations.

In the absence of a product line manager, and often as an initial organizing step, a clinical manager or nurse manager will take the role of cancer program coordinator. This role differs from the product/service line manager primarily in the diminished scope of service components

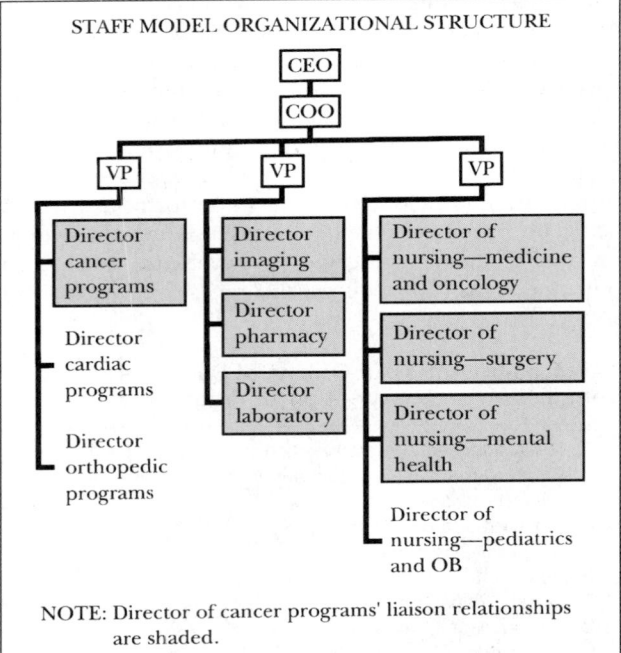

NOTE: Director of cancer programs' liaison relationships are shaded.

**FIGURE 51-2**   Staff model organizational structure option provides less control by oncology leadership and greater need for collaboration.

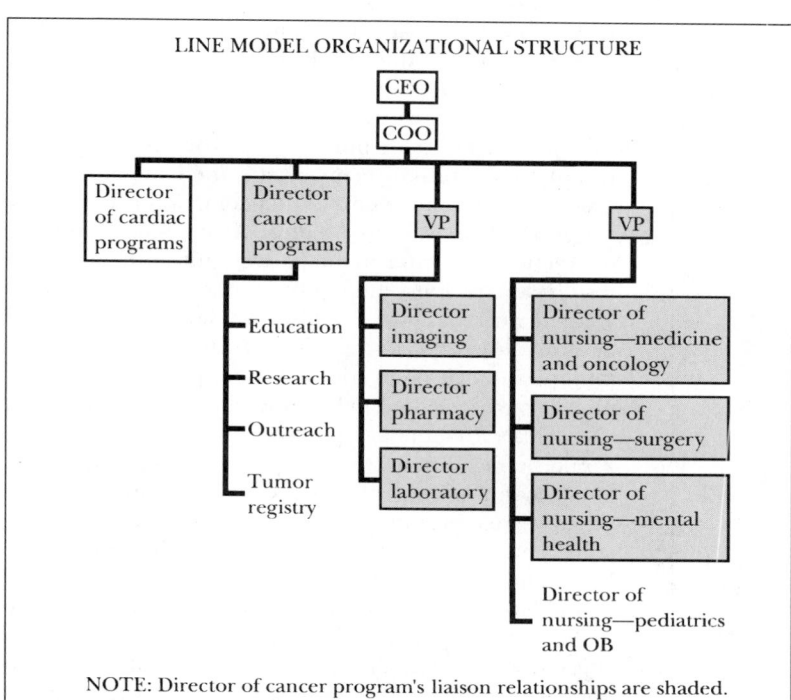

LINE MODEL ORGANIZATIONAL STRUCTURE

NOTE: Director of cancer program's liaison relationships are shaded.

**FIGURE 51-3**   Line model organizational structure grants control to oncology leadership for areas other than direct patient care.

they are expected to coordinate. The role of the coordinator is frequently added to a full-time job with clinical, managerial, or even direct patient care responsibilities. Tasks other than cancer program responsibilities compete for the coordinator's attention.

It is important to note that in 1990, the American Hospital Association reported that fewer than one-third (27%) of hospitals with cancer programs had one individual coordinating the service.[66] In 1991, Naidu et al[67] conducted a survey on product line management in hospitals. Slightly more than one-third (34.4%) of the responding organizations indicated they were implementing the PLM concept.[67] Analysis of respondents characterized these facilities as likely to be larger hospitals located in high-density population centers and facing intense competition, often proactive, and quick to recognize the importance of the marketing function. Study data confirmed that hospitals adopting PLM show a higher net income per bed, a higher gross revenue per bed, a higher return on equity, and a lower salary-to-revenue ratio.[67]

***Program leadership***   Cancer programs that achieve their goals do so because leaders provide the vision, strategy, motivation, and organization to support the multidisciplinary cancer care team members, as they achieve their objectives.[68] Many cancer programs are built around the reputation and dynamic leadership of one or two individuals. Frequently, one of these individuals is a physician. Ideally, program leadership is shared by a physician director and an administrative director.

The administrative director is charged with coordination and direction, and serves as the leader and facilitator of a group of professionals typically representing departments or delivery sites. The professionals interface with one another to deliver a continuum of oncology services in an effort to achieve clinical and educational outcomes and results that lead to patient and payer satisfactions, all within a system of cost accounting that tracks both benefits and costs. Primary duties of the administrative director include program/service planning, budget allocation and monitoring, clinical services planning (e.g., spearheading and providing administrative support for developing and implementing clinical pathways), data analysis and reporting, marketing, staff and community education, fundraising, and construction and renovation (see Table 51-7). The new structures of health care are likely to be built around processes, not function, and may call for a process flow manager rather than a product line manager.[60]

The medical director is responsible for ensuring treatment of patients, coordinating clinical care among distinct oncology specialties, and helping align physician and hospital incentives. Brady[69] asserts that the medical director plays a key role in consensus-building, within both the administrative and medical staffs.

The physician executive's role is to assist the health care organization to deliver its core business (clinical medicine), help strengthen physician loyalty and participation, and bring a medical perspective to the team.[70] Specific medical director's duties include physician relations, research protocol interface, networking, visionary

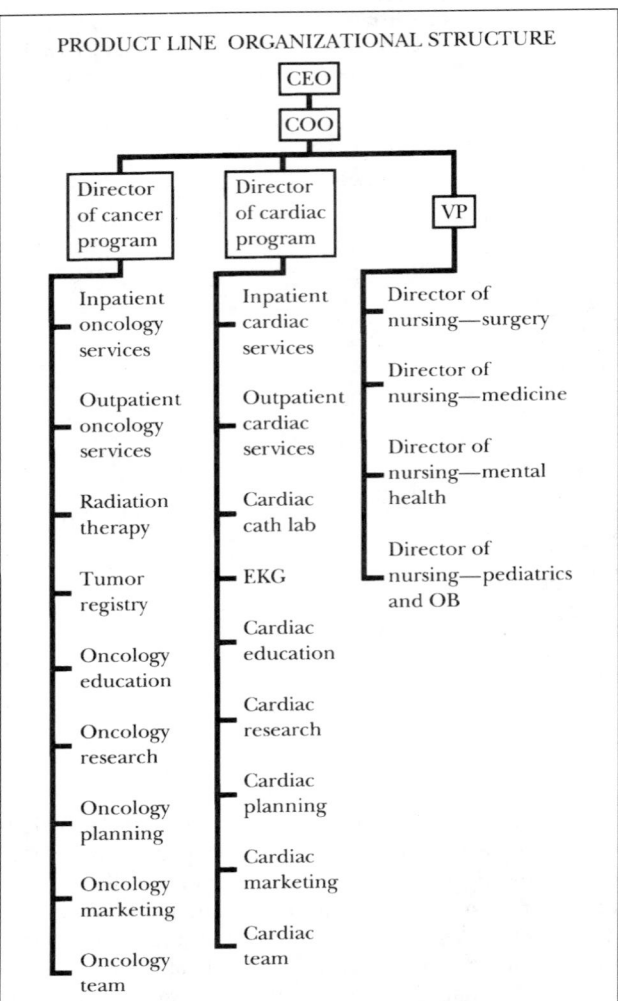

PRODUCT LINE ORGANIZATIONAL STRUCTURE

**FIGURE 51-4** Product line management organizational structure offers broad control by oncology leadership.

forecasting, medical education, clinical quality improvement, fundraising, and product differentiation.[64,71] (See Table 51-8.)

While the director's medical specialty may vary, the successful medical director invariably displays specific characteristics, including energy, zealousness, a desire for perfection, the ability to work with a high degree of chaos and ambiguity, strong clinical negotiating and leadership skills, and excellent communication skills.[64] An often overlooked quality is the ability to relate to members of the multidisciplinary team. The director must bring the medical perspective to team meetings and integrate that perspective into patient care plans, clinical pathways, marketing activities, and continuous quality improvement efforts. The ideal director is an individual who understands medical politics, the corporate environment, and the group's vision, and who remains current about the issues surrounding state-of-the-art cancer management.[72] A medical director who can build consensus, overcome ob-

stacles, and anticipate physician reaction and response when planning around sensitive issues during care delivery and payer negotiation strategy sessions is critical.[68]

Several decisions must be made when planning for this position and recruiting the individual who will fill the role of medical director. First is the issue of full-time versus part-time position, and its companion issue—the private practice decision. Medical directors who continue to practice medicine in the community can engender hostility and jealousy among the very colleagues they are charged with leading.[69,71] Other physicians may see the medical director's position as affording a former peer unfair advantage when competing for patients and referrals. Clearly, the issue can be mitigated, since the majority of medical directors are part-time.[73] However, the issue should be faced prior to hiring for the position.

A second issue concerns recruiting from inside the system versus recruiting external candidates. There may be internal candidates who are ideally suited for promotion to this position. On the other hand, conflicts within the medical staff may be exacerbated by promoting "one of the group," rather than hiring an outsider after a national search.[69] Again, this issue can be solved; a large number of cancer programs operate successfully under either scenario. What is important is to evaluate the costs and benefits of each decision when planning and budgeting for the position.

Scope of authority is a third major issue. To be successful, a medical director must be empowered to act.[69] There are times when the role of mediator (during conflict resolution) and/or consensus builder (when opposing opinions are solidifying) results in the physician administrator feeling estranged from both administration and medical staff members. This distancing and the potential isolation it causes for the medical director have some positive aspects, but all parties must be aware of the phenomena and be proactive in dealing with it.[69]

Clearly, the medical director and the administrative director must foster an open, collaborative relationship. If there is no synergy between the leaders, there can be

**TABLE 51-7** Administrative Director Responsibilities

- Develop and implement oncology strategic and business plans.
- Develop and assist in implementing oncology programs and departments.
- Oversee information systems (and data collection), analysis, and reporting of quality and financial data.
- Provide marketing, education, and research activities for the cancer program.
- Serve as the communication link and liaison between oncology services, hospital administration, and community agencies.
- Develop and maintain cancer program budgets.
- Develop and monitor product pricing and contracts.
- Manage specific departments.

**TABLE 51-8**   Medical Director Responsibilities

- Establish positive alliances between physicians and administration.
- Develop consensus, resolve conflicts, and mediate differences when administration and physician positions differ.
- Plan new oncology services and budget for adequate human and financial resources.
- Participate in payer/managed care contract negotiations.
- Assist in public education and community relations efforts.
- Oversee facility construction (cancer-related).
- Provide team leadership and vision during strategic planning.
- Access new technology and facilitate technology transfer to the institution/program.
- Develop, implement, and monitor quality improvement programs (including outcome-based clinical pathways).
- Oversee and support oncology-related research.
- Initiate creative alignments among physicians, other health care providers (e.g., hospice, home care agencies), acute care hospitals, and between networks.

no synergy within the program.[68] The most successful programs are predicated upon a peer relationship between the administrative director and the medical director. A harmonious effective working relationship is based on the different skills and perspectives these individuals bring to project tasks.

Brady[69] asserts that successful outcomes within the program depend on the ability of the two directors to collaborate on strategic planning, program development, marketing, community outreach, and systems designed to coordinate care. Finally, the medical director should be capable of promoting and stimulating enthusiasm that culminates in excellent cancer care.

## Financial Analysis

A primary goal of business is to sustain positive revenues and control costs while providing a high-quality product or service. A program's ability to achieve prominence and viability depends upon the leadership's ability to judge, monitor, and plan the quality of patient services and the program's costs and revenues. Financial reporting and cost-control measures are unquestionably the basis for utilization trends that will shape the future.[74]

The cancer program's strategic plan sets overall goals for volume and income growth. Individual departments and services will have similar growth projections or goals. One method of supporting nonreimbursable services is to ensure that aggregated oncology revenue and expenses are reported. Tumor registries, community education, and support groups are important qualitatively, but typically result in little or no revenue. It is only through careful evaluation of total revenues that these support

programs can be maintained. As inpatient revenues decline, who or what entity will rise to absorb the costs? How will such services fare in an integrated, accountable health care system?

The importance of an integrated data system has previously been noted. The ability to correlate clinical trial, clinical pathway experience, and outcomes with cost data is imperative, not only for accurate clinical and financial decision making but also for contracting purposes.[75] Financial success is based on cost containment and revenue enhancement. To assess cost containment, actual costs (direct/indirect, fixed/variable) must be available for all inpatient and outpatient services. It must be feasible to aggregate data by specific product lines (e.g., oncology services). Then this data must be available by physician provider and by specific diseases. Table 51-9 details a list of parameters to be collected and reviewed periodically for trends. Cost analysis sophistication varies among organizations.[76] Fortunately, cost data are of utmost importance to the finance department of all organizations and therefore usually hold a high organizational priority. The process of identifying costs is a laborious task for managers and requires constant updating. This also brings up turf issues. For example, who owns mammography revenue: the functional department (radiology) or the oncology product line?

Inpatient data are usually more easily attainable than outpatient data. Both are needed. As late as 1993, Lewis et al stated that "hospitals receive the bulk of cancer revenues from inpatient services and this should be the driving force in terms of measuring the success of the hospitals' cancer program in the future."[74] Today, reliance upon inpatient revenue could be problematic. Teaching centers with clinic-based medical practices may find that outpatient services overshadow inpatient in both revenue and expense.[77]

Outpatient data, especially comparable outpatient data, are much more difficult to determine in most facilities. By using a relative value scale to assign cost weights

**TABLE 51-9**   Financial Parameters for Review

Parameters should be measured for oncology in the aggregate including inpatient and outpatient services. Outpatient data should be separated by diagnostic (e.g., lab, radiology) and treatment (e.g., radiation therapy). It is helpful to be able to delineate each parameter by physician and by disease.

Inpatient, outpatient, home care, and hospice volume
Inpatient length of stay
Cost
  direct variable
  indirect variable
  direct fixed
  indirect fixed
Charges
Actual revenue
Cost to revenue ratio by payer
Payer mix
Productivity measures

to services and procedures regardless of whether they were provided on an inpatient or outpatient basis, Young et al[78] developed a framework for integrating inpatient and ambulatory payment systems. Using a different approach, Ford[79] created the composite patient encounter to equate outpatient care to inpatient care by measuring the production cost associated with each. He found the production-cost-per-outpatient-visit was about 10% of similar costs for one inpatient discharge in a 338-bed community hospital.

An effective integrated information system should be able to identify that a patient having an outpatient procedure (e.g., laboratory blood work or x-ray) is part of the cancer service line. Combining inpatient and outpatient data by individual patient allows for measurement of actual resource consumption and real profitability of the total service line. Ideally, outpatient statistics would include (by ICD-9 code): outpatient visit volume, outpatient visit cost, outpatient visit charge, outpatient visit revenue, payer mix, productivity measure, and percent change in each. See Table 51-9.

When tracking resource utilization, it is helpful to sort data by attending physician and by procedure. However, since many physicians are involved in each patient's care, these data may not accurately reflect only cancer care, especially for outpatient encounters. Because outpatient procedures vary greatly by charge and complexity (e.g., MRI versus complete blood count), aggregate outpatient figures may not mean much by themselves. These data will uncover trends in patient volume and profit. A grand total for all oncology care revenue, in excess of cost, is probably the critical figure that will allow for future program development or will necessitate that the program determine what services are to be eliminated.

Plotting volume growth and income for oncology services can prove enlightening. Figure 51-5 is an example

in which support group volume in a hypothetical hospital is growing but contributes negatively to the overall income, while surgical oncology admissions are growing slightly in volume and are profitable. Folger and Gee[80] provide formulas to develop such a graph as well as strategies for services positioned in each quadrant. For example, a high-growth, high-income program may develop a strategy to invest additional capital, market the program further, and identify markets outside the service area. A high-growth, low-income service (e.g., research in this scenario) may cause the oncology management to rethink their commitment to research, identify new funding sources, concentrate on cost-cutting measures, or consider an increase in prices for other services to support research.

In today's environment, the most effective method for maximizing revenues is negotiating favorable contracts with payers. Other avenues do exist, such as closely controlled medical records coding. Savvy coders use cost optimization techniques when clinically coding procedures by ICD-9, DRG, and CPT codes. Physicians must be held to strict standards regarding their complete and timely documentation so that medical records coding can be most advantageous.

Other revenue maximizing opportunities lie in charge accumulation and reconciliation methods, charge description listings, and adequate pricing strategies.[74] Nurses and other caregivers must be held to strict standards regarding their responsibilities in beginning the charging process.

The most successful strategy for controlling costs is appropriate utilization of resources. As noted in the quality section of this chapter, many centers have been successful in adopting resource-sparing techniques via clinical care pathways. Katterhagen and Patton[48] showed extraordinary cost savings by eliminating emergency department

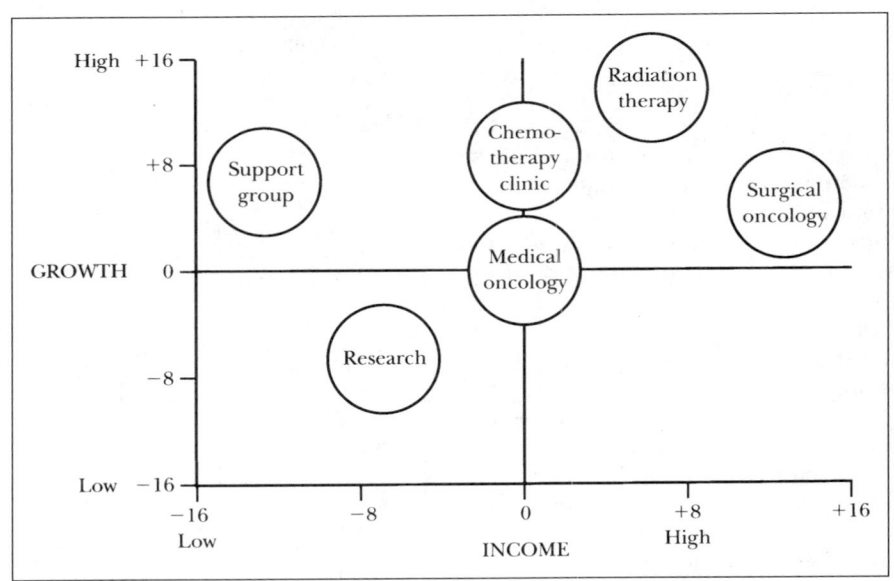

**FIGURE 51-5**  Sample graph measuring growth and income of oncology services.

admissions, eliminating care of oncology patients outside the oncology unit, and reducing ancillary services. They found that among medical respiratory neoplasm admissions 82% of lab results were normal. Reducing lab tests not only reduces the cost of care, but also reduces unnecessary discomfort for the patient.

Other cost-containment efforts relate to the judicious use of supplies purchased at discounted prices via purchasing cooperatives, reducing excessive hours of care, minimizing census fluctuations, and developing nursing units (e.g., transitional care units) that respond to the patient's level of care.

Irregularities in the Medicare payment systems presently reward some programs with cost-based reimbursement; those include home care, subacute nursing units, and rural and senior clinics. These favorable payment systems all have end points, and one could predict that entrepreneurial providers will drop programs as payment in these areas becomes less favorable. New Medicare legislation will support new programs (via financial reward) in the future. One might speculate that community-based case management, nurse-run symptom management clinics, and adult day care might be the new Medicare-supported initiatives.

Taking advantage of these irregularities to maximize Medicare reimbursement need not be seen as strictly financially driven. Having favorable reimbursement in one area allows for nonrevenue-producing services in another. The Resource Allocation section provides guidelines for selling "loss leaders" programs to administration, and examples of how to make difficult allocation decisions.

One component that is postponed year after year in many facilities is the oncology database. This is not surprising since sophisticated automation can be very expensive, does not have the emotional appeal that other cancer components offer, must usually be done in conjunction with other larger information service network decisions, and may become obsolete in a short time frame. However, a lack of integrated data will leave an otherwise excellent clinical program failing soon. Without data that link patient outcomes, cost, and satisfaction, health care providers cannot know the impact of interventions and certainly cannot convince third-party payers of their positive impact. The sophisticated public/patients are surfing the World Wide Web to find cancer support groups and advice regarding cancer treatment and drug interactions. A growing proportion of patients will want personal computer access to their caregivers and data at their convenience. Progressive cancer program leaders will be prepared to meet this need for data.

## COMPONENTS OF A CANCER PROGRAM

There are no specific answers to the questions: "How big must a hospital be to have a cancer program?" and "What are the necessary components of a hospital-based oncology program?" Across the country, hospitals from 100 beds to well over 1000 beds have varying components based upon the organizations' strategic plans, internal and external assessments, and human and financial resources. Table 51-10 lists some of the hundreds of components program designers may consider. The ability to move from "small" to "large" depends upon the market to be served, the resources available, and the emphasis to be placed upon oncology as a whole or upon a specific component of cancer care. Certainly, there are internationally recognized cancer centers that have few of the components listed because they have chosen to focus on one area. A long list of services or components should not be construed to equal quality.

A vast array of strategic initiatives should be considered when choosing the components for a specific program. The size of the organization and stage of the cancer program development are obviously to be considered. Another determining factor is whether the program stands alone or is part of a large network that has chosen to consolidate clinical programs. The obvious shift to ambulatory services has significantly reduced the need for inpatient-dedicated oncology units.

A cancer program's strategic plan should clearly dictate components. If the strategic plan calls for an emphasis on breast cancer then diagnostic technology, genetic counseling, mammography screening, and survivor groups are some of the components that support the focus on breast cancer.

The organization and operation of traditional oncology services are well known and documented. The components relating to support services, rehabilitation, screening, and detection are less well known, thus an emphasis is placed upon them here.

## Support Services

Table 51-11 is a list of potential supportive and continuing care services. Interest in psychosocial support has grown as advocacy movements for patients' rights have become strong.[81] Several studies indicate the prevalence of cancer patients' needs for concrete assistance. In a randomized survey of 629 cancer patients and 397 support individuals, Houts and colleagues found that 59% of the patients had at least one unmet psychosocial need during the first year of diagnosis.[82] The unmet need cited most often was for emotional support.[82]

Numerous studies suggest that the primary reasons patients have unmet needs is the lack of information and awareness that supportive care services exist, and/or they are unable to negotiate complex bureaucracies to obtain services in a timely manner.

The following decision structure may prove helpful to decide which supportive cancer services to offer, how to guarantee access to those services not offered within the system, and how to support needed out-of-system services:

**TABLE 51-10** Potential Components of a Cancer Program by Hospital Size or Stage of Development

| Component | Small | Medium | Large |
|---|---|---|---|
| Inpatient oncology units | Scattered oncology beds | Dedicated medical oncology and hematology unit<br>or<br>Dedicated medical-surgical oncology unit | Dedicated medical oncology and hematology unit<br>Surgical oncology unit<br>Pediatric oncology unit<br>Bone marrow transplant unit<br>Oncology ICU<br>On-unit pharmacy<br>Family room<br>On-unit library and patient education rooms |
| Ambulatory clinics | Chemotherapy infusion center | Chemotherapy and biotherapy center<br>Symptom management clinic<br>Day hospital<br>Breast health center<br>Pain management clinic<br>Second opinion clinics | Chemotherapy and biotherapy center<br>Symptom management clinic<br>Day hospital<br>Breast health center<br>Risk assessment center<br>Screening clinics<br>Disease-specific clinics<br>Treatment planning clinic<br>24-hour clinic<br>Rehabilitation center<br>Pain management<br>Patient library<br>Outpatient psychosocial support services<br>Outpatient nutritional support services<br>Transportation system to treatment<br>Second opinion clinics<br>Genetic counseling |
| Radiation therapy | External beam therapy<br>Simulation<br>Medical physics<br>Brachytherapy | External beam therapy<br>Simulation<br>Medical physics<br>Brachytherapy<br>Hyperthermia<br>High-dose afterloader brachytherapy<br>Extended service hours | External beam therapy<br>Simulation<br>Medical physics<br>Brachytherapy<br>Hyperthermia<br>High-dose afterloader brachytherapy<br>Intraoperative therapy<br>Conformation<br>Extended service hours |
| Surgery | Inpatient surgery<br>Outpatient surgery | Inpatient surgery<br>Outpatient surgery<br>Laser surgery<br>Stereotactic biopsy<br>Same day diagnosis<br>Cryosurgery | Inpatient surgery<br>Outpatient surgery<br>Laser surgery<br>Stereotactic biopsy<br>Same day diagnosis<br>Cryosurgery |
| Laboratory | Clinical and anatomical pathology<br>FNA cytology | Clinical and anatomical pathology<br>FNA cytology<br>Flow cytometry<br>Immunology<br>Cell analysis<br>Tumor markers | Clinical and anatomical pathology<br>FNA cytology<br>Flow cytometry<br>Immunology<br>Cell anlaysis<br>Cytogenetics<br>Monoclonal antibody<br>Cryopreservation<br>Histocompatibility<br>Tumor markers |

**TABLE 51-10**   Potential Components of a Cancer Program by Hospital Size or Stage of Development *(continued)*

| Component | Small | Medium | Large |
|---|---|---|---|
| Imaging | Mammography<br>Fluoroscopy<br>Ultrasound<br>Nuclear medicine | Mammography<br>Fluoroscopy<br>Ultrasound<br>Nuclear medicine<br>CT<br>MRI<br>Stereotactic capability | Mammography<br>Fluoroscopy<br>Ultrasound<br>Nuclear medicine<br>CT<br>MRI<br>PET<br>Stereotactic capability |
| Physicians | Medical oncologist<br>Radiation oncologist | Medical oncologists<br>Radiation oncologists<br>Hematologists<br>Surgical oncologist<br>Immunologist | Medical oncologists<br>Radiation oncologists<br>Hematologists<br>Surgical oncologists<br>Immunologists<br>Breast surgeons<br>Additional oncologists |
| American College of Surgeons | Accreditation | Accreditation with commendation | Accreditation with commendation |
| Support Services | Social services<br>Nutritionist<br>Clinical nurse specialist<br>Clergy<br>Financial counselor<br>Pharmacists<br>Oncology certified nurses | Social services<br>Nutritionist<br>Clinical nurse specialist<br>Clergy<br>Financial counselor<br>Pharmacists<br>Enterostomal therapists<br>Pain management<br>Psychologists<br>Protocol nurses<br>Oncology certified nurses<br>Library/patient education | Social services<br>Nutritionist<br>Clinical nurse specialist<br>Clergy<br>Financial counselor<br>Pharmacists<br>Enterostomal therapists<br>Pain management<br>Psychologists<br>Protocol nurses<br>Data managers<br>Patient educators<br>Group counselors<br>Oncology certified nurses<br>Library/patient education<br>Music therapy<br>Art therapy<br>Recreational therapy |
| Home care and hospice care | Contracted home care and hospice services | Hospital-based home care including chemotherapy<br>Hospital-based outpatient hospice<br>Infusion therapy | Hospital-based oncology home care including chemotherapy<br>Hospital-based inpatient and outpatient hospice<br>Infusion therapy |
| Rehabilitation services | Rehabilitation services with oncology focus | Oncology team of rehabilitation specialists | Expanded oncology team of rehabilitation specialists |
| Research | Cooperative group treatment protocols<br>Nursing research to practice forum<br>2% patients on clinical trials | Cooperative group treatment protocols<br>Cancer control protocols<br>Original treatment protocols<br>Nursing research to practice forum<br>Original nursing research<br>4% patients on clinical trials | Cooperative group treatment protocols<br>Cancer control protocols<br>Original treatment protocols<br>Nursing research to practice forum<br>Original nursing research<br>Epidemiological research<br>Basic science research<br>6% patients on clinical trials<br>Oncology research nurse and data collector |
| Oncology database | Tumor registry<br>Inpatient financial data | Integrated quality outcome and cost data—inpatient and outpatient | Integrated quality outcome and cost data—inpatient and outpatient |

*(continued)*

**TABLE 51-10**   Potential Components of a Cancer Program by Hospital Size or Stage of Development (continued)

| Component | Small | Medium | Large |
|---|---|---|---|
| | | Hospital-physician office information system<br>Participation in community information network<br>Product line cost/revenue accounting system<br>Computerized procedures, care paths, and variance analysis | Integrated quality outcome and cost data—inpatient and outpatient<br>Hospital-physician office information system<br>Participation in community information network<br>Product line cost/revenue accounting system<br>Computerized procedures, care paths, and variance analysis |
| Professional education | Staff competency-based continuing education<br>Team education programs<br>Chemotherapy certification classes | Staff competency-based continuing education<br>Team education programs<br>Outreach education<br>University affiliation<br>Chemotherapy certification classes | Staff competency-based continuing education<br>Team education programs<br>Outreach education<br>University faculty appointments<br>Regional conferences<br>National conferences<br>Chemotherapy certification classes |
| Community education | Speakers bureau<br>Focused education to employees and families<br>Cancer information brochures<br>Community advisory board | Speakers bureau<br>Focused education to employees and families<br>Work site program<br>Cancer information brochures<br>Community advisory board<br>Public/lending library for public, patient, family education | Speakers bureau<br>Focused education to employees and families<br>Work site program<br>School outreach efforts<br>Mass media<br>Cancer information hotline<br>Community advisory board<br>Public/lending library for public, patient, family education |
| Cancer screening | National screening participation annually | Continuing screening programs<br>Mobile vans | Ongoing cancer screening and risk assessment clinics<br>Mobile vans<br>Genetic screening and counseling |

1. Complete a patient needs-assessment annually, both within the system and within the community. Prioritize expenditures for services identified as needed and valuable.
2. Take the lead in developing a community-based (rather than a hospital-based) support services program, a community services network, and perhaps eventually a community services support facility.[83]
3. Use creative media efforts to publicize services available throughout the community. One hospital used its inpatient room and outpatient clinic televisions to operate a cancer learning and information channel.[84]
4. Involve and serve outpatients where cancer patients spend great amounts of time. Find ways to reach outpatients with supportive care services, such as nutritional support, transportation needs, and rehabilitation services.
5. Explore opportunities to establish a community-based (or system-based) foundation to assist with some of the costs associated with supportive care. Establishing a cancer fund as part of this foundation is one approach.

## Rehabilitation

Rehabilitation addresses the issues of function, quality of life, and independence in life routines.[85] Rehabilitation refers to the "process by which individuals, within their environments, are assisted to achieve optimal functioning, within the limits imposed by cancer."[86] The goals of rehabilitation are to improve the quality of life for those experiencing cancer and to assist the individual to regain wholeness.

While resource intensive, there is reason to believe that patient rehabilitation, and a patient's return to measurably improved functionality, may be seen as having value under a managed-care scenario. Since a return to functionality, and in particular a patient's own perception of his/her return to "wholeness" can be measured, rehabilitation is a concrete measurable outcome.

The following rehabilitation opportunities should be evaluated:

1. Organize and/or support a rehabilitation team.
2. Allow for early intervention (in proximity to diagnosis

**TABLE 51-11**   Suggested Supportive Care Services—The American College of Surgeons

Selected supportive and continuing care services include the following:
- Clinical nutrition
- Enterostomal therapy
- Home care
- Hospice
- Pain management
- Pastoral care
- Patient and family education
- Physical, rehabilitative, and occupational therapy
- Psychosocial counseling
- Support group(s)
- Survivorship program

Site-specific services may be available for patients diagnosed with the following cancers:
- Breast
- Colon
- Head and neck
- Lung
- Prostate

when possible) to ensure maximum recovery and minimum adaptation distress.

3. Design and monitor the rehabilitation process and transitions between caregivers and facilities for smooth coordination of care.

4. Incorporate care for outpatients into the rehab plan and budget.

5. Cancer survivors have needs immediately posttherapy and long-term. These issues often involve returning to the workplace.[86] Incorporate both physical and psychosocial rehabilitation services into the rehab program.

6. Develop and use outcome measures for rehabilitated patients.

7. Work with community agencies to form wider community rehab education, support, and exercise groups.

8. Network with community agencies to ensure patient access to rehab services if they are unavailable at the institution or within the system.

## Screening and Education

In the past decade, many cancer programs have increased their efforts in prevention and education (e.g., smoking cessation and skin cancer education efforts) and cancer screening (e.g., sponsoring reduced-rate mammograms, prostate-specific antigen tests, and skin and oral cancer screening).

Some experts now assert that screening for disease often is more expensive than treating it. The Office of Technology Assessment (OTA) notes that *unless limited to high-risk individuals*, screening for cancer costs more than therapy.[37] The key here, for program leaders, is to identify and serve high-risk individuals. In making decisions about which screening and prevention programs to offer, review the following factors:

1. Does the cancer program serve groups at high risk for site-specific cancers?

2. Can a consortium of providers unite to produce a community-sponsored and -financed screening and detection program?[88,89]

3. What does the community's needs assessment reveal about the importance of these activities to the public served? Does the community value these services in that they provide a halo, or image enhancement effect, on the system or program so that when patients need cancer care, they will tend to select the sponsoring organization?

4. Are these activities essential requirements to achieve the institution's mission?

5. What are the lost opportunity costs of providing certain site-specific activities?

6. When site-specific programs are selected, can adequate funds and personnel resources be allocated to achieve client satisfaction and to handle the necessary clinical follow-up tasks for individuals with abnormal test results?

## RESOURCE ALLOCATION

The need to carefully use our resources is more important today than ever, given the increasing cost of supplies, personnel, technology, and physical facilities and the decreasing revenue trends caused by managed care. There is a tendency among hospital managers to add programs and services, watch them grow, measure their activity in terms of volume, but rarely eliminate or completely refocus them. Perhaps the greatest attribute of the integrated oncology program managed jointly by a medical and administrative director is that responsibility and accountability for monitoring and annually revising services is clear. Product lines are intended to be based on strategic and business plans that can be measured and should be organized so that bureaucracy is held to a minimum and new opportunities can be grasped readily.

We tend to focus our annual review of the strategic plan on internal strengths and weaknesses. It is wise to also evaluate shifts in the service area's demographics. Decades ago mass migration from city centers to suburbs left inner-city hospitals caring for a primarily indigent population. Similar changes have been felt as the population ages faster than it grows in volume. It is also wise to evaluate neighboring service areas to determine if a market segment elsewhere can be encouraged to travel for integrated services or if a satellite can be established.

The challenge in resource allocation is, of course, the desire to implement new services as they emerge without reducing present services. Genetic counseling, facility renovation, music therapy, and patient education all vie for the same dollars. How these decisions should be made is debatable. The central issue is to determine which programs or services offer the greatest value to the users. In searching out these answers, it is important to revisit the organizational mission and the oncology strategic plan. For instance, do these plan documents help prioritize educational initiatives as well as wellness initiatives?

Clearly, taking good ideas from the bedside to the board room requires value analysis, champions, and a plan. It is important to rely upon the oncology database to evaluate the financial relative value of a service. Is the oncology contribution to the financial margin so significant that new nonrevenue producing activities can be introduced?

Competing initiatives can serve to splinter or solidify the oncology team. By involving the entire team in making service or purchase recommendations, team work is enhanced and stronger recommendations result. Table 51-12 is a simple method of initially prioritizing new service ideas.

This format requires an annual brainstorming session with the oncology team. Ideas are prioritized by the team, with relative expenses then identified. Some projects will require no infusion of financial resources, others will be moderately expensive, and others will need hundreds of thousands of dollars. Next, see how the ideas fit with the mission and strategic plan. A mobile screening van may fit with the organization's rural outreach initiative and may be combined with cardiac or diabetes service lines to make it most attractive. Regulatory agency requirements may boost some ideas, such as the need for nutritional assessment per JCAHO standards.

Be clear about who are the champions for specific services and recognize the political clout of certain members of your team. High-volume oncology surgeons have more political and financial influence with board members than do team members who do not attract patients into the system. Finally, draw general conclusions about a program's potential success. If a program appears to be doomed, either drop it and use your human resources to develop more viable programs or seek outside funding. Develop a cogent proposal for new services that meets, but does not exceed, the information needs of decision makers. Proposal formats are usually standard within organizations.

## Physical Facilities

Perhaps the biggest undertaking for any oncology program is the development of new facilities or the renovation of existing ones. A physical facility that is modern, visible, accessible, and has a comfortable ambience is advantageous in recruiting patients, physicians, and employees. The decision to develop or renovate is based upon the need for new space to meet projected volume of patients, new technology being introduced, or the need to consolidate present services in contiguous space.

After it is determined that new areas will be designed, small work groups are established to work with architects to perform functional analysis and help design the structure. The clinician's role is to tell the architect what will be done in the space (function), so the architect can design the space (form) in which to do the work safely and efficiently.[90] Work groups may include people from inpatient nursing units, ICUs or bone marrow transplant units, outpatient infusion service, radiation therapy, medical physics, 24-hour clinic, physician office space, research laboratory, and support space. As functions within the spaces become defined, integration of some services such as outpatient reception and medical records, or patient teaching may be considered. Functional issues to address are listed in Table 51-13.

A matrix is frequently used to determine how closely

**TABLE 51-12**   Oncology Program Prioritization

| Idea | Team Prioritization | Patient Prioritization | $ | Fits with Institutional Mission | Champion | Conclusion |
|---|---|---|---|---|---|---|
| Examples | | | | | | |
| Mobile Screening Van | 2 | 0 | $$$ | New business? One already in community | Breast center nurse | Poor probability |
| Nutritional Counseling | 4 | 3 | $ | JCAHO; reduces cost | Dietitian Surgeons Chemotherapy staff | Very good probability |
| Music Therapy | 3 | 3 | $ | Quality of life; no reimbursement | Psychiatric department | Look for outside funding |

**TABLE 51-13**   Functional Issues in Facility Planning

Department description
   Purpose
   Services
   Population served
   Educational programs
   Anticipated changes
   Current deficiencies

Statistical activity
   Historical (3 years)
   Workload
      Inpatient days or outpatient visits per day
      Average length of stay
      Number of discharges
      Number of special procedures (e.g., total body irradiation)
   Staff
      FTEs by job description
      Total number of people
      Greatest number of people on duty at one time, including
      students, physicians, etc.
   Projected (3 years)
   Workload
      Inpatient days or outpatient visits per day
      Average length of stay
      Number of discharges
      Number of special procedures
   Staff
      FTEs by job description
      Total number of people
      Greatest number of people on duty at one time

Relationships (spatial and communication)
   Intradepartmental
   Interdepartmental

Planning considerations
   Operational system (e.g., cart exchange, pneumatic tube)
   Major equipment and technology needs
   Unique design requirements

Reprinted with permission from Lamkin L: Assessment, development and evaluation of cancer programs. *Semin Oncol Nurs* 9:20, 1993. Used with permission.

adjacent new departments must be to each other and to existing departments within the facility.[34] For example, is it more important for the outpatient infusion center to be adjacent to the inpatient nursing unit, the pharmacy, or patient parking? Discussions regarding adjacent location will help determine if areas can be functionally related by use of computers or pneumatic tube systems in lieu of spatial contiguity.

It is important not to become so mired in space details that systems planning is neglected. The systems by which people, medical records, supplies, food, and drugs are moved, ordered, and returned are critical to the smooth functioning of all areas. There is no better time to realign systems and traffic flow than when planning new facilities.

Clinicians from each work group have the opportunity to design details within their areas. The nurse is in the best position to determine where the intravenous fluid control pump will stand, where oxygen can best be ac-

cessed, and where bathroom access is necessary. A friendly, comfortable environment and ambience are important to patients, visitors, and staff. Combining comfort and technology is a challenge, especially with constraints such as infection control and cost containment.

## Equipment and Technology

There is apparently a never-ending list of clinical innovations and new technology being developed in oncology. The more dynamic the oncology program team is, the more innovations they will be eager to implement. Because cancer itself, its diagnosis, its treatment, and its care are so complex, the innovations come from a variety of sources, and requests to the oncology program leadership are wide ranging. Most programs are not in a position of unlimited resources, either human or financial, and must make difficult and careful choices.

The most expensive components in an oncology program are still the capital investments necessary for radiation therapy equipment and diagnostic equipment (PET scanners, genetics laboratories) and the human and technical resources for bone marrow transplant programs.[91]

It helps to have a process and people in place to evaluate the relative merits of new technology. A simple process of evaluating new technology has five basic steps: (1) determining decision makers, (2) oncology team evaluation, (3) oncology team recommendations, (4) business planning, and (5) organizational approval. It is advantageous to build consensus among the oncology stakeholders before organizational approval is sought. The oncology leadership may be required to evaluate and prioritize a list of technology improvements. Before the financial analysis is undertaken, the oncology leadership should have evaluated its scientific merit, fit with the strategic plan, resources required, and relative benefit.

Another important issue to consider in capital expenditures is whether to lease or buy equipment. This is generally based upon the expected life of the equipment and the future internal rate of return.[92]

Another approach to managing special purchases involves assembling a capital acquisition team with a technical advisory committee using internal and external expertise as needed.[93] The process chosen for evaluating and adopting new technology or clinical innovations should be rigorous enough to ensure that funds are being wisely allocated, without being such a tedious process that team members are reluctant to suggest new ideas.

## Human Resources

Opportunities for reallocation of human resources within cancer programs abound. Reengineering, redesign, and retooling strategies are ten years old in health care and have now stabilized enough for evaluation.[94] Many organizations began their downsizing in the nursing departments and have met with varying success.

An organization usually will evaluate its entire work force and the processes used. Mergers and acquisitions forming giant health care systems have the opportunity to consolidate duplicative, nonpatient care areas such as human resource departments, payroll, physician credentialing, accounting, scheduling, referral services, marketing, finance, computer operations, materials management, and the executive staff.

The use of high technology also helps employees be more efficient so additional hours of direct care are available for patients. Computerized order entry, results reporting, charging, and inventory control result in greater human efficiency, more accurate billing, and better inventory systems. Point-of-care automation not only reduces human resource needs but also can result in: timely, legible documentation, reduction in medication errors and misbilling, easier dissemination of critical clinical information, reductions in costly transcription errors, and concomitant reduction in liability insurance premiums, clinical trends, flags, and variance analysis in clinical pathways.[95]

The use of fax machines, cellular phones and pagers, bar coding, voice mail, and magnetic sitters also reduces the paperwork staff are required to provide. Spurck et al reduced nonproductive time by 1500 annual nursing hours among 73 RNs by introducing cellular phones.[95]

One strategy that has met with mixed success is redesigning care to reduce registered nurse hours and increase nonprofessional hours of care. A variety of multiskilled workers have been used. Some examples include patient care associates or assistants who provide any combination of nursing assistant, housekeeping, transportation, and dietary support. Administrative support personnel may combine the roles of unit secretary, admitting, utilization review, insurance verification, medical record coding, and quality data collection. Other combination roles include phlebotomy, electrocardiogram, respiratory therapy, and pharmacy technician roles. There is no question that the versatile employee is a valuable one. Cross-training of staff throughout oncology can provide variable staffing and continuity of care between inpatient and outpatient areas.

The key to redesign among RNs and unlicensed assistive personnel (UAPs) is to maintain the RN's critical functions and to teach RNs how to manage UAPs. The American Nurses' Association has stated that "It is the nursing profession that defines and supervises the education, training and utilization of any unlicensed assistive role included in providing direct patient care and . . . is responsible and accountable for the provision of nursing practice and supervision of UAPs."[96] The Oncology Nursing Society has prepared a position paper on the use of UAPs in cancer care that suggests UAPs should not be used in those situations where the patient's disease or response are unpredictable or where specialized knowledge, judgment, or skills are necessary such as chemotherapy, pain management, symptom management plans,

grading of toxicity, and unstable patient assessment.[96] It is important for the oncology leadership to involve staff in planning and implementing redesign that meets the outcome and satisfaction needs of patients, and the professional satisfaction needs of the staff.

# CANCER PROGRAM MARKETING AND CONTRACTING

## Marketing

Marketing, traditionally disdained by those in the health care field, is now a topic of great concern for health care managers. Today, marketing is recognized as a needed management function in a highly competitive environment characterized by an excess capacity of inpatient beds and an oversupply of medical specialists.[97]

Successful marketing includes a well-designed product or service, appropriate pricing, communication methods, and a system for distributing the products/services (e.g., a hospital, affiliated physician's offices, a cancer center). The cancer program leadership needs to develop a marketing plan by determining the needs and wants of target markets and then designing, communicating, pricing, and delivering appropriate and competitively viable products and services.[97]

One of the peculiar situations faced by health care organizations is the scope and divergence of their markets. Patients, the worried-well, physicians, regulators, payers, HMOs, PPOs, government reimbursement agencies, employers, business roundtables, and other organizations are each seeking to change the way health care is organized, delivered, and financed.

Most believe medical services must be driven by the health care needs of the population. Assessing community health needs and resources is the first step for health care providers in identifying customer needs and requirements (such as price, quality, covered services). The next step is to translate these demands into desired or necessary services and programs that create value for community members.[98]

Health status indicators vary by community, and typically reflect the community's definition of health, whether that is defined as an individual's ability to function "normally" in daily activities, or practicing good habits to promote wellness. The CDC released a set of 18 indicators for the United States as a whole that include female breast cancer deaths, suicides, births to adolescents, and measles incidence.[99] A local community needs-assessment will no doubt yield indicators that reflect the concerns and values of its own population.

The needs-assessment will be useful to the cancer program leaders when evaluating which projects will be allocated funds. The assessment will help to ensure that money and resources support the most-needed program elements; that financial and social responsibilities are met; that providers recognize and understand critical community-wide health risks; and that products and services created have value for members, patients, and community citizens.[98] Marketing emerging health care systems offers new challenges. Rynne[100] notes that reaching the marketplace, in such a way that customers understand and are comfortable with an integrated product, is as difficult as creating the system in the first place.

Forming a marketing team can ensure a balance between clinical and sales initiatives. A marketing staff member assigned to the oncology service line should have a clearly delineated role and job function. That individual can use creative talents to tell the clinical story to the intended audience. The marketing team may consider using the talents and expertise of an advertising and/or public relations firm.[101] No matter how well cancer care professionals know the product and patients and their needs, most clinicians require assistance to formulate a message that audiences will hear, see, and respond to with enthusiasm. Using expert creative talent to design media campaigns and collaterals (e.g., brochures, media releases, annual reports) makes it easier to achieve marketing objectives.[102]

## Contracting

Historically, health care was reimbursed on a fee-for-service basis. Today a wide variety of contracting opportunities are available: discounted charge-basis, per diem rates, per visit or stay rates, global pricing, and capitation rates. Becoming a prudent and effective negotiator for oncology contracts requires first a willingness to take risks and be innovative and second a solid cost-accounting database.

To remain competitive in the marketplace and maintain cancer program prominence, skillful contracting is necessary. In many locales the insurers are so powerful that they choose a per diem or per visit rate and offer it to providers on a take-it or leave-it basis. Hospitals and physicians have found themselves being left out of major contracts or accepting contracts that barely cover the costs of care. Many insurers and employers are now selecting centers of excellence that will offer discounted rates. Delta Airlines recently directly negotiated cardiac care with six centers across the country for their 72,000 employees.[103] Over 60 programs applied for the privilege of discounting rates 35% to 50% off their standard rates.

Most per diem, per visit, or per stay rates are negotiated for an entire hospital organization. If an internal general managed-care contractor is responsible for system-wide rate negotiation, he or she should be cognizant of the proportion of care being delivered to oncology patients and the demographic shifts nationally and locally regarding cancer care. The risk the hospital accepts in per diem or per stay rates is that the population covered will maintain present illness and wellness patterns. With hospital per diem or per stay rate contracts, outpatient services usually remain fee-for-service.

A much greater risk is accepted by the organization that engages in managed-care contracts involving *global pricing* and *capitation*.[104] *Global pricing* is an all-inclusive price for the delivery of a discrete set of services.[105] This pricing strategy can be applied to a specific procedure (e.g., breast biopsy) or a course of treatment (e.g., diagnosis through one year of treatment for early-stage breast cancer). A clear definition of the boundaries of service is imperative to protect the provider. Because global pricing includes physician fees, inpatient and outpatient services, and frequently support services to add value, it is critical that all participants have and are willing to share cost data. The hospital must develop a formal, cooperative relationship with all providers. Physicians particularly must trust that the data they are providing to the hospital will be kept confidential and that the accounting of all revenues and expenses will be open to them.

Wodinsky et al report a successful global pricing strategy for first year treatment of early breast cancer.[105] Their average annual global charge is estimated to be $19,627 with 21.7% going to pretreatment planning, 14% for staging, 42.6% for surgical intervention, 10.7% for radiation, 4.9% for adjuvant systemic therapy, and 6.1% for hormonal and maintenance therapy. Models exist where the hospital receives the global rate and pays other providers a preestablished fee-for-service rate leaving the hospital at risk for shortfalls. Other models call for the creation of a physician-hospital organization (PHO) that receives the global fee and splits the revenues based upon prearranged formulas. This second method provides better-aligned incentives for all providers. The success of global pricing strategies lies in the standardized care of patients and contingency plans for clinical and financial outlier patients. If the PHO accepts responsibility for all patients, careful assessment of the population for potential outliers and planning for their care is necessary. Another technique is to detail in the contract that specific patient outliers will be excluded.

*Capitation* refers to the per capita payment amount managed care organizations or providers are paid to provide an enrollee (or member) with a specified package of medical services.[106] The capitation payment rate is expressed on a per member per month (PMPM) basis. This, too, can be negotiated on a procedural or time limited discrete package price. For example, Health Maintenance Organizations (HMOs) that purchase radiation services prefer to pay a PMPM rate to radiation therapy providers. If an HMO paid a provider $1 PMPM and had 100,000 members, the provider would receive $1,200,000 annually ($1 × 100,000 × 12 months) and for that would provide whatever radiation services the entire population required during that year. Some HMOs and managed-care organizations are now capitating all oncology services to specialized cancer centers on a PMPM basis. Again, the entity (hospital or PHO) that receives the revenue is at risk for providing all necessary services. So contractors must be intimately familiar with the demographics and health practices of the population they accept and their own cost of providing care.

Franklin[107] provides an excellent ten-step process for creating managed care products in oncology. Where the details of creating a managed care product and the associated risk may seem daunting, only those so prepared will survive the present and future health financing systems.

## CONCLUSION

As nurses move from clinical roles to program development roles, they have the opportunity to benefit a greater number of patients with their skill and knowledge. Nurses are in an excellent position to shape the future of integrated, full-service, technical yet caring, comprehensive cancer programs. Nurses must work with administrators and physicians using the planning and communication skills they have developed in previous positions. Many will be challenged to gain new knowledge of strategic and business planning as well as financial analysis so that they are as well respected in the boardroom as at the bedside.

Speedy changes in health care financing have resulted in a new urgency to carefully evaluate and plan the service components, maximize revenues, and control costs. The nurse who accepts the challenges of an administrative role must be prepared to champion quality patient care while articulating its financial ramifications.

This chapter suggests planning guidelines and explores new relationships among providers and between providers and payers. Specific management strategies for planning, structuring, ensuring quality and financial outcomes, and determining resource allocation and marketing are detailed. Possible cancer program components to maintain prominence are noted. Each nurse must evaluate the present situation, internally and externally, and the potential for growth in a particular setting. With the nurse administrator rests the responsibility to ensure that planning and implementation, at whatever level, remain patient-centered.

## REFERENCES

1. Yarbro CH, Yarbro JW: Historical development of cancer programs. *Semin Oncol Nurs* 9:3–7, 1993
2. Association of Community Cancer Centers: *Community Cancer Programs in the United States 1988–1989.* Rockville, MD, Association of Community Cancer Centers, 1989
3. Spallina JM: Planning for the future of cancer care: developing successful strategies for cancer care delivery. *J Oncol Manage.* 2:23–27, 1993
4. Jennings MC: Predicting managed care growth. *Healthcare Fin Manage.* 48:18–19, 1994
5. Weiss B: Managed care: there's no stopping it now. *Med Econ.* 72:26–43, 1995
6. Japsen B: Can NCI cancer centers still thrive under managed care? *Mod Healthcare.* 48:18–19, 1994
7. Gerber J, Wolff J, Klores W, et al: *Lifetrends.* New York, MacMillan, 1989
8. Dychtwald K, Flower J: *Age Wave.* New York, Bantam, 1990
9. Nathanson SN, Lerman D: Directions in cancer care, in Nathanson SN (ed): *Outpatient Cancer Centers Implementation and Management.* Chicago, American Hospital Publishing, 1988, pp 1–16
10. Conklin VK: Continuity of care issues for cancer patients and families. *Cancer* 64:290–294, 1989
11. Scheffler RM, Andrews NC (eds): *Cancer Care and Cost DRGs and Beyond.* Ann Arbor, MI, Health Administration Hospital Press Perspectives, 1989
12. Palmer P, Steiger N, Engleberg C: The cost of oncology care in a small community hospital. *Proc Am Soc Clin Oncol* 5:241, 1986 (abstr)
13. Flower J: The structure of organized change (a conversation with Kevin Kelly). *Healthcare Forum J* 38:24–41, 1995
14. Unland JJ: Hospital-physician relationships in the managed care environment. *Med Pract Management* 10:6–10, 1994
15. Shortell SM, Morrison EM, Friedman B: *Strategic Choices for America's Hospitals.* San Francisco, Jossey-Bass Publishers, 1992, pp 7, 297, 275
16. Luke RD, Begun JW, Pointer DD: Quasi firms: strategic interorganizational forms in the healthcare industry. *Acad Manage Rev* 14:9–19, 1989
17. Beckham JD: Big in the land of the giants, part 1. *Healthcare Forum J* 37:24–28, 1994
18. Goldsmith J: The illusive logic of integration. *Healthcare Forum J* 38:26–31, 1994
19. Burns LR, Thorpe DP: Trends and models in physician-hospital organization. *Health Care Manage Rev* 18:7–20, 1993
20. Hurley RE: The purchaser-driven reformation in healthcare: Alternative approaches to leveling our cathedrals. *Front Health Serv Manage,* 9:5–35, 1993
21. Coddington DC, Moore KD, Fischer EA: Integrating? Hang in there—the odds are in your favor. *Healthcare Forum J* 38: 72–76, 1995
22. Managed care: specialty doctors often sidelined by managed plans. *J Natl Cancer Inst* 87:864–868, 1995
23. Wodinsky HB, Bowing K: Oncology network development. *Cancer Manage* (in press)
24. American College of Surgeons: *Cancer Programs Approved.* Chicago, ACoS Commission on Cancer, 1995
25. Mortenson E, Kirkland C: *Community Cancer Program in the United States.* Rockville, MD, Association of Community Cancer Centers, 1996
26. National Cancer Institute: *Listing of National Cancer Institute P-30s.* Washington, DC, National Cancer Institute Cancer Centers Branch, 1995
27. Nash MG, Opperwall BC: Strategic planning: The practical vision. *J Nurs Admin* 18:12–18, 1988
28. Bookbinder NF: Strategic planning, in Nathanson SN (ed): *Outpatient Cancer Centers Implementation and Management.* Chicago, American Hospital Publishing, 1988, pp 17–32
29. Henderson JC: Aligning business and information technology domains: Strategic planning in hospitals. *Hosp Health Serv Admin* 37:71–87, 1992
30. Johnson L: Strategic management: A new dimension of nurse executive's role. *J Nurs Admin* 20:7–10, 1990
31. Buller PF, Timpson L: The strategic management of hospitals: Toward an integrative approach. *Health Care Manage Rev* 11:7–13, 1986

32. Beckman JD: Strategic thinking and the road to relevance. *Healthcare Forum J* 34:37–43, 1991

33. Aaker DA: *Developing Business Strategies*. New York, Wiley, 1988

34. Lamkin L: Assessment, development and evaluation of cancer programs. *Semin Oncol Nurs* 9:17–24, 1993

35. Mintzberg H: The rise and fall of strategic planning. *Harvard Bus Rev* 72:107–119, 1994

36. Waterman RH: The seven elements of strategic fit. *J Bus Strategy* Winter:69–73, 1982

37. Kassirer, JP: Managed care and the morality of the marketplace. *N Engl J Med.* 333:30–32, 1995

38. Feingold MG, Meyer JW, Briggs DS: Controlling costs and quality through clinical pathways: one cancer center's experience. *Oncol Issues* 6:24–28, 1991

39. Wiggers JG, O'Donovan KO, Redman S, et al: Cancer patient satisfaction with care. *Cancer* 66:610–616, 1990

40. Ogorzalek LL: Quality management issues. *Semin Oncol Nurs* 9:32–37, 1993

41. Patton MD: Action research and the process of continual quality improvement in a cancer center. *Oncol Nurs Forum* 20:751–755, 1993

42. Paris NM, Hines J: Payer and provider relationships: The key to reshaping health care delivery. *Nurs Admin Q* 19:13–17, 1995

43. Alsever RN, Ritchey T, Lima NP: Developing a hospital report card to demonstrate value in healthcare. *J Healthcare Qual* 17:19–28, 1995

44. Beddar SM, Aiken JL: Continuity of care: a challenge for the ambulatory oncology nurse. *Semin Oncol Nurs* 10:254–263, 1994

45. O'Hare P, Terry M: *Discharge Planning: Strategies for Ensuring Continuity of Care*. Rockville, MD, Aspen, 1988

46. Clark CM, Steinbender A: Implementing clinical paths in a managed care environment. *Nurs Econ* 4:230–234, 1994

47. Hawkins J, Goldberg PB: Planning, implementing and evaluating a chemotherapy critical path. *J Oncol Manage* 3:24–29, 1994

48. Katterhagen JG, Patton MD: Critical pathways in oncology: balancing the interest of hospitals and physicians. *J Oncol Manage* 3:20–26, 1993

49. Patton MD, Katterhagen JG: Critical pathways in oncology: aligning resource expenditures with clinical outcomes. *J Oncol Manage* 2:20–26, 1993

50. Micheletti JA, Shlala TJ: Case management can reduce costs and protect revenues. *Healthcare Fin Manage* 49:64–70, 1995

51. Lamkin L: Outpatient oncology settings: a variety of services. *Semin Oncol Nurs* 10:229–236, 1994

52. Joint Commission on Healthcare Accreditation Organizations: Appendix B, Joint Commission indicators for the indicator measurement system, beta-phase testing, and hospital internal use, in *Comprehensive Accreditation Manual for Hospitals*. Oakbrook Terrace, IL, 1995, pp 531–540

53. Association of Community Cancer Centers: *Standards for Cancer Programs*. Rockville, MD, Association of Community Cancer Centers, 1993

54. Commission on Cancer: *Cancer Program Standards*. Chicago, IL, American College of Surgeons, 1996

55. O'Kane ME: The National Committee for Quality Assurance. *Group Pract J* 41:44–49, 1992

56. Oncology Nursing Society: *Resource Manual for Oncology Nurse Managers and Administrators*. Pittsburgh, PA, Oncology Nursing Press, 1991

57. Davidson S: The metamorphosis of the modern physician, the theory to practice time warp. *Healthcare Forum J* 38:66–73, 1995

58. Spallina J: Cancer program integration: back to basics—Part 1. *Cancer Manage* 1:24–28, 1996

59. Spallina J: Cancer program integration: back to basics—Part 2. *Cancer Manage* 1:20–27, 1996

60. Beckham JD: Building the high performance accountable health plan. *Healthcare Forum J* 37:60–67, 1994

61. Charns MP, Smith LJ: Product line management and continuity of care. *Health Matrix* 7:40–49, 1989

62. Nackel PD, Kues JG, Irvin W: Product line management: systems and strategies. *Hosp Health Serv Admin* 31:109–122, 1986

63. Zelman WN, Parham DL: Strategic, operational and marketing concerns of product line management in healthcare. *Health Care Manage Rev* 15:25–35, 1990

64. Fountain M: A survey of cancer program administrators. *Oncol Issues* 6:20–22, 1991

65. Conklin A: Product/service line management, the basics. *Oncol Issues* 10:12–14, 1995

66. Sandrik K: Oncology: who's managing outpatient programs? *Hospitals* 64:32–37, 1990

67. Naidu GM, Kleimenhagen A, Pillari GD: Is product line management appropriate for your facility? *Health Care Mktg* F:6–17, 1993

68. MacDonald SA: Organizational approaches to cancer program development. *Semin Oncol Nurs* 9:8–16, 1993

69. Brady AM: The physician as leader of the oncology program, part II. *J Oncol Manage* 1:22–25, 1992

70. Joseph T: Greater future roles seen for physicians, physician executives. *Physician Executive* 17:3–7, 1991

71. Brady AM: The physician as leader of the oncology program, part I. *J Oncol Manage* 1:32–34, 1992

72. Coile RC: Cancer #1 center of excellence for the 21st century. *Hosp Strategy Rep* 2:7, 1990

73. Mannisto MM, Ney MS: Cancer program and medical directors: growing in number and importance. *Oncol Issues* 4:15–22, 1989

74. Lewis GW, Taylor RB, Mealor RS: What cancer program managers must know: the fiscal and regulatory challenge. *Semin Oncol Nurs* 9:59–67, 1993

75. Giles K: Using clinical financial pathways to capitate cancer. *Oncol Issues* 10:14–17, 1995

76. Gipe BT, Harris SC, Rosenberg M: A new method for direct cost analysis. *Cost and Quality* 1:13–20, 1995

77. Carson KD, Carson PP, Authenment J, et al: Strategic options for hospitals based on ownership types. *Hospital Topics* 72:21–29, 1994

78. Young WW, Joyce DZ, Bivens GD, et al: Incorporating the cost of ambulatory care into case mix-based hospital reimbursement. *J Ambulatory Care Manage* 11:54–67, 1988

79. Ford RL: What we do and how we measure it. *Hosp Health Serv Admin* 32:399–407, 1987

80. Folger JC, Gee EP: *Product Management of Hospitals, Organizing for Profitability*. Chicago, American Hospital Publishing, 1987

81. Lederberg MS, Massie MJ: Psychosocial and ethical issues in the care of cancer patients, in DeVita VT, Hellman S, Rosenberg SA (eds): *Cancer Principles and Practice of Oncology* (ed 4). Philadelphia, Lippincott, 1993, pp 2448–2464

82. Houts PS, Yasko JM, Kahn B, et al: Unmet psychological, social and economic needs of persons with cancer in Pennsylvania. *Cancer* 58:2355–2361, 1986

83. Horton JR, Gosey M, Fay A: Cancer support services: a working prototype. *J Oncol Manage* 3:34–43, 1994

84. Siegal M, Patyk M: A new approach to cancer education: the cancer information channel. *J Oncol Manage* 2:29–33, 1993

85. Gerber LH, Levinson S, Hick J, et al: Evaluation and management of disability: rehabilitation aspects of cancer, in DeVita VT, Hellman S, Rosenberg SA (eds): *Cancer Principles and Practice of Oncology* (ed 4). Philadelphia, Lippincott, 1993, pp 2538–2569

86. Frymark SL, Mayer DK: Rehabilitation of the person with cancer, in Groenwald SL, Frogge MH, Goodman M, Yarbro C (eds): *Cancer Nursing: Principles and Practice* (ed 3). Boston, Jones and Bartlett, 1993, pp 1361–1369

87. Leutwyler K: The Price of Prevention. *Sci Am* 272:124–129, 1995

88. Deisher R: Multiple benefits of cancer prevention and early detection programs. *Oncol Issues* 10:14–15, 1995

89. Horton JR, Gosey M, Fay A: Cancer support services: a working prototype. *J Oncol Mgt* 3:34–38, 1994

90. Davis PB: Facility design, in Nathanson SN (ed): *Outpatient Cancer Centers Implementation and Management*. Chicago, American Hospital Publishing, 1988, pp 63–91

91. Jewler D, Egan C: Revisioning Oncology. *Oncol Issues* 10: 23–28, 1995

92. Gipe BT: To lease or buy: a clinicians's guide for making the decision. *Cost and Quality* 1:4, 1995

93. Abdallah DO: Using acquisition teams and managing special purchases. *J Oncol Manage* 2:36–40, 1993

94. Barrett MW: Downsizing: doing it rationally. *Nurs Manage* 26:24–29, 1995

95. Spurck PA, Hohr ML, Seroka AM, et al: The impact of a wireless communication system on time efficiency. *JONA* 25:21–26, 1995

96. Oncology Nursing Society: *Position paper on the use of unlicensed assistive personnel in cancer.* Pittsburgh, Oncology Nursing Press, 1996

97. Kotler P, Clark RN: *Marketing for Healthcare Organizations.* Englewood Cliffs, NJ, Prentice Hall, 1989

98. Hospital Association of Pennsylvania: *A Guide for Assessing and Improving Health Status.* Hospital Association of Pennsylvania, 1993

99. Posten P: *Action Kit for Assessing Community Health.* Charlotte, NC, Sun Health Alliance, 1994

100. Rynne TJ: Bringing an integrated system to market. *Healthcare Forum J* 52–59, 1995

101. Luther WM: *The Marketing Plan, How To Prepare It and Implement It.* New York, Amacom, 1982

102. Gilden KM: The challenge of cancer care marketing. *Semin Oncol Nurs* 9:51–58, 1993

103. Leavenworth G: Four cost-cutting strategies. *Business and Health* 12:26–34, 1994

104. Horowitz JL, Kleinman MA: Advanced pricing strategies for hospitals in contracting with managed care organization. *J Ambulatory Care Manage* 17:8–17, 1994

105. Wodinsky HB, Stein MV, Friedman NS: Global pricing for cancer care: one hospital's preliminary report. *J Oncol Manage* 3:18–22, 1994

106. Grimaldi PL: Capitation savvy a must. *Nurs Manage* 26: 33–35, 1995

107. Franklin MA: Creating a managed care product for cancer services. *J Oncol Manage* 3:19–26, 1994

# Chapter 52

# Ambulatory Care

**Diane M. Otte, RN, MS, ET, OCN®**

## AMBULATORY CARE OVERVIEW

Ambulatory services continue to play a major role in the provision of care to individuals with cancer. This shift to ambulatory care will continue into the next century, with ambulatory care emerging as a subspecialty of oncology nursing.[1] Ambulatory care is synonymous with outpatient care and includes services such as diagnostic testing; screening and detection; treatment modalities such as chemotherapy, biotherapy, radiation therapy, blood component therapy, and surgical procedures; patient and family education; rehabilitation; nutritional support; psychosocial intervention; symptom management; procurement of prescriptions and supplies; and survivor services.[2,3]

Advances in cancer treatment and technology and the influences of economics and quality-of-life issues have promoted ambulatory services as a method for providing cancer patient and family care.[1] Health care reform, the increasing interest in health promotion practices, the demographics of advancing age, and a greater number of cancer survivors will further influence the development of outpatient oncology care.[4,5]

It is estimated that 80%–90% of all cancer care is delivered in outpatient settings, such as physicians' offices, freestanding oncology centers, and outpatient departments.[6] *Nursing's Agenda for Health Care Reform*[7] calls for a restructured health care system that enhances consumer access by delivering care in community-based settings, fosters consumer responsibility for self-care and informed decision making, and facilitates utilization of the most cost-effective providers in appropriate settings. Additional steps suggested to reduce health care costs include the use of a managed care approach, incentives for consumers and providers who are cost-effective, outcome-based health care policy development, and the implementation of a case management system to reduce fragmentation of care.[7]

## Ambulatory Care Settings

A wide variety of ambulatory care settings are available, including comprehensive cancer centers, community cancer centers, freestanding cancer centers, 23- to 24-hour clinics, chemotherapy and infusion centers, day surgery centers, physicians' offices, outreach and network programs, and other specialty centers that focus on screening, rehabilitation, and symptom management.

Cancer centers can be classified according to stated purpose, organizational structure (freestanding, joint venture, departmental, matrix, consortium) or source of funding (federal, state, private).[8] However, there is no consensus about what constitutes a cancer center. Shingleton defines a cancer center in the following way: "composed of a multidisciplinary group of research scientists and/or physicians who are bound together with a unity of purpose, who share concepts, facilities, and other resources, and who have developed an organizational structure that fosters effective management practices to achieve the desired goals of the group."[8,p.44]

The distinction between models or types of cancer centers and ambulatory settings is not always clear. A variety of services can generally be provided in all settings.

Comprehensive cancer centers, authorized by the National Cancer Act of 1971 and designated by the National Cancer Institute (NCI), are dedicated to conducting clinical research, training physicians in oncology subspecialties, maintaining data for new diagnoses, and providing clinical care to cancer patients.[8]

Community cancer centers have increased in number over the past two decades and are found in many areas of the country. They may have been established as part of a university system or as part of a community hospital. Lokich et al[9] describe three components that typically constitute a cancer center. First, a multiplicity of services is provided, including chemotherapy, radiation therapy, and surgical services (usually limited to minor procedures); programs for patient and staff education; and support services and diagnostic services. Second, such centers provide access to clinical trials to make new therapies available. Finally, cancer centers offer programs (not typical to the traditional office setting) such as blood transfusions and prolonged chemotherapy infusions. These community cancer centers have provided a way for patients to receive cancer care close to home with a "one-stop service" approach. Most patients no longer need to travel long distances to see an oncologist or receive treatment. In many situations the oncologist and nurses travel to satellite sites to see cancer patients.

### Freestanding centers

A freestanding cancer center (FSCC) may be a facility separate from an existing medical care delivery center such as a hospital, or it may be contiguous with or within a hospital facility. Freestanding centers may be joint ventures between health care providers or may be corporately owned and operated. The movement toward FSCCs resulted from the shift in medical care delivery from inpatient to outpatient settings and from patient demand for sophisticated therapies in the local community. FSCCs are usually based within the community, do not incorporate training of oncologists, and are not involved with on-site basic research.[9] The FSCC may provide a multitude of services or may be focused on only one service, for example, radiation oncology. Freestanding radiation oncology practices often are located within close proximity to a hospital (across the street) to enable easy transport of hospitalized patients for treatment. The center may also provide service to a number of hospitals in the area.

Affiliations of community programs with university-based cancer centers are occurring. Cancer networks are stretching across wide geographic areas. For example, Outreach Corporation, a not-for-profit group formed by the M. D. Anderson Cancer Center (MDACC) at the

University of Texas, is developing, marketing, and operating oncology programs in partnership with community institutions around the country.[10,11] Orlando Regional Medical Center entered into a formal agreement with MDACC to construct and operate a freestanding cancer center in central Florida. This partnership was formed to improve cancer care and enhance market share of the Orlando Cancer Center. The management team is made up of employees of the MDACC Outreach Corporation. The medical director for the center was selected from the Orlando community. With this affiliation, a multidisciplinary approach to cancer treatment is used. A major shift to outpatient care occurred within the Orlando community. Compatible values, goals, and the management and staff members' ability to communicate with each other are essential components of success for this type of affiliation.[11]

### Twenty-three– and twenty-four–hour clinics

The need for ambulatory services on a continuous basis has precipitated the development of a number of 24-hour services across the country. Lamkin[12] describes two categories of service: urgent oncology care and traditional infusion therapies given during expanded hours. Salick Health Care, Inc. operates several 24-hour centers for the provision of diagnostic services, chemotherapy, radiation therapy, and psychosocial support programs. Even though the centers may not be open 24 hours a day initially, health care professionals are on call to meet the needs of patients seeking therapy during nontraditional hours.[12] The Ambulatory Treatment Center of the University of Texas MDACC operates 24 hours per day. Urgent care visits and outpatient procedures—as well as chemotherapy and blood component therapy—are available.[3]

Such settings are specifically designed to deal with side effect management and unpredictable changes in the patient's condition following therapy. Many visits to hospital emergency rooms can be avoided since the patient has access to highly trained individuals to manage the specific oncology-related problems and implement the necessary interventions.

Twenty-three–hour clinics usually refer to a maximum length of stay for individuals rather than to the hours of operation. Individuals who require observation for potentially acute situations (e.g., reactions to blood components or chemotherapy, postoperative complications) are cared for in this type of setting, generally because insurers may not reimburse for an inpatient stay.[3] Frequently, individuals are classified as 23-hour observation patients and are on an inpatient unit of a hospital for this 23-hour stay.

### Day surgery

Moskowitz describes the increase in ambulatory surgery as "one of the most significant trends in health care."[13,p.166] Many types of cancer-related surgical procedures are performed in an ambulatory setting, including biopsy, bronchoscopy, gastrostomy, sigmoidoscopy, marrow harvest, lumpectomy, thyroidectomy, colonoscopy, insertion or removal of venous access devices, and many others. Advantages of ambulatory surgery include reduced cost, fewer complications, less disability, more individualized attention, and less anxiety for the individual undergoing the procedure. Disadvantages include situations in which individuals have not followed proper preoperative instructions, and difficulty with transportation home and with appropriate aftercare.[13] As health care continues to change, the oncology nurse has many opportunities to expand involvement in the development and implementation of quality care in these settings.

### Outpatient clinics and treatment centers

Outpatient clinics and treatment centers are found in a variety of settings, ranging from large medical centers and university settings to community hospitals. Clinics may specialize in treatment of specific disease sites, such as lung or breast, with highly specialized physicians and nurses.[3] Individuals may also seek second opinions from clinicians in these settings. Treatment centers can offer chemotherapy, blood component therapy, infusions, biotherapy, symptom management, rehabilitation services, radiation, and bone marrow transplant services.[3] Typically these environments offer a greater range of hours of service and support than the physician office setting where similar treatment may be offered. Increasingly, bone marrow transplant preparation and care is being provided in an outpatient setting.[3,14] Undoubtedly, the trend for procedures to move to the ambulatory setting will continue.

Another trend that continues is the development of site-specific cancer centers, such as breast clinics or centers. Brady and Foster[15] suggest that breast cancer may be an ideal choice for a site-specific program because of the increasing utilization of breast cancer screening services and the large number of breast cancer patients seen in most programs. Lee et al[16] provide an overview of the development of a comprehensive breast cancer program. Table 52-1 highlights the operational and programmatic components.

Two styles of breast centers are commonly seen: diagnostic breast centers and comprehensive breast centers. Diagnostic centers offer a variety of imaging services, education about breast self-examination, and clinical examination by a physician. In contrast, comprehensive centers offer these services as well as a full range of treatment and rehabilitative services in one setting with a multidisciplinary team approach. The critical component of success for a breast center is broad-based medical staff acceptance.[17] Incorporating a surgical practice within a comprehensive breast center requires adequate space, extensive planning, and a committed group of physicians with an expressed interest to make it happen.[18]

Community partnerships are commonly established as a way to develop breast health improvement projects.

**TABLE 52-1** Components of a Comprehensive Breast Center

| Operational | Programmatic |
|---|---|
| ACR accreditation | Breast self-examination instruction |
| Dedicated clinical, technical, and clerical staff | Clinical history and breast exam |
| Ongoing training/in-service: physicians, technologists, nurses | Sophisticated breast imaging/diagnostic procedures with dedicated equipment |
| Criteria-based physician-referral panels and physician-approved triage protocols for "unassigned" women; primary care (asymptomatic) and surgeons (symptomatic) | Fine-needle aspiration for both palpable and nonpalpable masses if appropriate cytopathology available (otherwise large-core biopsy) |
| Quality assurance protocols: procedures, equipment, patient flow, and follow-up | Second opinion and breast consultation service |
| Effective relationships with hospital-based tumor registry, finance, medical records, information systems, and diagnostic/therapeutic departments | Interdisciplinary pretreatment planning conferences: weekly sessions for all diagnosed patients |
| Well-researched marketing plan/evaluation: internal and external | Risk analysis and counseling |
| Computer-based information and tracking system: financial and clinical | Psychosocial assessment, crisis intervention, support group, and referral for long-term care |
| Clearly defined charge codes for all procedures: screening and diagnosis | Access to local, regional, and national clinical and behavioral research trials |
| | Community outreach: public, professional, and patient education |

Reprinted with permission from the *Journal of Oncology Managements*. Lee CZ, Coleman C, Link J: Developing comprehensive breast centers. Part one: Introduction and overview. *J Oncol Manage* 1:20–23, 1992.

Table 52-2 details action points to be addressed in establishing these innovative partnerships.[19] In Indiana, a breast health awareness program was developed and implemented with community African-American women who provided input to the program. A Minority Health Task Force was formulated with the goal of increasing participation in screening and education for this population. Successful programs can be developed in other communities by committed oncology nurses in partnership with the community.[20]

Site-specific cancer programs offer a number of advantages: patient convenience, improved medical decision making, and, ultimately, improved quality of care.[15,21] Services not generally available in the community can be offered in site-specific cancer centers, such as risk assessment, screening for the disadvantaged and minorities, and educational programs for both professionals and the public. Specialized programs for all major cancers (breast, lung, prostate, gastrointestinal, gynecologic) may eventually be developed, most likely in areas where there is a large population of patients.[15]

**TABLE 52-2** Development of Community Partnerships: Action Points

- Establishment of partnerships and empowerment of natural community leaders
- Promotion of partnerships with primary-care physicians
- Enhancement of collegial relationships with other providers and health care organizations
- Education of participants about the wellness model
- Recognition of cultural diversity
- Acknowledgment of priority differences and providers and community members
- Careful development of outreach and cancer prevention and control
- Consideration of the costs of outreach
- Targeted interventions
- Knowledge of the plan before proceeding

Adapted with permission from the *Journal of Oncology Management*. Tobin E: Assessing needs and developing community partnerships for breast healthcare services. *J Oncol Manage* 3:31–37, 1994.

## Outreach and satellite centers

Since individuals often want to remain in their own communities to receive cancer treatment, linkages between tertiary and rural hospitals are being developed. Harvey and Walker[22] describe a successful networking program in South Carolina. Through this program, patients are treated by oncologists at a tertiary setting and then return to rural or community hospitals for continued treatment. Staff in the rural or community setting were trained to provide the specialized care. Physician, patient, and family satisfaction with care in the outreach area was consistently evaluated as high.

Indiana Community Cancer Care (ICCC) is another example of a networking program, with multiple cancer clinics throughout Indiana that are established in hospitals to provide chemotherapy. A medical oncologist from ICCC makes the visits and is available to the local site clinic coordinator. ICCC also provides education for the satellite nurses and assists in the development of standards, procedures, protocols, quality activities, and documentation systems.[12]

Many community oncologists also perform outreach services through satellite centers in clinics within 20–100 miles of their base practice. Communication and professional relationship skills are critical for successful care in outreach service arrangements. Katterhagen et al[23] describe the Rural Illinois Cancer Consortium (RICC), an organization formed between the Regional Cancer Center of Memorial Medical Center in Springfield, Illinois, and five rural hospitals. The goal of the organization was to improve access to state-of-the-art cancer care. A study was conducted comparing breast cancer treatment in rural hospitals affiliated with the RICC (prior to the initiation of the outreach program and then after the program had been operating for two years) and those without the RICC program. The outreach program demonstrated improved access to breast cancer care. Statistically significant changes were seen for the use of diagnostic bilateral mammography and tumor staging. All variables changed in the desired direction of improving care.[23] This model could certainly be replicated in other settings.

Smith et al[24] developed the Rural Cancer Outreach Program to provide comprehensive cancer care and professional education to individuals in rural Virginia. In the program's first two years of operation, more than 350 individuals with cancer or related hematologic problems were treated in their own communities. Rural practitioners were educated and safely administered cancer care and demonstrated that rural cancer care is revenue-neutral or positive.

Tracy et al[25] describe advantages and disadvantages to visiting consultant clinics in rural hospital communities in Iowa. These opportunities may be a way to retain and enhance specialty referral bases. Travel time, time away from the central operation, increased communication demands, care plan coordination challenges, and logistical and system problems associated with practicing in multiple sites are among disadvantages for the specialists providing the services. Benefits to rural physicians and hospitals include increased availability of specialty services, increased outpatient revenues, reduced professional isolation, and heightened clinical reputation. Disadvantages to rural hospitals and physicians include the increased administrative efforts necessary to monitor care and review credentials, possible disruption of existing referral patterns, risk of losing patients to urban areas, and an increase in expenditures to accommodate the specialists.

The use of telemedicine to bring physicians and/or patients together through two-way interactive video conferencing has great potential for future rural health care settings. In this situation the referring physician in a rural community presents a patient to the consulting physician, who may be many miles away. Routine examinations (with the exception of palpation) can be performed and medical records can be accessed through the computer system. Lab reports, electrocardiograms, radiographs, and other diagnostic tests may be read via the system. Telemedicine sites can also be used for distance learning opportunities. Benefits of telemedicine include retention of patients in the rural community, increasing health care access, attraction of physicians to rural communities, and cost savings.[26]

### Office practices

Office practices continue to expand their scope of services. Many office practices administer chemotherapy and provide a number of other care services for patients, including laboratory, x-ray, nutritional counseling, education, and support groups. Office practice locations include urban, suburban, and rural settings. Each location will have population-specific issues to address and meet. The infrastructure of the office practice may influence the type of treatment offered. Practices affiliated with academic centers may be able to offer patients experimental drug regimens, unlike the solo practitioner in a rural setting, who may not be able to offer the same treatment.[27] Increasingly, care of the bone marrow transplant patient is being provided in the office setting. This may include actual delivery of high-dose chemotherapy prior to the transplant as well as posttransplant care. Many patients also return to their home communities (and oncologists) to receive follow-up posttransplant care. It is critical that collaborative relationships be established between these practice settings.[14]

Pearce and Feingold[28] describe a model hospital–medical oncology alliance that is becoming more common in this era of reimbursement changes and the need for integrated oncology programs to provide seamless care. Goals of this model include improved patient care, shared financial risk, and elimination of duplication in equipment, services, and supplies. A number of issues—encompassing clinical, financial, administrative, legal and political concerns—must be confronted when pursuing this type of alliance. Greater physician loyalty, improved case management, enhanced contracting ability, and management of reimbursement risk are all potential benefits of this type of alliance for the hospital. Benefits to the physician are freedom from administrative concerns, a greater financial base, and the opportunity to provide more integrated care.

### Other ambulatory centers (screening, rehabilitation, genetic)

Individuals participating in cancer screening programs prefer convenient, nonhospital facilities with a warm, friendly atmosphere.[29] The basic focus of these programs is to provide low-cost cancer detection services. Many centers established initially for cancer screening and detection are being redesigned without rebuilding to add screening programs for other diseases, including heart disease. One obstacle to the establishment of these centers is physician support. Involvement and investment by primary care physicians in the formation of the center is ideal; otherwise, physicians typically view screening centers as competitive entities and refrain from referrals or support. Among the factors contributing to a successful screening center are convenience and visibility, adequate volume to keep the cost affordable, and an approach directed at screening programs outside the usual programs.[29]

Screening services are being taken to rural environments as well. Walker et al[30] describe the West Virginia Rural Cancer Prevention Project, designed to improve the health of rural county residents by preventing cancer or diagnosing it earlier. The focus for the interventions were breast and cervical cancer. Community-based education, on-site mammography and colposcopy, improved breast and cervical screening and education programs, improving patient compliance and tracking within the local community health center, cessation of tobacco usage, and timely compliance were all selected for implementation. Although not all project outcomes were achieved, the concept of a broad-based program with multiple interventions to increase use of prevention and early diagnosis services in rural communities can be applied to other rural settings.

A realignment of financial incentives is encouraging practitioners to prevent illness or detect it earlier, and thus there is increased support for cancer prevention and early detection programs. In this era of managed care delivery, there is greater motivation for institutions to educate individuals about how to take better care of themselves and change harmful health behaviors.[31] The NCI is funding a number of programs dealing with smoking cessation, chemoprevention, and early detection.[31] Deisher[31] cites a study done by the Cancer Institute of Health Midwest with a potential cost savings of at least $12,700–$23,000 for each early-stage breast cancer detected in a coordinated multisite, high-volume mammography screening program. A multihospital screening and early detection program for breast, colorectal, prostate, and skin cancers is in place and includes up to 11 different screening sites for each of the eight to ten programs conducted each year. More than 35,000 asymptomatic people were screened from 1991 to 1995, with 427 cancers detected. More than 74% of these cases were early-stage cancers. Expenses of the program have been offset by the activities and reimbursement generated by the screenings and direct referrals.[32]

With millions of cancer survivors in America, a great potential exists for interventions and programs to meet the needs of this group. Promoting new behaviors that enhance early detection of recurrent disease and reduce risk factors for second malignancies should be addressed as part of the rehabilitation of patients with cancer.[33] Kliban developed a Cancer Survivors Resource Center (CSRC) to serve as a link between the community and the treatment facility.[33] The CSRC does one-to-one matching of survivors with newly diagnosed individuals, offers telephone support and community resource information,

has planned and conducted a forum for cancer survivors, and is staffed by volunteers who are cancer survivors.[33]

Cancer rehabilitation services, symptom control clinics, pain management centers, and cancer psychosocial clinics are also offered in a variety of settings.[12] Satterwhite et al[34] describe the development of a primary care HIV/AIDS clinic within a large university teaching hospital to meet the growing needs of this patient population. As certain patient care needs become more complex, specialized centers designed to meet these needs will likely develop.

Genetic screening will likely be an essential component of cancer screening in the future.[3,35] A number of cancer centers already offer hereditary cancer screening programs. It is anticipated that oncology nurses will become an integral part of genetic counseling programs.[35] Peters provides a review of the development of cancer risk counseling programs.[36,37] There are no formal, published cost-benefit analyses for cancer risk counseling available and no standardized billing codes or fee schedules.[37] Ethical, legal, social, consent, privacy, and confidentiality issues must all be thoroughly examined with policies and procedures in place prior to establishing a cancer risk counseling and genetic screening program.[37]

Engelking states that we will eventually be capable of "creating individual genetic profiles that provide clues about the relative risk for developing specific cancers."[38,p.63] Genetic subgrouping (groups of healthy but high-risk individuals) will lead to the acceptance of the "addition" method of cancer prevention described as the utilization of interventions designed to inhibit cancer promotion or prevent cancer initiation. Gene transfer technology will become a preventive strategy as well as a treatment strategy.[38]

## Planning Issues

Detailed discussions about planning ambulatory care services and facility design are available in the literature.[2,12,39–41] A functional development plan should be written using information elicited from both external and internal surveys. Table 52-3 describes an external and internal analysis utilizing a multidisciplinary planning process prior to beginning clinic planning.[3] Determining present services, physician referral patterns, patient population, financial and human resources, as well as local reimbursement policies is a critical element of the plan.[12]

Making site visits to other centers and interviewing physicians and staff can be helpful. Involving the individuals who will be utilizing the space is important. Conducting patient focus groups to identify issues may also prove valuable.[41] Depending upon the relationships that exist between the services that will occupy the center, planning may be sensitive and require knowledge of any particular issues that could possibly "derail" the entire project.

Space requirements are primarily determined by the services that will be provided. If all treatment modalities

**TABLE 52-3** Assessment for Clinic Planning

### EXTERNAL ANALYSIS

1. What is the total pool of cancer patients being treated in the geographic area? Where are patients cared for now?
2. Is the number of cancer patients growing? What is the case mix of the growing or underserved population?
3. Are patients satisfied with their present care?
4. What programs do competitors have in place? What expansion plans do they have?
5. What changes in oncology care are predicted?
6. Is the shift to ambulatory care complete in this region or will it continue? How far, how soon?
7. What impact will health care reform have on oncology care?
8. Of the core benefits, which are underprovided in this region? Which are well provided by a competitor?
9. What alliances can be made in oncology that will benefit other major service lines?

### INTERNAL ANALYSIS

1. What programs, clinics, and departments presently exist? What services do they provide?
2. What populations are served? Are volume trends increasing or decreasing?
3. What are the strengths and weaknesses of the present programs?
4. What is the financial performance of individual programs? Are the reimbursement trends positive or negative? Is the case mix changing?
5. Are the physician, nursing, and technical staff experts in their field? Are they well respected in the community?
6. Do patients report satisfaction? What trends exist in quality management?
7. Is the physical facility adequate? What could improve the facility?
8. What is the present market share? Is that trend positive or negative?
9. What services are patients and staff requesting?
10. What internal trends will shape future referrals (e.g., physicians leaving or joining the staff, new capitation contracts)?
11. How can we prepare for health care reform changes?

Reprinted from *Seminars in Oncology Nursing* with permission from Lamkin L: Outpatient oncology settings: A variety of services. *Semin Oncol Nurs* 10:229–236, 1994.

will be administered, space is provided for each area, as well as room for education of the public, patients, and health professionals. Space for the oncologists' office practices is often contained within the facility and leased to physicians.[12] If renovation of existing space is needed, great attention must be given to the phasing plan, temporary staff relocation, and patient inconvenience.

Provisions are made in all areas to ensure privacy of the patient while undergoing treatment. Careful consideration is given to the nursing station, support space, and waiting areas. Overall, the goal is to provide a friendly, warm atmosphere. Easy access to parking is essential. Equipment decisions will be based upon the services provided.

Marketing the cancer product line, center, or services is critical to patient referral patterns. The marketing approach should reflect the mission of the program.[2] A variety of methods are used to market cancer services, including media promotion, targeted mailings to specific population groups, billboards, newspaper inserts, speakers' bureaus, traveling vans, health fairs, screening programs, direct contact with referring physicians, and special sponsored events.

## THE ROLE OF THE NURSE IN AMBULATORY CARE

### Overview

The nurse's role in ambulatory care is complex and varied. Inherent in the role is provision of direct nursing care, education, counseling, health maintenance, preventive care, coordination of services, and continuity of care.[12] Three challenges commonly encountered by ambulatory oncology nurses are (1) the use of the telephone in successful delivery of patient care, (2) the time frame for conducting assessments and meeting patient needs, and (3) assisting with patient transition from one setting to another.[42]

#### Standards of care

The American Academy of Ambulatory Care Nursing (AAACN) is a professional organization whose members believe that ambulatory care nursing is essential for high-quality, cost-effective patient care. Shaping professional practice and environments, building collaborative relationships, and providing innovative thinking and vision are identified as goals of the organization.[43] Table 52-4 provides a summary of the nine standards developed by the AAACN. These standards can be adopted in most ambulatory care settings. The American Nurses' Association and the Oncology Nursing Society (ANA/ONS) Statement on the Scope and Standards of Oncology Nursing Practice were developed for the generalist in oncology nursing and have applicability to the ambulatory care nurse.[44] ONS has also developed Standards of Advanced Practice in Oncology Nursing.[45] Given the dynamic nature of the role of the advanced practice nurse (APN) in ambulatory settings, these standards provide a benchmark and framework for role delineation. The Joint Commission on Accreditation of Healthcare Organizations (JCAHO) requires that ambulatory care settings meet the same standards of quality as the inpatient setting.[46] In addition, the JCAHO publishes an accreditation manual for ambulatory health care that specifies standards specific to these settings.[47] Many oncology practices are using accreditation as a competitive strategy to win managed care contracts.[48] The Association of Community Cancer

**TABLE 52-4**  American Academy of Ambulatory Care Nursing: Administration and Practice Standards

| | |
|---|---|
| Standard I: Structure and Organization of Ambulatory Care Nursing | Ambulatory care nursing is based on a philosophy committed to the delivery of efficient, cost-effective, and quality nursing care. |
| Standard II: Staffing | Sufficient numbers of qualified nursing staff are available to meet patients' nursing care needs. |
| Standard III: Competency | Nursing staff demonstrate knowledge and skills necessary to complete their assigned responsibilities. |
| Standards IV: Ambulatory Nursing Practice | Registered nurses use the nursing process as a framework to determine the allocation and delivery of nursing care in the ambulatory setting. |
| Standard V: Continuity of Care | Ambulatory care nurses facilitate continuity of care through the nursing process, interdisciplinary collaboration, and coordination of all appropriate health care services, including available community resources. |
| Standard VI: Ethics and Patient Rights | Ambulatory care nurses recognize the dignity and worth of individuals, respect cultural, spiritual, and psychosocial differences, and apply philosophical and ethical concepts that promote equality and continuity of care. |
| Standard VII: Environment | Ambulatory care nurses facilitate the creation and maintenance of a hazard-free, safe, comfortable, and therapeutic environment for patients, visitors, and staff. |
| Standard VIII: Research | Ambulatory care nurses conduct and participate in clinical and health care systems research. Research findings are disseminated and used to improve patient care and organizational effectiveness. |
| Standard IX: Quality Management | The quality and appropriateness of ambulatory care nursing services are continuously assessed, evaluated, and improved. Ambulatory care nursing's quality management process is coordinated and integrated with that of the organization. Ambulatory care nursing leaders set expectations, provide resources and training, foster communication and coordination, and participate in improvement activities. |

Adapted from the *1996 Edition of Ambulatory Care Nursing Administration and Practice Standards.* Permission granted from the American Academy of Ambulatory Care Nursing, East Holly Avenue, Box 56, Pittman, NJ 08071-0056; phone 800.AMB.NURS; FAX 609.589.7463; aaacn@mail.ajj.com; http://www.inurse.com/~AAACN.

Centers also has standards that specifically detail ambulatory oncology services.[49]

### Responsibilities of the nurse

There are multiple roles and responsibilities for nurses in ambulatory care settings, including that of staff nurse, nurse manager (head nurse), clinical nurse specialist, nurse practitioner, nurse data manager or research nurse, and cancer program director.[50] The staff nurse is the professional who consistently interacts with the patient and family at every visit. Staff nurses have an integral role in assessing patients and developing a plan of care. Clinical nurse specialists and nurse practitioners are increasingly being utilized in ambulatory settings. These individuals are likely to be primary caregivers for groups of patients and function in collaborative relationships providing patient assessment, care planning, patient and family education and counseling, symptom management, coordination of services, and involvement in the community. Oncology nurses have also expanded their roles into

prevention/detection, symptom management, and survivorship activities. Nurses with strong administrative values and skills may find positions in the corporate world. Partnerships with physicians and nurse-directed multispecialty clinics are also on the horizon.

Several research studies have been conducted to more clearly delineate the responsibilities of nurses in ambulatory settings.[51,52] Tighe et al[52] studied 68 nurses representing both oncology and nononcology settings in ambulatory care to determine the frequency with which they performed certain tasks and activities. Oncology nurses reported most frequent involvement in (1) health care maintenance activities, followed by (2) counseling and (3) communication. There was also a statistically significant finding of greater involvement in communication and therapeutic care by the oncology nurses.[52]

Hastings and Muir-Nash[53] surveyed 33 ambulatory nursing administrators about the roles and responsibilities of nurses in ambulatory care settings. This study involved a revision of Verran's[51] original taxonomy that resulted in nine responsibility areas and 61 activities (in contrast to the seven areas and 47 activities of Verran's original taxonomy). All nine areas of responsibility were confirmed as components of nursing practice in ambulatory care by over 50% of the sample, with the exception of three activities—"forms preparation," "transporting," and "maintenance."

A survey of 606 ambulatory nurses by Hackbarth et al[54] provides a wealth of information about current and future ambulatory nursing practice. The purpose of the study was to describe the scope and dimensions of current ambulatory nursing practice; to project future ambulatory nursing roles; and to identify the dimensions and activities of the future role that should be retained by the professional nurse or delegated to others. University hospital outpatient nurses (n = 190), community hospital outpatient nurses (n = 197), physician group practice nurses (n = 127) and health maintenance organization (HMO) nurses (n = 92) were the respondents in the study. Table 52-5 describes dimensions of the current staff nurse role as identified by the study participants. Staff nurses in this study reported more frequently performing the lower-level dimensions such as enabling operations and technical procedures and less frequently performing dimensions requiring critical thinking and disciplinary knowledge. The study also identified significant factors that attract and retain nurses in ambulatory care: client and family contact, hours and schedules, the challenging nature of the job, seeing the outcomes of care, and autonomy. A lack of time, lack of support staff, excessive paperwork, and administrative blocks to clinical practice were identified as barriers.

These authors found significant differences in the model of care between settings (Figure 52-1).[55] Nurses with bachelor's and master's degrees were more common in university hospital outpatient departments. Nurses with the most education were more likely to belong to a professional nursing organization, chose a specialty area of practice such as oncology, and chose to practice in a primary or "other" model of nursing care. Oncology nurses in the study were more highly educated, consistently above the mean for performance of the teaching dimension, and showed a high frequency of the care coordination,

**TABLE 52-5**  Dimensions of the Current Staff Nurse Role in Ambulatory Care

| EIGHT CORE DIMENSIONS OF THE CURRENT CLINICAL PRACTICE ROLE | | |
|---|---|---|
| I. **Enabling Operation**<br>Maintain safe work environment<br>Maintain traffic box<br>Search for space/equipment<br>Set up room<br>Locate records<br>Order supplies<br>Transport clients<br>Provide emotional support<br>Take vital signs | II. **Technical Procedures**<br>Assist with procedures<br>Prepare client for procedures<br>Chaperone during procedures<br>Inform client about treatment<br>Witness signing consent forms<br>Administer oral/IM medications<br>Collect specimens | III. **Nursing Process**<br>Develop nursing care plan<br>Use nursing diagnosis<br>Complete client history<br>Assess client learning needs<br>Conduct exit interview<br>Evaluate client care outcomes<br>Chart each client encounter |
| IV. **Telephone Communications**<br>Telephone triage<br>Call pharmacy with prescription<br>Call client with test results | V. **Advocacy**<br>Make clients aware of rights<br>Promote positive public relations<br>Act as a client advocate<br>Triage client to appropriate provider | VI. **Teaching**<br>Instruct client on medical/nursing regimen<br>Instruct client on home and self-care |
| VII. **Care Coordination**<br>Long-term supportive relationship<br>Act as a resource person<br>Coordinate client care<br>Assess needs and initiate referrals<br>Find resources in the community<br>Instruct on health promotion | VIII. **Expert Practice within Setting**<br>Expertise in advanced nursing practice<br>Function as advanced nurse resource<br>Serve as preceptor for students<br>Design and present in-service education | |
| THREE CORE DIMENSIONS OF THE CURRENT QUALITY IMPROVEMENT/RESEARCH ROLE | | |
| I. **Quality Improvement**<br>Implement professional standards<br>Participate in preparation of QI plan<br>Collect and analyze QI data<br>Use QI plan in practice<br>Participate in interdisciplinary QI teams<br>Develop expected client outcomes | II. **Research**<br>Participate in research of others<br>Follow guidelines to protect human subjects | III. **Continuing Education**<br>Participate in on-site continuing education<br>Participate in off-site continuing education |

Adapted with permission from *Nursing Economics* and with permission from Janetti Publications, Inc. Hackbarth DP, Haas SA, Kavanagh JA, et al: Dimensions of the staff nurse role in ambulatory care: Part I. Methodology and analysis of data on current staff nurse practice. *Nurs Econ* 13:89–98, 1995.

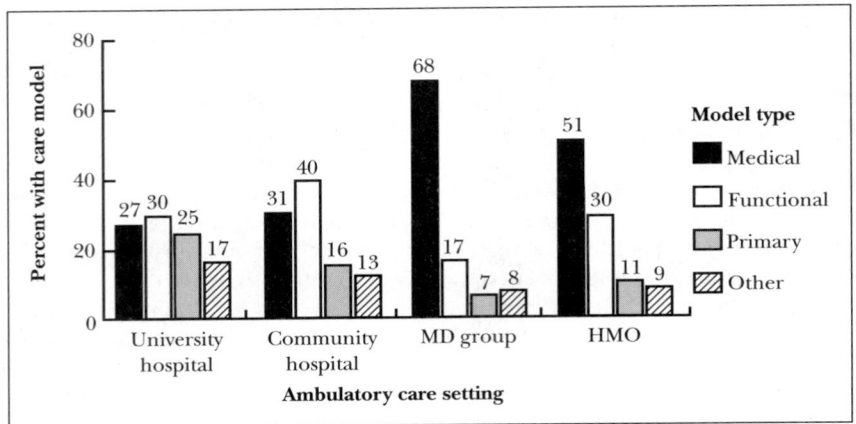

*Medical* = assist physician as needed; carry out nursing aspects of medical plan;
*Functional* = provide nursing care as needed during client visits to a random group
of clients; *Primary* = provide nursing care to the same clients within a specified
group during each ambulatory visit; *Other* = includes case management, community
nursing and open-ended.

**FIGURE 52-1** Model of nursing care by setting. Reprinted with permission from
Janetti Publications, Inc. Haas SA, Hackbarth DP, Kavanagh JA, et al: Dimensions
of the staff nurse role in ambulatory care: Part II. Comparison of role dimensions
in four ambulatory settings. *Nurs Econ* 13:152–165, 1995.

expert practice, and research dimensions regardless of
setting and model of care.

Shaw[56] describes a variety of roles for nurses in a comprehensive breast center. Although still controversial,
advanced practice nurses (APNs) (specifically nurse-practitioners) can provide cost-efficient, primary breast health
care that is high in clinical quality and consumer satisfaction. Lamkin[3] also suggests that the development of
integrated delivery systems will result in a greater appreciation for the APN. It is anticipated that APNs will be
involved in specialty practices as well as with primary
practice physicians. Research should be done to measure
outcomes, especially those related to cost, patient satisfaction, and replacement of direct medical intervention by
the APN.[3]

The role of the oncology nurse in the office practice
has expanded greatly with the shift of health care to the
ambulatory setting; it now encompasses a variety of roles,
including clinical, administrative/business, academic,
and consultative.[27] Highly developed assessment and organizational skills are essential to handle the large patient
population, in which patient care is intermittent and
brief. These assessments must be ongoing and include
treatment response, nutrition, pain, psychosocial, home
care, and resource assessments.

The office oncology nurse frequently is the liaison
between providers of each phase of the patient's care.
Many individuals receive continuous long-term treatment
while remaining in their community. These individuals
may benefit from a home care referral or may be able,
with thorough education, to manage their own care.[27]
Communication among all concerned is critical and facilitates the exchange of information. Implementation of a
"nurse exchange" program where nurses from hospital,
ambulatory, and home care settings trade places for a
period may lead to increased cooperation and coordination across the continuum of care.[27]

The office nurse also plays a key role in prevention
and detection activities and long-term follow-up of cancer
survivors. Cancer survivors have many concerns, and the
office nurse is in the unique position of addressing how
the survivor is adapting to life after treatment. Psychosocial assessments are particularly critical. The nurse's role
is that of an educator, supporter, counselor, coordinator,
and referral source.[27]

The office nurse is assuming a role in the management
of clinical trials in the office setting. These responsibilities
may include assisting the physician with obtaining informed consent, assessing patient responses to the research treatments, completing protocol forms, and
working with other nurse data managers to ensure appropriate care.[27]

Continuity of care and quality improvement activities
are also growing concerns in the office practice setting.
The development of communication channels between
the office practice and the hospital oncology unit is essential to ensure continuity of patient care. Behrend[27] suggests that the office oncology nurse is in a key position
to organize a team effort that assures quality care across
the continuum from office to hospital to home.

Nurse practitioners and oncology clinical nurse specialists are increasingly assuming roles in the radiation
oncology setting.[57] Comprehensive care, symptom management, management of patients receiving treatment,
follow-up care, community education, professional development, standards and policy development and research

activity coordination can all be done by these individuals.[57] The reader will find an extensive discussion of radiation therapy, including the role of the nurse and management of care, in chapter 13.

Given this expansion of roles in the ambulatory setting, oncology nurses must be an integral part of the team designing innovative care plans that provide not only cost-effective care delivery but also the best opportunity for cure. Clinical pathways have great potential for improving quality, eliminating waste, and optimizing resource utilization.[58] The pathways can also be used as a template for contracting services in managed care programs.

## Nursing Process

Nursing care delivered in the ambulatory setting follows the constructs of the nursing process and includes patient assessment, patient and caregiver teaching, telephone management, and documentation. Increasingly, the nurse in the ambulatory setting is regarded as the clinical expert and functions quite independently.

### Admission and assessment

The patient's first visit to the ambulatory setting provides an opportunity to establish what may be a long-term relationship. Every attempt is made to help the patient and accompanying significant other feel welcome and comfortable. The first visit can be utilized to give important logistical details about parking facilities, how to find the department, the routine at the time of the visit, and how long to plan to be there. Giving this information can demonstrate concern and alleviate some of the fear and anxiety associated with the experience since many patients are newly diagnosed.[12]

Knowing as much as possible about the patient prior to the first visit is ideal. Obtaining reports and old charts is helpful. Most ambulatory settings require that the patient complete the routine admission procedure, at least on the first visit. Thereafter, patients may be "part of the system," and additional, time-consuming stops in the admitting area are not necessary. For some patients, entering a door clearly marked "Cancer Center" (or some equivalent) is very difficult; thus, immediately putting the patient at ease is critical. Welcoming the patient and introducing the team and staff members is a common courtesy too often overlooked in the busy pace of the ambulatory setting. Simple things like offering refreshments or something to read while waiting are much appreciated. With increasing competition for managed care contracts and patient choice between insurance plans still likely, offering something to the patient that another setting does not offer may be critical.

Many settings provide patient education material and support groups.[59] A "questions and concerns form" may also be helpful for patients to use to record any of their concerns between appointments.[60] The use of volunteers in ambulatory settings can also facilitate comfort and reduce anxiety while patients are waiting. Touch-screen computer systems in waiting rooms that allow access to cancer educational material may also be beneficial.

Many excellent assessment forms exist, and most ambulatory settings have developed one specific to their setting. These forms should be brief but inclusive of pertinent physical, social, and psychological data and contain an indication of where detailed information can be found in the medical record.[12] Lin and Rigby[61] described a patient assessment tool tested with 232 patients in an ambulatory cancer referral center. They noted a high level of patient acceptance with the tool. Patients did not feel uncomfortable with the questions and felt that the form actually helped them get their thoughts in order and remind them of concerns they wanted to bring up. This approach can maximize the nurse's time and efficiency. Skinn and Stacey[62] also developed a self-reporting health history that is partially completed by patients and then utilized by the nurses to complete the interview. They too found a high level of patient acceptance with the tool and eventually developed an outpatient oncology record that provides documentation of all patient assessment findings and subsequent care.

Once the assessment has been completed, a discussion with the patient about the financial implications of the treatment plan is initiated and appropriate referrals are made to the oncology social worker or patient financial services representative. An explanation of future visits for ongoing assessments and to receive treatment is reviewed with the patient and family. There should be clear communication that the patient will occasionally be seen only by the nurse but that the patient's condition will be reviewed with the physician.

### Planning and evaluation

Planning and evaluation are important components of the nursing process and include activities such as development of the nursing care plan, use of nursing diagnoses, and evaluation of patient outcomes. These activities are still less developed and utilized in the ambulatory setting than in the inpatient setting.[55] More highly educated nurses tend to routinely initiate planning and evaluation component of care. Ambulatory care managers may want to seek a mix of staff with some baccalaureate-prepared nurses and implement models of care that foster more professional practice and autonomy.[55] This high-level dimension of nursing practice is an activity that should not be delegated and must remain an integral role of nurses in the ambulatory setting.[63]

### Documentation

Documentation is a major challenge facing nurses in ambulatory settings. Greater complexity of care and higher patient-nurse ratios demand accurate, concise, clear, and objective documentation. Documentation includes the nursing process, fulfills legal requirements, describes the nursing care delivered, and reflects the quality of nursing care. Documentation has become a major tool to promote continuity of care among multiple providers and settings. Nurses in the ambulatory setting may dictate (rather than write) progress notes and use an integrated chart that moves with the patient to increase their communication and impact on care both internally and externally.[27] Charting by exception, with the premise that only any unexpected response to the plan of care is documented, is a method of documentation that may be used effectively in the ambulatory care setting.[64] Multidisciplinary chart documentation is also becoming more common.

Flow sheets are used to fulfill a number of documentation needs. Oncology settings use flow sheets to record side effects, laboratory data, treatment administration information, and patient teaching. A number of flow sheets have been developed and reported in the literature.[27,64–67]

***Self-report tools*** Another approach to documentation is patient self-report.[64] Patients are usually asked to complete the tool at home and bring it on the day of treatment. The nurse then reviews the self-assessment, identifies concerns, and discusses interventions. Patients feel that completing the form gives them something constructive to do and allows them to share concerns in their own words. Nurses using self-report forms found that their documentation was less time-consuming and that objective assessments improved.

Youngblood et al[68] compared the number of symptoms identified by a patient report instrument with those documented in the patient's medical record. The relationship between the number of self-reported symptoms and quality of life was also examined in this study. Results showed that patients more comprehensively identified their symptoms as compared with assessments by others that were documented in the medical record. Commonly reported side effects included feeling sluggish, difficulty sleeping, dry mouth, skin and taste changes, loss of appetite, depression, hair loss, and nausea.

***Computerized patient record*** Use of point-of-care computer terminals has the potential for simplifying documentation issues.[65] These systems enable the nurse to immediately enter data into the computer, thus decreasing documentation time and improving accuracy. Using the computer in the ambulatory setting may decrease paper flow problems; allow for greater efficiency in documentation and more timely retrieval of patient information; and decrease frustration over inaccessible charts. Voice-activated systems are increasingly utilized in the medical setting. Specific portions of the medical record are prompted, and information is dictated to fill the field. Spoken commands can be formatted to include more lengthy descriptions. Forms can also be programmed to prompt the user if information is omitted.[65] Implementation of a computer-based patient record system is a challenging opportunity for information systems and nursing departments to collaborate.[69] The computerized patient record has the potential to decrease fragmentation, improve the quality and continuity of care and be integral to successful managed care.[70]

A computerized version of the ONS radiation therapy care record called *ONSET* is available from IMPAC Oncology Management Systems (415-254-4700). This software is a computerized documentation tool incorporating assessments, medications, teaching, planning, intervention, and outcomes.

At present, nurses are not widely using electronic information sources such as the Internet and bulletin boards, but this is another technology that holds potential for use in the ambulatory setting.[71,72] Barriers to use include not having access to a linked-up computer, intimidation by the technology, and concerns about security. Computers and networks will become essential conduits.[72] Patients and families are also increasingly "surfing the Net" to find cancer-related information. Health providers need to become familiar with these resources to assist patients in finding reliable information.[73]

For assessing quality of care, complying with regulations, communicating with other health care providers, and a multitude of other reasons, documentation will remain a significant component of care provided to the patient in the ambulatory setting. The expanding use of computers in this setting may simplify and expedite the process during the next decade.

## Technical Procedures

Nurses in the ambulatory setting frequently assist with technical procedures. This can involve preparing the patient to have the procedure through education as well as the physical preparation of the patient, being present and offering support during the procedure, and actually performing the procedure. Among the many types of care settings, community hospital outpatient nurses had the highest frequency of performance of technical procedures.[55] Surgical, ob/gyn, and family practices were the most common settings in which the ambulatory nursing staff were performing technical procedures. These may be areas in which assistive workers could be utilized, allowing the nursing staff to perform higher-level dimensions of nursing care.[55]

Nurses in ambulatory oncology settings are more likely to be performing high-tech procedures such as complex chemotherapy/biotherapy administration, blood and blood product administration, monitoring patients before and after procedures such as bone marrow biopsy and aspiration, lumbar punctures, stereotactic radiosurgery, and high-dose brachytherapy. These high-tech procedures are more risky and require highly educated nursing staff. Oncology certified nurses are in demand to assure appropriate knowledge and practice. Nurses functioning in these settings should check state and federal regulations to determine the scope of practice that is allowed. Maintenance of competencies is critical to avoid liability issues. It is not appropriate to delegate these activities to assistive personnel. This area is clearly one in which the APN has a role. The ability of the nurse to function independently in this setting is essential.

## Teaching and Advocacy

Patient education is a key component of the nurse's role in the ambulatory setting. Challenges involve determining the appropriate time to teach and having specific materials available. This was confirmed in a study done by Griffiths and Leek,[74] who assessed educational needs of patients with cancer and evaluated available resources. All of those responding expressed a strong need for educational materials and felt that written information was more effective than other types of information, such as that gathered from seminars, media, etc., with one-on-one conversations between the nurse and patient reported as the most effective source of information. Availability of materials was the most frequently mentioned problem in addressing patient needs. Each patient and family requires an individualized approach. In an extremely busy ambulatory setting, this may be difficult to accomplish.

Nurses in the ambulatory setting are fortunate that there is printed material available related to cancer, cancer treatment, and management of side effects. Educational materials can be obtained from the American Cancer Society, the National Cancer Institute, the Leukemia Society, pharmaceutical companies, and many other related organizations. In addition, some hospitals and health care organizations have developed their own materials, many of which are available for purchase. This written material can be used to reinforce or supplement patient education efforts. A variety of audiovisual materials are also available for purchase, but, unfortunately, many videotapes or slide programs are too expensive for many ambulatory departments to purchase.

It is important to assess the patient's desired method of learning rather than use the same approach for all patients. Some patients prefer to see a demonstration, while others prefer a one-to-one teaching approach. Still others may benefit from a videotape that can be taken home, watched at leisure, and reviewed many times. Siegel and Patyk[75] reported on the use of a Cancer Information Channel to provide programming of special interest to cancer patients and their families. Even though this approach was used with inpatients, it could have some applicability in the ambulatory setting as patients are waiting to be seen or undergoing lengthy treatments. Facilitation of patient-nurse-family discussions and open communication can be enhanced with this methodology.

Nurses should be involved with the planning, development, and testing of educational materials. It is important to pay special attention to the reading level of materials distributed to patients or available in display areas. Formulas have been developed that can be used to calculate reading levels.[76] A discrepancy exists between the reading level of the average adult and the reading level of many printed materials.[76-79] Meade et al[77] evaluated 51 booklets produced by the American Cancer Society. Using the SMOG formula, the reading level of the booklets ranged from grade 5.8 to 15.6 (SD = 2.2), with a mean reading level of grade 11.9. The median reading level of most Americans is closer to grades eight to ten. Only 6 of the 51 publications sampled were written at a grade nine or lower reading level. A lack of non-English publications was also noted.

Michielutte et al[78] did a similar analysis of the readability level of educational literature on cancer prevention and early detection. Reading level (SMOG) scores were computed for 159 brochures and pamphlets obtained from the American Cancer Society, the NCI, private companies, public nonprofit agencies, and state health departments. The average reading level found was between the 10th and 11th grade. Since low-income, low-education subgroups are at high risk for cancer, much of the available literature may be of limited value in providing information.[78]

Cooley et al[79] conducted a study with outpatients who had cancer and found that the majority of pamphlets were written at higher reading levels than those of the participants. Patients in this study also indicated that receiving multiple types of educational materials would be helpful to them. Nurses must be the leaders in developing creative, innovative, and comprehensive programs that are then studied to evaluate effectiveness on patient comprehension, self-care behaviors, and satisfaction.

Suggestions for improving readability include determining the medical terms that need definition and substituting simpler terms whenever possible. Illustrations may improve understanding of the material.[78] More intensive one-on-one discussions or use of picture cards, flip charts, and videos rather than the written material may help in the education process.[77]

It is also important to assess the patient's reading level using informal cues. A lack of interest in the material, lack of reading speed, expressions of frustration, inability to answer questions about the material, or the desire to let another person read the text may all be cues to the patient's inability to read at the needed level.[77]

Houts et al[80] conducted a literature review of information needed by family members of cancer patients and suggested strategies for meeting their needs (Table 52-6). The movement of patient care to the ambulatory setting has resulted in the family playing an increasingly important role in the patient's care. Family members often find themselves in shock and unfamiliar with who to ask and what to ask.[80] Unfortunately, many family members' needs for information are not being met. Family members can be confused by the complexities of today's health care system. Limited contact with health care professionals, uncertainty about when to contact physicians, what questions to ask and how to ask them, and fear that they will not understand the answer compounds problems of obtaining information.[80]

Nurses are an important source of information for family members. Frequently, family members receive filtered information, either from the patient or from an-

**TABLE 52-6** Information Needs of Families of Cancer Patients

| |
|---|
| Understandable medical information about cancer |
| Specific information about:<br>  Patient's current medical status<br>  Ongoing and future treatment plans<br>  Expected side effects<br>  Individual results |
| Best way to meet patient's physical and emotional needs |
| Emotional reactions to anticipate during various stages of treatment |
| Physical caregiving skills |
| Services available to help with coping |

Adapted with permission from *Journal of Cancer Education* 6:255–261. Houts PS, Rusenas I, Simmonds MA, et al: Information needs of families of cancer patients: A literature review and recommendations, 1991, Pergamon Press.

other health care professional. Strategies for meeting information needs of families are described in Table 52-7.

Gyauch described an educational program for family caregivers that was created to benefit cancer patients being sent home earlier and sicker. This program addressed physical care concerns, provided access to information about supportive community organizations and agencies, and identified and taught individuals about psychosocial needs of caregivers and cancer patients. Bilingual educators and outreach workers are also involved in delivering and promoting the program.

Weaver[82] reported an innovative approach with the development of computerized patient education material. The "how to" teaching sheets include general information, descriptions of procedures, the patient's/caregiver's responsibilities, possible problems, what to do, and who to contact for questions or information. The reading level of the computer-generated teaching sheets is rated at an eighth-grade level.

**TABLE 52-7** Strategies for Meeting Families' Information Needs

| |
|---|
| Use of generic information sources including booklets, tapes, videos, computer programs, and group education programs |
| Individualized communication of information |
| Demonstration of skills needed to care for the patient at home |
| Greater use of the nurse to convey information about the patient's health status |
| Greater assertiveness by family members |
| Willingness of health care professionals to be available and provide needed information |
| Referral to appropriate community organizations |

Adapted with permission from *Journal of Cancer Education* 6:255–261. Houts PS, Rusenas I, Simmonds MA, et al: Information needs of families of cancer patients: A literature review and recommendations, 1991, Pergamon Press.

Patient teaching in the ambulatory setting has changed, with increased emphasis on prevention and management of problems. Factors affecting patient and caregiver education include patient acuity; psychosocial issues and resources (including family support and financial resources); and the health care provider issues of time, money, and environment.[83]

The level of illness of patients is often a barrier to learning. Education can be accomplished only after the patient has achieved symptom relief. Psychosocial factors may either help or hinder the patient's ability to learn about the disease, treatment, and self-care. With more complicated therapies, such as continuous infusions and total parenteral nutrition, is the need for more in-depth patient education. One must determine the patient's financial and personal resources prior to beginning complex therapies.[83] The appropriate location for teaching is sometimes constrained due to space limitations, but any area that provides privacy, adequate seating and lighting, and patient comfort can be utilized. Preferably, the ambulatory setting would have designated space to be utilized for this purpose.[83]

Promoting effective patient education includes active involvement by the nurse in planning and presenting material and evaluating learning. A trusting relationship is built on effective communication skills, such as introducing oneself, a firm handshake, good eye contact, and a friendly demeanor.[83]

Hinds et al[84] reported a study of 36 patients undergoing radiation therapy. Patients were asked about the importance of receiving information about their cancer and cancer treatment, why the information was important, in what format they preferred to receive information, and whether there were any disadvantages to receiving information. The study results showed that patients want information for purposes of participation, preparation, and anxiety reduction. Patients felt that information offered a sense of control over the situation. Almost 75% of the sample stated there was no disadvantage to receiving information. Written communication in conjunction with verbal one-on-one communications (with their physician) was mentioned as the preferred method of receiving information. The study also suggested that there is a small group of individuals that does not want any information. This must be kept in mind as ambulatory care nurses assess patient and family educational needs.

Poroch[85] compared two groups of 25 patients undergoing radiation therapy for the first time. The experimental group received two structured teaching interventions that incorporated sensory and procedural information prior to the patient's beginning treatment. This group was significantly less anxious and more satisfied than the control group who received the standard information. Patients in the study wanted to be given information at the beginning of treatment and without having to ask questions. They also wanted to be able to ask the physician and nurse questions when needed.

Informational audiotapes are a cost-effective strategy for teaching self-care practices to patients undergoing radiation therapy. Hagopian[86] randomized 75 adult patients receiving radiation therapy to receive either standard care or standard care with the addition of the informational audiotapes. Patients in the experimental group were more knowledgeable about their treatment and practiced more self-care behaviors than the control-group subjects. The audiotapes covered information about radiation therapy, skin care, nutrition, fatigue, mouth care, diarrhea, and other topics and suggested self-care to deal with these side effects. The tapes were inexpensive to produce and could be utilized by the patient and family when convenient.

Newsletters can be valuable for patient education. Hagopian's[87] study of subjects reading a weekly radiation therapy newsletter showed that these individuals scored significantly higher on the knowledge test, but no significant differences were seen in the helpfulness or number of self-care behaviors or the severity of side effects. Further study is suggested to determine the benefits to be derived from a newsletter.

Group teaching is another approach utilized in a variety of settings. One ambulatory treatment center holds a two-hour class on chemotherapy prior to the patient's starting treatment.[12] Many other settings offer structured, ongoing weekly or monthly educational sessions for patients. Group classes provide opportunities for patients to interact with each other and share common experiences. It is also a time-efficient approach for the health professional. However, the opportunity for one-to-one consultation should always be available to supplement group classes.[12]

The ONS standards provide a guideline for patient and family education as well as for public education.[88] Self-care guides can assist both patient and caregiver education. These self-care guides are handy references that provide basic information about how to manage the side effects of treatment and can serve as a source of security and control to families and patients when unexpected questions or anticipated side effects eventually occur.[89] Figure 52-2 is an example of a self-care guide.

Still another approach is the development of a "learning center" or laboratory environment for learning, practicing, and demonstrating skills necessary for self-care.[89,90] A variety of learning or skill units can be offered, including administration of intravenous (IV) or intramuscular (IM) medications, caring for ostomies and wounds, providing home IV nutrition, placing feeding tubes and administering feedings, and caring for venous access devices. Goldstein[90] reports that attendance at a learning center results in patients and families achieving more learning outcomes as well as fewer hospital readmissions for reinsertion or treatment of complications.

Numerous teaching booklets have been published in the literature and can be duplicated, adapted, and used as models for ambulatory care nurses in their own settings.[91-94] Straw and Conrad[95] have compiled a listing of patient education resources related to biotherapy and the immune system.

It is anticipated that future changes in patient education will occur as research findings and new technologies direct patient teaching and patient learning needs change. The large number of cancer survivors, the aging population, changing reimbursement, socioeconomic demographics, and literacy will also affect ways of providing information.[74]

## Telephone Communications and Management

Triaging phone calls appropriately and efficiently is a major and time-consuming role of the nurse in the ambulatory setting.[96] Telephone activities include assessing patients' responses to the treatment given, providing information about prevention of side effects and symptoms, and evaluating patient outcomes. Phone calls from patients may relate to symptom complaints, clarification of information, prescription refills, crisis management, reporting and interpreting lab tests, referrals to community resources, assistance with reimbursement, and counseling. Calls can also come from family members, other health care professionals, referral sources, or business-related persons.[27]

Patient care–oriented calls can have multiple purposes: communication of changes in the care plan, reassurance of the patient and family about side effects, instructions to lessen the severity of the side effects, and assessment of supportive services. Phone calls may also be made by the nurse for follow-up purposes and provide an opportunity to reinforce symptom management and preventive actions. Confidentiality must be considered when dealing with patients' diagnoses, test results, and treatment decisions. Keeping a log of tests ordered is a way of tracking patients and written reports.[96] Documentation of phone calls and interventions is done as a standard of care. Using a duplicate form allows for appropriate distribution of the information to the chart, physician, etc.[27] Figures 52-3 and 52-4 are examples of two forms that can be used for this purpose. It is also critically important to document prescription refills.[96] Nurses also make calls to obtain insurance company approvals for the ongoing delivery of care and review of patient outcomes.

Many nursing hours are consumed by the time spent on each telephone call, the time necessary to obtain and review the chart and then write a note, and the time to locate and discuss a problem with the consultant (physician, nurse, etc.). Establishing specific times for nurses to make and receive routine phone calls may be helpful. Standard protocols for frequently occurring problems may facilitate nursing care delivery by telephone. Educational programs on the use of the telephone for care delivery may also be useful for the ambulatory nurse new to the setting.

Another use of the telephone in ambulatory oncology care is the "hot line," a toll-free 800 number that patients can call to make appointments or ask questions about their treatment or side effects. The hot line also lends itself to calls from the general public about screening or

## SELF-CARE GUIDE: CONSTIPATION

Patient Name: _____

*Symptom and description*   Constipation means being unable to move your bowels, having to push harder to move your bowels, or moving them less often that usual. Bowel movements will be small, dry, and hard. Constipation happens when you get less exercise, or when you eat and drink less than usual. Some medicines cause constipation. Constipation can cause pain and discomfort. Keeping your bowel routine regular and your bowel movements easy to pass is important. Your bowels should move every day with little or no strain.

You are at risk for constipation if you have a

- Decrease in the amount you eat and drink each day

- Decrease in your activity or exercise

- Medication that causes constipation

- Cancer that causes pressure on your bowel or changes in the way your bowel works

*Learning Needs*   You need to know how to prevent constipation and, if constipation happens, to manage it before it gets severe. You are at risk for constipation because of:

1. _____

2. _____

3. _____

4. _____

You should call _____ if you have not moved your bowels in _____.

Write down when you move your bowels and if there are changes in your normal bowel movements. Have the notes with you when you call or come for care. Try to prevent constipation by following the directions given next.

*Prevention*   You can help prevent constipation if you:

- Drink at least _____ glasses of fluid each day.

- Eat foods that are high in dietary fiber, especially _____
  _____

- Exercise daily. If you are unable to increase your exercise, tighten and relax the muscles in your abdomen and move your legs often while sitting or in bed.

- Take medications as instructed to prevent constipation.

- Try to move your bowels at your usual times. Many people find that after breakfast is a good time to try to have a bowel movement.

- Avoid using the bedpan if possible. A natural position on the toilet or on a commode is best.

- Tell your doctor or nurse about things that have worked for you in the past to prevent constipation.

*Management*   You can treat mild constipation by following the steps just listed in prevention. When your bowels have not moved for _____ or if you are at risk for severe constipation, you will need to use medications to help your bowels move regularly.

1. *Using medications to prevent constipation:* Preventing and managing constipation are easy when you work together with your health care provider. You may need to increase or decrease doses of medicine to achieve easy and regular bowel movements. Please follow these directions carefully, and feel free to call to ask questions or to let us know if your bowels are not regular.

2. *Goal:* To have a bowel movement every _____ day(s)

- Take _____ at bedtime.

**FIGURE 52-2**   Self-Care Guide: Constipation. Reprinted with permission from Jones and Bartlett. Curtiss CP: Constipation, in Groenwald SL, Frogge MH, Goodman M, Yarbro CH (eds): *Cancer Symptom Management*. Boston, Jones and Bartlett, 1996. © Jones and Bartlett Publishers.

- If you do not have a bowel movement in the morning,

  take _____ after breakfast.

- If you do not have a bowel movement by evening,

  take _____ at bedtime.

- If you do not have a bowel movement by the following morning,

  take _____ after breakfast.

3. If your bowels have not moved in 48 hours, call your doctor or nurse.

- Add _____ after breakfast, while continuing to

  take _____ as above.

4. Once you begin to have regular bowel movements, use the morning and evening doses of medicines you were taking when you had a bowel movement as your regular dose of medicine for your bowels.

5. If you are unsure of what to do, please call.

**Follow-Up**

If you are having trouble with your bowel movements, call your doctor or nurse. Be ready to tell them the following:

1. When you last had a bowel movement.

- Was it normal in size, color, and firmness?

- Was it difficult to pass?

- Have you had diarrhea?

2. The amount and kinds of fluid and food you are eating and drinking

3. The names and amounts of medicine you are taking for your bowels

4. Any changes in your health

5. Any new medications or treatments since your last visit

6. What you are doing to manage your bowels on your own

It is important to call your doctor or nurse if your pain medications are increased, so your bowel management plan can be checked. If you need help in learning about foods that help prevent constipation, call the nutritionist.

**Phone Numbers**

Nurse: _____  Phone: _____

Physician: _____  Phone: _____

Nutritionist: _____  Phone: _____

**Comments**


Patient's Signature: _____  Date: _____

Nurse's Signature: _____  Date: _____

**FIGURE 52-2**   Self-Care Guide: Constipation (continued).

```
┌─────────────────────────────────────────────────────────────────────────┐
│                        PATIENT CALL-IN RECORD                             │
│  ┌──────────────┬───────────────────────────┬──────────────────────────┐ │
│  │ Date:        │ Patient name:             │ Patient phone:           │ │
│  ├──────────────┼───────────────────────────┼──────────────────────────┤ │
│  │ Diagnosis:   │ Current therapy: Chemo ☐ Rad ☐ │ Being seen at: ☐ E ☐ N ☐ S IRCC │ │
│  ├──────────────┼───────────────────────────┴──────────────────────────┤ │
│  │ Next appt:   │ Physician:                                            │ │
│  ├──────────────┴───────────────────────────────────────────────────────┤ │
│  │ Reason for call:                                                      │ │
│  ├───────────────────────────────────────────────────────────────────────┤ │
│  │ Instructions:                                                         │ │
│  │                                                                       │ │
│  │                                                                       │ │
│  ├───────────────────────────────────────────────┬───────────────────────┤ │
│  │ Nurse signature:                               │ Time:                 │ │
│  ├────────────────────────────────────────────────┴──────────────────────┤ │
│  │ Physician comments:                                                   │ │
│  │                                                                       │ │
│  ├───────────────────────────────────────────────────────────────────────┤ │
│  │ Physician signature:                                                  │ │
│  └───────────────────────────────────────────────────────────────────────┘ │
└─────────────────────────────────────────────────────────────────────────┘
```

**FIGURE 52-3**   Patient call-in record. Reprinted with permission from the Oncology Nursing Press. Barhamand BA: Optimizing the use of the telephone for oncology nurses in office practices, in Carroll-Johnson RM (ed): *Meeting the Expanding Needs of the Office-Based Oncology Nurse.* Pittsburgh, Oncology Nursing Press, 1992, pp 8–14.

educational programs being offered in the community or general questions about problems or symptoms a person may be experiencing. Unless a particular staff member is identified to take these calls, it may be difficult to incorporate this activity into the daily routine. Before implementing such a program, consider this staffing issue as well as the expense of the toll-free number. In larger ambulatory settings, it is common for a telephone triage nurse to be identified.[12] These large settings may also benefit from the use of a wireless telecommunication system that has been used in inpatient settings. This portable phone system can result in time efficiency and enable nurses to stay with patients while contacting physicians, thus increasing staff and patient satisfaction.[97]

Providing patients with instructions and a way to reach someone after routine hours is critical and can be accom-

```
┌─────────────────────────────────────────────────────────────────────────────┐
│                      PHONE CALL DOCUMENTATION FORM                           │
│                                                                              │
│  (Patient Name, etc.)        │          Call Initiated by:      Urgency:    │
│                              │  Allergies_____  ☐ PT          ☐ Emergency │
│                              │  Time of call_____ ☐ Family_____ ☐ ASAP    │
│                              │  Time call returned__ ☐ MD_____   ☐ Today    │
│                              │  Length of call_____   Phone #_____          │
│                              │  ┌Purpose of call┐                            │
│                              │  ☐ Pt problem____  ☐ Pharmacy #_____       │
│  _____                 │  _____   ☐ Visiting RN #_____     │
│  ┌Additional notes:┐         │                                              │
│                              │  ☐ Drug refill     Name_____            │
│  _____                 │    Test results___ ┌Disposition of call┐      │
│                              │                    ☐ See orders  ☐ Medication change │
│  _____                 │  ☐ Questions about appt/tests  ☐ Drug refill  ☐ Test results given: │
│                              │  ☐ Update on pt status  ☐ TLH     ☐ By RN per MD OK │
│  _____                 │  ☐ Special         ☐ Called    ☐ To be given by MD │
│                              │    instructions___ ☐ Script     Notified_____ │
│                              │                      mailed                   │
│                              │  ☐ F/U required____                           │
│  _____                 │                                              │
│  Nurse signature  Date       │  ☐ Other          ┌Phone call documentation┐ │
└─────────────────────────────────────────────────────────────────────────────┘
```

**FIGURE 52-4**   Phone call documentation form. Reprinted with permission from the Oncology Nursing Press. Barhamand BA: Optimizing the use of the telephone for oncology nurses in office practices, in Carroll-Johnson RM (ed): *Meeting the Expanding Needs of the Office-Based Oncology Nurse.* Pittsburgh. Oncology Nursing Press, 1992, pp 8–14

plished in a variety of ways. Arrangements can be made to have the inpatient unit take phone calls from patients after routine hours and on weekends. In most situations, however, this is not desirable. Even though the patients may be known to the inpatient nurses, it is unlikely that these nurses will be thoroughly informed about the latest treatment or problem the patient is experiencing. An answering machine or a voice mail system on the ambulatory setting telephone can provide a detailed message about how to handle a problem or to reach someone.[27] An example of this might be a patient who calls to report a fever or another side effect. The patient would call the department phone and get a message directing him or her to contact the physician on call through the physician's answering service. Often, patients are calling to check on blood work, reschedule appointments, and so forth. In this case, they are able to leave a message so the nurse can respond.

Hagopian and Rubenstein[98] studied the effects of routine, planned telephone call interventions on 55 subjects undergoing radiation therapy. No significant differences were noted between the experimental group (who received the weekly telephone call) in anxiety, severity of side effects, helpfulness of self-care strategies, and coping strategies. The telephone calls did, however, demonstrate a caring attitude toward patients and allowed patients to talk about any concerns.

Follow-up phone calls after treatment has been completed are a routine practice in many settings. This practice provides an excellent opportunity for patient assessment and further self-care instructions. Phone calls to patients may be perceived as supportive. When patients know they have someone to call, anxiety may be relieved.

Patients receiving chemotherapy through an infusion pump should be given precise instructions about how to handle a problem after routine office hours. The clinic or office might contract with a local home health agency to provide this service. The home health agency may be willing to troubleshoot any minor problems with patients over the phone and, if necessary, make a home visit. Not every patient will need or want a specific home care referral, but many are reassured to know that someone to handle a problem is "only a phone call away." A key component of successful implementation of this approach is communication of important and current information about the patient. A form can be utilized for this communication (Figure 52-5). It is completed when the patient is started on chemotherapy that will continue at home and transmitted to the home health agency and updated when any changes occur. The home health agency's "on-call" nurse carries a notebook of these forms at all times. If a problem occurs, the referring ambulatory oncology nurse receives feedback on the next working day. In the meantime, the situation is handled by the home health nurse. This particular arrangement has the potential for meeting patients' and families' needs as well as ensuring continuity of care.

Telephone triage through the utilization of computer-ized on-line guidelines is also becoming more common and requires careful consideration. Ambulatory settings considering this technology should thoroughly evaluate the vendor and the computerized guidelines for facility adaptability, product support, tracking records, report capability, management of technological issues, and ease of use. In the future, telephone management will involve computer systems, coordinated total care, and a greater prevention focus, and will be an essential component of managed care contracts. The telephone is an important communication tool that will continue to play an integral role in the continuity of care of ambulatory oncology patients.[42]

## Care Coordination

The development and implementation of critical pathways and guidelines will have a significant impact on cost and outcomes in cancer care. Many authors have detailed their efforts in this arena.[99–115] Critical paths consist of a series of interventions specific to a group of patients with common attributes that are designed to promote the attainment of specific patient outcomes within a specific time frame.[99] Katterhagen and Patton describe the key leadership role that physicians play in the development of critical paths. They believe that critical pathways hold the potential to "dramatically alter the hospital culture."[99,p.25] A clear delineation of team member roles and staff education is essential for successful implementation.[99] Burns et al[100] have described a critical pathway for administering high-dose chemotherapy followed by peripheral blood stem cell rescue in the outpatient setting. They found several benefits to using the critical pathway in the outpatient setting, including enhanced communication between departments; a systematic flow of treatment; decreased variation in physician practice; timely insurance authorization; and team members understanding the feasibility of outpatient care.

A chemotherapy pathway for inpatients that moves the patient from preadmission to postdischarge with guidelines for daily interventions, treatments, and consultations has been developed by Hawkins and Goldberg.[101] Variances are tracked and compare the projected activities and outcomes to the documented activities and outcomes. In this way, trends can be identified that affect length of stay, resource consumption, or patient outcomes. In addition, variances direct revisions necessary in the pathway and identify quality improvement initiatives.[101] Pathways for oncology sepsis and outpatient chemotherapy have also been developed.[102]

Stanfill[103] suggests that the development of appropriate critical pathways based on fiscal impact is one strategy oncology program administrators can use to contribute to cost efficiency without compromising clinical outcomes. Prioritizing pathway development should be done by determining which diagnoses generate profitability and which do not. Taban and Cesta[104] evaluate the effectiveness of case management on the provision of

# INTERAGENCY REFERRAL FORM

Patient name _____ Primary caretaker _____ Insurance _____

Address _____ Relationship _____ SS# _____

Phone _____ Pharmacy _____ DOB _____

Primary MD _____ Phone _____ Surgeon _____ Phone _____

Oncologist _____ Phone _____ Oncology nurse _____ Phone _____

Diagnosis _____ Onset _____ Primary hospital _____ Treatment modalities _____

Secondary DX _____ Last hospitalization _____ Last chemo _____

_____ Last XRT _____

Mets _____ Referral to _____ Date _____

Services Requested: SN ___ PT ___ OT ___ ST ___ ET ___ MSW ___ HHA ___ Chaplain _____ Other _____

## Ability to Maintain Ventilation & Circulation

| BP | | SOB | | Edema | | MEDS | |
|----|----|-----|----|-------|----|------|----|
| P | | DOE | | | | | |
| WBC | | Cough | | Fatigue | | | |
| CRIT | | Chest pain | | Trans-fusion | | | |
| PLT | | Breath sounds | | VAD | | Last flush ___ | |

## Ability to Maintain Fluid Status

| Oral intake | | Skin | | MEDS | |
|-------------|----|------|----|------|----|
| Mucosa | | Wound ___ | | | |
| Thrush | | Drainage | | | |
| Stomatitis | | NG tube | | | |
| BUN ___ | Creat ___ | Fistulae | | | |

## Ability to Maintain Food Intake

| Current weight | | Nausea | | MEDS | |
|----------------|----|--------|----|------|----|
| Weight change | | Vomiting | | | |
| Appetite | | Dysphagia | | | |
| Diet | | Dry mouth | | | |
| Dentures | | | | | |

## Ability to Maintain Elimination

| Bowel habits | | Colostomy | | MEDS | |
|--------------|----|-----------|----|------|----|
| Constipation | | | | | |
| Diarrhea | | | | | |
| Bladder habits | | Foley | | | |
| Incontinent | | | | | |

## Ability to Maintain Comfort

| Pain description | Mild Mod Severe | PAIN REGIMEN |
|------------------|-----------------|--------------|
| Location | | |
| Control | Good Poor | |
| Bone mets | | |
| XRT | Calcium ___ | |

## Ability to Prevent Hazards & Achieve Safety

| Mental status | | MEDS | |
|---------------|----|------|----|
| Ambulation | | | |
| Sensory status | | | |
| Brain mets | | | |

## Ability to Cope with Illness & Treatment

| Anxiety | | MEDS | |
|---------|----|------|----|
| Depression | | | |
| Self-esteem | | | |
| Role changes | | | |
| Family support | | | |

Anticipated Teaching Needs

1. Dressing
2.
3.
4.

Anticipated DME Needs    Co _____

1. Hospital bed
2. Oxygen @ _____ L/m oximetry _____ PO2 _____
3. Wheelchair
4.

OTHER:

**FIGURE 52-5** Interagency referral form. Reprinted with permission from the Oncology Nursing Press. Shuster SA: The oncology office nurse's role in the coordination and continuity of care, in Carroll-Johnson RM (ed): *Meeting the Expanding Needs of the Office-Based Oncology Nurse*. Pittsburgh, Oncology Nursing Press, 1992, pp 15–20.

care through variance analysis, outcomes measurement, and outcomes management.

Stahl[105] discusses the necessity of critical pathway use in subacute care as one way to meet the challenge of the public's demand related to quality and cost-effectiveness. Micheletti and Shlala[106] describe clinical criteria screens that may dictate payment for patient care. Meister et al[107] describe the implementation and development of Home Care Steps™ protocols for use in the home care setting. They hope to eventually integrate the system to link with other projects across the health care continuum.

Clinical practice guidelines are being developed by many different commissions and professional societies.[108,109] Stair[109] provides general suggestions for the development of guidelines, including use of a multidisciplinary approach; incorporating a literature search; including a method of measuring compliance; determining how outcomes will be measured; defining topic and scope in a broad perspective across the continuum of care; developing a process for reviewing and updating the guidelines and continually evaluating the use and outcomes of the guidelines with the users.

White[110] describes the Patterns of Care Study (PCS) in radiation oncology. The PCS has developed guidelines for patients treated with radiation therapy for carcinoma of the prostate, breast, testes, cervix, uterus, nasopharynx, larynx, bladder, and tongue and for Hodgkin's disease. The Association of Community Cancer Centers[111] is also in the process of developing guidelines in cooperation with national and state oncology societies. The intent is that the guidelines will describe primary approaches to manage patients as well as serve as mechanisms that can be used in several ways. These include managed care providers using guidelines as standards for care, physicians and hospitals using them to assess the baseline cost of standard cancer care, critical path development, and evaluation of care. These guidelines are anticipated to be one-page faxable formats that illustrate standard therapeutic approaches (complete with literature citations) that will deliver the best outcomes for patients with cancer requiring standard care.

Kurowski[112] describes the development of guidelines for metastatic colon cancer, including antiemetics, growth factors, chemotherapy site care, febrile neutropenia, and total parenteral nutrition. These guidelines include measures related to mortality, morbidity, patient and physician satisfaction, quality of life, overall effectiveness, and availability of services.[112]

Regardless of the methodology used for clinical guideline evaluation, benchmark development is crucial. The use of benchmark comparisons to improve services in health care is relatively new. Sources of benchmarking information include the local community, hospital utilization data, state governments, comparison with similar communities, research literature, health care vendor studies, and health care associations.[114] Benchmark development in health care will promote creativity and present challenges for many years.

## NURSING ISSUES

Nurses face a variety of issues in the ambulatory care setting. These include models of nursing care delivery, productivity and classification systems, reimbursement, quality improvement, occupational hazards, continuity of care, and research.

### Models of Nursing Care Delivery

The evolution of the role of the ambulatory nurse, the complexity of care, and impending changes in health care legislation are challenging health care leaders to design cost-effective and efficient care delivery models.[116] A model of care delivery is a generic term to describe a method of organizing resources for the provision of patient care.

The compelling reasons for introducing a model specific for ambulatory nursing include the provision of more holistic care to patients with complex needs; introduction of quality initiatives; measurement of patient outcomes; better utilization of resources and the implementation of cost-containment measures.[116] Most nurses employed in ambulatory settings practice in a medical or functional model transplanted from the hospital.[63] Haas and Hackbarth[63] conducted a study of 606 ambulatory nurses that provided information about the current role of ambulatory nurses and delineated nine dimensions for future clinical practice and three dimensions for future quality improvement/research (Table 52-8; see also Table 52-5). When comparing current and future roles, several elements were similar, but the client teaching and expert practice/community outreach dimensions expanded in the future role. High-tech procedures are an entirely new dimension of future clinical practice.[63]

Models of care proposed by Haas and Hackbarth[63] include primary prevention, primary health care, primary nursing, case management, and paired partners. *Primary prevention* includes activities that either promote health in general or prevent the occurrence of diseases or injuries. Examples include health and nutrition education, health counseling, inoculations, and use of vitamin supplements. There are limitless opportunities for ambulatory nurses to play a key role in the delivery of these activities. A *primary health care* model constitutes the first level of contact of individuals, the family, and the community with the health system. Advanced practice nurses provide primary care in existing models.[42,63,117] *Primary nursing*, distinctly different from primary prevention or primary health care, is a model for nursing care delivery that has been utilized for years. Well suited for ambulatory care, primary nursing is designed to improve the quality of nursing care; recognize the patient and family as the unit of care, with the care designed accordingly; improve coordination of care between specialties; and ensure con-

**TABLE 52-8** Dimensions of the Future Staff Nurse Role in the Ambulatory Setting

### NINE CORE DIMENSIONS OF THE FUTURE STAFF NURSE CLINICAL PRACTICE ROLE

I. **Enabling Operations**
Order supplies
Locate records
Set up room
Search for space/equipment
Schedule appointments
Transport clients
Witness consent forms
Maintain traffic flow
Enter data in computer

II. **Technical Procedures**
Assist with procedures
Prepare client for procedures
Chaperone during procedures
Inform client about treatment
Administer oral/IM medications
Measure vital signs
Collect specimens

III. **Nursing Process**
Develop nursing care plan
Use nursing diagnosis plan
Conduct exit interview

IV. **Telephone Communications**
Telephone triage
Call pharmacy with prescription
Call client with test results

V. **Advocacy**
Make clients aware of rights
Promote positive public relations
Act as a client advocate
Triage client to appropriate provider

VI. **Client Teaching**
Assess client learning needs
Instruct client on medical/nursing regimen
Instruct client on home and self-care
Evaluate client care outcomes

VII. **High-Tech Procedures**
Administer blood/blood products
Perform complex treatments
Monitor clients before and after procedures

VIII. **Care Coordination**
Long-term supportive relationship
Act as a resource person
Coordinate client care
Assess needs and initiate referrals
Instruct on health promotion

IX. **Expert Practice/Community Outreach**
Expertise in advanced nursing practice
Function as advanced nurse resource
Design and present in-service education
Serve as preceptor for students
Independently provide primary care
Organize and conduct group teaching
Participate in community outreach
Follow up with clients in the home

### THREE CORE DIMENSIONS OF THE FUTURE QUALITY IMPROVEMENT/RESEARCH ROLE

I. **Quality Improvement**
Implement professional standards
Participate in preparation of QI plan
Collect and analyze QI data
Use QI plan in practice
Participate in interdisciplinary QI teams
Develop expected client outcomes
Utilize client classification system

II. **Research**
Facilitate nursing research
Participate in research of others
Follow guidelines to protect human subjects
Serve on research review board
Identify researchable questions
Evaluate nursing research findings
Conduct own nursing research

III. **Continuing Education**
Participate in on-site continuing education
Participate in off-site continuing education

Reprinted from *Nursing Economic,* 1996, Volume 14, Number 1, p. 17. Reprinted with permission of the publisher, Jannetti Publications, Inc., East Holly Avenue Box 56, Pitman, NJ 08071-0056; phone (609) 256-2300; FAX (609) 589-7463. (For a sample issue of the journal, contact the publisher.)

tinuity of care between settings. The primary nurse is accountable for coordinating a comprehensive plan of care that is continually reassessed, evaluated, modified, and implemented.[118]

*Case management* is an important model for nursing care delivery.[42,63,116–120] Health care literature has given this model much attention. It is loosely defined as a means of organizing care throughout the episode of illness, regardless of location.[116] The origins of case management can be traced to public health nurses from the turn of this century and to social work case management models.[119] Lamb[119] discusses three distinct models of nurse case man-

agement: hospital-based models in which coordination of care for high-risk individuals is done by nurses within the hospital; hospital-to-community models in which nurses work with high-risk individuals across settings; and community-based models in which case managers work with individuals primarily in their homes or other community settings. Patient populations who respond most favorably to a case management approach are those with complex problems who are seen frequently over a long period of time and have the potential for complications. Recommended tools for case managers include assessment and diagnostic skills, defined critical paths, understanding of community resources, collegial relationships with other health care providers, a tickler file, and computerized records.[63] Case management research needs to be conducted utilizing both qualitative and quantitative design if this innovative nursing care delivery model is to flourish.[119]

The collaborative nurse-physician model or joint practice has been implemented in all types of ambulatory settings.[12,116] This model usually has five components: (1) primary nursing, (2) increased clinical decision making by the nurse, (3) a collaborative practice committee of nurses and physicians, (4) joint record review, and (5) an integrated medical record.[121] This model allows nurses to manage resources so that triage occurs appropriately and there are designated appointment systems, easy access, and long-term follow-up. Enhanced communications occurring between the health care professionals on behalf of the patient may offer a more comprehensive health care experience.[116]

Another model of care that might be useful in some ambulatory settings is a *paired-partners approach*. In this model a professional nurse and other health care providers divide the nursing work. The registered nurse delegates and supervises the work done by providers, including licensed practical nurses, nurse aides, or technicians. This approach implies that the RNs work closely with their partners, including hiring, orienting, coaching, evaluating, and even firing them.[63]

## Productivity and Classification Systems

The increasing scope and intensity of nursing care provided in the ambulatory setting has resulted in the need for and use of classification systems and tools. Patient classification systems are a method of sorting individuals into levels for the purpose of predicting the demand for nursing care time.[122] Developing a system for ambulatory care is complex due to the many variables affecting the nursing role as well as the variety of facilities and types of clinics. Important differences between inpatient and ambulatory care that affect productivity and workloads include the following: (1) brief patient visits; (2) single visits involving multiple encounters; (3) patients returning for visits at irregular intervals; (4) patient needs varying significantly from one visit to another; (5) telephone management and screening as major components of ambulatory services; and (6) visits with a limited focus or purpose.[123]

In the outpatient setting, classification systems are typically used for retrospective analysis of patient characteristics, justification of resources, use of monitored trends for program planning, nursing workload analysis, patient care charges, validation of the nursing care provided, and quality assurance.[124] Goldfield[125] describes ambulatory encounter systems as the services provided during a visit of a patient to a health care professional. The development of these systems is occurring not only to classify encounters but also to determine payment and

measure quality. Patient needs must be linked with provider activities, resource use, and patient outcomes. Figure 52-6 identifies multiple purposes for patient classification systems.[123] Prescott and Soeken[126] propose a conceptual model for classification that includes concepts from both medical and nursing approaches; The Patient Intensity for Nursing: Ambulatory Care (PINAC) was designed and tested for use in the ambulatory setting. The structure of the PINAC reflects the factors of patient need for care and complexity of care. Each patient is evaluated and given a score. The PINAC was determined to be reliable, practical, and clinically meaningful to nurses in practice. Data from the PINAC can be used for staffing, budgeting, quality improvement, research, and other administrative purposes.

Many states have already implemented various ambulatory encounter systems. It is anticipated that the federal government will do so as well; thus it is critical to continue to find systems that truly encompass the scope of care provided to patients in the ambulatory setting.[125]

Medvec[124] offers suggestions for developing an ambulatory patient classification or workload analysis: (1) determine the present situation and develop patient care goals and objectives; (2) clarify what is to be accomplished; (3) examine present methods and develop a plan specific to the organization's needs; (4) involve staff and enlist organizational support; (5) educate staff and pilot the methodology, redefine the work if necessary; (6) provide feedback and allow input and opportunity for improvement planning; (7) design measures to test validity and reliability; and (8) compare data with other institutions when possible.

Riley and Seidner[127] have developed an ambulatory care productivity and patient charge system for their outpatient oncology and treatment center that is reanalyzed every two to three years because of changes in practice, reimbursement, and environment; this Patient Care Unit (PCU) System provides both a financial and a statistical database. The system is also based on clinical practice and patient care and allows for equitable charges, a delineation of standards of care, collaboration among the team members, and inclusion of professional practice within ambulatory payer codes. A bundling of all charges into treatment categories will eventually be done to prepare for the initiation of ambulatory patient groups.

Duval and Finn[5] developed a protocol-based staffing and scheduling model using a low-intensity time segment (LITS) or a high-intensity time segment (HITS) approach. Once the treatment protocol time frame is determined and assigned an LITS or a HITS, staffing determinations can be made. Room availability and operating hours need to be considered as well.[5]

Haas and Hackbarth[122] warn of the danger of using present inpatient classification systems. The systems cannot capture such information as the level of nursing judgment, complexity of care, activities performed simultaneously, time devoted to coordination of services in ambulatory care.

A major concern in the ambulatory area is maximizing

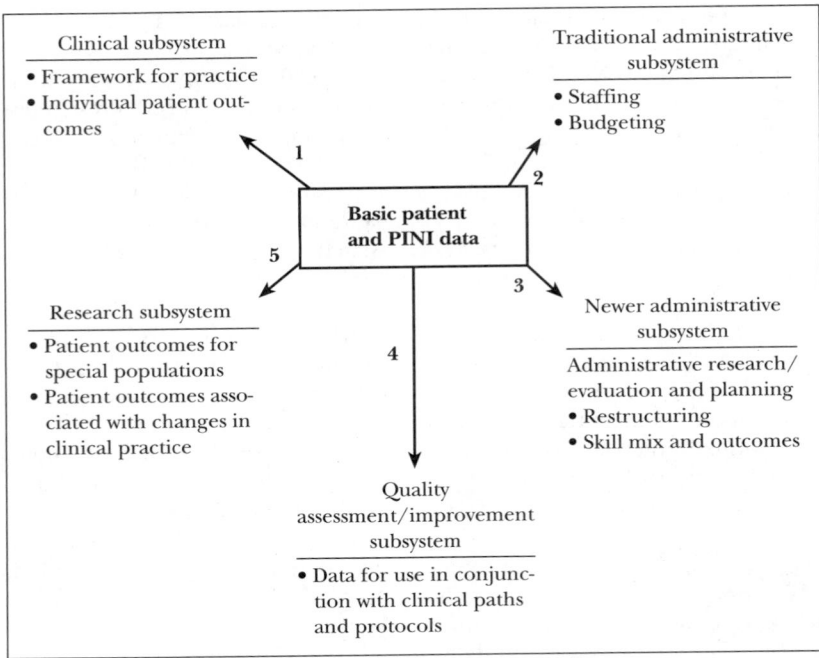

PINI = Patient Intensity for Nursing Index

**FIGURE 52-6**   Uses for patient classification systems. Reprinted from *Nursing Economic$*, 1996, Volume 14, Number 1, p. 17. Reprinted with permission of the publisher, Jannetti Publications, Inc., East Holly Avenue Box 56, Pitman, NJ 08071-0056; phone (609) 256-2300; FAX (609) 589-7463. (For a sample issue of the journal, contact the publisher.)

productivity. Effectively utilizing resources can result in improved profitability. Five techniques suggested to improve productivity are improving scheduling; staffing only for current workload; improving functional design of facilities; ensuring employee motivation; and increasing patient volume. It requires great skill to improve productivity without sacrificing quality. Reassessment of job functions and redesign of work patterns may be necessary to maximize the productivity of the workforce. Integration of inpatient and outpatient nursing services may facilitate continuity of care and cost-effectiveness.[128]

The introduction of the Resource-Based Relative Value Scale in 1992 changed many aspects of outpatient reimbursement.[129] It is anticipated that both medical and radiation oncologists will see decreases in reimbursement through this system. Hospitals will increasingly seek to employ physicians in order to contain costs when ambulatory encounter systems are initiated, resulting in a bundling of physician costs with hospital outpatient costs and drugs.[129] Wodinsky et al[130] developed outpatient cancer visit groups that were disease-specific rather than body system–specific. It was felt that these groups were clinically meaningful and easily understood by oncologists. Goldfield and Averill[131] discuss the use of clinical and charge data used in the development of approximately 275 ambulatory patient groups (APGs). These APGs are a "visit-based" system based on CPT-4 procedure codes. The APG

system may be viewed by managed care organizations and government entities as flexible and a good method for institutional and physician profiling of patterns of care. Under- or overutilization of procedures, tests, and visits will be readily apparent.

## Quality and Outcomes

An increased emphasis on cost reduction, improved clinical outcomes, and service quality has created new pressures on health delivery systems to demonstrate effectiveness throughout a continuum of care.[132,133] Consumers are now reviewing institutional report cards to compare health systems. The National Committee on Quality Assurance has joined the JCAHO in developing standards for accreditation. A transformation of the old quality system into a visible tool that is data based and incorporated into marketing and contracting efforts has resulted in the need to develop these programs in all settings.[132]

Historically, the focus of care has been on inpatient care, partly because ambulatory care delivery systems, roles, and procedures have been poorly understood. Measuring quality and outcomes in ambulatory care is accomplished utilizing the same concepts. Key principles include measuring what is done; measuring what is important to the customers; measuring what is feasible to collect and report and is meaningful to clinicians; and assuring that the measures selected are operational and concrete.[132] Table 52-9 provides sample indicators for the oncology ambulatory setting.

Miller and Flanagan[133] suggest beginning with one indicator relating to high volume, one indicator relating to high risk, and one indicator relating to a problem-prone aspect of care. Since most ambulatory services are concerned with prevention, diagnosis, and treatment, meaningful indicators are readily defined if a multidisciplinary approach is used. They suggest a reasonable target for a quality project as one for every 3000 outpatient encounters. Hardy and Forrer[134] describe the use of a value analysis and shared governance concept resulting in a comprehensive quality management approach.

The Quality Improvement in Ambulatory Care project was a national demonstration project undertaken in Minnesota.[135] This collaborative effort between three organizations encompassing clinics and physician office practices was implemented in a variety of settings. Program components included weekly meetings of the project team, monthly meetings of the quality improvement (QI) committee, and monthly meetings of the clinic QI representatives and the clinic QI medical directors. Reinforcement of quality activities at the various sites, provision for education about quality, and introduction of new QI tools were all goals of the project. The demonstration project broadened the perspective of quality as defined by providers, patients, and payers. Through this program, resources to develop worthwhile quality programs were

**TABLE 52-9**  Ambulatory Cancer Care Indicators for Quality

- Medication errors per month
- Patients very satisfied with clinic wait time
- Average turnaround time to retrieve unscheduled patient record
- Walk-ins per clinic session
- Average cost per visit
- Average supply cost per visit
- Average patient/family satisfaction with information received
- Number of complaints about staff skill with venipuncture
- Number of patients able to correctly demonstrate operation of self-managed infusion device on return visit
- Average time to schedule visit
- Infection rate after ambulatory procedure
- Number of patients experiencing blood transfusion reaction
- Self-report of pain on visual analogue scale

Reprinted from *Nursing Economic$,* 1996, Volume 14, Number 1, p. 17. Reprinted with permission of the publisher, Jannetti Publications, Inc., East Holly Avenue Box 56, Pittman, NJ 08071-0056; phone (609) 256-2300; FAX (609) 589-7463. (For a sample issue of the journal, contact the publisher.)

developed and implemented with a direct effect on patient care.[135]

Another approach to quality improvement may be the development of indicators that are standard to all oncology settings, with reports given to the cancer committee.[12] Clinical indicators for oncology developed by the JCAHO are expected to be implemented no sooner than 1997.[46] There are indicators for breast, colon, and lung cancer, with a primary focus on the diagnosis and treatment of the primary tumor. These indicators are not inclusive of many other important aspects of care but are important in defining quality care for the patient with cancer.[136] Reporting data regarding these indicators will be mandated and will allow for comparison of cancer programs across the state, region, and country. Lamkin[12] suggests that a major focus for quality measures in ambulatory settings should be geared toward an examination of the effectiveness of education since that is a primary function of the ambulatory care nurse.

The current struggles with health care financing and the use of developing technological advances in oncology care will provoke major conflicts related to cost containment versus the quality of care.[137] Many of these advances are equated with improved quality of care but also increased costs. The consumer focus will change health care professionals' evaluation of quality. Traditionally, end points such as morbidity and mortality rates have been the measurable standards to reflect quality of care. The consumer focus will force health care providers to determine new standards of measurement. Miaskowski[137] suggests that nurses are in a unique position to evaluate and emphasize a broad perspective of quality issues that focus on patient satisfaction, quality of life, and cost. Assessing the quality of care across multiple settings, with specific attention to the areas of education, symptom management, home care, and psychological support, will be important. It will be critical to examine the quality of care provided to patients as they make transitions across settings in the health care system. Patient-developed criteria will be necessary to evaluate quality and improve the patient's quality of life in the future.[137]

Patient satisfaction should be integrated with other quality measures to improve service. Malone and Pollock[138] offer specific recommendations in the development of a patient satisfaction survey. The Foundation for Accountability, an alliance of public and private health care purchasers and consumer organizations, is compiling performance measures the public can use to compare health plans.[139] Multiple groups and agencies including HMOs, group practices, medical practices, and employers are surveying patient satisfaction with their health care.

It is obvious that the emphasis on quality will remain. Oncology nurses have a tremendous opportunity to focus their efforts on providing and evaluating quality cancer care in the areas of education, symptom management, home care, and psychological support.[137] Nurse executives are challenged to create strategies to further develop nurses' clinical expertise and problem identification and problem-solving skills to facilitate QI teams.[122]

## Occupational Hazards

Oncology nurses working in ambulatory settings face occupational hazards—specifically, the safe handling of antineoplastic agents, radioactive materials, and blood and body fluids. Guidelines for protection in handling antineoplastic agents were revised by the Occupational Safety and Health Administration (OSHA) in 1995.[140] The ONS has also published guidelines and recommendations for practice related to chemotherapy.[141] Unfortunately, wide variations in practice still exist. Ambulatory oncology nursing administrators are challenged to establish protective measures in their settings.

The growth of continuous infusion administration of chemotherapy in the home setting necessitates considering these same issues for the home. Many patients receiving continuous infusions at home are not referred to home health agencies for in-home evaluations. One should question if patients have received adequate instruction about how to change drug delivery cassettes or handle drug spills.

Implementation of a facility-wide chemotherapy and radiotherapy task force to establish standards, protocols, procedures; recommend protective equipment purchases; and evaluate compliance with the accepted standards is highly desirable. This group should represent all departments involved with chemotherapy or radiotherapy preparation, handling, and administration. Physicians' offices and home care agencies should be included in this task force to encourage consistent approaches and continuity of care.

Exposure of staff to patients' blood and body fluids is common in oncology settings. Strict adherence to the OSHA guidelines is essential for protection of both staff and patients. To comply with the recommendations, personal protective equipment is to be provided at no cost to the employee. This includes but is not limited to gloves, gowns, laboratory coats, face shields or masks, eye protection, and similar items.[142]

Nurses in ambulatory oncology settings have a responsibility to be informed and adhere to current practices to avoid occupational hazards. Patients and families should also be protected from unnecessary exposure to hazardous situations. Education and compliance are critical factors for safe care. Use of standardized forms developed to facilitate consistent surveillance of health care workers who handle cytotoxic drugs should be considered.[143] Shortridge et al[144] conducted a cross-sectional study exploring the relationship between low-dose occupational exposure to antineoplastic drugs and menstrual dysfunction. This study compared female nurses in two national organizations and found an association between menstrual dysfunction and handling of cancer drugs in subjects between 30 and 45 who were currently administering antineoplastic drugs. Additional comparative studies are needed to examine effects of toxic chemicals in the workplace. The menstrual cycle may serve as a measure of potential health effects related to these toxic exposures.

## Continuity of Care

The oncology nurse in the ambulatory setting frequently maintains continuity of care with the patient and family. This results because hospitalization is utilized only for acute care and home or hospice care is usually required only for a limited time. Ambulatory nurses may follow patients for weeks, months, or even years. As third-party payers scrutinize care and consumers demand more, the necessity for continuity is even greater. The question remains as to how this continuity can best be accomplished. One might also ask the question: How do we define continuity of care in oncology? Beddar and Aikin offer the following definition: "Continuity of care is a philosophy and standard of care that involves patient, family, and health care providers working together to provide a coordinated, comprehensive continuum of care."[145,p.255] A continuum of care facilitates transitions between settings, results in improved patient outcomes, and contributes to cost-effectiveness.[145] To achieve a continuity of care that is integrated and comprehensive, several key components are essential. These components are highlighted in Table 52-10.

Case managers and clinical care coordinators are now utilized to oversee the continuum of care for specific patient populations.[145–147] Other strategies to enhance continuity of care have been reported in the literature.[14,27,145–147] Case and Jones[148] describe an Inpatient/Outpatient Data Flow Sheet that was developed and converted into a computerized program that could be initiated and/or accessed by oncology nurses in multiple areas to obtain and update information on shared patients. Most nurses questioned after the implementation of the system could give examples of how continuity of care had been improved. The use of this type of flow sheet continues to be a goal in many settings to enhance continuity of care.[65]

Use of the computer for information flow and retrieval of clinical databases is fully functional in many settings. The technical capability of the computer to integrate

---

**TABLE 52-10    Key Components of Continuity of Care**

- Interdisciplinary approach to care
- Comprehensive assessment of patient and family needs and strengths
- Patient and family education and involvement in decision making
- Development of measurable goals and a plan of care
- Identification and coordination of supplemental resources
- Integration of care through each transition
- Evaluation

Reprinted from *Seminars in Oncology Nursing* with permission from Beddar SM, Aikin JL: Continuity of care: A challenge for ambulatory oncology nursing. *Semin Oncol Nurs* 10:254–263, 1994.

information from multiple sources, store, and then later transmit the data to another location is especially advantageous for care of patients with cancer.[149] Laptop computers promote timely documentation. Decision-support capabilities are also available with more advanced computer systems. This is an ideal way to enhance continuity; thus, it is essential that oncology nurses become familiar with computers. In many settings, critical pathways and patient records are computerized and allow for access to the health care delivery system from multiple entry points.

Another approach to enhancing continuity of care is through multidisciplinary patient care conferences. Kerstetter[150] discusses the oncology multidisciplinary conference as a tool to increase communication and knowledge among departments providing oncology services. The Association of Community Cancer Centers emphasizes the importance of continuity of care and collaboration through a multidisciplinary team approach.[49] The goals of multidisciplinary conferences are twofold:

1. to provide a forum for education and communication among those involved in the care of the patient
2. to develop and evaluate individualized multidisciplinary care plans for oncology patients.[150]

Team members attending the conference include oncologists, oncology staff nurses, the oncology dietitian, social worker, the home health care coordinator, hospice nurse, oncology clinical nurse specialist, pharmacist, research nurse, radiation therapist, pastoral care coordinator, pain management specialist, oncology director, and rehabilitation therapists.[150] The particular setting may suggest others who should be part of the team. In some situations family meetings including the patient and appropriate team members may provide a forum for direct and supportive interaction.[146]

Another important aspect of continuity of care involves defining who the patient should call if a question or concern comes up after traditional working hours. The answer to this question varies according to setting. However, the patient and family must clearly understand who should be called and when to call.

Another method for ensuring improved continuity of care is a daily morning conference to discuss new patients on a given day, problems that have arisen, or general issues. This short meeting can include only the physician and the nurse or can be expanded to include the research nurse, radiation oncology/chemotherapy nurse, pharmacist, and others.

Development of communication channels between acute care settings and office practices can also enhance continuity of care for patients.[27] Including the office nurse in unit meetings as well as discharge planning can ensure smoother transitions. This concept also extends to home care teams. The office nurse is in a unique position to organize this team effort.[27]

Barriers to continuity of care have been identified.

Territoriality may become an issue with increased competition for patients and little incentive for cooperation with other agencies. Reimbursement issues also affect the scope of services available and may impact quality and continuity. Minimal collaboration due to a lack of knowledge about resources may also occur. Inadequate communication between caregivers and settings may also impede continuity of care.[145]

Continuity is critical to providing quality care to patients with cancer and will continue to be an essential component of a cancer program. The ambulatory oncology nurse is a key player in facilitating this continuity. Development of the concept of continuity of care in nursing curricula of basic and continuing education programs will help strengthen awareness. An expectation of professional accountability will also encourage greater attention to this issue.[145]

## Research

Research protocols are commonly offered to patients in outpatient settings and mandate that ambulatory nurses are familiar with the careful documentation essential to the clinical trials. Nurses in ambulatory settings may serve as data managers or may work closely with these individuals. Training to prepare staff for these roles is recommended.[12,128]

Nursing research in the ambulatory setting is now more common and is expected to be a major focus of future research efforts.[12,122,151] Haas and Hackbarth[122] documented ambulatory staff nurses' view of their future role as including research activities such as facilitating nursing research, serving on review boards, identifying research questions, evaluating research findings for practice application, and conducting research. Fitch and Thompson[152] describe the development of a research-based oncology nursing practice in an ambulatory cancer treatment and research facility. Table 52-11 details research-related roles and expectations of staff nurses in a comprehensive cancer program. They delineate the challenges of fostering a research-based oncology nursing practice. These challenges are trying to find a balance between the pressures of clinical practice and research, helping other health care professionals see the value of nursing research, trying to obtain funding, and determining what happens to projects that are not funded.[152] Ambulatory nurse managers must provide opportunities for participation in research activities. Standards developed by the American Academy of Ambulatory Care Nursing also address research and encourage active participation in conducting and participating in clinical and health care systems research.[43]

Haberman[151] looked at previous research or concept development in the area of ambulatory care oncology nursing and found that care delivery advances have outpaced the scientific basis for this practice. He provides an extensive review of suggestions for writing research

**TABLE 52-11**  Research-Related Roles and Expectations of Staff Nurses in a Comprehensive Cancer Program

| Research-Related Role | Expectations |
|---|---|
| Consumer | • Be aware of research conducted in one's field of practice |
| | • Critically analyze research conducted in one's field of practice |
| | • Incorporate valid research findings into one's own practice |
| | • Respond appropriately to patients' questions regarding research reported in the lay press |
| Facilitator | • Assist with the implementation of research studies<br>—Identify potential study subjects<br>—Implement a study intervention<br>—Record data for study purposes |
| Contributor | • Generate ideas from practice for research |
| | • Engage in dialogue with researchers regarding the clinical implications of study findings and future study ideas |
| Advocate | • Question the research knowledge base for existing policy/protocols |
| | • Advocate that new policies and protocols are based on current research knowledge where it exists |
| | • Respond appropriately to patients' questions about participation in or withdrawal from research studies |

Reprinted with permission from Oncology Nursing Press with permission from Fitch MI, Thompson L: Fostering the growth of research-based oncology nursing practice. *Oncol Nurs Forum* 23:631–637, 1996.

**TABLE 52-12**  Ambulatory Care Nursing Research Problems

- Classification systems for nursing and patient activities
- Models for the delivery of cost-effective nursing care
- Patient's satisfaction with care
- Care of patients at risk for special problems
- Strategies for cancer pain management
- Quality of life
- Survivorship
- Management of progressive disease
- Management of febrile episodes
- Management of immunosuppressed or immunocompromised patients, including individuals with AIDS
- Comfort, fatigue, nausea, and vomiting
- Ethics of care, clinical decision making, participation in clinical trials
- Personal and professional power
- Elements of successful multidisciplinary collaborative practices
- Computer-smart systems as an aide to assessment and charting

Adapted with permission from Jones and Bartlett with permission from Haberman MR: Research in ambulatory care settings: The need for and how to do research, in Buchsel PC, Yarbro CH (eds): *Oncology Nursing in the Ambulatory Setting: Issues and Models of Care*. Boston, Jones and Bartlett, 1993, pp 307–340.

questions, design options, an overview of research variables, measurement levels, statistical analysis plans, and strategies to optimize designs.[151] Table 52-12 is a listing of ambulatory care nursing research problems that nurses may want to consider pursuing. Given the unique aspects of ambulatory care nursing, multiple opportunities are available for the interested and resourceful ambulatory care nurse.[151]

## PATIENT-RELATED ISSUES

A number of patient-related issues are dominant in the ambulatory care setting. Self-care, ethical issues, and care of the disadvantaged are among the major issues that will be addressed in this section.

## Self-Care

Transition of patient care from the hospital to ambulatory and home settings has resulted in a shift in responsibility for family members caring for patients receiving treatment. *Self-care* is defined as how individuals care for themselves or alter conditions or objects in their environment in the interest of their own lives, health, or well-being.[153] Applying this definition to oncology, actions initiated by patients and families to prevent cancer, detect cancer, and manage the side effects of cancer treatment can be defined as self-care. Since the vast majority of oncology patients now receive treatment in the ambulatory care setting, there are a number of important considerations for the patient and the health care provider regarding self-care.

Fieler et al[154] conducted a study to describe self-care behaviors for prevention and early detection of chemotherapy side effects. The Prevention Behaviors Questionnaire (PBQ) was utilized with 46 participants and consisted of 17 items derived from standard patient education resources that focused on side-effect prevention and early detection. Results showed that trying to think positively, eating well-balanced meals, drinking more fluid, and taking naps were the most frequently reported behaviors.[154] Further research is needed to determine the links between self-care behavior and health outcomes.

A self-care diary in which patients recorded side effects including severity and reported the use and efficacy of self-care activities revealed a variety of self-care activities being used to manage the side effects, resulting in little to some relief.[155] This diary mechanism was effective for obtaining patients' reports of the side effects experienced and the usefulness of self-care activities. Diary entries can form the basis for evaluating the effectiveness of self-care activities and adjusting as necessary for future treatments.[155] Figure 52-2 is an example of a self-care guide that can be developed and utilized in any ambulatory setting.

Brinkman et al[156] developed a self-report form (Figure 52-7) related to chemotherapy toxicity for patients participating in clinical trials. Patients require no more than 15 minutes to complete the form, which they do while waiting to see their physician. The information is then reviewed by the nurse and physician and used in patient management. The self-report form becomes a permanent part of the patient record.

Brandt[157] conducted a study with 22 patients undergoing brachytherapy. Frequently identified learning needs included (1) how to manage side effects, (2) activity restrictions during implant, (3) pain management and comfort measures, (4) cause of current symptoms, and (5) how the implant could affect symptoms. Nurses caring for this population of patients should be aware of the benefits of patients' knowledge and active participation in their own care to help alleviate anxiety.

Goodman et al[158] describe two self-care kits developed for patients. The "new patient" kit contains general information that the patient needs to perform self-care as well as discount coupons for medications and information about community resources and wellness centers. A "survivor" kit is given to patients finishing chemotherapy. Self-care is an important behavior for cancer survivors also, since they need to be motivated to take an active role in their health care. Participating in health-promoting activities may help to lessen their feelings of hopelessness.

Giving emotional support was identified in a study as the most time-consuming and difficult task for family members.[159] Assisting with household tasks, errands, and transportation were also reported as time-consuming. Dependency was identified as the main contributor to caregiver burden.[159] It is important for the ambulatory care nurse to establish a relationship with the family caregiver as well as the patient in order to facilitate assessment, intervention, and support. A baseline of information about communication patterns, caregiver health, and family resources is critical.[159]

Yeager et al[160] conducted a study to compare knowledge about pain and the perception of the pain experience between outpatients experiencing cancer-related pain and their family caregivers. No significant differences in the knowledge scores were seen, but there was a significant difference in the perception of the pain experience, with family caregivers viewing the experience of pain more negatively than the patients did.

Cancer resource libraries are another method of empowering cancer patients and encouraging self-care. Libraries can provide information that may be otherwise unavailable or inaccessible; teach patients self-care, self-management, and coping skills; reduce stress and anxiety; emphasize the importance of prevention; and reinforce the hospital's interest in the patient's well-being.[161]

Montbriand[162] developed and tested a decision tree model outlining patients' decision strategies that has applicability in a wide variety of settings and suggests new and innovative ways for nurses to communicate with and assist patients through their cancer experience. Kristjanson and Ashcroft[163] completed an extensive literature review of the family cancer experience and were able to identify four major themes: developmental stage of the family, cancer illness trajectory, family responses to cancer, and health care provider behaviors. Since care of the cancer patient at home by families will increase in magnitude, future research and intervention studies are suggested based on this review.

The ambulatory care setting is increasingly being utilized for follow-up care after major cancer treatments, such as for bone marrow or peripheral stem cell transplant patients who may be seen entirely in an ambulatory setting or be discharged within a few days yet have to face long, stressful, and expensive recovery periods. A smooth transition throughout the continuum of care is essential. Self-care teaching and written guidelines for patients and families about care of venous access lines, administration of parenteral fluids, and symptom management are critical to effective management of these patients in an ambulatory environment.[164]

For optimal self-care behavior, patients and families need to be adequately taught about the specific treatment modality and side effect management. Safety issues, safe handling of drugs, and infection control are addressed. Lifestyles, distance from treatment centers, and financial and family issues may make compliance with treatment regimens difficult or impossible. Often the patient will turn to the nurse to discuss the situation. Encouraging and supporting self-care is a critical component of the nurse's role in the ambulatory oncology setting.

## Ethical Issues

Ethical issues encountered in ambulatory care are similar to those that arise in other settings. Whether patients are making informed decisions and how best to provide high-quality care are ever-present issues. Unfortunately, even today some patients sign informed consents for participation in clinical trials or other research without having a good understanding of what they will be experiencing. The ambulatory care nurse faced with this dilemma should alert other health team members. At times, decisions may have to be referred to administrators or an ethics committee. In an office or small setting, discussion and resolution of ethical dilemmas can be particularly difficult. Open and honest professional dialogue is usually an effective approach.

## MIDWEST COOPERATIVE GROUP OUTREACH PROGRAM
## PATIENT REPORT OF CHEMOTHERAPY SIDE EFFECTS

Patient's Name: _____  Date: _____

Date of last chemotherapy treatment: _____

Please list the names and dates of other chemotherapy drugs taken by mouth since your last chemotherapy treatment:

_____

_____

Below is a list of possible side effects. Please circle only the ones that apply and circle the amount.

| Side Effect | | | | Duration* |
|---|---|---|---|---|
| Nausea | Able to eat | Decreased intake | No intake | _____ |
| Vomiting | Once/24 hours | 2–5 times/24 hours | 6–10 time/24 hours | _____ |
| Diarrhea | Increase of 2–3 times/ 24 hours over normal | Increase of 4–6 times/24 hours or moderate cramping | Increase of 7–9 times/24 hours or severe cramping | _____ |
| Mouth Soreness | Tender/red mouth | Mouth sores (able to eat) | Mouth sores (unable to eat) | _____ |
| Fatigue | Mild (normal activity) | Moderate (decreased activity) | Severe (confined to bed/ chair 50% of awake time) | _____ |
| Constipation | Mild (hard stools) | Moderate (requires a laxative) | Severe (requires enema/ removal) | _____ |
| Loss of Appetite | Yes    No | Weight loss (in pounds): _____ | | _____ |
| Hair Loss | Mild | Pronounced | Total | _____ |
| Fever | 98.7°–100.4° | 100.5°–104.0° | Over 104.0° | _____ |
| Infection | Yes    No | Hospitalization required: Yes  No | | |
| Numbness/Tingling in the Hands or Feet | Explain: _____ | | | |
| Skin Changes | Explain: _____ | | | |
| Other | Explain: _____ | | | |

Medication required for any of the above           Yes    No        Name of medication: _____

*Duration of side effects should be described as less than (<) 24 hours; 2–3 days; 4–7 days; or more than (>) one week.

Patient's Signature: _____

**FIGURE 52-7**  Sample self-report form for chemotherapy side effects. Reprinted with permission from Oncology Nursing Press, Inc. Brinkman P, Hay D, Laubinger P: Chemotherapy toxicity assessment using a self-report tool. *Oncol Nurs Forum* 21:1731–1733, 1994.

As reimbursement becomes more limited, health care providers will face increasingly difficult decisions about who and how to treat, when to stop treatment, the aggressiveness of treatment, who is making decisions about treatment, and so on.[57] Ambulatory nurses will find themselves involved with these dilemmas and need to prepare themselves to face them with a knowledge base and a professional approach.

## Economic Issues

Access to health care has become a major concern for many Americans. Poverty has been shown to correlate with poor prognosis for all types of cancer.[165] Current reimbursement for health care is increasingly being reduced. Refusal by insurers to pay for research treatments limits participation in cancer research studies.[165] Unfortunately, many people are being denied care not only because they cannot afford to pay or are uninsured or underinsured but also because they do not have input into the politically controlled decision-making systems in society.[166] Denials for care occur if individuals do not obtain necessary approvals prior to beginning treatment. This presents dilemmas for all involved and usually additional burdens for the health care providers to assist patients with this process. Many insurance plans have restrictions that limit or prohibit care as well. Managed care approaches will continue to impact cancer care and force the development of new philosophies about care to be adopted in order for cancer programs to survive.[167] Those organizations that are poised to quickly respond to requests from third-party payers will have a competitive edge.

Direct reimbursement for nursing services continues to be a goal within nursing. Presently, reimbursement for nursing services varies significantly depending on the location of the practice setting, the insurance carrier and state, as well as the type of practitioner.[168] Patient outcomes are adversely impacted when reimbursement is denied for the proposed treatment. Patients have a need and right to be informed of the financial issues related to their cancer treatment, especially if the treatment involves investigational therapy.[168] Porter has conducted a retrospective comparative study identifying economic and outcome differences between two models of care—complement (compliance) and substitute (collaboration).[169,170] The research sites were two ambulatory cancer care agencies in central Canada: an oncology outpatient clinic in a community hospital and a regional cancer center.[169] Results showed significant differences in ambulatory nursing practice between the two settings. The *nurse complement model* is defined as a model in which the nurse complies with the medical directives and functions as a complement to the oncologist. The *nurse substitute model* is one in which the oncology nurse is in a collaborative relationship with the oncologist and regularly acts as a physician substitute.[169] The substitution of care by the nurse for the oncologist in outpatient settings may relate directly to health resource use by ambulatory cancer patients. In the substitute model, care normally provided by the oncologist (patient teaching, chemotherapy administration, and ongoing assessment and monitoring) is performed by the nurse.[169] These findings have implications for administrators who are hoping to reduce the number of nurses in outpatient settings in order to cut operating costs.[170] Further studies need to be done on the economic effectiveness of nursing before decisions are made based on inadequate information. An extensive discussion of the economics of cancer care and its impact on patients, families, and cancer nursing practice can be found in chapters 49 and 56.

## CONCLUSION

The ambulatory care setting will be the primary future setting for oncology services. To remain competitive in the marketplace and to meet the growing needs of health care consumers, ambulatory care centers will be providing a multitude of cancer services. The implementation of prospective payment for ambulatory care will present challenges for health care organizations. Increased computer capabilities will positively impact the ambulatory setting by simplifying documentation as well as assisting in decision making.

Miaskowski[137] challenges ambulatory care nurses to "create the preferred future" by examining the projections for the health care system of the twenty-first century. She delineates four components of this system: activities related to health promotion; management of chronic illness; traumatic injury and life-threatening illness care; and care of the frail and physically limited elderly and the terminally ill. Cross-training in pediatrics and geriatrics will be necessary for oncology nurses caring for these patient populations. Nurses will also need training in genetic counseling to help individuals understand all the implications of genetic screening tests. Having a broader view of health care economics and ethical decision-making principles will also allow nurses to be in the forefront of discussions and policy making at all levels. Developing skills in understanding and controlling new technologies such as robotics and telematics will demonstrate the critical "human" link between patients and machines.[137]

Engelking[38] and Boyle[171] have identified projections for future cancer care as detailed in Table 52–13. A proactive response is needed to meet the challenges ahead. New opportunities for nurses will include roles as genetic-risk analysts, health education media designers, patient readiness evaluators, technology accessors, partners in a holistic care center, treatment options advisers,[38] minority needs specialists, facilitators of intergenerational support teams, multispecialty nursing care providers, and cancer care policy activists.[171]

The impact of large numbers of cancer survivors will be especially felt in the ambulatory care area. Preparing patients and family members to assume 24-hour responsibility for self-care with intensive treatment regimens will continue to challenge the health care team.

Implementation of clinical pathways, standard treatment protocols, and algorithms[172-174] has become a reality and is projected to result in more thorough patient assessment,[174] decreased costs, enhanced quality of care, im-

**TABLE 52-13    Projections for Future Cancer Care**

> **PROJECTION:** Tomorrow's consumers of cancer care will be dramatically different from those of today, predominantly people of advanced age and diverse ethnic backgrounds, people living in poverty, and those willing to assume a greater role in health care–related decision making.
>
> **PROJECTION:** Social support dilemmas will be addressed by family mobilization and by unique intervention programs.
>
> **PROJECTION:** New "hybrids" of oncology nurses will emerge, evidenced by where and how they practice.
>
> **PROJECTION:** Cancer prevention, diagnosis, and treatment will be customized for and targeted to select patient subgroups.
>
> **PROJECTION:** Cancer management will be characterized by rapid technology transfer, emphasis on prevention, and aggressive multimodality treatment.
>
> **PROJECTION:** The "self-care movement" will drive a reintegration of a holistic healing and recovery orientation into cancer care.
>
> **PROJECTION:** Ethical responsibilities will become an accentuated component of oncology nursing.

From Boyle DM: New identities: The changing profile of patients with cancer, their families, and their professional caregivers. *Oncol Nurs Forum* 21:55–61, 1994; and Engelking C: New approaches: Innovations in cancer prevention, diagnosis, treatment, and support. *Oncol Nurs Forum* 21:62–71, 1994. Adapted with permission from Oncology Nursing Press, Inc.

proved communication,[172] and greater autonomy for nurses.[173]

Nurses in all settings must consider the special needs of the elderly. The ambulatory care setting provides an ideal setting to sponsor age-specific cancer prevention and early detection activities, perform age-specific assessments, evaluate treatment side effects, refer to established support networks, ensure continuity of care, modify patient education programs and strategies, serve as patient advocates, and influence health care policy.[128,175]

Issues in ambulatory care that will challenge all nurses include "growth, reimbursement, managing volumes, greater patient acuities, care standards, fewer dollars, billing and coding, delivery systems, managing margins, physician and employee compensation systems, recruitment and retention, incentives, governance, and coordination of multi-disciplinary providers and support staff."[176] These issues and others present tremendous opportunities to impact the care of cancer patients for nurses in ambulatory care settings.

# REFERENCES

1. Nevidjon BM: Ambulatory care services, in McCorkle R, Grant M, Frank-Stromborg M, Baird SB (eds): *Cancer Nursing: A Comprehensive Textbook* (ed 2). Philadelphia, Saunders, 1996, pp 1279–1286

2. Houston DA, Houston GR: Administrative issues and concepts in ambulatory care, in Buchsel PC, Yarbro CH (eds): *Oncology Nursing in the Ambulatory Setting: Issues and Models of Care.* Boston, Jones and Bartlett, 1993, pp 3–19

3. Lamkin L: Outpatient oncology settings: A variety of services. *Semin Oncol Nurs* 10:229–236, 1994

4. Sandrik K: Oncology: Who's managing outpatient programs? *Hospitals* 64(3):32–37, 1990

5. Duval AC, Finn TR: Development and application of an outpatient protocol-based staffing and scheduling model. *J Oncol Manage* 4:19–23, 1995

6. Sandrik K: Outpatient programs for oncology. *Trustee,* April 1990, p 19

7. *Nursing's Agenda for Health Care Reform.* Kansas City, MO, American Nurses Association, 1991

8. Shingleton WW: Cancer centers: Origins and purpose. *Arch Surg* 124:43–45, 1989

9. Lokich JJ, Silvers S, Brereton H, et al: Free-standing cancer centers: Rationale for improving cancer care delivery. *Am J Clin Oncol* 12:402–406, 1989

10. Mannisto MM: The emergence of cancer specialty centers. *Oncol Issues* 5:11–14, 1990

11. Otte DM: Report from the annual ACOA meeting, 1994: Mergers, affiliations and networks. *J Oncol Manage* 3:16–17, 1994

12. Lamkin L: The new oncology ambulatory clinic, in Buchsel PC, Yarbro CH (eds): *Oncology Nursing in the Ambulatory Setting: Issues and Models of Care.* Boston, Jones and Bartlett, 1993, pp 107–131

13. Moskowitz R: Day surgery for oncology patients, in Buchsel PC, Yarbro CH (eds): *Oncology Nursing in the Ambulatory Setting: Issues and Models of Care.* Boston, Jones and Bartlett, 1993, pp 165–183

14. Buchsel PC: Ambulatory care for the bone marrow transplant patient, in Buchsel PC, Yarbro CH (eds): *Oncology Nursing in the Ambulatory Setting: Issues and Models of Care.* Boston, Jones and Bartlett, 1993, pp 185–208

15. Brady AM, Foster J: The development of site-specific centers: The breast clinic. *Oncol Issues* 7:12–14, 1994

16. Lee CZ, Coleman C, Link J: Developing comprehensive breast centers: Part one. Introduction and overview. *J Oncol Manage* 1:20–23, 1992

17. Rabinowitz B: Comprehensive breast centers: Engendering physician involvement. *J Oncol Manage* 3:52–55, 1994

18. Robinson CB, Otte DM: Surgical practice within a comprehensive breast center. *J Oncol Manage* 3:38–40, 1994

19. Tobin E: Assessing needs and developing community partnerships for breast healthcare services. *J Oncol Manage* 3:31–37, 1994

20. Verfurth M: Initiating a breast health awareness program with community African-American women. *J Oncol Manage* 3:24–30, 1994

21. American Hospital Association: *Why Care about Breast Care.* Chicago, American Hospital Association, 1992

22. Harvey CD, Walker JR: Clinical linkages: A model for providing cancer care in a rural setting. *Oncol Issues* 5:11–12, 17, 1990

23. Katterhagen JG, Howe HL, Lehnherr M: Effectiveness of an oncology outreach program. *J Oncol Manage* 2:32–37, 1993

24. Smith TJ, Desch CE, Simonson CJ, et al: Teaching specialty cancer medicine in rural hospitals: The cancer outreach program as a model. *J Cancer Educ* 6:235–240, 1991

25. Tracy R, Saltzman KL, Wakefield DS: Considerations in

establishing visiting consultant clinics in rural hospital communities. *Hosp Health Serv Adm* 41:255–265, 1996

26. Dawson LJ: Telemedicine and its benefits to rural communities. *J Oncol Manage* 4:22–27, 1995

27. Behrend SW, Sklaroff RB: The evolving profile of the office oncology nurse, in Buchsel PC, Yarbro CH (eds): *Oncology Nursing in the Ambulatory Setting: Issues and Models of Care.* Boston, Jones and Bartlett, 1993, pp 73–106

28. Pearce D, Feingold MG: A model hospital-medical oncology alliance: One cancer center's experience. *J Oncol Manage* 2:26–30, 1993

29. Humphrey LJ, Lester P: Cancer prevention and detection centers: An overview and critique. *Semin Surg Oncol* 5:211–218, 1989

30. Walker R, Lucas W, Crespo R: The West Virginia Rural Cancer Prevention Project. *Cancer Pract* 2:421–426, 1994

31. Deisher RD: Multiple benefits of cancer prevention and early detection programs. *Oncol Issues* 10:14–15, 1995

32. Deisher RD: A multihospital screening and early detection program in Kansas City. *Oncol Issues* 10:16–19, 1995

33. Kliban MG: Differentiating a cancer center with programming for cancer survivors. *J Oncol Manage* 2:28–32, 34, 1993

34. Satterwhite BE, Settle JT, Cushnie PB, et al: Ambulatory care for patients with HIV/AIDS: Creating a specialty clinic. *Oncol Nurs Forum* 18:555–558, 1991

35. Loescher LJ: Genetics in cancer prediction, screening, and counseling: Part II. The nurse's role in genetic counseling. *Oncol Nurs Forum* 22:16–19, 1995 (suppl)

36. Peters JA: Familial cancer risk: Part I. Impact on today's oncology practice. *J Oncol Manage* 3:18, 20–26, 28–30, 1994

37. Peters JA: Familial cancer risk: Part II. Breast cancer risk counseling and genetic susceptibility testing. *J Oncol Manage* 3:14–22, 1994

38. Engelking C: New approaches: Innovations in cancer prevention, diagnosis, treatment, and support. *Oncol Nurs Forum* 21:62–71, 1994

39. Uhlenhake R: Is patient-focused outpatient cancer care on target? *J Ambulatory Care Manage* 18:32–42, 1995

40. Reed RA: Creating a healing environment by design. *J Ambulatory Care Manage* 18:16–31, 1995

41. Campbell B, Gries M: Facility design and construction. *Oncol Issues* 10:23–25, 1995

42. Cooley ME, Lin EM, Hunter SW: The ambulatory oncology nurse's role. *Semin Oncol Nurs* 10:245–253, 1994

43. American Academy of Ambulatory Care Nursing: *Ambulatory Care Nursing Administration and Practice Standards.* Pitman, NJ, Janetti, 1993

44. American Nurses' Association, Oncology Nursing Society: *Statement on the Scope and Standards of Oncology Nursing Practice.* Kansas City, MO, American Nurses' Association, 1996

45. Oncology Nursing Society: *Standards of Advanced Practice in Oncology Nursing.* Pittsburgh: Oncology Nursing Press, 1990

46. Joint Commission on Accreditation of Healthcare Organizations: *1996 Comprehensive Accreditation Manual for Hospitals.* Oakbrook Terrace, IL, JCAHO, 1995

47. Joint Commission on Accreditation of Healthcare Organizations: *1996 Comprehensive Accreditation Manual for Ambulatory Care.* Oakbrook Terrace, IL, JCAHO, 1995

48. Tappert TN: Joint commission accreditation for freestanding oncology practices. *Cancer Manage* 1:22–25, 1996

49. Association of Community Cancer Centers: *Standards for Cancer Programs.* Rockville, MD, ACCC, 1993

50. Nevidjon BM: The changing roles of oncology nurses in ambulatory care settings, in Buchsel PC, Yarbro CH (eds): *Oncology Nursing in the Ambulatory Setting: Issues and Models of Care.* Boston, Jones and Bartlett, 1993, pp 21–34

51. Verran JA: Delineation of ambulatory care nursing practice. *J Ambulatory Care Manage* 4:1–13, 1981

52. Tighe MG, Fisher SG, Hastings C, et al: A study of the oncology nurse role in ambulatory care. *Oncol Nurs Forum* 12:23–27, 1985

53. Hastings C, Muir-Nash J: Validation of a taxonomy of ambulatory nursing practice. *Nurs Econ* 7:142–149, 1989

54. Hackbarth DP, Haas SA, Kavanagh JA, et al: Dimensions of the staff nurse role in ambulatory care: Part I. Methodology and analysis of data on current staff nurse practice. *Nurs Econ* 13:89–98, 1995

55. Haas SA, Hackbarth DP, Kavanagh JA, et al: Dimensions of the staff nurse role in ambulatory care: Part II. Comparison of role dimensions in four ambulatory settings. *Nurs Econ* 13:152–165, 1995

56. Shaw SLJ: The role of the nurse in a comprehensive breast center. *J Oncol Manage* 3:49–51, 1994

57. Iwamoto R, Gough S: Radiotherapy: Ambulatory care models, in Buchsel PC, Yarbro CH (eds): *Oncology Nursing in the Ambulatory Setting: Issues and Models of Care.* Boston, Jones and Bartlett, 1993, pp 133–164

58. Giles K: Using clinical financial pathways to capitate cancer. *Oncol Issues* 10:14–17, 1995

59. Neese PY: Organization, updated communications systems, and personal responsibility facilitate patient flow. *Oncol Nurs Forum* 21:1091–1092, 1994

60. Leyden R: Keeping patients informed and involved helps to improve patient flow. *Oncol Nurs Forum* 21:1092, 1994

61. Lin EM, Rigby BJ: A structured self-reporting new patient assessment tool: Guide to oncology nursing practice. *Can Nurs J* 4:72–75, 1994

62. Skinn B, Stacey D: Establishing an integrated framework for documentation: Use of a self-reporting health history and outpatient oncology record. *Oncol Nurs Forum* 21:1557–1566, 1994

63. Haas SA, Hackbarth DP: Dimensions of the staff nurse role in ambulatory care: Part III. Using research data to design new models of nursing care delivery. *Nurs Econ* 13:230–241, 1995

64. Behrend SW: Documentation in the ambulatory setting. *Semin Oncol Nurs* 10:264–280, 1994

65. Barhamand BA: Documentation issues in cancer nursing, in McCorkle R, Grant M, Frank-Stromborg M, Baird SB (eds): *Cancer Nursing: A Comprehensive Textbook,* (ed 2). Philadelphia, Saunders, 1996, pp 1356–1365

66. Davis ME, DeSantis D, Klemm K: A flow sheet for follow-up after chemotherapy extravasation. *Oncol Nurs Forum* 22:979–983, 1995

67. Pfeifer P: Documentation of care in an oncology outpatient setting. *Oncol Nurs Forum* 19:809–818, 1992

68. Youngblood M, Williams PD, Eyles H, et al: A comparison of two methods of assessing cancer therapy–related symptoms. *Cancer Nurs* 17:37–44, 1994

69. Simpson RL: Trends in health-care computing according to CIOs. *Nurs Manage* 26:20–21, 1995

70. Fritz AG: The fragmented cancer record: How did we get to this point? *Oncol Issues* 10:17–20, 1995

71. Tietze MF, Huber JT: Electronic information retrieval in nursing. *Nurs Manage* 26:36–37, 41–42, 1995

72. Simpson RL: "Surfing" the Internet. *Nurs Manage* 26:18–19, 1995

73. Woodworth M, Loochtan A: A road map to cancer resources on the Internet. *Cancer Pract* 4:160–163, 1996

74. Griffiths M, Leek C: Patient education needs: Opinions of oncology nurses and their patients. *Oncol Nurs Forum* 22:139–144, 1995

75. Siegel M, Patyk M: A new approach to cancer education: The Cancer Information Channel. *J Oncol Manage* 2:29–33, 1993

76. Stephens ST: Patient education materials: Are they readable? *Oncol Nurs Forum* 19:83–85, 1992

77. Meade CD, Diekmann J, Thornhill D: Readability of American Cancer Society patient education literature. *Oncol Nurs Forum* 19:51–55, 1992

78. Michielutte R, Bahnson J, Beal P: Readability of the public education literature on cancer prevention and detection. *J Cancer Educ* 5:55–61, 1990

79. Cooley ME, Moriarty H, Berger MS, et al: Patient literacy and the readability of written cancer educational materials. *Oncol Nurs Forum* 22:1345–1350, 1995

80. Houts PS, Rusenas I, Simmonds MA, et al: Information needs of families of cancer patients: A literature review and recommendations. *J Cancer Educ* 6:255–261, 1991

81. Gyauch TM: Implementing a cancer education program for family and friend caregivers. *J Oncol Manage* 4:18–22, 1995

82. Weaver J: Patient education: An innovative computer approach. *Nurs Manage* 26:78–80, 83, 1995

83. DeMuth JS: Patient teaching in the ambulatory setting. *Nurs Clin North Am* 24:645–654, 1989

84. Hinds C, Streater A, Mood D: Functions and preferred methods of receiving information related to radiotherapy: Perceptions of patients with cancer. *Cancer Nurs* 18:374–384, 1995

85. Poroch D: The effect of preparatory patient education on the anxiety and satisfaction of cancer patients receiving radiation therapy. *Cancer Nurs* 18:206–214, 1995

86. Hagopian GA: The effects of informational audiotapes on knowledge and self-care behaviors of patients undergoing radiation therapy. *Oncol Nurs Forum* 23:697–700, 1996

87. Hagopian GA: The effects of a weekly radiation therapy newsletter on patients. *Oncol Nurs Forum* 18:1199–1203, 1991

88. Oncology Nursing Society: *Standards of Oncology Education: Patient/Family and Public.* Pittsburgh, Oncology Nursing Press, 1995

89. Dodd MJ: Self-care and patient/family teaching, in Groenwald SL, Frogge MH, Goodman M, Yarbro CH (eds): *Cancer Symptom Management.* Boston, Jones and Bartlett, 1996, pp 19–26

90. Goldstein NL: Patient learning center reduces patient readmissions. *Patient Educ Couns* 17:177–190, 1991

91. Walker FE, Roethke SK, Sandman V, et al: Guiding patients and their families through peripheral stem cell transplantation with the help of a teaching booklet. *Oncol Nurs Forum* 21:771–773, 1994

92. Mayer DK, Linscott E: Information for women: Management of menopausal symptoms. *Oncol Nurs Forum* 22:1567–1570, 1995

93. Neumark DE: Providing information about advance directives to patients in ambulatory care and their families. *Oncol Nurs Forum* 21:771–773, 1994

94. Mahon SM: Educating women about early detection of gynecologic cancers using a brochure. *Oncol Nurs Forum* 23:529–535, 1996

95. Straw LJ, Conrad KJ: Patient education resources related to biotherapy and the immune system. *Oncol Nurs Forum* 21:1223–1228, 1994

96. Barhamand BA: Optimizing the use of the telephone for oncology nurses in office practices, in Carroll-Johnson RM (ed): *Meeting the Expanding Needs of the Office-Based Oncology Nurse.* Pittsburgh, Oncology Nursing Press, 1992, pp 8–14

97. Spurck PA, Mohr ML, Seroka AM, et al: The impact of a wireless telecommunication system on time efficiency. *J Nurs Adm* 25:21–26, 1995

98. Hagopian GA, Rubenstein JH: Effects of telephone call interventions on patients' well-being in a radiation therapy department. *Cancer Nurs* 13:339–344, 1990

99. Katterhagen JG, Patton M: Critical pathways in oncology: Balancing the interests of hospitals and the physician. *J Oncol Manage* 2:20, 23–26, 1993

100. Burns JM, Tierney K, Long GD, et al: Critical pathway for administering high-dose chemotherapy followed by peripheral blood stem cell rescue in the outpatient setting. *Oncol Nurs Forum* 22:1219–1224, 1995

101. Hawkins J, Goldberg PB: Planning, implementing and evaluating a chemotherapy critical pathway. *J Oncol Manage* 3:24–29, 1994

102. Stair J: Oncology critical pathways. *Oncol Issues* 10:17–21, 1995

103. Stanfill PH: Cost-efficiencies in the oncology program: Strategies for survival. *J Oncol Manage* 4:18, 23–25, 1995

104. Taban HA, Cesta TG: Evaluating the effectiveness of case management plans. *J Nurs Adm* 25:58–63, 1995

105. Stahl DA: Critical pathways in subacute care. *Nurs Manage* 26:16–18, 1995

106. Micheletti JA, Shlala TJ: Understanding and operationalizing subacute services. *Nurs Manage* 26:49, 51–52, 54–56, 1995

107. Meister S, Rodts B, Gothard J, et al: Home Care Steps℠ protocols: Home care's answer to changes in reimbursement. *J Nurs Adm* 25:33–42, 1995

108. Hagland, M: Interview with Richard Doyle. *Hosp Health Netw,* Dec. 5, 1995 p. 47

109. Stair J: The present and future of guideline development. *Oncol Issues* 10:26–28, 1995

110. White RL: The Patterns of Care Study in radiation oncology. *Oncol Issues* 10:29, 1995

111. Mortenson LE, Harrigan EE: ACCC's guideline initiative. *Oncol Issues* 10:30–31, 1995

112. Kurowski B: Cancer carve-outs: Can they fulfill the promise of managed care. *Oncol Issues* 9:10–13, 1994

113. Association of Community Cancer Centers: *Oncology Critical Pathways.* Rockville, MD: Association of Community Cancer Centers, 1995

114. Aspling DL, Lagoe R: Benchmarking for clinical pathways in hospitals: A summary of sources. *Nurs Econ* 14:92–97, 1996

115. Comried LA: Cost analysis: Initiation of HBMC and first CareMap℠. *Nurs Econ* 14:34–39, 1996

116. Walter JM, Robinson SH: Nursing care delivery models in ambulatory oncology. *Semin Oncol Nurs* 10:237–244, 1994

117. Schaffner JW, Ludwig-Beymer P, Wiggins J: Utilization of advanced practice nurses in healthcare systems and multi-specialty group practice. *J Nurs Adm* 25:37–43, 1995

118. Farley B: Primary nursing in the oncology ambulatory setting. *Nurs Adm Q* 6(4):44–53, 1981

119. Lamb GS: Conceptual and methodological issues in nurse case management research. *Adv Nurs Sci* 15:16–24, 1992

120. Zander K: Nursing case management: Resolving the DRG paradox. *Nurs Clin North Am* 23:503–520, 1988

121. Koerner BL: Clarifying the role of nursing in ambulatory care. *J Ambulatory Care Manage* 10:1–7, 1987

122. Haas SA, Hackbarth DP: Dimensions of the staff nurse role in ambulatory care: Part IV. Developing nursing intensity measures, standards, clinical ladders, and QI programs. *Nurs Econ* 13:285–294, 1995

123. Prescott PA, Soeken KL: Measuring nursing intensity in ambulatory care: Part I. Approaches to and use of patient classification systems. *Nurs Econ* 14:14–21, 33, 1996

124. Medvec BR: Productivity and workload measurement in ambulatory oncology. *Semin Oncol Nurs* 10:288–295, 1994

125. Goldfield N: Ambulatory encounter systems: Implications for payment and quality. *J Ambulatory Care Manage* 16:33–49, 1993

126. Prescott PA, Soeken KL: Measuring nursing intensity in ambulatory care: Part II. Developing and testing PINAC. *Nurs Econ* 14:86–91, 116, 1996

127. Riley MA, Seidner S: Developing an ambulatory care productivity and patient charge system. *Oncol Issues* 9:14–16, 1994

128. Martin VR: Administrative issues in ambulatory oncology care. *Semin Oncol Nurs* 10:296–305, 1994

129. Mortenson LE, Miller CS: Economic considerations in ambulatory care, in Buchsel PC, Yarbro CH (eds): *Oncology Nursing in the Ambulatory Setting: Issues and Models of Care*. Boston, Jones and Bartlett, 1993, pp 35–48

130. Wodinsky H, Lion J, Elliott J: Outpatient cancer visit groups: A preliminary report on work in progress in Ontario, Canada. *Oncol Issues* 7:12–16, 1992

131. Goldfield NI, Averill RF: The development of an outpatient prospective payment system for oncologic services in America. *Oncol Issues* 7:10–11, 1992

132. Androwich I, Hastings C: A practical approach to developing system performance indicators. *Nurs Econ* 14:174–179, 1996

133. Miller ST, Flanagan E: The transition from quality assurance to continuous quality improvement in ambulatory care. *Qual Rev Bull* 19:62–65, 1993

134. Hardy VS, Forrer J: A comprehensive quality management approach. *Nurs Manage* 27:35, 38–39, 1996

135. Wiklund M, Sedin JL, Hill TJ: Quality improvement in ambulatory care: A network approach to quality improvement. *J Healthc Qual* 14:16–22, 1992

136. Marder RJ: Measuring the quality of care for the cancer patient. *Cancer* 67:1753–1758, 1991

137. Miaskowski C: Future trends in ambulatory care nursing, in Buchsel PC, Yarbro CH (eds): *Oncology Nursing in the Ambulatory Setting: Issues and Models of Care*. Boston, Jones and Bartlett, 1993, pp 341–351

138. Malone MP, Pollock EL: Monitoring patient satisfaction. *Oncol Issues* 10:19–21, 1995

139. Kertesz L: Patient is king: Studies define customers' satisfaction and the means to improve it. *Modern Healthc* 69(23):107–108, 112–114, 116, 118, 120, 1996

140. *Occupational Safety and Health Administration Technical Manual*. Section V: Health-Care Facilities. Chapter 3: Controlling Occupational Exposure to Hazardous Drugs. OSHA Instruction TED 1.15, Sept. 22, 1995. Washington, DC, Bureau of National Affairs, 1995

141. Oncology Nursing Society: *Cancer Chemotherapy Guidelines and Recommendations for Practice*. Pittsburgh: Oncology Nursing Press, 1996

142. Occupational Safety and Health Administration: Occupational exposure to bloodborne pathogens, final rule (29 CFR Part 1910.1030). *Federal Register* 56 (Dec. 6): 1991

143. Parillo VL: Documentation forms for monitoring occupational surveillance of healthcare workers who handle cytotoxic drugs. *Oncol Nurs Forum* 21:115–120, 1994

144. Shortridge LA, Lemasters GK, Valanis B, et al: Menstrual cycles in nurses handling antineoplastic drugs. *Cancer Nurs* 18:439–444, 1995

145. Beddar SM, Aikin JL: Continuity of care: A challenge for ambulatory oncology nursing. *Semin Oncol Nurs* 10:254–263, 1994

146. Pluth NM: Continuity of cancer care for patients and families through health care systems, in Buchsel PC, Yarbro CH (eds): *Oncology Nursing in the Ambulatory Setting: Issues and Models of Care*. Boston, Jones and Bartlett, 1993, pp 49–70

147. Winstead-Fry P, Bormolini S, Keech RR: Clinical care coordination program: A working partnership. *J Nurs Adm* 25:46–51, 1995

148. Case CL, Jones LH: Continuity of care: Development and implementation of a shared patient data base. *Cancer Nurs* 12:332–338, 1989

149. Hendrickson G, Kelly JB, Citrin L: Computers in oncology nursing: Present use and future potential. *Oncol Nurs Forum* 18:715–723, 1991

150. Kerstetter NC: A stepwise approach to developing and maintaining an oncology multidisciplinary conference. *Cancer Nurs* 13:216–220, 1990

151. Haberman MR: Research in ambulatory care settings: The need for and how to do research, in Buchsel PC, Yarbro CH (eds): *Oncology Nursing in the Ambulatory Setting: Issues and Models of Care*. Boston, Jones and Bartlett, 1993, pp 307–340

152. Fitch MI, Thompson L: Fostering the growth of research-based oncology nursing practice. *Oncol Nurs Forum* 23:631–637, 1996

153. Orem DE: *Nursing: Concepts of Practice* (ed 3). New York, McGraw-Hill, 1985

154. Fieler VK, Nail LM, Greene D, et al: Patients' use of prevention behaviors in managing side effects related to chemotherapy. *Oncol Nurs Forum* 22:713–716, 1995

155. Nail LM, Jones LS, Greene D, et al: Use the perceived efficacy of self-care activities in patients receiving chemotherapy. *Oncol Nurs Forum* 18:883–887, 1991

156. Brinkman P, Hay D, Laubinger P: Chemotherapy toxicity assessment using a self-report tool. *Oncol Nurs Forum* 21:1731–1733, 1994

157. Brandt B: Informational needs and selected variables in patients receiving brachytherapy. *Oncol Nurs Forum* 18:1221–1229, 1991

158. Goodman M, Blendowski C, Stewart I, et al: Kits help with patient care. *Oncol Nurs Forum* 21:1250, 1994

159. Carey PJ, Oberst MT, McCubbin MA, et al: Appraisal and caregiving burden in family members caring for patients receiving chemotherapy. *Oncol Nurs Forum* 18:1341–1348, 1991

160. Yeager KA, Miaskowski C, Dibble SL, et al: Differences in pain knowledge and perception of the pain experience between outpatients with cancer and their family caregivers. *Oncol Nurs Forum* 22:1235–1241, 1995

161. Klein-Alexander C: Cancer resource libraries: A way to empower cancer patients. *J Oncol Manage* 2:28–30, 32–35, 1993

162. Montbriand MJ: Decision tree model describing alternate

health care choices made by oncology patients. *Cancer Nurs* 18:104–117, 1995

163. Kristjanson LJ, Ashcroft T: The family's cancer journey: A literature review. *Cancer Nurs* 17:1–17, 1994

164. Buchsel PC: Administrative issues of an ambulatory care setting, in Buchsel PC, Whedon MB (eds): *Bone Marrow Transplantation: Administrative and Clinical Strategies.* Boston, Jones and Bartlett, 1995, pp 19–38

165. Merrill JM: Access to high-tech health care. *Cancer* 67: 1750–1752, 1991

166. Bal DG: Prevention and changing demographics: The underserved and cancer. *Cancer* 67:1814–1816, 1991

167. Franklin MA: Creating a managed-care product for cancer services. *J Oncol Manage* 3:19–26, 1994

168. Xistris DM, Houlihan NG: Impact of reimbursement and health care reform on the ambulatory oncology setting. *Semin Oncol Nurs* 10:281–287, 1994

169. Porter HB: The effect of ambulatory oncology nursing practice models on health resource utilization: Part 1. Collaboration or compliance? *J Nurs Adm* 25:21–29, 1995

170. Porter HB: The effect of ambulatory oncology nursing practice models on health resource utilization: Part 2. Different practice models—Different use of health resources? *J Nurs Adm* 25:15–22, 1995

171. Boyle DM: New identities: The changing profile of patients with cancer, their families, and their professional caregivers. *Oncol Nurs Forum* 21:55–61, 1994

172. Feingold MG, Meyer JW, Briggs DS: Controlling cost and quality through clinical pathways: One cancer center's experience. *Oncol Issues* 6:24–28, 31, 1991

173. Rudolf VM: Oncology nursing protocols: A step toward autonomy. *Oncol Nurs Forum* 16:643–647, 1989

174. Shackelford-Akers PA: An algorithmic approach to clinical decision making. *Oncol Nurs Forum* 18:1159–1163, 1991

175. Boyle DM, Engelking, C, Blesch KS, et al: Oncology Nursing Society position paper on cancer and aging: The mandate for oncology nursing. *Oncol Nurs Forum* 19:913–933, 1992

176. Curran CR: An interview with Mary Ann Moore. *Nurs Econ* 10:87–93, 1992

# Chapter 53

# Home Care

Joan C. McNally, RN, MSN, OCN®, CRNH

## OVERVIEW OF HOME HEALTH CARE

The dramatic changes occurring in the health care delivery system have significantly impacted home health care. Home health care is one of the most rapidly growing and changing fields in health care. The Health Care Financing Administration (HCFA) reports that the number of persons receiving Medicare home health services increased from 49 per 1000 enrollees in 1988 to 79 per 1000 enrollees in 1993. Visits also increased from 24 to 57 per person during this same five-year period, which resulted in a 400% increase in Medicare program expenditures for home health services totaling to $9.7 billion in 1993.[1] The National Association for Home Care (NAHC) reported a 12.3% increase in the number of home health agencies, from 5785 in 1988 to approximately 6497 in 1993.[2] In addition, HCFA projects that Medicare program expenditures will be $20.8 billion in the year 2000 and $29.4 billion in 2005.[3] This precipitous growth occurred after revisions in the *Medicare Home Health Agency Manual* (HAM) in 1989 expanded eligibility and coverage of home health services.[4] Other factors that have influenced the consumption of health care services include enactment of the prospective payment system (PPS) for hospital care in 1982, which resulted in shortened hospital stays, discharge of acutely ill patients, and the shift from hospital- to community-based care; the increase in the elderly population and their increased life span; changes in family structure with more women working outside the home; and decreasing support from family members who traditionally have provided the care needed to enable the elderly to remain at home. Efforts by payers to control national health expenditures have resulted in the emergence of managed care organizations to reduce unnecessary utilization and control costs of health care.[5] Although only 11.2% of Medicare beneficiaries were enrolled in managed care plans in June 1996, the Medicare program is expected to expand their program of cost containment.[6]

As defined by insurance eligibility guidelines, care at home can be preventive, diagnostic, therapeutic, rehabilitative, or long-term maintenance care. Home health care is an extension of the medical care system in which a physician oversees the care and the nurse is a primary provider and care manager through collaboration with the patient's physician. From the patient's point of view, home care seems to be the most efficient, effective, and least traumatic form of care, supported by the full range of multidisciplinary services.[7]

## Home Care Services

The goals of home health care are to promote, maintain, or restore health; to minimize the effects of illness and disability; or to allow for a peaceful death. Home health care provides short-term intermittent services to enhance the knowledge and skill of the patient and family in managing care. The services provided depend on the needs of the individual and the family. The traditional services covered by Medicare reimbursement and provided by certified home health agencies include nursing, physical therapy, speech and language pathology, medical social work, occupational therapy, home health aide services, and nutrition therapy.

### Nursing

Nursing is the foundation of home health care. Historically, nursing was the first health service to be provided in the home, and it remains the one most frequently utilized. Federal legislation has reinforced the position of nursing in home health care by requiring that nursing services be available in all home health agencies certified to receive Medicare or Medicaid funds. The nurse is the coordinator of all home care provided to the patient. Home care nursing responsibilities include assessment, direct physical care, evaluation of patient progress, patient and family teaching, supervision and coordination of patient care, and provision of psychosocial support. In 1989, nursing services were expanded to include assessment of patients who were likely to have a change in their health status and for management and evaluation of the plan of care for patients with multiple diagnoses.[4] Home health care nursing differs from private duty nursing in that care is provided on an intermittent basis rather than daily or for extended time periods. Previously, home nursing care was available only during daytime hours; however, 24-hour availability of home nursing care is now the norm.

### Homemaker–home health aide

The availability of homemaker–home health aide service is often the factor that determines whether a patient and family can opt for home care. The National Council for Homemaker–Home Health Aide Services defines responsibilities of the home health aide to include assistance with personal hygiene and homemaking tasks. The home health aide must have successfully completed a home health aide training course or have passed the home health aide competency evaluation written and skills test. The aide is supervised by the home health nurse, who is responsible for developing a plan of care with specific instructions for services to be provided by the home health aide to the patient. Under the direction of the nurse, the home health aide may assist the patient and family to perform treatments (e.g., wound care or ambulation exercises). The aide may perform personal care activities for the patient such as feeding, bathing, and grooming.

### Physical therapy

Physical therapists provide therapy for patients at home to treat their illness or injury or for restoration or maintenance of function that has been affected by the illness or injury. For example, physical therapy can be effective in restoring function compromised by brain tumor or pathological bone fracture or in developing a maintenance program of therapy to ensure medical safety of cancer patients in the home and prevent further deterioration. The physical therapist also instructs patients and caregivers in implementation of maintenance therapies.

### Occupational therapy

Occupational therapists assist patients to achieve their highest functional level and to be as self-reliant as possible. They can teach patients adaptive techniques and the use of adaptive equipment to improve their level of independence in activities essential to daily living. Occupational therapists provide preprosthetic and prosthetic training. They also assist in the selection or construction of splints to correct or prevent a deformity.

### Speech and language pathology

Speech and language pathologists provide therapy to individuals with communication problems of speech, language, or hearing or those with swallowing disorders. A major treatment goal is to facilitate maximum speech and language recovery and to enable patients to achieve a higher level of communicative abilities. The speech and language pathologist may also develop an effective maintenance therapy plan and instruct patients and caregivers in the implementation of the plan.

### Social work

Social workers in the home care setting have traditionally been considered referral agents who have knowledge of and access to the available community resources, particularly those involving money. Although this is one aspect of their role, equally important in home health are the social worker's roles as counselor and patient advocate. Counseling services to resolve social and emotional problems are often essential in promoting recovery and rehabilitation of the person with cancer.

### Nutrition services

The role of the nutritionist in home health care encompasses direct patient care through diet counseling and indirect care through staff consultation and education about dietary practices. In most instances, direct care is often secondary to consultation and staff education because few third-party insurers will reimburse for direct patient counseling by the nutritionist at home.

### Additional care services

In addition to the traditional services provided by certified home health agencies, a diverse assortment of services for the patient in the home are provided by physicians, dentists, chiropodists, respiratory therapists, vocational rehabilitation personnel, barbers, hairdressers, in-home companions, and homemaker/chore workers. Laboratory specimens can be obtained, radiographs taken, meals delivered, and transportation provided for the patient in the home. Home maintenance and repair services are also usually available.[8] Some supplemental services may require payment by the individual requesting them. However, some may be available from community service organizations at a reduced rate (e.g., Meals on Wheels from church groups, transportation from cancer societies) or covered by the patient's insurance if approved by the case manager.

## Types of Home Care Agencies

In a similar context, many types of organizations provide home care service. Selection of the most appropriate type of home care agency is based primarily on patient and family needs, the patient's financial arrangement or type of health insurance coverage, availability of family and community support, as well as the type of home care services available in the patient's community. Three classifications of agencies provide home care services: the official agency of the public health departments, Medicare-certified home health agencies, and private duty agencies.

### Official public health agencies

Official agencies are organized and administered within city, county, or multicounty health departments. Historically, the major focus of official health agencies has been preventive health care and infectious disease control. As such, home nursing care consists of biweekly or monthly home visits for patient teaching and supervision rather than direct physical care. State and local tax revenues fund the health department's traditional health promotion and disease prevention programs.

A number of official public health departments have

expanded the scope of their services and have developed Medicare-certified home health agencies. These operate as separate entities within their organizations.

### Medicare-certified home health agencies

Home health agencies, structured and operating within the specific guidelines defined by the HCFA in the Conditions of Participation, may be certified to participate in the federal health insurance program.[9] When certified, the home health agency is reimbursed for services provided to Medicare patients if those services are provided within their guidelines.

Medicare certification also authorizes the home health agency to provide and be reimbursed for services to Medicaid patients if those services are provided within the guidelines defined by each state for home care for the indigent. Medicare certification of a home health agency is also usually required by private insurance companies before reimbursement for home care services will be considered.

Medicare-certified home health agencies may be facility-based (i.e., hospital [27%], skilled nursing facility [2%]) or may be freestanding (i.e., visiting nurse association [7%], public [13%], proprietary [43%], private nonprofit [8%]).[2] Many health care systems have integrated home health agencies within the parent organization (e.g., the medical center and hospitals have a certified Medicare home health agency division to provide a continuum of care across several settings).

### Private duty agencies

Private duty agencies provide nursing care in the home by registered nurses, licensed practical nurses, home health aides, or companions for specific periods of time (e.g., 4, 8, 12, or 24 hours per day). The services may be contracted and paid by the patient or family or arranged through a case manager from the patient's health insurance company. These private duty agencies are often large, national, for-profit organizations.

### Other agencies

As home care agencies have become more comprehensive in scope, other agencies have emerged, such as durable medical equipment (DME) companies and infusion therapy agencies. DME companies provide medical equipment and supplies, including respiratory equipment, ostomy appliances, and parenteral feedings and supplies. Many DME companies have professional staff who teach and monitor the patient's ability to use equipment appropriately. Infusion therapy agencies provide parenteral medications (e.g., antibiotics, antineoplastics), total parenteral nutritional feedings, parenteral solutions, infusion devices, and equipment necessary for provision of infusion therapy at home. Most agencies

maintain a pharmacy and professional nursing staff to administer medications and fluids and to teach self-administration to the patient and family. Frequently the complex care requirements of the patient with cancer necessitate collaboration between the home health nurse and infusion therapy nurse to avoid fragmentation of care and to ensure comprehensive home care services.

## Continuity of Care

Continuity of care has been described as a complex interaction of the patient with a variety of health professionals, clinics, institutions, agencies, and systems with the objective of restoring bodily and psychosocial functions to an optimum potential and preventing additional dysfunction and inconvenience.[10] This multidisciplinary coordinated care must be provided throughout the continuum of disease if quality care is to be achieved. The most frequently used processes to ensure a comprehensive multidisciplinary approach to patient care are case management and discharge planning.

### Case management

Case management is a multidisciplinary approach to the process of identifying high-risk patients' needs and coordinating the appropriate use of resources to achieve identified patient care outcomes at a reduced cost across several settings of care.[11] Case management has been defined by the American Nurses' Association (ANA)[12] as a health care delivery process with the goals of providing quality health care, decreasing fragmentation, enhancing the patient's quality of life, and containing cost. The benefits of case management in the inpatient setting are a decrease in length of stay, coordination of resources for discharge, and facilitating communication among the disciplines.[13] A decrease in repeated hospitalization and an increase in the ability of patients to perform self-care and to access support when needed were noted in the home setting.[14] Increased patient and physician satisfaction was noted in both settings. The case manager may be a nurse from the hospital, clinic, insurance company, or home health agency who may follow the patient through the continuum of his or her illness or disease.[15]

### Discharge planning

Discharge planning is an interdisciplinary approach that centers on the family or significant other to facilitate the transition of the patient from one level of care to another, usually from the hospital to home. Discharge planning can enhance continuity of care through appropriate use of health care and community resources.[16]

The case management/discharge planning process begins with a comprehensive assessment of patient needs and the patient's and family's ability to comply with the treatment plans and cope with the disease. The patient's and family's perspective should be included as well as the observations and evaluations of professionals who have provided care to the patient. Assessment parameters include diagnosis, age, treatments, care requirements, functional limitations, cognitive abilities, interpersonal relationships with family members, concurrent illness of the patient or family members, usual coping mechanisms, financial and insurance resources, knowledge of disease and treatments, cultural factors, and social support systems.[10] The patient's diagnosis alone may not reflect the degree of illness, the complexity of care, or the number of support personnel required to assist the person at home. In some cases the physical facilities may be adequate and the family supportive, but the emotional adjustments and 24-hour commitment to provide care may overwhelm the patient and family, thus necessitating admission to an extended care facility. For others, caring for a loved one at home may be a positive experience that enables the family to function in its natural environment while providing ongoing patient care.

Cost-containment measures have resulted in the early discharge of cancer patients with highly complex treatment plans that must be managed in the home. It is expected that families will assume a significant increase in responsibility for the patient's care. Thus, in the current health care environment, patient and family involvement is essential for developing a plan for posthospital care and the successful implementation of posthospital treatment.[17] The majority of hospitalized patients with cancer whose situations are appropriate for home care have problems that include difficulty with eating, walking/ mobility, and breathing; complicated oral medication regimens; and pain.[18] Palliation of symptoms and pain control are major home care issues. Home care is indicated for patients with self-care difficulties (either temporary or long-term), those who lack knowledge in managing the direct effects and side effects of cancer treatments, or those who are homebound and require treatments (e.g., chemotherapy, antibiotics, or total parenteral nutrition).

Studies indicate that patients with inadequate or no support system, inadequate financial resources, poor environmental conditions, inability to carry out a treatment and medication regimen, inability to carry out activities of daily living, poor socialization, or anticipated problems resulting from one of these factors require posthospital care. The potential for success in home care is increased if the types of home health services necessary to assist with the supervision and management of the patient and adequate informal support are available.[19,20] Buehler and Lee[21] reported that in rural areas there are limited and inadequate health care resources available to support the patient with cancer and assist the family. O'Hare et al[22] noted that low-income, urban, black Americans with cancer were most likely to have unmet personal care and housekeeping needs and a high degree of distress from the symptoms of the disease. Family members can usually

manage well if they know that a home care nurse will be accessible to provide direction and assistance. The degree of informal support available also affects the family's ability to manage home care. *Informal support* refers to support systems such as friends, neighbors, and church groups. Assistance may range from check-in phone calls or running errands to providing the caregivers with respite by staying with the ill person.

The continuing care plan developed by the discharge planner or case manager in the acute care setting includes outcomes based on essential assessment data and interventions that address the patient's overall care needs. To promote continuity of care, it is essential to have effective communication between the referring professionals (e.g., discharge planner, case manager, clinic nurse) and the community service agency staff (e.g., home health nurse) who are caring for the patient during the next phase of care. In addition, timely reports of the patient's status promote quality patient care as the patient moves through the health care system.

## Unique Characteristics of the Home

The home is an important setting of care for the chronically or terminally ill, as well as for patients requiring sophisticated technological services. The home presents the nurse with conditions unlike those encountered in other health care settings. The protective environment and control the clinic or hospital provides the professional are absent. In the home the patient and family determine when and how the patient's plan of care will be implemented.

The patient and family are encouraged to assume responsibility for the care of the patient; this is the overall goal of home care. When an individual or family member states how things will be done, it reflects a desire to maintain independence. Lewis[23] examined the association between personal control and quality of life for individuals with late-stage cancer and demonstrated that greater personal control over an individual's life was associated with higher levels of self-esteem, lower self-reported anxiety, and more purpose in life.

It is critical that the home health nurse evaluate the physical and financial conditions to support the care required by the patient at home. Environmental barriers to safe care, including lack of utilities and equipment to provide for hygiene and the storage and preparation of food, or the presence of vermin are within the scope of the home health nurse's assessment. Inadequate health care coverage and financial limitations may prohibit leasing modern medical equipment or purchasing adequate medical supplies and pharmaceuticals. The nurse can assist the family in obtaining wheelchairs, walkers, and electric beds from community loan programs and teach the family aseptic techniques and proper handling of reusable medical supplies such as glass syringes and feeding tubes.

## ROLE OF THE NURSE IN HOME HEALTH

When home care nursing began in the 1890s, the role of the nurse was to provide nursing care to the sick and teach families cleanliness, proper care of the sick, and measures to promote health.[24] The advances in treatment of disease and changes in reimbursement of health care services have shifted the focus of home care nursing in the 1990s to one that emphasizes care of the acutely ill patient in the home. Nursing remains in the unique position to contribute to the care of the home health patient and the caregiver through advocacy, counseling, teaching, and direct care.[25]

### The Patient and Family as the Unit of Care

The cancer patient at home is an integral member of a unique system—the family. For home health nursing care to be successful, the nurse assesses the family's structure and processes, develops a plan of care that is congruent with the family's values and lifestyle, and includes the patient and family in the decision-making process.[26]

Speese-Owens[27] identified three types of family units: supportive, ambivalent, and hostile. The way a family functioned in the past is generally the way it will confront the current crisis of cancer. When a family member is faced with the threat of a potentially fatal disease, it is thought that people will forgive old behaviors, forget past misunderstandings, and band together for a common cause. This may occur in some families but not in many. Knowledge of the family's response to previous crises can provide insight into the family's basic coping patterns.[28] Family behavior can be described in terms of cohesion, adaptability, and communication. *Family cohesion* is the emotional bonding that members have with one another. *Family adaptability* is the ability of the system to change its power structure, role relationships, and relationship rules in response to situational and developmental stress. *Family communication* is a facilitator; it can enhance or restrict movement on the cohesion and adaptability dimensions. Family organization is influenced by communication processes, such as decision making and problem solving. Family coping is an indicator of family health.[29] Healthy family systems adjust to life changes and transitions by implementing functional strategies to utilize internal and external resources.

### Family assessment

As the communication link with the health care system, the home health nurse assesses family structure and processes to design interventions that mobilize a family's internal resources and receptivity to external resources. Assessment of the family begins with the patient's family of origin to obtain a history of family functioning. Family members' ages, geographic location, socioeconomic sta-

tus, cultural and ethnic background, roles, relationship to patient, developmental level, major stressors, alliances, and frictions are identified.[30]

The present living group, if different from the family of origin, is then assessed. In addition to the previous criteria, the assessment includes patterns of authority, level of family development, values, behavior, coping ability, health and functional status, stressors, support systems, and knowledge of the illness and health practices.

The following questions should be addressed during assessment of the family:

1. *Structure:* What is the composition of the family? Who is living in the household, and how are the household activities distributed? What family members live outside the home? Are there young children at home? Is the caregiver's role that of parent, requiring time and energy? The nurse can assist the family to redefine roles and redistribute household tasks or responsibilities.

2. *Pattern of authority:* Who is the decision maker? It is important to identify the persons in authority to facilitate patient care.

3. *Level of family development:* What is the level of family development that is being interrupted or affected? Families have certain developmental tasks that, if successfully completed, confer a sense of accomplishment and growth. For example, a young couple addresses the developmental tasks of establishing a household and planning for a family. A cancer diagnosis for either spouse disrupts the ability of the couple to achieve the identified tasks. Understanding and acknowledging the larger impact of a cancer diagnosis on the family can assist in the development of alternate acceptable goals for an intervening time period.

4. *Values:* What are the family's health care values? The caregiver who values health promotion is more likely to perform tasks to prevent problems than the individual whose orientation is that of illness or problem management. To promote optimal functioning of the patient, determine family activities that are important and will provide direction for care. For instance, if dinner taken together as a family is valued, nursing interventions are directed at facilitating this goal (e.g., obtaining necessary ambulation aids to enable the individual to get to the dining room).

5. *Behavior:* Do coordination and cohesion exist between various family members? Which members work together? What is the general pattern of family activities? Do family members do things together?

6. *Coping ability:* What are the strengths of the family and its individual members? What is the meaning of the cancer event to the family? How vulnerable is the family unit to a crisis event (such as cancer) related to the ability of family members to modify their respective roles, perform tasks essential for the continuity of family life, and redefine personal expectations and goals?[28] If a mo-

ther's cancer interferes with her adolescent daughter's autonomy and peer relationships because the teenager is depended upon to participate in care, the daughter may become a resentful or unwilling caregiver. The complexity of patient and family problems can sometimes overwhelm and immobilize the family. The nurse can assist members to identify measures to alter the experience and cope more effectively.

**7.** *Health and functional status:* What is the health and functional status of the caregiver(s)? Because 24-hour care of a loved one is physically and emotionally taxing, attention to the health of the caregiver(s) is imperative. Assessment also includes the caregiver's physical ability to perform the necessary tasks or procedures (such as lifting, moving, or transferring).

**8.** *Stressors:* Are there stressors outside of the individual's illness that may affect the family? Additional burdens that the family may be carrying are often overlooked by health care professionals in the face of a potentially fatal illness of one family member. However, these outside stressors may interfere with the delivery of care to the patient (e.g., a daughter who relieves the caregiver on weekends becomes ill) or with the energy level and emotional ability of the family to cope with the cancer experience.

**9.** *Support systems:* What outside support systems and assistance are available to the family? Patients and families are reluctant to ask for help or may not be aware of available community support or resources. The nurse can help the family identify and gather support in an attempt to prevent or diminish caregiver fatigue.

**10.** *Knowledge of illness and health practices:* What is the family's level of comprehension related to health practices? Because family members provide the majority of care, an assessment of their cognitive skills is necessary for the nurse to develop strategies to teach the caregivers the necessary patient care.

### Demands on caregivers

In several studies exploring the demands on primary caregivers of adult cancer patients, most caregivers reported that the patient's daily physical needs were being met by immediate relatives and close friends.[31–33] The problems most often identified were a lack of knowledge in management of the patient's physical symptoms and psychological needs as well as measures to assist the caregiver in coping with his or her role. Caregivers have reported a decrease in their abilities to cope when changes occur in the patient's health status. In addition, feelings of despair, isolation, vulnerability, and helplessness often negatively affect their coping abilities.

The financial burden on the family of a patient with cancer has increased significantly as patient care shifts from the acute care setting to the home setting.[33] Family costs include direct out-of-pocket cash expenditures for services, medications, and transportation that were either

not covered or only partially covered by third-party payers. The indirect costs of caring for a cancer patient at home include loss of caregiver earnings and cost of family labor expended to care for the patient at home. Stommel et al[34] reports that when cost of family labor is included, the average cost to the family caring for a patient with cancer at home for a three-month period is $4313. Table 53-1 lists the home care situations that have been identified as evoking the greatest stress for families and caregivers.

To enhance the family's ability to care for a patient at home, the home health nurse must function in two significant areas: nursing care that contributes to the physical well-being of the patient and nursing care that provides the patient and family with reassurance and practical and emotional support.[35] Nursing interventions that foster cohesion of the family and strengthen interaction, communication, cooperation, and emotional involvement will decrease isolation and enable the family to increase its autonomy and stability. Directing nursing intervention toward daily problem solving decreases the helplessness that families feel. Hohl[36] reported that patients cared for by a home health agency perceived their care as satisfactory in 95% of the surveys returned.

The nursing intervention most often cited by patients and caregivers as the most helpful is for the nurse to give excellent, knowledgeable, skilled, and personalized nursing care to the patient.[37–39] Other interventions reported to be helpful are listed in Table 53-2.

## Implementation of the Nursing Process

Today's home health nurse is expected to apply knowledge of the biological, social, and behavioral sciences to the nursing process, including a systematic assessment of patient and family needs, defining the characteristics of patient problems, formulating nursing diagnoses, developing and implementing the plan of care, and evaluating the outcomes of care.[40] The home health nurse often serves as the communication link in coordinating components of care.

### Assessment

The assessment of health problems in the home setting includes the patient's actual and potential health problems as well as relevant characteristics of the family and the environment (social, economic, and physical). The parameters for assessment of patients with cancer and their families at the time of admission to home care are listed in Table 53-3. The planning of interventions and the identification of patient outcomes should include the impact of the family and environment on the patient's health status and care needs.

A systematic approach to assessment of the specific physical tasks involved in the care of the patient will identify all potential aspects of care and will facilitate

**TABLE 53-1  Situations That Evoke the Greatest Stress for Caregivers**

| |
|---|
| Managing the patient's physical care and treatment regimen |
| Managing one's own home and the patient's home and finances |
| The need to be available 24 hours a day, 7 days a week |
| The fear of leaving the patient alone when the caregiver must leave the home |
| A change in the relationship or communications between the patient and caregiver |
| Disruption in the household routines; preparing different meals |
| Inability to spend time with one's own spouse and children, causing a strain in relationships |
| Often trying to balance the need to work outside the home with the care of the patient |
| The inability to meet the expectations of the health care system due to lack of time, knowledge, skill, or just being overwhelmed |

**TABLE 53-2  Most Helpful Nursing Interventions as Identified by Patients and Caregivers**

1. To give excellent, knowledgeable and skilled, personalized nursing care to the patient
2. Providing the patient with the necessary emergency measures if the need arises
3. Assuring the patient that nursing services will be available 24 hours a day, 7 days a week
4. Allowing the patient to do as much for himself/herself as possible
5. Teaching family members how to keep the patient physically comfortable
6. Answering questions honestly, openly, and willingly
7. Supporting the cohesion of the family by initiating and promoting interaction, communication, cooperation, and social and emotional involvement
8. Directing nursing intervention toward daily problem solving

planning and delegating responsibilities among caregivers.

## Planning

The high-incidence problem areas defined in the ANA/ONS *Standards of Oncology Nursing Practice*[41] provide the framework for assessment and planning for the patient's physical care requirements. These problem areas include comfort, nutrition, protective mechanisms, mobility, elimination, sexuality, ventilation, and circulation.

An assessment identifies specific care requirements to maintain the individual in the home setting; the assistance needed by the person who performs the identified care tasks; the equipment, assistive devices, and/or supplies required; and any associated factors that have an impact on the individual's ability to carry out identified care. These special care requirements are listed in Table 53-4.

## Nursing interventions

Nursing interventions in home health assist the patient and family by providing direct care and treatment, supervision of patient care, health and disease management teaching, counseling, and coordination of health care services. The home health nurse is responsible for observing and reporting changes to the patient's physician or other health care team members. The typical interventions, functions, and activities of the nurse in a cancer home health agency are listed in Table 53-5.

## Evaluation

Outcome measures can be used to assess the quality of nursing care in specific areas based on predictable results. Outcome measures may be based on the adequacy of patient teaching (e.g., patient/caregiver demonstrates Hickman catheter flush and dressing change), improve-

ment in physiological status (e.g., pain controlled, wound healing), improvement in functional status (e.g., patient transfers from bed to chair independently), improvement in compliance with treatments (e.g., medications are given as scheduled), and satisfaction with care as reported on patient and family surveys.[42,43]

However, outcomes are influenced by the multifactoral aspects of a patient's care environment and the natural history of the disease, which are beyond the nurse's control. Therefore, the potential limitations must be considered when outcome measures are used for quality assessment of home health care.[44]

## Coordination of Services

Coordination and collaboration skills are essential to promote continuity of care from the acute care setting, coordination of services in the home setting, and achievement of rehabilitation goals.[10,15] A multidisciplinary group of health care professionals from a variety of health care institutions and community service agencies may be involved with the home care of the person with cancer. The responsibility for coordinating these interventions and teaching the patient and family about the multitude of services is frequently undertaken by the home health nurse.[45] It is not unusual for the patient with cancer to be receiving care from an oncologist, radiologist, and family physician concurrently, in addition to having phlebotomists from laboratories, technicians from infusion therapy agencies, equipment vendors from medical equipment agencies, and therapists and home health aide visits to provide specific services. People with cancer may become alarmed and anxious about the number of "strangers" who enter their homes to provide care services. The nurse can provide reassurance to the patient and family by explaining the purpose of each service and coordinating the visits. The nurse also maintains and shares an awareness of the goals for rehabilitation for

**TABLE 53-3** Assessment Parameters on Admission of Cancer Patients to Home Care

A. Patient History:
  1. Primary tumor site and histology
  2. Metastatic site(s)
  3. Previous and current treatments
  4. Use of medications, vitamins not prescribed by physician
  5. Family cancer history
  6. Other health problems
  7. Patient's chief concern

B. Physical Assessment:
  All body systems (integumentary system; eyes, ear, nose, and throat; hematopoietic/lymphatic systems; respiratory system; cardiovascular system; gastrointestinal/abdominal areas; genitourinary system; nervous system; and musculoskeletal system)

C. Functional Status—ability to perform:
  1. Activities of daily living
  2. Instrumental activities of daily meal preparation, shopping, housekeeping, medication administration, communication

D. Physical Care Requirements of Patient (see Table 53-4)

E. Psychosocial Assessment:
  1. Patient's mood state or affect
  2. Causative factors/associated problems affecting the patient's mood state
  3. Impact of mood on the person's functioning (role performance, sexual functioning, functional performance status [IADL])
  4. Coping mechanisms
  5. Social supports
  6. Diversional activities

F. Caregiver Assessment:
  1. Health problems
  2. Functional status and physical stamina
  3. Knowledge of patient's illness, course of disease, and prognosis
  4. Knowledge of patient's physical care requirements
  5. Emotional ability to provide care
  6. Communications and relationship with patient
  7. Availability (caregiver's other roles and responsibilities)

G. Family Assessment:
  1. Structure (composition of members, roles, and responsibilities)
  2. Pattern of authority (who and how are decisions made)
  3. Level of development
  4. Values (important activities, characteristics)
  5. Behavior (cohesion, coordination, communication)
  6. Coping ability
  7. Health and functional status of members
  8. Stressors
  9. Support systems
  10. Knowledge of illness and health practices

H. Equipment and Supply Needs

I. Environment:
  1. Heat, ventilation, water
  2. Sanitation (waste disposal, vermin present)
  3. Safety factors in home (portable heaters, scatter rugs, lack of support rails)

**TABLE 53-3** (continued)

  4. Barriers in home (bulky furniture, clutter)
  5. Safety of location

J. Financial Assessment:
  1. Health insurance(s) for coverage of services, supplies, and equipment
  2. Family income available for out-of-pocket expenses

each patient in order to provide direction to the service providers.

A study by Shuster and Cloonan[46] of 24 home health agencies determined that nursing activities related to co-ordination of services (clinical case management) accounted for 12% of the nurse's time. Care coordination and collaborative activities of the home health nurse often expand to become case management, especially when caring for the patient with advanced metastatic disease or severe functional limitations. The home health nurse assumes responsibility for ongoing patient assessment, care planning, referrals for services, monitoring for appropriateness of services provided, routinely communicating the patient status with all service providers and payers, and evaluating the care provided based on patient and family goals and patient care outcomes.[47,48] Incorporating case management into the role of the home health nurse will achieve better patient care as described by the ANA, whose goals for case management are "the provision of quality health care along a continuum, decreased fragmentation of care across many settings, enhancement of the client's quality of life, and cost containment."[25]

## Documenting Nursing Care

Legal responsibilities of the home health oncology nurse include knowledge of and compliance with the nursing role as defined in the state Nurse Practice Act, the regulations that govern home health, and the standards of nursing practice for the nurse's community. The best evidence that the nurse has complied with these regulations and standards is the documentation of patient care.[49] Documentation must be complete, clear, accurate, objective, and timely to fulfill federal and state certification requirements and Medicare and third-party reimbursement requirements.[50] The written report of nursing activity provides the only concrete evidence of what occurred and can provide legal protection for the nurse and the home health agency. The guiding principle should be "more is better."[51] Principles of documentation include a comprehensive, accurate, and objective description of assessments, nursing actions, and the responses of the patient, family, and caregivers to interventions. The date and time of the occurrence and complete signature of the nurse must be included. Late entries are labeled as an "addendum," signed, and dated. Inadequate documentation implies inadequate nursing care, and it will

**TABLE 53-4** Patient Assessment—Physical Care Requirements

| Common Problem Areas | Specific Care Tasks (examples) | Assistance Required (examples) | Equipment/Supplies (examples) | Associated Factors |
|---|---|---|---|---|
| Comfort | Medication administration (oral, suppositories, injections, IV); positioning; odor control methods; distraction; massage | To what degree is the person able to meet comfort needs? Self-medication vs. minimal, moderate, or total assistance? | Hospital bed; medications; syringes; IV supplies | Anxiety; family conflict |
| Nutrition | Preparation of special diets; management of nausea/vomiting; preparation/ administration of tube feedings; hyperalimentation administration; measures to manage anorexia | To what degree is the person able to meet nutritional needs? Needs assistance with food purchase, preparation, feeding? | Blenders; food supplements, special foods; infusion pumps; gavage equipment; hyperalimentation supplies | Urine testing |
| Protective mechanisms | Personal hygiene needs; general measures to promote skin integrity; management of impaired skin/mucosal integrity (stomatitis, decubitus ulcers, wounds, radiation dermatitis); prevention/ management of infection (medication administration, cleansing/ care of equipment) | To what degree is the person able to accomplish activities of daily living; independent in activities of daily living vs. moderate or total assistance? Degree of assistance required with measures to maintain skin integrity? | Shower equipment (bars, chairs); dressings; irrigating syringes | Individual's mobility status |
| Mobility | Active/passive range-of-motion exercises; transferring, turning, positioning, application of braces; management of edema | To what degree is the person able to ambulate, turn, move, or transfer independently? How many assistants are needed? | Wheelchair; walker; trapeze; Hoyer lift; splints; braces | Individual's pain; fatigue; fractures; bone metastases; edema/ ascites; altered respiratory status |
| Elimination | Foley catheter care; self-catheterization; suprapubic catheter care; stoma management; ostomy bag changes; irrigations; skin care; management of constipation/diarrhea; use of bedpans; administration of enemas | To what degree is the person able to manage elimination needs? How much and what type of assistance is required? | Bedpan; urinal; bedside commode; enema equipment; laxatives; ostomy supplies | Individual's nutritional status; hydration; use of narcotic analgesics |
| Sexuality | Measures to maintain vaginal integrity (e.g., dilator); douching; intermittent catheterization | To what degree is the person able to perform tasks related to sexuality needs? | Foley catheters; straight catheters; douche equipment | Urinary elimination needs |
| Ventilation | Oxygen use; suctioning; tracheostomy care; postural drainage; medication administration | To what degree is the person able to perform tasks related to respiratory care? | Oxygen; suction catheters/ machine; humidifier; tracheostomy care sets | Modification of environmental temperature and humidity; removal of pollutants (smoke, chemicals, exhaust, dust) |
| Circulation | Increase fluid intake; prevent falls, injury, skin breakdown; encourage energy saving; perform activities of daily living; elevate extremities | To what degree is patient able to perform activities of daily living? What amount of assistance is needed? What activities are important to patient? | Hospital bed; wheelchair; walker; bedpan; shower rails and stool | Edema; ascites; postural hypotension; electrolyte imbalance |

McNally JC, Sumerville ET, Miaskowski C, et al: *Guidelines for Oncology Nursing Practice.* Philadelphia, Saunders, 1991.

**TABLE 53-5** Nursing Functions and Activities in Home Health

The Home Care Program nurse is especially prepared to offer the following services and support for patients with cancer and their families:

Direct nursing care
  Completes physical examination of the patient during each home visit
  Demonstrates all nursing care procedures being taught to the caregivers in the home
  Performs all procedures requiring the skill of a nurse (administration of intravenous fluid, insertion of a feeding tube, etc.)
  Administers chemotherapy prescribed by the physician
  Obtains laboratory specimens requested by the physician to monitor effects of the disease or disease treatment (specimens of blood, urine, sputum, or wound cultures)

Observation and reporting
  Assesses and reports signs and symptoms of an emergency medical problem resulting from side effects of medical treatment of the disease (e.g., bone marrow depression following chemotherapy)
  Assesses and reports potential signs and symptoms of an emergency medical problem resulting from the tumor (e.g., hypercalcemia)
  Assesses and reports signs and symptoms of disease progression
  Evaluates patient's response to prescribed medications and therapies
  Assesses patient's and family's emotional response to the course of the disease and/or the course of treatment of the disease

Supervision of patient care
  Identifies current and potential problems influencing the patient's care, including ability of patient to obtain needed care in the home
  Plans nursing care to correct, improve, or manage the identified patient problems
  Provides written instructions of medication schedules or patient care procedures for caregivers in the patient's home
  Supervises the care given to the patient in the home by the family, friends, volunteers, or home health aides
  Coordinates admission to the hospital if the need arises

Health and disease management teaching
  Instructs regarding actual and potential effects of the disease process based on the patient's or caregiver's readiness and ability to learn
  Teaches actual and potential effects of the disease treatment on the patient
  Teaches signs and symptoms requiring immediate notification of the nurse or physician
  Teaches purpose, side effects, amount, frequency, and method of administering each medication and treatment prescribed (e.g., analgesics, colostomy care, decubitus ulcer care)
  Instructs regarding nutrition and hydration requirements, including methods appropriate for the individual patient
  Instructs regarding rehabilitation and self-care techniques (e.g., ambulation with walker, range-of-motion exercises for lymphedema, energy saving, comfort measures)
  Instructs regarding prevention of complications and infections, including environmental safety and hygiene
  Instructs regarding health promotion and maintenance, with emphasis on prevention and early detection of disease

**TABLE 53-5** (continued)

Counseling
  Identifies emotional, spiritual, or social problems experienced by the patient and family
  Assists the patient and family to identify and express their feelings about effects of the disease or treatments
  Facilitates referral to appropriate resources for extended counseling

Coordination and collaboration
  Assists the patient and family to utilize formal and informal support services within the community
  Assesses and prioritizes patient and family needs; integrates and coordinates appropriate home health services into the plan of care (e.g., home health aide, medical social work, occupational therapy, physical therapy, speech therapy, nutrition consultation)

Michigan Cancer Foundation Services, Inc. (MCFSI) Home Care Program, Detroit, MI.

impact negatively on the agency's fulfillment of state licensure and certification requirements, delay or prohibit third-party reimbursement, place the agency at risk of a legal suit, and reflect a negative image of the agency and the quality of care provided.[50] Legally correct records include objective and subjective observations that are pertinent but avoid general terms (e.g., "patient doing well"), value judgments (e.g., "the change in the dose of phenytoin sodium apparently was not noted by nurse on previous visit"), opinions (e.g., "the confusion appears to be increasing"), or conclusions (e.g., "apparently the patient has bone metastasis").

The legal criteria for timeliness is the recording of an event at the time the care is given.[50] In the home health setting, this is within a day of the visit. Timely documentation is an essential component of nursing care. In addition to being a permanent record of the actions of the health care providers, the patient's clinical record communicates the patient's progress and health care services to other members of the health care team, quality assessment reviewers, and third-party payers.

## Rehabilitation Nursing

As treatment advances lead to increased survival for persons with cancer, rehabilitation has become an essential aspect of comprehensive cancer care. The Oncology Nursing Society position statement defines cancer rehabilitation as a "process by which individuals, within their environments, are assisted to achieve optimal functioning within the limits imposed by cancer."[52] Optimal functioning is attainment of the best degree of physical functioning, sustained nutritional adequacy, a practical level of independence in activities of daily living with self-care competence, a realistic outlook, and management of the cancer.[53] The goal of cancer rehabilitation is to improve the quality of life by maximizing functional ability and independence regardless of life expectancy and, when appropriate, reintroduction into the socioeconomic life of the community.[8] Factors to be considered in cancer rehabilitation include physical disabilities, psychological and social aspects, sexual functioning, nutrition, fitness and exercise, pain and symptom management, elimination, and skin care.[54] The underlying concepts of rehabilitation focus on interdisciplinary collaboration, comprehensive services, self-care, maximum function, prevention, family and cultural values, and the patient and family as a unit of care in the community.[55]

The impact of cancer is experienced by everyone involved in the life of the patient. Effective intervention requires the participation of the family in planning and implementing care. When patients and families become copartners with the rehabilitation team, they contract mutually agreeable goals, foster empowerment, educate for self-care, and enhance positive coping behaviors.[55]

The home care nurse plays a key role in cancer rehabilitation at home beginning with the initial assessment and progressing to coordination of all services provided, patient and family education, and referrals to community resources. Education is essential in enhancing patient independence and promoting self-care. Teaching plans should correlate with the patient's and family's learning needs and abilities. The plans incorporate interventions that emphasize activities the patient can perform. If patients cannot perform self-care activities themselves, they may benefit from learning techniques for directing others to perform the care according to their preferences. These teaching plans would include practical skills, assertiveness, and techniques for both giving instructions and problem solving. The greatest needs of patients with cancer and their caregivers have been found to be primarily psychological and informational.[56] Teaching stress reduction methods, communication and problem-solving skills, and information on disease process and care principles may facilitate patient and family coping.

The debilitating sequelae of cancer and treatment often necessitate the use of adaptive equipment to maintain the optimal level of independence and meaningful activity. Equipment such as ramps, rails, grab bars, and enlarged doorways can be constructed or modified for the home. Assistive devices such as universal cuffs for holding grooming devices promote patient independence and self-care.

Encouraging the patient and family to develop networks and supports in the community fosters independence and facilitates patient discharge from the home health agency. The discharge plan provides information on community agencies and services; the patient's health insurance coverage and contact persons; transportation services; vocational rehabilitation programs; and support groups identified by the rehabilitation nurse, patient, and family. To prevent fragmentation of care, referrals to appropriate agencies are carefully timed so they can begin their services when the patient is discharged from home health care. Insurers often limit payment for services to patients with chronic, debilitating disease and may terminate benefits before the patients have achieved

their rehabilitation potential and are educated about self-care. Introducing the discharge plan at time of admission to home care and revising it as needed may avert the negative effects of a premature discharge.

As the disease advances and the ability to maintain activities for independent functioning wanes, it is important to recognize that cancer patients are likely to need services such as personal care, meal preparation, shopping, housekeeping, and transportation. Failure to obtain these services may precipitate a family crisis. Recognizing these needs and initiating appropriate referrals will increase the quality of life for the patient and family.[57] In the home setting, the patient and family are in control; the family is an integral part of the patient's achievement of maximum rehabilitation potential.

## Role of the Advanced Practice Nurse

The complex care requirements of persons with cancer who are referred to home care, coupled with the need for highly specialized, cost-efficient, quality care, has created a role for the advanced practice nurse (APN) in home care. Several home health agencies have successfully integrated the APN, who functions in the traditional role of the oncology clinical nurse specialist (CNS) to improve the quality of care. However, the literature has few articles addressing the role of the APN in the home health setting.[58] Hamric[59] has defined the role of the CNS as an expert practitioner in a specific area of clinical nursing and as change agent within the health care system to improve the quality of patient care. The nursing activities of the APN in homecare include education, consultation, research, and administration, with the APN providing direct patient care and psychotherapy, developing nursing care protocols, teaching and consulting with health care professionals, and coordinating quality improvement activities.[60] The changing health care environment with the shift to managed care offers APNs an opportunity for professional growth in a variety of roles including case manager, primary care practitioner, education in managed care, quality improvement, and resource management.[61]

### Practitioner role

Direct care activities provided by the APN in home health care include advanced services and skills not usually available from the general nursing staff. Donley[62] reports that skills required in the new practice settings, including the home setting, are assessment of the family's health status, interpersonal relationships, lifestyles, and environment; provision of health education, preventative and primary care; evaluation of cultural, educational and religious values that deter persons from accessing or complying with health care; and skills in triaging, referrals, and ethical decision making. The APN is particularly adept in management of complex physical and psychological care requirements such as infusion therapy, extensive wounds, parenteral nutrition, intractable pain, and counseling and problem solving. Studies of CNSs in a hospital setting indicate that CNSs spend 47% of their time in direct care activities.[63] In home health care the percentage of time spent in these activities will vary with the agency's needs and resources.

The home health agency must consider the cost-effectiveness of the APN's provision of direct nursing care. Experienced community health nursing staff have been providing competent nursing care to patients with cancer prior to the advent of the APN. Staff nurses may feel frustrated by the loss of challenging cases, the lack of freedom to select cases, and the absence of recognition for services they have provided in the past. Restructuring the APN's role to include sharing complex cases with staff nurses provides the opportunity for the APN to increase the knowledge of agency staff in the new complex skills, fosters patient and family confidence when the APN is not available, and increases the availability of the APN to additional patients. Although this approach is more cost-effective over time for the home health agency, it can diffuse the bonding that occurs between the patient and the APN or staff nurse, and it can lessen rewards and satisfaction in nursing.[64]

### Educator role

Educational activities for both individual and group instruction of staff are usually included in the APN role. The APN has expertise in developing and implementing staff orientation, continuing education programs for the agency and community, and presenting patient care conferences to enhance staff knowledge and improve patient care.

### Consultant role

Consultative activities of the APN vary according to focus and goal. Consultation may include assisting staff with managing difficult cases or providing information to improve their skills, knowledge, self-assurance, or objectivity. The administration may ask the APN to develop or revise agency programs or assist with counseling problem staff. Frequent personal contact between the APN and staff will enhance the perception of the APN as a colleague with advanced knowledge and skills, facilitate sharing of goals and values in nursing, and promote collaboration between the APN and staff nurse in the provision of quality nursing care.

### Researcher role

Research activity for the APN varies from the basics of interpreting, evaluating, and communicating research findings to caregivers to the advanced level of research collaboration and actively generating or replicating research projects. The research activities of the APN in home health care are usually limited to reviewing research reports, communicating relevant data to agency staff, and incorporating research findings into nursing practice standards. Occasionally the opportunity arises for the APN to collaborate with colleagues in other settings on the implementation of relevant research studies and projects.

### Case management role

Case management is a process that plans, mobilizes, and monitors the resources that a patient uses over the course of an illness to achieve a balance between quality and cost.[65] APNs have effectively used case management in the acute inpatient setting to deliver quality patient care to achieve shorter lengths of stays while controlling use of human and material resources.[13,66,67] Balzer[14] identified specific high-risk situations in the home setting in which case management strategies were implemented by the APN to prevent multiple repeated hospitalizations or institutionalization of patients as well as to help the patient attain a higher level of independence in self-care.

The activities of the APN case manager in home care include assessment of patients with high acuity, complex care requirements, or high-risk status, and assessment of their family, environment, and health insurance benefits; establishment of nursing diagnosis; development of a multidisciplinary plan of care; implementation of the plan of care including delegation of specific interventions to the multidisciplinary team; coordination of services provided; collaboration with the multidisciplinary team and the health insurance worker; referral to community resources; and evaluation of outcomes. Some of these activities can overlap with the role of the home care nurse. The APN can avoid potential conflicts by respecting the professionalism and accountability of the home care nurse and supporting the relationship between the patient and the home care nurse.[68] The APN case manager can collaborate with the home care nurse in developing the plan of care, assist the nurse in goal setting, and delegate interventions to home care nurses based on their expertise. Consultation, education, and support should be made available to all home care staff, as well as backup for home care nurses when they are not available. An integrated approach to patient care through the case management process can be achieved in a home health agency with mutual respect and recognition of the expertise and contributions of the APN case manager and the multidisciplinary team.

### Evaluation of the APN role

Evaluation of the APN's role in home health is limited. Lamb and Stempel's[11] study demonstrated that long-term case management interventions enabled patients to gain confidence in their ability to care for themselves, accept greater responsibility for identifying their needs, select appropriate interventions, and use the health care system appropriately. Boyd et al[63] reported that the positive impact of the APN was predominantly in professional publication, revenue production, submission and acceptance of grant proposals, and assuring positive patient outcomes. The significance of improving care was evidenced by a decrease in staff errors and changes in clinical practice after the APN's review of occurrences or incidents. Further study is needed to evaluate the impact of the APN on patient outcomes.

In some home health agencies, APNs have provided education and support to staff nurses by sharing complex cases, presenting and participating in case conferences, developing patient educational materials, teaching orientation and in-service programs, distributing pertinent educational and research reports, and being available for consultation. APNs have produced revenues through home visits; participated in revisions of policies, procedures, and documentation forms; developed and conducted nursing process audits; served as home health liaisons to community health care organizations; and participated in professional oncology nursing activities in the community. As such, they have increased the credibility and recognition of the home health agency and improved the quality of home care services.

## ECONOMIC ISSUES

### Financing Home Health Care

In the current environment of cost containment, home health nurses struggle with issues such as who should have access to their care, what the quality of care should be, and who is worthy of care at the public's expense.[69] Advocates of home health care can demonstrate its desirability and potential cost-effectiveness in answering these questions. If comprehensive patient care is to be provided in a financially responsible manner, home health nurses need to be familiar with reimbursement guidelines defined by each reimbursement source, obtain the necessary approvals for care, and complete the required forms. Knowledge of the services, equipment, and supplies covered by the individual's insurance is essential.

The Medicare Act of 1965 included a home health benefit for the Medicare beneficiary living at home. Home health services available to Medicare recipients include nursing, physical therapy, speech therapy, occupational therapy, home health aide, and social work services. Eligibility requirements state that the beneficiary must be homebound and require skilled nursing, physical therapy, or speech and language pathology services ordered by a physician. *Homebound* means that leaving the home requires considerable effort. Services must be provided on a part-time, intermittent basis.[70] *Part-time* currently is defined as nursing and home health aide time totaling less than 8 hours per day or 35 hours per week. *Intermittent* currently is defined as services required at least every 60 days and daily visits limited to 21 consecutive days or having a predictable and finite end if daily visits

extend beyond 21 days. Many health insurance payers have incorporated portions of the Medicare regulations into their policies. Medicare reimburses at the lower end of reasonable cost or agency charge, on a per visit basis, up to a limit that is set annually by the U.S. Health Care Financing Administration (HCFA). The home health agency bills the Medicare program its established charges and is reimbursed a predetermined percentage of those charges. At the end of the agency's fiscal year, the agency files a cost report, from which a reasonable cost for providing services to Medicare beneficiaries is determined. A final settlement is determined based on the agency's costs for providing the service and the amounts billed by the agency and paid by the Medicare program.[71,72] Currently there are few limits placed on the number of visits made to Medicare patients, resulting in an extensive increase in expenditures. Federal legislators have proposed several measures to contain home health costs, including co-payments by beneficiaries, bundling of costs, and a prospective payment system that has been studied for several years.[73] Managed care organizations have entered the Medicare market slowly. Only 11.2% of Medicare beneficiaries were enrolled in a Medicare-managed care plan as of June 1996.[6]

Medicaid funding for home health services is a joint federal-state assistance program for the poor of all ages.[74] Federal regulations require states to provide a minimum range of home health services, including part-time nursing care, home health aides, medical supplies, and equipment. States receive matching funds for their expenditures and are allowed extensive flexibility in determining eligibility, services, and reimbursement. States may opt to provide additional services (e.g., physical, occupational, or speech therapy) or to reimburse home health agencies on a flat fee for service or agency cost. States may also offer waiver programs that are partially funded with federal funds and cover a broader range of services such as case management, long-term nursing, personal care, and homemaker or chore services. Lack of available state funds has limited state participation in these programs. Several proposals to decrease Medicaid expenditures are being reviewed by federal legislators. All proposals will restrict state home care programs.[74] In June 1995, 32% of Medicaid clients were enrolled in Medicaid managed care plans.[74]

Private insurance carriers (e.g., Blue Cross/Blue Shield, Aetna) vary significantly in their coverage for home health services. Most private carriers use managed care strategies to control utilization of services and contain cost. Individual plans may require partial payment (co-payments) by the beneficiary, may limit the number of visits, and may cover only specific services (e.g., nursing, home health aide services). Prior to admission, the home health agency will contact the carrier to determine the patient's specific coverage.

The oncology home care nurse must be aware of the services, equipment, and supplies covered for each patient and the documentation, authorizations, and approvals for care required by the reimbursement source in order to avoid nonpayment of services. A referral to the agency's social worker may be helpful in locating a community agency that will provide noncovered but needed service.

## Documentation for Reimbursement

Accurate descriptive documentation of home health nursing care is vital to reimbursement and continuation of home health services. Completing timely, appropriate documentation consumes a significant amount of staff time; a study of nursing activities in home health care showed that paperwork, charting, and completing recertifications accounted for 19% of nursing time.[46] Many articles have been published describing methods of documentation to ensure successful reimbursement,[75,76] and conferences on documentation techniques are usually well attended. The adage "If it wasn't charted, it wasn't done" has been expanded to "and if it wasn't charted in keeping with the regulations, it will not be reimbursed." It has been postulated that the rise in health care expenditures, including home health care, has led the government and fiscal intermediaries to enact regulations requiring specific documentation and has increased focused review in an effort to decrease costs by denial of payment for services designated as "noncovered" by the reviewer.[76]

If the nurse is able to document changes in the patient's physical status and changes in the treatment plan that correspond to the identified goals and outcomes, nursing service should be viewed as reasonable and necessary and therefore reimbursable.[51] Accurate and comprehensive nursing documentation, although time-consuming and requiring thoughtful deliberation, is essential for procuring reimbursement.

## Home Care for the Socially Disadvantaged

Health care expenditures for 1994 were $832.5 billion and absorbed 12.4% of the gross domestic product.[77] Despite these expenditures, Americans are not healthier than citizens of other countries of similar or lesser wealth.[78] Approximately 15% of Americans, or 37 million individuals, are not covered by any insurance plan, and another 20% have inadequate health insurance. The United States is one of only two large, industrialized nations that does not have a plan of universal health care for all citizens. The call for health care reform of the U.S. health system has gone unanswered by Congress, leaving more than one-third of the population with minimal or no health care insurance protection. However, concern over the rapid increases in health care spending, the serious financial difficulties of the government health care programs, and the crisis in employer-paid private financing of health care has sparked health care reform

at the state and local level.[79,80] State legislators, private health insurers, hospital administrators, and health care providers have taken the lead in implementing cost-containment measures that incorporate the concepts of managed care.[73] The state governors have submitted a proposal to Congress to give states control of the provision of health care services to Medicaid clients. The governors propose that greater flexibility would allow them to provide fewer benefits to the disabled and indigent and free up money to cover new populations, especially the working poor.[74] A prototype plan is being studied by the State of Oregon as a measure to ensure equitable and universal access to health care by prioritizing types of care.[81] Criticized as a dangerous rationing scheme when it was proposed, its progress is being closely watched by health care reform leaders, ethicists, health care providers, and insurers.

Since home health reimbursement by payers is based on cost, most home health agencies have limited funds available for services to persons without home health insurance. In some communities the United Way has allocated funds to voluntary home health organizations (e.g., the Visiting Nurses Association) for home health care of the indigent. The Medicare home health benefit does not cover long-term or chronic care. However, a growing number of elderly persons with cancer with functional limitations and chronic health problems live alone or with a spouse or sibling who may also be frail and elderly. A study of 1100 posthospitalization medical and surgical patients, aged 60 and older, demonstrated that females and black Americans had higher unmet personal care and housekeeping needs that were related to their living arrangements and health insurance coverage.[22]

During an acute exacerbation of an illness, patients are admitted to home health care after hospitalization for management of their skilled care needs and limited personal care. When the acute episode is resolved, the chronic problems continue. If a patient is kept beyond the need for skilled care, the home health agency faces a denial of payment for services provided. When a patient has a limited income, the social work home care staff are faced with the problem of locating a community service agency that provides follow-up monitoring and support services for personal care or homemaking without cost. Currently there are few publicly financed long-term care programs available for the needy.[74] Several bills to provide long-term personal care and support services to the elderly have been introduced in Congress, but to date none has passed.

The 1989 HCFA revisions to the *Medicare Home Health Agency Manual* recognized "management and evaluation of a beneficiary's plan of care" as skilled nursing care and thus reimbursable. This benefit expanded reimbursable home health services to include assessment, monitoring, teaching, and revisions of the plan of care for persons whose conditions have stabilized but who are at risk for complications or require frequent unskilled care from caregivers.

The use of public funds for wide-scale managed care services has focused on Medicaid recipients, a population that is least likely to understand the health care system and most in need of comprehensive, user-friendly health care services.[78] Reports of the increasing profit margin of managed care companies, the restrictions in choice of providers, and the increased responsibility on the enrollee in accessing managed care services have been a source of concern.[73,80] Kinsey[79] encourages local legislative, bureaucratic, and insurance planners, clinical providers, service administrators, and the targeted client group to initiate a planning forum to develop a core plan for a system of managing the care of diverse population groups while safeguarding individual and family well-being and improving their health.

## ETHICAL CONCERNS

The rapid growth and increased complexity of home health care have generated an increase of ethical concerns unique to the home care setting. Homes are shaped by the personal lifestyle and financial means of the cancer patient. Possessions, routines, and family structures may not be conducive to the provision of health care in the home.[82,83] For example, dirt or clutter in the home may create a safety hazard, obstruct movement, or impede provision of patient care. Family routines may not include accepted hygienic practices, and family activities may occur at any time of the night or day. Family structure may include aged parents, dependent spouses, young children, or estranged relatives with varied capabilities and motivation to learn and perform necessary treatments for patient care. Frequently, the cancer patient has been the primary caregiver of the family.

Reports of the type and incidence of ethical problems in home health care are limited.[84] A study by Young et al[85] demonstrated that the ethical concerns of home health providers were primarily maintaining agency solvency while not denying care to indigent patients, responding to conflicts between patients and families, providing care to abused or neglected patients, and candidly addressing decisions about treatment with the terminally ill. In another study, Aroskar[86] surveyed 319 home health nurses and identified their most frequently cited ethical problems as (1) patient decisions regarding treatment and health care that conflict with the health care provider's goals, (2) truth telling that reveals patient confidences or would lead to denial of needed patient care, and (3) provisions of health care benefits that are based on insurance reimbursement rather than patient need. Haddad[83] surveyed 30 health care providers to identify ethical concerns that are troublesome to role performance. Their concerns were categorized as problems with regulations that restricted services; incompetence of coworkers; and a broad category of various problems, including elder abuse, incompetent caregivers, abandonment, and racism. A study of ten patient-caregiver-nurse triads revealed that discrepant perceptions of pain among patients, caregivers, and home health nurses may potentiate ethical conflicts.[87] Home health nurses are usually familiar with the ethical principles of advocacy for patient autonomy (e.g., the right to make an informed decision regarding treatment and services) and the patient's right of self-determination to refuse treatment when incapacitated.[88,89] The Omnibus Reconciliation Act (OBRA) of 1989 and 1990 mandated home health agencies to inform patients of their rights and specifically of the right to be informed of advance directives and to have information about each patient's advance directives recorded in the patient's clinical record.

## Moral Values

Moral values are beliefs that are of ultimate importance to oneself, apply to all persons, guide our actions, and focus on promoting humankind. Values important to health care providers are respect for persons, patient advocacy, and accountability.[90] Respect for persons means respecting another person as one who shares the same human destiny as oneself.[91] Patient advocacy is the active support of the patient to be informed of his or her rights and options. Accountability is answerability for one's actions when one has agreed to provide a service. Moral values are described in the ANA *Code for Nurses with Interpretive Statements.*[92]

The values of the patient, family, and caregiver are not usually known when a patient is admitted to home care and not easily assessed during the initial visit. Their values have sometimes been formulated by cultural and societal beliefs that are different from those held by the nurse and may not include respect for handicapped, elderly, terminally ill, or mentally retarded persons. Families may be unwilling to purchase medical supplies or equipment needed by the patient because for them the value of money supersedes the value of new and sometimes expensive equipment for a terminally ill person. The nurse's efforts to advocate for the patient may also be rejected by the dependent patient who relies heavily on the family and caregivers to provide care. Thus, ongoing assessment of the values of the patient, family, and caregivers is essential to identify potential ethical conflicts and to plan for nursing care that is compatible with their needs and values.

## Ethical Principles

The ANA *Code for Nurses* identifies six principles that the nurse should use as moral guides to action. They are autonomy, beneficence, justice, veracity, confidentiality, and fidelity.[91,93]

*Autonomy* is the principle that gives patients the right to determine their actions based on their own decisions and implies that patients are independent and self-reliant. Conflicts arise in the home setting if a patient's decisions are detrimental to his or her health (e.g., refusing medications that are effective treatment for illness, choosing to remain at home when the care provided by the family/caregivers is substandard) or when patients are dependent on multiple caregivers with no designated primary decision maker.

The principle of *beneficence* directs the nurse to do good, to promote the welfare or well-being of others. A conflict may occur for the home care nurse if the patient lives in an apartment or neighborhood that is a risk to the personal safety of the nurse or when threats or attempts to do bodily harm may necessitate closing or not opening a case to home care service. The principle of *justice* guides the nurse to treat all persons equally and to give individuals what is owed to them by another person or society. However, limited health care coverage restricts compliance with this principle if needed services are not covered or are only partially covered and the patient does not have personal resources to purchase the service and supplies. The principle of *veracity* obligates the nurse to be truthful with the patient, peers, and other professionals and to avoid lying or deception. Conflicts may arise when the family or caregivers insist that the patient not be informed of specific information because it may be distressing. Truthfulness also requires the nurse to report a peer for poor performance that may not be observed by supervisors in the home care setting. The principle of *confidentiality* requires the nurse to respect and hold confidential all information shared by the patient. However, when innocent parties are in jeopardy, public law requires disclosure of this information, as in suspected cases of child abuse. Finally, the principle of *fidelity* requires the nurse to be faithful to his or her commitments and profession. When an agency is short-staffed, overtime work may create conflicts between the nurse's professional and personal life.

## Ethical Decision Making

When conflict occurs, the nurse must consider the patient, family, and caregivers as the unit of care and identify the moral values held by each person involved in the tasks of home care. A decision-making process can be used to assess the problem and potential courses of action and to consider what is right or good based on the values of the persons involved and ethical principles. Guidelines, similar to the nursing process, have been developed to assist the nurse (Table 53-6).[91,93–95] Many home health agencies are developing ethics committees to offer education in ethics to staff and patients and to serve as a forum for discussion of ethical conflicts identified by staff. The ethics committee can also develop agency policies and guidelines on ethical issues (e.g., informed consent, determination of competency, role of surrogate decision makers, withholding life-sustaining treatment, do-not-resuscitate decisions).[84]

**TABLE 53-6**  Process for Ethical Decision Making

1. Identify the ethical problem. Clarify the issues, including conflicting moral claims, the values of the involved persons, and their emotional responses.
2. Collect data from all involved in the problem. Identify the decision makers, listen to each person's perspective, and separate facts from emotions.
3. Identify all possible actions, the ethical principles that will be enhanced or negated by each action, and the projected outcome for each action.
4. Evaluate each action thoroughly. Consider the consequences of each action and its effect on each person. Attempt to prioritize the positive and negative outcomes for each action.
5. Make the decision. Select the action that most agrees with the values involved and has the most positive consequences. Inform all involved persons.
6. Act and then evaluate all aspects of the outcome.

Adapted with permission from DeWolf MS: Ethical decision-making, *Semin Oncol Nurs* 5:77–81, 1989; Andrew Jameton: *Nursing Practice: The Ethical Issues,* © 1984, pp. 66–69. Adapted by permission of Prentice-Hall, Englewood Cliffs, NJ.

## INFUSION THERAPY IN THE HOME

Infusion therapy is one of the most rapidly growing segments of home care. The growth of home infusion therapy has been stimulated by cost-containment pressure from third-party payers; the increase in the aging population; and advances in technology that have increased the safety, effectiveness, and availability of home infusion therapies.[96,97] In addition to cost reduction, home infusion therapy reduces the risk of complications from nosocomial infections, is convenient for patient and caregiver, and provides psychological benefits to patients who desire the comfort of their homes. The disadvantage to home infusion therapy is the burden placed on caregivers to learn and comply with treatment schedules and procedures.[98]

Advanced technology has produced an array of long-term central venous access devices (VADs) and infusion pumps that simplify parenteral administration of drugs in the home and have less risk for complications. The most frequently used central VAD for cancer therapies in the home are venous access ports. Infusion pumps have become smaller, more lightweight, simpler to program and adjust, and therefore easier to operate and maintain in the home.

The peripherally inserted central catheter (PICC), a soft, flexible silicone or polymer catheter, is used frequently in the home because it can be inserted by a nurse who is certified in the procedure.[98] Because the PICC is biocompatible and flexible, it can often remain in place for weeks or months. The PICC is inserted in the antecubital fossa and advanced until the catheter tip is in the axillary, subclavian, or brachiocephalic vein. Radiographic verification is required for placement beyond the axillary vein.[99] PICC lines require frequent flushing with heparin and dressing changes every three to seven days.

The advantages of the PICC as an alternative to a central VAD are the possibility of insertion in the home by a certified home health nurse, decreased cost, comfort to the patient, and long-term placement.

Home health management of the cancer patient receiving infusion therapy that incorporates sophisticated infusion pumps and VADs requires educated and experienced nurses, effective patient and caregiver education, clearly defined policies and procedures, and effective coordination of home care services.[98] Focus is on caring for the patient and family rather than on management of the equipment. Teaching self-care procedures for flushing a long-term central catheter is ineffective if the patient or caregiver is overwhelmed by a beeping infusion pump or manipulating a syringe and needle. An elderly spouse may expect the nurse to care for the VAD and refuse to learn the procedures. Counseling the patient, caregiver, and family regarding high-technology home care becomes the first priority. The home health nurse may need to discuss alternatives of nursing home or private duty nursing care if the spouse or caregiver is unwilling or unable to care for the patient.[85]

Communication between the infusion therapy personnel and the home health nurse for coordination of services and delineation of responsibilities will also decrease patient and family confusion and anxiety. A joint visit by the home health and infusion therapy nurses at the patient's home when home infusion therapy is initiated to review medical orders, set up and test equipment, review schedules and procedures for ordering supplies, and define each nurse's specific responsibilities promotes coordination of services. An Infusion Therapy/Home Health Coordination Record (Table 53-7) can be helpful in decreasing confusion and false expectations. After it is signed by both nurses, each agency receives a copy. A copy is left in the patient's home.

If risk of exposure to blood or other potentially infectious materials occurs during care of the patient receiving infusion therapy in the home, the nurse must comply with federal regulations for prevention of occupational exposure issued December 6, 1991.[100] In general, for home care these regulations mandate observation of universal precautions.

## Chemotherapy Administration

The demand for more cost-effective methods of treating cancer patients has stimulated the development of comprehensive home care services including administration of chemotherapy. For patients whose physical conditions preclude travel to an outpatient setting, intermittent bolus administration of chemotherapy in the home has become a viable option. Advanced technology not only has produced sophisticated drugs but also has provided methods to control the clinical side effects, promoting safe administration at home. Currently, continuous infusion of chemotherapeutic agents through an ambulatory infusion pump is the most frequently used delivery system in the home.

Continuous infusion and regional infusion of antineoplastic drugs increase exposure of tumor cells to higher total dose of drug, theoretically increasing tumor cell kill.[108] Nursing responsibilities may include changing the pump cassette containing the antineoplastic drugs, reprogramming the infusion pump, and monitoring and evaluating side effects of the therapy.

### Criteria for patient selection

Specific criteria must be met for intermittent, bolus administration of chemotherapy in the home. These include the following:

1. The patient meets the requirements for admission to home care as determined by the agency's licensing or certification agency.
2. The patient is stable and free of symptoms that preclude the safe administration of antineoplastic drugs.
3. The patient desires chemotherapy and is willing to pay for that portion of drugs and services not covered by medical insurance.
4. The patient has received the initial course of chemotherapy prior to administration in the home with no untoward effects.
5. The patient and family understand and are willing and able to assume related self-care activities.
6. The home must have a clean area, refrigerator, phone, electricity, and hot and cold running water.
7. Resources are available in the community for medications, supplies, laboratory services, and additional nursing or caregiving services.

Insurance reimbursement for antineoplastic drugs, equipment, supplies, and nursing services varies. The patient's medical insurance must be reviewed to determine coverage of both the home care nurse and the infusion therapy agency services prior to referring a patient for home chemotherapy since it may not be feasible for the patient to assume the costs.[101]

### Policies for chemotherapy administration

Home health agencies that offer chemotherapy as a service must develop specific policies and procedures. These usually include the following:

- patient eligibility requirements
- antineoplastic drugs approved for administration at home
- acceptable parameters of laboratory profiles and the schedule for obtaining laboratory studies
- procedures for each route of administration that include preparation, administration, and disposal of the drugs[102]
- specific criteria for withholding antineoplastic drugs
- educational requirements for nurses who administer antineoplastic drugs

**TABLE 53-7**  Infusion Therapy/Home Health Coordination Record

Patient Name _____   Date _____ ☐ Initial   ☐ Update

I.D. No. _____   H.I.T. Agency Involved _____

Start of H.I.T. Service _____   H.I.T. Contact _____

Type of H.I.T. _____   H.I.T. Phone _____

Pump Type _____

### RESPONSIBILITIES FOR SERVICE

| Activity | H.I.T. Agency | MCFSI |
|---|---|---|
| 1. Initial assessment of infusion therapy (Date _____ ) | | |
| 2. Initial teaching of infusion therapy (Date _____ ) | | |
| 3. Supplies management (ordering/delivery) | | |
| 4. Pharmaceuticals (preparation/delivery) | | |
| 5. Provision of medical equipment, pumps, supplies | | |
| 6. Ongoing assessment of equipment, supplies, etc. | | |
| 7. Ongoing assessment of patient's response to therapy | | |
| 8. Clinical monitoring, laboratory studies | | |
| 9. Catheter management | | |
| 10. Restarting IV | | |
| 11. Catheter repair | | |
| 12. Tubing/cassette changes<br>If MCFSI responsible, H.I.T. contact demonstrated procedure with MCFSI nurse ☐ Yes   ☐ No (If no, explain below) | | |
| 13. Dosage adjustment/pump reprogramming<br>If MCFSI responsible, H.I.T. contact demonstrated procedure with MCFSI nurse ☐ Yes   ☐ No (If no, explain below) | | |
| 14. Troubleshooting problems with pump | | |
| 15. Replacement of pump | | |
| 16. Pump Operations manual in home | | |
| 17. Physician contacts/reports | | |
| 18. 24-hour availability | | |
| 19. Other | | |

COMMENTS:

_____   _____
H.I.T. Representative (if available)        Date        MCFSI Home Care Program Nurse        Date

☐ Duplicate copy sent to agency                _____

                                               Beeper Number

H.I.T. = Home Infusion Therapy; *MCFSI* = Michigan Cancer Foundation Services, Inc.
Michigan Cancer Foundation Services, Inc. (MCFSI) Home Care Program, Detroit, MI.

Some agencies limit approved antineoplastic agents given at home to those that are nonvesicant or noncaustic. Many home health agencies will administer only drugs that can be infused within one to two hours. Home infusion therapy companies may administer antineoplastic drugs that require hydration and infusion over several hours, such as cisplatin. Investigational drugs should be considered for home administration only if the side effects have been identified and written information describing the drug's action and side effects has been provided to the agency. Although this information is readily available to the hospital or clinic nurse, it is more difficult for home care agencies to obtain. The use of VADs has facilitated the administration of chemotherapy at home. However, not all patients receiving chemotherapy have an existing intravenous line. An agency must determine whether the nurses will perform venipunctures. Some agencies require a patient to have an existing line if chemotherapy is to be given at home, while others require establishment of a free-flowing IV through which chemotherapy is administered rather than direct intravenous push administration. This ensures venous access and facilitates the flushing of the tubing.

Specific hematologic parameters must be designated at which chemotherapy will or will not be administered. A complete blood cell count (CBC), differential, and platelet count are obtained 36–48 hours prior to administration of each series of drug(s), and the physician is contacted to confirm, adjust, or withhold the dose of the antineoplastic agent. The Karmanos Cancer Institute Home Care Program's policy states that chemotherapy will not be administered when the white blood cell count is below 3000/mm$^3$ or the platelet count is below 75,000/mm$^3$. In the home, serial laboratory testing that may indicate bone marrow recovery is generally not available.

### Staff education

As in any setting, the nurse administering chemotherapy or caring for the person receiving continuous infusion chemotherapy must have the theoretical knowledge base and technical skills necessary to ensure the safety of the patient. Many agencies have developed a chemotherapy certification course based on the *Cancer Chemotherapy Guidelines* developed by the Oncology Nursing Society.[103] To be eligible to administer chemotherapy at home, the nurse should demonstrate

- knowledge of administration procedures and the purpose, action, and side effects of drugs as well as measures to manage untoward effects

- the ability to administer IV drugs via VADs, catheters, ports, pumps, and peripheral lines

- knowledge of appropriate preparation, transportation, and disposal of antineoplastic agents (a comprehensive review of this information is included in chapter 15).

### Safety considerations

Several studies have determined that mutagenic changes may occur in persons who handle chemotherapy drugs.[104,105] Potential hazards associated with the administration of antineoplastic agents have prompted the Occupational Safety and Health Administration (OSHA) to set guidelines for compounding, transporting, administering, and disposing of toxic chemotherapy agents.[106]

Potential risks to persons who come into contact with chemotherapy drugs and associated safety measures should be discussed with the patient and family prior to the initial home chemotherapy treatment.

Safety considerations include the following:

**1.** *Transport of drugs:* In the home setting, where infusion therapy service personnel are not available to prepare and deliver the drugs, the antineoplastic drugs may be obtained from the pharmacy by the family or nurse. The drugs should be labeled as cytotoxic, securely capped or sealed, and enclosed in an impervious packing material for transport. The family is cautioned to protect the package from breakage and is taught the necessary procedures should a spill occur.

**2.** *Preparation of drugs:* An area of the patient's home that is apart from frequent family activity and food preparation should be selected to prepare the drugs. If present, ceiling fans should be turned off. A work surface area that can be cleaned should be utilized (e.g., a card table). All family members should remain outside the rooms where the drugs are prepared and administered. If possible, the family should make arrangements for children to be cared for outside the home on the day of chemotherapy.

Supplies are assembled on a disposable, absorbent, plastic-backed pad that is taped over the work surface area. Only syringes, needles, and IV sets with Luer-lock fittings should be used. A plastic or metal tray can be lined with sterile gauze squares to catch and collect excess solution. A closable, puncture-resistant, shatter-resistant container is necessary for the disposal of contaminated sharp or breakable materials. Appropriate containers can be purchased from medical supply companies. Sealable 4-mil polyethylene or 2-mil polypropylene plastic bags with wire ties and labeled as "Biological Hazard" must be used for disposal of all supplies used in the preparation and administration of antineoplastic drugs.

Before donning the protective nonpenetrable gown, surgical latex gloves, mask, and goggles, the nurse reminds the patient and caregiver of the need for protection from exposure to the drugs. The patient or caregiver who participates in administering the drug should also wear protective garments. While preparing and administering the drugs, care is taken to prevent aerosolization; for example, sterile gauze should be wrapped around ampules prior to breaking and around needle tips while expelling air from syringes, priming IV lines, or inserting needles into vials or IV lines. While administering antineoplastic drugs, universal precautions for preventing transmission of human immunodeficiency virus, hepatitis B virus, and other blood-borne pathogens must be followed.[102] In the home the drugs (that require refrigeration) must be stored away from food, cosmetics, and areas of family activity.

**3.** *Spills:* Spills and breakages must be cleaned up immediately by a person wearing a protective gown, gloves, mask, and goggles. Liquids and solids are wiped up with absorbent pads or gauze, and the area is cleaned three times with detergent solution and rinsed with clean water. All contaminated materials should be placed in the plastic bag labeled "Biological Hazard."

**4.** *Patient care:* Blood, emesis, and excreta from patients who have received antineoplastic agents within 48 hours may be contaminated. The health care providers and caregivers must be informed of the need to wear protective garments if the potential exists to become contaminated, for example, when caring for the bedbound or incontinent patient. All contaminated linens should be prewashed separately once and then laundered again with the family laundry. All disposable bed pads, tissues, gowns, and gloves must be sealed in a plastic bag for disposal. Children should be discouraged from visiting the patient while chemotherapy is being administered.

**5.** *Disposal:* When administration is completed, all items that have been in contact with the drug are wrapped in an absorbent pad (including unused portions of the drug unless they are to be used in the future) and placed into the plastic bag labeled "Biological Hazard." A reusable drug vial should be cleaned with an alcohol pad, placed in a plastic bag, and stored according to the packaged directions regarding environmental temperature. The patient and family are warned that all persons must avoid contact with the drug (especially children). The nurse will transport the bag of contaminated waste to the home care agency for disposal. OSHA[106] recommends that all hazardous waste be disposed of in a licensed sanitary landfill. Therefore, home care agencies that administer antineoplastic drugs must have a contract for disposal of the hazardous wastes.

### Patient and family responsibilities

Some agencies require a caregiver to be present on the day(s) chemotherapy is administered to observe for problems and assist the patient in managing side effects. Written information about potential side effects is provided along with the descriptions of symptoms that need to be reported immediately to the physician or nurse. It is helpful to include the phone number of the health care providers on the written instructions. The patient and family is educated regarding management of side effects and self-care measures.[107] Many institutions have developed appropriate patient teaching guidelines. An excellent guideline, "Chemotherapy and You," is available without cost from the National Cancer Institute by phoning 1-800-4-CANCER.

Reimbursement for chemotherapy administration in the home varies according to the reimbursement policies of the third-party payers.[101,109] Reimbursement by Medicare and Medicaid programs has not been consistent for home health administration of antineoplastic drugs. Private insurances and health maintenance organizations (HMOs) may cover most of the cost. Each patient's coverage must be evaluated. Prior approval is typically necessary to ensure insurance coverage.

## Home Parenteral Nutrition

The administration of parenteral nutrition, one of the more complex therapies given in the home, is a rapidly growing option for cost-effective therapy for the malnourished patient with cancer.[110–112] A study by Howard,[113] indicated that only 20% of patients with cancer who received home parenteral nutrition (HPN) did well and experienced complete rehabilitation, a fact that should be considered in patient selection.

### Criteria for patient selection

Certain criteria are recommended for acceptance of a patient into an HPN program:

1. The patient's physical status is sufficiently stable to allow hospital discharge and safe home care for a reasonable period of time.
2. The patient has a central venous access device (VAD) and has received parenteral nutrition for a minimum of one week prior to discharge from the acute care facility.
3. The patient and/or a family member has good vision and manual dexterity, and is willing and able to learn and maintain the procedures necessary for HPN.
4. The amount and types of care requirements, as well as the benefits, risks, and financial considerations, have been evaluated and explained to the patient and caregiver prior to discharge.
5. Adequate resources are available in the community for obtaining medications and supplies as well as troubleshooting on a 24-hour basis. Additionally, laboratory services and home nursing care must be accessible. Most areas in the United States are currently serviced by home infusion therapy companies that provide necessary supplies, medications, and equipment.
6. The home environment is conducive to providing safe HPN, including running water, electricity, and a telephone.

The patient and family must assume primary responsibility for the administration of HPN. If the patient lives alone, a caregiver must be identified who will stay with the patient and administer the HPN until the patient is able to manage this care. Private duty nurses may be considered if a family member or willing caregiver is not available. Frequently the patient with cancer who requires HPN has additional complex care requirements, and the total amount of care required, especially at night, can impose a severe burden on the caregiver, who will therefore need occasional respite.

The financial costs of HPN vary according to locale and patient needs. Howard[113] reported that the cost of HPN is $6500 to $12,500 per month per patient for solutions and supplies, home nursing visits, and clinical follow-up with laboratory tests. Reimbursement from third-party payers has been inconsistent and restrictive. It is critical that the patient's medical insurance be reviewed by the discharge planner or home infusion company to determine HPN coverage. Frequently, the patient's insurance will cover a portion of the cost, with the patient responsible for the remainder. Infusion therapy companies usually bill the patient's medical insurance agency directly.

### Initial home assessment

The initial visit by the home care nurse should occur soon after the patient's arrival at home and should coincide with the arrival of supplies, equipment, medication, and home infusion therapy company personnel. This will allow time to review the medical orders for HPN with the patient and caregiver, test the infusion pump, review the schedule and procedures for ordering supplies, and define the specific responsibilities of the home care nurse and infusion therapy company personnel. It is essential that agencies administering HPN provide 24-hour service. Since HPN is usually infused at night, most problems occur at this time. Completing a patient assessment may take several visits because of the many essential activities required during the initial home visit related to the HPN. The initial assessment includes

1. the type and status of the VAD (VADs currently used include the tunneled single-, double-, and triple-lumen catheters, right atrial catheters, and ports for long-term administration)
2. the patient's and family's knowledge of the management of HPN and other caregiving needs
3. evaluation of the home environment for safety and cleanliness factors required for HPN (e.g., running water, electricity, working telephone)

Most acute care facilities have developed complete teaching programs that include catheter care, home monitoring techniques, solution preparation (if applicable), administration techniques, and emergency care. However, because the prospective payment system results in earlier discharges, patients may be sent home before they are fully knowledgeable of HPN management. Adequate refrigeration must be available in the home to store the two- to four-week supply of solutions. Most infusion therapy companies will provide a small refrigerator if needed. An electric infusion pump is necessary for safe administration of HPN.[111,114] Most infusion pumps have a battery backup that can operate the pump for several hours during an electrical outage. Thick carpeting or steps in multilevel homes may impede the patient's mobility during the infusion since the pumps are attached to portable IV poles.

### Nursing management

Twice-a-day home nursing visits are usually required initially. The nurse starts the infusion of HPN in the evening and discontinues it in the morning. The role of the nurse encompasses ongoing assessment and evaluation of the patient's status, direct patient care (e.g., HPN administration), supervision of the patient/family management of HPN, and patient/family education.

Written instructions for HPN procedures are usually given to the patient at the time of discharge from the acute care setting. It is helpful to adjust the HPN infusion time to the family's routine. HPN is often administered over 10–16 hours, including the patient's sleeping time. The infusion rate for the first and last hours is decreased to prevent hyperglycemia upon initiation and rebound hypoglycemia upon withdrawal of the HPN.

Clinical monitoring is critical initially. A flow sheet for documenting monitoring tasks is necessary. The patient and family are instructed to record the date, time, and results of the following:

- time of initiation/completion of HPN infusion
- daily temperature, pulse, respirations
- weight
- urine fractionals
- intake (HPN, additional IV fluids, oral fluids)
- output
- medications added to HPN; other medications given
- catheter care (heparin flush, cap change, dressing change)
- blood draws for laboratory tests

Although complications occur less frequently in the home than in the inpatient setting,[112] the patient and caregiver need oral and written instructions regarding symptoms requiring notification of the nurse or physician. The caregiver(s) and nurse should also observe the patient for depression or anxiety, which can occur with long-term HPN.[114,115]

## Intravenous Antimicrobial Therapy

Antimicrobial therapy is the most commonly used IV therapy at home.[98,112] Home parenteral antimicrobial therapy (HPAT) is a preferred method for delivering a course of therapy for many infectious diseases because of the significant cost savings compared with hospitalization costs.[116] It is the most appropriate therapy for infectious diseases that require either prolonged, repeated, or short-term antimicrobial agents with infrequent administration of drugs that are relatively safe. HPAT is also given in the home for low-risk cancer patients with fever and neutropenia.[117]

### Criteria for patient selection

Criteria for patient selection for HPAT include the following:[118]

1. Medical status is stable.
2. Other aspects of the patient's treatment plan can be monitored or performed at home; hospitalization continues for IV therapy only.
3. The patient and family understand and agree with the plan for home therapy.
4. The patient is psychologically stable, with no history of drug abuse.
5. The patient or caregiver has manual dexterity, basic mathematical and reading skills, the ability to comprehend and follow instructions, and the motivation to be educated to administer antibiotics.
6. The patient has a caregiver or support person available in the home to provide assistance.
7. The patient has peripheral veins suited for repeated cannulizations or has a central venous catheter in place.
8. The patient has a suitable home environment for therapy (e.g., refrigerator, freezer, telephone, transportation).
9. The arrangement of payment for supplies, medication, skilled nursing visits, laboratory tests, and clinic appointments is agreeable to the patient and family.

### Nursing management

As with any type of parenteral therapy, before the patient is discharged from the hospital, arrangements need to be made for the preparation and delivery of pharmaceutical supplies to the home. Infusion therapy agencies with pharmacies will prepare and deliver the antibiotics and the supplies on schedule. The patient is usually given enough supplies to last a week. If the antimicrobial agents are prepared in batches and sent to the patient for storage, frequent deliveries may be required depending upon the stability of the specific antibiotic agent.[119] During the active treatment phase, nursing visits may vary in frequency from three times a day to once a week. On each visit the nurse monitors vital signs, laboratory tests, equipment operation, supplies, adverse drug effects, and signs or symptoms of complications. Although the patient may prepare, store, and administer the HPAT, the home care nurse is responsible for ensuring that specific pharmaceutical guidelines are followed during the course of therapy (e.g., storage and mixing of drugs).

By far the simplest and least costly drug delivery system is gravity infusion adapted to the home. In those cases where the infusion rate is a critical factor in administration, it is preferable to use a mechanized infusion pump. The development of portable, programmable infusion pumps (such as the CADD-Plus® [Pharmacia Deltec]) that deliver a prescribed amount of drug intermittently over a 24-hour period have made HPAT feasible for persons who were ineligible in the past because of lack of caregiver support or dexterity.[120]

Factors such as dosing interval or adverse effects profile are important in selecting a drug. The antimicrobial agent of choice for home administration would be the safest, most effective, cost-efficient, and easily administered antimicrobial agent available. A drug that needs to be administered only once or twice daily is especially well suited for the home setting.[120] Consideration must be given to the stability of the medication and type of storage required. Recommended refrigeration temperature of 2°C–8°C (36°F–44°F) can be achieved in most home and commercial refrigerators. To prevent unnecessary freezing or warming, the temperature should be pretested before placing a supply of prepared parenteral bags in the refrigerator. It is advisable to purchase a refrigerator thermometer to monitor the temperature during active storage. Since some antimicrobial agents have a stability of 30 days or more, they are available as commercially frozen piggyback solutions as well as solutions prepared and frozen by pharmacies. If drugs are frozen, it is necessary to use proper thawing techniques to prevent inactivation or degradation. The drug is kept at room temperature until it is completely thawed (approximately one to three hours and four to six hours for 50-ml and 100-ml bags, respectively).[119] Except for certain drugs, a 24-hour supply of frozen, small-volume parenteral bags can be thawed in advance and then refrigerated to meet the next day's needs. Patient education is the key to safe administration of antimicrobial agents in the home. Content areas include venous access site care, signs and symptoms of drug side effects and recurrent infection, proper drug preparation procedures, drug administration techniques, catheter flushing and care, infusion pump operation (if applicable), and identification and resolution of problems. Instructions for patients in administration of antimicrobial agents in the home are listed in Table 53-8.

Reimbursement for HPAT has been inconsistent and varies according to the reimbursement policies of the individual third-party payer.[114] Since many insurers do

**TABLE 53-8**  Patient Teaching for Self-Administration of IV Antibiotics without a Pump

1. Remove bag with antibiotic solution from refrigerator and thaw according to directions (if applicable).
2. Wash hands thoroughly.
3. Insert needle with syringe attached into vial of heparin solution and withdraw prescribed amount. Replace needle on syringe. Keep capped.
4. Hang bag of antibiotic solution above arm on IV pole.
5. Fill chamber of IV tubing with fluid and purge air from tubing.
6. Cleanse venous access catheter cap with alcohol swab.
7. Connect IV tubing to catheter.
8. Establish IV flow rate as determined by physician.
9. When antibiotic is infused, disconnect tubing and inject heparin and flush venous access catheter.
10. Discard syringe and needles into a nonpenetrable container labeled "Infectious Wastes" for appropriate disposal.
11. Discard remaining used materials into double plastic bags. Seal and dispose with wastes.

Adapted from Brown RB: Selection and training of patients for outpatient intravenous antibiotic therapy. *Rev Infect Dis* 13:s147–s151, 1991 (suppl).

not cover HPAT, pretreatment approval from the insurer is usually necessary.

## Pain Management

Principles of pain management in the home setting include the following:

- an analgesic regimen that is the simplest to administer and provides sufficient pain relief to allow optimal functioning of the patient

- pain medications given around the clock, not PRN (continuous pain requires continuous treatment)

- measures other than analgesics to decrease pain employed consistently and effectively (e.g., relaxation techniques)

- interventions to prevent potential side effects of a narcotic analgesic regimen initiated concurrently (e.g., anticonstipation medications)

- ongoing comprehensive assessment of the patient's pain (identify the source of pain whenever possible and do not assume that the patient's pain is due to the malignant process)

- assessment of the patient and family misconceptions about the use and abuse of narcotic analgesics.

Chapter 20 provides a comprehensive review of pain management.

Oral analgesics such as concentrated solutions and sustained-release tablets of morphine are preferable for long-term cancer pain management for a number of reasons: effectiveness, ease of administration, increased compliance, allowance of uninterrupted sleep, no restriction of movement, and no equipment requirement.[121,122]

Intermittent or continuous infusion therapy for pain is given in the home setting via a variety of routes: subcutaneous, intravenous (IV), epidural, and subarachnoid.[123,124] For continuous infusions, use of ambulatory infusion pumps offers unimpeded mobility. Pain management via infusion therapy is associated with increased costs, risks related to an invasive procedure, anxiety, and care requirements necessitating a thorough evaluation of the patient and family prior to implementation.[125] A willing and able caregiver who can learn about pain control methods and equipment and cope with changes in the patient's pain status is essential. Patients and families are taught preparation and administration procedures, dressing change procedures, and catheter site care. The nurse is usually responsible for changing the medication cassette if the caregiver is unable to learn the procedure.

Patient-controlled analgesia (PCA) is an IV drug delivery system that delivers continuous dosing and allows patients to administer intermittent predetermined doses of analgesic. Small computerized, portable PCA pumps are available for home use. The ability to self-administer medication and manage pain produces a sense of control

for patients that seems to decrease feelings of powerlessness and vulnerability.[126,127] Citron et al[128] reported that PCA-administered morphine produced significant pain relief without undue sedation in severe cancer pain episodes.

Difficulty in obtaining narcotics for home use must be considered. Community pharmacies do not routinely stock potent narcotics and may require one or two weeks to obtain the drugs. Telephone-ordered prescriptions for potent narcotics are not accepted by a pharmacy. Therefore, analgesic requirements must be anticipated and methods of obtaining prescriptions planned. New prescriptions can be obtained from the hospital outpatient pharmacy until arrangements can be made with local pharmacies to order certain narcotics for the cancer patient. In addition, many patients may have difficulty paying for expensive analgesics. The home care social worker can be helpful in obtaining medications from pharmaceutical companies' indigent programs or community service agencies. Physicians may be reluctant to prescribe adequate doses of pain medication for patients in the home setting because of restrictive controlled substance laws in some states.[129] If this situation occurs, the home care nurse will discuss current pain management strategies with the physician and send references supporting adequate pain management approaches to physicians. If needed, a referral to a pain clinic will be requested or other physicians who have provided care can be contacted for assistance in managing the patient's pain.[130]

Measures to decrease pain other than narcotic analgesics may be more effective in the comfort of the patient's home. Behavioral coping strategies and noninvasive techniques can be taught to patients and families. These include distraction, relaxation,[131–133] and cutaneous stimulation. Other types of medications may be considered as adjunctive therapy. The emotional and psychological component of pain must be recognized. Tricyclic antidepressants are one group of drugs that most clinicians agree can play a role in pain management.[134] Other categories of medications include anticonvulsants (especially carbamazepine) and steroids for nervous system involvement. Over-the-counter medications such as hypnotics for insomnia, antitussives for cough, and antacids for dyspepsia are frequently found in home medicine cabinets and may be helpful.

Assessment of pain is ongoing. A change in the location, severity, or type of pain may indicate an acute problem that requires other interventions. For example, a home care patient with cancer of the prostate and diffuse bony metastases complained to the nurse that his pain was getting worse. A detailed pain assessment determined that the pain was now sharp rather than dull, localized to the center of his back, and became excruciating when he attempted to sit. He previously described his pain as more diffuse, regardless of position. No neurological deficits were noted. After a conference with the physician, the patient was transported by ambulance to the hospital, where radiological studies confirmed the presence of three vertebral compression fractures.

Patients and caregivers often negatively influence the treatment of pain as a result of their fears or beliefs about pain and potent narcotics. They may increase the dose interval, withhold doses, or refuse certain medications or certain routes of administration as they attempt to prevent dependence, addiction, somnolence, or sedation. Physiological dependence and tolerance are anticipated, but particular problems in the home can be managed both by adjusting the dose upward according to need or, conversely, by slowly decreasing the dose over time before discontinuing the narcotic. Twycross and Lack[135] note that experience with morphine and other opioid-like drugs shows that the dose usually increases over time, indicating the development of tolerance. Addiction (that is, psychological craving for a drug's psychic effects) is a phenomenon rarely seen in cancer pain management. This information is helpful to share with patients and families as they struggle to manage cancer pain at home.

## DISCHARGE FROM HOME HEALTH CARE

The overall goal of home health care is to facilitate the patient's and family's independence in managing daily life within the constraints imposed by the malignant disease. Home health services are discontinued or modified when the level of care required by the patient decreases; the family is willing, able, and knowledgeable in managing the patient's care; and the identified outcomes developed by the nurse, patient, and family have been achieved. For example, a person who is being followed for wound care may be discharged from services when it is apparent that the individual and family are demonstrating safe wound care and can identify signs or symptoms of potential problems. This does not necessarily mean that the wound is healed but rather that the patient can manage independently and safely. This is particularly true in the case of severely disrupted tissue integrity that is not expected to heal.

Patients will also be discharged from home health care when an exacerbation of the disease process produces symptoms that require management in an inpatient setting or when service needs change. For instance, when professional nursing is no longer required but assistance with household tasks or personal care is still necessary, the nurse should make a referral to a community service agency for homemaker/chore provider or personal care services.

Another reason for discharge is when the person's health status declines so that family members are physically, mentally, or emotionally unable to provide care at home. Patients and families need to be assisted and supported in their decision to move the patient to a long-term care setting. With increased emphasis on the home as the "ideal" (and financially advantageous) setting for care, families can often feel like failures when they decide to place the person in an extended care facility or to return the patient to the hospital. Guilt occurs even when families have provided excellent care for long periods of time.

An area of concern in patient discharge from home health care occurs when the patient and family desire to continue services but the nurse must discharge the patient because the patient's physical status has changed and no longer meets the requirements for reimbursable home health care. Potential liability may occur if the patient is subsequently injured as a result of precipitous termination of care.[136,137] The home health nurse may reduce the potential for liability with a thorough assessment of the patient's health status, nursing and health care needs, and the family and home situation prior to admission. If the nurse determines that the agency and staff cannot manage the patient and family service needs, the case should not be admitted to home health care. If the case is admitted to home health care, risk may be reduced by developing and implementing a comprehensive discharge plan at the time of admission. Table 53-9 lists the components of a discharge plan.

When evaluating the discharge process, important points to consider and document are (1) the patient's status on discharge, (2) evidence of planning for discharge, and (3) timeliness of the decision to discharge.

## QUALITY IMPROVEMENT IN HOME CARE

Quality improvement is essential in home health care in light of the changing health care environment to a managed care focus; increased competition; growth of advanced technological services; and the need to define the outcomes of home care service.[138] Quality improve-

**TABLE 53-9** Planning for Discharge from Home Care

1. Assess patient's physical, functional, psychosocial status prior to discharge and compare and evaluate with assessment at time of admission.
2. Identify patient outcomes and evaluate with goals identified at time of admission or as revised while receiving home health care.
3. Discuss plans and rationale for discharge with patient and family at time of admission, periodically during service, and 3 weeks prior to discharge.
4. Identify continuing patient care needs.
5. Assess patient and family knowledge and skill in performing continuing care needs.
6. Assist the patient and family to identify and form networks in the community.
7. If patient care needs exist, provide the patient and family with the names and addresses of community resources and assist with the referral if needed.

Adapted from Brent NJ: Avoiding patient abandonment charges: Balancing the legal and ethical issues. *Home Healthcare Nurse* 7:7–8, 1989.

ment is an ongoing process involving individual and group efforts. It requires a usable definition of quality; standards of quality as defined by the agency against which quality can be judged; collection, analysis, and dissemination of data and findings essential to processes and outcomes of service; and implementation of methods to initiate and evaluate subsequent planned changes.[139]

Home health agencies must define their philosophy, purpose, goals, and objectives as well as their policies and procedures for operations based on standards for home health care. The home health care regulatory bodies (e.g., Department of Public Health, HCFA), professional organizations (ANA, Oncology Nursing Society), and national organizations for home care have developed standards. Standards that are pertinent to home care for persons with cancer include the ANA and Oncology Nursing Society's *Standards of Oncology Nursing Practice*[41] and the ANA's *Standards of Home Health Nursing Practice*.[25]

Credentialing organizations (Joint Commission for Accreditation of Healthcare Organizations [JCAHO] and the National League of Nursing's Community Health Accreditation Program [CHAP]) have developed models for continuous quality improvement in home health agencies.[140] Many home health agencies now accredited by the JCAHO and the CHAP market their accreditation as an indicator of the quality of their services. Donabedian's[141] model for evaluation of quality embodies the home health agency's organizational structure, the process of service delivery, and the outcomes of care as interrelated dimensions of a system of care.

Quality improvement requires a commitment from senior management to support the concepts of the program and provide adequate financial and human resources. A quality improvement resource group with members from senior management and key departments can facilitate implementation of a quality improvement program.[142] To produce a change in the organization's culture to one of continuous, total quality performance in clinical, clerical, and financial functions, all agency staff must be educated in quality improvement theory and process and supported during the implementation program. The agency's customers, both internal and external, must be identified. The internal customers include the clinical, clerical, billing, and data entry staff, as well as supervisors and managers. External customers are the patients and their families; physicians, who are not only a referral source but also review and sign orders; hospital discharge planners; case managers; health insurance reimbursers; and suppliers of goods and equipment.

The process of service delivery is routinely evaluated by most home health agencies in quarterly utilization review committees, periodic process audits, and routine clinical record review by supervisors.[138] With quality improvement, processes of agency operations and service delivery that are essential to improving and achieving quality are targeted. Representatives of each department involved with a process form a team to examine its operations for flaws or redundancies and to discuss measures for improvement. The team may study how this process

functions in similar agencies to determine the goal and the strategies necessary to achieve the goal. Thus quality improvement is a new way of doing the work involving all staff in the process to produce quality service. It mandates doing things right every time.[139] The links between processes and outcomes of care are being studied by universities, home health professional organizations, providers, and payers to develop measurable outcomes that define quality.[143,144] However, the availability of consistent, reliable, and valid information from home health agencies is limited.

The National Association for Home Care has developed a uniform minimum data set of items of information with uniform definitions and categories that involve specific dimensions of home care services to guide health agencies in the collection of meaningful information. These data would be used in the development of measurable outcomes for home care. Shaughnessy et al[143] developed outcome measures of the quality of home care services for the Medicare program that are currently being field-tested in home health agencies. The outcomes being studied measure changes in the patient's ability to manage activities of daily living, participate in self-care, mobility, and morbidity (e.g., pain, dyspnea, depression, confusion). Data on hospital admission, visits to emergency departments, admissions to long-term care, and discharges to independent living—information frequently requested by managed care organizations— are also being collected.[145,146] These indicators will provide a framework for an outcome-based quality improvement program for home care. Service satisfaction surveys completed by service recipients are another measure of quality reflecting the home health agency's success in meeting the needs and expectations of the patient and the family's values and expectations. They often can serve to identify issues requiring improvement. A sampling of quality indicators is listed in Table 53-10. Additional studies and measures of quality of care are discussed in chapter 55.

## CONCLUSION

The home is an appropriate health care setting for individuals with cancer and other chronic or long-term illnesses. Home care agencies are expanding in numbers and variety of services. Advances in technology and cost-containment measures have shifted the focus of care from inpatient facilities to alternate delivery sources such as home care. Society's awareness of the scope of patient needs is increasing, as evidenced by the hospice movement, and families are becoming more willing to care for their members in the home. Individuals are living longer with a cancer diagnosis because of earlier detection and more effective treatment modalities. Today the majority of the life of an individual diagnosed with cancer is spent in the home setting. The patient and family living with cancer at home require a range of health care and

**TABLE 53-10** A Sampling of Quality Indicators

| Indicator | Example |
|---|---|
| Physiological status | Pain controlled |
| | Pressure ulcer(s) healed |
| Functional status | Transfers from bed to chair independently |
| | Ambulates without assistance |
| Health-related knowledge | Demonstrates wound care procedure |
| | Absence of wound infection |
| Treatment compliance | Follows medication schedule |
| | Absence of emergent care for disease-related problem |
| Satisfaction | High rate of satisfaction with care on survey |

Adapted from Shaughnessy PW et al: Outcome-based quality improvement in home care. *Caring* 44–49, 1995; and from Shaughnessy PW et al: Measuring and assuring the quality of home health care. *Health Care Financing Review* 16:35–67, 1994

social services to maintain optimal levels of physical, psychological, and social functioning. They also need help to support the patient through the continuum of illness. The nurse in the home setting is challenged to expand the quality of care provided to the patient and support for the family. Speaking on a very human level, the nurse has the privilege of entering the homes of individuals and families living with cancer at extremely critical times. The home setting provides an opportunity to fully understand the impact of the cancer experience on the lives of those involved and allows the nurse the opportunity to interact with patients and families on a level that is often difficult to achieve in other settings.

# REFERENCES

1. Department of Health and Human Services Health Care Financing Administration: Trends in Medicare home health agency utilization and payment: CYS 1974–93. *Health Care Financing Review: Statistical Supplement,* Washington, DC, pp 80–85, 1995
2. National Association for Home Care: Medicare certified home care agencies continue to show strong growth. *NAHC Bulletin* 636, 1995
3. Levit KR, Lazenby HC, Sivarajan L, et al: Data View: National health expenditures, 1994. *Health Care Financing Review* 17(3):205–242, 1996
4. Department of Health and Human Services Health Care Financing Administration: *Medicare Home Health Agency Manual.* Transmittal No. 222, Baltimore, MD, U.S. Department of Health and Human Services, April 1989
5. Fazzi RA, Agoglia RV: What home care executives should know about managed care organizations: Preliminary results from a national study. *Caring* 14(10):78–85, 1995
6. U.S. Department of Health and Human Services: Growth in Medicare Managed Care Enrollment, CYS 1985–96. *Health Care Financing Review, Statistical Supplement, 1996.* Baltimore, MD, U.S. Department of Health and Human Services, 126–127, 1996
7. Rose MA: Home care nursing practice: The new frontier. *Holistic Nurs Pract* 3:1–5, 1989
8. Council on Scientific Affairs, American Medical Association: Home care in the '90's. *JAMA* 263:1241–1244, 1990
9. Department of Health and Human Services Health Care Financing Administration: *Health Insurance for the Aged: Home Health Agency Manual.* Baltimore, DHHS, 1966
10. Conkling VK: Continuity of care issues for cancer patients and families. *Cancer* 64:290–294, 1989
11. Lamb GS, Stempel JE: Nurse case management from the client's view: Growing as insider-expert. *Nurs Outlook* 42:7–13, 1994
12. American Nurses' Association: *Nursing Case Management.* Kansas City, MO, ANA, 1988
13. Trella RS: A multidisciplinary approach to case management of frail hospitalized older adults. *J Nurs Adm* 23(2):20–26, 1993
14. Balzer J: The power to care: The positive aspects of case management. *J Home Health Care Prac* 6(2):12–16, 1994
15. Peters DA: A concept of nursing discharge. *Holistic Nurs Pract* 3(2):18–25, 1989
16. Koch MW: Synergy: Utilization management and discharge planning. *Continuing Care* 10(5):12–15, 1991
17. McNally JC, McEnroe LE: Home health care, in Buchsel PC, Yarbro CH (eds): *Oncology Nursing in the Ambulatory Setting.* Boston, Jones and Bartlett, 1993, pp 217–245
18. Yost LS: Cancer patients and home care: Extent to which required services are not received. *Cancer Pract* 3(2):83–87, 1995
19. Slevin AP, Roberts AS: Discharge planning: A tool for decision making. *Nurs Manage* 18(12):47–50, 1987
20. Siegal K, Raveis V, Houts P: Caregiver burden and unmet patient needs. *Cancer* 68:1131–1140, 1991
21. Buehler JA, Lee HL: Exploration of home care resources for rural families with cancer. *Cancer Nurs* 15:299–308, 1992
22. O'Hare PA, Malone D, Lusk E, et al: Unmet needs of black patients with cancer post hospitalization: A descriptive study. *Oncol Nurs Forum* 20:659–664, 1993
23. Lewis FM: Experienced personal control and quality of life in late-stage cancer patients. *Nurs Res* 31:113–119, 1982
24. Kalish PA, Kalish BJ: *The Advance of American Nursing.* Boston, Little, Brown, 1986, pp 259–289
25. American Nurses' Association: *Standards of Home Health Nursing Practice.* Kansas City, MO, ANA, 1986
26. Presznecker BL, Zerwekh JV, Horn BJ: The mutual-participation relationship: Key to facilitating self-care practices in clients and families. *Public Health Nurs* 6:197–203, 1989
27. Speese-Owens N: Psychological components of cancer nursing, in Bouchard-Kurtz R, Speese-Owens N (eds): *Nursing Care of the Cancer Patient* (ed 4). St. Louis, Mosby, 1981
28. Woodward W, Thobaben M: Special home health care nursing challenges. *Home Healthcare Nurse* 12(3):33–37, 1994
29. Denham S: Family routines: A construct for considering family health. *Holistic Nurs Pract* 9(4):11–23, 1995
30. DuFault K Sr, Firsich SC, Gardner A, et al: Ineffective family coping, in McNally JC (ed): *Guidelines for Oncology Nursing Practice.* Philadelphia, Saunders, 1991, pp 103–107
31. Stetz KM: Caregiving demands during advanced cancer: The spouse's needs. *Cancer Nurs* 10:260–268, 1987
32. Wingate AL, Lackey NR: A description of the needs of

noninstitutional cancer patients and their primary caregivers. *Cancer Nurs* 12:216–225, 1989

33. Hileman JA, Lackey NR, Hassanein RS: Identifying the needs of home caregivers of patients with cancer. *Oncol Nurs Forum* 19:771–777, 1992

34. Stommel M, Given CW, Given BA: The cost of cancer home care to families. *Cancer* 71:1867–1874, 1993

35. Hull MM: Coping strategies of family caregivers in hospice homecare. *Oncol Nurs Forum* 19:1179–1187, 1992

36. Hohl D: Patient satisfaction in home care/hospice. *Nurs Manage* 25(1):52–54, 1994

37. Hull MM: Hospice nurses: Caring support for caregiving families. *Cancer Nurs* 14:63–70, 1991

38. Skorupka P, Bohnet N: Primary caregiver's perceptions of nursing behaviors that best meet their needs in a home care hospice setting. *Cancer Nurs* 5:371–374, 1982

39. Giaquinta B: Helping families face the crisis of cancer. *Am J Nurs* 77:1585–1588, 1977

40. Van Ort S, Woodtli A: Home health care: Providing a missing link. *Gerontol Nurs* 15:4–9, 1989

41. American Nurses' Association and Oncology Nursing Society: *Standards of Oncology Nursing Practice*. Kansas City, MO, ANA, 1987

42. Shiber S, Larson E: Evaluating the quality of caring: Structure, process, and outcome. *Holistic Nurs Pract* 5:57–66, 1991

43. Leming T: Quality customer service: Nursing's new challenge. *Nurs Admin Q* 15:6–12, 1991

44. Kramer AM, Shaughnessy PW, Baumen MK, et al: Assessing and assuring the quality of home health care: A conceptual framework. *Milbank Q* 68:413–443, 1990

45. Cloonan PA, Shuster GF: Care coordination: A resource-intensive component of home health nursing practice. *Public Health Nurs* 7:204–208, 1990

46. Shuster GF, Cloonan P: Nursing activities and reimbursement in clinical case management. *Home Healthcare Nurse* 7:10–15, 1989

47. O'Hare PA, Terry MA: Community-based care management: A framework for delivery of services. *Home Healthcare Nurse* 9(3):26–32, 1991

48. Knollmueller RN: Case management: What's in a name? *Nurs Manage* 20(10):38–42, 1989

49. Creighton H: Legal significance of charting—Part 1. *Nurs Manage* 18(9):17–22, 1987

50. Connaway N: Documenting patient care in the home: Legal issues for home health nurses. *Home Healthcare Nurse* 3(5):6–8, 1985

51. Schulmeister L: Documentation in oncology nursing. *Current Issues in Cancer Nursing Practice Updates:* 1(9):1–8, 1993

52. Mayer D, O'Connor L: Rehabilitation of persons with cancer: An ONS position statement. *Oncol Nurs Forum* 16:433, 1989

53. Watson PG: The optimal functioning plan: A key element in cancer rehabilitation. *Cancer Nurs* 15:254–263, 1992

54. Blesch KS: Rehabilitation of the cancer patient at home. *Semin Oncol Nurs* 12:219–225, 1996

55. Hoeman SP: Community-based rehabilitation. *Holistic Nurs Pract* 6(2):32–41, 1992

56. Hileman JW, Lackey VR: Self-identified needs of patients with cancer at home and their caregivers: A descriptive study. *Oncol Nurs Forum* 17:907–913, 1990

57. Mor V, Guadagnoli E, Wool M: An examination of the concrete service needs of advanced cancer patients. *J Psychosoc Oncol* 5:1–7, 1987

58. Cyr LB: The clinical nurse specialist in a home health care setting. *Home Healthcare Nurse* 8(1):34–39, 1990

59. Hamric AB: Role development and functions, in Hamric AB, Spross J (eds): *The Clinical Nurse Specialist in Theory and Practice*. Orlando, FL, Grune and Stratton, 1986, pp 39–58

60. Moore SM: Promoting advanced nursing practice. *AACN* 4:603–608, 1993

61. Satinsky MA: Advanced practice nurse in a managed care environment, in Hickey IV, Quimette RN, Venegonski SL (eds): *Advanced Practice Nursing: Changing Roles and Clinical Applications*. Philadelphia, Lippincott-Raven, 1996, pp 126–145

62. Donley RSr: Advanced practice nursing after healthcare reform. *Nursing Economics:* 13(2):84–88, 1995

63. Boyd NS, Stasiowski SA, Catoe PT, et al: The merit and significance of the clinical nurse specialist. *J Nurs Adm* 21(9):35–43, 1991

64. Felder LA: Direct patient care and independent practice, in Hamric AB, Spross J (eds): *The Clinical Nurse Specialist in Theory and Practice*. Orlando, FL, Grune and Stratton, 1983, pp 59–72

65. Giuliano KK, Poirier CE: Nursing case management: Critical pathways to desirable outcomes. *Nurs Manage* 20(3):52–55, 1991

66. Etheridge P, Lamb GS: Professional nursing case management improves quality, access and cost. *Nurs Manage* 20(2):30–35, 1989

67. Cronin CJ, Maklebust J: Case-managed care: Capitalizing on the CNS. *Nurs Manage* 20(3):38–47, 1989

68. Benoit CB: Case management and the advanced practice nurse, in Hickey IV, Quimette RN, Venegoni SL (eds): *Advanced Practice Nursing: Changing Roles and Clinical Applications*. Philadelphia, Lippincott-Raven, 1996, pp 107–125

69. Pera MK, Gould EJ: Home care nursing: Integration of politics and nursing. *Holistic Nurs Pract* 3(2):9–17, 1989

70. Puig L: Health care comes home for savings. *Business Health* 7:10–20, 1989

71. Reif L: Making dollars and sense of home health policy. *Nurs Economics* 2:382–388, 1984

72. Simione WJ: Reimbursement for home care services. *Caring* 5:22–26, 1986

73. Seeber S, Baird SB: The impact of healthcare changes on home health. *Semin Oncol Nurs* 12:179–187, 1996

74. U.S. Department of Health and Human Services: Overview of the Medicaid Program. *Health Care Financing Review*. Statistical Supplement, Baltimore, MD, U.S. Department of Health and Human Services, 134–186, 1996

75. Della Monica E, Yuan J: Documentation in home care: Skilled observation. *Home Healthcare Nurse* 6(1):39–40, 1988

76. Omdahl DJ: Preventing home care denials. *Am J Nurs* 87:1031–1033, 1987

77. U.S. Department of Health and Human Services. Personal Health Care Expenditures: CYs 1960–2005. *Health Care Financing Review*. Statistical Supplement, Baltimore, MD, U.S. Department of Health and Human Services, 10–11, 1996

78. Rooks JP: Let's admit we ration health care—then set priorities. *Am J Nurs* 90(5):39–43, 1990

79. Kinsey KK: Risky business: Managing the health care of urban low-income families. *Holis Nurs Pract* 9(4):41–53, 1995

80. Hamill CT, Parver CP: Home health services: A vital component of managed care. *J Home Health Care Prac* 7(4):16–23, 1995

81. Capuzzi C, Garland M: The Oregon plan: Increasing access to health care. *Nurs Outlook* 38:260–286, 1990

82. Collopy B, Dubler N, Zuckerman C: The ethics of home care: Autonomy and accommodation. *Hastings Cent Rep* 20: 1–16, 1990 (suppl)

83. Haddad AM: Ethical problems in home health care. *J Nurs Adm* 22(3):46–51, 1992

84. Haddad AM: Ethical considerations in home care of the oncology patient. *Semin Oncol Nurs* 12(3):226–230, 1996

85. Young A, Pignatello CH, Taylor M: Who's the boss? Ethical conflicts in home care. *Health Prog* 69(11):59–62, 1988

86. Aroskar MA: Community health nurses: Their most significant ethical decision-making problems. *Nurs Clin North Am* 24:967–975, 1989

87. Taylor EJ, Ferrell BR, Grant M, et al: Managing cancer pain at home: The decisions and ethical conflicts of patients, caregivers, and home care nurses. *Oncol Nurs Forum* 20: 919–927, 1993

88. Veatch RM, Fry ST: *Case Studies in Nursing Ethics.* Philadelphia, Lippincott, 1987

89. Gadow S: An ethical case for patient self-determination. *Semin Oncol Nurs* 5:99–101, 1989

90. Beauchamp TL, Childress JF: *Principles of Biomedical Ethics* (ed 2). New York, Oxford University Press, 1983

91. Fry ST: Ethics and cancer care, in Baird S, McCorkle R, Grant M (eds): *Cancer Nursing: A Comprehensive Textbook.* Philadelphia, Saunders, 1991, pp 31–37

92. American Nurses' Association: *Code for Nurses with Interpretive Statements.* Kansas City, MO, ANA, 1985

93. DeWolf MS: Ethical decision-making. *Semin Oncol Nurs* 5: 77–81, 1989

94. Flaherty G: Ethics in nursing practice. *Today's Prof Nurse* 1: 10–12, 1990

95. Jameton A: *Nursing Practice: The Ethical Issues.* Englewood Cliffs, NJ, Prentice-Hall, 1984

96. Brown JM: Home care models for infusion therapy. *Caring* 9(5):24–26, 1990

97. Handy CM: Patient-centered high-technology home care. *Holistic Nurs Pract* 3(2):46–53, 1989

98. Steinheinheiser MM: Vascular access device choices for home care patients. *Caring* 14:14–26, 1995

99. Rountree D: The PIC catheter. *Am J Nurs* 91(8):22–26, 1991

100. Department of Health and Human Services Health Care Financing Administration Part II, 29 CRF 1910, 1030. Occupational exposure to bloodborne pathogens: Final rule. *Federal Register* 56:64175–64182, Dec. 6, 1991

101. Grace LA, Tomaselli BJ: Intravenous therapy in the home, in Terry J, Baronowski L, Lonsway RA (eds): *Intravenous Therapy: Clinical Principles and Practices.* Philadelphia, Saunders, 1995, pp 505–534

102. Gullo SM: Safe handling of antineoplastic drugs: Translating the recommendations into practice. *Oncol Nurs Forum* 15:595–601, 1988

103. Oncology Nursing Society: *Cancer Chemotherapy Guidelines and Recommendations for Practice.* Pittsburgh, ONS, 1996

104. Cloak M, Connor TH, Stevens KR, et al: Occupational exposure of nursing personnel to antineoplastic agents. *Oncol Nurs Forum* 12(5):33–39, 1985

105. Rogers B, Emmett EA: Handling antineoplastic agents: Urine mutagenicity in nurses. *Image: J Nurs Schol* 19: 108–113, 1987

106. Occupational Safety and Health Administration: *Work Practice Guidelines for Personnel Dealing with Cytotoxic (Antineoplastic) Drugs.* OSHA Instruction Publication 8–1. Washington DC, Office of Occupational Medicine, Jan. 29, 1986

107. Vega-Stromberg T: Chemotherapy administration, in Gorski LG (ed): *High Tech Home Care Manual.* Gaithersburg, MD, Aspen, 1994, pp 10:1–10

108. Graves T, Proemer J: New methods of chemotherapy administration-selected routes. *J Pharm Pract* 4:49–63, 1991

109. Balinsky W: Reimbursement for outpatient antibiotic therapy: Update. *Rev Infect Dis* 13:s193–195, 1991 (suppl 2)

110. Ford CD, Vizcarra C: Parenteral nutrition, in Terry J, Baronowski L, Lonsway RA (eds): *Intravenous Therapy: Clinical Principles and Practice.* Philadelphia, Saunders, 1995, pp 219–248

111. Konstantinides NW: Home parenteral nutrition: A viable alternative. *Oncol Nurs Forum* 12(1):23–29, 1985

112. Grace LA, Tomaselli BJ: Intravenous therapy in the home, in Terry J, Baronowski L, Lonsway RA (eds): *Intravenous Therapy: Clinical Principles and Practices.* Philadelphia, Saunders, 1995, pp 505–534

113. Howard L: Home parenteral nutrition in patients with a cancer diagnosis. *J Paren and Enteral Nutri* 16:935–995, 1992 (suppl)

114. Dudrick SJ, O'Connell JJ, Englert DM, et al: 100 patient years of ambulatory home total parenteral nutrition. *Ann Surg* 199:770–781, 1984

115. Bloch AS, Brown P: Methods of nutritional support in the home. *J Pain Symp Manage* 5:297–306, 1990

116. Grizzard MB, Harris G, Karns H: Use of outpatient parenteral antibiotic therapy in a health maintenance organization. *Rev Infect Dis* 13:s174–179, 1991 (suppl 2)

117. Telcott JA, Whalen A, Clark J, et al: Home antibiotic therapy for low-risk cancer patients with fever and neutropenia. *J Clin Oncol* 12:107–114, 1994

118. Brown RB: Selection and training of patients for outpatient intravenous antibiotic therapy. *Rev Infect Dis* 13:s147–151, 1991 (suppl)

119. Kasmer RJ, Hoisington LM, Yukniewicz S: Home parenteral antibiotic therapy: Part II. Drug preparation and administration considerations. *Home Healthcare Nurse* 5(1):19–29, 1987

120. Williams DN: Home intravenous antibiotic therapy: New technologies. *Recent Results Cancer Res* 121:215–222, 1991

121. Stoll HR: Effective pain control in cancer patients in the home care setting. *Recent Results Cancer Res* 121:36–42, 1991

122. Jacox A, Carr DB, Payne R, et al: Management of cancer pain. *Clinical Practice Guideline No. 9.* AHCPR publication No. 94-0592. Rockville, MD, Agency for Health Care Policy and Research, U.S. Department of Health and Human Services, Public Health Services, March 1994

123. Storey P, Hill HH, St. Louis RH, et al: Subcutaneous infusions for control of cancer symptoms. *J Pain Sympt Manage* 5:33–41, 1990

124. Wild L, Coyne C: The basics and beyond: Epidural analgesia. *Am J Nurs* 92:26–34, 1992

125. Whedon M, Ferrell BR: Professional and ethical considerations in the use of high-tech pain management. *Oncol Nurs Forum* 18(1):1135–1143, 1991

126. Rapsilber LM, Camp-Sorrell D: Ambulatory infusion pumps: Application to oncology. *Semin Oncol Nurs* 11: 213–220, 1995

127. Enck RE: Parenteral narcotics for pain control in the home care environment. *Caring* 9:38–41, 1990

128. Citron ML, Early AJ, Boyer M, et al: Patient controlled

analgesia for severe cancer pain. *Arch Intern Med* 146: 734–736, 1986

129. Shapiro RS: Legal bases for the control of analgesic drugs. *J Pain Symptom Manag* 9:153–159, 1994

130. Magrum L, Bentzen C, Landmark S: Pain management in home care. *Semin Oncol Nurs* 12:202–212, 1996

131. Mast D, Meyers J, Urbanski A: Relaxation techniques: A self-learning module for nurses, Unit I. *Cancer Nurs* 10: 141–147, 1987

132. Mast D, Meyers J, Urbanski A: Relaxation techniques: A self-learning module for nurses, Unit II. *Cancer Nurs* 10: 217–225, 1987

133. Mast D, Meyers J, Urbanski A: Relaxation techniques: A self-learning module for nurses, Unit III. *Cancer Nurs* 10: 279–285, 1987

134. American Cancer Pain Society: *Principles of Analgesic Use in the Treatment of Acute Pain and Cancer Pain* (ed 3). Skokie, IL, American Pain Society, 1992, pp 27–30

135. Twycross R, Lack S: *Oral Morphine in Advanced Cancer.* Bucks, United Kingdom, Beaconsfield Publishers, 1984

136. Brent NJ: Avoiding patient abandonment charges: Balancing the legal and ethical issues. *Home Healthcare Nurse* 7: 7–8, 1989

137. Fiesta J: Home care liability—Part II. *Nurs Manage* 26(12): 2, 1995

138. Chapman AH, Sebastian W: Selected issues in quality improvement and risk management. *Semin Oncol Nurs* 12: 231–237, 1996

139. Foreman JT: Continuous quality improvement in home care. *Caring* 12(10):32–37, 1993

140. Carefoot R: Total quality management implementation in home care agencies: Common questions and answers. *J Nurs Adm* 24(10):31–37, 1994

141. Donabedian A: Quality assessment and assurance: Unity of purpose, diversity of means. *Inquiry* 25:173–192, 1988

142. Bohnet NL, Ilcyn J, Milanovich PS, et al: Continuous quality improvement: Improving quality in your home care organization. *J Nurs Adm* 23(2):42–48, 1993

143. Shaughnessy PW, Crisler KS, Schlenker RE, et al: Measuring and assuring the quality of home health care. *Health Care Financing Review* 16(1):35–67, 1994

144. Pace KB: Data sets for home care organizations. *Caring* 14(2):38–42, 1995

145. Shaughnessy PW, Crisler KS, Schlenker RE, et al: Outcome-based quality improvement in home care. *Caring* 14(2): 44–49, 1995

146. Adams CE, Kramer S, Wilson M: Home health quality outcomes: Fee for services versus health maintenance organization enrollees. *J Nurs Adm* 25(11):39–45, 1995

# Chapter 54

# Hospice Care

**Jeanne Martinez, RN, MPH**

**Steven Wagner, RN, BSN**

## INTRODUCTION

Hospice care was developed to meet a simple objective: to facilitate a comfortable and natural death. However, the concept of a natural death runs counter to our society's values regarding youth, health, and technology, including medical technology. In our modern society, death is a taboo topic.[1] This has been reinforced by our current complex medical system, which errs on the side of technological intervention and overtreatment to prevent death.

### Development of the Hospice Concept

Developers of the hospice concept recognized that allowing a "natural death" requires preparation of the patient and family, changes in medical practice, and redesign or circumvention of some aspects of the existing health care system.[2] An analogy for the scope of the change can be made to birthing and medical care in American society. In the 1960s birthing was treated primarily as a medical problem. Change in the practice of obstetrics was instituted largely by consumer demand from the women's movement, which sought to view birth as a life process that involved the individual woman's right of control over her body and childbirth, as well as the importance of family participation. In response to this demand, obstetric medical practice changed to focus more on prenatal preventive care and education.[2] Attempts to deinstitutionalize the process included creating birthing centers that are more homelike and can facilitate family participation.

Hospice care in America was also influenced by consumer groups. Initially, hospice was likely to be described as a movement or as an "alternative" to mainstream medical care. When hospices first began to appear as organized programs, they were commonly volunteer programs with lay volunteers and a few nurses, organized from a church basement or around someone's dining room table. Today this model is all but extinct, except that hospice has kept the tenet of lay volunteers as part of the core team of interdisciplinary hospice services. The ideas for the American hospice were adapted directly from the English model at St. Christopher's Hospice, the world's first hospice, developed by Dame Cicely Saunders in 1968.

Today, the National Hospice Organization uses the following description to define the hospice philosophy: "Hospice care is specialized care for terminally ill people. Hospice care is a medically directed, interdisciplinary team managed program of services that focuses on the patient/family as the unit of service. Hospice care is palliative rather than curative, with an emphasis on pain and symptom control, so that a person may live the last days of life fully, with dignity and comfort, at home or in a home-like setting."[3]

## Role of Nurses in the Development of Hospice

The word *hospice*, or *hospitia*, was used during the Crusades in the Middle Ages to designate a place of temporary shelter for travelers or sick pilgrims.[2,4] In the late nineteenth century hospice was applied to the care of the dying by Sister Mary Aikenhead, a colleague of Florence Nightingale, who opened Our Lady's Hospice, in Dublin,[2,4] the first facility dedicated to care of the terminally ill.

Although Dame Cicely Saunders is best known as the medical director and founder of St. Christopher's Hospice, she began her career as a nurse and went on to become a medical social worker prior to attending medical school. Dame Saunders developed many of the current concepts in palliative care, including oral narcotic administration on a regular rather than on an as-needed basis.[2]

It was Dame Saunders's visit to Yale University in 1963 that precipitated the interest of Florence Wald, dean of the Yale School of Nursing, in the concept of hospice care. Wald subsequently resigned as dean to participate in the development of the first American hospice, Connecticut Hospice Inc. Connecticut Hospice began serving home care patients in 1974, and in 1979 opened an independent 44-bed inpatient facility, the first to be designed as a hospice.[4]

In 1984 the Joint Commission on Accreditation of Hospitals (JCAH) published its first standards manual for hospice programs.[5] Anne Rooney, RN, a former hospice director of Proviso-Leyden Hospice in Illinois and a former president of the Illinois State Hospice Organization, joined the JCAH in 1985 as associate director of Hospice and Home Care, to facilitate the nationwide accreditation process. In 1992 some of the original hospice standards were incorporated into the Joint Commission on Accreditation of Healthcare Organizations (JCAHO) standards applied to all dying patients in hospitals.[6] Dame Cicely Saunders, Florence Wald, and Anne Rooney are among the many who have made history and continue to make contributions in palliative and hospice care.

Another factor influencing the development of palliative care was the groundbreaking work in the 1960s of Elisabeth Kübler-Ross, a psychiatrist at the University of Chicago. Dr. Kübler-Ross pointed out that health care professionals, due largely to their own ineffectual coping with the subject of death, isolated dying patients. She helped to demystify the dying process by devising the radical teaching technique of interviewing dying patients in front of a group of health care professionals.[1] This not only provided an opportunity to learn firsthand from patients themselves but also provided role modeling for professionals on how to talk to patients. More than anyone else, Elisabeth Kübler-Ross opened the debate on care of the dying not only for the lay public but for health care professionals as well.

# PALLIATIVE CARE APPROACHES

Hospice care pivots around the idea of palliative medical management. Palliative management involves a shift in treatment goals from curative toward providing relief from suffering.[2] And relief of suffering in dying patients goes beyond merely identifying and treating physical symptoms. The emotional, spiritual, and existential components of suffering and pain must also be addressed. Our current health system consists largely of fragmented, specialized care episodes for specific problems rather than a holistic approach to illness.[2] Therefore, management of a patient with a palliative care approach will differ from an acute care approach.

## Principles of Palliative Care

The overall goal of treatment is to optimize quality of life; that is, the hopes and desires of a patient are fulfilled. Death is regarded as a natural process, to be neither hastened nor prolonged. Diagnostic tests and other invasive procedures are minimized, unless likely to result in the alleviation of symptoms. Use of "heroic" treatment measures is discouraged. When using narcotic analgesics, the right dose is the dose that provides pain relief without unacceptable side effects. The patient is the "expert" on whether pain and symptoms have been adequately relieved. Patients eat if they are hungry and drink if thirsty; hence, fluids and feeding are not forced. Care is individualized and based on the goals of the patient and family as the unit of care.

## Palliative versus Acute Care

The following example of a patient with shortness of breath illustrates the differences in approach if the goals of treatment are more palliative than curative. In an acute care situation, a patient with shortness of breath will have diagnostic studies to determine the etiology of the problem. These commonly include blood gas studies, a chest x-ray, complete blood count, and pulmonary function tests. The patient usually will be given supplemental oxygen for comfort. In addition, aggressive efforts to remove or reverse the etiology may be taken in acute care approaches.

When the goal of care is palliation, the etiology generally is either already known or could be unimportant if the patient has a short time to live. The diagnostic procedures for acute care result in some discomfort and often demand that a considerable amount of energy be expended by the patient, such as pulmonary function testing. Results of diagnostic studies still may not provide the information needed to determine which intervention will provide relief from shortness of breath. For example, a patient with chronic lung disease and abnormal blood gas studies may have symptomatically compensated and not feel as distressed as a patient with borderline blood gas studies, for whom shortness of breath is a new symptom.

When symptom management is the primary goal, first-line palliative treatment for shortness of breath is low-dose oral morphine given at regular intervals.[7,8] The low-dose morphine can be used concurrently with oxygen if needed but often is effective alone. Another important palliative measure is positioning the patient to maximize lung expansion. Many patients report that the use of a room fan provides significant relief.[9] Like pain, shortness of breath may be as closely related to psychological and social problems as it is to physical ones. These issues need to be identified, addressed, and treated. When anxiety is a significant factor, low-dose anxiolytic (e.g., a benzodiazepine) can be effective.[7,8]

## Patient Criteria for Hospice Care

Each program determines its own criteria for selecting patients to receive hospice care. For a patient to qualify for the Medicare Hospice Benefit, two physicians must certify that he or she is terminally ill and has less than six months to live.[10] This latter criterion is controversial for a number of reasons. Professionals who work with the dying know that accurate predictions of time of death cannot be made. It is therefore detrimental for physicians or nurses to attempt to give predictions about time of death to patients.[1]

It has proven to be even more difficult to predict prognosis in noncancer end-stage patients. This has prompted the development of more specific medical criteria to be required to admit noncancer patients into hospice care under the Medicare Hospice Benefit. At the urging of the Health Care Finance Administration (HCFA), initial guidelines were developed in 1995 by a national physician task force and revised in 1996 with more comprehensive criteria for eight categories of noncancer, end-stage illness. These include heart, pulmonary, and liver disease; dementia; and HIV. These criteria are currently being studied to assess their accuracy.[11]

Another criterion under Medicare and most state hospice regulations is that the patient sign a consent form or election statement declaring that hospice and palliative care are their choice of treatments and that they have the right to elect out of hospice at any time.[10] The following are additional criteria required by most hospice programs:

- The patient must have a primary caregiver, that is, friend or family member willing to be responsible for the patient's overall care.

- For home care, the patient needs to reside in the hospice program's geographic area.

- The patient must desire palliative, not curative, treatment.[2,4]

## HOSPICE CARE IN THE PRESENT

Development of a hospice program is not as simple as it was in the early phases of the hospice movement. Hospice programs have been affected by mandated guidelines of federal and state legislation. Currently, 34 states have their own licensing regulations, with licensure pending in an additional 7 states. In some states these regulations include a certificate-of-need review that can limit the number of hospices in a given area. Federal guidelines define the Hospice Medicare Benefit Plan used today. These guidelines were developed by hospice program planners to include cost incentives for encouraging home hospice care rather than hospitalization and cost control via a financial cap for all hospice care provided. These cost incentives were proposed for the federal legislature prior to the implementation of Medicare diagnostic related groups (DRGs).

### Models of Hospice Care

The present models for hospice care vary greatly in their size and the means by which they provide care. A recent National Hospice Organization (NHO) study indicated that 40% of all hospices were independent, community-based programs.[12] Though these independent community-based hospices contract with hospitals for inpatient care, their primary focus is care in the home. Funding, boards of directors, and policy decisions for the hospice are independent of the hospital or contracting agencies.

Thirty percent of hospices are owned by hospitals. The caseload is made up primarily of patients referred by physicians or staff from within the parent hospital.

Twenty-four percent of hospices are operated as part of a home health agency. The agency usually has a separate hospice component with at least one nurse coordinating hospice home care. The remaining 7% of hospices are coalition programs or operated in a nursing home setting.[12] Coalition programs are usually a negotiated care service contracted between long-term care facilities and hospice.

Acute care beds in the hospital for hospice patients may be scattered in the medical or oncology units. Some hospitals may have a unit specifically designed for inpatient care of hospice patients. These units attempt to simulate a comfortable, homelike atmosphere. Care is focused on symptom management and limitation of invasive or painful procedures. Visiting policies are less restrictive; for example, pets may be allowed to visit. Inpatient admission is principally for acute care management of pain or other symptoms that cannot be controlled easily in the home. Inpatient admission is also used for short-term respite care. Often patients return home after symptoms have been alleviated and the patient is medically stable. According to Medicare guidelines, at least 80% of an individual hospice's *aggregate* patient days of care under the Hospice Benefit must be provided at home. A maximum of 20% of aggregate days of care can be provided in the inpatient setting. If the maximum aggregate inpatient ratio of 20% is exceeded, the hospice can be denied reimbursement for the excess days.

The 1992 NHO study found that 72% of the 2503 U.S. hospice programs were Medicare-certified. These programs serve more than 340,000 patients annually. In this country, hospices care for an estimated one out of every three individuals who die of cancer and one out of every three individuals whose deaths are related to acquired immunodeficiency syndrome (AIDS).[12] The Medicare guidelines dictate that a full-service hospice be a medically directed program that incorporates home nursing care, social services, home health aid care, dietary counseling, occupational therapy, physical therapy, speech therapy, and counseling, along with trained volunteers to complete the nucleus of core services. The Medicare Hospice Benefit is the only federally funded health care program mandating the use of volunteers. Beyond the core services, the following may be included: art therapy, music therapy, psychologists, and bereavement coordinators (Figure 54-1). Under the Hospice Medicare Benefit, medical supplies, durable medical equipment, and medications are all paid for by the hospice. Since the aim of care is to keep patients at home, nursing and physician services, as well as medications, must be available 24 hours a day. In addition, the hospice must provide bereavement follow-up to the patient's family after death has occurred. The nurse assesses all needs on a continual basis and facilitates services and supplies for individual patients. This interdisciplinary team approach to hospice care accounts for the success of hospices in meeting the physical, emotional, and spiritual needs of patients within a holistic framework, at a time when the family system is experiencing crisis.

### Reimbursement and Funding Methods

Hospice care was a prototype for what is now commonly referred to as *case management*. Consistent with this case management approach is the Medicare Hospice Benefit's capitated per diem reimbursement structure. Per diem is a system of reimbursement that pays a flat daily rate for all services provided to a patient, rather than paying for individual services or items on the traditional fee-for-service basis. The advantages of the per diem system are that it allows the hospice the freedom and independence to provide a comprehensive approach to assess needs and prevent problems, and to provide additional team services as the patient's condition changes. This case management approach is the most efficient and effective way to keep a patient at home. Similarly, the annual per-patient reimbursement cap (which for 1995 was $13,369) is applied on an aggregate basis. For example, a hospice program can be reimbursed $16,000 within a year for one patient since this can usually be balanced out by another patient whose hospice reimbursement did not exceed $10,738 in the same year.

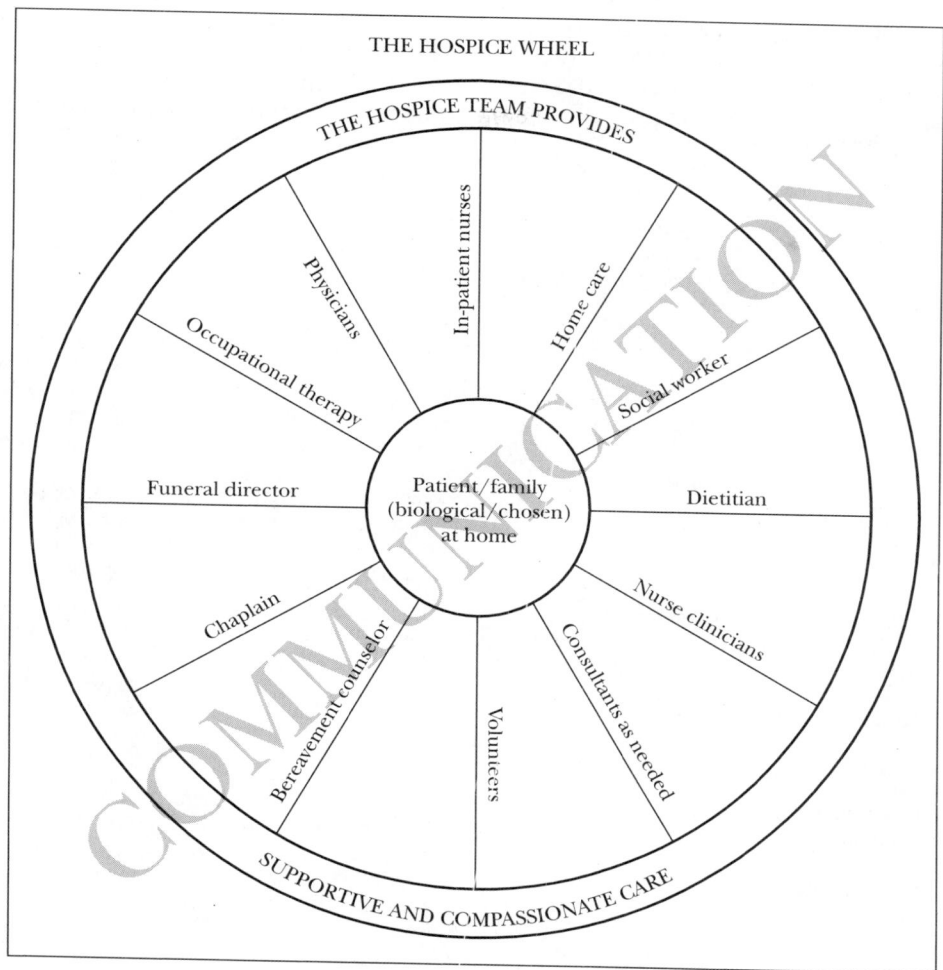

THE HOSPICE WHEEL

THE HOSPICE TEAM PROVIDES

Physicians

In-patient nurses

Occupational therapy

Home care

Social worker

Funeral director

Patient/family
(biological/chosen)
at home

Dietitian

Chaplain

Nurse clinicians

Bereavement counselor

Volunteers

Consultants as needed

COMMUNICATION

SUPPORTIVE AND COMPASSIONATE CARE

**FIGURE 54-1**   Many disciplines are involved in a coordinated effort to provide supportive and compassionate hospice care to the patient and family. (Reprinted with permission from Northwestern Memorial Hospice Program, Chicago, IL. Used by permission of John DeBerry.)

The per diem for the Medicare Hospice Benefit is reimbursed on four levels, as defined by the HCFA: (1) a routine rate, (2) a continuous rate for home care, (3) an inpatient rate for acute care, and (4) an inpatient rate for respite care.[4] For a patient to qualify for the Medicare Hospice Benefit, certification by two physicians of a prognosis of six months or less is required. Recertification of the patient's appropriateness for hospice care is required three times under the benefit. The first and second recertification periods are 90 days each. The third period is 30 days. The fourth benefit period is unlimited, so that after 210 days of care the patient does not need to be recertified for hospice services to continue. Only hospital care, pharmacy, or home care services contracted with the hospice program will receive reimbursement under the benefit. At any time the patient has the option to rescind the hospice benefit and return to regular Medicare Part A coverage.[10]

Eighty-nine percent of current hospices are operated not for profit.[12] Many hospice programs have made a commitment to provide basic hospice services of nursing visits, physician follow-up, social services, and volunteers, regardless of the patient's ability to pay. While the majority of hospice programs are Medicare-certified, Medicare accounted for only 68% of revenue to hospices in 1994. Medicaid provided 7%, private insurance provided 13%, and 12% came from a combination of donations, grants and private pay. Hospices have been successful in introducing per diem billing as the preferred means of reimbursement for private insurance hospice benefits, and today most private health insurance programs provide a hospice benefit of some sort.

## Patient Population

Of the patients who received hospice care in 1992, 78% were diagnosed with cancer, 4% had AIDS, 10% had end-stage heart disease, 1% had Alzheimer's disease, and 1% had renal diagnoses. The remaining 6% had "other" terminal conditions.[12] Of all these diagnoses, AIDS presents the greatest challenge to the health care system, including hospice programs.[2]

The principles of palliative care were originally developed by hospice to meet the needs of the elderly cancer patient. Hospice care is evolving to include patients of differing age-groups who have more complex physical and psychosocial concerns. Tables 54-1 and 54-2 demon-

**TABLE 54-1**  Interdisciplinary Team Care Plan—An Example

| INTERDISCIPLINARY CARE PLAN | | | |
|---|---|---|---|
| Problem | Persons Responsible | Goals/Outcome | Plan |
| Knowledge deficit related to home death | Nurse | Patient and family to express understanding of home death protocol, i.e., no heroic measures, no paramedics, no police; call hospice. Patient and family to demonstrate compliance with home infection control instructions. | Family meeting to discuss home death. Provide both written and verbal instructions as to signs and symptoms of home death and hospice protocol. Reinforce availability of hospice on 24-hour call. Observe the family for compliance with instructions. |
| Maintaining continuity of care | Nurse, hospice team, patient, family | Hospice coordinates patient's home care. | Establish care goals with patient and family. Weekly multidisciplinary meeting to review hospice plan of care. Send written plan of care to patient's physician on regular basis. |
| Altered comfort level related to advanced disease symptoms | Nurse, physician | Patient to express satisfaction with comfort level, i.e., describes pain as 2 or less on 0–5 comfort scale, with 0 being no pain and 5 being severe pain. Episodes of nausea and vomiting reduced. | Assess comfort level with each visit, at least twice weekly. Provide written and verbal instruction regarding analgesic regimen. Instruct family to contact hospice if discomfort increases. Hospice physician to visit monthly if patient is unable to visit clinic. |
| Alteration in physical mobility and safety related to progression of disease toward terminal phase | Physical or occupational therapist | Patient will be injury-free at home. Patient will prioritize functional activities desired. | Assess safety and mobility status at home. Promote activities of daily living. Assess need for assistive devices. Address work simplification and energy conservation measures. |
| Alteration in psychosocial status related to loss of independence, change in parenting role | Social worker, occupational therapist, volunteer, nurse | Patient will demonstrate adaptation to partial independence. Patient will complete legal arrangements for dependent children prior to death. | Social worker visits every week to assess patient's psychosocial status, financial concerns, and provide emotional support. Facilitate discussion and plans regarding choice of legal guardian for children after patient's death. Occupational therapist and volunteers to assist patient in creating a lasting remembrance that she can leave for her children after her death. |

**TABLE 54-1**  (continued)

| | INTERDISCIPLINARY CARE PLAN | | |
| --- | --- | --- | --- |
| Problem | Persons Responsible | Goals/Outcome | Plan |
| Alteration in family psychosocial status related to altered family process roles; anticipatory grieving of children | Social worker, bereavement counselor | Family to express feelings of increased support, ability to manage care at home. Patient and family will be able to verbalize good-byes to each other. Children will be able to express their feelings through verbal and/or nonverbal methods (i.e., art, play, or writing). | Notify school counselor of the stress the children are under so that the school can be helpful in providing support. Volunteers visit 8 hours per week to provide respite support. Social worker to visit every week and address anticipatory grieving based on the developmental age of each child. Team visits regularly to provide opportunity for family to express feelings. |
| Alteration in value/belief pattern related to spiritual distress | Chaplain | Patient and family to express feelings of enhanced spiritual support. | Assess patient and family spiritual needs. With family permission, identify community clergy and notify them of hospice involvement. Offer chaplain home visit to enhance spiritual support. |

**TABLE 54-2**  Aspects of Spiritual Care

The spiritual aspects of care encompass a person's relationship to things larger than the self: causes, principles, art, history, values, a higher power

- **Spiritual issues** include an individual's values, beliefs, religious practices, and concerns with the meaning of life.
- **Spiritual distress** may cause emotional or physical suffering.
- **Spiritual concerns** greatly affect the way someone grieves and the way someone dies.
- **Spiritual peace** leads to reconciliation with others and one's own self in the time of dying.

strate some of the unique challenges presented by a young patient whose care follows the multidisciplinary care management hospice model.

## NURSING AND HOSPICE CARE

### Nurse's Role

The nurse has a pivotal role on the multidisciplinary hospice team. It is imperative that the nurse be an experienced practitioner who develops skill in the specialized area of symptom management and support of the terminally ill. The nurse works cooperatively and communicates effectively within a multidisciplinary framework to actively promote holistic palliative care for hospice patients and their families. The nurse demonstrates self-direction and initiative in the role as practitioner, educator, and consultant. The nurse coordinates the care and services provided to the hospice patients and their families.[2] The education and experience required for hospice nurses vary among hospice programs. Many programs stipulate that nurses have a baccalaureate degree in nursing and have practiced for at least two years. Experience in the areas of oncology nursing, home care, or geriatrics is a definite advantage for a nurse considering a position in hospice.

The nurse has a strong leadership role within the multidisciplinary hospice team. Good communication skills, both verbal and written, enable the nurse to foster cooperation within the team and to fulfill federal and state medical record documentation requirements. As well as being technically competent, each nurse in hospice needs to be mentally healthy to provide adequate psychosocial care, support, and counseling.[13] The nurse individualizes the plan of palliative care to maximize the patient's physical and emotional comfort. When goals of care conflict, the nurse prioritizes care issues after consultation with the physician and team. Weekly team conferences help in resolving conflicts and developing a consistent approach.

The ability of the nurse to foster a relaxed, warm, personal relationship with the patient, family, and other team members helps to promote confidence in achieving the goals of care. Interpersonal skills are invaluable in enabling the nurse to discuss such difficult issues as preparation for home death and funeral arrangements. The stressful nature of terminal illness tends to bring out the best and the worst in the hospice staff and the patient and families. An unhurried approach to care gives the patient and family time and encouragement to address their concerns. When hospice nurses were compared with nonhospice nurses, nurses involved with hospice care were found to be higher in self-actualization, i.e., self-directing, possessing healthier internal values, demonstrating flexibility in the application of their values, exhibiting sensitivity to their own needs and feelings, and being able to express their needs and feelings freely to the hospice team.[14]

## Management of Care Issues

Direct patient care and physical assessment skills are important in the hospice nurse's role. The nurse often provides basic nursing care, such as skin care, care of central venous lines, checking compliance with medication regimens, and indwelling catheter management. The nurse also assesses the patient response to current care approaches and generally determines what and when changes need to be made. See Tables 54-3 and 54-4 for a summation of selected principles and approaches for symptom management in palliative care.

Pain management is one of the most common care challenges faced by the nurses and the team. Ongoing assessment of pain is an activity best accomplished with a formal assessment tool. Some hospice programs use a pain-intensity scale numbered 0–5, with 0 indicating no pain and 5 denoting maximum pain. Some nurses also utilize a visual analogue scale, with faces demonstrating emotional responses corresponding to the 0–5 number scale. In general, pain intensity of 0–2 represents adequate pain control. Pain intensity of 3 or above indicates a need for adjustment in the analgesic dosage. However, the patient should indicate at what level pain management is acceptable, and this should guide intervention. The nurse performs a general assessment of body systems with each home visit. It takes particular skill to make the assessment less obvious or less mechanical, to not interfere with the therapeutic rapport developed with the patient.

The goal of hospice is to provide palliative care in the home; therefore, effective physical assessment skills can make a difference in identifying a potential problem early enough for timely intervention to occur. A nurse on the hospice team is available to the patient on call 24 hours, 7 days a week, to address questions or concerns that develop between visits by the team. A physician also is available on a 24-hour basis to assist in consultation on medical issues.

Once the knowledge base and experience needed to function comfortably in the role of hospice nurse have been developed, the role of educator and consultant becomes more prominent. Initially, the nurse instructs the patient and family in the skills needed to provide safe and comfortable home care. Teaching tools should include written material to be left in the home whenever possible. The patient's and family's knowledge base is assessed, information is provided, and then understanding of the new information is confirmed. The experienced nurse also has the opportunity to educate peers and members of other disciplines in topics such as general hospice information, pain and symptom management, and the hospice approach to such terminal diseases as AIDS, Alzheimer's, end-stage heart disease, and lung disease. The consultative role comes into play when a patient is referred to hospice to be assessed for potential admission into the hospice program. The attending physician is contacted to determine reason for referral, do-not-resuscitate status, expected prognosis, and appropriate medical information. Other disciplines involved in patient care may also be contacted to obtain information on financial status, family dynamics, or home care support network. After eliciting the important referral information, the nurse approaches the patient and family to discuss the option of hospice care. Many hospice nurses find it takes about two years for a nurse to develop full expertise in the specialized assessments and skills needed to provide expert nursing care for a hospice patient.

**TABLE 54-3** Selected Principles and Approaches for Symptom Management

| Problem | Principles | Management Approaches |
|---|---|---|
| Pain | • Pain has both a sensory and an emotional component.<br>• Pain perception escalates with anxiety.<br>• Respiratory depression can be avoided by careful dose titration. Pain is a natural antagonist to narcotics. (Even patients with severe lung disease can tolerate large doses of narcotics if the dose is escalated gradually.)[8]<br>• Tolerance is rarely a problem due to the wide therapeutic range of narcotics. | • Explore patient and family perceptions of pain and usage of pain medication.<br>• Ask the patient how pain changes mood or contributes to fear and anxiety. Consider cultural influences on pain and its management.<br>• Instruct patient and family on positive effects of pain management, i.e., control of pain, improved mood and activity. |

**TABLE 54-3**  Selected Principles and Approaches for Symptom Management (continued)

| Problem | Principles | Management Approaches |
|---------|-----------|---------------------|

**Principles:**

- Addiction is extremely rare and unimportant in the terminally ill.
- Placebos are never appropriate.

**Constant pain requires constant medication:**
- Most short-acting narcotic analgesics are given every 4 hr.
- Sustained-release morphine is given every 12 hr, i.e., (MS Contin).
- Medicate to prevent pain. It takes less pain medication to keep pain away than to break acute pain cycles.
- Adequate pain control requires adequate dosing
- Oral route is preferable: easy to administer, economical, maintains therapeutic level of drug in blood plasma with regular dosing.

**Management Approaches:**

- Reinforce that addiction is not an issue.

- Assess/document patient's goal for pain management.
- Monitor/document pain level using 0–5 pain scale or visual analog scale.

| 0 | 1 | 2 | 3 | 4 | 5 |

0 No pain — 5 Worst possible pain

- Analgesic ladder
  I. *Mild pain:* Start with nonopioids (acetaminophen, aspirin, or NSAIDs), with or without adjuvant (see Table 54-4).
  II. *If pain persists:* Try weak opioid (codeine, oxycodone hydrocodone) with or without nonopioids, with or without adjuvant.
  III. *If pain still persists:* Try strong opioid, with or without nonopioid, with or without adjuvant.[7,8]

- Avoid:
  —meperidine—very low oral potency; toxic metabolite accumulation
  —pentazocine—no more potent than codeine; high incidences of hallucinations and agitation (30% in cancer patients)
  —methadone—extremely long half-life (48–72 hr); short duration of analgesia (6–8 hr); makes dose titration difficult in severely ill patients; however, may be the only affordable long-acting agent for your patient
  —IM/SQ injections—morphine 30 mg PO is as potent as 10 mg IM/SQ; can avoid pain and expense of injections with PO or SQ morphine

- **Commonly used drugs:** (Published tables vary in their suggested equianalgesic (equiv.) doses. Clinical response is the criterion that must be applied for each patient.)

| Drugs | Oral (approx. equiv. dose, mg) | Parenteral (approx. equiv. dose, mg) | Oral Dosing interval (hr) |
|-------|--------------------------------|--------------------------------------|---------------------------|
| Morphine | 30 | 10 | 3–4 |
| Hydromorphone (Dilaudid) | 4–6 | 1.5–2 | 4 |
| Levorphanol (Levo-Dromoran) | 4 | 2 | 6–8 |
| Codeine | 130† | 75 | 4–6 |
| Fentanyl patch (Duragesic) | 50 µg on skin | N/A | 72 |
| Methadone (Dolophine) | 20 | 10 | 6–8 |
| Meperidine* (Demerol) | 150 | 75 | 2.5–3.5 |

*Avoid use for chronic pain.

†Codeine doses above 65 mg usually are inappropriate due to diminishing incremental analgesia.

*(continued)*

**TABLE 54-3**  Selected Principles and Approaches for Symptom Management (continued)

| Problem | Principles | Management Approaches |
|---|---|---|
| | • According to WHO, morphine is the drug of choice for severe cancer pain. There is no ceiling to effective narcotic dosage.[8] | • Titrate dose as needed. |
| | • If PO medications are not possible, narcotics can be given by buccal, sublingual, rectal, or SQ routes without resorting to IV or IM administration. | • Utilize noninvasive comfort measures as appropriate, e.g., applications of ice, heat, gentle massage, relaxation techniques. |
| | • Continuous SQ infusions can be initiated at home with the help of home health or hospice nurses. | |
| | • If central line access is *already* established, IV infusion may be the route of choice and usually can be initiated at home. | • Evaluate effectiveness of analgesia at regular intervals. Teach the patient and family about the medications and alternate measures. |
| Dyspnea | • Defined as unpleasant awareness of increased need to ventilate. | • Oral morphine in low doses 5–10 mg every 4 hr. helps to decrease air hunger.[8] |
| | • Avoid high-dose bronchodilators. | • Help patient decrease anxiety through use of an anxiolytic, e.g., a benzodiazepine. |
| | • Theophylline toxicity is common as patients approach death. | • Position patient for maximum comfort by elevating head of bed. |
| | • Adrenergic agonists (metaproterenol, etc.) may exacerbate anxiety more than they help with dyspnea. | • Advise patient in methods to modify environment or activity to decrease physical exertion. |
| | | • Oxygen may be effective but more expensive than oral narcotics. |
| Seizures | • Patients with *recent history* of seizures should receive therapeutic doses of phenytoin, phenobarbital, carbamazepine, or valproic acid. | Options |
| | | • If patient cannot swallow phenytoin: |
| | | –midazolam—5–10 mg/day by SQ infusion |
| | | –phenobarbital—20–60 mg oral, sublingual BID |
| | | –carbamazepine—600 mg per rectum or SQ BID-TID |
| | | –valproic acid—250 mg QID per rectum |
| | | • Instruct caregiver on seizure precautions. Protect patient from injury in event of seizure. Remove or pad objects near head of body. Instruct patient and family regarding needs for regular dosing and side effects of seizure medication. |
| Diarrhea | • Rule out fecal impaction, bowel obstruction, laxative overuse, and other drug side effects.[8] | • Maintain hydration according to patient's comfort level and tolerance of fluids. Bland low-residue diet. Protect skin with barrier cream. |
| | | –ioperamide HCL—2–4 mg QID PRN |
| | | –diphenoxylate HCL, atropine sulfate—2.5–5 mg QID PRN |
| | | –natural psyllium fiber—1–3 tsp BID[8] |
| Constipation | • Nearly all patients on narcotics require a maintenance laxative regimen to prevent constipation. | • "Ladder" of increasing potency of laxatives: |
| | • As the dose of narcotic is increased, the dose of laxative must be increased. | a. standardized senna concentrate and docusate sodium or casanthranol and docusate sodium—1–2 tabs at hs |
| | • Patients who are not eating still may require laxatives as waste continues to be produced in the bowel in form of secretion, bacteria, and desquamation. | b. standardized senna concentrate and docusate sodium or casanthranol and docusate sodium—2 tabs BID |
| | | c. standardized senna concentrate and docusate sodium or casanthranol and docusate sodium—3 tabs BID |
| | | d. Lactulose—15cc BID |
| | | e. Lactulose—30cc BID |
| | | f. Lactulose—30cc TID-QID or along with b or c above. |
| | • Avoid | If a patient has not had a bowel movement in 24 hr, increase the laxative dose to the next higher level. |
| | –bulk laxatives—difficult for anorexic patients to take, and cause impaction if fluid intake is inadequate; *not* effective unless a patient is active and eating | If a patient has not had a bowel movement in 3 days, check for impaction and consider one of the following treatments once or twice daily until results are obtained: |
| | –frequent enemas—useful for severe cases of constipation; however, oral medications are better tolerated for prophylaxis. | a. Milk of magnesia 30cc at bedtime |
| | | b. 2 bisacodyl suppositories |
| | | c. Lactulose or sorbitol 30cc q 1 hr until results |

**TABLE 54-4**   Adjuvant Pain Therapy—Promote a Co-Analgesic

| Pain Source | Pain Character | Drug Class | Examples |
|---|---|---|---|
| Bone or soft tissue | Tenderness over bone or joint; pain on movement | NSAID | Ibuprofen 400 mg q4hr |
| Nerve damage or dysethesia | "Burning" or "shooting" pain radiating from spinal root or plexis | Tricyclic Anticonvulsant | Amitriptyline 10–50 mg q hs<br>Carbamazepine 200 mg q 6–12hr |
| Smooth muscle spasms | Colic-cramping, abdominal pain, bladder spasms | Anticholinergic | Diclomine 10 mg q 4–8hr<br>Oxybutynin 5–10 mg q 8hr |
| Anxiety | Generalized restlessness and discomfort | Antihistamine Benzodiazepine | Hydroxyzine 10–50 mg q 4hr<br>Lorazepam 0.5–1 mg q 6hr |
| Intracranial pressure | Headache | Steroids | Dexamethasone 6–10 mg q 6hr |

## DEATH IN THE HOME

Hospice philosophy is uniquely characterized by its approach to facilitating a person's death at home. It is common, if not universal, for patients and families to respond initially to the idea of death at home with fear and anxiety. Many adults in the United States have never seen anyone die.[15] In a society where death has been regarded as a medical problem requiring technological support, hospitalization, and professional care, we have lost the basic idea of death as a natural life event.[2] Patients' overriding concerns about death at home often revolve around being a burden to their family.[1] Family caregivers are concerned about their emotional ability to cope with a home death and the potential effects on other family members, particularly when children are in the home.

For most families, the ability to provide care for a home death will require teaching them about the death event itself, immediate signs of death, how to relieve symptoms and suffering, and how to access professional help when needed. When given enough time to work with a patient and family, hospice care is ideally structured to provide this support, education, and preparation. It is most satisfying for hospice nurses to provide a full spectrum of care that begins with a family that expresses much anxiety about caring for a patient at home and continues through the death event, where family members in bereavement cannot say enough about what a wonderful experience it was for them. In her book *Dying at Home,* Andrea Sankar relates her experience with the home death of her mother: "Home death is a powerfully significant experience despite the strain, exhaustion, and conflict that sometimes accompanies it. Its power lies in the fact that in the face of certain death, the caregiver can give the person life, that is, the continuation of life as a social being."[15]

### Advantages of Home Death

The approach of death evokes feelings of loss in a dying person.[16] Loss of control may be the most overwhelming and distressing feeling. This loss of control can be further intensified by hospitalization. Terminal care and death at home can afford the patient and family control over their environment, as well as the comfort of being in the midst of familiar surroundings. The patient at home maintains the opportunity to interact with neighbors, children, and pets. If children are living in the same home as the dying person, there is often concern that this experience will be detrimental to them. However, the opposite effect is often true. Rather than being protected from the illness and death, children can benefit from being involved in very concrete ways to better understand the dying process and facilitate their own grief.[15]

Another major loss for patients is diminishment of their role as contributing, social beings. Individuals have several roles that make up their identity. Loss of role in the workplace is one of the first major adaptations for a chronically or terminally ill person. However, being cared for at home can afford the opportunity for an alert patient to maintain his or her family role. When possible, this person will continue to be included in family events and in decision making as was previously the norm.[15]

A final and obvious advantage of home death is that unwanted medical intervention is much less likely to occur than for a patient in a hospital or nursing home setting. The greatest potential risk for a home patient to receive unwanted medical intervention arises if the emergency medical system (EMS) is accessed, since this can result in unplanned and unwanted resuscitation and, ultimately, ventilator care.

### Disadvantages of Home Death

Caregivers, particularly those lacking social outlets or family support, may find the physical and emotional task of home care and home death too difficult. Home death must be prepared for within the context of a realistic plan of care.

Although most anticipated deaths occur quietly without physical distress, the occasional patient may have symptoms too difficult to manage at home, such as uncontrolled hemorrhage. For such a patient, hospitalization may be the better option, as long as the care provided is according to the patient's goals, and the patient and family receive appropriate emotional and spiritual support. Lack of resources to provide adequate home care is another reason home death can prove too burdensome.

When hospice care is initiated, a psychosocial assessment is completed by interviewing the patient and family in the home environment. This assessment should address the emotional and physical health of the caregiver as well as the exploration of social and financial resources. Social resources include other family, friends, or neighbors willing to assume some of the patient care or other tasks. Financial resources include eligibility for the Medicare Hospice Benefit or hospice benefits available from commercial insurance plans. Often, life insurance policies can be accessed before death for a terminally ill patient to assist with the cost of home care or other needs.

This information, together with the nursing assessment of the patient, provides the basis for planning care and determining patient and family needs. However, even an in-depth assessment by experienced staff may not provide a reliable predictor for whether a patient will remain home to die. Hospices have provided care for a wide spectrum of families, from those with every resource who at the last minute access the EMS to those with limited finances and inadequate coping histories who are able to provide good care at home through the death event. Therefore, the hospice team generally will present the option of hospice home care to every patient and family if a safe plan of care can be established. At the same time, hospice staff should also discuss any other available options for care (e.g., an extended care facility). At each subsequent home visit, the hospice staff must reevaluate the patient/family situation and revise plans as necessary.

## Preparation of the Patient and Family

Once home death has been established as a desired goal, an individualized home care plan is developed with the patient and family. They need to know specifically what the hospice team can and will provide. Friends and other resources are also identified. The patient's primary caregiver may need permission and encouragement to ask for help from these other resources. It is emphasized with the primary caregiver that when a person is terminally ill, friends and neighbors may have difficulty coping with their feelings. This may be due to their discomfort with not knowing how to help. Many people are grateful to a patient or family caregiver who can assign specific tasks, enabling them to respond in a concrete, helpful way.

The primary caregiver is continually and carefully assessed to determine what he or she wants to and is capable of doing for direct care. Support to the primary caregiver and other family members includes acknowledging how physically and emotionally exhausting caring for someone ill at home can be. There are times when caregivers also need permission to take a break and to delegate care. The most effective hospice worker facilitates a series of informed choices and, as much as possible, allows patients and families to make their own decisions.

### Knowledge and preparation for the death event

Families need to be prepared for the actual time of the patient's death and the time immediately preceding it. The most difficult aspect of preparation is that each patient is an individual and each death occurs in a way that may not be completely predictable. However, there

---

**TABLE 54-5** Hospice Home Care Instruction Sheet: Signs and Symptoms of Approaching Death

The hospice team's goal is to help prepare you for some things that might occur close to the time of death. Although we can never predict exactly when a terminally ill person will die, we know when the time is getting close by a combination of signs and symptoms. Not all of these signs will appear at the same time, and some may never appear at all. All of the signs described are ways the body prepares itself for the final stages of life.

1. Your loved one may sleep more and might be more difficult to awaken. Hearing and vision may decrease.
    _What to do:_ Plan your time and activities for times when he/she is more alert. Always talk as if the person can hear you, even if he/she appears to be in a coma. When providing care, explain what you are doing as you do it.
2. There may be a gradual decrease in need for food and drink. Your loved one will say he/she doesn't have an appetite, isn't hungry. This is the body's natural response to the dying process. It is telling the person that eating and drinking are no longer helpful—that the body can't use food and fluid properly anymore.
    _What to do:_ Allow your loved one to choose when and what to eat or drink, even if this means little or nothing will be taken in. Liquids often are more easily tolerated than solid food.
3. Your loved one may become more confused or restless or experience visions of people and places.
    _What to do:_ Remind him/her of the time and the day and who is there with them. Be calm and reassuring when talking to him/her.
4. Hands, arms, feet, and legs may become cooler, and the skin may turn a bluish color with purplish splotches.
    _What to do:_ Use blankets for warmth. Do _not_ use an electric blanket or heating pad.
5. Irregular breathing patterns may occur. There might be a space of time (10–30 seconds) when there will be no breathing at all. This is called _apnea._ There may be phlegm in the throat that is difficult to cough.
    _What to do:_ Position the person on his/her side with head elevated.

Contact hospice team at any time for questions, or to discuss changes.

are some universal signs that families can anticipate and on which they can receive instruction. Table 54-5 is an example of a patient and family instruction sheet that lists many of the common signs seen in patients who are imminently dying. For family members who have cared for an ill person for a long time or are health care professionals themselves, it is important to emphasize that laboratory results and vital signs are unreliable indicators of the time of death.

Emotional care of the patient and family around the time of death occurs as the opportunity arises. The family is instructed to listen to the patient carefully, even if it appears that the patient is confused. Many times dying patients will speak in symbolic language.[17] A common example is a patient who talks about "going home." It may seem that the patient is confused if he or she already is home. Further conversation may indicate that "going home" refers to dying. It is not unusual for patients to report actually seeing or having conversations with a loved one who has died. Family members may be the most capable of interpreting some symbolic language for the patient. Patients may indicate when they feel they are ready to die. If this occurs, family members can be encouraged to allow the patient to "let go," that is, give the patient permission to die.[17] Although no one can be sure how much an individual has control over the time of his or her own death, having a family member tell the patient that it is all right to "let go" can add to the patient's peace of mind.[2]

### Funeral arrangements

In most situations a home death will go more smoothly if the patient and/or family chooses a funeral home before the death occurs. Although it can be most helpful for complete funeral arrangements to be made prior to the death of the patient, family members may find this action premature. Beyond choosing a funeral home, no other arrangements need be made prior to death.

The hospice team should be a resource to families as to different types of funeral homes available in their area. Important factors that differentiate funeral homes are religious affiliation, financial considerations, and policies about home death. The hospice team can also be a resource for information on organ and body donation and on autopsy as it relates to home death. These procedures usually are compatible with home death, as long as the wishes of the patient and/or family are known in advance so arrangements can be made with the funeral home. Finally, the hospice team needs to be a resource to ensure that the family is aware of local ordinances or laws surrounding an expected home death.

## Availability of the Hospice Team

Of utmost importance in supporting families through a patient's home death is instructing them on how to access the hospice team at any time on any day as needed.

Families should be encouraged to call about any changes in the patient's status or for what may seem like minor questions to them. For the hospice team, emotional support to exhausted and anxious family members is just as important an intervention as a change in pain medication for the patient. Family members also need to be instructed to call the hospice immediately should a home death occur. The time of instruction regarding accessing the hospice team is also a good time to remind families not to call the EMS, and to inform them of the possible consequences of such an action. This instruction often needs to be repeated because many people call 911 as a natural reaction to an "emergency."

## Facilitating Grief

As family members prepare for the death of a loved one at home, they are also preparing themselves for the loss. This is often referred to as *anticipatory grief*.[18] Family members who can give a dying person permission to "let go" are at the same time letting go themselves. Part of the hospice team's care is assisting loved ones in this grief phase. First, it may be helpful to explore with family members previous losses and coping mechanisms used. The family is encouraged to identify and discuss unresolved issues with the dying person. This can be an opportunity to resolve certain issues, so that after death there are no regrets on the part of the family. Even when conflict does not exist, family members can say things to the dying person that they may not have said or feel that they have not said enough previously.[2] The dying person and family members can honor the meaning of their relationship and their life together.[1] Asking a couple how they met or going through a family photo album with them is a good way to facilitate grieving and therapeutic life review. What follows is an example of one family's preparation for the death of their baby daughter and how it helped them work through their grief:

Mr. and Mrs. S were referred to a hospice program by their daughter's pediatric oncologist when they were told there was no more treatment available for the 2-year-old's cancer. The hospice nurse and a hospice volunteer were able to establish a good rapport with the parents early. The parents were concerned that their daughter no longer suffer, and they wished to care for her at home as long as possible. The parents had support from grandparents, friends, neighbors, and their local minister, who visited them at home. The parents described feeling much strength and love from all this support, until the hospice nurse talked to them about choosing a funeral home. Mrs. S was devastated. "I was so angry with that nurse. I thought, 'How dare she talk about such a horrible thing?' My daughter was still alive, and I wanted her with us as long as possible. I was so angry I almost called the hospice and told them never to send anyone out to see us again." However, after a few days, Mr. and Mrs. S talked for the first time about the inevitable death of their child. Rehearsing it in her mind, Mrs. S began to think about how she might feel if a stranger (the funeral director) would come into their home and remove her baby. She wondered if there was any reason she and her husband could not take the body to the funeral home themselves when death occurred. Mrs. S researched this and discovered there was no law in her state that would preclude this action. Mrs. S eventually was able to talk to the hospice nurse about her idea. The nurse contacted several area funeral homes to discuss the situation and gave Mr. and Mrs. S the names of the ones that would comply with this arrangement. The baby lived for another two months before she died quietly at home in her mother's arms. Mrs. S later recalled: "The nurse was wonderful. She came out and helped us wash and dress the baby and wrap her in a blanket. She understood that we needed time to do this. Our daughter died without any tubes or shots and we were able to take her to the funeral home ourselves. I think we did the best for her that we could."

This family had the time needed to experience the death event on their own terms. Preparing family members for the death of their loved one often means discussing issues the nurse assesses they may not yet be ready to hear. As in this situation, the nurse was not sure how much time was left prior to death. Ultimately, the parents were able to process their feelings and exert some choice and control in a very difficult situation.

## BEREAVEMENT CARE

Bereavement support is a required component of hospice care under Medicare and most state licensing regulations.[10] However, the specific structure of an individual hospice's bereavement program is not well defined. Each hospice program develops its own policies and mechanism for bereavement care and follow-up.

Grieving is a normal reaction to loss, with a wide variety of physical and emotional manifestations. Some of these are loss of appetite, sleeplessness, heart palpitations, lack of energy, sadness, and anger. J. William Worden[16] describes the following four tasks as necessary for the normal grief process to progress:

1. to accept the reality of the loss
2. to experience the pain of grief
3. to adjust to the environment in which the deceased is missing
4. to withdraw emotional energy and replace it in another relationship

The goal of bereavement care or counseling is to assist and support survivors to move through the loss and toward resolution.[16,18] Hospice programs generally follow survivors for one year, although there is no mandated standard time for follow-up. This period should be understood as the usual time frame in which the most acute grief occurs, not the period in which mourning is completed. Grief resolution is an individualized process that takes place gradually over varying periods of time.

Methods of bereavement care commonly include a bereavement assessment, contact of survivors at regularly scheduled intervals, and, as necessary, additional referrals for professional counseling for those with complicated or abnormal grief reactions. Bereavement support can also take the form of support groups, "socials" or "teas," educational classes on specific topics, and/or memorial services conducted by the hospice program.[2]

### Abnormal Grief

Survivors unable to progress through the tasks of mourning will develop some form of abnormal or complicated grief.[16] Generally, complicated grief will manifest itself in one of three ways. First, the grief reaction may be prolonged. Second, the grief reaction may be masked in behavioral or physical symptoms, even such seemingly unrelated symptoms as pain, sexual impotence, and behavioral "acting out." Finally, abnormal grief may be seen in exaggerated expressions of normal grief reactions, such as excessive anger, sadness, or depression.[16] For most hospice programs, therapy for abnormal grief extends beyond the scope of the bereavement care services provided. However, the hospice program staff should be able to identify and recommend competent referrals for abnormal grief syndromes.

Unresolved grief has been associated with multiple physical and emotional illnesses, including increased risk of suicide.[16,18] Therefore, facilitation of anticipatory grieving and bereavement can be viewed as preventive health care for survivors. Collin Murray Parkes, psychiatrist and consultant to St. Christopher's Hospice, came to the following conclusion after a review of the literature on the effectiveness of grief counseling. "The evidence presented here suggests that professional services and professionally supported voluntary and self-help services are capable of reducing the risk of psychiatric and psychoanalytic disorders resulting from bereavement."[18]

## STRESS AND THE HOSPICE NURSE

Providing compassionate care to the terminally ill and their loved ones can create unique stressors for the hospice team. Studies have shown that nurses and other hospice staff members tend to identify with younger patients (those under 40) and to feel a greater sense of injustice when these patients die. Staff attitudes toward death can be greatly influenced by unresolved grief issues in their own personal or professional life. Stress can be increased due to unrealistic expectations of ourselves, our coworkers, or the therapy we use to manage symptoms. The inability to relieve totally such symptoms as intractable pain and nausea can evoke feelings of impotence or helplessness. Supportive interactions with patients and their families can be emotionally draining, especially when long-standing problems in their interpersonal relationships are involved.[13]

Caregivers with high-stress jobs who cope successfully

are able to recognize when signs of stress are developing within themselves, acknowledge their own limits, and initiate self-help techniques or seek the help of others. Several methods for coping with stress have been used successfully by hospice staff members (Table 54-6).

## LEGAL AND ETHICAL ISSUES SURROUNDING HOSPICE CARE

Due to the population characteristics and specialized nature of terminal care, hospice programs have been innovators in encouraging patients to identify their own goals, particularly goals related to cardiopulmonary resuscitation (CPR), invasive procedures, and identification of family or friends to assist in decision making if the patient becomes incapacitated. However, the hospice nurse and other members of the team are directly affected by recent legislative and court decisions that can either hinder or enhance the ability to assist the family in meeting those goals.

### Advance Directives

The federal Patient Self-Determination Act, enacted in December 1991, requires hospices, hospitals, and other health care agencies to provide patients, on admission, with written information about two key areas: (1) their right to accept or refuse treatment under state law and (2) ways to execute advance directives such as a living will and a durable power of attorney for health care.[19] The purpose of this legislation is to ensure that patients' wishes are carried out in the event they become mentally incapacitated or are incapable of making or communicating their decisions. As with all other health care organizations receiving federal funds, hospice programs are mandated to provide information to facilitate completion of a living will or a durable power of attorney for health care. Hospice team members provide whatever information is needed to assist the patient in making an informed decision, especially when it affects the patient's decision not to have CPR, intravenous fluids, or tube feedings.

Patients with malignancy, sepsis, pneumonia, renal failure, diabetes, or advanced age have a low chance of survival after CPR. An average of 4% of patients receiving CPR in a general acute care setting survive. For those who do survive, quality of life afterward is compromised.[20] Hospice patients and families may need reassurance that their focus on comfort and quality of life is being reinforced by their decision not to have CPR. This same approach holds true when the decision not to have intravenous fluids or tube feedings is challenged. As death approaches, the patient may lose the ability to drink. Dehydration often occurs if death does not soon follow the inability to drink. However, fluid depletion has the following benign effects on quality of life:

- Urine output is decreased, so there is less incontinence.

- Gastric secretions lessen; therefore, episodes of vomiting decrease.

**TABLE 54-6**   Useful Methods for Coping with Stress

- Take responsibility for caring for yourself. Allow at least 15–20 minutes each day for quiet introspection. Assess your body for signs of stress, for example, muscle tension, headaches, insomnia, GI distress, and frequent illness. The body systems showing stress should be the focus for rejuvenation. For example, muscle tension may indicate a need for relaxation therapy.
- Reduce stress by prioritizing work. Make a conscious choice between those events worth your energy and those you need to delegate or otherwise not take on at all.
- Promote training and education not only for new staff but also for experienced team members. The continual development of our knowledge base promotes confidence. Special attention should be placed on identified stresses. If you are feeling overwhelmed, then dealing with family dynamics, reading, or attending a seminar on that subject could give you additional tools to improve future interactions.
- Take time off! Whenever possible get out of town, away from reminders of work.
- Take time for your hobby. Creative self-expression through arts, crafts, or hobbies can provide an additional outlet for release of stress.
- Focus on maintaining a healthy body through regular exercise and eating a balanced diet. Leave the clinical setting during lunch, and go for a long walk or do something not work-related.
- Seek supportive interactions with individuals or in a group. Regular involvement with a support group can be helpful in providing an environment to share with others on the team who are under similar pressures. Such interactions serve to promote team building and problem identification. For a group to be successful, trust and an open, nurturing environment must be established. An experienced facilitator can be invaluable in attaining this goal. Group members make a contract with each other to be supportive and nonjudgmental and to keep all conversation in strict confidence.
- Give yourself permission to find the humor in certain situations that otherwise may be tragic or depressing. Share this humor with other members of the hospice team, being careful to keep it respectful of patient and families involved.
- Focus on the positive satisfying aspects of the role of hospice caregiver. Assisting a patient in the last few days of life can be very rewarding. Promoting comfort and quality-of-life issues involves nursing skills and principles of the highest order.

- Pulmonary secretions lessen, resulting in less congestion.

- Peripheral edema secondary to tumor subsides, resulting in decreased pain from nerve compression.

- Although the sensation of dry mouth and thirst may increase, this can be relieved by good mouth care and small amounts of oral fluids.[21]

The U.S. Supreme Court's 1990 decision in the *Cruzon* case made it clear that life-and-death decisions depend on the availability of written evidence of the patient's wishes. Under the current Patient Self-Determination Act, individuals are not required to enact an advanced directive. However, failure to do so may later compromise their ability to limit aggressive medical treatment. In general, the power of attorney for health care is more useful than the living will. A living will is applicable only when it pertains to a terminal illness but not for a patient whose health is declining for medical reasons other than those that can be classified as terminal or if the patient is in a permanent vegetative state. The living will does not identify another person who can act as the agent for a disabled patient.[19]

Through the power of attorney for health care, the patient chooses an agent to act on the patient's behalf if the patient is no longer competent to make decisions. This is especially important for individuals who have diagnoses such as AIDS, cancer metastases to the brain, or other medical problems where eventual confusion or other mental status changes are an expected complication of the disease. By electing to use a power of attorney, the patient is able to make a statement as to his or her wishes regarding degree of removal of life support in the event of irreversible coma, use of artificial feeding if unable to swallow, and any limitation on the decision-making powers of the agent. A patient may also identify restrictions to care, such as those prohibiting blood transfusions for religious reasons.

The health care team caring for the patient in accordance with these documents usually is protected from liability if it follows the patient's wishes. A copy of the living will or health care power of attorney needs to be placed in the patient's medical record.

## Euthanasia and Suicide

The moral, ethical, and legal questions surrounding terminal illness and methods used to hasten death have their origins in ancient times. The English word *euthanasia* is taken from the Greek *euthanasias,* meaning "good or easy death." For the Greeks and other ancients, euthanasia did not necessarily denote an act or method of hastening death. It was important to the ancients that a person meet death voluntarily, with peace of mind and minimal suffering. This "good death" meant that the ill individual was meeting death in a condition of self-control. Toward this end, it was permissible to shorten a person's life intentionally.[22]

In modern times euthanasia has come to mean the intentional taking of the life of a terminally ill person for purposes of compassion. The modern concept is more accurately described as *active* euthanasia, for it is achieved by "doing something," such as giving the patient a lethal injection. *Passive* euthanasia can be described as "not doing something" that would preserve life, yet without being significantly burdensome.[22] Therefore, passive euthanasia has little bearing on our discussion of suicide and active euthanasia.

Euthanasia is quite different from refusing to receive medical treatment that will not contribute reasonably to improved quality of life and/or that proves to be gravely burdensome. Additionally, pain medication or other symptom management measures that are used in unusual quantity to improve comfort but could lead to an early death should not be considered euthanasia.[22] The operative and distinguishing concept is intent. If the intent is to relieve pain or manage symptoms and not to cause death, then the unintentional hastening of death by such care is not euthanasia.

In the past few years the issue of euthanasia, in the form of legalized physician-assisted suicide for the terminally ill, has emerged into a huge debate around the world, particularly in the United States. The issue of the "right" of a terminally ill individual to determine the timing and method of his or her own death came before the U.S. Supreme Court for the first time on January 8, 1997. As of this writing, a decision was still pending.

The NHO has taken a formal and firm position against physician-assisted suicide, arguing that optimal pain and symptom management, along with emotional support, are still not widely available to dying patients outside of hospice programs.[23] It has been the general experience of those who provide optimal palliative care that their patients do not need or desire euthanasia. However, even experts in palliative care acknowledge that there may always be some patients whose symptoms cannot be completely controlled or who may request euthanasia in spite of the availability of optimal terminal care. A concern is that the legalization of assisted suicide for this very small group might encourage the disabled, those with AIDS, those without caregivers, or the poor to seek the option of euthanasia.

Owing to this debate in our society, those in oncology, hospice care, and the care of other patients with end-stage diseases should be proactive in addressing euthanasia. Many hospice programs have addressed the issues of euthanasia, suicide, and requests for assisted suicide by preparing formal policies to provide staff with guidance in responding to these issues. When someone asks about, or expresses the desire for, euthanasia, the appropriate initial response from an individual nurse is a listening and caring attitude, followed by careful exploration of the patient's or family member's concerns or fears. It may become increasingly necessary to regularly assure dying patients in our care that we will continue to be there for them.

## FUTURE TRENDS AND CHALLENGES FOR HOSPICE CARE

### Underserved Populations

The earliest hospices in Connecticut, California, New Jersey, and Arizona were founded by and served a predominantly middle-class, white population. African-American and Hispanic populations historically have been underserved by health care agencies and hospice. The African-American population is better served than Hispanics, but not in proportion to their cancer-related death rates. Both of these minority populations are underrepresented or totally lacking among hospice staff and volunteers, even in urban hospice programs.[24] The reasons for this are complex but include the fact that African-American and Hispanic populations have less access to health care in general and are less likely to have medical insurance. Some religious beliefs and cultural values may also be a factor.[25]

Children represent another underserved population in the United States. Dedicated pediatric hospice services are rare. The 1992 NHO survey of hospice providers indicated that although most hospices will provide pediatric services, actual representation of children cared for by hospice was only about 2% of total patients served.[11] For example, in the Chicago metropolitan area, which is served by more than 20 hospice programs and four large children's hospitals, there are no dedicated pediatric hospice services.

Patients with AIDS represent a tremendous challenge to hospice. It is difficult to find a hospice program that will acknowledge denying services to those with an AIDS diagnosis. However, there remains the opinion among some in hospice leadership that AIDS does not "fit in" to current hospice practice. This is in spite of the evidence from the urban programs that successfully care for patients with AIDS, and from NHO support for AIDS care in hospice.[26]

AIDS patients utilize more resources than have been the norm for hospice patients. Their care is more complex and requires longer and more frequent nursing and social work visits. Patients with AIDS may require more attendant or custodial care due to the lack of primary caregivers and limited finances. The medications and supplies used are more varied and expensive, and their effectiveness may be unproven.

With AIDS, a more flexible interpretation of symptom management and an approach to quality-of-life issues are needed. Hospice programs differ as to what constitutes palliative care for AIDS patients. Treatments for AIDS often are double-edged, controlling some symptoms while in-

ducing others. No accepted standards for AIDS care in hospice have been firmly established. The course of AIDS is less predictable than that of most cancers, making prognostication within the six-month criterion difficult. The combined physical, psychosocial, spiritual, and financial needs of those with AIDS can tax the hospice team. Hospices, because of their commitment to compassionate care to all with a terminal disease, have a moral and ethical obligation to provide care to those who request it.[27]

There are other patient types who are considered "outliers," with diagnoses and social issues challenging hospice care. The Medicare Hospice Benefit was originally designed for the elderly cancer patient with an intact family available to provide most of the home care, supplemented by the support and resources of the hospice team.[2] However, we are rapidly facing an aging population with either no primary caregivers or immediate support persons who are too frail to provide care. The challenge for hospice is to broaden its scope to create effective care models for divergent populations. Residential and day care hospice components are two models currently being explored around the country.

### Research Issues

Empirical research is still needed in all areas of hospice and palliative care. Existing research focuses on pain and symptom management and psychosocial care. Areas least studied are volunteerism and spiritual care, the features most unique to hospice.[28] Other palliative care research topics could include suicidal ideation in the terminally ill, emotional factors hindering pain management, and long-term effectiveness of bereavement care. Both hospice models and hospice patient populations inherently make research difficult.[28] Limited funding and the relative lack of hospice and palliative care programs associated with academic institutions provide additional barriers to research.

### Integration into Health Care Practices

For years, Dame Cicely Saunders has believed that rather than creating a segregated system for the dying, hospice principles should be diffused throughout the health care system.[2] Hospice in the United States began as an anti–medical establishment and antiphysician movement. This antagonistic bias has unfortunately been a major factor preventing hospice and palliative care principles from being applied to dying patients on a broader scale. Terminal care should be integrated into all health care practice, particularly in the areas of oncology, geriatrics, and AIDS.

The JCAHO began to foster integration of hospice care with the revision of its hospital standards for 1992, which addressed needs of the dying patient under the patient rights section.[6] The regulations were greatly strengthened in 1996 with Standard RI.1.2.7 (Table 54-7). These regulations incorporate basic hospice standards of care for all dying patients in hospitals. The federal Patient Self-Determination Act also has played a role in furthering the ability of patients to forgo unwanted heroic treatment in the face of terminal illness.

In its short history, hospice has led the way in many health care trends, including case management, cost containment, home care utilization, and advance directives. Hospice now needs to integrate and adapt to the challenges facing our ever-changing health care system such as the following:

- health insurance plans promoting hospice as a cost-effective care approach

- accessing hospice care earlier

- delivering cost-effective care

- contracting with HMOs and managed care[29,p.87]

## CONCLUSION

Hospice is a program coordinated by nurses and staffed by professionals and volunteers, all striving to promote comfort and quality of life to those with a limited life span who wish such support. The thrust of this chapter has been to dispel the notion that hospice is a place for a dying person to spend his or her last hours without hope of enjoying life. Within hospice, the hope changes from that for a cure and a long life to hope for care and living for the moment. Death is no longer something to be avoided at all costs; rather, death is something as natural as birth, a doorway out of the suffering of this world. Home, family, and friends are not left behind but are included as an important part of hospice care. It is a privilege for health care professionals to be involved with human beings during the end of their lives. We hear their stories about what life was like for them. We help them toward what they would like the natural end of life to be.

---

**TABLE 54-7** Standard RI.1.2.7: The Hospital Addresses Care at the End of Life

| Intent of RI.1.2.7 |
| --- |
| Dying patients have unique needs for respectful, responsive care. All hospital staff are sensitized to the needs of patients at the end of life. Concern for the patient's comfort and dignity should guide all aspects of care during the final stages of life. |
| The hospital's framework for addressing issues related to care at the end of life provide for |
| • providing appropriate treatment for any primary and secondary symptoms, according to the wishes of the patient or the surrogate decision maker; |
| • managing pain aggressively and effectively; |
| • sensitively addressing issues such as autopsy and organ donation; |
| • respecting the patient's values, religion, and philosophy; |
| • involving the patient and, where appropriate, the family in every aspect of care; and |
| • responding to the psychological, social, emotional, spiritual, and cultural concerns of the patient and the family. |
| Effective pain management is appropriate for all patients, not just for dying patients. |

Copyright 1995 by the Joint Commission on Accreditation of Healthcare Organizations, Oakbrook Terrace, IL. Reprinted with permission from the 1996 *Comprehensive Accreditation Manual for Hospitals.*

## REFERENCES

1. Kübler-Ross E: *On Death and Dying.* New York, Macmillan, 1974
2. Amenta MO, Bohnet NL: *Nursing Care of the Terminally Ill.* Boston, Little, Brown, 1986
3. National Hospice Organization 1995, *NHO Newsline* 1, 1995
4. Paradis LF: *Hospice Handbook.* Rockville, MD, Aspen, 1985
5. Joint Commission on Accreditation of Hospitals: Chicago: The Commission, 1986
6. Joint Commission on Accreditation of Healthcare Organizations: *Accreditation Manual for Hospitals.* Oakbrook Terrace, IL, The Commission, 1992, pp 103–105
7. Kaye P: *Notes on Symptom Control.* Essex, England, Hospice Education Institute, 1991
8. Johanson G: *Symptom Relief in Terminal Care* (ed 3). Santa Rosa, CA, Home Hospice of Sonoma County, 1988, pp 18.1–18.4
9. Kerr D: A bedside fan for terminal dyspnea. *Am J Hospice Care* 6:23, 1989
10. *Hospice Surveyor Operation Manual.* Washington, DC, Hospice Association of America, 1989
11. Stuart B: *Medical Guidelines for Determining Prognosis in Selected Non-Cancer Diseases* (ed 2). Arlington, VA, National Hospice Organization, 1996
12. National Hospice Organization: 1992 Hospice statistics. *NHO Newsline* 1, 1995
13. Alexander D, Ritchie E: Stressors and difficulties in dealing with the terminal patient. *J Palliat Care* 6:28–33, 1990
14. Vincent PA: Do hospice nurses differ from non-hospice nurses? *Am J Hospice Care* 3:41–42, 1986
15. Sankar A: *Dying at Home.* Baltimore, Johns Hopkins, 1991, pp 1–15
16. Worden JW: *Grief Counseling and Grief Therapy.* New York, Springer, 1982
17. Pflaum MC, Kelley P: Understanding the final messages of the dying. *Nursing '86* 16(6):26–29, 1986
18. Parkes CM, Weiss RS: *Recovery from Bereavement.* New York, Basic Books, 1983
19. Wadill G: Advanced directives. *Hospice* 2:10–11, 1991
20. VonGunten C: CPR in hospitalized patients: When is it futile? *Am Fam Physician* 4:2130–2134, 1991
21. Musgrave C: Terminal dehydration. *Cancer Nurs* 13:62–66, 1990

22. O'Connell L: *Active Euthanasia, Religion and the Public Debate.* Chicago, Park Ridge Center Publishers, 1991, pp 18–22
23. Thal AE: *Proactive Responses to the Assisted Suicide/Euthanasia Debate.* Publication No. 713438. Washington, DC, National Hospice Organization, 1996
24. Machuca M: Marketing and minorities: Hospice in the Hispanic community. *Am J Hospice Palliat Care* 7:21–22, 1990
25. Gorden AK: Hospice and minorities: A national study. Ph.D. diss., University of Illinois, 1992
26. Foley FJ: AIDS palliative care: Challenging the palliative paradigm. *J Palliat Care* 11(2):9, 1995
27. Amento MO, Tahan CB: AIDS and the hospice community. *Hospice Journal* 7:1–2, 1991
28. Kristjonson LJ, et al: Research in palliative care populations: Ethical issues. *Palliat Care* 10(3):10–15, 1994
29. *The 1996 Comprehensive Accreditation Manual for Hospitals.* Oakbrook Terrace, IL, The Joint Commission on Accreditation of Health Organizations, 1995

# PART VIII

# Professional Issues
# in Cancer Care

# Chapter 55

# Quality of Care

**Diane Scott Dorsett, RN, PhD, FAAN**

## CONCEPTUAL FOUNDATIONS OF QUALITY CARE

### Historical Context and Origins

Well over a century ago, Nightingale[1] said that the prime objective in nursing was "to put the patient(s) in the best condition for nature to act." Since then, both conceptually and operationally, care has become the essence of nursing. Over the past 15 years, a science of caring has emerged as a discrete theme in the nursing literature,[2–6] but only recently has care been accorded the importance recognized by Nightingale so long ago.

The relevance of care to society's health is becoming increasingly evident as demographic trends, such as an expanding elderly population, accelerate the incidence of chronic disease and as an increasingly advanced treatment technology extends life. Cure, once an important concept in the history of illness, when disease was primarily acute and infectious, has been replaced by the notion of prolonged remission with maximal quality of life. As modern science ushers in a biological wave of modalities influencing prevention, detection, and treatment, clinical health care providers will continue to face the reality of increasingly rigorous treatments and more critically acute, morbid episodes superimposed on the chronic illness itself. Thus, as Benner[2] eloquently states, "In health care, caring sets up the possibility for cure."

As physicians attempt to master the rapidly changing complexities of cancer treatment in an increasing number of sicker patients, nursing care becomes a central issue. Quality of care is challenged by a health care system that contracts hospital stay time and health care cost coverage and by a health care environment in which large segments of the most vulnerable members of society (nonwhite, poor, less educated), who have greater than average health care needs, also have less than equal access to health care. Furthermore, those disadvantaged who do gain access often receive health care of lower quality—especially when measured in terms of appropriateness, timeliness, comprehensiveness, and continuity.[7] Documented in a publication of the President's Commission for the Study of Ethical Problems in Medicine and Biomedical and Behavioral Research, *Securing Access to Health Care*,[8] cancers of white Americans are detected earlier than those of nonwhites, and those of paying patients are found earlier than those of nonpaying ones.

Although the reasons for these trends are complexly interwoven into the social, political, and economic fabric of American society, the outcome places a heavy burden not only on the underserved population but on all other segments of the society as well. Given today's challenges of specialization, complex technology, patterns of chronic illness, and restrictive health care environment, the quality care of cancer patients and their families demands an interdisciplinary team approach and the extension of the role of nursing in its total management.

By the end of 1988, the Oncology Nursing Society had revised and expanded its scope-of-practice statement on the basis of a philosophical recognition that individuals with cancer and their families need to be fully informed and to participate actively in their care and treatment and, further, that competent, humane care demands a complementary team of specialty practitioners who communicate with one another and augment one another's efforts. Increasingly, the notion of the patient as the owner-manager of his or her total health, with the need for a head coach and a qualified, well-coordinated health care team, has been gaining acceptance.[9]

Recognizing the emerging health care system as possessing an ever-expanding place for the nurse as direct caregiver, educator, administrator, and researcher, the Oncology Nursing Society statement emphasized the importance of the oncology nurse as a *coordinator* of care, collaborating with other health care team members to make the best use of resources available to patients and families and, as their *advocate*, assessing and communicating the uniqueness of each patient's response to cancer, thereby promoting maximum independence and autonomy. In short, oncology nurses, by virtue of their knowledge, skills, and holistic (biopsychosocial) perspective of persons with cancer, are often viewed as the most qualified practitioners to assume the head coach role.

### Care and caring

To care is to respond to another in need because of pain, illness, or distress. Caring involves a sense of commitment and responsibility and, when taken to higher levels, can be considered a body of knowledge and skill known tacitly, empirically, or scientifically to accomplish change for the good. Although caring behavior is central to most public and private human activity, when defined for nursing, caring becomes a set of meaning-laden actions.[2,10] To wit, early in the education of most nursing students, Virginia Henderson's classic definition of nursing is introduced:

> Nursing is primarily assisting individuals (sick or well) with those activities contributing to health, or its recovery (or to a peaceful death) that they perform unaided when they have the necessary strength, will or knowledge; nursing also helps individuals carry out prescribed therapy and be independent of assistance as soon as possible.[11]

The definition of nursing as a profession, a discipline, and a practice, through such theaters of relevance, becomes public domain through the Nurse Practice Act. Nurse practice acts are state-determined but are remarkably similar in wording throughout the country. Most legislate nursing as the diagnosis and treatment of human responses in health and illness—a broad definition, further operationalized in the interest of public safety by a regulated and standardized system of education, registration, certification, standards of practice, and quality assurance.

Following the broad, formative brushstrokes of Nightingale,[1] who recognized "the fundamental needs of the sick and principles of good care," a concise, comprehensive definition of nursing by Harmer and Henderson,[11] and the more recent revisions that modernized nurse practice acts in this country, nursing began the establishment of a taxonomy of nursing diagnoses.[12–14] Nursing diagnoses operationalize the nurse practice act terminology, "human responses to an actual or potential health problem."[15]

Diagnostic taxonomies generally allow for a clear definition of professional purpose and for faster communication among the practitioners of a discipline, and they become the basis for a profession's research and development activity. As Herberth and Gosnell[13] advise, the next step is the integration of standards of practice and nursing diagnoses (Table 55-1) to foster relevant research, promote therapeutic interventions, and, ultimately, advance the quality of care.

Caring actions cannot be separated from intent, however, if the outcome is to be effective. It is not enough to practice according to a guiding set of rules and regulations. To achieve even an acceptable level of quality of care, one must have commitment, creativity, and a willingness to innovate at reasonable risk. Knowing one's craft well is not enough. Caring requires knowing our patients and their beliefs, values, and cultural norms and tailoring care accordingly. Thus understanding and defining quality of care in terms of practices that enable health promotion and recovery from illness requires that caring be intrinsic to the process. Leininger[5] defined caring as behavioral attributes characterized by empathy, support, compassion, protection, succor, and education, firmly grounded in a comprehension of the needs, problems, values, and goals of the person or group being assisted.

### Quality

The nature of quality is multifaceted and difficult to define, especially in relation to nursing care. Yet quality has emerged as the most important issue in patient care services in the final two decades of the twentieth century. The 1980s witnessed an integration of quality management, control, and assurance in nursing practice. To some observers, this integration has changed practice habits and promoted the individuation of care in innovative ways. These new ways of practice have led to the development of standards of care as the basic unit of analysis in the evaluation of quality in practice.[16]

Quality has become the focus of all cancer service

**TABLE 55-1**   Functional Health Pattern Categories and Nursing Diagnoses

| | |
|---|---|
| **Health perception—health management pattern** | **Elimination pattern** |
| Health maintenance alteration | Alteration in bowel elimination: constipation or intermittent |
| Health management deficit (total) | constipation pattern |
| Health management deficit (specify) | Alteration in bowel elimination: diarrhea |
| Health seeking behavior | Alteration in bowel elimination: incontinence or bowel |
| Noncompliance (specify) | incontinence |
| Potential noncompliance (specify) | Altered urinary elimination pattern |
| Potential for infection | Urinary incontinence: functional, stress, urge or total |
| Potential for physical injury | Stress incontinence |
| Potential for poisoning | Urinary retention |
| Potential for suffocation | |
| | **Self-perception—self-concept pattern** |
| **Nutritional-metabolic pattern** | Fear (specify focus) |
| Alteration in nutrition: potential for more than body requirements | Anticipatory anxiety (mild, moderate, severe) |
| or potential obesity | Anxiety |
| Alteration in nutrition: more than body requirements or exogenous | Mild anxiety |
| obesity | Moderate anxiety |
| Alteration in nutrition: less than body requirements or nutritional | Severe anxiety (panic) |
| deficit (specify) | Reactive depression (situational) |
| Ineffective breast feeding | Hopelessness |
| Impaired swallowing | Powerlessness (severe, low, moderate) |
| Potential for aspiration | Self-esteem disturbance |
| Alterations in oral mucous membranes | Body image disturbance |
| Potential fluid volume deficit | Personal identity confusion |
| Fluid volume deficit (actual) (1) | |
| Fluid volume deficit (actual) (2) | **Role-relationship pattern** |
| Fluid volume excess | Anticipatory grieving |
| Potential or actual impairment of skin integrity or skin breakdown | Dysfunctional grieving |
| Decubitus ulcer (specify stage) | Disturbance in role performance |
| Impaired skin or tissue integrity | Unresolved independence-dependence conflict |
| Altered body temperature | Social isolation |
| Ineffective thermoregulation | Social isolation (rejection) |
| Hyperthermia | Impaired social interaction |
| Hypothermia | Altered growth and development: social skills (specify) |

*(continued)*

**TABLE 55-1**   Functional Health Pattern Categories and Nursing Diagnoses (continued)

| | |
|---|---|
| Translocation syndrome<br>Altered family process<br>Weak mother-infant attachment or parent-infant attachment<br>Potential altered parenting<br><br>**Activity-exercise pattern**<br>Potential activity intolerance<br>Activity intolerance (specify level)<br>Fatigue<br>Impaired physical mobility (specify level)<br>Potential for disuse syndrome<br>Total self-care deficit (specify level)<br>Self-bathing—hygiene deficit (specify level)<br>Self-dressing—grooming deficit (specify level)<br>Self-feeding deficit (specify level)<br>Self-toileting deficit (specify level)<br>Self-care skills deficit<br>Diversional activity deficit<br>Impaired home maintenance management (mild, moderate, severe, potential, chronic)<br>Potential joint contractures<br>Ineffective airway clearance<br>Ineffective breathing pattern<br>Impaired gas exchange<br>Decreased cardiac output<br>Altered tissue perfusion<br>Dysreflexia<br>Altered growth and development<br><br>**Sleep-rest pattern**<br>Sleep-pattern disturbance<br><br>**Cognitive-perceptual pattern**<br>Pain<br>Chronic pain<br>Pain self-management deficit | Uncompensated sensory deficit (specify)<br>Sensory-perceptual alterations: input deficit or sensory deprivation<br>Sensory-perceptual alterations: input excess or sensory overload<br>Unilateral neglect<br>Knowledge deficit (specify)<br>Uncompensated short-term memory deficit<br>Potential cognitive impairment<br>Impairment of thought processes<br>Decisional conflict (specify)<br>Altered parenting<br>Parental role conflict<br>Impaired verbal communication<br>Altered growth and development: communication skills<br>Potential for violence<br><br>**Sexuality-reproductive pattern**<br>Sexual dysfunction<br>Altered sexuality patterns<br>Rape trauma syndrome<br>Rape trauma syndrome: compound reaction<br>Rape trauma syndrome: silent reaction<br><br>**Coping—stress tolerance pattern**<br>Coping, ineffective (individual)<br>Avoidance coping<br>Defensive coping<br>Ineffective denial<br>Impaired adjustment<br>Posttrauma response<br>Family coping: potential for growth<br>Ineffective family coping: compromised<br>Ineffective family coping: disabling<br><br>**Value-belief pattern**<br>Spiritual distress (distress of human spirit) |

Reproduced by permission from Gordon M: *Manual of Nursing Diagnosis 1988–1989*. St. Louis, Mosby.

provider groups, including the Commission on Cancer of the American College of Surgeons, the National Cancer Institute, the American Cancer Society, the College of American Pathology, the American College of Radiology, and, in joint affiliation, the American Nurses' Association and the Oncology Nursing Society.[17] Quality was, as Beyers[16] stated, "the banner of the 1980s" and will be the established base for the next major advance in clinical nursing during the 1990s and beyond.

Quality, by definition, is a set of properties, attributes, and capacities that are essential and unique to the focus of evaluation, be it nursing or a work of art. In a generic sense, quality connotes a degree of excellence as measured by recognized standards. Standards are characterized by utility, durability, stability, flexibility, and aesthetics and, in the health care environment, require the definition of correlates related to both clinical and organizational qualities. Beyers[16] defines these correlates of quality as cost, productivity, and risk.

Historically, approaches to quality management in the United States have gone through several "eras," from inspection and statistical accounting measures (time and motion studies), to quality assurance processes and procedures (chart audit), to the newest era of "strategic quality management."[18] Strategic quality management is based on the realities of market share and fiscal viability since health care is big business and the driving force has become patient satisfaction. The "new" approach to quality recognizes four important factors: (1) recognition of consumer need and response, (2) integrated service teams, (3) standards of practice, organization, and professional performance, and (4) data management systems that document structure, process, and outcome elements.[16]

Beyers[16] views these factors as interactive and as having the potential for a positive effect. When patient needs are understood, recognized, and met by a well-coordinated team of clinicians who are guided by high standards, the associated documentation will allow clinical outcomes to be "known," ultimately modifying patient response for the better.

Thus quality embraces the dimensions of structure (patient and environment norms), process (strategies of quality management), and outcome (documentation of clinical outcomes and patient satisfaction). For many experts, quality is driven by the profit motive. For nursing, quality must be powered both by its value as a public service and by the caring ethic for maximal effect.

The concept of quality of care is grounded in the integration of a sound body of knowledge and skill, standards of practice and performance that promote excellence, a coordinated team approach, and a built-in capacity for innovation (research), with all components fired by a deep sense of caring.

## Quality of Care Model

A model of quality of care (Figure 55-1) has been designed to represent the major goals in cancer care and treatment and those structural factors that ensure quality in terms of process and outcomes.

### Structure

In the 1980s, several critical components were set in place that allowed for a guiding definition of quality in cancer care. These structural elements include overall standards for oncology nursing practice and for the professional performance of the nurse who cares for patients with cancer and their families. These standards currently are undergoing integration with the classification of nursing diagnoses and further categorization into Gordon's

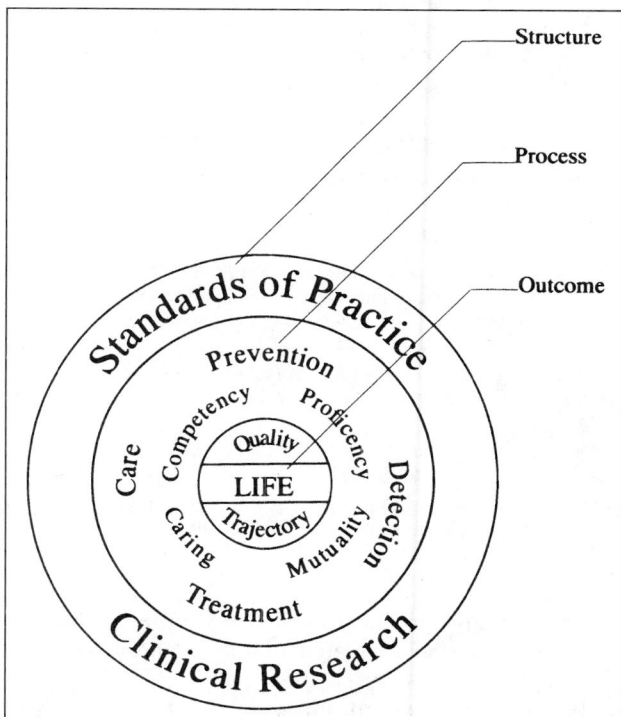

**FIGURE 55-1**   This model represents the major goals in cancer care and those structural factors that ensure quality of care in terms of process and outcome.

11 functional health pattern categories.[14] Another major structure that promotes quality of care is clinical research and the development of nursing technology to test and improve interventions and maximize positive results. Nursing research in cancer care can be built into every patient care environment on some level. For some, this might mean keeping up with the nursing research literature or participating in a journal club, or it might involve undertaking a small study of one's own or participating in a larger multisite research project. Research allows for the development of nursing technology as well: audiovisual patient teaching programs, drug dispensers that allow for safer self-administration of the many medications that cancer patients take at home, or measures that aid mobility, protect the skin and mucous membrane, or improve ventilation are examples of methods that achieve practical purposes toward the improvement or refinement of care. As these innovations are developed, they need to be tested and the results shared with others.

### Process

The second dimension of the quality-of-care model is represented by the process variables of cancer prevention, detection, treatment, and nursing care. This dimension brings together the nursing care–medical treatment complex because the components of this complex are mutually dependent in achieving the desired outcome. More often than not, nursing care revolves around medical treatment but, in the best sense, extends itself beyond the immediate goals of interest to the physician. Cell kill and reduced tumor size are important, but without attention to management of side effects and promotion of functional recovery, the effect is diminished at best and ineffective at worst. In this sense, cure and care are not dichotomous. Care augments and enhances cure and in the process humanizes the total outcome.

### Outcome

On a structural bed of sound standards and research innovation, the processes of prevention, detection, treatment, and care lead to patient outcome variables. The objectives of oncology care providers do not stop with the elimination of disease. Given the current status of cancer treatment, with a documented 50% cure rate in all patients with a diagnosis of cancer,[19,20] Paul Marks, president of Memorial Sloan-Kettering Cancer Center, placed the current climate in perspective:

> The implication of this [cancer biologic revolution] massive research effort is not that cancer will fade away in the next few years, or even decades. The discovery of oncogenes suggests that cancer may be an integral part of living, the result of interaction of our genes with the environment. Certainly, an understanding of the fundamental nature of carcinogenesis will transform the nature of clinical care. But it will not yield a magic bullet to cure the disease, nor a vaccine to prevent it. Cancer will not be eradicated like

smallpox or polio. Rather, what seems likely to emerge are new approaches to early diagnosis of cancers and new techniques to treat them, providing steady gains in our ability to cure and, more important, to prevent cancer.[20]

The bottom-line result of 30 years of massive biomedical scientific effort has been an extension of life for many patients with a diagnosis of cancer. Paralleling the work on this frontier, the biopsychosocial scientific effort in nursing has promoted advances in the quality of the lives that medical science has extended. The amalgamation of life extension and quality of life makes clear the ultimate and optimal outcome of cancer care: maximal quality of life for cancer patients and their families.

## Standards of Care

Nursing, as a science of caring, is based on a theoretical foundation for practice, continuously tested, refined, and verified by research, and a clearly articulated set of principles guiding that practice. Central to the concept of quality care is a set of standards that exists to guide practice by operationalizing its essence.

The publication of *Outcome Standards for Cancer Nursing Practice*[21] in 1979 and of its integration into the *Standards of Oncology Nursing Practice*[22] in 1987 were joint ventures of the Oncology Nursing Society (ONS) and the American Nurses' Association (ANA). Although the revision, *Standards of Oncology Nursing Practice,*[22] is rooted in the ANA published standards of nursing practice,[23] the former is a separate statement developed in recognition of cancer as a major health problem and of the importance of oncology nursing as a specialty practice devoted to the care of cancer patients and their families.

There are 11 standards of oncology nursing practice in the 1987 revision,[22] 6 that address professional practice and 5 that concern professional performance (Table 55-2). Practice standards focus on the process involved in patient care (theory, data collection, diagnosis, planning, intervention, and evaluation), with emphasis on 11 commonly occurring problem areas. Performance standards, in contrast, are criteria for professional development, interdisciplinary collaboration, quality assurance, ethics, and research in nursing as a discipline. To complement practice standards, the ONS published *Outcome Standards for Cancer Nursing Education,*[24] *Cancer Patient Education,*[25] and *Public Cancer Education.*[26] A summation of the oncology nursing practice standards follows.

### Standards of oncology nursing practice

I. The central core of oncology nursing is a logically articulated theoretical framework derived from the biological, social, behavioral, and physical sciences. There are at least a dozen major nursing theories that have been constructed to guide practice, but two of the most frequently used in oncology nursing are Orem's self-care deficit theory[27] and the Johnson behavioral system model.[28] With a sound theoretical base, the nursing pro-

**TABLE 55-2    Standards of Oncology Nursing Practice**

**Standards of Professional Practice**

I.    *Theory:* The oncology nurse applies theoretical concepts as a basis for decisions in practice.

II.   *Data collection:* The oncology nurse systematically and continually collects data regarding the health status of the client. The data are recorded, accessible, and communicated to appropriate members of the interdisciplinary team.

III.  *Nursing diagnosis:* The oncology nurse analyzes assessment data to formulate nursing diagnoses.

IV.   *Planning:* The oncology nurse develops an outcome-oriented care plan that is individualized and holistic. This plan is based on nursing diagnoses and incorporates preventive, therapeutic, rehabilitative, palliative, and comforting nursing actions.

V.    *Intervention:* The oncology nurse implements the nursing care plan to achieve the identified outcomes for the client.

VI.   *Evaluation:* The oncology nurse regularly and systematically evaluates the client's responses to interventions in order to determine progress toward achievement of outcomes and to revise the data base, nursing diagnoses, and the plan of care.

**Standards of Professional Performance**

VII.  *Professional development:* The oncology nurse assumes responsibility for professional development and continuing education and contributes to the professional growth of others.

VIII. *Multidisciplinary collaboration:* The oncology nurse collaborates with the multidisciplinary team in assessing, planning, implementing, and evaluating care.

IX.   *Quality assurance:* The oncology nurse participates in peer review and interdisciplinary program evaluation to assure that high-quality nursing care is provided to clients.

X.    *Ethics:* The oncology nurse uses the *Code for Nurses**
and *A Patient's Bill of Rights†* to guide ethical decision making in practice.

XI.   *Research:* The oncology nurse contributes to the scientific base of nursing practice and the field of oncology through the review and application of research.

*American Nurses' Association: *Code for Nurses with Interpretive Statements.* Kansas City, MO, The Association, 1985.

†American Hospital Association: *A Patient's Bill of Rights.* Chicago, The Association, 1972.

Reprinted with permission from *Standards of Oncology Nursing Practice,* © 1987, American Nurses' Association, Kansas City, MO.

cess is firmly grounded in established knowledge that can be constantly tested, evaluated, modified, and shared with colleagues.

II. Effective communication, assessment, and analytic skills are necessary to enable the oncology nurse to plan appropriate interventions for clients. The result is a sound database, available to the multidisciplinary team, that is maintained to reflect the most current and accurate clinical status of the patient.

III. The ability to make nursing diagnoses from the theoretical framework and the patient's database is essential to the plan of care. The diagnoses may emerge from actual or potential problems in 11 parameters: (1) prevention-detection, (2) information, (3) coping, (4) comfort, (5) nutrition, (6) protective mechanisms, (7) mobility, (8) elimination, (9) sexuality, (10) ventilation, and (11) circulation. Nursing diagnoses enable nurses to document problems and risks, planning, evaluation, and ultimately the research in care and collegial sharing that fosters continuity of care.

IV. Planning care is the first step in actively ensuring quality of care. During the planning process, goals are established and methods addressing the 11 parameters are selected.

V. The implementation of the plan uses independently and interdependently determined actions to achieve its goals. In most cases, however, the nurse should function autonomously but collaboratively with others. Intervention should be flexible and documented and should provide measurable evidence of effect in light of the plan.

VI. Finally, the evaluation of the plan and its outcomes allows for continuous update, revision, improvement, and refinements in the database and diagnoses and for resulting modifications in intervention. This evaluation is done in collaboration with the patient and family and the health care team, is fully documented, and ultimately leads to scholarly, scientific analysis through research.

## Standards of professional performance

VII. The first standard for professional performance makes clear (1) that the nurse is accountable for keeping abreast of advances in the field, maintaining current knowledge and skill, and incorporating them into practice and (2) that there is a commitment to the betterment of self, patients, colleagues, and the profession.

VIII. The complexity of cancer care today requires a multidisciplinary approach. Learning how to communicate effectively and to collaborate with team members is another indicator of professional development. There is considerable latitude in this standard in that the nurse may function effectively as participant, coordinator, and leader.

IX. Peer review and program evaluation have become mandated mechanisms in today's health care structure. Actively participating with an open, inquiring, and creative mind maximizes the possibility of quality improvement on individual, unit, and organizational levels.

X. The cancer care experience provides ample opportunity for ethical judgments. The rationale for the ethics standard spells out the profound ethical concerns in oncology nursing: right of self-determination, surrogate decision making, informed consent, treatment options, nontraditional treatment modalities, decisions about quality of life, confidentiality, distribution of resources, and matters of economics and value. Involvement with these issues can be demanding and challenging as well

as stressful and exhausting. Continuing education and peer support are important vehicles for professional growth in this area.

XI. The 1970s and 1980s ushered in a new era of research-based practice in nursing. Oncology nursing practice must be kept therapeutically effective through research. The latitude in this performance standard is substantial. Minimally, the practitioner should keep abreast of research-based studies published in the most relevant specialty journals and incorporate findings into practice. Through expanded education, the nurse might ultimately become the principal investigator of his or her own study and might cultivate a scholarly interest in research that becomes a lifelong pursuit and vehicle for the enhancement of quality care.

The most recent (1987) revisions of the *Standards of Oncology Nursing Practice* incorporated the separately published *Outcome Standards for Cancer Nursing Practice* published in 1979. The original outcome standards reflected ten high-incidence problem areas (Table 55-3) common to cancer as a major chronic disease with "intermittent acute episodes." When integrated with the 1987 revised practice standards concerned with data collection (II), nursing diagnoses (III), planning (IV), and evaluation (VI), the outcome assumes a patient-family-community focus, cuts across all phases of the cancer experience

**TABLE 55-3**  High-Incidence Problems in Cancer Nursing Practice

| | |
|---|---|
| I. | *Prevention and early detection:* Client and family possess adequate information about cancer prevention and detection. |
| II. | *Information:* Client and family possess knowledge about disease and therapy in order to attain self-management, participate in therapy, optimal living, and peaceful death. |
| III. | *Coping:* Client and family manage stress optimally according to their individual capacity and in accord with their value system. |
| IV. | *Comfort:* Client and family manage factors that influence comfort. |
| V. | *Nutrition:* Client and family manage nutrition and hydration optimally. |
| VI. | *Protective mechanisms:* Client and family possess knowledge to prevent or manage alterations in protective mechanisms. |
| VII. | *Mobility:* Client and family maintain optimal mobility. |
| VIII. | *Elimination:* Client and family manage problems with elimination. |
| IX. | *Sexuality:* Client and partner can manage threats to sexual function and satisfaction and maintain their sexual identity. |
| X. | *Ventilation:* Client and family can anticipate factors that impair ventilatory function and maintain optimal ventilatory capacity. |

Adapted from Oncology Nursing Society: *Outcome Standards for Cancer Nursing Practice.* Pittsburgh, The Society, 1979.

from prediagnosis to death, and recognizes the multiplicity of settings where patients are cared for today. These ten high-incidence areas provide an essential link between the operating practice standard and quality assurance.

# RESEARCH AND EVALUATION IN QUALITY OF CARE

## Background and Context

Research-based clinical practice and quality care are the hallmarks of professional nursing. These important processes are based on a theoretical body of knowledge, standards for practice, and valid and reliable measurements that allow for the evaluation of care and the expansion of the scientific foundation of practice.

The nursing literature of the 1970s saw a significant expansion in standardized approaches to measuring the quality of nursing care. As early as 1969, Donabedian[29] identified structure, process, and outcome variables in medicine as the three classic approaches to patient care evaluation.

One of the earliest studies of quality in nursing additionally tested the research tool "Patient Indicators of Nursing Care."[30] Seven physiological indicators reflecting nursing care–related complications were assessed. This study was a prototype of today's research evaluating patient outcome standards and nursing diagnosis–specific interventions. Majesky et al[30] chose three broad functional categories from Dorothy Johnson's theoretical framework—infection, immobility, and fluid imbalance—and operationalized them using 27 measurable indicators. The overall goal was to establish a reliable, valid, easy-to-use, clinically useful instrument to evaluate quality of nursing care.

Oncology nursing literature came of age with the beginning publication of two journals, *Cancer Nursing* and *Oncology Nursing Forum*. In a review[31] of research-based articles published in these journals through 1984, a total of 15 were found to evaluate nursing care programs. All interventions tested were educative or of a supportive, counseling nature, perhaps reflecting Herberth and Gosnell's finding[13] that over 40% of diagnoses involve knowledge deficit. Most of the studies did not allow for control-group comparisons. Nine articles described tools designed to evaluate patient outcomes. Rarely was care measured directly, and most measures were constructed by the investigator because of the lack of sound instrumentation at that time. Few were tested for accuracy or consistency.

A distinct shift in the cancer nursing literature, noted from 1985 onward, seemed to coincide with the establishment of oncology nursing standards and their clinically useful format (patient outcome standards and functional health classification). Clearly, more authors attempted

schema that integrated patients' clinical problems and deficits, nursing diagnoses, assessment parameters, causes, and interventions into plans for care that provided a useful guide for the practicing nurse and a methodical approach for quality assurance programs.

The following review of methods for measuring quality of cancer nursing care recognizes the seminal work of early researchers[32–36] but concentrates on studies published in the cancer nursing literature since 1985 that reflect more recent trends in the field (i.e., standards, nursing diagnoses, quality assurance, and measurement methods).

## Approaches to Measuring Quality of Care

There are three major approaches to measuring quality of care: (1) quality assurance programs, (2) clinical research that includes both program evaluation and experimental studies of interventions, and (3) measurement tool or instrument development that includes the construction of quantitative scales, questionnaires, and inventories and qualitative measures that include the establishment of clinical indicators, predictors, and guidelines for assessment.

### Quality assurance

The Joint Commission on the Accreditation of Health Care Organizations publishes standards used in the accreditation of hospitals and five other types of health care organizations (long-term care, psychiatric care, ambulatory health care, hospice care, and home care organizations) in this country.[37] These standards are concerned with the structures, processes, and outcomes of patient care activities in all services provided by the organization, including nursing services. There are eight standards that address the provision, management, and monitoring of nursing services regardless of location or institutional type. Four of the eight standards are concerned directly with the quality of nursing care: NR3 requires maintenance of established standards of nursing practice; NR5 mandates the use of the nursing process; NR7 delineates written documentation that care reflects optimal standards of practice; and NR8 provides for the monitoring and evaluation of care and the identification and resolution of problems.

The Joint Commission on the Accreditation of Health Care Organizations distinguishes between standards of care and standards of practice.[37] Whereas standards of care reflect expected patient outcomes of care activities, standards of practice are concerned with "the structure and process elements used by the nurse and nursing service to provide patient care."[38] Thus a standard of care focuses on the patient, and a standard of practice focuses on the nurse. Patterson[38] differentiates the two concepts further by explaining that a standard of care is what the patient outcome should be and what the patient can expect from nursing service, whereas standards of practice relate to what and how the nurse provides care to achieve the patient outcome. The outcomes of care generally are based on clinical criteria or well-defined indicators that are measurable and that reflect the quality and appropriateness of intervention. Quality, in this sense, depicts the degree of adherence between the standard of care and actual patient outcome, and appropriateness reflects the degree of congruence between what the patient needed to achieve in terms of a desired outcome and what the nurse provided.

Therefore, to operationalize a quality assurance program, the health care institution must maintain a sound system for documentation of nursing care activities and patient outcomes and must establish a system to review and assess regularly both quality and appropriateness. In addition to evaluation, there is the need for a system to rectify or resolve problems or breeches of quality in all aspects of care: diagnostic, preventive, therapeutic, rehabilitative, supportive, and palliative.

Depending on the nature and specialization of the nursing care unit, there may be a need for a more precise definition of both patient outcomes and nursing practices to achieve those outcomes, or what is known as *clinical functions*. Oncology nursing is a prime example of the need for care and practice standards to be tailored to the unique needs and problems of the cancer patient and for more precise operationalization of clinical functions such as assessment, evaluation of learning needs, provision of physical care, teaching, goal setting, nursing interventions based on nursing diagnosis, implementation of the medical plan of care and required medications and treatments, and the coordination of nursing goals and plans for care with those of other professional team members.[38]

In these specific cases, both health care institutions and accrediting organizations look to the professional specialty group to establish and promulgate those standards of nursing practice. Quality assurance structures look to organizations such as the ONS for current, state-of-the-art research-based standards.[38] On the basis of these published specialty guides, the hospital or agency customizes the standards further to be in line with the nature and character of its own caregiving environment. For example, nursing practice standards at one of the nation's five major cancer centers might differ from those in a small community hospital, where there may or may not be a discrete oncology unit or where there may or may not be a department of nursing research that focuses on oncology care. However, no matter how specialized or how large or small the institution might be, mandated quality assurance accords the *right* to quality of care as defined by the ONS standards of nursing practice to every oncology patient.

The literature is sparse in studies evaluating the quality of cancer nursing care by using patient outcomes as evidence. However, several articles stand out in their effort to improve the quality assurance process. This small body of literature reflects the complexities involved in studying quality and the many dimensions in focus and approach.

Five issues important to quality assurance were examined in nine studies reported in the period from 1985 to 1988: (1) quality assurance audit results for specific areas of care, (2) oncology patient classification systems, (3) Occupational Safety and Health Administration (OSHA) guidelines, (4) clinical database development, and (5) methods to identify and measure oncology nursing competencies and practice proficiency.

Oleske et al,[39] conducted a controlled study that measured the effects of both nurse specialist consultation and continuing education on the home care of cancer patients, using an audit measure documenting assessment, intervention, and evidence of outcomes for patients with breast and colon cancers. Findings revealed that improvement in nursing assessment and management performance occurred over time in all three intervention groups. However, only half the criteria for optimal nurse performance were achieved, with little increase in patient outcome scores. The greatest improvements were noted in patients' nutrition, and little improvement was noted overall in the management of pain and physiological complications. The authors recommend replication and offer the complete set of audit forms on request.

Similarly, Stephany[40] tested the reliability and validity of the Hope Hospice Quality Assurance Tool (HQAT), which assesses physical concerns, patient and caregiver education, and emotional and spiritual support, using operationally defined criteria. Test-retest stability and internal consistency of the tool were established. Content, criterion-related, and construct validities were tested and found to be high in the nurse group but only moderate for lay volunteers. The tool was modified, with subsequent improvement in reliability and validity scores. The report provides detailed descriptions of the quality assurance program, standards, and criteria of the assessment form. The rigor of the study produced an effective audit tool to measure the quality of hospice care.

Arenth[41] developed and validated an acuity classification of oncology patients based on the definition of four categories of emergent status. The system has served as the basis for calculating nursing hours per patient day, patient volumes, nursing utilization or productivity, and variable staffing in a large medical center.

Dudjak[42] described the Radiation Therapy Nursing Care Record, comprising six flow sheets designed to document the nursing care of patients undergoing radiation therapy. The record allows for baseline assessment of risk factors and problems and for nursing practices in assessment, teaching, and other interventions. The record has been used to justify staff needs and cost of nursing care and to further establish standards of practice.

Because safety is a cornerstone of quality assurance for both patients and health care providers, periodic updates such as Gullo's review[43] of safe handling of antineoplastic drugs are essential to the application of the OSHA guidelines to practice. Recommendations for avoiding exposure, for safe disposal, and for health evaluation and monitoring are given clearly according to a well-articulated knowledge framework. Gullo estimated that more than 60% of nurses were not using safe handling techniques, an important factor in quality assurance. Two articles by Williamson et al[44,45] reviewed the occupational risks of infection, musculoskeletal injury, exposure to antineoplastic agents, stress in the work environment, shift work, and reproductive health concerns of nurses. Their articles call for a greater intensity of clinically oriented research efforts in this area.

Two articles suggest methods of establishing a clinical database to provide a structured framework for the collection of critical data with which to formulate nursing diagnoses. Miaskowski and Nielsen[46] developed the Cancer Nursing Assessment Tool to evaluate the integrity of 15 functional systems at high risk because of cancer and its treatment. The assessment included teaching needs and discharge planning. Gray et al[47] published a clinical database that provides description and analysis of age, metastatic sites, diagnoses, and associated symptoms of hospitalized patients with advanced cancer. Their study of 1103 patients generated more than 400 variables and provided important information on problem areas related to cancer metastasis. Since symptom management is the "cornerstone of care" in this patient group, the database facilitated the identification of relevant nursing diagnoses and related nursing practices that improved the measurement of quality of care.

On another level, two separate studies by Moore et al[48] and McGee et al[49] sought to establish nurse competencies and to measure proficiency in cancer nursing practice. The Moore team constructed the Appraisal of Practice Behaviors Instrument, based on the five dimensions of the theoretical framework used by the ONS to develop the *Standards of Oncology Nursing Practice*. Three classes enrolled in a master's-level oncology nursing graduate program were tested before and after each of the two years of their educational program for both frequency and self-assessed proficiency in achieving the ONS outcome standards of oncology practice. The instrument consists of 92 items divided among six subscales. Findings revealed that frequency of practice and proficiency were positively related and that students significantly increased in self-assessed proficiency as their educational program progressed. The investigators suggest further evaluation of the instrument in both academic and clinical settings to expand the database.

In contrast, McGee et al[49] conducted a two-round Delphi survey to identify oncology clinical nurse specialist (OCNS) competencies. The initial pilot study amassed 363 competencies, which the investigators further divided into knowledge, skill, attitude, and human trait categories. Ranking by means for each category revealed that attitude and human traits were ranked highest in importance by the 47 respondents. Attitudes of greatest importance had to do with ethical practice, respect for humanity, responsibility for behavior, and commitment to continued learning. Identifying nursing diagnoses and commitment to cost-effective practices were ranked lowest in the category. The human traits most valued included accountability, common sense, caring, flexibility,

and resourcefulness. Of lower importance were sympathy and abstract thinking. The highest number of competencies, 173, were amassed in the "skills" category, and knowledge ranked second in number of competencies, totaling 137. The investigators, in interpreting their results, concluded that attitudes and human traits concerned with caring, commitment, and professionalism were ranked as those most important to OCNS functioning. They considered their results to be consistent with Yasko's survey[50] of 185 OCNSs, who reported a decided "care orientation" described as "keeping the client comfortable, maintaining a therapeutic environment, providing emotional support, personalized care, friendliness, emotional acceptance and ensuring that clients understand their medical problems."

The information generated from these key studies helps to expand and facilitate attempts to improve quality of care. By integrating findings from these and future studies on acuity, audit assessment tools, safety guidelines, clinical databases, and nursing competencies and practice proficiency, quality assurance will move into the era of strategic quality management predicted by Garven[18] and Beyers.[16]

### Clinical research

Research offers a means of improving and refining practice to ensure optimal outcomes. The desired result of practice usually is defined as a valuable change in the patient for the better. In most institutional settings, this means cost-effective patient outcomes and consumer satisfaction.

Clinical research, in the context of evaluating quality of care, includes two major categories: (1) experimental studies of nursing interventions and (2) evaluations of programs of care. The program of research in most disciplines is shaped by the intellectual and practical problems and challenges encountered in carrying out its objectives and by the diagnostic and functional categories that constitute its focus. For nursing, these areas for investigation can best be illustrated by the results of two Delphi surveys which examine research priorities in cancer nursing.

Oberst[51] polled a group of 575 oncology nurses throughout the United States, asking them what they thought was important to investigate systematically in order to improve their clinical practice. From those nurses giving the most direct care to cancer patients, Oberst's goal was to capture a heuristic force that would have an impact on patient welfare by using the research process as a catalyst. She asked nurses to identify the problems they confront every day in practice, the problems cancer patients have from the time of diagnosis, and how these problems arrange themselves in priority.

The results of Oberst's study determined ten priorities for cancer nursing research: (1) chemotherapy- or radiation-induced nausea and vomiting, (2) pain, (3) discharge needs, (4) grief, (5) stomatitis, (6) venipuncture in long-term therapy, (7) comfort and dignity of the terminally ill patient, (8) effective analgesia, (9) assistance with providing effective pain management, and (10) understanding the nurses' own attitudes toward pain and how it affects their ability to provide effective pain management. In addition, the oncology nurses responding to Oberst's survey reported that patient- and nurse-related research needs parallel one another. Optimal patient outcomes were inextricably tied to the reduction of deficits in nurse knowledge and skill in the ten patient-focused research priority areas.

Later, a partial replication of Oberst's work was conducted with 143 practicing oncology nurses from the four western provinces of Canada.[52] Results were similar but were expressed by requests for studies of specific interventions. Of the top 15 research priorities, the following areas emerged as most important: relaxation, imagery, and biofeedback techniques in the reduction of anticipatory nausea and vomiting and other side effects of treatment and in the enhancement of quality of life; ways to increase effectiveness of patient teaching in areas of patient compliance, self-care, and coping; approaches to improve discharge planning programs; methods of communicating diagnosis and prognosis to patients and families; approaches to strengthen effectiveness in primary care; ways to improve preceptorship programs; and therapeutic approaches to the relief of treatment- and disease-related symptoms and side effects. The emphasis of the Canadian results was clearly on studying nursing practices that improve the patient's condition, rather than on the problem itself. This shift may reflect the result of descriptive nursing research efforts and a more sophisticated practice during the years after Oberst's survey.[51]

In a review of research-based articles appearing in the cancer nursing literature between 1976 and 1984, Scott[31] found 122 articles representing 25% of all articles published. More than 60% of the studies were published after 1981, most concerned with side effects of treatment (26%) or with oncology nurses themselves (24%). Approximately 15% examined the impact of cancer on the family, and another 16% described phenomena about cancer patients. Only 12% were intervention-management studies, and fewer (7%) offered assessment-measurement approaches to evaluate care.

In a developmental sense, the era before 1985 may be viewed as a descriptive phase when the rich database that exists today was established. Clinical research, comprising both program evaluation and experimental studies of interventions, began slowly between 1980 and 1985, marked by the seminal work of Satterwhite et al,[53] Edlund,[55] Dodd and Mood,[54,55] Johnson,[56] Miller and Nygren,[57] Marty et al,[58] Watson,[59] and Henrich and Schag.[60] Since 1985, there has been an expansion of the cancer research literature addressing the priorities in the two Delphi surveys and testing the therapeutic effect of larger-scale programs of care.

Twenty-six experimental studies published since 1984 (Table 55-4)[61-86] addressed five of the ten (50%) outcome standards for cancer nursing practice. About half tested interventions to reduce treatment-induced side effects.

Nine studies (35%) tested interventions to reduce treatment-induced side effects. Nine studies (35%) tested interventions to optimize protective mechanisms by preventing infection or reducing skin and mucous membrane integrity deficits. Two studies (8%) evaluated educational programs to promote early cancer detection practices. As a whole, these studies reflected a growing sophistication in research design and measurement. Most were randomized, controlled investigations of the effect of a clearly defined intervention on a small, homogeneous sample. The instruments used to measure patient outcomes generally had been tested for reliability and validity or consisted of well-defined clinical indicators rated for construct validity by a panel of experts. All reports discussed study limitations, the generalizability of results, and implications for further research. Moreover, practically all made useful contributions to clinical knowledge.

From 1984 to 1996, a total of 18 program evaluation reports (Table 55-5)[87-103] covering a wider range of outcome standards were published. The largest number (eight, or 44%) evaluated programs designed to assist patients and families to cope with cancer. The next largest category (four, or 22%), comfort, described multidisciplinary pain management programs. The rest were divided among prevention-detection (one, or 6%), information (one, or 6%), protection (one, or 6%), and two economic feasibility studies (11%) of an adult day care hospital and a home transfusion program.

The therapeutic programs generally were well defined, as was the patient population. Most were service innovations based on the institution's database of patient needs and problems. In a majority of these studies, evaluation methods proved to be the weakest component. Although all programs were judged as valuable by the investigators, only half employed evaluation criteria developed before program initiation. Some measured quality by the number of clients seen or by unsolicited patient feedback. Others, however, made use of standardized surveys, questionnaires, interviews, and preprogram and postprogram comparisons of knowledge tests or needs assessments with baseline findings. Almost all investigative teams communicated willingness to share their programs with others but advised tailoring them to the unique needs of the institutions and their patient populations. Most suggested the need for further study and program modifications or refinements.

Although the program evaluations reflected significant effort in planning and execution by hardworking teams, it must be remembered that program evaluation is a mature methodology, generally requiring an expert team of outside investigators to conduct the study. Two noteworthy examples include the Brown University evaluation of the Adult Day Care Hospital, Memorial Sloan-Kettering Cancer Center[104] and the University of Washington study of the effect of the Planetree Unit, a primary-nursing, family-centered care facility at California Pacific Medical Center (Pacific campus), San Francisco.

The overall picture of 44 studies published over a 12-

**TABLE 55-4** Experimental Studies of Oncology Nursing Interventions and Patient Outcomes by Functional Pattern Category

| Author | Problem | Method | Findings | Implications |
|---|---|---|---|---|
| **PREVENTION AND EARLY DETECTION** | | | | |
| Rudolf and Quinn[61] | Education to promote TSE | N = 64 college men; Health Beliefs Survey for Testicular Cancer and Testicular Self-Examination Survey (modified by authors); pretest and posttest; educational program with film and silicone practice model | • Subjects lacked knowledge about testicular cancer and TSE<br>• Increased perception in benefits and decrease in barriers to TSE resulted<br>• Of "never performers," 63% did TSE at least once after program<br>• Perception of susceptibility and disease seriousness did not increase | • Need for education and for research testing of a variety of educational approaches<br>• Nurses should take lead<br>• Replication with time between testing and more controlled methods<br>• Further testing of instrument |
| Coleman et al[75] | BSE proficiency in older women (>50 years) | N = 79 women; random assignment 2-group design to compare women who were taught BSE using self-modeling as well as breast model methods with women taught by use of breast model only. Subjects evaluated using pre- and posttesting method. First posttest immediately after the teaching; second posttest 3 months later | • Women taught by both methods performed BSE significantly more proficiently than those taught by model only | • Performance is not always related to a woman's reported self-confidence<br>• Patients need to be evaluated directly to determine proficiency in BSE |
| **INFORMATION** | | | | |
| Hagopian[76] | Effect of weekly radiation therapy newsletter on knowledge, self-care, and severity of side effects | N = 103 radiation patients assigned to experimental (51) and control (52) groups. Experimentals had opportunity to read newsletter during treatment; controls did not. *Instruments:* Radiation Side Effects Profile, a knowledge test, and a demographics form; posttest-only design. | • Subjects who read newsletter scored significantly higher on knowledge test<br>• All other correlations nonsignificant | • Majority of patients found newsletter to be helpful source of information<br>• It cannot replace a caring professional |
| Hagopian[77] | Effect of informational audiotapes on knowledge and self-care behaviors in RT patients | N = 75 RT adults randomized into audiotape vs. standard care control groups using posttest measurement | • Experimental subjects were more knowledgeable and used more self-care measures and practiced more self-care behaviors than controls | • Audiotapes are a useful tool in radiation oncology patient teaching |

**TABLE 55-4**   Experimental Studies of Oncology Nursing Interventions and Patient Outcomes by Functional Pattern Category (continued)

| Author | Problem | Method | Findings | Implications |
|---|---|---|---|---|
| | | **INFORMATION** | | |
| Hughes[78] | Information amount and presentation in treatment selection and recall | $N = 71$ stage 1 & 2 breast cancer patients. Amount, location, and presentation determined by checklist observation with follow-up telephone survey | • Choice of treatment unrelated to amount and presentation during clinic visits<br><br>• Treatment selection related to amount of information received *before* clinic visit<br><br>• Patient recall of information about treatment and associated risks was poor | • Further research on both clinical implications and legal ramifications needed |
| Mansson et al[79] | Effect of demonstration-type preparation program on anxiety and cooperation during pediatric lumbar puncture | $N = 30$ children with leukemia/lymphoma, aged 4–17 years, divided into 3 groups of 10. Controls: no specific preparation; preparation using demo, doll, and book of photos of procedure. Preparation began 1 hour prior to LP. Child videotaped. Scales to measure anxiety and noncooperation | • Anxiety and noncooperation were strongly associated<br><br>• Children under 8 years exhibited higher anxiety, noncooperation, and self-rated pain<br><br>• Repeated preparations for subsequent LTs seemed effective<br><br>• No significant differences found among groups<br><br>• Children's self-reported pain ratings generally higher than anxiety and noncooperation | • Overall, children seemed to benefit from the attention. More research re clinical contacts with children needed |
| | | **COMFORT** | | |
| Beck[80] | Effect of music in decreasing cancer pain | $N = 15$ outpatients with cancer receiving scheduled analgesics for pain; experimental repeated measures crossover design using McGill Pain Questionnaire and analogue scales to measure mood and pain; from a menu of 7 types of music, subjects chose type of music preferred; controls listened to tape with low-frequency hum; tapes were 45 min in length; study conducted in 4 phases: baseline data for 3 days, randomized to E or C | • When listening to music, 75% had <20% response, 50% had <40% or >40% responses<br><br>• When listening to hum, 20% had <40% and >40% responses and 53% had no change in pain<br><br>• 60% listening to music reported some improvement in mood with music, with ⅓ responding with moderate to great improvement<br><br>• Mood and pain were found to be unrelated | • Music therapy has promise as a pain reducing modality, but further refinements in methods and research required |

*(continued)*

**TABLE 55-4** Experimental Studies of Oncology Nursing Interventions and Patient Outcomes by Functional Pattern Category (continued)

| Author | Problem | Method | Findings | Implications |
|--------|---------|--------|----------|--------------|
| | | COMFORT | | |
| | | group for 3 days, crossover to alternate group for 3 days, baseline repetition for all subjects for 3 days; pain ratings taken before and after listening to tape | • Although not statistically significant, overall music decreased pain 22%; hum decreased pain 11% | |
| Broome et al[81] | Effect of distraction and imagery on reducing pain during painful procedures in children and on reducing anxiety in child's mother | N = 14 children receiving lumbar punctures and their mothers; multiple case study design; children videotaped for first 3 visits to obtain baseline; distraction and imagery program not described; *instruments (child):* Child Medical Fear Scale, Observation of Behavioral Stress Scale, Baker-Wong FACES Scale; *instruments (mother):* Spielberger's State-Trait Anxiety Inventory (STAI), Parent Behavior Tool | • No change in children's fears or behavioral distress; children's pain ratings decreased significantly over time<br><br>• Mothers' state anxiety did not change<br><br>• Mothers' behaviors were nondistressed and stable over time | • Research control of ability of child to relax and use distraction and frequency of parent-child practice need to be improved<br><br>• Decrease in children's pain reports an important finding and corresponds with previous reports |
| Cotanch et al[62] | Self-hypnosis as antiemetic therapy | N = 20 children, aged 9–18 years, receiving chemotherapy; experimental and control groups; investigator-constructed visual analogue scale, self-report, nurse's charting; experimental subjects trained in relaxation and self-hypnosis | • Decrease in intensity and severity of nausea and vomiting in experimental group<br><br>• Increased oral intake in experimental group<br><br>• No difference in antiemetic administration between groups | • Further research in other age-groups |
| Frank[63] | Music and guided imagery as antiemetic therapy | N = 15 adults on variety of chemotherapy regimens—13 women, 2 men; single group; pretest and posttest STAI; Nausea and Vomiting Questionnaire; *intervention:* musical tapes and poster images during and after chemotherapy | • Decreased anxiety (STAI)<br><br>• Decreased intensity of vomiting<br><br>• No difference in perception of nausea, but duration showed nonsignificant downward trend | • Test intervention in other stressful, threatening situations (i.e., crisis and pain) |
| Scott et al[64] | Progressive Muscle Relaxation (PMR), guided imagery, and slow-stroke back massage vs. drug regimen as antiemetic therapy | N = 17 women with gynecologic cancer receiving chemotherapy; relaxation and drug groups; drug group received high-dose metaclopramide; Emetic Process Rating Scale (EPRS); relaxation group received 1-hr educational | • Relaxation group had reduced total duration<br><br>• Drug group had reduced peak vomiting phase<br><br>• No difference in intensity or amount of emesis between groups | • Testing interventions combining both methods<br><br>• Replication in other populations<br><br>• Continued testing of EPRS |

**TABLE 55-4**   Experimental Studies of Oncology Nursing Interventions and Patient Outcomes by Functional Pattern Category (continued)

| Author | Problem | Method | Findings | Implications |
|---|---|---|---|---|
| | | COMFORT | | |
| | | program with slide tape and were coached by nurse in relaxation | • Drug group experienced significantly increased diuresis unexplained by intake<br>• Content validity of EPRS established<br>• Verification of phase periodicity | • Data on norm phase periodicity for other chemotherapy regimens |
| Cotanch and Strum[65] | PMR as antiemetic therapy | N = 60; *3-group design:* experimental, placebo control (music), true control (no intervention); Dukes Descriptive Scale; Diary of Food Intake; STAI; upper skin-fold size; blood pressure; admission-discharge assessments | • PMR most effective in reducing frequency and duration of vomiting, general anxiety, and physiological arousal and in improving caloric intake in patients 48 hr after chemotherapy | • Replication |
| Parker[66] | Scalp hypothermia to reduce alopecia | N = 12 subjects receiving cyclophosphamide randomly assigned to 2 groups; experimental and control; SPENCO Hypothermia Cap; samples of hair loss for 7 days after treatment; scalp photographs | • Control subjects have significantly more hair loss than experimental subjects | • Clinical use |
| Dudjak[67] | Mouth care for mucositis therapy | N = 15 subjects receiving radiation therapy to head and neck area; random assignment of experimental and control groups; experimental subjects received hydrogen peroxide solution; control subjects received baking soda and water; oral examination guide; Oral Comfort Guide; subjects evaluated 8 times: once before radiation therapy and then once weekly for 5 weeks, at completion, and 1 month after completion | • Increase in perceived comfort in experimental group<br>• No difference in mouth condition between groups<br>• Hydrogen peroxide treatment judged more effective<br>• Both groups at lower incidence than published norms<br>• Rate of infection equal in both groups | • Replication<br>• Test other interventions<br>• Clinical use |
| Winningham and MacVicar[68] | Aerobic exercise as antiemetic therapy | N = 42 breast cancer patients; matched age and functional capacity; *3-group design:* experimental (stationary bike), placebo control (mild stretching), control (no treatment); | • Marked improvement in experimental compared with other groups in patient reports of nausea<br>• Increase in somatization scores in experimental groups | • Studies of other types of exercise, emetic treatment protocols, and studies to determine difference between exercise and relaxation |

*(continued)*

**TABLE 55-4** Experimental Studies of Oncology Nursing Interventions and Patient Outcomes by Functional Pattern Category (continued)

| Author | Problem | Method | Findings | Implications |
|---|---|---|---|---|
| | | **COMFORT** | | |
| | | *Treatment:* supervised 10-wk 3×/wk aerobic training on cycle ergometer; Symptom-Limited Graded Exercise Text (SLGXT); Symptom Checklist 90—Revised; Somatization Subscale; all tests given before and after treatment | | |
| Giaccone et al[69] | Scalp hypothermia to reduce alopecia | N = 39 patients receiving doxorubicin; randomly assigned to experimental (scalp hypothermia) or control (no treatment) group; SPENCO Hypothermia; evaluations after 2 full chemotherapy cycles; hair loss evaluated by nurse and physician using an operationalized scale | • Control subjects, 100% alopecia<br><br>• Experimental subjects, 37% prevention of hair loss<br><br>• No or slight hair loss in 7 of 19<br><br>• No instances of scalp metastasis in either group | • Clinical use |
| | | **COPING** | | |
| Mock et al[82] | Compare rehab treatment program results with usual-care group results of breast cancer patients: functional, physical, psychosocial adjustments | N = 14 women with breast cancer randomized into either treatment or usual-care control groups. Performance, functioning, psychosocial adjustment, self-concept, body image, and dysphoria were measured pre-, mid-, and postprogram. Experimental program included walking and support group attendance | • Selective measures of performance, psychosocial adjustment, and symptom intensity revealed improved adaptation in experimental group | • Patients benefit from an exercise and support group rehab program |
| | | **PROTECTIVE MECHANISMS** | | |
| Brandt et al[83] | Comparison of two CVC dressing protocols on catheter infections in ABMT patients | N = 101 patients, with long-term tunneled CVCs inserted in OR, randomized into two groups: (1) dry, sterile gauze changed every 24 hours; (2) Opsite 3000 ™ transparent moisture vapor permeable dressing changed weekly | • No statistical difference in infection rate between groups<br><br>• CVC sepsis occurred in 1 dry dressing and 5 Opsite subjects | • Both methods can be used safely |

**TABLE 55-4**   Experimental Studies of Oncology Nursing Interventions and Patient Outcomes by Functional Pattern Category *(continued)*

| Author | Problem | Method | Findings | Implications |
|--------|---------|--------|----------|--------------|
| | | PROTECTIVE MECHANISMS | | |
| Dodd et al[84] | Comparison of chlorhexidine with water in preventing mucositis | $N$ = 222 patients beginning mucositis-induced chemotherapy for 3 cycles. Randomized clinical trial of agents with results measured by Oral Assessment Guide with each chemotherapy cycle to determine any change in oral status | • No significant differences in incidence, days to onset, or severity | • Chlorhexidine is much less cost-efficient than water for preventing oral mucositis |
| Shivnan et al[85] | Comparison of transparent adherent dressing (TAD) and dry sterile gauze dressing (DSGD) in preventing infection in long-term central catheters | $N$ = 98; TAD (51); DSGD (47); randomized, stratified design with assignment to DSGD changed daily or TAD changed every 4 days; data collected with investigator-designed demographic and assessment forms for skin irritation and intactness, dryness of dressing, erythema, swelling, pain, and exudate; dressing comfort, ease of application, safety, change frequency, and satisfaction recorded | • DSGD group had significantly more skin irritation and wet dressings after showering, and had more exudate<br>• Exit site infection occurred in 2 TAD and 1 DSGD subjects<br>• No systemic infection occurred<br>• One catheter-related sepsis occurred in TAD group<br>• TADs required significantly fewer dressings and less nursing time and were significantly less costly<br>• Subjects reported greater satisfaction and comfort with TADs | • TADs provide a safe, comfortable, and cost-effective alternative to DSGDs |
| Yeoman et al[86] | Effect of chlorhexidene gluconate (CHG) in reducing perirectal infections in patients with acute leukemia | $N$ = 40 acute or chronic leukemia patients; 16 randomized to CHG group, 24 to nonmedicated skin cleanser group; chi-square and t-tests used to analyze (1) incidence of skin breakdown and rectal infections, and their correlation, (2) positive history of rectal infections, fissures, hemorrhoids, (3) presence of hemorrhoids, (4) severity of diarrhea, and (5) duration and severity of granulocytopenia; *instruments:* Perirectal Skin Assessment Tool (PSAT), perirectal clinical examinations conducted | • Treatment did not influence development of perirectal infections or degree or incidence of skin breakdown<br>• Severity and duration of granulocytopenia significantly related to development of rectal infections<br>• No other variable a statistically significant influence | • Due to small sample size, replication is advisable<br>• PSAT has some demonstrated validity and reliability<br>• Need for strategies to prevent rectal infection in immunocompromised patients is clear |

*(continued)*

**TABLE 55-4**  Experimental Studies of Oncology Nursing Interventions and Patient Outcomes by Functional Pattern Category (continued)

| Author | Problem | Method | Findings | Implications |
|---|---|---|---|---|
| | | PROTECTIVE MECHANISMS | | |
| | | by blinded evaluators for duration and severity of granulocytopenia, presence of hemorrhoids, severity of GI mucositis, signs of perirectal infection | | |
| Shell et al[70] | Dressings to treat radiation therapy skin reactions | N = 16 patients with moderate to severe radiodermatitis; comparison of moisture-permeable to conventional hydrous lanolin gauze; evaluation of healing time by use of 4 visual inspection parameters in number of days | • Healing time for MVP: 19 days vs. 24 days for lanolin gauze | • Warrants further study |
| Harwood and Bachur[71] | DMSO vs. local cooling in extravasation therapy | Animal study using 4 pigs; posttest-control experimental design; micromeasurements by primary investigator; measured time to healing DMSO vs. local cooling with ice vs. no-treatment control | • Local cooling more highly effective in preventing tissue necrosis after extravasation<br><br>• No difference between DMSO and control groups<br><br>• Time to healing increased with DMSO<br><br>• DMSO not recommended for treatment | • More studies to determine optimal schedule of cooling |
| Jones[72] | Catheter care procedures in central venous catheter infection | Evaluation of 2 catheter care procedures, one using fewer supplies and less time; assessment of observable evidence of infection, neutrophil count, and blood cultures | • No difference<br><br>• Only common factor connected with likelihood of infection: low neutrophil count at time of positive blood culture | • Conduct further studies to refine predictive risk factors |
| MacGeorge et al[73] | Mixing vs. reinfusion methods in drawing blood from Hickman catheter | N = 18 bone marrow transplant patients; hematocrit (Coulter counter); visual determination of hemolysis by expert laboratory technician | • No statistical difference in accuracy of laboratory values between 2 methods<br><br>• Mixing has advantage of less infection | • Replication in pediatric population with larger sample in variety of clinical settings |
| Petrosino et al[74] | Dressing to reduce central venous catheter infection | N = 52 patients with central venous catheters; random assignment to 4 dressing groups: Tegaderm transparent, Op-Site, gauze, no dressing; observation at 7 and 30 days for 5 indicators: skin culture, oral temperature, erythema, tenderness, drainage | • No difference among groups<br><br>• No dressing option seems simpler and less costly | • Further research on skin cleansing techniques |

*TSE,* testicular self-examination; *STAI,* State-Trait Anxiety Inventory; *PMR,* progressive muscle relaxation; *DMSO,* dimethyl sulfoxide.

**TABLE 55-5**   Care Program Evaluation Studies

| Program | Author | Method | Results |
|---|---|---|---|
| I. PREVENTION AND DETECTION | | | |
| Family High Risk Program | Beck et al[87] | Health Family Tree Questionnaire; Family health survey to assess satisfaction with program, health practices, health history, and behavior; includes retrospective data | • Evaluation ongoing<br>• No results as of publication |
| II. INFORMATION | | | |
| Patient Education Program | Nieweg et al[88] | Comparison of patient self-care of chemotherapy port infection rates with literature-based norms; weekly clinical assessments; no standardized evaluation methods used | • Empirically judged effective<br>• Takes considerable time<br>• Required teaching materials<br>• Greater social support involvement<br>• Less need for hospitalization<br>• Greater patient freedom |
| III. COPING | | | |
| I Can Cope | McMillan et al[101] | First national evaluation of ICC in 8 areas: demographics, format, objectives, content, audiovisual materials, training, implementation, evaluation | • Wide variations in comparison to official facilitator's guide<br>• Facilitators agreed with objectives and content<br>• Wide participant levels<br>• Topics most often requested include medical care, resources, emotional support, and stress management |
| Living with Cancer | Pillon and Joannides[102] | Based on anecdotal statements and empirical observation of a program conducted since 1979 | • Program needs to be comprehensive, addressing problems of the entire family from diagnosis to disease-free state or death<br>• Facilitators should include an oncology nurse and mental health clinician |
| We Can Weekend | Lane and Davis[89] | Postprogram participant evaluation; staff feedback; director evaluation of training sessions, staff, facilities, schedule, public relations, and supplies | • Recommended use of preprogram questionnaires to enable advance custom planning<br>• Also use a postprogram questionnaire |
| Living With Cancer | Fredette and Beattie[90] | Precourse and postcourse knowledge test; precourse and postcourse personal needs assessment; postcourse interviews; written comments of specialist-observer; end-of-class and end-of-program evaluations | • Coping skills can be taught<br>• Profiles "good coper" as one who pursues information and seeks opportunities to learn<br>• Adaptive, resilient, optimistic, and assertive<br>• Need further exploration into program design for those who desire less or differently structured programs |

*(continued)*

**TABLE 55-5** Care Program Evaluation Studies (continued)

| Program | Author | Method | Results |
|---|---|---|---|
| **III. COPING** | | | |
| Cancer Caregivers Program | Cawley and Gerdts[91] | Committee-constructed evaluation tool: evaluates 8 dimensions of care in terms of time, instructor, handouts | • Teaching skills of coping was primary value of program<br>• Provides steps in establishment of program<br>• Evaluation tool developed and provided<br>• Ongoing evaluation<br>• No results |
| I Can Cope | Diekmann[92] | Postprogram mail questionnaire | • Demographic characteristics<br>• Overall evaluation: valuable to help people learn about cancer<br>• More research to improve impact on coping |
| Bereavement Outreach Program | Mosely et al[93] | No formal means of evaluation | • Excellent client response<br>• Need to tailor program to institution |
| **IV. COMFORT** | | | |
| Home Pain Management Program | Coyle et al[94] | Evaluated 123 patients with advanced disease for pain management at home | • Nurse becomes primary liaison<br>• Successful pain management at home with use of analgesic and behavioral modes<br>• Team as expert information resource in community |
| Continuous SC Infusion Pain Management Program | Coyle et al[95] | Evaluated 15 patients for quality of pain management | • Avoids repeated injection, need for intravenous access, analgesia delay, pain breakthrough |
| Pain Management Team | Ferrell et al[96] | No evaluation of effect of interventions on pain | • Patients visits: 7500 (750 patients) over course of 5 years<br>• Community presentations: 300 |
| Patient-controlled Analgesia (PCA) Service | Kane et al[97] | Patient questionnaire on discharge; nurse evaluation of 2 pumps regarding safety, ease of use, saving of time; bedside flow sheets to rate pain and sedation; daily patient evaluation by PCA team | • Use of pump gives excellent control of pain in postsurgical patients, has few problems, and frees nurse to care for patient<br>• Further studies in chronic pain populations needed<br>• Choice of one pump over another |
| **V. NUTRITION** | | | |
| Home Parenteral Nutrition Program | Konstantinides[98] | Patient teaching flow sheet; no formal evaluation methods presented | • Cost estimated between $55,000 and $70,000 for nutritional solutions, supplies, home visits, clinic follow-up, and laboratory costs<br>• Guides for patient teaching, discharge planning, laboratory monitoring, and follow-up given |

**TABLE 55-5**   Care Program Evaluation Studies (continued)

| Program | Author | Method | Results |
|---|---|---|---|
| **VI. PROTECTION** | | | |
| Protocol for Venous Access Port | Long and Ovaska[103] | $N$ = 26 outpatients with venous access devices randomly assigned to sterile (12) or clean (14) group; sterile group used commercially prepared kit; compared occurrence of infection assessed by increase in WBC, febrile episode (>100.4), drainage, pain, redness, swelling, warmth at port site | • After 6 months, no documented infection in either group<br>• Institution changed to nursing protocol based on its cost-effectiveness |
| **VII. GENERAL FOCUS** | | | |
| Day Hospital for Cancer Patients | Clark[99] | Economic feasibility measures | • One-year pilot project<br>• Ongoing as of publication |
| Home Care Transfusion Program | Pluth[100] | Cost comparisons with patients receiving transfusions in different settings; client satisfaction; difficulties in implementation | • Cost-effective and beneficial to patients' quality of life |

year period suggests the beginning establishment of a clinical scientific base for practice. Clearly, much more research is needed in all standards-of-practice domains. Research that replicates or builds on the work of others and that refines established interventions may be the most economic ventures. However, to address meaningfully the issue of quality of care, longitudinal studies expanding the clinical database and testing effects of nursing intervention over time are critically needed. The oncology nursing research program, to have an impact on quality of care, will need not only to continue building the growing knowledge base in symptom management and patient education but also to turn attention to the issues of quality of life, recovery, transition, and the effect of a host of new modalities on patients' lives and health.

## Measurement tool development: Quantitative

As psychometric theory advances and the results of nursing research build over time, better methods for measuring quality of care will emerge. Hartshorn,[105] Duffy,[106] and Lynn[107] emphasize the importance of using reliable and valid instruments in clinical research. Duffy said that research-based practice should be precise enough to be replicable and to produce predictable patient outcomes. Hartshorn warned that results from studies employing poor instruments cannot be accepted or implemented. Indeed, many nursing studies that have required considerable time and effort conclude with a long list of limitations to the generalizability of their findings and with an underdeveloped interpretation of important data because of faulty design, inadequate sampling technique, and use of untested measurement tools.

The basic ingredients of sound quantitative measurement techniques include adequate reliability and validity of the instrument. Reliability tests both the stability (test-retest correlations) and the internal consistency (intercorrelations among items or alpha coefficient) of an instrument. Correlations of at least .8 in internal consistency and test-retest correlations ensure that the instrument is reliably measuring the construct it purports to measure and is stable in its ability to reproduce results in repeated testing of the sample. A third type of reliability, interrater reliability, is also important to ensure that all persons using a set of evaluation criteria have closely correlated results.[108]

Validity testing offers a way to assess the ability of the instrument to measure the construct of interest accurately and objectively. The three most important types of validity include construct, content, and criterion related (predictive or concurrent).[105,108] One of the most definitive signs of increasingly improved and sophisticated cancer nursing research is growing evidence that reliable and valid instruments were used.

Table 55-6 provides a partial list of cancer nursing measurement tools* grouped by functional category, including the construct measured and whether evidence of reliability and validity testing are given.[109–110] Note that most of these instruments quantify patient attributes. The

---

*For a current, inclusive discussion of clinical research tools in nursing, consult Frank-Stromberg's *Instruments for Clinical Nursing Research.*[111]

**TABLE 55-6** Tools to Measure Patient Outcomes

| Tool | Author | Construct | Findings | Implications |
|---|---|---|---|---|
| BMT Outpatient Nursing Treatment Record | Burns and Tierney[109] | Documentation method to enhance efficient and accurate communication in complex patient care environment | Reduction in written documentation time and verbal reports with easier assessment tracking | Staff satisfaction increased |
| Patient Assessment Record (PAR) | Allaster et al[110] | Nursing/toxicity assessment form for clinical trials | Form minimizes recording repetition while maintaining quality of toxicity data | Effective in enhancing toxicity documentation |
| Quality of Life Index (QLI) | Ferrans and Powers[112] | Quality of life | Likert scales (2) to determine importance and satisfaction in 18 life areas: life goals, general satisfaction, stress, physical health; reliability established; validity established; versions for normal, healthy adults and for kidney transplant, heart transplant, kidney dialysis, and cancer patients | Establishing norms in different populations |
| Cancer Malaise Scale | Kobashi-Schoot et al[113] | Physical fatigue, mental fatigue, malaise, psychological complaints in radiotherapy cancer patients; validity established | Malaise increased during course of treatment; physical symptoms increased late in course of treatment; malaise correlates with "feeling ill" or "not well" | Further correlation stratified by treatment level of radiation exposure |
| Quality of Life Index (QLI) | Padilla and Grant[114] | Linear analogue: psychological well-being, physical well-being, symptom control; 14 items; reliability established; validity established | | Further testing in variety of subject populations; use to test intervention effectiveness |
| Information Preference Questionnaire (IPQ) | Hopkins[115] | Information seeking; 5-point scale measuring preference for treatment information | Information seeking negatively related to age and severity of disease; reliability established; validity established | Needs additional testing to establish criterion and construct validities |
| Emetic Process Rating Scale (EPRS) | Scott et al[64] | Analogue scale: nausea, retching, vomiting, intake, output, vital signs, treatment; validity established | Evaluated antiemetic effect of clinical relaxation vs. drug intervention; scale found clinically useful | Further reliability and validity testing |
| Sexual Adjustment Questionnaire (SAQ) | Waterhouse and Metcalf[116] | Desire, activity level, relationship, arousal, techniques, orgasm | Persons with cancer significantly reduced scores on activity level, relationships, and techniques | Continued refinement and larger sample testing |
| Derdiarian Informational Needs Assessment (DINA) | Derdiarian[117] | Informational needs related to disease: personal, family, and social parameters | | Further instrument assessment and use in patient referral and follow-up |
| Patient Care Needs Survey | Fleming et al[118] | Comfort needs in advanced cancer patients: physiological, spiritual, psychosocial, patients' rights, dignity, self-worth | Identified 7 themes of comfort; decreased with severity of illness; calls for social support approach, including multidisciplinary | Further development and testing |
| Human Needs Assessment Scale | Lilley[119] | Likert scale of 35 human needs based on work by Yura and Walsh; modified to a 4-point scale; reliability established; evaluates importance of need | Instrument easy to use; nurses perceived patients' human needs similarly to patients' own assessment | Suggest development of nursing diagnosis and evaluation of nursing care to be based on this Human Need Model |

**TABLE 55-6**  Tools to Measure Patient Outcomes (continued)

| Tool | Author | Construct | Findings | Implications |
|---|---|---|---|---|
| Quality of Life Questionnaire (QLQ) | Young-Graham and Longman[120] | Likert-type brief scale: social dependency, symptom distress, behavior-morale, direction of life change; reliability established | Pilot study of patients with melanoma to test model of major hypothesized factors in quality of life | Further use in other populations; internal consistency confirmed |
| Derogatis Sexual Functioning Inventory (DSFI) (modified) | Blackmore[120] | Affect, body image, symptoms, drive, satisfaction, activity | Reduction in sexual activity postoperatively in orchidectomy cancer group | More research on sexuality of cancer patients |
| McGill Pain Questionnaire | Camp[122] | Location, quality, pattern, increase, intensity, verbal-nonverbal symptoms; reliability established; validity established | Compared patient perceptions and nurse documentation; less than 50% of patients' pain perceptions were documented | Replication and assessment of pain management protocols |
| Hypercalcemia Knowledge Questionnaire (HKQ) | Coward[123] | Hypercalcemia risk factors and knowledge | | Need for educational program to evaluate |
| Derdiarian Behavioral System Model | Derdiarian[124] | Achievement, affiliation, aggressive-protective, dependence, elimination, ingestion, restoration, sexuality; based on Johnson Behavioral Symptom Model; reliability established; validity established | Defines imbalance in behavioral subsystems caused by illness; predicts direction and quality of change; sensitive to age, site of cancer, and stage of cancer | Further studies in larger samples |
| Oral Assessment Guide | Eilers et al[125] | Stomatitis or oral mucositis and mucosal changes in radiotherapy and chemotherapy patients: voice, swallow, lips, tongue, saliva, mucous membranes, gingivae, teeth, and dentures | Clinical guide to evaluate oral care protocols and toxic effects of treatment protocols and persons at risk | Further clinical use |
| Breast Self-Examination (BSE) Belief and Attitude Questionnaire | Lauver[126] | Remembering, competence, comfort, interference, efficacy; reliability established | Positive relationship between frequency of BSE and competence, remembering, and comfort | Replication in larger, heterogeneous population with test-retrest reliability; further testing for methods to promote competence and remembering |
| Pain Assessment Tool (PAT) and Pain Flow Sheet (PFS) | McMillan et al[127] | Ongoing assessment of pain and its management | Pain intensity and level of sedation documented in 2-group study | Further research with both tools |
| Self-care and Symptom Report Interview | Rhodes et al[128] | Symptom distress, self-care activities, coping strategies regarding fatigue and weakness; based on Orem's self-care deficit theory | Lays foundation for tool to measure symptom occurrence and distress and to assess self-care efficacy | Ongoing development and testing |
| Linear Analogue Modification (LAM) of Profile of Mood States (POMS) | Sutherland et al[129] | Emotional distress; fatigue, anxiety, confusion, depression, energy, anger | Significant correlation between LAM and POMS in 29 subjects | To evaluate patients' ongoing emotional status as base for psychosocial interventions over time |
| Cancer Knowledge Test | Weinrich and Weinrich[130] | Belief in cancer myths, recall of American Cancer Society 7 warning signals, recognition of disease symptoms | Overall significant difference in cancer knowledge based on race, education, and income | Evaluation of health teaching on elderly, less educated, and low-income black persons |
| Champion's Instrument and Williams's Breast Inventory | Williams[131] | Likert scale of 5 constructs of Health Belief Model, health history, and personal knowledge | Health motivation represents 18% of variance; barriers, 8%; age differences | Further testing of variables |

aim is to establish further a normative database or to measure the qualitative outcomes of nursing practice, or both.

## Measurement tool development: Qualitative

During the past ten years, an increasing interest in qualitative methods of research has become evident in the nursing literature. Measuring quality of care quantitatively does not readily capture the contextual nature and natural richness of the situational and interpersonal data that compose the nursing care environment.

Nursing literature generally reflects attempts at establishing patient databases composed of qualitative sets of indicators, predictors, and assessment parameters that form the etiologic foundations of patient concerns and nursing practices. For example, if we review the available quantitative tools, most are based on the identification of indicators grouped to facilitate diagnostic reasoning. However, less precision is found in scoring instrument results. Few scoring systems are based on large amounts of normative data, particularly those established in healthy populations that allow clear comparisons and interpretation of new data.

The most recognized qualitative approaches include case study, grounded theory, phenomenology, and ethnography, among others (Ammon-Gaberson and Piantanida).[132] Qualitative research begins with carefully conceptualized and clearly articulated research questions to guide data collection and later interpretation. The motive is to understand an aspect of human experience and to shape a representation of it from the data. The results of the qualitative method may include (1) operationalizing a single concept, (2) developing a conceptual framework, (3) establishing guidelines for practice, (4) creating portraits, paradigm cases, or typologies, and (5) forming theory.

Although reliability testing and validity testing in the conventional sense do not have a place in the qualitative process, there are sound principles and methods to guide study design, data gathering, data analysis and management, data interpretation, and paradigm construction. These processes are no less rigorous than those of the quantitative approach. In many areas of quality-of-care research, the qualitative paradigm or a combination of the qualitative and quantitative paradigms may be the best approach.

The qualitative cancer nursing research literature represents a mixed bag of clinically relevant information that, for the purposes of a quality-of-care discussion, may be categorized according to format and content considerations. The research articles have been grouped as either indicators, predictors, or guidelines for care.

*Indicators* are sets of variables that describe empirically an important clinical manifestation. These sets are derived generally from a review of published work on the subject or a descriptive exploratory or qualitative study, or both. For example, Saunders and Valente's article[133] on suicide in cancer patients brings together their wealth

of empirical knowledge as well as general information about depression and suicide. One outcome is a useful "Brief Suicide Assessment Guide" for practitioners. In contrast, Thorne[134] reported the results of her phenomenological study of the family cancer experience, providing important insights into family perceptions and coping strategies when a member has cancer. Therefore, information in a wide variety of content areas produced sets of clues to facilitate better understanding of many common clinical issues.

*Predictors* are variables that have been tested to determine their ability to predict a future event with some degree of accuracy. Predictors are critical to nursing's role in health promotion and prevention. For example, Hays's article[135] on predictors of hospice utilization identified specific patient and family parameters that, when taken into consideration early enough in the nursing plan of care, have a good chance of strengthening the family unit so that the patient can be maintained at home under quality care conditions for longer periods. Another illustration of the establishment of predictors is the research that has identified clusters of variables predicting the occurrence of anticipatory nausea and vomiting.[136,137]

*Guidelines for care* are organized, integrated schemata for practice. These presentations are readily identifiable by title descriptors such as nursing care, nursing interventions, nursing implications, the nursing role, nursing assessments, nursing management, and nursing plans for a variety of patient problems, specialized treatments, or situations. In most cases, guidelines are in tabular format, resembling the traditional nursing care plan (problem, care, scientific rationale) with updated language such as nursing diagnoses, nursing etiology, nursing interventions, and nursing evaluations by outcome criteria.

Table 55-7 provides a list of indicators, predictors, and assessment guidelines used in recent studies addressing quality of care.[128,133–290] These articles report studies of cancer-related disease and treatment problems, psychosocial adjustment, risk factors, and family response and coping.

## QUALITY IN PERFORMANCE: APPLICATIONS IN PRACTICE

No discussion of care is complete without a look at process—the performance of nursing care and its meaning for both patient and nurse. Although patient outcome has become the basis for care evaluation, the multiple forces impinging on a patient's condition often make this method partially precise at best. Outcomes are relative, and frequently are only partly related to the quality of nurse performance. More often, quality is deeply embedded in the rich mutual interpretations of care and caring that constitute the nurse-patient bond. Measuring quality of care by documented patient outcome is only one aspect

**TABLE 55-7**  Indicators, Predictors, and Guidelines for Quality of Care

## Indicators

Adaptive strategies with cancer diagnosis[138]
Adjustment of children to mother's breast cancer[139]
Adolescent coping after cancer therapy[140]
Beliefs about breast cancer and mammography[141]
Brain tumor support group content and support[142]
Cancer fatigue[143]
Chemotherapy thoughts and images[144]
Children living with cancer[145]
Coagulation values in central venous catheters[146]
Cognitive dysfunction in BRMT[147]
Cognitive/emotional disruption in breast cancer patients after RT[148]
Expectations regarding breast cancer care[149]
Information and decisions in breast cancer[150]
Nurses' ethical/moral experiences[151]
Pain with mammography[152]
Quality of life and hospice care[153]
Research-based practices by oncology staff nurses[154]
Risk taking and decisions of adolescent cancer survivors[155]
Self-esteem in women receiving chemotherapy[156]
Sexuality of elders with cancer[157]
Voluntary physician-assisted dying[158]
Wire localizations for nonpalpable breast lesions[159]
Hypnosis for pain management in children[160]
Self-care and chemotherapy side effects[161]
Postchemotherapy quality of life in sarcoma patients[162]
Self-care and symptom distress in HIV seropositive men[163]
Quality of life after BMT[164]
Pain and psychological distress during ABMT[165]
Restrictions and obstacles in home care[166]
Quality of life and care during biological therapy[167]
Pain in children with cancer[168]
Family caregivers' descriptions of patients' pain[169]
Support and caring[170]
Maintaining hope during BMT[171]
Quest for meaning after BMT[172–174]
Treatment effect on male fertility and sexuality[175]
Breast self-examination techniques[176]
Nursing diagnosis in an oncology population[177]
Use of topical anesthetic to reduce pain in pediatric oncology patients[178]
Spiritual health of oncology patients[179]
Patient/significant other's response to detection program[180]
Nurse knowledge/teaching/performance of breast exams[181]
Fever patterns in neutropenic patients[182]
Psychological model of adjustment in gynecologic cancer patients[183]
Family cancer experience[134]
Sexual and reproductive issues for women with Hodgkin's disease[184,185]
Cancer-induced hypercalcemia[186]
Primary caregiver's perception of the dying trajectory[187]
Alterations in taste during cancer treatment[188]
Family responses to cancer hospitalization[189]
Characteristics of pain in hospitalized cancer patients[190]
Sexual changes after gynecologic cancer treatment[191]
Cisplatin-related peripheral neuropathy[192]
Weakness, fatigue, and self-care abilities[128]
Suicide in cancer patients[133]
Cancer pain control behavior[193]

## Predictors

Attribution, control, and adjustment[194]
Constipation and opioids[195]

Delayed complications of BMT[196]
Discard volumes from heparinized Hickman catheters[197]
Family experience in breast cancer[198]
Family caregiver needs in home hospice[199]
Laminar air flow vs. reverse isolation in BMT[200]
Lung cancer experience[201]
Nurses' cancer pain management[202]
Obstacles to cancer care in disadvantaged[203]
Oral gram-negative bacilli in BMT[204]
Patient/nurse perceptions of BMT symptomology[205]
Precancerous and cancerous cervical lesions[206]
PTSD in pediatric bone marrow recipients[207]
Side effects and self-care in patient chemotherapy[208]
Stress and development of breast cancer[209]
Strontium-89 treatment for prostate cancer[210]
Informational needs of patients receiving brachytherapy[211]
Impact of cancer pain on family caregivers[212]
Burdens of family members caring for chemotherapy patients[213]
Effect of granulocyte colony-stimulating factor on quality of life[214]
Biopsychosocial effects of interleukin-2[215]
Breast cancer detection behavior[216]
Amphotericin B–induced rigors[217]
Aerobic exercise and quality of life in women with breast cancer[218]
Life satisfaction and illness distress[219]
Protein deficiency, pressure sores, and cancer mortality[220]
Needs of home caregivers[221]
Fatigue mechanisms: tumor necrosis factor and exercise[222]
Sources of hope in chronic illness[223]
ARDS during interleukin-2 immunotherapy[224]
Precursors of cervical cancer[225]
Flushing protocols for central venous catheters[226]
Information seeking in HIV-positive homosexual/bisexual men[227]
Factors influencing successful return to workplace for cancer patients[228]
Effect of alkylating agent in acute nonlymphocytic leukemia[229]
Patterns of lung cancer dyspnea[230]
Anticipatory nausea and vomiting associated with cancer chemotherapy[136]
Patterns of hospice utilization[135]
Radiotherapy symptom profile[231]
Carotid artery rupture[232]
Colorectal cancer[233]
Glucocorticosteroid-induced depression[234]
Needs of family members of cancer patients[235]
Anticipatory nausea and vomiting[137]
Patterns of nausea, vomiting, and distress with antineoplastic drug protocols[236]

## Guidelines for Care

Acute myelogenous leukemia[237]
Acute tumor lysis syndrome[238]
Bacterial translocation with neutropenia[239]
Behavioral interventions in leukemia[240]
Bladder cancer[241]
Chronic myelogenous leukemia and acute promyelocytic leukemia[242]
Comforting children during RT[243]
Glial neoplasms[244]
Inpatient education and support programs[245]
Intravenous immunoglobulin[246]
Lambert-Eaton myasthenic syndrome[247]
Leukemia[248]
Patient involvement in treatment[249]
Producing videotapes for cancer education[250]
Social support and BSE[251]

*(continued)*

**TABLE 55-7**　Indicators, Predictors, and Guidelines for Quality of Care (continued)

| | |
|---|---|
| Strategies to improve cancer education[252] | Home care resources for rural families[273] |
| Testicular cancer[253] | Nursing of patient receiving antimitotics in chemotherapy[274] |
| Thyroid cancer[254] | Bereavement care[275] |
| Vena cava filters[255] | Handling of antineoplastic drugs[276] |
| VIPoma[256] | Prevention of chemotherapy-associated pneumonia in non-Hodgkin's lymphoma[277] |
| Nursing implications for photodynamic therapy[257] | |
| Care of patients with esophageal cancer[258] | Primary, secondary, and tertiary interventions for lymphedema[278] |
| Nursing of patients with multisystem organ failure[259] | Management of disseminated intravascular coagulation[279] |
| Care of families[260] | Care of patients treated with intrapleural tetracycline for malignant pleural effusion[280] |
| Nursing care of irradiated skin[261] | |
| Neurological assessment of cerebral edema[262] | The compromised host[281] |
| Spinal cord compression surgical care[263] | Management of venous access ports[282] |
| Care of patient with malignant ascites[264] | Morphine infusion for intractable cancer pain by implanted pump[283] |
| Care of patient with occult primary malignancy[265] | |
| Care of patient with Von Hippel–Lindau disease[266] | Care of head and neck cancer patients receiving myocutaneous flap reconstructive surgery[284] |
| Nursing management of cancer recurrence[267] | |
| Documentation of chemotherapy administration and patient teaching[268] | Care of patients receiving radiation therapy for rectal cancer[285] |
| | Care of patients receiving third-generation cephalosporins[286] |
| Chemotherapy flow sheet[269] | Assessment of gynecology patients[287] |
| Management of hypomagnesemia[270] | Needs of the spouse of the patient with advanced cancer[288] |
| Nursing during high-dose-rate brachytherapy[271] | Care of the family with cancer[289] |
| Diversion activity to enhance coping[272] | Skin care during radiotherapy[290] |

of the multipronged approach demanded, an important indication that evaluation must go beyond the standard.

Determining the quality of a process is tricky, and yet critical to the search for excellence. There are four important patterns to the process of giving and receiving care. The first is *mutuality*. Care behavior and the caring attitude forge a mutuality of response between two people that is characterized by reciprocity and complementarity. The experience is shared and cooperative, and the roles of caregiver and care receiver are complementary in that there is a degree of dissimilarity in the nature of the role relationship that works in a nondissonant way, allowing for harmony. However, the degree of dissimilarity is important in that the effect of care can be compromised if patient-nurse perceptions are either too much alike or radically different.

The nature of the mutual experience of caregiver and care receiver and their interacting perceptions are central to the quality of care. A growing literature focused on the congruity of nurse and patient perceptions reflects this phenomenon. In an early study by Jennings and Muhlenkamp,[291] caregivers' perceptions of their patients' affective states and the patients' self-reports of their anxiety, hostility, and depression were significantly different. Caregivers (i.e., physicians, nurses, nursing assistants) assessed patients as feeling significantly worse than patients reported feeling. Findings were interpreted in light of "Wright's requirement-of-mourning hypothesis" that caregivers may perceive patients as having negative feelings so that the caregivers' own value systems, which place emphasis on health, will be supported.[292]

In 1987 Verron et al[293] hypothesized that attitudes of health care providers, grounded in their values, influence the quality of patient care. The authors cited work linking learning, experience, and consequent changes in attitude with positively modified behavior that endured for long periods.[294] Further, they attempted to identify and measure attitude themes pertinent to caring for oncology patients. The Ideas About Oncology Patient Care Scale (IAOPC) resulted, generating four attitude-related factors: therapy, future outlook, terminality, and drug use. Through repeated instrument testing, the attitudes were found to be multidimensional, another indication of the complexities of measuring human responses to caregiving and care receiving.

Larson[3,295,296] laid a foundation for unraveling the intricacies involved in giving and receiving care. She interviewed two separate samples of patients and nurses to determine what nurse behaviors were most and least important in making cancer patients feel "cared for." Her assumption was that the optimal expectation of nursing care is for patients to feel cared for as a result of nursing actions. Feeling cared for was defined as a sensation of well-being and safety linked to the behavior of the nurse. Nurses and patients were asked to rank, in order of importance, 50 nurse caring behaviors categorized by six action themes: anticipation, accessibility, explanation-facilitation, provision of comfort, establishment of trust, and monitoring with follow-through. Findings revealed that patients and nurses held highly divergent opinions of what was most important. The highest-ranked behaviors reported by patients were those demonstrating competency, actions mostly concerned with monitoring and follow-through and with accessibility. Actions rated highest by nurses were more focused on meeting comfort and psychosocial needs, such as listening and touch. In an examination of the top ten responses of both groups, however, several mutual choices appeared: being quickly accessible, giving good physical care, putting the patient first, and listening. These choices indicated several important shared values.

Mayer[297] replicated Larson's study and found similar results. There was 100% agreement between samples of nurses in both studies regarding the most and least important caring behaviors. Comparisons of the two patient groups revealed 40% agreement for the most important behaviors and 80% for the least important. Across both studies and all samples, conventions of professional etiquette, such as appearance, cheerfulness, and polite social behavior, were viewed as least important. In Mayer's study, listening was again rated highest by nurses, and knowing how to give injections and intravenous infusions, and managing technical equipment remained most important to patients. Mayer concluded that patients seem to value the instrumental, technical caring skills and that nurses are more attuned to expressive caring behaviors.

These results might reflect understandable differences in perception between the two groups. Patients seemed to value those competencies and skills most concretely apparent and directly linked to their welfare. Nurses, on the other hand, may have perceived expressive and instrumental dimensions of care as inextricably connected, similar to the mutuality of care and cure. Who can deny the effect when patient preparation, technical skill, and gentleness are integrated during administration of an uncomfortable, intrusive procedure? To emphasize one aspect without the others decontextualizes care and strips it of its healing quality.

Several other comparison reports have documented discrepancies between patients' self-reports and their nurses' knowledge and understanding of patients' needs. Sodestrom and Martinson[298] found that 76% of a sample of nurses caring for hospitalized terminally ill patients considered spiritual needs low on the list of priorities because of the lack of time to incorporate spiritual assessment into care. Although the nurses correctly identified the meaning and purpose of their patient's relationship with God and the patient-nurse definitions of the term *spiritual* did not differ significantly, the nurses in this study did not view themselves as essential in meeting the spiritual needs of their terminally ill patients.

As the location of cancer care increasingly moves into the home, the concept of caregiver expands to include family members and others in charge of the patient's welfare. In light of this trend, congruence between caregiver and care recipient perceptions of quality of life was examined in 23 care dyads in a home hospice program.[299] The overall trend, although not statistically significant, was for patients to report a higher quality of life for themselves in comparison with their caregivers' assessments. Patients reported better sleeping and pain control than did caregivers, but much less fun and sexual satisfaction. Thus nurse caregivers are not alone in their struggle to interpret the patient's situation accurately.

The needs of family members as they care for their loved ones with cancer are emerging as an important dimension in quality of care. Dyck and Wright[300] found that almost half of their sample of next of kin said that nurses did not do anything for them as family members, nor did they expect anything. Their expectation, however, seemed to be a function of limitations in their knowledge of the role of the nurse and what was thought to be the appropriate focus—the patient. If the patient was competently cared for and the nurse kept the family accurately informed, families said they could not expect more. Yet a parallel analysis of their needs documented acceptance, support, and comfort as being very important to them. Furthermore, their rank-order of traits looked for in nurses differed depending on the stage of the patient's illness. Competence was number one in the early diagnostic stage, friendliness when the disease recurred, and compassion during the terminal stage. The authors concluded that appropriate emphasis of a trait is contextually determined and a significant way that nurses may express "caring for" patients.

The second major pattern in the caregiving and care-receiving process is *contextuality*. The contextual aspects of care have been highlighted repeatedly in these studies, with location of care and phase of illness emerging as two important determinants of the most appropriate clinical approach. Often, phenomenological studies provide the best look at contextuality.

For example, Thorne,[134] in studying helpful and unhelpful communications in care, refers to cancer as "a modern metaphor for human confrontation with existential uncertainty." She found that communication is important in shaping the illness experience. Patients in Thorne's study were able to recall communication with health care providers during their illness and distinguish between styles that were more and less helpful. She found that the more uncertain a patient's situation, the greater was the vulnerability to communication characterized by lack of concern. On the other hand, the providers' feelings of failure, vulnerability, and hopelessness were part of the total picture as well. Nurses did not figure prominently into this compilation of opinions about helpful and unhelpful communicators, although study subjects reported that physicians communicated more about the disease and illness and nurses provided advice about treatment and the illness. More often, a communication was perceived to be helpful if it was thought to be intentionally supportive. The most frequent unhelpful type was described as advice that was intentionally unhelpful, when the person withheld information or abused his power. Moreover, most important to the caring process was content, style, and a manner perceived by the patient as intentionally designed to be useful, encouraging, and supportive.

As a unit, these studies highlight the importance of mutuality and contextuality in determining the quality of nursing care performance. Yet two other patterns have emerged as major influences on quality of performance; these patterns are so mutually dependent that they must be considered as one: *competence and proficiency*.

Benner[301,302] says that the practical knowledge embedded in expert nursing needs to be understood and yet has not been fully elucidated. Since clinical practice involves constant interpretation and prediction based on complex, contextual information, expertise increases as the nurse becomes intuitively able to read the situation as a whole as a result of past experience. The experience of the nurse is central to proficiency, which Benner views as having five levels: novice, advanced beginner, competent nurse, proficient nurse, and expert. Experience is the vehicle by which the nurse passes through these phases.

Progress in the movement from novice to expert is reflected by three gradual changes in performance. Initially, rather than relying solely on abstract principles and procedures to guide nursing practice, the nurse acquires a personal knowledge rich in "paradigms" of various care issues. The paradigms emerge from past experience that not only challenges previously held perceptions but is powerful enough to change and refine those preconceptions and understandings. Later, as the nurse gains experience, situations are viewed holistically, with the nurse focusing only on the most relevant elements and having a deep sense of confidence in intuitive interpretations. Finally, there is full involvement in the situation as a confident, effective performer.

The fourth major pattern of the care process is *intentionality of caring*. Intentionality of caring represents the connecting pattern or matrix holding together mutuality, contextuality, and competence with proficiency. Intentionality of caring requires awareness and a determined effort to provide quality care in any setting or to facilitate others as they provide care for cancer patients. Intentionality of caring serves to enhance quality in practice by the following:

- recognizing that care is mutual—a cooperative venture between two human beings, based on a balanced complement of perceptions

- considering the context of the care environment on the basis of an understanding of the shared meaning of the circumstances

- encouraging pride in one's acquired competencies (knowledge, skills, attitudes, and traits) and having a desire to increase proficiency and become expert

Overall, intentionality of caring links the science and the art of nursing knowledge and skill. Its most overt manifestation in practice is known as *clinical judgment*.

## CONCLUSION

Every health care provider group today is struggling with the definition, provision, and evaluation of quality care. Nursing comes to the task from a long tradition of empirically established caring skills and a more recent scientific knowledge based on clinical research.

For two decades, experts in the quality assurance field have advocated a three-dimensional approach to the quality question based on structure, process, and outcome variables and their relatedness (see Figure 55-1). Structural elements are those grounding fundamentals that provide a sense of shared purpose and criteria against which effect can be measured. The structural elements include nursing's direction, definition, education, legislation, diagnostic taxonomy, standards of practice, research and technology, and programs of peer review and quality assurance.

Process is a much more elusive phenomenon in that it represents the individualized enactment of competencies characterized by knowledge, skills, human traits, and attitudes[49] under diverse and unique environmental conditions (contextuality) where the mutuality of caregiver and care receiver is central. Process is most manifest in the intentionality of caring of the care provider and in the proficiency with which competencies are revealed. Therefore, process is much more difficult to evaluate in comparison with the components of structure and outcome.

Oncology nursing has come closest to evaluating the process dimension by defining standards of performance that recognize several critical determinants of quality: continuously working to perfect the art, science, and skill of practice; participating as a contributing, valued member of the health care team; utilizing the problem-solving process in the planning, organization, and execution of care and in its evaluation through the conduct or utilization of research; and providing a health care service to patients on the basis of a host of both independent and interdependent interventions conducted in an autonomous way. The measurement of process is based generally on written documentation and periodic peer evaluation. Some attempts have been made to categorize[301] and to measure[48] proficiency, and the literature on caring as a science is expanding rapidly.

Outcome criteria have been defined in terms of patient outcomes, quality of life, and, for nursing to some degree, maximum life extension. These criteria are best represented by patient outcome standards and by a burgeoning literature focused on the quality of life of the individual with cancer and his or her family. As we gain knowledge about the quality of life, the purpose of nursing as a science of caring will more clearly be understood, and will further enable us to foster, nurture, and strengthen its quality.

## REFERENCES

1. Nightingale F: *Notes on Nursing.* New York, Appleton-Century-Crofts, 1859
2. Benner P: Nursing as a caring profession. Working paper for the Academy of Nursing Annual Meeting, Kansas City, MO, October 16–18, 1988
3. Larson P: Cancer nurses' perceptions of caring. *Cancer Nurs* 9:86–92, 1986

4. Gaut DA: A philosophic orientation to caring, in Leininger MM (ed): *Care: The Essence of Nursing and Health.* Thorofare, NJ, Slack, 1984, pp 17–26

5. Leininger MM (ed): *Care: The Essence of Nursing.* Thorofare, NJ, Slack, 1984

6. Watson J: *Nursing: The Philosophy and Science of Caring.* Boston, Little, Brown, 1979

7. Dougherty CJ: *American Health Care: Realities, Rights, and Reforms.* New York, Oxford University Press, 1988

8. President's Commission for the Study of Ethical Problems in Medicine and Biomedical and Behavioral Research: *Securing Access to Health Care,* vol. 1. Washington, DC, U.S. Government Printing Office, 1983

9. Oncology Nursing Society: Board approves revised scope of practice statement. *ONS News* 3:1–2, 1988

10. Taylor C: *Philosophic Papers,* vols. 1 and 2. Cambridge, Cambridge University Press, 1985

11. Harmer C, Henderson V: *Principles and Practices of Nursing.* New York, Macmillan, 1956

12. Mundinger L: Nursing diagnoses for cancer patients. *Cancer Nurs* 1:221–226, 1978

13. Herberth L, Gosnell DJ: Nursing diagnosis for oncology nursing practice. *Cancer Nurs* 10:41–51, 1987

14. Gordon M: *Nursing Diagnoses: Process and Application.* New York, McGraw-Hill, 1982

15. American Nurses' Association: *Nursing: A Social Policy Statement.* Kansas City, MO, The Association, 1980

16. Beyers M: Quality: The banner of the 1980s. *Nurs Clin North Am* 23:617–623, 1988

17. Winchester DP: The assurance of quality for the cancer patient. Paper presented at the American Cancer Society Symposium on Advances in Cancer Management, Los Angeles, December 1988

18. Garven DA: *Managing Quality: The Strategic and Competitive Edge.* New York, Free Press, 1988

19. National Cancer Institute: Five-year survival rates. *SEER Program.* Washington, DC, U.S. Government Printing Office, 1983

20. Henderson M: Introduction, in Roberts L (ed): *Cancer Today: Origins, Prevention, and Treatment.* Washington, DC, National Academy of Sciences Press, 1984

21. Oncology Nursing Society: *Outcome Standards for Cancer Nursing Practice.* Pittsburgh, The Society, 1979

22. Oncology Nursing Society and American Nurses' Association: *Standards of Oncology Nursing Practice.* Kansas City, MO, The Association, 1987

23. American Nurses' Association: *A Plan for Implementation of Standards of Nursing Practice.* Kansas City, MO, The Association, 1979

24. Oncology Nursing Society: *Outcome Standards for Cancer Nursing Education.* Pittsburgh, The Society, 1982

25. Oncology Nursing Society: *Cancer Patient Education.* Pittsburgh, The Society, 1982

26. Oncology Nursing Society: *Public Cancer Education.* Pittsburgh, The Society, 1983

27. Orem DE: *Nursing Concepts of Practice.* New York, McGraw-Hill, 1987

28. Johnson DE: The behavioral system model for nursing, in Riehl JP, Roy C (eds): *Conceptual Model for Nursing Practice* (ed 2). New York, Appleton-Century-Crofts, 1980

29. Donabedian A: Structure, process and outcome standards. *Am J Public Health* 59:1833, 1969

30. Majesky SJ, Brester MH, Nishio KT: Development of a research tool: Patient indicators of nursing care. *Nurs Res* 27:365–371, 1978

31. Scott DW: *The Research Connection: Practice, Research, Theory.* Keynote Address: American Cancer Society Nursing Research Conference, Honolulu, Hawaii, June 1985 Proceedings. Denver, American Cancer Society, 1986

32. Brown MH, Kiss ME: Cancer audit. *Cancer Nurs* 2:1–6, 1979

33. Legge JS, Reilly BJ: Assessing the outcomes of cancer patients in a home nursing program. *Cancer Nurs* 3:357, 1980

34. Valencius JC, Packard R, Widiss T: The ONS-ANA Outcome Standards for Cancer Nursing Practice: Two models for implementation—Implementation of the Nutrition Standard at City of Hope National Medical Center. *Oncol Nurs Forum* 7:137–140, 1980

35. Edlund BJ: Patient education: Determining the effectiveness of an ostomy care guide in facilitating comprehensive patient care. *Oncol Nurs Forum* 8:43–46, 1981

36. Wood HA, Ellerhorst JM: Using site-specific nursing algorithms as an adjunct to oncology nursing guidelines. *Oncol Nurs Forum* 10:22–27, 1983

37. Joint Commission on the Accreditation of Hospitals: *Accreditation Manual for Hospitals* (AMH/88). Chicago, The Commission, 1987

38. Patterson CH: Standards of patient care: The Joint Commission focus on nursing quality assurance. *Nurs Clin North Am* 23:625–638, 1988

39. Oleske DM, Otte DM, Heinze S: Development and evaluation of a system for monitoring the quality of oncology nursing care in the home setting. *Cancer Nurs* 10:190–198, 1987

40. Stephany TM: Quality assurance for hospice programs. *Oncol Nurs Forum* 12:33–40, 1985

41. Arenth LM: The development and validation of an Oncology Patient Classification System. *Oncol Nurs Forum* 12:17–27, 1985

42. Dudjak LA: Radiation Therapy Nursing Care Record: A tool for documentation. *Oncol Nurs Forum* 15:763–777, 1988

43. Gullo SM: Safe handling of antineoplastic drugs: Translating the recommendations into practice. *Oncol Nurs Forum* 15:595–601, 1988

44. Williamson KM, Selleck CS, Turner JC, et al: Occupational health hazards for nurses: Infection. *Image* 20:48–53, 1988

45. Williamson KM, Turner JC, Brown KC, et al: Occupational health hazards for nurses: Part II. *Image* 20:162–168, 1988

46. Miaskowski CA, Nielsen B: A cancer nursing assessment tool. *Oncol Nurs Forum* 12:37–42, 1985

47. Gray G, Adler D, Fleming C, et al: A clinical data base for advanced cancer patients: Implications for nursing. *Cancer Nurs* 11:77–83, 1988

48. Moore IM, Piper B, Dodd MJ, et al: Measuring oncology nursing practice: Results from one graduate program. *Oncol Nurs Forum* 14:45–49, 1987

49. McGee RF, Powell ML, Broadwell DC, et al: A Delphi survey of oncology nurse specialist competencies. *Oncol Nurs Forum* 14:29–34, 1987

50. Yasko JM: A survey of oncology clinical nursing specialists. *Oncol Nurs Forum* 10:25–30, 1983

51. Oberst MT: Priorities in cancer nursing research. *Cancer Nurs* 1:281–290, 1978

52. Western Consortium for Cancer Nursing Research: Priorities for cancer nursing research. *Cancer Nurs* 10:319–326, 1987

53. Satterwhite BA, Pryor AS, Harris MB: Development and evaluation of chemotherapy fact sheets. *Cancer Nurs* 3:277–284, 1980

54. Dodd MJ, Mood DW: Chemotherapy: Helping patients to know the drugs they are receiving and their possible side effects. *Cancer Nurs* 4:311–318, 1981

55. Dodd MJ: Self-care for side effects in cancer chemotherapy: An assessment of nursing interventions. Part II. *Cancer Nurs* 6:63–67, 1983

56. Johnson J: The effects of a patient education course on persons with a chronic illness. *Cancer Nurs* 5:117–123, 1982

57. Miller MW, Nygren C: Living with cancer: Coping behaviors. *Cancer Nurs* 1:297–302, 1978

58. Marty PJ, McDermott RJ, Gold RS: An assessment of three alternative formats for promoting breast self-examination. *Cancer Nurs* 6:207–211, 1983

59. Watson PJ: The effects of short-term postoperative counseling on cancer/ostomy patients. *Cancer Nurs* 6:21–29, 1985

60. Heinrich RL, Schag CC: A behavioral medicine approach to coping with cancer: A case report. *Cancer Nurs* 7:243–247, 1984

61. Rudolf VM, Quinn KL: The practice of TSE among college men: Effectiveness of an educational program. *Oncol Nurs Forum* 15:45–48, 1988

62. Cotanch P, Hockenberry M, Herman S: Self-hypnosis as antiemetic therapy in children receiving chemotherapy. *Oncol Nurs Forum* 12:41–46, 1985

63. Frank JM: The effects of music therapy and guided visual imagery on chemotherapy-induced nausea and vomiting. *Oncol Nurs Forum* 12:47–52, 1985

64. Scott DW, Donahue DC, Mastrovito RC, et al: Comparative trial of clinical relaxation and an antiemetic drug regimen in reducing chemotherapy-related nausea and vomiting. *Cancer Nurs* 9:178–187, 1986

65. Cotanch P, Strum S: Progressive muscle relaxation as antiemetic therapy for cancer patients. *Oncol Nurs Forum* 14:33–37, 1987

66. Parker R: The effectiveness of scalp hypothermia in preventing cyclophosphamide-induced alopecia. *Oncol Nurs Forum* 14:49–53, 1987

67. Dudjak LA: Mouth care for mucositis due to radiation therapy. *Cancer Nurs* 10:131–140, 1987

68. Winningham ML, MacVicar MG: The effect of aerobic exercise on patient reports of nausea. *Oncol Nurs Forum* 15:447–450, 1988

69. Giaccone G, DiGuilio F, Morandini MP, et al: Scalp hypothermia in the prevention of doxorubicin-induced hair loss. *Cancer Nurs* 11:170–173, 1988

70. Shell JA, Stanutz F, Grimm J: Comparison of moisture vapor permeable (MVP) dressings to conventional dressings for management of radiation skin reactions. *Oncol Nurs Forum* 13:11–16, 1986

71. Harwood KVS, Bachur N: Evaluation of dimethylsulfoxide and local cooling as antidotes for doxorubicin extravasation in a pig model. *Oncol Nurs Forum* 14:39–44, 1987

72. Jones PM: Indwelling central venous catheter–related infections and two different procedures of catheter care. *Cancer Nurs* 10:123–130, 1987

73. MacGeorge L, Steeves L, Steeves RH: Comparison of the mixing and reinfusion methods of drawing blood from a Hickman catheter. *Oncol Nurs Forum* 15:335–338, 1988

74. Petrosino B, Becker H, Christian B: Infection rates in central venous catheter dressings. *Oncol Nurs Forum* 15:709–717, 1988

75. Coleman EA, Riley MB, Fields F, et al: Efficacy of breast self-examination teaching methods among older women. *Oncol Nurs Forum* 18:561–566, 1991

76. Hagopian GA: The effects of a weekly radiation therapy newsletter on patients. *Oncol Nurs Forum* 18:1199–1203, 1991

77. Hagopian GA: The effects of informational audiotapes on knowledge and self-care behaviors of patients undergoing radiation therapy. *Oncol Nurs Forum* 23:697–700, 1996

78. Hughes KK: Decision making by patients with breast cancer: The role of information in treatment selection. *Oncol Nurs Forum* 20:623–628, 1993

79. Mansson ME, Bjorkhem G, Wiebe T: The effect of preparation for lumbar puncture on children undergoing chemotherapy. *Oncol Nurs Forum* 20:39–45, 1993

80. Beck SL: The therapeutic use of music for cancer-related pain. *Oncol Nurs Forum* 18:1327–1337, 1991

81. Broome ME, Lillis PP, McGahee TW, et al: The use of distraction and imagery with children during painful procedures. *Oncol Nurs Forum* 19:499–502, 1992

82. Mock V, Burke MB, Sheehan P, et al: A nursing rehabilitation program for women with breast cancer receiving adjuvant chemotherapy. *Oncol Nurs Forum* 21:597–605, 1994

83. Brandt B, DePalma J, Irwin M, et al: Comparison of central venous catheter dressings in bone marrow transplant recipients. *Oncol Nurs Forum* 23:829–836, 1996

84. Dodd MJ, Larson PJ, Dibble SL: Randomized clinical trial of chlorhexidine versus placebo for prevention of oral mucositis in patients receiving chemotherapy. *Oncol Nurs Forum* 23:921–927, 1996

85. Shivnan JC, McGuire D, Freedman S, et al: A comparison of transparent adherent and dry sterile gauze dressings for long-term central catheters in patients undergoing bone marrow transplant. *Oncol Nurs Forum* 18:1349–1356, 1991

86. Yeoman A, Davitt M, Peters CA, et al: Efficacy of chlorhexidene gluconate use in the prevention of perirectal infections in patients with acute leukemia. *Oncol Nurs Forum* 18:1207–1213, 1991

87. Beck S, Breckenridge-Patter S, Wallace S, et al: The Family High-Risk Program: Targeted cancer prevention. *Oncol Nurs Forum* 15:301–306, 1988

88. Nieweg R, Greidanus J, de Vries EGE: A patient education program for a continuous infusion regimen on an outpatient basis. *Cancer Nurs* 10:177–182, 1987

89. Lane CA, Davis AW: Implementation: We Can Week-end in the rural setting. *Cancer Nurs* 8:323–328, 1985

90. Fredette S, La F, Beattie HM: Living with cancer: A patient education program. *Cancer Nurs* 9:308–316, 1986

91. Cawley MM, Gerdts EK: Establishing a cancer caregiver's program: An interdisciplinary approach. *Cancer Nurs* 11:266–273, 1988

92. Diekmann JM: An evaluation of selected "I Can Cope" programs by registered participants. *Cancer Nurs* 11:274–282, 1988

93. Mosely JR, Logan SJ, Tolle SW, et al: Developing a bereavement program in a university hospital setting. *Oncol Nurs Forum* 15:151–155, 1988

94. Coyle N, Monzillo E, Loscalzo M, et al: A model for continuity of care for cancer patients with pain and neurooncologic complications. *Cancer Nurs* 8:111–119, 1985

95. Coyle N, Mauskop A, Maggard J, et al: Continuous SC infusions of opiates for cancer patients with pain. *Oncol Nurs Forum* 13:53–57, 1986

96. Ferrell BR, Wenzl C, Wisdom C: Evolution and evaluation of a pain management team. *Oncol Nurs Forum* 15:285–289, 1988

97. Kane NE, Lehman ME, Drugger R, et al: Use of patient-controlled anesthesia in surgical oncology patients. *Oncol Nurs Forum* 15:29–32, 1988

98. Konstantinides NI: Home parenteral nutrition: A viable alternative for patients with cancer. *Oncol Nurs Forum* 12:23–29, 1985

99. Clark M: A day hospital for cancer patients: Clinical and economic feasibility. *Oncol Nurs Forum* 13:41–45, 1986

100. Pluth NM: A home transfusion program. *Oncol Nurs Forum* 14:43–46, 1987

101. McMillan SC, Title MB, Hill D: A systematic evaluation of the "I Can Cope" program using a national sample. *Oncol Nurs Forum* 20:455–461, 1993

102. Pillon LR, Joannides G: An 11-year evaluation of a Living with Cancer program. *Oncol Nurs Forum* 18:707–711, 1991

103. Long MC, Ovaska M: Comparative study of nursing protocols for venous access ports. *Cancer Nurs* 15:18–21, 1992

104. Lewis PM: Implementing practice and organizational models. *Cancer Nurs* 8:75–78, 1985 (suppl 1)

105. Hartshorn JC: Research-based practice: The need for, use and reporting of instrument reliability and validity. *Heart Lung* 16:100–101, 1987

106. Duffy ME: Research in practice: The time has come. *Nurs Health Care* 6:127, 1985

107. Lynn MR: Reliability estimates: Use and disuse. *Nurs Res* 34:254–256, 1985

108. Nunally JC: *Psychometric Theory*. New York, McGraw-Hill, 1978

109. Burns JM, Tierney DK: A daily flowsheet for an outpatient bone marrow transplant treatment center. *Oncol Nurs Forum* 23:1313–1316, 1996

110. Allaster RM, Frayne BK, Malpage AS, et al: Development of a comprehensive nursing/toxicity assessment form. *Oncol Nurs Forum* 23:1317–1324, 1996

111. Frank-Stromborg M (ed): *Instruments for Clinical Nursing Research* (ed 2). Boston, Jones and Bartlett, 1997

112. Ferrans C, Powers M: Quality of Life Index: Development and psychometric properties. *Adv Nurs Sci* 8:15, 1985

113. Kobashi-Schoot JAM, Gerrit JFPH, Frits SAM, et al: Assessment of malaise in cancer patients treated with radiotherapy. *Cancer Nurs* 8:306–313, 1985

114. Padilla G, Grant M: Quality of life as a cancer nursing outcome variable. *Adv Nurs Sci* 8:45, 1985

115. Hopkins MB: Information seeking and adaptational outcomes in women receiving chemotherapy for breast cancer. *Cancer Nurs* 9:256–262, 1986

116. Waterhouse J, Metcalf MC: Development of the sexual adjustment questionnaire. *Oncol Nurs Forum* 13:53–59, 1986

117. Derdiarian AK: Informational needs of recently diagnosed cancer patients. *Cancer Nurs* 10:156–163, 1987

118. Fleming C, Scanlon C, D'Agostino NS: Patient care needs survey. *Cancer Nurs* 10:237–243, 1987

119. Lilley LL: Human need fulfillment alteration in the client with uterine cancer: The registered nurse's perception versus the client's perception. *Cancer Nurs* 10:327–337, 1987

120. Young-Graham K, Longman AJ: Quality of life and persons with melanoma: Preliminary model testing. *Cancer Nurs* 10:338–346, 1987

121. Blackmore C: The impact of orchidectomy upon the sexuality of the man with testicular cancer. *Cancer Nurs* 11:33–40, 1988

122. Camp LD: A comparison of nurses' recorded assessments of pain with perceptions of pain as described by cancer patients. *Cancer Nurs* 11:237–243, 1988

123. Coward DD: Hypercalcemia knowledge assessment in patients at risk of developing cancer-induced hypercalcemia. *Oncol Nurs Forum* 15:471–476, 1988

124. Derdiarian AK: Derdiarian Behavioral System Model (DBSM). *Scholarly Inquiry for Nursing Practice* 2(2):103–121, 1988

125. Eilers J, Berger AM, Petersen MC: Development, testing and application of the oral assessment guide. *Oncol Nurs Forum* 15:325–330, 1988

126. Lauver D: Development of a questionnaire to measure beliefs and attitudes about breast self-examination. *Cancer Nurs* 11:51–57, 1988

127. McMillan SC, Williams FA, Chatfield R, et al: Validity and reliability study of two tools for assessing and managing cancer pain. *Oncol Nurs Forum* 15:735–741, 1988

128. Rhodes VA, Watson PM, Hanson BM: Patients' descriptions of the influence of tiredness and weakness on self-care abilities. *Cancer Nurs* 11:186–194, 1988

129. Sutherland HJ, Walker P, Till JE: The development of a method for determining oncology patients' emotional distress using linear analogue scales. *Cancer Nurs* 11:303–308, 1988

130. Weinrich SP, Weinrich MC: Cancer knowledge among elderly individuals. *Cancer Nurs* 9:301–307, 1987

131. Williams RD: Factors affecting practice of BSE in older women. *Oncol Nurs Forum* 15:611–616, 1988

132. Amnon-Gaberson KB, Piantanida M: Generating results from qualitative data. *Image* 20:159–161, 1988

133. Saunders JM, Valente SM: Cancer and suicide. *Oncol Nurs Forum* 15:575–581, 1988

134. Thorne SE: Helpful and unhelpful communications in cancer care: The patient perspective. *Oncol Nurs Forum* 15:167–172, 1988

135. Hays JC: Patient symptoms and family coping. *Cancer Nurs* 9:317–325, 1986

136. Duigon A: Anticipatory nausea and vomiting associated with cancer chemotherapy. *Oncol Nurs Forum* 13:35–40, 1986

137. Coons HL, Leventhal H, Nerenz DR, et al: Anticipatory nausea and emotional distress in patients receiving cisplatin-based chemotherapy. *Oncol Nurs Forum* 14:31–35, 1987

138. Hagopian GA: Cognitive strategies used in adapting to a cancer diagnosis. *Oncol Nurs Forum* 20:759–763, 1993

139. Armsden GC, Lewis FM: Behavioral adjustment of school-age children of women with breast cancer. *Oncol Nurs Forum* 21:39–45, 1994

140. Weekes DP, Kagan SH: Adolescents completing cancer therapy: Meaning, perception and coping. *Oncol Nurs Forum* 21:663–670, 1994

141. Champion VL: Beliefs about breast cancer and mammography by behavioral stage. *Oncol Nurs Forum* 21:1009–1014, 1994

142. Leavitt MB, Lamb SA, Voss BS: Brain tumor support group: Content themes and mechanisms of support. *Oncol Nurs Forum* 23:1247–1256, 1996

143. Winningham ML, Nail LM, Burke MB, et al: Fatigue and the cancer experience: The state of the knowledge. *Oncol Nurs Forum* 21:23–36, 1994

144. Manson H, Manderino MA, Johnson MH: Chemotherapy: Thoughts and images of patients with cancer. *Oncol Nurs Forum* 20:527–532, 1993

145. Hockenberry-Eton M, Minick P: Living with cancer: Children with extraordinary courage. *Oncol Nurs Forum* 21:1025–1031, 1994

146. Pinto KM: Accuracy of coagulation values obtained from a heparinized central venous catheter. *Oncol Nurs Forum* 21:573–575, 1994

147. Bender CM: Cognitive dysfunction associated with biological response modifier therapy. *Oncol Nurs Forum* 21:515–523, 1994

148. Walker BL, Nail LM, Larsen L, et al: Concerns, affect and cognition disruption following completion of radiation treatment for localized breast or prostate cancer. *Oncol Nurs Forum* 23:1181–1187, 1996

149. Lauver D, Angerame M: Women's expectations about seeking care for breast cancer symptoms. *Oncol Nurs Forum* 20:520–523, 1993

150. Bilodeau BA, Degner LF: Information needs, sources of information and decisional roles in women with breast cancer. *Oncol Nurs Forum* 23:691–696, 1996

151. O'Connor KF: Ethical/moral experiences of oncology nurses. *Oncol Nurs Forum* 23:787–794, 1996

152. Nielsen B, Miaskowski C, Dibble SL: Pain and mammography: Fact or fiction? *Oncol Nurs Forum* 20:639–642, 1993

153. McMillan SC: The quality of life of patients with cancer receiving hospice care. *Oncol Nurs Forum* 23:1221–1228, 1996

154. Rutledge DN, Greene P, Mooney K, et al: Use of research-based practices by oncology staff nurses. *Oncol Nurs Forum* 23:1235–1241, 1996

155. Hollen PJ, Hobbie WL: Risk taking and decision making of adolescent long-term survivors of cancer. *Oncol Nurs Forum* 20:769–776, 1993

156. Carpenter JS, Brockapp DY: Evaluation of self-esteem of women with cancer receiving chemotherapy. *Oncol Nurs Forum* 21:751–757, 1994

157. Shell JA, Smith CK: Sexuality and the older person with cancer. *Oncol Nurs Forum* 21:553–558, 1994

158. Young A, Volker D, Rieger PT, et al: Oncology nurses' attitudes regarding voluntary, physician-assisted dying for competent, terminally ill patients. *Oncol Nurs Forum* 20:445–451, 1993

159. Kelly P, Winslow EH: Needle wire localization for nonpalpable breast lesions: Sensations, anxiety levels, and informational needs. *Oncol Nurs Forum* 23:639–645, 1996

160. Valente SM: Using hypnosis with children for pain management. *Oncol Nurs Forum* 18:699–704, 1991

161. Nail LM, Jones LS, Greene D, et al: Use and perceived efficacy of self-care activities in patients receiving chemotherapy. *Oncol Nurs Forum* 18:883–887, 1991

162. Arzouman JMR, Dudas S, Ferrans CE, et al: Quality of life of patients with sarcoma postchemotherapy. *Oncol Nurs Forum* 18:889–894, 1991

163. Lovejoy NC, Paul S, Freeman E, et al: Potential correlates of self-care and symptom distress in homosexual/bisexual men who are HIV seropositive. *Oncol Nurs Forum* 18:1175–1185, 1991

164. Belec RH: Quality of life: Perceptions of long-term survivors of bone marrow transplantation. *Oncol Nurs Forum* 19:31–37, 1992

165. Gaston-Johansson F, Franco T, Zimmerman L: Pain and psychological distress in patients undergoing autologous bone marrow transplantation. *Oncol Nurs Forum* 19:41–48, 1992

166. Maloney CH, Preston F: An overview of home care for patients with cancer. *Oncol Nurs Forum* 19:75–80, 1992

167. Rieker PP, Clark EJ, Fogelberg PR: Perceptions of quality of life and quality of care for patients with cancer receiving biological therapy. *Oncol Nurs Forum* 19:433–440, 1992

168. Sutters KA, Miaskowski C: The problem of pain in children with cancer: A research review. *Oncol Nurs Forum* 19:465–471, 1992

169. Ferrell BR, Cohen MZ, Rhiner M, et al: Pain as a metaphor for illness. Part II: Family caregivers' management of pain. *Oncol Nurs Forum* 18:1315–1321, 1991

170. O'Berle K, Davies B: Support and caring: Exploring the concepts. *Oncol Nurs Forum* 19:763–767, 1992

171. Ersek M: The process of maintaining hope in adults undergoing bone marrow transplantation for leukemia. *Oncol Nurs Forum* 19:883–889, 1992

172. Steeves RH: Patients who have undergone bone marrow transplantation: Their quest for meaning. *Oncol Nurs Forum* 19:899–905, 1992

173. Ferrell B, Grant M, Schmidt GM, et al: The meaning of quality of life for bone marrow transplant survivors. Part I: The impact of bone marrow transplant on quality of life. *Cancer Nurs* 15:153–160, 1992

174. Ferrell B, Grant M, Schmidt GM, et al: The meaning of quality of life for bone marrow transplant survivors. Part 2: Improving quality of life for bone marrow transplant survivors. *Cancer Nurs* 15:247–253, 1992

175. Smith DB, Babaian RJ: The effects of treatment for cancer on male fertility and sexuality. *Cancer Nurs* 15:271–275, 1992

176. Murali ME, Crabtree K: Comparison of two breast self-examination palpation techniques. *Cancer Nurs* 15:276–282, 1992

177. MacAvoy S, Moritz D: Nursing diagnoses in an oncology population. *Cancer Nurs* 15:264–270, 1992

178. Zappa SC, Nabors SB: Use of ethyl chloride topical anesthetic to reduce procedural pain in pediatric oncology patients. *Cancer Nurs* 15:130–136, 1992

179. Highfield MF: Spiritual health of oncology patients: Nurse and patient perspectives. *Cancer Nurs* 15:1–8, 1992

180. Vranicar-Lapka D, Barbour-Randall L, Trippon M, et al: Oncology patients' and their significant others' responses to a proposed cancer prevention/detection program. *Cancer Nurs* 15:47–53, 1992

181. Ludwick R: Registered nurses' knowledge and practices of teaching and performing breast exams among elderly women. *Cancer Nurs* 15:61–67, 1992

182. Henschel L: Fever patterns in the neutropenic patient. *Cancer Nurs* 8:301–305, 1985

183. Krouse HJ: A psychological model of adjustment in gynecologic cancer patients. *Oncol Nurs Forum* 12:45–49, 1985

184. Cooley ME, Cobb SC: Sexual and reproductive issues for women with Hodgkin's disease: I. Overview of issues. *Cancer Nurs* 9:188–193, 1986

185. Cooley ME, Yeoman AC, Cobb SC: Sexual and reproductive issues for women with Hodgkin's disease: Application of PLISSIT Model. *Cancer Nurs* 9:248–255, 1986

186. Coward DD: Cancer-induced hypercalcemia. *Cancer Nurs* 9:125–132, 1986

187. Holing EV: The primary caregiver's perception of the dying trajectory: An exploratory study. *Cancer Nurs* 9:29–37, 1986

188. Huldij A, Giesbers A, Poelhuis EHK, et al: Alterations in taste appreciation in cancer patients during treatment. *Cancer Nurs* 9:38–42, 1986

189. Lovejoy N: Family responses to cancer hospitalization. *Oncol Nurs Forum* 13:33–37, 1986

190. Donovan MI, Dillon P: Incidence and characteristics of pain in a sample of hospitalized cancer patients. *Cancer Nurs* 10:85–92, 1987

191. Jenkins B: Patients' reports of sexual changes after treatment for gynecological cancer. *Oncol Nurs Forum* 15:349–354, 1988

192. Ostchega Y, Donahue M, Fox N: High-dose cisplatin-related peripheral neuropathy. *Cancer Nurs* 11:23–32, 1988

193. Wilkie D, Lovejoy N, Dodd M, et al: Cancer pain control

behaviors: Description and correlation with pain intensity. *Oncol Nurs Forum* 15:723–731, 1988

194. Berckman KL, Austin JK: Causal attribution, perceived control and adjustment. *Oncol Nurs Forum* 20:23–30, 1993

195. Canty SL: Constipation as a side effect of opioids. *Oncol Nurs Forum* 21:739–745, 1994

196. Buchsel PC, Leum EW, Randolph SR: Delayed complications of bone marrow transplantation: An update. *Oncol Nurs Forum* 23:1305–1312, 1996

197. Mayo DJ, Dimond EP, Kramer W, et al: Discard volumes necessary for clinically useful coagulation studies from heparinized Hickman catheters. *Oncol Nurs Forum* 23:671–675, 1996

198. Hilton BA: Getting back to normal: The family experience during early stage breast cancer. *Oncol Nurs Forum* 23:605–614, 1996

199. Steele RG, Fitch MI: Needs of family caregivers of patients receiving home hospice care for cancer. *Oncol Nurs Forum* 23:823–828, 1996

200. Zerbe MB, Parkerson SG, Spitzer T: Laminar air flow vs. reverse isolation: Nurses' assessments of moods, behaviors and activity levels in patients receiving bone marrow transplants. *Oncol Nurs Forum* 21:565–568, 1994

201. Lindsey AM, Larson PJ, Sarna L, et al: The lung cancer experience: Nutritional intake, weight, functional status, and other factors—Comparison of variables and findings across three studies. *Oncol Nurs Forum* 20:465–493, 1993

202. O'Brien S, Dalton JA, Konsler G, et al: The knowledge and attitudes of experienced oncology nurses regarding the management of cancer-related pain. *Oncol Nurs Forum* 23:515–521, 1996

203. Underwood SM, Hoskins D, Cummins T, et al: Obstacles to cancer care: Focus on the economically disadvantaged. *Oncol Nurs Forum* 21:47–52, 1994

204. Raybould TP, Carpenter AD, Ferretti GA, et al: Emergence of gram-negative bacilli in the mouths of bone marrow transplant recipients using chlorhexidine mouthrinse. *Oncol Nurs Forum* 21:691–696, 1994

205. Larson PJ, Viele CS, Coleman S, et al: Comparison of perceived symptoms of patients undergoing bone marrow transplant and the nurses caring for them. *Oncol Nurs Forum* 20:81–88, 1993

206. Lovejoy NC: Precancerous and cancerous cervical lesions: The multicultural "male" risk factor. *Oncol Nurs Forum* 21:497–504, 1994

207. Heiney SP, Neuberg RW, Myers D, et al: The aftermath of bone marrow transplant for parents of pediatric patients: A post-traumatic stress disorder. *Oncol Nurs Forum* 21:843–847, 1994

208. Foltz AT, Gaines G, Gullotte M: Recalled side effects and self-care actions of patients receiving in-patient chemotherapy. *Oncol Nurs Forum* 23:679–683, 1996

209. Bryla CM: The relationship between stress and the development of breast cancer: A literature review. *Oncol Nurs Forum* 23:441–448, 1996

210. Altman GB, Lee CA: Strontium-89 for treatment of painful bone metastasis from prostate cancer. *Oncol Nurs Forum* 23:523–527, 1996

211. Brandt B: Informational needs and selected variables in patients receiving brachytherapy. *Oncol Nurs Forum* 18:1221–1229, 1991

212. Ferrell BR, Rhiner M, Cohen MZ, et al: Pain as a metaphor for illness. Part I: Impact of cancer pain on family caregivers. *Oncol Nurs Forum* 18:1303–1309, 1991

213. Carey PJ, Oberst MT, McCubbin MA, et al: Appraisal of caregiving burden in family members caring for patients receiving chemotherapy. *Oncol Nurs Forum* 18:1341–1348, 1991

214. Fazio MT, Glaspy JA: The impact of granulocyte colony-stimulating factor on quality of life in patients with severe chronic neutropenia. *Oncol Nurs Forum* 18:1411–1414, 1991

215. Jackson BS, Strauman J, Frederickson K, et al: Long-term biopsychosocial effects of interleukin-2 therapy. *Oncol Nurs Forum* 18:683–690, 1991

216. Champion VL: The relationship of selected variables to breast cancer detection in women 35 and older. *Oncol Nurs Forum* 18:733–739, 1991

217. Carney-Gersten P, Giuffre M, Levy D: Factors related to Amphotericin-B-induced rigors (shivering). *Oncol Nurs Forum* 18:745–750, 1991

218. Young-McCaughan S, Sexton DL: A retrospective investigation of the relationship between aerobic exercise and quality of life in women with breast cancer. *Oncol Nurs Forum* 18:751–757, 1991

219. Coward DD: Self-transcendence and emotional well-being in women with advanced breast cancer. *Oncol Nurs Forum* 18:857–863, 1991

220. Waltman NL, Bergstrom N, Armstrong N, et al: Nutritional status, pressure sores and mortality in elderly patients with cancer. *Oncol Nurs Forum* 18:867–873, 1991

221. Hileman JW, Lackey NR, Hassanein RS: Identifying the needs of home caregivers of patients with cancer. *Oncol Nurs Forum* 19:771–777, 1992

222. St. Pierre BA, Kasper CE, Lindsey AM: Fatigue mechanisms in patients with cancer: Effects of tumor necrosis factor and exercise on skeletal muscle. *Oncol Nurs Forum* 19:419–425, 1992

223. Raleigh EDH: Sources of hope in chronic illness. *Oncol Nurs Forum* 19:443–448, 1992

224. Farrell MM: The challenge of Adult Respiratory Distress Syndrome during interleukin-2 immunotherapy. *Oncol Nurs Forum* 19:475–480, 1992

225. Yoder L, Rubin M: The epidemiology of cervical cancer and its precursors. *Oncol Nurs Forum* 19:485–493, 1992

226. Kelly C, Dumenko L, McGregor SE, et al: A change in flushing protocols of central venous catheters. *Oncol Nurs Forum* 19:599–605, 1992

227. Lovejoy NC, Morgenrath BN, Paul S, et al: Potential predictors of information-seeking behavior by homosexual/bisexual (gay) men with a human immunodeficiency virus seropositive health status. *Cancer Nurs* 15:116–124, 1992

228. Berry DL, Catanzaro M: Persons with cancer and their return to the workplace. *Cancer Nurs* 15:40–46, 1992

229. Uhlenhopp MB: An overview of the relationship between alkylating agents and therapy-related acute nonlymphocytic leukemia. *Cancer Nurs* 15:9–17, 1992

230. Brown ML, Carrieri V, Janson-Bjerklie S, et al: Lung cancer and dyspnea: The patient's perception. *Oncol Nurs Forum* 13:19–24, 1986

231. King KB, Nail LM, Kreamer K, et al: Patients' descriptions of the experience of receiving radiotherapy. *Oncol Nurs Forum* 12:55–61, 1986

232. Lesage C: Carotid artery rupture: Prediction, prevention, preparation. *Cancer Nurs* 9:1–7, 1986

233. Messner RL, Gardner SS, Webb DD: Early detection: The priority in colorectal cancer. *Cancer Nurs* 9:8–14, 1986

234. Post-White J: Glucocorticosteroid-induced depression in the patient with leukemia or lymphoma. *Cancer Nurs* 9:15–22, 1986

235. Tringali CA: The needs of family members of cancer patients. *Oncol Nurs Forum* 13:65–70, 1986

236. Rhodes VA, Watson PM, Johnson MH, et al: Patterns of nausea, vomiting and distress in patients receiving antineoplastic drug protocols. *Oncol Nurs Forum* 14:35–44, 1987

237. Yeager KA, Miaskowski C: Advances in understanding the mechanisms and management of acute myelogenous leukemia. *Oncol Nurs Forum* 21:541–548, 1994

238. Stucky LA: Acute tumor lysis syndrome: Assessment and nursing implications. *Oncol Nurs Forum* 20:49–59, 1993

239. Carter LW: Bacterial translocation: Nursing implications. *Oncol Nurs Forum* 21:857–865, 1994

240. Caudell KA: Psychoneuroimmunology and innovative behavioral interventions in patients with leukemia. *Oncol Nurs Forum* 23:493–502, 1996

241. Kelly LP, Miaskowski C: An overview of bladder cancer: Treatment and nursing implications. *Oncol Nurs Forum* 23:459–468, 1996

242. Viele CS: Chronic myelogenous leukemia and acute promyelocytic leukemia: New bone marrow transplant options. *Oncol Nurs Forum* 23:488–493, 1996

243. Bucholtz JD: Comforting children during radiotherapy. *Oncol Nurs Forum* 21:987–1006, 1994

244. Armstrong TS, Gilbert MR: Glial neoplasms: Classification, treatment and pathways for the future. *Oncol Nurs Forum* 23:615–625, 1996

245. Grassman D: Development of inpatient oncology education and support programs. *Oncol Nurs Forum* 20:669–676, 1993

246. Timmerman PR: Intravenous immunoglobulin in oncology nursing practice. *Oncol Nurs Forum* 20:69–75, 1993

247. Struthers CS: Lambert-Eaton myasthenic syndrome in small cell lung cancer: Nursing implications. *Oncol Nurs Forum* 21:677–683, 1994

248. Wujcik D, Viele CS, Caudell KA: Leukemia management strategies: The next generation. *Oncol Nurs Forum* 23:477–487, 1996

249. Neufeld KR, Degner LF, Dick JAM: A nursing intervention strategy to foster patient involvement in treatment decisions. *Oncol Nurs Forum* 20:631–635, 1993

250. Meade CD: Producing videotapes for cancer education: Methods and examples. *Oncol Nurs Forum* 23:837–846, 1996

251. Lierman LM, Powell-Cope G, Benoliel JQ: Using social support to promote breast self-examination performance. *Oncol Nurs Forum* 21:1051–1056, 1994

252. Doak LG, Doak CC, Meade CD: Strategies to improve cancer educational materials. *Oncol Nurs Forum* 23:1305–1312, 1996

253. Hawkins C, Miaskowski C: Testicular cancer: A review. *Oncol Nurs Forum* 23:1203–1211, 1996

254. Baker KH, Feldman JE: Thyroid cancer: A review. *Oncol Nurs Forum* 20:95–104, 1993

255. Sticklin LA, Walkenstein M: Vena cava filters: A nursing perspective. *Oncol Nurs Forum* 20:507–515, 1993

256. Meriney DK: Pathophysiology and management of VIPoma: A case study. *Oncol Nurs Forum* 23:941–948, 1996

257. Dachowski LJ, DeLaney TF: Photodynamic Therapy. The NCI experience and its nursing implication. *Oncol Nurs Forum* 19:63–67, 1992

258. Held JL, Peahota A: Nursing care of patients with esophageal cancer. *Oncol Nurs Forum* 19:627–634, 1992

259. McFadden ME, Sartorius SE: Multiple system organ failure in patients with cancer. Part II: Nursing implications. *Oncol Nurs Forum* 19:727–737, 1992

260. Jassack PF: Families: An essential element in the care of the patient with cancer. *Oncol Nurs Forum* 19:871–876, 1992

261. Sitton E: Early and late radiation-induced skin alterations: Part II. Nursing care of irradiated skin. *Oncol Nurs Forum* 19:907–912, 1992

262. Saba MT, Magolan JM: Understanding cerebral edema: Implications for oncology nurses. *Oncol Nurs Forum* 18:499–505, 1991

263. Dyck S: Surgical instrumentation as a palliative treatment for spinal cord compression. *Oncol Nurs Forum* 18:515–521, 1991

264. Kehoe C: Malignant ascites: Etiology, diagnosis and treatment. *Oncol Nurs Forum* 18:523–530, 1991

265. Yeomans AC, Washington JB: Occult primary malignancies. *Oncol Nurs Forum* 18:539–544, 1991

266. Martz CH: Von Hippel–Lindau disease: A genetic condition predisposing tumor formation. *Oncol Nurs Forum* 18:545–551, 1991

267. Mahon SM: Managing the psychosocial consequences of cancer recurrence: Implications for nurses. *Oncol Nurs Forum* 18:577–583, 1991

268. Lynch M, Yanes L: Flowsheet documentation of chemotherapy administration and patient teaching. *Oncol Nurs Forum* 18:777–783, 1991

269. Moore JM, Knobf MT: A Nursing Flow Sheet for documentation of ambulatory oncology. *Oncol Nurs Forum* 18:933–939, 1991

270. McDermott KC, Almadrones LA, Bijorunas DR: The diagnosis and management of hypomagnesemia: A unique treatment approach and case report. *Oncol Nurs Forum* 18:1145–1152, 1991

271. Jordan LN, Mantravadi RVP: Nursing care of the patient receiving high-dose-rate brachytherapy. *Oncol Nurs Forum* 18:1167–1171, 1991

272. Radziewicz RM, Schneider SM: Using diversional activity to enhance coping. *Cancer Nurs* 15:293–298, 1992

273. Buehler JA, Lee HJ: Exploration of home care resources for rural families with cancer. *Cancer Nurs* 15:299–308, 1992

274. Lobert S: Antimitotics in cancer chemotherapy. *Cancer Nurs* 15:22–33, 1992

275. Cooley ME: Bereavement care: A role for nurses. *Cancer Nurs* 15:125–129, 1992

276. Valanis B, McNeil V, Driscoll K: Staff members' compliance with their facility's antineoplastic drug handling policy. *Oncol Nurs Forum* 18:571–576, 1991

277. Foote M: Nursing care of the patient with non-Hodgkin's lymphoma: Prevention of pneumonia associated with combination chemotherapy. *Cancer Nurs* 8:263–271, 1985

278. Getz DH: The primary, secondary and tertiary nursing interventions of lymphedema. *Cancer Nurs* 8:177–184, 1985

279. Rooney A, Haviley C: Nursing management of disseminated intravascular coagulation. *Oncol Nurs Forum* 12:15–22, 1985

280. Rossetti AC: Nursing care of patients treated with intrapleural tetracycline for control of malignant pleural effusion. *Cancer Nurs* 8:103–109, 1985

281. Gurevich I, Tafuro P: The compromised host: Deficit-specific infection in the spectrum of prevention. *Cancer Nurs* 9:263–275, 1986

282. Moore CL, Erickson KA, Yanes LB, et al: Nursing care and management of venous access ports. *Oncol Nurs Forum* 13:35–39, 1986

283. Paice JA: Intrathecal morphine infusion for intractable cancer pain: A new use for implanted pumps. *Oncol Nurs Forum* 13:41–47, 1986

284. Rodzwic D, Donnard J: The use of myocutaneous flaps in reconstructive surgery for head and neck cancer: Guidelines for nursing care. *Oncol Nurs Forum* 13:29, 1986

285. Hassay KM: Radiation therapy for rectal cancer and the implications for nursing. *Cancer Nurs* 10:311–318, 1987

286. Link DL: Antibiotic therapy in the cancer patient: Focus on third generation cephalosporins. *Oncol Nurs Forum* 14:35–41, 1987

287. Moreland BJ: A nursing form for gynecology patient assessment. *Oncol Nurs Forum* 14:19–23, 1987

288. Stetz KM: Caregiving demands during advanced cancer: The spouse's needs. *Cancer Nurs* 10:260–268, 1987

289. Lewandowski W, Jones SL: The family with cancer: Nursing intervention throughout the course of living with cancer. *Cancer Nurs* 11:313–321, 1988

290. Strohl RA: The nursing role in radiation oncology: Symptom management of acute and chronic reactions. *Oncol Nurs Forum* 15:429–434, 1988

291. Jennings BM, Muhlenkamp AF: Systematic misperception: Oncology patients' self-reported affective states and their care-givers' perceptions. *Cancer Nurs* 4:485–489, 1981

292. Wright BA: *Physical Disability: A Psychological Approach.* New York, Harper and Row, 1960

293. Verron JA, Longman A, Clark M: Development of a scale to measure undergraduate students' attitudes about caring for patients with cancer. *Oncol Nurs Forum* 14:51–55, 1987

294. Robb S: Attitudes and intentions of baccalaureate nursing students toward the elderly. *Nurs Res* 28:43–50, 1979

295. Larson P: Important nurse caring behaviors perceived by patients with cancer. *Oncol Nurs Forum* 11:46–50, 1984

296. Larson P: Comparison of cancer patients' and professional nurses' perceptions of important nurse caring behaviors. *Heart Lung* 16:187–192, 1987

297. Mayer DK: Oncology nurses' versus cancer patients' perceptions of nursing care behaviors: A replication study. *Oncol Nurs Forum* 14:48–52, 1987

298. Sodestrom KE, Martinson IM: Patients' spiritual coping strategies: A study of nurse and patient perspectives. *Oncol Nurs Forum* 14:41–46, 1987

299. Curtis AE, Fernsler JI: Quality of life of oncology hospice patients: A comparison of patient and primary caregiver reports. *Oncol Nurs Forum* 16:49–53, 1989

300. Dyck S, Wright K: Family perceptions: The role of the nurse throughout an adult's cancer experience. *Oncol Nurs Forum* 12:53–56, 1985

301. Benner P: *From Novice to Expert: Excellence and Power in Clinical Nursing Practice.* Menlo Park, CA, Addison-Wesley, 1984

302. Benner P, Wrubel J: *The Primacy of Caring: Stress and Coping in Health and Illness.* Menlo Park, CA, Addison-Wesley, 1989

# Chapter 56

# Impact of Changing Health Care Economics on Cancer Nursing Practice

**Valinda Rutledge, RN, MSN, MBA**

**Joy Stair, RN, MS**

## INTRODUCTION

During the last five years, multiple internal and external forces have converged to transform the health care industry. New terminology is being used, including words such as managed care, capitation, outcomes management, and virtual integration. Nursing is moving from a profession focused on caring for patients in the hospital to one concerned about the health of communities. The changes intensified with the Clinton administration's health care reform initiatives; however, the forces of change began much earlier in the 1980s with the advent of prospective payment models from government payers. Unfortunately, the prospective payment system did not bring the anticipated widespread decline in health care costs due to the cost shifting from the public to the private sector. As the Clinton health care reform debate intensified in the early 1990s, the marketplace accelerated the transition to managed care, and alternative payment models began to flourish. This market reform rather than legislative mandated reform resulted in a 4.7% reduction in health care costs in 1994.[1] Nurses must be cognizant of national health care trends to serve better as patient advocates. In this chapter market forces and their impact on nursing practice will be examined.

## CHANGING HEALTH CARE ECONOMICS

### Prospective Payment Model

Since the early 1970s the United States has experienced a 273% increase in per capita health care costs, yet the United States continues to rank seventh in developed countries for infant mortality.[2] The continual escalation of health care costs in the 1980s caused concern among business leaders and politicians. American businesses were declining in the global market and labor costs, in particular, were cited as a major factor for this decline. Benefit costs, with health care as the largest component, were also targeted as a concern. Business leaders were emphatic that to compete globally America's labor costs must change, or there would be a migration of businesses to other countries with lower costs.

At the same time, politicians were concerned about the impact of the growing federal deficit on long-term American growth. In an attempt to slow the growth of the federal deficit, diagnostic related groups (DRGs) were initiated by the federal government in the 1980s. There are 477 DRGs (based on diagnostic groupings and modified by severity indexes such as complications and comorbidity) for which payments are made to hospitals. The payment model is a "case rate" in which providers are reimbursed a predetermined amount based on a given illness or incident.

As hospitals began to lose money with the advent of DRGs, they attempted to shift their losses to businesses in the form of higher premiums. In response to these higher premiums, businesses began to examine other alternative health care plans that would control costs. Traditional health care plans attempted to control costs through strategies such as surgical second opinions and admission recertification. Unfortunately, these approaches were not successful and costs continued to rise. Some health care plans incorporated cost control systems to decrease resource consumption either by tightening utilization or through implementing plans in which the providers (hospital and physicians) would have a financial incentive to control cost for physicians and hospitals. Alternative delivery models such as health maintenance organizations (HMOs), preferred provider organizations (PPOs), and independent practice associations (IPAs) have risen in numbers as significant cost savings have been demonstrated by these models. It is clear that dramatic changes are coming that will have an impact on how care is rendered to patients.

### Health Care Delivery Models

Managed care health plans reduce costs through a variety of strategies by redesigning how patients are cared for. The major models are HMO, PPO, point of service (POS), and physician-hospital organization (PHO), which are differentiated by structure, provider risk-sharing, and degree of consumer choice of services, locations, and providers.[3]

#### Health maintenance organization (HMO)

HMOs (the oldest and largest type of managed care) contract to provide health care at a prenegotiated rate on a "per member per month" basis. The early success of HMOs was related to two major factors: the assumption of financial risk by physicians and the combining of the costs of all services (hospitals, ambulatory services, and physicians) into one charge. The first factor provided financial incentives to physicians for reasonable resource utilization. The second factor bundled the costs together and allowed the providers to determine the total cost of treating the patient. An additional factor that contributed to HMOs' early successes was the attraction of the healthy young consumer who required minimal services of the HMO, but the demographics have begun to shift to represent an older population. Initially, HMOs controlled costs through limiting access for their members to only a small set of participating providers. However, different models have developed as the public has demanded more choice.

The basis of the HMO model is a primary care physician (PCP) who is selected by the participant. All care must be authorized by this physician (frequently referred to as the "gatekeeper"), who is paid a fixed amount per patient to coordinate the care. The amount may either be a full capitation that includes both the costs for care provided by the PCP and the costs for referral to specialists, or it may be capitated for the PCP costs only. Clearly the savings are greatest with the total capitated model.

HMOs can be divided into three types based upon the structure of the relationship between the physician and health care facility: staff model, group model, and network models.[3,4] In a staff model HMO, all physicians are employed and salaried by the HMO. Because this model results in lower productivity (as determined by the number of patients seen per day) than other HMO models, financial incentives were added to physician compensation to enhance productivity.

In a group model HMO plan, the physicians are not salaried, but have a contractual arrangement with the HMO. The physician is compensated through the private practice, and there are incentives built into the arrangement for both quality and cost-effectiveness of care.

Both staff and group models are referred to as "closed models" due to the inability of community physicians to participate, with the care being rendered only by the HMO-designated physicians. Though these two models result in more cost savings than others, the number of enrollees is decreasing as consumers demand more choice in their health care plans.

The third plan, the network model, requires that physicians contract directly with the HMO, but the physicians continue to deliver care in their own private offices and also to treat non-HMO patients. This plan is referred to as an "open model" and is becoming a very popular option.

Forty-seven percent of Americans are currently enrolled in a traditional HMO, with the majority of the plans owned by for-profit organizations. In 1995, the *Wall Street Journal* reported multimillion dollar profits and huge executive salaries for some HMOs.[1] The public has responded negatively to these reports, which ultimately may result in erosion of enrollees and transferring into alternative health care plans.

Concerns regarding quality of care in HMOs continue to be raised in the media. To maintain confidence in the plans, and to differentiate plans from each other, quality of care must be documented through measurement of outcomes. To meet this challenge, HMOs' leadership has taken a proactive approach by developing methods to demonstrate the quality of their health plans. Employers review both cost and quality reports when making decisions about plan selection. The HMOs submit data that are checked by an outside audit company such as National Committee on Quality Assurance (NCQA), which also accredits HMOs and managed care plans. Not only is information gathered, such as length of wait time for an appointment, but the number and type of health screening tests administered, such as Pap smears or mammography, are also monitored. Two hundred and sixteen out of 500 HMOs (43%) elected to be surveyed by NCQA; only 36% received the full three-year accreditation. An alarming 13% did not pass the NCQA accreditation survey.[5]

Information about how various HMOs compare is also available from Health Plan Employer Data and Information Set (HEDIS). The HEDIS collects standard information, such as the rate of cesarean sections and percent of enrollees receiving screening tests, such as mammograms, which is used to compare HMOs. It is clear that once price is comparable among HMOs, they will be selected based on quality.

### Preferred provider organization (PPO)

In a PPO, contractual arrangements are negotiated between payers and health care providers (hospitals and/or physicians) to render care at a predetermined discounted amount (lower than the provider's customary fees). Members of PPOs have a greater variety of choices than are available in most HMOs because they have the option of choosing a non-PPO organization by agreeing to pay additional deductibles. PPOs have generated some cost savings, but controversy has developed over the practice of PPO physicians ordering more tests to compensate for lost income resulting from discounts provided to payers.[6]

### Point of service (POS) plans

The exponential growth of HMOs began to slow down as consumers became concerned about their ability to access care outside the plan if they required a treatment found in only a few academic centers. In response to consumer concern, the POS plan was devised, which allows members to access out-of-plan providers by agreeing to pay additional deductibles. This plan combines HMO utilization with fee-for-service–type freedom of choice and is one of the fastest-growing health care insurance plans. When POS plans were first introduced, they were seen as a strategy to transition back to HMOs. However, the reverse is actually true, as more HMOs are offering POS plans. The POS plan is very attractive for consumers who are asking for more choice and for employers looking for cost savings. It allows the consumer a wide choice of physicians within the plan, but imposes strict utilization strategies.

### Physician-hospital organization (PHO)

In a PHO, there is a contractual relationship between physicians and the hospital to accomplish several goals: to increase the opportunity to obtain managed-care contracts, to align the organizational structure with the financial incentives found in capitation, and to measure quality of care through outcomes.[7,8] Unfortunately, integration of hospitals and physicians into PHOs has not achieved the success that was predicted. The collaboration has led to enhanced relations between hospitals and physicians, but often has not led to significant cost reductions or increase in number of managed-care contracts. Lack of clarity involving regulatory issues of antitrust and licensure has limited PHOs' potential impact. It is unclear if PHOs will survive into the next century or if they will convert to organizations that can contract directly with the employer to provide health care services.

### Integrated delivery systems (IDSs)

PHOs often organize into integrated delivery systems (IDSs) to provide care more efficiently. IDSs can be both vertically and horizontally integrated. Vertical integration means that services such as inpatient, outpatient, radiation therapy, home care, physician office, and hospice oncology services are capable of being provided within the same system.[9] Horizontal integration is when these services are provided at different sites in the community. The recent high number of consolidations and mergers among health care organizations (hospitals, pharmaceutical companies, home care agencies, and even HMOs) are examples of horizontal integration. The two types of integration are also referred to as depth (vertical) and breadth (horizontal) of services.

During the last few years the number of IDSs has escalated in response to managed care growth. IDSs have been touted as the balance to the increasing influence of the growing numbers of large for-profit health care chains. The ability of large integrated systems to achieve their initial objectives (increased market share and decreased costs) remains in question.[10] Shortell[11] studied several multihospital systems from 1990 to 1996 to determine their changes in response to external market forces. He prefers the term "organized delivery system" instead of integrated delivery system because integration is a phase rarely achieved. Goldsmith[12] points out that IDSs tend to have more management layers contributing to higher costs and slower decision making. This increased bureaucracy also reduces communication and increases tension among clinical providers such as nurses/physicians and the health system executives, with potentially disastrous results. This is especially apparent in some areas of the country where unions have arisen as nursing staffs have reacted negatively to changes made by the organization in response to market forces. Goldsmith[13] also indicates that the growth of horizontally integrated systems has led to diminished profit margins, as profitable hospitals are burdened with dying and unsuccessful hospitals due to the reluctance of hospital boards of directors to close hospitals within a health care system. As cash reserves are used to bolster drowning facilities, the entire community suffers a loss of services.

Ownership of the assets by the health care system may not be the optimal method to achieve the goal of seamless delivery of care throughout the continuum. In fact, some systems have overpaid for certain components such as physician practices, which can dramatically decrease cash reserves for other capital projects. Several systems have begun to explore contractual arrangements in which information systems are linked (virtual integration), rather than merging entire systems.[12,14] The strength of a vertically and horizontally integrated system is not in ownership of facilities and services and large corporate offices, but rather in the ability to provide the optimal delivery

method (in both cost and quality) of care for the patients. It is also clear that fragmentation within health care with stand-alone hospitals will not enhance care of the patient. The key lies in developing formal collaborative arrangements between clinical providers and health care executives to provide mutual leadership in developing clinical systems to enhance the care not only to patients but to the community as a whole.

## Impact of Managed Care

The differences among HMOs, PPOs, and fee-for-service (indemnity) plans have begun to fade. HMOs are providing more choice of providers while indemnity plans have implemented case management programs for specific chronic diseases. Most employers offer a hybrid delivery model with a variety of strategies to manage care. Eric Wagner[4] suggests that managed care be viewed as a continuum, with one end being the traditional fee-for-service and the other typified by the closed-model HMO. In the middle are the hybrid types such as POS, PPO, and IPAs. Moving along this continuum will increase the type and complexity of controls utilized to decrease costs.

The public sector has demonstrated interest in promoting managed-care risk products for both Medicare and Medicaid programs in order to decrease their costs.[1] The Medicare HMO plans are attractive to seniors because of low copayments and enhanced prescription benefits. In fact, some programs are offering unusual benefits such as reimbursement for taxicab fees to health care appointments. Unfortunately, many organizations developing these Medicare risk programs target the healthy elderly who consume minimal health care resources, rather than enrolling the chronically ill patient. The benefit of these Medicare risk products will become more apparent when the artificial segmentation through selected enrollment is eliminated.

A few states have passed legislation to move Medicaid recipients into managed-care risk programs to reduce costs with varying success. Oregon generated widespread publicity in the early 1990s when the decision was made to deny reimbursement for bone marrow transplantation to Medicaid recipients. This stimulated much public outcry against "rationing" of health care.

## Payment Models

The type of payment model for hospitals and physicians can vary considerably based upon the health care plan strategies to control cost. It has been found that financial incentives change behavior more effectively than stringent utilization management strategies.[15] Thus the payment model selected will have a more significant impact on reducing costs than any other variable.

### Indemnity plans

Prior to the advent of DRGs, over 90% of all Americans were covered under indemnity plans (also referred to as "fee-for-service"). These plans allowed an incredible amount of freedom for the participant to choose providers, both physicians and hospitals. Tests and procedures could be ordered without consideration for cost or value. Providers received reimbursement for most tests, procedures, or services; thus, there were no financial incentives to conserve resources by either the hospital or physician. This was the major reason for escalating national health care costs. By the early 1990s, the number of people covered by fee-for-service plans had dropped to 22% while the numbers of enrollees in managed care exceeded those in traditional indemnity plans.[1]

### Discount from charges

Discount from charges is a modification of the fee-for-service model. The underlying premise of reimbursement for each service rendered remains unchanged, but a discount is negotiated from the provider. However, long-term savings are not achieved, because providers typically increase charges on a yearly basis to compensate for the discounting.

### Per diem payments

Per diem payment programs reimburse for each day of hospitalization; for example, $500 per day may be negotiated regardless of ancillary services used. However, this strategy has led to increased length of stay (LOS), as there are no incentives to shorten stay in acute-care settings. It does conserve resources utilized per day, but any savings achieved are offset by increased length of stay, particularly since resource consumption typically decreases on subsequent days in the hospital.

### Capitation

Capitation is an established dollar amount "per member per month," regardless of the services rendered by the providers; thus, providers have an incentive to keep enrollees healthy and prevent utilization of all services. A certain amount of money is often set aside by the contracting physician organization to give bonuses to physicians who exceed both quality and cost standards set for practice. Capitation generally includes both specialist and primary care services (full capitation) to prevent cost shifting to a noncapitated component. Earlier contracts capitated primary care, with specialist care remaining fee-for-service. Full capitation has raised ethical concerns regarding quality of care as a result of data indicating significant reductions in referrals to specialists. There are also reports of decreased use of diagnostic procedures in primary care, which may be an early warning of negative patient outcomes related to inappropriate withholding of care by the "gatekeeper."[15]

Although it is too early for definitive conclusions, nurses must be aware of the issue of economic incentives and their effects on health care. Quality measures must be developed and tracked consistently through the years.

Instruments such as HEDIS and NCDQ accreditation standards will assist in objectively evaluating quality of care. It is clear that as capitation becomes more prevalent, there will be an increasing need to have strict quality checkpoints to prevent personal financial gain from leading to withholding of care. Friedman[16] addresses the irony of providers' sudden interest in dealing with "inappropriate patient demand" for unnecessary services with the changing financial incentives. When reimbursement was the norm, health care professionals ordered procedures without consideration of the ultimate value of the service. Oncologists were trained to provide intervention at all costs, and this model was rewarded in a fee-for-service environment. Under a capitated system, however, there are financial incentives for controlling utilization of health care resources, and oncologists may find themselves in an ethical dilemma as the shift to withholding care gains momentum. Will the oncologist shift as much of the care as possible back to the primary care physician to decrease the number of patient visits to the specialist's office? Will the timing of the shift to hospice care be earlier for the patient under capitated care compared with fee-for-service plans?[17] Are these shifts in the best interest of the patient?

### Case rates

*Case rates* provide the institution with a set amount of money per procedure or service, such as $2000 for a mastectomy. Case rate is the model used for the Medicare DRG system. *Global rate* is a case rate that encompasses both the physician component and hospital costs for specific incidents, such as the total inpatient stay for a mastectomy and the corresponding follow-up physician visits. The global rate prevents cost shifting from physicians to the hospital.

Two major strategies that providers can use to maximize reimbursement when using noncapitated methods of physician payment are churning and upcoding.[18] *Churning* refers to the practice of increasing procedures and visits to enhance revenue as fees are discounted. Effective utilization management strategies will minimize the practice, but will require a strict physician review structure that is costly to maintain. *Upcoding* occurs when physicians report a more complex level of care or diagnosis to enhance reimbursement. Both of these practices are unnecessary with a capitated model. It is clear that the capitated model with the corresponding financial incentives has the greatest potential to decrease utilization over any other payment model. The impact of this financial incentive is very apparent in California where capitation is common and hospital occupancy averages around 40%.[13]

Even as the capitation payment model has shown the largest potential in reducing costs, the movement to a capitated model throughout the United States (with the exception of California, Arizona, and Minnesota) has been slow in the payer, provider, and consumer segments for a variety of reasons. Payers are reluctant to move quickly to the capitated model because of the incredible profits being realized with noncapitated plans such as case rates. Consumers are demanding more choice and are reluctant to relinquish control to the "gatekeeper." Though some providers are attempting to optimize profits during this transitional period by continuing acute-care admissions for services that can be done in the outpatient area (such as chemotherapy administration), many providers prefer capitated payment to facilitate the shift to a health-oriented/preventive model. The capitated model would allow funding of creative programs that meet the needs of patients, such as community programs focused upon prevention.

As we move along the health system continuum from fee-for-service/per diem/case rate/capitated payment model, many modifications will be necessary. In fee-for-service programs, there is a loose alignment of physicians and hospitals; in a capitated environment, the affiliation must be strong and collaborative. Organizational structures also will be modified to reflect the enhanced collaborative relationship between physicians and the organization. Additionally, information systems linking hospitals and physicians become paramount to survival in a capitated payment model.

## Determining Cost of Service

In the initial stages of the transition to a mature managed care market, price of the service becomes the single most important factor in obtaining contracts. In many markets, a cost-accounting system that is linked with the clinical system is essential for survival of the health system. These sophisticated financial systems allow for analysis of clinical resource utilization patterns so that timely strategies can be developed to decrease costs. Patient care cannot be redesigned by financial officers; only clinicians delivering care can reengineer the care. Physicians and nurses must lead the cost savings initiatives by collaborating in the analysis of the data and using tools such as critical pathways and case management to determine best practices. It is necessary for the nurse and physician to attain a basic understanding of costs and the associated terminology to determine the cost impact of proposed changes.

### Charges/cost

The first step in analyzing cost of service is to determine the costs of the specific diagnoses being examined. It is important not to confuse charge with cost. The charge is simply the price that is set initially for the service, while the cost is the actual dollar amount it takes to deliver the service. In the last few years hospitals have had to invest substantial dollars in cost-accounting systems to allow determination of "true" costs. Some organizations have attempted this analysis using a proxy of a cost-to-charge ratio that has skewed the data and can have an impact on the overall credibility of the analysis. With more sophisticated systems, the information is obtained from multiple sources and is transferred into data repositories where the integration is accomplished and a written or electronic report can be generated. The information collected includes the tests, procedures, and services used by the patient on a daily basis. The data are merged with the diagnoses abstracted by the medical records department. Nurses need to understand the components and the process of the electronic cost-accounting system to analyze the data and identify opportunities to enhance the system. For example, the decision to track services such as time on the ventilator in either block- or actual-time intervals may have an impact on the ability to determine the effects of a reengineering initiative. Understanding the system's process will allow for increased credibility and utilization of the data.

### Net revenue

In the era of fee-for-service, charges were interchangeable with revenue as payers reimbursed providers for full charges. However, payers are now routinely negotiating discounts from providers; thus net revenue (discounts subtracted from the charges) is the primary number to review when revenue is examined.

### Direct/indirect costs

Costs are classified from two different perspectives: behavior in relation to volume and ability to trace the service to a patient.[19] The latter is separated into two categories: direct and indirect. Direct costs can be traced clearly to a specific patient or service. Examples of direct costs are laboratory tests and medications. Indirect costs frequently are referred to as overhead costs and cannot be assigned directly to a specific patient, but need to be spread across all patients.

### Variable/fixed costs

The next two types of costs are variable and fixed. Variable costs change in relation to the number of patients cared for; for example, the amount of linen used will vary with the number of patients in the hospital. The fixed costs remain stable as the number of patients changes. An example of fixed costs is administrative salaries such as those for head nurses and educators. In most hospitals variable and fixed costs are divided into four major categories: variable direct labor, variable direct supplies, fixed direct labor, and overhead. Variable direct labor is represented by staff nurse salaries while fixed direct labor includes the head nurse or clinical nurse specialist. Variable direct supplies are those used in direct patient care, such as linen or medications. Overhead costs are not directly attributed to patients and include engineering services or human resources departments.

### Net operating income

Once the net operating revenue is determined (by subtracting the discount negotiated by the payer from the charges), total operating costs can be subtracted to obtain the net operating income. It is important to exclude any investment income to determine the measure of operating success. By dividing net operating income into the net revenue, the profit margin percent ratio can be obtained. Unfortunately, some hospitals are experiencing only a 2%–3% profit margin, thereby making it difficult to recapitalize operations with new technology or information systems necessary to succeed in a capitated environment. The same formula (total costs subtracted from net revenue) can be applied to specific programs, such as oncology programs, to determine their break-even point.

## INDUSTRY RESPONSE TO THE ECONOMIC ENVIRONMENT

As the health care industry attempts to define what it will be in the next century, hospitals, physicians, and other care providers scramble to position for the future. A complicating factor, to say the least, is that health care is in transition—we are caught in the transition from the fee-for-service model to a managed-care system. We are not sure what the delivery system will evolve into in order to meet future needs. However, some of the universal actions being taken are described briefly in the following sections.

### Move to Outpatient Care

By the year 2000, a multispecialty group of 40 physicians will be capable of performing in its offices 80%–90% of the procedures currently performed in a 300-bed community hospital.[20] The bottom line for hospitals is that a 50%–60% excess inpatient capacity in many markets is leading to brutal, unrelenting price competition and the necessity for massive downsizing.

### Implementation of Case Management

Case management is a collaborative process that promotes quality care for the individual and cost-effective results or outcomes for the health care coverage provider.[21] Typically, case managers are registered nurses who are responsible for managing care for patients with complex and potentially costly diseases such as cancer. Case managers act as advocates for both the patient and the program by assessing the patient's needs and determining what resources are appropriate for that particular patient. More importantly, the case manager follows treatment pathways and determines if outcome goals are being met.

### Development/Utilization of Critical Pathways and Guidelines

The development of critical pathways results in a plan of action that delineates the critical components or key indicators necessary to achieve a given outcome at the most efficient cost.[22] Programs that develop guidelines to effectively manage length of stay and resource consumption, manage utilization of services, integrate activities of both clinicians and management, and establish guidelines for variance management are in the forefront of positioning for change.

### Implications for Nursing

As both academic cancer centers and community programs position to remain competitive in the marketplace, personnel costs, especially costs of professional caregivers, have been the target of cost-cutting efforts. For example, in 1995, the Norris Cancer Center Hospital reported that RNs made up only 60% of the direct-care staff, down from 100% five years earlier, and the numbers are expected to fall as low as 40%.[23] Nursing positions have been replaced with lesser-trained individuals.

## NURSING APPROACHES TO THE CHANGING HEALTH CARE ENVIRONMENT

### Partnering with MDs

As resources become more scarce, the need to coordinate care among disciplines is essential since more than one profession cares for the patient. Inability to achieve collaboration in patient care will lead to fragmentation of care with increased costs and decreased patient satisfaction. Not only is coordination important in the clinical area to enhance patient care, but the participation of the physician leader on the administrative team will assist the organization in planning strategic objectives. Physicians have moved from being a customer of nursing to being a partner of nursing. This administrative partnership foreshadows the economic incentive alignment that is found with global capitated contracts. Once a capitated contract is in place, the PHO will drive the operational decisions because of the financial risk of both partners. Scrutiny of the costs per case (represented by clinical resource utilization) and cost per unit (department costs and productivity) should take place in the PHO to facilitate a collaborative approach. Shared positions between hospital and physician groups such as case managers and decision support analysts should be jointly funded by both hospital and physician groups to mutually support the programs. Until the financial incentives are aligned with global capitated contracts, administrative structures placing physicians and nurses into joint clinical leadership positions must be created to position the organization for the future. For-profit organizations are also exploring equity models in which physicians own a share of the for-profit corporation. Some hospitals have physician and nursing leaders as partners in providing day-to-day operational direction to specific service lines such as cancer. This strategy is successful in aligning physician-hospital partnerships in areas where capitation-type payment has not significantly penetrated the market.

## Benchmarking

Benchmarking identifies "best practice" in relation to current performance.[24] There are several indicators that are extremely helpful to benchmark: skill mix, nursing hours per patient day (NHPPD), cost per case, and length of stay. Sovie[25] suggests that we should never be satisfied with achieving the benchmark since it is a moving target in our fast-paced health care environment. It is also important that we understand the systems that support these best practices. For example, modifications to facilities may be necessary, such as changing an intensive care unit from private rooms to an open bed floor plan to support a proposed staff reduction of 25%. Electronic medical records may be required to achieve some of the outstanding reductions in NHPPD being quoted by some organizations. A question to be asked when benchmarking is: What systems and facilities are needed to support the benchmarked practices? Some hospitals have used commercial sources such as proprietary databases or consulting groups to obtain benchmarking data. The Internet can also provide easy access to benchmarking among different health care providers.

## Productivity Standards/Skill Mix

Since the cost of labor, particularly nursing, in most hospitals is the largest and most significant cost (usually in the range of 80%–85%), defining NHPPD for the specific units is critical to achieving financial targets and can be essential for a hospital's survival. Skill mix (percent of licensed to unlicensed staff) on a nonintensive care unit averages 55/45; however, in some hospitals under heavy price competition, the skill mix can be as low as 30/70. Involving the staff in collecting the benchmark data on the NHPPD promotes acceptance of the validity of the data more effectively than a "top-down" approach.

The nursing staff at St. Joseph Mercy Hospital in Ann Arbor, MI, embarked on a benchmark initiative with eight hospitals around the country to measure NHPPD and skill mix. The selected hospitals were similar to St. Joseph Mercy Hospital in acuity as measured by case mix and patient populations. These hospitals also were chosen because they differ from St. Joseph Mercy Hospital in terms of degree of managed care penetration in their area of the country and for-profit status. This allowed the staff to begin to plan for the future and not simply react to local changes. The distance between the hospitals allowed for frank and honest answers because the hospitals were noncompetitive. With the benchmarking data collected, it was evident that St. Joseph Mercy Hospital nursing units were generally functioning 5%–10% higher than the median NHPPD. Skill mix was in line with the hospitals surveyed.

The nursing profession continues to investigate in a variety of settings, both locally and nationally, the impact of downsizing on the quality of care rendered. In 1996 a report from the Committee on the Adequacy of Nurse Staffing in Hospitals and Nursing Homes from the Division of Health Care Services in the Institute of Medicine[26] concluded that insufficient data exist to support the concern that quality of care is negatively affected by the decrease in the ratio of licensed to unlicensed nursing personnel. Quality indicators are being developed by multiple professional organizations to begin measuring the impact of changes in registered nurse ratios and NHPPD upon care of the patient.

## Outcome Measurements

Clinical guidelines and outcome studies need to be coordinated rather than conducted on parallel tracks.[27] As guidelines are developed and implemented, the corresponding patient outcomes should be identified and monitored. Patient morbidity and mortality, patient satisfaction, and quality indicators such as medication errors and patient falls should be included in outcome data. Outcomes need to be retrieved electronically to decrease the time lag of data retrieval and facilitate a faster feedback loop. Guidelines should be modified to represent "best practice" as outcome data become available. In response to aggressively managed guidelines by HMOs and the advent of outcomes research[28–30] a new field has emerged: disease management. The underlying premise is that chronic diseases such as cancer or diabetes can be managed more effectively long term (lower costs and increased quality of life) by protocol-driven actions along the continuum of care. These protocols can encompass education and prevention as well as self-care activities. It is clear that nursing can provide a broad understanding of these initiatives and link the conceptual ideas with the financial-based realities.

# SPECIFIC ECONOMIC ISSUES IN CANCER CARE

In September 1994 the National Cancer Advisory Board (NCAB) Subcommittee to Evaluate the National Cancer Program presented the results of their evaluation undertaken to assess the achievements of the National Cancer

Program, to identify barriers to reducing the burden of cancer, and to make recommendations for future research and program directions.[31] The Subcommittee identified six major issues to be addressed if we are to prevail in our war on cancer:

1. Current *health care reform* proposals are devastating to the War on Cancer by denying resources for research and quality cancer care.
2. The National Cancer Program suffers from an *absence of national coordination* of cancer-fighting efforts in the public, private, and voluntary sectors.
3. Many people in this country, especially the poor, elderly, and uninsured, receive *inadequate cancer care.*
4. Current *laws, public policy, and governmental regulation* undermine cancer prevention, treatment, and control efforts.
5. Failure to support *translational research* hinders rapid development of cancer-fighting advances.
6. Current investment is insufficient to capitalize on *unprecedented opportunities in basic science research.*

The Subcommittee advised Congress to include in any health care reform plan as part of the core benefit package universal access to cancer care coverage that includes quality preventive, diagnostic, treatment, and rehabilitative/supportive services, including services provided in qualified clinical trials.

The issues identified by the Subcommittee summarize those areas to be addressed by cancer programs as they position for the future.

## Oncology Networks

It is clear that success in a managed-care environment will depend upon the ability to provide cost-effective, comprehensive care and to appropriately affiliate/align with physicians and other institutions. The concepts of *oncology networks and integrated systems* have emerged to respond to changes in payer relationships, reimbursement methods, contract requirements, provider affiliations, and changes in the status quo.[32] Ironically, yesterday's fierce competitors have become today's strategic partners.

The key components of value in integrated delivery systems include:[33]

1. Competitive position, based on increased efficiency and productivity rather than cost shifting
2. Standardized diagnostic/treatment protocols to decrease practice variances
3. Quality patient outcomes and survival rates that can be measured, documented, and communicated
4. Service level accessibility with appropriate geographic distribution

### Hospital alliances

A number of models for hospital alliances have been described[34] (Table 56-1). A simple alliance model aligns cancer programs at separate hospitals and retains separate day-to-day management of the two cancer programs. In this type of alliance, only a few functions tend to be centralized including some central purchasing, cancer education activities, and perhaps development of a global research function or alliance-wide guidelines/critical pathway development. There is little financial savings to this model, and there is duplication of overhead and some services.

A second structure identified as a "feeder" system aligns smaller hospitals offering fewer cancer services with larger centers that offer more specialized care. With this system, the entire spectrum of standard cancer care—from prevention to terminal care—is available. The smaller hospitals or "feeder" facilities have responsibility for primary detection, diagnosis, and surgery, with referral to the larger hospitals for tertiary and quarternary care needs.

The third model features a strong, centralized ownership of facilities. In this scenario, a number of poorly organized cancer programs form an alliance and decide to consolidate all of their programs at a single facility or at a few of their facilities. The benefits of this type of alliance are the elimination of redundant resources and the consolidation of best staff, physicians, and facilities at a central location.

The fourth model links a hospital or provider of care with an oncology "carve-out" organization. The carve-out may be a commercial firm, such as Caremark, American Oncology Resources, Salick Health Care, Inc., or Texas Oncology; it also may be a joint venture between several hospitals. In effect, the carve-out takes charge of all cancer care provided to alliance members. It capitates oncology patients, providing medical oncology and radiation oncology, and perhaps contracts for hospital beds and facilities as needed. The oncology carve-out organization assumes all risks for patient care, which may be a benefit to the hospital(s). On the other hand, the carve-out sets the quality for the hospital alliance.

### Physician/hospital alliances

While the preceding models describe various types of hospital alliances, fundamental to the concept of networks is the inclusion of physicians in any and all models.[35,36] Hospitals bring value to their physician partners, including access to capital, management and information system expertise, care continuity components, and education.

In a capitated environment, numerous services are typically provided by a network through its participants or through ancillary provider contracts:

*Office-based Services*

- Medical, radiation, and surgical oncology
- Malignant hematology
- Chemotherapy administration
- Selected drugs and supplies
- Office-based laboratory

**TABLE 56-1**   Models for Hospital Alliances

| Hospital Alliance Model | Key Features | Issues |
|---|---|---|
| Distributed Model | • Builds upon existing cancer programs at alliance institutions <br><br> • Supports separate administrative and medical directors <br><br> • Minimal centralized functions (e.g., educational planning, critical pathway development) | • Expensive and redundant overhead <br><br> • Duplication of services |
| Feeder System Model | • Alliance plays a much stronger centralized management role in system planning, monitoring, development. <br><br> • Smaller facilities perform diagnosis and surgery; "feed" patients to other hospitals for next level of care. <br><br> • Second-tier hospitals offer specialized cancer care (e.g., radiation oncology, chemotherapy). <br><br> • Third-tier hospitals provide tertiary care, full services including clinical trials, specialists (e.g., GYN oncology, BMT, pediatric oncology). <br><br> • Fourth tier (Alliance Level)—Full-time program administrative and physician leadership provide systemwide program development. | • Minimizes duplication of expensive overhead, allows for coordinated planning, and offers the potential for an integrated oncology organization attractive to MDs and purchasers of care <br><br> • Most facilities in this alliance model will take on a role that will not change in the future, since they will be locked in by corporate strategy dictated by the alliance. |
| Consolidation Model | • Strong, centralized ownership of facilities <br><br> • Consolidation of multiple cancer programs at a single facility or at a few of the alliance facilities | • Elimination of redundant resources <br><br> • Consolidation of the best staff, MDs, and facilities at a central location <br><br> • Alliance manages the financing, planning, and investment activities |
| Carve-out Model | • Relationship between an oncology "carve-out" organization and hospital(s) <br><br> • Carve-out organization capitates oncology patients, provides medical and radiation oncology, inpatient care. <br><br> • Carve-out organization sets the quality standards. | • Benefits to hospital are that the carve-out organization assumes all the risks for patient care; this may mean lower financial returns for hospital. |

Adapted from Mortenson LE.[34]

*Hospital-based services*
• Inpatient medical and surgical care

• Laboratory/pathology

• Diagnostic imaging

• Radiation oncology

*Ancillary provider-based services*
• Home care services

• Pain management

• Hospice

• Psychosocial counseling/supportive care

• Durable medical equipment

## Physician networks

Physician networks, both large and small, are also developing to bring together those physicians of varying specialties involved in the delivery of cancer care. This structure supports the physicians' abilities to contract with third-party payers to be the preferred or exclusive providers of care to an identified population of individuals.[37]

While oncology practices have traditionally consisted of only a few doctors, the past several years have witnessed the same networking in this area as in other specialties. One of the fastest-growing methods for grouping together is a physician practice management group, or PPM. The doctors sell their practices to a PPM. The PPM takes over the assets, administration, and nonmedical chores of cancer treatment. The doctors agree to practice exclusively in affiliation with the PPM. The PPM typically gets 10% of the practice revenues and 100% of the revenues from ancillary services like chemotherapy infusion.[38] The advantage to the physicians is that they do not have to deal with the administration of the practice, which has become increasingly complex and time-consuming.

### Academic center alliances

A number of alliances have occurred both among academic institutions and among academic institutions and community organizations. For example, the Dana-Farber Cancer Institute has consolidated its cancer services with Brigham and Women's Hospital and Massachusetts General Hospital (Partners' Health Care) in a pioneering joint venture. Managed care contract positioning was a primary factor driving this mega-networking venture. In 1996 the network had a combined total of over 6000 newly diagnosed cancer patients, 220,000 cancer outpatient visits, and $126 million in federal cancer center and research support.[39]

The University of Michigan Medical Center pioneered the development of radiation oncology professional services and joint venture networking with community hospitals. The UMMC faculty provide professional services at a number of teaching and community hospitals in southeastern Michigan.[39] This type of venture combines the strengths of each institution while reducing and/or sharing costs. It avoids service duplication while increasing regional cooperation and patient access to services close to home.

The City of Hope, a widely recognized cancer center in southern California, has developed a national network based upon the strategy of "virtual" integration. This network has been developed without the purchase of hospital facilities or physician practices. Network physicians and hospitals are credentialed by City of Hope, and care is provided under "stringent" guidelines. Much of the care is provided by network physicians in the community, and more complex cases are referred to City of Hope. This national network already holds contracts for 1 million covered lives in HMO carve-outs and center-of-excellence agreements with insurers.[1]

## Clinical Trials

Both the National Cancer Institute and the pharmaceutical industry sponsor clinical trials research. Trials sponsored by drug companies generally do not pose a financial concern for oncology programs, since the drug(s) being investigated are provided by the pharmaceutical company and funding is usually sufficient to cover the costs of conducting the research. A major barrier for both patients and institutions to participation in national studies is that third-party payers do not cover experimental treatment, which includes all research trials. The National Cancer Institute budget proposal for fiscal years 1997 and 1998,[40] states:

> Our ability to conduct clinical trials is in danger of being compromised by changes in the health care system. In the past, institutions have used surplus revenues from patient care services to supplement government research support. The growth of managed care has all but eliminated those discretionary funds. As a result, institutions can no longer sponsor research activities requiring capital expenditures and cannot support essential training for young investigators. These changes pose a very real danger for the continuation of cancer research and our ultimate success against cancer. University-based and NCI-designated comprehensive cancer centers traditionally have focused on research and education as their primary missions.

More recently, clinical services have become increasingly important because of the need for supplementing funding sources to support the primary missions of research and education. Conversely, the focus of community oncology programs has always been on clinical service, with research and education as secondary functions. Of significant importance, however, is that more than 50% of all patients accrued to cancer clinical trials are entered by community-based oncologists.[41]

From a community program perspective, the benefit to participation in clinical trials is the ability to provide patients access to state-of-the-art therapies for cancer treatment, control, and prevention. As institutions compete for managed-care contracts, the ability to offer comprehensive, cutting-edge care to populations of patients will become more crucial than at present. As an example of the growing focus on clinical research, the American College of Surgeons' Commission on Cancer now mandates participation in clinical research for accreditation of institutions with 750 cancer diagnoses per year.[42] Yet the challenge for hospitals and oncology program administrators is how to balance the additional costs of a research program infrastructure with the increasing pressures of cost containment and the threat of decreasing federal support.

From the third-party payers' standpoint, a very public and controversial battle has been waged over the use of high-dose chemotherapy autologous bone marrow transplants (HCD-ABMT) in women with advanced breast cancer. Insurers have, in many cases, refused to pay because this treatment is "experimental," "investigational," "not medically necessary," or "not medically accepted." An increase in litigation against insurers by women with breast cancer has forced courts to decide the experimental status of particular medical treatments. These decisions ultimately have broad implications for health care policy.

Insurers have developed various criteria for defining the experimental status of medical treatments and procedures that relate to one or more of the following categories:[43]

*Scientific criteria* In a scientific category insurers may require that the proposed treatment reach a certain percent success ratio, successfully complete various levels of clinical trial, be well received in peer-reviewed literature, or be superior to all existing procedures.

*Research criteria*   The research category focuses on the administration of the treatment, whereby insurers, when making coverage determinations, may consider consent forms, research protocols, or clinical trials as indicative of a treatment's experimental nature.

*Professional criteria*   In this category, great emphasis is placed on the consensus of medical professionals. Insurers may insist that the treatment be the standard, accepted practice among medical professionals either nationally or within a designated geographic area. Some insurers further require that the treatment be officially endorsed by a nationally recognized medical organization or governmental body.

More recently, a number of third-party payers have charged committees, composed of experts in the field, to assess which treatments are experimental under their policy's criteria. For example, Blue Cross/Blue Shield of Michigan has aligned with the Michigan Society of Hematology/Oncology to address these questions. Other states have enacted legislation specific to the approval of HDC-ABMT for women with breast cancer. Of greater encouragement is the action being taken by the National Association of Insurance Commissioners (NAIC) to work on model legislation regarding insurance coverage for experimental treatments, referred to as "new health services."[44] Support by NAIC is significant in that it represents suggested state legislation by the nation's state insurance commissioners.

In California, managed care has had a deleterious effect on clinical research. Within the community, the use of treatment protocols has diminished as HMOs have adhered strictly to the contract criterion of exclusion of payment for investigational care.[17] Partially as a result of this, the number of Community Clinical Oncology Programs (CCOPs) in California funded by NCI decreased from seven in 1983 to two in 1994. HMOs that succeed in the future likely will have a way of including clinical investigation protocols for willing patients and evaluating the pharmacoeconomic effect of newer types of technologies and newer types of drugs on total managed-care expenditures.

Of primary concern is whether oncology programs will be able to financially support participation in cancer prevention and control trials in the future. The NCI clearly is committed to research to prevent cancer as well as to improve the quality of life for those who develop cancer.[40] The breast cancer (Tamoxifen) and prostate cancer (Proscar) chemoprevention trials are hallmarks of this effort. A number of cancer control studies have led to improvements in the quality of life of cancer patients. Recent supportive care research has defined better clinical strategies to deal with cancer pain, allowing for better use of widely available pain medications and the development of more-effective, longer-acting antipain drugs. Today's health care environment does not offer financial support for these types of research.

## Cancer Drugs and Managed Care

There are two major concerns regarding cancer drugs in the managed-care environment. The first is whether or not new drug research will be slowed as the snowballing influence of managed care intensifies. The second is the long-standing need for approval of off-label usage of chemotherapeutic agents.

The first issue was partially addressed in March 1996 when the White House announced a plan to speed new drugs to the market. Under the FDA's new rules, anticancer drugs may be given early market approval before their effectiveness is proven conclusively, if drug companies can show that the drugs shrink tumors.[45] Furthermore, the FDA agreed to attempt to speed approval of drugs that have already been approved in other countries.

A survey entitled "New Medicines in Development for Cancer" by the Pharmaceutical Research and Manufacturers of America points optimistically to a vigorous lineup of oncology drugs in the pipeline.[46] The survey identifies 215 medicines in testing by 98 research-based pharmaceutical companies and the National Cancer Institute. In the period from 1993 to 1995, the number of medicines in development for cancer and cancer-related conditions increased dramatically (from 124 to 215) as the number of companies involved (from 49 to 98). Overall, U.S. pharmaceutical companies have increased their research and development spending from $12.7 billion in 1993 to $15 billion in 1995. The survey also shows that multiple agents are in development that target a broad range of cancers. Specifically, biotechnology is a leading focus of oncology research.

Off-label usage of antineoplastic drugs is becoming less of an issue as model legislation is being approved across the country on a statewide basis. In the 1980s, the government and insurance companies began to deny reimbursement for drugs used for indications outside of the package-insert indications approved by the FDA. In practice, once a drug has received FDA approval, the pharmaceutical company will not necessarily reapply to the FDA when additional indications for the drug's use are identified. Since the early 1990s the Association of Community Cancer Centers (ACCC) has led an effort to introduce model legislation requiring insurance companies to use the drug compendia and the peer-reviewed medical literature in making coverage determinations rather than using the FDA-labeled indication. In 1996 nineteen states had such a law in place. Furthermore, the National Association of Insurance Commissioners adopted a model act that seeks to prevent unfair discrimination among insured individuals; it is very similar to the ACCC bill in that it uses the drug compendia and peer-reviewed medical literature in making coverage determinations.[44]

## Critical Pathways/Care Guidelines

Activity in the area of development of oncology practice guidelines has paralleled that of the national (and international) movement in general and ranks as a priority for most hospitals and health care providers.[47,48] Guidelines are meant to improve the quality of care overall and achieve better outcomes by improving the consistency of care and identifying inappropriate care. Development of guidelines generally is prioritized according to those areas that are important to an organization, such as high-risk, high-volume, or high-cost diagnoses, procedures, or cases. Cancer care often meets all three criteria.

A number of national-level efforts to develop cancer treatment guidelines are underway. In 1994 the American Society of Clinical Oncology (ASCO) published a guideline on the use of hematopoietic colony-stimulating factors. The National Comprehensive Cancer Network, a consortium of NCI-funded comprehensive cancer centers, has published preliminary practice guidelines for breast cancer (noninvasive and invasive), small cell lung cancer, non-small cell lung cancer, and colon cancer; this group plans to develop treatment guidelines for 22 cancers that represent 90% of malignancies in the United States.

The Association of Community Cancer Centers (ACCC), with a large number of national and state oncology societies, has embarked on an effort to develop guidelines to ensure adequate reimbursement of appropriate care.[49] ACCC's intention is that the guidelines be descriptive of the primary approaches to manage patients and serve as mechanisms that can be used in several different ways. First, managed-care providers and other insurers can use the guidelines as a representation of current standard care. Physicians and hospitals can use the guidelines as a means of costing standard cancer care. Hospitals, alliances, and physician groups can use the guidelines as a starting point for critical pathway development. Additionally, guidelines will provide a framework for evaluating care.

Critical pathways usually describe a protocol specific for a particular organization or for a detailed patient management plan for a specific procedure. A critical pathway for DRG 410—chemotherapy is shown in Figure 56-1. This pathway was implemented in 1992 at the McAuley Cancer Care Center, St. Joseph Mercy Hospital, Ann Arbor, MI. Although most chemotherapy was administered in the outpatient clinic at that time, the length of stay (LOS) for those patients requiring admission was significantly higher at 4.2 days than the national average of 3.0. The care process was analyzed, and it was determined that the admitting process often added at least one day to the LOS, since patients were not admitted until late afternoon and orders for chemotherapy administration were not written until evening. By developing a pathway that allows patients to begin receiving chemotherapy in the outpatient clinic at 8:00 A.M. prior to a hospital bed being available, the LOS has been decreased to 2.2 days. The patient is transferred to the inpatient unit when a bed becomes available. Not only have these changes decreased LOS, but they have increased patient and family satisfaction as they no longer sit at home and wait to be called by the admitting department.

A clinical algorithm is a third type of guideline or pathway that clearly defines decision points in the care process and provides explicit directions to the caregiver. Figure 56-2 was developed for the management of sepsis-related hypotension on the oncology impatient unit, thereby eliminating the former practice of transferring all hypotensive patients to the intensive care unit.

Health reform, managed care, and computers will drive the use of guidelines in the years ahead. Some of the most significant reform plans being considered in Washington would require the widespread use of clinical practice guidelines. The reform plans being contemplated aim to reduce the practice of defensive medicine and improve health care quality by using best practices and reducing unwarranted and inappropriate care.[50] However, we must be careful to ensure that guidelines indeed reflect the best practice rather than only decreasing variation and focusing on the consensus of the majority.

Future guideline development will require definition of care across the continuum—not just for specific episodes of care. For example, as managed care or discounted fee-for-service plans further restrict use of ancillary services such as physical therapy, critical pathways must delineate the coordination of rehabilitation services including those that occur in the hospital, those provided by the home care agency, and continuing outpatient services if required. The rehabilitation plan must be viewed in its entirety with specific goals for each segment of the continuum.

Guidelines cannot be developed in and of themselves but must be developed in conjunction with collecting and analyzing outcomes data. The key to the future lies in the ability to improve clinical practice. Researchers at Johns Hopkins have demonstrated dramatic improvements in patient outcomes when guidelines have been developed from the clinical practice perspective—not the cost control perspective. With improvement in patient outcomes, costs have also been significantly reduced.[51]

## Continuum of Care

The move to a managed-care system presents to nursing some wonderful opportunities along with challenges. Coordinated care across the continuum is becoming a major focus driven by the need to be efficient in delivering the right care in the right setting. A number of initiatives hold promise for improvements in the provision of care and consumer outcomes:

**1.** Oncology care has long emphasized the diagnostic and treatment segments of the continuum of care. The shift to the left of the continuum with emphasis on prevention and keeping people healthy presents opportunities for oncology caregivers in the area of smoking prevention/cessation programs and dietary/nutritional counseling, among others. Employers across the country are incorporating into their employee health plans incen-

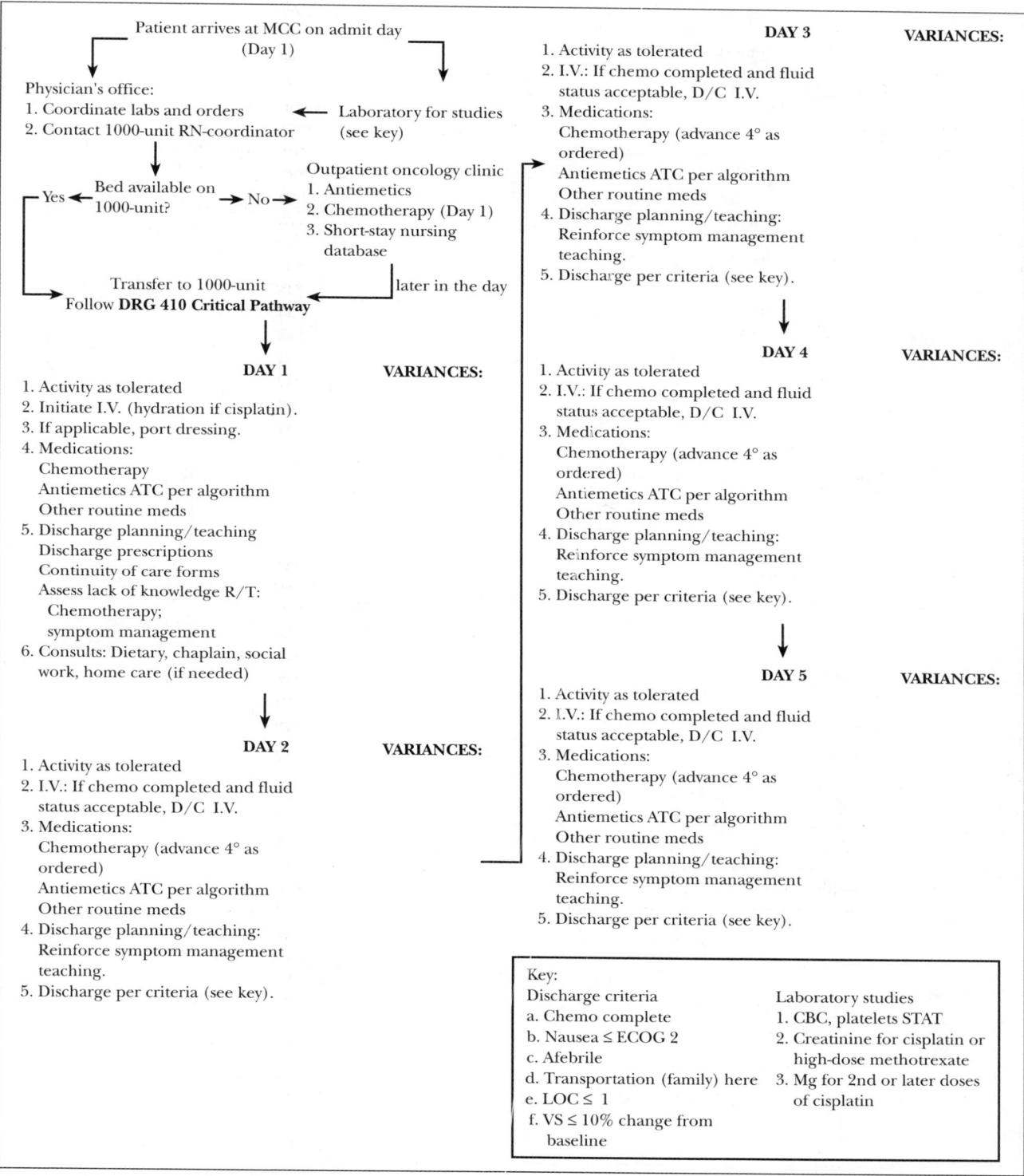

**FIGURE 56-1**  Critical pathway for DRG 410—chemotherapy.

tives for participating in wellness activities. Furthermore, HMOs and third-party payers are including clauses in their policies that allow different levels of coverage based upon the insured's health habits. The National Cancer Institute is placing greater emphasis on cancer prevention clinical trials. Together these efforts dictate to health care providers the need for greater emphasis on prevention programs.

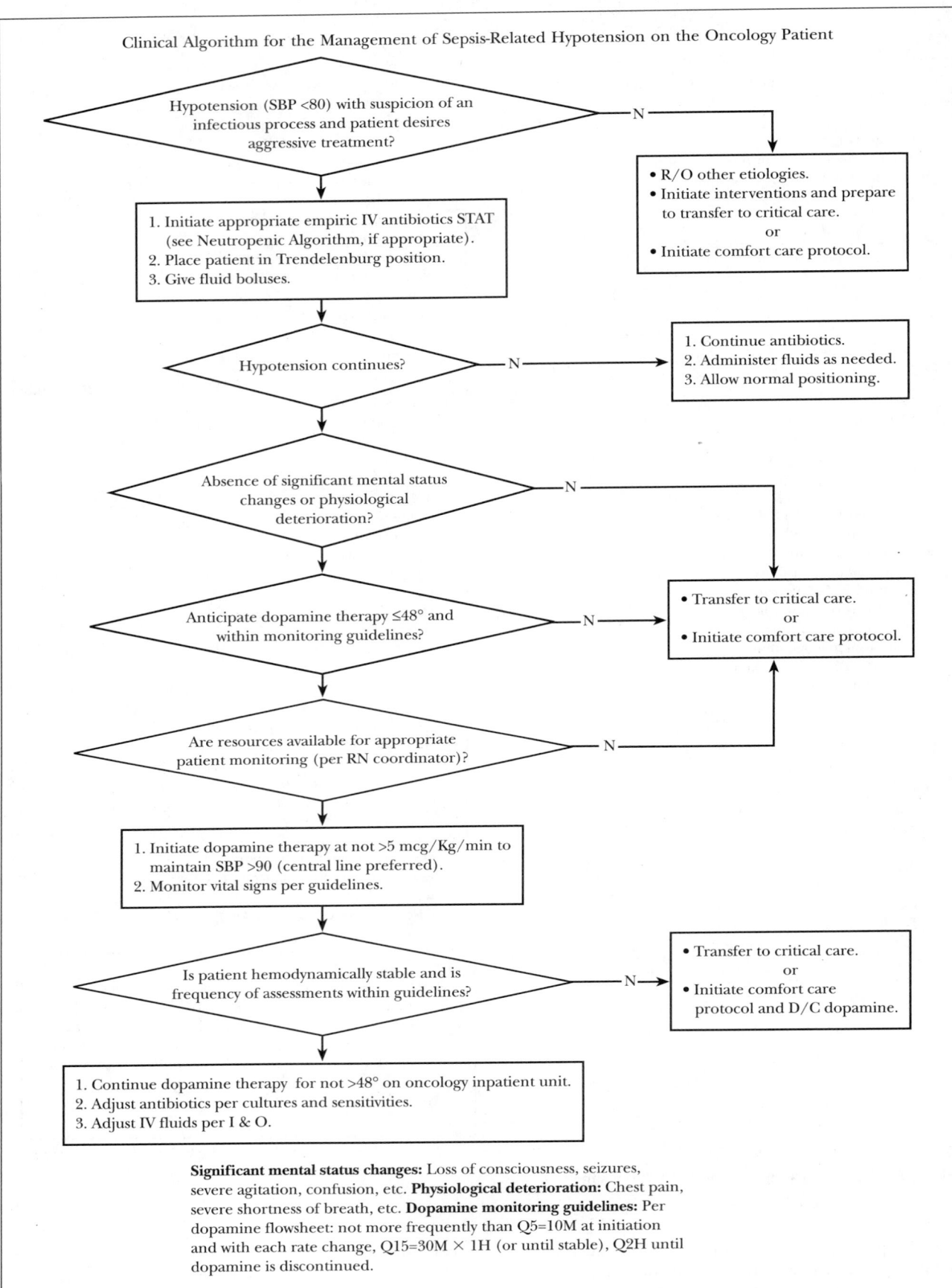

Clinical Algorithm for the Management of Sepsis-Related Hypotension on the Oncology Patient

Hypotension (SBP <80) with suspicion of an infectious process and patient desires aggressive treatment?

N →

- R/O other etiologies.
- Initiate interventions and prepare to transfer to critical care.
  or
- Initiate comfort care protocol.

1. Initiate appropriate empiric IV antibiotics STAT (see Neutropenic Algorithm, if appropriate).
2. Place patient in Trendelenburg position.
3. Give fluid boluses.

Hypotension continues?

N →

1. Continue antibiotics.
2. Administer fluids as needed.
3. Allow normal positioning.

Absence of significant mental status changes or physiological deterioration?

N →

Anticipate dopamine therapy ≤48° and within monitoring guidelines?

N →

- Transfer to critical care.
  or
- Initiate comfort care protocol.

Are resources available for appropriate patient monitoring (per RN coordinator)?

N →

1. Initiate dopamine therapy at not >5 mcg/Kg/min to maintain SBP >90 (central line preferred).
2. Monitor vital signs per guidelines.

Is patient hemodynamically stable and is frequency of assessments within guidelines?

N →

- Transfer to critical care.
  or
- Initiate comfort care protocol and D/C dopamine.

1. Continue dopamine therapy for not >48° on oncology inpatient unit.
2. Adjust antibiotics per cultures and sensitivities.
3. Adjust IV fluids per I & O.

**Significant mental status changes:** Loss of consciousness, seizures, severe agitation, confusion, etc. **Physiological deterioration:** Chest pain, severe shortness of breath, etc. **Dopamine monitoring guidelines:** Per dopamine flowsheet: not more frequently than Q5=10M at initiation and with each rate change, Q15=30M × 1H (or until stable), Q2H until dopamine is discontinued.

**FIGURE 56-2**  Sepsis-related hypotension algorithm.

**2.** Initiatives are expected to grow for screening of those cancers for which early diagnosis benefits patient outcomes. Although funding for screening is minimal at best, as more data are collected on the cost and outcomes of care for patients diagnosed at late-stage disease versus early-stage disease, it is expected that an increased screening initiative will result.

**3.** Diagnostic workup and treatment planning will become more efficient with the increase in the number and availability of multispecialty clinics in the community setting. Until more recently, clinics at which patients had the opportunity to be evaluated by all appropriate specialists at one visit were provided primarily by academic institutions. However, physicians in the community are joining together to establish methods of care delivery that are patient-friendly and efficient. Community multispecialty clinics for specific cancer sites (e.g., breast, prostate) are becoming the norm.

**4.** Efficient movement of the patient across the continuum will continue and improve as case management becomes refined.

**5.** As care shifts to the outpatient setting, home care and hospice services will become more fully integrated into the care-planning and guideline-development process.

## ONCOLOGY NURSING: POSITIONING FOR THE FUTURE

Within the nursing profession, several values and assumptions must be reassessed to meet the future demands of health care systems.[52] These are reflected in the following four paradigm shifts:

**1.** Our practice must evolve from a needs-driven model of care to one that is sensitive to limited resources.
**2.** Nurses believe that there is a direct correlation between manpower and quality. The true correlation is between critical thinking and quality.
**3.** Standardization and routines for patient care will be replaced by individualization and creativity.
**4.** Accountability, responsibility, and authority for clinical decision making will evolve from the manager to the practitioner, in partnership with the patient.

### Nursing Roles

There is strong consensus that the role of hospital nursing as traditionally defined in the past is changing and will continue to change as care moves to ambulatory settings. The diminishing role of hospitals within the health care continuum means the real future for nurses may lie elsewhere: in HMOs, ambulatory surgery centers, home care, nursing homes, etc.[53]

Positioning for the twenty-first century requires consideration of the forecasts for cancer at the turn of the millenium. Table 56-2 lists ten major forecasts for cancer in the twenty-first century. As this table reflects, new "hybrids" of oncology nurses will emerge, evidenced by where and how they practice. These roles will result from changes in sites of care, technological advances, change in work focus, and innovations in the education of nurses.[54]

McCaffrey-Boyle et al[54] project the following changes:

**1.** Nurses will take on the role of health care broker (case manager), matching patient needs to finite resources. They will have admitting privileges to nursing homes, home care agencies, and community nursing centers.
**2.** Nurses' work focus will include an intense orientation to wellness, and they will render health-prescriptive services at the worksite.
**3.** Critical care oncology nurses of the future will manage symptom distress in a growing population of patients receiving aggressive treatments who require intensive monitoring and support. These nurses will have prescriptive capabilities, including titration of biologics and supervision of complex ventilator weaning and extubation.

### Advanced Practice Roles

Health care reform has brought the role of advanced practice nurses to the forefront. To meet future challenges within the health care arena, a combination of physician and nonphysician providers will be required. The evolution to managed care creates the market conditions under which physician extender positions will flourish. Evidence suggests that advanced practice nurses (APNs) can provide much of the primary care and many other basic services currently performed by physicians.[56] Advanced practice nursing encompasses several categories of care providers, including nurse practitioners (NPs), clinical nurse specialists (CNSs), certified nurse midwives (CNMs), and certified registered nurse anesthetists (CRNAs).

The Oncology Nursing Society (ONS) endorses the title *advanced practice nurse* (APN) to designate clinical nurse specialist (CNS) and nurse practitioner (NP) roles in oncology nursing.[57] The ONS notes that the term advanced practice nurse does *not* imply the merger of the CNS and NP roles, nor does it exclude other master's-prepared nurses in education, administration, or research roles. The advanced practice oncology nurse, prepared at a minimum with a master's degree in nursing, has direct and indirect clinical foci in the care of individuals affected by cancer and works in collaboration with nurse colleagues in practice, education, administration, and research.

Nurses in advanced practice roles can make major impacts in the following areas:

**1.** Provision of direct patient care, as a physician extender
**2.** Assisting the staff nurse to develop critical thinking

**TABLE 56-2** Ten Major Forecasts for Cancer in the Twenty-first Century

**Patient/Family Profile**

1. Tomorrow's consumers of cancer care will be dramatically different from those of today, predominated by people of advanced age and diverse ethnic backgrounds, by people living in poverty, and by those willing to assume a greater role in health care-related decision making.

**Social Support**

2. Social support dilemmas will be addressed by family mobilization and by unique intervention programs.

**Oncology Nurse Profiles**

3. New "hybrids" of oncology nurses will emerge, evidenced by where and how they practice.

**Patient Subgroups**

4. Cancer prevention, diagnosis, and treatment will be customized for and targeted to select patient subgroups.

**Therapeutic Paradigm**

5. Cancer management will be characterized by rapid technology transfer, emphasis on prevention, and aggressive multimodality treatment.

**Mind-Body Renaissance**

6. The "self-care movement" will drive a reintegration of a holistic healing and recovery orientation into cancer care.

**Influence of Ethics**

7. Ethical responsibilities will become an accentuated component of oncology nursing.

**Cancer Care Economics**

8. The hallmarks of cancer care economics will be universal access, fewer payers, rationing of care, and salaried professionals.

**Practice Setting**

9. Team-directed cancer care will be delivered in multiple community-based sites.

**Language Reorientation**

10. Cancer care will be articulated through novel communication technologies and governed intensively by quality and cost outcomes.

Reprinted with permission from McCaffrey-Boyle D, Engelking C, Harvey C: Making a difference in the 21st century: Are oncology nurses ready? *Onc Nurs Forum* (21)1, 54, 1994.[55]

skills, raising the level of assessment and expanding the synthesis of information in the care provided at the bedside as the number of graduate medical education programs decrease

3. Monitoring and evaluating outcomes of care, which are defined by quality and cost-effectiveness[58]

A major issue facing advanced practice nurses is one of reimbursement for services. APNs can provide high-quality, cost-effective care, yet obtaining reimbursement from many HMOs and insurance companies has been difficult. While health care is moving toward a system of capitated payment, it has not yet been determined how APNs will be reimbursed for their services.[59] Historically, nurse practitioners have been reimbursed for care when provided in collaboration with a physician; clinical nurse specialists have been excluded from any type of reimbursement. As health care dollars tighten, it is imperative that APNs clearly define their contribution to care and develop the skills to negotiate reimbursement privileges within the various health plans.

## Setting Ethical Standards

"Caring" has been the hallmark of nursing practice, and many nurses are concerned that their ability to care is being compromised by the tumultuous changes taking place in today's health care environment.[60] In addition nurses come face-to-face on a daily basis with questions related to the ethics of health care situations resulting from pressures to streamline or limit the use of resources.[61]

A disturbing study published in the *New England Journal of Medicine*[62] reported that 16% of nurses in intensive care units who responded to a survey related they had taken independent measures to end patients' lives. It is alarming that individual practitioners have allowed their personal values to interfere with professional practice decisions. Additionally, these actions have major implications with respect to public trust, and they must be condemned by all health care professionals.

The American Nurses' Association outlined the precepts that form a values base for the entire nursing profession in the ANA's *Code for Nurses*.[63] This code delineates the fundamental ethical mandates that apply to all nursing roles and transcend varied practice settings and changing clinical realities. In 1994, the Ethics Advisory Council (EAC) of the Oncology Nursing Society considered the need to either develop a philosophy statement and a code of ethics for ONS or to continue endorsement of the ANA's *Code for Nurses;* the EAC concluded that developing a distinct code of ethics was not necessary and reaffirmed ONS' support of the ANA's document. The EAC believed it was important to articulate the values of ONS. The Oncology Nursing Society's five core values of *respectful care, quality of life, competence, collegiality, and fairness* speak from the shared experience of oncology nurses and provide a context for applying the *Code for Nurses* in oncology nursing practice.[64]

One of the major forecasts for cancer care in the twenty-first century (see Table 56-2) is that ethical responsibilities will become an accentuated component of oncology nursing. To meet this challenge, the need for nurses to be ethically grounded and discerning will continue to grow.

## A CONTROVERSIAL ISSUE IN CANCER CARE

### Use of Unlicensed Personnel

Budgetary constraints and the effects of the nursing shortage of the late 1980s–early 1990s have caused a restructuring of the delivery of nursing care in acute care hospitals by the addition of unlicensed assistive personnel (AP) as a clinical support service to the professional nursing staff.[65] As a general rule, unlicensed assistive personnel, including nursing or patient care assistants and technicians, are used in simple bedside care; some hospitals provide additional training for higher-level tasks such as performing phlebotomies, electrocardiograms, or respiratory therapy treatments.

There are widely diverse opinions regarding the use of unlicensed personnel and the implications for both nursing practice and the quality of patient care. One study found that overall, nurses' job satisfaction was negatively correlated with performing non-nursing functions.[66] However, nurses are often uncomfortable with the supervision and delegation functions required by the use of unlicensed staff.[67]

The Institute of Medicine Committee on the Adequacy of Nursing Staffing in Hospitals and Nursing Homes conducted a study to measure the quality of care provided by both licensed and unlicensed caregivers; the ANA was not able to demonstrate a difference in the quality of care or in patient outcomes.[26] The nursing profession consistently has defined itself according to the performance of certain tasks, whereas the value of the professional is in the coordination of care as the patient moves through the system. Nurses must be cognizant of the fact that until they are able to clearly define the value of the professional caregiver, there will always be less expensive personnel available to perform tasks.

In March 1996, the Oncology Nursing Society presented a position paper entitled *Assistive Personnel: Their Use in Cancer Care.*[68] ONS proposes "the oncology nurse who assesses, plans, implements, monitors, intervenes, evaluates, and coordinates the patient's plan of care, regardless of the patient's disease status or the setting in which care is provided, is accountable and responsible for all nursing care tasks delegated by her/him to an AP." This paper states:

> Patient care activities may be delegated to APs when the patient is stable, has a predictable disease trajectory, controlled symptoms and side effects, and predictable care outcomes. Activities that may be delegated with appropriate supervision include:

- Activities of daily living
- Vital signs
- Measuring intake and output
- Non-nursing tasks such as clerical work, stocking supplies, and errands
- Other limited, routine, patient care activities

Patient care activities should not be delegated to APs when the patient's condition is not stable or when care outcomes are not predictable. These situations include, but are not limited to:

- Complex patients with multiple, interrelated problems (e.g., patients with acute leukemia not in remission or superior vena cava syndrome)
- Patients who are symptomatic due to critical lab values
- Patients who are undergoing bone marrow transplant
- Patients who are critically ill or medically unstable (e.g., patients with sepsis or DIC)
- Patients with uncontrolled or poorly controlled pain
- Patients with or who are exhibiting early signs/symptoms indicative of oncologic emergencies
- Patients with complex disease processes and poorly controlled symptoms and treatment-related side effects

Finally, the Oncology Nursing Society states that the following list of nursing care functions, although neither exhaustive nor all inclusive, *should be performed* by oncology registered nurses (with appropriate education and experience) and *should not be delegated* to APs:

- Antineoplastic and biotherapy administration and management
- Assessment and management of patients receiving brachytherapy
- Pain assessment and management
- Wound assessment and management
- Symptom assessment, management, and toxicity grading
- Extravasation assessment and management
- Medication administration, assessment, and management
- Assessment and management of patient and family psychosocial needs
- Disease, treatment, and survivorship-related patient and family education
- Clinical trials education, administration, and documentation
- Assessment, management, and troubleshooting of intravenous catheters; venous, arterial, peritoneal, and intraventricular access devices; and ambulatory pumps (routine site care may be delegated)

- Assessment and management of long-term survivor issues

- Assessment and management of end-of-life care (components of care and/or comfort measures may be delegated)

- Facilitation of advanced directives

- Communication with multidisciplinary team members

- Development, assessment, and evaluation of patient care plans and discharge planning (in collaboration with others)

## CONCLUSION

As we approach the twenty-first century, the one constant on which we can count is that change—often swift and dramatic—will be a factor in the daily lives of health care professionals. In the field of oncology, new models and structures for care delivery will continue to evolve in an attempt to align state-of-the-art care with cost-effective systems. Guidelines for best oncology practice will remain a focus and may provide the framework for a reasonable approach to the allocation of resources and "rationing" of care. Technological advances will continue to stress the system, both in terms of capital costs of the new technology as well as its implementation in terms of location (nonduplication of equipment and the need to share among health centers) and appropriate utilization. As the pressure to contain health care costs continues, the community will become the major site of care.

As quickly and as dramatically as the health care environment changes, so must the nursing profession. Oncology nurses are key members of interdisciplinary teams that will develop and implement the guidelines that will direct all care. Nurses will be held accountable for patient outcomes and the ongoing improvement in care processes. The nurse's role will change from one of a task orientation to that of the coordinator and manager of care across settings and throughout a patient's health/illness trajectory.

These changes require new skills and a broader mindset for nursing. In addition to keeping up with advancing technology and remaining clinically astute, a solid financial framework is needed in order to understand the business of health care and its impact on care delivery. No longer can the nurse consider patient advocacy only in the context of clinical care; advocacy encompasses working with payers, employers, community agencies, and other components of delivery systems to facilitate and ensure quality, cost-effective care. As never before, nursing has a great opportunity to shape the future.

## REFERENCES

1. Coile RC, Jr: Assessing health care market trends and capital needs:1996–2000. *Health Care Fin Manage* 49:60–64, 1995
2. Everson LK: Cancer program development in the 1990s. *Oncol Issues* 8:8–10, 1993
3. Satinsky M: Advanced practice nurse in a managed care environment, in Hickey J, Oiumette R, Venegoni S (eds): *Advanced Practice Nursing* (ed 1). Philadelphia, Lippincott and Raven, 1996, pp 126–144
4. Wagner E: Types of managed care organizations, in Kongstvedt P (ed): *The Managed Care Handbook* (ed 2). Gaithersberg, MD, Aspen, 1993, pp 12–21
5. Mahar M: Time for a checkup. *Barron's* LXXVI 10:29–35, 1996
6. Alkire A, Stolz S: The employer's view of managed health care: From a passive to an aggressive role, in Kongstvedt P (ed): *The Managed Care Handbook* (ed 2). Gaithersberg, MD, Aspen, 1993, pp 255–264
7. Jacklevic MC: PHOs fall short of expectations. *Mod Health Care* 25:77–82, 1995
8. Abbey FB, Treash KM, Jr: Reasons providers form PHOs. *Health Care Fin Manage* 49:38–47, 1995
9. Ackerman FK, III: The movement toward vertically integrated regional health systems. *Health Care Manager Rev* 17:81–88, 1992
10. Walston SL, Kimberly JR, Burns LR: Owned vertical integration and health care: Promise and performance. *Health Care Manager Rev* 21:83–92, 1996
11. Shortell S: *Remaking Health Care in America* (ed 1). San Francisco, Jossey-Bass, 1996
12. Goldsmith JC: The illusive logic of integration. *Health Care Forum* 37:26–31, 1994
13. Goldsmith JC: Burning the seed corn. *Health Care Forum* 39:19–23, 1996
14. Coddington DC, Moore KD, Fischer EA: Integrating: Hang in there—the odds are in your favor. *Health Care Forum* 38:72–76, 1995
15. The Advisory Board: *Rewarding Cost-effective Medicine: Aligning Physician Incentives under Managed Care.* Washington, DC, The Advisory Board Company, 1995
16. Friedman E: Making choices, a demanding issue. *Health Care Forum* 39:9–11, 1996 (editorial)
17. Presant C: Oncology in a managed care environment. *Oncol Issues* 10:18–20, 1995
18. Kongstvedt P: Compensation of primary care physicians in open panels, in Kongstvedt P (ed): *The Managed Care Handbook* (ed 2). Gaithersberg, MD, Aspen, 1993, pp 55–69
19. Rutledge V, Bennett C: Cost containment initiatives: Analysis of clinical resource use, in Hickey J, Oiumette R, Venegoni S (eds): *Advanced Practice Nursing* (ed 1). Philadelphia, Lippincott and Raven, 1996, pp 225–252
20. Jewler D: Letting the future in: Highlights of ACCC's 12th Annual National Economics Conference. *Oncol Issues* 10:33–36, 1995
21. Kurowski B: Cancer carve-outs: Can they fulfill the promise of managed care? *Oncol Issues* 9:10–13, 1994
22. Stanfill PH: Cost-efficiencies in the oncology program: Strategies for survival. *J Oncol Manage* 4:18–25, 1995
23. McIntosh H: Managed care forces cancer centers to retrench. *J Nat Cancer Inst* 87:1204–1206, 1995

24. Aspling DL, Lagoe R: Benchmarking for clinical pathways in hospitals: A summary of sources. *Nurs Econ* 14:92–97, 1996

25. Sovie MD: Tailoring hospitals for managed care and integrated health systems. *Nurs Econ* 13:73–83, 1995

26. Wunderlich GS, Sloan FA, Davis CK: *Nursing staff in hospitals and nursing homes: Is it adequate?* Committee on the Adequacy of Nursing Staffing in Hospitals and Nursing Homes. Institute of Medicine. Washington DC, National Academy Press, 1996

27. Leavenworth G: The value of outcomes. Special Report on Guidelines. *Business & Health* 12:6–11, 1996 (suppl B)

28. Giles K: Disease management: A better alternative to the managed care process. *Oncol Issues* 11:15–20, 1996

29. Epstein RS, Sherwood LM: From outcomes research to disease management: A guide for the perplexed. *Ann Intern Med* 124:832–837, 1996

30. Harris JM: Disease management: New wine in new bottles? *Ann Intern Med* 124:838–842, 1996

31. Subcommittee to Evaluate the National Cancer Program, National Cancer Advisory Board: *Cancer at a Crossroads: AR report to Congress for the Nation.* Bethesda, MD, National Cancer Institute, 1994

32. Campbell B: Oncology networks: Genesis. *Oncol Issues* 10: 22–25, 1995

33. Spallina JM: The cancer program leadership challenge: Preparing for system integration. *J Oncol Manage* 3:30–33, 1994

34. Mortenson LE: Models for oncology within hospital alliances. *Oncol Issues* 10:15–17, 1995

35. Pearce D, Feingold M: A model hospital-medical oncology alliance: One cancer center's experience. *J Oncol Manage* 2: 26–30, 1993

36. Vandergrift T, Everson LK: Cancer program development in the 1990s: Survival in a managed care environment. *Oncol Issues* 8:14–16, 1993

37. Campbell B, Chandler C: Managed care, marketing & physician groups. *Oncol Issues* 11:19–21, 1996

38. Alpert B: Painful profits—cancer treatment firms may soon see their plump margins slashed. *Barron's* LXXVI 9:20–21, 1996

39. Bowing K: Regional report. *Cancer Manage* 1:21, 1996

40. National Cancer Institute, National Institutes of Health: *The Nation's Investment in Cancer Research; a Budget Proposal for Fiscal Years 1997/98.* National Cancer Institute, Bethesda, MD, 1996

41. Everson LE: The challenge for clinical research in community oncology programs. *Oncol Issues* 9:21–24, 1994

42. American College of Surgeon's Commission on Cancer: *Standards for Cancer Programs.* 1996

43. Wolf DS: Breast cancer patients versus their insurers. *Oncol Issues* 11:12–17, 1996

44. Young J: Off-label interest increases. *Oncol Issues* 11:6, 1996

45. Kessler D: FDA speeds up drug approval process. *The Washington Post* 30 March, 1996

46. Alexander W: Cancer drugs and managed care: The global picture. *Oncol Issues* 10:40–42, 1995

47. Stair J: Oncology critical pathways. *Oncol Issues* 10:17–21, 1995

48. Stair J: The present and future of guideline development. *Oncol Issues* 10:26, 1995

49. Mortenson LE, Harrigan EE: ACCC's guideline initiative. *Oncol Issues* 10:30–31, 1995

50. Strickland D: The future of guidelines. *Business & Health* 12:17–30, 1996 (suppl B)

51. Horn S: *Clinical Practice Improvement.* Presented at the national conference on outcomes, St. Lukes Episcopal Hospital, Houston, TX, April 1996

52. Wolf GA, Boland S, Aukerman M: A transformational model for the practice of professional nursing. *JONA* 24:51–57, 1994

53. Moore JD: Study seeks change in nursing staff uses. *Mod Health Care* 26:5, 1996

54. McCaffrey-Boyle D: New identities: The changing profile of patients with cancer, their families, and their professional caregivers. *Oncol Nurs Forum* 21:55–61, 1994

55. McCaffrey-Boyle D, Engelking C, Harvey C: Making a difference in the 21st century: Are oncology nurses ready? *Oncol Nurs Forum* 21:54, 1994

56. Schaffner JW, Ludwig-Beymer P, Wiggins J: Utilization of advanced practice nurses in health care systems and multi-specialty group practice. *JONA* 12:37–43, 1995

57. Hawkins R: Concluding remarks: Window to the future of advanced practice in oncology nursing. *Oncol Nurs Forum* 8: 43–45, 1995 (suppl)

58. Boyle DM: Documentation and outcomes of advanced nursing practice. *Oncol Nurs Forum* 8:11–17, 1995 (suppl)

59. Camp-Sorrel D, Spencer-Cisek P: Reimbursement issues for advanced practice. *Oncol Nurs Forum* 8:31–34, 1995 (suppl)

60. Miller KL: Keeping the care in nursing care, our biggest challenge. *JONA* 11:29–32, 1995

61. Moss MT: Principles, values, and ethics set the stage for managed care nursing. *Nurs Econ* 5:276–284, 1995

62. Asch DA: The role of critical care nurses in euthanasia and assisted suicide. *N Engl J Med* 21:1374–1379, 1996

63. American Nurses Association. *Code for nurses with interpretive statements.* Kansas City, MO, 1985

64. Scanlon C, Glover J: A professional code of ethics: Providing a moral compass in turbulent times. *Oncol Nurs Forum* 10: 1515–1521, 1995

65. Barter M, McLaughlin FE, Thomas SA: Use of unlicensed assistive personnel by hospitals. *Nurs Econ* 2:82–87, 1994

66. Hayes PM: Non-nursing functions: Time for them to go. *Nurs Econ* 3:120–125, 1994

67. Barger M, Furmidge ML: Unlicensed assistive personnel— issues relating to delegation and supervision. *JONA* 4:36–39, 1994

68. Oncology Nursing Society: *Assistive Personnel: Their use in Cancer Care.* Pittsburgh, ONS, 1996

# Chapter 57

# Ethical Issues in Cancer Nursing Practice

David C. Thomasma, PhD

# INTRODUCTION

Cancer care is challenging on many fronts. In addition to the many physical and emotional challenges faced by oncology nurses, many different ethical issues arise in caring for patients with cancer. Some of these issues are common to all branches of health care, some more specific to nursing, and some specific to cancer itself. This chapter will examine the issues in three broad categories: general issues, nursing issues, and cancer issues.

# GENERAL ETHICAL ISSUES

It is customary in every review of ethical theories to sketch the ethical principles of autonomy, beneficence, nonmaleficence, and justice.[1] To these are added alternative ethical analyses, including virtue theory, with a view toward suggesting the future of health care ethics.

## Autonomy

*Autonomy* is shorthand for a principle that compels us to respect the self-command of the individual. Since *autonomy* means quite literally self-rule, respect for the individual therefore includes not only the free choice a competent patient might make but also respect for the source of that freedom within the individual.[2] It would be contradictory to attempt to heal a patient while denying the patient's freedom and ability to make decisions about the healing process.

The idea of autonomy originated in the moral realm; that is, autonomy is part of what makes us moral. We are responsible for our own moral acts and must make our own moral rules. Therefore, autonomy should not be equated simply with patients' rights or even with the freedom to choose. It implies something deeper—that the core of what it means to be a person is moral responsibility to oneself and to others. This is not "pure" freedom but rather freedom to take responsibility for one's own actions and their consequences. In response to that level of responsibility, caregivers have a duty to respect the moral origins of the person, not just to respect the choices the person makes, as will be clarified later.

The notion of autonomy is foreign to traditional health care practice. For centuries, health care practitioners governed by the Hippocratic ethic practiced a form of paternalism, acting in the best interests of others without asking their preferences, or even explicitly acting against their preferences. An example would be refusing to acknowledge the wish of an elderly, competent but somewhat depressed woman to be "left alone" and allowed to die. Caregivers are often reluctant to accept the wishes of individuals with serious disease, especially if they think something still might be done to improve either longevity or quality of life. Another example might be a patient who, fearing the outcomes of cancer, decides to forgo not only any interventionist chemotherapy but also even a biopsy. Despite the right of individuals to determine their own treatment, this scenario would create a conflict between the caregiver's sense of duty to protect and prolong life and the autonomy and privacy rights of the individual patient.

## Beneficence

*Beneficence* is the principle of altruism, that is, to act in the best interests of others. It is the fundamental guiding force behind the helping professions, leading, for example, to the maxim "the patient comes first." Of course, it would be difficult to act at all times on the basis of this principle, since self-interest is a part of duty to oneself. Yet the principle creates an expectation in patients and in society as a whole that health professionals, who are often strangers to the patient, have promised and will take exceptional steps to place their patients' interests above their own.[3]

Sometimes a good thing like beneficence can run amok and lead to a paternalistic (maternalistic) form of "doing good" without attention to the wishes of the other person.[4] In some instances there is a necessary medical paternalism. For example, a patient may have executed the advance directive to refrain from putting her on a respirator due to advanced metastatic liver cancer but now finds herself in the emergency room due to an automobile accident. Her crushed rib cage is potentially treatable. Presumption would be to treat her, even with a respirator, for a reversible event she had not foreseen in her previous determinations about end-stage cancer. Most often, however, paternalism is regarded with moral opprobrium. Beneficence does not rule out trying to persuade patients and even sometimes to almost coerce them to overcome their fears and to help them choose what is in their best interests. But in the final analysis, it is unethical to act against the wishes of patients if they continue to refuse the offerings of modern health care.[5]

In cancer care it is frequently hard to determine what is in the patient's best interest. There may be conflicting courses of treatment, or only statistical or epidemiological information that may or may not apply to the circumstances.[6-8] Also, patients may become incompetent to speak for their own care in the later stages of the disease. In these instances, caregivers focus their efforts on trying to determine objective standards of care, avoiding making quality-of-life judgments by appealing to medical indications.[9] Yet these standards are not as objective as they might first appear. Often they are a combination of current practice, the best medical knowledge of the time, and attention to the context in which care is to be delivered. For instance, the patient's wishes are combined with a judgment about prognosis and weighed against the patient's condition, age, and reasons for treatment requests and refusals.

## Nonmaleficence

The third principle governing general health care ethical concerns is the principle of *nonmaleficence*. This principle covers the famous Hippocratic aphorism, "To help, or at least, to do no harm." When caregivers find that there is confusion or disagreement about what is in the patient's best interest, they must fall back to a position of trying, according to the Hippocratic oath, "at least, to do no harm."

In a way, nonharm is a minimalist beneficence position. Respecting the personhood of the patient requires an attempt to honor autonomy *and* to act in his or her best interests. At the very least, however, it means never harming intentionally.

The problem is to define harm. The definition scale can run from physical to psychological and even spiritual harm. Some examples will be discussed later in the context of dying. Since most cancer patients recover or stay in remission, however, it is appropriate here to consider a different example: A 42-year-old woman develops breast cancer metastases while being tried in court for running a prostitution ring under the guise of a high-class escort service. Her cancer now involves her spine and causes her intense pain. But an even greater problem for her is that her son is dying of AIDS, and she wants to care for him before succumbing to her disease and to her trial sentence.[10] Harm for her is the spiritual pain of not being able to nurture her son, rather than her physiological concerns (the spinal involvement of the cancer), or even her likely incarceration ("If the government wants me to go to jail, so be it," she said. "I'd like to spend my time now with my son, and after that they can have my life. I don't care"). This example demonstrates how harms ideally are determined by the patient in conjunction with caregivers, so that a mutually agreed-upon treatment plan can be developed.

## Justice

The principle of justice requires that we give each person his or her due. There are competing opinions of how to measure what is due.[11] Some thinkers argue for equity, trying to equalize the inequities of human life by taking from the rich and giving to the poor. Major social programs like Social Security, Medicare, Medicaid, and the income tax exemplify this method. Others argue that egalitarian methods are more appropriate; that is, everyone is entitled to exactly the same treatment (equality) regardless of the starting point.[12] Still others like libertarians argue that justice requires a fundamental respect for autonomy[13] and that one cannot alter the social situation

of rich and poor without the consent of the governed. For example, one cannot charge paying patients and their insurance companies more for cancer care than nonpaying patients, thus taking from those who have to help those who do not, without the express consent of the paying patients and their third-party payers.

The different views of justice have little bearing on clinical decisions at this time, although they do influence various proposals for access to care, and hover in the background of most of our social programs, which, as nurses are often aware, can do damage to individuals. As part of the principles of beneficence and nonmaleficence, efforts must be made to provide a better health care delivery system than that currently in place.

## Alternative Ethical Theories

The difficulty in clinical ethics is rooted in a confrontation between an abstracting tendency in the long and rewarding history of ethics and the concrete, individual problems encountered by professionals who must make quick decisions about very complex matters in order to benefit their patients. Ethical analysis must take careful note of numerous ethical theories, axioms, and other concerns in order to conduct a minimally decent conceptual and problematic analysis. This process takes time and, of necessity, becomes quite abstract. Health professionals and patients quickly lose interest in these abstractions and theoretical meanderings if they are not decisively and explicitly related to the realities of patient care. They must do ethics on the run.

Ethical principles appear abstract—or better, speculative—because they do not have as much social legitimacy as do the values of everyday life. Moral abstractions frequently are seen by nonphilosophers as devoid of the ingredients of moral concerns that people have in their day-to-day life. No doubt they can and do seep into that daily life, but the process of connecting theory to practice is long and subtle.[14] How often do we encounter physicians and patients who become impatient with "thinking" that has no practical consequence?[15]

Dissatisfaction with principle-based ethical theories has led to new proposals for moral analysis, such as casuistry, hermeneutics, and "ethics as story." *Casuistry* is an ancient methodology by which each case is analyzed on its own merits. No overarching principles will lead to a conclusion from one case to another. *Hermeneutics* is named after the Greek god Hermes, the messenger of the gods. It means interpreting the case in its whole context—the individual's life plans and values, the family's values, social and cultural factors, and the like. *Ethics as story* relies upon concrete narrative to ferret out the interests and values in each instance, especially with relationship to caregivers themselves. Each of these movements stresses the concreteness of the individual situation, the importance of interpreting values of those involved in the case, and the deeper moral drama and constraints that take place during the lives of individuals experiencing serious disease.

*Virtue theory* is also an alternative that may complement principle-based ethics. No principle could be implemented without the commitment of caregivers or patients to the good as they perceive it. Even the most rule-bound person must have virtues of interior commitment to the rules. On the other hand, relying solely on the virtuous caregiver and patient, without a set of objective moral guidelines or principles, leads to follies and foibles and opportunity for abuse.

A nursing philosophy goal to act *as if* the nurse were the patient and *as if* the nurse's values became the patient's values would require some limits. Clearly, the nurse could not carry out actions that would compromise her or his conscience. Further, sometimes disputes about care, like instituting or withdrawing fluids and nutrition for the dying patient,[16,17] limit the ability of some nurses to accomplish this nursing philosophy goal. This dynamic reveals the need for a relation between objective standards (the goal of nursing in this instance) and the virtue of the nurse (formed by his or her own conscience and personal standards).

Arguably the most important virtue for the nurse is compassion. This assertion is based on the view that of all the caregivers involved with the patient, the nurse is the one with the most "hands-on" duties. The implications of this virtue will be explored in the section on Nursing Ethical Issues.

## Reconciliation Efforts

The emphasis on personal autonomy in medical ethics is coming under greater scrutiny today. Thinkers concerned about libertarian assumptions implied by this emphasis have countered autonomy with the need for beneficence as well.[18,19] The implications of conflicts about medical ethics and ethics theory include the increased role of the health provider's values in caring for the dying patient;[20] greater attention to the relation between physician and patient, rather than exclusive focus on the needs and wants of the patient alone; and questions about the kind of society we ought to be.[21]

Pellegrino and Thomasma proposed that the goal of health care ought to be "beneficence-in-trust." By this we mean that the caregiver holds in trust the values of the patient in making joint decisions with the patient about best interests. It would not be appropriate to act in the best interests of the patient without paying attention to the autonomous decision making and values of the patient.[3] This is but one of a number of proposals to integrate the power of the healer's art with the autonomy of the patient.[22]

Another approach is that of libertarianism. Perhaps the most articulate spokesperson for a libertarian version of secular humanism is H. Tristram Engelhardt, Jr. In his *Bioethics and Secular Humanism*, he argues that secular humanism itself has no moral content. But as an ethical position it reigns supreme for moral argumentation among moral strangers, that is, individuals whose fundamental values are either unknown to one another, or, actually, whose moral values can be considered to be estranged from one another. Engelhardt bases his argument on a fundamental rationality all human beings share that can enlighten them in their pursuit of consensual agreements in bioethics.[23] Supporters of this view will be surprised by Engelhardt's revision of his *Foundations of Bioethics* (1996) in which more religious value systems find a role, and in which he argues that secular bioethics must, in principle, fail.[24]

No matter what approach is taken, it is important that individual moral commitments are not separated from ethical decision making. Further, schema for resolving ethical dilemmas must remain exceptionally sensitive to the concrete situation and particularities of both patient and nurse.[25] Finally, any doctrine of human rationality must be met with reservation: our own ineptitude at honoring others, our downright evil deeds, and the general violent nature of today's human society, in which individuals are treated as objects for the pleasure and good of others, call into question an unexamined view of human rationality. More important, a rationalistic approach to bioethical decision making ignores human beings' potentialities of nature and virtue to identify with a vulnerable, sick, or dying individual through compassion.

Let us look at two clinical management concepts in more detail, since they are closely related.

### Casuistry

Casuistry can be used as the basic model for how the good decision emerges in health care. Put simply, casuistry is the theory that each case is unique, and from that case are developed certain norms that may or may not be applicable in analogous cases. The goal of casuistry is to establish the paradigm case, in which most analysts would agree that a certain norm predominates—say, truth telling as an obligation to a cancer patient whose family is trying to protect the individual from the devastating news. Other cases are then related to this one and analyzed for the extent to which they "match" or "do not match" the paradigm case. Continuing the example of truth telling, an analogous case would be one in which the patient has had two heart attacks already and is prone to panic when hearing bad news. The family's desire to protect this patient is based on a different reason than in the paradigm case.

More theoretical work needs to be done on the assumptions of casuistry, however. This becomes apparent when we begin to delve into the ways in which we use clinical judgment to interpret experience by "mining" the good. By this I mean that we pay particular attention to patient and caregiver value systems, as well as the hierarchy of those values. Which values outrank others in the minds of the parties of the healing relationship?

The following discussion targets two major problems with casuistry.

The most difficult part of casuistry is that it presupposes a unified theory of human nature by which one case can be logically compared with another. This unified theory of human nature was provided by the *natural law* theory. But this theory, as it was employed in the past, is now as discredited as is traditional casuistry. Toulmin and Jonsen[26] argue that casuistry arose as a method at just that time in Western civilization when the metaphysical superstructure of Christianity began to collapse under the rise of the modern state, nationalism, and the age of reason. They therefore make the case that casuistry is eminently suitable for modern times, times of pluralism, times without a moral consensus.[27] Yet it is difficult to ignore the need for some mode of comparison by which one case is at the very least analogous to the other. Meaning is not wholly and completely individual. It arises in a context beyond or encompassing the individual case. The very basis for analogous cases is some lasting "something" that crosses the boundaries of each case.

There is a second, and related, problem. Casuistry was discredited by those who held that ethical theory was very important. The method of ethical analysis changed from case orientation to deducing practical conclusions from principles. Reinstituting casuistry as the model for both ethical and medical decisions neglects the importance of ethical theory and, analogously, of the relationship of individuals within the case and their values to the emergence of the good.

## Contextualism

Casuistry challenges the deductive model of ethical reasoning. It is closer to clinical judgment, it describes realistically (rather than ideally) how good decisions come about, and it is practical. Yet casuistry neglects the importance of theory and of the nexus of values that ethical theory seeks to protect. Is there a middle ground between deducing the good decision from abstract and theoretical principles that ignore clinical realities and educing the former entirely from the latter? Is there a middle ground between deduction and induction of the good?

A middle course between a generalist application of ethical theory and specialized case-by-case analysis is possible with a contextual grid for medical ethics.[28] Clinical ethics must address itself to contexts. Neither axioms nor standard moral rules are sufficient (although they are necessary, of course) to determine the validity of moral theory and ethical principles in resolving medical ethics problems.[29] Additional rules, or guidelines for relating theory and practice, must be developed according to this approach. Among these rules is that context serves as a way to analyze value hierarchies in concrete circumstances. Earlier it was emphasized that it is important to consider the particularities of a case, including its context,

for a properly compassionate analysis (to be discussed in more detail in the next section).

Thus, according to the contextualism theory, what is needed is a means by which to locate a moral problem and to exhibit the likely values and principles at issue within that locus. The context having been established by such a "grid," the discussion can proceed toward means for resolving the case by protecting the interests and values of those affected by it. But that is not all. The grid not only locates and focuses the moral discussion; it also hints at the cross-case commonalities that legitimize the acts of organizing similar cases, comparing them, and drawing conclusions about the new case.

A variability of contexts in the clinical resolution of cases is noticeable to all who work in the medical setting. This variability does not so much describe the relativity of values and principles as it does how the weight they bring to bear on a case is partially determined by the medical specialty involved; the personal values of the patient, family, or social group; the personal and professional values of the health care professionals involved; and the institutional setting in which the problem arises. Some principles and axioms will be given more weight than others in such a scheme, and one important component of the weighting will stem from the contexts. The good will arise out of the mix of these components.

Such a contextual grid is only one aspect, then, of what might be called *context-variable moral rules*. Other examples could be examined that do not fit the contextual grid pattern but are moral rules that in other ways vary with the context. Further, the contextual grid cannot encompass all of the variables in a case but only the ones most likely to be affecting the emphasis of some values or principles over others. This is precisely where deductive models of ethical reasoning fall short.

For example, the rule of protection of autonomy is more likely to be given prominent focus in a primary care context than in a tertiary care context, wherein one's autonomy is virtually always depressed and hence concern for autonomy is diminished in favor of a goal of preservation of life and/or restoration of health.[30] Furthermore, the rule of protection of autonomy is more likely to be emphasized in cases in which there is no threat to others than in cases wherein the common good must be considered. Finally, because the grid only *describes* most likely weights given to moral principles and rules in formulating an indicated course of action, one should not misconstrue the contextual grid as claiming that physicians in tertiary care settings do not care about protecting their patients' autonomy, or that public health officials stress social responsibility to the exclusion of individual well-being. All of these moral values bear upon a case. The grid only describes what values are most likely to take precedence over others.

The contextual grid theory rests on two distinctions. The first is the distinction between primary, secondary, and tertiary care settings, a standard distinction in medicine that forms one set of coordinates of the grid. Its importance for moral reasoning lies in the seriousness of the assault on personal wholeness brought about by the diseases in question.[31] Thus, a patient's wishes are more likely to be sought and respected in a primary care setting than in an emergency room after an attack of pulmonary insufficiency, where a paternalistic response may be more appropriate. The second distinction or coordinate of the grid is that between the individual and the number of persons affected by the problem. A good example would be the difference in moral analysis between an individual who refuses chemotherapy and wishes to die from cancer without "any fuss" and a mother of four whose children might still need her to help them cope with her impending death. The former wish might be respected almost immediately, whereas the latter's wish should be balanced with other duties she has as a mother.

The moral significance of this distinction is based on the increasing complexity that occurs when the values of different persons whose interests are affected by the outcome of the case enter our consideration and on our increased tendency to protect the common good the greater the number of affected persons. Recall again the grid's purpose to describe context-variable rules, that is, which principles and axioms are likely to be given more weight than others in a given circumstance in formulating a moral policy or in developing an indicated course of action.

With the increasing provision of patient care to managed care systems, the contextual grid distinctions between primary, secondary, and tertiary care may have to give way to a new set of categories of care, each with its own economic objective that sets the tone for moral analysis. First-level caregivers would have as their goal keeping individuals in a home environment as long as possible. Second-level caregivers would provide temporary institutional care, with the objective of returning the person home as soon as possible. Third-level caregivers would provide permanent institutional care with as little expense as is possible for the quality required. These objectives introduce quite different moral requirements of caregivers in each category of care, and would change the analysis provided by the contextual grid accordingly.

## Ethical Workup

An excellent tool developed for case analysis embodying the points raised so far is the Ethical Workup. The aim of this tool is to try to examine as many values as possible in the case and to reach a resolution that respects as many of these as possible. This is done through critical reflection on the importance of some values and principles over others in the context of the particular circumstances of the case. Thorough consideration of each step of the workup permits nurses and other health professionals to examine their own values as well as those of the patient, other caregivers, the hospital, and society as a whole. Furthermore, principles, rules, duties, and virtues

also come into play in the later steps during the resolution process. The following six-step workup for case-oriented bioethics courses has been developed. The health professional examining the case is addressed directly in the instructions:

---

**ETHICAL WORKUP GUIDE**

The workup is an attempt to distill from the discipline of ethics an essential process of moral reasoning that can be used to resolve cases. In other words, no attempt is made to force you to take one or another position in the history of ethical theory. Instead, you are asked to follow only one absolute: Come up with an ethically justifiable course of action for the patient. This meshes with your professional duty to act in the best interests of the patient.

*Step 1.* *What are the facts in the case?* Be sure to research any medical facts not presented in the case but possibly relevant to its outcome.

*Step 2.* *What are the values at risk in the case?* Describe all relevant values—that is, values of the physicians, patients, house staff, nurses, hospital administration, the institution, and society itself. This may not be an exhaustive listing of interests in the case.

*Step 3.* *Determine the principal conflicts between values and professional norms and between ethical axioms, rules, and principles.* Conflicts can occur among prima facie absolute values, norms, axioms, rules, and principles, and/or among each other. The principal clash, in the end analysis, is the one you determine it to be.

In determining this principal clash, you should explain if you think principles and values are absolute and whether to be ethical means to act on principles, or whether you hold that they are only at first glance, that is, prima facie absolute, and can yield to other important values and principles in the case. You should also note the difference between values, norms, axioms, rules, and principles.

*Step 4.* *Determine possible courses of action, and state which values and ethical principles each course of action would protect or infringe.* At this step you will grapple with fundamental moral theory. Are you willing to seek a solution that is based on a single principle? Or are you willing to note that each decision you might make will place some values, principles, etc., at risk? Would you then be satisfied with being utilitarian—that is, protecting as many values and principles as possible in the case?

*Step 5.* *Make a decision in the case.*

*Step 6.* *Defend this course of action. Why is X better than Y?* In defending this course of action, ask whether consensus ethics is appropriate. Is deciding on the basis of a majority or a consensus really the same as ethics? What makes it right? Should the decision rest on a single value or principle? Instead, should it protect as many values as possible? Or should it rest on the virtue of the caregivers or institutions in which it takes place?

Please respond to each of the following:

- Were any values, principles, norms, axioms, or rules weighted more heavily than others? If so, which values, principles, etc., were most important to protect and why? If not, was the case decided by protecting as many of the values in the case as possible?

**ETHICAL WORKUP GUIDE (continued)**

- Try to identify the type of moral reasoning applied in resolving the case (utilitarian, deontologic, virtue-ethic, care ethics, casuistic ethics, other) and state whether it was used because of your general preference in similar situations or because of its particular applicability to this specific case.

- Universality test: Would you be willing that your decision and its reasons become universal law and apply to every similar situation? To yourself? Is this test actually a valid way to determine what is ethical?

- What role does society play in making this decision palatable? Can you imagine a different society and different solution? Would the decision require you to change the political system or the way health care is delivered? Are social and political duties a feature of the nature of the profession and clinical judgment? Do you believe in cultural relativism?

- How does this decision relate to others you have made in your life, in courses, and in actuality as a professional?

# NURSING ETHICAL ISSUES

As we have seen, beneficence must go well beyond the minimalistic interpretation of avoiding harm. It entails helping others even when that involves inconvenience, sacrifice, and risk to self-interest. Conflicts occur between the obligation to help others and self-interest. At risk is the primary obligation of advocacy of the patient's interest, which is at the heart of any compassion-based medical ethic. If, as Loewy[32] contends, the possibility of suffering is the basis of a beneficent community, the compassion for the sick is one of the highest forms of virtue.

## The Virtue of Compassion

The community traditionally supported compassionate care of individuals by providing for individuals who were sick to be surrounded by those who loved them the most and knew their values. Decisions about health care were made within a context of compassion and respect for the values of the patient. Such care was impervious to marketplace economics. It was an act of mercy, not a commodity to be traded or delivered.

True compassion is more than emotion. It involves putting oneself imaginatively into the situation of another—a first step is sympathy.[33] For some, compassion is essential for health care; for others, it is an act of supererogation.[34] A number of bioethicists link an ability to be compassionate with increased moral judgment skills, with evidence that women are inherently less selfish than men in the healing professions.[35,36]

By contrast, today the community seems more concerned about the resources the sick divert from other projects. Rationing care appears to be more valued than providing it. The most vulnerable—the poor, the elderly, the chronically handicapped, the infants, the mentally ill, and the retarded—are the ones who will suffer the most from rationing. With concern about rationing comes a danger of shrinking from sacrifice—of time, emotions, energies, and money—that the care of the sick requires. So urgent has the economics of health care become that some traditional caregivers, like religious hospitals, contemplate withdrawing from this vital service.

But none of the changes in society or the technology of medical care can alter the call the sick themselves press upon caregivers so insistently, the call from fellow creatures in need.[37] Recognizing their need as persons can only be done if the caregiver's own self-perception is of being an agent of mercy and compassion.[38] What is the meaning of this compassion within the context of biomedical decisions?

Compassion is more than pity or sympathy. It transcends social work, philanthropy, and government programs. It is the capacity to feel, and suffer with, the sick person—to experience something of the predicament of illness, its fears, anxieties, temptations, its assault on the whole person, the loss of freedom and dignity, the utter vulnerability, and the alienation every illness produces or portends. And true compassion is more than feeling. It flows over in a willingness to help, to make some sacrifice, to go out of one's way. "No one can help anyone without entering with her whole person into the painful situation; without taking the risk of becoming hurt, wounded, or even destroyed in the process."[39]

Compassion entails a comprehension of the suffering experienced by another. Individuals who have themselves suffered are sometimes better able to understand others' suffering. As De Unamuno[40] says, "Suffering is the substance of life and the root of personality, for only suffering makes us persons." Compassion for the suffering of others thus enriches self-understanding, especially of what we too must someday pass through. Compassion helps us realize that sick brothers and sisters are not aliens; they are still very much part of the human family and are vital to one's own spiritual growth. The healthy need the sick to "humanize" them as much as the sick need the healthy to humanize their sickness.

For health professionals and the family or surrogates, compassion is the quality that keeps them from operating solely on the basis of objectivity and rationality. It enables them to recognize that, effective as our science and technology can be, they do not remove suffering. The sick cannot escape the confrontation with mortality that even a minor illness may entail. Human illness is always illness of the whole person—body, mind, and spirit. Hence, the illness and/or dying process is more than some aberration in an organ system. The illness transcends the biological to encompass the whole person and his or her value system. Illness fractures self-image, upsets the balance the patient has struck between aspirations and limitations. Illness is nothing less than a deconstruction of the self.

Compassion enables decision makers to assist in healing, if by healing we can mean the reconstruction of the person. Involved here is an effort to put back together a ruptured self that has separated into an ego and a body that has betrayed that individual.[31] Nurses help defend against the attack on the spirit as well as the attack on the body. The particularities of culture, ethnicity, and language make illness a unique experience for each person. True healing and appropriate decision making can only take place when all of the particulars and values of the individual and all the parties involved in the process of caring for the sick person are taken into account.[41] Compassionate care also means that the patient who cannot be cured by medical sciences—especially the dying cancer patient—may still be "healed" if we help him or her to express the meaning of a life in the final days of that life by respecting, insofar as possible, the patient's values and commitments.

## Clinical Ethics and the Relation to the Patient

Since the beginning of modern clinical ethics, it has been clear that the reasoning patterns of clinical judgment in medical care parallel those of ethical judgment. This realization is important for many reasons. For example, education programs in health professional schools have acquired a "clinical" focus of relevance and reality by stressing the similarities among nursing, medical, and ethical decision making.[42] Articles and books on the philosophy of health care have sometimes underscored the relation of the ethics of health care to clinical judgment.[14] More pointedly for our purpose, the nexus between clinical judgment and clinical ethics can help reveal structures of good decision making in patient care that are not simple products of contractual models of the provider-patient relationship. More is going on in that relationship than initially meets the eye.

Contrast a superficial view of the provider-patient relationship with one that digs more deeply into the humanity of caregiving. Some thinkers argue profoundly about traditional commitments to the value of human life within the patient care relationship as contrasted to respect for autonomy alone.[43] Thus, Leon Kass[44] presents a thoughtful articulation of what is owed a dying patient by health professionals. He argues that humanity is owed humanity, not just "humaneness" (i.e., being merciful by killing the patient). Kass suggests that the reason we are compelled to put animals out of their misery is that they are *not* human and thus demand from us some measure of humaneness. By contrast, human beings demand from us our humanity itself. This thesis, in turn, rests on the relationship "between the healer and the ill" as constituted, essentially, "even if only tacitly, around the desire of both to promote the wholeness of the one who is ailing."[46]

We might call the temptation to employ technology rather than one's personhood in the process of healing "the technological fix." The technological fix is not only easier to conceptualize and implement than the more difficult processes of human engagement but is also "suggested" by technology itself. The training and skills of modern health professionals are overwhelmingly nurtured within an environment of technological fixes. By instinct and proclivity, people in a modern civilization are tempted by technical rather than personal solutions to problems.

A responsible use of technological intervention with and for the sake of a patient requires not only rational analysis but also sensitivity to the particularities of the case and the emotional content of value commitments of the parties involved. The responsible use of power is a clinical ethics judgment about the best balance of interventions and outcomes. Such interactive concerns tend to present counterpressures to a straightforward honoring of patient wishes and autonomy.[45] The virtue of compassion requires an almost exquisite awareness of the physical condition of the patient (to assess outcomes) and the values of patients or of those speaking for them (to assess the quality of those outcomes measured against the patient's values).[46] In fact, compassionate virtue includes a sense of justice and love as well.[46]

The most dramatic examples of taking responsibility for the particularities of a case are culled from problems of withholding and withdrawing care from the dying. But compassion is also required to assess properly the interventions to be given to the weak and debilitated elderly, to the demented, to individuals with metastases, to other vulnerable people, and to individuals who wish to exercise their autonomy in ways that are clearly self-destructive.

## The Patient Self-Determination Act

The Patient Self-Determination Act went into effect in December 1991. The act requires all health care institutions, including home care and hospice, to notify patients upon admission to the institution or service of their rights under state law to execute an advance directive. Other provisions include asking patients whether they have issued an advance directive or wish to do so, asking for a copy if they have, putting that copy prominently in the patient record, and notifying the patient of the institution's commitment to honor the patient's wishes. Obtaining the wishes of individuals before they enter health care institutions or home health care should not be seen as yet another bureaucratic process. Instead, the Act should be used as an opportunity to evidence respect for the moral center of the person.

Part of the reason for the Act was surely to underscore the importance of patients' rights. But another was Congress's interest in controlling costs of health care, particularly during the last six months of a patient's life. Almost 40% of the Medicare budget covers this period. It would stand to reason that honoring patient wishes not only would show respect for individuals but also would help save critical health care funds.

Difficulties arise when the wishes expressed do not anticipate future events. Sometimes a patient agrees to a "do not resuscitate" (DNR) order regarding the primary disease of progressive, metastatic cancer but then develops sepsis that might be reversible. If the patient also had said earlier that she did not want to "be on a respirator," but that treatment is required to treat the sepsis, can her wishes be disregarded in this instance? Many health professionals are concerned that advance directives will artificially tie their hands in treatment decisions. Many patients agree, avoiding advance directives in favor of "letting the doctor decide." Nurses are usually caught in the middle on issues like this, as they find it difficult to interpret the treatment plan if the physician chooses to ignore advance directives for any reason. In such cases an ethics consult or patient-care discussion is recommended.

## Compassionate Analysis

The notion of "compassionate analysis" mentioned earlier embodies both the virtue of compassion and the various mechanisms available for protecting patient autonomy. Advances have occurred in emphasizing the rights of patients not only to determine the treatments they desire and do not desire during the dying process but also to choose treatments at any time during life, not just while dying. The efforts of patient advocacy groups in sponsoring and supporting legislation and court deliberations have been outstanding. As the use of living wills and advance directives, including the durable power of attorney, becomes more common, patient rights will be further clarified (e.g., how will they impact long-term care settings?).[47] What is important to note is that the underlying principle of such instruments is the prevention of suffering—that is, to increase the role of compassion in decisions about life-prolonging technology.[48] A logical extension of patient rights could be to allow even greater control over the dying process.

A living will gives advance directives for the final period of terminal illness. In most states where it has been approved, the living will covers only the terminal phase of an illness, interpreted to mean the last few weeks of a person's life. Most states explicitly rule out directives about fluids and nutrition. Consequently, the living will is a limited instrument. Much more favored is the durable power of attorney. This instrument gives another person authority to make health care decisions for an individual who becomes incompetent to do so. Not only would this person know the patient's wishes, but also he or she could communicate with the caregivers to discern the best treatment or nontreatment options during the course of temporary or permanent incompetency. The disease course changes, as do options along the way. Unforeseen events may occur.

The durable power, unlike the living will, covers any treatment decisions, formally anticipated or not, and at any stage in life, not just in a terminal situation. This is important because medical technology gives health care providers enormous power at all levels of life, especially at the end. Most often health care providers are concerned about the ethical issues in active, direct euthanasia, instead of being concerned with meeting a person's physical and social needs. The tendency of the "technofix" society is to prolong suffering in conditions of what has been defined as "hopeless injury":[49]

> a condition in which there is no potential for growth or repair; no observable pleasure or happiness from living . . . and a total absence of one or more of the following attributes of quality of life: cognition or recognition, motor activity, memory or awareness of time, consciousness, and language or other intelligent means of communicating thoughts or wishes.

Daily life is full of interactions with "things"—nonhuman and fundamentally incomprehensible to most persons. We sometimes get so used to technological processes that we behave as though they are substitutes for human and compassionate care. Eating for many elderly and dying patients has been replaced by tubes; participating in the spiritual and material values of human life has been replaced by "merely surviving," as a being subjugated to the products of human imagination. As Illich observes: "Medical civilization is planned and organized to kill pain, to eliminate sickness, and to abolish the need for acts of suffering and dying. . . . The new experience that has replaced dignified suffering is artificially prolonged, opaque, depersonalized maintenance."[50,p.106]

"Beings" subjected to such depersonalized maintenance may no longer be as human as the rest of us. This is no way to respect the value of human life. Is a permanently unconscious being without any ability to relate to its environment a "person"? Part of taking responsibility for our technology is to avoid this subjugation of human life to machinery in the first place, through more thorough discussions of possible outcomes and patient values regarding them.

## CANCER ETHICAL ISSUES

There is an increasing concern that medical technology impedes the search for meaning in life. This is especially true during serious illness, during its initial diagnosis, the hopeful process of recovery, and the anguished process of dying. Society's impediments to a search for meaning have been well described by thinkers such as MacIntyre.[27] The focus of this section will be on the concrete processes of decision making in caring for the cancer patient that reveal that same search for meaning. In other words, the primary ethical duty of compassionate cancer care is rooted in a mutual exploration of the human condition. The following are only a few of the specific ethical concerns related to cancer care.[51]

### The Dynamics of Cancer

The *dynamics of cancer* refers to the spiritual struggle of the patient to come to terms with the diagnosis of cancer.

The word *spiritual* is used deliberately to identify the intense inner realm of fundamental values each person possesses. The realm is often neglected in daily life because external matters and concerns so easily obscure it. Driving to the grocery store to select items for dinner, having the grandchildren at the house over the weekend, planning a vacation, and pursuing the myriad other events of daily living funnel our attention outside this spiritual dimension, though the values connected to the choices made in the external life are stored there. Periodically we may examine these values. Indeed, Socrates admonished that "the unexamined life is not worth living." But serious trauma in the external life is often necessary before people face their spiritual realm directly.

For a patient with cancer this spiritual struggle may be intensified by confusion about goals of treatment, longevity concerns, doubts about the most effective therapy, problems of cost and benefit, and the relation of these difficulties to the patient's long-standing system of values. Hence the examination of values that is forced on everyone with trauma and dreadful news is compressed in patients first hearing the news that they have cancer. Even though today advanced care can relieve the fear that to have cancer means to be sentenced to die, death is often the most immediate fear.

The dynamics of cancer has its own structure. At first, patients may feel guilty. Cancer is seen as self-destructive, almost as if the body is eating itself. One patient with colon cancer blamed herself, for example, because of her lengthy struggle with her son's alcoholism. She thought that she "took it out" on her own body, that she was bound to become seriously ill (and statistics bear her out). Another patient undergoing interleukin-2 therapy complained in tears that he could not spend another night with the nightmares he kept having, nightmares that acid he unleashed was destroying him and his family as it ate into the basement where they were hiding.

Later, patients usually arrive at a more peaceful stage. They come to see that they are not usually responsible for their cancer. Even if they risked cancer through smoking or other bad habits, they might forgive themselves. In this phase of the dynamic, cancer is made into an object, an "It,"[52] an invading army of cells. Because cancer, however, is an autocorporeal disease, conceptually it is inescapable to feel that one's own body has betrayed the person. For this reason, patients continue to view the body as a contributing factor to their disease, which contributes profoundly to the level of suffering they experience.

Depending on age and habits of resiliency, patients may choose to do battle with the "It" that is cancer. But the battle and the desire to fight it are complicated by the patient's own assessment of his or her life span. Regularly, patients refer to their own sense of impending end. Yet, as the data seem to indicate, caregivers treat cancer patients near the end of their lives more and more aggressively (and expensively).[53]

Guilt reemerges when individuals decide not to continue against the odds. This guilt is attached to the patient's worries about loved ones. Does my husband understand that I still love him, although I am no longer going to "fight" the cancer? Do my children perceive that I no longer find the odds of getting better while feeling worse on experimental therapy worth it? Families, in turn, seem to deny that their loved one could wind up like this, wasting away before their eyes.

The likelihood of participating in research therapies for cancer treatment may decline in elderly cancer patients due to lowered life span expectations; poorer prognosis due to more advanced stages of the disease; the body's inability to cope with the collateral effects; and, very importantly, a value hierarchy that places other factors, like the grandchildren's college education, over one's own continued life.

This, then, is the cancer dynamic: guilt, to objectification of the disease, to a sense of betrayal by the body, to struggles with the cancer, to relapse, and guilt about deciding to stop. The dynamic is a spiritual struggle. In the elderly it is compressed by their sense of the limitations on their life span. An important component at each step of the dynamic is the autonomous ranking of values, which is essential to grasp in the care of all patients, especially the elderly, who have had more opportunities to establish and hone their values through the challenges life has thrown their way.[54]

## Cancer and Autonomy

Autonomy is often identified with decision making, but patients themselves seldom make this identification. Given the complexity of the cancer dynamic, it is not surprising that caregivers might misjudge the role of autonomy in the spiritual struggles of their patients. The latter are engaged with at least three struggles:[55]

1. with the body, often leading to physical exhaustion
2. with the environment, their family, community, job, nursing home, etc.
3. with their own values, including their life plans, expectations, the hierarchy of their values, and so on

While the cancer dynamic continues, the patient identifies autonomy with reshuffling a hierarchy of values. These values are not communicated to caregivers as a general rule, and this is the challenge of creating a good therapeutic plan that does not deprive the patient of that which is most dear. The values can easily be missed in well-intentioned but ineffective efforts to respect the patient.

The importance of this value hierarchy for quality-of-life decisions cannot be overemphasized. By respecting this hierarchy we can best protect against paternalistic overtreatment against a patient's wishes[56] and any biased undertreatment of cancer patients. This point underlines the importance of finding out patients' values as part of the process of respecting them as persons. It is also the guiding principle in constructing a therapeutic plan.[57] If a patient chooses no therapy for prostate cancer in order to give his money to his grandchildren for their college education, this value is essential to the person he has chosen to become during his life. It makes no sense to strip his personhood from him.

## Cancer and Suffering

Pain is a major consideration in caring for any cancer patient. It can so preoccupy caregivers that concomitant suffering is masked. Yet it is the suffering of the patient that should appeal most to our compassion. The first source of suffering is the bifurcation of the person into an ego, often isolated and alone, and the body that has betrayed that person, the object taken over by the disease. This betrayal is bad enough for a person at any age, but in the elderly it is compounded by what are euphemistically called "the indignities of age." There is a documented disparity between patient and physician evaluation of the quality of life.[58,59] The patient's own judgment of his or her quality of life influences and predicts the patient's term of survival. Involving patients in decisions about the therapeutic plan can help heal the suffering caused by the division of the self into ego and body. This is an irony because patients' efforts to reconstitute the self tempt them to abandon decisions about their traitorous body to the doctors, turning instead to the ego and its values.

Attention to quality-of-life concerns can breach the gap and center the decisions about patient care.[60] In other words, concern for patient values, both making the effort to discover them and using them to design a humane treatment plan, is fundamental. Paying attention to patient decision making per se is structurally correct, but it is not enough to make a difference. Decision making is only a door through which higher forms of respect for persons pass. A good example would be how a "difficult patient," dying of breast cancer metastases, becomes less belligerent as soon as she is involved in the decisions yet to be made about her care. Once the offer to participate is accepted, the patient not only "accepts" the illness, either explicitly or implicitly, but also, by that very participation, becomes part of the healing relationship that was dysfunctional earlier.

The biggest danger a cancer patient faces is that of being stripped of his or her values in the face of the panoply of interventions we have available. The emotional roller coaster of promises and hopes versus outcomes and despairs can disrupt the relationships people have constructed all of their lives.[61] Letting go not only of one's life but also of one's social roles and relationships is part of this kind of care that only adds to the suffering the patient experiences. It is endemic to the goal of palliative medicine.

Suffering, then, is much more than personal disruption. Yet its base lies there, where the disease has shattered the human entity, at least for a time, until some synthesis can be effected. The primary task of caregivers is to aid

in this synthesis as much as possible. Some recommendations are:

- Minimize suffering, not only through pain control efforts but also by confronting one's own blockages to meeting the suffering person as a person. Training in pain control is essential to this step, but so is training in avoiding withdrawal and fears we have ourselves about dying.

- Make every effort to understand the patient's value system, so that it can be respected and employed in the treatment plan. This may include using values assessment tools.

- Implement the care plan as a means to minimize suffering. There is nothing worse for patients who are dying than having to wrestle with caregivers over the treatment plan.

- Even when the patient can no longer feel pain and is in a comatose state near the end of life, respecting his or her values is still essential so that the person he or she was, despite the current condition, is nonetheless respected.

## Termination of Treatment

All the preceding reflections are essential to a consideration of issues of termination of treatment. Such decisions involve the proportionality of the treatment to the expected and sometimes realized outcome for the individual in his or her specific circumstances.[62] The word *specific* is important. There is no absolute objective standard by which to measure this proportionality. Each instance must be judged on its own characteristics.

What might be deemed appropriate care for a younger patient, say an experimental chemotherapeutic regimen for a 36-year-old man newly diagnosed with pancreatic cancer, cannot be proposed for an older patient, for example, a 93-year-old previously healthy widow. The reasons for this difference may be broader than physical condition of the body alone. They may also be related to the individual's life plans.[63] The younger person may wish to buy some time to put his affairs in order, for little hope can be offered for improvement for a significant length of time in the face of pancreatic cancer. The elderly patient may have no such plans and may be quite willing to die despite any entreaties by the family to try to fight the disease. Her body may have given her so much pain by this point that she has come to consider it an impediment.

### Withholding and withdrawing

Most caregivers today seem more willing to withhold and withdraw major interventions deemed "heroic," but their reasons appear somewhat confused. Should this action be done with the goal of bringing about the patient's death (death induction[63])? In this analysis, death is seen as good and actions are taken to bring about that good.[64] We may be morally obligated to bring about what is perceived as the good in this regard.[65] Or, instead, should the goal be to remove treatments that prolong the patient's suffering, while not intending the patient's death? This intent is entirely different from the first. It assumes that death is either neutral or an evil, and that one cannot will such an evil and still maintain purity of heart. The action of withholding or withdrawing will be the same in either case, however.

The distinction in intent between aiming at the patient's death and aiming at reducing suffering originally was used to distinguish between active and passive euthanasia. The distinction has become essentially moot, since most of those who pay attention to it find that there is no moral difference between withholding and withdrawing on the one hand and actively bringing about death on the other, if the intent is that the patient's death would be a good thing.[66] This makes sense. If our intent in withdrawing care is to bring about death, then other more direct forms of euthanasia may seem much more appropriate. We do not want patients to suffer unduly, even if the pain itself is under control.

Currently Americans are hotly debating whether to legalize active euthanasia, aid in dying, and physician-assisted suicide.[67] In the majority of cases, pain control and addressing the suffering of patients as is done in hospice will be sufficient to properly care for patients. More effort must be made to confront and alleviate the patient's suffering, however. Having more dialogue about values will honor and support dying cancer patients. Use an interview format around values assessment, but do not confine the process to a single conversation. A continuing dialogue would be most appropriate. Although values do not change, attitudes about values do as the disease progresses.

Planning for a good death would lead to restraint of our technological interventions at various stages in the course of disease, depending on the patient's values, willingness to trade possible severe side effects for the chance of an improved, albeit temporary, quality of life, and the patient's self-definition.[68] Of major concern is allowing physicians to kill patients out of mercy in the context of a society that has so little respect for human life in other areas.

### Control of dying and life support

Our concerns should not be confined to dispatching persons too early by injections, if simultaneously little or no attention is paid to meeting their physical and social needs. One "technofix" solution to patient anguish is to prolong suffering in conditions of hopeless injury.[69] A good example, unfortunately all too common, is putting an 80-year-old senile and incompetent patient, dying of cancer, on renal dialysis. No family members are left to

protest. The patient is brought three times a week to the medical center from the nursing home.

Much of earlier technological intervention was not so much life-supporting but, as Albert Jonsen[70] suggests, organ-supporting. Now, increasingly, truly systematic efforts are made to prolong all the vital organ systems at once, getting the essential nutrients in and wastes out. We have moved not only from organ-specific technologies to systemic ones but also from temporary support to permanent support. Jonsen wonders just what exactly life support supports:

> We talk about the maintenance of life; we don't often talk about the maintenance of personhood. It interests me little, indeed, not at all, to be alive as an organism. In such a state I have no interests. It is enormously interesting for me to be a person. . . . It is the perpetuation of my personhood that interests me; indeed, it is probably my major and perhaps my sole real interest.[70,p.67]

The effect of employing life-prolonging technology on the dying without patient involvement in its application is to increase patient and family suffering. It may prolong the suffering of dying, and it provides social suffering by wasting resources that might benefit those with potentially reversible diseases.[71]

In order to protect human dignity, societies must maintain constant vigilance about protecting persons from both undertreatment and abandonment and inappropriate overtreatment. But how? Undertreatment occurs when the "bottom line" predominates over benefit to the patient. Only a national health coverage plan would eliminate this injustice. Overtreatment occurs through the technological enthusiasms of caregivers, the fear of "letting go," or appeals for unreasonable treatments from patients. Only institutional policies about appropriate treatment decisions coupled with compassionate analysis, as suggested earlier, will answer these problems. In both instances, we will be shepherding our technology for good human aims. This shepherding can be focused on an obligation to attempt to eliminate pain and to address suffering.

Control over one's own dying ought to be the focus of our public policy efforts. Decisions and choices patients make in this regard arise out of the context of their relationships with their loved ones and caregivers and of their own value history. Every effort should be made to help the caregivers and the dying maintain a personal and professional relationship.

### Nutrition and hydration

Those who oppose the withdrawal of nutrition and hydration do so on grounds that providing food and water to the dying is a special obligation not covered by our considerations so far, and that beneficence should overrule patient autonomy.[72,73] Specifically, they argue that such withdrawing or withholding leads directly to the death of the patient as much as does an injection, since the patient dies not of the underlying disease process but from starvation and dehydration.[74]

There are two problems with this contention. First, patients have a common-law right and probably a constitutional right to refuse treatment even if they are not dying. Second, patients may request aid in dying on the grounds we have just examined, namely, that death is a good and others have a duty out of compassion to bring about such a good. "Bringing it about" does not necessarily entail active, direct euthanasia, or even physician-assisted suicide. But it does require that all interventions, including fluids and nutrition, be examined for their impact on the desired goal of treatment.[75] If an earlier and less painful death, with less suffering for the patient, is the desired goal, then how does it make sense to provide medically delivered food and water unless the patient specifically requests it?

Nonetheless, those who support withholding or withdrawing fluids and nutrition may miss a main concern of opponents, that in the absence of expressed wishes, vulnerable persons may be "put to death" by such actions. For this reason some ethicists think that only objective criteria (medical indications presumably), not the context, life plans, or values of the individual, can be used in all withholding and withdrawing decisions.[74] Furthermore, they argue that anything else cannot be used to bring about death in patients who have made no advance directives or who have left only vague statements about not using heroic measures to prolong their lives. The family's expression of the values of the patient are regarded as insufficient reasons to remove such therapy.

## The role of the family

In light of the U.S. Supreme court decision in re *Cruzan*,[76] it is clear that the role of the family in speaking for patient values is confused. Recall that Nancy Cruzan was left in a permanent vegetative state after a car accident. For seven years she was fed through a feeding tube. After five years her parents sought to have the tube removed on the grounds that Nancy had mentioned before the accident that she would not want to live in such a condition. The State of Missouri argued that it had a Living Will law that required advance directives of this sort in writing. It interpreted the need for evidence of patient wishes very strictly. When the case reached the U.S. Supreme Court (the first and only termination-of-life-support case to do so), the Court affirmed the right of patients to control their medical interventions but seemed to place more emphasis on the right of the state to require evidence of patient wishes than on the right of families acting as guardians to speak for the values of patients. Although the case does not apply directly to persons with cancer, it does demonstrate that guardianship and family issues are still being worked out for incompetent patients.

Thus, it is very important to obtain advance directives from all patients, especially seriously ill ones. The preferred instrument in most states is the Durable Power of Attorney for Health Care. This document names ahead of time an individual who will speak for the patient when the patient is incompetent to make decisions about health care. It is limited in time to the duration of incompetence and in scope to decisions about health care only. Such an instrument often designates a family member to speak for the patient. Despite the cautions noted by the Supreme Court about family surrogacy, most persons feel comfortable about naming a family member to make decisions, since such a person knows them and their values best.

## Access to care

Callahan proposes, when patients are competent and can speak for themselves about medical care, that their options be limited past 80 years of age and that some interventions no longer be considered.[77] While we might conceivably agree with Callahan that there exists a certain point beyond which expensive medical technology should not be offered to elderly persons, this point should not be set by ageist limits but rather by the limits of medicine to provide any meaningful change in the outcome for patients during their last years.[78]

It may not be necessary to set such limits on the basis of age if we first try to respect a patient's value system.[79] Elderly persons will usually choose highly technical interventions less often than will younger cancer patients. Statistics show that when patients approach 80 years of age, we spend less on their care. So age and patient wishes apparently begin at that time to be "factored in." Does this mean that physicians ignore the patient's calculation of life span until one reaches "old old" age? Do these data suggest instead that there is a natural life span of about 80–85 years, after which it makes no sense, as Callahan has suggested, to employ major technological interventions to save lives?

Many patients over 80 are more ready to die than to fight cancer. It is not an instance of wanting to die, necessarily. Quite the contrary. Life is still regarded as precious. Instead, it is a matter of proportion. Patients over 80 are more accustomed to thinking that they will soon die anyway. One woman, 92 years old, refused to see a doctor for her suppurating breast cancer. She figured she would die soon and did not want to do so in a hospital where her little bit of savings would almost immediately vanish. She still lived at home, where neighbors and friends looked in on her. Yet when finally convinced to enter a hospital and have the breast removed, she was relieved to learn from her doctors that she would live for some time. ("Let's face it," they said, "you will most probably die of something else than the cancer because it grows so slowly in the elderly.") She was very happy that she would return home. Her plan? To go on a tour of Alaska!

So the post-80 syndrome cuts both ways. It may lead patients to give up too early on their care when they could achieve a significant quality of life. Or it may lead to age bias in offering and withholding care. On the other hand, it also may lead caregivers to sell patients a "bill of goods" that may bankrupt other patient values. A person from the Association of American Retired Persons in Nebraska wrote about a friend in another state who lost two premier family farms that had to be sold to pay for his care during his dying months. He had intended to bequeath them to his grandchildren. The end-stage "battle" with his disease was orchestrated and managed by his oncologist without attention to these primary values.

Among other important issues regarding access to cancer care are the problem of the rights of all persons to expensive interventions, the right to request experimental therapy (if any),[80] allocating scarce resources like interleukin-2, large-scale distribution of health care among competing health needs (e.g., the drain of caring for persons with AIDS on state and local health care budgets), and the distribution of funding for other human needs versus health care needs.

### Playing God

Modern medical technology empowers individuals beyond their normal capacities. Because technology is, by definition, an extension of human work, it tempts us to exceed the bounds of temperance. This leads to a kind of paternalism in which an individual comes to believe that he or she knows best what is good for another person due to superior technical knowledge. Medical technology adds to this traditional paternalism an even greater temptation, the temptation to "play God."[81] Usually a physician "god" is unrelenting in applying treatment interventions. Rarely, a pusillanimous abandonment of patients without sufficient intervention is found, as might occur when inappropriate judgments about either patient values or the patient's quality of life are made.[82]

It must be admitted that human beings have an incredible thirst for power. Surely this is one reason that humanity is perpetually dissatisfied with the status quo and constantly wants to change for the better. General Electric's slogan used to be "Progress is our most important product." Progress in what, one might ask? The answer cannot be just technological improvement. Leading a good life must include mastery of life's vicissitudes. There is nothing intrinsically wrong with our efforts to improve our lives; on the contrary, it is part of the mission of all human beings to use their facilities and propensities to bring about the good in their lives and in society. Yet it is important for health care that providers understand the risks and benefits of the technological interventions they propose.[83]

### Euthanasia

The problem of euthanasia, as well as the incredibly difficult questions about human reproduction and all the others in between the origin of life and the final moment of death, involves the question of dominion over life. Our technology makes the temptation to take control over life itself almost overwhelming. Inappropriate withdrawal and withholding of care is also a kind of "playing God" since it involves one individual, entrusted with the care of another, making judgments about the value of that person's life. It is important to distinguish here between objective evaluation of interventions and outcomes on the well-being of the patient and subjective quality-of-life judgments in which the physician and other caregivers judge that the life the patient is now living is not worthwhile for that person.

The danger in the United States today is in the economic sphere.[84] Will it be easier to use a simple method of dispatching those persons whose care costs too much or who are now considered to be a burden on society, like patients with advanced stages of cancer who require extensive care, than to address their suffering, which sometimes is overwhelming even for the most dedicated caregivers? The issue focuses attention on the importance of maintaining compassionate respect for human life in our society. For some, actions to eliminate burdensome life, even if requested by the patient him- or herself, are a form of "privatizing life," denying its social and communal dimensions as both a private and public good. These persons would argue strongly against direct euthanasia or physician-assisted suicide.[85] Others argue that euthanasia and/or assisted suicide are appropriate and important forms of caring for persons whose lives, by their own assessment, have become too burdensome to continue.[86–89]

## CONCLUSION

Some suggestions might therefore be as follows:

1. Consider that the duty to protect a patient's life lies primarily in protecting his or her autonomy and value hierarchy. It makes little sense to prolong a life if one does not respect the biography of that life as "written" by the patient. For this reason, I recommend paying more attention to discovering the patient's value system, through a values assessment interview and through constant discussion with the patient and the family throughout the course of treatment.

2. Require advance directives before one receives the first retirement check, enter that advance directive on a central computer, and update it whenever one enters a health care institution, nursing home, or hospice in accordance with current Patient Self-Determination Act procedures.[90] This suggestion differs significantly from the Patient Self-Determination Act of 1990 (implemented in December 1991), in that the latter requires only information and education, while my proposal requires executing an advance directive itself.[91,92] Current procedures for informing patients of their right to issue advance directives could be used with sample forms attached for their implementation. Home care nurses should be recruited for discussing

these instruments with all persons ready to retire as part of a national effort to prevent unnecessary and unwanted care.

3. Teaching guides should be developed for all health care professionals that would train them in the processes of implementing patient advance directives, since resistance to these directives is still encountered.

4. Change the current default mode of health care delivery in which it is assumed that everyone desires technological support of their life. Instead of assuming that during the last months of a patient's life everything possible should be done to prolong that life, the opposite assumption would be made unless the patient has issued advance directives to the contrary. Since some people's advance directive will be that they wish to make none, they will need to be warned that this means an assumption in favor of restraint rather than intervention.

5. Use a process like the Ethical Workup Guide to analyze and discuss cases that arise in one's service. By doing this, one not only gains greater critical awareness of one's own assumptions and values but also becomes more able to discuss the deepest commitments of one's profession.

# REFERENCES

1. Graber GC: Basic theories in medical ethics, in Monagle J, Thomasma DC (eds): *Medical Ethics: A Guide for Health Professionals.* Rockville, MD, Aspen, 1988, pp 462–475
2. Beauchamp T, Childress J: *Principles of Biomedical Ethics* (ed 3). New York, Oxford University Press, 1995
3. Pellegrino ED, Thomasma DC: *For the Patient's Good: The Restoration of Beneficence in Health Care.* New York, Oxford University Press, 1988
4. Thomasma DC: Beyond medical paternalism and patient autonomy: A model of physician conscience for the physician-patient relationship. *Ann Intern Med* 98:243–248, 1983
5. Thomasma DC: Some philosophical observations about autonomy in oncology, in Bergsma J, ed: *Autonomy and the Cancer Patient.* Utrecht, Netherlands, Department of Social Sciences and Medicine, Rijksuniversiteit Utrecht Medical School, 1985, pp 29–38
6. Thomasma DC: When healing involves risk to life: Risky medical procedures and experimentation. *New Catholic World* 230:163–167, July/Aug. 1987
7. Thomasma DC: High technology and dying. *New World Outlook* 46:256–258, 1986
8. Thomasma DC: Philosophical reflections on a rational treatment plan. *J Med Philos* 11:157–165, 1986
9. Thomasma DC: Quality of life judgments and medical indications. *Qual Life Cardiovasc Care* 2:113–118, 1986
10. Rossi R: Madam gets 1-yr house detention. *Chicago Sun-Times,* March 19, 1992
11. MacIntyre A: *Whose Justice? Which Rationality!* Notre Dame, IN, University of Notre Dame Press, 1988
12. Veatch R: *A Theory of Medical Ethics* (ed 2) New York, Basic Books, 1996
13. Engelhardt HT Jr: *The Foundations of Bioethics* (ed 2) New York, Oxford University Press, 1996
14. Graber G, Thomasma D: *Theory and Practice in Medical Ethics.* New York, Continuum, 1989
15. Thomasma D: Applying general medical knowledge to individuals: A philosophical analysis. *Theor Med* 9:187–200, 1988
16. Jansson L, Norberg A: Ethical reasoning concerning the feeding of terminally ill cancer patients: Interviews with registered nurses experienced in the care of cancer patients. *Cancer Nurs* 12:352–358, 1989
17. Davidson B: Ethical reasoning associated with the feeding of terminally ill elderly cancer patients: An international perspective. *Cancer Nurs* 13:286–292, 1990
18. Pellegrino ED, Thomasma DC: The conflict between autonomy and beneficence in medical ethics: Proposal for a resolution. *J Cont Health Law Policy* 3:23–46, 1987
19. Loewy E: The restoration of beneficence. *Hastings Cent Rep* 19:42–43, 1989
20. Thomasma DC: Ethical and legal issues in the care of the elderly cancer patient. *Clin Geriatr Med* 3:541–547, 1987
21. Thomasma DC: The basis of medicine and religion: Respect for persons. *Linacre Quart* 45:142–150, 1980
22. Brody H: *The Healer's Power.* New Haven, CT, Yale University Press, 1992, p 119
23. Engelhardt HT Jr: *Bioethics and Secular Humanism.* London/Philadelphia, SCM/Trinity Press International, 1991
24. Engelhardt HT Jr: *Foundations of Bioethics* (ed 2). New York: Oxford Univ Press, 1996
25. Walker MU: Moral particularity. *Metaphilosophy* 18:171–185, 1987
26. Toulmin S, Jonsen A: *The Abuse of Casuistry.* Berkeley, University of California Press, 1988
27. MacIntyre A: *After Virtue.* Notre Dame, IN, University of Notre Dame Press, 1981
28. Thomasma D: The context as moral rule in medical ethics, in Wright RA (ed): *Human Values in Health Care.* New York, McGraw-Hill, 1987, pp 142–156
29. Thomasma D: Decision making and decision analysis: Beneficence in medicine. *J Crit Care* 3:122–132, 1988
30. Thomasma D: Beyond medical paternalism and patient autonomy: A model of physician's conscience for the doctor-patient relationship. *Ann Intern Med* 98:243–248, 1983
31. Bergsma J, Thomasma D: *Health Care: Its Psychosocial Dimensions.* Pittsburgh, Duquesne University Press, 1982
32. Loewy E: *Suffering and the Beneficent Community: Beyond Libertarianism.* Buffalo, NY, SUNY Press, 1991
33. Welie JM: Sympathy as the basis of Compassion. *Cambridge Quarterly of Healthcare Ethics* 4:476–487, 1995
34. Thomasma DC, Kushner T: A dialogue on compassion and supererogation in medicine. *Cambridge Quarterly of Healthcare Ethics* 4:415–425, 1995
35. Loewy EH: Compassion, reason and moral judgment. *Cambridge Quarterly of Healthcare Ethics* 4:466–475, 1995
36. Self DJ, Gopalakrishnan G, Kiser WR, et al: The relationship of empathy to moral reasoning in first-year medical students. *Cambridge Quarterly of Healthcare Ethics* 4:448–453, 1995
37. John Paul II Pope: Humanize hospital work. Address to the Sixty-First General Chapter of the Hospital Order of St. John of God. *L'Osservatore Romano,* Jan. 24, 1983
38. Dougherty CJ, Purtilo R: Physician's duty of compassion. *Cambridge Quarterly of Healthcare Ethics* 4:426–433, 1995
39. Nouwen H: *The Wounded Healer.* New York, Doubleday, 1972, p 72
40. De Unamuno M: *The Tragic Sense of Life,* translated by Kerri-

gan A. Princeton, NJ, Princeton University Press, Bollingen Series, LXXXV, 4, 1972, p 224

41. Pellegrino ED, Thomasma DC: *Helping and Healing.* Washington DC: Georgetown University Press, 1997
42. McElhinney T, Pellegrino ED (eds): *Teaching Ethics, the Humanities, and Human Values in Medical Schools: A Ten-Year Overview.* Washington, DC, Institute on Human Values in Medicine, Society for Health and Human Values, 1982
43. Gaylin W, Kass L, Pellegrino ED, et al: Commentaries: Doctors must not kill. *JAMA* 259:2139–2140, 1988
44. Kass L: Arguments against active euthanasia by doctors found at medicine's core. *Kennedy Institute of Ethics Newsletter.* 3:1–3, Jan. 6, 1989
45. Marsden C: Caregiver fidelity in a pediatric bone marrow transplant team. *Heart Lung* 6:617–625, 1988
46. Rhodes R: Love thy patient: Justice, caring, and the doctor-patient relationship. *Cambridge Quarterly of Healthcare Ethics* 4:434–447, 1995
47. Rouse F: Living wills in the long-term care setting. *J Long-Term Care Adm* 17:14–19, Summer, 1988
48. Mehling A: Living wills: Preventing suffering or a deadly contract? *State Government News,* Dec. 1988, pp 14–15
49. Braithwaite S, Thomasma DC: New guidelines on foregoing life-sustaining treatment in incompetent patients: An anti-cruelty policy. *Ann Intern Med* 104:711–715, 1986
50. Illich I: *Medical Nemesis: The Expropriation of Health.* New York, Pantheon, 1976
51. Thomasma D: Ethics and professional practice in oncology. *Semin Oncol Nurs* 5:89–94, 1989
52. Cassell E: Disease as an "It." *Soc Sci Med* 10:143–146, 1976
53. Bried EM, Scheffler RM: The impact of healthcare financing on the quality of life of older cancer patients. *Oncology* 6:153–160, 1992 (suppl)
54. Thomasma D: The ethics of caring for the older patient with cancer: Defining the issues. *Oncology* 6:124–130, 1992 (suppl)
55. Slevin ML, Stubbs L, Plant HJ, et al: Attitude to chemotherapy: Comparing views of patients with cancer with those of doctors, nurses, and general public. *Brit Med J* 300:1458–1460, 1990
56. Cranford R: The care of the dying: A symposium on the case of Betty Wright—Going out in style, the American way, 1987. *Law, Med Health Care* 17:208–210, Fall 1989
57. Thomasma DC: Ethics and professional practice in oncology. *Semin Oncol Nurs* 5:89–94, 1989
58. Slevin ML, Stubbs L, Plant HJ, et al: Attitudes to chemotherapy: Comparing views of patients with cancer with those of doctors, nurses, and general public. *Brit Med J* 300:1458–1460, 1990
59. Ganz P: Does (or should) chronological age influence the choice of cancer treatment? *Oncology* 6:45–49, 1992 (suppl)
60. Walter JJ, Shannon TA (eds): *Quality of Life: The New Medical Dilemma.* New York and Mahwah, NJ, Paulist Press, 1990
61. Ferrell BR, Grant MM, Padilla GV, et al: Home care. *Oncology* 6:136–140, 1992 (suppl)
62. O'Rourke K: Should nutrition and hydration be provided to permanently unconscious and other mentally disabled persons? *Issues Law Med* 5:181–196, 1989
63. Thomasma DC: Caveat philosophus: Technology's abuse potential in the decision to terminate life. *J Am Geriatr Soc* 35:124–125, 1987
64. Bayles MD: Euthanasia and the quality of life, in Bayles MD, High DM (eds): *Medical Treatment of the Dying: Moral Issues.* New York, Schenkman Books, 1978, pp 128–152

65. Thomasma DC, Graber GC: *Euthanasia: Toward an Ethical Social Policy.* New York, Continuum, 1990
66. Rachels J: *Moral Problems.* New York, Harper and Row, 1971, pp 42–66
67. Doctor-aided suicide spurs ethics debate. *Chicago Tribune,* March 7, 1991, Sec. 1, 1
68. Bujorian GA: Clinical trials: Patient issues in the decision-making process. *Oncol Nurs Forum* 15:779–783, 1988
69. Luce EA, Frank AL, Kilner JF, et al: Lingering death from squamous cell carcinoma of the face. *Hosp Pract* 24:60–61, 65–66, 71–72, 1989
70. Jonsen A: What does life support support? in Winslade W (ed): *Personal Choices and Public Commitments: Perspectives on the Humanities.* Galveston, TX, Institute for the Medical Humanities, 1988, pp 61–69
71. Raffin TA, Shurkin JN, Sinkler W III: *Intensive Care: Facing the Critical Issues.* New York, Freeman, 1988, p 185
72. Callahan D: On feeding the dying. *Hastings Cent Rep* 13:22–23, 1983
73. Luce EA, Frank AL, Kilner JF, et al: Lingering death from squamous cell carcinoma of the face. *Hosp Practice* 24:65–66, 71–72, 1989
74. May W, et al: Feeding and hydrating the permanently unconscious and other vulnerable persons. *Issues Law Med* 3:203–211, Winter, 1987
75. Paris JJ, McCormick RA: The Catholic tradition on the use of nutrition and fluids. *America,* May 2, 1987, 356–360
76. Thomasma DC: The Cruzan decision and medical practice. *Arch Intern Med* 151:853–854, 1991 (editorial)
77. Callahan D: *Setting Limits: Medical Goals in an Aging Society.* New York, Simon and Schuster, 1987, pp 159–185, 241–242
78. Thomasma DC: Moving the aged into the house of the dead: A critique of ageist social policy. *J Am Geriatr Soc* 37:169–172, 1989
79. Thomasma DC: Ethical and moral issues in access to cancer care, in Scheffler RM, Andrews NC (eds): *Cancer Care and Cost: DRGs and Beyond.* Ann Arbor, MI, Health Administration Press, 1989, pp 211–223
80. Thomasma D, Micetich K: The ethics of patient requests in experimental medicine. Reprinted as monograph by the American Cancer Society, Oct., 1984
81. Taylor C: Ethics in health care and medical technologies. *Theor Med* 11:111–124, 1990
82. Wilkes E: Ethics in terminal care, in Dunstan GR, Shinebourne EA (eds): *Doctors' Decisions: Ethical Conflicts in Medical Practice.* New York, Oxford University Press, 1989, pp 197–204
83. Melski JW: Prices of technology: A blind spot. *JAMA* 267:1516–1518, 1992
84. Scitovsky AA, Capron AM: Medical care at the end of life: The interaction of economics and ethics. *Annu Rev Public Health* 7:59–75, 1986
85. Bernardin J Cardinal: Euthanasia: Ethical and legal challenge. Address to the Center for Clinical Medical Ethics, University of Chicago Hospital, May 26, 1988
86. Kevorkian J: A fail-safe model for justifiable medically-assisted suicide. *Am J Forensic Psych* 13:7, 41, 1992
87. Quill TE: Death and dignity—A case of individualized decision making. *N Engl J Med* 324:691–694, 1991
88. Humphrey D: *Final Exit: The Practicalities of Self-Deliverance and Assisted Suicide for the Dying.* Eugene, OR, Hemlock Society, 1991
89. *Trends Health Care, Law Ethics* 7: Winter, 1992
90. Thomasma DC: Advance directives and health care for the

elderly, in Hackler C Jr, Moseley R, Vawter D (eds): *Advance Directives in Medicine.* New York, Praeger, 1989, pp 93–109

91. Thomasma DC: From ageism toward autonomy, in Binstock R, Post S (eds): *Too Old for Health Care?* Baltimore: Johns Hopkins University Press, 1991, pp 138–163

92. PSDA well received in hospitals, despite early confusion. *Med Eth Advisor* 8:25–30, 1992 (editorial)

# Chapter 58

# Alternative Methods of Cancer Therapy

Connie Henke Yarbro, RN, MS, FAAN

## INTRODUCTION

Each year more than a million Americans are diagnosed as having cancer, and more than half will be cured with scientifically sound therapies. Each year thousands of cancer patients and many others who merely fear they might develop it will devote countless hours and invest billions of dollars in the use of alternative cancer remedies outside the realm of mainstream medicine. Others will use these methods as complementary techniques to help control symptoms of their disease or side effects from proven cancer therapy.[1] Additionally, thousands will seek information about such treatments.[2] Whether labeled "unconventional," "unsound," "unproven," "unorthodox," or "questionable," alternative treatments range from those that are both fraudulent and dangerous to those that are hazardous mainly to the pocketbook. Often, these treatments offer individuals a chance to participate in their own care, reflecting the naturalistic approaches so popular with the public today.[3]

The field of alternative and complementary therapies has become more visible and popular since Congress mandated the establishment of the Office of Alternative Medicine (OAM) in 1992 at the National Institutes of Health (NIH), which conducts alternative medicine research. Specialty centers have been established to conduct alternative medicine research and medical schools have established departments and courses on alternative medicine.[4] Health insurers are opening their doors to coverage of alternative health care. For example, Kaiser Permanente's Alternative Medicine Clinic at Vallejo, California offers acupuncture therapy, herbal medicine, and relaxation training based on referrals from primary care physicians.[5] And, communication via the Internet has provided the public with the latest information and sources of many alternative therapies.

The constant changes in terminology cause confusion for the public as well as for health care providers. Today, "alternative" is the popular lexicon for unconventional or questionable therapies. The American Cancer Society (ACS) has defined *alternative therapies* as unproven or disproven methods, whereas *complementary therapies* are supportive therapies that are used to complement standard mainstream therapy.[6] Oncology nurses are involved with complementary therapies that have been scientifically evaluated and proven to be helpful adjuncts in the care of patients with cancer (e.g., relaxation techniques, biofeedback, music therapy). However, in some situations complementary methods also can be used inappropriately.

Alternative methods of cancer management include diagnostic tests or therapeutic methods that have not shown activity in animal tumor models or in scientific clinical trials but are promoted for general use in cancer prevention, diagnosis, or treatment. Such methods may not be safe for the consumer, since they have not met the requirements of the U.S. Food, Drug, and Cosmetic Act. According to a 1984 report by the U.S. House of Representatives' Subcommittee on Health and Long-term Care, each year Americans spend $10 billion on unscientific remedies and $4 billion to $5 billion on fraudulent ones.[7,8] A national telephone survey of 1539 adults found that 34% used an unconventional therapy in 1990 spending almost $14 billion that year, of which $10.3 billion was paid out-of-pocket.[9] Questionable nutritional supplements alone are more than a $2 billion-a-year industry in the United States.[10] The exact number of cancer patients who try alternative therapies is unknown, but various studies have reported that 9%–94% of cancer patients admitted using alternative therapies.[11–17]

## HISTORICAL PERSPECTIVES

For thousands of years, individuals in need have turned to people offering what they hope will be an answer to their medical problems. Popular folk remedies for the treatment of cancer have been available for centuries. Only in relatively recent times has the scientific method, in conjunction with organized medicine and government, been able to provide a measure of confidence that a treatment is safe and effective.

### Legislation

Before the Food and Drug Act of 1906, thousands of unproven treatments were promoted to the American public. Often the treatments were not harmful in themselves. But as an anonymous physician noted in a letter to the *National Quarterly Review* in 1861, "Quackery kills a larger number annually than the disease it pretends to cure."[18]

In 1906 President Theodore Roosevelt signed into law the Pure Food and Drug Act, which forbade misleading or false statements on the labels of remedies. However, Janssen[19] reported that in 1910, in a crucial test of the new law, the U.S. Supreme Court ruled that the law involved only truthful labeling of ingredients used in drugs, not the false therapeutic claims on the drug label. Justice Oliver Wendell Holmes, Jr., concluded that individuals could not be prosecuted for what he termed "mistaken praise" of their treatments, even though the claims were false.

Noting the dangers of permitting unsafe and ineffective drugs on the market, President Taft exhorted the Congress, in 1911, to pass tougher legislation:

> There are none so credulous as sufferers from disease. The need is urgent for legislation which will prevent the raising of false hopes of speedy cures of serious ailment by misstatements of facts as to the worthless mixtures on which the sick will rely while their disease progresses unchecked.[20]

In 1912 Congress passed the Sherley Amendment, which made it a crime to make false or fraudulent claims regarding the therapeutic efficacy of a drug. However, this legislation was limited, in that it was still necessary to prove that the promoter intended to defraud the public. Mistaken claims could still be made, and patients could continue to be defrauded. In 1938 Congress eliminated this difficulty by passing legislation that required scientific proof of safety before a drug could be marketed.

In 1962 Congress clarified some of the language of the previous legislation and further added that drugs must demonstrate efficacy in addition to safety before they could be marketed. Thus, the process was created by which a substance became approved for prescription use by the Food and Drug Administration (FDA). The Food and Drug Commissioner[21] noted that the Food and Drug Act of 1962 means that "the absolute freedom to choose an ineffective drug was properly surrendered in exchange for the freedom from danger to each person's health and well-being from the sale and use of worthless drugs." This is, in fact, the same decision made over the years by those in government who have decided that only individuals certified by experts may practice medicine and are qualified to help the patients who would choose to seek their assistance. Although the Food and Drug Act of 1962 frequently has been challenged by those who promote questionable methods, the act was upheld by a decision of the U.S. Supreme Court in 1973.

## Past Unproven Methods

Questionable approaches to cancer treatment have existed for centuries, but a popular new alternative suddenly seems to develop and thrive almost every decade. Examples of unorthodox approaches, arranged according to their eras of popularity, are identified in Table 58-1. We have gone from the nineteenth century "holistic," or "natural," movement to the so-called drug approach of the early and mid-1900s, back to the holistic, natural, or diet-oriented regimens of today.[22] Many of the popular alternative methods of cancer treatment parallel the most promising developments in scientific clinical trials.[23] For example, during the 1960s and 1970s, when drugs were being developed as an effective treatment for cancer, spurious compounds (e.g., Krebiozen and laetrile) were being promoted to cancer patients. In the 1980s, the cancer clinical trials of immunotherapy and biologics corresponded with the unproven use of immunoaugmentative therapy and other compounds that purported to boost the immune system. The following discussion will review the alternative approaches from the era of the 1940s through the 1970s.

### Koch antitoxin therapy: 1940s–1950s

Koch antitoxin therapy, first mentioned in 1919[24] was a popular unproven cancer treatment during the 1940s and 1950s. The treatment consisted of pure distilled water

**TABLE 58-1**  Popular Alternative Treatments in the United States

| Era | Alternative Approaches and Treatments |
|---|---|
| 1800–1850 | Thompsonianism: emetics and hot baths |
| 1850–1900 | Homeopathy: use of highly distilled or diluted inorganic and organic substances |
| 1890s | Naturopathy: diets, massages, colonic irrigation<br>Early osteopathy and chiropractic: spinal manipulation |
| 1900s | Tablet, ointment, and tonic cancer cures |
| 1920s | "Energy" cancer cures: cosmic energy, radio waves, light therapy, psychic diagnoses and treatments |
| 1940s | Koch's glyoxylide |
| 1950s | Hoxsey's cancer treatment |
| 1960s | Krebiozen |
| 1970s | Laetrile |
| 1980s–1990s | Metabolic therapies: diet, megavitamins, minerals, enzymes, colonic irrigation<br>Macrobiotic diets<br>Pharmacological and biological therapies: antineoplastons, Cancell, dimethyl sulfoxide (DMSO), Greek cancer cure, live-cell therapy, megavitamins, herbal therapy, oxymedicine, immuno-augmentative therapy (IAT)<br>Electronic devices<br>Behavioral and psychological: mental imagery; spiritual, faith, or mind healing |

mixed with one part per trillion of a chemical called glyoxylide, which is merely glyoxylic acid (a normal body constituent) with water removed. Koch proposed that cancer was caused by a microorganism susceptible to the differential poison in his antitoxins. He also prescribed enemas and a special diet. Over 3000 health practitioners in the United States employed this regimen, paying $25 per ampule for it and charging patients as much as $300 for a single injection.[19] In 1942 the FDA held hearings across the United States in an effort to gather information regarding the promotion and use of Koch antitoxins. In 1943 the Canadian Cancer Foundation reported that no patients on a clinical trial using the Koch method benefited from the treatment.[25] Subsequently, the Federal Trade Commission issued a court order forbidding the promotion of Koch antitoxins because of their lack of therapeutic value. Although Koch antitoxins are illegal in the United States, they can still be obtained through the underground medical community or in Mexico.

### Hoxsey method: 1950s

The Hoxsey method has been around since the early 1920s. Hoxsey maintained that cancer was a result of a chemical imbalance in the body that caused healthy cells to mutate and become cancerous and that his therapy restored the chemical environment and killed the cancerous cells. Hoxsey's Herbal Tonic consisted of several different formulas: the "black medicine" was composed of cascara (a laxative) in an extract of licorice root, alfalfa, burdock root, red clover blossoms, buckthorn bark, barberry root, pokeweed, and prickly ash bark; the "pink medicine" contained potassium iodide and lactated pepsin.[26] Except for potassium iodide and the laxative, which are effective drugs but have no value in treating cancer, all the other ingredients have been discarded as medically ineffective.[19] Hoxsey also developed a tablet form of his medicines.

The FDA investigated nearly 400 cases of individuals who claimed to be cured of cancer through use of the Hoxsey method, and no legitimate case of a cure was discovered. In 1960 a federal court injunction declared sale of the treatment illegal.[19] At the time the Hoxsey clinics in Dallas, Texas and Portage, Pennsylvania were closed, over 10,000 individuals were enrolled as patients. The FDA estimated that over $50 million was spent for the Hoxsey drugs.[27] Today, Hoxsey's medicines are available at the BioMedical Center in Tijuana, Mexico.[28-30]

### Krebiozen: 1960s

Krebiozen allegedly was first produced by a Yugoslavian physician named Steven Durovic, who developed the substance from blood extracted from horses. In the mid-1950s Andrew C. Ivy, professor emeritus at the University of Illinois, endorsed Krebiozen as an effective cancer therapy. In 1961 the National Cancer Institute (NCI) obtained a sample of Krebiozen, and the substance was identified as creatine monohydrate, an amino acid found in all animal tissue.[31] Pre-1960 samples of Krebiozen actually contained mineral oil and small amounts of amyl alcohol and methylhydantoin.[32] The Krebiozen Research Foundation submitted 504 case records to the NCI in an effort to demonstrate therapeutic efficacy in justification of a clinical trial. A panel of 24 scientists reviewed these records and unanimously concluded that Krebiozen was an ineffective drug.[33] Although no clear scientific evidence of efficacy has been brought forward, the treatment was available until 1977.[19]

### Laetrile: 1970s

Laetrile is a general term for a group of cyanogenic glucosides, derived from several different seeds, e.g., apricot, peach, cherry, and almonds. It is also known as amygdalin and "vitamin B$_{17}$." Ernst T. Krebs, Sr., a physician, claimed to be the first individual to use a cyanogenic glucoside as an anticancer agent. In the 1940s he used amygdalin, derived from apricot kernels, and found it to be too toxic for use in humans, despite what he claimed were encouraging results. In 1952 his son, Ernst Krebs, Jr., reported that he had made an apricot formula that was safe for parenteral administration.

Laetrile's purported mechanism of action has changed over the years as scientific thinking has changed. Perhaps the most common hypothesis is that cancer cells possess an enzyme called β-glucosidase in larger quantities than healthy tissue, whereas normal tissue supposedly has greater quantities of the enzyme rhodanese, which is not present in cancerous tissue. The theory claims that the β-glucosidase in the cancerous tissues causes the laetrile to break down into glucose and mandelonitrile, which breaks down further into hydrogen cyanide (a toxic substance) and benzaldehyde (a mild anesthetic). The cyanide kills the cancer cells, so the theory goes, while the healthy tissue is protected by rhodanese, which converts cyanide into nontoxic sodium thiocynate. Most likely, the majority of the injected laetrile probably is excreted intact in the urine.[34]

Claims have been made that laetrile is a nontoxic form of "vitamin B$_{17}$" and that taking this vitamin can prevent cancer. No reputable scientist accepts the existence of vitamin B$_{17}$. Laetrile does not fulfill the requirements of a vitamin, because no disease state exists in its absence.[35] Evidence suggests that laetrile has toxic effects. The gastric lumen has enzymes capable of breaking laetrile down into hydrogen cyanide and mandelonitrile.[36] There are numerous reports of cyanide toxicity with the ingestion of fruits or seeds containing cyanogenic glucosides, including amygdalin.[33-37] Ingestion of laetrile with certain other foods, such as sweet almonds, lettuce, certain fresh fruits, and mushrooms, can potentiate the toxic reaction. In addition, a number of deaths attributed to cyanide poisoning from oral laetrile have been reported,[37-43] and laetrile by enema is also poisonous.[44,45]

Laetrile in the United States is either imported illegally or brought in under court order (exempting the substance from FDA supervision). This means the product is not required to meet standards of purity. There have been reports of fungal contamination of parenterally formulated laetrile, variations in dosage, and mislabeling of contents of laetrile exported from Mexican manufacturers.[46] For the cancer patient, whose immune system may already be compromised, an infection resulting from contamination could be fatal.

It is noteworthy that laetrile has been the most extensively tested unproven method of all time. Numerous animal studies[47-51] and two retrospective studies have shown no therapeutic benefit.[52,53] In the 1970s there was a movement to legalize laetrile in many states, and cancer patients were seeking laetrile therapy, many of them while discontinuing effective conventional therapy. Laetrile was a billion-dollar-a-year industry in 1979.[41] Thus, in 1980 the FDA gave approval to the NCI for the first prospective clinical trial of laetrile, and once again it was demonstrated that laetrile is ineffective against cancer.[54] The power of the proponent of questionable treatments over the public is illustrated by the fact that despite the proof published in 1982 that laetrile was worthless,[54] laetrile was still a billion-dollar-a-year industry in 1983.[55]

Laetrile's use as an anticancer drug has not ended. Today, many of the proponents of laetrile have changed their strategy of using it as a single agent and are combining it with vitamins, enzymes, or so-called metabolic therapy.[56]

# POPULAR ALTERNATIVE METHODS OF TODAY

Alternative methods of cancer treatment during the 1980s and the 1990s are primarily related to lifestyle, and as such cannot be regulated by the FDA. Many of the unproven methods place responsibility for a healthy lifestyle on the patient and have an aura of respectability in relation to conventional scientific medicine that is concerned with diet, environmental carcinogens, lifestyle, and relation between emotions and physiological responses.[57]

In a study of contemporary unorthodox cancer treatments, Cassileth and colleagues[12] reported that 13% of 304 patients being treated at the University of Pennsylvania Cancer Center have turned to practitioners of alternative methods at one time or another. An additional 365 patients who received alternative treatments were identified by contacting questionable practitioners and clinics. The total sample of 669 patients was interviewed. Among all the patients who had turned to alternative therapy, the most commonly used remedies were, in order, metabolic therapy, diet therapies, megavitamins, mental imagery, spiritual or faith healing, and "immune" therapy. The first three involved some form of nutritional therapy and were selected twice as frequently as the other regimens. This is supported by Read et al,[58] who found a high rate of vitamin/mineral/herbal supplementation in a group of 32 patients with cancer.

Thus nutritional therapy represents a major type of alternative cancer treatments. In part this may reflect public perceptions of the relationship of nutrition to health; in part it may reflect the fact that the FDA cannot regulate foods and vitamins in the same way it regulates drugs. In addition, other pharmacological and biological approaches and herbal approaches have gained popularity.[2] The following discussion will review dietary/metabolic therapy, pharmacological and biological approaches, immunoaugmentative therapy, and behavioral and psychological approaches as alternative methods of cancer management.

## Dietary Therapy/Metabolic Therapy

The goals of alternative dietary therapy overlap the goals of conventional nutritional support for cancer patients, since both try to counteract the nutritional and metabolic effects of the disease and its treatment.[2] However, alternative dietary methods go beyond scientifically accepted nutritional measures in that they claim to reverse the course of disease.

Many alternative cancer therapies emphasize natural cure through dietary manipulation or "metabolic" approaches. There are approximately 20 different types of metabolic regimens for the prevention of cancer and for cancer treatment, including restricted diets, specific dietary modification, enzyme therapy, cellular therapy, megavitamins, detoxification with colonic irrigations, and the development of an appropriate mental attitude.[59] The concepts of metabolic therapy are based on the theory that cancer is a result of impaired metabolism that causes a buildup of toxins in the body. Detoxification and manipulation of diet can remove these toxins, reestablish metabolic balance, and build the immune system to accomplish cure.[22,30,59]

### Gerson regimen

The Gerson treatment for cancer, developed by German physician Dr. Max Gerson in the 1920s, is the original "metabolic" therapy. It proposes that constipation or inadequate elimination of wastes from the body interferes with metabolism and healing.[60] Cure can be achieved through manipulation of diet and "detoxification," or purging the body of so-called toxins. There are many adaptations of Dr. Gerson's original program, but all have a consistent approach, which includes (1) avoidance of exposure to carcinogens, (2) positive mental outlook, and (3) eliminating wastes from the body. The daily schedule for the first three to four weeks includes 13 glasses of raw vegetable and fruit juices a day prepared in a specific way, five coffee enemas four hours apart, castor oil and castor oil enema every other day, and supplemental vitamins, minerals, and enzymes. Salt, water, coffee, berries, nuts, fish, meat, and dairy products are forbidden.[30,60,61] Other components that have been added to the regimen are oral and/or rectal hydrogen peroxide; rectal ozone gas treatments; "live-cell" therapy; IV glucose, insulin, and potassium; laetrile, and vaccines.[2]

The Gerson regimen, administered at Hospital de Baja California in Mexico costs approximately $2000 a week and lasts from three to six weeks.[30,60] There is an additional cost for a companion, since the patient will require help with the food preparation and enemas. Several reports[2,60] have noted that promotional brochures from the Gerson Institute claim to cure 90% of patients with early cancer and 50% of patients with advanced cancer; however, these claims are not supported by data or statistics. What has been reported is that repeated enemas and purgatives are more likely to lead to metabolic imbalance than to correct it, and coffee enemas have killed people.[45,62,63]

### Manner metabolic therapy

The late Harold Manner, PhD, a former professor of zoology at Loyola University, was another proponent of metabolic cancer therapy. He founded the Metabolic Research Foundation and supervised Clinica Manner in Tijuana, Mexico, up to his death in 1988. He claimed that "metabolic therapy" enhances the body's immune system so the tumor will disappear. The "Manner cocktail" consists of an intravenous solution of dimethyl sulfoxide (DMSO), and massive doses of vitamin C, vitamin A, and laetrile. There are various protocols for his metabolic therapy that may also include coffee enemas, fasting, a highly restricted diet that advocates raw milk, megavitamins, live-cell therapy, and enzymes.[64] The Manner regimen lasts 21 days and costs $6800.[30] More important, there is no objective evidence that the metabolic therapy of Harold Manner has any benefit in the treatment of cancer.[64]

### Macrobiotic diets

Over the years, a variety of diet therapies have been purported to be useful in the treatment of cancer. Today, the macrobiotic diet probably is the most popular, both for curing cancer and for preventing cancer. This diet has its origin in Zen mysticism, which proposes two antagonistic and complementary forces, yin and yang, that govern all things in the universe. Each food is classified as yin or yang, whereas each tumor is classified as being caused by an imbalance of either yin or yang. The diet is matched to the tumor to restore the balance between yin and yang, resulting in a cure or prevention, as the case may be.[55] In addition to diet, balance is also achieved through cooking techniques and attitude toward life.[65]

The original version of the diet, developed by George Ohsawa (1893–1966), involved ten macrobiotic diets ranging from diet −3 to diet 7. As an individual progresses from diet −3 toward diet 7, more and more foods are forfeited, until in diet 7 the diet consists exclusively of cereal grains.[65] In the 1970s, Michio Kushi[66] recommended a more "standard macrobiotic diet" that was less restrictive than diet 7. This consisted of 50%–60% whole cereal grains, 20%–25% vegetables, 5%–10% soups, 5%–10% beans and sea vegetables, occasional fish and fruits, and liquids sparingly. Some foods are not allowed because they are excessively yin or yang: meat, animal fat, poultry, eggs, dairy products, bananas, citrus fruits, potatoes, tomatoes, spinach, coffee, sugar, and vitamin supplements. Thus, the macrobiotic diet uses only plant proteins and is high in bulk and low in fat. The result is that a large quantity of macrobiotic foods must be eaten to meet the daily recommended energy allowance. For example, a healthy male who requires 2700 kilocalories would need 17 cups in volume.[67] At one time Kushi[66] recommended that modern medicine should be avoided except for emergency life-saving techniques; however, he is no longer against cancer patients' combining mainstream treatment with the macrobiotic diet.[2] He encourages patients to believe that since they had the power to create their illness, they also have the power to recover from it.

With adequate planning, vegetarian diets may be nutritionally sound; however, the diet recommended by Kushi is unsound. Macrobiotic therapy can result in malnutrition and cause a variety of serious health problems.[68] Of special note, cancer patients who follow the macrobiotic regimen should ensure adequate intakes of vitamins $B_{12}$ and D.[69] The American Cancer Society recently reviewed the literature and available information and found no objective evidence that macrobiotic diets are of benefit in the treatment of cancer.[69] There are also no valid data on the efficacy of the macrobiotic diet in the prevention of cancer; however, the cancer-preventive effects of the macrobiotic diet are being investigated.[1]

## Pharmacological and Biological Approaches

### Antineoplaston therapy

Antineoplastons were developed by Stanislaw R. Burzynski, MD, in the late 1960s. Burzynski originally isolated the antineoplastons from blood and then from the urine of individuals without cancer. He claims that antineoplastons are natural peptides and amino acid derivatives that cause cancer cells to change to normal cells, inhibit the growth of malignant cells, and are also useful in diagnosing cancer. However, his product is not a naturally occurring peptide. Also, he does not claim to cure cancer but reports complete remissions with minimal side effects.[2] He has numerous publications on antineoplastons in which he claims effectiveness; however, many of these publications are duplicates, published overseas and in non–peer-reviewed journals. Green[70] conducted an extensive review of Burzynski's publications between 1964 and 1990 and reported that none of the publications contained objective experimental evidence to support his hypothesis that a naturally occurring antineoplastic biochemical surveillance system exists in humans and that the urinary antineoplastons have not shown anticancer activity in experimental tumor systems. Yet other scientists believe that the compounds show some evidence of activity.[2,71]

Burzynski applied for an investigational new drug (IND) exemption in 1983, but it was put on "hold" because data were insufficient to justify its investigative use in humans. In 1989 the FDA released the hold to allow a study of the oral form (antineoplaston A10) in a small number of women with advanced refractory breast cancer. However, the study has not been initiated because the Burzynski staff reported that it is too costly to conduct a clinical trial in the United States.[2] To date, prospective, controlled clinical studies of antineoplastons have not taken place. Recently, an NCI site-visit team reviewed a best-case series of seven patients prepared for them by Burzynski. Based on their review, NCI encouraged a phase II study in patients with brain tumors.[70,71] However, the study failed to accrue patients and the clinical trial was closed.

Burzynski administers antineoplaston therapy at the Burzynski Research Institute in Houston, Texas, and uses different formulations for different forms of cancer. Duration of initial treatment is two to four weeks.[2] Antineoplastons are given orally or intravenously in regular, high, or megadoses.[72] A deposit of $3000–$5000 is required to start treatment, and this does not include the additional diagnostic tests or necessary equipment for administration. In November of 1995, Burzynski was indicted on 75 counts of mail fraud and violation of federal medical regulations.

### Cancell

Cancell, also known as Entelev, Jim's Juice, Croinic Acid, and Sheridan's Formula, is a mixture of synthetic chemicals created for their electrical properties. James Sheridan, a chemist, developed the formula as a result of what he describes as a dream and inspiration from God. In 1984 Edward J. Sopack acquired the formula for manufacturing Cancell after Sheridan was forced by the FDA to stop production.[73] The active ingredients include inositol, nitric acid, sodium sulfite, potassium hydroxide, sulfuric acid, and catechol, which are heated for most of the day, put in pint bottles, and refrigerated. According to Sopack[74] the formula reacts with the body electrically and lowers the voltage of the cell structure. Because cancer cells are weak, they convert directly to waste material when the voltage is lowered by Cancell, and the body then eliminates this waste material. The cancer cells are replaced with normal cells, and the cancer no longer exists.

According to Sopack[74] Cancell is more effective if taken internally and externally at the same time and must be taken for a minimum of 45 days. For internal usage, the liquid is given either orally (1/4 teaspoon every six hours, held under the tongue for five minutes, and then swallowed) or rectally (1/4 teaspoon injected into the rectum every six hours). For external usage, an area on the ball of the foot or the inside of the wrist is thoroughly cleaned with soap and water and several drops of DMSO are applied to that area. Then, 1/8 teaspoon of Cancell is placed on a cotton pad and the treated pad taped to the foot or wrist site. This process is repeated every 12 hours. In addition, Sopack recommends 3000 mg of Bromelain (pineapple enzyme) a day. If the patient has liver involvement, AIDS, or herpes virus, 1000 mg of glutathione should be taken before each meal. If the patient has AIDS, herpes, or EB virus, 2000 mg of butylated hydroxytoluline (BHT) should also be taken every night. Sopack advises patients that Cancell does not work if nicotine is in the blood; vitamins will interfere with function of Cancell; and it cannot be used with any other cancer therapy.[74]

Although the FDA obtained a permanent injunction prohibiting the distribution of Cancell in interstate commerce,[75] Sopack continues to distribute Cancell as "a gift" to anyone who requests it.

### Dimethyl sulfoxide (DMSO)

DMSO is an agent that has been used as an industrial chemical solvent and as a preservative for culture cells. It is rapidly absorbed through the intact skin. The use of a 50% solution of DMSO for bladder instillations is the only FDA-approved use of this agent in humans. However, the industrial form has been used alone or in combination with laetrile and other forms of "metabolic" therapy (e.g., Manner cocktail), with claims that it will restore the cancer cell to being a normal cell. A review of the literature by the American Cancer Society revealed no evidence that DMSO results in objective benefit in the treatment of cancer patients.[76]

### Live-cell therapy

Live-cell therapy—fresh-cell therapy, or cellular therapy—is the injection of cells from animal embryos or fetuses. The type of cells given supposedly matches the diseased tissue or organ in the patient. Proponents claim that the live cells contain active agents (not identified) that stimulate the immune system and repair and regenerate the host cells.[2,77] Cellular therapy is promoted for a variety of indications (e.g., menstrual disorders, premature aging, sterility, neoplastic conditions in early and advanced states.[78]

Live-cell therapy was developed by Dr. Paul Niehans of Switzerland. Currently, Dr. Wolfram Kuhnau, an associate of Dr. Niehans, heads the live-cell therapy program at the American Biologics Hospital in Tijuana, Mexico. Live-cell therapy is also offered at other Mexican clinics, usually is given in conjunction with metabolic therapy, and costs more than $20,000.[78] In a review of the literature, the American Cancer Society[77] found no scientific evidence that live-cell therapy was effective in the treatment of cancer. More important, serious side effects (brucellosis, encephalomyelitis, anaphylactic shock) have resulted from the injection of live-cell therapy.

### Megavitamins

The use of supplemental vitamins is another unproven approach that has been promoted as a treatment for cancer. Whereas certain cancers have been associated with low intake of some vitamins (e.g., lung cancer and vitamin A), there is no clear-cut evidence that high doses of vitamins prevent cancer. Studies are under way using retinoids (analogues of vitamin A) to reduce the incidence of cancer, but these studies have not yet demonstrated statistically significant reductions in incidence. Meanwhile, megadoses of vitamin C, vitamin A, and pangamic acid ("vitamin $B_{15}$") have been alleged to have antitumor properties and usually are combined with the metabolic/dietary regimens discussed earlier. However, excessive vitamin intake is useless against cancer and, more important, may be toxic.

***Vitamin C***   Megadose vitamin C probably is the most popular self-administered vitamin supplement. It has been promoted as a remedy for conditions ranging from the common cold to arthritis. It gained popularity when Cameron and Pauling[79] published a study claiming that terminal cancer patients who received massive doses of vitamin C survived much longer and had an improved quality of life. However, their study was not valid, because they selected the patients who received vitamin C whereas control subjects were selected from files, making the groups not comparable.[80] Widespread interest among cancer patients prompted a series of three NCI-funded randomized trials of vitamin C. These three prospectively randomized, placebo-controlled studies documented no consistent benefit from vitamin C in patients with advanced cancer.[81-83] There are theoretical reasons that ascorbic acid, acting as an antioxidant, might reduce the incidence of some cancers, and studies of the role of vitamin C in cancer continue.[84] However, megadoses of vitamin C can cause severe kidney damage,[85] release cyanide from laetrile,[86] and may cause death if administered intravenously.[87-89]

***Vitamin A***   Megadoses of vitamin A have also become popular for the treatment of cancer, either alone or in combination with other agents. Doses of vitamin A supplements, as low as five times the recommended dietary allowance (RDA), may be toxic and have no clear value in the treatment of cancer.[90] Studies of retinoids in cancer prevention are under way.

***Pangamic acid ("vitamin $B_{15}$")***   Pangamic acid, or "vitamin $B_{15}$," is not a vitamin. It has no standards for use and is not recognized by the FDA as a drug.[55] Even though it is illegal to sell it as either a drug or a food supplement in the United States, it is still available in many health food stores.[91] There is evidence that the chemicals in products labeled "$B_{15}$" or "pangamate" may promote the development of cancer.[92,93]

## Oxymedicine

Oxygen treatments (hydrogen peroxide, ozone gas, antioxidant enzymes) have gained popularity among the promoters of alternative cancer regimens. Hydrogen peroxide is administered by various routes: oral, rectal, intravenous, and vaginal. It is used by Donsbach as a part of the cancer cure at the Hospital Santa Monica in Tijuana, Mexico, where patients receive dilute infusions of 35% food-grade hydrogen peroxide during their stay at the clinic.[2] Promoters claim that it stimulates immunity, oxidizes toxins, and kills bacteria and viruses.[2] Ozone gas can be administered by rectal infusion, intramuscularly, or in blood transfusion. Ozone enemas are a part of the Gerson regimen at the Hospital de Baja California in Tijuana. Published information on ozone therapy in the treatment of cancer is minimal. Oxidizing agents such as hydrogen peroxide and ozone can be harmful, causing oxygen emboli and death.[94-97]

## Shark cartilage

Coverage by the media has generated much interest in the use of shark cartilage in the prevention and treatment of cancer. Proponents claim that shark cartilage is a protein that inhibits angiogenesis; however, no well-designed clinical trials have been done. The molecules of the active ingredients in the shark cartilage sold in health food stores are too large to be absorbed and the ingested product decomposes into inert ingredients.[1] Yet, many Americans are taking shark cartilage and paying $155.00 for a bottle of pills that lasts only ten days. Attempts were made by the OAM to investigate the effectiveness of shark cartilage; however, the shark cartilage received was contaminated.[1]

## Herbal remedies

Herbal concoctions such as chapparal tea, taheebo tea (pau d'arco), iscador, and essiac tea are popular alternative cancer therapies.[1,98] Herbs and plant products are the source of effective cancer chemotherapeutic agents, such as vincristine and taxol, that have been scientifically tested. However, herbal concoctions are not examined for safety and efficacy by the FDA and they can be harmful. For example, the FDA issued a warning in December 1992 that chapparal tea, which has been promoted as a "cancer remedy" and "blood purifier," has caused liver damage.[99]

# Immunologic Approach: Immunoaugmentative Therapy (IAT)

Dr. Lawrence Burton, PhD (doctor of zoology), is the originator of immunoaugmentative therapy (IAT) for cancer; treatment is given at his Immunology Research Centre located in the Bahamas. IAT is based on the theory that stimulation of the immune system will enable the body's normal defenses to destroy tumor cells. Several reviews of the therapy[2,23,100,101] describe the following theory of IAT:

> Normally the body produces "tumor antibody" that destroys tumor cells. There are two conditions where the protective system fails: if there is not enough "tumor complement" to signal the body to produce antibody, or if there is a "blocking protein" that blocks the antibody effect on the tumor. There is also a "deblocking protein" that opposes the action of the "blocking protein."

Burton's treatment regimens are based on the determination of the individual's daily or twice-daily blood levels of "tumor antibody," "tumor complement," "blocking protein factor," and "deblocking protein factor." Based on these results, Burton determines dosages for daily injections of "tumor complement," obtained from patients with cancer, and "tumor antibody" and "deblocking protein factor," which are obtained from the serum of persons without cancer.

Burton has not conducted any controlled trials of his treatment. An NCI analysis of the IAT materials revealed that the materials were dilute solutions of blood plasma, with no biological activity and none of the components that Burton suggests.[102] Scientific documentation of this therapy is lacking.[2,22,101,103]

In addition to the Bahamas facility, Dr. Burton recently opened facilities in Mexico and Germany. IAT treatment lasts from 6 to 12 weeks. The basic cost of treatment is $5000–$5200 for the first four weeks and $500 per week for additional weeks and $50–$85 for home maintenance.[101]

Safety concerns have arisen over the years: The unopened vials of treatment materials examined by NCI were found to be unsterile and contaminated with various bacteria;[104] skin abscesses at the injection site of IAT materials have been reported,[105] and in 1985 antibodies to hepatitis B and acquired immunodeficiency syndrome (AIDS) were found in the IAT serum.[102] Numerous attempts have been made to design a scientific clinical trial so IAT could be evaluated, but final agreements could not be reached.[2] IAT remains a hazardous approach to the treatment of cancer, with no documented clinical activity or scientific rationale.

## Behavioral and Psychological Approaches

### Mind body interventions

Mind body techniques are popular alternative methods used by cancer patients.[11,15] Proponents of mental imagery believe that attitude and stress are crucial in causation and cure of cancer and that relaxation and imagery will enhance the immune system and alter the course of malignancy.[106] Cancer patients and their partners are taught to use mental imagery and relaxation techniques to visualize cancer cells as weak and sick and to imagine body defenses as a powerful army that attacks and eliminates the cancer cells.[106]

Bernie Siegel also places responsibility on the individual by emphasizing a positive attitude toward survival.[107] He believes that medical treatment is only as effective as the patient's unconscious mind allows. Positive reinforcement and stress reductions can allow healing to take place. However, evaluation of his organized "exceptional cancer patients" (ECaP) versus non-ECaP patients revealed no difference in length of survival.[108]

Although the scientific and medical communities support the notion that a positive mental attitude can increase patient comfort and promote a sense of control and well-being, the methods may be harmful, in that individuals may be made to feel guilty because their particular personality type was responsible for the development of cancer.

Clearly, these approaches allow individuals' participation in care; however, they suggest that those patients who do not survive may not have been strong enough or had a good attitude. The ethical implications of these approaches should be a major concern. In counseling patients about available options, nurses can point out potential benefits of mind body techniques while stressing that the methods have no scientific documentation of effectiveness in tumor reduction or increased survival.

Many people find empowerment and comfort through various aspects of spiritual or faith healing. Cassileth and Brown[22] found that 71 of their 378 patients were attracted to this method of therapy, which involved use of prayer, "laying on of hands," incantation, or other ways of obtaining divine intervention to rid themselves of the disease. On the other hand, many patients resort to commercialized faith healers who defraud people of their money by claiming they can cure cancer. Other healers espouse self-love as a way to improve health.[109] Holland[110] notes that some methods that require patients to accept the idea that emotions contributed to their cancer may render patients vulnerable to guilt and depression. Thus, these methods may be more hazardous to the patients' well-being than is usually recognized.

## ALTERNATIVE TREATMENT FACILITIES

Unorthodox clinics are flourishing in Tijuana, Mexico, which has become a haven for promoters who treat cancer patients with alternative cancer therapies. Treatment for many other diseases as well as for AIDS are also promoted in many of these clinics. Most therapies are metabolic in nature, but combinations of numerous approaches exist.

Patients arriving at these clinics encounter not only unsound cancer treatments but also dubious diagnostic tests. Although most of the Tijuana clinics are unable to perform standard diagnostic biopsies and complicated tests, they often perform SMAC-24 and the carcinoembryonic antigen (CEA) test but use the tests inappropriately.[30,111] Useless tests that patients will encounter are the metabolic tolerance test and hair analysis, which are used to determine a patient's metabolic status. A "blood crystallization test" and "live-cell analysis" are others. There are tests to determine whether an individual is susceptible to or has cancer. These include Navarro Urine Test; Radionics analysis of energy from the blood; iridology, in which markings, discolorations, and textures of the iris reflect problems in the body[112]; applied kinesiology, which involves testing various muscles to determine if the cancer is responding, improving, or gone; and Kirlian photography, which takes a picture of an individual's fingers.[30] Table 58-2 provides information on the major Tijuana clinics.[28,30,111]

## PROMOTERS AND PRACTITIONERS OF ALTERNATIVE METHODS

### Strategies Used by Promoters

Promoters of alternative cancer remedies survive, thrive, and grow rich. Much effort and money are devoted to

**TABLE 58-2** Cancer Clinics in Tijuana, Mexico

| Clinic | Type of Facility | "Special" Diagnostic Tests | Major Treatment Regimens |
|---|---|---|---|
| American Biologics—Mexico SA. Medical Center | Small, modern clinic; inpatient and outpatient | *RLB blood test:* detects effects of "reactive oxygen toxic species" which signifies metabolic disruption <br><br> *Live-cell analysis:* cells and debris viewed by patient and practitioner <br><br> *Metabolic intolerance test:* blood on slide is mixed with food extracts; patient is allergic if white cells break | Individualized metabolic programs, "fresh" live-cell therapy injections, DMSO, oxymedicine, electromedicine |
| BioMedical Center | Large mansion; outpatient treatment | | Hoxsey's herbal preparations, vitamins, dietary instructions |
| Hospital de Baja California (Gerson Therapy Hospital) | Converted motel; outpatient | | Gerson therapy, coffee enemas, pressed liver juice, vegetable and fruit juices |
| Hospital Ernesto Contreras | Small, modern hospital; inpatient and outpatient | *Navarro Urine Test* (a chorionic gonadotropin quantitative test): supposedly can find "precancer" | Laetrile, enzymes, detoxification, live-cell therapy, interferons, low-dose chemotherapy, iscador, Bible study, sing-along sessions |
| Hospital Santa Monica | Hotel-like clinic; inpatient | Nutrient Deficiency Test | Hydrogen peroxide (intravenous, oral, ear drops, nasal spray, enemas); DMSO, live-cell therapy, colonics |
| Manner Clinic | Large, motel-like facility; inpatient | *Kirlian photography:* patient's finger placed on film in a little black box, and a picture is taken <br><br> Manner Normal Blood Profile | Manner cocktail, colonics, special enzymes, DMSO, "electroacuscope 80" (patient hooked up via electrodes and machine electronically manipulates patient's tissue to boost regeneration process), live-cell therapy |
| St. Jude International Clinic | Three rooms in back of a rundown building, outpatient | *Applied kinesiology:* pressing down on patient's arm and leg muscles to tell when cancer is gone or responding to treatment. <br><br> *Radionics:* various gadgets to detect cancer by analyzing energy radiating from blood, a picture of the person, or even a copy of patient's signature | Amino acid therapy, cobra venom, oxymedicine, herbal therapy |

Data from Kreiger L,[28] Lowell JA,[30] and the American Cancer Society.[111]

public relations and media presentations that use scientific words or phrases in a misleading and deceptive manner while retaining their emotional impact. Not mentioned are the facts that their remedies have never been objectively tested and found valid. They never acknowledge that any patients have failed to benefit from their regimen. Instead, they rely heavily on testimonials and anecdotes that do not separate fact from fiction, coincidence, or the natural history of the disease.[55] They also claim that a conspiracy exists within organized medicine or the government to keep "cures" from the American public so the "establishment" does not lose the money and business generated from cancer patients.

As with all advertising, the strategies used by the promoters of alternative treatment methods have become very sophisticated. Their claims are attuned to the times: (1) at a time when nutrition and mental attitude are being emphasized by the public, this reasonable interest is being exploited for personal profit; (2) at a time when society is emphasizing prevention, prevention of cancer is represented by advocates of alternative methods as achievable with their remedies; (3) there has been a tendency to combine many alternative methods to make objective evaluation difficult; and (4) a rising distrust of health professionals is being exploited.[55,113] It is a paradox that highly motivated and better-educated individuals are more likely to turn to questionable methods because of the promise that "you control your disease."[12,114]

## Organized Advocates of Alternative Cancer Therapy

The organizations most active in promoting alternative methods of cancer treatment are the International Association of Cancer Victors and Friends, Inc.;[115] the National Health Federation;[116] the Cancer Control Society; the Foundation for Advancement in Cancer Therapies (FACT); Coalition for Alternatives in Nutrition and Healthcare; American Quack Association; Project Cure and the Center for Alternative Cancer Research; Committee for Freedom of Choice in Medicine; and patient organizations associated with specific therapies (e.g., IAT).[2] Most of these organizations have journals or newsletters (which emphasize the antimedical establishment), hold seminars, and assist patients with information on unconventional treatments and provide lists of "recovered" patients. Some organizations take a more political stance by supporting legislation in deregulation of practitioners and promoting "freedom of choice."

## WHO SEEKS ALTERNATIVE CANCER TREATMENTS, AND WHY

Limited studies have shown that patients who seek questionable therapies are more likely to be Caucasian, have a higher income, and are better educated.[11–13,15,117] In addition, many patients seek alternative therapy to relieve symptoms and for a sense of control and comfort. Most patients learn about unconventional treatments by word of mouth, through the mass media (books, newspapers, television, radio), from advocacy groups, and at health food stores. Although many patients using alternative therapies continue with standard conventional treatment, the majority of patients did not inform their doctor that they were taking an alternative treatment.[98]

## Motivations and Reasons for Use

There are a variety of reasons why cancer patients pursue questionable therapy.

### Fear

Cancer creates many fears: fear of treatment, of death, of an uncertain future, of pain, of disfigurement, of loss of family, of loss of self-control and independence, of alienation, and of costly medical care. Given these fears, it is not difficult to understand why many individuals with cancer are in great need of hope and may seek alternative therapies that are offered as "nontoxic" therapies that will "cure" their disease. Most individuals want a treatment without risks or pain and with a good probability of cure. Resorting to some dietary or enzyme therapy

that promises no side effects or uses "the body's natural defenses" may coincide with the person's fantasies about being cured. That is, by utilizing unconventional therapy, the patient hopes for an unconventional cure.

### Desire for self-control

Use of an alternative method may provide an individual with a greater sense of self-control. This desire for control may result from feeling like a passive recipient of treatments designated by the health care team rather than like a partner in treatment decision making. Patients dissatisfied with their doctors and with conventional therapy feel they have control over their health, thus more confidence and a sense of well-being, since conventional therapy is often passive. Better-educated and highly motivated patients are more likely to turn to alternative methods, because the methods falsely promise to give the patient control over the disease.[12,114,118]

### Isolation/antiestablishment

The promoters of alternative methods frequently suggest that the government and organized medicine are in a conspiracy against curing cancer. They often appear as the underdog in battling the medical system in order to make a new risk-free treatment available to individuals with cancer. The isolation that is projected by the advocates of alternative treatment methods may be easy for the cancer patient to identify with, since they too feel isolated.

Additionally, today's health care delivery system of managed care does not allow much time for physicians to spend with patients. Thus, many patients turn to alternative practitioners because they will spend more time with them.

### Social pressures

Other reasons to use alternative methods can come via pressures exerted by family or friends.[110] The family has many of the same fears as the patient, and they often assist the patient in making treatment decisions. This responsibility can be overwhelming and frightening in and of itself. The family may feel that the best course is to try everything, with the hope that something will work; and it may also help them feel less guilty if the treatment does not work or the patient does not recover. In turn, the patient may feel obligated to meet the family's expectation to submit to these treatments so as not to alienate his or her support system. On the other hand, cancer patients might want to try whatever treatments are available, and, thus, the family might feel pressured to discover "cancer cures." Friends are also a source of information and may influence the patient and family.

Even with the best intentions of all parties, the overall outcome can be torturous for those involved. How difficult these times will be depends greatly on the personalities and relationships that existed before the cancer was diagnosed, the quality of communication that takes place, the availability of accurate information on treatment options and outcomes, and the effects of disease and therapy.

## CONTROL OF ALTERNATIVE METHODS

Any claim for a new method of cancer management in the United States must meet certain scientific standards and be capable of confirmation before it receives approval by the federal government for interstate distribution. However, most alternative approaches for the treatment of cancer lack scientifically interpretable data.[2]

Recently, the National Institutes of Health (NIH) were congressionally mandated to establish the NIH Office of Alternative Medicine (OAM).[119] Hawkins and Friedman,[120] from the NCI Cancer Therapy Evaluation Program, Division of Cancer Treatment, note that the pivotal question for the NCI in trying to improve cancer therapy is whether the treatment in question is effective, regardless of the source. Thus, the best way for NCI to resolve the controversies surrounding unconventional treatment approaches is to identify potential approaches for further evaluation by advising investigators in the preparation of best-case series and the conduct of pilot clinical trials.

The federal and state governments participate in the regulation of alternative treatment methods. The FDA has regulatory authority over the manufacturing and marketing of food, drugs, devices, and cosmetics so safety and efficacy are ensured. The FDA regulations do not apply to treatment regimens or practices but only to specific substances used in treatment (e.g., laetrile, antineoplastons, IAT). The Federal Trade Commission (FTC) monitors the advertising of foods and over-the-counter drugs and prohibits false or deceptive advertising. The U.S. Postal Service has authority to monitor for false advertising of mail order products. State laws regulate commerce within states (intrastate). For example, it is legal to manufacture and prescribe treatments that are not approved by the FDA, but only in the state in which the manufacture of the treatment takes place (e.g., Cancell in Michigan). It is illegal to transport unapproved drugs across state lines; however, such transport continues via underground networks. Some states have enacted laws that exempt questionable treatments from state regulation. For example, Oklahoma and Florida enacted provisions to legalize the use of IAT, although they later repealed the laws.

In addition to scientific investigation and legislative regulation, education plays a major role in the control of alternative cancer treatment. Private and government organizations provide information to health professionals and the public. The American Cancer Society maintains a continual, accurate record of alternative methods for cancer management. The Cancer Response System, a tele-

phone information service, allows the American Cancer Society to keep a record of inquiries regarding questionable methods. Other private organizations involved with the control of questionable methods are the American Society of Clinical Oncology, American Medical Association, and the National Council Against Health Fraud (NCAHF). The National Cancer Institute also receives inquiries through their Cancer Information Service. Table 58-3 identifies sources of information on alternative cancer remedies.

## ROLE OF NURSES/NURSING INTERVENTIONS

The progress in cancer care as a result of advances in science and technology over the last 20 years has been tremendous. In fact, it has become a major challenge just to maintain one's knowledge on the numerous drug combinations, biological therapies, and treatment protocols for the different types of cancer. Along with this progress has come the continued development of alternative cancer remedies and combinations of these treatment regimens. As nurses, we provide support, care, and comfort for patients within a health care system with rapidly changing and complex scientific treatment modalities. How can we sort through the confusing array of facts and choices available? How can we separate fact from fiction?

**TABLE 58-3  Sources of Information on Questionable Cancer Remedies**

American Cancer Society
Medical Affairs Subcommittee on Alternative and Complementary Methods
1599 Clifton Road, N.E.
Atlanta, GA 30329
(404) 329-7607

American Cancer Society (Cancer Response System)
1-800-ACS-2345

Consumer Health Information & Research Institute
3521 Broadway
Kansas City, MO 64111
(816) 753-8850

Food and Drug Administration
Office of Consumer Affairs—(301) 443-5006
Office of Health Affairs—(301) 443-5470
Rockville, MD 20852

National Cancer Institute (Cancer Information Service)
1-800-4-CANCER

National Council Against Health Fraud, Inc.
P.O. Box 1276
Loma Linda, CA 92354
(714) 824-4690

Some nurses are vulnerable to the simplicity of "holistic" medicine. The movement away from high technology is evident in several recent articles[121–123] in which nurses in England discussed the use of reflexology, aromatherapy, massage, herbalism, and dietary practice—all "complementary therapies." Reflexology on the feet is supposed to correspond to specific organs and to balance the body's energy. The NCAHF newsletter considers it "fringe nursing" and notes that it is unfortunate that nurses undermine their credibility by promoting such therapies.[124] Several state boards of nursing even award continuing education credits for nonscientific seminars on such topics as crystal healing, firewalking, reflexology, therapeutic touch, applied kinesiology, and aromatherapy.[125,126]

Behavioral methods (mental imagery, biofeedback, and even humor, which some clinicians and patients are using more systematically) are of major interest to nurses. How does a nurse sort through the beneficial or detrimental aspects of some methods. What about nutritional interventions, such as vitamin supplements? Many patients want to do something for themselves. How can nurses help them develop a plan of self-care, and when does that cross over into promoting ineffective cancer remedies?

Two recent articles highlight the problem that nurses face. Spiegel et al[127] reported that psychosocial intervention significantly increased survival in patients with metastatic breast cancer. (Reportedly, Spiegel never conceived such an outcome when he began the study. In fact, the study was undertaken to disprove the effect.)[128] However, it must be noted that a larger randomized study is needed to verify their results. A second study, by Cassileth et al,[117] further confuses the situation by providing convincing evidence that for patients with extensive cancer, there is no difference in survival between patients who received a particular unorthodox treatment regimen versus conventional therapy. However, they noted that quality of life was better among conventionally treated patients. Deprived of our conventional wisdom regarding unorthodox treatments, how are we to respond to patients who say, "Why not? It can't hurt, and it might help!"

The responsible position requires that nurses avoid simplistic cliches and deal realistically with the complexities and limitations of modern cancer care as well as the subtlety and seductiveness of the alternative cancer treatment industry. Four specific steps will assist in this difficult task.

## Identification of Alternative Therapies (Legitimate vs. Fringe Care)

The health professional must be informed both of the most frequently encountered alternative methods and of the particular aims of a given individual's therapy. The health professional should be able to explain the risks of unproven methods, such as toxicity, or, in instances where the unproven method is being used as a sole form of therapy, the risk of further progression of disease. For individuals using an unproven method in combination with standard therapy, it is still important to know what side effects to look for. A drug analysis may prove valuable for any substances the patient has been given by an unproven methods clinic. The risks of adverse effects can be increased when drugs are mixed with unorthodox substances, and the patient must be informed that all risks may not be known.

The Subcommittee on Unorthodox Therapies of the American Society of Clinical Oncology[129] has listed ten questions to ask in making a decision as to whether a treatment should be suspected of being questionable (Table 58-4). Although these questions were developed as a guide for the layperson, they are an excellent resource for the health professional.

## Assessment of Communication Channels and Patient Motivations

Communication patterns between the patient and family must be evaluated. The family may become preoccupied with seeking different therapies as a means of coping with stress. Such a situation may be intense enough to cause the family to engage in a conspiracy to exclude the patient from the decision-making process. Thus the patient is separated from the family's communication system and from the psychological and physical support that is so important. In this case, the family must be made aware of the impact of their actions on the patient. A social worker, chaplain, or patient-family support group might facilitate more effective intrafamily communication.

**TABLE 58-4**  Ten Questions to Ask in Deciding Whether a Treatment Is Unproven

1. Is the treatment based on an unproven theory?
2. Is there a purported need for special nutritional support?
3. Is there a claim for painless, nontoxic treatment?
4. Are claims published only in the mass media and not in reputable, peer-reviewed scientific journals?
5. Are claims for benefit merely compatible with a placebo effect?
6. Are the major proponents recognized experts in cancer treatment?
7. Do proponents claim benefit for use with proven methods of treatment? for prolongation of life? for use as a cancer preventative?
8. Is there a claim that only specially trained physicians can produce results with the drug, or is the preparation secret?
9. Is there an attack on the medical and scientific establishment?
10. Is there a demand by promoters for "freedom of choice" regarding drugs?

Subcommittee on Unorthodox Therapies, American Society of Clinical Oncology: Ineffective cancer therapy: A guide for the layperson. *J Clin Oncol* 1:154–163, 1983

## Maintenance of Positive Communication Channels

It is important for the physician and health care professional to discuss alternative methods of cancer management with patients, since patients are likely to hear about a variety of methods. By initiating such a discussion, the health care professional helps keep communication channels open for further inquiry by the patients and/or family. Table 58–5 identifies some potential questions to ask in order to assess a patient's risk and possible motivations for seeking alternative methods of cancer therapy. These questions provide an opportunity to discover unmet needs of the patient and family, assess their understanding of the therapies they have been receiving, assess their potential interest in unproven methods, and provide reinforcement to the patient and family that discussion of alternative treatment methods will not cause rejection or impair their communication with the health care team. A nonjudgmental attitude facilitates the assessment of the patient's and family's motivations for wanting to try an unproven method. In turn, the patient and family likely will be more receptive to the information provided by a health care professional who offers no negative response or moral judgment.

## Maintenance of Patient Participation in Their Health Care

Many patients turn to alternative cancer remedies because they do not feel like an active participant in their care and have lost hope that their conventional therapy

**TABLE 58-5** Questions That May Be Helpful in Assessing a Patient's Risk and Possible Motivation for Seeking Alternative Cancer Remedies

- Do you feel like an active participant in your health care?
  *If not:* How would you like to play a more active role?
- Are you having difficulty accepting your diagnosis?
- Do you feel a sense of helplessness and hopelessness?
- Do you feel depressed?
- Do you feel anxious?
- What type of diet do you follow?
- Do you take supplemental vitamins?
  *If so:* What kind?
- Do you frequent health food stores?
- Have you received any information regarding alternative methods of cancer treatment?
  *If so:*
  - Are you considering using this therapy?
  - What benefits do you perceive you will derive from this therapy?
  - Is your family encouraging you to pursue this therapy?
  - Would you like us to review the information?

will work. It is important for patients and family to participate in health care. Patients will be less likely to seek questionable cancer remedies if such needs are met.[3] Patient education can increase patient satisfaction, increase patient knowledge, and enhance self-care. For example, information on diet and nutrition provided in a positive context will help the patient feel a part of the therapeutic effort and may prevent the use of questionable dietary therapies. In the event of advancing illness or when conventional treatment modalities have been exhausted, hope and a sense of participation can sometimes be generated if we offer the patient participation in a clinical trial of investigative therapy.

If the patient pursues alternative methods, health care professionals should communicate that they will continue to provide care and would like to be kept informed of the treatments the patient is going to pursue. The patient should be urged to continue standard medical care.

## CONCLUSION

The health professionals caring for patients with cancer must be kept informed of alternative methods. The terms *questionable, unconventional, quackery, alternative,* and *complementary* suggest that the substance or method is being promoted even though it has not been proven effective. Just because a therapy is being promoted that has not been proven effective does not necessarily mean that it has no therapeutic value. It must be tested to determine its safety and efficacy. The present system relies on the scientific method to determine what therapies will be on the market, and improvements are continually being made in methods of evaluation. In this way the health care consumer is protected from unsafe therapies. As nurses we have the responsibility to stay informed, in order to help patients make educated health care choices. The challenge for health care professionals is to remain nonbiased and accept the patient's choice of treatment.

## REFERENCES

1. Cassileth BR, Chapman CC: Alternative and complementary cancer therapies. *Cancer* 77:1026–1033, 1996
2. Office of Technology Assessment: *Unconventional Cancer Treatments.* OTA-H-405. Washington, DC, U.S. Government Printing Office, 1990
3. Holland JC, Geary N, Furman A: Alternative cancer therapies, in Holland JC, Rowland JH (eds): *Handbook of Psychooncology.* New York, Oxford University Press, 1989, pp 508–515
4. Auer T: Training in alternatives: The next revolution in medicine. *Alt Ther Health Med* 1:16–17, 1995
5. Special Report: Alternative medicine gaining acceptance in managed care circles. *Med Utilization Manage* 6:4–7, 1996

6. American Cancer Society: *Mission Statement: Medical Affairs Subcommittee on Alternative and Complementary Methods.* Atlanta, GA, American Cancer Society, 1995

7. House Subcommittee on Aging: *Quackery: A 10-Billion-Dollar Scandal* (report). Committee publication No. 98-435. Washington, DC, U.S. Government Printing Office, 1984

8. House Subcommittee on Aging: *Quackery: A 10-Billion-Dollar Scandal* (hearing). Committee publication No. 98-463. Washington, DC, U.S. Government Printing Office, 1984

9. Eisenberg DM, Kessler RC, Foster C, et al: Unconventional medicine in the United States. *N Engl J Med* 328:246–252, 1993

10. Herbert V, Barnett S: *Vitamins and "Health" Foods: The Great American Hustle.* Philadelphia, George F. Stickley, 1981

11. Lerner IJ, Kennedy BJ: The prevalence of questionable methods of cancer treatment in the United States. *CA Cancer J Clin* 42:181–191, 1992

12. Cassileth B, Lusk E, Strouse T, et al: Contemporary unorthodox treatments in cancer medicine. *Ann Intern Med* 101:105–112, 1984

13. Cassileth BR: Unorthodox cancer medicine. *Cancer Invest* 4:591–598, 1986

14. Louis Harris and Associates: Health information and the use of questionable treatments: A study of the American Public. U.S. Department of Health and Human Services, study number 833015, 1987

15. Downer SM, Cody MM, McCluskey P, et al: Pursuit and practice of complementary therapies by cancer patients receiving conventional treatment. *BMJ* 309:86–89, 1994

16. Sawyer MG, Gannoni AF, Toogood IR, et al: The use of alternative therapies by children with cancer. *Med J Aust* 160:320–322, 1994

17. Montbriand MJ: Decision tree model describing alternative health care choices made by oncology patients. *Cancer Nurs* 18:104–117, 1995

18. Janssen WF: The cancer "cures": A challenge to rational therapeutics. *Analytical Chem* 50:197A–202A, 1978

19. Janssen WF: Cancer quackery—The past in the present. *Semin Oncol* 6:526–536, 1979

20. Message from President Taft. Congressional Record, 62 Cong., I Sess 2380 (June 21, 1911)

21. Kennedy D: Commissioner decision on status. *Federal Register* 42:39806–39967, 1977

22. Cassileth B, Brown H: Unorthodox cancer medicine. *CA Cancer J Clin* 38:176–186, 1988

23. Curt GA: Unsound methods of cancer treatment. *PPO Updates.* 4:1–10, 1990

24. Koch WF: A new and successful treatment and diagnosis of cancer. *Detroit Med J,* 1919

25. Letter to the Editor: Senator Langer abuses franking privilege by circulation of propaganda for Koch's cancer quackery. *JAMA* 137:1333, 1948

26. Hoxsey HM: *You Don't Have to Die—The Amazing Story of the Hoxsey Cancer Treatment.* New York, Milestone Books, 1956

27. Food and Drug Administration: Press release HEW-020. Washington, DC, U.S. Department Health, Education and Welfare, 1960

28. Kreiger L: Unorthodox clinics flourishing in Tijuana. *Am Med News* 3:25–27, 1985

29. American Cancer Society: Unproven methods of cancer management: Hoxsey method/BioMedical Center. *CA Cancer J Clin* 40:51–55, 1990

30. Lowell JA: Mexican cancer clinics, in Barrett S, Cassileth BR (eds): *Dubious Cancer Treatment.* Tampa, FL, American Cancer Society, Florida Division, 1991, pp 53–62

31. Holland JF: The Krebiozen story—Is cancer quackery dead? *JAMA* 200:213–218, 1967

32. American Cancer Society: *Unproven Methods of Cancer Management.* New York, American Cancer Society, 1971

33. Food and Drug Administration: Report of Director, National Cancer Institute, to Secretary Department of Health, Education and Welfare concerning decision of the Institute not to undertake clinical testing of Krebiozen. Washington, DC, FDA Records, 539.1.PX, 1963

34. Greenberg DM: The vitamin fraud in cancer quackery. *West J Med* 122:345–348, 1975

35. Greenstein JP, et al: Quantitative nutritional studies with water-soluble chemically defined diets. I. Growth, reproduction and lactation in rats. *Arch Biochem Biophysics* 72:396–416, 1957

36. Everly RC: Laetrile: Focus on the facts. *CA Cancer J Clin* 26:50–54, 1976

37. Sayre JW, Kaymakcalan S: Cyanide poisoning from apricot seeds among children in central Turkey. *N Engl J Med* 270:1113–1115, 1964

38. Gunders AE, Abrahamov A, Weisenberg E: Cyanide poisoning following the ingestion of apricot (*Prunas armeniaca*) kernel. *J Israel Med Assoc* 76:536–538, 1969

39. Humbert JR, Tress JH, Braico KT: Fatal cyanide poisoning: Accidental ingestion of amygdalin. *JAMA* 238:482, 1977 (letter)

40. Sadoff L, Fuchs K, Hollander J: Rapid death associated with laetrile ingestion. *JAMA* 239:1532, 1978

41. Herbert V: *Nutrition Cultism: Facts and Fictions* (ed 3). Philadelphia, George F. Stickley, 1981

42. Herbert V: Laetrile: The cult of cyanide. Promoting poison for profit. *Am J Clin Nutr* 32:1121–1158, 1979

43. Vogel SN, Sultan TR: Cyanide poisoning. *Clin Toxicol Exp Ther* 18:367–383, 1981

44. Ortega JA, Creek J: Acute cyanide poisoning following administration of laetrile enemas. *J Pediatr* 93:1059, 1979

45. Eisele JW, Reay DT: Deaths related to coffee enemas. *JAMA* 244:1608–1609, 1980

46. Food and Drug Administration: Toxicity of laetrile. *FDA Drug Bull* 7:25–32, 1977

47. Wodinsky I, Swiniarsky JK: Antitumor activity of amygdalin as a single agent and with beta-glucosidase on a spectrum of transplantable rodent tumors. *Cancer Chemo Rep* 59:939–950, 1975

48. Hill GJ, Shine TE, Hill HZ, et al: Failure of amygdalin to arrest B16 melanoma and BW5147 AKR leukemia. *Cancer Res* 36:2102–2107, 1976

49. Stock CC, Tarnowski GS, Schmid FA, et al: Antitumor tests of amygdalin in transplantable animal tumor systems. *J Surg Oncol* 10:81–88, 1978

50. Stock CC, Martin DS, Suguira K, et al: Antitumor tests of amygdalin in spontaneous animal tumor systems. *J Surg Oncol* 10:89–123, 1978

51. Ovejira AA, Houchens DP, Barker AD, et al: Inactivity of DL-amygdalin against human breast and colon tumor xenografts in athymic (nude) mice. *Cancer Treat Rep* 62:576–578, 1978

52. California Medical Association, Cancer Commission: The treatment of cancer with "Laetriles," *Calif Med* 78:320–326, 1953

53. Ellison NM, Byar DP, Newell GR: Special report on laetrile: The NCI laetrile review. *N Engl J Med* 299:549–552, 1978

54. Moertel CG, Fleming TR, Tubin J, et al: A clinical trial of amygdalin (laetrile) in the treatment of human cancer. *N Engl J Med* 306:201–207, 1982

55. Herbert V, Yarbro CH: Nutrition quackery. *Semin Oncol Nurs* 2:63–69, 1986

56. American Cancer Society: Unproven methods of cancer management: Laetrile. *CA Cancer J Clin* 41:187–191, 1991

57. Cassileth BR: Historical trends and patient characteristics, in Barrett S, Cassileth BR (eds): *Dubious Cancer Treatment*. Tampa, FL, American Cancer Society, Florida Division, 1991, pp 27–34

58. Read MH, St. Jeor S, Seymour K, et al: Supplementation practices of a group of patients with cancer. *J Am Diet Assoc* 90:278–279, 1990

59. Miller NJ, Howard-Ruben J: Unproven methods of cancer management. Part I: Background and historical perspectives. *Oncol Nurs Forum* 10:46–52, 1983

60. American Cancer Society: Unproven methods of cancer management: Gerson Method. *CA Cancer J Clin* 40:252–256, 1990

61. Gerson M: The cure of advanced cancer by diet therapy: A summary of 30 years of clinical experimentation. *Physiol Chem Phys* 10:449–464, 1978

62. Istre GR, Kreiss K, Hopkins RS, et al: An outbreak of amebiasis spread by colonic irrigation at a chiropractic clinic. *N Engl J Med* 307:339–342, 1982

63. Markman M: Medical complications of "alternative" cancer therapy. *N Engl J Med* 312:1640–1641, 1985 (letter)

64. American Cancer Society: Unproven methods of cancer management: The metabolic cancer therapy of Harold W. Manner, PhD. *CA Cancer J Clin* 36:185–189, 1986

65. Ohsawa G: *Cancer and the Philosophy of the Far East*. Binghamton, NY, Swan House Publishing, 1971

66. Kushi M: *Macrobiotic Approach to Cancer*. Wayne, NJ, Avery Publishing, 1982

67. Arnold C: The macrobiotic diet: A question of nutrition. *Oncol Nurs Forum* 11:50–53, 1984

68. Bowman BB, Kushner RF, Dawson SC, et al: Macrobiotic diets for cancer treatment and prevention. *J Clin Oncol* 2:702–711, 1984

69. American Cancer Society: Unproven methods of cancer management: Macrobiotic diets for the treatment of cancer. *CA Cancer J Clin* 39:248–251, 1989

70. Green S: "Antineoplastons": An unproved cancer therapy. *JAMA* 267:2924–2928, 1992

71. NCI plans trials of Burzynski's "Antineoplaston"; JAMA Report says no antitumor activity in tests. *Cancer Letter* 18:1–4, 1992

72. Burzynski Research Institute: Patient brochure on antineoplaston treatment. Houston, TX, The Institute, 1989

73. Lowell J: Cancell. *National Council Against Health Fraud Newsletter.* 14:3, 1991

74. Sopack E: *Important Information About Cancell* (promotional literature). Howell, MI, November 1988

75. *U.S. vs. James V. Sheridan and Edward J. Sopack.* Complaint for permanent injunction filed in the U.S. District Court of the Eastern District of Michigan. February 21, 1989

76. American Cancer Society: Unproven methods of cancer management: Dimethyl sulfoxide (DMSO). *CA Cancer J Clin* 33:122–125, 1983

77. American Cancer Society: Unproven methods of cancer management: Fresh-cell therapy. *CA: Cancer J Clin* 41:126–128, 1991

78. Alvarez G: Live-cell therapy at the Manner Clinic. *Manner and Metabolic Research Foundation Newsletter* 1:2–3, 1992

79. Cameron E, Pauling L: Supplemental ascorbate in the supportive treatment of cancer, prolongation of survival time in terminal human cancer. *Proc Natl Acad Sci USA* 73:3685–3689, 1976

80. Sampson WI: When the big C is a vitamin. *Coping* 2:35, 1988

81. Creagan ET, Moertel CG, O'Fallon JR, et al: Failure of high-dose vitamin C to benefit patients with advanced cancer. *N Engl J Med* 301:687–690, 1979

82. Moertel CG, Fleming TR, Creagan ET, et al: High-dose vitamin C versus placebo in the treatment of patients with advanced cancer who have had no prior chemotherapy. *N Engl J Med* 312:137–141, 1985

83. Tschetter L, Creagan ET, O'Fallon JR, et al: A community-based study of vitamin C (ascorbic acid) therapy in patients with advanced cancer. *Proc Am Soc Clin Oncol* 2:92, 1983 (abstr)

84. Marwick C: Cancer institute takes a look at ascorbic acid. *JAMA* 264:1926, 1990

85. Swartz RD, Wesley JR, Somermeyer MG, et al: Hyperoxaluria and renal insufficiency due to ascorbic acid administration during total parenteral nutrition. *Ann Intern Med* 100:530–531, 1984

86. Backer RC, Herbert V: Cyanide production from laetrile in the presence of megadoses of ascorbic acid. *JAMA* 241:1891–1892, 1979

87. Herbert V: The rationale of massive-dose vitamin therapy. (Megavitamin therapy: hot fiction vs cold facts), in Whilte PL, Selvey N (eds): *Proceedings: Western Hemisphere Nutrition Congress IV.* Acton, MA, Publishing Sciences Group, 1975, pp 84–91

88. Hodges RE: *Nutrition in Medical Practice*. Philadelphia, Saunders, 1980

89. Marshall CW: *Vitamins and Minerals: Help or Harm?* Philadelphia, George F. Stickley, 1983

90. Herbert V: Toxicity of 25,000 IU vitamin A supplements in "Health" food users. *Am J Clin Nutr* 36:185–186, 1982

91. Herbert V: Pangamic acid (vitamin $B_{15}$). *Am J Clin Nutr* 32:1534–1540, 1979

92. Colman H, Herbert V, Gardner A, et al: Mutagenicity of dimethyglycine when mixed with nitrite: Possible significance in human use of pangamates. *Proc Soc Exp Biol Med* 164:9–12, 1980

93. Gelernt MD, Herbert V; Mutagenicity of diisopropylamine dichloroacetate, the "active constituent" of vitamin $B_{15}$ (pangamic acid). *Nutr Cancer* 3:129–133, 1982

94. Sleigh JW, Linter SPK: Hazards of hydrogen peroxide. *Br Med J* 291:1706, 1985

95. Bassan NM, Dudai M, Shaley O: Near-fatal systemic oxygen embolism due to wound irrigation with hydrogen peroxide. *Postgrad Med J* 58:448–451, 1982

96. American Cancer Society: Questionable methods of cancer management: Hydrogen peroxide and other "hyperoxygenation" therapies. *CA Cancer J Clin* 43:47–55, 1993

97. Giberson TP, Kern JD, Pettigrew DW III, et al: Near-fatal hydrogen peroxide ingestion. *Ann Emer Med* 18:778–779, 1989

98. Montbriand MJ: An overview of alternate therapies chosen by patients with cancer. *Oncol Nurs Forum* 21:1547–1554, 1994

99. Gordon DW, Rosenthal G, Hart J, et al: Chapparal ingestion: The broadening spectrum of liver injury caused by herbal medications. *JAMA* 273:489–490, 1995

100. Zavertnik JJ: Immuno-augmentative therapy, in Barrett S, Cassileth BR (eds): *Dubious Cancer Treatment*. Tampa, FL, American Cancer Society, Florida Division, 1990, pp 63–72

101. American Cancer Society: Questionable methods of cancer management: Immuno-augmentative therapy (IAT). *CA Cancer J Clin* 41:357–364, 1991

102. Curt GA, Katterhagen G, Mahaney FX: Immunoaugmentative therapy: A primer on the perils of unproved treatments: *JAMA* 255:505–507, 1986

103. Easy cures for cancer still find support. *JAMA* 246:714–716, 1981

104. Curt GA: Warning on immunoaugmentative therapy. *N Engl J Med* 311:859, 1984

105. Centers for Disease Control: Cutaneous nocardiosis in cancer receiving immunotherapy injections—Bahamas. *MMWR* 33:471–477, 1984

106. Simonton OC, Simonton SM, Creighton JL: *Getting Well Again: A Step-by-Step, Self-Help Guide to Overcoming Cancer for Patients and Their Families*. New York, Bantam, 1980

107. Siegel B: *Love, Medicine & Miracles*. New York, Harper & Row, 1986

108. Gellert GA, Maxwell RM, Siegel BS: Survival of breast cancer patients receiving adjunctive psychosocial support therapy: A 10-year follow-up study. *J Clin Oncol* 11:66–69, 1993

109. Irish AC: Maintaining health in persons with HIV infection. *Semin Oncol Nurs* 5:302–307, 1989

110. Holland JC: Why patients seek unproven cancer remedies: A psychological perspective. *CA Cancer J Clin* 32:10–14, 1982

111. American Cancer Society: Questionable cancer practices in Tijuana and other Mexican border clinics. *CA Cancer J Clin* 41:310–319, 1991

112. Curt GA: Unsound methods of cancer treatment, in DeVita VT Jr, Hellman S, Rosenberg SA (eds): *Cancer: Principles and Practice of Oncology* (ed 4). Philadelphia, Lippincott, 1993, pp 2734–2747

113. King M: Falling victim twice. *Cancer News* 39:8–11, 1985

114. Hiratzka S: Knowledge and attitudes of persons with cancer toward use of unproven treatment methods. *Oncol Nurs Forum* 12:36–41, 1985

115. American Cancer Society: Unproven methods of cancer management: International Association of Cancer Victors and Friends, Inc. *CA Cancer J Clin* 39:58–59, 1989

116. American Cancer Society: Unproven methods of cancer management: National Health Federation. *CA Cancer J Clin* 41:61–64, 1991

117. Cassileth BR, Lusk EJ, Guerry D, et al: Survival and quality of life among patients receiving unproven as compared with conventional cancer therapy. *N Engl J Med* 324:1180–1185, 1991

118. Montbriand MJ: Freedom of choice: An issue concerning alternate therapies chosen by patients with cancer. *Oncol Nurs Forum* 20:1195–1201, 1993

119. Senate gives NIH director authority to permit research by unconventional MDs. *Cancer Letter* 18:3–4, 1992

120. Hawkins MJ, Friedman MA: Commentary: National Cancer Institute's evaluation of unconventional cancer treatments. *J Natl Cancer Inst* 84:1699–1702, 1992

121. Passant H: A holistic approach in the ward. *Nurs Times* 86:26–28, 1990

122. Evans M: Reflex zone therapy for mothers. *Nurs Times* 86:29–31, 1990

123. Smith M: Healing through touch. *Nurs Times* 86:31–32, 1990

124. National Council Against Health Fraud: Fringe nursing. *National Council Against Health Fraud Newsletter* 13:4, 1990

125. National Council Against Health Fraud: Registered nurses get CE credit for crystal healing coursework. *National Council Against Health Fraud Newsletter* 13:3, 1990

126. National Council Against Health Fraud: Colorado RN confronts pseudoscience in nurses continuing education. *National Council Against Health Fraud Newsletter* 15:3, 1992

127. Spiegel D, Bloom JR, Kraemer HC, et al: Effect of psychosocial treatment on survival of patients with metastatic breast cancer. *Lancet* 2:888–890, 1989

128. Barinaga M: Can psychotherapy delay cancer deaths? *Science* 246:448–449, 1989

129. Subcommittee on Unorthodox Therapies, American Society of Clinical Oncology. Ineffective cancer therapy: A guide for the layperson. *J Clin Oncol* 1:154–163, 1983

# Chapter 59

# Patient Education and Support

**Rose Mary Padberg, RN, MA, OCN®**

**Lawrence F. Padberg, PhD**

# INTRODUCTION

Nearly all health care professionals place a high value on patient education. In recent years the importance of patient education has been stated and reinforced many times, but nearly always with an emphasis on the content to be taught. For example, the *Guidelines for Oncology Nursing Practice*[1] include patient teaching directives in each section. These directives outline in detail the *content* to be taught. Such treatment of patient education is appropriate within each of the segments. The overall guidelines for practice, however, do not include directives for the oncology nurse to understand the *processes* of teaching and learning that underlie the patient teaching directive. With this in mind, it is not unreasonable for the oncology nurse to place an emphasis on *what* to teach rather than on understanding *how* to teach. And yet cancer nurses, often with little or no formal preparation in teaching theory or processes, regularly perform patient teaching and most often perform it well, guided by common sense, colleagues' examples, trial and error, and their own good judgment.

Even so, it is important to consider that the area of patient teaching is dependent not only on special expertise in terms of the information to be given but also on understanding the different ways in which individuals learn, the variety of strategies for patient teaching that are available, how to match appropriate strategies to specific content and specific learners, and much more.

The primary focus of this chapter is on patient education and the related area of patient support programming. Issues to be addressed will include understanding what patient education is and is not; understanding the many forms of patient support; a rationale for patient education and support drawn from an understanding of the multiple purposes assigned to them; theoretical perspectives and practical guidelines for patient teaching; difficulties in assuring continuity of teaching and support across settings; key factors to be considered in developing materials or in conducting patient education; resources available for patient teaching and support and how they can be accessed.

# A DEFINITION OF PATIENT EDUCATION

*Patient education* is "a planned learning experience using a combination of methods such as teaching, counseling, and behavior modification techniques which influence patients' knowledge and health behavior."[2] Though simply stated, this definition identifies three important elements. Patient education involves *planned* learning experiences. It is not haphazard or accidental. Patient education uses a *combination of methods*. There is no single way to conduct patient education. Rather, the health care provider involved in patient education has a variety of resources and techniques legitimately available for effective teaching. The methods can be shaped and tailored to best meet the needs, style, and capabilities of the learner and the educator, or particular conditions in the teaching-learning setting. Finally, patient education seeks to influence or modify a patient's knowledge and/or health behavior. The goal of patient education is *to effect some change in the learner*. While the health care provider serving as educator cannot always ensure that learning has occurred, that is the goal. To complete a teaching activity and confidently check off that the patient education responsibility has been fulfilled without assessing whether any change has occurred in the patient at best misses valuable information; at worst, it may falsely assume efficacy.

# PATIENT SUPPORT

The literature on cancer patient support includes a varied set of activities, programs, and groups. Some writers define support in terms of small-group mutual aid structures,[3] while others discuss support within the context of other forms of psychosocial interventions, including psychotherapy.[4,5] There is a distinction between psychotherapy groups, which seek to effect individual change through personal exploration and reflection, though done within the context of a group, and social support groups, which seek to help the group members find meaning and a sense of belonging through participation in the group.[6] Group psychotherapy may have social support outcomes, though these are not the primary purpose. Similarly, social support groups may assist some members to achieve personal changes through personal exploration and reflection flowing from the participation in the social group, but again such outcomes are not the purpose of the social support group.

The phenomenon of social support groups used in health care originated early in this century,[3] and recent estimates indicate that up to 15 million Americans participate in various types of support groups to deal with physical and emotional distress.[7] Support group objectives include sharing information that assists members in coping with cancer, finding inspiration or hope from the experiences of others, and the catharsis of being able to express strong emotions within a supportive setting.[3,6] The ability to express emotions helps in managing intense, negative feelings; it may also help by assisting the individual to move from coping with the emotions to beginning to resolve some of the causes.[5]

Educational and psychosocial programming are closely linked. Some patient education programs designed for groups have social support purposes. And even programs designed only for educational purposes may have social support outcomes and may be seen by many health care professionals and many participants as support programs.[3] For example, the "I Can Cope" program of the American Cancer Society (ACS) is designed as a patient education program. In the evaluation of the program when it was first developed, however, two of the three patient outcomes assessed were in the psychosocial area (state of anxiety, and purpose and meaningfulness in life),[8] and "I Can Cope" is often discussed among cancer care providers as a support program. Often programs are developed to combine both clear educational and social support/psychosocial purposes.[9–11]

Support programs may be tailored for people with a specific type of cancer, or for those in a particular stage of the illness, or for family members alone. There are concerns that some groups of people are less likely to join support groups or programs, and that special effort is needed to reach such audiences. In general, women and individuals of higher socioeconomic standing are most likely to participate in support programs. It has been suggested that men join programs that are identified as informational, and that programs designed to provide education and skill training, along with having support purposes, may be more effective in attracting men.[6] Once recruited to support programs, men may benefit more than women since men in our society have fewer opportunities for expressing emotions and receiving supportive response.[5] Efforts to better serve people from lower socioeconomic backgrounds require special considerations; issues in the area of serving culturally diverse audiences are discussed later in this chapter.

## UNDERSTANDING THE PURPOSES OF PATIENT EDUCATION

At first the purposes of patient education seem clear: that patients understand their diagnoses, their treatment options, their responsibilities as part of treatment; that they understand symptoms that need to be reported; that they comply with treatment procedures; and ultimately that they do all they can to promote a return to health, to adapt to ongoing limitations, or to cope with the reality of a terminal condition.

The possible intended outcomes of patient education are numerous. The purposes just stated reflect a care provider's perspective of those actions for which the patient should be responsible in order to maximize the positive benefits of treatment. Another perspective is that of a patient and family who want to understand the diagnosis and treatment options in order to make autonomous decisions regarding treatment—including the option to accept no further treatment. Still another perspective might be to ensure the care provider's compliance with a professional standard, or to fulfill an obligation or responsibility to the patient. From an organizational perspective, the purpose of patient education

might be stated in terms of meeting an accreditation standard, fulfilling a legal responsibility, or even avoiding any legal liability for leaving a patient uninformed.

A difficulty in thinking about patient education and in planning programs and activities is the complexity of the purposes attributable to patient education. Rather than trying to assign a narrower purpose to patient education, the health care provider should understand the complexity and think critically when attempting to define goals for any patient education activity.

Five rationales or perspectives supporting the need for patient education have been identified: patients' rights, professional standards, legal and agency mandates, benefits to patients, and benefits to society and/or health care agencies.[12] Of these, two are traditional views supporting patient education: first, benefit to patients, that is, providing the patient with certain knowledge and understanding necessary for beneficial treatment; second, satisfying professional standards, the duty of the health care provider to share information with the patient. Of course the view of what information is appropriate to share with the patient has changed over time. Notions of patients' rights to information and to autonomy in decision making, legal standards and questions of legal liability, and the broader view of societal gain through the cumulative impact of effective and efficient health care decisions resulting from patient education have developed only more recently as perspectives in health care. Whether traditional or recent, all five of these rationales support the importance of patient education.

## Patients' Rights

The idea of patients' rights as a basis for patient education flows from philosophical principles recognizing individual autonomy and the right to self-determination. It might be assumed that in a democratic society such as the United States, with our societal understanding of individual freedoms, the perspective of individual autonomy as a basis for patients' rights should be a long-standing condition. This perspective, however, has developed only in the latter half of the twentieth century.

It was only in 1972 that the American Hospital Association developed its formal statement on the rights of patients.[13] These include rights to information about diagnosis, treatment, prognosis, procedures and their medical consequences, and other areas. Over the past 20 years the rights of patients have become a cornerstone for contemporary health care, replacing the former paternalistic perspective that the health care professional knew what was best for the patient based on specialized knowledge and expertise. The recognition of patients' rights is reflected today in professional standards, in organizational standards and policies, and in laws related to health care practice.

In recent years issues related to cancer patients' rights have been broadened beyond the arena of treatment and direct health care. Cancer survivorship often leads to problems of discrimination. In 1989 the National Coalition for Cancer Survivorship developed a statement of the rights of cancer survivors, *The Cancer Survivor's Bill of Rights.*[14] This statement includes areas that have direct implications for patient education. The first section discusses responsibilities of health care professionals, but the statement also deals with issues of employment opportunity, insurability, and the personal expectations and pressures often placed upon cancer survivors.

## Professional Standards

The development of professional standards has reflected the changing perspectives regarding patients' rights. While professional standards in health care have long expressed the underlying philosophy of the Hippocratic oath—to do good and do no harm—recognition of and respect for a patient's right to full knowledge and self-determination have developed only more recently in conjunction with changing perspectives in the larger society. If the individual has the right to full knowledge regarding health status and a right to make self-determining health care decisions, then the health care professional has a responsibility to ensure that the patient has the knowledge base and appropriate support for such autonomy.

Clear guidelines regarding patient education responsibilities as part of professional standards, therefore, are relatively new. Fernsler and Cannon note that various American Nurses' Association documents that provide guidelines for the scope of professional practice give direction for nurses' responsibilities in patient education more through implication than through explicit statement.[12] The Oncology Nursing Society's *Outcome Standards for Cancer Patient Education* were first published in 1982.[15] A complementary set of standards on public education was produced in 1983, and the two were brought together into a single updated document in 1989. The current guidelines[16] provide descriptive criterion statements organized around five areas: the responsibilities and qualifications of the oncology nurse; patient and family educational resources; the content of patient and family education; the teaching-learning process and application of theory; and the anticipated learning outcomes for patients and family.

## Legal and Accreditation Requirements

States are responsible for establishing guidelines for professional practice through state law. State nursing practice acts, which delineate the responsibilities of and limitations on nursing practice, may include specific requirements for patient and family education or, more typically, may imply an obligation for patient teaching as a necessary part of fulfilling the duties and responsibilities of nursing practice.[12,17]

A specialized issue in legal responsibility for patient education is the area of informed consent. This concept has its roots in post–World War II reactions to the human

experimentation conducted by the Nazis, leading to the development of the Nuremberg Code to provide standards for use by the Nuremberg military tribunal.[18] Central to this code is the use of voluntary consent to protect human subjects in experimentation. Such consent assumes not only the ability to consent and freedom from coercion but also that there is an understanding of the risks and benefits, that the subject is giving an informed consent.

The codification of informed consent can be traced through several well-known landmark documents, including the Declaration of Helsinki, adopted by the World Medical Association in Helsinki, Finland, in 1964, and the Belmont Report, developed by the National Commission for the Protection of Human Subjects of Biomedical and Behavioral Research in 1978.[18] General acceptance of informed consent principles has extended over time beyond human subjects in research settings to broader expectations for informed consent by patients for participation even in standard treatment.

In addition to legal obligations for patient education, a variety of accreditation or other certifying standards have developed specific requirements for patient education, with responsibilities assigned to nurses and other health professionals. In 1993 the Joint Commission for the Accreditation of Healthcare Organizations (JCAHO) reorganized its standards for accreditation to bring stronger focus to the area of patient and family education. Combining standards previously found in many department-specific chapters, the 1993 accreditation manual included for the first time a chapter on patient and family education. This chapter has been retained through two subsequent rounds of further reorganization of the *Accreditation Manual for Hospitals.*[19,20]

Other agencies and organizations have joined this call for patient education as an integral part of health care. The Health Care Financing Administration (HCFA), which regulates Medicare and Medicaid reimbursement, mandates discharge planning and the patient and family education this implies.[21] In recognition of the JCAHO patient and family education standards, the HCFA accepts JCAHO-accredited institutions as also having met HCFA requirements.

The Association of Community Cancer Centers' *Standards for Cancer Programs* includes standards on patient and family education, as well as specific statements regarding the oncology nurse's responsibilities for patient and family education.[22]

## Patient Benefits

Patient education goals obviously include increasing patients' knowledge and understanding of the disease and their own diagnoses. Patient education and support seek to ensure compliance with treatment, appropriate self-care, attention to symptoms or change of status, and timely and accurate reporting of symptoms or health changes. A major focus of much patient education and of most support programs is improving psychological status by reducing anxiety, relieving depression, and maintaining self-concept or self-esteem. The ultimate goal is that education and support can contribute to improved physical status, defined in various ways when confronting an illness that has the high mortality rates associated with many forms of cancer.

While improved patient outcomes are the most readily acknowledged goals of patient education, empirical evidence for such outcomes is difficult to establish. Clinical research often faces difficulties in establishing control groups, avoiding confounding factors, and attaining sufficient sample size. Much of the literature on patient outcomes for education and support interventions deals primarily with aspects of psychosocial status. For example, among recently reported studies, education and orientation programs designed to prepare individuals for beginning treatment have been shown to reduce anxiety and overall stress and to improve satisfaction during the course of treatment.[23,24] A group program providing both psychosocial support and training in coping skills resulted in improved mood status and enhanced quality of life.[9] A group psychotherapy program for cancer patients experiencing depression helped to reduce anxiety and maladaptive somatic preoccupation as well as reducing depression.[4] An inpatient education and support program that included informational, emotional, and spiritual components increased knowledge of symptom management, decreased anxiety, reduced patients' sense of isolation, and increased their sense of control and comfort.[10] A computer-based educational and support system helped produce feelings of acceptance, motivation, understanding, and relief.[25,26]

There is less empirical information regarding education and support outcomes related to enhanced physical health status. Educational programs clearly serve to increase patient knowledge regarding self-care, symptom management, and monitoring and reporting changes in health status. As patient information needs are met, increased compliance with treatment regimens and reduced medical complications are achieved, thus contributing to reductions in preventable hospital readmissions and similar health benefits.[27] Emotional gains from education and support programs may influence the experience of physical symptoms. For example, a group psychotherapy program reduced physical symptoms of anorexia, nausea and vomiting, and fatigue. The investigators noted that such symptoms may be attributed to emotional sources and speculated on possible explanations for the effects of psychotherapy: that the symptoms are of emotional origin; or that one's emotional state can influence perceptions of symptoms and thus the reporting of them; or that these two factors combine in some way.[28]

It is difficult, however, to demonstrate that the benefits of patient educational and support programs seen in the psychosocial area translate into medical gains. An association between participation in education and support programs and survival has been shown.[3] It is not clear, however, what factors contribute to the links between support and survival. In addition to the potential direct effect of emotional state on physical state, other explanations might be that individuals who have an improved emotional outlook as a result of therapy or other support programs will monitor symptom changes more carefully; seek additional medical attention in a more timely manner; comply with treatment regimens more fully; or more easily manage difficult treatment regimens and thereby receive more rigorous treatment.

## Benefits to Society and to Health Care Organizations

The benefits to society and to health care organizations represent a fifth broad purpose for patient education,[12] an area of benefit not often considered. While patient and family education contributes to the improved physical and psychosocial health status of individuals experiencing illness, benefits accruing to organizations or individuals beyond the patient and family include reduced hospital stays, reduced utilization of health care materials and resources, and reduced absenteeism from school or work. Health care agencies may see significant benefits from avoiding extending hospital stays beyond reimbursable limits, reduced need for expensive forms of care, satisfied patients providing referrals, and increasing patient volume.

# THE TEACHING-LEARNING PROCESS: THEORY AND PRACTICE

While patient education literature is extensive, many of the reports in the nursing literature provide information on specific teaching activities or teaching materials developed and used in a specific practice setting. It has been noted that the majority of such reports are atheoretical.[29,30] A theoretical base is important because it provides the clinician with a guide for approaching individual patients and their needs, for selecting materials or methods when planning patient education activities, and for assessing the effectiveness or outcomes of those activities.

Although much of the patient education information is presented without linkage to theory, there are a number of theoretical perspectives and behavioral models that have been proposed to explain human behavior and behavioral change decisions related to coping and adaptation responses to illness and its treatment. Several will be reviewed here.

## The Health Belief Model

Several proposed models draw from a value expectancy perspective; that is, an individual's actions are shaped or determined by expectations of outcomes and the value placed upon those expected outcomes. A widely used value expectancy model is the Health Belief Model, originally developed in the 1950s to explain choices made for participating or not participating in tuberculosis screening programs.[31]

The Health Belief Model is based on several simple principles.[32] First, the individual must perceive a threat, and such perception is itself based upon a belief or recognition both that the threat is significant or severe and that the individual is in fact susceptible to the threat. Second, there must be an expectation that something can be done regarding the threat. The expectation includes three components: that a behavior change or an action taken will be beneficial in reducing either the severity of or the susceptibility to the threat; that benefits of the behavior change or action to be taken outweigh barriers or negative outcomes; and an expectation that one can accomplish the behavior change or action required.

The Health Belief Model is often used in considering public education strategies for health promotion and early detection of health problems. Health care professionals working in the area of public education can use the model in considering interventions that emphasize to target audiences their susceptibility to particular illnesses or the severity of the illness, or to stress the ease of taking certain health promotion actions. The model identifies the issues to address in order to create effective health education interventions.

Though often discussed within the context of health education, the general principles of the Health Belief Model also are useful in thinking about patient education. An individual who is a patient already has experienced illness and therefore readily acknowledges individual susceptibility. The patient may not understand the severity of the illness, although in cancer patient education more typically individuals anticipate that any cancer experience is serious and life-threatening. Thus, patients usually are already aware of the "threat" represented by their illness. However, to assist patients in making decisions about how to respond to the acknowledged threat, the expectation principles of the Health Belief Model still must be addressed. The patient must come to believe that possible actions are of value. The patient needs to be able to weigh the benefits of the actions compared with the barriers— are the potential benefits of treatment likely to be of greater value than the disadvantages such as the likely levels of pain, the disruptions of personal or family life, side effects of treatment, and costs to self or family? Finally, patient education must address the issue of efficacy, that the patient believes he or she can accomplish the actions required in order to undertake treatment. Thus the Health Belief Model can guide patient education—by understanding the issues, the patient makes a treatment decision and complies with the treatment regimen; and the health care provider identifies the education interventions needed to address these issues.

## The PRECEDE Model

The PRECEDE Model (the acronym is derived from Predisposing, Reinforcing, and Enabling Causes in Educational Diagnosis and Evaluation) attempts to provide a comprehensive consideration of factors predisposing, reinforcing, and enabling targeted health behaviors. Predisposing factors include knowledge, attitudes, beliefs, and values about health behaviors. If an individual has had a relative die quickly from cancer in spite of extensive treatment and then is diagnosed with the same type of cancer, the individual may simply believe that his or her fate is to repeat the course of events leading to death in the same way. Interventions to assist the person in learning specific information about diagnosis, options for treatment, and potential outcomes may be wasted unless some action is taken to address and change the predisposing belief.

Predisposing factors may be positive or negative. The PRECEDE model assists the clinician in understanding potential predisposing factors that may support or inhibit patient readiness and motivation to learn.

Reinforcing factors support the continuation of the intended health behavior or reinforce resistance to the targeted behavior. Patient education interventions that help the patient to see progress, that strengthen understanding and respond to questions or concerns, that provide reminders for continuing intended behaviors, and that continue providing support are reinforcing factors.

Enabling factors are resources or other structures within an individual's environment that may impact the target health behavior, enabling or facilitating or, conversely, inhibiting or serving as barriers to the intended behavior. For example, adverse side effects of treatment may become significant inhibitors of patient compliance. Eliciting information from the patient regarding any possible side effects being experienced and appropriately intervening to manage those effects are important steps to ensure continued compliance with the treatment regimen. The PRECEDE model helps in directing attention to enabling factors, acting to best utilize positive factors and to minimize or eliminate negative factors.

## Control Theory

A number of theories advanced in patient education are variations of personal control theory. The primary underlying perspective of control theory is an individual's perception or belief that specific outcomes are contingent upon the individual's own action or, alternately, other sources. Social learning theory,[33] or self-efficacy theory, is one widely utilized control theory. Perception of self-efficacy will affect the individual's decisions regarding behavior, level of effort, and persistence.

A sense of self-efficacy derives from four sources of information: personal mastery, vicarious experiences, verbal persuasion, and physiological feedback. Mastery learning, contract learning, and modeling are teaching techniques that are suggested as useful in working from this theoretical perspective.[30,32] For example, development of personal mastery in teaching skills can be accomplished by teaching in small increments with repetitions at each level until mastery is achieved. An attempt to present a complex task in its entirety, thus allowing the patient to experience unsuccessful attempts to demonstrate the behavior, would diminish a sense of self-efficacy and make learning more difficult.

Another theoretical perspective in the general area of control theory is locus of control, that is, a view that behavior is a function of expectancy and reinforcement, with expectancy defined along an internal control–external control continuum. Variations of this perspective define locus of control in three domains: personally controlled, controlled by chance, or controlled by powerful others.[29] Patient education interventions based on a locus of control theory perspective need to assess patient beliefs regarding control.

## Coping Theory

Another general category of theories applied to patient education is coping theory. Coping involves behavioral and/or cognitive responses to perceived stressors or threats intended to mediate or manage those stressors or threats. Lorig, drawing from the work of Lazarus and Folkman,[34] notes a variety of coping strategies used by individuals: confronting, distancing, self-control, seeking social support, accepting responsibility, escape-avoidance, problem solving, positive reappraisal, activity, distraction, self-talk, and prayer.[32] Lorig discusses approaches for patient education, or ways of understanding and interpreting patient actions, within each of these types of coping strategies. For example, confronting is a coping strategy that may be useful to patients experiencing difficulties caused by a nonsupportive spouse. A suggested approach consistent with a confronting coping strategy would be to provide the patients with teaching focused on reporting their own feelings, that is, confronting the stress or negative feelings they have, and moving them away from focusing on the question of spousal support.

Understanding coping strategies may help the health care professional to provide appropriate teaching to give the patient tools to deal with the issues being faced, or to provide teaching strategies that respond well to the coping style of the patient. Miller identified two coping styles for dealing with cancer or other major health threats—monitoring and blunting—that have implications for patient teaching.[35] *Monitors* are individuals who give high levels of attention to threatening health information. They tend to seek a great deal of information, to be more active in understanding their health condition, and to seek greater participation in decisions regarding their health status and treatment. In contrast, *blunters* are individuals who avoid information that presents threatening health information. They tend not to seek additional information and take less responsibility for health decisions. The phenomenon of differentiating patients as information seekers and nonseekers, and linking information seekers to more active involvement in care decisions, has been noted by other researchers.[36,37]

Health care professionals may tend to react in less than optimal ways when presenting information to monitors and blunters or information seekers and nonseekers.[35,38] Because monitors display greater agitation and concern in response to threatening information, providers may tend to avoid giving more information in an attempt to avoid further distress for the patient. On the other hand, because blunters tend to exhibit disinterest and take little initiative to seek more information, the health care professional may tend to extend or increase the presentation of information regarding a negative health condition, trying to ensure that the person has heard the relevant and important information. In both cases the health professional's actions may not be well suited to the coping styles of the patients. Monitors may benefit from more complete and extensive information; more information may increase understanding and certainty and help the individual to process the information and thus cope with the diagnosis. Blunters appear to cope with the threat by avoidance and distraction; forcing them to hear and confront threatening information may increase their anxiety and emotional distress. Thus the monitor-blunter coping style framework may be helpful to the health professional in guiding how to react to individual patients, how to best provide information that is most helpful to the individual.

## Adult Learning Theory

Another source of information and theoretical perspective that can inform patient education is the field of adult education and adult learning theory.[39] While there are a variety of learning theories that may be useful to draw from, much of adult education in recent years has been influenced by the work of Malcolm Knowles and the principles of *andragogy*, or adult education, that he proposed.[40] Knowles's principles of adult education can be helpful in considering the role of the nurse as an educator and the patient as a learner.[30] Adult learning theory also emphasizes task- or problem-oriented learning relevant to the needs and interests of the learner, a viewpoint that fits well with patient education.[27]

Knowles's perspective can be especially effective to assist in moving away from a paternalistic viewpoint, which assumes the health care professional has total responsibility for determining goals and process for patient teaching, and in moving toward a position that respects patient autonomy and rights of self-determination; shares responsibility in setting educational goals by responding to needs as identified by the patient/learner; and utilizes the resources represented by the knowledge and experience that the patient/learner brings to the learning setting. Table 59-1 provides a summary of Knowles's four assumptions regarding adult learners and their implications for patient education.

## Guidelines for Patient Teaching Practice

The nurse in clinical practice confronted with immediate patient education needs and seeking to respond as effectively as possible often looks first to practical guidelines rather than to a study of underlying theory. In response, much of the professional literature emphasizes practice tips and techniques either through case presentations or easy-to-use guides for practice. Morra provided a set of techniques for patient teaching that, combined with consideration of underlying principles drawn from theory, can assist the nurse in thinking about effective ways of meeting patients' needs (Table 59-2).[41]

Basic steps for conducting patient education include assessing educational needs, planning the teaching process, implementation, and evaluation. Assessing educational needs too often is done from the health care professional's perspective alone.[39] That is, the professional care provider can readily identify information about diagnosis, or treatment regimen, or potential side effects, or complications—all important information that should be conveyed to the patient and family. In addition, the experienced care provider is knowledgeable of typical psychosocial difficulties and can suggest resources for social and personal support. Effective needs assessment, however, must involve the patient, seeking to identify needs as seen from the patient's perspective too.

Involvement of the patient in needs assessment can be complex. As Morra notes, patients often are not sufficiently knowledgeable even to formulate meaningful questions.[41] The care provider needs to be attentive to indications of knowledge gaps expressed by patients, be ready to ask questions, and give patients ample time to think through their concerns and questions. The period immediately following diagnosis can be an especially difficult time emotionally, complicating the process of giving important information. McGinn, an oncology nurse who has experienced cancer, noted the initial shock of hearing a cancer diagnosis—and not hearing nearly everything else.[42] Complicating matters further, the patient later may feel too embarrassed to admit that he or she cannot remember the information given earlier and may be even less willing to ask questions in spite of feeling a loss of control and a need for information.

Assessing patient needs must be an ongoing process, recognizing that information often needs to be repeated and that new needs and questions will arise as the individual progresses through treatment. Similarly, psychosocial needs vary from one person to another and change over time. Reassessing support needs at various points, therefore, should be done in the same way as reassessing educational needs.

Information and support needs change substantially as different stages of living with cancer are experienced.[43] It is important to note that the new challenges and issues

**TABLE 59-1   Principles of Adult Learning and Their Implications for Practice**

| Principles | Assumptions and Implications |
|---|---|
| Adults are independent learners. | The process of moving from childhood to adulthood is a process of moving from dependence to increasing independence. There is a deep psychological need for adults to see themselves, as well as to have others see them, as generally independent or self-reliant. The educator working with adult learners must respect this independence and ability of the adult learner to control his/her own learning. Adults are responsible for what is to be learned and take an active role in their learning. The learning takes place between the learner and the material; the teacher is there only to facilitate the exchange. |
| Adults' past experiences are resources for learning. | Unlike children, adults have a reservoir of past experience that can be a resource for learning. Whenever possible, adults' past experiences should be drawn upon to enhance the learning process. Further, adults' self-images are often defined, at least in part, by their past experiences, and they have a deep investment in their value. Ignoring these past experiences in current learning can be interpreted as essentially rejecting a large part of the adult learner. |
| Adults' readiness to learn emerges from life's developmental stages. | The adult learner's readiness to learn develops from life's tasks and problems. As the adult years progress, there is a shift in career, social roles, personal responsibilities, etc. The transitions that evolve during life create opportunities for learning as the individual strives to better understand and cope. Such phases have been labeled as "teachable moments." The individual is both more highly motivated to learn, and the information is more readily understood when presented within this context. |
| Adults' learning is task- or problem-oriented | Adults will seek out various resources for specific learning (information or skills) to help them in answering a question or dealing with a problem. They are motivated in their learning to find answers or solve problems. Learning experiences will be most effective when they respond to adult learners' perceived needs. |

Reprinted with permission from Padberg RM and Padberg LF: Strengthening the effectiveness of patient education: Applying principles of adult education. *Oncol Nurs Forum* 17:65–69, 1990. Adapted from Knowles MS: *The Modern Practice of Adult Education: From Pedagogy to Andragogy* (ed 2). Upper Saddle River, NJ, Globe Fearon/Cambridge, 1980.

**TABLE 59-2   Guidelines for Patient Teaching**

| | |
|---|---|
| 1. Present the most important material first. | The first material presented is best remembered. Stress the important because people remember best the information they believe is most important. |
| 2. Offer information. | Do not wait for patients to ask before giving information. Make it easy for the person to start a conversation. Open the door by asking a question such as "Is there anything going on right now you'd like to talk about?" |
| 3. Combine sight and sound when presenting materials. | Most of the information a listener has stored in the brain has been received *visually*. Use printed explanations to accompany what you say. Remember that people respond to different methods of presenting printed materials, so combine different forms—questions and answers, pictures, charts, questions to ask, quizzes—all reinforcing one another. |
| 4. Ask patients and family members what they want to know about their illness. | People remember best the information they are most interested in knowing. |
| 5. Categorize. | Tell people the categories of information that you are going to discuss with them, then follow those categories. People remember better when the information is organized into parts that make sense and can be remembered as a set. |
| 6. Don't be afraid to repeat information. | Patients forget about a third of what is said to them. Recall of instructions and advice is less than 50%. Remember that a person's intelligence seems to show no relation to ability to recall and remember. |
| 7. Give information in small amounts whenever possible. | The proportion of information forgotten increases with the amount of information presented. |
| 8. Involve family members and supportive friends as completely as possible. | Encourage family/friends to share and discuss information, to participate in care, and to support the patient. Share with them appropriate sources of information. |
| 9. Try to give information when people are relatively calm. | Recall of information is related to level of anxiety, being poorest when anxiety is particularly high or low, and best when there is moderate anxiety. It is important to let people get over the initial shock of a cancer diagnosis before giving detailed information. |
| 10. Speak plainly and use short sentences. | Many people find long sentences, fast speech, and unfamiliar terms hard to understand. Don't speak "medicalese." Words such as *palpate* or *palliate* are not everyday household words, no matter the age or education of your audience. |
| 11. Ask for questions. | Encourage patients and family members to write down questions as they think of them for you to answer when you see them. Help them understand that you expect questions, no matter how simple or complex they might be. Stress that there is no such thing as a "stupid" question if it is bothering the patient. |
| 12. Help the patient and family understand there are choices from the beginning. | Some are simple such as choosing the time for treatment. Others are more complex such as different therapies. However, there are choices, and if the patient and family are not involved, someone else is making the choices. |
| 13. Be responsive to even the most searching and difficult question, such as second opinions or alternative treatments. | Answer them freely and fully. Make it known that seeking a second opinion is an accepted practice and that the majority of physicians respect an individual's right to further consultation. |
| 14. Encourage patients and family members to ask the doctor questions that only the doctor can answer. | Many people, particularly many older people, have problems asking doctors questions; and often people have problems recalling what the doctor has said. Encourage them to ask questions, and ensure them that the doctor wants them to ask anything about which they are confused or worried. Encourage them to write down the answers and keep them in a notebook or tape-record them to review when they get home and for future reference. Suggest that patients bring someone with them when they meet with the physician; different people hear different things. |
| 15. Ask questions yourself. | Ask patients to explain back to you what you have presented. Such feedback helps check whether they have heard the information as you intended. |
| 16. Use silence. | Don't try to keep the conversation moving. Wait to allow the questions or comments that will advise you where to go next. |
| 17. Take time to sit down. | Patients perceive a visit in which a health professional sits down as much longer than when the person is standing. Sitting close and at the person's level adds warmth to the visit. |
| 18. Maintain eye contact. | It signals that you are willing to talk. Not looking at a person gives the sense that you don't want a conversation. |
| 19. Body language affects communication. | Inappropriate facial expressions, nuances of body positions, and nervous habits can all convey impressions of disinterest or create barriers for open conversation. Often physical contact, such as holding a hand, can be appropriate and can help dissipate feelings of isolation or fear that cancer patients say they experience. |
| 20. Don't worry about not saying the right thing. | The simple, sincere gesture of one person reaching out to another communicates comfort, hope, and support. You—the nurse—are in a unique position to offer it. |

Morra ME: Making choices: The consumer's perspective. Adapted from *Cancer Nurs* 8:54–59, 1985 (suppl 1). Used with permission.

that arise at each stage create new needs for knowledge, understanding, and coping. Once needs are identified, plans for patient teaching activities to meet these needs can be developed. Several of the guidelines shown in Table 59-2 relate to how educational activities should be planned. The plan should include several relatively short teaching sessions that focus on a single area or small amount of related information. Family members or others who are providing assistance and support to the individual are included in all teaching sessions. Multimedia approaches are used whenever possible.

Planning allows for selection of resources and identification of specific activities to address all of the needs identified; for approaching these teaching activities in an ordered and prepared manner; for identifying who will be responsible for various teaching tasks; for establishing strategies to monitor or track the completion of teaching activities; and for planning how the achievement of learning outcomes will be assessed. Patient teaching responsibilities and activities should be included as components of any patient management planning tool or process. It is important to build into the plan easy access to care providers so that patients and families may readily ask questions, clarify information, and seek assistance when questions, concerns, and needs arise.

Patient teaching is not complete unless patient learning has been verified. Ongoing assessment incorporated in each teaching activity guides the teaching process: what information will need to be repeated, what concepts still need clarification, what new needs or questions have arisen. Evaluation is ongoing, a part of the teaching-learning process.

Much of patient-family teaching at the time of treatment focuses on aspects of self-care and, therefore, includes skill development as well as sharing knowledge. Competency in performing skills often is easier to assess than other learning since direct observation of skill performance can be used. Assessment of skill performance may require specialized resources such as skills labs or special demonstration models. For example, to provide a hands-on opportunity for mastectomy patients to practice caring for incisions and emptying drains, staff at a military medical center modified a CPR mannequin to simulate mastectomy surgery.[44]

Whether knowledge- or skill-oriented, the primary issue is that the level of learning needs to be assessed if there is to be any confidence that patient education has met its goals. When deficiencies are identified or new learning needs are identified as a result of assessment, this information serves as the new needs assessment findings for planning ongoing patient teaching activities.

## CONTINUITY ACROSS CARE SETTINGS

An important issue for consideration in patient education is providing effective patient teaching across multiple care settings. While this is not a new issue, changing patterns of health care delivery have introduced a greater need for addressing how patient education is coordinated and communicated across settings. Efforts to decrease length of stay in acute care settings, the increased use of outpatient services for initial treatment as well as follow-up care, expanded use of home health agencies, and the growth in new health care systems such as health maintenance organizations (HMOs) are all major contributors to these changes. Patient education needs also have increased as larger numbers of people are living with cancer as a chronic illness and as greater attention is given to their psychosocial needs. With earlier discharge and increased use of outpatient treatment and follow-up care, families and patients often are expected to perform technical and monitoring procedures previously done only by professionals and to take greater responsibility for coordinating care.[45] Attention must be given to preparing patients and families for these responsibilities and to the coordination of ongoing support during the period of self-care.

Continuity in care and patient education typically is considered from the view of linkage between the initial treatment setting and ongoing contact through the physician's office, the outpatient clinic, or the home health agency. The accreditation standards for hospitals address this interrelationship of patient and family education, discharge planning, and continuity of care, calling for the sharing of discharge plans and instructions with all health care providers working with the patient.[20]

The concept of continuity of care includes not only coordination and consistency across multiple settings but also the ongoing availability of or access to care services. Typically, comprehensive care is provided during the period of hospitalization or initial outpatient treatment, but the availability of care often drops quickly after discharge. Yet care needs, including medical, psychosocial, and daily living, extend throughout the illness and recovery experience.[27] Informational needs often change, thus making reassessment of patient teaching needs important at various points during the continuum of care.[46] Benefits of effective patient teaching, referrals, and follow-up processes include shortened hospitalizations, a decrease in preventable hospital readmissions, increased compliance with medical regimens, decreased medical complications, and improved psychosocial status (decreased anxiety, improved coping, increased sense of competency in self-care, and increased knowledge of therapy).[27]

There are a variety of models available for strengthening continuity of care. A recent review of continuity of care strategies looked both at studies focusing on effective approaches for inpatient teaching and discharge planning and at studies looking at teaching and planning interventions across the continuum of care.[27] For example, a visiting nurse service has successfully implemented a nursing practice model in which a nurse specialist from the home health agency serves as the primary contact and case manager for the patient. This individual is available to the patient and family on a 24-hour basis. In addition to providing direct care, the nurse assists in making treatment decisions and facilitates contacts for the patient and family across various care settings.[47,48]

Effective continuity of care and patient education are most dependent on strong communication among health care providers across all care settings.[49,50] Ultimately, standardization of discharge planning, patient education, and outpatient and community follow-up processes is needed in order to ensure continuity of care.[27]

# DEVELOPING PATIENT EDUCATION AND SUPPORT MATERIALS AND PROGRAMS

Though patient education and support resources from government agencies, nonprofit organizations, health care institutions, and commercial sources are extensive, there are times when it is appropriate to develop materials or programs designed to meet special needs within a specific health care setting. Material and program development has been described as a six-step process that should continually repeat itself; that is, evaluation of the implemented program should provide feedback that can then be used to refine the program, progressing again through the development steps. The process described here has been adapted from the developmental process presented in the National Cancer Institute Office of Cancer Communication's publication, *Making Health Communication Programs Work: A Planner's Guide.*[51] This process is shown graphically in Figure 59-1.

## Step 1: Planning and Strategy Selection

This is the basic planning stage for educational materials development. Several key issues are included in this stage:

1. Clearly identify the issues, problems, or patient education goals that need to be addressed. It should be clear why a decision is made to develop materials or a program for a particular setting or purpose and that existing materials are not sufficient to address the need.

2. Identify the target audience. This might be answered in many ways: by type of cancer or particular stage of the illness; whether the target group will be diverse or more narrowly defined in terms of factors such as age, gender, or ethnic or socioeconomic factors; the setting in which the audience will be found for the program or materials. Understanding the audience is important to guide decisions later regarding strategies to be used and to identify individuals for pretesting the materials.

3. Identify the intended outcomes, the goals of the materials or program. Measurable objectives should be established. Identify how they will be evaluated to determine the success of the materials or program.

4. Identify constraints—financial, time, personnel, setting—placed upon the development process and on the use of the materials once developed. These constraints will limit or guide later decisions.

## Step 2: Selecting Processes and Materials

This is the stage in which the purposes, characteristics of the audience, and constraints identified in step 1 will guide decisions about the types of materials or program structure that will be used. Decisions must be made about the processes or channels for delivering the materials or program; about the specific structure or format of the program or materials; whether some existing materials will be used (within a program) or modified (in developing new materials to meet a specific need), or all new materials will be developed. Consider what program structures or material formats work best for the target audience or within the setting or location in which the program will occur.

## Step 3: Developing Materials and Pretesting

At this stage the process moves from planning to development. The work of drafting and producing the actual materials must be done, with ongoing testing throughout the process. Involvement of expert reviewers to provide suggestions as development begins or to critique early materials can be especially useful both for shaping the content and for the style of presentation to be most effective. Also, those health care professionals who will use the materials or implement the program, or those who control decisions about adopting new materials or programs, should be involved. For example, if developing a new brochure for assisting patients in understanding a particular self-care technique, nurses who are involved in teaching these patients can provide guidance not only on the information that is needed but also on the types of questions that patients have, the time that is available for presenting the materials, the likely settings for this presentation, the opportunities for demonstration, and other particular conditions that will help guide the content and format.

### Serving special populations

Other considerations during development include making materials or programs responsive to diverse populations or, if the materials are targeted for a particular audience, making them appropriate for that target group. For instance, examples and illustrations in culturally sensitive materials should reflect diversity in racial and ethnic character, age, socioeconomic and occupational identification, and religious identification.

If the materials are being developed for use with a specific target audience, care must be taken to ensure

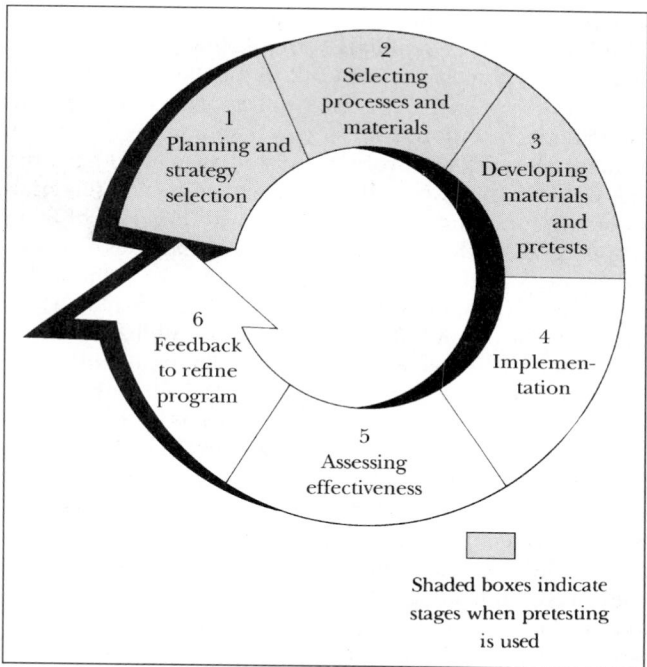

**FIGURE 59-1**  Steps in the development of patient education materials and resources. (Office of Cancer Communications, National Cancer Institute: *Making Health Communication Programs Work: A Planner's Guide.* NIH publication No. 92-1493. Washington, DC, U.S. Department of Health and Human Services, National Institutes of Health, 1992.)

that elements of the audience's standards and practices are properly presented and respected.

A special target audience may be defined in many ways, and tailoring materials for a special audience similarly may take many forms. Print materials developed for use with an elderly target group, for example, need to be sensitive to factors affecting readability such as font size and style. Programs for older persons need to consider issues such as the setting in which the program will be conducted and potential difficulties with acoustics and accessibility. Elders seeking to participate in education and support programs may be hampered by transportation problems; daytime programs held in settings linked to other programs and services for older persons enhance participation. In general, materials and programs designed for older people need to be developed with an awareness of the physiological changes associated with aging that may reduce or limit hearing, vision, motor function, and cognitive processes. Possible economic and psychosocial changes that may affect older persons' ability to participate and benefit also should be considered.[52,53] At the same time, health care professionals must avoid thinking of older people, or any special population, in stereotypical terms. Again considering older people as a target group, while there are general patterns that the care provider should be aware of, variability among the elderly reflects the diversity of the overall population. The

health professional should acknowledge the potential for individuals to experience cancer and their responses to cancer in divergent ways.[53,54]

Nurses whose practice settings serve people of diverse cultural backgrounds, and most practice settings do, need to be sensitive to cultural differences and to respond appropriately. Too often cultural diversity is described and discussed in the literature only in terms of racial or ethnic minority status. Culture, however, is a complex concept that includes a mix of beliefs, values, modes of dress, social relationships, behavioral norms, and other factors.[55] Cultural differences may affect many aspects of the interaction between health care professionals and their clients. The lack of common cultural background between health care professionals and clients has been suggested as a major contributor to problems in compliance.[56]

Strategies for effective culturally sensitive approaches to patient education and support are varied. Health care professionals serving populations from cultural backgrounds different from their own need to make linkages with key members of the target community, involving members of the community in the development of educational materials, programs, and community outreach strategies.[57,58] Placing programs in the community, in locations that reach the target audience, is important.[6,59] The Oncology Nursing Society's *Cancer Prevention in Minority*

*Populations*[60] is a helpful resource for understanding cultural perspectives within many ethnic minority populations and the implications of these cultural views for effective health care.

In spite of the large volume of patient education materials available today from government agencies, nonprofit organizations, and commercial vendors, materials designed to reach special populations are often difficult to find. This is an area in which nurses and other health care professionals may find the greatest need for developing local materials. For example, health care organizations serving large numbers of persons for whom English is not their first language or who have little or no ability to speak or read English may find bilingual or non-English materials difficult to obtain. Only a small portion of publications from the National Cancer Institute or the American Cancer Society are available in non-English versions. Developing such materials requires special attention to cultural differences as well as a sophisticated understanding of the language of the target audience. Translating materials from English should be done by individuals who are sufficiently fluent to fully understand connotations of words, common expressions and colloquial terms, and the application of formal and familiar forms of address.

## Readability

One aspect of printed patient education materials that has received considerable attention in the nursing literature is reading level. It is estimated that 20% of Americans read below the fifth-grade level.[61] A fifth-grade reading level has been identified as the minimum reading level for making good use of basic written materials;[62] individuals with reading skills below this level are functionally illiterate, lacking the reading and writing skills needed for daily activities in contemporary society. Many adults, while not illiterate, still have low literacy skills. The 1992 National Adult Literacy Survey found that 90 million adult Americans, or 47%, demonstrated low literacy.[63] Although the reading level of print materials can be easily evaluated, and though the literacy issue has been discussed in the literature, the use of reading levels that are barriers for many within the general public still occurs.

A review of 137 consent forms for clinical oncology protocols in use at a major university medical center found that reading levels of the forms varied from grade 6 to grade 16.[64] The mean grade level was 11.1, and only 6% of the forms had a reading level at grade 6 or lower. A 1992 study of 51 publications provided by the American Cancer Society found that only one publication was written below the sixth-grade level.[65] Over half of the publications were written at the 12th-grade level or higher, up to a level equivalent to graduate study. A more recent study assessed the reading levels of 30 commonly used patient education pamphlets provided by the ACS and the National Cancer Institute (NCI) and the educational attainment and actual reading levels of a group of cancer patients.[66] The 30 booklets ranged from grades 6 to 16 in reading level, with a mean grade level of 9.8. Only 27% of the patient group tested could be expected to understand all of the printed materials.

It should be noted that both the ACS and the NCI, as well as many other organizations that provide cancer patient education materials, are actively addressing problems with the level of literacy required for comprehending their materials. Currently, the ACS and the NCI review reading levels and modify materials to reach as broad an audience as possible as new materials are developed or as older publications are revised and updated. Both organizations also offer some publications specifically designed for use with low-literacy audiences.[61]

A variety of readability assessment scales are available. The readability formula used by the NCI's Office of Cancer Communication is the SMOG, selected because it provides ease of use with a high level of accuracy. Guidelines for using the SMOG readability test and a table for conversion of SMOG scores to approximate grade levels of reading ability are provided in Table 59-3. Readability scales generally assess the difficulty of vocabulary and sentence length and complexity. Readability tests designed for use on computers also may assess grammar, style, word usage, and punctuation as indicators of reading difficulty.[63]

Much of the literature addressing readability of materials is focused on reading level. Other factors, however, also contribute to the readability or the reader's likelihood of comprehending information being presented. Beyond the level of the text itself, comprehension is enhanced by how blocks of text are placed on the page, the use of open space and wide margins, the use of headings and other organizers, choice of typeface, the use of graphics and illustrations, and other design factors. For example, low-literate women exhibited better comprehension of information on cervical cancer and condyloma when given a pamphlet with illustrations and a narrative text rather than a pamphlet with no illustrations and a bulleted text, even though the pamphlet with illustrations had a slightly more difficult reading level (grade 8.4 versus 7.7).[67] Tables 59-4 and 59-5 provide guidelines for both reducing the reading difficulty and enhancing comprehension through design, illustrations, and other visual effects. If possible, using the assistance of a professional graphic designer can contribute to a design that maximizes the ease of reading and comprehension. An excellent resource for developing materials that work well with persons with low literacy is *Teaching Patients with Low Literacy Skills* by Doak et al.[62] Reducing the complexity of the text and using an effective format, graphics, and illustrations improves the readability for all readers, not just for those with low literacy.

The discussion here, and much of the discussion in the nursing literature regarding development of patient education materials, focuses on printed materials. In general, locally produced materials make less use of more complex technologies such as audio and video tapes,

**TABLE 59-3** The SMOG Readability Formula

To calculate the SMOG reading grade level, begin with the entire written work that is being assessed, and follow these four steps:

1. Count off 10 consecutive sentences near the beginning, in the middle, and near the end of the text.
2. From this sample of 30 sentences, circle all of the words containing three or more syllables (polysyllabic), including repetitions of the same word, and total the number of words circled.
3. Estimate the square root of the total number of polysyllabic words counted. This is done by finding the nearest perfect square, and taking its square root.
4. Finally, add a constant of 3 to the square root. This number gives the SMOG grade, or the reading grade level that a person must have reached if he or she is to fully understand the text being assessed.

A few additional guidelines will help to clarify these directions:

- A sentence is defined as a string of words punctuated with a period (.), an exclamation point (!) or a question mark (?).
- Hyphenated words are considered as one word.
- Numbers which are written out should also be considered, and if in numeric form in the text, they should be pronounced to determine if they are polysyllabic.
- Proper nouns, if polysyllabic, should be counted, too.
- Abbreviations should be read as unabbreviated to determine if they are polysyllabic.

Not all pamphlets, fact sheets, or other printed materials contain 30 sentences. To test a text that has fewer than 30 sentences:

1. Count all of the polysyllabic words in the text.
2. Count the number of sentences.

3. Find the average number of polysyllabic words per sentence as follows:

$$\text{Average} = \frac{\text{Total \# of polysyllabic words}}{\text{Total \# of sentences}}$$

4. Multiply that average by the number of sentences *short of 30*.
5. Add that figure on to the total number of polysyllabic words.
6. Find the square root and add the constant of 3.

Perhaps the quickest way to administer the SMOG grading test is by using the SMOG conversion table. Simply count the number of polysyllabic words in your chain of 30 sentences and look up the approximate grade level on the chart.

| SMOG Conversion Table* | |
| --- | --- |
| Total Polysyllabic Word Counts | Approximate Grade Level (+ 1.5 Grades) |
| 0–2 | 4 |
| 3–6 | 5 |
| 7–12 | 6 |
| 13–20 | 7 |
| 21–30 | 8 |
| 31–42 | 9 |
| 43–56 | 10 |
| 57–72 | 11 |
| 73–90 | 12 |
| 91–110 | 13 |
| 111–132 | 14 |
| 133–156 | 15 |
| 157–182 | 16 |
| 183–210 | 17 |
| 211–240 | 18 |

*Developed by Harold C. McGraw, Office of Educational Research, Baltimore County Schools, Towson, Maryland.

Office of Cancer Communications, National Cancer Institute: *Making Health Communication Programs Work: A Planner's Guide*. NIH publication No. 92-1493. Washington, DC, U.S. Department of Health and Human Services, National Institutes of Health, 1992.

computer programs, or computer technologies that provide interactive video capabilities. Just as in the development of print materials, there are many factors that distinguish effective audio-visual programs from ineffective ones. Some are much the same as those that affect print materials—culturally sensitive content, use of vocabulary and sentence structures that are appropriate for the literacy level of the audience. Many of the guidelines for use of format, illustrations and visual effects in print materials have comparable guidelines applicable to video or computer programs. But other factors also come into play; for example, the pace of presentation is very important since, unlike the pace of print materials, which is set by the reader, the pace of an audio or video program is not directly controlled by the listener or viewer. Production of materials using such technology usually will benefit greatly by having knowledgeable professionals who work with these media participate in the development.

### Pretesting

The development stage for patient education and support materials and programs can also be enhanced by pretesting draft materials with selected groups that are representative of the intended target audience. A variety of techniques can be used for pretesting, and a variety of characteristics or qualities of the materials can be evaluated. Are the materials attractive so that people will try to read them? Is the format easily followed? Is the information organized in a logical pattern or sequence? Most important, is the material understood? Are the learning goals achieved? Individual interviews, focus groups, surveys, and pilot testing of materials are all mechanisms that can be used for pretesting.

It is important again at this stage to use feedback from health care professionals who will use the materials. Both health care professionals and representatives from the target audience can provide important, though

**TABLE 59-4**  Reducing Reading Difficulty of Written Patient Education Materials

1. Pick short words—2 syllables or less.
2. Use common words. For instance, replace the word *physician* with the word *doctor.*
3. Write in the active voice. Instead of writing, "The patient should," say, "You should."
4. Create short sentences—5 to 7 words.
5. Write in conversational style, as if you were talking to the person.
6. Give information in small amounts—one idea at a time.
7. Do not use initials and abbreviations. Even simple ones, such as days of the week and months of the year, can be a problem for this audience.
8. Do not change a word just for variety. If you start using the word *cancer,* do not change to *tumor.*
9. Avoid lists. They present a problem in comprehension for adults with low literacy skills. If you use them, break them up with easily understandable visual effects.

Reprinted with permission from Morra ME, Varricchio C: Teaching patients with limited reading skills. *Cancer Pract* 1:154–156, 1993.

**TABLE 59-5**  Improving Readability with Pictures and Visual Effects

1. Make illustrations simple, direct, and lifelike. Use sketches and line drawings with heavy, clean lines. Make people look as human as possible.
2. When showing parts of the body, include sections that people will recognize, such as legs and arms. Do not show drawings only of the inside parts of the body.
3. Use visuals to show desired behavior. Show only the correct way to accomplish a task. Using visuals to demonstrate both right and wrong can be confusing.
4. Comic books that tell stories of real people, using human figures, can be useful teaching tools. Make sure the messages are short, with no more than 15 words in each balloon area.
5. Stylized visuals and abstract forms are not appropriate for this audience.
6. Do not use charts with many columns. Cut down the amount of statistical data.
7. Cartoons usually are not useful ways of communicating with low-literacy people. Cartoons often confuse, introducing figures that are irrelevant to the message.
8. Present one idea on a single page—or two pages if they are face-to-face. Simple ideas should not need more than two facing pages.
9. Two columns on a page are preferable. This ensures that the line will not be too long for a person to comprehend.
10. When using a series of steps, make them few. Place the steps in left-to-right order, down the page in the normal reading order. Number each step and place related text next to the visual, so that the reader does not need to move back and forth to other parts of the page.
11. Use an action title or caption to direct the reader on what to do. Make it brief—no more than 10 words. Tie captions directly into the visuals.
12. If you wish to emphasize something, underline it. Or use circles, arrows, larger print, or color to help the eye focus on critical points.
13. Do not use all capital letters, italics, or script. Avoid fancy typefaces. Avoid stylized symbols whenever possible. All of these are difficult for this audience to read. If possible, select 14-point type.
14. Have a clear idea in your mind why you are using a visual, and make sure the visual fits that objective. Make sure each visual has a distinct focus point.

Reprinted with permission from Morra ME, Varricchio C: Teaching patients with limited reading skills. *Cancer Pract* 1:154–156, 1993.

different, types of feedback. The health care professionals serve as the gatekeepers for this information—they are the individuals who will deliver the information or programs to patients. Their comments may have less to do with the appropriateness of language, style, or literacy level, focusing instead on factors that will affect practical usefulness. Are materials too lengthy to be presented in the time available? Will the materials complement other resources being used? Are they organized into categories of information or topical groupings that clinicians typically use as they speak with patients and families? Do clinicians have available any special equipment required (if the program or materials use audiotapes, videotapes, or computers)? Will they consider using the materials or program in their practice setting?

An excellent resource for guiding development of patient education materials is the NCI's publication *Clear & Simple: Developing Effective Print Materials for Low-Literate Readers.*[63] Although intended for assisting in developing materials for low-literacy audiences, the processes outlined and most of the issues discussed are applicable to any program or materials development activities.

## Step 4: Implementation

At this point the educational and support material or program is ready for use with the target group in the settings for which it was designed. Close monitoring of the implementation, especially in the early stages, might address several issues. Are the materials being provided to those for whom they were intended? Are enough copies available? Are the materials being used in the settings and for the purposes for which they were designed? Is there any initial feedback indicating major problems that need to be addressed? And, of special importance for future assessment and improvement of the materials or program, are evaluation procedures being followed as designed?

## Step 5: Assessing Effectiveness

At this stage, evaluation information collected during program implementation is reviewed to understand the level of effectiveness of the program or materials. Possible actions for addressing weaknesses and improving the program or materials are considered. The evaluation should be based upon information gathered as designed in step 1. The primary question to be addressed is whether the program or materials met the objectives. If materials were used in a manner different from that for which they were intended, or if the program was implemented differently than designed, what caused the changes? How did the changes impact effectiveness? What can be changed to improve the materials or program?

## Step 6: Program Refinement

The final step is to use the results of the evaluation to revise and refine the materials or program. The development cycle in effect becomes a spiral, with the evaluation findings of one cycle being used as the starting point to again look at objectives and strategies, and strengthen evaluation procedures; to update, revise, or replace materials; to use feedback from users and target audience representatives to test the revised materials or program; to once again implement or use the materials or program, including reevaluating outcomes; and to collect the evaluation information to plan for further refinement and a new cycle. The ongoing cycle also allows the materials or program to be continually updated with new information, or to meet new needs within the target audience, or to adjust to changes in the professional settings in which the materials or programs are used.

Developing materials or programs locally can be challenging. Using a careful sequence of developmental steps assures that the special effort and resources committed to the challenge are used well for the maximum gains possible.

## RESOURCES FOR PATIENT EDUCATION AND SUPPORT

The resources for patient education and patient support in oncology have expanded tremendously in recent years. Some resources are of long standing—the Cancer Information Service of the NCI has been in existence since 1975, and the ACS began its work of providing a wide range of public and patient education materials many years earlier. The past five to ten years, however, have seen rapid growth in new materials, information services, and support programs. In part, new resources reflect changes in technology, particularly the opportunities for rapid data retrieval and response as well as widespread access to electronic databases through computer technology. In part, the growth in resources and programs reflects the success in treatment of cancer and the resulting change in perspective, from viewing cancer as a fatal illness to a chronic illness. The increased numbers of people living with cancer have created a need for a wide range of both information and support resources. Public demand for information and support programs also reflects a growth in a consumer-oriented perspective throughout our society. And in part, the growth of resources reflects increased awareness of the need for information and the ongoing efforts by many organizations to provide better information and easier access for larger audiences.

In spite of the growth in resources and specialized systems for obtaining information, in a recent Oncology Nursing Society–sponsored study of nurses in clinical practice[68] nurses reported inadequate resources in many areas and difficulty in locating or accessing information when it is available. Nearly half of the nurses responding indicated that they often meet the gap between available resources and resource needs by using self- or institution-developed materials. Both nurses and their patients indicated a need for a central clearinghouse on available information. The researchers noted that it is unclear whether information is unavailable or instead nurses are unable to access available information.

Effective patient teaching is dependent not only upon process but also content. Accurate, effective instructional materials are essential. The following section reviews some of the major sources of information available for patients and their caregivers, both professional and nonprofessional, as well as the growing array of support materials, programs, and organizations.

### American Cancer Society

The ACS is a nationwide, community-based organization that offers a wide range of programs and services focused on public understanding about cancer; research on treatment, prevention, and early detection of cancer; and education and support for both health professionals and cancer patients and their families. The ACS provides many public education efforts, through public service advertising and other forms, seeking to enhance public understanding of cancer, cancer prevention and treatment, and cancer survivorship issues. In addition, the ACS provides direct information to individuals—cancer patients, families, or any individual from the general public seeking information—through two primary inquiry routes: the Resources, Information and Guidance (RIG) system operated by the division or local unit offices of the ACS, and the Cancer Resource Service (CRS) provided by the national ACS office. The national CRS program functions with paid staff, while the local RIG system is staffed by volunteers.

CRS staff can provide information regarding ACS publications, video programs, and other such material resources, and can arrange for such materials to be provided to the inquirer. In addition, the CRS staff can inform the person inquiring about resources available at the local level through the RIG system, and can provide information on how to make contact at the local level.

Complementing the national CRS, the local-level, volunteer-staffed RIG system can provide access to print and audiovisual materials provided by the ACS. In addition, the RIG provides information regarding locally offered ACS programs such as "I Can Cope," "Reach to Recovery," "CanSurmount," and "Look Good . . . Feel Better." The ACS also works in cooperation with other organizations and provides referrals to programs such as "lost cord clubs" and "ostomy support groups", and to specialized services such as those for families of children with cancer offered by the "Candlelighters Childhood Cancer Foundation."

The CRS and the RIG are complementary services, with the national service focused primarily on access to a wide variety of specialized informational materials and the local service intended to make links to the many direct services and programs available at the local level. At the present, the ACS is working to provide an improved integration of the two services, providing links between the national, divisional, and local offices so that an individual who accesses ACS services at any level need make only one contact. As noted in an ACS document, the ACS seeks to "produce a high quality, customer oriented, seamless system for delivering cancer disease and resource information to the public, cancer patients and their families."[69] In addition to making linkages between the various levels of the ACS and providing one-contact service, the ACS also seeks to develop two databases to provide rapid searches for information: a national resource directory to identify pamphlets or brochures, videos, and other information and teaching materials for both professional health care personnel and the general public; and a database providing detailed information, designed for cancer patients and their families, on standard treatments for all cancer types.

The ACS provides extensive resources for health care professionals as well as for public and patient education. These include over 250 publications for health care pro-

fessionals, research grant programs, scholarship and fellowship programs, and many types of support provided through the national, division, and local offices to professional groups. As one example of the ongoing support provided by local ACS offices for professional development, the Northern Virginia ACS office cosponsors with local nurses' organizations, and in recent years the local chapter of the Oncology Nursing Society, an annual institute for oncology nurses. This cooperative effort is now in its 38th year. The ACS provides staff logistical support, mailing services, and other types of assistance to this annual program, which serves over 400 nurses in the northern Virginia region. Similar cooperative efforts exist in many communities across the country.

Oncology nurses should be familiar with the information and support services available from the ACS for themselves and their patients. The national CRS can be contacted through a toll-free number: 1-800-ACS-2345 (1-800-227-2345). The numbers for contacting local and state offices of ACS can be found through local telephone directories.

Several of the ACS programs designed for education and support of cancer patients and their families are widely used and should be understood more thoroughly. Four, mentioned earlier, are described briefly here.

### "I Can Cope"

"I Can Cope" is an eight-session, 12-hour structured patient education program originally developed by oncology nurses with support from a local ACS office.[8] The success of the local program led to adoption by the ACS on the national level in 1979. The ACS currently provides a full packet of program materials as well as local training sessions for health care professionals to serve as program leaders.

"I Can Cope" is designed primarily as an educational program, but it also provides support for patients and families through group discussions and socialization.[3] It was extensively evaluated in 1991 and was revised based on the evaluation findings.[70]

### "Reach to Recovery" and "CanSurmount"

"Reach to Recovery," begun in 1973, and "CanSurmount," started in 1976 in Colorado and adopted nationally by the ACS in 1979, are similar programs offered by the ACS. Through these programs, cancer patients are put in contact on a one-on-one basis with ACS volunteers with similar backgrounds who are survivors of cancer. Typically individuals making contact with the ACS for such referrals have been newly diagnosed. "Reach to Recovery" was initiated as a program designed for breast cancer patients, giving them the opportunity to talk with another person who had experienced breast cancer. "CanSurmount" soon followed as a broad program designed to make similar personal contacts possible for people with other types of cancer.

## "Look Good . . . Feel Better"

This national program is designed to help women undergoing cancer treatment to address ways of maintaining grooming and appearance. Changes in personal appearance can be important factors affecting self-esteem, psychosocial well-being, and quality of life. "Look Good . . . Feel Better" was developed by the ACS in 1989 in cooperation with the Cosmetics, Toiletry and Fragrance Association Foundation and the National Cosmetology Association.

## National Cancer Institute

As the primary federal agency with responsibility for research on cancer causes, treatment, and prevention, the NCI is heavily involved in providing the most recent, up-to-date information to both health care professionals and the general public. Two offices within the NCI are especially assigned these responsibilities—the Office of Cancer Communication (OCC), established in 1974, and the International Cancer Information Center (ICIC), established in 1983. In recent years, the NCI has emphasized work to develop systems that allow easy access to comprehensive, state-of-the-art information, increasing the emphasis on quality-of-life issues, and strengthening information resources and access for underserved and hard-to-reach audiences. The major resource programs or systems established by the NCI to accomplish these purposes are described here.

### Physician Data Query

Developed in 1984, Physician Data Query (PDQ) is the NCI's most up-to-date source of cancer information. PDQ provides three types of information: cancer information summaries, clinical trial and standard protocols, and directories.[71]

Cancer information summaries are concise statements on the prognosis, staging, and treatment of more than 80 types of cancer, with statements on assessment and management of commonly encountered problems, screening summaries of evidence for selected types of cancer, summaries on selected investigational or newly approved drugs for treatment, and references and abstracts to key papers in the medical literature. The cancer information summaries are updated by five editorial boards; new and updated information is added to the database monthly.

While PDQ was initially developed for use by physicians and other health care professionals, a patient-intended component, the Patient Information File (PIF), has been added. As a result, cancer information summaries are available both for health care professionals and for the general public; the versions for the general public are written in lay language.

The second major component of PDQ is the clinical trial and standard protocol reports. This component provides information on over 1500 active treatment, supportive care, screening, and prevention studies with objectives, entry criteria, regimen information, and participating investigators. NCI-funded studies, non-NCI studies that have been reviewed by a PDQ editorial board, and European studies approved by the European Organization for Research and Treatment of Cancer or the United Kingdom Cancer Research Campaign are included in this database. A small number of standard therapy protocols also are listed.[72]

Finally, PDQ provides directories of physicians in clinical oncology practice, members of selected professional societies for physicians in oncology practice, clinical investigators for those protocols in the PDQ database, NCI grantees, and members of the NCI clinical trials cooperative groups. Over 21,000 physicians and 8000 organizations active in cancer care are included.[73]

The NCI has licensed a number of information distributors to provide direct access to PDQ; both on-line and CD-ROM versions are available. PDQ can be accessed through the MEDLARS system of the National Library of Medicine. In 1992 the NCI introduced an electronic service, CancerNet, allowing access to PDQ and some other information services free to users with access to Internet E-mail (cancernet@icicb.nci.nih.gov). Cancer-Net access was expanded through Internet gopher servers in 1993, and as of late 1995 over 55,000 requests were being received monthly through the CancerNet E-mail and gopher server links.[71]

PDQ also can be accessed indirectly by submitting requests for information through the OCC's Cancer Information Service (described later) and through Cancer-Fax. CancerFax, established in 1991, can be contacted at 301-402-5874 by use of a fax machine with a touch-tone telephone. Once connected, various voice prompts allow the caller to indicate the information being requested with numbered touch-tone responses. Most CancerFax information is available in both English and Spanish forms.[74] As of late 1995, CancerFax was fulfilling over 7000 requests monthly.[71]

In 1992–1993 the NCI initiated an assessment of the PIF of PDQ by conducting interviews with physicians, nurses, patient educators, librarians, and social workers.[75] Based on the findings regarding the flow of patient information and how PDQ/PIF was being used, eight NCI-designated comprehensive clinical cancer centers were funded as demonstration sites to expand the project. These sites collected baseline data over a ten-month period; each site then outlined proposed interventions and evaluation strategies for enhancing patient education, and health care professionals' and patients' access to and use of PDQ/PIF. As of late 1996, the NCI was working with the eight centers to define the details of the next phase of the project.[76]

### Cancer Information Service

The Cancer Information Service (CIS) is a national network of 19 regional offices funded and coordinated by the NCI's OCC. Established in 1975, the service currently receives and responds to 2400 inquiries daily across its 19 offices, or a total of over 600,000 inquiries annually. The CIS is contacted through the toll-free number 1-800-4-CANCER (1-800-422-6237); calls are routed to the appropriate regional center. The CIS centers are staffed by certified information specialists prepared to provide a wide variety of services and information.

The CIS is responsible for three types of services; the first is to provide up-to-date information in response to inquiries. Each CIS office can access the NCI's PDQ/PIF database and can provide information on treatment, detection, supportive care, and the full range of information available through PDQ/PIF. In addition, each center in the network is responsible for maintaining a directory of cancer-related services and programs in the region it serves—such as local and regional cancer education programs, speakers, regional cancer centers, and voluntary health organizations. Thus they help link individuals to specific services. Finally, each center's staff includes an outreach coordinator who is responsible for an outreach program designed to serve as a catalyst for cancer education initiatives in the region and for providing technical assistance for activities related to those initiatives. Such assistance might include providing state or regional statistical information, review of materials, program planning and evaluation assistance, or referral to appropriate individuals or organizations that can provide the particular expertise that is needed.[77]

As part of its information responsibilities, the CIS handles requests for NCI printed materials produced or developed by the OCC. These materials are sent primarily to health care professionals and organizations, which in turn distribute such information to the general public. In 1994, the OCC provided 23 million items for distribution to health care professionals, cancer patients and their families, and other individuals in the general public. The CIS also is the largest user of the PDQ, drawing information from PDQ in fulfilling its role of providing cancer diagnosis and treatment information, including clinical trial research options, to the public.[78]

### CancerLit

CancerLit is a comprehensive bibliographic database of published cancer research. CancerLit is designed for health care professionals, not the general public, and will not be discussed further here; however, oncology nurses should be aware of CancerLit as a valuable professional resource. Information on CancerLit can be obtained from either the OCC or the ICIC.

### Cancer Patient Education Network

As part of its ongoing efforts to enhance patient education, in 1989 the OCC established a network of patient education specialists representing all of the NCI-designated comprehensive clinical cancer centers to improve communication among health care professionals on cancer education needs and advances. The Cancer Patient Education Network (CPEN) has three prime goals: "(1) to increase cancer patient educators' access to the materials, services, and technical expertise of NCI's Patient Education Section (PES); (2) to encourage networking and sharing of information and resources among cancer patient educators; and (3) to provide PES staff with a direct link to the issues and concerns of cancer patients."[79]

The CPEN has developed several resources such as the *Resource Guide to Cancer Patient Education Programs,* a complete listing of planned educational programs of the NCI-designated centers. An annual conference offers members the opportunity to share information and to explore new developments in patient education. For further information about the CPEN, contact the NCI's Office of Cancer Communication, Patient Education Section (301-496-6792).

## Combined Health Information Database

The Combined Health Information Database (CHID) is a computer-based bibliographic database developed and maintained cooperatively by several health-related federal government agencies. Initiated in 1982, the CHID became available to health care professionals outside the federal government and to the public in 1985. At the present there are 25 subfiles within the CHID, including one devoted to cancer patient education and another for cancer prevention and control. The cancer patient education subfile is maintained by the NCI; the cancer prevention and control subfile is found in a database maintained by the Centers for Disease Control and Prevention. In addition to journal articles and books, the database includes bibliographic citations and abstracts for a variety of special reports, pamphlets, audiovisuals, product descriptions, "hard-to-find information sources," and health promotion and education programs at state and local levels. The CHID provides source and availability information for many of these materials to help users obtain materials directly.[80]

The CHID currently is available through a commercial vendor (OVID) and can be accessed through medical and university libraries or other organizations subscribing to this service. The CHID anticipates having the database accessible free through the World Wide Web beginning in Spring 1997.

## Advocacy and Support Groups

A large number of specialized organizations have been developed that focus on providing education and support programs for cancer patients and their families, particularly in the area of cancers affecting women.[81] Some of these organizations—such as the American Lung Association and the Leukemia Society of America—have long and well-known records of work in the field of advocacy and support for cancer research, public education, and patient education and support. There are, however, many such groups, some of national prominence, some with more regional impact. For example, Morra and Potts list more than 60 organizations—beyond the services and programs of the ACS and the NCI already discussed here—that provide various direct services, referrals, or advocacy programs for cancer patients and their families.[82]

This list of major resource organizations is in addition to several other resource lists provided by Morra and Potts, including professional organizations that provide referrals or listings of health providers; 55 NCI-designated cancer centers; six associations providing services or information on pain control; five home care organizations; ten national groups that can provide information regarding insurance and financial matters; cancer information databases and publication sources; and several other resource lists. A similar set of lists of cancer resources, with extended annotations, that is readily available to oncology nurses is provided annually by the Education Committee of the Oncology Nursing Society in the *Oncology Nursing Forum*.[83]

The National Hospice Organization is a national organization of local or regional hospice care provider groups. It seeks to promote hospice care and to encourage support for patients needing hospice care and their families. Another group, Hospice Link, provides a computerized database on hospice programs nationwide.

Many organizations and programs have focused on support for children with cancer and their families. Specialized information services are available on needs ranging from locating camps for children with cancer to understanding the limitations and opportunities for health insurance for these children. One of the most widely known organizations that concentrates on childhood cancer issues is the Candlelighters Childhood Cancer Foundation. Candlelighters focuses on assisting families to cope with the emotional stresses of dealing with childhood cancer.

The National Coalition for Cancer Survivorship (NCCS) was founded in 1986 based on a view that all persons who experience cancer are cancer survivors from diagnosis onward, experiencing different stages or "seasons" along the continuum of survivorship. The NCCS seeks to be both an organization of individuals and a coalition of organizations working in the field of cancer services, research, and advocacy. It focuses on a wide range of issues related to quality of life for cancer survivors: providing referral to appropriate local support services; addressing barriers to employment and access to health insurance; and advocating for changes in health care delivery and policy to maximize cancer survivors' access to optimal treatment and support. The NCCS responds to individual inquiries, provides free consultation services to survivors on employment and insurance issues, is developing a clearinghouse referral service called *Survivor Lifeline*, and publishes information materials, especially in the areas of employment rights and health insurance. The coalition is particularly active as an advocacy group, testifying and advocating at local, state, and national levels on public policy issues affecting cancer survivors.

The NCCS has been a powerful voice, among both the general public and health care professionals, in changing views about cancer. The perspective of survivorship that underlies the philosophy of the NCCS was first outlined and promoted by Fitzhugh Mullan, a physician and cancer survivor.[43] The concept of survivorship is conveyed in a simple statement often cited in materials provided by NCCS: "From the time of discovery and for the balance of life, an individual diagnosed with cancer is a survivor." Mullan described "seasons" along the continuum of survivorship. At the medical or acute stage, which begins with diagnosis, the focus is on efforts to contain the illness. From the view of patient education and support, emphasis is on understanding the illness, treatment and treatment options, self-care, and quality-of-life issues, and particularly on fostering an understanding that people can and do survive a cancer diagnosis.

When the course of treatment has been completed, or a period of remission occurs, the season of watchful waiting emerges. The person with cancer must reintegrate into a life pattern more like that which preceded diagnosis. It is not unusual for there to be a letdown or loss as a result of being less actively involved with the medical personnel who were regularly available during active treatment. Educational and support needs address a return to routine activities, coping with the fears of recurrence, the need for appropriate medical surveillance, and promoting wellness and healthy behaviors.

In the longer term, the individual moves to the season of permanent survival or cure. At this stage concerns about long-term effects of treatment, as well as social stigma and policy barriers that affect employment and insurability, become very important. Educational and support issues relate to these problems, seeking to empower cancer survivors to speak out for their rights. This activism for the rights of cancer survivors also builds support and understanding for other individuals at all stages of survivorship.

The view of cancer patients as survivors can be an effective strategy for thinking about the needs of patients at various stages of their experience with cancer. It is an important perspective for changing society's views of cancer, replacing unreasonable fears with understanding, and working to remove biases that place limits on the rights and opportunities of people with cancer.

## New Technologies and the Growth of Patient Education and Support

As noted earlier, the growth in recent years of patient education and support resources can be attributed in part to the development of new technologies that allow for rapid data retrieval from large computerized databases combined with widespread access to such electronic databases. The convergence of consumer telecommunications, electronic mass media, and computer systems is creating information service opportunities unimagined by most people even a few years ago.[84] The new technologies have made possible systems and services such as PDQ and the opportunity for users, including health care professionals and patients and families, to access such systems. Developing technologies such as the CD-ROM have created the possibility of interactive video programming that far exceeds the capabilities of older computer-based instructional programs.[85]

Nurses need to keep informed about new resources and how these might be utilized in their clinical practice. But it is also important to be aware of the resources available to patients and families who seek information on their own. As noted throughout the descriptions of various services presented here, most are available directly to the general public as well as to health care professionals. Of course, some services have been available to the public for many years; for example, many of the services, support programs, and information resources provided by the ACS were accessible through a telephone call to the local ACS office well before the widespread use of computer-based systems. But many of the new services, providing the most up-to-date and complete information, have been made possible through more recently developed computer and telecommunication technologies. And a growing phenomenon that appears to have the potential for transforming information gathering and support activities is public access to electronic networks such as the Internet. Such networks present new opportunities not only for the general public but also for nurses and other health care professionals.

The growth in the usefulness of electronic networks is rapidly increasing as the numbers of organizations and institutions placing information services on such networks increases. One aspect of electronic networks with tremendous potential for cancer patient support is the network bulletin board. A presentation at the 1995 Cancer Patient Education Network annual conference included a series of exchanges occurring through an Internet group titled Caregivers and Stress.[86] The participants were primarily family members caring for cancer patients, sharing their concerns and frustrations and offering one another consolation and empathy. Pilot studies of women with breast cancer have shown that access to a computer-based support system, including a bulletin board discussion group as well as various types of information, resulted in high usage of the system, favorable ratings of the value of the information component, and positive emotional responses including feelings of acceptance, motivation, understanding, and relief.[25,26]

The increasing availability and use of information drawn from electronic networks, and of talk groups as a source of nonprofessional information and support, raise a variety of questions regarding impact, the potential for benefit but also for misinformation and nonbeneficial contact, and changes that may result in the role of health care professionals in patient education.

The electronic networks provide new, expanding opportunities for patient and family education and support. They may serve to empower cancer patients to be more active and in control of their search for information and support.[84] The health care professional in cancer needs to be aware of the growth of these resources and to continue to seek information and understanding regarding the best use of such resources.

## FUTURE CONSIDERATIONS FOR PATIENT EDUCATION AND SUPPORT

Identifying future trends or long-term projections is difficult in any field. Yet engaging in some futurist speculation is important and necessary if we seek to prepare for the changes and new developments that will shape the realities of future practice. Others have noted trends in demographics, the influences of technology, and changing social patterns as factors affecting future patient education and cancer practice patterns.[87,88] Based on the review of literature and discussions with professionals working in patient education and support programs, the following emerge as four key areas of future change and challenge for education and support in oncology nursing practice.

### Demographic Patterns and Their Implications

Some future aspects not only of patient education but also of many other areas of our society will be determined by demographics. It is clear that the population of the United States is shifting to a larger percentage of older people based on the aging of the "baby boom" cohort. It is also clear that the United States' future population will be more diverse than the current population due both to differences in birth rates across various ethnic and racial groups and to patterns of immigration. These two known demographic trends point to the likelihood of increases in cancer incidence since many types of cancer are closely linked to aging, and to an increasing need for culturally sensitive and appropriate public education programs, medical care delivery systems, and patient education and support programming and materials.

These demographic patterns, in conjunction with changing socioeconomic patterns—themselves caused in part by demography—have implications for patient support structures and economic factors affecting education and support opportunities. For example, smaller family sizes and the mobility of our society contribute to a loss of extended family structures supporting people experiencing cancer. The reduced ratio of younger workers to older nonworking people will put greater economic burdens on those working adults and reduce resources for older persons experiencing cancer or other illnesses. A higher growth rate seen in low-income populations, persons less likely to receive preventative health care or early diagnosis, raises the likelihood of increased health problems, greater need for health care services, and economic pressure on health systems serving such populations.

These changes will present challenges for creating effective support structures, for meeting these needs with limited economic resources, and for creating effective outreach activities to reach disadvantaged and underserved populations.

## Changes in Technology

The potential benefits of new technologies, especially the advances in computer and telecommunications technology, have been discussed previously. The primary benefits that are readily seen are the tremendously expanded access to large amounts of information and the potential for bringing education and support programs to individuals without regard to physical barriers or distance. In addition, technological developments may make possible much wider use of more effective media, especially as developments in video technology bring down the cost of video communications and increase flexibility for continually updating such materials.

Caution may be raised about creating systems that provide information but lose a human dimension. The effective use of technology, however, may provide opportunities for even greater personal communications among individuals experiencing cancer and between health care providers and those needing assistance. The opportunities for communication among people from many different settings without regard to geographic barriers through computer bulletin board technology has tremendous potential for providing certain types of social support.

Special challenges in the area of using technology will be keeping pace with new developments, assisting those who find use of computers or other electronic equipment stressful or perplexing, and simply finding ways to assess, select, and manage the vast amount of resources that become available.

## The Changing Patterns of Health Care Delivery Systems

Much has been written in recent years regarding the changes in health care systems. Efforts to reduce both frequency and duration of hospitalizations; restrictions imposed by third-party payers; emphasis on cost reduction; an increasing role played by for-profit organizations in an area formerly dominated by nonprofit organizations; growth in outpatient and home health services; the diversity of roles played by nurses and many other health professionals; and the creation of new delivery systems such as health management organizations are all among the many changes that have been experienced.

The changing health care delivery system presents two major challenges from a patient education and support perspective. First, nurses need to be alert to the need to be advocates for strong education and support programming to ensure that these services are retained and appropriately incorporated within newly evolving forms of health care delivery. Second, particular attention is needed to ensure continuity in patient education and support services across the diverse components of the delivery system.

## Demonstrating Effectiveness of Patient Education and Support

This last area for consideration is related to each of the three already discussed. As changes in our population and social patterns call for new approaches in patient education and support, as technology provides new opportunities and new challenges, and as the health care system itself changes, there will be an ongoing need for research, development of new approaches, and careful evaluation to understand, document, and promote effective patient education and support.

Research and development in patient education and support obviously flow directly from the changes that have been described. There will be a need to find effective strategies to respond to new social conditions and to reach new and diverse audiences of people experiencing cancer. There will be a need to find the best ways to use new technologies. And there will be a need to create patient education and support approaches that fit within the new delivery systems. Most important, the ongoing financial pressures that all of health care will continue to experience will create a demand for solid evidence that patient education and support are important components of the health care system that result in measurable positive outcomes. Patient education and support must be shown to be essential elements of the health care system, and the system must be built in a way that will ensure the time, the resources, and the financial support for these critical elements.

## REFERENCES

1. McNally JC, Somerville ET, Miaskowski C, Rostad, M (eds): *Guidelines for Oncology Nursing Practice* (ed 2). Philadelphia, Saunders, 1991
2. Barlett EE: At last, a definition. *Patient Educ Counsel* 7: 323–324, 1985 (editorial)
3. Johnson J, Lane C: Role of support groups in cancer care. *Support Care Cancer* 1:52–56, 1993
4. Evans RL, Connis RT: Comparison of brief group therapies for depressed cancer patients receiving radiation treatment. *Public Health Rep* 110:306–311, 1995
5. Spiegel D: How do you feel about cancer now? Survival and psychosocial support. *Public Health Rep* 110:298–300, 1995 (commentary)

6. Cella DF, Yellen SB: Cancer support groups: The state of the art. *Cancer Pract* 1:56–61, 1993

7. Hermann JF, Cella DF, Robinovitch A: Guidelines for support group programs. *Cancer Pract* 3:111–113, 1995

8. Johnson J: The effects of a patient education course on persons with a chronic illness. *Cancer Nurs* 5:117–123, 1982

9. Cunningham AJ, Lockwood GA, Edmonds CV: Which cancer patients benefit most from a brief, group, coping skills program? *Int J Psychiatry Med* 23:383–398, 1993

10. Grassman D: Development of inpatient oncology educational and support programs. *Oncol Nurs Forum* 10:669–676, 1993

11. Gustafson DH, Taylor JO, Thompson S, et al: Assessing the needs of breast cancer patients and their families. *Qual Manage Health Care* 2:6–17, 1993

12. Fernsler JI, Cannon CA: The whys of patient education. *Semin Oncol Nurs* 7:79–86, 1991

13. American Hospital Association: *Statement on a Patient's Bill of Rights*. Chicago, American Hospital Association, 1973

14. Spingarn ND, Chasen NH: Working with your doctor and hospital system: Becoming a wise consumer, in Hoffman F (ed): *A Cancer Survivor's Almanac: Charting Your Journey*. Minneapolis, Chronimed, 1996, pp 55–65

15. Oncology Nursing Society Education Committee: *Outcome Standards for Cancer Patient Education*. Pittsburgh, Oncology Nursing Society, 1982

16. Oncology Nursing Society: *Standard of Oncology Education: Patient/Family and Public*. Pittsburgh, Oncology Nursing Society, 1995

17. Whitman NI, Graham BA, Gleit CJ, et al: *Teaching in Nursing Practice: A Professional Model* (ed 2). Norwalk, CT, Appleton and Lange, 1992

18. Office for Protection from Research Risks, National Institutes of Health: *Protecting Human Research Subjects: Institutional Review Board Guidebook*. Washington, DC, U.S. Government Printing Office, 1993

19. Joint Commission for the Accreditation of Healthcare Organizations: AMH completes transition to important functions. *Perspectives: The Joint Commission Newsletter* 14(3): 1, 7–8, 1994

20. Joint Commission for the Accreditation of Healthcare Organizations: *1995 Accreditation Manual for Hospitals*. Oakbrook, IL, Joint Commission for the Accreditation of Healthcare Organizations, 1994

21. *Conditions of Participation for Hospitals*, 59 Fed. Reg. 238, 64152–64153 (1994) (to be codified at 42 C.F.R. § 482)

22. Association of Community Cancer Centers: *Standards for Cancer Programs*. Rockville, MD, Association of Community Cancer Centers, 1993

23. Poroch D: The effect of preparatory patient education on the anxiety and satisfaction of cancer patients receiving radiation therapy. *Cancer Nurs* 18:206–214, 1995

24. Wells ME, McQuellon RP, Hinkle JS, et al: Reducing anxiety in newly diagnosed cancer patients: A pilot program. *Cancer Pract* 3:100–104, 1995

25. Gustafson D, Wise M, McTavish F, et al: Development and pilot evaluation of a computer-based support system for women with breast cancer. *J Psychosoc Oncol* 11:69–93, 1993

26. McTavish F, Gustafson DH, Owens BH, et al: CHESS: An interactive computer system for women with breast cancer piloted with an under-served population. *Proc Annu Symp Comput Appl Med Care* 599–603, 1994

27. O'Hare PA, Yost LS, McCorkle R: Strategies to improve continuity of care and decrease rehospitalization of cancer patients: A review. *Cancer Invest* 11:140–158, 1993

28. Forester B, Kornfeld DS, Fleiss JL, et al: Group psychotherapy during radiotherapy: Effects on emotional and physical distress. *Am J Psychiatry* 150:1700–1706, 1993

29. Padilla GV, Bulcavage LM: Theories used in patient/health education. *Semin Oncol Nurs* 7(2):87–96, 1991

30. Rankin SH, Stallings KD: *Patient Education: Issues, Principles, Practices* (ed 2). Philadelphia, Lippincott, 1992

31. Hochbaum GM: *Public Participation in Medical Screening Programs: A Sociopsychological Study*. Public Health Service publication No. 572. Washington, DC, US Government Printing Office, 1958

32. Lorig K: *Patient Education: A Practical Approach*. St. Louis, Mosby-Year Book, 1992

33. Bandura A: *Social Foundation of Thoughts and Actions: A Social Cognitive Theory*. Englewood Cliffs, NJ, Prentice-Hall, 1986

34. Lazarus RS, Folkman S: *Stress Appraisal and Coping*. New York, Springer, 1984

35. Miller SM: Monitoring versus blunting styles of coping with cancer influence the information patients want and need about their disease. *Cancer* 76:167–177, 1995

36. Manfredi C, Czaja R, Price P, et al: Cancer patients' search for information. *Monogr Natl Cancer Inst* 14:93–104, 1993

37. Hack TF, Degner LF, Dyck DG: Relationship between preferences for decisional control and illness information among women with breast cancer: A quantitative and qualitative analysis. *Soc Sci Med* 39:279–289, 1994

38. Howe KG: Approaches (and possible contraindications) to enhancing patients' autonomy. *J Clin Ethics* 5:179–188, 1994

39. Padberg RM, Padberg LF: Strengthening the effectiveness of patient education: Applying principles of adult education. *Oncol Nurs Forum* 17:65–69, 1990

40. Knowles MS: *The Modern Practice of Adult Education: From Pedagogy to Andragogy* (ed 2). Upper Saddle River, NJ, Globe Fedron/Cambridge, 1980

41. Morra ME: Making choices: The consumer's perspective. *Cancer Nurs* 8:54–59, 1985 (suppl 1)

42. McGinn KA: It's all in the timing. *ONS Patient Education SIG Newsletter* 6(1):1, 3, 1995

43. Mullan F: Seasons of survival: Reflections of a physician with cancer. *N Engl J Med* 313:270–273, 1985

44. Young-McCaughan S: Care path and CPR manequin have new roles in early discharge teaching. *Oncol Nurs Forum* 22: 149–150, 1995 (letter)

45. Stevenson E, Crosson K: Patient education: History, development, and current directions of the American Cancer Society and the National Cancer Institute. *Semin Oncol Nurs* 7: 135–142, 1991

46. Harrison-Woermke DE, Graydon JE: Perceived informational needs of breast cancer patients receiving radiation therapy after excisional biopsy and axillary node dissection. *Cancer Nurs* 16:449–455, 1993

47. Saunders JM, McCorkle R: Models of care for persons with progressive cancer. *Nurs Clin North Am* 26:365–377, 1985

48. Tornberg M, McGrath BB, Benoliel JQ: Oncology transition services: Partnership of nurses and families. *Cancer Nurs* 7: 131–137, 1984

49. Meili L: The community hospital perspective of clinical trials and the role of the nurse educator. *Semin Oncol Nurs* 7: 280–287, 1991

50. Ferrell BR, Grant M, Chan J, et al: The impact of cancer pain education on family caregivers of elderly patients. *Oncol Nurs Forum* 22:1211–1217, 1995

51. Office of Cancer Communication, National Cancer Institute: *Making Health Communication Programs Work: A Planner's Guide*. NIH publication No. 92-1493. Washington, DC, U.S.

Department of Health and Human Services, National Institutes of Health, 1992

52. McDermott MK: Patient education and compliance issues associated with access devices. *Semin Oncol Nurs* 11:221–226, 1995

53. Boyle DM: Realities to guide novel and necessary nursing care in geriatric oncology. *Cancer Nurs* 17:125–136, 1994

54. Boyle DM, Engelking C, Blesch KS, et al: Oncology Nursing Society position paper on cancer and aging: The mandate for oncology nursing. *Oncol Nurs Forum* 19:913–933, 1992

55. Habayeb GL: Cultural diversity: A nursing concept not yet reliably defined. *Nurs Outlook* 43:224–227, 1995

56. Charonko K: Cultural influences in "non-compliant" behavior and decision making. *Holistic Nurs Pract* 6:73–78, 1992

57. Dignan M, Sharp P, Blinson K, et al: Development of a cervical cancer education program for Native American women in North Carolina. *J Cancer Educ* 9:235–242, 1994

58. Freeman WL: Making research consent forms informative and understandable: The experience of the Indian Health Service. *Camb Q Health Ethics* 3:510–521, 1994

59. Yancey AK, Tanjasiri SP, Klein M, et al: Increased cancer screening behavior in women of color by culturally sensitive video exposure. *Prev Med* 24:142–148, 1995

60. Frank-Stromborg M, Olsen SJ (eds): *Cancer Prevention in Minority Populations: Cultural Implications for Health Care Professionals.* St. Louis, Mosby-Year Book, 1993

61. Morra ME, Varricchio C: Teaching patients with limited reading skills. *Cancer Pract* 1:154–156, 1993

62. Doak CC, Doak LG, Root JH: *Teaching Patients with Low Literacy Skills* (ed 2). Philadelphia, Lippincott, 1996

63. National Cancer Institute, National Institutes of Health: *Clear and Simple: Developing Effective Print Materials for Low-Literate Readers.* NIH publication No. 95-3594. Washington, DC, U.S. Department of Health and Human Services, National Institutes of Health, 1994

64. Grossman SA, Piantadosi S, Covahey C: Are informed consent forms that describe clinical oncology research protocols readable by most patients and their families? *J Clin Oncol* 12:2211–2215, 1994

65. Meade C, Diekmann J, Thornhill DG: Readability of American Cancer Society patient education literature. *Oncol Nurs Forum* 19:51–55, 1992

66. Cooley ME, Moriarty H, Berger MS, et al: Patient literacy and the readability of written cancer educational materials. *Oncol Nurs Forum* 22:1345–1351, 1995

67. Michielutte R, Bahnson J, Dignan MB, et al: The use of illustrations and narrative text style to improve readability of a health education brochure. *J Cancer Educ* 7:251–260, 1992

68. Griffiths M, Leek C: Patient education needs: Opinions of oncology nurses and their patients. *Oncol Nurs Forum* 22:139–144, 1995

69. Black BL: Comprehensive, seamless, integrated program for cancer resources, information and guidance. Unpublished material, American Cancer Society, Sept. 1995

70. McMillan SC, Tittle MB, Hill D: A systematic evaluation of the "I Can Cope" program using a national sample. *Oncol Nurs Forum* 20:455–461, 1993

71. Hubbard SM, Martin NB, Thurn AL: NCI's Cancer Information Systems: Bringing medical knowledge to clinicians. *Oncology* 9:302–307, 1995

72. National Cancer Institute, International Cancer Information Center/Office of Cancer Communications: Information about PDQ. Unpublished material, Dec. 1993

73. National Cancer Institute, NCI Information Associates Program: About PDQ. *ProtoCall: The Newsletter of the NCI Information Associates Program* 1:8, 1995

74. National Cancer Institute, National Institutes of Health: *CancerFax. Anyday. Anytime. Cualquier día y a cualquier hora.* Washington, DC, U.S. Department of Health and Human Services, National Institutes of Health, 1993

75. National Cancer Institute, International Cancer Information Center and Patient Education Section of Office of Cancer Communications: *PDQ Patient Information Interview Project: Final Report.* Bethesda, MD, National Cancer Institute, 1994

76. National Cancer Institute, International Cancer Information Center/Office of Cancer Communications: PDQ/PIF Demonstration Project. Unpublished material, May 1995

77. Thomsen C: Updates from the National Cancer Institute: Cancer Information Service update. Cancer Patient Education Network Conference, Washington, DC, September, 1995

78. Morra ME, Van Nevel JP, Nealon EO, et al: History of the Cancer Information Service. *Monogr Natl Cancer Inst* 14:7–33, 1993

79. National Cancer Institute, Office of Cancer Communications, Patient Education Section: *Guidelines for Establishing Comprehensive Cancer Patient Education Services.* Washington, DC, National Cancer Institute, 1993

80. National Cancer Institute, Office of Cancer Communications: Combined Health Information Database. General Information about CHID. Unpublished material, National Cancer Institute. March 1995

81. McCabe MS, Varricchio CG, Padberg RM, et al: Women's health advocacy: Its growth and development in oncology. *Semin Oncol Nurs* 11:137–142, 1995

82. Morra ME, Potts E: *Choices: Realistic Alternatives in Cancer Treatment* (ed 2, rev). New York, Avon Books, 1994

83. Education Committee of the Oncology Nursing Society: Cancer resources in the United States. *Oncol Nurs Forum* 22:1421–1432, 1995

84. Bartlett EE: The digital revolution and patient self-empowerment. *Patient Educ Counsel* 20:1–3, 1993 (editorial)

85. Agre P: Interactive computer technology. *Cancer Pract* 2:74–76, 1994

86. Sletten J: Computer technology in cancer patient education. Cancer Patient Education Network Conference, Washington, DC, Sept. 1995

87. Morra ME: Future trends in patient education. *Semin Oncol Nurs* 7:143–145, 1991

88. Boyle DM: New identities: The changing profile of patients with cancer, their families, and their professional caregivers. *Oncol Nurs Forum* 21:55–61, 1994

# Chapter 60

# Advancing Cancer Nursing Through Nursing Education

Gloria A. Hagopian, RN, EdD

## INTRODUCTION

In this chapter the history of cancer nursing education and some of the major influences on its development will be discussed. The current state of cancer nursing education at the generalist, advanced, and continuing education levels will be highlighted. Critical issues facing cancer nursing education today and in the future will be discussed.

## HISTORY OF CANCER NURSING EDUCATION

Specialized education in oncology nursing began in the 1940s. Day-long, then week-long continuing education programs were offered, often under the sponsorship of the American Cancer Society (ACS). Efforts to incorporate cancer nursing content at the baccalaureate level began in 1954 when the National Cancer Institute (NCI) funded four schools for this purpose.[1] There were several outcomes of this project, including the development by Diller of a cancer nursing test to measure students' knowledge, a cancer curriculum, and evaluation tools for faculty.[2] In 1982, *Outcome Standards for Cancer Nursing Education at the Fundamental Level* was written by the Oncology Nursing Society in cooperation with the American Nurses' Association, giving faculty guidelines for integrating oncology content into the curriculum at the fundamental or generalist level.[3] This document also served as the impetus to develop other guidelines for practice and graduate education.

The first graduate-level course with both theoretical and clinical components in cancer nursing was offered at Teachers' College in New York in 1946 by Nelson.[1,4,5] This course, two semesters in length, provided 16 credits toward a Master of Arts degree. The course focused on the nature of cancer as a biological phenomenon, patient needs, and nursing care measures. Public health aspects, such as early detection, home care, and community resources also were emphasized. The clinical part of the course was held at Memorial Hospital in New York. The program was supported in part by a grant from the ACS, New York Division. In 1950 a course for credit in cancer nursing and chronic disease was offered by the University of Minnesota School of Public Health.[1]

One of the first surveys of graduate programs to identify those that offered cancer nursing in the curriculum was done by the ACS in 1958.[1] Of the 22 programs responding to the questionnaire, only two indicated that cancer nursing was included in the curriculum. With specialization in other fields of nursing such as coronary care, dialysis, burns, and intensive care, interest in specializing in oncology nursing followed naturally, and university courses were soon developed. The first graduate oncology track leading to a master's degree was started at the University of Pittsburgh in 1968.[5]

Continuing education (CE) has always played an important part in cancer nursing and has been the most widely used method to increase the knowledge and skill of nurses.[6] Because of the lack of consistent preparation of nurses at the generalist level, CE programs were the most convenient way to provide the expertise needed to practice cancer nursing. The ACS was an early provider of educational programs for practicing nurses. Several cancer centers also have offered CE programs for nurses through the years, including Memorial Sloan-Kettering Cancer Center, Roswell Park Memorial Hospital, Ellis Fischel State Cancer Center, and City of Hope National Medical Center.[4] One of the first institutional CE programs to teach nurses cancer screening procedures was developed by White at M.D. Anderson Hospital.[1] This unique program, sponsored by the NCI, still offers one-week modules of site-specific cancer screening procedures.

## IMPORTANT INFLUENCES ON CANCER NURSING EDUCATION

### Organizations

Several very important cancer organizations have had a powerful impact on education in cancer nursing. They include the ACS, the Oncology Nursing Society (ONS), the NCI, and the Association of Pediatric Oncology Nurses (APON).

#### American Cancer Society

The ACS, organized in 1913, is a nationwide voluntary health agency dedicated to eliminating cancer as a health problem by preventing cancer, saving lives, and decreasing suffering through research, education, and service. It has more than 3000 units and 2.2 million volunteers. Among its activities are publications, continuing education programs, conferences, scholarships, professorships, and programs for students.[7] It sponsors several publications, *CA: A Journal for Clinicians, Cancer, Cancer News, Cancer Nursing News,* and the newest, *Cancer Practice.* The *Cancer Source Book for Nurses,* first published in 1950, has undergone several revisions, the latest in 1991.[8] The ACS distributes thousands of publications and audiovisual materials to nurses each year. National conferences for health professionals focusing on topics relevant to cancer control are held yearly, a nursing research conference is held every two to three years, and many (CE) programs are held at the local level.

The ACS professorship program was established to improve the care of the patient and the quality of nursing education in cancer. ACS professors are doctorally prepared experts in cancer nursing engaged in teaching, practice, and research whose salaries and research are funded by local divisions of the ACS. The professorship program was initiated in 1981, and since that time ten ACS local divisions have funded 20 ACS professors. In 1996, ten professors were receiving financial support through a grant to their school of nursing for further development and enhancement of the school's oncology nursing program.[9]

### Oncology Nursing Society

The ONS was incorporated in 1975. It was conceived and organized under the leadership of Marino, Yarbro, and others because they wanted to define their roles in cancer care, communicate with oncology nurses in similar roles, and develop continuing education programs.[1,10] The ONS mission today is to promote excellence in oncology nursing by setting standards, studying ways to improve oncology nursing, encouraging nurses to specialize in oncology nursing, fostering the professional development of oncology nurses, and maintaining an organizational structure responsive to the needs of its members.[11] In 1996, the ONS had 185 chapters and over 25,000 members; over 6000 members attended the Annual Congress and Fall Institute.[12] Activities of the ONS include the Annual Congress, the Fall Institute, coordination of 29 special interest groups (SIGs), and publication of *Oncology Nursing Forum, Oncology Nursing News,* and *ONS Nursing Scan.* Under the leadership of the Board of Directors, there are a number of active councils, task forces, and committees. The ONS offers several monetary awards to distinguished nurses to recognize outstanding contributions to the organization, to research, and to patient and public education. In addition, it recognizes public figures who have positively influenced the public perception.

The Education Committee of the ONS has been active over the years in developing standards of education that have had a significant impact on cancer nursing education. The standards developed for the generalist and advanced levels have provided guidelines for curriculum development.

### National Cancer Institute

The NCI, established in 1976, has made major contributions to oncology nursing education in a number of ways, including educational programs, work-study programs, fellowship programs, funding for research, predoctoral and postdoctoral research training grants, publications, and providing access to current reliable information through the Cancer Information Service (CIS).

Some of the educational programs in cancer for nurses that are funded by the NCI are: a short course in research training for postmaster's, doctoral, and postdoctoral nurses engaged in research; a short course in cancer prevention, detection, and screening for minorities; re-

gional workshops for African-American, Hispanic, and Native American nurses; and a short course for nurses in developing countries in prevention and early detection.

The NCI also has been instrumental in providing funding for faculty education. In 1950 a three-week institute on cancer nursing was offered to 30 nursing instructors.[4] Later, surveys by Oberst,[13] Miller and Herbst,[14] and VanScoy-Mosher[15] indicated there was a shortage of programs to prepare nurses to teach in oncology education programs. Because the rapidly expanding knowledge in cancer care required strengthening of oncology programs, and because there was concentration of educational programs in large urban areas, a unique project was funded by the NCI. This five-year project to develop a model for postmaster's fellowship programs in oncology nursing education was intended to increase the number of oncology nurse educators.[16] San Jose State University and the University of Alabama at Birmingham were awarded funds to develop the model curriculum. Thirty-four fellows completed the year-long program, that included clinical nursing, educator, and change agent roles.

Today, under the Cancer Nurse Training Program, the NCI offers a nine-month clinical training program for new baccalaureate graduates. The graduates work and attend classes on current cancer nursing practice and receive a monthly stipend.[17]

### Association of Pediatric Oncology Nurses

Another important organization is the Association of Pediatric Oncology Nurses (APON), established in 1973. Among its objectives are to promote excellence in the care of children with cancer, provide communication for nurses, disseminate information about care of patients, encourage publication in professional and lay literature, and support research in pediatric oncology. The activities of the organization include the publication of the *Journal of the Association of Pediatric Oncology Nurses (JAPON),* a newsletter, and an annual meeting. The organization has more than 900 members.[7]

## Scholarships

The existence of a large number of scholarships, fellowships, and other forms of financial assistance has had an important influence on attracting qualified students into cancer nursing programs. In 1981 scholarships for master's-level preparation were established by the ACS, and in 1986 scholarship support at the doctoral level began.[5,18,19] To date, 329 ACS scholarships, in the amount of $8000 per year, have been awarded at the master's level, while 49 students have received doctoral scholarships. This scholarship program represents a significant investment in cancer nursing education.

The ONS also offers scholarships at both the bachelor's and the master's levels. Since this program has been in existence, many recipients have benefited from the opportunity to attend school.

As mentioned earlier, the NCI offers fellowships at the predoctoral, doctoral, and postdoctoral levels. In addition to scholarships and fellowships, there have been other efforts in the past by the NCI and ACS to encourage nursing students to enter cancer nursing. The ACS sponsored a six-week summer course for senior students, and in 1971, the NCI, in conjunction with the ACS, offered a ten-week work-study program for baccalaureate students to increase their skills in caring for individuals with cancer in the areas of prevention, early detection, diagnosis, treatment, and rehabilitation.[20]

Many hospitals have tuition reimbursement programs that allow students to attend school and pay back the loan in work. If it were not for programs such as these, many nurses would have been unable to get advanced degrees.

## Certification

Certification has had a positive influence on cancer nursing. Certification acknowledges nurses' additional education or experience. The level of knowledge of certified nurses is above the level required for licensure, thus protecting the public by demanding a certain level of excellence in those who are certified. The mission of the Oncology Nursing Certification Corporation (ONCC) is to advance oncology nursing through the certification process.[21] Ultimately, the goal of certification is to promote the health and well-being of those diagnosed with or at risk for experiencing cancer.

In 1984 the ONCC contracted with the Educational Testing Service (ETS) to develop a test to assess the general oncology knowledge of the professional nurse.[21] Questions were written by oncology nurses and reviewed by the ONCC Test Development Committee and staff of the ETS. Questions for the 1986–1990 examination were based on the Oncology Nursing Society Core Curriculum. The current examination is based on a study sponsored by the ONCC. This study defined the dimensions of practice of oncology nursing and identified the knowledge required for practice as a competent oncology nurse. This Role Delineation Study, based on the responses of 1297 oncology nurses, formed the blueprint for the new generation of certification examinations in oncology nursing.

The certification examination is open to nurses who have the following:

- a current license

- two and one-half years of experience as a registered nurse over the 5-year period prior to application

- at least 1000 hours of oncology nursing practice within two and one-half years prior to application

The three-hour examination consists of 300 multiple-choice questions and covers seven subject areas: cancer nursing practice, major cancers, treatment, issues and trends in cancer care, prevention and detection, pathology, and epidemiology.[21]

Oncology-certified nurses have the opportunity to renew their certification at four-year intervals. To date, over 22,000 nurses have taken the certification examination. There are 15,450 oncology-certified nurses. The 1995 pass rate for the generalist exam was 77% for first-time candidates, with an overall pass rate of 82%.

The first Advanced Oncology Nursing Certification examination was offered in 1995 to nurses with a master's or higher degree and experience in administration, education, practice, or research. Of the 256 candidates, 219 (86%) passed the exam. In a number of states, Advanced Oncology Nursing Certification is recognized for the licensure of advanced practice nurses.

It is expected that computer-based testing will replace the current paper and pencil tests in a linear format. With computer adaptive testing, the candidates only answer as many questions as needed to determine a pass or fail score.

## CANCER NURSING EDUCATION TODAY

### Conceptual Framework

A conceptual framework consistent with the *Outcome Standards for Cancer Nursing Practice* has been developed by the Education Committee of the ONS consisting of four concepts: individual and family, health–illness, health care system, and community–environment.[3] Central to oncology nursing practice is the individual–family concept. The health–illness concept is the adaptation of the individual and family along a continuum. The practice of cancer nursing occurs in the health care system. The community–environment concept provides the resources and support necessary for individuals with cancer. The methods used to organize the knowledge necessary for cancer nursing practice is the nursing process and the research process.

### Standards of Oncology Nursing Education

The *Outcome Standards for Cancer Nursing Education at the Fundamental Level* were first published in 1982.[22] The ultimate outcomes of the standards are to enhance the quality of oncology nursing education and to improve the health care for the public. In 1987 the *Scope of Advanced Oncology Practice* was developed and laid the foundation for the development of *Standards for Oncology Nursing Education: Advanced Level.*[22,23] Guidelines for all levels of educational preparation are published in the *Standards of Oncology Nursing Education: Generalist and Advanced Practice Levels.* The purpose of the standards is to provide guidelines to:[22]

- plan and evaluate generalist education encompassing diploma, associate, and baccalaureate programs

- plan and evaluate advanced education at the master's, doctoral, and postdoctoral levels

- plan and evaluate continuing education programs at all levels

- assess individual knowledge of oncology nursing care

At both the generalist and specialist levels, five categories of standards with general descriptive statements relate to faculty, resources, curriculum, the teaching–learning process, and the learner.

### Generalist level

The generalist level of cancer nursing, originally referred to as the fundamental level, provides a core of knowledge, skill, and attitudes for beginning practice in cancer nursing. Although the generalist level encompasses diploma, associate, and baccalaureate educational programs, the literature deals only with baccalaureate education. There are several significant studies that have examined the oncology content at the undergraduate level and have contributed to our understanding of existing problems. In 1983 Brown, Johnson, and Groenwald sent a questionnaire to determine the status of cancer education to 982 NLN-accredited schools of nursing.[24] The study was undertaken because of concern that the fundamental education for nurses in cancer care was inadequate. Questions pertained to the content included in the curriculum, educational resources, preparation of faculty, and areas needing improvement. Responses from 672 schools (68%) were obtained. The investigators found that an average of 14.5 classroom hours were devoted to cancer nursing. The content areas inadequately covered included prevention, detection, oncological emergencies, late effects of treatment, unorthodox treatment, attitudes toward cancer, home care, social issues, political issues, resources, legal implications, and educational resources for nurses. The study suggested that an examination of the undergraduate curriculum was in order.

Pope reports on a similar study conducted in Switzerland by Stoll and Fellinger to identify the place of oncology education in basic programs.[25] Their questionnaire was sent to 50 schools, and 32 (64%) responded. The results were strikingly similar to the study by Brown and her colleagues. The average amount of time devoted to oncology nursing was 14 hours. The investigators concluded that cancer nursing education was inadequate in Switzerland in both quality and quantity. One of the recommendations of this study was to incorporate the practicing oncology nurse specialist into teaching.

Pope surveyed the wishes and needs of oncology students in six basic education programs in Switzerland. She questioned if some oncology content was too well integrated, thereby frustrating students. She suspected integration caused some students to forget that the programs had certain oncology content. Students responding to the survey could not agree as to what areas in oncology were most important in preparing them for care of patients with cancer. The students agreed that clinical experience is helpful and that content should be taught by an oncology nurse active in the field.[25]

Another European study, by Copp, reports the findings of the European commission about the state of cancer nursing in western Europe.[26] Again, the investigator came to the conclusion that cancer nursing education in western Europe follows the medical model, the faculty is without oncology experience, there is a paucity of teaching materials, and there is little connection between theory and practice.

Others have argued about the importance of the professional in developing a positive, empathetic attitude toward the patient and family. Fanslow suggested that a lack of educational preparation in oncology led to negative attitudes of both students and nurses.[27] Pope's study confirms the findings that suggest lack of oncology content leads to negative attitudes on the part of students.[25] Welch-McCaffrey[28] suggested that the development of an empathetic attitude toward the care of the patient with cancer is developed at the undergraduate level of nursing education.

Many creative ways to improve curricula in cancer nursing and promote positive attitudes about cancer care at the baccalaureate level have been attempted. Nevidjon and Deatrich[29] offered an intensive eight-week elective course that included lecture, patient care, seminar, skills lab, and individual supervision for senior students. The ONS/ANA *Outcome Standards* provided the organizing framework for the course. Horvitz and Trigg[30] developed a ten-week in-depth cancer course for senior students that included content on the physiological and psychological impact of cancer on the patient, family, and nurse. Mooney and Dudas[31] offered a two-credit ten-week independent course in cancer nursing for eight selected students. Content included the roles and responsibilities of nurses, psychosocial reactions of patients, critical knowledge needed by the oncology nurse, the purposes and activities of the ONS and other cancer organizations, and specialized skills needed to care for patients. Classes were held for two hours each week. A field experience at an ACS office, a support group, or observation experience in a hospital was included.[31]

Quinn-Casper and Holmgren, also believing that the highly specialized skills needed to care for patients with cancer were not consistently addressed at the baccalaureate level, tried a different approach.[32] Their belief that undergraduate curricula were deficient was based on the results of the survey by Brown and her colleagues.[24] Quinn-Casper and Holmgren developed a program with the ACS to provide supplementary cancer education programs for nursing students. After the first highly successful and well-attended one-day workshop was held, yearly workshops were instituted. Over 800 students have attended the annual one-day sessions over a four-year period. Local ACS chapters throughout the country now offer such programs for students.

Daly and Eardmann reported on the use of what they called an oncology search.[33] A study guide consisting of 12 items was used to provide opportunities for students to learn about a variety of topics beyond their assigned readings in an undergraduate course. Participating students became more aware of oncology resources and more interested in cancer nursing.

Although these efforts are commendable, these programs are scarce, and only limited numbers of students are able to benefit. In many other programs, glaring deficiencies still exist. Guidelines for curriculum content have been written, standards exist, teaching materials from the ONS and ACS are available, but many undergraduate curricula still are inadequate in content.

As part of a five-year federally funded project to increase and improve oncology nursing content in undergraduate programs, Longman and her colleagues initiated several activities.[34] First was the development of two tools, an attitude inventory and a knowledge test. A 30-item test was developed based on the *Outcome Standards*. The results indicated that students in the first semester scored lower than in other semesters, but scores increased as the students progressed through the program. The improvement of scores suggested a better incorporation of essential oncology content by faculty and increased knowledge on the students' parts due to participation in the activities of the project. Longman et al also offered an elective course on cancer care for students, provided opportunities for students to participate in ongoing oncology research, instituted a research symposium, and provided seminars to faculty about latest therapies and care to update their knowledge.[35]

### Advanced level

The advanced level of cancer nursing education encompasses graduate education. Education at this level is concerned with the development of a broader scope of practice, coordination, continuity, and evaluation of care. Most of the literature at this level is concerned with master's programs.

The *Master's Degree with a Specialty in Advanced Practice in Oncology Nursing* is an invaluable tool for faculty of all graduate oncology programs.[36] Its purpose is to provide a role definition and curriculum guide for educators in planning educational offerings as well as a program selection guide for students. The guide encompasses the six content areas of clinical practice, education, consultation, administration, research, and professionalism. Each area is organized by steps of the nursing process, suggested content, and outcome objectives.

At the end of 1995, there were 41 colleges and universities with graduate oncology programs listed by the Education Committee of the ONS.[37] Each program has its unique qualities, and any program should be carefully

examined before an applicant selects a school.[38] Many questions need to be asked by potential students to assess and choose the appropriate program, including: What is the reputation of the school? Who are the faculty? What are the resources of the school? What will the clinical experiences be like? Will oncology clinical nurse specialists be clinical preceptors? What is the tuition? Are sources of funding or research or teaching assistantship positions available?

As part of a feasibility study to determine the need to develop new graduate programs in oncology nursing, Piemme[5] identified the most significant problems of graduate oncology programs. Of the 21 programs responding, recruitment of students was listed by seven schools and was the most frequently cited problem. Six schools listed lack of financial support, four listed pressures on faculty time, and four listed a need for faculty prepared in oncology nursing as the most significant problem of their graduate oncology programs.[5] Although this study has not been replicated, many of these same problems continue to exist today.

There have been several reports of the development of instruments to test graduate student knowledge, attitudes, and skills. As part of their program evaluation, Piper, Moore, and Dodd studied changes in knowledge and attitudes in two cohorts of graduate students in oncology nursing.[39] Significant improvements were obtained in the knowledge domain, while there was lack of significant changes on the attitude instrument. The faculty also used the test scores to recommend remedial work.

A follow-up study evaluated the students' ability to apply their knowledge to clinical practice during the two-year master's program.[40] Using the ONS Conceptual Framework as the basis for the Appraisal of Practice Instrument, 39 students were asked to rank the frequency of use and degree of proficiency of each clinical behavior on subscales of individual–family, health–illness, health care system, community–environment, cancer nursing process, and cancer nursing research process. The results showed that students rated themselves more proficient in the more frequently used behaviors, gained in proficiency over time, and were more proficient in subject matter that was emphasized in the program.

In a survey of 185 clinical nurse specialists (CNSs) who were ONS members employed in oncology, Yasko found that 69% of the specialists reported they did not have theoretical content or planned experiences in oncology nursing in their graduate programs.[41] Sixty percent of the sample did not have planned contact with a CNS role model in the curriculum. At first, this lack of preparation in oncology theory and practice during their master's program appears shocking, but it may be explained by the fact that the respondents received their master's degrees from 60 different colleges. Since there were only 45 oncology graduate programs in 1990 and far fewer in 1983 when the study was reported, many of the nurses in the sample must have graduated from schools that did not have oncology programs. In any event, one could question if these specialists met the qualifications for the job at the time they were hired.

## Continuing Education

That nurses should participate in CE to maintain and enhance special knowledge and skills unique to oncology nursing seems to be universally accepted. Many CE programs are sponsored by the ONS and ACS, at both the national and the local levels. The content for CE programs in oncology nursing can be identified from many sources, including the ONS publications *Cancer Nursing Education at the Fundamental Level, Standards of Oncology Nursing Education,* and *Scope of Advanced Oncology Practice.*[3,22,23]

The *Standards for Continuing Education,* published by the American Nurses Association (ANA), may be useful as a general guide for those who plan CE programs.[42] Since 1987 the ONS has been an ANA-accredited approver and provider of CE programs and can provide assistance for planning CE materials and programs. In 1990 the ONS reviewed more than 50 applications for approval of CE programs.[12] Annually the *Oncology Nursing Forum* publishes a list of long-term CE programs, prepared by the Education Committee of the ONS.

Another helpful resource is a series of articles by Fernsler,[43] Volker,[44] Itano,[45] Belcher,[46] and McMillan[47] that describe how to develop and implement a CE program incorporating adult learning principles. The articles take the novice through the steps of doing a needs assessment, developing objectives, defining content and methods, and evaluating a program.

The ONS has a responsibility to provide CE to its members to help them acquire the knowledge and skills necessary for competent practice. In order to ensure successful CE program planning, the ONS conducted a needs assessment of its membership to determine learning needs.[48] A questionnaire was developed and mailed to one-half of the membership, or approximately 6500, and 38% responded. The top five topics about which the members said they definitely would attend a seminar were the clinical practice issues of oncological emergencies, pain, critical care, legal issues, and advanced practice roles.

Donaldson and his colleagues also tried to identify content areas as priorities for planning CE programs.[49] They developed an 87-item knowledge test based on the proposed core curriculum for certification examination. The results indicated that the topics labeled as the highest priority for CE program planning included nursing management of spinal cord compression, electrolyte imbalance, hypercalcemia, susceptibility to depression, treatment modalities such as chemotherapy and safe handling of drugs, prevention and early detection of cancer, characteristics of cancer, ONS standards, and patient advocacy. The nurses who participated in the study were nurses who provided cancer management care and did not designate themselves as oncology specialists.

Bushy and Kost confronted the issue of inaccessibility of CE programs in rural North Dakota and came up with a novel but successful model of delivering CE programs.[50] Recognizing that either hiring a consultant or bringing a prepared program to a small institution is a costly solution, the program planners decided to use Knowles' model of adult learning and place the responsibility for learning in the realm of the learners. The nurses decided on a topic they were interested in, listed objectives, and made active learning assignments. For a CE program on breast cancer the nurses gathered information from community resources, had mammograms, visited radiation therapy departments, interviewed patients about mastectomies, went to stores that sold prostheses, visited support groups, participated in other action activities, and then shared their information. The new CE model was thought to be successful, based on increased attendance and active participation. The model encourages peer discussion and getting to know the community and its resources.

## CRITICAL ISSUES AND CHALLENGES

### Invitational Conference on the Clinical Nurse Specialist Role

There are a number of critical issues and challenges in cancer nursing that educators must consider and make decisions about. Some of these issues have been raised by clinical specialists. Two invitational conferences on the role of the oncology clinical nurse specialist were held.[51,52] The first conference was held in 1984, and the recommendations, intended primarily for individuals, were widely read. A study on burnout among oncology clinical specialists was an outgrowth of the conference. The second conference was held in 1991. Among the recommendations for oncology education at the undergraduate level were the following:

- Cancer nursing content needs to be emphasized in classroom and clinical settings using the *Standards of Oncology Nursing Practice and Education.*

- Faculty needs updates.

- Hospitals need to use the *Standards of Nursing Practice.*

Specific recommendations to achieve these goals included closer cooperation between the National League for Nursing and the ONS Education Committee; distribution of *Standards of Oncology Nursing Practice and Education* and *Standards of Nursing Practice* to all faculty; and identification of model programs. Elective course offerings were encouraged, along with work-study programs, and the use of innovative teaching strategies, including computer-assisted interactive video.

Recommendations also were made for oncology nursing education at the graduate level. It was suggested that the following be more strongly emphasized at the time of the next revision of the standards:

- physical assessment

- clinical decision making

- prevention, screening, and early detection

- care of high-risk and underserved clients, such as the elderly and socioeconomically disadvantaged

- public health policy

- basic sciences, especially immunology

- developing skills for proposal development

- role immersion

- state-of-the-art communication systems

- alternative health care settings

- marketing the role

- mandatory clinical component

Graduate educators considered, discussed, and have worked to implement these ideas.

## State-of-the-Knowledge Conference on Advanced Practice in Oncology Nursing

Participants (clinical nurse specialists, nurse practitioners, educators, and administrators) at this invitational conference, held in 1994, discussed titling, reimbursement, documentation, prescriptive authority, education, licensure, certification, and credentialing. Their recommendations included the following:

- adopt the term Advanced Practice Nurse (APN) as a designation for clinical nurse specialists and nurse practitioners

- explore ramifications for second licensure for advanced practice

- develop a core graduate oncology curriculum

- support funding for postgraduate education

- explore the possibility of a joint APN certification examination with other organizations

- increase opportunities to expand the knowledge and involvement of APNs in the regulatory and legislative process

- revise the ONS *Standards of Practice*

- Incorporate advanced practice nurse outcomes into the ONS research priorities

- encourage APNs to seek opportunities for involvement in health care setting decision-making groups[53]

Graduate educators in oncology nursing have been discussing these ideas, and many have been implemented.

Some ideas deserve further thinking before implementation.

## Continuing Education

The invitational conference on the role of the oncology clinical nurse specialist did not specifically address CE and its role in meeting some of the recommendations. Since baccalaureate and master's educational programs do not always have the time or the flexibility to include all things, continuing education must be relied on to provide some of the content that cannot be dealt with within the confines of a curriculum. It may be necessary to establish separate, more definitive standards for informal and formal educational levels.

## Recruitment of Students

Much effort needs to go into recruitment of highly qualified students at all levels, especially at the master's and doctoral levels, to ensure an adequate supply of clinicians, specialists, teachers, and researchers in oncology nursing. Because admissions to nursing programs at both the undergraduate and graduate levels have decreased over the past few years, effort must be made to try to attract the traditional as well as the older, nontraditional student, an often untapped source. In order to do so, more flexibility may be needed in programs and course offerings, for more students may need to study part-time, due to high tuition costs and family responsibilities.

Recruitment of minority nurses is crucial. A critical mass of minority nurses who can work with minority populations to encourage prevention and early-detection practices is needed to make an impact on cancer care in this group of patients and to reduce high mortality rates. Studies have suggested that someone from the same culture is the best provider for the socioeconomically disadvantaged.[54] Creative clinical placements and experiences may need to be explored in order to reach the target population of patients. Some nontraditional settings that might be used are screening programs in food pantries, feeding centers, or storefront free health clinics, and church- or school-sponsored screening programs. Once enrolled in nursing programs, financial, academic, and other supportive services must be provided to ensure student success.

More students from other countries are studying in schools in the United States. Many of these students need assistance with socialization and language skills and other types of support. It is important that resources be identified to help foreign students with the transitions needed.

## Prevention and Early Detection

More emphasis must be placed on prevention, risk reduction, and early-detection activities. Most authorities believe that a large number of cancers could be prevented if people would choose healthier lifestyles. It is estimated that one in four individuals could be saved through early detection. The NCI has proposed that cancer mortality be reduced by 50% by the year 2000. Much of the activity in prevention and early detection is concentrated on breast, cervical, and lung cancer, with the majority of activity related to breast cancer. Nurses can have a powerful impact on patients in prevention and early-detection activities for the major sites of cancer. The nurse's role in primary and secondary prevention of cancer has been well documented by Frank-Stromborg and Rohan.[55]

## Practitioner or Specialist

In order to provide the care necessary to meet the challenges of the twenty-first century, highly knowledgeable, highly skilled advanced practice nurses (APN) who can function in multiple roles and settings are crucial. Advanced practice nurses with clinical nurse specialist, nurse practitioner, or blended roles are essential to meet future challenges. Most oncology programs traditionally have prepared clinical nurse specialists, who have provided exemplary care, made extraordinary contributions, and moved the nursing profession ahead. However, in today's health care arena, different skills are required to meet the varied needs of individuals with cancer and their families in a variety of settings. The roles of the APN are diverse and are expanding and evolving rapidly.

## Standards and the Curriculum

Faculty should be familiar with the recommended curriculum and follow the guidelines set forth in the *Standards*. As mentioned earlier, efforts began in the 1950s to incorporate cancer nursing into the curriculum. Now, over 40 years later, we are still struggling to incorporate cancer nursing content at the undergraduate level. It is crucial that basic information about oncology be included in baccalaureate programs. We have the tools and faculty, but curricula vary greatly in cancer content. Perhaps more definitive guidelines at the undergraduate level need to be written, similar to the master's degree guidelines.

While still in school students should be encouraged to share their knowledge, skills, and expertise with others. The nursing curriculum should include content on publishing. Practicing nurses at all levels need to share ideas to improve the oncology nursing practice. Craytor reported that the *Nursing Studies Index* listed only three articles by nurses about oncology nursing between 1900 and 1930.[4] The first oncology nursing textbook was not published until 1967, by Bouchard.[56] Today there are several journals devoted to oncology nursing and numerous textbooks. Although there has been exponential growth in the number of publications by oncology nurses, still more creative work needs to be shared.

Students also need public-speaking skills and media awareness training and should be well-versed in the legislative process and public policy issues. A working knowledge of nursing informatics and hospital information systems is essential. *Nursing informatics* is the science of the properties, structure, storage, and transmission of nursing knowledge. Hospital information systems involve the dedicated use of computers to collect, store, process, retrieve, and communicate patient care and administrative information to support those who provide care. It is imperative that graduates of nursing programs be computer literate and knowledgeable about using information by way of electronic networks.

Students should be encouraged to participate in local and national ACS and ONS activities or, if in pediatrics, APON activities. Participation should be mandatory, particularly at the graduate level. The meetings and conferences held by these organizations offer many opportunities to participate on committees, speak at meetings, and hold office. The opportunities to network with others, share ideas, and interact with the leaders in oncology nursing abound in these organizations, and can enhance one's career.

A model core graduate curriculum for the advanced practice nurse must be established. This should be done in conjunction with the American Academy of Colleges of Nursing.

## Teaching Approaches

Adult learning principles must be employed in our curricula. Reed Ash reminds us that we live in an ever-changing health care environment that requires us to change not only the way patient care services are provided but also the way we educate nurses to provide these services.[57] She cites the rising cost of health care, the increasingly sophisticated technologies, the increase in complex treatment protocols, and the demand for more and better health care as catalysts for change in our educational approaches. It is essential to develop program content and structure learning experiences at all levels that acknowledge the nurse as an adult learner. Adult learning concepts—including problem-centered approaches to teaching, immediate application of knowledge, recognition of individual experience, flexible scheduling, and self-directed learning—must be incorporated into educational offerings. In addition, computer-assisted instruction (CAI) needs to be incorporated into curricula.

## Faculty Competence

Faculty at all levels need to be prepared in oncology nursing. In addition, faculty need to be both knowledgeable in the latest trends and clinically competent as both clinical specialists and nurse practitioners. Attendance at oncology continuing education programs or required certification may help, but this will not completely solve the problem. The clinical doctorate (DNS and DNSc) is not a solution to clinical competence unless the graduates of these programs find ways to keep their skills and expertise current. Although some schools allow faculty to have joint appointments, this is not feasible for all faculty. New and different ways to ensure competency must be explored.

New forms of collaboration between faculty and clinical staff could be developed to provide faculty entrance and exposure to the clinical arena. A faculty consultation service in clinical sites could be developed that could provide benefits to all involved. Faculty have much theoretical knowledge that could be shared with clinical staff, while the faculty could get an update on current clinical practice. Another innovation might be joint research projects between faculty and clinical specialists that would allow faculty exposure to current clinical problems. Faculty collaboration with the nursing staff on clinical papers could also help keep faculty abreast of current practice issues. Faculty could assist staff with publication while keeping up to date on the latest in practice. Other ways to update faculty may already exist, but these need to be shared in the literature so others can benefit.

## Program Evaluation

Evaluation of oncology programs should be an ongoing process. However, very few program evaluation studies have been published.[24–26,34,35,39,40] The outcomes of the advanced practice nurse must be evaluated. Results of studies and evaluation tools need to be shared so our programs can continue to develop.

## Preceptors and Clinical Facilities

Nursing educators must continue to nurture clinical preceptors to act as role models for students in clinical agencies. Faculty need to assume responsibility for preparing clinical preceptors to work with students. Seminars devoted to adult learning principles, evaluation, and how to deal with the difficult student may be helpful in preparing preceptors for their roles. It is essential to recognize the contributions made by preceptors to our clinical programs and to give recognition for their time and commitment to student learning. Such recognition could take the form of appointment as adjunct faculty, which allows library privileges and attendance at school functions, or editorial assistance with manuscripts, which encourages publication.[58] Close cooperation between teachers and clinicians is essential to dispel the old dichotomy between education and practice.

## Doctoral Education

Well-qualified students and graduates of master's programs should be encouraged to continue their education in doctoral programs. Doctorally prepared oncology nurses are needed to ensure high-quality education, research, and practice in the future.

## Complex Care

Advances in technology and early-discharge practices have changed both inpatient and outpatient care. The use of ambulatory services has greatly escalated because of technological advances, changes in reimbursement, and consumer choice. It is estimated that nearly 90% of cancer care is delivered in the outpatient setting. Patients cared for in the home today are far sicker, with many more complex needs, than hospital patients of yesterday. This calls for changing roles and responsibilities of nurses in ambulatory and home settings, and more emphasis on these roles must be given in the curriculum.

## Certification and Recertification

Certification offers many benefits to the individual: increased visibility, peer recognition, self-satisfaction, and sometimes an edge in the job market. Sixty percent of the nurses who were certified in 1986 took the generalist recertification examination. This is comparable to other specialty organizations.[12] However, less than half of ONS members are certified. Efforts need to continue to increase the numbers of members who are certified. The question of recertification may need to be explored further to determine if reexamination is the best alternative for keeping the knowledge and practice of the membership current.

## Care of the Elderly

By the year 2020, the elderly population will double, providing new challenges and opportunities for creative approaches to prevention, early detection, and provision of care to elderly persons. Curricula in schools of nursing must include information on how to plan programs to incorporate healthy behaviors into lifestyles, and information specific to teaching and providing care to the elderly.

## Health Care Reform

In the rapidly changing health care environment that involves restructuring, redesign, and reengineering of the health care delivery system, nurses must be kept well-informed and involved in the decision-making process. *Restructuring* is dedicated to reducing waste while cutting costs. *Reengineering* is involved with examining the process of what and how things are accomplished. *Redesign,* or decision making about who does what, should assure the most appropriately trained and educated are doing the work they are best suited to do.[59] Restructuring and reengineering, for the most part, are positive. However, redesign has resulted in layoffs of nurses, decreased staffing, or a change in the mix of workers that can create unsafe conditions. Registered professional nurses have been replaced with unlicensed and ill-trained personnel who are performing skills at the bedside, hospital staff are being cross-trained to streamline care, and new graduates are having difficulty obtaining positions.[59] Nurses have been protesting with rallies, picketing, strikes, negotiation, and arbitration, and are taking the necessary steps to assure that high-quality care is delivered by registered nurses. Oncology nurses need to demonstrate that they are committed to professional competency through credentialing, educating consumers about the profession, and conducting research to demonstrate that specialized care and credentialing improves the quality of care.[60]

## Meeting New Health Care Challenges

Today more than 6 million Americans are survivors of cancer, and it is expected that by the twenty-first century over 65% of individuals diagnosed with cancer will survive longer than five years. This will have an enormous impact on delivery of services, rehabilitation, and quality-of-life issues. While more people are living with cancer, more and more people are becoming infected with HIV and dying of AIDS. It is expected that 20,000 children will have AIDS by the year 2000. Patient care will become increasingly community-based, home-centered, and self-care will be an expectation. Nurses must be prepared to meet the challenges of a diverse spectrum of patients and problems. The content of our educational programs must reflect the current and future problems and concerns of the health care arena. We can never become complacent about what we do in cancer education or practice, for new challenges continually arise, requiring innovative solutions and application of new knowledge and skills.

As Craytor wrote in 1982, oncology nurses face complex problems.[4] It is necessary to nurture and support all members of the specialty, for competition and jealousy can interfere with a powerful, united front. Craytor added that collaboration on the health care team is essential, and suggested that we focus on cost-effective practices and maintain adaptability to changing scientific, social, and economic conditions. Baird in 1995[61] states that we are practicing at a time when future directions have never been less clear. She challenges oncology nurses to look carefully at the major paradigms of change and ask how we can use our experience and skills to continue to make a difference.

## SUMMARY

Much has been accomplished in oncology nursing. Many fine educational programs exist at all levels of undergraduate, graduate, and continuing education. Oncology nursing has enjoyed strong support from many organizations. Many nurses have been certified in oncology nursing at the generalist level and now at the advanced level. A large number of highly motivated, highly effective, highly productive advanced practice oncology nurses have made numerous contributions to the specialty. Many more doctorally prepared oncology nurses are available than ever before, and they have made numerous contributions to practice, education, and research. Craytor said, "We owe much to the bold, intelligent, persuasive, and clinically able nurses who pioneered in the field. They were and are a truly remarkable group."[4,p.57]

As oncology nurses we should be proud of our accomplishments, but at the same time we must recognize the continual need to update knowledge, skills, and competence. We cannot abandon the good things that have been achieved over the years, such as the certification program, the development of standards, curriculum guides, scholarships, ACS professorships, and high-quality meetings, conferences, and congresses; nor can we rest on our laurels. We need to continue to evaluate, change, improve, and think in new and creative ways and always be prepared to meet new challenges as they arise.

## REFERENCES

1. Hilkemeyer R: A historical perspective in cancer nursing. *Oncol Nurs Forum* 9:47–56, 1982
2. Diller D: *An Investigation of Cancer Learning in Ninety Selected Schools of Nursing. Third Report.* Saratoga Springs, NY, Skidmore College, 1957
3. Oncology Nursing Society: *The Outcome Standards for Cancer Nursing Education at the Fundamental Level.* Pittsburgh, Oncology Nursing Society, 1982
4. Craytor JC: Highlights in education for cancer nursing. *Oncol Nurs Forum* 9:51–59, 1982
5. Piemme JA: Oncology clinical nurse specialist education. *Oncol Nurs Forum* 12:45–48, 1985
6. Longman AJ: Cancer nursing education, in Groenwald SL, Frogge MH, Goodman M, Yarbro CH (eds): *Cancer Nursing: Principles and Practice.* Boston, Jones and Bartlett, 1990, pp 1256–1269
7. Greene PA, Ades T: Cancer organizations, in Baird SB, McCorkle R, Grant M (eds): *Cancer Nursing: A Comprehensive Textbook.* Philadelphia, Saunders, 1991, pp 1162–1172
8. Baird SB (ed): *A Cancer Source Book for Nurses* (ed 6). Atlanta, American Cancer Society, 1991
9. American Cancer Society: Three nursing professorships approved. *Cancer Nurs News* 10:3, 1992
10. Yarbro CH: The history of cancer nursing, in Baird SB, McCorkle R, Grant M (eds): *Cancer Nursing: A Comprehensive Textbook.* Philadelphia, Saunders, 1991, pp 10–20
11. Oncology Nursing Society: *ByLaws.* May 1991
12. Candidates find advanced exam difficult but fair. *Oncology Nursing Certification Corporation News,* 9:1,3, 1995
13. Oberst M: Priorities in cancer nursing research. *Cancer Nurs* 1:281–290, 1978

14. Miller S, Herbst S: Summary of ONS membership survey. *Oncol Nurs Forum* 5:22–23, 1978

15. VanScoy-Mosher C: *Oncology Nursing Survey.* Pittsburgh, Oncology Nursing Society, 1979

16. Siegele D: Longitudinal evaluation of a model postmaster's program in oncology nursing education. *Oncol Nurs Forum* 11:61–62, 1984

17. National Cancer Institute: *Cancer Nurse Training Program.* Washington, DC, National Institutes of Health, 1987

18. American Cancer Society: *Master's degree students: Scholarships in cancer nursing.* ACS publication No. 0306. New York, American Cancer Society, 1992

19. American Cancer Society: *Doctoral degree students: Scholarships in cancer nursing.* ACS publication No. 0351. New York, American Cancer Society, 1992

20. Barckley V: Work-study program in cancer nursing. *Nurs Outlook* 19:328–330, 1971

21. Oncology Nursing Certification Corporation: *Oncology Nursing Certification Bulletin.* Pittsburgh, Oncology Nursing Society, 1992

22. Oncology Nursing Society Education Committee: *Standards of Oncology Nursing Education: Generalist and Advanced Practice Levels.* Pittsburgh, Oncology Nursing Society, 1989

23. Oncology Nursing Society: *Scope of Advanced Oncology Practice.* Pittsburgh, Oncology Nursing Society, 1987

24. Brown JK, Johnson JL, Groenwald SL: Survey of cancer nursing education in U.S. schools of nursing. *Oncol Nurs Forum* 10:82–83, 1983

25. Pope S: Fundamentals for a new concept of oncology nursing in the professional nursing education program. *Cancer Nurs* 15:137–147, 1992

26. Copp K: Education and training in cancer: A European perspective. *Cancer Nurs* 11:255–258, 1986

27. Fanslow J: Attitudes of nurses toward cancer and cancer therapies. *Oncol Nurs Forum* 12:42–45, 1984

28. Welch-McCaffrey D: Promoting the empathetic development of nursing in the care of the patient with cancer. *J Nurs Ed* 23:37, 1986

29. Nevidjon B, Deatrich J: Oncology clinical elective. *Oncol Nurs Forum* 12:57–59, 1985

30. Horvitz I, Trigg JM: Registered nurses and nursing students learn together in a cancer nursing course. *Nurs Educ* 12:6, 18, 42, 1987

31. Mooney M, Dudas S: Undergraduate independent study in cancer nursing. *Oncol Nurs Forum* 14:51–53, 1987

32. Quinn-Casper P, Holmgren C: Enhancing cancer nursing concepts in undergraduate curricula. *Cancer Nurs* 10:274–278, 1987

33. Daly J, Eardmann W: Oncology search: An innovative teaching method. *Nurs Educ* 13:28–30, 1988

34. Longman AJ, Verran JA, Clark M: Oncology knowledge inventory for undergraduate students. *Oncol Nurs Forum* 18:107–111, 1991

35. Longman A, Verran J, Clark L: Improving oncology nursing content in an undergraduate program. *J Nurs Ed* 27:42–44, 1988

36. Oncology Nursing Society, American Nurses Association: *The Master's Degree with a Specialty in Oncology Nursing.* Pittsburgh, Oncology Nursing Society, 1988

37. ONS Education Committee: Survey of graduate programs in cancer nursing. *Oncol Nurs Forum* 22:1273–1282, 1995

38. ONS Education Committee: Assessing Masters' programs in oncology nursing. *Oncol Nurs Forum* 22:1273–1274, 1995

39. Piper B, Moore I, Dodd M: Changes in cancer-related knowledge and attitudes: One graduate curriculum's experience. *Cancer Nurs* 8:272–277, 1985

40. Moore IM, Piper B, Dodd MJ, et al: Measuring oncology nursing practice: Results from one graduate program. *Oncol Nurs Forum* 14:45–49, 1987

41. Yasko J: A survey of oncology clinical nursing specialists. *Oncol Nurs Forum* 10:25–30, 1983

42. American Nurses Association: *Standards for Continuing Education in Nursing.* Kansas City, MO, The Association, 1984

43. Fernsler J: Developing continuing education programs in cancer nursing: An overview. *Oncol Nurs Forum* 14:59–60, 1987

44. Volker DL: Learning needs assessment. *Oncol Nurs Forum* 14:60–62, 1987

45. Itano J: Developing educational objectives. *Oncol Nurs Forum* 14:62–65, 1987

46. Belcher A: Defining content and methods. *Oncol Nurs Forum* 14:65–67, 1987

47. McMillan S: Program evaluation. *Oncol Nurs Forum* 14:67–70, 1987

48. Itano J, Miller CA: Learning needs of Oncology Nursing Society members. *Oncol Nurs Forum* 17:697–706, 1990

49. Donaldson WS, Glass EC, Helmick F, et al: Determining continuing education priorities in cancer management for nurses. *Oncol Nurs Forum* 15:625–630, 1988

50. Bushy A, Kost S: A model of continuing education for rural oncology nurses. *Oncol Nurs Forum* 17:207–211, 1990

51. Donoghue M, Spross J: Report from the First National Conference. *Oncol Nurs Forum* 12:35–73, 1985

52. Spross JA, Gallagher J, Powel LL: Conference recommendations: Practice administration research education and health care policy. *Oncol Nurs Forum* 19:32–41, 1992 (suppl)

53. Carroll-Johnson RM: Proceedings of the state-of-knowledge conference on advanced practice in oncology nursing. *Oncol Nurs Forum* 22:3–45, 1995 (suppl)

54. American Cancer Society: *Special Report on Cancer in the Economically Disadvantaged.* New York, The Society, 1986

55. Frank-Stromborg M, Rohan K: Nursing's involvement in the primary and secondary prevention of cancer. *Cancer Nurs* 15:79–108, 1992

56. Bouchard R: *Nursing Care of the Cancer Patient.* St. Louis, Mosby, 1967

57. Reed Ash C: Education: A case for change. *Cancer Nurs* 8:A15, 1985 (editorial)

58. Hagopian GA, Ferszt GA, Jacobs LA, et al: Preparing clinical preceptors to teach master's level students in oncology nursing. *J Prof Nurs* 8:295–300, 1992

59. Ketter J: Restructuring: Affecting the workforce and workplace for the new graduate. *Am Nurs* 10:4, 1995, (suppl)

60. Erickyon J: Editors' message. *OCCN News* 9:2, 1995

61. Baird SB: The impact of changing health care delivery on oncology practice. *Oncol Nurs* 2:1–13, 1995

# Chapter 61

# Advancing Cancer Nursing Through Nursing Research

**Mel Haberman, RN, PhD, FAAN**

## INTRODUCTION

Oncology nurses are poised to lead the transformation of cancer care in the new millennium. Quality of care is being championed by oncology nurses as the delivery of cancer services is restructured in a cost-driven, managed-care environment. Oncology nurses are ensuring the humanization of care in a biomedical culture that is mystified by technology. Nurses are playing a critical role in monitoring the ethical conduct of cancer research, and are vocal advocates for access to clinical trials by a diverse population that includes the poor and underserved. Moreover, nurses are assuming a pivotal role in the surveillance of people at genetic predisposition to cancer and in the delivery of genetic services.

The diversity of roles performed by oncology nurses requires a broad and in-depth theory base for practice. Despite recent advances in oncology nursing research, new mechanisms must be instituted to facilitate multi-institutional studies, nursing-effectiveness trials, and outcomes research. Promising clinicians and graduate students must be encouraged to enter a career in research. However, recruiting a new generation of nurse scientists and generating more theory will not be sufficient to actually change practice. Novel strategies for research dissemination and utilization must be developed and tested to ensure that practice becomes progressively evidence-based.

The purpose of this chapter is to explore some of the trends in health care and cancer care that provide the context for future advances in nursing science and research. Some priorities and topics for oncology nursing research are identified along with a brief discussion of nursing outcomes. Opportunities for clinicians and advanced practice nurses to become involved in research are described along with tips for making a study feasible, preparing a grant application, and securing funding. The components of research critique are presented as an aid to evaluating grant proposals, manuscripts, and research protocols. Guidelines for monitoring the ethical conduct of research are discussed and the chapter concludes with an overview of future directions for oncology nursing research.

## TRENDS IN HEALTH CARE AND ONCOLOGY

Advances in oncology nursing science occur within a broader social and political context. The current climate for health care reform in the United States follows a convoluted path. Federal and state governments, business, labor, cancer advocacy groups, and cancer specialists all have different opinions about the best way to deliver cancer care services. Furthermore, oncology care is currently more politicized and under greater public scrutiny than at anytime in history. Systems that guarantee access to comprehensive cancer care and to long-term follow-up are in a quandary as the provision of care shifts from the specialized oncology nurse and oncologist to the generalist. Moreover, in a managed-care environment, cancer care is all too often driven by reimbursement issues. Although managed care organizations and nurse scientists share the common goal of improving the wellness of individuals with cancer, nurse scientists are concerned with discovering a scientific foundation for practice while managed care corporations regard research as an investment to drive down the costs of care.[1]

Another trend in oncology care is the changing way researchers, clinicians, and consumers communicate with each other. Computer platforms are proliferating exponentially in conjunction with the development of new medical application software. Health care institutions are installing integrated computerized systems that include quality improvement monitoring, fiscal and operations management, electronic medical records, laboratory data banks, diagnostic imaging tools, and bibliographic reference software. Cancer organizations, research funding agencies, cancer advocacy groups, as well as volunteer and professional societies are now on the Internet's World Wide Web. All of these factors provide people with virtually instantaneous access to vast repositories of cancer-related information.

Cancer advocacy groups and consumers will perform a key role in shaping the future direction of cancer care and research. Consumers will demand legislation that ensures the timely clinical application of new cancer therapies, just as the HIV/AIDS community has successfully diminished the time it takes for new drugs to move from the bench to practice. Early in the twenty-first century, the Human Genome Project will lead to predictions of likely cancers. The ability to forecast potential cancers in entire populations of healthy people will revolutionize cancer prevention, screening, and detection activities; systems for monitoring people with a positive genetic profile for cancer; and health care ethics.

Future advances in nursing therapeutics will parallel new trends in cancer therapy. New applications are proliferating rapidly for biological response modifiers; blood cell and genetic transplants; aggressive ablative therapies; antiemetic, antibiotic, and pain therapies; cancer markers; tumor-suppressor genes; and oncogenes. The magnitude, scope, and pace of scientific discovery is pushing oncology nursing practice beyond the edge of existing theory.[2] As the specialty realigns itself to ensure the delivery of quality care in the midst of health care reform, advances in clinical practice will continue to outpace the development of new nursing theory for the near future. A clear set of research priorities is needed to focus nurse scientists' efforts to fill existing gaps in practice knowledge.

## TOPICS AND PRIORITIES FOR ONCOLOGY NURSING RESEARCH

Oncology nursing research focuses on the human experience of wellness and illness, the clinical therapeutics under the control of nurses, the systems designed to deliver cancer care, and the patient outcomes directly attributed to nursing intervention. By definition, clinical studies may examine the natural history of cancer and survivorship, nursing interventions targeted at improving health or ameliorating suffering, nursing staffing patterns and models of care, and quality of life outcomes that are sensitive to the caring actions of nurses. Many avenues exist for selecting a suitable research topic within the broad scope of oncology nursing practice.

McCorkle[3] identifies four methods for choosing a research topic: (1) the nurse's direct observation or clinical experience, (2) talking with other nurses about gaps in practice knowledge or clinical problems, (3) reading the literature and recognizing discrepancies in research findings or existing knowledge, and (4) examining a published theory and its suitability for practice. Topics for study also can be derived from guidelines for practice and care pathways, and written standards for total or continuous quality improvement. Another source of research topics is the critical evaluation of daily practice. Nurses can readily discover a lack of evidence-based support for many nursing interventions. A potential topic for research is often embedded in the statement, "I do not know why we do it this way. We have always done it this way as long as I can remember."

Topics for research can be identified from the results of research priority surveys. Oncology nurses have participated in five research priority surveys conducted by the Oncology Nursing Society (ONS) since 1981. Topics continuously ranked among the top ten research priorities from 1981 to 1994 include stress, coping, and adaptation; pain; patient education; prevention and early detection; and cost containment and economic issues.[4,5] Quality of life emerged as a leading research priority in both the 1991 and 1994 surveys. Three topics were ranked in the top ten priorities for the first time in the 1994 survey: risk reduction and screening, neutropenia and immunosuppression, and ethical issues.

Topics for research can be identified by looking at the types of studies conducted by other cancer researchers. In addition to conducting bibliographic searches on selected topics, many sites on the Internet have databases that contain compilations of currently funded projects as well as announcements for new grants. One of the most comprehensive clearinghouses for cancer information is OncoLink at the University of Pennsylvania (http://cancer.med.upenn.edu/). OncoLink is a gateway to dozens of cancer-related databases, including the Computer Retrieval of Information on Scientific Reports (CRISP). The CRISP biomedical database contains information by topic area on all grants funded by the National Institutes of Health (NIH), including the NCI's clinical trials and studies funded by the National Institute for Nursing Research (NINR). Other home pages on the Internet include:

NINR (http://www.nih.gov:80/ninr/)

NIH Office of Grants and Contracts (http://www.nih.gov:80/grants/)

NIH Division of Research Grants (http://www.drg.nih.gov/)

NCI's International Cancer Information Center (http://icicc.nih.gov/)

Oncology Nursing Society (http://www.ons.org)

The American Cancer Society (http://www.cancer.org) (includes information about the ACS's extramural grants program)

Another source of potential topics for research is a historical look at the small grants funded by the Oncology Nursing Foundation. From 1984 to 1996, the Oncology Nursing Foundation funded 137 oncology nurse investigators for a total of $1.1 million. Table 61-1 shows the funded projects categorized by topic area and the number of studies conducted in each area.

In summary, there is an abundance of topics that need further study by oncology nurses. Moreover, a focused research agenda for the specialty must be developed and articulated to funding agencies, volunteer cancer societies, other cancer care providers, and cancer advocacy groups. Reaching consensus on a common research agenda will require nurse scientists, clinicians, administrators, educators, and cancer survivors to work together to create a new spirit of cooperative science.

## OUTCOMES FOR NURSING RESEARCH

There is an urgent need to link caring behaviors, care pathways, and guidelines for practice to measurable, biopsychosocial outcomes of nursing care. Oncology nurse outcome managers and researchers must identify outcomes that provide informative data for understanding the effects of nursing therapeutics.[6,7] Some agreement must be reached on how to define nurse-sensitive outcomes and measure them in a standardized manner. Brooten and Naylor[6] warn us that the search for nurse-sensitive outcomes must not ignore the reality that nurses provide care within a broader culture of care. Consequently, studies of nursing outcomes must include system and organizational variables as well as outcomes that may be influenced more by other care providers or by the family.

Individuals with cancer, nurses, physicians, payers, managed care corporations, researchers, and health policy makers have different opinions about which outcomes are most salient.[1,8] In an effort to define and set a direc-

**TABLE 61-1** Oncology Nursing Research Funded by the Oncology Nursing Foundation from 1984–1996

| Topic Areas | Number of Projects |
|---|---|
| **1994 ONS Research Priorities** | |
| 1. Pain | 21 |
| 2. Cancer prevention | 1 |
| 3. Quality of life | 31 |
| 4. Risk reduction/screening | 6 |
| 5. Ethical issues | 0 |
| 6. Neutropenia/immunosuppression | 1 |
| 7. Patient education | 6 |
| 8. Stress, coping, and adaptation | 54 |
| 9. Cancer detection | 5 |
| 10. Cost containment/cost of care | 1 |
| **Other Topics** | |
| Intervention studies | 34 |
| Symptom management | 20 |
| Biophysical variables | 14 |
| Social support | 12 |
| Nausea and vomiting | 10 |
| Fatigue | 9 |
| Home care | 6 |
| Exercise | 5 |
| Health beliefs | 5 |
| HIV/AIDS | 4 |
| Hospice/terminal care | 3 |
| Therapeutic touch | 3 |
| Sexual functioning | 3 |
| Mucositis | 3 |
| Spiritual well-being | 2 |
| Vascular access devices | 1 |
| Informed consent | 1 |
| **Cancer Treatments** | |
| Chemotherapy | 25 |
| Biological response modifiers | 9 |
| Marrow and blood cell transplant | 9 |
| Surgical therapy | 6 |
| Radiation therapy | 5 |
| Intravesical therapy | 2 |
| **Types of Cancer** | |
| Breast | 42 |
| Hematologic | 6 |
| Gynecologic | 5 |
| Prostate | 4 |
| Colorectal | 3 |
| Head and neck | 2 |
| Bladder | 2 |
| Melanoma | 1 |
| Neurological | 1 |
| **Populations Studied** | |
| Family and caregivers | 18 |
| Children | 14 |
| Minority and multicultural | 14 |
| Survivors | 10 |
| Nurses | 9 |
| Animals | 4 |
| Elderly | 3 |

tion for outcomes research, the National Center for Nursing Research held a landmark conference in 1991 on patient outcomes research. The proceedings of this conference are available in a free publication from the U.S. Department of Health and Human Services.[9] As an aid to identifying general categories of nursing outcomes, Table 61-2 lists some of the common outcomes previously used for nursing research and quality assurance studies[10], nursing effectiveness studies,[6] and cancer-related quality of life.[11,12]

Several definitions of nursing outcomes exist in the literature. Lang and Marek define an outcome as "an end result of a treatment or intervention."[10, p.27] According to Lasker-Hertz and Houston,[7] outcomes research focuses on the end results of care and linking the process of care delivery with patient outcomes. The American Society of Clinical Oncology (ASCO) recently convened an advisory panel to develop guidelines for the assessment of cancer treatment outcomes.[8] ASCO makes a distinction between cancer treatment and patient outcomes. Cancer treatment outcomes measure the effect of therapy on the disease of cancer (e.g., complete or partial tumor response, response duration, time to progression, and tumor markers). Patient outcomes measure the direct effect of therapy on patients (e.g., mortality, quality of life, and treatment-related toxicities).

Many questions about nursing outcomes remain unanswered. How should outcomes be defined and measured in different settings and patient populations? What is the relationship between biophysical and psychosocial outcomes? Can nursing therapeutics be linked to predictions of cancer survival and quality of life outcomes? Can consensus be reached on a minimum set of core outcomes that are relevant to nurse clinicians, managers, administrators, and researchers?

Nursing effectiveness trials eventually will provide outcome data to substantiate the ways oncology nurses make a difference in the delivery of care and in improving patient outcomes. Eventually, clinicians and consumers alike will have access to these databases just as they currently have access to databases on the NCI's ongoing clinical trials.

## MECHANISMS FOR ONCOLOGY NURSING RESEARCH

### Research Conducted by Nurse Clinicians and Advanced Practice Nurses

Many opportunities exist for oncology nurses to participate in research. Although nurses with advanced graduate preparation in research are more likely to participate in research than nurses with little formal research preparation, staff nurses historically have been successful in obtaining small grant funding to conduct pilot and feasibility studies. Since it is difficult, if not impossible at

**TABLE 61-2**  Oncology Nursing Outcomes

| | |
|---|---|
| Biophysical Outcomes | Temperature, pulse, respiration, blood pressure, lung sounds, cardiac output<br>Laboratory tests: WBC, RBC, creatinine, serum glucose<br>Skin integrity, body surface area, abdominal girth<br>Sleep patterns, nutritional status, weight<br>Nosocomial infections, wound healing, renal and hepatic functioning |
| Psychosocial Outcomes | Cognitive status: attention span, memory, concentration, orientation<br>Moods: anxiety, depression, anger, hope, happiness<br>Coping skills, social support, beliefs in personal control<br>Social power, communication styles, interpersonal skills<br>Will-to-live, adaptation to illness, meaning of illness |
| Behaviors and Safety | Adherence to treatment protocols<br>Health- and illness-related knowledge, understanding and perceptions<br>Health beliefs, attitudes and motivation<br>Caregiving and self-care skills<br>Problem-solving and decision-making skills<br>Safety interventions, prevention of falls, use of access devices, ventilators |
| Quality of Life | Physical functioning: activities of daily living, mobility, sexuality<br>Social functioning: social support, social roles, family functioning<br>Emotional functioning: mood states, well-being, life-satisfaction<br>Symptoms: pain, nausea, fatigue, diarrhea, graft-versus-host disease<br>Spirituality: religiosity, self-transcendent experiences, faith<br>Economic status: out-of-pocket expenses, insurability, employment or school status, income |
| Delivery of Care and Utilization | Staffing patterns and mix, generalist vs. specialist care<br>Patient acuity<br>Length of stay, readmissions, cost-of-care, access to care, referral patterns<br>Goal attainment for care pathways, guidelines for care, quality improvement<br>Caregiver issues and burdens<br>Models of care: managed care, transition services, continuity models<br>Inpatient, ambulatory care, critical care, and home care services<br>Patient and staff satisfaction |

times, to conduct a research study while holding down a full-time clinical position, nurses can choose different types of research involvement. Table 61-3 identifies some of the ways nurses can participate in research depending on their level of education, formal research preparation, and the willingness of their employer to support research.

Research occurs within a context of critical inquiry. A climate for research can be fostered by initiating different activities that raise the level of critical thinking. Practice settings can be evaluated for their potential to support research by asking a series of questions. Do the nurses in the care setting talk about research? Do they identify gaps in practice and make statements like, "Somebody needs to study why we do. . . ."? Does the setting have a nursing research committee or someone designated to facilitate nursing studies? Do nurses have the same access as other staff to electronic databases and bibliographic search software? Does the setting hold journal clubs or regularly present research findings at inservice education programs or during staff meetings? Are there any graduate students or nursing faculty conducting research in the setting? Are there any rewards for participating in research (e.g., promotion or merit raises based on research and publication or funding to support travel to conferences to present research findings)? It is often

easier to conduct a study in a setting that encourages and rewards research than to struggle with institutional barriers or a lack of commitment to research.

## How to make a project feasible

Many staff nursing projects are doomed to failure from the beginning because the aim of the study is too broad and is unattainable without major funding and a dedicated research staff. Furthermore, new investigators may have been misled about the realities of conducting a well-designed study. Even with the support of grant funding and a project staff, researchers spend evenings, weekends, holidays, and vacation time conducting their studies, writing progress reports, seeking additional funding, mentoring project members, and preparing manuscripts or presentations. The old adage, "something always takes more time than originally intended," must have been first voiced by a sleep-deprived researcher. Moreover, research is as much a political process as a journey of scientific discovery. The nurse investigator must be prepared for bouts of discouragement and disillusionment, and for the territorial wars that commonly occur in multidisciplinary settings.

Despite the daily frustrations that are a natural facet

**TABLE 61-3**  Types of Research Involvement

| | |
|---|---|
| AA, Diploma, and BSN | Act as study monitors, data collectors, and project managers<br>Help develop projects and review for clinical feasibility<br>Conduct pilot/feasibility studies with assistance of research mentor<br>Participate in journal clubs<br>Conduct electronic literature searches<br>Prepare research-based guidelines for practice and care pathways |
| Master's Degree | Conduct independent projects or collaborate with a nurse scientist<br>Act as research mentor to staff nurses<br>Serve as project director or study monitor<br>Coordinate research dissemination and utilization activities<br>Provide research critique |
| Doctorate | Orchestrate a research career<br>Generate new knowledge: concept definition, theory development, instrumentation, and methodologic research<br>Serve on grant review study sections<br>Review proposals for scientific merit, clinical feasibility, and budget issues<br>Lead multi-institutional studies<br>Mentor graduate students and postdoctorate fellows<br>Provide expert testimony for health policy formation and funding priorities<br>Serve on advisory panels to evaluate the state-of-the-science<br>Study quality of care, cost and access, delivery models, and outcomes |

of conducting research, there are many ways to ensure that the experience is both successful and enjoyable. The investigator should make sure that the specific aim of the project is narrow, focused, and attainable in a realistic time period. It is a good idea to assemble a team of nurses who are interested in the same topic and to pool resources. Each member of the team can be responsible for developing a specific component of the research proposal. For instance, one person may write the review of the literature while others prepare a draft of the design and methods section, analysis plan, and so forth.

Another way to design a feasible study is to keep the timeline for completing the study realistic and flexible. It is not uncommon for a small study with a single research question to take one to two years to complete. It may be beneficial to join forces with oncology nurses at other sites in the community to obtain a larger and more diverse sample in a shorter period of time. Whenever possible, the investigator can apply for small grant funding to buy some paid release time to conduct the study and to obtain funding for word processing, photocopying, travel, supplies, consultation, computer time, and telephone expenses. Sometimes it is more efficient to tag a small study onto an existing protocol than to initiate a new project. Research nurses who manage projects for physician researchers often add a nursing component to an existing medical protocol. This type of adjunct study is called a companion study.[13]

Many design options exist for developing a feasible study and choosing the most suitable method of inquiry. Although the complexities of research design are beyond the scope of this chapter, several excellent nursing textbooks are available as references.[14–18] As an aid to outlining a research proposal or evaluating a grant application, Fig. 61-1 identifies the major components of a research protocol and grant application.

### Research consultation

Expert consultation from colleagues, a nurse scientist, and a statistician is essential. A consultant is chosen based on his or her publications, presentations, or track record of funded research in the proposed content area. The consultant should read and critique the proposal or grant application in the early, formative stages. Many cancer centers have an active nursing research committee that either conducts studies as a group or offers consultation and critique. If there is no committee in the setting, consider starting one. Written guidelines that describe how to start a clinical nursing research committee can be obtained from the Oncology Nursing Society.

Another source of research consultation is a local chapter of the Oncology Nursing Society. Every ONS chapter has been grouped by geographic region by the ONS Research Committee. Each chapter has an assigned volunteer nurse scientist who has agreed to offer research consultation to chapter members. Other sources of consultation include the research committee of the state nurses' association, local chapters of nursing specialty organizations, and the faculty of local schools of nursing. Many faculty members have clinical or research affiliations with cancer centers and other community agencies.

- Sign-off signatures from all institutional officials and research sites
- Abstract of study
- Specific aims, research questions, or hypotheses
- Significance of project
- Literature review, theoretical, or conceptual framework
- References
- Description of quantitative research design
  Historical
  Descriptive
  Correlational
  Causal comparative
  True experimental
  Quasi-experimental
  Clinical trials
  Instrument development and testing
- Description of qualitative research design
  Ethnography
  Grounded theory
  Hermeneutics
  Phenomenology
- Methodology and procedures
  Sample inclusion and exclusion criteria
  Power analysis to justify sample size
  Accrual, randomization, and sampling strategies
  Sample replacement due to attrition
  Theoretical sampling for qualitative designs
  Description of instruments, scoring, and reliability and validity
  Protocol adherence and stopping rules
  Control or minimize sources of random or systematic measurement error
  Data collection and data management
  Data analysis plan
  Assurances for obtaining informed consent, maintaining anonymity, and confidentiality of data
  Monitoring scientific integrity and ethical conduct
- Timeline for study
- Biosketches for all investigators, consultants, research staff
- Description of facilities, office space, lab equipment, computer resources
- Letters of support from program directors, research sites, consultants
- Itemized budget and budget narrative that justifies all expenses
- Other sources of funding and/or pending grants
- Consent form and letter of approval from Institutional Review Board or animal welfare committee
- If resubmitting a grant, a cover letter that addresses how the grant was modified based on an earlier review.

**FIGURE 61-1**  Sections of a research proposal or grant.

Staff nurses should not be hesitant to ask for consultation from faculty members who are engaged in research. The nurse researcher, in turn, may want to negotiate for some type of recognition for their contribution to the project or they may ask the nurse researcher for help with one of their studies. If a doctorate-prepared nurse scientist is not available, find out which nurses in the setting or community have conducted research and ask for assistance. Research nurses who conduct clinical trials for the NCI's cooperative research groups can often provide excellent research consultation, especially on the design and implementation of multi-institutional projects.

### Tips for grant preparation

Obtaining research funding is more competitive than ever. The chances of being successfully funded will improve if some basic tips for grant preparation are followed. The Oncology Nursing Society's Research Committee has developed many of the following tips for preparing a better grant application.

- Identify your strengths and weaknesses as a researcher. Find ways to overcome deficiencies. For instance, if you do not have preliminary data to support an application for major funding, plan a phased program of study that begins with a small-scale pilot study.

- If you do not have a track record of publications or funded research in your area of interest, get one or more consultants to improve your competitive edge. In addition to their expert advice, consultants act as an insurance policy to the funding agency. Funding sources want some type of guarantee that the investigator will do what is promised in the grant application and that their investment is buying the best science for the dollar. Having a consultant gives them these assurances and shows the grant reviewers that you recognize your limitations and have taken steps to strengthen the content areas beyond your expertise.

- The grant application and instructions are the road map. Follow the rules and suggested guidelines carefully. If the application says the funding agency is interested in projects that study x, y, and z, be sure the specific aims of your proposal address x, y, and z.

- Do not propose a full-scale study if a feasibility study is more appropriate. Pilot studies are useful to determine the effect size of an intervention; assess the feasibility of a research design or procedures for data collection; pretest an instrument in the population of interest; and to evaluate the risk, side effects, and compliance with a new nursing therapy.

- Try to anticipate how the reviewer will respond to your application. Make the application pleasant to look at and easy to read and understand. Follow the requirements for font style and size, margins, and printing. Use subheadings, tables, and graphs, if applicable. Adhere rigidly to the page limitations.

- Never assume the reviewers will understand your proposal as well as you do. Introduce new ideas incrementally. Move from the general to the specific. Start with basic definitions and explanations and finish with a full synthesis or complex explanation. Provide an immediate definition or explanation whenever you identify a new concept, theory, or research methodology for the first time. Have a deliberate strategy for educating the reviewers so they will understand every nuance of your study by the time they have finished reading the proposal.

- Use an editor to help you with writing style, use of grammar, and punctuation. Write clearly in an active voice using nonsexist language. Typographical errors and misspelled words reflect poorly on your attention to detail.

- Use the appendices to support your application rather than as a catch-all for everything that could not be squeezed into the body of the application. It is not the weight or thickness of the proposal that matters, but its quality.

- Support letters should be written specifically for the proposal and project. Avoid submitting generic letters that show the writer has little knowledge of the study. Provide letters that document access to clinical sites and patient populations, release time to perform the research, the availability of space and equipment, and so forth. Consultants should submit a letter that discusses their role and other contributions to the study.

- Budgets should never be inflated. Only request allowable expenses and justify why each budget item is essential to the project. Show how cost calculations were reached (e.g., a transcriptionist will be hired for 10 hours at $12 per hour for a total cost of $120).

- Check the application for any fatal flaws such as an inadequate sample size, low significance to the goals of the funding agency, or a project that is under- or over-ambitious for the funding level and desired time frame for the study.

- Check the overall integrity and logical consistency of the application by drawing a diagram that shows the interrelationships among the specific aims, design, sample, variables, instruments, and analysis plan. Does each section flow logically from the other? Are there any gaps in the project that may result in a fatal flaw? Has anything necessary been lost or has something been added that does not relate to the aims of the study?

### Funding for research

Many options exist for beginning researchers to obtain funding for preliminary and small-scale studies. Generally speaking, nurse scientists who have a previous track record of funded research have a better chance of obtaining major funding than a new investigator. If you do not have the qualifications to be competitive for major funding, look for funding sources that give special awards for new investigators and novice researchers and that support small grants, pilot, and feasibility studies.

A good fit between your study and the goals of the funding agency is essential to successful funding. Some funding sources restrict their grants awards to certain topics or high priorities while others provide relatively unrestricted funding. The American Nurses' Foundation, a subsidiary of the American Nurses' Association, funds approximately 20 small grants each year for new researchers or researchers entering a new area of study. Many of these awards are for unrestricted topics of study. The majority of the 28 small grants awarded by the Oncology Nursing Foundation are unrestricted, only requiring that the investigator study some aspect of oncology. However, some of the pharmaceutical companies that sponsor grants for the American Nurses' Foundation and the Oncology Nursing Foundation stipulate that the investigator must study specific symptoms, topics, or nursing therapeutics. If you are seeking funding from a national or local pharmaceutical company, be sure to find out if the funding is unrestricted or if the company requires you to study one of their products or the side effects associated with the use of a product.

Other sources of funding often can be found in the investigator's agency or local community. Many cancer centers have core program grants that provide seed money for start-up research projects. Nurses can often qualify for these monies especially if their protocol is tagged onto an existing medical protocol as a companion study. Many directors of nursing often try to protect small pockets of money to support seed money for nursing research projects. Guilds that sponsor fund-raising events for most comprehensive and community cancer centers are another potential source of research funding.

Chapters of the Oncology Nursing Society or other nursing specialty organizations, like the American Association of Critical-Care Nurses, are additional sources of local funding. Some societies require the grant applicant to be a member while others do not. The national nursing honorary society, Sigma Theta Tau, has local chapters at almost all university schools of nursing. Many local chapters, as well as the national organization of Sigma Theta Tau, give grant awards. Some state divisions of the American Cancer Society and the Leukemia Society of America have funding for research on the local level. Another source of potential funding for research is local fraternities and sororities. Most fraternal organizations have yearly fund-raising projects as a part of their community service mission. At the Fred Hutchinson Cancer Research Center, nurses were able to raise $20,000 by asking a local fraternity to donate the proceeds of their "Run for Cancer" to nursing research.

It is important to be aware of the various funding bulletins that are published locally by the grants and contracts offices of universities and cancer centers. These bulletins are usually published monthly or bimonthly and list all of the potential sources of funding and application deadline dates for dozens of funding agencies. The addresses for all federal and private foundations that support research can be obtained from a health science library or a grants and contracts office.

Health science libraries, cancer center libraries, and grants and contracts offices usually subscribe to a variety of weekly or monthly research funding publications. The *NIH Guide for Grants and Contracts* is the federal government's premier vehicle for announcing new grants. The *NIH Guide* is also available on the Internet (gopher://gopher.nih.gov:70/11/res/nih-guide). Another publication that identifies many opportunities for oncology research funding is the *Health Grants and Contracts Weekly: Selected Federal and Private Opportunities,* published weekly by Capital Publications, Inc. A bimonthly publication called *Research Activities,* published by the Agency for Health Care Policy and Research, gives updates of currently funded projects and features new funding opportunities for specific topic areas. Another publication entitled *The Blue Sheet: Health Policy and Biomedical Research News of the Week,* is published by F-D-C Reports, Inc. This publication identifies opportunities for clinical research funding and presents feature articles on research ethics and scientific integrity, to name a few.

## RESEARCH CRITIQUE

All nurses must be critical consumers of research even if they choose not to become involved in the actual conduct of research. Clinicians are often asked to evaluate the clinical feasibility of a study, the potential of the project to burden staff and patients, and the relevance of the research to daily practice. Of course, there is no perfect research study or gold standard for evaluating the merit of a study. Designing and implementing a study always involves a series of compromises.

Using a systematic tool or set of guidelines to evaluate the scientific merit of a study will allow the nurse to gauge the value of the study's findings for practice. Research critique involves asking a set of questions about the study and then evaluating the overall rigor and feasibility of the study. Many of the following components of a formal research critique are derived from the score sheet used by the grant reviewers for the Oncology Nursing Foundation. These evaluation criteria are geared more for quantitative research designs than for qualitative designs. Criteria for evaluating qualitative studies can be found elsewhere.[19–21]

### Components of Research Critique

#### Qualifications of investigators and staff

What are the qualifications of the principal investigator, consultants, and project staff? Have they conducted

prior research, published, or obtained grants in the area under study? Is a biographical sketch included for all key personnel?

### Abstract

Does the abstract accurately reflect the proposed research? A 200–250 word abstract should contain the following sections, if applicable: purpose, specific aims, significance, research design, setting, sample, methods, main research variables, analysis plan, and implications for practice.

### Specific aims

Are the aims clear and understandable? Do the aims flow logically from the purpose of the study? Are the aims consistent with any hypotheses or research questions?

### Significance of study

Is the study relevant to oncology nursing practice? Does it have potential to lead to further research, methodologic advances, or theory development?

### Background and review of literature

Is the conceptual or theoretical framework for the study identified? Is the review succinct, focused, and current? Does it include the appropriate classic studies on the topic? Is the literature simply reported verbatim or is it synthesized and interpreted by the investigator? Is what is known and not known about the topic logically linked to the aims of the current study? Are the findings of any pilot or feasibility study reported as preliminary data?

### Design and methods

There are several components to this section of a research proposal, including:

**Design**  Does the investigator clearly state the research design? Commonly used designs for quantitative and qualitative studies are listed in Figure 61-1.

**Sample and setting**  Is the sample described (i.e., the number of participants and the eligibility and exclusion criteria)? Are all random sampling and assignment procedures to either an experimental or control group explained? Has a power analysis been conducted to determine what sample size is needed to detect a significant difference between groups? Are the facilities and institutional resources needed to carry out the study described?

**Experimental variables**  If the study is using an experimental or quasi-experimental design, such as a nursing effectiveness trial, is the independent variable described in sufficient detail to allow for an evaluation of its clinical soundness and operational definition? Is a manipulation check or pretest of the independent variable (nursing intervention) described in the proposal? A manipulation check is the only way to demonstrate that the experimental intervention actually "takes or works" in the population being studied.

Are the outcome or dependent variables clearly identified and do the instruments actually measure the outcome variables of interest? Do the independent and dependent variables relate to the theoretical framework and review of literature? Are any potential threats to the internal validity of the study controlled for, so the investigator can conclude with confidence that it was the experimental therapy that actually made the difference between groups rather than some spurious or confounding factor?

***Instruments and measurement*** What concepts are being measured (e.g., symptoms of fatigue or pain)? If repeated measurement is planned, is evidence presented to show the instrument is capable of detecting changes over time? Has the instrument been used previously in the population under study? Are the instruments appended to the proposal? Has permission been obtained to use any copyrighted tools? If a tool has been modified, has a pilot study been conducted to test the reliability/validity of the adapted instrument?

Is there a discussion of the reliability and validity of the instruments, the weight given to individual items and subscales, and the scoring procedures? Common forms of validity include face and content validity, concurrent and predictive validity as types of criterion-related validity, and construct validity. Reliability tests include test-retest, inter-rater, internal consistency, and parallel or alternative forms reliability.[22]

***Data collection schedule and procedures*** Is there a description of how and when data will be collected and any training that is necessary to standardize data collection? Are the procedures realistic in terms of the clinical setting, treatment trajectory, and expected side effects of therapy? Will the procedures result in lower accrual or higher attrition rates? Does the instrument packet place undue burden on the participant, family, or staff? Are potential sources of random or systematic measurement error identified and, if possible, controlled for or minimized?

***Data analysis*** Is the statistical or analytic technique identified and is the analysis plan capable of answering each specific aim of the study?

***Study limitations*** Are the limitations identified and described?

***Protection of human participants*** Has approval been obtained from an Institutional Review Board (IRB) and is a copy of the IRB assurance letter appended? Has IRB approval been granted from all participating research sites? Are the procedures for obtaining informed consent and maintaining confidentiality described and are they adequate?

## Statement of scientific integrity

Is a plan included for monitoring the scientific integrity of the study across all performance sites? This section should include, if applicable, a discussion of the procedures that are necessary to monitor the recruitment of participants and the informed consent process. Procedures for maintaining the accuracy of data, adhering to IRB guidelines, ensuring the confidentiality of data, and the standardization of data collection should be described. Moreover, data entry and coding issues should be discussed (e.g., procedures for maintaining an audit trial of coding decisions, verifying the accuracy of electronically transmitted data, and safeguarding the security of data). Data analysis and reporting procedures should be described as well as steps taken to ensure the veracity of all products of analysis. The procedures adopted by the project team to safeguard against plagiarism and the fabrication, falsification, or misrepresentation of all research-related activities should be discussed as well as the process to be followed in the event of any inquiries, allegations, or confirmed acts of misconduct. Procedures for reporting adverse effects should be identified.

## Additional sections

The proposal should also contain a reference list, time table for accomplishing the study, and letters of support from agency personnel and consultants. Do the letters of support document access to performance sites, research participants, institutional facilities and resources committed to the study as well as matching research funds, if any? Is a line-item budget included in addition to a budget narrative that justifies why the itemized expenses are essential to the conduct of the study? Are any cost calculations described? Some grant applications require the investigator to list all sources of research funding and the percentage of salary support received from each source, including all pending grant support.

In summary, all nurses should have at least a beginning knowledge of research critique. The components of a formal critique are useful for evaluating the suitability of a published study for practice. Nurse investigators should ask their colleagues to critique the preliminary drafts of a proposal as many times as necessary to identify and fix any potential problems.

# SCIENTIFIC AND ETHICAL CONDUCT OF RESEARCH

Monitoring the scientific integrity of a project is an integral aspect of all nursing research. Confirmed incidents of misconduct have direct legal consequences and they jeopardize the reputation, future funding eligibility, and employability of the researcher. The public's confidence in research is justifiably eroded when reports of misconduct appear in the lay or scientific press. In some cases, the potential health of individuals with cancer may be at risk if adverse reactions go unreported, protocol-stopping rules are ignored, or falsified data are reported in the literature.

The U.S. Department of Health and Human Services published a booklet in 1995 entitled *Integrity and Misconduct in Research: Report of the Commission on Research Integrity*.[23] Research misconduct, as defined by the commission, is any "significant misbehavior that improperly appropriates the intellectual property or contributions of others, that intentionally impedes the progress of research, or that risks corrupting the scientific record or compromising the integrity of scientific practices."[23, p.13] Research misconduct does not involve honest errors of judgment, the stating of hypotheses that ultimately prove to be false, differences in the interpretation of data, or making scientific observations and analyses that may eventually prove to be in error.[23]

The misappropriation and misrepresentation of intellectual property are common examples of research misconduct. Misappropriation refers to an intentional or reckless act of plagiarism or a violation of the confidentiality associated with the review of scientific manuscripts or grants.[23] Misrepresentation is defined as a deliberate attempt to deceive or commit a reckless disregard for the truth by stating or presenting a falsehood, omitting facts, or the fabrication of data and findings.[23] Additionally, research misconduct may include the obstruction of inquiries or investigations of misconduct or noncompliance with regulations that govern the conduct of federal or privately funded research.

Other examples of research misconduct may include intentionally enrolling certain types of participants in a study to bias the findings in the hypothesized direction, entering participants that fail to meet eligibility criteria, administering an experimental treatment despite severe adverse reactions, fabricating data, reporting findings of a study that was never conducted, or substituting falsified data for legitimate data.[24]

Oncology nurses who witness an intentional act of research misconduct or who are asked to falsify data should follow the local institution's policies and regulations for reporting and handling incidents of misconduct. All cancer institutions that receive federal funding for research must have written policies for handling inquiries and allegations of misconduct. Assistance in developing institutional policies can be obtained from many sources: the literature,[23,25–27] the grants and contracts office of any university or cancer center, or health science libraries. The American Nurses' Association recently published *Guidelines on Reporting Incompetent, Unethical, or Illegal Practices*.[28] These guidelines can be used to develop institutional values and practices that discourage acts of scientific misconduct and foster ethically-based inquiry.

The principal investigator is ultimately responsible for establishing procedures to monitor the scientific integrity of a specific project. These procedures will depend on the unique aspects of the study (e.g., the number of research sites and geographic location of project staff, the potential risk posed by the experimental therapy, and the conditions under which the study will be prematurely terminated due to unacceptable risk). As an aid to developing a grant application or participating in research as a project staff member, Table 61-4 lists the types of generic activities that are needed to monitor scientific integrity and the ethical conduct of research. These activities are adapted from the Oncology Nursing Foundation's *Guidelines for the Responsible Conduct of Research*.

## FUTURE DIRECTIONS FOR RESEARCH

Oncology nursing research will increasingly shape health policy formation, cancer advocacy, the media's image of nursing, and the health of all people. Nursing research findings will be used to design and implement cancer public awareness and educational campaigns where nurses are identified as experts in cancer care. For example, the Fatigue Initiative through Research and Education (FIRE® Project) sponsored by the Oncology Nursing Foundation and Ortho Biotech, Inc., includes a national public awareness campaign to promote oncology nurses as leaders in the management of cancer-related fatigue.

Leading the transformation of cancer care, oncology nurses will set the research agenda on cancer-related women's health, access to affordable and comprehensive care by a diverse population, the assessment of symptom distress, and the management of disease symptoms and regimen-related toxicities. Moreover, nurses will be the preeminent clinical researchers in the areas of cancer pain, quality of life, spirituality, cancer-related fatigue, families' responses to cancer, and caregiver issues. Nurses will continue to study the delivery of humanistic care to individuals with HIV/AIDS.

Because of the broad domain of nursing science and the holistic nature of nursing practice, nurse investigators must begin to design nursing trials that integrate the many facets of the natural history of cancer. Models that synthesize the personal, environmental, and genetic risks for cancer are needed to guide research. Efforts must be made to synthesize several divergent literatures: (1) studies of cancer prevention, detection, screening, and diagnosis; (2) research on cultural beliefs about cancer; and (3) studies of the decision-making processes used by people undergoing traditional, experimental, or alternative therapy. Models that explain the economics of cancer care for different cancer diagnoses, therapeutic options, phases of survival, and quality of life outcomes are needed.

New descriptive and explanatory models of cancer must include a variety of contextual variables such as beliefs in personal control, the meaning given to the cancer experience, the decision-making processes of families, communication styles, social power, race and ethnicity, and the will-to-live, to name a few. For example,

**TABLE 61-4**    Activities to Monitor the Scientific Integrity of Research

| | |
|---|---|
| Data Collection Issues | Participant eligibility requirements: monitor all accrual procedures, the ongoing accuracy of inclusion and exclusion criteria, document actual accrual rates and all reasons for refusal or early withdrawal from study<br>Accuracy of data: choice of instruments, data entry or transcription reliability, procedures to audit and verify the accuracy of raw data extracted from medical records<br>Reliability of measurement and analysis: reliability of instruments, inter-rater agreement when more than one individual is collecting or coding data, sources of potential and/or actual measurement error<br>Staff training: standardized participant recruitment, data collection and entry procedures; ensure the confidentiality of data; use accepted practices for translating instruments into other languages<br>Institutional Review Board or animal welfare committee approval: adhere to policies of host institution regarding protection of human participants or the welfare of animals used for research, follow procedures for responding to adverse effects, maintain institutional approval for the duration of the study |
| Data Entry and Storage | Maintain a written audit trail of coding decisions<br>Verify the accuracy of data entry including electronically transmitted data<br>Safeguard the security of data and protect against unauthorized access to files |
| Data Analysis and Reporting | Monitor the accuracy of data during all phases of analysis<br>Ensure the veracity of all products of analysis<br>Safeguard against the fabrication, falsification, plagiarism, or misrepresentation of all aspects of research |
| Multi-institutional Projects | Monitor all aspects of scientific integrity and ethical conduct across all research sites |

how do individuals with cancer and their families make decisions all along the cancer trajectory (e.g., when nursing care is shifted from curative therapies to palliation and comfort measures and eventually to end-of-life care)? Future models of cancer also must identify which quality of life outcomes are meaningful to cancer survivors at various points in the cancer care continuum.

Oncology nurses are leading the current effort to establish cancer genetic services. With the advent of the genetics revolution, models are urgently needed to guide holistic research and practice. For instance, how will the experience of genetic testing, notification, counseling, and long-term monitoring influence the quality of life of healthy people who are at genetic risk for developing cancer? What are the ethical issues that will guide research in the field of cancer genetics? What are the elements of informed consent? How will confidentiality be protected and what security measures are needed to safeguard access to computer databases that identify people at risk? What is the potential for work and insurance discrimination by people and families carrying the genes for specific cancers? What roles are oncology nurses assuming in providing genetic counseling and implementing genetic therapies?

Other types of studies are needed to examine systems of care and models of nursing care delivery (e.g., advanced practice and certification issues and the care given by generalists, specialists, and unlicensed personnel). A focused effort is needed to conduct studies on the delivery of cost-effective nursing care by cancer consortiums, jointly affiliated institutions, managed care organizations, and by nurses who own an independent clinic or practice. Patient acuity systems for oncology are needed to guide the prediction of staffing patterns and mix, cost predictions, quality improvement outcomes, and morbidity and mortality outcomes. Instrumentation studies are needed to standardize the clinical assessment of regimen-related toxicities and the assessment of symptoms like fatigue, pain, nausea, vomiting, and quality of life, to name only a few. Additional instrumentation studies must focus on the translation of existing questionnaires into other languages or the initial development of multilingual instruments.

New mechanisms for conducting research must be established to gather data that are trustworthy and generalizable to large segments of cancer survivors. Research designs will need to become more complex and rigorous. Expert panels, composed of nurse investigators, clinicians, administrators, and educators, will need to examine the state-of-the-science of high priority research topics and form a research agenda for the specialty. The future will see the routine implementation of nursing effectiveness trials, multi-institutional studies conducted by nurses, instrumentation studies to develop clinical assessment tools, and formal programs for research dissemination and utilization. Nursing outcomes will be a focal point for virtually all oncology nursing research.

## CONCLUSION

Oncology nursing research will drive all facets of practice in the modern era of oncology nursing. As the largest group of cancer care professionals, oncology nurses must explore their own therapeutics and identify superior outcomes of holistic care. As vocal advocates for optimal quality of care, oncology nurses must continue to align themselves with cancer survivors and their quest to humanize care. Our challenge is to design theories of oncology nursing that embrace the best traditions of the art of nursing and give voice to the emerging science of nursing.

## ACKNOWLEDGMENTS

The author wishes to acknowledge the assistance of Kelli Wisdom and Linda Eaton, MN, RN, OCN® in the preparation of this manuscript. Mel Haberman is an employee of the Oncology Nursing Society (ONS). ONS does not assume any responsibility for the content of this publication.

## REFERENCES

1. Vessey J, Gennaro S: The bottom line. *Nurs Res* 45:67, 1996
2. Winters G, Miller C, Maracich L, et al: Provisional practice: The nature of psychosocial bone marrow transplant nursing. *Oncol Nurs Forum* 21:1147–1154, 1994
3. McCorkle R: Development of the research question, in Grant MM, Padilla GV (eds): *Cancer Nursing Research: A Practical Approach*. Norwalk, CT: Appleton and Lange, 1990, pp 27–42
4. Mooney KH, Ferrell BR, Nail LM, et al: 1991 Oncology Nursing Society research priorities survey. *Oncol Nurs Forum* 18:1381–1388, 1991
5. Stetz KM, Haberman MR, Holcombe J, et al: 1994 Oncology Nursing Society research priorities survey. *Oncol Nurs Forum* 22:785–789, 1995
6. Brooten D, Naylor MD: Nurses' effect on changing patient outcomes. *Image: J Nurs Sch* 27:95–99, 1995
7. Lasker-Hertz S, Houston S: Facilitating outcomes research. *Nurs Invest* 2:1–2, 1995
8. American Society of Clinical Oncology: Outcomes of cancer treatment for technology assessment and cancer treatment guidelines. *J Clin Oncol* 14:671–679, 1996
9. National Center for Nursing Research: *Patient Outcomes Research: Examining the Effectiveness of Nursing Practice*. NIH publication No. 93–3411. Rockville, MD, Department of Health and Human Services, 1992
10. Lang NM, Marek KD: Outcomes that reflect clinical practice, in National Center for Nursing Research: *Patient Outcomes Research: Examining the Effectiveness of Nursing Practice*. NIH publication No. 93–3411. Rockville, MD, Department of Health and Human Services, 1992, pp 27–38
11. Whedon M, Ferrell BR: Quality of life in adult bone marrow transplant patients: Beyond the first year. *Semin Oncol Nurs* 10:42–57, 1994
12. Bush NE, Haberman M, Donaldson G, et al: Quality of life of 125 adults surviving 6–18 years after bone marrow transplantation. *Soc Sci Med* 40:479–490, 1995
13. Ferrell BR, Cohen MZ: Companion studies. *Semin Oncol Nurs* 7:252–259, 1991
14. Grant MM, Padilla GV: *Cancer Nursing Research: A Practical Approach*. Norwalk, CT, Appleton and Lange, 1990
15. Mateo MA, Kirchhoff KT: *Conducting and Using Nursing Research in the Clinical Setting*. Baltimore, Williams & Wilkins, 1991
16. Woods NF, Catanzaro M: *Nursing Research: Theory and Practice*. St. Louis, Mosby, 1988
17. Haberman MR: Research in ambulatory care settings: The need for and how to do research, in Buchsel P, Yarbro C (eds): *Oncology Nursing in the Ambulatory Setting: Issues and Models of Care*. Boston, Jones and Bartlett, 1993, pp 307–340
18. Haberman MR: Nursing research, in Buchsel PC, Whedon MB (eds): *Bone Marrow Transplantation: Administrative and Clinical Strategies*. Boston, Jones and Bartlett, 1995, pp 365–402
19. Lincoln YS, Guba EG: *Naturalistic Inquiry*. Beverly Hills, CA, SAGE Publications, 1985
20. Denzin NK, Lincoln YS: *Handbook of Qualitative Research*. Thousand Oaks, CA, SAGE Publications, 1994
21. Haberman MR, Lewis FM: Selection of research design—Section I: Qualitative designs, in Grant MM, Padilla GV (eds): *Cancer Nursing Research: A Practical Approach*. Norwalk, CT, Appleton and Lange, 1990, pp 77–93
22. Haberman MR: The measurement of symptom distress, in Groenwald SL, Frogge MH, Goodman M, Yarbro CH (eds): *Cancer Symptom Management*. Boston, Jones and Bartlett, 1996, pp 10–18
23. Commission on Research Integrity: *Integrity and Misconduct in Research: Report of the Commission on Research Integrity*. Rockville, MD, U.S. Department of Health and Human Services, 1995; U.S. Government Printing Office, 1996
24. Mooney KH, Haberman MR: Cancer nursing research today, in McCorkle M, Grant M, Frank-Stromborg M, Baird S (eds): *Cancer Nursing: A Comprehensive Textbook* (ed 2). Orlando, Saunders, 1996, pp 1261–1276
25. Chop RM, Cipriano-Silva M: Scientific fraud: Definitions, policies, and implications for nursing research. *J Prof Nurs* 7:166–171, 1991
26. Grady C: Ethical issues in clinical trials. *Semin Oncol Nurs* 7:288–296, 1991
27. Hawley DJ, Jeffers JM: Scientific misconduct as a dilemma for nursing. *Image: J Nurs Sch* 24:51–55, 1992
28. Silva, M: *Ethical Guidelines in the Conduct, Dissemination, and Implementation of Nursing Research*. Washington, DC, American Nurses Publishing, 1995

# Chapter 62

# Cultural Diversity Among Individuals with Cancer

Karen N. Taoka, RN, MN, AOCN

Joanne K. Itano, RN, PhD, OCN®

# INTRODUCTION

Culture is a fundamental element that uniquely shapes each individual. It influences how we think, speak, act, and simply live our lives. As the United States becomes increasingly culturally diverse, there is an obvious need to realize the importance of culture in our lives, to acknowledge the diversity in values, and to embrace this diversity creating a truly culturally rich nation.

Cultural diversity encompasses more than just ethnic diversity. It is multifaceted and can include diversity in many forms such as sexual orientation, nontraditional lifestyle, age, socioeconomic status, and/or religious beliefs. In this chapter, the focus of cultural diversity is on ethnic diversity. (See Table 62-1 for definitions of selected terms.)

## Overview

As a nation, the United States historically has taken pride in its multicultural composition of peoples from many nations. However, until recently, this cultural diversity was largely limited to Caucasian immigrants from Europe who represented the majority of the population. Immigration in the twentieth century from areas such as southeast Asia, China, Japan, Korea, the Philippines, Mexico, and the Caribbean and a long overdue recognition of native Americans are factors that are rapidly redefining, the population composition of the United States. This is clearly evident when comparing the population composition in the 1950s when nine out of ten Americans were of European descent, with the composition in the 1990s, when one out of every four adults and one out of every three children are of African, Latin American, or Asian origin.[7]

Furthermore, current trends indicate that these ethnic minority populations are growing at rates that are surpassing the rest of the population. For example, Asian/Pacific Islander (API) Americans are the fastest growing minority in the United States. Between 1980 and 1990, the API population increased by 107.8 percent.[8] Projections by the U.S. Census Bureau predict that by the year 2050, the U.S. population will include the following distribution: whites 52.5%, Hispanic 22.5%, blacks 14.4%, APIs 9.7%, and native American 0.9%. These projections reflect a steady decrease in the white population from 76% in 1990 to the projected 52.5% in 2050, as compared to steady growth in the minority populations.[9] In addition, ethnic minority populations will not be distributed uniformly across the United States. For example, it is projected that in 2020 nearly two-thirds (62%) of the API population will be concentrated in California, New York, Texas, Hawaii, and Washington.[10]

Unfortunately, this trend of growing ethnic minority populations is not matched in the composition of health care professionals. In particular, data from the 1990 census revealed the underrepresentation of ethnic minority registered nurses where 3% of registered nurses were Hispanic, 4.4% API, and 8.1% African-American.[11] In 1994 the Institute of Medicine reported that minorities in the health professions were more underrepresented than 15 years ago.[7] Several reasons are identified for this underrepresentation and include inadequate math and science education for minorities, a lack of scholarships, and a lack of qualified students.[7] Underrepresentation is of concern since it has been shown that one of the more successful interventions in targeting health promotion activities and interventions for ethnic minorities is when health care professionals of the same ethnic group are directly involved.

A fundamental challenge for health care providers is that the health care beliefs and practices of many ethnic groups may not be congruent with mainstream, Westernized medicine. The use of traditional healers and folk medicine, for example, often plays a major role in the provision of holistic care for African-Americans, APIs, Hispanics, and native Americans.

This chapter provides an introduction to culture and cancer and the potential for oncology nurses to have a positive impact on the cancer experience for ethnic minority individuals and their families. A brief overview of cancer epidemiology in ethnic minorities is provided, followed by the value of transcultural nursing and a discussion of six phenomena that exist in every culture. A tool for cultural assessment is also provided. Because ethnic minorities are composed of a large percentage of immigrant groups, a section on heritage assessment is included that will assist the nurse in determining the degree of patient acculturation. An additional tool on

**TABLE 62-1** Definition of Selected Terms

|  |  |
|---|---|
| Acculturation: | Process by which an individual identifies with, and adapts to another culture; often adopts the other culture's values but still retains a part of his/her original culture; occurs on a continuum; leads to biculturalism |
| Culturally Competent Care: | Care that is provided with an awareness and appreciation of the cultural differences between the caregiver and patient; is individualized and respects the patient's cultural background. |
| Cultural Relativity: | Refers to the attempt to view or interpret the behavior of culturally different individuals within the context of those individuals' cultures; acknowledges that behavior that is appropriate in one culture may not be acceptable in another culture.[1] |
| Culture: | "Culture refers to the learned, shared, and transmitted values, beliefs, norms, and lifeways of a particular group that guides their thinking, decisions, and actions in patterned ways."[2,p.47] |
| Enculturation: | "The process by which an individual assumes the traits and behaviors of a given culture, adapting to it, adopting its values, and taking on that particular cultural identity."[3,p.36] Generally refers to the culture into which an individual is born. |
| Ethnicity: | "A sense of identification associated with a cultural group's common social and cultural heritage. . . . A person is born into an ethnic group but may also adopt characteristics of another ethnic group."[4,p.98] These characteristics include language, race, food preferences, religious faith, values, traditions, folklore, and many traits relevant to physical appearance.[4,5] |
| Ethnocentrism: | The tendency to view people unconsciously by using one's group and one's own customs as the standard for all judgments.[1] |
| Generalization: | Common patterns for beliefs and behaviors that are shared by a group; may be inaccurate when applied to specific individuals of that group.[6] |
| Race: | "A physical, not a cultural, differentiator based on a common heredity, using as identifiers characteristics such as skin color, head shape, and stature."[3,p.36] |
| Stereotype: | A fixed conception of a group allowing for no individuality; assumes all members of a group are alike. |
| Worldview: | "Refers to the way people tend to look out on the world or their universe to form a picture or a value stance about their life or world around them."[2,p.47] |

self-assessment will increase the reader's awareness of his or her perceptions and responses to people of varying backgrounds.

Specific cultural information and nursing considerations for four ethnic minority groups (African-American, API, Hispanic, and native American) follows. Last, broader issues that have an impact on culture and cancer nursing are presented.

The discussion on the four specific ethnic minority groups is limited by several factors. Foremost is the diversity within each group. Hispanics, African-Americans, APIs, and native Americans are composed of several subgroups, each with its own subculture. For example, the subgroups under the term Hispanic include Mexican American, Puerto Rican, Cuban American, and Central and South American. Added to the existence of subgroups and their unique cultures is the inherent heterogeneity due to intragroup differences such as socioeconomic status, education attainment level, and degree of acculturation. Most important is the individual within the group. Although profiles of ethnic minority groups are provided in this chapter, each patient is an individual with unique needs, regardless of his/her cultural background.

## Epidemiology

In 1996, of the estimated 1,359,150 new cases of cancer, approximately 136,380 (about 10%) were projected to be diagnosed in African-Americans and 38,000 (2.8%) among other ethnic minority groups.[12]

African-Americans, on the whole, have higher cancer incidence and mortality rates than do white Americans.[12] Comparison data in other ethnic minority groups are limited because they only recently have been collected and then on a somewhat limited basis. Kagawa-Singer[13] reports that the National Cancer Institute Surveillance, Epidemiology, and End Results (SEER) tumor registry program has listed API's only since 1978; however, initially only 4 out of 60 groups were coded: Chinese, Japanese, Filipino, and native Hawaiian. Recently, coding for Koreans and Vietnamese was initiated. In addition, aggregate data in the recent past lumped major groups together, making it difficult to sift out specific information (e.g., data on Chinese were grouped with those reported for APIs).

From the latest national data that are available, there are obvious differences in cancer incidence, mortality, and survival rates when data are compared across all groups. Age-adjusted incidence rates (overall and selected cancer sites) for 1988–1992 are based on SEER data and are provided in Table 62-2.[14] These data represent 14% of the total U.S. population with the following percentages of the specific ethnic populations: native Hawaiian (78%), Japanese (60%), Filipino (49%), Chinese (43%), Korean (34%), Vietnamese (31%), American Indian (27%), and Hispanic (25%).[14] Mortality rates, age-adjusted for the same time period are shown in Table

**TABLE 62-2**   SEER Incidence Rates, 1988–1992, Selected Sites

| Cancer Site | Alaska Native M | W | American Indian M | W | Black M | W | Chinese M | W | Filipino M | W | Hawaiian M | W |
|---|---|---|---|---|---|---|---|---|---|---|---|---|
| All sites | 372 | 348 | 196 | 180 | 560 | 326 | 282 | 213 | 274 | 224 | 340 | 321 |
| Brain and nervous system | * | * | * | * | 4.5 | 3.4 | 3.1 | 2.1 | 3.6 | 2.8 | * | * |
| Breast, invasive | * | 78.9 | * | 31.6 | 1.2 | 95.4 | * | 55.0 | * | 73.1 | * | 105.6 |
| Cervix uteri | — | 15.8 | — | 9.9 | — | 13.2 | — | 7.3 | — | 9.6 | — | 9.3 |
| Colon and rectum | 79.7 | 67.4 | 18.6 | 15.3 | 60.7 | 45.5 | 44.8 | 33.6 | 35.4 | 20.9 | 42.4 | 30.5 |
| Corpus uteri | — | * | — | 10.7 | — | 14.4 | — | 11.6 | — | 12.1 | — | 23.9 |
| Esophagus | * | * | * | * | 15.0 | 4.4 | 5.3 | * | 2.9 | * | 9.4 | * |
| Kidney and renal pelvis | * | * | 15.6 | * | 12.8 | 6.0 | 4.6 | 2.3 | 5.8 | 2.8 | 9.8 | * |
| Larynx | * | * | * | * | 12.7 | 2.5 | 2.8 | * | 2.4 | * | * | * |
| Leukemias | * | * | * | * | 11.5 | 6.8 | 7.2 | 4.4 | 10.7 | 6.6 | 10.8 | 7.2 |
| Liver and intrahepatic bile duct | * | * | * | * | 6.9 | 2.4 | 20.8 | 5.3 | 10.5 | 3.4 | * | * |
| Lung and bronchus | 81.1 | 50.6 | 14.4 | * | 117.0 | 44.2 | 52.1 | 25.3 | 52.6 | 17.5 | 89.0 | 43.1 |
| Lymphomas: Non-Hodgkin's lymphoma | * | * | * | * | 13.2 | 7.6 | 12.4 | 6.8 | 12.9 | 9.0 | 12.5 | * |
| Lymphomas: Hodgkin's disease | * | * | * | * | 2.3 | 2.0 | * | * | * | * | * | * |
| Melanoma of the skin | * | * | * | * | 1.0 | 0.7 | * | * | * | * | * | * |
| Multiple myeloma | * | * | * | * | 11.3 | 7.4 | 2.3 | 1.8 | 4.8 | 2.6 | * | * |
| Nasopharynx | * | * | * | * | 1.0 | * | 10.8 | 3.9 | 3.9 | * | * | * |
| Oral cavity (excluding Nasopharynx) | * | * | * | * | 20.4 | 5.8 | 5.3 | 2.3 | 5.4 | 5.3 | 11.7 | * |
| Ovary | — | * | — | 17.5 | — | 10.2 | — | 9.3 | — | 10.2 | — | 11.8 |
| Pancreas | * | * | * | * | 14.0 | 11.5 | 8.0 | 4.9 | 6.5 | 6.0 | 10.9 | 8.7 |
| Prostate | 46.1 | — | 52.5 | — | 180.6 | — | 46.0 | — | 69.8 | — | 57.2 | — |
| Stomach | 27.2 | * | * | * | 17.9 | 7.6 | 15.7 | 8.3 | 8.5 | 5.3 | 20.5 | 13.0 |
| Testis | * | — | * | — | 0.8 | — | 1.7 | — | 1.3 | — | * | — |
| Thyroid | * | * | * | * | 1.4 | 3.3 | 2.1 | 6.5 | 4.1 | 14.6 | * | 9.1 |
| Urinary bladder | * | * | * | * | 15.2 | 5.8 | 13.0 | 3.7 | 8.3 | 2.1 | * | * |

62-3 and are based on cancer deaths for the entire U.S. population as provided by the National Center for Health Statistics.[14] Table 62-4 shows five-year relative survival rates for 1975–1984 based on data from the NCI Special Populations Studies Branch.[15]

In reviewing the incidence tables, the reader is advised that there are limitations in the SEER data and to interpret these data cautiously because (1) SEER data does not reflect the total U.S. population; (2) cancer rates in smaller populations (e.g., native Hawaiian, Japanese, Vietnamese) are less precise than rates in larger populations (e.g., African-Americans, white Americans); (3) the native American population is represented by two separate groups: Alaska native (composed of individuals who identified themselves as Aleut, Eskimo, or American Indian) and American Indian (New Mexico); and (4) individuals who classify themselves as being of Hispanic ethnicity may be of any race, resulting in some overlap between the Hispanic classification and the other ethnic groups. However, the SEER data are helpful in identifying general ethnic patterns of cancer. In the following paragraphs, several key cancer incidence, mortality, and survival data unique to each ethnic group will be presented.

*African-American* men have the highest overall cancer incidence rates. The particular sites for which high incidence and mortality rates have been identified in both African-American men and women include esophagus (almost three times that of white Americans), prostate, uterine cervix, liver, larynx, multiple myeloma, and stomach.[12] Their five-year survival rate, based on data collected from African-Americans diagnosed with cancer from 1986–1991, was approximately 42% as compared to 58% for white Americans.[12]

*Hispanics* are composed of several diverse subgroups including Mexican American, Cuban American, Puerto Rican American, and people from the Caribbean and

**TABLE 62-2** SEER Incidence Rates, 1988–1992, Selected Sites (continued)

| Cancer Site | Japanese M | Japanese W | Korean M | Korean W | Vietnamese M | Vietnamese W | White M | White W | Hispanic† (Total) M | Hispanic† (Total) W |
|---|---|---|---|---|---|---|---|---|---|---|
| All sites | 322 | 241 | 266 | 180 | 326 | 273 | **469** | **346** | 319 | 243 |
| Brain and nervous system | 2.1 | * | * | * | * | * | 7.8 | 5.4 | 5.2 | 3.8 |
| Breast, invasive | * | 82.3 | * | 28.5 | * | 37.5 | 0.9 | 111.8 | 0.6 | 69.8 |
| Cervix uteri | — | 5.8 | — | 15.2 | — | **43.0** | — | 8.7 | — | 16.2 |
| Colon and rectum | **64.1** | **39.5** | 31.7 | 21.9 | 30.5 | 27.1 | 56.3 | 38.3 | 38.3 | 24.7 |
| Corpus uteri | — | 14.5 | — | 3.8 | — | 8.4 | — | 22.3 | — | 13.7 |
| Esophagus | **5.6** | * | * | * | * | * | 5.4 | 1.7 | 4.4 | 0.9 |
| Kidney and renal pelvis | 7.3 | 2.3 | 6.3 | * | * | * | 11.9 | 5.9 | 10.0 | 5.5 |
| Larynx | 2.5 | * | * | * | * | * | 7.5 | 1.5 | 5.1 | 0.7 |
| Leukemias | 6.6 | 4.5 | 6.5 | 4.7 | 9.5 | 8.3 | 13.5 | 7.9 | 9.4 | 6.4 |
| Liver and intrahepatic bile duct | 6.3 | **3.9** | 24.8 | **10.0** | 41.8 | * | 3.7 | 1.5 | 6.7 | 2.6 |
| Lung and bronchus | 43.0 | 15.2 | 53.2 | 16.0 | 70.9 | 31.2 | 76.0 | 41.5 | 41.8 | 19.5 |
| Lymphomas: Non-Hodgkin's lymphoma | 11.6 | 7.8 | 5.8 | 6.0 | 15.8 | * | 18.7 | 12.0 | 14.1 | 9.1 |
| Lymphomas: Hodgkin's disease | * | * | * | * | * | * | 3.3 | 2.6 | 2.5 | 1.6 |
| Melanoma of the skin | * | * | * | * | * | * | 14.5 | 10.1 | 2.7 | 3.2 |
| Multiple myeloma | 1.6 | * | * | * | * | * | 5.0 | 3.2 | 4.2 | 3.0 |
| Nasopharynx | * | * | * | * | 7.7 | * | 0.6 | 0.2 | 0.6 | * |
| Oral cavity (excluding nasopharynx) | 7.0 | **3.3** | * | * | 11.6 | * | 14.6 | 5.8 | 8.9 | 2.7 |
| Ovary | — | 10.1 | — | 7.0 | — | 13.8 | — | 15.8 | — | 11.4 |
| Pancreas | 8.7 | 7.3 | * | **7.6** | * | * | 9.8 | 7.4 | 8.0 | 6.9 |
| Prostate | 88.0 | — | 24.2 | — | 40.0 | — | 134.7 | — | 89.0 | — |
| Stomach | **30.5** | **15.3** | **48.9** | **19.1** | 25.8 | **25.8** | 10.2 | 4.4 | 15.3 | 8.0 |
| Testis | 2.3 | — | * | — | * | — | 5.0 | — | 2.9 | — |
| Thyroid | 1.6 | 5.4 | * | 7.8 | * | 10.5 | 2.6 | 6.5 | 2.0 | 6.2 |
| Urinary bladder | 13.7 | 4.1 | 10.4 | * | * | * | 31.7 | 7.8 | 15.8 | 4.3 |

(Note: Rates are "average annual" per 100,000 population, age-adjusted to 1970 U.S. standard; — = not applicable; * = rate not calculated when fewer than 25 cases.)

Numbers in boldface = Top three rates, as applicable.

†These figures are for **general comparison** only as this group may overlap the other ethnic populations in this table.

Miller BA, Kolonel LN, Bernstein L, et al[14]

South and Central America. The latest SEER data incidence rates that are available for Hispanic Americans primarily reflect Mexican Americans from the Los Angeles, San Francisco/Oakland, San Jose/Monterey, and New Mexico areas. Hispanics rank overall in the middle for incidence and mortality rates when compared to other ethnic groups. However, Hispanics have high incidence rates for cervical, prostate, and urinary bladder cancers.[14]

Much like Hispanics, several subgroups are included under the term *Asian/Pacific Islanders.* Among these subgroups are the Chinese, Japanese, Filipino, Korean, Vietnamese, Laotian, Cambodian, Hmong, Thai, native Hawaiian, Samoan, and Micronesian. The latest SEER data provide information only for the Chinese, Japanese, Filipino, native Hawaiian, Korean, and Vietnamese groups. Within these subgroups alone, the data are also very diverse. Native Hawaiians have the highest overall cancer incidence and mortality rates among the API. When compared to all racial/ethnic groups, native Hawaiian women have the highest incidence rate for uterine cancer.[14] Japanese, Chinese, Filipino, and Korean Americans, on the other hand, have overall lower incidence and mortality rates as compared to African-Americans, Alaskan natives, whites, and native Hawaiians. However, there are specific sites for which each of these subgroups

**TABLE 62-3** United States Cancer Mortality Rates, 1988–1992

| Cancer Site | Alaska Native M | W | American Indian M | W | Black M | W | Chinese M | W | Filipino M | W | Hawaiian M | W |
|---|---|---|---|---|---|---|---|---|---|---|---|---|
| All sites | 225 | 179 | 123 | 99 | 319 | 168 | 139 | 86 | 105 | 63 | 239 | 168 |
| Brain & nervous system | * | * | * | * | 3.1 | 2.1 | 2.1 | 1.4 | 1.6 | 1.4 | * | * |
| Breast, invasive | * | * | * | * | 0.4 | 31.4 | * | 11.2 | * | 11.9 | * | 25.0 |
| Cervix uteri | — | * | — | * | — | 6.7 | — | 2.6 | — | 2.4 | — | * |
| Colon and rectum | 27.2 | 24.0 | * | * | 28.2 | 20.4 | 15.7 | 10.5 | 11.4 | 5.8 | 23.7 | 11.4 |
| Corpus uteri | — | * | — | * | — | 6.0 | — | 2.2 | — | 1.3 | — | 8.4 |
| Esophagus | * | * | * | * | 14.8 | 3.7 | 4.2 | * | 2.2 | * | * | * |
| Kidney and renal pelvis | * | * | * | * | 5.1 | 2.2 | 1.3 | 0.9 | 1.9 | * | * | * |
| Larynx | * | * | * | * | 5.6 | 0.9 | 0.9 | * | * | * | * | * |
| Leukemias | * | * | * | * | 8.0 | 4.6 | 3.6 | 2.4 | 5.7 | 2.9 | 7.8 | * |
| Liver and intrahepatic bile duct | * | * | * | * | 6.6 | 2.7 | 17.7 | 4.6 | 7.8 | 2.3 | 9.2 | * |
| Lung and bronchus | 69.4 | 45.3 | * | * | 105.6 | 31.5 | 40.1 | 18.5 | 29.8 | 10.0 | 88.9 | 44.1 |
| Lymphomas: Non-Hodgkin's lymphoma | * | * | * | * | 5.8 | 3.4 | 5.2 | 2.3 | 5.0 | 3.0 | 8.8 | * |
| Lymphomas: Hodgkin's disease | * | * | * | * | 0.7 | 0.4 | * | * | * | * | * | * |
| Melanoma of the skin | * | * | * | * | 0.5 | 0.4 | * | * | * | * | * | * |
| Multiple myeloma | * | * | * | * | 7.3 | 5.0 | 1.2 | 1.3 | 2.2 | 1.0 | * | * |
| Nasopharynx | * | * | * | * | 0.6 | 0.2 | 4.6 | 1.2 | 1.7 | * | * | * |
| Oral cavity (excluding nasopharynx) | * | * | * | * | 8.7 | 2.1 | 1.6 | 0.7 | 1.2 | 1.3 | * | * |
| Ovary | — | * | — | * | — | 6.6 | — | 4.0 | — | 3.4 | — | 7.3 |
| Pancreas | * | * | * | * | 14.4 | 10.4 | 6.7 | 5.1 | 4.5 | 3.5 | 12.8 | 9.1 |
| Prostate | * | — | 16.2 | — | 53.7 | — | 6.6 | — | 13.5 | — | 19.9 | — |
| Stomach | * | * | * | * | 13.6 | 5.6 | 10.5 | 4.8 | 3.6 | 2.5 | 14.4 | 12.8 |
| Testis | * | — | * | — | 0.1 | — | * | — | * | — | * | — |
| Thyroid | * | * | * | * | 0.3 | 0.4 | * | * | * | 1.1 | * | * |
| Urinary bladder | * | * | * | * | 4.8 | 2.4 | 2.0 | 1.0 | 1.2 | * | * | * |

have high incidence rates. For example, Japanese Americans have high incidence rates for stomach and colorectal cancers.[14,16] Chinese Americans have high incidence rates for oral cavity (in particular, nasopharyngeal cancer) and liver cancers.[8,14] Filipino Americans have the highest incidence rates for thyroid cancer.[14] However, Filipinos have the lowest mortality rates and have among the lowest incidence rates along with Koreans and American Indians (New Mexico). Vietnamese women have the highest incidence rates for cervical cancer while Vietnamese men have the highest incidence rates for liver and intrahepatic bile duct cancers. Other sources similarly report a high incidence of liver cancer in southeast Asian groups that has been attributed primarily to hepatitis B infection.[8,17,18]

Composed of many tribes and more than 400 federally recognized nations, *native Americans* are yet another group that is made up of diverse subgroups. However, the SEER data is limited to only a portion of this large group and, as mentioned earlier, reflects separate coding for Alaskan natives and American Indians living in New Mexico. Although native Americans (New Mexico American Indians) have the lowest cancer incidence rates and rank mid to low in cancer mortality rates, these rates may reflect their shorter life span rather than a true lower incidence and mortality rate.[14,19] Native Americans (New Mexico American Indians), in fact, have the lowest five-year relative survival rates.[15] Colon, rectum, and lung are high incidence sites for Alaska natives while cancers of the ovary and kidney and renal pelvis are high-incidence sites for the American Indians of New Mexico.[14]

Possible factors that contribute to these variations in cancer incidence and mortality in different ethnic

**TABLE 62-3**   United States Cancer Mortality Rates, 1988–1992 (continued)

| Cancer Site | Japanese M | Japanese W | White M | White W | Hispanic† (Total) M | Hispanic† (Total) W |
|---|---|---|---|---|---|---|
| All sites | 133 | 88 | 213 | 140 | 129 | 85 |
| Brain and nervous system | 1.3 | 1.1 | **5.4** | **3.7** | **3.0** | **2.0** |
| Breast, invasive | * | 12.5 | 0.2 | **27.0** | 0.1 | 15.0 |
| Cervix uteri | — | 1.5 | — | 2.5 | — | **3.4** |
| Colon and rectum | 20.5 | 12.3 | 22.9 | 15.3 | 12.8 | 8.3 |
| Corpus uteri | — | 1.9 | — | 3.2 | — | 2.3 |
| Esophagus | **4.8** | **0.9** | 5.3 | 1.2 | 3.4 | 0.7 |
| Kidney and renal pelvis | 2.4 | 0.8 | 5.0 | 2.3 | 3.7 | 1.7 |
| Larynx | * | * | 2.3 | 0.5 | 1.9 | 0.2 |
| Leukemias | 4.4 | 2.2 | 8.5 | 5.0 | 5.1 | 3.4 |
| Liver and intrahepatic bile duct | 6.2 | **4.0** | 3.8 | 1.8 | 5.9 | 2.8 |
| Lung and bronchus | 32.4 | 12.9 | **72.6** | **31.9** | 32.4 | 10.8 |
| Lymphomas: Non-Hodgkin's lymphoma | 4.8 | 3.9 | 8.1 | 5.3 | 5.3 | **3.6** |
| Lymphomas: Hodgkin's disease | * | * | 0.7 | 0.4 | 0.6 | 0.3 |
| Melanoma of the skin | * | * | 3.4 | 1.7 | 0.8 | 0.5 |
| Multiple myeloma | * | * | 3.4 | 2.2 | 2.7 | 1.8 |
| Nasopharynx | * | * | 0.3 | 0.1 | 0.3 | 0.1 |
| Oral cavity (excluding nasopharynx) | 2.1 | 0.8 | **3.8** | 1.5 | 2.7 | 0.7 |
| Ovary | — | 5.0 | — | 8.1 | — | 4.8 |
| Pancreas | 8.5 | 6.7 | 9.7 | 6.9 | 7.1 | 5.2 |
| Prostate | 11.7 | — | **24.1** | — | 15.3 | — |
| Stomach | **17.4** | **9.3** | 6.1 | 2.8 | 8.4 | 4.2 |
| Testis | * | — | 0.3 | — | 0.2 | — |
| Thyroid | * | * | 0.3 | 0.3 | 0.2 | 0.5 |
| Urinary bladder | 2.0 | **1.2** | 5.8 | 1.7 | **2.8** | 0.9 |

(Note: Rates are "average annual" per 100,000 population, age-adjusted to 1970 U.S. standard; — = not applicable; * = rate not calculated when fewer than 25 cases. No mortality data available for Korean and Vietnamese groups.)

**Numbers in boldface = Top three rates, as applicable.**

†These figures are for **general comparison** only as this group may overlap the other ethnic populations in this table.

Miller BA, Kolonel LN, Bernstein L, et al[14]

groups include environmental and/or socioeconomic factors; access to health care; cultural values, beliefs, and health practices; and genetic predisposition. These factors are often interdependent and interrelated. For example, low socioeconomic status (SES) in ethnic minorities has a major impact on cancer incidence and mortality. This impact was noted by the American Cancer Society in 1989 when the survival rate of socioeconomically disadvantaged Americans with cancer was estimated at 10%–15% lower than for other Americans.[20] However, low SES is usually not the only variable that is involved. Other associated variables may include environmental exposure to carcinogens in the workplace or home, higher smoking rates, and personal fatalistic attitudes regarding cancer. An in-depth discussion of these factors can be found elsewhere.[13] Table 62-5 provides a brief summary.

# TRANSCULTURAL NURSING AND ASSESSMENT

## Transcultural Nursing

The aim of transcultural nursing is to understand and assist diverse cultural groups and members of such groups

**TABLE 62-4**  Five-Year Relative Survival Rates (%) by Race/Ethnic Group, 1975–1984

| Cancer Site | White | Black | Chinese | Japanese | Filipino | American Indian | Mexican American | Native Hawaiian |
|---|---|---|---|---|---|---|---|---|
| All sites | 51.9 | 39.6 | 47.5 | 53.1 | 46.1 | 35.4 | 48.4 | 43.2 |
| Oral cavity | 54.0 | 33.0 | 55.7 | 44.4 | 46.6 | 38.6 | 60.7 | 42.8 |
| Esophagus | 6.5 | 4.2 | 11.5 | 5.8 | 3.4 | — | 0.0 | 0.0 |
| Stomach | 15.3 | 17.5 | 21.6 | 29.8 | 18.8 | 8.9 | 17.8 | 12.9 |
| Colon and rectum | 53.2 | 46.7 | 53.1 | 61.7 | 44.8 | 39.7 | 45.0 | 58.4 |
| Liver | 3.8 | 3.1 | 2.0 | 1.5 | 6.7 | 0.0 | 0.0 | 6.6 |
| Gallbladder | 9.2 | 8.9 | — | 16.2 | — | 2.8 | 8.5 | 26.2 |
| Pancreas | 2.7 | 3.2 | 0.0 | 2.6 | 5.2 | 0.0 | 1.2 | 0.0 |
| Lung | 13.2 | 11.7 | 15.1 | 14.3 | 13.2 | 0.0 | 10.8 | 13.0 |
| Melanoma (skin) | 81.2 | 57.5 | — | 81.0 | — | — | 82.1 | — |
| Breast | 76.1 | 63.2 | 80.8 | 85.4 | 73.7 | 46.2 | 70.6 | 68.0 |
| Cervix uteri | 68.2 | 61.6 | 74.6 | 70.2 | 73.0 | 63.5 | 70.5 | 67.7 |
| Corpus uteri | 86.0 | 54.9 | 86.1 | 84.1 | 79.9 | 82.7 | 77.0 | 74.6 |
| Ovary | 37.6 | 40.9 | 43.3 | 43.5 | 44.7 | 42.9 | 38.7 | 46.8 |
| Prostate | 72.6 | 63.4 | 72.5 | 80.5 | 71.7 | 54.2 | 72.4 | 72.0 |
| Urinary bladder | 76.6 | 53.4 | 78.5 | 80.8 | 58.4 | — | 64.6 | 51.4 |
| Kidney | 51.9 | 56.3 | 60.7 | 63.1 | 47.0 | 49.7 | 51.4 | 59.0 |
| Brain and CNS | 23.3 | 28.5 | 35.9 | 40.6 | 29.6 | 37.6 | 32.2 | 38.9 |
| Hodgkin's disease | 74.7 | 71.0 | — | — | 43.5 | — | 69.0 | 74.1 |
| Non-Hodgkin's lymphoma | 50.2 | 47.9 | 50.3 | 41.1 | 33.8 | 31.1 | 41.1 | 40.2 |
| Leukemia | 35.5 | 28.0 | 19.8 | 26.0 | 22.3 | 21.4 | 25.7 | 21.1 |

Reprinted with permission from the American Cancer Society, Inc., *Cancer Facts and Figures for Minority Americans*, 1991.

with their nursing and health care needs. A thorough assessment of the cultural aspects of an individual's lifestyle, health beliefs, and health practices will enhance the nurse's decision making and judgment when providing care. Nursing interventions that are culturally relevant and sensitive to the needs of the patient decrease the possibility of stress or conflict arising from cultural misunderstandings. There are often problems when individuals from two cultural backgrounds with conflicting values meet unless at least one is willing to recognize and adapt to the values of the other. One method is to sensitize nurses to their own cultural biases and behaviors as well as to those of their patients.[21]

Culture affects how patients are viewed by health care professionals and the care that is rendered. Each individual is culturally unique. It is essential that nurses avoid stereotyping or projecting onto patients their own "cultural uniqueness" or "world views" if culturally appropriate care is to be provided. Stereotyping is a simplified, generally inflexible conception of the members of a group or subgroup. It is an end point in that no attempt is made to learn whether the individual in question fits the statement. Generalizations and stereotypes may appear similar but function differently. Generalizations are starting points. They indicate common trends but further information is needed to ascertain whether the statement is appropriate to a particular individual. Generalizations are developed when looking for common patterns to beliefs and behaviors that are shared by a group. It is hoped that the nurse will use generalizations about specific ethnic minorities in planning culturally competent care. Regardless of the ethnic minority group, there are always differences among those within the group. Each individual is unique and a product of past experiences, beliefs, and values that have been learned and passed down from one generation to the next.

A nurse must carefully identify his or her personal cultural beliefs and values to separate them from the patient's beliefs and values. It is natural to view people unconsciously by using one's own group and customs as the standard for all judgments. A nurse with this tendency will gather data only selectively in accordance with personal standards, values, and judgment, and may not be able to see what the patient has to offer or the different way in which the patient views the world. This ethnocentric view may limit the data the nurse gathers,

**TABLE 62-5**   Major Variables Identifed in the Discrepancy of Cancer Incidence and Mortality in Ethnic Populations

| | |
|---|---|
| Physiological and biochemical differences | Genetic differences |
| |   Consanguinity |
| |   Mutation rates |
| |   Genetic predisposition or protective factors |
| | Environmental factors such as exposure to toxic elements and dietary influences |
| | Exposure to infectious agents |
| |   Hepatitis B → hepatoma |
| |   Schistosomiasis → bladder cancer |
| Socioeconomic factors | Poverty |
| |   Differential access to diagnostic facilities and medical treatment |
| |   Work exposure to toxic chemicals |
| |   Availability and affordability of health-promoting food sources in adequate quantities |
| |   Educational base |
| |     Knowledge about current treatment and value of early detection |
| |   Discrimination |
| | Insurance—underinsured and uninsured |
| | Costs of family and home care—direct and indirect |
| |   Shift from hospital to home for semiacute care and long-term care |
| Structural aspects of the health care system | Documentation |
| |   Errors of measurement |
| |   Completeness of morbidity and mortality data |
| |   Lack of completeness and detail in coding categories |
| |   Lack of representatives in the ethnic samples |
| | Availability issues |
| |   Lack of facilities within reasonable distances |
| | Accessibility |
| | Practitioner/patient interactions |
| |   Time restrictions in clinical encounters |
| |   Clinic setting in which different doctor is seen at each visit |
| |   Focus on chief complaint by practitioners so that if it is not cancer-related, screening is not recommended |
| | Institutional racism |
| Cultural factors | Misconceptions about culture |
| | Definition of culture |
| | Acculturation and assimilation |
| | Acceptability |
| | Differential use of available facilities |
| | Late stage of presentation |
| | Attitudes and beliefs about cancer |
| | Attitudes, beliefs, and practices associated with early detection and treatment of cancer |
| | Social stigma |
| | Lifestyle differences in personal customs or habits |
| |   Reproductive and nursing habits |
| |   Sexual practice |
| |   Smoking |
| |   Alcohol use |
| |   Diet |
| | Response to racism |

Reprinted with permission from Kagawa-Singer M.[13]

distort the assessment of the patient's behavior, and lead to conflicts between the nurse and the patient. The nurse must be aware of his or her own ethnicity as well as the Western health care culture of which she or he is a part. Cultural relativity, the attempt to view or interpret the behavior of culturally different individuals within the context of their own culture, is the nurse's goal. This perspective acknowledges that behavior that is appropriate in one culture may not be so in another culture. It provides meaning to patient or family behaviors that caregivers might otherwise consider negative or confusing.[1]

There are a few assumptions and propositions basic to the practice of transcultural nursing. One is the belief that caring is a universal phenomenon that varies only in form and manifestations. Caring for others exists in all cultures but the methods by which it is carried out and the meanings that caring conveys are as diverse as the groups that define them.

Another assumption is what is valued and judged as "good" care is culturally determined, culturally based, and culturally validated. Members of a cultural group can identify and define what is good care but outsiders probably cannot do so in the same way. The closer the nursing care matches the patients' values and expectations, the more likely that patients will accept it. Patient satisfaction with nursing care is linked to the extent that expectations are shared and met.

Thus, transcultural nursing is concerned with shared meanings and the degree to which the nurse and patient agree or disagree about the cultural symbols of health, healing, illness, disease, and caring. How cultural groups define and treat various illnesses, promote and maintain health, prevent illness, and structure their health care

system are basic knowledge requirements for effective transcultural nursing care.[21]

## Cultural Assessment

Nurses need knowledge to provide culturally appropriate care that is free of gender, race, or religious bias. Culturally appropriate care is based on an accurate assessment, a systematic appraisal or examination of individuals, groups, and communities as to their cultural beliefs, values, and practices. Using this assessment, patient needs and nursing interventions are identified within the cultural context of the people being evaluated.

One useful assessment model is Giger and Davidhizar's Transcultural Assessment Model, outlined in Figure 62-1.[22] In this model six essential cultural phenomena are identified that the nurse considers in providing culturally competent nursing care. These phenomena are evident in all cultural groups and include communication, space, social organization, time, environmental control, and biological variations.

The culturally unique individual is a significant component of this model. The model illustrates that each individual is a product of past experiences, cultural beliefs, and cultural norms and that there is diversity within

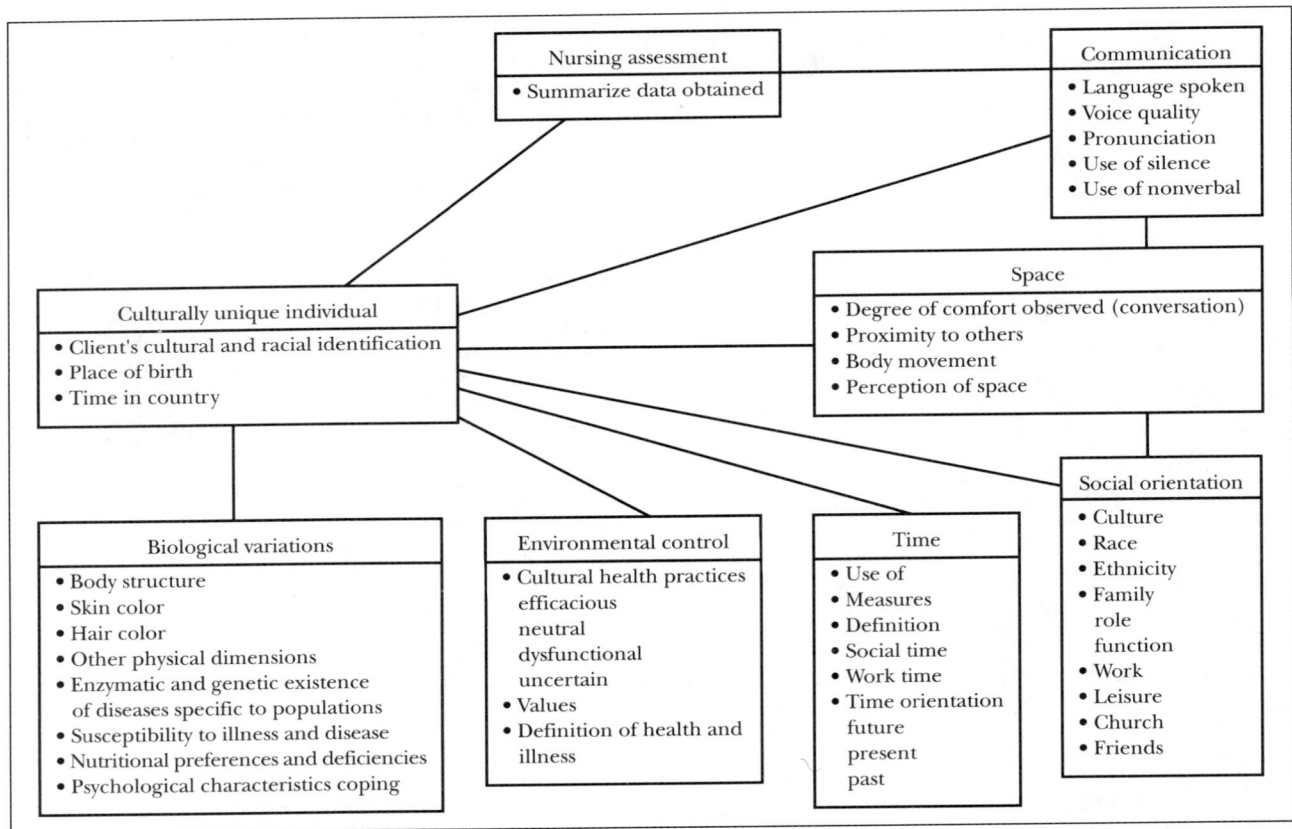

**FIGURE 62-1**   Giger and Davidhizar Transcultural Assessment Model. (Reprinted with permission from Giger JN and Davidhizar RE.[22])

cultural groups. However, knowledge of general baseline data relative to a specific cultural group is an excellent starting point to provide culturally appropriate care.

## Communication

Communication is the means by which culture is transmitted and preserved. Culture influences how feelings are expressed and what verbal and nonverbal expressions are appropriate. Cultural patterns of communication are embedded early and found in childrearing practices.

Verbal communication consists of both the spoken and written word. It includes vocabulary, grammatical structure, voice qualities, intonation, rhythm, speed, pronunciation, and use of silence. Language is basic to communication. Without it, the higher-order cognitive processes of thinking, reasoning, and generalizing cannot be conducted. Words are tools or symbols used to express ideas and feelings or to identify or describe objects. Words also shape experiences and influence cultural perceptions, convey interpretations, and influence relationships.

Developing familiarity with the patient's language is one of the best ways to gain insight into the individual's culture. Every language has a unique way of looking at the world and at experiences as well as a set of unconscious assumptions about the world and life.

The most obvious cultural difference among people is language. If the nurse does not speak the patient's language, a translator may be necessary. More often, however, the patient speaks the nurse's language with limited ability or uses language with denotative or connotative meanings different from the nurse's meaning.

The meaning of silence varies among cultural groups. Many native Americans and some traditional Chinese and Japanese people value silence and view it as essential to understanding an individual's needs. For people from Russia, France, or Spain silence may indicate agreement.[22,23]

Nonverbal communication includes touch, facial expressions, eye movement, and body posture. Through body language or motions, an individual conveys what cannot or may not be said in words. For a message to be accurately communicated, not only must words be translated but also the meaning held by nuances, intonation patterns, and facial expressions. Just as verbal behavior may undo nonverbal behavior, nonverbal behavior may repeat, clarify, contradict, modify, emphasize, or regulate the flow of communication.[24]

To communicate effectively with culturally diverse patients, the nurse needs to be aware of what nonverbal behaviors mean to the patient and what specific nonverbal behaviors mean in the patient's culture. It is not wise to assign meaning to nonverbal behaviors without validating their meaning with the patient.

In the United States, the mainstream culture views a firm, lengthy handshake as a symbol of good character and a sign of strength. For some native American groups, there is a light touch or grasp and just a passing of hands.

A vigorous handshake is viewed as an aggressive action.[24] Some societies believe that touch is magical and that the soul can leave the body on physical contact; therefore, casual touching is forbidden. In the southeast Asian Hmong culture, only certain elders are permitted to touch the head of others and children are never patted on the head.[25,26]

Communication is an essential part of establishing a relationship with a patient and family. Strategies for effective communication are outlined in Table 62-6.[24]

## Space

Space is a relative concept that includes the individual, the body, the surrounding environment, and objects within that environment. The relationship between the individual's own body, the objects, and people within the space is learned and influenced by one's culture. In Western cultures, spatial distances are defined as the intimate zone, the personal zone, and the social and public zones. The intimate zone is the smallest area of space around the individual, while the public zone is the largest area. The size of these areas varies with specific cultures. Americans, Canadians, and the British require more personal space while Latin Americans, Japanese, and Arabic individuals need the least amount of personal space and have a higher tolerance for crowding in public spaces.[27]

Personal space is the area that surrounds a person's body and includes space and objects within the space. An individual's comfort level is related to his or her personal space and discomfort is experienced when this personal space is invaded. Spatial behavior most often is described as a universal need for territoriality.

Territoriality is a state characterized by possessiveness, control, and authority over an area of physical space.[28] For the needs of territoriality to be met, the individual must be in control of some space, be able to establish rules for the space, and be able to defend it against invasion or misuse by others.[29] The use of restraints may increase the resistance by the patient since it involves physical invasion of personal space.

Nurses move through all spatial zones. Thus, the nurse must be sensitive to patients' reactions to movement toward them. A patient may physically withdraw or back away if the nurse is perceived as being too close. Explaining why there is a need to be close and asking permission to do so are helpful interventions.[4]

Objects in the environment may affect communication differently in different cultures. For example, positioning chairs at a 90-degree angle can communicate a cooperative stance whereas a side-by-side arrangement of chairs can decrease communication with Americans. Asians may feel more comfortable with a formal setting with the nurse behind a desk as they view health professionals as authority figures. The nurse's clothing, hair, jewelry, and fragrance also affect the message that the patient perceives. Symbols such as the stethoscope around the nurse's neck, name pins, uniforms, and caps

**TABLE 62-6**   Guidelines for Relating to Patients from Different Cultures

| Goal | Specific Actions |
|---|---|
| Assess your personal beliefs surrounding patients from different cultures. | • Review your personal beliefs and past experiences;<br>• Set aside any values, biases, ideas, and attitudes that are judgmental and may negatively affect care. |
| Assess communication variables from a cultural perspective. | • Determine the ethnic identity of the patient, including generation in America;<br>• Use the patient as a source of information when possible;<br>• Assess cultural factors that may affect your relationship with the patient and respond appropriately. |
| Plan care based on the communicated needs and cultural background. | • Learn as much as possible about the patient's cultural customs and beliefs;<br>• Encourage the patient to reveal cultural interpretation of health, illness, and health care;<br>• Be sensitive to the uniqueness of the patient;<br>• Identify sources of discrepancy between the patient's and your own concepts of health and illness;<br>• Communicate at the patient's personal level of functioning;<br>• Evaluate effectiveness of nursing actions and modify nursing care plan when necessary. |
| Modify communication approaches to meet cultural needs. | • Be attentive to signs of fear, anxiety, and confusion in the patient;<br>• Respond in a reassuring manner in keeping with the patient's cultural orientation;<br>• Be aware that in some cultural groups discussion concerning the patient with others may be offensive and may impede the nursing process. |
| Understand that respect for the patient and communicated needs is central to the therapeutic relationship. | • Communicate respect by using a kind and attentive approach;<br>• Learn how listening is communicated in the patient's culture;<br>• Use appropriate active listening techniques;<br>• Adopt an attitude of flexibility, respect, and interest to help bridge barriers imposed by culture. |
| Communicate in a nonthreatening manner. | • Conduct the interview in an unhurried manner;<br>• Follow acceptable social and cultural amenities;<br>• Ask general questions during the information-gathering stage;<br>• Be patient with a respondent who gives information that may seem unrelated to the patient's health problem;<br>• Develop a trusting relationship by listening carefully, allowing time, and giving the patient your full attention. |
| Use validating techniques in communication. | • Be alert for feedback that the patient is not understanding;<br>• Do not assume meaning is interpreted without distortion. |
| Be considerate of reluctance to talk when the subject involves sexual matters. | • Be aware that in some cultures sexual matters are not discussed freely with members of the opposite sex. |
| Adopt special approaches when the patient speaks a different language. | • Use a caring tone of voice and facial expression to help alleviate the patient's fears;<br>• Speak slowly and distinctly, but not loudly;<br>• Use gestures, pictures, and play acting to help the patient understand;<br>• Repeat the message in different ways if necessary;<br>• Be alert to words the patient seems to understand and use them frequently;<br>• Keep messages simple and repeat them frequently; |

**TABLE 62-6**  Guidelines for Relating to Patients from Different Cultures (continued)

| Goal | Specific Actions |
|---|---|
| Use interpreters to improve communication. | • Avoid using medical terms and abbreviations that the patient may not understand;<br>• Use an appropriate language dictionary.<br>• Ask the interpreter to translate the message, not just the individual words;<br>• Obtain feedback to confirm understanding;<br>• Use an interpreter who is culturally sensitive. |

Reprinted with permission from Giger JN and Davidhizar RE.[24]

may indicate to the patient that the nurse is a knowledgeable professional. In some cultures, the lack of these symbols may be viewed as a lack of competency or professionalism of the nurse.

Certain clothing or objects may be worn reflecting cultural beliefs. For example, a native American patient may wish to wear a medicine bundle.[30] Patients may wish to arrange their space differently and control the placement of objects on their bedside cabinet or over-bed table. These actions help establish the patient's personal space within which he/she feels a sense of control.

### Social organization

Cultural behavior or how one acts in certain situations is socially acquired. Patterns of cultural behavior are learned through enculturation that involves acquiring knowledge and internalizing values. Children learn cultural behavior by watching adults and making inferences about the rules of behavior. Patterns of cultural behavior are important to the nurse because they provide explanations for behavior related to life events. Life events that are significant transculturally include birth, death, puberty, childbearing, childrearing, illness, and disease.

Significant components of social organization include knowledge of family structure and organization, religious values and beliefs, and how ethnicity and culture relate to role and role assignment within group settings.[31]

The family is the basic unit of society. Cultural values can determine communication within the family, the norm for family size, and the roles of specific family members. In the Hispanic family the man is usually the provider and decision-maker. The woman may need to consult her husband prior to making decisions about her medical treatment or treatment of the children.[32] In native American and African-American families the mother or grandmother is viewed as the leader of the family and is usually the decision-maker. It is useful for the nurse to identify who has the "authority" to make decisions in a patient's family.

The value placed on children and elderly is also culturally determined. In some Scandinavian and native American cultures, children are not disciplined by physi-

cal punishment. They are allowed to interact with and to learn from their environment while caregivers provide subtle direction to prevent harm or injury. In Asian cultures, the elderly are considered the holders of the culture's wisdom and are highly respected. Responsibility for caring for elder relatives is dictated by cultural practices.

Gender roles are often culturally determined. In many cultures the woman is expected to maintain the home and raise the children. The man provides for and protects his family. In cultures in which women have little status and men dominate, as in many Middle Eastern and African countries, teaching from a female health provider may not be accepted.

The extent of the family's involvement in a hospitalized patient's care may be dictated by the culture. In some cultures, visits for long periods of time and participation in care is seen as a family responsibility. Personal and family information may be viewed as private and not to be shared even with health professionals. Patients from the Chinese culture may be offended by a nurse's questions during a proper assessment and may consider them to be invasive.[27]

Religions have an influence on the lifestyles of most cultures and may affect health care practices. Most religions have rituals that mark important events like birth, the entrance into adulthood, marriage, and death. Religious practices may prohibit eating certain foods (e.g., no pork for Jews and Muslims), eating a food on certain days (e.g., no meat on Good Friday for Roman Catholics), or accepting particular types of health care interventions (e.g., no blood transfusions for Jehovah's Witnesses). Religion may influence a patient's perception of the cause of an illness, its severity, and the type of healer required. As always, it is important not to assume that membership in a particular ethnic or cultural group is equated with a specific religion. Although many Hispanics are Catholics, assuming that a Mexican American patient is Catholic and offering to contact a priest may add to the patient's stress if he or she is not a Catholic.[1]

### Time

Time orientation refers to an individual's focus on the present or the future.[33] The American focus on time tends to be directed to the future, emphasizing planning and schedules. Long-range goals are important and health care measures in the present are often undertaken to prevent occurrence of illness in the future. Some African, Spanish, and southern European Americans are oriented more to the present than to the future. They may be late for appointments not because of their reluctance to make the appointment or lack of respect for the nurse but because they are more concerned about the activity in which they are currently engaged than about planning ahead to be on time. The present-oriented perspective is that time is flexible and events will begin when the person arrives.[4]

### Environmental control

Environmental control refers to the ability of members of a particular cultural group to plan activities that control nature or direct environmental factors. Since health is a balance between the individual and the environment, beliefs about causes of illness, health behaviors, and actions taken when illness or disease occur are all influenced by the individual's perception of the environment. This perception is in turn influenced by the individual's culture.

Herberg[34] describes three health belief views. In the magico-religious health belief view, health and illness are controlled by supernatural forces. Illness is seen as the result of being bad or opposing God's will. Thus, getting well also may be viewed as dependent on God's will. Some cultures believe magic can cause illness. For example, people from the West Indies may believe illness is the result of voodoo, while those from the Hispanic culture may believe that illness is caused by the evil eye or *mal ojo*. If a patient believes illness is due to a spell, then he or she may not recover until the spell is removed.

The scientific or biomedical health belief view is that life and life processes are controlled by physical and biochemical processes that can be manipulated by humans. Illness is caused by microorganisms or the breakdown of the body. The patient will expect medication, a treatment, or surgery to cure the health problem.

The holistic health view is that the forces of nature must be in balance or harmony. Human life is one aspect of nature and must be in harmony with the rest of nature. When the natural balance is disturbed, illness results. The Medicine Wheel is an ancient symbol used by native Americans of North and South America to express health and wellness. The four aspects of the individual's nature—the physical, the mental, the emotional, and the spiritual—must be in balance for the individual to be healthy. The concept of *yin* and *yang* from the Chinese and the hot/cold theory of illness in Hispanic cultures are other examples of holistic beliefs.[27]

Folk medicine is defined as those beliefs and practices relating to illness, prevention, and health that derive from cultural traditions rather than from modern medicine's scientific base. Folk medicine is thought to be more humanistic. The consultation and treatment take place in the community of the recipient, frequently in the home of the healer. The healer often prepares the treatment and frequently either the healer or patient performs some ritual practice. Because folk healing is culturally based, patients often find it more comfortable and less frightening than traditional Western medicine.

### Biological variations

Biological variations include differences in skin, eye, and hair color; facial characteristics; the amount of body hair; and body size and shape. Enzymatic and genetic variations may result in differences in the metabolism of drugs such as isoniazid, succinylcholine, caffeine, antihypertensives, and psychotropic drugs. Alcohol metabolism differs in European Americans from Asians because of different levels of the enzymes necessary for alcohol metabolism. The result is often facial flushing and palpitations in Asians after alcohol ingestion.

Some cultural groups are more susceptible to certain diseases. The increased or decreased incidence of a particular disease may be genetically determined. Nutritional preferences may also predispose certain cultural groups to particular diseases.[35]

Table 62-7 outlines a brief cultural assessment tool based on the Transcultural Assessment Model, which the nurse will find useful in gathering cultural data on patients and families.

## Heritage Consistency

People tend to assume the characteristics of the dominant culture where they reside via schools, television, radio, and motion pictures. The values and beliefs of a Vietnamese adolescent raised in the United States may be less traditional than his parents who immigrated to the United States. The heritage consistency theory views acculturation on a continuum and aids in assessing the degree to which people identify with the dominant or traditional cultures. It is possible to assess health beliefs by determining an individual's ties to traditional beliefs and his or her stage of acculturation. A relationship exists between strong personal identity with either a person's heritage or his or her level of acculturation, and the individual's health beliefs. Estes and Zitzow[36] developed a tool to assess and counsel alcoholic native Americans within a cultural context. It describes the degree to which lifestyle reflects tribal culture. The tool (Figure 62-2) has been expanded in an attempt to study the degree to which lifestyle reflects traditional culture.[37,38]

## Self Assessment

A major factor in working successfully with ethnic minorities is the nurse's knowledge about an ethnic group and

**TABLE 62-7   Cultural Assessment Tool**

| | |
|---|---|
| Culturally unique individual | Does the patient identify with a particular ethnic/racial/cultural group?<br>Where was the patient born?<br>How long has the patient lived in this country? |
| Communication | What language is spoken?<br>Can the patient communicate in English? If yes, both spoken and written?<br>Does the patient speak for self or defer to another?<br>What nonverbal communication behaviors are observed (e.g., touching, eye contact)? What significance do these behaviors have for the nurse-patient interaction? |
| Space | Observe the patient's proximity to other people and objects within the environment.<br>How does the patient react to the nurse's movement toward the patient?<br>Assess the patient's physical environment (especially important in home health nursing, community nursing, and long-term care nursing).<br>What cultural objects within the environment have importance for health promotion/health maintenance? |
| Social organization | What are the patient's roles? Is the patient the primary decision-maker for health care behaviors?<br>Must the patient consult another to make health decisions? If yes, who?<br>What other family members are important to the patient's decision making?<br>Are there cultural or religious leaders who are important in the client's health decision making?<br>Is there a religious affiliation linked with cultural affiliation (e.g., Jewish, Latino Catholic?) |
| Time | What is the patient's time orientation: past, present, or future?<br>What is the significance of time for the patient?<br>Does the patient talk about time in specific, such as dates or times, or in generalities, such as "a long time" or "a short time"? |
| Environmental control | How is health defined by the culture?<br>What does the patient believe to be the cause of the illness or health concern?<br>Has the patient used the services of cultural healers?<br>What healing practices has the patient used? Have folk healing behaviors been used?<br>Is the patient wearing or carrying any amulets or artifacts that are believed to have healing properties? |
| Biological variations | Are there normal variations in anatomic characteristics (e.g., body structure or size, skin color, facial characteristics)?<br>What are the dietary preferences of the patient? Are the dietary preferences related to the patient's ethnicity?<br>Is the patient at risk for nutritional deficiencies because of ethnicity (e.g., pernicious anemia, lactose intolerance)?<br>Are there variations in physiological functioning related to the patient's ethnicity or race (e.g., drug metabolism, alcohol metabolism)?<br>Are there illnesses or diseases that the patient is at risk for because of ethnicity or race (e.g., hypertension, diabetes mellitus, sickle-cell anemia)? |

From *Fundamentals of Nursing,* Fifth Edition, by Kozier, et al. Copyright (©) 1995 by Addison-Wesley Publishing Company. Reprinted by permission.

comfort in working with diverse populations. Figure 62-3[39] provides a simple tool for nurses to use in exploring their anticipated responses to 30 types of individuals representing five general categories: ethnic/racial, social issues/problems, religious, physically/mentally handicapped, and political. Completing the survey can assist the reader in identifying potential conflicts that could hinder effective professional care of specific categories of individuals.

# ETHNICITY AND CANCER

Spector[4] has summarized data for four major ethnic minority groups using the six cultural phenomena of the Transcultural Assessment Model. (See Table 62-8.[4,40]) In this section, the impact of ethnicity on responses to the cancer experience will be explored. For each of the four major ethnic groups, information about health beliefs and practices, healing practices, social organization, communication, space and time, death and dying, and biological variations will be presented. This information provides only a guideline for practice; each person is culturally unique. Nursing interventions that consider the patient and family's cultural background must be based on a sound assessment and validation of the role culture plays in the life of the patient and family.

There are many subgroups within the four major ethnic groups (African-American, API, Hispanic, and native American). It is beyond the scope of this chapter to provide an in-depth description of each subgroup's cultural

## Ethnic, Cultural, Religious Background

This set of questions is to be used to describe a given patient's—or your own—ethnic, cultural, and religious background. In performing a *heritage assessment* it is helpful to determine how deeply a given person identifies with his or her traditional heritage. This tool is most useful in setting the stage for assessing and understanding a person's traditional health and illness beliefs and practices and in helping to determine the community resources that will be appropriate to target for support when necessary. The greater the number of positive responses, the greater the degree to which the person may identify with his or her traditional heritage. The one exception to positive answers is the question about whether or not a person's name was changed.

1. Where was your mother born? _____
2. Where was your father born? _____
3. Where were your grandparents born? _____
   a. Your mother's mother? _____
   b. Your mother's father? _____
   c. Your father's mother? _____
   d. Your father's father? _____
4. How many brothers _____ and sisters _____ do you have?
5. What setting did you grow up in? Urban _____ Rural _____
6. What country did your parents grow up in?
   Father _____
   Mother _____
7. How old were you when you came to the United States? _____
8. How old were your parents when they came to the United States?
   Mother _____
   Father _____
9. When you were growing up, who lived with you? _____

10. Have you maintained contact with
    a. Aunts, uncles, cousins? (1) Yes _____ (2) No _____
    b. Brothers and sisters? (1) Yes _____ (2) No _____
    c. Parents? (1) Yes _____ (2) No _____
    d. Your own children? (1) Yes _____ (2) No _____
11. Did most of your aunts, uncles, cousins live near your home?
    (1) Yes _____ (2) No _____
12. Approximately how often did you visit family members who lived outside of your home?
    (1) Daily _____ (2) Weekly _____ (3) Monthly _____
    (4) Once a year or less _____ (5) Never _____
13. Was your original family name changed?
    (1) Yes _____ (2) No _____
14. What is your religious preference?
    (1) Catholic _____ (2) Jewish _____
    (3) Protestant _____ Denomination _____
    (4) Other _____ (5) None _____
15. Is your spouse the same religion as you?
    (1) Yes _____ (2) No _____
16. Is your spouse the same ethnic background as you?
    (1) Yes _____ (2) No _____
17. What kind of school did you go to?
    (1) Public _____ (2) Private _____ (3) Parochial _____
18. As an adult, do you live in a neighborhood where the neighbors are the same religion and ethnic background as yourself?
    (1) Yes _____ (2) No _____
19. Do you belong to a religious institution?
    (1) Yes _____ (2) No _____
20. Would you describe yourself as an active member?
    (1) Yes _____ (2) No _____
21. How often do you attend your religious institution?
    (1) More than once a week _____ (2) Weekly _____ (3) Monthly _____
    (4) Special holidays only _____ (5) Never _____
22. Do you practice your religion in your home?
    (1) Yes _____ (2) No _____ (if yes, please specify)
    (3) Praying _____ (4) Bible reading _____ (5) Diet _____
    (6) Celebrating religious holidays _____

**FIGURE 62-2** Heritage Assessment Tool.

23. Do you prepare foods special to your ethnic background?
   (1) Yes _____   (2) No _____
24. Do you participate in ethnic activities?
   (1) Yes _____   (2) No _____ (if yes, please specify)
   (3) Singing _____   (4) Holiday celebrations _____
   (5) Dancing _____   (6) Festivals _____
   (7) Costumes _____   (8) Other _____
25. Are your friends from the same religious background as you?
   (1) Yes _____   (2) No _____
26. Are your friends from the same ethnic background as you?
   (1) Yes _____   (2) No _____
27. What is your native language? _____
28. Do you speak this language?
   (1) Prefer _____   (2) Occasionally _____   (3) Rarely _____
29. Do you read your native language?
   (1) Yes _____   (2) No _____

**FIGURE 62-2**   Heritage Assessment Tool (continued).

Reprinted with permission from Spector RE: *Cultural Diversity in Health and Illness* (ed 4). Stamford, CT, Appleton & Lange, 1996.

beliefs and practices. Instead relevant group characteristics to the cancer experience are presented. Various sources are available that further explore the individual subgroups.[41–47]

## African-Americans

Most African-Americans were brought to the United States as slaves between 1619 and 1860 from the west coast of Africa. Many have also immigrated to the United States from other African countries, the West Indies, the Dominican Republic, Haiti, and Jamaica.[4] African-Americans constitute about one-tenth of the total U.S. population, but are disproportionately represented among the poor. They represent about one-third of the population below poverty level, and one-fourth are unemployed. Individuals in a lower socioeconomic group are at greater risk for illness because seeking health care for early symptoms and preventive care are not priorities for those who struggle with day-to-day survival.

Many African-Americans worked or continue to work in occupations that place them at risk for certain cancers. African-Americans were employed disproportionately in jobs involving coke ovens with greatest exposure to benzo-(a)-pyrene and other carcinogens. Years later, these workers had ten times the lung cancer rates, elevated skin cancer rates, and increased nonmalignant lung diseases. Compared to other races, more African-Americans worked in the rubber industry and developed increased rates of stomach, lung, blood, bladder, lymphatic, and prostate cancers.[48]

In general, the overall cancer incidence rate for African-American males is about 16% higher than that for Caucasian males. Among the different ethnic groups, African-Americans have the highest incidence and mortality rates for cancers of the esophagus, larynx, pancreas, and prostate, and for multiple myeloma. African-American women have the highest mortality rate for cervical cancer and African-American men have the highest incidence and mortality rates for lung cancer. African-American women experience significantly more cervical cancer and early-age breast cancer than Caucasians. The five-year survival rate from all cancers is about 16% lower for African-Americans than that for Caucasians.[49]

### Health beliefs and practices

The health beliefs of African-Americans include a tendency to categorize events as either desirable or undesirable. Illness is just another undesirable event along with bad luck, poverty, and unemployment. Some believe illness results from their failure to live according to or to accept God's will. An individual may believe that cancer is an unnatural illness, caused by supernatural or sinful behavior, and that it cannot be treated by Western medicine.

There is a strong relationship between faith and healing. All blessings come from God and only God can heal the sick. Illness may be perceived as a natural occurrence resulting from disharmony and conflict in some aspect of an individual's life, generally falling into one of three main areas: divine punishment, impaired social relationships, and environmental hazards. Divine punishment attributes illness to sin. An example of an impaired social relationship may be a spouse leaving or parents disowning a child. Environmental hazards include being struck by lightning or bitten by a snake.

Another belief among some African-Americans is that everything has an opposite. For every birth, there is a death; for every marriage, there is a divorce. Some may not distinguish between physical and mental illness and spiritual problems and may present themselves for treatment with a combination of somatic, psychological, and spiritual complaints. The nurse must acknowledge the patient's health belief system if the nurse expects the patient to participate in Western practices.

## How Do You Relate to Various Groups of People in Society?

Described below are different levels of response you might have toward a person.

**Levels of Response**
1. *Greet:* I believe I can *greet* this person warmly and welcome him or her sincerely.
2. *Accept:* I believe I can honestly *accept* this person as he or she is and be comfortable enough to listen to his or her problems.
3. *Help:* I believe I would genuinely try to *help* this person with his or her problems as they might relate to or arise from the label-stereotype given to him or her.
4. *Background:* I believe I have the *background* of knowledge and/or experience to be able to help this person.
5. *Advocate:* I believe I could honestly be an *advocate* for this person.

The following is a list of individuals. Read down the list and place a checkmark next to anyone you would *not* "greet" or would hesitate to "greet." Then move to response level 2, "accept," and follow the same procedure. Try to respond honestly, not as you think might be socially or professionally desirable. Your answers are only for your personal use in clarifying your initial reactions to different people.

| | Level of Response | | | | |
|---|---|---|---|---|---|
| | 1 | 2 | 3 | 4 | 5 |
| **Individual** | **Greet** | **Accept** | **Help** | **Background** | **Advocate** |
| 1. Haitian | ☐ | ☐ | ☐ | ☐ | ☐ |
| 2. Child abuser | ☐ | ☐ | ☐ | ☐ | ☐ |
| 3. Jew | ☐ | ☐ | ☐ | ☐ | ☐ |
| 4. Person with hemophilia | ☐ | ☐ | ☐ | ☐ | ☐ |
| 5. Neo-Nazi | ☐ | ☐ | ☐ | ☐ | ☐ |
| 6. Mexican American | ☐ | ☐ | ☐ | ☐ | ☐ |
| 7. IV drug user | ☐ | ☐ | ☐ | ☐ | ☐ |
| 8. Catholic | ☐ | ☐ | ☐ | ☐ | ☐ |
| 9. Senile, elderly person | ☐ | ☐ | ☐ | ☐ | ☐ |
| 10. Teamster Union member | ☐ | ☐ | ☐ | ☐ | ☐ |
| 11. Native American | ☐ | ☐ | ☐ | ☐ | ☐ |
| 12. Prostitute | ☐ | ☐ | ☐ | ☐ | ☐ |
| 13. Jehovah's Witness | ☐ | ☐ | ☐ | ☐ | ☐ |
| 14. Cerebral palsied person | ☐ | ☐ | ☐ | ☐ | ☐ |
| 15. ERA proponent | ☐ | ☐ | ☐ | ☐ | ☐ |
| 16. Vietnamese American | ☐ | ☐ | ☐ | ☐ | ☐ |
| 17. Gay/lesbian | ☐ | ☐ | ☐ | ☐ | ☐ |
| 18. Atheist | ☐ | ☐ | ☐ | ☐ | ☐ |
| 19. Person with AIDS | ☐ | ☐ | ☐ | ☐ | ☐ |
| 20. Communist | ☐ | ☐ | ☐ | ☐ | ☐ |
| 21. Black American | ☐ | ☐ | ☐ | ☐ | ☐ |
| 22. Unmarried expectant teenager | ☐ | ☐ | ☐ | ☐ | ☐ |
| 23. Protestant | ☐ | ☐ | ☐ | ☐ | ☐ |
| 24. Amputee | ☐ | ☐ | ☐ | ☐ | ☐ |
| 25. Ku Klux Klansman | ☐ | ☐ | ☐ | ☐ | ☐ |
| 26. White Anglo-Saxon | ☐ | ☐ | ☐ | ☐ | ☐ |
| 27. Alcoholic | ☐ | ☐ | ☐ | ☐ | ☐ |
| 28. Amish person | ☐ | ☐ | ☐ | ☐ | ☐ |
| 29. Person with cancer | ☐ | ☐ | ☐ | ☐ | ☐ |
| 30. Nuclear armament proponent | ☐ | ☐ | ☐ | ☐ | ☐ |

**Scoring Guide:** The previous activity may help you anticipate difficulty in working with some patients at various levels. The 30 types of individuals can be grouped into 5 categories: ethnic/racial, social issues/problems, religious, physically/mentally handicapped, and political. Transfer your checkmarks to the following form. If you have a concentration of checks within a specific category of individuals or at specific levels, this may indicate a conflict that could hinder you from rendering effective professional help.

| | 1 | 2 | 3 | 4 | 5 |
|---|---|---|---|---|---|
| **Individual** | **Greet** | **Accept** | **Help** | **Background** | **Advocate** |
| **Ethnic/racial** | | | | | |
| 1. Haitian American | ☐ | ☐ | ☐ | ☐ | ☐ |
| 6. Mexican American | ☐ | ☐ | ☐ | ☐ | ☐ |
| 11. Native American | ☐ | ☐ | ☐ | ☐ | ☐ |
| 16. Vietnamese American | ☐ | ☐ | ☐ | ☐ | ☐ |

**FIGURE 62-3** Self-Assessment Tool.

*(continued)*

| | Level of Response | | | | |
|---|---|---|---|---|---|
| | 1 | 2 | 3 | 4 | 5 |
| **Individual** | Greet | Accept | Help | Background | Advocate |
| 21. Black American | ☐ | ☐ | ☐ | ☐ | ☐ |
| 26. White Anglo-Saxon | ☐ | ☐ | ☐ | ☐ | ☐ |
| **Social Issues/Problems** | | | | | |
| 2. Child abuser | ☐ | ☐ | ☐ | ☐ | ☐ |
| 7. IV drug user | ☐ | ☐ | ☐ | ☐ | ☐ |
| 12. Prostitute | ☐ | ☐ | ☐ | ☐ | ☐ |
| 17. Gay/lesbian | ☐ | ☐ | ☐ | ☐ | ☐ |
| 22. Unmarried expectant teenager | ☐ | ☐ | ☐ | ☐ | ☐ |
| 27. Alcoholic | ☐ | ☐ | ☐ | ☐ | ☐ |
| **Religious** | | | | | |
| 3. Jew | ☐ | ☐ | ☐ | ☐ | ☐ |
| 8. Catholic | ☐ | ☐ | ☐ | ☐ | ☐ |
| 13. Jehovah's Witness | ☐ | ☐ | ☐ | ☐ | ☐ |
| 18. Atheist | ☐ | ☐ | ☐ | ☐ | ☐ |
| 23. Protestant | ☐ | ☐ | ☐ | ☐ | ☐ |
| 28. Amish person | ☐ | ☐ | ☐ | ☐ | ☐ |
| **Physically/Mentally Handicapped** | | | | | |
| 4. Person with hemophilia | ☐ | ☐ | ☐ | ☐ | ☐ |
| 9. Senile elderly person | ☐ | ☐ | ☐ | ☐ | ☐ |
| 14. Cerebral palsied person | ☐ | ☐ | ☐ | ☐ | ☐ |
| 19. Person with AIDS | ☐ | ☐ | ☐ | ☐ | ☐ |
| 24. Amputee | ☐ | ☐ | ☐ | ☐ | ☐ |
| 29. Person with cancer | ☐ | ☐ | ☐ | ☐ | ☐ |
| **Political** | | | | | |
| 5. Neo-Nazi | ☐ | ☐ | ☐ | ☐ | ☐ |
| 10. Teamster Union member | ☐ | ☐ | ☐ | ☐ | ☐ |
| 15. ERA proponent | ☐ | ☐ | ☐ | ☐ | ☐ |
| 20. Communist | ☐ | ☐ | ☐ | ☐ | ☐ |
| 25. Ku Klux Klansman | ☐ | ☐ | ☐ | ☐ | ☐ |
| 30. Nuclear armament proponent | ☐ | ☐ | ☐ | ☐ | ☐ |

**FIGURE 62-3**  Self-Assessment Tool (continued).

Reproduced with permission of the Association for the Care of Children's Health, 7910 Woodmont Avenue, Suite 300, Bethesda, MD 20814, from Randall-David E.: *Strategies for Working with Culturally Diverse Communities and Clients.* Bethesda, Association for the Care of Children's Health, 1989, pp. 7–9.

Some African-Americans may respond to pain stoically out of a desire to be a perfect patient; others may view pain as God's will. These individuals may need to be taught that pain retards healing and is medically undesirable.

African-Americans tend to be less knowledgeable about cancer than Caucasians and tend to underestimate the prevalence of cancer and the significance of the common warning signs for cancer. They are less likely to see a physician when experiencing warning signs or symptoms and less aware of the benefits of specific cancer screening methods. African-Americans are often more fatalistic about cancer and are less likely to believe that early detection or treatment can make a difference in the outcome of the disease. These factors lead to diagnosis at a later stage of illness, a poorer prognosis, and higher mortality rates for cancer.[49]

African-Americans are more likely than Caucasians to prefer to remain ignorant of their own cancer diagnosis. They are also less likely than Caucasians to regard surgery, chemotherapy, and radiation as effective cancer treatment measures and less optimistic about the chances of surviving cancer. In one study 64.3% of African-Americans believed that cancer was a death sentence, and 65.3% believed that treatment is worse than the disease. Eighty percent believed that cancer was spread by surgical treatment, and 20% indicated that they would rather not know that they had cancer.[50] Thus, nurses may find African-American patients unwilling, uncooperative, or what may appear to be noncompliant, partners in their treatment.[49]

African-American attitudes about the U.S. health care system may be explained partially by history. During slavery, African-Americans received inconsistent and often barbaric health care treatment and developed a deep mistrust of their white master and his harsh remedies and prescriptions. Even after slavery was abolished, African-Americans often received poor health care and inferior treatment in hospitals and clinics, that only reinforced their negative view of Western medicine, and led to a

**TABLE 62-8** Cross-Cultural Examples of Cultural Phenomena That Have an Impact on Nursing Care

| Nations of Origin | Environmental Control | Biological Variations* | Social Organization | Communication | Space | Time Orientation |
|---|---|---|---|---|---|---|
| **Asian**<br>China<br>Hawaii<br>Philippines<br>Korea<br>Japan<br>Southeast Asia (Laos, Cambodia, Vietnam) | Traditional health and illness beliefs<br>Use of traditional medicines<br>Traditional practitioners: Chinese doctors and herbalists | Liver cancer<br>Stomach cancer<br>Coccidioidomycosis<br>Hypertension<br>Lactose intolerance | Family: hierarchial structure, loyalty<br>Devotion to tradition<br>Many religions, including Taoism, Buddhism, Islam, and Christianity<br>Community social organizations | National language preference<br>Dialects, written characters<br>Use of silence<br>Nonverbal and contextual cuing | Noncontact people | Present |
| **African**<br>West Coast (as slaves)<br>Many African countries<br>West Indian Islands<br>Dominican Republic<br>Haiti<br>Jamaica | Traditional health and illness beliefs<br>Folk medicine tradition<br>Traditional healer: root-worker | Sickle cell anemia<br>Hypertension<br>Cancer of the esophagus<br>Stomach cancer<br>Coccidioidomycosis<br>Lactose intolerance | Family: many female, single parent<br>Large, extended family networks<br>Strong church affiliation within community<br>Community social organizations | National languages<br>Dialect: Pidgin, Creole, Spanish, and French | Close personal space | Present over future |
| **Europe**<br>Germany<br>England<br>Italy<br>Ireland<br>Other European countries | Primary reliance on modern health care system<br>Traditional health and illness beliefs<br>Some remaining folk medicine tradition | Breast cancer<br>Heart disease<br>Diabetes mellitus<br>Thalassemia | Nuclear families<br>Extended families<br>Judeo-Christian religions<br>Community social organizations | National languages<br>Many learn English immediately | Noncontact people<br>Aloof<br>Distant<br>Southern countries: closer contact and touch | Future over present |
| **Native American**<br>170 Native American Tribes<br>Aleuts<br>Eskimos | Traditional health and illness beliefs<br>Folk medicine tradition<br>Traditional healer: medicine man | Accidents<br>Heart disease<br>Cirrhosis of the liver<br>Diabetes mellitus | Extremely family oriented<br>Biological and extended families<br>Children taught to respect traditions<br>Community social organizations | Tribal languages<br>Use of silence and body language | Space very important and has no boundaries | Present |
| **Hispanic countries**<br>Spain<br>Cuba<br>Mexico<br>Central and South America | Traditional health and illness beliefs<br>Folk medicine tradition<br>Traditional healers: *Curandero, Espiritista, Partera, Senora* | Diabetes mellitus<br>Parasites<br>Coccidioidomycosis<br>Lactose intolerance | Nuclear family<br>Extended families<br>Compadrazgo: godparents<br>Community social organizations | Spanish or Portuguese primary language | Tactile relationships<br>Touch<br>Handshakes<br>Embracing<br>Value physical presence | Present |

*Indicates a high morbidity incidence.

Adapted with permission from Spector RE.[4]

high level of caution and mistrust.[51] African-Americans may choose not to seek care if they perceive that values will be compromised. To work effectively with African-American patients and families, the nurse will need to convey caring and understanding.

### Healing practices

A variety of folk healers are used by African-Americans. These healers are well-respected individuals and can be a powerful resource to the health care team. The healers understand the beliefs and needs of the people they serve. Symptoms may be of minor importance. Cure may involve self-treatment, consultation with a neighbor knowledgeable in home remedies, a physician, or someone regarded to have unusual powers. Religion is incorporated as part of therapy and is a means to a cure. There is a lay referral system that services the health needs of the community, and determines whether Western practitioners can be trusted and incorporated into the treatment. Openness, acceptance, and cooperation with this referral system by health care professionals may enhance acceptance and use of Western health care providers by African-Americans.

Help may be sought from the "old lady," a woman in the community who acts as a local consultant. She is knowledgeable about different home remedies made from spices, herbs, and roots used to treat common illnesses. She also gives advice and makes appropriate referrals to another type of practitioner when an illness or a particular medical condition extends beyond her practice.[52] The spiritualist has received the gift from God for healing incurable diseases or solving personal problems. This practitioner combines rituals, spiritual beliefs, and herbal medicines and is the most prevalent and diverse type of folk practitioner. There is a root doctor who meets the needs for herbs, oils, candles, and ointments. The Voodoo priest/priestess may inherit this title only by birthright and is perceived to have a special gift. Voodoo, which combines African, Christian, and magical beliefs related to religion and health care, is practiced by some African-Americans. It is believed to cause, as well as prevent, the action of malevolent forces. Awareness of what home remedies have been used would help the nurse understand cultural practices and determine if they are helpful, harmful, or neutral.[49,53]

A treatment plan that is congruent with the patient's own beliefs has a better chance of being successful. Cultural health practices that are helpful should be encouraged. For example, use of herbal teas in place of water can serve both traditional and Western practices.

### Social organization

Because of legalized segregation, African-Americans were isolated from mainstream society. Even today, many African-Americans have not assimilated into mainstream society, maintaining separate and often unequal lifestyles as compared to other Americans.

Under slavery, the role of the African-American male as husband and father was obliterated. He was not the head of the household or provider or protector of his family. He was someone's property. This history likely contributes to the large number of female-headed households among African-Americans today. The number of female-headed households has doubled between 1950 and 1991 to represent 46% of all African-American families.[54]

The African-American family is often oriented around women, and the wife or mother generally is charged with the responsibility for protecting the health of family members. The woman is expected to assist each family member in maintaining good health and in determining treatment if a family member is ill. Family members may enter the health care system at the advice of the matriarch of the family. Thus, the importance of the African-American woman in sharing information and helping the patient in decision making is important for the nurse to recognize.[53,55]

Some families have large social networks that are very supportive during times of illness. The added numbers may be helpful in provision of care and support but also may delay seeking help outside the network while consultation among the various members takes place. Including the members of the network in planning care may decrease the possibility of conflicting messages between the nurse and members of the network.[53]

Most African-Americans have a strong religious orientation and most belong to the Protestant faith, often Baptist or one of a number of other smaller fundamentalist denominations. Many African-Americans find it impossible to separate religious beliefs from health beliefs.[56] The most common and frequently cited method of treating illness remains prayer.[1]

The church plays an important role in the lives of African-Americans by championing their interests and providing tangible assistance during periods of economic and social instability. African-American churches meet not only the spiritual, but also the educational, physical, and social needs of their members. The church has been in a position to help African-Americans cope with and overcome the social and political barriers of unequal access to resources.[57,58]

The church is also a source of social identity, and allows escape from the harsh realities of life. It promotes self-esteem among its membership and serves as a curator for maintaining the cultures of many African-Americans. Given the importance of the church in the lives of many African-Americans, inclusion of the clergy in the health care team may be very helpful.

### Communication

The dialect that is spoken by many African-Americans is sufficiently different from standard English in pronunciation, grammar, and syntax as to be classified as "black English." The use of standard English versus black English varies among African-Americans and is sometimes related to educational level and socioeconomic status. Black English is a unifying factor for African-Americans in maintaining their cultural and ethnic identity. It is not uncommon for some African-Americans to speak standard English when in a professional capacity or when socializing with Caucasians, and then revert back to black English when in African-American settings. Some African-Americans who have not mastered standard English may become very quiet in settings in which they believe that standard English is required. This may be incorrectly interpreted as hostility, submissiveness, or agreement.[53]

Black English may be viewed from both linguistic and stylistic perspectives. Grammatical structure and word usage is the focus of the linguistic aspect. For example, there is no "th" sound in West African languages; thus words ending in "th" becoming "f" as in *mouf* for mouth and words beginning with "th" become "d" as in the words *dese, dat,* and *dem* for these, that, and them. The stylistic aspect refers to the communication power of black English. Black English is highly oral, stylized, rhythmic, and spontaneous. It is not an exact science, how it is spoken makes it black. The meanings of words are conveyed by how they are said (intonation and inflections), where they are placed in relation to each other, and how fast they are spoken. The power is seen in the various rituals, forms, or modes; and in sermons, raps, spirituals, and soul songs. The language reflects cultural attitudes toward time, nature, the universe, death, and evil.[59] African-Americans live with black English and dictate what happens to it. Black English means more than its words and is often only partially translatable. Words and expressions are not always meant to be defined and may not be understood by nonAfrican-Americans because many times they are meant to convey hardship, hope, reality, and possibilities.[60]

For more effective communication, the nurse who works with African-Americans must understand as much of the context of the dialect as possible. Viewing black English as an unacceptable form of English may lead to labeling and stereotyping the patient. Chiding and correcting the speech of African-Americans may result in the patient becoming quiet, passive, aggressive, or hostile. On the other hand, attempting to use words common to the patient's vocabulary and mimicking the language may be interpreted as dehumanizing.

Slang is also used and may have different meanings among individuals and among cultural groups. Clarifying the meaning of the slang terms is useful to prevent miscommunication. Words used by patients may be the same as those used by the nurse but may have different, idiosyncratic meanings for the patient. Using words commonly understood by African-Americans in place of more sophisticated medical terms might make the patient more receptive to teaching and more cooperative. Examples of such words include "miseries" for pain, "tired or low blood" for anemia, "throw up" for vomit, and "pass water, tinkle, or peepee" for urinate.

According to Sue,[61] some African-Americans may place a great deal of importance on nonverbal elements of communication. When working with African-American patients, keep in mind that eye contact, nodding, and smiling do not necessarily mean that the African-American patient is paying attention. Validation of the message is very important in improving communication. Nurses may find it difficult to communicate with African-American patients who speak loudly and seem hostile and aggressive. However, it is the expressive quality of black English that is often responsible for this behavior.[60]

Bigham[62] suggests a variety of ways to lessen the communication barrier between African-American patients and the nonAfrican-American nurse:

- treat African-Americans as you would normally treat others;

- use titles such as "Mr., Mrs., or Miss" unless your acquaintance is on a first name basis;

- do not patronize an African-American merely because of his or her race; and

- do not attempt to impress African-Americans by telling them about other members of their race who you know.

### Space and time

Many African-Americans have a "today" or "present" health orientation and their approach to the prevention of cancer may be to work out problems as they occur, rather than trying to prevent them from occurring. This approach is based on the belief that planning for the future is hopeless and is based on previous experiences with racism and discrimination. Many African-Americans believe that their future will be the same as their present and past.[63] This attitude about time and future may be translated as an acceptable lateness of 30 minutes to an hour. In planning nursing care for individuals with such time orientation, plan to explain when flexibility of time is acceptable and when a delay might result in a serious problem. Acceptance of lateness in appointments is helpful when possible.

African-Americans are highly involved people who tend to have several activities going on at the same time. This may create conflict for the nurse, who, in an effort to complete his or her nursing care, may be interrupted often by these activities. Negotiating with the patient and family to meet the needs of both the nurse and the patient may be helpful.

### Death and dying issues

In African language the primary time frames are past and present. No word exists for the distant future, as it has not yet happened. Consequently the future and the past are merged into the present. Life is viewed as cyclical in nature, beginning with conception and birth, and evolving to marriage, adulthood, old age, and death. All events are given by God. Death is a natural part of the cycle of life and is unavoidable. It is familiar and near and evokes no great fear or awe.[64]

The strong family network of African-Americans is called into action when a family member is seriously ill. Care of the terminally ill is a public rather than a private undertaking. Neighbors and friends share resources. The family develops plans for the care of the patient, identifies tasks, and assigns family members to assume them. The home is usually viewed as the place for the ill person to spend his/her final days. Frequent visitors are most common. The patient generally remains an active and vital force within the family until he or she can no longer do so. The decision as to whether to inform the patient of his or her terminal illness is made on an individual basis.[64]

Death may be viewed as a passage from the evils of this world to another state. It is a "going home" to be reunited with loved ones. It is not uncommon for African-Americans to plan their funerals and purchase grave plots long before their own deaths. Public and communal grief are openly expressed at traditional African-American funerals, which are termed "home-goings." People in the congregation respond spontaneously and out loud to the sermon. The choir may sing softly in the background during the sermon and prayers. There is a gradual increase in emotion as the funeral progresses and many of those attending express deep emotion. Music provides a means of sending the deceased joyfully on to the next leg of his or her journey.[27,64,65]

### Biological variations

A major biological variation in African-Americans is skin color. Some African-Americans may erroneously believe this darkness protects them from burning from the sun and from skin cancer. There is great variation in the darkness of skin color and those who are fairer-skinned have a greater risk for developing skin cancers from sun exposure. A darker skin color makes more difficult the assessment of pallor, jaundice, ecchymosis, or erythema. Assessing areas of lighter melanin pigmentation such as the sclera, conjunctiva, soles of feet, and palms of the hands may be useful.

The diet of many African-Americans contains little fresh produce, is highly seasoned, and includes frequent use of smoked and fatty meats as seasoning for vegetables and soups. Pork is often a staple meat because it is inexpensive. Thus, saturated fat intake may be high. In comparison to Caucasian women, African-American women are more likely to be obese, while African-American men are more likely to be underweight. The eating habits and compromised nutritional status of African-Americans could be a factor in the higher incidence and mortality rates from cancer.[49]

Lactose intolerance affects 75% of African-Americans. They lack the enzyme to convert lactose to glucose and galactose resulting in gastrointestinal symptoms of bloat-

ing, cramping, and diarrhea after the ingestion of milk and other products containing lactose. The intolerance tends to occur primarily in infancy shortly after weaning and in the teen years or early twenties. Treatment is to avoid milk products. As milk products are often suggested to improve nutrition for patients with cancer, awareness of possible lactose intolerance in the African-American population is significant for the nurse in patient and family teaching.[53]

Alcoholism is a major health problem in the African-American community and a risk factor for cancers of the mouth, larynx, tongue, esophagus, lung, and liver.[66] The causes of alcohol abuse include unemployment, the availability of the substance, peer pressure, escape from personal problems, and the prevalence of taverns as social centers in the African-American communities. Thus, the causes are complex social issues and difficult to treat.[67,68]

## Asian/Pacific Islanders

APIs are the fastest growing ethnic minority group in the United States. In 1990, this group was a little over seven million or about 3% of the total population. By 2050, the number of APIs in the United States is projected to increase by more than five times that of 1990 to approximately 41 million (9.7% of the total population).[9] A very heterogeneous group, the API are composed of individuals "originating from 28 Asian countries and 25 identified Pacific Island cultures."[8] Some of the API subgroups include Chinese, Japanese, Filipino, East Indian, Korean, Vietnamese, native Hawaiian, Samoan, Guamanian, Tongan, Laotian, Cambodian, Hmong, Thai, Burmese, and Indonesian. This marked ethnic diversity is further compounded by inherent variations within each subgroup such as degree of acculturation and socioeconomic status. Although often characterized as the "model minority," APIs are, in fact, bipolar in socioeconomic status and educational attainment. Many have good incomes but approximately one out of eight APIs live in poverty. Similarly, many APIs have a college degree or postgraduate education, but there is a significant number who are functionally illiterate.[8,69]

The differences in levels of acculturation, educational attainment, and socioeconomic status can be partly attributed to the large number of foreign-born APIs, estimated in 1990 at approximately 74% of the total API population. In addition, many of these foreign-born APIs were recent immigrants and refugees.[8]

Because approximately 95% of APIs are Asian Americans compared to 5% who are Pacific Islander Americans,[8] this section of the chapter will primarily address Asian Americans.

### Health beliefs and practices

Common among the APIs are the traditional health beliefs and practices that are carried out in varying degrees within each group. Nevertheless, because of the common influence of Chinese culture, there is much similarity in beliefs and practices among Asian groups. For example, one of the most common beliefs is that health is a state of harmony in body, mind, and spirit with nature and the universe.[4] Although native Hawaiians are not of Asian descent, harmony with nature is also an important health belief in this culture.[70]

Many APIs believe that a balance between hot and cold elements is essential for good health. In the Chinese, Japanese, and Korean cultures, in particular, this balance is defined as *yin* (cold) and *yang* (hot).[71-75] *Yin* and *yang* are life forces in which *yin* (cold) is characterized as female, dark, negative energy and *yang* (hot) is male, light, positive energy. Illness is believed to result from an imbalance of these two forces. The Chinese believe that the human body, illnesses, and foods possess *yin* or *yang* characteristics and treatment is aimed at reestablishing the balance.[72,73,76-79] For example, cancer is a *yin* or cold illness and would be treated with foods, herbs, and healing ceremonies that possess "hot" properties. The Filipino,[80] East Indian,[81] and Southeast Asian cultures[25,26] also have similar beliefs in hot and cold balance and health. Other explanations for illness include an imbalance of humoral elements, an obstruction of *chi* (an essential life energy), a curse by a spirit, spiritual imbalance, punishment for immoral behavior, or an imbalance in the body caused by exposure to wind or air.[72,81-85]

There exists a widespread belief among some API groups that suffering is part of life, a philosophy that may result in postponement in seeking medical treatment, either traditional or Western.[8,83] Fatalism is found in the Filipino culture where the attitude of "*bahala na*—it's in the hands of God" exists, especially when illness and pain are seen as punishment.[84,86] The belief among some southeast Asians in the inevitability of suffering and that an individual's lifespan is predetermined may inhibit them from seeking medical treatment.[83] In the Japanese culture, the term *shoganai* is used when misfortune strikes, such as an illness. Its translation: "it can't be helped," reflects an almost fatalistic view. Chinese Americans also have a fatalistic outlook on life in their belief that they lack control over nature.[73]

Many APIs believe that blood is a life force that cannot be replaced or, if taken, will disrupt the body's balance causing weakness and even death.[25,26,81] Therefore, many APIs fear venipunctures. The Hmong may be reluctant to receive blood transfusions since their perception is that the donor's spirit may enter their body via the transfusion.[25] The Chinese and Vietnamese may not agree to surgery when organs or body parts are to be removed because of their belief that the human body must be intact at the time of death to avoid potential adverse consequences in the afterlife.[26,87] The Vietnamese also avoid surgery since it is perceived as a last resort and associated with death.[26,88] The Hmong may refuse surgery because of their belief that cutting into the body releases spirits, causing an imbalance.[25]

## Healing practices

Included in their traditional health beliefs, APIs practice the use of herbal medications, seek traditional healers, and perform healing ceremonies. Because APIs often use herbal preparations concurrently with Western medicine, it is important to ascertain if, and what, herbal preparations are being used in order to anticipate possible drug interactions. For example, *ma huang* is a Chinese herb that contains ephedrine. Complications can arise if, in addition to the *ma huang*, the patient takes ephedrine via a Western practitioner's prescription.[87] Ginseng, another popular herb, is considered a stimulant and has hypertensive effects. Undesirable side effects can result if the patient takes ginseng in conjunction with Western antihypertensive medication.[73,77]

Traditional healers among the API include shamans (Laotian, Hmong), Chinese herbalists, *kahuna la'au lapa'au* (native Hawaiian), and *Hilot* (Filipino). These healers are often consulted before Western medical practitioners. In some cases, the perceived cause of the illness determines who is consulted first. For example, if southeast Asians believe that an illness is organic in origin, they may seek a Western physician. However, if the cause of illness is thought to be supernatural, a traditional healer would be consulted. If the illness persists after consulting with traditional healers, then they might seek Western treatment.[83] At this point, however, the disease may be at an advanced stage and untreatable. Then, because Western medicine cannot cure the illness, it is seen as ineffective. This may reinforce the use of traditional healers. For many APIs, the Western health care system is foreign. There is comfort in consulting a healer who understands, with whom one can communicate, and whose practice is familiar to the patient. Other explanations for why healers are often preferred over Western medical practitioners include that they are inexpensive and have a reputation for being effective for specific conditions.

Healing ceremonies or practices vary considerably across API groups. Some of these practices include moxibustion, cupping, acupuncture, massage, and skin scraping or coining.[73,79,82]

Moxibustion, used to restore the *yin-yang* balance, involves a deeply penetrating heat treatment. Small pellets or cones made of the herb *Artemesis vulgaris* (moxa) are placed at acupuncture points on the body and burned. The pellets/cones are removed when the patient feels the heat. This treatment leaves small, rounded or asymmetrical superficial burn marks. It is used in the treatment of ailments of the joints, muscles, bones, and back.[73,74,89]

Cupping also uses heat but in a different fashion. A material, such as alcohol-soaked cotton, is placed in a special cup and set on fire to create a vacuum in the cup. When the flame is extinguished, the cup is then placed immediately on the treatment area of the body where suction is created. The cup is kept there for 15–20 minutes or until it is easily removed. Cupping is used to treat pain, body aches, and headaches. It is a painful procedure that leaves circular burn marks approximately two inches in diameter. These burn marks have been misinterpreted as child abuse in southeast Asian children who have been treated with cupping.[79,90]

Skin scraping or coining involves the application of a special menthol oil or ointment to the symptomatic area. With the edge of a coin, the area is then rubbed in a firm, downward motion.[72] This procedure is used to treat a cold, heatstroke, headache, pain, vomiting, and indigestion.[90]

In the native Hawaiian culture, healing includes special rituals, prayers, and chants as well as the use of special herbs and plants.[91]

## Social organization

The APIs have very strong, family-centered systems.[73,86,92] The family exerts an extremely powerful force in an individual's life. The family or social network is of primary importance and the needs of the individual are often secondary to the larger group.[93,94] Health care decisions are often made by the family or social network rather than by the individual.

In many API groups, patrilineal authority along with filial piety and respect for elders often means that the eldest son or male head of the clan is the spokesperson for the patient.[95] This individual is the designated family spokesperson for medical practitioners to speak to when information about the patient's condition is given or when treatment decisions need to be made.

Because of the strong value placed on the family, API family members are more likely to actively participate in the patient's daily care. In the Chinese culture, caring for the patient is an expectation, that if not met, brings shame to the family.[73] Japanese and Filipino families also play significant roles in providing support and care for their family members. It is not unusual to have family members hovering about the patient and maintaining a bedside vigil.[92,93] Health care professionals need to be sensitive to these cultural needs, and also to support the family to prevent caregiver exhaustion, especially if one member is the sole caregiver.

## Communication

In many API groups, communication patterns are influenced by values that emphasize politeness, respect for authority, and avoidance of shame. These values prevent many APIs from asking health professionals questions or challenging a proposed diagnostic workup and/or treatment plan.[78,83,86,93] Instead, an API may nod his or her head, in what is interpreted as agreement. However, the patient may not necessarily agree or understand what the practitioner has said.[25,65] Thus, poor communication can occur between the API and the Western practitioner. This may have a detrimental effect for follow-up care if the

API patient, in frustration and confusion, does not return for further Western health services.[83]

In communicating with some API groups, Western practitioners may need to avoid or limit engaging in direct eye contact, as such eye contact may be perceived as being rude, challenging, or just culturally unacceptable.[25,26,96] For example, in the Filipino culture, direct eye contact between an older man and a young woman usually implies seduction or anger.[86,92] In the East Indian culture, eye contact between a woman and a man other than her husband can have sexual significance.[97] Avoiding eye contact by the South Vietnamese is a sign of respect when talking with someone perceived to be of different rank in education, social status, age, or gender.[26]

Many APIs prefer limited or no contact.[26,73,93] In some API groups the head is sacred and touching or patting the head is perceived as a rude gesture.[25,73] For some southeast Asians, crossing the legs and pointing the foot at the individual is also considered to be insulting.[83] Similarly, directing the sole of the shoe or foot toward Koreans is offensive to them.[96]

Many APIs do not speak English, or have limited proficiency in English as their second language. Because of this language barrier, interpreters are often used. However, communication via a third party presents challenges in ensuring that the literal meaning of the conversation is translated correctly along with the interpretation of nonverbal messages. When possible, use professional interpreters who can facilitate and ensure communication among the patient, family, and health professional.

In selecting an interpreter, first ascertain the specific dialect spoken by the patient and family. For example, a Filipino patient does not necessarily speak Filipino. There are several dialects spoken by Filipinos including Visayan, Tagalog, Ilocano, or Cebuano. Family interpreters are often used; however, the message relayed may not always be accurate.[98] For example, if the message is regarding a poor prognosis, the family member may modify it in an attempt to protect the patient. In addition, if interpreters are of the opposite sex, patients may not bring up symptoms or concerns that they perceive as either embarrassing or culturally unacceptable to discuss in the presence of the opposite sex. The traditional hierarchy in many API families where power and influence run from elders to youths is another potential pitfall when using family interpreters. In some instances, especially with recent immigrants, children may be used as interpreters since they usually have a better command of English. However, this reverses the rank of the child in the family and may put undue stress on the family.[81,99]

## Space and time

APIs value privacy and many are also very modest.[25,72,86,100] When physical examinations or procedures necessitate exposure of the body, exposure should be minimized by revealing only that part of the body that needs to be examined. Female API patients, such as East

Indian and Chinese women, may feel more comfortable being examined by female practitioners.[81,101,102]

The concept of time varies among the API groups. For example, the Japanese, who are present and future oriented, are usually prompt and adhere to fixed schedules.[93] On the other hand, Chinese are more present oriented, do not necessarily adhere to fixed schedules, and may be late for appointments.[73] Filipinos are past and present oriented and may disregard health-related matters. This time orientation is closely linked to their *bahala na* philosophy of leaving things in God's hands.[92]

## Death and dying issues

There are many issues regarding death and dying in the API groups. Bioethics, truth telling, patient's right to know, and advance directive decisions are based in Western culture. It is important to be aware that patient autonomy and self-determination in API groups may not be culturally acceptable or valued. As previously discussed, the family or family spokesperson frequently makes decisions about the patient's care rather than the patient.

The initiation and continuation of life-support measures also may vary from group to group. For example, many Filipinos are Catholic and may view discontinuing life support as morally wrong.[95] A similar viewpoint is shared by many Koreans who consider stopping life support as interfering with God's will; however, the initiation of life support is not.[95]

Conflict may arise between the value in Western medicine of open disclosure of a terminal illness and the value shared by many API groups that "to tell someone he or she is dying is not only rude but dangerous."[103, p. 325] For example, East Indians prefer not to tell patients the seriousness of their condition or the possibility of death. They believe that "speaking of possibilities may render them too real, and a traditional Indian does not speak lightly of death; . . . if a patient knows the gravity of the illness, he or she will give up hope and die."[81, p. 269] This is also seen in the Hmong culture where the disclosure of prognosis to a terminally ill patient "is the same as wishing death upon that person and may in fact bring about that person's death."[104, p. 426] Muller and Desmond[103] further note that in many Asian groups, "people fear that openly acknowledging an impending death is like casting a death curse upon the person; it will make the person despair and die even sooner. Thus, to engage in discussions of code status or the possibility of hospice care, interventions that can be seen as explicit preparation for death, is courting bad luck."[103, p. 325]

On the other hand, although hospice care discussions may not always be encouraged, some APIs prefer to die at home rather than the hospital.[87,95,96] This preference is due, in large part, to the value placed on the family and "the belief that the unfortunate who die among strangers and away from their familiar dwelling are forever condemned to wander in pain, so-called orphan souls, endlessly searching in vain for the family and home they missed when they died."[105, p. 24]

With the potential for conflict and frustration between the values of Western health care and the cultural values of various API groups, exploring life-support decisions with the patient and family is critical. Klessig suggests that the following information be determined.[95, p. 321]

What do they think about the sanctity of life?

What is their definition of death?

What is their religious background, and how active are they currently?

What do they believe are the causal agents in illness, and how do these relate to the dying process?

What is the patient's social support system?

Who makes decisions about matters of importance in the family?

By facilitating communication about these issues between the patient/family and the health care team, oncology nurses can assist in narrowing the gap between these two value systems and support the patient/family through this phase of the cancer experience.

## Biological variations

The incidence rate for liver cancer is exceptionally high in API groups, particularly the southeast Asian groups. This increased rate for liver cancer is linked to the high incidence of hepatitis B infection in these groups, largely due to the fact that these groups originate from areas where hepatitis B is endemic.

Japanese, Koreans, and Vietnamese all have high rates of stomach cancer.[14,71] This is attributed in part to genetic factors as well as environmental factors including the high ingestion of sodium, hot and spicy foods, and nitrates.[71]

Lactose intolerance is also common in APIs. Milk and cheese, common foods in the mainstream American diet, may therefore be unacceptable to this group. When providing oral supplements that are nonmilk containing but have the appearance of a milk product, the patient and family must be reassured that the supplement is not a milk product.

The physical characteristics of APIs may necessitate adjusting the dosage of certain medications. For example, Zhou et al[106] reported that in Chinese men, the propranolol dose may need to be decreased due to the greater sensitivity among Chinese to the effects of propranolol on heart rate and blood pressure when compared to Caucasians. The exact mechanism for these effects has not been determined; however, decreased protein binding may play a role.

Many APIs also have the distinguishing yellow cast to their skin that ranges in tone. This yellow cast can make the recognition of jaundice more challenging. In order to assess for jaundice, the sclera and excreta need to be checked.

Although not a biological variation, the higher smoking rates among southeast Asian men as compared to the general population deserves mention.[8] This is a prime area for health promotion activities. Another area of concern is the 1990 report showing that APIs had the lowest participation rate in Pap smears, mammography, breast examination, or smoking cessation counseling when compared to all other ethnic groups.[18] Possible reasons for this low participation rate include lack of health education programs targeted specifically for this group, fatalism belief, and decreased access to health care. See Table 62-9 for comparative percentages of participation among the different ethnic groups.

## Hispanics

"Hispanic" is an umbrella term for several subgroups in the United States including people of Mexican, Puerto Rican, Cuban, Caribbean, and Central and South American origin.[107] The Hispanic population has been growing five times as fast as the rest of the country's population. In 1989, the Hispanic population totaled 20 million in the 50 states and the District of Columbia. It increased 39% between the 1980 census and the 1990 census with half the growth attributable to immigration and the rest to birth. By the year 2050, this population is expected to be the largest U.S. minority.[108]

Nearly 63% of Hispanics live in the southwestern states of California, Texas, Arizona, New Mexico, and Colorado. Another 25% live in New York, New Jersey, Illinois, and Florida and the remaining 12% are scattered throughout the country.[109]

Generally, the cancer incidence rate among Hispanics ranks in the middle when compared to other ethnic groups. Many Hispanics delay seeking treatment for symptoms and continue to use folk remedies as their first choice in health care.[110] The largest concentrated population of Hispanics in the United States lives in Los Angeles, CA. In this group there is a high risk of gallbladder, cervical, and stomach cancers; an intermediate risk of pancreatic and prostate cancers; and a low risk of melanoma and colorectal, lung, and reproductive cancers.[111]

There appears to be a genetic predisposition and higher incidence of gallbladder cancer among Hispanic men and women in New Mexico. A similar pattern was found for biliary cancer in Hispanics in Los Angeles County.[112,113] Liver cancer rates after the age of 50 in Hispanic males and females increases dramatically.[114] A 1986 study found that compared to Caucasian women, Hispanic women with cervical cancer were younger, less educated, and had fewer sexual partners but were younger when they first had sex and had more children. They also had fewer visits to physicians and fewer Pap tests. These results may account for the advanced disease at diagnosis and the increased cervical cancer rates recorded.[115] Although the incidence rate of breast cancer is low, the mortality rate is high for Hispanic women. Cultural factors are thought to be responsible for delays in seeking health care and for larger, more advanced tumors at diagnosis of breast cancer.[116]

### Health beliefs and practices

Health is often believed to be the result of good luck or a reward from God for good behavior. The concept that a disease is God's will is widely accepted. Terminal illnesses especially are seen as the result of some indiscretion against God. Thus, health and illness in Hispanic groups have a strong religious association.

There is often a fatalistic belief that one is at the mercy of the environment and has little control over what happens. Personal efforts are unlikely to influence the outcome of a situation. Thus, Hispanics often do not believe that they are personally responsible for present or future successes or failures.[117]

Hautman[118] identifies several categories of disease in the Hispanic culture. The concept of hot and cold imbalance resembles the *yin* and *yang* in the Chinese culture. An equilibrium exists between hot and cold elements in a healthy body. To ensure good health, individuals must ingest both hot and cold foods.[119] Internal factors such as a change in body temperature and external factors such as the foods eaten can affect the hot/cold balance.

**TABLE 62-9**  Comparative Percentages of Participation in Clinical Preventive Services, 1990 Data

| | Pap Smears | Mammograms | Breast Exams | Nutrition Counseling | Smoking Counseling |
|---|---|---|---|---|---|
| APIs | 68* | 45 | 74* | 33 | 28* |
| Blacks | 83 | 47 | 84 | 44 | 39 |
| Hispanics | 76 | 45 | 79 | 34 | 33 |
| Native Americans | 80 | 41* | 80 | 32 | 44 |
| Whites | 78 | 54 | 83 | 31* | 52 |
| All races | 79 | 53 | 83 | 33 | 50 |

*Lowest rate for all groups

Adapted with permission from Chen MS Jr., A 1993 status report on the health status of Asian Pacific Islander Americans: Comparisons with Healthy People 2000 objectives. *Asian American and Pacific Islander Journal of Health* 1(1):45, 1993.

Many of the disorders caused by hot and cold imbalances are digestive in nature. A stomach ulcer is a "hot illness" caused by eating too much hot food. Excesses of heat developed from within the body and extending outward are believed to be related to cancer, rheumatism, tuberculosis, and paralysis.[120] The effort to balance hot and cold forces in the Hispanic belief system reflects the relationship between the individual and the environment.

Another common health disorder is believed to be caused by the dislocation of organs. *Empacho* or a blocked intestine occurs when undigested food sticks to the walls of the intestine. This is caused by eating improperly cooked foods or eating foods at the wrong times.[121]

Another group of illnesses is believed to be caused by magical interventions. *Mal ojo* or evil eye occurs when someone with a powerful glance looks improperly at a child. This is believed to be a manifestation of witchcraft. The child is affected by evil spirits. Treatment is a ceremonial ritual that includes passing an egg over the affected person's body while reciting prayers. *Susto* or sudden fright occurs when an individual experiences a stressful event at some time prior to the onset of symptoms. The stressors may be the death of a significant person, a child's nightmare, or the inability to adequately fulfill social role responsibilities. *Mal Puesto* (evil) is an illness caused by a hex bestowed by a *brujo* (witch), *curandero* (folk healer), or other person knowledgeable about witchcraft.[121,122]

There are two types of emotional diseases: mental and moral illnesses. Mental illness is seen as inevitable and the affected person is viewed as a victim of consequence. It is considered a disruption of a person's equilibrium by some supernatural force that requires traditional medical attention. Moral illness such as alcoholism is caused by the individual and the treatment is the responsibility of family members.[123]

The last category includes scientific diseases that cannot be treated by traditional health practices and must be diagnosed and treated by the Western health care system.

Since many Hispanics believe that external forces determine health and illness, they may not comply with suggested interventions or participate in wellness programs. There are a few accepted prevention practices such as being good, praying, and eating well to maintain balance, but these often are not practiced. Religious medals or amulets may be worn for protection.

Cancer is seen fatalistically as God's will and it goes against principle to aggressively treat the disease.[124] Family members, especially elders, should not be informed of their diagnosis as it will only worsen the illness. Cancer is viewed as deadly and engenders great fear. A stigma surrounds cancer and the disease is often seen as God's punishment for sins. Patients often say "I deserve to suffer." Cancer is viewed as contagious and hard to prevent because it is caused by many things. Thus, going to see the doctor early serves no useful purpose. Many Hispanic patients believe that chemotherapy does not work, that radiation may cause cancer, and that cancer will remain even after surgery to remove it. Some believe that certain cancer treatments may have side effects that can be passed on to family members (e.g., that family members may become radioactive if the patient is receiving radiation therapy).[109]

Hispanic individuals may believe that there is no need to see a physician unless a person is very ill. Hospitals are seen as places where people die. Therefore, medical attention may be sought only after symptoms develop or the individual is too ill to be cared for by the family.

One in four Hispanics lives at or below the poverty level. The cost of being sick includes not only the amount of money needed for care but also the loss of money in time missed from work.[125] Many Hispanics fear that because of their economic status and ethnicity, they may receive inferior care in the U.S. medical system.[126] Some believe they should only receive health care they can afford. So if they cannot afford to pay, some Hispanic individuals may not seek care. In general, Hispanics are less likely to have medical insurance than any other group. In 1988 13% of the U.S. population lacked health insurance: 10.2% Caucasian, 20% African-American, and 32% Hispanic.[127] The outcome in relation to cancer is late diagnosis and higher mortality rates despite the lower overall incidence of cancer in the Hispanic population.[109] The high percentage of Hispanics who are migrant farm workers also contributes to the overall decreased access to health care for that group.[128]

Individuals of Hispanic origin often believe that it is not appropriate to question those giving care because of the fear of retaliation. Since some Hispanics believe that physical touch can promote healing, if Western providers do not touch during their visit, some Hispanics may believe that they did not derive any benefit from that visit.

Martaus[129] offers six suggestions for assimilating Hispanic individuals to the U.S. health care system. First, health care providers must communicate their acceptance of the person's value system to establish trust. Second, providers should include a culturally relevant interview into the admission process. This defines the individual's perception of illness and allows the health care provider to establish a workable treatment plan. Third, the treatment plan must include a family focus as illness intensifies the need for family involvement. Fourth, many Hispanics are very religious and may view treatment without prayer as ineffective. Fifth, the health care workers must take responsibility for finding a common ground that incorporates traditional beliefs and modern health care. Finally, many Hispanics have a great fear of authority. They may believe that disease occurs because it is God's will and also may place great emphasis on treating doctors with respect.

### Healing practices

Home remedies are the first line of treatment. To cure a hot or cold imbalance, the opposite quality of the causative agent is applied. For example, if the causative agent for a headache is thought to have a hot quality, cold herbs may be placed on the temples to absorb the heat. If the cause has a cold quality, hot herbs are applied.[130] If the stool is green or yellow, the diarrhea is hot and the remedy is cold tea. If the stool is white, the diarrhea is cold and the remedy is hot tea.

There is usually a family folk healer, someone respected for her knowledge of folk medicine. The healing practices are passed down in the family from mother to daughter. If home remedies do not work, Mexican Americans send for the *curandero* or *herbalista*, a traditional folk medicine healer. This person receives his or her skills through an apprenticeship or as a gift from God and is knowledgeable in the use of herbs, diet, massage, prayer, and ritual.[131] Puerto Ricans seek the *espiritismo*, a folk healer with the gift of contacting the spirit world and healing through the powers of spirits. They analyze dreams, foretell the future, and use medals, prayers, and amulets as part of their treatment approach.[118] The Cuban population may seek medical help from a *santero*, a medicine man who works with the spirits of good within a system to promote wellness. Animal sacrifices, rituals, chanting, and prayers are used to aid in healing.[131] A *jerbero* is a healer that uses herbs and spices for prevention of illness and for healing. A *brujo* uses witchcraft for healing illnesses that may be related to jealousy or envy (*envidia*). If these fail, then Western physicians may be sought out for help.[121]

It is essential that the nurse demonstrate acceptance of the spiritual and folk basis of Hispanic people's health beliefs. Once this acceptance is conveyed, there is hope of influencing acceptance and understanding of the rationale for modern health care practices and thereby gaining the community's confidence.

### Social organization

The nuclear family (parents and children) are the foundation of the Hispanic community. Men are the breadwinners, assume the dominant role in Hispanic families, and are considered big and strong (*macho*). The hesitancy of a woman or child to make a decision may be due to the need to inform and obtain approval of the husband and father.[132] Women have always been the primary caretakers. The extended family is valued and the family's needs supersede those of the individual members. When a family member's illness is too serious for the wife and mother to handle alone, she may ask the extended family to help care for the sick individual. Family members often spend a lot of time in attendance when a family member is sick as their role is to protect, assist, care, and support. Family members may also speak for the patient.

Because of the value of the family in the patient's treatment and recovery, the family should be used to help with the patient's care. Suggesting family consultation when experiencing difficulty in getting a patient to follow a particular medical regimen will demonstrate that the nurse understands the importance of the family in regard to health matters.

Roman Catholicism is the predominant religion of Hispanics. Since it is such an important factor in the health beliefs of Hispanics, the patient may turn to religious practices to help overcome the illness. These include praying, making promises, visiting shrines, or offering medals and candles to a patron saint. During hospitalization, allowing time and providing privacy for the family to carry out these religious practices will be helpful to many Hispanics.[133]

### Communication

Spanish is the primary language with many dialectal differences. Many Hispanics are bilingual but will have a strong preference for their native language and during times of illness, they often revert to it. There is some mistrust of Anglo Americans and Western medicine, especially when the health care provider does not speak Spanish. Language may be a barrier and Hispanics may not let the provider know that they do not understand. Translators may be necessary.

The traditional Hispanic approach to communication requires the use of much diplomacy and tactfulness. Concern and respect for another's feelings dictate that a screen always be provided to preserve the patient's dignity. The manner of expression is likely to be elaborate and indirect to make personal relationship at least appear harmonious since respect of each person's individuality is important. Politeness and courtesy is highly regarded. Even if the Hispanic individual disagrees with another's point of view, direct argument or contradiction is considered rude and disrespectful. On the surface, he or she may seem agreeable but only because manners dictate that his or her genuine opinions are not openly expressed. This apparent agreement may lead to a false assumption that the patient understands and will follow through with whatever is proposed. In practice this may not be true.

Body language may be dramatic when expressing pain or emotion. Hispanics in pain may groan and moan to let those around them know they are uncomfortable and suffering.[134]

### Space and time

Adult Hispanics may be described as tactile in their relationships but there is a high degree of modesty. This is one reason why Hispanics do not enter the U.S. health care system. They generally do not like being touched by others or having to touch themselves and are not comfortable being examined by health care professionals of the opposite sex. Embarrassment is a common reaction to invasive procedures or body exposure during an examination.[109]

Despite the fact that Hispanics like consistent, close relationships and physical touching, female nurses should always assist a male physician in examining a female patient and vice versa, and guard against exposing body parts other than those that are the focus of the examination.[135] Male patients may refuse a complete examination because of their modesty. However, providing for close contact between family members and the ill patient is important for Hispanics.

Hispanics generally have a relaxed concept of time—a present orientation—and may be late for appointments. The patient may be more concerned with a current activity than with the activity of planning ahead to be on time. This action implies that future-oriented activities can be recovered but present-oriented activities cannot. The present time orientation helps explain why Hispanics often seek out the most accessible and affordable care first (folk healing and the folk practitioner). It is useful for the nurse to focus on short-term problems. For example, if a medication is not taken in a timely manner, the immediate effects should be emphasized.[117]

### Death and dying issues

The afterlife of heaven and hell exists in the Hispanic culture. As many Hispanics are Catholic, religious practices like baptism of the dying and the administration of the sacrament of the sick are important.

As expected, the family serves as a protective network for helping the dying and their survivors handle the emotional problems associated with death. The terminally ill patient is often not told directly by the family of his or her condition but demonstrates awareness of death's likelihood. Although there is a preference to remain at home to die, dying in a hospital is an acceptable alternative.[136] Public expression of grief is expected, especially among women.[137]

### Biological variations

The traditional Hispanic diet is high in fiber and carbohydrates from staples such as rice, beans, and corn. It contains few leafy green vegetables. Beans are a source of protein and daily intake tends to be small. The use of lard and the common practice of frying foods contribute to the high fat content of the Hispanic diet.[109]

Among the high-risk behaviors in the Hispanic population are obesity, alcohol consumption, and sexual practices. Obesity is a common problem among Hispanics in the United States due to their diet and lack of physical activity. In general, the culture accepts obesity as part of the natural aging process and does not emphasize low body weight.[138] To older individuals obesity may mean health and wealth. Obesity is a risk factor in cancers of the breast, colon/rectum, uterus, and prostate. Hispanic men tend to drink at younger ages and consume larger amounts of alcohol more often than do Caucasians. Alcohol contributes to cancers of the esophagus and pancreas. Cigarette smoking is on the rise in Hispanic adolescents although adult Hispanics smoke less than Caucasians or African-Americans. There is a high risk for cervical cancer because of sexual promiscuity and infrequent use of condoms by males, predisposing females to sexually transmitted diseases. In addition, low socioeconomic status and low levels of education often result in infrequent Pap smears, infrequent use of barrier contraceptives, and lack of reporting of genital warts.[115]

Skin color can vary from a natural tan to dark brown. Those with lighter color have more Spanish ancestry while darker-skinned individuals have more Indian ancestry.

## Native Americans

The native Americans (once called American Indians) include natives of the continental United States, Aleuts, and Alaskan Eskimos. They are a very diverse group consisting of many tribes and over 400 federally recognized nations each with its own traditions and cultural heritage.[139] Until the 1800s they lived in loosely formed, often nomadic bands and tribes and spoke more than 100 languages with countless dialects.[140] This section focuses on the natives of the continental United States.

There are approximately 1.6 million original residents of North America that make up the smallest of the defined U.S. minority groups. There are 33 states with Indian reservations. The largest tribes are the Navajo, Cherokee, Sioux, Chippewa, and Pueblo Indians with the greatest numbers living in Oklahoma, Arizona, California, New Mexico, and Alabama. The 1990 census shows a significant increase in the native American population due to high birth rates, improved counting by the U.S. Bureau of the Census, and the increase in self-identification, particularly among urban native Americans who have little connection to a tribal organization.[141]

Many tribes gave up their land in exchange for treaty rights in attempts to survive as Europeans increased in numbers and moved into territorial lands. Reservations were established. Those who live on reservations tend to lead a more isolated, rural type of existence. Reservations have a high percentage of very young members and a growing number of members over 55 years of age. Since the reservation land cannot support a growing and increasingly concentrated population, poverty and welfare dependency are common. Native Americans who relocated from reservations tended to move to urban areas away from the security network of their family, community, and tribal lifestyle. Although lured by greater opportunities and better jobs, many experienced culture shock with the large differences in the environment. In the past 25 years there has been a migration to urban areas and now nearly two-thirds of all native Americans live in non-reservation communities.[142]

Cancer is ranked as the third leading cause of death among native Americans, preceded by accidents and heart disease. Native Americans (American Indians (New Mexico)) also have the lowest cancer incidence and rank mid to low in mortality rates of all U.S. minority populations. Incidence rates among both males and females are significantly lower than among the white population.[14] Incidence rates are the highest for cancers of the kidney and renal pelvis in native American men, and of the ovary in native American women.[14] Low rates of cancer of the lung, breast, and colon/rectum are evident in native Americans. Because native Americans are younger than the majority population and have a shorter life expectancy, they often do not live long enough to develop cancer. This group has high rates of obesity and diseases associated with alcohol and tobacco use that are risk factors for many types of cancers.[143]

Cervical cancer occurs primarily among older native American women.[144] Factors affecting the increased incidence of cervical cancer include infrequent or no history of Pap smear screening and lack of follow-up for abnormal results. Barriers to screening and follow-up include poverty, significant unemployment, underfunded and overburdened health care services, lack of local treatment, use of the health care system for treatment of acute illness rather than for preventive care, and the belief that the test is unnecessary due to "good health." [145,146]

Gallbladder cancer and gallbladder diseases are common in native Americans. The reasons for these high rates are unknown but diet and genetic factors are implicated.[147]

At least one-third of the native American population live in extreme poverty. The social condition of native American communities such as limited educational levels, substandard housing, poor sanitation, malnutrition, and inadequate health services all contribute to the high incidence of deaths by accident, suicide, alcoholism, and cirrhosis of the liver.[148]

The Indian Health Service, through the Public Health Service, provides inpatient facilities and outpatient clinics and serves native Americans residing on reservations in 25 states and the Aleut and Eskimo residents of Alaska. Although health care is available, barriers for native Americans to access it include poverty and the lack of transportation. Native Americans believe in living day-to-day rather than in planning for the future, and do not have savings or insurance to pay for health care. Many live long distances from health care facilities and are resistant to hospital treatment.[1,149]

## Health beliefs and practices

Tribes vary in their beliefs about health and illness, but most tribes link health beliefs and religion. In the Western world, religion is often perceived as a discrete body of knowledge practiced in a specific place. To the native American, religion is something that surrounds an individual at all times and has a profound influence on the entire being.[150] It is these beliefs that may have maintained the native American against all odds of survival.

Health is both a physical and a spiritual state. Wellness is harmony in body, mind, and spirit and resilience, the ability to survive under exceedingly difficult circumstances. It is the patient's response or attitude toward circumstances that creates harmony.[151]

Health reflects living in harmony with nature and humans have an intimate relationship with nature. The earth is considered a living being, the body of a higher individual with a will and desire to be well. The earth is periodically healthy or ill just as humans are. An individual is expected to treat both his or her body and the earth with respect. If an individual harms the earth, he or she harms him or herself and vice versa. Because of this relationship between humans and nature, native Americans believe that humans should respect their bodies and nature through proper treatment. If people harm themselves, they harm the earth. In order to maintain themselves, native Americans must maintain a relationship with nature.[152]

Unwellness is caused by the disharmony of mind, body, and spirit. Natural unwellness is caused by the violation of a sacred or tribal taboo. Taboos can be moral, religious, or cultural. Violations not only affect the offender but the family as well.[151]

Illness may also be caused by witchcraft. Evil or negative energy comes from "one who is on the bad side" or "a person who walks at night." It can be premeditated or not so native Americans must be careful how they think or talk since bad thoughts can cause illness.[151] The Hopi Indians associate illness with evil spirits. The Navajos believe that witches are able to interact with evil spirits and can bring sickness and other unhappiness to those who annoy them. Traditionally, illness, disharmony, and sadness are seen by Navajos as the result "of displeasing the holy people, annoying the elements, disturbing animal and plant life, neglecting the celestial bodies, misuse of a sacred Indian ceremony, or tampering with witches and witchcraft".[153, p. 21] The cause of disease, injury, damage to property, or continued misfortune of any kind can be traced back to an action that should not have been performed such as breaking a taboo or contacting a ghost or witch. Thus, the treatment of illness must be focused on external causative factors and not on the illness or injury itself.[154]

All causes of illness or disease are believed to have supernatural aspects.[154] Treatment depends on whether the origins of bodily ailments are internal or external. Vogel[155] states that external causes of illness are fractures, dislocations, wounds, and snake or insect bites. If the cause is not apparent, then it is attributed to a supernatural agency. The belief that illnesses are caused by germs, a malfunctioning body part, or poor nutritional intake are foreign and unacceptable to native Americans. Sickness indicates a discord with the laws of nature and is most often caused by sorcery or witchcraft, taboo violation, disease or object intrusion, spirit intrusion or being possessed by spirits, or loss of soul. Iroquois Indians also believe that unfulfilled dreams or desires can result in illness. Restriction violations are also thought to cause sickness. Most tribes have prescriptions and prohibitions governing behavior and daily activities, many of which pertain to the prevention of illness. For example, a Navajo boy was diagnosed as having urinary retention caused by his urinating on an ant hill. The boy caused the ants to suffer and the ants' revenge came in the form of an illness. The boy was out of harmony with living entities that share the universe. The cure was a healing ceremony involving chants, prayers, and herbs administered by a medicine man.[142]

Diseases of object intrusion refer to the invasion of

the body by a worm, snake, insect, or small animal. This may be a result of witchcraft. Navajos may orally suck out the foreign object using a hollow tube or bone. Spirit intrusion is being possessed by disease-causing spirits of humans and animals. The healing ceremony is an exorcism of the bad spirits.[155] Soul loss usually occurs during a dream when the soul leaves the body and travels about. Witches and evil spirits can steal a soul. It is believed that the individual is in danger of dying if the soul is not recovered.

Many native Americans believe that they are responsible for their own health and illness. From birth, each person is responsible for him- or herself. If one lives in harmony then taboos are not broken and negative energy cannot enter the individual.[151]

The most prevalent pattern for the native American is the alternate use of traditional medicine and Western medicine either independently of each other or simultaneously. A native American patient may consult both a medicine person and a Western doctor at the same time. One treats the physical disease while the other helps the individual heal himself by restoring harmony. To treat the spirit and mind, a healer must understand why the disease occurred and begin to resolve the conflict occurring in mind, body, and spirit. In most instances the two systems are complementary and should be encouraged.[156]

There are preventive measures practiced generally to ward off the effects of witchcraft, to reestablish harmony, or to prevent possession by an evil spirit. The medicine person may prescribe wearing a talisman, a buckskin or cloth herbal bag that has preventive or curative powers. Removal of such items by the nurse without permission could result in serious consequences for the patient.[156]

Some tribes are not receptive to invasive bodily procedures and only reluctantly will agree to surgery. Relatives may refuse to donate blood because of the fear that if the recipient dies, they may die as well. Native Americans should be asked if they wish a body part back after surgery as some tribes believe the body must be intact for burial or that body parts can be used as a means of entering the body and cause harm.[156]

Offering food to native American patients during appointments may be helpful. This is referred to as "the give away," a celebration that meets basic needs, and shows welcome, concern, caring, friendship, and neighborliness. Offering food is a tangible expression of the link in a relationship and serves as something always to be remembered about that individual.

Because of a history of inconsistent care and disrespectful treatment, native Americans often are not comfortable with Western health care providers. Long waits in clinics, separation from their families, the unfamiliar routines of the hospital, and the often demanding and demeaning attitudes of nurses and physicians result in a variety of responses by the native American patient that may include silence or even leaving without returning.[149]

The pain threshold of native Americans is often thought of as being high as stoicism is valued. This stems from their tendency to look at things in totality so that when sickness occurs, it is viewed as an ailment of the whole body. Many will "grin and bear" fever and pain until the physical condition becomes disabling. Asking a native American, "where does it hurt?" might commonly be responded to as "all over." It may be more useful to have them point to where it hurts the most. When treatment is sought, medication generally is expected. If none is given, the native American may be disappointed as his expectations for treatment were not met.[142]

Helpful interventions in working successfully with native American patients include conveying acceptance of the whole human being without judgment of physical appearance, beliefs, or practices; recognition of unique cultural beliefs and behaviors; and making staff and services available when the need arises rather than through scheduling appointments. A lack of willingness to accept traditional healing practices may discourage many native Americans from using the Western health care system.

### Healing practices

The traditional healer is the medicine person who is wise in the ways of the land and nature. This person is well versed in the interrelationships of human beings, the earth and the universe, and knows the ways of plants and animals, the sun, moon, and stars. He or she takes the time to determine first the cause of the illness, the proper treatment, and often performs special ceremonies that may take several days.[149] These medicine men and women are "chosen," that is, divinely inspired. They are gifted with extrasensory perception that allows them to make mythological associations. Medicine men and women spend many years learning their skills and serving as apprentices. To the native American, every physical thing in nature has a spiritual component because the whole is viewed as being essentially spiritual in nature. Thus, the medicine man or woman looks for spiritual causes of illness.[149]

There are different types of medicine men and women with specific roles. The first type is those who assume a purely positive role. They can transform themselves into other forms of life (birds, animals, divine spirits), have greater power than others, and possess truly altruistic personalities. They cannot use their powers in a negative way. Their main role is to maintain cultural integration at a time of great cultural stress. The second type are capable of both good and evil. They are expected to perform negative acts toward the tribe's enemies and have knowledge of witchcraft, poisoning, and other ways of doing evil to others. The diviner-diagnosticians are the third type. They diagnose the cause of the disharmony and may indicate a cure but do not have the power or skill necessary to implement treatment. They are called "crystal gazer" or "hand trembler" depending on the method used in diagnosing the patient. Fourth are the medicine men and women who specialize in the use of herbs for curative and nonsacred medical procedures. These roles often are assumed by older women who tend to pass on their roles to their daughters. Fifth are those medicine men and women whose primary concern is to care for souls. They send their guardian spirits to restore a soul that has been lost or captured by an evil spirit or by another medicine person.

Last are the singers who are usually male. The singer is the medicine man who treats illnesses and disharmony. He does it through laying on of hands, removal of disease-causing objects from bodies, massage, heat treatments, sweatbaths, and the use of herbs and roots. The main effects are psychological. During the chant the patient feels cared for in a very personal way as the center of the singer's attention. The singer is regarded as a distinguished authority and a person of eminence with the gift of learning from the holy people. He is seen as more than a mere mortal. The ceremony is considered prestigious, mystical, and powerful. The sick person is taken into a circle and the patient becomes one with the holy people. The patient then comes into harmony with the universe and becomes free of all ills and evil.[154]

A cure often requires the involvement of several medicine men and women. Medicine people may use medicine bundles (*jists*) containing symbolic and sacred items or small jars of medicinal solutions; they may leave red, grey, or black marks on the patient's skin; use tobacco; or burn cedar sage, grasses, or whatever is appropriate for that tribe. Bracelets of shells, seeds, beads, or arrowheads also may be used.

The goal of treatment is always to enhance total healing. If a herbalist treats a patient, prayers and songs are also offered for mental and spiritual renewal. An important component of the healing is the patient's motivation for recovery. Native Americans believe an individual gets back in equal proportion what he gives in words and actions to another.[142]

Healing ceremonies differ from tribe to tribe with varying degrees of complexity. Most of these ceremonies take place in the home with the participation of family members and other tribal members. Supporting the use of healing ceremonies in the hospital and providing space and privacy is helpful for the native American patient and family. Objects may be left in the room that were used in the ceremony. These objects are associated with elements identified with the cause of illness and should not be removed without the permission of the patient and his or her family.

Purification is often practiced to maintain harmony with nature and to cleanse the body and spirit. Many believe that for every natural disease, the earth provides a cure. Roots are often chewed on to relieve pain, clear the mind, or treat a toothache. Herbs are viewed as agents of nature.[149]

Traditional medicines include cedar incense for purification and corn pollen for blessings. A "seat" in a sweat lodge is a type of purging that is useful for preventing and treating illness. Monthly sweats may be used because it is believed that the body periodically builds up bad or negative spirits that block energy. Navajo women do not participate in sweats. Objects to guard against witchcraft may be carried by some tribes especially at nonfamily gatherings.[155]

Western physicians are regarded as a type of herbalist who can cure symptoms but cannot restore the individual's harmonious relationship with nature because they do not know the important rituals. Native Americans believe that a real medicine woman or man will know without being told what is wrong with a person. White doctors are seen as asking many questions and often are unable to determine what is wrong. Some native Americans believe that health care providers from the Indian Health Service come to the reservations to "practice" on the Indians, and that a white person should not tell the Indian about the illness if they have not experienced it previously.[149]

## Social organization

Traditional native American families are generally very involved in making decisions about the member's health care and may often make the decision for the patient. As members of a matrilineal society, native American patients may not give consent for anything until permission is obtained from the mother, grandmother, or aunt. Sometimes consent may be obtained only after a ceremony. If this cannot be done in the hospital, the patient may leave and return after the ceremony.[157]

Native Americans rely on their family, tribe, and land to cope with stress. The extended family is very important especially during periods of crisis. The family members provide a source of security, strength, and emotional support. When hospitalized, a variety of relatives will come expecting to visit with the hospitalized relative. Limiting visitors to only close relatives is not useful to native Americans as they do not distinguish between close and distant relatives. Family members may make great sacrifices traveling long distances to visit their family member. The hospitalized person expects the family to visit and the family expects to visit the patient.[156]

## Communication

Older native Americans may speak only their traditional language and often there are not comparable medical terms in the tribal language. Although translators are needed, they must understand the nature of social, cultural, and familial lines of communication and respect. Some tribes believe that a discussion with one individual about another is a sign of disrespect and could break a cultural taboo, leaving oneself or family vulnerable to harm. For the Navajo, special emphasis is on individual rights. Each person speaks for him- or herself and each individual's action should be self-initiated. In this case, trying to obtain information about another may be difficult. Limited ability to speak English may limit the understanding of the patient. It is common for native Americans to be silent rather than to admit to not understanding.

Making direct eye contact may be viewed as looking into one's soul and could result in its loss. Thus, native Americans who do not look directly at care providers should not be labeled as "inattentive" or "uninterested." Prolonged eye contact is considered a sign of disrespect and pointing is viewed as insulting.

Interpersonal relationships are carefully spelled out among Indian tribes. Who one speaks to, when the speaking occurs, how one speaks, and the sequence of speaking are very important. For example, a mother-in-law cannot speak to her son-in-law or be in the same room with him.[158] Awareness of these relationships is helpful to the nurse in communicating with native American patients and families.

The organization of thought processes behind the spoken word is taught early in childhood. The spoken word is considered an integral part of the sacred nature of humans. Native American communication generally emphasizes language that promotes the values of generosity, bravery, compassion, respect for elders, and concern for the tribal entity. The importance of observing periods of silence is a cultural trait. Silence helps formulate one's thoughts so that the spoken words will have significance. An individual who interrupts, interjects, or hurries toward abrupt conclusions is perceived as immature. Native American individuals are very sensitive to body language. If a health care provider appears hurried, nervous, or impatient, native Americans are quick to sense these cues, and blocks to communication may occur. Since native Americans are comfortable with silence, they do not feel a need to talk constantly and continual talking by the health care provider who is trying to obtain an adequate history may not be well received.[142]

Native Americans are private people who do not readily volunteer information. Excessive questioning by Western health professionals may be responded to by nods. Patients may actually not understand or may give responses they think the nurse wishes to hear, especially if the question is regarded as inappropriate. Some Navajos are shy in groups and individual counseling may be more effective.

Often the native American will be observing the provider and saying very little. The patient may expect the provider to deduce the problem through instinct rather than by extensive use of questions during history taking. This expectation is derived from the belief that direct questioning is intrusive to the individual's privacy. Making a declarative statement about an obvious symptom and allowing time for the patient to respond may be more helpful.

It is common for native Americans to speak in a very soft voice. It is expected that the listener will pay attention and listen carefully in order to hear what is being said. Asking for a repeat statement is considered rude. Speaking with a patient in a quiet setting so that they may be heard more easily is suggested.

Note taking is considered taboo for some native Americans since Indian history is passed on through verbal story telling.[149]

Some native Americans consider a firm handshake a sign of aggression. Navajos extend their hand and lightly touch the hand of the person they are greeting. Introducing oneself in the native language is often appreciated as well as knocking on the door before entering a room.

Using body language that is open without closing or crossing the arms is suggested. Loud speech may be viewed as rude or angry and speaking slowly may be perceived as condescending.

Initiating a visit with casual conversation about family, social functions, and about the tribe they are from may be helpful since native Americans are very private. This introductory period provides a gradual ease into discussions about personal and family health. Never use first person language when discussing risk factors such as "If you don't stop smoking, you will get cancer," as this may be viewed as putting a hex on the individual. Use of the first person in language is seen as involving one's spirit. Some may feel that talking with someone other than a family member about breasts, testicles, examining one's own body, or uterine bleeding is improper.

## Space and time

The busy atmosphere of a hospital or clinic may be uncomfortable for the native American whose tribal society is comfortable and warm. Personal space is very important to some native Americans who may have difficulty adapting to situations that place them in spaces that are not familiar such as clinics or hospitals. Hospitals may be viewed as a place to die and native Americans are hesitant to be admitted or put into a room where another person has died. Some tribes would welcome having the room purified before they enter it.

Modesty is very significant to the native American; limited exposure of body parts is suggested. Permission should be asked to perform a physical examination, and native American women may prefer a female practitioner.

Indian time typically runs from one hour to a few days later than standard time.[159] Indian homes often have no clocks. Time is casual, present oriented, and relative to present needs that must be accomplished in a given time frame. A present time orientation may cause a Navajo patient to eat two meals today, four meals tomorrow, no meals the next day, and three the following day. This would create difficulty if the patient was instructed to take a medication three times a day with meals. The present time orientation often can cause native Americans to be late for appointments.

Since Native Americans do not like standing out in a group and value privacy, individual rather than group counseling is likely to be preferred.

## Death and dying issues

Existence is circular and continuous for most traditional native Americans. They existed as spirit beings with the supreme creator before birth. At death their spirit joins the creator and eventually returns to the physical world in another form.[151] Death consists of joining one's ancestors and good or bad deeds have nothing to do with this reunion.

Generally Navajos will not touch a person who is dying because they must let the person go and touching could delay the soul's journey to the next world. There is also the fear that if they touch the dying person, the person's ghost will return and bother them. According to legend, the Navajo people originally emerged from the earth as fully formed humans. At that time, one female was missing. She was eventually found and became known as death, sickness, and witchcraft. Since her hair was unraveled and her body covered with dry red ochre, the Navajos today may unravel the hair of their dead and cover their bodies with red ochre.[153]

Attitudes and approaches to death and dying vary considerably among the tribes. Some are very accepting of death and others view dying people and death with fear. Some wish their family members to die at home, others prefer the hospital. Suffering is a major value in the native American culture and dying and grief may be met with stoicism and silence. The opportunity to share feelings may be rejected by the patient or family.[160] The family, including children, should be with the dying person even though they often may avoid touching the dead person or articles associated with that person.[27]

### Biological variations

There is a high incidence of obesity and alcohol abuse in native Americans. Some believe that the disruption and subsequent loss caused by the European settlement of North America left many native Americans feeling powerless and hopeless. These feelings may contribute to many of the social problems experienced today by native Americans.

The native American diet has changed over time. When they were nomadic, the diet was high in fiber and low in fat. Today the diets are likely to be high in refined carbohydrates, fat, and sodium and low in fiber, meat, eggs, cheese, and milk. Obesity is a major problem. Many native Americans are also lactose intolerant.

Native Americans are dark skinned and conditions such as jaundice or cyanosis will present differently than in fairer-skinned Americans.

## NURSING ISSUES

### Cancer, Poverty, and Ethnicity

In the late 1970s the question of the role of poverty in the differences in incidence, mortality, and survival of different ethnic groups was first raised. It appeared that poverty, not race, accounted for the 10%–15% lower survival rate from cancer in many ethnic groups. Baquet et al[161] found that when corrected for economic status, African-Americans had a slightly lower incidence and mortality for a number of cancers than did white Americans. The disproportionate number of African-Americans in the lower socioeconomic strata accounted for the increased incidence. Berg et al,[162] in a study that included only Caucasians who received the same level of care, found that indigent patients had poorer survival rates for each cancer type. Page and Kuntz[163] studied male Veteran's Administration patients with cancer and found similar survival rates between black and Caucasian Americans except for cancer of the bladder. All patients received the same treatment standard without regard to ability to pay for services. McWhorter and colleagues[164] analyzed SEER data from 1978 to 1982 and found that for cancers of the breast, cervix, esophagus, male lung, pancreas, and stomach, poverty accounted for most if not all of the differences. Poverty could not eliminate the ethnic differences in incidence rates for cancers of the bladder, prostate, uterus, and multiple myeloma.

The impact of poverty on cancer is felt in ethnic minorities since a disproportionate number of ethnic minorities comprises the poor of America. For example, in 1990, a large percentage of API families were below the poverty level as compared to Caucasian families. In 1989, African-Americans comprised approximately one-third of America's poor and 28.7% of all Hispanics were poor.[165,166]

The "culture of poverty" includes economic factors such as unemployment, unskilled occupations, no savings, no health insurance, and frequent daily food purchases in small amounts; social factors, such as crowded living quarters, women as single parents, low education, and critical attitudes toward the dominant class; and psychological factors such as feelings of helplessness, inferiority, fatalism and dependency, and a present time orientation with inability to defer gratification. These increase cancer incidence and mortality by increasing the risk factors of chronic malnutrition; occupational exposure through unskilled jobs; early initiation into sex and multiple partners; and smoking and alcoholism, contributing to cancers of the lung, oral cavity, prostate, cervix, or esophagus.[165] Secondary prevention may be absent because of a present orientation where survival needs take precedence over screening and early detection. A critical attitude toward the middle class and a sense of fatalism may decrease participation in screening programs. Delayed tertiary prevention is due to a lack of insurance, inability to pay for service, or limited care access. Emergency rooms are often used inappropriately and referral to clinics may result in fragmented care, impersonal service, long waiting hours, and transportation and child care problems.[167]

There are many common elements between the culture of poverty and the cultures of the four ethnic groups discussed. Poverty is overrepresented in these groups. Fatalism is a health belief of African-Americans, APIs, and Hispanics. Many African-Americans, Hispanics, some API groups, and native Americans tend to be present oriented.

The many recommendations made in the American Cancer Society report[168] on *Cancer in the Economically Disadvantaged* to reduce cancer incidence and mortality in the poor would be effective in many ethnic groups. These recommendations cluster around improving access by (1) establishing programs where the economically disadvantaged or ethnic minorities can gather in emergency rooms, neighborhood clinics, or churches; (2) developing culturally relevant educational materials that may be translated into different languages; (3) recruiting and training health care providers and volunteers from the targeted groups in the special needs of the poor or of a particular ethnic group. These issues are addressed in subsequent sections.

## Strategies to Enhance Access to Health Care

A primary barrier to cancer care for many of the ethnic minority populations is access to health care, especially among the socioeconomically disadvantaged. Since 1989 when attention was directed to this particular need, several programs have been developed. Many of these programs focus on providing effective cancer screening for ethnic minority populations using culturally sensitive strategies. These strategies include the involvement of trusted and respected members of the community in the planning and delivery of health care services,[70] provision of social support by women in the social network,[169] and development of culturally sensitive patient education materials.[170]

One of these programs, *The Witness Project,* consists of African-American women volunteers who are cancer survivors. By "witnessing" or talking about their cancer experience at churches and community centers, these volunteers help to increase breast and cervical cancer awareness and stress the importance of early detection among minority women in rural central and eastern Arkansas.[171]

Another program is the American Cancer Society's *Harlem Education and Detection Project* in New York City. The program uses the patient navigator model to assist individuals in overcoming health care access barriers. This model "attempts to guide the individual around and through the labyrinth of the health care system, through many of the social, community, health, and attitudinal barriers to ensure that patients receive timely diagnosis and treatment."[172,p.97] In addition, the navigator provides education and support to the individual.

The *Wai'anae Coast Cancer Control Project* in Hawaii also uses the navigator model. This project emphasizes community-driven cancer control as a means of improving breast and cervical cancer screening practices among native Hawaiian women. The navigators in this project are community members who provide information on cancer, and assist individuals in "navigating" the unfamiliar health care system by scheduling clinic appointments and patient follow-up services.[70]

*Mujer a Mujer: Woman to Woman* is an example of a successful, culturally sensitive patient education program targeting Hispanic women. It was developed to reduce the mortality from cervical cancer in this group.[170] Palos offers some of the culturally appropriate strategies used in the development of this and other effective cancer control programs:[170, p. 112]

- Follow basic rules when initiating interpersonal communication such as being courteous and respectful to establish trust or confidence.

- Use focus groups comprising grassroots (community) and professional individuals to validate promoters or barriers to attitudes, knowledge, and behavior related to cancer and its prevention.

- Use influential formal and informal leaders such as religious leaders, community gatekeepers, or opinion leaders.

- Integrate religious, cultural, and, when appropriate, traditional (folk) medicine and healing practices, beliefs, and taboos.

- Involve the family, friends, and members of other influential support systems.

- Determine a group's preferred communication process (verbal or nonverbal) as well as language preference.

- Determine an individual's degree of acculturation or assimilation, when appropriate.

- Involve paraprofessionals such as folk healers, when and if appropriate.

- Integrate cultural assessments into daily nursing practice.

The success of these culturally sensitive programs indicates that the targeted populations will utilize the services "if they are available, accessible, and acceptable" and provided in a humane and caring manner.[173] In addition, the American Cancer Society identified several successful strategies including:[172, p. 100]

- Hire outreach staff who are indigenous to the community.

- Piggyback onto other community program agendas.

- Avoid the "cancer only" approach.

- Develop materials that are culturally relevant and community specific.

- Keep educational messages simple.

- Fight fatalism by emphasizing the person's ability to affect health through action.

- Emphasize wellness and health, not cancer and fear.

Many other programs that target the socioeconomically disadvantaged and/or ethnic minority populations are reported in the literature.[102,174–177] However, this is just the beginning and additional programs are needed to continue the outreach efforts to the socioeconomically disadvantaged ethnic minority populations.

## Culturally Appropriate Public/Patient Education

Ethnic minority cancer patients are not much different from other cancer patients in their basic cancer information needs and in experiencing many of the learning barriers such as anxiety and feeling overwhelmed about the disease and treatment. However, ethnic minorities present certain unique challenges such as communicating in a language other than English and cultural values, beliefs, and practices that can affect the teaching/learning process.

### Strategies

Because of these challenges, several strategies have been identified to provide culturally sensitive patient education interventions. These strategies include:[98,170,172] (1) the development of culturally relevant and community-specific materials, (2) keeping educational messages simple, (3) determining the preferred language as well as learning process (e.g., video versus booklets; group versus one-on-one teaching), and (4) identification of the preferred communication style of the individual such as how to address him or her and acceptable nonverbal communication. For example, as mentioned in the description of the different ethnic groups, the appropriateness and acceptance of direct eye contact varies among the groups. In addition, determining decision-making patterns for the particular ethnic group is also important. An example of this is seen in many API groups where the family, instead of the patient, makes treatment decisions. In these situations, teaching the patient alone about a proposed chemotherapy treatment may not be appropriate if the educational effort needs to be directed to the family for subsequent decision making and consent to treatment.

***Use of interpreters*** Language is a frequent barrier to effective patient education. The use of professional interpreters, if available, is the optimal choice. Family and/or friends may be used but the correct or complete message may not be relayed. This distortion and/or omission of parts of the message may be due to the interpreter's own skill and fluency in the language, the interpreter's subjective editing (e.g., to "protect" the patient), or the patient's comfort level in discussing personal issues in the presence of the family member or friend. Recommendations for using interpreters and

what to do if there is no interpreter are listed in Table 62-10.[178,179]

***Translating written materials*** Although there are translated cancer information materials now available, additional resources still are needed. Just as professional interpreters are desirable, certain guidelines also exist for translating material. Translating material that is written in English into another language is not enough. The newly-translated material must be back-translated into English by independent translators.[180] This is to ensure that the content and tone is accurately captured and maintained throughout the translation. After making any corrections indicated from the back-translation, it also is helpful to pilot test the finished product with a sample of the target population for which the translated material was created.

Another key point to remember when translating existing materials is to assess the reading level of the original material. Analyses of the reading level of available cancer education materials have shown an average reading level that is much higher than the actual reading level of the general population.[181,182] Thus, the reading level of the material to be translated may need to be adjusted before being translated. Just as literacy has been identified as a barrier to cancer patient education for the general population, literacy is also a challenge faced by many ethnic minority groups. As mentioned earlier, there are a significant number of APIs who are functionally illiterate.[8] In addition, the literacy level of ethnic minority groups will be influenced by whether they are literate in their native language. For example, the Hmong culture is primarily an oral culture and many Hmong who immigrated to the United States are illiterate in Hmong.[183]

***Preferred styles of learning*** Determining an individual's preferred style of learning is also important. The different styles include one-to-one versus group, oral tradition, story telling, peer educators, and receiving information from "powerful others."[98] Some cultural groups may have preferences for one or more learning styles. For example, in a survey of Spanish-speaking patients and family members, one-to-one teaching was preferred by the majority (79%) versus other strategies such as videos (37%), print materials (32%), and group classes (16%).[184]

In another example, knowing the learning style of the targeted ethnic minority population helped in the development of a culturally sensitive cancer education video. Since story telling is used by many native Americans to relay information, this video, *Standing Strong Against the Cancer Enemy,* used the story format to convey its educational message on cancer prevention.[185]

Other successful educational strategies include the use of peer educators and "powerful others" to relay information. Enlisting fellow ethnic minorities to teach their peers is the basic principle behind the peer educator's strategy. The use of "powerful others" often involves the recruitment of respected community leaders who are

**TABLE 62-10** Overcoming Language Barriers

### USE OF AN INTERPRETER

- Before locating an interpreter, be sure that the language the patient speaks at home is known, since it may be different from the language spoken publicly (e.g., French is sometimes spoken by well-educated and upper-class members of certain Asian or Middle Eastern cultures).
- Avoid interpreters from a rival tribe, state, region, or nation (e.g., a Palestinian who knows Hebrew may not be the best interpreter for a Jewish client).
- Be aware of sex/gender differences between interpreter and patient. In general, same sex/gender is preferred.
- Be aware of age differences between interpreter and patient. In general, an older, more mature interpreter is preferred to a younger, less experienced one.
- Be aware of socioeconomic differences between interpreter and patient.
- Ask the interpreter to translate as closely to verbatim as possible.
- An interpreter who is a nonrelative may seek compensation for services rendered.

Recommendations for Institutions
- Maintain a computerized list of interpreters who may be contacted as needed.
- Network with area hospitals, colleges, universities, and other organizations that may serve as resources.
- Utilize the translation services provided by telephone companies (e.g., American Telephone and Telegraph Company).

### WHAT TO DO WHEN THERE IS NO INTERPRETER

- Be polite and formal.
- Greet the person using the last or complete name. Gesture to yourself and say your name. Offer a handshake or nod. Smile.
- Proceed in an unhurried manner. Pay attention to any effort by the patient or family to communicate.
- Speak in a low, moderate voice. Avoid talking loudly. Remember that there is a tendency to raise the volume and pitch of your voice when the listener appears not to understand. The listener may perceive that the nurse is shouting and/or angry.
- Use any words known in the patient's language. This indicates that the nurse is aware of and respects the client's culture.
- Use simple words, such as *pain* instead of *discomfort*. Avoid medical jargon, idioms, and slang. Avoid using contractions. Use nouns repeatedly instead of pronouns. Example: Do *not say*, "He has been taking his medicine, hasn't he?" Do say, "Does Juan take medicine?"
- Pantomime words and simple actions while verbalizing them.
- Give instructions in the proper sequence. Example: Do *not* say, "Before you rinse the bottle, sterilize it," Do say, "First, wash the bottle. Second, rinse the bottle."
- Discuss one topic at a time. Avoid using conjunctions. Example: Do *not* say, "Are you cold and in pain?" Do say, "Are you cold [while pantomiming]? Are you in pain?"
- Validate if the patient understands by having him or her repeat instructions, demonstrate the procedure, or act out the meaning.
- Write out several short sentences in English, and determine the person's ability to read them.
- Try a third language. Many Indo-Chinese speak French. Europeans often know three or four languages. Try Latin words or phrases, if the nurse if familiar with the language.
- Ask who among the patient's family and friends could serve as an interpreter.
- Obtain phrase books from a library or bookstore, make or purchase flash cards, contact hospitals for a list of interpreters, and use both formal and informal networking to locate a suitable interpreter.

Reprinted with permission from Andrews MM.[178]

recognized authorities people will listen to for information.[98]

Providing effective public and patient education for ethnic minority groups presents many challenges and opportunities for oncology nurses. Using the strategies presented in this section along with the knowledge of the individual's cultural background, oncology nurses can develop and implement successful culturally sensitive public and patient education interventions.

## Clinical Trials and Cancer Research

Historically, there has been underrepresentation of minorities in clinical trials. Two major barriers that have been identified are ethnic minorities' distrust of outsiders doing research in their communities (often referred to as "white-run research") and the lack of culturally sensitive and specific educational materials.

Brawley[171] cites a number of additional barriers to accrual of ethnic minorities in clinical trials including:

- difficulties in transportation

- inconvenient clinic hours

- lack of day care

- differences in language

- lack of understanding

- fear of being denied care because of inadequate financial support

- fear that researchers will take advantage

- not understanding the value of the research to the participant[171, p. 22]

In response to this underrepresentation of minorities and to recruit more minorities to National Cancer Institute (NCI)-sponsored clinical trials, NCI developed the Minority-Based (MB) Community Clinical Oncology Program (CCOP). Since its inception in 1990, one of the fundamental factors that has facilitated the progress of this program is the health care providers' respect for, and increased understanding of the unique cultures that they serve.[171]

Although progress has been made in accruing ethnic minority patients to cancer treatment trials, accrual to cancer prevention trials has not been as successful. For example, the number of ethnic minority patients enrolled in the NCI's breast and prostate cancer prevention trials is less than desired.[171] One of the reasons may be the disproportionate number of ethnic minorities who are socioeconomically disadvantaged. With immediate, day-to-day survival issues taking top priority, participating in a cancer prevention trial in which results may not be evident for years, would probably be unattractive and even meaningless to these individuals.[171,186]

Whether the issue is accrual of ethnic minorities to cancer treatment or cancer prevention trials, continued efforts directed toward overcoming the identified barriers are needed. McCabe et al[187] identified several factors that facilitate participation in clinical trials among ethnic minorities who are socioeconomically disadvantaged. These factors include:

- adequate information and education about the risks, benefits, costs, and time commitment required

- peer group norms that are supportive of the goals of the trial

- endorsement of the goals of clinical trials by church, the cultural or social group, and the employer

- improved access to the health care system and the specific location where the trial is being conducted

- a perceived benefit to the individual from participation

- minimal actual cost to the individual in terms of time lost from work, transportation, and child care[187, p. 126]

### Research studies

Conducting research involving ethnic minorities presents several unique challenges. One consideration is the selection of the study sample. Because of the heterogeneity of the major groups, study samples need to be selected carefully. For example, if the study sample was identified as native Americans, knowing which subgroups were studied would make a difference in interpreting the research findings and for whom the data are generalizable.

A second issue is that during the actual planning of a research study, knowing which particular ethnic group will be studied can make a difference in the development of appropriate instruments and the chosen research methodology.[188] For example, Munet-Vilaro[189] reports from personal experience that Latinos prefer to be interviewed rather than to take home a written test. Based on the findings that several ethnic minority groups had difficulty in using Likert scales, a concern has also been raised whether the Likert Scale is culturally biased.[189,190] Flaskerud[190] further proposes that "problems in using Likert scales cross-culturally could be due to education, faulty translation, irrelevant content, lack of semantic equivalence, the differing character of social interactions in various groups, or the nature of the response required. It is also possible that the degree of variation Likert scales attempt to measure is meaningless in some cultural groups."[190, p. 186]

Another concern is research instruments that are developed in English and translated into another language. When this occurs, subtle cultural nuances and conceptual equivalency may be compromised, leading to difficulties in retaining the validity of the instrument.[189] Strategies to overcome these potential problems include back-translation by professional translators with the primary objective of maintaining the essence of the meaning. Pilot testing the instrument with the appropriate population is also recommended to establish reliability.[189]

As the U.S. population becomes more culturally diverse, there is an obvious need for more cancer research involving ethnic minorities, as well as the expertise to incorporate cultural considerations in developing and conducting cancer research studies.

## Resources

In response to the increasing awareness of the needs of our culturally diverse populations and the health care professionals who care for them, specific resources have been created along with the ongoing development of new ones. These resources are available at the national and local levels, and include educational materials and professional organizations.

Three of the major resources available at the national level are the Office of Minority Health Resource Center (OMH-RC), the National Cancer Institute's Cancer Information Service (CIS), and the American Cancer Society (ACS). Information available at the federal, state, and local levels on health-related resources for African-Americans, APIs, Hispanics, and native Americans are maintained by the OMH-RC.[42] The CIS provides information on cancer for the general public, cancer patients/families, and health care professionals. This organization has a national toll-free number that provides access to Spanish- and English-speaking staff. The ACS also provides information on cancer to the general public, patients/families and health care professionals and has developed specific educational materials targeting ethnic minorities. (See chapter 66: Cancer Nursing Resources, for the addresses and telephone numbers of these organizations.)

Several professional organizations also exist to promote cultural awareness in nurses and to provide support for ethnic minority nurses. One of these is the national organization for oncology nurses, the Oncology Nursing Society (ONS). ONS originally had two specific groups devoted to multicultural issues with an oncology focus: the Multicultural Advisory Council and the Transcultural Nursing Issues Special Interest Group (TNI SIG). The Council no longer exists, but its past efforts and the ongoing work of the TNI SIG continue to assist the ONS in achieving its objective of becoming a culturally competent organization. Also, the Transcultural Nursing Society of Illinois provides support to nurses for the delivery of culturally competent care. Professional nursing organizations that specifically target ethnic minority nurses include the Asian American/Pacific Islander Nurses' Association, the Association of Chicana/Latina Nurses, the Council of Black Nurses, the National Association of Hispanic Nurses, the National Black Nurses' Association, the National Center for the Advancement of Blacks in the Health Professions, and the Philippine Nurses' Association of America. National minority organizations such as the American Indian Health Care Association offer other available resources.

At the local level, several ACS divisions and units have developed specific educational materials for ethnic minorities. The California Division has cataloged materials for underserved and ethnic populations that are available within its division and some of the other ACS divisions.

Specific local resources may vary in their availability from region to region as a reflection of the ethnic minority populations that are served. For example, Hispanic resources are probably more accessible in New Mexico than in Hawaii. Other organizations that are not specifically cancer-related, such as the American Lung Association or refugee services, also may be of assistance in providing educational materials and/or programs for ethnic minority populations.

These resources offer much needed assistance to oncology nurses in providing culturally competent care. As resource development continues at all levels in the United States, individuals with cancer, their families, and the health care professionals who serve them all will benefit.

## CONCLUSION

Cultural diversity is an inescapable phenomenon that we will continue to experience with the rapidly changing composition of the population of the United States. The impact of cultural diversity on the provision of cancer care is multilayered. At one level each ethnic group, with its unique values, health beliefs, and practices, responds to cancer somewhat differently. Additional factors such as degree of acculturation, socioeconomic status, and educational attainment add yet another layer of inter- and intragroup diversity. A third level is an underlying, often negative perception among many ethnic minorities of the mainstream culture and Western medicine. This is primarily due to their history and experience with this culture, that in turn influences their health behaviors, attitudes, and acceptance of mainstream health care.

In the midst of this diversity, there are also shared responses among the major cultural groups. Many of the ethnic minority groups believe in and practice folk healing, consult both traditional and Western practitioners, and use both traditional and Western medicine. Many groups also place a high value on the family.

However, individual variations make it inappropriate to generalize certain group characteristics to all subgroups and each member of each group. Regardless of ethnicity, the individual must come first.

The heterogeneity and marked cultural diversity of our population presents many challenges for oncology nurses. This chapter surveyed key cultural beliefs and practices and their impact on cancer care of several ethnic groups. Because of the inherent differences between mainstream and ethnic minority cultures and the potential for misunderstanding and conflict, continued efforts at increasing knowledge, appreciation, and understanding of each culture are needed. Our challenge is to facilitate these efforts within ourselves, among other health professionals, and in the community at large.

## REFERENCES

1. Barkauskas V, Stoltenberg-Allen K, Baumann L, et al: Cultural considerations in health assessment, in Barkauskas V, Stoltenberg-Allen K, Baumann L, et al: *Health and Physical Assessment.* St. Louis, Mosby-Year Book, 1994, pp 149–181
2. Leininger MM: The theory of culture care diversity and universality, in Leininger MM (ed): *Cultural Care Diversity and Universality: A Theory of Nursing.* New York, National League for Nursing Press, 1991, pp 5–68
3. Seidel HM, Ball JW, Dains JE, et al: Cultural awareness, in Seidel HM, Ball JW, Dains JE, et al (eds): *Mosby's Guide to*

*Physical Examination* (ed 3). St. Louis, Mosby-Year Book, 1995, pp 34–56

4. Spector RE: Culture, ethnicity, and nursing, in Potter PA, Perry AG (eds): *Fundamentals of Nursing: Concepts, Process, and Practice* (ed 3). St. Louis, Mosby-Year Book, 1993, pp 94–119

5. Spector RE: Cultural factors in health, in Potter PA, Perry AG (eds): *Basic Nursing: Theory and Practice* (ed 2). St. Louis, Mosby-Year Book, 1991, pp 338–351

6. Galanti G: Basic concepts, in Galanti G: *Caring for Patients From Different Cultures.* Philadelphia, University of Pennsylvania Press, 1991, pp 1–14

7. Lewin M, Rice B (eds): *Balancing the Scales of Opportunity: Ensuring Racial and Ethnic Diversity in the Health Professions.* Committee on Increasing Minority Participation in the Health professions, Institute of Medicine. Washington, DC, National Academy Press, 1994

8. Lin-Fu JS: Asian and Pacific Islander Americans: an overview of demographic characteristics and health care issues. *Asia Am Pac Islander J Health* 1:20–36, 1993

9. Day JC: *Population Projections of the United States, by Age, Sex, Race, and Hispanic Origin: 1993 to 2050,* U.S. Bureau of the Census, Current Population Reports, P25-1104, Washington, DC, U.S. Government Printing Office, 1993

10. Campbell PR: *Population Projection for States, by Age, Race, Sex, and Hispanic Origin: 1993–2020.* U.S. Bureau of the Census, Current Population Reports, P25-111. Washington, DC, U.S. Government Printing Office, 1994

11. U.S. Dept. of Commerce, Bureau of the Census: *1990 Census of Population and Housing.* Equal Employment Opportunity File, Computer File, CD ROM. Washington, DC, Data User Services Division, 1993

12. American Cancer Society: *Cancer Facts & Figures—1996.* Atlanta, American Cancer Society, 1996

13. Kagawa-Singer M: Socioeconomic and cultural influences on cancer care of women. *Semin Oncol Nurs* 11:109–119, 1995

14. Miller BA, Kolonel LN, Bernstein L, Young JL Jr., Swanson GM, West D, Key CR, Liff JM, Glover CS, Alexander GA, Coyle L, Hankey BF, Ries LAG, Kosary CL, Harras A, Percy C, and Edwards (eds): *Racial/Ethnic Patterns of Cancer in the United States 1988–1992.* NIH publication No. 96–4104. Bethesda, MD, National Cancer Institute, 1996

15. American Cancer Society: *Cancer Facts and Figures for Minority Americans 1991.* Atlanta, American Cancer Society, 1991

16. Frank-Stromborg M: Changing demographics in the United States: implications for health professionals. *Cancer* 67:1772–1778, 1991 (suppl)

17. Lin-Fu JS: Population characteristics and health care needs of Asian Pacific Americans. *Public Health Rep* 103:18–27, 1988

18. Chen MS: A 1993 status report on the health status of Asian Pacific Islander Americans: comparisons with *Healthy People 2000* objectives. *Asia Am Pac Islander J Health* 1:37–55, 1993

19. Young JL, Ries LG, Pollack ES: Cancer patient survival among ethnic groups in the United States. *J Natl Cancer Inst* 73:344–352, 1984

20. American Cancer Society: A summary of the American cancer society report to the nation: cancer in the poor. *CA Cancer J Clin* 39:263–265, 1989

21. Herberg P: Theoretical foundations of transcultural nursing, in Andrews MM, Boyle JS (eds): *Transcultural Concepts in Nursing Care* (ed 2). Philadelphia, Lippincott, 1995, pp 3–47

22. Giger JN, Davidhizar RE: Introduction to transcultural nursing, in Giger JN, Davidhizar RE (eds): *Transcultural Nursing: Assessment and Intervention* (ed 2). St. Louis, Mosby-Year Book, 1995, pp 3–18

23. Flaskerud JH: Transcultural concepts in mental health nursing, in Boyle JS, Andrews MM (eds): *Transcultural Concepts in Nursing Care.* Glenview, IL, Scott, Foresman/Little Brown College Division, 1989, pp 243–269

24. Giger JN, Davidhizar RE: Communication, in Giger JN, Davidhizar RE (eds): *Transcultural Nursing: Assessment and Intervention* (ed 2). St Louis, Mosby-Year Book, 1995, pp 19–41

25. Rairdan B, Higgs ZR: When your patient is a Hmong refugee. *Am J Nurs* 92:52–55, 1992

26. Stauffer RY: Vietnamese Americans, in Giger JN, Davidhizar RE (eds): *Transcultural Nursing: Assessment and Intervention* (ed 2). St. Louis, Mosby-Year Book, 1995, pp 441–472

27. Kozier B, Erle G, Blais K, et al: Ethnicity and culture, in Kozier B, Erle G, Blais K, et al (eds): *Fundamentals of Nursing* (ed 5). Redwood City, CA, Addison-Wesley, 1995, pp 291–310

28. Hayter J: Territoriality as a universal need. *J Adv Nurs* 6: 79–85, 1981

29. Giger JN, Davidhizar RE: Space, in Giger JN, Davidhizar RE (eds): *Transcultural Nursing: Assessment and Intervention* (ed 2). St Louis, Mosby-Year Book, 1995, pp 43–60

30. Galanti G: Folk medicine—Practices and perspectives, in Galanti G: *Caring for Patients From Different Cultures.* Philadelphia, University of Pennsylvania Press, 1991, pp 95–109

31. Giger JN, Davidhizar RE: Social organization, in Giger JN, Davidhizar RE (eds): *Transcultural Nursing: Assessment and Intervention* (ed 2). St Louis, Mosby-Year Book, 1995, pp 61–87

32. Galanti G: Men and women, in Galanti G: *Caring for Patients From Different Cultures.* Philadelphia, University of Pennsylvania Press, 1991, pp 63–78

33. Galanti G: Communication and time orientation, in Galanti G: *Caring for Patients From Different Cultures.* Philadelphia, University of Pennsylvania Press, 1991, pp 15–33

34. Herberg P: Theoretical foundations of transcultural nursing, in Boyle JS, Andrews MM (eds): *Transcultural Concepts in Nursing Care.* Glenview, IL, Scott, Foresman/Little Brown College Division, 1989, pp 3–65

35. Giger JN, Davidhizar RE: Biological variations, in Giger JN, Davidhizar RE (eds): *Transcultural Nursing: Assessment and Intervention* (ed 2). St Louis, Mosby-Year Book, 1995, pp 127–161

36. Estes G, Zitzow D: *Heritage Consistency as a Consideration in Counseling Native Americans.* Paper presented at the Convention of the National Indian Education Association, Dallas, 1980

37. Spector RE: Heritage consistency: a predictor of health beliefs and practices. *Recent Advances in Nursing* 23:23–35, 1989

38. Spector RE: Culture, health and illness, in Spector RE: *Cultural Diversity in Health and Illness* (ed 4). Stamford, CT, Appleton & Lange, 1996, pp 63–88,371–373

39. Randall-David E: *Strategies for Working With Culturally Diverse Communities and Clients.* Washington, DC, Association for the Care of Children's Health, 1989, pp 7–9

40. Giger JN, Davidhizar RE: *Transcultural Nursing.* St. Louis, Mosby-Year Book, 1991

41. Andrews MM, Boyle JE (eds): *Transcultural Concepts in Nursing Care* (ed 2). Philadelphia, Lippincott, 1995

42. Frank-Stromborg M, Olsen SJ (eds): *Cancer Prevention in*

*Minority Populations: Cultural Implications for Health Care Professionals.* St. Louis, Mosby-Year Book, 1993

43. Galanti G: *Caring for Patients From Different Cultures.* Philadelphia, University of Pennsylvania Press, 1991

44. Giger JN, Davidhizar RE (eds): *Transcultural Nursing: Assessment and Intervention* (ed 2). St. Louis, Mosby-Year Book, 1995

45. Orque M, Bloch B, Monrrou LSA (eds): *Ethnic Nursing Care: A Multicultural Approach.* St. Louis, Mosby, 1983

46. Palafox N, Warren A (eds): *Cross-Cultural Caring: A Handbook for Health Care Professionals in Hawaii.* Honolulu, John A. Burns School of Medicine, 1980

47. Spector RE: *Cultural Diversity in Health and Illness* (ed 4). Stamford, CT, Appleton & Lange, 1996

48. Michaels D: Occupational cancer in the Black population: the health effects of job discrimination. *J Nat Med Assoc* 75:1014–1018, 1983

49. Clarke-Tasker VA: Cancer prevention and early detection in African Americans, in Frank-Stromborg M, Olsen SJ (eds): *Cancer Prevention in Minority Populations: Cultural Implications for Health Care Professionals.* St. Louis, Mosby-Year Book, 1993, pp 142–185

50. Bloom JR, Hayes WA, Saunders F, et al: Physician induced and patient induced utilization of early cancer detection practices among Black Americans. *Adv Cancer Control: Innov Res* 293:279–296, 1989

51. Savitt TL: Care of urban and industrial slaves, the aged and free blacks, in Savitt TL (ed): *Medicine and Slavery: The Diseases and Health Care in Antebellum Virginia.* Urbana, IL, University of Illinois Press, 1978, pp 185–218

52. Jordan WC: Voodoo medicine, in Williams RA (ed): *Textbook of Black-Related Diseases.* New York, McGraw-Hill, 1975, pp 115–138

53. Cherry B, Giger JN: African-Americans, in Giger JN, Davidhizar RE (eds): *Transcultural Nursing: Assessment and Intervention* (ed 2). St. Louis, Mosby-Year Book, 1995, pp 165–203

54. U.S. Dept. of Commerce, Bureau of the Census: *The Black Population in the United States, March 1991.* Washington, DC, U.S. Government Printing Office, 1992

55. Queen SA, Habenstein RW: The contemporary black American family, in Queen SA, Habenstein RW (eds): *The Family in Various Cultures* (ed 4). Philadelphia, Lippincott, 1974, pp 345–375

56. Snow LE: Tradition health beliefs and practice among lower class Black Americans. *West J Med* 139:820–828, 1977

57. Eng E, Hatch J, Callan A: Institutionalizing social support through the church and into the community. *Health Educ Q* 12:81–91, 1985

58. Askey DB, Parker D, Alexander D, et al: Clergy as intermediary—an approach to cancer control, in Mettlin C, Murphy GP (eds): *Progress in Cancer Control, IV: Research in the Cancer Center.* New York, Alan R. Liss, 1983, pp 417–424

59. Smitherman G: White English in blackface or who do I be? *Black Scholar* 1:32–39, 1973

60. Bloch B: Nursing care of black patients, in Orque M, Bloch B, Monrrou LSA: *Ethnic Nursing Care: A Multicultural Approach.* St. Louis, Mosby Co., 1983, pp 81–114

61. Sue D: Cross-cultural communication/counseling styles, in Sue D (ed): *Counseling the Culturally Different: Theory and Practice.* New York, Wiley, 1981, pp 49–74

62. Bigham GD: To communicate with Negro patients. *Am J Nurs* 64:113–115, 1964

63. Poussaint A, Atkinson C: Black youth and motivation. *Black Scholar* 1:43–51, 1970

64. Brown JA: Social work practice with the terminally ill in the black community, in Parry JK (ed): *Social Work Practice With the Terminally Ill: A Transcultural Perspective.* Springfield, IL, Charles C Thomas, 1990, pp 67–82

65. Kemp C: Sociocultural care, in Kemp C (ed): *Terminal Illness: A Guide to Nursing Care.* Philadelphia, Lippincott, 1995, pp 63–74

66. Ronan L: Alcohol-related health risks among Black Americans. *Alcohol Health Res World* 11:36–39, 1986

67. Williams M: Alcohol and ethnic minorities: Native Americans—an update. *Alcohol Health Res World* 11:5–6, 1986

68. Parker D, Harman M: The distribution of consumption model of prevention of alcoholic problems: a critical assessment. *J Study Alcohol* 39:377–399, 1978

69. U.S. Bureau of the Census: *Current Population Reports, Population Characteristics. P.20–459. The Asian and Pacific Islander Population in the United States, March 1991 and 1990.* Washington, DC, U.S. Government Printing Office, 1992

70. Hussey LOL, Itano JK, Taoka KN, et al: Cancer prevention and early detection in Native Hawaiians, in Frank-Stromborg M, Olsen SJ (eds): *Cancer Prevention in Minority Populations: Cultural Implications for Health Care Professionals.* St. Louis, Mosby, 1993, pp 113–138

71. Sawyers JE, Eaton L: Gastric cancer in the Korean-American: cultural implications. *Oncol Nurs Forum* 19:619–623, 1992

72. Gould-Martin K, Ngin C: Chinese Americans, in Harwood A (ed): *Ethnicity and Medical Care.* Cambridge, MA, Harvard University Press, 1981, pp 130–171

73. Chang K: Chinese Americans, in Giger JN, Davidhizar RE (eds): *Transcultural Nursing: Assessment and Intervention* (ed 2). St. Louis, Mosby-Year Book, 1995, pp 395–414

74. Lee P, Takamura J: The Japanese Americans in Hawaii, in Palafox N, Warren A (eds): *Cross-Cultural Caring: A Handbook for Health Care Professionals in Hawaii.* Honolulu, John A. Burns School of Medicine, 1980, pp 105–135

75. Hashizume S, Takano J: Nursing care of Japanese American patients, in Orque M, Bloch B, Monrrou LSA (eds): *Ethnic Nursing Care: A Multicultural Approach.* St. Louis, Mosby, 1983, pp 219–243

76. Ludman EK, Newman JM: Yin and yang in the health-related food practices of three Chinese groups. *J Nutr Educ* 16:3–5, 1984

77. Campbell T, Chang B: Health care of the Chinese in America, in Henderson G, Primeaux M (eds): *Transcultural Health Care.* Menlo Park, CA, Addison-Wesley, 1981, pp 162–171

78. Chen-Louie T: Nursing care of Chinese American patients, in Orque M, Block B, Monrrou LSA (eds): *Ethnic Nursing Care: A Multicultural Approach.* St. Louis, Mosby, 1983, pp 183–218

79. Buchwald D, Panwala S, Hooton TM: Use of traditional health practices by Southeast Asian refugees in a primary care clinic. *West J Med* 156:507–511, 1992

80. Anderson JN: Health and illness in Filipino immigrants. *West J Med* 139:811–819, 1983

81. Ramakrishna J, Weiss MG: Health, illness, and immigration—East Indians in the United States. *West J Med* 157:265–270, 1992

82. Gilman SC, Justice J, Saepharn K, et al: Use of traditional and modern health services by Laotian refugees. *West J Med* 157:310–315, 1992

83. Uba L: Cultural barriers to health care for Southeast Asian refugees. *Public Health Rep* 107:544–548, 1992

84. Baysa E, Cabrera E, Camilon F, et al: The Filipinos, in Palafox N, Warren A (eds): *Cross-Cultural Caring: A Handbook for Health Care Professionals in Hawaii.* Honolulu, John A. Burns School of Medicine, 1980, pp 197–212

85. Hart DV: Bisayan Filipino and Malayan folk medicine, in Henderson G, Primeaux M (eds): *Transcultural Health Care.* Menlo Park, CA, Addison-Wesley, Inc., 1981, pp 148–161

86. Orque MS: Nursing care of Filipino American patients, in Orque M, Bloch B, Monrrou LSA (eds): *Ethnic Nursing Care: A Multicultural Approach.* St. Louis, Mosby, 1983, pp 149–181

87. Kunz K, Lam C, Siu K, et al: The Chinese, in Palafox N, Warren A (eds): *Cross-Cultural Caring: A Handbook for Health Care Professionals in Hawaii.* Honolulu, John A. Burns School of Medicine, 1980, pp 26–50

88. Nguyen MD: Culture shock—a review of Vietnamese culture and its concepts of health and disease. *West J Med* 142:409–412, 1985

89. Chow E: Cultural health traditions: Asian perspectives, in Branch MF, Paxton PP (eds): *Providing Safe Nursing Care for Ethnic People of Color.* New York, Appleton-Century-Crofts, 1976, pp 99–114

90. Andrews MM: Transcultural perspectives in the nursing care of children and adolescents, in Andrews MM, Boyle JS (eds): *Transcultural Concepts in Nursing Care* (ed 2). Philadelphia, Lippincott, 1995, pp 123–179

91. Krauss BH: Medicine and medicinal herbs, in Krauss BH: *Plants in Hawaiian Culture.* Honolulu, University of Hawaii Press, 1993, pp 100–104

92. Vance AR: Filipino Americans, in Giger JN, Davidhizar RE (eds): *Transcultural Nursing: Assessment and Intervention* (ed 2). St. Louis, Mosby-Year Book, 1995, pp 417–438

93. Ishida D, Inouye J: Japanese Americans, in Giger JN, Davidhizar RE (eds): *Transcultural Nursing: Assessment and Intervention* (ed 2). St. Louis, Mosby-Year Book, 1995, pp 317–345

94. Lasky EM, Martz CH: The Asian/Pacific Islander population in the United States: cultural perspectives and their relationship to cancer prevention and early detection, in Frank-Stromborg M, Olsen SJ (eds): *Cancer Prevention in Minority Populations: Cultural Implications for Health Care Professionals.* St. Louis, Mosby, 1993, pp 78–112

95. Klessig J: The effects of values and culture on life-support decisions. *West J Med* 157:316–322, 1992

96. Earp JB: Korean Americans, in Giger JN, Davidhizar RE (eds): *Transcultural Nursing: Assessment and Intervention* (ed 2). St. Louis, Mosby-Year Book, 1995, pp 555–572

97. Miller SW, Goodin JN: East Indian Hindu Americans, in Giger JN, Davidhizar RE (eds): *Transcultural Nursing: Assessment and Intervention* (ed 2). St. Louis, Mosby-Year Book, 1995, pp 475–499

98. Tripp-Reimer T, Afifi LA: Cross-cultural perspectives on patient teaching. *Nurs Clin North Am* 24:613–619, 1989

99. Haffner L: Translation is not enough—interpreting in a medical setting. *West J Med* 157:255–259, 1992

100. Jenkins CNH, McPhee SJ, Bird JA, et al: Cancer risks and prevention practices among Vietnamese refugees. *West J Med* 153:34–39, 1990

101. Mo B: Modesty, sexuality, and breast health in Chinese-American women. *West J Med* 157:260–264, 1992

102. Lovejoy NC, Jenkins C, Wu T, et al: Developing a breast cancer screening program for Chinese-American women. *Oncol Nurs Forum* 16:181–187, 1989

103. Muller JH, Desmond B: Ethical dilemmas in a cross-cultural context—a Chinese example. *West J Med* 157:323–327, 1992

104. Brotzman GL, Butler DJ: Cross-cultural issues in the disclosure of a terminal diagnosis: a case report. *J Fam Pract* 32:426–427, 1991

105. Tung TM: Death, dying, and hospice: an Asian-American view. *Am J Hosp Palliat Care* 7:23–25, 1990

106. Zhou H-H, Koshakji RP, Silberstein DJ, et al: Racial differences in drug response: altered sensitivity to and clearance of propranolol in men of Chinese descent as compared with American Whites. *N Engl J Med* 320:565–570, 1989

107. U.S. Bureau of the Census: *Current Population Reports, The Hispanic Population in the United States.* Washington, DC, U.S. Government Printing Office, March 1989

108. U.S. Bureau of the Census: *Current Population Reports, The Hispanic Population in the United States.* Washington, DC, U.S. Government Printing Office, 1991

109. Cohen RJ, Rohaly JA: Cancer prevention and screening among Hispanic populations, in Frank-Stromborg M, Olsen SJ (eds): *Cancer Prevention in Minority Populations: Cultural Implications for Health Care Professionals.* St. Louis, Mosby-Year Book, 1993, pp 203–238

110. Martin J, Suarez L: Cancer mortality among Mexican-Americans and other Whites in Texas, 1969–1980. *Am J Public Health* 77:851–853, 1987

111. Mack TM, Walker A, Mack W, et al: Cancer in Hispanics in Los Angeles County. *Monogr Natl Cancer Inst* 69:99–104, 1985

112. Devor EJ, Buechley RW: Gallbladder cancer in Hispanic New Mexicans: I. general population 1957–1977. *Cancer* 45:1705–1712, 1980

113. Menck HR, Mack TM: Incidence of biliary tract cancer in Los Angeles. *Monogr Natl Cancer Inst* 62:95–99, 1982

114. Suarez L, Martin J: Primary liver cancer mortality and incidence in Texas Mexican Americans 1969–1980. *Am J Public Health* 77:631–633, 1987

115. Peters RK, Thomas D, Hagan DG, et al: Risk factors in invasive cervical cancer among Latinas and non-Latinas in Los Angeles County. *J Natl Cancer Inst* 77:1063–1077, 1986

116. Daly MB, Clark GM, McGuire WL: Breast cancer prognosis in a mixed Caucasian Hispanic population. *J Natl Cancer Inst* 74:753–757, 1985

117. Kuipers J: Mexican-Americans, in Giger JN, Davidhizar RE (eds): *Transcultural Nursing: Assessment and Intervention* (ed 2). St. Louis, Mosby-Year Book, 1995, pp 205–234

118. Hautman MA: Folk health and illness beliefs. *Nurse Pract* 4:23,26–27,31,34, 1979

119. Currier R: The hot-cold syndrome and symbolic medicine. *Ethnology* 5:251–263, 1966

120. Wilson H, Kneisl C: Cultural considerations, in Wilson H, Kneisl C (eds): *Psychiatric Nursing.* Reading, MA, Addison-Wesley, 1988, pp 1050–1077

121. Marsh WW, Hentges K: Mexican folk remedies and conventional medical care. *Am Fam Pract* 37:257–262, 1988

122. Foreman JT: Susto and the health needs of the Cuban refugee population. *Top Clin Nurs* 7:40–47, 1985

123. Gonzales-Swafford MJ, Gutierrez MG: Ethnomedical beliefs and practices of Mexican Americans. *Nurs Pract* 8:29–30, 32,34, 1983

124. Sugarek NJ, Deyo RA, Holmes BC: Locus of control and beliefs about cancer in a multi-ethnic clinic population. *Oncol Nurs Forum* 15:481–486, 1988

125. Rodriques J: Mexican Americans: factors influencing health practices. *J Sch Health* 53:136–139, 1983

126. Mardiros M: A view toward hospitalization: the Mexican-American experience. *J Adv Nurs* 9:469–478, 1984

127. Estrada A, Trevino F, Ray L: Health care utilization barriers among Mexican Americans: evidence from HHANES 1982–84. *Am J Public Health* 80:27–31, 1990 (suppl)

128. Kerr M, Ritchey D: Health promoting lifestyles of English-speaking and Spanish-speaking Mexican-American migrant farm workers. *Public Health Nurs* 7:80–87, 1990

129. Martaus TM: The health seeking process of Mexican-American migrant farm workers. *Home Health C Nurse* 4:32–36, 1986

130. Ingham J: On Mexican folk medicine. *Am Anthropologist* 72:76–87, 1970

131. Gomez GE, Gomez EA: Folk healing among Hispanic Americans. *Public Health Nurs* 2:245–249, 1985

132. Murillo N: The Mexican American family, in Martinez RA (ed): *Hispanic Culture and Health Care: Fact, Fiction and Folklore.* St. Louis, Mosby, 1978, pp 3–18

133. Logan B, Semmes C: Culture and ethnicity, in Logan B, Dawkins C (eds): *Family-Centered Nursing in the Community.* Reading, MA, Addison-Wesley, 1986, pp 112–113

134. Murillo-Rohde I: Hispanic American patient care, in Henderson G, Primeaux M (eds): *Transcultural Health Care.* Menlo Park, CA, Addison-Wesley, 1981, pp 224–238

135. Murillo-Rohde I: Care for all colors. *Imprint* 24:29–32, 50, 1977

136. Kalish RA, Reynolds DK: Mexican-Americans, in Kalish RA, Reynolds DK (eds): *Death and Ethnicity: A Psychocultural Study.* Farmingdale, NY, Baywood, 1981, pp 155–184

137. Salcido RM: Mexican-Americans: illness, death and bereavement, in Parry JK (ed): *Social Work With the Terminally Ill: A Transcultural Perspective.* Springfield, IL, Charles C Thomas, 1990, pp 113–127

138. National Coalition of Hispanic Health and Human Services Organizations: *Delivering Preventive Health Care to Hispanics: A Manual for Providers.* Washington, DC, The Coalition, 1988

139. Olsen SJ: Cancer prevention and early detection in Native Americans, in Frank-Stromborg M, Olsen SJ (eds): *Cancer Prevention in Minority Populations: Cultural Implications for Health Care Professionals.* St. Louis, Mosby-Year Book, 1993, pp 3–56

140. Emery G: Trail still tearful for Indian tribes. *Insight* 2:8–21, 1986

141. Vobejda B: More Americans declaring Indian identify. *The Washington Post*, February 11, 1991, A-1, col. 3

142. Wilson UM: Nursing care of American Indian patients, in Orque M, Bloch B, Monrrou LSA (eds): *Ethnic Nursing Care: A Multicultural Approach.* St. Louis, Mosby, 1983, pp 271–295

143. U.S. Dept. of Health and Human Services: *Report of the Secretary's Task Force on Black and Minority Health: Cancer, Vol. 3.* Washington, DC, U.S. Government Printing Office, 1989

144. Bivens MD, Fleetwood HO: A ten year survey of cervical carcinoma in Indians of the southwest. *Obstet Gynecol* 32:11–16, 1968

145. Skubi D: Pap smear screening and cervical pathology in an American Indian population. *J Nurse Midwife* 33:203–207, 1988

146. Horner RD: Cancer mortality in Native Americans in North Carolina. *Am J Public Health* 80:940–944, 1990

147. Weiss KM, Ferrell RE, Hanis CL, et al: Genetics and epidemiology of gallbladder disease in new world native peoples. *Am J Hum Genet* 36:1259–1278, 1984

148. American Indian Policy Review Commission: *Task Force Six: Indian Health.* Washington, DC, U.S. Government Printing Office, 1976

149. Spector RE: Health and illness in the American Indian, Aleut, and Eskimo communities, in Spector RE (ed): *Cultural Diversity in Health and Illness* (ed 4). Stamford, CT, Appleton & Lange, 1996, pp 215–240

150. Toelken B: Seeing with a native eye: How many sheep will it hold?, in Capps WH: *Seeing With a Native Eye: Essays on Native American Religion.* New York, Harper & Row, 1976, pp 9–24

151. Locust CS: *American Indian Beliefs Concerning Health and Unwellness.* Native American Research and Training Center, Monograph Series. Tucson, AZ, University of Arizona, 1985

152. Boyd D: *Rolling Thunder.* New York, Random House, 1974

153. Bilagody H: An American Indian looks at health care, in Feldman R, Buch D (eds): *Ninth Annual Training Institute for Psychiatrist-Teachers of Practicing Physicians.* Boulder, CO, WICHE, 1969

154. Kluckhohn C, Leighton D: The supernatural: Power and danger, in Kluckhohn C, Leighton D (eds): *The Navajo* (rev ed). Garden City, NJ, Doubleday, 1962, pp 178–199

155. Vogel VJ: Indian theories of disease and shamanistic practices, in Vogel VJ (ed): *American Indian Medicine.* New York, Ballantine Books, 1979, pp 13–35

156. Primeaux M, Henderson G: American Indian patient care, in Henderson G, Primeaux M (eds): *Transcultural Health Care.* Menlo Park, CA, Addison-Wesley, 1981, pp 239–254

157. Antle A: Ethnic perspectives of cancer nursing: the American Indian. *Oncol Nurs Forum* 14:70–73, 1987

158. Lammers PK: How they view you, themselves, and disease. *AORN J* 45:1211–1216, 1987

159. Yuki T: Cultural responsiveness and social work practice: an Indian clinic's success. *Health Soc Work* 11:223–229, 1986

160. Lewis R: Death and dying among the American Indians, in Parry JK (ed): *Social Work Practice With the Terminally Ill: A Transcultural Perspective.* Springfield, IL, Charles C Thomas, 1990, pp 23–32

161. Baquet CR, Horm JW, Gibbs T, et al: Socioeconomic factors and cancer incidence among blacks and whites. *J Natl Cancer Inst* 83:551–557, 1991

162. Berg JW, Ross R, Latourette HB: Economic status and survival of cancer patients. *Cancer* 39:467–477, 1977

163. Page WF, Kuntz AJ: Racial and socioeconomic factors in cancer survival: a comparison of Veteran's Administration results with selected studies. *Cancer* 45:1029–1040, 1980

164. McWhorter WP, Schatzkin AG, Horm JW, et al: Contribution of socioeconomic status to black/white differences in cancer incidence. *Cancer* 63:982–987, 1989

165. Freeman HP: Cancer in the socioeconomically disadvantaged. *CA Cancer J Clin* 39:266–288, 1989

166. U.S. Bureau of the Census: *U.S. Bureau of the Census Statistics.* Washington, DC, Government Printing Office, 1991

167. Lewis O: The culture of poverty. *Sci Am* 215:19–25, 1966

168. American Cancer Society: *Cancer in the Economically Disadvantaged: A Special Report.* Atlanta, American Cancer Society, 1989

169. Wilkes G, Freeman H, Prout M: Cancer and poverty: breaking the cycle. *Semin Oncol Nurs* 10:79–88, 1994

170. Palos G: Cultural heritage: cancer screening and early detection. *Semin Oncol Nurs* 10:104–113, 1994

171. Brawley OW: Minority accrual and clinical trials. *Oncol Issues* 10:22–24, 1995

172. Black BL, Ades TB: American Cancer Society urban demonstration projects: models for successful intervention. *Semin Oncol Nurs* 10:96–103, 1994

173. Black BL, Schweitzer R, Dezelsky T: Report on the American Cancer Society workshop on community cancer detection, education, and prevention demonstration projects for underserved populations. *CA Cancer J Clin* 43:226–233, 1993

174. Mack E, McGrath T, Pendleton D, et al: Reaching poor populations with cancer prevention and early detection programs. *Cancer Pract* 1:35–39, 1993

175. Eng E: The save our sisters project: a social network strategy for reaching rural Black women. *Cancer* 72:1071–1077, 1993

176. Dignan M, Sharp P, Blinson K, et al: Development of a cervical cancer education program for Native American women in North Carolina. *J Cancer Educ* 9:235–242, 1994

177. Robinson KD, Kimmel EA, Yasko JM: Reaching out to the African American community through innovative strategies. *Oncol Nurs Forum* 22:1383–1391, 1995

178. Andrews MM: Transcultural nursing care, in Andrews MM, Boyle JS (eds): *Transcultural Concepts in Nursing Care* (ed 2): Philadelphia, Lippincott, 1995, pp 49–96

179. Andrews MM: Transcultural considerations: Cross-cultural communication, in Jarvis C (ed): *Physical Examination and Health Assessment*. Philadelphia, Saunders, 1992, p 75

180. Marshall P: Cultural influences on perceived quality of life. *Semin Oncol Nurs* 6:278–284, 1990

181. Stephens ST: Patient education materials: are they readable? *Oncol Nurs Forum* 19:83–85, 1992

182. Cooley ME, Moriarty H, Berger MS, et al: Patient literacy and the readability of written cancer educational materials. *Oncol Nurs Forum* 22:1345–1351, 1995

183. Shadick KM: Development of a transcultural health education program for the Hmong. *Clin Nurs Spec* 7:48–53, 1993

184. Villejo L: Patient education for Hispanic cancer patients, in Jones LA (ed): *Minorities and Cancer*. New York, Springer-Verlag, 1989, pp 295–300

185. Brant J: Video review: standing strong against the cancer enemy. *Transcultural Nursing Issues Special Interest Group Newsletter* 4:3, 1994

186. Millon-Underwood S, Sander E, Davis M: Determinants of participation in state-of-the-art cancer prevention, early detection/screening, and treatment trials among African-Americans. *Cancer Nurs* 16:25–33, 1993

187. McCabe MS, Varricchio CG, Padberg RM: Efforts to recruit the economically disadvantaged to national clinical trials. *Semin Oncol Nurs* 10:123–129, 1994

188. Porter CP, Villarruel AM: Nursing research with African American and Hispanic people: guidelines for action. *Nurs Outlook* 41:59–67, 1993

189. Munet-Vilaro F: Methodologic issues in the implementation of a Latino population. *Proceedings of the Third National Conference on Cancer Nursing Research*. Atlanta, American Cancer Society, 1994, pp 39–43

190. Flaskerud JH: Is the Likert scale format culturally biased? *Nurs Res* 37:185–186, 1988

# Chapter 63

# Policy, Politics, and Oncology Nursing

Pamela J. Haylock, RN, MA, ET

Katherine McDermott, RN, MPA, OCN®

## INTRODUCTION

The implications for patient care and clinical nursing practice that have resulted from the health care debate, budgetary initiatives, and policy decisions of the 1990s are unprecedented. Nurses, physicians, and, most important, patients are lost in market metaphors that describe the current health care delivery system. Multimedia technology, commercial delivery care networks, corporate-medical conglomerates, and vertically integrated hospitals have radically changed the delivery of health care services. The marketplace is redefining how care will be provided well into the next century. Political agendas are shifting from a 30-year history of government-sponsored health care benefits to a system that employs market forces to allocate medical resources.[1,2] The short- and long-term implications of congressional efforts in the late 1990s to redefine the role of the federal government in the delivery of health care services are, to date, unknown.

Access to care and services, the way services are delivered, and the types and quality of services that are available are inherently linked to the politics of the culture and the policies of the country in which nurses work. It is a country's values, its dominant political forces and resulting policies that define nursing practice. To assume key roles as consumers and providers of health care, nurses must understand how these forces come together and the evolution of the changes taking place, and they must be active participants in systems that create and implement health care policy, programs, and services.

Policy encompasses the choices that society, a segment of society, or an organization makes regarding goals and priorities and how resources are allocated.[3] Policies are developed in many sectors: health, social, organizational, public, and institutional. Politics is a process of influence and exertion of control over situations and events through dealing effectively with other individuals and/or groups using compromise, consensus, and negotiation.[3,4] Politics arise in any diverse culture or society when conflicting values are present.

Policy and politics promote the value system of a society, prioritize its political agendas, and dictate legislative initiatives. The dominant values of American society that relate to health care policy include individuality, competition, consumer choice, entrepreneurship, low taxation, the Protestant work ethic, limited governmental intrusion, and a cohesive family unit. The existing socioeconomic environment influences the triad of policy, politics, and values. Together, these factors dictate future directions of both private and public health care sectors in the country. In turn, legislation and regulation arising from the political process influence how nursing is practiced.

The future of health care and nurses' roles are anticipated with a mixture of grief, fear, anxiety, and hope. Many nurses grieve for the loss of the "way things used to be." Fears and anxieties are engendered as a result of uncertainties, the necessity of change, and diminished job security. Finally, there is hope that out of the chaos characteristic of today's health care environment will come opportunity. For nursing, opportunity exists to expand nursing knowledge, the scope of nursing practice, professional recognition, and interdisciplinary collaboration, and ultimately to incorporate nursing's values into a more holistic health care policy. These outcomes can be achieved through political power exerted by nurses and their advocates who hold positions of influence and power.

Political activism is a logical extension of the nurse's traditional role as patient advocate. For example, political activism allows nurses to assume a critical role in helping members of the lay public accurately assess proposals for health care reform, new public and private insurance plans, or the quality of services offered within a health care plan. Individual nurses or groups of nurses can create or participate in partnerships and coalitions that foster quality nursing care and/or advocate for the public good.

This chapter provides information that can strengthen one's ability to assume a proactive role in policy-making and political processes. Historical and social factors affecting policy, political processes, and initiatives that relate to health care are reviewed, followed by discussions specific to politics affecting health care delivery, nursing, and cancer care services. A final section provides information about political approaches and resources for nurses to enhance their effectiveness in the political arena.

## NURSING'S POLITICAL LEGACY

Although modern-day nurses have not been particularly visible in the political arena, nursing is not without political role models. Florence Nightingale was intensely political. She used knowledge, experience, communication, analytic skills, and connections with powerful people to realize her political agenda. The American Civil War revolutionized nursing care in the United States. The use of political power by individual Civil War nurses—among them Clara Barton, described as a "battlefield activist"[5] and later a "lobbyist,"[6] Dorothea Dix, Superintendent of the Union's nurses, Juliet Hopkins, Superintendent of Hospitals in Richmond,[5] and Phoebe Yates Pember, Matron at Chimborazo Hospital in Richmond,[7]—introduced astonishing changes to the care of hospitalized soldiers. The political success of these women is amazing when viewed within the social mores of the time. Women were not regarded as intellectually capable of comprehending the intricacies of the political system, and concern for political issues threatened "womanly honor." Women did not have the right to vote. Each of these nurses, however, did have supporters in executive and legislative branches of the government. Their appeals to government authorities were successful strategies for improving patient welfare and removing barriers to the practice of nursing. Although each of these nurses varied in ways of establishing contact with officials, they shared the approach of personally connecting with political figures whose help they needed to enlist.

Lillian Wald and Lavinia Dock used political activism to attack social conditions that threatened public health and established the Henry Street Settlement House in New York City at the turn of the century. From 1915 on, Margaret Sanger challenged America's attitudes and approaches to family planning. She was jailed for her efforts and for a time fled to England.

The political successes of nurses like Nightingale, Barton, Wald, Sanger, and others who came after them required a thorough firsthand knowledge of the facts and a commitment to patients. So armed, these nurses discovered they could influence politicians and make a difference for patients. Florence Nightingale, who advocated outcomes-oriented research, continues to influence the health care revolution nearly 100 years after her death.[8]

Contemporary American nurses have been called the "untapped resource" of political activism.[9] Even though there are over 2 million registered nurses in the United States, nurses as a group have not harnessed or wielded political power. There is evidence that political participation of baccalaureate nurses is comparable to that of female teachers and engineers.[10] The political participation of nurses with associate degrees and diplomas is lower than that of their baccalaureate-prepared colleagues.[10] It has been suggested that nurses resist participation in political activities, contending that their role is to provide patient care, not to become embroiled in politics.[5] There are other reasons why nurses have not been major participants in the political arena. Politics is not something most nurses expect to include in their nursing careers. Only recently have professional nursing education programs incorporated political science courses into curricula, and thus few nurses have been involved in politics to serve as contemporary role models.

Additionally, the role of women in the political arena has been limited. Consider the fact that it took from 1916, the year women were granted the right to vote, until 1992 to place just ten women into the U.S. Senate—out of 100 seats. In 1995 there were 8 women in the Senate and 48 women in the House of Representatives. State political environments are more "friendly" toward women, but women are still outnumbered by men in state legislatures. An especially encouraging note is the increasing number of nurses who have won elected seats in state legislatures. Table 63-1 lists states in which nurses hold elected legislative positions.

Recent evidence indicates that nurses are increasingly using political power and lobbying efforts to improve patient welfare and nurses' working conditions.[11] Labor and delivery nurses provided political support for state

**TABLE 63-1** Nurse State Legislators in 1996

| State | Nurses Holding State Office |
|---|---|
| Alabama | 1 |
| Arkansas | 2 |
| Arizona | 2 |
| Connecticut | 4 |
| Georgia | 1 |
| Idaho | 3 |
| Indiana | 2 |
| Iowa | 2 |
| Kansas | 2 |
| Kentucky | 1 |
| Maine | 3 |
| Maryland | 5 |
| Massachusetts | 3 |
| Michigan | 2 |
| Minnesota | 3 |
| Mississippi | 1 |
| Missouri | 1 |
| Montana | 2 |
| Nevada | 3 |
| New Hampshire | 8 |
| New Jersey | 2 |
| North Dakota | 1 |
| Ohio | 2 |
| Oregon | 1 |
| Pennsylvania | 1 |
| Rhode Island | 2 |
| South Dakota | 1 |
| Texas | 1 |
| Vermont | 4 |
| Washington | 4 |
| West Virginia | 1 |
| Wisconsin | 2 |
| Wyoming | 2 |

American Nurses' Association State Government Affairs Office, 1996

measures that require third-party payers to cover a minimum of 48 hours of inpatient care for mothers and newborns after a vaginal birth and 96 hours following cesarean section.[12] Similar legislation is being considered at the federal level.[13] Lobbying by enterostomal therapy nurses helped derail legislation that would end reimbursement for disposable medical equipment, including ostomy and wound care supplies. Exercising political power is an essential strategy for safeguarding patient welfare in contemporary nursing practice. The responsibility for exercising political power remains with individual nurses committed to improving patient care.[5]

## SCOPE OF NURSING PRACTICE AND STATE BOARDS OF NURSING

Professional nursing's existence can be credited to individual nurses and groups of nurses determined to safeguard patient welfare. Whether or not this mission remains central to professional nursing depends on the definition of the scope of nursing practice. Nurses of today and the future must realize and guard this responsibility. The most influential public authorities over nursing practice, holding regulatory and disciplinary responsibility within the profession of nursing, are each state's Board of Nursing (BON).

In the United States a BON exists in all 50 states and the five territories. Even though North Carolina enacted the first law to regulate the practice of nursing in 1903,[14] it was not until 1938 that New York state legally mandated licensing for nurses.[15] Regulations vary from state to state but in general are promulgated in Nursing Practice Acts that define the scope of nursing practice. Nursing Practice Acts outline minimum requirements for providing safe, skilled nursing care to the public. Although the composition of a BON membership differs from state to state, boards share distinct functions and duties: regulation of practice and educational programs, licensing of individual nurses, and disciplinary review. Nominees to boards can be members of professional nursing organizations or members of the public at large. Most often, members are appointed at the discretion of state governors: BON members are political appointees. The number of registered nurse members on the 55 boards of nursing ranges from one to nine. Government representatives, commissioners, hospital administrators, physicians, and pharmacists are often appointed as board members.[15] Many states do not require that BON members be either U.S. citizens or residents of the state in which they serve.

In 20 states, nurses have exclusive control of the BON; in the remaining 30 states, multidisciplinary boards, commissions, and nonnursing review committees can develop legislation or make recommendations on nursing practice–related legislation.[16] The significance of the composition of a state BON is exemplified by actions occurring in Delaware. In July 1994, Delaware's governor signed a bill giving advanced practice nurses (APNs) prescriptive authority. The regulations were written by a joint practice committee (five APNs, two physicians, one pharmacist, and one member of the general public) before being submitted to the Board of Medicine for final approval.[17]

The political appointees to this committee, including five APNs, had powerful influence over the regulation of nursing. On the other hand, a state with a diverse BON and minimal nursing representation or members who lack knowledge regarding professional nursing practice could influence legislative initiatives that adversely affect nursing practice.

In an increasingly competitive environment, nurses are encountering growing efforts by the American Medical Association (AMA) and state Boards of Medicine to limit or diminish the scope of nursing practice. The medical community, especially state medical associations, exerts political influence through lobbying and political fund-raising in support of positions at state and national levels. Nurses, especially APNs, are vulnerable to these political maneuvers. For example, a private practice group in Florida exerted pressure on a member physician to replace an oncology APN with a newly graduated physician.[17] The Pennsylvania Board of Medicine used political influence to promote a change in the state's Professional and Vocational Standards to reflect a more restrictive practice environment for nurse-practitioners.[18] It developed restrictive regulations that failed to recognize nurse-practitioners' advanced education and preparation, their accountability by double licensure, or documented proof with regard to quality care provided by these APNs. This action did not change the Nursing Practice Act itself, but the BON, and consequently the scope of nursing practice, were adversely affected by the political climate in which the Board of Medicine held political control.[18]

As states negotiate new fiscal responsibilities, organized physicians' groups will most likely increase lobbying activities. Even though recommendations have been put forth that "states redesign health professional boards to reflect the interdisciplinary and public accountability demands of the changing health care delivery system,"[19] physicians are unlikely to willingly forfeit their mandated supervision over APNs.[17] In accordance with the predominant federalist philosophy of the late 1990s, that of returning more political power and decision making to the states, boards of nursing will be pressured to fulfill the political expectations of the political party in power.

Regulatory changes could expand the role of unlicensed assistive personnel, eliminate mandates to inform patients of their rights, and eliminate hospitals' requirements for discharge planning and social work support. Nurses can expect to encounter difficulties in providing services with diminished funding. Organized physician lobbying could threaten the traditional nursing roles of educating patients and families, serving as advocates, and enhancing quality patient care. Nurses must recognize that state health care reform initiatives are neither inherently good nor bad, and they must therefore be prepared to analyze, monitor, respond to, and perhaps initiate reform efforts. This political influence will promote the vision and voice of nursing in the policy debates, sustain the role of nurse as patient advocate, and strengthen nursing's image in the political arena.

## POLITICAL ISSUES AFFECTING CANCER CARE

The influence of politics on health care policy related to cancer care issues is exemplified in the types of services available in communities, access to evidence-based treatment modalities, supportive or adjuvant medications and supplies, and qualified providers. The following discussions on pain management, reimbursement for medications used off-label, reimbursement for clinical trials, and tobacco-related issues exemplify the impact of politics and policy on the services and care available to individuals affected by cancer.

### Pain Management

Policy and legislative issues surrounding proper pain management provide compelling examples of the impact of politics on cancer care and cancer nursing practice. State Cancer Pain Initiatives group the most critical barriers to optimal pain management into three major categories: (1) inadequate knowledge about cancer pain and improper management strategies among professionals and the lay public; (2) attitudes and misinformation about addiction, tolerance, and opioid analgesics among professionals and the lay public; and (3) regulatory restrictions that relate to storage, handling, prescribing, and payment.[20,21] Even though all three categories of barriers must be addressed in policy-making agendas, education of policy makers, professionals, and the public is essential. A common perception among legislators is that this country's drug problem is advanced by the diversion of legally prescribed drugs. If drugs are better controlled, the logic follows, the drug problem will be better controlled. A second myth is that there is a standard formula for pain management. A third myth arises from misinformation about what addiction and tolerance really mean. These assumptions are commonly held by legislators, policy makers, the public, and health care professionals.[22] However, the regulatory restrictions relating to storage, handling, prescribing, and payment need to be addressed through regulatory and/or legislative action.

#### Cost issues

Third-party reimbursement strategies sometimes seem to favor expensive, "high-tech" forms of pain management. Third-party payers, including Medicare, currently reimburse for intravenous (IV) morphine delivered in an inpatient setting and via patient-controlled analgesia (PCA). Costs of outpatient prescriptions of sustained-release opioid tablets and suppositories, or absorbable fentanyl are not usually reimbursed by third-party payers. Patients are sometimes prescribed parenteral morphine to justify professional home care visits or inpatient hospitalizations. Ferrell[23] calculated the costs of con-

tinuous infusion morphine to be between $2000 and $4000 per month per patient. In a 12-month period, 255 unscheduled admissions to one hospital (among a total of 2795 scheduled and 2977 unscheduled hospital admissions) had a primary admit diagnosis of "uncontrolled pain." The average length of stay for these admissions was 12 days. Ferrell estimated a cost of $20,000 for an average inpatient stay of 12 days. Based on these estimates, 255 admissions for uncontrolled pain cost this one institution over $5 million over a one-year period. The American Pain Society's Committee on Regulatory Affairs has made attempts, some of them successful, to influence pharmaceutical and durable medical equipment (DME) companies to cease lobbying that perpetuates unwarranted use of expensive, high-tech interventions.

#### Monitoring opioid analgesics

In the United States the Controlled Substances Act regulates production and distribution of opioids, stimulants, and sedative hypnotics—agents that are subject to controlled-substances laws because of their potential for abuse. These agents are divided into five categories or "schedules." Agents that have no accepted medical use are placed in schedule I but are available for scientific use. Agents that have been approved for medical use are placed in schedules II–V, depending on their potential for abuse; the agents commonly used in cancer pain protocols, such as morphine, hydromorphone, and fentanyl, are schedule II drugs. It has been shown that regulatory controls placed on Schedule II agents reduce prescribing of these medications. One regulatory control mechanism is the multiple copy prescription program (MCPP), which mandates use of duplicate or triplicate prescription forms, special prescribing privileges, controls, and monitoring of providers. Research indicates that the MCPP hampers the prescribing of schedule II opioids for terminally ill patients with chronic pain.[24] There was a 64% reduction in the prescribing of schedule II controlled substances, mainly opioid analgesics, after a MCPP was introduced in Texas, as well as a 57% reduction in Rhode Island, a 54% reduction in New York, and a 50% reduction in Idaho.[25] The MCPP seems to encourage substitution of weaker opioids in lower schedules for more potent schedule II opioids,[26,27] resulting in less effective management of pain.

Access to health care providers and adequate insurance coverage make a difference in the management of pain. One study involving a hematology and oncology patient population found significant differences in the amount and type of pain medications prescribed between patients with prescription drug coverage (Medicaid) and those without.[28] Access to medications, including analgesic medications, is subject to various political influences determining pharmacies' ability to stock medications, their ability to compound different formulations, or a pharmacist's likelihood of filling a prescription for a controlled substance.[21] Limited access to medications can influence patient compliance. If medication is difficult to procure—for example, requires physician visits for refill prescriptions, requires additional trips to a pharmacy, is expensive and not reimbursable, or is not available at all—patients are unable to follow even the simplest pain management plan.

In 1991, legislation was drafted that would increase federal regulations related to monitoring the prescription and use of opioid analgesics. Pain management advocates, including the American Pain Society's Regulatory Affairs Committee, the State Cancer Pain Initiatives, and the Oncology Nursing Society (ONS), voiced clear, consistent, and persistent opposition to this legislation. It was never introduced in Congress. More recently, the U.S. Drug Enforcement Administration (DEA) drafted a bill, the Controlled Substances Monitoring Act of 1994, which proposes requirements that pharmacists report schedule II and III dispensing, limits schedule III refills to two within 120 days, and requires states to implement electronic monitoring systems.[29] The Department of Health and Human Services and Congress expressed concerns that this legislation would have a negative impact on patients being treated with controlled substances and could violate patient confidentiality. Though this legislation has yet to pass, the fact that similar ideas with potential negative outcomes resurface even when one proposal is blocked makes it clear that continued monitoring and thoughtful consideration of all such proposals are warranted.

Other initiatives that indicate a move toward eliminating regulatory barriers to optimal pain management are state and federal intractable pain treatment laws and regulations[30] and state medical board guidelines for treatment of intractable pain.[31] State legislatures are increasingly including the use of drugs to treat pain in their definitions of the practice of medicine.[32] In 1989 Texas became the first state to approve an Intractable Pain Treatment Act (IPTA), followed by California in 1994. Other state medical boards have published guidelines that address the use of opioids for intractable pain.[33]

A federal legislative response to pain-related issues is exemplified by a bill introduced in 1996 that would establish a National Center for Pain Research within the National Institutes of Health (NIH). The center would identify, coordinate, and support research, training, health information dissemination, and activities related to acute pain, cancer- and human immunodeficiency virus (HIV)–related pain, back pain, headache pain, facial pain, and other painful conditions. The bill's sponsor, Senator Orrin Hatch (R-Utah), specifically referred to cancer pain in his introductory remarks and highlighted NIH data that indicate that the NIH spends $54 million (out of a $12 billion annual budget) per year on pain-related research, or .5% of its budget. According to Senator Hatch, pain research is spread across many of the Institutes, with little coordination of research activities.[34] The introduction of this bill and its numerous cosponsors indicate that some legislators acknowledge "serious problems associated with our Government campaign against pain."[34]

Signs of declining regulatory restrictions over opioids are viewed as a trend in the right direction by pain experts. The Department of Health and Human Services prevented the introduction of a national MCPP. The Agency for Healthcare Policy and Research has published clinical practice guidelines that recognize the need to improve the regulatory environment for prescribing opioids.[22] States are less inclined to start new MCPPs, and some states have taken action to disband existing MCPPs.[29] Even though it might seem that progress has been made, there are crucial questions yet to be addressed through policy-making, regulatory, and political processes. For example, "What should the law and medical board guidelines say about opioid prescribing?"[33] "What knowledge base, skills, and credentials prepare a nurse to prescribe controlled substances?" "In what settings should a nurse be allowed to prescribe controlled substances?" The answers to these questions may provide direction for nurses to influence regulation that supports optimal pain management.[35,36]

## Reimbursement for "Off-label" Use of Drugs

It has been estimated that one of every eight individuals with cancer do not get preferred therapy.[37] Most third-party payers, including Medicare and Medicaid, have used the federal Food and Drug Administration (FDA) package insert as a guide for determining what use of the drug in question is reimbursable. The FDA label is created during the FDA approval process, in which a drug is proved to be effective for one disease entity. Since the FDA approval process is both lengthy and expensive, most pharmaceutical companies that have successfully evaluated drugs for other indications do not put these agents through a second approval process. Instead, once a drug has received FDA approval, it is available for prescription based on an individual physician's discretion. There are drastic reimbursement differences in various regions, even within one state. Some payers follow the guide very strictly; others are more lenient. Even though a physician prescribes the drug, an insurance company may deny reimbursement.

A clear example of this is demonstrated in the history of interferon, which was released in the late 1980s. According to its initial FDA approval, interferon was indicated for treatment of hairy-cell leukemia, a relatively rare disease. Immediately after its approval, interferon was widely prescribed in the management of other forms of cancer, most notably acquired immunodeficiency syndrome (AIDS)–related malignancies such as Kaposi's sarcoma and lymphoma. The expense of interferon and the numbers of people for whom it was being prescribed caused payers to look for ways to avoid financial liability for its use. The FDA label provided a convenient way to circumvent costly reimbursement claims.

It is estimated that 56% of cancer drugs are used "off-label"—in the treatment of diseases other than the one indicated on the FDA label.[37] In many situations physicians select less effective protocols to avoid conflicts with third-party payers over reimbursement for off-label use; hence the statistic that one of every eight individuals with cancer does not get the preferred, most effective therapy. Uniform Coverage of Anticancer Drugs legislation was drafted in several states in collaboration with the Association of Community Cancer Centers.[38] According to the language in this legislation, payers must pay for drugs if their efficacy is outlined according to FDA approval, is supported by one or more citations included in at least one of the three compendiums (the *American Hospital Formulary Service Drug Information*, the *AMA Drug Evaluations,* or the *U.S. Pharmacopoeia Drug Information*), or is supported by clinical evidence reported in peer-reviewed medical literature. This legislation has been introduced and passed by several states, and nurses have figured prominently in moving these initiatives forward. Using language similar to the Uniform Coverage of Anticancer Drugs legislation adopted by several states, Congress included off-label provisions in legislation involving Medicare and Medicaid that became law in 1994.

## Reimbursement for Clinical Trials

The future of specialty practice and the advancement of treatment offered to individuals with cancer depends on research. The ability to do high-quality, meaningful research is dependent on researchers' abilities to enter adequate numbers of patients in a clinical trial. Most third-party payers currently do not pay for care or treatment that falls into the vaguely defined category of "experimental" care. This caveat prohibits many potential subjects from participating in clinical trials and sometimes forces physicians to recommend standard therapy when an investigational therapy might be more promising.[38]

Clinical research is impacted by the reconfiguration of health care funding. Leveling of NIH funding has resulted in greater scrutiny of the kinds of research being conducted, who is doing the research, how funding is allocated, and the government's role in supporting research. Existing divisions in the research community, including different disease groups, are made even more prominent by this scrutiny. Support for research in academic health centers is hampered by their expansive missions and higher patient care costs. Managed care plans and pharmaceutical companies are assuming roles in clinical research, leading to a set of new concerns, including an exodus of researchers from universities to the private sector and the perception that research directions are influenced by for-profit business strategies.

The dominance of managed care in the delivery of health care has created a growing concern within the oncology community that clinical trials will suffer from competing interests, particularly profit margins. Many oncologists are concerned that research trials and the educational training necessary to produce future generations of researchers will be affected by decreased funding. Funding sources for clinical and basic research have traditionally come from federal and state grants and industry support. In the managed care environment, public funding sources are diminishing. The major cutbacks introduced by the 104th Congress exert pressure on hospitals and academic medical centers. In the future, the primary funding source for oncology research will most likely be through the private sector.[39]

The federal budget funds several sources of medical- and health-related research, including the NIH and the Veterans Administration. The NIH awarded $5.8 billion to universities for research in fiscal year 1994, of which $1.8 billion (30.8%) funded administrative and facilities expenses associated with the conduct of research.[40] Concerns expressed by members of Congress and other bodies regarding the quality, appropriateness, size, and cost of NIH research programs make the NIH vulnerable to loss of support from influential legislators, organizations, and interest groups, resulting in decreased funding or outright elimination of programs.[41]

In 1996 the National Cancer Institute (NCI) initiated meetings with key professional and lay groups, including the ONS, the American Society of Clinical Oncologists, and the National Coalition for Cancer Survivorship, to discuss joint development of a comprehensive plan to assure access to cancer clinical trials in the managed care environment. Identified strategies fell into three categories: (1) patient/family and public education; (2) promotion of clinical trials to public, health maintenance organizations, and self-insured corporations; and (3) legislation. Participating organizations agreed to consider methods through which they might enhance the public's recognition of the usefulness of clinical trials and, subsequently, consumers' abilities to advocate for participation in appropriate clinical trials.[42]

In the legislative arena, a Senate bill was introduced in 1996 that would mandate Medicare to establish a five-year demonstration project to study and provide coverage of routine patient care costs for Medicare beneficiaries with cancer who are enrolled in an approved chemotherapy program. At least in its introductory phase, the bill does not provide reimbursement for investigational drugs and devices. The bill's sponsor contends that the demonstration project would produce the "information and experience needed to then modify Medicare's policy toward clinical trials."[43] Even if this bill does not become law, the discussion it generates could pressure the Health Care Financing Agency (HCFA) to be more receptive to a demonstration project with the NCI. An additional element is the fact that the HCFA is America's largest third-party payer. If the HCFA compares the costs and outcomes of clinical trials with those associated with standard care, other payers could hardly resist creating similar partnerships.

## Tobacco-Related Issues

Oncology nurses, through the collective voice created by the ONS and other health advocacy groups, continue to pursue strategies to decrease tobacco-related illnesses and premature deaths in the United States. During the society's more than 20-year history, its members have adopted several tobacco- and smoking-related resolutions that bind the organization to continued work in this direction.[44] Meetings of the ONS have been smoke-free since 1985, and members continue to support smoking cessation efforts such as the American Cancer Society's annual Great American Smokeout. The ONS maintains a formal liaison with the Coalition on Smoking OR Health, and as a result of coalition efforts the 101st Congress banned smoking on U.S. commercial flights lasting six hours or less, virtually eliminating smoking on all domestic flights. Subsequently, the 103rd Congress passed legislation banning smoking on international flights originating in the United States. In 1995, legislation was introduced to raise the tax on cigarettes and to bar tobacco companies from deducting advertising and promotional expenses from tax liability. Other legislation introduced in 1995 would force the tobacco industry to contribute to Medicare and Medicaid, ostensibly to cover costs associated with tobacco-related illnesses.

In 1996 President Clinton endorsed new rules that declare nicotine an "addictive" drug, making nicotine-containing products subject to FDA regulation. Tobacco companies have filed lawsuits to block implementation of these regulations; thus implementation may be delayed for years. Republicans, particularly those in tobacco-growing regions, accused the president of neglecting the interests of tobacco farmers and other tobacco-related industries. Tobacco lobbyists charge that FDA regulation will lead to regulatory overload. Nevertheless, according to the press, the move was declared a "major political plus" for President Clinton and fellow Democratic politicians during the 1996 election since Republicans are often accused (rightly or wrongly) of favoring monied tobacco interests.[45]

# POLITICS, SOCIAL POLICY, AND THE AMERICAN HEALTH CARE SYSTEM

Even though most people under the age of 50 cannot recall major political discussions around health care issues, the debate over a national health care plan actually began shortly after the turn of the twentieth century. Despite nearly 100 years of political skirmishing, the spectrum of health care issues is monumental in its complexity, and politicians and health care experts have not or cannot come to a consensus on how to address these issues. Table 63-2 outlines the chronology of health care reform initiatives in the United States.[46–49] The following

**TABLE 63-2** The Chronology of Health Care Reform in the United States

| Year | Action or Initiative |
| --- | --- |
| 1916 | The American Association for Labor Legislation proposes a standard bill for compulsory medical care and sickness benefits insurance. |
| 1927 | The Committee on the Costs of Medical Care meets to address the problems of health care delivery. |
| 1934 | Blue Cross is started under the direction of the American Hospital Association. |
| 1938 | First formal prepaid comprehensive health plan is developed: the Kaiser-Permanente Medical Care Program. |
| 1939 | Blue Shield is created by state medical societies. |
| 1946 | Congress enacts the Hospital Survey and Construction (Hill-Burton) Act. |
| 1949 | President Truman proposes a compulsory national health insurance system. |
| 1951 | President Truman withdraws his support for a national health insurance plan because of McCarthyism and Antisocialist sentiment. |
| 1965 | The Medicare and Medicaid laws are enacted. |
| 1970s | Five major health care proposals are placed before Congress. None is voted out of subcommittee. |
| 1971 | The National Cancer Program is established with passage of the National Cancer Act. |
| 1982 | The Tax Equity and Fiscal Responsibility Act (TEFRA) is passed to address inflationary cost-based reimbursement for Medicare providers largely through implementation of diagnosis-related groups (DRGs) to classify reimbursement. |
| 1990 | The Americans with Disabilities Act is passed, providing equal opportunity to disabled citizens. |
| 1993 | President Clinton proposes the Health Security Act. |
| 1994 | The Health Security Act fails. |
| 1996 | The Health Insurance Reform Act of 1995 is passed. It increases access to and security of health care benefits, and provides for increased portability of health care benefits. Limits exclusions of preexisting conditions. Allows for 4-year experimental inclusion of Medical Savings Accounts available to self-employed workers and workers in small businesses. Changes the IRS tax code to allow deductions for long-term and home health care. |
| 1996 | The Personal Responsibility and Work Opportunity Act is passed. Reforms the Welfare program. The Federal government sets terms for states to shift Medicaid recipients to managed care programs. |

Data from McDermott 1994;[46] Clinton 1993;[47] Jonas 1986;[48] Watson 1990.[49]

section illustrates how the current political environment, one that emphasizes a market approach, is shaping the future of health care delivery.

## The Current National Health Care Reform Debate

"The United States has the best system of health care in the world. Something needs to be done about this."[50] This seemingly contradictory statement by humorist Dave Barry captures the essence of the national health care reform debate. The American health care system has been described as a paradox of excess and deprivation.[51] Although technologically outstanding, the American health care system is expensive, does not provide universal coverage or basic services to all citizens, lacks the essentials of primary care, and emphasizes acute care. Health care costs have risen significantly since the mid-1960s, and estimates indicate that 40 million Americans are without health insurance; millions more lack adequate coverage.[52,53]

Strategies for health care reform pit the two major political parties in a debate revolving around a critical philosophical difference. A core Democratic value is that government should be the guarantor of the common good. Conversely, Republicans advocate minimal government involvement.[54]

Democratic candidates have historically played a large part in health care issues.[55] Political candidates choose issues that resonate with what they perceive to be voters' fundamental concerns at the time. Health care issues have not figured prominently in most presidential elections, with the most recent exception being the 1992 presidential campaign. Lack of focus on health care in presidential campaigns relates to the fact that, historically, American voters have not attached significant importance to health care issues. Opinion polls conducted between 1966 and 1987 reveal that Americans have not perceived health care as one of the nation's most important problems.[56] Although most Americans can cite problems with the health care system, 85% are insured and have (or believe they have) access to a system that works for them.[56]

Whether or not health care is a right has been, at the least, a topic of debate and, at most, a central and polarizing issue between political factions. The U.S. Constitution has no provision to support a claim to the right of all Americans to a minimal level of health care services. In contrast, this entitlement is found in the constitutions of a large number of nations in the Western hemisphere.[57]

In September 1993 President Clinton outlined the American Health Security Act of 1993.[47] The plan, described as an amalgam of regulation and market competition, was designed to placate those who favor a global cap on spending and those who prefer to rely on market forces. A National Health Board would oversee the activities of states within a budget designed to bring costs into line with inflation by 1999. The reform effort failed.

Several explanations for the failure of this reform effort have been advanced, none of them mutually exclusive. First, the Clinton administration did not provide the political leadership and managerial competence to take advantage of existing public support for health care reform. When the plan was revealed after a costly, lengthy, and secretive drafting process, it was criticized for its complexity, leading to charges that it would create a bureaucratic nightmare. Special-interest groups, including the Health Insurance Association of America and the National Federation of Independent Businesses, manipulated Congress to block legislative consideration and action. Second, voter surveys indicated that President Clinton's image as a "big-government proponent" resulted not only in a failed reform plan but also in the subsequent landslide victory that placed the Republican party in control of the House and the Senate for the first time in 40 years. Congressional Republicans soon adopted a legislative agenda, coined the "Contract with America," reflecting a "less government" and "balanced budget" philosophy. In accordance with this philosophy, market forces assumed a major role in redefining the delivery of health care in the United States.

Although none of the items in the "Contract with America" focused exclusively on health care issues, Medicare and Medicaid spending and other entitlement programs were targets for major budget reductions. To accomplish this, Congress approved the transfer of nearly all federal welfare programs, in the form of block grants, to the states.[58]

When funds are transferred to the states, governors and state legislators allocate these resources by eliminating or consolidating many small public health programs. However, the ramifications of shifting these allocations raise concerns of conflict of interest in state legislatures and the cost shifting from states to the private sector. For example, a study conducted by the Consumer Federation of America and Common Cause suggests that regulation of the insurance industry may be hampered by legislators who serve on insurance committees, who are themselves insurance agents or have other ties to the industry.[59] The process of setting standards for the insurance industry, a state responsibility, is therefore susceptible to lobbying and political influence. On the employer side, the National Leadership Coalition on Health Care, representing 93 companies including Chrysler, Ford, and labor unions, suggested that the proposed Medicaid cuts would cause states to cut 7.2 million people from eligibility.[60] This would result in hospitals and other providers treating uninsured people, shifting costs to employer-sponsored health insurance plans.[60] Medicare and Medicaid have been an integral part of health care in the United States for the last 30 years. Proposals for major budgetary reductions in these programs have provoked debates in both political philosophy and economics.

### Medicaid

Medicaid, created in 1965, is a federal-state matching entitlement program that provides medical assistance and long-term care to low-income individuals, the uninsured, and the disabled.[61] The Medicaid component represents nearly 40% of federal aid to states. Because of the escalating costs of this program (from $51.3 billion in 1988 to $157 billion in 1995) and the increasing number of recipients (from 22.3 million in 1989 to 32.1 million in 1993), the managed care concept has grown rapidly as an alternative to the variety of existing Medicaid state policies.[61] Many states' governors believe that enrolling Medicaid recipients into managed care plans will stem the growth of these costs and provide comprehensive care within political, social, and economic constraints.[62]

As of June 1994, over 40 million recipients were enrolled in Medicaid programs, with 7.8 million of these in managed care programs.[61] The predominant groups enrolled in Medicaid managed care programs include children and adults in poor, single-parent families. The biggest change has been the expanded role of Medicaid in long-term care.[63] Because poverty is associated with an increased incidence of cancer and lower survival rates, decreased access to care and lack of education present major challenges for nurses caring for indigent patients in isolated rural areas, those in depressed inner-city neighborhoods, and patients with disabilities.[64–66]

Medicaid recipients, unlike Medicare beneficiaries, lack a powerful political constituency to advocate for their needs. The long-term implications of converting Medicaid to separate state-run programs are, of course, unknown. Sure to ignite passionate debate are cutbacks in Medicaid funding, ethical issues raised by the rationing of care,[67] and the philosophical differences between the involved political and special-interest factions.

### Medicare

The second major restructuring initiative taking place at the federal level involves the Medicare program, which provides health care insurance for 95% of the nation's elderly. Medicare was enacted in 1965 and is sometimes referred to as the "world's largest insurance company."[68] Since its inception, Medicare has been based on the principle of social insurance. Social insurance is "the mandatory contributions that employees make to dedicated trust funds during their working years with the promise of receiving benefits (income or services) after they retire."[69] To date, the 36 million Medicare recipients, 65 years old and over, are generally pleased with the program. As currently run, Medicare offers benefits that include choices of physician, hospital, or home care provider and adheres to its original mission of providing appropriate and adequate care to the elderly. Criticisms of Medicare arise from the fact that few restraints on consumption of services are built into the program. Medicare has always been a fee-for-service plan under which physicians have incentives to order or perform more, not fewer, services. In 1995, $183 billion was spent to provide these services. Costs are projected to reach $222 billion in 1997.[63] These escalating costs have raised congressional concerns that the Medicare fund will be depleted by the year 2002. As the American population is increasingly living to an age where the incidence of cancer is higher, there is an increased demand for cancer care services associated with increased costs.[9,70]

America's elderly use medical specialists to a greater extent than their younger counterparts. When elders have a chronic illness, they develop relationships with a set of physicians (Blendon RJ, personal communication March 1996). This is especially significant in the elderly oncology patient population; more than 60% of all cancer deaths occur in patients 65 and older, and approximately 12% of people over 70 have a prior history of malignancy.[70] In fact, the median age for individuals who develop cancer is 67. The elderly, who have higher cancer mortality rates, are often socioeconomically disadvantaged.[70] Seventy-eight percent of Medicare beneficiaries have average annual incomes below $25,000 and spend approximately $3000 annually for out-of-pocket health care costs.[71] For this reason, many Medicare beneficiaries are being encouraged to join health maintenance organizations or other managed care entities that provide comprehensive services for fixed monthly premiums.

Additionally, the outcome of proposed Medicare changes is critical for Americans living in rural settings where health care facilities are scarce. Other proposed strategies will ask Medicare recipients to pay more. Hospitals and physicians will assume additional financial burdens.[72] At risk in budget-cutting maneuvers are Area Health Education Centers, the Rural Health Education Center, telemedicine grants, and all 50 state Offices of Rural Health.[72]

As rural hospitals decrease in number, or reduce bed capacity, it will be necessary to expand and improve community-based, ambulatory, and home care services, and to develop better methods of educating patients, families and caregivers who do not have access to oncology care. Issues and opportunities for nurses fall into four major categories: (1) access to services, (2) communication among providers, patients, and families, (3) professional and public education, and (4) access to and use of state-of-the-art technology, including telemedicine, teleconferencing, and other forms of electronic linkages.[73,74]

Republicans are seeking options to control the growth of Medicare spending and look to health maintenance organizations and other forms of managed care to control and coordinate care. Additional managed care choices, better information about them, and an improved reimbursement system will most likely accelerate the integration of managed care into Medicare.

## THE HEALTH CARE DELIVERY SYSTEM

The real reform in health care is evolving from private-sector employers and insurance companies who believe that the restructuring of the trillion-dollar health care industry will occur only through the development of managed care delivery networks. These organizations use a variety of approaches and incentives to influence decisions of health care providers and are transforming medical practice away from traditional settings to corporate entities.

The majority of Americans have health insurance coverage as an employer-sponsored benefit. The steady rise in the cost of providing these benefits since the early 1970s is causing employers to shift from fee-for-service plans to lower-cost managed care plans. Employers of both large and small companies are seeking ways to provide less costly, more efficient, reasonably good-quality medical services at discounted fees.[75] Extensive variations among employers' approaches to selecting health care benefits have led corporate benefit managers to become "proactive purchasers" of managed care plans. Identified trends that have resulted from these changes include the development of shared practices, negotiated price structures, and concessions from health care providers that include increasing employee deductions, limited dependent coverage, altering employee provider or plan choices, and increased participant accountability.[76] These practices, once unthinkable, are commonplace in today's health care market.

The evolution of a market-oriented health care delivery system that features for-profit hospital chains and ambulatory facilities, freestanding radiological units, and "vertically" integrated health maintenance organizations defines the culture of practice.[77] Because some managed care networks are created hastily and seek to reduce costs or create a profit at the expense of patient care, oncology nurses must educate themselves and advocate for patient and consumer needs in managed care networks and the benefits that are offered or eliminated. To successfully participate and practice within these complex structures and maintain the patient advocate role, oncology nurses must understand the basic concepts of managed care systems and the political environment that has fostered their development and implementation.

## Managed Care

*Managed care* is a recognized and accepted term that is synonymous with how millions of Americans receive health care services. As commonly defined, managed care refers to a "variety of methods of financing and organizing the delivery of comprehensive health care in which an attempt is made to control costs by controlling the provision of services."[78] This definition emphasizes the integration of health care financing with the delivery of medical care and cost containment.

Although an oft-stated goal of managed care plans is to limit expensive and inappropriate care without denying appropriate treatment, concerns have been raised by providers and patients about the emergence, rapid growth, and inherent restrictive practices of these plans.[79] Physicians are concerned about the limitations managed care places on clinical decision-making autonomy. Nurses express misgivings about the explicit or implicit rationing of certain services and potential restrictions in choices that could affect patients' well-being. Consumers, potential or actual patients, are troubled by contract regulations that mandate using only physicians, hospitals, or services that are part of the providers' network and subsequent restriction of choices. Consumer groups express concern about the lack of regulations and monitoring of managed care systems.

As the managed care industry expands, legislators are addressing deficiencies that have been reported by consumers, practitioners, and the media. The Health Insurance Reform Act, passed in August 1996, contains key insurance reforms that will have a significant impact on many Americans.[80] It addresses issues related to denial of coverage for preexisting conditions, makes eligibility for insurance "portable" from job to job, and allows small businesses and farmers to pool resources to buy insurance for employees and families across state lines. This legislation does not address the issue of the uninsured or the affordability of insurance. Although many of the reforms will be enacted at the state level, this legislation is the first step in revisiting the issues that brought the health care reform debate to the forefront in 1993.

Other legislation that has been proposed includes both House and Senate bills. One example is the Senate bill known as the Patient Communication Protection Act of 1996,[81] which prohibits health plans from interfering with health care provider–patient communications. Additional proposals would reform the health care liability system and establish quality improvement programs, prohibit insurers from offering monetary rewards to licensed health care practitioners who limit availability to appropriate services, and mandate full disclosure to enrollees of health maintenance organizations regarding physician credentials, services, and compensation paid to officers of the organization. The absence of a national reform plan or regulatory body that would monitor the managed care industry has prompted these legislative initiatives.

These examples of proposed legislation have implications for oncology care. Access to specialty care is a hallmark of the "old" health care delivery system. Managed care challenges traditional referral networks and systems. It has been estimated that health maintenance organization enrollment in the United States reached 50 million, or 16% of those Americans with health care insurance in 1994. For individuals with cancer, restricting access to oncology specialists, whether physicians or nurses, is a grave concern. In the process, patients lose an element of control over the kind of care they receive.

As a national trend, the number of specialty physicians is decreasing in proportion to the number of primary care physicians.[82] Primary care physicians, who may not be trained in oncology, are assuming the responsibility for managing the care of cancer patients as more Americans surrender third-party benefits to restrictive managed care plans. Within a capitated system, the managed care organization can decide to reduce the number of treatment visits or be pressured to shift office-based chemotherapy to a hospital setting where there is less financial risk to the organization. This shift in care settings appears to be the result of economic considerations rather than documented patient needs.

The "gatekeeping" phenomenon occurs when health maintenance organizations sharply limit access to specialists by interposing their own physicians between patients and oncology specialists. It also applies to employer purchasers of managed care plans who discourage their employees from accessing specialized care. They simply do not incorporate "carve-out" benefits for cancer care into benefit packages.[83] Other issues that may not be addressed adequately as a result of the rapid expanse of managed care systems include continuity of care, ethical considerations, and financial incentives for physicians and facilities to control costs.

Oncology nurses practicing in managed care settings should familiarize themselves with proposed state and national health care legislation. Although legislators attempt to appeal to all stakeholders, there is always a special-interest group, whether it is the state medical board, the insurance or pharmaceutical industry, or consumer advocacy group, that identifies the pros and cons of the legislation and lobbies aggressively to achieve its own goals. Oncology nurses must lobby for legislation that supports their values and promotes policies of quality care, choice of provider, and access to services.

## ENHANCING POLITICAL EFFECTIVENESS

Nurses have a vast amount of knowledge and experience to offer in health policy and legislative arenas at local, state, and federal levels. Legislation that is eventually enacted is usually initiated at the insistence of constituents. Legislative aides or assistants employed by legislators are assigned to research an issue and initiate a draft of possible legislation. At federal and state levels, legislative aides are usually young, generally under 25 years of age, with little or no health care background or experience. They are assigned to several, often quite diverse, topical areas and have little time to become expert in any one area.[84] In effect, people with the least amount of knowledge and experience are given the responsibility of writing legislation. While this might be a disadvantage of the system, it presents an opportunity for nurses. The expertise and experience of nurses regarding patient care is what legislators and their assistants do not know unless nurses tell them.

Just as Florence Nightingale and Clara Barton demonstrated, nurses can gain political power by increasing their own visibility. Regular and frequent contact with elected officials is important for establishing a working relationship that will benefit both the nurse and the official. Letters offering informed opinions, in support of an official's position as well as in opposition, can help build this symbiotic relationship. Identifying oneself as a constit-

uent, a voter, and an oncology nurse will enhance the impact of communication with elected officials.

## Communicating with Elected Officials

While communicating with elected officials need not be time-consuming, use of an accepted protocol will do much to foster a positive and productive relationship. Local offices of the League of Women Voters offer help in identifying state and federal elected officials. Local libraries usually maintain a list of current officials, officials' addresses, telephone numbers, and district maps. *The U.S. Congress Handbook,*[85] published for each congressional session, features members' pictures, biographies, committee membership, addresses, and phone and fax numbers, and names of key staff members. Internet resources provide similar sorts of information. Table 63-3 offers suggestions for effective written communications with elected officials.

A face-to-face meeting with an elected official to persuade her or him to support or sponsor legislation favorable to a particular cause or to repeal unfavorable legislation is a form of lobbying. The meeting is likely to be brief, with 15 minutes generally allotted for a constituent's visit. Given this limited opportunity, it is wise to

**TABLE 63-3**   Tips on Writing an Elected Official

1. Try to limit the letter to one typewritten page. If writing longhand, write legibly.
2. In a short first paragraph, state your purpose.
3. Stick to one issue or subject.
4. If a bill is the subject, cite it by its title and number.
5. Be factual and support your position with information about how legislation is likely to affect you and others. Avoid emotional, philosophical arguments.
6. If you believe legislation is wrong and should be opposed, say so. Indicate the likely adverse effects and suggest an alternative approach.
7. Ask for a response.
8. Do not start with a negative attitude: Set goals that facilitate compromise.
9. Provide support in obtaining information. Offer to contact expert resources. Offer to testify or find others who can testify.
10. Ask the legislator's views but do not demand support. Even if your position is not supported on one issue or bill, it may be the next time.
11. Be sure your name and return address are legible.
12. Say thank you.
13. The suggested address style is:
    The Honorable [first and last name]
    United States Senate
    Washington, DC 20510
    Dear Senator [last name]:
                        or
    The Honorable [first and last name]
    United States House of Representatives
    Washington, DC 20515
    Dear Representative [last name]:

prepare for and plan the visit. It is helpful to know about the official as a person, including his or her interests and concerns. For example, know the official's name, party affiliation, electoral history, committee assignments, personal information (e.g., education, previous employment, interests), general voting record and the record relating to the issue being considered, and the position on the specific issue. This information may help to determine whether the official is inclined to support or oppose a particular viewpoint or position, and whether actions on the part of constituents are likely to alter his or her position. Again, employing an acceptable protocol for meeting with legislators or legislative assistants will reflect positively on any constituent's influence. Table 63-4 offers tips for meeting with an elected official.[85]

Just as there is diversity in positions and people holding elected office, there is great diversity in how nurses might gain political influence. A small number of nurses have themselves achieved elected office. An increasing number of nurses have assumed roles as legislative assistants or other staff positions at state and federal levels. Any nurse, however, can achieve political influence without actually holding office or paid positions in an elected official's staff. Political success can come as a result of volunteer efforts. Nurses can offer volunteer services to a candidate, particularly during political campaigns.

Informally, nurses can take advantage of the esteem in which nurses are held by the public in general. A letter

**TABLE 63-4** Tips for Meeting With an Elected Official

1. Plan and prepare for the visit.
2. Make an appointment stating the subject to be discussed and the time needed, and identify the persons who will attend the meeting.
3. Select a spokesperson if others are going with you and agree on the presentation.
4. Know the facts, both legislative and related to your position. If a bill is being discussed, know the number and title.
5. Dress in business-style attire.
6. Arrive at the official's office on time, but do not be disappointed if the official is late.
7. Introduce yourself, including your name and title, and establish yourself as a constituent.
8. Present the facts in an orderly, concise, and positive manner.
9. Focus on one issue.
10. Relate the positive impact of legislation you support and the problems it corrects.
11. Relate the negative impact of legislation you oppose, and suggest, where appropriate, a different approach.
12. Leave fact sheets if possible.
13. Encourage questions. Discuss.
14. Ask for a favorable consideration.
15. Leave your business card.
16. Thank the official for his/her time and courtesy.
17. Leave promptly.
18. Send a "thank you" follow-up letter: Reiterate your point and send additional materials or information if available.

Adapted from Pullen: *The U.S. Congress Handbook;* Oncology Nursing Society, "Legislative Reference Handbook."

to the editor of a local paper about a health-related issue that is signed by an individual who acknowledges himself or herself as a registered nurse can hold considerable credence in a community. The likelihood of a letter being published seems to increase as the size of the community decreases, but nevertheless, letters can be influential in the social and political spheres in a targeted community. Along the same lines, letters to the editor of special-interest magazines or journals can sway constituents' opinions.

## Lobbying

Lobbying is a tactic of trying to influence policy through policy makers. Lobbying activities are proactive means of exercising group power and influencing constituents and legislators through analysis and persuasive communication.[86] The goal of lobbying for nursing and nurses is to effectively use those precious few moments when a legislator's attention is focused on issues pertinent to the nursing profession.[86] Lobbyists serve as a link between constituents (e.g., nurses, and public officials).

Effective lobbying is primarily related to three factors: (1) the amount of money spent by an organization, (2) the sophistication of the strategies used, and (3) the group's size, its geographic location, and the socioeconomic status of the members. These factors determine a lobbyist's level of access to decision makers.[86]

Lobbying is classified into two categories based on strategies used. *Inside lobbying* includes the formal and informal interactions that influence decision makers or their staffs. Historically, this took place in lobbies of legislative buildings—hence the term *lobbying*. Inside lobbying strategies include face-to-face interactions, providing oral testimony, networking with policy makers, drafting legislation, and developing and supplying target lists. Inside lobbying is often regulated and done by registered lobbyists but can be performed by volunteers as well. *Outside lobbying* refers to indirect, grassroots activities to mobilize support and educate constituents and/or legislators. Examples of indirect lobbying include providing campaign support, telephone contacts, telegrams, personal letters, E-mail communications, press conferences, letters to the editor, and other media activities.

In 1995 Congress redefined lobbyists as those persons who spend at least one-fifth of their paid work time engaged in meeting, conducting research, or working to influence federal policy makers and their aides.[87] This legislation is the outcome of congressional efforts to restructure the way government business is conducted and to convince skeptical voters that Congress can eliminate the conflicts of interest between lawmakers and wealthy benefactors. Under new regulations, lobbyists are required to register with Congress, disclose clients and policies they are attempting to affect, and disclose how much money they spend to influence federal officials.

Lobbying can occur at any stage in the legislative cycle and requires knowledge of the bill-to-law process to determine the most effective time to exert lobbying efforts. *Presession lobbying* begins months before a legislative session, when key issues are identified by the lobbyist's client. Preparation for presession lobbying requires prioritizing issues, research into the political, economic, and social positions of legislators, and analysis of political trends and issues. Presession is the ideal time to establish credibility and plan a legislative agenda.

*Lobbying during the session* requires monitoring and active networking with other like-minded special-interest groups. Even after the legislative session ends, *postsession lobbying* efforts continue. New legislation requires that new rules and regulations be authorized and drafted. Ad hoc committees, public hearings, written or verbal testimony, and letter-writing campaigns are important to postsession lobbying.

Correct timing is critical during the legislative cycle of a bill. Knowledge of the process of taking an issue from idea to a formal bill to law is therefore crucial in influencing policy and political processes. Figure 63-1 depicts this process.[88]

### Working with a lobbyist

The role of a lobbyist is to provide representation and expertise during legislative and decision-making processes. An individual's or group's ability to affect social policy and/or specific legislative initiatives will most often be enhanced by the guidance and assistance of a professional, skilled, and knowledgeable lobbyist. Throughout the legislative process, the lobbyist can offer suggestions, for example, in selection of the "right" author for the legislation—a legislator whose personality traits, level of commitment to the issue, and respect from legislative colleagues will increase the likelihood of proposed legislation being given due consideration. A skilled lobbyist can help devise strategies to activate "grassroots" support, including initiating letter-writing campaigns, assisting with development of written and oral testimony in support (or opposition) of the initiative, and identifying legislators who will consider the legislation.

## Coalitions

Coalitions are groups of people or associations that band together to pool resources, ideas, and expertise in pursuit of common goals.[89] The combined clout and credibility of a coalition allows it to exert far more power than that of an individual or an organization acting alone. Coalitions generally appoint a single spokesperson to present its message since legislative and regulatory bodies usually limit the number of speakers allowed to testify on a single issue.

Coalitions differ in organizational structure and purpose, ranging from informal and loosely structured to formal and regimented. The most common coalition is an informal group of interested entities created to allow participants to monitor an issue and network. Participants meet occasionally, and leadership is informal. For lobbying or public relations purposes, a loose coalition may adopt a formal identity and create a list of members, thus becoming a recognized "name" coalition. Name coalitions require little financial commitment on the part of participants.

Formal coalitions, created for active lobbying or public relations purposes, require monetary commitments and a staff. Formal coalitions exist to directly influence acceptance of an issue, for example, convincing the public to support a piece of legislation.

A productive relationship with a coalition can be established when individuals or organizations are familiar with how and why the coalition operates, and there are clear expectations about what the individual or group plans to contribute to the coalition. Considerations before an individual or organization decides to participate in a coalition include the following:[89]

- ability and willingness to assume the workload and responsibility expected by the coalition

- willingness or ability to candidly share information

- ability to offer financial support to the coalition

- willingness and ability to attend meetings and coalition functions

- degree to which the coalition's cause is perceived as worthwhile

- level of knowledge about who belongs to the coalition

- level of knowledge about who underwrites the coalition

Oncology nurses are quite often designated as representatives of the ONS to various coalitions, and through these roles they actively participate in strategies that influence social policy and legislation. The ONS is a member of several coalitions, including the Coalition on Smoking OR Health, the National Coalition for Cancer Research, the National Alliance of Breast Cancer Organizations, and the Nursing Organizations Liaison Forum of the American Nurses Association (ANA). Participation in these coalitions requires the ONS Board of Directors to regularly reflect and consider its role in the coalition, the current level of activity and directions of the coalition, and the fiscal priority setting that allows the ONS to support designated members' positions as organizational liaisons between the ONS and the coalition.[90]

## FUTURE TRENDS

"Change is not what it used to be. The status quo will no longer be the best way forward."[91] No one can accurately predict the future. But by analyzing trends, it is possible to make fairly accurate guesses to plan for the future. Trends point to the increasing age of the American population; the growing importance of technological innova-

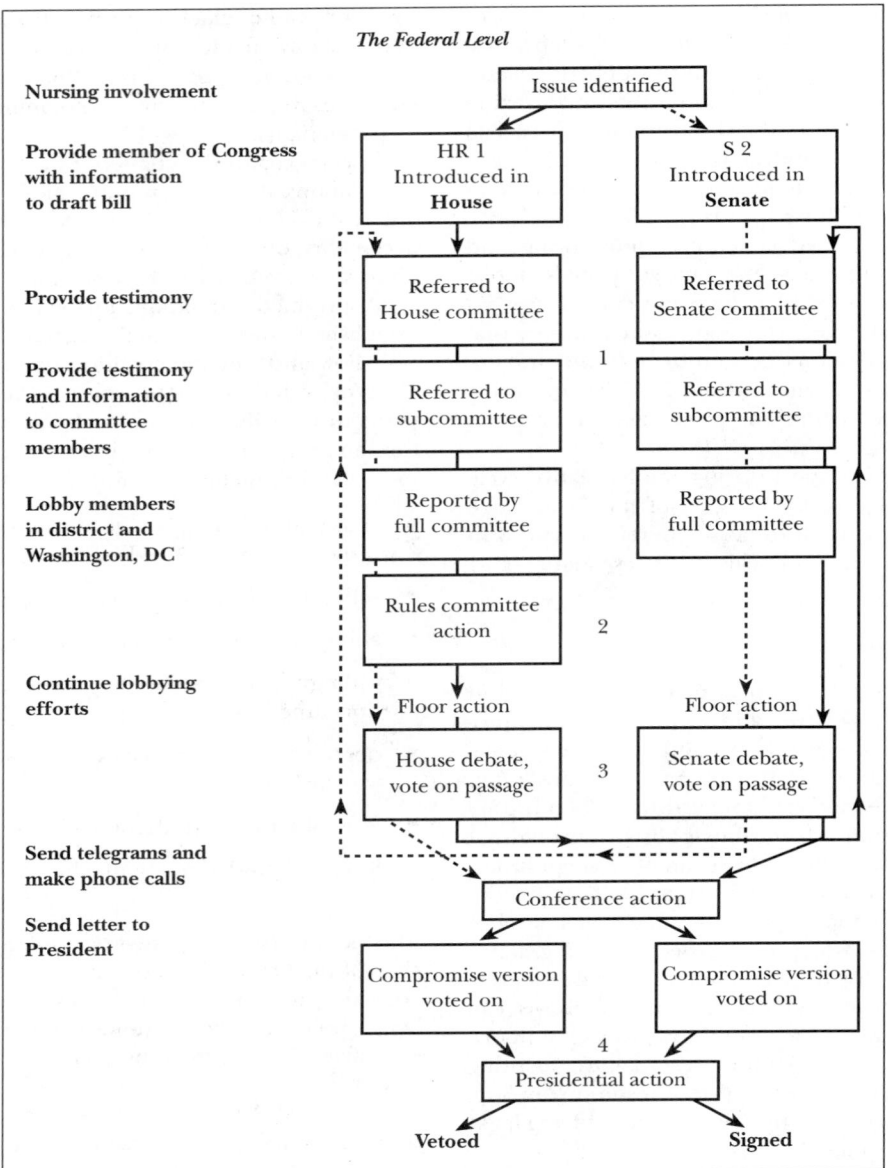

**The Federal Level**

Nursing involvement — Issue identified

Provide member of Congress
with information
to draft bill

HR 1 — Introduced in **House**

S 2 — Introduced in **Senate**

Provide testimony — Referred to House committee / Referred to Senate committee

Provide testimony
and information
to committee
members — Referred to subcommittee / Referred to subcommittee

Lobby members
in district and
Washington, DC — Reported by full committee / Reported by full committee

Rules committee action

Continue lobbying
efforts — Floor action / Floor action

House debate, vote on passage / Senate debate, vote on passage

Send telegrams and
make phone calls — Conference action

Send letter to
President — Compromise version voted on / Compromise version voted on

Presidential action

**Vetoed**  **Signed**

**FIGURE 63-1**  The process of how a bill becomes a law. Reprinted with permission from Mittelstadt PC and Hart MA: Legislative and regulatory processes, in Mason DJ, Talbot SW, Leavitt JK: *Policy and Politics for Nurses.* Philadelphia, Saunders, 1985.
[1]A bill goes to full committee first, then to special subcommittees for hearings, debate, revisions, and approval. The same process occurs when it goes to full committee. It either dies in committee or proceeds to the next step.
[2]Only the House has a Rules Committee to set the "rule" for floor action and conditions for debate and amendments. In the Senate, the leadership schedules action.
[3]The bill is debated, amended, and passed or defeated. If passed, it goes to the other chamber and follows the same path. If each chamber passes a similar bill, both versions go to conference.
[4]The President may sign the bill into law, allow it to become law without his signature, or veto it and return it to Congress. To override the veto, both houses must approve the bill by a ⅔ majority vote.

tion in oncology, including diagnostics and treatment; increased demand for cancer treatment in general; the importance of genetics and genetic therapy in cancer prevention, diagnosis, and treatment; an increase in the cancer cure rate; movement of treatment to outpatient and home care settings; decreased length of stay for the few treatment modalities that remain inpatient; and increased competition between physicians and hospitals for cancer services.[92,93]

For the nursing profession to ensure its vitality into the next century, it must assess trends and devise proactive strategies that allow nurses to take advantage of opportunities as they unfold. Changes, issues, and ethical questions will be set in motion, and individual or collective values will be challenged by scientific discoveries and technological advancements. At present, there is an incomplete understanding of the implications of many of the advances already made, let alone those yet to come, and therefore there is no defined direction or roles for nurses. A few individual nurses may be able to meet these challenges and find opportunities independently. Most nurses, however, would be more effective acting in collaboration with a like-minded group, coalition, or professional nursing organization.

## Challenges

Numerous challenges lie ahead for oncology nurses. For example, genetic research and the resulting identification of genes responsible for some diseases, including various forms of cancer, have altered the management of some individuals with cancer or at risk for malignant disease. We have only begun to see the potential of genetic research. Despite the sophistication of these findings, there is no research that addresses physical, psychosocial, and ethical outcomes of these scientific advances.[94] Issues arising from this research include psychosocial ramifications of access to genetic information, questions about who should have access to genetic information and potential violations of privacy and confidentiality, insurability and genetic potential for disease, and other ethical issues. Even though some of these issues come into conflict with traditional values—particularly those of privacy and confidentiality—public policy does not yet address these concerns. Legislation that begins to address gaps in current public policy is being introduced in the U.S. Congress,[95-97] but genetic science has advanced beyond current policy, the current system of checks and balances, and definition of safe, effective, and ethical practice in light of genetics knowledge and technology. The evolution of such policy is certain to engender political debate—and the oncology nurse can bring invaluable experience and the values of nursing to the policy-making process. To do so, experienced, knowledgeable, and prepared oncology nurses must be an integral part of the policy-making process.[94]

Demographers describe the advancing age of the American population. The traditional American values of "family" and "respect for elders" and current trends that disconnect families and isolate the elderly cause conflicts between values and current public policy. Advancing age is the greatest risk factor in the development of cancer and other diseases. Issues relating to the elderly, sick, and physically and mentally challenged, including questions of who gets care and what type of care older people should receive, have surfaced in ongoing political maneuvering relating to Medicaid and Medicare benefits, long-term care, and end-of-life issues. Legislative initiatives affecting Medicaid and Medicare benefits have been hotly debated, and such debate will escalate as funding cuts are made and resources are overtly or covertly rationed. Nursing organizations, including the ANA and the ONS, have voiced support for universal access to care for all citizens[98,99] and a health care delivery system designed to include, maintain, and improve access to long-term care, and to improve outcomes, costs, and quality of care in these facilities.[99,100] Although organizational position statements are useful tools for presentation of facts and issues, it is constituent and interest-group pressures that ultimately determine the success or failure of legislative initiatives. Nurses can and must play active constituent roles for these initiatives to survive the legislative process.

At the request of Congress, in and of itself the result of political processes, the Institute of Medicine (IOM) compiled the report *Nursing Staff in Hospitals and Nursing Homes: Is It Adequate?*[101] Conclusions have far-reaching implications for nurses currently in practice and those yet to enter the profession. According to the study, the quantity of registered nurses in the United States was determined to be adequate to meet national needs for the near future. The educational and skill mix was questioned in light of the changing health care system. The IOM recommends many changes, including training more APNs and more broadly trained nurses, increased use of APNs, increased numbers of nurses prepared to work in community-based and ambulatory care settings, increased presence of professional nurses in nursing homes on all shifts, and strengthening the leadership of directors of nursing. The report calls the lack of information about whether or not current delivery system redesign actually increases patient-centered care and reduces costs "shocking," and recommends that such data be collected.[101]

The report *Critical Challenges: Revitalizing the Health Professions for the Twenty-first Century* was released by the Pew Health Professions Commission in 1995.[102] The Pew Commission's recommendations for fewer professional nurses sharply conflicts with the ANA's projections for nursing personnel requirements. Statements released by the ANA suggest that the report is based on assumptions made by managed care organizations using economic criteria rather than exploration of actual consumer needs.[103] These two reports can have tremendous impact on the future of nursing. Legislators looking for data on which to base future policies, legislative initiatives, or decisions about health care and/or nursing roles will accept the reports of these influential entities in lieu of anything else. Unless nurses offer an alternative view, these recommendations will stand as fact. The ANA and nursing specialty organizations, including the ONS, collaborating through the network provided by the National Federation of Specialty Nursing Organizations, mounted a collective response to the Pew report that openly challenges the recommendations.

Managed care systems are influencing the role of the nurse and the scope of nursing practice. Some commentators propose a change in clinicians' ethical focus—from that of patient advocacy to being responsible stewards of society's resources.[104] Nurses, according to nurse ethicist Leah Curtin, should be concerned that managed care is undermining all aspects (choice, competence, communication, compassion, continuity, and no-conflict of interest) of the provider-patient relationship.[104]

## Nursing Opportunities

Porter-O'Grady[105] identifies five areas of opportunity in which nurses, especially APNs, can play a significant role: (1) primary care provider, (2) gatekeeper, (3) provider of cost-effective services, (4) case manager and practitioner in the emerging areas of family care, women's health, and rural health, and (5) wellness advocate and educator in geriatric services. Competencies specific to continued oncology nursing excellence connect oncology to gerontology, clinical trial processes, genetics, case management, ethics, wellness, prevention and early detection of disease, community-based skills, physical assessment skills, quality care, business and economics, epidemiology, anthropology, and patient, family, and community education.[106]

Nursing roles in patient care will continue to evolve as society and health care organizations address questions surrounding cost of care, where and how care is provided, and who should provide it.[107] The nurses' advocacy role might be enhanced. Nurses need to acquire knowledge to prepare patients and families to be effective advocates for their own needs. As policy shifts toward more self-reliance, measures implemented by Medicare and Medicaid will surely be adopted by other payers. Federal legislation, for example, the Health Insurance Reform Act of 1996, will be subject to interpretation and variable influences of special interests in each of the 50 state legislatures. Nurses, as providers, educators, and consumers, need to have a working knowledge not just of the clinical aspects of care but of the administrative regulations, financial components, and policy implications of what care is available and how care is provided.

## CONCLUSION

Whether acting alone, participating in a community coalition, or collaborating with a professional organization, nurses need to be aware of market, biomedical, and technological trends and the potential influence of these developments on policy and legislation. For most of the last century, health care has been seen as a service. Today, health care is both a service *and* a business. Health care services are increasingly encased in a business environment that, as yet, has few federal regulatory controls. It is nurses who provide many of the services, but they cannot ignore the business side of health care.

Technological improvement; fiscal assessments of delivery systems and health care plans (as opposed to quality indicators); closure of hospitals in rural areas and consolidation and merger of urban and suburban facilities; and the ever-increasing presence of for-profit systems provide opportunities for business to influence legislators and/or policy makers. Nurses must use national and state professional nursing organizations and specialty nursing organizations to keep abreast of these influences and resulting legislative priorities and initiatives. Information technology offers nurses increased opportunities for communication, information sharing, and networking among themselves as well as with consumers and patients. Communication technology such as the Internet offers limitless avenues through which nurses, other providers, and consumers can discuss issues, share concerns, access helpful resources, develop consensus on strategies for action, and communicate with elected officials and policy makers.

Annual membership satisfaction surveys conducted by the ONS indicate that its members want a proactive role in shaping their future through political processes that affect health care–related legislation and public policy, and regulations defining the scope of nursing practice.[108] With the trend of transferring the management of public health care programs to the states, the continuing evolution of the private sector in health care, and the widespread implications these trends portend, it is critical that nurses advocate for the needs of the population they serve and the profession of nursing. Nurses who are politically astute and proactive can influence change and be prepared for roles in the health care system of the future.

## REFERENCES

1. Richmond JB, Fein R: The health care mess: A bit of history. *JAMA* 273:69–71, 1995
2. Iglehart JK: The American health care system: Medicaid. *N Engl J Med* 328:896–900, 1993
3. Hanley BE: Policy development and analysis, in Mason DJ, Talbot SW, Leavitt JK (eds): *Policy and Politics for Nurses* (ed 2). Philadelphia, Saunders, 1993, pp 71–87
4. Fisher R, Ury W, Patton B (eds): *Getting To Yes* (ed 2). New York, Penguin Books, 1991
5. Rogge MM: Nursing and politics: A forgotten legacy. *Nurs Res* 36:26–30, 1987

6. Pryor EB: *Clara Barton, Professional Angel.* Philadelphia, University of Pennsylvania Press, 1987

7. Wiley BI (ed): *1862—1865—A Southern Woman's Story: Phoebe Yates Pember.* St. Simons Island, GA, Mockingbird Books, 1959

8. Noble H: Linking technology and health groups to find best cure. *New York Times,* Sept. 24, 1995, p A18

9. Hayes E, Tritsch R: An untapped resource: The political potential of nurses. *Nurs Adm Q* 13:33–39, 1988

10. Hanley BE: Political participation: How do nurses compare with other professional women? *Nurs Econ* 5:179–185, 1987

11. Campbell-Heider N, Hanna ND: Nursing's new political era. *Holistic Nurs Pract* 8:78–87, 1993

12. Lepler M: Nursing leadership meets managed care. *NURSEweek* 8(19):22–23, 1995

13. HR 3101: The Mother and Child Protection Act of 1996. *Congressional Record,* March 14, 1996, E359–E360

14. Greenlaw J: Definition and regulation of nursing practice: An historical survey. *Law Med Health Care* 13:117–121, 1985

15. Dalton JA, Speakman M, Duffey M, et al: The evolution of a profession: Where do boards of nursing fit in? *J Prof Nurs* 10:319–325, 1994

16. American Nurses Association: Report on legislative issues related to nursing practice. *Institute of Nursing Practice Agenda Item No. 4.* Washington, DC, American Nurses Association, 1994

17. Pearson LJ: Annual update of how each state stands on legislative issues affecting advanced nursing practice. *Nurse Pract* 19:11–21, 1994

18. Family Health Council of Central Pennsylvania: *Summary of Title 49: Professional and Vocational Standards.* Wormleysberg, PA, Family Health Council of Central Pennsylvania, Inc., 1994

19. Finocchio LJ, Dower CM, McMahon T, et al: *Reforming Health Care Workforce Regulation: Policy Considerations for the 21st Century.* San Francisco, Pew Health Professions Commission, December 1995

20. Hill CS: Relationship among cultural, educational, and regulatory agency influences on optimum cancer pain treatment. *J Pain Symptom Manage* 5:s37–s45, 1990 (suppl)

21. Rabon PG, Linette DC, Gonzalez MF, et al: Limited availability of medications for cancer patients. *South Med J* 86:914–918, 1993

22. Jacox A, Carr DB, Payne R et al: *Management of Cancer Pain: Clinical Practice Guideline No. 9.* Agency for Health Care Policy & Research, publication No. 94-0592. Rockville MD, U.S. Department of Health and Human Services, March 1994

23. Ferrell BR: Cost issues surrounding the treatment of cancer related pain. *J Pharmaceutical Care in Pain & Symptom Control* 1:9–23, 1993

24. Berina LF, Guernsey BG, Hokanson JA, et al: Physician perception of a triplicate prescription law. *Am J Hosp Pharm* 42:857–859, 1985

25. United States Department of Justice, Drug Enforcement Administration: *Multiple Copy Prescription Program Resource Guide.* Washington, DC, U.S. Government Printing Office, 1987

26. Sigler KA, Guernsey BG, Ingrim NB, et al: Effect of a triplicate prescription law on prescribing of Schedule II drugs. *Am J Hosp Pharm* 41:108–111, 1984

27. Von Roenn JH, Cleeland CS, Gonin R, et al: Physician attitudes and practice in cancer pain management: A survey from the Eastern Cooperative Oncology Group. *Ann Intern Med* 119:121–126, 1993

28. Holcombe R, Griffin J: Effect of insurance status on pain medication prescriptions in a hematology/oncology practice. *South Med J* 86:151–156, 1993

29. Angarola RT: DEA proposes Controlled Substances Monitoring Act. *APS Bull* 5(3):5, 22, 1995

30. Joranson D: Intractable pain treatment laws and regulations. *APS Bull* 5(2):1–3, 15–17, 1995

31. Joranson D: State medical board guidelines for treatment of intractable pain. *APS Bull* 5(3):1–5, 1995

32. Joranson D: Intractable pain treatment laws and regulations. *APS Bull* 5(2):1–3, 15–16, 1995

33. Joranson D: State medical board guidelines for treatment of intractable pain. *APS Bull* 5(3):1–4, 1995

34. Hatch O: *Congressional Record:* Senate, July 16, 1996, p S7889

35. Foley KM: Pain relief into practice: Rhetoric without reform. *J Clin Oncol* 13:2149–2151, 1995 (editorial)

36. McDermott KC: Prescriptive authority for advanced practice nurses: Current and future perspectives. *Oncol Nurs Forum* 22:25–30, 1995 (suppl)

37. Government Accounting Office: Report to Senate Committee on Labor and Human Resources, Sept. 1991, GAO/PEMD-91-14

38. Young J: Off-label drug scorecard. *Oncology Issues* 10(2):6, 30, 1995

39. Everson LK: Cancer program development in the 1990's. *Oncology Issues* 8(4):8–10, 1993

40. Toner R: Medicare target could be exclusive, many experts say. *New York Times,* Oct. 15, 1995, p A1

41. Ad Hoc Working Group of the National Cancer Advisory Board: *A Review of the Intramural Program of the National Cancer Institute.* Bethesda, MD, National Cancer Institute June 26, 1995

42. Oncology Nursing Society, Minutes of meeting, Board of Directors, June 25–28, 1996, Pittsburgh, PA

43. Boyd K (ed): *The Cancer Letter* 22(30):1–3, 1996

44. Piemme JA: Tobacco-related issues continue. *ONS News* 10(7):6, 1995

45. *USA Today,* Aug. 22, 1996, 1-A

46. McDermott KC: Health care reform: Past and future. *Oncol Nurs Forum* 21:827–831, 1994

47. Clinton WJ: *The President's Health Security Plan.* New York, Random House, 1993

48. Jonas S: *Health Care Delivery in the United States* (ed 4). New York, Springer, 1986

49. Watson PG: The Americans with Disabilities Act: More rights for people with disabilities. *Rehabil Nurs* 15:325–328, 1990

50. Barry D: This city is nothing like the planet earth: An outsider's guide to Washington. *Washington Post Magazine,* Aug. 14, 1994, pp 7–11, 24–27

51. Enthoven A, Kronick R: A consumer-choice health plan for the 1990s: Universal health insurance in a system designed to promote quality and economy. *N Engl J Med* 320:29–37, 1989

52. Specture P: Failure, by the numbers. *New York Times,* Sept. 24, 1994, p A19

53. Blendon RJ, Brodie M, Benson J: What should be done now that national health system reform is dead? *JAMA* 273:243–244, 1995

54. Staples B: The man who wouldn't be President. *New York Times Book Review,* Nov. 19, 1995, p 7

55. Blumenthal D, Berenson R: Health care issues in presidential campaigns. *N Engl J Med* 321:908–912, 1989

56. Blendon RJ: The public's view of the future of health care. *JAMA* 259:3587–3593, 1988

57. Curran WJ: The constitutional right to health care: Denial in the court. *N Engl J Med* 320:788–789, 1988

58. Families USA: White House, Congress begin crucial negotiations: Fate of Medicaid, Medicare at stake in budget battle. *ASAP Newsletter*, Washington, DC, December 1995 (web site address: //epn.org/families.html)

59. Verhovek SH: With power shift, state lawmakers see new demands. *New York Times*, Sept. 24, 1995, p 1, 24

60. Chronical News Service: Business group doubts GOP budget plan. *San Francisco Chronicle*, Dec. 6, 1995, A3

61. Iglehart JK: Medicaid and managed care. *N Engl J Med* 332:1727–1731, 1995

62. Grogan CM: Hope in federalism? What can the states do and what are they likely to do? *J Health Polit Policy Law* 20:477–484, 1995

63. Waid MO: Brief summaries of TITLE XVIII and TITLE XIX of the Social Security Act. *Soc Secur Bull* 56(4):1–3, 1993

64. Freeman H: The impact of clinical trial protocols on patient care systems in a large city hospital: Access for the socially disadvantaged. *Cancer* 72:2834–2838, 1993 (suppl)

65. Katz SJ, Hoffer TP: Socioeconomic disparities in preventive care persist despite universal coverage: Breast and cervical cancer screening in Ontario and the United States. *JAMA* 272:530–534, 1994

66. Geller AC, Miller DR, Lew RA, et al: Cutaneous melanoma mortality among the socioeconomically disadvantaged in Massachusetts. *Am J Public Health* 86:538–544, 1996

67. Wachter RM: Rationing health care: Preparing for a new era. *South Med J* 88:25–32, 1995

68. Wilensky GR: Incremental health system reform: Where Medicare fits in. *Health Affairs* 14(10):173–181, 1995

69. Iglehart JK: The American health care system: Medicare. *N Engl J Med* 327:1467–1472, 1992

70. Byrne A, Carney DN: Cancer in the elderly, in Ozols RF, Steele G, Kinsella TJ (eds): *Current Problems in Cancer* 17(3): St. Louis, Mosby, 1993, pp 150–204

71. Toner R: Medicare target could be elusive, many experts say. *New York Times*, May 16, 1995, pp A1, A20

72. Gorham M: Congressional rescissions mean big cuts for rural health programs. *Rural Health FYI* 17:3, 28–30, 1995

73. Haylock PJ, Cantril CA: Rural cancer care think tank uncovers significant issues/concerns. *ONS News* 10(10):10, 1995

74. Jenkins S: The future of rural communities: Mobilizing local resources, in Bushy A (ed): *Rural Nursing*, vol 2. Newbury Park, CA, Sage, 1991, pp 16–28

75. Freudenhiem M: Health costs paid by employers drop for first time in a decade. *New York Times*, Feb. 14, 1995, D9

76. Hurley RE, Thompson JR: The harsh realities of a managed care world. *Med Group Manage J* Sept/Oct:96, 1993

77. Clancy CM, Brody H: Managed care: Jekyll or Hyde? *JAMA* 273:338–339, 1995 (editorial)

78. Iglehart JK: Physicians and the growth of managed care. *N Engl J Med* 331:1167–1171, 1994

79. Mechanic D: Managed care: Rhetoric and realities. *Inquiry* 31:124–128, 1994

80. Star P: The signing of the Kennedy-Kassenbaum Bill, Aug. 22, 1966 (http://epn.org/library/signing.html)

81. Kassenbaum N: *Congressional Record*, Sept. 11, 1996, p S10330

82. Wennberg JE, Goodman DC, Nease RF, et al: Finding equilibrium in U.S. physician supply. *Health Affairs* 12:89–103, 1993

83. Kassirer JP: Access to specialty care. *N Engl J Med* 331:1151–1153, 1994

84. Grupenhoff JT: Profile of congressional health legislative aides. *Mt Sinai J Med* 50:1–7, 1983

85. Pullen D: *The U.S. Congress Handbook*. McLean, VA, Barbara Pullen, Publisher, 1974–1995

86. Bushy A, Smith TO: Lobbying: The hows and wherefores. *Nurs Manage* 21(4):39–41, 44–45, 1990

87. House OKs bill to reform lobbying. *San Francisco Chronicle* Nov 30, 1995, pp A1, A17

88. Mittelstad PC, Hart MA: Legislative and regulatory processes, in Mason DJ, Talbott SW, Leavitt JK (eds): *Policy and Politics for Nurses* (ed 2). Philadelphia, Saunders, 1993, pp 399–411

89. Hunt FD: How coalitions work. *Association Management*, June 1993, pp 93, 94, 108

90. Oncology Nursing Society: *Oncology Nursing Society Policy Manual*. Pittsburgh, Oncology Nursing Society, 1996

91. Handy C: *The Age of Unreason*. Boston, Harvard Business School Press, 1989

92. Stepnick L, Pagnani E (eds): *The Future for Oncology; New Technologies and Their Impact on the Competitive Marketplace*. Washington, DC, Advisory Board Company, 1994

93. Boyle DM, Engelking C, Harvey C: Making a difference in the 21st century: Are oncology nurses ready? *Oncol Nurs Forum* 21:53–79, 1994

94. Strauss ST, Calzone K, Jenkins J, et al: Genetics Project Team Report to the Oncology Nursing Society Board of Directors, Pittsburgh, PA, Oncology Nursing Society, June 17, 1996

95. Solomon GBH: *Congressional Record*, Aug. 2, 1996, p E1468

96. Slaughter LM: *Congressional Record*, March 27, 1996, p E476

97. Domenici PV: *Congressional Record*, June 24, 1996, p S6719

98. Oncology Nursing Society: *Fact Sheet: Universal Access to Health Care*. Pittsburgh, Oncology Nursing Society, 1996

99. American Nurses Association: *Nursing's Agenda for Health Care Reform*. Washington, DC, American Nurses Association, 1990

100. Oncology Nursing Society: *Fact Sheet: Long Term Care and Cancer*. Pittsburgh, Oncology Nursing Society, 1996

101. Institute of Medicine: *Nursing Staff in Hospitals and Nursing Homes: Is It Adequate?* Washington, DC, National Academy Press, 1996

102. Pew Health Professions Commission: *Critical Challenges: Revitalizing the Health Professions for the Twenty-first Century*. San Francisco, Pew Health Professions Commission, 1995

103. Keepnews D: ANA Challenges Pew Health Professions' findings. *Am Nurse* 28(1):3, 1996

104. Curtin LL: The ethics of managed care: Part I. Proposing a new ethos? *Nurs Manage* 27(8):18–19, 1996

105. Porter-O'Grady T: What an exciting time. *Advanced Practice Nursing Quarterly* 1:68–69, 1995

106. Haylock PJ, Boyle DM: Think tank held to ensure a preferred future for oncology nurses and the Oncology Nursing Society. *ONS News* 10(7):5, 1995

107. Parkman C: The staff nurse's role in the changing health-care scene. *NURSEweek* 8:(23), 8–9, 1995

108. Oncology Nursing Society: *Annual Membership Survey*. Pittsburgh, Oncology Nursing Society, 1995

# Chapter 64

# Role of the Oncology Advanced Practice Nurse

Annette Galassi, RN, MA, CANP, AOCN

## INTRODUCTION

This is an exciting time to be an oncology advanced practice nurse. Barriers to practice are collapsing and paradigms are shifting. The title "nurse practitioner" is no longer synonymous with primary care just as the title "clinical specialist" is no longer synonymous with specialty-based practice. This chapter will explore the history of advanced practice nursing, describe the educational preparation required for oncology advanced practice, and review critical issues including the regulation of advanced practice and third-party reimbursement. Finally, a vision of oncology advanced practice nursing for the twenty-first century will be painted through a description of emerging roles.

## HISTORY OF ADVANCED PRACTICE NURSING

### The Nurse Practitioner Movement

A nurse practitioner (NP) is a registered nurse who has advanced education and clinical training in a specialty area such as adult health or women's health. Nurse practitioners obtain medical histories, perform physical examinations, make medical and nursing diagnoses, and treat common health problems and chronic diseases. Since nursing practice is regulated by the nurse practice act of the state in which the NP is employed, the amount of autonomy the NP has in performing these functions varies from state to state.

The NP role originated in 1965 with a demonstration project at the University of Colorado to prepare pediatric nurse practitioners.[1] A perceived shortage of physicians, attributed to the siphoning of physicians to specialty practice, was the major impetus for the development of the NP role. The goal of the project by Lorretta Ford was to "develop a new educational and training experience (for professional nurses) to prepare them to assume an expanded role in child health as practitioners of nursing."[1,p.43] Shortly thereafter, family nurse practitioner programs were begun at the University of Washington, Cornell–New York Hospital, and the University of California, Davis. Most of these early NP programs were continuing education offerings or certificate programs affiliated with medical schools. The programs varied in length, quality, and content. Admission criteria also varied, with some programs requiring only that one be a registered nurse with a current license to practice.[2] Upon completion, the graduate might alternatively receive nothing, a certificate, a baccalaureate degree, or a master's degree.

In 1974, the American Nurses' Association (ANA) Congress on Nursing Practice published the first definitions of the roles of the NP. This was followed by the publication of guidelines for the preparation of adult and family nurse practitioners in continuing education programs. Guidelines for NP preparation subsequently have been developed by the Association of Women's Health, Obstetric, and Neonatal Nurses; the American College of Nurse Midwives; and the National Association of Pediatric Nurse Associates and Practitioners. Graduates of programs that adhere to the guidelines are eligible to take certification examinations sponsored by these organizations.

In 1979 the National League for Nursing, the agency that accredits schools of nursing, declared in their position statement on NP education that the NP should hold a master's degree in nursing. As of 1992 the American Nurses' Credentialing Center has required a master's degree or higher in nursing for certification as an adult, family, pediatric, school, or gerontological NP. Master's level education for NPs also is supported by the American Academy of Nurse Practitioners and the American Association of Colleges of Nursing.[3,4] As a result, NP education has shifted away from certificate programs and today encompasses graduate level programs in schools of nursing.

The trend towards master's degree preparation for NPs is noted in the following statistics. In 1979 there were 124 certificate programs and 74 master's degree programs preparing NPs.[5] As of 1996, the American Association of Colleges of Nursing identified 255 master's-level and/or post-master's NP programs.[6] It is estimated that there are only 15–20 certificate programs for NPs currently in existence.[7]

### The Development of the Clinical Nurse Specialist Role

While the NP role evolved with a strong focus on the medical model, the clinical nurse specialist (CNS) role was based on nursing models.[8] A CNS is a master's prepared registered nurse who has expert knowledge and skill in caring for a population of patients within a given specialty. Most authors agree on a core of four functional components of the CNS role including clinical practice, education, consultation, and research.[9] Administration and change agent have also been cited as functional components.

The first master's degree program with a clinical specialty was developed by Hildegard Peplau at Rutgers University in 1954.[10] Factors that led to the development of nurse specialists included a rapid expansion in scientific knowledge, an increasingly complex health care system, a shortage of health care personnel, and a heightened focus on public health care needs.[11] Nurse educators proposed the role of the CNS to counter the impersonal, fragmented, authoritarian, and tradition-based nursing practice that had developed following World War II.[12] The role was seen as a clinical option to the more traditional educator and administrator roles of graduate level nursing education.

Specialization in health care was the trend in the

1970s fostered by dramatic increases in knowledge and technology. Specialty-focused patient care areas were developed within the hospital and the expectation was that a CNS could provide expert bedside care, function as a role model for nursing staff, improve the quality of nursing care, and implement clinical nursing research in these areas. Initially, there was debate about the title and educational preparation of these nurses in expanded roles. Nurses with and without graduate degrees in nursing were using the title CNS or nurse clinician. In 1965 the ANA published a position paper stating the CNS title could be used only by nurses with a master's degree in nursing.[2,8] The ANA Social Policy Statement (1980) further defined the title CNS as an expert in a defined area of knowledge and practice with advanced preparation at the graduate level.[13] The ANA Council of Clinical Nurse Specialists, formed in 1980, was instrumental in developing the statement on the role of the CNS that established the four functional role components of expert practitioner, educator, consultant, and researcher.[14] Unlike the initial proliferation of certificate programs for the preparation of NPs there were no such programs for CNSs. Almost all CNS programs were developed at the master's degree level.

## The Trend Toward Merged Roles

NP practice traditionally has focused on primary care in an ambulatory setting while specialty-focused acute care has been within the domain of the CNS. Mundinger proposed that nurse practitioners care for patients while they are standing up and clinical nurse specialists care for patients while they are lying down.[15] This is no longer true. The boundaries that have traditionally existed between the NP and CNS are becoming less distinct and practice settings can no longer be used to distinguish one group of advanced practice nurses from another. Some NPs are specialty-focused or practice in an acute care setting, and some CNSs practice in an ambulatory setting.

Several research studies have been published that support the notion that the CNS and NP roles are more similar than different.[16–20] Elder and Bullough, in a survey of NP and CNS alumni from a master's of nursing program, found that both CNS and NP participated in patient and family teaching, counseling, psychosocial assessments, and use of the nursing process related to treatment regimens. The major difference between the two groups was that NPs spent more time in direct care and CNSs spent more time in indirect care.[16]

Forbes and colleagues conducted a survey of core curricula of graduate nursing programs that prepare clinical nurse specialists and nurse practitioners. The results of this survey suggested that the major difference in the preparation for these roles lies not in the curricula content but in the practice setting in which the role is operationalized.[17] This was also borne out in a comparative analysis of the CNS and NP role by Fenton and Brykczyn-

ski. The authors found that there was an advanced practice role for both the CNS and the NP and that much of the knowledge, skills, and competencies are shared. As a result, the authors have suggested that graduate schools of nursing consolidate the core curriculum for the advanced practice nursing programs.[18]

In Schroer's model of case management the roles of the CNS and NP are fully integrated.[19] The results of Williams and Valdivieso's survey of advanced practice nurses in South Carolina also supported the similarities of the CNS and NP roles. Differences were primarily related to relative emphasis on direct practice. NPs spent more time in direct practice whereas CNSs spent more time in the indirect roles of educator and consultant.[20]

The educational preparation of NPs and CNSs also is becoming more similar. With the shift of NP preparation to the graduate level, NP education includes nursing theory, research, and education principles. Likewise, CNS education has expanded to include health assessment.[21] Additionally, nurses with master's degrees in other nursing specialty areas have returned to post-master's nurse practitioner programs to obtain additional education.

## Advanced Practice Nursing Defined

The research cited previously supports the current trend in education and practice toward a merged role of advanced practice nurse. According to the American Nurses' Association, "Advanced practice registered nurses have acquired the knowledge base and practice experiences to prepare them for specialization, expansion, and advancement in practice."[22] This knowledge and skill is obtained at the master's or doctoral level in nursing. The National Council of State Boards of Nursing's definition of advanced practice nursing includes nurse practitioners, nurse anesthetists, nurse-midwives, and clinical nurse specialists with a graduate degree and a major in nursing or a graduate degree with a concentration in an advanced nursing practice category.[23] The National League for Nursing (NLN) has recommended the merging of the CNS and NP roles under the title APN.[24]

The Oncology Nursing Society in its position statement on advanced practice has endorsed the title "Advanced Practice Nurse" to designate both clinical nurse specialist and nurse practitioner roles. According to ONS's position statement, APNs are prepared, at a minimum, with a master's degree in nursing. The statement does not exclude other master's-prepared nurses in administration, education, or research.[25] The inclusion of other nonclinically focused, master's-prepared nurses is not consistent with the generally accepted use of the term APN.

In contrast, the ANA states that "The term advanced practice is used to refer exclusively to advanced clinical practice . . . Although nursing educators, administrators, and researchers are prepared educationally at the master's or doctoral level, they are not considered advanced practice registered nurses . . ."[22,p.15] The ANA

Council of Clinical Nurse Specialists and Council of Primary Health Care Nurse Practitioners were merged in 1990 to form the Council of Nurses in Advanced Practice.[26] Since that time, both CNSs and NPs who pass the American Nurses' Credentialing Center certification examination may use the credential CS (certified specialist).

The American Association of Colleges of Nursing's (AACN) position statement on the certification and regulation of advanced practice nurses states that "advanced practice nurse is an umbrella term appropriate for a licensed registered nurse prepared at the graduate degree level as either a CNS, NA, NM or NP."[4] AACN's position statement on nursing education's agenda for the twenty-first century states, "Advanced nursing practice requires graduate preparation which may focus on primary health care, case management, specialization, education, or administration across health settings."[27]

## The Evolution of the Oncology Advanced Practice Nurse

The evolution of oncology advanced practice nursing was similar to that of the clinical nurse specialist role. The first course in oncology nursing at the graduate level was offered by Teachers' College, Columbia University and Memorial Hospital in New York City in 1947. It consisted of an academic and clinical component and was 16 credit hours.[28] The first specialty tract in oncology nursing was begun at the University of Pittsburgh in 1968 as part of the medical-surgical master's degree in nursing.[29] The first graduate program in oncology nursing was developed at Rush University in Chicago in 1974–1975 under Myra Levine and Sue Hegyvary.

In 1978 the American Cancer Society invited a group of nurse educators, researchers, practitioners, and administrators involved with cancer nursing to meet. The purpose of the meeting was to reach consensus about the role and educational preparation of the specialist in cancer nursing. It resulted in the publication by the American Cancer Society of the first role definition and curriculum guidelines for the master's degree in nursing with a specialization in oncology nursing.[30] The focus was on the educational preparation of the oncology CNS. This guide was revised in collaboration with the Oncology Nursing Society in 1986 and most recently in 1994. The third edition, entitled *The Master's Degree with a Specialty in Advanced Practice Oncology Nursing*, has a significantly different focus than previous editions. The current curriculum guide has been broadened to support a blended role of an advanced practice oncology nurse that combines both CNS and NP skills. The authors believe this broad preparation will allow for the greatest flexibility in employment in a variety of cancer practice settings.[31] The course content of the curriculum guide includes clinical practice, education, consultation, collaboration, systems, role competency, research and outcomes evaluation, program development, and leadership.

There are currently over 40 master's degree programs in oncology nursing. Some programs are designed as a separate specialty while others are a tract or focus area within a nursing major. These programs vary in length, number of courses specific to oncology nursing, and credit hours in clinical oncology nursing.[32] Historically, the vast majority of these programs focused on the preparation of the oncology CNS. Currently, the specialty title of several of these programs, "advanced practice oncology nursing," reflects preparation in a blended or merged CNS/NP role.

McMillan et al conducted a role delineation study to determine the elements that make up the role of the oncology advanced practice nurse. They used a 190-item survey that consisted of five subscales: direct caregiver, consultant, administrator/coordinator, researcher, and educator. Six hundred thirty-seven master's-prepared oncology nurses responded for a 47% return rate. Fifty-eight percent identified their job title as CNS while only 7% identified their job title as NP. A comparative analysis of the advanced practice behaviors of the oncology CNS and NP was not done. Given the relatively small number of respondents who identified themselves as an NP such an analysis was likely to have been impossible. The study results were used by the Oncology Nursing Certification Corporation to design the Advanced Oncology Nursing Certification Examination.[33]

# REGULATION OF ADVANCED PRACTICE NURSING

"The purpose of any regulation of nursing practice is the protection of public health, safety and welfare."[34,p.617] The legal regulation of nursing, including advanced practice, is the responsibility of state boards of nursing. Each state's board of nursing is vested with this authority by the state legislature that enacts the state's nurse practice act. This approach has resulted in tremendous variability among states and a "patchwork quilt" of regulation surrounding advanced practice nursing. There is a great deal of inconsistency from state to state in the educational/ certification requirements, scope of practice, physician oversight, prescriptive authority, and level of regulatory oversight. There is even inconsistency regarding the definition of an advanced practice registered nurse. For example, some states include NPs, CNMs, CRNAs, and CNSs in the definition, others include NPs, CNMs, CRNAs, and only psychiatric-mental health CNSs, and still others include NPs, CNMs, and CRNAs only. These inconsistencies significantly limit the mobility of APNs and create confusion for the public, legislators, and other health care providers.[35]

An advanced practice nurse must obtain information regarding the regulatory requirements in the jurisdiction where the APN intends to practice. The applicant must then provide documentation of eligibility to meet the requirements. The board of nursing evaluates the applicant's credentials against the established criteria and grants authority to practice to those individuals meeting the criteria.

## Levels of Regulation

There are four levels of regulation—designation/recognition, registration, certification, and licensure. Designation/recognition is the least restrictive method of regulation and consists of recognition of credentials by a state's board of nursing. It does not involve an inquiry into competence of the APN by the board. Registration is the placement of names of APNs on an official board roster. It also does not involve an inquiry into competence nor does it define the scope of practice. Certification involves title regulation. The APN must meet specified, predetermined requirements and only those who meet the requirements may use the title. Certification attempts to measure competence. Licensure specifies scope of practice and applications for licensure are evaluated to ensure that predetermined requirements are met. Licensure also allows the grantor, such as the board of nursing, to take disciplinary action for violation of laws or rules.[36]

## Certification Versus Second Licensure

The regulation of advanced practice nursing has become a topic of increasing concern for the profession and one for which there is no consensus. The issue is whether certification or second licensure is the appropriate regulatory mechanism for advanced practice. Professional nursing organizations including the ANA have supported voluntary certification while state boards of nursing have favored second licensure. There are difficulties associated with both approaches.

Certification has been used by the ANA and various specialty organizations including ONS for a range of purposes, from recognizing excellence or professional achievement to denoting minimum competency to practice a specialty. There are more than 30 specialty nursing organizations that grant certification to nurses with training beyond the entry level.[37] The Oncology Nursing Certification Corporation is one such organization and offers both a basic and an advanced oncology nursing certification examination.

The term certification is confusing since it is used to refer to both specialty certification and advanced practice certification. Advanced practice certification requires education beyond the entry level, usually at the graduate level. However, not all professional organizations that offer advanced practice certification require a master's degree. NPs with a baccalaureate degree are eligible to take the advanced oncology nursing examination until the year 2000. After that time, a master's degree in nurs-

ing will be required. The eligibility criteria for the advanced oncology nursing certification examination is as follows:

- RN license

- Master's degree or higher in nursing (NPs with bachelor's degree may take examination until the year 2000)

- At least 30 months of experience as an RN within the five years prior to application*

- At least 2000 hours of oncology nursing experience within the five years prior to application

The American College of Nurse Midwifery and the Council on Certification for Nurse Anesthetists use certification to denote minimum competency to practice these specialties but do not require a master's degree. Practice and experience requirements and recertification requirements also vary among organizations (see Table 64-1).

There are no standard criteria used by professional organizations that offer certification examinations to ensure that the examination has a clinical focus. Yet in many states, national certification is used to regulate advanced nursing practice.[38]

The National Council of State Boards of Nursing's (NCSBN) initial position on advanced clinical nursing practice supported designation/recognition as the preferable method of regulation. This position has changed over time with the NCSBN currently favoring second licensure.[23] The NCSBN does not favor certification since many certification examinations are not designed to measure ability for regulatory purposes. The examination may not be psychometrically constructed for the purpose of legal regulation. Additionally, the subject matter of the examination may not be consistent with the scope of

**TABLE 64-1**  Professional Organizations Offering Advanced Practice Certification Examinations

| Organization | Master's Degree |
|---|---|
| American Academy of Nurse Practitioners | No |
| American College of Nurse Midwifery Certification Council, Inc. | No |
| American Nurses' Credentialing Center | Yes, since 1992 |
| The Council on Certification for Nurse Anesthetists | No |
| National Certification Board of Pediatric Nurse Practitioners and Nurses | No |
| The National Certification Corporation for the Obstetric, Gynecologic and Neonatal Nursing Specialties | No |

Experience may be in nursing administration, clinical practice, education, or research

practice being regulated. The NCSBN has agreed that professional certification, along with graduate education, may be used as a qualification for licensure as long as the board of nursing has established criteria for accepting the certification and maintains control of the licensure process.[36]

The feasibility of a second licensure examination was recently explored by an NCSBN task force, the Advanced Practice Nursing Coordination Task Force. This task force recommended the development of such an examination; however, the NCSBN has delayed action on this recommendation. Instead, the NCSBN Board of Directors was directed by its Delegate Assembly to collaborate with advanced practice certification organizations to ensure that current examinations are "legally defensible and psychometrically sound" for regulatory purposes. If progress is not made toward this goal, the NCSBN has stated that it will move forward on the creation of an examination for second licensure.[39]

Many professional nursing organizations, including the ANA, have supported the regulation of advanced practice through the mechanism of voluntary certification. This mechanism was established and is operated by professional nursing specialty organizations. Through certification, the profession maintains autonomy and responsibility for the regulation of advanced practice whereas through second licensure that control is assumed by state boards of nursing.[40]

A *standardized* certification process for advanced practice nursing would eliminate much of the criticism of the current certification process and potentially abolish the need for a second license to regulate nursing practice. Movement toward such a standardized certification process has begun. In 1991, the American Nurses' Credentialing Center and other certification boards formed the American Board of Nursing Specialties (ABNS). Membership in the ABNS is limited to those advanced practice nursing certification bodies that meet ABNS standards. This board is analogous to the American Board of Medical Specialties and other professional boards that certify individuals to specialize in a particular practice area.

The ANA supports the following features to be included within a regulatory system for advanced practice: a definition of an APN, an educational standard of a graduate degree, recognition of professional certification, and a description of scope of practice. According to personal communication with D. O'Neill (November 1995), the ANA does not support the inclusion of any reference to physician collaboration, supervision, or protocols as the authority to regulate advanced practice should reside solely with the state board of nursing.

Licensure, credentialing, and certification were topics discussed at the State-of-the-Knowledge Conference on Advanced Practice in Oncology Nursing sponsored by ONS in October 1994. The recommendation to explore the ramifications of second licensure for APNs and the feasibility of a joint certification examination with other organizations such as the ANA was accepted and included in ONS's position statement on advanced practice in oncology nursing.[25]

# PRESCRIPTIVE AUTHORITY

The authority for the APN to prescribe is regulated on the state level. Forty-seven states currently provide for some level of prescriptive authority.[38] The level of authority varies from independent prescriptive authority including controlled substances to dependent authority excluding controlled substances (see Table 64-2). The dependent statutes indicate that the APN is under supervision of a physician when performing this task.

## Controlled Substances

In states where APNs are allowed to prescribe controlled substances, Drug Enforcement Administration (DEA) registration numbers are required. The DEA has established a mid-level practitioner registration category under which APNs, physician assistants, and others are given individual DEA registration numbers.[41] These numbers begin with the letter M to allow responsible parties in the controlled substance distribution chain (e.g., pharmacists) to contact appropriate state officials to verify the authority the practitioner has been granted. DEA registration allows a wide variety of acts including purchasing, storing, administering, dispensing, and prescrib-

**TABLE 64-2**   Level of Prescriptive Authority by State

| | |
|---|---|
| Independent Prescriptive Authority including controlled substances | Alaska, Arizona, District of Columbia, Iowa, Montana, New Mexico, Oregon, Vermont, Washington, Wisconsin, Wyoming |
| Dependent Prescriptive Authority including controlled substances | Arkansas, Connecticut, Georgia, Indiana, Louisiana, Massachusetts, Maryland, Minnesota, Mississippi,* North Carolina, North Dakota, Nebraska, New York, Pennsylvania, Rhode Island, South Carolina,* South Dakota, Utah, West Virginia |
| Dependent Prescriptive Authority excluding controlled substances | Alabama, California, Florida, Hawaii, Idaho, Kansas, Kentucky, Michigan, Missouri, New Jersey, Nevada, Ohio,* Tennessee, Texas, Virginia |
| No Prescriptive Authority | Illinois, Oklahoma |

*In specific situations

ing controlled substances; however, the advanced practice nurse may engage in only those activities authorized by the state in which they practice.[42] Figure 64-1 provides information on obtaining a DEA registration number.

## Research Related to Prescriptive Authority

As regulatory changes are made that grant APNs prescriptive authority, implementation of these changes and their effects on access to care, clinical practice, and patient outcomes need to be evaluated. A small, pilot study done by Mahoney suggests that employers and administrators may be resistant to NPs prescribing medications even after a state has granted NPs this authority.[43] Such an arbitrary restriction on practice reduces the NPs efficiency, devalues the role, and limits the ability to provide a full range of health care services. Sekcenski et al evaluated state practice environments for PAs, NPs, and CNMs. The investigators used legal status, reimbursement, and prescriptive authority to identify states with favorable practice environments. Lack of prescriptive authority was an important factor in states with generally unfavorable practice environments. State practice environment scores for NPs were lowest (least favorable) for Ohio and Illinois and highest (most favorable) for Oregon, Montana, and North Dakota.[44]

## REIMBURSEMENT OF ADVANCED PRACTICE NURSING SERVICES

The effective utilization of an APN is, in part, tied to reimbursement of services provided. Reimbursement is provided through federal and state programs such as Medicare, Medicaid, or through private insurers includ-

---

An application for registration may be obtained along with the *Mid-level Practitioner's Manual* by mailing or telephoning a request to:

United States Department of Justice
Drug Enforcement Administration
Central Station
P.O. Box 28083
Washington, DC 20038-8083
(202) 307-7255

Some states require state-issued controlled substance registration numbers in addition to a DEA registration number. The state number must be obtained prior to applying for a DEA registration number. Contact the DEA for further information.

---

**FIGURE 64-1**  DEA registration information.

ing Health Maintenance Organizations (HMOs) and Preferred Provider Organizations (PPOs). Figure 64-2 provides information on obtaining provider numbers.

## Medicare Payment

Medicare is a federal health insurance program for individuals who are disabled or over the age of 65. It is funded through payroll deductions from Social Security. Part A of the program pays for costs incurred during hospitalizations; part B pays for physician services and for APN services under the following circumstances:

- Service is usually furnished by an MD/DO.

- Service is performed by a person who meets the Medicare definition of NP or CNS.

- NP or CNS is legally authorized to perform the service in the state in which it is performed.

- Service is performed in collaboration with an MD/DO.

Reimbursement for APNs varies considerably by the type of APN, the health care setting, and the payment rate.[45]

NPs and CNSs are eligible to receive direct reimbursement for nonhospital services only in rural settings, defined as counties that are in nonmetropolitan statistical

---

To receive direct reimbursement for services covered by Medicare or Medicaid, an advanced practice nurse must have a billing or provider number.

*Medicare Provider Number*

Contact the local Medicare carrier to obtain the registration form to apply for a Medicare billing number or contact the Social Security Office at 1-800-772-1213.

*Medicaid Provider Number*

To obtain a registration form to apply for a Medicaid provider number, contact the local Medicaid office within the state health department.

*CHAMPUS Provider Information*

To obtain a CHAMPUS provider application, write to the following address:

CHAMPUS
Provider File Operations
Post Office Box 100558
Florence, SC 29501-0558

Telephone numbers for CHAMPUS area offices:
Mid-Atlantic Region 1-800-467-8500
Western Region 1-800-225-4816
MN, WI, IA, WV, KY, OH 1-800-471-0704

---

**FIGURE 64-2**  Obtaining provider numbers.

areas. Services must be provided in "collaboration" with a physician and are reimbursed at 85% of the Medicare physician fee schedule. Hospital outpatient services provided in a rural setting are paid directly to the hospital at 75% of the Medicare physician fee schedule.

NPs are indirectly reimbursed when services are provided independently in a nursing home or "incident to" physician services. When provided in a nursing home, the NP's services are reimbursed at 85% of the physician rate and payment is made to the NP's employer (i.e., the nursing home). NP services provided "incident to" physician services means that the physician must be present in the same office suite in which services are provided. When provided in a hospital-based outpatient clinic, the presence of a physician is presumed since a physician is always available in the hospital. The physician generally must initiate the patient's care and maintain ongoing, direct involvement. "Incident to" services are considered physician services even if provided by an APN. They are billed as if the physician performed the service and are therefore reimbursed at the physician rate. The drawback to this arrangement is that it results in the APN being an "invisible provider."

APN services provided in the inpatient setting are included in the general payment made to the hospital by Medicare. Home visits made by the APN employed by a physician are not covered by Medicare if the physician is not present at the time the services are provided.

### Medicaid Payment

Medicaid is a joint state and federally funded health care program for lower income Americans. Direct reimbursement to pediatric and family nurse practitioners for services provided to children is federally mandated. Other health care services provided by other APNs may be reimbursed at the discretion of the state. The reimbursement rate is determined by each state.

### Payment by Other Providers

Health maintenance organizations may have contracts with Medicare to provide care to enrollees at a capitated annual rate regardless of the type of provider or the level of services provided. APNs who work in collaboration with a physician are eligible for reimbursement. The HMO receives a fixed, monthly payment per enrollee. The APN contracts directly with the HMO to provide services and is paid by the HMO.

The Civilian and Medical Program of the Uniformed Services (CHAMPUS) is a federal program that provides services to members of the uniformed services and their families when these services cannot be provided by a military hospital. NPs as well as psychiatric and mental health CNSs are eligible for direct reimbursement under CHAMPUS.

The Federal Employee Health Benefit Plan (FEHBP) offers health insurance plans to federal employees and retirees. Coverage of APN services is mandated and direct reimbursement of services is provided; however, there is a loophole. Prepaid health insurance plans that are part of the FEHBP network are not required to include APNs in their provider network. If APNs are part of the provider network, the specific health insurance plan determines the level of payment for APN services.

## COLLABORATION AND CONSULTATION—HALLMARKS OF ONCOLOGY ADVANCED PRACTICE

It is assumed that the OAPN possesses outstanding clinical skills that serve as the foundation for practice. The OAPN is expert in the process of patient and family education, skilled in the utilization of nursing research, and savvy in negotiating complex organizational structures. In addition to this clinical expertise, the OAPN also must be an expert consultant and skilled in the process of collaboration. The OAPN is on the cutting edge of practice, an often tenuous location. These skills are required to maintain that edge.

Madden and Pointe describe three consultative advanced practice role components—process, resource, and expert.[46] The process consultant is expert in a process required for practice such as the development of case management models, critical pathways, or documentation processes. The resource consultant is expert at meeting complex patient care needs through the effective utilization of resources. This may include implementing patient and family education groups and utilizing nursing research. The expert practitioner has specialized, in-depth knowledge that is utilized to care for a select group of patients.

Oncology and oncology advanced practice nursing lends itself to a collaborative model of practice. In this model, care is provided based on competence.[47] The skills of the provider are matched with the needs of the patient, thereby maximizing the strengths of each provider. The components necessary for successful collaboration include collegiality, communication, mutual goals, and interdependence of tasks.[48] Characteristics of a collaborative practice include mutual trust and understanding, as well as shared problem solving, decision making, and authority.[49]

There are several descriptions of collaborative practices in the literature. Shay and colleagues list specific requirements for the development of a collaborative oncology nurse practitioner practice:[50]

- detailed job description
- written collaborative practice agreement detailing scope of practice
- documentation of certification to perform invasive

procedures (e.g., bone marrow aspiration and biopsy, lumbar puncture)

- documentation of credentials as required by the institution and/or state (e.g., NP licensure, advanced practice certification, cardiopulmonary resuscitation certification)

- malpractice coverage

In this practice, NPs function independently in caring for a caseload of patients, whether in the ambulatory or acute care setting. When the patient's care needs extend beyond the NP's scope of practice, the care is transferred to a physician. The patient's care is transferred back to the NP when the patient's condition becomes stable and when mutually agreed upon by the physician and NP. Davis describes similar collaborative practices between psychiatric CNSs and physicians in private practice.[51] The author recommends evaluating the legal and financial aspects, and developing marketing and cost-justification strategies as integral to the successful implementation of such a practice.

## ONCOLOGY ADVANCED PRACTICE NURSING ROLES

The clinical nurse specialist role has been conceptualized as integrating the subroles of expert practitioner, educator, consultant, researcher, and manager/leader. In contrast, the nurse practitioner role always has emphasized the role of direct care provider. Most often, the CNS's primary responsibility is to the employing organization whereas the NP's primary responsibility is to the patient.

As the roles of the CNS and NP are reconceptualized, it becomes more useful to shift the focus away from role components and toward practice focus when describing the oncology advanced practice nurse (OAPN). Although the OAPN specializes in the care of individuals and families with cancer, the OAPN also often develops a practice focus. For example, the focus can be in a particular area of oncology advanced practice such as prevention and early detection or symptom management, or it can be in the care of individuals with a specific malignancy such as breast cancer.

Many of today's OAPN roles involve performing behaviors that traditionally have fallen within the realm of medicine. However, when performed by an OAPN these activities ". . . are transformed by a nursing perspective based on concepts of health promotion, disease prevention, and client advocacy."[52] The OAPN does not leave behind the nursing cap when s/he dons a stethoscope and enters the examination room.

Successful advanced practice is the expansion of nursing's traditional boundaries while preserving the essence of nursing. It is not only the ability to perform a physical examination and write chemotherapy orders. It is also the ability to translate to the patient and family the impact the treatment will have on their lives. It is the ability to identify trends, predict outcomes, and anticipate needs. Appendix A, which follows the references for this chapter, provides a sample of a position description for an oncology nurse practitioner.

### The OAPN in Primary Care

#### Prevention and early detection

The role of the nurse in cancer screening was described in the literature as early as 1978.[53] Although this role was not initially described as an advanced practice role, White et al noted that the physical examination for cancer screening and defining an individual's risk profile required specialized and continuing education.[54] This continues to be true today.

The OAPN is involved in many aspects of cancer screening from the identification of "at risk" individuals to performing physical examinations focusing on cancer screening. The OAPN also develops and implements educational programs in schools, community, and employment settings on cancer risk factors, prevention, and early detection practices. OAPNs teach self-examination, counsel on life style and risk-factor modification, and sponsor programs aimed at risk reduction such as nutritional and smoking cessation programs. They develop educational materials and conduct research in the area of prevention and early detection.[55]

#### Cancer genetic counseling

The rapid expansion of knowledge regarding the role of genetics in the development of cancer and the identification of cancer susceptibility genes has led to a role for the OAPN in cancer genetics. Cancer genetic screening and counseling currently focuses on individuals and families with a hereditary predisposition to cancer.[56] However, as genetic testing for certain cancers becomes commercially available, the demand for testing and for individuals qualified to conduct genetic counseling will increase.

OAPNs with knowledge and expertise in medical genetics and counseling are in an excellent position to provide screening, counseling, and education of individuals undergoing cancer genetic testing.[57] Research efforts in this area are still in their infancy. There is a need for research on attitudes regarding genetic testing, disclosure of results, coping with results, and impact on quality of life.[57,58]

### The OAPN in Secondary Care

#### Active treatment

OAPNs are involved in the care of patients receiving treatment for cancer as either direct care provider or consultant. As direct care provider, the OAPN obtains the initial history and performs the physical examination. Results of radiological and laboratory studies including pathology are reviewed in collaboration with the oncologist and a treatment plan is devised. The treatment plan and expected outcomes are discussed with the patient and family.[59] Side effects and self-care management strategies are reviewed in detail. In jurisdictions where OAPNs have prescriptive authority, orders for laboratory and radiological studies and treatment are written by the OAPN.

During the phase when the patient is receiving active treatment, the OAPN meets both the patient's medical and nursing needs. The OAPN manages the concomitant medical problems such as diabetes mellitus and hypertension, as well as any treatment-related side effects. Educational and psychosocial needs also are addressed.[50]

As a consultant, the OAPN in secondary care is involved in planning and implementing initiatives aimed at patient and family education and support. Educational initiatives usually focus on helping patients and families understand the disease process, its treatment, and potential side effects. The OAPN's expertise is also utilized in symptom management and they are often an important member of a multidisciplinary pain and symptom management team. They also may act as a consultant to the institution in establishing standards for oncology practice and developing critical pathways. These services are provided in a variety of settings—private practices, comprehensive cancer centers, hospital-based outpatient clinics, the patient's home.

### Follow-up care

At the conclusion of initial treatment, the patient enters the follow-up phase of care. The focus shifts to returning the patient to their premorbid condition, identifying and managing the long-term effects of therapy, and monitoring for disease recurrence. Many oncologists have limited time to spend caring for patients during this phase of their disease; their focus is on caring for patients receiving active treatment. OAPNs have assumed care for this patient population in many settings. In some organizations, the physician refers the patient to a nurse-managed clinic for follow-up.[60] In others, the patient is collaboratively cared for by the oncologist and OAPN with the OAPN assuming the role of primary provider when the patient moves into the follow-up phase. The OAPN is responsible for performing physical examinations, ordering and interpreting laboratory and radiological studies, and referring patients for diagnostic studies as needed.[50,60] Additionally, the OAPN maintains communication with the patient's primary care provider and referring physician. The OAPN also helps the individual become a cancer survivor, cope with fears related to recurrence, and manage long-term effects of therapy. The individual is referred to a wide variety of services in the community as needed, from apparel shops that specialize in mastectomy swimwear to attorneys who specialize in health discrimination.

## The OAPN in Tertiary Care

### Acute care

The OAPN long has been involved in the management of patients in the acute care setting. In most organizations, this role has been filled by the oncology CNS; however, in recent years organizational needs have changed and the role of the acute care NP has developed.[61] The two major trends that have led to the development of the acute care NP role are changes in medical residency training programs and the shift from fee-for-service to capitated payment plans for health care.

Medical education is placing a renewed emphasis on primary care, shifting the focus of training away from the inpatient setting and to the ambulatory setting. In recent years, some states have placed legal limits on the number of hours worked by medical residents. There have been cutbacks in the federal funding of residency training programs, leading to a downsizing of such programs. The shift away from fee-for-service-based care and the reduced levels of reimbursement for physician services have resulted in physicians caring for more patients for less revenue. The net result is that the physician has become less available to the patient and family. These forces have combined to create the need for qualified providers in the acute care setting.

While both the CNS and NP are advanced practice nursing roles with a similar goal—ensuring the provision of outstanding patient care—their means differ. The CNS affects care indirectly by working through the organization and the nursing staff facilitate changes that improve patient care. The NP affects care directly by managing the medical and nursing needs for a specific caseload of patients. Since the trend is toward using the singular title of OAPN, this term will be used for the remainder of this discussion.

The needs of the organization and the practice milieu determine whether the OAPN role is more similar to that of a CNS or an NP. Complex organizations such as academic medical centers and comprehensive cancer centers that traditionally have relied on medical residents to provide acute care services have been most affected by changes in medical residency programs. These organizations utilize both types of OAPNs in the acute care setting. The OAPN with a direct care emphasis is responsible for the management of a caseload of patients from admission through discharge. The OAPN has medical staff privileges and obtains the patient's health history, performs a physical examination, interprets laboratory and radiological studies, prescribes medications including chemotherapy, and coordinates discharge and follow-up care.[62] Invasive procedures such as bone marrow aspiration and biopsy, lumbar puncture, thoracentesis, and paracentesis also may be the responsibility of the OAPN. In essence, this OAPN is responsible for the minute-to-minute care of the patient in collaboration with the attending physician. The OAPN with an organizational focus performs functions such as acting as a mentor to nursing staff, consulting with nursing staff on the care of patients with complex needs, developing staff and patient educational programs, facilitating support groups, and implementing research-based changes in practice. This OAPN often has nursing department and hospital responsibilities such as committee representation.

### Blended role

Changes in physician payment have led to the attending physician being less available to patients, medical, and nursing staff. The OAPN role in this setting may incorporate components of both the traditional CNS and NP roles into one "blended" role.[19,63–65] Descriptions of these blended roles vary in the literature, but have one common theme—the delivery of coordinated, comprehensive, and cost-effective care. The OAPN serves as the link between the attending physician, the patient and family, the inpatient medical and nursing staff, and, increasingly in today's fiscal climate, the insurer. The OAPN in this role may facilitate the patient's admission to the hospital by performing the admission history and physical examination and writing the admission orders. The OAPN may examine the patient daily during hospitalization, triage patient problems by telephone, and coordinate the patient's discharge including making arrangements for home care services. Additionally, the OAPN sees patients in the ambulatory care setting, provides education related to the disease and treatment, and manages treatment-related side effects and toxicities. The OAPN also acts as a liaison between the nursing staff and the physician, bridging the gap in communication that often exists between the disciplines. The OAPN in this role may also actively participate in the education of nursing and medical staff and serve on hospital and nursing departmental committees.[63,64] The difference between this OAPN role and that of the direct care OAPN or organizational OAPN in tertiary care is the accountability for care across practice settings and the links with community providers including the insurer.

### Case manager

Another OAPN role that has emerged in tertiary care, primarily due to changes in health care reimbursement, is that of the case manager. Although the ANA recommends a minimum of a baccalaureate degree in nursing and three years of appropriate clinical experience, the economic and clinical demands of case management in tertiary care require a master's degree.[66] Many descriptions of case manager practice can be found in the literature.[19,69–72] Again, the emphasis is on "the three Cs"—coordinated, comprehensive, and cost-effective care. In most models, the case manager's practice is inpatient-based with little crossover into other practice settings. The case manager usually does not provide direct care but rather coordinates the care provided by others. The case manager keeps patients from "falling through the cracks" in a fragmented health care system. The focus is on ensuring the effective use of resources and meeting outcomes within an appropriate length of stay. Trends in patient outcomes are identified and measures are implemented to correct variances.

## The OAPN in Hospice and Bereavement Care

When the primary focus of treatment has shifted from cure to care, the services of an OAPN with an expertise in supportive care becomes important. These services can be provided through community resources such as hospice or the local visiting nurse service. Direct care is provided by a home health assistant while assessments are performed by a registered nurse with experience in hospice and home care as needed. Since OAPNs are not eligible for direct reimbursement of home visits, they usually are employed by the agency and utilized as a consultant for complex patients and families with difficult management issues. These financial constraints limit the OAPN's ability to practice independently in the home.

## The OAPN in Industry and Research

### Industry

OAPNs fill a multiplicity of roles in the health care industry. They are employed by insurers as case managers, by consulting firms as health care consultants, and by pharmaceutical and biotechnology firms in roles ranging from company sales representatives to educational consultants. They bring to these positions an "insider's" knowledge of health care. This, coupled with clinical expertise, makes them a valuable asset to an organization.

### Research

The OAPN is involved in research through utilizing research results, by implementing an independent research agenda, and in collaborating on medical research.

## ADVANCED PRACTICE NURSING—INTO THE TWENTY-FIRST CENTURY

There are three forces that will continue to influence changes in nursing practice in the coming years—the health care insurance industry, medical education, and scientific advances. The failure of government-initiated health care reform has precipitated a major restructuring in the health care system by the private sector. The traditional fee-for-service system of payment is being replaced by managed care systems in which providers agree to render services to a given group of patients for a predetermined fee. The insurer decides what services, medications, physicians, and hospitalizations will be covered. The primary motivator behind these decisions is cost and not necessarily quality. Physicians are receiving lower fees for their services and are being required to spend a larger amount of time on administrative issues related to patient care such as justifying a hospital admission to an insurer. To compensate, physicians are seeing more patients in less time. The result is a physician/patient interaction that is limited to what is medically essential. This type of limited care is especially difficult to provide to individuals with cancer whose informational, social, and emotional needs are tremendous. Oncology advanced practice nurses long have excelled in meeting these needs, but in a way that has been invisible. Restructuring of reimbursement offers OAPNs many opportunities to change this.

There are several ways OAPNs can continue to meet the needs of patients but in ways that are creative and cost-effective. The OAPN can directly market services to insurers, oncologists, and patients. The addition of an OAPN to an oncology practice can result in a larger volume of patients being seen and more comprehensive care being provided. The OAPN can assume the follow-up care of patients, enabling the practice to increase volume without significant cost. Alternatively, the OAPN can give the oncology practice an "edge" in a competitive market by offering a variety of educational and support services to patients.

Changes in medical education with its renewed emphasis on the preparation of primary care providers ultimately will result in fewer subspecialists, including oncologists. However, as the population ages, it is expected that the number of individuals with cancer will increase. The result will be fewer oncologists to care for these patients. This, too, will open new avenues to the OAPN. One opportunity will be in the care of the elderly person with cancer. It is predicted that OAPNs soon will be eligible for direct reimbursement for home visits under Medicare. This will dramatically change the face of home and hospice care. The OAPN no longer will be confined to the practice settings of the hospital, the outpatient clinic, or office setting. The OAPN will be able to make house calls, performing physical examinations and therapeutic procedures in the home.

Perhaps the most exciting change is the rapid scientific advances that are occurring and are having an impact on clinical practice. The discovery of genes linked to the development of malignancies has already led to innovations in diagnosis and treatment that were unheard of only a short time ago. AOPNs are in an ideal position to prepare patients, staff, and organizations for these changes.

## CONCLUSION

Advanced practice nurses have made important contributions to oncology care in the past. Studies have shown that APNs improve patient outcomes and deliver cost-effective, quality care with a high degree of patient satisfaction. The changes that are taking place in the health care system and in oncology practice will provide new opportunities and challenges for OAPNs in the twenty-first century.

## REFERENCES

1. Ford LC, Silver HK: The expanded role of the nurse in child care. *Nurs Outlook* 15:8, 43–45, 1967
2. Fenton MV, Brykczynski KA: Qualitative distinctions and similarities in the practice of clinical nurse specialists and nurse practitioners. *J Prof Nurs* 9:313–326, 1993
3. American Academy of Nurse Practitioners: *Standards of Practice.* Austin, TX, American Academy of Nurse Practitioners, 1993
4. American Association of Colleges of Nursing: *Position statement: Certification and Regulation of Advanced Practice Nurses.* Washington, DC, American Association of Colleges of Nursing, 1994
5. Hawkins JW, Thibodeau JA: *The Nurse Practitioner and Clinical Nurse Specialist: Current Practice Issues.* New York, Tiresias Press, 1983
6. American Association of Colleges of Nursing: *1995–1996 Enrollment and Graduations in Baccalaureate and Graduate Programs in Nursing.* Washington, DC, American Association of Colleges of Nursing, 1996 (suppl)
7. Pew Health Professions Commission: *Nurse Practitioners—Doubling the Graduates by the Year 2000.* San Francisco, UCSF Center for the Health Professions, 1994
8. Belcher A, Shurpin KM: Education of the advanced practice nurse in oncology. *Oncol Nurs Forum* 22:19–24, 1995
9. Naylor MD, Brooten D: The roles and functions of clinical nurse specialists. *Image* 25:73–78, 1993
10. Smoyak SA: Specialization in nursing: From then to now. *Nurs Outlook* 24:676–681, 1976
11. Camp-Sorrell D: Historical aspects of the CNS role. The future of Advanced Practice Nursing. *Oncology Nursing Society Joint Newsletter of the CNS and NP Special Interest Groups.* 4:2, 4, 1994
12. Reiter F: The nurse clinician. *Am J Nurs* 66:274–280, 1966
13. American Nurses' Association: *Nursing: A social policy statement.* Kansas City, Mo, American Nurses' Association, 1980
14. American Nurses' Association: *Role of the Clinical Nurse Specialist.* Kansas City, Mo, American Nurses' Association 1986
15. Mundinger MO: Health care reform: The best of times or worst of times. Speech at the American Academy of Nursing Annual Conference, October 21, 1994, Phoenix, AZ
16. Elder RG, Bullough B: Nurse practitioners and clinical nurse specialists: Are the roles merging? *Clin Nurse Specialist* 4:78–84, 1990
17. Forbes KE, Rafson J, Spross JA, et al: The clinical nurse specialist and nurse practitioner: Core curriculum survey results. *Clin Nurse Specialist* 4:63–66, 1990
18. Fenton MV, Brykczynski KA: Qualitative distinctions and similarities in the practice of clinical nurse specialists and nurse practitioners. *J Prof Nurs* 9:313–326, 1993
19. Schroer K: Case management: Clinical nurse specialist and nurse practitioner, converging roles. *Clin Nurse Specialist* 5:189–194, 1991

20. Williams C, Valdivieso GC: Advanced practice models: A comparison of clinical nurse specialist and nurse practitioner activities. *Clin Nurse Specialist* 8:311–318, 1994

21. Hawkins JW, Holcombe JK: Titling for advanced practice nurses. *Oncol Nurs Forum* 22:5–9, 1995 (Suppl.)

22. American Nurses' Association: *Nursing's Social Policy Statement*. Washington, DC, American Nurses' Association 1995

23. National Council of State Boards of Nursing, Inc.: *Position paper on the regulation of advanced nursing practice*. Chicago, National Council of State Board of Nursing, 1993

24. Reading BA: Titling and the advanced practice nurse. *Advanced Practice Nurse* Spring/Summer:7–8, 1994

25. Oncology Nursing Society: Position statement on advanced practice in oncology nursing. *Oncol Nurs Forum* 22:45, 1995 (suppl)

26. Mirr MP: Advanced clinical practice: A reconceptualized role. *AACN Clin Issues* 4:599–602, 1993

27. American Association of Colleges of Nursing: *Nursing education's Agenda for the 21st Century*. Washington, DC, American Association of Colleges of Nursing, 1995

28. Craytor JK: Highlights in education for cancer nursing. *Oncol Nurs Forum* 12:19–27, 1985 (suppl)

29. Piemme J: Oncology clinical nurse specialist education. *Oncol Nurs Forum* 12:45–48, 85, 1985

30. American Cancer Society: *The master's degree with a specialty in cancer nursing: Curriculum guide and role definition*. New York, American Cancer Society, 1978

31. American Cancer Society and Oncology Nursing Society: *The Master's Degree with a Specialty in Advanced Practice Oncology Nursing*. Atlanta, American Cancer Society, 1994

32. Brown J, Hinds P: Assessing master's programs in oncology nursing. *Oncol Nurs Forum* 22:1273–1282, 1995

33. McMillan SC, Heusinkveld KB, Spray J: Advanced practice in oncology nursing: A role delineation study. *Oncol Nurs Forum* 22:41–50, 1995

34. Hohman M, Vander Woude D: Regulation of advanced practice nursing: One state's approach. *AACN Clin Issues* 4:617–623, 1993

35. Safriet B: Health care dollars and regulatory sense: The role of advanced practice nursing. *Yale J Reg* 9:417–487, 1992

36. Greco K: Regulation of advanced nursing practice: Part one-second licensure. *Oncol Nurs Forum* 22:35–38, 1995 (suppl)

37. Fickeissen JL: Fifty-six ways to get certified. *Amer J Nurs* 90:50–57, 1990

38. Pearson LJ: Annual update of how each state stands on legislative issues affecting advanced nursing practice. *Nurse Pract* 21:10, 12–14, 16, 21, 22, 25, 26, 28–30, 33, 34, 36, 39, 40, 43–45, 49, 50, 52–54, 57, 58, 60–62, 65, 66, 68–70, 1996

39. *NP News*. Nov/Dec 1995

40. Steel JE: Advanced nursing practice. *AACN Clin Issues* 5:71–76, 1994

41. Minarik: Legislative and regulatory update: DEA registration for midlevel practitioners. *Clin Nurse Specialist* 7:319, 329, 1993

42. Midlevel Practitioner's Manual and Informational Outline of the Controlled Substances Act of 1970. Washington, DC, U.S. Government Printing Office, Document #351-29, 1993.

43. Mahoney DF: Employer resistance to state authorized prescriptive authority for NPs: Results from a pilot study. *Nurse Pract* 20:58–61, 1995

44. Sekscenski ES, Sansom S, Bazell C, et al: State practice environments and the supply of physicians assistants, nurse practitioners and certified nurse-midwives. *N Engl J Med* 331(19):1266–1277, 1994

45. Mittelstadt PC: Federal reimbursement of advanced practice nurses' services empowers the profession. *Nurse Pract* 18:43–49, 1993

46. Madden MJ, Pointe PR: Advanced practice roles in the managed care environment. *J Nurs Admin* 24:56–62, 1994

47. Sparacino PSA: Opportunities for the advanced practice nurse: Encroachment or collaboration? *Clin Nurse Specialist* 8:122, 1994

48. Hughes AM, Mackenzie CS: Components necessary in a successful nurse practitioner-collaborative practice. *J Am Acad Nurse Pract* 2:54–57, 1990

49. Burchell RC, Thomas DA, Smith L: Some considerations for implementing collaborative practice. *Am J Med* 74:9–13, 1983

50. Shay LE, Goldstein JT, Matthews D, et al: Guidelines for developing a nurse practitioner practice. *Nurse Pract* 21:72–81, 1996

51. Davis EA: Factors influencing the implementation of the CNS role in a private practice. *Clin Nurse Specialist* 8:42–46, 1994

52. Gee F: Letter to the editor. *Nurs Sci Q* 8:45–46, 1995

53. White LN, Cornelius JL, Judkins AF, et al: Screening of cancer by nurses. *Cancer Nurs* 1:15–20, 1978

54. White LN: Cancer prevention and detection: From twenty to sixty-five years of age. *Oncol Nurs Forum* 13:59–64, 1986

55. Frank-Stromborg M, Rohan K: Nursing's involvement in the primary and secondary prevention of cancer. *Cancer Nurs* 15:79–108, 1992

56. Mahon SM, Casperson DS: Hereditary cancer syndrome: Part 1—Clinical and educational issues. *Oncol Nurs Forum* 22:763–771, 1995

57. Loescher LJ: Genetics in cancer prediction, screening and counseling: Part II, the nurse's role in genetic counseling. *Oncol Nurs Forum* 22:16–19, 1995 (suppl)

58. Lerman C, Daly M, Balshem A: Attitudes about genetic testing for breast-ovarian cancer susceptibility. *J Clin Oncol* 12:843–850, 1994

59. Elmore E, Austin EO, Hodges S, et al: NPs help develop comprehensive primary care for patients with cancer. *Oncology Nursing Society Nurse Practitioner Special Interest Group Newsletter* 6(1):1, 1995

60. Judkins AF: Advanced practice nurses for follow-up care of breast cancer patients. *M.D. Anderson Case Reports and Review* 7:17–20, 1995

61. Keane A, Richmond T, Kaiser L: Critical care nurse practitioners: Evolution of the advanced practice nursing role. *Am J Critical Care* 3:232–237, 1994

62. Lynch MP: Inpatient oncology nurse practitioner's role evolves. *Oncology Nursing Society Nurse Practitioner Special Interest Group Newsletter* 6(1):2, 1995

63. Sawyers JE: Defining your role in ambulatory care: Clinical nurse specialist or nurse practitioner? *Clin Nurse Specialist* 7:4–7, 1993

64. Lin EM: A combined role of clinical nurse specialist and coordinator: Optimizing continuity of care in an autologous bone marrow transplant program. *Clin Nurse Specialist* 8:48–55, 1994

65. Soehren PM, Schumann LL: Enhanced role opportunities available to the CNS/Nurse Practitioner. *Clin Nurse Specialist* 8:123–127, 1994

66. Cronin CJ, Maklebust J: Case-managed care: Capitalizing on the CNS. *Nurs Manage* 20:38–39, 42–47, 1989

67. Zander K: Nursing case management: Strategic management of cost and quality outcomes. *J Nurs Admin* 18:23–30, 1988

68. Trinidad EA: Case management: A model of CNS practice. *Clin Nurse Specialist* 7:221–223, 1993

69. Lynn-McHale D, Fitzpatrick ER, Shaffer RB: Case management: Development of a model. *Clin Nurse Specialist* 7: 299–307, 1993

70. Sherman JJ, Johnson PK: CNS as unit-based case manager. *Clin Nurse Specialist* 8:76–80, 1994

71. Brubakken KM, Janssen WR, Ruppel DL: CNS roles in implementation of a differentiated case management model. *Clin Nurse Specialist* 8:69–73, 1994

72. Sterling YM, Noto EC, Bowen MR: Case management roles of clinicians: A research case study. *Clin Nurse Specialist* 8: 196–201, 1994

## APPENDIX A: ONCOLOGY NURSE PRACTITIONER POSITION DESCRIPTION

### General Description

A nurse practitioner (NP) is a registered nurse who has completed an accredited NP MS program. NP practice includes health supervision of well individuals, episodic care of individuals with acute, commonly occurring illnesses, and the long-term management of individuals with chronic conditions. NPs work collaboratively with physicians and other members of the health care team.

The oncology NP cares for individuals with cancer who are either receiving treatment or being monitored for disease progression, relapse, or for long-term side effects of therapy. Only those individuals whose disease, treatment, and side effects can be managed primarily in an ambulatory care setting are cared for by the oncology NP.

### Major Duties

The oncology NP functions independently as the care provider for a select group of individuals with cancer under the general supervision of an attending physician. Major duties fall into three broad categories: clinical practice, research, and education.

### Clinical Practice

The oncology NP:

1. Obtains a health history and assesses the patient's physical status through performance of a physical examination.
2. Assesses psychosocial situation, coping strategies, and learning needs of patients and significant other.
3. Develops and implements a plan of care based on clinical findings and disease process. This includes a plan for treatment, counseling, and education.
4. Communicates the plan of care to other members of the health care team.
5. Evaluates patient response to treatment and revises the plan of care as necessary and in collaboration with the attending physician.
6. Prescribes medications, laboratory, and diagnostic tests.
7. After successful performance of three supervised diagnostic procedures (i.e., bone marrow biopsies, thoracentesis, or paracentesis) the NP will independently perform these procedures on his or her patient population according to written guidelines.
8. Coordinates patient care with other departments and disciplines.
9. Requests consultation and/or initiates referrals for complex problems or specialized care as necessary.
10. Maintains complete and current medical record and flow sheets.
11. Dictates follow-up letters to primary care and referring physicians.

### Research

1. Assists with the design and implementation of clinical trials.
2. Acts as coinvestigator on medical clinical trials and as primary investigator on nursing research studies.
3. Acts as a patient advocate.
4. Evaluates and reports adverse effects and complications of treatment.

### Education

1. Serves as an expert resource in cancer to nursing staff, medical staff, patients, and families.
2. Conducts professional and patient educational programs.
3. Participates in patient care rounds and care conferences.
4. Acts as a preceptor for graduate students in NP and oncology nursing programs.
5. Acts as a role model and consultant to other members of the nursing staff.

### Qualifications

1. Graduate from an accredited NP program.
2. Current licensure as a registered nurse and NP.
3. A minimum of five years of oncology nursing experience. Advanced oncology nursing certification preferred.
4. Clinical expertise in caring for individuals with cancer.
5. Knowledge of current nursing and medical practice and research related to medical oncology.
6. Demonstrated commitment to continued professional growth as evidenced by membership in professional organizations and attendance at continuing education offerings.
7. Demonstrated strong written and verbal communication skills. Public speaking and publishing experience strongly preferred.

# Chapter 65

# Thriving as an Oncology Nurse

Mary Cunningham, RN, MS

## STRESS

Stress is a pervasive human problem that is associated to some degree with all the major institutions with which we are involved daily. That stress is associated with work is almost a given in our society, and this is no less true for nurses than for anyone else. Indeed, as shown throughout this chapter, cancer nursing has the potential for very high levels of stress.

The cost of not dealing with stress effectively (coping) can be high. As will be shown, patient care may be compromised, job burnout can be experienced, and even physical and psychological deterioration can result. It is therefore important for the nurse to recognize potential sources of stress and to implement coping strategies that permit continued job and life effectiveness.

*Stress* has been variously defined as a response, as a stimulus, and as a transaction. Selye[1] defined stress as a response to events in the environment, a response that is physiological and therefore unrelated to the nature of the stressor, the individual's thoughts and beliefs, or the situational context. Others have characterized stress as the potential residing within the stimulus or as something that results because of the event itself, again unmediated by personal factors or variations in the setting.[2-4]

Both of these definitions of stress can be criticized for being too simplistic and not reflecting what is known from empirical evidence. People respond differently to external events, both interpersonally (between people) and intrapersonally (within individuals), at different times. Thus, stress does not reside solely in the event or in the response of the person; it must instead reflect some *transaction* between the two that is modified by a third factor or set of factors.

The transactional model on which the discussion in this chapter is based views stress as the tension that results when the perceived demands of a situation (whether imposed from within the person or by the environment) are out of balance with (particularly, exceeded by) the perceived resources (again, both internal and external) available to the individual.[5,6] The individual is the focal mediator between stimulus and response, for stress lies in the individual's appraisal of events and not necessarily in the events themselves.[5] The use of the word *perceived* is deliberate; in the case of stress it is not so important that the resources ("supplies," in economic terms) are inadequate for the demands as it is that the person experiencing the stress believes this to be true.

## INDIVIDUAL APPRAISAL

The central focus of Lazarus' transactional model of stress is the nature of the transactions between the person and

the environment[5-7] (Figure 65-1). The individual appraises the events to which he or she is exposed as well as his or her own behavior in response to those events. An individual's appraisal of events and actions plays a determining role in the psychological stress experience. Stress arises from a transaction between the individual and the environment when the individual judges the stimuli as damaging, threatening, or challenging in relation to whether the demands tax or exceed appraised available resources.[6] Stress is the perceived imbalance between demands and abilities or resources. These appraisals and judgments determine stress reactions, the intensity and quality of the emotional response, and the outcomes of attempts to adapt to perceived stressors.[7] Therefore, stress lies in the perception of the event and not in the event itself.

*Cognitive appraisal* refers to evaluations and judgments of events and one's reactions to those events. Lazarus[5] described two types of cognitive appraisals: primary and secondary. *Primary* appraisal refers to a person's judgment about the significance of a stressor. It determines "what is at stake" in the situation and whether the individual is in trouble or deriving benefit. Primary appraisals of the transaction take three forms: irrelevant, positive (benign), or stressful. The encounter is *irrelevant* if it carries no implications for an individual's well-being, and it is *positive* if it preserves or enhances well-being. *Stressful* appraisals involve judgments of harm or loss, challenge, and threat. In *secondary* appraisal, judgments are made about resources and options available for coping, constraints on using these resources, and consequences. Primary and secondary appraisals differ in content but are interdependent processes. If the individual believes he or she can handle most stressful situations (secondary

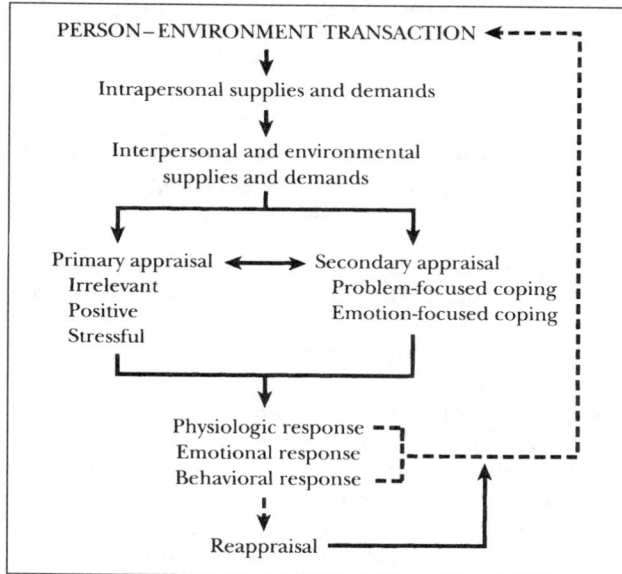

**FIGURE 65-1**  Lazarus' transactional model of stress.

appraisal), then most transactions will be judged as non-threatening (primary appraisal).[6]

Individuals cope with stress by continuously evaluating their relationship with the environment and with events in their lives.[5,6] This *reappraisal* alters an individual's perspective on demand and supplies and leads to the individual's adaptational coping.

## PERSON–ENVIRONMENT FIT

The transactional model of stress, that focuses on the relationship between the person and the environment, is furthered by the person–environment-fit model developed by French et al.[8] This model is based on a model of supplies and demands. French et al conceived of adaptation as a function of the "goodness of the fit" between the person and the environment. Fit is determined by the extent to which environmental supplies are available to meet individual needs (demands) as well as the ability (supplies) of the person to manage the demands imposed by the environment.[8,9] If the demands exceed supplies, or vice versa, adjustment is required to create a good fit.[8]

The person–environment-fit model is useful in understanding the relation between job satisfaction and occupational stress and that between a person's interacting roles and environment. "A job is stressful to the extent that it does not provide supplies to meet the individual's motives and to the extent that the ability of the individual falls below the demands of the job, which are prerequisite to receiving supplies."[10,p.178] The extent to which there is a discrepancy between supplies and demands is based in part on the individual's appraisal of self and environment. Clearly, it is important that individuals have an accurate understanding of their own personal resources and limitations as well as of environmental resources and demands.[7,9,11]

## DEMANDS—SOURCES OF STRESS

How can you work with dying patients? How can you give so much of yourself to perfect strangers? How can you work in today's health care environment? How do you stay calm in an emergency? Is your caring codependent? Most cancer nurses have been asked variations of these questions. Perceptions of self, role, coworkers, recipients of care, and work situations are key to the answers. The supplies and demands inherent in each area influence the amount of stress the nurse experiences. In general, stress in nursing generates from mismatches between efforts and results,[11,12] mismatches between nurse and environment[13] leading to role ambiguity and conflict, and mismatches between people[11,12] leading to interpersonal conflict.

In the transactional model of stress, the stress experienced by cancer nurses (and, indeed, everyone) involves an interplay between intrapersonal (self-concept, motivations, and personal needs), interpersonal (relationships with recipients of care and coworkers and the nature of cancer care), and environmental factors. These factors provide the demands and supplies that are appraised as satisfying or discrepant.

## Intrapersonal Factors

Lazarus,[5] Appley and Trumball,[14] and McGrath[15] emphasized that reactions to stress vary from person to person. Individuals bring into relationships and situations personal characteristics that influence their perceptions of other people and events as well as their reactions. Assessing personal characteristics is not about placing blame; rather, examining personal variables aids in understanding an individual's transaction with other people and events. Self-concept, personal needs, and motivations have the potential both of providing interpersonal demands and supplies and of playing a significant role in the mediation of a stress response.

### Self-concept

How we see ourselves plays an important role in our relationships with other people and our appraisal of events. Self-concept is developed through self-appraisal as well as through appraisal by others.[16] The self is made known by listening to self and to others. People think and engage in self-talk that affects self-concept and self-esteem.[17] Negative self-talk ("People don't like me," "I'm incompetent," "I can't do that procedure," "She's better than me") inadvertently can encourage an individual to meet the expectation of the negative statement. Pearlin and Schooler found that "freedom from negative attitudes toward self, the possession of a sense that one is in control of the forces impinging on oneself, and the presence of favorable attitudes towards oneself" were helpful in coping.[18,p.12] Likewise, self-concept can be threatened by the demands and negative input from coworkers and recipients of care as well as from the environment. In the supply-and-demand model of stress, people and environmental demands can be overwhelming if a person has little self-confidence or becomes too dependent on the explicit or implicit messages of others.

### Personal needs

Most people want approval, praise for accomplishments, love, and respect. These are basic human needs. The strength of an individual's motivation to fulfill these needs and where the individual looks to have them fulfilled have implications in helping relationships and work environments. Fulfillment of personal needs is a demand an individual brings to the environment.

***Approval and affection***  Individuals with intense need for approval and affection may work exceedingly hard to be pleasing and to satisfy the demands of recipients of care, coworkers, and employers. Meeting the demands of others in order to gain approval and be liked can lead to a reluctance to say "no," the sabotage of self-needs, disappointment, a sense of betrayal, and resentment if one's efforts are not appreciated or approved. Until recently, in exchange for long-term service and loyalty, employees trusted employers to fulfill approval and affection needs. But commitment to an employer no longer may be a reciprocal relationship.

***Autonomy and control***  People vary in their expectations about the extent to which they have control over their lives. An *internal* locus of control is the tendency to perceive that actions and outcomes are correlated and that one is in control of one's life.[19] Individuals with an *external* locus of control tend to expect little control over events. This perception of control is created through interaction with the environment, where actions and outcomes are either related (producing a sense of control) or unrelated (producing a sense of powerlessness).[20]

Clearly, the need to be independent and self-determining is a hallmark of personal growth and maturity.[21] Yet an excessive need to control, to refuse to share or delegate power, or to take on responsibility for everything and everyone is a perfect setup for a *mea culpa* reaction,[11] that is, the sense that "It's me," "I'm responsible," "It's my fault," and then overlooking the interpersonal and situational factors that influence the outcomes. The externally controlled individual bends at the demands of other people and the environment. Disappointments, blaming, and resentments can develop as personal needs go unfulfilled and the individual feels no power in affecting outcomes. DuCette and Wolk[22] argued that the critical element in this perception is for the person to distinguish where control is possible and where it is impossible.

Current health care environments require that professionals learn to work interdependently with a variety of disciplines, in a "model of community" environment in which collaborative practice is recognized as essential.[23] Interdependent models are evolving. Inherent in this evolution is both opportunity and uncertainty. Redesigning the way in which health care is planned and delivered magnifies issues of trust, control, self-esteem, intimacy, and interdependence.[24] Uneasiness with shared responsibility and accountability can result in the nurse continuing to "do it all" while complaining about being overworked, too busy, or terribly stressed.

### Personal motivations

*Motivation* has been defined as "the process of arousing or initiating behavior."[25,p.55] Behavior is incited by a desire for satisfaction of needs.[26] An individual's behavior is influenced by the expectation that behavior will bring about need fulfillment. One might question, for instance, "What leads people to enter a helping career?" or "Why

did I choose cancer nursing?" For many cancer nurses, a fundamental motivation is to make a difference, to be helpful. This motivation to be helpful is not predicated on characteristics of the patient requiring our professional efforts; for that reason, a dilemma exists when care is withheld to uninsured or underinsured. Clinicians may be stifled in their efforts to be helpful by payer sources that encourage less, rather than more service. With shortened hospital stays, staff may be unable to see the impact of their care on outcomes.[27] Failure to fulfill the motivation that prompted the decision to enter a helping profession can generate a great amount of stress. Vachon[28] explored the idea that motivation influences the nature of the stress experienced by professionals working with terminally ill patients. To illustrate, individuals motivated out of past personal experiences with cancer may expose previous, unresolved guilt, resulting in an overidentification with dying patients that can lead to emotional depletion and conflicts with other staff. Vachon found that if working with the dying happened by accident, emotional involvement with patients was minimal and the stress experienced stemmed from a lack of knowledge and feelings of professional impotence.

There are also self-centered reasons for choosing a helping profession.[11] Some may look for approval and affection through expressions of appreciation. Some may be involved in helping relationships to boost self-esteem and feelings of self-worth, or to fulfill the need for intimacy. Feeling good about oneself and feeling good about being helpful are reasonable outcomes in helping professions. Yet danger may rest in attempting to get personal needs met in a helping relationship, for often neither the recipients of care nor coworkers are able or expected to fulfill these needs.

Motivation or drive for need fulfillment influences how an individual appraises situations (whether or not needs will be fulfilled); so as a result, motivations influence stress reactions (behavior).[5] Motivations are modified by the expectations of self and others. If expectations are unrealistic, needs often go unmet. Smythe[29] identified unrealistic expectations stereotypically associated with nurses, such as: "A good nurse cares for all patients equally and is concerned about people all of the time, "A nurse's worth, whether or not she does a good job, is related to patient compliance, patient outcome, patient improvement, and patient happiness," and "Patients and supervisors and coworkers should appreciate us and our work."[29,p.30] The expectation that nurses can provide the care to which they are accustomed is unrealistic. Cost containment and limited resources have changed health care delivery and nurses are challenged to provide care differently than they have in the past. This is compounded by an increase in consumer and employer expectations. Expectations modify motivations and influence appraisal; if expectations are unrealistic, then feelings of anger and hostility (external expressions of unmet needs) can result, as can depression, a sense of failure, and low self-esteem (internal expressions of unmet needs). Cullen[27] recommends that nurses be honest with themselves about what they can and cannot do and that they take stock in their accomplishments rather than focusing on uncompleted tasks.

## Interpersonal Factors

Cancer nursing is a person-to-person profession that at the same time involves deeply rewarding and very demanding work.[30] "It takes a lot of energy to be calm in the midst of crisis, to be patient in the face of frustrations, and to be understanding when surrounded by fear, pain, anger, or shame."[11,p.17] To understand the interpersonal demands inherent in cancer nursing, one must understand the dynamics of nurse–patient relationships and the nature of cancer care.

### Helping relationships

Knowing one has been helpful often is the essence of the critical incidents described by cancer nurses.[31] Yet, according to Maslach,[11] the very structure of the helping relationship can promote a negative view of people or a shift from a positive to a negative view. This shift tends to frustrate the helper, dampen the helper's sensitivity, diminish the helper's sense of accomplishment, and generate emotional and physical exhaustion. As well, the quality of the interaction with the recipient in the helping relationship suffers. Four aspects of the helping relationship are pivotal in this positive-to-negative shift: focus on the problem, lack of positive feedback, level of emotional stress, and perceived possibility of change or improvement.[11]

***Focus on problems*** By definition, the recipient of care in a helping relationship has a problem (weakness, deficiencies, illness) that is the focus of the relationship.[11] The negative part of an individual or the individual's life is what the nurse sees. Although most of us have been taught to evaluate the strengths and resources of patients and families, what is normal or healthy (supplies) is secondary to the problems presented. The language or practices in most health care environments promote this problem-focused orientation: we make problem lists and nursing diagnoses such as "self-care deficit" and "knowledge deficit;" we use quality assurance measures that track deficiencies; we provide "salvage" treatment to cancer "victims." Helpers have no choice but to focus on the most urgent or acute problems in environments where time, money, and human resources (supplies) are scarce; as a result, supporting human assets necessarily becomes a secondary consideration. In most helping relationships, when the problem is resolved, the recipient goes away;[11] the relationship is over. It is easy to see how helpers can shift to a negative view of people in such settings.

***Lack of positive feedback*** The motivation for helping is to make a difference. Most helpers want both feedback about the quality of their efforts and appreciation. If

complaints or criticism from recipients and coworkers are the norm, a negative view of helping can result.[11] What kind of feedback is implied in the death of a patient? Do you hear from coworkers and managers when things go smoothly, or only when things go wrong? How do you feel when a patient complains about your failure to return a phone call when you are now doing the work of two people and staying late without pay in order to return the call?

Moreover, recipients may take for granted what the helper does well. Society, professional organizations, institutions, accrediting bodies, peers, and self can set up no-win situations by establishing very high standards that are difficult or nearly impossible to achieve. If the nurse is able to meet these expectations, recognition and appreciation still may not be forthcoming because recipients may not feel the need to provide feedback when the nurse is "merely doing her job." Feedback may only come if the expectations are not met. Lack of positive feedback is a source of stress, and helping relationships that offer no positive feedback over time are viewed negatively.

***Level of emotional stress*** Society upholds the belief that cancer inevitably means pain, suffering, and death. As a consequence, the diagnosis of cancer often is regarded with more fear and viewed as more threatening than other diagnoses.[32] The diagnosis of cancer generates a great deal of emotional distress. Helpers may attempt to decrease the emotional distress of recipients by encouraging the disclosure of feelings, facilitating coping by providing for a catharsis of the tension and anxiety connected with emotions while allowing for feedback and enhancing problem solving.[33] Yet what is the consequence to the helper of being on the receiving end of emotional disclosure or catharsis?

Larson described the helper's pit: The person we are trying to help is in the pit, and the helper is standing above, on the edge of the pit, reaching in to help.[30] If the nature of contact with people is especially upsetting, depressing, or difficult, the helper may fall into the pit. To avoid this, the helper may develop a negative, even dehumanized, perception of the recipient.[11,27] Nurses may claim immunity in order to deal with the threatening realities of being confronted with extreme distress, the threat inherent in being confronted repeatedly with one's own mortality, the inhumanity of others, and the threat of pain and disfigurement.[21] Another way to handle the feelings is by distancing oneself emotionally and/or physically, creating a shelter by adding a layer of callus. This strategy, however, often only adds to the nurse's distress.[30,33]

***Possibility of change or improvement*** The recipient's responsiveness to the helper influences the helper's view of the recipient. Lack of responsiveness dehumanizes. If the helper feels dehumanized, it is much easier to dehumanize the recipient and to view the recipient in a negative light. Helpers can react not only to a lack of personal responsiveness but also to a lack of change or improvement in the recipient's condition.[11] Evidence of making a difference often requires change or improvement. In its absence, the helper may have feelings of personal failure and ineffectiveness. Dealing with problems of a chronic nature, like cancer, where signs of change or improvement evolve slowly (or not at all) can magnify this sense of failure. To diminish these feelings, the helper may blame other people. The blame may be explicitly or implicitly expressed toward coworkers ("If you weren't so lazy," "Why didn't you give him a transfusion?") or patients ("You smoked cigarettes for 30 years and see what happened," "You ignored the lump"). This shift in blame to "it's you" contrasts with the *mea culpa* reaction, but both reactions place blame on people and fail to acknowledge the environment as a source of stress.[11,30]

### Cancer trajectory

Cancer poses unique challenges to care providers as well as to patients. Each cancer diagnosis and resulting illness has a unique trajectory.[9,34] Some patients will be cured, others will live with a chronic illness with periods of remission and recurrence, still others will die quickly.[35] Trajectory variability creates demands on care providers as variability creates uncertainty.[36] The demands are magnified when the nurse has to juggle numerous trajectories simultaneously. To deal with uncertainty, care providers often develop expectations regarding a patient's trajectory.[35] Although intended to diminish uncertainty, this too can serve as a stressor if the predictions are incorrect. If a patient dies sooner than predicted or unexpectedly, a crisis ensues. Stress is acute but short-lived. On the other hand, if a patient's death takes "too long," chronic stress develops. Anger and resentment can develop in response to a feeling of powerlessness at being unable to change the trajectory. The unpredictability of cancer leaves the cancer nurse with the dilemma of what messages to convey to patients and family members. The juxtaposition of hope and truth is stressful. The care provider may feel as though he or she is conspiring against the patient, feeling hypocritical by "seeing the handwriting on the wall" yet continuing to participate in providing treatment that is believed ineffective in changing the cure trajectory. "This helplessness is a product of the conflict between the helping person's concept of himself as a restorer and the patient's inability to be restored."[37,p.43]

### Prolonged involvement

Cancer nurses often are involved with patients and their families for extended periods of time. "Being present throughout the continuum" in part distinguishes cancer nursing from other nursing specialties. The ensuing nurse–patient-family relationship is one of the reasons cancer nurses are cancer nurses; yet it is paradoxical, as prolonged involvement provides both rewards for and demands on cancer nurses. In general, nurses "live with" patients and their families, whereas other health care professionals merely make episodic visits. Strength of identification with the patient and family is directly proportional to the intensity and extent of contact.[38] During sustained relationships (in many cases, from diagnosis through death), patients and families may manifest a kaleidoscope of emotions, including anger, frustration, grief, and fear.[39] The demands increase exponentially as the nurse cares for multiple patients and families experiencing different emotions, for there is no reaction among patients that cannot also occur in caregivers.[40] This sense of emotional liability is stressful.[34,35,37,38]

Fagin and Diers[41] describe nursing as a metaphor for intimacy. "Nurses are involved in the most private aspects of people's lives, and they cannot hide behind technology or a veil of omniscience as other practitioners or technicians in hospitals may do. Nurses, as trusted peers, are there to hear secrets, especially the ones born of vulnerability."[41,p.11] Patients and family members may view the nurse as "safe" for the expression of fears and feelings of sadness, isolation, helplessness, anger, or profound grief. Being faced with human suffering and distress of the spirit places the listener in a vulnerable position. "To sympathize is to give part of ourselves to others, and in giving and sharing to become vulnerable."[42,p.69]

One way to lessen the intensity of the relationship is to withdraw physical and emotional support. Withdrawal can take many forms: "becoming emotionally distant, ignoring patients' needs, avoidance, holding a part of oneself back, feeling cold and unsympathetic,"[33,p.24] and task orientation.[43] Paradoxically, these attempts to withdraw physical and emotional support tend to increase rather than reduce stress for the care provider. A stress-avoidance-guilt sequence develops, for distancing often leads to feelings of betrayal of the patient or family, doubt about one's helping ability and motivation, and guilt.[33]

### Treatment sequelae

The nurse often is responsible for the administration of treatments that induce distress and illness,[44] creating iatrogenic illness. Feeling as though one, as a nurse, is contributing to the suffering of patients is distressing, because it is not in keeping with an idealized image of the nurse as a professional provider of comfort and help.[45]

An assortment of stressors emerge at the start of aggressive treatment. If the treatment is curative, the staff may feel hopeful and rally to support patient compliance. Hope is felt by staff and patients. If the treatment fails, doubt surfaces. To deal with repetitive treatment failures, the caregiver may shift the responsibility for failure: from "the treatment failed" to "Mr. Smith failed treatment X" or "He's a treatment failure." If the therapies are causing significant morbidity, ambivalence or cynicism may develop ("We may be trying to cure his sarcoma, but he'll need a heart transplant if he survives the treatment"). The nurse administering investigational therapies may feel incompetent in predicting and managing side effects. The values and ethics of research may be questioned, especially if the staff is exposed only to patients who die from the treatment or who experience intolerable side effects.

Radical surgery often causes dramatic adverse changes in a patient's appearance and serves as a stressor to nurses. Radical neck dissections, hemipelvectomies, or radical vulvectomies were among the stressors categorized by nurses as disfiguring or difficult illnesses in a study conducted by Vachon.[35] The stress to the care provider associated with disfiguring surgeries stems from the disfigurement itself and, as with other therapies, questioning whether or not the surgery will actually have a positive impact on the quantity and/or quality of the individual's life.

Lack of consensus among health providers and patients regarding treatment goals is a source of stress for cancer nurses. Patients may request continuation of aggressive treatment, creating a dilemma for the nurse who believes palliation is the reasonable choice ("How can I support his decision when I know what's coming?"). When palliation is the goal, if caregivers are unable to provide the expected relief from symptoms, particularly if they view symptom management as a mandate ("It's the least we can do"), they experience great stress. Staff may feel impotent, guilty, helpless, and even that they are part of a conspiracy that let the patient down.

### Death

We are a death-denying society.[21] Yet in 1996 it was estimated that 554,770 people living in the United States would die of cancer.[46] Cancer nurses will encounter physical death; and, in a broader context, loss of social worth, value, control, energy, relationships, role, life's work, or hopes for the future.

Death calls the living into action.[47] Confrontation or repeated exposure causes us to face our own fears about death and contemplate our own mortality. Zilboorg[48] suggests that continual consciousness of the fear of death impairs functioning; in defense, the fear is repressed. Repression is more than simply putting it away; it means "constant psychological effort to keep the lid on."[48,p.467] Continual psychological efforts to repress fear of death or feelings associated with death of a patient demands energy. Losses do not occur in a vacuum; rather, they interact with, modify, and augment the other stresses in our personal and professional lives.[49] When we don't share each experience of death with significant others, the feelings or distress associated with each death accumulate.[33]

### Social nature of nursing practice

*Nurse* is derived from the Latin word for "nourish." Caring is the essence, the core of nursing.[50] Fagin and Diers considered *nursing* a metaphor for "mothering" that shares links with "nurturing, caring, comforting, laying on of hands."[41,p.6]

Leininger states "caring is one of the most crucial and essential ingredients for health, human development, human relatedness, well-being, and survival."[51,p.46] Caring includes "those assistive, supportive, or facilitative acts toward or for another individual or group . . .

[meant] to ameliorate or improve a human condition or lifeway."[51,p.45] Caring and feeling cared for are basic human needs that promote personal and societal health. Yet many of the activities associated with caring are seen in our society as essentially "mundane and hardly worth noticing."[21] Pearson wrote "caregiving is, at this moment in history, humble and invisible work, often unappreciated or underappreciated."[52,p.117]

Nurses historically have differentiated their service from other providers by focusing on caring. However, the importance of caregiving (caring) and the time required for the interpersonal work involved have not been systematically incorporated into reimbursement and health care redesign strategies.[23] Activities used by nurses to respond to caregiving needs of patients and families are not readily amenable to standard measurements.[53] Consequently "nurses increasingly experience moral distress when they are unable to provide high quality care."[23,p.9] Often our caregiving is thwarted by cost accounting systems that do not take caregiving into full account. White and Begun advocate that contemporary profession building must focus on knowledge and skills as well as quality and outcomes.[54] (See Table 65-1.)

Caring is devalued in our society in part because it is associated with "women's work" and subservience. American society is dominated by the constructs of a white male system in which individualism, independence, one-upmanship, logic, and rational thought are prized.[55] Consequently, bonding, consensus-making, comforting, empowering of others, generativity, and caring are suspect and are subordinated to individual desires and needs.[21,55] If the essence of nursing is caring, a major source of stress in nursing lies in the devaluation of caring and the lack of recognition and rewards given to the caregiver.[21] Most nurses can provide experiential data about the value patients place on caring. Nurses can create leverage by measuring "customer" values and satisfaction with fulfillment of these valued services.

Another societal devaluation of caring stems from the proliferation of codependency theory that calls into question the motive for caregiving.[56] Caring may be perceived as an illness when popularized by definitions such as "any suffering and/or dysfunction that is associated with or results from focusing on the needs and behaviors of others."[57] The damage of such labeling may include viewing caring as a symptom of a disease, self-blame for the stress experienced in caring work, doubting caring motivations, and cutting off social support.[56]

## Environmental Factors

Forces that contribute to demands include health care regulations, reimbursement issues, and institutional systems (short staffing, faulty equipment, changing care standards to meet employers' financial agendas). Some suggest that we work in "toxic environments" referring to the organizational forces that determine work pressures.[27] Role stressors (e.g., ambiguity, conflict, overload), health

**TABLE 65-1**   Contemporary Profession Building in Nursing

| Traditional Profession Building in Nursing | Contemporary Profession Building in Nursing |
| --- | --- |
| Concentrated on identifying unique nursing activities; independent and dependent nursing functions. | Interdependence, collaboration, teamwork |
| Profession self-regulation | Accountability to stakeholder—purchasers of nursing care; shared regulation rather than self-regulation |
| Rigid professional boundaries | Flexible boundaries responsive to change in health care needs of society |
| Focus on caring; contrasted to curing | Focus on knowledge and skills; focus on quality and outcomes |
| Nursing as an oppressed group | Nursing in a position of leadership |
| Nursing as a female profession; femaleness viewed as a distinguishing characteristic; contrasted to the male 'oppressors' | Recruitment of men into the profession; diversity of profession key to innovation and creative problem solving |
| Focus on job security based on longevity of employment within an organization | Job security based on contribution to organization; less emphasis on tasks; greater emphasis on outcome |
| Development of nursing science and nursing theory | Development of multidisciplinary health care theories |
| Focus on acute care setting | Focus on diverse settings |

Data from White K, Begun J[54]

care organizational changes, environmental climates, and professional relationships will be discussed.

### Role stressors

*Role ambiguity*   An individual must understand the expectations that others have of a particular role, as well as the duties, rights, responsibilities, and activities of the role, in order to adequately perform the role. Role ambiguity is the extent to which role expectations are not clearly communicated.[35] Role ambiguity experienced by nurses stems from a lack of clear definition of professional nursing as well as the diversity of roles currently performed by nurses.[58] In general, the greater the perceived role ambiguity, the greater the perceived stress.

Health care reengineering has compounded role ambiguity. Crossing training, multiskilled workers, multidisciplinary teams, and unlicensed assistive personnel are part of the reengineering vocabulary. Stable job descriptions are no longer the norm. Formation of multidisciplinary teams with shared responsibilities for patient outcomes creates uncertainty about "what particular piece of the process am I responsible for?" Lack of trust and respect in working relationships limits the flexibility often necessary to deal with role ambiguity. In the past, use of unlicensed assistive personnel (UAP) was to extend or complement the care provided by a professional nurse.[59] Besieged with fiscal constraints, a paradigm shift has occurred from using UAP as a complement to nursing care to substituting them for care by a professional nurse, even though there is no empirical evidence to confirm that nursing support personnel improve quality or decrease cost.[59,p.108] Many nurses trained within the past 15 years learned primary care nursing and now must learn supervisory and delegation skills perhaps without any clear-cut authority.

*Role conflict*   Role conflict is the extent to which the expectations of various others are in conflict or incompatible. Vachon[35] found role conflict to be a major stressor for nurses. The evolving role of the nurse may cause conflicts, particularly with physicians and social workers who feel that nurses are infringing on their traditional roles. Likewise, the evolving roles of other professionals or the addition of assistive personnel can create conflict by infringing on the traditional roles of nursing (e.g., pharmacists involved with patient teaching or social workers coaching patients regarding symptom management). "Carving out activities unique to nursing" (i.e., emphasizing rigid boundaries between the domain of nursing and that of other professionals) "has been the quest of nursing leaders and theorists"[54,p.80] (Table 65-1). Partnerships, collaborative teams, interdependence, and flexible boundaries are the mandates of health care reform. As roles change shape, role conflict is inevitable. Kahn found that "persons subjected to high role conflict report greater job-related tensions, lower job satisfaction, less confidence in the organization itself, and more intense experience of conflict."[60,p.5]

*Role overload*   Role overload is the extent to which a person is incapable of meeting multiple expectations,[35] and may result in physical and emotional exhaustion, negative feelings about patients, coworkers, and the organization, and a diminished sense of accomplishment.[11] French and Kaplan[61] distinguished between quantitative and qualitative overload. *Qualitative* overload implies that the job skills and knowledge exceed those of the individual. *Quantitative* overload implies that there is more work than can be done in a given period of time.[12] It has been estimated that the "cumulative real case mix change in hospitals has been on the order of a 20 percent growth in complexity between 1982–1991."[62,p.31] Therefore attempts to provide care with fewer professional staff seem especially ill-timed.[63] Yet the messages are clear: give quality care but conserve resources; give quality care but do it for an unmanageable number of acutely ill patients. There are emotional and professional consequences of doing more with less and being legally accountable.

As the size (quantitative) or acuity (qualitative) of overload increases, "burnout" manifests among health care professionals.[64,65] Larson[30,33] and Arena and Page[66] wrote about the stress of the "imposter phenomenon" experienced by nurses: the feeling of inadequacy and incompetence that can be attributed to both quantitative and qualitative role overload. Feelings of inadequacy and incompetence can evolve from rapidly changing medical technologies, defining *competence* as "perfection," "terror of error" or accountability overload, and excessive demands.[33]

The experience of overload can be aggravated by the imposition of tasks that have a high priority for the organization but a lower priority for the nurse.[67] In many HMOs, the quality of and access to services is secondary to profit.[68] Nurses' priorities are access, quality, and costs.[69] Role overload puts nurses in no-win situations, for if the nurse complies with the organizational demand for quantity service (one nurse for ten patients) the nurse may be unable to provide quality service ("It's impossible to provide quality care for ten patients on this unit!").[64] Rather than compromising quality of care, nurses tend to work overtime, often without compensation, and perpetuate the perceived stress. A shift in thinking must occur because "we know now that demonstrating how *much* we can do for the person with cancer has to be replaced with demonstrating how little we can do and still meet necessary needs."[70,p.2] Nurses must redefine nursing responsibilities, not tasks.

## Control issues: autonomy and authority

Job control is associated with autonomy and authority, that is, the sense that one has control of one's time and activities.[71] Pines and Aronson[12] found that stress increased as autonomy, a sense of control, and discretionary time decreased. Organizational characteristics such as "circumscribed authority, downward channels of commands, specialization, and formal accountability and hierarchy contribute to a sense of lack of autonomy and control."[12,p.106] A lack of autonomy engenders feelings of frustration, victimization, and helplessness. Nurses are most prone to this experience, for they are charged with tremendous responsibility but are given no real power or authority.[7] Nursing carries with it a high-risk element in the delivery of service; this, coupled with limited authority, can result in a feeling of accountability overload or the dilemma of being accountable yet not having the requisite power or authority to balance the demand.

Nurses can develop feelings of powerlessness as they discover that what happens is independent of their input, expressed concern, or verbal complaint.[72] Nurses are experiencing what some call a crisis in professional identity as

the locus of decision making has moved from the professional to the payer, leaving nurses feeling less autonomous and less in control.[73] As a consequence, estrangement from the work environment can occur ("I am going to put in my eight hours and then get the hell out of here!"). On the other hand, the need for autonomy can be so great that nurses will blame themselves for problems, errors, and the like just to maintain a sense of control.

## Physical work environment

Research in organizational psychology has demonstrated that the physical quality of the work environment has an effect on performance.[7,p.84] Claus and Bailey[13] found that overcrowded units, noise, poor lighting, poor ventilation, and malfunctioning equipment were physical stressors identified by health care professionals. Noise in health care environments tends to be intermittent, unexpected, and reverberant. In response, stress accumulates via a constant low level of arousal of the autonomic nervous system.[13] Many work environments were not designed to accommodate the people, equipment, or supplies that are required to care for people today. Many care areas were designed around open work stations creating continuous visual availability of staff. Space often is not appropriated for confidential conversations or team meetings. Staff need physical space in which to think and talk without fear of being overheard or interrupted.

## Intragroup and intergroup conflict

Conflict seems inevitable in the dealings of any two autonomous persons whose interests or relationships are interdependent.[74] Wise said,

It is naive to bring together a highly diverse group of people and expect that, by calling them a team, they will in fact behave as a team. It is ironic indeed to realize that a football team spends 40 hours a week practicing teamwork for the two hours on Sunday afternoon when their teamwork really counts. Teams in organizations seldom spend 2 hours per week practicing when their ability to function as a team counts 40 hours per week.[75,p.73]

Factors that influence intragroup and intergroup conflicts are varied: scarcity of, or competition for resources (time, money, people, skills), divergent goals, and group interdependence for work sequencing. Where team concepts are employed, the greater the interrelatedness and dependence on one another, the greater the potential for conflict.[74] The size of the organization, levels of authorities, and specialized roles influence the amount of conflict: as each increases, so does the conflict. In hierarchical structures, the suppression of conflict is often the norm.[75] As hierarchical structures within hospitals are broken down and team management environments are developed, the suppression of conflict must be addressed as it will inhibit functioning of the team. Group cohesiveness, compatibility, and group attitude about conflict influences whether and the means by which conflicts are addressed.[60,73] Nurses have overused avoidance as a technique for conflict resolution, diminishing their effectiveness in a team.[76–79]

Among the basic commitments for nurses who practice in accordance with generally accepted standards is that they participate as members of the health care team.[80] The Oncology Nursing Society's *Standards of Oncology Nursing Practice* state: "The oncology nurse collaborates with the multidisciplinary team."[81,p.18] This involves intergroup and intragroup relationships. Much has been written about physician–nurse conflict. Conflict is rooted in historical antecedent, power and status inequity, mutual lack of knowledge of and respect for unique contributions of each role, personality conflicts, and lack of communication regarding treatment goals.[29] The perception that one group has power over another leads to behaviors reflecting low self-esteem (manifested as trying to do more and more in order to prove worth), horizontal violence (directing anger, negativity, sarcasm towards peers rather than at "oppressor"), and passive–aggressive behavior.[27] Unresolved intragroup conflicts (nurse to nurse) seem to represent losing sight of the basic idea of nursing as a caring profession that includes care for and of not only patients but also fellow nurses.[80] Intragroup conflicts disrupt team stability, isolate team members, and lessen the likelihood that nursing staff will share feelings related to work experiences. Intragroup conflicts potentially rob the individual of the valuable resource of other nurses who can provide technical support and appreciation of one's work, facilitating the realization that one's feelings are not unique.[33,36,82] Maslach[67] showed that the incidence of burnout was lower for health care workers who actively expressed and shared their feelings with coworkers. But who are these individuals with whom we can share feelings? Our health care culture has changed. We are in competition with one another for a limited supply of jobs and group membership fluctuates daily through downsizing, cross-training, attrition, or addition of assistive personnel. Collaboration and team work can create stress given this culture shift and the diversity of group skills team members bring to the group.

## Organizational climate

Size, structure, goals, and organizational climate are organizational factors that can serve as sources of stress. Investigations reveal that the size of the organization is related directly to organizational tension.[71] One can only speculate about the impact of hospital mergers. Our employee "families" have in some cases grown to huge conglomerates with CEOs and headquarters off-site. Hospitals have inherent characteristics that foster stress: multiple levels of authority, heterogeneity of personnel, work interdependence, and specialization.[83] Ambiguity of organizational structure, procedures, and policies and, conversely, overregulation can both be perceived as stressful. Precise organizational charts, a chain of command, and detailed job descriptions and procedures can create stress due to perceived inflexibility and lack of individual con-

trol.[75] Organizational structure has been described as a major determinant of job performance, satisfaction, and burnout.[12]

Goals of the organization are both explicit and implicit. For instance, the organization may state that direct patient care services are top priority yet cut staff who provide direct patient services. The mission statement of the organization may espouse quality care *but* the implicit mission is one of cost containment, utilization control, and profit. Organizational goals may stand in opposition to professional ethics. In a survey conducted by the ANA,[84] Scanlon reported that 58% of the nurse respondents identified "cost containment issues that jeopardize patient welfare as a priority ethical issue." "Nursing is a moral enterprise."[85,p.1516] A core value of nursing is respect for the individual. Inherent are the principles of autonomy, beneficence, nonmaleficence, veracity, confidentiality, fidelity, and justice.[84,85] Much of the emerging health care system and organizational goals and objectives challenges the nurse's ability to uphold the central moral tenets articulated in the Code of Ethics.[85] Benoliel[23] referred to this as "moral distress," knowing the right thing to do and being blocked by institutional restraints. Consequently, the caregiver may experience stress when stated goals differ from reality[49] or conflict with core values.

Menzies[86] found that organizational climate can support or diminish nurse–patient relationships. At times it seems that organizations have lost sight of the fact that "the quality of interactions between patients and staff underlies the patient's evaluation of the overall quality of care."[24,p.12] Matthews[87] rated hospital administrations on a continuum from technological orientation to social-process (person) orientation. The degree of patient-centered nursing increased as social-process orientation increased and decreased as technological orientation scores increased. How this translates into nursing, which is a people-oriented profession, is that nurses who work in an organization that places a higher value on technology would be expected to experience job stress due to the devaluation of their patient-centered orientation.

## Management strategies—rewards

Reward, recognition, praise, encouragement, expressions of appreciation, and clear feedback are extremely powerful incentives. Pines and Aronson[12] found that employees were better equipped to handle work stress when these kinds of rewards were available. Health care professionals often experience increased stress when there is a noticeable lack of these rewards.[7,12,88]

Organizations that fail to differentiate compensation based on effort serve as a source of stress. Health care professionals partly gauge their relative worth in the organization by making inferences about the extent to which they are compensated for their contributions.[12] Lack of reward differentiation does not encourage the high-contributor while the low-contributor, seeing that the high-contributor gets equal reward, concludes that hard work does not pay off. Nurses now are faced with the recognition that long-term service, commitment, and loyalty are not rewarded. In fact, experience that brings with it financial compensation may be viewed as a liability. As a result, organizations run the risk of employees being merely compliant rather than committed.

Recognition and appreciation often are more important than dollars. Feedback from managers regarding work performance, negative and positive, is vital. People who receive recognition, appreciation, satisfaction, and a sense of significance from their work are more likely to be content with their income.[65] Lack of feedback, as well as a mismatch of work performance expectations between nurses and managers, can create conflict. Managers' ideas about how to evaluate work performance may differ from the nurse's ideas.[9] Managers may base their evaluation on criteria such as keeping patients on a critical path, size and acuity of patient caseload, patient classification systems, cost savings, shortened length of stay, efforts to keep patients out of the emergency room or hospital. On the other hand, the clinicians may place a higher value on the quality of the care rendered. Clearly, clinicians and administrators can create stress by setting up a "we-they" or "service versus business" mentality. Performance criteria must shift to patient outcomes as well as contribution to the organizational goals, including cost containment. Clinicians must team with managers in being proactive. Clinicians are challenged to measure the value of the "intangibles" provided to patients and families, to define and measure quality, and to systematically evaluate patient outcomes. Otherwise, clinicians will be frustrated by the criteria managers and organizations use to measure contributions of the clinician.

## SUPPLIES—STRESS MANAGEMENT STRATEGIES

Stress results from a mismatch or discrepancy between environmental demands and individual supplies or between environmental opportunities and individual needs and goals. Efforts to reduce stress then must alter one or both elements—environment or self—by either reducing demands or increasing supplies or altering one's interpretation of demands and supplies.[89] Coping embraces actions to reduce the mismatch between self and environment. Lazarus[5] suggested two general types of coping: problem-focused and emotion-focused. *Problem-focused* coping targets the environment or self for direct action by changing one's behavior or environmental conditions. *Emotion-focused* coping attempts to palliate or eliminate distressing emotions elicited by the stressor.[90] Emotion-focused coping does not change the self or environment, only the way one feels. Both direct and indirect actions call for a reappraisal of environment and self.[89] When a situation is assessed as having the potential for change, a person typically will use problem-focused coping, whereas emotion-focused coping is employed if the harmful or threatening

situation holds little potential for change. The challenge is to learn to manage effectively those things that can be controlled, to accept the things that cannot be controlled, and to recognize the difference.[7,18]

Caplan[91] identified characteristics of effective coping strategies. These characteristics can be useful criteria in evaluating coping behaviors.

1. *There is an active exploration of reality issues and a search for information.* Effective coping involves looking for realities without denial, repression, avoidance, or projection. The individual examines the role he or she plays in the situation as well as his or her response. Information is sought in order to gain an accurate appraisal.
2. *There is a free expression of positive and negative feelings. Feelings are mastered where possible; and where mastery is not possible, the inevitable is accepted.* Identifying what can be controlled decreases the frustration and energy drain in trying to control uncontrollable situations.
3. *There is an active effort to engage the help of others.* The individual realizes that it is okay to ask for information and support from other people.
4. *Problems are broken down into manageable bits and worked through one at a time.*
5. *There is a fundamental trust in oneself and others and a sense of optimism that something can be done to bring about a positive outcome.*

Because stress is a personal experience, stress prevention and management strategies begin with the individual. This is not to suggest that the experience of work stress is a sign of weakness or deficiency. Rather, the effects of self-regulation enable nurses to reappraise self and environment, evaluate the supplies and demands of the work environment, and develop problem- or emotion-focused coping strategies. Self-regulation involves knowing one's self and one's personal values, priorities, and beliefs.

Pines and Aronson[12] suggested several concrete coping strategies to manage stress: reappraisal of goals, time management, acknowledging vulnerabilities, compartmentalizing life and work, self-reinforcement, change in attitudes, creating balance, accentuating the positive, adopting a wellness philosophy, relaxation, and establishing a sense of control over one's practice. Several of the strategies will be presented in the following section.

### Intrapersonal Coping Strategies

#### Recognizing stress responses

"To thine own self be true." It is imperative that an individual begin to recognize the triggers and signs of physical, emotional, and mental stress (Figure 65-2). Self-understanding begins with self-observation. Maslach[11] suggests keeping a daily stress and tension log (Table 65-2). Recording this type of information can provide very helpful insight into emotional and cognitive responses, the precipitator of responses, and styles of coping. This

---

### PHYSICAL, BEHAVIORAL, AND INTELLECTUAL MANIFESTATIONS OF STRESS

**Physical**

Feelings of exhaustion and fatigue
Weight change
Insomnia
Gastrointestinal disturbances
Cool, clammy skin
Sweating
Trembling; tics; twitches
Muscle tension
Rapid, uncontrolled speech
Loss of libido; impotence
Frequent headaches
Increased use of food, nicotine, alcohol, tranquilizers
Repetitive accidents
Frequent illness

**Behavioral/Emotional**

Lability of mood; mood swings
Suspiciousness; mistrust
Anger; antagonistic attitude toward others; hostility
Depression
Defensive behavior; blaming; scapegoating
Feelings of helplessness, inadequacy
Loss of sense of humor
Irritability
Distancing from others; reduced personal involvement
Nail biting; habitual teeth gritting
Critical of self and others
Panic; feeling pressured
Increasing expression of dissatisfaction

**Intellectual**

Increased rigidity in thinking
Increased use of intellectualization as defense
Lack of initiative
Forgetfulness
Preoccupation
Lack of attention to detail
Diminished concentration
Increased depersonalization
Dreams laden with conflict
Absenteeism
Frequent job change or feeling stuck in job
Frequent excuse making

---

**FIGURE 65-2**   Adapted from Muldary,[7] Maslach,[11] Haber et al,[16] Vachon,[35] Mount,[49] Maslach,[67] and Cox et al.[82]

exercise is not about enumerating faults; rather, it allows one to recognize patterns of behavior and self-talk and thus to become able to make choices about how one will think and feel or appraise self and the environment.

### Setting realistic goals

Unrealistic self-expectations are a formula for defeat and a major cause of "self-doubt, self-blame, and lowered self-esteem."[33,p.25] It is imperative to examine self-expectations and goals. Covey suggests that we formulate our personal mission statements and "begin with the end in mind."[92,p.97] Establishment of goals involves values clarification, in which those things of greatest value are given highest priority. It involves knowing what can be changed and what cannot. Goals need to be specific, realistic, and measurable. Setting realistic goals improves the probability of success.

### Time management

Time is a scarce resource. Time management is vital to self-management[93] and essentially involves structuring time in order to meet goals. The first step in time management is knowing how time is used. Be aware of the outcomes of time spent. Is the time spent directed toward a goal or particular objective? Maintenance of a time log helps to distinguish time use directed toward a goal from time waste or time problems. Time waste is caused by self, by others, and by the organization. Self-generated time wasters include lack of self-discipline, worry, always saying "yes," procrastination, disorganization, and an unwillingness to delegate. Interruptions, phone calls, delays due to tardiness, interdependency of work effort (lab results not available = delay in clinic patient appointment), and group meetings to communicate information that could have been handled via memo or E-mail are examples of time wasters generated by other people. Other time wasters generated by the organization and the nature of nurses' work include ambiguity of roles, lack of clarity regarding organization's goals, redundancy of effort, frequent changes (mid-stream), failure to plan, and engaging nurses in non-nursing tasks.[92] An unwillingness to share in the responsibility of providing care or trying to "do it all" is not an effective time management strategy. Does the increased use of unlicensed assistive personnel actually free professional staff time to plan and evaluate care?[94,p.647] Not only must we document the patient outcomes when utilizing unlicensed assistive personnel but we also must pay close attention to professional staff time required for delegating and supervisory activities.

The overriding principle in time management is knowing how time is spent and being methodical in planning time in order to accomplish goals. Flexibility must be incorporated into the time blueprint. Keeping a record of how time is spent can be helpful and is the initial step in planning to utilize time effectively. Time documentation with associated time and motion cost estimates can provide leverage in promoting change for time directed toward goal fulfillment.

### Tuning into inner dialogue

A critical variable in what is experienced as stressful is one's perception or interpretation of the stressor.[5] These perceptions and interpretations are given voice in an ongoing dialogue we have with ourselves. Our beliefs about reality and about ourselves underlie our self-talk. Self-talk can be rational or irrational. Self-talk based on

**TABLE 65-2   Daily Stress and Tension Log**

Daily incidents of stress are recorded using the following categories:

| Description of Physical Signs of Stress | Time | Where? What? Who? | Thoughts? Feelings? | Response |
|---|---|---|---|---|
| Wake late; tired from working late on special project | 6:30 AM | DK calls to invite me to dinner; DK sounds happy and care-free | DK never takes on extra projects; she knows I am under a deadline; I feel like she does not understand | Feel defensive; feel guilty about never initiating contact with DK; feel angry; refuse invitation; know I need some fun |
| Tight shoulder muscles, fatigue; grit teeth | 1:30 PM | At work, in the middle of lunch and get paged with a new consult | I will never get home on time; feel anger and resentment at coworkers who all seemed to take vacations; I feel abandoned | Ate dessert; abrupt with secretary |
| Racing pulse; feel breathless; thoughts disorganized; difficult to concentrate | 3:30 PM | At work, meeting with new section chief; I want him to like and respect me | Resent that he has not met with me and now only at my request; I do not feel heard | Last minute preparation; did not communicate clearly; beat myself up after meeting, with a lot of negative messages |
| Insomnia; cannot turn off thoughts | 11:30 PM | At home, trying to fall asleep | Thinking about work day; fearing work load and what I need to get done in the next two days before vacation | Get up and make a list; decide to read |

Adapted from Maslach C[11]

rational thoughts promotes self-respect and goal attainment. Self-talk based on irrational thoughts tends to sabotage self-esteem, results in negative emotions, and inhibits the realization of goals.[29]

Ellis and Harper[17] developed the A-B-C model for examining the relationship between thoughts, feelings, and behaviors. Event A is the activating event; B involves the beliefs we have about the event (our self-dialogue); and C is the consequence (behaviors or feelings). For example: A—Patient is angry that you were delayed in returning his phone call requests for a prescription refill. B—You assume complete responsibility for the patient's anger and in turn become angry at your boss for cutting the clinic staff from eight professional staff to five staff and two assistive personnel. C—You confront your boss and question the soundness of her decision making, "They (assistive personnel) can't do telephone triage." Many believe that A, the activating event, directly causes C, the consequence. But something happens between A and C. Our self-talk (B) rather than the activating event (A) influences our feelings and behavior. Following the patient–nurse conversation, the nurse may say to herself "it's all my fault," "If Mary and Joan still worked here I could have returned the phone call sooner," "Administration is nuts," "I'd like them (administrators) to get those angry patient phone calls," "If the patient complains, will I be the next one to lose my job?" The consequence (C) may have looked differently if the conversation the nurse had with herself had been revised to "Mr. Jones and I have a good enough relationship that this incident will not change our future interactions,"

"He is concerned about the turn-around-time with his mail order prescription service," "Mr. Jones knows he can count on me," "I am going to keep track of patient complaints regarding wait time and provide this documentation to my boss."

The technique called *cognitive restructuring* involves learning to listen to self-talk and changing unwanted or irrational thoughts in order to change emotional response.[17,95] The first step in cognitive restructuring is to look at the event or individuals as objectively as possible in order to gain a clearer perspective on the event and any irrational thinking and to consider different responses. Although it is unrealistic to expect to make a positive response to all stressful situations, a sense of mastery and control comes from knowing that one has a choice in how situations are perceived, in addition to choosing the response.

### Accentuating the positive

Helping relationships often have a negative bias, for the recipients of care have problems for which they seek help from the caregiver.[11] The negatives in helping relationships can be countered by actively emphasizing what is good, pleasant, or satisfying about the helping relationship. We need to develop cheerleaders, people in our work environments who know when we have made a positive contribution and who are willing to tell us. Measuring patient outcomes is another strategy to accentuate the positives. Make the outcomes public. Larson recommends that nurses reflect on their "greatest moments;"

those times "when you make a difference, when you see the real impact of your caring."[30,p.862] Keeping a journal, maintaining a file of letters from patients and families or simply sharing the "moment" with a colleague helps to lessen the negative bias that can creep into helping relationships (Figure 65-3).

## Compartmentalizing work and life

Pines and Aronson[12] recommend making a clear distinction between home and work, including finding a balance between the energy expended at work and home activities. One form of compartmentalization is not discussing work-related issues at home, and vice versa. Although talking about work-related stress with family members or friends may provide catharsis and support, reliving work stress at home or with friends causes a reexperiencing of the distress.[7] Work-related stress is best discussed with someone who does the same kind of work, someone who can immediately empathize. Colleagues provide technical support and technical challenge and are in a unique position to understand the sense of loss and grief experienced in the midst of health care reform.[30,33] Another strategy to create a sense of separation between work and home is to allow for decompression time.[12] A decompression routine is a ritual that signals that one part of daily life is ending and another is beginning, that is, the passage from work life to personal life. One sequence of decompression activities might include: making a to-do list for the next day's activities before leaving work, listening to music on the way home, exercising, meditating, showering immediately on arriving home, or changing from work uniform into at-home clothes.

## Creating balance

"Every helper needs to find a way to be involved emotionally as a caregiver without burning out. . . . Em-

---

### GREATEST MOMENTS

The following are examples of "greatest moments" shared by colleagues:

I have known Cindi for only one year. I did her initial assessment when she came to the brain tumor clinic for the first time. I knew that Dr. S. was going to tell Cindi that there wasn't anything else to do so I went into the exam room with him. Cindi and her parents were devastated. I couldn't help it, but my eyes filled with tears. Her parents saw the tears in my eyes and later told me "We appreciate how much you care. You're really good at what you do." —JB

I was a brand new nurse and new to the unit. Nita was a 67-year-old woman with three or four primary malignancies. Nita was essentially living in the hospital. She had been labeled LTC, or long-term care. People treated her like she looked: bad body—bad brain. She was extremely dependent on the staff for physical care. I heard a lot of stories. She was very isolated. I began to question "What are we doing?" The tenured staff rolled their eyes at me, but my head nurse was very supportive. I went to Nita and told her that I was going to be her primary nurse and that I needed her help in developing a care plan. I will never forget coming out of report about two or three weeks later to find that Nita had showered, washed her hair, and made her own bed. Although she died at the hospital, she was able to make several visits home. I know that I had helped to make it possible. —MS

This is a card I got from Willard at Easter ("Happy Easter. God bless and watch over you. Your friend, Willard"). Willard is in a wheelchair and lives in a housing project. His girlfriend was a GYN patient. She died 12 years ago, and at Christmastime that year, several other staff and I took Willard fruit and gifts. We've been doing it ever since. In his own way, I know he loves us. —DS

Mr. Smith was being sent home to die, and he knew it. He had just spoken with his doctor. It was rough because he was such a fighter. He had trouble communicating because of the multiple head and neck surgeries. I will never forget this. He put on his call light and, in his garbled voice, asked the clerk to find me. He held my hand and told me how much it had meant to him that I had been part of his ammunition. We cried together. —GW

A patient was referred to the pain clinic. She questioned how she could continue in light of the amount of pain she was having. She had had radiation therapy and had terrible esophageal pain. As a consequence, she hadn't been able to eat. We gave her 10 mg of intravenous morphine, and it gave her complete relief. Only 10 mg! With the relief, she wanted to eat something. Someone had brought donuts to the clinic that morning, so I offered her one. I will never forget her saying: "Eating this donut is like having an orgasm." I think we all need to eat more donuts. —DT

Gloria is a 42-year-old woman diagnosed with breast cancer. At the time I met her, she had bone metastasis and had excruciating pain due to C4-C6 bone disease with cord compression. Gloria and I had developed a professional friendship. I went into her room to inquire about her degree of pain relief. She told me that her pain was under control, but she was quiet, not acting like herself, and looked really down. I took a risk by asking her if she wanted me to stay for a while. I told her that I thought she looked upset and sad. That was all the permission she needed. Up from the depths came pent-up anguish. It would have been easier to have been satisfied that her pain was relieved and not address the suffering. As she cried and I held her, my eyes filled with tears. The next day, as I walked by her room, Gloria called out to me. She asked me to come close to her bedside. There she was in her hard cervical collar reaching up to embrace me. She said, "I know you care. I saw the tears in your eyes. You really helped me." I needed to hear that because I was afraid that all I had done was contribute to her suffering by being the catalyst. It felt good to know that I had helped. —MC

**FIGURE 65-3**  Adapted from Larson D.[30]

pathy is a double-edged sword; it is simultaneously [the nurse's] greatest asset and point of real vulnerability."[30,p.857] Most nurses move along a continuum between overinvolvement and underinvolvement. Creating a balance between overinvolvement and depersonalization involves finding a blend of compassion and objectivity: detached concern.[7,11,30,96] With detached concern, the nurse has an honest concern for the patient's well-being but is able to maintain emotional and psychological distance.

So how does one learn detached concern? Most nursing educational programs stress the importance of empathy, but few balance that recommendation with the importance of maintaining emotional and physical distance.[21] Experienced practitioners typically learn detached concern through experience, most likely only after experiencing both ends of the involvement continuum. Weisman[40] recommends making the least possible contribution, sharing concerns, or calling on an absent witness. Making the least possible contribution does not mean doing as little as possible; rather, it means making a contribution that has the best chance for success with the least amount of strain. Another way to learn about detached concern is through sharing of experiences and seeking the feedback of peers regarding involvements with patients and families. "Coping well is aided by having something to measure our efforts (involvements) against and someone to derive support from."[40,p.167] The absent-witness technique involves asking a former patient, in absentia, to evaluate the care received. Questions couched in pragmatic terms provide feedback as to whether expectations regarding the level of involvement were desired or unrealistic.[40]

Intellectualization is another way of trying to achieve detached concern. It involves dealing with emotionally stressful situations in the abstract or as technical realities.[7] It serves as a defense mechanism in creating psychological or emotional distance from distressing situations. Given the intensity and intimacy of contact nurses have with patients, this process of dealing with people and events in one's head rather than in one's heart can serve as a buffer. A word of caution: exclusive use of intellectualization creates imbalance as one becomes increasingly underinvolved. This underinvolvement creates stress, since most nurses are dissatisfied with underinvolvement. Additionally, suppression of one's emotional experiences requires energy and at some point will require attention.

### Creating control of one's practice

This coping strategy involves developing and maintaining competency, setting limits, and organizing one's work to minimize stress and enhance satisfaction.[35] Developing and maintaining competence evolves through a series of stages. Nurses gain competency by developing professional skills through formal education programs, establishing goals, and testing competencies in clinical situations. Competency continues to be refined in ongoing professional experiences to the point that nurses feel secure in their work environment. Competency and control are nurtured through ongoing professional experiences, feedback, development of more complex skills through continuing education, refinement of personal and professional goals, and professional affiliations.

Mount stated that "reasonable limits of personal giving must be established if sustained, effective functioning is to be ensured."[49,p.1132] Limit setting helps to create a sense of mastery over one's work. This involves knowing and respecting one's limits and deciding what one can and cannot do and what one will and will not do. Working overtime and being on call while off duty are prime examples of areas where limit setting is required. Changing on-call status by rotating responsibility is another. The individual can do a lot to set limits, but individual effort can be greatly strengthened by organizational policies that establish limits for overtime, provide a mechanism for equal sharing of on-call responsibility, and give adequate compensation for overtime and on-call work.

Strategies to foster a sense of control over one's work include reorganization of work and development of specialized roles.[9] Organizing work assignments so the work is varied can counterbalance emotionally draining work with task-oriented work. Strategies to restructure work assignments could include job sharing (e.g., research nurse and staff nurse job sharing), changing the context of the contact with patients (e.g., cross-training staff to work in inpatient and outpatient settings), sharing responsibility for difficult patient care assignments (e.g., two to three staff nurses serve as patient's primary care nurses and rotate direct care responsibilities), and creating a balanced mix of patients (e.g., chemotherapy nurse cares for the newly diagnosed patient, the patient in remission, and the patient receiving relapse therapy).

In the last five to ten years, Americans' attitudes about jobs, security, and career have changed significantly, especially in health care.[96] A *then and now* perspective is captured in Table 65-3. To gain a sense of control over one's work is to be cognizant of one's marketability and the changing health care environment. Enumerate the skills and knowledge you currently possess. How could you use them differently? What additional skills and knowledge do you need? How will you obtain these additional skills

**TABLE 65-3** Changes in Americans' Attitudes Toward Employment

| Then | Now |
| --- | --- |
| Job security | Intense competition |
| Specialization | Cross-train |
| Stick with one job | Broaden skills and experience |
| Title matters | What title? |
| Career ladder | Career paths |
| Qualifications | Skills |

From Gary H[97]

and knowledge? How can the use of your skills and knowledge save the organization or payer source money? Demonstrate that your team provides care that improves patient outcomes. It is critical to stay informed about organizational change, to seek increased involvement with planning and implementing organizational strategies, and to demonstrate the value of your contributions to the organization. Remain current in health care trends. Consider how your skills and knowledge could address the realities of an aging and ethically diverse population, an increase in health care complexity, alternative practice settings, continued growth of managed care, limitation on reimbursement, shortened lengths of stay, and higher acuity.

Nurses can gain a sense of control by watching for employment opportunities as well as maintaining a current resume. A number of services are available to nurses changing or seeking different work. Internet™, America Online™, and CompuServe™ provide on-line career management help. Services include career counseling options, resume and cover letter templates, an employment agency database, and an employer contacts database. The Oncology Nursing Society has developed an *ONS Career Resource Kit* that includes job search tips, career development resources, and opportunities in alternative settings.

### Relaxation

Chronic stress often produces tense muscles, increased blood pressure, and fatigue. Relaxation brings mental and physical restoration. Relaxation is based on the mind–body connection and the premise that a relaxed body is the antithesis of a stressed mind. There are many forms of relaxation techniques: progressive deep-muscle relaxation, biofeedback, guided imagery, meditation, yoga, and autogenic training.[98] The key to the effectiveness of any technique is practice. Practice requires a commitment to self-care. Regular use of relaxation techniques can yield a state of relaxation that is incompatible with stress. Stress symptoms signal a warning; recognizing the symptoms requires learning to listen to one's body. Relaxation treats the symptoms, not the cause, but provides renewal to face the next challenge.

### Adopting a wellness philosophy

A wellness philosophy promotes healthy behavior. Healthy choices include eating a balanced diet, limiting alcohol and caffeine intake, ceasing smoking, practicing preventive health care (e.g., mammography, Pap smear, annual physical, dental care, eye exam), exercise, rest, recreation, socialization, and development of intimate relationships. The principal benefit of actively adopting a wellness philosophy is conditioning the body to withstand the deleterious effects of stress. Nurses are taught to train their minds for professional lives; likewise we must train and care for our bodies and spirits.

## Environmental Strategies

Opportunities for personal achievement, recognition, growth, responsibility, and advancement mean work satisfaction. Organizations must be responsive to supplying these opportunities. Allen and Kraft[99] described six principles that lead to a more satisfying work environment: involvement with establishing work objectives and methods, clarity of organization and structure, feedback and information, orientation and training, rewards, and supportive culture. The initial organization-based stress management strategy requires an assessment of the nurse's perceptions of the following: discrepancies between accountability and authority, extent to which the job provides variety and challenge, extent to which the nurse's role is clearly defined, extent to which the nurse's role conflicts with purported roles of others of different status and position, opportunities for continued training and development, adequacy of supplies/equipment/space, amount of actual freedom and independence, and extent to which the nurse is receiving feedback concerning performance.[7]

### Nurse–patient ratios

Nurses have a right to work in an environment that minimizes physical and emotional stress. Employers have a legal responsibility to provide sufficient staff to meet the care needs of patients.[100] The quality of nurse–patient interactions is influenced by the number as well as the acuity of the people for which the nurse is responsible.[12] As the number increases, so does role overload for the nurse. Staff–patient ratios that support the provision of quality patient care and equalization of demands with supplies decrease work load stress.[36] In an effort to contain costs, some organizations attempt to provide care with fewer professional staff and employ unlicensed assistive personnel (UAP). Assigning care tasks to non-professionals while decreasing professional staff seems ill-timed given the increase in patient complexity.[63] UAPs were originally intended to extend or complement professional nursing care. Presently the emphasis seems to be on lowering costs and providing substitutes for professional staff. However, it is questionable whether assistive personnel yield cost savings.[59] Prescott[101] provided an important review of the literature addressing the links between nursing/skill mix staffing and patient outcomes as it affects cost. Professional nurses need to redefine nursing responsibilities, demonstrating the impact on outcomes and patient satisfaction.[102] Utilize position papers prepared by the American Nurses' Association[103] and Oncology Nursing Society[94] regarding the use of UAPs. In order to be proactive, keeping current with the literature is pivotal. Consider creating a multidisciplinary journal club to discuss current literature.

Within your organizations, when changes are proposed ask "will the change ensure the protection of the quality of care delivered?"[70] Identify how the intended change responds to the needs of patients, payer sources, organization, and employees. Capitalize on consumer movements such as the *Foundation for Accountability* that represents about 80 million insured. At the conclusion of a July 1995 meeting of the *Foundation for Accountability,* the clear message was "more attention to quality."[104] Direct your attention to legislative action where debate is being held to "rein in managed care."[105,p.69] Bills calling for direct access to specialty care, mandated point of service options, and establishment of quality standards are being advanced. U.S. Rep. Edward Markey has introduced legislation to ban gag rules in contracts with providers.[105]

### Organizational flexibility

Kahn[60] wrote of organizational strategies to bring the organization more in line with the needs and abilities of the employee. A key strategy is organizational flexibility that implies concern for the individual. Often this involves giving the individual freedom, the permission to exert some control over her or his practice, and providing variability in routines. Distrust and failure to recognize the needs and abilities of the individual employee create an inflexible and myopic system. A decentralized management system that puts the authority and responsibility for decision making at the level of the front-line practitioner is a means of providing flexibility and control. "Giving the employee both the responsibility and accountability to use the [employee's] expertise more fully, enhances [employee] satisfaction, and usually results in a better product."[70,p.4] Porter-O'Grady[106] encourages managers to "empower the center," the individual closest to the customer. "The fundamental tenet in worker empowerment is the worker closest to the task . . . is usually in the best position to make change related to the task."[70,p.4] Worker empowerment also can serve to decrease the stress associated with feeling that those who make decisions are out of touch with the realities of providing care.

### Creating opportunities for withdrawal

Pines and Aronson[12] emphasized the importance of time out from stressful situations. This concept of "time out" is important to any work that involves emotional, physical, or mental stress. Time-out activities include providing not only for meal breaks but also for breaks from stressful work. Staff could share the direct care responsibilities for a particularly tedious or arduous patient care situation. A change in routine, perhaps working on a special project or attending continuing education programs away from the work site, could provide a needed time out. Strict attention must be paid to adhering to the rule that time away from work is truly time away from work. Organizations need to establish policies that guarantee protected time off and regular vacations. In addition, mental health days without penalty can provide emotional breathing space.

### Social support

John Donne wrote, "No man is an island, entire to himself." The presence or absence of social support plays a major role in stress. Caplan[9] defined social support as "enduring interpersonal ties" to a group of people who can be relied on to provide emotional sustenance, assistance, and resources; who provide feedback; and who share standards and values. Social support systems serve a number of functions. Most people need someone to listen actively to them, to listen without offering advice or making judgments. Technical appreciation and affirmation of competence can really only come from people who understand our work; nonexpert family members and friends are important for other types of emotional support and challenge that require someone who cares on a human-to-human level.[30]

Social support is crucial to nurses' well-being in today's complex health care system.[107] For nurses, receiving support often is difficult, for many nurses view themselves as caregivers, not as care receivers. Fear often keeps nurses from seeking support or expressing emotions: fear of not being accepted, fear of being seen as incompetent or inadequate, fear of being misunderstood, or fear of betrayal. Pines and Aronson[12] and Larson[33] refer to the phenomenon of the "fallacy of uniqueness," in which individuals falsely assume they are the only one feeling, thinking, or behaving in a particular way. By expressing feelings and experiences, nurses can learn that others share similar experiences—the nurse is no longer alone and isolated. These fears underscore the pivotal first step in the giving and getting of support: the development of trust and mutual respect. Larson[30,33] believes that, when helpers (nurses) talk about their stress and begin to see that much of how they feel, think, and behave is an inevitable part of their work, much of the distress in work can be ameliorated.

It is important to build work-based sources of support, because these seem to be more potent than individual efforts at reducing occupational stress.[107] In nursing, work-based supports not only provide for individual support but also provide a mechanism for institutional change through group problem solving. Staff meetings that give individuals opportunities to express themselves and to be involved with group problem solving can be a catalyst for the development of social support systems, as can task sharing and informal socialization.[12] Formalized support groups also can provide social support. They communicate a strong message of administrative support; it is important for staff to feel that administration recognizes the stress that staff can experience and that it is willing to provide the extra resources necessary.[99,107]

### Work team development

Vachon found that an important organizational coping mechanism was the "sense of belonging to a team that knew what it was doing, knew how to get members to work towards defined professional and personal goals, and knew how to support one another through professional and personal stressors."[35,p.212] Beckard[108] identified the characteristics of an effective team: clarity of objectives, goals, and priorities that are agreed on by team members; role expectations that are realistic and clearly defined; problem-solving and decision-making skills; group rules that support the objectives, goals, and priorities; concern for group members; and the ability to maximize group resources for the good of the group and the individual. These characteristics can be used as criteria for the periodic assessment of overall team functioning and effectiveness.

The organizational conditions of scarcity of or competition for resources, ambiguity (in procedures, policies, roles), overregulation, and exceptions ("The rules do not apply equally to everyone") provide rich fuel for conflict.[75] Effective group functioning can do much to manage or resolve conflict. When people in conflict are able to approach the conflict in an atmosphere of trust and mutual support, the energy that normally would be diverted to defensiveness is freed up for use in resolving the conflict.

## Maintaining Professional Integrity

"The moral basis of nursing exists in (a) the nurse–patient relationship and the patient's expectations that he or she will receive compassion and competent care, as well as protection of basic human rights, and (b) expectations by society that the practice of professional nursing is guided by ethical ideals, virtues, principles, and standards."[23,p.5] Nursing is a moral enterprise; consequently, an evolving source of stress experienced by nurses stems from an apprehension about our ability to uphold these moral tenets.[85] Nurses struggle with the ethical dilemmas associated with health care reform. Benchmark ethical principles and core values asserted in the *Code for Nurses*[109] and the ONS *Statement of Core Values*[85] serve as a guide for cancer nurses. It is critical that nurses be ethically grounded and discerning in their evaluation of patient care. We have a fiduciary relationship with patients who are reliant on our promise to help as well as on our professional integrity. Increasing our knowledge of the language and intent of ethical principles and core values will empower us to advocate for patients and challenge the unethical practices encountered at times in health care. This is critical to the effectiveness of our conversations with team members, administrators, and payers. Scanlon and Glover[85] recommend steps in making reliable moral judgments including: (1) identify the ethical issue, (2) gather relevant information, (3) describe the values at stake, (4) identify a range of options, (5) make a choice, (6) give reasons to support choices and (7) evaluate how the dilemma could be prevented. Creating a structure in order to discern the issues can help to mitigate the "moral distress." (See chapter 57.)

## CONCLUSION

Stress is pervasive to the human condition. Stress is the perceived imbalance between person–environment demands and abilities, or supplies. The reality-based and perception-based appraisals of intrapersonal, interpersonal, and environmental supplies and demands influence the amount and intensity of stress an individual experiences. The potential demands encountered and supplies available to cancer nurses have been described. Given the consequences to both individual and environment, it is imperative that cancer nurses and the organizations that employ them be committed to decreasing demands and increasing supplies where possible. To do otherwise is to jeopardize our "business," that is providing quality care to individuals diagnosed with cancer and their families.

## REFERENCES

1. Selye H: *Physiology and Pathology of Exposure to Stress*. Montreal, ACTA Medical Publishers, 1950
2. Derogatis L: Self-report measures of stress, in Goldberger L, Breznitz S (eds): *Handbook of Stress: Theoretical and Clinical Aspects*. New York, Free Press, 1982, pp 270–294
3. Holmes T, Masuda M: Magnitude estimates of social readjustments. *J Psychosom Res* 11:219–255, 1966
4. Holmes T, Rahe R: The social readjustment rating scale. *J Psychosom Res* 12:213–218, 1976
5. Lazarus R: *Psychological Stress and Coping Process*. New York, McGraw-Hill, 1966
6. Lazarus R, Folkman S: *Stress, Appraisal, and Coping*. New York, Springer, 1984
7. Muldary T: *Burnout and Health Professionals: Manifestations and Management*. Norwalk, CT, Appleton-Century-Crofts, 1983
8. French J, Rodgers W, Cobb S: Adjustment as person–environment fit, in Coelho GV, Hamburg DA, Adams JE (eds): *Coping and Adaptation*. New York, Basic Books, 1974, pp 213–222
9. Vachon M, Stylianos S: Caring for the caregiver: A person-centered framework, in Baird S, McCorkle R, Grant M (eds): *Cancer Nursing. A Comprehensive Textbook*. Philadelphia, Saunders, 1991, pp 1084–1093
10. Harrison R: Person–environment fit and job stress, in Cooper CL, Payne R (eds): *Stress at Work*. New York, Wiley, 1979, pp 175–205
11. Maslach C: *Burnout: The Cost of Caring*. Englewood Cliffs, NJ, Prentice-Hall, 1982
12. Pines A, Aronson E: *Career Burnout. Causes and Cures*. New York, Free Press, 1988
13. Claus K, Bailey J: *Living with Stress and Promoting Well Being*. St. Louis, Mosby, 1980
14. Appley M, Trumball R: On the concept of psychological stress, in Appley M, Trumball R (eds): *Psychological Stress: Issues in Research*. New York, Appleton-Century-Crofts, 1967, pp 1–13

15. McGrath JE: Stress and behavior in organization, in Dunnette M (ed): *Handbook of Industrial and Organizational Psychology*. Chicago, Rand McNally, 1976, pp 1351–1396

16. Haber J, Leach A, Schudy S, et al: *Comprehensive Psychiatric Nursing*. New York, McGraw-Hill, 1982

17. Ellis A, Harper R: *A New Guide to Rational Living*. Hollywood, CA, Wilshire Book, 1975

18. Pearlin L, Schooler C: The structure of coping. *J Health and Soc Behavior* 19:2–21, 1978

19. Rotter J, Seeman M, Liverant S: Internal vs. external locus of control of reinforcements: A major variable in behavior therapy, in Washburne N (ed): *Decisions, Values and Groups*. London, Pergamon, 1962, pp 76–99

20. Keane A, DuCette J, Adler D: Stress in ICU and non-ICU nurses. *Nurs Res* 34:231–236, 1985

21. Benner P, Wrubel J: *The Primacy of Caring. Stress and Coping in Health and Illness*. Menlo Park, CA, Addison-Wesley, 1989

22. DuCette J, Wolk S: Cognitive and motivational correlates of generalized expectancies for control. *J Pers Soc Psychol* 22:420–426, 1973

23. Benoliel J: The moral context of oncology nursing. *Oncol Nurs Forum* 20:5–12, 1993

24. del Bueno D: Ready, willing, able? Staff competence in the workplace redesign. *J Nurs Admin* 25:14–16, 1995

25. Benton D, White D: Satisfaction of job factors for registered nurses. *J Nurs Admin* 11:55–63, 1972

26. Maslow A: *Motivation and Personality*. New York, Harper & Row, 1954

27. Cullen A: Burnout. Why do we blame the nurse? *Am J Nurs* 95:23–27, 1995

28. Vachon ML: Motivation and stress experienced by staff working with the terminally ill. *Death Educ* 2:113–122, 1978

29. Smythe E: *Surviving Nursing*. Menlo Park, CA, Addison-Wesley, 1984

30. Larson D: The challenge of caring in oncology nursing. *Oncol Nurs Forum* 19:857–861, 1992

31. McDonnell K, Ferrell B: Oncology Nursing Society Life Cycle Task Force report: The life cycle of the oncology nurse. *Oncol Nurs Forum* 19:1545–1550, 1992

32. Silverman R, Wortman C: Coping with undesirable life events, in Garber J, Seligman M (eds): *Human Helplessness: Theory and Applications*. New York, Academic Press, 1980, pp 279–341

33. Larson D: Helper secrets. *J Psychosoc Nurs* 25:20–27, 1987

34. Larson P, Jennings B: The generation of stress in the provision of care, in Baird S, McCorkle R, Grant M (eds): *Cancer Nursing. A Comprehensive Textbook*. Philadelphia, Saunders, 1991, pp 1076–1083

35. Vachon ML: *Occupational Stress in the Care of the Critically Ill, the Dying, and the Bereaved*. Washington, DC, Hemisphere Publishing, 1987

36. McElroy A: Burnout—A review of the literature with application to cancer nursing. *Cancer Nurs* 5:211–217, 1982

37. Holsclaw P: Nursing in high emotional risk areas. *Nurs Forum* 4:36–45, 1965

38. Newlin N, Wellisch D: The oncology nurse: Life on an emotional roller coaster. *Cancer Nurs* 1:447–449, 1978

39. Ehlke G: The psychological aspects of cancer, in Burkhalter P, Donley D (eds): *Dynamics of Oncology Nursing*. New York, McGraw-Hill, 1976, pp 211–226

40. Weisman AD: Understanding the cancer patient: The syndrome of caregiver's plight. *Psychiatry* 44:161–168, 1981

41. Fagin C, Diers D: Nursing as metaphor. *N Engl J Med* 309:116–117, 1983

42. Travelbee J: "What's wrong with sympathy?" *Am J Nurs* 64:68–71, 1964

43. Wegmann J: Avoidance behaviors of nurses as related to cancer diagnosis and/or terminality. *Oncol Nurs Forum* 6:8–14, 1979

44. Stewart B, Meyerowitz B, Jackson L, et al: Psychological stress associated with outpatient oncology nursing. *Cancer Nurs* 5:383–387, 1982

45. Steeves R, Kahn D, Benoliel J: Nurses' interpretation of the suffering of their patients. *West J Nurs Res* 12:715–731, 1990

46. Parker S, Tong T, Bolden S, et al: Cancer statistics, 1996. *CA Cancer J Clin* 46:1–32, 1996

47. Becker E: *Denial of Death*. New York, Macmillan, 1973

48. Zilboorg G: Fear of death. *Psychoanal Q* 12:465–475, 1943

49. Mount B: Dealing with our losses. *J Clin Oncol* 4:1127–1134, 1986

50. Larson P: Important nurse caring behaviors perceived by patients with cancer. *Oncol Nurs Forum* 11:46–50, 1984

51. Leininger M: Caring: A central focus of nursing and health services, in Leininger M (ed): *Care: The Essence of Nursing and Health*. Thorofare, NJ, Slack, 1984, pp 45–58

52. Pearson C: *Awakening the Heroes Within*. San Francisco, Harper Collins, 1991

53. MacPherson K: A new perspective on nursing and caring in a corporate context. *Adv Nurs Sci* 11:32–39, 1989

54. White K, Begun J: Profession building in the new health care system. *Nurs Admin Q* 20:79–85, 1996

55. Schaef A: *Women's Reality*. San Francisco, Harper & Row, 1985

56. Larson D: The codependent caregiver: A dangerous myth? *Hospice* 6:17–19, 1991

57. Whitfield C: *Healing the Child Within*. Deerfield Beach, FL, Health Communication, Inc., 1967

58. Gunning C: The profession itself as a source of stress, in Jacobson S, McGrath H (eds): *Nurses Under Stress*. New York, Wiley, 1983, pp 113–126

59. Krapohl G, Larson E: The impact of unlicensed assistive personnel on nursing care delivery. *Nurs Economic$* 14:99–110, 1996

60. Kahn R: Conflict, ambiguity and overload: Three elements in job stress. *Occup Mental Health* 3:2–9, 1973

61. French J, Kaplan R: Organizational stress and individual strain, in Marrow A (ed): *The Failure of Success*. New York, AMACOM, 1973, pp 89–103

62. Aiken L, Salmon M: Health care workforce priorities: What nursing should do. *Inquiry* 31:318–329, 1994

63. Keepnew D, Marullo G: Policy imperatives for nursing in an era of health care restructuring. *Nurs Admin Q* 20:19–31, 1996

64. Maslach C, Pines A: The burnout syndrome in the day-care setting. *Child Care Q* 6:100–113, 1977

65. Pines A, Kafry D: Occupational tedium in the social services. *Social Work* 23:499–507, 1978

66. Arena D, Page N: The imposter phenomenon in the clinical nurse specialist role. *Image: J Nurs Scholar* 24:121–125, 1992

67. Maslach C: The burn-out syndrome and patient care, in Garfield C (ed): *Stress and Survival*. St. Louis, Mosby, 1980, pp 43–56

68. Finnerty J, Pinkerton J: Ethical considerations of managed care. *Obstet Gynecol Surv* 48:699–706, 1994

69. American Nurses' Association: *Nursing's Agenda for Health Care Reform*. Washington, DC, American Nurses' Association, 1991

70. Baird S: The impact of changing health care delivery on oncology practice. *Oncol Nurs: Patient Treat Support* 2:1–13, 1995

71. Kahn R, Wolfe D, Quinn R, et al: *Organizational Stress: Studies in Role Conflict and Ambiguity*. New York, Wiley, 1981

72. Seligman M: *Helplessness: On Depression, Development and Death*. San Francisco, William Freeman, 1975

73. Dunham-Taylor J, Marquette P, Pinczuk J: Surviving capitation. *Am J Nurs* 96:26–29, 1996

74. Wise H: Preface, in Wise H, Beckhard R, Rubin I (eds): *Making Health Teams Work*. Cambridge, MA, Ballinger, 1974, p 73

75. Pneuman R, Bruehl M: *Managing Conflict*. Englewood Cliffs, NJ, Prentice-Hall, 1982

76. Baker K: Improving staff nurse conflict skills. *Nurs Economics$* 13:295–298, 1995

77. Marriner A: Managing conflict. *Nurs Manage* 13:29–32, 1982

78. Hightower T: Subordinate choice of conflict handling modes. *Nurs Admin Q* 11:29–34, 1986

79. Barton A: Conflict resolution by nurse managers. *Nurs Manage* 22:83–86, 1991

80. Curtin L, Flaherty M: The nurse–nurse relationship, in McCorkle R, Hongladarom G (eds): *Issues and Topics in Cancer Nursing*. Norwalk, CT, Appleton-Century-Crofts, 1986, pp 24–40

81. American Nurses' Association and Oncology Nursing Society: *Standards of Oncology Nursing Practice*. Kansas City, MO, American Nurses' Association, 1987

82. Cox A, Andrews P: The development of support systems on oncology units. *Oncol Nurs Forum* 8:31–35, 1981

83. Calhoun G, Calhoun J: Occupational stress—implications for hospitals, in Selye H (ed): *Selye's Guide to Stress Research* vol 3. New York, VanNostrand Reinhold, 1983, pp 99–110

84. Scanlon C: Survey yields significant results. *Communiqué* (ANA Center for Ethics and Human Rights) 3:1–3, 1994

85. Scanlon C, Glover J: A professional code of ethics: Providing a moral compass in turbulent times. *Oncol Nurs Forum* 22:1515–1521, 1995

86. Menzies I: A case study in the function of social systems as a defense against anxiety. *Human Relat* 13:13–19, 1960

87. Matthews P: A study of the effect of administrative climate on the nurses' psychological orientation toward the hospitalized patient. Unpublished doctoral dissertation. University of California, Berkley, 1962

88. Lavandero R: Nurse burnout: What can we learn? *J Nurs Admin* 11:17–23, 1981

89. Menaghan E: Individual coping efforts: Moderators of the relationship between life stress and mental health outcomes, in Kaplan H (ed): *Psychosocial Stress*. New York, Academic Press, 1983, pp 157–191

90. Auerbach S: Stress management and coping research in the health care setting: An overview and methodological commentary. *J Consult Clin Psych* 57:388–395, 1989

91. Caplan G: *Principles of Preventative Psychiatry*. New York, Basic Books, 1964

92. Covey S: *The 7 Habits of Highly Effective People*. New York, Simon & Schuster, 1989

93. Smith C: Principles in time management, in Jacobson S, McGrath H (eds): *Nurses Under Stress*. New York, Wiley, 1983, pp 226–236

94. Medvic B, Pelusi J, Camp-Sorrell D, et al: Assistive personnel: Their use in cancer care—An Oncology Nursing Society position paper. *Oncol Nurs Forum* 23:647–651, 1996

95. Ellis A: *Reason and Emotion in Psychotherapy*. New York, Lyle Stuart, 1962

96. Lief H, Fox D: Training for "detached concern" in medical students, in Lief H, Lief V, Lief N (eds): *The Psychological Basis of Medical Practice*. New York, Harper & Row, 1963, pp 56–65

97. Gray B: How to prepare and plan for the career that suits your needs: Assess yourself, assess the market, sharpen your skills, go for it! *Nurs Allied Healthweek—Houston/San Antonio* 1:20–23, 1996

98. Charlesworth E, Nathan R: *Stress Management*. New York, Atheneum, 1985

99. Allen R, Kraft C: From burnout: Improving the quality of hospital work life. *Hosp Forum* 24:18–28, 1981

100. Jacobson S, McGrath M: *Nurses Under Stress*. New York, Wiley, 1983

101. Prescott P: Nursing: An important component of hospital survival under a reformed healthcare system. *Nurs Economic$* 11:192–199

102. American Nurses' Association: *Nursing Care Report Card for Acute Care*. Washington, DC, American Nurses' Association, 1995

103. American Nurses' Association: *RN Utilization of Unlicensed Assistive Personnel Position Statement*. Washington, DC, American Nurses' Association, 1992

104. Winslow R: Major purchasers of health services form alliance to evaluate HMO care. *Wall Street J* July 3: A3, 1995

105. Brider P: AJN Newsline. *Am J Nurs* 96:61–64, 1996

106. Porter-O'Grady T: The seven basic rules for successful redesign. *J Nurs Admin* 26:46–53, 1996

107. Schmitt M: Social support, occupational stressors, and health in cancer nursing, in Baird S, McCorkle R, Grant M (eds): *Cancer Nursing. A Comprehensive Textbook*. Philadelphia, Saunders, 1991, pp 1065–1075

108. Beckard R: Organizational implications of team building, in Wise H, Beckard R, Rubin I, Kyte A (eds): *Making Health Care Teams Work*. Cambridge, MA, Ballinger, 1974, pp 69–94

109. American Nurses Association: *Code for Nurses with Interpretative Statements*. Washington, DC, American Nurses' Association, 1985

# Chapter 66

# Cancer Nursing Resources

Barbara A. Barhamand, RN, MS, AOCN

# ALPHABETICAL INDEX

## How to Use This Chapter

These Cancer Nursing Resources were compiled from a recent survey of a variety of health- and oncology-related organizations and resources that responded in varying lengths and formats. This compilation is the latest information the author has received, but the accuracy and timeliness of membership information, prices for publications, and other data remain the responsibility of the respondents.

If you know the name of the resource you are looking for:

Refer to the Alphabetical Index, keeping in mind that many organizations change their names as they restructure or reprioritize. Each resource is followed by a bracketed number (its numerical listing) and a page reference.

If you are looking for a resource by subject (i.e., pain):

Refer to the Cross-Referencing Index where subjects are listed alphabetically. After each subject are numerical listings (in brackets) of resources that can be perused for appropriateness. Some resources are cross-referenced more than once; some are not cross-referenced at all if they are a resource of a more general nature.

## CROSS-REFERENCING SUBJECT INDEX

# ORGANIZATIONS

## Patient Assistance and Support Organizations

### 1. American Academy of Dermatology
P.O. Box 681069
Schaumburg, IL 60168
(708) 330-0230

The American Academy of Dermatology offers a catalogue of brochures that are available by writing the above address and enclosing a self-addressed, stamped envelope. The brochures are free of charge unless requested in quantities. The Academy gives physician referrals for patients in their geographic location.

Sample brochure titles include:

The Sun and Your Skin
Skin Cancer: An Undeclared Epidemic

### 2. American Brain Tumor Association
2720 River Road
Des Plaines, IL 60018
(formerly Association for Brain Tumor Research)
(847) 827-9910; FAX (847) 886-2282
E-mail: ABTA@aol.com
(800) 886-2282 Patient Services

The American Brain Tumor Association is a national organization that provides written information about brain tumors and their treatment. Services include patient education materials, listings of brain tumor support groups, referrals to support organizations, and information about treatment facilities. A complimentary triannual newsletter, the *Message Line*, describes research advances and announces updates to publications. Single copies of all materials are available to patients and health care professionals at no cost; the ABTA charges a nominal fee per each for multiple copies.

Publications from the American Brain Tumor Association:

**Basic information:**
A Brain Tumor—Sharing Hope (English and Spanish)
A Primer of Brain Tumors
Dictionary for Brain Tumor Patients
**Tumor information:**
About Ependymoma
About Glioblastoma and Anaplastic Astrocytoma
About Medulloblastoma/PNET
About Meningioma
About Metastatic Tumors to the Brain and Spine
About Oligodendroglioma and Mixed Glioma
About Pituitary Tumors
**Treatment information:**
Chemotherapy of Brain Tumors
Immunotherapy of Brain Tumors
Radiation Therapy of Brain Tumors, Part I: A Basic Guide
Radiation Therapy of Brain Tumors, Part II: Background and Research Guide
Shunts

**Information for and about children:**
ALEX'S JOURNEY: The Story of a Child with a Brain Tumor
When Your Child Is Ready to Return to School
**Help and resources:**
Coping With a Brain Tumor, Part I: From Diagnosis to Treatment
Coping With a Brain Tumor, Part II: During and After Treatment
Organizing a Support Group
Using a Medical Library

### 3. American Cancer Society (ACS)
1599 Clifton Road, NE
Atlanta, GA 30329-4251
(404) 320-3333; (800) ACS-2345

Each local unit or division has an extensive assortment of booklets, videos, slides, reprints, posters, audiotapes, programs, and proceedings available at no charge covering all aspects of the cancer experience. Many also are available in Spanish. Some states have a computer response system for approved information. The caller can request information on most cancer-related topics (e.g., unproven methods of cancer treatment) and receive a written synopsis with the "ACS's official opinion."

Sample pamphlet titles include:
First Aid for Laryngectomees
First Steps: Helping Words (for laryngectomees)
Your New Voice
Rehabilitating Laryngectomees
Finding a Lump in Your Breast
Back to School (for parents of children with cancer)
Caring for the Patient with Cancer at Home
Chemotherapy: What It Is, How It Helps
It Helps to Have Friends (when Mom or Dad has cancer)
Talking with Your Doctor
Talking with the Cancer Patient: Listen with Your Heart
When Your Brother or Sister Has Cancer
Colostomy—A Guide
Ileostomy—A Guide
Urostomy—A Guide
Sexuality and Cancer (for the woman who has cancer)
Sexuality and Cancer (for the man who has cancer)

### 4. ACS–I Can Cope

This course addresses the educational needs of people facing cancer—patients, family members, and friends. In a series of classes, often conducted in cooperation with a local hospital, participants learn about the diagnosis and treatment of cancer as well as self-care strategies for coping with the challenges that cancer presents. Physicians, nurses, social workers, and community representatives serve as guest speakers. The program has been recently revised and updated to incorporate information about advances in cancer control and to better utilize principles of adult learning and up-to-date audiovisual technologies.

### 5. ACS–Loan Closets

Many ACS units have loan closets that supply sickroom equipment for home cancer patients that is not otherwise covered by health insurance. Equipment may include wheelchairs, walkers, surgical dressings, bedpans, hospital beds, shower chairs, etc. This equipment can be borrowed for as long as needed. Contact your local unit for this free service.

### 6. ACS–Reach to Recovery

The American Cancer Society's Reach for Recovery program provides support and information about breast cancer and its treatment to women with a personal concern about the disease. Its goal is to help breast cancer patients deal with the physical, emotional, and cosmetic needs related to the disease and/or treatment. The program has more than 13,000 volunteers and is available in over 30 other countries. Reach to Recovery volunteers are women who have adjusted successfully to their own breast cancer experience and offer a positive role model to patients. They are carefully selected and trained to visit patients in the hospital, at home or another mutually agreed upon site, or by telephone. In some areas, visits are also made with partners of breast cancer patients and their family members. Empathetic, knowledgeable, and responsible volunteers provide objective medical information, but no medical advice. Originally, the program was limited to in-hospital volunteer visits with post-mastectomy patients. In recent years, Reach to Recovery has expanded in many communities to include specialized volunteer visits for early support and information on lumpectomy, breast reconstruction, and recurrence. Any hospital visit made by a Reach to Recovery volunteer first must be approved by the patient's attending physician. However, a hospital visit can be requested by another health professional such as a nurse or social worker. A family member, friend, or the patient herself may request a visit at home or away from the hospital. All visits made through the Reach to Recovery program are offered at no charge.

### 7. ACS–Road to Recovery: Man to Man Prostate Cancer Education and Support Program

This new program educates and supports men facing prostate cancer by providing them an opportunity to talk openly with each other and with health care professionals about their disease and related concerns. It consists of two primary components. The first is a presentation by a health care professional on a topic relevant to prostate cancer followed by questions and answers. The other component is a supportive sharing session facilitated by a trained ACS volunteer.

### 8. American Foundation for Urologic Disease, Inc.

300 West Pratt Street
Suite 401
Baltimore, MD 21201
(410) 727-2908; FAX (410) 528-0550

The American Foundation for Urologic Disease, Inc. is a national not-for-profit organization dedicated to the prevention and cure of urologic diseases through the expansion of medical research and the education of the public and health care professionals about urologic diseases and dysfunctions, including prostate and bladder cancer.

The foundation's health education councils are the nationally recognized clearinghouse for accurate and informative patient education materials for men, women, and children. More than 5 million patient education brochures have been published. Participation in national awareness programs help patients to work together with their physician to make an informed decision about treatment options.

The foundation's research scholars program has been the catalyst for the expansion of research funding to the best and brightest urologic investigators across the nation. More than $1 million each year is provided to fund urologic research.

The prostate cancer support group network facilitates intergroup communications and program development for individual prostate cancer survivor support groups. The network enhances quality of life for patients and their families and provides a forum for them to share ideas and feelings. The foundation offers a membership to patients, the public, and medical professionals. The periodical *Family Urology* is published quarterly.

### 9. American Lung Association (ALA)

1740 Broadway
New York, NY 10019-4374
(212) 315-8700; (800) LUNG-USA

The ALA is a nonprofit organization, devoted to conquering lung disease. The ALA promotes lung health by conducting educational programs, as well as sponsoring symposia, conferences, publications, films, fellowships, and research grants. Local chapters can provide smoking literature, posters, buttons, and smoking cessation materials.

Call for a free catalogue of public education materials that includes:

**Pamphlets:**
Cigarette Smoking: The Facts About Your Lungs
Facts About Asthma
Facts About Lung Cancer
Facts About Radon
Facts About Second-Hand Smoke
Lung Hazards on the Job: Occupational Lung Cancer
A No Smoking Coloring Book (for children)
Occupational Lung Diseases

**Posters:**
Thanks for Not Smoking
Brooke Shields: Smoking Spoils Your Looks

**Films:**
*Breathing Easy Film*—for fifth- through eighth-graders
*As We See It*—made for preteens

**Anti-smoking programs:**
Freedom from Smoking Booklets: a self-help book shows you how to quit smoking in 20 days
Freedom from Smoking Home Video Program *In Control*

**Puzzles:**
Have Fun!! Figure Out the Smoking Puzzle

### 10. American Self-Help Clearinghouse

Northwest Covenant Medical Center
Denville, NJ 07834-2995
(201) 625-7101 group information; TDD (201) 625-9053
(201) 625-9565 Administrative; FAX (201) 625-8848

**Consultation service**
The Clearinghouse staff and volunteers provide current information and contacts for any national self-help groups that address the caller's particular concern. If no appropriate national groups exist and the caller is interested in the possibility of joining with others to start a local group, information is available on model groups operating in other parts of the country, or individuals who are attempting to start such networks. Specific interests and concerns can also be

listed on the computer database that cross-references with over a dozen other self-help clearinghouses in the United States and Canada.

**Free handouts** (send a stamped, self-addressed envelope with request):

Ideas for Starting a Self-Help Group

Listing of phone contacts for self-help clearinghouses

**Print resource book**

*The Self-Help Sourcebook* is a comprehensive national guide to finding and forming mutual aid and self-help groups.

Updated contacts and descriptions for over 700 national and model self-help groups, that cover a broad range of disabilities, specific illnesses, parenting concerns, bereavement, and many other stressful life situations. Also included are general ideas and suggestions for starting a mutual-aid self-help group, contacts for dozens of self-help clearinghouses worldwide, a listing of over 100 national toll-free helplines, resources for rare and genetic illnesses, on-line computer networks, and an easy-to-use index.

Cost per copy postage-paid is $9.00 (book rate postage) or $11.00 (first-class mail). Prepayment required. ISSN:8756-1425. Paperback, 270 pages; May 1995.

**Other helpful organizations**

O.D.P.H.P. National Health Information Clearinghouse (800) 336-4797 in U.S.

National Organization for Rare Disorders (800) 999-N.O.R.D. in U.S.

Alliance of Genetic Support Groups (genetic illnesses) (800) 336-GENE in U.S.

### 11. Aplastic Anemia Foundation of America (AAFA)

P.O. Box 22689
Baltimore, MD 21203
(410) 955-2803

The AAFA was founded in 1984 to promote the need for furthering research into the causes and cures of aplastic anemia. In addition to educating the public about the disease, the AAFA assists those who have the disease and their families. Board and family support meetings are held.

### 12. Association for Research of Childhood Cancer

P.O. Box 251
Buffalo, NY 14225-0251
(716) 689-8922

The Association for Research of Childhood Cancer is composed of parents who have lost children to cancer and of people who support cancer research. The association funds the expansion and continuation of research in pediatric cancer centers and provides money for pilot projects in cancer research. The association meets six times per year to support parents of children with cancer and also publishes a quarterly newsletter and the *Parent/Child Handbook*.

### 13. CAnCare

Cancer Partners: A Supportive Network
2929 Selwyn Avenue
Charlotte, NC 28209
(704) 372-1232; FAX (704) 372-6910

CAnCare is a one-on-one psychosocial support service for cancer patients and their families. Volunteers have experienced cancer either as patient or family member. After completing a required training course, volunteers are matched with cancer patients with whom they build sup-portive relationships that last throughout the trauma. Volunteers, men and women, represent some 30 different cancers, and range in age from the 20s to the 80s. Listening to the concerns of the cancer patient, they help defuse fears and build hope. The link between volunteer and patient is a win-win situation, helping both as healing energy flows between them. CAnCare has been in service for 11 years. It is supported by churches, corporations, and grass-roots contributions.

### 14. Cancer Care, Inc.

1180 Avenue of the Americas
New York, NY 10036
(212) 221-3300; (800) 813-HOPE

Cancer Care is a nonprofit, nonsectarian, social service agency founded in 1944 to help cancer patients and their families and friends cope with the impact of cancer. Cancer Care is separate and apart from any other cancer organization. They are the largest agency in the nation solely dedicated to providing psychosocial support to cancer patients and their families and community education programs for the general public. They treat people at all stages of the illness and provide help to both patient and family.

Cancer Care provides the following services:

- professional counseling for cancer patients and their families, both on an individual basis and in groups

- supplementary financial assistance to help families meet certain home care costs such as homemakers, home health aides, housekeepers, transportation to radiation and chemotherapy treatments, and pain medication expense (only available in NY, NJ, and CT)

- bereavement counseling to help surviving family members cope with their loss

- information and referral to homemaking services, hospices, child care services, hospitals, and other resources in the community

- guidance to develop a plan for care for the patient at home

- volunteer program where volunteers act as friendly visitors to homebound or frail cancer patients

- education and training regarding psychosocial aspects of cancer for professionals and allied health care providers

Cancer Care has offices in:

New York City
1180 Avenue of the Americas
New York, NY 10036
(212) 302-2400

Long Island
20 Crossways Park North
Suite 304
Woodbury, NY 11797
(516) 364-8130

New Jersey Central office
241 Millburn Avenue, Suite 241-C
Millburn, NJ 07041
(201) 379-7500

Bergen County office
141 Dayton Street
Ridgewood, NJ 07450
(201) 444-6630

Connecticut
120 East Avenue
Norwalk, CT 06851
(203) 854-9911

Services are available at other part-time offices in the tri-state area. For information call (212) 302-2400 or 1-800-813-HOPE.

**15. Cancer Connection**
H & R Block Building
4410 Main
Kansas City, MO 64111
(816) 932-8453

The Cancer Connection was founded in 1980. It sponsors the Cancer Hot Line, a support group that matches cancer victims with volunteers who have the same type of cancer and have either been cured, are in remission, or are being treated. Volunteers describe treatments they have received and provide information referrals to persons newly-diagnosed with cancer. Cancer Hotlines operate in St. Louis, Kansas City, Ft. Lauderdale, Ft. Worth, Oklahoma City, Cleveland, and Pittsburgh. Long distance counseling is also available.

**16. Cancer Information Service**
NCI-Office of Cancer Communications
Building 31, Room 10A 16
Bethesda, MD 20892
(800) 4-CANCER

The Cancer Information Service (CIS) is a nationwide network of 19 regional field offices supported by the NCI that provides up-to-date information on cancer to patients and their families, health care professionals, and the general public. The CIS can provide specific information in English and Spanish about particular types of cancer, as well as information on how to obtain second opinions and the availability of clinical trials. Each CIS office has access to the NCI treatment database PDQ, which offers callers the most current state-of-the-art treatment and clinical trial information. Through the outreach program, the CIS serves as a resource for state and regional organizations by providing printed materials and technical assistance for cancer education, media campaigns, and community programs.

NCI publications are available on a wide variety of topics including prevention and detection, treatment, survivorship, and research. Many are also available for Spanish or pediatric clientele. All are free, but quantities may be limited per monthly order. Allow four to six weeks for delivery of large orders. A catalogue listing or specific booklets are available by phone order. Examples include:

Chemotherapy and You
Radiation Therapy and You
Eating Hints
Facing Forward
Get Relief from Cancer Pain
Taking Time
Advanced Cancer: Living Each Day
Talking with Your Child About Cancer
What Are Clinical Trials All About
When Cancer Recurs: Meeting the Challenge Again
When Someone in Your Family Has Cancer
Young People with Cancer
Cancer Survivorship: An Annotated Bibliography

Site-specific booklets address individual cancers in the series:
What you need to know about:

| | |
|---|---|
| Bladder | Lung |
| Bone | Melanoma |
| Brain and Spinal Cord | Multiple Myeloma |
| Breast | Non-Hodgkin's Lymphoma |
| Cervix | Head or Neck |
| Colon and Rectum | Ovary |
| Esophagus | Pancreas |
| Hodgkin's Disease | Prostate |
| Kidney | Skin |
| Larynx | Stomach |
| Adult Leukemia | Testis |
| Childhood Leukemia | Uterus |

**17. Cancer Support Network**
802 E. Jefferson
Bloomington, IL 61701
(309) 829-2273

The Cancer Support Network is a not-for-profit organization formed to provide personal support and encouragement to cancer patients in a number of ways. They do not provide medical advice or make referrals. Although not funded by the American Cancer Society or the National Cancer Institute, they do network with them and a variety of support groups across the country to get answers to questions asked by people with cancer. Cancer Support Network has a lending library, support groups, and hotline manned by volunteers—(309) 829-CARE.

**18. Candlelighters Childhood Cancer Foundation**
7910 Woodmont Avenue, Suite 460
Bethesda, MD 20814
(301) 657-8401 or (800) 366-CCCF; FAX (301) 657-8319

Candlelighters is an organization for children and the parents of children with cancer, as well as adult survivors of childhood cancer. There are presently 250 chapters in the United States. Candlelighters has two primary goals: to obtain consistent and adequate federal support for cancer research, and to help parents and other family members who share the particularly difficult experience of living with a child with cancer. A national newsletter is published quarterly, which serves as a communication link among parents and parents' groups and concerned professionals. A quarterly youth newsletter, *Candlelighters Childhood Cancer Foundation Youth Newsletter*, is written by and for adolescent cancer patients and teenage siblings to provide information to young cancer patients. The free newsletters include information about research in childhood cancer, bibliography materials, and group activities. A third newsletter for adult survivors of childhood cancers is also available. Local groups usually have their own newsletter. Candlelighters also publishes a resource list of childhood cancer education materials. All the above information is available free on request. The Ombudsman Program provides free legal help to those having difficulties with insurance, employment, or school.

**19. Children's Hospice International**
1850 M Street NW, Suite 900
Washington, DC 20036
(703) 684-0330; (800) 242-4453; FAX (703) 684-0226

Children's Hospice International provides a network of support for dying children and their families. It serves as a clearinghouse for research programs, support groups, and education and training programs for the care of terminally ill children. It also offers publications on topics such as home care for seriously ill children and pain management.

**20. Choice in Dying**
200 Varick Street, 10th Floor
New York, NY 10014-4810
(212) 366-5540; (800) 989-9455; FAX (212) 366-5337

CID is a national, not-for-profit organization dedicated to serving the needs of dying patients and their families. The organization developed the first living will 25 years ago and has distributed approximately 10 million living wills to date. CID is the nation's largest provider of state-specific advance directives—the general term for two types of legal documents: a living will and a durable power of attorney for health care. Individuals can receive one free set of their state's advance directive by calling (800) 989-9455. CID advocates the right of patients to participate fully in decisions about their medical treatment at the end of life. CID is the only organization that deals broadly and practically with end-of-life issues and provides substantial free public and professional education and counseling about the preparation and use of advance directives. CID provides reasonably priced educational videotapes, programs, speakers, and published materials to the general public, health care professionals, and lawmakers about the needs of people who are dying. A price list of materials, including bulk price/quantity discount information, are available upon request.

**21. Coping**
Media America, Inc.
P.O. Box 682268
Franklin, TN 37068-2268
(615) 790-2400

*Coping* magazine is the only nationally-distributed consumer magazine for people whose lives have been touched by cancer. Its primary purpose is to empower the readers (be they patients or professionals) by providing the knowledge they need to cope with the many issues confronting their daily lives. *Coping* aims to inspire patients and survivors to assume greater responsibility for, and participation in, the many facets of their disease. *Coping* is published bimonthly (six times a year) and the subscription cost is $18 annually ($24 Canadian/foreign) or $32 ($44 Canadian/foreign) for two years.

**22. Corporate Angel Network, Inc.**
Westchester County Airport, Building One
White Plains, NY 10604
(914) 328-1313; FAX (800) 328-4226

The Corporate Angel Network (CAN) is a nonprofit organization designed to arrange free air transportation for cancer patients. This nationwide program uses available seats on corporate aircraft being flown on business trips. CAN enables patients to obtain optimum treatment for their life-threatening disease. CAN permits patients to travel in comfort and dignity, spared the stresses of commercial air travel. CAN has already flown over 4300 patients through the cooperation and generosity of more than 500 participating corporations. Financial need is *not* a requirement.

Patient criteria include:
   Going to or from recognized treatment, consultation, or
      check-up.

Be able to walk onto the aircraft unassisted.
Not require life support systems or special services.
Provide doctor's name, address, and telephone number.
May be the bone marrow or blood platelet donor.
May be accompanied by someone, if space permits. Both
   parents may accompany a child patient.
Patients should make back-up commercial transportation plans.

CAN cannot guarantee to find an appropriate flight.

**23. Gilda Radner Familial Ovarian Cancer Registry**
Roswell Park Cancer Institute
New York State Department of Health
Elm and Carlton Streets
Buffalo, NY 14263
(800) OVARIAN; FAX (716) 845-7608

Individuals can register, and the registry has a newsletter.

**24. Histiocytosis Association of America**
302 N. Broadway
Pitman, NJ 08071
(800) 548-2758

The Histiocytosis Association of America is a nonprofit organization which supports the emotional and educational needs of families of children and the adult patients who have any of the histiocytoses. The Association has developed two free brochures:
   The Facts about Langerhans Cell Histiocytosis
   The Facts about Diabetes Insipidus and LCH

**25. Hospice Education Institute**
190 Westbrook Road
Essex, CT 06426-1511
(860) 767-1620; (800) 331-1620; FAX (860) 767-2746

The Hospice Education Institute is an independent, nonprofit organization founded in 1985. It serves a wide range of individuals and organizations interested in hospice and palliative care throughout the United States and around the world. Its toll-free referral service directs over 21,000 callers a year to local hospice programs. Further, by working with health and caring professionals and with educators who teach courses on dying, grief, and bereavement, the Hospice Education Institute disseminates information about hospice care at many levels.

The services of the Hospice Education Institute include:

- HOSPICELINK, which maintains a computerized and continually updated directory of hospice programs in the United States, and operates a toll-free telephone number (800-331-1620) to refer callers to local hospice and palliative care programs. HOSPICELINK also provides general information about the principles and practice of hospice care. Staff members will listen sympathetically and give limited, informal support to callers who wish to discuss immediate personal problems relating to terminal illness and bereavement. (HOSPICELINK does not offer medical advice, answer insurance questions, or provide psychological counseling.) There is no charge for any HOSPICELINK service.

- Regional seminars on many aspects of caring for dying and the bereaved are organized for health and caring professionals and qualified hospice volunteers. Since 1986, seminars have been offered in 24 states. Faculty members for these seminars are international multiprofessional experts on hospice care. The Institute also sponsors the annual Hospice Study Seminar in Britain—a two-week workshop for hospice professionals from all over the world.

- Advice and assistance are freely given to people working to begin or improve hospice care in their communities. Books and pamphlets are available from the Hospice Education Institute on hospice-related subjects. The Hospice Education Institute's *Notes on Symptom Control in Hospice and Palliative Care* is the definitive work to date on symptom control. ($28.95, plus $4.25 for shipping and handling)

Other publications are:
*Loss and Bereavement* (Cook/Phillips) ($12.95)
*Being There: Pastoral Care in Time of Illness* (Speck) ($13.95)
*Letting Go: Caring for the Dying and Bereaved* (Ainsworth-Smith/Speck) ($13.95)
*Hospice Movement* (Vintage) $13.00
*Good Friday People* (Orbis) $10.95
*Sharing the Darkness* (Orbis) $10.95
*How Many Times Can You Say Goodbye* (Liturgical Press) $6.95

### 26. International Association of Laryngectomees

c/o American Cancer Society
1599 Clifton Road, NE
Atlanta, GA 30329-4251
(404) 320-3333

The International Association of Laryngectomees (IAL) is a voluntary, nonprofit organization dedicated to the total rehabilitation of laryngectomees. The IAL promotes and supports the total rehabilitation of laryngectomees through the exchange and dissemination of ideas and information to laryngectomee clubs and to the public. These clubs encourage and help laryngectomees improve their quality of life by providing a supportive environment to help them make the adjustments associated with laryngectomy surgery.

The IAL works to upgrade the minimum standards for teachers of alaryngeal speech; to foster improvement in hospital laryngectomee programs; and to increase awareness about the appropriate first-aid techniques for laryngectomees. With support from the American Cancer Society, the IAL publishes educational materials and a tri-annual newsletter, maintains a registry of post-laryngectomy speech instructors, and sponsors an annual voice rehabilitation institute and an annual general meeting for laryngectomees.

The IAL was formed in 1952 by representatives of a number of laryngectomee clubs to answer the need for coordinating the activities of the clubs. The IAL consists of nearly 300 member clubs located throughout the United States and in several foreign countries. These clubs usually meet once or twice a month for informational programs and support. Most clubs also maintain a patient visitation program coordinated with medical professionals in local hospitals and clinics.

### 27. Let's Face It

A network for people with facial difference.
P.O. Box 29972
Bellingham, WA 98228-1972
(360) 676-7325

Let's Face It is the U.S. branch of an international self-help network dedicated to helping people with facial difference,

their loved ones, the professionals who care for them, and the communities in which they live, to understand and to solve the problems of living with this disability.

The goals of the organization are:

- To link and educate family, friends, and professionals.

- To educate the public to value the person behind every face.

- To assist facially different people to share their experiences, strengths, and hopes. Sharing experiences through a mutual help network often speeds adjustment to disabilities.

- To educate and provide continuing education to medical, nursing, and allied health professionals.

The organization has an annual directory, *Resources for People with Facial Difference*, that provides information on a variety of organizations the individual with a facial difference could utilize. For a free copy of this 40 page booklet, send a 9" × 12" self-addressed envelope, stamped with $3.00 postage, and a short note explaining the request.

### 28. Leukemia Society of America

National Headquarters
600 Third Avenue
New York, NY 10016
(212) 573-8484; (800) 955-4LSA (Hotline for Information)

The Leukemia Society of America, Inc. is a national voluntary health agency dedicated solely to seeking the cause and eventual cure of leukemia and allied diseases. The Society supports five major programs: research, patient aid, public and professional education, and community service.

**Research:**
The Society's research program is based on the belief that all medically sound approaches toward a cure or control of leukemia should be encouraged on a worldwide basis. To this end, almost $7.5 million was allocated in 1995 to support about 200 researchers working at 80 accredited institutions in the United States and throughout the world

**Education:**
The Society pursues an aggressive program to provide current information on leukemia and related diseases to the general public. It alerts the public to disease danger, treatment, and therapy through literature and posters, films and other audiovisual materials, speaking engagements, seminars and educational programs, news and feature releases, and public service advertising in all media. Information is available from each local chapter and from the Society's national headquarters in New York City.

**Patient aid:**
Financial assistance up to $750 a year per person is given by the Society to outpatients being treated for leukemia, lymphoma, multiple myeloma, and preleukemia. Outpatients are those not confined to a hospital, although they may be treated at various times at a hospital. They do not remain there for continuous management of their illnesses. In 1994, more than 6000 patients received $1.6 million supplementary financial aid from the Society.

**Community service:**
The Society conducts a two-way communications program established with the social service agencies and

treatment facilities in the area. Information is collected for the benefit of patients and families who may need to know about resources available to them. Chapters interact with government health departments and many varied family assistance organizations. The compilation and maintenance of resource and referral material is a high-priority item on our list of services so that assistance is available to all leukemia patients at all times.

**Sample of publications from the Leukemia Society of America:**

Facts About the Leukemia Society of America (English and Spanish)
Leukemia
Lymphomas
Hodgkin's Disease
Multiple Myeloma
Patient-Aid Program (English and Spanish)
What Everyone Should Know About Leukemia (English and Spanish)
Emotional Aspects of Childhood Leukemia
Bone Marrow Transplantation (English and Spanish)
Forty Years of Progress: The Story of the Leukemia Society Research Report
Chronic Myelogenous Leukemia (CML)
Acute Myelogenous Leukemia (AML)
Acute Lymphocytic Leukemia (ALL)
Chronic Lymphocytic Leukemia (CLL)
Coping with Survival

**Videotapes (VHS):**

*A Sense of Hope*
*Must Win*
*What It Is That I Have, Don't Want. . .*
*A Critical Decision*
*Otteau Christiansen; Victory Story*
*Closing in on a Cure*
*I'm Still Me*

**29. Look Good . . . Feel Better (LGFB)**
The CTFA Foundation
1101 17th St., N.W.
Suite 300
Washington, DC 20036
(800) 395-LOOK

Look Good . . . Feel Better is a free nationwide public service program that helps women cancer patients learn to overcome the appearance-related side effects associated with cancer treatment. Trained volunteers offer guidance and instruction to women in a supportive environment, helping them regain their confidence and self-esteem. Look Good . . . Feel Better is a nonmedical, product-neutral program made possible by a partnership between the Cosmetic, Toiletry & Fragrance Association (CTFA) Foundation, the American Cancer Society (ACS), and the National Cosmetology Association (NCA). The CTFA Foundation provides the complimentary makeup and free educational materials, such as videotapes and pamphlets, and secures financial support for LGFB. The ACS administers the program and the NCA organizes the volunteer cosmetologists.

Look Good . . . Feel Better is available to patients in one of three ways. The first, and most popular LGFB format, is a structured group session consisting of six to ten patients. This group session usually is offered in a hospital and

includes a group of trained cosmetologists who instruct the patients in how to use makeup, wigs, scarves, turbans, and accessories to camouflage the appearance changes resulting from their treatments. Each patient receives a complimentary bag of assorted cosmetics that are used in the session, with guidance from the cosmetologists. The goal is to teach the patients cosmetic techniques they can take home and use every day, allowing them to gain some control over their lives.

The second format available is a free, private consultation with a trained cosmetologist in a salon or other private setting. The techniques taught are the same as in a group session. We have found that the group session is the more popular of the two formats, because it tends to serve as an informal support group for the women by allowing them to discuss a part of their treatment that no one else understands quite as well as other patients and cosmetologists.

In locations where group or one-on-one Look Good. . . Feel Better sessions are not available, a patient brochure and self-help video are available through the ACS. Materials are available in English and Spanish.

**30. LymphEdema Foundation**
P.O. Box 834
San Diego, CA 92014-0834
(800) LYMPH-DX or (800) 596-7439

This organization provides information and resources to people with lymphedema and to health care professionals who treat the condition. Membership and the quarterly publication *LymphEdema Digest* are free of charge.

**31. Make-A-Wish Foundation of America**
100 W. Clarendon, Suite 2200
Phoenix, AZ 85013-3518
(602) 279-9474; (800) 722-9774

The Make-A-Wish Foundation of America is a nonprofit organization whose main purpose is to fulfill the wishes of children with life-threatening or terminal illnesses. The foundation will consider the wish of any child under the age of 18 anywhere in the world and covers all expenses related to granting the wish.

**32. Medic Alert Foundation**
2323 Colorado Ave.
Turlock, CA 95382
(800) 432-5378; (800) ID ALERT

Medic Alert's three-part life-protecting system consists of:

- A metal alerting emblem worn as a bracelet or necklace. The emblem bears the staff of Aesculapius, the internationally recognized insignia of the medical profession, and the words "Medic Alert." On the reverse side are engraved the special medical conditions of the wearer such as "hypertension," "takes beta blocker," "allergic to penicillin," or "wearing contact lenses." Also engraved on the back are the member's identification number and the number for Medic Alert's Emergency Response Center.

- The 24-hour-a-day Emergency Response Center provides detailed data to emergency personnel via a collect telephone call from anywhere in the world. Medic Alert's emergency hotline number engraved on the back of the emblem and printed on the wallet card provides vital information that aids diagnosis and speeds life-saving treatments.

- Each member receives a wallet card with personal and medical information in addition to that engraved on the emblem. Each year, the members receive a wallet card copy of the information listed on their computerized medical record. This serves as a reminder to members to keep their record up-to-date. The record may be updated at any time by phone or mail. Whenever the record is updated, a new wallet card is prepared with the new information and sent immediately to the member.

Medic Alert serves about 45 countries from a network of affiliate offices worldwide. Initial membership is $35 with annual renewals of $15. This includes a free update of medical records. Free memberships are provided to individuals with special economic needs on the written request of a physician or a social worker. Membership in the United States now totals approximately 2.3 million people.

### 33. National Alliance of Breast Cancer Organizations (NABCO)
1180 Avenue of the Americas
2nd Floor
New York, NY 10036
(NABCO prefers written inquiries.)
(212) 719-0154

NABCO is a central resource for information on breast cancer. Membership contributions are tax-deductible and entitle the member to receive the NABCO *Resource List*, a copy of the *NABCO News* (published quarterly), and special mailings on breast cancer issues. Individual–$40; Nonprofit group–$75; Business–$150.

The following is a list of publications developed from the 1994/95 edition of the National Alliance of Breast Cancer Organizations' (NABCO) Breast Cancer Resource List.

**General information about breast cancer:**
Breast Cancer: Risk, Protection, Detection, and Treatment
    Order from: DES Action, 1615 Broadway, Oakland, CA 94612 (31 pp; $2.50 each)
Early Detection Brochure
    Order from: NABCO (Up to 25 copies are free; $8.00 per 100)
*Dr. Susan Love's Breast Book*
    Susan Love, MD with Karen Lindsey. Reading, MA, Addison-Wesley (455 pp, paperback, $17; 1995). Available in bookstores.
*If You've Thought About Breast Cancer . . .*
    Order from: Rose Kuschner Breast Cancer Advisory Center, PO Box 224, Kensington, MD 20895, (301) 949-2531 (44 pp; single copies available free from Y-Me)
*Make Sure You Do Not Have Breast Cancer*
    Philip Strax, MD. New York, St. Martin's Press (118 pp, paperback, $8.95; 1991). Available in bookstores.
*The Breast Cancer Digest: A Guide to Medical Care, Emotional Support, Educational Programs, and Resources*
    NCI (84-1691) (212 pages, free; 1991)
*The Race Is Run One Step at a Time: My Personal Struggle and Every Woman's Guide to Taking Charge of Breast Cancer*
    Nancy Brinker with Catherine McEvily Harris. New York, Simon & Schuster (219 pp, hardcover, $18.95; 224 pp, paperback, $10). Available in bookstores or from the Komen Foundation.
*What You Need to Know About Breast Cancer*
    NCI (Catalogue # 91-1556); free; 33 pages

### 34. National Association of People with AIDS (NAPWA)
1413 K Street, N.W., 10th Floor
Washington, D.C. 20005
(202) 898-0414

The National Association of People With AIDS (NAPWA) is dedicated to improving the lives of people with HIV disease at home, in the workplace, and in the community. Since 1983, NAPWA has served as the "voice" for the needs and concerns of all people infected and affected by HIV/AIDS in the United States. NAPWA works to focus national attention on the realities faced by people living with HIV disease.

NAPWA seeks to accomplish its mission in four ways:
**Information services**

NAPWA provides access to a wealth of HIV/AIDS prevention, education, treatment, medical and psychosocial resources. NAPWA's information programs provide clear and useful answers to the diverse questions of those seeking information about HIV/AIDS. NAPWA-FAX, a fax-on-demand service, provides up-to-date information on topics such as funding opportunities for AIDS service providers, legal issues, nutrition, opportunistic infections, and treatments. This service is free and is available by calling 202-789-2222. The National Speakers Bureau utilizes speakers from across the country to present the perspectives and experiences of people living with HIV disease. This unique and successful peer-to-peer educational program reaches millions of people each year. The Bureau has specific programs targeting women, adolescents, communities of color, and people in the workplace. *Medical Alert*, NAPWA's free bimonthly publication, addresses the latest in treatments and alternative therapies. Subscriptions are provided to individuals and organizations around the United States and Puerto Rico.

**Treatment development**

The Treatment Development Partnership facilitates the exchange of medical information among people with HIV, federal regulatory agencies, biotechnology, and pharmaceutical companies. Coordinated by a medical doctor, this unique partnership works to accelerate the approval of life-sustaining pharmaceuticals and therapeutics for people living with HIV.

**Conference**

NAPWA conducts the largest gathering of individuals and AIDS service providers working on the front lines of the fight against HIV/AIDS at the annual National Skills Building Conference. Through a unique collaboration with the National Minority AIDS Council and AIDS National Interfaith Network, service providers and people living with HIV disease learn skills in financial management, service delivery, community relations, and fundraising.

**Public policy and education**

The focus of NAPWA's public policy and education activities is to consistently bring the perspective and experience of people living with HIV disease to national AIDS policy and to educate the public on these issues. The public policy and advocacy program teaches empowerment to people with HIV/AIDS and others affected by the epidemic to create appropriate action at the national, state, and local level. NAPWA's policy staff works at both the national and grassroots level to negotiate responsible public policy by disseminating information on its public policy positions, meeting with members of Congress and other decision makers, and by providing community advocacy training. *The Active Voice*, NAPWA's public policy and education publication, is aimed at providing individuals and advocates with information on significant AIDS issues. Readers also learn about successful advocacy strategies that they can in turn employ in their communities.

### General membership

Student $25; Basic $40; Friend $75; Advocate $100; AIDS service organization $150; Business $500.

Members receive all NAPWA publications, reduced rates and scholarship consideration at the National Skills Building Conference.

## 35. National Brain Tumor Foundation

785 Market Street, Suite 1600
San Francisco, CA 94103
(415) 284-0208; (800) 934-CURE; FAX (415) 284-0209

### Research

The National Brain Tumor Foundation has funded basic and applied laboratory research and clinical trials of new treatments at major institutions in the United States. The Foundation has also supported research into quality-of-life issues that regularly face brain tumor patients.

### Recovery

The National Brain Tumor Foundation refers patients and family members to a network of support groups throughout the United States. A volunteer-staffed SUPPORT LINE connects brain tumor patients with professional caregivers and those who have survived the disease. Further, the SUPPORT LINE serves as a link for friends, family members, and others involved in the lives of brain tumor patients.

### Resources

A comprehensive GUIDE is available for patients and families who want to learn about brain tumors, often in a very short period of time, in order to make informed decisions. *SEARCH*, the Foundation's newsletter, keeps readers in touch with advances in treatment and psychosocial support.

### Publications available from the National Brain Tumor Association

*Brain Tumors, A Guide.* 72 pages of up-to-date information on the diagnosis, treatment, and classification of brain tumors. Examples of current research into causes and cures. A special section on pediatric brain tumors. How to be a survivor; what are your rights as a patient; how to join a support group; and more. One free copy to a patient or family member/review copy for organizations; 2–10 copies $6.50 each; 11–50 copies $5.75 each; 51 or more copies $5.50 each.

*Brain Tumor Support Groups in North America.* Published annually by the American Association of Neurological Surgeons, Joint Section on Brain Tumors, and sponsored by NBTF, this is the most up-to-date listing of patient/family brain tumor support groups. This publication also includes a list of national resources for those with central nervous system neoplasms. One free copy to a patient or family member/review copy for organizations; additional copies $1.50 each.

*Gathering a Life—A Journal of Recovery*, by Jeanne Lohmann. When Jeanne Lohmann's husband was diagnosed as having a brain tumor, she responded as a wife and as a writer. These short prose pieces are a tribute to Hank's life and the manner in which he left it, and to their marriage. Sixty-one pages. Each copy $8.75.

"Short- and Long-Term Disability Income Synopsis." One free copy with any order.

## 36. National Cancer Survivors Day Foundation, Inc. (NCSF)

P.O. Box 682285
Franklin, TN 37068-2285
(615) 794-3006; FAX (615) 794-0179

National Cancer Survivors Day (NCSD) is America's nationwide annual celebration of life for cancer survivors, their families, friends, and oncology teams. Each celebration is an annual milestone in a survivor's fight against cancer, and there are 8 million cancer survivors in America. National Cancer Survivors Day was founded by cancer survivor Richard Bloch (H & R Block) and his wife, Annette, who serve each year as the Founding Co-Chairs. NCSD is celebrated on the first Sunday in June of each year in communities throughout America and Canada. It is the world's largest cancer survivor event.

## 37. National Chronic Pain Outreach Association, Inc. (NCPOA)

7979 Old Georgetown Road, Suite 100
Bethesda, MD 20814-2429
(301) 652-4948; FAX (301) 907-0745

The National Chronic Pain Outreach Association, Inc. (NCPOA) is a nonprofit organization established in 1980. Its purpose is to lessen the suffering of people with chronic pain by educating pain sufferers, health care professionals, and the public about chronic pain and its management.

The benefits of joining include:

- an information clearinghouse that offers books, pamphlets, cassettes, and videotapes for both pain sufferers and health care professionals. (Nonmembers can also purchase these pamphlets, books, cassettes, tapes, and videotapes.)

- *Lifeline*, a quarterly magazine which provides information on pain management and coping methods.

- lectures and seminars to increase public awareness of chronic pain.

- "do-it-yourself kit" for people who want to start their own local chronic pain support groups.

- referrals to NCPOA member health care professionals and medical facilities nationwide.

- a computerized registry of chronic pain support groups in the United States and Canada (although NCPOA does not directly sponsor any groups).

## 38. National Coalition for Cancer Survivorship (NCCS)

1010 Wayne Ave., 5th Floor
Silver Springs, MD 20910
(301) 650-8868; FAX (301) 565-9670

The National Coalition for Cancer Survivorship (NCCS) represents grassroots organizations throughout the United States of over 10,000 cancer survivors. The NCCS was founded in 1986 by 24 cancer experts and Dr. Fitzhugh Mullan, a cancer survivor, to promote an understanding of cancer survivorship and provide advocacy to improve the quality of living for cancer survivors.

Through the national organization and a network of local organizations, the NCCS fosters the following goals:

- to promote programs that will empower survivors as informed consumers

- to operate a clearinghouse that disseminates survivorship articles, literature, and information on local and national survivorship activities and programs

- to act as a voice for cancer survivors to the media, medical establishment, and government

NCCS publications highlight issues vital to survivors such as locating resources, communicating with the health care team, being a savvy consumer of medical services, and fighting job and insurance discrimination.

*NCCS Networker,* a quarterly publication offering the latest news of people, events, and issues that impact survivors' lives.

*Charting the Journey,* an almanac of resources for survivors published by Consumer Reports Books.

*Facing Forward,* a guide for those finishing treatment, published by the National Cancer Institute in collaboration with NCCS.

*Teamwork: The Cancer Patient's Guide to Talking with Your Doctor.* Published by NCCS through an educational grant from Lederle Laboratories.

### 39. National Leukemia Research Association, Inc.

585 Stewart Avenue, Suite 536
Garden City, NY 11530
(516) 222-1944; FAX (516) 222-0457

The National Leukemia Association, Inc. was founded in 1965 as a not-for-profit organization dedicated to raising funds to support research into the causes and cure of leukemia and to provide patient aid to those families in need while meeting the expenses incurred in leukemia treatment. The Association is a voluntary agency that is totally supported by public contributions.

The National Leukemia Association provides aid to leukemia patients and their families. The Board of Trustees, in conjunction with its Patient Aid Committee, sets the policies and standards for administering this program. The National Leukemia Association will assist patients not covered by existing medical policies with laboratory fees, radiation therapy treatment, drugs, and blood transfusions. Unusual and extraordinary expenses not covered above will be considered based upon need and availability of funds.

### 40. National Lymphedema Network

2211 Post Street, Suite 404
San Francisco, CA 94115
(800) 541-3259; FAX (415) 921-2911

Established in 1988, the Network is a nonprofit organization that disseminates information on the prevention and management of primary and secondary lymphedema to the general public as well as to health care professionals. Their services include a computer data bank, educational course offerings and a quarterly newsletter containing educational articles, a resource guide, "penpals," and updates on conferences and professional training courses.

### 41. National Marrow Donor Program

Coordinating Center
3433 Broadway Street, N.E.
Minneapolis, MN 55413
(612) 627-5844; FAX (612) 627-5899
Office of Patient Advocacy: (800) 526-7809
Potential Marrow Donor: (800) MARROW-2

The National Marrow Donor Program, that is funded by the federal government, was created to improve the effectiveness of the search for bone marrow donors so that a greater number of bone marrow transplants could be carried out. It keeps a registry of potential bone marrow donors and provides a free packet of information on bone marrow transplantation. Patients who need resources in this area can obtain help from the Office of Patient Advocacy within the National Marrow Donor Program.

### 42. Oley Foundation

A-23 Hun Memorial
Albany Medical Center
Albany, NY 12208-3478
(518) 262-5079; (800) 776-6539 (OLEY); FAX (518) 262-5528

The Oley Foundation is a nonprofit, tax-exempt organization established in 1983 to address the special needs of consumers (patients) home parenteral and/or enteral nutrition (homePEN). Since then, Oley has worked to build a homePEN community that fosters the sharing of information between consumers, clinicians, home care services, and third-party payers. By providing information and emotional support to consumers, Oley enhances the lives of those requiring home nutritional support. All of Oley's programs are provided at no charge to consumers and their caregivers.

Specific projects include:

- *LifelineLetter*—a bimonthly newsletter written for home PEN consumers, families, clinicians, researchers, and home care services

- A grassroots network of volunteers who provide information and emotional support to fellow homePEN consumers and caregivers

- An annual conference for homePEN consumers and clinicians

- A clearinghouse for information on homePEN therapy issues

### 43. Project Inform

1965 Market Street, Suite 220
San Francisco, CA 94103
(415) 558-8669; FAX (415) 558-0684

Fighting HIV/AIDS takes knowledge, strength, and dedication. Founded in 1985, Project Inform is an independent, nonprofit, community-based AIDS service organization, dedicated to providing direct services to persons infected with HIV or at risk for infection. The Project has a singular national reputation for effectively providing the public with clear and trustworthy information about early intervention strategies, and treatments for HIV-related problems. Project Inform also advocates at the Food and Drug Administration and the National Institutes of Health on behalf of those infected. The Project's work has strongly influenced the direction of national AIDS policy.

Services include:

- a national toll-free hotline

- fact sheets and bulletins

- a periodic journal, *PI Perspective*

- a local and national speakers bureau

- the Treatment Action Network.

Their hotline for HIV positive, AIDS, and ARC family and friends, medical and service providers is (415) 558-9051 (local and international) and (800) 822-7422 (USA).

Their in-depth discussion papers include:

Day One—After you've tested positive, Doctor, Patient and HIV: Building a cooperative relationship
Antivirals A–Z
Preventing PCP
Management of Opportunistic Infections
Acyclovir

### 44. Ronald McDonald House

Kroc Drive
Oak Brook, IL 60521
(630) 623-7418

Ronald McDonald House is a "home away from home," a temporary lodging facility, for the families of seriously ill children being treated at nearby hospitals. The Houses provide an environment for emotional support to parents and siblings of sick children through a loving, caring, stable place they can call "home."

People helping people in times of serious need have made the Ronald McDonald House program what it is today. Each of the 165 Houses in 12 countries is owned and operated by a local not-for-profit corporation composed of members of the medical community, McDonald's owner/operators, businesses and civic organizations, and parent volunteers. Each House raises money locally, as well as benefits from a general Ronald McDonald House fund. Families staying at Ronald McDonald House are asked to make a donation ranging from $5 to $15 per day; if that is not possible, their stay is free.

### 45. Skin Cancer Foundation

245 Fifth Avenue, Suite 2402
New York, NY 10016
(212) 725-5176; FAX (212) 725-5751

The Skin Cancer Foundation, a nonprofit foundation, is the only national organization concerned solely with the world's most prevalent malignancy—cancer of the skin. The Foundation conducts public and medical education programs and provides support for medical training and research to help reduce the incidence, morbidity, and mortality of skin cancer.

The Skin Cancer Foundation has a variety of booklets, posters, slide presentations, and a video available regarding a multitude of issues. A contribution of $25 pays for a one-year subscription to *Sun & Skin News* (four issues, for public education) or *The Melanoma Letter* (four issues, for professional education). Write or call for a free catalogue, or send a self-addressed, stamped envelope for a sample of a specific brochure. Bulk orders for distribution are available for a fee.

Their booklets include:

Sunproofing Your Baby
Basal Cell Carcinoma—The Most Common Cancer
The Many Faces of Malignant Melanoma
Squamous Cell Carcinoma
For Every Child Under the Sun: A Guide to Sensible Sun
The ABCD's of Moles and Melanomas
Dysplastic Nevi & Malignant Melanoma—A Patient's Guide
Sun Sense

### 46. Sunshine Foundation

2001 Bridge Street
Philadelphia, PA 19124
(215) 535-1413 inside Philadelphia; (800) 767-1976 outside Philadelphia; FAX (215) 535-8397

The Philadelphia-based organization was founded by former police officer, Bill Sample in 1976, to grant the dreams and wishes of chronically ill, terminally ill, and handicapped children all over the country suffering from illnesses such as cancer, spina bifida, muscular dystrophy, sickle cell anemia, cystic fibrosis, AIDS, progeria, and many others too numerous to mention. The Sunshine Foundation is a registered, nonprofit organization with 29 all-volunteer chapters throughout the United States.

### 47. Sunshine Foundation

Dream Village Site
5400 C.R. 547 North
P.O. Box 255
Loughman, FL 33858
(941) 424-4188; (800) 457-1976; FAX (941) 424-4360

On a 22-acre site just 15 minutes from the Magic Kingdom, the Sunshine Foundation has constructed a Village where the dreams and wishes of chronically and terminally ill children are answered. Over 2000 special children have enjoyed this unique Village, which is specifically designed with them in mind. Each of the seven cottages has a fantasy theme in the child's bedroom. Special features include a pool with a ramp for wheelchair-dependent children, a handicapped accessible playground, and a game room. Since its inception in 1976, Sunshine Foundation has fulfilled the dreams and wishes of more than 21,000 very special children.

### 48. Susan G. Komen Breast Cancer Foundation

5005 LBJ Freeway
Suite 370
Dallas, TX 75244
(214) 450-1777; (800) 462-9273; FAX (214) 450-1710

The Susan G. Komen Breast Cancer Foundation was established in 1982 by Nancy Brinker to honor the memory of her sister, Susan G. Komen, who died of breast cancer. The Foundation is a national organization with a network of volunteers working through local chapters and Race for the Cure events in over 60 cities throughout the United States, fighting to eradicate breast cancer as a life-threatening disease by advancing research, education, screening, and treatment. The Komen Foundation is the largest private funder in the country of research dedicated solely to breast cancer.

The Foundation has a national toll-free Breast Care Helpline that is answered by trained, caring volunteers who provide timely and accurate information (in English and Spanish) to callers with breast health and breast cancer concerns.

A sample of pamphlets available (single copies are free):

Breast Self-Exam Shower Card
Caring for Your Breasts
Mammography. . .A Picture Can Save Your Life
Questions about Breast Health, What You Need to Know
Questions to Ask the Doctor About Breast Cancer:
    When going for a mammogram
    If you find a lump in your breast
    About breast biopsy

When breast cancer is diagnosed
Before breast surgery
After breast surgery
About treatment choices
About radiation therapy
About breast cancer chemotherapy
About hormone therapy
About bone marrow transplant
About reconstructive breast surgery
About lymphedema
If someone you love has breast cancer

**Book:**

Brinker, Nancy and Harris, Catherine M: *The Race is Run One Step at a Time* (ed 3) 1995. Available by calling the Foundation. $13.95.

**Videos:**

*Breast Cancer: A common risk.* A series of short vignettes highlighting issues related to breast cancer risk, breast health, fear and misconceptions, accessing medical services, the family's role in medical care and breast cancer treatment. $10.00 (English and Spanish) 14 minutes.

*El Auto Examen Del Seno: Un Habito Saludable (Breast Self-Exam: A healthy habit).* This video addresses some common myths, beliefs, and behaviors that create barriers to performing breast self-examination. The technique of breast self-examination is demonstrated. $10.00 (Spanish) 13 minutes.

### 49. United Ostomy Association

36 Executive Park, Suite 120
Irvine, CA 92714
(714) 660-8624; (800) 826-0826

Local chapters are composed primarily of ostomates who provide aid, moral support, and education to those who have a colostomy, ileostomy, or urostomy surgery. The chapter supplements the work of the surgeon by offering rehabilitation through follow-up by people who have learned to live with an ostomy. Trained members make visits to homes and hospitals, on request, with the prior consent of the patient's physician. Chapters have medical advisory boards consisting of nonsurgeon physicians, surgeons, and enterostomal therapists trained in ostomy care and the use of equipment. At regular monthly meetings, open to anyone who is interested, members can exchange practical, personal experiences about their ostomies, see ostomy equipment displayed, and hear speakers who are knowledgeable about ostomy. All local chapters are volunteer organizations. A list of the chapters is available on request from the UOA. Annual chapter dues vary from no fee to $30. Each member of the UOA receives the *Ostomy Quarterly* magazine and is eligible to participate in the UOA insurance programs. The UOA has both publications and slide programs, which cover every aspect of ostomies.

A sample of publications available from the United Ostomy Association:

The Ostomy Book for Nurses
Coping with an Ostomy
Ostomy Dietary Guidelines
Anatomy of Ostomy Brochure
So You Have/Will Have an Ostomy
About Ostomy
Colostomy: A Guide (English)
Ileostomy: A Guide
Urostomy: A Guide
Transverse Colostomy: A Guide
Sex/Courtship/Single Ostomate
Sex and the Female Ostomate

### 50. US TOO! International, Inc.

930 North York Road, Suite 50
Hinsdale, IL 60521-2993
(630) 323-1002; (800) 808-7866; FAX (630) 323-1003

US TOO!, a not-for-profit organization incorporated in the state of Illinois was created through the efforts of a small group of prostate cancer survivors. Since its inception, US TOO! has been organized to be run for and by men with prostate disease. US TOO! is an autonomous support organization dedicated to working in harmony with professional, business, and lay groups involved with prostate cancer to provide information and support for survivors and their families. US TOO! has initiated over 400 support groups in the United States, Canada, Turkey, Europe, and Australia. The primary objective of US TOO! is to give participants a forum where they can compare experiences and discuss matters of interest relating to prostate cancer and prostate disease. At most meetings a medical professional speaks on some phase of the diagnosis, staging and/or treatment of prostate cancer or BPH topics. Participants also have the opportunity to discuss individual experiences that may be of interest to the group. All meetings are free of charge. Annual membership includes a $25 donation and a subscription to their quarterly newsletter, *The Prostate Cancer COMMUNICATOR.*

### 51. Wellness Community

National Office
2716 Ocean Park Blvd., Suite 1040
Santa Monica, CA 90405
(310) 314-2555; FAX (310) 314-7586

The Wellness Community provides free psychosocial support services for adults with cancer and their families. There are 14 Wellness Communities throughout the United States. The Wellness Community is a tax-exempt, charitable corporation, and serves as an adjunct to conventional medical treatment.

The following services are provided:

**Sharing groups**
These are informal, drop-in groups held twice a week and led by people who have or have had cancer.

**Participant groups**
Licensed psychotherapists lead two-hour group sessions once a week.

**Family groups**
Licensed psychotherapists lead two-hour weekly group sessions composed of significant others of people with cancer in a participant group.

**Relaxation/Visualization**
Twice per week there are sessions where participants are taught how to involve themselves in the self-help procedures.

**Education**
During the month, lectures and dialogues are presented by authorities in fields of interest to cancer patients.

**Workshops**
Each week, there are workshops presented by experts in matters such as voice dialogue, use of humor, moderate exercise, art therapy, journal writing, etc.

**Special groups**

Special groups are presented on an ongoing basis to consider specific areas of concern to cancer patients such as breast, prostate, and brain cancer networking; problems of parents with cancer; groups for couples to look at the problems of intimacy brought on by cancer.

**The Wellness Connection**

Twice during the month, members of The Wellness Community who wish to remain connected to the community come together for support and socializing.

**Open forum**

Every two months, participants meet with staff members to present new ideas and suggestions for optimizing their use of the program.

**Clubs**

Groups of participants meet on their own at the facility to carry on activities such as the Nutrition Club, where a highly trained nutritionist leads discussions on selected topics of interest to the participants where diet can be used in the fight for recovery.

**Social events**

At least once a month, there are social gatherings such as seasonal parties, potlucks, charade nights, joke fests, sing-a-longs, and other events that bring participants together to laugh and play.

**52. Women's AIDS Network (WAN)**

584 Castro Street, Suite 321
San Francisco, CA 94114
(415) 621-4160; FAX (415) 863-4740

The Women's AIDS Network (WAN), established in June 1983 at the Second National AIDS Forum in Denver, is the oldest nonprofit organization catering to women infected or affected by HIV/AIDS. In March 1984, women involved with AIDS services in the San Francisco Bay Area began meeting monthly. WAN's membership includes women in medical, mental health, and social services, women living with HIV/AIDS, community activists, and social and political advocates.

WAN advocates and provides for the development and improvement of public policies, education, and services for the diverse population of women infected and affected by HIV/AIDS. WAN distributes monthly newsletters, holds monthly education forums, maintains a resource library, and offers information and referrals to individuals and organizations.

**53. Y-ME**

212 W. Van Buren, 4th Floor
Chicago, IL 60607-3908
(312) 986-8338 Business & 24 hour Hotline; (312) 986-9505 (Hispanic Hotline)
(800) 221-2141 National Hotline (weekdays, 9–5); FAX (312) 986-0020

Founded in 1978 by Ann Marcou and Mimi Kaplan, two mastectomy patients, Y-ME has become the largest breast cancer support program in the USA. It provides hotlines (staff and volunteers who have personally experienced breast cancer), presurgery counseling, open door meetings, early detection workshops, a speakers bureau, resource library, wigs and prosthesis bank, and inservice workshops for health care professionals. Volunteers are professionally supervised, and the information provided to patients is monitored by a medical advisory board. Contributing members receive a bimonthly newsletter.

**54. YWCA of the U.S.A. ENCORE*plus***

Office of Women's Health Initiatives
624 Ninth Street, NW 3rd Floor
Washington, DC 20001
(800) 95E-PLUS; FAX (202) 783-7123

ENCORE*plus* is a system of health promotion through education, clinical service delivery, and patient "navigation" and advocacy. The community-based program targets women over 50 in need of early detection education and breast and cervical cancer screening and support services. It also provides women in treatment for and recovering from breast cancer a unique combined peer support group and exercise program.

## Professional Organizations and Resources

**55. AIDS Action Council**

1875 Connecticut Avenue, N.W., Suite 700
Washington, DC 20009
(202) 986-1300; FAX (202) 986-1345; E-mail: HN3384@handsnet.org

Established in 1984, AIDS Action Council is the only national organization solely dedicated to shaping federal HIV/AIDS policy. Cited by *The New York Times* as "among the country's most powerful advocacy groups," AIDS Action represents more than 1000 community-based HIV/AIDS organizations across the nation. AIDS Action Foundation, the council's sister organization, is a nonprofit 501(c)(3) organization. It supports and promotes the work of the council through policy research, media advocacy, information dissemination, and grassroots outreach and education. Also, AIDS Action houses the Pedro Zamora Memorial Fund and convenes the coalition National Organizations Responding to AIDS (NORA), that includes more than 150 organizations advocating on a wide range of HIV/AIDS issues.

**56. American Academy of Pain Medicine**

4700 West Lake Avenue
Glenview, IL 60025-1485
(847) 375-4731

AAPM is the official organization representing physicians in the field of pain in the United States. It is a specialty society recognized by the American Medical Association. Our mission is to enhance the practice of pain medicine in the United States. In working to achieve this mission, AAPM's goals are to promote a socioeconomic and political climate conducive to the practice of pain medicine in an effective and efficient manner, and to ensure quality and comprehensive medical care by physicians specializing in chronic pain medicine to patients in need of such services. The benefits of membership in AAPM include the following:

- Membership directory, listing primary care and specialty physicians with an interest in pain medicine

- Subscriptions to *The Clinical Journal of Pain*, the official AAPM journal

- Special rates on all AAPM activities and products, such as annual meetings, regional seminars, and the *Directory of Pain Management Facilities* (not available to trainee members)

- AAPM awards recognition program

**57. American Association for Cancer Education, Inc.**

Robert M. Chamberlain, PhD
Department of Epidemiology, University of Texas
MD Anderson Cancer Center
1515 Holcombe Boulevard, P.O. Box 189
Houston, TX 77030-4095
(713) 792-3020; FAX (713) 792-0807
E-mail: RCHAMBERLAIN
@REQUEST.MDA.UTH.TMC.EDU

The purpose of the AACE has been "to provide a forum for those concerned with education of groups who attempt to advance the cause of early cancer detection, promote individualized multimodality therapy, or develop programs of rehabilitation for cancer patients." This multidisciplinary organization brings together basic scientists, surgeons, internists, oncology nursing educators, pediatricians, pathologists, gynecologists, dentists, and radiation oncologists. They hold an annual fall meeting.

The official journal of the Association is the *Journal of Cancer Education* and is listed in *Index Medicus*. The Association has occasionally sponsored other publications such as *Concepts in Cancer Medicine*, edited by S. Benham Kahn, MD et al, and *Self-Assessment of Current Knowledge in Oncology*, edited by John Foley, MD. The Association also distributes a President's Newsletter, and abstracts accepted for presentation at the annual meeting are published as a Supplement to the *Journal of Cancer Education*.

The American Association for Cancer Education does not produce or distribute cancer education materials.

**58. American Association for Cancer Research**

Margaret Foti, Executive Director
Public Ledger Building
620 Chestnut Street, Suite 816
Philadelphia, PA 19106
(215) 440-9000; FAX (215) 440-9313

The American Association for Cancer Research (AACR) is the world's largest professional society of scientists specializing in both basic and clinical cancer research. Its 7600 members are experts in the areas of molecular biology and genetics of cancer, tumor biology, virology, carcinogenesis, toxicology and risk assessment, endocrinology, epidemiology and prevention, pharmacology and therapeutics, immunology, and all aspects of clinical investigations pertaining to human cancer. The publications of the association include: *Cancer Research, Cell Growth and Differentiation, Cancer Epidemiology, Biomarkers and Prevention, Directory of Members*, and *Proceedings of the American Association for Cancer Research*.

**59. American Cancer Society**

Terri Ades, RN, HSN, OCN®
Director, Nursing Programs
1599 Clifton Road, NE
Atlanta, GA 30329-4251
(404) 329-7617; (800) ACS-2345

The American Cancer Society is the nationwide voluntary health organization dedicated to eliminating cancer as a major health problem by preventing cancer, saving lives from cancer, and diminishing suffering from cancer through research, education, and service.

The Society offers scholarships to interested oncology nurses at both the Master's and Doctoral level. The scholarships provide a stipend of $8000 per year for a maximum of two years for a Master's degree in nursing and $8000

per year for a maximum of four years for a Doctoral degree in nursing or related area.

**60. American Foundation for AIDS Research (AmFAR)**

1515 Broadway, Suite 3601
New York, NY 10036-8901
(212) 682-7440; and
5900 Wilshire Boulevard
2nd Floor East Satellite
Los Angeles, CA 90036-5032
(213) 857-5900

The American Foundation for AIDS Research is the nation's leading private-sector funding organization dedicated to AIDS research, education, and public policy. AmFAR serves as a catalyst to identify major gaps in AIDS biomedical and social science research and education, and provides funding to support innovative projects designed to fill the gaps. Since it started in late 1985, AmFAR has awarded $32 million in seed or start-up grants to more than 530 research teams and education projects. Eighty percent of AmFAR's grants underwrite a broad range of scientific research to find a vaccine and effective treatments for AIDS. Twenty percent of the grants go to experimental educational programs designed to prevent the spread of the disease. AmFAR is dedicated to mobilizing the good will, energy, and generosity of caring Americans to end the AIDS epidemic.

AmFAR sponsors a number of major publications, including:

- *AIDS/HIV Experimental Treatment Directory*, published quarterly, that tracks the testing of promising AIDS treatments

- *AIDS Information Resources Directory*, published annually, that lists and critically evaluates most AIDS-related educational materials available in the United States

- *AIDS Clinical Care*, published monthly by the *New England Journal of Medicine*, that contains the latest AIDS clinical management information for physicians

- *AIDS Education, A Business Guide*, a blueprint for developing AIDS education

- *AIDS Targeted Information Newsletter*, published monthly, that lists, with editorial comments, all major AIDS-related scientific, medical, social science, and public policy research papers published worldwide.

**61. American Hospital Association Resource Center**

1 N. Franklin
Chicago, IL 60606
(312) 422-2000; FAX (312) 422-4700

The AHA publishes an annual catalogue of monographs and AV products available, with a section designated for nursing resources.

**62. American Organization of Nurse Executives (AONE)**

1 N. Franklin
Chicago, IL 60606
(312) 422-2800; FAX (312) 422-4503
E-mail: http://www.aone.org

The American Organization of Nurse Executives (AONE) is the voice of nursing leadership in health care. With 5000 members, AONE is the national professional organization for nurses who design, facilitate, and manage care. AONE initiatives at the national level are reinforced through the activities of more than 60 chapters at the state and metropolitan levels. AONE is dedicated to the stewardship of health policy and to the professional development of nurse leaders operating in a dynamic environment. The organization achieves its objective through a spirit of collaboration. Benefits of AONE membership include education, networking, and information exchange, a comprehensive membership and resource directory, website, and a career development and referral center. The organization publishes a newsletter, *AONE Updates*, every three weeks. Annual membership is $200.

### 63. American Pain Society
5700 Old Orchard Road, First Floor
Skokie, IL 60077-1057
(847) 966-5595; FAX (847) 966-9418

The American Pain Society, a national chapter of the International Association for the Study of Pain (IASP), is a multidisciplinary, not-for-profit educational and scientific organization consisting of clinicians and researchers. The mission of APS is to serve people in pain by advancing research, education, treatment, and professional practice. We recognize that this goal can best be accomplished as a joint and interactive effort among basic scientists and health care professionals. APS was founded in 1979 and has grown to more than 2000 members. Over the years, the American Pain Society has expanded its programming and publications to meet the needs of its membership.

Publications of the American Pain Society:
*APS Journal*, a quarterly publication, provides a forum for the scholarly presentation and discussion of issues.
*APS Bulletin* offers feature articles on clinical and basic science topics, organizational news, and a calendar of events.
*APS Membership Directory* features a complete listing of all APS members—geographically, alphabetically, and by specialty.
*Principles of Analgesic Use* (ed 3) is a concise, compact, easily accessible reference guide. ($2.00/nonmembers)

Benefits of membership include reduced fees on education programs:
Annual Scientific Meeting features plenary sessions, workshops, symposia, posters, and exhibits—more than 200 presentations in all. Network with the 1000 people who attend.
Pain Update programs offer a series of in-depth half-day clinical sessions dealing with the latest in pain research and professional practice.
Educational programs offer continuing education credits.

### 64. American Society for Parenteral and Enteral Nutrition (ASPEN)
8630 Fenton Street, Suite 142
Silver Spring, MD 20910
(301) 587-6315; FAX (301) 587-2365
E-mail: http://www.peak.com/clinnut.org

ASPEN's mission is to serve as a preeminent, interdisciplinary, research-based, patient-centered clinical nutrition society throughout the world. ASPEN is a scientific society whose members are health care professionals dedicated to assuring that every patient receives optimal nutrition care. ASPEN firmly believes that a multidisciplinary approach works best for the delivery of nutrition support services. The physician's medical background, together with the knowledge and expertise of the dietitian, the nurse, and the pharmacist will ensure that the patient receives optimum nutritional care.

ASPEN offers the following membership categories:
**Active member**
Must hold an MD, DO, PhD or equivalent degree, PharmD, or MS in nutrition, or be a registered dietitian, registered nurse, or registered pharmacist, who is engaged in or actively related to any phase of clinical or laboratory use of parenteral/enteral nutrition.
**Affiliate member**
May be a trainee of disciplines qualifying for active membership or an industry sales/marketing representative or others involved or supportive of parenteral and enteral nutrition who are not eligible for active membership.
**Emeritus member**
Any active or affiliate member who has at least five years of continuous membership in the society, and is 65 years of age and retired.

To receive membership applications or other ASPEN services, call the FAX on Demand service at 800-905-7781 and request an index.

### 65. American Society for Therapeutic Radiology and Oncology (ASTRO)
1891 Preston White Drive
Reston, VA 22091
(703) 716-7588; FAX (703) 476-8167

The American Society for Therapeutic Radiology and Oncology (ASTRO) consists of American Board of Radiology certified physicians, radiation therapists, and radiation biologists whose professional practice is therapeutic radiology.

The objectives of the Society are:

* to extend the benefits of radiation therapy to cancer patients

* to advance the scientific basis of radiation therapy

* to provide for the education and professional fellowship of its members

### 66. American Society of Clinical Oncology (ASCO)
225 Reinekers Lane, Suite 650
Alexandria, VA 22314
(703) 299-0151; (888) 282-2552; FAX (703) 299-1044; or
Director of Government Relations
American Society of Clinical Oncology
750 17th Street, NW, Suite 1100
Washington, DC 20006
(202) 778-2396; FAX (202) 778-2330

The Society promotes and fosters the exchange of information related to neoplastic diseases (with particular emphasis on human biology, diagnosis, and treatment) for physicians who are academically based or in private practice throughout the United States and other countries. ASCO publishes the *Journal of Clinical Oncology*, and sponsors two conferences annually.

### 67. American Society of Hematology (ASH)

Michael Payne, Executive Director
1200 19th Street, NW, Suite 300
Washington, DC 20036-2412
(202) 857-1118; FAX (202) 857-1164

The American Society of Hematology (ASH) is a professional organization that devotes its efforts to charitable, scientific, and educational activities and endeavors including specifically but not limited to promoting and fostering, among the many scientific and clinical disciplines, the exchange and diffusion of information and ideas relating to blood and blood-forming tissues and encouraging investigations of hematologic matters. ASH was founded in 1958 and has played an active role in bringing together clinical practitioners and scientists, and in the development of hematology as a discipline through the establishment of standards for certification. The ASH newsletter, produced for Society members three times per year, offers relevant articles on a variety of topics related to the field of hematology and Society activities. In addition, membership includes a subscription to *BLOOD*, the official Journal of the American Society of Hematology, which is published 24 times a year.

### 68. Association for the Care of Children's Health

7910 Woodmont Avenue
Suite 300
Bethesda, MD 20814
(301) 654-6549; FAX (301) 986-4553

The Association for the Care of Children's Health (ACCH) is an educational and advocacy organization with a multidisciplinary membership structure. ACCH membership totals over 4000, representing health and social service professionals, educators, researchers, parents, and community leaders. ACCH members work within their institutions, organizations, and communities to promote improved systems of health care for children and their families.

Beyond this service of advocacy, ACCH:

- produces educational materials that provide greater understanding of psychosocially sound, developmentally supportive, family-centered care and practical knowledge to make it a reality

- holds an annual conference, bringing together members and others to share knowledge, skills, and experiences

- plans and coordinates Children and Hospitals Week each year to focus community attention on the unique needs of children and families as they interact with the health care system

- publishes *Children's Health Care*, a quarterly journal, along with five newsletters, *ACCH News, ACCH Network, Affiliate Update, Canadian Connections,* and *Child Health Design*

- assists a North American parent network in working collaboratively with professionals in shaping systems of health care

- convenes periodic meetings of families caring for children with HIV infection

- provides services to designers and architects to ensure that planning, space allocation, construction, renovation, and design are responsive to the unique needs of children, families, and other care providers

- provides information, referral, and support through a clearinghouse for professionals and families of infants with disabilities and special health needs.

ACCH publishes many educational resources for professionals, children, and families. ACCH also educates and supports its members and others through an annual conference, Children and Hospitals Week, and several award and grant programs. Through four major program areas, the National Center for Family-Centered Care, Pediatric AIDS: Commitment to Caring, the Design Resource Center, and the National Information Clearinghouse for infants with disabilities and life-threatening conditions, ACCH offers significant support for greater understanding and improved systems of health care for children and their families.

Selected publications that are available from the Association for the Care of Children's Health include:

*Parent Resource Directory* (4th Edition; C. Schmitt [ed], 1991) A networking resource for those caring for children with chronic illnesses or disabilities. Listings by state/province of over 400 parents of children with special needs. Included addresses, child's condition, and parents' particular interests and skills. 121 pp. $7.00

*Pediatric AIDS: The Challenge of HIV Infection in Infants, Children, and Adolescents* (P. A. Pizzo and C. M. Wilfert [eds], 1990) Comprehensive, authoritative text on pediatric HIV infection covering many perspectives: evolving epidemiology; biology, pathogenesis, and transmission; diagnostic issues; clinical manifestations; treatment; and prevention, education, and public policy. 813 pp. $84.95

*You and HIV: A Day at a Time* (L.S. Baker, 1991) This easy-to-read, illustrated book guides children with HIV and their families through the medical and psychological whats and whys of HIV transmission, diagnosis, treatment, home care, and emotional responses. Strongly emphasizes living with the disease, with room to write personal notes or information. 258 pp. $16.95

*Seasons of Caring* (Film/Videotape, 1986) Reveals the concerns and priorities of families caring for children with special health needs. Addresses issues encountered by parents, teachers, social workers, school administrators, physicians, nurses, and others caring for these children and their families. 40 minutes, color. (16 mm–$245.00; VHS–$140.00; Preview–$60.00)

### 69. Association of American Cancer Institutes (AACI)

c/o Roswell Park Cancer Institute
Dr. E.A. Mirand, Secretary-Treasurer
666 Elm Street
Buffalo, NY 14263
(716) 845-3028; FAX (716) 845-8178

The Association of American Cancer Institutes (AACI) was originally established in 1959 as the Association of Cancer Institute Directors. In 1973 the organization was incorporated as the AACI. Today, 78 cancer centers throughout the United States are members of the AACI; six cancer centers throughout the world are corresponding members.

The AACI provides an organization structure to carry out the following objectives:

- to afford an opportunity for the leadership of cancer institutes and centers throughout the world to meet and discuss mutual problems

- to foster collaboration via state, regional, national, and international programs for the control of cancer through research, education, and service

- to support investigations into the causes, nature, prevention, and treatment of cancer and the rehabilitation of cancer patients by encouraging the exchange of ideas, information, personnel, and the provision of special facilities and training opportunities

- to foster educational and training opportunities in the related biomedical sciences

- to provide guidance to federal, state, and local governments, private and civic organizations concerning cancer research, diagnosis, treatment and prevention, and the rehabilitation of cancer patients

### 70. Association of Community Cancer Centers (ACC)
Lee Mortenson, Executive Director
11600 Nebel Street, Suite 201
Rockville, MD 20852
(301) 984-9496; FAX (301) 770-1949

The ACCC acts as the national voice of community multidisciplinary cancer care professionals. It serves as a forum on national issues and a source of information on policy, management, and financing issues related to oncology. Members include institutions and individuals.

The Association publishes *Oncology Issues*, a bimonthly publication devoted to information on the economic and programmatic issues of community cancer programs and their components. The Association issues updates on federal legislation and regulation affecting cancer care providers' ability to deliver quality care.

In addition, the association publishes *Community Cancer Programs in the United States*, the annual ACCC Roster. This volume provides detailed information on each member institution, including program components, personnel, and history. The names and addresses of general members are also listed.

Each year, ACCC publishes the most recent comparative data on current cancer-related DRGs. These reports contain analyses of average reimbursement, average cost, average profit/loss, and total reimbursement by hospital size and region. The report is titled "Cancer DRGs: A Comparative Report on Key Cancer DRGs."

### 71. Association of Freestanding Radiation Oncology Centers (AFROC)
2755 Bristol Street, Suite 110
Costa Mesa, CA 92626
(714) 545-2087

AFROC is a nonprofit organization composed of physicists, physicians, administrators, technicians, and clinical personnel working in freestanding, fully equipped radiation centers. It acts as a forum for addressing concerns and as an advocate for reimbursement and legislative policies affecting the centers. Full membership is $500, and benefits include a quarterly newsletter, *Source*; legislative information; reduced rates at the annual meeting; and current information on reimbursement, economic issues, practice development/marketing ideas, financial management, quality assurance, and more.

### 72. Association of Nurses in AIDS Care (ANAC)
1555 Connecticut Avenue NW, Suite 20
Washington, DC 20036
(202) 462-1038

The Association of Nurses in AIDS Care is a national association with members all over the United States and Canada plus members in Australia, France, the Netherlands, Taiwan, Panama, England, and the Philippines.

"The mission of ANAC is to promote the individual and collective professional development of nurses involved in the delivery of health care to people infected or affected by the Human Immunodeficiency Virus (HIV) and to promote the health and welfare of infected individuals by:

- creating an effective network among nurses in AIDS care

- studying, researching, and exchanging information, experiences, and ideas leading to improved care for persons with HIV infection

- providing leadership to the nursing community in matters related to AIDS/HIV infection

- promoting social awareness concerning issues related to HIV/AIDS

Inherent in these goals is the abiding commitment to the prevention of further HIV infection."

The Association of Nurses in AIDS Care was founded in September of 1987, held its first formal meeting in New York City in May 1988, and now has grown to a membership of over 1400 nurses. Membership in ANAC entitles members to the following benefits:

*Journal of the Association of Nurses in AIDS Care,* that is published quarterly;

*Newsletter of the Association of Nurses in AIDS Care,* that is also published quarterly;

Monographs and position statements on issues affecting health professionals;

Discounted educational meetings.

### 73. Association of Pediatric Oncology Nurses (APON)
4700 W. Lake Avenue
Glenview, IL 60025-1485
(847) 375-4724; FAX (847) 375-4777

APON has been in existence since 1973. Membership in the organization is open to all registered nurses who are either interested in or engaged in pediatrics or pediatric oncology. Annual dues are $65, which entitles the member to receive a copy of the quarterly journal, *J.A.P.O.N.*, *A.P.O.N. Newsletter,* and other pertinent publications; attend all business meetings and programs at a reduced rate; and vote on all issues concerning the organization.

The objectives of the organization are to:

- promote excellence in the specialty of pediatric oncology nursing

- provide opportunities for communication among all nurses who work with children who have cancer through quarterly newsletters and an annual seminar .

- encourage dissemination of information among nurses about the medical and nursing care of pediatric oncology patients that is used in various areas of the country

- encourage members to update professional and lay literature with regard to the care of children with cancer

- encourage and support research in nursing care of children with cancer.

APON has several publications for purchase by both members and nonmembers: *Chemotherapy Book, Scope of Practice and Outcome Standards of Pediatric Oncology Nursing,* and *Patient/Family Annotated Bibliography.*

### 74. Commission on Accreditation of Rehabilitation Facilities

101 North Wilmot Road, Suite 500
Tucson, AZ 85711
(602) 748-1212; FAX (602) 571-1601

The Commission on Accreditation of Rehabilitation Facilities' fundamental commitment is to provide quality services to people with disabilities and others in need of rehabilitation. Through the mechanism of standards setting, field participation and review, and accreditation, the Commission is the recognized authority for a wide range of habilitation/rehabilitation organizations and programs in the areas of Medical Rehabilitation, Behavioral Health (Alcohol and other Drug and Mental Health), and Employment and Community Support. The goal of these programs is to make a positive difference in the lives of people with disabilities and others in need of rehabilitation as they strive to attain optimal self-sufficiency, independence, and productivity.

The Commission began in 1966. It is a private, not-for-profit organization that has had the benefit of a broad base of support and involvement on the part of consumers, providers, and purchasers of specialized services for people with disabilities and others in need of rehabilitation. The Commission's success is directly attributed to the profound impact it has had on the provision of quality-oriented rehabilitation services.

**The following materials can be purchased from the Commission:**

*Standards Manual and Interpretive Guidelines for Medical Rehabilitation* ($90)
*Self-Study Questionnaire for Medical Rehabilitation* ($45)
*Directory of Accredited Organizations Serving People with Disabilities* ($45)
*Survey Checklist for Medical Rehabilitation* ($15)
*Market-Based Planning* document ($16)
A variety of resource publications on Program Evaluation ($16 each)

**Other resources:**
**CARF 101s**
Two day seminars designed to familiarize organizations with the accreditation process, the standards and their utilization in day-to-day operations, and how the standards will be applied during the survey process.
**Medical Conferences**
Three to four day conferences designed to address topics of relevance to the field of rehabilitation and the accreditation process. These are conducted in February and July of each year.

### 75. Gynecologic Cancer Foundation

401 N. Michigan Avenue
Chicago, IL 60611
(312) 644-6610; FAX (312) 527-6640

The foundation's primary goal is to disseminate information to the medical community and the public at-large about current trends and techniques in gynecologic cancer. The foundation provides a liaison with the National Cancer Institute and other cancer-based health and medical agencies to promote and initiate education and research in the field and to report findings related to gynecologic oncology. The foundation also supports research in the area of gynecologic oncology.

### 76. International Association for the Study of Pain (IASP)

909 NE 43rd St., Suite 306
Seattle, WA 98105
(206) 547-6409; FAX (206) 547-1703; Telex: 265214
E-mail: IASP@locke.hs.washington.edu
www: http://weber.u.washington.edu/~crc/IASP.html

IASP was founded in 1973 and was incorporated in 1974 as a nonprofit organization to:

- foster and encourage research of pain mechanisms and pain syndromes and to help improve the management of patients with acute and chronic pain by bringing together basic scientists, physicians, and other health professionals of various disciplines and backgrounds who have interest in pain research and management.

- promote education and training in the field of pain.

- promote and facilitate the dissemination of new information in the field of pain, including sponsorship of a journal, *PAIN.*

- promote and sponsor a triennial World Congress of the Association and such other meetings as may be useful or desirable for the advancement of the purposes of IASP.

- encourage formation of national associations for the study and treatment of pain.

- encourage the adoption of a uniform classification, nomenclature, and definition regarding pain and pain syndromes.

- encourage the development of a national and international data bank and to encourage the development of a uniform records system with respect to information relating to pain mechanisms, syndromes, and management.

- inform the general public of results and implications of current research in the area.

- advise international, national, and regional agencies of standards relating to the use of drugs, appliances, and other procedures in the therapy of pain.

- engage in such other activities as may be incidental to or in furtherance of the aforementioned purposes.

**Membership**

Active membership in IASP is open to scientists, physicians, dentists, psychologists, nurses, physical therapists, and other health professionals actively engaged in pain research and those who have special interest in the diagnosis and treatment of pain syndromes. The Association currently has 5800 members in 85 countries, and independent chapters in 50 countries. IASP holds a world congress every three years (abstracts, proceedings, and refresher course syllabi are published). The Association is a nongovernmental organization affiliate (NGO) of the World Health Organization. IASP has established a program of Special Interest Groups (SIGs) designed to enable members to have a forum to discuss specific interests in the pain field in depth. Five SIGs are currently functioning: central pain, pain in childhood, clinical-legal aspects of pain, pain and the sympathetic nervous system, and rheumatic pain.

IASP Press was established in 1994 and is dedicated to providing members and others with timely, high-quality, attractive, low-cost publications relevant to the problem of pain.

### Publications and books:

The monthly journal, *PAIN*, begun in 1975 and published by Elsevier, is the official journal of IASP and contains review articles, original research articles in both the clinical and basic sciences, book reviews, and letters to the editor.

A newsletter is published bimonthly and mailed to all members; contains general information about IASP activities, a technical corner, new books section, and an international meetings calendar.

*Pain: Clinical Updates* is published three times a year; contains state-of-the-art information on various clinical topics in the pain field.

Membership directory is published annually and mailed to all members.

*Classification of Chronic Pain: Description of Chronic Pain Syndromes and Definitions of Pain Terms.* Prepared by the Committee on Taxonomy, this is a detailed, comprehensive classification of pain syndromes and a minimum standard vocabulary (terms and definitions) for the field of pain. (240 pp; $20.00; second edition, 1994)

*Core Curriculum for Professional Education in Pain.* Prepared by the Task Force on Professional Education to identify the core of common knowledge necessary to best serve the patient and to communicate across disciplinary lines. In outline form with an extensive bibliography. (152 pp; $25.00; second edition, 1995)

*Ethical Guidelines for Investigations of Experimental Pain in Conscious Animals.* (Free to members; 1983)

*Curricula on Pain for Schools of Dentistry, Medicine, Nursing, Occupational/Physical Therapy, and Pharmacy.* Outlines of model pain courses for listed specialties. A psychology curriculum is in preparation. (1988, 1992, 1993, 1994)

*Desirable Characteristics for Pain Treatment Facilities.* Prepared by the Task Force on Guidelines for Desirable Characteristics for Pain Treatment Facilities to serve as a guideline for both practitioners and governmental and professional organizations involved in the establishment of pain treatment facilities. (Free to members; 1990)

*Standards for Physician Fellowship in Pain Management.* Prepared by an IASP Task Force to serve as a guideline for physicians who seek further training. Includes prerequisites for both trainee and training facility. (1990)

*Refresher Course Syllabus.* Refresher Courses are held at the time of IAS's triennial world congresses. A syllabus is available for purchase. (approx. 140 pp; $15.00)

*Congress Abstracts.* Abstracts of all papers to be presented at an IASP Congress are mailed to all IASP members in advance of the Congress and are available for all registrants. Additional copies are available for purchase. (approx. 500 pp; $15.00)

*Proceedings of the 7th World Congress on Pain.* Held in Paris, France, 1993. (949 pp; $65.00; 1994)

*Back Pain in the Workplace.* Prepared by the Task Force on Pain in the Workplace, it addresses back pain disability, worksite-based interventions to minimize disability, job-change flexibility, early medical management of disability, and early and long-term disability management and return to work. (90 pp; $25.00; 1995)

*Pharmacological Approaches to the Treatment of Chronic Pain: New Concepts and Critical Issues.* (326 pp; $55.00; 1994)

*Touch, Temperature, and Pain in Health and Disease: Mechanisms and Assessment.* (548 pp; $69.00; 1994)

*Temporomandibular Disorders and Related Pain Conditions.* (506 pp; $67.00; 1995)

*Visceral Pain.* (528 pp; $69.00; 1995)

**Books in preparation include:** *Reflex Sympathetic Dystrophy, Pain in the Elderly, Pain Centers at a Crossroads*

**77.   International Myeloma Foundation**
2120 Stanley Hills Drive
Los Angeles, CA 90046
(800) 452-CURE

The International Myeloma Foundation promotes education for both physicians and patients regarding myeloma, its treatment, and management. The foundation funds research, holds clinical and scientific conferences, and publishes a quarterly newsletter, *Myeloma Today.*

**78.   International Society of Nurses in Cancer Care (ISNCC)**
The Royal College of Nursing
20 Cavendish Square
London W1M 0AB Great Britain
01-71-495-6119; FAX 01-71-495-6104

Established in 1984, this society's goal is "to enable cancer nurses to share their knowledge and problems on a worldwide basis." Members of the society are required to pay an annual fee based on the size of the active membership of their organization, institution, or agency. Societies, interest groups, and clinical or educational institutions are able to join the Society in their own right. Members receive the newsletter *International Cancer Nursing News.* The International Society of Nurses in Cancer Care has *A Core Curriculum for a Post-Basic Course in Palliative Nursing* which is available for purchase.

Every two years the Society hosts an International Conference. This conference attracts approximately 2000 nurses from over sixty countries to gain knowledge, and share expertise and skills tailored to their own level of experience. ISNCC is a nongovernmental organization affiliate of the World Health Organization (WHO).

**79.   International Union Against Cancer**
(Union Internationale Contre Le Cancer—UICC)
Rue de Conseil—General 3
1205 Geneva, Switzerland
(4122) 809 18 11; FAX (4122) 809 18 10
E-mail: UICC@atge.automail.com

UICC is a nongovernmental, independent association composed of multidisciplinary cancer organizations. Its purpose is to encourage the fight against cancer worldwide, promoting communication internationally in cancer research, treatment, prevention, and patient support. Membership dues are based on an organization's ability to pay. Congresses are held biennially.

Department Directory:
Director          (4122) 809 1820
    uicc@atge.automail.com
Education         (4122) 809 1830
    imortara@atge.automail.com
Fellowships       (4122) 809 1840
    bbaker@atge.automail.com
Finance           (4122) 809 1860
    wbill@atge.automail.com
GLOBALink         (4122) 809 1850
    isreal@atge.automail.com
Publications      (4122) 809 1875
    ehansen@atge.automail.com

### 80. Intravenous Nurses Society

Fresh Pond Square
10 Fawcett Street
Cambridge, MA 02138
(617) 441-3008; FAX (617) 441-3009

The Intravenous Nurses Society is the national nonprofit professional association for nurses involved in the delivery of intravenous therapies. Membership fee is $90 (1996). Founded in 1973, the Society exists to promote excellence in intravenous nursing through standards, education, public awareness, and research. INS's ultimate goal is to insure access to the highest quality, cost-effective care for all individuals requiring intravenous therapies in all practice settings worldwide. The Society holds two major educational meetings each year in May and November. Membership benefits include:

Subscriptions to the Society's publications, including the *Journal of Intravenous Nursing* and the membership newsletter, *Newsline*

Reduced registration fee at INS Annual Meeting and November National Academy

Reduced rate for *Intravenous Nursing Standards of Practice*, the nationally recognized standards of IV nursing care

Reduced rate for *Implantable Ports* videotape

### 81. Johanna's On Call To Mend Esteem, Inc.

Cancer Rehabilitation Nurse Consultants
199 New Scotland Avenue
Albany, New York 12208
(518) 482-4178

Johanna's On Call To Mend Esteem is a nonprofit cancer rehabilitation nursing service that promotes preventive, restorative, supportive, and palliative nursing interventions for people with cancer. Educational services intended to enhance knowledge and promote the practice of self-examination are provided to the general public.

**Educational booklets** (written for patients and for use as an educational tool by nurses):

*Maintaining a Positive Image with Cancer Therapy* (a wellness workbook/journal) $4.50

Maintaining a Positive Image with Breast Cancer Surgery $2.00

Maintaining a Positive Image with Hair Loss and Cancer Therapy $3.50

Breast Health Diary—A Monthly Reminder to Keep an Eye on Your Breast Health $3.00

**Educational audiovisual tapes** (for combined audiences—patients/families/community/professional):

*Maintaining a Positive Image with Hair Loss and Cancer Therapy* (15 minutes) $19.95

*Maintaining a Positive Image with Breast Cancer Surgery* (15 minutes) for loan $19.95

*It's Your Body Check Yourself Out*—a teen breast self-exam program (6 minutes) $35.00

*BSE Rap*—an instructional music audio tape $8.00

### 82. National AIDS Fund

1400 I St. NW, Suite 1220
Washington, DC 20005
(202) 408-4848; FAX (202) 408-1818

The National AIDS Fund is in its eighth year of making grants to local communities for planning and service provision in response to America's HIV epidemic. The National AIDS Fund is dedicated to eliminating HIV disease as a major health and social problem. We work in partnership with the public and private sectors to provide care and to prevent new infections—through advocacy, grantmaking, research, and education—in communities and in the workplace.

### 83. National Cancer Registrars Association (NCRA)

P.O. Box 15945-295
Lenexa, KS 66285-5945
(913) 438-6272; FAX (913) 541-0156

The National Cancer Registrars Association (NCRA), chartered in 1974 and incorporated in 1976, is a nonprofit professional organization whose purposes are to establish standards of education for cancer registrars and to inform its members of the latest methods of cancer diagnosis, treatment, and current trends in incidence and survival. NCRA has over 2000 members. NCRA offers a certification examination semi-annually. Applicants must meet specific qualifications. Individuals who pass the examination become Certified Tumor Registrars (CTRs). Inquiries regarding certifications should be directed to NCRA's Home Office.

### 84. National Coalition for Cancer Research

c/o Capitol Associates Incorporated
426 C Street, NE
Washington, DC 20002
(202) 544-1880; FAX (202) 543-2565

The NCCR was founded in 1986 to support and strengthen the purposes of the National Cancer Act through public education and communication about the value of cancer research, treatment, and prevention. Today, the Coalition is composed of twenty national lay and professional organizations committed to the eradication of cancer.

The NCCR represents more than:

10,000 cancer survivors and their families

40,000 children with cancer as well as their parents and brothers and sisters

65,000 cancer researchers, nurses, physicians, and health care workers

82 specialized care cancer centers and institutions

over two million voluntary advocates united in conquering cancer

The watchwords of the NCCR epitomize its mission—Research Cures Cancer. The collaborative actions of the key organizations in the cancer community are designed to:

- communicate the value of research to progress against cancer

- make clear the contributions that the National Cancer Program has made to the reduction of cancer morbidity and mortality as well as to the quality of life experienced by cancer patients and survivors

- ensure adequate funding for research that will improve cancer diagnosis, treatment, and prevention

- cooperate with other organizations in support of public health policies that will lead to the eradication of cancer

The Coalition's mission is to provide a forum for a group of diverse cancer-concerned organizations to advance cancer research through collaborative action in such areas as public education and advocacy, leading to the eradication of cancer and its effects. Therefore, membership comprises a diverse group of individuals that are patient-focused as well as research-focused. The bylaws of the organization stipulate that only an organization or institution is able to participate as members and therefore no individual members are accepted.

### 85. National Hospice Organization (NHO)

1901 North Moore Street
Suite 901
Arlington, VA 22209
(703) 243-5900; (800) 658-8898 (Hospice helpline);
FAX (703) 525-5762

Established in 1978, NHO is a nonprofit organization, promoting quality care to the terminally ill and their significant others. NHO has worked over the past decade to establish hospice as a part of the health care delivery system in the United States. As a result of its efforts, hospice is now included as a Medicare/Medicaid benefit and as an employee benefit for 80% of American workers in medium- and large-sized business. The number of hospices also has increased from one in 1974 to over 2500 in 1995. Most hospices are members of NHO and receive NHO's technical assistance, education programs and events, publications, and advocacy and referral services. Membership has several categories and includes *The Hospice Journal* among numerous other publications and workshops. NHO membership includes 2000 hospices and 3400 individuals.

### 86. National League of Nursing (NLN)

350 Hudson Street
New York, NY 10014
(800) 669-1656; FAX (212) 989-3710

The National League of Nursing (NLN) is a leader in advancing the health of diverse communities through nursing. Its broadbased mission is to improve education and health outcomes by linking communities and information.

In pursuit of this mission, NLN provides leadership in several areas:

- redesigning the delivery of nursing education and health care services through community-focused models

- developing quality educational strategies for emerging health care needs and services

- expanding nursing research to include state-of-the-art interdisciplinary qualitative and quantitative community-focused agendas

- forging alliances and like-thinking knowledge-based institutions and community groups

NLN is also a leader in making available to the professional and lay public an array of knowledge tools from NLN Press, NLN video, and the prestigious *NNHC: Perspectives on Communities.*

Significant publications related to oncology concerns include:

**Publications:**
*Breast Cancer: Twenty Women's Stories*
*The Light around the Dark*
*Annual Review of Women's Health* (vol 1, 2,& 3)
*Through the Northern Native Looking Glass: Breast Cancer Stories from Northern Native Women*
*In Women's Experiences* (vol 1 & 2)

**Videos:**
*Therapeutic Touch: Healing through Human Energy Fields*
*Meet NIC: The Nursing Interventions Classification*
*Nursing Research: A Comprehensive Approach*

NLN and its subsidiary, Community Health Accreditation Program (CHAP), that ensures the quality of community and home health agencies are at the core of national and international efforts to transform health care. Effective dependable health care available and accessible for all communities, whatever the economic or social status of its members, is of paramount concern.

In 1991 the Field Institute for Technology in Nursing Education (FITNE) and NLN published the fourth edition of the *Directory of Educational Software for Nursing,* that provides information for anyone interested in using a computer to teach nursing. There are complete descriptions and purchasing information for over 300 computer-assisted instruction (CAI) programs. Included are 100 new CAI programs for IBM and Apple Macintosh computers. Ratings were done by more than 2500 health care professionals; there are several oncology-related programs listed in this directory. Publication No. 41-2405 ($79.95).

### 87. Nursing Pain Association

Pain Study Office, N411Y, Box 0606
School of Nursing
University of California
San Francisco, CA 94143
(415) 476-4040

The purpose of the organization is to foster and promote education, research, and high standards of practice in the care of patients with pain.

To emphasize the application of pain research findings to nursing care by:

- improving the quality of nursing care provided to the patient in pain

- providing opportunities for members to continue their growth as pain specialists

- providing a forum for networking among members

- providing continuing pain education to nurse colleagues

- promoting nursing research related to pain

**Membership benefits:**
Pain Education Programs
Annual Bay Area Conference in California—reduced fee
Regular members' meetings—no charge
Dinners (informal, social/professional, networking)

**Referral service:**

Professional network—Identify local and national experts for a specific pain problem

Direct individuals to current literature on a specific pain topic

**Consultation bureau:**

Pain curricula, research, and client-based practice (fees negotiated by individual consultant)

**Speaker's bureau:**

Pain education programs for site-specific needs

**Publications:**

Membership directory

Newsletter

### 88. Oncology Nursing Society (ONS)

501 Holiday Drive
Pittsburgh, PA 15220-2749
(412) 921-7373; FAX (412) 921-6565

ONS was founded in 1975 to promote the highest professional standards of oncology nursing; study, research, and exchange information, experiences, and ideas leading to improved oncology nursing; encourage nurses to specialize in the practice of oncology nursing; identify resources within the group; and establish guidelines of nursing care for patients with cancer. Annual dues are $71 (1996), which entitles a member to the society's peer-reviewed journal, *Oncology Nursing Forum*, and a newsletter, *ONS News*, that are published 10 times 12 twelve times per year, respectively. Members also are entitled to reduced rates for the annual Congress, the annual Fall Institute, an opportunity to serve on society committees, and research and travel awards. In 1981 the Oncology Nursing Foundation, an allied organization of ONS, was established to enhance the quality of cancer nursing throughout the disease process. Annually, this national Foundation awards nursing research grants; presents undergraduate, graduate, and doctoral scholarships; and funds public education projects. Additional awards include the Mara Mogensen Flaherty Memorial Lecture and the Pearl Moore Career Development Award.

In 1984, ONS founded another allied organization, the Oncology Nursing Certification Corporation, whose purpose is to develop, administer, and evaluate a program for the certification of oncology nurses at both the generalist and advanced levels. The certification examinations test the general and advanced oncology nursing knowledge base of the professional nurse. The first exam, offered in 1986, resulted in 1384 oncology certified nurses. Testing for both exams is offered each year at the ONS Congress and the generalist exam is offered again in the fall at 50 permanent sites and other specially arranged sites throughout the United States. Presently, there are over 15,000 generalist oncology certified nurses and more than 200 advanced oncology certified nurses.

ONS publishes guidelines and standards for various aspects of oncology nursing and makes these publications available through its national office. In 1995 there were more than 185 chapters of ONS across the country.

Partial list of publications:

The *Oncology Nursing Forum*, the Society's official journal
The Society's newsletter, the *ONS News*
*Guidelines for Cancer Nursing Practice*
*Cancer Chemotherapy Guidelines* (module format)—Course

Content and Clinical Practicum, Acute Care Setting, Outpatient Setting, Home Care Setting, and Management of Extravasation of Anaphylaxis
*Biotherapy: Recommendations for Nursing Course Content and Clinical Practicum*
*Access Device Guidelines* (module format)—Catheters, Ports and Reservoirs, and Pumps
*Guidelines for Safe Handling of Cytotoxic Drugs: An Independent Study*
*Standards for Oncology Nursing Practice, Oncology Nursing Education, Oncology Patient Education, Public Oncology Education,* and *Advanced Practice in Oncology Nursing*
*Core Curriculum in Oncology Nursing*
Directory of Nurse Researchers
ONS Position Paper on Cancer Rehabilitation
ONS Position Paper on Cancer Pain
Oncology Nursing Review: A Computer-Assisted Instruction Program

### 89. Radiation Research Society

2021 Spring Rd., Suite 600
Oakbrook, IL 60521
(630) 571-2881; FAX (630) 571-7837

The Radiation Research Society (RRS) is a professional organization composed of basic and clinical researchers who have specialized expertise in the effects of environmental radiation exposure, including mutagenesis and oncogenesis. Research and clinical interests include the use of radiation in medicine and industry, mainly for the radiation therapy of cancer and for imaging in diagnostic tests. The Society publishes the *Radiation Research Journal* monthly, and the *Radiation Research Newsletter* quarterly.

The Radiation Research Society has set forth a number of objectives to meet the needs of its professional membership, such as:

- encouraging in the broadest manner possible the advancement of radiation research in all areas of the natural sciences

- facilitating cooperative research between the disciplines of physics, chemistry, biology, and medicine in the study of the properties and effects of radiation

- promoting the dissemination of knowledge in these and related fields through publications, meetings, and educational symposiums

### 90. Society of Gynecologic Oncologists

401 N. Michigan Avenue
Chicago, IL 60611
(312) 644-6610; FAX (312) 527-6640
E-mail: SGO@sbo.com

The Society of Gynecologic Oncologists (SGO) currently has over 700 members who devote their professional research and clinical expertise to cancers that affect the female reproductive organs.

The SGO includes physicians from all over the United States and directs its efforts to the following objectives:

- to improve the care of patients with gynecologic cancer

- to advance knowledge and raise standards of practice in gynecologic oncology

- to encourage research in gynecologic oncology

- to cooperate with other individuals and organizations interested in oncology and related fields

**91. Society of Surgical Oncology**

85 W. Algonquin Road, #550
Arlington Heights, IL 60005
(847) 427-1400; FAX (847) 427-1294

The Society of Surgical Oncology (SSO) is composed of over 1500 physicians whose mission is to ensure the highest quality of comprehensive cancer care possible.

To carry out this mission, the Society endorses and supports the following objectives:

- to develop and disseminate optimal standards for multidisciplinary cancer care, including screening, skilled operative management, adjuvant therapies, rehabilitation, and follow-up

- to promote the specialty of surgical oncology through continuing education and the training of medical students, surgical residents, and fellows

- to foster clinical and laboratory research and the dissemination of new information to its membership, the surgical and other professional cancer communities, and the public

Members must be board certified by the American Board of Surgery or an equivalent surgical board; and complete one year of surgical oncology training or six years of related oncology surgery to meet requirements. The Society's journal, *Annals of Surgical Oncology*, is published six times a year.

**92. Wisconsin Cancer Pain Initiative**

3675 Medical Sciences Center
1300 University Avenue
Madison, WI 53706
(608) 262-0978; FAX (608) 265-4014
E-mail: wcpi@facstaff.wisc.edu

The Wisconsin Cancer Pain Initiative is a multidisciplinary effort aimed at improving the management of cancer pain. It is a cooperative effort of clinical care facilities, higher education, government, and many health care professionals including physicians, nurses, pharmacists, social workers, and others throughout the state of Wisconsin. The Initiative is a World Health Organization demonstration program.

It is the goal of the Wisconsin Cancer Pain Initiative to:

- help health professionals acquire and apply cancer pain information and management techniques

- promote the use of existing drug and nondrug methods to alleviate suffering

- change attitudes about cancer pain management

- dispel fears about medications that relieve pain

- educate patients and families on available treatments

The Wisconsin Cancer Pain Initiative is working to improve the management of cancer pain in Wisconsin through the development of:

- a resource manual for making pain management a priority in all health care settings

- a handbook on cancer pain management for health professionals

- educational displays for the public and professionals

- educational booklets about cancer pain for adults and children

- a speakers' bureau

- a network of patient advocates and clinical consultants

- a clearinghouse of resource materials

- improved communication among health professionals

- media coverage to improve public information

- curriculum improvements in the schools of medicine, nursing, and pharmacy

- evaluation of laws and regulations that may be barriers to good pain management

Resource material available from the Wisconsin Cancer Pain Initiative:

*The Handbook of Cancer Pain Management* ($3.50 per copy plus postage)
Patient Education Booklets (50 cents per copy plus postage)
*Cancer Pain Can Be Relieved*—a guide for adult patients and families
*Children's Cancer Pain Can Be Relieved*—for parents of children with cancer
*The Wisconsin Cancer Pain Initiative: Helping Health Professional Help Cancer Patients in Pain*—this brochure presents the basic principles of cancer pain management and the goals of the Wisconsin Cancer Pain Initiative. It is available free of charge.

Displays are useful for showing at meetings and in clinics, hospitals, and shopping malls. Borrowers are asked to pay the UPS shipping fee and to return the display to the Initiative.

Teaming Up to Fight Cancer Pain (for health professionals)
Helping Patients and Families Improve Cancer Pain Management (for the general public)

Videos can be borrowed; borrowers are asked to pay the UPS shipping fee to return these materials to the Initiative.

*Cancer Pain Can Be Conquered* (Slide/tape set). An 11-minute presentation on cancer pain, targeted at the patient, family, and general public, available in a slide/tape and a video format.
*My Word Against Theirs*. Produced by the Texas Cancer Pain Initiative. Several cancer patients describe the barriers they faced as they tried to get adequate relief of their pain. There is particular emphasis on concerns about addiction. To order, write Dr. C. Stratton Hill, Jr., M.D. Anderson Hospital, 1515 Holcombe Boulevard, Houston, TX 77030 (713) 792-2824.
*Winning the Battle* and *Control Your Cancer Pain*. Both about 12 minutes. Produced in 1990 by the Marshfield Clinic. The first video addresses three common myths about cancer pain control; the second corrects common misconceptions about how pain medications work ($59 each; $99 the pair). Order from Marshfield Video Network, 1000 North Oak Avenue, Marshfield, WI 54449.

* A separate listing of each State Cancer Pain Initiative is listed on pages 1828–1830.

**93. Wound Ostomy Continence Nursing Society (WOCN)**
2755 Bristol Street, Suite 110
Costa Mesa, CA 92626
(714) 476-0268; FAX (714) 545-3643

The Wound Ostomy Continence Nursing Society is a professional association for Enterostomal Therapy nurses. The mission is to provide education, research, certification, and a collaborative atmosphere to support state-of-the-art health care management for individuals with wounds, ostomies, and incontinence. Some benefits of membership include: *Journal of ET Nursing, Standards of Care, WOCN News,* a Membership Directory, a Professional Practice Manual, scholarships, and research grants. The Society also accredits ET programs and offers certification by examination.

# GOVERNMENT AGENCIES AND RESOURCES

**94. Cancer Communications Pretesting**
National Cancer Institute
(800) 4-CANCER

The National Cancer Institute's Office of Cancer Communications has published a booklet that provides information and guidance about measuring the effectiveness of the health message. It is provided free of charge. One booklet, *Making Health Communication Programs Work: A Planner's Guide* (NIH publication No. 89-1493), discusses the purpose of pretesting, planning the health message, conducting pretesting research, conducting the pretest, and measuring the readability of the health message. It provides an extensive bibliography about pretesting and evaluating public service announcements and is provided free of charge.

**95. Center for Substance Abuse Prevention**
National Clearinghouse for Alcohol and Drug Information (NCADI)
P.O. Box 2345
11426 Rockville Pike, Suite 200
Rockville, MD 20852
(301) 468-2600; (800) 729-6686; TDD (800) 487-4889

The National Clearinghouse for Alcohol and Drug Information (NCADI) is a service of the U.S. Center for Substance Abuse Prevention (CSAP). As the national focal point for information on alcohol and other drugs, NCADI collects, prepares, classifies, and distributes information about alcohol, tobacco and other drugs, prevention strategies and material, research, treatment approaches and resources, and training programs for professionals, community education programs, parents, children, and virtually all interested individuals. The Clearinghouse also provides a variety of free printed material including pamphlets, booklets, posters, resource guides, and directories; a reference and referral service; and the use of the library. Services and most materials are available at no cost to the public; videotapes and disk-based products carry a small cost recovery fee. Information about materials and services is available by calling the toll-free number.

NCADI works closely with more than 700 state and associate clearinghouses and information centers through CSAP's Regional Alcohol and Drug Awareness Resource (RADAR) Network to bring prevention resources to local communities and refer interested people to these resources. *Prevention Pipeline*, a bimonthly publication, is available on a subscription basis through NCADI and provides news and features on prevention issues, strategies, and programs; research abstracts; funding source updates; and a calendar of upcoming conferences.

With a computer, modem, and phone line, anyone now can access the resources of CSAP's National Clearinghouse for Alcohol and Drug Information. Instant access is available through PREVline (PREVention on-line), an electronic communication system dedicated to exchanging information concerning ATOD prevention. After connecting to PREVline, for USER ID, type *new* to create your account.
**Computer and modem:** Dialup (301) 770-0850; Settings N-8-1; Speed Up to 1440 baud
**Internet** Telnet: ncadi.health.org  FTP: ftp.health.org
Gopher: gopher  Mosaic: www.health.org

**96. Consumer Information Center**
General Services Administration
Pueblo, CO 81009
(719) 948-4000

The Consumer Information Center, a federal mail order operation, distributes consumer publications on topics such as children, food and nutrition, health, exercise, and weight control. The *Consumer Information Catalog* is available free from the Center and must be used to identify publications being requested.

**97. Consumer Product Safety Commission**
Washington, DC 20207
(301) 492-6800; (800) 638-2772 (hotline);
E-mail: info@cpsc.gov

An independent federal regulatory agency with jurisdiction over consumer products used in and around the home, the Commission sets standards and conducts information programs on potentially hazardous products, among them carcinogens and other chronic hazards. Single copies of printed materials are available free of charge. The hotline number allows the caller via a touch tone system to obtain and report information on specific products.

Information on CPSC activities can be obtained in a number of ways including the agency's Internet, fax-on-demand and toll-free Hotline services. Through the Internet, CPSC news releases, public calendar and other information can be obtained using the agency's "gopher" service: cpsc.gov

**98. Critical Care, Heart, Lung, Blood, Neurology, and Cancer Nursing Service**
National Institutes of Health
10 Center Dr., MSC 1664, 10/7D50
Bethesda, MD 20892-1664
(301) 496-2987; FAX (301) 402-6941

Nurses from the Service provide care to patients entered on intramural clinical research trials evaluating cancer therapies.

**99. Division of Cancer Prevention and Control**
National Cancer Institute
Bethesda, MD 20892-4200
(301) 496-6616

The Division of Cancer Prevention and Control (DCPC) plans and conducts basic and applied research programs aimed at reducing cancer incidence, morbidity, and mortality. Activities are carried out across five phases of research: hypothesis development, methods testing, controlled intervention trials, defined population studies, and demonstrations relevant to the prevention and management of cancer. DCPC plans, directs, and coordinates the support of basic and applied research on cancer prevention and control at cancer centers and community hospitals. It also coordinates program activities with federal and state agencies and establishes liaisons with professional and voluntary health agencies, labor organizations, cancer organizations, and trade associations.

**100. Food and Nutrition Information Center**
National Agriculture Library Center/USDA
10301 Baltimore Blvd., Room 304
Beltsville, MD 20705-2351
(301) 504-5719; FAX (301) 504-6409
E-mail: fnic@nalusda.gov

The Center is a resource for the informational needs of professionals interested in nutrition education, food service management, and food technology. They acquire and lend books and audiovisual materials to answer questions on the topics of food and nutrition.

**101. National AIDS Clearinghouse**
P. O. Box 6003
Rockville, MD 20849-6003
(800) 458-5231; FAX (301) 738-6616
TDD (800) 243-7012

The National AIDS Clearinghouse was initiated in October 1987 by the U.S. Department of Health and Human Services, Public Health Service, Centers for Disease Control (CDC), as part of its national information and education plan to respond to the public health threat posed by the human immunodeficiency virus (HIV) and acquired immunodeficiency syndrome (AIDS). The Clearinghouse is a centralized source providing current information on HIV infection and AIDS programs, materials, and services to professionals.

The National AIDS Clearinghouse:

- identifies and responds to the information needs of professionals involved in the development and delivery of HIV-prevention programs

- distributes selected HIV prevention-oriented publications

- coordinates an information network among organizations involved in the fight against AIDS

- disseminates information about ongoing federally and privately sponsored HIV and AIDS clinical trials through the AIDS Clinical Trials Information Service (ACTIS). For more information about ACTIS call (800) TRIALS-A (800) 874-2572.

- provides information about funding opportunities for community-based and HIV and AIDS service organizations

The *Catalog of HIV/AIDS Materials for Professionals* lists publications and audiovisual materials distributed by the National AIDS Clearinghouse. The Clearinghouse offers a comprehensive information service for people working in the field of HIV and AIDS prevention including public health professionals, educators, social service workers, at-torneys, human resource managers, and employers. These professionals work in a variety of settings, including state AIDS programs, community-based organizations, service organizations, businesses, and associations. The materials in the *Catalog of HIV/AIDS Materials for Professionals* are produced by the Centers for Disease Control, other U.S. Public Health Service agencies, and other organizations. Most publications are free of charge and can be ordered easily by calling (800) 458-5231 or by returning the order form in the centerfold of the catalog.

**102. National Center for Chronic Disease Prevention & Health Promotion**
Centers for Disease Control
4770 Buford Hwy., NE, Mailstop K13
Atlanta, GA 30341-3724
(770) 488-5080; FAX (770) 488-5969

The Center provides assistance to state and local health departments in tracking risk factors/conditions in the population; coordinates a telephone-based survey, the Behavioral Risk Factor Surveillance System, on major risk factors such as smoking, alcohol, nutrition, hypertension, weight, seat belt use, and preventative health measures such as mammography, clinical breast examination, Pap smear, and colorectal cancer screening; implements the National Breast and Cervical Cancer Early Detection Program and the National Program of Cancer Registries; implements Comprehensive School Health Education programs; and maintains CDP File, a CD-ROM product that contains information on national health education efforts.

**103. National Center for Health Statistics**
Division of Epidemiology and Health Promotion
6525 Belcrest Road, Room 1064
Hyattsville, MD 20782

This agency provides informational assistance in the development of health measures for health researchers, administrators, and planners.

**104. National Health Information Center**
Office of Disease Prevention and Health Promotion
P.O. Box 1133
Washington, DC 20013-1133
(301) 565-4167

The National Health Information Center, a service of the Office of Disease Prevention and Health Promotion, is a central source of information and referral for health questions from the public and health care professionals. It maintains a computer database of government agencies, support groups, professional societies, and other organizations that can answer questions on specific health care topics. In addition, the Center offers a library containing medical and health reference books, directories, information files, and periodicals; database development on organizations that provide health information; and a number of publications including resource guides and bibliographies.

Some publications prepared by this office are:
Department of Health and Human Services (DHHS) *Prevention Reports,* which summarize prevention-oriented findings in the scientific literature in abstract form
*Healthfinder Series,* which provides resource lists on specific health topics and events

*Healthy People 2000*, the National Health Promotion and Disease Prevention's objectives and health goals for the year 2000. Included are over 300 objectives in 22 priority areas, such as nutrition, tobacco use, environmental health, cancer, and HIV infections.

### 105. National Heart, Lung, and Blood Institute Information Center

National Institutes of Health
P.O. Box 30105
Bethesda, MD 20824-0105
(301) 251-1222; FAX (301) 251-1223

The information center is a service of the NHLBI that provides health professionals and the general public with the most current information available about high blood pressure, cholesterol, asthma, obesity, heart attack, and heart disease. The Information Center disseminates educational, programmatic, and scientific materials and responds to inquiries. The Information Center database is also part of the Combined Health Information Database (CHID) available through OVID Technologies. Series publications include *Heart Memo* and *Asthma Memo*.

### 106. National Institute for Occupational Safety and Health (NIOSH)

U.S. Department of Health and Human Services
Office of the Director
200 Independence Avenue, SW
Humphrey Building, Room 715-H
Washington, DC 20201
(202) 401-6997

NIOSH is a federal research agency. The NIOSH provides technical information to the National Institute for Occupational research programs and supplies information to others on request. Of interest is its research in the area of handling cytotoxic drugs and laminar airflow hoods. It also has developed guidelines for health care workers in preventing the transmission of hepatitis B virus and HIV.

### 107. National Institute on Aging

Public Information Office
9000 Rockville Pike
Bldg. 31, Room 5C27
Bethesda, MD 20892
(301) 496-1752

The National Institute on Aging's Public Information Office carries out a legislatively mandated information and education program for the general public, mass media, physicians, health care workers, other government agencies, and service organizations. Free consumer materials are available on many topics pertaining to older adults, including cancer and smoking.

### 108. National Library of Medicine

National Institutes of Health
8600 Rockville Pike
Bethesda, MD 20894
(301) 496-6308 Public Information Office
(301) 496-6095 Reference Section

The National Library of Medicine collects, organizes, and disseminates both printed and audiovisual materials. The collection, technical and scientific in nature, is primarily for medical professionals. The Library offers an extensive computerized literature retrieval service. A list of bibliographies, catalogues, and indexes with specific ordering instructions is available from the Public Information Office.

### 109. National Technical Information Service

National Audiovisual Center
(703) 487-4650; FAX (703) 321-8547;
TDD (703) 487-4639; RUSH service (800) 553-NTIS
To order via the Internet: orders@ntis.fedworld.gov. (To avoid sending your account number with each Internet order, call (703) 487-4682 to register your credit card at NTIS.)

The National Technical Information Service is the central resource for U.S. government scientific, technical, engineering, and business-related information. The collection also contains similar information from foreign government and from domestic and foreign nongovernment sources. Each year, NTIS adds more than 85,000 new titles to its collection of approximately 2.5 million products. The collection includes technical reports, periodicals, databases, computer software, diskettes, CD-ROMs, audiovisuals, and on-line services.

**Sample listing:**

*Basic Medical Pathology—Neoplasia I: Nomenclature of Benign vs. Malignant States* (1994). This program uses photomicrographs of normal and neoplastic tissues and organs to define and describe changes that tissues go through when the normal cell cycle is interrupted and neoplasia occurs. (30-minute VHS videotape)

FedWorld is the NTIS's electronic access point to locate, order, and acquire health-related and other information from the results of government-conducted or sponsored research and development. Access is free of charge. Current FedWorld features include walk-you-through prompts, a simple on-line system, and electronic delivery of many products. The Preview Database allows immediate access to bibliographic citations for thousands of new information products that are available for purchase.

FedWorld subsystems to locate health-related information include:

- CancerNet, from the NCI—provides summaries of treatment, supportive care, screening, prevention, and investigational drug information written both in Spanish and English.

- The Agency for Health Care Policy and Research subsystem provides abstracts of electronic publications on subjects including home health care, hospitals, and health technology assessments.

FedWorld HEALTH Gateway Systems provides access to many bulletin board systems including:

- Food and Drug Administration (FDA) Information and Policies

- Health and Human Services (OASH) Health and AIDS Information and Reports

- National Institute of Health Grant Line (NIHGL)

- Health and Human Services Primary Health Care Information (PHC)

- Center for Substance Abuse Prevention (CSAP) Alcohol and Drug Information

FedWorld Marketplace is a resource for health-related information products including:

- Respiratory Health Effects of Passive Smoking: Lung Cancer and Other Disorders

- FDA Food Code (download, or in paper copy)

- America's Maturing Majority

- Blood Alcohol Content Estimator software program

- Handbook of Child & Elder Care Resources

To connect to the NTIS FedWorld On-Line Information Network:

**By modem,** set modem parity to none; data bits to 8; stop bit to 1. Set terminal emulation to ANSI; set duplex to full; set communication software to dial FedWorld at (703) 321-FEDW (3339).

**By internet,** Telnet to fedworld.gov. For internet file transfer protocol (FTP) services, connect to ftp.fedworld.gov. For World Wide Web services, point your web browser to open the URL http://www.fedworld.gov.

**FedWorld Marketplace,** once connected, select option M from Main Menu.

**NTIS Preview Database,** once connected, select option B (Locate and Reference Government Information), then choose option B.

### 110. National Toxicology Program
National Institute of Environmental Health Sciences
M.D. A0/01, Box 12233
Research Triangle Park, NC 27709
(919) 541-1371

The NTP coordinates and conducts toxicology and test method development research and provides information about potentially hazardous chemicals, including those that cause cancer. Information in the form of technical reports on particular chemicals, as well as the annual report on carcinogens, is available free of charge until supplies are exhausted.

### 111. Occupational Safety and Health Administration (OSHA)
U.S. Department of Labor
Office of Information and Consumer Affairs
200 Constitution Avenue, NW
Washington, DC 20210
(202) 219-8148

OSHA is a federal enforcement agency. The Publication Distribution Office responds to inquiries from the general public, health care professionals, industry, educational institutions, and other sources about a limited number of job-related carcinogens and toxic substances. The Regulatory Text of OSHA's Final Standard for Occupational Exposure to Bloodborne Pathogens is available through this office. It has published guidelines for handling antineoplastic drugs and other information related to health care worker safety.

A new service, OSHA FAX-ON-DEMAND, offers immediate information by dialing 1-900-555-3400. Callers can have a wide variety of OSHA information faxed to them (i.e., Bloodborne Facts Index) immediately. The database includes agency news releases (updated daily), fact sheets, publications listings, information on the Department of Labor's electronic bulletin board, OSHA listings, OSHA inspection statistics, and other information. The system offers more than 200 brief documents to the public for a nominal telephone charge of $1.50. Most documents are five pages or fewer, and the typical cost of faxing a two-page item is $3.00.

### 112. Office of Cancer Communications
National Cancer Institute
Bethesda, MD 20892
(301) 496-5583

The Office of Cancer Communications provides information on all aspects of the cancer problem to physicians, scientists, educators, Congress, the Executive Branch, the media, and the public. It fosters and coordinates a national cancer communications program designed to provide the public and health care professionals with information they need to take more responsible health actions. The Cancer Information Service CIS (800-4-CANCER) is located within this office, with a network of locations across the country.

### 113. Office of Consumer Affairs
Food and Drug Administration
5600 Fishers Lane
Rockville, MD 20857
(301) 443-3170

The Office of Consumer Affairs, Food and Drug Administration, responds to consumer inquiries and serves as a clearinghouse for consumer publications on a variety of topics including pregnancy, mammography, food and nutrition, proper use of drugs, and health fraud. Over 250 pamphlets are available free of charge; requests should be made in writing.

### 114. Office of Minority Health
Division of Information and Education
5600 Fishers Lane, Suite 1000
Rockville, MD 20857
(301) 443-5224; FAX (301) 443-8280

The mission of the Office of Minority Health (OMH) is to improve the health of racial and ethnic populations through the development of health policies and programs. Racial and ethnic minority communities served by the office are African-American, American Indian and Alaska Native, Asian American and Pacific Islander, and Hispanic/Latino. The OMH targets the health concerns responsible for most of the excess mortality suffered by racial and ethnic minority populations: alcohol and other drug use, cardiovascular disease and stroke, cancer, diabetes, infant mortality, violence, and HIV/AIDS. OMH also targets "cross-cutting" issues essential to health improvements: access to health care, cultural competency in health service delivery, improved health data, and the availability of health professionals to serve minority communities. Access to databases and publications are available through the Resource Center (see next entry).

### 115. Office of Minority Health Resource Center (OMH-RC)
P.O. Box 37337
Washington, DC 20013-7337
(800) 444-MHRC

The MHRC is a division of the Public Health Service, Department of Health and Human Services. The OMH-RC is the largest resource and referral service on minority health in the nation. Established in 1987, it facilitates the exchange of information. All resource center services are free and can be obtained by calling or visiting the library in Silver Spring, MD. When you call, an information specialist (English- or Spanish-speaking) will help you find what you need via database search, publication order, or organization referral.

**116. Office on Smoking and Health**
Centers for Disease Control
Mailstop K-50
4770 Buford Highway, NE
Atlanta, GA 30341
(800) CDC-1311; (770) 448-5705

The Office on Smoking and Health produces and distributes a number of informational and educational materials. It also offers bibliographic and reference services to researchers and others. The materials and services are available free of charge. In addition, the office produces pamphlets, posters, and public service announcements that contain various health messages.

**117. Patient Referral Service**
Warren Grant Magnuson Clinical Center
National Institutes of Health
Building 10, Room 1C255
10 Center Drive, MSC 1170
Bethesda, MD 20892-1170
(301) 594-5790

Numerous cancer trials take place at the Clinical Center, NIH's on-site hospital facility. Patients are admitted only on referral by a physician. The patient's condition must be under active investigation by NIH researchers at the time of admission. Submit the patient's medical history and diagnosis to the referral service or call for more information about our clinical trials. Patients accepted into a protocol are not charged for care but may be responsible for transportation costs.

# COOPERATIVE CLINICAL TRIAL GROUPS

Following are the U.S. Clinical Trials Cooperative Groups from which information can be obtained on clinical trials being conducted, eligibility criteria, treatment plan of the clinical trial, and how to refer a patient to one of these trials. Currently in the United States, fewer than 10% of eligible adult patients are entered on clinical trials. The result of this low percentage of patients is a delay in answering important therapeutic and scientific questions and in disseminating therapeutic advances to the general oncology community. There are multiple clinical trials conducted within each of the Cooperative Groups.

**118. Brain Tumor Cooperative Group (BTCG)**
William R. Shapiro, MD
Barrow Neurological Institute
St. Joseph's Hospital
350 West Thomas Road
Phoenix, AZ 85013
(602) 285-3895

**119. Cancer and Leukemia Group B (CALGB)**
Gini Fleming, MD
208 S. LaSalle Street, Suite 2000
Chicago, IL 60604-1104
(312) 702-9171; FAX (312) 345-0117

**Affiliations** (Community Clinical Oncology Programs):
Cancer Therapy Evaluation Program
Eastern Maine Medical Center CCOP

Hematology Oncology Associates of Central New York CCOP
North Shore University Hospital CCOP
Southeast Cancer Control Consortium CCOP
Southern Nevada Cancer Research Foundation CCOP
Medical Center of Delaware CCOP
San Diego Kaiser Permanente CCOP
Mount Sinai CCOP
New Jersey CCOP
Syracuse Hematology-Oncology CCOP
St. Michaels' Medical Center Tri-County CCOP
Green Mountain Oncology Group CCOP

**120. Children's Cancer Group (CCG)**
Anita Khayat, PhD, MBA
P.O. Box 60012
Arcadia, CA 91066-6012
(818) 447-0064

**Affiliations:**
Cancer Therapy Evaluation Program
Colorado Cancer Research CCOP
Duluth Clinic CCOP
Geisinger CCOP
Iowa Oncology Research Association CCOP
Marshfield Medical Foundation CCOP
North Shore University Hospital CCOP
Sioux Community Cancer Consortium CCOP
St. Luke's Hospitals CCOP
Medical Center of Delaware CCOP
Bay Area Tumor Institute CCOP
Southern Nevada Cancer Research Foundation CCOP

**121. Eastern Cooperative Oncology Group (ECOG)**
Frontier Science
303 Boylston Street
Brookline, MA 02146
(617) 632-3610; FAX (617) 632-2990

**Academic and Cancer Centers:**
Albany Medical College
Albert Einstein College
Case Western-MetroHealth Medical Center
Emory University
University of Florida (Gainesville)
Fox Chase Cancer Center
Indiana University Medical Center
Johns Hopkins University
Mayo Clinic
University of Miami
Moffitt Cancer Center
New York University Medical Center
Northwestern University
Medical College of Ohio
University of Pennsylvania
University of Pittsburgh
University of Pretoria
University of Rochester
Rush Presbyterian-St. Luke's Medical Center
Stanford University
Thomas Jefferson University
Tufts University-New England Medical Center
Vanderbilt University
Medical College of Wisconsin
University of Wisconsin

**Affiliations** (Community Clinical Oncology Programs):
  Cancer Therapy Evaluation Program
  Ann Arbor Regional CCOP
  Arizona Minority-Based CCOP
  Carle Clinic CCOP
  Cedar Rapids CCOP
  Colorado CA Research Program CCOP
  Duluth Clinic CCOP
  Evanston CCOP
  Fairfax Hospital CCOP
  Geisinger CCOP
  Grady Hospital CCOP
  Illinois Oncology Research Association CCOP
  Iowa CCOP
  Kalamazoo CCOP
  Main Line Health CCOP
  MeritCare Hospital CCOP
  Metro-Minnesota CCOP
  Missouri Valley Cancer Consortium CCOP
  Ochsner CCOP
  San Juan CCOP
  Scottsdale CCOP
  Sioux Community Cancer Consortium CCOP
  Toledo CCOP
  Tulsa CCOP

**122. European Organization for Research and Treatment of Cancer (EORTC)**
Celestina Arrigo
Francoise Meunier, MD
Avenue E Mounier 83—B11
B-1200 Brussels (Bruxelles), Belgium
32-2-774-16-11
32-2-774-16-30

**123. Gynecologic Oncology Group (GOG)**
Jack Kellner, Administrative Director
1234 Market Street, Suite 1945
Philadelphia, PA 19107-3798
(215) 854-0770; FAX (215) 854-0716

**Affiliation:**
  Cancer Therapy Evaluation Program

**124. Intergroup Rhabdomyosarcoma Study**
Harold Maurer, MD
University of Nebraska Medical Center
Omaha, NE 68198-6545
(402) 559-4204

**Affiliation:**
  Cancer Therapy Evaluation Program

**125. National Surgical Adjuvant Breast and Bowel Project (NSABP)**
Mary Ketner, RN
230 McKee Place, Suite 402
Pittsburgh, PA 15213
(412) 383-1400; FAX (412) 383-1388

**Affiliations** (Community Clinical Oncology Programs):
  Cancer Therapy Evaluation Program
  Alton Ochsner Medical Foundation CCOP
  Ann Arbor Regional CCOP
  Atlanta Regional CCOP
  Bay Area Tumor Institute CCOP
  Billings Interhospital CCOP

  Carle Cancer Center CCOP
  Cedar Rapids CCOP
  Central Illinois CCOP
  Colorado Cancer Research CCOP
  Columbia River CCOP
  Columbus CCOP
  Dayton CCOP
  Duluth Clinic CCOP
  Evanston Hospital CCOP
  Fairfax CCOP
  Grand Rapids CCOP
  Greater Phoenix
  Green Mountain CCOP
  Greenville South Carolina CCOP
  Illinois Oncology Research Association CCOP
  Iowa Oncology Research Association CCOP
  Kalamazoo CCOP
  Kansas City CCOP
  Marshfield CCOP
  Medical Center of Delaware CCOP
  Mercy Hospital CCOP
  Meritcare Hospital CCOP
  Metro-Minnesota CCOP
  Missouri Valley Cancer Consortium CCOP
  Mt. Sinai Medical Center CCOP
  Natalie Warren Bryant CCOP
  New Jersey CCOP
  North Shore University Hospital CCOP
  Northern New Jersey CCOP
  Northwest CCOP
  Ozarks Regional CCOP
  San Diego Kaiser Permanente CCOP
  Santa Rosa Memorial Hospital Regional CCOP
  Sioux Community Cancer Consortium CCOP
  Southeast Cancer Control Consortium CCOP
  Southern Nevada Cancer Research Foundation CCOP
  Spartanburg CCOP
  St. Louis, MO CCOP
  Syracuse Hematology Oncology CCOP
  Toledo CCOP
  Tri-County, Newark, NJ CCOP
  Virginia Mason Research Center CCOP
  Wichita CCOP

Minority-Based Community Clinical Oncology Programs (MBCCOP):
  Grady Hospital MBCCOP
  Kings County MBCCOP
  MCV/CMH of Virginia MBCCOP
  San Juan MBCCOP
  South Texas MBCCOP
  University of South Alabama MBCCOP

**126. National Wilms' Tumor Study Group (NWTSG)**
Daniel M. Green, MD
Roswell Park Cancer Institute
Pediatric Division
Elm & Carlton Streets
Buffalo, NY 14263
(716) 845-2334; FAX (716) 845-8003
E-mail: ROSDANGR@UBVMS.CC.BUFFALO.EDU

**Affiliation:**
  Cancer Therapy Evaluation Program

127. **North Central Cancer Treatment Group (NCCTG)**
Patricia Koenig, RN
200 First Street SW
Rochester, MN 55905
(507) 284-4642
**Affiliations:**
    Cancer Therapy Evaluation Program
    Carle Cancer Center CCOP
    Cedar Rapids CCOP
    Duluth Clinic CCOP
    Geisinger CCOP
    Illinois Oncology Research Association CCOP
    Iowa Oncology Research Association CCOP
    Mayo Clinic
    Ochsner CCOP
    Rapid City Regional CCOP
    Sioux Community Cancer Consortium CCOP
    St. Luke's Hospitals CCOP
    Toledo CCOP

128. **Pediatric Oncology Group (POG)**
Sue Giovannazi-Bannon, MS
645 N. Michigan Avenue, Suite 910
Chicago, IL 60611
(312) 482-9944; FAX (312) 482-9460
**Affiliations** (Community Clinical Oncology Programs):
    Cancer Therapy Evaluation Program
    Bergen-Passaic CCOP
    Columbia River CCOP
    Florida Pediatric CCOP
    Louisiana State University Minority Program CCOP
    Ochsner CCOP
    University of South Alabama CCOP
    US TEX PED CCOP
    Wichita CCOP

129. **Radiation Therapy Oncology Group (RTOG)**
Nancy W. Smith
1101 Market Street, 14th Floor
Philadelphia, PA 19107
(215) 574-3205; FAX (215) 928-0153
**Affiliations** (Community Clinical Oncology Programs):
    Cancer Therapy Evaluation Program
    Atlanta Regional CCOP
    Carle Cancer Center CCOP
    Catherine McAuley Health Center CCOP
    Columbia River CCOP
    Greenville SC CCOP
    Kaiser Permanente CCOP
    Main Line Health CCOP
    Medical Center of Delaware CCOP
    Metro-MN CCOP
    North Shore University Hospital CCOP
    Ochsner Clinic CCOP
    Southeast Cancer Control Consortium CCOP
    Southern Nevada Cancer Research Foundation CCOP
    South Jersey Oncology Group
    Spartanburg CCOP

130. **Southwest Oncology Group (SWOG)**
Operations Office
Charles Coltman, MD
14980 Omicron Drive
San Antonio, TX 78245-3217
(210) 677-8808; FAX (210) 677-0006

**Affiliations** (Community Clinical Oncology Programs):
    Cancer Therapy Evaluation Program
    Atlanta Regional CCOP
    Bay Area CCOP
    Billings Interhospital CCOP
    Central Illinois CCOP
    Columbia River CCOP
    Columbus CCOP
    Dayton CCOP
    Grand Rapids CCOP
    Greater Phoenix CCOP
    Greenville, South Carolina CCOP
    Kansas City CCOP
    Northwest CCOP
    Ozark Regional CCOP
    Spartanburg CCOP
    St. Louis-Cape Girardeau CCOP
    Virginia Mason Medical Center CCOP
    Wichita CCOP

Minority-Based Community Clinical Oncology Programs (MBCCOP):
    Hawaii MBCCOP
    Kings County MBCCOP
    LSU Medical Center MBCCOP
    San Antonio MBCCOP
    University of South Alabama MBCCOP

# NURSING EDUCATIONAL OPPORTUNITIES

## 131. Graduate Level Oncology Nursing Programs

Many nursing schools offer graduate education in oncology, and the potential student can choose from several types of programs. Some programs offer separate, distinct, oncology clinical specialist master's curricula, whereas others offer the oncology component within the graduate program in medical-surgical nursing. Nurse practitioner programs also are offered with Acute Health, Pediatrics, Adult Health, Gerontological, and Family Health focuses.

The Oncology Nursing Society publication, *The Master's Degree with a Specialty in Advanced Practice Oncology Nursing* (1994) serves a dual purpose as a guide for (1) nursing educators in establishing new oncology programs or evaluating current ones and (2) prospective students in selecting a program. Another excellent source is the article "Survey of Graduate Programs in Cancer Nursing" in *Oncology Nursing Forum* 22:1275–1282, 1995. This article details specific information about each program (clinical focus, program length, application deadline, NLN accreditation). The *1996 Peterson's Guide to Nursing Programs* (ed 2) is another resource for lists of undergraduate, graduate, and nurse practitioner programs and is available in most bookstores and medical libraries.

The following list provides a state-by-state guide to graduate level oncology nursing programs. Because curricula and programs change, the reader is advised to contact universities to determine if the school of nursing offers a graduate level program in oncology nursing and/or nurse practitionership.

**Alabama**

University of Alabama at Birmingham
School of Nursing
Birmingham, AL 35294
Judy Holcombe, RN, DSN
Associate Professor: Adult Oncology
(205) 934-6588
Penelope Wright, RN, PhD
Assistant Professor: Pediatric Oncology
(205) 934-6659

**Arizona**

University of Arizona
College of Nursing
Tucson, AZ 85721
Ida (Ki) Moore, RN, DNSc, FAAN
Associate Professor
(520) 626-6154

**California**

University of California, Los Angeles (UCLA)
School of Nursing
Los Angeles, CA 90024-6918
Linda Sarna, RN, DNSc, OCN®
American Cancer Society Professor of Oncology
Nursing
Assistant Professor
(310) 825-8690

University of California, San Francisco (UCSF)
School of Nursing
Department of Physiological Nursing
San Francisco, CA 94143-1060
Christine Miaskowski, RN, PhD
(415) 476-1942

**Colorado**

University of Colorado
School of Nursing
4200 East Ninth Avenue, Box C-288
Denver, CO 80262
Program Director: Paula Nelson-Marten, RN, PhD,
OCN®
Academic Dean: Peggy Chin, RN, PhD, FAAN
(303) 270-5592

**Connecticut**

Yale University
School of Nursing
New Haven, CT 06536-0740
Wendy Holmes, RN, MSN
Assistant Professor/Coordinator
Medical-Surgical Nursing Program
(203) 737-2355

**Delaware**

University of Delaware
College of Nursing
University of Delaware
Newark, DE 19716
Jayne Fernsler, RN, DSN, AOCN
Associate Professor
(302) 831-8673

**Florida**

University of Miami
School of Nursing
Miami, FL 33124
Judith Jezek, RN, EdD
Associate Dean
(305) 284-3666

University of South Florida
College of Nursing
Tampa, FL 33612
Susan McMillan, RN, PhD, FAAN
Chairperson, Oncology Nursing
American Cancer Society Professor of Oncology
Nursing
(813) 974-9188

**Georgia**

Emory University
Nell Hodgson Woodruff School of Nursing
Atlanta, GA 30322
Donna Owen, RN, PhD
Adult Oncology Assistant Professor
Rosalind Bryant, RN, MN, PNP
Pediatric Oncology Instructor
(404) 727-3931

Georgia State University
School of Nursing
College of Health Sciences
Atlanta, GA 30303
Sherry Gaines, RN, PhD
Associate Dean
(404) 651-3044

**Illinois**

Loyola University
Niehoff School of Nursing
Medical-Surgical Nursing
6525 N. Sheridan Rd.
Chicago, IL 60626-5385
Esther Matassarin-Jacobs, RN, PhD, OCN®
Associate Professor
(773) 508-3271

Rush University
College of Nursing
Chicago, IL 60612
Judith Paice, RN, PhD, FAAN
Assistant Professor
(312) 563-2045

**Indiana**

Indiana University
School of Nursing
Indianapolis, IN 46223
Cheryl Bean, RN, DSN, CS, OCN®
Associate Professor
(317) 274-2471

**Maryland**

Johns Hopkins University
1830 Monument Street
Baltimore, MD 21205
Patricia Grimm, RN, PhD, CS
Assistant Professor
American Cancer Society Professor of Oncology
Nursing
(410) 955-4280

University of Maryland
School of Nursing
Baltimore, MD 21201
Anne E. Belcher, RN, PhD, FAAN
Associate Professor
(410) 706-7407

**Massachusetts**

Massachusetts General Hospital Institute of Health
Professions
Boston, MA 02108-3402
Jean Leuner, RN, PhD
Interim Program Director
(617) 726-3163

**Minnesota**

University of Minnesota
School of Nursing
Health Sciences Unit F 6-101
308 Harvard Street SE
Minneapolis, MN 55455
Janice Post-White, RN, PhD
Assistant Professor
American Cancer Society Professor of Oncology
Nursing
(612) 624-1921

**Missouri**

St. Louis University
School of Nursing
St. Louis, MO 63104
Ramona M. Wessler, RN, PhD
(314) 577-8934

University of Missouri, Columbia
School of Nursing
Columbia, MO 65211
Rosemary J. Porter, RN, PhD
Associate Dean for Student Affairs
Director, Graduate Studies
(573) 882-0228

**Nebraska**

University of Nebraska
College of Nursing
Adult Health and Illness Department
Omaha, NE 68105-1065
Lani Zimmerman, RN, PhD
(402) 559-6627

**New York**

Columbia University
School of Nursing
New York, NY 10032
Marianne Glasel, RN, MS, MA
Director, Oncology and Accelerated Master's
Programs
(212) 305-4196

The Sage Colleges
Sage Graduate School
Troy, NY 12180
Ann M. Gothier, RN, PhD
Director, Graduate Program in Nursing
(518) 270-6878

State University of New York, Buffalo
School of Nursing
910 Kimball Tower
Buffalo, NY 14214
Katherine G. Wallace, RN, PhD
Assistant Professor
(716) 829-3271

University of Rochester
School of Nursing

Rochester, NY 14642
Linda S. Jones, RN, DNS
Associate Professor
Cancer Center Nursing
(716) 275-2371

**North Carolina**

Duke University
School of Nursing
Durham, NC 27710
Mary T. Champagne, RN, PhD
Dean
(919) 684-3786

University of North Carolina at Chapel Hill
School of Nursing
Chapel Hill, NC 27514
Barbara B. Germino, RN, PhD, FAAN
Chairperson, Adult and Geriatric Health
(919) 966-4269

**Ohio**

Case Western Reserve University
Frances Payne Bolton School of Nursing
Cleveland, OH 44106
M. Linda Workman, PhD, RN, FAAN, OCN®
Associate Professor of Nursing
American Cancer Society Professor of Oncology
Nursing
(216) 368-8855

Ohio State University
College of Nursing
Columbus, OH 43210-1289
Edna Menke, RN, PhD
Associate Dean
(614) 292-8045

**Pennsylvania**

Gwynedd-Mercy College
Gwynedd Valley, PA 19437
Patricia S. Bennett, RN, EdD, OCN®
Oncology Nursing
Graduate Nursing Division
(215) 646-7300, ext. 404

University of Pennsylvania
School of Nursing
Nursing Education Building
Philadelphia, PA 19104
Ruth McCorkle, RN, PhD, FAAN
American Cancer Society Professor of Oncology
Nursing
(215) 898-9134

University of Pittsburgh
School of Nursing
Pittsburgh, PA 15261
Margaret Rosenzweig, RN, MSN, CRNP-C, OCN®
Graduate Program Oncology Nursing
(412) 624-0072

**South Carolina**

University of South Carolina
College of Nursing
Columbia, SC 29208
Janet F. Nussbaum, RN, EdD
Oncology Nursing
(803) 777-4205

**Tennessee**

Vanderbilt University
School of Nursing
Nashville, TN 37240
James C. Pace, RN, DSN, MDiv, OCN®
Oncology Specialty
(615) 322-2815

**Texas**

University of Texas
School of Nursing
Health Science Center
Houston, TX 77030
Jeanette Adams, RN, DrPH, OCN®
Division Head: Oncology
(713) 792-7881

**Utah**

University of Utah
College of Nursing
25 South Medical Drive
Salt Lake City, UT 84112
Kathi Mooney, RN, PhD, FAAN
Professor
(801) 581-8272

**Virginia**

George Mason University
Fairfax, VA 22030
Jeanne Sorrell, DAEd
Coordinator, Advanced Clinical Nursing
(703) 993-1944

Virginia Commonwealth University
Medical College of Virginia
School of Nursing
Richmond, VA 23298
Mary Ropka, RN, PhD, FAAN
Chair, Adult Health
(804) 828-3347

**Washington**

University of Washington
Department of Physiological Nursing
Seattle, WA 98195
Betty Gallucci, RN, PhD
Professor
(206) 616-1961

**Wisconsin**

University of Wisconsin
School of Nursing
Madison, WI 53792
Sandra Ward, PhD, RN
Clinical Science Center
(608) 263-5277

## 132. Enterostomal Therapy Nursing Education Programs (ETNEP)

An enterostomal therapy (ET) nurse provides acute and rehabilitative care for people with select disorders of the gastrointestinal, genitourinary, and integumentary systems. The ET nurse offers direct patient care for patients with abdominal stomas, wounds, fistulas, drains, pressure ulcers, and incontinence. As a clinician, educator, consultant, researcher, and administrator,

the ET nurse plays a pivotal role in the guidance of optimum patient care. There are currently nine ETNEPs in the United States that are accredited by the Wound Ostomy Continence Nurses Society (WOCN). Accreditation by the WOCN guarantees the student that the program meets established criteria regarding course content, clinical experience, faculty, and student/faculty ratio.

Applicants must be RNs, have a baccalaureate degree with a major in nursing, and have one year of recent clinical experience (within five years in medical-surgical nursing). Program structure is diverse to meet the wide variety of needs of prospective students. Types of program structures include:

**Traditional:** Course is seven to eight weeks in duration. Theory and clinical experience are acquired at the ETNEP.

**Off-Site Clinical Experience:** Theory component is three to four weeks at the ETNEP; clinical component is arranged by the student at a facility closer to home under the supervision of a qualified board-certified ET nurse.

**Master's:** Course work and clinical experience are integrated into a Master's Degree program. The student receives graduate credit while completing the program.

**Specialty:** Course focuses on only one clinical area (wounds, ostomy, or continence) and is only three to four weeks in length.

Tuition varies for each program, and the student is also responsible for the expense of books, supplies, and room and board arrangements. Scholarships are available by competitive application through the WOCN, American Cancer Society, United Ostomy Association, and many of the ETNEPs. At the completion of a WOCN-accredited program, the graduate is awarded a certificate designating ET Nurse status, and is eligible to become Board Certified by passing the ET Board Certification examination. Information about certification can be requested from the WOCN.

WOCN-Accredited Enterostomal Therapy Nurse Education Programs (ETNEPs):

**California**

University of Southern California ETNEP
320 W. 15th Street, Leavey Hall
Los Angeles, CA 90015
(213) 743-2362
Program Director: Barbara Bates-Jensen, RN, MN, CETN

**Georgia**

Emory University WOCNEP
The Emory Clinic, Room 3610
1365 Clifton Road, N.E.
Atlanta, GA 30322
(404) 778-4067
Program Director: Dorothy Doughty, RN, MN, CETN
Medical Director: George Daneker, MD

**Minnesota**

Abbott Northwestern Hospital ETNEP
Department 14201
800 E. 28th Street at Chicago Avenue
Minneapolis, MN 55407
(612) 863-4601
Program Director: Brenda M. Kerschbaum, RN, MS, CETN

**New York**

Albany Medical Center ETNEP
A-73 New Scotland Avenue
Albany, NY 12208
(518) 262-3958 or (800) 829-3958
Program Director: Sharon A. Aronovitch
Program type: Independent study

**Ohio**

R.B. Turnbull, Jr. School of ET Nursing
Cleveland Clinic Foundation, Room KK-54
9500 Euclid Avenue
Cleveland, OH 44195-5161
(216) 444-5966
Program Director: Paula L. Erwin-Toth, RN, MSN,
CETN
Medical Director: John Oakley, MB, BS, FRACS

**Pennsylvania**

Harrisburg Area ETNEP
Wicks Educational Associates, Inc.
5012 Lenker Street, Suite 202
Mechanicsburg, PA 17055
(717) 737-2770; FAX (717) 737-7683
Program Development: Lucy J. Wicks, RN, MSN,
CETN

**South Carolina**

Medical University of South Carolina, Wound Care
Education Program
College of Nursing-Continuing Education
171 Ashley Avenue
Charleston, SC 29425-2401
(803) 792-2651
Program Director: Phyllis Bonham, RN, MS, CETN
Program Type: Wound Care only

**Texas**

University of Texas M.D. Anderson Cancer Center
ETNEP
Department of Nursing-82
1515 Holcombe Blvd.
Houston, TX 77030
(713) 745-0216
Program Director: Beverly Hampton, RN, MSN,
CETN, OCN®

# PRINT AND ELECTRONIC RESOURCES

There are a myriad of oncology-related journals and books available for reference, and the number of on-line services is rapidly increasing. This section of the chapter lists examples of each type of resource and is not intended to be all-inclusive.

## 133. Oncology Periodicals

*Medical and Health Care Books and Serials in Print,* found in most medical libraries, is an excellent bibliographic resource for periodicals. Each journal listing includes publisher, subscription price, frequency of publication, and indexing information. A partial list, specific to the needs of oncology nurses, includes:

*Acta Haematologica*
*Acta Oncologica*
*Advanced Practice Nurse*

*Advances in Cancer Research*
*AIDS Care*
*AIDS Patient Care*
*American Journal of Clinical Oncology*
*American Journal of Hematology*
*American Journal of Hospice and Palliative Care*
*American Journal of Pediatric Hematology-Oncology*
*Annals of Oncology*
*Anticancer Research*
*Blood*
*Breast Cancer Research and Treatment*
*British Journal of Cancer*
*British Journal of Haematology*
*CA—A Cancer Journal for Clinicians*
*Canadian Oncology Nursing Journal*
*Cancer*
*Cancer Chemotherapy and Pharmacology*
*Cancer Forum*
*Cancer Genetics and Cytogenetics*
*Cancer Immunology and Immunotherapy*
*Cancer Letters*
*Cancer Nursing*
*Cancer Practice*
*Cancer Research*
*Cancer Review*
*Cancer Treatment Reviews*
*Carcinogenesis*
*Clinical Oncology Alert*
*Clinical Data Management*
*Contemporary Oncology*
*Critical Review in Oncology-Hematology*
*Current Opinions in Oncology*
*Current Problems in Cancer*
*European Journal of Cancer and Clinical Oncology*
*European Journal of Gynecological Oncology*
*European Journal of Surgical Oncology*
*Hematology-Oncology Clinics of North America*
*International Journal of Cancer*
*Journal of American Academy of Nurse Practitioners*
*Journal of Cancer Education*
*Journal of Clinical Oncology*
*Journal of Experimental and Clinical Hematology*
*Journal of the National Cancer Institute*
*Journal of Neuro-Oncology*
*Journal of Pain Symptom Management*
*Journal of Palliative Care*
*Journal of Pediatric Oncology Nursing*
*Journal of Psychosocial Oncology*
*Journal of Tumor Marker Oncology*
*Journal of Wound, Ostomy and Continence Care*
*Leukemia Research*
*Medical and Pediatric Oncology*
*Medical Oncology and Tumor Pharmacotherapy*
*National Cancer Institute (NCI) Monographs*
*National Cancer Institute Journal*
*Neoplasma*
*Nurse Practitioner*
*Nurse Practitioner Forum*
*Nutrition and Cancer*
*Oncogene*
*Oncology*
*Oncology Nursing Forum*
*ONS Nursing Scan in Oncology*
*Ostomy Wound Management*
*Pediatric Hematology and Oncology*

*Progress in Cancer Research and Therapy*
*Recent Results in Cancer Research*
*Seminars in Hematology*
*Seminars in Oncology*
*Seminars in Oncology Nursing*
*Seminars in Surgical Oncology*
*Yearbook of Oncology*

The resource book *Medical and Health Care Books and Serials in Print* also lists books available on cancer-related topics for the public. It is updated annually and is available in most hospital and medical libraries. Many books are professional texts and deal with all aspects of oncology medicine and nursing, including the diagnosis and treatment of cancer; others are personal stories for public reading and deal with coping and side effects from treatment, and are anecdotal in style. There is also a wide variety available in bookstores and libraries.

## 134. Personal Assistance/Patient Stories

Benjamin H, Trubo R: *From Victim to Victor.* WAT Braille, 1990

Bloch A, Bloch R: *Cancer . . . There's Hope.* Cancer Connection, 1986

Bloch A, Bloch R: *Fighting Cancer.* Cancer Connection, 1987

Borysenko J: *Minding the Body, Mending the Mind.* Bantam, 1988

Brack P: *Moms Don't Get Sick.* Melius, 1990

Comfort G, Comfort P: *Dying to Live.* Tyndale, 1992

Cook JC: *Coping with Cancer One Day at a Time.* Woodland, 1988

Doan Noyes D, Mellody P: *Beauty & Cancer: A Woman's Guide to Looking Great While Experiencing the Side Effects of Cancer Therapy.* AC Press, 1988

Dollinger M, Rosenbaum E, Cable G: *Everyone's Guide to Cancer Therapy.* Andrews & McMeel, 1991

Dravecky D, Stafford T: *Comeback.* HarperCollins, 1990

Gaes J: *My Book for Kids with Cansur.* Melius Peterson, 1988

Harwell A: *Ready to Live, Prepared to Die.* Shaw, 1995

Harwell A, Tomasik K: *When Your Friend Gets Cancer: How You Can Help.* Shaw, 1987

Johnson J, Klein L: *I Can Cope: Staying Healthy with Cancer* (ed 2). DCI, 1994

Kauffman DG: *Surviving Cancer: A Practical Guide for Those Fighting to Win.* Acropolis, 1989

MacDonald JA: *When Cancer Strikes: A Book for Patients, Families and Friends.* Prentice-Hall, 1982

Morra M, Potts E: *Choices: Realistic Alternatives in Cancer Treatment.* Avon, 1987

Mullan F: *Vital Signs: A Young Doctor's Struggle with Cancer.* FS & G, 1983

Muraa A, Stewart B: *Man to Man: When the Woman You Love Has Breast Cancer.* St. Martin's Press, 1989

Siegel BS: *Love, Medicine, and Miracles.* Harper & Row, 1986

Siegel ME: *The Cancer Patient's Handbook: Everything You Need to Know about Today's Care and Treatment.* Walker & Co., 1986

Simonton C, Matthews-Simonton S, Creighton, J: *Getting Well Again.* Bantam, 1988

Snyder M: *An Informed Decision: Understanding Breast Reconstruction.* Little, Brown, 1989

Sturgeon-Day L: *A Slice of Life: A Personal Story of Healing Through Cancer,* Lifeways, 1991

Wadler J: *My Breast: One Woman's Cancer Story.* Addison-Wesley, 1992.

## 135. On-Line Library Retrieval Services

Library or electronic information services have become a convenient, timely, and cost-effective method of accessing information by computer. Most hospital and university libraries subscribe to specific on-line databases, or they can be accessed from personal computers via a modem.

**136. CancerFax—National Cancer Institute**
International Cancer Information Service
9030 Old Georgetown Road
Bldg. 82 Room 219
Bethesda, MD 20892
FAX (301) 402-5874; for assistance, (301) 496-8880

CancerFax was created by the NCI to combine the computer and the fax machine. The NCI sends current data on cancer treatment to any health care professional with a fax machine free of charge utilizing the PDQ database. There are two types of summaries, one for health professionals and one for the general public; the service is available 24 hours a day, seven days a week. There is no charge for the service itself; the user pays only for the cost of the call to the CancerFax computer in Maryland.

**137. Knightridder Information Services, Inc.**
2440 El Camino Real
Mountainview, CA 94040
(800) 334-2564; (415) 528-7709 in CA

Knightridder Information Service (formerly known as DIALOG) has a scope of 380 databases in the subject areas of science, business, technology, chemistry, law, medicine, engineering, social sciences, economics, current events, and more. Average costs are $6.00 to $16.50 for a ten-minute search, plus printing charges, if done off-line. MEDLINE, CIS, and NURSING & ALLIED HEALTH are all accessible with Knightridder Information Services.

**138. National Library of Medicine**
8600 Rockville Pike
Bethesda, MD 20894
(301) 496-6193; (800) 638-8480

The NLM's MEDLARS is a service that allows for cost-effective searching of specialized databases and is available 24 hours a day. The user pays only for the time spent making the search and how much information is actually downloaded. There is no fee to access the system. Citations can be printed on the user's printer, or printed at the NLM and mailed ("off-line"). An off-line print costs $0.18 per page, with a typical page containing eight citations without abstracts and two or three citations with abstracts. Specific databases include:

AIDSDRUGS (information about AIDS-related drugs)
AIDSLINE (AIDS-related references)
AIDSTRIALS (AIDS-related clinical trials)
AVLINE (records of audiovisuals)
BIOETHICSLINE (information about bioethics)
CANCERLIT (information relating to cancer literature)

CATLINE (records of books)
CHEMLINE (information about chemical substances)
CCRIS (chemical carcinogenesis research information)
DIRLINE (directory of 15,000 information resources)
HEALTH (information about health care services)
HSDB (hazardous substances data bank)
MEDLINE (abstracts to journal articles)
PDQ (advances in cancer treatment and clinical trials)
RTECS (registry of toxic effects and chemical substances)
TOXLINE (toxicological information)
TRI (toxic chemical release inventory)

The NLM developed GRATEFUL MED software to allow for easy access to the Library's vast collection of medical and health science information. Because it both formulates the search strategy and presents the results off-line, computer time is brief, productive, and cost-effective. An average search costs less than $3.00. The software is IBM- or Macintosh-compatible, available on five floppy disks or one diskette, and sells for $29.95. GRATEFUL MED software can be ordered from the National Technical Information Service (NTIS).

### 139. OVID Technologies
333 7th Ave.
New York, NY 10001
(800) 950-2035; (212) 563-3006; FAX (212) 563-3784
(800) 950-2371 (Technical Support Center in Utah)
WWW site: www.ovid.com

OVID Technologies is another comprehensive electronic information service. Over 80 databases are available in the areas of medicine/pharmacology, education, life sciences, physical/applied sciences, reference, business, and social sciences/humanities; costs are based on on-line time, document charges, and telecommunications (if applicable). OVID On-Line is a menu-driven service offering the most popular databases (including CANCERLIT, MEDLINE, PDQ and NURSING & ALLIED HEALTH). Cost of a search is specific to the database being used.

## STATE CANCER PAIN INITIATIVES

### 140. State Cancer Pain Initiatives Resource Center
1300 University Avenue, #3671
Madison, WI 53706
(608) 265-4013; FAX (608) 265-4014

The state pain initiative movement is one primarily of education, advocacy, and creation of a positive regulatory climate. Pain initiatives are developed at the state level in order to tailor their programs to the unique geographic, cultural, and political characteristics of their region. The focus is on cancer relief because it is a pain syndrome easily recognized and described. It is hoped that progress toward relief of cancer pain will bring new awareness of and skill in relieving pain of other etiology and disease states.

The Resource Center was established in January, 1993. Its goals are to:

- foster the growth and development of state cancer pain initiatives

- plan and organize the annual national meetings for state cancer pain initiatives

- provide information about cancer pain management to health professionals as well as to patients and families

- assist state cancer pain initiatives in working with the media and with other forms of communication and outreach to patients, families, and the general public

- collaborate with the NCI Office of Cancer Communications and the Agency for Health Care and Policy Research (AHCPR) in the dissemination of the Clinical Practice Guideline for the Management of Cancer Pain

- support individual and collective research efforts by state cancer pain initiatives

- act as an information exchange, referral source, and clearinghouse among initiatives

**State Contacts for Cancer Pain Initiatives**

**Arizona**
Eugenie A. Obbens, MD
Barrows Neurological Institute
350 West Thomas
Phoenix, AZ 85013
(602) 406-3390

**Arkansas**
Barbara Oberste, RN
Partners in Care, Inc.
5326 W. Markham, Suite 19
Little Rock, AR 72205
(501) 664-1600; FAX (501) 666-2916

**California (Northern)**
Christine Miaskowski, RN, PhD
Department of Physiological Nursing
University of California, SF
P.O. Box 0610 N611Y
San Francisco, CA 94143
(415) 476-9407; FAX (415) 476-8899

**California (Southern)**
Betty R. Ferrell, RN, PhD, FAAN
Department of Nursing Research and Education
City of Hope National Medical Center
1500 East Duarte Road
Duarte, CA 91010-0269
(818) 359-8111; FAX (818) 301-8941

**Colorado**
Kelly Ambler, RN, BSN
Director of Nursing
Hospice of Larimer County
5205 S. College Avenue
Ft. Collins, CO 80525
(303) 226-6533; FAX (303) 226-6999

**Connecticut**
Didi Loseth, RN, MSN
95 Peace Acre Lane
Stratford, CT 06497-1314
(212) 639-8708; (212) 717-3081

**Delaware**
Gretchen W. Jones, RN, MS, OCN®
P.O. Box 581
Hockessin, DE 19707
(302) 658-7468; FAX (610) 274-2082

**Florida**

Lori A. Ladd, RN, MSN
H. Lee Moffitt Cancer Center
12902 Magnolia Drive
Tampa, FL 33610-9497
(813) 972-8456; FAX (813) 979-3068

**Georgia**

Anne Marie McKenzie-Brown, MD
1719 Pine Ridge Dr. NE
Atlanta, GA 30324
(404) 616-5521; FAX (404) 616-9213

**Hawaii**

Hob Osterlund, RN, MS
The Queen's Medical Center
1301 Punchbowl Street
Honolulu, HI 96813
(808) 547-4726; FAX (808) 537-7822

**Idaho**

Darryl Denison, RN
Neuro Surgery Group
999 N. Curtis Road, Suite 405
Boise, ID 83706
(208) 378-3055; FAX (208) 378-2968

**Illinois**

Carol J. Swenson, RN, MS, OCN®
Swedish American Hospital
1400 Charles Street
Rockford, IL 61104-2298
(815) 968-4400; FAX (815) 961-2199

**Indiana**

Neil Irick, MD
Pain Resource Center
2020 W. 86th Street, Suite 310
Indianapolis, IN 46260
(317) 872-2332; FAX (317) 872-2889

**Iowa**

Peggy Christ, RN
Jennie Edmundson Hospital
933 E. Pierce St.
Council Bluffs, IA 51502
(712) 328-6000

**Kansas**

Connie Rundle, RN, MSN
Stormont Vail Regional Medical Center
1500 SW 10th St.
Topeka, KS 66604
(913) 354-5253; FAX (913) 354-5093

**Kentucky**

Lin Edwards, RN, MS
Director of Professional Relations
Hospice of Louisville
3532 Ephraim McDowell Drive
Louisville, KY 40205-3224
(502) 456-6200; FAX (502) 456-6655

**Louisiana**

Ginny Barden, Program Director
ACS—Louisiana Division
2200 Veteran's Memorial Highway, Suite 214
Kenner, LA 70062
(504) 469-0021; FAX (504) 469-0033

**Maine**

Kandyce Powell, RN, MSN
Executive Director

Maine Hospice Council
16 Winthrop St.
Augusta, ME 04330
(207) 626-0651

**Maryland**

Rebecca Finlely, PharmD
University of Maryland Cancer Center
22 South Greene St.
Baltimore, MD 21201
(410) 328-7683; FAX (410) 328-6896

**Massachusetts**

Margaret Barton Burke, RN, MS, OCN®
c/o ACS—Massachusetts Division
247 Commonwealth Avenue
Boston, MA 02116
(617) 267-2650; FAX (617) 563-3163

**Michigan**

Les Bricker, MD
2799 W. Grand Boulevard
Detroit, MI 48202
(313) 876-1859; FAX (313) 876-7911

**Minnesota**

Paula Sallmen, RN, BSN, OCN®
Virginia L. Piper Cancer Institute
800 E. 28th St. at Chicago
Minneapolis, MN 55407-3799
(612) 863-4633; FAX (612) 863-4689

**Mississippi**

Karen Koch, PharmD
N. Mississippi Medical Center
830 S. Gloster St.
Tupelo, MS 38801
(601) 841-3778; FAX (601) 841-3785

**Missouri**

Mary Ann Coletti, RN, OCN®
Director of Detection/Treatment and Medical Affairs
3322 American Avenue
Jefferson City, MO 65109
(573) 782-3932

**Nebraska**

Elaine J. Pohren, RN, MSN
University of Nebraska Medical Center
600 S. 42nd St.
Omaha, NE 68198-5640
(402) 559-4364; FAX (402) 559-9107

**Nevada**

Sherry Therrin, RN
3920 S. Eastern Ave., Suite 200
Las Vegas, NV 89119

**New Hampshire**

Paul Arnstein, RN
Concord Hospital
250 Pleasant St.
Concord, NH 03301
(603) 225-2751; FAX (603) 226-0016

**New Jersey**

Donna Bocco
2600 U.S. Hwy 1
P.O. Box 2201
New Brunswick, NJ 08902-0803
(908) 297-8000; FAX (908) 297-9043

**New Mexico**
Carol Dolan, RN, MSN
University of New Mexico Cancer Center
900 Camino de Salud NE
Albuquerque, NM 87131
(505) 277-8746; FAX (505) 277-2841

**New York**
Kim Calder, MPS
Cancer Care, Inc.
1180 Avenue of Americas
New York, NY 10036
(212) 221-3300; FAX (212) 719-0263

**North Carolina**
Jo Ann Dalton, RN, EdD
School of Nursing
University of North Carolina
7460 Carrington Hall
Chapel Hill, NC 27599
(919) 966-1582; FAX (919) 966-7298

**North Dakota**
LaRae Palmer, RN
Hospice of Red River Valley
702 28th Avenue North
Fargo, ND 58102
(701) 237-4629; FAX (701) 280-9069

**Ohio**
Pam Tolbert
Arthur G. James Cancer Hospital
300 W. 10th Ave.
Columbus, OH 43210
(614) 293-6274; FAX (614) 293-6027

**Oklahoma**
Barbara Bilderback, RN, MS
St. Francis Hospice
6161 S. Yale Ave.
Tulsa, OK 74136
(918) 494-6465; (918) 494-6460

**Oregon**
Alicia Super, RN, BSN, OCN®
P.O. Box 6313
Portland, OR 97228-6313
(503) 229-7760; FAX (503) 790-1208

**Pennsylvania**
Georgia Trosle, RN
P.O. Box 850 C2804B
Hershey, PA 17033
(717) 531-6849; FAX (717) 531-6221

**Rhode Island**
Phoebe Fernald, RN, MS, OCN®
Rhode Island Hospital
Department of Medical Oncology
593 Eddy Street
Providence, RI 02903
(401) 444-5248; FAX (401) 784-0318

**South Dakota**
Kris Gaster, RN, MS, OCN®
624 Wiswall Place
Sioux Falls, SD 57105
(605) 339-8000; FAX (605) 339-7543

**Tennessee**
Alvin Mauer, MD
University of Tennessee/Memphis
3 N. Dunlap, 3rd Floor
Memphis, TN 38163
(901) 448-5717

**Texas**
Chree Boydstun
P.O. Box 980185
Houston, TX 77098-1724
(713) 745-1468; FAX (713) 794-1724

**Utah**
Perry G. Fine, MD
Associate Professor
Department of Anesthesiology
University of Utah Health Sciences Center
50 N. Medical Drive
Salt Lake City, UT 84132
(801) 581-6393; FAX (801) 585-6160

**Vermont**
Jean Harkins, RN
Medical Center Hospital of Vermont
111 Colchester Avenue
Burlington, VT 05402
(802) 656-2415; FAX (802) 656-5324

**Virginia**
Susan Robinson, RN, MS, OCN®
Massey Cancer Center
Box 37
Richmond, VA 23298-0037
(804) 786-0450; FAX (804) 828-8453

**Washington**
Judy Kornell, RN, MN, OCN®
Fred Hutchinson Cancer Research Center
1124 Columbia Street, FB600E
Seattle, WA 98104
(206) 667-5021; FAX (206) 667-3531

**West Virginia**
Chris Zinn, RN, CRNH
Kanawha Hospice Care
1143 Dunbar Ave.
Charleston, WV 25064
(304) 768-8523; FAX (304) 768-8627

**Wisconsin**
June L. Dahl, PhD
Medical Sciences Center, Rm. 3675
1300 University Avenue
Madison, WI 53706
(608) 262-0978; FAX (608) 265-4014

# COMPREHENSIVE, CLINICAL, AND CONSORTIUM CANCER CENTERS

**141.** The National Cancer Act of 1971 authorized the development of new comprehensive research and demonstration centers known as comprehensive cancer centers and specialized cancer centers. Through community outreach activities, comprehensive cancer centers are to provide coordination and leadership within their geographic regions to ensure the availability of complete care for patients with cancer.

At present, there are 27 comprehensive (*) cancer centers and 13 clinical (**) cancer centers designated by the NCI. A treatment center must meet rigorous criteria set by the NCI, including the ability to perform advanced diagnostic and treatment methods; support a strong research program; and participate in an integrated nationwide system in prevention, diagnosis, and treatment. Information about referral procedures, treatment costs, and services available to patients can be obtained from the individual cancer centers listed below:

**Alabama**

University of Alabama at Birmingham Comprehensive Cancer Center*
Basic Health Sciences Building, Rm. 108
1918 University Boulevard
Birmingham, AL 35294
(205) 934-5077

**Arizona**

University of Arizona Cancer Center*
1501 North Campbell Avenue
Tucson, AZ 85724
(602) 626-6372

**California**

Kenneth Norris Jr. Comprehensive Cancer Center*
University of Southern California
1441 Eastlake Avenue
Los Angeles, CA 90033-0804
(213) 226-2370

Jonsson Comprehensive Cancer Center*
University of California at Los Angeles
200 Medical Plaza
Los Angeles, CA 90027
(213) 206-0278; (800) 825-2631

City of Hope National Medical Center**
Beckman Research Institute
1500 East Duarte Road
Duarte, CA 91010
(818) 359-8111, ext. 2292

University of California at San Diego Cancer Center**
225 Dickinson Street
San Diego, CA 92103
(619) 543-6178

**Colorado**

University of Colorado Cancer Center**
4200 East 9th Avenue, Box B190
Denver, CO 80262
(303) 270-3007

**Connecticut**

Yale University Comprehensive Cancer Center*
333 Cedar Street
New Haven, CT 06510
(203) 785-4095

**District of Columbia**

Lombardi Cancer Research Center*
Georgetown University Medical Center
3800 Reservoir Road, N.W.
Washington, DC 20007
(202) 687-2192

**Florida**

Sylvester Comprehensive Cancer Center*
University of Miami Medical School
1475 Northwest 12th Avenue
Miami, FL 33136
(305) 545-1000

**Illinois**

Robert H. Lurie Cancer Center**
Northwestern University
303 East Chicago Ave.
Olson Pavilion, Room 8250
Chicago, IL 60611
(312) 908-8400

University of Chicago Cancer Research Center**
5841 S. Maryland Avenue
Chicago, IL 60637
(312) 702-9200

**Maryland**

The Johns Hopkins Oncology Center*
600 North Wolfe Street
Baltimore, MD 21205
(301) 955-8964

**Massachusetts**

Dana-Farber Cancer Institute*
44 Binney Street
Boston, MA 02115
(617) 632-3476

**Michigan**

Meyer L. Prentis Comprehensive Cancer Center of Metropolitan Detroit*
110 East Warren Avenue
Detroit, MI 48201
(313) 745-4329

University of Michigan Cancer Center*
101 Simpson Drive
Ann Arbor, MI 48109-0752
(313) 936-9583

**Minnesota**

Mayo Comprehensive Cancer Center*
200 First Street Southwest
Rochester, MN 55905
(507) 284-3413

**New Hampshire**

Norris Cotton Cancer Center*
Dartmouth-Hitchcock Medical Center
One Medical Center Drive
Lebanon, NH 03756
(603) 646-5505

**New York**

Memorial Sloan-Kettering Cancer Center*
1275 York Avenue
New York, NY 10021
(800) 525-2225

Columbia University Comprehensive Cancer Center**
College of Physicians and Surgeons
630 West 168th Street
New York, NY 10032
(212) 305-6905

Roswell Park Cancer Institute*
Elm and Carlton Streets
Buffalo, NY 14263
(716) 845-4400; (800) ROSWELL

Albert Einstein College of Medicine**
1300 Morris Park Avenue
Bronx, NY 10461
(212) 920-4826

Kaplan Cancer Center*
New York University Medical Center
462 First Avenue
New York, NY 10016-9103
(212) 263-6485

University of Rochester Cancer Center**
601 Elmwood Avenue, Box 704
Rochester, NY 14642
(716) 275-4911

**North Carolina**

Duke Comprehensive Cancer Center*
P.O. Box 3814
Durham, NC 27710
(919) 684-2748

Lineberger Comprehensive Cancer Center*
University of North Carolina
School of Medicine
Chapel Hill, NC 27599
(919) 966-4431

Cancer Center of Wake Forest University at the
Bowman Gray School of Medicine*
300 South Hawthorn Road
Winston-Salem, NC 27103
(919) 748-4354

**Ohio**

Ohio State University Comprehensive Cancer Center*
Arthur C. James Cancer Hospital
410 West 10th Avenue
Columbia, OH 43210
(614) 293-8619; (800) 638-6996

Ireland Cancer Center at Case Western Reserve
University**
University Hospitals of Cleveland
2074 Abington Road
Cleveland, OH 44106
(216) 844-5432

**Pennsylvania**

Fox Chase Cancer Center*
7701 Burholme Avenue
Philadelphia, PA 19111
(215) 728-2570

University of Pennsylvania Cancer Center*
3400 Spruce Street
Philadelphia, PA 19104
(215) 662-6364

Pittsburgh Cancer Institute*
200 Meyran Avenue
Pittsburgh, PA 15213-2592
(800) 537-4063

**Tennessee**

Drew-Meharry-Morehouse Consortium Cancer
Center
1005 DB Todd Blvd.
Nashville, TN 37208
(615) 327-6927

St. Jude Children's Research Hospital**
322 North Lauderdale Street
Memphis, TN 38101-0318
(901) 522-0306

**Texas**

San Antonio Cancer Institute**
4450 Medical Drive
San Antonio, TX 78229
(210) 616-5798

University of Texas*
M.D. Anderson Cancer Center
1515 Holcombe Boulevard
Houston, TX 77030
(713) 792-3245

**Utah**

Utah Cancer Center**
University of Utah School of Medicine
50 North Medical Drive, Room 2C110
Salt Lake City, UT 84132
(801) 581-4048

**Vermont**

Vermont Regional Cancer Center*
University of Vermont
1 South Prospect Street
Burlington, VT 05401
(802) 656-4580

**Virginia**

Massey Cancer Center**
Medical College of Virginia
Virginia Commonwealth University
1200 East Broad Street
Richmond, VA 23298
(804) 371-5116

**Washington**

Fred Hutchinson Cancer Research Center*
1124 Columbia Street
Seattle, WA 98104
(206) 667-5000

**Wisconsin**

Wisconsin Clinical Cancer Center*
University of Wisconsin
600 Highland Avenue
Madison, WI 53792
(608) 263-8090

## PHARMACEUTICAL RESOURCES

A valuable resource for nurses and other health care professionals seeking information for professional and patient use are the pharmaceutical companies. Most offer educational information that is product-specific, but most also offer a variety of other complimentary products and services. Nurses are encouraged to check with their area sales representative for specific requests, or call the company headquarters.

## 142. Pharmaceutical Product and Educational Assistance

**Amgen, Inc.**
1840 Dehavilland Dr.
Thousand Oaks, CA 91320
(800) 944-5100

All products available by phone, or from local sales representative.

**Patient education booklets:**
> How to Give Yourself a Subcutaneous Injection
> The First Step in Chemotherapy is Overcoming Your Fear
> The Most Important Part of Your Treatment is You
> Neupogen (Filgrastim)—Part of the Good News about Today's Chemotherapy

**Patient education videos:**
> *How to Give Yourself a Subcutaneous Injection*
> *What I Wish I Knew* (for breast cancer patients, hosted by Jill Eikenberry)

**Bristol-Myers Squibb**
P.O. Box 4500
Princeton, NJ 08543-4500
(609) 897-3440
Bristol-Myers Squibb Oncology has several patient and nurse education materials available. Please contact your local oncology sales representative for copies of the most recent information.

**Immunex Corporation**
51 University Street
Seattle, WA 98101
(800) IMMUNEX; FAX (800) 221-6820
All products available by mail, phone, or FAX request.

**Patient education booklet and video:**
> *Understanding Your Bone Marrow Transplant*

**Professional education booklet:**
> Cells of the Hematopoietic Cascade
> Older Patient Compendium
> ACS Textbook of Clinical Oncology

**Professional education video:**
> *Cells of the Hematopoietic Cascade*

**Janssen Pharmaceutica**
1125 Trenton-Harbourton Rd.
Titusville, NJ 08560
800 JANSSEN; (609) 730-2000; FAX (609) 730-3044
All products available from local sales representatives.
Pain Intervention Network (PIN) Resource Portfolio includes:
> Practice Approaches and Applications (professional monograph)
> Patient Discussion Card (professional education aid)
> Patient Leaflet
> Pain Assessment Slide Ruler
> Cancer Nutrition Facts—tear sheet
> PIN Newsletter (professional publication)

**Pharmacia-Upjohn, Inc.**
7000 Portage Rd.
Kalamazoo, MI 49001
(616) 323-4000
All products available from local sales representative.

**Patient education booklets**
(multiple copies available; for patient display):
> Tumor Markers
> Cancer Terms
> Blood Counts and Infection
> Record of Blood Counts
> You Are in Charge! Making the Most of Your Cancer Treatment

**Patient education video:**
> *Bone Marrow Transplantation—The Patient's Perspective*

**Purdue Frederick Company**
100 Connecticut Avenue
Norwalk, CT 06850-3590
(203) 853-0123
All products available by mail, phone, or from local sales representative.

**Patient education booklets:**
> Managing Cancer Pain: AHCPR Guidelines (English and Spanish)
> Comfort Assessment Journal (English and Spanish)
> Home Care of the Hospice Patient (English and Spanish)
> Up-to-date Answers to Questions about Measuring Pain (English and Spanish)

**Patient education videos:**
> *Partners Against Pain: Helping to Control Cancer Pain*
> *My Word Against Theirs. . .Narcotics for Cancer Pain Control*

**Professional education booklets:**
> T.I.M.E. Titration Principles
> Dispelling the Myths about Morphine
> American Pain Society Guide: Acute Pain and Cancer Pain
> First-Pass Effect Visual Aid
> Pain Assessment Scale

**Professional assistance products:**
> Partners Against Pain—Opioid Dosage Conversion (slide calculator)
> Cancer Pain Management: Defining New Standards of Care (Continuing Education program)

**TAP Pharmaceuticals**
2355 Waukegan Rd.
Deerfield, IL 60015
(800) 622-2011
All products available by phone.

**Patient education booklets:**
> Lupron Depot 7.5 mg: Your Choice for Treating Prostate Cancer
> Your Health & Your Prostate

**Patient education videos:**
> *Lupron Depot 7.5 mg: Your Choice for Treating Prostate Cancer*
> *LifeLines: A Guide to Life with Prostate Cancer*

**Zeneca Pharmaceuticals**
c/o Nolvadex Marketing
1800 Concord Pike
P.O. Box 15437
Wilmington, DE 19850-5437
All products available by mail or from local sales representative.

**Patient education booklet:**
> Progress for Life

**Patient education video:**
> *Progress for Life*
> *In Touch for Life (for Lumpectomy patients)*
> *In Touch for Life (for Mastectomy patients)*

## 143. Pharmaceutical Reimbursement & Financial Assistance

**Amgen, Inc.**
(800) 272-9376

Insurance billing guidance and information available to health care professionals.

Safety Net Program will provide Neupogen free of charge to medically needy patients.

## Amersham Healthcare
(800) 321-4669

Reimbursement hotline is a service available to health care professionals and patients that provides information on coverage, coding, claims submission, and reimbursement policies for Metastron (strontium-89).

## Berlex Inc.
(800) 473-5832

Hotline for health care providers for insurance claims assistance regarding Fludara.
Fludara Pact Program provides access to assistance for indigent patients.

## Bristol-Myers Squibb Oncology

Reimbursement Assistance Program (RAP)
(800) 872-8718
RAP assists health care professionals with information and assistance in insurance reimbursement.

Access Program
(800) 272-4878

This program provides Bristol-Myers Squibb Oncology products free of charge to uninsured or underinsured patients.

## Cerenex Pharmaceuticals
(800) 745-2967

Reimbursement hotline assists providers with insurance coverage and problem claims.
Cerenex will also provide Zofran free of charge to those who cannot afford the cost of therapy.

## Chiron Therapeutics
(800) 775-7533

Reimbursement hotline provides assistance with payment and coverage guidelines and will assist with appeals for denied claims regarding the use of Proleukin.

## Ciba-Geigy
(908) 277-5849

Patient Assistance Program
This program provides free Aredia and Tegretol to appropriate patients who are unable to afford the cost of therapy and who are not covered by third-party reimbursement.

## Glaxo-Wellcome Co.
3030 Cornwallis Rd.
Research Triangle Park, NC 27709

Reimbursement Hotline
(800) 270-0425
The Hotline is available to answer questions related to coverage and reimbursement of all Wellcome Oncology products. Reimbursement specialists will assist callers with claims submissions, appeals, and prior authorization.

Patient assistance
(800) 722-9294

This program is designed to provide financially disadvantaged individuals rapid access to any Burroughs Wellcome Co. product at no cost. Patients who cannot afford

therapy and who are uninsured, do not qualify for publicly funded medication assistance programs, or are in the process of applying for such programs are potential candidates.

## Janssen Pharmaceutica
Patient Assistance Program
1800 Robert Fulton Dr., Third Floor
Reston, VA 22091-4346
(800) 544-2987

This program will provide Ergamisol, Nizoral, Duragesic, Propulsid, Hismanal, and Imodium free of charge to persons who meet specific medical and financial criteria and lack third-party insurance necessary to obtain treatment.

## Ortho Biotech, Inc.
(800) 553-3851

The Reimbursement Hotline will provide reimbursement counsel, assistance in claims submissions and appeals, free carrier intervention services, and letters of "medical necessity," for health care professionals who are assisting patients receiving Procrit or Leustatin.
The Reimbursement Assurance Program will provide free Procrit to physicians' offices in amounts equal to that which a patient already received while appealing a reimbursement decision.
The Financial Assistance Program will provide Procrit and Leustatin free of charge to patients who meet medical and financial criteria, and do not have third-party coverage.
The Cost Sharing Program sets a maximum limit on out-of-pocket expense to a patient for the annual cost of therapy.

## Roche Laboratories
340 Kingsland Street
Nutley, NJ 07110-1199
(800) 443-6676

The Oncoline is a reimbursement support program that has access to the NCI databases and medical literature searches.
Cost Assistance Program (CAP) is a plan to limit the amount the patient must pay for Roferon-A out-of-pocket. They also provide Roferon-A free of charge for those without insurance coverage.

## Schering
Interactive Reimbursement Information Services
104 W. Anapamu St.
Santa Barbara, CA 93101
(800) 521-7157

This program will provide Intron and Eulexin free of charge to persons who meet specific medical and financial criteria and lack third-party insurance necessary to obtain treatment.

## Zeneca Pharmaceuticals Foundation
P.O. Box 15197
Wilmington, DE 19850-5197
(800) 424-3727

This program provides Nolvadex free of charge to patients who are financially unable to pay for them.

# Index

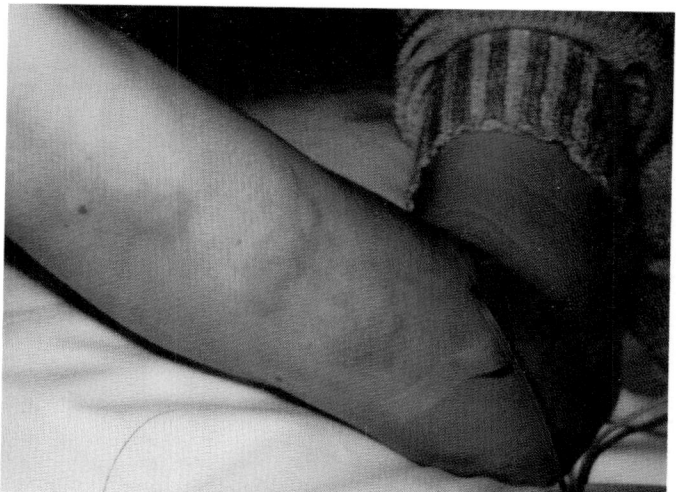

**PLATE 1** Venous flare (doxorubicin) (Figure 15-2).

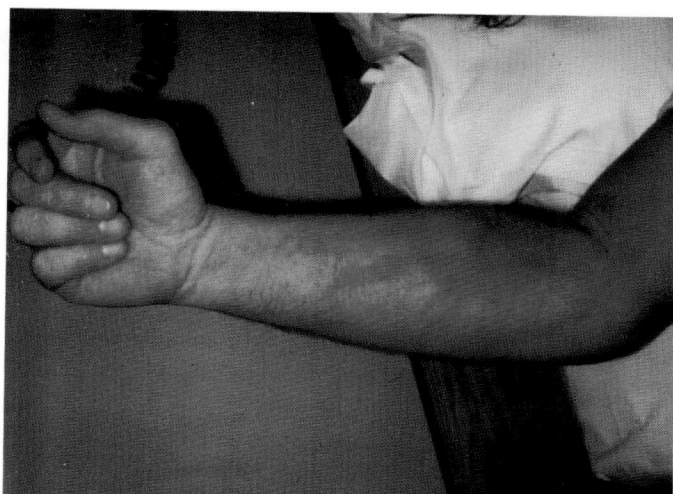

**PLATE 2** Venous extravasation 2½ weeks after doxorubicin extravasation (Figure 15-3).

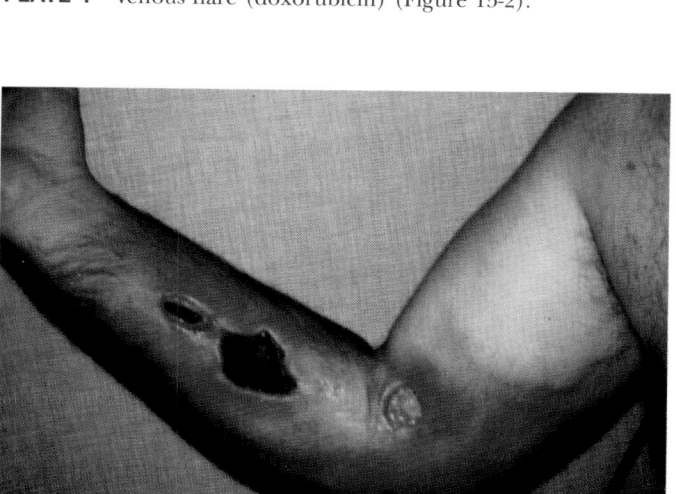

**PLATE 3** Same patient 4½ months after doxorubicin extravasation (Figure 15-4).

**PLATE 4** Doxorubicin extravasation after 12 days. No pain with movement. Healed spontaneously (Figure 15-7).

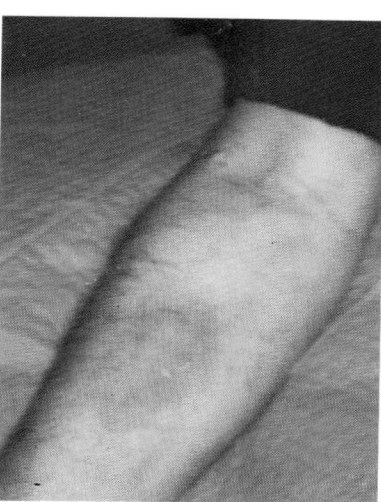

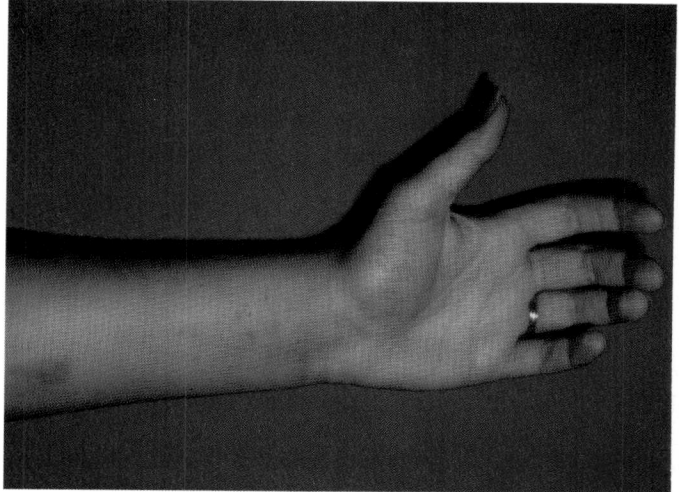

**PLATE 5** Erythema and edema at injection site one week after doxorubicin administration (Figure 15-8).

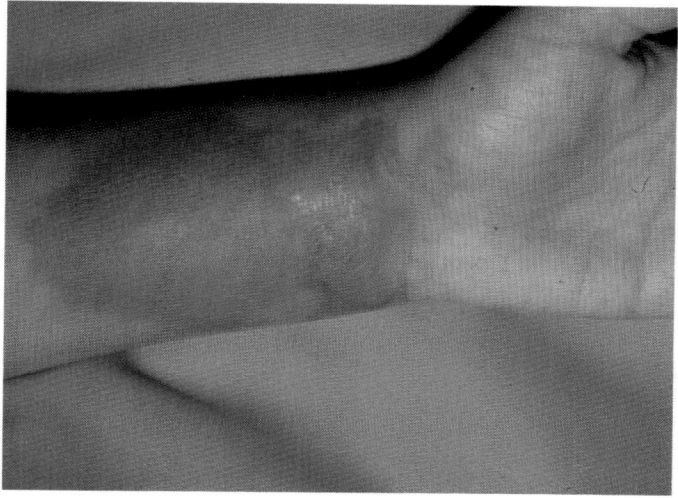

**PLATE 6** At three weeks, blister formation and demarcation are present (Figure 15-9).

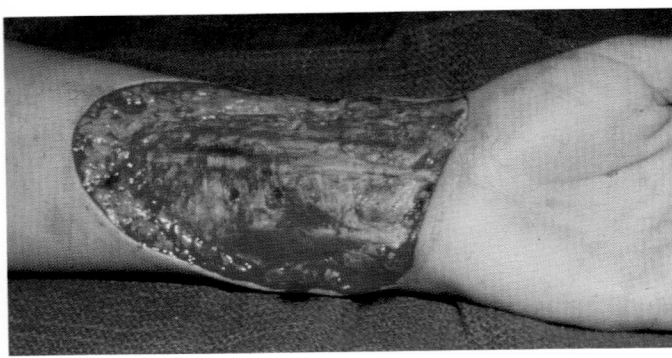

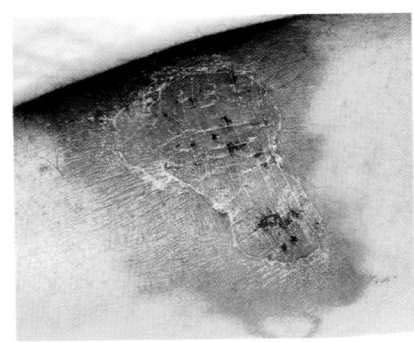

**PLATE 7** Tissue surgically excised after doxorubicin extravasation (Figure 15-10).

**PLATE 8** Docetaxel infiltration (Figure 15-11).

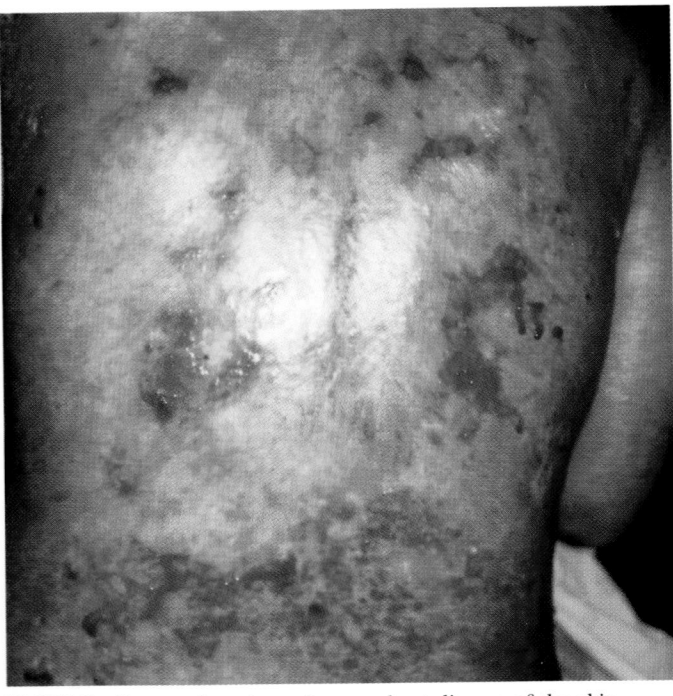

**PLATE 9** Severe chronic graft-versus-host disease of the skin (Figure 18-9).

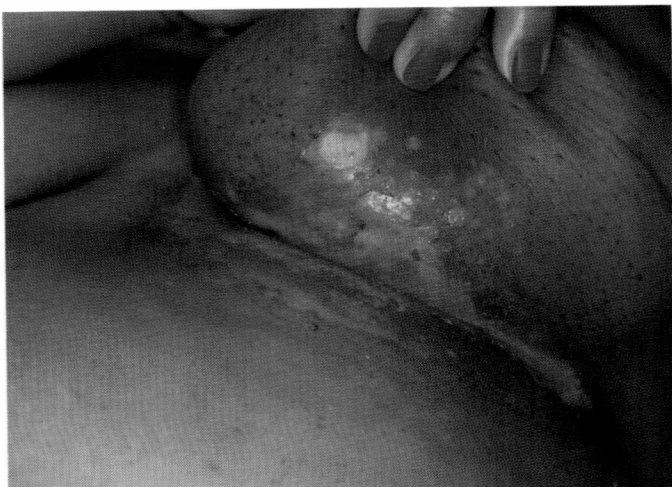

**PLATE 10** Moist desquamation with radiation therapy and concomitant methotrexate, 5-fluorouracil, and leucovorin (Figure 29-2).

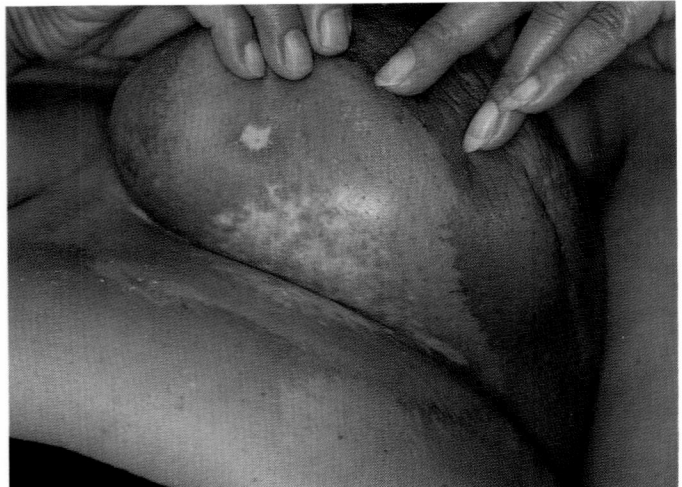

**PLATE 11** Two weeks after completion and treatment three times daily with domeboro soaks, wound cleanser, and epithelial stimulating wound gel (Figure 29-3).

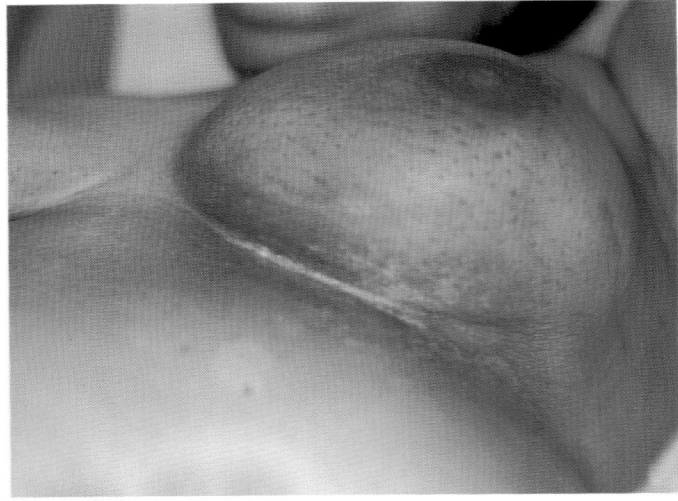

**PLATE 12** Three months after completing radiation (Figure 29-4).

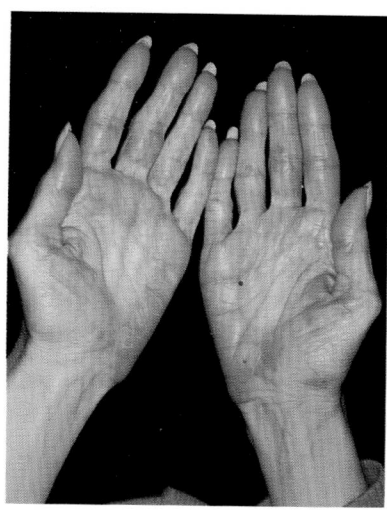

PLATE 13  Acral erythema following floxuridine infusion (Figure 29-9).

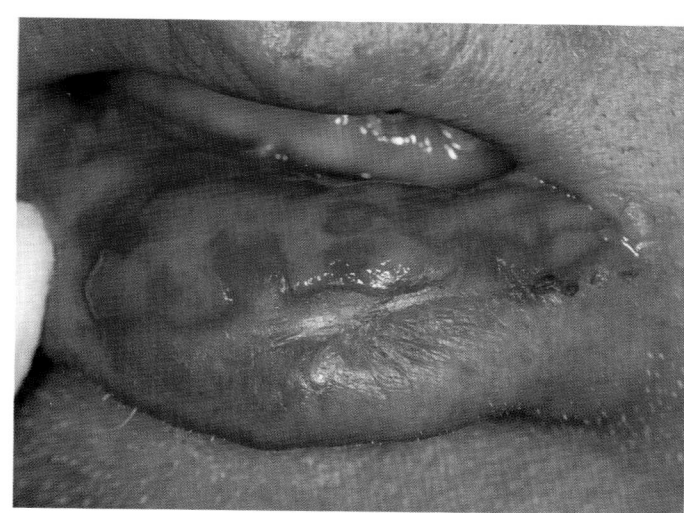

PLATE 14  Methotrexate-induced stomatitis, grade 3 (Figure 29-12).

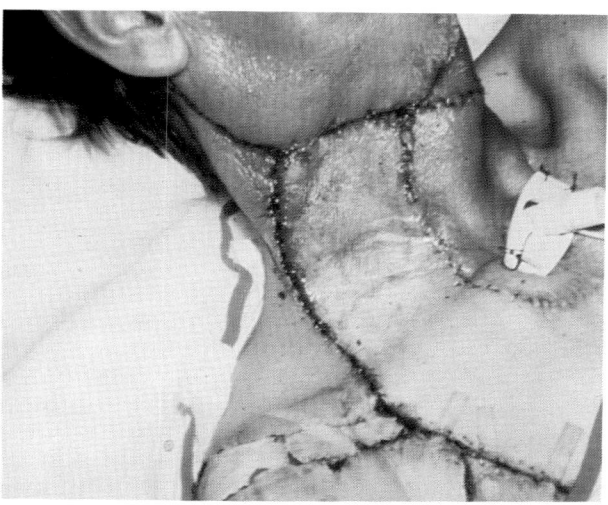

PLATE 15  Sequence of flap death. Immediate post-op. Line of demarcation evident (Figure 40-6).

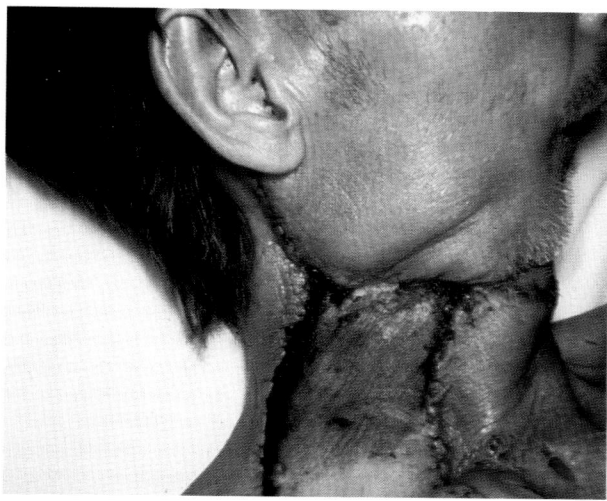

PLATE 16  Line of demarcation pronounced (Figure 40-7).

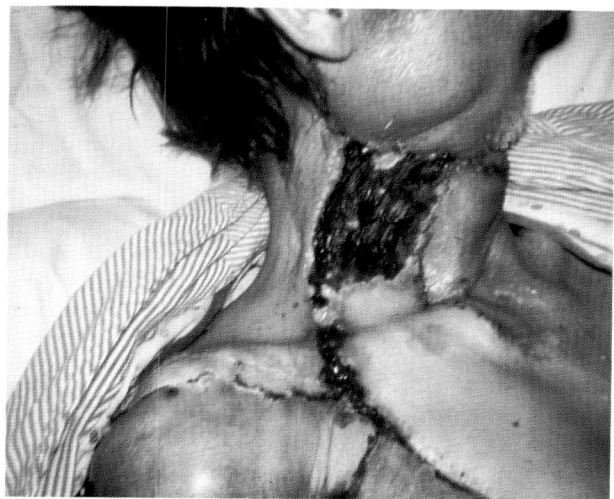

PLATE 17  Distal tip of flap necrosed (Figure 40-8).

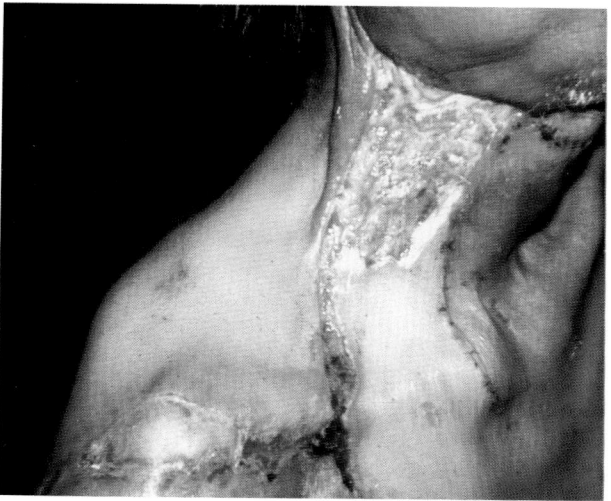

PLATE 18  Necrotic portion of flap debrided (Figure 40-9).

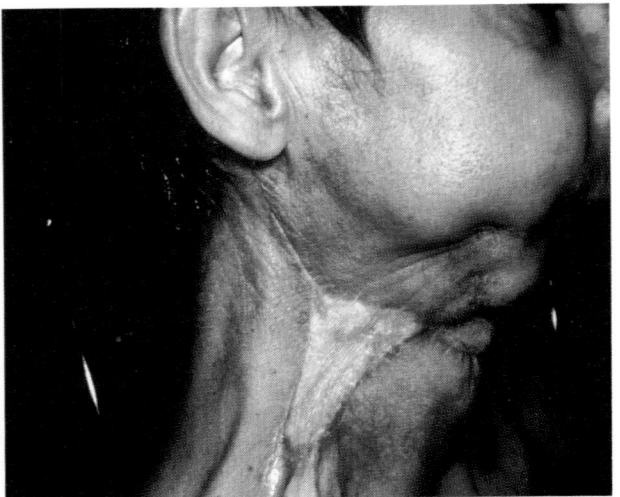

**PLATE 19**  Area reconstructed with skin graft (Figure 40-10).

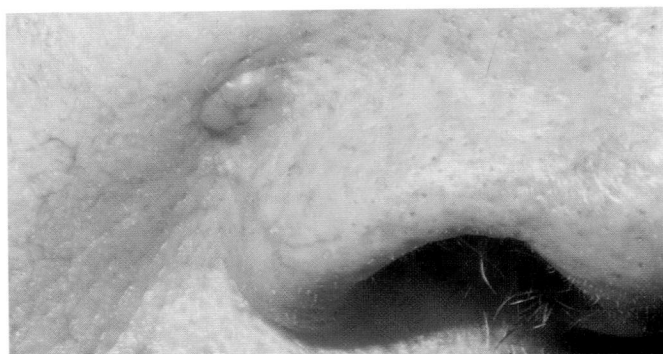

**PLATE 20**  Basal cell carcinoma (Figure 46-2).

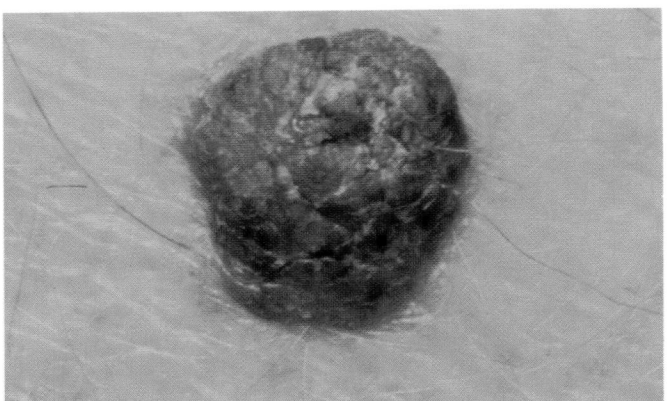

**PLATE 22**  Normal mole (Figure 46-4).

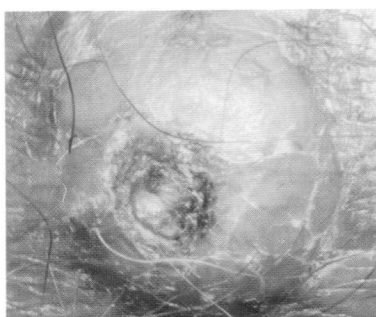

**PLATE 21**  Squamous cell carcinoma of the skin (Figure 46-3).

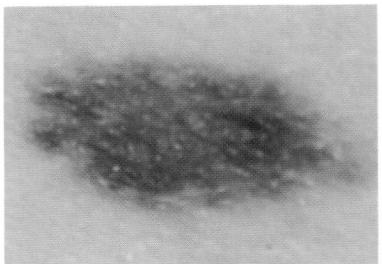

**PLATE 23**  Dysplastic nevus (Figure 46-5).

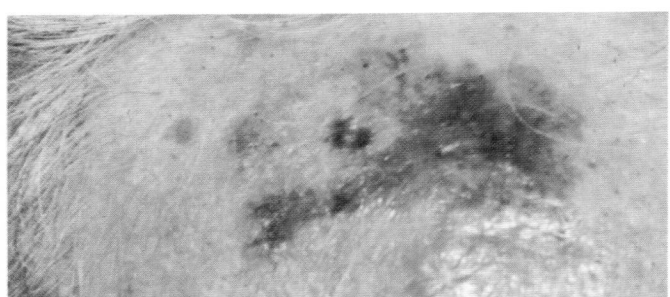

**PLATE 24**  Lentigo malignant melanoma (Figure 46-6).

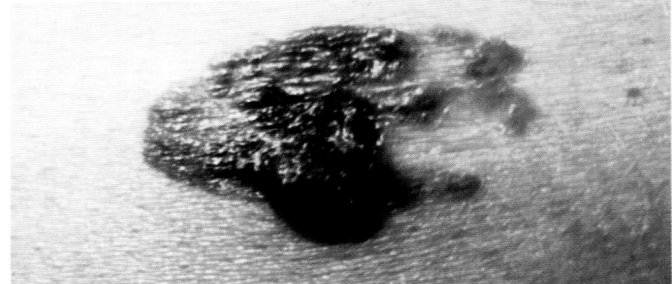

**PLATE 25**  Superficial spreading melanoma (Figure 46-7).

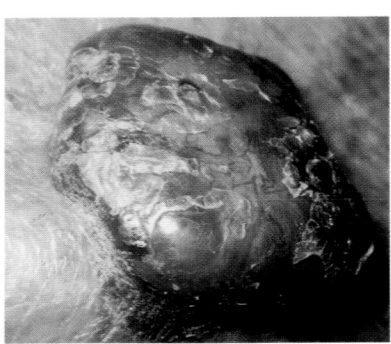

**PLATE 26**  Nodular melanoma (Figure 46-8).

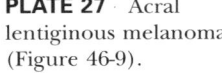

**PLATE 27**  Acral lentiginous melanoma (Figure 46-9).

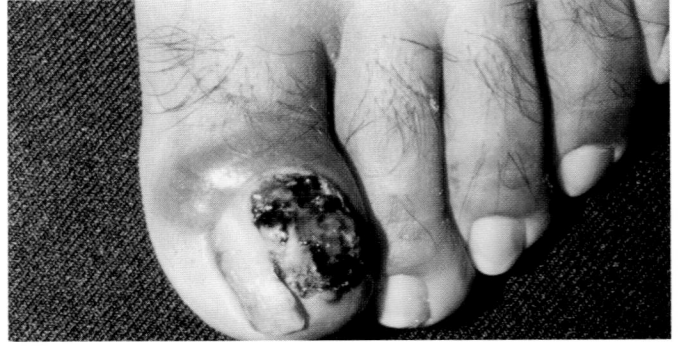

malignancy, 690–691,
694, 1272; *see also* Hypercalcemia
"Hungry bone syndrome,"
1063
HUS; *see* Hemolytic uremic syndrome
Hutchinson's melanotic
freckle, 1363; *see also*
Lentigo maligna
HVL; *see* Half-value layer
Hyaluronidase, 339
Hycamtin; *see* Topotecan
Hydration
in hypercalcemia treatment,
695–696, 707
termination of, ethics of,
1619–1620
Hydrazine sulfate, and appetite, 677
Hydrea; *see* Hydroxyurea
Hydrocarbon adducts, and carcinogenesis, 10, 41
Hydrocephalus, and brain
tumor surgery, 1018,
1027
Hydrocortisone, 303, 1072
drug interactions with, 299
in hypercalcemia treatment,
697–698
Hydromorphone, 557
administration of, 563, 564,
566–567
5 Hydroxyindoleacetic acid
(5 HIAA), 180
Hydroxyurea (Hydrea), 303,
310, 400
oral administration of, 323
Hydroxyzine, analgesic use of,
562
Hypercalcemia, 684–699
assessment of, 694, 707
breast cancer and, 685, 690,
691–692
calcium homeostasis and
normal, 686–688, 706
physiology of, 685–692
causes of, 685
clinical manifestations of,
692–694, 706
defined, 685
dehydration and, 695–696
1,25-dihydroxyvitamin D
and, 687, 690
diuretics and, 696
hematologic cancer and, 692
humoral, of malignancy,
690–691
incidence of, 685
laboratory studies in, 694
local osteolytic, 690, 691–692
multiple myeloma and, 692,
706, 1324
paraneoplastic, 704, 705
etiology of, 704
incidence of, 704

parathyroid tumors and,
1062, 1063–1064
pathophysiology of, 688–692,
706
treatment of, 694–698, 707
weight bearing and, 692
Hyperchromaticism, 21
Hypercoagulability, 619–623
paraneoplastic thromboembolism and, 712
Hyperfractionation (HFX),
266, 279, 1019
Hyperparathyroidism; *see also*
Parathyroid hormone
(PTH)
hypercalcemia and, 685; *see
also* Hypercalcemia
Hyperpigmentation, chemotherapy-induced, 780
Hypersensitivity reactions
(HSRs), cutaneous
chemotherapy-induced, 329,
780–782
Hypertension
pheochromocytoma and,
1074
portal, and hepatic resection,
1104, 1109
Hyperthermia, radiotherapy
modification with,
261–262, 817–818
bone and soft-tissue sarcoma
and, 879
brain tumors and, 1020–1021
head and neck cancer and,
1222
Hyperuricemia
multiple myeloma and, 1324
tumor lysis syndrome and,
416–417
Hyperviscosity syndrome, and
multiple myeloma, 1324
Hypnosis, in pain management, 241, 242, 570
Hypocalcemia, "hungry bone
syndrome" and, 1063
Hypocoagulation, 618–619
Hypogeusia, 657, 796; *see also*
Taste alterations
Hypoglossal nerve, 983
examination of, 1006
Hypoglycemia, and endocrine
neoplastic syndromes,
705
Hypokalemia, and adrenocortical tumors, 1072
Hyponatremia
brain tumor surgery and,
1018
ectopic ADH production
and, 707–708; *see also*
Syndrome of inappropriate antidiuretic hormone secretion
(SIADH)
Hypoparathyroidism, 1060

Hypopharyngeal carcinoma,
1204
anatomy and, 1211–1212
etiology of, 1211
rehabilitation needs after,
1213
staging of, 1212
treatment of, 1212–1213
Hypoplasia, and parenchymal
radiosensitivity, 260
Hyposmia, 657, 1215
Hypotension; *see also* Blood
pressure
pancreatic surgery and, 1130
Hypothalamic-inhibiting hormones, 743
Hypothalamic-releasing hormones, 743
Hypothalamus
hormones produced by, 743
pituitary tumor development
and, 1064
Hypothermia, scalp, 786
Hypothyroidism, 826–827
Hypovolemia, and pancreatic
surgery, 1130
Hypoxia, and apoptosis, 13
Hypoxic cells, and radiosensitivity, 260
Hysterectomy, radical, 759,
1187
total abdominal, 1149
total vaginal, 1172, 1176


IAOPC; *see* Ideas About Oncology Patient Care Scale
IASP; *see* International Association for the Study of
Pain
IAT (immunoaugmentative
therapy), 1632–1633
Iatrogenic secondary lymphedema, 738–739
IBD; *see* Inflammatory bowel
disease
IBMTR; *see* International Bone
Marrow Transplant Registry
Ibuprofen, in pain management, 556
"I Can Cope" program, 1644,
1658
ICI Pharma; *see* Goserelin acetate
ICIC; *see* International Cancer
Information Center
ICP; *see* Intracranial pressure
ICRF–159; *see* Razoxane
ICRF–187; *see* Dexrazoxane
Idarubicin (Idamycin), 302,
305
extravasation of, 332, 337
intravenous administration
of, 373
toxicity of, 405
Ideas About Oncology Patient

Care Scale (IAOPC),
1578
Idiopathic thrombocytopenic
purpura (ITP),
612–613, 615
IDSs; *see* Integrated delivery systems
IFNs; *see* Interferons
Ifosfamide (Ifex), 296, 298,
302, 304
drug interactions with, 300,
301
intravenous administration
of, 374
toxicity of, 400, 406, 409, 413,
414
IGF-I; *see* Insulinlike growth factor I
IGF-II; *see* Insulinlike growth
factor II
IHO; *see* Integrated health organization
IL; *see* Interleukin *entries*
Ileal conduit, 895–896
nursing care after, 899–901
Ileal reservoir, continent; *see*
Continent urinary diversion
Ileus, paralytic, and renal surgery, 912
Illness behavior, 78–79
Imagery, 1637
in pain management, 241,
242, 569–570, 571
Imaging, 179–189; *see also* specific disease, specific imaging technique
patient preparation for, 179,
183–185
preferred procedures in,
179, 182
Imipramine
analgesic use of, 560
drug interactions with, 300
Immobilization, in pain management, 569
Immune surveillance, 427
Immune system, 427–430; *see
also* Antigens
bone marrow transplantation and, 484
cervical intraepithelial neoplasia and, 859
effector mechanisms of,
427–430
infection and, 586, 589
Kaposi's sarcoma and, 849
lymphocytes in, 1295
metastasis and, 28
neoplasia and, 1292–1293
paraneoplastic syndromes
and, 708–709, 714
treatment effects on, late,
829
Immunex; *see* Sargramostim
Immunization, and prevention,
96–98, 494–495